Veterinary Pharmacology and Therapeutics

Ninth Edition

Veterinary Pharmacology and Therapeutics

Ninth Edition

Edited by

Jim E. Riviere
DVM, PhD, DSc (hon)

Mark G. Papich
DVM, MS

Consulting Editor

H. Richard Adams
DVM, PhD, Diplomate ACVECC (Hon)

WILEY-BLACKWELL
A John Wiley & Sons, Inc., Publication

Ninth Edition first published 2009

First through Eighth Editions first published 1954, 1957, 1965, 1977, 1982, 1988, 1995, 2001

Blackwell Publishing was acquired by John Wiley & Sons in February 2007. Blackwell's publishing program has been merged with Wiley's global Scientific, Technical, and Medical business to form Wiley-Blackwell.

Editorial Office
2121 State Avenue, Ames, Iowa 50014-8300, USA

For details of our global editorial offices, for customer services, and for information about how to apply for permission to reuse the copyright material in this book, please see our website at www.wiley.com/wiley-blackwell.

First, second, and third editions 1954, 1957, and 1965 edited by L. Meyer Jones; fourth edition 1977 edited by L. Meyer Jones, Nicholas H. Booth, and Leslie E. McDonald; fifth and sixth editions 1982 and 1988 edited by Nicholas H. Booth and Leslie E. McDonald; seventh and eighth editions 1995 and 2001 edited by H. Richard Adams.

Library of Congress Cataloguing-in-Publication Data

Veterinary pharmacology and therapeutics.—9th ed. / edited by Jim E. Riviere, Mark G. Papich ; consulting editor, H. Richard Adams.

p. ; cm.

Rev. ed. of: Veterinary pharmacology and therapeutics / edited by H. Richard Adams. 8th ed. 2001.

Includes bibliographical references and index.

ISBN 978-0-8138-2061-3 (alk. paper)

1. Veterinary pharmacology. I. Riviere, J. Edmond (Jim Edmond) II. Papich, Mark G.

[DNLM: 1. Drug Therapy–veterinary. 2. Pharmacology. 3. Poisoning–veterinary. SF 915 V587 2008]

SF915.V49 2009

636.089′5–dc22

2008025003

A catalog record for this book is available from the U.S. Library of Congress.

Set in 11/13pt Adobe Garamond by SNP Best-set Typesetter Ltd., Hong Kong
Printed in the United States

2 2009

CONTENTS

CONTRIBUTORS

H. Richard Adams, DVM, PhD
Diplomate ACVECC (Hon)
Dean Emeritus
College of Veterinary Medicine, University of Missouri
Carl B. King Dean of Veterinary Medicine
College of Veterinary Medicine and Biomedical Sciences
Texas A&M University
College Station, Texas 77843-4461

Luis I. Alvarez, Med Vet, PhD
Assistant Professor
Laboratorio de Farmacologis
Departamento de Fisiopatologia
Facultad de Ciencias Veterinarias
Universidad Nacional del Centro
Campus Universitario
Argentina

Ronald E. Baynes, DVM, PhD
Associate Professor
Department of Population Health and Pathobiology
Center for Chemical Toxicology Research and Pharmacokinetics
North Carolina State University
College of Veterinary Medicine
4700 Hillsborough Street
Raleigh, NC 27606

Melanie Berson, DVM
Director
Division of Therapeutic Drugs for NonFood Animals
Office of New Animal Drug Evaluation
Food and Drug Administration
Center for Veterinary Medicine
7500 Standish Place
FDA/CVM/HFV-110
Rockville, MD 20855

Margarita A. Brown, DVM, MS
Safety Review Coordinator
Office of Surveillance and Compliance
Center for Veterinary Medicine
U.S. Food and Drug Administration
7519 Standish Place
Rockville, MD 20855

Patrick Burns, BVSc, MACVSc
DACVA
College of Veterinary Medicine
The Ohio State University
601 Vernon L. Tharp Street
Columbus, OH 43210

Cynthia A. Cole, DVM, PhD
DACVCP
IDEXX Pharmaceuticals, Inc.
7009 Albert Pick Road
Greensboro, NC 27409

Gordon L. Coppoc, DVM, PhD
Professor and Head
Department of Basic Medical Sciences
School of Veterinary Medicine
Purdue University
625 Harrison Street
West Lafayette, IN 47907-2026

Arthur L. Craigmill, PhD
DABT
Environmental Toxicology Extension
University of California
One Shields Avenue
Davis, CA 95616

Gigi Davidson, RPh
Director of Clinical Pharmacy Services
VTH Pharmacy
North Carolina State University
College of Veterinary Medicine
4700 Hillsborough Street
Raleigh, NC 27606

Jennifer L. Davis, DVM, PhD
Diplomate ACVIM, Diplomate ACVCP
Department of Clinical Sciences
North Carolina State University
College of Veterinary Medicine
4700 Hillsborough Street
Raleigh, NC 27606

Ian F. DeVeau, PhD
Director
Veterinary and Radiopharmaceuticals Group
United States Pharmacopeia
Department of Standards Dev
12601 Twinbrook Parkway
Rockville, MD 20852-1790

Levent Dirikolu
Physiology and Pharmacology
College of Veterinary Medicine
501 DW Brooks Drive
Athens, GA 30602

Bernadette Dunham, DVM, PhD
Director
Center for Veterinary Medicine
U.S. Food and Drug Administration
MPN-IV, Room 181, HFV-1
7519 Standish Place
Rockville, MD 20855

Duncan Ferguson, VMD, PhD
Diplomate ACVCP, Diplomate ACVIM
Veterinary Biosciences
The University of Illinois College of Veterinary Medicine
Urbana, IL 61801

John Gadsby, PhD
Professor
Department of Molecular Biomedical Sciences
College of Veterinary Medicine
North Carolina State University
4700 Hillsborough Street
Raleigh, NC 27606

Jody L. Gookin, DVM, PhD
Diplomate ACVIM
Assistant Professor
Department of Clinical Sciences
College of Veterinary Medicine
North Carolina State University
4700 Hillsborough Street
Raleigh, NC 27606

Joan Gotthardt, DVM
Director
Division of Therapeutic Drugs for Food Animals
Office of New Animal Drug Evaluation
Division of Therapeutic Drugs for Food Animals
FDA Center for Veterinary Medicine
7500 Standish Place
FDA/CVM/HFV-110
Rockville, MD 20855

Victoria Hampshire, VMD
Senior Regulatory Veterinarian and Reviewer
CDRH/ODE/DCD/PVDB
9200 Corporate Boulevard
HFZ-450
Rockville, MD 20850

Mark C. Heit, DVM, PhD
DACVCP
Senior Director, Research and Development
Velcera Inc.
777 Township Line Road
Yardely, PA 19067

Margarethe Hoenig, DVM
Professor
Physiology and Pharmacology
College of Veterinary Medicine
501 DW Brooks Drive
Athens, GA 30602

Laura Hungerford, DVM, MPH, PhD
Senior Advisor for Science Policy
Center for Veterinary Medicine
Office of New Animal Drug Evaluation
U.S. Food and Drug Administration
7500 Standish Place
FDA/CVM/HFV-100
Rockville, MD 20855

Robert P. Hunter, MS, PhD
Elanco Animal Health
2001 West Main Street
P.O. Box 708
Greenfield, IN 46140

Fernanda A. Imperiale, Vet, PhD
Research Fellow
Laboratorio de Farmacologis
Departamento de Fisiopatologia
Facultad de Ciencias Veterinarias
Universidad Nacional del Centro
Campus Universitario
(7000) Tandil
Argentina

Deborah T. Kochevar, DVM, PhD
DACVCP
Henry and Lois Foster Professor
Dean
Cummings School of Veterinary Medicine
Tufts University
200 Westboro Road
North Grafton, MA 01536

Butch KuKanich, DVM, PhD
Diplomate ACVCP
Department of Anatomy and Physiology
College of Veterinary Medicine
Kansas State University
228 Coles Hall
Manhattan, KS 66506-5802

Cory Langston, DVM, PhD
Diplomate ACVCP
Professor
College of Veterinary Medicine
Box 6100
Spring Street
Mississippi State University
Starkville, MS 39762-6100

Carlos E. Lanusse, Med Vet Dr Cs Vet, PhD
Diplomate ECVPT
Professor
Laboratorio de Farmacologis
Departamento de Fisiopatologia
Facultad de Ciencias Veterinarias
Universidad Nacional del Centro
Campus Universitario
(7000) Tandil
Argentina

Peter Lees, PhD, DSc
Royal Veterinary College
Hawkshead Campus
London University
North Mymms
Hatfield, Hertfordshire, AL97TA
United Kingdom

Adrian L. Lifschitz, Vet, PhD
Lecturer
Laboratorio de Farmacologis
Departamento de Fisiopatologia
Facultad de Ciencias Veterinarias
Universidad Nacional del Centro
Campus Universitario
(7000) Tandil
Argentina

Marilyn Martinez, PhD
Senior Research Scientist
Center for Veterinary Medicine
U.S. Food and Drug Administration
7500 Standish Place
Rockville, Maryland 20855

Katrina L. Mealey, DVM, PhD
DACVIM, DACVCP
Department Veterinary Clinical Sciences
College of Veterinary Medicine
Washington State University
ABDF 1020
Pullman, WA 99164-6610

Matthew W. Miller, DVM, MS
Diplomate ACVIM (Cardiology)
Professor of Cardiology
Charter Fellow
Michael E. DeBakey Institute
Department of Small Animal Clinical Sciences
College of Veterinary Medicine and Biomedical Sciences
Texas A&M University
College Station, Texas 77843-4461

Maria L. Mottier, Vet, PhD
Research Fellow
Laboratorio de Farmacologis
Departamento de Fisiopatologia
Facultad de Ciencias Veterinarias
Universidad Nacional del Centro
Campus Universitario
(7000) Tandil
Argentina

Margaret Oeller, DVM
Office of Minor Use and Minor Species Animal Drug Development
Center for Veterinary Medicine
U.S. Food and Drug Administration
7500 Standish Place
Rockville, MD 20855

Luisito S. Pablo, DVM, MS
Diplomate ACVA
Department of Large Animal Clinical Sciences
College of Veterinary Medicine
University of Florida
PO Box 100136
Gainesville, FL 32610

Mark G. Papich, DVM
Diplomate ACVCP
Professor
North Carolina State University
Department of Molecular Biomedical Sciences
College of Veterinary Medicine
4700 Hillsborough Street
Raleigh, NC 27606

Peter J. Pascoe, BVSc
DACVA, DECVA
Professor
Department of Surgical and Radiological Sciences
School of Veterinary Medicine
University of California
Davis, CA 95616-8745

Lysa P. Posner, DVM
Diplomate ACVA
Associate Professor
Anesthesiology Section
Department of Molecular Biomedical Sciences
North Carolina State University
College of Veterinary Medicine
4700 Hillsborough Street
Raleigh, NC 27606

Srujana Rayalam, BVSc, MVSc
The University of Georgia
College of Veterinary Medicine
Athens, GA 30602

Doodipala Samba Reddy, R.Ph., Ph.D.
Associate Professor
Dept of Neuroscience and Experimental Therapeutics College of Medicine
Texas A&M Health Science Center
228 Reynolds Medical Building
College Station, Texas 77843

Jim E. Riviere, DVM, PhD DSc(hon)
Director and Distinguished Professor
Center for Chemical Toxicology Research and Pharmacokinetics
Department of Population Health and Pathobiology
North Carolina State University
College of Veterinary Medicine
4700 Hillsborough Street
Raleigh, NC 27606

Juan M. Sallovitz, Med Vet, PhD
Research Fellow
Laboratorio de Farmacologis
Departamento de Fisiopatologia
Facultad de Ciencias Veterinarias
Universidad Nacional del Centro
Campus Universitario
(7000) Tandil
Argentina

Sergio F. Sanchez Bruni, Med Vet, PhD
Associate Professor
Laboratorio de Farmacologis
Departamento de Fisiopatologia
Facultad de Ciencias Veterinarias
Universidad Nacional del Centro
Campus Universitario
(7000) Tandil
Argentina

Stefan Schuber, PhD
Director
Scientific Reports
United States Pharmacopeia
12601 Twinbrook Parkway
Rockville, MD 20852-1790

Maya Scott, DVM, PhD
4466 TAMU
Veterinary Physiology and Pharmacology
Texas A & M University
College Station, TX 77843-4466

Barbara L. Sherman, MS, PhD, DVM
DACVB
Clinical Associate Professor
Department of Clinical Sciences
College of Veterinary Medicine
North Carolina State University
4700 Hillsborough Street
Raleigh, NC 27606-1496

Geof W. Smith, DVM, PhD
Assistant Professor
Department of Population Health and Pathobiology
College of Veterinary Medicine
North Carolina State University
4700 Hillsborough Street
Raleigh, NC 27606

Eugene P. Steffey, MVD, PhD
Professor
Department of Surgical & Radiological Sciences
School of Veterinary Medicine
University of California
2112 Tupper Hall
Davis, California 95616

Stephen F. Sundlof, DVM, PhD
DABVT
Director
Center for Food Safety and Applied Nutrition
U. S. Food and Drug Administration
5100 Paint Branch Parkway
College Park, MD 20740

Lisa A. Tell, DVM
Professor
Diplomate ABVP, Diplomate ACZM
Food Animal Residue Avoidance Databank and National Research Project 7
Department of Medicine and Epidemiology
School of Veterinary Medicine
University of California
One Shields Avenue
Davis, CA 95616

Pierre-Louis Toutain, DVM, Dr Sci
Diplomate ECVPT
UMR 181 Physiopathologie et Toxicologie Experimentales
INRA/ENVT
Ecole Nationale Veterinaire de Toulouse
23 chemin des Capelles—BP 87614
31076 TOULOUSE cedex 03 FRANCE

Guillermo L. Virkel, Med Vet, PhD
Lecturer
Laboratorio de Farmacologis
Departamento de Fisiopatologia
Facultad de Ciencias Veterinarias
Universidad Nacional del Centro
Campus Universitario
(7000) Tandil
Argentina

Alistair Webb, BVSc, PhD
FRCVS, MRCA, DVA, Diplomate ACVA
Department Physiological Sciences
College of Veterinary Medicine
University of Florida
PO Box 100144
Gainesville, FL 32610-0144

Keith Zientek, PhD
Senior Scientist
Bioanalytical Systems, Inc.
3138 NE Rivergate, Bldg. 301C
McMinnville, OR 97128

PREFACE

Welcome to the ninth edition of *Veterinary Pharmacology and Therapeutics*, the first edition of which was authored some 6 decades ago by Dr. L. Meyer Jones, a father of American veterinary pharmacology. As with previous editions, this book remains dedicated to veterinary medical students enrolled in professional schools and colleges of veterinary medicine. However, this book also has a broader audience in that veterinary medicine interns and residents, graduate students in comparative biomedical sciences, laboratory animal specialists, and researchers using animals have adopted this as the standard source for information available on comparative pharmacology.

The present edition is both an outgrowth of, and extension to, the eighth edition edited by H. Richard Adams. The major changes are focused on integrating topics covered in the traditional drug-specific chapters to several new chapters covering their applications in areas such as minor species or racing animals. The chapters on treatment of clinical problems are also greatly expanded to integrate the basic concepts discussed in earlier sections of the book with management of clinical diseases. This allows a discussion of pharmacological concepts from a different perspective than basic pharmacology, because drugs that are used throughout veterinary medicine in applications under different clinical scenarios often need further explanation. To accomplish our goals, experts in the clinical specialty areas and pharmacologists with expertise in specific areas have contributed tremendously to this edition of the textbook. A number of "traditional chapters" were completely revamped and revised by new contributors and other previous chapters were updated. We have attempted to provide an international perspective to this new edition by adding international authors and including drugs that have been used all over the world.

Veterinary pharmacology is in the process of great change and advancement. For many years, veterinary pharmacology was simply an extension of human pharmacology as common human medications were extrapolated for use in animal diseases. However, in the new millennium, there has been a greater emphasis by the pharmaceutical companies toward developing animal-specific drugs for their unique indications. Many of these include treatment aimed at quality of life issues in companion animals. As in previous editions, many human drugs—used off-label in animals—also are discussed, with an emphasis on the importance of interspecies differences. Sophisticated therapeutic approaches are being developed and utilized on a routine basis. New drug entities are being used and a more precise utilization of existing medications is employed in clinical practice. Antimicrobial and antiparasitic drugs must be used in a more intelligent and prudent fashion to avoid development of resistance that can impact both animals and human public health. Human food safety concerns regarding drugs used in food-producing animals have taken on increased concern. All these developments lead to both growth and a broadening of this discipline, which is central to the practice of veterinary medicine.

One of the most important applications of this textbook will be as a supplement and reference source for instructors teaching veterinary pharmacology to professional veterinary students, graduate students, and veterinary technicians. To accommodate this use, the chapters have been organized logically in an order and format that will support the teaching of veterinary pharmacology to students. Whenever possible, helpful tables, diagrams, and charts are provided to facilitate learning. Teaching veterinary pharmacology to students has changed tremendously since the early editions of this textbook. Because of the tremendous explosion in the number of drugs available, it is no longer possible to cover every drug and every indication in a veterinary course. Therefore, this book is intended to be a supplement to a veterinary pharmacology course for the student to have access to more in-depth and comprehensive information than can be presented in course lectures.

In addition to the many authors that have contributed to this edition of *Veterinary Pharmacology and Therapeutics,* we owe a special thanks to the previous editor, and consulting editor for this edition, H. Richard Adams. We are proud to carry on as editors with the hope of continuing the excellence and quality that was a characteristic of the editions that he edited. We are also appreciative of the support of the publishers at Wiley-Blackwell. Among these individuals, special thanks go to Dede Andersen, Antonia Seymour, Jill McDonald, and Nancy Simmerman. We also thank Luann Kublin and especially Jeneal Leone, administrative assistants at CCTRP-NCSU, for their help in processing these chapters.

Jim E. Riviere
Mark G. Papich

Veterinary Pharmacology and Therapeutics

Ninth Edition

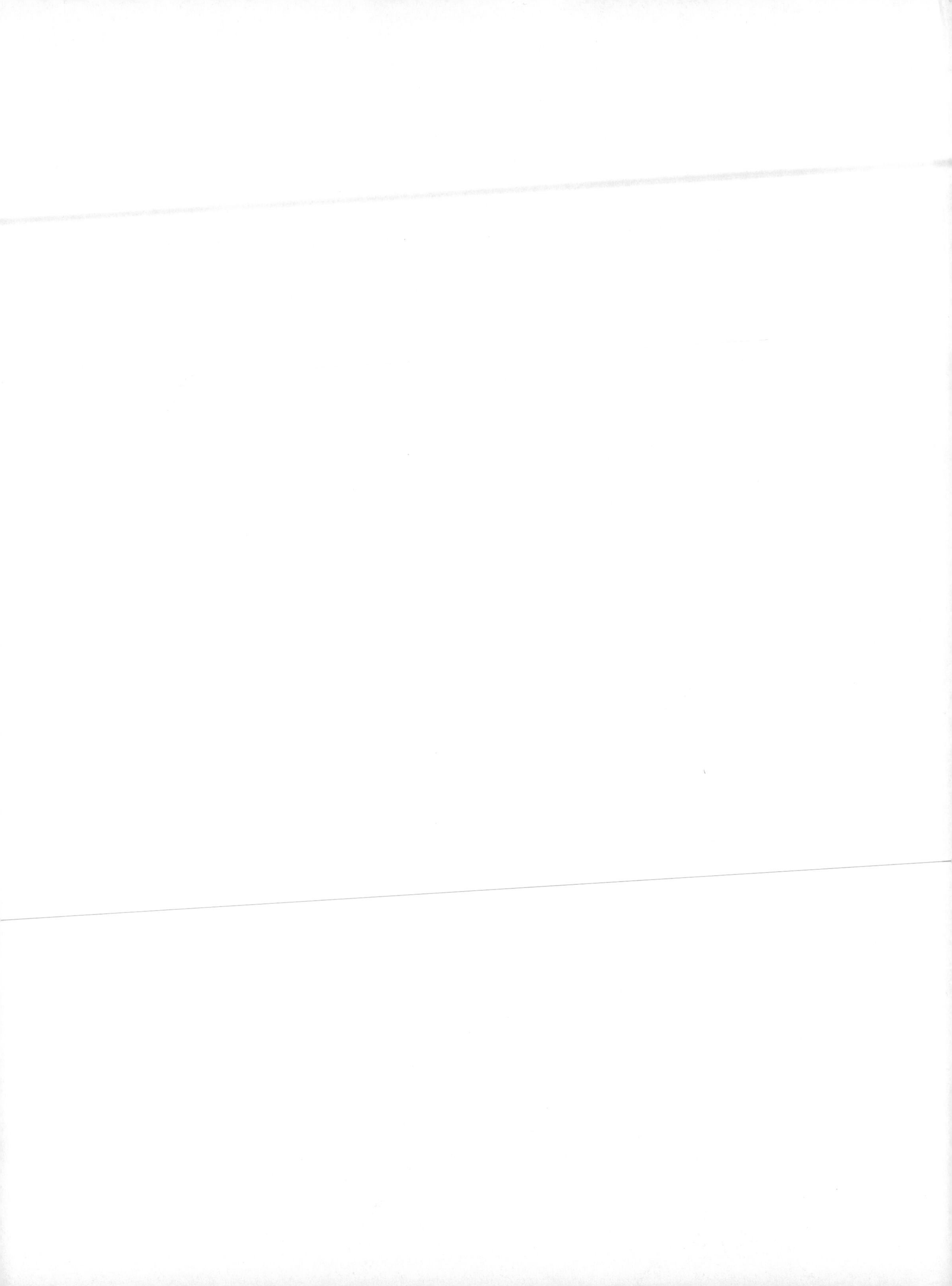

SECTION 1
Principles of Pharmacology

CHAPTER 1

VETERINARY PHARMACOLOGY: AN INTRODUCTION TO THE DISCIPLINE

JIM E. RIVIERE AND MARK G. PAPICH

Pharmacology is the science that broadly deals with the physical and chemical properties, actions, absorption, and fate of chemical substances termed *drugs* that modify biological function. It is a discipline that touches most areas of human and veterinary medicine and closely interfaces with pharmaceutical science and toxicology.

HISTORY OF PHARMACOLOGY

As long as humans and their animals have suffered from disease, chemical substances have played a role in their treatment. Substances obtained from plants and animals or their products were used according to precise prescriptions through antiquity. The mechanism attributed to why these substances worked are deeply rooted in the beliefs and mythologies of each culture, as were the rituals involved in their preparation.

The early history of pharmacology parallels human efforts to compile records of ailments and their remedies. The earliest recorded compilation of drugs, the *Pen Tsao*, consisted of a list of herbal remedies compiled in the reign of Chinese Emperor Shennung in 2700 B.C. Classic examples of medicinal use of chemicals, herbs, and other natural substances are found in the recorded papyri of ancient Egypt. The *Kahun papyrus*, written about 2000 B.C., lists prescriptions for treating uterine disease in women and specifically addresses veterinary medical concerns. The *Ebers papyrus*, written in 1150 B.C. is a collection of folklore covering 15 centuries of history. It is composed of over 800 prescriptions for salves, plasters, pills, suppositories, and other dosage forms used to treat specific ailments.

The ancient Greek philosopher-physicians of 500 B.C. taught that health was maintained by a balance of "humors," which were affected by temperature, humidity, acidity, and sweetness, rather than to the direct actions of gods or demons. Disease was treated by returning these humors to a proper balance. Hippocrates (460–370 B.C.) was an ancient Greek physician of the Age of Pericles. He is referred to as the "father of medicine" in recognition of his lasting contributions to the field as the founder of the Hippocratic school of medicine. He was a firm believer in the healing powers of nature, conducted systematic observations of his patients' symptoms, and began moving the practice of medicine from an art to a systematic clinical science. The first true *material medica*, a compilation of therapeutic substances and their uses, was compiled in 77 A.D. by Aristotle's student Dioscorides, while serving as a surgeon in Nero's Roman Legion traveling throughout the

Mediterranean. This served as the basis for the later works of Galen (131–201) that emerged as the authoritative material medica for the next 1,400 years! In fact, some pharmaceutical preparations consisting of primarily herbal or vegetable matter are still referred to as galenical preparations. As the Dark Ages descended upon Europe, such scholarship transferred to Byzantium, where in fact a veterinary compilation for farm animal treatments, *Publius Vegetius,* was compiled in the 5th century.

It took until the Renaissance to awaken the spirit of discovery in Europe. The Swiss physician Theophrastus Bombastus von Hohenheim (1492–1541), known as Paracelsus, introduced the clinical use of laudanum (opium) and a number of tinctures (extracts) of various plants, some of which are still in use today. He is remembered for using drugs for specific and directed purposes, and for the famous dictum "All substances are poisons; there is none which is not a poison. The proper dose separates a poison from a remedy." As these practices took root, official compilations of medicinal substances, their preparation, use, and dosages, started to appear in Europe. These publications, termed *pharmacopeia,* provided a unifying framework upon which the pharmaceutical sciences emerged. The first printed pharmacopeia, titled the *Dispensatorium* was published by Valerius Cordus in 1547 in Nuremberg, Germany. Local publications emerged in different European cities, with two pharmacopeias published in London in 1618. The *Edinburgh Pharmacopoeia* published in 1689 became the most influential during this period. It took until the mid-19th century before truly national pharmacopeias took hold, with the first *United States Pharmacopeia* published in 1820. The first *United States Pharmacopeia* has been given the title USP-0; the current edition of the *United States Pharmacopeia* is titled USP-30. There was also a British pharmacopeia published in 1864 and the *British Pharmacopeia* continues to be published today.

The history of pharmacology parallels the development of modern medicine and the realization that specific natural products and substances may cure specific diseases. The 16th and 17th centuries were marked by great explorations and the beginning of medical experimentation. In 1656, Sir Christopher Wren made the first intravenous injection of opium in a dog. The bark of the cinchona tree was brought by Jesuits from South America for use of treatment of malaria. In 1783, the English physician William Withering reported on his experience in the use of extracts from the foxglove plant to treat patients with "dropsy," a form of edema most likely caused by congestive heart failure.

In the early 1800s the French physiologist-pharmacologist Megendie, working with the pharmacist Pelletier, studied the effects of intravenous injections of ipecac, morphine, strychnine, and other substances on animals. Megendie was the first to prove that chemicals can be absorbed into the vascular system to exert a systemic effect. A prolific scientist, he also published a formulary that survived through eight editions from 1821–1836. The Spanish physician Orfila published the results of many experiments in a book entitled *Toxicologie Generale* in 1813. A student of Megendie, the famous physiologist Claude Bernard, and others showed in the mid-1800s that the active ingredient of foxglove botanical preparations was digitalis, and its action was on the heart. We continue to use digoxin today for the treatment of congestive heart failure in humans and animals. The important aspect of these early studies was that they used the experimental paradigm for demonstrating chemical activity, establishing both the philosophy and methods upon which the discipline of modern pharmacology is based.

The term *Pharmakologie* was applied to the study of material medica by Dale in London as early as 1692; however, it is generally regarded that the biochemist Rudolph Buchheim in the Baltic city of Dorpat established the first true experimental laboratory dedicated to pharmacology in the mid-18th century. He published some 118 contributions on a variety of drugs and their actions, and argued for pharmacology to be a separate discipline distinct from material medica, pharmacy, and chemistry. His work included in 1849 a textbook *Beiträge zur Ärzneimittellehre,* which classified drugs based on their pharmacological action in living tissue. He deleted traditional remedies if he could not demonstrate their action in his laboratory. This is the beginning of what we now know as *evidence-based pharmacology,* which requires that a chemical be termed a drug only if a specific action in living tissues can be demonstrated.

His student, Oswald Schmiedeberg, became a Professor of Pharmacology at the University of Strasbourg in 1872 and took upon himself the goal of making pharmacology an independent scientific discipline based upon precise experimental methodology that ultimately displaced material medica in medical school curriculums throughout Europe by the end of the 19th century and by the early 20th century in America. He studied the correlation between the chemical structure of substances and their effectiveness as narcotics. He published some 200 publications as well as an authoritative textbook in 1883 that went through seven editions. This text classified drugs by their actions and separated experimental pharmacology from therapeutics. In addition he founded and edited the first pharmacology journal *Archiv für experimentelle Pathologie und Pharmakologie* in 1875, which in 2007 published volume 375 as *Naunym-Schmiedeberg's Archives of Pharmacology.* His more than 150 students spread the discipline of pharmacology throughout Europe and America.

One of his students, Dr. John Abel, held the first full-time professorship in pharmacology at the University of Michigan and is considered by some to be the father of American pharmacology. Professor Abel then moved to Johns Hopkins Medical School where he continued his basic pharmacological research and founded the *Journal of Biological Chemistry* as well as the *Journal of Pharmacology and Experimental Therapeutics.* He was instrumental in founding the *American Society of Pharmacology and Experimental Therapeutics* in 1908.

From these origins, the various disciplines of pharmacology grew, the common factor being the focus in experimental methods to discover and confirm drug actions. Today, the basic philosophy remains unchanged, although modern techniques are grounded in analytical chemistry, mathematical models, and the emerging science of genomics.

VETERINARY PHARMACOLOGY

The development of veterinary pharmacology generally paralleled that of human pharmacology. However, there is archeological evidence of an Indian military hospital for horses and elephants from 5000 B.C., at which time there also existed an extensive medical education program at the Hindu university at Takkasila. The formal discipline of veterinary pharmacology has its origins in the establishment of veterinary colleges and hospitals in France, Austria, Germany, and the Netherlands in the 1760s as a response to epidemics of diseases such as rinderpest that decimated animal populations throughout Western Europe. The Royal College of Veterinary Surgeons was established in London in 1791 followed in 1823 by the Royal (Dick) School of Veterinary Studies in Edinburgh. The earliest veterinary colleges were established in the United States in 1852 in Philadelphia and in Boston in 1854; however, both were short-lived. Modern existing North American veterinary schools founded in the late 1800s, and which continue in operation, include those in Iowa, Ohio, Ontario, Pennsylvania, and New York.

In these early colleges, teaching of pharmacology in veterinary schools was essentially material medica, and remained closely aligned with parallel efforts occurring in medical schools, especially when colleges were colocated on the same campuses. This was evident in the European schools, with a separation really occurring in the 20th century. However, this linkage was not absolute. An early mid-19th century veterinary textbook *The Veterinarian's Vade Mecum* was published by John Gamgee in England. It was essentially a material medica and did not reflect the biological-based classification system for substances used by Professor Buchheim in the same period. The first American professor of therapeutics at the School of Veterinary Medicine at Iowa State was a physician, D. Fairchild. Similarly, a textbook of veterinary pharmacology *Veterinary Material Medica and Therapeutics* published by the School of Veterinary Medicine at Harvard was authored by Kenelm Winslow, a veterinarian and physician. This book, an 8th Edition of which was published in 1919, began to follow the modern thrust described earlier of relating drug actions to biological effects on tissues. It seems veterinary medicine's 21st-century preoccupation with the "one-medicine" concept has deep historical roots.

The important event, which fully shifted veterinary pharmacology from one focused on material medica to the actual science of pharmacology, was the publication by Professor L. Meyer Jones in 1954 of the 1st Edition of the textbook you are now reading. From this point forward, veterinary pharmacology positions have existed in Colleges of Veterinary Medicine throughout the world, the structure of which are often a reflection of local university history, priorities, and academic structure.

Organized veterinary pharmacology occurred rather simultaneously in Europe and the Americas. The American Academy of Veterinary Pharmacology and Therapeutics (AAVPT) was founded in 1977 and the European Association for Veterinary Pharmacology and Toxicology (EAVPT) in 1978. These two organizations, together with the British Association for Veterinary Clinical Pharmacology and Therapeutics, launched the *Journal of Veterinary Pharmacology and Therapeutics* (JVPT) in 1978. Its founder, Dr. Andrew Yoxall, hoped that the journal would improve coordination and communication among pharmacologists and veterinary clinicians, and designed it for the publication of topics relating both to the clinical aspects of veterinary pharmacology, and to the fundamental pharmacological topics of veterinary relevance. Now in its 30th year of publication, and also cosponsored by both the American College of Veterinary Clinical Pharmacology (ACVCP) and the Chapter of Veterinary Pharmacology of the Australian College of Veterinary Scientists, this journal remains the primary outlet for publication of veterinary-related science-based pharmacology investigations.

The discipline of clinical pharmacology is more directly related to applying pharmacological principles—particularly pharmacokinetics—to clinical patients. Fellows of the AAVPT formed the AVMA-recognized board certified specialty—the American College of Veterinary Clinical Pharmacology (ACVCP)—in 1991. The establishment of the ACVCP paralleled the establishment of the American Board of Clinical Pharmacology (ABCP)—the human medical counterpart—in the same year with the cooperation of the American College of Clinical Pharmacology.

REGULATIONS

A different perspective of the development of veterinary pharmacology over the last century is the development of regulatory bodies to insure that safe, effective, and pure drugs reach commerce. As discussed above, *material medica* and *pharmacopeia* were in large part the force that held pharmacology together as a discipline for centuries. Since 1820, the *United States Pharmacopeia (USP),* a private, not-for-profit organization, has endeavored to establish standards for strength, quality, purity, packaging, and labeling for all manufacturers of pharmaceutical substances in the United States. It took until 1990, under the pressure of Dr. Lloyd Davis, one of the founding fathers of AAVPT and ACVCP, to have USP specifically develop Committees to develop USP standards and information for veterinary drugs. Until this time, veterinary drugs whose manufacturers desired the "USP Label" processed drugs through committees that were largely populated by experts in human pharmaceutical sciences and medicine.

In the 20th century, due to the proliferation of charlatans and fraud in manufacture and distribution of so-called "pure" medicinal products, coupled with serious human health calamities due to nonregulated drugs reaching the market, Congress in 1927 established the Food, Drug and Insecticide Administration, which later became known as the Food and Drug Administration (FDA). In 1938, the pivotal Federal Food, Drug and Cosmetic Act was passed giving FDA the authority to regulate animal drugs by requiring evidence of product safety before distribution. In 1959, a veterinary medical branch was developed as a division and the Food Additive Amendments Act was passed, which gave FDA authority over animal food additives and drug residues in animal-derived foods. A Bureau of Veterinary Medicine, with Dr. M. Clarkson as its first director, was established in 1965 to handle the increasing regulatory responsibilities of animal drugs. Today, the FDA Center for Veterinary Medicine, directed by Dr. Bernadette Dunham, is the primary regulatory body for veterinary drugs in the United States. The interested reader should consult Chapters 54 and 55 of the present text for a more in-depth discussion of the current state of veterinary regulatory authority.

WHAT IS VETERINARY PHARMACOLOGY?

As can be appreciated from the breadth of material covered by the present textbook, veterinary pharmacology covers all aspects of using chemical and biological substances to treat diseases of animals. The basic principles of drug action are identical across veterinary and human pharmacology. Thus the principles of absorption, distribution, metabolism, and elimination covered here are the same as in any human pharmacology text, except for a focus on crucial species differences in anatomy, physiology, or metabolism that would alter these processes. The topics of pharmacodynamics, pharmacogenomics, and pharmacokinetics are also species-independent in basic concepts. These topics encompass what truly should be termed *comparative pharmacology*.

The subspecialties of veterinary pharmacology cover all those seen in human pharmacology, the classification of which can be seen from the division of the present text. These include classifying drugs as acting on the nervous, inflammatory, cardiovascular, renal, endocrine, reproductive, ocular, gastrointestinal, respiratory, and dermal systems as well as those used in chemotherapy of microbial, parasitic, and neoplastic diseases. Because of the potential exposure and heavy parasite load of both companion and production animals, antiparasitic drugs will get deeper coverage than seen in a human pharmacology text. There are a number of specialty areas that also reflect unique aspects of veterinary medicine, including aquatic and avian species, as well as aspects of regulations related to using drugs in food-producing animals with the resulting production of chemical residues and potential human food safety issues. This is simply not an issue in human medicine.

The discipline is often simply divided into basic and clinical pharmacology, the distinction being whether studies are conducted in healthy or diseased animals, studying experimental models or natural disease states, or involve laboratory or clinical studies in an actual veterinary clinical situation. However, the common denominator that separates a veterinary pharmacologist from his/her human pharmacology colleagues is dealing with species differences in both disposition and action of drugs.

Comparative pharmacology is the true common theme that courses through the blood of all veterinary pharmacologists, be they basic or clinical in orientation. How does a drug behave in the species being treated? Is the disease pathophysiology similar across species? Do dosages need to be adjusted? Are microbial susceptibilities for pathogens different? Is a drug absorbed, eliminated, or metabolized differently in this species or breed? Can the dosage form developed for a dog be used in an equine patient? Are there unique individual variations in the population due to pharmacogenomic variability that would alter a drug's effect in this patient? Are there unique species-specific toxicological effects for the drug in this patient? Is there a potential for drug-drug, drug-diet, or drug-environment interactions? Will this animal or its products be consumed by humans as food, and thus are potential residues from drug therapy a concern? All of these questions are addressed in the chapters that follow in this textbook.

The focus of veterinary pharmacology is to provide a rational basis for the use of drugs in a clinical setting in different animal species. These principles are fully discussed in the remainder of this text. The practicing veterinarian should appreciate every day that when a drug is given to a patient in his/her care, an experiment in clinical pharmacology is being conducted. The astute and successful practitioner will use principles of pharmacology to assure that the correct drug and dosage regimen is selected for the diagnosis in hand, that proper clinical outcomes will be assessed for both assuring efficacy and avoiding adverse effects, and finally that if a food-producing animal is being treated, proper caution is taken to insure the safety of animal-derived products to the human consumer.

REFERENCES AND ADDITIONAL READING

Andersen, L. and Higby, G.J. 1995. The Spirit of Voluntarism. A Legacy of Commitment and Contribution. The United States Pharmacopeia 1820–1995. Rockville, MD: The United States Pharmacopeial Convention.

Center for Veterinary Medicine, Food and Drug Administration. 2007. A Brief History of the Center for Veterinary Medicine. http://www/fda.gov/cvm/aboutbeg.htm.

Davis, L.E. 1982. Veterinary Pharmacology—An Introduction to the Discipline. In Booth, N.J. and McDonald, L.E. (eds.) Veterinary Pharmacology and Therapeutics, 5th Ed. Ames: Iowa State University Press, pp. 1–7.

Jones, L.M. 1977. Veterinary Pharmacology—Past, Present, and Future. In Jones, L.M., Booth, N.J., and McDonald, L.E. (eds.) Veterinary Pharmacology and Therapeutics, 4th Ed. Ames: Iowa State University Press, pp. 3–15.

Parascandola, J. 1992. The Development of American Pharmacology: John J. Abel and the Shaping of a Discipline. Baltimore: Johns Hopkins University Press.

USP 30-NF 25. United States Pharmacopeial Convention. 12601 Twinbrook Parkway, Rockville, Maryland 20852. (www.usp.org).

Van Miert, A.S.J.P.A.M. 2006. The Roles of EAVPT, ECVPT and EAVPT Congresses in the advancement of veterinary pharmacological and toxicological science. Journal of Veterinary Pharmacology and Therapeutics 29(Suppl. 1):9–11.

CHAPTER

2

ABSORPTION, DISTRIBUTION, METABOLISM, AND ELIMINATION

JIM E. RIVIERE

The four key physiological processes that govern the time course of drug fate in the body are absorption, distribution, metabolism, and elimination, the so-called *ADME processes.* Pharmacokinetics, the study of the time course of drug concentrations in the body, provides a means of quantitating ADME parameters. When applied to a clinical situation, pharmacokinetics provides the practitioner with a useful tool to design optimally beneficial drug dosage schedules for each individual patient. In the research and premarketing phase of drug development, it is an essential component in establishing effective yet safe dosage forms and regimens. An understanding of pharmacokinetic principles allows more rational therapeutic decisions to be made. In food animals, pharmacokinetics provides the conceptual underpinnings for understanding and utilizing the withdrawal time to prevent violative drug residues from persisting in the edible tissues of food-producing animals. A working knowledge of this discipline provides the framework upon which many aspects of pharmacology can be integrated into a rational plan for drug usage.

AN OVERVIEW OF DRUG DISPOSITION

To fully appreciate the ADME processes governing the fate of drugs in animals, the various steps involved must be defined and ultimately quantitated. The processes relevant to a discussion of the absorption and disposition of a drug administered by the intravenous (IV), intramuscular (IM), subcutaneous (SC), oral (PO), or topical (TOP) routes are illustrated in Figure 2.1. The normal reference point for pharmacokinetic discussion and analysis is the concentra-

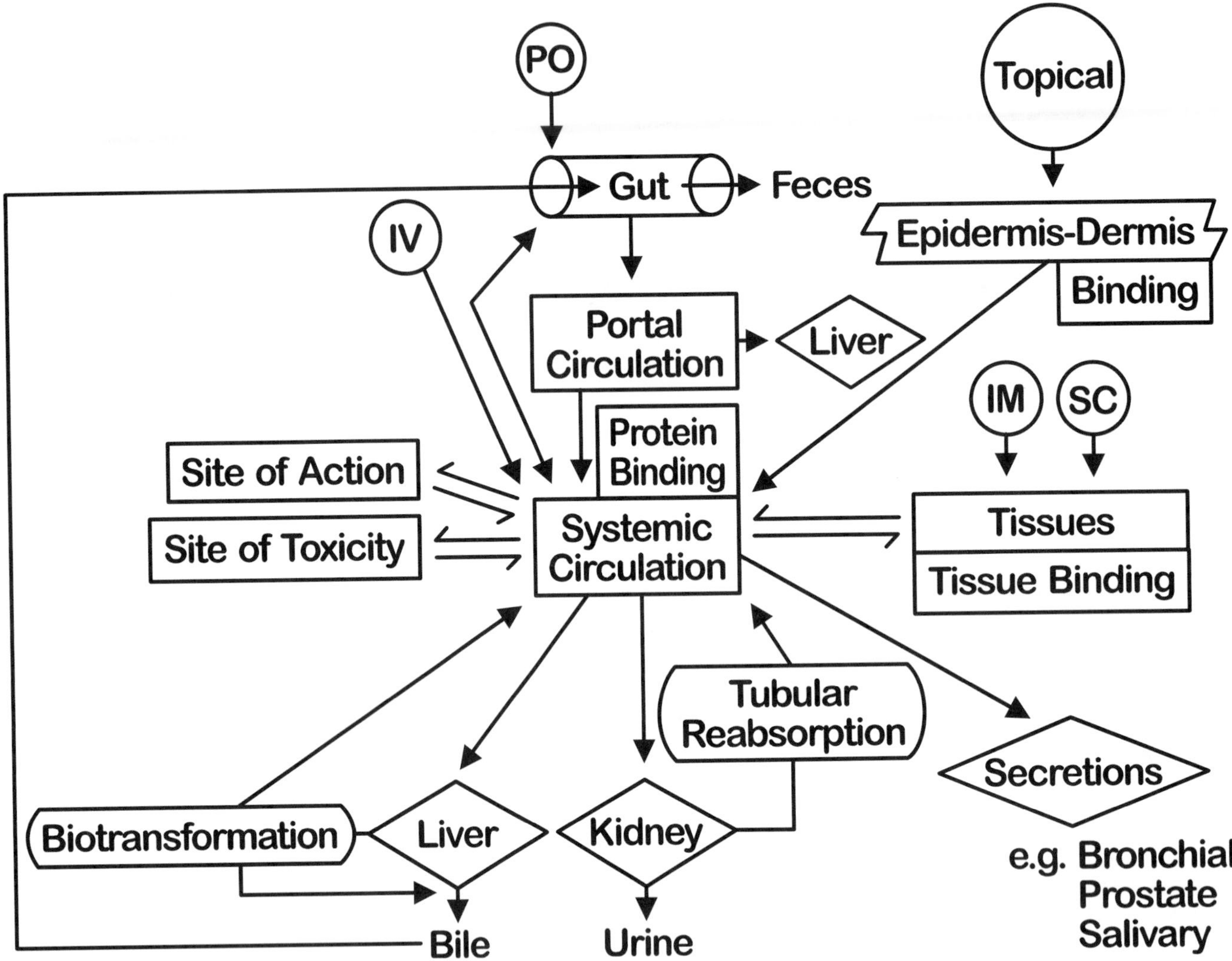

FIG. 2.1 Basic schema by which drug is absorbed, distributed, metabolized, and excreted from the body. These processes are those that form the basis for developing pharmacokinetic models.

tion of free, non–protein-bound drug dissolved in the serum (or plasma), because this is the body fluid that carries the drug throughout the body and from which samples for drug analysis can be readily and repeatedly collected. For the majority of drugs studied, concentrations in the systemic circulation are in equilibrium with the extracellular fluid of well-perfused tissues; thus, serum or plasma drug concentrations generally reflect extracellular fluid drug concentrations.

A fundamental axiom of using pharmacokinetics to predict drug effect is that the drug must be present at its site of action in a tissue at a sufficient concentration for a specific period of time to produce a pharmacologic effect. Since tissue concentrations of drugs are reflected by extracellular fluid and thus serum drug concentrations, a pharmacokinetic analysis of the disposition of drug in the scheme outlined in Figure 2.1 is useful to assess the activity of a drug in the in vivo setting.

This conceptualization is especially important in veterinary medicine where species differences in any of the ADME processes may significantly affect the extent and/or time course of drug absorption and disposition in the body. By dividing the overall process of drug fate into specific phases, this relatively complex situation can be more easily handled. It is the purpose of this chapter to overview the physiological basis of absorption, distribution, metabolism, (biotransformation) and elimination. This will provide a basis for the chapter on pharmacoki-

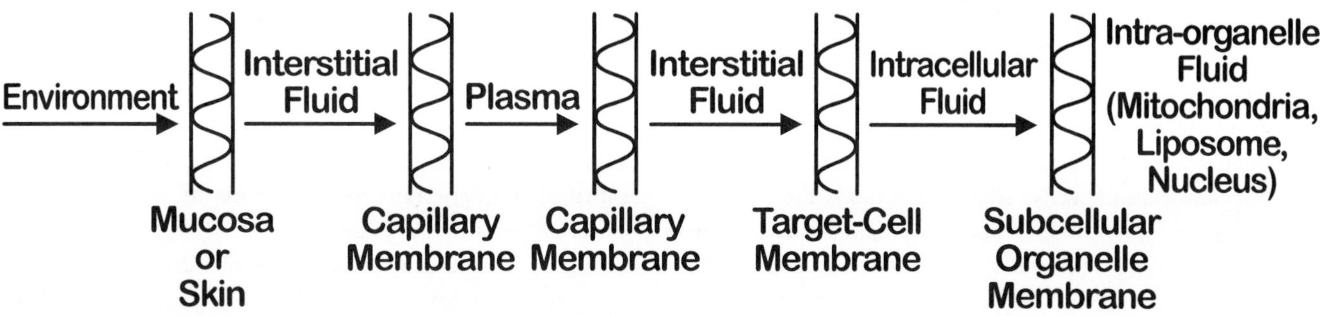

FIG. 2.2 Illustration of how absorption, distribution, and excretion is essentially a journey of the drug through various lipoidal membrane barriers.

netics that will deal with quantitating these processes in more detail.

Despite the myriad of anatomical and physiological differences among animals, the biology of drug absorption and distribution, and in some cases even elimination, is very similar in that it involves drug molecules crossing a series of biological membranes. As illustrated in Figure 2.2, these membranes may be associated with either several layers of cells (tissue) or a single cell, and both living and dead protoplasm may be involved. Despite the different biochemical and morphological attributes of each of these membranes, a unifying concept of biology is the basic similarity of all membranes, whether they be tissue, cell, or organelle. Although the specific biochemical components may vary, the fundamental organization is the same. This fact simplifies the understanding of the major determinants of drug absorption, distribution, and excretion.

These membrane barriers often directly or indirectly define the nature of compartments or other mathematical modules in pharmacokinetic models. Biological spaces are defined by the restrictions on drug movement imposed by these barriers. The most effective barriers are those that protect the organism from the external environment. These include the skin as well as various segments of the gastrointestinal and respiratory tract, which also protect the internal physiologic milieu from the damaging external environment. However, the gastrointestinal and respiratory barriers are modified deep within the body to allow for nutrient and gas exchange vital for life. The interstitial fluid is a common compartment through which any drug must transit either after absorption on route to the blood stream or after delivery by blood to a tissue on route to a cellular target. Capillary membranes interfacing with this interstitial fluid compartment are relatively porous due to the fenestrae that allow large molecules to exchange between tissues and blood. Membranes define homogeneous tissue compartments and membranes must be traversed in all processes of drug absorption and disposition.

All cellular membranes appear to be primarily lipid bilayers into which are embedded proteins that may reside on either surface (intra- or extracellular) or traverse the entire structure. The lipid leaflets are arranged with hydrophilic (polar) head groups on the surface and hydrophobic (nonpolar) tails forming the interior. The specific lipid composition varies widely across different tissues and levels of biological organization. The location of the proteins in the lipid matrix is primarily a consequence of their hydrophobic regions residing in the lipid interior and their hydrophilic and ionic regions occupying the surface. This is thermodynamically the most stable configuration. Changes in the fluidity of the lipids alter protein conformations, which then may modulate their activity. This is the primary mechanism of action for gaseous anesthetics. In some cases, aqueous channels form from integral proteins that traverse the membrane. In other cases, these integral proteins may actually be enzymatic transport proteins that function as active or facilitative transport systems. The primary pathway for drugs to cross these lipid membranes is by passive diffusion through the lipid environment.

Thus, in order for a drug to be absorbed or distributed throughout the body, it must be able to pass through a lipid membrane on some part of its sojourn through the body. In some absorption sites and in many capillaries, fenestrated pores exist, which allow some flow of small molecules. This is contrasted to some protected sites of the body (e.g., brain, cerebral spinal fluid) where additional membranes (e.g., glial cells) may have to be traversed before a drug arrives at its target site. These specialized membranes could be considered a general adaptation to further shelter susceptible tissues from hostile lipophilic chemicals. In this case, drug characteristics that promote transmembrane diffusion would favor drug action and effect (again unless specific transport systems intervene).

This general phenomenon of the enhanced absorption and distribution of lipophilic compounds is a unifying tenet that runs throughout the study of drug fate. The body's elimination organs can also be viewed as operating along a somewhat similar principle. The primary mechanism by which a chemical can be excreted from the body is by becoming less lipophilic and more hydrophilic, the latter property being required for excretion in the aqueous fluids of the urinary or biliary systems. When a hydrophilic or polar drug is injected into the bloodstream, it will be minimally distributed and rapidly excreted by one of these routes. However, if a compound's lipophilicity evades this easy excretion, the liver and other organs may metabolize it to less lipophilic and more hydrophilic metabolites that have a restricted distribution (and thus reduced access to sites for activity) in the body and can be more readily excreted. This basic tenet runs throughout all aspects of pharmacology and is a useful concept to predict effects of unknown compounds.

DRUG PASSAGE ACROSS MEMBRANES

Considerable evidence exists that lipid-based membranes are permeable to nonpolar lipid-soluble compounds and polar water-soluble compounds with sufficient lipid solubility to diffuse through the hydrophobic regions of the membrane. The rate of diffusion of a compound across a membrane is directly proportional to its concentration gradient across the membrane, lipid\water partition coefficient, and diffusion coefficient. This can be summarized by Fick's Law of Diffusion in Equation 2.1:

$$\begin{array}{l}\text{Rate of}\\ \text{diffusion}\\ \text{(mg/sec)}\end{array} = \frac{\text{D (cm/sec) P}}{\text{h (cm)}}(\text{X}_1 - \text{X}_2)(\text{mg}) \qquad (2.1)$$

where D is the diffusion coefficient for the specific penetrant in the membrane being studied, P is the partition coefficient for the penetrant between the membrane and the external medium, h is the thickness or actual length of the path by which the drug diffuses through the membrane, and $X_1 - X_2$ is the concentration gradient (ΔX) across the membrane. The diffusional coefficient of the drug is a function of its molecular size, molecular conformation and solubility in the membrane milieu, and degree of ionization. The partition coefficient is the relative solubility of the compound in lipid and water that reflects the ability of the penetrant to gain access to the lipid membrane. Depending on the membrane, there is a functional molecular size and/or weight cutoff that prevents very large molecules from being passively absorbed across any membrane. When the rate of a process is dependent upon a rate constant (in this case [DP/h] often referred to as the permeability coefficient P) and a concentration gradient, a linear or first-order kinetic process is evident (see Chapter 3 for full discussion). In membrane transfer studies, the total flux of drug across a membrane is dependent on the area of membrane exposed; thus the rate above is often expressed in terms of cm^2. If the lipid : water partition coefficient is too great, depending on the specific membrane, the compound may be sequestered in the membrane rather than traverse it.

Evidence also exists that membranes are more permeable to the nonionized than the ionized form of weak organic acids and bases. If the nonionized moiety has a lipid : water partition coefficient favorable for membrane penetration, it will ultimately reach equilibrium on both sides of the membrane. The ionized form of the drug is completely prevented from crossing the membrane because of its low lipid solubility. The amount of the drug in the ionized or nonionized form depends upon the pKa (negative logarithm of the acidic dissociation constant) of the drug and the pH of the medium on either side of the membrane (e.g., intracellular versus extracellular fluid; gastrointestinal versus extracellular fluid). Protonated weak acids are nonionized (e.g., COOH) while protonated weak bases are ionized (e.g., NH_3+). If the drug has a fixed charge at all pHs encountered inside and outside of the body (e.g., quarternary amines, aminoglycoside antibiotics), they will never cross lipid membranes by diffusion. This would restrict both their absorption and distribution and generally lead to an enhanced rate of elimination. It is the nonionized form of the drug that is governed by Fick's Law of Diffusion and described by Equation 2.1 above. For this equation to predict the movement of a drug across membrane systems in vivo, the relevant pH of each compartment must be considered relative to the compound's pKa; otherwise, erroneous predictions will be made.

When the pH of the medium is equal to the pKa of the dissolved drug, 50% of the drug exists in the ionized state and 50% in the nonionized, lipid soluble state. The ratio of nonionized to ionized drug is given by the Henderson-Hasselbalch equation (Equations 2.2 and 2.3).

For acids:

$$pKa - pH = \log\left[(H\ Acid)^0/(H\ Acid)^-\right] \quad (2.2)$$

For bases:

$$pKa - pH = \log\left[(H\ Base)^+/(H\ Base)^0\right] \quad (2.3)$$

These equations are identical as they involve the ratio of protonated (H) to nonprotonated moieties. The only difference is that for an acid, the protonated form $(H\ Acid)^0$ is neutral while for a base, the protonated form $(H\ Base)^+$ is ionized.

As can be seen by these equations, when the pH is one unit less or one unit more than the pKa for weak bases or acids, respectively, the ratio of ionized to nonionized is 10. Thus each unit of pH away from the pKa results in a tenfold change in this ratio. This phenomenon allows for a drug to be differentially distributed across a membrane in the presence of a pH gradient, an effect that often dwarfs that obtainable by increasing dose to increase drug delivery to a specific tissue. The side of the membrane with the pH favoring ionized drug (high pH for an acidic drug; low pH for an alkaline drug) will tend to have higher total (ionized plus nonionized) drug concentrations. This pH partitioning results in so-called "ion-trapping" in the area where the ionized drug predominates. Figure 2.3 illustrates this concept with an organic acid of pKa = 3.4 partitioning between gastric contents of pH = 1.4 and plasma of pH = 7.4. Assuming that the nonionized form of the drug (U) is in equillibrium across the membrane, then, according to Equations 2.1 and 2.2, there will be a 100-fold

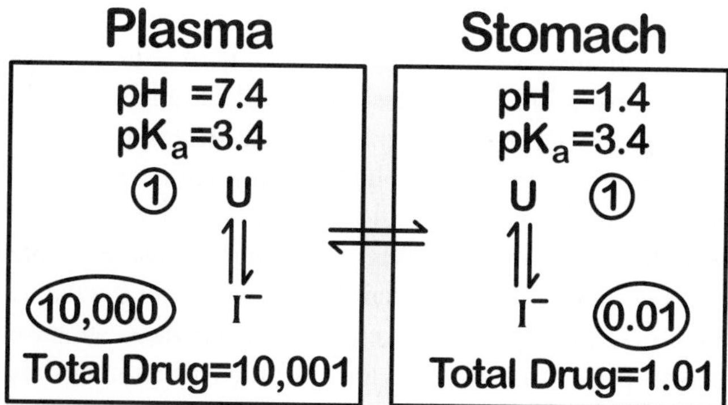

FIG. 2.3 The phenomenon of pH partitioning and ion-trapping of a weak acid.

(log 2; 3.4–1.4) difference on the gastric side and a 10,000-fold (log 4; 7.4–3.4) difference on the plasma side of the membrane, for a transmembrane concentration gradient of total drug (U plus I) equal to 10,001/1.01. Note that the unionized concentration on both sides of the membrane are in equillibrium. It is the total drug concentrations that are different. In this case, the gradient is generated by the difference in pH across an ion-impermeable barrier generated by the local milieu.

Such a gradient would greatly favor the absorption of this weak acid across the gastrointestinal tract into plasma. This is the situation that exists for weak acids such as penicillin, aspirin, and phenylbutazone. In contrast, a weak base would tend to be trapped in this environment and thus minimal absorption would occur. Examples of such weak bases are morphine, phenothiazine, and ketamine. Specific active transport systems may modify these predictions (e.g., beta-lactam transporters in intestines). With the weakly basic strychnine pH-dependent absorption is toxicologically significant. If strychnine were placed into the strongly acidic stomach, no systemic toxicity would be observed. However, if the stomach were then infused with alkali, most of this base would become nonionized, readily absorbed, and lethal. In summary, weak acids are readily absorbed from an acid environment and sequestered in an alkaline medium. In contrast, weak bases are absorbed in an alkaline environment and trapped in an acidic environment.

This pH partitioning phenomenon is not only important in understanding absorption (as illustrated above), but also in any situation where the pH of fluid compartments across a biological membrane is different. It will occur for a drug distributing from plasma (pH = 7.4), to milk (pH = 6.5–6.8), to cerebrospinal fluid (pH = 7.3), or to intracellular sites (pH = 7.0). Thus weakly acidic drugs will tend not to distribute into the milk after systemic distribution (e.g., penicillin) while weakly basic drugs (e.g., erythromycin) will. If a disease process alters the pH of one compartment (e.g., mastitis), the normal equillibrium ratio will also be perturbed. In mastitis, where pH may increase almost one unit, this preferential distribution of basic antibiotics will be lost. The relatively acidic pH of cells relative to plasma is responsible for the relatively large tissue distribution seen with many weakly basic drugs (e.g., morphine, amphetamine). Similarly, in the ruminant, many basic drugs tend to distribute into the rumen, resulting in distribution volumes much larger than those in monogastrics. In fact, a drug that distributes into this organ may then undergo microbial degradation resulting in its elimination from the body.

This phenomenon is also very important for the passive tubular reabsorption of weak acids and bases being excreted by the kidney. For carnivores with acidic urine relative to plasma, weak acids tend to be reabsorbed from the tubules into the plasma while weak bases tend to be preferentially excreted. This principle has been applied to the treatment of salicylate (weak acid) intoxication in dogs where alkaline diuresis promotes ion trapping of the drug in the urine and hence its rapid excretion. Disease-induced changes in urine pH will likewise alter the disposition of drugs sensitive to this phenomenon.

Movement across the fenestrated capillaries of the body from plasma to tissue areas generally allows movement of most drugs. In these cases, relatively small molecules (molecular weights <1,000) can pass through independent of their lipid solubility, but larger molecules are excluded. In all of these scenarios, drugs move through these tissues as a solute dissolved in water and essentially are transported wherever the water goes. This process is termed *bulk-flow* and is dependent on the concentration of drug dissolved in the plasma or tissue fluid. This is a linear process and thus is easily modeled by most pharmacokinetic systems. It is the subsequent uptake into cells and special tissue areas that are governed by the diffusion processes above.

There exists several specialized membranes that possess specific transport systems. In these cases, the laws of diffusion and pH partitioning do not govern transmembrane flux of drugs. These specializations in transport can best be appreciated as mechanisms by which the body can exert control and selectivity over the chemicals that are allowed to enter the protected domain of specific organs, cells, or organelles. Such transport systems can be rather nonspecific, as are those of the kidney and liver that excrete charged waste products.

In the gastrointestinal tract, relatively nonspecific transport systems allow for the absorption, and thus entrance to the body, of essential nutrients that do not have sufficient lipophilicity to cross membranes by diffusion. In specific tissues, they allow for select molecules to enter cells depending upon cellular needs, or allow compounds that circulate throughout the body to have a biological response only in a tissue possessing the correct transport receptor. The primary example is the protein carrier-mediated processes of active transport or facilitated diffusion. These systems are characterized by specificity and saturability. In the case of active transport, biological energy is utilized to move a drug against its concentration gradient. In facilitated diffusion, the carrier protein binds to the drug and carries it across the membrane down its concentration gradient. The drugs transported by these systems normally cannot cross the membrane by passive diffusion because they are not lipophilic. These systems are important for the gastrointestinal absorption of many essential nutrients and some drugs (e.g., beta-lactams), for cellular uptake of many compounds (e.g., glucose), for the removal of drugs from the cerebral spinal fluid through the choroid plexus, and for biliary and renal excretion of numerous drugs.

In some tissues, cells may absorb drugs by endocytosis or pinocytosis, processes where a compound binds to the surface of the membrane that then invaginates and interiorizes the compound. This is not a primary mechanism of transmembrane passage for most therapeutic drugs, although it can affect tissue residue profiles in food-producing animals. Most inorganic ions such as sodium and chloride are sufficiently small that they easily can cross aqueous pores and channels through membranes. The movement of these charged substances is generally governed by the transmembrane electrical potential maintained by active ion pumps.

Finally, active transport may also occur in the opposite direction to remove a drug after it has been absorbed into specific cells or tissue sites. This is called the *P-glycoprotein system,* a class of drug transporters originally associated with multiple drug resistance (MDR) encountered in cancer chemotherapy. MDR transporters have been identified in intestinal epithelial cells, the placenta, kidney tubules, brain endothelial cells, and liver bile canaliculus. These will be addressed throughout this text for specific drug classes.

In conclusion, an understanding of the processes that govern the movement of drugs across lipid-based biological membranes is important to the study of drug absorption, distribution, and excretion. Lipid-soluble drugs are easily absorbed into the body and well distributed throughout the tissues. In contrast, hydrophilic drugs are not well absorbed and have limited distribution but are easily eliminated. Metabolism converts lipophilic drugs to more easily excreted hydrophilic entities. If membranes separate areas of different pH, concentration gradients may form due to pH partitioning or ion trapping. Membranes are the building blocks of biological systems and play a central role in defining the complexity of pharmacokinetic models.

ABSORPTION

Absorption is the movement of the drug from the site of administration into the blood. There are a number of methods available for administering drugs to animals. The primary routes of drug absorption from environmental exposure in mammals are gastrointestinal, dermal, and respiratory. The first two are also used as routes of drug administration for systemic effects, with additional routes including intravenous, intramuscular, subcutaneous, or intraperitoneal injection. Other variations on gastrointestinal absorption include intrarumenal, sublingual, and rectal drug delivery. Many techniques are also used for localized therapy, which may also result in systemic drug absorption as a side effect. These include among others; topical, intramammary, intraarticular, subconjunctival, and spinal fluid injections.

GASTROINTESTINAL ABSORPTION. One of the primary routes of drug administration is oral ingestion of a pill or tablet that is designed to deliver a drug across the gastrointestinal mucosa. The common factor in all forms of oral drug administration is a method to deliver a drug such that it gets into solution in the gastrointestinal fluids from which it can then be absorbed across the mucosa and ultimately reach the submucosal capillaries and the systemic circulation. Examples of oral drug delivery systems include solutions (aqueous, elixirs) and suspensions, pills, tablets, boluses for food animals, capsules, pellets, and sustained release mechanical devices for ruminants. The major obstacle encountered in comparative and veterinary medicine is the enormous interspecies diversity in comparative gastrointestinal anatomy and physiology, which results in major species differences in strategies for and efficiency of oral drug administration. This is often appreciated but overlooked when laboratory animal data is extrapolated to humans. Rats and rabbits are widely utilized in preclinical disposition and toxicology studies, although many investigators fail to appreciate that these species' gastrointestinal tracts are very different from one another and from humans.

From a pharmacologist's perspective, the gastrointestinal tract of all species can be simply presented as diagrammed in Figure 2.4. The GI tract is best conceptualized as actually being part of the external environment, which, in contrast to the skin, is protected and whose microenvironment is closely regulated by the organism. Because of the gastrointestinal tract's central role in digestion and nutrient absorption, there are many evolutionary adaptations to this basically simple mucosa structure that allow for physical, chemical, enzymatic, and microbial breakdown of food for liberation and ultimate absorption of nutrients. This tract is further adapted such that these digestive processes do not harm the organism's own tissues, which in carnivores may be identical to the food being eaten.

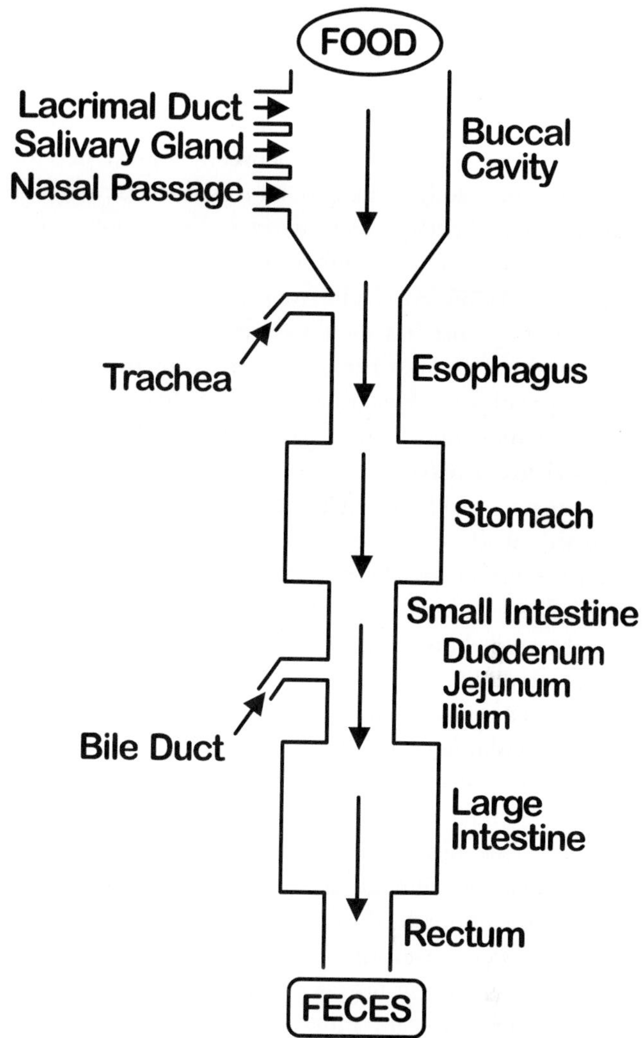

FIG. 2.4 Functional structure of the gastrointestinal tract.

The gastrointestinal tract presents a significant degree of heterogeneity relative to morphology and physiology that translates to great regional variations in drug absorption. In the oral cavity, where food is masticated, some absorption may occur in sublingual areas. In fact, this site is actually utilized as a route for systemic drug (e.g., nitroglycerin) and nicotine (e.g., oral tobacco) delivery. The esophagus and cranial portion of the stomach is lined by cornified epithelium, which provides an effective barrier that often decreases the chance of absorption for drugs formulated for intestinal drug delivery. A great deal of recent research activity has been focused on developing new transbuccal drug delivery systems. As mentioned, the prototype example was sublingual nitroglycerin tablets. Newer systems use novel adhesive technology which allow actual polymer patches to adhere to the buccal mucosa. Such products are also being considered for some therapeutic applications in veterinary medicine (e.g., feline oral sprays). Compared to oral gastrointestinal absorption, buccal delivery bypasses the portal vein and thus eliminates the potential for first-pass hepatic biotransformation, discussed later.

The simple mucosal lining of the stomach allows absorption; however, the presence of surface mucus, which protects the epithelium from self-digestion secondary to acid and enzyme secretion, may be a barrier for some drugs. The acidity and motility of the stomach also creates a hostile environment for drugs and even influences the absorption of drugs farther down the tract. For oral drug absorption to be successful, the drug must be capable of surviving this relatively harsh environment. For some drugs (e.g., penicillin G) susceptible to acid hydrolysis, minimal absorption by the oral route will occur unless they are administered in a formulation that protects them in an acid environment but liberates them in the more alkaline environment of the intestines. Release of the drug from the stomach, a process controlled by gastric emptying, is a major rate-determining step in the onset and duration of oral drug activity.

The primary site for most drug absorption is the small intestine. In this region of the gastrointestinal tract, the pH of the contents are more alkaline and the epithelial lining is conducive to drug absorption. The blood flow to this region is also much greater than to the stomach. The small intestine is lined by simple columnar epithelium resting on a basement membrane and a submucosal tissue bed that is very well perfused by an extensive capillary and lymphatic network. This capillary bed drains into the hepatic portal vein. One of the major anatomical adaptations for absorption in this region is the presence of microvilli, which increase the surface area of the small intestine some 600-fold over that of a simple tube. The second anatomical adaptation are the villi of the intestine, which can be easily appreciated by examining a cross section (Fig. 2.5). Since diffusion is the primary mechanism for drug absorption, the increase in area due to these two anatomical configurations significantly increases absorption, as can be seen from reviewing the area contribution to Equation 2.1. There are species differences in inherent permeability of the intestinal mucosa to chemicals, with the dog recently being recognized as having a higher permeability to many drugs than humans.

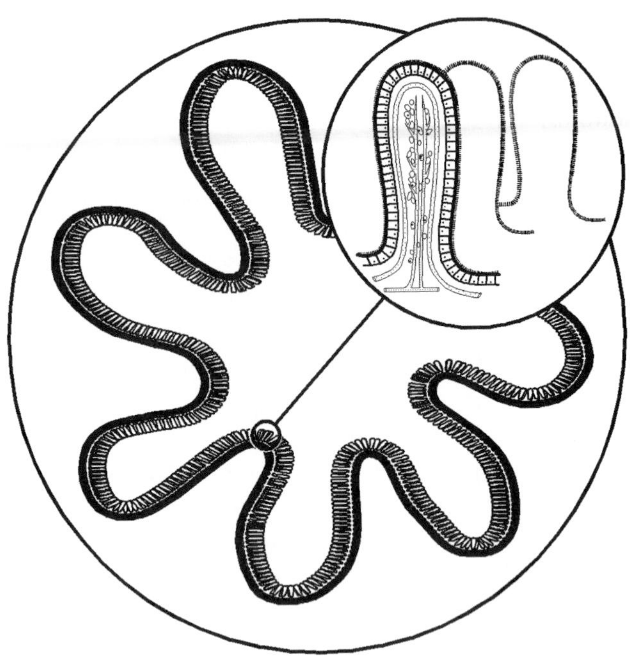

FIG. 2.5 Cross-section of the small intestine showing villi adaptations, which serve to increase surface area available for absorption.

The viable epithelial cells of the intestines are also endowed with the necessary enzymes for drug metabolism that contributes to a second "first-pass" effect. Recent research has also indicated that the mechanism and extent of absorption, and magnitude of local intestinal metabolism, varies between the tips and crypts of the villi. The final determinant of a drug's tortuous journey through the gastrointestinal tract is the resident microbial population that inhabits the intestinal contents. Many bacteria are capable of metabolizing specific drugs, resulting in a third component of the first-pass effect. This epithelial and bacterial biotransformation is generally categorized as *presystemic* metabolism to differentiate it from that which occurs following portal vein delivery of drug to the liver. However, from the perspective of pharmacokinetic analysis of plasma drug concentrations following oral drug administration, all three components are indistinguishable and become lumped into the aggregate process of oral absorption assessed as K_a.

Disintegration, Dissolution, Diffusion, and other Transport Phenomenon. In order for a drug to be absorbed across the intestinal mucosa, the drug must first be dissolved in the aqueous intestinal fluid. Two steps, disintegration and dissolution, may be required for this to occur. *Disintegration* is the process whereby a solid dosage form (e.g., tablet) physically disperses so that its constituent particles can be exposed to the gastrointestinal fluid. Dissolution occurs when the drug molecules then enter into solution. This component of the process is technically termed the *pharmaceutical phase* and is controlled by the interaction of the formulation with the intestinal contents.

Some dosage forms, such as capsules and lozenges, may not be designed to disintegrate, but rather to allow a drug to slowly elute from their surface. Dissolution is often the rate-limiting step controlling the absorption process and can be enhanced by formulating the drug in salt form (e.g., sodium or hydrochloride salts), buffering the preparation (e.g., buffered aspirin), or decreasing dispersed particle size (micronization) so as to maximize exposed surface area. Alternatively, disintegration and dissolution can be decreased so as to deliberately provide slow release of the drug. This strategy is used in *prolonged-release* or *controlled-release* dosage forms and involves complex pharmaceutical formulations that produce different rates of dissolution. This may be accomplished by dispersing the dosage form into particles with different rates of dissolution or by using multilaminated dosage forms, which delays release of the drug until its layer is exposed. All of these strategies decrease the overall rate of absorption. Similar strategies can also be used to target drugs to the distal segments of the gastrointestinal tract by using enteric coatings that dissolve only at specific pH ranges, thereby preventing dissolution until the drug is in the region targeted. This strategy has been applied for colonic delivery of drugs in humans for treatment of Crohn's disease.

In slow-release or long-acting formulations, the end result is that absorption becomes slower than all other distribution and elimination processes, making the pharmaceutical phase the rate-limiting or rate-controlling step in the subsequent absorption and disposition of the drug. When this occurs, as will be seen in the pharmacokinetic modeling chapters to follow, the rate of absorption controls the rate of apparent drug elimination from the body and a so-called *flip-flop* scenario becomes operative.

There are significant species differences in the ability to use controlled-release oral medications designed in humans, by far the largest market, in other species. The first limitation involves the inability to use cellulose-based systems in ruminants due to the ability of rumen microbes to digest the normally inert cellulose matrix that controls rates of drug delivery. The second arises because of shorter gastrointestinal transit times in small carnivores, such as domestic cats and dogs, compared to humans. In this instance, drug release is designed to occur in the longer transit times seen in humans (approx. 24 hours). In dogs and cats which have transit times half that of humans, drug release may still be occurring even after the tablet has been eliminated in the feces due to the shorter transit times. Other examples include the narrower pyloric opening in dogs, compared to humans, that may increase gastric retention of some larger dosage forms. These are but a few examples of significant species differences that, based on anatomical and physiological factors, prevent the ready transferability of complex dosage forms across species.

After the drug is in solution, it must still be in a nonionized relatively lipid-soluble form to be absorbed across the lipid membranes comprising the intestinal mucosa. For orally administered products, the pH of the gastrointestinal contents becomes very important, as is evident from the earlier discussion on pH partitioning. Specifically, a weak acid would tend to be preferentially absorbed in the more acidic environment of the stomach since a larger fraction would be in the nonionized form. However, the much larger surface area and blood flow available for absorption in the more alkaline intestine may override this effect. It is important to mention at this point why a weak acid such as aspirin is better absorbed in a bicarbonate buffered form, which would tend to increase the ionized fraction and thus decrease membrane passage. The paradox is that dissolution must first occur, a process favored by the ionized form of the drug. It is only the dissolved ionized aspirin that is available to the partitioning phenomenon described earlier. Thus, when more aspirin is dissolved in the buffered microenvironment, more is available for partitioning and diffusion across the mucosa. In contrast to the situation of a weak acid, a weak base would tend to be better absorbed in the more alkaline environment. However, it must be repeated that the very large surface area available in the intestines, coupled with high blood flow and a pH of approximately 5.3 in the immediate area of the mucosal surface makes it the primary site of absorption for most drugs (weak acids with pKa >3 and weak bases with pKa <7.8). Species differences in both gastric and intestinal pH further modulate this differential (e.g., canine gastric pH is much higher than humans). A further obstacle to absorption is that the compound must also be structurally stable against chemical or enzymatic attack. Finally, compounds with a fixed charge and/or very low (or very high) lipid solubility for the uncharged moiety, may not be significantly absorbed after oral administration. Examples include the polar aminoglycoside antibiotics, the so-called "enteric" sulfonamides, and quaternary ammonium drugs.

There are also specific active transport systems present within the intestinal mucosa of the microvilli that are responsible for nutrient absorption. However, these systems have a very high capacity and if a specific drug or toxicant has the proper molecular configuration to be transported, saturation is unlikely. There is some evidence that select therapeutic drugs (e.g., beta-lactams such as ampicillin) may be absorbed by active transport systems in the small intestine. There are also transport systems (p-glycoprotein) that expel absorbed drug back into the intestinal lumen. This system is beginning to be studied more closely in veterinary species and will be discussed later in this chapter under distribution and elimination.

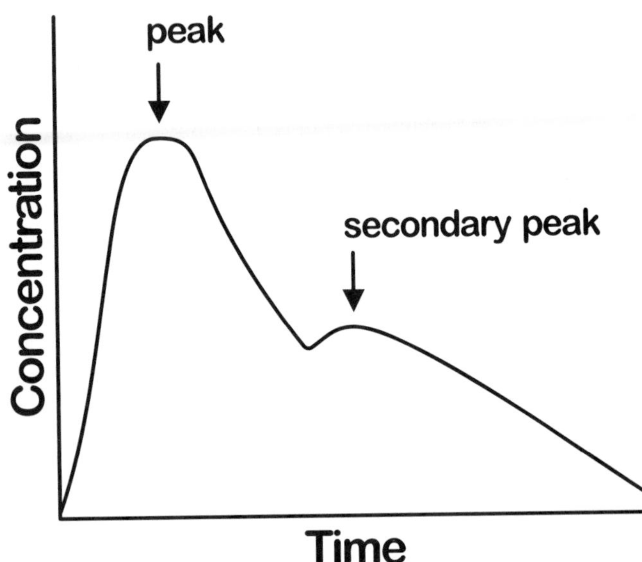

FIG. 2.6 Concentration versus time profile demonstrating a secondary peak that could result from enterohepatic recycling.

Enterohepatic Recycling. The gastrointestinal tract has also evolved into an excretory organ for elimination of nonabsorbed solid wastes and other metabolic byproducts excreted in the bile. The bile duct drains into the upper small intestine. For some drugs, this results in a phenomenon called *enterohepatic recycling* whereby a drug from the systemic circulation is excreted into the bile and is reabsorbed from the small intestine back into the bloodstream. In many cases, drugs that are metabolized by Phase II conjugation reactions are "unconjugated" by resident bacterial flora which generates free drug for reabsorption. Thus compounds that are excreted into the bile may have a prolonged sojourn in the body because of the continuous opportunity for intestinal reabsorption. The cardinal sign of this process is a "hump" in the plasma drug concentration-time profile after administration (Fig. 2.6). Bile also serves to emulsify fatty substances that are not capable of solubilizing in the primarily aqueous environment of the intestines. The result of this detergent-like action of bile is to form large surface area micelles having a hydrophilic surface and hydrophobic interior. These act as transport vehicles to deliver fat soluble drugs to the intestinal brush border surface for diffusion across the lipid membrane into the cell. Without the interaction of bile acids, fatty substances would not be available for absorption since they could not traverse this "dissolution" barrier. Thus unlike most drugs, compounds that are absorbed by this route often must be administered with a meal to promote bile acid secretion and associated micelle formation.

Species Effects on Gastrointestinal Transit Time and Food Interactions. Food may also interact with other aspects of oral drug absorption and have opposite effects for more hydrophilic drugs. Depending on the physicochemical properties of the specific drug, administration with food may significantly decrease absorption. Such effects are not only drug-dependent, but also are species-dependent due to the continuous foraging behavior of ruminants and some other omnivores compared to the periodic feeding habits of predatory carnivores. These variables are difficult to incorporate into formal pharmacokinetic models yet they add to the variability in parameters derived from these studies or in drug response between species.

The first potential interaction relates to the rate of drug delivery to the small intestine that is governed by the rate of drug release from the stomach, the *gastric emptying time*. This process is dependent upon the eating habits of the species, with continuous foraging animals (e.g., herbivores such as horses and ruminants) having a steady input of drug and a relatively stable gastric pH compared to periodic eaters (e.g., carnivores like dogs and cats and omnivores such as pigs) who have more variable eating patterns with large swings in gastric pH depending on the presence or absence of food. In addition, the drug may directly interact with the ingested food, as is the case of chelation of tetracyclines with divalent cations such as Mg^{++} in antacids or Ca^{++} in milk products. Thus, the decision to administer a compound with or without food is species- and drug-dependent and may significantly alter the bioavailability (rate and extent of absorption) of the drug.

The forestomachs of a ruminant provide a major obstacle to the delivery of an oral dosage form to the true stomach (abomasum) for ultimate release to the intestines, although a significant amount of drug absorption may occur from this site. The rumen is essentially a large fermentation vat (>50 liters in cattle, 5 liters in sheep) lined by stratified squamous epithelium, buffered at approximately a pH of 6 by extensive input of saliva, which maintains it in a fluid to soft consistency, designed primarily for the absorption of volatile fatty acids. If drugs dissolve in this medium and remain intact, they undergo tremendous dilution that decreases their rate of absorption. They then are pumped from the rumen and reticulum through the omasum for a rather steady input of drug into the true stomach. An understanding of the physiology of the ruminant has allowed for the development of some unique and innovative mechanical drug delivery technologies which essentially are encapsulated pumps which "sink" to the bottom of the rumen and become trapped, much as many unwanted objects tend to when ingested by a ruminant (e.g., nails and wire in hardware disease). These submarinelike devices then slowly release drug into the ruminal fluid for a true sustained-release preparation. In preruminant calves, a drug may bypass the rumen entirely through the rumen-reticulo groove and essentially behave as if administered to a monogastric. In contrast, fermentation in the horse occurs after drug absorption by the small intestine and thus has less impact than in ruminants. However, a nonabsorbed drug that reaches the equine large intestines and cecum, the site of fermentation, may have disastrous effects (e.g., colic) if digestive flora or function is perturbed.

First-Pass Metabolism. Another unique aspect of oral drug absorption is the fate of the absorbed drug once it enters the submucosal capillaries. Drug absorbed distal to the oral cavity and proximal to the rectum in most species enters the portal circulation and is transported directly to the liver where biotransformation may occur. This is a major cause for differences in a drug's ultimate disposition compared to all other routes of administration. This may result in a significant first-pass biotransformation of the absorbed compound. For a drug that is extensively metabolized by the liver, this first-pass effect significantly reduces absorption of the active drug even when it is absorbed across the mucosa. This occurs for many opiate medications in dogs, reducing their efficacy after oral administration. Finally, some drugs that are too polar to be absorbed across the gastrointestinal wall are formulated as ester conjugates to increase lipid solubility and enhance absorption. Once the drug crosses the gastrointestinal epithelium in this form, subsequent first-pass hepatic biotransformation enzymes and circulating blood and mucosal esterases cleave off the ester moiety releasing free drug into the systemic circulation.

There are selected drug administration sites that avoid first-pass hepatic metabolism by allowing absorption through gastrointestinal tract segments *not* drained by the portal vein. These include the oral cavity buccal and rectal routes of drug administration in some species, although this assumption hasn't been tested in many veterinary species.

Formulation Factors. The pharmaceutical literature is replete with formulation factors that may influence the dissolution and absorption of a drug preparation, assuming in the first place that one has an active component of known purity and potency. The issue then becomes what are the potential interactions that can occur between the active ingredients and the excipients that make up the formulation. Additionally, what are the effects of the practitioner's compounding techniques (materials used, mixing efficacy, etc.) on the amount of active ingredients ultimately appearing in the formulation. Although this discussion is the focus of a biopharmaceutics text, the strategies are often encountered in pharmacokinetics as they may affect the parameters estimated after oral administration.

Table 2.1 depicts the pharmaceutical processes involved in absorption that may be affected by formulation. Following oral administration of tablets, disintegration must first occur. The speed and efficacy of this process will determine how much drug is actually available for subse-

TABLE 2.1 Pharmaceutical factors affecting absorption

Disintegration
Excipients
Compaction pressure
Enteric coatings, capsules
Homogeneity
Dissolution
Particle size/Surface area
Binding
Local pH, buffers
Boundary layers
Barrier Diffusion
Solubility
Transit time

quent steps. The resulting particle size (and hence surface area) is an important determinant for the next dissolution phase where the drug enters solution, an absolute prerequisite for diffusion across the mucosal barrier. Dissolution also involves diffusion across the liquid boundary layers that are an interface between the particles and the absorption milieu. Many pharmaceutical factors may affect the efficiency of the disintegration and dissolution processes. For tablets, the nature and homogeneity of the excipients become important considerations. These factors are the primary determinants of differences in efficacy between so-called "pioneer" and generic drug products. Once the drug is in solution, binding or complexation to inert filler ingredients may occur. It is important to remember that all of this is happening while the particles are in transit through the gastrointestinal tract. Thus, if the formulation results in a decreased rate of disintegration or dissolution, the rate and extent of absorption may be decreased, especially in species with very short gastrointestinal transit times. Similar factors are involved with oral capsules and even liquid dosage forms where the drug may interact with the vehicle. In fact, these scenarios are probably most pertinent to practitioner compounding. For capsules, the breakdown of the capsule replaces tablet disintegration as the initial rate-determining step. After release of the capsule contents, all of the above factors come into play. It cannot be overstated that such pharmaceutical factors are critical determinants of the extent and rate of subsequent drug absorption.

TOPICAL AND PERCUTANEOUS ABSORPTION. The skin is a complex, multilayered tissue comprising 18,000 cm^2 of surface in an average human male. The quantitative prediction of the rate and extent of percutaneous penetration (into skin) and absorption (through skin) of topically applied chemicals is complicated by the biological variability inherent in skin. Mammalian skin is a dynamic organ with a myriad of biological functions. The most obvious is its barrier property that is of primary concern in the absorption problem. Another major function is thermoregulation that is achieved and regulated by three mechanisms in skin: thermal insulation provided by pelage and hair, sweating, and alteration of cutaneous blood flow. Other functions of skin include mechanical support, neurosensory reception, endocrinology, immunology, and glandular secretion. These additional biological roles lead to functional and structural adaptations that affect the skin's barrier properties and thus the rate and extent of percutaneous absorption.

The skin is generally considered to be an efficient barrier preventing absorption (and thus systemic exposure) of most topically administered compounds. It is a membrane that is relatively impermeable to aqueous solutions and most ions. It is, however, permeable in varying degrees to a large number of solid, liquid, and gaseous xenobiotics. Although one tends to think of most cases of poisoning as occurring through the oral or, less frequently, the respiratory route, the widespread use of organic chemicals has enhanced risk exposure to many toxicants that can penetrate the dermal barrier.

The gross features of mammalian skin are illustrated in Figure 2.7. Compared to most routes of drug absorption, the skin is by far the most diverse across species (e.g., sheep versus pig) and body sites (e.g., human forearm versus scalp). Three distinct layers and a number of associated appendages make up this nonhomogenous organ. The epidermis is a multilayered tissue varying in thickness in humans from 0.15 mm (eyelids) to 0.8 mm (palms). The primary cell type found in the epidermis is the keratinocyte. Proliferative layers of the basal keratinocyte (stratum germinativum) differentiate and gradually replace the surface cells (stratum corneum) as they deteriorate and are sloughed from the epidermis. A number of other cell types are also found interspersed in the epidermis including the pigmented melanocytes, Merkel cells which may play a sensory role, and Langerhans cells which probably play a role in cutaneous immunology.

In respect to drug penetration, the primary biochemical change is the production of fibrous, insoluble keratin that fills the cells, and a sulfur-rich amorphous protein that

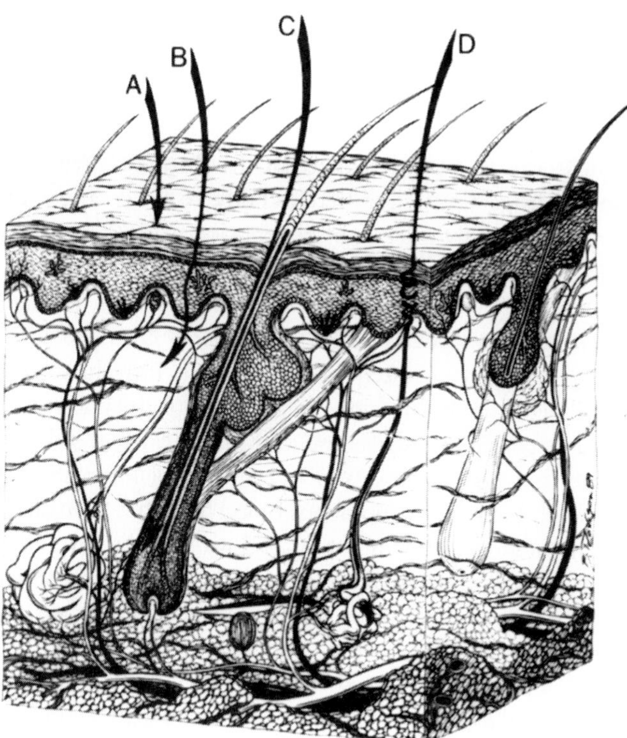

FIG. 2.7 Microstructure of mammalian skin showing potential routes of penetration (A) Intercellular, (B) Transcellular, (C) Intrafollicular, (D) Via sweat ducts.

comprises the cell matrix and thickened cell membrane. In addition, the keratinocytes synthesize a variety of lipids that form the distinguishing granules in the stratum granulosum that release their contents into the intercellular spaces. The end result in the stratum corneum is dead proteinaceous keratinocytes embedded in an extracellular lipid matrix, a structure referred to by Elias as the "Brick and Mortar" model.

The Stratum Corneum Barrier. It is this outermost layer, the stratum corneum, that provides the primary barrier to the penetration of foreign compounds. This barrier consists of flattened, stratified, highly keratinized cells embedded in a lipid matrix composed primarily of sterols, other neutral lipids and ceramides. Although highly water retarding, the dead, keratinized cells are highly water absorbent (hydrophilic), a property that keeps the skin supple and soft. A natural oil covering the skin, the sebum, especially present in some species such as sheep, appears to maintain the water-holding capacity of the epidermis but has no appreciable role in retarding the penetration of xenobiotics. Disruption of the stratum corneum removes all but a superficial deterrent to penetration.

Dermis and Appendages. The dermis is a highly vascular area, providing ready access for drug distribution once the epithelial barrier has been passed. The blood supply in the dermis is under complex, interacting neural and local humoral influences whose temperature-regulating function can have an effect on distribution by altering blood supply to this area. The absorption of a chemical possessing vasoactive properties would be affected through its action on the dermal vasculature; vasoconstriction would retard absorption and increase the size of a dermal depot, while vasodilation may enhance absorption and minimize any local dermal depot formation.

The appendages of the skin are found in the dermis and extend through the epidermis. The primary appendages are the sweat glands (eccrine and apocrine), hair, and sebaceous glands, all of which show great interspecies and interregional variability. Since these structures extend to the outer surface, they potentially play a role in the penetration of certain compounds.

Topical Drug Delivery and the Definition of Dose. From the perspective of pharmacokinetic models of transdermal and topical drug delivery systems, there are significant differences from other routes of administration (e.g., oral, injection) as to what constitutes a dose. For most exposures, the concentration applied to the surface of the skin exceeds the absorption capacity. However, for therapeutic transdermal patches with a fixed concentration of the drug and rate-controlled release properties, it is the contact surface area that more accurately reflects dose and thus dose is expressed not in mg/kg, but mg/cm^2 of dosing area. This surface area dependence also holds for any topical application even if absorption capacity is superseded. Yet, another source of nonlinearity results secondary to the effects of occlusive (water-impermeable) drug vehicles or patches. As the skin hydrates, a threshold is reached where transdermal flux dramatically increases (approximately 80% relative humidity). When the skin becomes completely hydrated under occlusive conditions, flux can be dramatically increased. Therefore, dose alone is often not a sufficient metric to describe topical doses, and application method and surface area become controlling factors.

Pathways for Dermal Absorption. Anatomically, percutaneous absorption might occur through several routes. The current consensus is that the majority of nonionized, lipid-soluble toxicants appear to move through the intercellular lipid pathway between the cells of the stratum corneum, the rate-limiting barrier of the skin. Very small and/or polar molecules appear to have more favorable penetration through appendages or other diffusion shunts, but only a small fraction of drugs are represented by these molecules. Simple diffusion seems to account for penetration through the skin whether by gases, ions, or nonelectrolytes.

The rate of percutaneous absorption through this intercellular lipid pathway is correlated to the partition coefficient of the penetrant. This has resulted in numerous studies correlating the extent of percutaneous absorption with a drug's lipid:water partition coefficient. Some workers further correlated skin penetration to molecular size and other indices of potential interaction between the penetrating molecule and the skin that are not reflected in the partition coefficient. For most purposes, however, dermal penetration is often correlated to partition coefficient. If lipid solubility is too great, compounds that penetrate the stratum corneum may remain there and form a reservoir. Alternatively, penetrated compounds may also form a reservoir in the dermis. For such compounds, slow release from these depots may result in a prolonged absorption half-life. Conditions that alter the composition of the lipid (harsh delipidizing solvents, dietary lipid restrictions, disease) may alter the rate of compound penetration by changing its partitioning behavior.

Recent studies have demonstrated that the skin may also be responsible for metabolizing topically applied compounds. Both Phase I and II metabolic pathways have been identified. For some compounds, the extent of cutaneous metabolism influences the overall fraction of a topically applied compound that is absorbed, making this process function as an alternate absorption pathway. Cutaneous biotransformation is used to promote the absorption of some topical drugs that normally would not penetrate the skin. Cutaneous metabolism may be important for certain aspects of skin toxicology when nontoxic parent compounds are bioactivated within the epidermis, e.g., benzo(a)pyrene to an epoxide. Finally, resident bacteria on the surface of the skin may also metabolize topical drugs, as was demonstrated with pentochlorophenol absorption in pig skin dosed in soil with and without antibiotics. This effect is potentiated under warm and wet occlusive dosing conditions that both promote bacterial growth and reduce skin barrier properties.

Variations in Species and Body Region. Penetration of drugs through different body regions varies. In humans, generally the rate of penetration of most nonionized toxicants is in the following order: scrotal > forehead > axilla = scalp > back = abdomen > palm and plantar. The palmar and plantar regions are highly cornified producing a much greater thickness that introduces an overall lag time in diffusion. In addition to thickness, the actual size of corneacytes and differences in hair follicle density may affect absorption of more polar molecules. Finally, differences in cutaneous blood flow that have been documented in different body regions may be an additional variable to consider in predicting the rate of percutaneous absorption. These factors are also important in animals.

Although generalizations are tenuous at best, human skin appears to be more impermeable, or at least as impermeable, as the skin of the cat, dog, rat, mouse, or guinea pig. The skin of pigs and some primates serve as useful approximation to human skin, but only after a comparison has been made for each specific substance. The major determinants of species differences are thickness, hair density, lipid composition, and cutaneous blood flow.

Factors that Modulate Absorption. Soaps and detergents are perhaps the most damaging substances routinely applied to skin. Whereas organic solvents must be applied in high concentrations to damage the skin and increase the penetration of solute through human epidermis, only 1% aqueous solutions of detergents are required to achieve the same effect. For a specific chemical, rate of penetration can be drastically modified by the solvent system used. In transdermal patches, specific chemical enhancers (e.g., solvents such as ethanol; other lipid-interacting moieties) are included in the formulation to reversibly increase skin permeability and enhance drug delivery. Alternatively, drug release is formulated to be rate-limiting from the patch system (membranes, microencapsulation, etc.) so that a constant (zero-order) release from the patch occurs, thereby providing controlled drug delivery. Since patches are designed with the permeability properties of specific species in mind, care must be taken when using a patch designed for one species in another.

There are a number of topical veterinary drugs routinely used to achieve long-acting systemic therapeutic endpoints in animals. These include the topical pesticides formulated as "spot-ons" and "pour-ons." These products are fully discussed in the Dermatopharmacology and Ectoparasiticides chapters of this text.

Another strategy for transdermal delivery, which has not widely been employed in veterinary medicine, is to overcome the cutaneous barrier by using electrical (iontophoresis) or ultrasonic (phonophoreses) energy, rather than the concentration gradient in diffusion, to drive drugs through the skin. These techniques hold the most promise for delivering peptides and oligonucleotide drugs that now only can be administered by injection. In these cases, dose is based on the surface area of application and the amount of energy required to actively deliver the drug across skin. In iontophoresis, this amounts to a dose being expressed in μAmps/cm^2. Formulation factors are also very different since many of the excipients used are also delivered by the applied electrical current in molar proportion to the active drug. Finally, a recent but related strategy is to use very short-duration, high-voltage electrical pulses (electroporation) to reversibly break down the stratum corneum barrier, allowing larger peptides and possibly even small proteins to be systemically delivered.

RESPIRATORY ABSORPTION. The third major route for systemic exposure to drugs and toxicants is the respiratory system. Since this system's primary function is gas exchange (O_2, CO_2), it is always in direct contact with environmental air as an unavoidable part of breathing. A number of toxicants are in gaseous (CO, NO_2, formaldehyde), vapor (benzene, CCl_4), or aerosol (lead from automobile exhaust, silica, asbestos) forms and are potential candidates for entry via the respiratory system. There are no approved inhalational drugs for use in veterinary medicine. Each mode of inhalational exposure results in a different mechanism of compound absorption and for the purposes of this text, a different definition of dose.

Opportunities for systemic absorption are excellent through the respiratory route since the cells lining the alveoli are very thin and profusely bathed by capillaries. The surface area of the lung is large (50–100 m^2), some 50 times the area of the skin. Based on these properties and the diffusion equation presented earlier (Equation 2.1), the large surface area, the small diffusion distance, and high level of blood perfusion maximize the rate and extent of passive absorption driven by gaseous diffusion.

The process of respiration involves the movement and exchange of air through several interrelated passages including the nose, mouth, pharynx, trachea, bronchi, and successive smaller airways terminating in the alveoli where gaseous exchange occurs. All of these anatomical modifications protect the internal environment of the air passages from the harsh outside environment by warming and humidifying the inspired air. The passages also provide numerous obstacles and baffles to prevent the inhalation of particulate and aerosol droplets. Thus the absorption of particulate and aerosolized liquids, such as those employed in nebulized drug therapy, is fundamentally different from that of gases. The absorption of such impacted solids and liquids along the respiratory tract has much more in common with oral and topical absorption, with the critical caveat that the precise dose of compound finally available for absorption is very difficult to determine. Great strides have been made in developing aerosol drug delivery devices for human use that take advantage of this mechanism of impaction; however, these may not be transferable to veterinary species since their efficacy is closely related to the geometry and physiology of the human respiratory tract.

Another unique aspect of respiratory exposure is the fact that the pulmonary blood circulation is in series with the systemic circulation. Thus, in contrast to cutaneous or oral exposure, compounds absorbed in the lung will enter the oxygenated pulmonary veins that drain to the systemic arterial circulation. Compared to oral administration, this reduces first-pass hepatic metabolism. However, the pulmonary circulation is adept at metabolizing peptides secondary to its role in inactivating peptide hormones.

Vapors and Gases. Since the rate of entry of vapor-phase toxicants is controlled by the alveolar ventilation rate, the toxicant is presented to the alveoli in an interrupted fashion whose frequency in humans is equal to the rate of breathing: about 20 times/min. Doses are generally discussed in terms of the partial pressure of the gas in the inspired air. Upon inhalation of a constant tension of a toxic gas, arterial plasma tension of the gas approaches its tension in the expired air. The rate of entry is then determined by the blood solubility of the toxicant. If there is a high blood : gas partition coefficient, a larger amount must be dissolved in the blood to raise the partial pressure. Gases with a high blood : gas partition coefficient require a longer period to approach the same tension in the blood as in inspired air than it takes for less soluble gases. Similarly, a longer period of time is required for blood concentrations of such a gas to be eliminated thus prolonging detoxification.

Another important point to consider in determining how much of an inhaled gas is absorbed into the systemic circulation is the relationship of the fraction of lung ventilated compared to the fraction perfused. Increased perfusion of the lung will favor a more rapid achievement of blood-gas equilibrium. Decreased perfusion will decrease the absorption of toxicants even those that reach the alveoli. Various "ventilation/perfusion mismatches" may alter the amount of an inhaled gas that is systemically absorbed. Similarly, pulmonary diseases that thicken the alveoli or obstruct the airways may also affect overall absorption.

Aerosols and Particulates. The absorption of aerosols and particulates is affected by a number of physiological factors specifically designed to preclude access to the alveoli. The upper respiratory tract, beginning with the nose and continuing down its tubular elements, is a very efficient filtering system for excluding particulate matter (solids, liquid droplets). The parameters of air velocity and directional air changes favor impaction of particles in the upper respiratory system. Particle characteristics such as size, coagulation, sedimentation, electrical charge, and diffusion are important to retention, absorption, or expulsion of airborne particles. In addition to these characteristics, a mucous blanket propelled by ciliary action clears the tract of particles by directing them to the gastrointestinal system (via the glottis) or to the mouth for expectoration. This system is responsible for 80% of toxicant lung clearance. In addition to this mechanism, phagocytosis is very active in the respiratory tract, both coupled to the directed mucosal route and via penetration through interstitial tissues of the lung and migration to the lymph, where phagocytes may remain stored for long periods in lymph nodes. Compared to absorption in the alveoli, absorption through the upper respiratory tract is quantitatively of less importance. However, inhaled toxicants that become deposited on the mucous layer can be absorbed into the myriad of cells lining the respiratory tract and exert a direct toxicologic response. This route of exposure is often used to deliver pharmaceutics by aerosol. If a compound is extremely potent, systemic effects may occur.

The end result of this extremely efficient filtering mechanism is that most inhaled drugs deposited in nasal or buccal mucous ultimately enter the gastrointestinal tract. This can best be appreciated by examining the respiratory drainages depicted in Figure 2.1. Therefore, the disposition of aerosols and particulates largely mirrors that of orally administered drugs.

Nasal administration is a preferred route for many inhalant medications in humans. In these cases, great care is made to deliver aerosols of the specific size for deposition on the nasal musosa and upper respiratory tract. The bioavailability of these compounds is assessed using the techniques developed for other routes, although a local effect is often desired. The problems with this strategy are the attainment of an accurately delivered dose and the inactivation and binding of administered drug by the thick mucous blanket. Drugs delivered by this route usually have a wide therapeutic window and large safety index. The final point to consider relates to some specific peculiarities of nasal absorption. In the region of the olfactory epithelium, there exists a direct path for inhaled compounds to be absorbed directly into the olfactory neural tissue and central nervous system, thereby bypassing both the systemic circulation and the blood-brain barrier. The mass of drugs involved in this uptake process is very small and thus would not affect a pharmacokinetic analysis. However, this route has obvious toxicological significance and unfortunately has not been carefully studied in veterinary species.

OTHER ROUTES OF ADMINISTRATION. In order to complete this discussion of absorption, it is important to realize that there are other extravascular drug administration routes that are often encountered. Relative to pharmacokinetic analysis, these are dealt with in the same fashion as the primary routes discussed above. The important difference is that in all cases, the barrier to absorption is less than that encountered in oral or topical delivery. Second, all of these routes involve an invasive procedure to inject drug into an internal body tissue, thereby bypassing the epithelial barriers of the skin and gastrointestinal tract.

The primary therapeutic routes of drug administration are subcutaneous (SC or SQ) and intramuscular (IM). In these cases, the total dose of drug is known and injected into tissue that is well perfused by systemic capillaries that drain into the central venous circulation. Both of these routes as well as intravenous administration are termed *parenteral* to contrast primarily with oral (*enteral)* and topical dosing, which are classified as *nonparenteral* routes of drug administration. A primary difference between these two classes is that parenteral routes bypass all of the body's defensive mechanisms. Parenteral dosage forms are manufactured under strict guidelines that eliminate microbial and particulate contamination resulting in sterile preparations that must be administered using aseptic techniques. This restriction does apply to oral or topical dosage forms. As with all methods of drug administration, there are numerous variables associated with SC and IM dosing that can be conveniently classified into pharmaceutical and biological categories.

Finally, there are other occasional routes of drug administration employed that require absorption for activity. Administration of drugs by intraperitoneal injection is often used in toxicology studies in rodents since larger volumes can be administered. Peritoneal absorption is very efficient, provided adequate "mixing" of the injection with the peritoneal fluid is achieved. The majority of drug absorbed after interperitoneal administration enters the portal vein and thus may undergo first-pass hepatic metabolism. The disposition of intraperitoneal drug thus mirrors oral administration.

Some drugs are administered by conjunctival, intravaginal, or intramammary routes. In these cases achievement of effective systemic concentrations are often not required for what is an essentially local therapeutic effect. Prolonged absorption from these sites may result in persistent tissue residues in food producing animals if the analytical sensitivity of the monitoring assay is sufficiently low. The systemic absorption of these dosage forms is quantitated using procedures identical to those employed for other routes of administration.

BIOAVAILABILITY. The final topic to consider is the assessment of the extent and rate of absorption after oral, topical, or inhalational drug administration. The extent of drug absorption is defined as absolute systemic availability and is denoted in pharmacokinetic equations as the fraction of an applied dose absorbed into the body (F). Although this topic will also be discussed extensively in Chapter 3, it is important and convenient at this juncture to introduce the basic concepts so as to complete the discussion of drug absorption. If one is estimating the extent of drug absorption by measuring the resultant concentrations in either blood or excreta, one must have an estimate of how much drug normally would be found if the entire dose were absorbed. To estimate this, an intravenous dose is required since this is the only route of administration that guarantees that 100% of the dose is systemically available (F = 1.0) and the pattern of disposition and metabolism can be quantitated. Parameters used to measure systemic availability are thus calculated as a ratio relative to the intravenous dose.

For most therapeutic drug studies, systemic absorption is assessed by measuring blood concentrations. The amount of drug collected after administration by the route under study is divided by that collected after intravenous administration. When drug concentrations in blood (or serum or plasma) are assayed, total absorption is assessed by measuring the area under the concentration-time curve (AUC) using the trapezoidal method. This is a geometrical technique that breaks the AUC into corresponding trapezoids based on the number of samples assayed. The terminal area beyond the last data point (a triangle) is estimated and added together with the previous trapezoidal areas. Absolute systemic availability then is calculated as in Equation 2.4:

$$F\ (\%) = \frac{AUC_{route}\ \ Dose_{iv}}{AUC_{iv}\ \ Dose_{route}} \tag{2.4}$$

Calculation of *F* provides only an estimate of the extent, and not rate, of drug absorption. To calculate rate, pharmacokinetic techniques are required and presented in Chapter 3. Finally, so-called relative systemic availability may be calculated for two nonintravenous formulations where the data for the reference product is in the denominator and the test formulation in the numerator.

DISTRIBUTION

A toxicant absorbed into the systemic circulation following any route of administration must reach its site of action at a high enough concentration for a sufficient period of time to elicit a biological response. Distribution processes determine this outcome. There are numerous tissues to which a chemical may be distributed, some of them capable of eliciting a pharmacologic or toxicologic (intended versus unintended) response while others serve only as a sink or depot for the chemical. Sinks may also be formed as a result of chemical binding to tissue or plasma proteins. The toxicologic significance of such sinks is that chemicals will be distributed to, and in some cases stored in, these tissues and only slowly released back into the systemic circulation for ultimate elimination. Such tissue binding may actually protect against acute adverse effects by providing an "inert" site for toxicant localization. Storage may, however, prolong the overall residence time of a compound in the body and promote accumulation during chronic exposure, two processes that would potentiate chronic toxicity.

If the animal is a food-producing species, such tissue storage may result in residues in the edible meat products. Tissue concentrations thus become an endpoint in themselves, devoid of a biological or toxicological relevance in the tissue they are found. Their relevance is set by regulations that legally establish safe tissue tolerances or maximum residue levels for specific tissues and species. These are based upon extrapolations of safety to the consuming human population and food consumption patterns.

Distribution of chemicals to peripheral tissues is dependent on four factors: 1) the physiochemical properties of the compound, 2) the concentration gradient established between the blood and tissue, 3) the ratio of blood flow to tissue mass, and 4) the affinity of the chemical for tissue constituents. The physiochemical properties of the chemical (pKa, lipid solubility, molecular weight) are most important in determining its propensity to distribute to a specific tissue. For most molecules, distribution out of the blood into tissue is via bulk flow through the capillary pores or by simple diffusion down a concentration gradient; hence distribution is generally described by first-order rate constants. One could consider distribution as "absorption" into the tissues from the blood. The complicating factors are that the driving concentration is now dependent upon blood flow, the surface area for "absorption into tissues" is dependent upon capillary density and tissue mass, the relevant partition coefficient is the blood/tissue ratio, and plasma/tissue protein binding complicates the picture. An understanding of distribution is a prerequisite to predicting pharmacologic response.

PHYSIOLOGICAL DETERMINANTS OF DISTRIBUTION. Body fluids are distributed between three primary compartments, only one of which, vascular fluid, is thought to have an important role in the distribution of most compounds throughout the body. Human plasma amounts to about 4% of the total body weight and 53% of the total blood volume. By comparison, the interstitial tissue fluids account for 13%, and intracellular fluids 41%, of body weight. Use of recently developed microdialysis and ultrafiltration probes and catheters allow the concentration of drug to be directly monitored in the interstitial fluid and thus further open the window for pharmacokinetic analysis. The concentration that a compound may achieve in the blood following exposure depends in part upon its apparent volume of distribution. If it is distributed only in the plasma, a high concentration could be achieved in the vascular system. In contrast, the concentration would be markedly lower if the same quantity of toxicant were distributed to a larger pool including the interstitial water and/or cellular fluids.

The next major consideration is the relative blood flow to different tissues. Two factors will potentiate chemical accumulation into a tissue: high blood flow per unit mass of tissue and a large tissue mass. Tissues with a *high blood flow/mass* ratio include the *brain, heart, liver, kidney,* and *endocrine glands*. Tissues with an *intermediate ratio* include *muscle* and *skin,* while tissues with a *low ratio* (indicative of poor systemic perfusion) include *adipose tissue* and *bone.* These ratios are generalizations and some tissues may actually be categorized in two disparate groups. An excellent example is the kidney where the renal cortex receives some 25% of cardiac output and thus has a very high blood flow/mass ratio. However, the renal medulla receives only a small fraction of this blood flow and thus could be categorized in the intermediate to low group. If the affinity of the chemical for the tissue is high, it will still accumulate in poorly perfused tissues (such as fat), although it will take a long period of time to "load" or "deplete" these tissues. A relatively low blood flow/mass ratio is a major physiologic explanation for depot formation.

TISSUE BARRIERS TO DISTRIBUTION. Some organs have unique anatomic barriers to xenobiotic penetration. The classic and most studied example is the blood-brain barrier, which has a glial cell layer interposed between the capillary endothelium and the nervous tissue. In the membrane scheme depicted in Figure 2.2, this amounts to an additional lipid membrane between the capillary and target tissue. Only nonionized lipid-soluble compounds can penetrate this barrier. Similar considerations apply to ocular, prostatic, testicular, synovial, mammary gland, and placental drug or toxicant distribution. In addition, pH partitioning phenomenon also may occur since the protected tissue (e.g., cerebrospinal fluid) may have a lower pH than the circulating blood plasma. Chemicals may also distribute into transcellular fluid compartments, which are also demarcated by an epithelial cell layer. These include cerebrospinal, intraocular, synovial, pericardial, pleural, peritoneal, and cochlear perilymph fluid compartments.

A few tissues possess selective transport mechanisms that accumulate specific chemicals against concentration gradients. For example, the blood-brain barrier possesses glucose, L-amino acid, and transferrin transporters. If the toxicant resembles an endogenous transport substrate, it may preferentially concentrate in a particular tissue. Recent work with the blood-brain barrier has demonstrated that some of these tissues also possess drug efflux transport processes that remove drug from the protected sites. Two such processes are p-glycoprotein associated with multidrug resistance (MDR) and the weak organic acid cell-to-blood efflux systems.

P-glycoprotein is a member of the so-called ATP-binding cassette proteins that include the cystic fibrosis transmembrane regulator and the sulfonyurea-sensitive ATP-dependent potassium channel. Drugs such as vinblastine, vincristine, or cyclosporine, which have the proper physiochemical characteristics (high lipophilicity) to enter the brain, do not achieve effective concentrations because of this active efflux mechanisms. This transport system has recently been shown to cause the unique breed sensitivity of Collies to ivermectin toxicity. These transporters are also responsible for decreased bioavailability of some drugs due to active pumping of absorbed drug back into the intestinal lumen. A number of drugs also inhibit p-glycoprotein transport (e.g., ketoconazole, cyclosporine), which forms the basis for some complex drug-drug interactions. Similar processes and transport systems for peptides, and other compounds are also found in other organs (e.g., liver). Chapter 50 in this text should be consulted for further details on Pgp.

PLASMA PROTEIN BINDING. Following entry into the circulatory system, a chemical is distributed throughout the body and may accumulate at the site of toxic action, be transferred to a storage depot, or be transported to organs that will detoxify, activate, or eliminate the compound. Although many toxicants have sufficient solubility in the aqueous component of blood to account for simple solution as a means of distribution, the primary distribution mechanism for insoluble toxicants appears to be in association with plasma proteins. Although cellular components (e.g., red blood cells) may also be responsible for transport of drugs, such transport is seldom the major route. The transport of compounds by lymph is usually of little quantitative importance for many drugs, although it may be very important in delivering some lipophilic drugs and potentially nanoparticles to select organs. Both erythrocytes and lymph can play roles in the transport of some lipophilic drugs and toxins, in some instances to an important extent.

Studies of plasma proteins have shown albumin to be particularly important in the binding of drugs. This is especially true for weak acids, with weak bases often binding to acid glycoproteins. For certain hormones, specific high-affinity transport proteins are present. Studies of toxicant binding have been more limited, but there is evidence of a significant binding/partitioning role for lipoproteins in carrying very lipophilic chemicals in the blood. In the case of most drug-protein interactions, reversible binding is established, which follows the Law of Mass Action and provides a remarkably efficient means whereby drugs can be transported to various tissues. The strength of this association may be quantitated through the use of the dissociation constant, K_{diss}. Among a group of binding sites on proteins, those with the smallest K_{diss} value for a given drug will bind it most tightly. In contrast to reversible binding seen with most therapeutic drugs, agents like cisplatin and some potentially carcinogenic metabolites that are formed from chlorinated hydrocarbons (such as CCl_4) are covalently bound to tissue proteins. In this case, there is no true distribution of the drug as there is no opportunity for dissociation.

Once a molecule binds to a plasma protein, it moves throughout the circulation until it dissociates, usually for attachment to another large molecule. Dissociation occurs when the affinity for another biomolecule or tissue component is greater than that for the plasma protein to which the toxicant was originally bound. Thus, forces of association must be strong enough to establish an initial interaction, and they must also be weak enough such that a change in the physical or chemical environment can lead to dissociation. Dissociation could occur by binding to proteins of greater affinity (lower K_{diss} values), binding with a higher concentration of proteins of lower affinity, or changes in K_{diss} with changes in ionic strength, pH, temperature, or conformational changes in the binding site induced by binding of other molecules. As long as binding is reversible, redistribution will occur whenever the concentration of one pool (i.e., blood or tissue) is diminished. Redistribution must occur when the concentration is diminished in order to reestablish equilibrium.

Proteins complex with drugs by a variety of mechanisms. Covalent binding may have a profound direct effect on an organism due to modification of an essential molecule, but it usually accounts for a minor portion of the total dose and is of no importance in further distribution of drugs since such compounds cannot dissociate. As previously mentioned, when metabolites of some compounds are covalently bound to proteins, there may be no opportunity for subsequent release of the drug apart from release upon breakdown of the protein itself. The cancer chemotherapeutic drug cisplatin covalently binds to albumin through an aquation reaction. In incubation studies, "aging" occurs after a short period of time independent of drug concentration and the majority of circulating cisplatin is covalently bound.

Noncovalent binding is of primary importance with respect to drug distribution because of the opportunities to dissociate after transport. In rare cases, the noncovalent bond may be so tight (K_{diss} extremely small) that a compound remains in the blood for very lengthy periods. For example, 3-hydroxy-2,4,4-triiodo-α-ethyl hydrocinnamic acid has a half-life of about 1 year with respect to its binding to plasma albumin. The new cephalosporin antimicrobial cefovecin similarly is approximately 97% bound in dogs and has a half-life of 5.5 days, very long for this class of drugs.

Charged drugs may be bound to plasma proteins by ionic interactions. Electrostatic attraction occurs between two oppositely charged ions on a drug and a protein. Proteins are thereby capable of binding charged metal ions. The degree of binding varies with the chemical nature of each compound and the net charge. Dissociation of ionic bonds usually occurs readily, but some members of the transition group of metals exhibit high association constants (low K_{diss} values) and exchange is slow. Ionic interactions may also contribute to binding of alkaloids with ionizable nitrogenous groups and other ionizable toxicants. Hydrogen bonds arise when a hydrogen atom, covalently bound to one electronegative atom, is "shared" to a significant degree with a second electronegative atom. As a rule, only the most electronegative atoms (O, N, and E) form stable hydrogen bonds. Protein side chains containing hydroxyl, amino, carboxyl, imidazole, and carbamyl groups can form hydrogen bonds, as can the N and O atoms of peptide bonds themselves. Hydrogen bonding plays an important role in the structural configuration of proteins and nucleic acids. Van der Waals forces produce weak interactions, which act between the nucleus of one atom and the electrons of another atom, i.e., between dipoles and induced dipoles. The attractive forces arise from slight distortions induced in the electron clouds surrounding each nucleus as two atoms are brought close together. The binding force is critically dependent upon the proximity of interacting atoms and diminishes rapidly with distance. However, when these forces are summed over a large number of interacting atoms that "fit" together spatially, they can play a significant role in determining specificity of toxicant-protein interactions. A final mechanism of binding is based on hydrophobic interactions. When two nonpolar groups come together, they exclude the water between them, and this mutual repulsion of water results in a hydrophobic interaction. The minimization of thermodynamically unfavorable contact of a polar grouping with water molecules provides the major stabilizing effect in hydrophobic interactions.

Methods for Assessing Protein Binding. A number of methods have been employed to study drug-protein interactions, including ultrafiltration, electrophoresis, equilibrium dialysis, solvent extraction, solvent partition, ultracentrifugation, spectrophotometry, and gel filtration. The most widely used techniques are ultrafiltration and equilibrium dialysis. The basic concept is that a semipermeable membrane is used which restricts passage of protein but allows unbound drug to cross the barrier according the diffusion. Bound drug is placed on one side of the membrane and samples are collected from the protein-free side. Ultrafiltration allows rapid protein-drug separation while equilibrium dialysis requires time for the separation to occur. The fraction of free drug is then calculated based on the amount of total drug used.

Protein-binding data are frequently expressed in terms of percent of drug bound. Although useful, the limitations should be recognized, for as drug concentration is lowered, the percentage of binding increases. When a compound has a high affinity for a protein (e.g., albumin), percent binding falls sharply when the total drug concentration exceeds a certain value that saturates the binding sites available.

Displacement. If a toxicant or drug is administered after binding sites on a protein are occupied by another chemical, competition for the site occurs, and a higher concentration of free drug may be available. Competition for the same site on plasma proteins may have especially important consequences when one of the potentially toxic ligands has a very high affinity. If compound A has low fractional binding (for example, 30%) and compound B displaces 10% of A from the protein, the net increase of free A is from 70% to 73%, a negligible increase. However, if A were 98% bound and 10% is displaced, the amount of free A increases from 2% to 12%, a sixfold increase in free toxicant. A change in binding may also occur when a second drug produces an allosteric effect resulting in altered affinity of the protein for the originally bound drug (noncompetitive binding). There is great debate as to the clinical significance of such drug-protein displacements that increase drug free fraction, since, as will be seen in the next sections, the increased free concentration of drug may result in its increased elimination from the body, negating any enhanced activity or toxicity secondary to the displacement.

Most pharmacokinetic models in both human and comparative medical literature assess only total drug concentrations. When the extent of protein binding differs dramatically between species, inappropriate extrapolations often occur if the drug is very highly protein bound in one species. Similarly, interpretation of the extent of tissue distribution when the extent of protein binding is not known may be misleading. The most precise predictions can often be made when the free fraction of drug is known over the concentration ranges of the study being conducted.

OTHER FACTORS AFFECTING DISTRIBUTION. Among the factors that affect distribution, apart from binding to blood macromolecules per se, are the route of administration, molecular weight, rate of metabolism, polarity, and stereochemistry of the parent compound or metabolic products, and rate of excretion. Molecular weight, charge, and/or polarity have been previously discussed. Stereoselectivity in the disposition of a drug is an often ignored phenomenon which could influence many studies. Its impact on metabolism is obvious; however, any receptor-mediated binding or transport process, including high-specificity protein binding could be affected. Propranolol and ibuprofen have been shown to demonstrate stereoselective distribution.

A major factor determining distribution is the extent of tissue binding, a process identical to that of serum protein binding except that the results on drug disposition are opposite. Tissue binding is governed by the same mechanisms as discussed above and tends to increase a drug's distribution, although not necessarily activity, if the drug is sequestered away from active drug receptors or target microorganisms. Covalent binding also occurs and is relevant to toxicology and tissue residue depletion. Depending on the pharmacokinetic model employed, irreversible covalent tissue binding may actually be mathematically detected as an increase in the drug's elimination, if only blood samples are used in the analysis, since there is no redistribution of drug back into the blood. For distribution to be quantitated, the basic assumption in most pharmacokinetic models is that the process is irreversible and thus ultimately an equilibrium will be achieved between drug movement into and out of tissue. When irreversible binding occurs, compound is extracted from blood and when excretory output (e.g., urine, feces, expired air) is not monitored, this is interpreted in many models as elimination. These model assumptions are often ignored.

As can be appreciated from this discussion, there are numerous factors that could affect distribution of a compound to tissues. Another is the methodology used to assess tissue distribution. Autoradiography is an excellent technique to anatomically localize distributed drug to the level of organs, cells, and even subcellular components. However, most pharmacokinetic studies rely on analytical techniques. When a tissue sample is collected from an animal, the sample is actually a homogenate of cells, extracellular fluid, and blood. The concentration measured cannot be uniquely assigned to any specific tissue or body fluid compartment. The use of microdialysis and ultrafiltration provides a direct estimate of extracellular fluid concentrations.

The extent of distribution of a compound is termed its volume of distribution (Vd) and is calculated by equations such as Equation 2.5:

$$\text{Vd (l)} = \text{Dose (mg)}/\text{Concentration (mg/l)} \quad (2.5)$$

The *Vd* is actually a proportionality constant relating the plasma concentration to administered dose. Actual approaches to determine this will be presented in Chapter 3.

RENAL ELIMINATION

The ultimate route for drug elimination from the body is the kidney. Drugs can also be eliminated in bile, sweat, saliva, tears, milk, and expired air; however, for most therapeutic drugs these routes are generally not quantitatively important as mechanisms for reducing total body burden of drug. The degree of lipid solubility and extent of ionization in blood determines how much of drug will be excreted by the kidney. For drugs that are first biotransformed by the liver, the more water-soluble metabolites are then ultimately excreted through the kidney into the urine. The kidney has also been the most widely studied excretory organ because of the accessibility of urine to collection and analysis. Many of the principles utilized by pharmacologists in quantitating excretory organ function, especially clearance, were originally developed by renal physiologists to noninvasively assess kidney function. Dr. Homer Smith's classic reference on renal physiology is still instructive for the determination of renal clearance.

There are two components relevant to any discussion of renal drug excretion: physiology and quantitation. Renal drug excretion can be considered using the same principles of membrane transport developed earlier, except in this case the movement is from the vascular system to outside the body. Generally, only drugs that are either dissolved in the plasma or bound to circulating blood proteins are available for excretion. The pharmacokinetic parameter estimated by most of these approaches is the renal clearance of the drug.

RENAL PHYSIOLOGY RELEVANT TO CLEARANCE OF DRUGS. For a perspective of drug excretion from the body, the kidney will be considered only as an excretory organ designed to remove foreign compounds (e.g., drugs) and metabolic by-products (e.g., creatinine, urea) from the blood. As will become evident, the major clinical indices of renal function such as blood urea nitrogen, serum creatinine, and creatinine clearance are actually pharmacokinetic parameters of creatinine and urea excretion!

The kidney receives approximately 25% of the cardiac output and thus processes a prodigious amount of blood. The kidney functions in a two-step manner to accomplish its function. The first step is passage through a filtering unit to retain formed cellular elements (e.g., erythrocytes, white blood cells) and proteins in the blood, only allowing the passage of plasma fluid into the remainder of the kidney. The second step utilizes a system of anatomically and physiologically segmented tubules to further modify the contents of the filtered fluid depending on a host of physiological needs including but not limited to fluid, electrolyte, and acid-base balance and the regulation of systemic blood pressure.

The primary functional unit of the kidney is the nephron depicted in Figure 2.8. Depending on the species, there may be 500,000 nephrons per kidney. The sum of their individual function is the observed organ function. Their specific anatomical arrangement is species-dependent, often determined by the evolutionary adaptation of the animal to its environment relative to the need to conserve body fluids. The filtration unit is the glomerulus, while

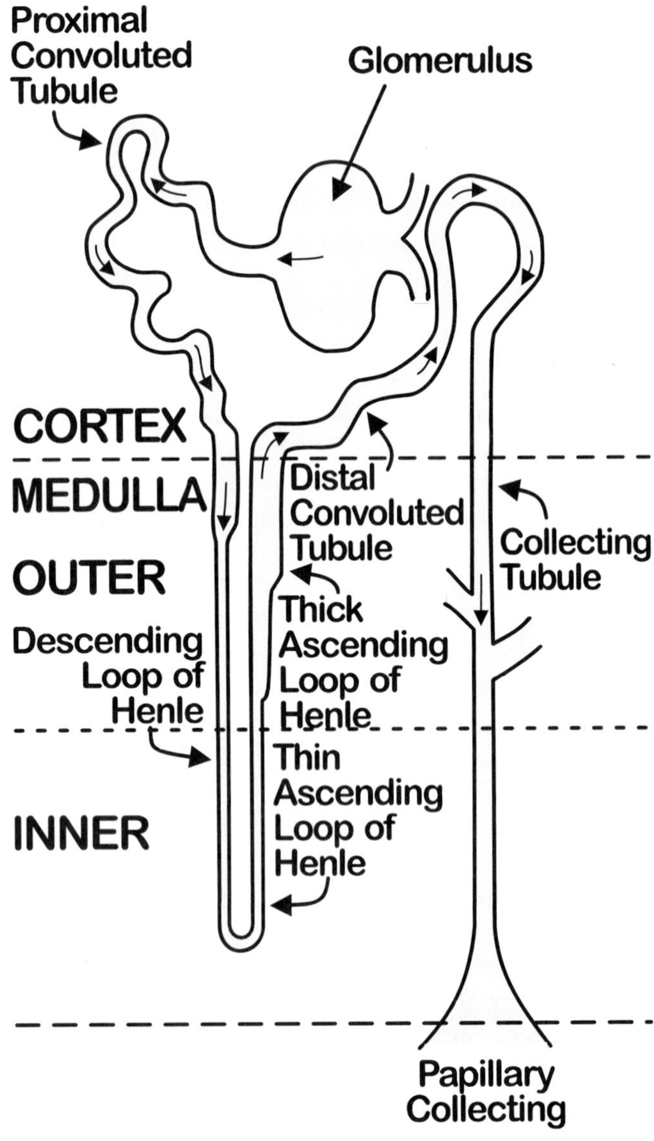

FIG. 2.8 Structure of a nephron.

the remainder of the fluid processing is accomplished by the extensive tubular system, whose segments are named in relation to their relative distance (proximal versus distal) measured *through* the tubules from the glomerulus. The junction between these is a unique anatomical adaptation called the Loop of Henle that is designed to use countercurrent exchangers to efficiently produce a concentrated urine since most of the water that is filtered by the glomerulus must be reabsorbed back into the body. The Loop of Henle also forces the distal tubules to return toward the surface of the kidney to interact with the glomeruli. Grossly, the region of the kidney containing the glomeruli as well as the proximal and returning distal tubules are on the outside toward the surface and comprise the renal cortex. This region of the kidney is very well perfused by blood and is primarily characterized by oxidative metabolic processes. The interior region is the medulla that is occupied by the penetrating Loops of Henle, is poorly perfused, and is characterized by anaerobic metabolism. The amount of tubular fluid filtered by the glomeruli is acted upon by the various nephron segments to reabsorb wanted materials (primarily water and sodium) back into the blood and to let the remainder be excreted into the urine.

The kidney is also the site where acid-base balance is metabolically tuned by controlling acid and base excretion. Some of these processes are coupled to electrolyte secretion (e.g., potassium and sodium) and thus are further modulated by hormones such as aldosterone. These nephron functions may inadvertently alter the amount of drug eliminated in the tubules by changing tubular fluid pH and consequently the ionized fraction of weak acids and bases according to the Henderson-Hasselbach equation presented earlier. This modification in tubular fluid may affect the value of renal clearance determined in pharmacokinetic studies.

There are specific tubular transport systems that excrete products directly into the tubular fluid, which are not filterable because of plasma protein binding. Other transport systems reabsorb essential nutrients (e.g., glucose) back into the blood that were filtered into the tubular fluid. Drugs are also processed by these same transport systems making drug excretion dependent upon the physiological status of the animal. This is especially true when a drug biochemically resembles an endogenous substrate. As is similar to all transport processes, saturation and competition may occur, which may impart nonlinear behavior on a drug's kinetics.

MECHANISMS OF RENAL DRUG EXCRETION. Drugs are normally excreted by the kidney through the processes of 1) glomerular filtration, 2) active tubular secretion and/or reabsorption, and/or 3) passive, flow-dependent, nonionic back diffusion. These processes can be considered as vectorial quantities, each possessing magnitude and direction relative to transport between tubular fluid and blood. Their sum determines the ultimate elimination of a specific drug by the kidney as illustrated in Figure 2.9. *The total renal excretion of a drug equals its rate of filtration plus secretion minus reabsorption.* If a drug is reabsorbed back from the tubular fluid into the blood, its net renal excretion will be reduced. In contrast, if a drug is secreted from the blood into the tubular fluid, its net excretion will be increased. These events will be subsequently quantitated.

Excretion by glomerular filtration is unidirectional with drug removal from the blood by bulk flow. Only non–protein-bound drugs are eliminated by this process, a characteristic that is important when predicting elimination pathways for drugs. The rate of drug filtration, therefore, is dependent upon both the extent of drug protein binding and the glomerular filtration rate (GFR) whose calculation will be developed below.

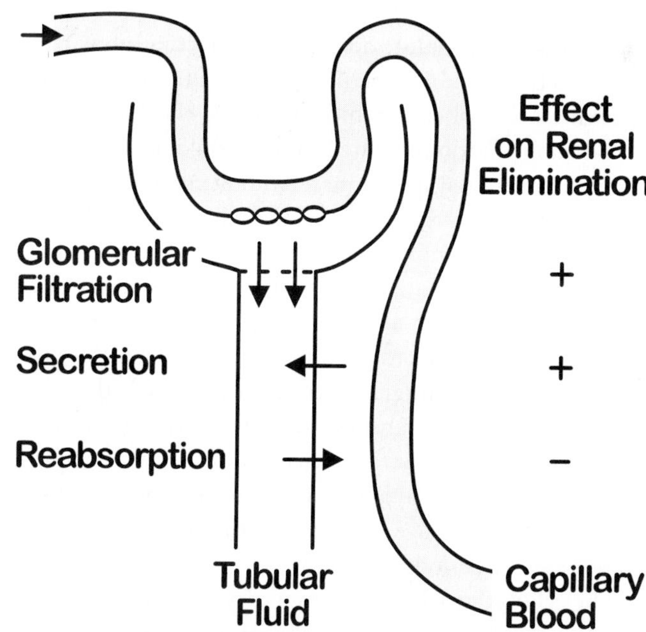

FIG. 2.9 Vectorial processes of nephron function and their net effect on overall renal drug elimination.

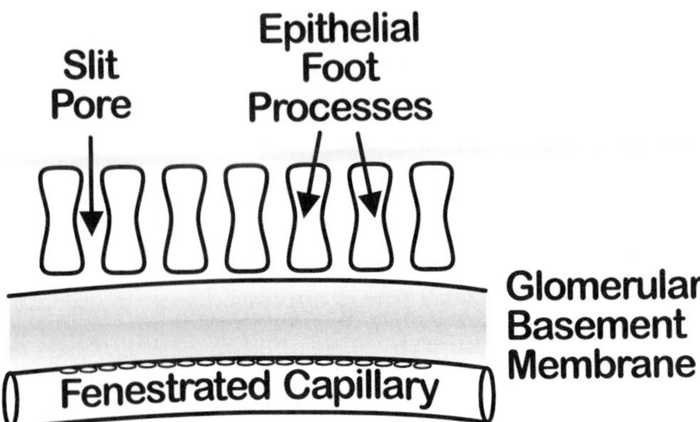

FIG. 2.10 The glomerular filtration barrier.

Glomerular filtration is essentially ultrafiltration through the relatively permeable glomerular filtration barrier, which consists of the epithelial cells of Bowman's capsule, the glomerular basement membrane, and the slit-pores formed from juxtaposing epithelial foot processes (Figure 2.10). These possess a fixed negative charge that is a major contributor to the rate-limiting aspect of this barrier. When damaged, filtration selectivity is impaired and proteins may pass into tubular fluid. This is the primary manifestation of glomerular diseases that affect drug excretion.

The magnitude of active tubular secretion is not affected by the extent of plasma drug protein binding. These saturable, carrier-mediated processes are energy dependent and described by the laws of Michaelis-Menton enzyme kinetics. In order to promote absorption from the tubular filtrate into blood, tubule cells have microvilli, much like the intestinal mucosal cells, which maximize the surface area to cell volume ratio presented to the tubule. For secretion from the interstitial space into the tubule lumen, the basolateral surfaces of these cells (side facing the capillaries) have intensive membrane invaginations that also increase the surface area for interaction with the perfusing capillaries to facilitate active secretion. To provide the energy to drive these processes, proximal tubule cells have high mitochondrial densities to generate ATP, which fuels the Na^+-K^+ ATPase-coupled transport systems. This high level of oxidative metabolism is the primary reason for the sensitivity of the kidney to hypoxic or anoxic conditions, which result in renal damage if blood perfusion is interrupted even for short periods of time.

The cellular structure of transport systems across tubule cells involves two separate pairs of transport proteins, which creates an overall "polarity" of tubule cell function relative to the interstitial fluid and tubular lumen (Figure

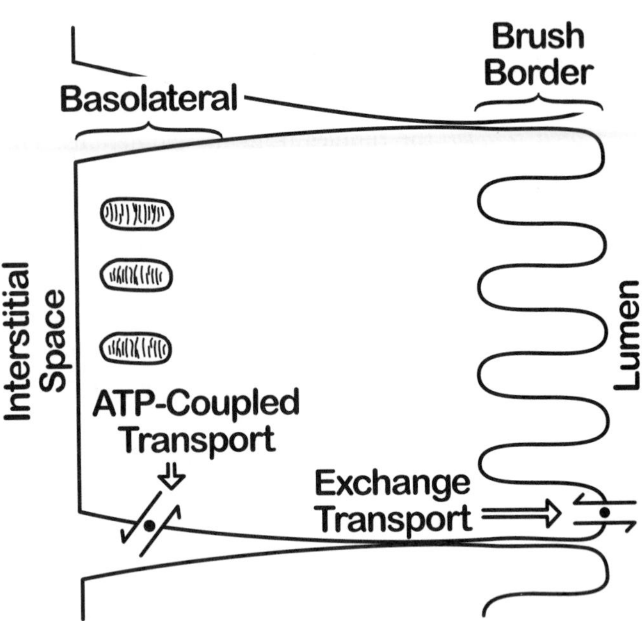

FIG. 2.11 Schematic of a renal tubular cell illustrating location of active and exchange transport systems.

2.11). One set is located in the brush border of the interface with tubular fluid and the other is located in the basolateral membrane. Energy coupling with ATP generally occurs in the basal portion of the cell (proximity to mitochondria), which, in secretion, builds up intracellular drug concentrations that are then transported to the tubular fluid by concentration-driven facilitated transport carriers. In reabsorption, the reverse occurs as the basolateral active "pumps" create low intracellular drug concentrations, which promote facilitated carrier-mediated reabsorption through the brush-border tubular membrane. Most transport systems are also stoichometrically coupled to the transport of an electrolyte (e.g., Na^+, K^+, Cl^-, H^+), which assures electrical neutrality and provides a mechanism for modulating the systemic concentrations of these elements. The primary ion, which drives these transporters and which regulates overall renal function, is sodium. Thus, all drug transport systems are usually coupled to a Na^+ ATPase transmembrane system whose structure and polarity will determine the nature and direction of drug movement.

There are two distinct secretory pathways in the later sections of the proximal renal tubule that are relevant to a discussion of drug and toxicant excretion: one for acidic and one for basic compounds. The primary orientation of this system is from blood to tubular filtrate, removing drugs and/or metabolite conjugates from the blood. Active reabsorption systems are also present that act on a drug already present in the filtered load. These systems are generally present to recover essential nutrients (e.g., glucose) that have been filtered by the glomerulus. Some drugs reach their target sites by this mechanism making their tubular fluid concentration more important for predicting activity than their blood concentrations. An excellent example is the diuretic furosemide that is first secreted by the tubules into the tubular fluid and then is actively reabsorbed back into the tubular cells to gain access to its receptors for activity. Thus, the best concentration-time profile to predict the diuretic action of furosemide is that of the urine rather than blood.

Drugs (and other endogenous substrates) may compete for tubular transport sites, thereby functioning as reversible, competitive inhibitors. This interaction has been classically studied with the organic acid transport system. Weak acids such as probenecid or phenylbutazone will inhibit secretion of the weak acid penicillin, thereby prolonging penicillin blood concentrations. Thus, when more than one drug in the same ionic class is administered, their rate and extent of renal excretion will be affected. Many drug metabolites are conjugates (e.g., glucuronides) produced by Phase II hepatic biotransformation reactions and secreted by the transport system for weak acids, which may further complicate the pattern of drug excretion.

There are direct pharmacokinetic implications to the carrier-mediated mechanism of renal tubular drug secretion. The limited capacity of carrier-mediated processes means that above certain blood drug concentrations, transport will proceed at a maximal rate independent of concentration in blood; that is, so-called *nonlinear zero order kinetics* will become controlling, which will have adverse effects on the utility of normal linear pharmacokinetic models. These factors may become more important in renal disease states where renal capacity is already diminished. Under these circumstances, drug renal clearance will approach the glomerular filtration rate because additional drug concentrations in blood will not now be secreted into the urine. At subsaturation concentrations, renal clearance of an actively secreted substance is dependent on and limited by renal plasma flow and thus flow-limited mechanisms discussed below will become important considerations.

The final determinant of a drug's renal disposition is the mechanism of nonionic passive tubular reabsorption, or back diffusion, a process dependent upon urine flow rate, lipid solubility of the nonionized drug moiety, and urine pH. At low urine flow rates, there is greater opportunity for diffusion of drug from the distal tubular fluid back into the blood. Diffusion is facilitated by the high concentration of drug in the tubular fluid. Polar compounds having low lipid solubility, such as many drug metabolites, are not reabsorbed since they cannot cross the lipid membrane. In contrast, lipid-soluble, nonionized drugs are reabsorbed into the blood. The ratio of ionized to nonionized molecules determines the concentration gradient that drives the drug into the fluid. The extent of reabsorption is again a function of the drug's pKa and the pH of the tubular fluid, as described by the Henderson-Hasselbach equations (see Equations 2.2 and 2.3). The pH of the urine can undergo drastic changes as a function of diet and coadministered drugs (e.g., urine acidifiers and alkalizers). Tubular reabsorption of organic acids occurs with pKa values between 3.0 and 7.5 and for basic drugs with pKa values between 7.5 and 10.5. Weak acids thus are reabsorbed at low urinary pH (acidic), while weak bases are reabsorbed at high urinary pH (alkaline). Therefore, the renal excretion of an acidic drug decreases in acidic urine but increases in alkaline urine.

This principle is employed in treating salicylate intoxication in dogs. A brisk, alkaline diuresis is induced to decrease salicylate reabsorption into the blood and hasten excretion into the urine by trapping the salicylic acid in an ionized form in the alkaline urine. Reabsorption is further decreased by the elevated urinary flow rate. In contrast, induction of an alkaline diuresis will enhance the toxicity of basic drugs by increasing the amount of tubular reabsorption. Drugs often employed in critical care situations, such as procainamide or quinidine, have increased reabsorption and thus systemic activity in this alkaline state.

Species differences in urinary pH can have a major influence on the rate of renal excretion of ionizable drugs. Carnivores tend to have a more acidic (pH 5.5–7.0) urine than herbivores (pH 7.0–8.0). Thus, with all other disposition factors being equal, a weakly acidic drug will have a higher renal excretion in herbivores than in carnivores and a weakly basic drug will have a greater renal excretion in carnivores than in herbivores. In healthy animals, small changes in urinary pH or urine flow rate do not significantly contribute to altered drug clearance. However, with decreased function in renal disease, there is a decreased tubular load of drug. Altered urinary pH theoretically could further decrease overall drug clearance.

There are two other peculiarities of renal tubular transport that must be discussed before quantitating these processes. Some drugs are reabsorbed into the tubules by pinocytosis. This occurs by interaction of filtered drug in the tubular fluid with the brush border membrane. This is a very low-capacity and slow process that is easily saturated. Pinocytozed drugs are then transferred to lysosomes and generally digested in the cell (e.g., peptides and filtered proteins such as β_2 microglobulin). However, for some compounds, such as the aminoglycosides, enzymatic breakdown does not occur and the drug is essentially stored in the kidney. Therefore, although the drug is reabsorbed from the tubular fluid, it is not transported through the cell into the blood. Thus unlike other tubular reabsorption processes, reabsorption with storage or metabolism does decrease elimination of drug from the body. Such reabsorption has toxicologic significance because the drug does accumulate in the tubular cells and could produce an adverse effect. Finally, this phenomenon has a major influence on the prediction of tissue residue profiles in the kidney resulting from drugs with prolonged elimination half-lives (e.g., aminoglycosides).

The final confounding influence on determination of renal drug clearance is when a drug is metabolized by the kidney. Most of the Phase I and Phase II enzymatic systems present in the liver also exist in the kidney, although different isozymes may be expressed. Oxidative processes generally occur within the proximal tubule cells. Two scenarios may occur. The first is when the drug is solely metabolized by the kidney and not the liver, or a combination of both processes occurs. The second is when *relay* metabolism occurs and the kidney further metabolizes a drug already biotransformed by the liver. These interactions are complex and generally are of toxicologic significance.

Renal drug biotransformation may also occur in the medulla by anaerobic metabolic processes (e.g., prostaglandin endoperoxide synthetase). This process is small relative to reducing overall body burden because only 1% of renal blood flow delivers compounds to this region, but it has toxicologic significance to the renal medulla where drug and/or metabolite may accumulate. Finally, brush border enzymes are present that metabolize peptides in the filtered tubular load to amino acids for reabsorption. Stereoselectivity in both active tubular secretion and metabolism in the kidney may occur with specific drugs (e.g., quinidine). The implications to assessment of renal drug excretion is similar to that of drugs metabolized by the kidney and is usually not taken into account.

THE CONCEPT OF CLEARANCE AND ITS CALCULATION. Clearance is a concept widely used to measure the efficiency of drug elimination from an organ or the whole body. The concept was developed for use in assessing kidney function by renal physiologists. The problem with simply measuring the concentration of drug in urine as an index of its renal excretion is that the kidney also modulates the volume of urine produced in association with its primary mission of regulating fluid balance. Thus, the concentration of drug alone may be higher or lower depending on the ultimate urine volume. To accurately assess how much drug is eliminated, the product of volume of urine produced and the concentration of drug in urine (mass/volume) must be determined to provide the amount excreted (mass). If timed urine samples are collected, an excretion rate (mass/time) is determined. Similarly, to assess how efficient this process is, one must know how much drug is actually presented to the kidney for excretion. This is related to the concentration of drug in the arterial blood. The physiological concept of clearance was developed by early workers to generate a parameter that measured the true efficiency of renal excretion processes by assessing the total mass of compound ultimately excreted and relating it to the concentration of drug presented to the kidney for excretion.

There are two definitions of renal clearance that are used to define equations to calculate this parameter from real data. The first is *the volume of blood cleared of a substance by the kidney per unit of time*, that is, the volume of blood required to contain the quantity of drug removed by the kidney during a specific time interval. This will be derived when we have developed pharmacokinetic parameters in Chapter 3 to quantitate Vd and fractional excretion rates. The second definition is *the rate of drug excretion relative to its plasma concentration*. In both cases, the actual value for a drug's renal clearance is the vectorial sum of {filtration + tubular secretion − tubular reabsorption}, making it a parameter that estimates the entire contribution of the kidney to drug elimination. Similarly, any change in renal drug processing will be reflected in renal clearance *if* it is not compensated for by more distal components of the renal tubules.

There are two types of data needed to calculate clearance: 1) an estimate of blood drug concentration presented to the kidney and 2) the amount of drug removed by the kidney. The latter can be estimated either by measuring the amount of drug excreted by the urine or comparing the difference between the renal arterial and venous drug concentrations to assess how much drug was extracted while passing through the organ.

To begin, we will use the classic approach (Equation 2.6), which directly measures extraction, based on Fick's Law:

$$\text{Cl (ml/min)} = (\text{Q})(\text{E}) = (\text{Q})\frac{(\text{C}_{\text{art}} - \text{C}_{\text{ven}})}{(\text{C}_{\text{art}})} \quad (2.6)$$

where Q is renal arterial blood flow (ml/min), E is the extraction ratio and C_{art} and C_{ven} are arterial and venous blood concentrations. The obvious difficulty with this approach is that arterial and venous blood samples must be collected. However, renal physiologists realized that this approach could be modified to more easily assess renal function if a few assumptions were made.

The first is that the amount of substance removed or extracted by the kidney is equivalent to that which is excreted into the urine. If one makes a timed collection of urine and measures the urine concentration and volume, the amount (X) of drug extracted by the kidney over a specific time interval, that is, its *rate* of renal excretion denoted $\Delta X/\Delta t$, is the following (Equation 2.7):

$$\Delta\text{X}/\Delta\text{t(mg/min)} = [\text{U}_\text{X}\text{ (mg/ml)}][\text{V (ml/min)}] \quad (2.7)$$

where U_x is the concentration of drug in urine and V is the urine production. Now the only component needed is the concentration presented to the kidney. Workers used constant rate intravenous infusion of chemicals to insure that so-called *steady state* blood concentrations were achieved. With this experimental design, the renal clearance of substance X is calculated as the following (Equation 2.8):

$$\text{Cl}_{(\text{renal})}\text{ (ml/min)} = (\Delta\text{X}/\Delta\text{t})/\text{C}_{\text{art}} = \text{U}_\text{X}\text{ V}/\text{C}_{\text{art}} \quad (2.8)$$

This expression is equivalent to the definition for clearance above that relates the rate of drug excretion to its plasma concentration. This expression serves as the basis for many of the pharmacokinetic techniques to be developed in subsequent chapters.

Some minor discrepancies may result when drug clearances are calculated by use of blood or plasma data alone versus techniques such as those that employ urine collection. As discussed earlier, tubular reabsorption with storage (e.g., aminoglycoside antibiotics) will result in a lower $\text{Cl}_{(\text{renal})}$ calculated from urine data rather than blood-based methods because tubular reabsorption would not be reflected in the venous blood concentrations since the substance is now trapped in the tubular cells. A similar discrepancy may occur with intrarenal drug metabolism since this process does not return parent drug to venous blood. In a research setting, the difference is often used as conclusive evidence that either of these two phenomena actually occur.

NONLINEARITY OF TUBULAR SECRETION AND REABSORPTION. The discussion thus far has been limited to determining clearances of substances that are primarily eliminated through glomerular filtration. The pharmacokinetics of this process are linear since saturation does not occur and only non–protein-bound drugs are filtered through the glomerular basement membrane complex. When the renal clearance of a drug eliminated by glomerular filtration is estimated, only the filtration of the free or unbound drug is assessed; thus changes in protein binding will change the net excretion of the drug. Drugs and toxicants that undergo passive tubular reabsorption obey Fick's Law of Diffusion since concentration gradients described again by linear first-order rate constants provide the driving force across the tubular epithelium. In contrast, compounds that are actively secreted from postglomerular capillaries across the renal tubules and into the tubular fluid show saturation at high concentrations, competition with drugs secreted by the same pathways, and dependence on the magnitude of renal blood flow; all hallmarks of nonlinear pharmacokinetic behavior. For such compounds, clearance will not be constant but rather will be dependent upon the concentration of drug presented to the kidney.

As tubular secretory pathways become saturated, a drug's clearance will decrease. To develop this concept, we will revisit our definition of a drug cleared by GFR and acknowledge that only the free or unbound drug concentration (C_f) is eliminated by filtration. Protein bound drug (C_b) cannot be filtered. Therefore, the rate of renal excretion ($\Delta X/\Delta t$) can be expressed as simply this (Equation 2.9):

$$\Delta\text{X}/\Delta\text{t} = \text{C}_\text{f} \times \text{GFR} \quad (2.9)$$

As C_f becomes greater, $\Delta X/\Delta t$ will increase in direct proportion (e.g., linearly increase). However recalling Equation 2.8, its clearance will be $\Delta X/\Delta t$ *divided* by C_{art}. In this case, C_{art} is the total blood concentration presented to the kidney ($C_f + C_b$). Clearance thus equals the following (Equation 2.10):

$$\text{Cl}_{(\text{renal})} = (\Delta\text{X}/\Delta\text{t})/\text{C}_{\text{art}} \quad (2.10)$$

These relations have two implications. The first is that as total blood concentrations of drug increase, so does $\Delta X/\Delta t$; however, $Cl_{(renal)}$ remains constant (Equation 2.11) because

$$Cl_{(renal)} = (C_f \times GFR)/(C_{art}) \tag{2.11}$$

and C_{art} will increase in direct proportion to $C_f + C_b$ as long as the fraction bound does not change. However, if the extent of protein binding of a drug is increased ($C_f \downarrow$, $C_b \uparrow$), its rate of renal excretion, $\Delta X/\Delta t$, will decrease as will its clearance since the C_{art} ($C_f + C_b$) will be constant. Therefore, drugs cleared by filtration have constant clearance with changing total drug concentrations but are sensitive to the extent of protein binding. This is one reason that displacement of a drug from protein binding that increases C_f will result in increased renal clearance, which then reduces its concentration to normal. For such a drug with high protein binding, only the small fraction presented for filtration can ever be extracted and cleared by the kidney. Since the total renal clearance of a compound is the sum of filtration plus secretion, a drug *solely cleared by filtration* will have a relatively low clearance compared to one that is also actively secreted. If one considers this in terms of the extraction ratio (E) defined above, Cl_B will always be less than the renal blood flow (Q) since the extraction ratio is less than one and dependent on the glomerular filtration fraction. Such drugs are termed *low extraction* drugs and their $Cl_{(renal)}$ will be sensitive to the extent of protein binding. Examples of such drugs include inulin, the aminoglycoside antibiotics, tetracyclines, digoxin, and furosemide.

In contrast, consider a drug that also undergoes active tubular secretion. In this case, even a drug that is protein bound (C_b) or distributed into red blood cells will be secreted into the urine since the affinity for specific tubular transport proteins will be greater than that for the relatively nonspecific protein-binding sites or partitioning in erythrocytes. The extraction ratio will thus approach 1.0 and $Cl_{(renal)}$ will approach the renal blood flow Q. Such drugs are termed *high extraction* or *perfusion-limited* to acknowledge the relationship of clearance to blood flow. The classic example is para-amino hippurate (PAH) because it is almost completely extracted as it passes through the kidney, making its clearance almost equal to renal plasma flow. In fact, PAH renal clearance had once been used in clinical situations to estimate renal blood flow. Other such drugs include many of the beta-lactam antibiotics (e.g., penicillin) and many sulfate and glucuronide conjugate products of hepatic drug biotransformation. Another implication of active tubular secretion is that at sufficiently high concentrations, saturation of the secretory pathways may occur. Finally, the maximal renal clearance possible is renal blood flow.

The final pathway modulating renal excretion is when a drug undergoes passive tubular reabsorption. The dependency of this process on urinary pH has already been discussed. In this case, C_{art} will be constant but $\Delta X/\Delta t$ and thus $Cl_{(renal)}$ will vary depending on the urinary pH. Since this is an equillibrium process, time is required for this diffusion to occur. Thus if the renal clearance of a drug is dependent on urine flow, it is presumed to undergo passive tubular reabsorption. When high tubular loads are presented, reabsorption is overloaded as equillibrium cannot be achieved and non-reabsorbed drug is eliminated into the urine.

We have focused this discussion on renal drug elimination. However, clearance is used throughout physiology and pharmacokinetics to quantitate drug elimination through any organ as well as from the body. The relevant equation (Equation 2.12) defining the whole body clearance (Cl_B) of a drug is the sum of all elimination clearances:

$$Cl_B = Cl_{(renal)} + Cl_{(hepatic)} + Cl_{(other)} \tag{2.12}$$

Calculation of Cl_B provides an efficient strategy for estimating how a drug or toxicant is eliminated from the body as it indirectly compares systemic clearance to renal and hepatic clearances.

HEPATIC BIOTRANSFORMATION AND BILIARY EXCRETION

Hepatic disposition is one of the final keys in the ADME scheme needed to describe the disposition of many drugs and chemicals in the body. The liver is responsible for both biotransformation and biliary excretion. In many ways, the liver should be considered as two separate organs, one encompassing metabolism and the other biliary excretion.

Drug localization and biotransformation in the liver are dependent on many factors associated with both the biological system and drug itself. These factors include the biological properties of the liver (chemical composition, relative activity of major drug metabolism enzymes, hepatic volume/perfusion rate, and drug accessibility to and extraction by hepatic metabolic sites) as well as the physicochemical properties of the drug (pKa, lipid solubility, molecular weight). In a quantitative sense, the liver is the major drug metabolism organ in the body.

Species differences in drug metabolic fate are, in most cases, the primary source of variation in drug disposition and, therefore, in drug activity or toxicity, across species. Extrapolation of metabolism data between animal species is an important issue as is the ability to correlate in vivo pharmacokinetic and metabolic data with in vitro metabolic findings.

Recalling our earlier discussion about the phenomenological role of metabolism in drug distribution and excretion, it would be hard to imagine what would happen in biological systems without xenobiotic metabolism. Absorbed compounds would stay in the body for a much longer period of time and have prolonged activity, tissue accumulation, and, potentially, toxicity. Metabolism is necessary for the animal or human body to rid itself of lipophilic xenobiotics as an effective defense mechanism against adverse effects. In general, the intensity of drug action is proportional to the concentration of the drug and/or its active metabolite(s) at the target site. On the other hand, drug-associated toxicity is also dependent on the chemical form (active or inactive) and concentration at the same or other relevant target site. Therefore, any process or factor that modifies the drug/metabolite concentration at a target site will cause an altered activity or toxicity profile. Drug metabolism may often result in metabolite(s) with altered chemical structures, which change the receptor type affected, drug-receptor affinity, or pharmacological effect. Most parent drugs can be deactivated to inactive metabolites. In contrast, some drugs can also be activated either from an inactive form (prodrug) to an active drug, or from an active form (e.g., meperidine) to an active metabolite (normeperidine) with similar activity/toxicity. Therefore, drug metabolism can either reduce or enhance parent drug's effect, create another activity, or even elicit toxicity, depending on both the drug and the biological system in question.

Therefore, the pharmacological and pharmacokinetic properties of a drug can be changed by metabolism in one or several of the following ways: pharmacological activation or deactivation; change in disposition kinetics of drug uptake (absorption from application site), distribution, and excretion (e.g., bile excretion, enterohepatic circulation, and renal excretion). The remainder of this chapter focuses on hepatic metabolism and drug hepatobiliary excretion in animal species and introduces some basic biochemical and pharmacokinetic concepts relevant to this role. Although these discussions are focused on the liver, the principles elucidated may also be applicable to extrahepatic sites of drug biotransformation.

PHASE I AND PHASE II REACTIONS. Various metabolic pathways are involved in drug metabolism including oxidation, reduction, hydrolysis, hydration, and conjunction. These processes can be divided into Phase I and Phase II reactions (Table 2.2). Phase I includes reactions introducing functional groups to drug molecules necessary for the Phase II reactions, which primarily involve conjugation. In other words, Phase I products act as substrates for Phase II processes, resulting in conjugation with endogenous compounds, which further increase their water solubility and polarity, thus retarding tissue distribution and facilitating drug excretion from the body. Specific examples of drug metabolism are included in chapters throughout this text. The focus of this introduction will be to briefly overview the general processes involved in drug metabolism relative to how they might affect pharmacokinetic parameters and the disposition of drugs in the body. Interested readers should consult standard texts in drug metabolism or biochemical pharmacology/toxicology for specific detailed examples illustrating the chemistry and genetic control of these processes.

Our knowledge regarding the molecular mechanisms of drug metabolism has been predominately gained from studies on the liver at different experimental levels including in vivo intact animals; ex vivo liver perfusion; and in vitro liver slices, hepatocyte cell cultures, isolated/purified subcellular hepatocyte organelles, and isolated enzyme or enzyme components. Two subcellular organelles are quantitatively the most important; the endoplasmic reticulum

TABLE 2.2 Drug metabolism reactions

Phase I	Phase II
Oxidation	Glucuronidation/glucosidation
-Cyt P-450–dependent	Sulfation
-Others	Methylation
Reduction	Acetylation
Hydrolysis	Amino acid conjugation
Hydration	Glutathione conjugation
Dethioacetylation	Fatty acid conjugation
Isomerization	

(ER) (isolated in the microsome fraction) and the cytosol (isolated in the soluble cell fraction). Phase I oxidation enzymes are almost exclusively localized in the ER, along with the Phase II enzyme of glucuronyl transferase. In contrast, other Phase II enzymes are mainly present in the cytoplasm. Microsomal fractions of the hepatocyte retains most, if not all, of the enzymatic activity in drug metabolism.

Phase I metabolism includes four major pathways: oxidation, reduction, hydrolysis, and hydration, among which oxidation is the most important. Attention is usually focused on oxidation mediated by the microsomal mixed-function oxidase system (e.g., cytochrome P450, etc.) due to its central role and significance in governing the metabolic disposition of many drugs and xenobiotics. An understanding of this pathway is often critical to making interspecies extrapolations.

Phase II conjugating enzymes play a very important role in the deactivation of the Phase I metabolites of many drugs as well as in direct deactivation of some parent compounds when their specific structure doesn't require Phase I modification. For example, the analgesic drug paracetamol can be deactivated directly by Phase II reactions using glutathione, glucuronide, and sulfate conjugation mechanisms. Phase II deactivation can be achieved by both gross chemical modification of the drug thereby decreasing their receptor affinity, and by enhancement of excretion from the body, often via the kidney.

Among the reactions catalyzed by drug metabolism enzymes in the hepatic ER, cytochrome (Cyt) P450-dependent mixed-function oxidation is the most intensively studied. This reaction catalyzes the hydroxylation of hundreds of structurally diverse drugs and compounds, whose only common feature appears to be a relatively high lipophilicity. The enzyme consists of a family of closely related isoenzymes embedded in the ER membrane. Its name is based on the fact that the cytochrome is a pigment that exhibits a maximal absorbance wavelength of 450 nm when reduced and complexed with carbon monoxide. With the advent of gene cloning and sequencing, and the application of molecular biology techniques to Cyt P450 structure analysis, tremendous progress was made in the last decade in the isolation and sequencing of the cDNAs encoding multiple forms of the hemoprotein. The rapid determination of full-length Cyt P450 amino acid sequences enabled the development of a coherent nomenclature system describing hundreds of different and unique Cyt P450s.

TABLE 2.3 Example of cytochrome P450 enzymes in the dog

Subfamily	Gene Code	Sample Substrates
1A	1A1, 1A2	Theophylline
2B	2B11	Phenobarbital, dextromethorphan
2C	2C21, 2C41	Testosterone
2D	2D15	β blockers
3A	3A12, 3A26	Macrolides, steroids, cyclosporine

A great deal of work has been fostered in this area through development of a nomenclature system for cytochrome P450 enzymes (CYP) based on DNA/amino acid sequence. This allows enzymes to be unambiguously classified. An enzyme is coded by its family (1,2, . . .) followed by subfamily (A–D) and then gene (1,2, . . .), and if necessary, allelic variant (*1, *2, . . .). Thus, a common enzyme found in dogs is termed CYP3A12, which is responsible for steroid oxidation. These enzymes are classified on the basis of sequence and not function. There is thus a great deal of overlap between substrate specificities and enzymes with different CYP identifications. The numbers are also species-specific, thus preventing direct comparison between species. Not surprisingly, most work has been done for human enzymes, although recently work has also begun to define the primary enzymes involved in veterinary species. Table 2.3 lists the cytochrome P450 enzymes identified in the dog.

IMPACT OF METABOLISM. One can precisely predict the impact of drug metabolism on therapeutic drug effect if one can identify the precise enzymes by which a drug is metabolized. The same enzymes are not involved in metabolizing the same drugs in different species, and in many cases, substrate specificities overlap, making precise prediction difficult. A variety of Phase I and Phase II reactions can take place simultaneously or sequentially in the body. For example, parathion can be catalyzed by Cyt P450 to an intermediate, which in turn can either be further oxidized to paraoxon or hydrolyzed to *p*-nitrophenol followed by conjugation reactions. Finally, as discussed earlier, a compound metabolized in the liver may be subsequently metabolized in the kidney prior to excretion, making it possible for these various metabolic steps to be carried out in multiple organs. Stereochemistry also plays a major role in drug metabolism since most enzyme system can be stereoselective. Examples include the enantiomers of amphetamine, cyclophosphamide, pentobarbitone, phenytoin, verapamil, and warfarin. Large differences in enzyme expression and function occur between species. Many of these were first identified in broad differences in the ability of some species studied to perform Phase II reactions (e.g., cats deficient in glucuronidation, pigs in sulfation). We now know that this is even more complex, especially in species differences in specific CYP isoenzymes.

To further complicate this scenario, there is often overlap between cytochrome P450 substrate specificities and those for P-glycoprotein. That is, the same drug may be handled by both systems, classic examples being cyclosporine and ketoconazole. Such phenomena are often detected by complex and species-specific drug-drug interactions. For compounds handled in such a fashion, one can be assured that large differences will be seen between animal species.

In summary, Phase I metabolism is primarily responsible for drug deactivation, although Phase II plays an important role in deactivation of some drugs. Phase I reactions prepare drugs or toxicants for Phase II metabolism; i.e., Phase I modifies the drug molecule by introducing a chemically reactive group on which the Phase II reactions can be carried out for the final deactivation and excretion. This increased water solubility after metabolism restricts a drug's metabolite distribution to extracellular fluids, thereby enhancing excretion. Specific pathways for drug metabolism and transport are discussed in the individual drug chapters as well as in Chapter 50.

HEPATIC CLEARANCE. As presented in our discussion on renal excretion, clearance of a drug by an organ (Cl_{org}) can be ultimately defined as a function of its blood flow (Q_{org}) and its extraction ratio (E_{org}) expressed in Equation 2.6 as $Cl_{org} = Q_{org} E_{org}$. The ability of the liver to remove drug from the blood, defined as *hepatic clearance,* is related to two variables: intrinsic hepatic clearance (Cl_{int}) and rate of hepatic blood flow (Q_h), as defined in Equation 2.13:

$$Cl_h = Q_h[Cl_{int}/(Q_h + Cl_{int})] = Q_h E_h \qquad (2.13)$$

where Cl_h is the hepatic clearance, Q_h is the hepatic blood flow, and $Cl_{int}/(Q_h+Cl_{int})$ is the hepatic extraction ratio or E_h. Intrinsic clearance (Cl_{int}) is conceptualized as the maximal ability of the liver to extract/metabolize drug when hepatic blood flow is not limiting. It represents the inherent metabolic function of all enzyme systems in the liver to metabolize the drug in question. As seen in Equation 2.13, when $Cl_{int} >> Q_h$, hepatic extraction ratio ≈ 1.0 (*flow-limited or high extraction*, usually seen with $E_h > 0.8$), Cl_h is dependent only on the blood perfusion rate Q_h. The more blood passing through the liver, the more drug molecules will be extracted by the liver for metabolic elimination. A hepatic blood perfusion-dependent hepatic clearance will then be seen. Drugs with such high extraction ratios will show significant first-pass metabolism after oral administration to the extent that this route of administration may not produce effective systemic drug concentrations. Finally, the highest hepatic Cl possible is Q_h.

In contrast, if $Cl_{int} << Q_h$, the E_h is close to zero and thus the Cl_h is dependent only on the Cl_{int}; i.e., the liver extracts as many drug molecules as it can from the blood flow presented (*metabolism-limited or low extraction*, usually with $E_h < 0.2$). These two extremes occur with propranolol and antipyrine, respectively. Intermediate values of extraction ratio of 0.2–0.8 give hepatic clearance rates that can be dependent to varying extents on both hepatic blood perfusion rate and intrinsic clearance. Based on earlier discussions, one can appreciate that such classifications are very species specific since they depend upon the presence of specific enzyme systems for the specific drug.

To estimate hepatic drug clearance, one must consider the drug's physicochemical properties, hepatic drug metabolism enzyme activity, and rate of hepatic blood perfusion. This relationship between hepatic clearance and liver blood perfusion rate for drugs with different extraction ratios can be appreciated when Equation 2.13 is plotted in Figure 2.12. With a lower hepatic extraction drug, the blood perfusion rate is less important to $Cl_{hepatic}$. For a high hepatic extraction drug, the $Cl_{hepatic}$ is proportional to the blood flow as discussed earlier. The reader should note the similarity of this discussion to that introduced earlier concerning capacity or flow-limited renal tubular clearance. The concepts are identical for both organs; however, they are more often employed when hepatic clearance is modeled due to the much greater difference in species-inherent metabolic capacities.

METABOLISM INDUCTION AND INHIBITION. Drug metabolism is substantially influenced by enzyme induction or inhibition that occurs secondary to the deliberate or passive intake of a number of chemicals that animals are increasingly exposed to either in the environment, for medical reasons, as dietary supplements, or in humans simply as a result of lifestyle (smoking, alcohol consump-

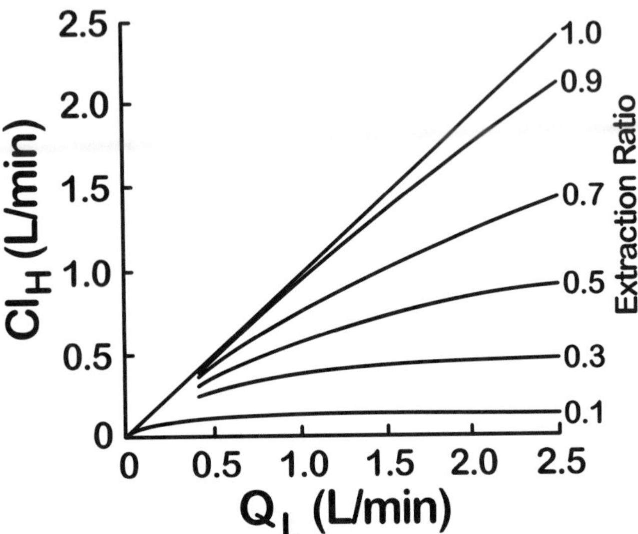

FIG. 2.12 Relationship between liver blood flow (Q) and hepatic clearance (Cl_H) for drugs with different hepatic extraction ratios. Extraction ratio values are at a blood flow of 1.5 l/min.

tion, etc.). In laboratory animals, contaminants and natural constituents of diet have been shown to affect the pattern of drug metabolism observed. In many cases, the compound itself may alter its own metabolic fate by induction or inhibition.

Induction. Many currently used drugs, food additives, household chemicals, and environmental contaminants (including pesticides) possessing diverse chemical structure, pharmacological or toxicological activity are well known to induce their own metabolism and/or that of other compounds in humans and animals. Induction of metabolism may arise as a consequence of increased synthesis (at different transcriptional/translational levels), decreased degradation, activation of preexisting components, or a combination of these processes. With so many compounds able to alter hepatic metabolism, a great deal of effort has been spent in recent years to understand the mechanisms behind these processes. This is important from a therapeutic perspective since the intrinsic hepatic clearance of a drug will change if the enzymes responsible for metabolizing it are induced, thereby increasing metabolic capacity. Similarly, the pattern of Phase I and Phase II metabolism may be changed if one enzyme component's activity has been modified by inducers. These interactions introduce a significant complexity to pharmacokinetic models describing the disposition of drugs extensively metabolized by the liver. However, they have also prompted research efforts aimed at elucidating the mechanisms behind these processes, which, when understood, should provide a strategy for developing mechanistically meaningful models for simulation of drug metabolic disposition.

Of particular importance to the overall hepatic metabolic clearance of a drug is the activity of the Cyt P450 system. In the mid-1960s, both Cyt P450 and its associated flavoprotein reductase were found to be induced by phenobarbitone pretreatment that was accompanied by induction of drug metabolism. Induction was generally accompanied by increases in liver microsomal Cyt P450 content. Diverse drug metabolism responses to different inducers, which all induce hepatic Cyt P450, can be dependent on the substrate of interest (substrate specificity) with stero- and regioselectivity, suggesting that subpopulations of Cyt P450 (isoenzymes) might be present. This now widely accepted concept has had a profound influence on drug discovery, design of metabolism studies, and the resulting structure of pharmacokinetic models. With the advent of the CYP nomenclature system discussed above, enzymes can now be classified both as to substrate specificity, but also as to which compounds induce or inhibit their function. Pharmacogenomic studies have begun to identify the specific genes responsible for isoenzyme induction and also identify species differences. Unfortunately, these studies are just beginning to be applied in veterinary species and a complete picture is lacking of their impact on clinical therapeutics. The important concept is that induction will occur and could have a significant impact on therapeutic efficacy.

Metabolism Inhibition. Similar to the induction of metabolism, inhibition is a well-recognized phenomenon secondary to serial drug dosing, coadministration of drugs, endogenous compounds, environmental xenobiotics, and complex multiple-ingredient drug formulations. Several mechanisms for metabolism inhibition have been noted, including the destruction of preexisting enzymes {by prophyrinogic drugs and xenobiotics containing olefinic (C = C) and acetylenic (C ≡ C) functions}, inhibition of enzyme synthesis (by metal ions), or complexing with the hemoprotein thereby inactivating enzymes. Many drug-drug interactions may be explained at the level of Cyt P450 destruction. In contrast to the prophyrinogic drugs, metal ions such as cobalt exert their inhibitory effects by modulating both the synthesis and degradation of the heme prosthetic group of Cyt P450. Formation of inactive Cyt

P450-inhibitor complex is another mechanism for drug metabolism inhibition. Inhibitors are usually substrates of Cyt P450 and require metabolic conversion to exert their full inhibitory effects, in a manner similar to prophyrinogic drugs and xenobiotics. However, inhibitors forming complexes with hemoprotein are metabolized by Cyt P450. These inhibitors can form metabolic intermediates or products that tightly bind to the hemoprotein, thereby preventing its further participation in drug metabolism. As can occur with induction, coadministration of inhibitor drugs may result in clinically important drug interactions. Specific examples of such interactions are presented within the drug-specific chapters of this text.

BILIARY DRUG ELIMINATION. As an exocrine function of the liver, bile excretion is thought to be present in almost all vertebrates. The three basic physiological functions of the bile are 1) to serve as the excretory route for products of biotransformation, 2) to facilitate the intestinal absorption of ingested lipids such as fatty acids, cholesterol, lecithin, and/or monoglycerides due to the surfactant properties of bile forming mixed micelles, and 3) to serve as a major route for cholesterol elimination in order to maintain normal plasma cholesterol levels. In addition to its physiological functions, bile is also pharmacologically and toxicologically important since some heavy metals and enzymes are also excreted via the biliary system. Bile secretion is very important to chemical/drug transport and elimination under both physiological and pathological conditions. However, bile secretion has proven difficult to study mainly due to the inaccessibility of the biliary tree for direct sampling.

The Mechanism of Bile Formation. Bile is continuously produced by liver cells and then stored in the gall bladder, except for those species (rat, horse) lacking it. The pH of bile ranges from 5.0–7.5 depending mainly on the animal species. Biliary excretion is a major route for some drugs with MW >300 and a high degree of polarity. This occurs by active transport of drug and metabolites into bile, thus saturation and competition are important issues to consider. Passive diffusion of drug into bile is insignificant. Most of the compounds secreted into bile are finally excreted from the body in feces where they may be subject to enterohepatic circulation and degradation by intestinal microflora.

Bile is formed at two sites: the ramifications of the bile duct within the portal triads and the anastomosing network of the narrow bile canaliculi in the hepatic parenchyma. The bile canaliculi are the primary secretory units of the liver. These small channels or furrows are lined by the apical membranes of the hepatocytes and thus do not have their own epithelium or basement membrane. Because hepatocytes form a canalicular lumen wherever they abut, most canaliculi communicate with each other, forming an anastomosing network. Similar to the relationship of the nephron to the kidney, the volume and composition of canalicular bile are often determined by the activity of several cords of hepatocytes.

The overall bile flow is in the opposite direction to sinusoidal blood flow and thus solute transfer from plasma to bile involves a counterflow process (Fig. 2.13). Such a blood-bile flow pattern reduces rediffusion of biliary solutes such as drugs and metabolites back into sinusoidal plasma in the portal area, which is richer in solute concentration, bathes periportal hepatocytes, and is exposed to higher canalicular concentration of any given solute. Three routes of fluid and drug transfer from the sinusoid to the bile canaliculus have been postulated: transcellular, paracellular, and vesicular. These multiple mechanisms con-

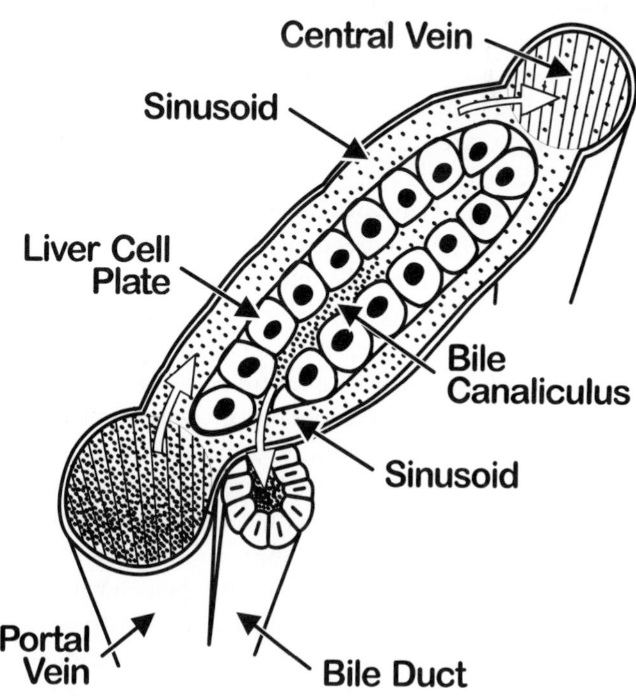

FIG. 2.13 Gradient concept of bile secretion in a liver lobule.

tribute to the large interspecies differences seen in biliary drug excretion.

Drug uptake into hepatocytes by passive diffusion is so efficient that it is rate-limited by the delivery of the drug to the liver (i.e., blood flow) rather than membrane transport per se, thereby exhibiting flow-dependent clearance. However, for highly polar molecules, passive diffusion is not an efficient mode of hepatocellular uptake, and there is an increased reliance on carrier-mediated transport systems. Drug metabolites, particularly conjugated metabolites (e.g., sulphates and glucuronides), are invariably more polar than their precursors and thus are more likely to experience hepatocyte membranes as diffusional barriers. With such a barrier, the hepatocellular export of a locally formed metabolite will depend on the presence and activity of carrier-mediated transport systems for sinusoidal efflux and biliary excretion. Transport systems of current interest include the P-glycoproteins, which are responsible for the biliary excretion of a range of organic cations, and the canalicular multispecific organic anion transporter. Intracellular trapping of metabolites formed in the liver, secondary to low membrane permeability, is clinically important because many are potentially hepatotoxic and/or capable of interfering with the hepatic transport of endogenous compounds or other drugs and metabolites. Again this phenomenon is conceptually similar to renal tubular sequestration and has similar pharmacokinetic implications. Finally, if the metabolite is unstable, intracellular accumulation can lead to the regeneration of the precursor and so-called "futile cycling" within hepatocytes.

Biliary Drug Transport. Some parent drugs and numerous drug metabolites derived from hepatic metabolism are excreted in the bile into the intestinal tract. The excreted metabolites can be excreted via feces although, more commonly, they are subject to reabsorption into the blood and are eventually excreted from the body via urine. There are at least three different biliary transport pathways for organic anions, cations, and neutral compounds, although metals may also have their own transport carriers/systems. Both *organic anions* and *organic cations* can be actively transported into bile by carrier systems again similar to those involved in the renal tubule. Such transport systems are nonselective, and ions with similar electrical charge may compete for the same transport mechanisms. Additionally, a third carrier system, whose activity is sex-dependent, may be involved in the active transport of *steroids* and *related compounds* into bile. In contrast to renal excretion, amphiphatic drugs (those having both polar and nonpolar properties) are preferentially excreted in the bile. The drug (or metabolite) excreted into the small intestine can be reabsorbed into blood forming the so-called drug enterohepatic cycle. This is an important factor changing the blood : liver or liver : bile drug concentration ratios during studies of the hepatobiliary transport mechanisms and drug hepatic elimination.

The biliary excretion of weak acids is the most important mechanism in drug hepatic elimination. Bromosulfophtalein (BSP) and analogues are dyes used as diagnostic probes of liver function and model substances in studies of the hepatic uptake of organic anions. Antibiotics such as ciprofloxacin can be actively excreted into bile in the presence of a biliary tract obstruction. Tetracyclines, mainly excreted into urine via glomerular filtration, are also concentrated in the liver and accordingly excreted into the small intestine via the bile, and then partially reabsorbed.

Glucuronides of endogenous compounds and drugs can be actively transported from hepatocytes into bile via transport systems similar to those for organic anions. Glucuronide conjugates are very important in hepatic drug metabolism and biliary excretion. The effectiveness of biliary excretion for glucuronide conjugates can be greatly limited by enzymatic hydrolysis after the bile is mixed with the small intestine contents, thereby releasing the parent drugs to be reabsorbed and enter the enterohepatic cycle. The reabsorbed drugs and metabolites can be ultimately excreted in urine. Some drug metabolites further undergo either biotransformation in the liver or other organs or are subjected to microbiological and physicochemical degradation in the small intestine before being excreted in the feces.

Weak bases can be actively transported into bile via carrier systems similar to the renal transport processes. Atropine, isoproterenol, and curare are eliminated by this mechanism, with atropine being almost equally excreted by the kidney (unchanged form) and hepatic metabolism followed by biliary excretion. Organic cation transport is not as important as the organic anion pathway. Neutral compounds may employ the third transport systems. Ouabain, a cardiac glycoside, is used as a model uncharged and nonmetabolized (by rat liver) compound in hepatobiliary transport studies. Organic anions and neutral steroids such as ouabain may share common mechanisms in their excretory pathways.

TABLE 2.4 Mean bile flow in selected species

Species	Bile Flow (ml/min/kg Body Weight)
Cat	11
Chicken	20
Dog	4–10
Guinea pig	200
Hamster	50
Human	5–7
Monkey	10
Mouse	78
Opossum	20
Pig	9
Pony	19
Rabbit	90
Rat	50–80
Sheep	43

Molecular weight is a key determinant of the extent to which drug/metabolite molecules are transported into bile. The molecular weight cutoff required for biliary excretion is much greater than that for renal tubular secretion, being from 300–500 in most species. If the molecular weight is lower, the compound may be preferentially excreted in urine. Molecules with weights from 3–500 to 850 Da may be eliminated via both the renal and biliary routes. Excretion of molecules larger than 850 Da occurs mainly via the biliary active transport system. However, molecular weight is not the sole factor determining the route of drug excretion. Physicochemical properties of the drug (polarity/lipophilicity, structure) are also very critical to the extent of biliary excretion of a drug/metabolite, with amphiphatic drugs being well secreted by the biliary route.

The specific animal species being studied is also an important factor, as reflected in different molecular weight cutoff thresholds. Table 2.4 lists species differences in bile flow rate that may also contribute to the great species specificity seen in biliary drug transport. Such variations in both a species' enzyme profile for biotransformation and inherent ability to excrete drugs in bile result in great difficulty in predicting hepatic clearance across drugs in different species.

CONCLUSION

This chapter presents an overview of some essential principles of ADME that are needed to understand drug and species-specific behavior of drugs. The next chapter focuses on the pharmacokinetic tools used to quantitate these processes so that safe and effective dosages of drugs can be administered to animals.

SELECTED READING

Alberts, B., Bray, D., Lewis, J., Raff, M., Roberts, K., and Watson, J.D. 1989. Molecular Biology of the Cell, 2d Ed. New York: Garland Publishing Co.

Ariens, E.J., Soudijn, W., and Timmermans, P.B.M.W.M. 1983. Stereochemistry and Biological Activity of Drugs. Oxford: Blackwell Scientific Press.

Balimane, P.V., Han, Y.H., and Chong, S. 2006. Current industrial practices of assessing permeability and p-glycoprotein interaction. The AAPS Journal. 8:E1–13.

Barza, M. 1981. Principles of tissue penetration of antibiotics. Journal of Antimicrobial Chemotherapy, SuppC. 8:7–28.

Borchardt, R.T., Smith, P.L., and Wilson, G. 1996. Models for Assessing Drug Absorption and Metabolism. New York: Plenum Press.

Brodie, B.B., Gillette, J.R., and Ackerman, H.S.. 1971. Handbook of Experimental Pharmacology, Vol. 28, Part I, Concepts in Biochemical Pharmacology. Berlin: Springer.

Calabrese, E.J. 1991. Principles of Animal Extrapolation. Chelsea, MI: Lewis Publishers.

Chauret, N., Gauthier, A., Martin, J., and Nicoll-Griffith, D.A. 1997. In vitro comparison of cytochrome p450-mediated activities in human, dog, cat and horse. Drug Metabolism Disposition. 25:1130–1136.

Chiou, W.L., Jeong, H.Y., Chung, S.M., and Wu, T.C. 2000. Evaluation of using dogs as an animal model to study fraction of oral dose absorbed of 43 drugs in humans. Pharmaceutical Research. 17:135–140.

Chow, S.C., and Liu, J.P. 2000. Design and Analysis of Bioavailability and Bioequivalence Studies. 2nd Ed. New York: Marcel Dekker.

Davson, H., and Danielli, J.F. 1952. Permeability of Natural Membranes, 2d Ed. London: Cambridge University Press.

Edman, P. and Björk, E. 1992. Routes of delivery: Case studies. (1) Nasal delivery of peptide drugs. Advanced Drug Delivery Reviews 8:165–177.

Elmquist, W.F., and Sawchuck, R.J. 1997. Application of microdialysis in pharmacokinetic studies. Pharmaceutical Research 14:267–288.

Firth, E.C., Nouws, J.F.M., Driessenss, F., Schmaetz, P., Peperkamp, K., and Klein, W.R. 1986. Effect of injection site on the pharmacokinetics of procaine penicillin G in horses. American Journal of Veterinary Research 47:2380–2384.

Gibson, G.G., and Skett, P. 1994. Introduction to Drug Metabolism. 2d Ed. New York: Blackie A&P.

Hardee, G.E., and Baggot, J.D. 1998. Development and Formulation of Veterinary Dosage Forms, 2d Ed. New York: Marcel Dekker.

Hayes, A.W. 1994. Principles and Methods of Toxicology, 3d Ed. New York: Raven Press.

Illing, H.P.A. 1989. Xenobiotic Metabolism and Disposition. Boca Raton, FL: CRC Press.

Jenner, P., and Testa, B. 1981. Concepts in Drug Metabolism. New York: Marcel Dekker.

Kalow, W. 1992. Pharmacogenetics of Drug Metabolism. New York: Pergamon Press.

Klaasen, C.D. 2001. Casarett and Doull's Toxicology: The Basic Science of Poisons, 6th Ed. New York: McGraw-Hill.

Lee, V.H.L. and Yamamoto, A. 1990. Penetration and enzymatic barriers to peptide and protein absorption. Advanced Drug Delivery Reviews 4:171–207.

Lees, P. (editor). 2004. Special Review Issue: PK and PK-PD in veterinary medicine. Journal of Veterinary Pharmacology and Therapeutics. 27:395–535.

Mammarlund-Udenaes, M., Paalzow, L.K., and deLange, E.C.M. 1997. Drug equilibration across the blood-brain barrier: Pharmacokinetic considerations based on the microdialysis method. Pharmaceutical Research 14:128–134.

Martinez, M.N. and Riviere, J.E. 1994. Review of the 1993 Veterinary Drug Bioequivalence Workshop. Journal of Veterinary Pharmacology and Therapeutics 17:85–119.

Martinez, M.N., Papich, M.G., and Riviere, J.E. 2004. Veterinary application of in vitro dissolution data and the biopharmaceutics classification system. Pharmacopeial Forum 30:2295–2303.

Mealey, K.L. 2004. Therapeutic implications of the MDR-1 gene. Journal of Veterinary Pharmacology and Therapeutics. 27:257–264.

———. 2006. Pharmacogenetics. Veterinary Clinics of North America. 36:961–973.

Monteiro-Riviere, N.A., Bristol, D.G., Manning, T.O., Rogers, R.A., and Riviere, J.E. 1990. Interspecies and interegional analysis of the comparative histological thickness and laser Doppler blood flow measurements at five cutaneous sites in nine species. Journal of Investigative Dermatology 95:582–586.

Okey, A.B. 1990. Enzyme induction in the cytochrome P450 system. Pharmacology and Therapeutics 45:241–298.

Pang, K.S. and Rowland, M. 1977. Hepatic clearance of drugs. Journal of Pharmacokinetics and Biopharmaceutics. 5:625–653.

Patton, J.S. and Platz, R.M. 1992. Routes of delivery: Case studies. (2) Pulmonary delivery of peptides and proteins for systemic action. Advanced Drug Delivery Reviews 8:179–196.

Peterson L.R., and Gerding, D. 1980. Influence of protein binding of antibiotics on serum pharmacokinetics and extravascular penetration: Clinically useful concepts. Reviews of Infectious Diseases 2:340–348, 1980.

Pratt, W.B. and Taylor, P. 1990. Principles of Drug Action, 3d Ed. New York: Churchill Livingstone.

Qiao, G.L., Williams, P.L., and Riviere, J.E. 1994. Percutaneous absorption, biotransformation and systemic disposition of parathion in vivo in swine. I. comprehensive pharmacokinetic model. Drug Metabolism and Disposition 22:459–471.

Raub, T.J. 2006. P-glycoprotein recognition of substrates and circumvention through rational drug design. Molecular Pharmacology. 3:3–25.

Riviere, J.E. 1999. Comparative Pharmacokinetics: Principles, Techniques and Applications. Ames, IA: Blackwell.

———. 2006. Dermal Absorption Models in Toxicology and Pharmacology. Boca Raton, FL: Taylor and Francis.

———. 2006. Biological Concepts and Techniques in Toxicology: An Integrated Approach. New York: Taylor and Francis.

Riviere, J.E. and Heit, M.C. 1997. Electrically-assisted transdermal drug delivery. Pharmaceutical Research 14:691–701.

Rowland, M., Benet, L.Z., and Graham, G.G. 1973. Clearance concepts in pharmacokinetics. Journal of Pharmacokinetics and Biopharmaceutics 1:123–136.

Shou, M., Norcross, R., Sandig, G., Lu, P., Li, Y., Mei, Q., Rodrigues, A.D., and Rushmore, T.H. 2003. Substrate specificity and kinetic properties of seven heterologously expressed dog cytochromes p450. Drug Metabolism Disposition. 31:1161–1169.

Singer, S.J., and Nicholson, G.L. 1972. The fluid mosaic model of the structure of cell membranes. Science 175:720–731.

Smith, H.W. 1956. Principles of Renal Physiology. New York: Oxford University Press.

Tavoloni, N., and Berk, P.P. 1993. Hepatic Transport and Bile Secretion: Physiology and Pathophysiology. New York: Raven Press.

Teodori, E., Dei, S., Martelli, C., Scapecchi, S., and Gualteiri, F. 2006. The functions and structure of ABC transporters: Implications for the design of new inhibitors of Pgp and MRP1 to control multidrug resistance (MDR). Current Drug Targets 7:893–909.

Toutain, P.L., and Bousquet-Melou, A. 2002. Free drug fraction versus free drug concentration: A matter of frequent confusion. Journal of Veterinary Pharmacology and Therapeutics 25:460–463.

Toutain, P.L., and Koritz, G.D. 1997. Veterinary drug bioequivalence determination. Journal of Veterinary Pharmacology and Therapeutics 20:79–90.

Tozer, T.N. 1981. Concepts basic to pharmacokinetics. Pharmacology Therapeutics 12:109–131.

Upton, R.N. 1990. Regional pharmacokinetics I. Physiological and physiological basis. Biopharmaceutics and Drug Disposition 11:647–662.

Waterman, M.R., and Johnson, E.F. 1991. Cytochrome P450. Methods in Enzymology, Volume 206. New York: Academic Press.

CHAPTER 3

PHARMACOKINETICS

JIM E. RIVIERE

Pharmacokinetics is best defined as *the use of mathematical models to quantitate the time course of drug absorption and disposition in man and animals.* With the tremendous advances in medicine and analytical chemistry, coupled with the almost universal availability of computers, what was once an arcane science has now entered the mainstream of most fields of human and veterinary medicine. This discipline has allowed dosages of drugs to be tailored to individuals or groups to optimize therapeutic effectiveness, minimize toxicity, and avoid violative tissue residues in the case of food-producing animals. This subject and its concepts have become especially important as a consequence of the dramatic and almost radical changes that occurred at the end of the last decade relative to the regulations surrounding drug use in veterinary medicine in the United States. For most of the recent past, the operative concept was that a single dose of drug listed on a product label was optimal for all therapeutic uses. Recently, however, the legal concept of "flexible or professional labeling" and the passage by the U.S. Congress in 1994 of the Animal Medicinal Drug Use Clarification Act (AMDUCA) legalizing extralabel drug use challenged this simplistic ideal of a single optimal dose. The veterinarian must now select a drug dose based on numerous factors inherent to the therapeutic scenario at hand to maximize therapeutic efficacy and minimize the likelihood of drug-induced toxicity or induction of microbial resistance. Unlike human medicine and companion animal practices, food animal veterinarians face the further restriction that proper withdrawal times must be determined to ensure that drug residues do not persist in the edible tissues or by-products (milk, eggs) of treated animals long after they have left the care of the veterinarian (Fig. 3.1). As will be demonstrated, the "withdrawal time" is in reality a pure

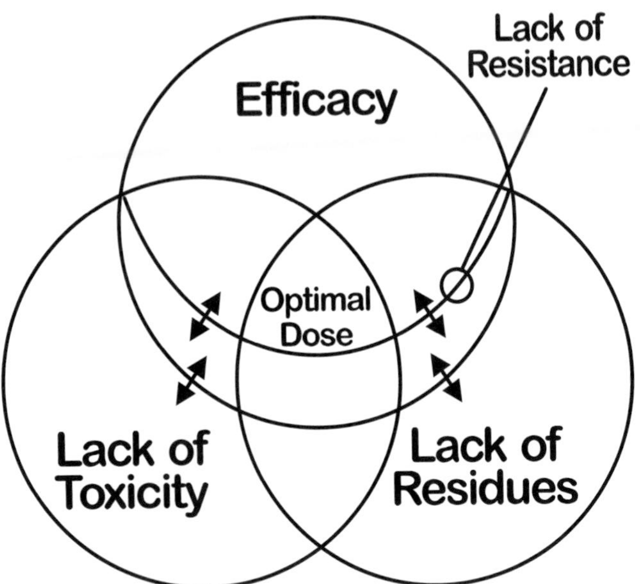

FIG. 3.1 The food animal veterinarian's dilemma in optimizing the dose of a therapeutic drug.

pharmacokinetic parameter since it can be calculated solely from a knowledge of the legal tissue tolerance and the drug's half-life or rate of decay in that tissue.

Yet it is not only the food animal veterinarian that faces these challenges. The laboratory animal and exotic/zoo animal worker must often extrapolate drug dosages across species with widely differing body sizes and physiology since there are very few approved drugs for the treatment of such animals. Pharmacokinetic principles and techniques are ideally suited for this application. Practitioners are often faced with disease processes (e.g., renal failure) that are known to affect the disposition of a drug. Knowledge of how such a pathological process affects a drug's clearance is sufficient knowledge to adapt a dosage regimen appropriate for this condition.

The previous chapter of this text presented the underlying physiology of drug fate. The processes involved in absorption, distribution, and elimination are the primary phenomena that must be quantitated to predict the fate of a drug or toxicant in an animal. The two primary characteristics needed to adequately describe these processes are their *rate* and *extent*. In fact, this can be appreciated in the origin of the word *kinetic,* which is defined as: "*of or resulting from motion.*" Many mathematical approaches to this problem have evolved over the course of the history of pharmacokinetics. In addition, hybrid as well as novel strategies are constantly being developed to quantitate these processes. However, all approaches share certain fundamental properties that are based upon estimating the rates of chemical movement.

A PRIMER ON THE LANGUAGE OF PHARMACOKINETICS

The roots of pharmacokinetics lie in the estimation of rates. The language is that of differential calculus. It is instructive to briefly overview the basic principles of rate determination since the logic imbedded in its syntax forms the basis of pharmacokinetic terminology.

To begin, a *rate* in pharmacokinetics is defined as *how fast the mass of a compound changes per unit of time,* which is expressed mathematically as the change (represented by the Greek letter delta, Δ) in mass per small unit of time (Δt). This is synonymous with the flux of drug in a system. Units of rate are thus mass/time. For the sake of convenience only, we will express this in terms of mg/min. We will begin this discussion using mass of a compound (X), which in clinical terms would be related to the dose, rather than using concentration. As will be developed shortly, mass and concentration are easily convertible using the proportionality factor of volume of distribution.

The rate of drug excretion ΔX/Δt actually has two components, a constant that reflects the rate of the process and the amount of compound available for transfer (Equation 3.1):

$$\Delta X/\Delta t = KX^n \tag{3.1}$$

where K is the fractional rate constant (1/min), X (mg) is the mass or amount of a compound available for transfer by the process being studied, and n is the order of the process.

For a first-order process, n = 1. Since $X^1 = X$, this equation simplifies to Equation 3.2:

$$\Delta X/\Delta t = KX \tag{3.2}$$

By definition, in first-order or linear processes, K is *constant* and thus *the actual rate of the process (ΔX/Δt) varies in direct proportion (and hence linearly) to X.* K can be viewed as the fraction of X that moves in the system being studied (absorbed, distributed, or eliminated) per unit of time. Therefore, as X increases, ΔX/Δt increases in direct proportion. In linear models, the rate constant is fixed but the rate of the process changes in direct proportion to the mass available for movement.

As can again be appreciated by examining the equation for Fickian diffusion (Equation 2.1 in Chapter 2), compounds that are either absorbed, distributed, or eliminated in direct proportion to a concentration gradient are by definition first-order rate processes. The rate constants (K_n) modeled in pharmacokinetics are actually aggregate constants reflecting all of the membrane diffusion and transfer processes involved in the disposition parameter being studied. This includes pH partitioning phenomena in the body, which exist when blood and a cellular or tissue compartment have a pH gradient that alters the fraction of drug available for diffusion. Recall that it is only the unionized fraction of a weak acid or base that diffuses down its gradient across a lipid membrane. The rate constant also reflects the degree of plasma protein binding since only the free fraction of drug is available for distribution. The actual value of a K in a pharmacokinetic model thus reflects all of these variables whose relationship defines the biological system that we are attempting to quantitate.

For a nonlinear or zero-order process, by definition n = 0. Since $X^0 = 1$, the rate equation now becomes

$$\Delta X/\Delta t = K_0 \tag{3.3}$$

In this scenario, the *rate of excretion is fixed and thus independent of the amount of compound available, X. K_0* now has the units of rate (mg/min) and is *not* a mass-independent fractional rate constant. Although this would appear to simplify the situation, in reality nonlinear kinetics actually complicate most models. Nonlinear behavior becomes evident when saturation of a process occurs. The focus of most pharmacokinetic studies is on drugs with linear pharmacokinetics since the majority of therapeutically active compounds are described by these models.

The use of $\Delta X/\Delta t$ to describe the rate of a process is experimentally and mathematically cumbersome, since $\Delta X/\Delta t$ changes as a function of concentration. Figure 3.2 graphically depicts this scenario. Calculus has been used to describe these same processes using the concept of a derivative. Instead of describing rates in terms of some small, finite time interval (Δt), differential equations express rate in terms of the change in compound mass over an infinitesimally small time interval termed dt. Equation 3.1 could now be written as the following (Equation 3.4):

$$dX/dt = -KX \tag{3.4}$$

The biological interpretation is identical. Note that *K* and *X* are the same in both equations; the only change is a conceptual one in that *dX/dt* now describes the instantaneous rate of change in mass over time. By convention, if the amount of drug is increasing, dX/dt is positive (e.g., absorption of drug into the blood); if it is declining (e.g., elimination or distribution from the blood), the rate is negative or −dX/dt.

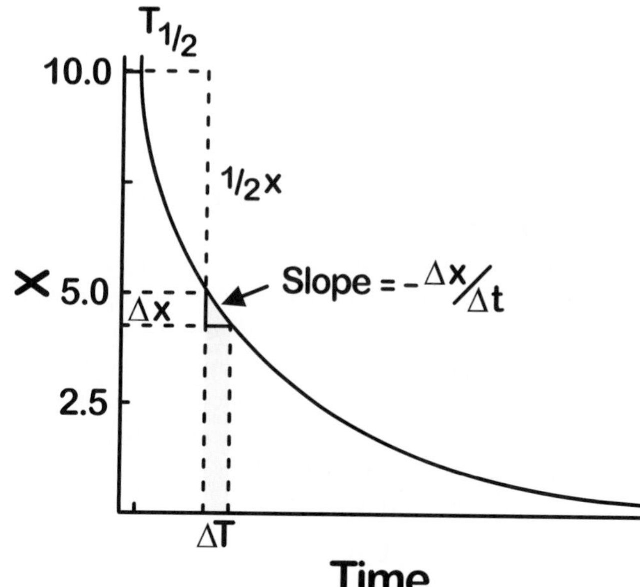

FIG. 3.2 Plot of the decay in drug (X) versus time. The T1/2 is defined as the time required for X to deplete to 1/2 X. Slope at any time is $\Delta X/\Delta T$.

One may solve a differential equation through the process of integration (∫), which transforms the equation back into terms of t rather than dt. Integration is in reality a process by which the area under the curve (AUC) defined by $\Delta X/\Delta t$ is taken. By repeatedly summing these areas for the entire experimental period, the area under the curve will be obtained. We introduced this concept in Equation 2.4 when the concept of AUC was introduced. Analogous to the relation of a derivative to a slope, integration sums the areas under infinitesimally small regions defined by dX/dt.

We can use the technique of integration to solve the rate Equation 3.4. We must integrate the equation from X at time zero (X_0) through X at time t (X_t) to obtain a formula for the mass of drug at any time (Equation 3.5):

$$\int_0^t \left(\frac{dX}{dt}\right) dt = \int_0^t (-KX)\, dt \tag{3.5}$$

There are numerous techniques to accomplish this integration and the interested reader should consult a calculus textbook for further details. The result is the following (Equation 3.6):

$$X_t = X_0 e^{-Kt} \tag{3.6}$$

where e is the base of the natural logarithm (e = 2.713). *It is important to realize that the process of integrating the differential equation describing rate generates the exponential term found in most linear pharmacokinetic models.* Exponentials can easily be eliminated from an equation by taking their natural logarithm (*ln*) since the logarithm is defined as the power to which a base (in this case *e*) is raised. Taking the natural logarithms of Equation 3.6 yields the following (Equation 3.7):

$$\ln X_t = \ln X_0 - Kt \tag{3.7}$$

If one plots the data, a straight line results as seen in Figure 3.3, which is much easier to deal with than the curve in Figure 3.2. Recalling the algebraic expression for a straight line on x-y coordinates, in this case the y intercept becomes X_0 and the slope of the line is –K. The equation has been linearized providing a simple graphical method to calculate the rate constant.

This equation can be linearized because it is a first-order rate function. This type of plot, which is widely used throughout pharmacokinetics, is termed a semilogarithmic plot (in contrast to the Cartesian plot) since the logarithm of mass is plotted against time. Again, *when a straight line results on a semilogarithmic plot, one can assume that a linear first-order process is operative and the slope of the line is the exponent of an exponential equation.* Alternatively, a linear regression program on a computer or pocket calculator could be used to calculate K by regressing the ln X against time; the slope is –K and the y intercept is $\ln X_0$. For those more comfortable with graph paper that uses logarithms to the base 10 (log x) $\{10^x\}$ rather than the base e (ln x) $\{e^x\}$ where x is the logarithm, the transformation of bases can be accomplished as the following (Equation 3.8):

$$\log X = \ln X / 2.303 \tag{3.8}$$

which transforms Equation 3.7 to

$$\log X_t = \log X_0 - Kt/2.303 \tag{3.9}$$

If base 10 semilogarithmic graph paper is used to plot Figure 3.3, the slope becomes –K/2.303. As this technique was in widespread use before the advent of digital computers, some workers and texts still occasionally use this approach.

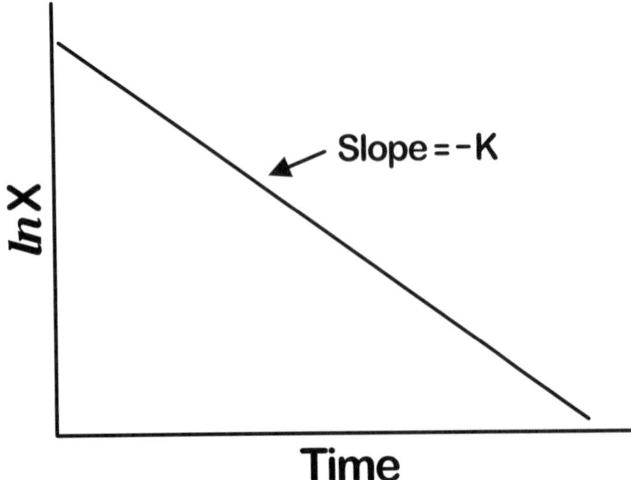

FIG. 3.3 Semilogarithmic plot of drug decay versus time with slope equal to –K.

THE CONCEPT OF HALF-LIFE

The exponential equations in pharmacokinetics have another property that is important to biological applications. This is the concept of half-life (T1/2) whose logic is central to all of this discipline. The astute biologist reading this text will have realized that Equation 3.6 is the same as that used to describe population doubling times in microbiology or ecology and used to generate population growth curves, defined as the time needed for a population of organisms to double their total numbers when they are in their so-called *logarithmic* growth phase. The only difference is that since growth is described, the exponent is positive in this application. In pharmacokinetics, our perspective is a T1/2, which is instead the time required for the amount of drug to decrease by one-half or 50%. The concept of T1/2 is applicable only to first-order rate processes.

Using Equation 3.7, one can derive a simple equation for T1/2. We first rearrange terms to solve for T, which yields

$$T = (\ln X_0 - \ln X_t)/K \tag{3.10}$$

We now solve for the time at which X_t is equal to 1/2 the initial amount X_0, that is, where T = T1/2. Substituting these values, the equation reduces to

TABLE 3.1 Relationship of T1/2 and amount of drug (A) in the body

Number of T1/2s	% of Drug Remaining	% of Drug Eliminated
1	50	50
2	75	25
3	87.5	12.5
4	93.75	0.625
5	96.88	0.312
6	98.44	0.156
7	99.22	0.078
8	99.61	0.039
9	99.80	0.019
10	99.90	0.0097

$$K = 0.693/T\,{}^{1}\!/_{2}. \qquad (3.11)$$

It is this transformation of *K* with T1/2 that introduces the ln 2 or 0.693 into many pharmacokinetic equations.

What does T1/2 really mean? Assume that we start with X, decrease it by half, and repeat this process 10 times. Table 3.1 compiles this data and lists how much drug is remaining and how much has been excreted over each Δt corresponding to one T1/2. Note that if you sum these columns, you would have accounted for 99.9% of the original dose X. After 10 T1/2s, 99.9% of the drug has been eliminated or the rate process being studied has been completed. This also illustrates the logic that must be used when dealing with doses. For example, if you double the dose to 2×, then after 1 T1/2 you would be back to the original dose! Many rules of thumb used in pharmacokinetics and medicine are based on this simple fact. For therapeutic drugs, most workers assume that after five T1/2s, the drug has been depleted or the process is over since 97% of the depletion has occurred. This also illustrates a very simple way to calculate T1/2, by simply determining the time required for drug concentration to decrease by 50%. This was depicted in Figure 3.2. Equation 3.11 can then be used to obtain K. It now is time to develop our first pharmacokinetic model using mathematical rather than physiological concepts.

ONE-COMPARTMENT OPEN MODEL

The most widely used modeling paradigm in comparative and veterinary medicine is the compartmental approach. In this analysis, the body is viewed as being composed of a number of so-called equilibrium compartments, each defined as representing nonspecific body regions *where the rates of compound disappearance* are of a similar order of magnitude. Specifically, the fraction or percent of drug eliminated per unit of time from such a defined compartment is constant. Such compartments are classified and grouped on the basis *of similar rates of drug movement* within a kinetically homogeneous but anatomically and physiologically heterogeneous group of tissues. These compartments are theoretical entities that allow formulation of mathematical models to describe a drug's behavior over time with respect to movement within and between compartments. Since pharmacologists and clinicians sample blood as a common and accessible biological matrix for assessing drug fate, most pharmacokinetic models are constructed with blood or plasma drug concentrations as the central reference to which other processes are related.

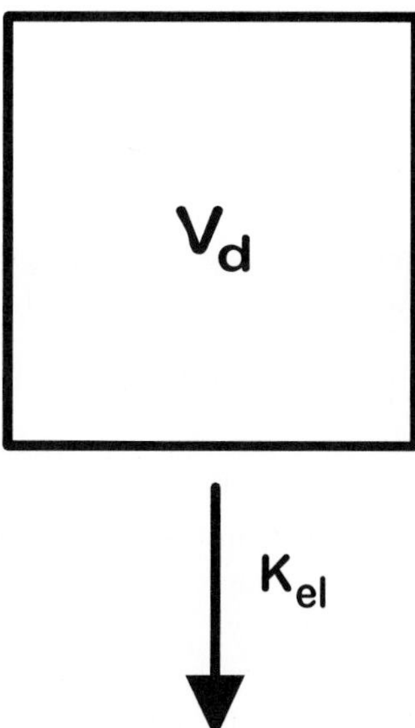

FIG. 3.4 One-compartment open pharmacokinetic model.

The simplest compartment model is when one considers the body as consisting of a single homogeneous compartment; that is, the entire dose X of drug is assumed to move out of the body at a single rate. This model depicted, in Figure 3.4, is best conceptualized as instantly dissolving and homogeneously mixing the drug in a beaker from which it is eliminated by a single rate process described by the rate constant K, now termed K_{el}. Since the drug leaves the system, the model is termed *open*. Equation 3.6 is the pharmacokinetic equation for the one-compartment open model. Although expressed in terms of the amount of drug remaining in the compartment, most experiments measure concentrations. This requires the development of the volume of distribution (Vd) (recall Equation 2.5 when distribution was discussed). In terms of the one-compartment model, this would be the volume of the compartment into which the dose of drug (D) instantaneously distributes. *Vd* thus becomes a *proportionality factor* relating *D* to the observed concentration *Cp* by

$$Vd(ml) = X(\cancel{mg})/Cp(\cancel{mg}/ml) = D/Cp \quad (3.12)$$

Using this relation, we can now rewrite Equation 3.6 in terms of concentrations, which are experimentally accessible by sampling blood, instead of the total amount of drug remaining in the body.

$$Cp = X_0/Vd\ e^{-Kelt} = Cp_0 e^{-Kelt} \quad (3.13)$$

A semilogarithmic plot seen after intravenous administration using this model is depicted in Figure 3.5. Vd quantitates the apparent volume into which a drug is dissolved, since, recalling the discussion in Chapter 2, the true volume is determined by the physiology of the animal, the relative transmembrane diffusion coefficients, and the chemical properties of the drug being studied. A drug that is restricted to the vascular system will have a very small Vd; one which distributes to total body water will have a very large Vd. In fact, it is this technique that is used to calculate the plasma and interstitial spaces.

From this simple analysis, and using the model in Figure 3.4, a number of useful pharmacokinetic parameters may be defined. Assuming that an experiment such as depicted in Figure 3.5 has been conducted using a dose of D and values for K_{el} and Vd have been determined, T1/2 can easily be calculated from Equation 3.11 above.

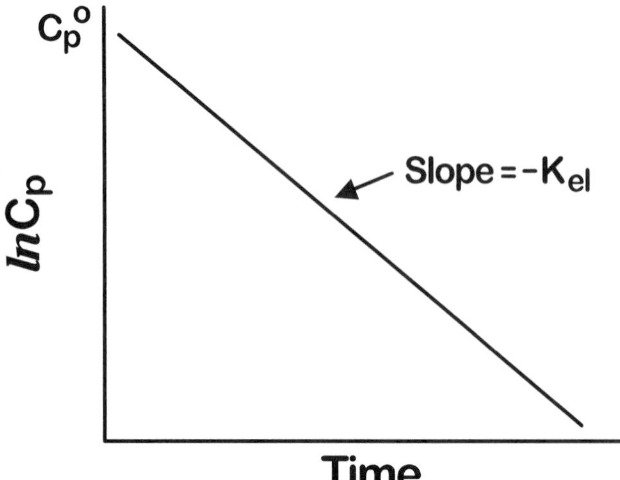

FIG. 3.5 Semilogarithmic concentration-time profile for a one-compartment drug with slope is $-K_{el}$ and intercept Cp_0.

CLEARANCE. Recalling the development of clearance concepts in Chapter 2, we now can easily determine Cl_B using this information. Clearance was defined as *the volume of blood cleared of a substance by the kidney per unit of time.* If one considers the whole body, this would read as *the volume of distribution of drug in the body cleared of a substance per unit of time.* Translating this sentence to the syntax of pharmacokinetic terminology and considering whole body elimination, Vd represents the volume and K_{el} the fractional rate constant (units of 1/time). Thus clearance is

$$Cl_B(ml/min) = Vd(ml)K(1/min) \quad (3.14)$$

There is another method available to calculate Cl_B. In Chapter 2, clearance was also defined in Equation 2.8 as *the rate of drug excretion relative to its plasma concentration.* We can also express this sentence in the syntax of pharmacokinetics and get this relation:

$$Cl_B = (dX/dt)/Cp \quad (3.15)$$

If we integrate both the numerator and denominator of this relation from time $0 \rightarrow \infty$, the numerator is the sum of the total amount of drug which has been excreted from the body; that is, the administered dose D. The denominator is the integral of the plasma concentration time profile the area under the curve (AUC). The relation thus becomes:

$$Cl_B = D/AUC \quad (3.16)$$

There are two approaches to calculate AUC. A common approach is to use the trapezoidal method depicted in Figure 3.6. However, for the one-compartment model that generates the semilogarithmic C-T plot depicted in Figure 3.5, the problem is simply determining the area of the right triangle. The area of this triangle (AUC) is height divided by the slope of the hypotenuse, or:

$$AUC = Cp_0/K_{el} \quad (3.17)$$

INTERPRETATION OF PHARMACOKINETIC PARAMETERS. With these equations, we now have the three so-called *primary pharmacokinetic* parameters describing drug disposition in the body: *T1/2*, Cl_B, and *Vd*. The data

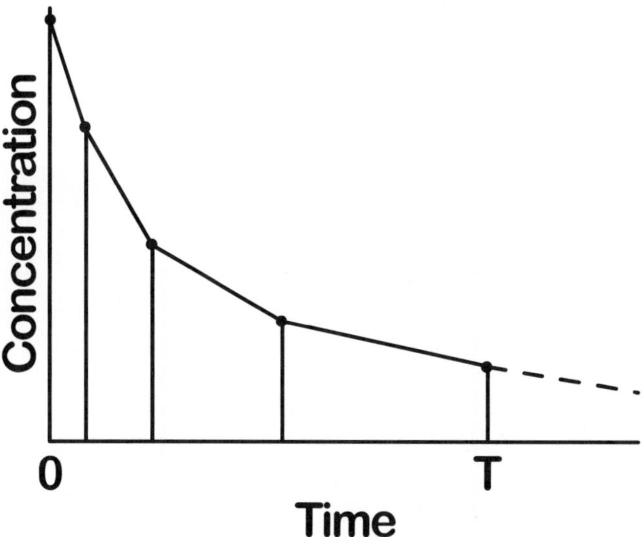

FIG. 3.6 Trapezoids formed from sampled concentration versus time data for calculation of areas. To estimate the total AUC, the curve must be extrapolated beyond the ultimate sample time, T, to infinity (----).

required to calculate them is a knowledge of dose and an experimental derivation of either K_{el} or T1/2.

This is a good place to discuss the limits of calculating parameters from such simple concentration-time profiles. Only two parameters are actually being "measured" from this analysis: the slope K_{el} and intercept Cp_0 of the semilogarithmic plot, which—using Equation 3.12 directly—determines Vd. The third parameter Cl is "calculated" from the two measured parameters. Based on the mathematical method used to calculate these, some workers suggested that K_{el} and Vd are the independent parameters in a pharmacokinetic analysis and Cl is a derived parameter. This assertion is usually made when the statistical properties of the parameters are being defined since errors for these can be easily obtained. However, this belief is an artifact of the use of a compartmental model as a *tool* to get at values for these physiological parameters. Biologically, the truly independent parameters are the Vd and Cl, with K_{el} and thus T1/2 becoming the dependent variables. From this biological perspective, the true relationship is

$$T1/2 = (0.693 \times Vd)/Cl \tag{3.18}$$

The observed half-life of a drug is dependent upon *both* the extent of a drug's distribution in the body *and* its rate of clearance. If the clearance of a drug is high (e.g., rapidly eliminated by the kidney), the T1/2 is relatively short. Logically, a slowly eliminated drug will have a prolonged T1/2. Not obvious at first is that if a drug is extensively distributed in the body (e.g., lipid soluble drug distributed to fat), Vd will be large *and* the T1/2 will also be relatively prolonged. In contrast, if a drug has restricted distribution in the body (e.g., only the vascular system), the Vd will be small and thus the T1/2 relatively short. In a disease state, T1/2 may be prolonged by either a diseased kidney, a reduced capacity for hepatic drug metabolism, or an inflammatory state, which increases capillary perfusion and permeability, thus allowing drug access to normally excluded tissue sites. Therefore, T1/2 is physiologically dependent on both the volume of distribution and clearance of the drug.

Cl_B is the sum of clearances from all routes of administration:

$$Cl_B = Cl_{Renal} + Cl_{Hepatic} + Cl_{other} \tag{3.19}$$

There is another strategy that can be used to estimate clearance in an intravenous study. This is based on the basic principle of mass balance. The strategy is to infuse a drug into the body at a constant rate R_o (mass/time) and then measure plasma drug concentrations. By definition, when a steady-state plasma concentration is achieved, C^{ss} (mass/volume), the rate of drug input must equal the rate of clearance from the body, Cl_B:

$$R_o(mg/min) = C^{SS}(mg/\cancel{ml}) \times Cl(\cancel{ml}/min) \tag{3.20}$$

Rearranging this equation gives a simple formula for determining Cl:

$$\begin{aligned} Cl(ml/min) &= R_o(\cancel{mg}/min)/C^{SS}(\cancel{mg}/ml) \\ &= R_o/C^{SS}(ml/min) \end{aligned} \tag{3.21}$$

The Cl calculated in this manner is identical to that determined using Equations 3.14 and 3.16 above, and requires only knowing the rate of infusion and assaying the achieved steady-state concentration. One may also calculate the Vd from an intravenous infusion study by the relation:

$$Vd = R_0/C^{SS}K_{el} \tag{3.22}$$

Many of the pharmacokinetic parameters above may also be obtained by analysis of urine data alone, an approach beyond the focus of the present introduction.

ABSORPTION IN A ONE-COMPARTMENT OPEN MODEL. The analysis above assumes that the drug was injected into the body, which behaves as a single space into which the drug is uniformly dissolved. The first real world

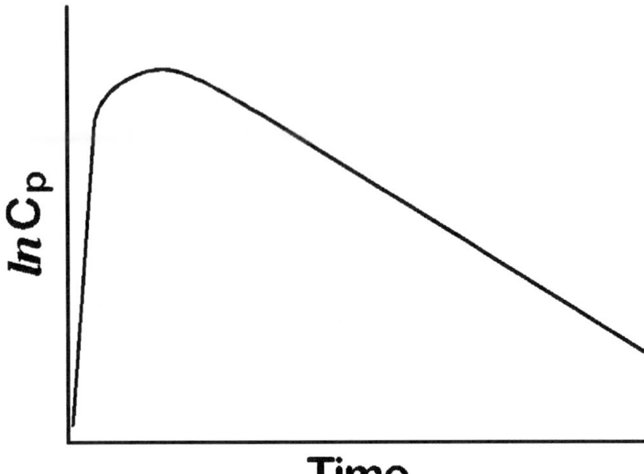

FIG. 3.7 Semilogarithmic plot of plasma concentration versus time with first-order absorption.

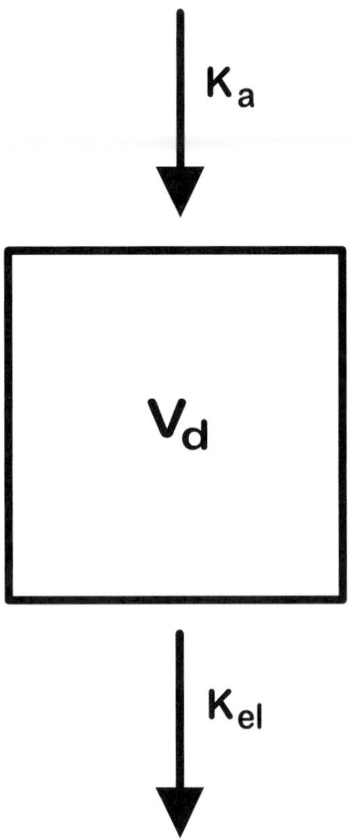

FIG. 3.8 One-compartment open pharmacokinetic model with first-order absorption.

complication is when the drug is administered by one of the extravascular routes discussed in Chapter 2. In this case, the drug must be absorbed from the dosing site into the bloodstream. The resulting semilogarithmic concentration-time profile, depicted in Figure 3.7, now is characterized by an initial rising component that peaks and then undergoes the same log-linear decline. The proper pharmacokinetic model for this scenario is depicted in Figure 3.8. The rate of the drug's absorption is governed by the rate constant K_a. When the absorption process is finally complete, elimination is still described by K_{el} as depicted in Figure 3.5. The overall elimination half-life can still be calculated using K_{el} if this terminal slope is taken after the peak (C^{max}) in the linear portion of the semilogarithmic plot (providing $K_a >> K_{el}$). However, calculation of Vd and Cl becomes more complicated since K_a is present and, unlike an intravenous injection, one is not assured that all of the drug has been absorbed into the body. In order to handle this, we must now write the differential equations to describe this process by including rate constants for absorption and elimination:

$$dX/dt = K_a D - K_{el} X \qquad (3.23)$$

where D is the administered dose driving the absorption process and X is now the amount of dose absorbed and available for excretion. The relationship between D and X is the absolute systemic availability F originally introduced in Equation 2.4 [X = FD]. In the language of differential equations, rates are simply additive, which allows the same data sets to be described in components reflecting the different processes. As above, integrating this equation and expressing it in terms of concentrations, gives the expression that describes the profile in Figure 3.9:

$$C = \frac{K_a FD}{Vd(K_a - K_{el})}[e^{-K_{el}t} - e^{-K_a t}] \qquad (3.24)$$

This is an excellent point in the discussion to appreciate the validity of the use of multiexponential equations to describe blood C-T profiles as the exponential terms, which, like the rates above from which they were derived, are simply additive. A C-T profile is the sum of the underlying exponential terms describing the rate processes involved. This property of superposition is the basis upon which observed C-T profiles may be "dissected" to obtain the component rates. Figure 3.9 illustrates this process where an observed semilogarithmic profile is plotted as a composite of its absorption phase (controlled by K_a) and the elimination phase (controlled by K_{el}). In contrast to the intravenous scenario, the time zero intercept is now a more complex function, which is dependent upon the

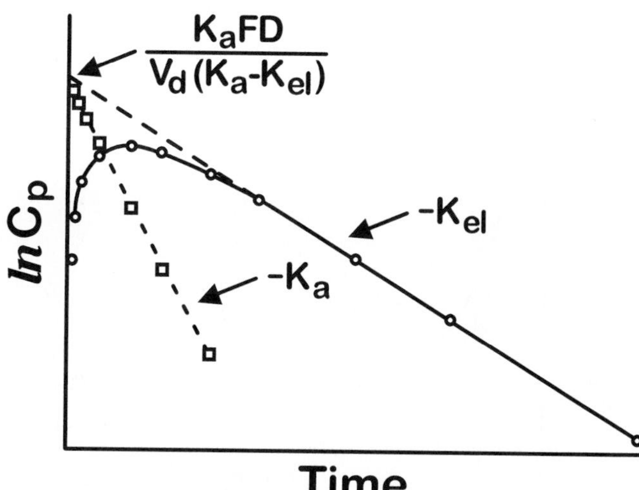

FIG. 3.9 Semilogarithmic plot of plasma concentration versus time using a one-compartment open pharmacokinetic model with first-order absorption. The profile is decomposed into two lines with slopes $-K_a$ and $-K_{el}$.

fraction of administered dose that is systemically available and thus able to be acted on by the elimination process described by the rate constant K_{el}. For this procedure to work, K_a must be greater than K_{el} so that at later time points e^{-Kat} approaches zero. If $K_a < K_{el}$, the same C-T profile will result; however, now the terminal slope will be K_a as it is the rate-limiting process! One just "flip-flopped" K_a for K_{el}. In fact, recalling the discussion in Chapter 2 on slow-release dosing formulations, we termed the resulting effect on disposition of drug in the body an example of the flip-flop phenomenon, the origin of which is this relation. When an extravascular route of administration is used, one can never be certain that the C-T profile is not dependent upon a slow, and thus rate-limiting, absorptive process secondary to a formulation factor. If a depot or slow-release formulation is administered such that $K_a < K_{el}$, the terminal slope will reflect the rate of absorption rather than the rate of elimination. T1/2 may be overestimated as it will now reflect $0.693/K_a$ rather than $0.693/K_{el}$. Complete absorption also cannot be assured (e.g., F = 1); thus one never truly knows the size of the absorbed dose. Accurate estimates of Cl and Vd, reflecting the true pharmacokinetic disposition of a drug, are required as input to determine these relations. These are best calculated after a complete intravenous injection. Finally, as discussed above for intravenous administration, urine analysis may also be used to estimate absorption parameters.

As we leave this section, it is a good time to underscore the relationship of some ADME processes as they translate to pharmacokinetic parameters; namely absorption, clearance, and volume of distribution, and further relate to the main determinants of a dosage regimen—namely, F and T1/2. This can be appreciated as

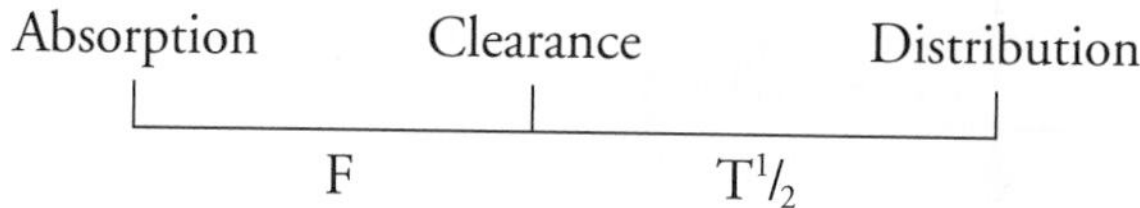

F was determined by Equation 2.4 as the ratios of AUC_{oral}/AUC_{iv}. The intravenous D is a function of Cl and AUC from Equation 3.16. Half-life was a function of Vd and Cl in Equation 3.18. This scheme shows how F is a function of absorption and clearance processes (AME) while half-life is a function of clearance and distribution (DME).

Why are these relationships important? One of the main clinical applications of pharmacokinetic principles is to construct dosage regimens, the approach that is fully presented below. Diseases that change any of these primary pharmacokinetic parameters would be expected to change the plasma concentrations achieved after dosing, and thus drug effect. For example, renal disease that reduced GFR, might reduce Cl_B for drugs primarily eliminated by the kidney. Similarly, liver disease might alter disposition of hepatically cleared drugs. In contrast, diseases that resulted in severe elimination and fluid accumulation could alter Vd. Both of these scenarios would increase T1/2 and alter plasma concentrations. The relationship between concentration and effect is extensively discussed in the next chapter on pharmacodynamics.

TWO-COMPARTMENT MODELS

Many drugs are not described by a simple one-compartment model since the plasma concentration time profile is not a straight line. This reflects the biological reality that for many drugs, the body is not a single homogeneous compartment, but instead is composed of regions that are defined by having different *rates* of drug distribution. Such a situation is reflected in the two-compartment model depicted in Figure 3.10. The drug initially is distributed in the central compartment and by definition is eliminated from this compartment. The difference comes because now the drug also distributes into other body regions at a rate that is different from that of the central compartment.

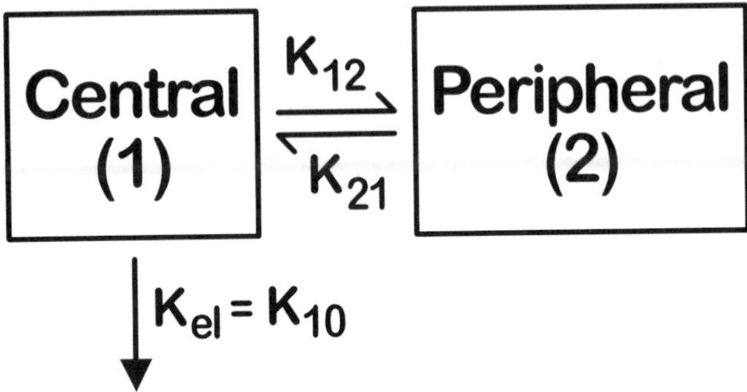

FIG. 3.10 Generalized open two-compartment pharmacokinetic model after intravenous administration with elimination (K_{el}) from the central compartment. K_{12} and K_{21} represent intercompartmental microrate constants.

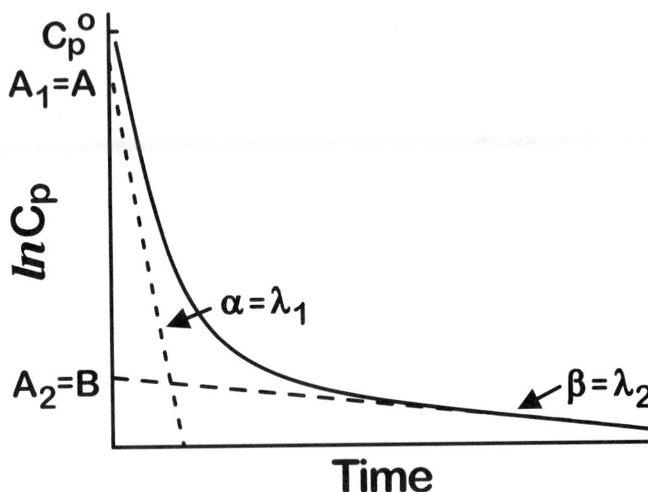

FIG. 3.11 Semilogarithmic plasma concentration versus time profile of a drug described by a two-compartment open model. Parameters are defined in the text.

As presented in Chapter 2, there are many factors that determine the rate and extent of drug distribution into a tissue (e.g., blood flow, tissue mass, blood/tissue partition coefficient, etc.). When the composite rates of these flow and diffusion processes are significantly different than K_{el}, then the C-T profile will reflect this by assuming a biexponential nature. For many drugs, the central compartment may consist of blood plasma and the extracellular fluid of highly perfused organs such as the heart, lung, kidneys, and liver. Distribution to the remainder of the body occurs more slowly, which provides the physiological basis for a two-compartment model. Such a peripheral compartment is defined by a distribution rate constant (K_{12}) out of the central compartment and a redistribution rate constant (K_{21}) from the peripheral back into the central compartment. As discussed in the distribution chapter, depots or sinks may also occur. This is a pharmacokinetic concept where the distribution rate constants are significantly slower than K_{el} and thus become the rate-limiting factor defining the terminal slope of a biexponential C-T profile, a situation analogous to flip-flop in absorption studies.

We will begin the discussion of multicompartmental models with the principles of analyzing a two-compartment model after intravenous administration (Fig. 3.11). This is the most common scenario encountered in comparative medicine and the principles easily translate to more complicated models. The fundamental principle involved is that the observed serum concentration time profile is actually the result of two separate pharmacokinetic processes that can be described by two separate exponential terms, commonly written as:

$$C_p = Ae^{-\alpha t} + Be^{-\beta t} \qquad (3.25)$$

Note the similarity of this biexponential equation to that presented for absorption in Equation 3.24. In this case we have terms with slopes (α and β) and corresponding intercepts (A and B). The C-T profile on semilogarithmic plots is depicted in Figure 3.11. By definition, $\alpha >> \beta$ and thus β is the terminal slope. If $\alpha \approx \beta$, the slopes of the two lines would be equal and we would be back to the single line of Figure 3.5 and a one-compartment model!

When dealing with multicompartmental models, it becomes necessary to introduce new nomenclature to denote the intercept terms and slopes of the C-T profile because, as will be shown shortly, the observed slopes are no longer synonymous with the elimination and distribution micro-rate constants as they were when we were analyzing absorption plots for K_{el} and K_a. When these models were constructed, the defining differential rate equations could be written in terms of the mass of drug in the central compartment (X). In the two-compartment model of Figure 3.10, this equation now must describe drug movement in terms of the mass of drug in compartment one and two. The solution to these differential equations are the slopes of the biexponential C-T profile giving α and β. Multicompartmental models have their own syntax: the slopes of the C-T profile are named using the Greek alphabet, starting with the most rapid rate α for distribution followed by β for elimination. The intercept terms are denoted using the Roman alphabet as A_n, in this example, A_1 being related to α and A_2 to β.

A preferred nomenclature carries less phenomenological context and uses the Greek letter λ_n, with n = 1, 2, 3, . . . progressing from the most rapid to the slowest rate process. The corresponding intercept terms are denoted as A_n. This nomenclature describes any multicompartmental model without implying a physiological basis to the underlying mechanism responsible for the different rates observed. The biexponential equation for a two-compartment model may now be written as

$$Cp = A_1 e^{-\lambda_1 t} + A_2 e^{-\lambda_2 t} \tag{3.26}$$

The actual rate constants describing flux between compartments are now termed micro-rate constants and denoted by k_{xy}, where compound moves from x → y. When the origin or destination of a compound is outside of the body, x or y is denoted as 0, respectively. K_a thus becomes k_{01} and K_{el} becomes k_{10}. With a two-compartment model, three Vds may be calculated; the volume of the central compartment V_c or V_1, the peripheral compartment V_p or V_2, and the total volume of distribution in the body V_t or $V_1 + V_2$. As will be seen below, the actual Vd calculated from the data is dependent upon the method used; however, the only estimate of V_t which can be broken into its component central and peripheral volumes is the volume of distribution at steady-state, Vd_{ss}.

Now that we have the appropriate nomenclature, it is instructive to derive the differential rate equations for λ_n and A_n based on the microconstants which define them. For a two-compartment model after intravenous injection of dose D with elimination occurring from the central compartment, the following differential equation describes the rate of drug disposition:

$$dC_1/dt = -(k_{12} + k_{10})C_1 + (k_{21})C_2 \tag{3.27}$$

Processes that remove compound from the central compartment (k_{10} and k_{12}) are grouped together and have a negative rate since they result in a descending C-T profile. The only process that adds chemical to the central compartment (k_{21})—that is, redistribution from the peripheral compartment—is assigned a positive rate and results in an ascending C-T profile. The rate of this process is driven by the concentration of compound in the peripheral compartment. Note the similarity of this equation to the differential equation for absorption in a one-compartment model (Equation 3.23). In this model, the only process that added drug to the central compartment was k_a, which therefore was assigned a positive sign, while the only process removing drug was $-K_{el}$. Similarly, as stressed throughout this text, the driving mass for this passive absorption process was the fraction of administered dose (F X) available for absorption. The power and essence of pharmacokinetic analysis is that the physiological processes driving drug disposition can be quantitated by using differential equations describing drug flux into and out of observable compartments, with most models structured to reflect the central compartment, which is monitored via blood sampling as the primary point of reference. Solution of the differential Equation 3.27 by integration yields Equations 3.25 or 3.26 describing the biexponential C-T profile characteristic of a two-compartment open model.

The observed slopes λ_1 and λ_2 and intercepts A_1 and A_2 are related to the microconstants as

$$k_{21} = (A_1\lambda_2 + A_2\lambda_1)/(A_1 + A_2) \tag{3.28}$$

$$k_{el} = \lambda_1\lambda_2/k_{21} \tag{3.29}$$

$$k_{12} = \lambda_1 + \lambda_2 - k_{21} - k_{10} \tag{3.30}$$

Similarly, each of the slopes now has a corresponding T1/2 calculated as

$$T1/2_{\gamma 1} = 0.693/\gamma_1\{Distribution) \tag{3.31}$$

$$T1/2_{\gamma 2} = 0.693/\gamma_2\{Elimination) \tag{3.32}$$

The slope of the terminal phase of the C-T profile reflects the elimination T1/2 and is the primary parameter used to calculate dosage regimens. Note that since $\gamma_1 >> \gamma_2$, $T1/2_{\gamma 1} << T1/2_{\gamma 2}$ and at later time points (recall the five T1/2 rule), distribution will be complete and the biexponential Equation 3.26 collapses to the monoexponential equation $Cp = A_2e^{-\lambda 2t}$. This equation is similar in form to the one-compartment Equation 3.13 except the intercept is now A_2 and not Cp_0 and the slope is $-\gamma_2$ and not K_{el}. This property of "disappearing" exponentials with large γs at later time points provides the basis for analyzing polyexponential C-T profiles using the curve "stripping" approach (technically called the method of residuals) discussed earlier.

It is often difficult to accurately estimate distribution parameters when γ_1 is very rapid since early blood samples must be collected, sometimes before blood has completely circulated. In a large animal such as a horse or cow, this requires a few minutes and thus very early samples (e.g.,

<5 minutes) will not have sufficient time for this mixing to occur. Secondly, small errors in sample timing result in a large % error (1 minute off for a 5-minute sample; error is 20%) and thus the data obtained at very early time points is often extremely variable. In contrast, 5 minutes off of a 6-hour sample is only a 1% error making estimates of terminal slopes much less variable.

VOLUMES OF DISTRIBUTION. There are now three volumes of distribution to contend with: V_c or V_1, V_p or V_2, and $V_t = (V_1 + V_2)$. These are again calculated by a knowledge of intercepts and administered dose (assuming intravenous administration). The relevant intercept is C_p^0, which is now simply $A_1 + A_2$:

$$V_1 = D/C_p^0 = D/(A_1 + A_2) \quad (3.33)$$

$$Vd_{ss} = V_1\{(k_{12} + k_{21})/k_{21}\} \quad (3.34)$$

$$V_2 = Vd_{SS} - V_1 \quad (3.35)$$

$$Vd(B) = D/B = D/A_2 \quad (3.36)$$

$$Vd_{area} = D/AUC\gamma_2 = D/(AUC\beta) \quad (3.37)$$

$$= Vd_\beta = (k_{10}\, V_1)/\gamma_2 \quad (3.38)$$

The relation between these estimates are

$$Vd(B) > Vd_{area} > Vd_{SS} > V_C \quad (3.39)$$

The easiest to discard is *Vd(B)*, the apparent volume of distribution by extrapolation, since it is often used when a complete analysis of the curve is avoided and only the terminal slope and its intercept A_2 is determined. As discussed above, this estimate completely ignores V_1. Similarly, V_c is defined as only the central compartment volume. It is the volume from which clearance is determined and is used in some infusion calculations.

The volume of distribution at steady-state, Vd_{ss}, is the most "robust" estimate since it is mathematically and physiologically independent of any elimination process or constant. It is the preferred Vd estimate for interspecies extrapolations and the study of the effects of altered physiology on Vd since it is independent of elimination. Theoretically, Vd_{ss} describes the Vd at only a single time point when the rate of elimination equals that of distribution. The point at which this occurs is the inflection point or bend in the C-T profile that occurs because the more rapid tissue distribution phase has now peaked. This is best appreciated in Figure 3.12 when the concentrations in the central and tissue compartments are plotted.

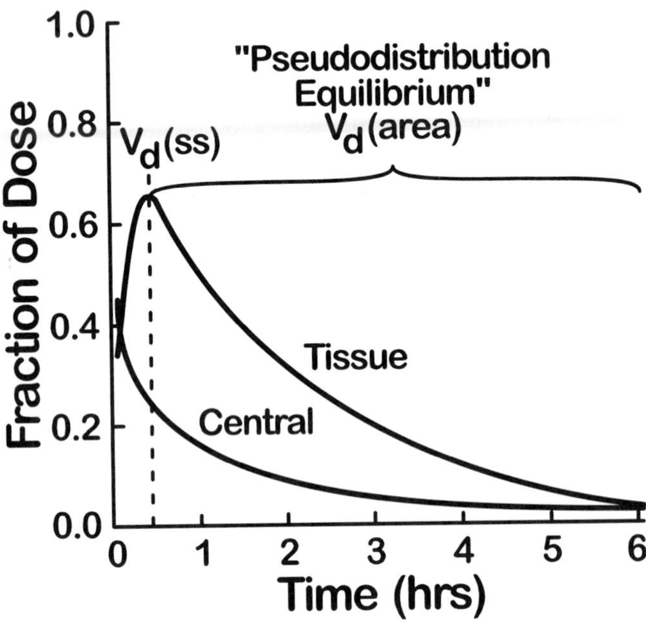

FIG. 3.12 Relationship between Vd_{ss} and Vd_{area} for a drug described by a two-compartment model. Note that Vd_{ss} is only descriptive of the volume of distribution at the peak of the tissue compartment concentration versus time profile, while Vd_{area} describes the volume throughout the terminal elimination phase.

Vd_{area} is often used when clinical dosage regimens are constructed because it reflects the area during the elimination phase of the curve which predominates in any dosage regimen (See Figure 3.12). This is absolutely equivalent to Vd_β, the so-called volume of distribution at pseudodistribution equilibrium. If the rate of elimination is very prolonged (slow), as seen in severe renal disease, the terminal slope of the concentration-time profile may approach zero (plateaus; T1/2 becomes very long), which effectively "stretches out" the curve's inflection due to a plateau in the peripheral tissue compartment. Under this scenario, Vd_{area} becomes equal in value to Vd_{ss}.

Physiologically, a way to conceptualize Vd is to compare the individual compartment volumes based on plasma versus tissue binding, as:

$$Vd = V_{plasma} + V_{tissue}(fu_{plasma}/fu_{tissue}) \quad (3.40)$$

This relationship nicely shows the effect that both plasma and tissue protein binding can have on volume of distribution. Note that V_{plasma} and V_{tissue} do not directly correspond to V_1 and V_2, respectively, as the latter are determined by relative rates since both volumes actually include plasma and tissue.

CLEARANCE. Knowing V_1, one can easily calculate the systemic clearance since Cl_B occurs from the central compartment and is essentially the same as a one-compartment model.

$$Cl = K_{10}V_1 \quad (3.41)$$

Alternatively, Cl_B may be calculated using the model-independent intravenous infusion Equation 3.21 presented earlier. The only difference is that with the more complex distribution kinetics present in a multicompartmental model, the time to reach C^{ss} may be significantly longer. Finally, Cl_B may also be determined using Equation 3.16 based on AUC. In a two-compartment model, AUC may be calculated using slopes and intercepts by the relation

$$AUC = (A_1/\gamma_1) + (A_2/\gamma_2) \quad (3.42)$$

which can be generalized for a multicompartmental model to

$$AUC = \sum A_i/\lambda_i \quad (3.43)$$

Using Vd_{ss} and Cl_B, Equation 3.18 can again be used to calculate the overall T1/2 of drug in the body. This T1/2 reflects both distribution and elimination processes and is very useful as input into an interspecies allometric analysis. This is not equivalent to the terminal elimination half-life, T1/2 (λ_2), and must be calculated from the Cl_B and Vd_{ss} parameters.

ABSORPTION IN A TWO-COMPARTMENT MODEL. When an extravascular dose is administered as input into a two-compartment model (Figure 3.13), the differential equation defining this model is

$$V_1\, dC_1/dt = -(k_{12} + k_{10})C_1V_1 + k_{21}C_2V_2 + k_{01}X \quad (3.44)$$

The movement of drug in the central compartment is now driven by three different concentrations; C_1, C_2 as well as the fraction of the administered dose D that is available for absorption (X). There are a number of approaches to solve this model. An example of the equation describing such a plasma profile would be

$$C_p = k_{01}D/V_1\left[A_1'e^{-\alpha\lambda 1t} + A_2'e^{-\lambda 2t} - A_3'e^{-K01t}\right] \quad (3.45)$$

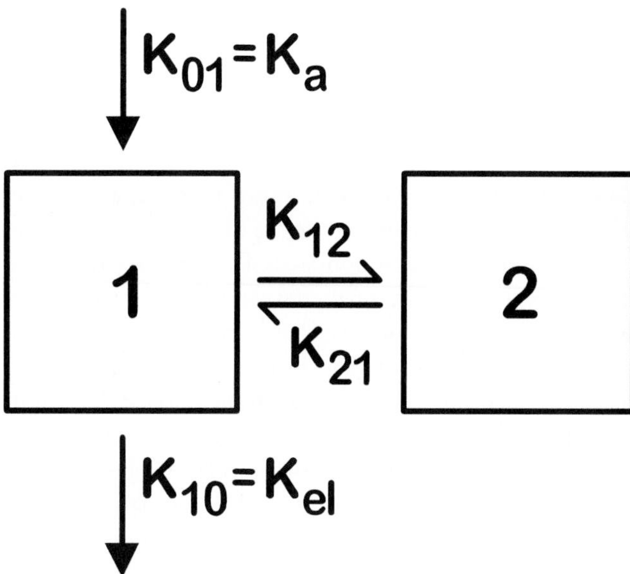

FIG. 3.13 Generalized open two-compartment pharmacokinetic model with first-order absorption (K_{01}) into and elimination (K_{el}) from the central compartment. K_{12} and K_{21} represent intercompartmental constants reflecting distribution.

In this case, the intercepts (A_n') are different than those obtained from an intravenous study (A_n) and significantly more complex since the "driving" concentrations in compartments one and two are now dependent upon the fraction absorbed in a fashion analogous to the terms of Equation 3.24 seen for absorption in a one-compartment model. However, in reality, it is difficult to separate k_{01} from λ_1 since the two are of a similar order of magnitude, coupled with the earlier discussed concern that early time points are often prone to large errors. Depending on the ratio of rate constants, the C-T profile may even appear monoexponential! The final complication is that absorption flip-flop may also occur making selection of k_{01} and λs very difficult. The only method to reliably address all of these problems is to conduct an independent intravenous bolus study using a two-compartment model and independently estimate λ_1 and λ_2 to arrive at an estimate of the absorbed dose. These equations are now easily analyzed using modern computer software.

DATA ANALYSIS AND ITS LIMITATIONS. Clearly, as pharmacokinetic models become more complex, one must question the wisdom of pursuing such analyses. In reality, there are mathematical limitations to the complexity of the model able to be fit to an experimental data set which is based on the "information density," that is, how many data points are analyzed relative to how many parameters need to be calculated. This is similar to the statistical concept of "degrees of freedom." In practice, there are better approaches to model complex absorption using noncompartmental strategies of residence times and linear system deconvolution analysis, which are discussed in advanced texts. The final consideration with two-compartmental models, and one that is even more serious for multicompartmental models, is the actual structure of the model studied. Up until now, we have *assumed* that input into (absorption) and output from (elimination) the model are via the central compartment (model A), and furthermore, all samples are taken from this compartment and expressed as differential equations based on dC_1/dt. However, other possible structures exist for the basic two-compartment model. For example, drug may be infused into a tissue bed, or drug could distribute to the organ before metabolism and thus elimination in that organ. Many of these latter type of problems occur when the rate of distribution is actually slower than elimination making the initial exponential term reflect elimination. Very lipophilic chlorinated hydrocarbon chemicals may initially distribute extensively throughout the body and then slowly (periods of months) redistribute to the blood where metabolism would then occur. The redistribution rate constant would be the rate-limiting process. All would generate C-T profiles described by the sum of exponential very similar to those discussed above. However, the equations which *link* these fitted parameters to the underlying microrate constants would be very different.

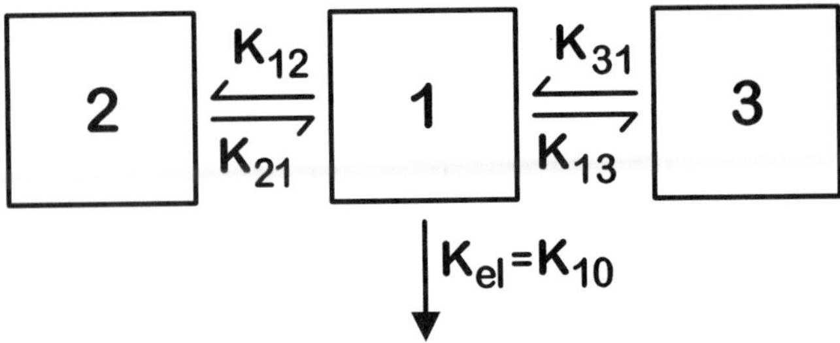

FIG. 3.14 Three-compartment pharmacokinetic model after intravenous administration. Parameters are defined in text.

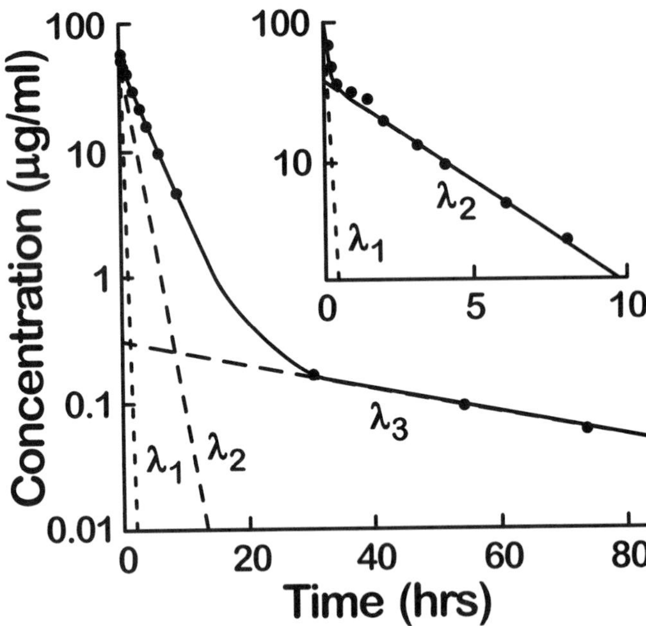

FIG. 3.15 Semilogarithmic plot of plasma concentration versus time for intravenous gentamicin in the dog. Disposition is described by a three-compartment model when samples are collected over 80 hours and a two-compartment model when samples are collected for only 10 hours (insert).

MULTICOMPARTMENTAL MODELS

The final level of compartmental model complexity to be dealt with in this chapter is the three-compartment model depicted in Figure 3.14 that generates the C-T profile in Figure 3.15. These data were obtained following intravenous gentamicin administration to dogs. In this case, gentamicin distributes into two different compartments from the central compartment, one with rates faster (k_{12}/k_{21}) and the other with rates slower (k_{13}/k_{31}) than k_{10}. The slopes of the C-T profile for λ_1 primarily reflects the contribution of rapid distribution while λ_3, the terminal slope, primarily reflects the contribution of slower distribution into the so-called deep compartment. This model is applicable to many three-compartment drugs encountered in veterinary medicine (e.g., aminoglycosides, tetracyclines, persistent chlorinated hydrocarbon pesticides). Drug elimination from the central compartment is primarily reflected in λ_2 or β and through general usage is termed the β *elimination phase*.

These types of models are generally employed when experiments are conducted over long time frames and C-T profiles monitored to low concentrations. If the data are truncated at earlier times as shown in the insert of Figure 3.15, a normal two-compartment model is adequate to describe the data. However, if the goal of a study were to describe the tissue residue depletion profile of a drug in a food-producing animal, the tissue C_3-T profile would be of interest since it is the tissue where legal tolerances are established. This makes such complicated models useful in food animal veterinary medicine.

Models consisting of more than three compartments have been used when the data are of sufficient quality (sensitive analytical method, sufficient samples) to warrant such an analysis. The polyexponential equation describing n-compartment models is

$$Cp = \sum_{i=1}^{n} A_i e^{-\lambda it} \tag{3.46}$$

The differential equations needed to link these slopes and intercepts to the micro-rate constants are exceedingly complex and will not be discussed further. These complex models are only presented to give an appreciation of the types of models encountered when tissue residue predictions are encountered.

In respect to prediction of tissue residues, when a tissue sample is taken, one is not measuring just concentrations in that tissue since the vascular and extracellular fluid components of that tissue are actually part of the central compartment. Similar arguments can be made for other components. When one is looking at deep compartment disposition, this may be satisfactory since release from these depots are rate-limiting, making this tissue component larger than any other phase that has already reached equilibrium. Equations are available to fractionate a tissue mass into vascular, extracellular, and cellular components based again on Vd estimates. Alternatively, tissue cages or microdialysis probes may be inserted into the tissue mass and extracellular kinetics modeled. These data are often presented in veterinary studies dealing with antimicrobial distribution to infected tissues.

Compartmental modeling concepts and techniques have defined the discipline of pharmacokinetics and continue to be extremely useful tools. One- and two-compartment analyses form the basis for most models used in human as well as veterinary and comparative medicine. These two models also serve as the foundation upon which many of the other techniques now to be briefly discussed are based. Modern computers have facilitated the analysis of these data to the point that the user no longer has to derive all of the relevant differential equations. Comprehensive software packages are available to effortlessly perform these calculations, even if the data does not support the model analyzed! Concerns such as these have led many clinical pharmacologists in both human and veterinary medicine to move away from complex multicompartmental models and adopt so-called *model-independent* approaches when their goal is to predict dosage regimens for clinical applications.

NONCOMPARTMENTAL MODELS

Over the last two decades, there has been generalized adoption of noncompartmental methods in veterinary and comparative pharmacokinetics. Noncompartmental models were first developed and applied to radiation decay analysis and remain dominant in the physical and biological science literature for general applications. Since their first application to problems in pharmacokinetics by Yamaoka in 1979, noncompartmental methods have grown steadily in use. This approach is for the most part actually an application of well-developed statistical moment theory, a full discussion of which is beyond the scope of this text. The approach involves primarily calculation of the Slopes, Heights, Areas and Moments (SHAM) of plasma concentration time curves. Statistical moment theory describes drug behavior based on the mean or average time an administered drug molecule spends in a kinetically homogeneous space, a concept identical to that of a compartment. The difference again is that no specific inferences are being made about the structure of these spaces.

Rather than being based on diffusion, these models are based on probability density functions that define drug disposition in terms of the probability of the drug being in a specific location. Instead of determining rates in terms of rate constants or half-lives, they describe processes in terms of statistical moments; the most useful is the mean residence time (MRT; τ). These are based on plasma concentration data and are determined by calculating areas under concentration versus time curves. MRT is calculated as

$$MRT = \frac{\int_0^\infty tC(t)dt}{\int_0^\infty C(t)dt} = \frac{AUMC}{AUC} \tag{3.47}$$

The denominator of this equation is the AUC we have discussed earlier in terms of calculating clearance and bioavailability. The numerator is known as the area under the [first] moment curve (AUMC), which is the CT-T profile. AUC and AUMC are depicted in Figure 3.16.

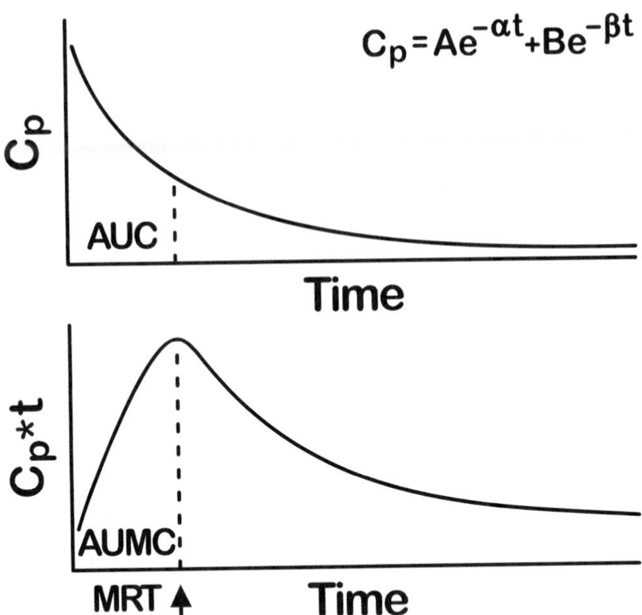

FIG. 3.16 Plasma concentration versus time (C-T) and its first-moment (CT-T) plots demonstrating AUC, AUMC, and MRT.

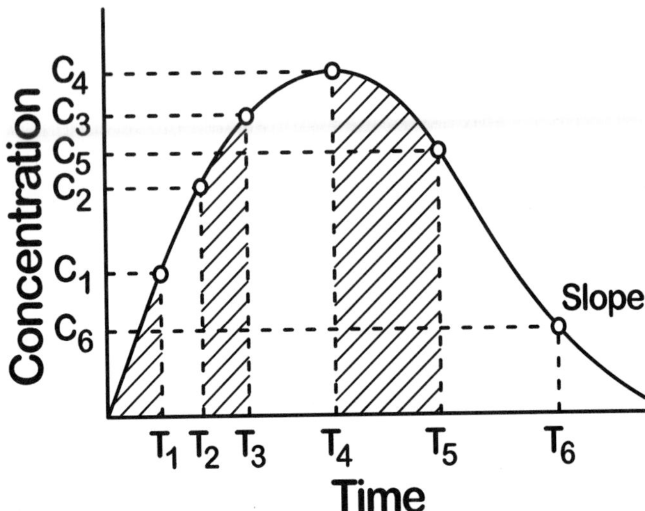

FIG. 3.17 Breakdown of a plasma concentration versus time curve into trapezoids used to calculate the area under the curve. The terminal area from T_6 to T_∞ is calculated from extrapolating the terminal slope.

The MRT could be thought of as the statistical moment analogy to the half-life (T1/2), and it is inversely related to the first-order elimination rate of a one-compartment open model:

$$MRT_{IV} = 1/K_{el} \qquad (3.48)$$

Rearranging demonstrates that $K_{el} = 1 / MRT_{iv}$. Recalling Equation 3.18 where $T1/2 = 0.693/K_{el}$, substitution gives us

$$T1/2 = 0.693\,(MRT) \qquad (3.49)$$

The MRT thus becomes an excellent parameter to describe the length of drug persistence in the body, much as the half-life is used in many compartmental pharmacokinetic models. The T1/2 used in this context is the elimination T1/2 in the body, and not that calculated from the terminal exponential phase for multicompartmental models. If the dose of drug is administered by intravenous infusion, the MRT_{iv} may be calculated as

$$MRT_{iv} = MRT_{infusion} - (Infusion\ Time)/2 \qquad (3.50)$$

where $MRT_{infusion}$ is simply calculated from the observed data using Equation 3.47.

The primary task to solve model–independent or non-compartmental models is the direct estimation of the moments from data. This essentially is determining the relevant AUCs and moments from the C-T profile. When the C-T profile is described by a polyexponential equation of the form $f(t) = A_i e^{-\lambda_i t}$, Equation 3.43 ($AUC = \Sigma A_i / \lambda_i$) can be generally used to determine AUC. The AUMC may then be calculated as

$$AUMC = \sum A_i / (\lambda_i)^2 \qquad (3.51)$$

The simplest and most commonly used method for estimating area under any curve is the trapezoidal rule. This technique is important since it is the primary method used to assess bioavailability by regulatory agencies. The approach is again illustrated in Figure 3.17.

$$AUC = \sum_{n=1}^{N} \frac{C_n + C_{n+1}}{2}(t_{n+1} - t_n) \qquad (3.52)$$

The summation is over N trapezoids, formed by N+1 data points. This algorithm is quick and, if enough data points are available, relatively accurate. It is also a simple algorithm to implement on a computer. The area under each pair of connected points describes a trapezoid (except when one of the points has zero value, in which case one of the legs of the trapezoid has zero length, making a triangle). The area under the entire curve is then the sum of the areas of the individual trapezoids, which can easily be calculated. The area under the final triangle is estimated by the AUC and must be estimated to infinite time. Generally, this portion of the AUC should be less than 20%

of the total. Many methods have been proposed for this, the most common being $AUC_{T\rightarrow\infty} = C_T / \lambda_n$, where λ_n is the terminal slope of the C-T profile. The estimation of the first moment for calculation of MRT is the summed trapezoids plotted on a CT-T graph. The attraction of statistical moment analysis to pharmacokinetics is the use of trapezoids to determine the relevant areas. No assumptions but the underlying mechanisms of drug disposition are made, and computer curve fitting is not required.

To complete this brief introduction to this area, one other residence time having general application in clinical pharmacology is the mean absorption time (MAT). Other residence times may be calculated but are not used in determining dosage regimens in clinical medicine. MAT is technically the mean arrival time into the systemic circulation of bioavailable absorbed molecules. MAT is the statistical moment theory equivalent of estimating K_a. MAT is a computationally straightforward method to characterize the rate of drug absorption in bioavailability studies. The simplicity of this approach is that transit times are additive. MAT is the mean time for drug molecules to remain unabsorbed. MAT is simply the difference in MRT following intravenous injection (MRT_{IV}) and another noninstantaneous administration (MRT_{Route}):

$$MAT = MRT_{Route} - MRT_{IV} \tag{3.53}$$

Assuming absorption is described by a first-order process with an apparent rate constant of k_a, then

$$MAT = k_a^{-1} \tag{3.54}$$

making the absorption half-life

$$T1/2_{[abs]} = ln\,2 \cdot MAT \tag{3.55}$$

On the other hand, when absorption is assumed to be a zero-order process (e.g., constant rate), then

$$MAT = T/2 \tag{3.56}$$

where *T* is the duration of the absorption. Note the similarity to the infusion Equation 3.50 above. In reality, a constant rate infusion is a zero-order absorption whose MAT is just one-half the length of the infusion.

The reader should recall that the determination of systemic availability expressed in Equation 2.4 [$F = (AUC_{Route})(Dose_{IV})/(AUC_{IV})(Dose_{Route})$] is a noncompartmental analysis. An AUC should be determined by the trapezoidal methods presented in this chapter. If the point of an analysis is to determine bioequivalence between two formulations, one is actually calculating relative systemic availability, a concept equivalent to determining whether two formulations are clinically interchangeable. In addition, the metrics time to peak concentration (T^{max}) and peak concentration (C^{max}) are often compared. Comparison of MATs would also shed light on the equivalence of two formulations. The reader should consult the references in the section "Selected Readings," later in this chapter for further approaches and the Food and Drug Administration website (www.fda.gov/CVM) for current bioequivalence guidelines for veterinary products.

The determination of Cl_B using statistical moment theory is easily obtained using the previously defined Equation 3.16 where $Cl_B = D/AUC$. Using the trapezoidal methods to estimate AUC makes this a robust estimate of clearance. The volume of distribution at steady-state (Vd_{ss}), according to statistical moment theory, is simply the product of MRT and CL:

$$Vd_{SS} = Cl_B\ MRT \tag{3.57}$$

This, incidentally, affords the expression for half-life as a function of clearance, by solving Equation 3.57 for MRT:

$$T_{1/2} = \frac{\ln 2 \cdot Vd_{SS}}{Cl_B} \tag{3.58}$$

which is the same as that presented in Equation 3.18. Substitution of the respective expressions for MRT (Equation 3.47) and CL (Equation 3.16) into Equation 3.57 yields

$$Vd_{SS} = \frac{D_{i.v.} \cdot AUMC}{AUC^2} \tag{3.59}$$

Another volume parameter also calculated using statistical moments sometimes encountered for dosage regimens is Vd_{area}:

$$Vd_{area} = \frac{D_{i.v.}}{k_{el} \cdot AUC} \tag{3.60}$$

Statistical moment methods provides a powerful tool for calculating many of the common pharmacokinetic parameters that are routinely encountered in veterinary medicine. This includes the concept of bioequivalance discussed above, as well as generating parameters that are used to construct dosage regimens and assess the effect of disease on drug effects. As can now be even more fully appreciated, Cl_B and Vd_{ss} are truly independent parameters that

TABLE 3.2 Noncompartmental equations for calculating common pharmacokinetic parameters

$Cl_B = Dose / AUC$

$Cl_D = V_c \lambda_1 - Cl_B$

$Vd_{ss} = (Dose \times AUMC) / AUC^2$

$V_c = Dose / Cp_0$

$MRT_{iv} = AUMC/AUC = V_d(ss) / Cl_B$

$MAT = MRT_{route} - MRT_{iv}$

$T1/2 = 0.693\ MRT = 0.693\ Cl_B / Vd_{ss}$

$T1/2\ (\lambda) = 0.693 / \lambda$

$F = (AUC_{route})\ (Dose_{iv}) / (AUC_{iv})\ (Dose_{route})$

$AUC = \Sigma A_i / \lambda_i$

$AUMC = \Sigma A_i / (\lambda_1)^2$

$Cp_0 = \Sigma A_i$

Note that AUC and AUMC could be calculated using trapezoidal analysis of areas rather than fitting curves to obtain estimates of A_i and λ_i.

quantitate distribution and excretion using computationally robust techniques based on minimal model-specific assumptions. We have presented this approach since it is the primary method by which pharmacokinetic parameters are now determined in veterinary medicine. Table 3.2 is a compilation of equations useful to calculate these parameters from an analysis of a C-T profile.

NONLINEAR MODELS

Most pharmacokinetic models incorporate the common assumption that drug elimination from the body is a first-order process, and the rate constant for elimination is assumed to be a true constant, independent of drug concentration. In such cases, the amount of drug cleared from the body per unit time is directly dose or concentration-dependent, the percentage of body drug load that is cleared per unit time is constant, and the drug has a single constant elimination half-life. Fortunately, first-order elimination (at least apparent first-order elimination) is typical in drug studies. First-order linear systems application greatly simplifies dosage design, bioavailability assessment, dose-response relationships, prediction of drug distribution and disposition, and virtually all quantitative aspects of pharmacokinetic simulation.

However, drugs most often are *not* eliminated from the body by mechanisms that are truly first-order by nature. Actual first-order elimination applies only to compounds that are eliminated exclusively by mechanisms not involving enzymatic or active transport processes (i.e., processes involving energy). As presented in Chapter 2, they are primarily driven by diffusion and obey Fick's Law. The subset of drugs not requiring a transfer of energy in their elimination is restricted to those that are cleared from the body by urinary and biliary excretion, and among those, only drugs that enter the renal tubules by glomerular filtration or passive tubular diffusion. All other important elimination processes require some form of energy-consumptive metabolic activity or transport mechanism. What is the impact of this on pharmacokinetic parameters?

The reason energy-involved processes are not strictly first-order is that they are generally *saturable,* or more specifically are *capacity-limited.* At clinical dosages, the majority of drugs do not reach saturation concentrations at the reaction sites, and follow first-order linear kinetics. Recalling for first-order processes, a constant percentage of remaining drug is cleared per unit time, and the drug has a discrete, concentration-independent elimination rate constant (K) and thus half-life. For drugs eliminated by zero-order kinetics or saturated pathways, however, a constant quantity of drug is eliminated per unit of time, and this quantity is drug concentration–independent and the drug does not have a constant, characteristic elimination half-life. The potential impact of saturable, leading to zero-order (versus first-order) elimination, can be profound, and its effects include altered drug concentration profiles, scope and duration of drug activity, and distribution and disposition among tissues. Saturable hepatic metabolism may markedly affect drug absorption due to reduced clearance (lower hepatic extraction) and altered first-pass activity after oral administration. Nonlinearity is associated with a nonconstant T1/2 at different doses or when a plot of dose versus AUC is not linear, indicating that Cl is reduced as dose increases.

The primary technique used to model saturable metabolic process employs the Michaelis-Menten rate law. This can be expressed as

$$\frac{dC}{dt} = \frac{V_{max} C}{K_m + C} \tag{3.61}$$

where V_{max} is the maximum velocity (rate) of the reaction, and K_m is the Michaelis constant that relates concentration to effect. There are two notable simplifying conditions of the Michaelis-Menten equation. If $K_m >> C$, then Equation 3.61 reduces to

$$\frac{dC}{dt} = \frac{V_{max} \cdot C}{K_m} \qquad (3.62)$$

This is equivalent to first-order elimination after IV administration in a one-compartment model where $dC/dt = -K_{el}C$. Thus, assuming elimination by a single biotransformation process, the first-order elimination rate constant K_{el} becomes V_{max}/K_m. If however, $K_m << C$, saturation is occurring and then Equation 3.62 collapses to

$$dC/dt = -V_{max} = -K_0 \qquad (3.63)$$

The rate in this case is independent of drug concentration (i.e., a constant), which describes a zero-order process, and the rate of drug elimination is now equal to $-K_0$.

Often, drugs are found to be eliminated by both first-order and nonlinear processes in parallel. In such cases, Equation 3.62 must be expanded to include the strictly first-order elimination processes:

$$\frac{dC}{dt} = -\frac{V_{max}C}{K_m + C} - k'_{el}C \qquad (3.64)$$

What is the impact of this on clinical veterinary pharmacology? The precise calculation of V_{max} and K_m is not done in clinical practice. However, values of Cl_B and T1/2 are assumed to be constant. When saturation occurs, Cl_B decreases and T1/2 increases, resulting in dosage regimens that accumulate with potential adverse effects. Recalling discussions in Chapter 2 on metabolism and saturation, the same phenomenon can also occur if enzyme inhibition occurs. In contrast, enzyme induction would increase clearance and reduce T1/2 resulting in decreased and potentially ineffective plasma concentrations.

SUMMARY OF MODELING APPROACHES

With the advent of modern computers, advanced software packages and sensitive and high-throughput analytical techniques, more comparative pharmacokinetic data are becoming available, and such data are being included in package inserts of approved products. The focus of this chapter is to develop basic pharmacokinetic concepts that serve as the foundation of dosage regimen construction in clinical practice. Obviously, many of the more complex models were only presented in order to illustrate these basic concepts. It is crucial that the practitioner know assumptions and limitations involved in a specific clinical case. However, there are additional pharmacokinetic approaches that are used in comparative medicine which in some cases complement the basic approaches above, and in others offer significant advantages. Two of these will be briefly introduced. Standard pharmacokinetic textbooks should be consulted for more detail.

POPULATION PHARMACOKINETICS. All of the models discussed to this point have been focused on predicting drug concentrations in the individual animal. However, in many cases populations are of interest. For example, it would be ideal to know the basic pharmacokinetic parameters for a drug in the population at large that would apply to all breeds, ages, and gender. More important would be knowledge of which subpopulation had significantly different parameters. This is normally achieved by collecting a large number of plasma samples in individual animals and averaging resulting pharmacokinetic data from small (4–6 animals) studies. Recently, techniques have been developed that allow one to conduct studies in large numbers of individuals with less individual sampling. The approach uses very simple pharmacokinetic models (e.g., Equation 3.13) or SHAM approaches, and collect more physiological data (body weight, age, creatinine) to solve the models. For example, instead of estimating Cl_B only from C-T data, one establishes a relation between GFR and Cl_B, and through statistical approaches, uses both data sets. The mathematics and statistical approaches in these so-called "mixed-effect" models (called *mixed* because kinetic and statistical models are combined) are beyond the scope of the present text. However, their adoption by scientists in drug development areas will ensure that better estimates of pharmacokinetic parameters, applicable to populations, will be available.

PHYSIOLOGICAL-BASED PHARMACOKINETIC (PBPK) MODELING. The second approach to studying pharmacokinetics in animals and humans is PBPK modeling. This approach is fundamentally different than discussed above as models are constructed by defining the body as a series of anatomical tissues connected by the vascular system (Fig. 3.18). Data is collected in plasma as well as tissue compartments, which are defined both on the basis of overall effect on drug disposition as well as

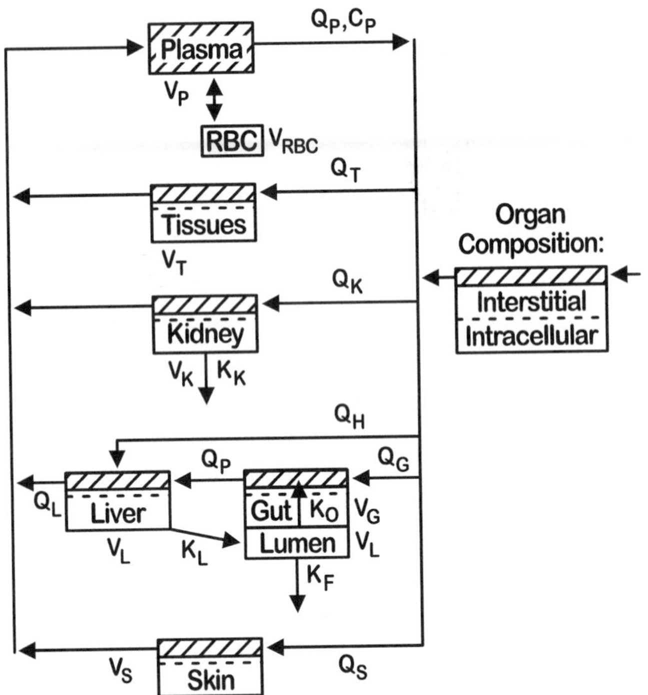

FIG. 3.18 Structure of a physiologically-based pharmacokinetic model (PBPK) incorporating disposition in plasma, liver, kidney, skin, and the gastrointestinal tract. Elimination from the body occurs from the kidney (K_K), liver (K_L) and gut lumen in feces (K_F). Oral absorption is allowed (K_O). V refers to organ volumes of distribution and Q to organ blood flows.

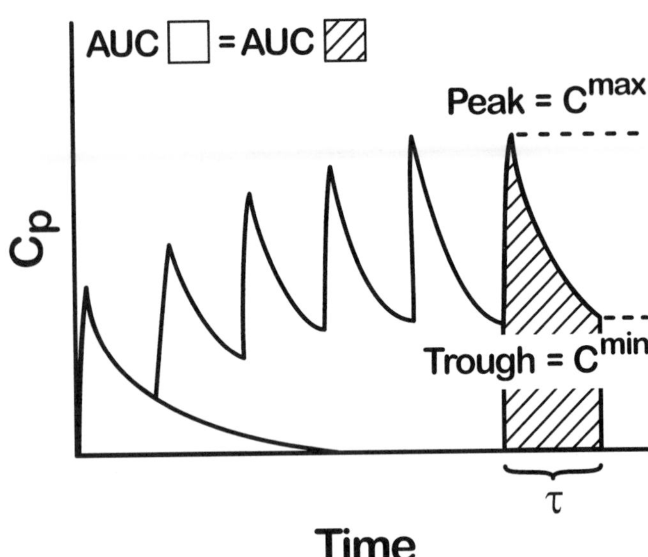

FIG. 3.19 Plasma concentration (Cp) versus time profile after multiple extravascular drug administration demonstrating accumulation. Peak and trough concentrations represent those after achievement of steady-state where the AUC under a dosing interval τ (hatched area) is equal to that after a single dose (shaded area).

sites of action or toxicity. Data input consists of blood flows into tissues as well as the partitioning coefficients for drug between blood and tissues. The model is solved in terms of a series of mass-balance equations defining input and output from each organ, very similar to that discussed when clearance was introduced in the last chapter (Equation 2.6). Advanced software packages facilitate solving these complex equations.

These models are extensively employed in the field of toxicology where data collected in laboratory animals are used to extrapolate to humans. In these cases, models may be defined in mice or rats, and then human physiological parameters inputted to estimate human disposition. The models are well suited to integrate in vitro laboratory data on toxicity or effect, as well as being able to simultaneously model parent drug and metabolite disposition. They have recently been used to study tissue residue depletion in food animals because they allow for predictions in the target tissues monitored by veterinary regulatory authorities.

DOSAGE REGIMENS

The primary use of pharmacokinetics in a clinical setting is to calculate safe and effective drug dosage regimens for patients. These are generally based on target plasma drug concentrations that are believed to be therapeutically effective. The dose required to achieve and then maintain these target concentrations must be calculated using a knowledge of the drug's pharmacokinetic parameters in these individuals.

This concept is best addressed by visualizing the drug's C-T profile after multiple dose administration as depicted in Figure 3.19. There are two descriptors of the dosage regimen that are important to describe a multiple dose regimen. These are the dose and dosage interval (τ). The dose is further classified as the initial or *loading dose* (D_L) required to rapidly achieve an effective plasma concentration and the *maintenance dose* (D_M) needed to sustain these concentrations. The resulting profile is characterized by *peak* (C^{max}) and *trough* (C^{min}) plasma concentrations, which result after the animal has achieved a steady-state condition.

The shape of such a multiple dosage regimen is dependent upon the relationship between the T1/2 of the drug and the length of the dosage interval, τ. Assuming that a single dose of drug is administered to an animal, the resulting C-T profile after extravascular administration will resemble that depicted in Figure 3.7 (plotted on a semilog C-T axis), which (plotted on a normal C-T axis) is the first hatched profile (----) in the left of Figures 3.19 and 3.20. The AUC of this C-T segment describes the quantity of drug cleared from the body (Equation 3.16). If a second dose of drug were given after the first dose were completely eliminated (e.g., approximately five T1/2s), then this profile would be repeated as depicted in Figure 3.20. This dosage regimen, where τ is >> five T1/2s, does not result in any drug accumulation in the body. The peak and trough plasma concentrations of this multiple dose regimen is the same as seen after a single dose and the equations presented earlier (Equation 3.13 for an intravenous dose and Equation 3.24 for an extravascular dose) may be used to describe the profile. The dose required to achieve a specific peak concentration or C^{max} after administering a very rapidly absorbed preparation is essentially obtained by rearranging the equation for volume of distribution (Equation 3.12) which becomes

$$Dose = (C^{max})Vd \tag{3.65}$$

If the drug is not completely bioavailable (e.g., F < 1), this equation is divided by the systemic availability F. Administering this dose at every τ will result in the same C-T

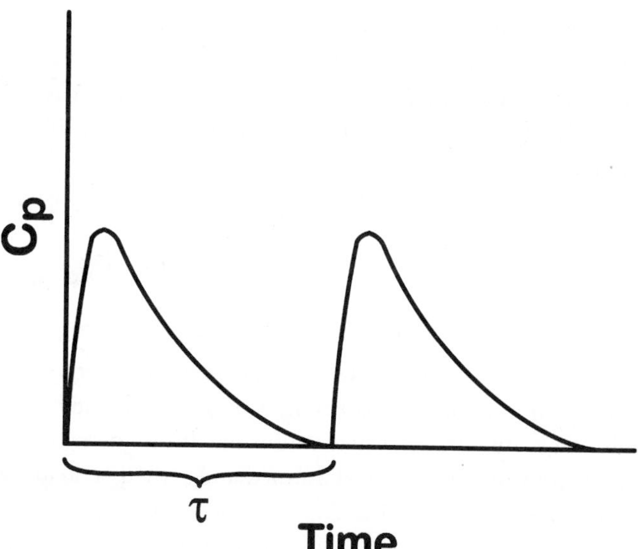

FIG. 3.20 Plasma concentration (Cp) versus time profile after multiple extravascular drug administration with no accumulation, resulting in independent pharmacokinetics described by two single-dose profiles.

profile characterized by C^{max} and a C^{min} of essentially zero.

However, the more likely scenario is that depicted in Figure 3.19 where a second dose is administered before the first dose is completely eliminated from the body. In this case, the drug concentrations will accumulate with continued dosing. This accumulation will stop or reach a *steady-state* when the amount of drug administered at the start of each dosing interval is equal to the amount eliminated during that interval. This can be appreciated since the AUC under one dosing interval is equal to that after a single dose administration. In fact, steady-state could be defined as the dosing interval where the AUC for that interval is equal to the single dose AUC. Administering repeated doses at a τ defined in this manner will continuously produce a C-T profile with the same peak and trough plasma concentrations.

There are a series of simple formulae derived from basic pharmacokinetic principles that can be used to precisely derive these profiles. The first is to determine C^{avg}, which is a function of the Vd and the ratio of the T1/2 and τ where

$$C^{avg} = \frac{(1.44)(F)(D)}{Vd_{area}} \cdot \frac{T1/2}{\tau} = \frac{C^{max} - C^{min}}{ln(C^{max}/_{p}{}^{min})} \tag{3.66}$$

Recalling the relationship between T1/2, Cl and Vd presented earlier in Equation 3.18, rearrangement yields *1/Cl = 1.44 T1/2/*Vd_{area}. It is instructive when studying these relations to recall that 0.693 is the ln 2 and 1.44 is 1/ln2. Substituting this into Equation 3.66 yields

$$C^{avg} = \frac{F}{Cl} \cdot \frac{D}{\tau} \tag{3.67}$$

Another relationship becomes evident from these formulae. We learned earlier that Cl is defined as D/AUC, which allows Equation 3.67 to be algebraically expressed as C^{avg} = (F) (AUC)/τ. This relation quantitates the observation presented earlier that the AUC under any dosing interval τ will always be the same when steady-state conditions are achieved.

Two factors that are important in designing dosage regimens emerge from Equations 3.66 and 3.67. The ratio D/τ can be defined as the *dosage rate* and is the major determinant under the control of the clinician that determines the amount of drug which will accumulate in the body. The ratio T1/2/τ is a proportion relating the relative length of the dosing interval to the half-life of the drug.

If the inverse of this ratio is taken, the *relative dosage interval* ε may be defined as: $\varepsilon = \tau/T1/2$. These two ratios provide useful parameters to gauge the shape and height of the C-T profile produced by a tailored dosage regimen, as well as adjust dosages in disease states with reduced clearances.

The primary factor governing the extent of drug accumulation in a multiple dose regimen is the fraction of a dose eliminated in one dosing interval, termed f_{el}. This can be easily calculated by first determining the amount of drug remaining at the end of a dosing interval, f_r. We showed earlier that the amount of drug in the body at any time t is given by the exponential (Equation 3.6) relation $X_t = X_0 e^{-kt}$. If one substitutes τ for t at the end of a dosing interval, then f_r is defined as

$$f_r = 1 - f_{el} = X_t / X_0 = e^{-k\tau} = e^{-\lambda\tau} \qquad (3.68)$$

where k is the fractional elimination constant or the relevant slope of the terminal phase of the C-T profile governing the disposition of the drug. Therefore,

$$f_{el} = 1 - f_r = 1 - e^{-\lambda\tau} = 1 - e^{-0.693/(\tau/T\frac{1}{2})} = 1 - e^{-0.693\varepsilon} \qquad (3.69)$$

Using f_{el}, the peak and trough concentrations may be calculated as

$$C^{max} \frac{(F)(D)}{(Vd_{area})(f_{el})} \qquad (3.70)$$

$$C^{min} = (C^{max})(1 - f_{el}) \qquad (3.71)$$

The ratio of the fluctuation in C_p^{max} and C_p^{min} can be determined as

$$C^{max}/C^{min} = e^{0.693(\tau/T1/2)} \qquad (3.72)$$

and

$$ln(C^{max}/C^{min}) = 0.693(\tau)/(T1/2) = 0.693\varepsilon \qquad (3.73)$$

This is an extremely powerful relationship that demonstrates that the magnitude of fluctuations in a C-T profile is directly related to the *relative* dosage interval ε. As either τ increases or T1/2 decreases, this ratio will get larger and result in a greater fluctuation in drug concentrations.

Using these relationships and rearranging Equation 3.70 to solve for dose, one can now derive the dosage formulae required to achieve a C-T profile with specified target peak and trough concentrations:

$$D_M = (f_{el})(Vd_{area})(C^{max})/F$$
$$= Vd_{area}(C^{max} - C^{min})/F \qquad (3.74)$$

$$D_L = (D_M)(f_{el})$$
$$= (Vd_{area})(C^{max})/F \qquad (3.75)$$

Thus to construct a dosage regimen, the only parameters that are required are the Vd_{area} and T1/2 (and hence λ or k_{el}) of the drug to calculate f_{el}. If one is targeting only the average plasma concentration, then Equation 3.66 can be solved for dose as

$$D_M = \frac{(C^{avg})(Vd_{area})}{(1.44)(F)} \times \frac{\tau}{T1/2}$$
$$= \frac{(0.693)(C^{avg})(Vd_{area})}{F} \times \frac{\tau}{T1/2} \qquad (3.76)$$
$$= \frac{(C^{avg})(C1)(\tau)}{F}$$

The magnitude of f_{el} is a good estimate of the degree of fluctuation that occurs between the peak and trough concentration at steady-state. As the ratio of τ/T1/2 or ε approaches zero, f_{el} approaches zero and the amount of fluctuation in a dosage interval is minimal. In contrast, when this ratio is large, f_{el} approaches one and the peak and trough concentrations have a large degree of fluctuation.

When f_{el} is very small, C^{max} approaches C^{min} since f_{el} approaches zero when τ approaches zero. The resulting C-T profile becomes characterized by C^{avg}. This occurs when the drug is given as an intravenous infusion. The rate of an intravenous infusion (R mg/min) is essentially an *instantaneous* dose rate and is equivalent to D/τ. When R is inserted in Equation 3.67 for D/τ and F is set equal to 1 (since an intravenous dose is be definition 100% systemically available),

$$C^{avg} = R/Cl \qquad (3.77)$$

and

$$R\,(mg/min) = (C^{avg})(Cl) \qquad (3.78)$$

which is identical to Equation 3.20 presented earlier for the steady-state plasma concentration (C^{ss}) obtained after administering an intravenous infusion. If one desires that concentration be achieved immediately, then a loading dose may be calculated as

$$D_L = (C^{avg})(Vd) \qquad (3.79)$$

Comparing Equations 3.66 and 3.77 is instructive since it demonstrates the dependence of the average steady-state concentration on the rate of drug input (R or D/τ) in mass/time and the rate of drug elimination exemplified by the clearance. When constructing and comparing dosage regimens, the C^{avg} of any two regimens will always be the same as long as D/τ is constant. This factor becomes very important when dosage regimens are constructed for patients with impaired clearance due to renal disease. The larger the f_{el} or ε is in a single dosage interval τ, the greater the fluctuation in plasma concentrations. To minimize fluctuation but maintain a constant C^{avg}, smaller maintenance doses (D_M) must be administered at shorter dosage intervals.

It is also important to stress at this point that the length of time required to achieve steady-state for any dosage regimen is solely based on the rate-controlling λ or T1/2 of the drug in the clinical situation. Thus with drugs having a prolonged half-life, a loading dose may often have to be administered to rapidly achieve therapeutically effective plasma concentrations.

The principles presented in this chapter may be widely applied for a number of therapeutic situations. For most drugs employed in a clinical setting, the relevant T1/2 will be that governing the elimination of the drug's C-T profile. If the drug exhibits nonlinear pharmacokinetic properties and accumulates, saturation may occur and the clearance operative at low concentrations may be reduced at the higher concentrations seen at steady-state, leading to further accumulation and potential toxicity. In contrast, if the drug induces its own metabolism, the disposition and thus required dosage regimen may be greater after chronic use to prevent relapse. This has been seen with certain anticonvulsant drugs.

Other considerations are operative when administering extravascular drugs with relatively slow rates of absorption. In many cases, the governing rate process may be the absorption phase (k_a) and a flip-flop situation will occur. In this case, it will take five *absorption* T1/2s to reach steady-state. These approaches to constructing dosage regimens are ideally suited when pharmacokinetic parameters are obtained from the noncompartmental models. In these cases, the same equations may be used.

COMMENTS ON EFFICACY AND SAFETY. The final point to consider is the relationship between the target C^{max} and C^{min} concentrations and therapeutic or toxic effect. This relation is best presented in Figure 3.21, which depicts a hypothetical C-T profile versus various target Cs for efficacy and toxicity. The precise manner by which a

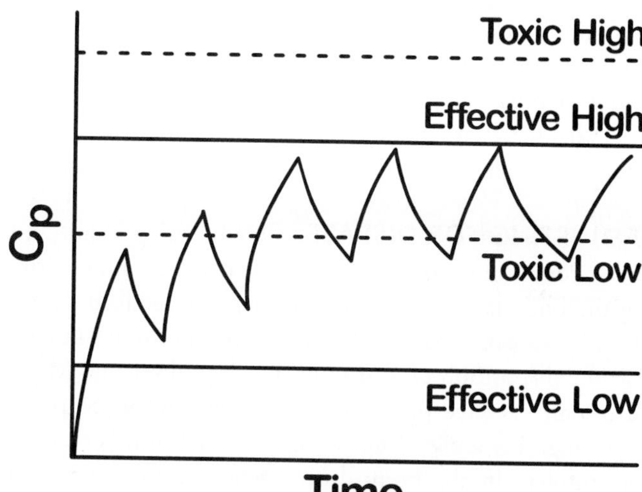

FIG. 3.21 Relationship between a multiple-dose plasma concentration versus time profile and thresholds for efficacy and toxicity, which define the therapeutic benefit/risk ratio for the drug.

pharmacokinetic profile is linked to its pharmacodynamic or toxicodynamic effects will be presented in Chapter 4. This relationship is very dependent upon the pharmacology of the drug itself, and cannot be easily generalized across all drugs. As will be discussed in the next chapter, drug potency, efficacy, sensitivity, and specificity define the mathematical nature of the link between the C-T profile and effect. Individual chapters of this text must be consulted for an overview of mechanism of drug action, that is, what biochemical receptors are targeted by the individual drug. If an antimicrobial is involved, the mechanism of bacteria killing is important.

It is instructive to realize that the form of a C-T profile is by itself only dependent upon the dosage regimen parameters (D/τ) and the pharmacokinetics of the drug in the patient. The resulting efficacy or toxicity of the profile is dependent upon the underlying pharmacology and toxicology of the drug. These biological effects are often, though not always, correlated to plasma concentrations. Thus, for a specific drug, one might have data that would indicate that efficacy would occur when C is maintained above the *effective low* concentration and toxicity would be expected to occur only if concentration exceeded the *toxic high* level plotted. In this case, the dosage regimen that produced this C-T profile would be considered optimal since at steady-state it is well within the *therapeutic window* defined by these two thresholds. However, if the efficacy of the drug were defined by the *effective high* threshold plotted, the regimen would not be therapeutically effective. Similarly, if the relevant toxicological threshold were the *toxic low* line in this figure, one would predict that this regimen would be unsafe to administer.

ADJUSTING FOR DISEASE. One of the primary and most common factors that affects the disposition of a drug in the body is disease-induced changes in renal function. It is no surprise that renal disease has a profound impact on the disposition of a drug in the clinical setting. Many drugs are excreted primarily in urine as unchanged pharmacologically active drug. Drugs excreted in this manner accumulate in the body during renal insufficiency as a direct result of decreased renal clearance and is the primary manifestation of renal disease, which is compensated for in clinical dosage adjustment regimens. Renal disease can also influence other aspects of drug disposition, including altered protein binding, volume of distribution, and hepatic biotransformation. All of these effects complicate the establishment of safe and efficacious regimens for drug therapy. The chapters on specific drugs should be consulted when considering their use in such patients.

Of course, the obvious choice for selecting a drug for a patient with renal disease is to use a drug not cleared by the kidney. If this is not possible, current approaches for constructing adjusted dosage regimens for renal insufficiency or failure compensate only for decreased renal clearance of the parent drug and are based upon the principles of dosage regimen construction discussed above. In this approach, we assume 1) a standard loading dose is administered; 2) drug absorption, volume of distribution, protein binding, nonrenal elimination, and tissue sensitivity (dose-response relation) are unchanged; 3) creatinine clearance is directly correlated to drug clearance; and 4) there is a relatively constant renal function over time.

The ultimate aim of dosage adjustment in renal disease is to fulfill the fundamental therapeutic postulate that the C-T profile should be as similar as possible to the normal situation. Recall above that ε, the ratio τ/T1/2, determines the fluctuation in a multiple dose C-T profile based on its influence on the value of f_{el} from Equation 3.69. The dose ratio, D/τ, determines the average steady-state plasma concentration (C^{avg}). If τ is not adjusted in the face of an increasing T1/2 in a patient with renal failure, C^{avg} will dramatically increase, as can be seen from revisiting Equation 3.66. This can be compensated either by reducing D or increasing τ in this equation, which is the basis of the dose modification methods introduced below. However, the fluctuations in these regimens is a function of f_{el} which in a renal disease patient is dependent upon ε. Thus τ must be increased to compensate for the prolonged T1/2 if f_{el} and thus fluctuations are to be dampened. When constructing dosage regimens for patients in renal disease which has fundamentally altered pharmacokinetic parameters, both D and τ must be modified to achieve C^{avg} and f_{el}, which are similar to the patient with normal renal function.

Let us assume that one has already defined a safe and effective dosage regimen for use in a normal patient. These normal dosage regimens are then adjusted according to the dose fraction by two basic procedures. The first method, termed *constant-interval, dose-reduction* (DR), reduces the dose (D) by a factor of the dose fraction. Dose interval (τ) is the same as that used in the healthy animal. The dose fraction K_f is calculated as the ratio of diseased/healthy drug Cl, GFR or creatinine clearance.

$$D_{reanal\ failure} = D_{normal} K_f, \quad \tau_{reanal\ failure} = \tau_{normal} \tag{3.80}$$

The second method, *constant-dose, interval-extension method* (IE), extends the dosage interval by the inverse of the dose fraction, a value referred to as the *dose-interval multiplier:*

$$\tau_{reanal\ failure} = \tau_{normal}(1/K_f), \quad D_{renal\ failure} = D_{normal} \tag{3.81}$$

This type of dose adjustment strategy may also be implemented through the use of a nomogram where the dosage interval multiplier for this IE regimen is simply read off a plot of creatinine clearance. A comparison of these two methods is presented in Figure 3.22.

The therapeutic goal is to maintain a constant product of (T1/2 × D/τ) in healthy animals and those with renal failure. When this product is constant, the average steady-state plasma concentration of drug will remain unchanged. This is the approach followed in the DR and IE methods. A constant steady-state plasma concentration is achieved by the use of the dose fraction to compensate for decreased T1/2 in the following manner:

$$(T\,{}^1\!/\!_2 \cdot D/\tau)_{normal} = K_f (T\,{}^1\!/\!_2 \cdot D/\tau)_{renal\ failure} \tag{3.82}$$

When repeated doses of a drug are administered, accumulation occurs until steady-state plasma concentrations are achieved, a process taking five half-lives. The

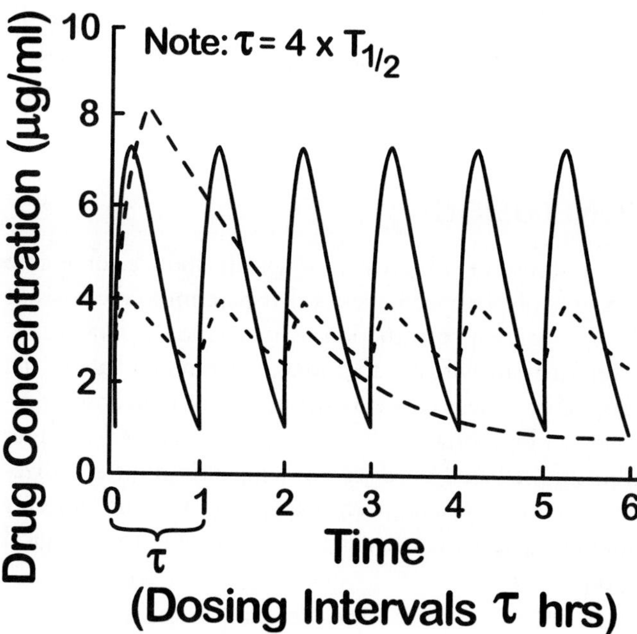

FIG. 3.22 Comparison of constant dose (– – –) and constant interval (- - - -) regimens in renal failure (Cl_{cr} = one-sixth usual) with a normal dosage regimen (——) in a healthy patient. τ is the dosage interval.

prolonged T1/2 present in patients with renal insufficiency would cause excessive delay in attaining steady-state concentration. Therefore, an appropriate loading dose should always be administered so that a therapeutic concentration of the drug is immediately attained. If the constant interval method is employed, this can be accomplished by giving the usual dose initially, followed by the calculated reduced dose. If the constant dose method is used, the initial two doses should be given according to the usual interval. The selection of which method to use is very drug dependent, both in terms of efficacy and potential toxicity.

The above equations hold for drugs that are excreted solely by the kidney, since the dose fraction adjusts dosages as if only renal elimination occurred. For drugs undergoing biotransformation, an estimate of the percent of nonrenal clearance is necessary. More detailed texts should be consulted for dealing with these cases. If hepatic disease is present, the same strategy holds if one has a marker for hepatic dysfunction. The problem is that there is no "creatinine" equivalent to assess the degree of functional hepatic impairment. One also must consider the hepatic extraction ratio and subsequent renal clearance of metabolites. Again, a specialty text in this area should be consulted.

INTERSPECIES EXTRAPOLATIONS

The ultimate aim of any interspecies extrapolation would be to predict drug activity or toxicity in a new species not previously studied. There are two sources of error inherent to such an extrapolation. The first is that a drug's pharmacokinetic profile (especially excretion, metabolism, and distribution) does not extrapolate across species without adjusting for some individual species characteristics. The second, which will always be problematic, is that the pharmacodynamic response of a drug may be very different between species and not at all related to pharmacokinetics. This latter concern may not be important for antimicrobial drugs since the pathogenic organisms being treated should have susceptibilities that are pathogen-dependent and host-independent. However, for drugs that interact with physiological functions that have species-specific receptor types and distributions, an estimate of pharmacokinetic parameters may not be sufficient to predict pharmacodynamic response.

There is a wealth of empirical observations that suggest that physiologic functions such as O_2 consumption, renal glomerular filtration, cardiac output, etc., are not linearly correlated to the mass of an individual animal, both within and between species. That is, if one expresses any physiologic function on a per kg body weight basis (e.g., GFR/kg), an *isometric* relationship would suggest that the parameter is constant. However, in the case of these physiologic functions, such a relationship does not hold since the parameter on a mg/kg basis still is species dependent and not constant. A knowledge of body weight does not allow one to determine the value of the parameter across species with different body weights. However, if these parameters are expressed on a per unit surface area basis, many parameters such as GFR will be equivalent across species. More refined analyses suggest that the optimal scaling factor would be to a species' Basal Metabolic Rate (BMR). Empirical observations suggest that BMR is a function of (body weight in Kg) raised to the 0.75 power [$GFR = f(BW_{kg})^{0.75}$]; when expressed on body surface area, the exponent is 0.67. An exponent of 0.75 is also theoretically predicted if metabolic functions are based on a model where substances in the body are transported through space-occupying fractal networks of branching tubes (e.g., the vascular system) that minimize energy dissipation and share the same size at the smallest level of structure (e.g., capillaries). Whatever the mechanism, these approaches are well suited for extrapolating drug disposition across species.

Equations where a parameter is related to a mathematical function (in this case, a power function) of a metric such as body weight is termed an *allometric* relationship. The extensive literature surrounding this question of how one "collapses" physiological parameters between species has created a field of study called *allometry*. Since most drug pharmacokinetic parameters are dependent upon some physiological function, they may also be scaled across species using these strategies. The method for doing this is to correlate the parameter of concern (e.g., GFR, Cl_B, T1/2 = most common) with body weight (BW) using the following allometric equation:

$$Y = a(BW)^b \quad (3.83)$$

where Y is the parameter of concern, a is the allometric coefficient and b the allometric exponent. The data is obtained using simple linear regression on $\log_{10}$ Y versus $\log_{10}$ BW, as depicted in Figure 3.23. The slope is the allometric exponent b and the intercept a. There is uniform agreement that for most physiologic processes, the allometric exponent b ranges from 0.67 to 1.0. Note that if the parameter being modeled is an inverse function of a physiologic process (e.g., T1/2), the exponent will be 1-b for that process. The coefficient a is actually the value of Y for a 1.0 kg BW animal (b = 0).

Numerous texts and research manuscripts deal with this topic in greater depth. The important clinical take-home message to the veterinarian is that for equivalent effects, the dose may be greater in a smaller animal on a body weight basis. In cancer chemotherapeutics, doses are often expressed on the basis of body surface area, an adjustment that essentially compensates for the allometric exponent.

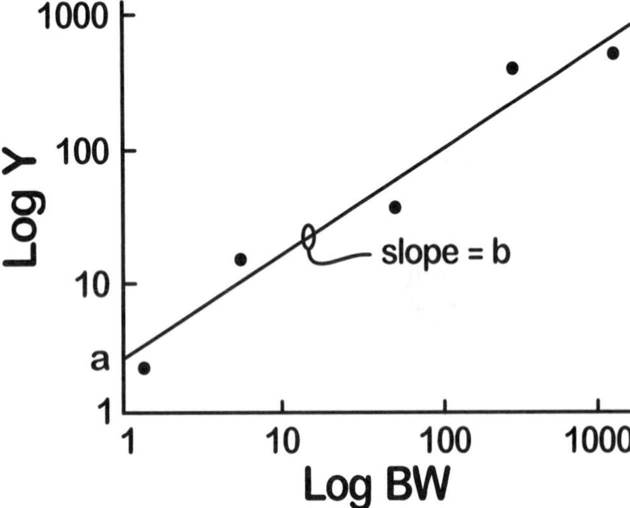

FIG. 3.23 Basic log-log allometric plot of a biological parameter (Y) versus body weight (BW) with slope b and intercept a.

CONCLUSION

The purpose of this chapter was to introduce some core concepts of pharmacokinetics that determine the basis of dosage regimen construction in medicine. In most cases, a veterinarian will use the dosage recommended on the drug label. These concepts define where that dose originates, and importantly, how the clinician should consider adjusting it based on disease, therapeutic nonresponsiveness, or toxicity. The next chapter will present concepts linking a plasma concentration time profile to biological effect.

SELECTED READING

Baggot, J.D. 1977. Principles of Drug Disposition in Domestic Animals: The Basis of Veterinary Clinical Pharmacology. Philadelphia: W.B. Saunders Co.

———. 1992. Clinical pharmacokinetics in veterinary medicine. Clinical Pharmacokinetics. 22:254–273.

Bourne, D.W.A. 1995. Mathematical Modeling of Pharmacokinetic Data. Lancaster, PA: Technomic Publishing Co.

Boxenbaum, H. 1982. Interspecies scaling, allometry, physiological time, and the ground plan for pharmacokinetics. Journal of Pharmacokinetics and Biopharmaceutics. 10:201–227.

Caines, P.E. 1988. Linear Stochastic Systems. New York: Wiley and Sons.

Chow, S.C., and Liu, J.P. 2000. Design and Analysis of Bioavailability and Bioequivalence Studies. New York: Marcel Dekker.

Craigmill, A.L., Riviere, J.E., and Webb, A.L. 2006. Tabulation of FARAD Comparative and Veterinary Pharmacokinetic Data. Ames, IA: Blackwell.

Dhillon, A., and Kostrzewski, A. 2006. Clinical Pharmacokinetics. London: Pharmaceutical Press.

Gibaldi, M., and Perrier, D. 1982. Pharmacokinetics, 2d Ed. New York: Marcel Dekker.

Hardee, G.E., and Baggot,D. 1998. Development and Formulation of Veterinary Dosage Forms, 2d Ed. New York: Marcel Dekker.

Mordenti, J. 1986. Man versus beast. Pharmacokinetic scaling in mammals. Journal of Pharmaceutical Sciences. 75:1028–1039.

Notari, R.E. Biopharmaceutics and Clinical Pharmacokinetics, 3d Ed. New York: Marcel Dekker.

Patterson, S. and Jones, B. 2006. Bioequivalence and Statistics in Clinical Pharmacology. Boca Raton, FL: Chapman and Hall/CRC.

Reddy, M.B., Yang, R.S.H., Clewell, H.J., and Andersen M.E. 2005. Physiologically Based Pharmacokinetic Modeling. Hoboken, NJ: Wiley.

Riviere, J.E. (1999). Comparative Pharmacokinetics: Principles, Techniques and Applications. Ames, IA: Blackwell.

Rowland, M., and Tozer, T.N. 1995. Clinical Pharmacokinetics: Concepts and Applications, 3d Ed. Philadelphia, PA: Lippincott, Williams and Wilkins.

Segre, G. 1982. Pharmacokinetics—Compartmental representation. Pharmacology and Therapeutics. 17:111–127.
———. 1988. The sojourn time and its prospective use in pharmacology. Journal of Pharmacokinetics and Biopharmaceutics. 16:657–666.
Special Reviews Issue: PK and PK-PD in Veterinary Medicine. 2004. Journal of Veterinary Pharmacology and Therapeutics. 27:395–535.
Teorell, T. 1937. Kinetics of distribution of substances administered to the body. Archives International Pharmacodynamics 57:205–240.
Wagner, J.G. 1975. Fundamentals of Clinical Pharmacokinetics. Lancaster, PA: Technomic Publishing Co.
Welling, P.G., and Tse, F.L.S. 1995. Pharmacokinetics: regulatory, Industrial, and Academic Perspectives. New York: Marcel Dekker.
West, G.B., Brown, J.H., and Enquist, B.J. 1997. A general model for the origin of allometric scaling laws in biology. Science 276:122–126.
Winter, M.E. 1988. Basic Clinical Pharmacokinetics, 2d Ed. Spokane, WA: Applied Therapeutics.
Yamaoka, K., Nakagawa, T. and Uno, T. 1978. Statistical moments in pharmacokinetics. Journal of Pharmacokinetics and Biopharmaceutics 6:547.

CHAPTER

4

MECHANISMS OF DRUG ACTION AND PHARMACOKINETICS/ PHARMACODYNAMICS INTEGRATION IN DOSAGE REGIMEN OPTIMIZATION FOR VETERINARY MEDICINE

PIERRE-LOUIS TOUTAIN

INTRODUCTION

Pharmacokinetics (PK) studies the fate of drugs in the animal whereas pharmacodynamics (PD) studies the action of a drug from its interaction with receptors, to the effect on animal populations. Pharmacokinetic/pharmacodynamic (PK/PD) integration consists of describing and explaining the time course of the drug effect (PD) via the time course of its concentration in the plasma (PK). A tenet in pharmacology is that the plasma concentration controls the concentration at the site of action (the so-called *biophase* where receptors are located) and that a proportional relationship exists between the plasma and biophase concentrations at equilibrium. This is why plasma concentration, which is easy to measure, can be used as an explicative variable of the in vivo drug effect when integrating PK and PD data in a PK/PD modeling approach (Fig. 4.1). Plasma concentration, unlike the biophase concentration, is also easy to control with an appropriate dosage regimen and one of the main goals of PK/PD analysis is to precisely determine the dosage regimen (dose, dosage interval). The ultimate goal in controlling the

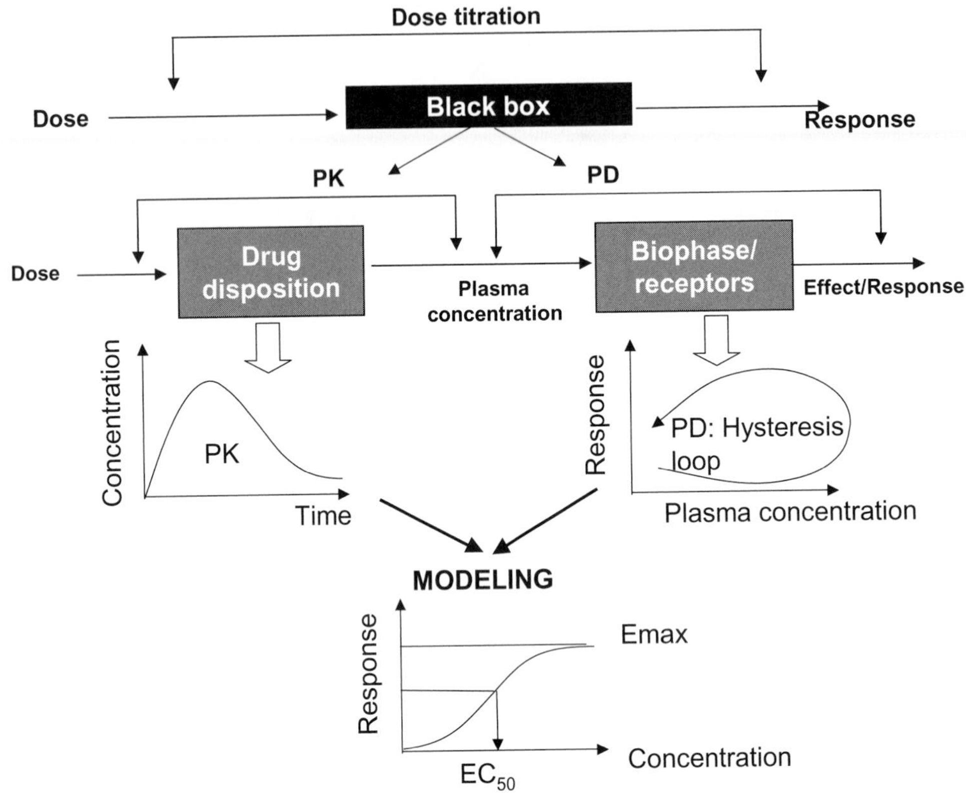

FIG. 4.1 Dose-effect relationship versus PK/PD modeling. Both approaches aim at documenting the same relationship between dose and drug response. A dose-effect relationship is a black-box approach in which the dose is the explicative variable of drug response. In a PK/PD approach, the black box is opened, thereby enabling the two primary processes that separate dose from response to be recognized. In the first step (PK), the dose is transformed into a plasma concentration profile. In the second step (PD), the plasma concentration profile becomes the variable, which explains the drug response. The difficulty with the PK/PD approach is that the development of effect and plasma concentrations over time is usually not in phase. This means that a hysteresis loop is observed when the response is plotted against plasma concentrations and data modeling is required to estimate the PD parameters (E_{max}, ED_{50}, and slope).

plasma drug concentration (also termed *drug exposure* or *internal dose*) is to achieve some expected endpoint in terms of drug efficacy and safety.

The first part of this chapter addresses the question of drug pharmacodynamics with special emphasis on the relationship between drug concentration and intensity of action at the receptor level. Recent reviews include Colquhoun 2006; Kenakin 2004; Lees et al. 2004a; Rang 2006. A glossary of pharmacodynamic terms and symbols is given in Lees et al. 2004a; Neubig et al. 2003. A series of articles devoted to receptor physiology was published in a special issue of the British Journal of Pharmacology (BPS 75th Anniversary Supplement, January 2006, vol.147(S1) pages S1–S308). The second part of this chapter is devoted to the in vivo situation and to the whole drug response. The classical dose-titration methods for dose determination and their limits are described with special emphasis on the alternative PK/PD approaches. The use of PK/PD modeling in studies of veterinary drugs has been reviewed (Toutain 2002; Toutain and Lees 2004) for antibiotics (Lees et al. 2006; McKellar et al. 2004; Toutain et al. 2002), ACE-inhibitors (Toutain and Lefebvre 2004) and NSAIDs (Lees et al. 2004b; 2004c).

TYPES OF DRUG TARGETS

Most drugs act via an interaction with certain proteins (Fig. 4.2). Exceptions are drugs in which the activity is based on physical properties. Examples include osmotic

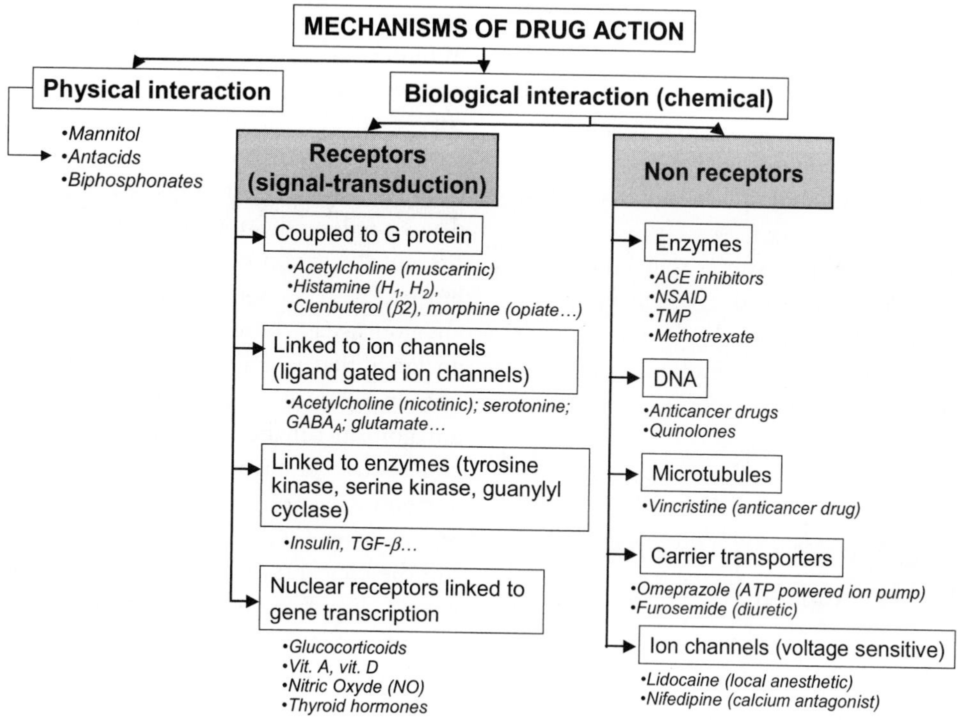

FIG. 4.2 Mechanisms of drug action. For most drugs, the drug action is mediated by some biological interaction with a macromolecule of the cell, often a protein. Different proteins are involved as drug targets and the term receptor is used only when the interaction triggers a cascade of events for signal transmission.

diuretics (e.g., mannitol) and antacids. Protamine can be injected as an antidote of heparin and acts as a physical antagonist by binding to it. General anesthetics were previously thought to produce their effect by simply dissolving in the lipid bilayer of the nerve membrane. It is currently acknowledged that anesthetics act by binding to some target protein. For certain intravenous anesthetics such as propofol, the target has been identified as the $GABA_A$ receptor but for inhalational anesthetics, the exact mechanism of drug action remains unknown.

Four types of protein are targeted by drugs: enzymes, carriers, ion channels, and receptors (Fig. 4.2). The term *receptor* should be reserved for regulatory proteins that play a role in intercellular communication. Thus, enzymes, ion channels, and carriers are not usually classified as receptors.

Enzymes such as cyclooxygenases are the target site for nonsteroidal anti-inflammatory drugs (NSAIDs), and their inhibition leads to the suppression of proinflammatory prostaglandins. Acetylcholine esterase, an enzyme that metabolizes acetylcholine at the receptor site, is a target site for cholinesterase inhibitors (neostigmine, physostigmine, . . .). Cholinesterase inhibitors act indirectly by preventing the enzyme from hydrolyzing acetylcholine. Other examples of enzymes serving as drug targets are dihydrofolate reductase for trimethoprim (an antibacterial) and angiotensin converting enzyme (ACE) for ACE-inhibitors such as benazepril and enalapril.

Carriers (also termed *membrane transport proteins*) are target sites for many drugs. The $Na^+/K^+/2Cl^-$ symport in the nephron is the site of action of furosemide. Furosemide acts at the luminal surface of the thick ascending limb of the loop of Henle to prevent sodium chloride reabsorption. ATP-powered ion pumps such as the sodium pump (Na^+/K^+ = ATPase) are the target sites for cardioactive digitalis and the Na^+/H^+ pump in the gastric parietal cell is the target site for proton pump inhibitors such as omeprazole.

Some drugs, such as local anesthetics, produce their effects by directly interacting with ion channels. They inhibit voltage-gated Na^+ channels in sensory neurons by binding to some specific site within the Na^+ channel and produce a direct effect by incapacitating the protein molecule. This mechanism of drug action on ion channels should not be confused with that of ligand-gated ion channels, i.e., which function as ionotropic receptors (see the later section "Macromolecular Nature of Drug Receptors").

Other nonreceptor/nonprotein targets that function as sites of action are nucleic acids for drugs such as actinomycin D, an antineoplastic antibiotic. DNA is also the target for a number of antibiotics (quinolones) as well as mutagenic and carcinogenic agents.

DRUG RECEPTOR AND LIGAND AS AGONIST OR ANTAGONIST

A receptor is a molecule or a polymeric structure on the surface or inside a cell that specifically recognizes and binds an endogenous compound. Binding sites are 3D structures forming pockets or grooves on the surface of protein that allow specific interactions with compounds known as ligands, which are molecules of complementary shape to the protein-binding site (lock-and-key analogy). Receptors possess an effector system (also termed *signal-transduction pathways*). In this they differ from acceptors that are molecules without signal-transduction pathways (e.g., serum albumin) characterized by a binding process that is not followed by a physiological response.

Endogenous neurotransmitters, such as hormones, act as molecular messengers and are endogenous ligands. Drugs may be viewed as exogenous ligands. After attachment to a receptor site, a drug may produce a cascade of biochemical events that results in drug action. A drug is said to be an agonist when it produces a measurable physiological or pharmacological response characteristic of the receptor (contraction, relaxation, secretion, enzyme activation, etc.). A *full agonist* produces a maximal effect under a given set of conditions, whereas a *partial agonist* produces only a submaximal effect regardless of the amount of drug applied. For opioid receptors, morphine and fentanyl are full agonists able to initiate strong analgesia while buprenorphine is a partial agonist (Lees et al. 2004a). Even if buprenorphine is unable to achieve the same level of analgesia provided by a maximally effective dose of full agonists, it may be preferred for postsurgical analgesia because its effect is of long duration and adverse effects are minimal.

In contrast to an agonist, some drugs may be unable to trigger any action on their own, after attachment to a receptor site, but are able to block the action of other agonists. These "silent drugs" are termed antagonists; most drugs used in therapeutics are receptor antagonists and prevent the action of natural agonists (neurotransmitters, hormones, . . .). Some drugs may be both agonist and antagonist e.g., butorphanol, a central-acting morphinic analgesic that is mainly an antagonist at the *mu* receptor but an agonist at the *kappa* receptor. Two forms of antagonism can be distinguished: competitive and noncompetitive antagonism. In competitive antagonism, antagonists act on the same receptor as the agonist; this is said to be reversible when it can be surmounted by increasing the concentration of the agonist. Examples of therapeutic agents acting by competitive antagonism are atropine (an antimuscarinic agent) and propranolol (a beta blocker). In irreversible (competitive) antagonism, a net displacement of the antagonist from its binding site cannot be achieved by increasing the agonist concentration, and, operationally, it resembles noncompetitive antagonism. This occurs when the antagonist is bound covalently and irreversibly to its receptor binding site. Although there are few drugs of this type, irreversible antagonists are used as experimental probes for investigating receptor function. Noncompetitive antagonism refers to the situation wherein a drug blocks the cascade of events normally leading to an agonist response, at some downstream point. This is the case of Ca^{2+} channel blockers, such as nifedipine, which prevent the influx of calcium ions through the cell membrane and nonspecifically block any agonist action requiring calcium mobilization, as in smooth muscle contraction. The concept of physiological antagonism refers to the interaction of two drugs whose opposing actions on a physiological system tend to cancel each other out. For example, histamine acts on receptors of the parietal cells of the gastric mucosa to stimulate acid secretion, while omeprazole blocks this effect by inhibiting the proton pump.

Antagonists were viewed solely as "silent ligands" until the discovery of the so-called "inverse agonists." An inverse agonist is a drug that acts at the same receptor as that of an agonist, yet produces an opposite effect (see later for the mechanism of inverse agonist action). Figure 4.3 summarizes the spectrum of activities that ligands can display.

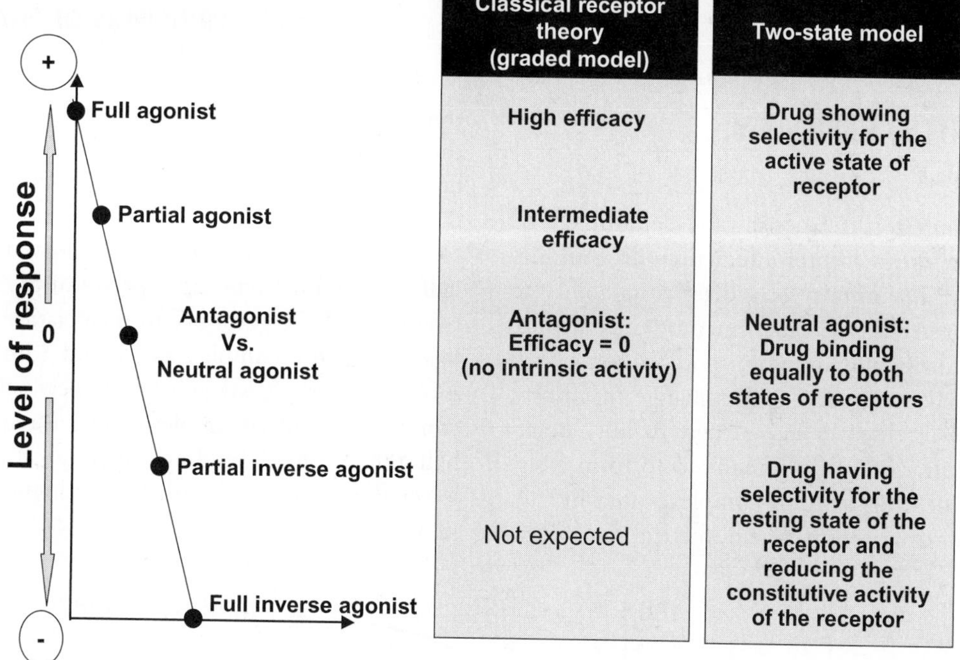

FIG. 4.3 Schematic representation of the spectrum of drug effect from full agonist (maximum positive effect) to full inverse agonist (maximum negative effect). Such a spectrum is seen only if a constitutive receptor activity exists that can be inhibited by an inverse agonist (see Fig. 4.9 for explanation). According to the "receptor theory," drugs may be agonists or antagonists. A full agonist produces full receptor activation leading to a maximal response; a partial agonist produces a submaximal response and possible blockade of a full agonist activation. An antagonist does not produce any physiological response but is able to block the response of an endogenous ligand or exogenous agonist. In the framework of the two-state model, any drug is viewed as an agonist, and an antagonist is a neutral agonist producing no response. According to this model, efficacy is genuinely explained by the relative affinity of the drug for one of the states of the receptor (activated or resting state), and inverse agonists are drugs showing selectivity for the resting state of the receptor. An inverse agonist acts as an antagonist but has the supplementary property over a classical antagonist of reducing receptor-mediated constitutive activity.

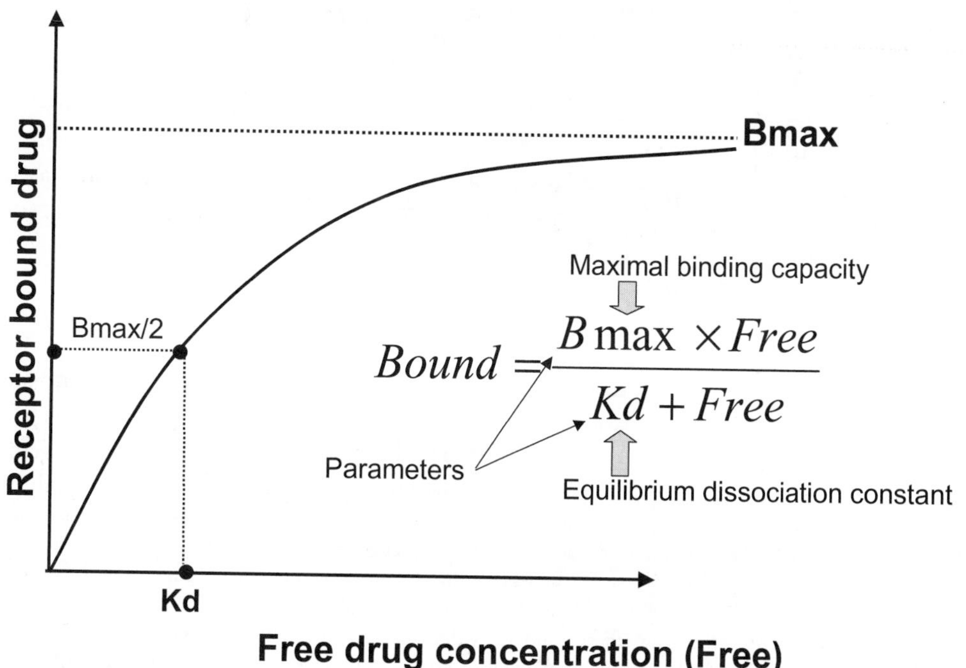

FIG. 4.4 Relationship between free drug concentration (*Free*) (independent variable) i.e., the driving concentration, and receptor-bound drug (dependent variable). Affinity of a drug for its receptor is expressed by Kd (a low Kd means a high affinity). B_{max} indicates the maximal binding capacity of the receptor.

DRUG AFFINITY, EFFICACY, AND POTENCY

The concentration-effect relationship is determined by two features of the drug-receptor interaction: drug affinity and drug efficacy. The affinity of a drug is its ability to bind to a receptor. Affinity is determined by the chemical structure of the drug, and minimal modification of the drug structure may result in a major change in affinity. This is exploited to discover new drugs. Affinity determines the concentration of drug required to form a significant number of drug-receptor complexes that in turn are responsible for drug action. The numerical representation of affinity for both an agonist and an antagonist is the constant of affinity denoted Ka (dimension M^{-1}, i.e., liter per mole). A Ka of 10^7 M^{-1} means that one mole of the ligand must be diluted in 10^7 liters of solvent to obtain a concentration of the free ligand able to saturate half the maximal binding capacity of the system. It is the reciprocal of the equilibrium dissociation constant of the ligand-receptor complex noted Kd (dimension M, i.e., mole per liter). A Kd of 10^{-7} M means that a free ligand concentration of 10^{-7} mole per liter is required to saturate half the maximal binding capacity of the system. The lower the Kd value of a drug, the higher the affinity for its receptor.

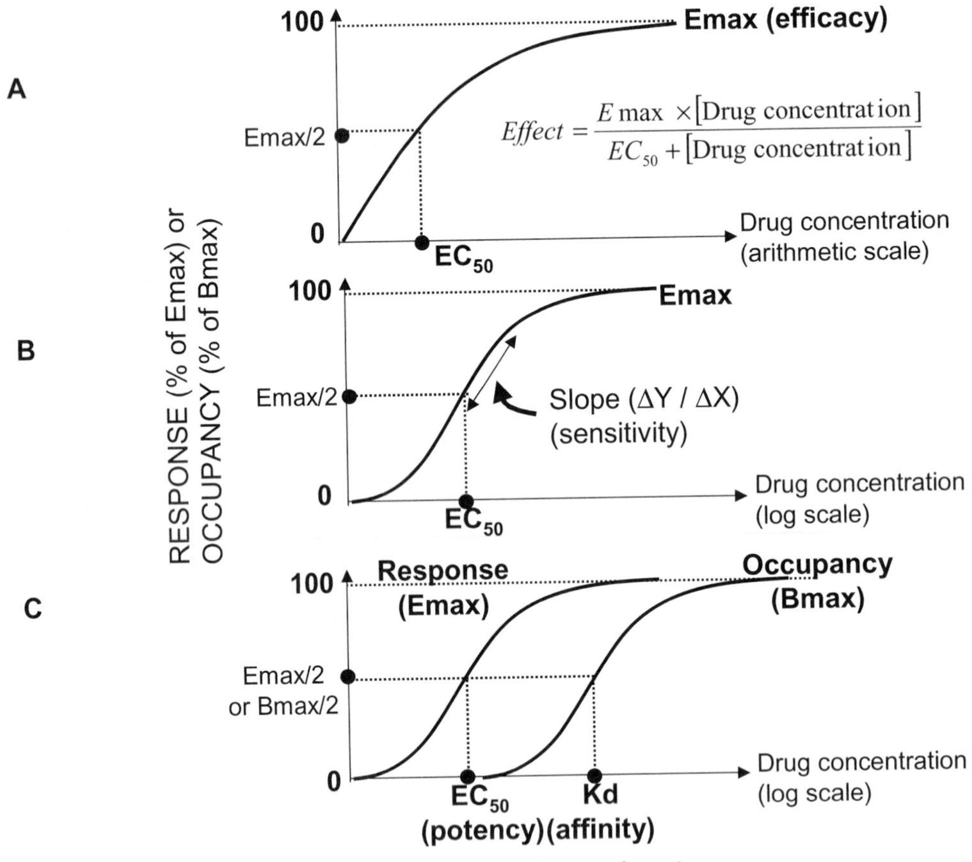

FIG. 4.5 The dose-response relationship and definition of the three main pharmacodynamic parameters.
(A) When the drug response (arithmetic Y axis) is plotted against the tested dose (arithmetic X axis), a hyperbolic relationship is often observed with a maximal effect noted E_{max}. EC_{50} is the concentration that produces an effect equal to half E_{max}.
(B) When the same data are represented using an X log scale, the relationship becomes sigmoidal with a more or less steep slope. The advantage is to compress the dose scale and to visualize the slope more easily. A sigmoidal curve allows the definition of three drug parameters, namely E_{max}, ED_{50}, and the slope ($\Delta Y/\Delta X$). E_{max} describes the drug efficacy and EC_{50} describes the drug potency. The slope (measured by the *n* of the Hill equation; see Equation 4.4 in the text) indicates the sensitivity of the dose-effect curve. The slope of the curve is involved in the drug selectivity (see Fig. 4.11).
(C) This plot shows that the concentration effect curve is situated to the left of the free concentration (occupancy)-bound curve with EC_{50} generally $\ll$ Kd.

Radioactive receptor ligands (radioligands) or fluorescent probes are used to accurately determine receptor affinity. The relationship between bound and free ligand may be described by a hyperbolic equation (Fig. 4.4) corresponding to the Michaelis Menten equation, i.e., Equation 4.1:

$$Bound = \frac{B\max \times Free}{Kd + Free} \tag{4.1}$$

Where B_{max} (a parameter) represents the maximal binding capacity (the total number of receptors), *Free* is the molar concentration of the free ligand, *Bound* is the bound ligand concentration, and *Kd* (a parameter) is the equilibrium constant of dissociation.

From this equation, the receptor occupancy (i.e., the fraction of receptor occupied) can be described by Equation 4.2:

$$fraction\ occupied = \frac{Bound}{B\max} = \frac{Free}{Free + Kd} \tag{4.2}$$

This is known as the Hill-Langmuir equation.

The generation of a response for the drug-receptor complex is governed by a property named *efficacy*. Efficacy is the drug's ability, once bound, to initiate changes that lead to the production of responses. It is a property of the ligand/receptor pair. This term is used to characterize the level of maximal response (E_{max}) induced by an agonist. In contrast, a pure antagonist has no intrinsic efficacy because it does not initiate a change in cell functions. This concept of efficacy is not to be confused with the drug's "clinical efficacy" whereby an antagonist may be fully efficacious. This is because blocking the binding of an endogenous agonist to the receptor by an antagonist may be clinically useful.

Potency corresponds to the concentration of drug required to achieve a given effect. It is expressed by the EC_{50} (or the IC_{50} if the effect is an inhibition), i.e., the concentration of an agonist that produces 50% of the maximum possible response for that agonist (Fig. 4.5). Potencies of drugs vary inversely with the numerical value of their EC_{50}, and the most potent drug is the one with the lowest EC_{50}. When different drugs within a series are compared, the most potent drug is not necessarily the most clinically efficacious (Fig. 4.6). A low potency is only a disadvantage when the effective dose is too large to be convenient; e.g., for a spot-on or an eye drop, the volume to be administered must be small and only relatively potent drugs can be administered in this way.

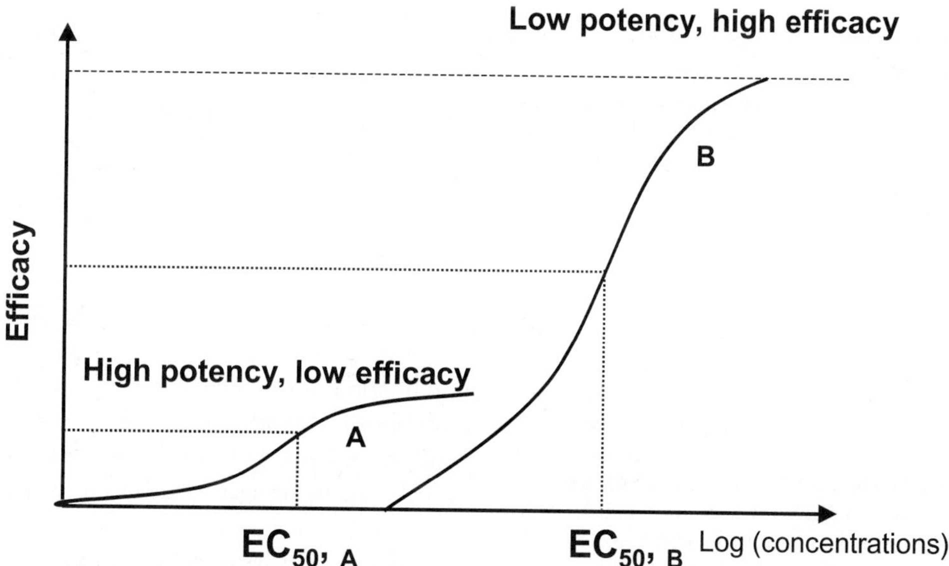

FIG. 4.6 Drug potency versus drug efficacy. These two terms are often confused. Potency is expressed in terms of concentration (X axis) and EC_{50} is the parameter measuring drug potency. Efficacy (Y axis) expresses the level of response with a maximal possible effect (E_{max}). Efficacy is the parameter of interest for a clinician but potency may be a limiting factor if the drug has to be administered in a small volume. Here, drug A has a higher potency than drug B but has a lower efficacy.

DRUG SPECIFICITY AND SELECTIVITY

The drug receptor interaction is responsible for the specificity and selectivity of drug action. When the drug acts only on a single target (enzyme, receptor, . . .), it is said to be "specific." Specificity is linked to the nature of the drug-receptor interaction and more precisely to the macromolecular structure of the receptors (or enzymes). As receptors are generally proteins, the diversity in 3D shape required for ligand specificity is provided by the polypeptide structure. The recognition of specific ligands by receptors is based on the complementarity of the 3D structure of the ligand and a binding pocket on the macromolecular target. The shapes and actions of receptors are currently being investigated by x-ray crystallography and computer modeling.

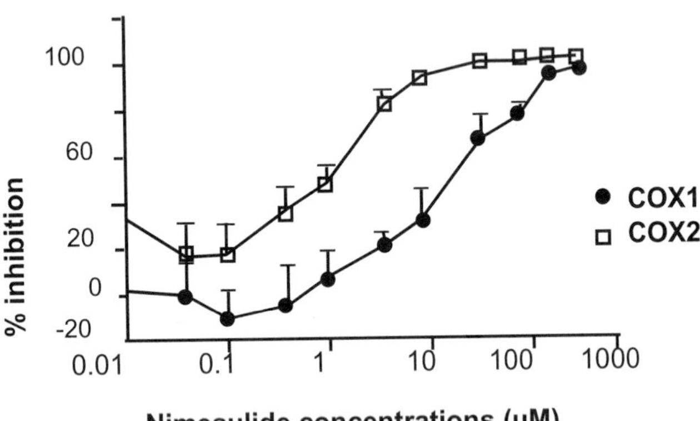

FIG. 4.7 Drug selectivity. For a nonsteroidal antiinflammatory drug (NSAID) such as nimesulide, the antiinflammatory properties are linked to the inhibition of cyclo-oxygenase (COX). There are two isoforms of COX: COX-1 and COX-2. COX-2 is an inducible enzyme formed at the site of inflammation and producing proinflammatory prostaglandins such as PGE_2, whereas COX-1 is a constitutive enzyme that performs a range of housekeeping functions. The selective inhibition of COX-2 is considered the primary action to be achieved for a NSAID and the nonselective inhibition of COX-1 is considered detrimental especially for the digestive tract (ulceration). This COX-2/COX-1 selectivity can be explored ex vivo using a whole blood assay (Toutain et al. 2001b). When this assay was conducted using canine blood, the production of TxB_2 by platelets was used to measure COX-1 inhibition and the production of PGE_2 from LPS-stimulated leucocytes was used to measure COX-2 inhibition. The IC_{50} values were 1.6 ± 0.4 µM for COX-2 and 20.3 ± 2.8 µM for COX-1 indicating that nimesulide is about 12 times more potent for COX-2 than for COX-1 isoenzymes. Nevertheless, nimesulide cannot be considered as a selective COX-2 inhibitor but only as a preferential COX-2 inhibitor. COX-2 would need to be almost totally inhibited to obtain a full antiinflammatory effect, and this is impossible to achieve without any COX-1 inhibition.

Specificity is rare. Most drugs can display activity toward a variety of receptors and are more often selective than specific. For example, histamine antagonists produce several effects, such as sedation and prevention of vomiting, which do not depend on histamine antagonism. Selectivity is related to the concentration range. The drug may be specific at a low concentration if it activates only one type of target, whereas several targets may be involved simultaneously (activated, inhibited, . . .) if the drug concentration is increased. This is the case with nonsteroidal antiinflammatory drugs and inhibition of the different subtypes of cyclooxygenases (COX-1 versus COX-2 isoenzymes) (Fig. 4.7). Lack of selectivity in vivo may lead to an overall complex and unpredictable pharmacological response and even undesirable side effects. Assessing the therapeutic usefulness of a new drug requires the determination of its full spectrum of biological activities toward a variety of relevant targets. The next task is then to explore this in vivo and select an appropriate dosage regimen that maintains the plasma drug concentration within the range in which only the desired response is expressed (i.e., within the so-called *therapeutic window*).

CHEMICAL FORCES AND DRUG BINDING

Several chemical intermolecular forces such as ionic bonds, hydrogen bonds, and Van der Waals forces may be involved in reversible binding of the drug to the receptor. In contrast, drug-receptor interactions involving covalent bond formation (very tight) are generally irreversible. Covalent binding to receptors is relatively rare. However covalent binding is more frequent for drugs acting on enzymes. COX-1 inhibitors are generally reversible although aspirin acts as a noncompetitive inhibitor of platelet COX-1 through a covalent binding mechanism. This is achieved by irreversible acetylation and explains the duration of the action of aspirin on blood coagulation. Because platelets have no nucleus, the effect of aspirin is reversed by the production of new platelets. Omeprazole (a proton pump inhibitor) is another example of irreversible binding to enzyme (H^+,K^+-ATPase). Drugs that bind covalently to DNA (alkylating agents) are extensively used as anticancer drugs.

Since many drugs contain acid or amine functional groups that are ionized at physiological pH, ionic bonds are formed by the attraction of opposite charges in the receptor site. Ionic bonds are the strongest non-covalent bonds. The attraction of opposite charges is brought about by polar-polar interactions as in hydrogen bonding. Although this electrostatic interaction is weaker than the ionic bond, an important feature of hydrogen bonding is the structural constraint. Thus the formation of hydrogen bonds between a drug and its receptor provides some information about the 3D structure of the resulting complex. The same forces are responsible for the shape of the protein and for its binding properties, so shape influences binding and, in turn, binding can influence protein shape. The ability of protein to change shape is called *allostery*.

MACROMOLECULAR NATURE OF DRUG RECEPTORS

Many receptors are transmembrane proteins embedded in the lipid bilayer of cell membranes. They have two functions: ligand binding and message transduction. Transmembrane receptors include metabotropic and ionotropic receptors (Fig. 4.8). The four superfamilies of receptor proteins include 1) ligand-gated ion channels, which are membrane-bound receptors, directly linked to an ion channel; 2) G-protein coupled receptors, which are membrane-bound receptors coupled to G-proteins; 3) tyrosine kinase-linked receptors, which are membrane-bound receptors containing an intrinsic enzymatic function (tyrosine kinase activity) in their intracellular domain; and 4) transcription factor receptors that are intracellular receptors regulating gene transcription.

The activation of metabotropic receptors (tyrosine kinase receptors and G-protein–coupled receptors) leads to some changes in metabolic processes within the cell, whereas ionotropic receptors directly open or close an ion channel. When an ionotropic receptor is activated, it opens a channel that immediately allows ions such as Na^+, K^+, or Cl^- to flow. In contrast, when a metabotropic receptor is activated, a series of intracellular events is first triggered that may also subsequently result in ion channel opening.

G-protein-coupled receptors (GPCRs), also known as *seven transmembrane receptors (7TM receptors),* transduce an extracellular signal (ligand binding) into an intracellular signal (G-protein activation). The signal is transferred via conformational alterations to a member of the family of G-proteins. GP may act directly on an ionic channel or activate an enzymatic system (adenylyl cyclase, guadenylyl cyclase, phospholipase C, . . .) to release a range of second messengers (cAMP, cGMP, IP3, etc.), which ultimately permits certain ions to enter or leave the cell. Muscarinic acetylcholine receptor, adrenoceptors (alpha-1, alpha-2, beta), dopamine, histamine, opioids, ACTH, and other receptors are examples of 7TM receptors.

The *receptor tyrosine kinase (RTK)* family is also a class of metabotropic cell surface receptors, which exert their regulatory effect by phosphorylating different effector proteins. An RTK consists of an extracellular binding site and an intracellular portion with enzymatic activity (tyrosine kinase, serine kinase) and usually spans the cell membrane once only. TK enzymes can transfer a phosphate group from ATP to a tyrosine residue in an intracellular protein to increase its phosphorylation. Protein phosphorylation is one of the underlying mechanisms regulating protein function. It can alter the biological properties or the interaction of proteins with other proteins or peptides. This family of receptors includes insulin, IGF-1, cytokines, epidermal growth factor, etc. The hormones and growth factors that act on this class of receptors are generally growth-promoting and function to stimulate cell division.

Ionotropic receptors activate transmembrane ion channels. They contain a central pore that functions as a ligand-gated ion channel. Nicotinic cholinergic receptor, $GABA_A$ receptor, glutamate, aspartate, and glycine receptors are ligand-gated ion channels.

Transcription factor receptors, such as those for steroid hormones, thyroid hormone, vitamin D, or retinoids receptors are intracellular proteins serving as transcription factors. After binding the ligand, e.g., a steroid hormone, the activated receptors translocate to the nucleus and bind to a DNA sequence called the *response element* and initiate the transcription of specific gene(s).

RECEPTOR TYPES AND SUBTYPES

Endogenous neurotransmitters (acetylcholine, norepinephrine, . . .) often bind to more than one type of receptor. This allows the same signaling molecule to produce a variety of effects in different tissues. For example, acetylcholine acts via both G-protein receptors (e.g., M2 muscarinic receptors in the heart) and ligand-gated channels (nicotinic muscle receptors). Historically, the classification of receptors has been based on their effect and relative potency toward selective agonists and antagonists. Now the association of molecular biology and cloning techniques has led to the discovery of novel receptor subtypes,

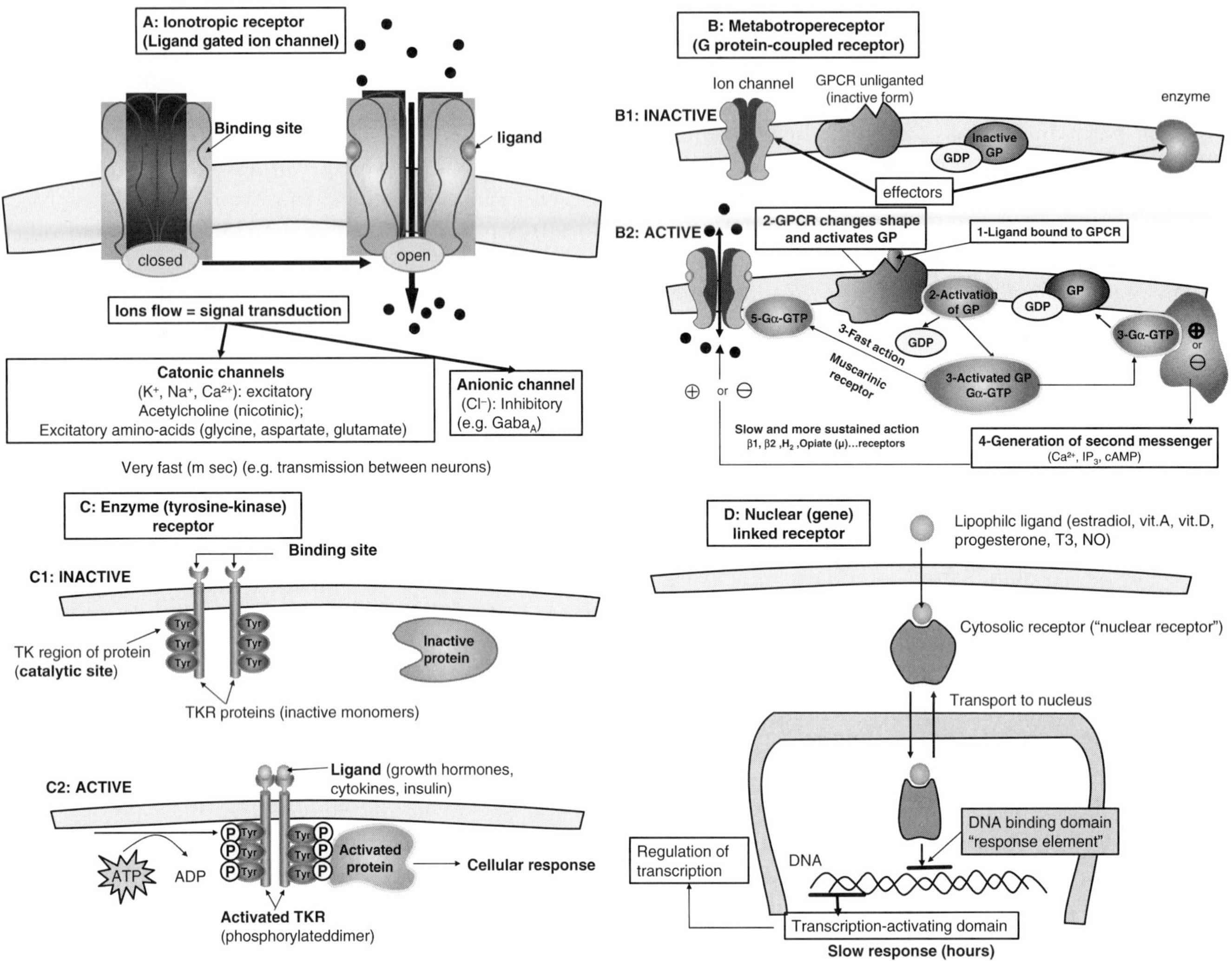

FIG. 4.8 Types of receptors and signaling mechanisms.

(A) Ion channels receptors. Ion channels inhibitors or ligand-gated receptors (ionotropic receptors) are protein forming on aqueous pores in the plasma membrane. Ligand binds at a specific site on the receptor. This leads to conformational changes, which open the channel and allow ions to flow into the cell. The change in ion concentration within the cell triggers cellular response. These receptors react in milliseconds. This type of receptor is not to be confused with voltage-gated ion channels that are not considered to be receptors (no signal transduction).

(B) G protein–coupled receptors. G protein–coupled receptors (GPCR) are single polypeptide chains forming seven transmembrane domains within the membrane with a segment able to interact with G proteins.

B1 (inactive state): G protein (GP) is attached to the cytoplasmic side of the membrane and is inactive as long as a ligand binds to GPCR. An ion channel or enzymes are possible terminal effectors of GPCR.

B2 (active state) steps 1 to 4:

step-1: Binding of a ligand changes the shape of the GPCR that interacts with a GP.

step-2: Interaction causes activation of GP with guanosine diphosphate (GDP) being exchanged against guanosine triphosphate (GTP).

step-3: The activated GP (Gα-GTP) moves either towards an enzyme, or directly modulates the conductance of an ionic channel (e.g., muscarinc receptor).

step-4: When an enzyme is activated (adenylyl cyclase, guanylyl cyclase, . . .) a second messenger (Ca^2+, cAMP, cGMP . . .) is generated and can mediate an action. Then G protein hydrolyses GTP back to GDP.

The advantage of this signal transduction pathway is twofold: signal amplification and signal specificity.

(C) Tyrosine kinase receptors

C1 (inactive state): tyrosine kinase receptors (TKR) are transmembrane receptors consisting of individual polypeptides each with a large extra-cellular binding site and an intracellular tail with an enzyme (tyrosine (Tyr) kinase, serine kinase).

C2 (active state): When a ligand binds to both receptors, the 2 receptor polypeptides aggregate to form a dimmer. This activates the tyrosine kinase part of the dimmer. Each uses ATP to phosphorylate the tyrosines on the tail of the other polypeptide as well as other down stream signaling proteins. The receptor proteins are now recognized by relay proteins inside the cell. Relay proteins bind to the phosphorylated tyrosines and may activate different transduction signals.

(D) Nuclear receptors. Intracellular receptors are located in the cytoplasm or the nucleus (NO, thyroid hormones, steroids . . .) the signal molecule (lipophilic) must be able to cross the plasma membrane. The ligand binds to a receptor called a nuclear receptor although some are located in the cytosol (e.g., glucocorticoid receptors) and migrate to the nucleus after binding a ligand. This activation pathway leads to a long lasting effect usually over several hours.

and their expression as recombinant proteins has facilitated the discovery of more selective drugs. IUPHAR (the International Union of Basic and Clinical Pharmacology) has a committee on receptor nomenclature and drug classification and regularly publishes updated reviews and a compendium in its journal (*Pharmacological Reviews*; see www.iuphar.org).

DRUG RECEPTOR THEORIES: FROM THE OCCUPANCY THEORIES TO THE TWO-STATE MODEL.

Drug receptor theories consist of a collection of evolving models that correspond to the historical progression of knowledge and permit qualitative and quantitative description of the relationship between drug concentrations and their effect. Before the advent of molecular biology, the various effects of agonists and antagonists were described by operational mathematical modeling, i.e., with no or minimal mechanistic considerations (black-box approach). Effects were measured on isolated tissue in an organ bath chamber and the collected data were modeled using relatively simple equations derived from the law of mass action, as in Equation 4.1.

Occupancy Theory was the first model and was proposed by Clark in 1923 (Rang 2006). The receptor–ligand interaction was described as a bimolecular interaction and the receptor–ligand complex was considered responsible for the generation of an effect. This model assumes that drug response is a linear function of drug occupancy at the receptor level. Consequently, the drug has to occupy all receptors to achieve a maximal effect (E_{max}), and the response is terminated when the drug dissociates from the receptor. Thus, in the equation for receptor binding (see Equation 4.1) the terms B and B_{max} can be replaced with E (effect) and E_{max}, leading to Equation 4.3:

$$Effect = E_{max} \times \frac{[Drug]}{Kd + [Drug]} \qquad (4.3)$$

in which *Effect* (the dependent variable) is the observed effect, E_{max} (a parameter) is the maximal possible effect for that system, *Kd* is a parameter measuring affinity, and *Drug* is the drug concentration, i.e., the independent variable. In this simple occupancy model of drug action, the concentration of drug required to produce 50% of the maximal effect (i.e., the EC_{50}) is numerically equal to the dissociation constant (i.e., Kd).

This equation describes the classical hyperbolic agonist–effect relationships. These relationships are often presented on a log-scale, in which case they are sigmoidal (see Fig. 4.5). It should be noted that some drugs do not follow the classical monotonic dose-effect relationship but rather a U-shaped relationship. Here, drugs may cause low dose simulation and high dose inhibition of response (or the inverse) leading to the concept of Hormesis (for details, see Calabrese and Baldwin 2003), a challenging concept to apply in toxicology.

The occupation model of Clark was only confirmed in a limited number of cases. As a rule, the physiological response produced by a ligand is not directly proportional to occupancy and it was evident that some drugs acting at the same receptor could elicit different maximal effects at maximal receptor occupancy leading to the notion of partial agonist versus full agonist. To account for these discrepancies, which could not be explained by the occupation theory, Ariens (1954) suggested the existence of a proportionality factor, termed the *intrinsic activity*, between the amount of ligand-receptor complex and the observed effect. At almost the same time, Stephenson (1956) introduced the terms of affinity for the binding step and the concept of (molecular) efficacy for the production of a response. In this concept, a maximal response did not necessarily correspond to 100% receptor occupancy but could occur when only a few receptors were occupied. This led to the concept of spare receptors or a receptor reserve; thus activation of fewer than 1% of receptors at the skeletal neuromuscular junction, for example, is enough to elicit an action potential and maximal contraction of muscle fiber. According to Stephenson's concept the final effect of a drug is not directly proportional to the number of receptor–ligand complexes but is linked to the generation of an intermediary step, termed *stimulus*, and it is the stimulus that is proportional to the amount of receptor-ligand complex. Finally, the stimulus is translated by the tissue into a more-or-less amplified response. Thus, the efficacy of an agonist according to Stephenson is the parameter that indicates its ability to generate the stimulus instead of the final response in Ariens's theory. These concepts of intrinsic activity and efficacy have been historically important to our understanding of the mechanism of drug action because they acknowledge two different properties of molecules: the affinity of the ligand for the receptor (as measured by its Kd) that determines the receptor occupancy, and a second property that is the ability to activate the receptor once bound. Thus a partial agonist may show higher affinity than a full agonist but be less effective in generating a biological response because its intrinsic activity is lower than that of a full agonist (see Fig. 4.6). Currently, with the advent of molecular biology and the availability of recombinant receptor systems, it is possible to better understand how an agonist actually works, and physiologically based models rather than the black-box approach are used to explain the concept of efficacy. Currently the most generic model is known as the *two-state model* (Fig. 4.9).

The two-state model of drug action is consistent with most observations of agonists and antagonists and is genuinely able to explain the nature of inverse agonists and the existence of a spontaneous (constitutive) activity of receptors. Briefly, this model assumes that the receptor molecule exists in two extreme conformations, with the active and inactive forms in dynamic equilibrium. It is the conformational change (i.e., isomerization) of the receptors from an inactive to active state that initiates the pharmacological response. This spontaneous equilibrium may be shifted by the binding of ligands to the receptor. For example, the GABA–benzodiazepine receptor exists in two

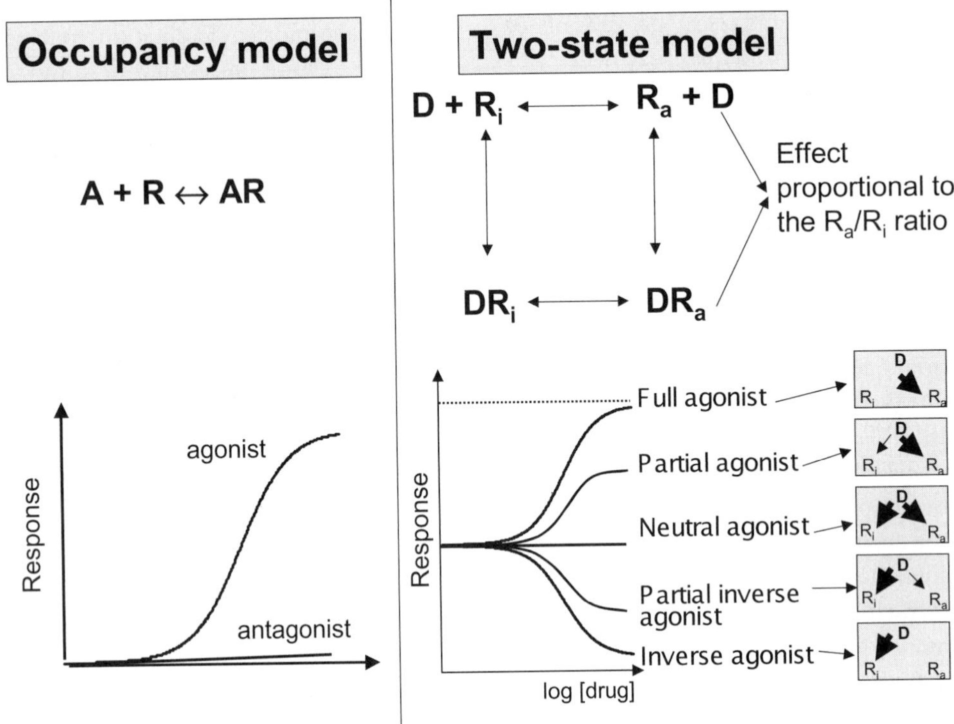

FIG. 4.9 Model of receptor activation: the graded activation model (left) vs. the simple two-state model (right). The graded activation model implies that agonists can induce different degrees of conformational changes in the receptor (R) and thus different levels of response. In this model, the unliganted receptor is silent (no basal activity) while in the two-state model there is a pre-existing resting and an active state. For the occupancy model, the level of response is explained by the concept of efficacy (see Fig. 4.3) and an antagonist is a drug with a null (molecular) efficacy but that blocks access to the receptor of other ligands. In the two-state model, a receptor can switch between two conformational states that are in equilibrium: an active state (Ra) and an inactive state (Ri). When no drug (D) is present, a constitutive basal signal output (the existing physiological or biochemical response) is more or less high depending on the actual Ra/Ri ratio. Drug binding to R may shift the equilibrium in either direction. The extent to which the equilibrium is shifted toward Ra or Ri is determined by the relative affinity of the drug for the two conformational states. A drug with a higher affinity for Ra than for Ri will drive the equilibrium to Ra and thereby activate the receptor. Such a drug is called an *agonist* and a full agonist is a drug selective enough regarding Ra to drive all the receptor in its active state and get a maximal response. When a drug has only a moderately greater affinity for Ra than for Ri, its effect will be lower than for a full agonist and such a drug is termed a *partial agonist* because it cannot produce a full effect. A drug that binds Ra and Ri with equal affinity will not alter the equilibrium between Ra and Ri, will have no net effect of its own and will act as a competitive antagonist. Finally, a drug with a higher affinity for Ri than for Ra will shift the equilibrium toward Ri and will produce an effect opposite to that of an agonist and is termed an *inverse agonist*. For example cimetidine and ranitidine are inverse agonists of H_2-receptors. Under conditions where the conformational equilibrium of the unliganted receptors is strongly in favor of Ri (i.e., no constitutional spontaneous activity), the model is operationally equivalent to the graded model.

conformations, an active open channel conformation with high affinity for GABA, and an inactive closed conformation with low affinity for GABA. The two forms are in equilibrium. In this scheme diazepam (an agonist) shows high affinity for the active conformation stabilizing the binding of GABA to the activated conformation. The inactive conformation would be favored in the presence of inverse agonists.

In the framework of this model, an agonist is a ligand that preferentially binds to the active state of the receptor and thus shifts the equilibrium in the direction of the active state. A full agonist is selective for the active form, whereas a partial agonist has only a slightly higher affinity for the active receptor than for the inactive form. An inverse agonist is a ligand for which a response may be observed only if there is a preexisting level of receptor activity, as with $GABA_A$ receptors. The two main sources of tone result from either the presence of endogenous ligand or from constitutive receptor activity. These active receptors display a basal effect even if there are no agonist ligands binding to them. A decrease in physiological or biochemical response may be observed if an inverse agonist with a preference for the inactive receptor is added.

In the framework of this biologically based theory, the classical receptor theory has to be revisited. For instance, the measured Kd no longer represents the affinity for either active or inactive receptor but lies in between and Kd is a function of both affinity and efficacy (for details, see Rang 2006). Many compounds previously identified as antagonists appear to act as (partial) inverse agonists, i.e., they actually diminish the constitutive activity of the receptor. This is the case of cimetidine, which was previously considered an H_2 antagonist. Although the therapeutic relevance of inverse agonists needs to be confirmed, the ligand of choice may be an inverse agonist for some receptors with high constitutional activity. Finally the last type of ligand to be considered in the two state model paradigm is the neutral competitive antagonist that has equal affinity for both conformations and does not affect the equilibrium.

The two-state model has given rise to more advanced models such as the ternary complex model or the extended ternary complex model to take into account our knowledge of the signal transduction associated with G-protein–coupled receptors.

Currently, our concepts are still evolving and new descriptive terms such as functional selectivity, agonist-directed trafficking, biased agonism, protean agonism, etc., are being introduced to explain what were previously viewed as artifacts (see Urban et al. 2007, Kenakin 2007).

DOWN- AND UP-REGULATION

The effect of a drug often diminishes when it is given repeatedly. The term used to describe a gradual decrease in responsiveness to chronic drug administration (days, months) is *tolerance*. Tachyphylaxis is an acute form of tolerance. Several pharmacodynamic mechanisms (desensitization, loss of receptor, exhaustion of mediator, . . .) and pharmacokinetic mechanisms (metabolism induction, active extrusion of the drug, . . .) may explain tachyphylaxis and tolerance. Chronic stimulation of receptors with a drug results in a state of long-term desensitization, also termed *down-regulation*. This is often due to a decrease in the number of receptors, whereas understimulation leads to up-regulation due to an increase in the number of receptors and a functional supersensitivity. Receptor expression is a dynamic process with equilibrium between the synthesis and destruction of receptors. For example, the binding of a hormone such as insulin to its receptors on the surface of a cell initiates endocytosis of the hormone-receptor complex and its destruction by intracellular lysosomal enzymes. This internalization regulates the number of sites that are available for binding on the cell surface. Although receptor desensitization is generally an unwanted effect complication, it can provide a way of controlling certain physiological systems. For example, long-term contraception by means of GnRH agonist-induced down-regulation of pituitary secretion of LH and FSH has been explored in dogs and cats. The advantage of this nonsurgical method is its reversibility when the treatment is discontinued.

AN OVERVIEW ON THE DETERMINATION OF AN EFFECTIVE AND SAFE DOSAGE REGIMEN

The determination of a safe and effective dose or dosing regimen (i.e., dose and dosage interval) is essential for an appropriate exposure of receptors and optimal use of drugs. Dose-response analysis consists of using appropriate scientific tools to answer the following questions (Ruberg 1995):

1) Is there any drug effect? 2) Which doses exhibit a different response to the control? 3) What is the nature (shape) of the dose-response relationship? 4) What is the optimal dose? In addition, an optimal dosage regimen in veterinary medicine must not only be safe and effective when administered to a single animal in well-controlled conditions but also when administered collectively to food-producing animals. It also needs to be optimized to avoid any public health concerns regarding the questions of drug residues, pollution of the environment, or antimicrobial drug resistance.

Various scientific tools are available to answer these different questions, and the choice of a given approach will be dictated by the therapeutic area, the phase of drug development, the availability or not of surrogate endpoints with good metrological properties, and the ease with which the clinically relevant outcomes can be assessed.

In veterinary medicine the most well-established approach is the *dose-titration trial.* This consists of testing different dose levels and selecting the one that achieves some preestablished regulatory requirement in terms of cure rate (as for antiparasitic drugs).

Although this dose-titration approach has its attractions, it also has limitations and these led to the investigation of alternatives such as the PK/PD approach. The plasma concentration profile is generally the driving force controlling the time course of drug concentration at the site of action (biophase for systemically acting drugs). This led to integration of the PK and PD information by means of a link model, and production of a versatile tool that could be used to determine the optimal dosage regimen. In PK/PD, the variable selected to explore the dose-effect relationship is the plasma concentration profile (not the nominal administered dose).

PK/PD modeling enables the numerical values of the three key PD parameters characterizing any drug: maximal efficacy (E_{max}), potency (EC_{50}), and sensitivity to be determined in vivo. The sensitivity is assessed from the slope of the concentration-effect relationship and is a major determinant of the drug's selectivity (see Fig. 4.5). Once these different PD parameters have been established, the dose-effect relationship and the time-to-effect relationships corresponding to different possible PK profiles can easily be explored by simulations to predict the time course of drug effects under different physiological and pathological conditions. These different scenarios may then be given to clinicians to assist them in designing future confirmatory clinical trials.

DESIGNS FOR DOSE TITRATION AND THE DETERMINATION OF AN EFFECTIVE DOSE

The selection of a dose should be based on well-controlled studies and the accepted statistical methodology. A simple parallel design is often selected in veterinary medicine. In this case the animals (healthy, spontaneously or experimentally infected or infested, . . .) are randomly allocated to a few predetermined dose groups (often including a placebo, low dose, medium dose, and high dose, i.e., four dose levels), and the endpoints of interest are compared using some appropriate statistical test of the hypothesis (Fig. 4.10). The parallel design has the advantage of being straightforward in design and analysis but has several serious limits: Because each subject receives only one dose level, it provides only a group mean (population average) dose response, not an individual dose response. This design leads to biased parameter estimates and poor or no estimates of variability and is unable to provide information on the shape of the individual dose-response relationship (Verotta et al. 1989), which is needed to determine drug selectivity. More importantly, the dose selected as the most effective dose is unlikely the optimal dose. The selected dose is obligatorily one of the tested doses and is highly dependent on the power of the design (number of tested animals), so trials with a small sample size generally lead to the selection of an excessively high dose.

The parallel design is used in studies of antiparasitic and antimicrobial drugs as the pivotal outcome is eradication of the pathogen (an irreversible drug effect). In contrast, drugs acting on physiological systems (e.g., cardiovascular, nervous system, kidney, . . .) almost invariably act reversibly so that a crossover design becomes possible.

In a crossover design each animal is tested with a range of dose levels so that individual dose-response curves are generated. So long as the number of tested doses is sufficient, the dose-effect relationship for a given animal can then be modeled using a classical sigmoidal relationship of the form (Equation 4.4)

$$Effect = E_0 \pm \frac{E\max \times Dose^n}{ED_{50}^n + Dose^n} \tag{4.4}$$

where *Effect* (dependent variable) is the predicted effect of a given dose (independent variable), E_0, the effect without the drug (i.e., a placebo effect or the base line response of the system); E_{max} is the maximum possible effect; and ED_{50} is the dose producing half E_{max}. E_{max} is a measure of the

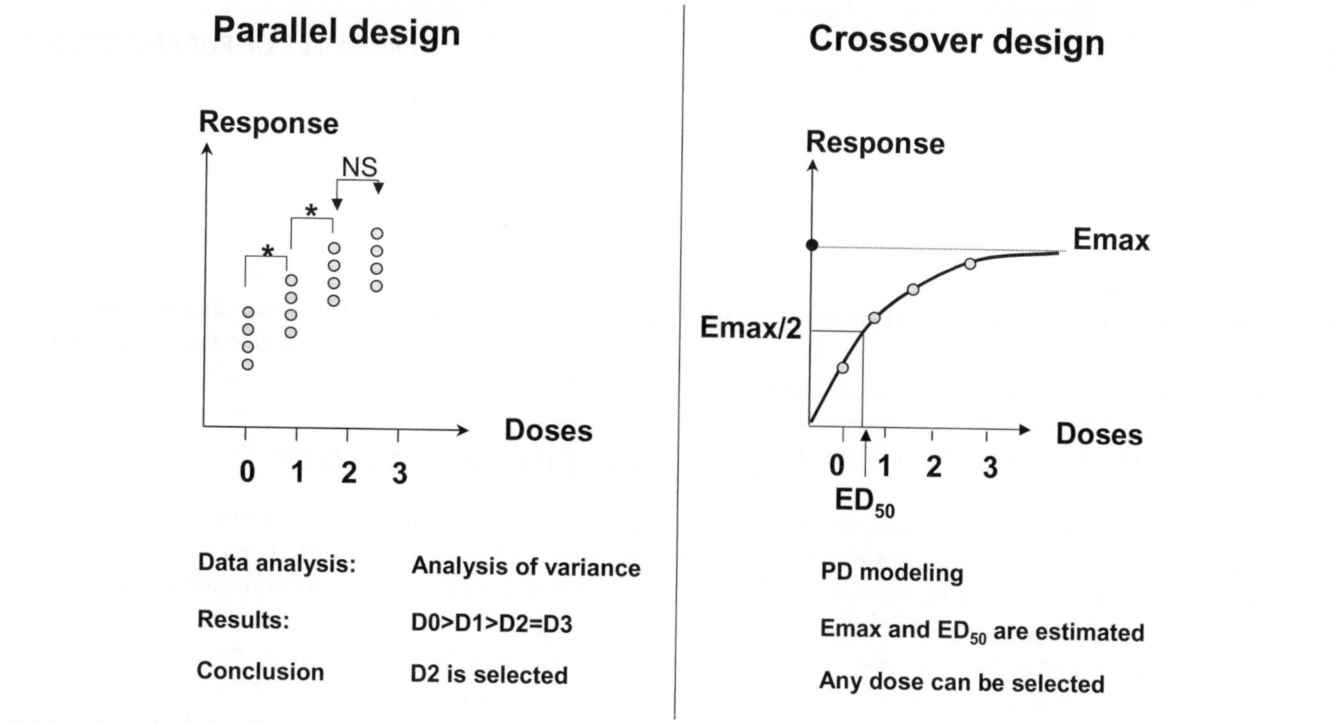

Parallel design

Response

NS

0 1 2 3 Doses

Data analysis: Analysis of variance

Results: D0>D1>D2=D3

Conclusion D2 is selected

Crossover design

Response

Emax

Emax/2

0 1 2 3 Doses

ED_{50}

PD modeling

Emax and ED_{50} are estimated

Any dose can be selected

FIG. 4.10 Parallel vs. crossover design for a dose-titration study. In a parallel design the animals (here n = 4 per group) are randomly assigned to one of the tested doses (0, 1, 2 or 3). Data analysis is performed by a test of the hypothesis (ANOVA), the selected dose being one of the tested doses (no interpolation). Here D2 would be selected because it gives a significantly higher response (*) than D1 but is not significantly (NS) different from D3. In a crossover design, all the animals receive all the tested doses and individual dose-effect curves are generated. For each individual curve, PD parameters (E_{max}, ED_{50}) can be computed and any dose over the tested range can be selected. With a crossover design, but not in a parallel design, information is obtained about the shape of the dose-response relationship and on variability within the population.

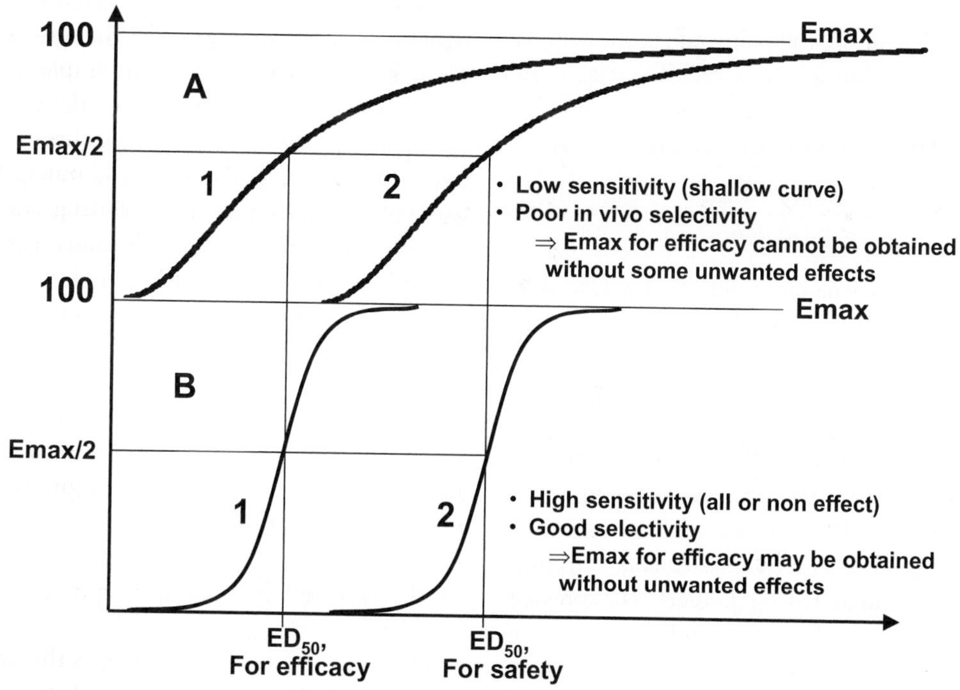

FIG. 4.11 In vivo drug selectivity is related to both the therapeutic index (i.e., the ratio $ED_{50,safety}/ED_{50,efficacy}$) and to the slope of the concentration effect relationship. Drugs A (top) and B (bottom) have the same potency (ED_{50}) and the same efficacy (same E_{max}) for the desired effect (curve 1) and unwanted effects (curve 2) i.e., the same therapeutic index. However, they differ in terms of sensitivity (slope) (shallow for drug A and steep for drug B). Only with drug B can the full effect (i.e., E_{max}) be obtained without any significant side effect despite the fact that drugs A and B have the same $ED_{50,safety}/ED_{50,efficacy}$ ratio. Definition of therapeutic index by $ED_{10,safety}/ED_{90,efficacy}$ does not take into account the differences in sensitivity of dose-response curves.

drug (physiological) efficacy whereas ED_{50} is a measure of the drug potency (see Fig 4.10). It should be stressed that although the two terms *efficacy* and *potency* are often confused and used interchangeably within scientific and pharmaceutical communities, the most potent drug may not always offer the most clinically effective dose (see Fig. 4.6).

When an exponent (n) is included in the model, it reflects the slope of the dose-effect relationship and can provide information about drug selectivity for the tested effect (see below) (Fig. 4.11).

This relationship can then be used to define the minimum effective dose, the maximum effective dose, and the maximum tolerated dose. The fundamental difference between parallel and crossover designs is that with a crossover design, any dose within the range of doses tested can be selected as the optimal dose because interpolation is possible, whereas this is not the case for a parallel design (see Sheiner et al. 1991, for details).

THE DIFFERENCE BETWEEN DOSE TITRATION AND THE PK/PD MODELING APPROACH IN DETERMINING A DOSE

It should be noted that in the following equation, ED_{50} is not a true PD parameter but a hybrid PK/PD variable. In fact ED_{50} is the product of three separate determinants, as indicated by the following relationship (Equation 4.5):

$$ED_{50} = \frac{Clearance \times EC_{50}}{Bioavailability} \tag{4.5}$$

where *Clearance* is the plasma clearance, *Bioavailability* is the extent of the systemic bioavailability (for the extravascular route of drug administration) and EC_{50} is the plasma concentration providing half E_{max}.

Figure 4.1 illustrates the fundamental differences between a dose-ranging trial and a PK/PD trial. Both aim at documenting the same relationship between dose and drug response but in a PK/PD analysis, the effect is explained by replacing dose with the plasma concentration profile so that the estimated drug potency is expressed as an EC_{50}, not an ED_{50}. The EC_{50}, unlike ED_{50}, is a true PD parameter. There is only one EC_{50} for a given endpoint and this EC_{50} value is not influenced by PK parameters, administration route, or formulation. This means that if a new formulation of the drug is to be developed, there is no need to run a new PK/PD trial. All that is required is a PK study to establish the influence of the new bioavailability on the effect. Hence, EC_{50} has a much wider application than ED_{50}, and the determination of EC_{50} is a primary objective of PK/PD studies. Furthermore, because the plasma concentration–time data include temporal information, PK/PD modeling is appropriate not only for establishing a suitable dose but also the dosage interval.

BUILDING PK/PD MODELS

In general three different models are considered when building a PK/PD model: a PK model transforming the dose into a concentration versus time profile, a link model describing transfer of the drug from the plasma into the biophase, and a PD model relating the biophase concentration to an effect (Holford and Sheiner 1981).

The PK model is generally a traditional compartmental model and the PK parameters are estimated in the conventional way. The PK model is used to provide concentration data for the PD model.

The plasma concentration profile and the effects are usually not in phase, and plasma concentration cannot directly be incorporated into a PD model. The effect of most drugs lags behind the plasma concentration. This can easily be visualized by plotting the effects (Y axis) against plasma concentrations (X axis). A loop is observed when the data points are in chronological order. This is known as a *hysteresis loop* from the Greek word meaning "coming late" (Fig. 4.12). When a hysteresis loop is observed, the cause of the delay must be identified to select the appropriate modeling strategy. When the delay is of PK origin (e.g., slow rate of drug distribution at the biophase, . . .), and when the drug effect is directly related to the drug concentration at the biophase level, a so-called "effect compartment model" can be chosen. A link model is interposed between the PK and PD model to account for the delay. Generally, this consists of describing drug transfer into the biophase by a first-order rate constant, which is the parameter of the link model. The first-order rate constant (generally noted K_{e0}) can be estimated from the time course of the drug effect (see Holford and Sheiner 1981, for details).

For most drugs, the combination of the drug with its receptor is followed by a cascade of time-dependent biochemical, physiological, and/or pathophysiological events (see Fig. 4.8). Thus the delay between plasma concentration and the response is due to the intrinsic temporal

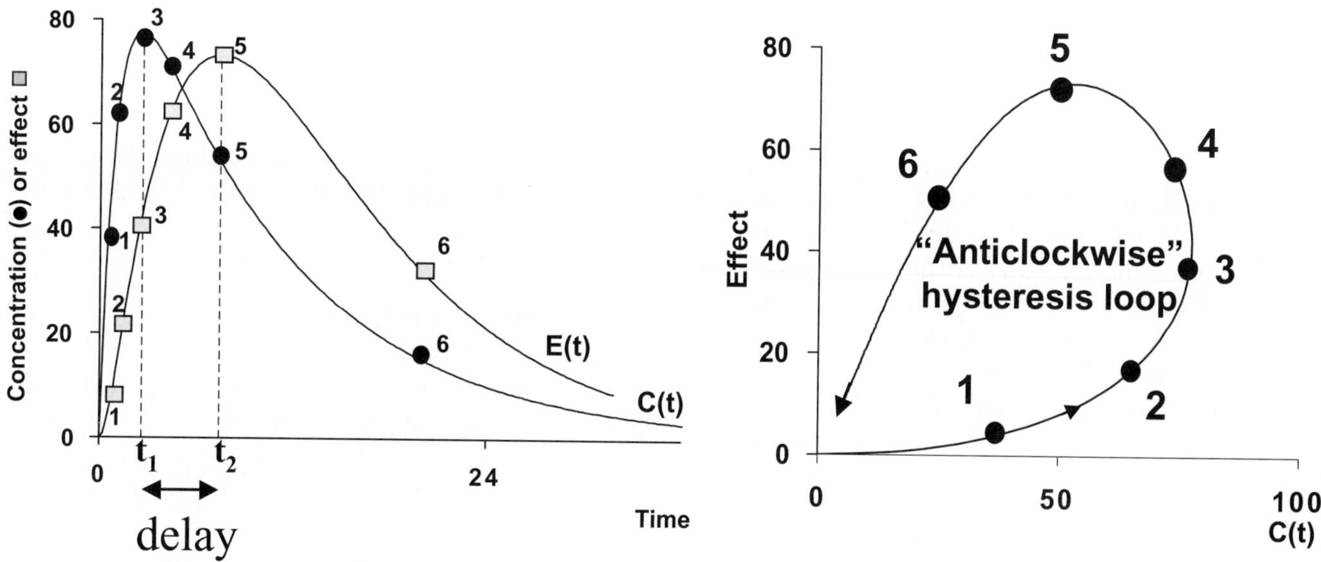

FIG. 4.12 In general, plasma concentration–time and effect-time relationships are not in phase. The peak concentration occurs at time t_1 and peak effect occurs at a later time t_2. An arithmetic plot of effect versus time reveals a hysteresis loop. For any given concentration, two different levels of effect are possible.

responsiveness of the system. The so-called indirect response models are used for this type of response.

Four basic indirect response models have been proposed (Dayneka et al. 1993), based on Equation 4.6, which describes the rate of change of response over time with no drug present:

$$\frac{dR}{dt} = K_{in} - K_{out}R \tag{4.6}$$

where dR/dt represents the rate of variation in the response variable (R). The model assumes that the measured response is being formed at a constant rate (K_{in}) but disappears in a first-order manner (K_{out}). For the variation in body temperature during fever, K_{in} is the thermogenesis and K_{out} expresses the rate of thermolysis. It can then be assumed that the indirect drug action consists of inhibiting or stimulating physiological factors that control production or dissipation of the measured effect as described in Equation 4.7:

$$\frac{dR}{dt} = K_{in} \times \{\text{stimulation or inhibition function}\} - K_{out} \times \{\text{stimulation or inhibition function}\} \times R \tag{4.7}$$

where the *stimulation or inhibition function* can be the classical E_{max} model.

The final model to consider in the PK/PD modeling approach is the PD model. There are two main types of PD models, describing either a graded concentration-effect relationship or a quantal concentration-response relationship. A graded model is used when the response to different drug concentrations can be quantified on a scale (e.g., body temperature, survival time). On the other hand, in a quantal model (also known as a *fixed-effect model*), the described effects are nominal (categorical) (e.g., dead or alive, cured of parasites or not, appearance of unwanted effects or not, . . .). The dose or exposure in quantal dose-response (or exposure-response) relationships is not related to the intensity of the effect but to the frequency of an all-or-none effect. Quantal responses are often clinical endpoint outcomes, whereas graded responses are often surrogates.

The most general model for a graded effect relationship is the Hill model, also known as the sigmoidal E_{max} model (Equation 4.8):

$$E(t) = E_0 \pm \frac{E\max \times C^n(t)}{EC_{50}^n + C^n(t)} \tag{4.8}$$

where *E(t)* is the effect observed for a given concentration at time *t* [*C(t)*], E_{max} is the maximal effect attributable to the drug, EC_{50} is the plasma concentration producing 50% of E_{max}, and *n* is the Hill coefficient, representing the slope of the concentration-effect relationship. When $n = 1$, the Hill model reduces to the E_{max} model, which corresponds to a hyperbolic function. Many drug effects involve the modulation of a physiological variable (e.g., blood pressure). In this case, inclusion of the term E_0 in Equation 4.8 indicates the presence of a baseline effect. E_0 can also represent a placebo effect.

When the drug effect corresponds to the inhibition of a biological process, the drug effect is subtracted from the baseline (E_0) and EC_{50} is often expressed as an IC_{50}, that is, the concentration producing 50% of the maximum inhibition effect (E_{max}). (For other PD models, see Holford and Sheiner 1981.)

Equation 4.8 contains several parameters (E_0, E_{max}, EC_{50} or IC_{50}, and *n*). The ultimate goal of PK/PD modeling is to evaluate the means and variances of these parameters from the in vivo observations of *E(t)* obtained over a range of *C(t)* values.

In a quantal concentration response relationship, i.e., when the outcome is binary (e.g., cure or no cure) or when the results of drug effect are provided as scores (responder/nonresponder), the link between the measure of drug concentration exposure and the corresponding probability is given by a logistic equation of the form (Equation 4.9):

$$P = \frac{1}{1 + e^{-(a+bX)}} \tag{4.9}$$

where *P* is the probability (e.g., of cure from 0 to 1), *a* is a parameter for baseline (e.g., a placebo effect) and *b* is an index of sensitivity (similar to a slope), and X is the independent variable and may be the exposure (rather than the instantaneous concentration) or a quantitative index predicting efficacy (ex. AUC/MIC for a concentration-dependent antibiotic). Figure 4.13 shows a logistic curve for the probability of cure of an antibiotic. In logistic regression, the dependent variable is termed a *logit,* which is the natural log of the odds (Equation 4.10):

$$\log(odds) = \text{logit}(P) = Ln\frac{P}{(1-P)} \text{ and } odds = \frac{P}{1-P} \tag{4.10}$$

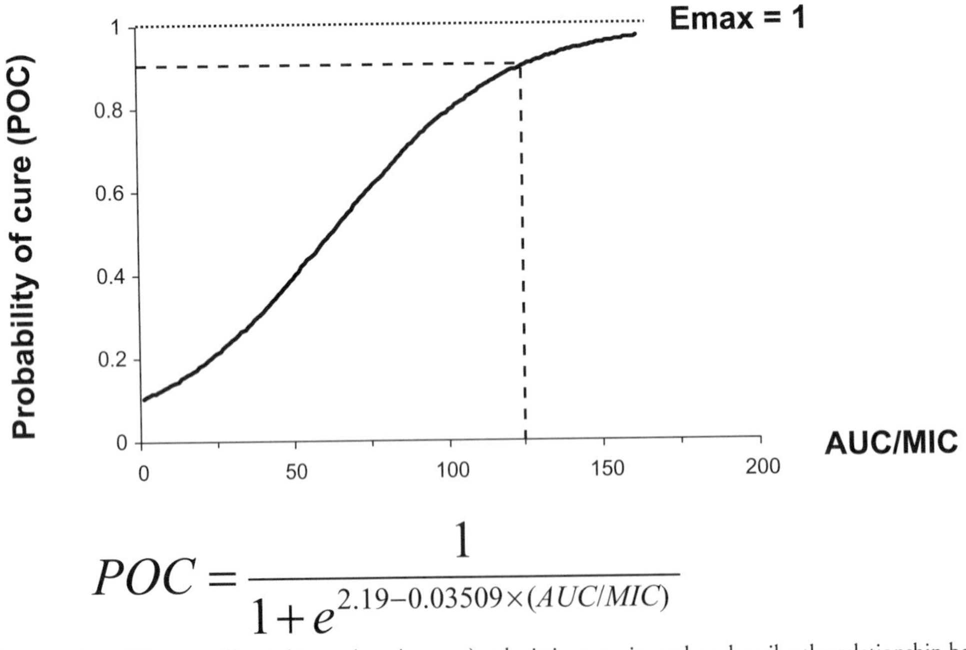

$$POC = \frac{1}{1+e^{2.19-0.03509\times(AUC/MIC)}}$$

FIG. 4.13 Logistic regression. When an effect is binary (cure/no cure), a logistic curve is used to describe the relationship between the independent variable (often dose, exposure, or any explicative variable) and the dependent variable (a probability between 0 and 1). This quantal dose-response curve does not relate dose to intensity of effect but to the frequency in a population of individuals in which a drug produces an all-or-nothing effect. Here, the probability of cure (POC) for a hypothetical concentration-dependent antibiotic has been plotted against the value of a PK/PD index generally selected for this class of antibiotics (i.e., AUC/MIC). The value 2.19 yields P = 0.1 when *X* is zero (placebo effect) and b = 0.035 gives the "sensitivity," i.e., the slope of the response. Here, for an AUC/MIC of 125 h, the POC is 0.9 (90%).

SELECTION OF THE DOSE AND DOSAGE REGIMEN

The next step, after estimating all the relevant PD parameters, is to select a dose level and a dosage interval. When the PD parameters have been estimated with a direct effect model and the investigated endpoint has a clinical meaning, Equation 4.5 can be used directly. Often, in the case of NSAIDs, a dose that is close to the ED_{50} is selected and this can easily be computed by incorporating the corresponding EC_{50} into Equation 4.5. For example, in the horse, the estimated potency of phenylbutazone, determined from its effects on stride length in an experimental carpitis, indicated an EC_{50} of 3.6 μg/ml (Toutain et al. 1994). As the plasma clearance of phenylbutazone in the horse is 991 ml/kg per day, the calculated dose required to achieve half the maximal effect is 3.6 mg/kg/day. This is slightly below the manufacturer's recommended daily dosage of 4.4 mg/kg. However, if the investigated endpoint for an NSAID is the PGE_2 inhibition, i.e., a biochemical surrogate, the EC to incorporate into Equation 4.5 may differ from the EC_{50}. It has been shown that at least 90–95% of the magnitude of COX-2 inhibition is clinically relevant. In this case, it is an EC_{95} that should be incorporated in Equation 4.5. In calves treated with tolfenamic acid, for instance, 95% PGE_2 inhibition is obtained with a plasma concentration of 0.245 μg/ml. When this EC_{95} is incorporated into Equation 4.5 together with the plasma clearance of tolfenamic acid in calves (7.2 l/kg per day) a dose of 1.76 mg/kg/24 h is obtained. This is approximately equal to the manufacturer's recommended daily dose of 2 mg/kg.

When the PD parameters have been established using an indirect effect model, the relationship between the clinical response and the EC_{50} is not straightforward. This is also true when the goal is to select the optimal dosage regime to achieve a particular plasma concentration profile (e.g., to maintain plasma concentrations above the MIC for a time-dependent antibiotic) or to determine the most appropriate time interval between two administrations (i.e., to optimize efficacy while minimizing unwanted side effects). In these cases the best approach is to perform simulations. The PK/PD model can be used to simulate a large number of dose and dosage interval scenarios and screen for those dosage regimens with the best efficiency or safety margins. Such analysis requires no additional time or cost during drug development. For example, it was shown for nimesulide in dogs that a PK/PD model predicted a better antipyretic efficacy for nimesulide at a dosage regimen of 2.5 mg/kg twice a day rather than at

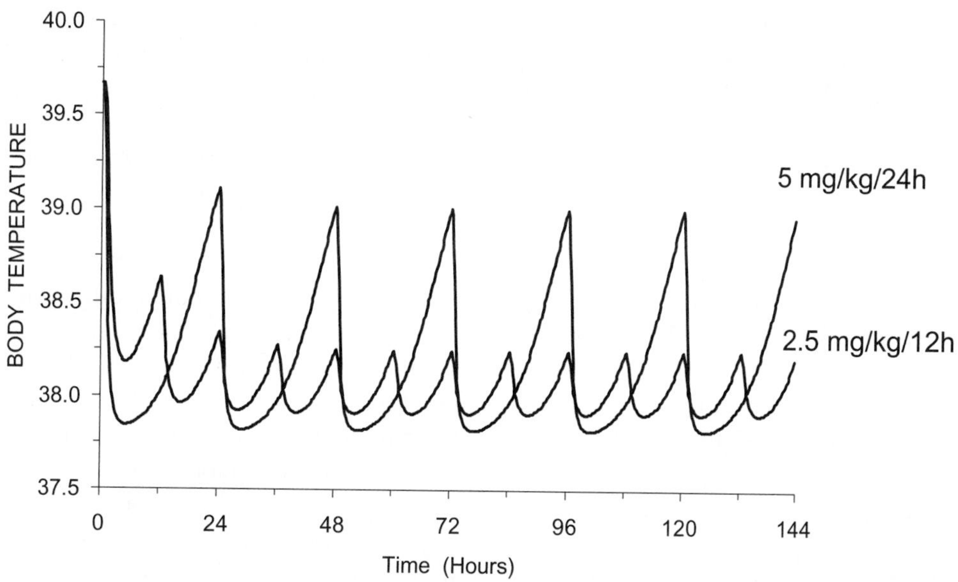

FIG. 4.14 Plot of predicted body temperature (°C) versus time (h) after administration of nimesulide in dogs at two different dosage regimens (2.5 mg/kg/12 h and 5 mg/kg/24 h, for 6 consecutive days). Visual inspection of the figure suggests the superiority of the 2.5 mg/kg/12 h dosage regimen (from Toutain et al. 2001a).

5 mg/kg per day, although both dosage regimens were equivalent in terms of lameness suppression (Toutain et al. 2001a) (Fig. 4.14).

The PK/PD approach may also be used to determine an optimal dosage regimen for antibiotics. The objectives of rational antibiotic therapy are dual, i.e., optimization of clinical efficacy, and minimization of the selection and spread of resistant pathogens (Lees and Shojaee Aliabadi 2002; Toutain et al. 2002). The poor sensitivity of clinical outcomes in indicating the best dosage regimen in terms of bacteriological cure, has prompted investigation of the value of PK/PD surrogate indexes to establish an optimal dosage for antibiotics. Three PK/PD indices appear to be sufficient to predict antibiotic effectiveness: The AUC/MIC ratio, an index used for quinolones, the C_{max}/MIC ratio (where C_{max} is the maximum plasma concentration), an index selected for aminoglycosides, and T > MIC (the time during which plasma concentrations exceed MIC, expressed as a percentage of the dosage interval), an index selected for the so-called time-dependent antibiotics such as beta-lactams. All three indices are surrogate markers of what is ultimately expected, i.e., clinical recovery and bacterial eradication.

It should be noted that these PK/PD predictive indices of in vivo efficacy are built on free plasma antibiotic concentrations, and not on total plasma concentration or total tissue antibiotic level. Indeed, most pathogens of clinical interest are located extracellularly and the biophase for antibiotics is the extracellular fluid.

Once a PK/PD surrogate index has been selected, its breakpoint values (critical values) need to be considered in relation to the clinical objectives. For quinolones, it is generally reported that the plasma concentration should be five times higher than the limiting MIC (generally the MIC_{90}, i.e., the MIC covering 90% of the bacterial population). This is equivalent to saying that the PK/PD breakpoint, for the index predictive of quinolone efficacy (i.e., AUC/MIC) calculated over 24 h, should be 125 h.

Taking the example of a quinolone, the expected daily dose can easily be computed from Equation 4.11:

$$\textit{Daily Dose} \text{ for a quinolone} = \frac{\text{Plasma clearance} \times \left(\dfrac{AUC}{MIC}\right) \text{breakpoint value} \times MIC_{90}}{fu \times \text{Bioavailability}} \quad (4.11)$$

with *fu*, the free fraction. The *(AUC/MIC)* breakpoint value in Equation 4.11 is, for example, 125 h and in this case, the plasma clearance of the quinolone under investigation should be expressed per hour (not per day) if the daily dose has to be computed. More simply, the daily dose can be computed using the following equation that is actually Equation 4.11 with EC_{50} equated to $5 \times MIC_{90}$ (Equation 4.12):

$$\textit{Daily Dose} \text{ for a quinolone} = \frac{\text{Plasma clearance} \times 5 \times MIC_{90}}{fu \times \text{Bioavailability}} \quad (4.12)$$

Here, *Plasma clearance* is the daily clearance and *5* is the scale factor equivalent to the breakpoint value of 125 h (5 is the roundup of 125 h/24 h) and by which the MIC_{90} should be multiplied to guarantee an appropriate efficacy (for further explanation of Equations 4.11 and 4.12, see Toutain 2003; Toutain et al. 2007).

POPULATION PK/PD

One important advance has been to separate the two main sources (PK and PD) of variability through the use of population PK/PD approaches. In this way, population analysis can explain the variation between animals (or groups of animals) not only in terms of drug exposure but also in terms of drug responsiveness. This is especially true in the case of antibiotics, where clinical response is affected not only by the ability of the drug to reach the site of infection but also by the PD variability (host response to the invading pathogen and bacterial susceptibility). In the case of antibiotics, if both the PK and PD (MIC) variabilities are known from relevant population investigations, the statistical distribution of the selected PK/PD index that is predictive of clinical efficacy can readily be established using Monte Carlo simulations. *Monte Carlo* is a term applied to a numerical method with a built-in random process. It involves combining the variability of antimicrobial drug exposure with the variability in pathogen susceptibility according to the corresponding probability density functions. With Monte Carlo simulations, a large hypothetical population of animals (or outcomes) may be generated to determine the probability of attaining a given PK/PD breakpoint in a given proportion of the population (Fig. 4.15). This allows selection of a dosage regimen based on attaining the recommended PK/PD target breakpoint in most animals. (For more details, see Lees et al. 2006.)

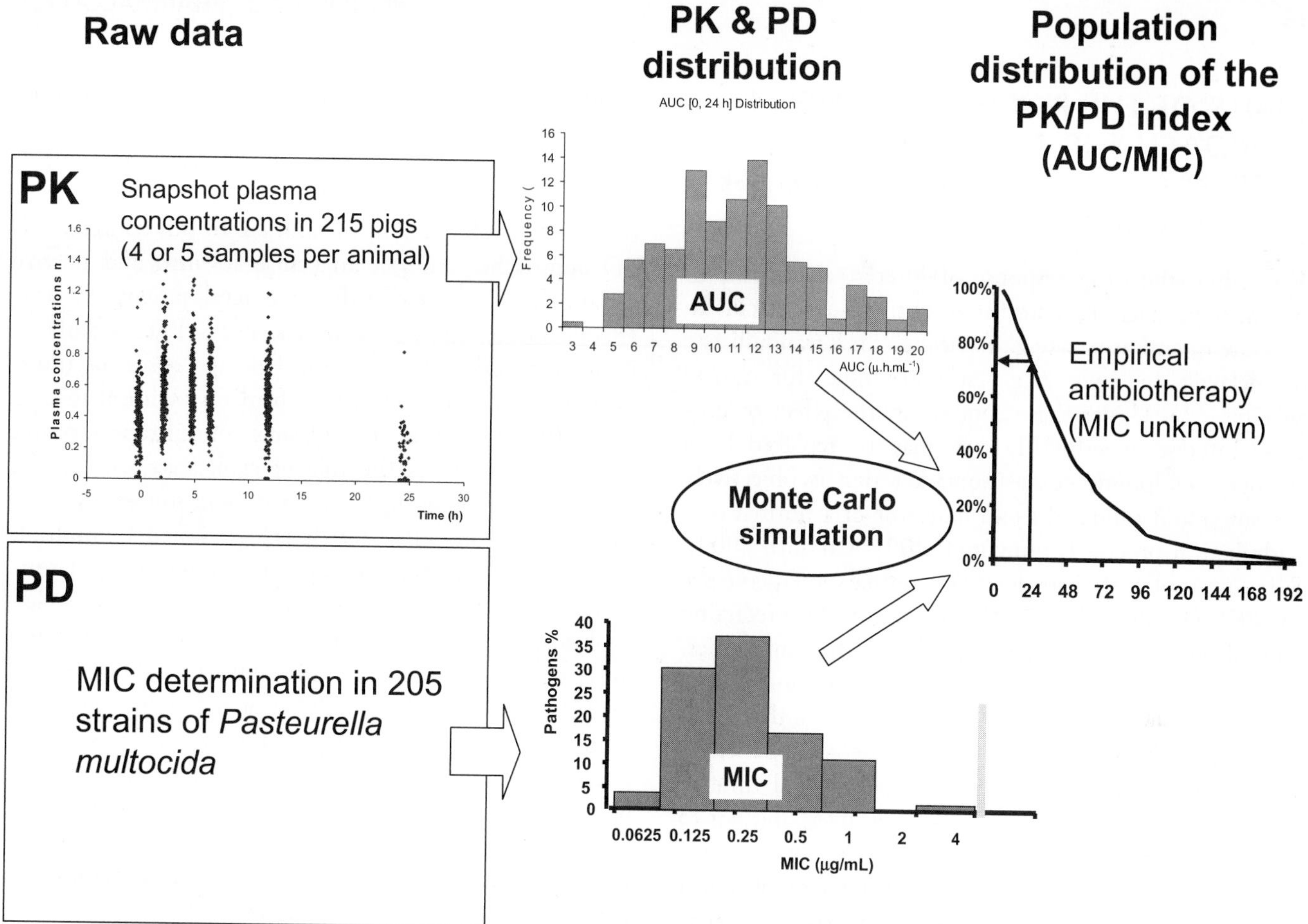

FIG. 4.15 Monte Carlo simulation and the PK/PD index population distribution for doxycycline in pigs.
Left top panel: plasma concentrations of doxycycline were measured in 215 pigs under field conditions (4 or 5 samples per pig) after metaphylactic treatment by oral route. The plasma concentrations were obtained with a second doxycycline dose of 5 mg/kg administered approximately 14 h after an initial 5 mg/kg dose.
Left bottom panel: Minimum Inhibitory Concentration (MIC) was determined in 205 strains of *Pasteurella multocida.*
Middle panel: This shows exposure distribution as AUC(0–24 h) and the MIC distribution. These two distributions were used for Monte Carlo simulations. The application of Monte Carlo simulation accounts in a balanced manner for variability in drug exposure (AUC) as well as pathogen susceptibility data (MIC distribution) to establish the population distribution of the relevant PK/PD index (AUC/MIC).
Right panel: The curve gives the percentage of pigs in a population attaining a given value of the PK/PD predictor (AUC/MIC). The curve was generated for an empirical antibiotherapy (MIC distribution known, but MIC for the involved pathogen unknown) based on an administered dose of doxycycline of 10 mg/kg i.e., the recommended daily dose regimen. Visual inspection of the curve indicates that a PK/PD index of 24 h (i.e., a daily mean plasma concentration equal to the corresponding MIC) would be attained in 72% of the pigs with an empirical antibiotherapy. If it is assumed that only the free drug is active, the achieved breakpoint should be divided by approximately 10, as the extent of plasma protein binding for doxycycline is about 90%.

LIMITS OF THE PK/PD MODELING APPROACH FOR A DOSE DETERMINATION: CLINICAL RESPONSE VERSUS SURROGATE

Very often the drug response of interest is difficult to obtain (e.g., bacterial cure for an antibiotic), difficult to measure quantitatively (e.g., demeanor for a tranquilizer), or delayed in time (e.g., survival time for cancer therapy, . . .). Under these conditions, the effect of ultimate interest in a PK/PD trial may be replaced by a surrogate endpoint, i.e., a biomarker that is objectively measured and validated as an indicator of a normal or a pathological process (Anonymous 2001; Colburn 2000). Some examples of surrogates in veterinary medicine are the PK/PD indices that have been proposed for predicting clinical success and bacteriological cure for antibiotics. Angiotensin converting enzyme (ACE) inhibition is used as a surrogate to evaluate ACE inhibitors, although it should be kept in mind that the ultimate goal of therapy with ACE inhibitors is to increase the survival time of diseased animals and the quality of their lives, and not to inhibit an enzymatic activity. Indeed, a drug may have a favorable effect on a biomarker and an unfavorable effect on the disease and any biomarker believed to be a surrogate of clinical relevance needs to be validated. The CAST trial in human medicine is an appropriate illustration (Ruskin 1989). It was initially thought that pharmacological suppression of premature ventricular contractions (PVCs) identified by postmyocardial infarct monitoring could reduce the incidence of subsequent arrhythmias. The abilities of different antiarrhythmic drugs to prevent cardiac death (class I antiarrhythmic) were tested against a placebo. It was finally shown that drug therapy was not only associated with a reduction of PVC but also with an increase in the incidence of arrhythmic deaths. This trial illustrates that any surrogate needs to be validated for its clinical relevance even when it has a strong mechanistic link with the condition under treatment.

CONCLUSION

A drug action is first expressed at a target site (receptor, enzyme, transporter, . . .) where it produces a biochemical or a cellular event such as enzyme inhibition or depolarization. This primary drug action then leads rapidly to some physiological and observable changes such as smooth muscle contraction, a decrease of blood pressure or an inhibition or stimulation of the secretion of some endogenous substance. This is the primary drug effect. Ultimately these short time effects are collectively responsible for the delayed overall clinical response such as the survival time or the well-being of the animal. In this context, PK/PD approaches are able to bridge in vitro and in vivo situations, i.e., to predict the time-development of a drug effect from some in vitro drug action. PK/PD is a tool that is mainly used to select rational dosage regimens (dose, dosing interval) for pivotal confirmatory clinical testing. In PK/PD modeling, the plasma concentration profile (not the dose) plays the role of explicative variable for effect. Because it separates the two main sources of interspecies variability (PK/PD) it is well suited to multiple species drug development and interspecies extrapolation. The PK/PD approach offers many advantages over a classical dose titration, especially the possibility of determining a dosage regimen by testing only a single dose. The main limitation of the PK/PD approach is that surrogate biomarkers are used to judge efficacy, i.e., some drug effects rather than the overall clinical response, the risk being to determine a dose that is effective against the biomarker but does not improve the disease. This is particularly true in chronic disease where the clinical outcome may take months or years to occur.

REFERENCES

Anonymous (2001) Biomarkers and surrogate endpoints: Preferred definitions and conceptual framework. Clin Pharmacol Thera, 69, 89–95.

Ariens, E.J. (1954) Affinity and intrinsic activity in the theory of competitive inhibition. I. Problems and theory. Arch Int Pharmacodyn Ther, 99, 32–49.

Calabrese, E.J. and Baldwin, L.A. (2003) Hormesis: the dose-response revolution. Annu Rev Pharmacol Toxicol, 43, 175–197.

Colburn, W.A. (2000) Optimizing the use of biomarkers, surrogate endpoints, and clinical endpoints for more efficient drug development. J Clin Pharmacol, 40, 1419–1427.

Colquhoun, D. (2006) The quantitative analysis of drug-receptor interactions: a short history. Trends Pharmacol Sci, 27, 149–157.

Dayneka, N.L., Garg, V. and Jusko, W.J. (1993) Comparison of four basic models of indirect pharmacodynamic responses. J Pharmacokinet Biopharm, 21, 457–478.

Holford, N.H. and Sheiner, L.B. (1981) Pharmacokinetic and pharmacodynamic modeling in vivo. CRC Crit Rev Bioeng, 5, 273–322.

Kenakin, T. (2004) Principles: receptor theory in pharmacology. Trends Pharmacol Sci, 25, 186–192.

Kenakin, T.P. (2007) Pharmacological Onomastics: What's in a name? Br J Pharmacol.

Lees, P., Concordet, D., Shojaee Aliabadi, F. and Toutain, P.L. (2006) Drug selection and optimisation of dosage schedules to minimise antimicrobial resistance, In: Aarestrup, F.M. (Ed.) Antimicrobial Resistance in Bacteria of Animal Origin. ASM Press, Washington, DC, USA.

Lees, P., Cunningham, F.M. and Elliott, J. (2004a) Principles of pharmacodynamics and their applications in veterinary pharmacology. J Vet Pharmacol Thera, 27, 397–414.

Lees, P., Giraudel, J., Landoni, M.F. and Toutain, P.L. (2004b) PK-PD integration and PK-PD modelling of nonsteroidal anti-inflammatory drugs: principles and applications in veterinary pharmacology. J Vet Pharmacol Ther, 27, 491–502.

Lees, P., Landoni, M.F., Giraudel, J. and Toutain, P.L. (2004c) Pharmacodynamics and pharmacokinetics of nonsteroidal anti-inflammatory drugs in species of veterinary interest. Journal of Veterinary Pharmacology and Therapeutics, 27, 479–490.

Lees, P. and Shojaee Aliabadi, F. (2002) Rational dosing of antimicrobial drugs: animals versus humans. Int J Antimicrob Agents, 19, 269–284.

McKellar, Q.A., Sanchez Bruni, S.F. and Jones, D.G. (2004) Pharmacokinetic/pharmacodynamic relationships of antimicrobial drugs used in veterinary medicine. J Vet Pharmacol Ther, 27, 503–514.

Neubig, R.R., Spedding, M., Kenakin, T. and Christopoulos, A. (2003) International Union of Pharmacology Committee on Receptor Nomenclature and Drug Classification. XXXVIII. Update on terms and symbols in quantitative pharmacology. Pharmacol Rev, 55, 597–606.

Rang, H.P. (2006) The receptor concept: pharmacology's big idea. Br J Pharmacol, 147 Suppl 1, S9–16.

Ruberg, S.J. (1995) Dose response studies. I. Some design considerations. J Biopharm Stat, 5, 1–14.

Ruskin, J.N. (1989) The cardiac arrhythmia suppression trial (CAST). N Engl J Med, 321, 386–388.

Sheiner, L.B., Hashimoto, Y. and Beal, S.L. (1991) A simulation study comparing designs for dose ranging. Stat Med, 10, 303–321.

Stephenson, R.P. (1956) A modification of receptor theory. Br J Pharmacol Chemother, 11, 379–393.

Toutain, P.L. (2002) Pharmacokinetics/pharmacodynamics integration in drug development and dosage regimen optimization for veterinary medicine. AAPS Pharm Sci, 4, article 38 (www.aapspharmsci.org/view.asp?art=ps040438).

Toutain, P.L. (2003) Guest Editorial—Antibiotic treatment of animals—A different approach to rational dosing. The Vet J, 165, 98–100.

Toutain, P.L., Autefage, A., Legrand, C. and Alvinerie, M. (1994) Plasma concentrations and therapeutic efficacy of phenylbutazone and flunixin meglumine in the horse: pharmacokinetic/pharmacodynamic modelling. J Vet Pharmacol Ther, 17, 459–469.

Toutain, P.L., Bousquet-Melou, A. and Martinez, M. (2007) AUC/MIC: A PK/PD index for antibiotics with a time dimension or simply a dimensionless scoring factor? J Antimicrob Chemother, accepted.

Toutain, P.L., Cester, C.C., Haak, T. and Laroute, V. (2001a) A pharmacokinetic/pharmacodynamic approach vs. a dose titration for the determination of a dosage regimen: the case of nimesulide, a Cox-2 selective nonsteroidal anti-inflammatory drug in the dog. J Vet Pharmacol Ther, 24, 43–55.

Toutain, P.L., Cester, C.C., Haak, T. and Metge, S. (2001b) Pharmacokinetic profile and in vitro selective cyclooxygenase-2 inhibition by nimesulide in the dog. J Vet Pharmacol Ther, 24, 35–42.

Toutain, P.L., del Castillo, J.R.E. and Bousquet-Mélou, A. (2002) The pharmacokinetic-pharmacodynamic approach to a rational dosage regimen for antibiotics. Res Vet Sci, 73, 105–114.

Toutain, P.L. and Lees, P. (2004) Integration and modelling of pharmacokinetic and pharmacodynamic data to optimize dosage regimens in veterinary medicine. J Vet Pharmacol Ther, 27, 467–477.

Toutain, P.L. and Lefebvre, H.P. (2004) Pharmacokinetics and pharmacokinetic/pharmacodynamic relationships for angiotensin-converting enzyme inhibitors. J Vet Pharmacol Ther, 27, 515–525.

Urban, J.D., Clarke, W.P., von Zastrow, M., Nichols, D.E., Kobilka, B., Weinstein, H., Javitch, J.A., Roth, B.L., Christopoulos, A., Sexton, P.M., Miller, K.J., Spedding, M. and Mailman, R.B. (2007) Functional selectivity and classical concepts of quantitative pharmacology. J Pharmacol Experim Ther, 320, 1–13.

Verotta, D., Beal, S.L. and Sheiner, L.B. (1989) Semiparametric approach to pharmacokinetic-pharmacodynamic data. Am J Physiol, 256, R1005–1010.

SECTION 2

Drugs Acting on the Autonomic Nervous System

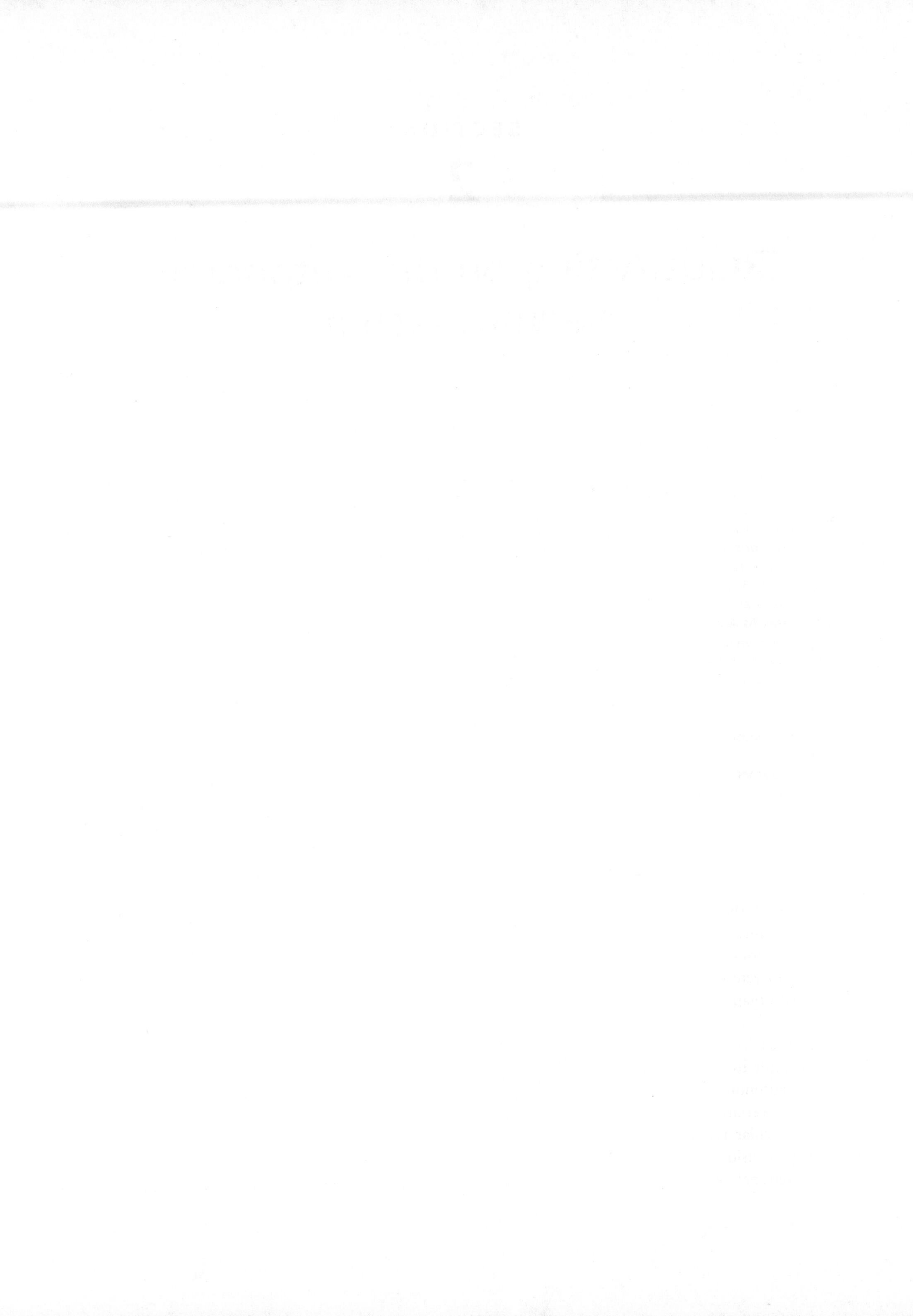

CHAPTER

5

INTRODUCTION TO NEUROHUMORAL TRANSMISSION AND THE AUTONOMIC NERVOUS SYSTEM

H. RICHARD ADAMS

Primary diseases of the autonomic nervous system are infrequently encountered in domestic animals, and yet drugs that alter autonomic activity are used daily in the clinical practice of veterinary medicine. Physiologic functions of diseased organs often are still responsive to their nervous supply and may favorably respond to drugs that induce autonomic effects. Also, autonomic blocking drugs are often used prior to anesthesia to prevent inadvertent stimulation of autonomic influences on visceral tissues and, furthermore, certain autonomic drugs are life-saving antidotes to particular types of chemical intoxicants. A thorough comprehension of autonomic pharmacology is required for a rational approach to therapeutic management of a wide variety of clinical disorders in animals (Freeman and Miyawaki 1993; Westfall and Westfall 2006).

ORGANIZATION OF THE AUTONOMIC NERVOUS SYSTEM

The autonomic nervous system is a peripheral complex of nerves, plexuses, and ganglia that are organized to modulate the involuntary activity of secretory glands, smooth muscles, and visceral organs. This system functions to sustain homeostatic conditions during periods of reduced physical and emotional activity and, equally important, to assist in internal bodily reactions to stressful circumstances. The autonomic nervous system also has been termed the *visceral, involuntary,* or *vegetative nervous system* (Low 1993; Brunton et al. 2006).

In relation to clinical pharmacology, the most important components of the autonomic nervous system are the outflow (efferent) nerve tracts. Efferent autonomic tracts supply motor innervation to visceral structures. The efferent segment of the autonomic nervous system is divided into two principal components: the sympathetic nervous system and the parasympathetic nervous system. Sympathetic and parasympathetic outflow tracts comprise preganglionic neurons and postganglionic neurons. The cell body of a preganglionic neuron is located within the central nervous system (CNS). The synapse (junction) of a preganglionic axon with a ganglionic neuronal body occurs outside the CNS within an autonomic ganglion. An axon of a ganglionic cell passes peripherally and innervates its effector organ or organ substructure. The junction of a postganglionic axonal terminal with its effector cell is termed a *neuroeffector junction.*

SYMPATHETIC NERVOUS SYSTEM. The sympathetic nervous system is often synonymously referred to as the *thoracolumbar outflow* because of its anatomic origin (Fig. 5.1). Sympathetic preganglionic fibers (axons) originate from cell bodies localized within the intermediolateral columns of the thoracic and lumbar regions of the spinal cord. These fibers exit the spinal cord with the ventral (anterior) nerve roots and enter the paravertebral chain of sympathetic ganglia. Paravertebral (or vertebral) ganglia are located bilaterally to the ventral aspects of the vertebral column. Ganglia on each side are interconnected by nerve fibers to form sympathetic ganglionic chains that extend into the cervical and sacral regions; however, ganglia in these areas receive fibers only from the thoracolumbar spinal cord.

Prevertebral ganglia are located more peripherally than the vertebral chain and include the celiac, cranial (anterior) mesenteric, and caudal (posterior) mesenteric ganglia. They supply fibers to abdominal and pelvic viscera. Sympathetic control to the head and neck arises from cranial (anterior or superior), middle, and caudal (posterior or inferior) cervical ganglia. Fibers from the cervical ganglia and the anterior thoracic ganglia innervate the thoracic organs.

The adrenal medulla is an extremely important component of the sympathetic nervous system. It is embryologically and functionally homologous to a sympathetic ganglion but does not contain postsynaptic neuronal cells. Instead, secretory chromaffin cells are present. They are innervated by typical preganglionic fibers that issue from the midthoracic spinal cord. Adrenal chromaffin cells release epinephrine and norepinephrine from the adrenal gland into the circulatory system.

PARASYMPATHETIC NERVOUS SYSTEM. Parasympathetic outflow tracts originate from the midbrain, medulla oblongata, and sacral spinal cord (Fig. 5.2). The parasympathetic component of the autonomic nervous system is referred to anatomically as the *craniosacral outflow.*

The vagus nerve (the 10th cranial nerve) is the most important parasympathetic nerve trunk. It arises from the medulla oblongata and sends efferent fibers to all thoracic and abdominal viscera from the caudal pharyngeal region to the cranial portions of the large colon. The sacral portion of the parasympathetic system comprises nerve fibers arising from the sacral spinal cord. These fibers form the pelvic nerves; they terminate in ganglion cells located in the colon, bladder, and sex organs.

Parasympathetic ganglia are localized more peripherally than sympathetic ganglia and usually are close to innervated structures. In many cases, parasympathetic ganglia are within innervated organs. Parasympathetic discharge usually is discrete and affects specific effector systems individually.

GENERAL CONCEPTS OF AUTONOMIC FUNCTION

AUTONOMIC INTERRELATIONSHIPS. Most visceral organs are innervated by both parasympathetic and sympathetic divisions (see Figs. 5.1 and 5.2), often producing contrasting effects on the same structure. For example, parasympathetic fibers of the vagus nerve elicit a decrease in heart rate, whereas sympathetic cardiac nerves accelerate heart rate. Such reciprocating relationships allow varying degrees of qualitative, as well as quantitative, changes in organ function, depending upon the relative needs of the organism (Low 1993; Brunton et al. 2006). Principal

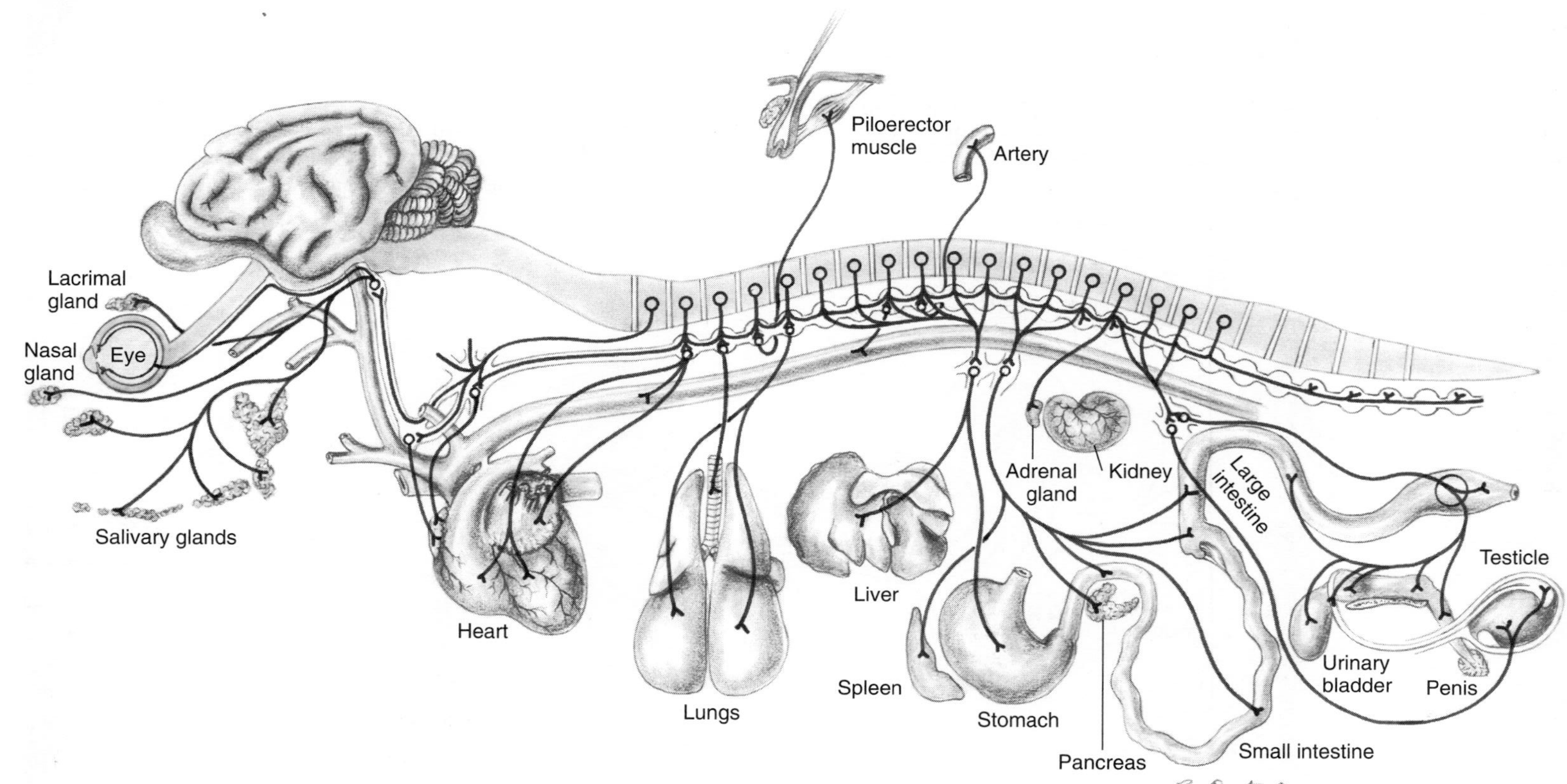

FIG. 5.1 Anatomical representation of motor innervation from the sympathetic nervous system to various body organs and tissues. Preganglionic sympathetic neuron bodies within the thoracolumbar region of the spinal cord send axons peripherally to synapse with ganglionic neuron bodies comprising the sympathetic ganglionic chains located along each side of the vertebral column. Postganglionic axons exit the sympathetic ganglionic chains and pass peripherally to innervate those cells regulated by the sympathetic (thoracolumbar) division of the autonomic nervous system. Preganglionic fibers are dark gray; postganglionic fibers are light gray. Drawn by Dr. Gheorghe M. Constantinescu, University of Missouri.

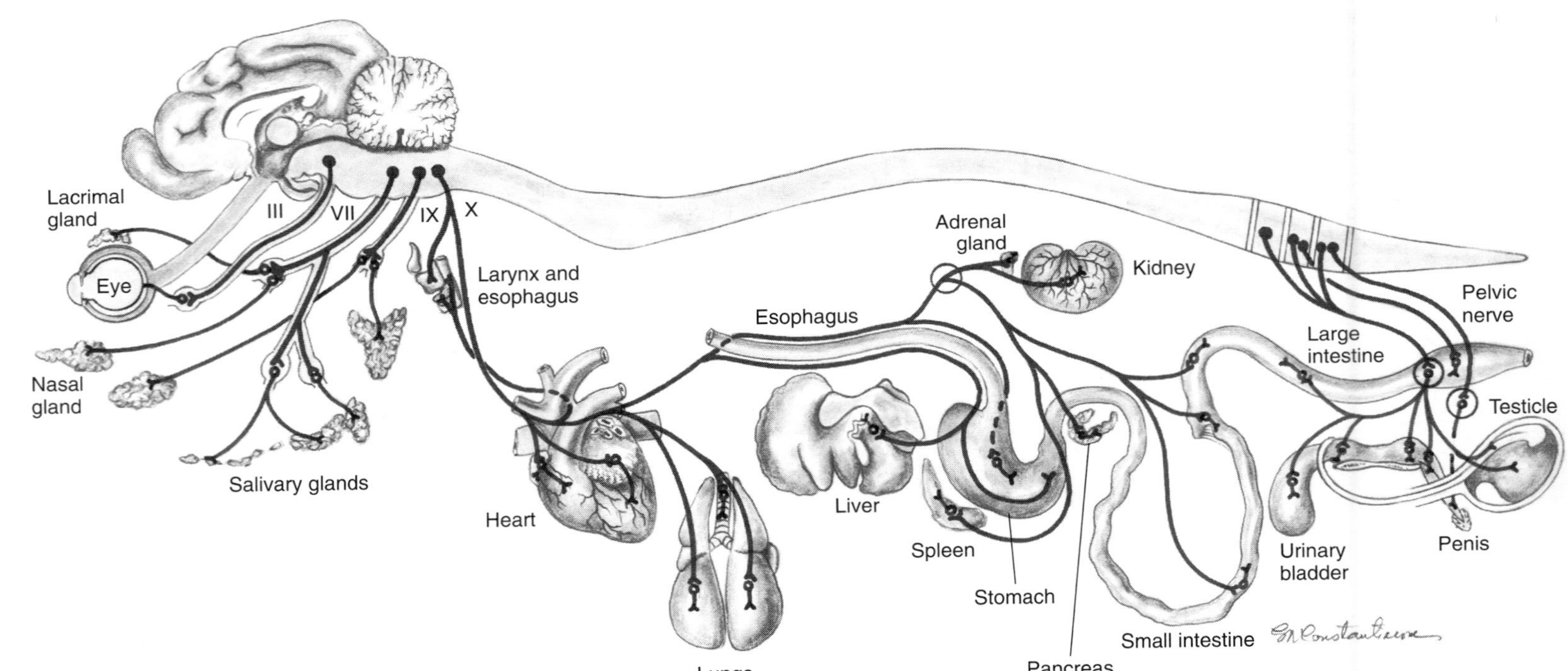

FIG. 5.2 Anatomical representation of motor innervation from the parasympathetic nervous system to various body organs and tissues. Preganglionic parasympathetic neuron bodies within cranial and sacral zones of the central nervous system send axons peripherally to synapse with ganglionic neuron bodies localized within or adjacent to visceral tissues. Postganglionic axons exit parasympathetic ganglia and innervate those cells regulated by the parasympathetic (craniosacral) division of the autonomic nervous system. Roman numerals depict cranial nerves carrying parasympathetic neurons. Preganglionic fibers are dark gray; postganglionic fibers are light gray. Drawn by Dr. Gheorghe M. Constantinescu, University of Missouri.

organ responses mediated by sympathetic and parasympathetic discharge are summarized in Table 5.1 (Freeman and Miyawaki 1993; Westfall and Westfall 2006).

ORGAN RESPONSES TO AUTONOMIC DISCHARGE. The sympathetic outflow tract and closely associated adrenal medulla are often referred to as the *sympathoadrenal* (or *sympathoadrenomedullary*) *axis*. This axis is extremely reactive. Activity varies discretely on a moment-to-moment basis consistent with the needs of the organism. Thus small changes required for homeostasis are readily accomplished. The sympathoadrenal axis can also discharge in a mass action affecting virtually all sympathetically innervated structures. Such a unitary sympathoadrenal discharge occurs in response to severe rage or fear and readies the organism for "fight or flight." Accordingly, cardiovascular activity is accelerated; an increase in heart rate, myocardial contractile strength, cardiac output, and blood pressure is observed. Blood is redistributed from splanchnic and cutaneous beds to voluntary skeletal muscles; bronchioles dilate and respiration increases; pupils enlarge; and blood glucose concentration increases. The organism is now better prepared to effectively react to the stimulus that instigated the sympathetically mediated fight-or-flight reaction (Saper 2002).

Conversely, the parasympathetic nervous system functions mainly to regulate localized organ changes and is not organized for mass action. Whereas sympathetic activation results in expenditure of energy, the parasympathetic system reacts to generate and maintain biologic energy.

TABLE 5.1 Typical responses of effector tissues to sympathetic and parasympathetic nerve impulses

Effector tissues	Sympathetic-mediated responses[1]	Parasympathetic-mediated responses[2]
Heart	General excitation	General inhibition
Sinoatrial (SA) node	β_1-increase heart rate	Decrease heart rate
Atria	β_1-increase contractile force, conduction velocity	Decrease contractile force
Atrioventricular (AV) node	β_1-increase automaticity, conduction velocity	Decrease conduction velocity; AV block
His-Purkinje system	β_1-increase automaticity, conduction velocity	. . .
Ventricles	β_1-increase contractile force, conduction velocity, irritability[3]	Decrease contractile force[4]
Blood vessels		
Coronary	α_1-constriction; β_2-dilation[5]	Dilation[6]; constriction[6]
Cutaneous, mucosal	α_1-constriction	Dilation[7]
Cerebral	α_1-constriction; β_2-dilation	Dilation[7]
Skeletal muscle	α_1-constriction; β_2-dilation[8]	Dilation[7]
Splanchnic	α_1-constriction; β_2-dilation[9]	Dilation[7]
Renal	α_1-constriction; β_2-dilation[9]	Dilation[7]
Genital	α_1-constriction	Dilation[10]
Veins	α_1-constriction	
Endothelium	α_2-dilation	
GI tract	General inhibition	General excitation
Smooth muscle	β_1-relaxation; α-relaxation[11]	Increase motility and tone
Sphincters	α-contraction	Relaxation
Secretions	Decrease (usually)	Increase
Gallbladder and ducts	Relaxation	Contraction
Bronchioles		
Smooth muscle	β_2-relaxation	Contraction
Glands	Inhibition (?)	Stimulation
Eye		
Radial muscle, iris	α_1-contraction (mydriasis)	. . .
Sphincter muscle, iris	. . .	Contraction (miosis)
Ciliary muscle	β-relaxation; far vision	Contraction; near vision
Urinary bladder	Urinary retention	Urination
Fundus	β_1-relaxation	Contraction
Trigone, sphincter	α-contraction	Relaxation

TABLE 5.1—***continued***

Effector tissues	Sympathetic-mediated responses[1]	Parasympathetic-mediated responses[2]
Splenic capsule	α-contraction, β_2-relaxation	. . .
Sweat glands	Secretion (cholinergic);[12] β_2-secretion (horse)	
Salivary glands	α_1-scant, viscous secretion	Profuse, watery secretion
Piloerector muscles	α-contraction	. . .
Kidney renin release	α_2-decrease; β_1-increase	. . .
Uterus[13]	α_1-contraction; β-relaxation (nonpregnant > pregnant)	Contraction[14]
Genitalia		
Male	α-ejaculation	Erection[15]
Female	. . .	Erection[15]
Adrenal medulla	Secretion of epinephrine > norepinephrine (cholinergic)	. . .
Autonomic ganglia	Ganglionic discharge (cholinergic)	Ganglionic discharge[16]
Liver	β_2-glycogenolysis and gluconeogenesis (α in some species)	. . .
Pancreas		
Islet cells	α_2-decrease secretion; β_2-increase secretion	. . .
Acini	α-decrease secretion	Increase secretions
Fat cells	β_1-lipolysis	. . .
Adrenergic nerve terminals	α_2-decrease release of norepinephrine; β_2-increase release of norepinephrine	± Release of norepinephrine[17]
Platelets	α_2-aggregation	. . .

Note: Superscript numbers are defined as follows: (1) α and β designate the principal adrenoceptor type subserving a tissue response. α_1, α_2, β_1, and β_2 designate the receptor subtype. The usual receptor types are presented; considerable interspecies variation exists, particularly with reference to subtypes. (2) Except when otherwise designated (e.g., ganglia), parasympathetic responses are subserved by muscarinic receptors. (3) Catecholamine-induced irritability of the myocardium may be associated with β_1 and α receptors; systemic pressor response may contribute. (4) Muscarinic receptors subserving decreased contractility are demonstrable in ventricular muscle, but the significance is not definitely known. (5) In small coronary arteries, β receptors are more numerous, more sensitive, and/or more responsive than α receptors. In large coronary arteries α receptors can be demonstrated. β_1 and β_2 subtypes differ depending upon species. (6) Depending upon experimental conditions, cholinergic effects on coronary blood vessels have been reported as both constriction and dilation (Kalsner 1989). (7) Arterial smooth muscle generally is not innervated by the parasympathetic nervous system (exceptions include blood vessels of genitalia). Thus cholinergic receptors in most arterial beds are not associated with parasympathetic nerves. In certain regions (e.g., arteries of skeletal muscles) sympathetic cholinergic vasodilator fibers are present, but their physiologic importance is poorly understood. (8) In skeletal muscle arteries β receptors are more sensitive than α receptors. (9) β receptors of visceral blood vessels seem less important than α receptors. (10) Parasympathetic-induced dilation of genital blood vessels (which contributes to erection) is not mediated by ACh; the neurotransmitter is believed to be nitric oxide; see (15) below. (11) β-inhibitory receptors may be localized on smooth muscle cells, whereas α-inhibitory receptors may be localized on parasympathetic cholinergic (excitatory) ganglionic cells of Auerbach's plexus. (12) In humans, sweat glands are innervated by postganglionic sympathetic axons that release ACh (i.e., cholinergic) rather than norepinephrine (i.e., adrenergic). In domestic animals, however, sweat glands are regulated by adrenergic (e.g., horse) or cholinergic mechanisms, depending upon species and type of gland (Robertshaw 1980). (13) Uterine responses vary depending on species and stage of estrus, pregnancy, and menstrual cycle (when present). (14) Contractile responses dominate; cholinergic drugs can induce severe myometrial contractions and abortion. (15) Smooth muscle erectile tissue is relaxed by parasympathetic impulses, thereby leading to vascular space engorgement and erection. The neurotransmitter at these sites is not ACh but is believed to be nitric oxide. (16) Ganglionic transmission is subserved predominantly by nicotinic receptors. (17) See Chapter 6 for distribution of α_1 and α_2 receptor subtypes in arteries. In many blood vessels endothelial α_2 receptors mediate vasodilation through the release of endothelium-derived nitric oxide. In contrast, α_2 receptors of vascular smooth muscle subserve vasoconstriction.

Parasympathetic activity therefore has been referred to as a "live-and-let-live" type of response (Adams 1977). Digestive breakdown of nutrients, e.g., is enhanced by increased parasympathetic activity to the GI system. Myocardial oxygen consumption and energy utilization are decreased by vagal-mediated decreases in heart rate and contractile strength of the heart.

How an individual organ will respond to sympathetic or parasympathetic impulse traffic can be predicted by considering whether a particular physiologic activity would benefit the fight-or-flight response (sympathetic) or the live-and-let-live response (parasympathetic). This physiologic concept is important to the pharmacology student because an understanding of how tissues respond to autonomic nervous activity often can be extrapolated to understanding how tissues will respond to autonomic drugs. This can save much memorization work; e.g., it is logical that an increase in heart rate, myocardial contractile strength, and cardiac output would be beneficial to an effective fight-or-flight reaction to rage or fear. Conversely, cardiac rest would be consistent with the sedentary condition of the live-and-let-live state. Thus activation of the heart would be a result of sympathetic discharge, whereas diminished cardiac activity would be a result of parasympathetic discharge (Wang and Wang 2004). Accordingly, a sympathomimetic drug would increase cardiac function, and a parasympathomimetic drug would reduce cardiac function.

INFORMATION TRANSMISSION. Information is communicated from nerve to nerve and from nerve to effector organ by a process termed *neurohumoral transmission*. This process involves release from a nerve terminal of a chemical neurotransmitter that reacts with specialized receptor areas on the innervated cell. Activation of the receptor instigates characteristic physiologic responses in the effector cell (Westfall and Westfall 2006).

The neurotransmitter at all ganglia (both parasympathetic and sympathetic) and at most parasympathetic neuroeffector junctions is acetylcholine (ACh). In a few regions (e.g., erectile tissue of genitalia) the neurotransmitter at parasympathetic neuroeffector junctions is not ACh (Klinge and Sjöstrand 1974; Klinge et al. 1978). Norepinephrine (noradrenalin) is the transmitter released at the majority of sympathetic neuroeffector junctions and is considered to be "the" sympathetic neurotransmitter. At a few sympathetic neuroeffector junctions (e.g., sweat glands in humans) ACh is the transmitter.

Nerves that release ACh are classified chemically as cholinergic nerves. Nerves that release norepinephrine are classified chemically as adrenergic or noradrenergic nerves. A third type of nerve is classified as nonadrenergic-noncholinergic (NANC) since these neurons release neither norepinephrine nor ACh. Instead, these NANC neurons release nitric oxide as their neurotransmitter substance (Adams 1996; Galligan 2002). It now seems clear, e.g., that nitric oxide is the NANC neurotransmitter responsible for penile erection (see the section "Nitric Oxide," later in this chapter).

Preganglionic and postganglionic relationships of sympathetic and parasympathetic efferent fibers are shown schematically in Figure 5.3, which should be studied

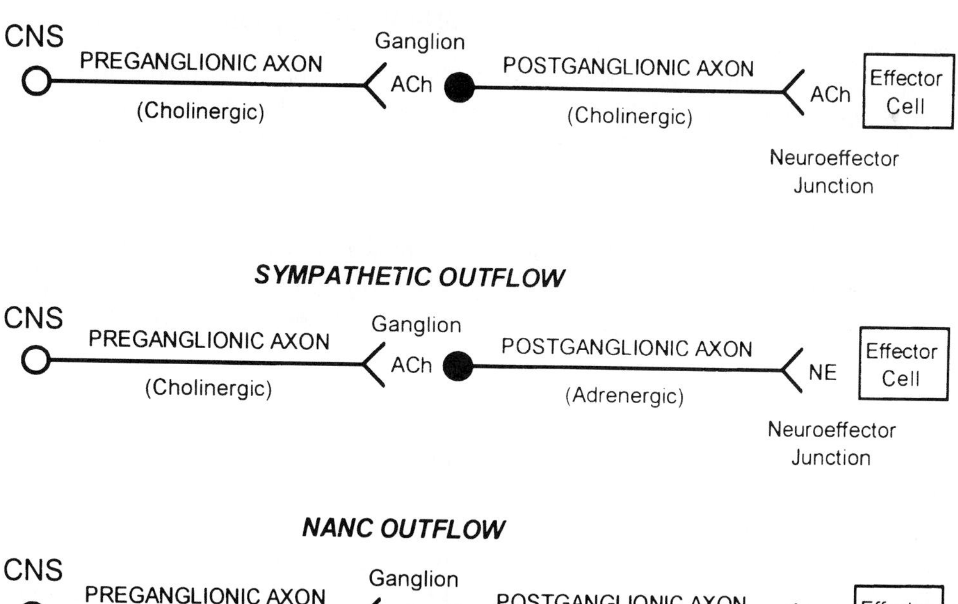

FIG. 5.3 Schematic representation of the preganglionic and postganglionic relationships of sympathetic and parasympathetic outflow tracts. ○ = CNS preganglionic nerve bodies; ● = ganglionic cell bodies. ACh is the neurotransmitter released at sympathetic and parasympathetic ganglia and at most parasympathetic neuroeffector junctions. Norepinephrine (NE) is the neurotransmitter released at adrenergic sympathetic neuroeffector junctions. (See text for exceptions.) Cholinergic fibers release ACh. Adrenergic fibers release NE. Some autonomic nerves are classified as nonadrenergic-noncholinergic (NANC) neurons; they release nitric oxide (NO), which diffuses into effector cells without the necessity of cell surface receptors. Pre- and postganglionic relationships for NANC nerves are putative. ? = the ganglionic transmitter serving NANC neurons is believed to be ACh.

thoroughly. Often, difficulty is encountered in correlating classifications of sympathetic and parasympathetic nerves with chemical classifications of adrenergic and cholinergic nerves. An adrenergic nerve releases norepinephrine and is a sympathetic postganglionic nerve. A cholinergic nerve releases ACh but can be a parasympathetic preganglionic nerve; a parasympathetic postganglionic nerve; a sympathetic preganglionic nerve; and, in a few regions, a sympathetic postganglionic nerve. The proposed relationships for NANC nerves, which release nitric oxide, are also included in Figure 5.3 (Änggard 1994; Adams 1996; Galligan 2002).

CENTRAL INTEGRATION OF AUTONOMIC ACTIVITY. Afferent fibers and brain nuclei that influence peripheral motor function are important when physiologic interactions of the autonomic nervous system are considered. Afferent fibers transmit information concerning visceral pain, cardiovascular activity, respiration, and numerous other organ functions from peripheral receptive areas to the CNS (Lang and Szilagyi 1991; Saper 2002).

Afferent fibers are usually nonmyelinated and pass into the CNS along autonomic nerve trunks such as the vagus, pelvic, and splanchnic nerves. Sensory fibers often make up a considerable portion of autonomic nerve trunks. An autonomic reflex arch involves passage of information along an afferent pathway, reaction of CNS sites to the received impulse, and resulting change in efferent discharge. Well-known examples involve the baroreceptor (pressure- or stretch-sensitive) areas localized in the aortic arch and carotid sinus and the chemoreceptive cells localized in the aortic arch and carotid bodies. Information concerning blood pressure, blood O_2 and CO_2, and respiration is relayed from these sites via afferent fibers to CNS areas.

The hypothalamus is the principal supraspinal site involved in modulation of both sympathetic and parasympathetic outflow traffic. Autonomic participation in regulation of blood pressure, body temperature, carbohydrate metabolism, water-electrolyte balance, sexual responses, emotions, and sleep is mediated through hypothalamic pathways. The medulla oblongata contains nuclei that integrate blood pressure and respiration, often interacting with hypothalamic regions.

Cerebral cortical foci may also influence autonomic activity. The Pavlovian experiments are classic examples of conscious and emotional brain centers affecting peripheral autonomic activity. In these experiments, a dog was repeatedly fed only after the ringing of a bell. Eventually, ringing a bell would evoke an increase in secretory activity of the GI tract in anticipation of a meal. Such basic experiments led numerous research workers to subsequently propose that certain disorders of body viscera may actually represent psychic influence on central autonomic sites rather than organic disease.

The pharmacologic activity of certain drugs is characterized by dominant CNS effects rather than peripheral-mediated responses. Amphetamine, e.g., affects peripheral adrenergic neuroeffector junctions; however, the overall response to amphetamine in an intact animal is characterized by CNS stimulation. Conversely, some drugs used for their CNS effects (tranquilizers) may also have profound peripheral autonomic actions. The phenothiazine tranquilizers, e.g., may depress blood pressure rather markedly by blocking the interaction of norepinephrine with adrenergic receptor sites in blood vessels. Such peripheral and central interactions should always be kept in mind when the total pharmacologic profile of a drug is evaluated prior to its clinical use.

NEUROHUMORAL TRANSMISSION

Most autonomic drugs used clinically exert primary pharmacologic activities by altering some essential step in the neurohumoral transmission process. In the remaining portions of this chapter, the physiologic steps involved in neurohumoral transmission will be summarized. In subsequent chapters, autonomic drugs that affect the neurohumoral transmission process in the parasympathetic and sympathetic nervous systems will be examined.

GENERAL CONCEPTS. Although numerous investigators have provided various relevant information, the first definitive evidence of chemical neurotransmission seems to have been obtained by Loewi (1921) and co-workers. In these simple but scientifically elegant experiments, Loewi electrically stimulated the vagus nerve of an isolated perfused frog heart. The perfusate leaving this preparation was perfused through another frog heart. Upon stimulation of the vagus nerve to the first heart, Loewi observed that this heart was immediately depressed. Within a few seconds, the second heart was also depressed. Certainly, the most logical explanation for this finding was that stimulation of the vagus nerve liberated a chemical "myocardial inhibitory" substance that was carried in the perfusate to the second heart. This substance, referred to as *Vagusstoff* (*vagus substance*), was later identified as ACh.

The basic techniques proved by Loewi have been modified and utilized by numerous investigators to map other adrenergic and cholinergic pathways. ACh was found to be the chemical released from all (parasympathetic and sympathetic) autonomic preganglionic fibers and most postganglionic parasympathetic fibers. Norepinephrine is the neurotransmitter released at the majority of sympathetic neuroeffector junctions (see Fig. 5.3). Nitric oxide is the neurotransmitter discharged by certain NANC neurons innervating regions of the GI tract, the vasculature, and the external genitalia (Änggard 1994; Lowenstein et al. 1994).

Several criteria should be met before a chemical can be accepted as a neurotransmitter: 1) stimulation of a nerve should markedly increase the concentration of the active substance in the effluent, 2) the proposed mediator should be chemically and pharmacologically identified and characterized, 3) exogenous administration of the chemical should identically simulate nerve stimulation, 4) other drugs should have basically similar effects on responses to nerve stimulation and the proposed transmitter substance, and 5) cellular mechanisms capable of manufacturing, storing in an inactive form, and inactivating the neurotransmitter should be demonstrable (Lefkowitz et al. 1990).

PHYSIOLOGIC EVENTS. Events involved in neurohumoral transmission at neuroeffector junctions can be subdivided into axonal conduction, synthesis and release of the neurotransmitter, receptor events, and catabolism of the neurotransmitter.

Axonal Conduction. Axonal conduction refers to the passage of an impulse along a nerve fiber. An action potential reflects a reversal of the polarization state present at rest and is the result of permeability changes that occur at the axonal surface as an impulse is propagated along a nerve fiber. A suprathreshold stimulus initiates a localized change in the permeability of the axonal membrane. Suddenly, permeability of the fiber to Na^+ is greatly increased in relation to K^+; Na^+ moves inward in the direction of its large electrochemical gradient. This movement is detected by an instantaneous change in the membrane potential in a positive direction. The positively charged Na^+ increases in concentration within the axon; the membrane potential moves from ~85 mV toward zero and then overshoots to the extent that momentarily the inside of the fiber is positive in relation to the exterior of the cell.

Repolarization of the membrane occurs rapidly as the selective permeability characteristics of the axonal membrane are quickly reestablished. The axon once again becomes relatively impermeable to Na^+ and relatively more permeable to K^+, and the negativity of the interior of the cell is quickly reestablished. A schematic representation of axonal conductance and resulting neurohumoral transmission events is presented in Figure 5.4.

Although the localized permeability changes associated with an action potential are extremely short-lived, they elicit similar alterations in membrane function in immediately adjacent quiescent areas of the axon. Thus the action potential is self-propagating, and in this manner an action potential is conducted along an axonal fiber. Axonal conduction is insensitive to most drugs. Even local anesthetics must be used in high concentrations in immediate contact with the nerve before excitability is blocked. However, subsequent events in neurohumoral transmission are quite susceptible to drug actions.

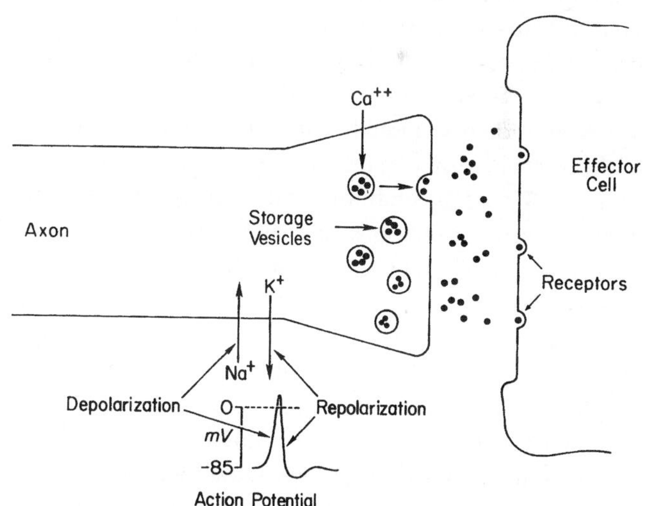

FIG. 5.4 Schematic representation of neurohumoral transmission. The axonal action potential represents a self-propagating depolarization-repolarization of the axon that is characterized by an influx of Na+ and an efflux of K+. As the action potential arrives at the nerve terminal, it facilitates an inward movement of Ca++, which triggers the discharge of neurotransmitter (•) from storage vesicles into the junctional cleft. Neurotransmitter reacts with specialized receptor areas on the postjunctional membrane and initiates a physiologic response in the effector cell.

Neurotransmitter Release. Release of neurotransmitter substance is triggered by arrival of the axonal action potential at the nerve terminal (see Fig. 5.4) (Klein 1973). Ca^{++} acts to link or couple the excitation of the membrane (action potential) with discharge of neurotransmitter from the axon terminal. The action potential initiates an inward movement of Ca^{++} into the nerve terminal from the interstitial space and/or superficial membrane binding sites at the axon terminal. Inward movement of Ca^{++} triggers exocytotic discharge of neurotransmitter from the vesicles into the junctional cleft (Jahn et al. 2003). Nitric oxide is not stored in synaptic vesicles. Instead, the increase in cytosolic Ca^{++} activates a Ca^{++}-dependent enzyme: nitric oxide synthase. The activated form of this enzyme utilizes molecular oxygen and a nitrogen moiety from the amino acid l–arginine to yield nitric oxide. The latter is highly lipophilic and it rapidly diffuses to effector cells (Adams 1996).

Receptor Events. After rapid migration of neurotransmiter across the cleft, the mediator substance bonds with receptive areas on the postsynaptic membrane. Cell surface receptors are specialized macromolecular structures of the cell that a neurotransmitter interacts with to elicit a response (Hein and Schmitt 2003; Kohout and Lefkowitz 2003). Many types and subtypes of receptors have now been isolated and cloned. The clinical utility of all such discoveries remains to be defined.

Receptor events caused by interaction of neurotransmitter substance with the receptor may be of two general types: excitatory or inhibitory. If the neurotransmitter initiates an excitatory response in the cell, receptor activation triggers a general increase in permeability of the postsynaptic membrane to all ions. Electrically, these changes are characterized as an excitatory postsynaptic potential, which then propagates localized permeability changes in adjacent portions of the cell membrane, and an action potential is conducted along the remainder of the innervated cell.

An inhibitory postsynaptic potential occurs when the neurotransmitter initiates a selective increase in permeability of the postsynaptic membrane to only smaller ions (e.g., K^+, Cl^-). Thus outward movement of K^+ and inward movement of Cl^- along their respective concentration gradients increase the net negative charge within the cell and actually hyperpolarize the postsynaptic membrane. The resulting hyperpolarization of the membrane increases the threshold to stimuli and, in effect, elicits an inhibitory response in the cell.

Catabolism of Neurotransmitter. Termination of the duration of action of the adrenergic neurotransmitter norepinephrine is through metabolism by both intraneuronal and extraneuronal enzymes. However, the uptake of norepinephrine back into the adrenergic nerve terminal and diffusion of norepinephrine away from receptor sites are probably more important pathways for termination of norepinephrine activity. Extraneuronal ACh is rapidly hydrolyzed by acetylcholinesterase (AChE), a quite specific enzyme localized in close proximity to the synaptic cleft. Nitric oxide is a highly reactive free radical, and it undergoes oxidation to nitrites and nitrates within seconds.

ADRENERGIC NEUROHUMORAL TRANSMISSION

For critical examination of adrenergic mechanisms, the interested reader is referred to the detailed bibliographies accumulated by Lefkowitz et al. (1990), Ma and Huang (2002), and Phillipp and Hein (2004).

CATECHOLAMINES. Norepinephrine, epinephrine, and dopamine are endogenous catecholamines; they are the sympathetic neural and humoral transmitter substances in most mammalian species. Norepinephrine and dopamine are believed to transmit impulse information in specific areas within the CNS; norepinephrine is also the neurotransmitter at most peripheral sympathetic neuroeffector junctions. Epinephrine is the major hormone released from the adrenal medulla. Catecholamines are stored in an inactive form within granular structures in nerve terminals and chromaffin cells.

Synthesis. Norepinephrine is synthesized from the amino acid phenylalanine in a stepwise process summarized in Figure 5.5. The aromatic ring of phenylalanine is hydroxylated by action of an enzyme, phenylalanine hydroxylase. This reaction yields tyrosine, which is converted to dihydroxyphenylalanine (dopa) by the enzyme tyrosine hydroxylase. This reaction involves additional hydroxylation of the benzene ring, and it is believed to represent the rate-limiting step in catecholamine synthesis (Vulliet et al. 1980).

Dopa is decarboxylated by the enzyme l–aromatic amino acid decarboxylase (dopa decarboxylase) to dihydroxyphenylethylamine (dopamine). Conversion of

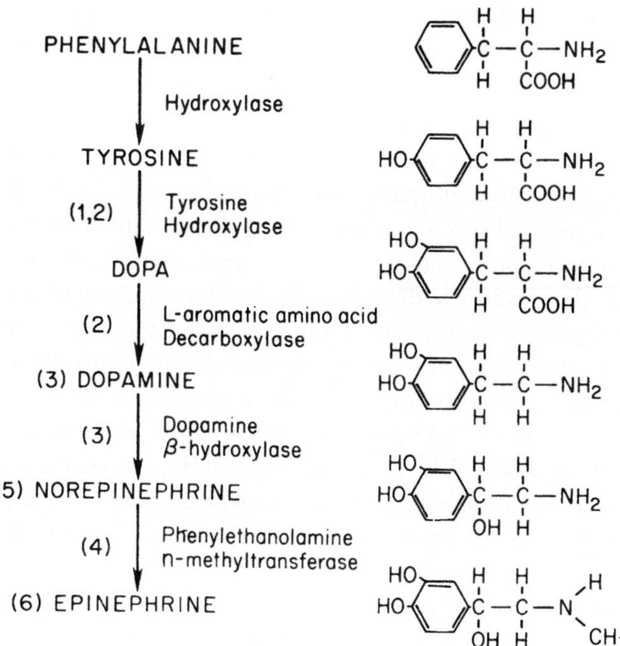

FIG. 5.5 The biosynthetic pathway of norepinephrine and epinephrine. (1) = the rate-limiting step, (2) = occurs within axoplasm, (3) = occurs within amine storage granule, (4) = occurs primarily within cytoplasm of adrenal medullary chromaffin cells, (5) = stored primarily within amine storage granule of adrenergic neurons, (6) = stored within amine storage granule of chromaffin cells.

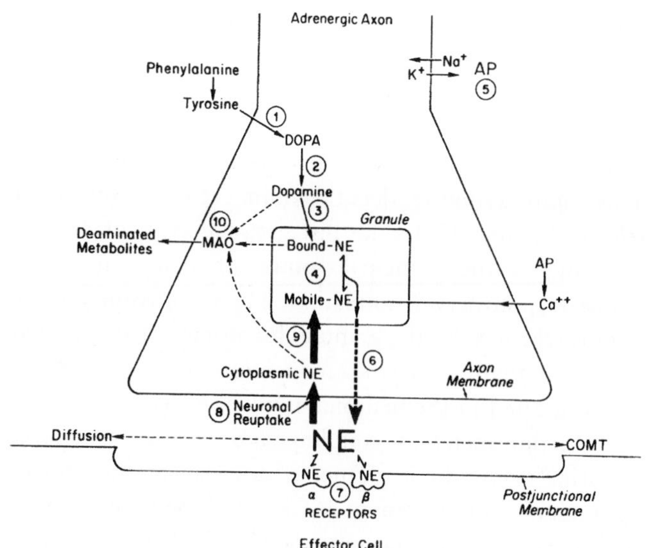

FIG. 5.6 Neurohumoral transmission at the adrenergic neuroeffector junction: proposed physiologic pathways and sites of action susceptible to modification by pharmacologic agents. (1) Tyrosine is hydroxylated to dopa. This reaction, considered to be the rate-limiting step in catecholamine synthesis, is inhibited by a-methyl-p-tyrosine. (2) Dopa is decarboxylated to dopamine. Dopa decarboxylase inhibitors (e.g., a-methyldopa) inhibit this step. (3) Dopamine is taken up into the storage granules and oxidized to norepinephrine (NE). a-Methyldopamine inhibits conversion of dopamine to NE and is converted to a-methylnorepinephrine. a-Methyl NE is then stored in the granule and upon nerve stimulation may be released as a "false neurotransmitter." (4) NE is stored in the granule in a bound and free (mobile) form. Tyramine-like drugs release NE from adrenergic neurons. (5) The axonal action potential is a self-propagating depolarization process that upon reaching the nerve terminal increases influx of Ca++, which then triggers the discharge of NE from the nerve terminal. Bretylium inhibits NE release. (6) NE is released from the neuron via exocytotic emptying of the contents of storage granules into the junctional cleft. Newly synthesized NE may be preferentially released. (7) Released NE reacts with receptor sites on the postjunctional membrane of the effector cell. This step is blocked by adrenergic blocking agents (e.g., α-phentolamine, β-propranolol). Receptive areas (that modify NE release) may also be located on the prejunctional membrane of the nerve terminal (see Fig. 5.7). (8) Extraneuronal NE can be taken back up into the nerve terminal by an active Na+-dependent uptake process. This step is inhibited by cocaine and imipramine-like drugs. Extraneuronal NE may also diffuse from the junction or be catabolized by catechol-O-methyltransferase. (9) Cytoplasmic NE may be taken up into the granule by a Mg++-ATP-dependent uptake process. Reserpine-like drugs inhibit this step. (10) Monoamine oxidase (MAO) can deaminate cytoplasmic NE and dopamine. MAO inhibitors (e.g., pargyline) suppress this step. The bold dashed line = release of NE from the granular pool into the junctional cleft. Small dashed lines = catabolic pathways. Bold solid lines = uptake processes. Double-headed arrows = reversible pathways.

tyrosine to dopa to dopamine is believed to occur within the cytoplasm. Dopamine is taken up into the storage granule. In some central anatomic sites (e.g., mammalian extrapyramidal system), dopamine seems to act as the primary neurotransmitter rather than its metabolites, norepinephrine and epinephrine (Aghajanian and Bunney 1973; Bartholini et al. 1973).

In peripheral adrenergic neurons and adrenal medullary chromaffin cells, intragranular dopamine is hydroxylated in the β position of the aliphatic side chain by dopamine-β-hydroxylase to form norepinephrine. In the adrenal medulla, norepinephrine is released from the granules of chromaffin cells and is *N*-methylated within the cytoplasm by phenylethanolamine *N*-methyltransferase to form epinephrine. Epinephrine is subsequently localized in what seems to be another type of intracellular storage granule prior to its release from the adrenal medulla.

Storage, Release, Reuptake, and Metabolism. Physiologic events involved in adrenergic neurotransmission and susceptibility of these events to pharmacologic agents are outlined schematically in Figure 5.6. Catecholamines are taken up from the cytoplasm into granules by an active transport system that is adenosine triphosphate (ATP) and Mg^{++} dependent. Storage within the granular vesicles is accomplished by complexation of the catecholamines with ATP and a specific protein, chromogranin. This complexation renders the amines inactive until their release (Shore 1972). The intragranular pool of norepinephrine is the principal source of neurotransmitter released upon nerve stimulation. The cytoplasmic amine pool is taken up by the granules for storage or inactivated by a deaminating enzyme, monoamine oxidase (MAO), that is located in the neuronal mitochondria.

Excitation-secretion coupling and release of norepinephrine from adrenergic nerve terminals are dependent upon an inward movement of Ca^{++}. Released norepinephrine migrates across the synaptic cleft and interacts with specific adrenergic receptor sites on the postjunctional membrane of the innervated cell.

A very active amine uptake system is present in the axonal membrane of postganglionic sympathetic nerve terminals. This transport system is Na^{+} and energy dependent, and it functions to recapture or reuptake catecholamines that have been released from the nerve (Iverson 1973).

The adrenergic neuronal uptake mechanism is referred to as *Uptake$_1$*. Uptake$_2$ signifies the extraneuronal uptake of catecholamines into surrounding tissue.

The duration of action of norepinephrine can be terminated by active reuptake via Uptake$_1$ into the nerve across the axoplasmic membrane (the amine reuptake pump), diffusion from the cleft via extracellular fluid, or metabolic breakdown by an extraneuronal enzyme, catechol-*O*-methyltransferase (COMT). Activity of COMT involves methylation of one of the ring hydroxyl groups (3-OH).

Norepinephrine that has been taken back into the nerve may be restored in granules or deaminated by MAO. Deamination of norepinephrine or epinephrine by MAO initially yields the corresponding aldehyde, which in turn is further oxidized to 3,4-dihydroxymandelic acid. Alternatively, the 3-hydroxyl group of norepinephrine and epinephrine can first be methylated by COMT to yield normetanephrine and metanephrine, respectively. The *O*-methylated or deaminated metabolites can then be acted upon by the other enzyme to yield 3-methoxy-4-hydroxymandelic acid. The deaminated *O*-methylated metabolites can then be conjugated with sulfate or glucuronide prior to excretion by the kidneys.

Pharmacologic Considerations. Many drugs exert their pharmacologic activity by altering the synthesis, storage, and release mechanisms of catecholamines. Most of these agents are used in humans to control hypertension or affect central autonomic centers (e.g., tranquilization, antidepression, antiparkinsonism).

Certain drugs act as false substrates for the catecholamine-synthesizing enzymes; e.g., α-methylpara-tyrosine inhibits tyrosine hydroxylase, the rate-limiting step in norepinephrine formation. Thus norepinephrine stores are not replenished by newly synthesized norepinephrine. Alpha-methyldopa may be converted to α-methyldopamine to α-methylnorepinephrine by dopa decarboxylase and dopamine-β-hydroxylase, respectively. The α-methylnorepinephrine is active at CNS α_2 receptors, which reduce sympathetic efferent nerve traffic to the cardiovascular system.

Reserpine-like drugs block the granular uptake process (Shore 1972). Catecholamine stores are depleted and adrenergic functions are markedly altered by prolonged treatment with even small doses of reserpine (Adams et al. 1971, 1972). Guanethidine can slowly deplete norepinephrine and interfere with its release. Bretylium blocks the neuronal release of neurotransmitter. The experimental drug 6-hydroxydopamine produces a functional peripheral sympathectomy by destroying adrenergic nerve terminals (Gauthier et al. 1974).

Other drugs (e.g., cocaine, imipramine) inhibit the neuronal reuptake process so that released norepinephrine is available for a longer period for reaction with receptor sites. Inhibition of MAO by drugs result in accumulation of catecholamines. Drugs like tyramine and amphetamine release intraneuronal stores of catecholamines. Most adrenergic drugs important to clinical veterinary medicine act primarily by activating or blocking postjunctional adrenergic receptors in peripheral tissues or the CNS.

ADRENERGIC RECEPTORS. The interaction of neurohormone with an adrenergic receptor (i.e., adrenoceptor) may elicit either an excitatory or an inhibitory response. Following isolation and identification of norepinephrine as the adrenergic neurotransmitter, attention was directed to differences in postjunctional events that might explain such contrasting results. In his classic paper, Ahlquist (1948) proposed that there were two basic types of adrenergic receptors: α and β. Epinephrine is the most potent α-receptor stimulant, norepinephrine is intermediate, and isoproterenol is the least active. On the other hand, isoproterenol is the most potent β-receptor agonist, epinephrine is intermediate, and norepinephrine is least active. Epinephrine is therefore classified as a mixed α-β agonist, whereas isoproterenol is virtually a pure β agonist with few, if any, α-receptor effects. Norepinephrine is primarily an α agonist; however, it does activate the excitatory β receptors in the heart.

RECEPTOR SUBTYPES. The concept of dissimilar adrenoceptors has been strongly supported by observations that certain adrenergic antagonists block only α or β receptors (Moran 1973). Furthermore, studies with selective antagonists and agonists have demonstrated that β receptors can be divided into two subtypes: β_1 and β_2 (Lands et al. 1967). Beta receptors in the heart are β_1; they are associated with excitatory responses. Isoproterenol, epinephrine, and norepinephrine activate β_1 adrenoceptors. $Beta_2$ receptors are localized in vascular smooth muscle and bronchiolar smooth muscle; they instigate inhibitory (relaxant) effects. Norepinephrine has little effect on β_2 receptors, whereas epinephrine and isoproterenol are very active at β_2-receptor sites.

Alpha receptors located at adrenergic nerve terminals show a somewhat different responsiveness to drugs when compared to the classic α receptors of effector cells, leading to their designation as α_2 (Starke et al. 1977; Langer 1980). Other studies have supported the existence of different α-receptor populations but indicate that α_1 and α_2 subtypes are not necessarily restricted to postjunctional and prejunctional localizations, respectively (U'Prichard and Snyder 1979).

Designation of adrenoceptors as either α_1, α_2, β_1, or β_2 is now well accepted. A summary of the different adrenergic receptor types in various sympathetically innervated tissues is given in Table 5.1. Numerous studies have now established that classification of receptor types and subtypes is far more complex than Ahlquist (1948) envisioned. Indeed, there are many types of α receptors, β receptors, muscarinic receptors, nicotinic receptors, and others (Robidoux et al. 2004; Salminen et al. 2004; Brown and Taylor 2006). Because the clinical importance of such complexities remains to be established, this textbook will consider clinically relevant receptor nomenclatures.

CHOLINERGIC NEUROTRANSMISSION

ACh is the neurotransmitter substance at most parasympathetic neuroeffector junctions, autonomic ganglia, the adrenal medulla, somatic myoneural junctions, and certain CNS regions (Brimblecombe 1974; Waser 1975; Goldberg and Hanin 1976). Neurohumoral transmission processes seem to be basically similar at all cholinergic junctions. Autonomic ganglionic and somatic myoneural transmission will be discussed in greater detail in subsequent chapters.

SYNTHESIS, STORAGE, RELEASE, AND CATABOLISM OF ACH. ACh is synthesized within cholinergic nerves by the enzymatic transfer of an acetyl group from acetyl coenzyme A to choline. This reaction is catalyzed by the enzyme choline acetylase (also referred to as *choline acetyltransferase*) and is summarized in Figure 5.7. The acetyl coenzyme A is formed by the action of an enzyme, acetyl kinase, which mediates the transfer of an acetyl group from adenylacetate (formed from acetate and ATP) to the coenzyme A molecule. Choline is transported from the extracellular fluid into the cholinergic nerve by an energy-requiring axoplasmic uptake process (Ferguson and Blakely 2004). ACh is stored within axonal vesicular structures in a concentrated solution or bound to membranes or both.

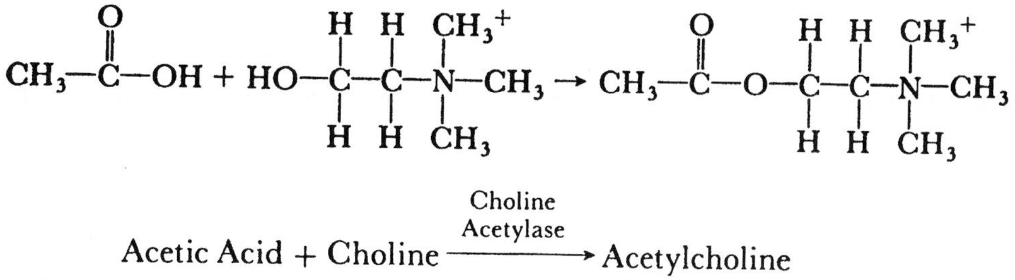

$$CH_3-\overset{\overset{\displaystyle O}{\|}}{C}-OH + HO-\underset{\underset{\displaystyle H}{|}}{\overset{\overset{\displaystyle H}{|}}{C}}-\underset{\underset{\displaystyle H}{|}}{\overset{\overset{\displaystyle H}{|}}{C}}-\underset{\underset{\displaystyle CH_3}{|}}{\overset{\overset{\displaystyle CH_3^+}{|}}{N}}-CH_3 \rightarrow CH_3-\overset{\overset{\displaystyle O}{\|}}{C}-O-\underset{\underset{\displaystyle H}{|}}{\overset{\overset{\displaystyle H}{|}}{C}}-\underset{\underset{\displaystyle H}{|}}{\overset{\overset{\displaystyle H}{|}}{C}}-\underset{\underset{\displaystyle CH_3}{|}}{\overset{\overset{\displaystyle CH_3^+}{|}}{N}}-CH_3$$

$$\text{Acetic Acid} + \text{Choline} \xrightarrow{\text{Choline Acetylase}} \text{Acetylcholine}$$

FIG. 5.7 Formation of ACh involving choline acetylase, choline, and acetic acid. Source of the acetic acid moiety is acetyl coenzyme A.

ACh is released from the nerve terminal upon arrival of an axonal action potential (Jahn et al. 2003). ACh within the junctional space is rapidly inactivated by hydrolysis by a specific enzyme, AChE. AChE is present in cholinergic nerves, autonomic ganglia, and neuromuscular and neuroeffector junctions. A somewhat similar enzyme, pseudocholinesterase (butyrocholinesterase), is present in serum and other body tissues.

CHOLINERGIC RECEPTORS. There are two basic types of cholinergic receptors within the peripheral efferent autonomic nerve tracts: nicotinic and muscarinic. The nicotinic responsive sites were found to be present in autonomic ganglia, adrenal medullary chromaffin cells, and also the neuromuscular junction of the somatic nervous system. Accordingly, these sites have been referred to as *nicotinic cholinergic receptors.*

Nicotine does not, however, simulate or block the action of ACh at the parasympathetic neuroeffector junctions in heart muscle, smooth muscle, or secretory glands. The plant alkaloid muscarine was found to simulate the activity of ACh at these sites but not at the previously described nicotinic receptors. Muscarinic receptors therefore designate the type of receptor present at cholinergic neuroeffector junctions in muscle and glands.

A nicotinic response usually denotes an excitatory response, whereas muscarinic receptor activation may elicit an excitatory or inhibitory response, depending on the tissue. This seems to be related to either a general increase in permeability to all ions (depolarization-excitatory) or a selective increase in permeability to small ions like K^+ (hyperpolarization-inhibitory), respectively. Nicotinic and muscarinic cholinergic receptors have been placed into different subtypes (Birdsall et al. 1983; Chassaing et al. 1984; DeBiasi 2002), but the relevance of these subclassifications to clinical veterinary medicine is unclear at this time.

PHARMACOLOGIC CONSIDERATIONS. A wide variety of chemical and biologic agents affect cholinergic neurotransmission. The synthesis of ACh is inhibited by hemicholinium, which blocks the entrance of choline into the cholinergic nerve. Botulinum toxin interferes with the release of ACh. The plant alkaloids nicotine and muscarine have been mentioned in preceding paragraphs. Atropine and related alkaloids block muscarinic receptors, whereas curare blocks nicotinic receptor sites. The activity of endogenous and exogenous ACh is markedly augmented by many chemicals that act as cholinesterase inhibitors (anticholinesterase agents). The therapeutic importance of cholinergic and anticholinergic agents will be discussed in Chapter 7.

AUTONOMIC RECEPTOR SITES ON NERVE TERMINALS

Release of autonomic transmitters from nerve terminals can be influenced by other transmitters interacting with specific receptor sites present on the nerve terminal (for reviews, see Adams 1983, 1984; Boehm and Kubista 2002).

Muscarinic cholinergic receptors at adrenergic nerve endings mediate an inhibition of the neuronal release of norepinephrine (Muscholl 1973). Such receptors may well explain the reduced cardiac responses to sympathetic nerve activity when vagal influence is increased (Stuesse et al. 1979). Several unrelated autacoids (e.g., histamine, prostaglandins) also inhibit norepinephrine release from adrenergic nerves, evidence for inhibitory presynaptic receptors specific for certain autacoids (Horton 1973).

There also is evidence for α_2- and β_2-adrenoceptive sites on adrenergic nerve terminals. Prejunctional α_2 receptors mediate a decrease in the amount of norepinephrine released upon nerve stimulation. The function of these α_2 sites has been envisioned as a local feedback control mechanism through which norepinephrine can inhibit its own release once a threshold concentration has been obtained in the junctional space. Conversely, the prejunctional β_2 receptors subserve increased release of norepinephrine (Adams 1984).

It is tempting to speculate on the physiologic significance and implications of such local inhibitory-facilitatory feedback mechanisms. However, although these extremely complex interrelationships most likely exist, neither the complete physiologic nor the complete pharmacologic significance of all presynaptic receptors has been definitely established (Boehm and Kubista 2002; DeBiasi 2002; Fetscher et al. 2002). The clinical relevance of the α_1- and α_2-receptor subtypes and β_1- and β_2-receptor subtypes is considered in Chapter 6.

PUTATIVE NEUROHUMORAL SUBSTANCES

Biologic substances other than ACh and the catecholamines have been proposed as probable (putative) neurotransmitter substances. Histamine, e.g., has been suggested as a potential neurotransmitter at certain peripheral and CNS sites, as have different neuropeptide substances. There is even evidence now that certain peptides coexist in the same neuron as primary neurotransmitters (Iverson et al. 1983; Hokfelt et al. 2000). It remains unclear whether these peptides serve as primary neurotransmitters themselves or, more likely, modulate either the axon or the effector cell process in the neurohumoral communication event.

Considerable evidence has revealed that serotonin (5-hydroxytryptamine) acts as a neurotransmitter in specific brain centers and some peripheral nerves. The functional consequences of tryptaminergic transmission have not been completely defined, but it is likely that 5-hydroxytryptamine participates in thermoregulation, sleep cycles, and extrapyramidal influences on motor control of skeletal muscles. Gamma-aminobutyric acid has been shown to be an inhibitory neurotransmitter at certain CNS sites.

Although several putative neurotransmitter substances are involved in information transfer in the central and peripheral nervous systems (Luetje 2004), the pharmacologic activity of most autonomic drugs and numerous centrally acting agents can often be explained best by actions on cholinergic or adrenergic pathways (Westfall 2004; Wess 2004).

NITRIC OXIDE

Nitric oxide is an unlikely candidate for an endogenously synthesized messenger for physiologic and pathophysiologic communications in living organisms (Lowenstein et al. 1994; Adams 1996). Compared to classical neurotransmitters and polypeptides, nitric oxide is an exceptionally small and simple molecule comprising a single atom each of nitrogen and oxygen and existing under atmospheric conditions as a gas. With an unpaired electron in its outer orbit, nitric oxide is a radical species with a biological half-life of only a few seconds; it reacts rapidly with oxygen or with iron moieties of heme-containing proteins. Nitric oxide also is a combustion product generated in cigarette smoke, smog, and jet engine exhaust.

Despite considerable interest in nitric oxide as an environmental pollutant, it gathered little notice from biomedical scientists until the recent discovery that this compound is actively synthesized by different cell types, where it serves as a key regulator of a wealth of different bodily functions. These include immunomodulation, antimicrobial defenses, tumoricidal activity, neurotransmission in both the central and peripheral nervous systems, respiration, intestinal peristalsis, penile erection, and cardiovascular dynamics. The idea that a small molecule of gas can be synthesized by mammalian cells and then serve as a key controller of physiologic functions truly represents a new frontier in medicine (Adams 1996).

The surge of biomedical interest in nitric oxide can be traced directly to several lines of investigation involving the biochemistry of carcinogenesis, immunomodulatory and antimicrobial characteristics of activated macrophages, and control of hemodynamics (Änggard 1994; Langrehr et al. 1993). Relative to vascular effects, the discovery of endothelium-derived relaxing factor (EDRF) by Furchgott and Zawadzki (1980) unquestionably was a pivotal step in the recognition that mammalian cells can synthesize nitric oxide. These investigators observed that ACh produced vasodilation in isolated blood vessels only when the vascular endothelium was intact. This classical observation prompted an explosion of interest in vascular endothelium as a necessary intermediary in the vascular smooth muscle relaxation induced not only by ACh but also by many other vasodilators, including bradykinin, thrombin, oxytocin, adenosine diphosphate, and substance P. It became clear that when such agents interacted with vascular endothelium, the latter released an endogenous factor responsible for vasorelaxant responses to the former—hence, the discovery of EDRF (Furchgott and Zawadzki 1980). Depending on species and vascular bed, some vasodilator agents exert both endothelium-dependent and endothelium-independent actions as part of their pharmacodynamic profiles (Cogswell et al. 1995).

It is now widely accepted that EDRF is in fact either authentic nitric oxide, a closely related nitrosothiol that releases nitric oxide to target cells, or both. Nitric oxide migrates from the endothelium and activates the cytosolic form of guanylyl cyclase in adjacent vascular smooth muscle cells. This activation accelerates conversion of guanosine triphosphate (GTP) to cyclic guanosine monophosphate (cGMP), with the latter leading in turn to relaxation of vascular smooth muscle and its accompanying vasodilation.

Endothelium-derived nitric oxide was not simply an experimental curiosity of isolated blood vessels. Indeed, pharmacologic inhibition of nitric oxide biosynthesis in intact animals elicits a pronounced systemic hypertensive response owing to a substantial increase in peripheral vascular resistance. Because this peripheral vasoconstriction is expressed under basal conditions, it became clear that EDRF is an important modulator of normal vasodilator tone regulated by a dynamic release of endothelium-derived nitric oxide on a moment-to-moment basis. These remarkable findings revolutionized long-held concepts about control of peripheral vasomotion, prompting robust searches for different agents that would selectively modulate the biosynthesis of nitric oxide.

NITRIC OXIDE BIOSYNTHESIS. Details of the complex biochemical and electron-transfer steps culminating in the formation of nitric oxide have been reviewed (Änggard 1994; Langrehr et al. 1993; Lowenstein et al. 1994; Schulz and Triggle 1994). In brief, nitric oxide is synthesized from an N^G-guanidino nitrogen of the amino acid L–arginine. The D–enantiomer of arginine is inactive. The enzyme family responsible for nitric oxide biosynthesis is nitric oxide synthase (NOS).

Several different isoforms of NOS have been characterized, and the identifying nomenclatures are still undergoing modification as new molecular and cofactor requirements are discovered. The two original isoforms described were the constitutive NOS (cNOS) and the inducible NOS (iNOS).

The NOS prototypically present in endothelium and neurons is cNOS; this enzyme is constitutively present under basal conditions, and its activation is dependent on calmodulin and Ca^{++}. Nitric oxide synthesis from cNOS is activated within seconds to minutes after intracellular Ca^{++} is increased in response to classical cell surface receptors and affiliated signal-transduction mechanisms that culminate in elevated cytosolic Ca^{++}. The cNOS synthesizes nitric oxide in relatively small amounts; synthesis dynamically ceases as cellular Ca^{++} falls to basal concentrations. The biosynthesis of endothelium-derived nitric oxide and its subsequent role as an activator of guanylyl cyclase in vascular smooth muscle are schematized in Figure 5.8.

The iNOS is prototypically induced in macrophages and hepatocytes, but it is not present in these or other cell types under basal conditions. When macrophages are exposed to LPS and/or certain cytokines such as tumor necrosis factor-α or interleukin-1, de novo synthesis of nascent iNOS is initiated by transcriptional regulation. Several hours are required for maximal expression of iNOS, which produces amounts of nitric oxide large enough to destroy pathogenic microorganisms. Although calmodulin is an integral subunit component of iNOS, its regulatory role is unknown in that Ca^{++} does not seem to be required for iNOS activity.

Recent experiments have provided evidence that iNOS is not restricted to macrophages and hepatocytes; it can also be induced in a rather impressive spectrum of different cell types including vascular smooth muscle, endothelium, Kupffer cells, neutrophils, and possibly cardiac myocytes (Schulz and Triggle 1994).

Nitric oxide is a nonpolar gas and it readily crosses cellular membranes, providing access to intracellular structures in nearby cells. Unlike classical neurotransmitters and hormones, nitric oxide does not seem to require a specific macromolecular protein for its receptor site. Nitric oxide is oxidized rapidly upon contact with oxygen, yielding the much less active nitrites and nitrates. Alternatively, nitric oxide can interact with the heme constituent of iron-containing enzymes, leading to configurational modifications that adjust catalytic activity of the affected enzyme.

Activation of cytosolic guanylyl cyclase through nitrosation of its heme moiety is considered a cardinal mechanism of action of nitric oxide in platelets and smooth muscles. The resulting increase in cGMP is the intracellular messenger subserving the physiologic response to nitric oxide (see Fig. 5.8). Smooth muscle relaxation and anti–platelet-aggregating actions of nitric oxide are mimicked by cell-permanent forms of cGMP and are potentiated by inhibitors of the cGMP phosphodiesterase enzyme. Activation of guanylyl cyclase by nitric oxide not only is responsible for dilation of blood vessels and inhibition of thrombogenesis but is involved in neuronal signaling and cytotoxicity responses to nitric oxide as well.

Because of amino acid heterogenicity in the structural motif of the different isoforms of NOS, the following nomenclature modification has been proposed: the neuronal cNOS has been referred to as *NOS-I,* the macrophage iNOS as *NOS-II,* and the endothelial cNOS as *NOS-III.* This nomenclature will no doubt continue to evolve as new discoveries are made.

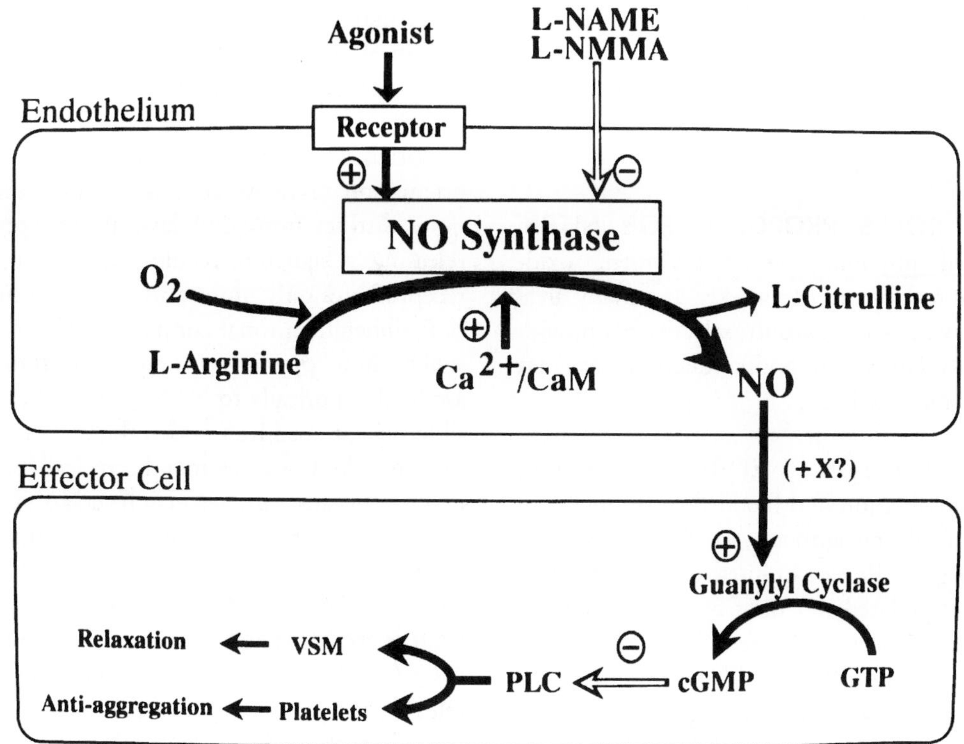

FIG. 5.8 The biosynthetic pathway for nitric oxide (NO) in vascular endothelial cells. Increased intracellular Ca++ activates the Ca++-calmodulin (CaM)-dependent enzyme NO synthase, which utilizes O_2 and l-arginine to form NO. NO activates guanylyl cyclase in nearby platelets and vascular smooth muscle (VSM), leading to increased formation of cyclic guanosine monophosphate (cGMP). The latter inhibits phospholipase C (PLC) and exerts other effects that lead to changes in cellular functions, e.g., vasodilation and antiaggregation of platelets. l-arginine analogs such as l-nitroarginine methylester (L-NAME) and l-nitro-monomethyl arginine (L-NMMA) inhibit NO synthase. (+X?) = possible biological carrier of NO. + = activates; – = inhibits.

PHARMACOLOGIC MODULATION OF NITRIC OXIDE SYNTHESIS AND ACTION. Organic compounds containing nitrate or nitroso moieties such as nitroglycerine, nitroprusside, *S*-nitroso-*N*-acetylpenicillamine, $NaNO_3$, and sydnonimines undergo tissue-catalyzed metabolism or spontaneous breakdown to yield exogenous-source nitric oxide. These and related compounds serve as nitric oxide donors, and their pharmacodynamic actions mimic in many respects the physiologic effects of endogenously synthesized nitric oxide.

There are several different types of NOS inhibitors, including congeners of the substrate L–arginine. The N^G-substituted L-arginine analogs include *N*-nitro-L–arginine methylester (L–NAME), *N*-nitro-L–arginine, and *N*-methyl-L–arginine (L–NMA). These inhibitors generally are competitive when administered concomitantly with L–arginine, and studies are under way to identify arginine analogs that are more selective for either iNOS or cNOS. Arginine analogs are routinely described as "specific" inhibitors of NOS, and yet few studies have systematically tested whether these agents also possess pharmacologic actions unrelated to NOS inhibition. In this regard, for instance, recent studies have indicated that L–NAME is a muscarinic receptor antagonist and may therefore inhibit effects of ACh by muscarinic receptor blockade. As another example, apparently L–NMMA can be metabolized to L–arginine and actually accelerate NOS activity under some circumstances. Such pharmacologic limitations should be considered when drugs are assumed to be "specific" inhibitors of NOS.

Other inhibitors of NOS include calmodulin antagonists for cNOS, flavoprotein binders for iNOS and cNOS, heme binders such as carbon monoxide for iNOS and cNOS, and inhibitors of iNOS induction. Inhibitors of iNOS induction include corticosteroids and certain cytokines such as transforming growth factor-α and interleukins-4 and -10. Although tumor necrosis factor-α is a strong inducer of iNOS, recent experiments indicate this cytokine may inhibit synthesis or accelerate breakdown of cNOS.

PHYSIOLOGIC ROLES PROPOSED FOR NITRIC OXIDE. Proposed physiologic roles for nitric oxide undergo dynamic revision almost weekly, and many areas overlap. The following points are quite selective but provide a brief glimpse of the wealth of bodily functions that may be modulated by nitric oxide.

Circulation. Basal release of EDRF is a primary determinant of vasodilation and blood flow through vascular networks, including coronary, cerebral, renal, and skeletal muscle arteries. Release of nitric oxide from endothelial cNOS is stimulated not only by certain receptor agonists but also by shear stresses exerted over the intimal surface by flowing blood. Nitric oxide from endothelial cNOS participates in vascular autoregulatory control mechanisms, e.g., in hypoxia-induced vasodilation and metabolic demand–induced vasodilation associated with ischemia-reperfusion.

Recent studies have shown that immunomodulatory-inflammatory stimuli can induce an iNOS in both endothelium and vascular smooth muscle. Thus, nitric oxide derived from both the intimal layer and the blood vessel wall may play important pathophysiologic roles in the local circulatory response to infection and inflammation (Parker and Adams 1993).

Nitric oxide exerts antiaggregating actions in platelets, thereby eliciting thrombolytic or antithrombogenic effects. Inhibition of aggregation is not restricted to platelets; nitric oxide also slows leukocyte adhesion and aggregation onto the vascular intimal surface. Inhibition of platelet aggregation and adhesion by nitric oxide is believed to be an important constituent of the antithrombogenic characteristic of the intimal surface of the blood vessel lumen. Impaired synthesis of nitric oxide has been implicated in the formation of atherosclerosis and the affiliated loss of vasodilator function.

Neurotransmitter. Nitric oxide is believed to act as a neuronal messenger in both the central and peripheral components of the nervous system. In the brain, nitric oxide participates in experience-driven synaptic plasticity that may control learning and memory retention. Nitric oxide may well be the mediator of neuronal responses to certain excitatory amino acids. And because of its ability as a gas to be "broadcast" and diffuse from a single neuron to large numbers of nearby cells, nitric oxide may be an important controller of neuronal development and spatial orientation of neuronal centers. This exciting theory is quite distinct from the classical concept of one neuron releasing a signal molecule that interacts with specific receptor sites only on one adjacent neuron.

Peripheral neuronal control of intestinal peristalsis and synchronous opening-closing of GI sphincters has been ascribed historically to NANC nerves because the responsible neurotransmitter was unknown. It now seems that certain NANC nerves may be reclassified as nitric oxide neurons because this gas may be a NANC neurotransmitter in the alimentary tract, external genitalia, and the respiratory tract.

Respiratory Tract. There is increasing evidence that NANC nerves innervating bronchiolar smooth muscle release nitric oxide, which serves as a mediator of neurogenic bronchodilator tone. End-stage chronic obstructive pulmonary disease has been associated with decreased nitric oxide production, and it has been proposed that oxidation of nitric oxide may be accelerated in inflamed airways, leading to loss of bronchodilator reserves. Hypoxia-induced pulmonary vasoconstriction is an important compensatory reaction diverting or shunting blood flow away from nonperfused pulmonary zones and toward selective perfusion of oxygenated alveoli. Loss of this reflex may be an important component of acute respiratory distress syndrome (ARDS) and may also occur during prolonged periods of general anesthesia. Because of its conjoint bronchodilator and vasodilator activities, nitric oxide has not escaped the attention of pulmonary care centers. Inhalation of exogenous nitric oxide is undergoing evaluation as a selective vasodilator in oxygenated alveoli since inhaled gas would be delivered only to ventilated regions of the lung; this would selectively enhance perfusion only of oxygenated alveoli, thereby improving ventilation-perfusion matching.

Penile Erection. Neurogenic control of penile erection is issued through the sacral division of the parasympathetic nervous system, and yet drugs that block receptors for the classical parasympathetic neurotransmitter ACh fail to prevent erection. This decades-old perplexity was resolved by the discovery of NANC neurons containing NOS in pelvic nerve plexuses. These nitric oxide neurons extend into the cavernous nerve and affect processes in the corpus cavernosum and its affiliated penile blood vessels. Nitric oxide is the final chemical mediator controlling relaxation of corpus cavernosum smooth muscle and its supplying blood vessels, leading to vascular tumescence necessary for erection. This basic mechanism is controlled by the NO-mediated increase in cyclic GMP, which is in turn metabolized by the type 5 phosphodiesterase enzyme. Phosphodiesterase 5 inhibitors such as sildenafil (Viagra), tadalafil (Cialis), and vardenafil (Levitra) allow cyclic GMP to accumulate in the corpus cavernosum of the penis, thereby enhancing and prolonging penile erection. These drugs are used commonly in humans to treat erectile dysfunctions.

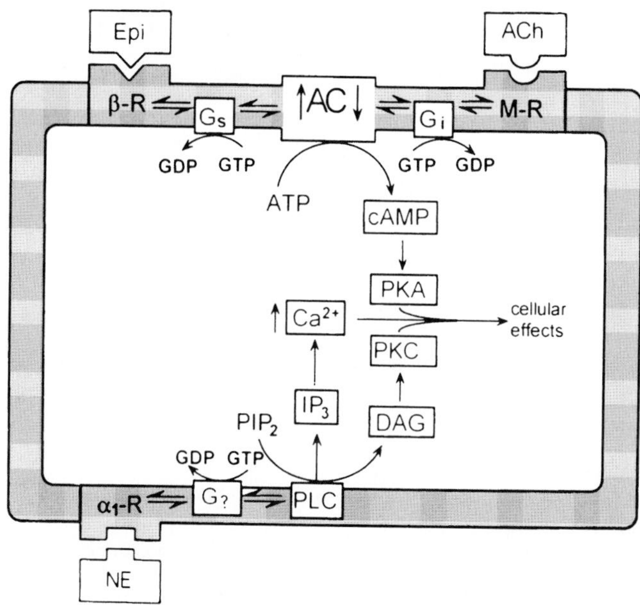

FIG. 5.9 Signal transduction pathways involving cell surface receptors (R), guanine nucleotide-binding regulatory proteins (G), and intracellular Ca++. Activation of β-R by epinephrine (Epi) involves a stimulatory G (Gs), which serves as a GTPase (converting GTP to GDP) and activates the enzyme adenylyl cyclase (AC). The latter converts ATP to cyclic adenosine 3′,5′monophosphate (cAMP), which activates protein kinase A (PKA). Acetylcholine (ACh) binds with a muscarinic-R (M-R) linked to an inhibitory G (Gi), which reduces catalytic activity of AC and hence PKA. Activation of α1-R by norepinephrine (NE) activates another G (G?), which in turn activates phospholipase C (PLC). PLC hydrolyzes a membrane phospholipid phosphatidylinositol-4,5-bisphosphate (PIP2), releasing inositol-1, 4,5-trisphosphate (IP3) and diacylglycerol (DAG), which release endoplasmic reticulum Ca++ and activate protein kinase C (PKC), respectively. PKA and PKC phosphorylate various cellular constituents that, in concert with elevated cytosolic Ca++, elicit characteristic changes in cellular functions.

Their concomitant use with nitrovasodilators must be carefully monitored owing to the likelihood of synergistic effects on blood vessels leading to profound vasodilation and hypotension.

Gastrointestinal Function. Peristalsis of the alimentary tract and synchrony of GI sphincter functions are believed to be regulated by nitric oxide released from neurons. Nitric oxide production and NOS have been localized to the enteric nerve plexuses formerly classified as intestinal NANC neurons. Nitrate concentration is elevated in diarrhea, and colonic production of nitric oxide is increased in patients with ulcerative colitis. Abnormalities of nitric oxide production have been implicated in esophageal motility disorders associated with esophageal achalasia and pyloric motility dysfunction in infantile hypertrophic pyloric stenosis. These interrelations between nitric oxide and GI function suggest more than an incidental role for nitric oxide in regulation of intestinal smooth muscle function.

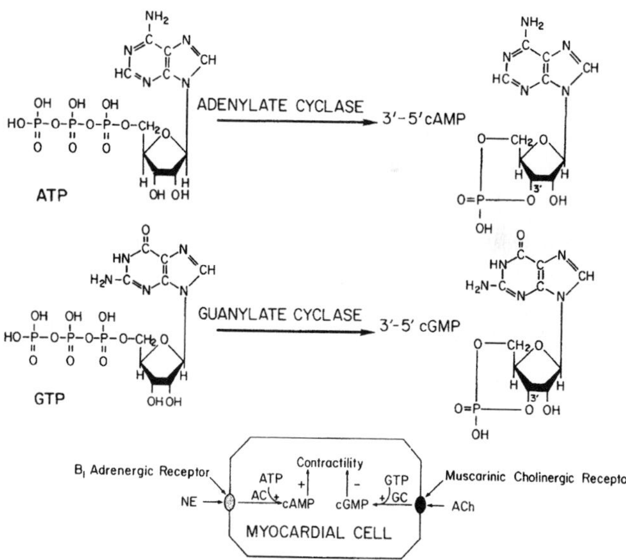

FIG. 5.10 Structures and biosynthetic pathways of cyclic AMP (cAMP) and cyclic GMP (cGMP) and a schematic of their potential roles as intracellular messengers for autonomic neurotransmitters. Activation of β-adrenergic receptors by NE increases activity of adenylate cyclase (AC), an enzyme that catalyzes (+) the conversion of ATP to cAMP. Increased intracellular cAMP leads to increased (+) contractility (via several mechanisms) of the myocardial cell. ACh activates muscarinic receptors, which leads to activation of guanylate cyclase (GC), an enzyme that catalyzes (+) the conversion of guanosine triphosphate to cGMP. Increased intracellular concentration of cGMP leads (via several mechanisms?) to decreased myocardial contractility.

G PROTEINS AND CYCLIC NUCLEOTIDES

Cyclic adenosine 3′,5′-monophosphate (cAMP), a cyclic nucleotide, acts as a "second messenger" to link certain agonist-receptor interactions with cellular responses (Sutherland and Rall 1960; Robison et al. 1967; Robison 1971; Rall 1972). Cyclic AMP is formed from ATP by the catalytic action of the enzyme adenylyl cyclase. It is broken down to 5′-adenosinemonophosphate by another enzyme, phosphodiesterase. Phosphodiesterase in turn represents a large family of related isoenzymes that have preferential action on either cyclic AMP or cyclic GMP in different tissues. Adenylyl cyclase is believed to be localized in the cell membrane in mammalian cells that contain the cAMP system (Gilman 1984). Adenylyl cyclase is closely linked to numerous hormonal receptor sites, and changes in intracellular concentration of cAMP explain the pharmacologic activity of certain autonomic drugs and hormones (Baillie and Housley 2005).

Alteration of adenylyl cyclase and resultant change in cAMP by various adrenergic drugs have been demonstrated in numerous mammalian tissues, including spleen; kidney; brain; adipose cells; and cardiac, skeletal, and smooth muscles. An increase in the tissue concentration of cAMP is generally associated with β-receptor activation, whereas a decrease in cAMP seems to be mediated in some tissues by α_2 receptors. Numerous endocrine hormones may also act via alteration of tissue levels of cAMP. In contrast, the inositol triphosphate pathway is the intracellular mechanism linked to α_1-receptor activation. The

TABLE 5.2 Classification of autonomic drugs

Classification	Other Terms	Pharmacologic Effects	Mechanisms and Examples
Sympathomimetic	Andrenergic*	Resemble effects caused by stimulation of adrenergic neurons	Direct acting—α,β-adrenergic receptor agonists (α-phenylephrine; β-isoproterenol; α,β-epinephrine)
	Adrenomimetic*	Simulate effects of epinephrine and norepinephrine	Indirect acting—release endogenous stores of catecholamines (tyramine, amphetamine) Increase sympathetic discharge (nicotinic cholinergic agonists)[†]
Sympatholytic			
Receptor blocking effects	Adrenergic blocking drugs	Inhibit effects of sympathomimetic drugs; inhibit responses caused by stimulation of adrenergic neurons	Block α or β receptors (α blocker—phentolamine; β blocker—propranolol)
Neuronal blocking effects	Adrenolytic	Inhibit responses caused by stimulation of adrenergic neurons	Deplete endogenous catecholamines (reserpine) Inhibit release of morepinephrine from nerve terminals (bretylium)
Parasympathomimetic	Cholinergic[§]	Resemble effects caused by stimulation of postganglionic parasympathetic neurons	Direct acting—cholinergic receptor agonists (ACh, carbachol)
	Cholinomimetic[§]	Simulate effects of ACh	Indirect acting—cholinesterase inhibitors (neostigmine, organophosphates)
Parasympatholytic			
Receptor blocking effects	Cholinergic[§] blocking drugs	Inhibit effects of ACh; inhibit responses caused by stimulation of postganglionic parasympathetic neurons	Block nicotinic[§] or muscarinic receptors (muscarinic blocker—atropine; nicotinic blocker—hexamethoruum)
Neuronal blocking effects	Anticholinergic[§]	Inhibit responses caused by stimulation of postganglionic parasympathetic neurons	Inhibit release of ACh from nerve terminals (botulinum toxin)

*These terms refer specifically to activities at adrenergic synapses, adrenergic neuroeffector junctions, and adrenergic receptors.

[†]Sympathomimetic effects may be produced by nicotinic cholinergic agents by their excitatory action on sympathetic ganglia, the adrenal medulla, and adrenergic nerve terminals, causing sympathetic discharge and release of epinephrine and norepinephrine. However, these activities should be considered as secondary when broad-based classifications of autonomic drugs are considered.

[§]These terms also refer to nonautonomic sites (e.g., somatic neuromuscular junction, CNS). Thus the terms parasympathomimetic and parasympatholytic are reserved to describe activities at the parasympathetic neuroeffector junction (i.e., in relation to muscarinic receptors; see text).

cellular pathways linking hormone receptors to guanine nucleotide-binding regulatory proteins (i.e., G proteins), cyclic nucleotides, and associated enzymes are schematized in Figure 5.9 (also see Lambert 1993; Schwinn 1993; Levitzki et al. 1993; Palczewski et al. 2000).

The interrelationship of β adrenoceptors and cAMP has been intensely studied in heart muscle. Catecholamines increase the concentration of cAMP in the myocardium by activating adenylyl cyclase secondary to their agonist effects at the cardiac β_1 adrenoceptors. Increases in cAMP correspond with an increase in heart rate and contractile strength, and effects of catecholamines in the heart are mediated by the formation of cAMP.

Several groups of drugs have been known to elicit autonomic-like activity in various tissues, but attempts to associate these effects with change in neurohumoral transmission have failed. It now seems that certain of these drugs bypass receptor sites and act on the same cAMP system as the catecholamines. The methylxanthines (caffeine, theobromine, theophylline), e.g., elicit changes in heart function reminiscent of β-receptor activation in that they elicit positive inotropic and chronotropic responses. However, β blockers do not prevent the cardiac actions of the methylxanthines. These drugs are phosphodiesterase inhibitors. By inhibiting the phosphodiesterase enzyme, the catabolism of cAMP is impaired and the cellular concentration of this nucleotide increases. Furthermore, the methylxanthines potentiate the effect of catecholamines and other drugs that activate adenylyl cyclase (Samir Amer and Kreighbaum 1975).

Another related nucleotide, cyclic guanosine 3′,5′-monophosphate (cGMP), is also important as an intracellular messenger in many cell types (Robison 1971). Specifically, cGMP is the second messenger for the effects of ACh mediated through activation of the muscarinic receptor. The structures and biosynthetic pathways of cAMP and cGMP are presented in Figure 5.10 along with a model of their potential antagonistic actions on myocardial contractility (George et al. 1975; Nawrath 1976).

AUTONOMIC DRUGS

Drugs that exert pharmacologic effects simulating activation, intensification, or inhibition of either the sympathetic or the parasympathetic nervous system have been historically referred to as *autonomic drugs*. As a rule, autonomic drugs are classified according to the physiologic activity they mimic. Table 5.2 summarizes the classification of the basic types of autonomic drugs that will be discussed in subsequent chapters.

REFERENCES

Adams, H. R. 1977. In L. M. Jones, N. H. Booth, and L. E. McDonald, eds., Veterinary Pharmacology and Therapeutics, 4th ed., p. 86. Ames: Iowa State Univ Press.

———. 1983. Pharmacologic problems in circulation research: alpha adrenergic blocking drugs. Circ Shock 10(3):215–223.

———. 1984. New perspectives in cardiopulmonary therapeutics: receptor-selective adrenergic drugs. J Am Vet Med Assoc 185(9):966–974.

———. 1996. Physiologic, pathophysiologic, and therapeutic implications for endogenous nitric oxide. J Am Vet Med Assoc 209:1297–1302.

Adams, H. R., Smookler, H. H, Clarke, D. E., Jandhyala, B. S., Dixit, B. N., Ertel, R. J., and Buckley, J. P. 1971. Clinicopathologic effects of chronic reserpine administration in mongrel dogs. J Pharm Sci 60(8):1134–1138.

Adams, H. R., Dixit, B. N., Smookler, H. H., Buckley, J. P. 1972. Clinical and biochemical effects of chronic reserpine administration in mongrel dogs. Am J Vet Res 33(4):699–707.

Aghajanian, G. K., and Bunney, B. S. 1973. In E. Usdin and S. Snyder, eds., Frontiers in Catecholamine Research, p. 643. Elmsford, NY: Pergamon.

Ahlquist, R. P. 1948. A study of the adrenotropic receptors. Am J Physiol 153:586–600.

Änggard, E. 1994. Nitric oxide: mediator, murderer, and medicine. Lancet 343:1199–1206.

Baillie, G., and Houslay, M. 2005. Arrestin times for compartmentalized cAMP signalling and phosphodiesterase-4 enzymes. Curr Opin Cell Biol 17:129–134.

Bartholini, G., Stadler, H., and Lloyd, K. G. 1973. In E. Usdin and S. Snyder, eds., Frontiers in Catecholamine Research, p. 471. Elmsford, NY: Pergamon.

Birdsall, N. J., Hulme, E. C., and Stockton, J. M. 1983. Muscarinic receptor subclasses: allosteric interactions. Cold Spring Harbor Symp Quant Biol 48, pt. 1:53–56.

Boehm, S., and Kubista, H. 2002. Fine tuning of sympathetic transmitter release via ionotropic and metabotropic presynaptic receptors. Pharmacol Rev 54:43–99.

Brimblecombe, R. W. 1974. Drug Actions on Cholinergic Systems. Baltimore: University Park Press.

Broadley, K. J. 1996. Autonomic Pharmacology. London: Taylor and Francis.

Brown, J. H. P., and Taylor, P. 2006. Muscurinic receptor agonists and antogonists. In L. L. Brunton, J. S. Lazo, and K. L. Parker, eds., The Pharmacological Basis of Therapeutics, 11th ed., pp. 183–200. New York: McGraw Hill.

Brunton, L. L., Lazo, J. S., and Parker, K. L. 2006. The Pharmacologic Basis for Therapeutics, 11th ed. New York: McGraw Hill.

Chassaing, C., Dureng, G., Baissat, J., and Duchene-Marullaz, P. 1984. Pharmacological evidence for cardiac muscarinic receptor subtypes. Life Sci 35(17):1739–1745.

Cogswell, A. M., Johnson, P. J., and Adams, H. R. 1995. Evidence for endothelium-derived relaxing factor/nitric oxide in equine digital arteries. Am J Vet Res 56:1637–1641.

DeBiasi, M. 2002. Nicotinic mechanisms in the autonomic control of organ systems. J Neurobiol 53:568–579.

Ferguson, S., and Blakely, R. 2004. The choline transporter resurfaces: New roles for synaptic vesicles? Mol Interv 4:22–37.

Fetscher, C., Fleichman, M., Schmidt, M., Krege, S., and Michel, M. C. 2002. M_3 muscarinic receptors mediate contraction of human urinary bladder. Br J Pharmacol 136:641–643.

Freeman, R., and Miyawaki, E. 1993. The treatment of autonomic dysfunction. J Clin Neurophysiol 10:61–82.

Furchgott, R. F., and Zawadzki, J. V. 1980. The obligatory role of endothelial cells in the relaxation of arterial smooth muscle by acetylcholine. Nature 288:373–376.

Galligan, J. J. 2002. Pharmacology of synaptic transmission in the enteric nervous system. Curr Opin Pharmacol 2:623–629.

Gauthier, P., Nadeau, R. A., and de Champlain, J. 1974. Cardiovascular reactivity in the dog after chemical sympathectomy with 6-hydroxydopamine. Can J Physiol Pharmacol 52(3):590–601.

George, W. J., Busuttil, R. W., Paddock, R. J., White, L. A., and Ignarro, L. J. 1975. Opposing regulatory influences of cyclic guanosine monophosphate and cyclic adenosine monophosphate in the control of cardiac muscle contraction. Rec Adv Stud Cardiol Struc Metab 8:243–250.

Gilman, A. G. 1984. Guanine nucleotide-binding regulatory proteins and dual control of adenylate cyclase. J Clin Invest 73(1):1–4.

Goldberg, A. M., and Hanin, I., eds. 1976. Biology of Cholinergic Function. New York: Raven.

Hein, L., and Schmitt, J. P. 2003. α_1-Adrenoceptors in the heart: Friend or foe? J Mol Cell Cardiol 35:1183–1185.

Hokfelt, T., Broberger, C., Xu, Z. Q., Sergeyev, V., Ubink, R., and Diez, M. 2000. Neuropeptides: An overview. Neuropharmacology 39:1337–1356.

Horton, E. W. 1973. Prostaglandins at adrenergic nerve-endings. Br Med Bull 29(2):148–151.

Iverson, L. L. 1973. In E. Usdin and S. Snyder, eds., Frontiers in Catecholamine Research, p. 403. Elmsford, NY: Pergamon.

Iverson, L. L., Iverson, S. D., and Snyder, S. H. 1983. Handbook of Psychopharmacology, vol. 16, pp. 519–556. New York: Plenum.

Jahn, R., Lang, T., and Sudhof, T. 2003. Membrane fusion. Cell 112:519–533.

Kable, J. W., Murrin, L. C., and Bylund, D. B. 2000. In vivo gene modification elucidates subtype-specific functions of $\alpha(2)$-adrenergic receptors. J Pharmacol Exp Ther 293:1–7.

Kalsner, S. 1989. Cholinergic constriction in the general circulation and its role in coronary artery spasm. Circ Res 65:237–257.

Klein, R. L. 1973. In E. Usdin and S. Snyder, eds., Frontiers in Catecholamine Research, p. 423. Elmsford, NY: Pergamon.

Klinge, E., Fränkö, O., and Sjöstrand, N. O. 1978. Cholinergic and adrenergic innervation of the penis artery of the bull: transmitter concentrations and synaptic vesicles. Experientia 34(12):1624–1626.

Klinge, E., and Sjöstrand, N. O. 1974. Contraction and relaxation of the retractor penis muscle and the penile artery of the bull. Acta Physiol Scand Suppl 420:1–88.

Kohout, T. A., and Lefkowitz, R. J. 2003. Regulation of G protein-coupled receptor kinases and arrestins during receptor desensitization. Mol Pharmacol 63:9–18.

Lambert, D. G. 1993. Signal transduction: G proteins and second messengers. Br J Anaesthesia 71:86–95.

Lands, A. M., Arnold, A., McAuliff, J. P., Luduena, F. P., and Brown, T. G., Jr. 1967. Differentiation of receptor systems activated by sympathomimetic amines. Nature 214(88):597–598.

Lang, E., and Szilagyi, N. 1991. Significance and assessment of autonomic indices in cardiovascular reactions. Acta Physiol Hung 78:241–260.

Langrehr, J. M., Hoffman, R. A., Lancaster, J. R., and Simmons, R. L. 1993. Nitric oxide—a new endogenous immunomodulator. Transplantation Overview 55:1205–1212.

Levitzki, A., Marbach, I., and Bar-Sinai, A. 1993. The signal transduction between β-receptors and adenylyl cyclase. Life Sci 52:2093–2100.

Loewi, O. 1921. Pfluegers Arch Ges Physiol 189:239.

Low, P. A. 1993. Autonomic nervous system function. J Clin Neurophysiol 10:14–27.

Lowenstein, C. J., Dinerman, J. L., and Snyder, S. H. 1994. Nitric oxide: a physiologic messenger. Ann Intern Med 120:227–237.

Luetje, C. W. 2004. Getting past the asterisk: The subunit composition of presynaptic nicotinic receptors that modulate striatal dopamine release. Mol Pharmacol 65:1333–1335.

Ma, Y. C., and Huang, X. Y. 2002. Novel signaling pathways through the β-adrenergic receptors. Trends Cardiovasc Med 12:46–49.

Moran, N. C. 1973. In E. Usdin and S. Snyder, eds., Frontiers in Catecholamine Research, p. 291. Elmsford, NY: Pergamon.

Muscholl, E. 1973. In E. Usdin and S. Snyder, eds., Frontiers in Catecholamine Research, p. 537. Elmsford, NY: Pergamon.

Nawrath, H. 1976. Cyclic AMP and cyclic GMP may play opposing roles in influencing force of contraction in mammalian myocardium. Nature 262(5568):509–511.

Palczewski, K., Kumasaka, T., Hori, T., Behnke, C. A., Motoshima, H., Fox, B. A., Le Trong, I., Teler, D. C., Okada, T., Stenkamp, R. E., Yamamoto, M., and Miyano, M. 2000. Crystal structure of rhodopsin: A G protein-coupled receptor. Science 289:739–745.

Parker, J. L., and Adams, H. R. 1993. Selective inhibition of endothelium-dependent vasodilator capacity by *E. coli* endotoxemia. Circ Res 72:539–551.

Philipp, M., and Hein, L. 2004. Adrenergic receptor knockout mice: Distinct functions of 9 receptor subtypes. Pharmacol Ther 101:65–74.

Rall, T. W. 1972. Role of adenosine 3′,5′-monophosphate (cyclic AMP) in actions of catecholamines. Pharm Rev 24(2):399–409.

Robertshaw, D. 1980. Handb Exp Pharmacol 53:345.

Robidoux, J., Martin, T. L., and Collins, S. 2004. β-Adrenergic receptors and regulation of energy expenditure: A family affair. Annu Rev Pharmacol Toxicol 44:297–323.

Robison, G. A. 1971. Cyclic AMP. New York: Academic Press.

Robison, G. A., Butcher, R. W., and Sutherland, E. W. 1967. Adenyl cyclase as an adrenergic receptor. Ann NY Acad Sci 139(3):703–723.

Salminen, O., Murphy, K. L., McIntosh, J. M., Drago, J., Marks, M. J., Collins, A. C., and Grady, S. R. 2004. Subunit composition and pharmacology of two classes of striatal presynaptic nicotinic acetylcholine receptors mediating dopamine release in mice. Mol Pharmacol 65(6):1526–1535.

Samir Amer, M., and Kreighbaum, W. E. 1975. Cyclic nucleotide phosphodiesterases: properties, activators, inhibitors, structure-activity relationships, and possible role in drug development. J Pharm Sci 64(1):1–37.

Saper, C. B. 2002. The central autonomic nervous system: Conscious visceral perception and autonomic pattern generation. Annu Rev Neurosci 25:433–469.

Schulz, R., and Triggle, C. R. 1994. Role of NO in vascular smooth muscle and cardiac muscle function. TIPS—July 15:255–259.

Schwinn, D. A. 1993. Adrenoceptors as models for G protein–coupled receptors: structure, function and regulation. Br J Anaesthesia 71:77–85.

Shields, R. W., Jr. 1993. Functional anatomy of the autonomic nervous system. J Clin Neurophysiol 10:2–13.

Shore, P. A. 1972. Transport and storage of biogenic amines. Ann Rev Pharm 12:209–226.

Smyth, E. M., Burke, A., and Fitzgerald, G. A. 2006. Lipid-derived autacoids: eicosanoids and platelet-activating factor. In L. Brunton, J. S. Lazo, and K. L. Parker, eds., The Pharmacological Basis of Therapeutics, 11th ed. New York: McGraw Hill.

Starke, K., Taube H. D., and Browski, E. 1977. Presynaptic receptor systems in catecholaminergic transmission. Biochem Pharm 26(4): 259–268.

Sutherland, E. W., and Rall, T. W. 1960. In J. R. Vane, F. E. W. Wolstenholme, and M. O'Conner, eds., Adrenergic Mechanisms, p. 295. Boston: Little, Brown.

U'Prichard, D. C., and Snyder, S. H. 1979. Distinct alpha-noradrenergic receptors differentiated by binding and physiological relationships. Life Sci 24(1):79–88.

Vulliet, P. R., Langan, T. A., and Weiner, N. 1980. Tyrosine hydroxylase: a substrate of cyclic AMP–dependent protein kinase. Proc Natl Acad Sci USA 77(1):92–96.

Wang, Z., Shi, H., and Wang, H. 2004. Functional M_3 muscarinic acetylcholine receptors in mammalian hearts. Br J Pharmacol 142:395–408.

Waser, P. G., ed. 1975. Cholinergic Mechanisms. New York: Raven.

Wess, J. 2004. Muscarinic acetylcholine receptor knockout mice: Novel phenotypes and clinical implication. Annu Rev Pharmcol Toxicol 44:423–450.

Westfall, T. C. 2004. Prejunctional effects of neuropeptide Y and its role as a cotransmitter. Exp Pharmacol 162:138–183.

Westfall, T. C., and Westfall, D. P. 2006. Neurotransmission: The autonomic and somatic nervous systems. In L. L. Brunton, J. S. Lazo, and K. L. Parker, eds., The Pharmacological Basis of Therapeutics, 11th ed., pp. 137–200. New York: McGraw Hill.

CHAPTER

6

ADRENERGIC AGONISTS AND ANTAGONISTS

H. RICHARD ADAMS

Amine substances that cause physiologic responses similar to those evoked by the endogenous adrenergic mediators epinephrine and norepinephrine are known as adrenergic drugs (Westfall and Westfall 2006). They are referred to as sympathomimetic agents because their pharmacologic effects mimic sympathetic nervous system activity. Sympathetic neurons and affiliated receptors of innervated cells are depicted in Figure 6.1. Most clinically relevant adrenergic agonists exert their principal pharmacodynamic actions through receptor activation. Just the opposite, adrenergic receptor antagonists prevent receptor activation and thereby reduce sympathetic activity. "Sympatholytic," "adrenolytic," and "adrenergic blocking" are terms used to describe pharmacologic effects that, in general, simulate a decrease in adrenergic nerve activity. These terms are not synonymous, and they have been used to describe different types of antiadrenergic actions, as will be discussed later in this chapter.

ADRENERGIC (SYMPATHOMIMETIC) DRUGS

Pharmacologic effects of sympathomimetic amines are mediated by activation of adrenergic receptors of effector cells innervated by the sympathetic nervous system (Fig. 6.1). Noninnervated adrenoceptors also are present in some cell types. In general, therefore, pharmacologic effects of adrenergic agonists can be equated to physiologic effects resulting from increased sympathoadrenal discharge. A thorough understanding of basic adrenoceptor concepts is important to the future practitioner because this

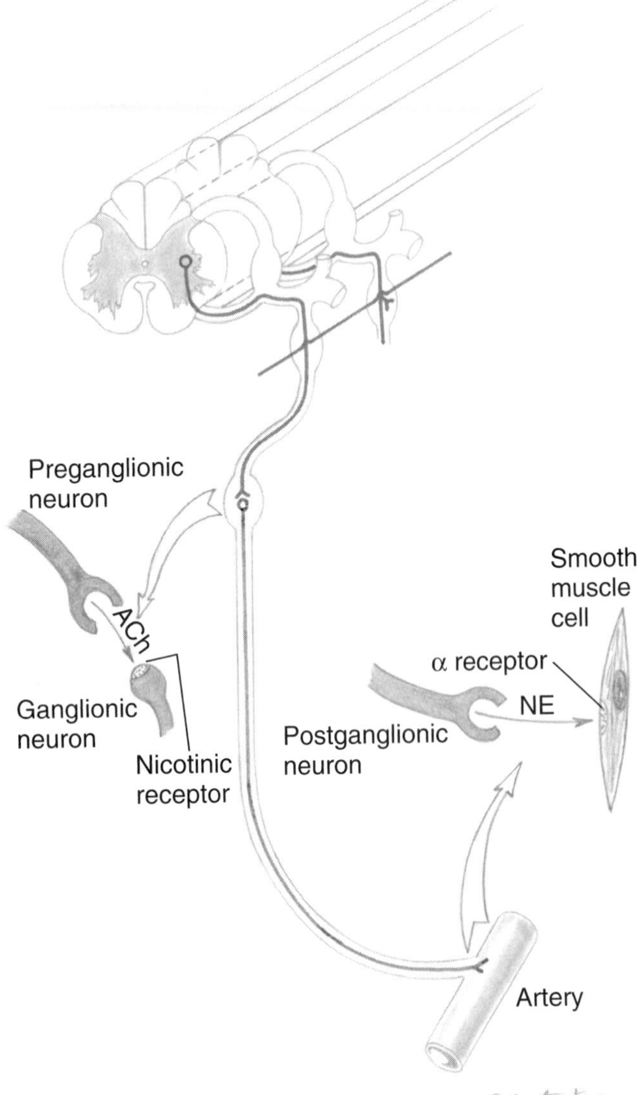

FIG. 6.1 Anatomical relationships of sympathetic neuronal outflow tracts and affiliated receptors of innervated cells. Sympathetic preganglionic axons exit the thoracolumbar region of the spinal cord and synapse with ganglionic neurons in an adjacent ganglion, or pass through the latter to synapse with a neuron within a distant ganglion (shown). The preganglionic axon terminal releases the neurotransmitter acetylcholine (ACh), which activates nicotinic cholinergic receptors on the ganglionic neuron body. The resulting stimulation of the ganglionic neuron promotes release of the neurotransmitter norepinephrine (NE) from the axon terminal at the postganglionic sympathetic neuroeffector junction at blood vessels (shown) or other tissues innervated by sympathetic neurons. NE activates α- (shown) or β-adrenergic receptors present on cells innervated by the sympathetic division of the autonomic nervous system. Preganglionic fibers are dark gray; postganglionic fibers are light gray. Drawn by Dr. Gheorghe M. Constantinescu, University of Missouri.

information has direct application to the clinical use of all adrenergic agonists and antagonists (Adams 1984).

ADRENERGIC RECEPTORS. Adrenergic receptors (i.e., adrenoceptors) are macromolecular structures localized on or within the surface membrane of cells innervated by adrenergic neurons (and certain noninnervated cells). The basic physiologic function of the adrenergic receptor is to recognize and interact with the endogenous adrenergic mediators norepinephrine and epinephrine. This interaction triggers a series of complex intracellular events that yield a characteristic change in effector cell activity.

A classic simplification of the complex field of adrenergic receptors was formulated by Ahlquist in 1948; he proposed the existence of two basic types of adrenergic receptors, which he designated as alpha (α) and beta (β). This classification system is based on the relative potencies of several adrenergic agonists to elicit excitatory and inhibitory effects in different tissues.

STRUCTURE-ACTIVITY RELATIONSHIPS. Several factors have complicated determination of optimal structural requirements for adrenergic drugs. Most adrenergic drugs affect both α and β receptors, and the ratio of α and β activity varies tremendously between drugs and species. Some adrenergic agents cause indirect effects mediated by release of endogenous norepinephrine. Despite these various and often conflicting interrelationships, some general and some rather specific aspects of the structure-activity relationship of sympathomimetic amines have been determined.

The basis for sympathetic-like activity of various drugs depends upon the similarity of their chemical structure to that of the endogenous adrenergic mediators norepinephrine and epinephrine. The nucleus of this chemical structure, β-phenylethylamine, is a benzene ring and an ethylamine side chain. Substitution may be made on the aromatic ring, on the α and β carbons of the side chain, and on the amine moiety. (The α and β nomenclature of the carbon atoms represents organic chemical terminology and has no relationship to the α- and β-receptor classification.)

The chemical structures and related pharmacologic characteristics of several adrenergic drugs are summarized in Table 6.1. Epinephrine, norepinephrine, dopamine, and isoproterenol have a hydroxyl group on both the 3 and 4

TABLE 6.1 Chemical structures and related pharmacologic activities of some commonly used sympathomimetic amines

Drug	Ring (3 6 / 4 1 / 3 2)	β CH	α CH	NH	Activity	Clinical use
β-phenylethylamine	. . .	H	H	H	. . .	. . .
β-phenylethanolamine	. . .	OH	H	H	. . .	. . .
Catecholamines						
Dopamine	3-OH, 4-OH	H	H	H	α, $β_1$, D	P, C, K
Norepinephrine	3-OH, 4-OH	OH	H	H	α, $β_1$	P, C
Epinephrine	3-OH, 4-OH	OH	H	CH_3	α, β	P, C, A, B
Isoproterenol	3-OH,4-OH	OH	H	$CH(CH_3)_2$	β	C, B
Noncatecholamines						
Metaraminol	3-OH	OH	CH_3	H	α	P
Phenylephrine	3-OH	OH	H	CH_3	α	P, Rb
Tyramine	4-OH	H	H	H	I	. . .
Hydroxyamphetamine	4-OH	H	CH_3	H	I	CNS
Amphetamine	. . .	H	CH_3	H	I	CNS
Methamphetamine	. . .	H	CH_3	CH_3	I	CNS
Ephedrine	. . .	OH	CH_3	CH_3	I, α, β	P, C, CNS

Note: α = α receptor; β = β receptor; A = allergic reactions; B = bronchodilator ($β_2$ receptor); C = cardiac stimulation ($β_1$ receptor); CNS = central nervous system excitation; D = dopamine may interact with α, $β_1$, and dopaminergic receptors; I = indirect-acting, causes release of endogenous norepinephrine that acts on α and β receptors; K = renal vasodilation (dopaminergic receptors); P = pressor activity; Rb = reflex bradycardia from pressor activation of baroreceptor-vagal reflex.

positions of the benzene ring. Because 3,4-dihydroxybenzene is also known as catechol, sympathomimetic amines containing this nucleus are termed catecholamines. In general, the catechol nucleus is required for maximum α and β potencies. Removal of one or both hydroxyl groups from the aromatic ring especially reduces β activity; e.g., phenylephrine is identical in structure to epinephrine except for the lack of one hydroxyl group on the ring (Table 6.1). Phenylephrine is almost exclusively an α agonist, whereas epinephrine is a mixed α-β agonist. Substitution of a ring hydroxyl group similarly reduces potency and may actually yield an antagonist (i.e., an adrenergic blocking drug such as the β blocker dichloroisoproterenol).

Substitution on the β-carbon atom of the side chain results in less active central actions in relation to peripheral effects. Substitution on the α-carbon atom yields a compound that is not susceptible to oxidation by monoamine oxidase (MAO).

Alkyl substitutions on the amino moiety affect the ratio of α- and β-agonistic properties. Within limits, increasing the size of the aliphatic substitution increases β activity. Epinephrine (*N*-methylnorepinephrine) is a more potent β agonist than norepinephrine. Isoproterenol (*N*-isopropylnorepinephrine) is a more potent β agonist than epinephrine or norepinephrine. Naturally occurring norepinephrine and epinephrine are in the levo configuration at the β-carbon atom. Dextrorotatory substitution on the β carbon yields the many times less potent *d*-isomers.

ADRENERGIC RECEPTOR SUBTYPES: PHARMACOLOGIC APPLICATIONS. Historically, the principal events responsible for information transmission across noradrenergic neuroeffector junctions were believed to include only the following: biosynthesis and storage of norepinephrine in the neuron terminal; exocytotic discharge of norepinephrine from the neuron; activation of effector cell α- or β-adrenergic receptors by released norepinephrine; and active "reuptake" of a portion of the free norepinephrine back into the axon terminal, thereby decreasing transmitter availability at the postjunctional receptors. We now know, however, that α- and β-adrenergic receptors of effector cells exist as subclasses and, furthermore, that several types of receptor-linked mechanisms operate within the adrenergic nerve endings themselves (Langer 1980; Adams 1984; Breit et al. 2004).

Prejunctional α Receptors. The α-adrenergic receptors on the sympathetic neuron are believed to be important physiologically and pharmacologically; they subserve an autoinhibitory regulation of norepinephrine release mechanisms. The physiologic role of α-receptor prejunctional events is envisioned as a local servomechanism through which norepinephrine can govern its own release once a threshold concentration of transmitter has been exceeded within the junction (Saeed et al. 1982).

Prejunctional β Receptors. Epinephrine also can activate the prejunctional autoinhibitory α receptors, with potency about equal to that of norepinephrine. Interestingly, however, low concentrations of epinephrine actually accelerate norepinephrine release. This facilitatory action is shared by the β agonist isoproterenol and prevented by β-blocking drugs. These findings indicate that noradrenergic nerve endings possess β receptors that subserve a stimulatory effect on transmitter release mechanisms, an action opposite to that of the prejunctional α receptor.

Norepinephrine itself seems to have little influence on the prejunctional β-autostimulatory receptors, perhaps because this receptor population is more representative of β_2 rather than β_1 subtype. Thus the α-controlled autoinhibitory cycle probably dominates during usual communication between neuron and effector cell. A model of noradrenergic neurohumoral transmission incorporating prejunctional α and β receptors is presented in Figure 6.2, along with representative effector cells, their prototypical receptor classes, and associated physiologic responses (Adams 1984).

Adrenergic Receptor Classification. The original differentiation of adrenergic receptors into the two main classes, α and β, was based mainly on the relative potencies of the agonists norepinephrine, epinephrine, and isoproterenol in eliciting excitatory or inhibitory effects in a series of tissues (e.g., heart, vasculature, lungs) (Ahlquist 1948). Excitatory responses were generally designated as α-receptor events, and, for the most part, inhibitory responses were designated as β-receptor events. The excitatory β receptors of the heart represented an important exception to this rule and pointed toward different types of β receptors, named β_1 and β_2. Later, α-receptors were likewise separated into α_1 and α_2 subtypes. Since then,

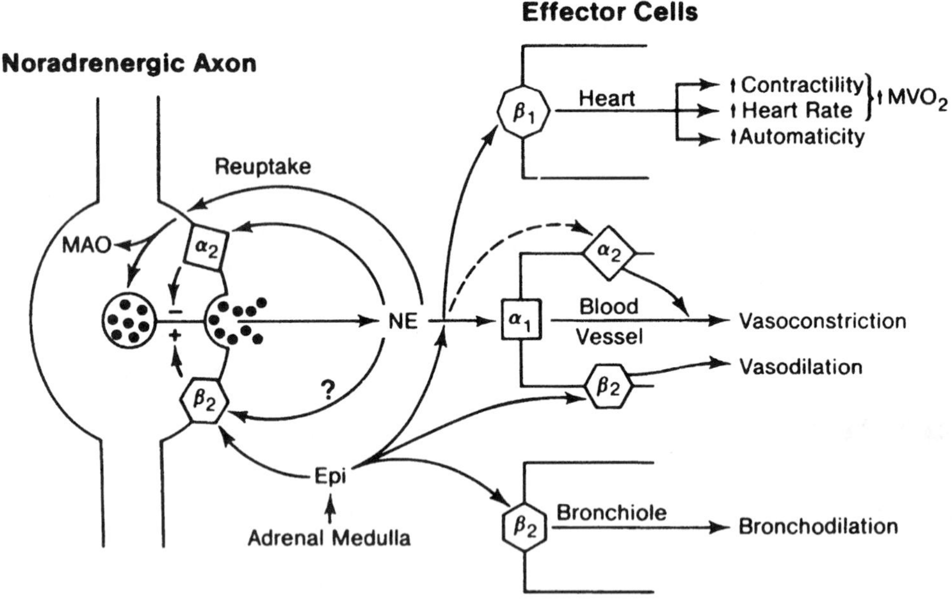

FIG. 6.2 Schematic diagram of peripheral noradrenergic neuroeffector junctions with a model axon terminal varicosity on the left and typical effector cells on the right. The predominant adrenoceptor subtypes and associated physiologic responses of the heart, blood vessel, and bronchiole are depicted. Norepinephrine (NE) released from the neuron can interact postjunctionally with innervated α_1 or β_1 receptors of effector cells and perhaps overflow (dashed line) to other nearby postjunctional receptors. NE also can activate prejunctional α receptors (α_2 subtype) to inhibit further release of NE. NE is removed from the junctional cleft by diffusion, extraneuronal uptake, and active uptake (reuptake) into the neuron, where it is metabolized by monoamine oxidase (MAO) or reincorporated into storage vesicles. Prejunctional β receptors (β_2 subtype) subserve a facilitatory effect on NE release, but it is questionable (?) whether NE itself activates this β_2-autostimulatory feedback loop. NE also has little β_2-agonist activity in blood vessels or bronchioles, whereas epinephrine (Epi) can activate all types of α and β adrenoceptors. MVO_2 = myocardial oxygen demand (Adams 1984).

virtually all receptor types have been categorized into many receptor subclasses with somewhat different pharmacodynamic profiles. This text will focus on the primary receptor types until clinical relevance has been determined for the plethora of receptor subtypes now discovered (Morimoto et al. 2004; Osborne et al. 2004; Robidoux et al. 2004; Westfall and Westfall 2006).

β_1-β_2 Adrenergic Receptor Subtypes. Partly because of the potent β-stimulatory properties of norepinephrine in some tissue (e.g., the heart), but not others (e.g., the lungs), it was suggested that β receptors actually comprised a heterogeneous population of two distinct subtypes: β_1 and β_2 (Lands et al. 1967). Many tissues contain both β_1 and β_2 receptors in various ratios, depending on species and other variables (Sun et al. 2002). One subtype usually dominates and provides the tissue and organ with their functional classification as being under either β_1- or β_2-receptor control. A compilation of the predominant β-receptor subtype in several tissues is included in Table 5.1.

Cardiac β_1 Receptors. The functionally prevalent β receptor in the myocardium of most if not all mammalian species is the β_1 subtype. These receptors are activated in the following order of potency: isoproterenol > epinephrine > norepinephrine. Activation of cardiac β_1 receptors leads to the characteristic sympathomimetic response of the heart as schematized in Figure 6.3. In brief, this entails positive inotropic effects (increased contractility), positive chronotropic effects (increased heart rate), positive dromotropic effects (accelerated conduction of the cardiac impulse), and emergence of latent pacemaker activity. Increased heart rate and contractility lead in turn to increased myocardial oxygen demand and metabolic coronary vasodilation.

Pulmonary and Vascular Smooth Muscle β_2 Receptors. The β-adrenergic receptors of the pulmonary airways and peripheral vascular beds are mainly the β_2 subtype (Fig. 6.2). These receptors are activated potently by isoproterenol and epinephrine but quite poorly by norepinephrine. The β_2-pulmonary receptors subserve relaxation of bronchiolar smooth muscle and its accompanying bronchodilation, leading to an improvement in airway conductance. Vascular smooth muscle β_2 receptors are present in various tissues, where they mediate vasodilation and reduced vascular resistance. Although there is some

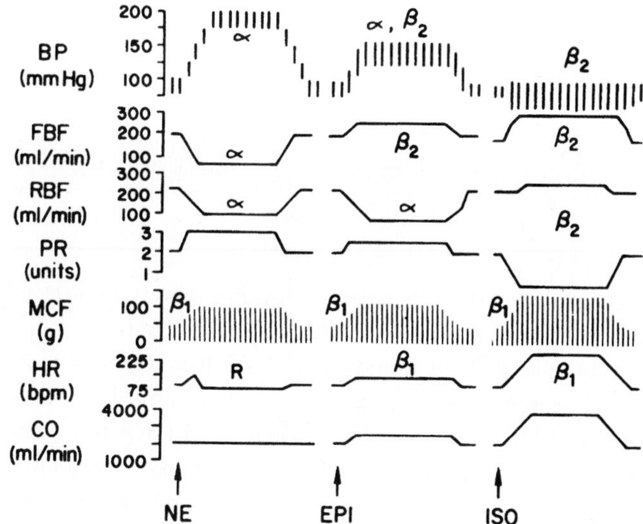

FIG. 6.3 Cardiovascular effects of intravenously administered norepinephrine (NE), epinephrine (Epi), and isoproterenol (ISO) in a dog. Schematic representations of effects of equivalent doses of these amines on blood pressure (BP), femoral blood flow (FBF), renal blood flow (RBF), peripheral vascular resistance (PR), myocardial contractile force (MCF), heart rate (HR), and cardiac output (CO). α = response mediated primarily by α-adrenergic receptor; β = response mediated primarily by β-adrenergic receptor (β_1 or β_2 subtype); R = reflex mediated. Characteristics of cardiovascular excitation evoked by these agents are due to differences in their α-β agonistic properties (Table 6.2). See text for explanation of each response.

uncertainty, most β_2-vascular receptors are probably noninnervated and, as with the pulmonary β_2 receptors, depend mainly on circulating epinephrine for activation and basal adrenergic tone (Fig. 6.2).

α_1-α_2 Receptor Subtypes. Alpha receptors also can be divided into two distinct subpopulations: α_1 and α_2. This nomenclature began with the realization that the prejunctional α-receptor population responded to drugs somewhat differently than did the usual α receptors of effector cells. This led to classification of the typical effector cell α receptor as α_1 subtype, while the nerve terminal receptor was designated as α_2 (Fig. 6.2).

Alpha$_2$ receptors are not restricted anatomically to neuronal elements. They also are located on some noninnervated cell types, e.g., thrombocytes. Moreover, α_2 receptors also share certain tissue and functions with the α_1 subgroup. Pressor responses mediated by norepinephrine and epinephrine, e.g., involve activation of α_1- and α_2-receptor types in vascular smooth muscle. The α_1 receptor represents the innervated vascular receptors, whereas the α_2

TABLE 6.2 Adrenergic receptor activation by catecholamines

Receptor Type	Tissue	Response	Potency of Agonists
α	Blood vessels	Vasconstriction	Epinephrine > norepinephrine >>> isoproterenol
β_1	Heart	Positive inotropic and chronotropic effects	Isoproterenol > epinephrine ≧ norepinephrine
β_2	Blood vessels	Vasodilation	Isoproterenol > epinephrine >>> norepinephrine

Note: > = greater than; ≧ = greater than or equal; >>> = many times greater.

type in this tissue is believed to localize predominantly in extrasynaptic regions of vascular smooth muscle cells. Endothelial cells of blood vessels also have α_2 receptors, which subserve release of endothelium-derived relaxing factor (EDRF) leading to vasodilation. EDRF has been identified as nitric oxide or a closely related compound that releases nitric oxide (see Chapter 5; Lowenstein et al. 1994; Änggard 1994).

Based on the foregoing summary of α_1-α_2 and β_1-β_2 receptor subtypes and respective tissue responses, it should be apparent that all adrenergic drugs do not necessarily produce identical effects. Their pharmacologic profiles vary depending upon their basic chemical structure and resulting activities as α, β, or mixed α-β agonists. Nevertheless, sympathomimetic amines exhibit many similar pharmacodynamic properties. Therefore, only representative adrenergic drugs will be examined in detail; other agents will be compared in relation to differences they may exhibit in agonistic properties (i.e., activity at α or β receptors) and in mechanisms of action (i.e., direct- or indirect-acting sympathomimetic activity).

It also is important to realize that the α_1-α_2 and β_1-β_2 classification of receptors is an oversimplification of receptor subtypes as mentioned previously. There are multiple subtype divisions of α_1, α_2, β_1, and β_2 receptors (Alberts 1993; Feldman 1993; Barnes 1993; Westfall and Westfall 2006). However, the clinical relevance in veterinary medicine of adrenergic receptor classifications beyond α_1-α_2 and β_1-β_2 remains to be clarified.

CATECHOLAMINES

Catecholamines are direct-acting sympathomimetic amines. They activate receptors of effector cells; therefore, adrenergic nerves are not required for their effects.

EPINEPHRINE, NOREPINEPHRINE, AND ISOPROTERENOL. Epinephrine (adrenaline) and norepinephrine (noradrenaline, levarterenol, arterenol) are endogenous biogenic amines; isoproterenol (isopropylarterenol) is not found in the body but is chemically synthesized. Subtle differences in the pharmacologic effects of structurally related adrenergic drugs can be demonstrated by comparing cardiovascular effects of these three agents, as shown schematically in Figure 6.3.

Different cardiovascular responses seen with epinephrine, norepinephrine, and isoproterenol in Figure 6.3 are due to differences in the ratios of their α- and β-agonistic properties. Classification of adrenergic receptors in the heart and blood vessels, related effects, and the order of potency of epinephrine, norepinephrine, and isoproterenol are shown in Table 6.2.

Norepinephrine, because of its α-agonist properties, activates the α-vascular receptors, resulting in intense vasoconstriction; peripheral resistance increases and femoral and renal blood flows decrease (Fig. 6.3).

Although epinephrine is a potent α stimulant, it also is very active at β receptors. Beta$_2$ receptors in blood vessels subserve vasodilation. In response to epinephrine, vasoconstriction occurs in vascular beds that have predominantly α receptors (e.g., abdominal viscera); however, vasodilation can occur in beds that contain β_2 receptors (e.g., skeletal muscle). Blood flow increases in areas in response to regional vasodilation (e.g., femoral flow) but decreases if vasoconstriction dominates (e.g., renal flow) (Fig. 6.3).

Because isoproterenol is a selective β agonist, it causes vasodilation, fall in diastolic blood pressure, decrease in peripheral resistance, and increase in blood flow to areas containing β receptors (e.g., femoral blood flow). The renal vasculature has few β receptors and is therefore little affected by isoproterenol (Fig. 6.3).

The heart is activated by epinephrine, norepinephrine, and isoproterenol (Fig. 6.3). Isoproterenol is the most potent of the three and causes a relatively greater increase in myocardial contractile force, heart rate, and cardiac output than the similarly acting epinephrine. Norepinephrine also increases myocardial contractile force, but bradycardia occurs at the peak pressor effect of this amine. This is due to an increase in vagal tone reflexly instigated by the pronounced norepinephrine-induced increase in mean blood pressure. Norepinephrine-mediated peripheral vasoconstriction may decrease venous return so cardiac output does not increase, although the heart is activated.

These examples demonstrate differences in selective cardiovascular effects of these closely related catecholamines. Nevertheless, it should be apparent that all three agents elicit the same basic result, a net increase in cardiovascular activity.

Pharmacologic Effects

Blood Pressure. Norepinephrine administered intravenously either by slow infusion or bolus injection causes a dose-related increase in systolic and diastolic blood pressures due to bodywide vasoconstriction. Mean blood pressure increases accordingly; little change is seen in pulse pressure.

Slow intravenous (IV) infusion of small amounts of epinephrine usually causes a fall in diastolic blood pressure that may or may not be accompanied by a slight increase in systolic pressure. This response is due to regional vasodilation (β_2-receptor–mediated), which causes a decrease in peripheral resistance. However, a bolus IV injection of a large amount of epinephrine (e.g., 1–3 µg/kg) causes a pronounced increase in blood pressure that is as remarkable as that produced by norepinephrine. It should be appreciated that epinephrine is an extremely potent pressor agent. This pressor response depends upon vasoconstriction, myocardial stimulation, and tachycardia. Bradycardia can occur at the peak pressor response as a result of reflex vagal activity. A depressor effect may be observed after the pressor response to a large dose of epinephrine. This secondary response is related to residual activation of β_2 receptors in blood vessels.

Following a single bolus injection of norepinephrine or epinephrine, the pressor response lasts for several minutes, then gradually decreases and returns to normal within 5–10 minutes. Isoproterenol increases pulse pressure predominantly by lowering diastolic pressure. This effect is due to β_2-receptor–mediated vasodilation.

Vascular Smooth Muscle. This type of tissue can contain both α_1- and α_2-receptor subtypes (which subserve vasoconstriction) and β_2 receptors (which subserve vasodilation). Epinephrine and norepinephrine are very potent constrictors of cutaneous and mucosal blood vessels in mammalian species. Adrenergic receptors in these vessels are almost exclusively α. Intense vasoconstriction, increased vascular resistance, and decreased blood flow occur in these regions in response to norepinephrine and epinephrine. This is often seen as a blanching type response in skin or mucosal membranes.

Since epinephrine is a more potent α agonist than norepinephrine, it is 2–10 times more active than norepinephrine in constricting cutaneous and mucosal vessels. Smaller arterioles and precapillary sphincters are particularly responsive to the vasoconstrictor catecholamines. They are active regardless of whether they are applied topically to blood vessels, sprayed upon mucosal surfaces, injected perivascularly, or administered systemically. Isoproterenol has little if any effect on cutaneous and mucosal vessels, because of the relative lack of β receptors in these tissues.

The renal vasculature has predominantly α receptors. Epinephrine and norepinephrine cause vasoconstriction in the kidney and a generalized increase in vascular resistance in this organ. Renal blood flow is decreased even in the presence of an elevated systemic blood pressure (Fig. 6.3). Large doses of α-agonistic catecholamines may actually induce a functional renal shutdown caused by decreased perfusion of the kidney. During this period, urinary output is substantially decreased from lowered glomerular filtration rate.

Isoproterenol has little effect on renal arteries because of the small number of β receptors in kidney vasculature. However, direct injection of the drug into the renal artery increases renal blood flow. In addition, there are β_1 receptors in the kidney, which upon activation cause a release of renin into the circulation for angiotensin formation.

Mesenteric arteries are constricted by norepinephrine and epinephrine as a result of activation of α receptors. Mesenteric arterial resistance is markedly increased and splanchnic blood flow decreases proportionately. In some circumstances, i.e., with small doses, epinephrine may cause slight vasodilation of splanchnic arteries because of the presence of β_2 receptors.

Skeletal muscle blood vessels have both α and β receptors. Vasoconstriction or vasodilation can be induced, depending upon the α- and β-agonistic profiles of a vasostimulatory amine. Norepinephrine, because of its relative lack of effect on β-vascular receptors, elicits vasoconstriction in skeletal muscles caused by activation of α receptors. Vascular resistance increases and blood flow decreases proportionately.

Beta receptors in skeletal muscle blood vessels are more sensitive to epinephrine than are the α receptors. Therefore, small amounts of epinephrine actually cause a decrease in vascular resistance and an increase in blood flow to voluntary muscles through vasodilation. However, large doses of epinephrine cause vasoconstriction in skeletal muscles from the α-receptor–mediated contraction overriding β-mediated relaxation. If α receptors are blocked, the response to epinephrine is converted to vasodilation from unmasking of the β effect. If a β blocker is used, the α-mediated constrictor effects of epinephrine are accentuated.

Isoproterenol causes relaxation of skeletal muscle blood vessels, increased blood flow to voluntary muscle masses, and decreased vascular resistance in these structures caused by activation of the vascular β receptors. Since isoproterenol has little effect on α receptors, β blockade abolishes the vasodilator effect of isoproterenol but does not convert the response to vasoconstriction.

Coronary arteries dilate in response to catecholamines (isoproterenol > epinephrine ≥ norepinephrine). The major portions of this vasodilator response are secondary to increased myocardial contractility and heart rate and resulting metabolic demands of the heart. Alpha receptors that subserve vasoconstriction can be demonstrated in the coronary vasculature; however, they are more prevalent in larger vessels than in smaller nutrient arteries. Beta receptors dominate, causing vasodilation and increased coronary blood flow in response to catecholamines. Studies with isolated vessels suggest that coronary receptors are either the β_1 subtype (Cornish and Miller 1975) or the β_2 subtype (Sun et al. 2002), while in vivo studies indicate the β_2 subtype (Moreland and Bohr 1984). This is different from most other vasodilator β receptors that have generally been characterized as β_2, irrespective of in vivo or in vitro setting.

Cerebral arteries are less responsive to adrenergic agonists than most other vascular beds. This is compatible with the concept that cerebral blood flow, like coronary blood flow, is controlled principally by local metabolic needs rather than by the nervous system. Nevertheless, both α-vasoconstrictor and β-vasodilator receptors can be demonstrated in cerebral blood vessels.

Vascular Mechanisms. Mechanical function of a vascular smooth muscle cell depends upon the availability of free intracellular Ca^{++} in the vicinity of contractile proteins. Norepinephrine and epinephrine produce vascular contraction by initially causing release of an intracellular (sequestered) source of Ca^{++} to the contractile proteins in response to activation of α_1 receptors. The signal-transduction mechanism linking α_1 receptors to vasoconstriction involves the G protein, phospholipase C, and inositol triphosphate pathway (Brodde and Michel 1992).

Cyclic adenosine 3′,5′-monophosphate (cAMP) is increased in response to β_2-receptor activation; this mechanism utilizes the stimulatory G protein (G_s) and adenylyl cyclase pathway (Feldman 1993; Schwinn 1993; Levitzki et al. 1993) (Fig. 5.9).

Myocardial Effects. Isoproterenol, epinephrine, and norepinephrine are potent myocardial stimulants. They increase the strength of myocardial contractile force and accelerate heart rate. These changes represent direct effects that are not dependent upon changes in venous return (preload), afterload, or other hemodynamic variables. Contractile and rate effects of catecholamines are mediated via direct activation of β receptors of the myocardial and pacemaker cells. Myocardial β receptors are subtyped predominantly as β_1. Isoproterenol is 10–20 times more active in the heart than epinephrine; norepinephrine is somewhat less potent than epinephrine.

The increase in myocardial contractility (positive inotropic effect) seen with each of the three agents is produced in both atrial and ventricular muscles. The positive inotropism in the whole heart is characterized by more rapid and forcible systolic ejection. The rate of pressure changes in the ventricular chambers is increased. The systolic interval is shortened and diastolic relaxation takes place more quickly. Oxygen consumption is accelerated to a relatively greater extent than the heart work is increased. Therefore, cardiac efficiency is sacrificed at the expense of absolute increase in myocardial contractility produced by catecholamines.

Acceleration of heart rate (positive chronotropism) induced by catecholamines is due to changes in the automaticity of pacemaker cells. The spontaneous depolarization process in the sinoatrial node cells is accelerated; velocity of the action potential is enhanced in these and other conduction system cells. Purkinje fibers are similarly affected by epinephrine and norepinephrine. Latent or normally inactive pacemaker cells are activated by these agents; they become more excitable and fire more easily or even spontaneously.

Norepinephrine, epinephrine, and isoproterenol increase myocardial irritability, resulting in serious tachyarrhythmias, especially in sensitized animals or with large doses. This can be partially blocked by an α blocker (Benfry 1993). However, pure α agonists such as phenylephrine and methoxamine are weak arrhythmogenic agents. Also, a β blocker such as propranolol is more active than an α blocker in decreasing the arrhythmias evoked by epinephrine and norepinephrine. Certain halogenated anesthetics (halothane, chloroform) increase the sensitivity of the heart to cardiac rhythm irregularities induced by catecholamines.

Bradycardia often occurs during the peak pressor response seen after administration of epinephrine or norepinephrine to intact animals. This can be blocked by vagotomy or atropine; it is dependent upon the hypertensive response causing an increase in vagal discharge via the baroreceptor reflex mechanisms. It is usually more pronounced with norepinephrine than with epinephrine because of the relatively greater increase in mean blood pressure seen with the former. Tachycardia is invariably produced by isoproterenol.

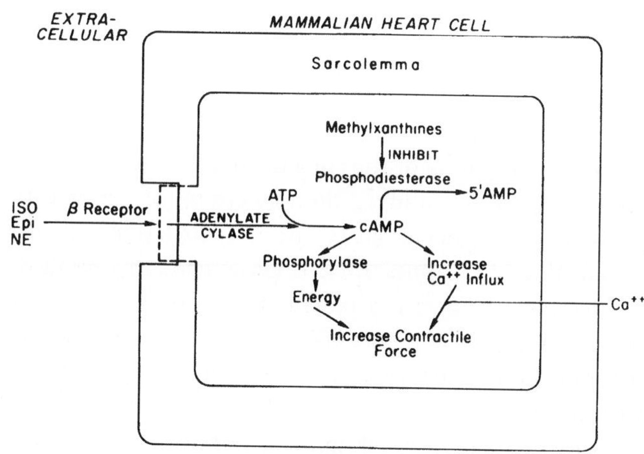

FIG. 6.4 Representation of proposed involvement of cyclic adenosine monophosphate (cAMP) in the myocardial effects of catecholamines. ISO = isoproterenol; Epi = epinephrine; NE = norepinephrine; ATP = adenosine triphosphate; 5′AMP = 5-adenosine monophosphate. The intracellular receptor for cAMP is protein kinase A, which phosphorylates different cellular substrates, resulting in changes in cell function. The stimulatory G protein (Gs) links the β-receptor recognition site to the catalytic component of adenylyl (adenylate) cyclase; see Fig. 5.9. Phosphorylase represents this and other biochemical reactions influenced by cAMP (see text).

Myocardial Mechanisms. In a heart muscle cell, contractile Ca^{++} is believed to originate in part from superficial sarcolemmal sites. Calcium bound at these sites is in rapid equilibrium with Ca^{++} within the extracellular space (Langer 1974; Parker and Adams 1977). Ca^{++} influx from superficial sites links membrane excitation (i.e., the cardiac action potential) to contraction of the myofibers. Catecholamines enhance the influx of Ca^{++} into the myocardial cell, due to increased intracellular concentrations of cAMP.

Activation of the cardiac β_1 receptor by epinephrine, norepinephrine, and isoproterenol increases the activity of a G_s-protein–linked adenylyl cyclase (Brodde and Michel 1992; Feldman 1993). This enzyme catalyzes the conversion of adenosine triphosphate (ATP) to cAMP. Cyclic AMP causes an increased Ca^{++} influx through the slow Ca^{++} channels of the sarcolemma, resulting in increased availability of Ca^{++} at the contractile proteins (Watanabe and Besch 1974). Cyclic cAMP activates protein kinase A, which phosphorylates various substrates, culminating in changes in cellular functions responsible for positive inotropic and chronotropic responses to β_1-receptor activation.

Several drugs alter the cAMP system in complementary ways; e.g., the methylxanthines inhibit the enzyme (phosphodiesterase) that inactivates cAMP (Figure 6.4). These drugs, termed phosphodiesterase inhibitors, cause increase in cAMP concentrations and a positive inotropic effect in heart muscle. They potentiate inotropic activity of the catecholamines.

Respiratory Effects. Epinephrine is a potent bronchodilator as a result of relaxation of bronchial smooth muscle. This effect is particularly pronounced if bronchial muscle is contracted by other drugs (e.g., acetylcholine, histamine) or by anaphylactoid or asthmatic conditions. Adrenergic receptors in bronchiolar muscle are of the β_2 type. Isoproterenol is therefore a potent bronchiolar dilator, whereas exogenous norepinephrine has relatively less effect. Epinephrine and isoproterenol have been used clinically to dilate bronchiolar passageways during episodes of allergic reactions. As bronchodilators, however, selective β_2 agonists such as terbutaline and salbutamol have advantages over conventional catecholamines. The former drugs relax bronchiolar smooth muscle (β_2) with less cardiac excitatory effects (β_1) than seen with epinephrine (α-β_1-β_2 agonist) or isoproterenol (β_1-β_2 agonist), as discussed later in this chapter.

Gastrointestinal System. Adrenergic drugs inhibit gastrointestinal (GI) activity in a manner similar to that seen upon stimulation of the sympathetic nerves. The frequency and amplitude of peristaltic contractions in the gut are decreased as a result of relaxation of the intestinal smooth muscle. These effects are from activation of β-adrenergic receptors of the smooth muscle cells. Adrenergic drugs also inhibit the function of excitatory parasympathetic nerves via α_2 effects. This action contributes further to GI quiescence. Isoproterenol, as a result of β effects, exerts a rather potent inhibitory effect on GI smooth muscle. GI sphincters are generally contracted by α-sympathomimetic agents. This is in basic agreement with the overall slowing down of GI activity produced by sympathetic nerve stimulation.

Secretion of digestive juices is also decreased by α-sympathetic agents. Although salivary glands are activated in response to sympathetic activity, the saliva produced is scant and viscous, in contrast to the profuse and watery salivation seen with parasympathetic activity.

Catecholamines can exert both an inhibitory and a stimulatory effect on secretion of insulin by β cells of the pancreatic islets. The facilitatory effect is mediated via β-receptor activation, the inhibitory effect via α-receptor activation. The α-inhibitory effect is strongly predominant in vivo in most species. Since insulin is antagonistic to many of the metabolic actions of adrenergic mediators (e.g., gluconeogenesis, hyperglycemia), inhibition of insulin release by the catecholamines reinforces their metabolic effects.

Adrenergic drugs have no application as GI inhibitory agents in clinical situations. Cardiovascular effects are usually concurrently produced by dosages required to inhibit GI function. Also, parasympathetic activity in the GI system can quickly override the depressant effects exhibited by most sympathomimetic drugs.

Uterine Muscle. Both α and β receptors are present in the uterus. Responses of uterine smooth muscle to catecholamines are quite variable, depending on species and stage of the estrous and gestational cycles; e.g., in the cat, epinephrine relaxes the nongravid uterus but contracts the uterus during late pregnancy. In the rabbit, epinephrine contracts the gravid and nongravid uterus. In humans, epinephrine contracts the pregnant or nonpregnant uterus when examined in vitro. In situ, however, responses vary; epinephrine may cause relaxation of the uterus during late pregnancy. Isoproterenol usually exerts relaxant effects in uterine muscle even in the presence of epinephrine-induced contraction. The presence of circulating hormones such as estrogen and progesterone modify responses of the uterus to other agents. There is presently little clinical application of catecholamines as effectors of uterine motility. However, selective β_2 agonists (e.g., salbutamol, ritodrine) have been used in human obstetrics to relax the uterus and delay premature labor.

Spleen. Smooth muscle of the splenic capsule is contracted by epinephrine and norepinephrine via α effects. The size of the spleen decreases and blood is discharged into the circulation. This response is probably functional in physiologic states such as acute hypoxia, severe fear or rage, hemorrhage, or other conditions that elicit a generalized activation of the sympathoadrenal axis.

The splenic effects of catecholamines are easily and decisively demonstrable in dogs anesthetized with pentobarbital. Under these circumstances, the spleen is enlarged and engorged with blood. Injection of small amounts of norepinephrine or epinephrine into the splenic artery causes a pronounced contraction of the spleen and a remarkable diminution of its size. Injection of these agents directly under the splenic capsule causes intense localized contraction of the capsule. These effects are associated with α receptors. Relaxation of the splenic capsule via β receptors also has been demonstrated.

Pilomotor Effects. Norepinephrine and epinephrine cause contraction of piloerector muscles; hairs become erect. This effect is mediated by α receptors; it is often seen in animals during severe reaction to fear or rage.

Ocular Effects. Mydriasis occurs in response to stimulation of the sympathetic innervation to the eye. IV administration or topical application of epinephrine or norepinephrine causes pupillary dilation via α effects. Parasympathetic activity easily overrides adrenergic activity in the eye, however, and responses to adrenergic drugs may vary considerably. The nictitating membrane, or third eyelid, is contracted by norepinephrine and epinephrine; conjunctival and scleral blood vessels are constricted. Intraocular pressure may decrease slightly upon local instillation of epinephrine; this effect is sometimes useful in treating wide angle glaucoma and is believed to depend upon β-receptors (Osborne et al. 2004).

Central Nervous System Effects. Catecholamines do not readily cross the blood-brain barrier. Therefore, epinephrine and norepinephrine have little effect on the central nervous system (CNS). Certain noncatecholamine adrenergic agents, like amphetamine, readily cross the blood-brain barrier and elicit pronounced stimulation of the CNS.

Metabolic Effects. Catecholamines exert several rather striking effects on anabolic and catabolic activities in different organs and tissues. In mammals, there is an overall calorogenic effect (increase in general metabolism) associated with a 20–30% increase in oxygen consumption. Glycogenolysis occurs in the liver and skeletal and cardiac muscles following exposure to epinephrine, norepinephrine, or isoproterenol. There is also an acceleration of fatty acid mobilization and lactic acid formation. Accordingly, concentrations in the blood of glucose, free fatty acids, and lactic acid are increased. The order of potency of catecholamines in eliciting these metabolic changes varies in different tissues and species. In general, the glycogenolysis effect in muscles and liver follows the potency order of that associated with β receptors.

The metabolic activities of catecholamines have been associated with alterations of tissue concentration of cAMP. In hepatic and muscle tissue, e.g., adenylyl cyclase activity is increased by catecholamines, resulting in an accelerated conversion of ATP to cAMP, which in turn activates protein kinase A; the latter accelerates conversion of the inactive phosphorylase enzyme (phosphorylase b) to an active form (phosphorylase a) that then catalyzes the catabolism of glycogen to glucose. Similarly, the catecholamines have been associated with changes in the relative activities of other protein kinases, lipases, and phosphofructokinases by increases in cAMP formation (Schmid-Schonbein and Hugli 2005).

Absorption and Biotransformation. Epinephrine and norepinephrine are not absorbed to any appreciable extent following oral administration because of destruction within the GI tract. The liver rapidly inactivates by oxidative deamination and conjugation any norepinephrine or epinephrine that is absorbed into the portal system. Isoproterenol is absorbed following oral or sublingual administration but often in such an erratic manner as to be therapeutically nonuseful. Catecholamines are readily absorbed from aerosolized sprays or after parenteral administration. Subcutaneous (SC) dosages are more slowly absorbed than intramuscular (IM) injections.

Injected norepinephrine and epinephrine are metabolized by MAO and COMT (catechol-*O*-methyltransferase) enzymes; the inactive metabolites are excreted in urine. A portion of the *O*-methylated and deaminated metabolites are conjugated prior to excretion. MAO and COMT are present in many tissues; breakdown of catecholamines does not depend entirely upon the liver or kidney. Uptake of norepinephrine and epinephrine into adrenergic neurons away from their active receptor sites is an important pathway for termination of their pharmacologic activities (see Chapter 5). This is demonstrated by injecting a drug that blocks the amine uptake pump, e.g., cocaine, which potentiates the pressor response to norepinephrine and epinephrine. Inhibition of MAO and COMT has little effect on responses to single injections of catecholamines.

Preparations. *Epinephrine*, USP, the free base, is obtained from adrenal medullary extracts of domestic farm animals or is chemically synthesized. It is a white or light brown crystalline powder that is relatively insoluble in water but readily forms the water-soluble salt epinephrine hydrochloride upon addition to dilute hydrochloric acid. Solutions are unstable in alkaline mediums or upon exposure to light or heat and discolor to pink and eventually brown. Discoloration indicates oxidation of epinephrine to an inactive form; such solutions should be discarded.

Epinephrine Injection, USP, and *Epinephrine Solution*, USP, are aqueous solutions of epinephrine hydrochloride (adrenaline hydrochloride) prepared in a 1 : 1000 (1 mg/ml; 0.1%) solution; they are probably the most commonly used preparations of epinephrine. The former solution is sterile. Addition of small amounts of sodium bisulfite retards oxidative breakdown of epinephrine.

Sterile Epinephrine Suspension, USP, is a sterile suspension of epinephrine, usually 2 mg/ml, in sesame or peanut oil for IM injection only. This product is used when prolonged activity is desired.

Epinephrine Bitartrate, USP, is available in aerosol and ophthalmic solutions.

Norepinephrine (levarterenol) Bitartrate, USP (*l*-norepinephrine bitartrate), is a white crystalline powder (monohydrate salt) that readily dissolves in water. Solutions turn pink upon exposure to light, heat, or air and should be discarded if discoloration occurs.

Norepinephrine (levarterenol) Bitartrate Injection, USP, is a sterile aqueous solution usually containing 0.2% (2 mg/ml) of the salt (equivalent to 0.1% or 1 mg/ml of norepinephrine base). Bisulfite is included to delay oxidation.

Isoproterenol Hydrochloride, USP (Isuprel hydrochloride), is the water-soluble hydrochloride salt. Solutions of this compound also oxidize when exposed to light or air.

Isoproterenol Hydrochloride Injection, USP, is a sterile aqueous solution of isoproterenol hydrochloride for parenteral injection. Available preparations usually contain 0.2 mg/ml (0.02%).

Isoproterenol Hydrochloride Tablets, USP, are available in 10 mg and 15 mg sizes.

Clinical Use

With Local Anesthetics. Epinephrine is commonly used in concentrations of 1:100,000 to 1:20,000 in local anesthetic solutions. It causes pronounced local vasoconstriction and thereby localizes the action and delays the absorption of the infilterable anesthetic. Since norepinephrine is a less potent α agonist than epinephrine, it is infrequently used in local anesthetic solutions.

Local Hemostatic. Vasoconstrictor effects of epinephrine (1:100,000 to 1:20,000 solution) may be used to control superficial bleeding of mucosal and SC surfaces by application of moistened gauze sponges or by aerosol sprayed directly onto the damaged region. Epinephrine solutions have been used topically during ophthalmic surgery to control hemorrhage. Epistaxis and dental extractions are other indications. Epinephrine is effective only against hemorrhage from capillaries and arterioles and should not be used in attempts to control bleeding from larger vessels. Although smooth muscle of large vessels contracts in response to amines, this effect is by no means sufficient to occlude the lumen. During surgery, topical application of epinephrine should be considered only as a temporary aid for controlling bleeding to assist in visualization of the operative field. Serious bleeding may well recur subsequent to termination of activity of this catecholamine if routine ligation of blood vessels is disregarded.

Hypotension. Pressor amines are often used to maintain blood pressure during spinal surgery, and epinephrine is quite effective in treating hypotension associated with anaphylactic shock. The peripheral vasoconstrictor effects of norepinephrine, epinephrine, and other adrenergic drugs have also been used in attempts to treat and prevent hypotension occurring during other shock syndromes. However, blood pressure elevation due to peripheral vasoconstriction is not an adequate substitution for correcting serious underlying problems such as hypovolemia, undetected hemorrhage, and electrolyte and fluid imbalances. Some shock states are characterized by peripheral vasoconstriction secondary to a generalized sympathoadrenal discharge. Under such circumstances, administration of epinephrine or norepinephrine may serve to compound the problem by causing further intensification of vasoconstriction in vital areas (e.g., splanchnic and renal vascular beds) (Adams and Parker 1979). In some cases, the exact opposite effect (blockade of α-adrenergic receptors) has been proposed as a treatment in shock. These factors should always be considered when use of sympathomimetic amines during shock therapy is considered.

In shock cases characterized by loss of vascular tone, use of pressor amines has been suggested. Also, reestablishment of normal blood volume in some shock patients does not seem to correct the vascular complications, and blood pressure remains seriously depressed. Pressor agents may be of some use. Norepinephrine has been used under these circumstances. Usually, a 4 ml vial of 0.2% norepinephrine bitartrate (0.1% of free norepinephrine base; 1 mg/ml) is added to 1 L of sterile isotonic saline solution or 5% dextrose solution, which gives a final concentration of norepinephrine base of 4 μg/ml of solution. This solution is slowly infused intravenously until blood pressure is maintained somewhat lower than normal. Usually, an infusion rate of 0.1–0.2 μg/kg/min proves effective; however, administration should be to effect. The pressor response to norepinephrine can be readily controlled since it disappears within 1 or 2 minutes after stopping the infusion. Blood pressure should be closely monitored during the infusion process. An attempt should always be made to closely monitor cardiovascular function during treatment with any of the catecholamines. Isoproterenol has been used in some low cardiac output stages of shock. Soma et al. (1974) recommend a slow IV infusion of a 0.1–0.2 μg/ml solution of isoproterenol.

Cardiac Effects. Catecholamines are indicated in treatment of certain cardiac disorders: cardiac arrest, partial or complete atrioventricular (AV) block, and Stokes-Adams syndrome (Adams 1981). With cardiac arrest, an attempt is first made to restore heartbeat by mechanical means such as a precordial blow, electrical shock, or external cardiac massage. If the heart starts contracting, isoproterenol or epinephrine can be given by slow IV drip to maintain heart rate and cardiac output after circulation is restored. Care should be taken with IV infusion, since epinephrine may precipitate ventricular fibrillation if prefibrillatory rhythm is presented.

If asystole persists, norepinephrine or epinephrine (0.5–1.0 ml of a 1 : 10,000 solution; i.e., 50–100 μg) may be administered directly into the left ventricular chamber in an attempt to restore contraction. Larger doses may be required in some instances. The heart should then be massaged to ensure circulation of the catecholamine through the coronary vasculature. Peripheral circulation should be maintained by cardiac massage until myocardial contraction is restored.

Isoproterenol is used for treating heart block. Complete AV heart block in a dog was treated with 0.05 mg (approximately 3.5 μg/kg) of isoproterenol administered intravenously; the heart rate increased almost immediately from 44 beats/minute to 68 beats/minute (Buchanan et al. 1968). Because of its potency, isoproterenol should be administered by slow IV infusion rather than rapid bolus injection. Slow IV drip of a dilute solution can be instituted until the heart rate is maintained at 80–100 beats/minute. Thereafter, IM injections of 0.1–0.2 mg isoproterenol every 4 hours may prove effective. Isoproterenol tablets (15–30 mg) have been given every 4 hours; however, patients should be closely monitored because absorption after oral administration is erratic. Buchanan et al. (1968) found that orally administered isoproterenol (30 mg twice daily) was ineffective in treating complete AV block in a dog. Ettinger (1969) infused isoproterenol (5 μg/ml in dextrose and water) intravenously at a rate (usually 1 ml/minute) sufficient to maintain the ventricular rate at 80/minute. Isoproterenol was then administered subcutaneously every 6 hours at the dose of 0.2 mg. Oral administration of an isoproterenol tablet (30 mg) every 6 hours was prescribed for several weeks. Catecholamines should not be used in the presence of acute or chronic heart failure. These agents decrease efficiency of myocardial contraction by increasing oxygen demands of the heart muscle and compound the heart failure syndrome.

Anaphylactic and Allergic Reactions. Epinephrine is extremely effective and often lifesaving in treatment of acute anaphylactic shock. It quickly reverses the precipitous fall in blood pressure and cardiac irregularities associated with this type of syndrome. Histaminelike constriction of bronchiolar smooth muscles occurs during anaphylaxis; these effects are rapidly antagonized by epinephrine. Bronchiolar passageways are dilated by epinephrine as a result of relaxation of the smooth muscle, and dyspnea is quickly counteracted. Care should be taken that allergic signs do not recur after epinephrine activity has terminated.

Bronchial Asthma. Isoproterenol and epinephrine have been useful for providing immediate relief from bronchial asthma. These agents activate the β_2 receptors of the bronchial smooth muscle cells, causing relaxation and prompt relief by dilating the airways. Norepinephrine is ineffective in dilating passageways even though it may transiently decrease mucosal congestion by constricting mucosal blood vessels. For systemic relief from allergic and anaphylactoid reactions, epinephrine can be administered subcutaneously or intramuscularly, because with these routes effective blood levels are quickly achieved. However, if a patient is presented in late stages of anaphylactic shock or other similar life-threatening situations, IV administration may be required.

In large domestic animals (cattle, horses) 4–8 mg epinephrine can be given intramuscularly or subcutaneously by injection of 4–8 ml of a 1 : 1000 dilution of epinephrine solution. Sheep and swine may be administered 1–3 ml of the 1 : 1000 dilution. Dogs and cats are usually given 1–5 ml of a 1 : 10,000 (0.1 mg/ml) dilution. Based on a body weight range of approximately 5–25 kg, this represents a dosage schedule of approximately 20 μg/kg. A dose this large should be administered only by IM or SC injection. Response of animals to adrenergic drugs may vary considerably; therefore, repeat injections or somewhat larger doses may be required in some cases. If IV administration is necessary, one should proceed cautiously and give no more than 0.25–0.5 μg/kg. In experimental animals, 1–2 μg/kg epinephrine or norepinephrine administered by IV bolus injection causes a pronounced increase in cardiovascular activity, and even slightly larger doses may well lead to serious arrhythmias. Selective β_2 agonists (e.g., terbutaline, metaproterenol) may supplant epinephrine and isoproterenol as bronchodilators (see β_2-selective bronchodilators).

Toxicity. As implied in the preceding discussion, toxicity of the catecholamines is usually characterized by untoward cardiovascular responses. In particular, cardiac dysrhythmias such as tachycardia and even fatal ventricular fibrillation may occur following inadvertent overdosage. Hyperthyroid conditions, thyroid therapy, digitalis therapy, halogenated hydrocarbon anesthetics, and thiobarbiturates predispose a patient to the myocardial toxicity of catecholamines. The influence of anesthetics on the arrhythmogenicity of catecholamines is believed to be due to sensitization of the heart muscle. Myocardial sensitization to catecholamines is evoked by trichlorethylene, ethyl chloride, cyclopropane, halothane, chloroform, methoxyflurane, and fluroxene (listed in order of decreasing effect) (Katz and Katz 1966). Thiobarbiturates increase the incidence of epinephrine- and norepinephrine-induced arrhythmias in chloroform-anesthetized dogs (Claborn and Szabuniewicz 1973; Wiersig et al. 1974).

Hypertensive crises occur from norepinephrine or epinephrine overdosage; cerebral vascular accidents and ruptured aneurysms may result. The latter represents a potential problem in horses because of a fairly common incidence of undiagnosed verminous aneurysms. Large or repeated dosages of epinephrine and isoproterenol have been associated with myocardial ischemia and necrosis; these effects are prevented by β-blocking agents. Local necrosis and sloughing of tissue may occur at injection sites because of intensive vasoconstriction and resulting ischemia.

In short, the catecholamines are extremely potent agents; under no circumstances should they be considered innocuous. Therapeutic use of these drugs should always be carefully monitored by a trained individual familiar with their indications, limitations, and toxicities.

DOPAMINE. Dopamine (3,4-dihydroxyphenylethylamine) was thought to be important only as the immediate biochemical precursor to norepinephrine. Dopamine itself is now known to have important physiologic functions in mammalian species and is receiving attention in certain clinical circumstances in humans (Caccavelli et al. 1992). Parkinson's disease, e.g., has been related to decreased concentrations of dopamine in the basal ganglia, and treatment with l-dopa has proved effective in controlling motor disorders in some Parkinsonism patients. l-dopa crosses the blood-brain barrier (dopamine does not in significant quantities) and is decarboxylated to dopamine.

Dopamine receptors of vascular smooth muscle are categorized as dopamine$_1$ (DA_1), and the inhibitory dopamine receptors of peripheral sympathetic neurons are DA_2 subtype (Murphy et al., 2001; Goldberg and Rajfer 1985). Experimental hemodynamic studies indicate that dopamine also has use as a selective cardiovascular agent. In anesthetized dogs, IV injection of 1–9 μg/kg dopamine induces a slight depressor response associated with a decrease in total peripheral resistance, a decrease in renal vascular resistance, an increase in renal blood flow, and an increase in cardiac output. Large amounts, 9–81 μg/kg, produce pressor responses and a more pronounced increase in myocardial contractile force (Setler et al. 1975). Cardiovascular effects of dopamine depend on activation of different types of catecholaminergic receptors. The pressor response is blocked by an α blocker (e.g., phenoxybenzamine), and the cardiac stimulatory effects are blocked by a β blocker (e.g., propranolol). Part of the myocardial effects of dopamine are thought to be indirect and mediated by release of norepinephrine from cardiac sympathetic nerves (Fig. 6.5).

The cardiovascular actions of dopamine depend on the dose administered (Fig. 6.5): At a low dose, (0.5–2 μg/kg/min effects on dopaminie (D_2) predominate. At a medium dose (2–5 μg/kg/min) β-receptor effects occur. At high doses (5–10 μg/kg/min) α-receptor effects (vasoconstriction) are observed. Dopamine infusions will increase both blood pressure and cardiac output. These effects are caused by stimulating cardiac contractility and heart rate via the action on α_1-adrenergic receptors. In addition, dopamine increases the release of norepinephrine from nerve terminals because dopamine is a precursor for norepinephrine. It produces a greater chronotropic effect than dobutamine (discussed below). At the low doses listed above, effects on dopamine receptors causes vasodilation in renal and splanchnic vessels, whereas at the high dose, dopamine will stimulate the α-adrenergic receptors on vessels and produce vasoconstriction.

Clinical Use. Because dopamine's actions are dose-dependent, the rate administered is adjusted to reach the desired clinical effect. Dopamine has been administered at doses of 2–10 μg/kg/min for the acute management of heart failure, and cardiogenic shock. Like dobutamine, dopamine has a very short half-life and must administered via continuous intravenous infusion (CRI). When preparing intravenous solutions, one may admix 200–400 mg of dopamine with 250–500 ml of fluid. Dopamine is unstable in alkaline fluid solutions, such as those containing bicarbonate.

Use in renal failure: It has been proposed that dopamine dilates renal arterioles, increases renal blood flow, and glomerular filtration rate. This effect is proposed to occur via activation of renal dopamine-1 (DA_1) receptors. Because of this proposed effect, the use for treating acute renal

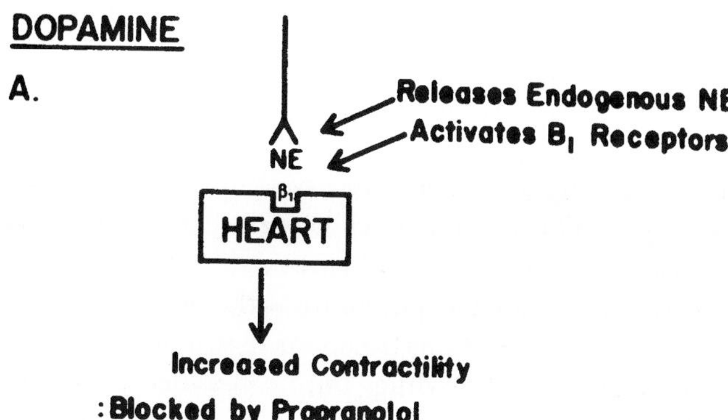

B. Activates Alpha Adrenoceptors (>10 μg/kg)

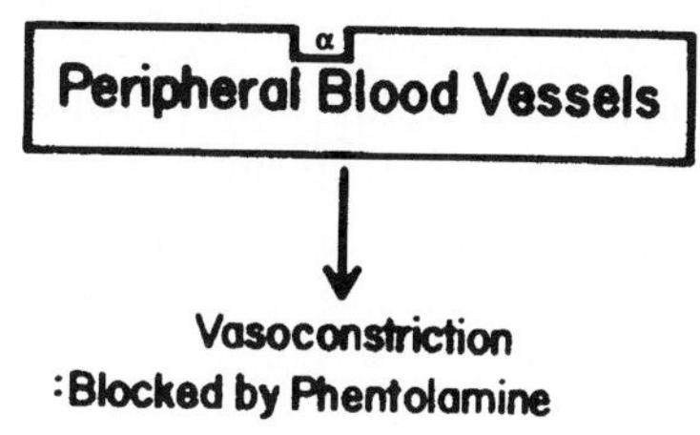

C. Activates Dopaminergic Vascular Receptors (<10 μg/kg)

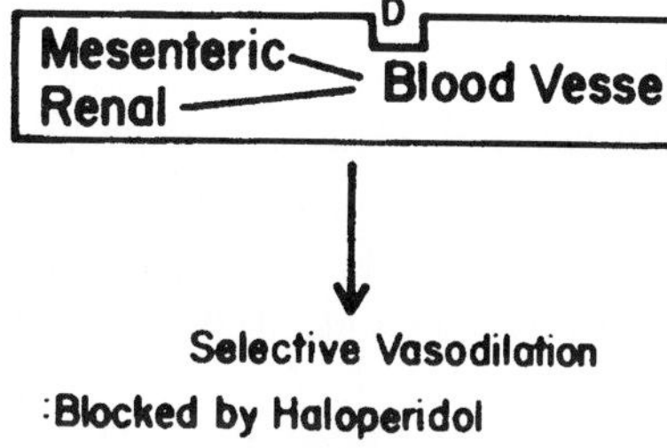

FIG. 6.5 Cardiovascular activities of dopamine. (A) Dopamine increases heart rate and myocardial contractility by directly activating β_1 adrenoceptors and releasing neuronal stores of endogenous norepinephrine (NE); these activities are blocked by the β-blocking agent propranolol. (B) Dopamine in large doses activates α adrenoceptors of blood vessels, resulting in vasoconstriction and a pressor response. This is blocked by the α-blocking agent phentolamine. (C) Dopamine in low doses can selectively dilate mesenteric and renal arterial beds (and perhaps cerebral and coronary arterial beds) by activation of dopamine-response (dopaminergic) receptors. It is not blocked by an α- or β-blocking agent but is blocked by the CNS dopamine antagonist haloperidol (Adams and Parker 1979).

failure has been described in older literature (Hosgood 1990). However, recent evaluation of the effects (Sigrist 2007, Rosati et al, 2007; Wohl et al. 2007) have raised doubts about the clinical effectiveness of dopamine for treatment of acute renal failure. Cats do not have as many DA_1 receptors as other animals; therefore it has not been effective in cats (Wohl et al. 2007). In addition, evaluation in people and other animals has not produced desired effects (Sigrist 2007). Therefore, the use for this indication is now discouraged.

Adverse Effects: Excessive doses can cause tachycardia and vasoconstriction. Avoid leakage of drug outside the vein because it can cause tissue necrosis.

One study indicated that dopamine (about 5 μg/kg/min) was effective in terminating advanced AV heart block in four ill foals that were refractory to atropine (Whilton and Trim 1985).

FENOLDOPAM. Fenoldapam (Corlopam injection) is a selective dopamine-receptor agonist (Murphy et al. 2001). It is specific for the dopamine DA_1 receptor, and therefore has been used in investigations to determine the action of dopamine on vascular beds and between species. Because of its action on the DA_1 receptor of vascular beds—causing vasodilation—uses of fenoldopam in people has included treatment of severe hypertension, improvement in tissue perfusion to the gastrointestinal tract, and renal protection from vasoconstriction. In veterinary medicine, it has produced delayed diuresis in cats at a dose of 0.5 μg/kg/min IV (Simmons et al., 2006), but has only been used experimentally in dogs.

DOBUTAMINE. Dobutamine hydrochloride (Dobutrex) is a synthetic catecholamine that evokes a positive inotropic response in the heart. Importantly, dobutamine elicits this activity via an activation of β_1 receptors subserving increased myocardial contractility, with less activity at β_1 receptors subserving chronotropic effects and β_2 receptors subserving peripheral vasodilation. There are some effects on cardiac α-receptors, which may play a role in heart rate control. In dogs (Rosati et al. 2007), dobutamine had effects on both β_1 and β_2 receptors, which produced increased cardiac contractility (β_1) and also vasodilation of skeletal muscle vessels (β_2). This compound was formulated and synthesized by Tuttle and Mills (1975) in a search for agents that would selectively increase cardiac contractility without affecting heart rate, cardiac rhythmicity, or blood pressure. The net cardiovascular response to dobutamine actually comprises different effects of its sterioisomers as well as important reflex adjustments (Swanson et al. 1985).

Potential advantages of dobutamine over conventional catecholamines relates to the relative multiplicity of actions of the latter agents. Dobutamine, because of its relative inotropic cardioselectivity, may have advantages over other adrenergic amines in the therapy of low-output cardiac failure. However, in anesthetized dogs, it did not have an advantage over dopamine (Rosati et al. 2007) in this regard.

The hemodynamics of dobutamine were studied in dogs by Hinds and Hawthorne (1975) and Willerson et al. (1976). Dobutamine produces a dose-related increase in myocardial contractility, velocity of myocardial fiber shortening, ejection fraction, and stroke work. Importantly, these increments in cardiac contractility occur without changes in ventricular preload or heart rate when dobutamine is infused in doses of 5–20 μg/kg/min; cardiac output increases and total peripheral resistance is slightly decreased. After cardiopulmonary bypass in dogs, mortality rate and cardiovascular function were improved by dobutamine infusion (5 μg/kg/min); an increase in automaticity or arrhythmia was not detected (Eyster et al. 1975).

In dogs anesthetized with pentobarbital, Willerson et al. (1976) found increased ST-segment elevation during infusion of dobutamine after coronary artery ligation; heart rate also increased under these conditions. Tachycardia, arrhythmia, and blood pressure changes are likely if optimal dosage levels are exceeded. At high doses of 6 and 8 μg/kg/min there was a precipitous increase in heart rate and onset of arrhythmias in anesthetized dogs (Rosati et al. 2007). More information is needed about the cardiac and hemodynamic actions of dobutamine, particularly in different species and under clinical conditions. However, dobutamine is an important adrenergic agent because of its relative inotropic cardioselectivity when the desired goal of therapy is to improve ventricular function by direct inotropic stimulation (Loeb et al. 1977).

NONCATECHOLAMINES

Although the 3,4-dihydroxybenzene structure yields maximum potency, many drugs lacking the catechol nucleus have proved to be clinically useful. As with the catecholamines, the end effects of these drugs are mediated by the adrenergic receptors of effector cells. However, the mechanism of obtaining receptor activation varies considerably from one drug to another. Surgical sympathetic denervation abolishes or markedly reduces the effects of some agents (e.g., tyramine, an experimental sympathomimetic amine) but does not reduce effects of epinephrine. Reserpine causes a functional sympathectomy by depleting adrenergic neurons of their stores of norepinephrine. Pretreatment with reserpine markedly decreases the response to tyramine but does not decrease effects of epinephrine. An α-blocking agent, however, prevents effects of tyramine, epinephrine, and norepinephrine. These findings indicate that tyramine acts presynaptically to cause a release of endogenous norepinephrine from the nerve, which in turn acts on postjunctional receptors. Based on these types of findings, adrenergic drugs can be classified into three groups: direct-acting (effects not decreased by denervation), mixed-action (effects partially reduced by denervation), and indirect-acting (effects markedly reduced by denervation) (Fig. 6.6).

Despite these complex interrelationships, the peripheral effects of adrenergic drugs can be explained by activation, whether direct or indirect, of the α and/or β receptors. Therefore, effects of these drugs can be compared with the previously discussed pharmacologic effects of the direct-acting agents norepinephrine, epinephrine, and isoproterenol.

EPHEDRINE. *Ephedrine*, USP, was originally isolated from the Chinese shrub *Ma huang (Ephedra)* but is now chemically synthesized. The natural product has been used in oriental medicine for centuries and was introduced into

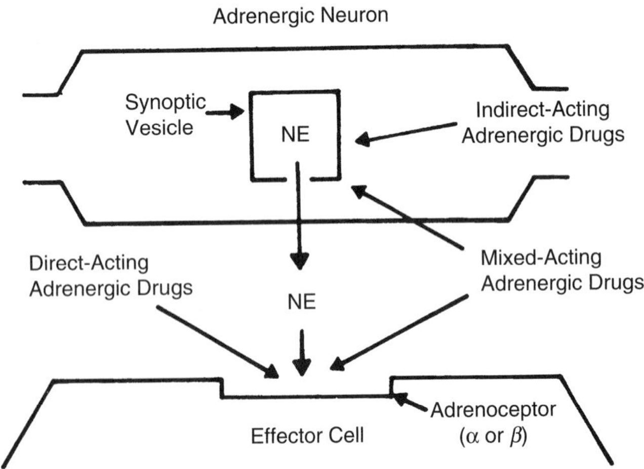

FIG. 6.6 Pathways of adrenoceptor activation by adrenergic drugs. Norepinephrine (NE) is stored in neuronal vesicles. Direct-acting adrenergic drugs activate the receptors of the effector cell; indirect-acting agents evoke release of endogenous NE. Arrows point to sites of action (Adams and Parker 1979).

modern therapeutics during the 1920s (Chen and Schmidt 1930). The structure of ephedrine and related pharmacologic effects are shown in Table 6.1. The levo isomer is the most active form of this component. Ephedrine exerts its sympathomimetic effects by direct activation of adrenergic receptors and release of endogenous norepinephrine.

There are no commercial brands of ephedrine marketed currently, but some herbal supplements still exist.

Pharmacologic Effects

Cardiovascular. IV administration of ephedrine produces hemodynamic changes similar to those caused by bolus injection of epinephrine. Systolic and diastolic blood pressures increase, myocardial contractile force increases, heart rate increases if vagal reflexes are blocked, and cardiac output increases if venous return is adequate. Vasoconstriction occurs in kidney, mesenteric, and cutaneous circulations; blood flow to these regions decreases. Blood flow may increase, however, through coronary, cerebral, and skeletal muscle vascular beds. Ephedrine is many times less potent a pressor agent than epinephrine, but its effects last 7–10 times longer. Cardiovascular effects are obtained after oral administration of ephedrine, whereas epinephrine is inactive if given by mouth.

In contrast to epinephrine and norepinephrine, repeated injections of ephedrine evoke progressively smaller pressor responses in intact animals. This condition, tachyphylaxis, is probably dependent upon different factors. First, because ephedrine causes a release of endogenous amines, stores of norepinephrine may eventually be depleted, so less and less is available for release. The long duration of action of ephedrine may also contribute to development of tachyphylaxis. During long courses of cardiovascular stimulation, reflex mechanisms attempt to return hemodynamic function toward normal. Blood pressure may return to somewhat normal values, although ephedrine, because of its delayed elimination, is still present at receptor sites. Repeated injections therefore prove less effective if occupation of the receptors by prior administration of ephedrine still exists.

Central Nervous System. Ephedrine is a CNS stimulant. It stimulates corticomedullary regions and, in large doses, causes excitement, apparent anxiety, and muscular tremors. Respiratory centers of the medulla oblongata are activated by appropriate doses of ephedrine. This effect has been used clinically to reverse respiratory depression, particularly if respiratory problems are associated with barbiturate overdosage. Ephedrine is infrequently used for this purpose now, since other central stimulants have proved more effective or more reliable. Other adrenergic drugs such as amphetamine stimulate the CNS to a greater extent than ephedrine.

Ocular. Mydriasis occurs after local or systemic administration of ephedrine as a result of active stimulation of the radial muscle of the iris. A 10% solution has been used to enlarge the pupillary space to facilitate ophthalmic examination.

Bronchial Smooth Muscle. Ephedrine is effective in causing relaxation of bronchial smooth muscle and increasing the diameter of bronchiolar passageways; these effects are believed to be due to direct activation of β receptors.

Clinical Use. *Ephedrine hydrochloride*, is used rarely in veterinary medicine. Veterinarians should be cautious about so-called herbal products that may be given inadvertently to animals. The products that contain ephedra alkaloids (also known as *ma huang*), produce a similar effect as the drug ephedrine. Side effects are possible and fatal cardiac events and seizures have occurred in young adults consuming high doses. The adverse cardiovascular and central nervous system effects have been reported (Haller & Benowitz, 2000).

Ephedrine solution, 1–1.5%, can be applied topically onto congested mucosal membranes to evoke vasoconstriction and decongestion. Ephedrine is effective in reducing allergic responses, but the onset of action is slower than with epinephrine. Ephedrine is sometimes included in cough suppressant preparations for relief from bronchiolar congestion and vascular constriction.

AMPHETAMINE. *Amphetamine Sulfate*, USP, or β-phenylisopropylamine, induces pronounced stimulation of the CNS as well as causing marked peripheral α and β effects. A considerable portion of the pharmacologic effects of amphetamine is due to release of endogenous norepinephrine. Cardiovascular effects of amphetamine are somewhat similar to those produced by ephedrine. An increase of systolic and diastolic blood pressures is observed. Heart rate is reflexly slowed and cardiac output is not affected to any appreciable extent. Cardiovascular effects are observed after the drug is given by the oral route. The l-isomer is a somewhat more active pressor agent than the d-isomer. The chemical structure of amphetamine is shown in Table 6.1.

Amphetamine is active if given by mouth; CNS effects persist for several hours. The entire CNS is affected, but effects on the cerebrum are most evident in humans: increased alertness, loss of fatigue, euphoria, and a sense of exhilaration. The performance of athletes is improved; this is attributed to improvement of activities requiring mental and physical coordination. After effects of amphetamine have dissipated, pronounced depression may occur. In humans amphetamine is most often used in treatment of neuropsychiatric disorders such as mild but chronic depression, narcolepsy, alcoholism, and in some cases of hyperkinesis in children.

Amphetamine is no longer available for use in veterinary medicine in the USA and is subject to strict control under the 1970 Controlled Substances Act. Prior to the strict control of amphetamine it was used in veterinary therapeutics for its stimulatory effects on the respiratory centers in the medulla oblongata. The entire cerebrospinal axis is affected, but particularly the brain stem and cortex. The *d*-isomer, dextroamphetamine, is the most centrally active. Its analeptic potency is similar to that of pentamethylenetetrazol. Amphetamine increases both the rate and depth of inspiration in anesthetized animals. It was used intravenously (4–4.5 mg/kg) in the dog to overcome respiratory depressant effects of barbiturate overdose.

In dogs, the drug selegiline (l-Deprenyl, Eldepryl, Anipryl) is registered for treatment of canine hyperadrenocorticism and cognitive dysfunction in older dogs. It is discussed in more detail in Chapter 21. The action of selegiline is to inhibit MAO type B (and other MAOs at higher doses) and it is proposed to inhibit the metabolism of dopamine in the central nervous system. However, it also inhibits the metabolism of phenylethylamine (Milgram et al. 1993; Milgram et al. 1995). (Phenylethylamine in laboratory animals produces amphetaminelike effects.) In addition, there are two active metabolites, which are l-amphetamine and l-methamphetamine. In dogs, even though there were increases in amphetamine concentrations, (Milgram et al. 1993) they were not high enough to produce adverse effects. However, at high doses (>3 mg/kg) the authors proposed that increased amphetamine concentrations could explain the observed behavioral changes. As noted above, the l-isomer metabolites are not as active as their d-forms and studies have not supported a potential for amphetaminelike abuse or dependency from selegiline, compared to other amphetaminelike drugs.

PHENYLEPHRINE. *Phenylephrine Hydrochloride*, USP (Neosynephrine), is similar in structure to epinephrine except that it lacks the 4-OH group on the benzene ring; the chemical structure and pharmacologic characteristics of phenylephrine are shown in Table 6.1. Phenylephrine is a direct-acting sympathomimetic amine at α_1 receptors and does not depend upon release of endogenous norepinephrine for its effects. Similar to norepinephrine, phenylephrine causes peripheral vasoconstriction by direct activation of α_1 receptors of blood vessels. However, dissimilar to norepinephrine, it has very little effect at cardiac β receptors. Systolic and diastolic blood pressures are increased by phenylephrine; reflex bradycardia usually occurs. The predictable reflex-mediated slowing of the heart rate by phenylephrine has led to use of this agent in human patients to control episodes of paroxysmal atrial tachycardia.

Phenylephrine is a less potent pressor agent than norepinephrine but has a longer duration of action. The IV dose for dogs is 0.088 mg/kg; approximately twice this amount should be given if administered by the SC or IM route.

Short-acting topical agents often include phenylephrine a common ingredient in over-the-counter nasal sprays (e.g., NeoSynephrine®). These products also have been applied topically to decrease bleeding associated with some surgical procedures.

PHENYLPROPANOLAMINE (PPA). *Phenylpropanolamine* was first approved in 1959 and has been widely available over-the-counter (OTC) as a nonprescription drug for many years for humans. Familiar brand names are Dexatrim, Acutrim (appetite suppressants), and Propagest and Rhindecon (decongestants). A study from Yale University suggested that phenylpropanolamine in appetite suppressants, and possibly decongestants, is a risk factor for hemorrhagic stroke in women. *Because of the risk of hemorrhagic stroke in women, the Food and Drug Administration (FDA), announced on November 6, 2001 that it was taking steps to remove phenylpropanolamine from all drug products and has requested that all drug companies discontinue marketing products containing phenylpropanolamine.* However, phenylpropanolamine is still available for veterinary use to treat urinary incontinence in dogs. The effect of phenylpropanolamine (PPA) and other sympathetic agonists, such as pseudoephedrine, for treating urinary incontinence arise from their stimulation of the alpha-receptor—to increase the tone of the urinary sphincter, and its beta-receptor effects—to relax the detrussor muscle of the bladder wall and allow more urine filling.

The most common drug used for this purpose has been phenylpropanolamine (PPA). There is a registered formulation of phenylpropanolamine available in the U.K. for treatment of urinary incontinence in dogs, (Propalin syrup), which has now been marketed in the U.S. Dose is approximately 1–2 mg/kg q8 to 12 h. Dosage forms include: PROIN ppa: 75, 50, 25 mg liver-flavored tablets and 25 mg flavored syrup and Propalin syrup: 50 mg/ml syrup.

Phenylpropanolamine, ephedrine, and pseudoephedrine also are used as raw ingredients to illegally manufacture methamphetamine for "street use" in so-called "Meth Labs." Therefore, the control of these drugs is much greater in recent years. Pseudoephedrine is no longer available over-the-counter in many states in the U.S.

METHOXAMINE AND METARAMINOL. The chemical structure of *Methoxamine Hydrochloride*, USP (Vasoxyl), is β-hydroxy-β-(2,5-dimethoxyphenyl)-isopropylamine. The chemical structure and related pharmacologic effects of *Metaraminol Bitartrate*, USP (Aramine), are included in Table 6.1. Like phenylephrine, these drugs act almost exclusively as direct-acting sympathomimetic amines at peripheral α receptors. They have minimal detectable myocardial stimulatory properties. Their pressor effects on systolic and diastolic blood pressures can be explained by peripheral vasoconstriction and increased peripheral resistance. Reflex bradycardia usually results. These drugs are used as pressor agents. After IV injection, the pressor response to methoxamine occurs rapidly and may persist for 1 hour. With IM administration, 15 minutes is usually required for the pressor response to take effect and it usually lasts 1–1.5 hours.

α_2-SELECTIVE AGONISTS

The CNS contains α_2 receptors on neurons involved in control of blood pressure and heart rate. CNS α_2 receptors also modulate CNS perception of pain as well as levels of sedation. Activation of CNS α_2 receptors by α_2 agonists can lower systemic blood pressure, explaining their role as antihypertensive agents in human medicine. In veterinary medicine, α_2 agonists are used for their sedative and analgesic properties, thereby gaining chemical restraint and relief from pain (for more in-depth discussion, see Chapter 13).

β_2-SELECTIVE BRONCHODILATORS

The bronchodilators for treating respiratory disease will be discussed in more detail in Chapter 49. β_2-agonist effects of isoproterenol have been used successfully to improve airway diameter and conductance in obstructive pulmonary disorders such as bronchitis, emphysema, and asthmatic-like syndromes. Because of equipotent β_1 activity, however, cardiac excitation and tachydysrhythmias represent limiting side effects of isoproterenol when only β_2-bronchodilator action is sought. Similar limitations apply to epinephrine, although it is still the drug of choice for treating acute anaphylaxis when a combination of β_2 bronchodilation, β_1-cardiac stimulation, and α vasoconstriction is needed. Cardiac side effects with epinephrine or isoproterenol can develop after any route of administration but are more pronounced after parenteral injection than with aerosol inhalation. For these reasons, considerable effort has been expended in the development of drugs with more selective β_2 activity and therefore less propensity for β_1-cardiac excitation.

Metaproterenol, albuterol, isoetharine, terbutaline, pirbuterol, bitolterol, fenoterol, formoterol, procaterol, salmeteral, and clenbuterol are newer drugs that meet the requirements for high β_2- and relatively less β_1-agonist activity. Indeed, these drugs are generally classified as β_2-selective bronchodilators. Most of these compounds are absorbed after oral administration and have prolonged duration of bronchodilator action, other distinct advantages over the short-lived response to isoproterenol and epinephrine.

Clenbuterol (Ventipulmin®) was approved in 1998 for use in horses to treat recurrent airway obstruction (RAO, formerly called COPD), but use in food animals is illegal. Its use has not been reported in small animals. In horses, it was shown to improve airway conductance in horses for several hours after a single IV injection at a dose of 0.8 μg/kg; heart rate increased dramatically but for less than 2 minutes (Shapland et al. 1981). The brief tachycardia may have been reflexly mediated due to transient β_2

vasodilation and hypotension. Unanticipated blood pressure responses may therefore represent a concern after systemic administration of β_2 bronchodilators. Blood pressure changes should be less pronounced after aerosol inhalation. However, untoward side effects, including β_1-cardiac stimulation, can be expected with any route of administration if optimal dosage ranges of the β_2 bronchodilators are exceeded.

Patients often become refractory to bronchodilator effects of adrenergic agonists during long-term therapy, and this is believed to reflect down-regulation or agonist-induced loss of the β_2-pulmonary receptor population. An alternative approach involves concomitant administration of a methylxanthine, such as aminophylline, along with the β_2 agonist. Methylxanthines are discussed in more detail in Chapter 49. Methylxanthines inhibit the intracellular enzyme known as phosphodiesterase. This enzyme is responsible for the metabolism of cAMP, which is the intracellular messenger for β-receptor activation and mediates the resulting cellular reactions that culminate in bronchodilation. Because the results of β-receptor stimulation are mediated through an increase in cAMP synthesis and because methylxanthines inhibit the breakdown of cAMP and prolong its intracellular sojourn, combined therapy with a β_2 agonist and aminophylline can result in accentuated bronchodilator effects.

ANTIADRENERGIC DRUGS

Numerous agents have been discovered that prevent either the pharmacologic effects of sympathomimetic drugs, the physiologic responses evoked by stimulation of adrenergic nerves, or both (Westfall 2004). The terms *adrenolytic* and *sympatholytic* have been used to describe such activities; however, more precise terminology is presently in use. Adrenergic antagonists interact with adrenergic receptors and by occupying these sites do not allow an adrenergic agonist access to the receptor (Bolger and Al-Nasser 2003; Westfall and Westfall 2006). Adrenergic neuron blocking drugs do not block receptors; instead, they act presynaptically at the nerve terminal to cause a decreased release of the endogenous neurotransmitter norepinephrine.

ADRENERGIC ANTAGONISTS. In 1906 Dale reported that pretreatment of cats with ergot alkaloids prevented some of the hemodynamic effects of epinephrine. These studies presented the first evidence of the drug action now commonly referred to as adrenergic blockade. Adrenergic blocking drugs exert their pharmacologic effects by interlocking with and occupying adrenergic receptors. In this manner, adrenergic agonists are prevented from affixing to the receptor site; effects of the agonist are abolished or markedly decreased.

The adrenergic blocking effects of ergot alkaloids (and some drugs like phentolamine that were subsequently synthesized) were identified as being present only at those adrenergic receptors designated by Ahlquist (1948) as α. In fact, for over 50 years the only adrenergic blocking agents identified inhibited α-receptor–mediated effects. This problem delayed full acceptance of Ahlquist's (1948) differentiation of α- and β-receptor sites. However, Powell and Slater (1958) and Moran and Perkins (1958) demonstrated that the 3,4-dichlorophenyl analog of isoproterenol selectively inhibited those responses ascribed by Ahlquist (1948) to be mediated by β receptors. This drug, dichloroisoproterenol, blocked the vasodilation, cardiac stimulation, and bronchial smooth muscle relaxing effects of catecholamines but had no effect on α-mediated effects. *Propranolol Hydrochloride*, USP (Inderal), was subsequently identified as a β-blocking agent, and it serves as the prototype for this drug group.

PHARMACOLOGIC CONSIDERATIONS

Receptor Blockade. The α- or β-inhibitory effects of representative adrenergic blocking drugs (e.g., α blockade with phentolamine and β blockade with propranolol) on the blood pressure and myocardial effects of sympathomimetic drugs are shown in Figure 6.7. Alpha blockade abolishes the pressor response to norepinephrine. Epinephrine is a mixed α-β agonist; α blockade by phentolamine not only prevents the pressor response to epinephrine, it actually converts it to a depressor response. This is called epinephrine reversal. Since the α receptors are occupied by phentolamine, only the vasodilator β_2 receptors are available for interaction with epinephrine. Thus epinephrine causes a fall in blood pressure. Alpha blockade does not affect the α_2-receptor–mediated depressor effect of isoproterenol nor does it affect the cardiac stimulant effects of the catecholamines.

Propranolol, a nonselective β_1-β_2 blocker, inhibits the β_1-cardiac stimulant effects of isoproterenol, epinephrine, and norepinephrine (Fig. 6.7). It also blocks the β_2-depressor response to isoproterenol but does not prevent the α-receptor–mediated pressor response to norepinephrine.

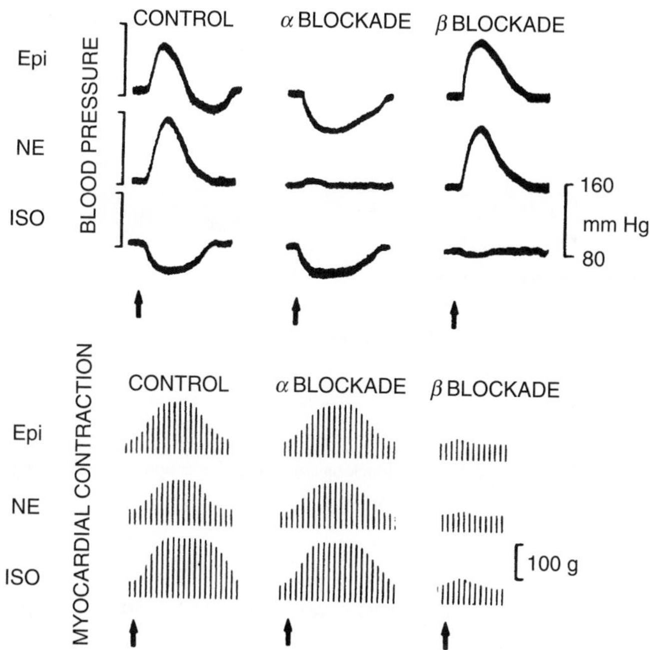

FIG. 6.7 Effects of α- and β-adrenergic blockade on the blood pressure and myocardial effects of epinephrine (Epi), norepinephrine (NE), and isoproterenol (ISO) in a dog. Control = effects of amines in the absence of an adrenergic blocking drug. α blockade = effects of amines after administration of an α blocker (e.g., phentolamine); β blockade = effects of amines after administration of a β blocker (e.g., propranolol). Epi, NE, or ISO was injected intravenously at arrow. a blockade inhibits the pressor response to NE, does not affect the depressor effect of ISO, converts the pressor effect of Epi to a depressor effect (Epi reversal), and does not affect the cardiac stimulant effects of the amines. β blockade does not affect pressor responses to NE, inhibits depressor effect of ISO, inhibits the secondary depressor effect of Epi, and inhibits myocardial stimulant effects of all three amines (see text for details).

The secondary depressor effect of epinephrine seen in the control situation is due to residual β_2-receptor–mediated vasodilation; this too is inhibited by propranolol.

Pharmacologic Effects. The degree of autonomic nervous system activity at any one time plays an important role in determining the extent of pharmacologic effects that will be produced by an adrenergic blocking agent. For example, administration of a β-blocking drug to a trained quiescent patient does not cause profound cardiovascular effects because at rest the heart is not under pronounced sympathetic influence. Upon physical exertion, however, an increase in heart rate and cardiac output is produced as a result of increased sympathetic nervous system activity. If the patient is required to exercise during treatment with propranolol, these characteristic cardiac responses are not obtained since the β-adrenergic receptors of the heart are blocked by this drug.

Effects of an α-blocking agent are similarly influenced by the existing state of autonomic nervous system activity. If the cardiovascular system is under pronounced sympathetic dominance (e.g., during fright or severe hypovolemia), an α-blocking drug will cause a decrease in blood pressure. This occurs because the α receptors of blood vessels are occupied by the α-blocking agent and are no longer available to norepinephrine or to circulating epinephrine.

Pharmacologic effects of adrenergic blocking agents can be reliably predicted by considering the distribution of α and β receptors in the body and the respective physiologic functions they subserve. Distribution of α and β receptors in various organs and tissues and their pharmacologic characteristics are summarized in Tables 5.1 and 6.3.

α-Adrenergic Blocking Agents

Ergot Alkaloids. Ergot alkaloids are not used clinically in humans or lower animals for α-blocking effects. They affect a variety of organs at concentrations less than those required for α blockade. Therefore, they are not truly prototypical α blockers; however, they were the first adrenergic blocking agents identified (Dale 1906).

Ergot is a fungus (*Claviceps purpurea*) that parasitizes rye and other grains. Ingestion of contaminated grain products has caused outbreaks of ergotism in humans and domestic animals throughout the world. Ergot is a mixture of different types of alkaloids that have biologic effects. The ergonovine group lacks a polypeptide side chain; it does not cause adrenergic blockade but has potent oxytocic activity. The ergotamine group causes adrenergic blockade but has little effect on nonvascular smooth muscle.

The predominant vascular effect of ergot is not α blockade but is related to intense peripheral vasoconstriction. These compounds cause a direct stimulation of smooth muscle, including that of peripheral blood vessels. Because of peripheral vasoconstriction, ergot initially causes a pressor response that may persist for a fairly long time. Larger doses eventually block the α-adrenergic receptors; α-receptor–mediated effects of norepinephrine, epinephrine, and other agonists are inhibited. Beta receptors are not affected.

TABLE 6.3 Classification and characteristics of catecholaminergic receptors

	Receptor Types			
Characteristics	α	β_1	β_2	Dopamine
Potency of agonists	E > NE > D > I	I > E ≥ NE > D	I > E > NE > D	D > E, NE, I
Antagonists				
α blockers (PHEN)	Block	No	No	No
β blockers				
General (PROP)	No	Block	Block	No
β_1 (PRACT)	No	Block	Weak block	No
β_1 (BUT)	No	Weak block	Block	No
Dopamine antagonist (HAL)	No	No	No	Block

Note: E = epinephrine; NE = norepinephrine; D = dopamine; I = isoproterenol; PHEN = phentolamine; No = no blocking effect; PROP = propranolol; PRACT = practolol; BUT= butoxamine; HAL = haloperidol. See Table 6.4 for further breakdown of α receptors into $\alpha_1 - \alpha_2$ subtypes.

Because of α-blocking effects, ergot produces epinephrine reversal as previously described (Fig. 6.7). In ergot-treated animals, vasodilation and hypotension occur after administration of epinephrine (or other mixed α-β agonists) resulting from β-receptor dominance in the presence of α blockade. Although this is not the most prominent effect of ergot, it is the most interesting, since it led to identification of other, more selective α blockers. Large doses of ergot cause serious circulatory disturbances because of intense and persistent vasoconstriction of peripheral vessels. This is characterized by stasis of blood in the capillaries and arterioles, thrombosis, and eventually obliterative endarteritis, leading to gangrene of the extremities. Sloughing of portions of the feet, hooves, tails, ears, and tongues have occurred in ergot-poisoned animals.

Synthetic α-Blocking Agents. The synthetic α blockers fall into several classes of structurally unrelated chemical compounds; structure-activity relationships have not been clarified. There are several groups of α blockers such as the haloalkylamine derivatives (phenoxybenzamine, dibenamine), the imidazoline derivatives (phentolamine, tolazoline), the benzodioxans (piperoxan, dibozane), and the dibenzazepine derivatives (azapetine); see Figure 6.8 for chemical structures.

Members of the phenothiazine derivative tranquilizers also have α-adrenergic blocking properties. These drugs are discussed in detail in relation to their CNS effects in a later chapter; their peripheral vascular actions are also of interest. Chlorpromazine and several other related compounds can cause blockade of α receptors. These agents alter pressor effects of catecholamines (they can cause epinephrine reversal) but it seems likely that the total cardiovascular effects are from a variety of factors such as concomitant antihistaminic, antiserotonergic, and anticholinergic effects.

Inhibition of pressor responses to catecholamines by the other synthetic α blockers, however, can be ascribed almost entirely to α-receptor blockade. Phentolamine and phenoxybenzamine are older α-blocking drugs. Their site of action is the α receptor; β responses are not blocked. *Phenoxybenzamine Hydrochloride*, USP (Dibenzyline), and other related haloalkylamines such as dibenamine produce a noncompetitive block; increasing the dosage of an α agonist will not overcome the α blockade produced by phenoxybenzamine. This characteristic seems to be due to the drug binding in a very stable manner to the receptor or nearby structures. *Phentolamine Hydrochloride*, USP (Regitine hydrochloride), and *Tolazoline Hydrochloride*, USP (Priscoline hydrochloride), however, cause a competitive blockade of α receptors that can usually be antagonized by increasing the availability of agonist.

Cardiovascular Effects. Slow IV infusion of phenoxybenzamine or phentolamine to a normal patient usually does not cause a remarkable change in blood pressure. Usually, a slight to moderate fall in pressure occurs; however, these drugs will cause a marked hypotensive response if a patient's cardiovascular system is under pronounced sympathetic tone. This is particularly evident during hypovolemia, since in this state sympathetic discharge increases to maintain adequate blood pressure in the presence of low circulating blood volume.

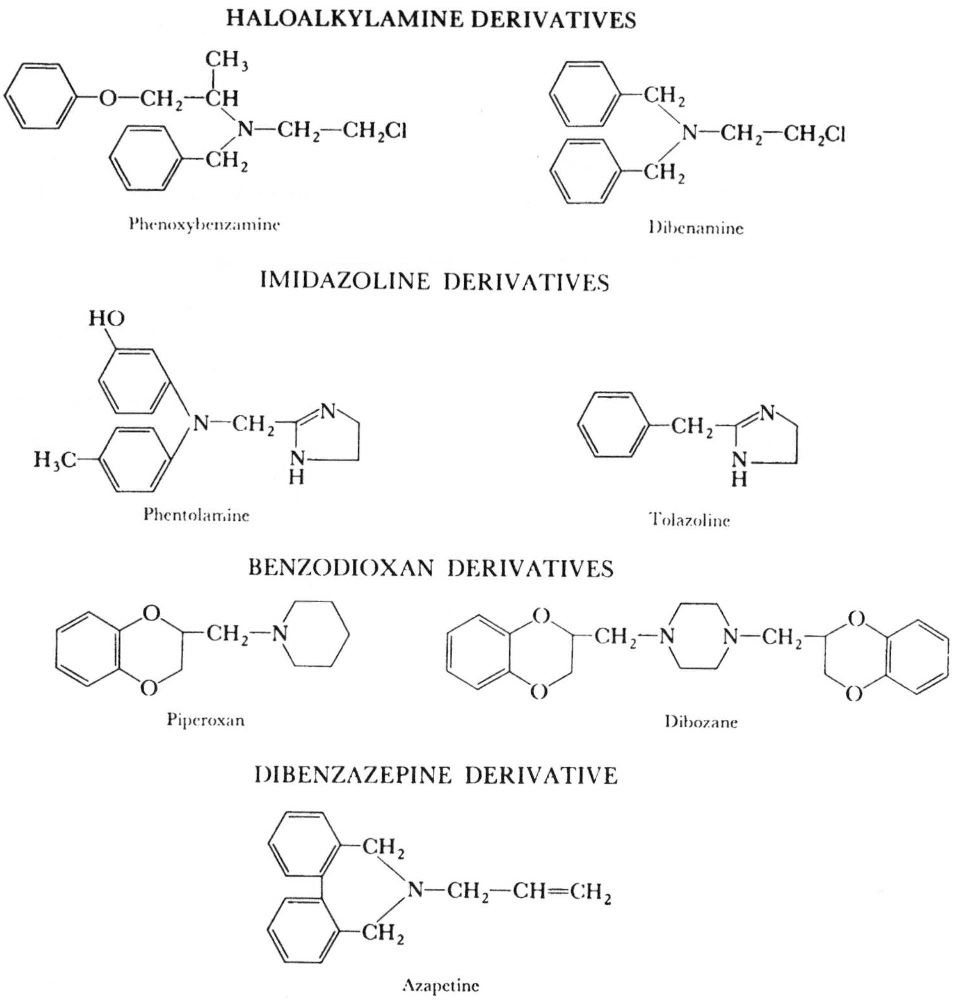

HALOALKYLAMINE DERIVATIVES

Phenoxybenzamine

Dibenamine

IMIDAZOLINE DERIVATIVES

Phentolamine

Tolazoline

BENZODIOXAN DERIVATIVES

Piperoxan

Dibozane

DIBENZAZEPINE DERIVATIVE

Azapetine

FIG. 6.8 Chemical structures of some α-adrenergic blocking drugs.

If phenoxybenzamine or other potent α blockers are given by rapid IV injection, severe hypotension and other adverse cardiovascular effects are seen; however, these effects probably involve factors other than α blockade.

In humans, α blockade evokes little change in blood pressure if the patient is supine, but pronounced hypotension occurs when the patient stands. This response is called postural or orthostatic hypotension. It is due to blockade of the vascular α receptors that are normally active in the efferent limb of reflex blood pressure pathways.

Other reflex changes are also altered. Reflex hypertension caused by anoxia is prevented by α blockade, as is the pressor response to occlusion of the carotid arteries (the bilateral carotid artery occlusion reflex depends upon increased sympathetic vasoconstrictor tone and increased release of epinephrine from the adrenal gland). Because of their occupation of α receptors, α-blocking agents prevent transmission of the nerve impulse to the α receptors of blood vessel cells and also block interaction of circulating epinephrine with α receptors. In this manner, reflex pressor responses are inhibited. Alpha-blocking agents increase blood flow through capillaries and arterioles as a result of α-receptor blockade and perhaps some direct relaxing effect on vascular smooth muscle.

Positive inotropic and chronotropic effects of catecholamines in heart muscle are not prevented by phentolamine or phenoxybenzamine. However, studies have shown that drugs having α-blocking effects decrease arrhythmias caused by catecholamines (Claborn and Szabuniewicz 1973; Wiersig et al. 1974; Benfry 1993). This has been demonstrated in nonanesthetized subjects and after sensitization of the myocardium by halogenated hydrocarbon anesthetics. It is not known if this is mediated entirely by α blockade. The haloalkylamines have a slight direct depressant effect on the heart that may be involved. Also, inhibition of the pressor effects of catecholamines (known to contribute to sensitization of the myocardium to arrhythmias) may also contribute (Katz and Katz 1966).

Under certain conditions, α-blocking agents partially decrease the inotropic effects of catecholamines in isolated heart muscle. This response varies from species to species, and in some cases it is demonstrable only during abnormally low temperatures. Although heart muscle contains α_1 receptors that increase myocardial contractility, the positive inotropic and chronotropic effects of catecholamines are predominately β-receptor–mediated events.

Other Effects. Phentolamine and phenoxybenzamine cause relaxation of the nictitating membrane (3rd eyelid); contractile responses caused by stimulation of sympathetic nerves or administration of an α agonist are blocked in this structure. The ocular effects of epinephrine and norepinephrine are inhibited by α blockers, as are pilomotor effects. The GI tract is variably influenced by α blockers, caused in part by the presence of β receptors in this system that also subserve relaxation.

Pharmacokinetics. The haloalkylamines and the imidazolines are effective whether administrated by mouth or injection. However, the former group is absorbed inefficiently after oral administration; only 20–30% of the drug is absorbed in active form from the GI tract. The onset of action of phenoxybenzamine and dibenamine is prolonged even after IV administration. These drugs may be converted to active intermediates, which then exert α-blocking effects. Their local irritating properties restrict their clinical use to oral or IV administration. Effective blood levels of tolazoline may not be obtained after oral administration, since it is slowly absorbed from the GI tract and is rapidly excreted by the kidneys. Phentolamine is less than 30% as active when given by mouth as when injected. Biotransformation pathways of the α-adrenergic blocking agents have not been clarified. Several of these drugs may localize in body adipose tissue because of their relatively high fat solubility.

Clinical Use. The α-receptor blocking drugs have been used with varying degrees of success in attempts to reduce vasoconstriction in the treatment of peripheral vasospasm, hypertension, pheochromocytoma, and visceral ischemia during circulatory shock syndromes. Early members of the α-antagonist group have not achieved appreciable cardiovascular application in veterinary practice and they have proved only slightly more useful in human medicine.

Certain types or stages of shock syndromes have been reported to respond favorably to an α-blocking agent. This is believed to be due to antagonism of catecholamine-induced peripheral vasoconstriction in vital visceral regions (e.g., renal and splanchnic circulation). Phenoxybenzamine (0.44–2.2 mg/kg diluted in 500 ml isotonic saline or glucose) administered by slow IV infusion has been suggested as a treatment procedure for preventing ischemia of the microcirculation during shock in animals. If hypotension occurs upon administration of an α-blocking agent during shock, adequate fluid replacement has not been achieved. It is essential that additional administration of blood or plasma expanders be instituted prior to continuing the infusion of the α-blocking agent. Currently, α-blocking agents are used infrequently, if at all, during the management of circulatory shock.

Nonselective α_1-α_2 Blockers. An important limitation to therapy with the older α blockers such as phentolamine and phenoxybenzamine is their paradoxic sympathomimetic activity, especially in the heart. Administration of α blockers can result in cardiac excitation and increased plasma concentrations of epinephrine and norepinephrine (Saeed et al. 1982). Historically, these effects were attributed to a triphasic adjustment in autonomic nerve activity instigated reflexly by the hypotensive response to inhibition of α-vasoconstrictor tone. These three phases are increased sympathetic efferent traffic over the cardioaccelerator nerves, decreased vagal impulses to the sinoatrial pacemaker, and increased sympathetic firing to the adrenal medulla. Study indicates, however, that the cardiac response to α-blocking agents is even more complex than originally surmised and involves yet a fourth pathway that incorporates the α_2-adrenergic neuronal receptors.

It is now known that phenoxybenzamine and especially phentolamine can block both α_1- and α_2-receptor subtypes (Table 6.4). Thus these drugs not only inhibit the α receptors of the vascular smooth muscle cell but can likewise block the α_2 receptors of the noradrenergic nerve endings (Fig. 6.2). Since the prejunctional α_2-receptor subtype controls the previously discussed feedback inhibition of norepinephrine and epinephrine release mechanisms, α_2 blockade would thereby free the noradrenergic neuron and adrenal chromaffin cell from a resident suppressor system (Saeed et al. 1982). An important consequence of such action would be an augmentation of the

TABLE 6.4 Relative order of selectivity of several α antagonists for α_1- and α_2-adrenergic receptor subtypes

Prazosin	α_1
Trimazosin	
Corynathine	
WB 4101	
Phenoxybenzamine	
Clozapine	
Phentolamine	
Piperoxan	
Tolazoline	
Yohimbine	
Rauwolscine	α_2

Source: Adams 1984.

Note: α_1-blocking activity diminishes and α_2-blocking activity increases as the list is traversed from top to bottom. Drugs in the middle are nonselective blockers of both receptor subtypes.

net quantity of catecholamines mobilized and released by reflex mechanisms. This sequence would not be manifested at either α_1- or α_2-vasoconstrictor receptors, owing to the original nonselective α-receptor blocking action of the drug. In the heart, however, the increased availability of catecholamines can explain the β_1-receptor stimulation and accentuated cardiac responses that can be associated with use of nonselective α antagonists.

Selective α_1 Blockers. Prazosin is an α antagonist with selectivity for the α_1-receptor subtype (Table 6.4). Since it leaves the prejunctional α_2 receptors operational, prazosin should exert less reflex sympathomimetic response than would a nonselective α_1-α_2 antagonist. Confirming this theory is a study that compares the hemodynamic effects of prazosin and phentolamine in conscious dogs (Saeed et al. 1982). Both drugs induced equivalent reductions in peripheral vascular resistance and blood pressure. Phentolamine also evoked significant increases in heart rate, cardiac output, oxygen consumption, and plasma concentrations of norepinephrine and epinephrine. Prazosin did not elicit these sympathomimetic side effects despite equivalent reduction in systemic blood pressure. The differences between prazosin and phentolamine can be explained by the α_1-receptor selectivity of the former, leaving intact the α_2-autoinhibitory mechanisms for catecholamine release (Fig. 6.2).

In addition, since extrasynaptic α_2 receptors of vascular smooth muscle also remain unblocked during therapy with prazosin, these vasoconstrictor receptors are available to help maintain vasomotor tone in the resistance and capacitance beds. Thus orthostatic hypotension seems to be less of a problem with α_1-selective blockers such as prazosin than with nonselective α_1-α_2 blockers such as phentolamine.

Because of reduced frequency of reflex cardiac excitation and orthostatic hypotension, prazosin and other α_1-selective antagonists have established an important niche in antihypertensive therapy in humans. These agents may also prove useful as peripheral vasodilators for reducing cardiac workload without reflex tachycardia in heart failure syndromes. Indeed, a study indicated that peripheral vasodilation with prazosin was effective in four dogs with congestive heart failure that were refractory to digoxin (Atwell 1979). However, digoxin was continued at reduced dosage in three of the dogs. It is unclear whether the beneficial responses in these patients were attributable to unloading of the heart by prazosin, to improvement in digoxin dosage management, or to both.

Selective α_2 Blockers. Yohimbine and rauwolscine are experimental drugs that have prominent blocking actions at α_2 receptors with little or no activity at α_1 receptors. These drugs are used commonly to investigate α_2-receptor–dependent mechanisms in different tissues. Also, there is considerable interest in yohimbine as an antidote to CNS depressant drugs that have α_2-receptor agonist activity in the brain. Table 6.4 ranks the order of selectivity of several α blockers relative to their antagonistic activity at α_1- and α_2-receptor subtypes.

β-Adrenergic Blocking Agents. Dichloroisoproterenol was the first drug demonstrated to cause a specific blockade of β-adrenergic receptors. Because it also caused an initial stimulation of the same receptors, subsequent studies were directed to identification of other β-blocking agents that lacked agonistic properties. Propranolol is structurally related to its precursors; it is many times more potent than pronethalol and has very minimal agonistic effects. Propranolol and related β antagonists are somewhat similar in structure to the β agonist isoproterenol, as seen in Figure 6.9. These compounds have an isopropyl-substituted secondary amine on the carbon side chain; this moiety appears to be important for effective interaction with the β receptor. The levoconfiguration of the asymmetric carbon atom on the side chain of propranolol yields the many times more potent β-blocking isomer than does the *d*-configuration. A large number of β blockers has been

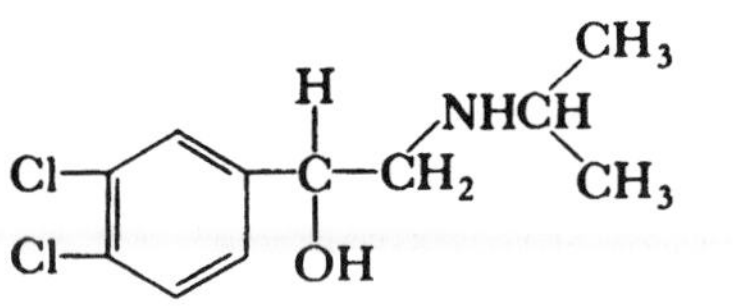

Dichloroisoproterenol

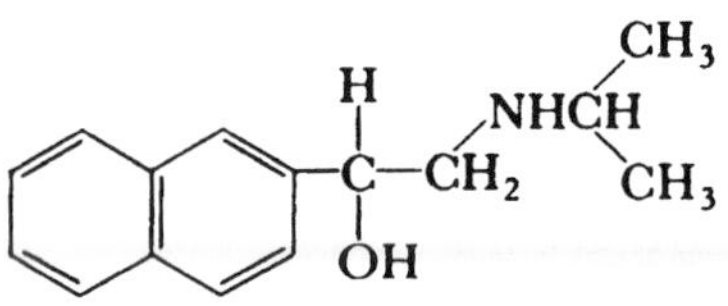

Pronethalol

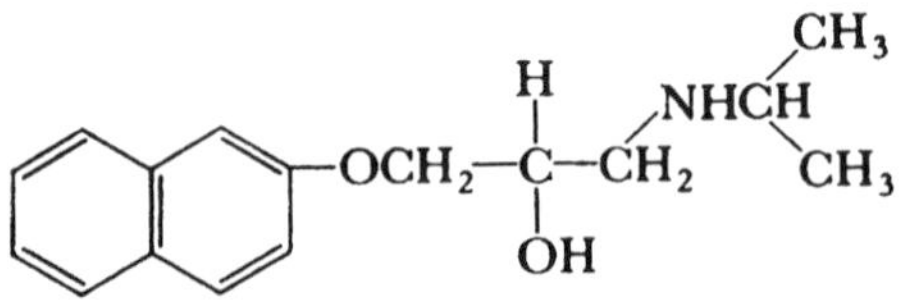

Propranolol

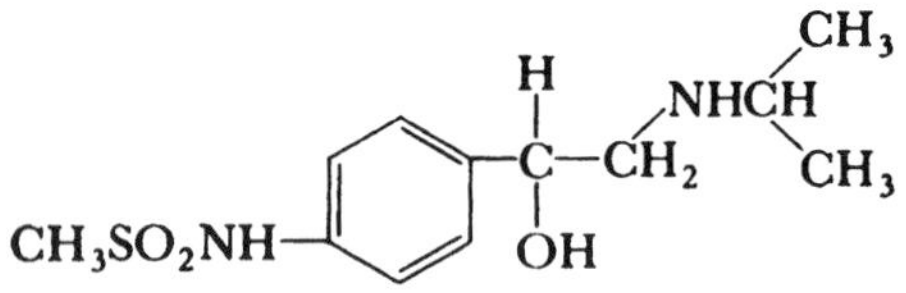

Sotalol

FIG. 6.9 Chemical structures of some β-adrenergic blocking drugs.

discovered with disparate pharmacodynamic actions, indicating a rather large group of β receptor subtypes (Gauthier et al. 2000; Ignarro et al. 2002; Maggioni et al. 2003). The clinical relevance of all these receptor subtypes to clinic veterinary medicine is unclear at this time.

Cardiovascular Pharmacologic Effects. Propranolol causes minimal depression of heart rate, myocardial contractile force, and cardiac output during normal conditions, because at rest the heart is not under pronounced sympathetic tone. However, if the heart is functioning under sympathetic nervous system dominance (e.g., during exercise), a relative bradycardia and a rather pronounced decrease in myocardial contraction and cardiac output will be produced. This drug prevents the positive inotropic and chronotropic effects of catecholamines in the heart as a result of β_1-receptor blockade and antagonizes the arrhythmogenic actions of the catecholamines.

Under most physiologic conditions, β_2-vascular receptors participate only in a limited manner to homeostatic regulation. Thus β-blocking agents affect blood pressure primarily through their effects on cardiac output rather than by peripheral vascular effects. Vasodilation produced by isoproterenol or epinephrine is blocked by propranolol, however, and the vasoconstrictor response to epinephrine (α response) may be somewhat accentuated. The vasoconstrictor effects of norepinephrine or other α agonists are not blocked by propranolol.

Bronchiolar airways are under sympathetic dominance, resulting in an active state of relaxation of the bronchiolar smooth muscle. By blocking β_2 receptors, propranolol inhibits sympathetic bronchodilator activity and causes bronchiolar constriction. This effect is especially prominent during episodes of allergic reactions and bronchiolar asthma; nonselective β_1-β_2–blocking drugs are contraindicated in these and related conditions.

Pharmacokinetics. Effective blood concentrations of propranolol are obtained after oral administration, but a large dose is required when given by this route. Biotransformation takes place primarily within the liver, and several active metabolites have been identified. In some species, 4-hydroxypropranolol is as active a β-adrenergic blocking agent as the parent compound. Propranolol causes a competitive blockade of β receptors. Therefore, large doses of β agonists can overcome the β-blocking effects of this drug. Pharmacokinetic features of propranolol and other β blockers were reviewed by Muir and Sams (1984).

Clinical Use. In human medicine, the β-receptor antagonists are used rather extensively to help manage several important medical problems, including hypertension, angina, cardiac dysrhythmias, hypertrophic obstructive cardiomyopathies, hyperthyroidism, anxiety-related muscle tremors, glaucoma, and myocardial reinfarction (Keating et al. 2003; Maggioni et al. 2003). The β blockers are utilized considerably less in veterinary practice but have application for controlling cardiac dysrhythmias provoked by overactivity of the sympathetic nervous system. Controlled clinical trials are generally lacking; however, β blockers also have potential benefit in domestic animals for reducing cardiac work effort in obstructive cardiomyopathies and perhaps for lowering myocardial oxygen demand in chronic heart failure syndrome. By blocking the β_1 receptors of the heart, the drugs decrease the inotropic, chronotropic, and arrhythmogenic effects of the endogenous catecholamines and other β-adrenergic agonists.

Wiersig et al. (1974) reported that 1 mg/kg racemic propranolol administered intravenously to dogs markedly decreased the incidence of ventricular fibrillation induced by epinephrine and norepinephrine during halothane and thiobarbiturate anesthesia. In this respect, propranolol was more effective than chlorpromazine or acepromazine. Adrenergic antagonists should be infused very slowly when given by the IV route, since cardiovascular depression may occur if they are administered by bolus IV injection.

Beta-blocking drugs are frequently effective in decreasing AV conduction and thereby controlling ventricular rate in patients with atrial fibrillation or flutter. Propranolol has been shown to be effective in controlling atrial and ventricular arrhythmias induced by digitalis excess and in treating paroxysmal arrhythmias that prove resistant to digitalis and quinidine. In dogs, slow IV infusion of propranolol (1–3 mg) has been proposed for treatment of digitalis-induced supraventricular tachycardia, idiopathic sinus tachycardia, and supraventricular tachycardia. The oral dose is 10–40 mg every 8 hours. Other nonselective β_1-β_2 blockers that have found use in clinical medicine include nadolol, timolol, and pindolol (Westfall and Westfall 2006).

β_1-Selective Antagonists. The preceding clinical uses of β antagonists depend on their block of the β_1-receptor subtype. Thus a drug with selective β_1-blocking action would have therapeutic capabilities equivalent to propranolol or other nonselective β_1-β_2 antagonists, but with reduced risk for loss of important β_2-receptor events as unwanted side effects (Morimoto et al. 2004). Propranolol and other β_1-β_2 blockers, e.g., are potentially harmful in certain patient populations owing to β_2-receptor inhibition in lung airways, leading to bronchoconstriction; in vascular smooth muscle, leading to changes in blood pressure and distribution of cardiac output; and in hepatocytes, leading to disruption of glucose metabolism. The latter condition is especially important in insulin-dependent diabetics, while loss of bronchodilator tone obviously is critical in patients with reduced respiratory reserve (Goldsmith and Keating 2004).

Some of the newly discovered β antagonists were found to be relatively more selective for the β_1- than for the β_2-receptor subtype (Nodari et al. 2003). Metoprolol is prototypical for this group. These drugs are commonly referred to as cardioselective β blockers because the mainstay of their clinical uses pertains to antagonism of the cardiac β_1 receptors. Some β blockers and associated affinities for receptor subtypes are included in Table 6.5, along with approximate biologic half-life values. Some of these compounds are lipophilic and undergo rather rapid biotransformation by liver enzymes, while others are lipophobic and depend upon renal excretory mechanisms for a longer half-life (Muir and Sams 1984). Metoprolol has found extensive use in human cardiovascular conditions wherein the β_1 receptors are the target (Westfall and Westfall 2006).

β Blockers and Reduced Cardiac Reserves. It should be remembered that β-blocking drugs, whether of the β_1-selective or β_1-β_2–nonselective group, should be administered cautiously in patients with preexisting heart disease (Felix et al. 2001). Under such conditions, cardiac performance may well depend on increased dominance of sympathetic activity as part of the compensatory attempt to maintain hemodynamics (Moniotte et al. 2001). Blockade of sympathetic input to the β_1 receptors of the heart, especially if sudden, can precipitate cardiac decompensation and failure (Fung et al. 2003). As a good example, Kittleson and Hamlin (1981) reported that propranolol caused cardiac decompensation in a dog with congestive heart failure that had been responding favorably to a vasodilator (hydralazine). If β blockade is attempted in the setting of reduced myocardial contractile reserves, it should be implemented cautiously with strict scrutiny of the patient's hemodynamic status (Cleland 2003; Czuriga et al. 2003; de Groot et al. 2004).

Intrinsic Sympathomimetic Activity. An interesting facet of the pharmacodynamic profile of certain β blockers is their intrinsic sympathomimetic activity (ISA) (Table 6.5). This means that these agents exert partial agonist effects; hence, they maintain a slight basal stimulation of the β receptors while also preventing further receptor activation through their primary antagonistic action. An advantage of ISA might be that basal tone to the cardiac β_1 receptors and pulmonary β_2 receptors may forestall cardiac depression and bronchoconstriction, respectively. Another advantage of low-grade β-receptor stimulation might be a reduced tendency for the up-regulation of β-receptor numbers that can follow long-term therapy with β antagonists. Administration of any of the β blockers should be discontinued gradually after chronic treatment

TABLE 6.5 Pharmacodynamic characteristics and empiric dosage schedules for several β-adrenergic-blocking drugs

Drug	β_1-Receptor Block	β_2-Receptor Block	ISA*	Half-Life† (hr)	Oral Dose (mg, TID)	IV Dose‡ (mg)
Propranolol	Yes	Yes	No	1–2	5–40	1–5
Timolol	Yes	Yes	No	1–2	0.5–1	0.4–1
Nadolol	Yes	Yes	No	3–8	5–40	. . .
Oxprenolol	Yes	Yes	Yes	.2	5–40	1–12
Alprenolol	Yes	Yes	Yes	.2	20–80	5–10
Pindolol	Yes	Yes	Yes	2–4	1–4	0.4–2
Metoprolol	Yes	No§	No	1–2	5–40	. . .
Atenolol	Yes	No§	No	3–6	20–80	. . .
Practolol	Yes	No§	Yes	No longer used	. . .	. . .

Sources: Adams 1984; Muir and Sams 1984.

Note: The biologic half-life values and dosage ranges for all β-blocking drugs have not been determined for domestic animals under clinical conditions. This table represents an empiric extrapolation based on data from either experimental studies in dogs or clinical studies in humans. Dosage schedules should be considered only as fundamental guidelines, and actual therapy should be implemented with lower dosages while patient response is closely monitored.

*ISA = intrinsic sympathomimetic activity.

†Biologic half-life values vary considerably, and variations among patients regarding therapeutically effective plasma concentrations reach four- to twentyfold.

‡Intravenous therapy with β blockers to control cardiac dysrhythmias should be done slowly and cautiously with dilute solutions while the electrocardiogram is monitored.

§β_1 selectivity is lost with higher dosages.

to prevent supersensitivity to agonists secondary to the receptor up-regulation or antagonist-induced receptor sensitivity phenomenon.

Additional β-receptor antagonists have been discovered that express additional complex effects. Labetalol, for example, is a competitive antagonist at α_1 and both β-receptor subtypes; it has been used as an oral antihypertensive agent in humans (Westfall and Westfall 2006). Carvedilol not only blocks α_1 and β_{-1}-β_2 receptors, but it also exerts antioxidant effects, which justifies its testing in heart failure patients. Other multiaction "third-generation" blockers include bucindolol, celiprolol, nebivolol, and several others; their clinical utility remains questionable.

In human medicine, many questions remain about the clinical relevance of ISA, receptor up-regulation, and even cardioselective blocking profiles with the β-receptor antagonists (Brexius et al. 2001). Even less is known about the practical relevance of these aspects in veterinary medicine. Until more data are available, metoprolol or other β_1-selective antagonists should be considered when β-blocking effects are deemed necessary in patients with preexisting pulmonary disease or diabetic-related disorders.

ADRENERGIC NEURON-BLOCKING DRUGS AND CATECHOLAMINE-DEPLETING AGENTS. These drugs act presynaptically at the adrenergic nerve terminal and prevent release of norepinephrine; they do not block the postsynaptic adrenergic receptor. Therefore, responses to direct-acting sympathomimetic amines are not prevented. However, effects of indirect-acting sympathomimetic amines (agents that cause release of endogenous norepinephrine) are attenuated by neuron-blocking and amine-depleting drugs, since the latter agents affect neuronal mechanisms that are active in the norepinephrine release process. For example, reserpine is a catecholamine-depleting agent that causes a severe reduction of the neuronal stores of norepinephrine. Therefore, less is available for release by an indirect-acting amine such as tyramine. Pressor effects of tyramine are thereby attenuated. Adrenergic neuron-blocking and amine-depleting drugs have not been used in clinical veterinary medicine to any appreciable extent.

Reserpine has been used for treating hypertension and psychic disorders in humans and is extensively used in research as a pharmacologic tool to deplete endogenous catecholamines from peripheral and CNS adrenergic pathways. Chronic daily treatment of dogs with reserpine (approximately 26 μg/kg, administered orally) induces a marked decrease in the concentration of norepinephrine in the hypothalamus, pons-medulla oblongata, and heart (Adams et al. 1971, 1972). Pronounced disturbances in peripheral and central sympathetic functions occur, and myocardial damage has been suspected. The mechanism of action of reserpine is related to an impairment of the

Mg^{++}- and ATP-dependent capacity of intraneuronal vesicles to accumulate and store catecholamines. After treatment with reserpine, amines are released from granular storage sites into the neuronal cytoplasm, where they are metabolized by MAO (Shore 1972).

Guanethidine is another agent that depletes catecholamines from adrenergic nerves. However, responses to adrenergic nerve stimulation are inhibited by guanethidine before detectable amine depletion occurs. A local anestheticlike effect at the adrenergic nerve terminal is thought to be involved. Guanethidine does not effectively pass the blood-brain barrier and has relatively less effect on central adrenergic pathways than reserpine. Guanethidine is used in antihypertensive therapy in humans; propranolol is sometimes given concurrently to block the reflex tachycardia resulting from guanethidine-induced hypotension.

Bretylium is an adrenergic neuron-blocking drug originally used in attempts to control hypertension. Side effects such as postural hypotension precluded the extensive use of this drug in clinical situations. Bretylium is often used in research to prevent the release of norepinephrine from adrenergic nerves. This drug does not deplete adrenergic neurons of their catecholamine stores; in this respect, it is dissimilar to reserpine and guanethidine. Bretylium seems to exert a local anesthetic-like effect at the adrenergic nerve terminal and, by this mechanism, decreases the amount of norepinephrine discharged from the nerve. Interestingly, because of its direct prolonging effect on refractoriness of ventricular tissue, bretylium has been approved for control of certain types of cardiac arrhythmias.

MISCELLANEOUS AGENTS. A chemical sympathectomy is produced by 6-hydroxydopamine. This compound is taken up into adrenergic nerves and causes anatomic destruction of the nerve terminal. Several weeks are required for regeneration of these structures after treatment with 6-hydroxydopamine.

Alpha-methyldopa is taken up into the adrenergic nerves, where it is biotransformed by the catecholamine-synthesizing enzymes into α-methylnorepinephrine, which is then stored in the amine granules. The α-methyl group protects this compound from oxidation by MAO. Therefore, endogenous norepinephrine may be displaced from the granule, metabolized by MAO, and replaced by α-methylnorepinephrine. The α-methylnorepinephrine is a potent α_2 agonist, thereby decreasing sympathetic efferent outflow from the CNS.

Alpha-methyl-para-tyrosine inhibits tyrosine hydroxylase, the rate-limiting enzyme in the synthesis of norepinephrine. Norepinephrine stores are not replenished, and depletion of this amine occurs after cessation of synthesis.

MAO inhibitors are used in humans as mood elevators or antidepressants. These drugs interfere with the oxidative deamination of catecholamines; these amines accumulate in the neuron after treatment with a MAO inhibitor. Responses to peripheral nerve stimulation do not seem to be markedly augmented by MAO inhibitors; however, effects of indirect-acting sympathomimetic amines are markedly potentiated by pretreatment with them. This is due partly to the increased concentration of amine that is available for release by the indirect-acting agent. Hypertensive crises and cerebral vascular accidents have occurred in human patients who ingested tyramine-containing foods (e.g., cheese, wine) while they were taking MAO inhibitors.

Cocaine inhibits the neuronal amine uptake pump of adrenergic nerves. This pump functions to take norepinephrine back up into the nerve. Other amines (e.g., tyramine) gain access into the neuron by this uptake mechanism. Thus cocaine potentiates the effect of norepinephrine but blocks the effect of tyramine. Imipramine and desmethylimipramine are tricyclic antidepressants; they, too, block the neuronal amine uptake mechanism.

REFERENCES

Adams, H. R. 1981. Cardiovascular emergencies: drugs and resuscitative principles. Vet Clin North Am 11:77–102.

———. 1984. New perspectives in cardiopulmonary therapeutics: Receptor-selective adrenergic drugs. J Am Vet Med Assoc 185(9):966–974.

Adams, H. R., Dixit, B. N., Smookler, H. H., Buckley, J. P. 1972. Clinical and biochemical effects of chronic reserpine administration in mongrel dogs. Am J Vet Res 33(4):699–707.

Adams, H. R., Parker, J. L. 1979. Pharmacologic management of circulatory shock: cardiovascular drugs and corticosteroids. J Am Vet Med Assoc 175:86–92.

Adams, H. R., Smookler, H. H., Clarke, D. E., Jandhyala, B. S., Dixit, B. N., Ertel, R. J., Buckley, J. P. 1971. Clinicopathologic effects of chronic reserpine administration in mongrel dogs. J Pharm Sci 60(8):1134–38.

Ahlquist, R. P. 1948. A study of the adrenotropic receptors. Am J Physiol 153:586–600.

Alberts, P. 1993. Subtype classification of presynaptic α_2-adrenoceptors. Gen Pharmac 24:1–8.

Änggard, E. 1994. Nitric oxide: mediator, murderer, and medicine. The Lancet, 343:1199–1206.

Atwell, R. B. 1979. The use of alpha blockade in the treatment of congestive heart failure associated with dirofilariasis and mitral valvular incompetence. Vet Rec 104:114–16.

Barnes, P. J. 1993. β-Adrenoceptors on smooth muscle, nerves and inflammatory cells. Life Sci 52:2101–9.

Benfry, B. G. 1993. Antifibrillatory effects of α_1-adrenoceptor blocking drugs in experimental coronary artery occlusion and reperfusion. Can J Physiol Pharmacol 71:103–11.

Bolger, A. P., and Al-Nasser, F. 2003. β-Blockers for chronic heart failure: Surviving longer but feeling better? Int J Cardiol 92:1–8.

Breit, A., Lagace, M., and Bouvier, M. 2004. Hetero-oligomerization between β_2 and β_3 receptors generates a β-adrenergic signaling unit with distinct functional properties. J Biol Chem 279:28756–28765.

Brixius, K., Bundkirchen, A., Bolck, B., Mehlhorn, U., and Schwinger, R. H. 2001. Nebivolol, bucindolol, metoprolol and carvedilol are devoid of intrinsic sympathomimetic activity in human myocardium. Br J Pharmacol 133:1330–1338.

Brodde, O. E., Michel, M. C. 1992. Adrenergic receptors and their signal transduction mechanisms in hypertension. J Hypertens 10(Suppl 7): S133–S145.

Buchanan, J. W., Dear, M. G., Pyle, R. L., et al. 1968. Medical and pacemaker therapy of complete heart block and congestive heart failure in a dog. J Am Vet Med Assoc 152:1099–109.

Caccavelli, L., Cussac, D., Pellegrini, I., Audinot, V., Jaquet, P., Enjalbert, A. 1992. D_2 dopaminergic receptors: normal and abnormal transduction mechanisms. Horm Res 38:78–83.

Chen, K. K., Schmidt, C. F. 1930. Ephedrine and related substances. Medicine 9:1–117.

Claborn, L. D., Szabuniewicz, M. 1973. Prevention of chloroform and thiobarbiturate cardiac sensitization to catecholamines in dogs. Am J Vet Res 34:801–4.

Cleland, J. G. 2003. β-Blockers for heart failure: Why, which, when, and where. Med Clin North Am 87:339–371.

Cornish, E. J., Miller, R. C. 1975. Comparison of the beta-adrenoceptors in the myocardium and coronary vasculature of the kitten heart. J Pharm Pharmacol 27:23–30.

Czuriga, I., Riecansky, I., Bodnar, J., Fulop, T., Kruzsicz, V., Kristof, E., and Edes, I. For the NEBIS Investigators. NEBIS Investigators Group. 2003. Comparison of the new cardioselective β-blocker nebivolol with bisoprolol in hypertension: The nebivolol, bisoprolol multicenter study (NEBIS). Cardiovasc Drugs Ther 17:257–263.

Dale, H. H. 1906. On some physiological actions of ergot. J Physiol (Lond) 34:163–206.

de Groot, A. A., Mathy, M. J., van Zwieten, P. A., and Peters, S. L. 2004. Antioxidant activity of nebivolol in the rat aorta. J Cardiovasc Pharmacol 43:148–153.

Ettinger, S. 1969. Isoproterenol treatment of atrioventricular block in the dog. J Am Vet Med Assoc 154:398–405.

Eyster, G. E., Anderson, L. K., Bender, G., et al. 1975. Effect of dobutamine in postperfusion cardiac failure in the dog. Am J Vet Res 13:1285–89.

Feldman, A. M. 1993. Modulation of adrenergic receptors and G-transduction proteins in failing human ventricular myocardium. Circulation 87(Suppl IV):IV27–IV34.

Felix, S. B., Stangl, V., Kieback, A., Doerffel, W., Staudt, A., Wernecke, K. D., Baumann, G., and Stangl, K. 2001. Acute hemodynamic effects of β-blockers in patients with severe congestive heart failure: Comparison of celiprolol and esmolol. J Cardiovasc Pharmacol 38:666–671.

Fung, J. W., Yu, C. M., Kum, L. C., Yip, G. W., and Sanderson, J. E. 2003. Role of β-blocker therapy in heart failure and atrial fibrillation. Cardiac Electrophysiol Rev 7:236–242.

Gauthier, C., Langin, D., and Balligand, J. L. 2000. β_3 adrenoceptors in the cardiovascular system. Trends Phamacol Sci 21:426–431.

Goldberg, L. I., Rajfer, S. I. 1985. Dopamine receptors: Applications in clinical cardiology. Circulation 72:245–48.

Goldsmith, D. R., and Keating, G. M. 2004. Budesonide/fomoterol: A review of its use in asthma. Drugs 64:1597–1618.

Haller, C. A., Benowitz, N. L. 2000. Adverse cardiovascular and central nervous system events associated with dietary supplements containing ephedra alkaloids. New Engl J Med 343:1833–1838.

Hinds, J. E., Hawthorne, E. W. 1975. Comparative cardiac dynamic effects of dobutamine and isoproterenol in conscious instrumented dogs. Am J Cardiol 36:894–901.

Hosgood G. 1990. Pharmacologic features and physiologic effects of dopamine. J Am Vet Med Assoc 197:1209–1211.

Ignarro, L. J., Byrns, R. E., Trinh, K., Sisodia, M., and Buga, G. M. 2002. Nebivolol: A selective β_1 adrenergic receptor antagonist that relaxes vascular smooth muscle by nitric-oxide and cyclic GMP-dependent mechanism. Nitric Oxide 7:75–82.

Katz, R. L., Katz, G. J. 1966. Surgical infiltration of pressor drugs and their interaction with volatile anaesthetics. Br J Anaesth 38:712–18.

Keating, G. M., and Jarvis, B. 2003. Carvedilol: A review of its use in chronic heart failure. Drugs 63:1697–1741.

Kittleson, M. D., Hamlin, R. L. 1981. Hydralazine therapy for severe mitral regurgitation in a dog. J Am Vet Med Assoc 179:903–4.

Lands, A. M., Arnold, A., McAuliff, J. P., Luduena, F. P., Brown, T. G., Jr. 1967. Differentiation of receptor systems activated by sympathomimetic amines. Nature 214(88):597–98.

Langer, G. A. 1974. Calcium in mammalian myocardium: localization, control, and the effects of digitalis. Circ Res 35(Suppl 3):91–98.

Langer, S. Z. 1980. Presynaptic regulation of the release of catecholamines. Pharm Rev 32(4):337–62.

Levitzki, A., Marbach, I., Bar-Sani, A. 1993. The signal transduction between β-receptors and adenylyl cyclase. Life Sci 52:2093–2100.

Loeb, H. S., Bredakis, J., Gunner, R. M. 1977. Superiority of dobutamine over dopamine for augmentation of cardiac output in patients with chronic low output cardiac failure. Circulation 55:375–78.

Lowenstein, C. J., Dinerman, J. L., Snyder, S. H. 1994. Nitric oxide: a physiologic messenger. Ann Intern Med 120:227–37.

Maggioni, A. P., Sinagra, G., Opasich, C., Geraci, E., Gorini, M., Gronda, E., Lucci, D., Tognoni, G., Balli, E., and Tavazzi, L. 2003. β Blockers in patients with congestive heart failure: Guided use in clinical practice investigators. Treatment of chronic heart failure with β adrenergic blockade beyond controlled clinical trials: The BRING-UP experience. Heart 89:299–305.

Milgram, N. W., Ivy, G. O., Murphy, M. P., et al. 1993. The effect of L-deprenyl on behavior, cognitive function, and biogenic amines in the dog. Neurochemical Research 18: 1211–1219.

———. Effects of chronic oral administration of l-deprenyl in the dog. Pharmacol Biochem and Behav 51: 421–428.

Moniotte, S., Kobzik, L., Feron, O., Trochu, J. N., Gauthier, C., and Balligand, J. L. 2001. Upregulation of β_3-adrenoceptors and altered contractile response to inotropic amines in human failing myocardium. Circulation 103:1649–1655.

Moran, N. C., Perkins, M. E. 1958. Adrenergic blockade of the mammalian heart by a dichloro analogue of isoproterenol. J Pharmacol Exp Ther 124:223–37.

Moreland, R. S., Bohr, D. F. 1984. Adrenergic control of coronary arteries. Fed Proc 43:2857–61.

Morimoto, A., Hasegawa, H., Cheng, H-J., Little, W. C., and Cheng, C. P. 2004. Endogenous β2-adrenoceptor activation contributes to left ventricular and cardiomyocyte dysfunction in heart failure. Am J Physiol Heart Circ Physiol 286:H2425–H2433.

Muir, W. W., Sams, R. S. 1984. Clinical pharmacodynamics and pharmacokinetics of beta-adrenoceptor blocking drugs in veterinary medicine. Comp Cont Ed Prac Vet 6:156–67.

Murphy M. B, Murray C, Shorten G. D. 2001. Fenoldopam—A selective peripheral dopamine receptor agonist for the treatment of severe hypertension. N Eng. J Med 345:1548–1557.

Nodari, S., Metra, M., and Dei Cas, L. 2003. β-Blocker treatment of patients with diastolic heart failure and atrial hypertension. A prospective, randomized comparison of the long-term effects of atenolol vs. nebivolol. Eur J Heart Failure 5:621–627.

Osborne, N. N., Wood, J. P. M., Chidlow, G., Casson, R., DeSantis, L., and Schmidt, K-G. 2004. Effectiveness of levobetaxolol and timolol at blunting retinal ischaemia is related to their calcium and sodium blocking activities: Relevance to glaucoma. Brain Res Bull 62:525–528.

Parker, J. L., Adams, H. R. 1977. Drugs and the heart muscle. J Am Vet Med Assoc 171:78–84.

Powell, C. E., Slater, I. H. 1958. Blocking of inhibitory adrenergic receptors by a dichloro analog of isoproterenol. J Pharmacol Exp Ther 122:480–88.

Robidoux, J., Martin, T. L., and Collins, S. 2004. β-Adrenergic receptors and regulation of energy expenditure: A family affair. Annu Rev Pharmacol Toxicol 44:297–323.

Rosati, M., Dyson, D. H., Sinclair, M. D., et al. 2007. Response of hypotensive dogs to dopamine hydrochloride and dobutamine hydrochloride during deep isoflurane anesthesia. Am J Vet Res 68:483–494.

Saeed, M., Sommer, O., Holtz, J., et al. 1982. Alpha-adrenoceptor blockade by phentolamine causes beta-adrenergic vasodilation by increased catecholamine release due to pre-synaptic alpha-blockade. J Cardiovasc Pharmacol 4:44–52.

Schmid-Schonbein, G., and Hugli, T. 2005. A new hypothesis for microvascular inflammation in shock and multiorgan failure: Self-digestion by pancreatic enzymes. Microcirc 12:71–82.

Schwinn, D. A. 1993. Adrenoceptors as models for G protein-coupled receptors: structure, function and regulation. Br J Anaesthesia 71:77–85.

Setler, P. E., Pendleton, R. G., Finlay, E. 1975. The cardiovascular actions of dopamine and the effects of central and peripheral catecholaminergic receptor blocking drugs. J Pharmacol Exp Ther 192:702–12.

Shapland, J. E., Garner, H. E., Hatfield, D. G. 1981. Cardiopulmonary effects of clenbuterol in the horse. J Vet Pharmacol Ther 4:43–50.

Shore, P. A. 1972. Transport and storage of biogenic amines. Annu Rev Pharmacol 12:209–26.

Sigrist N. E. 2007. Use of dopamine in acute renal failure. J Vet Emerg Crit Care 17:117–126.

Simmons J. P., Wohl J. S., Schwartz D. D., et al. 2006. Diuretic effects of fenoldopam in healthy cats. J Vet Emerg Crit Care 16:96–103.

Soma, L. R., Burrows, C. F., Marshall, B. E. 1974. In R. W. Kirk, ed. Current Veterinary Therapy, V: Small Animal Practice, p. 26. Philadelphia: W. B. Saunders.

Sun, D., Huang, A., Mital, S., Kichuk, M. R., Marboe, C. C., Addonizio, L. J., Michler, R. E., Koller, A., Hintze, T. H., and Kaley, G. 2002. Norepinephrine elicits β_2-receptor–mediated dilation of isolated human coronary arterioles. Circulation 106:550–555.

Swanson, C. R., Muir, W. W., Bednarski, R. M., et al. 1985. Hemodynamic responses in halothane-anesthetized horses given infusions of dopamine or dobutamine. Am J Vet Res 46:365–70.

Tuttle, R. R., Mills, J. 1975. Dobutamine: development of a new catecholamine to selectively increase cardiac contractility. Circ Res 36:185–96.

Watanabe, A. M., Besch, H. R., Jr. 1974. Cyclic adenosine monophosphate modulation of slow calcium influx channels in guinea pig hearts. Circ Res 35:316–24.

Westfall, D. P. 2004. In C. R. Craig and R. E. Stitzel, eds. Modern Pharmacology, Adrenoceptor antagonists. pp. 109–120. Baltimore: Lippincott Williams & Wilkins.

Westfall, T. C. and Westfall, D. P. 2006. Adrenergic agonists and antagonists. In L. L. Brunton, J. S. Lazo, and K. L. Parker, eds. The Pharmacologic Basis of Therapeutics, 11th ed. New York: McGraw Hill.

Whilton, D. L., Trim, C. M. 1985. Use of dopamine hydrochloride during general anesthesia in the treatment of advanced atrioventricular heart block in four foals. J Am Vet Med Assoc 187:1357–61.

Wiersig, D. O., Davis, R. H., Jr., Szabuniewicz, M. 1974. Prevention of induced ventricular fibrillation in dogs anesthetized with ultrashort acting barbiturates and halothane. J Am Vet Med Assoc 165:341–45.

Willerson, J. T., Hutton, I., Watson, J. T., et al. 1976. Influence of dobutamine on regional myocardial blood flow and ventricular performance during acute and chronic myocardial ischemia in dogs. Circulation 53:828–33.

Wohl J. S., Schwartz D. D., Flournoy W. S. et al. 2007. Renal hemodynamic and diuretic effects of low-dosage dopamine in anesthetized cats. J Vet Emerg Critical Care 17:45–52.

CHAPTER 7

CHOLINERGIC PHARMACOLOGY: AUTONOMIC DRUGS

H. RICHARD ADAMS

Acetylcholine (ACh) is the messenger between nerve endings and innervated cells of autonomic ganglia, parasympathetic neuroeffector junctions, some sympathetic neuroeffector junctions, somatic neuromuscular junctions, the adrenal medulla, and certain regions of the central nervous system (CNS). It has been recognized for many years that considerable therapeutic benefit could be derived from drugs that would selectively mimic the action of ACh only at certain of these sites or, alternatively, that could selectively prevent only unwanted effects of this biogenic substance. Although ideal drugs have yet to be identified, some agents have been found to be relatively more active at certain cholinergic sites than at others. In this chapter, drugs that influence postganglionic parasympathetic neuroeffector junctions and autonomic ganglia by ACh-like or ACh blocking effects will be examined (Brown and Taylor 2006; Westfall and Westfall 2006). Parasympathetic neurons and affiliated receptors of innervated cells are depicted in Figure 7.1.

PARASYMPATHOMIMETIC AGENTS

Cholinergic is used to describe an ACh-like effect without distinction as to anatomic site of action. *Parasympathomimetic* is used specifically to describe an ACh-like effect on effector cells innervated by postganglionic neurons of the parasympathetic nervous system (Fig. 7.1). Most of the cholinergic drugs considered here are used clinically for their parasympathomimetic activities. However, the scope of pharmacologic activity of several of these compounds is not restricted to parasympathomimetic effects but includes cholinergic actions throughout the body (Barnes and Hansel 2004).

Based on mechanism of action, drugs that cause parasympathomimetic effects can be divided into two major groups: direct-acting agents, which like ACh activate cholinergic receptors of the effector cells, and cholinesterase inhibitors, which allow endogenous ACh to accumulate and thereby intensify and prolong its action (Brown and Taylor 2006).

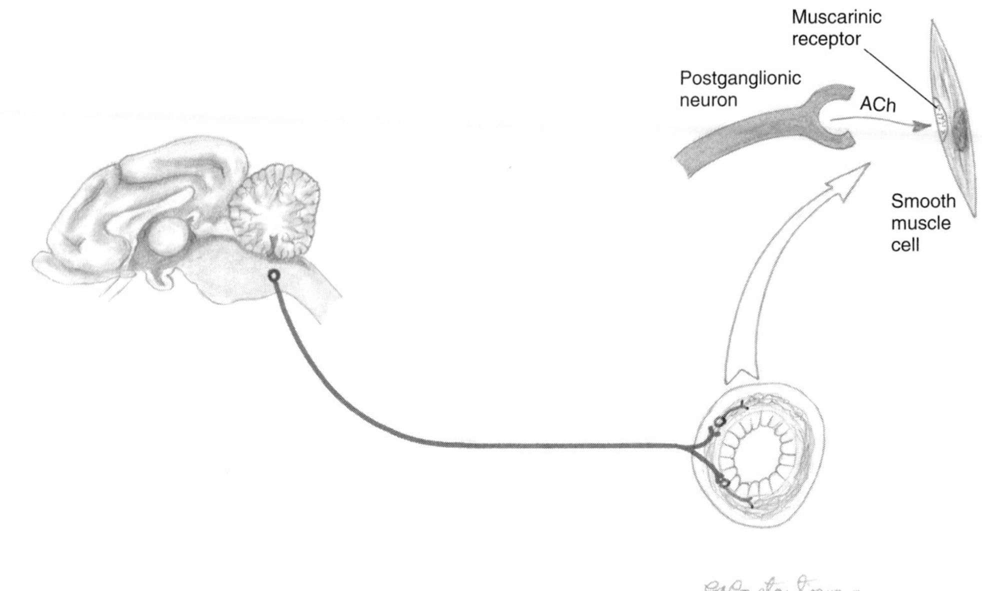

FIG. 7.1 Anatomical relationships of parasympathetic neuronal outflow tracts and affiliated receptors of innervated cells. Parasympathetic preganglionic axons exit cranial (shown) or sacral zones and pass peripherally to synapse with a neuron body located within (shown) or adjacent to innervated tissue. The preganglionic neuron releases the neurotransmitter acetylcholine (ACh), which activates nicotinic cholinergic receptors on the ganglionic neuron body. The resulting stimulation of the ganglionic neuron promotes release of ACh from the axon terminal at postganglionic parasympathetic neuroeffector junctions within the intestinal tract (shown) or other tissues innervated by parasympathetic neurons. ACh activates muscarinic cholinergic receptors present on cells innervated by the parasympathetic division of the autonomic nervous system. Preganglionic fibers are dark gray; postganglionic fibers are light gray. Drawn by Dr. Gheorghe M. Constantinescu, University of Missouri.

DIRECT-ACTING PARASYMPATHOMIMETIC AGENTS

Direct-acting parasympathomimetic agents consist of esters of choline and naturally occurring cholinomimetic alkaloids.

CHOLINE ESTERS. Choline, a member of the B vitamin group, possesses the characteristic depressor action of a cholinergic drug when injected intravenously in large unphysiologic amounts; however, its potency is multiplied thousands of times when it is esterified with acetic acid to yield ACh.

ACh, although essential for maintenance of body homeostasis, is not used therapeutically for two important reasons. First, it acts simultaneously at various tissue sites and no selective therapeutic response can be achieved. Second, its duration of action is quite brief because it is rapidly inactivated by the cholinesterases. Several derivatives of ACh are more resistant to hydrolysis by cholinesterase and have a somewhat greater selectivity in their sites of action. Of several hundred choline derivatives that have been synthesized, carbachol, bethanechol, and methacholine have proved effective for certain clinical uses and will be discussed here.

Mechanism of Action. Pharmacologic effects of ACh and related choline esters are mediated by activation of specific ACh-responsive sites (i.e., cholinergic receptors or cholinoceptors) located on cells innervated by cholinergic nerves and, in some cases, on cells that lack cholinergic innervation. Choline esters act directly on postsynaptic receptors and do not depend upon endogenous ACh for their effects. Based on differential responsiveness to cholinergic agonists and antagonists, two basic types of cholinoceptors have been identified within the peripheral efferent pathways of the mammalian autonomic nervous system (Fig. 7.1).

Nicotinic Receptors. Beginning with the early studies by Dale (1914), it was known that nicotine in small doses mimics certain actions of ACh and in larger doses blocks these same cholinergic effects. As summarized in Chapter

5, nicotinic responsive sites are present in autonomic ganglia, adrenal medullary chromaffin cells, and neuromuscular junctions of the somatic nervous system. Accordingly, receptors at these sites are called nicotinic cholinergic receptors, and effects of cholinergic drugs at these sites are described as nicotinic effects. Nicotinic receptors at ganglia are different subtypes from those localized to voluntary skeletal muscle.

Muscarinic Receptors. Nicotine does not mimic ACh at postganglionic parasympathetic neuroeffector junctions, i.e., parasympathetic innervation to heart muscle, smooth muscle, and exocrine glands. The mushroom alkaloid muscarine was found to selectively mimic activity of ACh at these sites, but not at the previously mentioned nicotinic receptors (Chapple et al. 2002). Muscarinic receptors, therefore, designate the type of cholinoceptors present at postganglionic parasympathetic neuroeffector junctions (Fig. 7.1; Eglen et al. 2001). Muscarinic receptors are also present in some blood vessels that lack cholinergic innervation and at neuroeffector junctions of the sympathetic nervous system that are cholinergic (see Chapter 5). The parasympathomimetic, or muscarinic, effects produced by drugs examined in this chapter are equivalent to the physiologic changes evoked by postganglionic parasympathetic nerve impulses, as listed in Table 5.1 (Lewis et al. 2001).

Atropine is a cholinergic blocking agent that selectively blocks muscarine receptors without blocking nicotinic sites; whereas hexamethonium, d-tubocurarine, and large doses of nicotine block nicotinic but not muscarinic receptors. Multiple subtypes of muscarinic receptors have been identified by molecular biology technology, but the clinical implications of such discoveries have yet to be defined for veterinary medicine (Wess 2004; Willmy-Matthes et al. 2003; Matsui et al. 2000).

ACh evokes an excitatory response in some tissues, e.g., smooth muscle of the gastrointestinal (GI) tract, but causes inhibitory responses in other tissues, e.g., myocardium. In general, excitatory effects of ACh are due to depolarization of the postsynaptic membrane characterized by an increase in permeability of the membrane to both Na^+ and K^+ ions. Inhibitory effects have been associated with an inhibitory G protein (i.e., G_i) linked to diminution of adenylyl cyclase and resulting decreased formation of cAMP and protein kinase A (Lambert 1993). In some tissues, muscarinic receptors are linked to activation of guanylyl cyclase with increased formation of cGMP (Lambert 1993).

Structure-Activity Relationships. Direct-acting cholinergic agonists contain structural groupings that allow interaction of the agent with cholinergic receptors and result in similar changes in membrane configuration and thus ion permeability as caused by ACh. Choline esters contain a quaternary nitrogen atom to which three methyl groups are attached. Except for some naturally occurring cholinomimetic alkaloids, a quaternary nitrogen moiety is usually required for a direct potent action on cholinergic receptors. Like its counterpart the ammonium ion, the quaternary nitrogen group carries a positive charge; this cationic group electrostatically binds with a negatively charged (anionic) site of the cholinergic receptor. The anionic site is believed to be the main determinant of receptor events, and interaction of the cationic head of ACh with the anionic site is the primary instigator of conformational changes that lead to alterations in membrane permeability.

Receptive macromolecules (i.e., cholinergic receptors and cholinesterases) that recognize and bind ACh have, in addition to the anionic site, a region that combines with the ester component of ACh (Fig. 7.2) (Hucho et al. 1991). In cholinesterase, this region is called the esteratic site and its combination with the carboxyl group results in hydrolysis of the ester (see discussion later in this chapter). Hydrolysis of ACh does not occur upon its interaction with a receptor, however, and the ester-attracting region of the receptor is called the esterophilic site (Inestrosa and Perelman 1990; Massoulie et al. 1993; Taylor 2006a, 1991).

ACh is ideally arranged structurally so that it combines with the esterophilic and anionic sites of both nicotinic and muscarinic receptors and acetylcholinesterases (Hucho et al. 1991). When both components of the ester moiety of ACh (i.e., the carbonyl group and the ether oxygen) are replaced by methylene molecules, agonistic properties at both muscarinic and nicotinic sites are reduced. If only the ether oxygen of ACh is substituted by a methylene group, the muscarinic potency is markedly decreased but nicotinic properties are little affected. Introduction of a methyl group on the β-carbon atom of the choline segment considerably reduces nicotinic properties but does not reduce muscarinic activities. These findings indicate that the esterophilic sites are arranged somewhat differently in muscarinic than in nicotinic receptors and therefore influence specificity of agonistic and antagonistic properties of different drugs. The esterophilic region may contain subunits that individually attract either the ether oxygen or

A. $CH_3-C(=O)-O-CH_2-CH_2-N^{+}(CH_3)_3$ (2) (1)

3 3 3 3 − 3

Esterophilic Site   Anionic Site

Receptor

δ^+ δ^- — (−)

B.

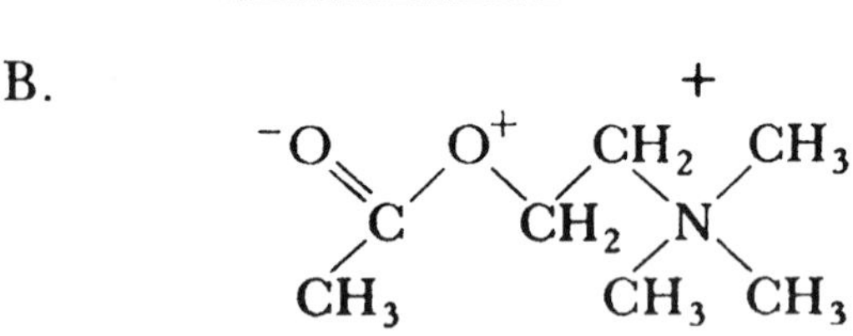

FIG. 7.2 Interaction of ACh and its receptor. **A.** (1) = electrostatic bond between cationic (quaternary N+) group of ACh and the anionic site of the receptor. (2) = dipolar binding of ester of ACh with the esterophilic site of the receptor [*note:* in ACh-cholinesterase interaction, (2) = covalent bonding of carboxyl carbon to a protonated acidic group of the esteratic site of the enzyme]. (3) = probable existence of hydrophobic bonds between the various methyl groups and adjacent proteins of the receptor surface. Based on the postulated interaction of ACh and cholinesterase (modified from Eldefrawi 1974). **B.** Electrical charge distribution of ACh and its receptor (Khromov-Borisov and Michelson 1966).

the carbonyl oxygen by hydrogen bonding and dipole-dipole interaction, respectively (Fig. 7.2B) (Khromov-Borisov and Michelson 1966).

ACh is the prototypical cholinergic agent; it acts at all cholinoceptor sites and therefore evokes both nicotinic and muscarinic effects. Acetyl-β-methylcholine (methacholine) is identical in structure to ACh except for the substitution of a methyl group on the β-carbon atom of the choline group. This structural change yields a compound that is primarily a muscarinic receptor agonist lacking significant nicotinic effects when given in usual dosages. Further, it is more active on the cardiovascular system than on the GI tract. Duration of action of methacholine is considerably longer than that of ACh because the former drug is hydrolyzed by acetylcholinesterase (AChE) at a much slower rate than is ACh and methacholine is almost totally resistant to breakdown by pseudocholinesterase.

Carbachol and bethanechol each have a carbamyl (NH_2COO-) group substituted for the acetic moiety of ACh, and bethanechol also has a β-methyl group. Both of these agents are almost completely resistant to inactivation by the cholinesterases. Their duration of action is therefore considerably longer than that of ACh. Carbachol is active at both muscarinic and nicotinic receptor sites (therefore it is cholinomimetic and not just parasympathomimetic), whereas bethanechol is primarily a muscarinic agonist. Unlike methacholine, both these drugs are somewhat more active on smooth muscles of the GI tract and urinary bladder than on cardiovascular function. Chemical structures of these choline esters and their related pharmacologic characteristics are shown in Table 7.1.

Acetylcholine. Although ACh is not used clinically, it is the prototypical cholinergic agonist, and an understanding of its activity is imperative for a comprehension of the pharmacologic effects of other cholinomimetic drugs. The biosynthesis, neuronal release, cellular activities, and inactivation of endogenous ACh are examined in Chapter 5 and should be reviewed in conjunction with this chapter.

Since ACh is a mixed nicotinic-muscarinic agonist, different effects can be produced by administration of this agent, depending upon the relative dominance of muscarinic (parasympathomimetic) or nicotinic actions. These effects can be differentiated by use of small and large doses of ACh and by using selective cholinergic blocking drugs. In general, parasympathomimetic effects dominate with small doses, whereas with large doses cholinergic effects at other tissue sites are also produced. Therefore, muscarinic receptors seem to be more susceptible than nicotinic receptors to ACh. Use of cholinergic blocking drugs and small and large doses of ACh to differentiate muscarinic and nicotinic effects of ACh is shown in Figure 7.3. This figure is discussed in greater detail in the following sections.

Pharmacologic Effects. *Cardiovascular Effects of Small Doses of ACh.* Intravenous (IV) administration of small amounts of ACh (5–10 μg/kg) produces a brief but rapid fall in systolic and diastolic blood pressures. This is due to a decrease in peripheral resistance resulting from dilation of blood vessels. Most blood vessels receive little or no parasympathetic innervation (see Chapter 5). Therefore, most vascular smooth muscle is different from other smooth muscle in that its muscarinic receptors are noninnervated.

TABLE 7.1 Chemical structures (A) and scope of cholinergic receptor activating properties (B) of some choline esters

A.

Compound	Structure
Choline	$(CH_3)_3N^+ \cdot CH_2 \cdot CH_2 \cdot OH$
Acetylcholine	$(CH_3)_3N^+ \cdot CH_2 \cdot CH_2 \cdot O \cdot COCH_3$
Methacholine	$(CH_3)_3N^+ \cdot CH_2 \cdot CH_2 \cdot O \cdot COCH_3$
Carbachol	$(CH_3)_3N^+ \cdot CH_2 \cdot CH_2 \cdot O \cdot CONH_2$
Bethanechol	$(CH_3)_3N^+ \cdot CH_2 \cdot CH(CH_3) \cdot O \cdot CONH_2$

B.

	Susceptibility to Cholinesterase		Agonistic Properties				
			Muscarinic Receptors				
	True	Pseudo	CV	GI	UB	E	Nicotinic Receptors
Choline							
Acetylcholine	+++	+++	+++	+++	++	+	+++
Methacholine	+	–	+++	++	++	+	±
Carbachol	–	–	+	+++	+++	++	+++
Bethanechol	–	–	±	+++	+++	++	–

Note: CV = cardiovascular; GI = gastrointestinal; UB = urinary bladder; E = eye.

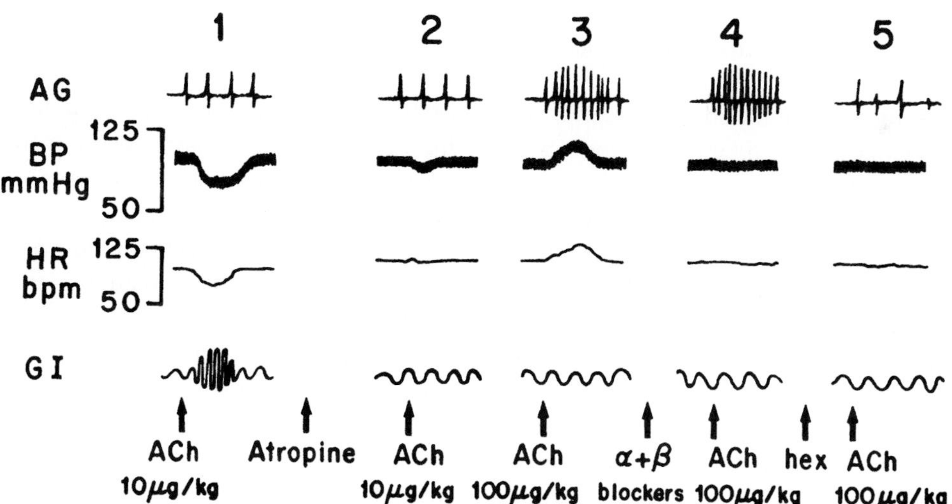

FIG. 7.3 Muscarinic and nicotinic effects of ACh on blood pressure, heart rate, intestinal motility, and autonomic ganglionic action potentials in an anesthetized dog. Schematic reproductions: 1. A small dose of ACh (10 mg/kg) administered intravenously causes hypotension, bradycardia, and intestinal contractions caused by direct stimulation of muscarinic receptors of blood vessels, heart, and intestinal smooth muscle, respectively. These effects are brief because of rapid destruction of ACh by cholinesterase. 2. Atropine blocks the muscarinic receptors and thereby prevents the effects seen in (1). 3. Large doses of ACh (100 mg/kg) stimulate, in addition to muscarinic receptors, nicotinic receptors of parasympathetic and sympathetic ganglionic neurons, causing an increase in frequency and amplitude of ganglionic action potentials. Although all autonomic ganglia are activated, impulses arising from parasympathetic ganglia do not reach their effector cells because of blockade of parasympathetic postganglionic neuroeffector junctions by atropine. Sympathomimetic responses (pressor effect and tachycardia) result. 4. Impulses arising from sympathetic ganglia are prevented from reaching their effector cells by adrenergic blocking drugs; however, ganglionic nicotinic receptors are still activated by ACh. 5. Hexamethonium (hex) blocks nicotinic receptors of ganglia and thereby inhibits the nicotinic ganglionic stimulating effect of ACh and reduces ganglionic action potentials. AG = action potentials of autonomic ganglionic neuron; BP = systemic blood pressure; HR = heart rate; GI = intestinal peristaltic waves.

Interestingly, muscarinic receptors subserving dilation of blood vessels are located on the endothelium rather than on the smooth muscle itself. Activation of endothelial muscarinic receptors by ACh causes the endothelial cells to release endothelium-derived relaxing factor (EDRF) (Furchgott and Zawadzki 1980), identified as nitric oxide (Lowenstein et al. 1994). Nitric oxide transfers to the vascular smooth muscle cells and therein activates cytosolic guanylyl cyclase; the resulting increase in cGMP provokes vascular smooth muscle relaxation and vasodilation, as summarized in Figure 5.8 (Adams 1996; Toda and Okamura 2003).

Somewhat larger doses of ACh (10–30 μg/kg) produce pronounced muscarinic effects; therefore, a pronounced decrease in peripheral resistance and blood pressure is produced. In addition to the hypotension response, a slowing of the heart rate occurs after administration of ACh (a transient tachycardia may initially occur from the hypotensive response affecting baroreceptor reflex activity). Atrial myocardial cells contain muscarinic receptors associated with vagal fibers that mediate negative chronotropic and inotropic effects. The chronotropic effects predominate; they are due to a decreased slope of phase 4 (spontaneous depolarization) of the pacemaker action potential of the sinoatrial (SA) node.

ACh, in addition to its pronounced slowing effect on heart rate, exerts important effects on impulse conduction. In the atria, cholinergic activation slows conduction velocity but shortens action potential duration and the effective refractory period. These actions reinforce atrial dysrhythmias and lead to atrial flutter and fibrillation. In the atrioventricular (AV) node, however, ACh slows conduction velocity but prolongs the refractory period. Thus, although cholinergic drugs can exacerbate atrial tachyarrhythmias, the number of aberrant impulses that effectively traverse the AV junction into the ventricular cells can be decreased concomitantly by the same agent. The net effect is a slowing of ventricular rate; this mechanism has pharmacologic importance, because the beneficial slowing effects of digitalis on ventricular rate in patients with atrial fibrillation or flutter is mediated in part by increased vagal tone.

Different arrhythmias that can result from use of cholinergic drugs include sinus arrest, severe bradycardia, incomplete and complete heart block, notching and decreased amplitude of the P wave, momentary ventricular asystole, and atrial fibrillation and flutter.

Smooth Muscle. GI motility and secretions are enhanced by ACh in a manner identical to that seen upon stimulation of the parasympathetic innervation to the alimentary tract. These effects may be difficult to detect with small doses because duration of action of ACh is brief owing to rapid destruction by cholinesterase. Larger doses markedly increase secretions and peristaltic movements of the GI tract.

ACh stimulates smooth muscle of the urinary bladder and uterus to contract (Chapple et al. 2002). Bronchiolar smooth muscle is also contracted by ACh, resulting in decreased diameter of airways (Barnes and Hansel 2004; Fisher et al. 2004). The smooth muscle effects of ACh are blocked by atropine and therefore are due to muscarinic receptor activation.

Central Nervous System. Because of its highly charged quaternary nitrogen group, ACh is lipophobic and poorly penetrates cell membranes and the blood-brain barrier. Thus CNS effects are not observed when usual dosages are administered. However, intraarterial injection into cerebral arteries of large amounts of ACh or its direct application into the CNS produces increased electrical activity, excitation, and possibly convulsions. Both muscarinic and nicotinic receptors are present in the CNS (Krnjevic 2004).

Muscarinic and Nicotinic Effects of Large Doses of ACh. With high doses (50–100 μg/kg), muscarinic effects of ACh on postganglionic effector cells are accentuated. Profound hypotension is caused by extensive peripheral vasodilation. Duration of this effect is prolonged. Heart rate slows dramatically and momentary asystole can occur. The GI tract and other visceral smooth muscles are markedly activated; defecation, urination, and vomiting may result.

Large doses of ACh produce, in addition to the muscarinic (i.e., parasympathomimetic) effects described above, stimulation of the nicotine receptors of autonomic ganglia (both parasympathetic and sympathetic) and the adrenal medulla. These effects are particularly evident when the muscarinic receptors of the parasympathetic neuroeffector junctions are blocked by atropine. Under these circumstances large doses of ACh stimulate nicotinic receptors of both sympathetic and parasympathetic ganglia. However, because the muscarinic receptors of the parasympathetic neuroeffector junctions are blocked by atropine, impulses originating from parasympathetic ganglia will not reach their effector cells. Only impulses originating from sympathetic ganglia will do so; therefore, only sympathomimetic responses will be evident. These are characterized by an increase in blood pressure, tachycardia, and other typical sympathetic-mediated effects, which can be blocked by use of appropriate adrenergic blocking drugs (see Chapter 6) or by use of a ganglionic blocking agent (Fig. 7.3).

Adrenal Medulla. The adrenal medulla is functionally analogous to autonomic ganglia, and nicotinic receptors of adrenal medullary chromaffin cells are innervated by typical preganglionic cholinergic fibers. These receptors are stimulated by ACh to cause release of epinephrine and norepinephrine from chromaffin cells into the circulation. This effect contributes to the overall nicotinic-mediated sympathomimetic effect evoked by large doses of ACh in the presence of muscarinic blockade.

Skeletal Muscle. Intraarterial injection of significant quantities of ACh will produce skeletal muscle fasciculations caused by penetration of some of the agent to motor end-plates and resulting activation of nicotinic receptors of skeletal muscle cells. Continued exposure to excessive amounts of ACh causes severe fasciculations and asynchronous contractions and terminates in a depolarizing paralysis. Also, if an atropinelike drug has not been given, an increase in blood flow to the injected muscle occurs as a result of vasodilation from stimulation of the muscarinic receptors of blood vessel endothelial cells and the resulting release of EDRF.

Methacholine, Carbachol, and Bethanecol. The pharmacologic effects of these choline esters are equivalent to the previously outlined parasympathomimetic effects of ACh and thus are similar to the physiologic changes evoked by stimulation of postganglionic parasympathetic nerves as listed in Table 5.1. Carbachol also has marked nicotinic agonistic characteristics; however, differences between the parasympathomimetic actions of these choline esters are primarily quantitative and vary principally in relative selectivity for one organ system or another (Table 7.1).

Methacholine (acetyl-β-methylcholine) is a synthetic choline ester used occasionally in human therapeutics but infrequently employed in veterinary medicine. Methacholine causes muscarinic effects on cardiovascular function similar to those produced by ACh, but it is considerably less active on the GI system and has few agonist properties at nicotinic receptors.

Carbachol (Lentin, carbamylcholine chloride, Doryl) is an extremely potent choline ester that is active at both muscarinic and nicotinic receptors and therefore causes pharmacologic effects similar to changes evoked by ACh. These are particularly prominent on the nicotinic receptors of autonomic ganglia; however, this drug is also very potent at muscarinic sites. For example, IV injection of doses as small as 2 μg/kg causes a transient slowing of heart rate and hypotension owing to muscarinic effects.

Bethanecol (Urecholine, carbamylmethylcholine) is somewhat similar to methacholine and carbachol in scope of pharmacologic activity. Unlike carbachol, however, it is primarily a muscarinic agonist and has little stimulant effects on nicotinic receptors.

Pharmacologic Effects. *Cardiovascular Effects.* Methacholine is more active on the cardiovascular system than on the GI or urinary tracts. The opposite selectivity is seen with carbachol and bethanechol. IV administration of methacholine, like ACh, produces a depressor response and slowing of heart rate caused by activation of muscarinic receptors of blood vessels and the heart, respectively. Cardiac rhythm is altered by methacholine, and the AV node is particularly sensitive to this agent. Conduction velocity through the AV node is decreased. Various degrees of heart block, including complete AV disassociation, can occur with large doses. IV administration of methacholine to normal nonanesthetized animals can produce atrial fibrillation, as can ACh. These effects are blocked by atropine. Carbachol evokes blood pressure changes similar to those seen with methacholine except relatively less pronounced, whereas bethanechol is considerably less active on cardiovascular function.

GI Tract. Carbachol and bethanecol are relatively more active on the GI and urinary tracts than on the cardiovascular system. Methacholine is also active on the alimentary canal but only in large doses. Carbachol is a potent GI stimulant. It evokes profuse salivation and an increase in peristaltic movements of the gut resulting in increased fluidity of feces and defecation. These responses are due to activation of muscarinic receptors. GI stimulant effects of choline esters are relatively well defined in simple-stomached animals, but responsiveness of ruminants may vary. Effects of carbachol and various other autonomic drugs on the GI tract of ruminants are summarized in previous editions of this text.

Other Smooth Muscle. Uterine musculature, in in vitro strips and the intact animal, is contracted by carbachol. This response is more evident during the latter stages of gestation. Carbachol should not be used during pregnancy, because abortion or uterine rupture might result. After parturition, carbachol may be useful in expelling uterine contents.

Similar to ACh, carbachol causes contraction of bronchiolar smooth muscle, resulting in a decreased airway. The urinary bladder is contracted by carbachol and bethanechol, and frequent urination results. Effects of carbachol and bethanechol on these as on other smooth muscles are muscarinic and blocked by atropine.

Skeletal Muscle. Carbachol does not discernibly affect skeletal muscle when usual dosages are employed. If a high dose is inadvertently given, muscle fasciculations and even paralysis may occur. This is a nicotinic effect due to carbachol causing a persistent depolarization block of the postjunctional membrane of the neuromuscular junction. Because of relative lack of agonistic effects at nicotinic sites, bethanechol and methacholine have little effect on voluntary muscles.

Sweating. Profuse sweating in the horse is evoked by carbachol. It is not known if this is due to a direct effect on sweat glands, a ganglionic stimulating effect, an increase in circulating catecholamines (as a result of adrenal medullary stimulation), or local release of catecholamines from adrenergic neurons. Because sweat gland mechanisms in the horse seem to be β_2 adrenergic (Bijman and Quinton 1984), either of the latter two mechanisms could be involved.

Other Effects. Carbachol, like ACh, is a mixed nicotinic-muscarinic agonist. It therefore has a potent stimulating effect on autonomic ganglia and the chromaffin cells of the adrenal medulla. Such an effect on the adrenal medulla would cause an increased discharge of epinephrine and norepinephrine into the bloodstream, which in turn could produce diffuse sympathomimetic effects. This relationship may explain why adrenergic-like effects have occasionally been encountered during the use of carbachol. Nicotinic effects of carbachol on autonomic ganglia can be demonstrated by the hypertensive response obtained with large doses after the postganglionic muscarinic receptors have been blocked with atropine (Fig. 7.3).

Clinical Uses. Methacholine and bethanechol are not used frequently in clinical veterinary medicine. Methacholine has been used in humans and animals to produce peripheral vasodilation in treating different vascular disorders such as Raynaud's disease and ergot poisoning, respectively. It has been used in human medicine to control tachycardia of supraventricular origin. Ventricular tachycardia and nodal paroxysmal tachycardia (in which the origin is in the AV node) are not amenable to methacholine therapy. Bethanechol, 1 mg administered subcutaneously twice daily, has been used to treat urinary bladder atony in cats after incidences of urolithiasis; however, care should be taken to ensure that the urethra is completely patent.

Carbachol is a potent drug, and care should be taken to avoid overstimulation of the GI tract and uterus during its clinical use. It has been used for treatment of colic and impactions of the intestinal tract; however, its use in such cases should be closely monitored. If excessive peristaltic movements are induced in a patient suffering from intestinal obstruction, rupture or intussusception may occur. Before resorting to a potent cholinomimetic compound such as carbachol, consideration should first be given to more conservative approaches to GI therapy such as the use of mineral oil, saline cathartics, water, or other stool softeners. If these measures are not successful, carbachol may be cautiously added to the therapeutic regimen. Repeated small subcutaneous (SC) doses of 1–2 mg carbachol at 30- to 60-minute intervals have been used in treating colic in mature horses after treatment with oils and saline cathartics had been instituted. Dosages should be decreased to 0.25–0.5 mg in foals.

When administered during the middle of farrowing, carbachol (2 mg subcutaneously) has been reported to decrease the incidence of stillbirths in litters from sows and gilts by increasing uterine contractions (Sprecher et al. 1975). However, severe salivation, vomiting, diarrhea, and frequent urination were adverse side effects.

Carbachol has been used in treatment of rumen atony and impaction in cattle. After conservative treatment with stool softeners, repeated doses of 1–2 mg have proved effective in stimulating rumen motility. However, single doses greater than 4 mg may be ineffective and in some cases may actually inhibit ruminoreticular activity. Carbachol should not be given by IV or, probably, intramuscular (IM) injection because of its potency. It is given by the SC route; however, the dosage is still critical. Fatalities have occurred in human patients after IM injection of carbachol.

NATURALLY OCCURRING CHOLINOMIMETIC ALKALOIDS. Pilocarpine, muscarine, and arecoline are plant alkaloids that exert parasympathomimetic effects with minimal activity at nicotinic sites. Although all three agents are used in research, only pilocarpine has been used to any appreciable extent in clinical medicine.

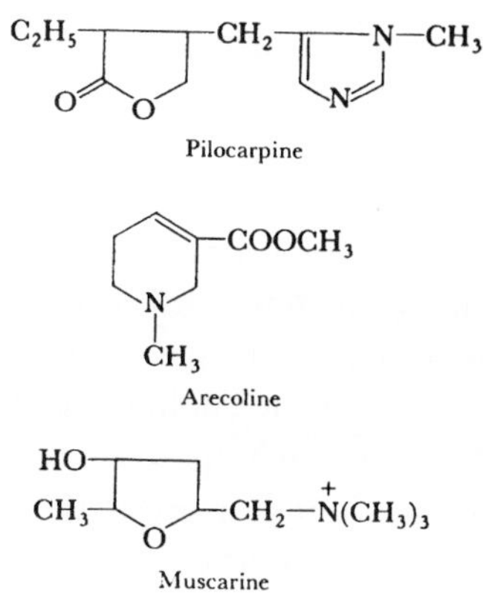

Pilocarpine

Arecoline

Muscarine

FIG. 7.4

Pilocarpine nitrate is the water-soluble salt of the alkaloid pilocarpine, obtained from leaves of the Brazilian shrubs *Pilocarpus jaborandi* and *P. microphyllus.* Arecoline is an alkaloid found in the betel nut, the seed of the betel palm *(Areca catechu).* Muscarine is found in the poisonous mushrooms *Amanita muscaria.* The chemical structures of these three compounds are given in Figure 7.4.

Pharmacologic Mechanisms and Effects. Pilocarpine, arecoline, and muscarine are rather selective parasympathomimetic agents; i.e., their cholinomimetic activity is exerted primarily at muscarinic sites with minimal nicotinic effects. Even the slight ganglionic-stimulating effects of pilocarpine and arecoline are believed to be from activation of the secondary muscarinic pathway involved in ganglionic transmission (see latter part of this chapter). These cholinomimetic alkaloids evoke their parasympathomimetic effects by direct stimulation of the muscarinic receptors of cells innervated by postganglionic cholinergic nerves. They do not inhibit cholinesterase. Also, because their effects are produced in chronically denervated tissue, they are not dependent upon release of endogenous ACh.

Pilocarpine is particularly effective in stimulating flow of secretions from exocrine glands, including salivary, mucous, gastric, and digestive pancreatic secretions. As with ACh it causes contraction of GI smooth muscle, thereby increasing smooth muscle tone and peristaltic activity. Of considerable importance, pilocarpine has a potent constrictor effect on the pupil.

Arecoline activates muscarinic receptors of cholinergically innervated effector cells of glands, smooth muscles, and myocardium and therefore produces the usual parasympathomimetic effects. It is similar to pilocarpine in scope of activity but is considerably more potent. Arecoline depresses heart rate and blood pressure and may produce dyspnea by constricting the bronchioles. Dyspnea generally is not marked except in cases where the dose is toxic or the animal has previously been affected with a respiratory ailment such as acute pulmonary emphysema. Arecoline stimulates secretion of the glands of the digestive tract and increases peristaltic movements of the gut. Increased flow of saliva, occurring within 5 minutes following a SC injection and lasting for an hour, is particularly noticeable. Arecoline contracts the urinary bladder.

Muscarine has been employed experimentally for many years because it has a selective excitatory effect on the effector cells of tissues innervated by postganglionic cholinergic nerves. It does not stimulate the nicotinic receptors of autonomic ganglia or skeletal muscle as does ACh.

Clinical Uses. Pupillary constriction (miosis) occurs when pilocarpine is administered systemically or applied topically to the eye. Clinically, solutions of 0.5–2% are used for instillation into the conjunctival sac for treatment of glaucoma. Pilocarpine stimulates the sphincter muscle of the iris and the ciliary muscle of the lens, causing pupillary constriction and spasm of accommodation. Intraocular pressure momentarily increases, followed by a persistent decrease. Fixation of the lens for near vision lasts only 1–2 hours; however, miosis, which develops within about 15 minutes after instillation, persists 12–24 hours. Pilocarpine is also used alternately with mydriatics to prevent synechiation, but it is contraindicated in patients with iridocyclitis.

Toxicology. Toxic doses of the cholinomimetic alkaloids evoke severe colic and diarrhea and exocrine gland secretions. The pupil is markedly constricted. Dyspnea occurs because of constriction of the bronchioles and accumulation of mucus in the airways. Hypotension and extreme cardiac slowing, complicated by excessive bronchoconstriction and bronchial secretions, lead to death. Arecoline or systemic exposure to pilocarpine is contraindicated in animals with heart failure, depression or disease of the respiratory tract, and spasmodic colic and during gestation. Atropine is a specific antidote to toxic doses of arecoline, pilocarpine, and muscarine. Toxic action of the poisonous mushroom in humans results from the parasympathomimetic action of muscarine.

CHOLINESTERASE INHIBITORS

The function of AChE in terminating the transmitter action of endogenous ACh at cholinergic synapses and neuroeffector junctions is discussed in Chapter 5. Cholinesterase inhibitors (anticholinesterase agents) inactivate or inhibit AChE and pseudocholinesterase and thereby intensify activity of endogenous ACh. In addition, the activity of drugs that are biotransformed by cholinesterase (e.g., succinylcholine) is also prolonged by cholinesterase inhibitors. Because these drugs magnify the actions of endogenous ACh at all cholinergic receptors, their scope of activity is not limited to parasympathomimetic effects but includes cholinomimetic actions throughout the body (Taylor 2006b).

Physostigmine, neostigmine, and edrophonium are examples of the type of anticholinesterase agent that produces a reversible inhibition of cholinesterase, whereas organophosphate compounds such as diisopropyl fluorophosphate (DFP) produce an irreversible inhibition. Although there is considerable distinction between these two groups of anticholinesterases, their pharmacologic effects are similar because of a common basic mechanism of action.

PHARMACOLOGIC CONSIDERATIONS

Mechanism of Action. The pharmacologic effects of cholinesterase inhibitors can be explained almost entirely by their characteristic inhibitory action on AChE. This results in decreased hydrolysis of neuronally released ACh and intensification of its action at cholinergic receptors. This is particularly true with the irreversible organophosphate compounds and can be demonstrated by lack of miotic effect of topically applied DFP in a chronically denervated eye, where there is no source of ACh. Neostigmine and other quaternary nitrogen anticholinesterase agents exert some direct effects (either agonistic or antagonistic) on cholinergic receptors in addition to inhibition of cholinesterase. At the somatic neuromuscular junction, e.g., muscle twitch stimulant effects of neostigmine are attributed to direct receptor activation as well as to cholinesterase inhibition. The direct effect is not uniform throughout the body. Neostigmine, like DFP, is miotically inactive in the denervated eye. Effects of physostigmine, a tertiary amine, can be explained almost entirely by its anticholinesterase activity.

Molecular. The enzymatic interactions of AChE, ACh, and cholinesterase inhibitors are shown schematically in Figure 7.5 and can be summarized as follows (Taylor 1991, 2006a; Inestrosa and Perelman 1990; Massoulie et al. 1993). AChE contains two active sites that recognize specific parts of the ACh molecule: an anionic (negatively charged) region where electrostatic binding occurs with the cationic nitrogen of the choline moiety, and an esteratic site where the carboxyl portion of the acetyl ester binds to it by covalent bonding. After ACh–AChE interaction occurs, the choline portion is split off, leaving the acetylated esteratic site. Acetic acid is rapidly formed as water reacts with the acetyl group, and the enzyme is thereby reactivated (Wilson 1954).

Neostigmine, physostigmine, and other carbamate derivatives interact with the anionic and esteratic sites of the enzyme, thereby preventing ACh from affixing to the enzyme. Neostigmine and physostigmine are believed to be hydrolyzed in a manner similar to but much slower than that of ACh (Wilson et al. 1960); i.e., the alcoholic portion of the anticholinesterase compound is split off, leaving a carbamylated esteratic site. A carbamic acid is then formed upon reaction with water, and the enzyme is regenerated (Fig. 7.5). Although the rate of combination of inhibitor with AChE is only a few times slower than the analogous combination of ACh with the enzyme, the rate of hydrolysis is probably over 10^6 times faster for ACh. Therefore, neostigmine and related drugs are reversible cholinesterase inhibitors as a result of their acting as competitive substrates hydrolyzed at a much slower rate than the endogenous substrate ACh (Taylor 1991, 2006a; Massoulie et al. 1993).

Edrophonium and tetraethylammonium ions are complex and simple quaternary nitrogen compounds, respectively, that interact with the anionic site of cholinesterase. Therefore, they are not hydrolyzed but act as simple competitive reversible inhibitors. Accordingly, the duration of action of edrophonium is much shorter than that of neostigmine or physostigmine.

Organophosphate compounds interact with AChE at the esteratic site and form an extremely stable enzyme-inhibitor complex that does not undergo significant spontaneous disassociation. The esteratic site is persistently phosphorylated, and recovery of cholinesterase activity is dependent upon de novo synthesis of new enzyme. Some organophosphates (e.g., echothiophate) may interact with both the anionic and esteratic sites. Because cholinesterase

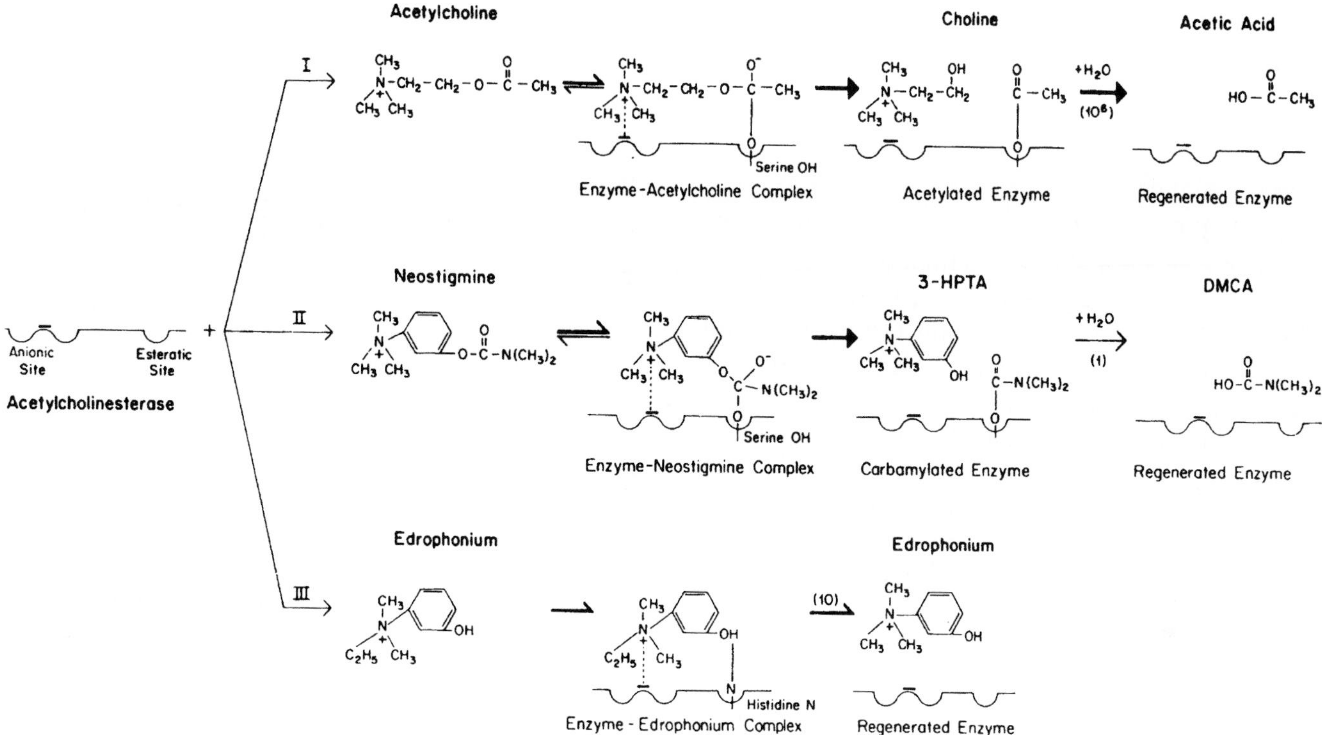

FIG. 7.5 Interaction of ACh, neostigmine, and edrophonium with AChE. I. ACh complexes with AChE via electrostatic binding of the quaternary (cationic) N+ of the choline group with the anionic site of the enzyme and by interaction of the carbonyl group with a serine hydroxyl group of the esteratic site. Choline is split off, yielding the acetylated enzyme, which interacts with H_2O to yield acetic acid and the reactivated enzyme. II. Neostigmine complexes with AChE to yield 3-hydroxyphenyltrimethylammonium (3-HPTA) and carbamylated enzyme, which then react with H_2O to give N,N-dimethylcarbamic acid (DMCA) and the reactivated enzyme; this reaction is $\cong 10^6$ slower than the comparable reaction involving ACh and AChE. III. Edrophonium complexes with AChE via electrostatic interaction at the anionic site and by H bonding to the imidazole N atom of histidine at the esteratic site; this complex is reversible, yielding reactivated AChE and edrophonium. The numbers in parentheses refer to relative rates of reaction (Taylor 1990a; Inestrosa and Perelman 1990; Massoulie et al. 1993).

synthesis requires days, organophosphates cause an irreversible inhibition. As discussed below, however, certain oxime compounds exhibit such high affinity for the organophosphate that they can actually cause detachment of the inhibitor from the esteratic site, resulting in cholinesterase reactivation (see Fig. 7.8, later in this chapter).

Pharmacologic Effects. Effects of cholinesterase inhibitors can be reliably predicted by considering the anatomic location of cholinergic nerves and the respective physiologic processes they modulate in their innervated cells. Parasympathomimetic (muscarinic) effects of these agents are equivalent to the effects associated with postganglionic parasympathomimetic nerve impulses. Cholinesterase inhibitors also cause intensification of ACh activity at nicotinic sites. Therefore, these drugs can cause the following effects: stimulation of postganglionic muscarinic receptors of effector cells, resulting in typical parasympathomimetic activity; stimulation of adrenal chromaffin cells to discharge catecholamines into the circulation; initial stimulation and subsequent depolarization block of nicotinic receptors of autonomic ganglia and skeletal muscle fibers; and marked CNS cholinergic effects.

Although all these activities can be seen with excessive doses, therapeutic doses usually result in more selective actions; e.g., neostigmine and other quaternary nitrogen compounds do not easily penetrate the blood-brain barrier and therefore exert little CNS activity. These compounds are relatively more active at nicotinic receptors of the skeletal neuromuscular junction than at muscarinic sites of autonomic effector cells. Tertiary amines and organophosphates are less lipophobic and can cross the blood-brain barrier and evoke CNS effects. These compounds are relatively more active with low doses at autonomic receptor sites than on voluntary muscles.

REVERSIBLE INHIBITORS. *Physostigmine,* USP (Eserine), is an alkaloid extracted from the dried ripe seed of a vine, *Physostigma venenosum,* which grows in tropical West Africa. This seed, also called the Calabar or "ordeal" bean, was used by tribal Africans in witchcraft ordeals. A person accused of a crime was forced to eat the bean. If vomiting occurred, the accused did not die and was considered innocent. If there was no vomiting, however, death resulted and the suspect was declared guilty.

Neostigmine Bromide, USP (Prostigmine), is the salt of a synthetically produced substance discovered in a research investigation of compounds structurally related to physostigmine. Physostigmine also can be synthesized. *Edrophonium Chloride,* USP (Tensilon), is a synthetically derived agent that produces pharmacologic effects similar to neostigmine except that its duration of action is considerably shorter. It is used primarily as an anticurare agent. *Pyridostigmine Bromide,* USP (Mestinon, Regonol), and *Ambenonium Chloride,* USP (Mytelase, Mysuran), are moderately long acting, chemically synthesized cholinesterase inhibitors used primarily in management of myasthenia gravis and curare overdosage. The chemical structures of physostigmine, neostigmine, and edrophonium are shown in Figure 7.6.

CH_3NHCOO — CH_3 — N — N — CH_3 CH_3

Physostigmine

$(CH_3)_2NCOO$ — $\overset{+}{N}(CH_3)_3$

Neostigmine

HO — $\overset{+}{N}$ — CH_3, C_2H_5, CH_3

Edrophonium

FIG. 7.6

Mechanism of Action. These agents produce their effects by combining with cholinesterase and thereby preventing the enzyme from hydrolyzing ACh. ACh released during normal cholinergic nerve impulses has a prolonged and uninterrupted action upon cholinergic receptors. The interaction with cholinesterase is reversible, so as the inhibitor-enzyme complex breaks down, the enzyme is reactivated and it will now hydrolyze ACh and terminate its activity. At certain sites, neostigmine may act directly on receptors and evoke release of ACh from nerve endings; however, these are considered to be secondary actions.

Pharmacologic Effects

Digestive Tract. Physostigmine and neostigmine cause contraction of smooth muscle, thereby increasing motility and peristaltic movements of the gut. Frequency and strength of peristaltic waves are increased, and movement of intestinal contents is accelerated. Physostigmine has been used in animals for initiating peristaltic movements and evacuating the digestive tract. Excessive peristalsis leading to intestinal spasm and colic complicates use for this purpose. Physostigmine is given by SC or IM injection; its action after oral administration is unreliable. Neostigmine is not absorbed effectively after oral administration because of its quaternary nitrogen structure.

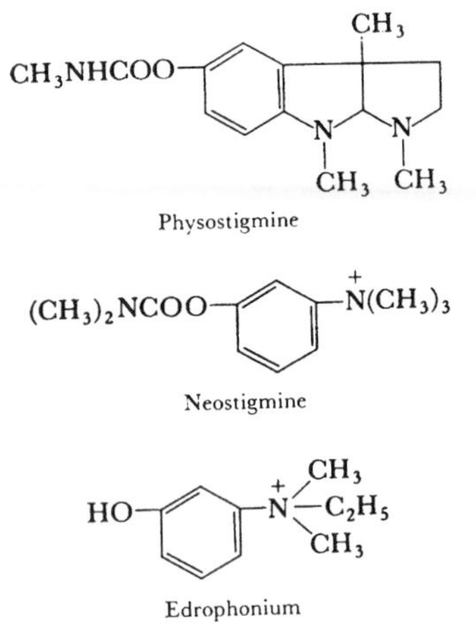

Ocular Effects. Physostigmine causes pupillary constriction and spasm of accommodation when applied locally to the eye or when injected for systemic effect. Intraocular pressure decreases, and physostigmine has been used in treating glaucoma to relieve elevated intraocular pressure.

Skeletal Muscle. Besides its major action of inactivating AChE at the somatic myoneural junction, neostigmine is believed to directly stimulate nicotinic receptors of skeletal muscle fibers. Physostigmine is not active in denervated muscle. The skeletal muscle effects of neostigmine are relatively more pronounced at low doses than the smooth muscle effects of this agent. Twitching of skeletal muscles may be observed when a large dose of physostigmine or neostigmine is injected.

Physostigmine, neostigmine, pyridostigmine, and edrophonium are anticurare agents; they are antagonists to *d*-tubocurarine and other nondepolarizing (competitive) neuromuscular blocking agents at the somatic myoneural junction. These drugs can be used clinically to counteract an excessive dose of true curarimimetic agents but should not be used in attempts to antagonize the depolarizing neuromuscular blocking agents (e.g., succinylcholine), since synergism may actually occur (see Chapter 8).

Other Effects. A therapeutic dose of physostigmine or neostigmine does not produce pronounced effects on cardiovascular function. Effects of higher doses are complicated by concurrent ganglionic stimulation and muscarinic effects on the heart and blood vessels. Usually, hypotension and a bradycardia leading to arrhythmias are produced. Smooth muscle of the bladder is cholinergically innervated and therefore is contracted by cholinesterase inhibitors. Bronchiolar smooth muscle is also contracted by these agents.

Clinical Uses. *Physostigmine Salicylate*, USP (Isopto Eserine), or *Physostigmine Sulfate*, USP, can be used to produce miosis of the pupil and reduce intraocular pressure in the treatment of glaucoma. A solution of 0.5–1% physostigmine salicylate can be applied topically three times a day. The maximum miotic effect is obtained within an hour and may persist 12–24 hours, depending upon the dosage. Physostigmine may also be used alternately with atropine to prevent or break down synechia formed between lens and iris, such as occurs with periodic ophthalmia in horses.

Physostigmine has been used in a SC dose of 30–45 mg in cattle to stimulate ruminal activity in treatment of simple impaction or nonobstructive atony. Physostigmine, neostigmine, pyridostigmine, and edrophonium can be used to overcome the effects of true curarelike drugs in voluntary muscles, but the latter two agents are used more commonly for this purpose (Chapter 8).

Neostigmine has been used extensively in treating myasthenia gravis in humans. In myasthenialike syndromes in dogs, neostigmine has also proved beneficial (Hall and Walker 1962). Marlow (1977) reported problems in controlling signs of myasthenia gravis in a dog treated with 60 mg neostigmine administered orally twice daily; difficulty was encountered in differentiating myasthenia crisis from cholinergic crisis. The former indicates an exacerbation of muscle weakness disease, whereas the latter refers to overdosage of the cholinesterase inhibitor with its attendant muscle weakness caused by excessive accumulation of ACh at the neuromuscular junction. Edrophonium, because of its brief duration of action, has been used to differentiate cholinergic and myasthenic crises in humans. If IV injection of this agent improves muscle function, myasthenia crisis is indicated and the dose of cholinesterase inhibitor used in maintenance therapy should be increased. However, if muscle weakness is accentuated by edrophonium, a cholinergic crisis is indicated and the dose of the cholinesterase inhibitor used in maintenance therapy should be reduced accordingly.

Impaction or other obstructions of the alimentary tract constitute a contraindication to the systemic use of cholinesterase inhibitors. Violent peristalsis produced by these drugs can cause rupture or intussusception of the gut. These drugs should not be used during pregnancy, particularly late in term, because of the danger of producing abortion.

Toxicology. Large doses of physostigmine first stimulate and then depress the CNS; small to moderate doses have little effect, whereas massive doses can produce convulsions. Neostigmine does not cross the blood-brain barrier to an appreciable extent. Toxic doses of these agents produce marked skeletal muscle weakness, nausea, vomiting, colic, and diarrhea. The pupil is markedly constricted and fixed. Dyspnea is characteristically seen from constriction of the bronchiolar musculature. Bradycardia and lowered blood pressure are also characteristic signs. Respiratory paralysis caused by depolarization block of the neuromuscular junction and compounded by excess bronchiolar secretions is the usual cause of death. Atropine is the most effective pharmacologic antagonist for physostigmine or neostigmine toxicity.

ORGANOPHOSPHORUS COMPOUNDS. Diisopropyl fluorophosphate (diisopropyl phosphorofluoridate, DFP) is the prototypical organophosphate anticholinesterase agent. Related compounds include the alkyl pyrophosphates such as hexaethyltetraphosphate, tetraethylpyrophosphate (TEPP), and octamethyl pyrophosphortetramide (Taylor 2006a). Organophosphates were originally introduced as pesticides by German scientists prior to and during World War II; however, there was considerable speculation by many scientists as to the potential use of these highly toxic substances as antipersonnel devices in chemical warfare. Subsequently, a wide variety of organophosphorus compounds has been synthesized and extensively investigated. Some of the more important of these used as pesticides are parathion [Thiophos, diethyl *O*–(4-nitrophenyl) phosphorothioate]; malathion [*O,O*–dimethyl

TABLE 7.2 Structural formulas of several organophosphate anticholinesterase agents

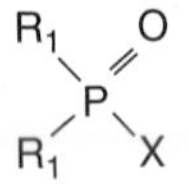

General formula

R_1	R_2	X	Agent
Isopropyl	Isopropyl	Fluoride	DFP
Pinacolyl	Methyl	Fluoride	Soman
Dimethylamino	Ethoxyl	Cyanide	Tabun
Isopropylamino	Isopropylamino	Fluoride	Mipafox
Ethoxyl	Ethoxyl	*S*-(2-Trimethylaminoethyl)	Echothiophate

Source: Modified from Volle 1971, p. 602.

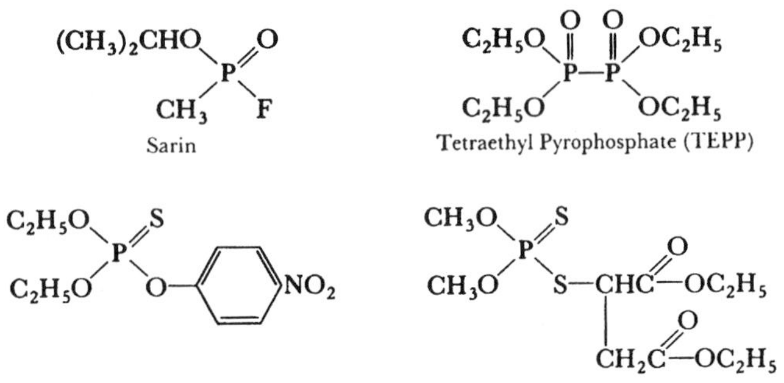

Sarin

Tetraethyl Pyrophosphate (TEPP)

Parathion

Malathion

FIG. 7.7 Representative structural formulas for organophosphate compounds.

S–(1,2-dicarbethoxyethyl) phosphorodithioate]; ronnel [*O,O*–dimethyl *O*–(2,4,5-trichlorophenyl) phosphorothioate]; and Co-ral. Soman, tabun, and sarin are extremely potent synthetic compounds that have been referred to as nerve gases. Dichlorvos (*O,O*–dimethyl-2,2-dichlorovinyl phosphate or 2,2-dichlorovinyl dimethyl phosphate) has been used as an oral anthelmintic in veterinary medicine and impregnated in flea collars as a pesticide.

Although the chemical structures of organophosphate compounds vary considerably, the basic moiety is a phosphate with various organic groups attached to it, as described in Table 7.2. Representative structural formulas are shown in Figure 7.7.

Mechanism of Action, Effects, and Toxicity. Organophosphates irreversibly phosphorylate the esteratic site of both AChE and the nonspecific or pseudocholinesterase throughout the body (Fig. 7.8). Endogenous ACh is not inactivated, and the resulting effects are due to the excessive preservation and accumulation of endogenous ACh (Taylor 2006a, 1991; Gutman and Besser 1990). Organophosphate poisoning produces diffuse cholinomimetic effects: profuse salivation, vomiting, defecation, hypermotility of the GI tract, urination, bradycardia, hypotension, severe bronchoconstriction, and excess bronchial secretions. These signs reflect excess activation of muscarinic receptors of postganglionic parasympathetic neuroeffector junctions with typical parasympathomimetic actions.

In addition to the muscarinic effects, skeletal muscle fasciculations, twitching, and, subsequently, muscle paralysis occur. These effects are due to persistent excessive stimulation of the nicotinic receptors of skeletal neuromuscular junctions, resulting in the depolarizing type of striated muscle paralysis (Gutman and Besser 1990). Convulsions and frequently death are seen in organophosphate poisoning, caused by penetration of the agent into the CNS and subsequent intensification of the activity of ACh at CNS sites (Gutman and Besser 1990).

Antagonists and Antidotes

Atropine. Because atropine blocks muscarinic receptors, it not only lessens severity of the parasympathomimetic effects but also increases the quantity of organophosphate required to produce death; e.g., the ratio of the median lethal dose (LD_{50}) of sarin in atropine-treated dogs to the LD_{50} in nonatropinized dogs may be 150 : 1 (DeCandole and McPhail 1957). These ratios vary with the animal species and organophosphate, but atropine is almost invariably beneficial. In addition, because atropine is a competitive antagonist to ACh, large doses are effective even if administered after exposure to an organophosphate.

Cholinesterase Reactivators. Although phosphorylation of the esteratic site of cholinesterase by organophosphates yields a normally irreversible complex, certain compounds cause a disassociation of the enzyme bondage. Pralidoxime (pyridine-2-aldoxime-methiodide, 2-PAM) was synthesized based on structural requirements postulated by Wilson (1958) to be necessary for a selective antidote to organophosphate-cholinesterase interaction. This compound causes an effective removal of the phosphate group from the enzyme, so the enzyme is reactivated (Fig. 7.8). This and related oxime compounds are undoubtedly the most valuable adjunct to atropine therapy in treating organophosphate poisoning; e.g., pretreatment of animals with 2-PAM increases by several times the LD_{50} of various organophosphates. If atropine is given in conjunction with 2-PAM, the lethal dose is increased many more times.

Similarly, animals previously exposed to toxic doses of organophosphates experience considerable improvement after treatment with 2-PAM. In dogs, 10–20 mg/kg 2-PAM administered by slow IV injection is usually effective; this dose may have to be repeated. In horses and cattle, 20 mg/kg and 10–40 mg/kg, respectively, are used. Since 2-PAM significantly reverses the combination of organophosphate with cholinesterase, the reactivated enzyme can then perform its normal function. The phosphorylated enzyme complex tends to age with time and to become resistant to reactivation by oximes. Thus treatment with 2-PAM should not be delayed once organophosphate intoxication is diagnosed. Although treatment with 2-PAM alone has been used successfully in human incidences of organophosphate poisoning, atropine should always be used first to block muscarinic receptor sites.

Various other reactivator oximes such as pyridine-2-aldoxime dodecaiodide (designed for CNS effects), monoisonitrosoacetone, and diacetylmonoxime have also been investigated. Oxime reactivators are probably ineffective in antagonizing the carbamate cholinesterase inhibitors and in some cases apparently can act synergistically.

Clinical Uses of Organophosphates. Organophosphorus compounds have achieved widespread use as anthelmintics and pesticides because they are highly toxic to a wide variety of internal and external parasites. Their introduction in the late 1940s and 1950s had considerable impact on pest control. Concurrent with their widespread use, however, is the potential for immediate and/or delayed damage to humans, domestic animals, and wildlife. The ecologic impact of organophosphate pesticides has received considerable attention from various conservation organizations, and there is some evidence that certain of the compounds may be tumorigenic when given in large doses to experimental animals. Dichlorvos-impregnated collars can occasionally cause hypersensitivity skin reactions on the animal's neck and, less frequently, on pet owners.

Organophosphates such as DFP and TEPP have been used locally to constrict the pupil in human patients for treatment of glaucoma; DFP (0.1% in peanut oil) and echothiophate (phospholine iodide, 0.03–0.25% solutions) are sometimes used for this purpose in dogs. Effects

FIG. 7.8 Interaction of organophosphate diisopropyl fluorophosphate (DFP) with AChE and reversal by pralidoxime (2-PAM). DFP interacts irreversibly with the esteratic site of AChE to yield a phosphorylated enzyme complex with virtually no spontaneous release of diisopropylphosphoric acid (DIPPA) and regeneration of active enzyme. However, 2-PAM and other oximes can interact with the phosphorylated enzyme complex via electrostatic binding at the anionic site of AChE and binding at the P atom; the oxime-phosphonate is split off, yielding a regenerated enzyme. The numbers in parentheses refer to relative rates of reactions (Taylor 1990a; Inestrosa and Perelman 1990; Massoulie et al. 1993).

of these compounds are relatively long lasting and the dosage must be carefully controlled.

Precautionary Note about Clinical Uses of Cholinesterase Inhibitors. As repeatedly emphasized, cholinesterase inhibitors are highly reactive molecules capable of influencing functions of cholinergic nerves throughout the body. This is particularly true with the organophosphates. At no time should their clinical use be considered as an innocuous procedure. Care should always be taken by the clinician to insure that the patient is not exposed either to drugs that are metabolized by cholinesterase (e.g., succinylcholine) or to other cholinesterase inhibitors (e.g., pesticide dips or sprays) for several days before and after administering either a reversible or irreversible anticholinesterase agent. If not, serious and even fatal synergistic interactions can occur (Hines et al. 1967). Other types of drugs (e.g., phenothiazine tranquilizers) may decrease cholinesterase activity as a potential side effect; their concurrent use with anticholinesterase drugs should be avoided or closely monitored.

Severely ill, debilitated animals should not be exposed to a cholinesterase inhibitor except in emergency situations. If hepatic disease is presented, synthesis of cholinesterase may be markedly reduced and effects of cholinesterase inhibitors can be intensified and/or prolonged. Respiratory illness may be exacerbated by excessive bronchiolar constriction and secretion. Abortion may occur, particularly during the latter gestational periods. Because of the potency of cholinesterase inhibitors, especially organophosphate compounds, care should always be taken to closely follow the manufacturer's individual dosage recommendations and procedural directions.

PARASYMPATHOLYTIC AGENTS

Parasympatholytic drugs prevent ACh from producing its characteristic effects in structures innervated by postganglionic parasympathetic nerves. They also inhibit effects of ACh on smooth muscle cells that respond to ACh but lack cholinergic innervation; i.e., these drugs inhibit the muscarinic actions of ACh and related cholinergic agonists. In fact, "muscarinic blocking" or "antimuscarinic" is actually more completely descriptive of the effects of this group of drugs than is "parasympatholytic," because muscarinic receptors are blocked irrespective of whether they are innervated by a parasympathetic nerve. Clinically, however, these drugs are used almost exclusively for their parasympatholytic activities. This group of drugs includes atropine and related alkaloids and numerous synthetically derived compounds.

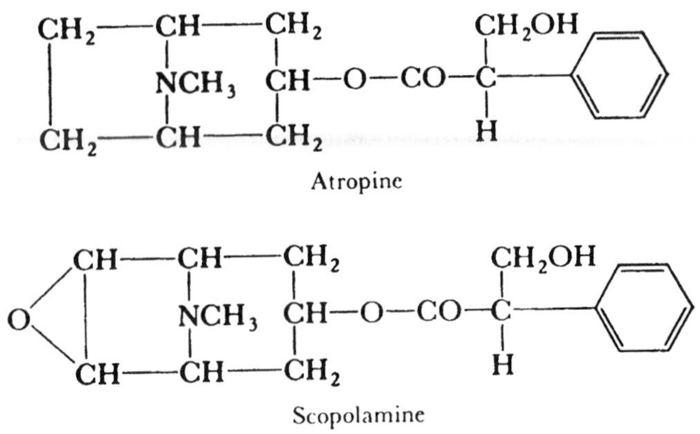

Atropine

Scopolamine

FIG. 7.9

ATROPINE AND SCOPOLAMINE. Atropine, the prototypical muscarinic blocking agent, is an alkaloid extracted from the belladonna plants that belong to the Solanaceae (potato family) and include *Atropa belladonna* (deadly nightshade), *Datura stramonium* (jimsonweed), and *Hyoscyamus niger* (henbane). Alkaloids obtained from *Atropa belladonna* are atropine (which is a racemic mixture of *d*-hyoscyamine and *l*-hyoscyamine, racemization occurring during the extraction procedure), scopolamine (*l*-hyoscine), and others of lesser significance. Because atropine is actually an equal mixture of *d*- and *l*-hyoscyamine and the dextro form of hyoscyamine is biologically inactive, a given quantity of atropine is about one-half as potent as the same quantity of *l*-hyoscyamine. Despite the inactive dextrorotatory component, atropine is nevertheless effective in very small doses. Chemically, the atropine molecule consists of two components joined through an ester linkage: tropine, which is an organic base, and tropic acid. Other related alkaloids also contain the aromatic tropic acid moiety combined by ester linkage to either tropine or another organic base, scopine. The chemical structures of atropine and scopolamine are given in Figure 7.9.

Mechanism of Action. *Atropine Sulfate*, USP, *Scopolamine Hydrobromide*, USP (Hyoscine), and other related alkaloids interact with muscarinic receptors of effector cells and by occupying these sites prevent ACh from affixing to the receptor area. Physiologic responses to parasympathetic nerve impulses are thereby attenuated. Pharmacologic effects of exogenously administered ACh and other muscarinic agonists are similarly blocked by atropine and scopolamine. Although muscarinic receptors have been divided into M_1, M_2, M_3 and other subtypes (Chassaing et al. 1984; Brown and Taylor 2006), the utility of this nomenclature to clinical veterinary medicine is unclear at this time.

Blockade of muscarinic receptors of smooth muscle, cardiac muscle, and glands by atropinelike drugs involves a competitive antagonism. Therefore, large doses of ACh or other cholinomimetic drugs (e.g., carbachol, cholinesterase inhibitors) can overcome or surmount inhibitory effects of atropine at these sites.

Although atropine and related compounds act immediately distal to all postganglionic cholinergic nerve endings, this block is not equally effective throughout the body. Salivary and cholinergic sweat glands are quite susceptible to small doses of atropine, whereas somewhat larger doses are required for a vagolytic effect upon the heart. GI and urinary tract smooth muscles are less sensitive to atropine, and even larger dosages are required to inhibit gastric secretion. Except for effects on salivation and cholinergic sweating, it is difficult to achieve a selective action on targeted structures without concurrently inducing side effects on other, more susceptible sites. Net pharmacologic effects of atropinic drugs in a particular organ are influenced by the relative dominance of parasympathetic or sympathetic tone in that structure. After cholinergic impulses are blocked, adrenergic nerves become dominant and sympathomimetic-like effects may contribute to the final effect.

Pharmacologic Effects

Cardiovascular System. The usual therapeutic doses of atropine do not markedly affect blood pressure; however, pulse rate is altered. Tachycardia is the dominant effect, and large doses of atropine invariably produce an increased heart rate. Small doses may initially produce a slight slowing of heart rate, but this effect is believed to be due to transient stimulation of vagal nuclei of the medulla oblongata and perhaps to transient stimulation of peripheral receptors prior to their block (Averill and Lamb 1959; Ashford et al. 1962). The ease with which atropine produces tachycardia is dependent in part upon the degree of vagal tone of the individual patient. Because atropine blocks transmission of vagal impulses to the heart, animals with a preexisting high vagal tone would show a relatively greater tachycardia than those with low vagal tone.

Cardiac output tends to increase with atropine primarily because of increase in heart rate. Arterial blood pressure either remains unchanged or increases slightly in a normal animal. In animals exposed to exogenous ACh or other cholinomimetics (e.g., cholinesterase inhibitors), atropine can cause a relative increase in blood pressure, because muscarinic effects of the agonists will be blocked. Also, atropine unmasks the hypertensive response to high experimental doses of cholinergic agonists resulting from their nicotinic effects (see Fig. 7.3).

Because atropine blocks the cardiac vagus, it markedly reduces or abolishes cardiac inhibitory effects of drugs acting through a vagal mechanism and will attenuate vagal-mediated reflex responses. Accordingly, the pressor effects of epinephrine and norepinephrine are accentuated in atropinized animals by blockade of the cardiac limb of vagal-baroreceptor reflexes. Large doses of atropine are directly depressant to the myocardium and also cause cutaneous dilation as a result of a direct vascular smooth muscle effect.

GI System. Atropine causes relaxation of GI smooth muscle by inhibiting contractile effects of cholinergic nerve impulses. Thus, atropine and related drugs can be helpful in treatment of intestinal spasm and hypermotility. Inhibition of smooth muscle motility extends from stomach to colon, although the degree of blockade may not be uniform. Insofar as rumen motility is concerned, adequate doses are consistently inhibitory, and atropine is one of the few agents that can be relied upon to produce cessation of rumen motility.

Secretions of the GI tract are also blocked by atropine. Salivation is reduced quite markedly. Similarly, secretions of intestinal mucosa are inhibited; however, gastric secretions are reduced only with exceedingly high doses that also block virtually all other muscarinic sites.

Bronchioles. Cholinergic innervation to the bronchioles modulates secretion of mucus and contraction of bronchiolar smooth muscle. Atropine and other drugs of the belladonna group block effects of cholinergic impulses and thereby decrease secretions and increase luminal diameter of the bronchioles. The dilator action of atropine is valuable in counteracting constriction of bronchioles following overdosage of a parasympathomimetic drug.

Atropine often will give temporary symptomatic relief from the dyspnea of "heaves" in horses, and it has been used by unscrupulous individuals for this purpose. A SC dose of atropine (30 mg) may produce immediate relief in the horse lasting 1–3 hours; however, dyspnea worsens after effect of the drug has terminated. A crude form of the drug, such as belladonna leaves, administered orally produces its effect within 30 minutes, with a duration of about 24 hours. When atropine medication is suspected, the following signs should be detectable: dry oral mucosa, dilated and relatively fixed pupils, and tachycardia.

Ocular Effects. Atropine blocks the cholinergically innervated sphincter muscle of the iris and the ciliary muscle of the lens, resulting in mydriasis and cycloplegia after topical or systemic administration. Because atropine blocks cholinergic effects, adrenergic nerve impulses dominate and the pupil actively dilates. Atropine is contraindicated in the presence of increased intraocular pressure from acute angle glaucoma because the drainage system of the anterior chamber of the eye is impeded during mydriasis.

Urinary Tract. Atropine relaxes smooth muscle of the urinary tract. The spasmolytic effect on the ureters may be of some benefit in treatment of renal colic. Atropine tends to cause urine retention because it inhibits smooth muscle tone. This effect may be of some use in reducing frequency of micturition that accompanies cystitis; however, the deleterious effects of only partially emptying the bladder should be considered.

Sweat Glands. Atropine has a definite anhydrotic action in species such as humans, who have a cholinergic mechanism in control of sweat secretion, and a large dose may cause a hyperpyrexic response. Atropine does not directly affect sweating in species that have adrenergic mechanisms in control of sweating (e.g., equines) and has minimal effect in species that do not use cholinergic sweating as an important component of thermoregulation.

Central Nervous System. Therapeutic doses of atropine produce minimal effects on the CNS (Fisher et al. 2004). Excessive doses may cause hallucinations and disorientation in humans and mania and excitement in domestic animals. Excessive motor activity followed by depression and coma is the usual sequence of events. Scopolamine has a slight sedative effect; when combined with morphine it produces analgesia and amnesia (referred to as "twilight sleep") in human patients. These effects of scopolamine usually are not detectable in domestic animals. While small doses may be depressant in dogs and cats, larger doses produce delirium and excitement in these species and also in horses.

Toxicology. There is considerable interspecies variation in the toxicity of belladonna and atropine; the route of administration is also important. Herbivora are usually more resistant than Carnivora. Certain strains of rabbits are quite resistant to a diet of belladonna leaves, because an esterase (atropinase) of the liver hydrolyzes and thus inactivates atropine. However, rabbits fed on such a diet may prove toxic if eaten by dogs, cats, or humans because of the large amount of alkaloid present in muscle tissues. Horses, cattle, and goats are relatively resistant to belladonna when it is administered orally; however, these species are quite susceptible to atropine when it is injected parenterally. Swine are not resistant to belladonna ingested from eating the deadly nightshade plant.

Signs of atropine poisoning are similar in all mammalian species. Dry mouth, thirst, dysphagia, constipation, mydriasis, tachycardia, hyperpnea, restlessness, delirium, ataxia, and muscle trembling may be observed; convulsions, respiratory depression, and respiratory failure lead to death. A drop of urine obtained from a patient suspected of atropine toxicosis causes mydriasis when placed in the eye of a cat. Also, the tested pupil will not constrict when exposed to light, while the untreated eye will. This simple procedure may prove helpful in the differential diagnosis of belladonna intoxication.

Clinical Uses. Parasympatholytic drugs are used to control smooth muscle spasm as antispasmodics or spasmolytics. Antispasmodics can be used to decrease or abolish GI hypermotility and depress hypertonicity of the uterus, urinary bladder, ureter, bile duct, and bronchioles. Parasympatholytics are not as effective as epinephrine or other adrenergic amines in dilating the bronchioles, but atropine is effective in antagonizing excessive cholinergic stimulation at these sites.

Atropine is used routinely as an adjunct to general anesthesia, particularly with inhalant anesthetics, to decrease salivary and airway secretions. Also, atropine is frequently given in conjunction with morphine to reduce salivary secretions that may be produced by the latter drug. When used prior to anesthesia, the dose of atropine in dogs is 0.045 mg/kg, administered subcutaneously.

The newer inhalant anesthetics produce minimal respiratory irritation, and bronchiolar secretions are considerably less pronounced than with older agents like ether. Thus the routine preoperative use of atropine in all patients has been questioned, especially because this drug may increase the potential for certain cardiac arrhythmias. Moreover, use of atropine in cattle often results in several days of inappetence concomitant with postoperative rumen stasis (Garner et al. 1975). In the horse, use of atropine is sometimes questioned because of the possibility of reducing intestinal motility to the degree that colic develops (Klavano 1975). However, some clinicians cautiously use IV atropine (0.01 mg/kg) to prevent the second degree heart block induced by xylazine in horses. Because of the incidence or potential for anesthesia-associated tachyarrhythmias with atropine, glycopyrrolate (see below) has been advocated as an alternative to atropine for muscarinic blockade in routine preanesthetic medication.

Atropine is used routinely to facilitate ophthalmoscopic examination of internal ocular structures and functions and also for treatment of various ocular disorders. Homatropine hydrobromide, because of its shorter duration of action, has largely replaced atropine for ophthalmoscopic purposes in human patients. Application of a few drops of 1–2% solution of atropine into the conjunctival sac causes mydriasis within 15–20 minutes. Maximum pupillary dilation occurs in about 2 hours and may be detectable for several days. The time course of the cycloplegic action of atropine is similar to that of mydriatic action. Mydriatics like atropine are helpful in preventing or breaking down adhesions between the iris and the lens when used alternately with miotics.

Atropine is an essential antidote to anticholinesterase overdosage or poisoning.

SYNTHETIC MUSCARINIC BLOCKING AGENTS.

Synthetic muscarinic blocking agents were chemically synthesized in attempts to find atropine substitutes that would act selectively at certain muscarinic sites and therefore would have fewer undesirable side effects than the alkaloids.

Glycopyrrolate. *Glycopyrrolate*, NF, is a quaternary nitrogen anticholinergic agent that has received attention for preanesthetic use in veterinary medicine. It exerts potent antimuscarinic activity but reportedly has some benefits when compared to atropine. The tachycardia response associated with muscarinic block at the SA node, e.g., seems to be somewhat less of a problem with glycopyrrolate. In dogs this compound effectively diminishes the volume and acidity of gastric secretions and reduces intestinal motility; it also reduces and controls excessive secretions of the respiratory tract. Similar control of respiratory secretions by glycopyrrolate has been reported in cats, and its duration of action exceeds that of atropine. Also, because of its more polar nitrogen moiety, glycopyrrolate penetrates the blood-brain barrier less effectively than atropine, with less propensity for unwanted CNS side effects. The muscarinic blocking action of glycopyrrolate is evident within minutes after IV injection. After SC or IM administration, maximal effects generally develop within 30–45 minutes, and vagal blocking action can be demonstrated for 2–3 hours, while the antisialagogue response is evident for up to 7 hours. The glycopyrrolate dose is approximately 10 μg/kg by SC, IM, or IV routes, administered 15 minutes or so prior to anesthetic induction (Short et al. 1974; Short and Miller 1978).

Homatropine. *Homatropine Hydrobromide*, USP, is similar in structure to atropine except that it is an ester of mandelic acid rather than of tropic acid. Homatropine closely resembles atropine in most of its pharmacologic actions, particularly the ocular effects. Mydriasis and cycloplegia are produced in the eye by topical application of a 2–5% solution of homatropine, but these effects last for a shorter duration than those resulting from atropine. Homatropine produces fewer side effects on cardiovascular and GI functions than atropine and is considerably less toxic than the parent drug.

Methantheline, Propantheline, Methylatropine, and Others. *Methantheline Bromide*, USP, *Propantheline Bromide*, USP, and *Methylatropine Nitrate*, INN, are quaternary amines used primarily as smooth muscle relaxants. Because of the charged quaternary group, these compounds do not cross the blood-brain barrier to an appreciable extent. Accordingly, they are considerably less effective than atropine as antagonists to organophosphates, since the CNS effects of the latter agents would not be blocked. In addition to muscarinic blocking effects, these drugs act as autonomic ganglionic blockers, which most likely contributes to their antispasmodic effect on GI smooth muscle. Other newer muscarinic receptor antagonists include Mepenzolate Bromide, Pirenzepine and its analog Telanzepine, Ipratropium, and Tiotropium;

however, their clinical application in veterinary medicine is uncertain (Brown and Taylor 2006).

AUTONOMIC GANGLIONIC BLOCKING DRUGS

MECHANISMS. Following Langley's investigations in 1889, it has been known that small doses of nicotine stimulate autonomic ganglion cells, and larger doses block the transmitter function of ACh at these same sites. Therefore, the cholinergic receptors of ganglion neurons have been classified as nicotinic. Considerable evidence is now available indicating that impulse transmission within autonomic ganglia is much more complicated than originally believed. Studies have demonstrated a secondary excitatory cholinergic pathway in autonomic ganglia that is apparently muscarinic, and an inhibitory catecholaminergic mechanism has also been recorded (Eccles and Libet 1961; Libet 1970; Akasu 1992). The different putative pathways involved in synaptic transmission in sympathetic autonomic ganglia are shown schematically in Figure 7.10.

The physiologic purposes of these different ganglionic pathways are poorly understood. Evidence for participation of different types of receptors has been gained primarily from studies of sympathetic ganglia. Parasympathetic ganglia are studied less frequently because of their poor accessibility. The nicotinic receptor represents the primary ganglionic transmission pathway present in all autonomic ganglia. The muscarinic receptors on the postganglionic neuron may facilitate impulse transmission events that are normally dominated by the nicotinic mechanisms. The adrenergic component may act as a modulator to prevent excessive impulse traffic.

NICOTINE. Nicotine is an alkaloid obtained from leaves of the tobacco plant. Nicotine sulfate, the most commonly produced salt, is available commercially in an aqueous solution that contains 40% alkaloidal nicotine. This solution long has been designated by the proprietary name of Blackleaf 40. Nicotine was the original autonomic ganglionic blocking agent; however, it is not used clinically for this purpose. Nicotine first stimulates and then in higher doses blocks nicotinic receptors by producing a persistent depolarization of the receptor area.

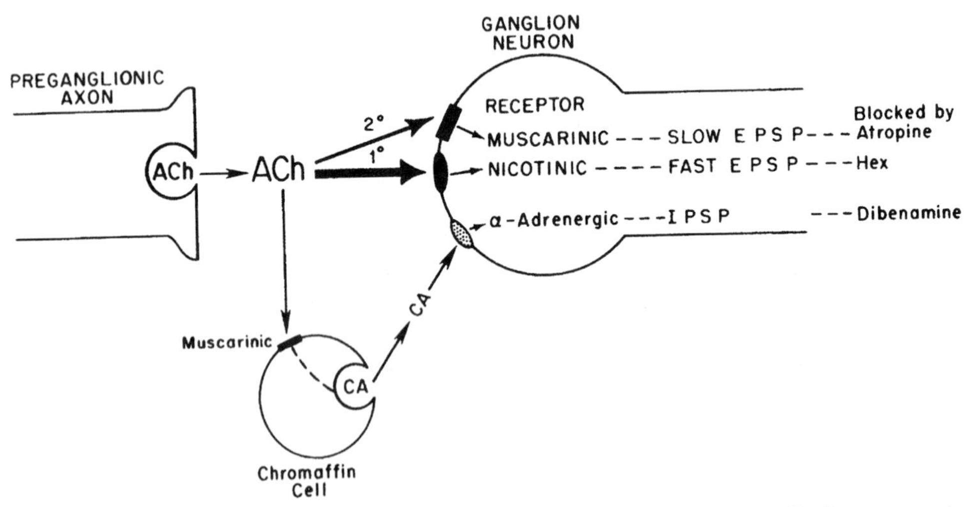

FIG. 7.10 Impulse transmission in sympathetic autonomic ganglia. ACh is discharged from the preganglionic nerve terminal and interacts with a nicotinic receptor on the ganglionic neuron to cause a rapid depolarization measured electrically as a fast excitatory postsynaptic potential (EPSP). ACh also interacts with a muscarinic receptor on the ganglionic neuron to cause a delayed depolarization measured electrically as a slow EPSP. In addition, ACh activates nearby chromaffin cells through a muscarinic receptor, which results in a release of catecholamine (CA: dopamine or epinephrine). CA interacts with an α receptor on the ganglionic neuron to cause an inhibitory (hyperpolarization) response measured electrically as an inhibitory postsynaptic potential (IPSP). 1° and 2° indicate primary (nicotinic) and secondary (muscarinic) pathways of excitatory ganglionic impulses, respectively; hex = hexamethonium (Eccles and Libet 1961; Libet 1970; Nishi 1974; Akasu 1992).

Pharmacologic Effects

Central Nervous System. Alkaloidal nicotine is an extremely toxic substance that transiently stimulates and then severely depresses the CNS. Death is from respiratory paralysis of the diaphragm and chest muscles resulting from descending paralysis and depolarization block of the nerve-muscle junction of skeletal muscle. Nicotine is absorbed through the chitinous shell of insects after a direct spraying or after contacting a sprayed surface and kills by paralysis of the CNS.

Cardiovascular System. Both cardioaccelerator and cardioinhibitor nerves are activated by small amounts of nicotine, which cause stimulation of all autonomic ganglia. Since the cardioinhibitor nerve (vagus) is predominant, the response to a small dose, or the initial response to a large dose of nicotine is a decreased pulse rate. Because of paralysis of all autonomic ganglia, the heart rate returns toward normal after a large dose has taken full effect, and a relative tachycardia may result. Similarly, small doses of nicotine can cause a pressor response, by stimulation of the predominating sympathetic ganglia that furnish post-ganglionic vasoconstrictor fibers to arterioles. However, peripheral vasodilation results from ganglionic block after large doses.

Gastrointestinal. Nicotine activates the smooth muscles and secretory glands of the digestive tract with the following clinical signs: excessive salivation, increased gastric secretion, vomiting, increased peristalsis, and defecation.

Skeletal Muscle. Nicotine initially stimulates nicotinic receptors of the motor end-plate and in large doses produces a depolarizing muscle paralysis. This effect has been used in attempts to immobilize wild animals for capture.

Acute Nicotine Poisoning. Accidental ingestion of the 40% solution of nicotine sulfate results in acute toxicosis characterized by excitement, hyperpnea, salivation, pulse rate irregularities, diarrhea, and emesis in species that vomit. After this transient stimulatory phase, a depressed state occurs and is characterized by incoordination, tachycardia, dyspnea, coma, and death from respiratory paralysis.

SYNTHETIC GANGLIONIC BLOCKING AGENTS.

Nicotine is not used clinically in animals or humans as a ganglion blocker, since it activates nicotinic sites before blockage occurs and affects functions of various tissues throughout the body. However, several drugs have been discovered that preferentially block autonomic ganglia by a nondepolarizing (competitive) mechanism. These drugs are bis-quaternary compounds, i.e.,

$$(CH_3)_3\overset{+}{N}(CH_2)_n\overset{+}{N}(CH_3)_3$$

In cases where the methonium groups are separated by five or six methylene groups (i.e., $n = 5$ or 6), a selective site of action at autonomic ganglia is obtained. These compounds interact with nicotinic receptors of the ganglion cells and thereby block impulse transmission across the ganglionic synapse. Dissimilar to nicotine, they do not cause initial depolarization. Members of this group of ganglionic blocking agents include hexamethonium (n = 6; *C*-6), pentamethonium (n = 5; *C*-5), chlorisondamine, pentolinium, trimethidinium, and azamethonium. In addition, there are several other ganglionic blocking drugs that are not bis-quaternary compounds, such as tetraethylammonium ions, mecamylamine, and pempidine.

Pharmacologic Effects and Uses. Because of the blockade of impulse transmission at the ganglia, effects of ganglionic blocking agents are manifested on effector organs innervated by the postganglionic fibers of the sympathetic or parasympathetic nervous system. The overall effects of these agents on various functions are dependent upon the predominance of sympathetic or parasympathetic tone in a particular structure, as indicated in Table 7.3 (Taylor 2006b). Because the GI system functions predominantly under parasympathetic tone, ganglionic blockade will result in a relative parasympatholytic effect; decreased motility and secretions and constipation result. Similarly, because heart rate is under dominant vagal tone, a relative tachycardia may result. However, because tone of peripheral blood vessels is dominated by sympathetic impulses, vasodilation and hypotension occur after ganglionic block. Similarly, the output of catecholamines by the adrenal medulla is also reduced. Severe postural hypotension and even syncope may result. The hypotensive effect has occasionally been utilized in surgery to decrease the chance of hemorrhage in highly vascular areas; however, ganglionic blocking agents have achieved no significant purpose in clinical veterinary medicine.

TABLE 7.3 Usual predominance of sympathetic or parasympathetic tone in various tissues and consequent effects of autonomic ganglionic blockade

Structures	Predominant Tone	Effects of Ganglionic Blockade
Cardiovascular		Overall depression; block reflexogenic changes
Arterioles	Sympathetic	Vasodilation: increased peripheral blood flow; hypotension
Veins	Sympathetic	Vasodilation: pooling of blood; decreased venous return
Heart	Parasympathetic	Tachycardia
Gastrointestinal	Parasympathetic	Decreased tone and motility; constipation
Eye		
Iris	Parasympathetic	Mydriasis
Ciliary muscle	Parasympathetic	Cycloplegia
Urinary bladder	Parasympathetic	Urinary retention
Salivary glands	Parasympathetic	Dry mouth
Sweat glands	Sympathetic	Annidrosis

Source: Taylor 1990b.

REFERENCES

Adams, H. R. 1996. Physiologic, pathophysiologic, and therapeutic implications of endogenous nitric oxide. J Am Vet Med Assoc 209:1297–1302.

Akasu, T. 1992. Synaptic transmission and modulation in parasympathetic ganglia. Japan J Physiol 42:839–64.

Ashford, A., Penn, G. B., Ross, J. W. 1962. Cholinergic activity of atropine. Nature 193:1082–83.

Averill, K. H., Lamb, L. E. 1959. Less commonly recognized actions of atropine on cardiac rhythm. Am J Med Sci 237:304–18.

Barnes, P. J., and Hansel, T. T. 2004. Prospects for new drugs for chronic obstructive pulmonary disease. Lancet 364:985–996.

Bijman, J., Quinton, P. M. 1984. Predominantly beta-adrenergic control of equine sweating. Am J Physiol 15:R349–R353.

Brown, J. H. and Taylor, P. 2006. Muscarinic receptor agonists and antagonists. In L. L. Brunton, J. S. Lazo, and K. L. Parker, eds., The Pharmacologic Basis of Therapeutics, 11th ed., New York: McGraw Hill.

Brunton, L. L., Lazo, J. S., and Parker, K. L., eds. 2006. The Pharmacologic Basis of Therapeutics. New York: McGraw Hill.

Chapple, C. R., Yamanishi, T., and Chess-Williams, R. 2002. Muscarinic receptor subtypes and management of the overactive bladder. Urology 60:82–89.

Chassaing, C., Dureng, G., Baissat, J., Duchene-Marullaz, P. 1984. Pharmacological evidence for cardiac muscarinic receptor subtypes. Life Sci 35(17):1739–45.

Dale, H. H. 1914. The action of certain esters and ethers of choline, and their relation to muscarine. J Pharmacol Exp Ther 6:147–90.

De Candole, C. A., McPhail, M. K. 1957. Sarin and paraoxon antagonism in different species. Can J Biochem Physiol 35:1071–83.

Eccles, R. M., Libet, B. 1961. Origin and blockade of the synaptic responses of curarized sympathetic ganglia. J Physiol (Lond) 157:484–503.

Eglen, R. M., Choppin, A., and Watson, N. 2001. Therapeutic opportunities from muscarinic receptor research. Trends Pharmacol Sci 22:409–414.

Eldefrawi, M. E. 1974. In J. I. Hubbard, ed., The Peripheral Nervous System, p. 181. New York: Plenum.

Fisher, J. T., Vincent, S. G., Gomeza, J., Yamada, M., and Wess, J. 2004. Loss of vagally mediated bradycardia and bronchoconstriction in mice lacking M_2 or M_3 muscarinic acetylcholine receptors. FASEB J 18:711–713.

Furchgott, R. F., Zawadzki, J. V. 1980. The obligatory role of endothelial cells in the relaxation of arterial smooth muscle by acetylcholine. Nature 288:373–76.

Garner, H. E., Mather, E. C., Hoover, T. R., et al. 1975. Anesthesia of bulls undergoing surgical manipulation of the vas deferentia. Can J Comp Med 39:250–55.

Gutmann, L., Besser, R. 1990. Organophosphate intoxication: pharmacologic, neurophysiologic, clinical, and therapeutic considerations. Sem Neurology 10:46–51.

Hall, L. W., Walker, R. G. 1962. Suspected myasthenia gravis in a dog. Vet Rec 74:501–3.

Hines, J. A., Edds, G. T., Kirkham, W. W., et al. 1967. Potentiation of succinylcholine by organophosphate compounds in horses. J Am Vet Med Assoc 151:54–59.

Hucho, F., Jarv, J., Weise, C. 1991. Substrate-binding sites in acetylcholinesterase. Trends Pharmacol Sci 12:422–26.

Inestrosa, N. C., Perelman, A. 1990. Association of acetylcholinesterase with the cell surface. J Membr Biol 118:1–9.

Khromov-Borisov, N. V., Michelson, M. J. 1966. The mutual disposition of choline receptors of locomotor muscles, and the changes in their disposition in the course of evolution. Pharmacol Rev 18:1051–90.

Klavano, P. A. 1975. Proc Am Assoc Equine Pract, p. 149.

Krnjevic, K. 2004. Synaptic mechanisms modulated by acetylcholine in cerebral cortex. Prog Brain Res 145:81–93.

Lambert, D. G. 1993. Signal transduction: G proteins and second messengers. Br J Anaesth 71:86–95.

Lewis, M. E., Al-Khalidi, A. H., Bonser, R. S., et al. 2001. Vagus nerve stimulation decreases left ventricular contractility in vivo in the human and pig heart. J Physiol 534:547–552.

Libet, B. 1970. Generation of slow inhibitory and excitatory postsynaptic potentials. Fed Proc 29:1945–56.

Lowenstein, C. J., Dinerman, J. L., Snyder, S. H. 1994. Nitric oxide: a physiologic messenger. Ann Intern Med 120:227–37.

Marlow, C. A. 1977. Myasthenia gravis in a dog [letter]. Vet Rec 101:123.

Martyn, J. A. J., White, D. A., Gronert, G. A., Jaffe, R. S., Ward, J. M. 1992. Up-and-down regulation of skeletal muscle acetylcholine receptors. Anesthesiology 76:822–43.

Massoulie, J., Pezzementi, L., Bon, S., Krejci, E., Vallette, F. M. 1993. Molecular and cellular biology of cholinesterases. Prog Neurobiol 41:31–91.

Matsui, M., Motomura, D., Karasawa, H. et al. 2000. Multiple functional defects in peripheral autonomic organs in mice lacking muscarinic acetylcholine receptor gene for the M_3 subtype. Proc Natl Acad Sci USA 97:9579–9584.

Nishi, S. 1974. In J. I. Hubbard, ed., The Peripheral Nervous System, p. 225. New York: Plenum.

Short, C. E., Miller, R. L. 1978. Comparative evaluation of the anticholinergic agent glycopyrrolate as a preanesthetic agent. Vet Med Small Anim Clin 73(10):1269–73.

Short, C. E., Paddleford, R. R., Cloyd, G. D. 1974. Glycopyrrolate for prevention of pulmonary complications during anesthesia. Mod Vet Pract 55:194–96.

Sprecher, D. J., Leman, A. D., Carlisle, S. 1975. Effects of parasympathomimetics on porcine stillbirth. Am J Vet Res 36:1331–33.

Taylor, P. 2006a. Anticholinesterase agents. In L. L. Brunton, J. S. Lazo, and K. L. Parker, eds., The Pharmacological Basis of Therapeutics, 11th ed. New York: McGraw Hill.

———. 2006b. Agents acting at the neuromuscular junction and autonomic ganglia. In L. L. Brunton, J. S. Lazo, and K. L. Parker, eds., The Pharmacological Basis of Therapeutics, 11th ed. New York: McGraw Hill.

———. 1991. The cholinesterases. J Biol Chem 266:4025–28.

Toda, N., and Okamura, T. 2003. The pharmacology of nitric oxide in the peripheral nervous system of blood vessels. Pharmacol Rev 55:271–324.

Volle, R. L. 1971. In J. R. DiPalma, ed., Drill's Pharmacology in Medicine, 4th ed., p. 584. New York: McGraw-Hill.

Wess, J. 2004. Muscarinic acetylcholine receptor knockout mice: Novel phenotypes and clinical implications. Annu Rev Pharmacol Toxicol 44:423–450.

Westfall, T. C., and Westfall, D. P. 2006. Neurotransmission: The autonomic and somatic nervous systems. In L. L. Brunton, J. S. Lazo, and K. L. Parker, eds., The Pharmacological Basis of Therapeutics, 11th ed. New York: McGraw Hill.

Willmy-Matthes, P., Leineweber, K., Wangemann, T., Silber, R. E., and Brodde, O. E. 2003. Existence of functional M_3-muscarinic receptors in the human heart. Naunyn Schmiedebergs Arch Pharmacol 368:316–319.

Wilson, I. B. 1954. In W. D. McElroy and B. Glass, eds., Symposium on the Mechanism of Enzyme Action, p. 642. Baltimore: Greenwood.

———. 1958. A specific antidote for nerve gas and insecticide (alkylphosphate) intoxication. Neurology 8:41–43.

Wilson, I. B., Hatch, M. A., Ginsburg, S. 1960. Carbamylation of acetylcholinesterase. J Biol Chem 235:2312–15.

SECTION 3

Anesthetics and Analgesics

CHAPTER

8

INTRODUCTION TO DRUGS ACTING ON THE CENTRAL NERVOUS SYSTEM AND PRINCIPLES OF ANESTHESIOLOGY

PETER J. PASCOE AND EUGENE P. STEFFEY

Drugs that act in the central nervous system (CNS) are of fundamental importance to health care delivery. Some agents are administered to animals to directly improve their well-being. For example, without general anesthesia, modern surgery would not be possible. Some drugs alter behavior and improve animal-human interaction. They may induce sleep or arousal or prevent seizures. Drugs that act in the CNS are sometimes administered in an attempt to understand the cellular and molecular basis for CNS actions (i.e., physiology and pathophysiology) and/or identify the sites and mechanisms of action of other drugs. Finally, CNS actions of some drugs come as unwanted "side effects" when those drugs are used to treat conditions elsewhere in the body. For example, seizures may result from the injection of too much local anesthetic.

The first purpose of this chapter is to review principles of organization and function of the CNS. The intent is to lay a foundation from which later discussion on principles and applied aspects of CNS pharmacology can meaningfully follow. Behavior-altering drugs and anesthetics are routinely administered to animals by veterinarians and allied personnel. Appropriate use of these drugs is an important application of our knowledge of CNS pharmacology. Therefore, this chapter will conclude with a review of the principles of contemporary veterinary anesthesiology.

INTRODUCTION TO CNS DRUGS

NEUROANATOMY AND NEUROPHYSIOLOGY. The CNS is largely the same anatomically across mammalian species. The brain and spinal cord have evolved to collect information about external and internal changes and to provide integration of this information in such a way as to promote the survival and reproduction of the animal. The information is gathered by sensory neurons that transduce a stimulus (e.g., light, sound, gas in the intestine) to an electrical signal (neuronal depolarization) that is transmitted to the central nervous system. The CNS then interprets this signal, computes a response, and initiates an output to effect an appropriate action (if needed). This response may need very little CNS integration or may need much greater interpretation. For example, an animal that steps on a red hot object stimulates a reflex arc to initiate an immediate withdrawal reflex without any conscious perception that the object was hot. On the other hand a cat faced with a juicy steak sitting on a kitchen counter must first recognize the steak for what it is, and then compare that with its memory for what such an object might taste like and balance this with the memory of the punishment it received the last time it tried to steal such an object from that location. These latter computations involve complex integration in the CNS, and the neuronal involvement is largely controlled by chemical substances that cause, modify, or inhibit the depolarizations that lead to the final outcome.

Although the CNS of most mammals has the same basic organization, it is not surprising that evolutionary pressures have created differences in the relative size of certain components. This is easily demonstrated by examining the olfactory lobes of the brain in a human being and a dog, the latter having a much greater relative size than in people. There are also chemical differences in the CNS of different species that are not as readily explainable but clearly have an impact on our use of drugs to modify CNS activity. It is well known that opioids can cause excitation in horses and sedation in dogs and the distribution of mu and kappa receptors is very different between the two species (Hellyer et al. 2003).

In order to understand how drugs may modify activity within the CNS it is necessary to understand the normal processes that are used to alter interactions between cells within the CNS. To modulate incoming signals mechanisms are necessary that allow acceptance or rejection of a particular impulse. In a few areas within the mammalian CNS there are neurons that are joined by electrical synapses. These synapses are characterized by tight connections between the two cells with ion channels that are aligned between the two cells. This arrangement does not allow the receiving cell to change the signal since depolarization of the first cell will result in depolarization of the second cell. However, this arrangement is useful where it is important that a number of cells fire simultaneously to produce a coordinated response and, since the signal can travel in either direction, it enhances the capability of this system to function in this way. The signal is also transmitted much more quickly between the cells (0.1 ms) so it can generate a very rapid response. Brainstem neurons involved in the coordination of breathing have this type of synapse and so do some neurons involved in the secretion of hormones from the hypothalamus This electrical coordination allows them to produce a "pulse" of hormone by all firing simultaneously.

The vast majority of the neurons in the mammalian CNS, however, communicate by means of chemical signals. The depolarization of the first neuron travels down its axon by virtue of the opening of voltage gated sodium channels (Fig. 8.1). At the synapse this wave of depolarization activates voltage gated calcium channels that allow calcium to flow down the concentration gradient (approximately 10^{-3}M outside the cell to 10^{-7}M inside the cell) into the cytosol of the synapse. The presence of this increased concentration of calcium activates the discharge of vesicles containing a chemical messenger (neurotransmitter) into the synaptic cleft. This neurotransmitter diffuses across the small gap between the neurons and attaches to receptors on the postsynaptic membrane where it might produce one or more of four changes. It might cause a slight depolarization, but not enough to trigger an action potential; it might cause enough depolarization for the generation of an action potential (excitation); it might cause modifications to the internal milieu of the cell such that it could be more or less receptive to further signals (modulation); or it might cause an ionic shift resulting in hyperpolarization of the cell (inhibition). It is then necessary to have some mechanism to terminate that signal so that the postsynaptic neuron can return to its resting state to allow further signals to be received. This can occur by destruction of the neurotransmitter or its uptake into the presynaptic terminal or other surrounding cells.

PRESYNAPTIC PROCESSES. The cellular mechanisms that occur to allow these events to happen are complex and involve many steps. The neurotransmitters involved can be classed into three basic groups: the amino acids, the amines, and the peptides. Amino acids can be absorbed from the extracellular fluid but usually involve active transport molecules to achieve this and some are immediately ready to use in this form. The amines and γ-amino-butyric acid (GABA) need to be synthesized from smaller building blocks that require the presence of enzymes. These enzymes are generally made in the cell body and diffuse slowly down the length of the axon to the axon terminal (Fig. 8.1). This slow axonal transport occurs at 0.5–5 mm/day. Once an amino acid or amine is present in the nerve terminal it is packaged into synaptic vesicles (40–60 nm in

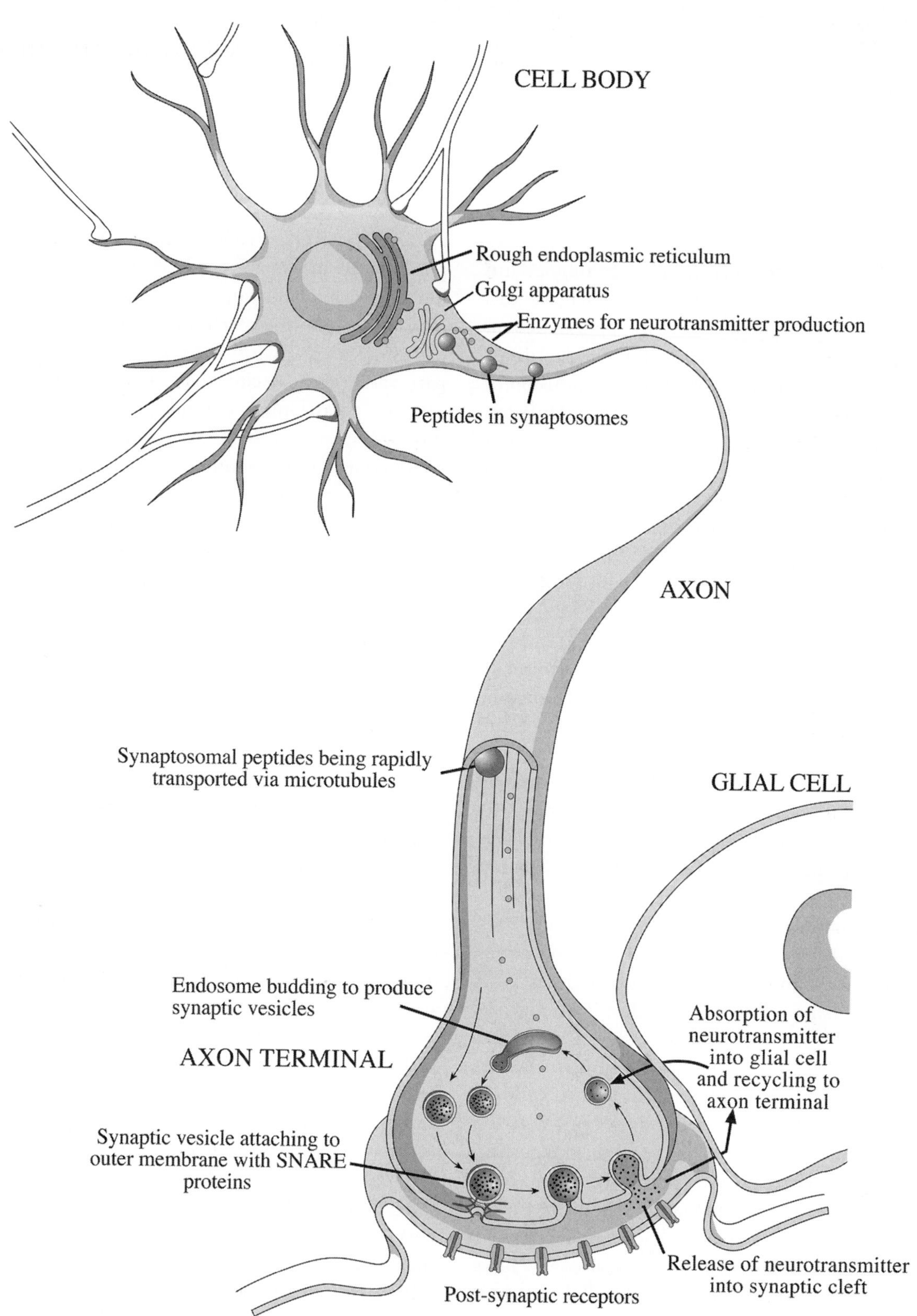

FIG. 8.1 Neuron that is involved in chemical transmission. Enzymes and peptides are made in the cell body and transported to the axon terminal. The transport of enzymes is slow, whereas peptide synaptic vesicles are transported actively down the microtubules. Neurotransmitters are packaged into synaptic vesicles and these accumulate near the synaptic cleft. When the cell depolarizes the synaptic vesicles merge with the outer cell membrane and release neurotransmitter into the synaptic cleft. This chemical acts on the receptors on the postsynaptic membrane to alter postsynaptic cell function. Some neurotransmitters are destroyed in the cleft, some are reabsorbed into the axon terminal and some may be absorbed by neighboring glial cells and destroyed or recycled into the axon terminal.

diameter) using an active transporter system. For these small molecules the synaptic vesicles are seen as small clear-core vesicles on electron microscopy. The peptides, on the other hand, are manufactured in the cell body and packaged into larger vesicles at this site. They are actively transported to the axon terminal using microtubules and ATP-requiring proteins such as kinesin to achieve this (Fig. 8.1). These large dense-core vesicles (appearance on electron microscopy) move at about 400 mm/day down the axon, so this occurs much faster than the diffusion of the enzymes needed for GABA and amine production. The synaptic vesicles tend to cluster around dense areas of the synaptic membrane (called *active zones*) that contain the necessary proteins to achieve transmitter release. The active zones have calcium channels that provide the stimulus for activation of the cascade required for docking and exocytosis of the synaptic vesicle. One family of these proteins, referred to as the SNARE proteins (Soluble N-ethylmaleimide Attachment protein Receptors) form complexes between the synaptic vesicle and the cell membrane (docking) and help promote the next step in the process (fusion of the membranes) so that the contents of the vesicle can be ejected into the synaptic cleft (exocytosis). These proteins are cleaved by botulinum and tetanus toxin, thus preventing neurotransmitter release (Breidenbach and Brunger 2005). In the case of botulinum toxin this effect remains peripheral at the neuromuscular junction whereas tetanus toxin is transported to the CNS where its effects occur mainly in inhibitory neurons, thus explaining the different manifestations of the two diseases (paralysis with botulinum and muscular rigidity with tetanus). The synaptic vesicles may then be reformed (endocytosis) with the aid of proteins called *clathrins* and recycled to be filled again with more neurotransmitter. The whole process from formation, exocytosis to endocytosis, and refilling of these synaptic vesicles can be carried out in about 1 minute, thus enabling frequent signaling from the terminal. Many synaptic terminals contain both small clear-core (amino acids and amines) and large dense core vesicles (peptides). The peptide-containing vesicles are not usually released as readily as the clear-core vesicles and require a greater concentration of intracellular calcium for their release (usually the result of rapid repetitive depolarization of the neuron), thus providing the potential for a different signal to be associated with a more intense stimulus. Many presynaptic terminals have receptors on them that respond to the neurotransmitter being released (autoreceptors). This is usually presented as a feedback loop, which results in the inhibition of further release of the neurotransmitter.

POSTSYNAPTIC PROCESSES. The receptors on the postsynaptic membrane can be divided into two types: the ionotropic or ligand-gated receptors and the metabotropic receptors. Ionotropic receptors allow the immediate passage of an ion across the cell membrane. For the most part these are proteins that allow passage of sodium, calcium, potassium, or chloride. The metabotropic receptors activate a process inside the cell that may alter ionic conduction through another channel or they may alter the production of other substances within the cell that could change how the cell reacts to further stimulation. This process is very powerful because it can amplify the initial signal received. One receptor might activate a cellular enzyme that then catalyzes the production of many molecules, and each of these may further amplify the effect by activating further reactions. Normally the signal from an ionotropic receptor is seen almost immediately, whereas the effect from a metabotropic receptor may take longer and may last longer after the stimulus.

In the CNS an individual neuron may receive input from hundreds of other neurons. Each synapse with its neurotransmitter can either excite (increase the resting membrane potential toward 0) or inhibit (decrease the resting membrane potential to a more negative value). The final effect on that individual neuron will be a result of the type of input it receives and the relative timing of that input. If there is simultaneous input from several excitatory neurons at the same time, it is likely that the neuron will depolarize and send a signal on to the next cell in the pathway. This is referred to as spatial summation. On the other hand if a single input kept on firing it might achieve enough depolarization to trigger an action potential. This is referred to as temporal summation. If this neuron had received several signals from inhibitory neurons during this period the magnitude of the excitatory signal would have to be greater in order for the neuron to achieve a threshold for the action potential. Note, however, that inhibition under these conditions is not normally absolute and that if a strong enough stimulus is applied it will overcome the inhibition.

The attachment of a neurotransmitter to a receptor could be followed by a number of events. The receptor could have an effect and then the neurotransmitter and the receptor could be absorbed into the cell, thus terminating this effect (receptor internalization). The neurotransmitter could be destroyed by a chemical reaction catalyzed by an enzyme located nearby in the synaptic cleft. Some of the fragments of the molecule could then be absorbed again into the presynaptic terminal and reassembled into the original neurotransmitter while some fragments diffuse into the surrounding extracellular fluid. Lastly, the molecule could diffuse off the receptor as the concentration gradient reverses and it could be taken up into the presynaptic terminal or into surrounding glial cells for further transport back into the presynaptic terminal. These actions usually require the presence of transporter proteins for maximal efficiency.

THE NEUROTRANSMITTERS AND THEIR RECEPTORS. There are a number of criteria for establishing a chemical as a neurotransmitter and a great deal of effort has been taken to ensure that these criteria are met by potential candidates. Just finding a chemical in the CNS does not mean that it is a neurotransmitter.

The substance must be present in the presynaptic terminal.

The substance must be released into the synaptic cleft when the presynaptic terminal depolarizes. In most instances this should be dependent on the intracellular release of calcium.

There should be receptors for the substance on the postsynaptic membrane that can be activated by exogenous placement of the substance on those receptors.

In the past this kind of proof was difficult to obtain because an individual synapse is so small and being able to record from it so technically challenging. Even with molecular biologic techniques it is not simple but there have been a number of instances where a receptor has been discovered before the neurotransmitter that binds to it.

The Amino Acids

Glutamate. Glutamate is generally considered to be an excitatory neurotransmitter and is used in about half of the synapses in the brain. It is a nonessential amino acid that does not cross the blood brain barrier so it has to be synthesized by the neuron (Table 8.1). Once it has been released into the synaptic cleft it is removed via a high-affinity uptake process on the presynaptic terminal and local glial cells involving excitatory amino acid transporters (EAATs). So far five of these EAATs have been identified and their locations in the brain and relative activities vary (Bridges and Esslinger 2005). The glutamate taken up in glial cells is converted to glutamine, which can then be absorbed by the presynaptic terminal and converted back to glutamate. Both EAATs and VGLUTs have become targets for pharmacological manipulation. Glutamate acts on three families of ionotropic receptors and three classes of metabotropic receptors. The ionotropic receptors are named after the agonists that were first shown to activate them: N-methyl D-aspartate (NMDA receptor); α-amino-3-hydroxy-5-methylisoxazole-4-propionate (AMPA receptor); kainate (kainate receptor). As with most of these receptors they are composed of four or five subunits of membrane-spanning proteins and this gives rise to the possibility of many forms for each receptor (Table 8.1). These variations provide a basis for pharmacological targeting of individual receptors. The metabotropic receptors are divided into three classes with class I (mGluR1&5) acting via $G_{q/11}$ proteins to increase phospholipase C (excitatory) and classes II (mGluR2–3) and III (mGluR4, mGluR6–8) acting via G_i/G_o proteins to inhibit adenylyl cyclase activity (inhibitory). So although the major effects of glutamate are excitatory there are parts of the brain where it can act as an inhibitory neurotransmitter. The NMDA receptors are important in the practice of anesthesia and analgesia because drugs that are antagonists at this receptor (cyclohexanones such as ketamine and tiletamine) are commonly used. At least six binding sites have been identified on the NMDA receptor for pharmacological activity. The site that binds glutamate (1) opening the channel to the entry of sodium and calcium into the cell. This site appears to need glycine to be bound to the receptor (2) for the glutamate to be fully effective. A third site within the channel binds phencyclidine and other cyclohexanones (3). There is also a voltage-gated magnesium binding site (4) within the channel—the ejection of magnesium from this site with depolarization opens the channel for further activity. There are also an inhibitory divalent site that binds zinc (5) near the mouth of the channel and a polyamine regulatory site (6) that potentiates the currents generated from the receptor when it is activated. The NMDA receptor is thought to affect long-term potentiation, memory, and plasticity of the nervous system. Long-term potentiation is likely involved with the modulation of nociceptive input. Activation of the receptor is also involved in the process of excitotoxicity leading to neuronal death.

TABLE 8.1 Small molecule neurotransmitters with their origins, transport proteins, method of catabolism, and receptors

Neurotransmitter	Synthesized From	Transport of Raw Material into Presynaptic Terminal	Rate-Limiting Step in Synthesis	Vesicle Transport	Reuptake	Catabolism	Ionotropic Receptors	Metabotropic Receptors and Associated G Protein
Glutamate	Glutamine or α-oxoglutarate	Excitatory amino-acid transporter (EAAT)		Vesicular glutamate transporter (VGLUT)	EAAT1–5	Glutamine synthetase	NMDA (NR1, NR2A–D)	Class I (mGluR1&5) $G_{q/11}$
							AMPA (Glu R1–4)	Class II (mGluR2–3) G_i/G_o
							Kainate (Glu R5–7, KA1–2)	Class III (mGluR4, mGluR6–8) G_i/G_o
Glycine	Serine?		Serine trans-hydroxymethylase & D-glycerate dehydrogenase		Glycine transporter (GLYT1–2)		Glycine (α_{1-4}, β subunits)	None
GABA	L-glutamic acid	EAAT	Glutamic acid decarboxylase ($GAD_{65\ \&\ 67}$)	Vesicular GABA transporter (VGAT)	GATs	GABA transaminase	$GABA_{A\ \&\ C}$	$GABA_B$ G_i
Acetylcholine	Choline and acetyl CoA	High affinity transporter	Choline transport	Vesicular acetylcholine transporter	High affinity transporter of choline	Acetylcholinesterase (AChE)	Nicotinic AChRs (α_{2-9}, β_{1-4}, γ, δ subunits)	Muscarinic (M1–5) $G_{q/11}$ – M1, M3, M5 G_i – M2, M4
Dopamine	Tyrosine	Diffusion	Tyrosine hydroxylase (TH)	Vesicular monoamine transporter (VMAT)	Dopamine transporter (DAT)	Monoamine oxidase (MAO) and catecholamine-o-methyl-transferase (COMT)	None	D1 & D5 G_s D2, D3, D4 G_i
Norepinephrine & epinephrine	Tyrosine	Diffusion	Tyrosine hydroxylase (TH)	Vesicular monoamine transporter (VMAT)		Monoamine oxidase (MAO) and catecholamine-o-methyl-transferase (COMT)	None	α_{1A-D} G_q α_{2A-C} G_i β_{1-3} G_s
Histamine	Histidine	Diffusion	Histidine decarboxylase	Vesicular monoamine transporter (VMAT)	?	Monoamine oxidase (MAO) and catecholamine-o-methyl-transferase (COMT)		H_1 G_q H_2 G_s H_3 G_i
5-HT, Serotonin	Tryptophan	Active transport across the BBB	Tryptophan-5-hydroxylase	Vesicular monoamine transporter (VMAT)	Specific 5-HT transporter (SERT)	Monoamine oxidase (MAO)	$5\text{-}HT_3$	$5\text{-}HT_{1A-E,5}$ G_i $5HT_2$ G_q $5HT_{4,6,7}$ G_s

Glycine. This is an inhibitory neurotransmitter, which is found in high concentrations in the medulla and spinal cord. Because glycine is found in all tissues in the body it has been difficult to isolate its activity in the CNS. The glycine receptor is a pentameric structure, and four α-subunits and one β-subunit have been identified. It is a ligand gated chloride channel allowing the ingress of chloride ions, making the inside of the cell more negatively charged (hyperpolarization). The glycine and strychnine binding sites are located on the α_1 subunit. Once released into the synaptic cleft glycine is taken back up into the presynaptic terminal or into surrounding glial cells by an active transporter for glycine (GLYT1-2) with GLYT-2 being the version mainly expressed on neurons. As indicated above, glycine interacts with glutamate at the NMDA receptor and GLYT is found in those neurons despite a lack of glycine receptors.

GABA. This is the major inhibitory neurotransmitter within the CNS and is present in as many as one-third of all synapses in the CNS. By comparison with its concentrations in the CNS it is found only in trace amounts elsewhere in the body. GABA is made from L-glutamic acid and this reaction is catalyzed by glutamic acid decarboxylase (GAD); this irreversible reaction needs a cofactor—pyridoxal phosphate (PLP a form of vitamin B_6). There are two forms of GAD (GAD_{65} and GAD_{67}) and GAD_{65} has a higher affinity for PLP, making its activity more easily regulated. GABA is broken down to succinic semialdehyde by GABA-transaminase (GABA-T), which also requires PLP and this can then enter the Krebs cycle via further breakdown to succinic acid. Since both GAD and GABA-T are dependent on PLP a diet deficient in vitamin B_6 can lead to a decreased level of GABA in the brain with resulting seizures. GABA may be broken down into a number of other metabolites including γ-hydroxybutyric acid (GHB). There is some evidence that the breakdown to GHB is a reversible response and that GHB might be used in the brain to make GABA. GHB has been used in anesthesia and is now an abused street drug; part of its action might be to promote the production of GABA, although a specific GHB receptor is proposed, and GHB is also a partial agonist at the $GABA_B$ receptor.

Once GABA is released into the synaptic cleft its action is terminated mainly by reuptake into the presynaptic terminal using GABA transporters (GATs). Some GABA is taken up into surrounding glial cells using the same mechanism but there does not appear to be a mechanism for transfer of this GABA back to the neuron, so the latter must synthesize more GABA to make up for the amount lost. The GABA receptors are divided into an ionotropic group ($GABA_A$, $GABA_C$) and a metabotropic group ($GABA_B$). The $GABA_A$ receptor (Fig. 8.2) is a ligand gated chloride channel and when activated will tend to hyperpolarize the cell. It contains four subunits, and at least 21 proteins (α_{1-7}, β_{1-4}, γ_{1-4}, δ, ε, θ, ρ_{1-3}) have been identified that can be used to make up this receptor giving it a great deal of structural diversity. It has been shown that some of these variations have different relative sensitivities to GABA providing the potential for different levels of response to release of the same neurotransmitter. The inhalant anesthetics may activate the $GABA_A$ receptor but this is unlikely to be the only site of action. Propofol and etomidate enhance the action of GABA at the receptor at low concentrations and directly activate the $GABA_A$ receptor at higher concentrations while barbiturates are much less selective for this receptor. The benzodiazepines have a separate binding site on the receptor that enhances the opening of the channel when natural GABA attaches to

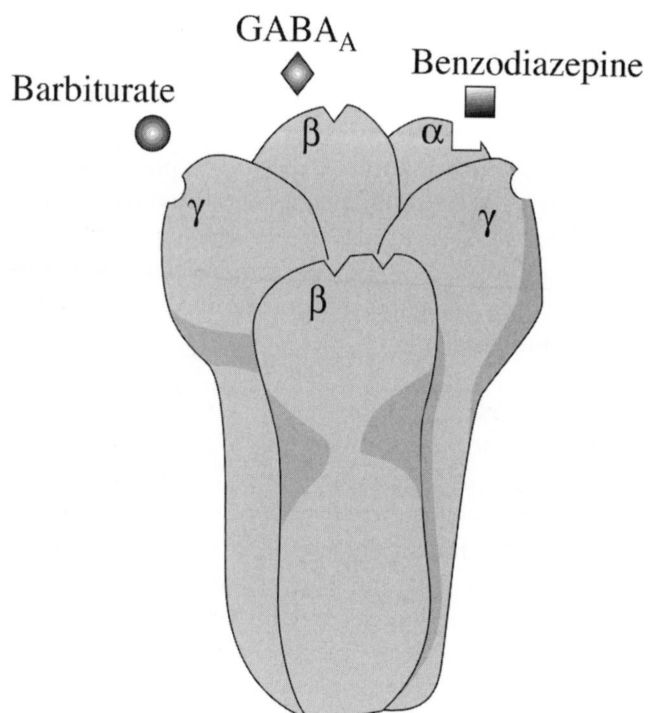

FIG. 8.2 $GABA_A$ receptor showing the pentameric structure and protein subtypes that make up the receptor. Neurotransmitters and drugs attach to different subunits on the receptor.

its binding site (Fig. 8.2). The $GABA_B$ receptor is coupled to G_i proteins that are indirectly linked to potassium channels (increased conductance) and calcium channels (decreased conductance). The latter effect is important for $GABA_B$ receptors located on the presynaptic membrane since this will decrease the amount of calcium released into the cell following an action potential and therefore decrease the release of GABA from the terminal (autoinhibitory response). It is thought that baclofen reduces GABA release via this mechanism.

The Amines

Acetycholine. Acetylcholine (ACh) is synthesized from choline and acetyl coenzyme A (acetyl CoA) in a reaction catalyzed by choline acetyltransferase (ChAT). Choline is mainly derived from the blood and from the phospholipid, phosphatidylcholine, and is transported into cells by a high-affinity transporter. Acetyl CoA is derived from glucose or citrate in the mammalian CNS. The synthesized ACh is packed into vesicles via a vesicular acetylcholine transporter. Once released into the synaptic cleft the ACh attaches to a receptor. In the CNS most of these are nicotinic receptors (nAChRs), another group of pentameric proteins with multiple possible subunits (α_{2-9}, β_{1-4}, γ, δ). These are nonspecific ion channels that are excitatory. Some areas of the CNS, especially the forebrain and striatum, also contain muscarinic receptors that are metabotropic G protein coupled receptors (M1–5). Activation of these receptors has an inhibitory effect on dopamine-mediated motor responses. The synaptic cleft also contains acetylcholinesterase (AChE), which is a highly efficient enzyme (5,000 molecules of ACh hydrolyzed/sec/molecule AChE) that promotes the breakdown of ACh to choline and acetic acid. The choline is taken back up into the nerve terminal for remanufacture to ACh. Atropine acts on central muscarinic receptors but is not specific to any one subtype. Organophosphates block the action of AChE, thus allowing accumulation of ACh in both the PNS and CNS. This leads to typical signs of parasympathetic activation—salivation, lacrimation, urination, diarrhea, and bradycardia—but may also be accompanied by convulsions and eventually coma and death.

Dopamine. Dopamine (DA) is synthesized from tyrosine with tyrosine hydroxylase (TH) catalyzing the conversion of tyrosine to L-DOPA and DOPA decarboxylase catalyzing the conversion to dopamine. The production of an activated phosphorylated TH is dependent on calcium ion concentration, cyclic AMP and a tetrahydrobiopterin (BH_4). The latter binds to a site on TH that can also bind DA, so increasing concentrations of DA will inhibit the production of more DA. Dopamine is packed into synaptic vesicles by a vesicular monoamine transporter (VMAT) and can then be released into the synapse from these vesicles. Termination of the action of dopamine is mainly by reuptake into presynaptic terminals by a DA transporter (DAT). The resorbed dopamine is converted to dihydroxyphenylacetic acid (DOPAC) by monoamine oxidase in the nerve terminal. Dopamine taken up by surrounding glial cells is converted to homovanillic acid by catecholamine-o-methyl-transferase (COMT). There are species differences in the relative importance of these reactions.

Dopamine receptors can be divided into two forms, D1 and D2-like. Dopamine1 and D5 are classed together and D2–4 are the D2-like receptors. These are all metabotropic G protein coupled receptors. The D1 receptors are linked to a G_s protein that increases the cellular concentration of cAmp while the D2 receptors are linked to a G_i protein having the opposite effect. D1 receptors are generally found on postsynaptic membranes and while D2 receptors are present on some postsynaptic sites they are more commonly found as autoreceptors on the presynaptic membrane. At this site they seem to be able to affect both synthesis and release of dopamine from the nerve terminal.

Dopamine is found in a number of regions of the brain but its presence in the corpus striatum is thought to play a major role in motor coordination and locomotion. Dopamine is also involved with reward, reinforcement, and motivation, and it is this aspect that contributes to its role in drugs of addiction. For example, cocaine inhibits DAT, thus prolonging the presence of dopamine in the synaptic cleft and prolonging its action on the postsynaptic membrane. Phenothiazines are thought to be dopamine antagonists and hence they reduce motivation and action while monoamine oxidase inhibitors will increase dopamine release and are used in the treatment of depression. Drugs that block D2 receptors will decrease the release of dopamine and at high enough doses will produce catalepsy.

Norepinephrine and Epinephrine. These are much less important neurotransmitters within the CNS compared with dopamine (about one-quarter to one-third of the number of neurons containing dopamine) but are also involved in wakefulness, attention, and feeding behavior. Norepinephrine (NE) is produced from DA with the aid of dopamine-β hydroxylase and epinephrine is further synthesized with the aid of phenylethanolamine-N-methyltransferase. The latter is found in a discrete number of neurons that are different from those secreting NE. Both neurotransmitters are packed into vesicles using VMAT and are metabolized by MAO and COMT when taken back up into the cell. Norepinephrine is removed from the synaptic cleft by norepinephrine transporter (NET) and this will also transport epinephrine—no specific epinephrine transporter has been identified.

The alpha- and beta-adrenergic receptors for these neurotransmitters are G protein coupled metabotropic receptors and are further divided into α_{1A-D}, α_{2A-C}, and β_{1-3}. The α_{1A-D} are associated with a G_q protein that results in a slow depolarization due to the inhibition of K^+ channels while the α_{2A-C} receptors are associated with a G_i protein that results in hyperpolarization. The α_2 receptors are found on both presynaptic and postsynaptic terminals. They act as autoreceptors on the presynaptic terminal to decrease the release of NE. Since wakefulness is dependent on tonic activity on these neurons it follows that the inhibition of this activity would tend to lead to sedation and lack of movement. This is the principle behind the use of alpha-2 agonists, which decrease the release of NE and may hyperpolarize the postsynaptic cells as well. Alpha-2 antagonists have the opposite effect and can cause central excitation when administered alone.

Histamine. Histamine is produced from the amino acid, histidine catalyzed by the enzyme histidine decarboxylase. It is transported into vesicles using VMAT and released into the synaptic cleft where it can act on one of three histamine receptors (H_{1-3}). No plasma membrane transporter has been identified for histamine but it is metabolized by histamine methyltransferase and MAO. The histamine receptors are G protein coupled metabotropic receptors. H1 is coupled with a G_q protein affecting inositol phospholipase, H2 is coupled with a G_s protein that increases the cAmp concentrations while the H3 receptor is coupled with a G_i protein with opposing effects. It is thought that the H3 receptor is the autoreceptor on the presynaptic terminal involved in decreasing the release of histamine and possibly other neurotransmitters present in the same cells.

Histamine is also thought to be involved in aspects of wakefulness and is strongly associated with the vestibular apparatus, explaining the use of antihistamines in the control of motion sickness and that drowsiness is a common effect with antihistamines that cross the blood-brain barrier.

5-Hydroxytryptamine or Serotonin. 5-Hydroxytryptamine (5-HT) is synthesized from tryptophan via 5-hydroxytryptophan catalyzed by the enzymes tryptophan-5-hydroxylase and then aromatic L-amino acid decarboxylase. Tryptophan is transported into the brain via an active process that also transports other large neutral amino acids. This means that the production of 5-HT is dependent not only on the concentration of tryptophan in the diet but also on the relative amounts of tryptophan. Dietary restriction of tryptophan depletes 5-HT production while increased dietary tryptophan increases 5-HT production up to a point where the tryptophan-5-hydroxylase enzyme system becomes saturated. As with many biologic systems a treatment that alters one component may be compensated for by changes in another component. For example, increased dietary tryptophan could be compensated for by a decrease in tryptophan-5-hydroxylase. Once synthesized 5-HT is packed into vesicles using VMAT and once released, it is transported back into the cell by a specific 5-HT transporter (SERT). This protein is the target for a number of therapeutic agents called the *selective serotonin reuptake inhibitors (SSRIs)*, of which fluoxetine (Prozac) is one. Once taken up, 5-HT is mainly broken down using MAO.

At least 12 5-HT receptors have been identified (5-HT_{1A-E}, 5-HT_{2A-C}, 5-HT_{3-7}), with the majority being G protein coupled metabotropic receptors. The exception to this is 5-HT_3, which is a ligand gated ionotropic receptor that allows influx of cations to cause excitation of the postsynaptic membrane. The 5-HT_1 receptors are coupled with G_i proteins and 5-HT_2 with G_q proteins, and the others are thought to be associated with G_s proteins (with the exception of 5HT_5, which is probably associated with a G_i protein).

5-HT is also involved in the regulation of sleep and attention and it plays a role in nociception and the control of emesis. Some potent antiemetics such as ondansetron and granisetron are 5-HT_3 antagonists. Recent work suggests that the 5-HT_3 receptor may be involved in the mechanism of action of inhaled anesthetics (Solt et al. 2006; Stevens et al. 2005). Serotonin syndrome is a condition described in people that presents with multiple signs, including alterations in conscious state (agitation, anxiety, seizures to lethargy and even coma), autonomic dysfunction (central and peripheral actions of 5-HT—hyperthermia, sweating, tachycardia, hypertension, dyspnea, dilated pupils), and neuromuscular changes (myoclonia, hyperreflexia, and ataxia). This syndrome is being reported more commonly because of the many drugs being prescribed that affect the 5-HT system. Amitriptyline, tramadol, meperidine, and St John's wort all reduce 5-HT uptake while selegeline and St John's wort reduce 5-HT catabolism. Combinations of these drugs or excessive doses of a single agent can lead to this syndrome (Jones and Story 2005). In dogs a similar syndrome has been described following ingestion of 5-hydroxytryptophan (Gwaltney-Brant et al. 2000).

Peptides. Many peptides have been identified as playing a part in neurosignaling. These substances are synthesized in the cell body as a prepropeptide that may contain a number of different peptide molecules. Proopiomelanocortin (POMC) is a good example since it contains ACTH, α- and γ-melanocyte stimulating hormone (MSH), γ-lipotropic hormone, and β-endorphin. The final peptide neurotransmitter is generated by peptidases cleaving the prepropeptide into its component parts and this cleavage may be tissue-specific. In the anterior lobe of the pituitary, POMC is converted mainly to ACTH, whereas the output from the intermediate lobe consists mainly of β-endorphin and MSH. Most of the peptides are colocalized in synaptic terminals with smaller molecule neurotransmitters (Table 8.2) and their release may be dependent on a different signal strength than with the smaller molecules. Typically it takes a greater amount of calcium in the synaptic vesicle to get the peptide to be released. Once the peptide has been released it attaches to receptors on the postsynaptic membrane and it generally takes lower concentrations of these molecules, compared with the smaller neurotransmitters, to have an effect. A peptide may also diffuse more broadly to influence neurons further away as suggested by the fact that receptors for some peptides are in separate anatomical locations to the neurons producing the peptidergic agonist. As for the other neurotransmitters, peptide receptors often come in a variety of subtypes and these may be found in different locations of the CNS and subserve different signaling purposes. They are all G protein metabotropic receptors. Once released into the synaptic cleft the peptides are catabolized by peptidases that are present in the extracellular matrix.

TABLE 8.2 Colocalization of some small molecule neurotransmitters with peptides

Neurotransmitter	Peptides Found in the Same Terminals
Glutamate	Substance P Orexin Enkephalin
GABA	Somatostatin Cholecystokinin (CCK)
Acetylcholine	VIP 5-HT
Dopamine	CCK Neurotensin
Norepinephrine	Somatostatin Enkephalin NPY Neurotensin
Epinephrine	NPY Neurotensin
5-HT	Substance P TRH Enkephalin

The peptides can be divided into several groups that have more to do with their discovery than their function within the CNS: the gut/brain peptides, the pituitary hormones, the hypothalamic releasing factors, the opioid peptides, and others (Table 8.3). Of these, the tachykinins (specifically Substance P) and the opioids are the most important with regard to nociception. Substance P is colocalized with glutamate in many of the small fiber afferents that are involved with sensing hot/cold and noxious stimulation and it attaches to one of the neurokinin receptors (NK_{1-3}). Opioid peptides (β-endorphin, dynorphin, leu-enkephalin, met-enkephalin, α and β neoendorphin, orphanin FQ) act at the mu, kappa, delta, or orphanin FQ receptors (MOP, KOP, DOP, and NOP). These peptides are present in the dorsal horn of the spinal cord and throughout the CNS and are largely involved in the modulation of nociception. The relative abundance and location of these peptides and their receptors varies between species.

Other Neurotransmitters

Purines. ATP, adenosine, and adenine dinucleotides (ApnA) are released into the synaptic cleft of some neurons. These differ from classic neurotransmitters in that ATP and ApnA may be in the same synaptic vesicle as other

TABLE 8.3 Peptide neurotransmitters

Neuropeptide	Receptors
Gut/brain peptides	
Substance P, Neurokinin A & B	NK_{1-3}
Vasoactive intestinal peptide (VIP)	$VPAC_{1\&2}$, PAC_1
Neuropeptide Y	Y_{1-5}
Cholecystokinin (CCK)	$CCK_{1\&2}$
Orexin A & B	$OX_{1\&2}$
Pituitary peptides	
Vasopressin	$V_{1\&2}$
Oxytocin	OT
Adrenocorticotrophic hormone (ACTH)	MC1–5R
α-melanocyte stimulating hormone (α-MSH)	MC1–5R
Prolactin	
Hypothalamic releasing peptides	
Thyrotropin releasing hormone (TRH)	$TRH_{1\&2}$
Luteinizing hormone-releasing hormone (LHRH)	
Somatostatin	SST_{1-5}
Growth hormone releasing hormone (GHRH)	
Gonadotropin releasing hormone (GnRH)	GnRHR
Opioid peptides	
Leu-enkephalin	MOP, DOP
Met-enkephalin	MOP, DOP
Endorphin	MOP, DOP
Dynorphin	MOP, KOP
α and β4 neoendorphin	MOP, KOP, DOP
Orphanin FQ	NOP
Others	
Angiotensin	$AT_{1\&2}$
Neurotensin	$NTS_{1\&2}$
Corticotropin releasing factor (CRF)	$CRF_{1\&2}$
Calcitonin gene-related peptide (CGRP)	$CGRP_1$, $AM_{1\&2}$
Bradykinin	$B_{1\&2}$

small molecule neurotransmitters, while adenosine is not stored in vesicles. Further ATP can be converted to adenosine in the synaptic cleft to act on its receptors separately from the ATP. Adenosine attaches to P_1 receptors (A_1, A_{2A-B}, A_3), which are all G protein coupled receptors; ATP can attach to P_{2X1-5} (ionotropic) or $P_{2Y1,2,4,6,11}$ (metabotropic) receptors. Adenosine has hypnotic and anxiolytic effects and is involved in the modulation of nociception.

Endocannabinoids. Anandamide and 2-arachidonylglycerol (2-AG) are thought to act on cannabinoid receptors (CB1-2). This is an unusual signaling pathway because the ligands are released from the postsynaptic cell and have an effect on the presynaptic terminal. The current hypothesis is that the increase in postsynaptic cytoplasmic calcium, triggered by depolarization, stimulates the release of the cannabinoid neurotransmitter and this attaches to CB1 receptors on the presynaptic terminal resulting in an inhibitory effect. The CB1 receptors are located on GABA terminals so the inhibition of GABA release reduces the inhibitory effect of GABA and causes stimulation (e.g., increased appetite associated with cannabis administration).

Agmatine. Agmatine is a decarboxylated arginine that has been found as an endogenous neurotransmitter and has been proposed as a natural agonist at the imidazoline receptor. These receptors are of interest to the clinician because many of the α_2 agonists used in practice are imidazolines (e.g., medetomidine, detomidine, romifidine). However, investigations with this substance have also shown that it interacts with the glutmatergic system and acts as an antagonist at the NMDA receptor and inhibits nitric oxide synthase. It has been shown to be able to decrease pain resulting from inflammation, neuropathy and spinal cord injury (Fairbanks et al. 2000).

Role of Nonneuronal Cells. The normal development and activity of the CNS is dependent on the glial cells. The three types of glial cells—oligodendrocytes, astrocytes, and microglia—are all intimately associated with neurons. The oligodendrocytes form myelin sheaths for neurons in the CNS (equivalent to the Schwann cells in the PNS), the astrocytes ensheath synaptic junctions, provide a scaffolding within the CNS, and ensheath the capillaries as part of the blood-brain barrier. Microglia are present throughout the CNS and were thought to be relatively quiescent until needed to provide clean-up duties by engulfing foreign materials and pathogens. It is now clear that all of these cells also have a function in cell-to-cell signaling even though they do not have the ability to depolarize. As indicated in the section above, astrocytes that surround the synaptic junctions play a role in absorbing neurotransmitters and, in some cases, metabolizing them and/or transferring them back to the presynaptic terminal. Some of these molecules may also activate the glial cells—substance P, ATP, and excitatory amino acids have all been shown to do this. Other substances that may be released from the neuron to activate the glia include nitric oxide and fractalkine. Disturbingly, it has also been shown that morphine can activate glial cells and so the administration of an opioid analgesic may be enhancing the transmission of nociceptive information (Watkins et al. 2005)! However, the depolarization of the synaptic terminal itself may also activate the astrocyte and open calcium channels. An influx of calcium into the astrocyte may induce increased production of factors that can feed back to the synapse or this change may be transmitted to other astrocytes via the tight junctions that connect these cells. Factors released by glia that might alter synaptic transmission include prostaglandins, nerve growth factor (NGF), brain-derived neurotrophic factor (BDNF), the neurotrophins NT-3 and NT-4/5, and the proinflammatory cytokines interleukin-1 (IL-1) and tumor necrosis factor (TNF). As an example it has been shown that BDNF activates a specific sodium channel on some neurons and this plays a role in long-term potentiation. Thus the glial cells may release factors into their local environment that affect the activity of a number of neurons adding an amplifying effect to signals being processed through this network. Using drugs that modify the activation of glial cells (e.g., minocycline) or drugs that block cell signaling pathways internally (e.g., p38 MAP kinase inhibitors) or the production of activators (e.g., antiprostaglandins) has the potential to alter pain perception.

Interactions Between Neurotransmitter Systems. The descriptions above are overly simplistic in many areas since there are multiple interactions between the neurotransmitters and the processes that control them. The colocation of neurotransmitters within the same presynaptic terminals means that even the signal produced from a single terminal can be modified by the intensity of the incoming signal or other chemicals in the local environment. It is also being shown that receptor proteins can interact directly to modify the signal being received. For example, D5 interacting with $GABA_A$ and D1 with NMDA. In the latter case activation of D1 receptors decreases the cell-surface localization of NMDA receptors, whereas activation of the NMDA receptor increases the number of D1 receptors on the cell surface (Lee and Liu 2004).

BLOOD-BRAIN BARRIER. In order for any drug to produce an effect on the CNS it has to gain access to the neurons and other cells in the brain. Neuronal function relies on having a very stable extracellular ionic content and limiting the number of "foreign" substances to a minimum, such that exposure of neurons to nanomolar concentrations of some neurotransmitters can produce an effect. In order to achieve this, animals have developed a barrier from the blood that allows the passage of small molecules but restricts the passage of ionic compounds and most larger molecules (Abbott 2005; Hawkins and Davis 2005). This barrier is formed by tight junctions between endothelial cells, pericytes, a basement membrane, and by astrocytes that encase the capillaries (Fig. 8.3). As well as the tight junctions the endothelial cells have an increased content of mitochondria, a lack of fenestrations, and minimal pinocytotic activity compared with capillaries in other parts of the body. The barrier is not present in some areas of the brain, namely, the circumventricular organs (CVOs). These include the subfornical organ at the roof of the third ventricle, the median eminence and the organum vasculosum of the lamina terminalis (OVLT) in the floor of the third ventricle, the pineal gland and the subcommissural organ at the back of the third ventricle, and the area postrema near the fourth ventricle. The chemoreceptor trigger zone (CTZ) is in the area postrema and its lack of a BBB may be part of the explanation for the rapid onset of emesis with some opioids (e.g., morphine). These drugs produce an antiemetic effect at the vomiting center, which is behind the BBB, and so the resultant effect is dependent on the rate at which the drug activates these two areas. With hydrophilic drugs, penetration to the vomiting center is slower than the effect on the CTZ with resulting emesis. More lipophilic opioids (e.g., fentanyl) inhibit the vomiting center at about the same time as they excite the CTZ, giving a much lower incidence of emesis. These CVOs have a comparatively small surface area and are thought to be separated from the rest of the brain by a glial barrier, thus limiting the spread of material taken up through the CVOs. The choroid plexus is comparatively leaky, but substances that gain access to the CSF have relatively limited access to neuronal tissue. The surface area of the choroid plexus is about 1/1000 of the area of the BBB.

The transfer of molecules across the BBB under normal physiologic conditions is regulated by three factors. There are carrier proteins that are used to carry essential molecules such as glucose, amino acids, amines, adenine, adenosine, and thyroid hormones across the barrier. There are receptor-mediated methods involved in the transcytosis of some peptides. Insulin, transferrin, and leptin are examples of peptides that are transferred by receptor-mediated transcytosis. There are also active efflux systems to eject

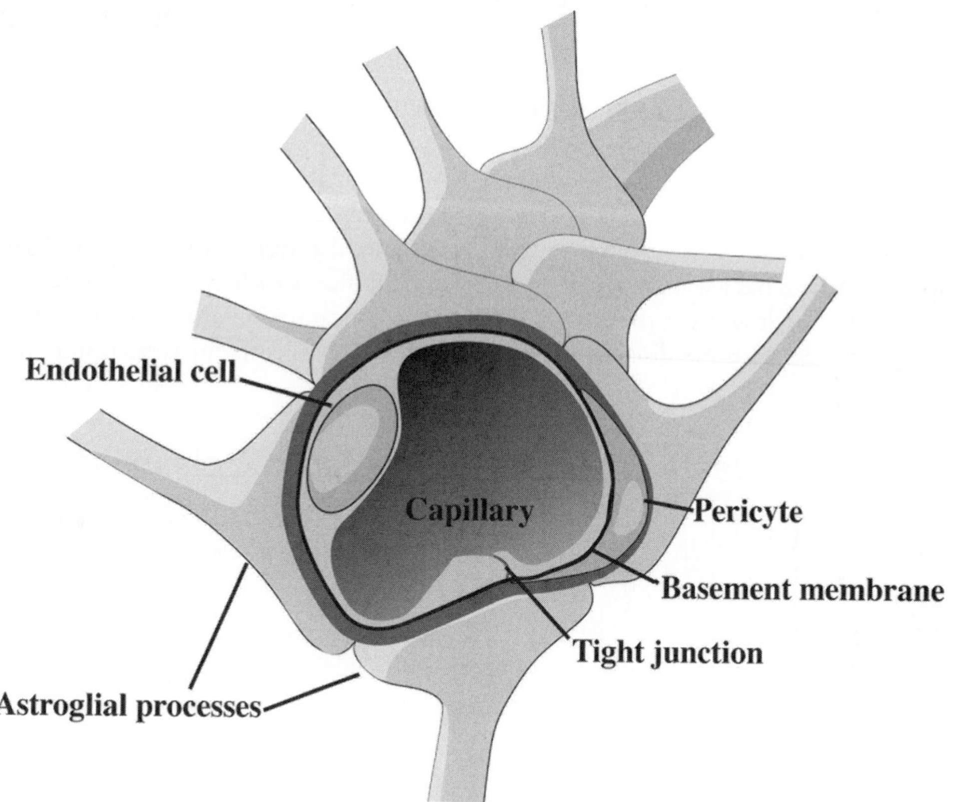

FIG. 8.3 Blood-brain barrier. The endothelial cells have tight junctions that link the cells in such a way as to minimize passage of material through the cells. These cells also have fewer pinocytotic vesicles and more mitochondria than capillary endothelial cells elsewhere in the body. These cells are surrounded by a basement membrane and there are pericytes in this location. Astroglial foot processes surround the outside of the capillary.

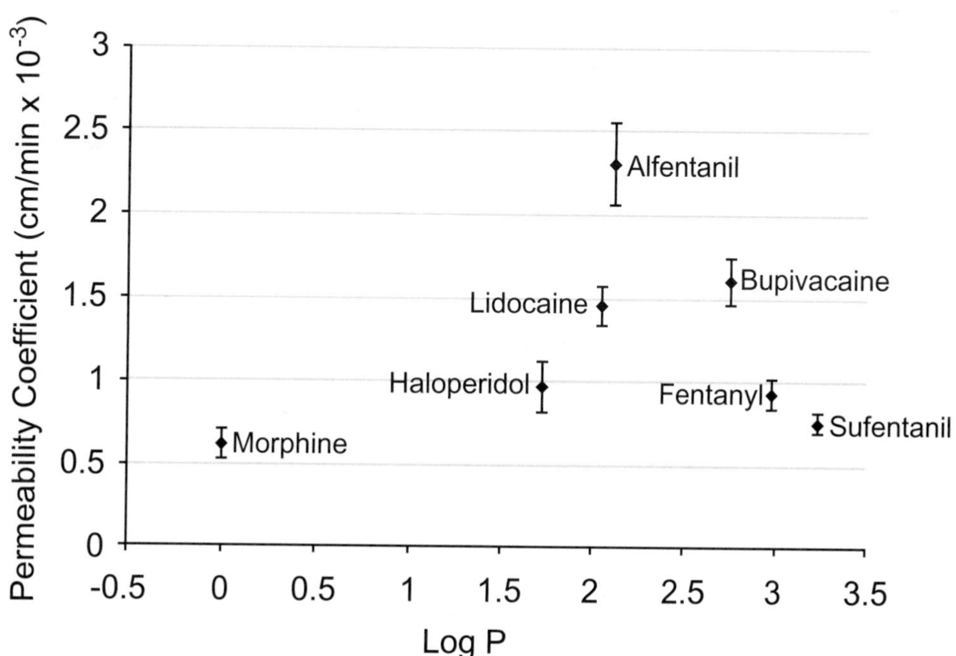

FIG. 8.4 Permeability of dural membranes to various drugs used in anesthesia versus their octane: buffer partition coefficient, expressed here as Log P. (Data drawn from Bernards and Hill 1992.)

substances from the brain. These carrier-mediated efflux systems are designed to eject unwanted metabolites from the extracellular space in the brain and have now been shown to have significant effects on the access of some drugs to the CNS. One of the proteins involved in this process is P-glycoprotein, which has a wide substrate specificity and transports a range of drugs from the CNS. This has become of clinical interest with the discovery of the MDR-1 gene that is responsible for the production of P-glycoprotein. In some herding breed dogs (Collies and Australian Shepherds) a polymorphism of this gene results in increased toxicity to a number of drugs that was first recognized as ivermectin toxicity (Mealey 2004). It is now evident that a lack of P-glycoprotein may also alter the brain concentration of a number of other drugs. In MDR-1 deficient mice brain concentrations of morphine and

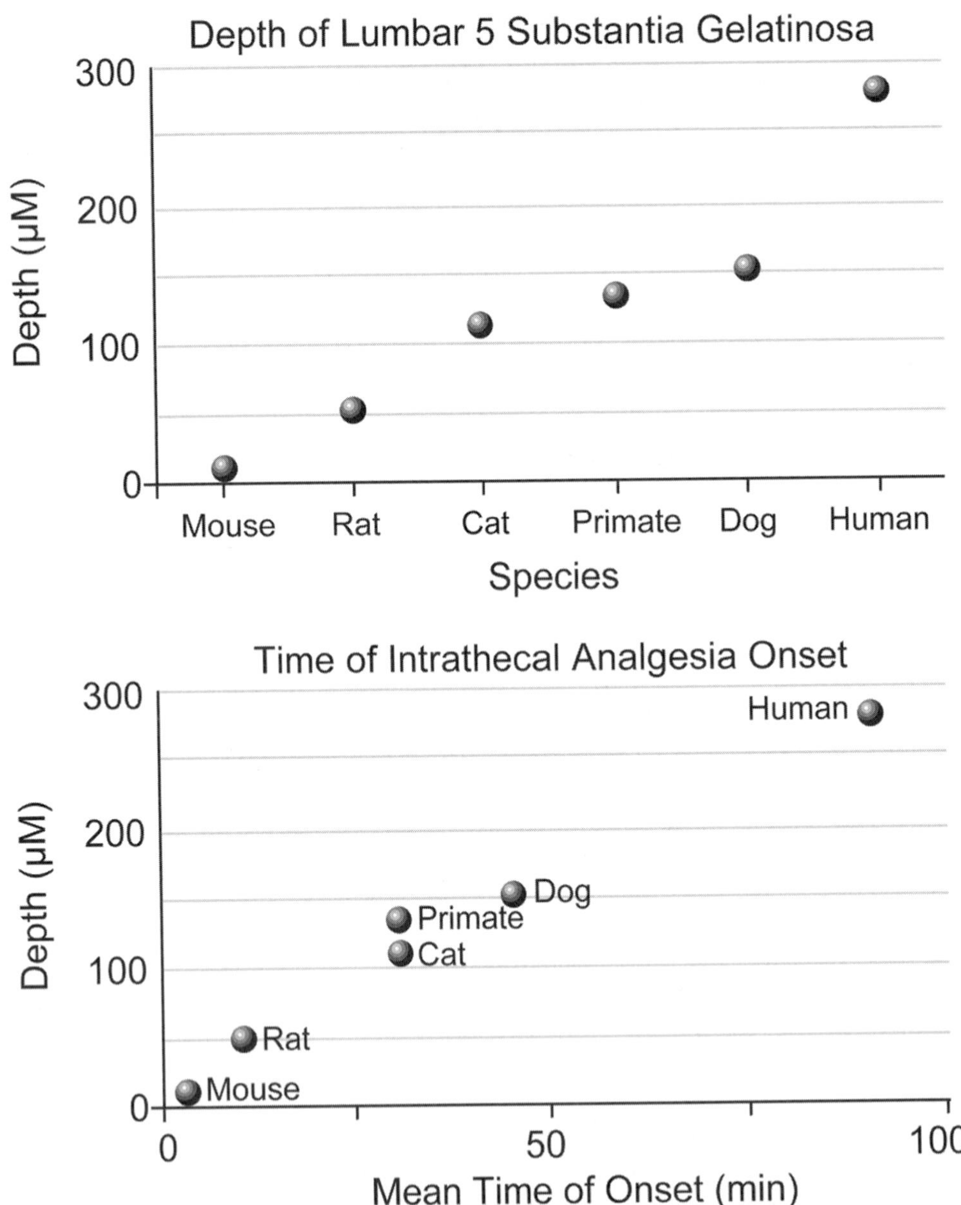

FIG. 8.5 Relationship of the distance from the surface of the spine to the substantia gelatinosa at the fifth lumbar segment in various species (top) and the rate of onset of morphine (intrathecal at minimally effective doses) in these different species (bottom). Drawn from Yaksh TL, Spinal Analgesic Mechanisms. In *Pain 2005—An Updated Review.* International Association for the Study of Pain, 909 NE 43rd St, Suite 306, Seattle, WA 98105-6020.

fentanyl were increased by 25% and the uptake of methadone was increased by 200–1500% (Dagenais et al. 2004; Wang et al. 2004). Butorphanol may have a more profound effect in MDR-1 deficient dogs. Phenothiazines have been shown to have an inhibitory effect on P-glycoprotein and may thus alter the uptake of other drugs into the brain. Acepromazine seems to have a more profound effect in these dogs (Mealey 2006).

The rate at which drugs cross the BBB is governed by the above activities and also the physicochemical properties of the drug itself. Molecular size, lipid solubility, hydrogen bond donor sites, and external oxygen and nitrogen affect the passage across the BBB. Polar molecules are not able to cross the BBB, so the drug needs to be present in an unionized form in order to get into the brain. Lipid solubility is measured in a number of ways but one of the most common is to measure the octanol/buffer partition coefficient and express this as a log value, usually given as Log P. Molecules that are less likely to penetrate the BBB would have a molecular weight >450 g/mol, a Log P >4, >5 hydrogen bond donors and the sum of nitrogen and oxygen atoms >10. On the other end molecules with low Log P values (<2) also have low penetrance leading to a sigmoid shaped curve when Log P is plotted against brain uptake. This can be illustrated by the pharmacodynamics of morphine (Log P = 0.1), alfentanil (log P = 2.1) and sufentanil (Log P = 3.24), where the peak effects of the drugs are approximately at 2–3 hours, 1 minute, and 6 minutes, respectively (Lotsch 2005).

EPIDURAL BARRIER. Drugs administered into the epidural space must diffuse through the dural membranes in order to reach the spinal cord where they might have an effect (Bernards and Hill 1990, 1991). This diffusion is dependent on many of the usual factors (concentration gradient, molecular size, polarity, lipid solubility, and distance) but the same sigmoid effect of lipid solubility is seen here as well (Bernards and Hill 1992). This is demonstrated in Figure 8.4 where Log P is plotted against meningeal permeability measured in vitro. Epidural fat plays a role in that very lipid-soluble drugs tend to get absorbed here thus limiting their uptake into the spinal cord. The main meningeal barrier to diffusion is the pia-arachnoid membrane with its complex mix of aqueous fluids (CSF and extracellular fluid) and lipid membranes. The distance effect is illustrated in Figure 8.5 where the time to onset is plotted against depth across a number of species following intrathecal administration (Yaksh 2005).

PRINCIPLES OF ANESTHESIOLOGY

Anesthesiology is defined as the art and science of administration of anesthesia. The term also describes a clinical specialty of medicine (including veterinary medicine) that emerged during the early 1900s when a few physicians began devoting full time to the clinical administration of anesthetics. Anesthesiology was officially recognized as an organized specialty in medicine with the establishment in 1938 of a peer-certifying body of physicians, the American Board of Anesthesiologists (ABA). Initially, the ABA was an affiliate board of the American Board of Surgery but in 1941 it became an independent board. In addition, in 1940 a section of anesthesiology was formed within the American Medical Association. In 1975 the American College of Veterinary Anesthesiologists was officially recognized by the American Veterinary Medical Association as the body to certify veterinarians as specialists in veterinary anesthesia. Broader summaries of the development of anesthesiology are available elsewhere (Smithcors 1971; Larson 2005; Weaver 1988; Weaver and Hall 2005). The central role of the anesthetist is 1) to apply methods to minimize or eliminate pain, relax muscles, and facilitate patient restraint during surgical, obstetrical, and other medical, diagnostic, and therapeutic procedures and 2) to monitor and support life functions in patients during the operative period as well as in critically ill, injured, or otherwise seriously ill patients. The skills and knowledge that have developed in the field have extended the clinical practice of anesthesiology into intensive care, cardiac and pulmonary resuscitation, and the control of pain problems unrelated to surgery. The word *anesthesia* is derived from the Greek for "insensible" or "without feeling." The word does not necessarily imply loss of consciousness. In the realm of veterinary anesthesiology, anesthesia, and anesthetics are used for a variety of reasons (Table 8.4).

TABLE 8.4 Use of anesthetics in animals

Elimination of sensibility to noxious stimuli
Humane restraint (e.g., protect animal, facilitate diagnostic or surgical procedure)
Technical efficiency (e.g., protect personnel, facilitate diagnostic or surgical procedure)
Specific biomedical research tool (e.g., sleep time)
Control convulsions
Euthanasia

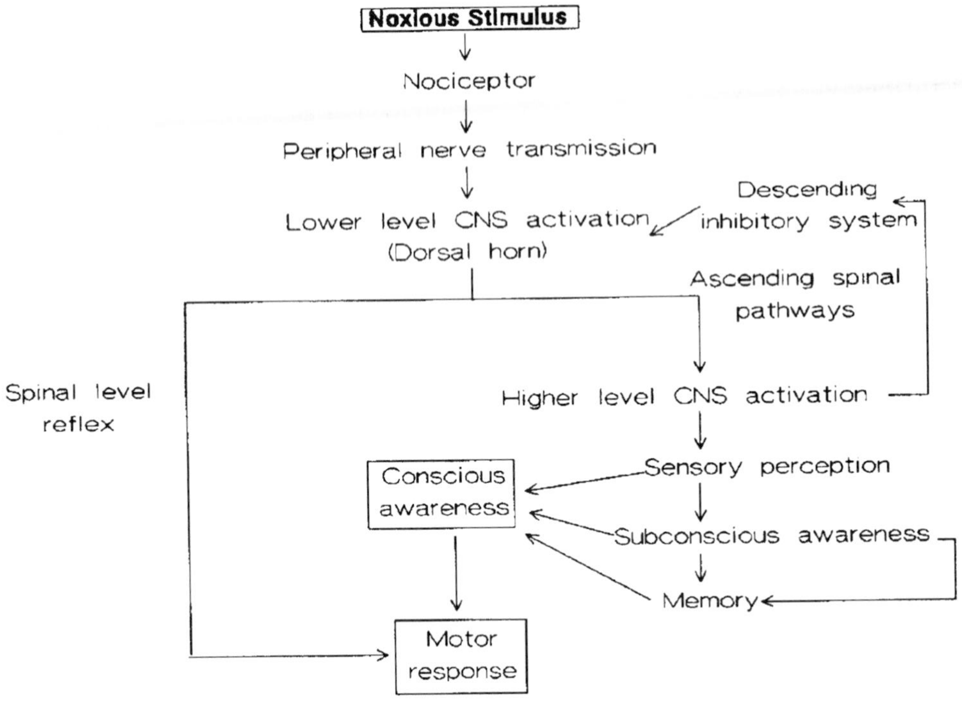

FIG. 8.6 Events in the reaction to a noxious stimulus.

ANESTHETIC USE

Perception of Noxious Stimuli (Pain). Prevention of the perception of a noxious stimulus during surgery is the primary justification for anesthesia. A noxious stimulus is defined as a stimulus that is potentially damaging to body tissue. Nociception has no emotional or perceptional connotation. Pain is an unpleasant sensory and emotional experience; it is a perception, not a physical entity. The perception of pain depends on a functioning cerebral cortex. The concept of pain includes several interdependent dimensions: the sensory/discriminative and motivational/affective.

It is not the intent to sidetrack here into semantic issues or to belabor what are to some fine points, but it is necessary for completeness to stress that contemporary reasoning holds that pain is a subjective response in conscious human beings. When considering "pain" in animals, it is important to recognize that our knowledge of pain in animals is largely inferential. We approach the subject with "the tacit assumption . . . that stimuli are noxious and strong enough to give rise to the perception of pain in animals if the stimuli are detected as pain by human beings, if they at least approach or exceed tissue damaging proportion and if they produce escape behavior in animals" (Kitchell and Erickson 1983).

Classical Approach to Mechanisms of Pain. Before further discussion of methods by which insensitivity is produced, it is helpful to briefly review the mechanisms whereby an individual becomes aware of and reacts to a noxious stimulus (Fig. 8.6). This inclusion here is justified on the basis that knowledge of these mechanisms offers the clinician targets for single or multiple attacks in an attempt to abolish or minimize pain.

Acute pain that is provoked by disease or injury (planned or unplanned) is the net effect of many interacting and complex anatomic paths and physiological mechanisms. The stimulus excites a specialized receptor organ, the nociceptor. Nociceptors are distributed throughout the body but are frequently grouped as somatic (cutaneous, muscle, bone, joint, fascia) or visceral. Nociceptors are located at the termination of free nerve endings of small poorly myelinated or nonmyelinated A-delta and C afferent nerves. The nociceptors transduce the stimuli into nociceptive impulses that are transmitted to the CNS. Impulses that originate from areas below the head are transmitted via fibers that synapse with interneurons or second-order neurons in the dorsal horn of the spinal cord. Impulses from the head travel via fibers within the cranial nerves to the medulla, where they synapse with neurons in the trigeminal nuclei (medullary dorsal horn). In the spinal cord, the signal is subjected to a variety of potential modulating influences in the dorsal horn. For a long time the dorsal horn was considered to perform simply as a relay station. More recent evidence indicates it contains an incredibly complex circuitry and rich biochemistry that permits not only reception and transmission of nociceptive impulses but also a large degree of signal processing. After being subjected to these modulating influences, some of the impulses may then stimulate somatomotor and preganglionic sympathetic neurons and provoke nocifensive reflex responses. Nociceptive impulses also activate other neurons making up the ascending systems that pass to the brain stem and brain. Supraspinal systems that are probably involved in processing nociceptive information to progressively higher levels of awareness include the reticular formation, limbic system, hypothalamus, thalamus, and cortex.

Activation of the reticular formation results in abrupt awakening, diffuse alertness, and initiation of protective homeostatic responses. In turn, affective (emotional) alertness is obtained through cortical arousal. The animal is now fully knowledgeable regarding the cause and strength of the noxious stimulus and its relationship to the environment. The animal in turn reacts with a coordinated response.

For more detailed information the reader is referred elsewhere (McMahon and Koltzenburg 2006; Loeser 2001).

Immobility. Although the primary reason for anesthetic delivery is to render the animal insensible to pain, restraint and technical efficiency are also long-recognized important considerations. Although viewed as an extreme in approach today, Alexandre Liautord, a Frenchman, noted in his 1892 *Manual of Operative Veterinary Surgery:* "In veterinary surgery, the indication for anesthesia has not, to the same extent as in human, the avoidance of pain in the patient for its object, and though the duties of the veterinarian include that of avoiding the infliction of *unnecessary* pain as much as possible, the administration of anesthetic compounds aims principally to facilitate the performance of the operation for its own sake, by depriving the patient of the power of obstructing, and perhaps even frustrating its execution, to his own detriment, by the violence of his struggles, and the persistency of his resistance. To prevent these, with their disastrous consequences, is the prime motive in the induction of the anesthetic state" (quoted in Smithcors 1971). More in keeping with contemporary thought are the words of George H. Dadd written in 1854 in *The Modern Horse Doctor:* "We recommend that, in all operations of this kind, the subject be etherized, not only in view of preventing pain, but that we may, in the absence of all struggling on the part of our patient, perform the operation satisfactorily, and in much less time after etherization has taken place than otherwise. So soon as the patient is under the influence of that valuable agent, we have nothing to fear from his struggles, provided we have the assistance of one experienced to administer it" (quoted in Smithcors 1971 (Smithcors 1971). Many of these same clinical principles can and should also be applied directly to the research environment.

ANESTHESIA CLASSIFIED. Anesthesia is produced by both chemical (i.e., drugs) and physical (e.g., sensory nerve destruction) means. Anesthetic drugs are frequently classified according to their route of administration (Table 8.5). Some drugs are only suited for common delivery via one route, e.g., the inhalation anesthetics, while many of the injectable agents may be administered in a variety of different manners depending on the drug and the desired endpoint of effect.

TABLE 8.5 Routes by which anesthetic or anesthetic adjuvant drugs are administered in animals

1. Topical
   a. Cutaneous
   b. Mucous membrane
2. Injection
   a. Intravenous
   b. Subcutaneous
   c. Intramuscular
   d. Intraperitoneal
   e. Intraosseous
3. Gastrointestinal tract
   a. Oral
   b. Rectal
4. Respiratory system (e.g., inhalation)

TABLE 8.6 Techniques of anesthesia based on extent of loss of sensation

1. Local/regional: drugs placed in close proximity to nerve membranes, causing conduction block
   a. Topical or surface
   b. Area infiltration
      i. Subdermal
      ii. Intravenous regional
   c. Perineural (i.e., nerve trunk)
   d. Peridural (i.e., epidural or caudal)
   e. Subarachnoid (i.e., spinal)
2. General anesthesia: state of controlled, reversible CNS depression (including unconsciousness) produced by one or multiple drugs
   a. Injectable
   b. Inhalation
   c. Balanced

Local and Regional Anesthesia. Anesthetics are also classified according to the region of the body influenced (Table 8.6). For example, a local anesthetic is administered, usually to conscious or mildly sedated animals, to desensitize a localized or regional area of the body. It is deposited in close proximity to a nerve membrane, causing nerve conduction blockade.

General Anesthesia. General anesthesia is a condition induced by pharmacological or other means that results in controlled, reversible CNS depression. It is true that some drugs in the process of producing anesthesia cause excessive stimulation and activity in the brain, but all anesthetic agents ultimately reduce and stop electrical activity in the brain and decrease brain oxygen consumption. On this basis it is proper to characterize anesthetic agents as CNS depressants.

There is no consensus about the essential elements that comprise the behavioral state that we term *general anesthesia*. Further complication is added by trying to match human and animal studies. For example, sedation is sometimes defined as loss of appropriate responsiveness to verbal command—relatively easy for use with human subjects, more difficult or not possible with animals. For this introductory overview and further discussion, basic elements of general anesthesia will, in addition to reversibility, include absence of awareness (unconsciousness), no recall of events at the conscious level (amnesia), conscious insensitivity to pain (analgesia), and muscle relaxation and diminished motor response to noxious stimulation (immobility). In recent years the importance of minimal autonomic nervous system response to noxious stimulation has been also emphasized by some in clinical applications.

General anesthesia has traditionally been considered a dose-related continuum of a series of events passing into each other (Fig. 8.7), from alert wakefulness through lethargy and drowsiness (sedation), unconsciousness (with and without somatic and visceral response to external stimuli), coma, and death. The wakefulness to coma series implies progressive loss of higher CNS (cortical) function followed by depression of brain stem functions. While portions of this scheme have been challenged, its use is generally acceptable and offers a convenient method to set the stage for further discussion of introductory level understanding or principles of general anesthesia.

Techniques of General Anesthesia. General anesthesia is pharmacologically induced and maintained in animals via one of two general methods. The oldest approach, which is still used in certain animal applications, is the single-agent technique. With this technique, an agent such as pentobarbital, thiopental, or ketamine (or perhaps two agents such as xylazine and ketamine given simultaneously or in close time proximity) is administered at sufficient dose to provide the complete spectrum of characteristics of general anesthesia. This method is simple but may be more life threatening, especially under adverse circumstances, including animal ill health. Because *all* anesthetic agents have some undesirable effects when used alone (the LD_{50}/ED_{50} is commonly no more than 2–4), modern anesthetic practice increasingly involves the use of combinations of drugs. This technique is known as *balanced anesthesia*. With this technique, multiple drugs in low dosage are used, each drug for a specific purpose. The ultimate intent is to take advantage of the desirable features of selected drugs while minimizing their potential for harmful depression of homeostatic mechanisms. This technique is especially advantageous when used with physiologically compromised individuals. An example of such an approach is the combined use of a low dose of a hypnotic-sedative drug for unconsciousness and amnesia, an opioid for profound analgesia with little cardiovascular insult, a neuromuscular blocking drug for muscle relaxation, and intermittent positive pressure ventilation with oxygen to facilitate respiratory gas exchange in the face of total skeletal muscle paralysis. Unfortunately, the balanced technique is complex, and inexperienced or careless use of a drug combination may aggravate undesirable drug

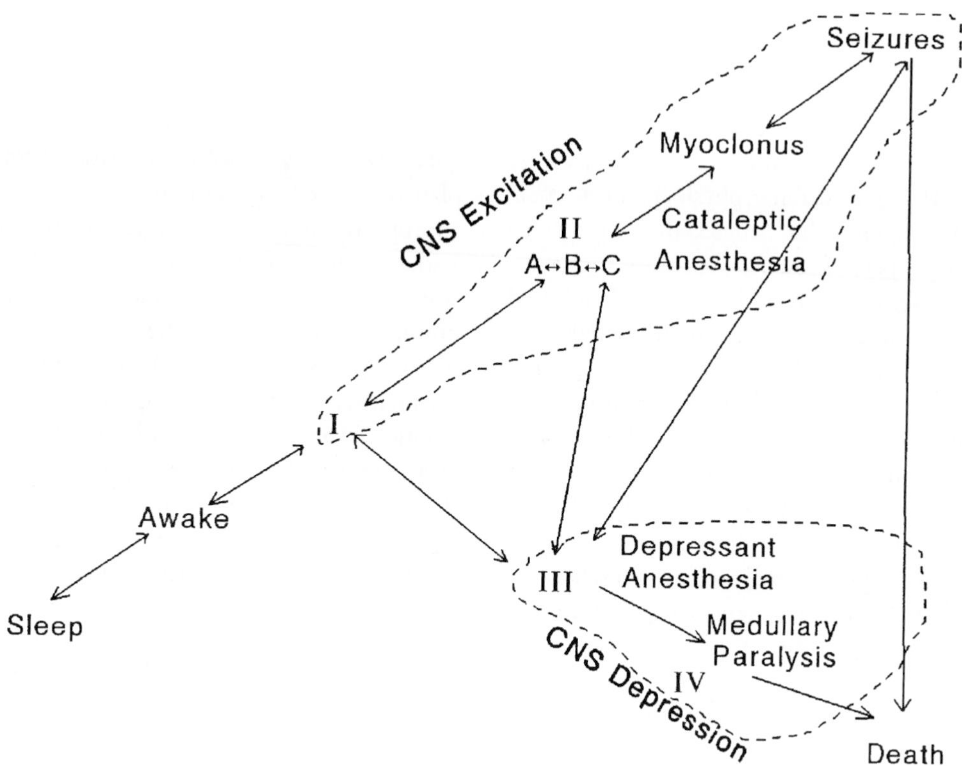

FIG. 8.7 Schematic representation of the stages of anesthesia according to Winters et al. (1972) and Winters (1976). The schematic has been modified slightly from its original description. I–IV refer to the classic stages of anesthesia.

actions and/or other common difficulties encountered by the anesthetist.

Mechanism of Action Causing General Anesthesia. There have been many attempts to explain the mechanism of general anesthesia at a molecular level. Three simple observations limit possible explanations. The rate at which anesthesia can be induced and wakefulness resumed effectively rules out long-term biochemical events and focuses attention on drug-induced alterations of short-term biochemical events. In addition, the diverse chemical structures of anesthetic agents also pose a problem in arriving at a common theory of action. For example, anesthetic drugs range from inert gases such as xenon, relatively simple inorganic (nitrous oxide) and organic (chloral hydrate and chloroform) compounds, to progressively more complex molecules such as pentobarbital, ketamine, and alphaxalone. The absence of a common chemical structure reduces the possibility of a specific-receptor–mediated action. Finally, explanation of their anesthetic action must in some way be linked with their ability to cause superimposed selective and specific anesthetic "side effects," such as reductions in myocardial contractility.

An important neurophysiological action common to most general anesthetics is to depress both spontaneous and evoked neuronal activity in many regions of the brain and spinal cord. Actions exerted on synaptic transmission seem most sensitive while nerve conduction is little influenced. Anesthetics may reduce synaptic transmission by interfering with neurotransmitter release from presynaptic nerve terminals, altering reuptake of neurotransmitter after release, by altering binding of neurotransmitter to postsynaptic receptor sites or by influencing ionic conduction following activation of postsynaptic receptors. The varied nature of these sites does not preclude a specific action at the molecular level. At this point in time ionic mechanisms are the focus of extensive study. The transfer of ions underlies the transmission of neuronal impulses and occurs at the plasma membranes of neurons. Thus synaptic or axonal membranes are favored sites for anesthetic action.

For more than a century, two concepts have dominated thinking about the mechanism of action of general anesthetics. Since a wide range of structurally unrelated agents caused anesthesia, Claude Bernard postulated that all of them did so by a common mechanism; the *unitary theory of narcosis* (Leake 1971). A striking physiochemical characteristic of inhalation anesthetic drugs is their lipid solubility—a physical property shown to correlate best with anesthetic potency. This correlation is commonly referred to as the *Meyer-Overton rule* after the two individuals who independently (1899 and 1901, respectively) noted that the potency of anesthetics increased directly in proportion to their partition coefficient between olive oil and water (i.e., the concentration ratio of the agent in oil and water at equilibrium). Because inhalation anesthetic molecules are hydrophobic and therefore distribute to sites in which they are removed from aqueous environments, and because of the close correlation between potency and lipophilicity, it is theorized that these anesthetics act in the cell membrane lipid layer. It is thought that their presence somehow distorts the membrane structure, which in turn causes occlusion of the pores through which ions pass. These two concepts formed the basis of the long-held notion that at least inhalation anesthetics act nonspecifically on hydrophobic lipid components of cell membranes.

During the past 10–15 years there has been increasing evidence that specific neuronal membrane proteins that permit translocation of ions during membrane excitation are the primary targets for anesthetic action. This is a dramatic departure from the classic view that all general anesthetics act in a common but nonspecific way. Debate is ongoing whether, at least inhalation anesthetics disrupt ion flow through membrane channels by an indirect action on surrounding lipids or via a second messenger, or alternatively, and the increasingly favored view, that they link directly to membrane channel proteins. More specifically, recent work suggests that γ-aminobutyric acid type A ($GABA_A$) receptors are most likely involved in the actions of many, but not all general anesthetics. Some inhaled anesthetics may also act by inhibiting such excitatory ion channels as neuronal nicotinic and glutamate receptors. Regardless, the molecular mechanism of action of general anesthetic drugs is still far from clear, and there is much to learn regarding this phenomenon. Readers are referred elsewhere for more in-depth, timely analysis of this topic and from which some of this discussion was summarized (John and Prichep 2005; Campagna et al. 2003; Koblin 2005).

BASICS OF CLINICAL ANESTHESIA. A favorable anesthetic course begins with a good plan—a plan based on sound pharmacological and physiological principles. There is no rigid format. *No anesthetic technique is unequivocally the best for all animals under all circumstances.* Each plan is adapted to prevailing circumstances. Accordingly, appropriate anesthetic management requires a broad understanding of the physiology of bodily life support systems (e.g., respiratory, circulatory, central and autonomic nervous systems), the pathology and pathophysiology of the condition(s) necessitating anesthesia and surgery, the pharmacology and principles and techniques of administration of anesthetic and adjuvant drugs, and monitoring and support of vital organ function. The rationale that underlies the selection of an appropriate anesthetic protocol is outlined in Table 8.7.

Drug selection for anesthetic management is accomplished by considering the pharmacological requirements for the individual case, reviewing and selecting major drug classes that are appropriate for the specific needs, and then reviewing characteristics and selecting the specific drug(s) within the desired drug class(es). Frequently, the best drug and technique are those with which the clinician is most experienced; i.e., there is an art to the clinical administration of potent, life-threatening drugs such as those used in anesthetic management.

Drugs used in anesthetic management can be conveniently classified according to time frame of use: the preanesthetic, perianesthetic, and immediate postanesthetic periods.

Preanesthetic Period. Drugs are usually administered to animals (usually 15–45 minutes) before induction of general anesthesia. The primary aims of preanesthetic medication are to calm the animal, facilitate handling, and relieve preoperative pain. These along with secondary goals are listed in Table 8.8. Unfortunately, preanesthetic medication is not without its complications, which also

TABLE 8.7 Considerations in the selection of appropriate anesthetic protocol and drugs

1. Animal characteristics (e.g., species, age, physical status)
2. Capabilities and confidence of anesthetist
3. Capabilities of surgeon and surgical requirements
4. Available drugs, facilities, and ancillary personnel
5. Wishes of client

TABLE 8.8 Goals for preanesthetic medication

1. Alleviate or minimize pain
2. Allay apprehension
3. Facilitate handling
4. Minimize undesirable reflex autonomic nervous system activity
   a. Parasympathetic
      i. Vagal nerve
      ii. Secretions: salivary, bronchial
   b. Sympathetic
      i. Arrhythmic
      ii. Arterial blood pressure alterations
5. Supplement general anesthesia
   a. Add to level of analgesia, sedation
   b. Reduce anesthetic requirement
6. Minimize undesirable postanesthetic recovery complications
7. Prevent infection
8. Continue treatment of intercurrent disease

TABLE 8.9 Complications of preanesthetic medication

1. Depressed vital organ function
   a. Direct effects
   b. Interaction with anesthetic and other adjuvant drugs
2. Antianalgesia
3. Prolonged sedation influencing recovery from anesthesia
   a. Prolonged recumbency
   b. Ataxia

TABLE 8.10 Major classes of drugs (and specific drug examples) commonly considered for preanesthetic medication

1. Tranquilizer-sedative
   a. Acepromazine
   b. Azaperone
   c. Benzodiazepines
      i. Diazepam
      ii. Midazolam
2. Hypnotic-sedative
   a. Pentobarbital
   b. Chloral hydrate
3. Opioid
   a. Agonist
      i. Morphine
      ii. Meperidine
   b. Agonist-antagonist
      i. Butorphanol
4. α-adrenergic agonist
   a. Xylazine
   b. Detomidine
   c. Romifidine
   d. Medetomidine
5. Dissociative
   a. Ketamine
6. Commercially prepared combinations of sedating drugs
   a. Telazol (tiletamine + zolazepam)
7. Parasympatholytic
   a. Atropine
   b. Glycopyrrolate

must be considered in formulating the anesthetic management plan (Table 8.9). The concurrent use of two or three drugs is usually required to accomplish the desired preanesthetic conditions in the patient. These are selected from a variety of major drug classes (Table 8.10). The extent of drug combinations advocated by individuals attests to the variety of circumstances commonly encountered clinically and to the lack of agreement on optimal drug effects.

Tranquilizer-Sedatives. Tranquilizers (ataractics or neuroleptics) are frequently administered to animals to produce a calming effect, i.e., tractability or "chemical restraint." This group of drugs includes the phenothiazine, the butyrophenone, and the benzodiazepine subclasses. They are frequently used in combination with other preanesthetic drugs (e.g., opioids), because lower doses can be used than would be the case if each drug were used alone and the degree of sedation accomplished by the drug combination is often potentiated without causing further severe circulatory and respiratory depression.

The phenothiazines have received widespread use for many years. Their potency facilitates easy administration, and favorable tranquilization is usually realized. They have antiarrhythmic, antihistaminic, and antiemetic effects that may be particularly desirable. The α_1-adrenergic blocking action of the phenothiazines is likely to be of special concern in some patients because it may result in arterial hypotension.

The butyrophenones also have α_1-adrenergic blocking activity, but appear to be less potent in this regard. Largely on the basis of cost and the lack of broad-based, clear advantages, the butyrophenones are less frequently used for anesthetic management of veterinary patients than other drugs in the tranquilizer grouping.

Although benzodiazepines are increasingly used with other drugs to induce and maintain general anesthesia, especially in some animals their use in the preanesthetic period is, like the butyrophenones, very limited. Pain and occasional erratic absorption after intramuscular injection are characteristic of some benzodiazepines (e.g., diazepam). Also, sedative actions in otherwise healthy animals are quite variable across animal species commonly encountered in veterinary practice. Sedation caused by benzodiazepines can be reliably reversed by a specific antagonist at least in some species.

Hypnotic-Sedatives. Drugs of this class, including the barbiturates and chloral hydrate, cause a dose-dependent spectrum of CNS depression, sedation, sleep, anesthesia, coma, and death. They produce minimal ventilatory and circulatory depression in sedative doses. Disadvantages of their use include a lack of analgesia and the absence of specific antagonists. Use of drugs from this class have largely been replaced in the preanesthetic period by the α_2-adrenergic agonist drugs.

α_2-Adrenergic Drugs. Drugs such as xylazine cause dose-related sedation and analgesia. They are widely used across species lines singly and in combination with, especially, opioids and dissociative agents. Bradycardia, mild arterial hypertension followed by more prolonged hypotension, hyperglycemia, and increased urine volume are commonly attendant effects. Direct antagonists of varying purity and effectiveness are now available.

Opioids. Potent analgesia, sedation, and the absence of direct myocardial depression are important advantages of the use of opioids in the preanesthetic period. Patients with preexisting preoperative pain or who will require painful diagnostic or therapeutic procedures before anesthetic induction are likely candidates for opioid preanesthetic medication. Opioid premedication is also appropriate prior to anesthetic management techniques that use opioids as a predominant component (i.e., a balanced technique, see above). Predominant adverse effects of opioids when used prior to anesthesia include depression of medullary ventilatory control centers resulting in decreased responsiveness to carbon dioxide and in turn hypoventilation. Opioids commonly induce a vagotonic effect so heart rate may also be decreased to variable degrees depending on agent, dose, and animal species. In some species (e.g., the dog) opioids commonly cause CNS sedation, while in others (e.g., the horse) excitement or CNS arousal are predominant concerns. Opioid-induced vomition in some species (e.g., dog) may be wanted (e.g., a newly presented patient with a full stomach requiring anesthesia for a diagnostic or minor surgical procedure) or unwanted (e.g., risk of pulmonary aspiration of vomitus in elderly or depressed patients). They also decrease intestinal propulsive and ruminal activity.

Dissociative Drugs. Drugs such as ketamine reliably cause a state of somatic analgesia and sedation in some species (e.g., cat) and may be of benefit in special clinical situations (e.g., highly fractious animals under conditions of limited management choices). Its relatively wide margin of safety in otherwise healthy animals is of special benefit under conditions of limited patient control or knowledge base.

The most prominent disadvantage of their use is that, depending on dosage, this class of drugs may cause CNS arousal in some species (e.g., horse) leading to animal excitement or frank convulsions.

Drug Combinations. Sometimes drug combinations are marketed to provide ready access to clinical benefits of two drugs while attempting to minimize their individual disadvantages. For example, Telazol® is a combination of tiletamine, a dissociative agent, and zolazepam, a benzodiazepine tranquilizer-sedative. The combination improves the reliability of the sedative properties of either drug used alone without adding extensively to further vital organ depression (e.g., cardiopulmonary depression). However, as a consequence of the fixed combination, a prolonged duration of effect may be an unwanted result.

Parasympatholytic (Anticholinergic) Drugs. The most common reason for administering drugs such as atropine or the more potent, longer-acting glycopyrrolate before induction of general anesthesia is to reduce upper-airway and salivary secretions (antisialagogue effect) and counteract reflex bradycardia occurring with, for example, concurrent opioid use or certain surgical manipulations (e.g., ocular).

In years past it was routine to use anticholinergics as part of the premedication scheme. Although modern inhalation anesthetics tend to decrease airway secretions it is very common in clinical management of small companion animals to administer opioids as part of anesthetic premedication so anticholinergics may still be considered beneficial in preventing bradycardia. Some argue that heightened vagal tone is best treated just prior to its anticipated occurrence or at first sign of its presence. Sparing use of anticholinergic drugs reduces the risk of other unwanted effects such as tachycardia or reduced gastrointestinal motility. Avoidance of gastrointestinal stasis is of special importance in herbivorous animals, for whom preanesthetic gastrointestinal emptying is almost never desired or accomplished. Mydriasis is another effect (e.g., of atropine) that is often undesirable because it confounds interpretation of some clinical signs of anesthesia and/or exposes the patient to potential retinal damage in some uncontrolled postanesthetic circumstances.

Anesthetic Period. The administration of anesthesia requires a combination of knowledge, skill, and ingenuity. The anesthetic drugs selected and their doses and methods of delivery will largely depend on the animal, the facilities available, and the skill of the individual who will administer them.

General anesthetics are usually given by inhalation or injection; on rare occasions anesthetic drugs may be given orally or per rectum. More specific information on anesthetic delivery is given later in this volume and in cited references (Hall et al. 2001; Dorsch and Dorsch 1999; Tranquilli et al. 2006).

Drugs of several classes of injectable agents (Table 8.11) are commonly used for general anesthesia. These are preferably given intravenously (IV); however, because of the varied circumstances associated with clinical conditions in veterinary medicine, the intramuscular (IM) route is also widely used. The IV route is the preferred means of inducing general anesthesia because anesthetic induction with the loss or reduction of many of the patient's life-protecting reflexes is consistently the most crucial maneuver in managing general anesthesia. The IV administration permits incremental dosing and thus titration of the level of anesthetic to a desired end point. This technique is often desired especially in critically ill patients or in unfamiliar circumstances because of the likelihood of unpredictable animal responses to a "routine" dose of drug. Drugs of a single class are used alone or in combination with other drugs listed in Table 8.11 (e.g., inhalation anesthetics and neuromuscular blocking drugs) to achieve suitable anesthetic conditions. Many of the drugs from the classes listed in Table 8.11 are also used at lower dosage for preanesthetic medication (Table 8.10).

TABLE 8.11 Major classes of CNS drugs (and examples) commonly considered for general anesthesia

1. Hypnotic-sedatives
   a. Ultrashort-acting (i.e., Thiopental)
      i. Short-acting (e.g., Pentobarbital)
2. Dissociative
   a. Ketamine
3. Opioid
   a. Morphine
   b. Oxymorphone
   c. Fentanyl
   d. Alfentanil
4. Drug combinations (i.e., Telazol®)
5. Others
   a. Guaifenesin
   b. Propofol
   c. Etomidate
   d. Alphaxalone
6. Tranquilizer-sedatives*
   a. Benzodiazepines
      i. Diazepam
      ii. Midazolam

*Use as an anesthetic adjuvant in conjunction with others on the list, e.g., opioids or ketamine.

The barbiturates likely continue as overall the most popular intravenous anesthetic for animals. They have universal (or at least nearly so) geographic and species application. Accurate information is not readily available but likely the dissociative class of drugs has become a close second choice in popularity to the barbiturates. For example, ketamine may be used alone in some species or combined with other drugs to produce a state that enables restraint and surgery and can be administered via a variety of routes, a decided advantage for fractious animals and/or treatment outside the controlled hospital environment. Propofol, especially in small companion animals (i.e., dogs) also has become very popular to induce and maintain especially short term intravenous anesthesia.

Opioids in large doses are the basis for balanced anesthetic techniques for human patients, especially those patients with circulatory system instability or those undergoing cardiac surgery. This method is also applicable to some veterinary patients (e.g., dogs) and is presently used to varying degrees. An important point to keep in mind is that opioids, even in large doses, do not predictably produce unconsciousness, so other drugs are used concurrently to accomplish the individualized goals of general anesthesia. Also, some animal species (e.g., horses) are excited by even moderate (by comparison to other species, e.g., dogs) opioid doses.

Immediate Postanesthetic Period. The immediate postanesthetic period is also known as the *anesthetic recovery period.* It begins with the discontinuation of the administration of anesthetic drugs. Recovery of healthy animals from routine anesthetic techniques is usually, but not always, uneventful and routine. Circumstances such as compromised physical status and unfamiliar anesthetic techniques heighten the likelihood of recovery problems. The immediate goal of this period is the rapid return of the patient's independent, uncompromised ability to maintain normal respiratory and circulatory systems function and to return sensory and motor abilities to preanesthetic levels as soon as possible. Despite this overriding philosophy, when the needs of different species and circumstances are considered, the actual broad plan is less clear. For example, most of the contemporary inhalation anesthetics do not have potent or persistent analgesic properties at alveolar concentrations associated with awakening. The sooner a patient recovers following surgery, the sooner there is potential for pain and discomfort for the patient. Consequently, the question arises, is it better for a patient to awaken quickly following surgery and then receive, as needed, analgesic drugs, or is it more desirable and beneficial for the patient to receive analgesic drugs toward the end of the anesthetic period and as a result have a slower recovery from general anesthesia and transition to sensation? The same therapeutic dilemma applies to the patient who may emerge from anesthesia excited and risk a particularly "stormy" recovery with attendant physical injury. The various combinations of drugs used in anesthetic management coupled with unique species characteristics make it impossible to describe here all of the patterns of recovery that occur and appropriate therapeutic schemes. In the end, individualized therapy is the most desirable plan.

Hazards of the recovery period that may require therapeutic intervention are listed in Table 8.12.

TABLE 8.12 Hazards of the immediate postanesthetic period

1. Circulatory system complications
   a. Arterial hypotension
   b. Arterial hypertension
   c. Cardiac dysrhythmias
2. Respiratory system complications
   a. Hypoxemia
   b. Hypercapnia (hypoventilation)
3. Pain
4. Emergence excitement (physical trauma)
5. Hyperthermia/hypothermia
6. Vomiting
7. Delayed awakening

EVALUATION OF THE RESPONSE TO ANESTHESIA. Since very early in the history of general anesthesia attempts have been made to correlate observations of the effects of anesthetics with "depth" of anesthesia. To be able to define the depth of anesthesia is important for a number of reasons. For example, too little or too much anesthesia is a threat to life. Consequently, if one can determine the magnitude of anesthesia with reasonable accuracy, patient safety is improved and optimal operating conditions are facilitated for the health care providers. Furthermore, specific guidelines help the novice anesthetist provide appropriate anesthetic conditions. Finally, in investigative circumstances an accurate means for describing and comparing anesthetic levels within or between studies is essential so that we may account for the effects of the anesthetic in our overall understanding versus other variables that may be operant and of interest at the time of study. It would be very helpful to be able to precisely define the depth of anesthesia in every animal from moment to moment regardless of the anesthetic technique. Unfortunately, this is presently not possible, so we rely on estimates.

More than 50 years ago Guedel (Guedel 1920, 1927) published his classic description of the four stages of anesthesia. The traditional classification is based on a progressive depression of a continuum of CNS function. Guedel extended the descriptions of earlier workers such as Plomley (1847) and Snow (1847) to divide the state of anesthesia into distinct "packages," each correlating with a particular set of physiological responses or reflexes, i.e., clinical signs. The organizational scheme includes four stages of anesthesia and subdivides the third stage into four strata (i.e., planes) (see earlier editions of this text for a broader description). Guedel's system has been prominent in pharmacology texts (including earlier editions of this text) and anesthesia texts for more than 6 decades. The concept is included here in only abbreviated form because with newer drugs and changes in clinical practice its importance in the discussion of fundamental principles of anesthesia is limited.

The classic signs and stages are partly recognizable with many general anesthetics (e.g., the barbiturates), but they are incomplete or are obscured when using modern anesthetics (e.g., ketamine) and/or techniques. It is important to remember that Guedel's description was based on his observation of the actions of diethyl ether administered to otherwise unmedicated human patients who were breathing spontaneously. This is a situation far different from contemporary clinical practice (including veterinary), in

TABLE 8.13 Useful signs in clinical assessment of anesthetic depth

1. Cardiovascular system
   a. Heart rate and rhythm[a]
   b. Arterial blood pressure[b]
   c. Mucous membrane color
   d. Capillary refill time
2. Respiratory system
   a. Breathing frequency[a]
   b. Ventilatory volumes (tidal and minute ventilation)[a]
   c. Character of breathing[a]
   d. Arterial or end-tidal CO_2 partial pressure[b]
3. Eye
   a. Position and/or movement of eyeball[b]
   b. Pupil size[a]
   c. Pupil response to light
   d. Palpebral reflex
   e. Corneal reflex
   f. Lacrimation
4. Muscle
   a. Jaw or limb tone[a]
   b. Presence or absence of gross movement[a]
   c. Shivering or trembling[a]
5. Miscellaneous
   a. Body temperature
   b. Laryngeal reflex[a]
   c. Swallowing[a]
   d. Coughing[a]
   e. Vocalizing[a]
   f. Salivating
   g. Sweating
   h. Urine flow

Source: Steffey 1983.
[a]Moderate or [b]high specificity in assessment of anesthetic depth for various animal species and anesthetic agents.

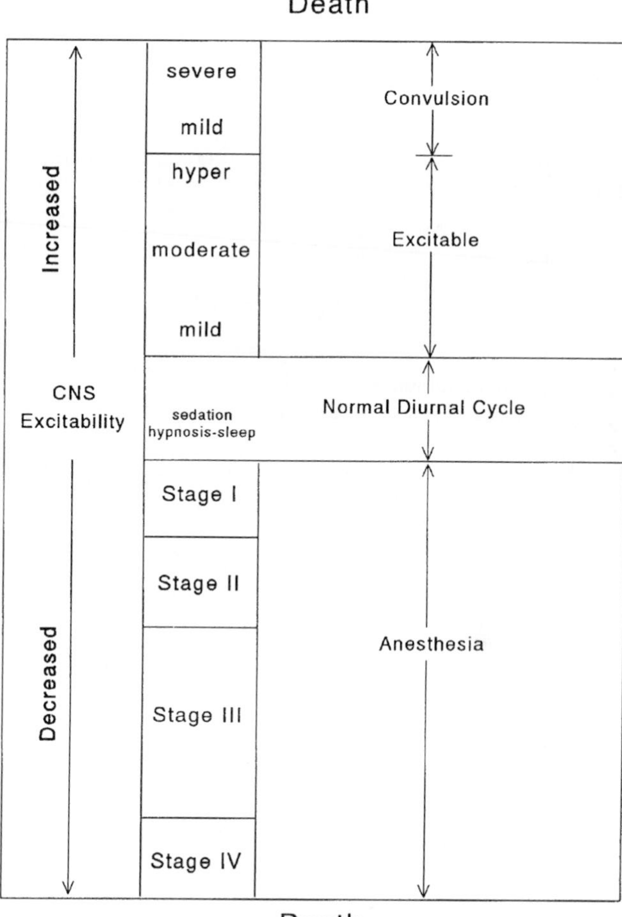

FIG. 8.8 The classic unidimensional schema of CNS excitation and depression. (Modified from Winters 1976.)

which controlled mechanical ventilation is common and newer and multiple anesthetic and adjuvant drugs are an important part of the anesthetic plan. There are unique differences in the way different species react to conditions of general anesthesia that also must be taken into consideration. Because of diethyl ether's characteristics and the methods of delivery, the onset and "deepening" of anesthesia were slow. This situation facilitated a slow (relative to today's standards) unfolding. In addition, numerous physiological responses to anesthetics that are widely monitored today (Table 8.13) are not included in the classic description.

With the emergence of anesthetics such as ketamine and enflurane (absent from veterinary practice for more than a decade) the concept that all anesthetics are depressants required reconsideration. Winters et al. (1967) proposed replacement of the classic, unidirectional schema (Fig. 8.8) of CNS excitation and depression with a new schema that included a description of progressive states of both CNS depression and excitation (Fig. 8.9). The new schema recognized bidirectional influences of drugs acting on the CNS and was based on results of electrophysiological studies of anesthetic, excitatory, hallucinogenic, and convulsive agents in cats (Winters et al. 1967, 1972; Winters 1976).

Guedel's scheme also does not take into consideration the modifying influences of such things as duration of anesthesia (Dunlop et al. 1987; Steffey et al. 1987a,b) or varying magnitudes of surgical stimulus intensity on the signs of anesthesia (Eger et al. 1972; Steffey 1983). In modern clinical anesthetic practice it is recognized that no single observation is always reliable as a sign indicating a

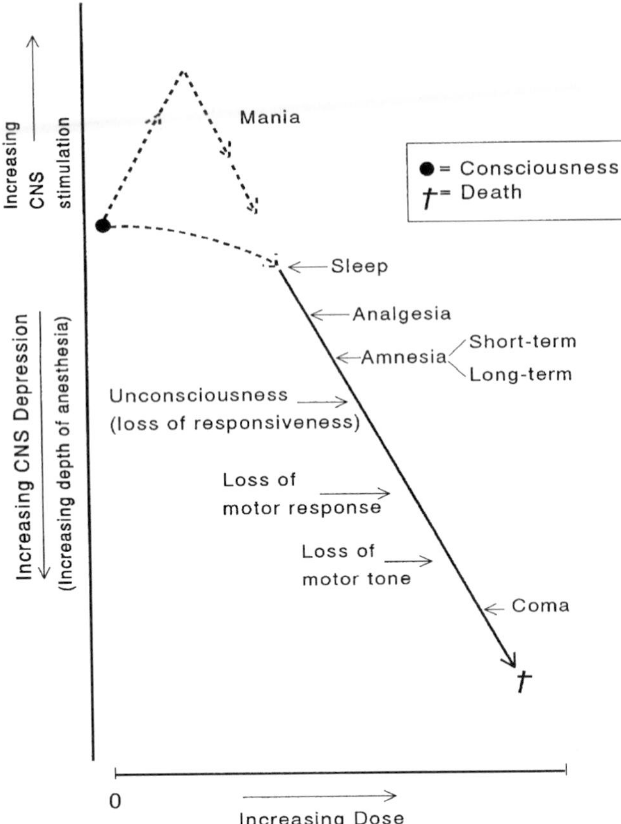

FIG. 8.9 The anesthetic continuum as viewed clinically in a healthy subject.

specific magnitude of anesthesia. Accordingly, anesthetists are encouraged to develop a basic background knowledge of both the individual to be anesthetized and the selected drugs. Current advice for anesthetic management under clinical conditions is to use an initial anesthetic loading dose just necessary to suppress purposeful movement and to observe all signs possible in each patient (Table 8.13) and then to manipulate further anesthetic dose in relation to continual stimulus-patient response assessment. If the level of anesthesia is in doubt, err on the side of an animal that is too lightly anesthetized.

Stimulus assessment is of special importance since the intensity of stimulus applied to an anesthetized animal may rapidly and markedly alter the observed signs (Eger et al. 1972; Steffey 1983). A quiet animal with reasonable vital signs may quickly show evidence of light to moderate anesthesia in the presence of intense visceral stimulation despite no change in anesthetic delivery. Common responses to anesthetic dose-stimulus interaction are given in Table 8.14.

TABLE 8.14 Common responses to anesthetic dose stimulus interaction

1. Signs of presurgical anesthesia
   a. Bradycardia, tachycardia, arrhythmia
   b. Arterial hypertension
   c. Pupillary dilation, lacrimation, globe rotation
   d. Tachypnea or breath holding
   e. Deep breathing
   f. Reduced alveolar/arterial PCO_2
   g. Limb/body movement
   h. Salivation, vomition
   i. Swallowing
   j. Laryngeal spasm
   k. Phonation
2. Signs of deep surgical anesthesia
   a. Bradycardia, tachycardia, arrhythmia, cardiac arrest
   b. Arterial hypotension
   c. Pupillary dilation, dry cornea, centrally fixed eye
   d. Shallow breathing, Respiratory arrest (*not* breath holding)
   e. Elevated alveolar/arterial PCO_2
   f. Muscle flaccidity

Source: Steffey 1983.
Note: Importance of a given sign in a specific species and/or individual varies.

More precise quantitative measures of anesthetic depth are of obvious interest for the clinician and essential in research. Measurement of end-expired (alveolar) concentration of inhaled anesthetics is a more precise indication of anesthetic level than clinical signs when this type of anesthetic agent is used. In addition, there is continued interest in using electrophysiological approaches to measure depth of anesthesia in both the laboratory and the operating room. For example, it is long known that anesthetic drugs alter the spontaneous electroencephalogram and other electrophysiologic measures of CNS function. Recent notable use of this information is the development of bispectral EEG signal processing for monitoring anesthetic depth (Rampil 1998). The bispectral (BIS) index is a complex, proprietary EEG parameter that was approved by the U.S. Food and Drug Administration for commercial availability about 10 years ago as a monitor of anesthetic effect in human patients. Studies using such technology have shown good correlations with clinical signs in a number of animal species but its general application will have to await more detailed information and a decrease in the cost of the equipment. For a more complete review of central nervous system–focused electrophysiological technology applied to anesthetic management of human patients, see Stanski and Shafer (2005).

REFERENCES

Abbott, N.J. 2005. Dynamics of CNS barriers: evolution, differentiation, and modulation. Cell Mol Neurobiol 25: 5–23.

Bernards, C.M. and Hill, H.F. 1990. Morphine and alfentanil permeability through the spinal dura, arachnoid, and pia mater of dogs and monkeys. Anesthesiology 73: 1214–1219.

———. 1991. The spinal nerve root sleeve is not a preferred route for redistribution of drugs from the epidural space to the spinal cord. Anesthesiology 75: 827–832.

———. 1992. Physical and chemical properties of drug molecules governing their diffusion through the spinal meninges. Anesthesiology 77: 750–756.

Breidenbach, M.A. and Brunger, A.T. 2005. New insights into clostridial neurotoxin-SNARE interactions. Trends Mol Med 11: 377–381.

Bridges, R.J. and Esslinger, C.S. 2005. The excitatory amino acid transporters: pharamacological insights on substrate and inhibitor specificity of the EAAT subtypes. Pharmacol Ther 107: 271–285.

Campagna, J.A., Miller, K.W., and Forman, S.A. 2003. Mechanisms of actions of inhaled anesthetics. N Engl J Med 348: 2110–2124.

Dagenais, C., Graff, C.L., and Pollack, G.M. 2004. Variable modulation of opioid brain uptake by P-glycoprotein in mice. Biochem Pharmacol 67: 269–276.

Dorsch, J.A. and Dorsch, S.E. 1999. Understanding Anesthesia Equipment. Williams & Wilkins, Baltimore.

Dunlop, C.I., Steffey, E.P., Miller, M.F., and Woliner, M.J. 1987. Temporal effects of halothane and isoflurane in laterally recumbent ventilated male horses. Am J Vet Res 48: 1250–1255.

Eger, E.I., II, Dolan, W.M., Stevens, W.C., Miller, R.D., and Way, W.L. 1972. Surgical stimulation antagonizes the respiratory depression produced by Forane. Anesthesiology 36: 544–549.

Fairbanks, C.A., Schreiber, K.L., Brewer, K.L., Yu, C.G., Stone, L.S., Kitto, K.F., Nguyen, H.O., Grocholski, B.M., Shoeman, D.W., Kehl, I.J., Regunathan, S., Reis, D.J., Yezierski, R.P., and Wilcox, G.L. 2000. Agmatine reverses pain induced by inflammation, neuropathy, and spinal cord injury. Proc Natl Acad Sci 97: 10584–10589.

Guedel, A.E. 1920. Third stage ether anesthesia: a sub-classification regarding the significance of the position and movements of the eyeball. Am J Surg 24, Suppl: 53–57.

———. 1927. Stages of anesthesia and reclassification of the signs of anesthesia. Anesth Analg 6: 157–162.

Gwaltney-Brant, S.M., Albretsen, J.C., and Khan, S.A. 2000. 5-Hydroxytryptophan toxicosis in dogs: 21 cases (1989–1999). J Am Vet Med Assoc 216: 1937–1940.

Hall, L.W., Clarke, K.W., and Trim, C.M. 2001. Veterinary Anaesthesia. Bailliere Tindall, London.

Hawkins, B.T. and Davis, T.P. 2005. The blood-brain barrier/neurovascular unit in health and disease. Pharmacol Rev 57: 173–185.

Hellyer, P.W., Bai, L., Supon, J., Quail, C., Wagner, A.E., Mama, K., and Magnusson, K.R. 2003. Comparison of opioid and alpha-2 adrenergic receptor binding in horse and dog brain using redioligand autoradiography. Vet Anaesth Analg 30: 172–182.

John, E.R. and Prichep, L.S. 2005. The anesthetic cascade: A theory of how anesthesia suppresses consciousness. Anesthesiology 102: 447–471.

Jones, D. and Story, D.A. 2005. Serotonin syndrome and the anaesthetist. Anaesth Intensive Care 33: 181–187.

Kitchell, R.L. and Erickson, H.H. 1983. Introduction: What is pain? *In* Animal Pain: Perception and Alleviation. Edited by R.L. Kitchell and H.H. Erickson. American Physiological Society, Bethesda p. vii–viii.

Koblin, D.D. 2005. Mechanisms of action. *In* Miller's Anesthesia. Edited by R.D. Miller. Elsevier Churchill Livingstone, Philadelphia pp. 105–130.

Larson, M.D. 2005. History of anesthetic practice. *In* Miller's Anesthesia. Edited by R.D. Miller. Elsevier Churchill Linvingstone, Philadelphia pp. 3–52.

Leake, C.D. 1971. Claude Bernard and anesthesia. Anesthesiology 356: 112–113.

Lee, F.J. and Liu, F. 2004. Direct interactions between NMDA and D1 receptors: a tale of tails. Biochem Soc Trans 32: 1032–1036.

Loeser, J.D. 2001. Bonica's Management of Pain. Lippincott Williams & Wilkins, Philadelphia.

Lotsch, J. 2005. Pharmacokinetic-pharmacodynamic modeling of opioids. J Pain Symptom Manage 29: S90–103.

McMahon, S.B. and Koltzenburg, M. 2006. Wall and Melzack's Textbook of Pain. Elsevier Churchill Livingstone, London.

Mealey, K.L. 2004. Therapeutic implications of the MDR-1 gene. J Vet Pharmacol Therap 27: 257–264.

———. 2006. Adverse drug reactions in herding-breed dogs: The role of P-glycoprotein. Compend Contin Ed Pract Vet 2006: 23–33.

Plomley, F. 1847. Stages of anaesthesia. Lancet 1: 134.

Rampil, I.J. 1998. A primer for EEG signal processing in anesthesia. Anesthesiology 89: 980–1002.

Smithcors, J.F. 1971. History of veterinary anesthesia. *In* Textbook of Veterinary Anesthesia. Edited by L.R. Soma. Williams & Wilkins Co., Baltimore pp. 1–23.

Snow, J. 1847. On the Inhalation of the Vapour of Ether in Surgical Operations: Containing a Description of the Various Stages of Etherization, and a Statement of the Results of Nearly Eighty Operations in which Ether has been Employed in St. George and University College Hospitals. Churchill, London.

Solt, K., Stevens, R.J., Davies, P.A., and Raines, D.E. 2006. General anesthetic-induced channel gating enhancement of 5-hydroxytryptamine type 3 receptors depends on receptor subunit composition. J Pharmacol Exp Ther 315: 771–776.

Stanski, D.R. and Shafer, S.L. 2005. Measuring depth of anesthesia. *In* Miller's Anesthesia. Edited by R.D. Miller. Elsevier, Churchill Livingstone, Philadelphia pp. 1227–1264.

Steffey, E.P. 1983. Concepts of general anesthesia and assessment of adequacy of anesthesia for animal surgery. *In* Animal Pain: Perception and Alleviation. Edited by R.L. Kitchell and H.H. Erickson. American Physiological Society, Bethesda pp. 133–150.

Steffey, E.P., Farver, T.B., and Woliner, M.J. 1987a. Cardiopulmonary function during 7 h of constant-dose halothane and methoxyflurane. J Appl Physiol 63: 1351–1359.

Steffey, E.P., Kelly, A.B., and Woliner, M.J. 1987b. Time-related responses of spontaneously breathing, laterally recumbent horses to prolonged anesthesia with halothane. Am J Vet Res 48: 952–957.

Stevens, R., Rusch, D., Solt, K., Raines, D.E., and Davies, P.A. 2005. Modulation of human 5-hydroxytryptamine type 3AB receptors by volatile anesthetics and n-alcohols. J Pharmacol Exp Ther 314: 338–345.

Tranquilli, W.J., Thurmon, J.C., and Grimm, K.A. 2006. Veterinary anesthesia and analgesia. Lippincott Williams & Wilkins, Baltimore.

Wang, J.S., Ruan, Y., Taylor, R.M., Donovan, J.L., Markowitz, J.S., and DeVane, C.L. 2004. Brain penetration of methadone (R)- and (S)-enantiomers is greatly increased by P-glycoprotein deficiency in the blood-brain barrier of Abcb1a gene knockout mice. Psychopharmacology (Berlin) 173: 132–138.

Watkins, L.R., Hutchinson, M.R., Johnston, I.N., and Maier, S.F. 2005. Glia: novel counter-regulators of opioid analgesia. Trends Neurosci 28: 661–669.

Weaver, B.M.Q. 1988. The history of veterinary anaesthesia. Vet Hist 5: 43–57.

Weaver, B.M.Q. and Hall, L.W. 2005. Origin of the association of veterinary anaesthetists—Editorial. Vet Anaesth Analg 32: 179–183.

Winters, W.D. 1976. Effects of drugs on the electrical activity of the brain: Anesthetics. Annu Rev Pharmacol Toxicol 16: 413–426.

Winters, W.D., Ferrar-Allado, T., Guzman-Flores, C., and Alcaraz, M. 1972. The cataleptic state induced by ketamine: a review of the neuropharmacology of anesthesia. Neuropharmacology 11: 303–315.

Winters, W.D., Mori, K., Spooner, C.E., and Bauer, R.O. 1967. The neurophysiology of anesthesia. Anesthesiology 28: 65–80.

Yaksh, T. L. Spinal analgesic mechanisms. Justins, D. M. 369–380. 2005. Sydney, IASP. World Congress on Pain.

CHAPTER 9

NEUROMUSCULAR BLOCKING AGENTS

H. RICHARD ADAMS

Neuromuscular blocking agents used clinically act by interfering with the effectiveness of the endogenous neurotransmitter acetylcholine (ACh) to activate nicotinic cholinergic receptors of skeletal muscle cells, thereby inhibiting receptor-coupled transmembrane ion movements necessary for muscle contraction (Bouzat et al. 2004; Unwin 2005). The end results of this action are skeletal muscle paralysis and muscular relaxation (Kita and Goodkin 2000). Neuromuscular blocking agents are most often used as adjuvants to anesthesia to facilitate tracheal intubation, abdominal muscle relaxation, and orthopedic manipulations, and as part of balanced anesthesia procedures to reduce the amount of general anesthetic required in high-risk patients (Taylor 2006b).

DEVELOPMENT

Development of neuromuscular blocking drugs originated with the discovery of curare, a tarlike mixture of plant material used as a poison by South American Indians. The actual ingredients of the poison for arrows, blowgun darts, and spears were known only to the local "pharmacist," who was often the tribal medicine man or witch doctor. Thus the botanical preparations obtained by explorers could not be identified as to content; they were simply classified according to the containers in which they were packaged. Tubo-, para-, or bamboo-curare was contained in cutoff bamboo tubes; this mixture was usually obtained from southern Amazon tribes. The plant origin of tube-curare preparations was primarily Menispermaceae (*Chondodendron tomentosum*). Calabash-curare was packaged in hollow gourds or calabashes; it was the most active preparation. Pot-curare came in small earthenware pottery from the central part of the Amazon basin; this concoction often contained plants other than Menispermaceae. The most important constituent isolated from curare is *d*-tubocurarine. Complete discussions of the colorful and interesting history of curare have been presented by McIntyre (1972) and Waser (1972).

Original studies in the nineteenth century by Claude Bernard (1856) demonstrated that curare prevented the muscle contraction elicited by stimulation of the motor nerve. It did not, however, affect the central nervous system (CNS), prevent response to direct stimulation of the muscle, or depress axonal conductance. It was proposed that curare acted at the nerve-muscle junction. Reports since then have substantiated, clarified, and extended observations concerning the neuromuscular blocking properties of curare alkaloids. Early results stimulated active research into the chemical structural requirements of curarelike compounds, leading to the discovery of other types of neuromuscular blocking agents.

THE NICOTINIC RECEPTOR AND STRUCTURE-ACTIVITY RELATIONSHIPS

Neuromuscular blocking agents possess chemical structural groups that allow interaction of the agent with the nicotinic cholinergic receptor (Brejc et al. 2001). However, these drugs cause distinctly different effects from the endogenous mediator ACh. One group of neuromuscular blocking drugs, competitive agents, occupies the receptor so that ACh cannot act. The other group, depolarizing agents, acts in a more complicated manner and initially causes depolarization before blockage occurs (Taylor 2006b).

Based on general chemical structural characteristics, Bovet (1951) placed neuromuscular blocking agents into two large categories. One group is characterized by large, bulky, and nonflexible molecules; members of this group include *d*-tubocurarine, dimethyl (or trimethyl) tubocurarine, gallamine, and pancuronium, all of which produce a competitive (nondepolarizing) block. The other group is characterized by long, slender, flexible molecules that allow free bond rotation. Decamethonium and succinylcholine are in this group; these agents cause a depolarizing block. The dichotomy in basic structural arrangement of competitive and depolarizing agents has been offered as a partial explanation for dissimilar effects evoked by interaction of these agents with the nicotinic cholinergic receptor.

The proposed charge distribution of the cholinergic receptor was shown in Chapter 7, and a schematic of the nicotinic cholinergic receptor is illustrated in Figure 9.1. Among other requirements, receptors contain anionic (negatively charged) binding sites separated by set distances. These negative sites are essential for electrostatic bonding of the cationic (positively charged) nitrogen moiety of ACh (and exogenous chemicals) to the receptors (Brejc et al. 2001).

Occupation of negative binding sites by ACh activates influx of Na^+ and efflux of K^+ along their respective concentration gradients, resulting in membrane excitation. Occupation of these sites by the molecularly rigid competitive agents stabilizes the receptors so that the membrane pores are not easily affected. Depolarizing agents initially act similarly to ACh. Because of their flexible structure, they allow initial channel activation but for some reason cause a persistent short-circuiting of the receptor so that additional changes in electrical potential are not achieved.

Different investigative groups have now isolated the nicotinic cholinergic receptor from the electric eel and electric ray (Taylor 2006a,b; Unwin 2005) and also from mammalian skeletal muscle (Dolly and Barnard 1977). The cobra neurotoxin, α-bungarotoxin, binds irreversibly and with high specificity to ligand recognition sites of the nicotinic receptor. This toxin, when radiolabeled, has allowed remarkable achievements in isolating and characterizing the nicotinic receptor (Kistler et al. 1982).

The nicotinic cholinoceptor is a pentameric asymmetric molecule (8 × 14 nm) of about 250 kilodaltons that spans the bilayer of the postjunctional membrane (Fig. 9.1). The receptor comprises five individual subunits in a stoichiometric ratio of $\alpha_2\beta\gamma\delta$; the γ-subunit is replaced by an ε-subunit in muscle from adult animals. Each subunit has

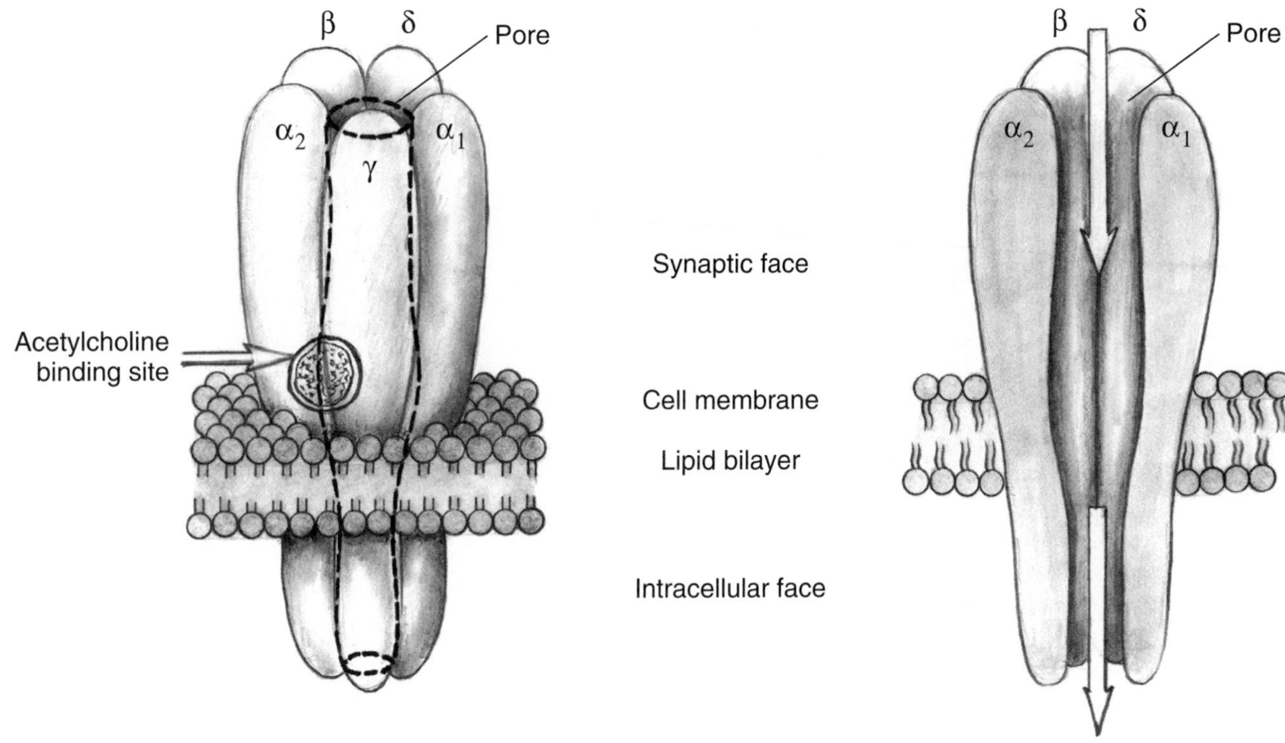

FIG. 9.1 Schematic representation of the nicotinic cholinergic receptor. The receptor is embedded across the cell membrane lipid bilayer, presenting a synaptic face to the neuroeffector junction between the neuron and innervated cell, and an intracellular face within the cytoplasm. The receptor comprises a pentameric configuration of four separate subunits with a stoichiometric ratio of $\alpha_2\beta\gamma\delta$; in adult muscle $\alpha_2\beta\varepsilon\delta$. The α subunits contain the primary ligand binding sites for recognition of acetylcholine and related agents. Subunit arrangement forms an internal pore that allows passage of select ions upon receptor activation and resulting membrane depolarization (see text). Redrawn from Unwin et al. (1988) by Dr. Gheorghe M. Constantinescu, University of Missouri.

an extracellular and intracellular exposure and also contains sequences of hydrophobic amino acids that are the likely regions embedded within the membrane bilayer (Taylor 2006b). In vivo, the pentamerous receptor complex occurs as a dimer or couplet, with two adjacent receptors connected via a disulfide bond between two δ-subunits. The five subunits of each monomere receptor complex are elongated perpendicular to the postjunctional membrane and are arranged circumferentially to form a rosette around a central lumen (Fig. 9.1). This central transmembrane channel of the receptor complex represents the previously discussed membrane pore for ion fluxes instigated by agonist activation of the receptor (Unwin 2005). Agonist and antagonist binding sites are believed to be restricted to the α-subunits (Kistler et al. 1982). Whereas acetylcholine evokes receptor activation upon binding to the α-subunits, occupation of these same sites by antagonists prevents effective receptor activation (Karlin 2002). The muscle becomes paralyzed, whether in response to a competitive blocking agent or to transient activation by a depolarizing blocking agent. Chemical structures of several commonly used neuromuscular blocking agents are shown in Figure 9.2 to demonstrate structural differences of the competitive and depolarizing types.

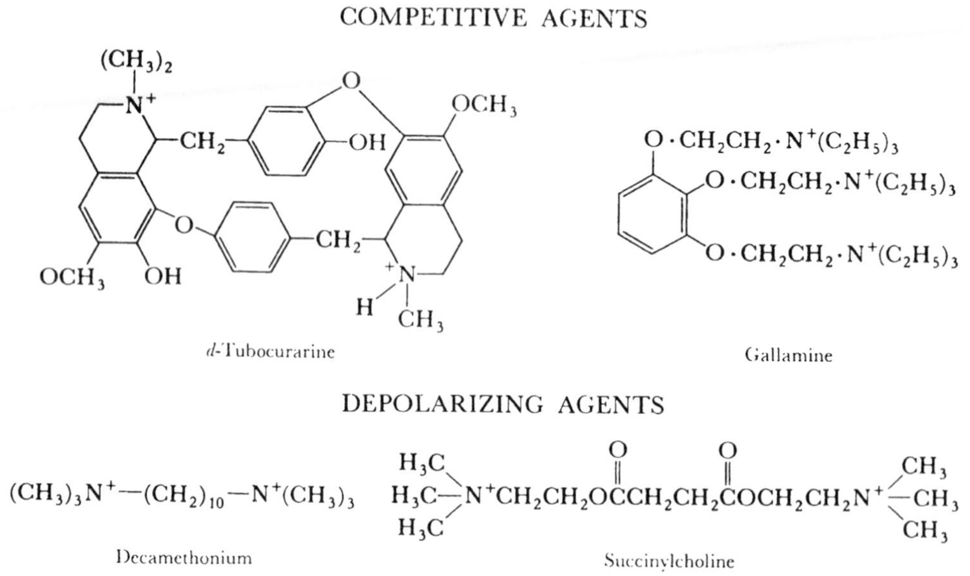

COMPETITIVE AGENTS

d-Tubocurarine

Gallamine

DEPOLARIZING AGENTS

$(CH_3)_3N^+—(CH_2)_{10}—N^+(CH_3)_3$

Decamethonium

$(H_3C)_3N^+CH_2CH_2OCOCH_2CH_2COOCH_2CH_2N^+(CH_3)_3$

Succinylcholine

FIG. 9.2 Chemical structures of some commonly used neuromuscular blocking agents.

IMPULSE TRANSMISSION AT THE SOMATIC NEUROMUSCULAR JUNCTION

Prior to discussing neuromuscular blocking agents, impulse transmission at the somatic neuromuscular junction will be reviewed in relation to sites of action of different drugs. General concepts of cholinergic transmission were mentioned in Chapters 5 and 7.

PHYSIOLOGIC AND ANATOMIC CONSIDERATIONS. The majority of investigations aimed at identifying cholinergic transmission mechanisms have utilized the somatic myoneural junction because of its accessibility in relation to other cholinergic synapses. Although the term synapse was originally proposed to describe a nerve-nerve junction, it is commonly used in reference to neuroeffector junctions. A representation of a somatic neuromuscular junction (synapse) and proposed sites of drug actions are shown in Figure 9.3.

Terminal branches of a motor axon lose their myelin sheath and embed within invaginations of the cell membrane of the skeletal muscle cell; these invaginations are termed synaptic gutters. A synaptic gutter, in turn, has many microinvaginations or infoldings called either junctional folds or subneural folds. The space within the synaptic gutter between the nerve ending and the muscle cell is called the synaptic cleft. *Presynaptic* refers to axonal elements, whereas *postsynaptic* refers to constituents of the muscle cell.

Vesicular structures localized within cholinergic nerve terminals represent storage sites for ACh (see Chapter 5). As an axonal action potential arrives at the nerve terminal, it increases the release of ACh from the storage vesicles into the synaptic cleft. This step (excitation-secretion coupling) is dependent upon mobilization into the neuron of extracellular Ca^{++} and/or Ca^{++} bound to superficial membrane areas of the nerve terminal. Released ACh reacts with the specialized receptor sites of the subsynaptic membrane and causes depolarization of this structure. Cholinergic receptors of somatic myoneural junctions are classified as nicotinic; they are located on the outer membrane of the muscle cell and are almost exclusively confined to the postsynaptic membrane. After denervation, sensitivity to ACh spreads over the entire muscle cell.

Extraneuronal ACh is rapidly metabolized by acetylcholinesterase (AChE) enzyme, which is localized in the end-plate region. Although it may be bound in part to presynaptic elements, it is concentrated at the postsynaptic membrane (Inestrosa and Perelman 1990; Hucho et al. 1991).

PHARMACOLOGIC CONSIDERATIONS. The neuromuscular junction is quite susceptible to alteration by selective pharmacologic agents. Various drugs, toxins, electrolytes, and other agents alter in different manners the synthesis, storage, release, receptor interactions, and catabolism of ACh. Several important factors affecting cholinergic transmission are outlined in Figure 9.3.

Hemicholinium and triethylcholine compete with choline for choline uptake into cholinergic neurons; ACh synthesis is prevented by lack of choline (Ferguson and Blakely 2004). Existing vesicular stores of ACh are exhausted upon nerve stimulation, and a gradual weakening and eventual paralysis result.

Nerve conduction is affected by only a few substances. The local anesthetics, when in high concentration and immediate contact with the axon, act to stabilize the nerve by inactivating both Na^+ and K^+ channels so that axonal action potential propagation is halted. The pufferfish poison tetrodotoxin and the shellfish poison saxitoxin decrease the permeability of excitable membranes to Na^+ (but not K^+); thus axonal action potentials are not generated, and paralysis results. These toxins do not cause an initial depolarization of nerves; they act noncompetitively, are approximately 100,000 times more potent than cocaine or procaine, and are frequently used in research. Clinical cases of fatal food poisoning have been attributed to ingestion of these substances.

Botulinum toxin is an extremely potent substance (lethal dose for a mouse is 4×10^7 molecules) produced by *Clostridium botulinum.* It is ingested occasionally by humans and lower animals and often is fatal. It decreases the amount of ACh released from cholinergic nerves (Davis and Barnes 2000).

Magnesium ions (Mg^{++}) interfere with release of ACh from the nerve terminal by competing for the transport mechanisms responsible for mobilization of Ca^{++} into the nerve. Mg^{++} uncouples the excitation-secretion coupling process. An insufficient concentration of Ca^{++} produces

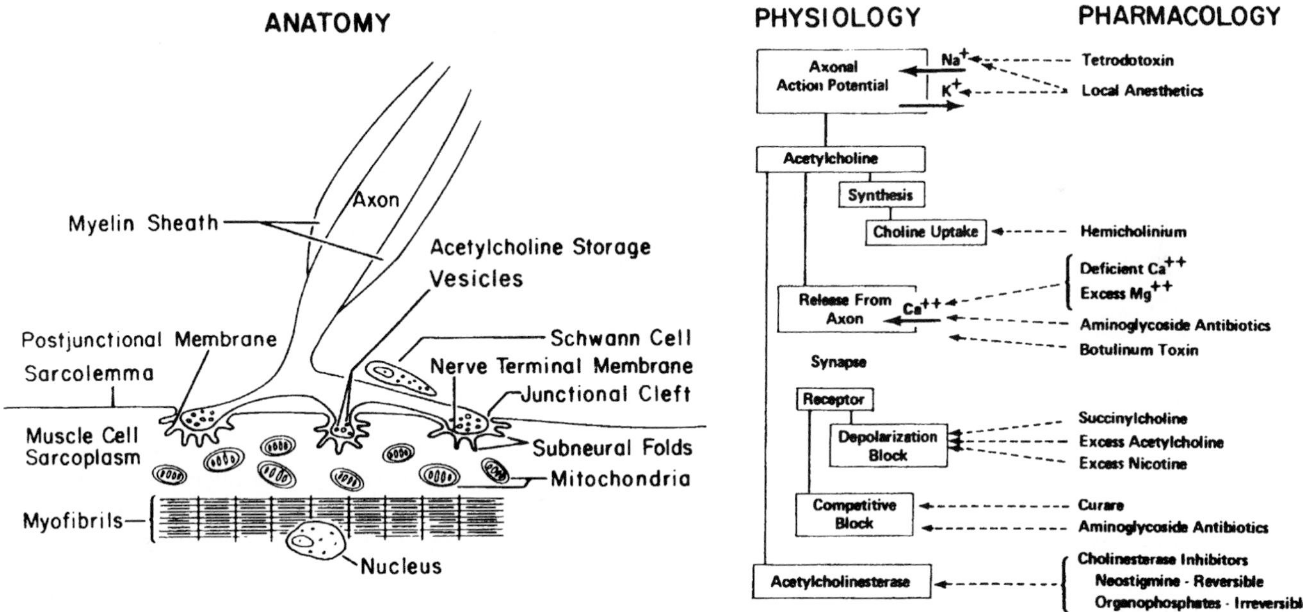

FIG. 9.3 Schematic representation of a somatic neuromuscular junction (synapse), related physiologic pathways, and proposed sites of action of various pharmacologic agents. An axonal action potential (AP) is characterized by an influx of Na+ and an efflux of K+. Tetrodotoxin and saxitoxin inactivate Na+ pathways. Local anesthetics block Na+ and K+ pathways. Choline uptake into the neuron is blocked by hemicholinium; synthesis of ACh is prevented. As the AP arrives at the nerve terminal, it instigates inward movement of Ca++; this triggers discharge of ACh into the junctional cleft. A lack of Ca++ or an excess of Mg++ decreases release of ACh. Aminoglycoside antibiotics also interfere with Ca++-dependent release of ACh. Botulinum toxin inhibits ACh release. Decamethonium and succinylcholine (depolarizing neuromuscular blocking agents) cause persistent depolarization block of the motor end-plate region, as do excess ACh and nicotine. Curare, gallamine, and pancuronium (competitive neuromuscular blocking agents) compete with ACh for postjunctional receptors but do not cause depolarization. Aminoglycoside antibiotics decrease sensitivity of the postjunctional membrane to ACh. Catabolism of ACh by acetylcholinesterase is inhibited by reversible and irreversible anticholinesterase agents; ACh accumulates. (Modified from Taylor 2006b; Couteaux 1972.)

similar effects. Mg^{++} also acts postsynaptically to decrease the effectiveness of ACh to activate receptors.

Aminoglycoside antibiotics (i.e., neomycin-streptomycin group) inhibit release of ACh from motor nerves by decreasing availability of Ca^{++} at superficial membrane binding sites of the axonal terminal, thereby inhibiting the excitation-secretion coupling process. These antibiotics also reduce sensitivity of the postsynaptic membrane to ACh (Adams 1984).

Cholinesterase inhibitors (see Chapter 7) decrease the hydrolytic activity of AChE and pseudocholinesterase (Taylor 1991, 2006a). ACh rapidly accumulates at receptor sites. Muscle fasciculations, spasms, convulsions, and eventually apnea occur after overdosage with cholinesterase inhibitors.

POSTJUNCTIONAL MECHANISMS OF NEUROMUSCULAR BLOCKADE

The pharmacologic effects of clinically useful neuromuscular blocking drugs can best be explained by a direct alteration of the effectiveness of ACh to activate postjunctional (postsynaptic) receptors (Taylor 2006b). According to the mechanisms of postjunctional action, neuromuscular blocking agents are classified as either a competitive (nondepolarizing) or a depolarizing agent.

COMPETITIVE (NONDEPOLARIZING) AGENTS. These drugs compete with ACh for available cholinergic receptors at the postsynaptic membrane and, by occupying these receptors, prevent the transmitter function of ACh. A prototype of this group of drugs is *d*-tubocurarine (*Tubocurarine Chloride,* USP, Tubarine). Other similarly acting agents include *Metocurine Iodide,* USP (Metubine) (previously referred to as dimethyl tubocurarine iodide), gallamine (*Gallamine Triethiodide,* USP, Flaxedil), and pancuronium (*Pancuronium Bromide,* Pavulon). Newer competitive agents include fazadinium, a rapidly acting drug that undergoes hepatic biotransformation; alcuronium; atracurium, a synthetic compound that undergoes spontaneous and enzymatic degradation to inactive metabolites; and vecuronium, a derivative of pancuronium (Taylor 2006b; Agoston et al. 1992). Pharmacologic characteristics of several neuromuscular blocking agents are summarized in Table 9.1.

TABLE 9.1 Characteristics of neuromuscular blocking agents

Generic Name	Trade Name	Chemical Class	Duration properties	Onset (min)	Duration (min)	Biotransformation
Depolarizing Agents						
Succinylcholine	Anectine	Choline ester	Ultrashort	<2	6–8	Hydrolysis by plasma cholinesterases
Nondepolarizing (Competitive) Agents						
d-Tubocurarine		Natural alkaloid (cyclic benzylisoquinoline)	Long	4–6	80–120	Renal elimination; liver clearance
Atracurium	Tracrium	Benzylisoquinoline	Intermediate	2–4	30–40	Spontaneous degradation; hydrolysis by plasma cholinesterases
Doxacurium	Nuromax	Benzylisoquinoline	Long	4–6	90–120	Renal elimination; liver metabolism and clearance
Mivacurium	Mivacron	Benzylisoquinoline	Short	2–4	12–18	Hydrolysis by plasma cholinesterases
Pancuronium	Pavulon	Ammonio steroid	Long	4–6	120–180	Renal elimination; liver metabolism and clearance
Pipecuronium	Arduan	Ammonio steroid	Long	2–4	80–100	Renal elimination; liver metabolism and clearance
Rocuronium	Zemuron	Ammonio steroid	Intermediate	1–2	30–40	Liver metabolism; renal elimination
Vecuronium	Norcuron	Ammonio steroid	Intermediate	2–4	30–40	Liver metabolism and clearance; renal elimination

Source: Modified from Taylor 2006b.

Ultrarefined experimental techniques (e.g., measurement of single-cell electrical activity and microionophoretic application of drugs) have verified the primary site of action of competitive blocking agents as the subsynaptic membrane (Bowen 1972; Hubbard and Quastel 1973). At this region, *d*-tubocurarine is believed to have the same or similar affinity as ACh for cholinergic receptors; i.e., *d*-tubocurarine can interact with these sites as well as ACh. However, *d*-tubocurarine does not exhibit receptor activating properties. Although *d*-tubocurarine binds to or in some way interlocks with the cholinoceptors, it has no depolarizing activity and therefore does not cause an end-plate potential. Moreover, the *d*-tubocurarine-receptor interaction renders affected receptors unavailable for interaction with ACh. ACh-induced end-plate potentials are reduced to subthreshold levels or abolished in curarized muscles. In the absence of induced end-plate potentials and subsequent muscle action potentials, the muscle relaxes and is, in fact, paralyzed.

Based on competitive interaction between nondepolarizing agents and ACh, cholinesterase inhibitors were found to be effective in antagonizing effects of these blocking agents (Taylor 2006a). Cholinesterase inhibitors prevent the enzymatic catabolism of ACh. More ACh is available for interaction with cholinoceptors and thereby decreases effectiveness of competitive blocking agents. This relationship has been exploited clinically in successful efforts to terminate effects of nondepolarizing agents. However, cholinesterase inhibitors do not antagonize effects of the other class of neuromuscular blockers, the depolarizing drugs.

DEPOLARIZING AGENTS. *Succinylcholine Chloride,* USP (Quelcin, Anectine, Sucostrin, Suxamethonium), and *Decamethonium Bromide,* USP (Syncurine, C-10), are members of this group of agents. These drugs exert their skeletal muscle paralyzing effects by interfering with ACh-mediated depolarization of the postsynaptic membrane. In contrast to the well-defined mechanism of the competitive agents, certain aspects of the mechanism(s) of depolarizing neuromuscular blockers are continually debated.

Succinylcholine and related drugs interact with postsynaptic cholinergic receptors but cause distinctly different effects than curarelike drugs. Initially, an end-plate potential and a corresponding muscle action potential are elicited upon exposure to succinylcholine. These depolarization changes in membrane potential are similar to those produced by the endogenous mediator ACh. However, ACh is immediately hydrolyzed by cholinesterase; the postsynaptic membrane repolarizes and is prepared for subsequent activation by additional quanta of ACh. Succinylcholine elicits a prolonged depolarization of the end-plate region that does not allow the subsynaptic membrane to completely repolarize and renders the motor end-plate nonresponsive to the normal action of ACh.

Because of the initial depolarizing action, transient contraction of muscle cells occurs after administration of succinylcholine and related agents. This is characterized in vivo as momentary asynchronous muscle twitches and fasciculations. Because of the persistent depolarization of the postsynaptic membrane, however, subsequent impulse transmissions are blocked and a flaccid type of paralysis ensues. The molecular mechanism(s) of depolarizing neuromuscular blocking agents is not completely understood but may be biphasic.

Phase I Block. Depolarization of the motor end-plate region by ACh is characterized by increased permeability of the subsynaptic membrane to Na^+ and K^+. As ACh is catabolized by AChE the selective permeability characteristics of the postsynaptic membrane are rapidly reestablished. Repolarization occurs. Succinylcholine, however, causes a persistent increase in permeability of the postsynaptic membrane to Na^+ and K^+. ACh cannot act as a transmitter, and impulse transmission fails. It should be remembered that ACh, when in excess, also causes persistent depolarization block of cholinergic synaptic junctions.

Phase II Block. Phase II block occurs in some instances after prolonged exposure to a depolarizing agent and is characterized by a change from the depolarizing block to one that in some ways resembles that caused by curare. The actual mechanisms involved are poorly understood and opinion is contradictory as to this transition. Zaimis (1959) believes, e.g., that confusion has occurred because in some species some blocking agents have a "dual mechanism"; i.e., they cause some effects that resemble depolarization block and cause other effects that resemble competitive blockade.

After exposure of isolated nerve-muscle preparations to succinylcholine, the initial peak level of depolarization subsides. Subsequently, the end-plate becomes transiently sensitive to depolarizing agents. Gradually, a competitive-like blockade results and seems to be at least partially susceptible to reversal by cholinesterase inhibitors. Tachyphylaxis to depolarizing agents quickly develops and the receptors now appear to be insensitive to ACh. However, the importance of Phase II has not been clearly defined for each depolarizing neuromuscular blocking agent.

As a group the depolarizing neuromuscular blocking agents cause depolarization of receptor areas of muscle fibers sometime during their course of action. Increasing availability of ACh by administration of a cholinesterase inhibitor has no effect or in some cases may actually intensify the neuromuscular block of a depolarizing agent. Just the opposite, cholinesterase inhibitors can be quite effective in antagonizing the competitive block produced by nondepolarizing curaremimetic agents.

PHARMACOLOGIC EFFECTS OF NEUROMUSCULAR BLOCKING AGENTS

SKELETAL MUSCLE

Competitive Neuromuscular Blocking Agents. Nondepolarizing curarelike drugs interact with nicotinic cholinergic receptors of skeletal muscle cells and render them inaccessible to the transmitter function of ACh. Flaccid paralysis occurs. Neither axonal conductance nor response to direct stimulation of muscle is blocked by curare agents.

A schematic representation of an in vivo nerve-muscle preparation is shown in Figure 9.4. This sciatic nerve-gastrocnemius muscle preparation of anesthetized cats is often used to examine actions and interactions of neuromuscular blocking agents. In this preparation, stimulation of the sciatic nerve causes contraction (kg of isometric tension) of the gastrocnemius muscle.

Figure 9.5 demonstrates the neuromuscular blocking effect of *d*-tubocurarine on indirectly stimulated muscle twitch of the sciatic nerve-gastrocnemius muscle preparation of a cat, as described in Figure 9.4. In this example, muscle twitch quickly decreases after intravenous (IV) injection of *d*-tubocurarine, reaches peak depression within a few minutes, and then gradually returns to normal in approximately 15 minutes. Tubocurarine does not evoke an initial increase in muscle twitch; this lack of facilitation is a consistent finding with nondepolarizing agents. Gallamine, metocurine, and pancuronium produce similar characteristics of neuromuscular paralysis. Metocurine is

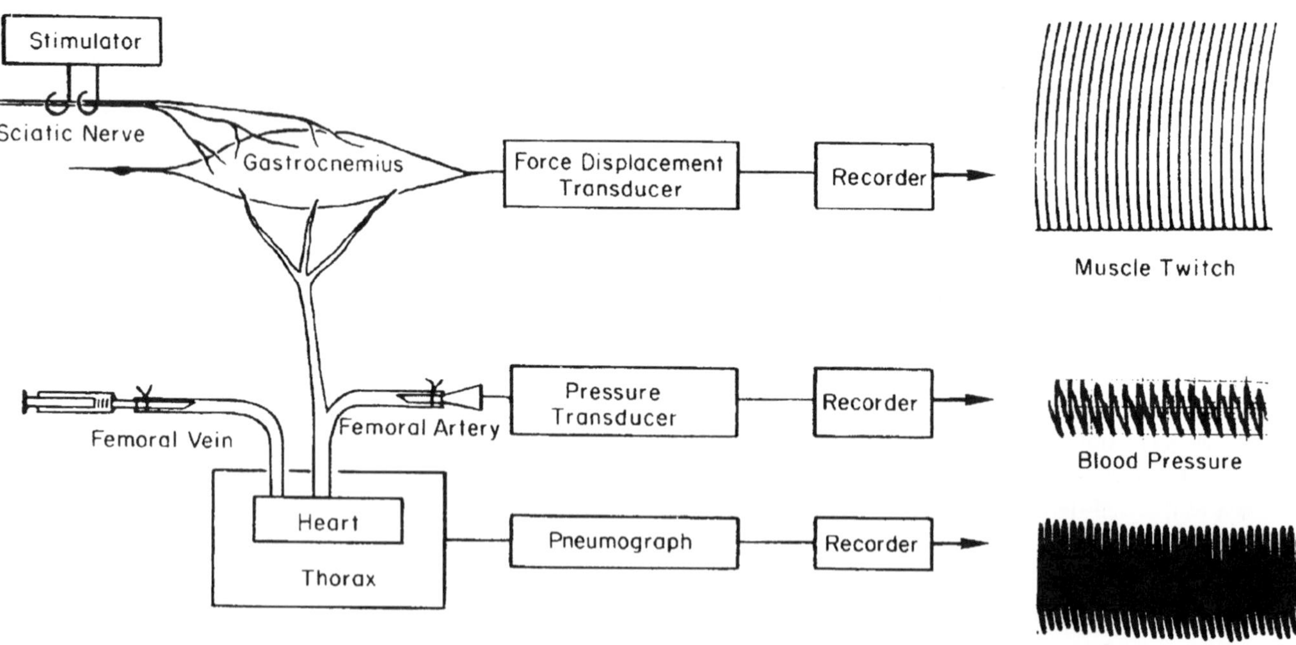

FIG. 9.4 Schematic representation of a sciatic nerve-gastrocnemius muscle preparation in an anesthetized cat. Stimulation of the isolated and decentralized sciatic nerve evokes contraction (muscle twitch) of the gastrocnemius muscle. Femoral arterial blood pressure and respiratory movements can be measured concurrently. Neuromuscular blocking drugs can be administered intravenously and changes in muscle twitch height observed.

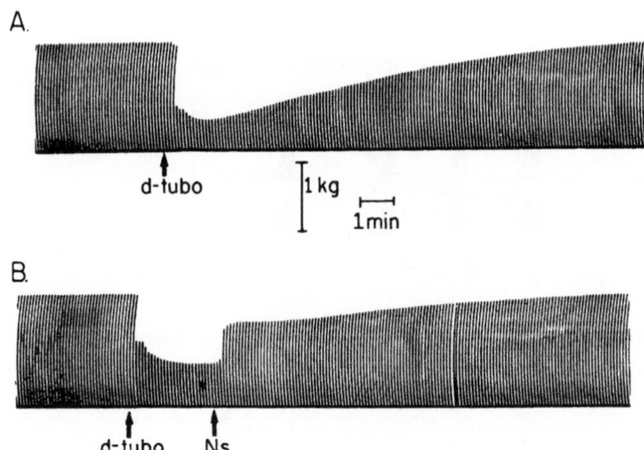

FIG. 9.5 Neuromuscular blocking effect of *d*-tubocurarine (*d*-tubo) and reversal of the *d*-tubo by neostigmine in a sciatic nerve-gastrocnemius muscle preparation of a cat. The cat was anesthetized with pentobarbital; muscle twitch was monitored as described in Figure 9.4. (A) Typical depression of muscle twitch by *d*-tubo (0.2 mg/kg) administered intravenously at designated arrow. (B) Antagonism of *d*-tubo (0.2 mg/kg) induced depression of muscle twitch by neostigmine (Ns; 0.1 mg/kg). Agents were administered intravenously at arrow. Notice rapid antagonism of the neuromuscular blocking effect of *d*-tubo by Ns. Compare this with the lack of antagonism by Ns of the muscle twitch depressant effect of succinylcholine in Figure 9.6.

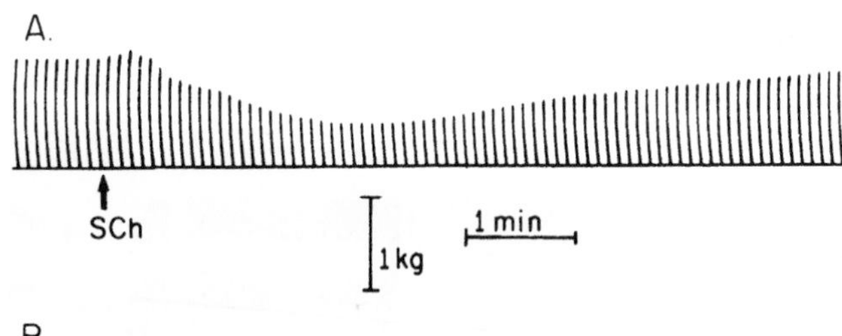

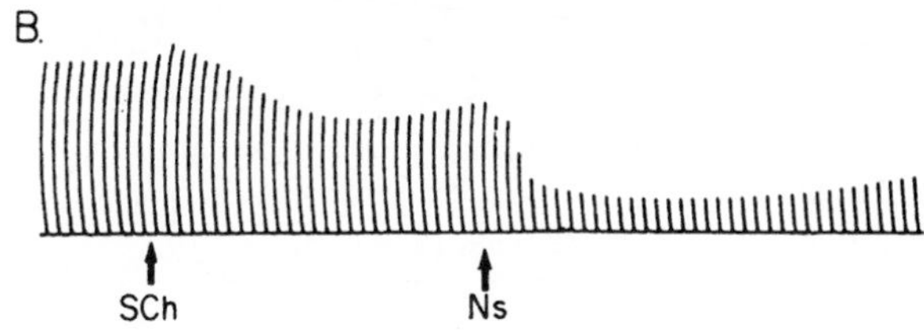

FIG. 9.6 Neuromuscular blocking effect of succinylcholine (SCh) and augmentation of its effect by neostigmine (Ns) in a sciatic nerve-gastrocnemius muscle preparation of a cat. The cat was anesthetized with pentobarbital; muscle twitch was monitored as described in Figure 9.4. (A) Typical depression of muscle twitch by SCh (0.04 mg/kg) administered intravenously at designated arrow. (B) Augmentation of the muscle twitch depressant effect of SCh (0.04 mg/kg) by Ns (0.1 mg/kg). Agents were administered intravenously at designated arrows. Notice augmentation of the degree and duration of effect of SCh by Ns. Compare this with the antagonism by Ns of the neuromuscular blocking effect of *d*-tubo in Figure 9.5.

3–10 times more active than *d*-tubocurarine, pancuronium is 5–7 times more potent than *d*-tubocurarine, and gallamine is somewhat less active.

Antagonism of the neuromuscular blocking effects of *d*-tubocurarine by administration of a cholinesterase inhibitor, neostigmine, is shown in Figure 9.5. By comparing the two tracings in this figure, it is readily apparent that neostigmine markedly hastens recovery from the muscle twitch depression caused by *d*-tubocurarine. This antagonistic interaction is primarily attributed to the anticholinesterase activity of neostigmine. Inhibition of cholinesterase delays the catabolic breakdown of ACh and allows its accumulation at receptor sites. Newly available ACh, now in increased concentration at the postsynaptic membrane, effectively competes with *d*-tubocurarine for the cholinoceptors. ACh-mediated depolarization of the end-plate, muscle action potentials, and muscle contraction are restored; muscle twitch quickly returns to normal.

Depolarizing Neuromuscular Blocking Agents. Succinylcholine and decamethonium elicit transient muscle fasciculations prior to causing neuromuscular paralysis. This is due to initial depolarization of the motor end-plate and is characterized in the intact animal by asynchronous muscular contractions of the head, body trunk, and limbs. Fasciculation does not always occur in anesthetized animals.

The in vivo neuromuscular blocking effect of a small dose of succinylcholine in a cat nerve-muscle preparation is shown in Figure 9.6. Initially, there is a slight and transient facilitory effect of succinylcholine on neuromuscular transmission; muscle twitch height momentarily increases by a small increment as a result of the initial depolarizing effect of the drug. Subsequently, however, muscle twitch rapidly decreases and within 1–2 minutes maximum depressant effect is obtained. Shortly thereafter, the neuromuscular effects of succinylcholine subside and muscle twitch returns to normal within an additional 5–8 minutes. The magnitude and duration of neuromuscular paralysis is dependent upon the dosage of succinylcholine. The relatively short duration of succinylcholine activity is from rapid biotransformation of this drug by plasma pseudocholinesterase. Decamethonium causes similar characteristics of neuromuscular blockade, but the duration of action of this drug is considerably longer than that seen with succinylcholine.

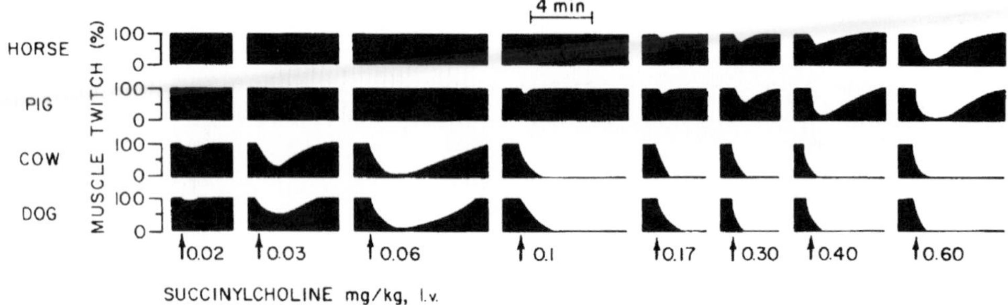

FIG. 9.7 Schematic representations of the neuromuscular blocking effect of succinylcholine iodide in nerve-muscle preparations of different species during barbiturate anesthesia. Notice interspecies differences in degree and duration of paralysis caused by succinylcholine. (Modified from Hansson 1956, after Lumb and Jones 1973.)

The effects of a cholinesterase inhibitor, neostigmine, on the neuromuscular paralysis produced by succinylcholine are demonstrated in Figure 9.6. By comparing the two tracings in this figure, it is apparent that neostigmine potentiated the muscle twitch depression evoked by succinylcholine and prolonged recovery from the effects of this agent. This synergistic interaction is primarily attributed to the anticholinesterase activity of neostigmine, resulting in decreased biotransformation of both succinylcholine and endogenous ACh. Thus succinylcholine and ACh are available at receptor sites for longer periods and the duration of depolarizing neuromuscular paralysis is prolonged.

The potency of neuromuscular effects of succinylcholine varies in different species (Hansson 1958), as shown schematically in Figure 9.7. Bovine and canine species are quite sensitive to succinylcholine, whereas horses and pigs are considerably less responsive. This difference is probably dependent upon species differences in the activity of pseudocholinesterase, the enzyme that biotransforms succinylcholine (Radeleff and Woodard 1956; Palmer et al. 1965). Cattle and sheep, e.g., have considerably less detectable pseudocholinesterase activity than horses and pigs. Administration of purified pseudocholinesterase preparation to dogs increases resistance to succinylcholine (Hall et al. 1953).

AUTONOMIC EFFECTS. Synaptic transmission at autonomic ganglia involves activation by ACh of nicotinic receptors of the postganglionic nerve body (see Chapter 7). It is not surprising, therefore, that neuromuscular blocking agents (which act at somatic nicotinic sites) may also alter ganglionic transmission.

Tubocurarine is an excellent example of a drug selected for site of action at nicotinic receptors of the somatic myoneural junction that as a side effect also acts at ganglionic nicotinic receptors. Tubocurarine interacts with ganglionic receptors, renders them inaccessible to ACh, and thereby increases the threshold of the postganglionic nerve to ACh. However, as a general rule, autonomic ganglia are less sensitive to curare than are the myoneural junctions. Ganglionic impulse transmission involves, at least partially, a muscarinic pathway (see Chapter 7); *d*-tubocurarine has little blocking effect on muscarinic receptors. Thus in most cases it would be anticipated that ganglionic transmission is functional during treatment with curarelike drugs. Nevertheless, hypotension believed to be partly dependent upon ganglionic blockade can occur after administration of *d*-tubocurarine.

Other neuromuscular blocking drugs, both competitive and depolarizing types, have been shown experimentally to alter ganglionic transmission, but in clinically insignificant amounts. Succinylcholine induces transient ganglionic stimulation prior to blockade evoked by larger doses. The former effect may partially explain hypertension that has occurred subsequent to succinylcholine administration.

Parasympathetic effects of neuromuscular blocking agents are usually minimal. Pancuronium has anticholinesterase activity. Succinylcholine and decamethonium are approximately 1,000 times and 100 times less potent, respectively, than ACh in eliciting contraction of guinea pig ileum. In dogs, large doses of succinylcholine induce salivation; this is antagonized by pretreatment with atropine (Hansson 1956).

HISTAMINE RELEASE. Tubocurarine causes release of histamine. The magnitude of this response varies, depending on species, dosage, and rate and route of administration. Intraarterial infusion of *d*-tubocurarine evokes histamine release in the perfused hindlimb preparation of dogs, and histaminelike wheals can be produced by subdermal and intraarterial administration of *d*-tubocurarine. In vivo, increased respiratory tract secretions and bronchospasm seen after administration of *d*-tubocurarine have been attributed to histamine release, as has the hypotensive effect of *d*-tubocurarine. Pretreatment with antihistamine drugs antagonizes these side effects; they are not inhibited by atropine or neostigmine.

Metocurine, succinylcholine, decamethonium, and gallamine are very weak histamine-releasing agents.

CENTRAL NERVOUS SYSTEM. Although synaptic transmission in the brain is altered by direct application of neuromuscular blocking drugs into the brain, CNS effects are nondetectable when these drugs are administered by other routes. Neuromuscular blocking agents do not gain entry into the CNS to any appreciable extent because of the presence of the highly charged quaternary ammonium moieties. Therefore, neither CNS depression nor tranquilization is produced by neuromuscular blocking agents. Nonambulation results only from peripheral myoneural paralysis. This was decisively confirmed when Smith (Smith et al. 1947) allowed himself to be paralyzed with *d*-tubocurarine. At no time during the experiment did he experience hypnosis, tranquilization, amnesia, anesthesia, or analgesia. He simply could not voluntarily breathe or move, an experience described as quite frightful.

CARDIOVASCULAR EFFECTS. As outlined above, *d*-tubocurarine often induces hypotension, particularly if rapidly administered to dogs. Slight increases in heart rate and cardiac output have been observed after administration of gallamine, apparently from a vagolytic effect on the heart (Longnecker et al. 1973). Others have reported no significant cardiovascular changes after IV administration of gallamine to anesthetized dogs (Evans et al. 1977). In cats, mild atropinelike effects on the heart were observed after injection of gallamine, pancuronium, and alcuronium chloride (Alloferin) (Hughes and Chapple 1976).

Studies with pancuronium in humans and dogs indicated that this agent evokes slight increases in heart rate, blood pressure, and cardiac output during thiobarbiturate anesthesia (Coleman et al. 1972; Reitan and Warpinski 1975). Cardiovascular effects of this agent were absent if patients were pretreated with atropine. Others have reported no significant cardiovascular changes with pancuronium (Brown et al. 1973). Similarly, studies have indicated that neither pancuronium nor gallamine significantly altered heart rate or blood pressure in anesthetized horses (Klein et al. 1983). Atracurium (up to 0.6 mg/kg) and vecuronium (up to 0.2 mg/kg) were reported to have negligible effects on arterial blood pressure in dogs (Jones 1985).

Succinylcholine usually evokes minimal cardiovascular changes in horses or dogs if administered during general anesthesia; blood pressure remains fairly constant if artificial breathing is provided (Evans et al. 1977; Benson et al. 1979).

Subparalytic doses of succinylcholine increase the arrhythmogenicity of epinephrine during light halothane anesthesia in dogs (Tucker and Munson 1975). In dogs not treated with succinylcholine, an average dose of 4.15 μg/kg epinephrine was required to evoke premature ventricular contractions, whereas an average dose of 1.6 μg/kg epinephrine was the arrhythmogenic dose in dogs pretreated with 0.25 mg/kg succinylcholine. However, *d*-tubocurarine provides a slight protection against epinephrine-induced arrhythmias. Mechanisms involved in these drug interactions have not been clarified. If deemed essential, catecholamines should be used cautiously in patients treated with depolarizing neuromuscular blocking agents.

Also, succinylcholine has been reported to increase susceptibility to the myocardial irritant effects of digitalis preparations, and it has been suggested that succinylcholine may be contraindicated in digitalized patients (Dowdy et al. 1965).

Pronounced cardiovascular side effects have been reported in horses after administration of succinylcholine (Larson et al. 1959; Hofmeyer 1960; Lees and Tavernor 1969). In general, these effects seem to be more pronounced in unanesthetized and nontranquilized animals than during general anesthesia. Severe hypertension, initial bradycardia followed by tachycardia, atrioventricular conduction disturbances, and extrasystoles have been reported, and myocardial damage has been suspected. Early institution of artificial respiration has been reported to block the blood pressure effect. The hypertensive response seems to be at least partially mediated by the succinylcholine-induced dyspnea and the accompanying blood PO_2-PCO_2 disturbances, causing a reflexogenic increase in blood pressure. Direct activation of autonomic ganglia by succinylcholine may also be involved.

It should be remembered that neuromuscular blocking agents do not depress the brain unless or until apnea-induced hypoxia actually causes syncope. Prior to hypoxic states, skeletal muscle paralysis affords no depression whatsoever of conscious centers of the brain of nonanesthetized animals. It seems likely, then, that the novel sensations experienced by conscious animals as they are being paralyzed evoke profound fright. This can cause activation of autonomic centers within the brain. Autonomic discharge may be altered markedly resulting in cardiovascular side effects. Autonomic blocking agents (ganglionic block with hexamethonium, β-adrenergic block with propranolol) substantially decrease the cardiovascular side effects of succinylcholine.

OCULAR EFFECTS. Clinically important ocular effects depend upon the pronounced contracture of ocular muscles that occurs after treatment with depolarizing neuromuscular blockers. These agents are contraindicated in glaucoma, since intraocular pressure may be increased.

SERUM POTASSIUM. Depolarizing neuromuscular blocking agents cause a release of K^+ from skeletal muscle. Elevation of serum K^+ may result, particularly if repeated injections are given.

PHARMACOKINETICS. Neuromuscular blocking agents with quaternary nitrogen groups are ionized at all levels of physiologic pH. Therefore, they are highly charged, lipophobic compounds and cross lipoprotein membrane barriers poorly. Little if any absorption occurs after oral administration of these drugs. South American Indians were well aware of this, since they ingested flesh of curare-poisoned animals without concern. Inefficient absorption after oral administration has little importance to modern medicine, however, because these agents should be given by the IV route so that muscle relaxation can be quickly evaluated. Whereas South American Indians were concerned only with one end point, death, and were worried only about underdosage, practitioners are concerned with facilitating muscle relaxation and are extremely concerned with overdosage. Administration of neuromuscular blocking agents should be closely monitored and correlated at all times, with effects observed in the patient.

Intramuscular (IM) injection of neuromuscular blocking agents is occasionally used to immobilize nondomestic animals. Absorption occurs rapidly after IM injection, and effective blood concentrations are obtained shortly thereafter.

Tubocurarine is distributed primarily in the extracellular space throughout body tissues, but it concentrates at myoneural junctional regions (Waser 1967). It penetrates cells poorly because of the charged state of the molecule. The liver and kidney participate in the biologic fate of *d*-tubocurarine; however, duration of action of this agent normally does not depend upon biotransformation. Rather, redistribution of *d*-tubocurarine away from the neuromuscular junction and into nonspecific body compartments is believed to account for the short duration of action of a single dose of this drug. Repeated treatment or excessive amounts of *d*-tubocurarine tends to saturate nonspecific sites. Under these circumstances, renal excretion becomes important as a mechanism for termination of activity of *d*-tubocurarine. If injection must be repeated, less drug is needed to evoke muscle relaxation. Cumulative neuromuscular blockade occurs when injections are repeated, since *d*-tubocurarine is excreted rather slowly by the kidneys.

Gallamine and metocurine are probably handled similarly to *d*-tubocurarine. Gallamine is excreted virtually unchanged in the urine, as are decamethonium and pancuronium. These agents are thought to bind only minimally to tissues. Renal failure markedly prolongs their duration of action.

Atracurium is one of a series of new competitive agents that was developed to overcome pharmacokinetic disadvantages of the older drugs. Atracurium is rapidly inactivated by plasma esterases and also, importantly, by a spontaneous chemical degradation instigated at physiologic pH and body temperature (Table 9.1). Atracurium is therefore noncumulative, and the duration of action of the same dose does not increase with repetitive injections (Agoston et al. 1980). In dogs, Jones (1985) recommended that atracurium be administered initially at 0.5 mg/kg, followed by increments of 0.2 mg/kg. The duration of neuromuscular blocking action of vecuronium, another new agent, is similar to that of atracurium and is about one-third to one-half that of pancuronium. Vecuronium undergoes hepatic biotransformation and is excreted predominantly in the bile; it is somewhat cumulative, and this characteristic can be expected to be more pronounced in the presence of hepatic disease (Jones 1985). Because of its short duration of action and affiliated ease of control, atracurium has become a frequently used neuromuscular blocking agent in veterinary anesthesiology.

Succinylcholine is rapidly disposed of by the body, since it is a suitable substrate for plasma pseudocholinesterase. This enzyme quickly hydrolyzes succinylcholine to the considerably less active metabolite succinylmonocholine. This metabolite is more slowly broken down by pseudocholinesterase to succinic acid and choline, natural body constituents. The interspecies potency of succinylcholine varies considerably. This has been attributed to species differences in activity of pseudocholinesterase.

INTERACTIONS

Various drugs influence the pharmacologic effects of muscle relaxants. Neuromuscular blocking agents themselves alter activity of other neuromuscular agents. As would be expected, competitive agents summate with each other. Similarly, depolarizing agents also interact synergistically with one another. However, tubocurarine decreases the muscle twitch depressant effects of succinylcholine and decamethonium. This is related to persistent occupation of a certain portion of receptors by tubocurarine, although muscle twitch may have recovered (see margin of safety of neuromuscular transmission below). Depolarization of the end-plate by succinylcholine or decamethonium is partially impeded by the stabilizing effects of tubocurarine. Succinylcholine antagonizes the effects of curare as a result of the partial agonistic characteristics of the former agent. These complex antagonistic interactions, however, have no clinical application, since they depend upon complicated treatment and time and dosage schedules. During clinical situations, neuromuscular blocking agents should not be used in attempts to reverse the effects of other types of neuromuscular blocking agents, since potentiation may occur despite experimental results to the contrary.

The interaction of cholinesterase inhibitors with neuromuscular blocking agents has been discussed above. Cholinesterase inhibitors decrease responsiveness to the competitive agents, while they tend to increase intensity and duration of action of depolarizing agents (Sunew and Hicks 1978). Organophosphate pesticides and anthelmintics, carbamates, and any other cholinesterase inhibitor may cause interactions. The phenothiazine family of tranquilizers has some anticholinesterase activity. Use of succinylcholine in a patient exposed to an organophosphate may be particularly hazardous if a phenothiazine tranquilizer has also been administered.

Many general anesthetics, in addition to depressing the CNS, depress impulse transmission at somatic myoneural junctions. Halothane acts synergistically with curarelike drugs but to a lesser extent than ether. Methoxyflurane and pentobarbital also have depressant effects on myoneural transmission events.

Aminoglycoside antibiotics (neomycin, streptomycin, dihydrostreptomycin, kanamycin, gentamicin) decrease the release of ACh from the nerve and also the sensitivity of the end-plate to ACh (Pittinger and Adamson 1972; Adams et al. 1976a). They do not cause depolarization. Their effects in many ways resemble those of low Ca^{++} or excess Mg^{++}. The presynaptic effect of antibiotics is believed to be due to interruption of Ca^{++}-dependent events at the axonal membrane (Adams 1984). Cholinesterase inhibitors such as neostigmine antagonize the postsynaptic depressant effect of these antibiotics. Ca^{++} antagonizes the presynaptic action and is usually more effective than neostigmine in reversing the neuromuscular paralyzing effects of aminoglycoside antibiotics. These antibiotics interact synergistically at the myoneural junction with neuromuscular blocking agents, anesthetics, and other antibiotics. The clinical significance of neuromuscular interactions of antibiotics and other drugs has been well established in humans and has been suggested in lower animals (Adams and Bingham 1971). These subjects have been reviewed (Pittinger et al. 1970; Adams et al. 1976b; Keller et al. 1992).

Different disease states influence pharmacologic effects of neuromuscular blocking agents. Hepatic synthesis of pseudocholinesterase is decreased in the presence of liver disease. The duration of succinylcholine activity will be prolonged if the liver is seriously affected. Administration of purified pseudocholinesterase preparation hastens recovery from effects of succinylcholine (Scholler et al. 1977).

Renal problems delay excretion of *d*-tubocurarine, gallamine, pancuronium, and decamethonium. Anand et al. (1972) successfully reversed persistent gallamine-induced neuromuscular paralysis in a renally incompetent human patient by use of artificial diuresis.

CLINICAL USE

Muscle paralysis proceeds at different rates in different body regions after administration of a neuromuscular blocking agent. Usually, head and neck muscles are affected first, often within 0.25–1 minute after injection. This characteristic is employed in a biologic assay (i.e., head-drop test in rabbits) for determining potency of an unknown concentration of curare. The tail is usually affected with the head and neck. Subsequently, muscles of the limbs are paralyzed, then the deglutition and laryngeal muscles. Abdominal muscles, intercostal muscles, and the diaphragm are then paralyzed in this order. Recovery usually proceeds in the reverse of this sequence (Hall 1971).

Attempts have been made in clinical practice to use the sequential development of muscle paralysis by administering doses of neuromuscular blocking agents adequate to paralyze ambulatory muscle but insufficient to affect the diaphragm. This has not always proved effective, because respiratory insufficiency may still occur, although the diaphragm is seemingly spared. Therefore, it is imperative that apparatus for administering artificial respiration be available when neuromuscular blocking agents are used clinically. To circumvent the need for immediate establishment of an adequate airway and other emergency procedures, it would seem wise to routinely perform tracheal intubation and institute artificial respiration whenever a neuromuscular blocking agent is used.

Muscle relaxants have been used in clinical practice for several purposes: to facilitate tracheal intubation; to paralyze respiratory muscle so that artificial respiration can be easily controlled; to increase muscle relaxation to facilitate surgical access to difficult anatomic regions; to evoke muscle relaxation to facilitate orthopedic manipulations and, particularly, fracture reduction; and as part of balanced anesthesia procedures to reduce the amount of general anesthetic required.

Tracheal intubation may be performed in a nonanesthetized animal immediately after a paralyzing dose of neuromuscular blocking agent has taken effect. Prior administration of a sedative or tranquilizer is advisable for humane reasons and to circumvent potential side effects that may be precipitated by fear reaction to paralysis.

A wide range of dosages of neuromuscular blocking agents has been reported for use of these drugs during anesthesia (Hansson 1956; Tavernor 1971; Lumb and Jones 1973). Often this variance reflects differences in investigative procedures of the original studies, e.g., the use of different anesthetics and sedatives, different salts of the neuromuscular blocking agent, different nerve-muscle preparations, and in some cases the use of nonanesthetized subjects. Neuromuscular blocking agents should be given to effect rather than by bolus administration of a set pre-calculated dose. It is advisable for these drugs to be administered by titration during anesthesia and to be continuously correlated with muscle relaxation much in the way that barbiturates are administered for induction of general anesthesia.

In dogs, 0.4–0.5 mg/kg *d*-tubocurarine administered intravenously will cause generalized skeletal muscle relaxation, but hypotension frequently occurs as a side effect in this species. In pigs, 0.2–0.3 mg/kg *d*-tubocurarine will usually afford acceptable muscular relaxation; blood pressure effects are less in this species than in the dog. Tubocurarine is somewhat more potent in ruminants; doses of 0.05–0.06 mg/kg have been suggested for use in young lambs and goats.

Approximately 1 mg/kg gallamine causes complete muscle paralysis in both dogs and cats within 1–2 minutes after IV injection and lasts 15–20 minutes. A hypotensive response may be induced in cats with gallamine but is infrequently observed in dogs. In young ruminants (lambs and calves), 0.4 mg/kg gallamine is effective, whereas the dose in horses is 0.5–1 mg/kg.

Solutions of succinylcholine should always be refrigerated and kept on ice in the field, since this agent undergoes spontaneous hydrolysis. Hansson (1956) reported that the IV ED_{50} (dose that reduced muscle twitch by 50%) of succinylcholine in the sciatic nerve-gastrocnemius muscle preparation of anesthetized dogs was 0.045–0.060 mg/kg. This dose did not effectively paralyze the respiratory muscles, however, and 0.085 mg/kg was required to induce transient apnea, whereas 0.11 mg/kg and 0.22 mg/kg were needed to cause apnea for 18–21 minutes and 23–27 minutes, respectively. In unanesthetized dogs, IM administration of 0.12 mg/kg succinylcholine caused ataxia in 5 minutes and forced abdominal respiration in 7 minutes; recovery was apparently complete in 30 minutes. In clinical situations, 0.3 mg/kg succinylcholine administered intravenously will usually afford good muscle relaxation in dogs, whereas in the cat, 1 mg/kg may be required. In dogs, Hansson (1956) reported that 0.15 mg/kg succinylcholine was effective in paralyzing the diaphragm during thoracotomy procedures. However, Eyster and Evans (1974) suggested the use of 0.5 mg/kg succinylcholine for muscle relaxation in dogs during thoracotomy for open-heart surgery. This dose was also reported to control muscle twitches evoked by inadvertent stimulation of nerves during use of electrocautery. Duration of paralysis varies and should be closely monitored.

In rhesus monkeys, 1–2 mg/kg succinylcholine administered intravenously has been used for restraint for tuberculosis testing and endotracheal intubation (Lindquist and Lau 1973). In pigs, approximately 2 mg/kg succinylcholine is effective. Much smaller amounts (0.01–0.02 mg/kg) are required in cattle and sheep. Hansson (1956) reported that 0.13–0.18 mg/kg succinylcholine is required to immobilize nonanesthetized horses. However, the generally accepted dose of succinylcholine in horses, when used alone, is 0.088 mg/kg (Lumb and Jones 1973).

Succinylcholine has been used without anesthesia in horses for casting and restraint during brief surgical procedures such as castration. This practice should not be condoned, because no anesthesia is afforded for painful procedures, severe fright is seemingly evoked, and pronounced cardiovascular disturbances and even myocardial damage may result. Succinylcholine should not be used as a sole restraining agent during surgical procedures but only in conjunction with a general or local anesthetic.

Moreover, care should always be taken during the use of neuromuscular blocking agents to ensure that the patient does not simply remain paralyzed after recovery from the anesthetic. This has occurred in human patients and has led to successful lawsuits by patients and receipt of monetary compensation. Although lower animals cannot complain, it behooves us as veterinarians to ensure that our patients are not inadvertently subjected to such excruciatingly painful incidents.

MARGIN OF SAFETY OF NEUROMUSCULAR TRANSMISSION. The concept of a margin of safety of neuromuscular transmission bears discussion in relation to clinical use of these drugs. It has been estimated that a relatively large percentage of the cholinergic receptors must be occupied by a curare agent before muscle twitch fails. In the cat diaphragm, e.g., muscle twitch is not affected until about 80% of the receptors are blocked by *d*-tubocurarine, and twitch is not completely abolished until about 90% of the receptors are occupied (Waud and Waud 1972). A somewhat greater margin of safety was found in dogs. Accordingly, for recovery of the diaphragm from the effects of a previous injection of *d*-tubocurarine, only a small percentage (5% in dogs, 18% in cats) of the receptors need to be free. Therefore, and most important, although to all outward signs recovery seems complete, over 80% of the receptors can still be blocked.

Recognition of this aspect becomes clinically important in the postoperative recovery room and should be considered in patients that have been exposed to neuromuscular blocking drugs and/or other myoneural depressants such as anesthetics. As a patient regains some control of voluntary muscles, spontaneous respiration returns and may seem completely normal. However, it must be remembered that at this time an extremely small margin of safety of neuromuscular transmission exists. That is, only a small percentage of the postsynaptic receptors are available for interaction with ACh; this small fraction of receptors is now responsible for maintaining muscle contraction. Therefore, if the patient is then exposed to another drug that as a side effect depresses neuromuscular function (even though it may be minimal or even nondetectable normally), disastrous complications may result. Anesthetic mortality has occurred in humans that can be attributed to such interactions. For example, Pridgen (1956) reported the anesthetic deaths of two children who were given neomycin intraperitoneally immediately after completion of successful laparotomies under ether anesthesia. Initially, respiration was adequate, but within a short time after administration of the antibiotic, persistent apnea occurred. Death followed several hours later. It seems likely that the margin of safety of neuromuscular transmission was reduced in these infants by ether, resulting in marked augmentation of the neuromuscular blocking properties of neomycin. Pittinger et al. (1970) estimated a 9% death rate in human patients experiencing antibiotic-induced respiratory problems in conjunction with anesthetics and neuromuscular blocking agents. Apnea and eventual death in a traumatized dog were attributed to antibiotic (dihydrostreptomycin)-induced neuromuscular paralysis (Adams and Bingham 1971).

These examples illustrate potential problems that may be inadvertently introduced in a patient that seemingly is recovering quite well from anesthesia and surgery. The margin of safety of neuromuscular transmission should be considered any time that anesthetics, neuromuscular blocking agents, or any other drug that depresses myoneural function are used in multiple drug regimens.

CLINICAL REVERSAL OF NEUROMUSCULAR PARALYSIS. Treatment of persistent neuromuscular paralysis and/or treatment of inadvertent overdosage of neuromuscular blocking agents should be approached conservatively (Bevan et al. 1992). The initial step should be immediate artificial respiration and withdrawal of administration of the involved agent. Often, artificial respiration will allow adequate time for the drug to be disposed of by the patient's system. Exposure to other drugs that may synergistically interact with neuromuscular blocking agents should be avoided. If a competitive neuromuscular blocking agent was used, paralysis can usually be effectively antagonized by administration of a cholinesterase inhibitor such as neostigmine or edrophonium (Hildebrand and Howitt 1984). Neostigmine can be administered to small and large animals by slow IV injection at the dose of 0.022 mg/kg. It should be remembered that cholinesterase inhibitors will cause intensification of ACh activity at both muscarinic and nicotinic receptors. Atropine (0.04 mg/kg) should be administered prior to or in conjunction with neostigmine to circumvent the muscarinic effects of the latter drug (Klein et al. 1983; Jones 1985). Care should be taken to ensure that paralysis does not recur after antagonism by neostigmine; additional injection of neostigmine may be required.

Because cardiovascular complications occasionally occur after treatment with atropine and neostigmine, new ideas have evolved in management of persistent paralysis in patients treated with nondepolarizing neuromuscular blocking drugs. These include substitution of quaternary ammonium muscarinic antagonists in place of atropine (to avoid potential CNS effects of atropine) and substitution of pyridostigmine and edrophonium for neostigmine. Pyridostigmine in combination with propantheline or glycopyrrolate, e.g., produced less abrupt changes in heart rate than combined therapy of either atropine-neostigmine or atropine-pyridostigmine. Pyridostigmine (0.05–0.08 mg/kg), a moderately long-acting drug, and edrophonium (0.2–0.4 mg/kg), a short-acting agent, when combined with either propantheline (0.03–0.06 mg/kg) or glycopyrrolate (0.004–0.006 mg/kg), were reported to produce a rapid and effective reversal of pancuronium-induced neuromuscular block in humans, with minimal changes in heart rate and almost no incidence of arrhythmias (Gyermek 1977). The clinical effectiveness of the above regimen in reversing neuromuscular paralysis produced by competitive agents other than pancuronium or in other species should be examined.

A new drug, 4-aminopyridine, was found to antagonize curare-induced neuromuscular block; however, this agent is not a cholinesterase inhibitor. Instead, it evokes release of ACh from the somatic nerve terminal. Advantages of 4-aminopyridine over cholinesterase inhibitors include longer duration of action without muscarinic side effects. Thus concurrent therapy with atropinelike drugs is unnecessary. The CNS excitatory effects of 4-aminopyridine limit its use in doses adequate to completely antagonize curare block. However, this agent markedly potentiates the anticurare activity of cholinesterase inhibitors. This combined therapy of low doses of 4-aminopyridine and a cholinesterase inhibitor has considerable potential application to clinical reversal of the nondepolarizing type of neuromuscular blocking agents (Miller 1979).

Neostigmine or other cholinesterase inhibitors should not be used in attempts to reverse the effects of a depolarizing agent (Sunew and Hicks 1978). Reliable chemical antidotes are not available for this group of agents. Artificial respiration may be required for a prolonged period. Injection of purified pseudocholinesterase preparation has been shown to hasten recovery from the effects of succinylcholine (Scholler et al. 1977).

Because of the small therapeutic index of neuromuscular blocking agents, their clinical use should always be supervised by qualified experienced personnel who are thoroughly familiar with the indications, limitations, hazards, and methods of administration of these highly active drugs.

REFERENCES

Adams, H. R. 1984. Pharmacodynamic actions of antimicrobial agents in host cell membranes. J Am Vet Med Assoc 185:1127–30.

Adams, H. R., Bingham, G. A. 1971. Respiratory arrest associated with dihydrostreptomycin. J Am Vet Med Assoc 159:179–80.

Adams, H. R., Mathew, B. P., Teske, R. H., et al. 1976a. Neuromuscular blocking effects of aminoglycoside antibiotics on fast- and slow-contracting muscles of the cat. Anesth Analg (Cleve) 55:500–507.

Adams, H. R., Teske, R. H., Mercer, H. D. 1976b. Anesthetic-antibiotic interrelationships. J Am Vet Med Assoc 168:409–12.

Agoston, S., Salt, P., Newton, D., et al. 1980. The neuromuscular blocking action of ORG NC 45, a new pancuronium derivative, in anaesthetized patients: a pilot study. Br J Anaesth 52:53S–59S.

Agoston, S., Vandenbrom, R. H. G., Wierda, J. M. K. H. 1992. Clinical pharmacokinetics of neuromuscular blocking drugs. Clin Pharmacokinet 22:94–115.

Anand, J. S., Mehta, R. K., Munshi, C. A., et al. 1972. Reversal of neuromuscular blockade by artificial diuresis: case report. Can Anaesth Soc J 19:651–53.

Benson, G. J., Hartsfield, S. M., Smetzer, D. L., et al. 1979. Physiologic effects of succinylcholine chloride in mechanically ventilated horses anesthetized with halothane in oxygen. Am J Vet Res 40:1411–16.

Bernard, C. 1856. C R Acad Sci (Paris) 43:825.

Bevan, D. R., Donati, F., Kopman, A. F. 1992. Reversal of neuromuscular blockade. Anesthesiology 77:785–805.

Bouzat, C., Gumilar, F., Spitzmaul, G., et al. 2004. Coupling of agonist binding to channel gating in an ACh-binding protein linked to an ion channel. Nature 430:896–900.

Bovet, D. 1951. Some aspects of relationship between chemical constitution and curare-like activity. Ann NY Acad Sci 54:407–37.

Bowen, J. M. 1972. Estimation of the dissociation constant of d-tubocurarine and the receptor for endogenous acetylcholine. J Pharmacol Exp Ther 183:333–40.

Brejc, K., van Dijk, W. J., Klaassen, R. V., et al. 2001. Crystal structure of an ACh-binding protein reveals the ligand-binding domain of nicotine receptors. Nature 411:269–276.

Brown, E. M., Smiler, B. G., Plaza, J. A. 1973. Cardiovascular effects of pancuronium. Anesthesiology 38:597–99.

Coleman, A. J., Downing, J. W., Leary, W. P., et al. 1972. The immediate cardiovascular effects of pancuronium, alcuronium and tubocurarine in man. Anaesthesia 27:415–22.

Couteaux, R. 1972. In J. Cheymol, ed., Neuromuscular Blocking and Stimulating Agents, vol. 1, p. 7. Elmsford, NY: Pergamon.

Davis, E., and Barnes, M. P. 2000. Botulinum toxin and spasticity. J Neurol Neurosurg Psych 68:141–147.

Dolly, J. O., Barnard, E. A. 1977. Purification and characterization of an acetylcholine receptor from mammalian skeletal muscle. Biochemistry 16:5053–60.

Dowdy, E. G., Duggar, P. N., Fabian, L. W. 1965. Effect of neuromuscular blocking agents on isolated digitalized mammalian hearts. Anesth Analg (Cleve) 44:608–17.

Evans, A. T., Anderson, L. K., Eyster, G. E., et al. 1977. Cardiovascular effects of gallamine triethiodide and succinylcholine chloride during halothane anesthesia in the dog. Am J Vet Res 38:329–31.

Eyster, G. E., Evans, A. T. 1974. In R. W. Kirk, ed., Current Veterinary Therapy, V: Small Animal Practice, p. 255. Philadelphia: W. B. Saunders.

Ferguson, S., and Blakely, R. 2004. The choline transporter resurfaces: New roles for synaptic vesicles? Mol Interv 4:22–37.

Gyermek, L. 1977. Clinical pharmacology of the reversal of neuromuscular block. Int J Clin Pharmacol 15:456–62.

Hall, L. W., ed. 1971. Wright's Veterinary Anaesthesia and Analgesia, 7th ed., p. 1. Baltimore: Williams & Wilkins.

Hall, L. W., Lehman, H., Silk, E. 1953. Response in dogs to relaxants derived from succinic acid and choline. Br Med J 1:134–36.

Hansson, C. H. 1956. Succinylcholine iodide as a muscle relaxant in veterinary surgery. J Am Vet Med Assoc 128:287–91.

———. 1958. Studies on the effect of succinylcholine in domestic animals. Nord Vet Med 10:201–16.

Hildebrand, S. V., Howitt, G. A. 1984. Antagonism of pancuronium neuromuscular blockade in halothane-anesthetized ponies using neostigmine and edrophonium. Am J Vet Res 45:2276–80.

Hofmeyer, C. F. B. 1960. Some observations on the use of succinylcholine chloride (suxamethonium) in horses with particular reference to the effect on the heart. J S Afr Vet Med Assoc 31:251–59.

Hubbard, J. I., Quastel, D. M. 1973. Micropharmacology of vertebrate neuromuscular transmission. Annu Rev Pharmacol 13: 199–216.

Hucho, F., Jarv, J., Weise, C. 1991. Substrate-binding sites in acetylcholinesterase. Trends Pharmacol Sci 12:422–26.

Hughes, R., Chapple, D. J. 1976. Effects of non-depolarizing neuromuscular blocking agents on peripheral autonomic mechanisms in cats. Br J Anaesth 48:59–68.

Inestrosa, N. C., Perelman, A. 1990. Association of acetylcholinesterase with the cell surface. J Membr Biol 118:1–9.

Jones, R. S. 1985. New skeletal muscle relaxants in dogs and cats. J Am Vet Med Assoc 187:281–82.

Karlin, A. 2002. Emerging structures of nicotinic acetylcholine receptors. Nature Rev Neurosci 3:102–114.

Keller, R. S., Parker, J. L., Adams, H. R. 1992. Cardiovascular toxicity of antibacterial antibiotics. In D. Acosta, ed., Cardiovascular Toxicology, 2d ed. New York: Raven Press.

Kistler, J., Stroud, R. M., et al. 1982. Structure and function of an acetylcholine receptor. Biophys J 37:371–83.

Kita, M., and Goodkin, D. E. 2000. Drugs used to treat spasticity. Drugs 59:487–495.

Klein, L., Hopkins, J., Beck, E., et al. 1983. Cumulative dose responses to gallamine, pancuronium, and neostigmine in halothane-anesthetized horses: neuromuscular and cardiovascular effects. Am J Vet Res 44:786–92.

Larsen, L. H., Loomis, L. N., Steel, J. D. 1959. Muscle relaxants and cardiovascular damage: with special reference to succinyl-choline chloride. Aust Vet J 35:269–75.

Lees, P., Tavernor, W. D. 1969. The influence of suxamethonium on cardiovascular and respiratory function in the anaesthetized horse. Br J Pharmacol 36:116–31.

Lindquist, P. A., Lau, D. T. 1973. The use of succinylcholine in the handling and restraint of rhesus monkeys (*Macaca mulatta*). Lab Anim Sci 23:562–64.

Longnecker, D. E., Stoetling, R. K., Morrow, A. G. 1973. Cardiac and peripheral vascular effects of gallamine in man. Anesth Analg (Cleve) 52:931–35.

Lumb, W. V., Jones, E. W. 1973. Veterinary Anesthesia, p. 343. Philadelphia: Lea & Febiger.

Martyn, J. A. J., White, D. A., Gronert, G. A., Jaffe, R. S., Ward, J. M. 1992. Up-and-down regulation of skeletal muscle acetylcholine receptors. Anesthesiology 76:822–43.

Massoulie, J., Pezzementi, L., Bon, S., Krejci, E., Vallette, F. M. 1993. Molecular and cellular biology of cholinesterases. Prog Neurobiol 41:31–91.

McIntyre, A. R. 1972. In J. Cheymol, ed., Neuromuscular Blocking and Stimulating Agents, vol. 1, p. 187, Elmsford, NY: Pergamon.

Miller, R. D. 1979. Recent developments with muscles relaxants and their antagonists. Can Anesth Soc J 26:83–93.

Palmer, J. S., Jackson, J. B., Younger, R. L., et al. 1965. Normal cholinesterase activity of the whole blood of the horse and angora goat. Vet Med 58:885–86.

Pittinger, C., Adamson, R. 1972. Antibiotic blockade of neuromuscular function. Annu Rev Pharmacol 12:169–84.

Pittinger, C. B., Eryasa, Y., Adamson, R. 1970. Antibiotic-induced paralysis. Anesth Analg (Cleve) 49:487–501.

Pridgen, J. E. 1956. Respiratory arrest thought to be due to intraperitoneal neomycin. Surgery 40:571–74.

Radeleff, R. D., Woodard, C. T. 1956. Vet Med 51:512.

Reitan, J. A., Warpinski, M. A. 1975. Cardiovascular effects of pancuronium bromide in mongrel dogs. Am J Vet Res 36:1309–11.

Scholler, K. L., Goedde, H. W., Benkmann, H. 1977. The use of serum cholinesterase in succinylcholine apnoea. Can Anaesth Soc J 24:396–400.

Smith, S. M., Brown, H. O., Toman, J. E. P., et al. 1947. Lack of cerebral effects of *d*-tubocurarine. Anesthesiology 8:1–14.

Sunew, K. Y., Hicks, R. G. 1978. Effects of neostigmine and pyridostigmine on duration of succinylcholine action and pseudocholinesterase activity. Anesthesiology 49:188–91.

Tavernor, W. D. 1971. In L. Soma, ed., Textbook of Veterinary Anesthesia, p. 111. Baltimore: Williams & Wilkins.

Taylor, P. 2006a. Anticholinesterase agents. In L. L. Brunton, J. S. Lazo, and K. L. Parker, eds., The Pharmacological Basis of Therapeutics, 11th ed. New York: McGraw Hill.

———. 2006b. Agents acting at the neuromuscular junction and autonomic ganglia. In L. L. Brunton, J. S. Lazo, and K. L. Parker, eds., The Pharmacological Basis of Therapeutics, 11th ed. New York: McGraw Hill.

———. 1991. The cholinesterases. J Biol Chem 266:4025–28.

Tucker, W. K., Munson, E. S. 1975. Effects of succinylcholine and d-tubocurarine on epinephrine-induced arrhythmias during halothane anesthesia in dogs. Anesthesiology 42:41–44.

Unwin, N. 2005. Refined structure of the nicotinic acetylcholine receptor at 4Å resolution. J Mol Biol 346:967–989.

Unwin, N., Toyoshima, C., Kublaek, E. 1988. Arrangement of the acetylcholine receptor subunits in the resting and desensitized states determined by cryvelectromicroscopy of crystalized Torpedo postsynaptic membranes. J Cell Biol 107:1123–38.

Waser, P. G. 1967. Receptor localization by autoradiographic techniques. Ann NY Acad Sci 144:737–55.

———. 1972. In J. Cheymol, ed., Neuromuscular Blocking and Stimulating Agents, vol. 1, p. 205. Elmsford, NY: Pergamon.

Waud, B. E., Waud, D. R. 1972. The margin of safety of neuromuscular transmission in the muscle of the diaphragm. Anesthesiology 37:417–22.

Whittaker, V. P. 1990. The contribution of drugs and toxins to understanding of cholinergic function. TIPS 11:8–13.

Zaimis, E. J. 1959. In D. Bovet, F. Bovet-Nitti, G. B. Marini-Mettolo, eds., International Symposium on Curare and Curare-like Agents, p. 191. Amsterdam: Elsevier.

CHAPTER

10

INHALATION ANESTHETICS

EUGENE P. STEFFEY

Inhalation anesthetics are unique among the anesthetic drugs because they are administered, and in large part removed from the body, via the lungs. They are used widely for the anesthetic management of animals in part because their pharmacokinetic characteristics favor predictable and rapid adjustment of anesthetic depth. In addition, a special apparatus is usually used to deliver the inhaled agents. This helps minimize patient morbidity or mortality because it facilitates accurate and controlled anesthetic delivery, lung ventilation, and improved arterial oxygenation.

The search for anesthetic agents with ever greater safety and fewer side effects is ongoing. Over the nearly 150 years that inhalation anesthesia has been used in clinical practice fewer than 20 agents have actually been introduced and approved for general use with patients (Fig. 10.1). Fewer than 10 of these have had any history of widespread clinical use in veterinary medicine, and only 5 are of current clinical importance in North America. This chapter will focus on this last group of anesthetics (Table 10.1). The oldest two members of this group are nitrous oxide (N_2O) and halothane. Isoflurane is currently the most widely used inhaled anesthetic. Sevoflurane, the most recently introduced volatile agent has gained a notable share of the commercial market in veterinary medicine and is about to replace halothane (if it has not already done so) as the

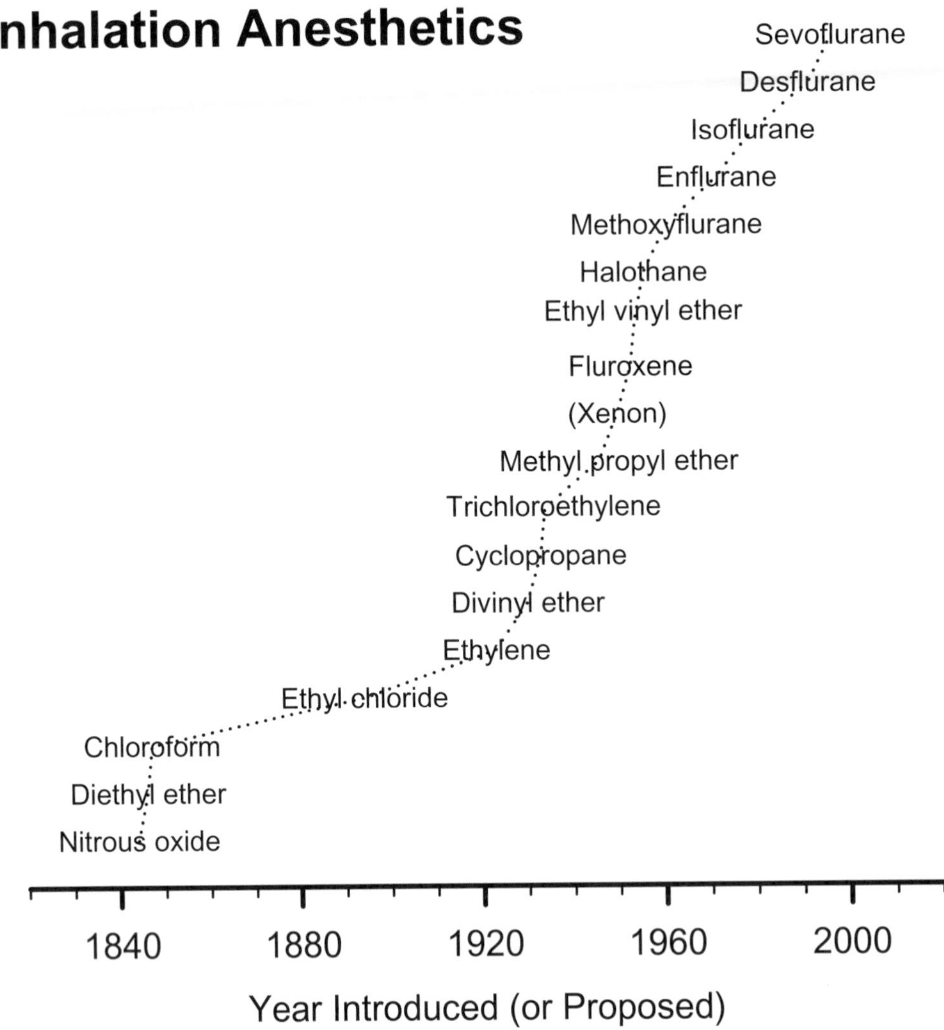

FIG. 10.1 Inhalation anesthetics introduced or proposed (xenon) for clinical practice (modified from Eger 1985).

TABLE 10.1 Inhalation anesthetic agents

Group 1: Agents in current use for animals	
Volatile	Gas
Halothane	Nitrous oxide (N_2O)
Isoflurane	
Desflurane	
Sevoflurane	
Group 2: Gaseous agent under investigation	
Xenon	
Group 3: Volatile agents of immediate past use/interest	
Enflurane	
Methoxyflurane	
Diethyl ether	

second most commonly used inhalation anesthetic for animal patients in North America. Finally, desflurane, the other newly introduced agent, like sevoflurane, is expensive and requires a unique vaporizer for delivery. As a result it presently has only very limited direct impact on the anesthetic management of animal patients. Unfortunately, none of these is the ideal inhalation anesthetic. An ideal agent would have characteristics that include a stable shelf life without preservatives and compatibility with existing delivery equipment. It would be inexpensive to purchase, nonflammable, and easily vaporized under ambient conditions. Such an agent would have a low blood solubility to foster rapid changes in anesthetic depth and permit rapid, controlled recovery from anesthesia. The ideal agent would be very potent, thereby allowing anesthesia at low inspired concentrations and maximizing flexibility of adjustments of inspired oxygen concentration. There would be no cardiopulmonary depression; the agent would not be irritating to airways and would be compatible with catecholamines and other vasoactive drugs. Finally, it would produce good skeletal muscle relaxation, resist degradation in the body, and be nontoxic to kidneys, liver, and gut.

The search for the ideal agent continues; however, with the possible exception of xenon, the author is unaware of any new agents near clinical introduction at this time. Xenon, a noble gas whose anesthetic properties were first described more than 50 years ago (Fig. 10.1) is once again being considered for clinical use with human patients (Lawrence et al. 1946; Lynch, III et al. 2000). However, despite its many advantages, improved manufacturing techniques, and development of more efficient systems to deliver it, the predictably high cost associated with its use will likely still discourage clinical application to veterinary practice.

A third group of inhalation anesthetics is comprised of agents that once enjoyed variable popularity for veterinary application (Table 10.1). These agents are no longer broadly used in clinical circumstances or are commercially unavailable so they will not be discussed beyond brief mention of examples here. Data of typical contemporary interest regarding their action in species of clinical importance to veterinary medicine are generally lacking, but readers interested in further information on agents in this group are referred to early editions of pharmacology (Booth and McDonald 1988) and veterinary anesthesia textbooks (Hall 1971; Soma 1971; Lumb and Jones 1973; Short 1987a). This third group of anesthetics includes agents like chloroform and cyclopropane. These agents have long been discarded for general use in human and veterinary medical practice because they cause liver failure (chloroform) or are explosive (cyclopropane). Diethyl ether, on the other hand, was widely used for clinical anesthetic management of human patients and a variety of animals up to about 20 years ago but then was largely replaced by newer agents because it is flammable (Duncalf 1982). This characteristic negates its use in the environment of the modern operating room, which ordinarily includes a variety of electrical surgical support (e.g., electrocautery), anesthetic delivery and patient monitoring and ventilating devices. In this edition, enflurane and methoxyflurane have been moved from the previous edition's listing of minor agents of clinical use for animals to the listing of agents of historical interest (Table 10.1). Accordingly, their review in this edition's chapter has been downplayed to an only occasional mention in various sections. Readers interested in more veterinary-related review of these drugs are directed elsewhere (Steffey 1996, 2001).

PHYSIOCHEMICAL CHARACTERISTICS

The chemical structure of inhalation anesthetics and their physical properties are important determinants of their actions and safety of administration. Consequently, brief discussion of aspects of Figure 10.2 and Table 10.2 is appropriate because physiochemical characteristics determine and/or influence practical considerations such as how the agents are supplied by the manufacturer (e.g., as a gas or as a liquid), the stability of the anesthetic molecule to degradation by physical factors (e.g., heat, light) and by substances it contacts during use (e.g., metal, soda lime). The equipment necessary to safely deliver the agent to the patient (e.g., vaporizer, breathing apparatus) is influenced by some of these properties as are the agent's uptake by the patient and its distribution within and elimination

TABLE 10.2 Some physiochemical properties of volatile anesthetics

Property	Desflurane	Halothane	Isoflurane	Sevoflurane	Enflurane	Methoxyflurane
Molecular weight	168	197	185	200	185	165
Liquid specific gravity (20°C) (g/ml)	1.47	1.86	1.49	1.52	1.52	1.42
Boiling point (°C)	23.5	50	49	59	57	105
Vapor pressure						
20°C (68°F)	664	244	240	160	172	23
24°C (75°F)	798	288	286	188	207	28
ml of vapor/ml of liquid at 20°C	209.7	227	195	183	198	207
Preservative necessary	No	Yes	No	No	No	Yes
Stability in soda lime	Yes	Decomposes	Yes	Decomposes	Yes	Decomposes

Sources: Wallin et al. (1975), Lowe and Ernst (1981), Eger, II (1985a, 1993), Jones (1990), Miller and Greene (1990), Laster et al. (1994).

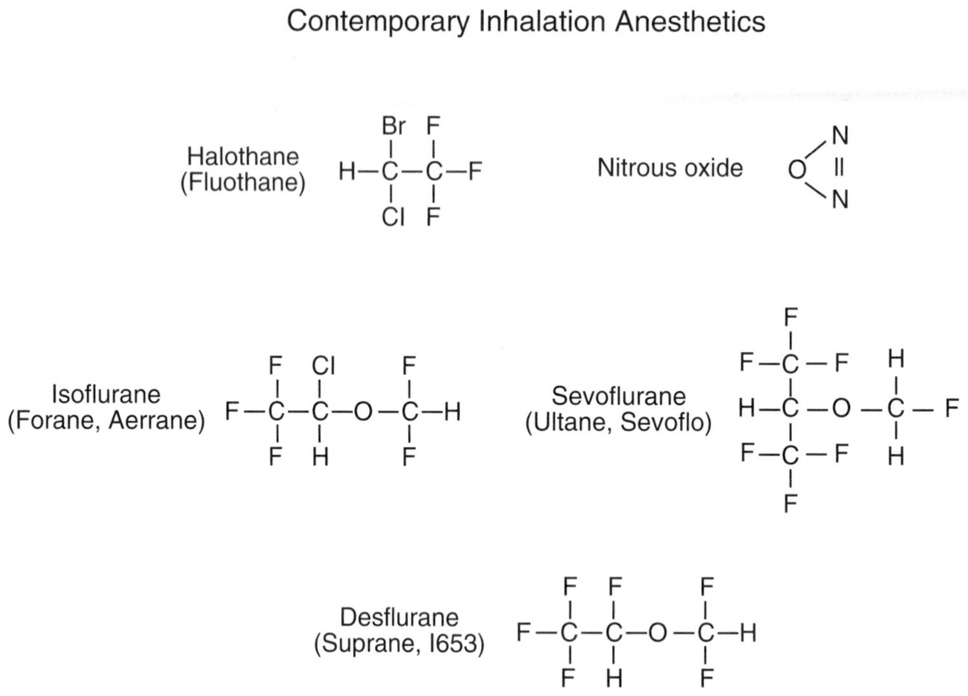

Contemporary Inhalation Anesthetics

Halothane (Fluothane)

Nitrous oxide

Isoflurane (Forane, Aerrane)

Sevoflurane (Ultane, Sevoflo)

Desflurane (Suprane, I653)

FIG. 10.2 Chemical structure of contemporary inhalation anesthetics. Trade names are in parentheses.

(including potential for metabolic breakdown) from the patient.

CHEMICAL CHARACTERISTICS. All contemporary inhalation anesthetics are organic compounds except nitrous oxide (N_2O) (Fig. 10.2). Agents of current interest are further classified as either aliphatic (i.e., straight or branch chained) hydrocarbons or ethers (i.e., two organic radicals [R] attached to an atom of oxygen; the general structure is RCOCR).

In the continued search for a less reactive, more potent, nonflammable inhalation anesthetic, focus on halogenation (i.e., addition of fluorine, chlorine, or bromine; iodine is least useful) of these compounds has predominated. Chlorine and bromine especially convert many compounds of low anesthetic potency to more potent drugs. Historically, interest in fluorinated derivatives was delayed until the 1940s because of difficulties in synthesis, and thus quantities available for study were limited. Methods of synthesis, although difficult, have improved considerably and have facilitated discovery of currently used agents (Fig. 10.1). Interestingly, organic fluorinated compounds are a group of extreme contrasts: some are toxic, others are not; some are extremely inert, others are highly reactive. In some anesthetics fluorine is substituted for chlorine or bromine to improve stability but at the expense of reduced anesthetic potency and solubility.

Halothane (Fig. 10.2) is a halogenated aliphatic saturated hydrocarbon (ethane). Predictions that halogenated structure would provide nonflammability and molecular stability encouraged the development of halothane in the early 1950s. However, soon after clinical introduction it was observed that the concurrent presence of halothane and catecholamines increased the incidence of life-threatening cardiac arrhythmias in human patients. An ether linkage in the molecule favors a reduced incidence of cardiac arrhythmias. Consequently, this chemical structure is a predominant characteristic of all agents developed or proposed for clinical use since the introduction of halothane (Fig. 10.2).

Despite many favorable characteristics and improvements over earlier anesthetics (Fig. 10.1), including improved chemical stability, halothane is susceptible to decomposition. Accordingly, halothane is stored in dark bottles, and a very small amount of a preservative, thymol, is added to it to retard breakdown. Thymol is much less volatile than halothane and over time collects within the

TABLE 10.3 Partition coefficients at 37°C

Agent	Blood/Gas	Oil/Gas	Brain/Blood	Heart/Blood	Liver/Blood	Kidney/Blood	Muscle/Blood	Fat/Blood
Desflurane	0.45	19	1.2	1.2	1.5	0.9	1.7	29
N_2O	0.46	1.4	1.1	1.0	—	—	1.2	2.4
Sevoflurane	0.65	47	1.7	1.7	2.0	1.2	2.6	52
Isoflurane	1.4	98	1.6	1.6	1.9	1.0	2.6	50
Enflurane	2.0	96	1.4	—	1.9	1.0	1.1	42
Halothane	2.4	224	1.9	1.7	2.3	1.3	2.9	57
Methoxyflurane	15	970	1.3	—	1.9	0.7	1.0	60
Xenon	0.12	1.8	1.6	—	—	0.9	0.9	—

Values summarized from direct measurements of human tissue or derived from measurements, both cited in Eger, II (1985a), Eger, II et al. (2003). Values for xenon from Goto et al. (1998), Lynch, III et al. (2000).

devices used to control delivery of the volatile anesthetic (i.e., vaporizers) and causes them to malfunction. To achieve greater molecular stability, fluorine is substituted for chlorine or bromine in the anesthetic molecule. This chemical manipulation adds shelf life to the substance and negates the need for additives such as thymol. Unfortunately, the fluorine ion is also toxic to some tissues (e.g., kidneys), which is of substantial concern if the parent compound (e.g., methoxyflurane, enflurane, sevoflurane; Fig. 10.2) is not resistant to metabolism.

PHYSICAL CHARACTERISTICS. In simplest form the administration of inhalation anesthetics requires a carrier gas that must include oxygen, a source of anesthetic, and a patient breathing circuit. For very small animals (e.g., laboratory rodents or small birds) this may mean nothing more than placing the animal in a closed air-filled chamber that contains a cotton pledget saturated with liquid anesthetic (e.g., isoflurane). With larger animals and/or to provide more controlled delivery of anesthetic and O_2 it is more appropriate to use specialized equipment. Such equipment, though more complex, greatly improves the safety of the anesthetic technique. It includes what is commonly referred to as an anesthetic machine, one or more vaporizers, and a patient breathing circuit. Extensive reviews of basic and advanced anesthetic equipment are available elsewhere (Short 1987b; Hartsfield 1996; Dorsch and Dorsch 1999; Brockwell and Andrews 2005).

The chain of events whereby anesthetic is transferred under control from a container to sites of action in the central nervous system (CNS) involves many physical characteristics that can be quantitatively described (Tables 10.2–10.4). The practical clinical applications of these quantitative descriptions will be briefly reviewed here.

TABLE 10.4 Rubber or plastic/gas partition coefficients at room temperature

Agent	Rubber	Polyvinyl chloride	Polyethylene
Desflurane	19	35	16
N_2O	1.2	—	—
Sevoflurane	29	68	31
Isoflurane	62	110	2
Enflurane	74	120	2
Halothane	120	190	26
Methoxyflurane	630	—	118

Values summarized from direct measurements cited in Eger, II (1985a), Eger, II et al. (2003).

More in-depth background information is available elsewhere (Hill 1980; Lowe and Ernst 1981; Eger, II 1990).

The physical characteristics of importance to this review are divided into two general categories; those that determine the means by which the agents are administered and those that help determine their kinetics in the body. This information is applied in the clinical manipulation of anesthetic induction and recovery and in facilitating changes in anesthetic levels in timely fashion.

PROPERTIES DETERMINING METHODS OF ADMINISTRATION

A variety of physical properties determine the means by which inhalation anesthetics are administered. These include molecular weight, boiling point, liquid density (specific gravity), and vapor pressure.

GAS VERSUS VAPOR. Inhalation anesthetics are either gases or vapors. In relation to inhalation anesthetics the term *gas* refers to an agent, like N_2O (or xenon), that exists in its gaseous form at room temperature and sea-level pressure. The term *vapor* indicates the gaseous state of a substance that at ambient temperature and pressure is a liquid. With the exception of N_2O and xenon, all the contemporary anesthetics fall into this category. Desflurane (Table 10.2), one of the newest volatile liquids, comes close to the transition stage and has some properties unique among the inhalation anesthetics and these will be discussed later in this chapter.

Regardless whether inhalation agents are supplied as a gas or volatile liquid under ambient conditions, the same physical principles apply to each agent when in the gaseous state.

METHODS OF DESCRIPTION. Quantities of inhalation anesthetic agent are usually characterized by one of three methods: pressure (e.g., in mmHg), concentration (in volumes %), or mass (in mg or g). The form most familiar to clinicians is that of concentration (e.g., *X*% of agent A in relation to the whole gas mixture). Modern monitoring equipment samples inspired and expired gases and provides concentration readings for inhalation anesthetics. Precision vaporizers used to control delivery of inhalation anesthetics are calibrated in percentage of agent, and effective doses are almost always reported in percentages. Pressure is also an important way of describing inhalation anesthetics and will be discussed next. Finally, the molecular weight and agent density are used in many calculations to convert from liquid to vapor volumes and mass (Hill 1980).

VAPOR PRESSURE. The vapor pressure of an anesthetic is a measure of its ability to evaporate; i.e., it is a measure of the tendency for molecules in the liquid state to enter the gaseous (vapor) form. The vapor pressure of a volatile anesthetic must at least be sufficient to provide enough molecules of anesthetic in the vapor state to produce anesthesia at ambient conditions. The *saturated vapor pressure* represents a maximum concentration of molecules in the vapor state that can exist for a given liquid at each temperature. The *saturated vapor concentration* can be easily determined by relating the vapor pressure to the ambient pressure. Using halothane and associated information from Table 10.2 as an example, we see that a maximal concentration of 32% halothane is possible under usual operating-room conditions; that is, $244/760 \times 100 = 32\%$, where 244 mmHg is the vapor pressure at 20C and 760 mmHg is the barometric pressure at sea level. Thus, other variables considered constant, the greater the vapor pressure, the greater the concentration of the drug deliverable to the patient. Therefore, again from Table 10.2, halothane, for example, is more volatile than sevoflurane and less volatile than desflurane under similar conditions.

BOILING POINT. The boiling point of a liquid is defined as the temperature at which the vapor pressure of the liquid is equal to the atmosphere pressure. Customarily, the boiling temperature is stated for the standard pressure of 760 mmHg. The boiling point decreases with increasing altitude since the vapor pressure does not change but the barometric pressure decreases.

The boiling point of N_2O is −89°C at 1 atmosphere pressure, sea level. It is thus a gas under operating-room conditions. Because of this it is distributed for clinical purposes in steel tanks compressed to the liquid state at about 750 psi (pounds per square inch; 750 psi/14.9 psi [1 atmosphere] = 50 atmospheres). As the N_2O gas is drawn from the tank, liquid N_2O is vaporized, and the overriding gas pressure remains constant until no further liquid remains in the tank. At that point only N_2O gas remains, and the gas pressure decreases from this point as remaining gas is vented from the tank. Consequently, the weight of the N_2O plus tank rather than the gas pressure within the tank is a more accurate guide to the remaining contents of the tank (Haskins and Sansome 1979).

Desflurane, one of the two newest clinically available volatile anesthetics, poses an interesting problem since its boiling point (Table 10.2) is near room temperature. This characteristic accounted for an interesting engineering challenge in developing an administration device (i.e., vaporizer) for routine use in the relatively constant environment of the operating room and limits its use to a narrow range of circumstances commonly encountered in veterinary medical applications. For example, because of its low boiling point, even evaporative cooling has large influences on the vapor pressure and thus on the vapor concentration of gas mixtures delivered to the patient.

PROPERTIES INFLUENCING DRUG KINETICS: SOLUBILITY

Anesthetic gases and vapors dissolve in liquids and solids. The solubility of an anesthetic is a major characteristic of the agent and has important clinical ramifications. For example, anesthetic solubility in blood and body tissues is a primary factor in the rate of uptake and distribution within the body. It is therefore a primary determinant of the speed of anesthetic induction and recovery. Solubility in lipid bears a strong relationship to anesthetic potency, and the tendency to dissolve in anesthetic delivery components such as rubber influences equipment selection and other aspects of anesthetic management.

The extent to which a gas will dissolve in a given solvent is usually expressed in terms of its *solubility coefficient* (Table 10.3). With inhalation anesthetics solubility is most commonly expressed as a partition coefficient (PC). Other expressions of solubility include the Bunson and Ostwald solubility coefficients (Eger, II 1974; Hill 1980).

The PC is the concentration ratio of an anesthetic in two solvent phases, for example, blood and gas. It thus describes the affinity or capacity of an anesthetic for one solvent phase relative to another, that is, how the anesthetic will *partition* itself between two phases after equilibrium has been reached. Anesthetic gas movement occurs because of a partial pressure difference in the two phases so that when there is no longer any anesthetic partial pressure difference between the two phases, there is no longer any net movement of anesthetic in either phase direction, and equilibrium has been achieved. Solvent/gas PCs are summarized in Table 10.3. Values noted in this table are for human tissues since they are the most widely valued and thus the data are readily available in the anesthesia literature. Incomplete listings for some other species such as, for example, the pig are also available (Yasuda et al. 1990) and show some differences compared to listings for humans. Rubber/gas and plastic/gas PCS are given in Table 10.4. It is important to emphasize that many factors besides species can alter anesthetic agent solubility (Mapleson et al. 1972; Eger, II 1974; Eger and Eger, II 1985; Lerman et al. 1986). Perhaps most notable after the nature of the solvent is that of temperature.

Of all the PCs that have been described or are of possible interest, two are of particular importance in the practical understanding of anesthetic management. They are the blood/gas and the oil/gas solubilities.

BLOOD/GAS PARTITION COEFFICIENT. The blood/gas solubility (Table 10.3) is a measure of the speed of anesthetic induction, recovery, and change of anesthetic levels. For example, other factors considered constant, the lower the blood/gas PC, the more rapid the anesthetic induction or rate of change of anesthetic level in response to a stepwise change in anesthetic delivery. Further information regarding the influence of anesthetic blood solubility on practical aspects of anesthetic management is presented in the section on pharmacokinetics.

OIL/GAS PARTITION COEFFICIENT. The oil/gas PC is another solubility characteristic of clinical importance (Table 10.3). This PC describes the ratio of concentration of an anesthetic in oil (in this case olive oil is the generally agreed upon standard) and gas phases at equilibrium. The oil/gas PC correlates inversely with anesthetic potency (see section in this chapter titled "Anesthetic Dose: The Minimum Alveolar Concentration") and describes the capacity of lipids for anesthetic.

OTHER PARTITION COEFFICIENTS. Solubility characteristics for tissues (Table 10.3) and other media like rubber and plastic (components of anesthetic delivery equipment; Table 10.4) are also important. For example, tissue solubility determines in part the quantity of anesthetic removed from the blood to which it is exposed. The higher the tissue solubility, the longer it will take to saturate the tissue with anesthetic agent. Thus, other things considered equal, agents very soluble in tissues will require a longer period for induction and recovery. If the rubber goods are of substantial amount in the apparatus used to deliver the anesthetic to the patient (e.g., an anesthetic delivery apparatus for horses versus one used for dogs) and anesthetic agent solubility in rubber is large (see Table 10.4), the amount of uptake of anesthetic agent by the rubber may be of clinical significance because these things delay anesthetic induction. As noted in Table 10.4, the newest volatile agents, desflurane and sevoflurane, are not very soluble in rubber.

PHARMACOKINETICS: UPTAKE AND ELIMINATION OF INHALATION ANESTHETICS

The aim in administering an inhalation anesthetic to a patient is to achieve an adequate partial pressure or tension of anesthetic (P_{anes}) in the CNS to cause a desired level of anesthesia. Anesthetic depth varies directly with P_{anes} in the CNS. The rate of change of anesthetic depth is of obvious clinical importance and is directly dependent upon the rate of change in anesthetic tensions in the various media in which it is contained before reaching the CNS. This section will not provide an extensive review of these principles. If more information is desired, readers are directed to reviews by Eger, II (1974, 2005), Eger, II et al. (2003), Mapleson (1989), and Steffey (1991, 1994, 1996).

Movement of molecules of inhalation anesthetics, like O_2 and CO_2, occurs down partial pressure gradients (Fig. 10.3). Gases move from regions of higher tension to those of lower tension until equilibrium (i.e., equal pressure in the two media) is established. Thus, during anesthetic induction, the P_{anes} at its source, say in the vaporizer, is high (which, in turn as we recall, is dictated by the vapor pressure) and is progressively less as anesthetic travels from vaporizer to patient breathing circuit, from circuit to lungs, from lungs to arterial blood, and, finally, from arterial blood to body tissues (e.g., brain; Fig. 10.3). Of these, the alveolar partial pressure (P_A) of anesthetic is most crucial to our further understanding. The reasoning for this is as follows. The brain (and spinal cord) is very rich in blood supply, and the anesthetic in arterial blood (P_aAnes) rapidly equilibrates with brain (P_{brain}Anes). Usually gas exchange at the alveolar level is sufficiently efficient when the P_aAnes is close to P_AAnes. Thus, the P_{brain}Anes closely follows P_AAnes, and controlling the P_AAnes is a reliable indirect way for controlling P_{brain}Anes and anesthetic depth.

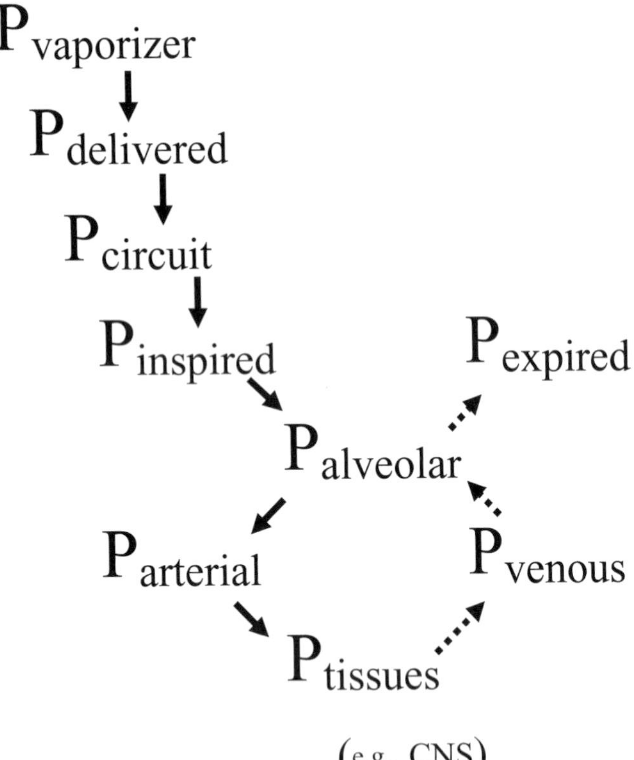

FIG. 10.3 The flow pattern of inhaled anesthetic agents during anesthetic induction and recovery. Inhalation anesthetics may be viewed as the development of a series of partial pressure (tension) gradients. During induction there is a high anesthetic tension in the vaporizer that decreases progressively as the flow of anesthetic moves from its source to the CNS. Some of these gradients are easily manipulated by the anesthetist while others are not or are done so with difficulty.

At this point it may also be helpful to recall that although the partial pressure of anesthetic is of primary importance, we frequently define clinical dose of an inhaled anesthetic in terms of concentration (C; i.e., volumes %). As previously noted, this is because it is common practice for the clinician to regulate and/or measure respiratory and anesthetic gases in volumes %. In addition, in the gaseous phase the relationship between the P_{anes} and the C_{anes} is a simple one:

$$P_{anes} = \text{fractional anesthetic concentration} \times \text{total ambient pressure}$$

The fractional anesthetic concentration is of course $C_{anes}/100$. However, as we reviewed in the section above, in the blood or tissue phases, for example, the actual quantity of anesthetic vapor contained in this solvent phase depends on both the P_{anes} and the anesthetic solubility (or PC) in the solvent phase. Consequently, at equilibrium, the partial pressure in all phases will be equal, but the concentration will vary.

The P_A of anesthetic is a balance between anesthetic input (i.e., delivery to the alveoli) and loss (uptake by blood and body tissues) from the lungs (Fig. 10.3). A rapid rise in P_A of anesthetic is associated with a rapid anesthetic induction or change in anesthetic depth. Factors that contribute to a rapid change in P_A of anesthetic are summarized in Figure 10.4.

DELIVERY TO THE ALVEOLI. Delivery of anesthetic to the alveoli and therefore the rate of rise of the alveolar concentration or fraction (F_A) toward the inspired concentration or fraction (F_I) depends on the inspired anesthetic concentration itself and the magnitude of alveolar ventilation. Increasing either one of these or both increases the rate of rise of the P_A of anesthetic; that is, other things considered equal, there is an increase in speed of anesthetic induction or change in anesthetic level.

A. Increased alveolar delivery of anesthetic
   1. Increased inspired anesthetic concentration
      a. Increased vaporization of agent
      b. Increased vaporizer dial setting
      c. Increased anesthetic-laden fresh gas inflow to the patient breathing circuit
      d. Decreased gas volume of patient breathing circuit
      e. Vaporizer positioned in a patient rebreathing circuit
   2. Increased alveolar ventilation
      a. Increased minute ventilation
      b. Decreased ventilation of respiratory system dead space
B. Decreased removal of anesthetic from the alveoli
   1. Decreased blood solubility of anesthetic
   2. Decreased cardiac output
   3. Decreased alveolar-venous anesthetic gradient

FIG. 10.4 Factors related to a rapid change in alveolar anesthetic tension.

Inspired Concentration. The inspired concentration has a number of variables controlling it. First of all, the upper limit of inspired concentration is dictated by the agent vapor pressure, which in turn is dependent on temperature. This may be especially important considering the breadth of veterinary medical application of inhaled anesthesia and methods of vaporizing volatile anesthetics under widely diverse conditions (e.g., some environmental conditions are quite hostile).

Characteristics of the patient breathing system in use can also be a major factor in generating a suitable inspired concentration under usual operating-room conditions. Characteristics of special importance include the volume of the system, the amount of rubber or plastic in the system, the position of the vaporizer relative to the breathing circuit (i.e., within or outside the circuit), and the fresh gas inflow to the patient breathing circuit.

Though of less concern with contemporary inhalation anesthetics, the solubility of some anesthetics (methoxyflurane was an extreme clinically important example; Table 10.4) in rubber and plastic will also delay development of an appropriate inspired anesthetic concentration. The loss of anesthetic to these equipment "sinks" serves to increase the apparent volume of the anesthetic circuitry and may, in some cases, be clinically important (e.g., use of rubber hoses and a large rubber rebreathing bag on circuits designed for anesthetic management of horses and other large animals).

Alveolar Ventilation. An increase in alveolar ventilation increases the rate of delivery of inhalation anesthetic to the alveoli. If unopposed, alveolar ventilation would rapidly increase the alveolar concentration of anesthetic so that within minutes the alveolar concentration would equal the inspired concentration. However, in reality the input created by alveolar ventilation is initially countered by the volume of the lung's functional residual capacity (FRC) and through a greater portion of the anesthetic period by absorption of anesthetic into blood. Predictably, hypoventilation reduces the rate at which the alveolar concentration increases over time compared to the inspired concentration; that is, anesthetic induction is slowed. Alveolar ventilation is altered by changes in anesthetic depth (increased depth usually means decreased ventilation), mechanical ventilation (usually increases ventilation), or changes in dead-space ventilation (i.e., for constant minute ventilation, a decrease in dead-space ventilation results in an increase in alveolar ventilation).

REMOVAL FROM ALVEOLI: UPTAKE BY BLOOD. As noted by Eger (Eger, II 1974) anesthetic uptake is the product of three factors: solubility (S; the blood/gas solubility, Table 10.3), cardiac output (CO), and the difference in the anesthetic partial pressure between the alveoli and venous blood returning to the lungs ($P_A–P_v$; expressed in mmHg); that is,

$$\text{Uptake} = S \times CO \times [(P_A - P_v)/P_{bar}]$$

where P_{bar} = barometric pressure in mmHg. Note that if any of these three factors equals zero, there is no further uptake of anesthetic by blood.

Solubility. The solubility of an inhalation anesthetic in blood and tissues is characterized by its partition coefficient (PC; Table 10.3).

Compared to an anesthetic agent with high blood solubility (PC), an agent with low blood solubility should be associated with a more rapid equilibration between tissue phases because a large amount of the highly soluble anesthetic must be dissolved in the blood before equilibrium is reached with the gas phase. In the case of the agent with a high blood/gas PC, the blood acts like a large "sink" into which the anesthetic is poured, and accordingly blood is "reluctant" to give up agent to other tissues (like the brain). For purposes of the present discussion, the blood only serves as a conduit for drug delivery to brain and spinal cord and as such can be visualized as a large or small pharmacologically inactive reservoir that is interposed between the lungs and the agent's site of desired pharmacological activity (i.e., brain and spinal cord). Therefore, an anesthetic agent with a low blood/gas PC is usually more desirable than a soluble agent, because it is associated with 1) a more rapid anesthetic induction (i.e., more rapid rate of rise in alveolar concentration during induction; Fig. 10.5), 2) more precise control of anesthetic depth (i.e., alveolar concentration during the anesthetic maintenance phase of anesthesia), and 3) a more rapid elimination of anesthetic and recovery from anesthesia (i.e., a rapid decrease in alveolar concentration during the anesthetic recovery phase).

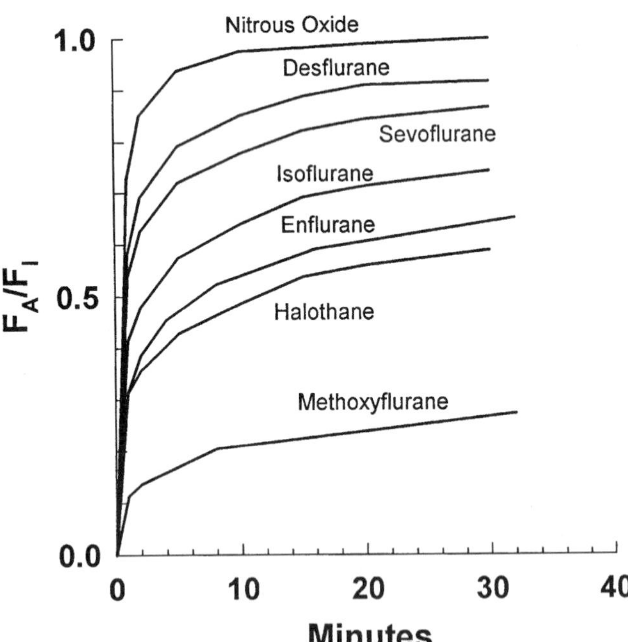

FIG. 10.5 The rise in the alveolar (F_A) anesthetic concentration toward the inspired (F_I) concentration. Note the rise is most rapid with the least soluble anesthetic, N_2O, and slowest with the most soluble anesthetic, methoxyflurane. All data are from studies of humans. The curves are redrawn from Eger and Eger, II (1985); Eger, II (1992).

Cardiac Output. The amount of blood flowing through the lungs and on to body tissues (cardiac output, or CO) also influences anesthetic uptake from the lungs. The greater the CO, the more blood passing through the lungs carrying away anesthetic from the alveoli. Thus, a large CO, like increased anesthetic agent blood solubility, delays the alveolar rise of P_{anes}. Patient excitement is an example in which a relatively large CO is anticipated. Conversely, a reduced CO should be anticipated with a patient in shock. Such a situation is associated with a relative increase in the rate of rise of the P_A of anesthetic and makes anesthetic induction more risky.

Alveolar to Venous Anesthetic Partial Pressure Difference. The magnitude of difference in anesthetic partial pressure between the alveoli and venous blood is related to the amount of uptake of anesthetic agent by tissues. Not surprisingly, the largest gradient occurs during induction. Once the tissues no longer absorb anesthetic (i.e., equilibrium between the two phases is reached), there is no longer any uptake of anesthetic agent from the lungs (i.e., the venous blood returning to the lungs contains as much agent as when it left the lungs). The changes in gradient in between these extremes result from the relative distribution of CO. In this regard it is important to recognize that roughly 70–80% of the CO is normally directed to only a small volume of body tissues in a lean individual (Table 10.5) (Eger, II 1974; Staddon et al. 1979; Webb 1985; Yasuda et al. 1990). That is, tissues such as brain, heart, hepatoportal system, and kidneys represent only about 10% of the body mass but normally

TABLE 10.5 Blood flow characteristics to tissue groups (Eger, II 1974)

	Tissue Group*			
	Vessel-Rich	Muscle	Fat	Vessel-Poor
% of body mass	10	50	20	20
% of cardiac output	75	19	5	<1

*Brain, heart, hepatoportal, kidney are examples of components of the "vessel-rich" grouping; ligaments, tendons, bone are examples within the "vessel-poor" tissue grouping.

receive about 75% of the total blood flow each minute. As a result these highly perfused tissues equilibrate with arterial anesthetic tension fairly rapidly (actual timing is influenced by agent solubility). Since the venous anesthetic tension equals that in the tissue within 10–15 minutes, about 75% of the blood returning to the lungs is the same as the alveolar tension. This presumes there has been no change in the mean time in arterial tension. Thus uptake is reduced. Skin and muscle compose the major bulk of the body (about 50% in humans) but at rest receive only about 15–20% of the CO, so saturation of this tissue group takes up to a few hours to accomplish. Fat is a variable component of body bulk and receives only a small proportion of blood flow. Consequently, anesthetic saturation of this tissue group is very slow, especially given that all anesthetics are considerably more soluble in fat than in other tissue groups (Table 10.3).

Other factors can further influence the magnitude of the alveolar-to-arterial anesthetic partial pressure gradient. They include abnormalities of lung ventilation/perfusion (Eger, II and Severinghaus 1964), loss of anesthetic via the skin (Stoelting and Eger, II 1969; Fassoulaki et al. 1991; Lockhart et al. 1991b) and into closed gas spaces (Eger, II 1974, 1985b, 2005), and metabolism (Eger, II 1974, 2005). These influences are special and/or are of lesser degree and therefore will not be further discussed here.

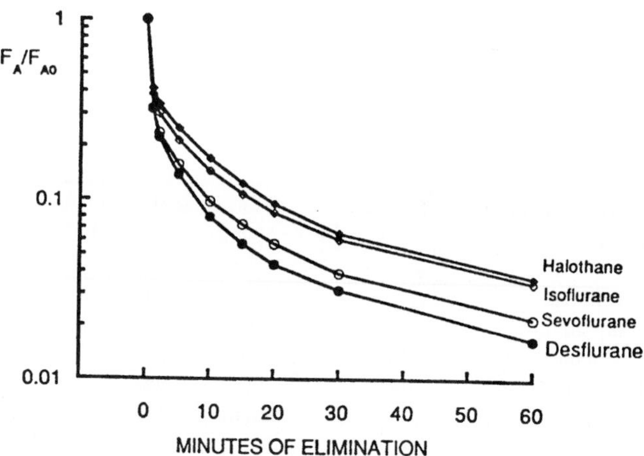

FIG. 10.6 The fall in alveolar (F_A) concentration relative to the alveolar concentration at the end of anesthesia (F_{A0}). Note that the newest, most insoluble volatile anesthetic, desflurane, is eliminated in humans more rapidly than the other contemporary potent anesthetics. Not shown is information for methoxyflurane; if present, the curve for methoxyflurane would appear above that for halothane (from Eger 1992; reprinted with permission).

ANESTHETIC RECOVERY. Recovery from inhalation anesthesia results from the elimination of anesthetic from the CNS. This requires a decrease in alveolar anesthetic partial pressure (concentration), which in turn fosters a decrease in arterial and then CNS anesthetic partial pressure (Fig. 10.3). Prominent factors accounting for recovery are the same as those for anesthetic induction. Therefore, factors such as alveolar ventilation, CO, and especially agent solubility play prominent roles in recovery from inhalation anesthesia. Indeed, the graphic curves representing the washout of anesthetic from the alveoli versus time (Fig. 10.6) are essentially the inverse of the wash-in curves seen earlier (Fig. 10.5). That is, the washout of the less soluble anesthetics is high at first, then rapidly declines to a lower output level that continues to decrease but at a slower rate.

The output with the more soluble agent is also high at first, but the magnitude of decrease in alveolar anesthetic concentration is less and only more gradually decreases with time (Fig. 10.6). Thus recovery from the two newest agents, desflurane and sevoflurane is faster than with isoflurane and even more so than the older agents (Eger, II et al. 1987; Frink, Jr. et al. 1992b).

A factor that is important in the rate of recovery but not during the induction period is the duration of anesthesia. Because there is a greater reserve in the body of more soluble agents like halothane (even more so for methoxyflurane) after a prolonged administration, its alveolar concentration will be slow to fall in comparison to a less soluble agent like sevoflurane or desflurane (Eger, II and Johnson 1987; Eger, II 1993; Eger et al. 1998). Similarly, dose of anesthetic also influences recovery rate following anesthesia; a longer recovery time follows a higher alveolar dose of a given anesthetic and among anesthetics the magnitude of influence is directly related to agent's blood/gas partition coefficient (Eger, II 1993).

Other factors that are important to varying but smaller degrees to inhalation anesthetic elimination from the body include percutaneous loss (Stoelting and Eger, II 1969; Cullen and Eger, II 1972; Fassoulaki et al. 1991; Lockhart et al. 1991b) and intertissue diffusion of agents (Carpenter et al. 1986a, 1987). Metabolism may also play a small role with some inhalation anesthetic agents (e.g., methoxyflurane and perhaps even halothane;) (Cahalan et al. 1981; Carpenter et al. 1986b, 1987; Baden and Rice 2000), especially in cases of clinically unusual, prolonged

TABLE 10.6 Biotransformation of inhalation anesthetics in humans

Anesthetic	Anesthetic Recovered as Metabolites (%)	Reference
Methoxyflurane	50	Holaday et al. (1970)
Halothane	20–25	Rehder et al. (1967), Cascorbi et al. (1970)
Sevoflurane	3	Eger, II (1994)
Enflurane	2.4	Chase and Holaday (1971)
Isoflurane	0.17	Holaday et al. (1975)
Desflurane	0.02	Eger, II (1994)
Nitrous oxide	0.004	Hong et al. (1980b)

TABLE 10.7 The minimum alveolar concentration (MAC) of inhalation anesthetics

Anesthetic	Cat	Dog	Horse	Human
Methoxyflurane	0.23	0.29	0.28	0.16
Halothane	1.04	0.87	0.88	0.74
Isoflurane	1.63	1.30	1.31	1.15
Enflurane	2.37	2.06	2.12	1.68
Sevoflurane	2.58	2.36	2.31	2.05
Desflurane	9.79	7.20	8.06	7.25
Xenon[a]	—	119	—	71
Nitrous oxide	255	222	205	104

[a]Lynch, III et al. (2000).

anesthesia. No appreciable effect on recovery by metabolism is expected for agents such as isoflurane and the newer agents desflurane and sevoflurane.

BIOTRANSFORMATION. Inhalation anesthetics are not chemically inert (Van Dyke et al. 1964). They undergo varying degrees of metabolism (Table 10.6), primarily in the liver but also to lesser degrees in the lung, kidney, and intestinal tract (Stier et al. 1964; Rehder et al. 1967; Holaday et al. 1970; Mazze and Fujinaga 1989; Martin, Jr. and Njoku 2005). The importance of this is twofold. First, in a very limited way with older anesthetics, metabolism may facilitate anesthetic recovery (supra vide). Second and more important is the potential for acute and chronic toxicities by intermediary or end metabolites of inhalation agents on, especially, kidneys, liver, and reproductive organs (Mazze and Fujinaga 1989; Martin, Jr. and Njoku 2005).

For further information on the biotransformation of inhalation anesthetics in general and for specific details regarding individual anesthetic agents, see reviews by Mazze and Fujinaga (1989) and Martin, Jr. and Njoku 2005).

ANESTHETIC DOSE: THE MINIMUM ALVEOLAR CONCENTRATION. In 1963 Merkel and Eger described what has become the standard index of anesthetic potency for inhalation anesthetics: MAC (Merkel and Eger, II 1963). MAC is the minimum alveolar concentration of an anesthetic that prevents gross purposeful movement in 50% of subjects exposed to a supramaximal noxious stimulus. Thus, MAC corresponds to the effective dose-50, or ED_{50}; half of the subjects are anesthetized and half are not. The dose that corresponds to the ED_{95} (95% of the individuals are anesthetized), at least in humans, is 20–40% greater than MAC (deJong and Eger, II 1975); and 2.0 times the MAC (i.e., 2 MAC) represents a deep level of anesthesia, in some cases even an anesthetic overdose. MAC values for contemporary inhalation anesthetics for a variety of animals commonly encountered in clinical veterinary medicine and humans are summarized in Table 10.7.

The anesthetic potency of an inhaled anesthetic is inversely related to MAC (i.e., potency = 1/MAC). From information presented above it also follows that MAC is inversely related to the oil/gas PC. Thus, a very potent anesthetic (e.g., methoxyflurane) has a low MAC value and a high oil/gas PC; an agent of low anesthetic potency (e.g., N_2O) has a high MAC and a low oil/gas PC.

A number of characteristics of MAC deserve emphasis (Eger, II 1974). MAC is defined in terms of a percentage of 1 atmosphere and therefore represents an anesthetic partial pressure at the anesthetic site of action (i.e., remember $P_x = C/100\ C\ P_{bar}$, where P_x stands for the partial pressure of the anesthetic in the gas mixture, C is the anesthetic concentration in volumes %, and P_{bar} is the barometric, or total, pressure of the gas mixture). Thus, although the concentration at MAC for a given agent may vary depending on ambient pressure conditions (e.g., sea-level versus high-altitude locations), the anesthetic partial pressure at MAC would be the same.

Second, the A in MAC represents *a*lveolar concentration, not the inspired or delivered (as, e.g., from a vaporizer) concentration. This is important because as we reviewed above (Fig. 10.3), after sufficient time for equilibration (i.e., minutes), alveolar partial pressure represents arterial and brain anesthetic partial pressures. In addition, the alveolar concentration is easily monitored with contemporary technology.

Finally, it is important to note that MAC is normally determined in healthy animals under controlled laboratory conditions in the *absence* of other drugs and other circumstances common to clinical use that may modify the requirements for anesthesia. There are many factors that may influence MAC (anesthetic requirement); some increase and some decrease MAC. This subject is beyond the scope of this chapter and readers are referred to reviews by Quasha et al. (1980) and Stoelting and Hillier (2006a).

PHARMACODYNAMICS: ACTIONS AND TOXICITY OF THE INHALATION ANESTHETICS

Inhalation anesthetic agents influence vital organ function. Some actions are associated with the use of all agents while other actions are a special or prominent feature of one or a number of the agents. The differences in actions, and in particular undesirable actions, of specific anesthetic agents are major considerations when selecting one agent over another for clinical use. Undesirable actions also provide important impetus for development of new agents and/or anesthetic techniques.

The following review of the actions and toxicity of inhaled anesthetics draws from results of studies of many different species, including humans (in some cases humans are the most completely studied species). Readers are encouraged to seek further information about species- and/or agent-specific from other notable reviews (Eger, II 1985a,b, 1993; Steffey 1991, 1994, 1996; Haskins and Klide 1992; Eger, II et al. 2003; Stoelting and Hillier 2006b).

It is important to stress that many variables commonly accompany anesthetic management of animals in both clinical and laboratory settings. These variables influence drug pharmacodynamics and may cause individuals to respond differently from test subjects that were studied under standardized conditions. Examples of such confounding variables include species, duration of anesthesia, noxious (surgical) stimulation, mechanical ventilation, coexisting disease, concurrent medications, and extremes of age. This subject is further discussed in the reviews noted above.

CENTRAL NERVOUS SYSTEM. Inhalation anesthetics produce a reversible generalized CNS depression for which the degree of depression is often described as depth of anesthesia. The components of general anesthesia have traditionally been considered to include unconsciousness, amnesia, analgesia, and immobility. Some also include in this concept suppression of autonomic reflexes. Most recently in attempting to better define the site(s) and mechanism(s) of action of inhalation anesthetics this list has been distilled to just two reversible qualities applying to all inhalation agents: amnesia and immobility in response to a noxious stimulus (Eger, II et al. 2003). Action within the spinal cord prevents movement in response to noxious stimulus (Antognini and Schwartz 1993; Rampil et al. 1993; Rampil 1994; Rampil and King 1996), while the higher CNS centers (exact locations not yet identified) mediate amnesia.

The cellular and molecular mechanisms of how inhalation agents act to produce general anesthesia remains unanswered. However, our understanding has increased substantially in the past decade as focused investigative activity to provide explanation has intensified. The mechanism of action of the inhalation anesthetics may or may not be similar to the mechanisms of action of injectable anesthetics.

Inhalation anesthetics disrupt nervous conduction of signals (transfer electrical activity). They do so by disrupting transfer of ions. As a result synaptic or axonal membranes or both are most often assumed to be the primary site of anesthetic action (Koblin 2005). Inhalation anesthetics considered broadly are structurally diverse, suggesting they do not act directly on a simple specific receptor. However, any plausible hypothesis identifying a site of action must account for the strong correlation between the effects of anesthetics at a site and the partition coefficient of the anesthetic, i.e., the Meyer-Overton rule (Fig. 10.7) (Meyer 1899; Overton 1901; Koblin 2005). A current ongoing debate is whether lipids or proteins are the primary sites of anesthetic action within the membrane (Overton 1901; Dilger 2001). Additional sources of review of our rapidly evolving understanding of this important topic appear briefly in Chapter 8 and in greater depth elsewhere (Antognini et al. 2003; Eger, II et al. 2003; Koblin 2005; Rubin et al. 2006).

Several anesthetic agents in contemporary use have epileptogenic potential, especially in predisposed individuals. Concern is that seizure activity may result in CNS (neuronal) injury if cerebral metabolic rate (substrate supply)

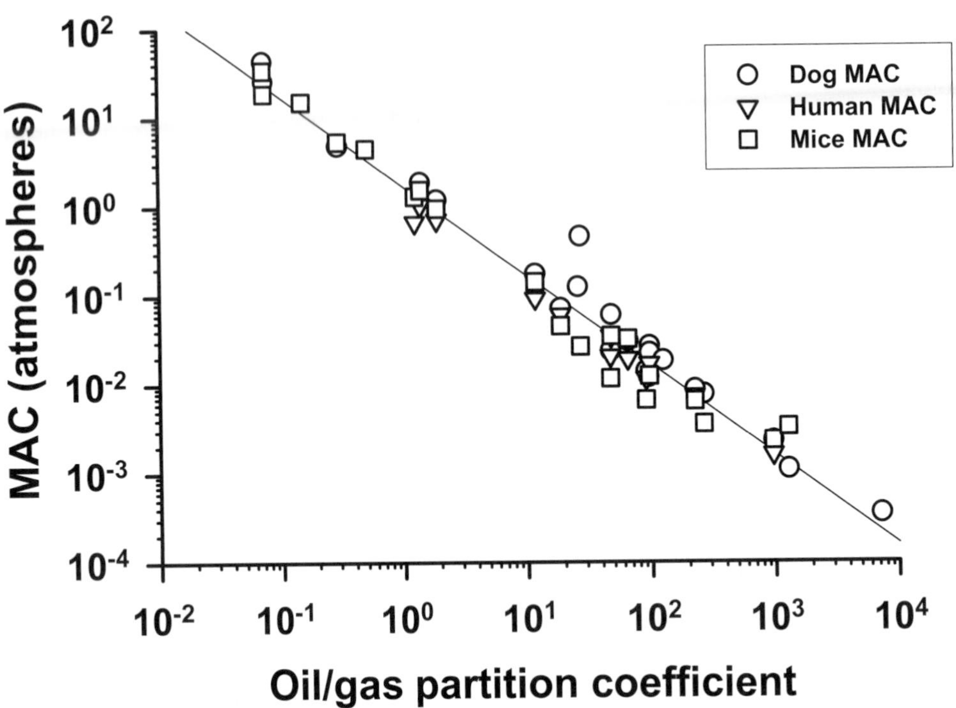

FIG. 10.7 Oil/gas partition coefficients versus potency (MAC) of inhalation anesthetics in dogs, humans, and mice (data from Koblin 2005).

exceeds supply. Both enflurane (Joas et al. 1971; Neigh et al. 1971) and sevoflurane (Adachi et al. 1992; Komatsu et al. 1994; Osawa et al. 1994; Woodforth et al. 1997; Newble 2000; Zhou et al. 2000) can predispose the brain to convulsive activity. Isoflurane (Koblin et al. 1981; Fukuda et al. 1996; Murao et al. 2000), sevoflurane (Karasawa 1991; Fukuda et al. 1996; Murao et al. 2000), and desflurane (Fang et al. 1997) can suppress convulsive activity induced by such drugs as bupivacaine, lidocaine, and penicillin.

The fragile relationship between cerebral blood flow, intracranial pressure, and cerebral metabolic rate for oxygen is an especially important consideration in some types of patients. For example, an increase in intracranial pressure can reduce cerebral perfusion pressure to the extent that cerebral blood flow is reduced. This situation may in turn result in a reduction of oxygen delivery below that of metabolic oxygen demands required for brain vitality.

Inhalation anesthetics are potent cerebral vasodilators and tend to increase cerebral blood flow. Anesthetic-induced cerebral vasodilation and associated increases in cerebral blood flow increase intracranial pressure usually to a trivial extent in normal individuals but perhaps to a life-threatening extent in patients with preexisting reduced intracranial compliance (e.g., tumor, hemorrhage). In such cases isoflurane with hyperventilation (changes in arterial carbon dioxide tension, P_aCO_2, result in corresponding directional changes in cerebral blood flow [Patel and Drummond 2005]) is preferred over a similar anesthetic management plan incorporating halothane.

RESPIRATORY SYSTEM. All contemporary inhalation anesthetics depress alveolar ventilation. As a consequence, the P_aCO_2 is increased in direct relation to anesthetic dose (MAC multiple; Fig. 10.8). The magnitude of P_aCO_2 is also species related (Fig. 10.9). In addition, the normal stimulation to ventilation caused by an increased P_aCO_2 and/or a low arterial oxygen tension (P_aO_2) is reduced (Knill and Gelb 1978; Knill et al. 1983; Dahan et al. 1994, 1996; Pavlin and Su 1994; Sarton et al. 1996; Sjogren et al. 1998, 1999).

Bronchospasm is associated with some diseases and other patient conditions and contributes to increased airway resistance. Among the earlier available volatile

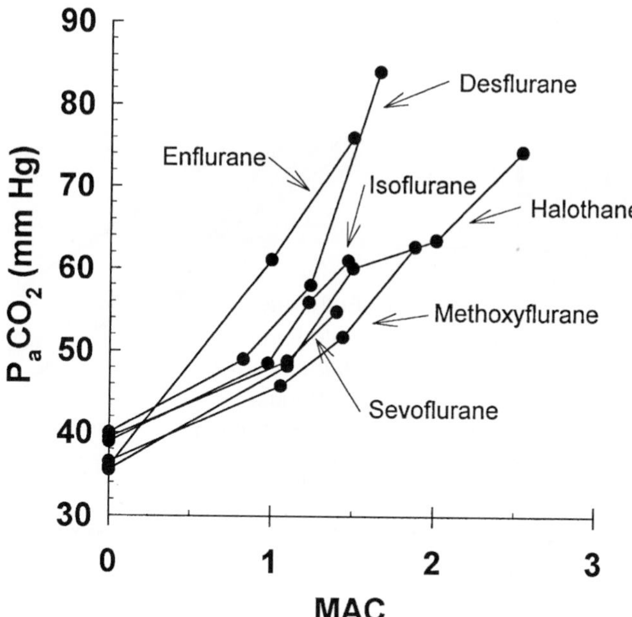

FIG. 10.8 A summary of the effects of contemporary volatile anesthetics on P_aCO_2 in humans, the species for which data are most complete (data from Munson et al. 1966; Larson, Jr. et al. 1969; Calverley et al. 1978; Rorabeck 1978; Doi and Ikeda 1987; Lockhart et al. 1991a).

anesthetics, halothane was the most effective bronchodilator (Klide and Aviado 1967; Coon and Kampine 1975). More recent work with isoflurane, sevoflurane, and desflurane indicate the relaxation of constricted bronchial muscles by these agents are equal to or exceed that caused by halothane (Hirshman and Bergman 1978; Lunam et al. 1983; Mazzeo et al. 1996; Habre et al. 2001).

Volatile inhalation anesthetics may inhibit reflex hypoxic pulmonary vasoconstriction and thereby contribute to a maldistribution of ventilation to perfusion and an increase in the alveolar-to-arterial partial pressure of oxygen and decrease in P_aO_2 (Marshall et al. 1984; Pavlin and Su 1994). However, results of in vivo studies of clinically relevant concentrations of volatile anesthetics suggest minimal or no inhibitory effects (Mathers et al. 1977; Fargas-Balyak and Forrest 1979; Domino et al. 1986; Lesitsky et al. 1998; Kerbaul et al. 2000; Kerbaul et al. 2001). Airway irritation caused by inspiring an inhalation anesthetic is undesirable. Airway irritation has not been generally recognized as a problem associated with induction of anesthesia in animals. However, human patients commonly react by breath-holding, coughing, and laryngospasm when exposed to concentrations of 7% or more desflurane early in the course of anesthesia (Eger, II 1993;

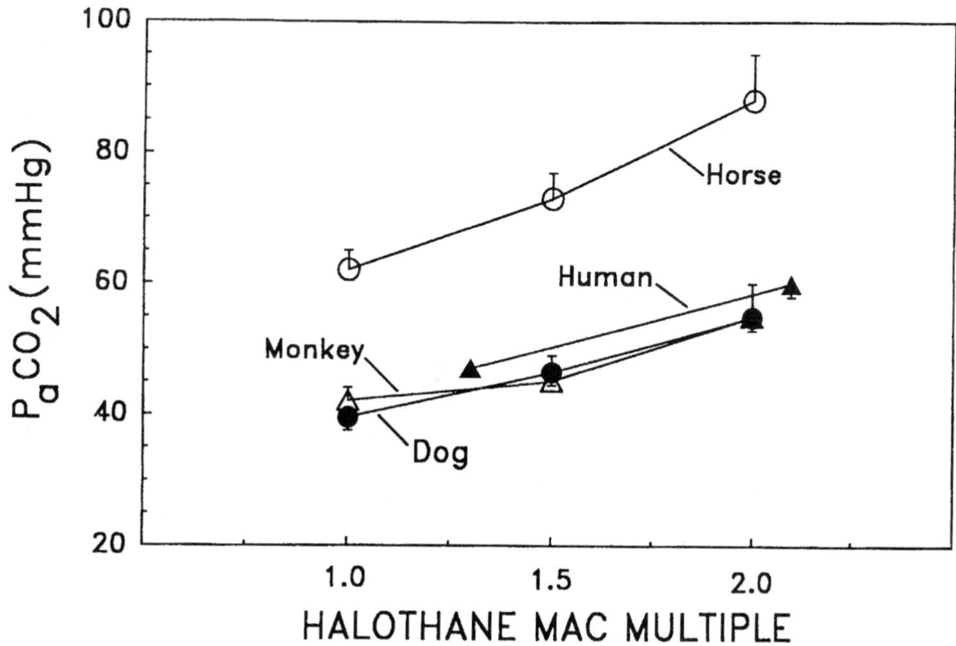

FIG. 10.9 The P_aCO_2 (mean ± SE; mm Hg) in spontaneously breathing, healthy dogs, horses, humans, and monkeys during halothane-oxygen anesthesia. The anesthetic dose is expressed as a multiple of the minimum alveolar concentration (MAC) for each species. Reproduced from Steffey (1991) with permission.

Terriet et al. 2000). As a result, desflurane is not commonly used for anesthetic induction in human patients.

CARDIOVASCULAR SYSTEM. Inhalation anesthetics may produce drug-specific and/or dose-related effect. Such effects may manifest as changes in arterial blood pressure, cardiac output, stroke volume, heart rate, and/or rhythm of heartbeat. Such changes may be caused by effects on myocardial contractility, peripheral vascular smooth muscle, and/or autonomic nervous system tone. Effects imposed by inhalation anesthetics may be further impacted by controlled versus spontaneous ventilation, concurrently administered drugs with direct or indirect hemodynamic actions, and preexisting cardiovascular disease.

All of the volatile anesthetics decrease cardiac output, usually via a decrease in myocardial contractility (Eisele, Jr. 1985; Eger, II 1985a; Pagel et al. 1991b, 1993; Boban et al. 1992; Warltier and Pagel 1992) and, in turn, stroke volume. The magnitude of change is dose related and dependent on agent (Klide 1976; Steffey and Howland, Jr. 1978a, 1980; Eger, II 1985a, 1994; Merin et al. 1991; Warltier and Pagel 1992; Swanson 1996; Mutoh et al. 1997). Arterial blood pressure is also decreased in a dose-related manner (Steffey et al. 1974a,b; Steffey and Howland, Jr. 1977, 1978a; Merin et al. 1991; Frink, Jr. et al. 1992c; Mutoh et al. 1997) (Fig. 10.10). The decrease in arterial blood pressure is usually related to a decrease in cardiac output, but in some cases (agent or species related) a decrease in peripheral vascular resistance may also play an important but lesser role.

All volatile anesthetics depress myocardial contractility via alterations of intracellular calcium homeostasis at several subcellular locations in normal cardiac muscle. The rank order of depression of contractile function is halothane = enflurane > isoflurane = desflurane = sevoflurane (Pagel et al. 2005). Volatile anesthetics can provide important beneficial effects on mechanical function during myocardial ischemia and myocardial reprofusion injury. For more complete review of mechanisms of action of volatile anesthetics on myocardial function readers are referred to the recent review by Pagel et al. (2005).

Inhalation anesthesia may alter the normal distribution of blood flow to organs. Specific effects are agent, dose, and time related (Vatner and Smith 1974; Manohar and Parks 1984a,b; Manohar and Goetz 1985; Bernard et al. 1991; Merin et al. 1991; Hartman et al. 1992; Eger, II et al. 2003). For example, volatile anesthetics cause a dose-dependent increase in cerebral blood flow (Patel and Drummond 2005) similar circumstances may decrease blood flow to liver and kidneys (Gelman et al. 1984a,b; Sladen 2005).

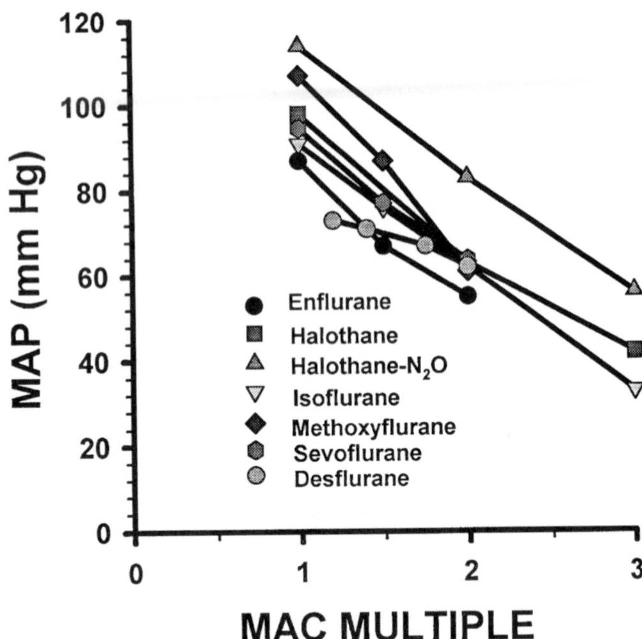

FIG. 10.10 Inhalation anesthetics cause a dose-dependent (expressed as multiples of MAC) decrease in mean arterial blood pressure (MAP) in dogs whose ventilation is mechanically controlled to produce eucapnia (data from Steffey et al. 1974b, 1984; Steffey and Howland 1978; Merin et al. 1991; Frink, Jr. et al. 1992c).

Temporal changes in cardiovascular function have also been reported in a variety of animals during inhalation anesthesia (Vatner and Smith 1974; Dunlop et al. 1987; Steffey et al. 1987b,c,d; Steffey et al. 1993a).

Cardiac Rhythm and Catecholamines. Inhalation anesthetics may increase the automaticity of the myocardium (Price 1966). This effect is exaggerated by adrenergic agonists (Katz and Epstein 1968). Inhalation anesthetics, especially halothane, also may sensitize the heart to arrhythmogenic effects of catecholamines (Raventos 1956; Joas and Stevens 1971; Munson and Tucker 1975; Johnston et al. 1976; Eger, II 1985a; Weiskopf et al. 1989; Moore et al. 1993; Navarro et al. 1994; Pagel et al. 2005).

LIVER. Hepatocellular injury may result as a general consequence of a reduction in hepatic blood flow or by direct volatile anesthetic agent toxicity (O'Connor et al. 2005).

Of the contemporary volatile agents, the metabolites of halothane are most often associated with direct hepatotoxicity (Kenna et al. 1988; Pohl et al. 1989). Direct hepatic injury from volatile anesthetics has decreased with each new generation of agent. The minimal degradation and rapid elimination of desflurane supports prediction of its improved safety (Eger, II et al. 1987; Jones et al. 1990c; Weiskopf et al. 1992; Steffey et al. 2005b).

KIDNEYS. All of the volatile anesthetics reduce renal blood flow and glomerular filtration rate in a dose-related manner (Malhotra et al. 2005). As a consequence, during anesthesia even healthy animals produce small volumes of concentrated urine. This response is a common finding regardless of the species studied. A transient increase in serum urea nitrogen, creatinine, and inorganic phosphate also may accompany inhalation anesthesia, especially if prolonged (Steffey et al. 1979, 1980, 2005a,b; Eger II 1985a). In most cases the effects of inhalation anesthesia on renal function are rapidly reversed after anesthesia. Beyond these general responses, methoxyflurane is notable with regard to its potential for causing nephrotoxicity (Mazze et al. 1971; Mazze 2006) (see below).

SKELETAL MUSCLE. The volatile anesthetics are associated with some small amount of skeletal muscle relaxation, likely a direct result of their CNS depression. They also enhance the muscle relaxation induced by the nondepolarizing neuromuscular blocking drugs that are sometimes used as adjuvants in the anesthetic management of patients.

Malignant hyperthermia, is a rare (except in certain strains of pigs and human family lines), life-threatening pharmacogenetic myopathy, that has been associated with all modern inhalation anesthetics. It is most commonly associated with halothane anesthesia. While both sevoflurane and desflurane can trigger induction of malignant hyperthermia, available data indicates these two more newly available volatile anesthetics are less potent triggers than halothane (Wedel et al. 1993; Allen and Brubaker 1998; Kudoh and Matsuki 2000). This topic will be further discussed below.

ACTIONS BY AGENT. Actions by agent will be discussed in this section. The volatile agents will be reviewed first, followed by the gaseous agent, N_2O. Despite some renewed interest in focused limited clinical use for human patients, xenon is not likely to see clinical use for veterinary patients and will therefore not be discussed further (Cullen and Gross 1951; Kennedy et al. 1992; Dingley et al. 1999; Lynch, III et al. 2000). The agents for further focal review are halothane, isoflurane, desflurane, and sevoflurane, and then, N_2O. Since the last edition of this textbook, isoflurane remains the most popular inhalation anesthetic in veterinary practice in North America, while the clinical use of halothane has further declined in favor of the two new volatile anesthetics. Likely, use of sevoflurane is presently at least about equal to halothane use in the U.S. Coverage of methoxyflurane, enflurane, and diethyl ether has been substanially downgraded here from previous editions of this text because of more limited worldwide availability and use with animals. For additional information on these three inhalation anesthetics and others such as chloroform, see previous editions of this textbook.

Halothane. *Halothane*, USP (Fluothane), a multihalogenated ethane, is a clear, volatile liquid. Introduction of halothane into clinical practice in 1957 represented a significant advance in anesthesia pharmacology, since the drug possessed characteristics of rapid induction and recovery, potency, and nonflammability, with minimal side effects (Brown and Sipes 1977). By 1960 halothane was the most popular potent anesthetic agent used in humans in the Western world. In present day its common use with both human and animal patients has been largely replaced by the newer volatile anesthetics and as a result its commercial availability is becoming more limited.

Biotransformation. About 60–80% of administered halothane is eliminated unchanged in the exhaled breath (Table 10.6). The remainder is eliminated via other routes either unchanged or as metabolites. Biotransformation of halothane occurs primarily in the liver; most as a result of the cytochrome P450 system in the endoplasmic reticulum of the hepatocytes. It has been well established that a major metabolite of halothane biotransformation in humans and animals is trifluoroacetic acid (Van Dyke and Wood 1975; Neubauer 2004). Other metabolites resulting from oxidative metabolism via the cytochrome P450 pathway are inorganic chloride (Cl^-) and to a lesser extent bromine (Br^-). Since the bond for fluorine (F^-) is much stronger than for Cl^- or Br^-, little F^- is released. In humans, Br^-

from halothane breakdown will induce headache, ataxia, lethargy, and EEG alterations (Tinker et al. 1976). In the dog (Pedersoli 1980) and horse (Rice and Steffey 1985a), serum bromide concentrations increase significantly during and following a period of halothane anesthesia.

An alternative route of halothane metabolism is via a reductive pathway requiring anaerobic conditions and the presence of an electron donor. Both Br^- and F^- are metabolites of this pathway (Neubauer 2004). An increase in halothane metabolism occurs in experimental animals when inducing agents such as phenobarbital and isoniazid are given prior to halothane (deGroot et al. 1982; Rice et al. 1987). Prolonged administration of low-dose halothane can also result in increased drug metabolism (Linde and Berman 1971; Ross and Cardell 1978). Such circumstances may have clinical consequences.

Central Nervous System. Halothane depresses CNS function in a dose-related fashion until respiratory and cardiovascular collapse and death. The MAC for halothane in the dog is 0.9%; values for some other species are given in Table 10.7.

Cerebral blood flow usually increases during halothane anesthesia and may result in an accompanying increase in cerebrospinal fluid pressure (Patel and Drummond 2005). Halothane is the most potent of the contemporary volatile anesthetics in this regard, making it a less desirable anesthetic for animals with preexisting space-occupying intracranial lesions and/or increased cerebrospinal fluid pressure. The cerebral metabolic oxygen consumption is reduced in dose-related fashion.

Shivering during recovery from halothane is common. Its cause is related to heat loss associated with general anesthesia and other ill-defined mechanisms (Sessler et al. 1988; Sessler 2006). Some drowsiness remains evident for several hours after halothane anesthesia even in ambulatory animals.

Cardiovascular System. Halothane depresses circulatory system function. Studies of a variety of mammals, including humans, indicate that cardiac output, stroke volume, and arterial blood pressure are less during halothane anesthesia compared to the awake, unmedicated individual. Further decreases in cardiovascular function accompany increasing alveolar doses of halothane (Eger, II et al. 1970; Steffey et al. 1974a,b, 1977; Steffey and Howland 1978; Steffey and Howland, Jr. 1980; Ingwersen et al. 1988; Grandy et al. 1989; Pavlin and Su 1994). For example, as halothane dose is increased, mean arterial blood pressure decreases because cardiac output decreases. Total peripheral vascular resistance changes very little; thus peripheral vasodilation is not the primary cause of hypotension in many of the species common to veterinary medicine. The reduction in cardiac output is caused by a decrease in stroke volume as a result of a direct drug-induced depression in myocardial muscle contractility.

Effects on heart rate vary widely depending on species and associated conditions. Often there is little change in heart rate over a range of clinical anesthetic doses. The rhythm of the heartbeat may vary during halothane anesthesia. Especially at light levels of anesthesia spontaneous arrhythmias may appear. There is some evidence that deeper levels of halothane anesthesia decrease this incidence (Muir et al. 1959; Purchase 1966).

Halothane is especially well noted for its likelihood to predispose the heart to premature ventricular extrasystoles in the presence of catecholamines (Purchase 1966; Pavlin and Su 1994). It is the most potent of the contemporary volatile anesthetics in this regard. Increased endogenous release of catecholamines may occur as a result of surgical stimulation and insufficient anesthesia or from an elevation in P_aCO_2 secondary to hypoventilation. Catecholamines (e.g., epinephrine) and other sympathomimetic amines are sometimes injected during anesthesia and surgery to facilitate patient management or reduce localized bleeding. Thus, anesthetic influence on heartbeat rhythm is not a trivial matter. Some anesthetic adjuvant drugs may increase (e.g., xylazine, thiopental, and thiamylal [Bednarski et al. 1985; Tranquilli et al. 1986]), and others may decrease (e.g., acepromazine, lidocaine; [Muir, III et al. 1975; Horrigan et al. 1978]), the arrhythmogenic dose of epinephrine during halothane anesthesia.

The baroreceptor reflex is a short-term central mechanism to aid in arterial blood pressure homeostasis. Halothane depresses the sensitivity of the baroreceptor reflex (Pavlin and Su 1994).

The cardiovascular effects of halothane change with duration of anesthesia. A time-related increase in arterial blood pressure, stroke volume, and cardiac output has been a common finding in studies of dogs (Steffey et al. 1987b), horses (Dunlop et al. 1987; Steffey et al. 1987d, 1990a,b, 1993a), and humans (Price et al. 1970; Bahlman et al. 1972).

Respiratory System. Halothane depresses respiration in a dose-related manner. As a result, the P_aCO_2 increases and there is less efficiency in oxygenating arterial blood and perhaps hypoxemia (Steffey et al. 1974a, 1975, 1977; Dobkin et al. 1976; Steffey and Howland 1978; Grandy et al. 1989). The volume of expired minute ventilation decreases initially as a result of a decrease in tidal volume; respiratory frequency also tends to decrease from awake conditions but the extent is species and condition variable. As anesthetic depth is increased, breathing rate also decreases. In otherwise unmedicated healthy dogs and horses the alveolar halothane concentration that is associated with complete respiratory arrest is 2.9 MAC (Regan and Eger, II 1967) and 2.6 MAC (Steffey et al. 1977), respectively.

Because halothane has bronchodilator action (Colgan 1965; Klide and Aviado 1967), it has been long considered the anesthetic agent of choice for patients with either a history of asthma or upon anticipated or real bronchospasm during induction or maintenance of anesthesia (Pavlin and Su 1994).

Liver. Hepatic blood flow is decreased during halothane anesthesia, mostly as a passive consequence of reduced cardiac output and decreased liver perfusion pressure. The reduced blood flow per se, unless extreme, is not usually of a magnitude to result in clinical consequences.

Hepatic dysfunction that sometimes occurs following inhalation anesthesia is most often associated with halothane. The etiology is unknown but the syndrome is likely actually multiple entities (Pohl and Gillette 1982; O'Connor et al. 2005). One entity is a mild transient form of hepatic dysfunction that is associated with all of the inhaled (or other) anesthetics and may result from hepatocyte hypoxia (perhaps as a result of reduced tissue oxygen delivery) (Ross, Jr. and Daggy 1981; Harper et al. 1982a,b; Shingu et al. 1982a,b). Another entity, "halothane hepatitis," is rarer but far more severe and often fatal. The most frequently invoked theories regarding its etiology include the metabolism of halothane to a (hepatic) reactive metabolite (Plummer et al. 1982) and the occurrence of an immune-mediated hypersensitivity (allergic) reaction, a process that is more directly hepatocellularly damaging. The immunological basis for halothane hepatitis has recently been extensively reviewed (Pohl and Gillette 1982; Hubbard et al. 1988).

Laboratory and clinical studies of some clinically important veterinary species (e.g., horses and ponies) indicate there are alterations in hepatic function and cellular integrity associated with halothane anesthesia (Gopinath et al. 1970; Gopinath and Ford 1976; Joyce et al. 1983; Engelking et al. 1984; Steffey et al. 1993c).

Kidney. Halothane is not known to have a direct nephrotoxic effect. However, diminution of renal function may occur secondary to an anesthetic reduction in renal blood flow and glomerular filtration rate. The effects reverse rapidly after anesthesia is discontinued (Steffey et al. 1980, 1991, 1993c).

Skeletal Muscle. Halothane causes some relaxation of skeletal muscle via its action on the CNS. It also increases the magnitude and duration of muscle relaxation induced by nondepolarizing neuromuscular blocking drugs (e.g., pancuronium).

Rarely, induction of anesthesia triggers a rapidly developing hypermetabolic reaction in the skeletal muscle of susceptible individuals. The syndrome was originally described as associated with halothane, but other inhaled anesthetics have also since been implicated. The resultant syndrome of malignant hyperthermia is characterized by muscle rigidity, a rapid rise in body temperature, large consumption of oxygen, and consequent production of CO_2. Death rapidly ensues in most cases unless very aggressive therapy is instituted. Dantrolene is currently the drug of choice for specific therapy.

It is most commonly reported in susceptible swine (Landrace, Pietrain, and Poland China) and human patients and is caused by an acute loss of intracellular control of calcium. The subject was recently reviewed by Gronert et al. (2005).

Undoubtedly malignant hyperthermia has been wrongfully diagnosed in the past as a cause for hyperthermia in some veterinary patients when a more detailed investigation would have revealed other causes.

Isoflurane. *Isoflurane*, USP (Forane, Aerrane), is a halogenated methyl ethyl ether. Isoflurane and enflurane are structural isomers. Both compounds contain the same number of atoms of fluorine, chlorine, carbon, hydrogen, and oxygen.

Isoflurane was first synthesized in 1965, and its widespread clinical use for human patients began in 1981. At least in North America, it is now the most widely used volatile anesthetic agent for human patients. Isoflurane is now also in widespread clinical use in veterinary patients. It is probably the most commonly used inhaled agent for dogs, cats, horses, and birds.

Biotransformation. In humans and animals isoflurane resists biodegradation. In humans less than 0.2% of the isoflurane taken up by the body is metabolized (Holaday et al. 1975); this rate of metabolism is far less than for halothane, methoxyflurane, and enflurane (Table 10.6). Both inorganic fluoride and trifluoroacetic acid have been identified as end products of isoflurane metabolism (Martin, Jr. and Njoku 2005). The resistance of isoflurane to metabolism accounts for the very small increase in serum fluoride concentration even after prolonged isoflurane administration (Cousins et al. 1973; Dobkin et al. 1973; Mazze et al. 1974).

Isoflurane is defluorinated by cow, dog, lamb, and rat hepatic microsomes (Rice and Steffey 1985b). In contrast to adult horses, it is not significantly metabolized by neonatal horses (Rice and Steffey 1985a).

The small quantities of degradation products account for the lack of direct renal or hepatic toxicity. Isoflurane also does not appear to be a mutagen, teratogen, or carcinogen (Eger, II et al. 1978; Eger, II 1985a).

Central Nervous System. Isoflurane, unlike its isomer enflurane, does not produce seizure activity. Cats given isoflurane display "sharp waves" (isolated spiking) on the EEG. This activity is also seen in cats with halothane, enflurane, and methoxyflurane and may be a species peculiarity (Julien and Kavan 1974; Kavan and Julien 1974).

Isoflurane has become the agent of choice for critically ill animal patients. The MAC for isoflurane is in the range 1.2–1.7% depending upon the species of focus (Table 10.7).

Isoflurane has anticonvulsant effects (Koblin et al. 1981). Electrical silence is seen on the EEG at 2 MAC (Clark and Rosner 1973).

Most studies in animals have shown that isoflurane causes less cerebral vasodilation than halothane (Eger, II 1985a; Drummond et al. 1986). Cerebral circulation autoregulation is maintained with isoflurane but is impaired by halothane (Miletich et al. 1976; Todd and Drummond 1984). For these reasons isoflurane is usually preferred over halothane for neurosurgery.

Cardiovascular System. Isoflurane depresses cardiovascular function in a dose-related fashion (Steffey and Howland, Jr. 1977; Steffey et al. 1977, 1987a; Eger, II 1985a; Ludders et al. 1989). The magnitude of its effect on arterial blood pressure is similar to halothane, although with isoflurane the cause is more related to a decrease in the systemic vascular resistance. Also like halothane it decreases cardiac contractility and stroke volume, resulting in a decrease in cardiac output. However, results of studies in a number of species indicate that isoflurane, especially at light and moderate levels, affects cardiac output less than halothane does. Isoflurane thus affords a wider margin of patient safety.

Heart rate tends to be better maintained during isoflurane and may be increased from awake conditions. It remains relatively constant over a range of alveolar isoflurane doses. Heart rhythm is usually little affected by isoflurane, and the incidence of dysrhythmias after injection of vasoactive substances (including catecholamines) is substantially reduced in comparison to halothane (Joas and Stevens 1971; Tucker et al. 1974; Johnston et al. 1976; Eger, II 1985a; Bednarski and Majors 1986).

As with halothane, duration of isoflurane anesthesia influences the magnitude of cardiovascular function, at least in some species (Dunlop et al. 1987; Steffey et al. 1987c).

Respiratory System. Isoflurane, like halothane, depresses respiration and increases P_aCO_2 (Steffey and Howland, Jr. 1977, 1980; Steffey et al. 1977; Eger, II 1985a; Pavlin and Su 1994). The magnitude of depression is dose and time related and is at least equal to or often greater than that caused by halothane under similar conditions (Cromwell et al. 1971; Steffey and Howland, Jr. 1977; Rorabeck 1978; Steffey et al. 1985; Eger, II 1985a; Hodgson et al. 1985a; Steffey et al. 1987c; Pavlin and Su 1994; Brosnan et al. 2003).

In some species, like the horse, during light and moderate levels of anesthesia respiration is characterized by large tidal volume and low breathing rate (Steffey et al. 1977; Hodgson et al. 1985a,b; Brosnan et al. 2003). Respiratory depression accompanying isoflurane anesthesia may be increased in magnitude by concurrent administration of opioids (Ossipou and Gebhart 1984; Steffey et al. 1993b), a common practice in clinical circumstances.

The alveolar concentration that causes apnea is 2.5 MAC for the dog (Steffey and Howland, Jr. 1977) and 2.3 MAC for the horse (Steffey et al. 1977).

The work of Hirshman in dogs sensitized to ascaris antigen suggests that isoflurane (and enflurane) is as effective in decreasing the constrictive ability of airway smooth muscle as halothane (Hirshman et al. 1982). Thus, isoflurane may serve as an acceptable alternative to halothane in animals with elevated airway resistance (Englesson 1974; Hirshman et al. 1982).

Liver. Blood flow to the liver is altered less by isoflurane than halothane, so isoflurane might be preferable to halothane in patients at risk for hepatic injury (Lunam et al. 1983; Seyde and Longnecker 1984; Gelman et al. 1984a,b; Gelman 1987). Results of tests of hepatic function and cellular integrity show only minimal changes following isoflurane anesthesia, and the changes are only transient in nature (Steffey et al. 1979; Eger, II 1985a; Daunt et al. 1992). Transient hepatic insult has been reported with hypoxemia and halothane but not isoflurane anesthesia (Whitehair et al. 1996).

Kidney. As with halothane, renal blood flow and urine volume are depressed with isoflurane. Changes in blood components related to renal function and/or injury are not seen or are small in magnitude and are rapidly reversed following anesthesia (Steffey et al. 1979; Eger, II 1985a; Daunt et al. 1992).

Isoflurane resists metabolism and the release of F^- is small, so direct renal toxicity by this drug is unlikely and this prediction has been supported by long-term, widespread clinical use in many species.

Skeletal Muscle. Isoflurane is more potent than halothane in its ability to enhance the neuromuscular blocking effect of nondepolarizing neuromuscular blocking drugs (Miller et al. 1972; Eger, II 1985a).

Isoflurane is among the anesthetic drugs reportedly able to trigger malignant hyperthermia (Gronert et al. 2005).

Muscle blood flow was better maintained in rats, dogs, and humans anesthetized with isoflurane than with halothane (Seyde and Longnecker 1984; Gelman et al. 1984b; Eger, II 1985a).

Desflurane. *Desflurane*, USP (Suprane), is one the two newest inhalation anesthetics released for general clinical use. Its actions have been investigated in humans and in a variety of animal species, including dogs, horses, and pigs. Broad reviews of its actions are available elsewhere (Eger, II 1993; Clarke 1999).

Desflurane, formally known as I-653, was first synthesized in the 1960s along with similar agents such as enflurane and isoflurane. It was not actively investigated at that time because it was difficult to produce and its greater anesthetic potency compared to other prospects was considered undesirable (Eger, II 1993). Its first reported use in humans was in 1990 (Jones 1990; Jones et al. 1990a,b).

Desflurane has a high vapor pressure (Table 10.2) and requires a newly designed, temperature-controlled, pressurized vaporizer for predictable delivery (Andrews et al. 1993). It has a very low solubility (Eger, II 1987) in blood (Table 10.3), and other tissues (Yasuda et al. 1989), contributing to greater precision of control over the maintenance of anesthesia and a very rapid emergence from anesthesia (Eger, II and Johnson 1987; Yasuda et al. 1990, 1991a,b; Jones et al. 1990a; Steffey et al. 2005b).

Biotransformation. Desflurane resists degradation by the body to a greater degree than any of the other volatile anesthetics (Koblin et al. 1988; Koblin 1992); actual amounts of degradation are too small to measure accurately. Results to date do not indicate any toxicity associated with its use in a variety of species. Although the magnitude of breakdown is different, desflurane is expected to be metabolized in a manner similar (parallel) to that for isoflurane (Neubauer 2004). Resulting products are free fluoride ions, trifluoroacetic acid, CO_2 and water (Eger, II 1993).

Central Nervous System. Desflurane is less potent than other contemporary volatile agents (Table 10.7). For example, MAC for the dog, horse, and pig is 7.2%, 8.1%, and 10.0%, respectively (Doorley et al. 1988; Eger, II et al. 1988; Steffey et al. 2005b).

Desflurane causes dose-related depression of EEG activity comparable to effects seen with an equipotent dose of isoflurane (Rampil et al. 1988, 1991). Epileptiform EEG activity is not reported.

Desflurane causes dose-dependent decreases in cerebrovascular resistance (vasodilation) and cerebral metabolic rate of oxygen consumption similar to actions by halothane and isoflurane (Lutz et al. 1990). As is the case with isoflurane, desflurane may also result in an increase in brain volume and associated intracranial pressure increase (Young 1992). Although these effects are trivial in animals without intracranial pathology (Lutz et al. 1990, 1991), the agent must be used carefully in patients with decreased intracranial compliance. Desflurane is similar to isoflurane in that cerebrovascular responsiveness to carbon dioxide is maintained (Lutz et al. 1991).

Cardiovascular System. The cardiovascular actions of desflurane are similar to those of isoflurane (Weiskopf et al. 1988, 1989, 1991; Warltier and Pagel 1992; Clarke et al. 1996; McMurphy and Hodgson 1996; Mutoh et al. 1997; Santos et al. 2005; Steffey et al. 2005b). Like isoflurane and halothane, desflurane decreases mean arterial blood pressure and stroke volume in dose-related fashion. But cardiac output during desflurane, as with isoflurane, is better maintained compared to conditions during halothane anesthesia. Heart rate is usually higher and peripheral vascular resistance less with desflurane compared to the other volatile agents (Pagel et al. 1991a). Myocardial contractility is depressed (Pagel et al. 1991b; Boban et al. 1992). Desflurane does not predispose the heart to ventricular arrhythmias, nor does it sensitize it to arrhythmogenic effects of epinephrine (Weiskopf et al. 1989; Moore et al. 1993).

Respiratory System. Desflurane, like other contemporary volatile anesthetics, causes a dose-related respiratory depression (Lockhart et al. 1991a; Mutoh et al. 1997; Santos et al. 2005; Steffey et al. 2005b). Its effects in this regard in humans are most comparable to those of enflurane (i.e., more depressing than isoflurane). Apnea occurs in pigs at alveolar desflurane concentrations between 1.2 and 1.6 MAC, while the apneic threshold in dogs is 2.38 MAC (Warltier and Pagel 1992).

Liver. Desflurane depresses hepatic blood flow only minimally. In a reported study of dogs, total hepatic blood flow (portal plus hepatic arterial) was significantly decreased by desflurane only at the two highest anesthetic concentrations (1.75 and 2.0 MAC) (Merin et al. 1991). These actions were not significantly different from isoflurane.

Desflurane is not associated with hepatic toxicity in humans (Jones et al. 1990c; Weiskopf et al. 1992), swine (Holmes et al. 1990), horses (Steffey et al. 2005b), or rats (Eger, II et al. 1987).

Kidney. Renal blood flow is not substantially altered by desflurane (Merin et al. 1991). Because desflurane is extremely resistant to degradation, it is not expected to possess, and has not to date shown, nephrotoxic potential (Jones 1990c; Weiskopf et al. 1992; Neubauer 2004).

Skeletal Muscle. Desflurane, like isoflurane and enflurane, causes muscle relaxation and enhances the action of neuromuscular blocking drugs (Caldwell et al. 1991). Desflurane is also a trigger of malignant hyperthermia in susceptible swine (Wedel et al. 1991).

Sevoflurane. *Sevoflurane* was synthesized in the early 1970s, and its characteristics were first described in 1975 (Wallin et al. 1975). It was difficult and expensive to synthesize at the time, and was known to be degradable. As a result it was not introduced until the late 1980s, first in Japan (Doi and Ikeda 1987; Katoh and Ikeda 1987) and then in the U.S. in 1995.

Its physical characteristics were noted earlier in this chapter. Briefly, sevoflurane has a vapor pressure similar to enflurane (Table 10.2). Its blood solubility is less than isoflurane but greater than desflurane (Wallin et al. 1975; Strum and Eger, II 1987). It is degraded in the presence of soda lime and Baralyme, commonly used CO_2 absorbents in anesthetic delivery circuits (Wallin et al. 1975; Strum et al. 1987; Liu et al. 1991; Frink, Jr. et al. 1992a). to $CH_2F\text{-}O\text{-}C{=}CF_2(CF_3)$ (known as Compound A). Compound A is lethal in 50% of animals (LD_{50}) at a concentration of 400 ppm (Morio et al. 1992). For further discussion of concerns of levels of Compound A in human patients, see Mazze (1992) and Neubauer (2004).

Biotransformation. Like all fluorinated volatile anesthetics, sevoflurane is biotransformed to organic and inorganic fluoride metabolites (Kharasch 1995). The in vitro rate of defluorination of sevoflurane is about the same as for methoxyflurane (Cook et al. 1975a,b). In vivo, however, the serum F^- concentration associated with sevoflurane is much less than with methoxyflurane (Cook et al. 1975b; Holaday and Smith 1981; Martis et al. 1981; Neubauer 2004). Likely this difference is related to sevoflurane's reduced tissue solubility. Sevoflurane defluorination is increased by prior induction of microsomal enzymes with drugs such as phenobarbital (Cook et al. 1975a; Neubauer 2004). Serum F^- concentrations from anesthetized horses are similar to those from humans under similar conditions (Aida et al. 1996; Steffey et al. 2005a).

Central Nervous System. Like desflurane and other commonly used inhalation anesthetics, sevoflurane decreases cerebral vascular resistance and cerebral metabolic rate, and increases intracranial pressure in a dose-related manner (Manohar 1986; Scheller et al. 1988; Patel and Drummond 2005). Its cerebral vasodilating potency is considered a little less than isoflurane and desflurane (Patel and Drummond 2005). It does not cause EEG or gross motor evidence of seizure activity in dogs (Wallin et al. 1975; Scheller et al. 1990).

Cardiovascular and Respiratory Systems. Sevoflurane's actions on the circulatory and respiratory systems are qualitatively and quantitatively similar to those of isoflurane (Manohar and Parks 1984b; Bernard et al. 1990; Eger, II 1994; Lerman et al. 1994; Ebert et al. 1995a,b; Pypendop and Ilkiw 2004). Sevoflurane does not increase the arrhythmogenicity of the heart (Wallin et al. 1975), and the arrhythmogenic dose of epinephrine in dogs anesthetized with sevoflurane is similar to that during isoflurane anesthesia (Hayashi et al. 1988).

Liver and Kidney. Overall information to date suggests that sevoflurane, or its degradation products, does not produce hepatic or renal injury (Frink, Jr. 1995; Kenna and Jones 1995; Malan, Jr. 1995; Hikasa et al. 1996; Obata et al. 2000; Conzen et al. 2002; Malhotra et al. 2005; O'Connor et al. 2005; Steffey et al. 2005a). However, caution is warranted since the biodegradation of sevoflurane to F^- occurs and degradation by soda lime or Baralyme produces another renal toxic agent, Compound A (Mazze 1992). The concentration threshold for renal toxicity in rats could be reached in clinical practice (Eger, II 1994; Gonsowski et al. 1994a,b). Indeed, recognition for possible renal damage from Compound A led to the present package labeling for sevoflurane that warns physicians against its use for human patients at fresh gas flow rates (from the anesthetic delivery apparatus) of less than 2 l/min. It has been recommended (Mazze and Jamison 1995) that sevoflurane not be used in patients with impaired renal function.

Skeletal Muscle. Sevoflurane enhances the action of neuromuscular blocking drugs and can trigger malignant hyperthermia in susceptible animals (Schulman et al. 1981; Gronert et al. 2005).

Methoxyflurane. *Methoxyflurane*, USP (Metofane, Penthrane), was first synthesized in 1958 and was introduced clinically a few years later (Artusio et al. 1988). It was a popular inhalation anesthetic for anesthetic management of small companion and laboratory animals throughout most of the 1970s and 1980s. Its use for human patients rapidly declined following discovery of its ability to cause vasopressin-resistant polyuria renal failure (Crandell et al. 1966; Mazze et al. 1971; Mazze 2006). Despite its limited reported toxicity in species of clinical importance in veterinary medicine, its use in clinical practice declined markedly throughout the 1990s as newer anesthetic agents and anesthetic techniques appeared. Its commercial availability is extremely limited if at all and it is therefore not further discussed in this edition. Interested readers are referred to the chapter on inhalation anesthetics in earlier editions of this text for further information.

Enflurane. *Enflurane*, USP (Ethrane), was synthesized in 1963, introduced for clinical trial in human patients in 1963, and released for general clinical human use in 1972 (Dobkin et al. 1976). It is a chemical isomer of isoflurane (Fig. 10.2). Its introduction was encouraged because of the clinical need for an alternative inhalation anesthetic to halothane, especially for human patients. The epileptogenic nature of enflurane at moderate levels of anesthesia was noted early in its introduction in both humans and animals (Joas et al. 1971; Neigh et al. 1971; Julien and Kavan 1972; Clark and Rosner 1973; Klide 1976; Steffey et al. 1977; Steffey 1978; Steffey and Howland, Jr. 1978a; Bassell et al. 1982). Although it was investigated for use with small companion animals and horses it received only early and brief clinical exposure in clinical veterinary practice. Interested readers are referred to the corresponding chapter in earlier editions of this text for further information.

The Gaseous Anesthetic: Nitrous Oxide. The pharmacology of N_2O and its scope in the clinical practice of anesthesiology (human and animal patients) have been reviewed by Eger, and readers are advised to consult his text as the next step for information beyond the brief summary given here (Eger, II 1985b).

Nitrous oxide, USP (N_2O), is a colorless, nonirritant, slightly sweet-smelling, nonflammable gas. Nitrous oxide is commercially available as a gas stored in steel cylinders at a pressure of about 750 psi or nearly 50 atmospheres. Since its introduction into clinical practice more than 150 years ago, its use has formed the basis for more general anesthetic techniques of human patients than any other single inhalation agent. Its widespread use resulted from many desirable properties, including low blood solubility (Table 10.3), limited cardiovascular and respiratory system depression, and minimal toxicity (Eger, II 1985b). Its use in the anesthetic management of animals became a natural extension of its use for humans.

An overview of uptake and distribution (pharmacokinetics) of inhalation anesthetics including brief insight into some relatively unique ways the physical properties of N_2O influence its movement into, within, and from the body was given above and because of space limitations will not be further addressed here. Readers are referred to the works of (Eger, II 1974, 1985b) for more information on such clinically important subjects as "the second gas effect," "diffusion hypoxia," and movement of N_2O into closed gas spaces.

Biotransformation. Nitrous oxide is metabolized (reductive pathway) by intestinal anaerobic bacteria to molecular nitrogen (N_2) and free radicals (Hong et al. 1980a,b; Neubauer 2004). Unlike other inhalation anesthetics, N_2O is not believed to be directly metabolized by animal tissues.

Central Nervous System. Nitrous oxide is not a potent anesthetic (Table 10.7) and under ambient conditions will not anesthetize a fit, healthy individual. Consequently, to get important benefits of N_2O it is necessary to use it in high inspired concentrations but at the same time remembering that as the concentration of N_2O is increased there is a change in the proportion and partial pressure of the various other constituents of the inspired breath, notably O_2. Consequently, to avoid hypoxemia, 75% of the inspired breath is the highest concentration that can be safely administered (at sea level to healthy individuals, less at altitude or in the face of, especially, cardiopulmonary disease). The potency of N_2O in animals important to clinical veterinary medicine is only about one-half the anesthetic potency of that found for humans. Thus, the value of N_2O in veterinary clinical practice is further compromised. When used it serves as an anesthetic adjuvant; that is, it is used in conjunction with an injectable and/or another inhalation anesthetic. Since its depression of other vital organs such as the heart, lungs, kidneys, etc., is small in comparison, its purpose in this case is to reduce the amount of the primary, more potent inhaled or injectable anesthetic drug for anesthesia and thereby lessen overall harmful effects on vital organ function.

The effects of N_2O on the EEG are similar to those produced by the volatile anesthetics. At low subanesthetic levels (about 30%, inspired), N_2O increases EEG frequency and lowers voltage, and at higher subanesthetic concentrations (e.g., 60%), N_2O increases voltage. Adding N_2O to a light level of anesthesia produced by other drugs tends to increase voltage and decrease frequency (Frost 1985).

N_2O causes an increase in cerebral blood flow, cerebral metabolic rate, and intracranial pressure. The magnitude of change seems to depend upon whether it is administered alone or in conjunction with other anesthetics. Dramatic increases in intracranial pressure occur in animals when N_2O is used alone (Theye and Michenfelder 1968; Pelligrino et al. 1984; Patel and Drummond 2005).

Cardiovascular and Respiratory Systems. Under ambient conditions the effects of N_2O on the cardiovascular and respiratory function (other than reducing the inspired O_2 concentration) are small compared to those of the other inhalation anesthetics. Nitrous oxide is a direct myocardial depressant. However, it also causes sympathetic nervous system stimulation and the release of catecholamines. The sympathetic stimulation, coupled with the mild, direct depressant properties of N_2O, results in comparatively little cardiovascular depression (Steffey et al. 1974a,b; 1975; Steffey and Howland, Jr. 1978b; Eisele, Jr. 1985; Penicaud et al. 1987; Pypendop et al. 2003). This end result is one of the distinguishing factors of N_2O relative to the other inhalation anesthetics.

In some circumstances N_2O may contribute to an increased incidence of cardiac arrhythmias (Liu et al. 1982; Lampe et al. 1990a). There is some evidence to suggest that its use contributes to an increased incidence of myocardial ischemia in some circumstances (Philbin et al. 1985; Leone et al. 1988; Nathan 1988; Diedericks et al. 1993).

Liver and Kidney. Nitrous oxide has little or no effect on liver or kidney function in patients exposed under most clinical circumstances (Brodsky 1985; Lampe et al. 1990b; Lampe et al. 1990c). Nitrous oxide interferes with several vitamin B_{12}–dependent reactions. The result is an irreversible inactivation of the enzyme methionine synthase that in turn results in a reduced amount of thymidine, an essential DNA base. The subsequent interference with DNA synthesis prevents production of both leukocytes and red blood cells by bone marrow. Similarly, exposure to N_2O can produce a polyneuropathy ("nitrous oxide neuropathy") that is indistinguishable from that associated with pernicious anemia, that is, subacute degeneration of the spinal cord (Brodsky 1985; Martin, Jr. and Njoku 2005). The bone marrow changes would be expected to be seen only in the sickest of patients and after about 10 hours or more of N_2O anesthesia (O'Sullivan et al. 1981). The neurologic disease is most commonly associated with rare, long-term exposure in a grossly contaminated work environment or with chronic abuse of N_2O (a potential consideration in the management of the veterinary practice) (Layzer et al. 1978; Layzer 1978; Brodsky 1985; Martin, Jr. and Njoku 2005). Both forms are described in humans and animals.

Skeletal Muscle. Nitrous oxide is at best only a weak trigger to the development of malignant hyperthermia in susceptible subjects (Gronert et al. 2005).

TRACE CONCENTRATIONS OF INHALATION ANESTHETICS: OCCUPATIONAL EXPOSURE

In 1968, Bruce and coworkers (1968) published a retrospective study of the causes of death among anesthesiologists over a 20-year period. Their work revealed a trend toward higher than normal incidences of death from reticuloendothelial and lymphoid malignancies. The possibility that chronic exposure to low levels of waste inhalation anesthetic agents constitutes a health hazard to medical personnel attracted worldwide interest among health workers (Linde and Bruce 1969; Cohen 1971; Whitcher et al. 1971; Millard and Corbett 1974; Cohen et al. 1975; Manley and McDonell 1980; Milligan et al. 1980; Dreesen et al. 1981; Manley et al. 1982). Of particular concern are reports that inhalation anesthetics are potential mutagens, carcinogens, and/or teratogens and that fetal death, spontaneous abortion, birth defects, or cancer in exposed workers might result (Cohen et al. 1971; Ad Hoc Committee on Effects of Trace Anesthetic Agents on Health of Operating Room Personnel. 1983). To date, the overwhelming conclusion from both animal and human studies is that there is no carcinogenic risk either from exposure to the currently used inhaled anesthetics (Neubauer 2004). Further, modern fluorinated inhalation anesthetics are not mutagenic although a 1990 and 1992 study have shown cytogenic damage in operating room personnel exposed to waste anesthetic gases (Natarajan and Santhiya 1990; Sardas et al. 1992; Martin, Jr. and Njoku 2005). Data to date regarding human reproduction effect remain equivocal; a firm cause-and-effect relationship between chronic exposure to trace levels of anesthetics and human health problems does not exist. Nevertheless, interest in this topic remains high and supported by results of a study in which reduced fertility was reported among dental assistants exposed to high levels of nitrous oxide (Rowland et al. 1992). Recent reviews of investigations of operating room pollution include Boivin (1997), Hoerauf et al. (1997), Berry (1999), Wiesner et al. (2000), Berry et al. (2005).

The risk of long-term exposure to trace concentrations of inhalation anesthetics for those in operating-room conditions seems minimal. However, even if anesthetics have low potential for causing long-term toxicity, exposure of a large population may represent a considerable public health hazard as anesthesiologists, surgeons, dental personnel, and veterinarians and their technical assistants have a variable but sometimes heavy exposure to inhalation anesthetics. Accordingly, current knowledge is suggestive enough to encourage practices to reduce the contamination by inhalation anesthetics of operating-room personnel. More information on scavenging waste inhalation anesthetic gases is available in anesthesiology texts (Dorsch and Dorsch 1999; Brockwell and Andrews 2005; Tranquilli et al. 2006). For more in-depth review of potential hazards to health care providers, readers are referred to Martin and Njoku's recently updated chapter in *Miller's Anesthesia* (especially pp. 256–263) (Neubauer 2004), which summarizes, "There appears to be no risk associated with brief periods of low-level occupational exposure to waste anesthetic gases in the operating room, PACU [Post-Anesthetic Care Unit], or ICU [Intensive Care Unit]. Occupational exposure to high concentrations (10^3 ppm) may be correlated with an increased incidence of abortions and decreased fertility. Individuals with vitamin B_{12} deficiencies may be at risk of neurologic injury from N_2O."

REFERENCES

Ad Hoc Committee on Effects of Trace Anesthetic Agents on Health of Operating Room Personnel. 1983. Waste anesthetic gases in operating room air: a suggested program to reduce personnel exposure. American Society of Anesthesiologists, Park Ridge, Illinois.

Adachi, M., Ikemoto, Y., Kubo, K., and Takuma, C. 1992. Seizure-like movements during induction of anaesthesia with sevoflurane. Br J Anaesth 68: 214–215.

Aida, H., Mizuno, Y., Hobo, S., Yoshida, K., and Fujinaga, T. 1996. Cardiovascular and pulmonary effects of sevoflurane anesthesia in horses. Vet Surg 25: 164–170.

Allen, G.C. and Brubaker, C.L. 1998. Human malignant hyperthermia associated with desflurane anesthesia. Anesth Analg 86: 1328–1331.

Andrews, J.J., Johnston, R.V., Jr., and Kramer, G.C. 1993. Consequences of misfilling contemporary vaporizers with desflurane. Can J Anaesth 40: 71853–76.

Antognini, J.F., Carstens, E., and Raines, D.E. 2003. Neural mechanisms of anesthesia. Humana Press, Totowa, NJ.

Antognini, J.F. and Schwartz, K. 1993. Exaggerated anesthetic requirements in the preferentially anesthetized brain. Anesthesiology 79: 1244–1249.

Artusio, J.F., Vanpoznak, A., Hunt, R.E., Tiers, F.M., and Alexander, M. 1988. A clinical evaluation of methoxyflurane. Anesthesiology 21: 512–517.

Baden, J.M. and Rice, S.A. 2000. Metabolism and toxicity of inhaled anesthetics. *In* Anesthesia. Edited by R.D.Miller. Churchill Livingstone, New York pp. 147–173.

Bahlman, S.H., Eger, E.I., II, Halsey, M.J., Stevens, W.C., Shakespeare, T.F., Smith, N.T., Cromwell, T.H., and Fourcade, H. 1972. The cardiovascular effects of halothane in man during spontaneous ventilation. Anesthesiology 36: 494–502.

Bassell, G.M., Cullen, B.F., Fairchild, M.D., and Kusske, J.A. 1982. Electroencephalographic and behavioral effects of enflurane and halothane anaesthesia in cats. Br J Anaesth 54: 659–665.

Bednarski, R.M. and Majors, L.J. 1986. Ketamine and arrhythmogenic dose of epinephrine in cats anesthetized with halothane and isoflurane. Am J Vet Res 47: 2122–2126.

Bednarski, R.M., Majors, L.J., and Atlee, J.L. 1985. Epinephrine-induced ventricular arrhythmias in dogs anesthetized with halothane: Potentiation by thiamylal and thiopental. Am J Vet Res 46: 1829–1832.

Bernard, J.M., Doursout, M.-F., Wouters, P., Hartley, C.J., Cohen, M., Merin, R.G., and Chelly, J.E. 1991. Effects of enflurane and isoflurane on hepatic and renal circulations in chronically instrumented dogs. Anesthesiology 74: 298–302.

Bernard, J.-M., Wouters, P.F., Doursout, M.-F., Florence, B., Chelly, J.E., and Merin, R. 1990. Effects of sevoflurane and isoflurane on cardiac and coronary dynamics in chronically instrumented dogs. Anesthesiology 72: 659–662.

Berry, A., McGregor, D.G., Baden, J.M., Bannister, C., Domino, K.B., Ehrenwerth, J., Eisenkraft, J.B., Mazze, R.I., and Spence, A.A. 2005. Waste Anesthetic Gases: Information for management in anesthetizing areas and the postanesthetic care unit (PACU). American Society of Anesthesiologists.

Berry, A.J. 1999. Recommended exposure limits for desflurane and isoflurane. Anesth Analg 88: 1424.

Boban, M., Stowe, D.F., Buljubasic, N., Bampine, J.P., and Bosnjak, Z.J. 1992. Direct comparative effects of isoflurane and desflurane in isolated guinea pig hearts. Anesthesiology 76: 775–780.

Boivin, J.-F. 1997. Risk of spontaneous abortion in women occupationally exposed to anaesthetic gases: a meta-analysis. Occup Environ Med 54: 541–548.

Booth, N.H. and McDonald, L.E. 1988. Veterinary Pharmacology and Therapeutics. Iowa State University Press, Ames.

Brockwell, R.C. and Andrews, J.J. 2005. Inhaled anesthetic delivery systems. *In* Miller's Anesthesia. Edited by R.D.Miller. Elsevier, Churchill Livingstone, Philadelphia pp. 273–316.

Brodsky, J.B. 1985. Toxicity of nitrous oxide. *In* Nitrous Oxide/N_2O. Edited by E.I.Eger, II. Elsevier, New York pp. 259–279.

Brosnan, R.J., Steffey, E.P., LeCouteur, R.A., Imai, A., Farver, T.B., and Kortz, G.D. 2003. Effects of ventilation and isoflurane end-tidal concentration on intracranial and cerebral perfusion pressures in horses. Am J Vet Res 64: 21–25.

Bruce, D.L., Eide, K.A., Linde, H.W., and Eckenhoff, J.E. 1968. Causes of death among anesthesiologists: a 20-year survey. Anesthesiology 29: 565–569.

Cahalan, M.K., Johnson, B.H., and Eger, E.I., II 1981. Relationship of concentrations of halothane and enflurane to their metabolism and elimination in man. Anesthesiology 54: 3–8.

Caldwell, J.E., Laster, M.J., Magorian, T., Heier, T., Yasuda, N., Lynam, D.P., Eger, E.I., II, and Weiskopf, R.B. 1991. The neuromuscular effects of desflurane, alone and combined with pancuronium or succinylcholine in humans. Anesthesiology 74: 412–418.

Calverley, R.K., Smith, N.T., Jones, C.W., Prys-Roberts, C., and Eger, E. I., II 1978. Ventilatory and cardiovascular effects of enflurane anesthesia during spontaneous ventilation in man. Anesth Analg 51: 610–618.

Carpenter, R.L., Eger, E.I., II, Johnson, B.H., Unadkat, J.D., and Sheiner, L.B. 1986a. Pharmacokinetics of inhaled anesthetics in humans: measurements during and after the simultaneous administration of enflurane, halothane, isoflurane, methoxyflurane, and nitrous oxide. Anesth Analg 65: 575–583.

———. 1986b. The extent of metabolism of inhaled anesthetics in humans. Anesthesiology 65: 201–206.

———. 1987. Does the duration of anesthetic administration affect the pharmacokinetics or metabolism of inhaled anesthetics in humans? Anesth Analg 66: 1–8.

Cascorbi, H.F., Blake, D.A., and Helrich, M. 1970. Differences in the biotransformation of halothane in man. Anesthesiology 32: 119–123.

Chase, R.E., Holaday, D.A., Fiserova-Bergerova, V., Saidman, L.J., and Mack, F.E. 1971. The biotransformation of ethrane in man. Anesthesiology 35: 262–267.

Clark, D.L. and Rosner, B.D. 1973. Neurophysiologic effects of general anesthetics. 1. The electroencephalogram and sensory evoked responses in man. Anesthesiology 38: 564–582.

Clarke, K.W. 1999. Desflurane and sevoflurane: new volatile anesthetic agents. Vet Clin North: Am Small Anim Pract 29: 793–810.

Clarke, K.W., Alibhai, H.I.K., Lee, Y.-H.L., and Hammond, R.A. 1996. Cardiopulmonary effects of desflurane in the dog during spontaneous and artificial ventilation. Res Vet Sci 61: 82–86.

Cohen, E.N. 1971. Metabolism of the volatile anesthetics. Anesthesiology 35: 193–202.

Cohen, E.N., Bellville, J.W., and Brown, B.W. 1971. Anesthesia, pregnancy, and miscarriage: a study of operating room nurses and anesthetists. Anesthesiology 35: 343–347.

Cohen, E.N., Brown, B.W., Jr., Bruce, D.L., Cascorbi, H.F., Corbett, T. H., Jones, T.W., and Whitcher, C.E. 1975. A survey of anesthetic health hazards among dentists. Journal of the American Dental Association 90: 1291–1296.

Colgan, F.J. 1965. Performance of lungs and bronchi during inhalation anesthesia. Anesthesiology 26: 778.

Conzen, P.F., Kharasch, E.D., Czerner, S.F.A., Artru, A.A., Reichle, F.M., Michalowski, P., Rooke, G.A., Weiss, B.M., and Ebert, T.J. 2002. Low-flow sevoflurane compared with low-flow isoflurane anesthesia in patients with stable renal insufficiency. Anesthesiology 97: 578–584.

Cook, T.L., Beppu, W.J., Hitt, B.A., Kosek, J.C., and Mazze, R.I. 1975a. A comparison of renal effects and metabolism of sevoflurane and methoxyflurane in enzyme-induced rats. Anesth Analg 54: 829–835.

———. 1975b. Renal effects and metabolism of sevoflurane in Fischer 344 rats: an in-vivo and in-vitro comparison with methoxyflurane. Anesthesiology 43: 70–77.

Coon, R.L. and Kampine, J.P. 1975. Hypocapnic bronchoconstriction and inhalation anesthetics. Anesthesiology 43: 635–641.

Cousins, M.J., Mazze, R.I., Barr, G.A., and Kosek, J.C. 1973. A comparison of the renal effects of isoflurane and methoxyflurane in Fischer 344 rats. Anesthesiology 38: 557–563.

Crandell, W.B., Pappas, S.G., and Macdonald, A. 1966. Nephrotoxicity associated with methoxyflurane anesthesia. Anesthesiology 27: 591–607.

Cromwell, T.H., Stevens, W.C., Eger, E.I., II, Shakespear, T.F., Halsey, M.J., Bahlman, S.H., and Fourcade, H.E. 1971. The cardiovascular effects of compound 469 (Forane) during spontaneous ventilation and CO2 challenge in man. Anesthesiology 35: 17–25.

Cullen, B.F. and Eger, E.I., II 1972. Diffusion of nitrous oxide, cyclopropane, and halothane through human skin and amniotic membrane. Anesthesiology 36: 168–173.

Cullen, S.C. and Gross, E.G. 1951. The anesthetic properties of xenon in animals and human beings, with additional observations on krypton. Science 113: 580–582.

Dahan, A., Sarton, E., vandenElsen, M., vanKleef, J., Teppema, L., and Berkenbasch, A. 1996. Ventilatory response to hypoxia in humans: Influences of subanesthetic desflurane. Anesthesiology 85: 60–68.

Dahan, A., vandenElsen, M., Berkenbosch, A., DeGoede, J., Olievier, I. C.W., Burm, A.G.L., and Vankleef, J.W. 1994. Influence of subanesthetic concentration of halothane on the ventilatory response to step changes into and out of sustained isocapnic hypoxia in healthy volunteers. Anesthesiology 81: 850–859.

Daunt, D.A., Steffey, E.P., Pascoe, J.R., Willits, N., and Daels, P.F. 1992. Actions of isoflurane and halothane in pregnant mares. J Am Vet Med Assoc 201: 1367–1374.

deGroot, H., Harnisch, U., and Noll, T. 1982. Suicidal activation of microsomal cytochrome P-450 by halothane under hypoxic conditions. Biochem Biophys Res Commun 107: 885.

deJong, R.H. and Eger, E.I., II 1975. MAC expanded: AD_{50} and AD_{95} values of common inhalation anesthetics in man. Anesthesiology 42: 408–419.

Diedericks, J., Leone, B.J., Foex, P., Sear, J.W., and Ryder, W.A. 1993. Nitrous oxide causes myocardial ischemia when added to propofol in the compromised canine myocardium. Anesth Analg 76: 1322–1326.

Dilger, J.P. 2001. Basic pharmacology of volatile anesthetics. *In* Molecular Bases of Anesthesia. Edited by E. Moody and P. Skolnick. CRC Press, New York pp. 1–35.

Dingley, J., Ivanova-Stoilova, T.M., Grundler, S., and Wall, T. 1999. Xenon: recent developments. Anaesthesia 54: 335–346.

Dobkin, A.B., Heinrich, R.G., Israel, J.S., Levy, A.A., Neville, J.F., Jr., and Ounkasem, K. 1976. Clinical and laboratory evaluation of a new inhalation angent: Compound 347 (CHF2-O_CF2-CHF-Cl). Anesthesiology 29: 275–287.

Dobkin, A.B., Kim, D., Choi, J.K., and Levy, A.A. 1973. Blood serum fluoride levels with enflurane (Ethrane) and isoflurane (Forane) anaesthesia during and following major abdominal surgery. Can Anaesth Soc J 20: 494–498.

Doi, M. and Ikeda, K. 1987. Respiratory effects of sevoflurane. Anesth Analg 66: 241–244.

Domino, K.B., Borowec, L., Alexander, C.M., Williams, J.J., Chen, L., Marshall, C., and Marshall, B.E. 1986. Influence of isoflurane on hypoxic pulmonary vasoconstriction in dogs. Anesthesiology 64(4): 423–430.

Doorley, M.B., Waters, S.J., Terrell, R.C., and Robinson, J.L. 1988. MAC of I-653 in beagle dogs and New Zealand white rabbits. Anesthesiology 69: 89–92.

Dorsch, J.A. and Dorsch, S.E. 1999. Understanding Anesthesia Equipment. Williams & Wilkins, Baltimore.

Dreesen, D.W., Jones, G.L., Brown, J., and Rawlings, C.A. 1981. Monitoring for trace anesthetic gases in a veterinary teaching hospital. J Am Vet Med Assoc 179: 797–799.

Drummond, J.C., Todd, M.M., Scheller, M.S., and Shapiro, H.M. 1986. A comparison of the direct cerebral vasodilating potencies of halothane and isoflurane in the New Zealand white rabbit. Anesthesiology 65(5): 462–468.

Duncalf, D. 1982. Flammable anesthetics are nearing extinction. Anesthesiology 56: 217–218.

Dunlop, C.I., Steffey, E.P., Miller, M.F., and Woliner, M.J. 1987. Temporal effects of halothane and isoflurane in laterally recumbent ventilated male horses. Am J Vet Res 48: 1250–1255.

Ebert, T.J., Harkin, C.P., and Muzi, M. 1995a. Cardiovascular responses to sevoflurane: a review. Anesth Analg 81: S11–S22.

Ebert, T.J., Muzi, M., and Lopatka, C.W. 1995b. Neurocirculatory responses to sevoflurane in humans: a comparison to desflurane. Anesthesiology 83: 88–95.

Eger, E.I., II 1974. Anesthetic Uptake and Action. Williams & Wilkins, Baltimore.

———. 1985a. Isoflurane (forane); A compendium and reference. Anaquest.

———. 1985b. Nitrous Oxide/ N_2O. Elsevier, New York.

———. 1987. Partition coefficients of I-653 in human blood, saline, and olive oil. Anesth Analg 66: 971–974.

———. 1990. Uptake and distribution. *In* Anesthesia. Edited by R.D.Miller. Churchill Livingstone, New York pp. 85–104.

———. 1992. Desflurane animal and human pharmacology: aspects of kinetics, safety, and MAC. Anesth Analg 75: S3–S9.

———. 1993. Desflurane (Suprane): A Compendium and Reference. Healthpress Publishing Group, Rutherford.

———. 1994. New inhaled anesthetics. Anesthesiology 80: 906–922.

———. 2005. Uptake and distribution. *In* Miller's Anesthesia. Edited by R.D.Miller. Elsevier, Churchill Livingstone, Philadelphia pp. 131–153.

Eger, E.I., II, Eisenkraft, J.B., and Weiskopf, R.B. 2003. The Pharmacology of Inhaled Anesthetics. Dannemiller Memorial Educational Foundation, San Francisco.

Eger, E.I., Gong, D., Koblin, D.D., Bowland, T., Ionescu, P., Laster, M.J., and Weiskopf, R.B. 1998. The effect of anesthetic duration on kinetic and recovery characteristics of desflurane versus sevoflurane, and on the kinetic characteristics of compound A, in volunteers. Anesth Analg 86: 414–421.

Eger, E.I., II and Johnson, B.H. 1987. Rates of awakening from anesthesia with I-653, halothane, Isoflurane, and sevoflurane—A test of the effect of anesthetic concentration and duration in rats. Anesth Analg 66: 977–983.

Eger, E.I., II, Johnson, B.H., Strum, D.P., and Ferrell, L.D. 1987. Studies of the toxicity of I-653, halothane, and isoflurane in enzyme-induced, hypoxic rats. Anesth Analg 66: 1227–1230.

Eger, E.I., II, Johnson, B.H., Weiskopf, R.B., Holmes, M.A., Yasuda, N., Targ, A., and Rampil, I.J. 1988. Minimum alveolar concentration of I-653 and isoflurane in pigs: definition of a supramaximal stimulus. Anesth Analg 67: 1174–1177.

Eger, E.I., II and Severinghaus, J.W. 1964. Effect of uneven pulmonary distribution of blood and gas on induction with inhalation anesthetics. Anesthesiology 25: 620–626.

Eger, E.I., II, Smith, N.T., Stoelting, R.K., Cullen, D.J., Kadis, L.B., and Whitcher, C.E. 1970. Cardiovascular effects of halothane in man. Anesthesiology 32: 396–409.

Eger, E.I., II, White, A.E., Brown, C.L., Biava, C.G., Corbett, T.H., and Stevens, W.C. 1978. A test of the carcinogenicity of enflurane, isoflurane, halothane, methoxyflurane and nitrous oxide in mice. Anesth Analg 57: 678–694.

Eger, R.R. and Eger, E.I., II 1985. Effect of temperature and age on the solubility of enflurane, halothane, isoflurane, and methoxyflurane in human blood. Anesth Analg 64: 640–642.

Eisele, J.H., Jr. 1985. Cardiovascular effects of nitrous oxide. *In* Nitrous Oxide / N_2O. Edited by E.I.Eger, II. Elsevier, New York pp. 125–156.

Engelking, L.R., Dodman, N.H., Hartman, G., Valdez, H., and Spivak, W. 1984. Effects of halothane anesthesia on equine liver function. Am J Vet Res 45: 607–615.

Englesson, S. 1974. The influence of acid-base changes on central nervous system toxicity of local anesthetic agents. I. an experimental study in cats. Acta Anaesthesiol Scand 18: 79.

Fang, Z.X., Laster, M.J., Gong, D., Ionescu, P., Koblin, D.D., Sonner, J., Eger, E.I., and Halsey, M.J. 1997. Convulsant activity of nonanesthetic gas combinations. Anesth Analg 84: 634–640.

Fargas-Balyak, A. and Forrest, J.B. 1979. Effect of halothane on the pulmonary vascular response to hypoxia in dogs. Can Anaesth Soc J 26: 6–14.

Fassoulaki, A., Lockhart, S.H., Freire, B.A., Yasuda, N., Eger, E.I., II, Weiskopf, R.B., and Johnson, B.H. 1991. Percutaneous loss of desflurane, isoflurane, and halothane in humans. Anesthesiology 74: 479–483.

Fourcade, H.E., Stevens, W.C., Larson, C.P.J., Cromwell, T.H., Bahlman, S.H., Hickey, R.F., Halsey, M.J., and Eger, E.I., II. 1971. The ventilatory effects of Forane, a new inhaled anesthetic. Anesthesiology 35: 26–31.

Frink, E.J., Jr. 1995. The hepatic effects of sevoflurane. Anesth Analg 81: S46–S50.

Frink, E.J., Jr., Malan, T., Morgan, S., Brown, E., Malcomson, M., and Brown, B.R., Jr. 1992a. Quantification of the degradation products of sevoflurane in two CO_2 absorbents during low-flow anesthesia in surgical patients. Anesthesiology 77: 1064–1069.

Frink, E.J., Jr., Malan, T.P., Atlas, M., Dominguez, L.M., DiNardo, J.A., and Brown, B.R., Jr. 1992b. Clinical comparison of sevoflurane and isoflurane in healthy patients. Anesth Analg 74: 241–245.

Frink, E.J., Jr., Morgan, S.E., Coetzee, A., Conzen, P.F., and Brown, B.R., Jr. 1992c. The effects of sevoflurane, halothane, enflurane, and isoflurane on hepatic blood flow and oxygenation in chronically instrumented greyhound dogs. Anesthesiology 76: 85–90.

Frost, E.A.M. 1985. Central nervous system effects of nitrous oxide. *In* Nitrous Oxide / N_2O. Edited by E.I.Eger, II. Elsevier, New York pp. 157–176.

Fukuda, H., Hirabayashi, Y., Shimizu, R., Saitoh, K., and Mitsuhata, H. 1996. Sevoflurane is equivalent to isoflurane for attenuating bupivacaine-induced arrhythmias and seizures in rats. Anesth Analg 83: 570–573.

Gelman, S. 1987. General anesthesia and hepatic circulation. Can J Physiol Pharmacol 65: 1762–1779.

Gelman, S., Fowler, K.C., and Smith, L.R. 1984a. Liver circulation and function during isoflurane and halothane anesthesia. Anesthesiology 61: 726–731.

———. 1984b. Regional blood flow during isoflurane and halothane anesthesia. Anesth Analg 63: 557–566.

Gonsowski, C.T., Laster, M.J., Eger, E.I., II, Ferrell, L.D., and Kerschmann, R.L. 1994a. Toxicity of compound A in rats: effect of a 3-hour administration. Anesthesiology 80: 556–565.

———. 1994b. Toxicity of compound A in rats: effect of increasing duration of administration. Anesthesiology 80: 566–573.

Gopinath, C. and Ford, E.J. 1976. The influence of hepatic microsomal amidopyrine demethylase activity on halothane hepatotoxicity in the horse. J Pathol 119: 105–112.

Gopinath, C., Jones, R.S., and Ford, E.J.H. 1970. The effect of repeated administration of halothane on the liver of the horse. J Pathol 102: 107–114.

Goto, T., Suwa, K., Uezono, S., Ichinose, F., Uchiyama, M., and Morita, S. 1998. The blood-gas partition coefficient of xenon may be lower than generally accepted. Br J Anaesth 80: 255–256.

Grandy, J.L., Hodgson, D.S., Dunlop, C.I., Curtis, C.R., and Heath, R.B. 1989. Cardiopulmonary effects of halothane anesthesia in cats. Am J Vet Res 50: 1729–1732.

Gronert, G.A., Pessah, I.N., Muldoon, S.M., and Tautz, T.J. 2005. Malignant hyperthermia. *In* Miller's Anesthesia. Edited by R.D. Miller. Elsevier Churchill Livingstone, Philadelphia pp. 1169–1190.

Habre, W., Petak, F., Sly, P.D., Hantos, Z., and Morel, D.R. 2001. Protective effects of volatile agents against methacholine-induced bronchoconstriction in rats. Anesthesiology 94: 348–353.

Hall, L.W. 1971. Wright's Veterinary Anaesthesia and Analgesia. Bailliere Tindall, London.

Harper, M.H., Collins, P., Johnson, B., Eger, E.I., II, and Biava, C. 1982a. Hepatic injury following halothane, enflurane, and isoflurane anesthesia in rats. Anesthesiology 56: 14–17.

———. 1982b. Postanesthetic hepatic injury in rats: influence of alterations in hepatic blood flow, surgery and anesthesia time. Anesth Analg 61: 79–82.

Hartman, J.C., Pagel, P.S., Proctor, L.T., Kampine, J.P., Schmeling, W.T., and Warltier, D.C. 1992. Influence of desflurane, isoflurane and halothane on regional tissue perfusion in dogs. Can J Anaesth 39: 877–887.

Hartsfield, S.M. 1996. Anesthetic machines and breathing systems. *In* Lumb & Jones' Veterinary Anesthesia. Edited by J.C.Thurmon, W. J.Tranquilli, and G.J.Benson. Williams & Wilkins, Baltimore pp. 366–408.

Haskins, S. and Sansome, A.L. 1979. A time-table for exhaustion of nitrous oxide cylinders using cylinder pressure. Vet Anesth 6: 6–8.

Haskins, S.C. and Klide, A.M. 1992. Opinions in small animal anesthesia. Vet Clin North Am Small Anim Pract 22: 381–411.

Hayashi, Y., Sumikawa, K., Tashiro, C., Yamatodani, A., and Yoshiya, I. 1988. Arrhythmogenic threshold of epinephrine during sevoflurane, enflurane, and isoflurane anesthesia in dogs. Anesthesiology 69: 145–147.

Hikasa, Y., Kawanabe, H., Takase, K., and Ogasawara, S. 1996. Comparisons of sevoflurane, isoflurane, and halothane anesthesia in spontaneously breathing cats. Vet Surg 25: 234–243.

Hill, D.W. 1980. Physics applied to anaesthesia. Butterworth & Co (Publishers) Ltd, London.

Hirshman, C.A. and Bergman, N.A. 1978. Halothane and enflurane protect against bronchospasm in an asthma dog model. Anesth Analg 57: 629–633.

Hirshman, C.A., Edelstein, H., Peetz, S., Wayne, R., and Kownes, H. 1982. Mechanism of action of inhalational anesthesia on airways. Anesthesiology 56: 107–111.

Hodgson, D.S., Steffey, E.P., Woliner, M., and Grandy, J. 1985a. Ventilatory effects of isoflurane anesthesia in horses. Veterinary Surgery 14: 74. Ref Type: Abstract

Hodgson, D.S., Steffey, E.P., Woliner, M.J., and Miller, M.F. 1985b. Alteration in breathing patterns of horses during halothane and isoflurane anesthetic induction. *In* Proceedings of the Second International Congress of Veterinary Anesthesia. Edited by J. Grandy, S. Hildebrand, W. McDonell, et al. Veterinary Practice Publishing Co., Santa Barbara, CA pp. 195–196.

Hoerauf, K., Funk, W., Harth, M., and Hobbhahn, J. 1997. Occupational exposure to sevoflurane, halothane and nitrous oxide during paediatric anaesthesia. Anaesthesia 52: 215–219.

Holaday, D.A., Fiserova-Bergerova, V., Latto, I.P., and Zumbiel, M.A. 1975. Resistance of isoflurane to biotransformation in man. Anesthesiology 43: 325–332.

Holaday, D.A., Rudofsky, S., and Treuhaft, P.S. 1970. The metabolic degradation of methoxyflurane in man. Anesthesiology 33: 579–593.

Holaday, D.A. and Smith, F.R. 1981. Clinical characteristics and biotransformation of sevoflurane in healthy human volunteers. Anesthesiology 54: 100–106.

Holmes, M.A., Weiskopf, R.B., Eger, E.I., II, Johnson, B.H., and Rampil, I.J. 1990. Hepatocellular integrity in swine after prolonged desflurane (I-653) and isoflurane anesthesia: evaluation of plasma alanine aminotransferase activity. Anesth Analg 71: 249–253.

Hong, K., Trudell, J.R., O'Neil, J.R., and Cohen, E.N. 1980a. Biotransformation of nitrous oxide. Anesthesiology 53: 354–355.

———. 1980b. Metabolism of nitrous oxide by human and rat intestinal contents. Anesthesiology 52: 16–19.

Horrigan, R.W., Eger, E.I., II, and Wilson, C. 1978. Epinephrine-induced arrhythmia during enflurane anesthesia in man: A nonlinear dose-response relationship and dose-dependent protection from lidocaine. Anesth Analg 57: 547–550.

Hubbard, A.K., Gandolfi, A.J., and Brown, B.R., Jr. 1988. Immunological basis of anesthetic-induced hepatotoxicity. Anesthesiology 69: 814–817.

Ingwersen, W., Allen, D.G., Dyson, D.H., Pascoe, P.J., and O'Grady, M.R. 1988. Cardiopulmonary effects of a halothane/oxygen combination in healthy cats. Can J Vet Res 52: 386–392.

Joas, T.A. and Stevens, W.C. 1971. Comparison of the arrhythmic doses of epinephrine during forane, halothane, and fluroxene anesthesia in dogs. Anesthesiology 35: 48–53.

Joas, T.A., Stevens, W.C., and Eger, E.I., II 1971. Electroencephalographic seizure activity in dogs during anaesthesia: studies with Ethrane, fluroxene, halothane, chloroform, divinyl ether, diethyl ether, methoxyflurane, cyclopropane and forane. Br J Anaesth 43: 739–745.

Johnston, R.R., Eger, E.I., II, and Wilson, C. 1976. A comparative interaction of epinephrine with enflurane, isoflurane and halothane in man. Anesth Analg 55: 709–712.

Jones, R.M. 1990. Desflurane and sevofluranel Inhalation anaesthetics for this decade. Br J Anaesth 65: 527–536.

Jones, R.M., Cashman, J.N., Eger, E.I., II, Damask, M.C., and Johnson, B.H. 1990a. Kinetics and potency of Desflurane (I-653) in volunteers. Anesth Analg 70: 3–7.

Jones, R.M., Cashman, J.N., and Mant, T.G.K. 1990b. Clinical impressions and cardiorespiratory effects of a new fluorinated inhalation anaesthetic, desflurane (I-653), in volunteers. Br J Anaesth 64: 11–15.

Jones, R.M., Koblin, D.D., Cashman, J.N., Eger, E.I., II, Johnson, B.H., and Damask, M.C. 1990c. Biotransformation and hepato-renal function in volunteers after exposure to Desflurane (I-653). Br J Anaesth 64: 482–487.

Joyce, J.T., Roizen, M.F., and Eger, E.I., II 1983. Effect of thiopental induction on sympathetic activity. Anesthesiology 59: 19–22.

Julien, R.M. and Kavan, E.M. 1972. Electrographic studies of a new volatile anesthetic agent: enflurane (Ethrane). J Pharmacol Exp Ther 183: 393–403.

———. 1974. Electrographic studies of isoflurane (Forane). Neuropharmacology 13: 677–681.

Karasawa, F. 1991. The effects of sevoflurane on lidocaine-induced convulsions. J Anesth 5: 60–67.

Katoh, T. and Ikeda, K. 1987. The minimum alveolar concentration (MAC) of sevoflurane in humans. Anesthesiology 66: 301–304.

Katz, R.L. and Epstein, R.A. 1968. The interaction of anesthetic agents and adrenergic drugs to produce cardiac arrhythmias. Anesthesiology 29: 763–784.

Kavan, E.M. and Julien, R.M. 1974. Central nervous systems' effects of isoflurane (forane). Can Anaesth Soc J 21: 390–402.

Kenna, J.G. and Jones, R.M. 1995. The organ toxicity of inhaled anesthetics. Anesth Analg 81: S51–S66.

Kenna, J.G., Satoh, H., Christ, D.D., and Pohl, L.R. 1988. Metabolic basis for a drug hypersensitivity: antibodies in sera from patients with halothane hepatitis recognize liver neoantigens that contain the trifluoroacetyl group derived from halothane. J Pharmacol Exp Ther 245: 1103–1109.

Kennedy, R.R., Stokes, J.W., and Downing, P. 1992. Anaesthesia and the "inert" gases with special reference to xenon. Anaesth Intensive Care 20: 66–70.

Kerbaul, F., Bellezza, M., Guidon, C., Roussel, L., Imbert, M., Carpentier, J.P., and Auffray, J.P. 2000. Effects of sevoflurane on hypoxic pulmonary vasoconstriction in anaesthetized piglets. Br J Anaesth 85: 440–445.

Kerbaul, F., Guidon, C., Stephanazzi, J., Bellezza, M., LeDantec, P., Longeon, T., and Aubert, M. 2001. Sub-MAC concentrations of desflurane do not inhibit hypoxic pulmonary vasoconstriction in anesthetized piglets. Can J Anaesth 48: 760–767.

Kharasch, E.D. 1995. Biotransformation of sevoflurane. Anesth Analg 81: S27–S38.

Klide, A.M. 1976. Cardiovascular effects of enflurane and isoflurane in the dog. Am J Vet Res 37: 127–131.

Klide, A.M. and Aviado, D.M. 1967. Mechanism for the reduction in pulmonary resistance induced by halothane. J Pharmacol Exp Ther 158: 28–35.

Knill, R.L. and Gelb, A.W. 1978. Ventilatory responses to hypoxia and hypercapnia during halothane sedation and anesthesia in man. Anesthesiology 49: 244–251.

Knill, R.L., Kieraszewicz, H.T., Dodgson, B.G., and Clement, J.L. 1983. Chemical regulation of ventilation during isoflurane sedation and anaesthesia in humans. Br J Anaesth 49: 957–963.

Koblin, D.D. 1992. Characteristics and implications of desflurane metabolism and toxicity. Anesth Analg 75: S10–S16.

———. 2005. Mechanisms of action. *In* Miller's Anesthesia. Edited by R.D. Miller. Elsevier Churchill Livingstone, Philadelphia pp. 105–130.

Koblin, D.D., Eger, E.I., II, Johnson, B.H., Collins, P., Terrell, R.C., and Speers, L. 1981. Are convulsant gases also anesthetics. Anesth Analg 60: 464–470.

Koblin, D.D., Eger, E.I., II, Johnson, B.H., Konopka, K., and Waskell, L. 1988. I-653 resists degradation in rats. Anesth Analg 67: 534–539.

Komatsu, H., Tale, S., Endo, S., Fukuda, K., Ueki, M., Nogaya, J., and Ogli, K. 1994. Electrical seizures during sevoflurane anesthesia in two pediatric patients with epilepsy. Anesthesiology 81: 1535–1537.

Kudoh, A. and Matsuki, A. 2000. Sevoflurane stimulates inositol 1,4,5-trisphosphate in skeletal muscle. Anesth Analg 91: 440–445.

Lampe, G.H., Donegan, J.H., Rupp, S.M., Wauk, L.Z., Whitendale, P., Fouts, K.E., Rose, B.M., Litt, L.L., Rampil, I.J., Wilson, C.B., and Eger, E.I., II 1990a. Nitrous oxide and epinephrine-induced arrhythmias. Anesth Analg 71: 602–605.

Lampe, G.H., Wauk, L.Z., Donegan, J.H., Pitts, L.H., Jackler, R.K., Litt, L.L., Rampil, I.J., and Eger, E.I., II 1990b. Effect on outcome of prolonged exposure of patients to nitrous oxide. Anesth Analg 71: 586–590.

Lampe, G.H., Wauk, L.Z., Whitendale, P., Way, W.L., Murray, W., and Eger, E.I., II 1990c. Nitrous oxide does not impair hepatic function in young or old surgical patients. Anesth Analg 71: 606–609.

Larson, C.P., Jr., Eger, E.I., II, Muallem, M., Buechel, D.R., Munson, E.S., and Eisele, J.H. 1969. The effects of diethyl ether and methoxyflurane on ventilation: II. A comparative study in man. Anesthesiology 30: 174–184.

Laster, M.J., Fang, Z., and Eger, E.I., II 1994. Specific gravities of desflurane, enflurane, halothane, isoflurane, and sevoflurane. Anesth Analg 78: 1152–1153.

Lawrence, J.H., Loomis, W.F., Tobias, C.A., and Turpin, F.H. 1946. Preliminary observations on the narcotic effect of xenon with a review of values for solubilities of gases in water and oils. J Physiol (London) 105: 197–204.

Layzer, R.B. 1978. Myeloneuropathy after prolonged exposure to nitrous oxide. Lancet 2: 1227–1230.

Layzer, R.B., Fishman, R.A., and Schafer, J.A. 1978. Neuropathy following abuse of nitrous oxide. Neurology 28: 504–506.

Leone, B.J., Philbin, D.M., Lehot, J.J., Foex, P., and Ryder, W.A. 1988. Gradual or abrupt nitrous oxide administration in a canine model of critical coronary stenosis induces regional myocardial dysfunction that is worsened by halothane. Anesth Analg 67: 814–822.

Lerman, J., Schmitt-Bantel, B.I., Gregory, G.A., Willis, M.M., and Eger, E.I., II 1986. Effect of age on the solubility of volatile anesthetics in human tissues. Anesthesiology 65: 307–312.

Lerman, J., Sikich, N., Kleinman, S., and Yentis, S. 1994. The pharmacology of sevoflurane in infants and children. Anesthesiology 80: 814–824.

Lesitsky, M.A., Davis, S., and Murray, P.A. 1998. Preservation of hypoxic pulmonary vasoconstriction during sevoflurane and desflurane anesthesia compared to the conscious state in chronically instrumented dogs. Anesthesiology 89: 1501–1508.

Linde, H.W. and Berman, M.L. 1971. Nonspecific stimulation of drug-metabolizing enzymes by inhalation anesthetic agents. Anesth Analg 50: 656–667.

Linde, H.W. and Bruce, D.L. 1969. Occupational exposure of anesthetists to halothane, nitrous oxide and radiation. Anesthesiology 30: 363–368.

Liu, J., Laster, M.J., Eger, E.I., II, and Taheri, S. 1991. Absorption and degradation of sevoflurane and isoflurane in a conventional anesthetic circuit. Anesth Analg 72: 785–789.

Liu, W.S., Wong, K.C., Port, J.D., and Aridriano, K.P. 1982. Epinephrine-induced arrhythmia during halothane anesthesia with the addition of nitrous oxide, nitrogen or helium in dogs. Anesth Analg 61: 414–417.

Lockhart, S.H., Rampil, I.J., Yasuda, N., Eger, E.I., II, and Weiskopf, R.B. 1991a. Depression of ventilation by desflurane in humans. Anesthesiology 74: 484–488.

Lockhart, S.H., Yasuda, N., Peterson, N., Laster, M.J., Taheri, S., Weiskopf, R.B., and Eger, E.I., II 1991b. Comparison of percutaneous losses of sevoflurane and isoflurane in humans. Anesth Analg 72: 212–215.

Lowe, H.J. and Ernst, E.A. 1981. The quantitative practice of anesthesia; use of closed circuit. Williams & Wilkins, Baltimore.

Ludders, J.W., Rode, J., and Mitchell, G.S. 1989. Isoflurane anesthesia in sandhill cranes (*Grus canadensis*): minimal anesthetic concentration and cardiopulmonary dose-response during spontaneous and controlled breathing. Anesth Analg 68: 511–516.

Lumb, W.V. and Jones, E.W. 1973. Veterinary Anesthesia. Lea & Febiger, Philadelphia.

Lunam, C.A., Hall, P.M., and Cousins, M.J. 1983. Cardiovascular and hepatic effects of halothane and isoflurane in a guinea-pig model of "halothane hepatitis." Clin Exp Pharmacol Physiol 10: 726–730.

Lutz, L.J., Milde, J.H., and Milde, L.N. 1990. The cerebral functional, metabolic, and hemodynamic effects of desflurane in dogs. Anesthesiology 73: 125–131.

———. 1991. The response of the canine cerebral circulation to hyperventilation during anesthesia with desflurane. Anesthesiology 74: 504–507.

Lynch, C., III, Baum, J., and Tenbrinck, R. 2000. Xenon anesthesia. Anesthesiology 92: 865–868.

Malan, T.P., Jr. 1995. Sevoflurane and renal function. Anesth Analg 81: S39–S45.

Malhotra, V., Sudheendra, V., and Diwan, S. 2005. Anesthesia and the renal and genitourinary system. *In* Miller's Anesthesia. Edited by R.D. Miller. Elsevier Churchill Livingstone, Philadelphia pp. 2175–2207.

Manley, S.V. and McDonell, W.N. 1980. Anesthetic pollution and disease. J Am Vet Med Assoc 176: 515–518.

Manley, S.V., Taloff, P., Aberg, N., and Howitt, G.A. 1982. Occupational exposure to waste anesthetic gases in veterinary practice. California Veterinarian 36: 14–19.

Manohar, M. 1986. Regional brain blood flow and cerebral cortical O2 consumption during sevoflurane anesthesia in healthy isocapnic swine. J Cardiovasc Pharmacol 8(6): 1268–1276.

Manohar, M. and Goetz, T.E. 1985. Cerebral, renal, adrenal, intestinal, and pancreatic circulation in conscious ponies and during 1.0, 1.5, and 2.0 minimal alveolar concentrations of halothane-O2 anesthesia. Am J Vet Res 46: 2492–2498.

Manohar, M. and Parks, C. 1984a. Porcine regional brain and myocardial blood flows during halothane-O2 and halothane-nitrous oxide anesthesia: comparisons with equipotent isoflurane anesthesia. Am J Vet Res 45: 465–474.

Manohar, M. and Parks, C.M. 1984b. Porcine systemic and regional organ blood flow during 1.0 and 1.5 minimum alveolar concentrations of sevoflurane anesthesia without and with 50% nitrous oxide. J Pharmacol Exp Ther 231: 640–648.

Mapleson, W.W. 1989. Pharmacokinetics of inhalational anaesthetics. *In* General Anaesthesia. Edited by J.F. Nunn, J.E. Utting, and B.R. Brown, Jr. Butterworths, London pp. 44–59.

Mapleson, W.W., Allott, P.R., and Steward, A. 1972. The variability of partition coefficients for halothane in the rabbit. Br J Anaesth 44: 650.

Marshall, C., Lindgren, L., and Marshall, B.E. 1984. Effects of halothane, enflurane and isoflurane on hypoxic pulmonary vasoconstriction in rat lungs in vitro. Anesthesiology 60: 304–309.

Martin, J.L., Jr. and Njoku, D.B. 2005. Metabolism and toxicityy of modern inhaled anesthetics. *In* Miller's Anesthesia. Edited by R.D. Miller. Elsevier Churchill Livingstone, Philadelphia pp. 231–272.

Martis, L., Lynch, S., Napoli, M.D., and Woods, E.F. 1981. Biotransformation of sevoflurane in dogs and rats. Anesth Analg 60: 186–191.

Mathers, J., Benumof, J.L., and Wahrenkrock, E.A. 1977. General anesthesia and regional hypoxic pulmonary vasoconstriction. Anesthesiology 46: 111–114.

Mazze, R.I. 1992. The safety of sevoflurane in humans. Anesthesiology 77: 1062–1063.

———. 2006. Methoxyflurane revisited: Tale of an anesthetic from cradle to grave. Anesthesiology 105: 843–846.

Mazze, R.I., Cousins, M.J., and Barr, G.A. 1974. Renal effects and metabolism of isoflurane in man. Anesthesiology 40: 536–542.

Mazze, R.I. and Fujinaga, M. 1989. Biotransformation of inhalational anaesthetics. *In* General Anaesthesia. Edited by J.F. Nunn, J.E. Utting, and B.R. Brown. Butterworths, London pp. 73–85.

Mazze, R.I. and Jamison, R. 1995. Renal effects of sevoflurane. Anesthesiology 83: 443–445.

Mazze, R.I., Trudell, J.R., and Cousins, M.J. 1971. Methoxyflurane metabolism and renal dysfunction: clinical correlation in man. Anesthesiology 35: 247–252.

Mazzeo, A.J., Cheng, E.Y., Bosnjak, Z.J., Coon, R.C., and Kampine, J.P. 1996. Differential effects of desflurane and halothane on peripheral airway smooth muscle. Br J Anaesth 76: 841–846.

McMurphy, R.M. and Hodgson, D.S. 1996. Cardiopulmonary effects of desflurane in cats. Am J Vet Res 57: 367–370.

Merin, R.G., Bernard, J.M., Doursout, M.F., Cohen, M., and Chelly, J.E. 1991. Comparison of the effects of isoflurane and desflurane on cardiovascular dynamics and regional blood flow in the chronically instrumented dog. Anesthesiology 74: 568–574.

Merkel, G. and Eger, E.I., II 1963. A comparative study of halothane and halopropane anesthesia: including method for determining equipotency. Anesthesiology 24: 346–357.

Meyer, H.H. 1899. Theorie der alkoholnarkose. Arch Exptl Pathol Pharmakol 42: 109–118.

Miletich, D.J., Ivankovich, A.D., Albrecht, R.F., Reimann, C.R., Rosenberg, R., and McKissic, E.D. 1976. Absence of autoregulation of cerebral blood flow during halothane and enflurane anesthesia. Anesth Analg 55: 100–109.

Millard, R.I. and Corbett, T.H. 1974. Nitrous oxide concentrations in the dental operatory. J Oral Surg 32: 593–594.

Miller, E.D.J. and Greene, N.M. 1990. Waking up to desflurane: The anesthetic for the 90s? Anesth Analg 70: 1–2.

Miller, R.D., Way, W.L., Dolan, W.M., Stevens, W.C., and Eger, E.I., II 1972. The dependence of pancuronium- and d-tubocurarine-induced neuromuscular blockades on alveolar concentrations of halothane and Forane. Anesthesiology 37: 573–581.

Milligan, J.E., Sablan, J.L., and Short, C.E. 1980. A survey of waste anesthetic gas concentrations in U.S. Airforce veterinary surgeries. J Am Vet Med Assoc 177: 1021–1022.

Moore, M.A., Weiskopf, R.B., Eger, E.I., II, Wilson, C., and Lu, G. 1993. Arrhythmogenic doses of epinephrine are similar during desflurane or isoflurane anesthesia in humans. Anesthesiology 79: 943–947.

Morio, M., Fujii, K., Satoh, N., Imai, M., Kawakami, U., Mizuno, T., Kawai, Y., Ogasawara, Y., Tamura, T., Negishi, A., Kumagal, Y., and Kawai, T. 1992. Reaction of sevoflurane and its degradation products with soda lime. Anesthesiology 77: 1155–1164.

Muir, B.J., Hall, L.W., and Littlewort, M.C.G. 1959. Cardiac irregularities in cats under halothane anaesthesia. Br J Anaesth 31: 488–489.

Muir, W.W., III, Werner, L.L., and Hamlin, R.L. 1975. Effects of xylazine and acetylpromazine upon induced ventricular fibrillation in dogs anesthetized with thiamylal and halothane. Am J Vet Res 36: 1299–1303.

Munson, E.S., Larson, C.P., Jr., Babad, A.A., Regan, M.J., Buechel, D.R., and Eger, E.I., II 1966. The effects of halothane, fluroxene and cyclopropane on ventilation: a comparative study in man. Anesthesiology 27: 716–728.

Munson, E.S. and Tucker, W.K. 1975. Doses of epinephrine causing arrhythmia during enflurane, methoxyflurane and halothane anesthesia in dogs. Can Anaesth Soc J 22: 495–501.

Murao, K., Shingu, K., Tsushima, K., Takahira, K., Ikeda, S., Matsumoto, H., Nakao, S., and Asai, T. 2000. The anticonvulsant effects of volatile anesthetics on penicillin-induced status epilepticus in cats. Anesth Analg 90: 142–147.

Mutoh, T., Nishimura, R., Kim, H., Matsunaga, S., and Sasaki, N. 1997. Cardiopulmonary effects of sevoflurane, compared with halothane, enflurane, and isoflurane, in dogs. Am J Vet Res 58: 885–890.

Natarajan, D. and Santhiya, S.T. 1990. Cytogenic damage in operating theatre personnel. Anaesthesia 45: 574–577.

Nathan, H.J. 1988. Nitrous oxide worsens myocardial ischemia in isoflurane-anesthetized dogs. Anesthesiology 68: 407–416.

Navarro, R., Weiskopf, R.B., Moore, M.A., Lockhart, S., Eger, E.I., II, Koblin, D.D., Lu, G., and Wilson, C. 1994. Humans anesthetized with sevoflurane or isoflurane have similar arrhythmic response to epinephrine. Anesthesiology 80: 545–549.

Neigh, J.L., Garman, J.K., and Harp, J.R. 1971. The electroencephalographic pattern during anesthesia with Ethrane: effects of depth of anesthesia, $PaCO_2$ and nitrous oxide. Anesthesiology 35: 482–487.

Neubauer, J.A. 2004. Comroe's study of aortic chemoreceptors: a path well chosen. J Appl Physiol 97: 1595–1596.

Newble, D.I. 2000. Assessment of clinical competence. Br J Anaesth 84: 432–433.

O'Connor, C.J., Rothenberg, D.M., and Tuman, K.J. 2005. Anesthesia and the hepatobiliary system. *In* Miller's Anesthesia. Edited by R.D. Miller. Elsevier Churchill Livingstone, Philadelphia pp. 2209–2229.

O'Sullivan, H., Jennings, F., Ward, K., McCann, S., Scott, J.M., and Weir, D.G. 1981. Human bone marrow biochemical function and megaloblastic hematopoiesis after nitrous oxide anesthesia. Anesthesiology 55: 645–649.

Obata, R., Bito, H., Ohmura, M., Moriwaki, G., Ikeuchi, Y., Katoh, T., and Sato, S. 2000. The effects of prolonged low-flow sevoflurane anesthesia on renal and hepatic function. Anesth Analg 91: 1262–1268.

Osawa, M., Shingu, K., Murakawa, M., Adachi, T., Kurata, J., Seo, N., Murayama, T., Nakao, S., and Mori, K. 1994. Effect of sevoflurane on central nervous system electrical activity in cats. Anesth Analg 79: 52–57.

Ossipou, M.H. and Gebhart, G.F. 1984. Light pentobarbital anesthesia diminishes the antinocieptive potency of morphine administered intracranially but not intrathecally in the rat. Eur J Pharmacol 97: 137–141.

Overton, E. 1901. Studien über die narkose, zugleich ein beitrag zur allgemeinen pharmakologie. Gustav Fischer Jena: 1–195.

Pagel, P.S., Kampine, J.P., Schmeling, W.T., and Warltier, D.C. 1991a. Comparison of the systemic and coronary hemodynamic actions of desflurane, isoflurane, halothane, and enflurane in the chronically instrumented dog. Anesthesiology 74: 539–551.

———. 1991b. Influence of volatile anesthetics on myocardial contractility in vivo: Desflurane versus isoflurane. Anesthesiology 74: 900–907.

———. 1993. Evaluation of myocardial contractility in the chronically instrumented dog with intact autonomic nervous system function: effects of desflurane and isoflurane. Acta Anaesthesiol Scand 37: 203–210.

Pagel, P.S., Kersten, J.R., Farber, N.E., and Warltier, D.C. 2005. Cardiovascular pharmacology. *In* Miller's Anesthesia. Edited by R.D. Miller. Elsevier Churchill Livingstone, Philadelphia pp. 191–229.

Patel, P.M. and Drummond, J.C. 2005. Cerebral physiology and the effects of anesthetics and techniques. *In* Miller's Anesthesia. Edited by R.D. Miller. Elsevier Churchill Livingstone, Philadelphia pp. 813–857.

Pavlin, E.G. and Su, J.Y. 1994. Cardiopulmonary pharmacology. *In* Anesthesia. Edited by R.D. Miller. Churchill Livingstone, New York pp. 125–156.

Pedersoli, W.M. 1980. Serum bromide concentrations during and after halothane anesthesia in dogs. Am J Vet Res 41: 77–80.

Pelligrino, D.A., Miletich, D.J., Hoffman, W.E., and Albrecht, R.F. 1984. Nitrous oxide markedly increases cerebral cortical metabolic rate and blood flow in the goat. Anesthesiology 60: 405.

Penicaud, L., Ferre, P., Kande, J., Leturque, A., Issad, T., and Girard, J. 1987. Effect of anesthesia on glucose production and utilization in rats. Am J Physiol 252: E365–E370.

Philbin, D.M., Foex, P., Drummond, G., Lowenstein, E., Ryder, W.A., and Jones, L.A. 1985. Postsystolic shortening of canine left ventricle supplied by a stenotic coronary artery when nitrous oxide is added in the presence of narcotics. Anesthesiology 62: 166–174.

Plummer, J.L., Beckwith, A.L.J., Bastin, F.N., Adams, J.F., Cousins, M.J., and Hall, P. 1982. Free radical formation in vivo and hepatotoxicity due to anesthesia with halothane. Anesthesiology 57: 160–166.

Pohl, L.R. and Gillette, J.R. 1982. A perspective on halothane-induced hepatotoxicity. Anesth Analg 61: 809–811.

Pohl, L.R., Kenna, J.G., Satoh, H., and Christ, D. 1989. Neoantigens associated with halothane hepatitis. Drug Metab Rev 20: 203–217.

Price, H.L. 1966. The significance of catecholamine release during anesthesia. Br J Anaesth 38: 705–711.

Price, H.L., Skovsted, P., Pauca, A.L., and Cooperman, L.H. 1970. Evidence for b-receptor activation produced by halothane in man. Anesthesiology 32: 389–395.

Purchase, I.F. 1966. Cardiac arrhythmias occurring during halothane anaesthesia in cats. Br J Anaesth 38: 13–22.

Pypendop, B.H. and Ilkiw, J.E. 2004. Hemodynamic effects of sevoflurane in cats. Am J Vet Res 65: 20–25.

Pypendop, B.H., Ilkiw, J.E., Imai, A., and Bolich, J.A. 2003. Hemodynamic effects of nitrous oxide in isoflurane-anesthetized cats. Am J Vet Res 64: 273–278.

Quasha, A.L., Eger, E.I., II, and Tinker, J.H. 1980. Determination and applications of MAC. Anesthesiology 53: 315–334.

Rampil, I.J. 1994. Anesthetic potency is not altered after hypothermic spinal cord transection in rats. Anesthesiology 80: 606–610.

Rampil, I.J. and King, B.S. 1996. Volatile anesthetics depress spinal motor neurons. Anesthesiology 85: 129–134.

Rampil, I.J., Lockhart, S.H., Eger, E.I., II, Yasuda, N., Weiskopf, R.B., and Cahalan, M.K. 1991. The electroencephalographic effects of desflurane in humans. Anesthesiology 74: 434–439.

Rampil, I.J., Mason, P., and Singh, H. 1993. Anesthetic potency (mac) is independent of forebrain structures in the rat. Anesthesiology 78: 707–712.

Rampil, I.J., Weiskopf, R.B., Brown, J.G., Eger, E.I., II, Johnson, B.H., Holmes, M.A., and Donegan, J.H. 1988. I-653 and isoflurane produce similar dose-related changes in the electroencephalogram of pigs. Anesthesiology 69: 298–302.

Raventos, J. 1956. The action of fluothane: a new volatile anaesthetic. Br J Pharmacol 11: 394–409.

Regan, M.J. and Eger, E.I., II 1967. Effect of hypothermia in dogs on anesthetizing and apneic doses of inhalation agents. Determination of the anesthetic index (apnea/MAC). Anesthesiology 28: 689–700.

Rehder, K., Forbes, J., Alter, H., Hessler, O., and Stier, A. 1967. Halothane biotransformation in man: a quantitative study. Anesthesiology 28: 711–715.

Rice, S.A., Maze, M., Smith, C.M., Kosek, J.C., and Mazze, R.I. 1987. Halothane hepatotoxicity in Fischer 344 rats pretreated with isoniazid. Toxicol Appl Pharmacol 87: 411–420.

Rice, S.A. and Steffey, E.P. 1985a. Metabolism of halothane and isoflurane in horses. Vet Surg 14: 76. Ref Type: Abstract

———. 1985b. Metabolism of three inhaled anesthetics by cow, dog, lamb and rat hepatic microsomes. *In* Proceedings of the Second International Congress of Veterinary Anesthesia. Edited by J. Grandy, S. Hildebrand, W. McDonell, et al. Veterinary Practice Publishing Co., Santa Barbara, CA pp. 164–165.

Rorabeck, C.H. 1978. Pathophysiology of the anterior compartment syndrome: an experimental investigation. J Trauma 18: 299–303.

Ross, W.T. and Cardell, R.R. 1978. Proliferation of smooth endoplasmic reticulum and induction of microsomal drug-metabolizing enzymes after ether or halothane. Anesthesiology 48: 325–331.

Ross, W.T., Jr. and Daggy, B.P. 1981. Hepatic blood flow in phenobarbital pretreated rats during halothane anesthesia and hypoxia. Anesth Analg 60: 306–309.

Rowland, A.S., Baird, D.D., Weinberg, C.R., Shore, D.L., Shy, C.M., and Wilcox, A.J. 1992. Reduced fertility among women employed as dental assistants exposed to high levels of nitrous oxide. N Engl J Med 327: 993–997.

Rubin, E., Miller, K.W., and Roth, S.H. 2006. Molecular and cellular mechanisms of alcohol and anesthetics. The New York Academy of Sciences, New York.

Santos, M., Lopez-Sanroman, J., Garcia-Iturralde, P., Fuente, M., and Tendillo, F.J. 2005. Cardiovascular effects of desflurane in horses. Vet Anaesth Analg 32: 355–359.

Sardas, S., Cuhruk, H., Karakaya, A.E., and Atakurt, Y. 1992. Sister-chromatic exchanges in operating room personnel. Mutat Res 279: 117–120.

Sarton, E., Dahan, A., Teppema, L., vandenElsen, M., Olofsen, E., Berkenbosch, A., and vanKleef, J. 1996. Acute pain and central nervous system arousal do not restore impaired hypoxic ventilatory response during sevoflurane sedation. Anesthesiology 85: 295–303.

Scheller, M.S., Nakakimura, K., Fleischer, J.E., and Zornow, M.H. 1990. Cerebral effects of sevoflurane in the dog: comparison with isoflurane and enflurane. Br J Anaesth 65: 388–392.

Scheller, M.S., Tateishi, A., Drummond, J.C., and Zornow, M.H. 1988. The effects of sevoflurane on cerebral blood flow, cerebral metabolic rate for oxygen, intracranial pressure, and the electroencephalogram are similar to those of isoflurane in the rabbit. Anesthesiology 68: 548–552.

Schulman, M., Braverman, B., Ivankovich, A., and Gronert, G. 1981. Sevoflurane triggers malignant hyperthermia in swine (letter). Anesthesiology 54: 259–260.

Sessler, D.I. 2006. Temperature monitoring. *In* Miller's anesthesia. Edited by R.D. Miller. Elsevier Churchill Livingstone, Philadelphia pp. 1571–1597.

Sessler, D.I., Israel, D., Pozos, R.S., Pozos, M., and Rubinstein, E.H. 1988. Spontaneous post anesthetic tremor does not resemble thermoregulatory shivering. Anesthesiology 68: 843–850.

Seyde, W.C. and Longnecker, D.E. 1984. Anesthetic influences on regional hemodynamics in normal and hemorrhaged rats. Anesthesiology 61: 686–698.

Shingu, K., Eger, E.I., II, and Johnson, B.H. 1982a. Hypoxia may be more important than reductive metabolism in halothane-induced hepatic injury. Anesth Analg 61: 824–827.

———. 1982b. Hypoxia per se can produce hepatic damage without death in rats. Anesth Analg 61: 820–823.

Short, C.E. 1987a. Inhalant anesthetics. *In* Principles & Practice of Veterinary Anesthesia. Edited by C.E. Short. Williams & Wilkins, Baltimore pp. 70–90.

———. 1987b. Principles and Practice of Veterinary Anesthesia. Williams & Wilkins, Baltimore.

Sjogren, D., Lindahl, S.G.E., Gottlieb, C., and Sollevi, A. 1999. Ventilatory responses to acute and sustained hypoxia during sevoflurane anesthesia in women. Anesth Analg 89: 209–214.

Sjogren, D., Lindahl, S.E., and Sollevi, A. 1998. Ventilatory responses to acute and sustained hypoxia during isoflurane anesthesia. Anesth Analg 86: 403–409.

Sladen, R.N. 2005. Renal physiology. *In* Miller's Anesthesia. Edited by R.D. Miller. Elsevier Churchill Livingstone, Philadelphia pp. 777–811.

Soma, L.R. 1971. Textbook of Veterinary Anesthesia. Williams & Wilkins Co., Baltimore.

Staddon, G.E., Weaver, B.M.Q., and Webb, A.I. 1979. Distribution of cardiac output in anaesthetized horse. Res Vet Sci 27: 38–45.

Steffey, E.P. 1978. Enflurane and isoflurane anesthesia: a summary of laboratory and clinical investigations in horses. J Am Vet Med Assoc 172: 367–373.

———. 1991. Inhalation anesthetics and gases. *In* Equine Anesthesia; Monitoring and Emergency Therapy. Edited by W.W. Muir, III and J.A.E. Hubbell. Mosby Year Book, St. Louis pp. 352–379.

———. 1994. Inhalation anesthesia. *In* Feline Anaesthesia. Edited by L.W. Hall and P.M. Taylor. Bailliere Tindall Ltd., London pp. 157–193.

———. 1996. Inhalation anesthetics. *In* Lumb & Jones' Veterinary Anesthesia. Edited by J.C. Thurmon, G.J. Benson, and W. Tranquilli. Lea & Febiger, Philadelphia pp. 297–329.

———. 2001. Inhalation anesthetics. *In* Veterinary Pharmacology and Therapeutics. Edited by H.R. Adams. Iowa State University Press, Ames pp. 184–212.

Steffey, E.P., Dunlop, C.I., Cullen, L.K., Hodgson, D.S., Giri, S.N., Willits, N., Woliner, M.J., Jarvis, K.A., Smith, C.M., and Elliott, A.R. 1993a. Circulatory and respiratory responses of spontaneously breathing, laterally recumbent horses to 12 hours of halothane anesthesia. Am J Vet Res 54: 929–936.

Steffey, E.P., Dunlop, C.I., Farver, T.B., Woliner, M.J., and Schultz, L.J. 1987a. Cardiovascular and respiratory measurements in awake and isoflurane-anesthetized horses. Am J Vet Res 48: 7–12.

Steffey, E.P., Eisele, J.H., Baggot, J.D., Woliner, M.J., Jarvis, K.A., and Elliott, A.R. 1993b. Influence of inhaled anesthetics on the pharmacokinetics and pharmacodynamics of morphine. Anesth Analg 77: 346–351.

Steffey, E.P., Farver, T., Zinkl, J., Wheat, J.D., Meagher, D.M., and Brown, M.P. 1980. Alterations in horse blood cell count and biochemical values after halothane anesthesia. Am J Vet Res 41: 934–939.

Steffey, E.P., Farver, T.B., and Woliner, M.J. 1984. Circulatory and respiratory effects of methoxyflurane in dogs: comparison of halothane. Am J Vet Res 45: 2574–2579.

Steffey, E.P., Farver, T.B., and Woliner, M.J. 1987b. Cardiopulmonary function during 7 h of constant-dose halothane and methoxyflurane. J Appl Physiol 63: 1351–1359.

Steffey, E.P., Gillespie, J.R., Berry, J.D., and Eger, E.I., II 1974a. Cardiovascular effects with the addition of N2O to halothane in stump-tailed macaques during spontaneous and controlled ventilation. J Am Vet Med Assoc 165: 834–837.

Steffey, E.P., Gillespie, J.R., Berry, J.D., Eger, E.I., II, and Rhode, E.A. 1974a. Cardiovascular effect of halothane in the stump-tailed macaque during spontaneous and controlled ventilation. Am J Vet Res 35: 1315–1319.

———. 1974b. Circulatory effects of halothane and halothane-nitrous oxide anesthesia in the dog: controlled ventilation. Am J Vet Res 35: 1289–1293.

———. 1975. Circulatory effects of halothane and halothane-nitrous oxide anesthesia in the dog: spontaneous ventilation. Am J Vet Res 36: 197–200.

Steffey, E.P., Giri, S.N., Dunlop, C.I., Cullen, L.K., Hodgson, D.S., and Willits, N. 1993c. Biochemical and haematological changes following prolonged halothane anaesthesia in horses. Res Vet Sci 55: 338–345.

Steffey, E.P., Hodgson, D.S., Dunlop, C.I., Miller, M.F., Woliner, M.J., Heath, R.B., and Grandy, J. 1987c. Cardiopulmonary function during 5 hours of constant-dose isoflurane in laterally recumbent, spontaneously breathing horses. J Vet Pharmacol Therap 10: 290–297.

Steffey, E.P., and Howland, D, Jr. 1977. Isoflurane potency in the dog and cat. Am J Vet Res 38: 1833–1836.

———. 1978a. Potency of enflurane in dogs: comparison with halothane and isoflurane. Am J Vet Res 39: 673–677.

———. 1978b. Potency of halothane-N_2O in the horse. Am J Vet Res 39: 1141–1146.

———. 1980. Comparison of circulatory and respiratory effects of isoflurane and halothane anesthesia in horses. Am J Vet Res 41: 821–825.

———. 1978. Cardiovascular effects of halothane in the horse. Am J Vet Res 39: 611–615.

Steffey, E.P., Howland, D.J., Giri, S., and Eger, E.I., II 1977. Enflurane, halothane and isoflurane potency in horses. Am J Vet Res 38: 1037–1039.

Steffey, E.P., Kelly, A.B., Hodgson, D.S., Grandy, J.L., Woliner, M.J., and Willits, N. 1990a. Effect of body posture on cardiopulmonary function in horses during five hours of constant-dose halothane anesthesia. Am J Vet Res 51: 11–16.

Steffey, E.P., Kelly, A.B., and Woliner, M.J. 1987d. Time-related responses of spontaneously breathing, laterally recumbent horses to prolonged anesthesia with halothane. Am J Vet Res 48: 952–957.

Steffey, E.P., Mama, K.R., Galey, F., Puschner, B., and Woliner, M.J. 2005a. Effects of sevoflurane dose and mode of ventilation on cardiopulmonary function and blood biochemical variables in horses. Am J Vet Res 66: 606–614.

Steffey, E.P., Willits, N., Wong, P., Hildebrand, S.V., Wheat, J.D., Meagher, D.M., Hodgson, D., Pascoe, J.R., Heath, R.B., and Dunlop, C. 1991. Clinical investigations of halothane and isoflurane for induction and maintenance of foal anesthesia. J Vet Pharmacol Therap 14: 300–309.

Steffey, E.P., Woliner, M.J., and Dunlop, C. 1990b. Effects of five hours of constant 1.2 MAC halothane in sternally recumbent, spontaneously breathing horses. Equine Vet J 22: 433–436.

Steffey, E.P., Woliner, M.J., Puschner, B., and Galey, F. 2005b. Effects of desflurane and mode of ventilation on cardiovascular and respiratory functions and clinicopathologic variables in horses. Am J Vet Res 66: 669–677.

Steffey, E.P., Wong, P., Hildebrand, S.V., Hodgson, D., Meagher, D.M., Pascoe, J.R., Wheat, J.D., et al. 1985. Halothane and isoflurane anesthesia in foals. *In* Proceedings of the Second International Congress of Veterinary Anesthesia. Edited by J. Grandy, S. Hildebrand, W. McDonell, et al. Veterinary Practice Publishing Co., Santa Barbara, CA pp. 102–103.

Steffey, E.P., Zinkl, J., and Howland, D.J. 1979. Minimal changes in blood cell counts and biochemical values associated with prolonged isoflurane anesthesia of horses. Am J Vet Res 40: 1646–1648.

Stier, A., Alter, H., Hessler, O., and Rehder, K. 1964. Urinary excretion of bromide in halothane anesthesia. Anesth Analg 43: 723–728.

Stoelting, R.K. and Eger, E.I., II 1969. Percutaneous loss of nitrous oxide, cyclopropane, ether and halothane in man. Anesthesiology 30: 278–283.

Stoelting, R.K. and Hillier, S.C. 2006a. Pharmacokinetics and pharmacodynamics of injected and inhaled drugs. *In* Pharmacology & Physiology in Anesthetic Practice. Edited by R.K. Stoelting and S.C. Hillier. Lippincott Williams & Wilkins, Philadelphia pp. 3–41.

———. 2006b. Pharmacology & Physiology in Anesthetic Practice. Lippincott Williams & Wilkins, Philadelphia.

Stoelting, R.K. and Miller, R.D. 1989. Basics of Anesthesia. Churchill Livingston, New York.

Strum, D.P. and Eger, E.I., II 1987. Partition coefficients for sevoflurane in human blood, saline, and olive oil. Anesth Analg 66: 654–657.

Strum, D.P., Johnson, B.H., and Eger, E.I., II 1987. Stability of sevoflurane in soda lime. Anesthesiology 67: 779–781.

Swanson, C.R. (*Editor*). 1996. Anesthesiology update. Vet Clin North Am: Food Anim Pract 12.

Terriet, M.F., Desouza, G.J.A., Jacobs, J.S., Young, D., Lewis, M.C., Herrington, C., and Gold, M.I. 2000. Which is most pungent: isoflurane, sevoflurane or desflurane? Br J Anaesth 85: 305–307.

Theye, R.A. and Michenfelder, J.D. 1968. The effect of nitrous oxide on canine cerebral metabolism. Anesthesiology 29: 1119–1124.

Tinker, J.H., Gandolfi, A.J., and Van Dyke, R.A. 1976. Elevation of plasma bromide levels in patients following halothane anesthesia: time correlation with total halothane dosage. Anesthesiology 44: 194–196.

Todd, M.M. and Drummond, J.C. 1984. A comparison of the cerebrovascular and metabolic effects of halothane and isoflurane in the cat. Anesthesiology 60: 276–282.

Tranquilli, W.J., Thurmon, J.C., Benson, G.J., and Davis, L.E. 1986. Alteration in the arrhythmogenic dose of epinephrine (ADE) following xylazine administration to halothane-anesthetized dogs. J Vet Pharmacol Therap 9: 198–203.

Tranquilli, W.J., Thurmon, J.C., and Grimm, K.A. 2006. Veterinary anesthesia and analgesia. Lippincott Williams & Wilkins, Baltimore.

Tucker, W.K., Rackstein, A.D., and Munson, E.S. 1974. Comparison of arrhythmic doses of adrenaline, metaraminol, ephedrine, and phenylephrine, during isoflurane and halothane anesthesia in dogs. Br J Anaesth 46: 392–396.

Van Dyke, R.A., Chenoweth, M.B., and Van Poznak, A. 1964. Metabolism of volatile anesthetics. I. conversion *in vivo* of several anesthetics to $^{14}CO_2$ and chloride. Biochem Pharmacol 13: 1239–1247.

Van Dyke, R.A. and Wood, C.L. 1975. *In vitro* studies on irreversible binding of halothane metabolite to microsomes. Drug Metab Dispos 3: 51–57.

Vatner, S.F. and Smith, N.T. 1974. Effects of halothane on left ventricular function and distribution of regional blood flow in dogs and primates. Circ Res 34: 155–167.

Wallin, R.F., Regan, B.M., Napoli, M.D., and Stern, I.J. 1975. Sevoflurane: a new inhalational anesthetic agent. Anesth Analg 54: 758–766.

Warltier, D.C. and Pagel, P.S. 1992. Cardiovascular and respiratory actions of desflurane: is desflurane different from isoflurane? Anesth Analg 75: S17–S31.

Webb, A.I. 1985. The effect of species differences in the uptake and distribution of inhalant anesthetic agents. *In* Proceedings of the Second International Congress of Veterinary Anesthesia. Edited by J. Grandy, S. Hildebrand, W. McDonell, et al. Veterinary Practice Publishing Co., Santa Barbara, CA pp. 27–32.

Wedel, D.J., Gammel, S.A., Milde, J.H., and Iaizzo, P.A. 1993. Delayed onset of malignant hyperthermia induced by isoflurane and desflurane compared with halothane in susceptible swine. Anesthesiology 78: 1138–1144.

Wedel, D.J., Iaizzo, P.A., and Milde, J.H. 1991. Desflurane is a trigger of malignant hyperthermia in susceptible swine. Anesthesiology 74: 508–512.

Weiskopf, R.B., Cahalan, M.K., Eger, E.I., II, Yasuda, N., Rampil, I.J., Ionescu, P., Lockhart, S.H., Johnson, B.H., Freire, B., and Kelley, S. 1991. Cardiovascular actions of desflurane in normocarbic volunteers. Anesth Analg 73: 143–156.

Weiskopf, R.B., Eger, E.I., II, Holmes, M.A., Rampil, I.J., Johnson, B.H., Brown, J.G., Yasuda, N., and Targ, A.G. 1989. Epinephrine-induced premature ventricular contractions and changes in arterial blood pressure and heart rate during I-653, isoflurane, and halothane anesthesia in swine. Anesthesiology 70: 293–298.

Weiskopf, R.B., Eger, E.I., II, Ionescu, P., Yasuda, N., Cahalan, M.K., Freire, B., Peterson, N., Lochhart, S.H., Rampil, I.J., and Laster, M. 1992. Desflurane does not produce hepatic or renal injury in human volunteers. Anesth Analg 74: 570–574.

Weiskopf, R.B., Holmes, M.A., Eger, E.I., II, Johnson, B.H., Rampil, I.J., and Brown, J.G. 1988. Cardiovascular effects of I-653 in swine. Anesthesiology 69: 303–309.

Whitcher, C.E., Cohen, E.N., and Trudell, J.R. 1971. Chronic exposure to anesthetic gases in the operating room. Anesthesiology 35: 348–353.

Whitehair, K.J., Steffey, E.P., Woliner, M.J., and Willits, N.H. 1996. Effects of inhalation anesthetic agents on response of horses to three hours of hypoxemia. Am J Vet Res 57: 351–360.

Wiesner, G., Harth, M., Hoerauf, K., Szulc, R., Jurczyk, W., Sobczynski, P., Hobbhahn, J., and Taeger, K. 2000. Occupational exposure to inhaled anaesthetics: a follow-up study on anaesthetists of an eastern European university hospital. Acta Anaesthesiol Scand 44: 804–806.

Woodforth, I.J., Hicks, R.G., Crawford, M.R., Stephen, J.H., and Burke, D.J. 1997. Electroencephalographic evidence of seizure activity under deep sevoflurane anesthesia in a nonepileptic patient. Anesthesiology 87: 1579–1582.

Yasuda, N., Lockhart, S.H., Eger, E.I., II, Weiskopf, R.B., Johnson, B.H., Freire, B.A., and Fassoulaki, A. 1991a. Kinetics of desflurane, isoflurane, and halothane in humans. Anesthesiology 74: 489–498.

Yasuda, N., Lockhart, S.H., Eger, E.I., II, Weiskopf, R.B., Liu, J., Laster, M.J., Taheri, S., and Peterson, N.A. 1991b. Comparison of kinetics of sevoflurane and isoflurane in humans. Anesth Analg 72: 316–324.

Yasuda, N., Targ, A.G., and Eger, E.I., II 1989. Solubility of I-653, sevoflurane, isoflurane, and halothane in human tissues. Anesth Analg 69: 370–373.

Yasuda, N., Targ, A.G., Eger, E.I., II, Johnson, B.H., and Weiskopf, R.B. 1990. Pharmacokinetics of desflurane, sevoflurane, isoflurane, and halothane in pigs. Anesth Analg 71: 340–348.

Young, W.L. 1992. Effects of desflurane on the central nervous system. Anesth Analg 75: S32–S37.

Zhou, T.J., White, P.F., Chiu, J.W., Joshi, G.P., Dullye, K.K., Duffy, L.L., and Tongier, W.K. 2000. Onset/offset characteristics and intubating conditions of rapacuronium: a comparison with rocuronium. Br J Anaesth 85: 246–250.

CHAPTER

11

INJECTABLE ANESTHETIC AGENTS

LYSA P. POSNER AND PATRICK BURNS

Injectable anesthetics provide a rapid means of producing sedation or anesthesia in veterinary patients. The four stages of anesthesia used to define central nervous system (CNS) depression are similar in a patient regardless of whether the anesthetic is injected or administered by inhalation. An advantage of injectable anesthetics, particularly when administered intravenously (IV); is the ability to proceed more rapidly through Stage II anesthesia (the excitement stage). This allows a more rapid, smooth induction of anesthesia, which is more pleasant in the small animal and safer in the large animal.

There is no anesthetic agent that produces ideal anesthesia under all circumstances. When evaluating an injectable anesthetic agent, it is important to evaluate both the pharmacokinetics (absorption, distribution, metabolism, and excretion) and the pharmacodynamics (the physiologic effects) of a particular drug in order to select the agent most suited to a particular clinical condition, in a particular species.

INDICATIONS FOR INJECTABLE ANESTHESIA

There are many situations where injectable anesthesia has advantages over inhalation anesthesia. Intravenous induction of anesthesia allows for rapid control of the airway, which can prevent aspiration and allows for the administration of oxygen, with or without an inhalant anesthetic. Injectable anesthetics allow for unobstructed visualization of the upper airway for examination or surgical procedures as well as endoscopic access to the upper and lower airways. Similarly, IV anesthetics can provide rapid control and reduction in CNS activity. This is important in patients that are actively having a seizure or who have elevated intracranial pressure. Injectable anesthetics are less stressful for most patients compared with an inhalant induction and can attenuate the excitement seen during Stage II anesthesia. For large animals (e.g., horses), preventing the excitement stage is paramount for the animal's safety as well as the medical personnel. Total intravenous anesthesia (TIVA) has become popular in human and veterinary medicine because it can decrease the stress response, is associated with better recoveries, provides cardiovascular stability, and maintains cerebral autoregulation better than inhalants.

Intramuscular injection (IM) of anesthetics can be advantageous for fractious animals, or for wildlife or exotic animals, where injectable agents can be administered remotely (e.g., dart or syringe pole). Finally, injectable anesthesia decreases the exposure of people and the environment to inhalant gases.

DISADVANTAGES OF INJECTABLE ANESTHESIA

In general, injectable anesthetic agents have a large volume of distribution and wake-up is associated with redistribution and then metabolism of the drug. Thus, it can be hard to fine-tune anesthetic depth and wake-up compared with the inhalant drugs that are generally excreted unchanged through the lungs quite rapidly. However, some of the currently available intravenous agents (e.g., propofol, remifentanil) have such short durations of action that depth of anesthesia can be readily adjusted by changing the administration rate. These types of drugs have made it possible for safe and satisfactory anesthesia without the use of inhalation agents.

Another potential disadvantage of injectable anesthetics is the potential for human abuse. Therefore, many injectable anesthetic agents, as well as agents commonly used concurrently with them, are classified as controlled substances under the 1970 USA Controlled Substances Act. This places restrictions on purchase, storage, record keeping and use of these drugs.

PROPERTIES OF AN IDEAL INJECTABLE ANESTHETIC DRUG

There is no ideal injectable (or inhalation) anesthetic drug available at this time. One can, however, hypothesize what properties such a drug would have. These can be divided into physiological and pharmacological properties.

IDEAL PHYSIOLOGICAL PROPERTIES. The ideal injectable anesthetic agent should produce unconsciousness and amnesia, as well as provide analgesia and muscle relaxation. The ideal drug would produce those qualities while maintaining physiological homeostasis; that is, there should be no adverse changes in cardiovascular, respiratory, gastrointestinal, CNS, or endocrine functions.

IDEAL PHARMACOLOGICAL PROPERTIES. An ideal injectable anesthetic should have a wide margin of safety (high therapeutic index) in a variety of species. It should have a short duration of action and be noncumulative. The drug should be readily metabolized and/or excreted, ideally by more than one route. A specific and complete reversal agent should be available. The ideal drug would be chemically stable, have a long shelf life, have a physiologic pH, have a nontoxic vehicle, and would be inexpensive.

BARBITURATES

HISTORY. Barbituric acid was first synthesized in 1864 by Adolph von Baeyer, but the compound was considered clinically useless (Short 1983). By the early 1900s, the barbiturates or drugs derived from barbituric acid were shown to produce sleep and prevent seizures, and an anesthetic revolution took place. Barbiturates are CNS depressants and can be used at increasing doses to produce sedation, hypnosis, anesthesia, coma, and even death (euthanasia solutions). The two major uses for barbiturates in modern veterinary medicine are as induction agents for anesthesia and as anticonvulsants.

CLASSIFICATION

Chemistry. Barbiturates are derivatives of barbituric acid, which is a combination of malonic acid and urea (Fig. 11.1). The addition of alkyl or aryl group at position 5 of the barbituric acid ring imparts CNS depressant effects. Further modification of the molecule by substituting sulfur (thio) for oxygen (oxy), at position 2 of the barbiturate acid ring, increases the lipid solubility (thiobarbiturates versus oxybarbiturates) (Fig 11.2). Lipid solubility can also be enhanced by increasing the number of side chains at position 5a and 5b of the barbituric acid ring (Fig. 11.2). Increasing solubility results in a decreased duration of action (shorter acting), an increased metabolic degradation, and an increased hypnotic potency (Fig. 11.3). Longer side chains at position 5 increases anticonvulsant activity (Figs. 11.4, 11.5).

Barbiturates are often classified by either their duration of action (e.g., long, intermediate, short, or ultrashort) or by their chemical structure. The chemical structure (e.g.,

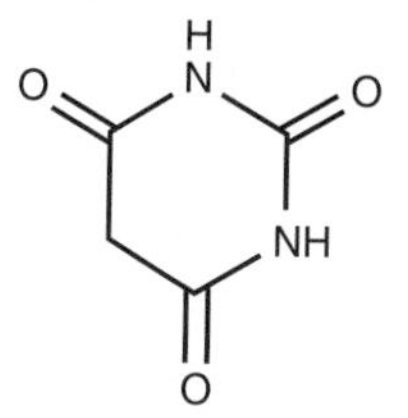

FIG. 11.1 Barbituric acid.

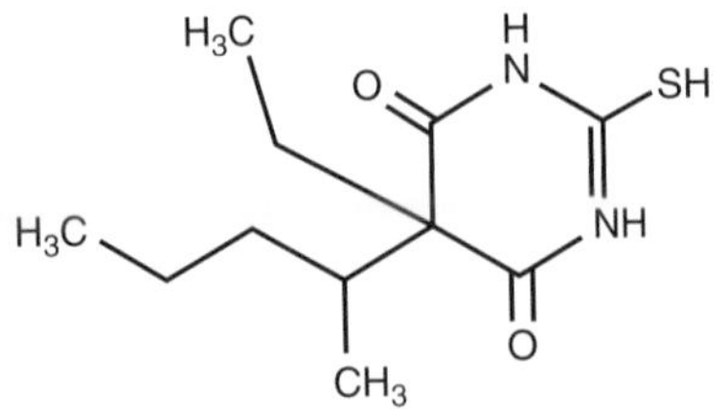

FIG. 11.2 Thiopental.

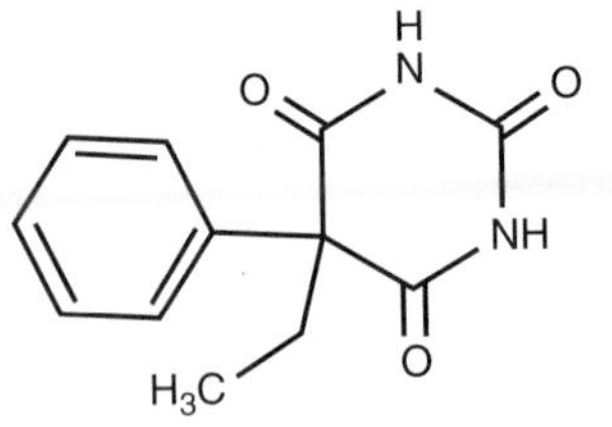

FIG. 11.4 Phenobarbital.

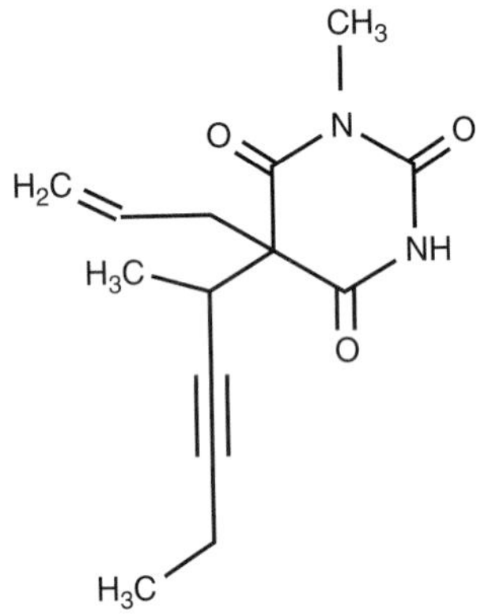

FIG. 11.3 Methohexital.

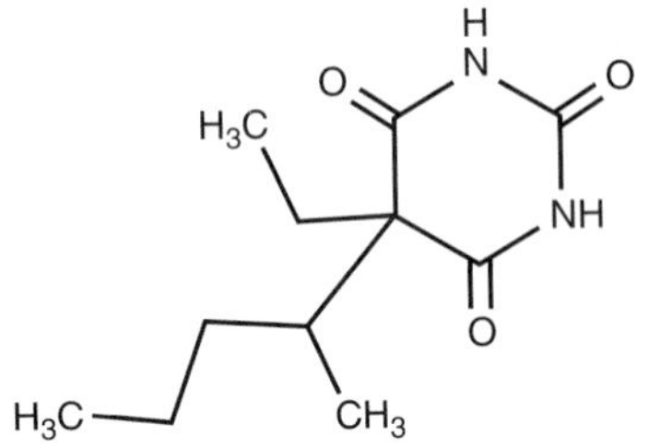

FIG. 11.5 Pentobarbital.

TABLE 11.1 Type of barbiturate, durations of action, and common use

Drug	Oxygen/Sulfur at Position 2	Duration of Action	Common Use
Phenobarbital	Oxybarbiturate	~12 hr	Anticonvulsant
Pentobarbital	Oxybarbiturate	1–2 hr	Anesthesia/euthanasia
Thiopental	Thiobarbiturate	~20 min	Anesthesia
Thiamylal	Thiobarbiturate	~20 min	Anesthesia
Methohexital	Oxybarbiturate	~10–15 min	Anesthesia

oxybarbiturates, thiobarbiturates) of barbiturates determines the time of onset and duration of action which, in turn, determines their use. (Table 11.1).

How Supplied. Barbiturates are sparingly soluble in water. Aqueous solutions are weakly acid and will combine with sodium or other fixed alkalis to form water-soluble salts that can be delivered IV. The sodium atom joins the oxygen atom attached to carbon 2. These salts hydrolyze in water to form very alkaline solutions with a pH usually between 9 and 10. Thus, although barbiturates are acids they are prepared as salts that are bases. The high alkalinity of the solution makes it caustic if given perivascularly (can cause sloughing of tissue) but makes the solution fairly bacteriostatic. Barbiturates are delivered as a racemic mixture with their L-isomers nearly twice as potent as their D-isomers.

MECHANISM OF ACTION. Barbiturates depress the reticular activating system (RAS), which controls arousal and inhibits the development or spread of epileptiform activity. The RAS system is particularly sensitive to barbiturates (Harvey 1975) and animals are unable to be aroused or to maintain the wakeful state following administration.

Barbiturates work by potentiating inhibitory effects and inhibiting excitatory effects. They increase γ-aminobutyric acid (GABA) binding (main inhibitory neurotransmitter) by decreasing the rate of dissociation of GABA from its receptor. Activation of the GABA receptors increases transmembrane chloride conductance resulting in hyperpolarization of the postsynaptic cell membrane, which causes inhibition of the postsynaptic neuron. Barbiturates also block glutamate binding (main excitatory neurotransmitter) at AMPA receptors.

Furthermore, at high doses, barbiturates can decrease transmission of nerve impulses at nicotinic acetylcholine receptors in the neuromuscular junction. These effects occur because barbiturates decrease the sensitivity of polysynaptic junctions to the depolarizing action of acetylcholine, which results in muscle weakness.

SPECIFIC BARBITURATES

Thiopental Sodium (Pentothal Sodium, Thiopentone Sodium). Thiopental is the most commonly used barbiturate in veterinary medicine. It is an ultrashort-acting thiobarbiturate and differs from pentobarbital only at the number 2 carbon where a sulfur molecule has replaced the oxygen. It is a yellow crystalline powder that is unstable in aqueous solutions. Thiopental is dispensed as a powder buffered with sodium carbonate, which is commonly reconstituted with sterile water or sterile saline. Once reconstituted, thiopental has a pH between 9 and 10. The high alkalinity of the solution results in thiopental having a long shelf life, but as the solution ages it becomes less potent (Lumb and Jones 1996). Although supplied in an alkaline pH, thiopental is a weak organic acid with a pK_a value of 7.6; and has a relatively low ionization (39%) at plasma pH (Brandon and Baggot 1981). The nonioned moiety is highly lipid soluble, which allows it to quickly penetrate the blood-brain barrier and thus be a rapidly acting anesthetic.

In general the 2.5% solution is used with small animals and the 2.5% or 5% solution is used with larger animals. Thiopental can been mixed with propofol in a 1 : 1 (vol: vol) ratio which is chemically stable (Paw and Garrood 1998). The combination of the two GABA agonists produces a synergistic clinical effect and improves the induction and recovery profile of thiopental to more resemble that of propofol (Ko et al. 1999).

Thiamylal (Surital). Thiamylal was an ultrashort-acting thiobarbiturate commonly used in veterinary medicine, but it is no longer commercially available. Its chemistry, pharmacokinetics and pharmacodynamics were similar to thiopental; however, the incidence of bigeminy was more common with thiamylal (~65–85%) than it is with thiopental (~40%) (Plumb 1999).

Pentobarbital Sodium (Nembutal Sodium). Pentobarbital is a short-acting oxybarbiturate that has been used in veterinary medicine since the early 1930s. Although commonly used in the past for clinical anesthesia, its current use is primarily as a euthanasia solution and for anesthesia in laboratory rodents. Pentobarbital is effective when given intraperitoneally as well as intravenously and thus can be used successfully in small rodents. It undergoes extensive hepatic metabolism and is totally dependent on the liver for biotransformation and elimination. Animals can show excitement during induction and recovery, which can be prevented by concurrent use of tranquilizers or sedatives. It is recommended to administer $^1/_3$ to $^1/_2$ the calculated dose of pentobarbital intravenously as a bolus to quickly get through the Stage II (excitement) anesthesia and then to titrate the remainder of the dose to reach the desired depth of anesthesia.

The duration of action of pentobarbital is much longer (4–8×) than thiopental in most animals and therefore is much less commonly used for anesthesia. However, its long duration of action makes it clinically useful for long-term anticonvulsant treatment.

Euthanasia Solutions. Pentobarbital is the primary ingredient in most commercially available euthanasia solutions. Lidocaine and phenytoin are often added to increase cardiovascular depression as well as change the solution from a Schedule II controlled drug to a Schedule III controlled drug (Plumb 1999). The lethal dose of pentobarbital in the dog is 85 mg/kg orally and 40–60 mg/kg intravenously. Toxicosis, including death, has been reported in dogs fed uncooked meat from a horse euthanized 8 days previously with pentobarbital (Polley and Weaver 1977). Cooking does not inactivate pentobarbital in meat, as animals euthanatized with pentobarbital and rendered at a commercial plant showed virtually no degradation of the drug (O'Connor 1985). The recommended dose for euthanasia is 87 mg/kg IV.

Phenobarbital Sodium (Luminal, Phenobarbitone). Phenobarbital was first synthesized in Germany in 1912 and was marketed as Luminal. It is a long-acting oxybarbiturate, currently, whose primary use is as an anticonvulsant or for long-term sedation (e.g., for treatment of animals with strychnine poisoning or tetanus). For more information on the anticonvulsant use of phenobarbital, see Chapter 20.

Methohexital Sodium (Brevital). Methohexital is a unique oxybarbiturate in that it is ultrashort-acting. Methohexital is twice as potent as thiopental (Turner and Ilkiw 1990) but has a higher incidence of CNS excitatory effects. Methohexital activates abnormal EEG tracings in epilepsy-prone subjects. Methohexital should not be used in patients with increased CNS excitation (e.g., strychnine poisoning) or with seizure disorders.

Methohexital should be administered intravenously; however, perivascular injection does not produce tissue irritation. Administration of methohexital should be fairly rapid since slow injection rates can be associated with muscular tremors and excitement. Excitement and muscle tremors can be reduced by prior administration of sedatives or tranquilizers.

The duration of action of methohexital is short, with dogs and cats attaining sternal recumbency within 5–10 minutes of administration (Sams et al. 1985). Although methohexital is metabolized 4–5× faster than thiopental, awakening is due to redistribution rather than metabolism. In greyhounds, recovery from methohexital anesthesia is significantly faster than from thiopental (Sams et al. 1985) and until the introduction of propofol to veterinary practice, methohexital was considered the induction agent of choice for greyhounds.

PHYSIOLOGIC EFFECTS

CNS. Barbiturates are administered to produce anesthesia (short-acting barbiturates), or as anticonvulsants (long-acting barbiturates). However, they possess properties that are favorable to cerebral physiology. Barbiturates decrease cerebral blood flow (CBF) (Albrecht et al. 1977) and cause a dose-dependent depression of the electroencephalogram (EEG) eventually resulting in a flat EEG (Kiersey et al. 1951). They decrease cerebral oxygen consumption ($CMRO_2$) particularly in cortical areas by up to 55%, which parallels the depression of the neuronal activity. Metabolic needs of the brain remain constant: only hypothermia will decrease cerebral metabolic needs (Steen et al. 1983). Furthermore, they decrease intracranial pressure (Bedford et al. 1980) and similarly decrease intraocular pressure (Mirakhur and Shepherd 1985). Since ICP decreases more than MAP, cerebral perfusion pressure is preserved. Thus barbiturates like thiopental are often chosen to anesthetize patients with CNS disease or trauma.

Methohexital, is an ultrashort-acting barbiturate, but is an exception to the cerebro-friendly status of barbiturates. Methohexital has been associated with generalized excitement and activation of epileptic foci (Stoelting 1999) and is not recommended for patients with a seizure history.

Cardiovascular. Barbiturates cause changes in the cardiovascular system that are dependent on the dose and the physiologic status of the patients. In healthy dogs, there is a decrease in stroke volume and contractility with an increase in heart rate (HR) and systemic vascular resistance (Turner and Ilkiw 1990). In healthy dogs, there is a minimal change to cardiac output as the reflex tachycardia compensates for the decrease in stroke volume, but mild hypotension is often seen.

It is generally accepted that in compromised dogs, barbiturates result in an exaggerated cardiovascular depression. However, healthy dogs that suffered from acute blood loss did not show a depression in cardiovascular parameters (Ilkiw et al. 1991). Dogs and pigs do, however, need a smaller induction dose following severe hemorrhage (Weiskopf and Bogetz 1985). Caution should be used when administering barbiturates to patients with dehydration, hypovolemia, anemia, blood loss, or underlying cardiac disease.

Thiopental can precipitate ventricular arrhythmias; particularly bigeminy (Muir 1977) as well as potentiate epinephrine-induced arrhythmias (Atlee and Malkinson 1982). Lidocaine can be administered with thiopental. This allows less thiopental to be administered (reduces cardiovascular depression) and protects against ventricular arrhythmias (Rawlings and Kolata 1983). Caution should be used when administering thiopental to patients with high sympathetic tone or who are already arrhythmic.

There is a dose dependent affect of the vasomotor center by barbiturates. Rapid IV injection of an induction dose of a thiobarbiturate causes a sharp but transitory fall in arterial pressure because of the high concentration briefly depressing the vasomotor center. Venodilation results in splenic sequestration of RBCs and a concomitant drop in packed cell volume (PCV). For this reason barbiturates are often avoided for anesthesia of patients scheduled for a splenectomy. Furthermore, the vasodilation contributes to heat loss. With a decline in heat production during anesthesia and an increase in heat loss owing to peripheral vasodilation, anesthetized patients can quickly become hypothermic.

Barbiturates do not block the autonomic responses to pain or intubation and thus should be administered with drugs that will attenuate those responses (e.g., opioids).

Respiratory. When used at induction doses, barbiturates produce central respiratory depression. There is a decrease in respiratory rate and minute ventilation, with apnea in some patients (Quandt et al. 1998). In addition to causing respiratory depression, the barbiturates decrease the reflex responses to hypercapnia and hypoxemia (Hirshman et al. 1975). Following induction with a barbiturate, patients should be intubated and assisted with breathing as necessary. The blood concentration inhibiting the respiratory center is considerably less than that arresting the heart, so patients that are apneic may be stable cardiovascularly. The occurrence of bigeminy appears to be decreased in well-oxygenated patients. Oral barbiturates have minimal or no effect on respiratory function, probably due to lower plasma concentrations.

Muscular. Barbiturates provide good muscle relaxation and generally produce favorable intubating conditions. Laryngeal reflexes are preserved with barbiturate anesthesia (Jackson et al. 2004) facilitating better evaluation of laryngeal function. The increased sensitivity of laryngeal and bronchial reflexes can lead to laryngospasm (Barker et al. 1992). Although laryngeal reflexes are preserved, all patients induced with a barbiturate should be intubated.

Gastrointestinal. No important effects such as diarrhea or intestinal stasis have been routinely noted following standard use of thiobarbiturates.

Kidney. The thiobarbiturates appear to have no direct effect upon the kidney, but can decrease urine output because of decreased blood flow and glomerular filtration rate resulting from hypotension. Patients with uremia have decreased plasma binding of barbiturates (more physiologically available drug) and thus need lower induction doses (Ghoneim and Pandya 1975). Approximately 25% of phenobarbital is excreted unchanged by the kidney (Plumb 1999) and thus patients with impaired renal function are at risk for prolonged and or exaggerated effects.

Fetus/Neonate. Most barbiturates easily cross the placenta, and equilibrium between maternal and fetal circulations is established within a few minutes. While in utero, most fetuses are slightly acidemic when compared to the mother. Since barbiturates are more active in acid environments, it is possible that the neonate will have a greater concentration of active drug. In humans, anesthesia with thiopental for cesarean sections resulted in neonates with depressed reflexes, altered acid-base status, and delayed suckling when compared to epidural anesthesia (Sener et al. 2003.) Similarly, neurologic function was depressed in puppies following cesarean sections where the dam was administered thiopental (Luna et al. 2004). Pentobarbital has been associated with slow neonatal recovery, delayed nursing and increased morbidity (Lumb and Jones 1996).

Miscellaneous. Doses of thiobarbiturates that produce surgical anesthesia depress basal metabolism so that less body heat is produced during anesthesia concurrently with excessive heat loss as a result of vasodilation. It is important that surgical patients anesthetized with barbiturates be kept warm.

The decrease in vasomotion associated with barbiturates also leads to splenic sequestration of red blood cells (RBCs). Since the spleen can become quite large and a significant amount of blood can be stored in the spleen, barbiturates are not recommended for patients having a splenectomy.

Glucose effect is a term used to describe a reanesthetizing action seen in animals recovering from barbiturate anesthesia that are administered glucose solutions. Glucose decreases microsomal metabolism and thus can decrease barbiturate metabolism (Peters and Strother 1972). A similar event can occur with administration of epinephrine; however, little clinical effect is seen at routine barbiturate doses (Hatch 1966).

Analgesia. Barbiturates do not provide analgesia. While anesthetized, nociceptive input is not perceived by the brain, but the pain pathways are activated. In patients where pain will continue following anesthesia, alternative analgesics should be used. At subanesthetic doses, barbiturates may cause hyperalgesia, but this effect is controversial and probably not clinically relevant when barbiturates are used as induction agents.

INDICATIONS. The most common use of barbiturates in veterinary medicine is for rapid induction of general anesthesia. They are also used for the prevention and treatment of seizures, and for euthanasia (see Chapters 16 and 18).

PHARMACOKINETICS

Thiopental. Thiopental is highly protein bound (>70%) (Brandon 1981) and has a pKa near 7.6. After IV administration, thiobarbiturates are initially present in high concentrations in highly perfused tissues (e.g., the brain), resulting in rapid induction of general anesthesia. Thiobarbiturates then redistribute to the moderately perfused body tissues (e.g., muscle). This redistribution to moderately perfused tissues decreases the concentration in the plasma in brain tissues, allowing the animal to regain consciousness. Further redistribution to adipose tissue from both highly and moderately perfused tissues results in the complete recovery from thiobarbiturate anesthesia. Animals with lower percentages of fat and/or muscle tissue have a smaller percentage of area for the barbiturates to redistribute to. Thus, normally lean patients (e.g., sight hounds), neonates, or cachetic patients might have prolonged recoveries from thiobarbiturates. Similarly, since awakening depends on redistribution, repeated dosing is not recommended because of cumulative effects and prolongation of recovery.

Pharmacokinetics of thiopental in rabbits, sheep, and dogs showed an initial volume of distribution of 38.6 ± 10 ml/kg, 44.5 ± 9.1 ml/kg, and 38.1 ± 18.4 ml/kg, respectively (Ilkiw et al. 1991) Elimination half-life was longest in the sheep (251.9 ± 107.8 min) shorter in the dog (182.4 ± 57.9 min) and shortest in the rabbit (43.1 ± 3.4 min) (Ilkiw et al. 1991).

The activity of a drug is dependent on the percentage of the drug that is unbound and unionized. Since thiopental is an acid it is nonionized in an acid environment. It is also highly protein bound. Many ill patients are both acidemic and hypoproteinemic and thus may have greater percentage of active drug available to them. Thus, the therapeutic index may be smaller in sicker animals making them easier to overdose.

Phenobarbital. Phenobarbital is readily absorbed from the GI tract with bioavailability ~90% in dogs (Pedersoli et al. 1987) and ~99% in horses (Plumb 1999).

Pharmacokinetics of an IV bolus dose of phenobarbital in horses showed a volume of distribution at steady state of 0.803 ± 0.07 l/kg, terminal phase elimination of 18.3 ± 3.65 hr, and total body clearance 30.8 ± 6.2 ml/kg/hr (Duran et al. 1987). In the dog, volume of distribution is ~0.75 l/kg (Plumb 1999), the mean half-life was 92.6 ± 23.7 hours, mean total clearance 5.6 ± 2.31 ml/kg/hr (Pedersoli et al. 1987). In the goat, the volume of distribution for pentobarbital (30 mg/kg) administered intravenously is 0.72 l/kg; the first-order disappearance rate kinetic constant is 0.76 hour and the half-life is 0.91 hour (Boulos et al. 1972).

Pentobarbital. Pentobarbital is well absorbed from the GI tract. It is 35–45% protein bound. In dogs, the elimination-phase half-life of pentobarbital is 8.2 ± 2.2 hr. The steady-state volume of distribution is 1.08 ± 0.21 liters/kg and the elimination clearance is 0.0013 ± 0.0004 liters/min (Frederiksen et al. 1983). Comparatively, ruminants, especially sheep and goats, metabolized pentobarbital much faster; elimination half-life for the goat is ~1 hr compared to dogs which is ~8.0 hr (Plumb 1999).

METABOLISM. Barbiturates are almost completely biotransformed in the liver and eliminated by the kidney. Most barbiturates are metabolized principally by the hepatic microsomal enzyme system and cause microsomal enzyme induction (P450 system). This can result in altered metabolism of other drugs as well of the barbiturate itself if given repeatedly. Alternatively, neonates, cachetic, or hypothermic animals can have decreased microsomal metabolism and thus these drugs may have a prolonged effect in these animals. Recovery times for patients with hepatic dysfunction can be markedly prolonged, but they are fairly normal in patients with renal dysfunction.

Although awakening from thiobarbiturates is generally more rapid than from oxybarbiturates (except for methohexital), the former is due to rapid redistribution rather than from rapid metabolism.

Greyhounds are deficient in oxidative enzymes needed for metabolism of thiobarbiturates (Robinson et al. 1986). Thus, along with having low fat stores, metabolism is extremely prolonged and awakening may be >8 hours. Thiobarbiturates should not be used in greyhounds.

Tolerance has been reported with multiple or frequent use of barbiturates. It can occur as a sequela to the induction of microsomal enzyme activity (i.e., increased metabolism) or as a general neurological adaptation to chronic barbiturate effects.

ADVERSE EFFECTS/CONTRAINDICATIONS. Barbiturates can cause sequestration of red blood cells (RBCs) in the spleen from venodilation. Thus, these drugs are often avoided for a splenectomy.

Thiobarbiturates should not be used in greyhounds (see above).

Perivascular administration of thiobarbiturates can result in tissue damage and necrosis (sloughing). If accidental perivascular administration occurs, the affected area should be infiltrated with either saline or lidocaine. Lidocaine has the benefit of providing pain relief, but using both, when infiltrated in sufficient doses to dilute the thiopental, will prevent tissue damage.

DOSE. Table 11.2 shows dose ranges to produce anesthesia for common barbiturates in different species. Lower doses are generally used when patients are premedicated with other CNS depressants or have serious concurrent disease, and higher doses are generally needed when no other drugs are given. The use of premedicants with barbiturate anesthesia allows for a smoother induction and recovery.

The pH of thiopental is ~10 and therefore should be given only by IV injection, as any injection outside of the vein can lead to pain and skin sloughing. Intraarterially, barbiturates, in particular thiopental, produce spasms of the arterial wall, which can lead to thrombosis and poor perfusion if collateral circulation is not present (e.g., pinnae of ear, digits). Thiopental should not be administered into body cavities.

Thiopental should be administered "to effect." That is, a dose is calculated but given slowly until the desired effect is present; usually the endpoint is a patient that can be easily intubated. The slower-acting barbiturates need to have a portion of the dose "bolused" to prevent seeing the excitement stage. If thiopental is given after premedication, this quick bolus is unnecessary.

Most barbiturates have a similar but small therapeutic index (lethal dose/therapeutic dose); however, the shorter acting barbiturates have fewer postanesthetic complications because of their shorter duration of action.

It should be remembered that barbiturates are acids and therefore are nonionized (in an active form) in the acidemic patient. Uremia can decrease protein binding and further increase the percentage of active drug. Many ill patients present acidemic (e.g., lactic acidosis) and hypoproteinemic. These patients are at risk for a relative overdose of barbiturate drugs.

TABLE 11.2 Doses of common barbiturates in various species

	Thiopental mg/kg IV	Pentobarbital mg/kg IV*	Phenobarbital mg/kg IV	Methohexital mg/kg IV
Dog	8–22	2–30	6.0	3–11
Cat	8–22	2–15	6.0	3–11
Horse	4–15		1.0–10.0	5
Cow	4–22			
Sheep	8–15	20–30		
Goats	8–20	20–30		
Llamas	6–15			
Pigs	5–12	10–30		5–8
Mice		30–90 (IP)		
Rats		20–40 (IP)		
Rabbits	20–50	15–40		10
Chickens	20			
Primates	2–20	37		2

*Dose of pentobarbital for euthanasia is 87 mg/kg.
IP = Intraperitoneal.

DURATION OF ACTION. Duration of action of thiopental in dogs is fairly short, with extubation occurring 25.2 ± 15.7 minutes after an induction dose and ability to walk unaided at 72.8 ± 26.1 minutes (Quandt et al. 1998). Since all of the barbiturates require extensive liver metabolism, it should be expected that neonates and animals with hepatic dysfunction would have a prolonged duration of action. There is also significant individual variation based on sex, weight, nutritional status, body temperature, and breed as well as the type of barbiturate used. For example, thiobarbiturates have a longer duration in greyhounds than in mixed breeds (Robinson et al. 1986). Alternatively, methohexital, an oxybarbiturate, induces a shorter period of anesthesia in the greyhounds than thiopental, a thiobarbiturate (Robinson et al. 1986).

Chloramphenicol can double the duration of action of pentobarbital due to depression of microsomal enzyme activity. Since awakening from thiobarbiturates is due to redistribution and not metabolism, the concurrent administration of chloramphenicol with thiopental does not prolong awakening when both drugs are used at clinically relevant doses (Reiche and Frey 1981).

SPECIES DIFFERENCES

Dogs

Sight Hounds. Since awakening from anesthesia is due to redistribution of barbiturates to fat and muscle, lean breeds with small fat stores (e.g., whippet, Irish wolfhounds) can show an exaggerated effect to barbiturates. With little area to redistribute the drug, these breeds also have an increased risk of prolonged duration of action and overdose.

Greyhounds. Greyhounds are classified as sight hounds and are at risks as discussed above. In addition, greyhounds are deficient in oxidative enzymes needed for metabolism of thiobarbiturates and thus can have extremely prolonged recoveries (Robinson et al. 1986). Although not fatal, the increased risk of overdose coupled with the prolonged recovery makes thiopental not recommended for use with greyhounds.

In greyhounds, recovery from methohexital anesthesia is significantly faster than from thiopental (Sams et al. 1985).

Ruminants. Barbiturates can be successfully used for anesthesia in ruminants, but due to the propensity for ruminants to regurgitate, the airway needs to be protected by placement of a cuffed orotracheal tube.

In cattle, a congenital condition ("pink tooth") that increases porphyrin concentrations can occur, which can lead to neurologic disturbances from demyelination of peripheral and cranial nerves. In the liver, barbiturates stimulate production of an enzyme that increases porphyrin production, potentially making the disease worse (Mees and Frederickson 1975). Animals afflicted with a known or suspected disturbance in porphyrin metabolism should not be administered barbiturates.

Sheep and goats, metabolized pentobarbital up to eight times faster than dogs (Plumb 1999).

Swine. Many pigs may have prolonged recoveries from thiopental administration (~1 hr) versus other animals (~15 min). It is possible that redistribution of thiopental to the increased fat stores may contribute to the prolonged effect of the drug. Barbiturates do not trigger malignant hyperthermia.

Horses. The administration of thiopental to horses without prior sedation is not recommended as there is significant excitement and incoordination. Rather, horses should be administered thiopental following sedation with an alpha-2 agonist (e.g., xylazine) and/or guaifenesin, and/or a benzodiazepine (e.g., diazepam). Induction of anesthesia in horses with thiopental causes horses to become recumbent by the flexion of all four legs, as compared to ketamine where most horses will flex their hind legs first and assume a dog-sitting posture before complete recumbency. Care should be taken to prevent horses from injuring themselves during induction and recovery.

Methohexital should not be used alone in horses because of excitation during induction and/or recovery.

Birds. Thiopental has been successfully used in birds interosseously (Valverde et al. 1993), but because of prolonged recoveries and increased mortality, it is not recommended.

Reptiles. Barbiturates are metabolized very slowly in reptiles, resulting in a prolonged recovery. Therefore, they are rarely used in this group of animals.

DRUG INTERACTIONS. All CNS depressants (e.g., opioids, alpha-2 agonists, phenothiazine sedatives) can potentiate the effects of barbiturates, reducing the required induction dose. Long-acting barbiturates induce hepatic microsomal enzymes, which increases the metabolism of other drugs metabolized by the same system (e.g., chloramphenicol, beta blockers, and metronidazole).

OVERDOSE/ACUTE TOXICITY. Treatment for an overdose with short-acting barbiturates should center on supportive treatment of respiratory and cardiovascular depression. This may include positive pressure ventilation, fluid therapy, and inotropic support.

Clearance of long-acting barbiturates is considerably greater in alkaline than in acid urine. Thus alkalinization of urine with sodium bicarbonate increases the elimination rate and is clinically useful in treatment of intoxication from long-acting barbiturates.

If a known perivascular injection occurs, the area should be infiltrated with saline for dilution and acidification and a local anesthetic to decrease pain.

REGULATORY INFORMATION

Controlled Drug Status

Thiopental: Schedule II controlled drug
Phenobarbital: Schedule IV controlled drug
Pentobarbital: Schedule II controlled drug
Methohexital: Schedule III controlled drug

Withdrawal Times

Thiopental: Extralabel use: At least 1 day for meat; 24 hr for milk
Phenobarbital: No regulatory information available
Pentobarbital: No regulatory information available

VETERINARY PRODUCTS

Thiopental is approved by the FDA for use in dogs and cats
Thiopental: Sodium thiopental 2.5% solution, Fort Dodge Animal Health, Wyeth
Pentobarbital is approved by the FDA for use in dogs and cats.
Pentobarbital: Pentobarbital Sodium for injection, 64.8 mg/ml, Schering-Plough
Phenobarbital: None

HUMAN PRODUCTS

Thiopental: Pentothal Abbot Laboratories, 2.5% solution
Pentobarbital: Pentobarbital Sodium (Nembutal Sodium), 50 mg/ml, Ovation Pharmacy
Phenobarbital: Phenobarbital sodium for injection (Generic), 30, 60, and 130 mg/ml

PROPOFOL

HISTORY. Propofol is an intravenous anesthetic used for sedation, induction of anesthesia, and maintenance of anesthesia, when administered as a constant rate infusion (CRI). It has been approved for human use since 1989 and is popular in veterinary medicine due to its smooth induction and recovery. It is unusual in that it is supplied in a milky white emulsion, which is administered intravenously.

CLASSIFICATION

Chemistry. Propofol (2,6-diisopropylphenol) is an alkyl-phenol derivative that is water insoluble but a highly lipid soluble (Fig. 11.6).

How Supplied. Propofol is available as an aqueous emulsion containing propofol (10 mg/ml), soybean oil (100 mg/ml), glycerol (2.5 mg/ml), egg lecithin (12 mg/ml), and sodium hydroxide (to adjust pH to 7.0). It is stable at room temperature and not light sensitive. The formulation available contains no preservatives and will support bacterial growth (Wachowski et al. 1999). Since propofol is an emulsion, it should be shaken well before using.

Aquafol is a water soluble form of propofol, but is not available or licensed for use in the U.S.

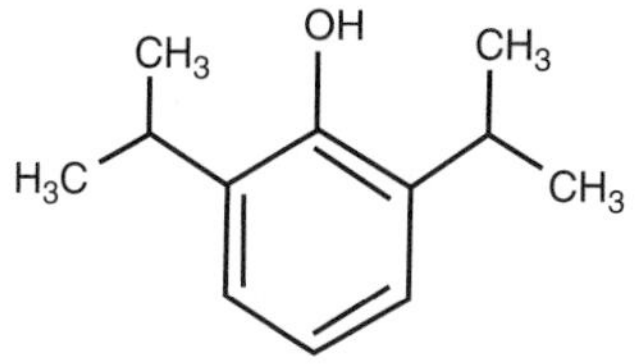

OH, CH_3, CH_3, H_3C, CH_3

FIG. 11.6 Propofol.

MECHANISM OF ACTION. Propofol produces hypnosis by its effect on the inhibitory $GABA_A$ receptor (Ying and Goldstein 2005). Propofol decreases the rate of GABA dissociation from its receptors, thus increasing the opening of chloride channels. Increased chloride conductance results in hyperpolarization of postsynaptic cell membranes and inhibition of the postsynaptic neurons resulting in hypnosis and amnesia.

INDICATIONS. Clinical uses of propofol include induction of general anesthesia, short-term sedation, long-term sedation (e.g., ventilator patients), maintenance of anesthesia (via constant rate infusion), and treatment of status epilepticus. Propofol should only be administered intravenously; however, extravasation does not cause skin sloughing.

PHYSIOLOGIC EFFECTS

CNS. Propofol induces CNS depression by enhancing the effects of GABA, an inhibitory neurotransmitter, providing a rapid, smooth induction of general anesthesia.

Propofol produces a favorable neurologic status as it decreases intracranial pressure (ICP), decreases cerebral perfusion pressure, and decreases cerebral metabolic oxygen consumption (Pinaud et al. 1990). Intracranial pressure is reduced in patients with both normal and elevated ICP. Propofol has also been shown to maintain cerebral autoregulation in pigs (Lagerkranser et al. 1997) and increase cerebral autoregulation in humans (Harrison et al. 2002); thus, propofol has become a popular anesthetic for patients with CNS disease.

Similar to its effects on intracranial pressure, propofol causes an acute decrease in intraocular pressure by 30–40% when administered at anesthetic doses. (Neel et al. 1995).

Myoclonus has been reported following propofol administration and some have hypothesized that propofol might lower the seizure threshold. However, propofol has been shown to be anticonvulsant and does not produce seizure activity in patients with documented epilepsy (Cheng et al. 1996). Propofol has been used successfully in both dogs and humans for long-term control of status epilepticus.

Following propofol anesthesia, many human patients report a feeling of euphoria as well as having had amorous dreams (Canaday 1993). Many domestic animals recover from propofol clear headed, coordinated and seemingly feeling well.

Cardiovascular. Induction doses of propofol are associated with systemic hypotension (Reich et al. 2005). Although propofol causes negative inotropy, the decrease in blood pressure is primarily via a decrease in systemic vascular resistance (vasodilation); systemic vascular resistance decreased by 21% in dogs following an induction dose of propofol (5 mg/ml) (Wouters et al. 1995). Following an induction dose of propofol, the heart rate is often decreased or unchanged, even with systemic hypotension (Whitwam et al. 2000). This is in contrast to the barbiturates where there is often an increased heart rate in response to the decrease in blood pressure.

Propofol can enhance the ability of epinephrine to induce cardiac arrhythmias but does not appear to be inherently arrhythmogenic (Kamibayashi et al. 1991).

Respiratory. Apnea is a commonly seen following bolus administration of propofol. The apnea associated with propofol is rate related; that is, the faster the administration the more likely the incidence of apnea (Musk et al. 2005). Respiratory depression resulting in mild hypercapnia and acidosis are also seen in spontaneously breathing dogs following induction doses (Robertson et al. 1992) and in dogs administered propofol as a constant rate infusion. Patients given propofol should be monitored for hypoxemia and hypercapnia, and if necessary the patient should be intubated and provided supplemental oxygen. Propofol should be given cautiously in patients where securing an airway may be difficult (e.g., laryngeal masses, guinea pigs, etc.).

Muscular. Propofol provides excellent muscle relaxation, but occasionally results in short- and long-term myoclonic movements in humans and dogs (Nimmaanrat 2005). Signs resolve spontaneously, but severity of movement can interfere with surgical procedures. Anecdotal treatment with ketamine at 1 mg/kg IV has resulted in the resolution of signs (author's personal experience). Laryngeal reflexes are decreased and result in a favorable intubating environment, but might increase the risk of aspiration in patients without a protected airway.

Miscellaneous

Fetal. Propofol does cross the placenta and enter the fetal circulation, but it appears to be readily removed from the fetal circulation after birth and produces minimal effects on healthy, newborn, human infants (Dailland et al. 1989) or puppies (Luna et al. 2004).

Neuroendocrine. Propofol does not cause histamine release (Mitsuhata and Shimizu 1993) and results in a diminished stress response compared with inhalant anesthetics (Ledowski et al. 2005).

Antiemetic. Propofol has been shown to decrease post anesthetic nausea and vomiting in people at both anesthetic and subanesthetic doses (Apfel et al. 2004); however, this effect has not been documented in domestic animals.

Antipruritic. Subanesthetic IV doses of propofol have been shown to decrease the pruritus seen following spinally administered opioids in humans (Horta et al. 2006).

Analgesia. Propofol does not provide any analgesia or produce hyperalgesia, as has been reported with barbiturate anesthesia (Wilder-Smith et al. 1995).

PHARMACOKINETICS. The pharmacokinetics of propofol in dogs is best described using a two-compartment open model (Zoran et al. 1993). Initially the drug is extensively taken up by the CNS, resulting in rapid CNS depression and induction of anesthesia. It is then rapidly redistributed from the brain to other tissues and removed from the plasma by metabolism. Propofol's lipophilic nature results in a large apparent volume of distribution (Vd) (17.9 l/kg in mixed-breed dogs) and steady-state volume of distribution (Vd_{ss}) (9.7 ml/kg). The initial distribution half-life ($t_{1/2\alpha}$) is short, as is the plasma disappearance ($t_{1/2\beta}$), due to rapid redistribution of the drug from the brain to other tissues and extensive metabolism. The Vd and Vd_{ss} are smaller in greyhounds, 11.2 l/kg and 6.3 ml/kg, respectively, suggesting they have slower recoveries (Zoran et al. 1993). Geriatric dogs (>8.5 years) have also been shown to have a slower clearance than what has been reported for younger dogs (Reid and Nolan 1996).

The pharmacokinetics of propofol in cats has not been fully determined; however, cats appear to have a similar response to, and dose requirement as, dogs for propofol. Interestingly, it has been shown that in cats there is a significant pulmonary uptake of propofol (Matot et al. 1993).

Propofol does not accumulate (noncumulative) after repeated doses and/or prolonged infusions (Adam et al. 1980; Mandsager et al. 1995).

METABOLISM. The total body clearance of propofol is rapid and exceeds hepatic blood flow, suggesting extrahepatic metabolism (Veroli et al. 1992). Indeed, in one study done on human patients undergoing liver transplantation, the amount of propofol metabolite excreted did not decrease when the liver was excluded from the circulation (Veroli et al. 1992), and the pharmacologic effects are not different in patients with cirrhosis (Servin et al. 1990). The site of extrahepatic metabolism is unclear, but pulmonary tissue has been shown to contribute to propofol metabolism in cats (Matot et al. 1993). There may be significant species differences in the site and amount of extrahepatic metabolism.

Although awakening is generally attributed to redistribution, the termination of the effect of propofol is largely attributed to rapid and extensive biotransformation by the liver to inactive metabolites, which are excreted in the urine. In the dog the two major urinary metabolites of propofol are the glucuronide and sulfate conjugates of 4-hydroxypropofol (2,6-diisopropyl-1,4-quinol) (Hay Kraus et al. 2000). The formation of this intermediate derivative appears to be a critical initial step in the biotransformation and elimination of propofol in dog (Hay Kraus et al. 2000). It has also been shown that there are breed differences in metabolic enzyme pathways, which would account for the slower drug clearance seen in greyhound and geriatric dogs (Reid and Nolan 1996; Court et al. 1999; Hay Kraus et al. 2000).

ADVERSE EFFECTS/CONTRAINDICATIONS. Propofol can cause local pain on injection, which is often worse in small peripheral veins. Some anesthetists will preferentially choose larger veins, administer through a running IV line, or administer a small volume of 2% lidocaine before administering propofol to prevent the pain on injection.

Propofol has been associated with increased wound infection. Retrospective analysis of dogs and cats with clean wounds showed an almost four times greater risk of postoperative infection in animals administered propofol (Heldmann et al. 1999). Strict aseptic technique should be used when preparing and administering propofol and unused drug should be discarded within 24 hr.

Because of the lipid emulsion, propofol has been suggested as a cause of postanesthetic pancreatitis. Pancreatitis associated with propofol has been reported, albeit rarely, in humans; it has not been reported in veterinary species (Gottschling et al. 2005).

Propofol syndrome is a rare but often lethal complication following a prolonged continuous administration of propofol. Patients can develop a metabolic acidosis, rhabdomyolysis, renal failure, cardiac arrhythmias, and cardiac failure. The pathophysiology of this syndrome appears to involve a disturbance of mitochondrial metabolism induced by propofol (Trampitsch et al. 2006). Neonates and septic patients appear to have a greater risk of developing the syndrome. Any patient on a prolonged infusion of propofol should be monitored for these potential adverse signs.

SPECIES DIFFERENCES

Dogs. Propofol can be used for short or long-term sedation, induction of general anesthesia and continuous rate infusions. The induction dose required for greyhounds is not different from that required for mixed-breed dogs; however, the recovery time was longer for greyhounds (see above).

Cats. Propofol can induce oxidative injuries to feline red blood cells if used repeatedly over several days. This can result in Heinz body formation, anorexia, diarrhea, and malaise (Andress 1995). Thus, cats should not be administered propofol more frequently than 3–4 consecutive days and caution should be used with extended propofol infusions.

Horses. Following sedation with an alpha-2 agonist some horses showed excitement at induction, but have smooth well-coordinated recoveries (Mama et al. 1996). Although good recovery characteristics are important for horses, the presence of induction excitement and the prohibitive cost for large patients make it unlikely that propofol will be routinely used in equine patients.

Swine. Propofol does not trigger malignant hyperthermia in susceptible animals (Fruen et al. 1995). However, good sedation is necessary to provide reasonable venous access. Respiratory depression and apnea have been reported with propofol administration in pigs (Tendillo et al. 1996); thus, propofol should be used with caution unless intubation can be readily accomplished.

Birds. Propofol produces significant respiratory depression in red-tailed hawks and great horned owls (Hawkins et al. 2003). It is reasonable to presume that all birds may need ventilatory assistance when anesthesia is maintained with propofol. CNS excitement has been noted at recovery (Hawkins et al. 2003).

DOSE. Propofol should be administered slowly to effect. The dose needed will depend on the type and dose of premedication, the health of the patient, and how painful the procedure will be. Premedicants that add CNS depression can decrease induction doses by more than 50%. Time of unconsciousness depends on premedicants and dose of propofol administered. Generally, unconsciousness last from 2–8 minutes. The doses in Table 11.3 have been reported for the listed species; however, each patient is different and the total dose should be titrated for a particular patient.

TABLE 11.3 Doses of propofol in various species

Species	Induction Dose (mg/kg IV)	CRI* Dosage (mg/kg/min IV)	Reference
Dog	3–7	0.2–0.6	
Cat	5–8	0.5–1.0	
Horse-Adult	4–8		Mama et al. 1996
Horse–Foal	2.0	0.33	
Donkey	2	0.21	
Pig	2–3	0.1–0.2	Tendillo et al. 1996
Llama	2	0.4	Duke et al. 1997
Ferret	2–4		
Rabbit	2–10		

*CRI: constant rate infusion.

DRUG INTERACTIONS. Propofol is compatible with 5% dextrose, which can be used to dilute propofol for constant rate infusion. Dilution should not be less than 2 mg/ml.

Propofol can be mixed with thiopental in a 1:1 solution. The mixture has been shown to be stable and provided smooth inductions that were similar to thiopental but better recoveries (more like propofol) (Ko et al. 1999).

OVERDOSE/ACUTE TOXICITY. Accidental overdose of propofol can result in severe cardiovascular and respiratory depression. Treatment is supportive: fluid therapy, intubation and ventilation, positive inotrope, and/or vasoactive drugs. Fortunately, the duration of effect is short.

REGULATORY INFORMATION

Controlled Drug Status. Propofol is a noncontrolled drug.

Withdrawal Times. Withdrawal times have not been established for animals that produce food.

VETERINARY PRODUCTS. Rapinovet (Schering-Plough) 10 mg/ml in 20 ml vials.

PropoFlo (Abbot Laboratories) 10 mg/ml in 20 ml vials

HUMAN PRODUCTS. Diprivan (Zeneca) 10 mg/ml in 20, 50 and 100 ml vials.

DISSOCIATIVES

HISTORY. Dissociative anesthetics (e.g., ketamine) have been extensively used in veterinary medicine and may still be the most common class of anesthetics in use. The first dissociative anesthetic was phencyclidine hydrochloride (PCP, "Angel Dust"), which, due to side effects and abuse in humans, is no longer available. Newer phencyclidine derivatives include ketamine hydrochloride and tiletamine hydrochloride. Ketamine is also a drug of abuse in humans ("Special-K") and tiletamine is marketed only in combination with zolazepam under the trade name, Telazol® or Zolatel®.

The term *dissociative anesthetic* originated from the use of ketamine in human patients. When anesthetized with ketamine, patients appeared to feel dissociated from or unaware of their environment, but did not always appear asleep (cataleptic). Later it was determined that these drugs did indeed dissociate the thalamocortical and limbic systems causing the change in awareness.

CLASSIFICATION

Chemistry

Ketamine. Ketamine (Fig. 11.7), 2-(o-chlorophenol)-2-(methylamino)-cyclohexanone hydrochloride, is a phencyclidine derivative that exists as a racemic mixture with the S (+) isomer producing four times the potency of the R (–) isomer.

Tiletamine. Tiletamine (Fig. 11.8), 2-[ethylamino]-2-[2-thienyl]-cyclohexanone hydrochloride, is a phencyclidine (Fig. 11.9) derivative.

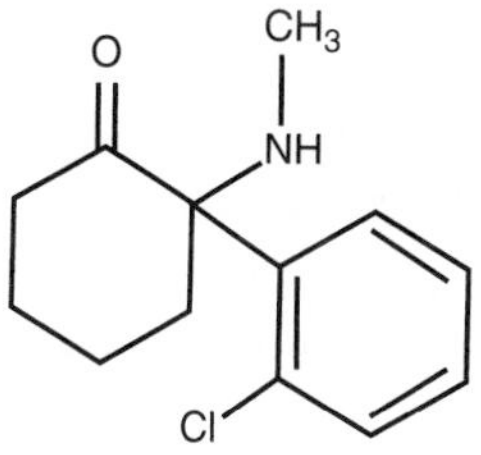

FIG. 11.7 Ketamine.

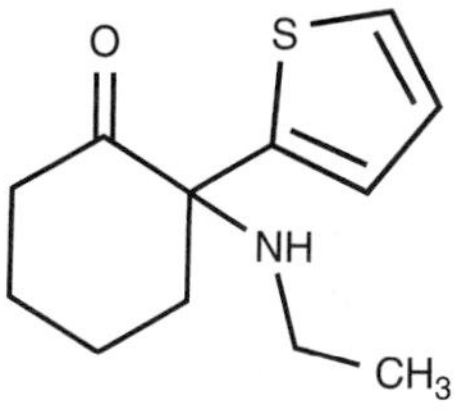

FIG. 11.8 Tiletamine.

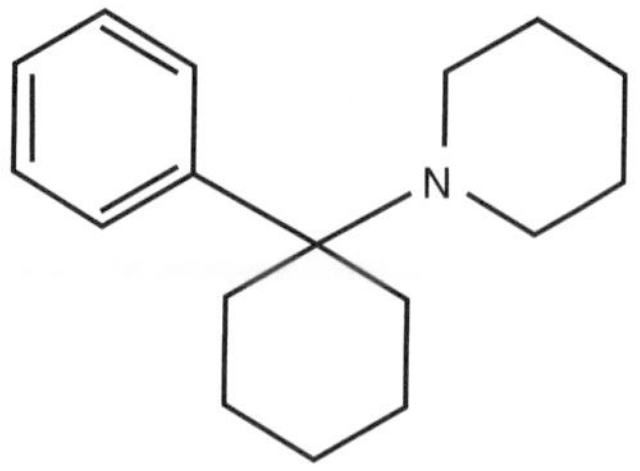

FIG. 11.9 Phencyclidine.

How Supplied

Ketamine. Ketamine is supplied as a 10%, aqueous solution (pH 3.5–5.5). It is preserved with benzethonium chloride.

Tiletamine. Tilematine is supplied only in combination with zolazepam as a white powder. The addition of 5 ml diluent produces a solution containing the equivalent of 50 mg tiletamine base, 50 mg zolazepam base, and 57.7 mg mannitol per milliliter. This solution has a pH of 2 to 3.5.

MECHANISM OF ACTION. Dissociative anesthetics are noncompetitive antagonists at *N*-methyl-D-aspartate (NMDA) receptors and bind to the NMDA receptor at the phencyclidine binding site. Thus, these drugs prevent the binding of the excitatory neurotransmitter, glutamate, at the NMDA receptor, resulting in depressed activity at the thalamocortical and limbic systems and depression of nuclei in the reticular activating system. Dissociatives also have some effect at opioid receptors, monoaminergic receptors, muscarine receptors, and voltage-sensitive calcium channels, but unlike other induction agents do not interact with GABA receptors (Annetta et al. 2005).

Anesthesia with dissociatives produces an altered consciousness or catalepsy. Human patients report that these drugs make them "not care" about what is going on around them.

Unlike other induction agents, dissociative anesthetics produce analgesia, which is likely at least partially mediated through activation of mu and kappa opioid receptors. The NMDA receptor is also involved in pain processing, including central and peripheral sensitizations and visceral pain.

PHYSIOLOGIC EFFECTS

CNS. Based on EEG findings, the antagonism of NMDA receptors produces a dissociation of the thalamocortical and limbic systems (Reich and Silvay 1989). This produces an altered consciousness or catalepsy, where the patient does not appear asleep but does not react to noxious or nonnoxious stimuli. Although the patient may not look asleep, NMDA antagonists are effective at producing amnesia (Haas and Harper 1992). When used alone, the dissociative anesthetics rarely produce a surgical depth of anesthesia, but when combined with other CNS depressants they produce adequate relaxation and immobility.

The CNS effects of dissociatives are different than most other anesthetics. They increase cerebral blood flow (CBF), which is coupled with an increase in cerebral glucose metabolism and oxygen demand ($CMRO_2$) (Dawson et al. 1971). The increased CBF is caused by vasodilation of cerebral vessels and an increase in blood pressure, which results in an increase in intracranial pressure (ICP). Hypercapnia contributes to the rise in ICP and controlling ventilation can attenuate the rise in ICP. Thus, these drugs should not be used in any patient having or suspected of having elevated ICP, or where cerebral metabolic demands may not be being met.

Ketamine causes the development of EEG patterns that are epileptiform (Kayama 1982) and is used to elicit more robust seizures during electroconvulsive therapy (Krystal 2003 et al.). Consequently, some anesthesiologists have recommended against its use in patients with a seizure history (Lumb and Jones 1996). However, there is also mounting evidence that ketamine is anticonvulsive (Reder et al. 1980) as well as neuroprotective (Himmelseher and Durieux 2005). Consequently, ketamine should not be used in patients with elevated ICP, but may be used cautiously in patients with other neurologic diseases.

Dissociative anesthetics cause an increase in norepinephrine via central adrenergic stimulation and a decreased reuptake, resulting in an increase in sympathetic tone (Stoelting 1999). The increase in norepinephrine affects all systems under adrenergic control (e.g., cardiovascular, respiratory, endocrine, etc.).

Emergence delirium (e.g., anxiousness, vocalization, thrashing) is a concern whenever dissociative anesthetics are used. This may be merely unpleasant in smaller animals, but can be dangerous when used in larger animals (e.g., horses). Emergence delirium can be attenuated or prevented by administering dissociative anesthetics with sedatives or tranquilizers (e.g., xylazine, diazepam, acepromazine).

Awakening from ketamine is primarily due to redistribution of drug, although some effects are from metabolism.

Cardiovascular. Ketamine has direct myocardial depressant effects (Diaz et al. 1976), but its administration is generally associated with increase in cardiac output, mean aortic pressure, pulmonary arterial pressure, central venous pressure, and heart rate (Haskins et al. 1985). The stimulatory effects likely result from both directly stimulating the central adrenergic centers (i.e., increased sympathetic tone) and inhibiting the neuronal uptake of catecholamines, especially norepinephrine (Annetta et al. 2005). The cardiovascular stimulation is associated with an increase in myocardial work and myocardial oxygen demands (Haskins et al. 1985), thus ketamine should be used with caution in patients with severe cardiovascular disease. Although the sympathetic stimulation overrides the direct cardiovascular depressant effects of ketamine (Adams 1997), a patient that is catecholamine depleted (i.e., critically ill) may show more of the cardio-depressive effects.

The increased sympathetic tone also may cause tachycardia; however, dysrhythmias are uncommon clinically. Caution should be used with patients that are already tachycardic or dysrhythmic.

Ketamine preserves cardiovascular function and oxygen balance during experimentally produced septic shock (Van der Linden et al. 1990). This cardiovascular sparing effect may be due to the ability of ketamine to block the inflammatory cascade caused by endotoxins that depress cardiovascular function (Taniguchi and Yamamoto 2005), as well as by increasing levels of norepinephrine that may attenuate the inappropriate peripheral vasodilation seen in septic patients.

Respiratory. Dissociative anesthetics generally have a mild effect on minute ventilation and therefore usually cause a mild increase in carbon dioxide concentrations. This is in contrast to many other anesthetics that are potent respiratory depressants. However, when other CNS depressants are administered with ketamine, significant respiratory depression can be seen. Ketamine also can cause an *apneustic* pattern of breathing, which is characterized by a rapid sequence of breaths followed by breath holding on inspiration. This occurs more commonly with rapid IV administration of ketamine. Although apneustic breathing is unusual to watch, minute ventilation and carbon dioxide levels are generally normal.

Ketamine has bronchodilating properties and decreases airway resistance (Durieux 1995). This makes it useful as an induction drug for patients with clinical asthma as well as patients with obstructive airway disease (e.g., chronic obstructive pulmonary disease).

When ketamine is used as a sole anesthetic, pharyngeal and laryngeal reflexes remain active (Robinson and Johnston 1986). Preservation of these reflexes, however, leads to an increased risk of laryngospasm and coughing secondary to secretions or manipulation in the oropharynx. These complications make ketamine a poor drug for use in endoscopy or oropharyngeal surgery. Although laryngeal reflexes are preserved they can be uncoordinated, and thus aspiration is possible. Endotracheal intubation should be used to maintain and protect the airway.

Additionally, ketamine stimulates salivation, which can be copious at times. The administration of an anticholinergic (e.g., glycopyrrolate) for its antisialagogue properties can attenuate the amount of salivation. Caution should be used when using anticholinergics in patients with small airways as the antisialagogue properties can make for viscous secretions that can occlude the airways or endotracheal tube.

Muscular. Dissociative anesthetics provide little muscle relaxation and may cause muscle rigidity, myoclonus, and/or uncoordinated muscle movements. Muscle relaxation is generally provided by the coadministration of sedatives or tranquilizers (e.g., benzodiazepine, alpha-2 agonists).

Upper airway muscle tone and reflexes are preserved when dissociatives are used alone. However, since these drugs are generally administered with muscle relaxants, laryngeal control is then diminished or absent. Endotracheal intubation is recommended for all anesthetized patients to maintain and protect the airway.

Miscellaneous. The appearance of patients anesthetized with dissociative anesthetics is different than with most other anesthetics. Many patients do not close their eyes, can have muscle tone and muscle movement, and often do not look "asleep." It is important to protect the corneas of patients with adequate lubrication and prevent objects from rubbing on the cornea. Coadministration of sedatives or tranquilizers can attenuate these signs.

Analgesia. NMDA antagonists provide a significant amount of analgesia, particularly when used in conjunction with other analgesics. For many years the dogma has been that ketamine provided greater somatic, compared with visceral, analgesia. However, this view is too simplistic to explain the varied analgesic effects and should be discarded. The mechanism for antinociception is complex and likely involves interactions at more than one type of receptor. Ketamine provides a use-dependent (i.e., works better when the nerves are stimulated) blockade of the NMDA receptor as well as inhibiting neurotransmitter release, both of which has been shown to mediate nociception (Annetta et al. 2005). Analgesia is also likely mediated by the action of ketamine on mu and kappa opioid receptors (Annetta et al. 2005). Opioid receptors extend beyond the CNS and spinal cord and occur in many peripheral tissues.

When used at subanesthetic doses, NMDA antagonists are effective in supplying analgesia for acute surgical pain and have opioid sparing effects (Annetta et al. 2005). Additionally, NMDA antagonists are effective at treating chronic pain associated with central sensitization (wind-up pain), neuropathic pain, (Guirimand et al. 2000) and likely other types of inflammatory pain. When ketamine is used at subanesthetic doses, behavioral changes are not seen.

INDICATIONS. Dissociative anesthetics are used for chemical restraint, for rapid induction of anesthesia, and to provide analgesia. They can safely be used in most species and can be administered intramuscularly and intravenously.

PHARMACOKINETICS. Pharmacokinetic values for ketamine in various species are summarized in Table 11.4.

Both ketamine and tiletamine are highly lipid soluble, so absorption is rapid from the intramuscular (IM) route with peak plasma concentration reached in ~10 minutes (Baggot and Blake 1976). Ketamine can also be absorbed through oral or rectal mucous membranes. This makes it possible to administer by spraying the drug in the mouth of fractious/feral animals or to administer rectally (Hanna et al. 1988). Cats administered ketamine orally often salivate profusely, presumably from the bitter taste or low pH or both. Cats administered ketamine rectally showed a slow smooth induction, no pain during administration and a ~43% availability of drug (Hanna et al.1988).

METABOLISM. Ketamine is biotransformed by the liver by *N*-demethylation to norketamine, which then undergoes hydroxylation to form a water-soluble glucuronide derivative that is eliminated in urine (White et al. 1982; Stoelting 1999). Norketamine is an active metabolite of ketamine and has 10–30% activity of the parent drug (Leung and Baillie 1986). In the cat, ketamine only undergoes transformation to norketamine, which is excreted largely unchanged in the urine (Hanna et al. 1988). Since the active metabolites are excreted by the kidneys, decreased renal excretion may prolong the effects of the drug.

Telazol® is an equal mixture of tiletamine and zolazepam (a benzodiazepine), so the metabolism of this drug needs to be discussed in terms of the two drugs. In cats, the duration of effect of zolazepam exceeds that of tiletamine so that with time, the pharmacodynamic effect is that of the benzodiazepine; tranquilization (Product-Label 2004). In dogs, the duration of effect of tiletamine exceeds that of zolazepam so that with time, the pharmacodynamic effects reflect the dissociative, including muscle rigidity, sympathetic stimulation, and emergence delirium (Product-Label 2004). Other species have similar disparities in metabolism and recoveries from Telazol. Pigs awaken slowly and calmly, whereas horses can have an

TABLE 11.4 Pharmacokinetics of ketamine in various species

Species	Dose (mg/kg IV)	Distribution Phase (min)	Elimination Half-Life (min)	Protein Binding %	Clearance (ml/min/kg)	Reference
Dog	15	1.95	61	53.5	32.2	Kaka et al. 1980
Cat	25	2.7	78.7	53	21.3	Hanna et al. 1988
Horse	2.2	2.9	42	50	26.6	Kaka and Klavano 1979
Calf	5.0	6.9	60.5		40.4	Waterman 1984
Humans	2.2	4.68	130	60		Domino et al. 1984

agitated recovery if not provided with additional sedation. Reversal of the zolazepam in animals with prolonged recoveries can lead to an anxious recovery if sufficient plasma levels of tiletamine are still present.

ADVERSE EFFECTS/CONTRAINDICATIONS

CNS. Ketamine should not used in animals with elevated intracranial pressure.

Cardiovascular. Ketamine should be use with caution in patients with coronary artery disease, uncontrolled arterial hypertension, cardiomyopathy, or heart failure.

Emergence Delirium. Caution should be used in patients where emergence delirium could be injurious to the patient or to medical personnel (e.g., horse). Emergence delirium can be prevented or attenuated by coadministration of sedatives or tranquilizers. In general, dissociative anesthetics should not be administered as sole agents.

Ocular Disease. Ketamine should not be used animals with elevated intraocular pressure or with an open globe injury due to the rise in intraocular pressure following administration.

Increased Sympathetic Tone. Dissociatives should be avoided in patients with high sympathetic tone, such as hyperthyroidism or pheochromocytoma, since administration of these drugs can increase norepinephrine levels and exacerbate the side effects of these diseases.

Urethral Obstruction or Renal Insufficiency. Caution should be used in patients where excretion of the active metabolites may be decreased, such as cats with urethral obstruction or anuric renal failure.

DOSE. Dose ranges for ketamine and tiletamine in various species are listed in Table 11.5.

The pH of ketamine is 3.5, which can cause some irritation and pain during IM injections. The volume per kg of body weight of Telazol is less than an equipotent amount of ketamine. This makes it attractive for work with exotic animals where the volume may be important (e.g., darts or syringe poles).

TABLE 11.5 Dose of ketamine and tiletamine in various species

Species	Dosage of Ketamine (mg/kg)*	Dosage of Telazol® (mg/kg)[&]
Dog	5–10 IV	3–6 IM
Cat	5–10 IV: 10–20 mg/kg PO 25 mg/kg rectally	4–7 IM
Cattle	2–4 IV	2–4 IV
Camelid	2–4 IV	0.5–2 IV; 2–4 IM
Ferret	5–10 IV	
Horses	2 IV	1–3 IV (following alpha-2 agonist)
Rat	40–80 IM	30–60
Pigs	10 IM	6 IM (following alpha-2 agonist) 0.01–0.02 ml/kg as TKX[+]
Rabbits	20–50 IM	30–60 IM[#]
Primates	2–4 IV; 10–15 IM	3 IM

*Following sedation with benzodiazepine, alpha-2 agonist, or phenothiazine.
[&]Dose for Telazol is for combination of drugs at 100 mg/ml.
[#]Telazol® should not be used in New Zealand White rabbits.
[+]TKX = 500 mg Telazol® (as powder) + 250 mg ketamine + 250 mg xylazine.

SPECIES DIFFERENCES

Horses. Horses should not be administered dissociative anesthetics as single agents due to the lack of muscle relaxation and recovery delirium. Telazol® in particular can be associated with rough anesthetic recoveries and should be balanced with the use of additional sedatives or tranquilizers.

Tigers. Great controversy occurs over the use of Telazol® in the large cats and in tigers specifically. Although there is little published evidence, many anesthesiologists and zoo medicine specialists caution against the use of Telazol® in the large cats (Tilson et al. 1995; Muir et al. 2000; Morris 2001). Reported complications have ranged from slow ataxic recoveries to delayed (2–4 days after anesthesia) neurologic dysfunction, including hindlimb weakness, drowsiness, hyperreflexia, hyperresponsive behavior, twitches, seizures, and death (Tilson et al. 1995; Klein 2007; Lewis 2007).

Rabbits. At clinical doses, tiletamine (the dissociative part of Telazol®) causes lethal renal tubular necrosis in New Zealand White rabbits (Doerning et al. 1992). Other rabbit species appear unaffected.

Swine. A combination known as TKX (Telazol, ketamine, xylazine) is commonly used to anesthetize pigs. The mixture is composed of 500 mg (as powder) Telazol®, 250 mg ketamine and 250 mg xylazine (TKX). Due to slow zolazepam metabolism, pigs can have prolonged recoveries after TKX.

Use of ketamine in animals susceptible to malignant hyperthermia (MH) has been controversial; however, ketamine did not induce MH in 76 susceptible pigs (Dershwitz et al. 1989).

DRUG INTERACTIONS. The concurrent administration of other CNS depressants can increase respiratory and cardiovascular depression. Chloramphenicol can prolong recovery times from ketamine (Amouzadeh et al. 1989) as well as from Telazol (Plumb 1999).

OVERDOSE/ACUTE TOXICITY. Ketamine has a large therapeutic index, so treatment of an overdose is primarily supportive care and addressing side effects, such as respiratory or cardiovascular depression, muscle rigidity, emergence delirium, or adrenergic stimulation.

REGULATORY INFORMATION

Controlled Drug Status. Ketamine is a Schedule III controlled drug.

Telazol® is a Schedule III controlled drug.

Withdrawal Times. Ketamine: Extralabel use: at least 3 days for meat and 48 hr for milk.

VETERINARY PRODUCTS. Ketamine is approved by the FDA for IM use in the cat and nonhuman primates.

KetaFlo; Abbot Laboratories 100 mg/ml.

Telazol is approved by the FDA for IM use in dogs and cats (restricted during pregnancy).

Telazol; Fort Dodge Animal Health, Division of Wyeth 50 mg/ml Tiletamine and 50 mg/ml zolazepam/ml of solution.

HUMAN PRODUCTS. Ketalar; Parkedale Pharmaceuticals, 10 mg/ml, 50 mg/ml, 100 mg/ml.

ETOMIDATE

HISTORY. Etomidate was first introduced into human anesthesia practice in 1972. At the time it was considered close to the "ideal anesthetic" due to its ability to maintain hemodynamic stability, minimally depress the respiratory centers, and because it has a large therapeutic index (the lethal dose/effective dose). However, the ideal anesthetic has yet to be found, and etomidate also has untoward side effects.

CLASSIFICATION. Etomidate is a noncontrolled, nonbarbiturate compound suitable for rapid intravenous anesthetic induction.

Chemistry. Etomidate is an ethyl ester of a carboxylated imidazole compound with a chemical formula of *R*-(+)-pentylethyl-1*H*-imidazole-5 carboxylate sulfate (Fig. 11.10). The imidazole component allows for differing solubility at different pH concentrations. At a low (acidic) pH, etomidate is water soluble, but it becomes lipid soluble at physiologic pH. There are two isomers, but only the (R)(+) isomer has anesthetic properties.

How Supplied. Etomidate is poorly water soluble, but highly soluble in alcohol; thus, it is supplied as a 2% solution in 35% propylene glycol at a pH of 6.9. When supplied in propylene glycol, etomidate has an osmolarity of ~4620 osmole.

MECHANISM OF ACTION. Etomidate is an agonist at the gamma-amino-butyric-acid (GABA) receptor ($GABA_{A\beta3}$) producing hypnosis and CNS depression by enhancing the effects of the inhibitory neurotransmitter GABA (O'Meara et al. 2004). Binding of GABA to the receptors increases chloride conductance, resulting in hyperpolarization of the postsynaptic neuron.

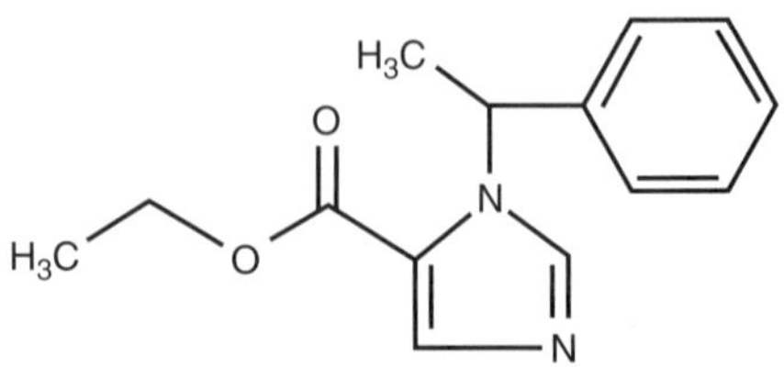

FIG. 11.10 Etomidate.

PHYSIOLOGIC EFFECTS

CNS. Etomidate is considered cerebral-friendly because it results in decreased intracranial pressure (ICP), decreased cerebral blood flow (CBF), and decreased cerebral metabolic rate for O_2 ($CMRO_2$). Since the mean arterial pressure (MAP) is essentially unchanged, this results in a favorable metabolic state for the CNS; the cerebral perfusion pressure is increased as is the cerebral oxygen supply: demand ratio. The EEG quiets (similar to the barbiturates), but there can be increased EEG activity at epileptogenic foci. Grand mal seizures have been reported, and some anesthetists argue against its use in patients with a known seizure history (Bergen and Smith 1997).

Due to similar mechanisms, the intraocular pressure (IOP) is also decreased. Intraocular pressure can decrease by up to 60%, but the effect lasts only for ~5 minutes.

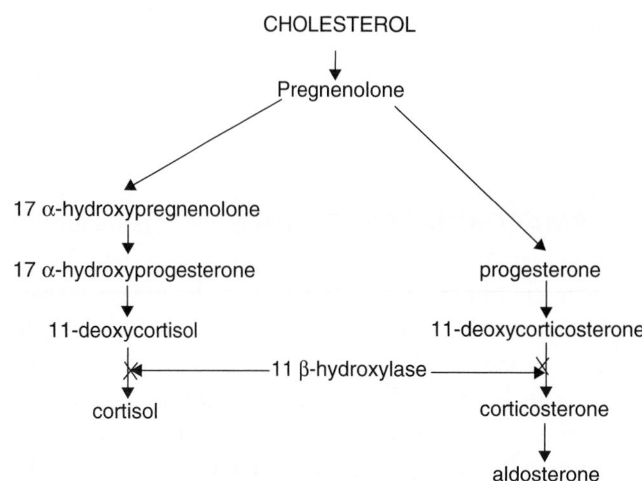

FIG. 11.11 Pathway for cortisol and aldosterone production.

Cardiovascular. Etomidate is unique among most intravenous injectable anesthetics in that it causes minimal hemodynamic changes and thus maintains cardiovascular function. At routine induction doses, etomidate causes minimal changes in stroke volume (SV), mean arterial pressure (MAP), cardiac index (CI), pulmonary artery pressure (PAP), pulmonary arterial wedge pressure (PAWP), central venous pressure (CVP), or systemic vascular resistance (SVR) (De Hert et al. 1990). In addition to causing minimal CV derangements, the baroreceptor and sympathetic nervous system reflexes remain intact, which also contributes to hemodynamic stability. Etomidate is not arrhythmogenic, does not sensitize the heart to catecholamine, and does not cause histamine release.

Respiratory. Etomidate has minimal respiratory effects. Induction doses can result in brief periods of apnea, but generally arterial carbon dioxide partial pressure ($PaCO_2$) is only slightly increased if affected at all. Arterial oxygen (PaO_2) is generally unaffected. However, when etomidate is administered with other drugs that can affect CNS function, more respiratory depression can be seen. Since etomidate has limited effect on muscle relaxation, airway reflexes are generally maintained. Intubation, however, is highly recommended.

Endocrine. In the early 1980s it was noted that there was increased morbidity and mortality in patients sedated long term (e.g., patients on ventilators) with etomidate due to a decreased cortisol production (Wagner et al. 1984). Etomidate causes a reversible inhibition of the enzyme 11-beta-hydroxylase (Fig. 11.11), which is an integral part of the pathway that converts cholesterol to glucocorticoids and mineralocorticoids. The resultant decrease in cortisol, corticosterone, and aldosterone production raises concern for patients' ability to respond to stress. Following induction with etomidate, suppression of the adrenal-cortical axis is depressed for up to 6 hours in dogs and 3 hours in cats (Dodam et al. 1990; Moon 1997). Single induction doses do not cause clinical problems associated with steroid production, but care should be taken with patients with preexisting adrenal-cortical diseases (e.g., hypoadrenocorticism). Furthermore, extended periods of use (e.g., constant rate infusions) are not recommended.

Muscular. Etomidate does not provide significant muscle relaxation. Muscle rigidity and myoclonus can be seen at and following induction, but is not associated with seizurelike EEG activity. The use of muscle relaxants (e.g., benzodiazepines) can minimize the incidence and intensity of the muscle movements (Doenicke et al. 1999). Etomidate can potentiate the effects of nondepolarizing neuromuscular blockers.

Analgesia. Etomidate does not provide any analgesia. If patients are anesthetized to facilitate surgery or painful procedures, analgesia must be provided separately (e.g., opioids, alpha-2 agonist).

INDICATIONS. Etomidate is indicated for the rapid intravenous induction of anesthesia, particularly in patients with cardiovascular instability.

PHARMACOKINETICS. Following intravenous administration, etomidate is rapidly distributed into the CNS to produce anesthesia. Etomidate is 75% bound to plasma proteins. Etomidate fits a three-compartment pharmacokinetic model with a short redistribution half-life (29 min in humans; 22 min in cats) and a large steady-state volume of distribution (2.5–4.5 l/kg in humans; 4.9 l/kg in cats). The elimination half-life varies from 2.9 to 5.3 hours in humans and is 2.9 hours in cats (Wertz et al. 1990). Redistribution of etomidate into body tissues is responsible for awakening, and recovery time from anesthesia is similar to thiopental, but slower than propofol.

METABOLISM. In humans, etomidate is 98% metabolized by liver (2% excreted unchanged in urine) by hydrolysis or glucuronidation via plasma esterases and hepatic microsomal enzymes. Metabolites are inactive and excreted in the urine (85%) and bile and feces (15%). Etomidate should be used cautiously in patients with liver disease as metabolism can be prolonged.

ADVERSE EFFECTS/CONTRAINDICATIONS. Adverse effects of adrenocortical suppression and myoclonus have been discussed above.

Other adverse effects of etomidate arise from the propylene glycol vehicle. The intravenous injection of propylene glycol can be painful. Pain can be minimized by administering etomidate through a running IV line or by injecting lidocaine (0.1–.05 mg/kg [dog]) through the catheter before induction. Furthermore, propylene glycol causes the solution to be hyperosmotic (~4620 Osm) compared to plasma (~300 Osm), and thus etomidate has been associated with intravascular hemolysis (Moon 1994). Clinically relevant hemolysis has been reported following prolonged administration (i.e., constant rate infusions) in dogs (Ko 1993). Etomidate is available in a lipid vehicle (Lipuro) instead of propylene glycol, but it is not available in the United States.

DOSE. Etomidate has wide safety margin, due to a large therapeutic index (16) (i.e., lethal dose is 16 times the hypnotic dose) compared to the therapeutic indexes for propofol and thiopental (3 and 5, respectively). Etomidate should be titrated intravenously "to-effect." The wide dose range reflects the additive and sometimes synergistic effects of many premedications (e.g., opioids, benzodiazepines, phenothiazines). As discussed previously, etomidate should be administered following adequate premedication. Duration of anesthesia is directly related to dose. Constant rate infusions (CRI) are not recommended due to the potential for adrenocortical suppression and hemolysis (see above):

Dogs: 0.5–4.0 mg/kg IV
Cats: 0.5–4.0 mg/kg IV
Pigs: 2–4 mg/kg IV
Mice: 11 mg/kg IV; 24 mg/kg IP

SPECIES DIFFERENCES

Cats. Due to the extensive liver metabolism of etomidate and fragility of feline red blood cells; cats may be more likely to have clinical hemolysis following etomidate administration.

Dogs. Clinical hemolysis has been seen following constant rate infusions.

Swine. Etomidate did not trigger malignant hyperthermia in susceptible pigs (Suresh and Nelson 1985).

DRUG INTERACTIONS. Concurrent use of other drugs that depress the CNS (e.g., barbiturates, opioids, general anesthetics, etc.) can potentiate the effects of etomidate.

OVERDOSE/ACUTE TOXICITY. Acute overdoses would be expected to cause enhanced pharmacologic effects of the drug. Treatment would be supportive (i.e., mechanical ventilation) until the effects of the medication are diminished.

STORAGE/STABILITY/COMPATIBILITY. Unless otherwise labeled, store etomidate injection at room temperature and protect from light.

REGULATORY INFORMATION

Controlled Drug Status. Etomidate is a noncontrolled drug.

VETERINARY PRODUCTS. None.

HUMAN PRODUCTS. Etomidate Injection 2 mg/ml in 10 ml, 20 ml ampules, single use vials and 20 ml Abboject Syringes; Amidate® (Hospira); generic (Bedford); (Rx).

GUAIFENESIN

HISTORY. Guaifenesin (glyceryl guaiacolate, GG), has been used as a therapeutic agent for more than 80 years. It has been used as an adjunct to anesthesia in the horse since 1949 and has been used in the U.S. since 1965. It is still commonly used in people as an expectorant, but is used for its sedation and muscle relaxation properties in veterinary medicine.

CLASSIFICATION

Chemistry. Guaifenesin, 3-(0-methoxy-phenoxy)-1,2-propanediol, is chemically similar to the muscle relaxant mephenesin (Fig. 11.12).

How Supplied. Guaifenesin is supplied as a 5% solution or as a white powder that is reconstituted to a 5% solution with water. It is not readily water soluble and partially precipitates out of solution at 22°C (72°F) or cooler (Funk 1973). Warming and agitation usually eliminate the precipitate.

MECHANISM OF ACTION. Guaifenesin is a central-acting skeletal muscle relaxant, but its exact mechanism of action is unknown. It selectively depresses or blocks nerve impulse transmission at the internuncial neuron level of the spinal cord, brainstem, and subcortical areas of the brain causing sedation and muscle relaxation.

OH O CH_3

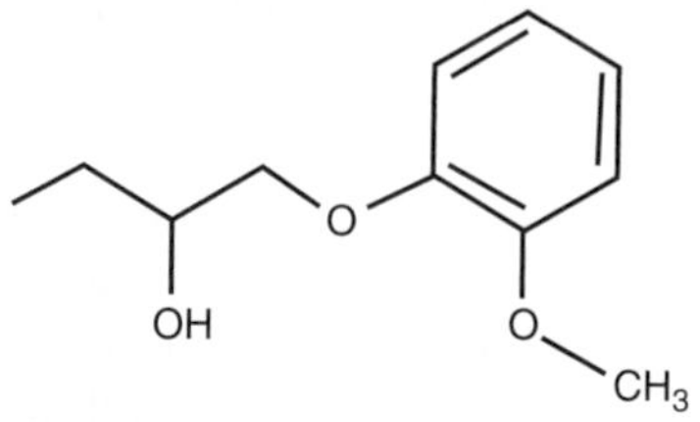

FIG. 11.12 Guaifenesin.

INDICATIONS. In veterinary medicine guaifenesin is used as an adjunct anesthetic in equine and ruminant patients, both during induction and as a form of total intravenous anesthesia. It is used to smooth induction and recovery as well as for decreasing the amount of induction drug needed (Brouwer 1985). When used alone, animals may obtain recumbency, but surgical anesthesia is not attained.

PHYSIOLOGIC EFFECTS

CNS. Guaifenesin is a central-acting skeletal muscle relaxant. It selectively depresses or blocks nerve impulse transmission at the internuncial neuron level of the spinal cord, brainstem, and subcortical areas of the brain causing sedation and muscle relaxation (Plumb 1999; Muir et al. 2000).

Cardiovascular. In the horse, initially there is a transient decrease in arterial blood pressure, which returns to normal, but myocardial contractile force and heart rate are relatively preserved (Hubbell and Muir 1980). Many studies, in many species, have looked at the effects of guaifenesin on cardiac function when used in conjunction with other anesthetics such as ketamine, thiopental and xylazine (Muir et al. 1978; Thurmon et al. 1986; McMurphy et al. 2002; Picavet et al. 2004). It is difficult to interpret the cardiovascular effects with respect to guaifenesin alone. However, it is likely that the additional CNS depression and muscle relaxation of guaifenesin allows for smaller doses of more cardiovascular depressing drugs such as thiopental or xylazine to be used. Thus, guaifenesin may be useful in preserving cardiovascular function when used with other anesthetic drugs.

Respiratory. Even though guaifenesin is a skeletal muscle relaxant, in therapeutic amounts, it does not cause paralysis of the respiratory muscles (intercostal and diaphragm). Often respiratory rate is increased but minute ventilation is unchanged (Lumb and Jones 1996; Muir et al. 2000; Hubbell et al. 1980). At doses greater than needed to obtain recumbency, respiratory depression might become significant.

Muscular. Guaifenesin produces generalized skeletal muscle relaxation. At recommended doses, it does not affect respiratory muscles enough to significantly alter ventilation. The laryngeal and pharyngeal muscles are relaxed, which facilitates intubation of the trachea. At excessive doses, guaifenesin can produce a paradoxical increase in muscle rigidity (Muir et al. 2000).

Miscellaneous. Guaifenesin crosses the placenta and can be detected in the plasma of the fetus (Hubbell et al. 1980). Adverse effects of guaifenesin in newborns have not been reported.

Analgesia. Previous editions of this book have suggested that guaifenesin is analgesic, but there is little evidence to support that claim.

PHARMACOKINETICS. Extensive evaluation of the pharmacokinetics of guaifenesin has not been performed. When administered to horses as a single agent, recumbency occurs in ~2 minutes and can last ~6 minutes. Sedation from a single dose may last 15–30 minutes. There is gender difference in the half-lives of ponies; where males have a T1/2 of ~85 minutes whereas the female T1/2 is ~60 minutes (Davis and Wolff 1970).

METABOLISM. Guaifenesin undergoes biotransformation in the liver to a glucuronide, which is then excreted in the urine.

ADVERSE EFFECTS/CONTRAINDICATIONS. The manufacturer cautions against administration with physostigmine, but does not explain the interaction. The use of guaifenesin in cows at concentrations exceeding 5% has been associated with red blood cell hemolysis (Wall and Muir, 3rd 1990).

DOSE. Guaifenesin has a moderately high therapeutic index as three to four times the dose required to produce recumbency of the horse can be administered before death occurs (Funk 1973). The primary disadvantage in the use of guaifenesin is the large volume of solution required to produce relaxation.

Horse: The approved dose is 2.2 ml/kg (110 mg/kg). This dose is reduced when administered with other CNS depressants (75–100 mg/kg).

SPECIES DIFFERENCES

Horses. Horses are still routinely sedated and anesthetized using guaifenesin. Generally it is combined with or given immediately prior to other anesthetic drugs, such as xylazine, ketamine, or thiopental (see the next section, "Triple Drip"). Guaifenesin aids in producing a smooth induction and recovery as well as minimizing the amount of other drugs needed to produce the desired effect. The administration of xylazine (1.1 mg/kg) prior to guaifenesin reduces the IV dose necessary to induce lateral recumbency in adult horses (Hubbell et al. 1980). When using guaifenesin for sedation immediately prior to induction with ketamine or thiopental, it should be administered until the horse begins to knuckle the fore- or hindlimbs. At that point, the guaifenesin should be discontinued and the induction agent immediately given. Hemolysis of red blood cells (as seen in cattle) has not been associated with guaifenesin concentrations up to 10% (Grandy and McDonell 1980).

Cattle. The use of guaifenesin in cattle and small ruminants is similar to that of horses. The use of guaifenesin in concentrations exceeding 5% has been associated with a dose-dependent red blood cell hemolysis (Wall and Muir, 3rd 1990).

Dogs. Guaifenesin has been used to treat strychnine poisoning in dogs (Bailey and Szabuniewicz 1975), but it is generally no longer used for sedation or anesthesia of dogs.

TRIPLE DRIP. Guaifenesin has been extensively used in combination with ketamine and xylazine. In horses the mixture is commonly comprised of guaifenesin (50 mg/ml), ketamine (1–2 mg/ml), and xylazine at (0.5–1.0 mg/ml). In cattle and small ruminants, guaifenesin (50 mg/ml) has been combined with ketamine (1–2 mg/ml) and xylazine (0.05–0.1 mg/ml). These combinations can be administered as induction agents, but they are more routinely administered following anesthesia induction for maintenance of anesthesia. They should be administered "to effect" but generally are administered ~1–2 ml/kg/hr. Guaifenesin has similarly been combined with detomidine (40 ug/ml) and ketamine (4 mg/ml) and administered at a continuous infusion rate of 0.8 ml/kg/min (Taylor et al. 1998).

Guaifenesin (50 mg/ml) can also been mixed with thiopental (2 mg/ml) and similarly used for maintenance of anesthesia at ~1.5 ml/kg/hr (Muir et al. 2000).

DRUG INTERACTIONS. Guaifenesin is often mixed with ketamine and xylazine (triple drip) and with barbiturates with apparent stability. The manufacturer cautions against administration with physostigmine, but does not explain the interaction.

OVERDOSE/ACUTE TOXICITY. Guaifenesin has a wide therapeutic margin. Overdose can be associated with respiratory depression and muscle rigidity. Treatment should be based on supportive care until plasma levels decrease.

The use of guaifenesin in cows at concentrations exceeding 5% has been associated with red blood cell hemolysis (Wall and Muir, 3rd 1990).

REGULATORY INFORMATION. Guaifenesin is approved as a skeletal muscle relaxant for use in horses, but not for use in meat production animals. Guaifenesin is approved for use in people as an expectorant.

Controlled Drug Status. Guaifenesin is not a controlled drug.

Withdrawal Times. Extralabel use in food animals: 3 days for meat and 48 hours for milk.

VETERINARY PRODUCTS. Guailaxin: Fort Dodge Animal Health. Sterile Powder 50 gm.

Gecolate/Glycodex Injection: Summit Hill Laboratories. 5% solution.

HUMAN PRODUCTS. There are no parenteral formulations approved for people. There are many oral, OTC formulations such as Mucinex: Adams Respiratory Lab. 600 mg tablets.

NEUROSTEROIDS

HISTORY. Synthetic neuroactive steroids have been intermittently popular in human and veterinary anesthesia for more than 30 years. The two most popular formulations, Althesin and Saffan®, are mixtures of two neurosteroids; alphaxalone and alphadolone. Although these drugs have been widely used in Canada and the U.K., they have never been approved for use in veterinary medicine and are rarely if ever used in the U.S.

CLASSIFICATION

Chemistry. Alphaxalone (3-alpha-hydroxy-5-alpha-pregnane-11,20-dione) (Fig. 11.13) and alphadolone (3-alpha,21-dihydroxy-5-alpha-pregnane-11,20-dione) (Fig. 11.14) are steroid compounds.

How Supplied. Althesin/Saffan: Each ml contains 12 mg of neurosteroid as a mixture of 9 mg alphaxalone and 3 mg alphadolone in a 20% polyoxyethylated castor oil–based surfactant (cremophor).

Alfaxan-CD: Each ml contains 10 mg alfaxalone in 2-hydroxypropyl-beta cyclodextrin.

MECHANISM OF ACTION. Neuroactive steroids are agonists at the γ-aminobutyric acid ($GABA_A$) receptor. Activation of the GABA receptors increases transmembrane chloride conductance resulting in hyperpolarization of the postsynaptic cell membrane, which causes inhibition of the postsynaptic neuron. This results in inhibition of pathway activation controlling arousal and awareness.

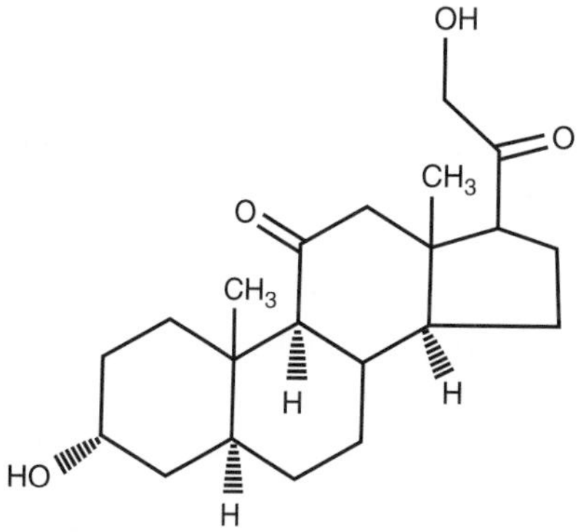

FIG. 11.13 Alphadolone.

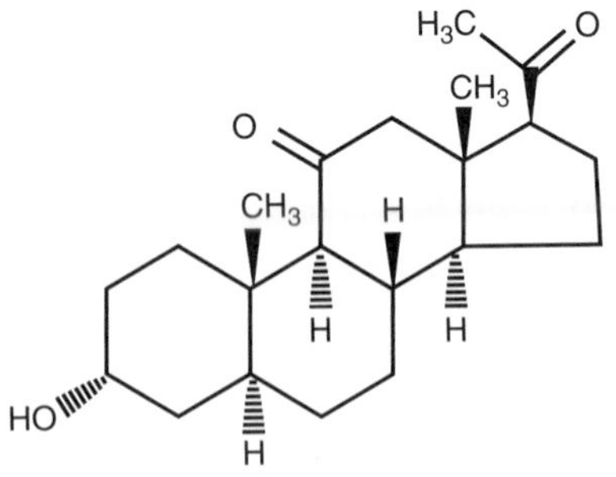

FIG. 11.14 Alphaxalone.

INDICATIONS. Neuroactive steroids are indicated for the intramuscular or intravenous induction of anesthesia in dogs and cats.

PHYSIOLOGIC EFFECTS

CNS. Neurosteroids produce unconsciousness and anesthesia along with a dose dependent decrease in EEG activity (Zattoni et al. 1980). They produce a favorable neurologic environment by decreasing cerebral blood flow, intracranial pressure, and cerebral metabolic demands (Rasmussen et al. 1978).

Cardiovascular. Althesin administration to cats at moderate doses (<9 mg/kg) produces a transient drop in systemic arterial blood pressure with an increase in heart rate. At doses of 12 mg/kg, cats had a decrease in cardiac output of ~43%, mostly through a decrease in stroke volume (Dyson et al. 1987). This conflicts with prior reports that Althesin has less of a negative inotropic action on the myocardium of the cat than thiopental (Gordh 1972). Alfaxalone decreases epinephrine-induced arrhythmias in cats anesthetized with alpha chloralose (Al-Khawashki et al. 1980).

Severe hypotension and cardiovascular collapse has been associated with neurosteroid administration. The vehicle cremophor, as well as both steroids, have been implicated in histamine release. (Read more in the section "Allergic Reactions.")

Respiratory. Neurosteroids generally preserve respiratory function, although some animals may have a brief period of apnea (Dyson et al. 1987).

Muscular. Neurosteroids provide good muscle relaxation when used alone, but may cause muscle tremors, paddling, and hyperesthesia during the recovery phase (Lumb and Jones 1996).

Miscellaneous. Perivascular injection causes tissue damage or appears to sting.

Neurosteroids produce minimal hormonal effect; Althesin possesses less than 1/60 the activity of betamethasone and is slightly less active than hydrocortisone. There is no evidence that it clinically interferes with mineralocorticoid or glucocorticoid production.

Allergic Reactions. Neurosteroids are associated with allergic reactions ranging from erythema and edema to life-threatening anaphylaxis. Approximately 25% of cats will have edema of feet, ears, and muzzle, which resolves usually within 2 hours (Lumb and Jones 1996). Dogs have been reported to have allergic responses that release histamine and result in significant hypotension. The vehicle (polyoxyethylated castor oil) is generally considered the major factor in the histamine release and, although possible, it is less likely that either steroid would elicit the reaction (Lumb and Jones 1996). A formulation of alphaxalone in a noncremophor vehicle (cyclodextran) has recently been marketed in Australia and does not appear to cause an allergic reaction in dogs or cats (Ferre et al. 2006).

Analgesia. There is little literature on the analgesic effects of alphaxalone or alphadolone in veterinary patients. However, there is strong evidence that neurosteroids produce analgesia mediated through $GABA_A$ receptors (Nadeson and Goodchild 2000).

PHARMACOKINETICS. Minimal information is available on the pharmacokinetics of the neurosteroids in veterinary patients. In cats, relaxation occurs ~10 seconds after IV injection and surgical anesthesia is produced in ~30 seconds (Lumb and Jones 1996). Following IM injection in cats, onset of anesthesia occurs in 6–12 minutes (Lumb and Jones 1996). Depth and duration of action is dependent on dose. Neither alphaxalone nor alphadolone acetate is extensively protein bound and neither appears cumulative.

METABOLISM. In the rat, alphaxalone is metabolized rapidly by the hepatic mixed function oxygenase system.

Induction of cytochrome P450 caused a decrease in the duration of the anaesthetic affect of Althesin (Sear and McGivan 1981). In humans, radio-labeled alphaxalone was biotransformed and 70% was excreted through the bile and 30% excreted in the urine (Strunin et al. 1977).

ADVERSE EFFECTS/CONTRAINDICATIONS. Previous authors of this chapter have cautioned against the use of barbiturates with Althesin with little explanation. It is possible that since both are GABA receptor agonists their effects are synergistic and led to an anesthetic overdose. An alternative reason may involve histamine release from Althesin coupled with the depressant cardiovascular effects of both drugs leading to cardiovascular collapse.

DOSE

Althesin:
- Cat: 9 mg/kg IV 12–18 mg/kg IM
- Dog: not recommended

Alfaxan-CD RTU:
- Cat: 0.5–2 mg/kg IV
- Dog: 0.5–2 mg/kg IV

SPECIES DIFFERENCES

Dogs. Due to the risk of anaphylactic reaction, neurosteroids prepared in a cremophor vehicle should not be used in dogs.

Horses. Intravenous Althesin can cause CNS excitation including violent paddling, galloping movement, and poor muscle relaxation (Lumb and Jones 1996). Although prior sedation with xylazine can attenuate these reactions, the use of Althesin is not recommended for use in horses.

OVERDOSE/ACUTE TOXICITY. Neurosteroids have a large therapeutic index, when allergic reactions do not occur, and a short duration of action (Ferre et al. 2006). Therefore, treatment of an overdose should focus on supportive care.

For animals with an allergic reaction, treatment should focus on the vasodilating effects of histamine release (e.g., fluid therapy, inotropic support, vasoconstrictors, antihistaminics, and steroids).

REGULATORY INFORMATION

Controlled Drug Status. Not controlled.

VETERINARY PRODUCTS. There are no neurosteroids manufactured or approved for use in animals in the United States. Saffan is available in the U.K., and Alfaxan-CD is approved for use in dogs and cats in Australia.

Saffan: Schering Plough Animal Health: U.K. 12 mg/ml solution

Alfaxan-CD RTU: Jurox Pty. Ltd. Rutherford Australia. 10 mg/ml solution

HUMAN PRODUCTS. There are no human products.

MISCELLANEOUS INTRAVENOUS ANESTHETICS

CHLORAL HYDRATE

History. Chloral hydrate is the ingredient in the notorious "Mickey Finn" named after a Chicago bartender who used the sedative properties combined with alcohol to rob his victims. It was introduced into medicine as a hypnotic in 1869 (Gauillard and Cheref 2002) and was among the first CNS depressants to be used in veterinary medicine. Chloral hydrate is rarely used to treat insomnia in people and for sedation in children, but is no longer used in conjunction with human anesthesia. It is a mutagen and a potential carcinogen and is rarely if ever used in veterinary medicine. This drug is discussed in greater detail in the 7th Edition of this text.

Classification

Chemistry. Chloral Hydrate, 1,1,1-Trichloro-2,2-dihydroxyethane, is the end product of chlorination of acetic aldehyde and addition of water (Fig. 11.15). Chloral hydrate volatilizes on exposure to air and has an aromatic, penetrating odor. One gram of chloral hydrate is soluble in 0.25 ml water and in 1–2 ml of fat solvents.

How Supplied. Presently, chloral hydrate is approved only for use in combination with pentobarbital and magnesium sulfate. Each ml contains 42.5 mg of chloral hydrate, 8.86 mg of pentobarbital, and 21.2 mg of magnesium sulfate in 33.8% propylene glycol and 14.25% ethyl alcohol.

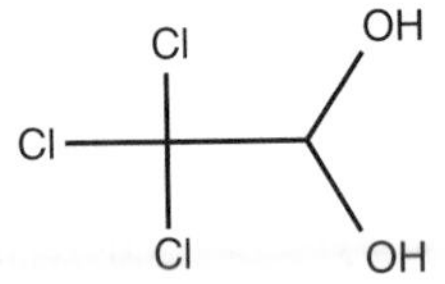

Cl Cl Cl OH OH

FIG. 11.15 Chloral hydrate.

Mechanism of Action. The mechanism of action is unknown, but the synergy of chloral hydrate with other GABA agonists (ethanol, benzodiazepines) makes it likely that it has a binding site at the GABA receptor (Gauillard and Cheref 2002). Additionally, flumazenil, a benzodiazepine antagonist has been successfully used to treat chloral hydrate overdose in people (Gauillard and Cheref 2002).

Indications. Chloral hydrate has been used for general sedation and as an adjunct to anesthesia primarily in horses and cattle. It is rarely used in modern veterinary practice.

Physiologic Effects. Chloral hydrate is a sedative hypnotic drug. It produces a dose-dependent sedation with a wide margin of safety when used at sedative doses. It is, however, a poor anesthetic and when administered at anesthetic doses, the margin of safety is narrow. At anesthetic doses (compared with sedative doses), chloral hydrate produces significant respiratory and cardiovascular depression. Although chloral hydrate produces CNS depression, it does not provide analgesia, and muscle relaxation is poor.

When administered IV, the sedative effects are seen almost immediately. Following oral administration, sedation occurs in 30 to 60 minutes. Choral hydrate is metabolized by alcohol dehydrogenase into trichloroethanol (TCE) and trichloroacetic acid. TCE is an active metabolite (Gauillard and Cheref 2002). The half-life of chloral hydrate is short (minutes), but the half-life of TCE is greater than 8 hours in humans (Gauillard and Cheref 2002).

The effects of chloral hydrate can be intensified when administered with other CNS depressants. Interestingly, chloral hydrate slows ethanol metabolism, thereby enhancing the effects of ethanol.

Chloral hydrate is irritating to the esophagus and GI tract, when administered orally, and should be administered in a diluted solution or following a meal. When administered intravenously, chloral hydrate can cause tissue necrosis and sloughing when administered perivascularly. When administered intraperitoneally, pain, ileus, and fibrosis may occur.

Dose. Chloral hydrate in solution can be injected intravenously or administered orally in solution or by capsule. It should not be administered intraperitoneally.

Cattle. For intravenous use only. For sedation: 0.025–0.05 ml/kg IV. For general anesthesia: 0.1–0.025 ml/kg IV until the desired effect is produced. Cattle usually require a lower dosage on the basis of body weight compared to horses. Oral administration is not recommended due to GI irritation.

Horses. For intravenous use only. For sedation: 0.025–0.05 ml/kg IV. For general anesthesia: 0.1–0.025 ml/kg IV until the desired effect is produced. Oral administration is not recommended due to GI irritation.

Chloral Hydrate with Magnesium Sulfate. The addition of magnesium (mixture of 12% chloral hydrate and 6% magnesium sulfate) to a chloral hydrate solution increases the muscle relaxation and duration of action of chloral hydrate. The primary effect of magnesium is its neuromuscular blocking action, similar to the curariform agents. From this standpoint, magnesium is beneficial in producing skeletal muscle relaxation, which chloral hydrate does poorly. Inasmuch as magnesium sulfate alone produces only neuromuscular blockade and death due to asphyxia, it is inhumane to use it in euthanasia.

Chloral Hydrate with Magnesium and Pentobarbital. The combination of chloral hydrate, magnesium sulfate, and pentobarbital sodium (previously marketed as Chloropent and Equithesin) provides some of the desirable depressant actions of each compound but minimizes the adverse effects of each by using smaller doses of each individual drug.

Regulatory Information. Chloropent is approved for use in cattle and horses.

Controlled Drug Status. Schedule IV controlled drug.

Withdrawal Times. There is no regulatory information available.

Veterinary Products. Chloropent (Fort Dodge Animal Health) is approved for use in horses and cattle. It contains chloral hydrate, pentobarbital, and magnesium sulfate. Each ml contains 42.5 mg of chloral hydrate, 8.86 mg of pentobarbital, and 21.2 mg of magnesium sulfate in 33.8% propylene glycol and 14.25% ethyl alcohol.

Human Products. There are no human products.

CHLORALOSE

Classification

Chemistry. Chloralose, 1,2-O-(2,2,2-trichloroethylidene)-alpha-D-glucofuranose, is prepared by condensing anhydrous glucose with chloraldehyde (chloral) in the presence of sulfuric acid (Fig. 11.16). A mixture of α-chloralose and β-chloralose is formed, of which the α-chloralose form is the active form. Chloralose is difficult to dissolve in an aqueous medium without simultaneous heating, but the solution should not be boiled.

How Supplied. Chloralose is generally prepared and administered intravenously in 1% concentration.

Indications. As an anesthetic agent, chloralose is restricted to laboratory animals in which recovery from anesthesia is not necessary. It is used primarily in physiologic experimentation because it purportedly does not interfere with respiratory and cardiac reflexes, e.g., baroceptor and chemoceptor activities.

Mechanism of Action. The mechanism of action has not been identified. An active metabolite of chloralose, trichloroethanol, is the same as for chloral hydrate. It is likely that both have interaction at the GABA receptor (see the previous section "Chloral Hydrate").

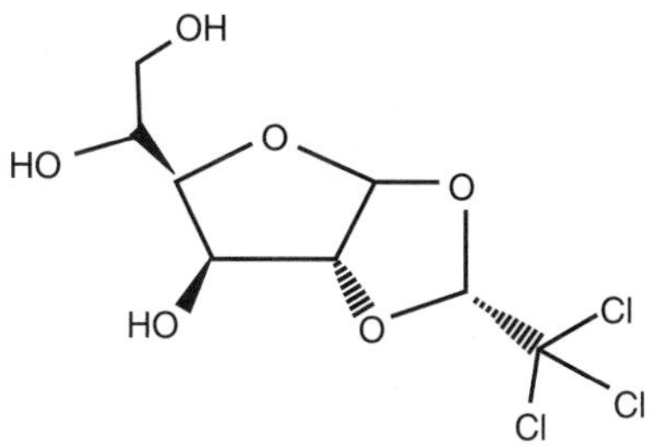

OH
HO
O
O
HO
O
Cl
Cl
Cl

FIG. 11.16 Chloralose.

Physiologic Effects. Chloralose induces prolonged hypnosis, lasting up to 8–10 hours. It is metabolized to chloraldehyde or chloral, which is mainly transformed into trichloroethanol (a metabolite of chloral hydrate). Hypnosis and anesthesia produced by chloral hydrate and chloralose are quite similar because of the formation of trichloroethanol.

Chloralose was considered an ideal drug for sedation/anesthesia of research animals due to its purported ability to provide CNS depression while not depressing baroreceptor reflexes, vasomotor centers, or spinal reflexes. However, spinal reflex activity may increase to the degree that muscle activity ("convulsions") similar to those of strychnine poisoning develops in the dog and cat (Lees 1972). Paddling movements and muscle fasciculations have been seen in pigs, sheep, and other species. Surgical anesthesia cannot be reached by administration of chloralose alone.

Concern exists about how much CNS depression occurs. People with alpha-chloralose overdose show marked CNS depression, with depressed-to-flat EEG waves (Manzo et al. 1979). Furthermore, people showed respiratory depression, muscle fasciculations, and seizurelike activity, similar to what had been reported in the dog (Manzo et al. 1979; Lees 1972). Its effectiveness as an anesthetic varies among species, and it is least effective in the dog. It is not recommended for survival procedures because of rough induction, prolonged recovery, and seizurelike activity. There is little indication that these drugs provide analgesia and they should not be used as single agents for surgical interventions.

Intraperitoneal injections produce pain and inflammation and are not recommended.

Dose

Dogs: 40–110 mg/kg IV
Cats: 40–80 mg/kg IV
Sheep: 45–55 mg/kg IV
Pigs: 55–86 IV

URETHANE

History. Urethane was a popular anesthetic for laboratory animals. It was primarily used for nonsurvival surgery due to its long duration of action, but is no longer recommended because it is carcinogenic.

Classification

Chemistry. Urethane (ethyl carbamate) is the ethyl ester of carbamic acid. It is chemically related to urea and is readily soluble in water and alcohol (Fig. 11.17).

Mechanism of Action. The mechanism of action of urethane has been poorly studied. Recently it has been shown in rats that urethane selectively alters potassium currents to depress neuronal excitability (Sceniak and MacIver 2005). This is a unique mechanism for an anesthetic.

Physiologic Effects. Urethane produces long-lasting unconsciousness of 8–10 hours duration. Spinal reflexes, neural transmission, and cardiopulmonary function are minimally affected. Unlike chloralose, urethane appears to induce analgesia and muscle relaxation. Urethane has been administered by most routes including topically to frogs.

Urethane is metabolized slowly into carbamic acid and ethyl alcohol. Liver injury is produced by urethane. The rate of elimination is slow and it is associated with long difficult recoveries.

Carcinogenic. Urethane is on the National Institute of Health (NIH) list of drugs that are "reasonably anticipated to be a human carcinogen" (U.S. Department of Health and Human Services 2005). Exposure can be by inhalation, ingestion, or dermal contact. Strict precautions should be taken to prevent exposure to personnel.

Dose. Urethane is not recommended for use due to its potential as a carcinogen and because there are safer anesthetics available.

Rodents: 1 g/kg IV: 1–2 g/kg IP

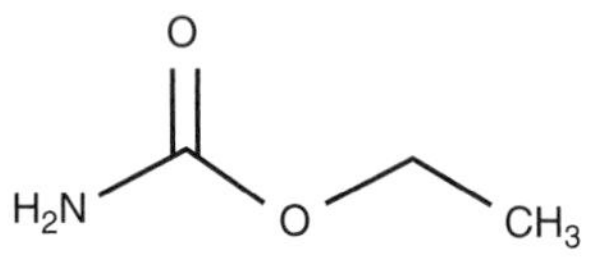

FIG. 11.17 Urethane.

PROPANIDID

History. Propanidid was introduced in human anesthesia by Bayer but anaphylactic reactions caused it to be withdrawn shortly afterward. It is now widely believed that these reactions were caused by the Cremophor-EL vehicle rather than the active molecule itself.

Classification

Chemistry. Propanidid (3-Methoxy-4-((N,N-diethylcar bamido)methoxy)phenyl)acetic acid n-propyl ester, is phenylacetate, nonbarbiturate, general anesthetic (Fig. 11.18).

Mechanism of Action. Propanidid produces its action by interaction at the GABA receptor.

Physiologic Effects. Anesthesia with propanidid has been associated with CNS excitatory side effects (rigidity, myoclonus) and with seizures. Reaction with the vehicle, Cremophor, has been associated with anaphylactic reactions.

Dose. Rats: sedation: 17.7 mg/kg IV; anesthesia: 50 mg/kg IV.

METOMIDATE

History. Metomidate is a nonbarbiturate anesthetic that is in the same family as etomidate. It had been used as an anesthetic in mammals and birds, but is primarily used today as a fish anesthetic.

Classification

Chemistry. Metomidate (methyl 1-(alpha-methylbenzyl) imidazole-5-carboxylate) is an imidazole compound (Fig. 11.19).

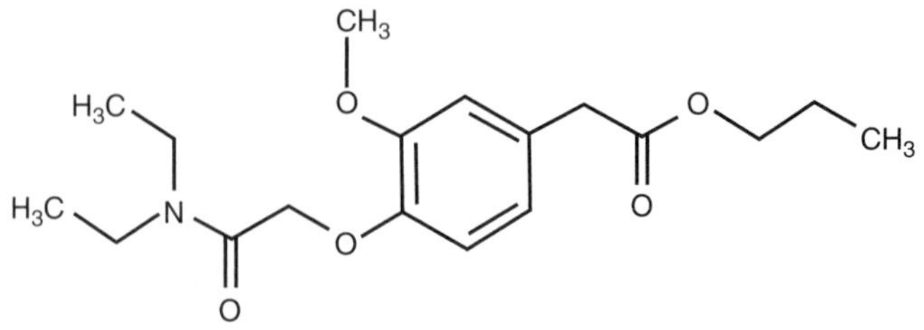

FIG. 11.18 Propanidid.

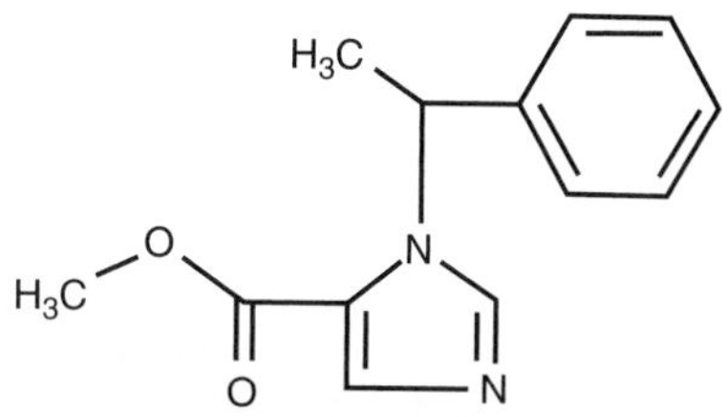

FIG. 11.19 Metomidate.

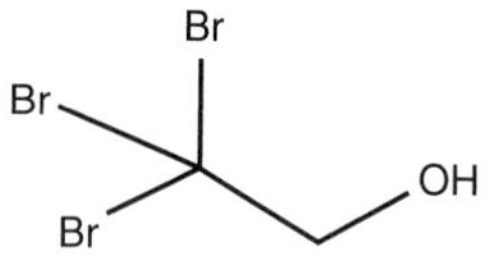

FIG. 11.20 Tribromoethanol.

How Supplied. Metomidate is a white powder, soluble in water and ethanol. It is generally reconstituted to 1% or 5% solutions, which are acidic: pH ~3.

Mechanism of Action. Imidazole anesthetics are gamma-aminobutyric acid (GABA) receptor agonists that produce anesthesia and amnesia (Stoelting 1999).

Physiologic Effects. Metomidate produces hypnosis, anesthesia, and muscle relaxation. Cardiovascular function is generally preserved, but respiratory depression and apnea can occur. They are poor muscle relaxants and provide no analgesia.

Imidazoles (metomidate and etomidate) have been credited with providing complete anesthesia and decreasing the stress response. Unfortunately, the stress-free aspects attributed to these drugs are not accurate. Metomidate blocks the 11-beta hydroxylation of cortisol both in mammals and in fish. This seriously perturbs the complex positive and negative feedback pathways for control of the neuroendocrine cascade. The fish are experiencing the same stress, but are not able to respond to it by producing cortisol. Researchers should be cautious in interpreting stress response in fish exposed to imidazole anesthetics.

Fish exposed to metomidate can have dark skin discoloration after exposure. Because cortisol inhibits the release of ACTH, and ACTH stimulates melanocyte-stimulating hormone, it is hypothesized that the decrease in cortisol production that occurs with the use of these drugs results in an increase in melanocyte-stimulating hormone (Harms and Bakal 1994).

Dose. Fish: Immersion agent: 0.5–10 mg/l.
Injection: 3 mg/kg IV

TRIBROMOETHANOL

History. Tribromoethanol is a popular injectable anesthetic agent used in mice. It was manufactured as Avertin®, but this product is no longer available. Investigators who want to use tribromoethanol as an anesthetic must make their own solutions.

Classification

Chemistry. 2,2,2-Tribromoethanol is a powder that is formed from the reduction of tribromoacetaldehyde and aluminum isopropylate (Fig. 11.20).

Mechanism of Action. Tribromoethanol produces generalized CNS depression but its direct mechanism of action is unknown.

Physiologic Effects. Tribromoethanol produces generalized CNS depression including the cardiovascular and respiratory centers. It undergoes hepatic conjugation and the glucuronide is excreted in the urine. Tribromoethanol produces repeatable anesthesia, but sleep times can be variable in young or sick animals (Meyer and Fish 2005).

Adverse Effects. Tribromoethanol is an irritant, especially at high doses, high concentrations, or with repeated use (Meyer 2005). Anesthesia with tribromoethanol can result in ileus, abdominal adhesions, increased generalized morbidity, and increased mortality (Meyer and Fish 2005). Tribromoethanol has been associated with impaired fertility (Meyer and Fish 2005). Tribromoethanol degrades in the presence of heat or light to produce toxic byproducts. Degraded solutions can be both nephrotoxic and hepatotoxic. Administration of degraded tribromoethanol solutions has been associated with death, often 24 hours after surgery.

Dose. Due to the increased morbidity and mortality following anesthesia, and repeated anesthetics, tribromoethanol is recommended only for terminal studies (Meyer and Fish 2005).

Mouse: 250 mg/kg IP

REFERENCES

Adam, H. K., J. B. Glen, et al. 1980. Pharmacokinetics in laboratory animals of ICI 35 868, a new i.v. anaesthetic agent. Br J Anaesth 52(8): 743–6.

Adams, H. A. 1997. [S-(+)-ketamine. Circulatory interactions during total intravenous anesthesia and analgesia-sedation]. Anaesthesist 46(12): 1081–7.

Al-Khawashki, M. I., H. A. Ghaleb, et al. 1980. Pharmacological effects of althesin and its steroidal components on the cardiovascular system. Middle East J Anaesthesiology 5(7): 457–69.

Albrecht, R. F., D. J. Miletich, et al. 1977. Cerebral blood flow and metabolic changes from induction to onset of anesthesia with halothane or pentobarbital. Anesthesiology 47(3): 252–6.

Amouzadeh, H. R., S. Sangiah, et al. 1989. Effects of some hepatic microsomal enzyme inducers and inhibitors on xylazine-ketamine anesthesia. Vet Hum Toxicol 31(6): 532–4.

Andress, J. L., T. K. Day, et al. 1995. The effects of consecutive day propofol anesthesia on feline red blood cells. Vet Surg 24(3): 277–82.

Annetta, M. G., D. Iemma, et al. 2005. Ketamine: new indications for an old drug. Curr Drug Targets 6(7): 789–94.

Apfel, C. C., K. Korttila, et al. 2004. A factorial trial of six interventions for the prevention of postoperative nausea and vomiting. N Engl J Med 350(24): 2441–51.

Atlee, J. L., 3rd, and C. E. Malkinson. 1982. Potentiation by thiopental of halothane–epinephrine-induced arrhythmias in dogs. Anesthesiology 57(4): 285–8.

Baggot, J. D. and J. W. Blake. 1976. Disposition kinetics of ketamine in the domestic cat. Arch Int Pharmacodyn Ther 220(1): 115–24.

Bailey, E. M. and M. Szabuniewicz. 1975. Use of glyceryl guaiacolate ether in treating strychnine poisoning in the dog. Vet Med Small Anim Clin 70(2): 170–4.

Barker, P., J. A. Langton, et al. 1992. Movements of the vocal cords on induction of anaesthesia with thiopentone or propofol. Br J Anaesth 69(1): 23–5.

Bedford, R. F., J. A. Persing, et al. 1980. Lidocaine or thiopental for rapid control of intracranial hypertension? Anesth Analg 59(6): 435–7.

Bergen, J. M. and D. C. Smith. 1997. A review of etomidate for rapid sequence intubation in the emergency department. J Emerg Med 15(2): 221–30.

Boulos, B. M., W. L. Jenkins, et al. 1972. Pharmacokinetics of certain drugs in the domesticated goat. Am J Vet Res 33(5): 943–52.

Brandon, R. A. and J. D. Baggot. 1981. The pharmacokinetics of thiopentone. J Vet Pharmacol Ther 4(2): 79–85.

Brouwer, G. J. 1985. Use of guaiacol glycerine ether in clinical anaesthesia in the horse. Equine Vet J 17(2): 133–6.

Canaday, B. R. 1993. Amorous, disinhibited behavior associated with propofol. Clin Pharm 12(6): 449–51.

Cheng, M. A., R. Tempelhoff, et al. 1996. Large-dose propofol alone in adult epileptic patients: electrocorticographic results. Anesth Analg 83(1): 169–74.

Court, M. H., B. L. Hay-Kraus, et al. 1999. Propofol hydroxylation by dog liver microsomes: assay development and dog breed differences. Drug Metab Dispos 27(11): 1293–9.

Dailland, P., I. D. Cockshott, et al. 1989. Intravenous propofol during cesarean section: placental transfer, concentrations in breast milk, and neonatal effects. A preliminary study. Anesthesiology 71(6): 827–34.

Davis, L. E. and W. A. Wolff. 1970. Pharmacokinetics and metabolism of glyceryl guaiacolate in ponies. Am J Vet Res 31(3): 469–73.

Dawson, B., J. D. Michenfelder, et al. 1971. Effects of ketamine on canine cerebral blood flow and metabolism: modification by prior administration of thiopental. Anesth Analg 50(3): 443–7.

De Hert SG, KM Vermeyen, et al. 1990. Influence of thiopental, etomidate, and propofol on regional myocardial function in the normal and acute ischemic heart segment in dogs. Anesth Anal June; 70(6): 600–7.

Dershwitz, M., F. A. Sreter, et al. 1989. Ketamine does not trigger malignant hyperthermia in susceptible swine. Anesth Analg 69(4): 501–3.

Diaz, F. A., J. A. Bianco, et al. 1976. Effects of ketamine on canine cardiovascular function. Br J Anaesth 48(10): 941–6.

Dodam, J. R., K. T. Kruse-Elliott, et al. 1990. Duration of etomidate-induced adrenocortical suppression during surgery in dogs. Am J Vet Res 51(5): 786–8.

Doenicke, A. W., M. F. Roizen, et al. 1999. Reducing myoclonus after etomidate. Anesthesiology 90(1): 113–9.

Doerning, B. J., D. W. Brammer, et al. 1992. Nephrotoxicity of tiletamine in New Zealand white rabbits. Lab Anim Sci 42(3): 267–9.

Domino, E. F., S. E. Domino, et al. 1984. Ketamine kinetics in unmedicated and diazepam-premedicated subjects. Clin Pharmacol Ther 36(5): 645–53.

Duke, T., C. M. Egger, et al. 1997. Cardiopulmonary effects of propofol infusion in llamas. Am J Vet Res 58(2): 153–6.

Duran, S. H., W. R. Ravis, et al. 1987. Pharmacokinetics of phenobarbital in the horse. Am J Vet Res 48(5): 807–10.

Durieux, M. E. 1995. Inhibition by ketamine of muscarinic acetylcholine receptor function. Anesth Analg 81(1): 57–62.

Dyson, D. H., D. G. Allen, et al. 1987. Effects of saffan on cardiopulmonary function in healthy cats. Can J Vet Res 51(2): 236–9.

Ferre, P. J., K. Pasloske, et al. 2006. Plasma pharmacokinetics of alfaxalone in dogs after an intravenous bolus of Alfaxan-CD RTU. Vet Anaesth Analg 33(4): 229–36.

Frederiksen, M. C., T. K. Henthorn, et al. 1983. Pharmacokinetics of pentobarbital in the dog. J Pharmacol Exp Ther 225(2): 355–60.

Fruen, B. R., J. R. Mickelson, et al. 1995. Effects of propofol on Ca2+ regulation by malignant hyperthermia-susceptible muscle membranes. Anesthesiology 82(5): 1274–82.

Funk, K. A. 1973. Glyceryl guaiacolate: some effects and indications in horses. Equine Vet J 5(1): 15–9.

Gauillard, J., S. Cheref, et al. 2002. [Chloral hydrate: a hypnotic best forgotten?]. Encephale 28(3 Pt 1): 200–4.

Ghoneim, M. M. and H. Pandya. 1975. Plasma protein binding of thiopental in patients with impaired renal or hepatic function. Anesthesiology 42(5): 545–9.

Gordh, T. 1972. The effect of Althesin on the heart in situ in the cat. Postgrad Med J 48: Suppl 2:31–7.

Gottschling, S., R. Larsen, et al. 2005. Acute pancreatitis induced by short-term propofol administration. Paediatr Anaesth 15(11): 1006–8.

Grandy, J. L. and W. N. McDonell. 1980. Evaluation of concentrated solutions of guaifenesin for equine anesthesia. J Am Vet Med Assoc 176(7): 619–22.

Guirimand, F., X. Dupont, et al. 2000. The effects of ketamine on the temporal summation (wind-up) of the R(III) nociceptive flexion reflex and pain in humans. Anesth Analg 90(2): 408–14.

Haas, D. A. and D. G. Harper. 1992. Ketamine: a review of its pharmacologic properties and use in ambulatory anesthesia. Anesth Prog 39(3): 61–8.

Hanna, R. M., R. E. Borchard, et al. 1988. Pharmacokinetics of ketamine HCl and metabolite I in the cat: a comparison of i.v., i.m., and rectal administration. J Vet Pharmacol Ther 11(1): 84–93.

Harms, C. and B. Bakal. 1994. Techniques in Fish Anesthesia. Proceedings of the American Association of Zoo Veterinarians and Association of Reptilian and Amphibian Veterinarians.

Harrison, J. M., K. J. Girling, et al. 2002. Effects of propofol and nitrous oxide on middle cerebral artery flow velocity and cerebral autoregulation. Anaesthesia 57(1): 27–32.

Harvey, S. C. 1975. In L. S. Goodman and A. Gilman, eds., The Pharmacological Basis of Therapeutics, 5th ed., p. 60. New York: Macmillan.

Haskins, S. C., T. B. Farver, et al. 1985. Ketamine in dogs. Am J Vet Res 46(9): 1855–60.

Hatch, R. C. 1966. The effect of glucose, sodium lactate, and epinephrine on thiopental anesthesia in dogs. J Am Vet Med Assoc 148(2): 135–40.

Hawkins, M. G., B. D. Wright, et al. 2003. Pharmacokinetics and anesthetic and cardiopulmonary effects of propofol in red-tailed hawks (*Buteo jamaicensis*) and great horned owls (*Bubo virginianus*). Am J Vet Res 64(6): 677–83.

Hay Kraus, B. L., D. J. Greenblatt, et al. 2000. Evidence for propofol hydroxylation by cytochrome P4502B11 in canine liver microsomes: breed and gender differences. Xenobiotica 30(6): 575–88.

Heldmann, E., D. C. Brown, et al. 1999. The association of propofol usage with postoperative wound infection rate in clean wounds: a retrospective study. Vet Surg 28(4): 256–9.

Himmelseher, S. and M. E. Durieux. 2005. Revising a dogma: ketamine for patients with neurological injury? Anesth Analg 101(2): 524–34, table of contents.

Hirshman, C. A., R. E. McCullough, et al. 1975. Hypoxic ventilatory drive in dogs during thiopental, ketamine, or pentobarbital anesthesia. Anesthesiology 43(6): 628–34.

Horta, M. L., L. C. Morejon, et al. 2006. Study of the prophylactic effect of droperidol, alizapride, propofol and promethazine on spinal morphine-induced pruritus. Br J Anaesth 96(6): 796–800.

Hubbell, J. A., W. W. Muir, et al. 1980. Guaifenesin: cardiopulmonary effects and plasma concentrations in horses. Am J Vet Res 41(11): 1751–5.

Ilkiw, J. E., J. A. Benthuysen, et al. 1991. A comparative study of the pharmacokinetics of thiopental in the rabbit, sheep and dog. J Vet Pharmacol Ther 14(2): 134–40.

Ilkiw, J. E., S. C. Haskins, et al. 1991. Cardiovascular and respiratory effects of thiopental administration in hypovolemic dogs. Am J Vet Res 52(4): 576–80.

Jackson, A. M., K. Tobias, et al. 2004. Effects of various anesthetic agents on laryngeal motion during laryngoscopy in normal dogs. Vet Surg 33(2): 102–6.

Kaka, J. S. and W. L. Hayton. 1980. Pharmacokinetics of ketamine and two metabolites in the dog. J Pharmacokinet Biopharm 8(2): 193–202.

Kaka, J. S., P. A. Klavano, et al. 1979. Pharmacokinetics of ketamine in the horse. Am J Vet Res 40(7): 978–81.

Kamibayashi, T., Y. Hayashi, et al. 1991. Enhancement by propofol of epinephrine-induced arrhythmias in dogs. Anesthesiology 75(6): 1035–40.

Kayama, Y. 1982. Ketamine and e.e.g. seizure waves: interaction with anti-epileptic drugs. Br J Anaesth 54(8): 879–83.

Kiersey, D. K., R. G. Bickford, et al. 1951. Electro-encephalographic patterns produced by thiopental sodium during surgical operations; description and classification. Br J Anaesth 23(3): 141–52.

Klein, L. 2007. Experience with Telazol use in tigers. L. Posner. Raleigh, NC.

Ko, J. C. 1993. Acute haemolysis associated with etomidate-propylene glycol infusion in dogs. J Vet Aneaesth 20(December): 92–94.

Ko, J. C., F. J. Golder, et al. 1999. Anesthetic and cardiorespiratory effects of a 1 : 1 mixture of propofol and thiopental sodium in dogs. J Am Vet Med Assoc 215(9): 1292–6.

Krystal, A. D., R. D. Weiner, et al. 2003. Comparison of seizure duration, ictal EEG, and cognitive effects of ketamine and methohexital anesthesia with ECT. J Neuropsych Clin Neurosci 15(1): 27–34.

Lagerkranser, M., K. Stange, et al. 1997. Effects of propofol on cerebral blood flow, metabolism, and cerebral autoregulation in the anesthetized pig. J Neurosurg Anesthesiol 9(2): 188–93.

Ledowski, T., B. Bein, et al. 2005. Neuroendocrine stress response and heart rate variability: a comparison of total intravenous versus balanced anesthesia. Anesth Analg 101(6): 1700–5.

Lees, P. 1972. Pharmacology and toxicology of alpha chloralose: a review. Vet Rec 91(14): 330–3.

Leung, L. Y. and T. A. Baillie. 1986. Comparative pharmacology in the rat of ketamine and its two principal metabolites, norketamine and (Z)-6-hydroxynorketamine. J Med Chem 29(11): 2396–9.

Lewis, J. 2007. Telazol Use in Tigers. L. Posner. Raleigh, NC: E-mail.

Lumb and Jones. 1996. Lumb & Jones Veterinary Anesthesia. Baltimore, Williams & Wilkins.

Luna, S. P., R. N. Cassu, et al. 2004. Effects of four anaesthetic protocols on the neurological and cardiorespiratory variables of puppies born by caesarean section. Vet Rec 154(13): 387–9.

Mama, K. R., E. P. Steffey, et al. 1996. Evaluation of propofol for general anesthesia in premedicated horses. Am J Vet Res 57(4): 512–6.

Mandsager, R. E., C. R. Clarke, et al. 1995. Effects of chloramphenicol on infusion pharmacokinetics of propofol in greyhounds. Am J Vet Res 56(1): 95–9.

Manzo, L., P. Richelmi, et al. 1979. Electrocerebral changes in acute alpha-chloralose poisoning: a case report. Vet Hum Toxicol 21(4): 245–7.

Matot, I., C. F. Neely, et al. 1993. Pulmonary uptake of propofol in cats. Effect of fentanyl and halothane. Anesthesiology 78(6): 1157–65.

McMurphy, R. M., L. E. Young, et al. 2002. Comparison of the cardiopulmonary effects of anesthesia maintained by continuous infusion of romifidine, guaifenesin, and ketamine with anesthesia maintained by inhalation of halothane in horses. Am J Vet Res 63(12): 1655–61.

Mees, D. E., Jr. and E. L. Frederickson. 1975. Anesthesia and the porphyrias. South Med J 68(1): 29–32.

Meyer, R. E. and R. E. Fish. 2005. A review of tribromoethanol anesthesia for production of genetically engineered mice and rats. Lab Anim (NY) 34(10): 47–52.

Mirakhur, R. K. and W. F. Shepherd. 1985. Intraocular pressure changes with propofol ("Diprivan"): comparison with thiopentone. Postgrad Med J 61 Suppl 3: 41–4.

Mitsuhata, H. and R. Shimizu. 1993. Evaluation of histamine-releasing property of propofol in whole blood in vitro. J Anesth 7(2): 189–92.

Moon, P. F. 1994. Acute toxicosis in two dogs associated with etomidate-propylene glycol infusion. Lab Anim Sci 44(6): 590–4.

———. 1997. Cortisol suppression in cats after induction of anesthesia with etomidate, compared with ketamine-diazepam combination. Am J Vet Res 58(8): 868–71.

Morris, P. J. 2001. Chemical immobilization of felids, ursids and small ungulates. Vet Clin of North Amer: Exotic Anim Pract 4: 267–299.

Muir, W. W. 1977. Thiobarbiturate-induced dysrhythmias: the role of heart rate and autonomic imbalance. Am J Vet Res 38(9): 1377–81.

Muir, W. W., J. Hubbell, et al. 2000. Handbook of Veterinary Anesthesia. St. Louis, Mosby.

Muir, W. W., R. T. Skarda, et al. 1978. Evaluation of xylazine, guaifenesin, and ketamine hydrochloride for restraint in horses. Am J Vet Res 39(8): 1274–8.

Muir, W. W., 3rd, P. Lerche, et al. 2000. Comparison of four drug combinations for total intravenous anesthesia of horses undergoing surgical removal of an abdominal testis. J Am Vet Med Assoc 217(6): 869–73.

Musk, G. C., D. S. Pang, et al. 2005. Target-controlled infusion of propofol in dogs—Evaluation of four targets for induction of anaesthesia. Vet Rec 157(24): 766–70.

Nadeson, R. and C. S. Goodchild. 2000. Antinociceptive properties of neurosteroids II. Experiments with Saffan and its components alphaxalone and alphadolone to reveal separation of anaesthetic and antinociceptive effects and the involvement of spinal cord GABA(A) receptors. Pain 88(1): 31–9.

Neel, S., R. Deitch, Jr., et al. 1995. Changes in intraocular pressure during low dose intravenous sedation with propofol before cataract surgery. Br J Ophthalmol 79(12): 1093–7.

Nimmaanrat, S. 2005. Myoclonic movements following induction of anesthesia with propofol: a case report. J Med Assoc Thai 88(12): 1955–7.

O'Connor, J. J., C. M. Stowe, et al. 1985. Fate of sodium pentobarbital in rendered products. Am J Vet Res 46(8): 1721–4.

O'Meara, G. F., R. J. Newman, et al. 2004. The GABA-A beta3 subunit mediates anaesthesia induced by etomidate. Neuroreport 15(10): 1653–6.

Paw, H. G., M. Garrood, et al. 1998. Thiopentone and propofol: a compatible mixture? Eur J Anaesthesiol 15(4): 409–13.

Pedersoli, W. M., J. S. Wike, et al. 1987. Pharmacokinetics of single doses of phenobarbital given intravenously and orally to dogs. Am J Vet Res 48(4): 679–83.

Peters, M. A. and A. Strother. 1972. A study of some possible mechanisms by which glucose inhibits drug metabolism in vivo and in vitro. J Pharmacol Exp Ther 180(1): 151–7.

Picavet, M. T., F. M. Gasthuys, et al. 2004. Cardiopulmonary effects of combined xylazine-guaiphenesin-ketamine infusion and extradural (inter-coccygeal lidocaine) anaesthesia in calves. Vet Anaesth Analg 31(1): 11–9.

Pinaud, M., J. N. Lelausque, et al. 1990. Effects of propofol on cerebral hemodynamics and metabolism in patients with brain trauma. Anesthesiology 73(3): 404–9.

Plumb, D. C. 1999. Veterinary Drug Handbook. Ames, Iowa State University Press.

Polley, L. and B. M. Weaver. 1977. Accidental poisoning of dogs by barbiturates in meat. Vet Rec 100(3): 48.

Product-Label. 2004. Telazol Product Label. F. D. A. Health. Fort Dodge.

Quandt, J. E., E. P. Robinson, et al. 1998. Cardiorespiratory and anesthetic effects of propofol and thiopental in dogs. Am J Vet Res 59(9): 1137–43.

Rasmussen, N. J., T. Rosendal, et al. 1978. Althesin in neurosurgical patients: effects on cerebral hemodynamics and metabolism. Acta Anaesthesiol Scand 22(3): 257–69.

Rawlings, C. A. and R. J. Kolata. 1983. Cardiopulmonary effects of thiopental/lidocaine combination during anesthetic induction in the dog. Am J Vet Res 44(1): 144–9.

Reder, B. S., L. D. Trapp, et al. 1980. Ketamine suppression of chemically induced convulsions in the two-day-old white leghorn cockerel. Anesth Analg 59(6): 406–9.

Reich, D. L., S. Hossain, et al. 2005. Predictors of hypotension after induction of general anesthesia. Anesth Analg 101(3): 622–8, table of contents.

Reich, D. L. and G. Silvay. 1989. Ketamine: an update on the first twenty-five years of clinical experience. Can J Anaesth 36(2): 186–97.

Reiche, R. and H. H. Frey. 1981. Interactions between chloramphenicol and intravenous anesthetics. Anaesthesist 30(10): 504–7.

Reid, J. and A. M. Nolan. 1996. Pharmacokinetics of propofol as an induction agent in geriatric dogs. Res Vet Sci 61(2): 169–71.

Robertson, S. A., S. Johnston, et al. 1992. Cardiopulmonary, anesthetic, and postanesthetic effects of intravenous infusions of propofol in greyhounds and non-greyhounds. Am J Vet Res 53(6): 1027–32.

Robinson, E. P. and G. R. Johnston. 1986. Radiographic assessment of laryngeal reflexes in ketamine-anesthetized cats. Am J Vet Res 47(7): 1569–72.

Robinson, E. P., R. A. Sams, et al. 1986. Barbiturate anesthesia in greyhound and mixed-breed dogs: comparative cardiopulmonary effects, anesthetic effects, and recovery rates. Am J Vet Res 47(10): 2105–12.

Sams, R. A., W. W. Muir, et al. 1985. Comparative pharmacokinetics and anesthetic effects of methohexital, pentobarbital, thiamylal, and thiopental in greyhound dogs and non-greyhound, mixed-breed dogs. Am J Vet Res 46(8): 1677–83.

Sceniak, M. and B. MacIver. 2005. Urethane Anesthesia: A Novel and Specific Mechanism of Action. Anesthesiology 103: A141.

Sear, J. W. and J. D. McGivan. 1981. Metabolism of alphaxalone in the rat: evidence for the limitation of the anaesthetic effect by the rate of degradation through the hepatic mixed function oxygenase system. Br J Anaesth 53(4): 417–24.

Sener, E. B., F. Guldogus, et al. 2003. Comparison of neonatal effects of epidural and general anesthesia for cesarean section. Gynecol Obstet Invest 55(1): 41–5.

Servin, F., I. D. Cockshott, et al. 1990. Pharmacokinetics of propofol infusions in patients with cirrhosis. Br J Anaesth 65(2): 177–83.

Short, C. E. 1983. Pratical Use of the Ultrashort-Acting Barbiturates. Princeton Junction, Veterinary Learning Systems Co, Inc.

Steen, P. A., L. Newberg, et al. 1983. Hypothermia and barbiturates: individual and combined effects on canine cerebral oxygen consumption. Anesthesiology 58(6): 527–32.

Stoelting, R. 1999. Pharmacology and Physiology in Anesthetic Practice. Philadelphia, Lippincott-Raven.

Strunin, L., et al., 1977. Metabolism of 14C-labelled alphaxalone in man. Br J Anaesth 49(6): p. 609–14.

Suresh, M. S. and T. E. Nelson. 1985. Malignant hyperthermia: is etomidate safe? Anesth Analg 64(4): 420–4.

Taniguchi, T. and K. Yamamoto. 2005. Anti-inflammatory effects of intravenous anesthetics on endotoxemia. Mini Rev Med Chem 5(3): 241–5.

Taylor, P. M., J. J. Kirby, et al. 1998. Cardiovascular effects of surgical castration during anaesthesia maintained with halothane or infusion of detomidine, ketamine and guaifenesin in ponies. Equine Vet J 30(4): 304–9.

Tendillo, F. J., A. Mascias, et al. 1996. [Cardiorespiratory and analgesic effects of continuous infusion of propofol in swine as experimental animals]. Rev Esp Anestesiol Reanim 43(4): 126–9.

Thurmon, J. C., W. J. Tranquilli, et al. 1986. Cardiopulmonary responses of swine to intravenous infusion of guaifenesin, ketamine, and xylazine. Am J Vet Res 47(10): 2138–40.

Tilson, R., G. Brady, et al. 1995. Management and Conservation of Captive Tigers. Apple Valley, MN, Minnesota Zoo.

Trampitsch, E., M. Oher, et al. 2006. [Propofol infusion syndrome.]. Anaesthesist 55(11): 1166–1168.

Turner, D. M. and J. E. Ilkiw. 1990. Cardiovascular and respiratory effects of three rapidly acting barbiturates in dogs. Am J Vet Res 51(4): 598–604.

———. 1990. Potency of rapidly acting barbiturates in dogs, using inhibition of the laryngeal reflex as the end point. Am J Vet Res 51(4): 595–7.

U.S. Department of Health and Human Services, P. H. S., National Toxicology Program. January 31, 2005. 11th Report on Carcinogens.

Valverde, A., D. Bienzle, et al. 1993. Intraosseous cannulation and drug administration for induction of anesthesia in chickens. Vet Surg 22(3): 240–4.

Van der Linden, P., E. Gilbart, et al. 1990. Comparison of halothane, isoflurane, alfentanil, and ketamine in experimental septic shock. Anesth Analg 70(6): 608–17.

Veroli, P., B. O'Kelly, et al. 1992. Extrahepatic metabolism of propofol in man during the anhepatic phase of orthotopic liver transplantation. Br J Anaesth 68(2): 183–6.

Wachowski, I., D. T. Jolly, et al. 1999. The growth of microorganisms in propofol and mixtures of propofol and lidocaine. Anesth Analg 88(1): 209–12.

Wagner, R. L., P. F. White, et al. 1984. Inhibition of adrenal steroidogenesis by the anesthetic etomidate. N Engl J Med 310(22): 1415–21.

Wall, R. and W. W. Muir, 3rd. 1990. Hemolytic potential of guaifenesin in cattle. Cornell Vet 80(2): 209–16.

Waterman, A. E. 1984. The pharmacokinetics of ketamine administered intravenously in calves and the modifying effect of premedication with xylazine hydrochloride. J Vet Pharmacol Ther 7(2): 125–30.

Weiskopf, R. B. and M. S. Bogetz. 1985. Haemorrhage decreases the anaesthetic requirement for ketamine and thiopentone in the pig. Br J Anaesth 57(10): 1022–5.

Wertz, E. M., G. J. Benson, et al. 1990. Pharmacokinetics of etomidate in cats. Am J Vet Res 51(2): 281–5.

White, P. F., W. L. Way, et al. 1982. Ketamine—its pharmacology and therapeutic uses. Anesthesiology 56(2): 119–36.

Whitwam, J. G., D. C. Galletly, et al. 2000. The effects of propofol on heart rate, arterial pressure and adelta and C somatosympathetic reflexes in anaesthetized dogs. Eur J Anaesthesiol 17(1): 57–63.

Wilder-Smith, O. H., M. Kolletzki, et al. 1995. Sedation with intravenous infusions of propofol or thiopentone. Effects on pain perception. Anaesthesia 50(3): 218–22.

Wouters, P. F., M. A. Van de Velde, et al. 1995. Hemodynamic changes during induction of anesthesia with eltanolone and propofol in dogs. Anesth Analg 81(1): 125–31.

Ying, S. W. and P. A. Goldstein. 2005. Propofol suppresses synaptic responsiveness of somatosensory relay neurons to excitatory input by potentiating GABAA receptor chloride channels. Mol Pain 1(1): 2.

Zattoni, J., C. Siani, et al. 1980. [Effects of the intravenous infusion of althesin on intracranial pressure and related functions]. Minerva Anestesiol 46(2): 183–8.

Zoran, D. L., D. H. Riedesel, et al. 1993. Pharmacokinetics of propofol in mixed-breed dogs and greyhounds. Am J Vet Res 54(5): 755–60.

CHAPTER

12

OPIOID ANALGESIC DRUGS

BUTCH KUKANICH AND MARK G. PAPICH

INTRODUCTION

The opioids include drugs that are true opiates—derivatives of opium—and drugs that are synthetic agents but also affect opiate receptors. An opiate includes morphine, codeine, hydromorphone, and other chemically similar drugs. These drugs differ among one another primarily in potency, but also may have different pharmacokinetic and pharmacodynamic properties. Opioids include all the opiates, as well as synthetic drugs, such as fentanyl and meperidine (pethidine) that are not chemically related to opium or morphine, but act as opiate receptor agonists. Various types of opiate receptors will be discussed later in the chapter.

The opioids are valuable tools in the veterinarian's armamentarium of drugs. Although most of the drugs in this group are controlled substances because of their potential for abuse by humans, they can have profound effects for treatment of animals (Table 12.1). There are many overlapping areas with other therapeutic uses discussed in other chapters of this book (for example, Chapters 11, 12, 47, 49, and 59).

An important advantage of opioid analgesic drugs is their high efficacy and remarkable safety. If adverse effects are recognized, their short half-lives in animals usually produce a rapid lessening of clinical signs. If adverse reactions are severe (e.g., dysphoria or life-threatening respiratory depression) these drugs also have the benefit of reversibility, which is accomplished quickly with administration of the opiate antagonist naloxone. This lack of serious adverse effects allows clinicians to gradually escalate doses of opioid agonists in patients as needed for pain. (Opioid agonists/antagonists may have a ceiling effect limiting the effectiveness of high doses, as discussed later.)

TABLE 12.1 Therapeutic uses of opioids in animals

Analgesia (antinociception)
Sedation
Calming and euphoria
Immobilization and chemical restraint
Diarrhea, inhibition of gastrointestinal motility
Antitussive
Adjunctive use for general anesthesia
Increased locomotor activity (used illegally in performance horses for this)

BACKGROUND ON OPIOIDS

OPIOID ROLE IN ANALGESIA. A nociceptive stimulus produces an unpleasant sensation. Pain is the coupling of the unpleasant sensation with conscious perception and eliciting an emotional response. There is debate on whether animals have emotional responses, and whether they can feel pain, but there is no debate that nociception is present in animals. Nociceptive receptors are free nerve endings distributed throughout the body, which detect a nociceptive stimulus. Nociceptive stimuli are transmitted from peripheral nerves though the spinal cord to numerous areas within the central nervous system. For the discussions in this chapter, *pain* and *nociception* will be used synonymously.

Large strides have been made recently in the recognition and treatment of pain in animals. Treatment regimens used in people cannot be easily extrapolated to animal species treated by veterinarians. Therefore, several pharmacokinetic and pharmacodynamic studies have been performed in order to better our understanding of opioids in animals.

HISTORY OF OPIOIDS. Opioids are considered the prototypical analgesics by which other analgesics are compared. Opium was first imported into the United States in 1840, primarily from the country of Turkey. It was widely used to treat a variety of maladies, including pain, diarrhea, and coughing. In the 1870s, after the Civil War, opiate use and addiction was a recognized problem. Opiates are derivatives of opium, which is a group of alkaloids isolated from the pods of the poppy seed. There are over 20 opiate alkaloids in opium, and in the early 19th century, the chemist Sertürner isolated morphine, which he named after *Morpheus*, the Greek god of sleep and dreams. Heroin was also developed in the early 1900s by the same chemists at Bayer who developed aspirin. It was intended to be a safe and nonaddictive analgesic. There have been other attempts—none completely successful—during the next century to develop drugs as effective as the opiates, but without the abuse and addiction potential. The opioids are now controlled by regulatory authorities. In the United States, this body is the Drug Enforcement Agency (DEA) and drugs are scheduled on the basis of their addictive potential (Schedule I through IV). Schedule I drugs have no realistic medical benefit. Schedule II drugs can be highly addictive but have important therapeutic uses.

Morphine and most of the pure agonists are listed in Schedule II (Table 12.2). In veterinary medicine, the earliest recorded use of opium was in 1815, when it was considered important in the *Materia Medica* (Stalheim 1990) (See Chapter 1 for a discussion of the *Materia Medica*.) In 1930 morphine was first recommended in a veterinary pharmacology textbook for treatment of horses for colic, cough, and for analgesia. Although recommended for treatment of pain and colic in horses at that time, the adverse effects in horses were not recognized. Other drugs

TABLE 12.2 United States drug scheduling of the opioid narcotics

Substance	DEA Number	Other Names and Brand Names
Schedule I		
Acetyldihydrocodeine	9051	Acetylcodone
Benzylmorphine	9052	
Codeine methylbromide	9070	
Codeine-N-oxide	9053	
Desomorphine	9055	
Dihydromorphine	9145	
Etorphine (except HCl)	9056	
Heroin	9200	Diacetylmorphine, diamorphine
Morphine methylbromide	9305	
Morphine methylsulfonate	9306	
Morphine-N-oxide	9307	
Nicomorphine	9312	Vilan
Normorphine	9313	
Schedule II		
Alfentanil	9737	Alfenta
Carfentanil	9743	Wildnil
Dihydrocodeine	9120	Didrate, Parzone
Diphenoxylate	9170	
Diprenorphine	9058	M50-50
Ethylmorphine	9190	Dionin
Etorphine HCl	9059	M 99
Fentanyl	9801	Innovar, Sublimaze, Duragesic
Hydrocodone	9193	Dihydrocodeinone
Hydromorphone	9150	Dilaudid, dihydromorphinone
Levomethorphan	9210	
Levorphanol	9220	Levo-Dromoran
Meperidine	9230	Demerol, Mepergan, pethidine
Methadone	9250	Dolophine, Methadose, Amidone
Methadone intermediate	9254	Methadone precursor
Morphine	9300	MS Contin, Roxanol, Duramorph, RMS, MSIR
Opium extracts	9610	
Opium fluid extract	9620	
Opium poppy	9650	Papaver somniferum
Opium tincture	9630	Laudanum
Opium, granulated	9640	Granulated opium
Opium, powdered	9639	Powdered opium
Opium, raw	9600	Raw opium, gum opium
Oxycodone	9143	OxyContin, Percocet, Tylox, Roxicodone, Roxicet
Oxymorphone	9652	Numorphan
Racemethorphan	9732	
Racemorphan	9733	Dromoran
Remifentanil	9739	Ultiva
Sufentanil	9740	Sufenta

TABLE 12.2—*continued*

Substance	DEA Number	Other Names and Brand Names
Schedule III		
Buprenorphine	9064	Buprenex, Temgesic
Butabarbital	2100	Butisol, Butibel
Codeine combination product 90 mg/du	9804	Empirin, Fiorinal, Tylenol, ASA or APAP w/codeine
Hydrocodone & isoquinoline alkaloid 15 mg/du	9805	Dihydrocodeinone + papaverine or noscapine
Hydrocodone combination product 15 mg/du	9806	Tussionex, Tussend, Lortab, Vicodin, Hycodan, Anexsia
Nalorphine	9400	Nalline
Schedule IV		
Butorphanol	9720	Stadol, Stadol NS, Torbugesic, Torbutrol
Pentazocine	9709	Talwin, Talwin NX, Talacen, Talwin Compound
Schedule V		
Codeine preparations 200 mg/100 ml or 100 gm		Cosanyl, Robitussin A-C, Cheracol, Cerose, Pediacof
Dihydrocodeine preparations 10 mg/100 ml or 100 gm		Cophene-S, various others
Diphenoxylate preparations 2.5 mg/25 ug $AtSO_4$		Lomotil, Logen
Ethylmorphine preparations 100 mg/100 ml or 100 gm		
Opium preparations 100 mg/100 ml or gm		Parepectolin, Kapectolin PG, Kaolin Pectin P.G.

Complete list may be found at: http://www.usdoj.gov/dea/pubs/scheduling.html

used in the early 20th century by veterinarians included combinations of morphine and atropine for pain in dogs and the use of paregoric (tincture of opium) for treatment of flatulence. Early veterinary preparations included paregoric, laudanum (opium), ipecac and opium (Diver's powder), morphine, heroin (0.5 to 2 grains for a horse), codeine, and dionin (ethylmorphine) (Stalheim 1990).

Veterinary medicine has advanced considerably since those early years and it is common for modern veterinary hospitals to include morphine and other potent derivatives in their pharmacy. Injectable solutions, constant rate infusions, and transdermal delivery devices are common in most veterinary hospitals now to be used as preanesthetics, anesthetic adjuncts, and to provide analgesia. They also provide a sedating effect and are used for chemical restraint. Opioids include the derivatives of opium (opiates) as well as the synthetic drugs. The synthetic drugs include meperidine, fentanyl, and extremely potent derivatives such as carfentanil. These also interact with opiate receptors and are used by veterinarians.

PHYSIOLOGY OF OPIOIDS. Three classes of opiate receptors have been identified: μ, κ, and δ (Table 12.3). Numerous opiate receptor subtypes have also been identified. In some textbooks, a sigma (σ) receptor is listed, but the significance of this receptor is not understood and is not considered a true opiate receptor by many pharmacologists.

Endogenous opioids are natural chemicals in the body (peptides) that interact with opiate receptors to produce natural physiologic responses, including modulation of pain. Beta endorphin is the endogenous opioid peptide with the highest affinity for μ receptors and is derived from proopiomelanocortin. Leucine- and methionone-enkephalin are derived from proenkephalin and are the endogenous ligands for the δ receptor. Dynorphin A is the endogenous ligand for the κ receptor and is derived from prodynorphin. The role of dynorphins remains controversial because they induce sensitization of nociceptive transmission through activation of NMDA receptors.

An endogenous opioid peptide, termed *nociceptin* or *orphanin FQ* (N/OFQ), with similar homology to dynorphin has also been described (Meunier et al. 1995; Reinschied et al. 1995). Orphanin precursors have been identified in the hippocampus, cortex, and numerous sensory sites (Neal et al. 1999). Exogenous N/OFQ administration results in a variety of responses ranging from analgesia to antianalgesia and opioid antagonism. However, N/OFQ antagonists have consistent analgesic properties when administered supraspinally, which may

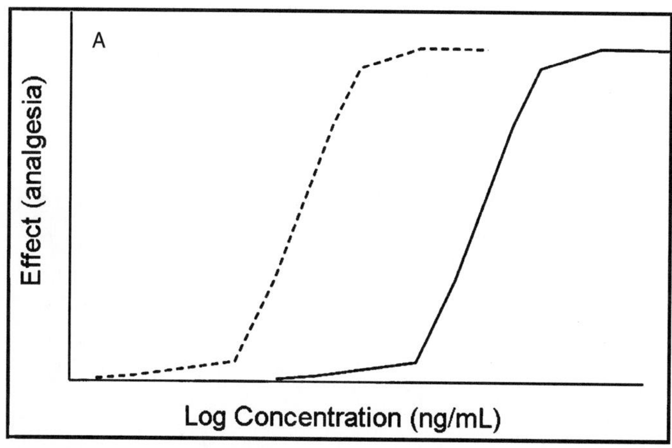

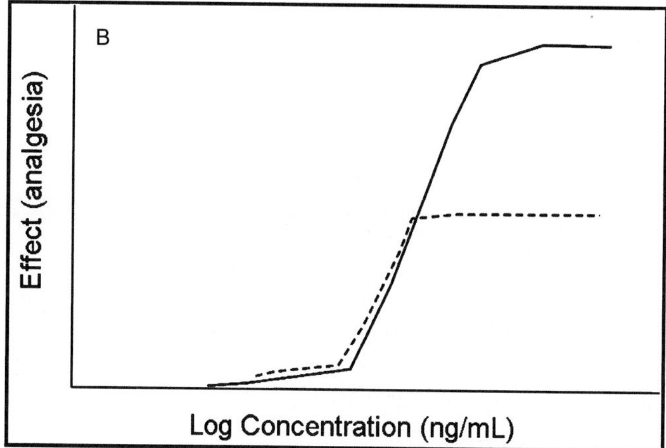

FIG. 12.1 Panel A demonstrates two drugs with equal efficacy but different potency, such as fentanyl and morphine. Panel B demonstrates drugs with equal potency, but different efficacy, such as fentanyl and buprenorphine.

prove to be a useful target for analgesics in the future (Heinricher 2005).

Opioids have been characterized by the type of interaction with the opiate receptor type(s) with which they interact (μ, κ, and δ), and by the effect elicited upon binding (Fig. 12.1). Opioids may be full agonists, partial agonists, antagonists, and combinations thereof. An agonist produces a dose-dependent effect, which eventually plateaus with unconsciousness and anesthesia. A partial agonist binds to the opiate receptor, but plateaus at a submaximum response (less than an agonist) despite increasing doses. The opioid antagonists are competitive antagonists, which displace the agonist from the opiate receptor, but do not result in receptor activation. Morphine is a full agonist at the μ receptor, whereas buprenorphine is a partial agonist. Nalbuphine is an antagonist at the μ receptor but an agonist κ at the receptor.

TABLE 12.3 Opiate receptor types and their associated effects

μ Receptor	κ Receptor	δ Receptor
Analgesia (spinal & supraspinal)	Analgesia (spinal & supraspinal)	Analgesia (spinal & supraspinal)
Respiratory depression	Decrease gastrointestinal motility	
Decrease gastrointestinal motility		
Decrease biliary secretions		
Increase appetite	Increase appetite	Increase appetite
Sedation		
Euphoria	Sedation	
Antidiuresis		
Decrease urine voiding reflex	Diuresis (decrease ADH release)	Immunomodulation
Decrease uterine contractions	Miosis/mydriasis	
Miosis/mydriasis		
Nausea/vomiting		
Immunomodulation		

ADH = antidiuretic hormone.

Note: Some textbooks also list the sigma-receptor, but this may not have any significance.

OPIOID PHARMACODYNAMICS

ANALGESIA. Opioids exert their primary analgesic effect by binding to spinal and supraspinal receptors (Tables 12.3, 12.4). When an opioid binds to receptors it produces activation of G-coupled proteins (which inhibit adenylyl cyclase), activation of receptor linked K^+ ion channels, and inhibition of voltage gated Ca^{2+} channels. Presynaptic μ, κ, and δ spinal receptors are present in the dorsal horn of the spinal cord, decreasing excitatory neurotransmitter release by decreasing the rate of calcium influx. Postsynaptic μ receptors are also present in the dorsal root ganglion, which hyperpolarize the neuron by increasing potassium channel conductance resulting in a decreased propagation of the nociceptive signal.

The supraspinal opioid pathways are poorly understood, but concurrent activation with spinal receptors result in analgesic synergism (Roerig et al. 1989; Yeung et al. 1980).

TABLE 12.4 The primary sites of action for opioid and associated drugs used in veterinary medicine

	μ	κ	δ	α-2	5-HT	NMDA	M1	M3	GABA
Morphine	++	+							
Hydromorphone	++								
Oxymorphone	++								
Hydrocodone	+								
Codeine	+								
Oxycodone	++								
Heroin	++	+*							
Methadone	++			+		–			
Meperidine	++				++			––	
Fentanyl	++								
Carfentanil	++								
Etorphine	++	++	++						
Propoxyphene	+								
Buprenorphine	+								
Butorphanol	+	++							
Tramadol	+**			+	++		–**		
Nalbuphine	––	++							
Pentazocine	+	++							
Nalorphine	––	+							
Naloxone	––	–	–						–
Naltrexone	––	––	––						
Nalmefene	––	–	–						
Diprenorphine	––	––	––						

5-HT serotonin. NMDA n-methyl-d-aspartate. M1 muscarinic M1. M3 muscarinic M3. ++ agonist. + submaximal agonist. – antagonist. –– submaximal antagonist. * via metabolism to morphine. ** via metabolism to o-desmethyltramadol.

Synergism also exists between supraspinal μ and δ receptors when concurrently activated. Opioid receptors are also located in various locations in the descending pain inhibitory pathways. Pain inhibitory pathways are activated by opioids producing an inhibition of GABA receptor-mediated inhibitory effects in the descending pathways.

RESPIRATORY DEPRESSION. Opioids produce a dose-dependent respiratory depression mediated via activation of the μ receptor. Respiratory depression is produced by a decreased response to increased carbon dioxide partial pressures (PCO_2). The respiratory depressant effects of opioids are well tolerated in healthy animals even when supratherapeutic doses are administered. Concurrent anesthesia may increase the respiratory depressant effects of opioids (Hug et al. 1981). These effects may be more problematic in animals with preexisting respiratory disease (asthma, bronchitis, cor pulmonale) or increased intracranial pressure. However, ordinarily in animals respiratory depression does not produce a clinical problem.

Opioids cross the placenta and respiratory depressant effects on the fetus can occur and should be monitored and treated appropriately. Naloxone administered sublingually (or parenterally) to newborns will reverse deleterious opioid effects.

CENTRAL NERVOUS SYSTEM EXCITATION. High doses of morphine and other opioids produce excitement and very high doses result in convulsions. In dogs, morphine, 180–200 mg/kg IV, produced grand mal seizures, but convulsive changes in electroencephalogram (EEG) tracings and excitement were seen in dogs administered morphine 20 mg/kg SC (Wikler and Altschul 1950; de Castro et al. 1979). Cats respond similarly to high doses of morphine where 20 mg/kg SC produced EEG tracings consistent with convulsive activity and generalized excitement (Tuttle and Elliot 1969). Cats are one of the species that is more sensitive to morphine-induced CNS excitation and dysphoria. Although, when morphine was administered to healthy cats at doses up to 2 mg/kg, without concurrent sedatives/tranquilizers, it was well tolerated and did not produce excitement (Barr et al. 2000). Nevertheless, doses used in cats are typically smaller than doses used in dogs to produce a similar analgesic effect.

Horses are also more sensitive to the excitement caused by this group of drugs. Dose-dependent excitation and increased locomotor activity has been observed in horses and may occur before maximum analgesia is obtained with the degree of excitation dependent on the specific opioid (Muir et al. 1978; Tobin et al. 1979). Excitement produced in horses from opioids has prevented the use of some of these drugs for use alone without other sedatives or tranquilizing agents. For example, buprenorphine, normally well-tolerated in dogs and cats, produced restlessness, excitement, head-shaking, pawing, and leg-shifting at a dose of 5 and 10 mcg/kg IV (Carregaro et al. 2006, 2007) that was dose-dependent. Increase in locomotor activity persisted for 3–4 hours. Increased locomotor activity has been observed with both mu-agonists and kappa-agonists (Mama et al. 1992). When morphine was investigated for its use as an anesthetic adjunct for horses at doses of 0.25 and 0.2 mg/kg with isoflurane anesthesia (Steffey et al. 2003), the authors concluded that undesirable and dangerous behavior during recovery from the high dose of morphine still persisted after 4 hours, and did not support the use of morphine as an anesthetic adjunct in this regimen. However, studies demonstrating excitement and increased locomotor activity in horses were performed predominantly in healthy pain-free horses. When opioids have been used in painful horses, fewer adverse reactions are observed (Mircica et al. 2003). Some protocols have been used in horses with pain when modest dosages are administered, often with a tranquilizer or sedative.

The explanation for increased susceptibility to these effects is probably related to the distribution of opiate receptors in certain regions of the brain independent of the drug's pharmacokinetics. The distribution of opiate receptors in brains of animals that are sedated from opioids (e.g., dogs) is greater than the animals that are more prone to excitement (horses, cats). Alternatively, the excitement may be due to a release of excitatory neurotransmitters. Some anesthesiologists suggest that the reaction may be dopaminergic, adrenergic, or caused by decreased activity of the inhibitory neurotransmitter gamma aminobutyric acid (GABA). Release of acetylcholine also has been suggested (Mullin et al. 1973). In another study, it was suggested that excitement in animals may be caused by histamine release. Morphine administration to dogs induced greater histamine release, and also more excitement compared to oxymorphone after administration of an equianalgesic dose (Robinson et al. 1988). When morphine was compared to hydromorphone in dogs (Guedes et al. 2007), morphine caused a transient increase in plasma histamine and most dogs also exhibited neuroexcitatory behavior. By contrast, hydromorphone did not cause increases in histamine and no dogs became excited.

CARDIOVASCULAR EFFECTS. Morphine depresses cardiac output in dogs, but increases it in horses (Muir et al. 1978; Lind et al. 1981). Opioids produce bradycardia in dogs, but they usually compensate well and treatment for the bradycardia is not routinely indicated (Copland et al. 1992). If necessary, the bradycardia can be reversed with atropine.

Opioids produce minimal cardiovascular effects when administered to animals in clinically relevant doses (Barnhart et al. 2000; Pant et al. 1983; Hug et al. 1981; Kayaalp and Kaymakcalan 1966; Priano and Vatner 1981). Changes in mean arterial pressure range from minimal increases to minimal decreases (~10% from baseline values). Increases in plasma histamine concentrations following morphine administration are often cited as producing hypotensive effects in dogs, but histamine release is short-lived (Guedes et al. 2007) and minimal effects on blood pressure are noted following IV morphine administration. The cardiovascular effects of opioids appear to be more pronounced in anesthetized animals in which supratherapeutic doses result in various degrees of hypotension.

The effects of opioids on myocardial blood flow are variable with some studies demonstrating increases in blood flow where others show decreases (Pant et al. 1983; Vatner et al. 1975). This is in contrast to the consistent effects in people, coronary vasodilation and increased myocardial perfusion. The use of morphine in animals with congestive heart failure cannot be routinely recommended due to the variable effects produced.

ANTITUSSIVE EFFECT. Opioids produce an antitussive effect through a central inhibition of the cough center independent of their respiratory depressant effects (Chou and Wang 1975). Both mu- and kappa-receptor agonists have been documented to produce antitussive effects (Takahama and Shirasaki 2007). The antitussive effect is more resistant to naloxone reversal than the analgesic effect of opioids (Chau et al. 1983). Morphine, butorphanol, methadone, and tramadol have demonstrated antitussive effects in dogs or cats (Rosierre et al. 1956; Cavanagh et al. 1976; Nosal'ova et al. 1991). Hydrocodone has antitussive properties in rats and people, and is commonly used in dogs for this purpose although studies definitively demonstrating its efficacy in dogs and cats are lacking (Hennies et al. 1988; Homsi et al. 2002). Although dextromethorphan—which does not affect opiate receptors—is used as an over-the-counter medication to treat coughing in people, these effects have recently been challenged. Dextromethorphan has not been shown to be an effective antitussive in small animals and oral absorption is questionable (discussed more specifically later in this chapter).

GASTROINTESTINAL EFFECTS

Emetic Properties. Emesis and nausea can occur following administration of opioids via stimulation of the chemoreceptor trigger zone (CRTZ) (Mitchelson 1992). Opioids also may stimulate central dopamine (D_2) receptors in the vomiting center to produce vomiting. Opioids appear to have differing emetic effects with morphine causing emesis more frequently than hydromorphone or oxymorphone in dogs (Valverde et al. 2004). The emetic response is complicated by the observation that opiates also act as antiemetics in the vomiting center (Scherkl et al. 1990). It is not unusual to observe that emesis occurs after the first initial dose to a patient, but not with subsequent doses. It is also observed that patients in pain experience less emesis than healthy research animals. These observations may be related to the antiemetic effects produced after an initial dose, or the antiemetic effects produced by endogenous opioids in painful patients.

Since the CRTZ is not protected by the blood-brain barrier, low plasma concentrations can produce emesis following oral morphine administration without producing an analgesic effect (KuKanich et al. 2005a). In cats, morphine appears to produce more of an emetic effect as compared to fentanyl, meperidine, buprenorphine, and butorphanol (Taylor et al. 2001; Robertson et al. 2003; Robertson et al. 2005). Hydromorphone produces signs of nausea (salivation and lip licking) in cats and may elicit emesis (Wegner et al. 2004).

Release of histamine or dopaminergic effects also may produce the emetic response. Apomorphine, one of the most reliable emetics in dogs, is a central-acting dopamine (DA_1, DA_2) agonist. Dopamine is one of the neurotransmitters in the vomiting center as well as in the CRTZ. Likewise, histamine is released for a short time after morphine administration to dogs (Guedes et al. 2007) and histamine is also known as one of the neurotransmitters involved in emesis.

Gastrointestinal Motility. Opioids produce a decrease in gastrointestinal motility via both central and peripheral mechanisms. The review by DeHaven-Hudkins et al., (2007) provided details on the distribution of the receptors in the gastrointestinal tract and effects associated with stimulation, either from endogenous opioids or exogenous opioids. Opioid-mediated effects in the gastrointestinal tract are through the μ-opiate receptor. Expression of μ-opiate receptors have been found in the submucosal plexus, myenteric plexus, and longitudinal muscle of the ileum. In healthy animals, the regulation of these receptors and their function helps to maintain gut homeostasis within the enteric nervous system by coordinating intestinal motility and intestinal secretions. Motility-induced changes are accomplished by inhibiting the release of intestinal acetylcholine (Ach) and/or Substance P. Intestinal secretion is also inhibited. Mu-opioid receptor–mediated stimulation of the gastrointestinal tract slows gastric emptying, decreases secretion and increases intestinal fluid absorption, reduces propulsive motility, and increases pyloric and other sphincter tone. The single most common clinical consequence is constipation.

After the initial emetic effect, opioids decrease gastric motility resulting in prolonged gastric emptying. Opioids can also increase the tone of the antrum and the duodenum resulting in difficult intubation with an endoscope. The small intestinal effects of opioids initially appeared to be limited to the proximal portions; however, additional studies demonstrated effects on the ileum as well. Decreased propulsive motility and decreased intestinal, pancreatic, and biliary secretions occur in the small intestine. There is increased tone of all gastrointestinal sphincters, including those of the pancreatic duct. However, increases in rhythmic, segmental, nonpropulsive contractions also occur. The reabsorption of water is increased due to delayed passage of the ingesta, and in combination with the decreased intestinal secretions the resultant effect is increased viscosity of the bowel contents.

Morphine initially stimulates large bowel motility, and defecation often occurs shortly after administration in dogs and cats (Tuttle and Elliot 1969; Barnhart et al. 2000; Lucas et al. 2001). Following initial defecation, opioids produce a decrease in colonic propulsive motility and secretions, but increases in nonpropulsive rhythmic contractions occur similar to that in the small intestine. Therefore the passage of colonic contents is delayed and the fluid content is decreased. The decreased gastrointestinal motility can result in constipation, an adverse effect, or be used therapeutically as a treatment for diarrhea.

URINARY TRACT. Opioids produce a variety of effects on the urinary tract. Mu-agonists increase the tone of urinary sphincters. Micturition is inhibited, which may result in urine retention and may be mediated by spinal, as opposed to local, mechanisms (Drenger et al. 1986, 1989).

Mu-receptor agonists cause decreased urine production. As discussed by Robertson et al. (2001), although it has been documented that morphine produces an antidiuretic effect and decrease in urine output, the exact mechanism is unclear. It is not known whether it is caused by a release of arginine vasopressin (AVP) (also known as antidiuretic hormone), or via some other mechanism. In contrast, κ opioid agonists produce a diuretic effect as a result of decreased AVP concentrations (Craft et al. 2000).

IMMUNE SYSTEM EFFECTS. The effects of opioids on the immune system are complex and poorly understood. The immune system effects are likely related to the specific opioid administered and the duration of treatment. A complex interaction of the immune system, sympathetic nervous system, and endocrine system (hypothalamic-pituitary-adrenal axis), and direct effects on leukocytes occur. Immunosuppressive and immunostimulant properties have been identified depending on the experimental conditions. However, studies have indicated withholding opioids in immunocompromised patients that are painful result in a worsening immune function (Page and Ben-Eliyahu 1997).

TOLERANCE AND DEPENDENCE. Although these traits are often associated with opioid use in humans, they have been well documented in animals. Tolerance and dependence can be demonstrated in animals, but these drugs are seldom used for a long-enough period of time in veterinary patients for this issue to have clinical consequences. The NMDA receptor may play a role in opioid tolerance and dependence as treatment with NMDA antagonists attenuates withdrawal symptoms in experimental settings (Yeh et al. 2002). The consequence of tolerance is that drug dosages may need to be increased with chronic administration of opioids.

Opioids administered for a period as short as 5–7 days may result in dependence in dogs. In one study, constant rate infusion to dogs at a rate of 1–5 mg/kg/day produced physical dependence by day 8 (Yoshimura et al. 1993). Withdrawal signs can be elicited in dogs after dependence with injections of naloxone. Signs of withdrawal in dogs include nausea, aggression, vocalization, vomiting, hyperactivity, hyperthermia, tremors, and salivation. Withdrawal can also be elicited from administration of a μ antagonist or partial agonist such as butorphanol or buprenorphine following short-term administration of a μ agonist (Yoshimura et al. 1993).

Therefore, if an animal has been receiving continuous opioid drugs for longer than 5–7 days, withdrawal signs may occur after discontinuing the drug, or after administration of an antagonist. The dose of the μ agonist should be decreased to wean a patient off of an opioid as opposed to switching to a partial agonist or antagonist.

Because of the potential for abuse, the distribution of pharmaceutical opioids is controlled by the Drug Enforcement Agency (DEA) in the United States. Drugs are scheduled on the basis of addiction potential and medical use (see Table 12.2) from Schedule I to Schedule IV. Schedule I drugs are highly addictive but have little medical use. Schedule II drugs are also highly addictive but have legitimate medical uses.

OPIOID PHARMACOKINETICS

Opioids tend to be well absorbed when administered orally, intramuscularly, or subcutaneously. However, due to substantial first-pass metabolism the oral administration of most opioids results in poor bioavailability and erratic plasma concentrations in animals. Administration of opioids per rectum to animals results in a minimal increase in bioavailability over per os administration, since the

TABLE 12.5 Pharmacokinetic parameters of opioids administered IV and PO bioavailability in dogs and cats

	Half-life (h)		Clearance (ml/min/kg)		Volume of Distribution (l/kg)		Oral Bioavailability	
	Dogs	Cats	Dogs	Cats	Dogs	Cats	Dogs	Cats
Morphine	1.2	1.3	60	24	4	2.6	5–20%	
Oxymorphone	0.8		52		3.7			
Hydromorphone	0.6–1.0	1.6	68–106	28	4.5–5.3	3.1		
Fentanyl	3–6	~2.5	35	20	10	2.6		
Meperidine	0.8	1.8	43	40	1.9	4.0	11%	
Methadone	2–4		30		3.5		<LOQ	
Oxycodone	1.9*						low*	
Hydrocodone	1.7		41		5.0		40–84%	
Codeine	1.5		36		3.2		6.5%	
Buprenorphine	5	6.9	16	16	17.5	7.1	3–6%	
Butorphanol	1.6**	6.6**	57**	12.7**	8.0**	7.7**		
Nalbuphine	1.2		46		4.6		5.6%	
Tramadol	0.8		55		3.0		65%	

*Oral dose data, no IV dose administered.
**Only IM data available clearance is per bioavailability, volume of distribution is per bioavailability.
<LOQ = no measurable plasma concentrations.

majority of drug absorbed by this route of administration is still subject to first-pass hepatic metabolism. Nasal and oral transmucosal administration of opioids can bypass first-pass hepatic metabolism. However, irritation, the volume of drug to be delivered, dosing frequency, and species-specific differences have limited the clinical effectiveness of transmucosal administration to buprenorphine in cats.

Opioids are well distributed throughout the body. Opioids are bound to plasma proteins in variable amounts from low to high protein binding depending on the individual drug. The opioids are lipophilic and weak bases. These physiochemical properties favor intracellular accumulation. Consequently, opioids have a large volume of distribution, which greatly exceeds total body water. Additionally, administration of opioids with high lipophilicity, such as fentanyl, can produce rapid redistribution from tissues that are highly perfused, such as the central nervous system, to tissues that are less perfused, such as muscle and fat. The result is a more rapid decrease in concentrations (and effect) in the target organs in comparison to total body elimination. Repeated doses or a constant rate infusion may result in drug accumulation with an increased effect and slow recovery. This phenomenon is similar to that seen with repeated doses of thiobarbiturates.

Most opioids are metabolized to polar compounds and subsequently excreted in the urine, but a small amount of unchanged drug may be eliminated in the urine. Conjugation reactions are the primary means of opioid metabolism, although cytochrome P450 (CYP) mediated metabolism can also occur. Extrahepatic metabolism of morphine occurs in dogs resulting in clearance rates exceeding the combined hepatic blood flow and glomerular filtration rates. Glucuronide conjugation is the primary conjugation pathway of morphine in most animal species except cats, which are a species relatively deficient in some glucuronidation mechanisms (Court and Greenblatt 1997). Sulfate conjugation is the primary means of morphine metabolism in cats. Despite differences in metabolic pathways, cats effectively metabolize morphine with total body clearance approximating the expected hepatic blood flow rate indicative of a high extraction drug. Oxidative metabolism, mediated by CYP, appears to be the primary mechanism of fentanyl (and derivatives), methadone, and meperidine metabolism. The pharmacokinetic parameters of opioids in dogs and cats are presented in Table 12.5.

CLINICAL PHARMACOLOGY

ANALGESIA. Opioids are commonly used for analgesia and to relieve pain. Severe pain, often associated with trauma, should be treated with μ opioid agonists with high intrinsic activity (i.e., morphine, hydromorphone, fentanyl). Although some references have stated opioids should not be administered to animals in shock, there is no basis for this recommendation. Pain can contribute markedly to the adverse effects associated with shock, and opioids improve the hemodynamics and tissue perfusion of painful patients. As previously stated, the hypotensive effects of intravenous opioids (including morphine) are minimal when administered in clinically relevant doses, and concurrent supportive measures, such as fluid therapy are essential to successful therapy in these patients. Mild to moderate pain (i.e., soft tissue surgery) has been managed with μ opioid agonists, partial agonists, mixed agonist-antagonists, or tramadol.

Preemptive analgesia, dose administration prior to surgery or a painful stimulus, has been shown to provide more effective analgesia than administration of opioids postoperatively (Lascelles et al. 1997). This is thought to occur by decreasing central sensitization (aka *the wind-up phenomenon*).

Chronic and neuropathic pain appear to be less responsive to opioid analgesia. Higher doses of opioids in people are needed for controlling neuropathic pain (Rowbotham et al. 2003). For neuropathic pain, it may be more effective to use a multimodal approach utilizing opioids in combination with other drug classes such as NMDA antagonists (ketamine infusion), and α-2 agonists (medetomidine infusion). This approach appears to be more effective in refractory cases.

ANTITUSSIVE. Butorphanol tablets (Torbutrol) are registered by the FDA for antitussive use in dogs. Hydrocodone is routinely prescribed for its antitussive effects in dogs. Codeine exhibits poor bioavailability in dogs and may not be effective when administered orally. Tramadol tablets have demonstrated effectiveness as an antitussive in experimental models, but have yet to be evaluated clinically. All of the opioids are expected to be effective antitussives when administered parenterally. As mentioned previously, dextromethorphan—a nonopiate that is a common ingredient in human over-the-counter cough medications—is not an effective antitussive in dogs.

CONGESTIVE HEART FAILURE. As mentioned under "cardiovascular effects" of the pharmacodynamic section, routine use of morphine is no longer recommended in treatment of congestive heart failure in animals due to variable effects on coronary blood flow.

ANTIDIARRHEAL. Opioids are effective antidiarrheal drugs as they decrease gastrointestinal secretions, decrease propulsive gastrointestinal contractions, and increase nonpropulsive segmental gastrointestinal contractions. Loperamide is the most commonly recommended opioid for the treatment of diarrhea because of reliable effects, availability over the counter (not a controlled substance), low cost, and safety profile. Loperamide is p-glycoprotein (p-gp) substrate and as a result is excluded from the CNS in normal animals. However, if concurrent p-gp inhibitors (cyclosporine, ketoconazole) are coadministered or the animal is deficient in p-gp (~30% of Collies are affected), sedation, dysphoria, and other CNS effects may be noted. Diphenoxylate is also marketed as an antidiarrheal, but is not used frequently as it has not demonstrated increased efficacy over loperamide, is a prescription drug, and is a Schedule V drug requiring special record keeping.

SEDATION AND ANESTHESIA. Opioids are commonly coadministered with sedatives, tranquilizers, and anesthetics. Additive or synergistic sedative and analgesic effects occur when opioids are used in combination with sedatives and anesthetics. Combinations of these drug classes result in decreased dosages of the individual drugs with the potential for decreased adverse effects. Additionally preemptive analgesia increases the effectiveness of postoperative analgesics, decreasing opioid consumption, adverse effects, and cost. A more thorough review of sedation and anesthesia drug combinations is presented in Chapters 11 and 13.

CONTRAINDICATIONS, WARNINGS, AND DRUG INTERACTIONS

Head Trauma. As a drug class opioids exhibit a wide safety margin. Cautious use of opioids in patients with head trauma is warranted as respiratory depression may increase blood carbon dioxide concentrations resulting in cerebral vasodilation and worsening effects of cerebral edema.

Temperature Regulation. Opioids have varying effects on temperature regulation depending on the species (Adler et al. 1988). Panting occurs after administration of opioids in some dogs. Hydromorphone and oxymorphone caused 60% of the dogs to pant in one study (Smith et al. 2001). Panting can be aggravating, especially in animals being induced with inhalant anesthetics, but is usually self-limiting. It is not related to effects on the respiratory center, but is a reaction to the effect of opioids on the thermoregulatory center of the hypothalamus, whereby the body's set point is decreased by 1–3°F and dogs pant to lower their temperature. The depression of a dog's body temperature is a consistent finding in published studies (Lucas et al. 2001).

In contrast, administration of opioids has produced an increase in body temperature in cats. Hydromorphone has been the best documented to produce this reaction (Posner et al. 2007; Niedfeldt and Robertson 2006), but butorphanol also has caused hyperthermia. In published studies hyperthermia associated with hydromorphone has been as high as 41–42°C (107–108°F) in cats for as long as 5 hours. The authors of these studies warn of high temperatures affecting postoperative recovery in cats when opioids are used for analgesia.

Interactions Between Opioid Drugs. There has been a controversy as to whether or not administration of opioid pure agonists with opioid agonist/antagonists will produce an interaction that diminishes the analgesic effect of the combination. There is a possibility that, because drugs such as butorphanol and pentazocine have antagonistic properties on the μ-receptor, these drugs will partially reverse some effects of pure agonists such as morphine if they are administered together. The clinical significance of this antagonism has been debated. There are few reports that have documented that such a combination is antagonistic. Reversal of the pure μ-opioids can occur and acute pain or signs of opioid withdrawal may be precipitated following concurrent administration (Lascelles and Robertson 2004).

In dogs, butorphanol can partially reverse the effects of oxymorphone (Lemke et al. 1996). Butorphanol may reverse some respiratory depression and sedation from pure agonists, but some of the analgesic efficacy is preserved. In dogs that received butorphanol for postoperative pain associated with orthopedic surgery, there was no diminished efficacy from subsequent administration of oxymorphone (Pibarot et al. 1997). However, in another study, some dogs that had not responded to butorphanol after shoulder arthrotomy responded to subsequent administration of oxymorphone, but the oxymorphone dose required to produce an adequate effect was higher than what would be required if oxymorphone was used alone (Mathews et al. 1996).

Other results have been observed in cats. Increased analgesia, decreased analgesia, or no effect has been observed from combinations of agonists and antagonists. When butorphanol and oxymorphone were administered to cats in combination, there was greater efficacy than either drug used alone, with no observed antagonistic effects (Sawyer et al. 1994; Briggs et al. 1998). On the other hand, the administration of hydromorphone with butorphanol may decrease the analgesic from either drug used alone (Lascelles and Robertson 2004). When butorphanol, buprenorphine, and the combination of both drugs were administered to cats all three treatments provided similar antinociceptive effects (Johnson et al. 2007). Although butorphanol is a kappa-receptor agonist/mu-receptor antagonist, and buprenorphine is a kappa-receptor antagonist/mu-receptor partial agonist, there was no antagonism detected. However, the design of the study may have prevented a more sensitive delineation of treatment effects.

The available reports in animals indicate that some antagonism may indeed occur in clinical patients, but in some patients—and perhaps in different species—there may also be a synergistic effect. Whether or not there may be differences in the antagonism versus synergism of butorphanol and pure agonists for different types of pain (that is, comparing analgesia for somatic pain versus visceral pain) has not been established for animals. One use of antagonistic qualities of the opioids has been to administer a mu-receptor antagonist, or partial agonist (for example, buprenorphine) to lessen some of the dysphoric effects caused occasionally from pure mu-receptor agonists such as morphine or fentanyl, while still providing some degree of analgesia.

Interactions with Drug Clearance. Opioids are high clearance drugs in animals; therefore, they rely more on hepatic blood flow than activity of liver enzymes for clearance. Interactions with hepatic microsomal Cytochrome P450 enzymes, protein binding, or loss of hepatic function are not expected to affect opioid drug clearance. However, impairment in hepatic blood flow may drastically affect opioid drug clearance.

Renal impairment decreases the clearance of morphine glucuronide metabolites with a resultant metabolite accumulation. However, the importance of opioid glucuronide metabolites has not been shown in animals and clinical consequence of metabolite accumulation has not been demonstrated in animals.

Interactions with Other Analgesics and Antidepressants. The most common drug-drug interactions with opioids occur when combined with tranquilizers/sedatives and this combination is often used clinically to increase sedation. There is a specific interaction described in people between monoamine oxidase inhibitors (MAO inhibitors) and meperidine. The use of these drugs together has caused an unpredictable, and sometimes fatal, reaction. The reaction includes excitation, sweating, rigidity, coma, and seizures. This reaction seems to be rather specific for meperidine (Demerol), but if animals receive MAO inhibitors and another opiate, it is suggested to first administer a test dose of the opiate and observe the animal carefully. If there is no adverse reaction, subsequent doses can probably be administered safely. Although nonspecific MAO inhibitors (e.g., types A and B MAO inhibitors) are rarely used in veterinary medicine for treatment of depression, as they are in people, other drugs with MAO-inhibiting qualities are used in animals. For example, selegiline, a specific MAO-type B inhibitor, (deprenyl, Anipryl) is used in dogs to treat canine hyperadrenocorticism and cognitive disorder (discussed in Chapter 21). Amitraz (Mitaban) is also a MAO-inhibitor and is found in pet collars and dips to prevent and treat mite infections in animals. Although no reactions in animals have been described between amitraz or selegiline and opioid analgesic drugs, one should administer these drug combinations cautiously, at least for the first dose.

USES IN FOOD-PRODUCING ANIMALS. Use of other opioids in food-producing animals is permitted by the Animal Medicinal Drug Use Clarification Act (AMDUCA) if an adequate withdrawal interval can be determined. Therefore the Food Animal Residue Avoidance Databank (FARAD) or a reliable reference (Papich 1996) should be consulted prior to opioid administration to food-producing species in order to obtain the most current withdrawal interval recommendations.

OPIOID AGONISTS

MORPHINE. Morphine is still commonly used, despite the development of newer opioids, due to its safety, efficacy, tolerability, and low cost. Current dosage recommendations are presented in Table 12.6. Morphine is effective for mild to severely painful conditions. Intravenous administration results in mast cell degranulation and histamine release, but the clinical consequences are minimal. Histamine release may possibly account for transient excitement, but it is short-lived (Robinson et al. 1988; Guedes et al. 2007). Morphine exhibits moderate protein binding in most species approximating 30%. Morphine is also produced endogenously in both humans and animals in response to inflammation and stress (Brix-Christensen et al. 2000; Yoshida et al. 2000.)

Dogs. Morphine exhibits a wide safety profile in dogs, with 40 mg/kg producing severe coronary perfusion effects, 180 mg/kg eliciting seizures, and death at doses higher

TABLE 12.6 Morphine dosages

	IV	IV Infusion	IM/SC	PO
Dog	0.25–0.5 mg/kg q 2–3 h	0.1–0.2 mg/kg/h	0.25–1 mg/kg q 2–4 h	NR
Cat	0.1–0.25 mg/kg q 2–3h	0.05–0.1 mg/kg/h	0.1–0.5 mg/kg q 2–4h	NR
Horse	0.1–0.2 mg/kg once	NR	0.1–0.2 mg/kg once	NR
Cattle				NR
Sheep			≤10 mg total dose	NR
Goat			≤10 mg total dose	NR
Swine			0.2–0.9 mg/kg	NR
Rat/mouse			2–5 mg/kg q 4 h	NR
Guinea Pig/Hamster			2–5 mg/kg q 4 h	NR
Rabbit			2–5 mg/kg q 4 h	NR
Primates			0.5–2 mg/kg q 4–6 h	NR
Ferrets			0.5 mg/kg q 4–6 h	NR

NR = not recommended.

than 200 mg/kg (de Castro et al. 1979). The pharmacokinetics of morphine were reported in several studies and are summarized in Table 12.5. Constant rate IV infusion of morphine has been reported in studies in which high clearance rates were reported (KuKanich et al. 2005c; Lucas et al. 2001; Guedes et al. 2007). Due to its poor oral and rectal bioavailability, morphine should be administered parenterally in order to achieve therapeutic concentrations. Morphine is minimally absorbed following transdermal administration of a pluronic lecithin organogel formulation; therefore, this route of administration is not recommended (Krotscheck et al. 2004). Morphine is primarily metabolized by hepatic and extrahepatic glucuronide conjugation to morphine-3- and morphine-6-glucuronide. Morphine-3-glucuronide (M3G) has little analgesic effect and may be responsible for some of the adverse effects. Morphine-6-glucuronide (M6G) has analgesic effects that are greater than the parent drug, morphine. However, little of the M6G metabolite was found in canine studies (KuKanich et al. 2005). A 30–45 minute lag time to maximum effect (0.5 mg/kg IV) occurs primarily due to slow penetration into the CNS, but clinically relevant analgesia occurs within 5–15 minutes. Duration of analgesia is from 1–4 hours following administration 0.25–1 mg/kg IV, IM, SC, with the length of effect proportional to the dose (KuKanich et al. 2005b,c). Due to the rapid and complete absorption of morphine administered IM and SC the dosing interval is the same as for IV administration. In addition to its analgesic effects, morphine is effective as an antitussive, antidiarrheal, and sedative. Adverse effects associated with morphine are typical of opioids and can include sedation, emesis, hypothermia, constipation, dysphoria, pain on injection, defecation, panting, miosis, respiratory depression, and decreased urine production. Morphine produced transient increases in histamine release in dogs compared to other opioids (Guedes et al. 2007). Neonates are more sensitive to the respiratory depressant effects of morphine, but dogs as young as 2 days old required doses of 1 mg/kg before significant respiratory depression occurred (Bragg et al. 1995). Morphine may elicit emesis more frequently than other opioids although rapid tolerance to this adverse effect develops and emesis rarely occurs with repeated administration (Valverde et al. 2004). A study examining the effect of ketoconazole on morphine pharmacokinetics in Greyhounds indicated no dose adjustments are needed for this breed or when ketoconazole is administered concurrently with morphine (KuKanich and Borum 2008a).

Cats. Morphine is well tolerated in cats, rarely producing CNS excitation when administered in clinically recommended doses. At a dose of 3 mg/kg in experimental cats it did not produce excitement, whereas 5–10 mg/kg produced signs of CNS excitation (Sturtevant and Drill 1957). Morphine, 2 mg/kg IM, was well tolerated with mydriasis, sedation, pacing, pouncing, emesis, and fascination with water being noted as adverse effects, but CNS excitation and "morphine mania" were not noted in the study (Barr et al. 2000). At clinically relevant doses of 0.2 mg/kg it produced vomiting in healthy cats, but otherwise did not produce dysphoria or excitement (Steagall et al. 2006). Instead, the cats exhibited euphoria with purring, kneading, and increased affection.

The primary mechanism of morphine metabolism in cats appears to be formation of sulfate conjugates in contrast to glucuronide conjugates produced by most other species (Yeh et al. 1971). The lack of glucuronide conjugate formation in cats is not unexpected, but the metabolism is still rapid in cats and indicative of a high extraction drug. Pharmacokinetic studies in cats have indicated a smaller volume of distribution and slower clearance as compared to dogs, with the elimination half-life being nearly identical (KuKanich et al. 2005a; Taylor et al. 2001). Assuming cats respond to the analgesic effects of morphine at similar concentrations as other animals, 0.2–0.3 mg/kg IV, IM, SC every 3–4 hours would produce similar plasma concentrations as other animal species. Adverse effects of morphine in cats are similar to those reported in dogs.

Studies examining the effects of morphine on FIV-infected cats produced unexpected results. Morphine, 1–2 mg/kg administered once daily subcutaneously on 2 consecutive days per week, significantly reduced the clinical signs associated with FIV infection, including delayed lymphadenopathy, CNS deterioration, and a trend toward decreased viral load (Barr et al. 2000, Barr et al. 2003). Clinical trials in naturally infected cats have not been conducted.

Horses. Morphine has been safely administered to horses under some conditions, but reports of excitement, behavior changes, and sustained increased locomotor activity have discouraged its routine use for pain control. Reports of excitement following morphine administration to horses may be caused by doses that were too high, and lack of concurrent sedatives (e.g., alpha-2 agonists or tranquilizers) administered. In comparison to other species, horses seem to be the most prone to excitation as an adverse effect. Morphine, 0.1–0.25 mg/kg IV, as a sole agent, has been administered with no reported excitement and resulted in decreased anesthetic consumption, produced minimal hemodynamic, and minimal blood gas effects (Clark et al. 2005; Bennet et al. 2004; Steffey et al. 2003; Combie et al. 1983; Muir et al. 1978). However, higher doses, 0.66 mg/mg and above, resulted in adverse effects of blood gas measurements, dysphoria, and excitement, and therefore should be avoided (Brunson and Majors 1987; Kalpravidh et al. 1984). Coombie et al. (1983) recommended that morphine should not be administered less than 7 days prior to a race as it is detectable in the urine at 144 hours (6 days). (Regulation of drugs in racing animals is discussed in more detail in Chapter 59.) Repeated doses of morphine should be used extremely cautiously in horses due to its constipating effect and the potential for impaction and colic.

Ruminants. The clinical use of morphine in ruminants in rare. The lack of residue depletion studies and the potential to decrease rumen contractions have limited its use.

Swine. Morphine has been associated with CNS excitation in swine, but like other species, this is likely to be related to the dose administered. The clinical use of morphine in swine is limited by the lack of residue depletion studies, but with increasing numbers of swine as companion animals (e.g., pot-bellied pigs) morphine use in this species may increase.

Small Mammals. Morphine has been used in rats, mice, guinea pigs, and ferrets as an analgesic, preanesthetic, and sedative. Analgesic effects are rapid following IM and SC administration, typically occurring within 15 minutes and lasting up to 4 hours, similar to other species.

Rabbits. Morphine has been previously reported to produce profound sedation in rabbits when administered 8 mg/kg IM as a preanesthetic. However, pharmacokinetic studies indicate analgesic dosages are probably in the range of 2–4 mg/kg IM or SC every 4–6 hours.

Fish. Morphine has been used in fish to control pain (Sneddon 2003). Fish not only feel pain (Sneddon et al. 2003), but they also appear to have opiate receptors. However, one study in which morphine was administered at high doses also reported that there were significant adverse cardiovascular effects (Newby et al. 2007).

Fish appear to have slower clearance rates than mammals. In one study (Newby et al. 2006) clearance rates were 25 to 50 times slower than dogs, and mean residence times were 7 hr and 27 hr in two species of fish.

Nonhuman Primates. Nonhuman primates require relatively large doses of morphine, 1–2 mg/kg, for sedation. However, nonhuman primates also appear to be relatively resistant to respiratory depression at these dosages despite high plasma concentrations (Lynn et al. 1991). Analgesic dosages are more likely in the range of those recommended for dogs.

HYDROMORPHONE. Hydromorphone is a morphine derivative with greater lipophilicity and potency as compared to morphine (Murray and Hagen 2005) (Table 12.7). Hydromorphone is approximately 7 times more potent than morphine with a similar duration of effect. Due to a greater lipophilicty, hydromorphone is expected to have a slightly quicker onset of action than morphine (5–10 minutes) and maximum effect (20–30 minutes) following IV administration. Hydromorphone has high intrinsic activity at the μ-opioid receptor. The effectiveness for mild to severe pain is similar to morphine when doses are used that are of equal potency. It was equally effective as oxymorphone in dogs when administered at equally potent doses (Smith et al. 2001) (0.11 mg/kg for oxymorphone; 0.22 mg/kg for hydromorphone). Hydromorphone produces less of an emetic effect than morphine, but

TABLE 12.7 Comparable potency of opioids

Drug	Brand Name	Potency*
Morphine	Generic	1
Codeine	Generic	0.1
Meperidine	Demerol	0.16
Propoxyphene	Darvon	0.16–0.3
Butorphanol	Torbugesic	1–7
Hydrocodone	Vicodin	6
Oxycodone	Percocet, Oxy-Contin	3–6
Oxymorphone	Numorphan	10–15
Hydromorphone	Dilaudid, generic	8
Buprenorphine	Buprenex	25
Fentanyl	Sublimaze	100

*Potency is based on relative potency in comparison to morphine.

emesis and nausea still occur relatively frequently. Hydromorphone produced less histamine compared to morphine when doses were administered that had equal potency (Guedes et al. 2006). In dogs, hydromorphone was studied at two doses, 0.1 and 0.2 mg/kg IV (Guedes et al. 2008). The pharmacokinetics were similar to what has been reported for morphine in dogs (see Table 12.5), with a short half-life, high volume of distribution, and high clearance that exceeded hepatic blood flow. There were no significant differences in pharmacokinetics between doses. However, significant differences in the pharmacokinetics of hydromorphone occurred between 0.1 and 0.5 mg/kg, with the higher dose resulting in significantly decreased clearance and prolonged half-life (KuKanich et al. 2008a). Antinociception was detected for 2 hours (Guedes et al. 2008).

The pharmacokinetics and pharmacodynamics of hydromorphone have been investigated in cats (see Table 12.5) in which a rapid clearance and short half-life were determined, similar to morphine (Wegner et al. 2004; Wegner and Robertson 2007). Although analgesic effects produced had a duration of up to 8 hours in the experimental model, it is unlikely these correlate with clinical analgesia. The recommended dosage interval for hydromorphone is the same as morphine, every 2–4 hours in dogs and cats.

Hydromorphone is available as oral syrup and tablets as hydromorphone hydrochloride. Although the pharmacokinetics of the oral formulations have not been reported for dogs, it is expected to be small or negligent because of the high first-pass clearance. Hydromorphone hydrochloride injection is widely available and is popular in veterinary medicine. Current dose recommendations for hydromorphone are presented in Table 12.8.

OXYMORPHONE. Oxymorphone is a morphine derivative with 10 times the potency of morphine (see Table 12.7) and similar lipophilicity. Oxymorphone produces less emesis, nausea, and sedation than morphine and hydromorphone when administered at equianalgesic doses to dogs and cats. Oxymorphone also causes less histamine release in dogs (Robinson et al. 1988). Oxymorphone is primarily eliminated as drug conjugates (56% of total dose) with small amounts eliminated unchanged in the urine (5.3%) or as 6-keto reduction metabolites (1.6%) in dogs. The pharmacokinetics of oxymorphone in dogs are similar to other opioids, such as morphine and hydromorphone with a large volume of distribution, rapid clearance, and short half-life (KuKanich et al. 2008b). The maximum concentration, 21.5 ng/ml, occurred at approximately 10 minutes, after 0.1 mg/kg SC with an elimination half-life of 1 hour.

Oxymorphone, 0.03 mg/kg IV, produced similar effects in horses as morphine. Although a veterinary formulation is FDA approved, it is not currently available. Intermittent availability problems with the human-approved products have also occurred. Oxymorphone is not used commonly due to intermittent supply problems and cost. Current dose recommendations for oxymorphone are presented in Table 12.9.

HYDROCODONE. Hydrocodone is a morphine derivative effective for mild to moderate pain and as an antitussive. The analgesic efficacy of hydrocodone has not been evaluated in dogs, but it appears to have the highest oral bioavailability of the opioids although it has not been extensively evaluated. The efficacy of hydrocodone is in part due to metabolism to hydromorphone, which occurs

TABLE 12.8 Hydromorphone dosages

	IV	IV Infusion	IM/SC	PO
Dog	0.1 mg/kg q 2–4 h	0.02–0.04 mg/kg/h	0.1 mg/kg q 2–4 h	NR
Cat	0.05–0.1 mg/kg q 2–4 h	0.02–0.03 mg/kg/h	0.05–0.1 mg/kg q 2–4 h	NR
Horse	0.01–0.02 mg/kg once	NR	0.01–0.02 mg/kg once	NR
Rat/mouse			0.3–0.7 mg/kg q 4 h	NR
Guinea Pig/Hamster			0.3–0.7 mg/kg q 4 h	NR
Rabbit			0.3–0.7 mg/kg q 4 h	NR
Primates			0.1–0.3 mg/kg q 4–6 h	NR
Ferrets			0.05–0.1 mg/kg q 4–6 h	NR

NR = not recommended.

TABLE 12.9 Oxymorphone dosages

	IV	IV Infusion	IM/SC	PO
Dog	0.05–0.1 mg/kg q 2–4 h	0.005–0.01 mg/kg/h	0.05–0.1 mg/kg q 2–4 h	NR
Cat	0.025–0.05 mg/kg q 2–3 h	0.01–0.02 mg/kg/h	0.025–0.11 mg/kg q 2–4 h	NR
Horse	0.01–0.02 mg/kg once	NR	0.01–0.02 mg/kg once	NR
Rat/mouse			0.2–0.5 mg/kg q 4 h	NR
Guinea Pig/Hamster			0.2–0.5 mg/kg q 4 h	NR
Rabbit			0.2–0.5 mg/kg q 4 h	NR
Primates			0.05–0.2 mg/kg q 4–6	NR
Ferrets			0.05 mg/kg q 4–6 h	NR

NR = not recommended.

TABLE 12.10 Opiates combined with nonsteroidal antiinflammatory drugs (NSAIDs)

Opioid	NSAID	Common Brand Name
Hydrocodone	Acetaminophen	Vicodin, Hydrocet, Lorcet
Codeine	Acetaminophen	Tylenol with Codeine
Codeine	Aspirin	Empirin
Hydrocodone	Aspirin	Damason
Oxycodone	Aspirin	Percondan
Oxycodone	Acetaminophen	Percocet, Tylox, Roxicet

in dogs (Findlay et al. 1979; Barnhart and Caldwell 1977). Demethylation of hydrocodone to hydromorphone is more prominent in dogs than the demethylation of codeine to morphine (Findlay et al. 1979). Hydrocodone is also much better absorbed orally in dogs than codeine (6–7% versus 34–44%) (Findlay et al. 1979). This may explain why many veterinarians prefer oral hydrocodone as an antitussive treatment over codeine in dogs.

Hydrocodone is available for oral use (syrup and tablets) as hydrocodone bitartrate. Preparations that contain hydrocodone for oral use in people in the United States also contain homatropine (Hycodan). In other countries oral formulations may contain only hydrocodone. Hydrocodone also is available with nonsteroidal antiinflammatory drugs (Table 12.10). Oral absorption or efficacy of these formulations has not been reported in animals.

When administered as an antitussive, the atropine is not expected to have therapeutic or adverse effects on coughing. The recommended dose for dogs as an antitussive is 0.22 mg/kg every 4–8 hours; for analgesia higher doses are likely to be needed, 0.44 mg/kg every 6–8 hours. However, the efficacy and safety of hydrocodone at the higher dosages have not been evaluated.

CODEINE. Codeine is a naturally occurring alkaloid similar in structure to morphine. In humans the oral bioavailability is 60% and approximately 10% of the dose is metabolized to morphine, which may be responsible for the majority of the analgesic effects because codeine has low affinity for opiate receptors. However, in more recent studies, the amount of morphine produced in people may be much lower than previously assumed (Shah and Mason 1990). In dogs the oral bioavailability is poor (6–7%) and minimal demethylation to morphine occurs (Findlay et al. 1979). Therefore the clinical effectiveness of oral codeine is questionable. There are oral formulations of codeine combined with acetaminophen (Table 12.10) but the analgesic efficacy has not been examined in dogs.

There are multiple metabolites of codeine, for example, 6-glucuronide, norcodeine, and morphine. In people, approximately 10% of codeine is metabolized to morphine, via o-demethylation, which is further metabolized to other compounds that may be active (e.g., morphine-6-glucuronide). It has always been assumed that the activity of codeine was produced by morphine or its metabolites; thus it would have approximately 10% of the efficacy of morphine. However, more recent evidence suggests that other metabolites (for example, codeine-6-glucuronide) may be responsible for codeine's analgesic activity (Lötsch et al. 2006). In dogs, morphine is a minimal metabolite of codeine, but there is substantial codeine glucuronidation in dogs (Findlay et al. 1979). However, clinical effectiveness of codeine in animals has not been reported.

Parenteral codeine administration results in weak analgesic effects due to it lack of conversion to morphine and is expected to be effective only for mild pain. Due to the availability of other opioids codeine is rarely indicated for use in veterinary medicine.

OXYCODONE. Oxycodone is a morphine derivative with mild-to-moderate analgesic effects. In humans oxycodone has a 50–70% oral bioavailability and is available as an extended release tablet (Table 12.10). Clinical use of oxycodone in animals has not been evaluated. Similar to the pattern observed for other opiates in dogs, oral systemic absorption is low. A dose of 0.5 mg/kg resulted in a C_{MAX} of only 6.5 ng/ml at 15 min and was below LOQ by 3 hours. However, only two dogs were evaluated. Nevertheless, the low oral systemic availability would likely result in poor efficacy; therefore, its use is not recommended. It also has high abuse potential in people and would be a risk if stocked in veterinary hospitals (Weinstein and Gaylord 1979).

HEROIN. Heroin is the diacetyl congener of morphine and is widely abused by humans. Heroin is available for medical use in some countries, but does not possess greater analgesic activity than morphine. The lipophilicity of heroin is greater than that of morphine, resulting in a faster onset of action and the rapid euphoric effect following IV administration. Heroin is rapidly metabolized to morphine in most species. Although there is some historical use of heroin in veterinary medicine, current administration of heroin in veterinary medicine is not recommended due to the high abuse potential, and it is listed as a Schedule I drug by the United States DEA (Table 12.2).

APOMORPHINE. Apomorphine will reliably induce vomiting in dogs. It is used to treat poisoning in dogs if administered shortly after a dog has ingested a poison. It is not effective as an emetic in cats, which illustrates the interspecies differences in distribution and response of opiate receptors. (In cats, xylazine, an alpha-2 agonist, is a more reliable emetic.)

Apomorphine's action is presumably via direct stimulation of the chemoreceptor trigger zone (CRTZ) in the area postrema (Mitchelson 1992). Alternatively, it acts as a dopamine (D_2) agonist, which is a neurotransmitter in both the CRTZ and vomiting center. At high concentrations it acts as an *antiemetic,* presumably via action on central opiate μ-receptors (Scherkl et al. 1990). Naloxone increases, rather than decreases, the emetic effects because naloxone blocks the μ-receptor–mediated antiemetic effects. The route of administration can also influence the effect. Rapid increases in blood concentrations such as from IV or rapid IM absorption can produce antiemetic effects by opposing the emetic action in the CRTZ. This explains why lower concentrations produced by SC and mucosal administration may be more effective for producing emesis.

The dose used in dogs has covered a wide range, with the ED_{95} reported to be 0.02 mg/kg IV, to 4 mg/kg orally. The most reliable doses listed in review papers are 0.1 mg/kg SC or 0.05 mg/kg IV. After IV injection of 0.1 mg/kg it produces vomiting reliably in dogs. However, it was more effective if administered SC than if given IM, probably because of rates of absorption as mentioned above (Scherkl et al. 1990). In these studies doses of 0.04 and 0.1 mg/kg were studied. Alternatively, a 6 mg tablet of apomorphine hydrochloride can be mixed with sterile water or saline solution. A few drops of this solution can be placed in the conjunctival sac. When vomiting occurs, the solution should be promptly rinsed out of the eye. The pH of this hydrochloride solution is low, so it can be irritating to the ocular membranes if not rinsed.

The half-life of apomorphine in dogs is 48 minutes after IV injection and it is highly absorbed from IM and SC injection (Scherkl et al. 1990). Apomorphine is much less active orally because of high first-pass metabolism. Adverse effects are attributed to the dopaminergic effects (e.g., hypotension, drowsiness, dyskinesia).

Apomorphine hydrochloride can be obtained from some sources as a 6 mg tablet, or a 2 ml ampule (Apokyn) at a concentration of 10 mg/ml for IV, SC, or IM use. For people, a 3 ml cartridge (10 mg/ml, Apokyn) injectable formulation is administered SC—usually 2 to 6 mg per injection—to treat episodes of severe Parkinson's disease (to be coadministered with an antiemetic) (Lees 1993). This is a disease in which there is a deficiency of dopamine, and apomorphine's dopaminergic effects can be helpful. A sublingual formulation is also used to treat erectile dysfunction in men.

METHADONE. Methadone has traditionally been used in humans to treat opiate addiction (Kosten and O'Connor 2003). It was first shown to have this property in 1948 and was adopted as one of the principal treatments for opiate addiction in 1965. The advantage of methadone in this use is that the severity of withdrawal signs from methadone is much less than from heroin. It also has a much longer half-life (approximately 24 hrs) than morphine or heroin and is orally absorbed. Therefore, addiction treatment programs can administer methadone once-a-day orally to avoid intravenous injections and achieve good compliance rates. At one time, methadone's only common use was for treatment of opiate addiction. However, it is now considered a valuable analgesic drug as well.

Methadone is a μ-receptor opiate agonist with high intrinsic activity. Methadone also has some activity as an antagonist at NMDA receptors and inhibits reuptake of norepinephrine and serotonin, all of which contribute variably to its analgesic activity. As a result, pain that is poorly controlled with other opioids (morphine, hydromorphone, and fentanyl), such as chronic and neuropathic pain, may be controlled more effectively with methadone (Foley 2003). Activity on the NMDA receptor inhibits tolerance from developing to the opiate effects. Additionally, methadone has demonstrated synergistic analgesic effects when coadministered with morphine and additive effects when administered in combination with oxymorphone, oxycodone, fentanyl, alfentanyl, or meperidine (Bolan et al. 2002). Methadone is a 50 : 50 racemic mixture with the L-chiral isomer (L-*enantiomer*) primarily responsible for the opioid pharmacologic effect and both isomers, L-and D-methadone, capable of binding to the NMDA receptor. Levomethadone contains only the active enantiomer; therefore, the administered dose should be 1/2 of the racemic formulation. Although oral formulations of methadone are inexpensive and readily available, the oral bioavailability is low, and detectable plasma concentrations are not achieved in dogs dosed orally (KuKanich et al. 2005d).

Despite poor oral absorption, methadone appears to be well tolerated following IV administration, with nausea, vomiting, defecation, and dysphoria not reported in dogs. Sedation was a prominent adverse effect and, as with other μ-receptor agonists, dose dependent respiratory depression occurs (KuKanich et al. 2005d, KuKanich and Borum 2008b). Minimal cardiovascular effects are noted in healthy dogs following clinically relevant methadone dosages, but increased systemic vascular resistance and coronary vascular resistance have been documented. Therefore methadone should be used cautiously in animals prone to congestive heart failure, with underlying cardiac disease, or with hypertension.

The analgesic potency of methadone is similar to that of morphine (Table 12.7) and as a result the administered dose range is similar. However, the elimination of methadone is slower, resulting in longer dosing intervals as compared to morphine. The recommended dose of methadone for dogs is 0.5 mg/kg IV every 6 hours or 0.5–1 mg/kg every 6–8 hrs IV, IM, SC. A study of methadone in Greyhounds indicated methadone is rapidly eliminated after IV administration in this breed, with a higher dose and more frequent administration recommended 1 mg/kg q 3–4 hours (KuKanich and Borum 2008b). Repeated IM and SC injections may result in tissue irritation and inflammation. In cats, methadone, 0.6 mg/kg IM, was well tolerated when administered as a preanesthetic (Bley et al. 2004) and was effective for postoperative pain at a dose of 0.5–0.6 mg/kg (Dobromylskyj 1993; Bley et al. 2004). Although repeated doses were not evaluated, a suggested dose interval based on pharmacokinetics and clinical observations is every 6–8 hours in cats. At a dose of 0.2 mg/kg SC to healthy cats, there were no adverse effects observed, euphoria was exhibited, and it was as effective against nociceptive stimuli as morphine (Steagall et al. 2006).

Methadone appears to be well tolerated in horses when administered up to 0.2 mg/kg IV in combination with an α-2 agonist (Schatzman et al. 2001; Nilsfors et al. 1988). It also has been used in horses with ketamine protocols. Minimal cardiovascular effects were observed and as expected there was an increase in sedation with the combination as compared to the α-2 agonist alone. Healthy, pain-free horses administered methadone (0.12 mg/kg IV) as a sole agent showed increases in heart rate, arterial blood pressure, and cardiac output, but only minimal effects on blood gas parameters. Euphoria and dysphoria was of approximately 15 minutes in duration, but was subjectively less than the same effects produced by morphine, meperidine, and oxymorphone, but similar to that of pentazocine (Muir et al. 1978). An advantage of methadone in horses is that at doses in the range of 0.1 mg/kg, IV, sedation occurs, but they will not become recumbent. The horses will remain in a sedated standing position without incoordination, allowing minor procedures to be performed.

Methadone is available as an oral cherry-flavored concentrate 10 mg/ml (Methadose) and an oral tablet (40 mg). It is also available as an injectable solution.

MEPERIDINE (PETHIDINE). The availability of newer opioids has resulted in a dramatic decrease in the use of meperidine in veterinary medicine. Meperidine (*meperidine* is the USAN terminology but *pethidine* is used in the

BAN) is a synthetic opioid with antimuscarinic and negative inotropic effects that differ from most of the other opioids. Meperidine appears to have the most cardiac depressant effects of the opioids. Similar to morphine, histamine release occurs following IV administration, but the clinical relevance appears to be minimal as adverse effects were not reported following intravenous meperidine administered to dogs (2 and 5 mg/kg) or cats (11 mg/kg) (Ritschel et al. 1987; Davis and Donnelly 1968). Meperidine is less potent than morphine (Table 12.7). It may be less constipating and cause less nausea than morphine. A meperidine metabolite, normeperidine, has CNS excitatory effects and accumulates following multiple doses in humans and can result in seizures. This metabolite in people has contributed to the *serotonin syndrome* that is associated with some drugs and drug combinations and is a precaution to its use in human medicine today. However, normeperidine appears to be a minor metabolite in dogs and cats. Meperidine as the parent drug can also exhibit some effects on serotonin receptors and can result in serotonin syndrome if combined with a monoamine oxidase inhibitor (selegiline), tricyclic antidepressant, serotonin reuptake inhibitor, or tramadol. Pharmacokinetics are summarized in Table 12.5. Meperidine is well absorbed following IM administration to dogs and cats, but the rate of absorption is variable. Meperidine has poor oral and transmucosal bioavailability in dogs.

Meperidine (1.1 mg/kg IV) produces similar adverse effects in horses as morphine (0.1 mg/kg). The duration of analgesia is approximately 1 hour as meperidine is rapidly redistributed following IV administration. The elimination half-life is 1 hour and multiple doses would be expected to result in drug accumulation and longer duration of effect, and increase the risk of altered gastrointestinal tract motility.

FENTANYL. Fentanyl is a synthetic opioid that is selective for the μ-opioid receptor. Its use has increased in veterinary medicine as an intravenous administration and transdermal preparation. Similar to other opioids, fentanyl has minimal cardiovascular effects at clinically relevant dosages in healthy animals, but results in dose-dependent respiratory depression (Grimm et al. 2005; Hug and Murphy 1979). Fentanyl has a wide safety profile with doses as high as 300 times the recommended dose not being lethal in spontaneously breathing dogs. Even when high-dose fentanyl transdermal delivery was administered to dogs undergoing surgery, fentanyl did not produce postoperative respiratory depression (Welch et al. 2002). It is highly lipophilic—approximately 1,000 times more lipophilic than morphine. As a result, the onset of action is rapid in comparison to the other opioids because of rapid diffusion into the CNS. Fentanyl CSF concentrations peak between 2.5 and 10 minutes following IV administration in comparison to morphine, which peaks at 15–30 minutes in dogs. Respiratory depression occurs immediately following IV fentanyl administration. Fentanyl is primarily eliminated by metabolism, with hydroxylation and dealkylation being the primary mechanisms, and less than 8% of the total dose is eliminated as unchanged drug. Pharmacokinetics are summarized in Table 12.5, and current dose recommendations for fentanyl are presented in Table 12.11.

As a very lipophilic molecule with high potency (see Table 12.7), fentanyl is ideally suited for transdermal penetration to produce systemic effects. Fentanyl is available in a transdermal delivery device, generally referred to as the "fentanyl patch," which bypasses first-pass hepatic metabolism resulting in therapeutic plasma concentrations.

Dogs. Fentanyl is well tolerated in dogs with a lower incidence of nausea, vomiting, and dysphoria as compared to some of the other opioids, but variable sedation has been observed. In dogs fentanyl is about 60% bound to plasma proteins, and protein binding is linear with plasma concentration. Pharmacokinetics are listed in Table 12.5. Following IV bolus administration, plasma fentanyl concentrations decrease rapidly primarily due to redistribution with a concurrent rapid decrease in the effects. The distribution half-life is approximately 45 minutes (Kyles et al. 1996). This phenomenon is similar to that seen with thiobarbiturates where redistribution from the CNS is primarily responsible for recovery from anesthesia. There is a more prolonged terminal phase with a mean elimination half-life in dogs of 6 hours (Kyles et al. 1996), indicating

TABLE 12.11 Fentanyl dosages

	IV	IV Infusion	IM/SC
Dog	5–10 μg/kg q 1–3 h	2–5 μg/kg/h	5–10 μg/kg q 1–3 h
Cat	5–10 μg/kg q 1–3 h	2–5 μg/kg/h	5–10 μg/kg q 1–3 h
Horse	2–4 μg/kg q 3–4 h	0.3–0.5 μg/kg/h	2–4 μg/kg q 3–4 h

Note: dosages are in μg/kg. 1,000 μg = 1 mg.

that steady-state plasma concentrations will be achieved at 18–24 hours if administered as an IV infusion. In order to rapidly achieve and maintain targeted plasma concentrations, loading doses (up to 2 μg/kg) of fentanyl may need to be administered at the beginning of an IV infusion (Fig. 12.2).

Fentanyl is well absorbed, but variably, in dogs when administered by a transdermal patch (Kyles et al. 1996), with patches requiring changing every 72 hours (3 days) to maintain a therapeutic effect. There is a 12–24-hour lag time before therapeutic effects are achieved following patch application, consistent with the time needed to achieve steady-state from an IV infusion as noted above. Although the fentanyl patches are not registered for animals, the human sizes are used. Fentanyl patches are available in sizes of 12, 50, 75, and 100 μg/hr delivery rates. Despite this range of sizes, there have been no differences observed in plasma concentrations in dogs when 50 μg/hr patches were compared with 100 μg/hr patches (Egger et al. 1998). High-dose patches were well-tolerated in dogs (Welch et al. 2002) and have been effective for treating both soft-tissue and orthopedic surgical pain in dogs (Robinson et al. 1999; Kyles et al. 1998).

Cats. Cats have tolerated fentanyl well with only mild adverse effects that have included sedation, purring, rubbing, kneading, and mydriasis. The total body clearance of fentanyl is similar to that of dogs, but due to a much lower volume of distribution, the elimination half-life is much shorter (~2.5 hr) (Lee et al. 2000). Fentanyl is also well absorbed, but variably, in cats from the transdermal patch (Lee et al. 2000). Doses most often used for fentanyl patches in cats are the 25 μg/hr patch. In very small cats, if one-half of the patch is covered (absorption is dependent on the exposed surface area of the patch), the rate of delivery is reduced by approximately one-half (Davidson et al. 2004). Twelve micrograms per hour patches are also available if lower dosages are needed.

In contrast to dogs, the drug concentrations persist longer in the skin of cats resulting in a longer terminal half-life after fentanyl patches are removed from the skin (Lee et al. 2000). Therapeutic plasma concentrations can

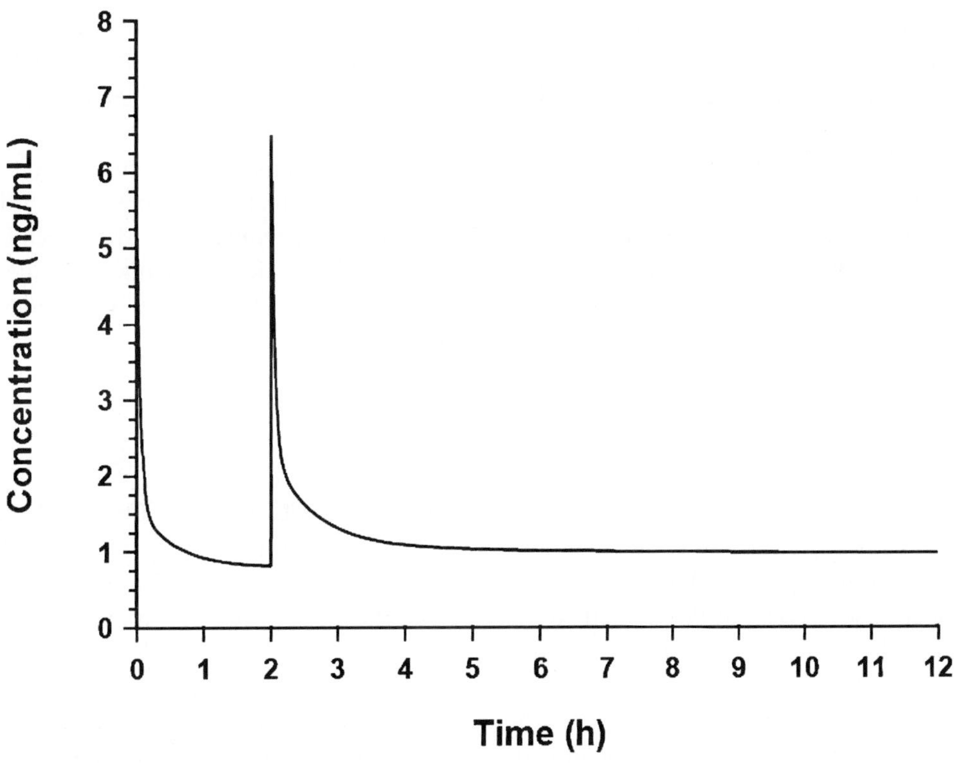

FIG. 12.2 The expected plasma profile of fentanyl administered as 2 loading doses, 5 μg/kg IV, at time 0 and 2 h and IV infusion 2 μg/kg/h starting at time 0 in dogs. The second IV loading dose is administered to prevent drug concentrations from dropping below 1 ng/ml. The targeted plasma concentration of fentanyl is 1 ng/ml for analgesia.

be maintained for 120 hours (5 days) in cats after administration of a 25 μg/hr patch. Because of the shorter half-life a 6–12-hour lag time to therapeutic effect occurs following application of fentanyl patches to cats, which is shorter than in dogs. Clinical studies have demonstrated efficacy of transdermal fentanyl in cats for pain from surgical onychectomy (Gellasch et al. 2002; Franks et al. 2002).

Horses. Although fentanyl has been administered IV in some analgesic and anesthetic protocols for horses, it is not used as often as other opioids. When fentanyl is administered IV to horses, it is relatively well-tolerated, but stimulation of locomotor activity has been well documented at 20 μg/kg (Mama et al. 1992) and at even lower doses of 5 μg/kg (Kamerling et al. 1985).

Acceptance of the fentanyl transdermal delivery has not been as good as in other animal species, however. Although fentanyl is well absorbed following application of transdermal patches in horse (Maxwell et al. 2003), concentrations are variable. In that study, the investigators applied two 100 μg/hr fentanyl patches to horses. They observed high absorption and plasma levels that were in a range considered to be therapeutic, but these levels were not as long-lasting as in small animals. In another study, after application of three 100 μg/hr patches to horses, the concentrations achieved levels that were in a therapeutic range, but were variable (Orsini et al. 2006). There was a peak at approximately 12 hours, but the concentration declined during the next 72 hours without attaining a steady-state plateau as seen in the smaller animals. These authors also observed high variability among horses, with some horses failing to achieve concentrations in the therapeutic range.

Application of fentanyl patches to horses for controlling pain has produced mixed results. Veterinarians that have used low doses (one or two of the 100 μg/hr patches) have not been impressed with the results. It was cited that fentanyl is capable of controlling visceral pain in horses without producing adverse effects, but that somatic musculoskeletal pain was less effectively controlled, or may require higher doses (Orsini et al. 2006). Thomasy et al. (2004) found that transdermal fentanyl controlled musculoskeletal pain in some horses that had not responded to nonsteroidal antiinflammatory drugs (NSAIDs) alone, but improvement was minimal. The study by Orsini et al. (2006) concluded that a minimum of three 100 μg/hr patches are necessary to control pain in horses, and some horses may not respond. To maintain effective levels, patches should be reapplied every 36 to 48 hours, in contrast to dogs, cats, and people. Alternatively, the authors propose that patches not be removed for 100 hours but that new ones be applied during treatment at 36 hours and every 24 hours thereafter.

Other Large Animal Species. Fentanyl also has been investigated as an anesthetic adjunct and analgesic in sheep, goats, and llamas. In the study by Grubb et al. (2005) the application of four 75 μg/hr fentanyl patches produced plasma fentanyl concentrations in a range judged to be therapeutic. It was well tolerated in these llamas.

Fentanyl was administered IV and via transdermal patch to goats (Carroll et al. 1999). Although the IV half-life was short (1.2-hour mean), it was otherwise well tolerated. A single 50 μg/hr transdermal patch produced plasma concentrations in an effective range, but the results were highly variable among goats. Plasma concentrations were not sustained at the steady-state level that has been observed in other animals.

SUFENTANIL, ALFENTANIL, REMIFENTANIL. Sufentanil, alfentanil, and remifentanil are fentanyl derivatives that exhibit similar pharmacodynamic effects as fentanyl. Sufentanil is 5 to 7 times more potent than fentanyl and eliminated metabolically similar to fentanyl. Alfentanil is a fentanyl derivative, which is less potent, but eliminated in a similar manner. Remifentanil is unique among the fentanyl derivatives as it undergoes nonhepatic metabolism (primarily muscle and intestinal) resulting in a short terminal half-life (~30 minutes) and a rapid clearance in dogs.

CARFENTANIL AND ETORPHINE. Carfentanil and etorphine are primarily used for sedation and capture of zoo and wild animals. For a complete discussion of the use of these drugs for this indication, the reader is referred to more detailed book chapters (Carpenter and Brunson 2007; Caulkett and Arnemo 2007). Carfentanil is a very potent fentanyl derivative. It is reported to be 8,000–10,000 times more potent than morphine. Carfentanil is a DEA Schedule II controlled substance with additional registration and storage requirements that must be met prior to obtaining it. The capture dose is 0.005–

0.02 mg/kg and carfentanil is available as 3 mg/ml solution. Its use for this purpose is facilitated by the extremely high potency that allows specialists in this field to administer small volumes via projectile dart.

Etorphine is also a very potent opioid used primarily for capture and restraint of zoo and wildlife species. The same precautions should be undertaken when handling etorphine as for carfentanil. The lethal dose of etorphine in humans is reported to be as low as 30 μg (0.03 mg) total dose.

Etorphine (M99) has a potency of as much as 3,000–4,000 times that of morphine. Like carfentanil, the high potency allows it to be used in the field by administration via small volumes in a projectile dart. As little as 8–10 mg, or less (total dose) can bring down a full-grown African elephant. It is usually reversed with the antagonist, diprenorphine (M 50–50). Because of the high potency of etorphine, it should only be used by trained and experienced individuals who are aware of the risks. A reversing agent (naloxone) should be on hand in the event of accidental human exposure.

After IM injection, the action of etorphine is prompt, within 20 minutes. The animals may then be easily restrained or brought to lateral recumbency. If the action is not antagonized, the immobilized state usually persists for 30 to 60 minutes. Used by itself in exotic species, the IM doses of etorphine that usually result in rapid immobilization, sedation, and analgesia are listed in Table 12.12. For most hoofed zoo animals, the dose is approximately 1–2 mg (total dose). For example, a zebra requires about 1.5 mg and the rhinoceros 1–1.5 mg (total dose).

For some animals, etorphine has been combined with the alpha-2 agonist xylazine. Hyaluronidase (150 iu) has also been added to etorphine and etorphine/xylazine mixtures to increase the absorption rate.

Etorphine or carfentanil should not be used in animals intended for food. There are restrictions on using such immobilizing agents near the hunting seasons. Currently the only opioids marketed in the United States for use in food-producing species are carfentanil and naltrexone, which are labeled for use in Cervidae. Carfentanil and naltrexone should not be administered within 30 and 45 days, respectively, of hunting season.

TABLE 12.12 Doses of etorphine in animals for immobilization

Family	Dose (mg/45 kg or 100 pounds)
Equidae (Mongolian horse, zebra)	0.44
Ursidae (black, grizzly, polar bear)	0.5
Cervidae (fallow deer, moose)	0.98
Bovidae (antelope, bighorn sheep)	0.09

Safe use of etorphine requires special precautions. Carfentanil or etorphine should never be used without an antagonist available (such as naltrexone) or be handled without training and experience. These are lipophilic drugs and there is the potential for exposure to lethal doses from skin contact and transdermal absorption. Domestic animals should be properly controlled and restrained prior to IV or IM administration to avoid accidental self-injection. For example, the lethal dose of etorphine for adult humans is small—only 30–120 mcg. Accidental injections of small amounts of etorphine-acepromazine have led to serious respiratory depression, coma, and death in people. In the event of an accidental injection of etorphine, administration of naloxone (0.8 mg) is necessary, to be repeated at 5-minute intervals if symptoms are not reversed. Naloxone, rather than diprenorphine should be used for reversal.

PROPOXYPHENE. Propoxyphene is a methadone congener, which is considered to possess less analgesic activity than codeine, but can cause marked respiratory depression. Due to the low efficacy of propoxyphene its use in veterinary medicine is not recommended.

PARTIAL AND MIXED RECEPTOR OPIOIDS

BUPRENORPHINE. Buprenorphine is a high-affinity partial agonist at the μ-opioid receptor, but an antagonist for the kappa receptor (Johnson et al. 2005). Its effects including analgesia, sedation, euphoria, gastrointestinal effects, and respiratory depression are attributed to the μ-opioid receptor activity. Buprenorphine exhibits a ceiling to its analgesic and respiratory depressant effects, in which increased doses do not produce a greater increase in response. It also appears to have a higher safety profile than full μ-receptor agonists. For example, the ratio of LD_{50} to ED_{50}—a measure of the therapeutic index—is 464 for morphine, but 12,313 for buprenorphine. The LD_{50} in dogs is 79 mg/kg, but therapeutic doses usually do not exceed 0.04 mg/kg. In cats, compared to full agonist μ-receptor agonists, it produces less dysphoria, excitement, vomiting, and nausea. It is a Schedule III narcotic (Table 12.2) and has less potential for abuse than pure μ-opioid receptor agonists.

The cardiovascular safety of buprenorphine has been evaluated (Carregaro et al. 2006; Martinez et al. 1997). The changes observed were not important enough to produce clinical significance.

Because buprenorphine is a μ-opioid receptor partial agonist, and a kappa-receptor antagonist, there is concern that it may inhibit the effects of coadministered opioids. Although theoretically it is possible that buprenorphine could antagonize the antinociceptive effects of other opioids, there is no clinical evidence of this property. In laboratory animals, preadministration of buprenorphine did not cause impairment of μ-receptor acceptability beyond the duration of antinociceptive activity (Englbeger et al. 2006). Nevertheless, buprenorphine binds to the μ-opioid receptor with higher affinity than other opioids. It will displace other opioids to elicit a withdrawal response in individuals with opioid dependence. Because of the high receptor affinity, it will require a much higher dose of naloxone to reverse respiratory depression and other opioid effects compared to doses used to reverse effects from morphine.

The high affinity of buprenorphine for the μ-opiate receptor may induce a longer duration of pain control in animals. This duration of analgesia in cats has been reported to be less than 4 hours (Taylor and Houlton 1984; Robertson et al. 2005; Stanway et al. 2002), up to 5 hours (Johnson et al. 2007), but suggested to be as long as 8 hours in some review papers. In dogs, the analgesic effects were not much longer than the effects from morphine (Brodbelt et al. 1997). The potency of buprenorphine is approximately 25 times that of morphine (Table 12.7). In some of the clinical studies of buprenorphine in people it had comparable efficacy to that of morphine. In animals, the efficacy of buprenorphine has been evaluated in some veterinary studies of surgical pain—primarily in cats. It was more effective than morphine in cats (Stanway et al. 2002), more effective than oxymorphone or ketoprofen (Dobbins et al. 2002), and equally as effective as butorphanol (Johnson et al. 2007). When administered subcutaneously in cats (0.02 mg/kg) it produced a minimum antinociceptive effect in comparison to morphine or methadone, but the route of administration may have limited its effect (Steagall et al. 2006). It was equally effective as morphine in dogs (Taylor and Houlton 1984). It is—at minimum—effective for treatment of mild to moderate pain and perhaps effective for more severe pain. In most of the studies in which the analgesic effects have been evaluated, doses of 10 μg/kg (0.01 mg/kg) and even as high as 40 μg/kg have been used in dogs, cats, and horses. This is higher than a typical standard dose for humans, which is 4–8 μg/kg.

The oral bioavailability of buprenorphine is poor due to its rapid clearance and first-pass metabolism. Buprenorphine has high lipophilicity (Log P > 3), consistent with a high volume of distribution (greater than 7 l/kg) and high brain-to-plasma tissue ratios. Buprenorphine is highly protein bound in whole blood. In dogs, buprenorphine glucuronide conjugates appear to be the primary metabolites, which are primarily eliminated via biliary secretion. The metabolism of buprenorphine in cats has not been reported.

Similar to other opioids clinically relevant cardiovascular changes are minimal, but increases in total peripheral resistance can occur. Buprenorphine is well tolerated in dogs and cats with sedation, mydriasis (cats), and euphoria occurring as adverse effects. Nausea and vomiting are possible, but occur rarely with buprenorphine. Excitement in horses after doses of 5 and 10 μg/kg IV have been observed (Carregaro et al. 2007), which was characterized as head-nodding, shifting, trotting, and restlessness. Excitement may be less in horses that have clinical pain.

Despite the lipophilicity of buprenorphine the onset of effect appears to be delayed following IV administration. Initially the lag in effect was thought to be due to slow binding to the opiate receptors, but recent studies in rats indicate the distribution into the CNS may be the rate-limiting step (Yassen et al. 2005). The effect of buprenorphine may also last longer than the plasma concentrations due to the slow diffusion out of the CNS.

Buprenorphine is rapidly and well absorbed following IM administration to cats with a peak concentration (T_{MAX}) of ~3 minutes. Subcutaneous absorption may be more delayed (Steagall et al. 2006). Although absorption from the gastrointestinal tract is small owing to first-pass effects, buccal or sublingual (mucosal) administration is well absorbed. In people, there are sublingual tablets used primarily for treatment of opiate addiction. The absorption in people from this route is 30% or higher. In cats, the oral-mucosal absorption is higher because the cat's saliva pH is higher than humans. The higher saliva pH favors higher lipophilicity for buprenorphine (pKa 8.3; Log P 4.98). Oral-mucosal absorption in cats was reported to be close to 100% (Robertson et al. 2003). Mucosal

TABLE 12.13 Buprenorphine dosages

	IV/IM/SC	Oral Transmucosal	PO
Dog	0.01–0.04 mg/kg q 4–8 h	NR	NR
Cat	0.01–0.02 mg/kg q 4–8 h	0.01–0.02 mg/kg q 4–12 h	NR
Horse	0.005–0.01 mg/kg	NR	NR
Rat/mouse	0.05–0.1 mg/kg q 4–12 h	NR	NR
Guinea Pig/Hamster	0.05–0.1 mg/kg 4–12 h	NR	NR
Rabbit	0.01–0.05 mg/kg q 4–12 h	NR	NR
Primates	0.005–0.01 mg/kg q 4–12 h	NR	NR
Ferrets	0.01–0.03 mg/kg q 4–12 h	NR	NR

NR = not recommended.

absorption has not been reported for dogs, but this route has been used successfully in horses (Walker 2007).

Oral bioavailability of buprenorphine is low (9.7%) and variable in rats, and less than 10% in people. In rats it was not effective by oral administration until high dosages (≥5 mg/kg PO) are administered (Martin et al. 2001; Brewster et al. 1981). The dose resulting in analgesia (5 mg/kg) was not voluntarily eaten in gelatin by the rats and needed to be administered via gavage. Current dose recommendations for buprenorphine are presented in Table 12.13.

Buprenorphine hydrochloride is available in Europe as a veterinary formulation (*Vetergesic*). In the U.S., the human formulation is used, (*Buprenex*, 0.3 mg/ml). The sublingual tablet used in people is administered to treat opiate addiction. There are two sublingual tablets: *Suboxone*, which contains 2 mg buprenorphine and 0.5 mg naloxone (4 : 1 ratio), and *Subutex*, a 2 mg tablet. Naloxone is present in *Suboxone* to discourage abuse; it is not absorbed systemically with sublingual administration to a significant degree and does not elicit a withdrawal response by this route. Transdermal administration of buprenorphine is being pursued by pharmaceutical sponsors. In Europe there is a buprenorphine transdermal delivery device available for human use. In the United States, a transdermal patch has been investigated (10 or 20 μg/hr sizes) but is not available at this time. Transdermal absorption of buprenorphine in dogs, cats, or horses has not been reported.

BUTORPHANOL. Butorphanol is a κ-opioid receptor agonist and either a partial agonist or antagonist at the μ-opioid receptor. The potency is often reported to be 5–7 times that of morphine, but unpublished data by the author (BK) indicates butorphanol is equipotent to morphine (Table 12.7). The efficacy of butorphanol is limited to mild and moderate pain, but it is one of the most commonly used analgesics and anesthetic adjuncts in veterinary medicine.

Butorphanol is a weak base with a pKa of 8.6, and is highly lipophilic with a Log P (octanol:water) of 3.68. The commercially available preparations of butorphanol are available as butorphanol tartrate. One mg of butorphanol tartrate is equivalent to 0.68 mg of butorphanol base. The commercially available injectable preparation (Torbugesic, Torbutrol, Stadol) is available in 0.5, 2, and 10 mg of butorphanol (base)/ml in a buffered solution (pH of 3.5 to 5.5). Tablets (Torbutrol) are available as 1, 5, and 10 mg of butorphanol (base).

Butorphanol has been commonly used in cats with a dose range of 0.1 to 0.8 mg/kg. Above 0.8 mg/kg there is a ceiling effect and no further beneficial effects occur with higher doses. The duration of effect is not increased with higher doses (Sawyer et al. 1991; Lascelles and Robertson 2004). Routes of administration include intramuscular, intravenous, subcutaneous, and oral. Pharmacokinetics are listed in Table 12.5. The comparison of clearance and terminal half-life between dogs and cats indicates substantially slower elimination in cats compared to dogs.

Compared to other opioids, butorphanol is reported to have a faster onset of effect (Lascelles and Robertson 2004), although in other studies the onset was longer (Johnson et al. 2007). The duration of antinociceptive activity of butorphanol is variable, depending on the report. It has generally been 3 hours or less in most studies (Lascelles and Robertson 2004; Sawyer and Rech 1987), and from less than an hour to 1.5 hours in dogs (Grimm et al. 2000; Sawyer et al. 1991). In a review of several studies spanning a 20-year period in cats (Wells and Papich 2008), the mean duration of analgesia for all dosages and routes was 160.3 minutes with a standard deviation of ± 130.8 min. The mean dosage administered was 0.4 mg/kg. The effective plasma concentration was above 45 ng/ml from the analysis of these studies, which is maintained for approximately 3 hours at a dose of 0.4 mg/kg.

Butorphanol is effective as an antitussive when administered per os to dogs (Gingerich et al. 1983) and cats, but due to its poor bioavailability, it is not an effective analgesic unless high doses are administered (1–2 mg/kg PO q2–4 h). The sedative effects of butorphanol are prominent and appear to occur at lower dosages than its analgesic effects. Therefore, sedation following butorphanol administration should not be interpreted as analgesia (Sawyer et al. 1991). Butorphanol is currently a DEA Schedule IV drug (Table 12.2) because of lower abuse potential compared to full μ-receptor agonists.

Butorphanol, like other opioids, causes minimal clinically relevant cardiovascular effects when administered at recommended dosages. Intramuscular and subcutaneous administration is painful. Adverse effects are similar to other opioids including sedation, dysphoria, mydriasis (cats), decreased GI motility, and constipation. The respiratory depressant effects of butorphanol appear to be less than that of opioid agonists.

In horses, butorphanol has been favored over other opioids because it is better tolerated. Excitatory effects, although possible, are less than with other opiates because these effects are primarily mediated via the μ-opioid receptor (see section on CNS excitement earlier in this chapter). Decreased fecal output was observed in horses (Sellon et al. 2001, 2004), but it was transient and not as severe as with other opioids. Less severe inhibition of gastrointestinal motility in horses is probably attributed to less stimulation of the μ-opioid receptor by butorphanol (see section on gastrointestinal effects of opioids earlier in this chapter; DeHaven-Hudkins et al. 2007).

Doses used in horses for treatment of visceral pain are in the range of 0.1 or 0.2 mg/kg IV as a bolus. After a bolus injection, ataxia, increased locomotor activity, and decreased intestinal motility may occur. In horses, the duration of effectiveness from a single dose is short—30 to 90 minutes in most studies. Therefore, to maintain analgesia without producing high peak concentrations that occur with intermittent boluses, a constant dose infusion protocol has been developed by Sellon et al. (2001, 2004). In those studies the half-life in horses was short (44 minutes) and the clearance was rapid (21 ml/kg/min). To maintain a plasma concentration in the effective range (judged to be 20–30 ng/ml) a loading dose of 18 μg/kg followed by a constant rate infusion of 24 μg/kg/hr. This treatment was well-tolerated with few adverse cardiovascular effects, but some ataxia. In a follow-up study (Sellon et al. 2004) a lower infusion dose of 13 μg/kg/hr was administered to patients that had undergone abdominal surgery. These horses had decreased fecal output, but it was only transient. There was less pain in treated horses, recovery from surgery was faster, and hospitalization time was less.

NALBUPHINE. Nalbuphine is a κ agonist and μ-receptor antagonist with similar pharmacologic effects as butorphanol. Nalbuphine is effective for mild to moderate pain and appears to be well tolerated in dogs and cats although it has not been extensively investigated. Very few studies have investigated nalbuphine in horses, but effects and adverse effects are expected to be similar to morphine and butorphanol. Advantages of nalbuphine over butorphanol is that nalbuphine is not currently a DEA scheduled drug; therefore, special record keeping is not necessary, and nalbuphine is less expensive. Nalbuphine exhibits similar potency and pharmacokinetics as morphine; therefore, dosage recommendations are the same as for morphine. Nalbuphine can be administered to antagonize the respiratory depressant effects of opioid agonists, but maintain some degree of analgesia.

PENTAZOCINE. Pentazocine is a κ agonist and μ-receptor partial agonist with similar pharmacologic effects as butorphanol and nalbuphine. Pentazocine is effective for mild to moderate pain with a 1–3-hour duration of effect. Pentazocine may cause less sedation as compared to other opioids, but similar to other opioids it can cause excitement and tremors at high doses.

NALORPHINE. Nalorphine is a partial κ agonist and μ-receptor antagonist that exhibits minimal analgesic effects. The efficacy of reversing opioid agonist–induced respiratory depression is variable and can exacerbate it in some cases. Therefore, the use of nalorphine is not recommended.

OPIOID ANTAGONISTS

The primary indication for opioid antagonists is for the treatment of an opioid agonist overdose if severe respiratory depression is present. The duration of antagonist effect is often shorter than that of the agonist and repeated doses are typically required. Opioid antagonists must be used extremely cautiously in animals that are painful as administration can result in acute exacerbation of pain leading to cardiovascular shock and even death. Nalbuphine and butorphanol can also be used to reverse the respiratory depressant effects of opioid agonists while maintaining some analgesia. Opioid antagonists not only reverse exogenously administered opioids, but also endogenous opioid peptides. Opioid antagonists are effective in controlling crib biting in horses, but due to the need for parenteral administration and efficacy limited to 6 hours or less, are not clinically useful.

NALOXONE. Naloxone is an opioid antagonist with greater activity at the μ receptor than at the κ and δ receptors. Naloxone also interacts at the GABA receptor as an antagonist and as a result can elicit seizures upon administration. Naloxone is typically administered 0.01–0.04 mg/kg IV and repeated as needed every 2–3 minutes to reverse respiratory depression. Careful titration can reverse the respiratory depressant effects of an opioid agonist while maintaining some degree of analgesia.

NALTREXONE. Naltrexone is an opioid antagonist with activity at the μ, κ, and δ receptors. Naltrexone is most commonly used to reverse carfentanil. It is administered at a dose of 100 mg naltrexone for 1 mg carfentanil, with 1/4 of the dose administered IV and the remaining 3/4 administered SC.

NALMEFENE. Nalmefene is an opioid antagonist with greater activity at the μ receptor than at the κ and δ receptors, similar to naloxone. However, the duration of effect is longer than that of naloxone. Nalmefene administered at 0.012 mg/kg/h was as efficacious as naloxone 0.048 mg/kg/h in antagonizing the respiratory depressant effects of fentanyl administered to dogs.

DIPRENORPHINE. Diprenorphine (M 50/50) is an antagonist at the μ, κ, and δ receptors, similar to naltrexone. Diprenorphine is used primarily to reverse the effects of etorphine. Two milligrams of diprenorphine will reverse the effects of 1 mg etorphine.

NEWER AGENTS Newer antagonists are being explored for use, primarily to limit the adverse effects of opioids on gastrointestinal motility. These agents are considered *peripheral* opioid antagonists, rather than *central* opioid antagonists. Such agents include alvimopan and methylnaltrexone. They are being investigated to be used as therapeutic agents to treat gastrointestinal motility problems associated with opioid analgesic use as well as other stress or pain syndromes that cause a decrease in gastrointestinal motility (for example, postoperative ileus) (DeHaven-Hudkins et al. 2007). These agents are capable of restoring gastrointestinal motility, but preserving opioid-mediated analgesia. Alvimopan has advantages over methylnaltrexone with respect to potency and duration of activity.

OTHER CENTRAL ANALGESIC DRUGS

TRAMADOL. Tramadol is a centrally acting analgesic eliciting its effects through a complex interaction at μ-opiate receptors and as serotonin (5-HT) reuptake inhibitor, noradrenergic reuptake inhibitor (α-2), and muscarinic (M1) antagonist. Tramadol is both highly lipophilic (Log P 2.5) and highly soluble (33 mg/ml), making it suitable for oral and IV administration. (There is no IV formulation commercially available in the U.S. at this time.)

Tramadol is administered as a racemic mixture (+ and –). It is metabolized to greater than 30 metabolites, with perhaps as many as 11 significant metabolites. The most important metabolite, with respect to pharmacologic activity is the active metabolite, o-desmethyltramadol (also referred to as the M1 metabolite), which is metabolized by the CYP2D isoenzyme. Concurrent administration of a CYP2D inhibitor (quinidine, fluoxetine, paroxetine, or sertraline) with tramadol significantly decreases the analgesic effects following tramadol administration. Additionally, CYP2D poor metabolizers (human) have poorly controlled pain in response to tramadol administration.

Tramadol's pharmacologic effects are complicated. The effects can be attributed to both the (+) and (–) isomer.

Tramadol (+) is a μ-opiate agonist (weak) and also inhibits serotonin (5-HT) uptake at the synapse. Tramadol (−) inhibits norepinephrine reuptake and can produce analgesic activity via alpha-2 receptors. The metabolite o-desmethyltramadol (M1) (+) is a μ-opiate agonist with potency of 200–300× tramadol. Taken together, the effects of tramadol may accomplish *multimodal analgesia* via these mechanisms. All three mechanisms described can produce analgesia, sedation, and other pharmacologic effects.

Tramadol is effective for mild to moderate pain and appears to be well tolerated in dogs. Tramadol has also demonstrated efficacy as an antitussive agent (Nosal'ova et al. 1991). Sedation, nausea, and vomiting are adverse effects that may be attributed to tramadol administration. Tramadol has less effect on GI motility as compared to opioid drugs. Tramadol may lower the seizure threshold; therefore, it should be used cautiously in patients prone to seizures, such as epileptics. Intravenous administration of o-desmethyltramadol to healthy dogs resulted in sedation, whereas IV tramadol did not (KuKanich and Papich 2004). Concurrent administration of tramadol and a serotonin agonist (tricyclic antidepressant, selective serotonin reuptake inhibitor, serotonin-norepinephrine reuptake inhibitor or meperidine) should be avoided due to the potential for serotonin syndrome (Mohammad-Zadeh et al. 2008).

The efficacy of tramadol as an analgesic in cats has been reported only in some research abstracts, but the results are consistent with opioid-mediated analgesia. There are important differences between cats and dogs (Table 12.14). Cats have slower clearance and a longer half-life compared to dogs. Most importantly, the clearance of the desmethylmetabolite (M1), which is conjugated to glucuronic acid for elimination in other animals, is much slower in cats. Because the clearance is lower in cats than in dogs, the ratio of M1 to tramadol is 1 : 1 or higher in cats (Table 12.14). Because the M1 metabolite is associated with greater opiate-mediated effects than the parent drug, opiate effects have been more often observed in cats. Because the clearance is slower in cats than dogs, the dose should be lower. In cats tramadol at a dose of 4 mg/kg IV produced a dose-dependent respiratory depression, which was partially reversed by naloxone in anesthetized cats (Teppema 2003). A dose of 4 mg/kg orally produced some dysphoria and mydriasis in some of the experimental cats (Papich and Bledsoe 2007). Tramadol, 10 mg/kg IP, significantly reduced the cough reflex in response to mechanical irritation in cats (Nosal'ova et al. 1991). Dose recommendations for cats have been in a range of 2–4 mg/kg PO q 12 hours, but further work is necessary to determine the optimum dose and frequency.

In dogs, tramadol is rapidly metabolized following oral and IV administration, with o-desmethyltramadol being one of the many metabolites (KuKanich and Papich 2004). The half-life of tramadol following IV and oral administration is 0.8 and 1.7 hours, respectively (Table 12.14). The half-life of o-desmethyltramadol is 2.2 hours following oral tramadol administration. The oral bioavailability of tramadol in fasted dogs is 65 ± 38%, indicating variable absorption. The current dose recommendation for tramadol use in dogs is 3–5 mg/kg PO q 6–8 hours.

In horses there is only very limited information available on tramadol effects and pharmacokinetics. When doses have exceeded 2–3 mg/kg, adverse effects have been observed that included tremors, muscle fasciculations, and head nodding. After IV administration the half-life in

TABLE 12.14 Tramadol pharmacokinetics in animals compared to people

	Dogs	Cats	People
Tramadol			
Half-life (hours)	0.8	2.5, 2.2	5–6
Peak concentration oral	1402 (11 mg/kg)	536 (4 mg/kg); 914 ng/ml (5.2 mg/kg)	200–400 ng/ml (1.4 mg/kg)
Volume of distribution	3 l/kg	3 l/kg	2.8, 3.4 l/kg
Clearance (ml/kg/min)	55	21	6–7
Systemic absorption from oral dose	65%	93%	70%
O-Desmethyltramadol (M1)*			
Half-life (hours)	1.7	4.5, 4.3	6–7
Peak concentration (ng/ml) oral	449	519 (4 mg/kg); 655 (5.2 mg/kg)	55–200 (1.4 mg/kg)
Ratio M1/tramadol	0.28	1–1.2	0.35

*All of the O-desmethyltramadol (M1) pharmacokinetic parameters were derived from administration of tramadol as the parent drug.
References: KuKanich and Papich (2004); Papich and Bledsoe (2007); Pypendop and Ilkiw (2007); Grond and Sablotzki (2004).

horses is short at 1–1.4 hours, and volume of distribution is 1.6–2.6 l/kg. Clearance is intermediate between dogs and cats, but higher than people (20–30 ml/kg/min). The half-life of the M1 metabolite is 3.6 hours. The ratio of M1/tramadol has been highly variable among horses and between routes of administration. It has ranged from less than 0.1 to 0.95. The half-life has been longer after oral administration, which may be caused by slow intestinal transit. Analgesic efficacy in horses has not been established.

The efficacy of tramadol for treating pain in animals has not been clearly established. It is considered a mild analgesic in people. In dogs and cats the anecdotal use has ranged from mild postsurgical pain to severe pain from cancer. It has been administered safely with anesthetics and NSAIDs. As mentioned previously, it should be used cautiously with other drugs (e.g., tricyclic antidepressants and serotonin reuptake inhibitors, Chapter 21) that affect serotonin metabolism. Because of the activity on serotonin metabolism, which is similar to other drugs (discussed in more detail in Chapter 21), tramadol has been explored for some behavior treatments.

Tramadol (Ultram, and generic) is available in 50 mg tablets. An extended release tablet (Ultram-ER) also has been examined in dogs (Papich et al. 2007). A single 300 mg tablet produces sustained plasma concentrations in dogs in excess of 24 hours. There are no commercially available injectable formulations in the U.S.

OTHER ROUTES OF ADMINISTRATION

In order to maximize analgesic effects and minimize adverse effects, other routes of opioid administration have been evaluated. The two routes most commonly utilized are epidural and synovial administration.

EPIDURAL. Opioids administered by the epidural route interact with spinal opiate receptors to elicit an analgesic response. Epidural opioid administration results in systemic absorption of the opioid, but at lower concentrations, due to the lower dose, than parenteral administration. The more lipophilic opioids, such as fentanyl and its derivatives, oxymorphone, and buprenorphine, are rapidly distributed to the plasma resulting in systemic drug exposure and minimal benefits compared to parenteral administration. Morphine is the most common opioid administered by the epidural route. Epidural administration results in decreased adverse effects such as sedation and dysphoria, but other adverse effects such as urine retention and constipation can still occur. The efficacy of epidural morphine administration appears to include mild to severe pain. The high efficacy is probably due to the very high concentrations of morphine interacting with the spinal receptors. Techniques for administering opioids via this route in veterinary species are provided in more detail in other chapters (Skarda and Tranquilli 2007).

PERIPHERAL. Opiate receptors have been identified in the synovial membranes of various species including the horse and dog (Sheehy et al. 2001; Keates et al. 1999). Intraarticular administration of morphine following endoscopic procedures produces a significant analgesic effect as compared to a placebo in humans (Lawrence et al. 1992). Low plasma concentrations are attained following intraarticular administration, presumably resulting in fewer adverse effects. Dose titration studies or placebo-controlled studies of intraarticular morphine in horses have not been reported. Intraarticular morphine 0.1 mg/kg diluted to a volume 0.5 ml/kg appears to decrease the need for supplemental analgesia following stifle surgery in dogs (Sammarco et al. 1996). Other techniques for local administration of opioids are provided in more detail in other chapters (Skarda and Tranquilli 2007).

THE USE OF OPIOIDS IN NONMAMMALIAN VERTEBRATES

The information available on the use of opioids in nonmammalian vertebrates is limited. The presence of opioid receptors is highly conserved among groups of vertebrates (mammals, birds, frogs, and fishes) (Li et al. 1996). Mu, κ, and δ opiate receptors have been identified in birds' brains as high affinity, but appear to be low in density as compared to mammals. The relative density of opioid receptors also appears to be dependent on the species of bird evaluated (Table 12.15). Therefore a drug effective in parrots may or may not be effective in doves, finches, waterfowl, ratites, etc. A wide range of opioid dosages are recommended in mammals. For example, the dose of morphine in mammals ranges from 0.1 mg/kg in horses to 5 mg/kg in rodents, a fiftyfold difference. It then seems reasonable that the efficacy and range of dosages would be similar for the multiple species of birds due to their diverse size and physiology.

TABLE 12.15 Relative supraspinal opiate receptor density in different species

	μ	κ	δ
Frog brain	37%	19%	44%
Chicken forebrain	58%	25%	17%
Pigeon brain	14%	76%	10%
Junco (passerine) brain	74%	22%	4%
Rat forebrain	41%	9%	50%
Mouse forebrain	25%	13%	62%
Guinea Pig forebrain	25%	50%	25%
Dog cortex	5%	58%	37%
Human cortex	29%	37%	34%

Few studies have evaluated the efficacy of opioids in companion birds. Butorphanol (1 mg/kg IM) decreased the MAC of isoflurane in cockatoos, which may be indicative of analgesic effects (Curro et al. 1994). The duration of effect or different doses were not evaluated. In a separate study, butorphanol (1 mg/kg IM) resulted in a greater effect than buprenorphine (0.1 mg/kg IM) in African Grey Parrots (Paul-Murphy et al. 1999). However, only a single dose for each drug was assessed, the birds were evaluated only out to 60 minutes, and neither drug was effective in greater than 50% of the animals assessed at 60 minutes. As a result of the sparse information available few opioid dosages are recommended in birds, and those are primarily anecdotal. Butorphanol 1–3 mg/kg q 4 h IM appears to be safe to administer to birds. Larger birds would be expected to require a lower dosage, whereas small birds would be expected to require a higher dosage.

The effects of various opioids have been studied in amphibians (grass frogs). A single study evaluated the analgesic effects of morphine, methadone, meperidine, fentanyl, and buprenorphine in an experimental model (Table 12.16). The opioids were administered SC into the dorsal lymph sac. The effective dose to elicit a 50% maximum analgesic response (ED_{50}) was determined as well as the lethal dose (LD) of some of the compounds (Stevens et al. 1994). The analgesic effects lasted for at least 4 hours, which was the last timepoint evaluated. In turtles, butorphanol did not provide an antinociceptive effect, even when administered at a high dose of 2.8 and 28 mg/kg, but it produced respiratory depression (Sladky et al. 2007). However, in the same turtles morphine at 1.5 or 6.5 mg/kg produced significant antinociceptive effects. Morphine at these doses caused long-lasting respiratory depression.

TABLE 12.16 The dose required to elicit a 50% maximum analgesic effect (ED_{50}) and lethal dose (LD) of opioids in tree frogs

	ED_{50} (mg/kg)	LD (mg/kg)
Morphine	24.6	ND
Fentanyl	0.47	30
Methadone	6.1	1000
Meperidine	31.7	ND
Buprenorphine	46.4	ND

ND = not determined.

At these doses the respiratory depression may limit clinical use. These studies in turtles indicate that the population of opioid receptors may be different in turtles compared to other vertebrates.

The analgesic effects of morphine and meperidine were evaluated in crocodiles (Kanui and Hole 1992). Morphine, 0.3 mg/kg IP, was the dose that produced the maximum analgesic effect in the experimental model. Morphine, 0.1 mg/kg IP, produced significant analgesic effects from 30 minutes to 2 hours. The analgesic effect following the higher dose, 0.3 mg/kg, would be expected to last longer, but the duration of the higher dose was not assessed. Meperidine produced a maximum response at a 2–4 mg/kg IP dose, and 2 mg/kg IP resulted in significant analgesia from 30 minutes to 3 hours.

The effects of butorphanol, 1 mg/kg IM on the minimum alveolar concentration of isoflurane were evaluated in green iguanas (Mosley et al. 2003). No significant reduction in the MAC occurred, but only a single dose was assessed. A separate study demonstrated butorphanol, 1 mg/kg, had no significant cardiovascular effects in iguanas when administered to isoflurane anesthetized animals (Mosley et al. 2004).

The effects of opioids have not been extensively evaluated in fish due to inherent difficulties evaluating pain in fish. Morphine 0.3 mg/g (300 mg/kg) appeared to produce an analgesic response in an experimental rainbow trout model, but the duration of the effect was not evaluated (Sneddon et al. 2003). The metabolism and analgesic effects of morphine in goldfish were evaluated following a bath administration (Jansen and Greene 1970). No metabolites were identified and recovery of unchanged morphine accounted for nearly 100% of the administered dose. A morphine bath consisting of 0.56 mg of morphine per 1,000 ml water resulted in maximal inhibition of an electrical stimulus model in 5/5 fish; however, tolerance was rapidly noted with repeated exposure every 3 days. Jansen and Greene reported apparent CNS excitement with higher doses similar to mammals. In winter flounder, morphine at high doses of 40 mg/kg IP or 17 mg/kg IV produced marked cardiovascular depression that lasted for 48 hours (Newby et al. 2007).

Harms et al. (2005) examined the effects of butorphanol and ketoprofen in postoperative Koi. Butorphanol, 0.4 mg/kg IM, produced a significant difference in postoperative behavior in Koi carp as compared to ketoprofen and saline, which may be indicative of an analgesic response.

REFERENCES

Adler MW, Geller EB, Rosow CE. Cochin, J, The opioid system and temperature regulation. Annu Rev Pharmacol Toxicol. 1988. 28:429–49.

Barnhart JW, Caldwell WJ. Gas chromatographic determination of hydrocodone in serum. J Chromatogr. 1977. 130:243–9.

Barnhart MD, Hubbell JA, Muir WW, Sams RA, Bednarski RM. Pharmacokinetics, pharmacodynamics, and analgesic effects of morphine after rectal, intramuscular, and intravenous administration in dogs. Am J Vet Res. 2000. 61:24–8.

Barr MC, Billaud JN, Selway DR, Osborn HG, Henriksen SJ, Phillips TR. Effects of multiple acute morphine exposures on feline immunodeficiency virus disease progression. J Inf Dis. 2000. 182;725–32.

Barr MC, Huitron-Resendiz S, Sanchez-Alavez M, Henriksen SJ, Phillips TR. Escalating morphine exposures followed by withdrawal in feline immunodeficiency virus-infected cats: a model for HIV infection in chronic opiate abusers. Drug Alcohol Depend. 2003. 72:141–9.

Bennett RC, Steffey EP, Kollias-Baker C, Sams R. Influence of morphine sulfate on the halothane sparing effect of xylazine hydrochloride in horses. Am J Vet Res. 2004. 65:519–26.

Bolan EA, Tallarida RJ, Pasternak GW. Synergy between mu opioid ligands: evidence for functional interactions among mu opioid receptor subtypes. J Pharmacol Exp Ther. 2002. 303:557–62.

Bragg P, Zwass MS, Lau M, Fisher DM. Opioid pharmacodynamics in neonatal dogs: differences between morphine and fentanyl. J Appl Physiol. 1995. 79:1519–24.

Brewster D, Humphrey MJ, Mcleavy MA. The systemic bioavailability of buprenorphine by various routes of administration. J Pharm Pharmacol. 1981. 33:500–6.

Briggs SL, Sneed K, Sawyer DC. Antinociceptive effects of oxymorphone-butorphanol-acepromazine combination in cats. Vet Surg. 1998. 27:466–472.

Brix-Christensen V, Goumon Y, Tonnesen E, Chew M, Bilfinger T, Stefano GB. Endogenous morphine is produced in response to cardiopulmonary bypass in neonatal pigs. Acta Anaesthesiol Scand. 2000. 44:1204–8.

Brodbelt DC, Taylor PM, Stanway GW. A comparison of preoperative morphine and buprenorphine for postoperative analgesia for arthrotomy in dogs. J Vet Pharmacol Ther. 1997. 20:284–289.

Brunson DB, Majors LJ. Comparative analgesia of xylazine, xylazine/morphine, xylazine/butorphanol, and xylazine/nalbuphine in the horse, using dental dolorimetry. Am J Vet Res. 1987. 48:1087–91.

Carpenter RE, Brunson DB. Exotic and zoo animal species. Chapter 31. 785–806. In: Tranquilli WJ, Thurmon JC, Grimm KA. Lumb and Jones' Veterinary Anesthesia and Analgesia. Fourth Edition. Blackwell Publishing, 2007.

Carregaro AB, Luna SP, Mataqueiro MI, de Queiroz-Neto A. Effects of buprenorphine on nociception and spontaneous locomotor activity in horses. Am J Vet Res. 2007. 68:246–50. Erratum in: Am J Vet Res. 2007 May;68(5):523.

Carregaro AB, Neto FJ, Beier SL, Luna SP. Cardiopulmonary effects of buprenorphine in horses. Am J Vet Res. 2006. 67:1675–80.

Carroll GL, Hooper RN, Boothe DM, Hartsfield SM, Randoll LA. Pharmacokinetics of fentanyl after intravenous and transdermal administration in goats. Am J Vet Res. 1999. 60:986–991.

Caulkett NA, Arnemo JM. Chemical immobilization of free-ranging terrestrial mammals. Chapter 32. pp. 807–832. In: Tranquilli WJ, Thurmon JC, Grimm KA. Lumb and Jones' Veterinary Anesthesia and Analgesia. Fourth Edition. Blackwell Publishing, 2007.

Cavanagh RL, Gylys JA, Bierwagen ME. Antitussive properties of butorphanol. Arch Int Pharmacodyn Ther. 1976. 220:258–68.

Chau TT, Carter FE, Harris LS. Antitussive effect of the optical isomers of mu, kappa and sigma opiate agonists/antagonists in the cat. J Pharmacol Exp Ther. 1983. 226:108–13.

Chou DT, Wang SC. Studies on the localization of central cough mechanism; site of action of antitussive drugs. J Pharmacol Exp Ther. 1975. 194:499–505.

Clark L, Clutton RE, Blissitt KJ, Chase-Topping ME. Effects of perioperative morphine administration during halothane anaesthesia in horses. Vet Anaesth Analg. 2005. 32:10–5.

Combie JD, Nugent TE, Tobin T. Pharmacokinetics and protein binding of morphine in horses. Am J Vet Res. 1983. 44:870–4.

Copland VS, Haskins SC, Patz JD. Cardiovascular and pulmonary effects of atropine reversal of oxymorphone-induced bradycardia in dogs. Veterinary Surgery. 1992. 21: 414–417.

Court MH, Greenblatt DJ. Biochemical basis for deficient paracetamol glucuronidation in cats: an interspecies comparison of enzyme constraint in liver microsomes. J Pharm Pharmacol. 1997. 49:446–449.

Craft RM, Ulibarri CM, Raub DJ. Kappa opioid-induced diuresis in female vs. male rats. Pharmacol Biochem Behav. 2000. 65:53–9.

Curro TG, Brunson DB, Paul-Murphy J. Determination of the ED50 of isoflurane and evaluation of the isoflurane-sparing effect of butorphanol in cockatoos (*Cacatua* spp.). Vet Surg. 1994. 23:429–33.

Davidson CD, Pettifer GR, Henry JD. Plasma fentanyl concentrations and analgesic effects during full or partial exposure to transdermal fentanyl patches in cats. Am J Vet Res. 2004. 224:700–705.

Davis LE, Donnelly EJ. Analgesic drugs in the cat. J Am Vet Med Assoc. 1968. 153:1161–67.

de Castro J, Van de Water A, Wouters L, et al. Comparative study on the epileptoid activity of the narcotics used in high and massive doses in curarised and mechanically ventilated dogs. Acta Anaesthesiol Belg. 1979. 30:55–69.

DeHaven-Hudkins DL, DeHaven RN, Little PJ. Techner LM. The involvement of the mu-opioid receptor in gastrointestinal pathophysiology: Therapeutic opportunities for antagonism at this receptor. Pharmacol Ther. 2008. 117:162–187. doi: 10.1016/j.pharmthera.2007.09.007.

Dobbins S, Brown NO, Shofer FS. Comparison of the effects of buprenorphine, oxymorphone hydrochloride, and ketoprofen for postoperative analgesia after onychectomy or onychectomy and sterilization in cats. J Am Anim Hosp Assoc. 2002. 38:507–514.

Dobromylsky JP. Assessment of methadone as an anesthetic premedicant in cats. J Sm Anim Pract. 1993. 34:604–608.

Drenger B, Magora F, Evron S, Caine M. The action of intrathecal morphine and methadone on the lower urinary tract in the dog. J Urol. 1986. 135:852–5.

Drenger B, Magora F. Urodynamic studies after intrathecal fentanyl and buprenorphine in the dog. Anesth Analg. 1989. 69:348–53.

Egger CM, Duke T, Archer J, Cribb PH. Comparison of plasma fentanyl concentrations by using three transdermal fentanyl patch sizes in dogs. Vet. Surg. 1998. 27:159–166.

Englberger W, Kögel B, Friderichs E, et al. Reversibility of opioid receptor occupancy of buprenorphine in vivo. Eur J Pharmacol. 2006. 534:95–102.

Findlay JW, Jones EC, Welch RM. Radioimmunoassay determination of the absolute oral bioavailabilities and O-demethylation of codeine and hydrocodone in the dog. Drug Metab Dispos. 1979. 7:310–4.

Foley KM. Opioids and chronic neuropathic pain. N Engl J Med. 2003. 348:1279–1281.

Franks JN, Boothe HW, Taylor L, Geller S, Carroll GL, Cracas V, Boothe DM. Evaluation of transdermal fentanyl patches for analgesia in cats undergoing onychectomy. J Am Vet Med Assoc. 2000. 217:1013–1018.

Gellasch KL, Kruse-Elliott KT, Osmond CS, Shih AN, Bjorling DE. Comparison of transdermal administration of fentanyl versus intramuscular administration of butorphanol for analgesia after onychectomy in cats. J Am Vet Med Assoc. 2002. 220:1020–4.

Gingerich DA, Rourke JE, Strom PW. Clinical efficacy of butorphanol injectable and tablets. Veterinary Medicine/Small Animal Clinician. February 1983; 179–182.

Grimm KA, Tranquilli WJ, Gross DR, Sisson DD, Bulmer BJ, Benson GJ, Greene SA, Martin-Jimenez T. Cardiopulmonary effects of fentanyl in conscious dogs and dogs sedated with a continuous rate infusion of medetomidine. Am J Vet Res. 2005. 66:1222–6.

Grimm KA, Tranquilli WJ, Thurmon JC, Benson GJ. Duration of nonresponse to noxious stimulation after intramuscular administration of butorphanol, medetomidine, or a butorphanol-medetomidine combination during isoflurane administration in dogs. Am J Vet Res. 2000 Jan;61(1):42–47.

Grisneaux E, Pibarot P, Dupuis J, Blais D. Comparison of ketoprofen and carprofen administered prior to orthopedic surgery for control of postoperative pain in dogs. JAVMA. 1999. 215:1105–1110.

Grond S, Sablotzki A. Clinical pharmacology of tramadol. Clinical Pharmacokinetics. 2004. 43:879–923.

Grubb TL, Gold JR, Schlipf JW, Craig AM, Walker KC, Riebold TW. Assessment of serum concentrations and sedative effects of fentanyl after transdermal administration at three dosages in healthy llamas. Am J Vet Res. 2005. 66:907–909.

Guedes AG, Papich MG, Rude EP, Rider MA. Pharmacokinetics and physiological effects of two intravenous infusion rates of morphine in conscious dogs. J Vet Pharmacol Ther. 2007. Jun;30(3):224–33.

Guedes AG, Rude EP, Rider MA. Evaluation of histamine release during constant rate infusion of morphine in dogs. Vet Anaesth Analg. 2006. 33:28–35.

Guedes AGP, Papich MG, Rude EP, and Rider MA. Comparison of plasma histamine levels following intravenous administration of hydromorphone and morphine in dogs. J Vet Pharmacol Ther. 2007. 30:516–522.

Harms CA, Lewbart GA, Swanson CR, Kishimori JM, Boylan SM. Behavioral and clinical pathology changes in koi carp (*Cyprinus carpio*) subjected to anesthesia and surgery with and without intra-operative analgesics. Comp Med. 2005. 55:221–6.

Heinricher MM. Nociceptin/orphanin FQ: Pain, stress and neural circuits. Life Sci. 2005. 77:3127–32.

Hennies HH, Friderichs E, Schneider J. Receptor binding, analgesic and antitussive potency of tramadol and other selected opioids. Arzneimittelforschung. 1988. 38:877–80.

Hersh EV, Lally ET, Moore PA. Update on cyclooxygenase inhibitors: has a third COX isoform entered the fray? Curr Med Res Opin. 2005. 21:1217–26.

Homsi J, Walsh D, Nelson KA, Sarhill N, Rybicki L, Legrand SB, Davis MP. A phase II study of hydrocodone for cough in advanced cancer. Am J Hosp Palliat Care. 2002. 19:49–56.

Hug CC, Jr, Murphy MR. Fentanyl disposition in cerebrospinal fluid and plasma and its relationship to ventilatory depression in the dog. Anesthesiology. 1979. 50:342–9.

Hug CC, Jr, Murphy MR, Rigel EP, Olson WA. Pharmacokinetics of morphine injected intravenously into the anesthetized dog. Anesthesiology. 1981. 54:38–47.

Jacqz, E, Ward, S, Johnson, R, Schenker, S, Gerkens, J, Brank, RA. Extrahepatic glucuronidation of morphine in the dog. Drug Metab Disp. 1986. 14:627–630.

Jansen GA, Greene NM. Morphine metabolism and morphine tolerance in goldfish. Anesthesiology. 1970. 32:231–5.

Johnson JA, Robertson SA, Pypendop BH. Antinociceptive effects of butorphanol, buprenorphine, or both, administered intramuscularly in cats. Am J Vet Res. 2007. 68:699–703.

Johnson RE, Fudala PJ, Payne R. Buprenorphine: considerations for pain management. J Pain Sympt Mgmt. 2005. 29:297–326.

Julius D, Basbaum AI. Molecular mechanisms of nociception. Nature. 2001. 413:203–10.

Kalpravidh M, Lumb WV, Wright M, Heath RB. Effects of butorphanol, flunixin, levorphanol, morphine, and xylazine in ponies. Am J Vet Res. 1984. 45:217–23.

Kamerling SG, Dequick DJ, Weckman TJ et al. Dose-related effects of fentanyl on autonomic and behavioral responses in performance horses. Gen Pharmacol. 1985. 16:253–258.

Kanui TI, Hole K. Morphine and pethidine antinociception in the crocodile. J Vet Pharmacol Ther. 1992. 15:101–3.

Kayaalp SO, Kaymakcalan S. A comparative study of the effects of morphine in unanaesthetized and anaesthetized cats. Br J Pharmacol Chemother. 1966. 26:196–204.

Keates HL, Cramond T, Smith MT. Intraarticular and periarticular opioid binding in inflamed tissue in experimental canine arthritis. Anesth Analg. 1999. 89:409–15.

Kosten TR, O'Connor PG. Management of drug and alcohol withdrawal. New Engl J Med. 2003. 348:1786–1795.

Krotscheck U, Boothe DM, Boothe HW. Evaluation of transdermal morphine and fentanyl pluronic lecithin organogel administration in dogs. Vet Ther. 2004. 202–11.

KuKanich B, Borum SL. Effects of ketoconazole on the pharmacokinetics and pharmacodynamics of morphine in healthy Greyhounds. Am J Vet Res. 2008a. 69:664–9.

———. The disposition and behavioral effects of methadone in Greyhounds. Vet Anaesth Analg. 2008b. 35:242–8.

KuKanich B, Hogan BK, Krugner-Higby LA, Smith LJ. Pharmacokinetics of hydromorphone hydrochloride in healthy dogs. Vet Anaesth Analg. 2008a. 35:256–64.

KuKanich B, Hogan BK, Krugner-Higby LA, Toerber S, Smith LJ. Pharmacokinetics and behavioral effects of oxymorphone after intravenous and subcutaneous administration to healthy dogs. J Vet

Pharmacol Ther. 2008b, *in press.* doi: 10.1111/j.1365-2885.2008.00987.x

KuKanich B, Lascelles BD, Aman AM, Mealey KL, Papich MG. The effects of inhibiting cytochrome P450 3A, p-glycoprotein, and gastric acid secretion on the oral bioavailability of methadone in dogs. J Vet Pharmacol Ther. 2005d. 28:461–6.

KuKanich B, Lascelles BD, Papich MG. Use of a von Frey device for evaluation of pharmacokinetics and pharmacodynamics of morphine after intravenous administration as an infusion or multiple doses in dogs. Am J Vet Res. 2005c. 66:1968–74.

KuKanich, B., Lascelles, B.D.X., Papich, M.G. Pharmacokinetics of morphine and plasma concentrations of morphine-6-glucuronide following morphine administration to dogs. J Vet Pharmacol Ther. 2005a. 28:371–376.

———. Assessment of a von Frey device for evaluation of the antinociceptive effects of morphine and its application in pharmacodynamic modeling of morphine in dogs. Am J Vet Res. 2005b. 66:1616–1622.

KuKanich B, Papich MG. Pharmacokinetics of tramadol and the metabolite O-desmethyltramadol in dogs. J Vet Pharmacol Ther. 2004. 27:239–46.

Kyles, A. E., Hardie, E.M., Hansen, B.D., and Papich, M.G. Comparison of transdermal fentanyl and intramuscular oxymorphone on post-operative behaviour after ovariohysterectomy in dogs. Res Vet Sci. 1998. 65:245–251.

Kyles, A.E., M.G. Papich, and E.M. Hardie. Disposition of transdermally administered fentanyl in dogs. Amer J Vet Res. 1996. 57:715–719.

Lascelles BD, Cripps PJ, Jones A, Waterman AE. Post-operative central hypersensitivity and pain: the pre-emptive value of pethidine for ovariohysterectomy. Pain. 1997. 73:461–71.

Lascelles BD, Robertson SA. Antinociceptive effects of hydromorphone, butorphanol, or the combination in cats. J Vet Intern Med. 2004. 18:190–5.

Lawrence AJ, Joshi GP, Michalkiewicz A, Blunnie WP, Moriarty DC. Evidence for analgesia mediated by peripheral opioid receptors in inflamed synovial tissue. Eur J Clin Pharmacol. 1992. 43:351–5.

Lee, D.D., Papich, M.G., Hardie, E.M. Comparison of pharmacokinetics of fentanyl after intravenous and transdermal administration in cats. Amer J Vet Res. 2000. 61:672–677.

Lees AJ. Dopamine agonists in Parkinson's disease: a look at apomorphine. Fundam Clin Pharmacol. 1993. 7:121–128.

Lemke KA, Runyon CL, Horney BS. Effects of preoperative administration of ketoprofen on anesthetic requirement and signs of postoperative pain in dogs undergoing elective ovariohysterctomy. JAVMA. 2002. 221:1268–1274.

Lemke KA, Tranquilli WJ, Thurmon JC, et al. Ability of flumazenil, butorphanol, and naloxone to reverse the anesthetic effects of oxymorphone-diazepam in dogs. J Am Vet Med Assoc. 1996. 209:776–779.

Li X, Keith DE, Evans CJ. Multiple opioid receptor-like genes are identified in diverse vertebrate phyla. FEBS Letters 1996. 397:25–29.

Lind RE, Reynolds DG, Ganes EM, Jenkins JT. Morphine effects on cardiovascular performance. Am Surg. 1981. 47:107–111.

Lötsch J, Skarke C, Schmidt H, Rohrbacher M, Hofmann U, Schwab M, Geisslinger G. Evidence for morphine-independent central nervous opioid effects after administration of codeine: Contribution of other codeine metabolites. Clin Pharmacol Ther. 2006. 79:35–48.

Lucas AN, Firth AM, Anderson GA, Vine JH, Edwards GA. Comparison of the effects of morphine administered by constant-rate intravenous infusion or intermittent intramuscular injection in dogs. J Am Vet Med Assoc. 2001. 218:884–91.

Lynn AM, McRorie TI, Slattery JT, Calkins D, Opheim KE. Pharmacokinetics and pharmacodynamics of morphine in infant monkeys. Dev Pharmacol Ther. 1991. 16:41–7.

Mama KR, Pascoe PJ, Steffey EP. Evaluation of the interaction of mu and kappa opioid agonists on locomotor behavior in the horse. Can J Vet Res. 1992. 57:106–109.

Markenson JA. Mechanisms of chronic pain. Am J Med. 1996. 101:6S–18S.

Martin LB, Thompson AC, Martin T, Kristal MB. Analgesic efficacy of orally administered buprenorphine in rats. Comp Med. 2001. 51:43–8.

Martinez EA, Hartsfield SM, Melendez LD, Matthews NS, Slater MR. Cardiovascular effects of buprenorphine in anesthetized dogs. Am J Vet Res. 1997. 58:1280–1284.

Mathews KA, Paley DM, Foster RA, Valliant AE, Young SS. A comparison of ketorolac with flunixin, butorphanol, and oxymorphone in controlling postoperative pain in dogs. Can Vet J. 1996. 37:557–567.

Maxwell LK, Thomasy SM, Slovis N, Kollias-Baker C. Pharmacokinetics of fentanyl following intravenous and transdermal administration in horses. Equine Vet J. 2003. 35:484–90.

Meunier JC, Mollereau C, Toll L, Suaudeau C, Moisand C, Alvinerie P, Butour JL, Guillemot JC, Ferrara P, Monsarrat B et al. Isolation and structure of the endogenous agonist of opioid receptor-like ORL1 receptor. Nature. 1995. 377:532–5.

Mircica E, Clutton RE, Kyles KW, Blissitt KJ. Problems associated with perioperative morphine in horses: a retrospective case analysis. Vet Anaesth Analg. 2003. Jul;30(3):147–155.

Mitchelson F. Pharmacological agents affecting emesis: A review. Drugs. 1992. 43:295–315.

Mohammad-Zadeh LF, Moses L, Gwaltney-Brant SM. Serotonin: a review. J Vet Pharmacol Ther. 2008. 31:187–99.

Mosley CA, Dyson D, Smith DA. Minimum alveolar concentration of isoflurane in green iguanas and the effect of butorphanol on minimum alveolar concentration. J Am Vet Med Assoc. 2003. 222:1559–64.

———. The cardiovascular dose-response effects of isoflurane alone and combined with butorphanol in the green iguana (*Iguana iguana*). Vet Anaesth Analg. 2004. 31:64–72.

Muir WW, Skarda RT, Sheehan WC. Cardiopulmonary effects of narcotic agonists and a partial agonist in horses. Am J Vet Res. 1978. 39:1632–5.

Mullin WJ, Phillis JW, Pinsky C. Morphine enhancement of acetylcholine release from the brain in unanesthetized cats. Eur J Pharmacol. 1973. 22:117–119.

Murray, A, Hagen, NA. Hydromorphone. J Pain Sympt Mgmt. 2005. 29: S57–66.

Neal CR Jr, Mansour A, Reinscheid R, Nothacker HP, Civelli O, Akil H, Watson SJ Jr. Opioid receptor-like (ORL1) receptor distribution in the rat central nervous system: comparison of ORL1 receptor mRNA expression with (125)I-[(14)Tyr]-orphanin FQ binding. J Comp Neurol. 1999. 412:563–605.

Newby NC, Gamperl AK, Stevens ED. Cardiorespiratory effects and efficacy of morphine sulfate in winter flounder (*Pseudopleuronectes americanus*). Am J Vet Res 2007. 68:592–597.

Newby NC, Mendonca PC, Gamperl K, Stevens ED. Pharmacokinetics of morphine in fish: winter flounder (*Pseudopleuronectes americanus*) and seawater-acclimated rainbow trout (*Oncorhynchus mykiss*). Comp Biochem Physiol Part C. 2006. 143:275–283.

Niedfeldt RL, Robertson SA. Postanesthetic hyperthermia in cats: a retrospective comparison between hydromorphone and buprenorphine. Vet Anaesth Analg. 2006 Nov;33(6):381–389. (Comment in: Vet Anaesth Analg. 2006. Nov;33(6):341–342.)

Nilsfors L, Kvart C, Kallings P, Carlsten J, Bondesson U. Cardiorespiratory and sedative effects of a combination of acepromazine, xylazine and methadone in the horse. Equine Vet J. 1988. 20:364–7.

Nosal'ova G, Strapkova A, Korpas J. Relationship between the antitussic and analgesic activity of substances. Acta Physiol Hung. 1991. 77:173–8.

Orsini JA, Moate PJ, Kuersten K, Soma LR, Boston RC. Pharmacokinetics of fentanyl delivered transdermally in healthy adult horses—Variability among horses and its clinical implications. J Vet Pharmacol Ther. 2006. 29:539–46.

Pant KK, Verma VK, Mishra N, Singh N, Sinha JN, Bhargava KP. Effects of morphine and pethidine on coronary vascular resistance, blood pressure, and myocardial infarction-induced cardiac arrhythmias. Jpn Heart J. 1983. 24:127–33.

Papich MG. Drug residue considerations for anesthetics and adjunctive drugs in food producing animals. Vet Clin N Amer (Food Anim Pract) C.R. Swanson (editor). 1996. 12:693–706.

Papich MG, Bledsoe DL. Tramadol pharmacokinetics in cats after oral administration of an immediate release tablet. ACVIM Ann Forum [abstract], Seattle, WA, 2007.

Papich MG, Davis JL, Chen AX, Bledsoe DL. Tramadol pharmacokinetics in dogs and an in vitro-in vivo correlation of an oral extended release tablet. ACVIM Annual Forum [abstract], Seattle WA, USA, 2007.

Paul-Murphy JR, Brunson DB, Miletic V. Analgesic effects of butorphanol and buprenorphine in conscious African grey parrots (*Psittacus erithacus erithacus* and *Psittacus erithacus timneh*). Am J Vet Res. 1999. 60:1218–21.

Pibarot P, Dupuis J, Grisneaux E, et al. Comparison of ketoprofen, oxymorphone hydrochloride, and butorphanol in the treatment of postoperative pain in dogs. J Am Vet Med Assoc. 1997. 211:438–444.

Posner LP, Gleed RD, Erb HN, Ludders JW. Post-anesthetic hyperthermia in cats. Vet Anaesth Analg. 2007. 34:40–47.

Priano LL, Vatner SF. Morphine effects on cardiac output and regional blood flow distribution in conscious dogs. Anesthesiology. 1981. 55:236–243.

Pypendop BH, Ilkiw JE. Pharmacokinetics of tramadol, and its metabolite O-desmethyl-tramadol, in cats. J Vet Pharmacol Ther. 2008. 31:52–9.

Reese CJ, Short CE, Hollis NE, Barlow LL. Assessing the efficacy of perioperative carprofen administration in dogs undergoing surgical repair of a ruptured cranial cruciate ligament. JAAHA. 2000. 36:448–455.

Reinscheid RK, Nothacker HP, Bourson A, Ardati A, Henningsen RA, Bunzow JR, Grandy DK, Langen H, Monsma FJ Jr, Civelli O. Orphanin FQ: a neuropeptide that activates an opioidlike G protein-coupled receptor. Science. 1995. 270:792–4.

Riedel W, Neeck G. Nociception, pain, and antinociception: current concepts. Z Rheumatol. 2001. 60:404–15.

Ritschel WA, Neub M, Denson DD. Meperidine pharmacokinetics following intravenous, peroral and buccal administration in beagle dogs. Methods Find Exp Clin Pharmacol. 1987. 9:811–5.

Robertson SA, Hauptman JG, Nachreiner RF, and Richter MA. Effects of acetylpromazine or morphine on urine production in halothane-anesthetized dogs. Am J Vet Res. 2001. 62:1922–1927.

Robertson SA, Lascelles BDX, Taylor PM and Sear JW. PK-PD modeling of buprenorphine in cats: intravenous and oral transmucosal administration. J Vet Pharmacol Ther. 2005. 28:453–460.

Robertson SA, Taylor PM, Lascelles BD, Dixon MJ. Changes in thermal threshold response in eight cats after administration of buprenorphine, butorphanol and morphine. Vet Rec. 2003. 153:462–5.

Robertson SA, Taylor PM, and Sear JW. Systemic uptake of buprenorphine by cats after oral mucosal administration. Vet Rec 2003. 152:675–678.

Robertson SA, Taylor PM, Sear JW, Keuhnel G. Relationship between plasma concentrations and analgesia after intravenous fentanyl and disposition after other routes of administration in cats. J Vet Pharmacol Ther. 2005. 28:87–93.

Robinson EP, Faggella AM, Henry DP, Russell WL. Comparison of histamine release induced by morphine and oxymorphone administration in dogs. Am J Vet Res. 1988. 49:1699–1701.

Robinson TM, Kruse-Elliott KT, Markel MD, Pluhar GE, Massa K, Bjorling DE. A comparison of transdermal fentanyl versus epidural morphine for analgesia in dogs undergoing major orthopedic surgery. J Amer Anim Hosp Assoc. 1999. 35:95–100.

Roerig SC, Fujimoto JM. Multiplicative interaction between intrathecally and intracerebroventricularly administered mu opioid agonists but limited interactions between delta and kappa agonists for antinociception in mice. J Pharmacol Exp Ther. 1989. 249:762–8.

Rosiere CE, Winder CV, Wax J. Ammonia cough elicited through a tracheal side tube in unanesthetized dogs: comparative antitussive bioassay of four morphine derivatives and methadone in terms of ammonia thresholds. J Pharmacol Exp Ther. 1956. 116:296–316.

Rowbotham M, Twillingi L, Davies PS, Reisner L, Taylor K, and Mohr D. Oral opioid therapy for chronic peripheral and central neuropathic pain. New Engl J Med. 2003. 348: 1223–1232.

Roher Bley, C, Neiger-Aeschbacher G, Busato A, Schatzmann U. Comparison of perioperative racemic methadone, levo-methadone and dextromoramide in cats using indicators of post-operative pain. Vet Anaesth Analg. 2004. 31:175–82.

Sammarco JL, Conzemius MG, Perkowski SZ, Weinstein MJ, Gregor TP, Smith GK. Postoperative analgesia for stifle surgery: a comparison of intra-articular bupivacaine, morphine, or saline. Vet Surg. 1996. 25:59–69.

Sawyer D, Briggs S, Paul K. Antinociceptive effect of butorphanol/oxymorphone combination in cats (abstract). In Proceedings of the 5th International Congress of Veterinary Anesthesiology 1994, 161.

Sawyer DC, Rech RH. Analgesia and behavioral effects of butorphanol, nalbuphine, and pentazocine in the cat. 1987. J Am Anim Hosp Assoc. 23:438–446.

Sawyer DC, Rech RH, Durham RA, Adams T, Richter MA, Striler EL. Dose response to butorphanol administered subcutaneously to increase visceral nociceptive threshold in dogs. Am J Vet Res. 1991. 52:1826–30.

Schatzman U, Armbruster S, Stucki F, Busato A, Kohler I. Analgesic effect of butorphanol and levomethadone in detomidine sedated horses. J Vet Med A Physiol Pathol Clin Med. 2001. 48:337–42.

Scherkl R, Hashem A, Frey H-H. Apomorphine-induced emesis in the dog—routes of administration, efficacy, and synergism by naloxone. J Vet Pharmacol Ther. 1990. 13:154–158, 1990.

Schumacher, MA, Basbaum, AI, Way, WL. Opioid Analgesics & Antagonists in: Basic and Clinical Pharmacology. Katzung BG ed. New York, NY; McGraw Hill. 2004. 497–516.

Sellon DC, Monroe VL, Roberts MC, Papich MG. Pharmacokinetics and adverse effects of butorphanol administered by single intravenous injection or continuous intravenous infusion in horses. Am J Vet Res. 2001. Feb;62(2):183–9.

Sellon DC, Roberts MC, Blikslager AT, Ulibarri C, Papich MG. Effects of continuous rate intravenous infusion of butorphanol on physiologic and outcome variables in horses after celiotomy. J Vet Intern Med. 2004. 555–63.

Shah JC, Mason WD. Plasma codeine and morphine concentrations after a single oral dose of codeine phosphate. J Clin Pharmacol. 1990. 30:764–766.

Sheehy JG, Hellyer PW, Sammonds GE, Mama KR, Powers BE, Hendrickson DA, Magnusson KR. Evaluation of opioid receptors in synovial membranes of horses. Am J Vet Res. 2001. 62:1408–12.

Skarda RT, Tranquilli WJ. Local and regional anesthetic and analgesic techniques (in dogs, cats, horses, ruminants and swine). Chapters 20–23, pp. 561–682. In: Tranquilli WJ, Thurmon JC, Grimm KA. Lumb and Jones' Veterinary Anesthesia and Analgesia. Fourth Edition. Blackwell Publishing, 2007.

Sladky KK, Miletic V, Paul-Murphy J, Kinney ME, Dallwig RK, Johnson SM. Analgesic efficacy and respiratory effects of butorphanol and morphine in turtles. J Amer Vet Med Assoc. 2007. 230:1356–1362.

Smith LJ, Yu J K-A, Bjorling DE, Waller K. Effects of hydromorphone or oxymorphone, with or without acepromazine, on preanesthetic sedation, physiologic values, and histamine release in dogs. J Am Vet Med Assoc. 2001. 218:1101–1105.

Sneddon LU. The evidence for pain in fish: the use of morphine as an analgesic. Appl Anim Behav Sci. 2003. 83:153–162.

Sneddon LU, Braithwaite VA, Gentle MJ. Novel object test: examining nociception and fear in the rainbow trout. J Pain. 2003. 4:431–40.

Stalheim OHV. Flowers in the blood: Opium and veterinary medicine. J Am Vet Med Assoc. 1990. 197:1324–1325.

Stambaugh JE Jr, Lane C. Analgesic efficacy and pharmacokinetic evaluation of meperidine and hydroxyzine, alone and in combination. Cancer Invest. 1983. 1:111–7.

Stanway GW, Taylor PM, Brodbelt DC. A preliminary investigation comparing pre-operative morphine and buprenorphine for postoperative analgesia and sedation in cats. Vet Anaesth Analg. 2002. 29:29–35.

Steagall PVM, Carnicelli P, Taylor PM, Luna SPL, Dixon M, Ferreira TH. Effects of subcutaneous methadone, morphine, buprenorphine, or saline on thermal and pressure thresholds in cats. J Vet Pharmacol Ther. 2006. 29:531–537.

Steffey EP, Eisele JH, Baggot JD. Interactions of morphine and isoflurane in horses. Am J Vet Res. 2003. 64:166–75.

Stevens CW, Klopp AJ, Facello JA. Analgesic potency of mu and kappa opioids after systemic administration in amphibians. J Pharmacol Exp Ther. 1994. 269:1086–93.

Sturtevant FM, Drill VA. Tranquilizing drugs and morphine-mania in cats. Nature. 1957. 179:1253.

Takahama K, Shirasaki T. Central and peripheral mechanisms of narcotic antitussives: codeine-sensitive and –resistant coughs. Cough. 2007. 3:1–8.

Taylor PM Houlton JEF. Post-operative analgesia in the dog: a comparison of morphine, buprenorphine, and pentazocine. J Sm Anim Pract. 1984. 25:437–451.

Taylor PM, Robertson SA, Dixon MJ, Ruprah M, Sear JW, Lascelles BD, Waters C, Bloomfield M. Morphine, pethidine and buprenorphine disposition in the cat. J Vet Pharmacol Ther. 2001. 24:391–8.

Teppema LJ, Nieuwenhuijs D, Olievier CN, Dahan A. Respiratory depression by tramadol in the cat: involvement of opioid receptors. Anesthesiology. 2003. 98:420–7.

Thomasy SM, Slovis N, Maxwell LK, Kollias-Baker C. Transdermal fentanyl combined with nonsteroidal anti-inflammatory drugs for analgesia in horses. J Vet Internl Med. 2004. 18:550–554.

Tobin T, Combie J, Shults T. Pharmacology review: actions of central stimulant drugs in the horse II. J Equine Med Surg. 1979. 3:102–109.

Tuttle WW, Elliott HW. Electrographic and behavioral study of convulsants in the cat. Anesthesiology. 1969. 30:48–64.

Valverde A, Cantwell S, Hernandez J, Brotherson C. Effects of acepromazine on the incidence of vomiting associated with opioid administration in dogs. Vet Anaesth Analg. 2004. 31:40–5.

Vatner SF, Marsh JD, Swain JA. Effects of morphine on coronary and left ventricular dynamics in conscious dogs. J Clin Invest. 1975. 55:207–17.

Walker AF. Sublingual administration of buprenorphine for long-term analgesia in the horse. Vet Rec. 2007. 160:808–809.

Wegner K, Robertson SA, Kollias-Baker C, Sams RA, Muir WW. Pharmacokinetic and pharmacodynamic evaluation of intravenous hydromorphone in cats. J Vet Pharmacol Ther. 2004. 27:329–36.

Wegner K, Robertson, SA. Dose-related thermal antinociceptive effects of intravenous hydromorphone in cats. Vet Anaesth Analg. 2007. 34:132–8.

Weinstein SH, Gaylord JC. Determination of oxycodone in plasma and identification of a major metabolite. J Pharm Sci. 1979. 68: 527–8.

Welch JA, Wohl JS, Wright JC. Evaluation of postoperative respiratory function by serial blood gas analysis in dogs treated with transdermal fentanyl. J Vet Emerg Crit Care. 2002. 12:81–87.

Wells S, Papich MG, et al. Pharmacokinetics of butorphanol in cats after intramuscular injection and buccal mucosal administration. 2008, *in press.*

Wikler A, Altschul S. Effects of methadone and morphine on the electroencephalogram of the dog. J Pharmacol Exp Ther. 1950. 98:437–46.

Yassen A, Olofsen E, Dahan A, Danhof M. Pharmacokinetic-pharmacodynamic modeling of the antinociceptive effect of buprenorphine and fentanyl in rats: role of receptor equilibration kinetics. J Pharmacol Exp Ther. 2005. 313:1136–49.

Yeh SY, Chernov HI, Woods LA. Metabolism of morphine by cats. J Pharm Sci. 1971. 60:469–71.

Yeh GC, Tao PL, Chen JY, Lai MC, Gao FS, Hu CL. Dextromethorphan attenuates morphine withdrawal syndrome in neonatal rats passively exposed to morphine. Eur J Pharmacol. 2002. 453:197–202.

Yeung JC, Rudy TA. Sites of antinociceptive action of systemically injected morphine: involvement of supraspinal loci as revealed by intracerebroventricular injection of naloxone. J Pharmacol Exp Ther. 1980. 215:626–32.

Yoshida S, Ohta J, Yamasaki K, Kamei H, Harada Y, Yahara T, Kaibara A, Ozaki K, Tajiri T, Shirouzu K. Effect of surgical stress on endogenous morphine and cytokine levels in the plasma after laparoscopic or open cholecystectomy. Surg Endosc. 2000.14:137–40.

Yoshimura K, Horiuchi M, Konishi M, Yamamoto K. Physical dependence on morphine induced in dogs via the use of miniosmotic pumps. J Pharmacol Toxicol Methods. 1993. 30:85–95.

CHAPTER

13

SEDATIVE AGENTS: TRANQUILIZERS, ALPHA-2 AGONISTS, AND RELATED AGENTS

LYSA P. POSNER AND PATRICK BURNS

PHENOTHIAZINE DERIVATIVES

GENERAL PHARMACOLOGIC CONSIDERATIONS

History/Introduction. Phenothiazines have been used in veterinary medicine since the 1950s as tranquilizers, but the class originally was used as an antipsychotic drug for the treatment of schizophrenia. The term *neuroleptic* was first used to describe the effects of phenothiazines on the central nervous system, although the term *major tranquilizer* is still used. The most commonly used phenothiazine in veterinary medicine is acepromazine (ACP).

Classification. Sedatives/Hypnotics/Anxiolytics, α-adrenergic antagonists.

Chemistry. Phenothiazine derivative.

How Supplied

Acepromazine 10 mg/ml

Promazine Granules: 27.5 mg/g

Mechanism of Action. Phenothiazines inhibit central dopaminergic receptors (D2), which produces sedation and tranquilization. Dopamine receptors are included in the family of G-protein–coupled receptors. Dopamine acts as a first messenger by interacting with the receptor proteins of the postsynaptic membrane. This interaction results in transduction of the signal by a guanine nucleotide-binding regulatory protein (G protein) to an appropriate intracellular effector system, or second messenger. Five mammalian dopamine receptor subtypes have been described and they are further subtyped as D1 and D2 based on their ability to inhibit or enhance adenylyl cyclase activity (Lachowicz 1997). Peripherally, the phenothiazines block norepinephrine at alpha adrenergic receptors.

Indications. Phenothiazines are commonly administered for general sedation. They are commonly used perianesthetically to reduce anxiety, reduce induction and maintenance drugs doses, and contribute to more balanced anesthesia. Phenothiazines are commonly administered with opioids (e.g., morphine) to produce *neuroleptic analgesia*; the combination produces synergic effects of each class (i.e., greater sedation and greater analgesia).

Phenothiazines can also prevent nausea and vomiting and some have antihistamine properties.

Pharmacodynamic Effects

CNS. All phenothiazines exert a sedative action by depressing the brain stem and connections to the cerebral cortex, but they may vary in potency and duration of action. The sedative effect does not appreciably affect coordinated motor responses, and arousal is easily accomplished. All phenothiazines decrease spontaneous motor activity in animals. Extrapyramidal symptoms (rigidity, tremor, akinesia) are also observed as side effects of phenothiazines in animals administered high doses.

Many textbooks and formularies consider phenothiazines, and particularly acepromazine, contraindicated for patients with seizure histories; however, there is little scientific evidence to support this, and a recent retrospective has disputed this and has even suggested that acepromazine may be anticonvulsant (Tobias et al. 2006).

Cardiovascular. In addition to blockade of the central effect of catecholamines (e.g., dopamine), phenothiazines are known to block peripheral actions of catecholamines. Alpha-adrenergic receptors are blocked by phenothiazine derivatives, which results in peripheral vasodilation. The vasodilation often produces arterial hypotension, and may induce shocklike conditions. Healthy animals show mild changes to arterial blood pressure; however, the hypotensive effects may be exaggerated in patients that are anesthetized, debilitated, or hypovolemic. Vasoconstrictors, such as phenylephrine, antagonize the hypotensive effects of phenothiazines (Ludders et al. 1983). Phenothiazines should be used cautiously with regional (epidural and intrathecal) anesthetic procedures because they potentiate the arterial hypotensive effects of local anesthetics.

Sedation and decrease in catecholamines generally result in a lowered heart rate, although a mild reflex tachycardia can be seen in patients with clinical hypotension. Phenothiazines prevent epinephrine-induced ventricular fibrillation during use of halogenated anesthetics (e.g., halothane) (Muir 1975).

Respiratory. Clinical doses of phenothiazines ordinarily have little effect upon respiratory activity. Respiratory rate is often depressed, but minute volume remains normal (i.e., no change in CO_2). However, respiratory depression may be seen or exaggerated when phenothiazines are administered with other CNS or respiratory depressants (e.g., opioids, isoflurane) or when used at high doses.

Musculoskeletal. Phenothiazines provide good muscle relaxation and are often used in conjunction with anesthetics that do not provide muscle relaxation or that result in muscle rigidity (e.g., ketamine). The phenothiazine, acepromazine, has been shown to decrease the incidence of malignant hyperthermia in pigs (see species differences).

Pharmacokinetics and Metabolism. Phenothiazines have a large volume of distribution (Vd) and are highly protein bound. In the horse, acepromazine has Vd = 6.6 l/kg and is >99% protein bound (Ballard 1982). Time to clinical effect is generally ~15 minutes after IV administration and ~30 minutes after IM administration. Phenothiazines are long acting in most species; elimination half-life is 3.1 hr in the horse and 7.1 hr in the dog (Ballard 1982; Hasham et al. 1992). Phenothiazines undergo extensive hepatic metabolism and metabolites are excreted in the urine (Maylin 1978). Bioavailability in dogs after oral administration is ~20% (Hasham et al. 1992).

Miscellaneous

Thermoregulation: Phenothiazines alter thermoregulation by decreased catecholamine binding in the hypothalamus (where thermoregulation is controlled centrally) as well as by altering vasomotor tone in the peripheral vessels that participate in heat retention and elimination. Following administration, patients should not be exposed to extreme temperature fluctuations for at least 8 hr.

Platelet aggregation: Acepromazine has been shown to decrease platelet aggregation (Barr et al. 1992). At clinically relevant doses the decrease in aggregation did not change coagulation times, however, acepromazine should be used with caution in patients with any coagulopathy or thrombocytopenia.

Hematocrit: Phenothiazines markedly reduce the hematocrit of animals. The decrease in packed-cell volume (PCV) by phenothiazines is due to splenic sequestration of red blood cells as well as translocation of fluids in response to hypotension. Blood samples drawn from phenothiazine-treated animals for diagnostic purposes should be interpreted accordingly.

Antiemetic: Phenothiazines are antiemetic, presumably from the blockade of dopamine receptors in the chemoreceptor trigger zone within the medulla (DiChiara 1978).

Phototoxicity: Experimental phototoxicity can be induced in laboratory animals following administration of chlorpromazine in the presence of black-light irradiation (Akin 1979). Although phototoxic reactions in animals do not appear to be an important clinical problem, those with scanty hair and white hair probably should not receive excessive exposure to sunlight during treatment with phenothiazines.

Analgesia. Phenothiazine derivatives have little or no analgesic activity. Tranquilization must be supplemented with analgesics and/or general anesthetics to block nociceptive responses during painful procedures.

PHENOTHIAZINES USED IN VETERINARY PRACTICE

Many phenothiazines are used to treat psychiatric problems in people and animals. The following sections discuss the three phenothiazines that are currently used in veterinary medicine to produce sedation.

ACEPROMAZINE MALEATE

Synonyms: Acetylpromazine, Vetranquil, Plegicil, Acepromazina, Acetopromazine, Azepromazine, Atsetozin, Notensil, Plivafen, Anergan, ACE, ACP; IUPAC Name: but-2-enedioic acid; 1-[10-(3-dimethylaminopropyl)phenothiazin-2-yl]ethanone (Fig. 13.1).

Acepromazine is the most commonly used phenothiazine in veterinary medicine. It is supplied in a yellow aqueous solution and in tablet form.

PROMAZINE HYDROCHLORIDE

Synonyms: 10H-Phenothiazine-10-propanamine, N,N-dimethyl-Dimethyl(3-phenothiazin-10-ylpropyl)amine (Fig. 13.2).

Promazine is phenothiazine similar to acepromazine. It is currently rarely used in the parenteral form, but is more popular as a granular oral medication that is mixed with feed.

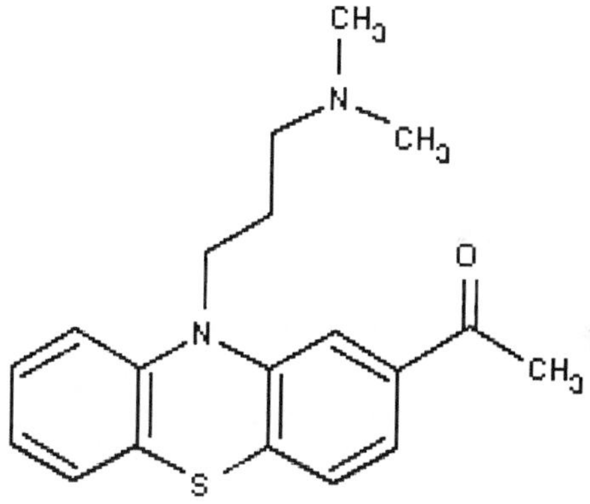

CH_3 N CH_3 O CH_3 N S

FIG. 13.1 Acepromazine.

CH_3 H_3C N N S

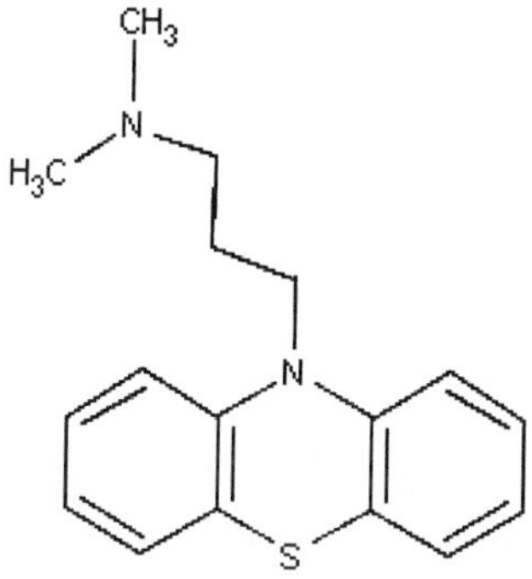

FIG. 13.2 Promazine.

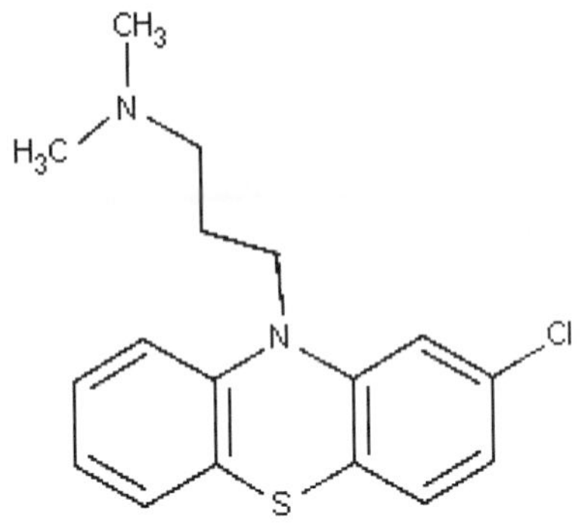

FIG. 13.3 Chlorpromazine.

CHLORPROMAZINE HYDROCHLORIDE

Synonym: IUPAC Name: 3-(2-chlorophenothiazin-10-yl)-N,N-dimethyl-propan-1-amine (Fig. 13.3).

Chlorpromazine is primarily used as an antiemetic in dogs and cats, but is occasionally used as a preanesthetic sedative. It is generally contraindicated for use with horses, due to a high incidence of ataxia and altered mentation.

Dose:

Acepromazine

Dogs and cats:
- 0.01 to 0.1 mg/kg IV, IM or SQ
- 0.5–2.0 mg/kg PO q 6–8 hrs

Horses:
- 0.01 to 0.05 mg/kg IV, IM or SQ

Swine:
- 0.03–0.2 mg/kg IV, IM, SQ

Cattle:
- 0.01–0.1 mg/kg IV, IM, SQ

Sheep and goats:
- 0.05–0.1 mg/kg

Rabbits:
- 1 mg/kg IM

Promazine

Dogs and cats:
- 2.2–4.4 mg/kg IV, IM

Horses:
- 0.44–1.1 mg/kg IV, IM
- Granules: 1–2 mg/kg PO (mixed in feed)

Cattle:
- Granules: 1.5–2.75 mg/kg PO (mixed in feed)

Chlorpromazine

Dogs and cats:
- 0.55–2.0 mg/kg IV, IM

Cattle:
- 0.2 mg/kg IM

Swine:
- 1.1 mg/kg IM

Species Differences

Horse: Phenothiazines have been associated with prolonged paraphimosis (penile prolapse) in the horse, particularly in stallions. Routine sedative doses are generally associated with paraphimosis, which generally resolves within 30 minutes. However, in some horses prolapse can remain for greater than 100 minutes causing swelling, trauma, and failure to retract normally. Anecdotal reports suggest pathologic paraphimosis does not occur when total dose does not exceed 10 mg/horse. It is generally recommended to not administer phenothiazines to breeding animals.

Chlorpromazine is not recommended in horses due to extreme ataxia and altered mentation.

Dog: Anecdotal reports suggest that a familial line of boxer dogs have an exaggerated reaction to the phenothiazine, acepromazine. In those dogs, sedation and hypotension are greater than expected and there have been reports of syncopal episodes presumably from hypotension. Aggressive treatment of hypotension has resulted in full recoveries. Therefore acepromazine may be avoided altogether in boxer dogs or used at much reduced doses.

Dogs with high vagal tone (bulldogs, boxers) have anecdotally been reported to have greater morbidity and mortality when administered acepromazine, presumably due to the adrenergic blocking effects of the drug. Similar recommendations for avoidance or reduced dosages have been made.

Pig: Acepromazine in IM doses of 1.1 and 1.65 mg/kg, respectively, prevents occurrence of halothane-induced malignant hyperthermia in 40% and 73% of susceptible pigs (McGrath 1981).

Drug Interactions. All phenothiazines should be used cautiously with any drugs that also produce vasodilation or hypotension.

All phenothiazines when administered with other CNS depressants can produce exaggerated CNS depression. Doses of one or both drugs may need to be reduced.

Overdose/Acute Toxicity. The phenothiazines have very high therapeutic index, particularly when used in conscious (nonanesthetized) animals (Stoelting 1999).

Dogs that received more than 100 times the recommended oral dose had no fatalities (Plumb 1999). This safety margin is diminished in anesthetized patients where many protective reflexes are attenuated.

Contraindications. Phenothiazines should not be used in patients that are dehydrated, hypovolemic, bleeding, or in shock because of the drugs' effect on vessel tone (vasodilation). Phenothiazines should not be used in patients with coagulopathies or thrombocytopenia due to their effect on platelet aggregation (see above). Phenothiazines should be used cautiously in boxer dogs, brachiocephalic dogs, breeding stallions, and debilitated animals.

Regulatory Information

Controlled Drug Status. Not controlled.

Withdrawal Times. No withdrawal times for the dog, cat, or horse; however, phenothiazines are not to be used in horses intended for human consumption.

Veterinary Products

Acepromazine

Acepromazine is approved by the FDA for use in dogs, cats, and horses.

Acepromazine Maleate Injection 10 mg/ml (Boehringer Ingelheim Vetmedica, Inc.)

Acepromazine Maleate 10 or 25 mg Tablets (Boehringer Ingelheim Vetmedica, Inc.)

Acepromazine Maleate Injection 10 mg/ml (IVX Animal Health, Inc.)

PromAce® Injectable 10 mg/ml (Fort Dodge Animal Health, Division of Wyeth)

PromAce® 5, 10, or 25 mg Tablets (Fort Dodge Animal Health, Division of Wyeth)

Promazine

Promazine is approved by the FDA for use in dogs, cats, and horses.

Promazine HCl Injectable 50 mg/ml (Fort Dodge Animal Health, Division of Wyeth)

Promazine HCl granules; 10.25 oz containers: 27.5 mg/gram (Fort Dodge)

Chlorpromazine

Chlorpromazine is used off-label in veterinary patients.

Human Products

Chlorpromazine

Chlorpromazine Hydrochloride Concentrate; Oral 100 mg/ml (Actavis Mid Atlantic)

Chlorpromazine Hydrochloride Injectable; Injection 25 mg/ml (Baxter Hlthcare)

Thorazine: Chlorpromazine Hydrochloride Syrup; Oral 10 mg/5 ml (Glaxosmithkline)

α_2-ADRENERGIC AGONISTS

GENERAL PHARMACOLOGIC CONSIDERATIONS

History/Introduction. The veterinary use of α_2-adrenergic agonists was first reported in the late 1960s (Clarke and Hall 1969) and revolutionized sedation and anesthesia particularly with large animals. Alpha-2-adrenergic agonists produce profound sedation, provide chemical restraint, and produce analgesia. Furthermore, α_2-adrenergic agonists reduce drug tolerance and act synergistically with opioids. Administration of alpha-2 agonists can be parenteral; intramuscular, and intravenous, as well as transdermal and neuraxial. Commonly used alpha-2 agonists in veterinary medicine include xylazine, detomidine, and medetomidine. The adrenergic agonists, which include the alpha-2 agonists, are also discussed in Chapters 5 and 6.

Classification. Alpha-2-adrenergic agonists are major tranquilizers that also possess significant analgesic properties and suppress the neuroendocrine stress response.

Chemistry. The basic structure of the alpha-2-adrenergic agonist is a benzene ring, which is attached to a dihydro-imidazole ring via either a hydrocarbon or amine cross-linkage. Xylazine is the only α_2-adrenergic agonist in clinical use that is not an imidazoline receptor ligand but has a thiazole ring instead of the dihydro-imidazole ring. One of the nitrogen atoms is substituted for a sulphur atom. The difference in receptor affinities between the different ligands is due to the degree of methylation of the benzene ring and halogenation of the dihydro-imidazole ring. The receptor selective affinities in Table 13.1 are based on the relative bindings of different ligands in the rat brain (Virtanen et al. 1988). The interaction between the hydroxyl substituted groups found on α_2-adrenergic agonists and the repositioning of the transmembrane helices of the α_2-adrenergic receptor determines the stability of the receptor/G-protein complex and therefore of agonist efficacy (Tian et al. 2000).

TABLE 13.1 Ratio of drug selectivity

Compound	$\alpha_2:\alpha_1$ Selectivity	I_2-Imidazoline Activity
Agonists		
Xylazine	160	No
Clonidine	220	Yes
Detomidine	260	Yes
Romifidine		Yes
Medetomidine	1620	Yes
Dexmedetomidine		Yes
Antagonists		
Idazoxan	27	Yes
Tolazoline		Yes
Yohimbine	40	No
Atipamezole	8526	No

TABLE 13.2 CNS anatomical location of alpha2-adrenoceptor subtypes

α_2-Adrenoceptor Subtype	Anatomical Location in the Central Nervous System
A	Brain
	Concentrated in the locus coeruleus but is also found in brainstem, cerebral cortex, septum, hypothalamus, hippocampus, and amygdala
	Spinal cord
	Central terminals of the nociceptive primary afferent fibers
B	Thalamus
C	Brain
	Basal ganglia, olfactory tubercle, hippocampus, cerebral cortex
	Spinal cord
	Axonal endings of the excitatory interneurons in the dorsal horn or lateral spinal nucleus
D (species variant of the human subtype A)	Brain stem of sheep
	Spinal cord

How Supplied. All the α_2-adrenergic agonists described come in an injectable form of varying strengths (see "Veterinary-Approved Products" below). Clonidine is the only drug that comes in oral and ophthalmic preparations as well as a transdermal patch. There is also a commerically available clonidine preparation for neuraxial administration.

Mechanism of Action. Alpha-2-adrenergic agonists exert their mechanism of action on the α_2-adrenergic and/or imidazoline receptors (Bousquet 1999; Head 1999). Anatomical locations of the α_2-adrenergic and imidazoline receptors are summarized in Table 13.2. The α_2-adrenergic receptors are classified into three main subtypes A, B and C, based on receptor cloning. The subtype D is considered a species variant of the human subtype A (Badino 2005; Calzada 2001).

The major sedative and analgesic effects of the α_2-adrenergic agonists are mediated via the activation of the α_{2A}-adrenergic receptor subtype found in the locus coeruleus (Scheinin and Schwinn 1992) and spinal cord (Lawhead 1992) (Table 13.2). These α_2-adrenergic receptors have seven transmembrane domains and are part of the serpentine class of receptors (Khan 1999). The third and fourth transmembrane domains appear to be the most important in determining receptor binding for the α_{2A}-adrenergic receptor (Matsui et al. 1989). In general these receptors are linked to G proteins that initiate the intracellular effector mechanism. These effector mechanisms will vary depending upon which G protein is activated. The activation of the α_2-adrenergic receptor will inhibit the positive feedback mechanism for the release of norepinephrine from the presynaptic nerve endings by reducing calcium conductance at N-type calcium channels (Cormack 2005). The attenuation of norepinephrine decreases arousal (causes sedation) and inhibits the afferent pain pathway.

The α_2-adrenergic agonists also have some agonistic activity on the α_1-adrenergic receptor. It is this action on the α_1-adrenergic receptor that causes some of the attenuation of effect mediated by the α_2-adrenergic receptors and many of the adverse side effects and possibly some of the paradoxical behavior seen. The ratio of α_2-adrenergic receptor binding to α_1 receptor binding is often denoted as $\alpha_2:\alpha_1$ ratio. Drugs with a high $\alpha_2:\alpha_1$ ratio are more specific for the sedative and analgesic effects of this class of drugs (Table 13.1).

Imidazoline receptors appear to play a major role in mediating the central hypotension and antiarrhythmogenesis of α_2-adrenergic agonists. Xylazine is not considered an imidazoline receptor agonist. Imidazoline receptors have not been reported to have any role in the development of sedation or anesthesia.

Indications. The α_2-adrenergic agonists are major tranquilizers that are used in veterinary patients for sedation, chemical restraint, and analgesia. Xylazine is also used as an emetic in feline patients.

General Pharmacodynamic Effects

CNS. Alpha-2 agonists produce profound reliable sedation by activation of receptors in locus coeruleus nucleus located in the brainstem (Scheinin et al. 1992). Different species react differently to alpha-2 agonists and these differences are due to different α_2-adrenergic receptor subtypes in the CNS. Ruminants, most notably, have α_{2D}-adrenergic receptors (Schwartz and Clark 1998), which makes them particularly sensitive to the sedative effects of α_2-adrenergic agonists (Scheinin et al. 1992).

The duration of the sedation and level of analgesia are dose-dependent. Smaller doses produce moderate sedation of a shorter duration while higher doses can produce profound sedation of a longer duration.

Activation of α_1-adrenergic receptors in the CNS will cause arousal, agitation, increased locomotor activity, and vigilance (Sinclair 2003). Although this is not a wanted effect, it explains why, in some animals, or with some drugs that have more α_1 receptor activity, an animal may show paradoxical excitement or movement.

Selective and nonselective α_2-adrenergic agonists show profound anesthetic sparing effects with both induction agents and inhalant agents (MAC-sparing of up to 90%) (Vickery 1989; Kauppila et al. 1992; Kuusela 2003; Savola 1991).

The α-2 agonist, medetomidine, does not raise intracranial pressure during isoflurane anesthesia in the dog (Keegan et al. 1995), and other α-2 agonists are routinely used in people with CNS disease to provide anxiolysis and blood pressure stabilization, minimize the sudden increases in intracranial pressure during the recovery period, and reduce postoperative opioids, which minimizes cerebral vasodilation caused by hypercapnia (Cormack 2005). Dexmedetomidine did not alter intracranial hemodynamics (e.g., cerebral blood flow) in patients with head trauma (Grille et al. 2005). The α-2 agonists, clonidine (Hoffman et al. 1991) and dexmedetomidine, (Hoffman 1991b) have been shown to improve neurologic outcome from incomplete cerebral ischemia models used in the rat and rabbit. Caution should be used in patients with CNS disease where vomiting is common, such as in cats administered xylazine, because vomiting can increase intracranial pressure.

In normotensive, nonglaucomatous dogs, intravenous medetomidine caused miosis and had little effect on intraocular pressure (Verbruggen et al. 2000). No change in intraocular pressure was seen in horses sedated with detomidine (Komaromy et al. 2006). The use of α_2-adrenergic agonists in animals suffering from ocular disease, needs to be done cautiously due to the propensity for vomiting or the lowering of the head in sedated large animals which can cause an increase in intraocular pressure (Komaromy et al. 2006).

Cardiovascular. Alpha-2-adrenergic agonists produce a biphasic cardiovascular response, which is due to differences in the centrally and peripherally mediated responses. Both the α_2-adrenergic and imidazoline receptors are involved in the centrally mediated effects of the α_2-adrenergic agonists (Bousquet 1999; Head 1999).

In the initial phase, activation of central α-2-adrenergic receptors reduce the sympathetic outflow (decreased norepinephrine) and thereby increase the parasympathetic tone, which will result in negative inotropic, chronotropic, and dromotropic effects on the heart as well as peripheral vasodilation. First- and second-degree atrioventricular heart block is commonly seen during this initial period. Peripherally, α-2- and α-1-adrenergic receptors are activated in the vascular endothelium, causing profound vasoconstriction. The increase in arterial blood pressure results in a baroreceptor-mediated reflex bradycardia. Most patients in this initial phase are hypertensive and bradycardic. During the second phase the heart rate remains low (likely due to decreased norepinephrine) despite the systemic vascular resistance decreasing (diminished effect at the peripheral α-2- and α-1-adrenergic receptors in the vasculature) (Bloor et al. 1992). This suggests a shift in the homeostasis set point of the baroreceptor reflex or inhibition of the baroreceptor reflex (Schmeling 1991). Patients during this phase may be hypotensive and bradycardic. The use of a selective peripheral α_2-adrenergic antagonist will nullify the initial vasoconstrictive effect; however, it does not reverse the long-term central effects of α_2-adrenergic agonists. These vasopressor effects are more intense if an intravenous bolus is used rather than the intramuscular route or a slow intravenous infusion (Dyck et al. 1993).

At therapeutic doses, alpha-2 agonists decrease cardiac output in most species by more than 50% (Pypendop 1998; Bueno 1999; Lamont 2001). Reduction in cardiac output is not only due to the baroreceptor reflex but also due to the concomitant reduction in stroke volume, increased afterload, low catecholamine levels, coronary vasoconstriction, and reduced myocardial oxygen consumption (Kuusela 2004). There appears to be a ceiling effect with the cardiovascular responses to α_2-adrenergic agonists (Kuusela 2000; Pypendop and Verstegen 2001; 1998), which occurs at the low end of the dosing range (~5 μg/kg of medetomidine) (Pypendop 1998). Higher doses produce more sedation and analgesia and increase the duration of action.

The use of anticholinergics prior to or at the same time as an α_2-adrenergic agonist is controversial as they will only partially prevent the decrease in cardiac output and increase the risk of dysrhythmia (Sinclair 2002) and hypertension (Bloor et al. 1992). Hypertension is more likely when the anticholinergic is administered during the initial vasoconstrictive phase than in the secondary hypotensive phase. Arrhythmias are more likely to occur when the anticholinergic is given after the cardiovascular effects (i.e., hypertension and bradycardia) are seen compared with prior to or concurrently with an alpha-2 agonist (Short 1991). Arrhythmias are likely due to increases in myocardial workload (increased heart rate and increased afterload) and oxygen consumption. Dexmedetomidine has been shown to be protective against the arrhythmogenic effects of the halothane-epinephrine interaction, and this protection is possibly due to decreased norepinephrine levels (Kamibayashi 1995). Alpha-1-adrenergic receptors have also been implicated in the formation of arrhythmias mediated via α_2-adrenergic agonists, especially with xylazine due to its relatively low $\alpha_2:\alpha_1$-adrenergic receptor affinity (Bozdogan and Dogan 1999).

Alpha$_2$-adrenergic agonists will redistribute blood flow from nonessential regions, such as the skin and visceral, to the central organs, such as the brain, heart, and kidneys (Lawrence 1996; Pypendop 1998).

Respiratory. Alpha-2-adrenergic agonists tend to cause a centrally mediated reduction in respiratory rate and minute ventilation, with no or with mild increases in $PaCO_2$ and mild reductions in PaO_2 (Kolliasbaker et al. 1993; Pypendop 1999; Sinclair 2002; Lerche 2004). The respiratory depression is not as great compared with other anesthetic drugs such as opioids (Sinclair 2003) or inhalational anesthetics (Bloor et al. 1989). Respiratory depression is exaggerated with the addition of other respiratory depressants or CNS depressants, which can result in respiratory acidosis, hypoxemia and cyanosis (Pypendop 1999; Vahavahe 1989). It is speculated that the cyanosis may also be due to slower blood flow through the peripheral capillary beds and an increased oxygen extraction (Sinclair 2003). It is therefore recommended to administer supplemental oxygen to animals, especially those that have received a combination of respiratory depressants.

The respiratory effects caused by α_2-adrenergic agonists appear to be somewhat species specific (Kastner 2006; Bloor et al. 1989). In sheep, xylazine can cause rapid increases in respiratory rate, airway pressures, and pulmonary elastance with slight changes in $PaCO_2$. Hypoxemia is frequently observed, culminating in fulminant pulmonary edema and death in some individuals (Celly et al. 1997). Within 3 minutes of administration, sheep have activation of pulmonary intravascular macrophages (PIM) that produce extensive damage to the capillary endothelium and alveolar type-I cells, intraalveolar hemorrhage, and interstitial and alveolar edema (Celly et al. 1997). These changes have also been observed after neuraxial administration of a lower dose of α_2-adrenergic agonists (Kinjavdekar 2006). Dexmedetomidine causes similar respiratory changes in the sheep and goat (Kutter 2006). Administration of an α_2-adrenergic antagonist reversed the sedation; however, the respiratory effects were not completely eliminated.

Musculoskeletal. Alpha-2-adrenergic agonists produce reliable muscle relaxation and are frequently administered for that effect and to balance drugs that do not provide good muscle relaxation (e.g., ketamine).

Muscle twitching has been noted in the dog with the use of several α_2-adrenergic agonists; however, this phenomenon disappears with intramuscular as opposed to intravenous administration (Sinclair 2003). Head bobbing and facial twitching has also been observed in the horse for a transient period after the administration of α_2-adrenergic agonists (Xylazine Package Insert 1988).

Dexmedetomidine with its sympatholysis, analgesia, and muscle-relaxing properties may prove to be a useful supportive therapy in tetanus. This muscle relaxation is mediated via its interaction with the interneurons in the spinal cord (Sinclair 2003).

Gastrointestinal. Alpha$_2$-adrenergic agonist (xylazine) may cause vomiting in up to 90% in cats and 30% in dogs (Cullen 1999). Xylazine acts on the area postrema in the cat to cause emesis. This appears to be a postsynaptic α_2-adrenergic receptor-mediated event, which can be antagonized by alpha-2 antagonist drugs yohimbine, tolazoline, and idazoxan (Jovanovic-Micic 1995).

Gastrointestinal motility and acid secretion is reduced and transit time is prolonged in a number of species, with the large bowel more sensitive to the effects of α_2-adrenergic agonists in ruminants, dogs, and horses (Sasaki 2000; Maugeri 1994). The depression in gastrointestinal motility can be reversed with the use of an alpha-2 antagonist.

Renal. Alpha-2-adrenergic agonists cause diuresis by multiple mechanisms. They reduce the production or release of antidiuretic hormone (ADH, arginine vasopressin) from the pituitary (Humphreys 1975; Reid 1979); inhibit the actions of ADH on the collecting tubules; and enhance the excretion of sodium (Gellai 1988; Smyth 1985a; Strandhoy 1982; Barr 1979). Renin levels are decreased by the direct activation of renal α_2-adrenergic receptors and indirectly by the initial hypertension produced by the α_2-adrenergic agonists (Smyth 1985b; Smyth 1987) further contributing to diuresis.

Alpha-2-adrenergic agonists also affect micturition by decreasing micturition pressure, bladder capacity, micturition volume, and residual volume via both spinal and peripherally mediated mechanism (Ishizuka et al. 1996). This combined with the diuresis will have animals produce large amounts of dilute urine that is frequently voided.

Endocrine Stress Response. The suppression of the stress response in association with anesthesia and surgery has been shown to decrease morbidity. Generally, α_2-adrenergic agonists cause a reduction in catecholamine levels, and suppresses the stress response in various species via their actions on both α_2-adrenergic and imidazoline receptors (Oharaimaizumi and Kumakura 1992). The combination of particular species and particular alpha-2 agonist results in differing effects on the neuroendocrine response. In the horse, detomidine will suppress catecholamine activity without suppressing cortisol activity (Raekallio et al. 1991), whereas in cattle, medetomidine will suppress catecholamine activity without suppressing cortisol activity (Ranheim et al. 2000). Interestingly, in the dog, clinical doses of medetomidine did not suppress cortisol levels (Ambrisko and Hikasa 2003). Dexmedetomidine is a potent inhibitor of steroidogenesis in the adrenal glands and therefore reduces cortisol production (Kharasch 1992).

Glucose. Xylazine causes a mild transient hyperglycemia. The effect of α_2-adrenergic agonists on glucose homeostasis is complex and depends on the species and which drug is being used. The hyperglycemia reported after the use of xylazine is due to a decrease in insulin release from the β cells and/or an increase glucagon release from the α cells (Angel 1990; Brockman 1981; Niddam 1990). Medetomidine causes a decrease in insulin without the resultant increase in glucose in dogs (Ambrisko and Hikasa 2003). Imidazoline receptors may play a role in the insulin suppression by activating ATP-sensitive K^+ channels in pancreatic β-cells (Jonas 1992). Both α_1- and α_2-adrenergic receptors have a role in the hyperglycemia seen after the administration of xylazine. Prazosin (α_1-adrenergic antagonist) was shown to attenuate this hyperglycemic response in cows. When hyperglycemia is present, it is rarely high enough to cause glucosuria.

Reproductive. The clinical effect of α_2-adrenergic agonists on uterine contractility and blood flow is influenced by the level of estrogen and progesterone. Estrogen leads to an up-regulation in α-adrenergic receptors while progesterone will cause a down-regulation. It appears that receptor numbers stay the same throughout the estrus cycle but there are changes to the transmembrane signal pathways that cause the differences in myometrial contractility (Re 2002). There have been case reports of cows going into premature labor after the administration of xylazine (Vanmetre 1992). Low doses of detomidine (<60 µg/kg IM) in the cow and horse and medetomidine (<20 µg/kg IV) in the dog, respectively, decreased myometrial contractions (Jedruch 1986; Jedruch 1989a; Jedruch 1989b). Higher doses of medetomidine in the dog did cause an increased myometrial contraction (Jedruch et al. 1989). Myometrial contractions in the nongravid uterus were observed at any equipotent dose of an α_2-adrenergic agonist (Jedruch 1989b; Schatzmann 1994). This biphasic response of the gravid uterus to α_2-adrenergic agonists may possibly be mediated by their effect on the α_1-adrenergic receptor (Ford 1995; Gaspar 2001; Kolarovszki-Sipiczki 2007).

The effects of medetomidine (40 µg/kg IM) (Sakamoto 1997) and xylazine (200 µg/kg IM) (Sakamoto 1996) on intrauterine pressure and uterine blood flow have been studied in the goat. Both agents crossed the placenta, reduced uterine blood flow for 120 minutes, and increased intrauterine pressure. The metabolic acidosis, mild hypoxemia and hypercapnia seen in the maternal circulation were also seen in the fetal circulation. These observations would suggest that the use of α_2-adrenergic agents in near-term pregnant animals be used with caution, especially if there is historical or physical evidence to suggest that fetal distress is already present.

Miscellaneous

Thermoregulation: Body temperature may fall in response to the administration of α_2-adrenergic agonists. This is presumed to be due to the CNS depression, reduction in muscle activity (reduction in shivering), and loss of vasomotor control. Clonidine and dexmedetomidine have been shown to decrease the vasoconstrictive and shivering thresholds (Talke et al. 1997). Animals may be cool to the touch and unable to thermoregulate their body temperature. Care must be taken during the recovery phase to prevent both cooling and overheating of these animals.

Equine recovery: The use of α_2-adrenergic agonists during the postoperative period following inhalant anesthesia of horses has been shown to improve the quality of the recovery and reduce the number of attempts to stand, at the expense of slightly prolonging the recovery period (Talke et al. 1997; Bienert 2003; Santos 2003). The dose of α_2-adrenergic agonists used during this postanesthesia period may be a little as 10–20% of the "usual" premedication dose (Santos et al. 2003).

Platelet activation: At very high doses, α_2-adrenergic agonists enhance catecholamine-potentiated platelet aggregation (Sjoholm 1992).

Analgesia. Alpha-2 agonists produce profound analgesia and can be administered parenterally and neuraxially (e.g., epidurally). Analgesia is produced by activation of alpha-2 receptors in the CNS in the locus coeruleus (Schwartz and Clark 1998) and in the substantia gelatinosa of the dorsal horn of the spinal cord (Hamalainen 1995; Savola 1996a; Kendig 1991; Savola 1990). There is also evidence to suggest that some of the analgesia is mediated via I_2-imidazoline receptors (Diaz 1997; Regunathan 2006) as imidazoline receptor agonist and antagonists can modulate the analgesia produced by morphine (Gentili 2006).

Alpha-2 agonists are synergistic with opioids, lidocaine and N-methyl D-aspartate (NMDA) receptor antagonists (e.g., ketamine) (Glynn and O'Sullivan 1996; Lee 1995; Regunathan 2006).

In people with tolerance to opioids, or chronic pain syndromes, α_2-adrenergic agonists are routinely used for rescue analgesia. A major limiting factor to using this class for analgesia is the concurrent sedation and ataxia.

Unwanted sedation can be minimized by administration of neuraxial α_2-adrenergic agonists. Epidural administration can produce potent analgesia with minimal sedative or cardiovascular effects compared with intravenous administration (Aminkov 1998; Greene 1995). The primary receptor subtypes found in the spinal cord are $\alpha_{2A/D}$ and α_{2C}. Due to the high lipophilicity of these drugs, there is some systemic absorption and systemic effect (e.g., sedation) after neuraxial administration. The use of α_2-adrenergic antagonists following neuraxially administered α_2-agonists can reduce the side effects while maintaining a good level of analgesia (Skarda 1990, 1991).

Pharmacokinetics Properties. The onset of action of most α_2-adrenergic agonists following intravenous administration is within minutes. Peak effect usually occurs within 10–15 minutes (Garcia-Villar et al. 1981; Pypendop and Verstegen 2001). Intramuscular administration of α_2-adrenergic agonists, will approximately double the time to peak effect; however, the bioavailability is variable (40–95%) depending upon the species (Kastner 2003; Garcia-Villar et al. 1981). Bioavailability of intramuscular xylazine in the horse and sheep is approximately 50% as compared to 75% in the dog (Garcia-Villar et al. 1981). Detomidine bioavailability was higher in the horse (66%) and cow (85%) following intramuscular administration (Salonen 1989). The onset of action of medetomidine in the cat appears to be slightly faster than in the dog, despite similar distributions and elimination rates. The bioavailability following intramuscular injection in both these species was close to 100% (Salonen 1989). The duration of action is probably the most significant difference between the α_2-adrenergic agonists. When evaluating equipotent doses of medetomidine and dexmedetomidine in the horse, it is interesting to note the differences in the elimination half-life in young ponies. The presence of the levomedetomidine prolongs the half life medetomidine (51 minutes) compared to dexmedetomidine (19 minutes) (Bettschart-Wolfensberger et al. 1999, 2005a). There also appears to be an age-related decrease in the elimination of dexmedetomidine in ponies; however, dexmedetomidine still has a shorter duration of action than medetomidine (for an overview of the pharmacokinetic parameters of the various α_2-adrenergic agonists in the common domestic species, see Table 13.3). There was no information available on the pharmacokinetics of romifidine in any species at the time of the writing of this chapter.

Interestingly, there is a lack of correlation between plasma levels and pharmacodynamic effects of medetomidine. Clinical effects can be seen for up to 7 hours despite

TABLE 13.3 Alpha2-adrenergic agonists pharmacokinetics

Drug	Species	Dose (mg/kg)	Mean Residence Time (mins)	Volume of Distribution (L/kg)	$Clearance_{Tot}$ (mL/kg/min)	Elimination Half-Life (mins)	Reference
Xyalzine							
	Dog	1.4 (IV)		2.52	81	30.1	(Garcia-Villar et al. 1981)
	Cat						
	Horse	0.6 (IV)		2.46	21	49.5	(Garcia-Villar et al. 1981)
	Cattle	0.2 (IV)		1.94	42	36.5	(Garcia-Villar et al. 1981)
	Sheep	1.0 (IV)		2.74	83	23.1	(Garcia-Villar et al. 1981)
Detomidine							
	Horse	0.08 (IV) [IM]		0.74 ± 0.25 [1.56]	7.1 ± 1.6 [10.1]	71.4 ± 16.2 [106.8]	(Salonen et al. 1989)
	Cattle	0.08 (IV) [IM]		0.73 ± 0.17 [1.89]	9.5 ± 1.9 [12.3]	79.2 ± 27 [153.6]	(Salonen et al. 1989)
Medetomidine							
	Dog	0.04 (IV)		1.28 ± 0.19	21.0 ± 7.3	57 ± 15	(Kuusela et al. 2000)
	Dog	0.08 (IV)		2.8	31.5	58.2	(Salonen 1989)
	Dog	0.08 (IM)		3.0	27.5	76.8	(Salonen 1989)
	Cat	0.08 (IM)		3.5	29.5	81	(Salonen 1989)
	Horse	0.007 (IV)	32.9 ± 7.21	2.2 ± 0.52	66.6 ± 9.9	51.3 ± 13.09	(Bettschart-Wolfensberger et al. 1999)
	Calf	0.04 (IV)	30.1 ± 4.0	1.75 ± 0.30	33.1 ± 5.5	44.4 ± 14.2	(Ranheim et al. 1998)
	Lactating dairy cows	0.04 (IV)	72.7 ± 30.7	1.21 ± 0.32	24.2 ± 6.5	52.7 ± 25.3	(Ranheim et al. 1999)
	Sheep	0.04 (IV)	37.2 ± 10	1.7 ± 0.26	44.2 ± 11.3	34.8 ± 7.3	(Ranheim et al. 2000)
	Sheep	0.03 (IM)	70 ± 17.4	3.9 ± 2.4	81.0 ± 21.5	32.7 ± 14.9	(Kastner et al. 2003)
Dexmedetomidine	Dog	0.02 (IV)		0.86 ± 0.22	20.1 ± 8.0	47 ± 14	(Kuusela et al. 2000)
	Young ponies	0.0035 (IV)				19.8 (28.9)	(Bettschart-Wolfensberger et al. 2005)
Levomedetomidine							
	Dog	0.02 (IV)		2.68 ± 0.57	67.8 ± 11.5	38 ± 18	(Kuusela et al. 2000)
Clonidine							
	Sheep	0.006 (IV)		~5 L		95	(Castro and Eisenach 1989)

the plasma levels being detectable for only 2 hours. This discrepancy implies either a long tissue-binding period or an active metabolite (Ranheim 1999, 2000a).

SPECIFIC ALPHA-2 AGONISTS

XYLAZINE HYDROCHLORIDE

Synonyms: Prestwick_962, Spectrum_001267, Xylazinum, Xilazina, Bay 1470, WH 7286; IUPAC Name: N-(2,6-dimethylphenyl)-5,6-dihydro-4H-1,3-thiazin-2-amine (Fig. 13.4).

Xylazine was the first α_2-adrenergic agonist used in veterinary medicine and its clinical use was first described in 1969 in a number of species (Clarke and Hall 1969; Keller 1969; Müller 1969). Xylazine is often thought of as the prototypical α_2-adrenergic agonist; however, it does have one of the lowest $\alpha_2:\alpha_1$ affinities (see Table 13.1) and does not bind to imidazoline receptors. This higher affinity for α_1-adrenergic agonists may account for some of the paradoxical aggression that may occasionally be seen with xylazine. It is also the least potent of any of the α_2-adrenergic agonists in clinical use. Cattle are particularly sensitive to the effects of xylazine and require approximately one-tenth the dose compared with other species. The dose rate of other α_2-adrenergic agonists in cattle is similar to that of other species. Conversely, swine require two to three times the dose of xylazine compared to the dog, cat, or horse. This species difference appears to be due to differences in G-protein signaling pathways rather than receptor subtype or receptor population (Torneke 2003). Xylazine is the alpha-2 agonist most likely to cause vomiting in the dog, whereas almost all alpha-2 agonists cause vomiting in cats (Jovanovic-Micic 1995; Hikasa 1992; Sinclair 2003).

Dose:

Dogs and cats:
  0.1–1 mg/kg IV, IM
Horses:
  0.02–1.0 mg/kg IV, IM
Bovine:
  0.01–0.1 mg/kg IV, IM
Ovine and Caprine (xylazine can induce respiratory distress (see “Respiratory”):
  0.05–0.2 mg/kg IV, IM
Cervidae (Deer):
  0.5–4 mg/kg IM

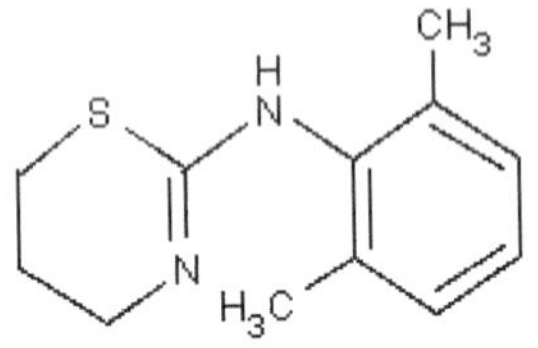

FIG. 13.4 Xylazine.

DETOMIDINE HYDROCHLORIDE

Synonyms: Detomidinum, Detomidina, 76631-46-4; IUPAC Name: 4-[(2,3-dimethylphenyl)methyl]-3H-imidazole (Fig. 13.5).

Detomidine is registered for use in the horse only; however, it is used in bovines and to a lesser degree in small ruminants (Singh 1994, 1991). It has a higher $\alpha_2:\alpha_1$ ratio than xylazine; however, the pharmacodynamic differences between the various α_2-agonists at equipotent doses are minimal except for the duration of action (England and Clarke 1996; Bueno 1999). Detomidine appears to have the longest duration of action (Yamashita 2000) and results in the longest duration of ataxia (Hamm 1995; England 1992). Although it has a long duration of action accompanied by ataxia, detomidine was one of the first α_2-adrenergic agonists to be administered as a constant rate infusion in horses for standing surgical procedures (Daunt 1993; Wilson 2002). Interestingly, when horses are stationary, they are less likely to weight-shift or lift their feet compared with horses sedated with xylazine.

Oral detomidine has been used with varying degrees of success in a number of species (Pollock 2003; Ramsay 2002; Grove 2000; Sleeman 1997). A combination of detomidine and ketamine administered orally in the cat proved more effective than a combination of ketamine and

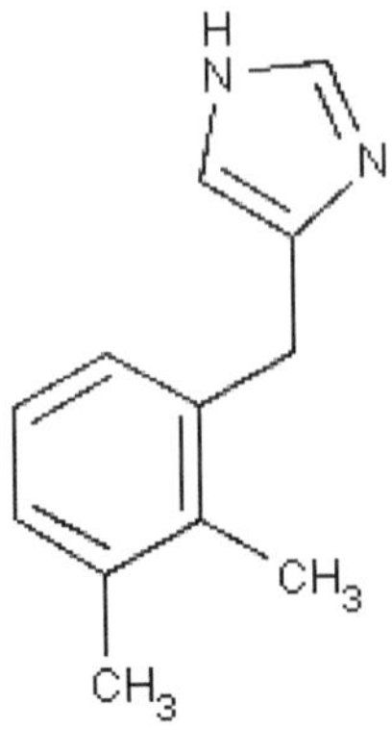

FIG. 13.5 Detomidine.

xylazine or medetomidine (Grove 2000). Oral detomidine in the horse produced maximal sedation 30 minutes post-administration (Ramsay 2002). There is limited information available about the use of detomidine in small animals (Jadon 1998).

Dose:

Horses:	Parenteral 5–40 μg/kg IV, IM
CRI:	Loading bolus 8.4 μg/kg IV
	1st 15 min 0.5 μg/kg/min IV
	2nd 15 min 0.3 μg/kg/min IV
	3rd 15 min 0.1 μg/kg/min IV
Oral:	60 μg/kg orally (Ramsay 2002)
Cats:	
Oral:	500 μg/kg detomidine + 10 mg/kg ketamine (Grove 2000)

MEDETOMIDINE HYDROCHLORIDE

Synonyms: Precedex, Domitor, Medetomidinum, Medetomidina, MPV-785, (RS)-4-(alpha,2,3-Trimethylbenzyl)imidazol; IUPAC Name: 4-[1-(2,3-dimethylphenyl)ethyl]-3H-imidazole (Fig. 13.6).

Medetomidine is a racemic mixture of two optical enantiomers, dexmedetomidine and levomedetomidine (1 : 1). The structure of these two enantiomers is a mirror image of each other, but each possesses different biological activity (Kuusela 2004). The active component of medetomidine is dexmedetomidine; however, medetomidine does not appear to have simply half the potency of dexmedetomidine (Kuusela 2000, 2001b). Levomedetomidine may act as a competitive inverse agonist against dexmedetomidine, resulting in a lower pharmacodynamic effect (Kuusela 2000, 2001b). Levomedetomidine, at clinical doses, has been shown to have little biological effect (Macdonald 1991; Savola 1991; Kuusela 2000), but has significant drug interactions and causes hepatic microsomal enzyme inhibition (Kharasch 1992; Pelkonen 1991).

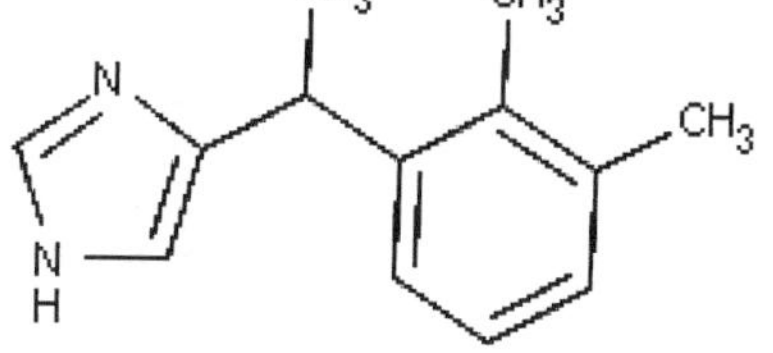

Medetomidine is used frequently to treat emergence delirium following anesthesia. Microdoses of 1–2 μg/kg are usually sufficient to quiet a patient and allow it to rest comfortably. Similarly, constant rate infusions of medetomidine have become popular in the ICU setting to provide similar sedation, anxiolysis, and analgesia.

Dose:

Dogs:	
Single injection:	1–20 μg/kg IV, IM
Constant rate infusion:	1–5 μg/kg/hour
Cats:	
Single injection:	1–40 μg/kg IV, IM
Constant rate infusion:	1–5 μg/kg/hour
Horses:	
Single injection:	2–10 μg/kg IV, IM
Constant rate infusion:	0.03–0.1 μg/kg/min

DEXMEDETOMIDINE

Synonyms: Dexmedetomidinum, Dexmedetomidina, MPV 1440; IUPAC Name: 4-[(1R)-1-(2,3-dimethylphenyl)ethyl]-3H-imidazole (Fig. 13.7).

Dexmedetomidine is the dextro-enantiomer of the racemate medetomidine. It has only recently (2007) been approved for use in the dog by the FDA. There appears to be a complex interaction between the dextro-enantiomer and levo-enantiomer to cause the resultant pharmacodynamic effects of the racemic mixture of medetomidine. Dexmedetomidine appears to be more potent than medetomidine.

Sedation and analgesia are similar to medetomidine; however, there is an apparent ceiling effect with sedation (Kuusela 2004).

Levomedetomidine appears to intensify the bradycardic effects of dexmedetomidine; therefore dexmedetomidine may be a safer preparation than medetomidine due to the higher heart rate and subsequent higher cardiac output (Kuusela 2004).

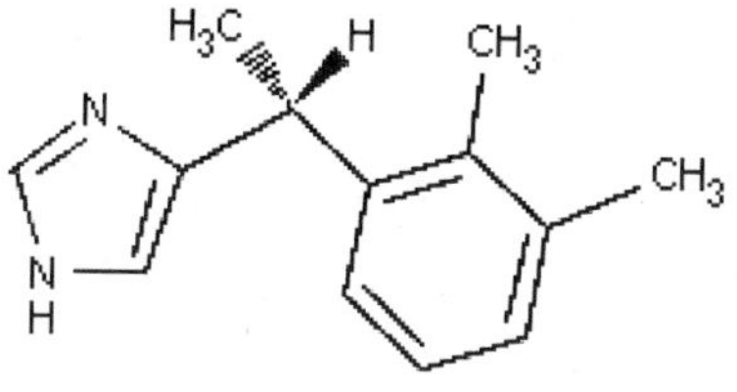

FIG. 13.6 Medetomidine.

FIG. 13.7 Dexmedetomidine.

Unlike other α_2-adrenergic agonists, dexmedetomidine does not inhibit ADH-induced increased permeability to urea in the medullary collecting tubules of rats (Rouch 2002).

Dose:

Dogs:
- Single injection: 1–20 µg/kg IM, IV
- Constant rate infusion: 0.5–3.0 µg/kg/hr IV (Pascoe 2006)

Cats:
- Single injection: 1–20 µg/kg IM, IV

ROMIFIDINE

Synonyms: Romifidinum, Romifidina, 2-(2-Bromo-6-fluoroanilino)-2-imidazoline, 65896-16-4; IUPAC Name: N-(2-bromo-6-fluoro-phenyl)-4,5-dihydro-1H-imidazol-2-amine (Fig. 13.8).

Romifidine is a more selective alpha-2 agonist than xylazine and in the horse produces less ataxia compared with equipotent doses of other α_2-adrenergic agonists (England 1992; Hamm 1995). Preoperative romifidine improved the quality of recovery in horses, (Jaugstetter 2002; Ramsay 2002), which may reflect the longer duration of action of romifidine compared to xylazine or less ataxia. Alpha-2-adrenergic agonist given during the anesthetic recovery period will prolong the recovery by approximately 10 to 15 minutes; however, it will result in fewer attempts to stand and a better quality of recovery (Bienert 2003; Santos 2003; Bettschart-Wolfensberger 2005b).

Romifidine causes similar cardiovascular depression in the cat (Selmi 2004; Selmi 2002) and dog (Sinclair 2002; Lemke 1999). There is a ceiling effect with respect to the cardiovascular changes induced by romifidine in the dog and horse (Freeman 2002; Pypendop 2001). A similar ceiling effect was reached for the level of sedation in the dog (<25–40 µg/kg IV) (Pypendop 2001).

The amount of analgesia romifidine produces in the horse is controversial, with some researchers finding no analgesic effects (Hamm 1995), while others have documented analgesia (Moens 2003; Spadavecchia 2005). Romifidine in the cat and dog has been shown to potentiate the effects of other anesthetic induction and inhalational agents (Gomez-Villamandos 2005; England 1997). Neuraxial romifidine potentiates the effects of epidural morphine and lidocaine (Kinjavdekar 2006; Fierheller 2004).

Dose:

Horses:
- Single injection: 40 to 120 µg/kg IV
- Constant rate infusion: 0.3 µg/kg/min IV (Kuhn 2004) MAC-sparing

Dogs:
- Single injection: 1–40 µg/kg IV

Cats:
- Single injection: 5–200 µg/kg IM

For the dog and cat, compared with xylazine (1 mg/kg): equipotent dose of romifidine in the cat is 200 µg/kg IM (Selmi 2004) and in the dog 40–60 µg/kg IV (England 1996; Lemke 1999).

CLONIDINE

Synonyms: Clonidine: Chlornidinum, Adesipress, Catarpresan, Catarpres, Clonidin, Duraclon, Catapresan, Catapressan, Catapres-TTS; IUPAC Name: N-(2,6-dichlorophenyl)-4,5-dihydro-1H-imidazol-2-amine) (Fig. 13.9).

In 1966, Clonidine was first identified as an antihypertensive agent (Frank 1966). Clonidine is classified as a partial agonist at the α_2-adrenergic receptor site (Tian 2000; Jasper 1998) and binds with both α_2-adrenergic and imidazoline receptors. The use of clonidine in veterinary medicine has increased recently with its use in neuraxial anesthesia and analgesia (DeRossi 2006). Like other α_2-adrenergic agonists it potentiates and prolongs the actions of lidocaine with an epidural blockade. Clonidine also has the potential for use as an adjunct analgesic therapy, especially with the transdermal preparations; further research

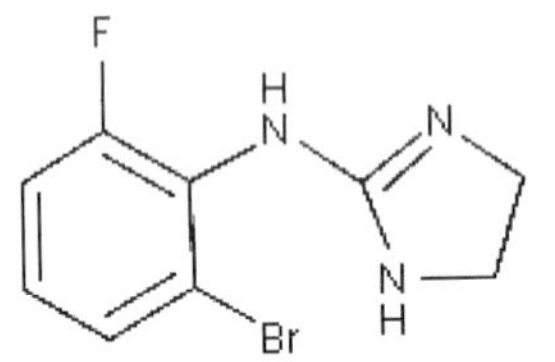

FIG. 13.8 Romifidine.

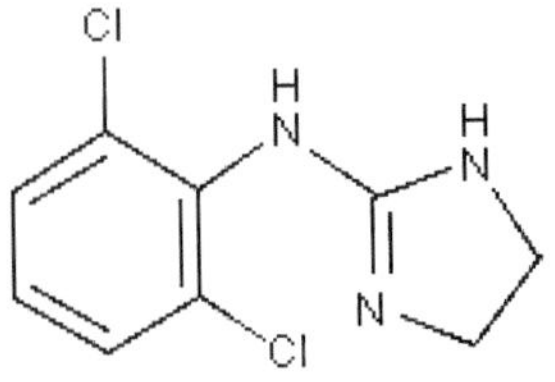

FIG. 13.9 Clonidine.

into this potential use needs to be undertaken (Dirikolu 2006).

Species Differences. There are species sensitivity differences to the α_2-adrenergic agonists. In general, from most sensitive to least sensitive are the following: bovine > camelids > small ruminants > cat, dog, and horse > porcine > small laboratory animals.

Cattle: Ruminants, most notably, have an α_{2D}-adrenergic receptor (Schwartz and Clark 1998), which makes them sensitive to the sedative effects of α_2-adrenergic agonists. In particular, cattle need ~1/10 the dose of xylazine compared with dogs.

Sheep: Xylazine causes the activation of pulmonary intravascular macrophages (PIM), which results in acute lung injury (see "Respiratory Effects").

Horse: Equipotent intravenous doses for sedation in the horse are considered as the following: xylazine (1 mg/kg), medetomidine (5–10 µg/kg), romifidine (40–80 µg/kg), and detomidine (20–40 µg/kg) (Bryant 1991; England 1992; Yamashita 2002).

Adverse Effects/Contraindications. It is possible to see sudden arousal from α2-adrenergic agonist–induced sedation that may proceed to aggression. Many individuals appear to be sensitive to sound and first touch (Clarke 1989). Ideally, agitated animals need to be allowed to calm down prior to the administration of α_2-adrenergic agonists.

Emesis is common with alpha-2 agonists in small animals and caution should be used with patients where vomiting is unwanted.

Alpha-2-adrenergic agonists should not be used in animals with compromised cardiac output, such as preexisting heart disease, especially those with bradydysrhythmia, poor myocardial contractility, obstructive valvular disease, dehydration, hypovolemia, or sepsis.

Caution should also be used in patients with diabetes mellitus. The decrease in insulin release and increase in glucose with this class of drug would also seem to preclude its use in diabetic patients until further investigations have taken place.

Drug Interactions. Alpha-2-adrenergic agonists potentiate the effects of other sedative agents, barbiturates, propofol, ketamine, etomidate, and inhalational agents due to their CNS depression and analgesic activity. The dosage of induction agents is greatly reduced and there is a profound MAC-sparing effect. The respiratory depression of α_2-adrenergic agonists is potentiated by other respiratory depressants, especially opioids. This combination is more likely to cause hypercapnia and hypoxemia compared to α_2-adrenergic agonists alone.

Overdose/Acute Toxicity. Treatment for the overdose of an α_2-adrenergic agonist is centered on the use of α_2-adrenergic antagonists titrated to effect. Careful monitoring of the cardiovascular system is required. Overzealous use of these antagonists may lead to full antagonism and adverse signs, as has been reported with the use of tolazoline in llamas (Read et al. 2000). Other supportive therapy may include external regulation of body temperature and monitoring of blood glucose levels.

Regulatory Information

Controlled Drug Status. Not controlled.

Withdrawal Times

Xylazine: Cattle: 4 days for meat; 24 hr milk
Detomidine: Cattle: 3 days meat; 72 hr milk

Veterinary Products

Medetomidine

Medetomidine is approved by the FDA for use in the dog.

Domitor®: Medetomidine HCl 1 mg/ml (Orion, Corp.)

Dexmedetomidine

Dexmedetomidine is approved by the FDA for use in the dog.

Dexdomitor®: Dexmedetomidine HCl 0.5 mg/ml (Orion, Corp.)

Detomidine

Detomidine is approved by the FDA for use in the horse.

Dormosedan™: Detomidine HCl 10 mg/ml (Orion, Corp.)

Romifidine

Romifidine is approved by the FDA for use in the horse.

Sedivet® 1% Injection: Romifidine HCl 10 mg/ml (Boehringer Ingelheim Vetmedica, Inc.)

Xylazine

Xylazine is approved by the FDA for use in the dog, cat, horse, and deer.

Rompun® Injectable: Xylazine HCl 20 mg/ml and 100 mg/ml (Bayer Healthcare LLC, Animal Health Division)

Anased® Injectable: Xylazine HCl 20 mg/ml and 100 mg/ml (Lloyd, Inc.)
Cervizine 300 Injectable: Xylazine HCl 300 mg/ml, (Lloyd, Inc.)
Xylazine HCl Injection 100 mg/ml (Boehringer Ingelheim Vetmedica, Inc.)

Clonidine

There are no veterinary-approved products for these drugs.

Human Products

Dexmedetomidine

Precedex® Injectable: Dexmedetomidine 100 μg/ml (Hospira, Inc.)

Clonidine

Duraclon: Clonidine Hydrochloride Injectable; Injection 0.1 mg/ml and 0.5 mg/ml (Xanodyne Pharm)
Catapres-Tts-1: Clonidine Film, Extended Release; Transdermal 0.1 mg/24 hr (Boehringer Ingelheim)
Clonidine Hydrochloride: Clonidine Hydrochloride Tablet; Oral 0.1 mg, 0.2 mg, 0.3 mg (Actavis Elizabeth)

α_2-ADRENERGIC ANTAGONISTS

GENERAL PHARMACOLOGIC CONSIDERATIONS

History/Introduction. Alpha-2-adrenergic receptor antagonists are used primarily in veterinary medicine to reverse the effects of the α_2-adrenergic agonists. The ability to reverse the α_2-adrenergic agonists increases their appeal for use, especially for the chemical restraint of exotic wildlife. Three antagonists are routinely available for use in veterinary medicine: yohimbine, atipamezole, and tolazoline.

Classification. Drugs in this class are all α_2-adrenergic receptor ligands that are competitive antagonists at the α_2-adrenergic receptor site. They all have varying degrees of antagonism at the α_1-adrenergic receptor site as well (Table 13.1). Tolazoline has the lowest affinity for all the α_2-adrenergic receptor subtypes A, B, C, and D, as compared to yohimbine and atipamezole. Tolazoline not only has activity on α_2-adrenergic and I_2-Imidazoline receptor sites (I_2-IR) but also has direct vasodilator effects (Lemke 1996) and histaminergic antagonistic activity (Tucker 1982). Yohimbine does have some activity on dopaminergic and serotonergic receptors but no activity on imidazoline receptors. It is moderately selective for the α_2 receptor with a binding ratio of 40:1 (Tranquilli 2007). Atipamezole is the most selective and specific for the α_2-adrenergic receptors with a binding ratio of 8526:1 (Tranquilli 2007). Atipamezole has very little activity on any other receptor class, unlike the other α_2-adrenergic antagonists.

Chemistry. Yohimbine (mw = 390.9 g/mol) is an alkaloid extracted from the bark of the *Pausinystalia yohimbe* tree and is found in a variety of botanical sources such as the Rauwolfia root (Tam 2001); it is chemically related to reserpine. Tolazoline (mw = 196.7 g/mol) and atipamezole (mw = 212.3 g/mol) are part of the imidazoline chemical family (Sargent 1994). Tolazoline is structurally related to phentolamine (α_1-adrenergic agonist). They are freely soluble in water or ethanol.

Alpha-2 agonists and antagonists are extraordinarily similar compounds; the difference between the cationic nitrogen and an aromatic ring plane, in the order of one angstrom, is what accounts for the differences between an α_2-adrenegic agonist and antagonist (Rouvinen 1993).

How Supplied

Yohimbine hydrochloride: Each ml contains 2.0 mg, methylparaben 0.9 mg, propylparaben 0.1 mg, citric acid 3.34 mg, and water for injection, pH-adjusted with sodium hydroxide. A higher strength formulation of yohimbine (5 mg/ml) is available for use in wildlife.

Tolazoline hydrochloride: Each ml contains equivalent to 100 mg base activity, chlorobutanol 5.0 mg, tartaric acid 7.8 mg, sodium citrate dihydrate 7.8 mg, and water for injection. The pH is adjusted with hydrochloric acid and sodium citrate. Tolazoline HCl injection is supplied as 100 mg/ml in a 100 ml multidose vial and should be protected from light.

Atipamezole: Atipamezole is supplied in 10 ml, multidose vials containing 5.0 mg of atipamezole hydrochloride per ml. Each ml of contains 5.0 mg atipamezole hydrochloride, 1.0 mg methylparaben (NF), 8.5 mg sodium chloride (USP), and water for injection

Mechanism of Action. Sedation, anxiolysis, analgesia, and the central and peripheral cardiovascular changes induced by α_2-adrenergic agonists are competitively inhibited by the α_2-adrenergic antagonists to varying degrees (Carroll 2005). Sedation may be reversed; however, there may be an incomplete reversal of the cardiovascular-induced changes (Lemke 2004; Hubbell 2006). The antagonism of the presynaptic α_2-adrenergic and I_2-imidazoline receptors blocks the negative feedback loop on the regulation of the norepinephrine release from the presynaptic nerve endings of the sympathetic nervous system (Gothert 1992; Molderings 1995).

Tolazoline is a nonselective α-adrenergic antagonist, which has more activity on the α_2-adrenergic receptor compared to the α_1-adrenergic receptor.

Yohimbine is a selective α_2-receptor antagonist with a specificity between tolazoline and atipamezole.

Atipamezole is the most specific α_2-adrenergic antagonist (Table 13.1) and is nonselective against the α_2-adrenergic receptor subtypes. It has approximately 100 times the affinity of the α_2-adrenergic receptor site compared to yohimbine (Schwartz 1998).

All three antagonists have the potential to cause CNS excitement and cardiovascular effects that include vasodilation and tachycardia. It is always recommended that α_2 receptor antagonist be given slowly and to effect to minimize these adverse effects. Alternatively, a fraction of the dose may be given slowly IV and the rest or all given IM to minimize side effects.

Indications. Alpha-2 receptor antagonists are routinely used to reverse the sedative or cardiovascular effect of alpha-2 agonist drugs. Generally, the antagonist with a similar specificity is chosen. For example, yohimbine is commonly reversed with yohimbine and medetomidine is reversed with atipamezole. In some species differences do exist. Cattle and small ruminants sedated with xylazine appear to have better reversal when treated with tolazoline compared with yohimbine.

Reversal of Analgesia. Abrupt and compete reversal of α_2-adrenergic agonists may lead to a sudden increase in sympathetic activity and nociception that may be deleterious as well as being inhumane. In various animal studies that used a sustained nociception model, the use of atipamezole to reverse the effects of α_2-adrenergic agonists increased the nociceptive response by blocking the norepinephrine feedback inhibition of the pain sensation (Pertovaara 2005). Following α_2 receptor antagonism, patients may be administered other analgesics such as opioids or NSAIDs.

YOHIMBINE

Synonyms: Yohimbine: Quebrachine, Quebrachin, Corynine, Yohimbin, Aphrosol, Johimbin, Aphrodine, (+)-Yohimbine, (+)-Yohimbin, (Fig. 13.10).

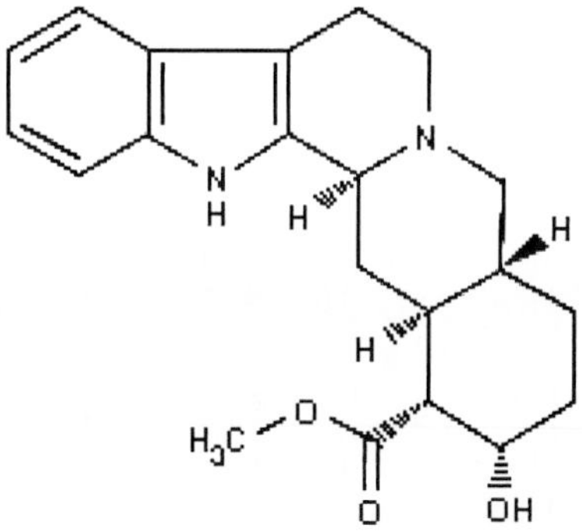

FIG. 13.10 Yohimbine.

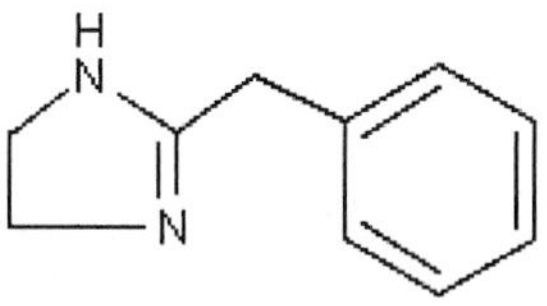

FIG. 13.11 Tolazoline.

Yohimbine is a moderately selective α_2-receptor antagonist. It is most commonly used to reverse the effects of the α_2 agonist xylazine in dogs, cats, horses, and exotic species. Pharmacokinetic data for various species are summarized in Table 13.4. Rapid IV administration can result in hypotension and excitement. Yohimbine has the potential to cause seizures at higher doses via GABA-ergic and NMDA-mediated pathways (Dunn 1992) although this is rarely seen clinically.

TOLAZOLINE

Synonyms: Vasodilatan, Benzidazol, Olitensol, Priscoline, Prefaxil, Artonil, Kasimid, Lambril, Priscol, Tolazine; IUPAC Name: 2-benzyl-4,5-dihydro-1H-imidazole (Fig. 13.11).

Tolazoline is a nonselective α_2 receptor antagonist. It is most commonly used to reverse the effects of xylazine in cattle, camelids, and exotic species. In addition to antagonism of the α_2 receptor, tolazoline has histaminergic and cholinergic effects (Tranquilli 2007) as well as direct effects on the vascular endothelium by decreasing systemic vascular resistance and increasing venous capacitance (Tranquilli 1984; Short 1987). As with all the antagonists, tolazoline should be administered slowly and to effect to prevent unwanted side effects.

TABLE 13.4 Alpha$_2$-adrenergic antagonists—pharmacokinetics

Drug	Species	Dose	Mean Residence Time (mins)	Volume of Distribution (l/kg)	Clearance$_{Tot}$ (ml/kg/min)	Elimination Half-Life (mins)	Reference
Yohimbine	Steer	0.25 mg/kg IV	86.7 ± 46.2	4.9 ± 1.4	69.6 ± 35.1	46.7 ± 24.4	(Jernigan 1988)
	Horse	0.075–0.15 mg/kg IV	106 ± 72.1 to 118.7 ± 35.0	2.7 ± 1.0 to 4.6 ± 1.9	34.0 ± 19.4 to 39.6 ± 16.6	52.8 ± 27.8 to 76.1 ± 23.1	(Jernigan 1988)
	Dog	0.4 mg/kg IV	163.6 ± 49.7	4.5 ± 1.8	29.6 ± 14.7	104.1 ± 32.1	(Jernigan 1988)
Tolazoline	Dog	6 mg/kg via ET tube*		1.65 ± 0.3	10.9 ± 4.8	156 ± 81	(Paret 1999)
	Horse					60	(Plumb 1999)
	Lamb	2 mg/kg IV		2.5 ± 0.7	27.1 ± 7.6†	70	(Ward 1984)
Atipamezole							
	Dog						
	Cat						
	Horse						
	Dairy cow	0.2 mg/kg IV	38.3 ± 15.7	1.77 ± 0.64	48.1 ± 13.1	35.2 ± 17.9	(Ranheim 1999)$
	Calf	0.2 mg/kg IV	48.1 ± 9.2	2.97 ± 1.4	42.9 ± 3.9	52.1 ± 7.0	(Ranheim 1998)$
	Sheep	0.2 mg/kg IV	34.4 ± 7.9	2.0 ± 0.54	56.3 ± 9.5	34.2 ± 11.9	(Ranheim 2000)$

*Following the use of xylazine and thiopental.
†In lambs 17 days of age. Clearance increased to 60 ml/kg/min by the age of 28 days.
$Following medetomidine 0.04 mg/kg IV.

Although tolazoline generally provides better reversal for cattle and camelid species, there have been reports of adverse effects and fatalities within those species with appropriate and inappropriate dosing (Reed 2000).

The pharmacokinetics for antagonists in several species are summarized in Table 13.4.

FIG. 13.12 Atipamezole.

ATIPAMEZOLE

Synonyms: Antisedan, Atipamezol, Atipamezolum, 4-(2-ethyl-2-indanyl)imidazole, MPV 1248; IUPAC Name: 4-(2-ethyl-1,3-dihydroinden-2-yl)-3H-imidazole (Fig. 13.12).

Atipamezole is a highly specific α_2 receptor antagonist that was designed to reverse the effects of medetomidine. It is most commonly used in dogs, cats, and exotic species. Along with its high specificity for the α_2 receptor, atipamezole does not bind at α_1-adrenergic, 5HT, histaminergic, muscarinic, or dopaminergic receptors (Tranquilli 2007), which decreases side effects with administration.

Regardless of the specificity, some animals require repeated dosing to get a full reversal, and some animals can become resedated later.

Pharmacokinetics for several species are summarized in Table 13.4.

Adverse Effects/Contraindications. Sudden death from cardiovascular collapse has been reported anecdotally in patients given α_2 receptor antagonist IV. One possible reason for acute cardiovascular collapse could be the preservative methylparaben; in atipamezole it can cause histamine release and therefore reduce blood pressure. However, it is more likely that when the antagonist is given in large doses IV to patients with peripheral vasoconstriction, reflex bradycardia, and high vagal tone; the rapid relaxation of vessel tone coupled with bradycardia induces the cardiovascular collapse. Caution should be used when quickly administering an antagonist while a patient is in the acute vasoconstrictive phase. Intramuscular administration is less likely to produce acute cardiovascular changes.

The safety of α_2-adrenergic antagonists has not been established in pregnant, lactating animals intended for breeding purposes, or metabolically unstable patients.

This class of drug is not intended for use in food-producing animals.

Some precautions need to be taken when using α_2-adrenergic antagonists to avoid an abrupt reversal of sedation and analgesia. This may cause delirium, apprehension and aggression during the reversal process. Animals should be monitored for the reversal of hypothermia, bradycardia, respiratory depression, and level of analgesia.

Dose:

Alpha-2 antagonists can produce side effects when administered alone or in concentrations greater than the agonist. Antagonists can be given to effect or in partial doses (e.g., 1/2 reversal).

Yohimbine

Dogs and cats:
 0.11 mg/kg IV; 0.25–0.5 mg/kg IM
Horses:
 0.075 mg/kg IV
Cattle and sheep:
 0.125–0.2 mg/kg IV

Tolazoline

Dogs and cats:
 4 mg/kg IV slowly
Horses:
 4 mg/kg IV slowly
Cattle:
 2–4 mg/kg IV slowly (calves 1 mg/kg IV slowly)
Llamas:
 2 mg/kg IM

Atipamezole

Many veterinarians administer atipamezole at an equal volume to the amount of medetomidine given. Given each drug's concentration, this is equivalent to reversing with five times the concentration of medetomidine. Although not very scientific, the method works and can easily be scaled back to do partial reversals.

Dogs and cats: 0.1–0.3 mg/kg IM (IV in emergencies)
Horses: 30–60 μg/kg IV, IM

It should be noted that atipamezole is licensed for intramuscular administration only. The preservative methylparaben causes histamine release in a small percentage of patients following intravenous administration, which may cause hypotension.

Species Differences. Llamas appear to be more sensitive to the adverse effects of tolazoline compared with other species. It has been recommended to administer tolazoline at 2 mg/kg intramuscularly to minimize these adverse effects (Hart 1985). The use of tolazoline in captive bears has proven to be ineffective for the reversal of α_2-adrenergic agonists and is therefore not recommended in this group of animals (Stoelting 1999).

Drug Interactions. There is little information regarding drug interactions between α_2-adrenergic antagonists and other drugs. Yohimbine administration is not recommended with antidepressants and other antipsychotic drugs due to potentiation of adverse effects of yohimbine and the possibility of death (Zhang 2002). It has been noted that when large doses of tolazoline have been administered with norepinephrine or epinephrine a biphasic response is seen that results in a sudden increase in blood pressure (Trevor 2001). The use of α_2-adrenergic antagonists with anticholinergics or positive chronotropes may cause excessive tachycardia.

Overdose/Acute Toxicity

Tolazoline: Gastrointestinal disturbances, agitation, muscle fasciculations, tachycardia, mild hypertension, and—at high doses—ventricular arrhythmias and death were seen with the administration of tolazoline alone. Overdoses of tolazoline at five times the recommended dose have been associated with fatalities in horses (Yeh 1988).

Atipamezole: Healthy dogs have tolerated up to 10 times the recommended dose of atipamezole. Clinical signs observed were dose-dependent and resembled a dog receiving a stimulant. Signs of an overdose included excitement, panting, trembling, vomiting, mild diarrhea, and scleral injection. There is the possibility of some local reaction at the site of injection. No significant clinical signs are seen following a regular dose of atipamezole in nonsedated dogs.

Regulatory Information

Controlled Drug Status. Not controlled. This class of drug is to be prescribed by a veterinarian only.

Withdrawal Times

Yohimbine: 7days for meat; 72 hr for milk.

They are not approved for use in food-producing animals.

Veterinary Products

Yohimbine

Yohimbine is approved by the FDA for use in the dog and cervidae (elk & deer).

Yobine® Injectable Solution: Yohimbine HCl 2 mg/ml (Lloyd, Inc.)

Antagonil®: Yohimbine HCl 5 mg/ml (Wildlife Laboratories, Inc.)

Tolazoline

Tolazoline is approved by the FDA for use in the horse.

Tolazine™ Injection: Tolazoline HCl 100 mg/ml (Lloyd, Inc.)

Atipamezole

Atipamezole is approved by the FDA for use in the dog and cat.

Antisedan®: Atipamezole HCl 5 mg/ml (Orion, Corp.)

BENZODIAZEPINE DERIVATIVES

GENERAL PHARMACOLOGIC CONSIDERATIONS

History/Introduction. The first benzodiazepine, chlordiazepoxide, was discovered accidentally in 1954 by Dr. Leo Sternbach. Diazepam (Valium®) is a simplified version of chlordiazepoxide and was marketed in 1963 for anxiety. Diazepam is on the World Health Organization's "Essential Drugs List," which is a list of minimum medical needs for a basic health care system. Although many benzodiazepines are used in people and animals for behavioral modification, only diazepam, midazolam, lorazepam, and zolazepam will be discussed as sedatives and adjuncts to anesthesia. This group of drugs is also discussed in Chapter 21 with the drugs that affect animal behavior, and with the anticonvulsants in Chapter 20.

Classification. Benzodiazepines are sedative-hypnotics due to their propensity to cause anxiolysis, sedation, and sleep. They are also classified as minor tranquilizers.

Chemistry. A benzodiazepine consists of a benzene ring, which is fused to a seven-member diazepine ring. All of the clinically useful benzodiazepines, and most of the active metabolites, contain an aryl substitute at the 5th position of the diazepine ring as well as N-substitutions at the 1st and 4th positions (5-aryl-1,4-benzodiazepine). The hypnotic-sedative action of these drugs is due to the substitution of a halogen or a nitro group at the 7th position of the benzodiazepine structure (Fig. 13.13; Table 13.5).

FIG. 13.13 Benzodiazepine structure with a halogen group on the 7th carbon.

TABLE 13.5 Benzodiazepine physiochemical properties

	Diazepam	Midazolam	Lorazepam
Molecular weight	284.7	325.8	321.1
Melting point °C	132	159	167
Water solubility @ 25°C	50 mg/l	1030 mg/l	80 mg/l
pKa	3.4	6.15	13
pH of commercial product	6.2–6.9	3–3.6	

How Supplied

Diazepam: Injectable formulations of diazepam consist of a 5 mg/ml solution with 40% propylene glycol, 10% ethanol, 5% sodium benzoate/benzoic acid buffer, and 1.5% benzyl alcohol as a preservative. The solution is buffered to a pH of 6.2–6.9. Propylene glycol and ethanol allow the diazepam to be dissolved into solution. The cloudy appearance of solutions does not alter the potency of diazepam; however, do not administer if a precipitate forms and does not clear. There is significant adsorption of diazepam onto the PCV (plastic) tubing when diazepam is administered as a constant rate of infusion (Daniell 1975).

Midazolam: The clinical preparations of midazolam are water-based (not in propylene glycol) and buffered to a pH of 3.5. This will result in stabilization of the diazepine ring and increasing water-solubility of the midazolam. As the pH increases to >4.0 (physiologic pH), the diazepine ring opens and thus increases the lipid-solubility of midazolam after administration (Prindle 1970). Therefore, at injection the drug is more water soluble, but quickly becomes more lipid soluble once in the body. However, if midazolam is going to be administered by the sublingual or rectal routes, the clinical preparation needs to be buffered to a pH >4.0 to increase the lipophilicity and subsequent transmucosal absorption (Cornick-Seahorn 1998). Midazolam is compatible with normal saline and lactated Ringer's solution.

Lorazepam: The vehicle of lorazepam consists of propylene glycol 79%, polyethylene glycol 18–20% and benzyl alcohol 2% (v/w %). Lorazepam may be diluted with sterile water, normal saline, or dextrose 5% prior to intravenous use because of the propensity to cause phlebitis (Ativan®, Baxter Health Care Group Package Insert). Intravenous administration should be slow.

Zolazepam: Zolazepam is supplied only with tiletamine as a powder that is reconstituted to 5 ml of solution. Each ml contains 50 mg zolazepam (and 50 mg tiletamine). The reconstituted solution has a pH of 2.2–2.8.

Mechanism of Action. Benzodiazepines bind to and activate the benzodiazepine receptor binding site (BZ receptor), which is located on the gamma subunit of the gamma-aminobutyric acid receptor subtype A ($GABA_A$) (Court and Greenblatt 1992). $GABA_A$ is a large macromolecule, which also contains a number of other binding sites for drug classes such as barbiturates and alcohols. This explains the synergistic effect of these drugs on $GABA_A$-mediated inhibition of the CNS. Agonism of the BZ binding site on $GABA_A$ receptors increases the frequency of the opening of the chloride ion channel leading to hyperpolarization of the postsynaptic neuron (Yeh 1988), producing decreased neuronal transmission. The heterogeneity of the $GABA_A$ subunits is in part responsible for the differing clinical actions of the various benzodiazepines (Upton 2001). The highest concentration of $GABA_A$ receptors is found in the cerebral cortex, with very few receptor sites found outside the CNS; hence the minimal cardiovascular effects of benzodiazepines (Cornick-Seahorn 1998).

Indications. Benzodiazepines are used in veterinary medicine as anticonvulsants, adjuncts to anesthetic induction agents, skeletal muscle relaxants, and for behavioral modification. In the healthy patient, behavioral effects are mild and may be paradoxical because the reduction in inhibitions can result in vocalization, excitement, and dysphoria. Sedation is more reliable in neonates, geriatrics, or ill patients or, as the authors would say, "very young, very old, or very sick." In small ruminants benzodiazepines are generally effective at causing sternal recumbency and sedation.

Pharmacodynamic Effects

CNS. The use of benzodiazepines alone to induce sedation can cause unpredictable results. This is especially true in young and healthy individuals. Paradoxical excitement, agitation, vocalization, and dysphoria may be seen after IV and IM administration. Benzodiazepines are commonly combined with other agents such as opioids, α_2-adrenergic agonists or ketamine to provide a more predictable sedation.

Benzodiazepines cause a reduction in cerebral blood flow and even greater reduction in oxygen consumption making them an excellent class of drug for central neurological disease (Reves 1985). Diazepam at a dose of 0.2 mg/kg IV caused a reduction in theta, delta, alpha, and beta-frequencies of the electroencephalogram of anesthetized dogs without any changes to the cardiovascular parameters (Court and Greenblatt 1992). Diazepam potentiates the opioid reduction in the MAC of inhalant anesthesia (Ilkiw 1996). Diazepam, like other benzodiazepines, is anticonvulsant.

Cardiovascular. Clinical doses of benzodiazepines cause minimal cardiovascular depression and are commonly administered to patients with cardiovascular disease. As the dose is increased there are reductions in both mean arterial blood pressure and systemic vascular resistance (Bishnoi 2005) while there is an increase in coronary flow and cardiac output, and reduction in myocardial oxygen consumption (Buhrer 1990). It appears these effects are centrally mediated since diazepam had little effect on isolate myocardial preparations (Loscher 1984). This reduction in preload and afterload may be beneficial in patients suffering from congestive heart failure. These cardiovascular depressant effects may be more profound in hypovolemic or debilitated patients.

Respiratory. Benzodiazepines produce a mild, but dose-dependent, respiratory depression (Scherkl 1989). Respiratory depression may be exaggerated when benzodiazepines are combined with other CNS depressants or when administered to debilitated patients.

Musculoskeletal. Benzodiazepines potentiate the GABA-ergic–mediated muscle relaxation of inhibitory neurons at the level of the spinal cord (Elliott 1976), which produces reliable muscle relaxation. This class of drug is often administered with other anesthetic drugs that do not provide muscle relaxation (e.g., ketamine). At the clinical doses, midazolam can cause ataxia and in some species is capable of causing recumbency (Platt 2000). In horses, midazolam can cause pacing, paddling, and agitation (Loscher 1984). These adverse effects tend to be transient. Benzodiazepines do potentiate non-depolarizing neuromuscular antagonists; however, there does appear to be a ceiling effect to this potentiation.

Miscellaneous

Pain on administration: The vehicle, propylene glycol, of diazepam may cause pain when administered intravenously or intramuscularly. Pain is reported to be worse when administered in small veins.

Appetite stimulation: Diazepam is an appetite stimulant, particularly in cats. However, diazepam also slows down gastric emptying and may produce profound sedation if used too frequently (Podell 1998).

Hemolysis: The propylene glycol vehicle of diazepam can cause lysis of red blood cells (RBC). Large volumes or constant rate infusion may cause clinical hemolysis and are therefore not recommended.

Analgesia. Benzodiazepines do not produce analgesia, but they may potentiate other analgesics (e.g., opioids, alpha-2 agonists).

DIAZEPAM HYDROCHLORIDE

Synonyms: Diazepam, Ansiolisina, Valium, Calmocitene, Ceregulart, Neurolytril, Tranquirit, Ansiolin, Apozepam, Atensine (Fig. 13.14).

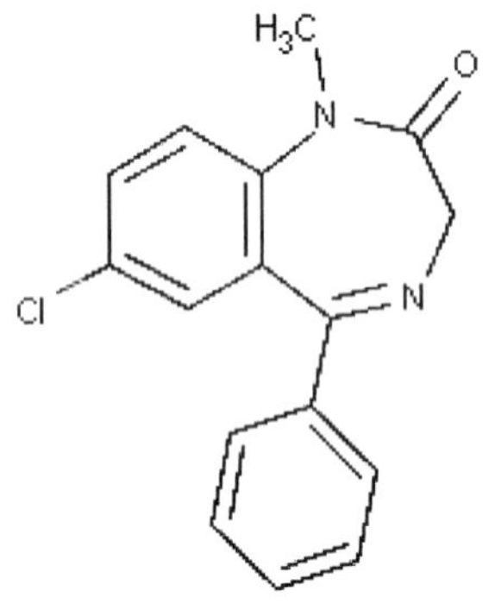

FIG. 13.14 Diazepam.

Diazepam has been used clinically since 1963 and is often the standard against which all other benzodiazepines are measured. Diazepam is a highly lipid-soluble benzodiazepine, which has a much shorter duration of action in dogs and cats compared with people. Many of the unwanted side effects of diazepam use are caused by the vehicle propylene glycol. Propylene glycol is hyperosmotic, which can lead to hemolysis of red blood cells; painful when injected IM or IV; can cause cardio-depression at high doses; and causes erratic absorption with any route other than IV. Diazepam can be administered rectally (Papich 1995).

MIDAZOLAM MALEATE

Synonyms: Versed, Dormicum, Hypnovel, Rocam, nchembio747-comp32, Midazolamum [INN-Latin], DEA No. 2884, EINECS 261-774-5, BRN 0625572, Ro 21-3981 (Fig. 13.15).

The water-soluble characteristic of midazolam is due to the presence of the imidazole ring structure (Podell 1998). Midazolam has approximately twice the potency and BZ receptor affinity as compared with diazepam, but has similar pharmacodynamics. It is largely replacing diazepam due to water solubility, a reduction in price, and relative availability. Lack of propylene glycol allows administration IV, IM, and SQ with reliable bioavailability. Midazolam can be administered intranasally (Henry 1998).

LORAZEPAM

Synonyms: Ativan, Temesta, Tavor, o-Chloroxazepam, o-Chlorooxazepam, Delormetazepam, Norlormetazepam,

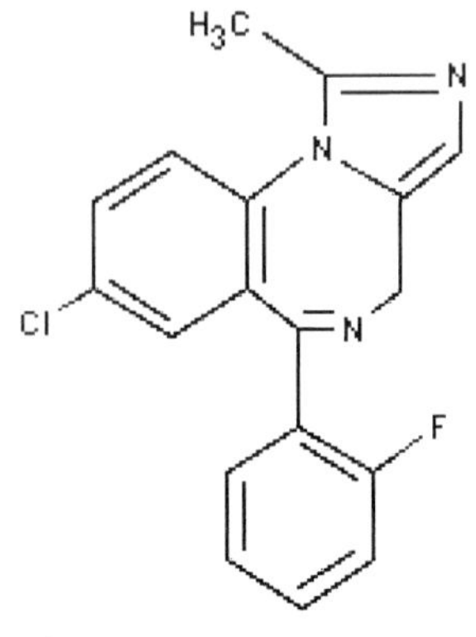

FIG. 13.15 Midazolam.

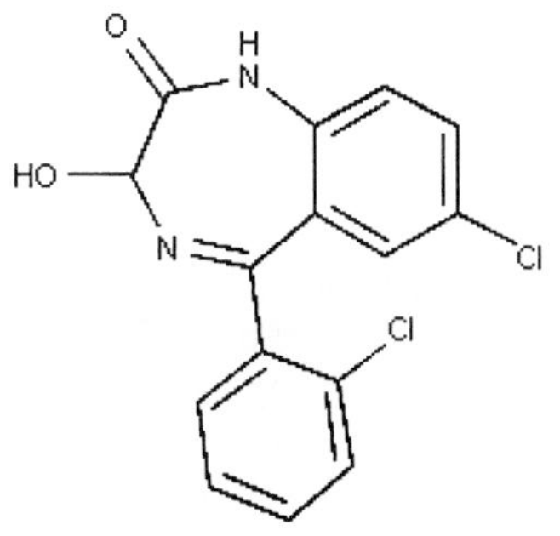

FIG. 13.16 Lorazepam.

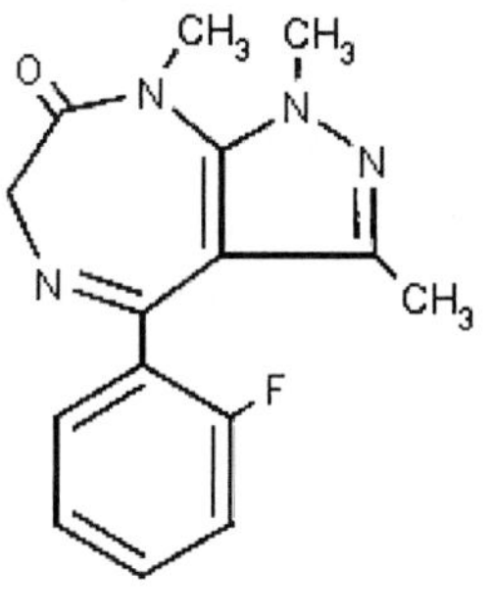

FIG. 13.17 Zolazepam.

Aplacassee, Bonatranquan; IUPAC Name: 10-chloro-2-(2-chlorophenyl)-4-hydroxy-3,6-diazabicyclo[5.4.0]undeca-2,8,10,12-tetraen-5-one (Fig. 13.16).

Lorazepam is approximately 10 times as potent as diazepam. Lorazepam is absorbed nearly completely by any route given (oral, sublingual, or IM) in small animals except for the rectal route (Scherkl 1986). Lorazepam brain levels last longer than the plasma; therefore the therapeutic effect may last longer than the apparent plasma half-life (Brown 1991). Lorazepam is replacing diazepam as a first-line treatment to status epilepticus in people due to better absorption from various administration routes, the lack of active metabolites, higher BZ receptor affinity, and longer receptor binding time compared to diazepam (Frey 1985). It has the greatest amnestic effect when compared to diazepam or midazolam in humans (Altahan 1984).

ZOLAZEPAM. Zolazepam is a benzodiazepine similar to diazepam. It is only available in combination with tiletamine, an NMDA antagonist (like ketamine), in the anesthetic drug Telazol® (Fig. 13.17). Little clinical information on exists on zolazepam alone. When used in combination with tiletamine, zolazepam has different metabolic rates in different species. In cats and pigs, zolazepam is more slowly metabolized and they awake slowly and calmly. In comparison, in dogs and horses, zolazepam is metabolized more rapidly and they awake more quickly and more agitatedly.

Pharmacokinetics Properties. Diazepam, midazolam, and lorazepam are the only benzodiazepines that are currently available in the U.S. in an injectable form (zolazepam is available with tiletamine) (Table 13.6). Benzodiazepines have been administered via a number of different routes, which include submucosal, sublingual, intranasal, and per rectum (McNicholas 1983), with varying degrees of bioavailability.

Since the plasma half-life of diazepam in the dog is only 14–16 minutes, most of the clinical effect of this benzodiazepine administered via the rectal route is caused by its metabolites: desmethyldiazepam and oxazepam (Podell 1998). In the dog, rectal administration of drugs does not obviate the first-pass effect by the liver. The rectal blood supply of the dog as compared to a human is such that a higher percentage of blood draining the rectum will indeed pass through the liver before going into the systemic circulation (Wagner 1998). This is the main reason why investigators have started to use other routes of administration, such as sublingual, transmucosal, and intranasal (Papich and Alcorn 1995). In fact, the T_{max} following intranasal administration of diazepam in the dog was only 90 seconds slower than by the intravenous route (Anika 1985). The bioavailability was 80%. A rapid onset of intranasal midazolam was also seen in rabbits using a drop technique (Brown 1993); however, it has a lower bioavailability in the dog (Ilkiw 1998). The transmucosal administration of midazolam may be improved theoretically by buffering the solution to a physiologic pH prior to administration, thereby improving its lipid solubility (Court 1992). Absorption could also be improved upon by the use of an atomizing device to increase the surface area in contact with the solution being administered compared to a drop technique (Court 1993).

The T_{max} for diazepam after IV administration in the dog is approximately 4 minutes (Stegmann 2001) compared to 15 minutes for midazolam (Zhang 2002). This does not necessarily correlate with the peak pharmacodynamic effect due to differences in metabolism and penetration of the drug into the CNS. It is the degree of lipid solubility rather than the amount of protein binding or

TABLE 13.6 Benzodiazepine pharmacokinetics in various species

	Species	Equivalent Dose (mg)	Volume of Distribution (l/kg)	Protein Binding (%)	Clearance (ml/kg/min)	Elimination Half-Life (mins)	Metabolites	Reference
Diazepam	Dog	0.5 mg/kg IV				14–16	Desmethyldiazepam*, Oxazepam*, Temazepam*	(Papich and Alcorn 1995)
	Dog	2 mg/kg IV	1.5–2.2‡		19 ± 4.2‡	126–294‡		(Loscher and Frey 1981)
	Cat				4.72 ± 2.45	330	Desmethyldiazepam*, Oxazepam*, Temazepam*	(Cotler et al. 1984)
	Human		0.7–1.7	98	0.2–0.5	1200–3000	Desmethyldiazepam*, Oxazepam*, Temazepam*	
Midazolam	Dog	0.5 mg/kg IV	3.0 ± 0.9	96		59–95	1-OH and 4-OH midazolam†	(Court et al. 1992)
	Dog	0.5 mg/kg IV			12.1 ± 2.24	27.8–31		(Brown et al. 1993)
	Human		1.1–1.7	94	6.4–11	102–156		
Lorazepam	Dog	0.3 mg/kg IV	100 ± 15 l				Lorazepam glucuronide, hydroxylorazepam	(Podell et al. 1998)
	Human		0.8–1.3	98	0.8–1.8	660–1320		
Flumazenil	Dog	0.008–0.01 mg/kg IV				40–80	Glucuronide forms of flumazenil	(Oliver et al. 2000)

ionization that determines the rate of entry into the CNS by benzodiazepine drugs (Gillis 1974). Other studies have found that midazolam causes a faster onset of change to the electroencephalograph compared to diazepam (Scherkl 1986). Midazolam does have some advantage over diazepam and lorazepam due to its shorter elimination and context-sensitive half-lives, making it the most ideal agent for constant rate infusions (Scherkl 1989).

Diazepam, chlordiazepoxide, and oxazepam are all metabolized by the same pathways in the dog and humans, but differently in the rat (Podell 1998). Benzodiazepines undergo biotransformation initially by reduction, such as diazepam and midazolam, chlordiazepoxide, and clorazepate, or they may simply undergo glucuronide conjugation such as lorazepam. Diazepam has a number of active metabolites such as desmethyldiazepam, oxazepam, and temazepam (Upton 2001). Desmethyldiazepam, the main metabolite in most species (Wala 1991), appears to have the most clinical effect due to its long half-life. Approximately 50% of diazepam is metabolized to desmethyldiazepam in the cat (Hoyumpa 1981). Following glucuronide conjugation, benzodiazepines are excreted in the urine (Martens 1990). Glucuronidation is possible in the cat albeit at a much slower rate of formation over a number of days (Syracuse Research Corporation 2007). The slower rate of glucuronidation and clearance of desmethyldiazepam may help explain why flumazenil administration to cats a day after a benzodiazepine has shown a clinical effect, especially in cats with impaired metabolism. Desmethyldiazepam and oxazepam reach their T_{max} within 2 hours postadministration of diazepam either IV or per os (Trevor 2001). The elimination half-lives of desmethyldiazepam and oxazepam are approximately 3.5 and 5.5 hours postadministration of diazepam, respectively, regardless of route of administration. These metabolites have only approximately 1/3 the anticonvulsant potency of diazepam (Morgan 2002).

In the dog, cat, and pig, lorazepam is metabolized by the liver to lorazepam glucuronide (Marty 1991), and to a lesser degree by other splanchnic organs (Driessen 1987). It is interesting that the main metabolite in the cat is lorazepam glucuronide. The main routes of excretion are via the urine and feces in approximately equal amounts (Morgan 2002).

Species Differences. *Cats:* There have been case reports of cats developing hepatic failure following repeated oral administration of diazepam. Caution should be used with repeated dosing in the species (Oliver 2000).

Adverse Effects/Contraindications. It is not uncommon to see a transient period of agitation, vocalization, excitement, muscle fasciculations, and ataxia in a number of species immediately after administration of a benzodiazepine. This is especially so in the cat, dog, and horse (Forster 1993). The high rate of occurrence of these abnormal behaviors makes the use of benzodiazepine alone in these species unpredictable. It is recommended to use other agents in combination with benzodiazepines to reduce these side effects and maintain the beneficial effects of the benzodiazepines.

In humans, diazepam has been implicated in causing congenital abnormalities when administered in the first trimester. Neonates born to mothers that have received a benzodiazepine immediately prior to parturition may require a benzodiazepine antagonist. The safe use of benzodiazepines in pregnant or lactating animals has not been investigated; however, the presence of a number of benzodiazepines and their metabolites has been documented in maternal milk, especially in the casein fraction (Artru 1991). Casein levels are highest in colostrum, and then decline over the course of lactation.

Caution should be used when sedating animals exhibiting fear-induced aggression, as the disinhibition caused by the benzodiazepines may provoke an attack. There are clinical reports of the development of hepatic failure in some cats after the oral administration of diazepam after only a few days (Oliver 2000).

Contraindications to benzodiazepines include patients with hypersensitivities to benzodiazepines, hepatic dysfunction, and acute narrow-angle glaucoma. Patients discontinuing a benzodiazepine require their dose to be tapered off to avoid abstinence syndrome from sudden cessation. Long-term use of benzodiazepines causes physical dependence in the dog and the use of flumazenil may precipitate abstinence syndrome (tremors, hotfoot walking twitches, tonic-clonic seizures, and occasional death) (Oliver 2000). The more severe signs are seen with diazepam use and are mainly attributed to the active metabolite of desmethyldiazepam (Klotz 1988). Signs of withdrawal are apparent as early as 24 hours after the cessation of diazepam. The severity of the withdrawal/abstinence syndrome is less with lorazepam (Oliver 2000).

Dose:

Diazepam

Dogs and cats:

Sedation:	0.1–0.5 mg/kg IV. (IM administration is no longer recommended since propylene glycol is painful on IM injection and absorption is erratic compared with IV dosing.) 0.2–2.0 mg/kg rectally

Adjunct induction agent: Diazepam is often used as an induction synergistic adjunct to thiopental, propofol, and etomidate at a rate of 0.1–0.2 mg/kg IV given immediately before the induction agent.

Anticonvulsant:	0.5–2 mg/kg IV (Carbajal 1996)
Appetite stimulant in cats:	0.05 mg/kg IV

Horses:

Neonatal sedation:	0.05–0.2 mg/kg IV
Adjunct to anesthesia induction:	0.1 mg/kg IV
Anticonvulsant:	0.02–0.4 mg/kg IV

Small ruminants:

Sedation:	0.1–1.0 mg/kg IV
Adjunct to anesthesia induction:	0.1–0.3 mg/kg IV
Appetite stimulation (goats):	0.04 mg/kg IV (Oliver 2000)

Midazolam

Midazolam is considered twice as potent as diazepam, so doses approximately half of that of diazepam are often given.

Dogs and Cats:

Sedation:	0.1–0.4 mg/kg IV, IM, SQ 0.2–1.0 mg/kg intranasal
Adjunct to anesthesia induction agent:	0.1–0.2 mg/kg IV
Anticonvulsant:	0.5–1.0 mg/kg IV

Ruminants:

Sedation:	0.1–1.0 mg/kg IV
Adjunct to anesthesia induction agent:	0.1 mg/kg IV

Horses:
 Neonatal sedation: 0.05–0.2 mg/kg IV
 Adjunct to anesthesia
  induction: 0.1 mg/kg IV
 Anticonvulsant: 0.02–0.4 mg/kg IV

Lorazepam

Dogs:
 Sedation: 0.2 mg/kg IV

Drug Interactions. The administration of other CNS depressants i.e., inhalant anesthetics, barbiturates, opioids, α_2-adrenergic agonists, etc., with a benzodiazepine often results in an additive CNS depressant effect. A reduction in benzodiazepine metabolism may be observed if coadministered with the following drugs: cimetidine, erythromycin, isoniazid, ketoconazole, propranolol, and valproic acid, whereas rifampin will increase the metabolic rate of benzodiazepines (Michenfelder 1971). This is true for benzodiazepines that first undergo oxidation as part of their hepatic metabolism (Ikeda 1983), i.e., diazepam and midazolam, but not lorazepam. Benzodiazepines reduce the metabolism of digoxin, thus requiring the patient to be monitored for digoxin serum levels to avoid toxicity. Thyroidal uptake of I^{123} or I^{131} may be reduced by benzodiazepines (Pettifer 1993).

After 24 hours in a polyvinylchloride (PVC) bag, approximately 55% of the diazepam in solution will be adsorbed onto the surface of the bag and tubing (Katherman 1985). This is not true for polyethylene, nylon, and polypropylene bags. This is not of a concern for midazolam or lorazepam.

Overdose/Acute Toxicity. Clinical signs of acute intoxication have included ataxia/disorientation, depression, agitation, gastrointestinal upset, weakness, tremors, vocalization, tachycardia, tachypnea, and hypothermia that developed within 10–30 minutes postingestion. Use standard decontamination procedures, such as emesis and activated charcoal for acute oral ingestion. Intravenous fluids, positive inotropes, vasopressors, and the specific benzodiazepine antagonist, flumazenil, may be used for severe CNS depression and cardiovascular instability (Ostheimer 1975).

Regulatory Information

Controlled Drug Status. Schedule IV controlled drug

Withdrawal Times. There are no established withdrawal times for benzodiazepines.

Veterinary Products. There are no FDA veterinary-approved products.

Human Products

Diazepam (DEA Schedule IV)

Diastat Acudial: Diazepam Rectal Gel 10 mg/2 ml, 20 mg/4 ml (5 mg/ml) (Valeant)
Diazepam Intensol: Diazepam Concentrate; Oral 5 mg/ml (Roxane)
Diazepam: Diazepam Injectable 5 mg/ml (Baxter Hlthcare)
Diazepam: Diazepam Solution; Oral 5 mg/5 ml (Roxane)
Diazepam: Diazepam Tablet 2 mg, 5 mg, 10 mg (Actavis Elizabeth)
Valium: Diazepam Tablet 2 mg, 5 mg, 10 mg (Roche)

Midazolam (DEA Schedule IV)

Midazolam: Midazolam HCl Injectable Eq 1 mg Base/ml, Eq 5 mg Base/ml (Abraxis Pharm)
Midazolam: Midazolam HCl Syrup; Oral Eq 2 mg Base/ml (Apotex Inc)

Lorazepam (DEA Schedule IV)

Intensol: Lorazepam Concentrate; Oral 2 mg/ml (Roxane)
Ativan: Lorazepam Injectable; Injection 2 mg/ml, 4 mg/ml (Baxter Hlthcare Corp.)
Lorazepam Injectable; Injection 2 mg/ml, 4 mg/ml, & Preservative Free 2 mg/ml, 4 mg/ml (Bedford)
Lorazepam Tablet; Oral 0.5 mg, 1 mg, 2 mg (Ivax Pharms)

BENZODIAZEPINE ANTAGONISTS

GENERAL PHARMACOLOGIC CONSIDERATIONS

History/Introduction. Flumazenil was introduced in 1987 by Hoffmann-La Roche under the trade name Anexate™. It is still the only benzodiazepine antagonist available in the U.S.

Classification. Flumazenil is a specific and exclusive benzodiazepine (BZ) competitive antagonist with a high affinity for the benzodiazepine receptor sites. Flumazenil has virtually no agonist activity at the BZ receptor sites.

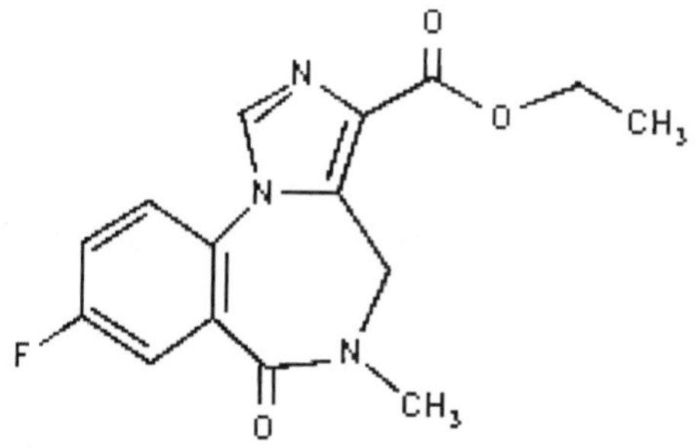

FIG. 13.18 Flumazenil.

Chemistry. Flumazenil is a 1,4-imidazobenzodiazepine derivative, which lacks the 5-aryl group that is normally attached to the diazepine ring (Fig. 13.18). The molecular weight of flumazenil is 303.3 g/mol. It is relatively insoluble in water (128 mg/l), which is only slightly improved by acidifying the solution (Grandy and Heath 1987).

How Supplied. Intravenous preparations of flumazenil are 0.1 mg/ml in a 5 ml vial. Each ml contains 0.1 mg of flumazenil compounded with 1.8 mg of methylparaben, 0.2 mg of propylparaben. 0.9% sodium chloride, 0.01% edetate disodium, and 0.01% acetic acid. The pH is adjusted to 4 using hydrochloric acid and or sodium hydroxide (Romazicon, Roche; Package Insert).

Mechanism of Action. Flumazenil competitively antagonizes the action of benzodiazepines on the benzodiazepine receptor (BZ) binding site on the $GABA_A$ receptor, thus preventing the resultant hyperpolarization of the postsynaptic membrane. Flumazenil does not, however, antagonize the CNS effects of other sedative-hypnotics, ethanol, opioids, or general anesthetics and their interaction with the $GABA_A$ receptor. There is some antagonistic interaction with endogenous benzodiazepine-like substances, which appear to be elevated in patients with hepatic encephalopathy. This effect appears to be transient (Vallance 1988). In some animals flumazenil has a weak partial agonist effect at low concentrations (Romazicon, Roche; Package Insert). The degree of reversal is a dose-dependent phenomenon of all the benzodiazepine agonist activity. The prevention of amnesia is less reliable (Nashan 1984).

Indications. The main indication for flumazenil is the competitive reversal of benzodiazepine agonists.

FLUMAZENIL

Synonyms: Romazicon, Flumazepil, Anexate, Lanexat, Mazicon, Flumazenilum [Latin], Flumazenilo [Spanish], nchembio747-comp37; IUPAC name: ethyl 8-fluoro-5,6-dihydro-5-methyl-6-oxo-4H-imidazo[1,5-a][1,4]benzodiazepine-3-carboxylate (Fig. 13.18).

Pharmacodynamic Effects

CNS. Flumazenil reverses the electroencephalographic changes induced by benzodiazepine in the dog and horse (Ward 1984). Flumazenil has been shown to produce either a transient (Grandy 1987) or no effect in reversing the effects of hepatic encephalopathy (Pettifer 1993).

Cardiovascular. Flumazenil has no effect on left ventricular function or coronary hemodynamics observed in human patients with coronary arterial disease (Stoelting 1999). In cats, however, flumazenil administered after diazepam or midazolam antagonized the fall in blood pressure caused by the benzodiazepines agonists (Gvozdenovic 1993).

Respiratory. Tidal volume and minute ventilation are restored to normal with the use of flumazenil following a benzodiazepine;, the CO_2 response curve of the respiratory center is still depressed (González 2001). Flumazenil does not exhibit any respiratory stimulatory effects even at ten times the dose (Statile 1988).

Miscellaneous. Flumazenil does not affect intraocular pressure in healthy human volunteers when given alone, but does reverse the decrease in intraocular pressure seen after the administration of benzodiazepines (Yamashita 2003).

Pharmacokinetics Properties. The recovery of cognitive function in people after the administration of flumazenil occurs within one arm-to-brain circulation time (Serrano 1976). The time for reversal in a model using midazolam-induced respiratory depression using flumazenil was 120 ± 25 seconds IV and up to 310 ± 134 seconds IM (Plumb 1999). In man, flumazenil is metabolized by the liver (99%) to the deethylated free acid and glucuronide conjugate (Sams 1996), both of which are excreted in the urine. None of the metabolites of flumazenil appears to be active (Chui 1994). The distribution phase is approximately 4 to 11 minutes and the elimination phase is 40 to 80 minutes. Hepatic diseases will approximately double the elimination phase. Flumazenil has a 50% binding, most of which is to albumin (66%). Sublingual and per rectal administration of flumazenil has been shown to be as effective as intramuscular administration. The per rectal dose used, however, was higher than the intramuscular dose (Adam 1999) since the bioavailability is much lower (Arneth 1985). Flumazenil has a high first-pass effect; therefore, the oral route is not recommended (Pettifer 1993). Submucosal administration of 0.2 mg flumazenil achieved a T_{max} in 4 minutes with a C_{max} of 8.5 ± 1.5 ng/ml declining to a level of 2 ng/ml over the next 2 hours (Fischler 1986). Levels of flumazenil >5 ng/ml are sufficient to reverse benzodiazepine-induced sedation (Roche package insert for flumazenil). The duration for which plasma levels were above this for both routes of administration was approximately 1 hour. Bioavailability was near 100% when administered via the mucosal route. Both the rectal (Stoelting 1999) and endotracheal (McLeish 1977) routes of administration are effective for the reversal of benzodiazepines in humans. The former may not be true for dogs unless a higher dose is used to counter the high first-pass effect that drugs will undergo with rectal administration (Dodman 1979).

Adverse Effects/Contraindications. The use of flumazenil in patients who have been treated chronically with benzodiazepine or have received an overdose of tricyclic antidepressants has the potential of precipitating seizures. This phenomenon of benzodiazepine abstinence syndrome has been seen in dogs experimentally (Radcliffe 2000). Arrhythmias and death have been observed after the use of flumazenil in patients that have received both benzodiazepines and tricyclic antidepressants (VMRCVM Drug Information Laboratory 2007). Flumazenil should be given slowly intravenously with close physiologic monitoring in patients who have received a benzodiazepine and a tricyclic antidepressant. In dogs that have never received a benzodiazepine, doses of flumazenil ranging from 18 mg/kg to 72 mg/kg resulted in a reduction in activity with no other effects seen (Grandy 1987).

To help reduce the pain or discomfort at the injection site, flumazenil may be diluted or administered into a large vein. Extravasation of flumazenil may result in local tissue inflammation and necrosis (Bustamante 1997). Other adverse effects reported in humans have been agitation, euphoria, hyperventilation, sweating, blurred vision, dizziness and headache, rash, nausea, and vomiting.

Flumazenil is contraindicated in patients with a known hypersensitivity to benzodiazepines or flumazenil, patients receiving a benzodiazepine for a life-threatening condition, or patients showing signs of a tricyclic antidepressant overdose. In such cases, supportive therapy should be instituted without the administration of flumazenil.

Dose:

Dogs:

0.008–0.04 mg/kg IV, IM, submucosal, endotracheal, rectal

Repeated doses of flumazenil may be required for the reversal of benzodiazepine-induced sedation, especially in patients with concurrent hepatic disease.

Horses:

0.01–0.02 mg/kg IV for both the foal and adult horse

Drug Interactions. The use of flumazenil in patients that have received tricyclic antidepressants may result in fatal arrhythmias. Theophylline and aminophylline potentiates the actions of flumazenil. There is some evidence to suggest that midazolam may affect the pharmacokinetics of flumazenil and vice versa. Repeat dosing of flumazenil may be required for the reversal of long acting benzodiazepines.

Overdose/Acute Toxicity. In the dog the LDL_o has been reported at >30 mg/kg IV; another study using 18–72 mg/kg IV showed only a slight reduction in activity in benzodiazepine naive dogs. An overdose of flumazenil may be treated with a benzodiazepine, barbiturate, or phenytoin.

Regulatory Information

Controlled Drug Status. Not controlled

Withdrawal Times. No withdrawal times have been formulated for flumazenil.

Human Products

Flumazenil

Romazicon: Flumazenil Injectable; Injection 0.1 mg/ml (HLR)

Flumazenil Injectable; Injection 0.1 mg/ml (Abraxis Pharm)

Flumazenil Injectable; Injection 0.1 mg/ml (Apotex Inc)

Flumazenil Injectable; Injection 0.1 mg/ml (Baxter Hlthcare)

Flumazenil Injectable; Injection 0.1 mg/ml (Bedford Labs)
Flumazenil Injectable; Injection 0.1 mg/ml (Sandoz)
Flumazenil Injectable; Injection 0.1 mg/ml (Sicor Pharms)

BUTYROPHENONE DERIVATIVES

GENERAL PHARMACOLOGIC CONSIDERATIONS

History/Introduction. Haloperidol was the first butyrophenone introduced in 1957, followed by droperidol in 1961. The use of butyrophenones in veterinary practice has declined over the past few decades with the introduction of other more predictable agents. Azaperone is now the most commonly used butyrophenones for veterinary practice today in the fields of swine and wildlife medicine.

Classification. The butyrophenones are one of the major classes of antipsychotic drugs in use in human medicine. They are a neuroleptic sedative, which has its main effect mediated via dopaminergic (D_2) antagonism. Butyrophenones also have antagonistic activity against α_1-adrenergic, histaminergic, and cholinergic receptors. The latter interactions are mild in effect.

Chemistry. Azaperone has a molecular weight of 327.4 g/mol. Azaperone is more water soluble than droperidol, with a solubility of 131 mg/l at 25°C. The log-partition coefficient (n-octanol/aqueous buffer at pH 9.9) is 3.3, which is a measure of lipid solubility.

Droperidol has a molecular weight of 379.44 g/mol. Droperidol is practically insoluble in water (4.2 mg/l) and only slightly soluble in ethanol or methanol. The log-partition coefficient (n-octanol/aqueous buffer at pH 9.9) is 3.58. It has a pKa of 7.64.

How Supplied. Azaperone comes as a clear, pale yellow, sterile, injectable solution with a concentration of 40 mg/ml in a 100 ml multidose bottle. Azaperone should be discarded 28 days after the multidose vial has been opened.

Droperidol plus fentanyl are combined and marketed in the preparation, Innovar-vet®, and is the only registered veterinary product. It comes in an injectable form only. Each milliliter of this preparation contains droperidol 20 mg and fentanyl 0.4 mg. The combination is used in people, but is no longer marketed for veterinary medicine.

Droperidol injection is prepared as a nonpyrogenic solution of droperidol in water for intravenous or intramuscular injection. The pH is 3.4 using lactic acid to adjust the pH to a range of 3.0–3.8. The concentration of the solution is 2.5 mg/ml. The solution is intended for single-dose only.

Mechanism of Action. The main CNS effects of butyrophenones are due to the antagonism of D_2 receptors and to a lesser degree the α_1-adrenergic receptor. Relative receptor binding affinities of haloperidol re $D_2 > D_1 = D_4 > \alpha_1 > 5\text{-}HT_2$. Butyrophenones also have some antihistaminergic effects. The relative reduced affinity for α_1-adrenergic antagonism is the reason why the butyrophenones do not cause the same degree of vasodilation when compared with the phenothiazines.

The dopaminergic receptors are broken up into two main groups, the D_1-like (D_1 and D_5 receptor subtypes) and D_2-like (D_2, D_3, and D_4 receptor subtypes) receptor groups. All dopaminergic receptors are a G protein coupled with seven transmembrane domains. The intracellular effects vary dramatically depending upon which subtype of dopaminergic receptor is being antagonized. The neurological effect of dopaminergic antagonism is based upon which subtype and anatomical location is being affected.

Indications. Azaperone is used mainly for the antipsychotic effect in swine for its calming effects when mixing weanlings and feeder pigs, transportation, or obstetrical conditions. It has also been used in sows to help prevent aggression directed toward piglets. Both azaperone and droperidol have been used as a preoperative sedative in a number of species including wildlife species. Droperidol is also a very effective antiemetic for any emetic or other response that involves the chemoreceptor trigger zone.

AZAPERONE

Synonyms: Stresnil, Fluoperidol, Azeperone, Eucalmyl, Suicalm, Sedaperone vet, Azaperon; IUPAC Name: 1-(4-fluorophenyl)-4-(4-pyridin-2-ylpiperazin-1-yl)butan-1-one, (Fig. 13.19). Molecular weight is 327.2 g/mol. The water solubility is 131 mg/l.

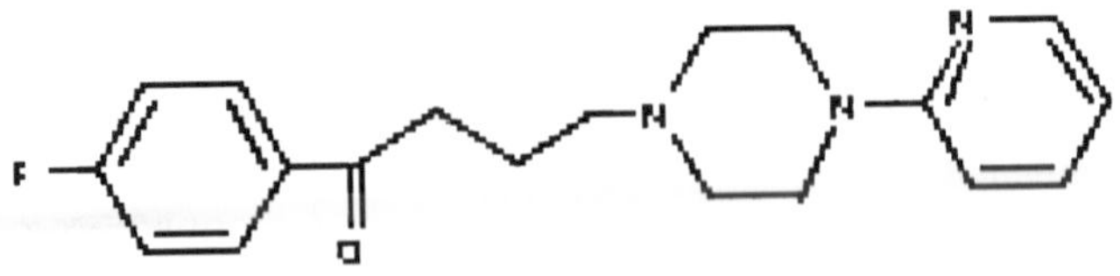

FIG. 13.19 Azaperone.

Pharmacodynamic Effects

CNS. Azaperone in most clinical situations will cause moderate to excellent levels of sedation for restraint. However, in the horse, there have been isolated reports of paradoxical excitement following IV administration of azaperone, which was not seen with IM administration.

Cardiovascular. In the horse and pig, azaperone will cause a reduction in mean arterial blood pressure for at least 4 hours following intramuscular administration. In young pigs, heart rate and cardiac output decrease by 20–40% (Tranquilli 2007). This is due to a reduction in systemic vascular resistance, which leads to a transient increase in heart rate and cardiac output. Other researchers have since shown the increase in heart rate is in part due to a central vagolytic effect and not as a consequence of changes in peripheral blood pressure. The cardiovascular changes lasted longer than the sedative effects of azaperone.

Respiratory. Butyrophenones generally have mild effects on ventilation. Azaperone (0.4–0.8 mg/kg) administered intramuscularly in horses caused only slight changes to the PaO_2, $PaCO_2$, and pH that were clinically insignificant; however, the hemoglobin level did fall by 5–10% for approximately 4 hours. The latter effect is assumed to be due to splenic sequestration of erythrocytes. It was noted in some individual horses an increase in respiratory rate following azaperone.

Musculoskeletal. Muscle tone is reduced with azaperone; however, the resultant ataxia is mild when compared to phenothiazines and α_2-adrenergic agonists.

Onset and Duration of Action. The onset of sedation in horses was apparent within 10 minutes with a maximal effect seen within 20–60 minutes following administration. The duration of sedation lasted from 2 to 6 hours.

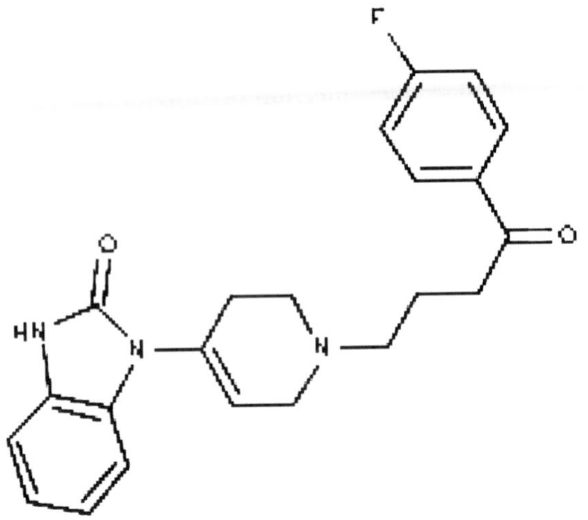

FIG. 13.20 Droperidol.

Miscellaneous. Butyrophenones can cause a mild reduction in body temperature.

Azaperone decreases the incidence of halothane-induced malignant hyperthermia in pigs.

Analgesia. Azaperone, like all butyrophenones, does not provide analgesia. Analgesia must be provided separately when butyrophenones are used perianesthetically.

DROPERIDOL

Synonyms: Droleptan, Innovar, Properidol, Sintodril, Sintosian, Inapsine, Vetkalm, Dridol, Halkan, Thalamonal®. IUPAC Name: 3-[1-[4-(4-fluorophenyl)-4-oxo-butyl]-3,6-dihydro-2H-pyridin-4-yl]-1H-benzoimidazol-2-one (Fig. 13.20). Molecular weight = 379.4. Droperidol has a pKa of 7.46 and has a water solubility of 4.2 mg/l at a neutral pH.

Droperidol with fentanyl (Innovar-vet®) is approved for dogs in the U.S., but is no longer marketed because of abuse potential and adverse behavioral effects in dogs.

Pharmacodynamic Effects

CNS. The sedative effects of butyrophenones are from the antagonism of dopamine (D2) receptors in the mesolimbic-mesocortical pathways of the brain. Adverse signs associated with large doses of butyrophenones, such as extrapyramidal signs, (dyskinesis, muscle tremors, and restlessness) are associated with dopaminergic antagonism of the nigrostriatal pathways.

Droperidol-fentanyl combination has been shown to have little effect on cerebral blood flow and metabolism; however, droperidol alone will cause cerebral vasoconstriction and reduction in cerebral flow without a reduction in cerebral metabolic rate. Droperidol alone or in combination with fentanyl does not increase cerebrospinal fluid production. Droperidol does not produce amnesia, nor does it have anticonvulsant effects.

The droperidol-fentanyl combination often leads to a quiet, tractable patient, which may become laterally recumbent depending upon the dose administered. Maximal sedation appeared to be approximately 30 minutes postadministration following subcutaneous injection (Grandy and Heath 1987). The butyrophenones do not produce the same degree of ataxia as compared to the phenothiazines. A low dose of the Innovar-Vet preparation (0.005 ml/kg IV) provided adequate sedation with minimal changes to the electroencephalogram, which is ideal for electrophysiological studies. Butyrophenones may reduce the seizure threshold.

Reports of severe aggressive behavior following sedation have been reported in dogs following the combination of droperidol and fentanyl.

Cardiovascular. The reduction in blood pressure caused by droperidol is a result of the central and peripheral α_1-adrenergic receptor antagonism. Vasodilation is mild in most circumstances with little to no depression of the myocardial contractility except at high doses of droperidol (1 mg/kg IV). An increase in heart rate without any significant change in blood pressure is seen when the droperidol-fentanyl combination is used in cats and dogs. The increase in heart rate seen with droperidol is due to the blockade of the central vagal activity, rather than changes to the peripheral blood pressure. Droperidol will antagonize the dopaminergic-mediated increase in renal blood flow caused by a dopamine constant rate infusion.

Antagonism of dopaminergic receptors in the adrenal medulla using low doses of droperidol may lead to an increase in release of catecholamines and a subsequent hypertensive crisis, especially in patients with a pheochromocytoma. At higher doses droperidol will inhibit the release of catecholamines from the adrenal medulla.

Similar to phenothiazines, the butyrophenones also possess protections against epinephrine-induced dysrhythmia effects due to the α_1-adrenergic receptor antagonism and local anesthetic qualities. Large doses of droperidol decrease the conduction of impulses along accessory pathways, and therefore have a protective mechanism against reentry arrhythmias. In 2001 the FDA issued a "Black Box Warning" for the use of droperidol causing torsades de pointes. Butyrophenones do prolong the QTc interval; however, that alone does not cause torsades de pointes. This warning has since been removed. This effect has not been reported in any veterinary patients.

Respiratory. Droperidol does not affect resting ventilation or the ventilatory response to carbon dioxide. There appears to be an augmented ventilatory response to arterial hypoxemia, thought to be due to the dopaminergic antagonism at the level of the carotid body. When droperidol is combined with fentanyl and administered to cats subcutaneously, a reduction in respiratory rate was seen, however without any significant change to PaO_2, $PaCO_2$, or pH. In the dog (Innovar-Vet, 0.05 ml/kg IV or 0.1 mg/kg IM) there are clinically insignificant changes to the arterial blood gases with a gradual reduction in respiratory rate over time.

Musculoskeletal. The butyrophenones will usually result in a reduction in muscle tone in the majority of patients. The dopaminergic antagonism of the butyrophenones may result in pacing, restlessness, and tremors in a small percentage of patients. (See Adverse Effects/Contraindications).

Miscellaneous

Antiemetic: Small doses of droperidol given at the time of induction have been shown to be an effective antiemetic. This potent antiemetic effect is due to the dopaminergic antagonism of the dopamine receptors in the chemoreceptor trigger zone of the medulla. Droperidol will antagonize the effects of apomorphine; however, it has no effect on motion-sickness (labyrinthine-induced).

Platelet aggregation: Droperidol has an antithrombotic effect, which appears to be mediated by attenuating platelet activation and aggregation.

Aggression: Severe postsedation aggression has been anecdotally reported in dogs and in particular Doberman Pinchers.

Analgesia. Droperidol in itself does not provide any analgesia; however, the droperidol-fentanyl preparation has substantial analgesic properties due to the opioid, fentanyl.

Pharmacokinetics Properties. There is little information regarding the pharmacokinetics of the butyrophenones used in veterinary practice. The onset time after intramuscular injection is less than 10 minutes in most species with a peak effect seen approximately 30 minutes postadministration. The duration of action is 2 to 4 hours in pigs. Azaperone in pigs is biotransformed in the liver with 13% excreted in the feces. The two main metabolites of azaperone in the horse are 5′-hydroxyazaperol and 5′-hydroxyazaperone, which are conjugated by glucuronidation. Metabolite residues are highest in the kidneys and are present in the urine for at least 3 days after administration; however, most of the drug is eliminated from the body within 16 hours.

The onset of droperidol-fentanyl combinations in the dog administered either IV or IM is 2 and 9 minutes, respectively. The duration of action is approximately 20 to 60 minutes depending on dose and route of administration. In humans, droperidol is biotransformed in the liver into two metabolites and its elimination is described using a two-compartment model. The volume of distribution at steady state is 2.0 l/kg. The clearance is relatively large at 14 ml/kg/min and the elimination half-life is relatively short at 103–134 minutes. This is similar to fentanyl. The CNS actions of droperidol last longer than this, which leads to speculation that droperidol has a longer receptor occupation than fentanyl.

Adverse Effects/Contraindications

Penile Prolapse: Doses of azaperone greater than 1 mg/kg IM may cause penile prolapse in boars, which may predispose to injury.

Hypothermia: The use in cold weather and the resultant vasodilation caused by azaperone may lead to hypothermia.

Behavioral effects: Butyrophenones may produce dysphoric effects, especially in patients with a high level of anxiety. It is also possible to induce a feeling of restlessness (akathisia) in humans, which may manifest as pacing and agitation in veterinary patients. Extrapyramidal signs are seen in 1% of human patients with the use of droperidol. For this reason droperidol should not be given to any patients receiving antiparkinsonian therapy such as selegiline. Muscle tremors, spasticity, and irritability have only been seen in the dog after the use of high doses in the range of 11–22 mg/kg IV. Salivation, sweating, muscle tremors, and vocalization have been reported in the horse following intravenous administration of azaperone at a dose of 0.29–0.57 mg/kg.

Catecholamine release: Droperidol can cause an increase in catecholamine release from the adrenal medulla, especially at low doses (0.006 mg/kg IV) in the dog. The use of droperidol in patients with a pheochromocytoma should be avoided.

ECG: The butyrophenones can cause a prolongation of the QT interval and their use in patients with bradydysrhythmia should be used with an anticholinergic or avoided where possible.

Contraindications: Contraindications for the use of butyrophenones include coma, severe CNS depression from other sedatives, hypersensitivities, preexisting use of antiparkinsonian drugs, prolonged QT interval, hypokalemia, epilepsy, and conditions with preexisting hypotension.

Dose:

Azaperone

Swine:

0.5–2 mg/kg IM

Horses:

0.4–0.8 mg/kg IM. Intravenous administration is not recommended due to the paradoxical excitement seen in a high percentage of horses.

Deer:

0.3 mg/kg IM in combination with xylazine 1 mg/kg IM.

Rhinoceroses:

0.04 mg/kg IM

Droperidol

Dogs:

0.6–2.2 mg/kg of droperidol IV, IM

0.030.11 ml/kg of Innovar–Vet® IV or IM

Cats:

2.2 mg/kg of droperidol

0.11 ml/kg Innovar–Vet® IM

Swine:

0.3 mg/kg IM

Species Differences

Guinea Pigs: Droperidol with fentanyl (Innovar-Vet) can cause muscle swelling, lameness, and self-mutilation and is not recommended (Thurman 1996).

Doberman Pincher Dogs: There are anecdotal reports of postsedation aggression and head bobbing.

Drug Interactions. Droperidol potentiates the effects of other anesthetic agents, which will necessitate a reduction in the dose of induction and inhalational agents.

Butyrophenones will inhibit the effect of dopamine on renal blood flow. The use of butyrophenones in patients receiving selegiline may precipitate extrapyramidal signs.

Overdose/Acute Toxicity. The successful reversal of droperidol-fentanyl–induced sedation has been described using 4-aminopyridine 0.5 mg/kg IV and naloxone 0.04 mg/kg IV following a fivefold overdose. Repeated doses were required due to renarcosis. Other supportive measures such as intravenous fluids, positive inotropes, and chronotropes, as well as respiratory support may be required to counteract the hypotension and respiratory depression.

Regulatory Information

Controlled Drug Status. Schedule IV veterinary prescription only.

Withdrawal Times. There is a 10-day withholding period prior to slaughter.

Veterinary Products

Azaperone

Stresnil: Azaperone 40 mg/ml (Schering-Plough Animal Health Corp.) Injection approved for use in pigs in the U.S.

Droperidol

Droperidol is approved by the FDA for use in the dog.

Innovar-Vet® Injection: Droperidol: Fentanyl 20 mg: 0.4 mg/ml (Schering-Plough Animal Health Corp.)

Human Products

Droperidol

Inapsine: Droperidol Injectable; Injection 2.5 mg/ml (Akorn)

Droperidol: Droperidol Injectable; Injection 2.5 mg/ml (Hospira)

Droperidol: Droperidol Injectable; Injection 2.5 mg/ml (Luitpold)

REFERENCES

Aantaa, R. & Scheinin, M. (1993) Alpha2-Adrenergic Agents In Anesthesia. Acta Anaesthesiologica Scandinavica, 37, 433–448.

Adam, L. A. (1999) Confirmation Of Azaperone And Its Metabolically Reduced Form, Azaperol, In Swine Liver By Gas Chromatography/Mass Spectrometry. Journal Of AOAC International, 82, 815–824.

Akin, F., Rose, A. 3rd, Chamness, T. & Marlowe, E. (1979) Sunscreen Protection Against Drug-Induced Phototoxicity In Animal Models. Toxicology Applied Pharmacology, Jun 30;49(2):219–24.

Altahan, F., Loscher, W. & Frey, H. H. (1984) Pharmacokinetics Of Clonazepam In The Dog. Archives Internationales De Pharmacodynamie Et De Therapie, 268, 180–193.

Ambrisko, T. D. & Hikasa, Y. (2003) The Antagonistic Effects Of Atipamezole And Yohimbine On Stress-Related Neurohormonal And Metabolic Responses Induced By Medetomidine In Dogs. Canadian Journal Of Veterinary Research-Revue Canadienne De Recherche Veterinaire, 67, 64–67.

Aminkov, B. & Pascalev, M. (1998) Cardiovascular And Respiratory Effects Of Epidural Vs Intravenous Xylazine In Sheep. Revue De Medecine Veterinaire, 149, 69–74.

Andrade, S. F., Sakate, M., Laposy, C. B. & Sangiorgio, F. (2006) Yohimbine And Atipamezole On The Treatment Of Experimentally Induced Amitraz Intoxication In Cats. International Journal Of Applied Research In Veterinary Medicine, 4, 200–208.

Angel, I., Niddam, R. & Langer, S. Z. (1990) Involvement Of Alpha2-Adrenergic Receptor Subtypes In Hyperglycemia. Journal Of Pharmacology And Experimental Therapeutics, 254, 877–882.

Anika, S. M. (1985) Diazepam And Chlorpromazine Stimulate Feeding In Dwarf Goats. Veterinary Research Communications, 9, 309–12.

Ansah, O. B., Raekallio, M. & Vainio, O. (1998) Comparison Of Three Doses Of Dexmedetomidine With Medetomidine In Cats Following Intramuscular Administration. Journal Of Veterinary Pharmacology And Therapeutics, 21, 380–387.

———. (2000) Correlation Between Serum Concentrations Following Continuous Intravenous Infusion Of Dexmedetomidine Or Medetomidine In Cats And Their Sedative And Analgesic Effects. Journal Of Veterinary Pharmacology And Therapeutics, 23, 1–8.

Arneth, W. (1985) Distribution Of Azaperone And Azaperol Residues In Swine. Fleischwirtschaft, 65, 945–950.

Artru, A. A. (1991) Intraocular Pressure In Anaesthetized Dogs Given Flumazenil With And Without Prior Administration Of Midazolam. Canadian Journal Of Anaesthesia—Journal Canadien D'anesthesie, 38, 408–14.

Aziz, M. A. & Martin, R. J. (1978) Alpha Agonist And Local Anaesthetic Properties Of Xylazine. Zentralblatt Fur Veterinarmedizin. Reihe A, 25, 181–8.

Badino, P., Odore, R. & Re, G. (2005) Are So Many Adrenergic Receptor Subtypes Really Present In Domestic Animal Tissues? A Pharmacological Perspective. Veterinary Journal, 170, 163–174.

Ballard, S., Shults, T., Kownacki, A., Blake, J. & Tobin T. (1982) The Pharmacokinetics, Pharmacological Responses And Behavioral Effects Of Acepromazine In The Horse. Journal Of Veterinary Pharmacology Therapeutics, Mar;5(1):21–31.

Barr, J. G. & Kauker, M. L. (1979) Renal Tubular Site And Mechanism Of Clonidine-Induced Diuresis In Rats: Clearance And Micro Puncture Studies. Journal Of Pharmacology And Experimental Therapeutics, 209, 389–395.

Barr, S. C., Ludders, J., Looney, A., Gleed, R. & Erb, H. (1992) Platelet Aggregation In Dogs After Sedation With Acepromazine And Atropine And During Subsequent General Anesthesia And Surgery. American Journal Of Veterinary Research, Nov;53(11):2067–70.

Bettschart-Wolfensberger, R., Clarke, K. W., Vainio, O., Aliabadi, F. S. & Demuth, D. (1999) Pharmacokinetics Of Medetomidine In Ponies And Elaboration Of A Medetomidine Infusion Regime Which Provides A Constant Level Of Sedation. Research In Veterinary Science, 67, 41–46.

Bettschart-Wolfensberger, R., Freeman, S. L., Bowen, I. M., Aliabadi, F. S., Weller, R., Huhtinen, M. & Clarke, K. W. (2005a) Cardiopulmonary

Effects And Pharmacokinetics Of I.V. Dexmedetomidine In Ponies. Equine Veterinary Journal, 37, 60–64.

Bettschart-Wolfensberger, R., Kalchofner, K., Neges, K. & Kastner, S. (2005b) Total Intravenous Anaesthesia In Horses Using Medetomidine And Propofol. Veterinary Anaesthesia And Analgesia, 32, 348–354.

Bienert, A., Bartmann, C. P., von Oppen, T., Poppe, T., Schiemann, V. & Deegen, E. (2003) Recovery Phase Of Horses After Inhalant Anaesthesia With Isofluorane (Isoflo (R)) And Postanaesthetic Sedation With Romifidine (Sedivet (R)) Or Xylazine (Rompun (R)). Deutsche Tierarztliche Wochenschrift, 110, 244–248.

Bishnoi, P. & Saini, N. S. (2005) Cardio-Respiratory Effects Of Midazolam In Calves. Veterinary Practitioner, 6, 1–5.

Bloor, B. C., Abdulrasool, I., Temp, J., Jenkins, S., Valcke, C. & Ward, D. S. (1989) The Effects Of Medetomidine, An Alpha2-Adrenergic Agonist, On Ventilatory Drive In The Dog. Acta Veterinaria Scandinavica, Suppl. 85, 65–70.

Bloor, B. C., Frankland, M., Alper, G., Raybould, D., Weitz, J. & Shurtliff, M. (1992) Hemodynamic And Sedative Effects Of Dexmedetomidine In Dogs. Journal Of Pharmacology And Experimental Therapeutics, 263, 690–697.

Boehringer Ingelheim Vetmedica, I. (2004) Romifidine Hydrochloride 1%. In Boehringer Ingelheim Vetmedica, I., Highway, N. B. & St. Joseph, M. (Eds.) Sedivet 1% Injection.

Bonfiglio, M. F., Fisherkatz, L. E., Saltis, L. M., Traeger, S. M., Martin, B. R., Nackes, N. A. & Perkins, T. A. (1996) A Pilot Pharmacokinetic-Pharmacodynamic Study Of Benzodiazepine Antagonism By Flumazenil And Aminophylline. Pharmacotherapy, 16, 1166–1172.

Booth, N. H., Hatch, R. C. & Crawford, L. M. (1982) Reversal Of The Neuroleptanalgesic Effect Of Droperidol-Fentanyl In The Dog By 4-Aminopyridine And Naloxone. American Journal Of Veterinary Research, 43, 1227–1231.

Bordet, R. (2004) Dopamine Receptors: General Aspects. Revue Neurologique, 160, 862–870.

Boronat, M. A., Olmos, G. & Garcia-Sevilla, J. A. (1999) Attenuation Of Tolerance To Opioid-Induced Antinociception By Idazoxan And Other I2-Ligands. Annals Of The New York Academy Of Sciences, 881, 359–363.

Bourin, M., Malinge, M., Colombel, M. C. & Larousse, C. (1988) Influence Of Alpha Stimulants And Beta Blockers On Yohimbine Toxicity. Progress In Neuro-Psychopharmacology & Biological Psychiatry, 12, 569–74.

Bousquet, P., Bruban, V., Schann, S., Greney, H., Ehrhardt, J. D., Dontenwill, M. & Feldman, J. (1999) Participation Of Imidazoline Receptors And Alpha2-Adrenoceptors In The Central Hypotensive Effects Of Imidazoline-Like Drugs. Annals Of The New York Academy Of Sciences, 881, 272–278.

Boyd, R. E. (2000) Alpha(2)-Adrenergic Agonists As Analgesic Agents. Expert Opinion On Therapeutic Patents, 10, 1741–1748.

Bozdogan, O. & Dogan, A. (1999) Effect Of Adrenergic Receptor Blockade With Yohimbin, Metroprolol Or Prazosin On Arrhythmogenic Dose Of Epinephrine In Xylazine-Kethamine Anesthetized Dogs. Turkish Journal Of Veterinary & Animal Sciences, 23, 327–332.

Bradshaw, E. G., Pleuvry, B. J. & Sharma, H. L. (1980) Effect Of Droperidol On Dopamine-Induced Increase In Effective Renal Plasma Flow In Dogs. British Journal Of Anaesthesia, 52, 879–83.

Briggs, G. M. & Meier, C. F., Jr. (1986) Effect Of Yohimbine On Action Potentials Recorded From Isolated Canine Ventricular Myocytes. European Journal Of Pharmacology, 127, 125–8.

Brockman, R. P. (1981) Effect Of Xylazine On Plasma Glucose, Glucagon And Insulin Concentrations In Sheep. Research In Veterinary Science, 30, 383–384.

Brown, S. A. & Forrester, S. D. (1991) Serum Disposition Of Oral Clorazepate From Regular-Release And Sustained-Release Tablets In Dogs. Journal Of Veterinary Pharmacology And Therapeutics, 14, 426–429.

Brown, S. A., Jacobson, J. D. & Hartsfield, S. M. (1993) Pharmacokinetics Of Midazolam Administered Concurrently With Ketamine After Intravenous Bolus Or Infusion In Dogs. Journal Of Veterinary Pharmacology And Therapeutics, 16, 419–425.

Bryant, C. E., England, G. C. W. & Clarke, K. W. (1991) Comparison Of The Sedative Effects Of Medetomidine And Xylazine In Horses. Veterinary Record, 129, 421–423.

Bueno, A. C., Cornick-Seahorn, J., Seahorn, T. L., Hosgood, G. & Moore, R. M. (1999) Cardiopulmonary And Sedative Effects Of Intravenous Administration Of Low Doses Of Medetomidine And Xylazine To Adult Horses. American Journal Of Veterinary Research, 60, 1371–1376.

Buhrer, M., Maitre, P. O., Crevoisier, C. & Stanski, D. R. (1990) Electroencephalographic Effects Of Benzodiazepines. 2. Pharmacodynamic Modeling Of The Electroencephalographic Effects Of Midazolam And Diazepam. Clinical Pharmacology & Therapeutics, 48, 555–567.

Bustamante, V. R. & Valverde, A. (1997) Determination Of A Sedative Dose And Influence Of Droperidol And Midazolam On Cardiovascular Function In Pigs. Canadian Journal Of Veterinary Research, 61, 246–250.

Calzada, B. C. & De Artinano, A. A. (2001) Alpha-Adrenoceptor Subtypes. Pharmacological Research, 44, 195–208.

Carbajal, R., Simon, N., Blanc, P., Paupe, A., Lenclen, R. & Olivermartin, M. (1996) Rectal Flumazenil To Reverse Midazolam Sedation In Children. Anesthesia And Analgesia, 82, 895–895.

Carroll, G. L., Hartsfield, S. M., Champney, T. H., Geller, S. C., Martinez, E. A. & Haley, E. L. (2005) Effect Of Medetomidine And Its Antagonism With Atipamezole On Stress-Related Hormones, Metabolites, Physiologic Responses, Sedation, And Mechanical Threshold In Goats. Veterinary Anaesthesia And Analgesia, 32, 147–157.

Carroll, G. L., Matthews, N. S., Hartsfield, S. M., Slater, M. R., Champney, T. H. & Erickson, S. W. (1997) The Effect Of Detomidine And Its Antagonism With Tolazoline On Stress-Related Hormones, Metabolites, Physiologic Responses, And Behavior In Awake Ponies. Veterinary Surgery, 26, 69–77.

Castro, M. & Eisenach, J. (1989) Pharmacokinetics And Dynamics Of Intravenous, Intrathecal, And Epidural Clonidine In Sheep. Anesthesiology, Sep;71(3):418–25.

Celly, C. S., Mcdonell, W. N., Young, S. S. & Black, W. D. (1997) The Comparative Hypoxaemic Effect Of Four Alpha(2) Adrenoceptor Agonists (Xylazine, Romifidine, Detomidine And Medetomidine) In Sheep. Journal Of Veterinary Pharmacology And Therapeutics, 20, 464–471.

Christina Haerdi-Landerer, M., Schlegel, U. & Neiger-Aeschbacher, G. (2005) The Analgesic Effects Of Intrathecal Xylazine And Detomidine In Sheep And Their Antagonism With Systemic Atipamezole1. Veterinary Anaesthesia And Analgesia, 32, 297–307.

Chui, J. W. & White, P. F. (2001) Nonopioid Intravenous Anesthesia. In Barash, P. G., Cullen, B. F. & Stoelting, R. K. (Eds.) Clinical Anesthesia. 4th Ed. Philadelphia, Lippincott Williams & Wilkins.

Chui, Y. C., Esaw, B. & Laviolette, B. (1994) Investigation Of The Metabolism Of Azaperone In The Horse. Journal Of Chromatography B-Biomedical Applications, 652, 23–33.

Cistola, A. M., Golder, F. J., Centonze, L. A., Mckay, L. W. & Levy, J. K. (2004) Anesthetic And Physiologic Effects Of Tiletamine, Zolazepam, Ketamine, And Xylazine Combination (Tkx) In Feral Cats Undergoing Surgical Sterilization. Journal Of Feline Medicine And Surgery, 6, 297–303.

Clarke, K. W. (1969) Effect Of Azaperone On The Blood Pressure And Pulmonary Ventilation In Pigs. Veterinary Record, 85, 649–651.

Clarke, K. W. & England, G. C. W. (1989) Medetomidine, A New Sedative-Analgesic For Use In The Dog And Its Reversal With Atipamezole. Journal Of Small Animal Practice, 30, 343–348.

Clarke, K. W. & Hall, L. W. (1969) Xylazine—A New Sedative For Horses And Cattle. Veterinary Record, 85, 512–517.

Cormack, J. R., Orme, R. M. & Costello, T. G. (2005) The Role Of Alpha2-Agonists In Neurosurgery. Journal Of Clinical Neuroscience, 12, 375–378.

Cornick-Seahorn, J. L. & Seahorn, T. L. (1998) Cardiopulmonary And Behavioral Effects Of Midazolam Hcl And Reversal With Flumazenil In Pony Foals. Veterinary Surgery, 27, 169.

Cotler, S., Gustafson, J. H. & Colburn, W. A. (1984) Pharmacokinetics Of Diazepam And Nordiazepam In The Cat. Journal Of Pharmaceutical Sciences, 73, 348–51.

Court, M. H., Dodman, N. H., Greenblatt, D. J., Agarwal, R. K. & Kumar, M. S. (1993) Effect Of Midazolam Infusion And Flumazenil Administration On Epinephrine Arrhythmogenicity In Dogs Anesthetized With Halothane. Anesthesiology, 78, 155–62.

Court, M. H. & Greenblatt, D. J. (1992) Pharmacokinetics And Preliminary Observations Of Behavioral Changes Following Administration Of Midazolam To Dogs. Journal Of Veterinary Pharmacology And Therapeutics, 15, 343–50.

Cullen, L. K. (1999) Xylazine And Medetomidine In Small Animals: These Drugs Should Be Used Carefully. Australian Veterinary Journal, 77, 722–723.

Daniell, H. B. (1975) Cardiovascular Effects Of Diazepam And Chlordiazepoxide. European Journal Of Pharmacology, 32, 58–65.

Das, D. K. & Murthy, G. S. (2005) Immobilization Of A Sloth Bear With Xylazine Ketamine And Reversal With Yohimbine. Indian Veterinary Journal, 82, 776–777.

Daunt, D. A., Dunlop, C. I., Chapman, P. L., Shafer, S. L., Ruskoaho, H., Vakkur, O., Hodgson, D. S., Tyler, L. M. & Maze, M. (1993) Cardiopulmonary And Behavioral-Responses To Computer-Driven Infusion Of Detomidine In Standing Horses. American Journal Of Veterinary Research, 54, 2075–2082.

Delehant, T. M., Denhart, J. W., Lloyd, W. E. & Powell, J. D. (2003) Pharmacokinetics Of Xylazine, 2,6-Dimethylaniline, And Tolazoline In Tissues From Yearling Cattle And Milk From Mature Dairy Cows After Sedation With Xylazine Hydrochloride And Reversal With Tolazoline Hydrochloride. Veterinary Therapeutics, 4, 128–134.

Derossi, R., Righetto, F. R., Almeida, R. G., Medeiros, U. & Frazilio, F. O. (2006) Clinical Evaluation Of Clonidine Added To Lidocaine Solution For Subarachnoid Analgesia In Sheep. Journal Of Veterinary Pharmacology And Therapeutics, 29, 113–119.

Diaz, A., Mayet, S. & Dickenson, A. H. (1997) BU-224 Produces Spinal Antinociception As An Agonist At Imidazoline I-2 Receptors. European Journal Of Pharmacology, 333, 9–15.

Dichiara, G. & Gessa, G. L. (1978) Dopamine Receptors And Phenothiazines. Advanced Pharmacology Chemotherapy, 15, 87.

Dirikolu, L., Mcfadden, E. T., Ely, K. J., Elkholy, H., Lehner, A. F. & Thompson, K. (2006) Clonidine In Horses: Identification, Detection, And Clinical Pharmacology. Veterinary Therapeutics, 7, 141–155.

Dodman, N. H. & Waterman, A. E. (1979) Paradoxical Excitement Following The Intravenous Administration Of Azaperone In The Horse. Equine Veterinary Journal, 11, 33–5.

Driessen, J. J., Van Egmond, J., Van Der Pol, F. & Crul, J. F. (1987) Effects Of Two Benzodiazepines And A Benzodiazepine Antagonist On Neuromuscular Blockade In The Anaesthetized Cat. Archives Internationales De Pharmacodynamie Et De Therapie, 286, 58–70.

Dunn, R. W. & Corbett, R. (1992) Yohimbine-Induced Seizures Involve NMDA And Gabaergic Transmission. Neuropharmacology, 31, 389–95.

Dyck, J. B., Maze, M., Haack, C., Vuorilehto, L. & Shafer, S. L. (1993) The Pharmacokinetics And Hemodynamic-Effects Of Intravenous And Intramuscular Dexmedetomidine Hydrochloride In Adult Human Volunteers. Anesthesiology, 78, 813–820.

Elliott, H. W. (1976) Metabolism Of Lorazepam. British Journal Of Anaesthesia, 48, 1017–23.

England, G. C. W. & Clarke, K. W. (1996) Alpha2 Adrenoceptor Agonists In The Horse—A Review. British Veterinary Journal, 152, 641–657.

England, G. C. W., Clarke, K. W. & Goossens, L. (1992) A Comparison Of The Sedative Effects Of 3 Alpha2-Adrenoceptor Agonists (Romifidine, Detomidine And Xylazine) In The Horse. Journal Of Veterinary Pharmacology And Therapeutics, 15, 194–201.

England, G. C. W., Flack, T. E., Hollingworth, E. & Hammond, R. (1996) Sedative Effects Of Romifidine In The Dog. Journal Of Small Animal Practice, 37, 19–25.

England, G. C. W. & Hammond, R. (1997) Dose Sparing Effects Of Romifidine Premedication For Thiopentone And Halothane Anaesthesia In The Dog. Journal Of Small Animal Practice, 38, 141–146.

Erne-Brand, F., Jirounek, P., Drewe, J., Hampl, K. & Schneider, M. C. (1999) Mechanism Of Antinociceptive Action Of Clonidine In Nonmyelinated Nerve Fibres. European Journal Of Pharmacology, 383, 1–8.

Fierheller, E. E., Caulkett, N. A. & Bailey, J. V. (2004) A Romifidine And Morphine Combination For Epidural Analgesia Of The Flank In Cattle. Canadian Veterinary Journal-Revue Veterinaire Canadienne, 45, 917–923.

Fischler, M., Bonnet, F., Trang, H., Jacob, L., Levron, J. C., Flaisler, B. & Vourch, G. (1986) The Pharmacokinetics Of Droperidol In Anesthetized Patients. Anesthesiology, 64, 486–489.

Fleischer (Ed), L. A. (2005) Miller's Anesthesia (Online). Miller's Anesthesia [Electronic Resource] / Edited By Ronald D. Miller; Atlas Of Regional Anesthesia Procedures Illustrated By Gwenn Afton-Bird. In Miller, R. D. & Llc, M. D. C. (Eds.) 6th Ed. St. Louis, Mo., Md Consult.

Ford, S. P. (1995) Control Of Blood Flow To The Gravid Uterus Of Domestic Livestock Species. Journal Of Animal Science, 73, 1852–1860.

Forster, A., Crettenand, G., Klopfenstein, C. E. & Morel, D. R. (1993) Absence Of Agonist Effects Of High Dose Flumazenil On Ventilation And Psychometric Performance In Human Volunteers. Anesthesia And Analgesia, 77, 980–984.

Fowler, M. E. (1989) Medicine And Surgery Of South American Camelids: Llama, Alpaca, Vicuña, Guanaco/Murray E. Fowler, Ames, Iowa State University Press.

Frank, H. & Von Loewenich-Lagois, K. (1966) Therapeutic Examination And Studies On Renal Function With A New Antihypertensive Agent (St 155). Deutsche Medizinische Wochenschrift, 91, 1680–6.

Freeman, S. L., Bowen, I. M., Bettschart-Wolfensberger, R., Alibhai, H. I. K. & England, G. C. W. (2002) Cardiovascular Effects Of Romifidine In The Standing Horse. Research In Veterinary Science, 72, 123–129.

Freeman, S. L. & England, G. C. W. (2000) Investigation Of Romifidine And Detomidine For The Clinical Sedation Of Horses. Veterinary Record, 147, 507–511.

Frey, H. H. & Loscher, W. (1985) Pharmacokinetics Of Anti-Epileptic Drugs In The Dog: A Review. Journal Of Veterinary Pharmacology And Therapeutics, 8, 219–33.

Garcia-Villar, R., Toutain, P. L., Alvinerie, M. & Ruckebusch, Y. (1981) The Pharmacokinetics Of Xylazine Hydrochloride An Interspecific Study. Journal Of Veterinary Pharmacology And Therapeutics, 4, 87–92.

Gaspar, R., Foldesi, I., Havass, J., Marki, A. & Falkay, G. (2001) Characterization Of Late-Pregnant Rat Uterine Contraction Via The Contractility Ratio In Vitro—Significance Of Alpha(1)-Adrenoceptors. Life Sciences, 68, 1119–1129.

Gellai, M. & Edwards, R. M. (1988) Mechanism Of Alpha2-Adrenoceptor Agonist-Induced Diuresis. American Journal Of Physiology, 255, F317–F323.

Gentili, F., Cardinaletti, C., Carrieri, A., Ghelfi, F., Mattioli, L., Perfumi, M., Vesprini, C. & Pigini, M. (2006) Involvement Of I-2-Imidazoline Binding Sites In Positive And Negative Morphine Analgesia Modulatory Effects. European Journal Of Pharmacology, 553, 73–81.

Gentili, F., Pigini, M., Piergentili, A. & Giannella, M. (2007) Agonists And Antagonists Targeting The Different Alpha2-Adrenoceptor Subtypes. Current Topics In Medicinal Chemistry, 7, 163–186.

Gerkens, J. F., Desmond, P. V., Schenker, S. & Branch, R. A. (1981) Hepatic And Extrahepatic Glucuronidation Of Lorazepam In The Dog. Hepatology, 1, 329–335.

Gillis, R. A., Thibodeaux, H. & Barr, L. (1974) Antiarrhythmic Properties Of Chlordiazepoxide. Circulation, 49, 272–82.

Gluckman, M. I. & Stein, L. (1978) Pharmacology Of Lorazepam. Journal Of Clinical Psychiatry, 39, 3–10.

Glynn, C. & O'Sullivan, K. (1996) A Double-Blind Randomised Comparison Of The Effects Of Epidural Clonidine, Lignocaine And The Combination Of Clonidine And Lignocaine In Patients With Chronic Pain. Pain, 64, 337–343.

Gomez-Villamandos, R. J., Redondo, J., Martin, E. M., Dominguez, J. M., Granados, M. M., Estepa, J. C., Ruiz, I., Aguilera, E. & Santisteban, J. M. (2005) Romifidine Or Medetomidine Premedication Before Propofol-Sevoflurane Anaesthesia In Dogs. Journal Of Veterinary Pharmacology And Therapeutics, 28, 489–493.

González Gil, A., Illera, J. C., Silván, G. & Illera, M. (2001) Plasma Glucocorticoid Concentrations After Fentanyl-Droperidol, Ketamine-Xylazine And Ketamine-Diazepam Anaesthesia In New Zealand White Rabbits. Veterinary Record, 148, 784–786.

Goodall, J., Hagan, R. M. & Hughes, I. E. (1984) A Contribution, From A Possible Local Anaesthetic Action, To The Effects Of Yohimbine On Evoked Noradrenaline Overflow. Journal Of Pharmacy And Pharmacology, 36, 278–80.

Gothert, M. & Molderings, G. J. (1992) Modulation Of Norepinephrine Release In Blood Vessels—Mediated By Presynaptic Imidazoline Receptors And Alpha2-Adrenoceptors. Journal Of Cardiovascular Pharmacology, 20, S16–S20.

Grandy, J. L. & Heath, R. B. (1987) Cardiopulmonary And Behavioral Effects Of Fentanyl-Droperidol In Cats. Journal Of The American Veterinary Medical Association, 191, 59–61.

Granholm, M., Mckusick, B. C., Westerholm, F. C. & Aspegren, J. C. (2006) Evaluation Of The Clinical Efficacy And Safety Of Dexmedetomidine Or Medetomidine In Cats And Their Reversal With Atipamezole. Veterinary Anaesthesia And Analgesia, 33, 214–223.

Greene, S. A., Keegan, R. D. & Weil, A. B. (1995) Cardiovascular Effects After Epidural Injection Of Xylazine In Isoflurane-Anesthetized Dogs. Veterinary Surgery, 24, 283–289.

Grille, P., Biestro, A., Fariña, G. & Miraballes, R. (2005) Effects Of Dexmedetomidine On Intracranial Hemodynamics In Severe Head Injured Patients. Neurocirugia.

Grove, D. M. & Ramsay, E. C. (2000) Sedative And Physiologic Effects Of Orally Administered Alpha(2)-Adrenoceptor Agonists And Ketamine In Cats. Journal Of The American Veterinary Medical Association, 216, 1929–1932.

Gvozdenovic, L. V., Popovic, M. R., Jakovljevic, V. S. & Lukic, V. (1993) Effect Of Fentanyl, Ketamine And Thalamonal On Some Biochemical Parameters In Ethanol-Treated And Untreated Dogs. Human & Experimental Toxicology, 12, 279–83.

Haapalinna, A., Viitamaa, T., Macdonald, E., Savola, J. M., Tuomisto, L., Virtanen, R. & Heinonen, E. (1997) Evaluation Of The Effects Of A Specific Alpha2-Adrenoceptor Antagonist, Atipamezole, On Alpha1- And Alpha2-Adrenoceptor Subtype Binding, Brain Neurochemistry And Behaviour In Comparison With Yohimbine. Naunyn-Schmiedebergs Archives Of Pharmacology, 356, 570–582.

Hall, J. A., Magne, M. L. & Twedt, D. C. (1987) Effect Of Acepromazine, Diazepam, Fentanyl-Droperidol, And Oxymorphone On Gastroesophageal Sphincter Pressure In Healthy Dogs. American Journal Of Veterinary Research, 48, 556–7.

Hall, L. W., Lagerweij, E., Nolan, A. M. & Sear, J. W. (1994) Effect Of Medetomidine On The Pharmacokinetics Of Propofol In Dogs. American Journal Of Veterinary Research, 55, 116–120.

Hamalainen, M. M. & Pertovaara, A. (1995) The Antinociceptive Action Of An Alpha2-Adrenoceptor Agonist In The Spinal Dorsal Horn Is Due To A Direct Spinal Action And Not To Activation Of Descending Inhibition. Brain Research Bulletin, 37, 581–587.

Hamm, D., Turchi, P. & Jochle, W. (1995) Sedative And Analgesia Effects Of Detomidine And Romifidine In Horses. Veterinary Record, 136, 324–327.

Hart, B. L. (1985) Behavioral Indications For Phenothiazine And Benzodiazepine Tranquilizers In Dogs. Journal Of The American Veterinary Medical Association, 186, 1192–4.

Hashem, A., Kietzmann, M. & Scherkl, R. (1992) The Pharmacokinetics And Bioavailability Of Acepromazine In The Plasma Of Dogs. Deutsch Tierarztl Wochenschr, Oct;99(10):396–8.

Head, G. A. (1999) Central Imidazoline- And 2-Receptors Involved In The Cardiovascular Actions Of Centrally Acting Antihypertensive Agents. Annals Of The New York Academy Of Sciences, 881, 279–286.

Hellyer, P. W., Mama, K. R., Shafford, H. L., Wagner, A. E. & Kollias-Baker, C. (2001) Effects Of Diazepam And Flumazenil On Minimum Alveolar Concentrations For Dogs Anesthetized With Isoflurane Or A Combination Of Isoflurane And Fentanyl. American Journal Of Veterinary Research, 62, 555–560.

Henry, R. J., Ruano, N., Casto, D. & Wolf, R. H. (1998) A Pharmacokinetic Study Of Midazolam In Dogs: Nasal Drop Vs. Atomizer Administration. Pediatric Dentistry, 20, 321–6.

Hikasa, Y., Abe, M., Satoh, T., Hisashi, Y., Ogasawara, S. & Matsuda, H. (1999) Effects Of Imidazoline And Non-Imidazoline Alpha-Adrenergic Agents On Canine Platelet Aggregation. Pharmacology, 58, 171–182.

Hikasa, Y., Ogasawara, S. & Takase, K. (1992) Alpha-Adrenergic Subtypes Involved In The Emetic Action In Dogs. Journal Of Pharmacology And Experimental Therapeutics, 261, 746–754.

Hiyoshi, Y., Miura, H., Uemura, K., Endo, H., Ozawa, K., Maeda, N., Tamagawa, T. & Iguchi, A. (1995) Effects Of Imidazoline Antagonists Of Alpha(2)-Adrenoceptors On Endogenous Adrenaline-Induced Inhibition Of Insulin Release. European Journal Of Pharmacology, 294, 117–123.

Hoffman, W. E., Cheng, M. A., Thomas, C., Baughman, V. L. & Albrecht, R. F. (1991) Clonidine Decreases Plasma-Catecholamines And Improves Outcome From Incomplete Ischemia In The Rat. Anesthesia And Analgesia, 73, 460–464.

Hoffman, W. E., Kochs, E., Werner, C., Thomas, C. & Albrecht, R. F. (1991b) Dexmedetomidine Improves Neurologic Outcome From Incomplete Ischemia In The Rat—Reversal By The Alpha2-Adrenergic Antagonist Atipamezole. Anesthesiology, 75, 328–332.

Hoyumpa, A. M., Patwardhan, R., Maples, M., Desmond, P. V., Johnson, R. F., Sinclair, A. P. & Schenker, S. (1981) Effect Of Short-Term Ethanol Administration On Lorazepam Clearance. Hepatology, 1, 47–53.

Hsu, W. H., Hanson, C. E., Hembrough, F. B. & Schaffer, D. D. (1989) Effects Of Idazoxan, Tolazoline, And Yohimbine On Xylazine-Induced Respiratory Changes And Central Nervous-System Depression In Ewes. American Journal Of Veterinary Research, 50, 1570–1573.

Hsu, W. H., Schaffer, D. D. & Hanson, C. E. (1987) Effects Of Tolazoline And Yohimbine On Xylazine-Induced Central-Nervous-System Depression, Bradycardia, And Tachypnea In Sheep. Journal Of The American Veterinary Medical Association, 190, 423–426.

Hubbell, J. A. E. & Muir, W. W. (2006) Antagonism Of Detomidine Sedation In The Horse Using Intravenous Tolazoline Or Atipamezole. Equine Veterinary Journal, 38, 238–241.

Hugnet, C., Buronfosse, F., Pineau, X., Cadore, J. L., Lorgue, G. & Berny, P. J. (1996) Toxicity And Kinetics Of Amitraz In Dogs. American Journal Of Veterinary Research, 57, 1506–1510.

Humphreys, M. H., Reid, I. A. & Chou, L. Y. (1975) Suppression Of Antidiuretic Hormone Secretion By Clonidine In The Anesthetized Dog. Kidney International, 7, 405–12.

Ikeda, S. & Schweiss, J. F. (1983) Failure Of Droperidol And Ketamine To Influence Cerebrospinal Fluid Production In The Dog. Acta Medica Okayama, 37, 511–7.

Ilkiw, J. E., Suter, C. M., Farver, T. B., Mcneal, D. & Steffey, E. P. (1996) The Behaviour Of Healthy Awake Cats Following Intravenous And Intramuscular Administration Of Midazolam. Journal Of Veterinary Pharmacology And Therapeutics, 19, 205–216.

Ilkiw, J. E., Suter, C., McNeal, D., Farver, T. B. & Steffey, E. P. (1998) The Optimal Intravenous Dose Of Midazolam After Intravenous Ketamine In Healthy Awake Cats. Journal Of Veterinary Pharmacology And Therapeutics, 21, 54–61.

Ishizuka, O., Mattiasson, A. & Andersson, K. E. (1996) Role Of Spinal And Peripheral Alpha(2) Adrenoceptors In Micturition In Normal Conscious Rats. Journal Of Urology, 156, 1853–1857.

Jadon, N. S., Kumar, A., Sharma, B. & Singh, S. P. (1998) Detomidine As A Preanaesthetic In Thiopentone Anaesthesia In Dogs. Indian Journal Of Animal Sciences, 68, 48–49.

Jasper, J. R., Lesnick, J. D., Chang, L. K., Yamanishi, S. S., Chang, T. K., Hsu, S. A. O., Daunt, D. A., Bonhaus, D. W. & Eglen, R. M. (1998) Ligand Efficacy And Potency At Recombinant Alpha(2) Adrenergic Receptors—Agonist-Mediated [S-35]Gtp Gamma S Binding. Biochemical Pharmacology, 55, 1035–1043.

Jaugstetter, H., Jacobi, R. & Pellmann, R. (2002) Comparison Of Romifidine And Xylazine As Premedicants Before General Anaesthesia In Horses Regarding The Postsurgical Recovery Period. Praktische Tierarzt, 83, 786–791.

Jedruch, J. & Gajewski, Z. (1986) The Effect Of Detomidine Hydrochloride (Domosedan) On The Electrical-Activity On The Uterus In Cows. Acta Veterinaria Scandinavica, 189–192.

Jedruch, J., Gajewski, Z. & Kuussaari, J. (1989a) The Effect Of Detomidine Hydrochloride On The Electrical-Activity Of Uterus In Pregnant Mares. Acta Veterinaria Scandinavica, 30, 307–311.

Jedruch, J., Gajewski, Z. & Ratajskamichalczak, K. (1989) Uterine Motor-Responses To An Alpha2-Adrenergic Agonist Medetomidine Hydrochloride In The Bitches During The End Of Gestation And The Post-Partum Period. Acta Veterinaria Scandinavica, Suppl. 85, 129–134.

Jernigan, A. D., Wilson, R. C., Booth, N. H., Hatch, R. C. & Akbari, A. (1988) Comparative Pharmacokinetics Of Yohimbine In Steers, Horses And Dogs. Canadian Journal Of Veterinary Research-Revue Canadienne De Recherche Veterinaire, 52, 172–176.

Jonas, J. C., Plant, T. D. & Henquin, J. C. (1992) Imidazoline Antagonists Of Alpha2-Adrenoceptors Increase Insulin Release In vitro By Inhibiting Atp-Sensitive K+ Channels In Pancreatic Beta-Cells. British Journal Of Pharmacology, 107, 8–14.

Jovanovic-Micic, D., Samardzic, R. & Beleslin, D. B. (1995) The Role Of Alpha-Adrenergic Mechanisms Within The Area Postrema In Dopamine-Induced Emesis. European Journal Of Pharmacology, 272, 21–30.

Kaivosaari, S., Salonen, J. S. & Taskinen, J. (2002) N-Glucuronidation Of Some 4-Arylalkyl-1h-Imidazoles By Rat, Dog, And Human Liver Microsomes. Drug Metabolism And Disposition, 30, 295–300.

Kalchofner, K. S., Ringer, S. K., Boller, J., Kastner, S. B. R., Lischer, C. & Bettschart-Wolfensberger, R. (2006) Clinical Assessment Of Anesthesia With Isoflurane And Medetomidine In 300 Equidae. Pferdeheilkunde, 22, 301.

Kamibayashi, T., Mammoto, T., Hayashi, Y., Yamatodani, A., Takada, K., Sasaki, S. & Yoshiya, I. (1995) Further Characterization Of The Receptor Mechanism Involved In The Antidysrhythmic Effect Of Dexmedetomidine On Halothane/Epinephrine Dysrhythmias In Dogs. Anesthesiology, 83, 1082–1089.

Kaplan, S. A., Lewis, M., Schwartz, M. A., Postma, E., Cotler, S., Abruzzo, C. W., Lee, T. L. & Weinfeld, R. E. (1970) Pharmacokinetic Model For Chlordiazepoxide—Hcl In The Dog. Journal Of Pharmaceutical Sciences, 59, 1569–74.

Karjalainen, A., Virtanen, R. & Karjalainen, A. (1986) Synthesis Of 4(5)-(2,3-Dihydro-1h-Inden-2-Yl) Imidazoles, A Novel Class Of Potent Alpha2-Adrenoceptor Antagonists. IX International Symposium On Medical Chemistry. Berlin.

Kastner, S. B. R. (2006) A(2)-Agonists In Sheep: A Review. Veterinary Anaesthesia And Analgesia, 33, 79–96.

Kastner, S. B. R., Wapf, P., Feige, K., Demuth, D., Bettschart-Wolfensberger, R., Akens, M. K. & Huhtinen, M. (2003) Pharmacokinetics And Sedative Effects Of Intramuscular Medetomidine In Domestic Sheep. Journal Of Veterinary Pharmacology And Therapeutics, 26, 271–276.

Katherman, A. E., Knecht, C. D. & Redding, R. W. (1985) Effects Of Fentanyl Citrate And Droperidol On Electroencephalographic Findings In Dogs. American Journal Of Veterinary Research, 46, 974–6.

Kauppila, T., Jyvasjarvi, E. & Pertovaara, A. (1992) Effects Of Atipamezole, An Alpha2-Adrenoceptor Antagonist, On The Anesthesia Induced By Barbiturates And Medetomidine. Anesthesia And Analgesia, 75, 416–420.

Kearns, K. S., Swenson, B. & Ramsay, E. C. (2000) Oral Induction Of Anesthesia With Droperidol And Transmucosal Carfentanil Citrate In Chimpanzees (*Pan Troglodytes*). Journal Of Zoo And Wildlife Medicine, 31, 185–189.

Keegan, R. D., Greene, S. A., Bagley, R. S., Moore, M. P., Weil, A. B. & Short, C. E. (1995) Effects Of Medetomidine Administration On Intracranial Pressure And Cardiovascular Variables Of Isoflurane-Anesthetized Dogs. American Journal Of Veterinary Research, 56, 193–198.

Keller, H. (1969) Clinical Experience With The New Sedative Rompun (Xylazine) In Horses. Berl. Müch. Tierärztl. Wschr., 82, 366–370.

Kendig, J. J., Savola, M. K. T., Woodley, S. J. & Maze, M. (1991) Alpha2-Adrenoceptors Inhibit A Nociceptive Response In Neonatal Rat Spinal-Cord. European Journal Of Pharmacology, 192, 293–300.

Khan, Z. P., Ferguson, C. N. & Jones, R. M. (1999) Alpha-2 And Imidazoline Receptor Agonists—Their Pharmacology And Therapeutic Role. Anaesthesia, 54, 146–165.

Kharasch, E. D., Herrmann, S. & Labroo, R. (1992) Ketamine As A Probe For Medetomidine Stereoisomer Inhibition Of Human Liver Microsomal Drug-Metabolism. Anesthesiology, 77, 1208–1214.

Kinjavdekar, P., Aithal, H. P., Amarpal, P., Pawde, A. M., Pratap, K. & Singh, G. R. (2006) Potential Effect Of Romifidine With Lidocaine Administration In Goats. Small Ruminant Research, 64, 293–304.

Kinjavdekar, P., Amarpal, G. R. S., Pawde, A. M., Aithal, H. P. & Gupta, O. P. (2003) Influence Of Yohimbine And Atipamezole On Haemodynamics And ECG After Lumbosacral Subarachnoid Administration Of Medetomidine In Goats. Journal Of Veterinary Medicine Series A—Physiology Pathology Clinical Medicine, 50, 424–431.

Klotz, U. & Kanto, J. (1988) Pharmacokinetics And Clinical Use Of Flumazenil (Ro 5-1788). Clinical Pharmacokinetics, 14, 1–12.

Ko, J. C. H. & Mcgrath, C. J. (1995) Effects Of Atipamezole And Yohimbine On Medetomidine-Induced Central-Nervous-System Depression And Cardiorespiratory Changes In Lambs. American Journal Of Veterinary Research, 56, 629–632.

Kolarovszki-Sipiczki, Z., Gaspar, R., Ducza, E., Paldy, E., Benyhe, S., Borsodi, A. & Falkay, G. (2007) Effect Of Alpha1-Adrenoceptor Subtype-Selective Inverse Agonists On Non-Pregnant And Late-Pregnant Cervical Resistance In Vitro In The Rat. Clinical And Experimental Pharmacology And Physiology, 34, 42–47.

Kolliasbaker, C. A., Court, M. H. & Williams, L. L. (1993) Influence Of Yohimbine And Tolazoline On The Cardiovascular, Respiratory, And Sedative Effects Of Xylazine In The Horse. Journal Of Veterinary Pharmacology And Therapeutics, 16, 350–358.

Komaromy, A. M., Garg, C. D., Ying, G. S. & Liu, C. C. (2006) Effect Of Head Position On Intraocular Pressure In Horses. American Journal Of Veterinary Research, 67, 1232–1235.

Kuhn, M., Kohler, L., Fenner, A., Enderle, A. & Kampmann, C. (2004) Isoflurane Sparing And The Influence On Cardiovascular And Pulmonary Parameters Through A Continuous Romifidine Hydrochloride Infusion During General Anaesthesia In Horses—A Clinical Study. Pferdeheilkunde, 20, 511.

Kutter, A. P. N., Kastner, S. B. R., Bettschart-Wolfensberger, R. & Huhtinen, M. (2006) Cardiopulmonary Effects Of Dexmedetomidine In Goats And Sheep Anaesthetised With Sevoflurane. Veterinary Record, 159, 624.

Kuusela, E. (2004) Dissertation: Dexmedetomidine And Levomedetomidine, The Isomers Of Medetomidine, In Dogs. Department Of Clinical Veterinary Sciences, Faculty Of Veterinary Medicine. Helsinki, Finland, University Of Helsinki.

Kuusela, E., Raekallio, M., Anttila, M., Falck, I., Molsa, S. & Vainio, O. (2000) Clinical Effects And Pharmacokinetics Of Medetomidine And Its Enantiomers In Dogs. Journal Of Veterinary Pharmacology And Therapeutics, 23, 15–20.

Kuusela, E., Raekallio, M., Vaisanen, M., Mykkanen, K., Ropponen, H. & Vainio, O. (2001a) Comparison Of Medetomidine And Dexmedetomidine As Premedicants In Dogs Undergoing Propofol-Isoflurane Anesthesia. American Journal Of Veterinary Research, 62, 1073–1080.

Kuusela, E., Vainio, O., Kaistinen, A., Kobylin, S. & Raekallio, M. (2001) Sedative, Analgesic, And Cardiovascular Effects Of Levomedetomidine Alone And In Combination With Dexmedetomidine In Dogs. American Journal Of Veterinary Research, 62, 616–621.

Kuusela, E., Vainio, O., Short, C. E., Leppäluoto, J., Huttunen, P., Ström, S., Huju, V., Valtonen, A. & Raekallio, M. (2003) A Comparison Of Propofol Infusion And Propofol/Isoflurane Anaesthesia In Dexmedetomidine Premedicated Dogs. Journal Of Veterinary Pharmacology & Therapeutics, 26, 199–204.

Lamont, L., Bulmer, B., Grimm, K., Tranquilli, W. & Sisson, D. (2001) Cardiopulmonary Evaluation Of The Use Of Medetomidine Hydrochloride In Cats. American Journal Of Veterinary Research, Nov;62(11):1745–9.

Lapin, I. P. (1980) Adrenergic Nonspecific Potentiation Of Yohimbine Toxicity In Mice By Antidepressants And Related Drugs And Antiyohimbine Action Of Antiadrenergic And Serotonergic Drugs. Psychopharmacology, 70, 179–85.

Lawhead, R. G., Blaxall, H. S. & Bylund, D. B. (1992) Alpha2a Is The Predominant Alpha2 Adrenergic-Receptor Subtype In Human Spinal-Cord. Anesthesiology, 77, 983–991.

Lawrence, C. J., Prinzen, F. W. & De Lange, S. (1996) The Effect Of Dexmedetomidine On Nutrient Organ Blood Flow. Anesthesia And Analgesia, 83, 1160–1165.

Lee, I., Yamagishi, N., Oboshi, K. & Yamada, H. (2003) Antagonistic Effects Of Intravenous Or Epidural Atipamezole On Xylazine-Induced Dorsolumbar Epidural Analgesia In Cattle. Veterinary Journal, 166, 194–197.

Lee, Y. W. & Yaksh, T. L. (1995) Analysis Of Drug-Interaction Between Intrathecal Clonidine And Mk-801 In Peripheral Neuropathic Pain Rat Model. Anesthesiology, 82, 741–748.

Lees, P. & Serrano, L. (1976) Effects Of Azaperone On Cardiovascular And Respiratory Functions In The Horse. British Journal Of Pharmacology, 56, 263–9.

Lemke, K. A. (1999) Sedative Effects Of Intramuscular Administration Of A Low Dose Of Romifidine In Dogs. American Journal Of Veterinary Research, 60, 162–168.

———. (2004) Perioperative Use Of Selective Alpha-2 Agonists And Antagonists In Small Animals. Canadian Veterinary Journal—Revue Veterinaire Canadienne, 45, 475–480.

Lemke, K. A., Tranquilli, W. J., Thurmon, J. C., Benson, G. J. & Olson, W. A. (1996) Ability Of Flumazenil, Butorphanol, And Naloxone To Reverse The Anesthetic Effects Of Oxymorphone-Diazepam In

Dogs. Journal Of The American Veterinary Medical Association, 209, 776.

Lemke, R. P., Alsaedi, S. A., Belik, J. & Casiro, O. (1996) Use Of Tolazoline To Counteract Vasospasm In Peripheral Arterial Catheters In Neonates. Acta Paediatrica, 85, 1497–1498.

Lerche, P. & Muir, W. W. (2004) Effect Of Medetomidine On Breathing And Inspiratory Neuromuscular Drive In Conscious Dogs. American Journal Of Veterinary Research, 65, 720–724.

Lloyd Laboratories. (April 19, 1996) Tolazoline Hcl. In Lloyd, I., 604 West Thomas Avenue, P. O. B. A. & Shenandoah, I., U.S.A. (Eds.) 100 mg/Ml In A 100 ml Multi-Dose Vial Ed.

———. (September 26, 1989) Yohimbine 2 mg/Ml. In Vet-A-Mix, I., 604 West Thomas Avenue, P. O. B. A. & Shenandoah, I. U. S. A. (Eds.).

Loscher, W. & Frey, H. H. (1981) Pharmacokinetics Of Diazepam In The Dog. Archives Internationales De Pharmacodynamie Et De Therapie, 254, 180–195.

———. (1984) Kinetics Of Penetration Of Common Antiepileptic Drugs Into Cerebrospinal Fluid. Epilepsia, 25, 346–52.

Ludders, J., Reitan, J., Martucci, R., Fung, D. & Steffey, E. (1983) Blood Pressure Response To Phenylephrine Infusion In Halothane-Anesthetized Dogs Given Acetylpromazine Maleate. American Journal Of Veterinary Research. Jun;44(6):996–9.

Luna, S. P. L., Aguiar, A. J. A. & Curi, P. R. (1988) Effects Of Midazolam On Blood Gas Tension And Acid-Base Balance In Dogs. Ars Veterinaria, 4, 9–14.

Macdonald, E., Scheinin, M., Scheinin, H. & Virtanen, R. (1991) Comparison Of The Behavioral And Neurochemical Effects Of The 2 Optical Enantiomers Of Medetomidine, A Selective Alpha2-Adrenoceptor Agonist. Journal Of Pharmacology And Experimental Therapeutics, 259, 848–854.

Mandema, J. W., Tukker, E. & Danhof, M. (1992) In Vivo Characterization Of The Pharmacodynamic Interaction Of A Benzodiazepine Agonist And Antagonist—Midazolam And Flumazenil. Journal Of Pharmacology And Experimental Therapeutics, 260, 36–44.

Martens, H. J., De Goede, P. N. & Van Loenen, A. C. (1990) Sorption [SIC] Of Various Drugs In Polyvinyl Chloride, Glass, And Polyethylene-Lined Infusion Containers. American Journal Of Hospital Pharmacy, 47, 369–73.

Martin, W. R., Sloan, J. W. & Wala, E. (1990) Precipitated Abstinence In Orally Dosed Benzodiazepine-Dependent Dogs. Journal Of Pharmacology And Experimental Therapeutics, 255, 744–55.

Marty, J., Nitenberg, A., Philip, I., Foult, J. M., Joyon, D. & Desmonts, J. M. (1991) Coronary And Left-Ventricular Hemodynamic-Responses Following Reversal Of Flunitrazepam-Induced Sedation With Flumazenil In Patients With Coronary-Artery Disease. Anesthesiology, 74, 71–76.

Matsui, H., Lefkowitz, R. J., Caron, M. G. & Regan, J. W. (1989) Localization Of The 4th Membrane Spanning Domain As A Ligand-Binding Site In The Human Platelet Alpha2-Adrenergic Receptor. Biochemistry, 28, 4125–4130.

Maugeri, S., Ferre, J. P., Intorre, L. & Soldani, G. (1994) Effects Of Medetomidine On Intestinal And Colonic Motility In The Dog. Journal Of Veterinary Pharmacology And Therapeutics, 17, 148–154.

Maylin, G., Dewey, E., Ebel, J., & Henion, J. (1978) The Metabolism Of Promazine And Acetylpromazine In The Horse. Drug Metababolic Disposition, Jan–Feb;9(1):30–6.

Maze, M., Hayward, E., Jr. & Gaba, D. M. (1985) Alpha 1-Adrenergic Blockade Raises Epinephrine-Arrhythmia Threshold In Halothane-Anesthetized Dogs In A Dose-Dependent Fashion. Anesthesiology, 63, 611–5.

McGrath, C., Rempel, W., Addis, P. & Crimi, A. (1977) Acepromazine And Droperidol Inhibition Of Halothane-Induced Malignant Hyperthermia (Porcine Stress Syndrome) In Swine. American Journal Of Veterinary Research, 1981 Feb;42(2):195–8.

McLeish, I. (1977) Skeletal Muscle Rigidity In A Dog Following Fentanyl/Droperidol Administration: A Case Report. Veterinary Anesthesia, 4, 2–4.

McNicholas, L. F., Martin, W. R. & Cherian, S. (1983) Physical Dependence On Diazepam And Lorazepam In The Dog. Journal Of Pharmacology And Experimental Therapeutics, 226, 783–9.

McNicholas, L. F., Martin, W. R. & Pruitt, T. A. (1985) N-Desmethyldiazepam Physical Dependence In Dogs. Journal Of Pharmacology And Experimental Therapeutics, 235, 368–76.

Mealey, K. L. & Boothe, D. M. (1995) Bioavailability Of Benzodiazepines Following Rectal Administration Of Diazepam In Dogs. Journal Of Veterinary Pharmacology And Therapeutics, 18, 72–4.

Med-Tech, I. (1988) Xylazine. Xylazine Hcl Injection. 100 mg/Ml Ed. 7410 Nw Tiffany Springs Parkway, Suite 260, Kansas City, Missouri 64153.

Meyer, H. P., Legemate, D. A., Van Den Brom, W. & Rothuizen, J. (1998) Improvement Of Chronic Hepatic Encephalopathy In Dogs By The Benzodiazepine-Receptor Partial Inverse Agonist Sarmazenil, But Not By The Antagonist Flumazenil. Metabolic Brain Disease, 13, 241–51.

Michenfelder, J. D. & Theye, R. A. (1971) Effects Of Fentanyl, Droperidol, And Innovar On Canine Cerebral Metabolism And Blood Flow. British Journal Of Anaesthesia, 43, 630–636.

Miksa, I. R., Cummings, M. R. & Poppenga, R. H. (2005) Determination Of Acepromazine, Ketamine Medetomidine, And Xylazine In Serum: Multi-Residue Screening By Liquid Chromatography—Mass Spectrometry. Journal Of Analytical Toxicology, 29, 544–551.

Moens, Y., Lanz, F., Doherr, M. G. & Schatzmann, U. (2003) A Comparison Of The Antinociceptive Effects Of Xylazine, Detomidine And Romifidine On Experimental Pain In Horses. Veterinary Anaesthesia And Analgesia, 30, 183–190.

Molderings, G. J. & Gothert, M. (1995) Inhibitory Presynaptic Imidazoline Receptors On Sympathetic-Nerves In The Rabbit Aorta Differ From I-1 And I-2 Imidazoline Binding-Sites. Naunyn-Schmiedebergs Archives Of Pharmacology, 351, 507–516.

Morgan, G. E., Mikhail, M. S., Murray, M. J. & Larson, C. P. (Eds.) (2002) Clinical Anesthesiology, New York, Lange Medical Books/McGraw-Hill, Medical Pub. Division.

Moyer, J. R. & Vincent, C. M. (2001) Preoperative Medication. In Barash, P. G., Cullen, B. F. & Stoelting, R. K. (Eds.) Clinical Anesthesia. 4th Ed. Philadelphia, Lippincott Williams & Wilkins.

Muir, W. W. & Gadawski, J. E. (2002) Cardiovascular Effects Of A High Dose Of Romifidine In Propofol-Anesthetized Cats. American Journal Of Veterinary Research, 63, 1241–1246.

Muir, W., Werner, L., & Hamlin, R. (1975) Effects Of Xylazine And Acetylpromazine Upon Induced Ventricular Fibrillation In Dogs Anesthetized With Thiamylal And Halothane. American Journal Of Veterinary Research, Sep;36(9):1299–1303.

Müller, A., Weibel, K. & Furukawa, R. (1969) Rompun (Xylazine) As A Sedative In The Cat. Berl. Münch, Tierärztl. Wschr, 82, 396–397.

Muller, J. M. V., Feige, K., Kastner, S. B. R. & Naegeli, H. (2005) The Use Of Sarmazenil In The Treatment Of A Moxidectin Intoxication In A Foal. Journal Of Veterinary Internal Medicine, 19, 348–349.

Mustonen, P., Savola, J. M. & Lassila, R. (2000) Atipamezole, An Imidazoline-Type Alpha(2)-Adrenoceptor Inhibitor, Binds To Human Platelets And Inhibits Their Adrenaline-Induced Aggregation More Effectively Than Yohimbine. Thrombosis Research, 99, 231–237.

Nashan, B., Inoue, K. & Arndt, J. O. (1984) Droperidol Inhibits Cardiac Vagal Efferents In Dogs. British Journal Of Anaesthesia, 56, 1259–66.

Niddam, R., Angel, I., Bidet, S. & Langer, S. Z. (1990) Pharmacological Characterization Of Alpha2 Adrenergic Receptor Subtype Involved In The Release Of Insulin From Isolated Rat Pancreatic-Islets. Journal Of Pharmacology And Experimental Therapeutics, 254, 883–887.

Nishimura, R., Kim, H., Matsunaga, S., Hayashi, K., Tamura, H., Sasaki, N. & Takeuchi, A. (1993) Comparison Of Sedative And Analgesic/Anesthetic Effects Induced By Medetomidine, Acepromazine, Azaperone, Droperidol And Midazolam In Laboratory Pigs. Journal Of Veterinary Medical Science, 55, 687–690.

Oharaimaizumi, M. & Kumakura, K. (1992) Effects Of Imidazole Compounds On Catecholamine Release In Adrenal Chromaffin Cells. Cellular And Molecular Neurobiology, 12, 273–283.

Oliver, F. M., Sweatman, T. W., Unkel, J. H., Kahn, M. A., Randolph, M. M., Arheart, K. L. & Mandrell, T. D. (2000) Comparative Pharmacokinetics Of Submucosal Vs. Intravenous Flumazenil (Romazicon) In An Animal Model. Pediatric Dentistry, 22, 489–93.

Orion Corp. (August 6, 1996) Atipamezole Hcl For Injection 5 mg/Ml In 10 ml Multidose Vial (Package Insert). In Pfizer Inc., E. N. S., New York, N.Y. 10017 (Ed.) Antisedan.

Ostheimer, G. W., Shanahan, E. A., Guyton, R. A., Daggett, W. M. & Lowenstein, E. (1975) Effects Of Fentanyl And Droperidol On Canine Left Ventricular Performance. Anesthesiology, 42, 288–91.

Paalzow, L. (1974) Analgesia Produced By Clonidine In Mice And Rats. Journal Of Pharmacy And Pharmacology, 26, 361–3.

Palmer, R. B., Mautz, D. S., Cox, K. & Kharasch, E. D. (1998) Endotracheal Flumazenil: A New Route Of Administration For Benzodiazepine Antagonism. American Journal Of Emergency Medicine, 16, 170–172.

Papich, M. G. & Alcorn, J. (1995) Absorption Of Diazepam After Its Rectal Administration In Dogs. American Journal Of Veterinary Research, 56, 1629–36.

Paret, G., Eyal, O., Mayan, H., Ben-Abraham, R., Vardi, A., Manisterski, Y., Barzilay, Z. & Ezra, D. (1999a) Pharmacokinetics Of Endobronchial Tolazoline Administration In Dogs. American Journal Of Perinatology, 16, 1–6.

Paret, G., Eyal, O., Mayan, H., Gilad, E., Ben-Abraham, R., Ezra, D. & Barzilay, Z. (1999b) Endotracheal Tolazoline: Pharmacokinetics And Pharmacodynamics In Dogs. Acta Paediatrica, 88, 1020–1023.

Pascoe, P. J., Raekallio, M., Kuusela, E., Mckusick, B. & Granholm, M. (2006) Changes In The Minimum Alveolar Concentration Of Isoflurane And Some Cardiopulmonary Measurements During Three Continuous Infusion Rates Of Dexmedetomidine In Dogs. Veterinary Anaesthesia And Analgesia, 33, 97–103.

Pelkonen, O., Puurunen, J., Arvela, P. & Lammintausta, R. (1991) Comparative Effects Of Medetomidine Enantiomers On In vitro And In vivo Microsomal Drug-Metabolism. Pharmacology & Toxicology, 69, 189–194.

Pertovaara, A., Haapalinna, A., Sirvio, J. & Virtanen, R. (2005) Pharmacological Properties, Central Nervous System Effects, And Potential Therapeutic Applications Of Atipamezole, A Selective Alpha(2)-Adrenoceptor Antagonist. CNS Drug Reviews, 11, 273–288.

Pettifer, G. R. & Dyson, D. H. (1993) Comparison Of Medetomidine And Fentanyl-Droperidol In Dogs: Sedation, Analgesia, Arterial Blood Gases And Lactate Levels. Canadian Journal Of Veterinary Research, 57, 99–105.

Pinthong, D., Songsermsakul, P., Rattanachamnong, P. & Kendall, D. A. (2004) The Effects Of Imidazoline Agents On The Aggregation Of Human Platelets. Journal Of Pharmacy And Pharmacology, 56, 213–220.

Pinthong, D., Wright, I. K., Hanmer, C., Millns, P., Mason, R., Kendall, D. A. & Wilson, V. G. (1995) Agmatine Recognizes Alpha2-Adrenoceptor Binding-Sites But Neither Activates Nor Inhibits Alpha2-Adrenoceptors. Naunyn-Schmiedebergs Archives Of Pharmacology, 351, 10–16.

Platt, S. R., Randell, S. C., Scott, K. C., Chrisman, C. L., Hill, R. C. & Gronwall, R. R. (2000) Comparison Of Plasma Benzodiazepine Concentrations Following Intranasal And Intravenous Administration Of Diazepam To Dogs. American Journal Of Veterinary Research, 61, 651–4.

Plumb, D. C. (1999) Veterinary Drug Handbook, Ames, Iowa, Iowa State University Press.

Podell, M., Smeak, D. & Lord, L. K. (1998) Diazepam Used To Control Cluster Seizures In Dogs. Journal Of Veterinary Internal Medicine, 12, 120–1.

Podell, M., Wagner, S. O. & Sams, R. A. (1998) Lorazepam Concentrations In Plasma Following Its Intravenous And Rectal Administration In Dogs. Journal Of Veterinary Pharmacology And Therapeutics, 21, 158–60.

Pollock, C. G. & Ramsay, E. C. (2003) Serial Immobilization Of A Brazilian Tapir (*Tapirus Terrestrus*) With Oral Detomidine And Oral Carfentanil. Journal Of Zoo And Wildlife Medicine, 34, 408–410.

Potter, W. Z. & Hollister, L. E. (2001) Antipsychotic Agents & Lithium. In Katzung, B. G. (Ed.) Basic & Clinical Pharmacology. 8th Ed. New York: London, McGraw-Hill.

Powell, J. D., Denhart, J. W. & Lloyd, W. E. (1998) Effectiveness Of Tolazoline In Reversing Xylazine-Increased Sedation In Calves. Journal Of The American Veterinary Medical Association, 212, 90.

Prindle, K. H. J., Gold, H. K., Cardon, P. V. & Epstein, S. E. (1970) Effects Of Psychopharmacologic Agents On Myocardial Contractility. Journal Of Pharmacology And Experimental Therapeutics, 173, 133–137.

Pypendop, B. & Verstegen, J. (1999) Cardiorespiratory Effects Of A Combination Of Medetomidine, Midazolam, And Butorphanol In Dogs. American Journal Of Veterinary Research, 60, 1148–1154.

Pypendop, B. H. & Verstegen, J. P. (1998) Hemodynamic Effects Of Medetomidine In The Dog: A Dose Titration Study. Veterinary Surgery, 27, 612–622.

———. (2001) Cardiovascular Effects Of Romifidine In Dogs. American Journal Of Veterinary Research, 62, 490–495.

Quan, N., Xin, L., Ungar, A. L. & Blatteis, C. M. (1992) Preoptic Norepinephrine-Induced Hypothermia Is Mediated By Alpha2-Adrenoceptors. American Journal Of Physiology, 262, R407–R411.

Radcliffe, R. W., Ferrell, S. T. & Childs, S. E. (2000) Butorphanol And Azaperone As A Safe Alternative For Repeated Chemical Restraint In Captive White Rhinoceros (*Ceratotherium Simum*). Journal Of Zoo And Wildlife Medicine, 31, 196–200.

Raekallio, M., Vainio, O. & Scheinin, M. (1991) Detomidine Reduces The Plasma-Catecholamine, But Not Cortisol Concentrations In Horses. Journal Of Veterinary Medicine Series A-Zentralblatt Fur Veterinarmedizin Reihe A-Physiology Pathology Clinical Medicine, 38, 153–156.

Ramsay, E. C., Geiser, D., Carter, W. & Tobin, T. (2002) Serum Concentrations And Effects Of Detomidine Delivered Orally To Horses In Three Different Mediums. Veterinary Anaesthesia And Analgesia, 29, 219–222.

Ramseyer, B., Schmucker, N., Schatzmann, U., Busato, A. & Moens, Y. (1998) Antagonism Of Detomidine Sedation With Atipamezole In Horses. Journal Of Veterinary Anaesthesia, 25, 47–51.

Ranheim, B., Arnemo, J. M., Ryeng, K. A., Soli, N. E. & Horsberg, T. E. (1999) A Pharmacokinetic Study Including Some Relevant Clinical Effects Of Medetomidine And Atipamezole In Lactating Dairy Cows. Journal Of Veterinary Pharmacology And Therapeutics, 22, 368–373.

Ranheim, B., Arnemo, J. M., Stuen, S. & Horsberg, T. E. (2000) Medetomidine And Atipamezole In Sheep: Disposition And Clinical Effects. Journal Of Veterinary Pharmacology And Therapeutics, 23, 401–404.

Ranheim, B., Horsberg, T. E., Soli, N. E., Ryeng, K. A. & Arnemo, J. M. (2000) The Effects Of Medetomidine And Its Reversal With Atipamezole On Plasma Glucose, Cortisol And Noradrenaline In Cattle And Sheep. Journal Of Veterinary Pharmacology And Therapeutics, 23, 379–387.

Ranheim, B., Soli, N. E., Ryeng, K. A., Arnemo, J. M. & Horsberg, T. E. (1998) Pharmacokinetics Of Medetomidine And Atipamezole In Dairy Calves: An Agonist-Antagonist Interaction. Journal Of Veterinary Pharmacology And Therapeutics, 21, 428–432.

Re, G., Badino, P., Odore, R., Zizzadoro, C., Ormas, P., Girardi, C. & Belloli, C. (2002) Identification Of Functional Alpha-Adrenoceptor Subtypes In The Bovine Female Genital Tract During Different Phases Of The Oestrous Cycle. Veterinary Research Communications, 26, 479–494.

Read, M. R., Duke, T. & Toews, A. R. (2000) Suspected Tolazoline Toxicosis In A Llama. Journal Of The American Veterinary Medical Association, 216, 227.

Read, M. R. & McCorkell, R. B. (2002) Use Of Azaperone And Zuclopenthixol Acetate To Facilitate Translocation Of White-Tailed Deer (*Odocoileus Virginianus*). Journal Of Zoo And Wildlife Medicine, 33, 163–165.

Regunathan, S. (2006) Agmatine: Biological Role And Therapeutic Potentials In Morphine Analgesia And Dependence. AAPS Journal, 8, E479–E484.

Reid, I. A., Nolan, P. L., Wolf, J. A. & Keil, L. C. (1979) Suppression Of Vasopressin Secretion By Clonidine: Effect Of Alpha-Adrenoceptor Antagonists. Endocrinology, 104, 1403–6.

Reves, J. G., Fragen, R. J., Vinik, H. R. & Greenblatt, D. J. (1985) Midazolam—Pharmacology And Uses. Anesthesiology, 62, 310–324.

Robertson, S. A. & Eberhart, S. (1994) Efficacy Of The Intranasal Route For Administration Of Anaesthetic Agents To Adult Rabbits. Laboratory Animal Science, 44, 159–165.

Rouch, A. J. & Kudo, L. H. (2002) Agmatine Inhibits Arginine Vasopressin-Stimulated Urea Transport In The Rat Inner Medullary Collecting Duct. Kidney International, 62, 2101–2108.

Rouvinen, J., Hoffren, A. M., Karjalainen, A. & Pakkanen, T. A. (1993) Modelling Of Alpha2-Adrenergic Ligands. Drug Design And Discovery, 10, 285–95.

Sakamoto, H., Kirihara, H., Fujiki, M., Miura, N. & Misumi, K. (1997) The Effects Of Medetomidine On Maternal And Fetal Cardiovascular And Pulmonary Function, Intrauterine Pressure And Uterine Blood Flow In Pregnant Goats. Experimental Animals, 46, 67–73.

Sakamoto, H., Misumi, K., Nakama, M. & Aoki, Y. (1996) The Effects Of Xylazine On Intrauterine Pressure, Uterine Blood Flow, Maternal And Fetal Cardiovascular And Pulmonary Function In Pregnant Goats. Journal Of Veterinary Medical Science, 58, 211–217.

Salonen, J. S. (1989) Pharmacokinetics Of Medetomidine. Acta Veterinaria Scandinavica, Suppl. 85, 49–54.

Salonen, J. S., Vahavahe, T., Vainio, O. & Vakkuri, O. (1989) Single-Dose Pharmacokinetics Of Detomidine In The Horse And Cow. Journal Of Veterinary Pharmacology And Therapeutics, 12, 65–72.

Salonen, J. S., Vuorilehto, L., Gilbert, M. & Maylin, G. A. (1992) Identification Of Detomidine Carboxylic-Acid As The Major Urinary Metabolite Of Detomidine In The Horse. European Journal Of Drug Metabolism And Pharmacokinetics, 17, 13–20.

Salonen, S., Vuorilehto, L., Vainio, O. & Anttila, M. (1995) Atipamezole Increases Medetomidine Clearance In The Dog—An Agonist-Antagonist Interaction. Journal Of Veterinary Pharmacology And Therapeutics, 18, 328–332.

Sams, R. A., Gerken, D. F., Detra, R. L., Stanley, S. D., Wood, W. E., Tobin, T., Yang, J. M., Tai, H. H., Jeganathan, A. & Watt, D. S. (1996) Identification Of Metabolites Of Azaperone In Horse Urine. Journal Of Pharmaceutical Sciences, 85, 79–84.

Santos, M., Fuente, M., Garcia-Iturralde, P., Herran, R., Lopez-Sanroman, J. & Tendillo, F. J. (2003) Effects Of Alpha2 Adrenoceptor Agonists During Recovery From Isoflurane Anaesthesia In Horses. Equine Veterinary Journal, 35, 170–175.

Sargent, C. A., Dzwonczyk, S. & Grover, G. J. (1994) The Effect Of Alpha2-Adrenoceptor Antagonists In Isolated Globally Ischemic Rat Hearts. European Journal Of Pharmacology, 261, 25–32.

Sarma, K. K. & Pathak, S. C. (2001) Cardio Vascular Response To Xylazine And Hellabrunn Mixture With Yohimbine As Reversal Agent In Asian Elephants. Indian Veterinary Journal, 78, 400–402.

Sasaki, N., Yoshihara, T. & Hara, S. (2000) Difference In The Motile Reactivity Of Jejunum, Cecum, And Right Ventral Colon To Xylazine And Medetomidine In Conscious Horses. Journal Of Equine Science, 11, 63–68, 5.

Savola, J. M. (1989) Cardiovascular Actions Of Medetomidine And Their Reversal By Atipamezole. Acta Veterinaria Scandinavica, Suppl. 85, 39–47.

Savola, J. M. & Virtanen, R. (1991) Central Alpha2-Adrenoceptors Are Highly Stereoselective For Dexmedetomidine, The Dextro Enantiomer Of Medetomidine. European Journal Of Pharmacology, 195, 193–199.

Savola, M., Savola, J. M. & Puurunen, J. (1989) Alpha2-Adrenoceptor-Mediated Inhibition Of Gastric-Acid Secretion By Medetomidine Is Efficiently Antagonized By Atipamezole In Rats. Archives Internationales De Pharmacodynamie Et De Therapie, 301, 267–276.

Savola, M. K. T., MacIver, M. B., Doze, V. A., Kendig, J. J. & Maze, M. (1991) The Alpha2-Adrenoceptor Agonist Dexmedetomidine Increases The Apparent Potency Of The Volatile Anesthetic Isoflurane In Rats In-Vivo And In Hippocampal Slice In-Vitro. Brain Research, 548, 23–28.

Savola, M. K. T. & Savola, J. M. (1996a) Alpha2a/D-Adrenoceptor Subtype Predominates Also In The Neonatal Rat Spinal Cord. Developmental Brain Research, 94, 106–108.

———. (1996b) [H-3] Dexmedetomidine, An Alpha(2)-Adrenoceptor Agonist, Detects A Novel Imidazole Binding Site In Adult Rat Spinal Cord. European Journal Of Pharmacology, 306, 315–323.

Savola, M. K. T., Woodley, S. J., Kendig, J. J. & Maze, M. (1990) Alpha2b Adrenoceptor Activation Inhibits A Nociceptive Response In The

Spinal-Cord Of The Neonatal Rat. European Journal Of Pharmacology, 183, 740–740.

Schatzmann, U., Josseck, H., Stauffer, J. L. & Goossens, L. (1994) Effects Of Alpha2-Agonists On Intrauterine Pressure And Sedation In Horses—Comparison Between Detomidine, Romifidine And Xylazine. Journal Of Veterinary Medicine Series A-Zentralblatt Fur Veterinarmedizin Reihe A-Physiology Pathology Clinical Medicine, 41, 523–529.

Scheinin, M. & Schwinn, D. A. (1992) The Locus Ceruleus. Site Of Hypnotic Actions Of Alpha2-Adrenoceptors Agonists? Anesthesiology, 76, 873–875.

Scherkl, R. & Frey, H. H. (1986) Physical Dependence On Clonazepam In Dogs. Pharmacology, 32, 18–24.

Scherkl, R., Kurudi, D. & Frey, H. H. (1989) Clorazepate In Dogs: Tolerance To The Anticonvulsant Effect And Signs Of Physical Dependence. Epilepsy Research, 3, 144–50.

Schillings, R. T., Sisenwine, S. F., Schwartz, M. H. & Ruelius, H. W. (1975) Lorazepam: Glucuronide Formation In The Cat. Drug Metabolism And Disposition: The Biological Fate Of Chemicals, 3, 85–8.

Schmeling, W. T., Kampine, J. P., Roerig, D. L. & Warltier, D. C. (1991) The Effects Of The Stereoisomers Of The Alpha2-Adrenergic Agonist Medetomidine On Systemic And Coronary Hemodynamics In Conscious Dogs. Anesthesiology, 75, 499–511.

Schwartz, A. E., Maneksha, F. R., Kanchuger, M. S., Sidhu, U. S. & Poppers, P. J. (1989) Flumazenil Decreases The Minimum Alveolar Concentration Isoflurane In Dogs. Anesthesiology, 70, 764–6.

Schwartz, D. D. & Clark, T. P. (1998) Selectivity Of Atipamezole, Yohimbine And Tolazoline For Alpha-2 Adrenergic Receptor Subtypes: Implications For Clinical Reversal Of Alpha-2 Adrenergic Receptor Mediated Sedation In Sheep. Journal Of Veterinary Pharmacology And Therapeutics, 21, 342–347.

Schwinn, D. A., Correasales, C., Page, S. O. & Maze, M. (1991) Functional-Effects Of Activation Of Alpha1-Adrenoceptors By Dexmedetomidine—In vivo And In vitro Studies. Journal Of Pharmacology And Experimental Therapeutics, 259, 1147–1152.

Selmi, A. L., Barbudo-Selmi, G. R., Mendes, G. M., Figueiredo, J. P. & Lins, B. T. (2004) Sedative, Analgesic And Cardiorespiratory Effects Of Romifidine In Cats. Veterinary Anaesthesia And Analgesia, 31, 195–206.

Selmi, A. L., Barbudo-Selmi, G. R., Moreira, C. F., Martins, C. S., Lins, B. T., Mendes, G. M. & McManus, C. (2002) Evaluation Of Sedative And Cardiorespiratory Effects Of Romifidine And Romifidine-Butorphanol In Cats. Journal Of The American Veterinary Medical Association, 221, 506–510.

Serrano, L. & Lees, P. (1976) The Applied Pharmacology Of Azaperone In Ponies. Research In Veterinary Science, 20, 316–23.

Short, C. (1991) Effects Of Anticholinergic Treatment On The Cardiac And Respiratory Systems In Dogs Sedated With Medetomidine. Veterinary Record, Oct 5;129(14):310–3.

Short, C. E. (Ed.) (1987) Principles & Practice Of Veterinary Anesthesia, Edited By Charles E. Short, Baltimore, Williams & Wilkins.

Sinclair, M. D. (2003) A Review Of The Physiological Effects Of Alpha(2)-Agonists Related To The Clinical Use Of Medetomidine In Small Animal Practice. Canadian Veterinary Journal-Revue Veterinaire Canadienne, 44, 885–897.

Sinclair, M. D., Mcdonell, W. N., O'Grady, M. & Pettifer, G. (2002) The Cardiopulmonary Effects Of Romifidine In Dogs With And Without Prior Or Concurrent Administration Of Glycopyrrolate. Veterinary Anaesthesia And Analgesia, 29, 1–13.

Singh, A. P., Peshin, P. K., Singh, J., Sharifi, D. & Patil, D. B. (1991) Evaluation Of Detomidine As A Sedative In Goats. Acta Veterinaria Hungarica, 39, 109–114.

Singh, J. T., Singh, A. P., Peshin, P. K., Sharifi, D. & Patil, D. B. (1994) Evaluation Of Detomidine As A Sedative In Sheep. Indian Journal Of Animal Sciences, 64, 237–238.

Singh, K., Sobti, V. K., Bansal, P. S. & Rathore, S. S. (1989) Studies On Lorazepam As A Premedicant For Thiopental Anesthesia In The Dog. Journal Of Veterinary Medicine Series A-Zentralblatt Fur Veterinarmedizin Reihe A-Physiology Pathology Clinical Medicine, 36, 750–754.

Sjoholm, B., Voutilainen, R., Luomala, K., Savola, J. M. & Scheinin, M. (1992) Characterization Of [H-3] Atipamezole As A Radioligand For Alpha2-Adrenoceptors. European Journal Of Pharmacology, 215, 109–117.

Skarda, R. T. (1991) Antagonist Effects Of Atipamezole On Epidurally Administered Detomidine-Induced Sedation, Analgesia And Cardiopulmonary Depression In Horses. Journal Of Veterinary Anaesthesia, 79–81.

Skarda, R. T., St Jean, G. & Muir, W. W. (1990) Influence Of Tolazoline On Caudal Epidural Administration Of Xylazine In Cattle. American Journal Of Veterinary Research, 51, 556–560.

Sleeman, J. M., Carter, W., Tobin, T. & Ramsay, E. C. (1997) Immobilization Of Domestic Goats (*Capra Hircus*) Using Orally Administered Carfentanil Citrate And Detomidine Hydrochloride. Journal Of Zoo And Wildlife Medicine, 28, 158–165.

Sleeman, J. M. & Gaynor, J. (2000) Sedative And Cardiopulmonary Effects Of Medetomidine And Reversal With Atipamezole In Desert Tortoises (*Gopherus Agassizii*). Journal Of Zoo And Wildlife Medicine, 31, 28–35.

Smyth, D. D., Umemura, S. & Pettinger, W. A. (1985a) Alpha2-Adrenoceptor Antagonism Of Vasopressin-Induced Changes In Sodium Excretion. American Journal Of Physiology, 248, F767–F772.

Smyth, D. D., Umemura, S., Yang, E. & Pettinger, W. A. (1985b) Alpha2-Adrenoceptor Stimulation And Inhibition Of Renin Release In The Isolated Perfused Kidney. Hypertension, 7, 841–841.

———. (1987) Inhibition Of Renin Release By Alpha-Adrenoceptor Stimulation In The Isolated Perfused Rat-Kidney. European Journal Of Pharmacology, 140, 33–38.

Sofia, R. D. & Harakal, J. J. (1975) Evaluation Of Ketamine Hcl For Anti-Depressant Activity. Archives Internationales De Pharmacodynamie Et De Therapie, 214, 68.

Spadavecchia, C., Arendt-Nielsen, L., Andersen, O. K., Spadavecchia, L. & Schatzmann, U. (2005) Effect Of Romifidine On The Nociceptive Withdrawal Reflex And Temporal Summation In Conscious Horses. American Journal Of Veterinary Research, 66, 1992–1998.

Stafford, K. J., Mellor, D. J., Todd, S. E., Ward, R. N. & Mcmeekan, C. M. (2003) The Effect Of Different Combinations Of Lignocaine, Ketoprofen, Xylazine And Tolazoline On The Acute Cortisol Response To Dehorning In Calves. New Zealand Veterinary Journal, 51, 219–226.

Statile, L., Puig, M. M., Warner, W., Bansinath, M., Lovitz, M. & Turndorf, H. (1988) Droperidol Enhances Fentanyl And Sufentanil, But Not Morphine, Analgesia. General Pharmacology, 19, 451–454.

Stegmann, G. F. & Bester, L. (2001) Sedative-Hypnotic Effects Of Midazolam In Goats After Intravenous And Intramuscular Administration. Veterinary Anaesthesia And Analgesia, 28, 49–55.

Stoelting, R. K. (1999) Pharmacology And Physiology In Anesthetic Practice / Robert K. Stoelting, Philadelphia, Lippincott-Raven.

Strandhoy, J. W., Morris, M. & Buckalew, V. M. (1982) Renal Effects Of The Antihypertensive, Guanabenz, In The Dog. Journal Of Pharmacology And Experimental Therapeutics, 221, 347–352.

Suzuki, T. (1984) [Action Of Benzodiazepines On Spinal Dorsal Root Reflex Potentials In Cats]. Nippon Yakurigaku Zasshi, 84, 99–108.

Sylvina, T. J., Berman, N. G. & Fox, J. G. (1990) Effects Of Yohimbine On Bradycardia And Duration Of Recumbency In Ketamine/Xylazine Anaesthetized Ferrets. Laboratory Animal Science, 40, 178–182.

Syracuse Research Corporation. (2007) Droperidol. Chemidplus Advanced (Electronic Database).

Syracuse Research Corporation. (2007) Flumazenil. Chemidplus Advanced (Electronic Database).

Talke, P., Tayefeh, F., Sessler, D. I., Jeffrey, R., Noursalehi, M. & Richardson, C. (1997) Dexmedetomidine Does Not Alter The Sweating Threshold, But Comparably And Linearly Decreases The Vasoconstriction And Shivering Thresholds. Anesthesiology, 87, 835–841.

Tam, S. W., Worcel, M. & Wyllie, M. (2001) Yohimbine: A Clinical Review. Pharmacology And Therapeutics, 91, 215–243.

Teng, B. Y. & Muir, W. W. (2004) Effects Of Xylazine On Canine Coronary Artery Vascular Rings. American Journal Of Veterinary Research, 65, 431–435.

Thompson, J. R., Kersting, K. W. & Hsu, W. H. (1991) Antagonistic Effect Of Atipamezole On Xylazine-Induced Sedation, Bradycardia, And Ruminal Atony In Calves. American Journal Of Veterinary Research, 52, 1265–1268.

Thurman J., Tranquilly W., Benson G. (1996) Lumb & Jones Veterinary Anesthesia. 3rd Edition. Baltimore, Williams & Wilkins.

Tian, W. N., Miller, D. D. & Deth, R. C. (2000) Bidirectional Allosteric Effects Of Agonists And Gtp At Alpha(2a/D)-Adrenoceptors. Journal Of Pharmacology And Experimental Therapeutics, 292, 664–671.

Tobias, K., Marioni-Henry, K., Wagner, R. (2006) A Retrospective Study On The Use Of Acepromazine Maleate In Dogs With Seizures. Journal Of The American Animal Hospital Association, Aug;42(4):283–9.

Torneke, K., Bergstrom, U. & Neil, A. (2003) Interactions Of Xylazine And Detomidine With Alpha2-Adrenoceptors In Brain Tissue From Cattle, Swine And Rats. Journal Of Veterinary Pharmacology And Therapeutics, 26, 205–211.

Tranquilli, W. & Thurmon, J. C. (1984) Alpha Adrenoceptor Pharmacology. Journal Of The American Veterinary Medical Association, 184, 1400–2.

Tranquilli W, Thurman J, Grimm K (2007) Lumb And Jones Veterinary Anesthesia. 4th Ed. Ames, Blackwell Publishing.

Trevor, A. J. & Way, W. L. (2001) Sedative-Hypnotic Drugs. In Katzung, B. G. (Ed.) Basic & Clinical Pharmacology. 8th Ed. New YorkLondon, Mcgraw-Hill.

Tucker, A., Brown, D. T. & Greenlees, K. J. (1982) Pulmonary And Systemic Vascular Actions Of Tolazoline In Anesthetized Dogs. Pediatric Pharmacology, 2, 231–243.

Uggla, A. & Lindqvist, A. (1983) Acute Pulmonary-Edema As An Adverse Reaction To The Use Of Xylazine In Sheep. Veterinary Record, 113, 42–42.

Upton, R. N., Ludbrook, G. L., Grant, C. & Martinez, A. (2001) In Vivo Cerebral Pharmacokinetics And Pharmacodynamics Of Diazepam And Midazolam After Short Intravenous Infusion Administration In Sheep. Journal Of Pharmacokinetics And Pharmacodynamics, 28, 129–53.

Vahavahe, T. (1989) Clinical Evaluation Of Medetomidine, A Novel Sedative And Analgesia Drug For Dogs And Cats. Acta Veterinaria Scandinavica, 30, 267–273.

Vallance, S. R., Fitzovich, D. E., Billman, G. E. & Randall, D. C. (1988) Effect Of Innovar Upon The Autonomic Control Of The Heart In Intact Dog. Journal Of The Autonomic Nervous System, 23, 47–54.

Vanmetre, D. C. (1992) A Case-Report Of The Treatment Of An Overdose Of Xylazine In A Cow. Cornell Veterinarian, 82, 287–291.

Vayssettes-Courchay, C., Bouysset, F., Cordi, A. A., Laubie, M. & Verbeuren, T. J. (1996) A Comparative Study Of The Reversal By Different Alpha(2)-Adrenoceptor Antagonists Of The Central Sympatho-Inhibitory Effect Of Clonidine. British Journal Of Pharmacology, 117, 587–593.

Verbruggen, A. M. J., Akkerdaas, L. C., Hellebrekers, L. J. & Stades, F. C. (2000) The Effect Of Intravenous Medetomidine On Pupil Size And Intraocular Pressure In Normotensive Dogs. Veterinary Quarterly, 22, 179–180.

Verstegen, J., Fargetton, X., Zanker, S., Donnay, I. & Ectors, F. (1991) Antagonistic Activities Of Atipamezole, 4-Aminopyridine And Yohimbine Against Medetomidine Ketamine-Induced Anesthesia In Cats. Veterinary Record, 128, 57–60.

Vickery, R. G. & Maze, M. (1989) Action Of The Stereoisomers Of Medetomidine, In Halothane-Anesthetized Dogs. Acta Veterinaria Scandinavica, Suppl. 85, 71–76.

Virtanen, R. (1989) Pharmacological Profiles Of Medetomidine And Its Antagonist, Atipamezole. Acta Veterinaria Scandinavica, Suppl. 85, 29–37.

Virtanen, R., Savola, J. M. & Saano, V. (1989) Highly Selective And Specific Antagonism Of Central And Peripheral Alpha2-Adrenoceptors By Atipamezole. Archives Internationales De Pharmacodynamie Et De Therapie, 297, 190–204.

Virtanen, R., Savola, J. M., Saano, V. & Nyman, L. (1988) Characterization Of The Selectivity, Specificity And Potency Of Medetomidine As An Alpha2-Adrenoceptor Agonist. European Journal Of Pharmacology, 150, 9–14.

Vmrcvm Drug Information Laboratory. (2007) Database Of Approved Animal Drug Products (Daad). Veterinary Medical Informatics.

Wagner, S. O., Sams, R. A. & Podell, M. (1998) Chronic Phenobarbital Therapy Reduces Plasma Benzodiazepine Concentrations After Intravenous And Rectal Administration Of Diazepam In The Dog. Journal Of Veterinary Pharmacology And Therapeutics, 21, 335–41.

Wala, E. P., Martin, W. R. & Sloan, J. W. (1991) Distribution Of Diazepam, Nordiazepam, And Oxazepam Between Brain Extraneuronal Space, Brain Tissue, Plasma, And Cerebrospinal Fluid In Diazepam And Nordiazepam Dependent Dogs. Psychopharmacology (Berl), 105, 535–40.

Walsh, V. P. & Wilson, P. R. (2002) Sedation And Chemical Restraint Of Deer. New Zealand Veterinary Journal, 50, 228–236.

Ward, D. S. (1984) Stimulation Of Hypoxic Ventilatory Drive By Droperidol. Anesthesia And Analgesia, 63, 106–110.

Wiese, A. J. & Muir, W. W. (2007) Anaesthetic And Cardiopulmonary Effects Of Intramuscular Morphine, Medetomidine And Ketamine Administered To Telemetered Cats. Journal Of Feline Medicine And Surgery, 9, 150–6.

Wildlife Laboratories Inc. (February 3, 1993) Yohimbine 5 mg/Ml. In Incorporated, W. L., 1401 Duff Drive, S. & Fort Collins, C. (Eds.).

Wilson, D. V., Bohart, G. V., Evans, A. T., Robertson, S. & Rondenay, Y. (2002) Retrospective Analysis Of Detomidine Infusion For Standing

Chemical Restraint In 51 Horses. Veterinary Anaesthesia And Analgesia, 29, 54–57.

Yamashita, K., Harada, K., Yokoyama, T., Tsuzuki, K., Maehara, S., Seno, T., Izumisawa, Y. & Kotani, T. (2003) Combination Of Droperidol And Butorphanol As Premedication For Inhalation Anaesthesia In Dogs. Journal Of The Japan Veterinary Medical Association, 56, 325–331.

Yamashita, K., Muir, W. W., Tsubakishita, S., Abrahamsen, E., Lerch, P., Hubbell, J. A. E., Bednarski, R. M., Skarda, R. T., Izumisawa, Y. & Kotani, T. (2002) Clinical Comparison Of Xylazine And Medetomidine For Premedication Of Horses. Journal Of The American Veterinary Medical Association, 221, 1144–1149.

Yamashita, K., Tsubakishita, S., Futaoka, S., Ueda, I., Hamaguchi, H., Seno, T., Katoh, S., Izumisawa, Y., Kotani, T. & Muir, W. W. (2000) Cardiovascular Effects Of Medetomidine, Detomidine And Xylazine In Horses. Journal Of Veterinary Medical Science, 62, 1025–1032.

Yeh, F. C., Chang, C. L. & Chen, H. I. (1988) Effects Of Midazolam (A Benzodiazepine) On Cerebral Perfusion And Oxygenation In Dogs. Proceedings Of The National Science Council, Republic Of China. Part B, Life Sciences, 12, 174–9.

Zhang, J., Niu, S., Zhang, H. & Streisand, J. B. (2002) Oral Mucosal Absorption Of Midazolam In Dogs Is Strongly Ph Dependent. Journal Of Pharmaceutical Sciences, 91, 980–2.

Zornow, M. H., Maze, M., Dyck, J. B. & Shafer, S. L. (1993) Dexmedetomidine Decreases Cerebral Blood-Flow Velocity In Humans. Journal Of Cerebral Blood Flow And Metabolism, 13, 350–353.

CHAPTER

14

LOCAL ANESTHETICS

ALISTAIR I. WEBB AND LUISITO S. PABLO

Local anesthetics are drugs that produce reversible loss of sensation in an area of an animal's body without the loss of consciousness or alteration of central nervous system activity (CNS). By convention, physical methods such as cold are not included in this definition even though various ethers sprayed on skin to produce numbness were the first recorded methods of producing local anesthesia. One advantage of local anesthesia is the avoidance of changes in physiological function that is associated with general anesthesia and the fact that animals don't lose their ability to ambulate except in spinal procedures. These advantages are most appreciated in horses and farm animals where recumbency itself presents significant risks of trauma, myositis, ruminal tympany, and regurgitation. This is not to say that local anesthetics are without risk (McIntyre 1999). However, such risk is mainly dose related and can be avoided with judicious techniques.

The origin of pharmacological local anesthesia starts with the use of cocaine, first as a surface analgesia in ophthalmology and then administered parenterally to block nerve conduction (Koller 1928). The local anesthetic produced by cocaine was successful but its faults (toxicity and abuse potential) drove chemists to develop compounds that could be as effective without those problems.

Other than compounds that have been shown serendipitously to have local anesthetic properties (amitripty-

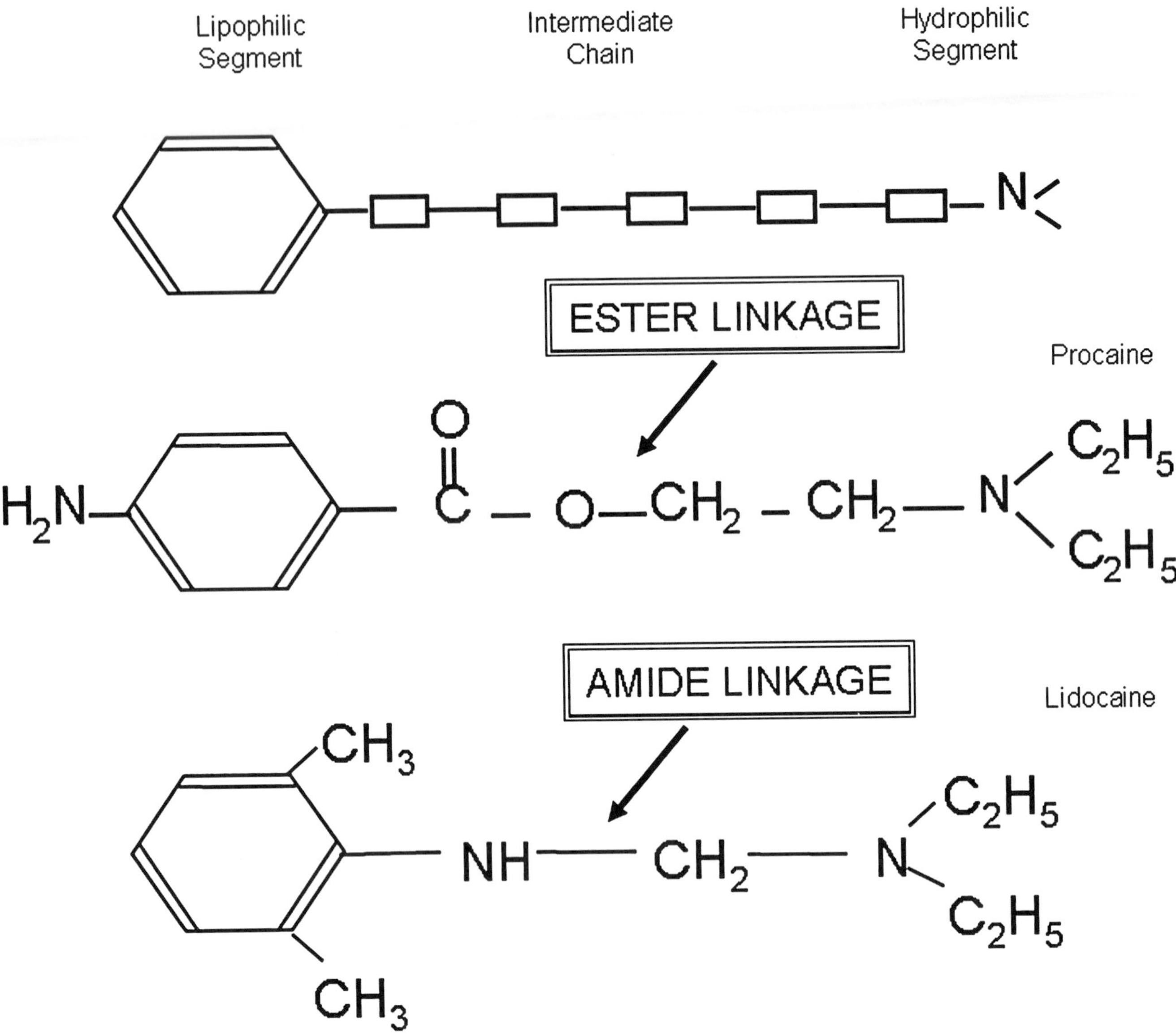

FIG. 14.1 Diagram showing basic structure of a typical local anesthetic alongside diagrams of procaine and lidocaine as examples of aminoester and amide local anesthetics.

line, opioids, and xylazine), the chemicals developed have similar chemical structures—i.e., a lipophilic end (aromatic sections) and an aminoalkyl hydrophilic side chain linked by an intermediate chain. A prototype is shown in Figure 14.1.

MECHANISMS

The key target of local anesthetics is the sodium channel in the membranes of excitable cells. Based on amino acid sequences, the channels can be sorted into two types: Na_v1 and Na_x (Ogata and Ohishi 2002). The Na_v1 group, which consists of 9 subtypes, acts as transmembrane voltage gated channels while the Na_x is concentration dependent. The opening of the Na_v1 channels is considered to be responsible for the action potential upstroke in excitable cells while the Na_x channels move sodium ions responses to concentration gradients across the membranes. Local anesthetics act at the sodium channels to prevent generation and propagation of nerve impulses or action potentials.

This is achieved by the local anesthetic decreasing and preventing the transient increase in the permeability of excited cell membranes to sodium ions.

The rate of rise of the action potential declines and impulse conduction slows, leading to a decrease in the probability of propagation occurring. Nerve conduction is eventually extinguished. Local anesthetics also interact with the potassium channels but require high concentrations of the drug, and blockade of conduction is not accompanied by any significant change in resting membrane potential.

The character of the conduction block a local anesthetic produces depends on the local anesthetic penetrating to the axoplasmic side of the nerve cell, the length of axon blocked, and the transiency of the block. In the case of myelinated nerves penetration is possible only at the nodes of Ranvier, and there the critical length is at least two nodes. Local anesthetics enter and leave the sodium channel when it is open (during the action potential) so that the more active a nerve is the greater the opportunities for the drugs to enter the channel. Thus a nerve cell that is repetitively stimulated is more sensitive to blocking. This is a *frequency-dependent block*.

Peak plasma concentrations of local anesthetics depend on the amount of drug injected, the drug's physical characteristics, the presence or absence of vasoconstrictors, and the site of injection. CNS effects are of progressive depression of electrical activity. Seemingly paradoxically, this can initially show as depression of inhibitory activity allowing frank displays of neuromuscular irritability and activity.

The effects of local anesthetics on the cardiovascular system (CVS) relate to changes to myocardial excitability and conduction. These are primarily decreases in the force of contraction and, except for bupivacaine, do not cause malignant electrical activity.

STRUCTURE AND CHEMISTRY

All of the local anesthetics are considered amphipathic. That is, they have opposing lipophilic and hydrophilic entities linked by an intermediate chain, which contains either an ester or an amide bond. The majority of the compounds have tertiary amines as the hydrophilic group and an unsaturated aromatic ring for the lipophilic end. The tertiary amines have ionic properties and are weak bases, which are poorly soluble in water. This means they have to be formulated for commercial packaging as salts (often hydrochloride). A key function for the hydrophilic moiety is its affinity for the axoplasmic side of the sodium channels in the nerve membrane. The intermediate linking chain serves to align the lipophilic amine group into the sodium channel. It has two forms: *ester-linked,* where there is an aminoester link derived from benzoic acid, and *amide-linked,* where the link is an aniline derivative.

The length of the chain is important as the peak potency for the tertiary amine blocking the sodium channel is optimal between three and seven carbon lengths.

The ester chain is relatively unstable and is broken down by plasma pseudocholinesterase. These local anesthetics have short plasma half-lives. Any condition or intoxication that limits or competes for the cholinesterases prolongs the activity of that group of local anesthetics and may increase risk of toxicity. Such agents include carbamyl and organophosphate insecticide and ophthalmic compounds.

The amide link is more stable than the esters and actually stands up to heat sterilization. Elimination of these molecules needs biotransformation with conjugation by the liver. The molecules' stability means longer plasma half-lives and increased risk of cumulation and toxicity. Bupivacaine, mepivacaine, and propivacaine are pipecoloxylidide (PPX) derivatives. They have an asymmetrical carbon atom linking the amide chain to the lipophilic tail. This asymmetry results in left- (s) or right- (r) handed configurations or enantiomers, which can have significantly different kinetic, dynamic, and toxicological properties. The importance of the differing enantiomers is demonstrated in the recent releases of two major local anesthetic compounds in monoisomeric formulations: levobupivacaine and ropivacaine (s-bupivacaine and s-propivacaine, respectively).

There are other structural features that influence a local anesthetic's action. Increased hydrocarbon substitution on the tertiary amine increases the compound's sodium channel blocking potency. This occurs when the butyl group substitutes for methyl on the piperidine ring and mepivacaine changes to bupivacaine. Bupivacaine is four times as potent as mepivacaine. Similarly, if the ester local anesthetic procaine is altered only by addition of a 4-aliphatic chain to the lipophilic end, it becomes tetracaine, which is 10–16 times more potent.

As mentioned above, local anesthetics are weak bases so they are prepared as salts to facilitate dissolution. When a local anesthetic is dissolved it establishes an equilibrium between its neutral or uncharged base form and the positively charged cationic form. The ratio between these two forms is a function of the drug's negative log of the acid dissociation constant (pK_a) and the pH or acidity of the solution. A compound's pK_a is defined as the pH when base and cation concentrations are equal. This can be seen inspecting a customized version of the Henderson-Hasselbalch equation:

$$pH = pK_a + \log \frac{[\text{B or local anesthetic}]}{[BH^+]}$$

When $[B]/[BH^+]$ is unity, the pK_a is equal to pH. By the same logic, as the pH falls (acidity increases) the $[B]/[BH^+]$ ratio must fall and the concentration of the cationic form of the local anesthetic increases. A pH shift of 0.1 can result in a 10% increase in the cation form. This change in pH is important if the local anesthetic must diffuse across cell walls or lipoprotein membranes and only the neutral base can cross. One example is injection of local anesthetic into inflamed (acidic) tissues. Another example is where local anesthetic diffuses across the placenta into a fetus whose blood is more acidic than in the maternal circulation. In that example, the cationic form of the local anesthetic in the fetus cannot equilibrate back across the placenta (Johnson et al. 1999). In this example, placental transfer is further complicated by differences in pK_a and protein binding (Biehl et al. 1978; Finster et al. 1972; Kuhnert et al. 1987; Thomas et al. 1976). The basic information and pK_as of the major local anesthetics are listed in Table 14.1 along with their other physicochemical characteristics. In considering this table, one must be aware how differences in values published in different sources reflect differences in methodology and reporting criteria (Strichartz et al. 1990).

The major clinical properties of local anesthetics are based on the following:

Potency. Potency relates to lipid solubility and amount of the neutral base available at the action site. Both lipid solubility and pK_a promote penetration of the drug to the site of action. Unfortunately, toxicity parallels increases of potency so the relative safety margin decreases. The potencies for the major local anesthetics are listed in Table 14.2.

Duration of action. The length of time a drug blocks sensory transmission depends on how well it penetrates into the axoplasm and reaches the sodium channel, how strongly it binds to the channel, and finally how quickly it is removed. The ease of penetration and amount of drug reaching the sodium channel is a function of lipid solubility. The second factor is the strength of the bond that the drug has with the sodium channel protein. Compounds such as etidocaine were especially noted for this property. Length of block duration is an eagerly sought-after property as it allows use of local anesthetics in relief of postoperative and chronic pain. The relief of pain with an unclouded sensorium confers a huge advantage to local anesthesia. The final factor affecting duration of blockade is the continued presence or absence of the local anesthetic drug at the site of action. The primary determinant is perfusion at the site of administration and the subsequent removal of the drug into the systemic circulation. Limiting perfusion or vasoconstriction is intrinsic with cocaine and to a lesser degree ropivacaine. With the other drugs it requires the addition of exogenous vasoconstrictors such as epinephrine.

Onset of action. The time a local anesthetic takes to produce a sensory block is determined by placement of the drug, the concentration used, the molecule size, and the proportion of cationic drug present. The latter is determined by the pK_a. The lower the pK_a, the more uncharged base available to penetrate into the axoplasmic space of the nerve. Lidocaine and mepivacaine have lower pK_as than bupivacaine (see Table 14.1) and therefore shorter onsets. In human dentistry a short onset is a highly sought-after characteristic and articaine has been developed to meet that demand. It has a lower pK_a than lidocaine and a quicker onset. Of course, if the pK_a is very low the local anesthetics will be mainly available in the insoluble base form. Benzocaine has a pK_a of 2.5 and is so sparingly soluble that it is limited to topical mucosal applications and fish anesthesia where the base's penetrative power is fully utilized. Lipophilicity and protein binding slow diffusion and delay onset.

Differential block. Sensitivity of different neural transmissions to local anesthetics is primarily a function of the physical characteristics of the nerves. The simplicity of this can be confounded by positioning of tracts within bundles of the spinal cord. The general order of decreasing sensitivity is pain and temperature first and then proprioception and motor functions. As the goal of local anesthesia is to obtund pain it would not require that motor function be blocked when the sensory component has been blocked. Therefore it is desirable that, when local anesthetics cease to block sensory nerve transmission ("wear off"), motor function and proprio-

TABLES 14.1A and 14.1B Basic information for major aminoester and amide local anesthetics that have been used in human and veterinary practice. The amides are subdivided as pipecoloxylidide (PPX) and aminoalkyl (AAX) derivatives (USP Expert Committee 2006; Specialized Information Services 2006)

Drug	Structure	Date of First Clinical Use	CAS	mw Base	Type
cocaine	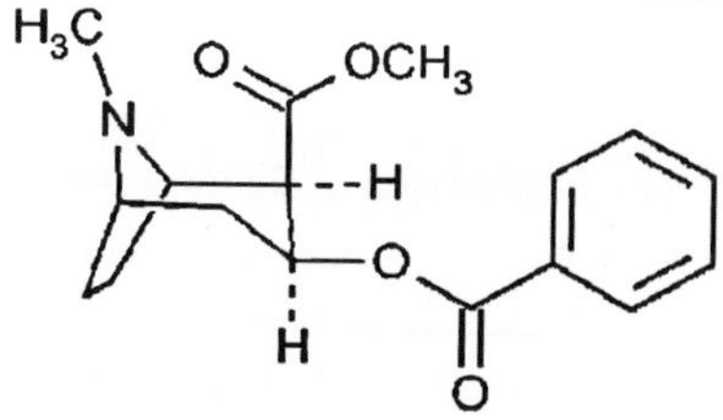	1884	50-36-2	303	ester
benzocaine	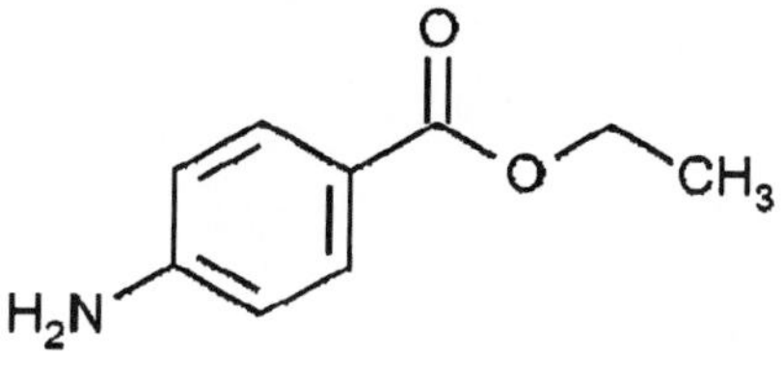	1900	94-09-7	166	ester
procaine	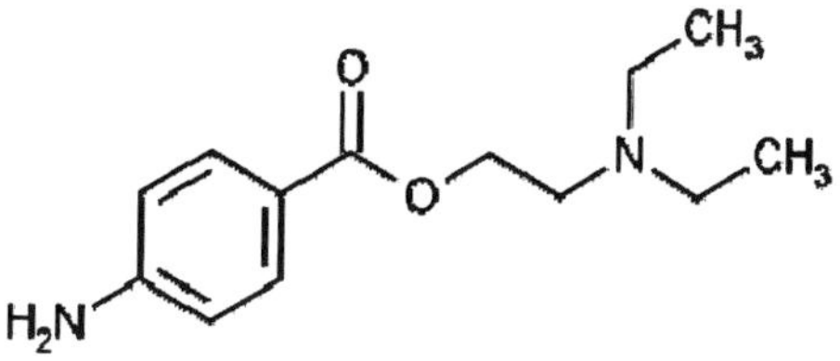	1904	59-46-1	236	ester
dibucaine	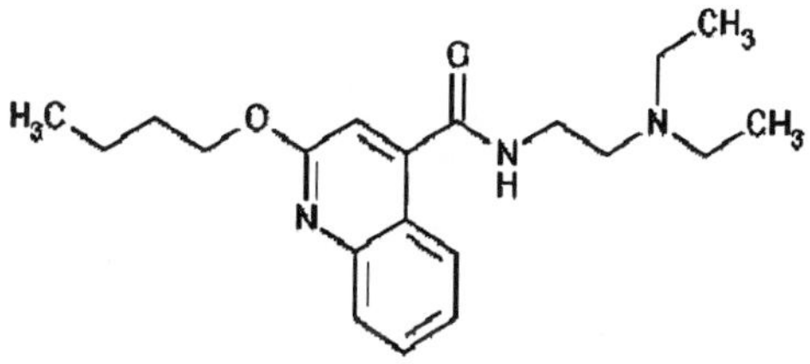	1929	85-79-0	343	ester
tetracaine	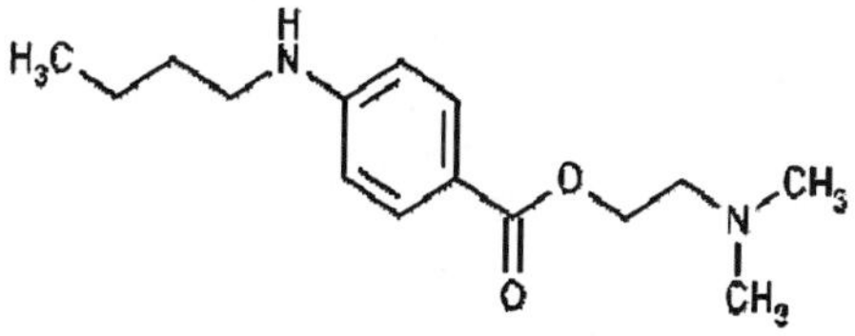	1930	94-24-6	264	ester
propracaine	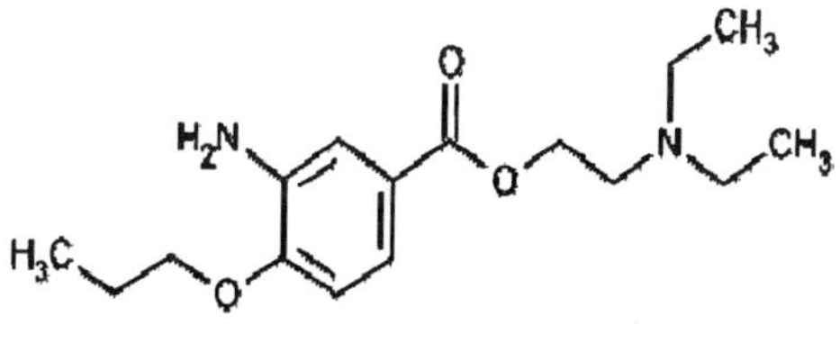	1953	499-67-2	294	ester

TABLES 14.1A and 14.1B—*continued*

Drug	Structure	Date of First Clinical Use	CAS	mw Base	Type	Subtype
lidocaine	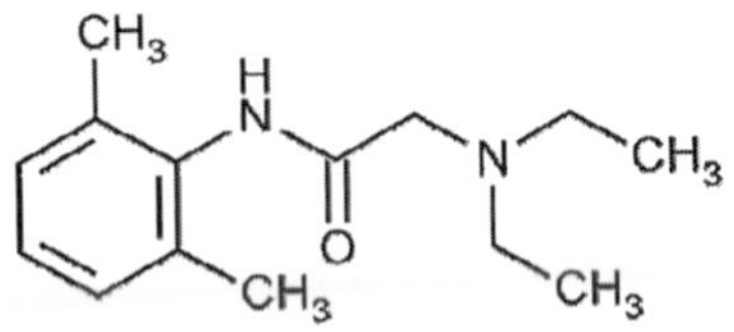	1948	137-58-6	234	amide	AAX
mepivacaine	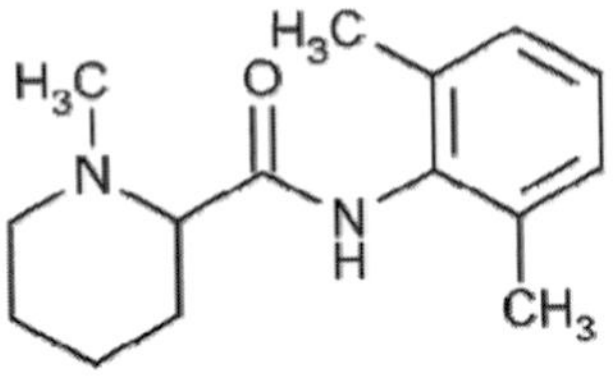	1957	96-88-8	243	amide	PPX
prilocaine	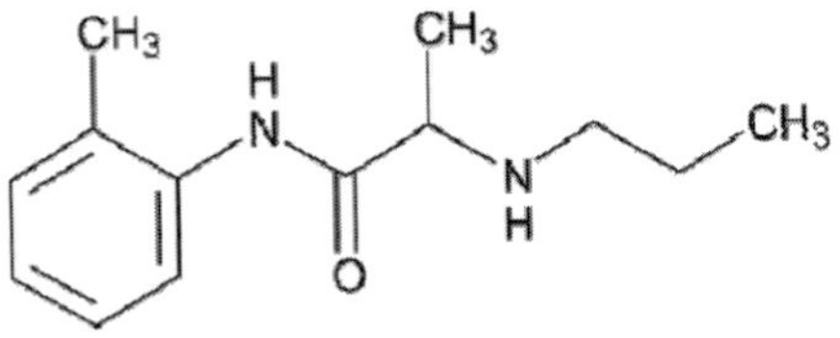	1960	721-50-6	220	amide	AAX
bupivacaine	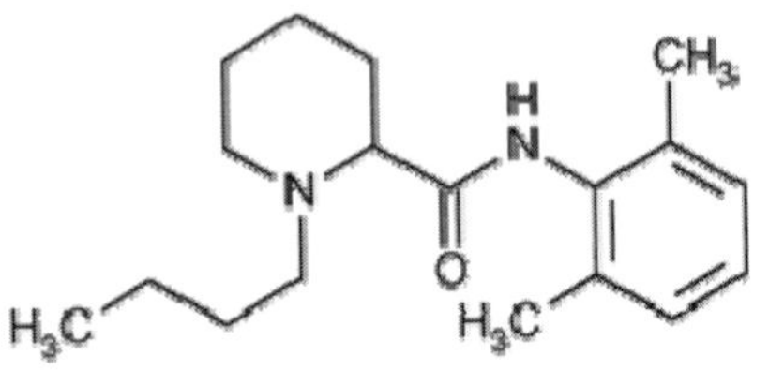	1963	38396-39-3	288	amide	PPX
etidocaine	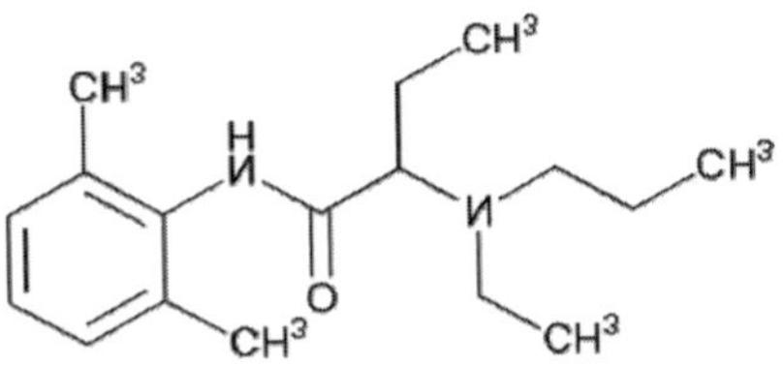	1972	36637-18-0	276	amide	AAX
articiane	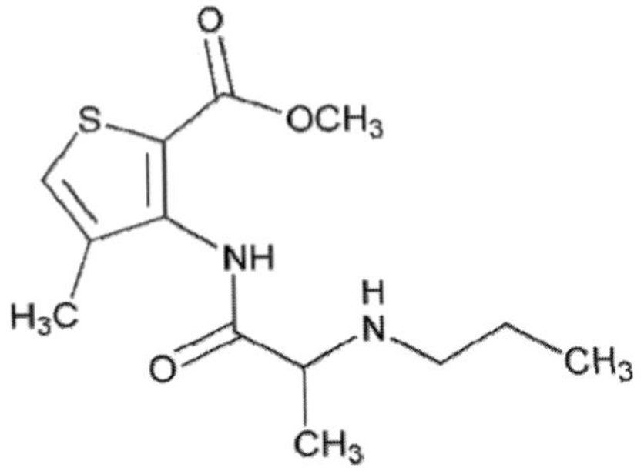	1975	23964-58-1	320	amide/ester	thiophene
ropivacaine	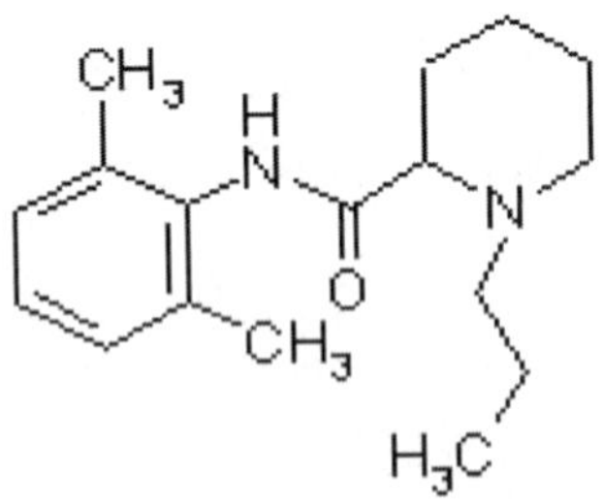	1996	84057-95-4	274	amide	PPX
levobupivacaine	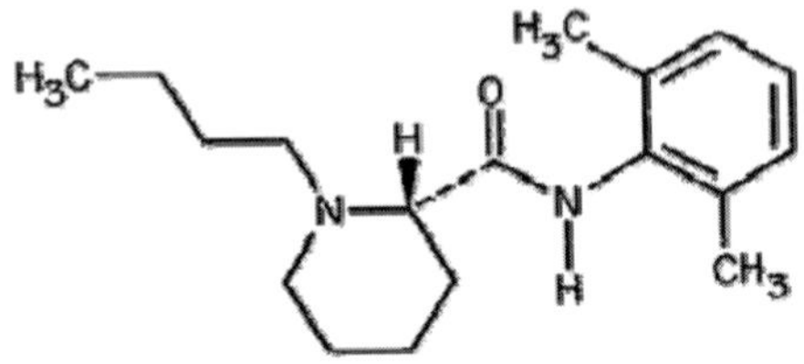	1999	27262-47-1	288	amide	PPX

TABLE 14.2 Basic physicochemical and pharmacodynamic characteristics of the major aminoester and amide local anesthetics that are currently used in veterinary practice (Rosenberg et al. 1986; Arthur 1987; Strichartz et al. 1990; Viscomi 2004; Leuschner and Leblanc 1999)

Drug	Potency [Rat Sciatic]	Onset	Duration	pK_a	Protein Binding	Oil Lambda	Log p (Octanol-water)
Esters							
benzocaine				2.5			132
tetracaine	8	slow	120	8.4	76	80	541
procaine	1	slow	50	8.9	5.8	1	3.1
Amides							
lidocaine	2	fast	90	7.8	64	2.5	110
mepivacaine	2	rapid	130	7.7	80	1	42
bupivacaine	8	slow	360	8.1	95	27.5	560
levobupivacaine	8	slow	360	8.1	>97	27.5	
ropivacaine	6	slow	360	8.2	94	6.1	115
articiane		fast	60	7.8	95	1.5	

ception have already returned to normal. A very important example in veterinary medicine is where limb nerve blocks have been performed in horses for therapeutic or diagnostic purposes and proprioception is still impaired. Allowed to move freely, the horse can injure itself with unguarded movement or foot placement. It is one reason racing authorities have banned the use of local anesthetics in competing animals. In human anesthesiology the use of local anesthetics in spinal and epidural techniques is optimized when there is no or only limited motor effects while sensory blocks are present allowing ambulation and better bladder function. The long-acting local anesthetic etidocaine was withdrawn from the market because of problems associated with persistent motor block.

Plasma protein binding. As local anesthetics are absorbed from their injection sites they enter the general circulation and are available for systemic effects. To be systemically active, a drug must be available to enter sites of potential activity and this requires it be both unbound and unionized. All of the local anesthetics have significant binding to plasma protein (commonly 1–2 μg/ml). There are two proteins involved with binding of local anesthetics—alpha-1 glycoprotein and albumin. Local anesthetics have high affinity for the former but it is very limited in capacity. In contrast albumin has a high capacity but low affinity. The binding is concentration and pH dependent with the percentage bound decreasing as concentration rises or rising as pH falls. In drugs such as bupivacaine, levobupivacaine, and ropivacaine where the amount bound is very high (over 95%), small changes in percent bound means big changes in unbound drug being available. For example, a drop in binding from 95% to 93% increases by 40% the amount being unbound (5% to 7% of total drug). Events that can change protein binding include drug interactions when drugs that have a higher affinity for the albumin binding sites are administered (barbiturate or phenylbutazone), pH changes, and diseases that lower plasma protein concentrations per se.

METABOLISM

The breakdown and elimination of local anesthetics is important because the balance of uptake from the site of injection and the drugs' elimination is a major determinant of their toxicity. Once a drug moves away from the injection site it is available for either metabolism or movement into sensitive sites of possible intoxication in the CNS and CVS. When injected intravascularly, either accidentally or as part of an IVRA procedure, the delay in reaching the circulation is eliminated unless appropriate time is allowed to elapse, as in the case of IVRA (Arthur 1987).

The initial metabolism of aminoesters (cocaine, benzocaine, procaine, and tetracaine) is the hydrolysis of the ester link by plasma esterases such as cholinesterase. There are differences between species in cholinesterase activity (Tecles and Ceron 2001; Kalow and Genest 1957; Reidenberg 1972) and, in humans, some intraspecies genetic variation as seen with dibucaine (Kalow and Genest 1957). In the case of injection into the intrathecal space, the CSF has no esterase activity and the drug's effect continues until the drug is resorbed into the general circulation. In the case of procaine, the products of the hydrolysis are diethlaminoethanol and para-aminobenzoic acid (PABA). The latter antagonizes sulfonamide antibiotics and shares that drug's ability to provoke allergic reactions.

Metabolism of the amide-linked local anesthetics requires biotransformation by the liver. The alternative metabolic paths have not been well differentiated for the common species with the most data being gathered from studies in rats. There are detailed studies of urinary metabolite production in horses generated by racing chemists (Harkins et al. 1995) but these do not necessarily cast light on the different mechanisms involved. Some local anesthetic is excreted in the urine unchanged. In humans it is less than 2% for lidocaine, 5% for bupivacaine, and over 10% for mepivacaine.

The initial steps in the metabolism of lidocaine are done in the liver by oxidative dealkylation by cytochrome P450 enzymes (CYPs) (Keenaghan and Boyes 1972). The dealkylation produces monoethylglycine xylidide (MEGX) and glycine xylidide (GX), with the MEGX being further broken down to monoethylglycine and xylidide. It should be noted that both MEGX and xylidide have sodium channel activity (MEGX's is about 75% that of lidocaine while xylidide's is only 10%). The xylidide is further metabolized and then excreted in the urine. Prilocaine, related to lidocaine, is the most rapidly metabolized amide-linked local anesthetic because it is a secondary amine. Its problem is that the hydrolysis produces O-toluidine, which is a potent oxidant of hemoglobin to methemoglobin.

The pipecolyl xylidides derivatives (mepivacaine, bupivacaine, and ropivacaine) also undergo cleavage of the amide bond but at a slower rate because of the bulky alkyl groups on the piperidine nitrogen. As the number of carbons increases from one (mepivacaine) to three (ropivacaine) to four (bupivacaine) so is amide cleavage resisted. Dealkylation is less important in this group with greater activity in N-demethylation to produce the less toxic metabolite pipcolylxylidine (PPX) with parahydroxylation of the xylidine ring. In humans more mepivacaine is excreted unchanged renally than for the other common local anesthetics.

Hepatic disease, by degrading microsomal enzyme capability, can prolong or even limit metabolism. Similarly, drugs that induce the enzymes (barbiturates) can increase drug breakdown while, in contrast, drugs that can inhibit the P450 system can prolong drug elimination (examples are chloramphenicol, clonidine, ketoconazole, macrolide antibiotics, midazolam, and verapamil).

FORMULATION

Local anesthetics come in an amazing variety of presentations and formulations. Lidocaine is a particular example as it comes as sterile injectable solutions for parenteral use, gels and ointments for topical use, aerosol sprays for airway application, and patches for transdermal application. A constant problem facing the compounding pharmacist is the base's poor solubility. A common technique used to achieve dissolution of local anesthetics is to use salts. This means the solution has a pH of around 6. The addition of epinephrine requires an even lower pH (below 3). An injectate with such a low pH causes stinging pain on injection. Efforts have been made to lessen this. For example, alkalinization with the addition of sodium bicarbonate has been used with mixed results (Sinnott et al. 2000). Unfortunately, there is precipitation over a short period of time, so the sodium bicarbonate has to be freshly added and the mixture used within 10–20 minutes. Paradoxically, carbonation (acidification) has been used to promote intracellular acidosis by diffusion of CO_2 into the axoplasm and thus promoting the cation form of the local anesthetic. The cation will then bind with the sodium channel receptors. There are no approved pH manipulated products in the USA.

BARICITY. Local anesthetics used in spinal anesthesia need to have a specific gravity that limits their ascension in the subaracnoid space. Normal formulations have specific gravities close to water and thus are hypobaric and will move upward in the subarachnoid space. To stop this and increase the specific gravity (hyperbaric) glucose is added.

CONCENTRATIONS. Careful attention must be paid to drug labels. Only there can one determine what concentration and form of local anesthetic is present. Especially one should note what the label unit is: the base or the salt? For example, 1 g of lidocaine HCl is equivalent to 0.83 g of lidocaine base. Another concentration difference that can confuse a person reading label data is whether the drug's concentration is cited for blood or plasma. Because local anesthetics are more soluble in the red cells the concentration in plasma is less than in whole blood, with the range being 70–90% less.

VASOCONSTRICTORS. Vasoconstrictors are often added to local anesthetic preparations to keep the drug at the injection site for a longer period. The most common vasoconstrictor is epinephrine. Vasoconstriction serves mainly to prolong the duration of the block and also to delay systemic uptake. The latter is important in that it reduces risk of toxicity. Vasoconstriction limits bleeding in an infiltration site area. An accidental intravascular injection of a solution containing epinephrine will alert the clinician through tachycardia produced. The common epinephrine formulation is a 1:2,00,000 concentration. Another agent that has been used is phenylephrine, which is very similar to epinephrine but has less potent CVS effects. Local anesthetics containing potent vasoconstrictors should not be used where endarterial blood supply might be compromised such as in a ring block in a cow's teat.

PRESERVATIVES. All multidose preparations contain preservatives. These include sodium metabisulphite, methylparaben, benzyl alcohol, and EDTA. All have been associated with complications. Bisulphite compounds are considered to be neurotoxic, especially under conditions of tissue acidosis and hypoxia. Methylparaben presents increased allergic reaction potential, and benzoic acid related compound can cause intoxication in cats. EDTA can cause local muscle tetany because of associated calcium chelation. The potential for local anesthetics to provoke allergic reactions is based on human case data and must be considered small. There are preparations that are preservative-free. These are indicated for intrathecal administration where presence of preservative can induce both acute and chronic neural damage and nerve root irritation syndromes.

It is interesting that local anesthetic formulations have been claimed to have bacteriocidal activity per se (Sakuragi et al. 1996, 1997). This property is not universally accepted. Differences between drugs and concentrations have been cited as reasons for these discrepancies (Chandan et al. 2005; Olsen et al. 2000; Parr et al. 1999; Stratford et al. 2002). Some investigators have studied this effect in propofol mixtures which are preservative-free and where the mixture does lessen the pain of injection (Aydin et al. 2002).

ONSET PROMOTORS. There are drugs that speed the rate the local anesthetic reaches and binds to the sodium channel receptor. Most are drugs that manipulate the pH of the preparation. The thought is that they promote penetration of the neural sheath by alkalinizing the solution. The agents are then used to provide an intracellular acidic media to promote the formation of the ionized cationic form that binds to the receptor. The efficacy of these additives is not clear, but the most common is carbonation. These formulations are not approved in the U.S. so their use involves compounding and would constitute extralabel drug use (ELDU).

POTENTIATING ADDITIVES. The major group of drugs used to increase the depth or duration of local anesthetic blocks is the alpha-2 sympathomimetics. In human medicine this has been clonidine and in veterinary medicine, xylazine. The alpha-2 agonists can be absorbed from the site of injection and have systemic effects that are most obvious in the ruminants, which have greater sensitivity to this group of drugs. Opioids and ketamine also have been added to local anesthetic formulations for intrathecal and epidural injection or to be used by themselves. Special care should be taken with these agents because only morphine and clonidine are available in preservative-free preparations at this time.

TOXICITY OF LOCAL ANESTHETICS

The major signs of local anesthetic toxicity involve the CNS and the CVS. Local anesthetic–induced CNS toxicity is usually seen at significantly lower plasma concentrations than that associated with CVS toxicity. For example, CVS effects of lidocaine at concentrations below 5 μg/ml depress only cardiac automaticity. Arteriolar relaxation starts to produce hypotension only as the concentration increases above that 5 μg/ml concentration (Fig. 14.2).

NEUROTOXICITY. Local anesthetics have neurotoxicity as their major side effect. The common type is generalized descending CNS depression that is proportional to circulating free and unbound drug. The signs are dose related. Initial signs are subjective in humans but in animals might show in minor behavioral changes. The first objective signs are of muscle twitching and tremors. These are initially

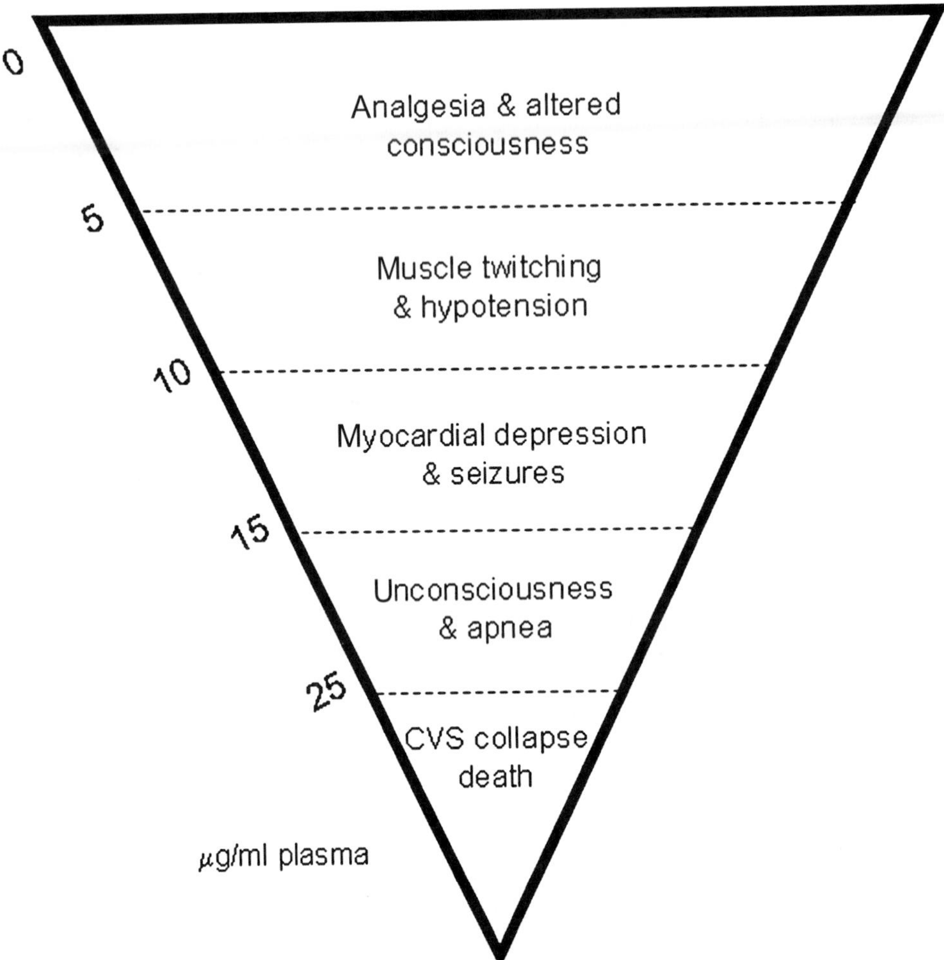

FIG. 14.2 Diagrammatic representation of the deepening CNS depression associated with increasing plasma concentrations of lidocaine.

seen around the head and face but rapidly spread, progressing to full tonic-clonic convulsions. Last, there is severe CNS depression with respiratory depression and death. The sequence is thought to be centered in the limbic area, which is highly vascular and therefore rapidly equilibrates with circulating levels of local anesthetic. The initial twitching and convulsions result from preferential blockade of inhibitory pathways. These excitatory effects should not be confused with cocaine's CNS effects, which uniquely affect neurotransmitters and delay uptake of norepinephrine. There are distinct differences between agents in the toxicity associated with a single bolus. This is because there are critical concentrations of the free drug that have penetrated into the CNS. Opposing reaching these concentrations are ease of penetrating the blood brain barrier, lipophilicity, bound versus free drug concentrations, and whether the rate of metabolism is fast enough to tip the equilibration. The ester-linked local anesthetics are an example of the latter point. They are so rapidly metabolized in the plasma that CNS toxicity is seen only when there are perturbations of cholinesterase activity. Similarly, highly lipid-soluble and protein-bound amides such as bupivacaine can have plasma peak concentrations too transient to provoke frank CNS signs before the CVS side effects appear.

Risk Factors. The prime risk factor is dose. Dose is the reason why toxicity is more often seen in smaller animals where the mg/kg restrictions often get overlooked or weight estimations are a source of error. The site of injection is important as vascularity means more rapid uptake into the systemic circulation and greater risk of accidental intravascular injection. There is intravenous regional anesthesia (IVRA) where there is deliberate intravascular injection, but it is withheld from the circulation with a tourniquet. With appropriate tourniquet administration and maintenance IVRA usually avoids toxic levels. The risk comes with premature release of the tourniquet. Such intravascular injection mishaps produce considerable blood level of the local anesthetics. It is for that reason that use of the racemic bupivacaine preparations is considered too risky for use in IVRA. A site that that is highly vascular and yields high circulating levels of local anesthetic is the intercostal space.

There is anecdotal information suggesting some species idiosyncrasies (examples: cats and goats) but there are no controlled data to support these reports. However given known species differences in plasma protein, drug metabolism and body composition such differences should be expected.

Drug Interactions. Drug interactions are potentially important considerations in changing how or when one would use local anesthetics. Example of potential interactions would be changes in convulsive threshold (CNS depressants and tranquilizers), competition for plasma binding sites, and induction or inhibition of microsomal enzymes responsible for breakdown of the amide local anesthetics. Not all interactions are problems because the interaction with epinephrine prolong sensory block and lowering toxicity is something planned and sought.

Other types of toxicity reported as being associated with local anesthetics but not commonly observed, are transient neurotoxicity and myotoxicity (Zink and Graf 2004). The neurotoxicity has been associated with spinal and epidural anesthesia and with high concentrations of lidocaine. No clear etiology has been established, but numerous factors have been considered: catheter design, preservatives, and direct cytotoxicity. The myotoxicity seems slow to develop and resolves well. A possible reason for why there are few clinical reports would be that the signs occur past clinical oversight.

CARDIOTOXICITY. The primary signs of local anesthetic cardiovascular toxicity are hypotension and dysrhythmias. The hypotension occurs from a number of causes that include depression of myocardial contractility, direct relaxation of vascular smooth muscle, and loss of vasomotor sympathetic tone.

Lidocaine is commonly used for stabilizing ventricular dysrhythmias, so ventricular tachycardia and fibrillation are infrequent consequences of most local anesthetics and are primarily associated with bupivacaine (Carpenter 1997). CVS sensitivity to bupivacaine stems from its lipophilicity facilitating a rapid entrance to open myocardial sodium channels during action potentials (systole). The drug does not move from the sodium channel as fast during diastole when binding and lipid solubility slow the exiting of bupivacaine allowing it to accumulate. Thus, as heart rate increases, accumulation is greater. This selective cardiotoxicity of bupivacaine is shared with etidocaine. The most serious manifestation of this is reentrant arrhythmias with consequent problems with resuscitation (Davis and de Jong 1982). This presents as bupivacaine induced cardiac collapse being the hardest of the common agents to resuscitate (Groban et al. 2001). Groban et al. dosed dogs with local anesthetic until cardiovascular collapse (mean blood pressure below 45 mm Hg) and then applied standard resuscitation protocol, including open chest cardiac massage. Less than half of the bupivacaine-dosed dogs survived and, although all of the lidocaine dogs survived, 80% required prolonged supportive therapy.

A recent report of how rats and dogs were resuscitated successfully after seemingly fatal doses of bupivacaine when they received intravenous boluses of the lipid emulsion Intralipid® shows great promise (Picard and Meek 2006; Weinberg et al. 1998, 2003). How this works is only conjecture at this time but in vitro data suggest highly lipid-soluble local anesthetics partition into lipid emulsions (Weinberg et al. 2006).

PREVENTION AND TREATMENT OF TOXICITY.

Prevention of local anesthetic toxicity is based on keeping the plasma concentration as low as possible. The first steps are to limit dose size and to keep the injectate concentration low. Once administered, the absorption of the local anesthetic has to be slowed. The latter can be achieved by combining vasoconstrictors with the local anesthetic, avoiding sites with high vascularity where practicable, and avoiding accidental intravascular administration. The latter can be accomplished by application of anatomical knowledge or use of a test dose. If a solution containing epinephrine is used in the test dose, intravascular administration will be detected by an almost instantaneous tachycardia.

Toxicity of local anesthetic manifested as seizure can be managed by providing a high concentration of supplemental oxygen and the intravenous administration of a benzodiazepine (diazepam or midazolam). In animals that develop cardiovascular depression or collapse, prompt ventilatory and cardiovascular support should be instituted. If the animal stops breathing, the trachea should be intubated and the ventilation controlled. A high concentration of oxygen should be used. With severe hypotension, epinephrine is given intravenously. Atropine is indicated if there is bradycardia. Dysrhythmia caused by bupivacaine is refractory to drug treatment. Intravenous boluses of the lipid emulsion Intralipid® may be tried.

STABILITY

Local anesthetics are very stable at room temperature (15–30°C). Solutions of amide local anesthetics that do not contain epinephrine can be autoclaved (15 psi at 121°C for 15 minutes). Solutions containing epinephrine need protection from sunlight and are usually sold in amber-colored containers for that reason. Any local anesthetic solution that is cloudy, contains precipitate, or is discolored should be discarded.

DRUG INTERACTIONS AND DISEASE

Drug interactions involving local anesthetics come in varied ways: potentiation of CNS depressants, altered metabolism, altered protein binding, and enhancement of toxicity.

Lidocaine's potentiation of inhalation anesthetics is well documented with reduction of isoflurane requirements in cats, dogs, and horses (Himes, Jr. et al. 1977; Doherty and Frazier 1998; Muir, III et al. 2003; Pypendop and Ilkiw 2005). The use of a local anesthetic in continuing mode like this needs the drug to be administered using a constant rate infusion (CRI). CRI has been also found useful as a prokinetic in treatment of ileus (Rimback et al. 1990; Malone et al. 2006) and neuropathic pain (Mao J. and Chen L.L. 2000).

Uremia is associated with alterations in protein binding. In the potent and highly bound amides, differences of a few percentages in plasma protein binding equal major increases in the amount of unbound active drug. Change in binding together with altered renal excretion cause increases in plasma concentrations of local anesthetic, as seen in the case of ropivacaine (Pere et al. 2003).

REGULATORY ISSUES

Local anesthetics have an unusual status in the United States regarding approval by the Food and Drug Administration (FDA). Only mepivacaine and proparacaine are approved for use as local anesthetics in animals (mepivacaine for horses only and proparacaine with the unusual approved species being "animals"). However, local anesthetics are incorporated in many FDA-approved proprietary formulations. The most important of these are otitic preparations and where procaine is compounded with penicillin G to create a slower releasing formulation of the antibiotic. The procaine-penicillin combination causes problems when horses and greyhounds are treated with the procaine containing antibiotic, and then they test positive for procaine when examined for drugs in association with racing or showing (Sundlof et al. 1983). Local anesthetics are considered to be Class 2 substances by the Association of Racing Commissioners International (ARCI), and their detection in postrace urine samples can result in substantial penalties.

The lack of an FDA approval could be problematic in food-producing animals but FDA regards the use of local anesthetics in those species to be of low regulatory concern. Because extralabel drug use (ELDU) requires an extended withdrawal time in food-producing animals, the Food Animal Residue Avoidance Databank (FARAD), recognizing the very short half-life of local anesthetics, has recommended a 24-hour withdrawal interval for both meat and milk (Craigmill et al. 1997).

INDIVIDUAL DRUGS

The structures, physical characteristics, and pharmacodynamic effects of the local anesthetics are set out in Tables 14.1, 14.2 and 14.3. References consulted for these data can differ slightly so, where there were multiple sources, the most common values are cited. The animal pharmacokinetic data (Tables 14.4A and B) are taken from the Food Animal Residue Avoidance Databank (FARAD) pharmacokinetic database (Craigmill et al. 2006). The individual references in that database have been evaluated and, in many cases, the data submitted to further analyses.

PROCAINE. Procaine was the first local anesthetic synthesized. Although it lacked the potency and ability to penetrate mucous membranes, procaine proved to be a

TABLE 14.3 The central nervous and cardiovascular toxicity for major local anesthetics. The CNS data are shown for those species reported in the literature while the CVS data are for the dog only (Liu et al. 1982, 1983; Phoenix Scientific 2005; Covino 1987).

Drug	Convulsant Dose—100% mg/kg						Reduction in Cardiac Output [dogs] Dose mg/kg IV			CVS LD_{100}
	Mice	Rabbits	Monkeys	Cats	Dogs	Sheep	25%	50%	100%	
procaine		15		35			80	100	240	
tetracaine		3			4		10	20	26	27
lidocaine	111	6	14–22	15	22	5.8	20	30	60	76
mepivacaine			18	18			25	40	80	
bupivacaine	57		4	5	5	2.7	5	10	20	20
etidocaine			5		8	2.2	10	20	40	27
prilocaine			18	22			25	40	80	

TABLE 14.4A The pharmacokinetic parameters in humans for lidocaine, mepivacaine, bupivacaine, and ropivacaine entaniomers [lidocaine is achiral and ropivacaine is available only as the S(–) isomer]. Where there was a significant difference between entaniomers for a particular parameter the value is marked with an asterisk (*) (Burm et al. 1997; Burm et al. 1994).

Drug	Lidocaine	Mepivacaine		Bupivacaine		Propivacaine
entaniomer	achiral	R(–)	S(+)	R(+)	S(–) levobupivacaine	S(–) ropivacaine
Vss [l]	73	103	54*	84	54*	54
CL [l/min]	1.2	0.8	0.4*	0.4	0.3*	0.5
terminal T1/2 [hr]	1.6	1.9	2.0*	3.6	2.6*	1.9

successful attempt to get away from cocaine's toxicity and abuse potential. It has low lipid solubility and thereby a low potency. It is rapidly metabolized by plasma cholinesterase to PABA and diethyl-amino ethanol. Procaine has the most noticeable incidence of allergic reactions and this is generally attributed to the PABA. In animals this seems to be manifested as urticaria. Although its original trade name Novocaine® is synonymous for local anesthetic for lay and professional people it is seldom used for local anesthesia today. Today procaine's major use in the combination with penicillin G where, when injected into muscle, it slows penicillin's release into the systemic circulation.

LIDOCAINE. Lidocaine is an amide local anesthetic that is the most widely used local anesthetic in medical and veterinary practice. In the United Kingdom was formerly called *lignocaine.* It has a relatively rapid onset (2–5 minutes), an intermediate duration of action (20–40 minutes), and a lower toxicity than the more potent and longer acting bupivacaine. Lidocaine toxicity shows initially as CNS toxicity and, when caused by a single bolus, is fairly transient and passes in 2–5 minutes. Higher doses can result in CVS toxicity with hypotension being the major sign. In normal concentrations (1–5 μg/ml) (Wilcke et al. 1983). Lidocaine has a significant role as a treatment for ventricular arrhythmias being classed as a IB antiarrhythmic. Lidocaine has the greatest diversity of routes of application of all of the local anesthetics. Although its topical uses are considered to be limited to mucous membranes, it has been combined with prilocaine in EMLA® ointment and lidocaine patches that do allow it to penetrate skin. The formulations for topical application include gels, ointments, viscous solutions and sprays. It is probably the best local anesthetic for infiltration. The

TABLE 14.4B The pharmacokinetic parameters for the major local anesthetics are listed by species. The data are abstracted from the FARAD Kinetic Database and chosen on the basis of both number of animals in the studies and the fullness of the data (Craigmill et al. 2006).

Drug/Species	Dose mg/kg	T1/2 hr	MRT hr	Vd ml/kg	Cl ml/kg/hr
cocaine					
NHP (rhesus)	1	0.63			
sheep	1	0.14		3.59	319
procaine					
horses	2.5	0.84		671	225
lidocaine					
camel	1	2.67	2.6	683	255
dog	6	0.87	1.06	2487	2326
guinea pigs	10	0.25	0.36	1420	65.3
horses	0.42	0.43	0.52	189	361
mice	10	0.37		1512	
NHP (rhesus)	10	0.3	0.47	760	400
rabbits	3.5	0.19	0.07	2320	162
rats	50	1.5		975	443
sheep	2	0.7	0.07	503	2578
swine	2	2.67	0.83	720	858
bupivacaine					
NHP (rhesus)	1	1.33	1.1	0.66	10
swine	2.5	0.79	1.15	390	340
ropivacaine					
swine	0.05		0.72		

addition of epinephrine assists in delaying its dispersion from the site of injection as well as helping limit bleeding. The same solutions are used in peripheral nerve blocks and IVRA. Lidocaine is used for short-duration spinal (subarachnoid or intrathecal) and epidural blocks where the formulation without preservatives should be used. Vials and bottles of lidocaine or the other local anesthetics that are preservative-free should be discarded after use as the combination of site of use and risk of contamination makes continued use unacceptable. The same is true when mixing other agents with the local anesthetic; first, there are very limited studies on the stability of these mixtures and, second, admixtures present significant risk of microbial contamination.

Lidocaine has a variety of uses. It suppresses cough associated with endotracheal tube insertion or removal. It has also been used in endotracheal intubation of cats. The larynx is sprayed to desensitize it and delay the onset of laryngospasm. Despite common belief, the larynx is not paralyzed, and often the initial reaction to the spray is to actually precipitate some spasm (Rex 1971). Cetacaine® is another preparation containing benzocaine and tetracaine that was used for the same purpose. However, it produces methemoglobin and its use has all but ceased. Lidocaine has also been used in human medicine to suppress the pain associated with intravenous injection of hyperosmolar solutions such as propofol.

MEPIVACAINE. Mepivacaine is an amide local anesthetic with potency and toxicity slightly above that of lidocaine. Although it is the only parenterally administered local anesthetic approved by the FDA (horses), it is not widely used in veterinary medicine. Its unique role has been its use in equine limb blocks where mepivacaine's apparent ability to diffuse though tissue surrounding its injection site creates less postinjection edema (Bishop 1996).

BUPIVACAINE. Bupivacaine is the most potent long-acting amide local anesthetic and is a member of the pipecoloxylidide (PPX) group. It was derived from mepivacaine by substitution of the methyl group by butyl. Along with its potency comes a long duration of action. With lidocaine it is one of the most popular local anesthetics in veterinary medicine. It is available in a racemic 50/50 mixture of S- and D-enantiomers. Toxicity is much lower in S-preparation so a mono-isomeric formulation of the S-enantiomer by itself has been released as levobupivacaine. It has a slow onset (large nerves can take up to 20–30 minutes for complete blockade), but it also is the longest lasting of the major available local anesthetics with sensory blocks lasting 5–8 hours. Both of these times depend on concentration and dose administered. The kinetics of these enantiomers are compared in Table 14.4A. Bupivacaine has a greater CVS toxicity. Free drug concentration rises rapidly once binding sites are filled, and the onset of CVS signs of toxicity often mask or overshadow the CNS signs. The greater risks involved with the CVS toxicity makes treatment of CNS toxicity with diazepam problematic as bupivacaine and diazepam may compete for binding sites. Such competition would liberate more bupivacaine and increase free plasma concentrations of the drug (Moore et al. 1979). Limiting the amount of local anesthetics injected systemically can prevent signs of frank intoxification. Suggested maximum doses for dogs are 6–10 mg/kg for lidocaine, 5–6 mg/kg for mepivacaine, 2–3 mg/kg for bupivacaine and 3 mg/kg for ropivacaine (Skarda 1996; Grimm 2002; Lamont 2002; Tranquilli et al. 2004). Doses one-half to three-quarters of these are recommended for cats. Higher doses are tolerated when using formulations containing a vasoconstrictor.

Bupivacaine's application include infiltration, nerve blocks, intrapleural administration and spinal and intrathecal techniques. Because of the risk of toxicity, its use in intravenous regional anesthesia is considered contraindicated. It does not work topically on skin or mucous membranes

ROPIVACAINE. Ropivacaine is a pure S(-)-enantiomer of propivacaine. It is a long-acting amide local anesthetic that has efficacy and potency nearly as high as bupivacaine and levobupivacaine but has lower CNS and CVS toxicity. If there are any differences between bupivacaine and ropivacaine it is the slightly shorter period of activity in spinal and epidural applications and a lowered ability to penetrate large motor nerves. It is the reduced lipophilicity that contributed to the lowered penetration of the motor nerves, combined with its stereoselective properties that allows ropivacaine to have significantly reduced CVS toxicity compared to bupivacaine (Simpson et al. 2005). Ropivacaine has a diphasic effect on peripheral vasculature—it is vasoconstrictive when injected at a concentration below 0.5 w/v% and there is dilation at concentrations over 1 w/v% (Cederholm et al. 1992).

TOPICAL USE: SKIN AND MUCOUS MEMBRANES

BENZOCAINE. Benzocaine is a unique local anesthetic as it has the lowest pK_a. It is unionized and has very low solubility. Benzocaine's use is limited to applications where topical absorption is needed. For this reason it is a common ingredient of throat lozenges. Benzocaine has an important role in handling fish because it is unionized and thus readily absorbed by the fish's gills to produce general anesthesia. The anesthesia can progress to death and benzocaine is also used for euthanasia in fishes.

Benzocaine used to be a laryngeal spray for intubation in cats, but not only is its metabolite benzoic acid poorly handled by cats, the spray was reported to cause methemoglobin. It has been withdrawn.

Benzocaine is metabolized by ester hydrolysis at about the same speed as procaine producing PABA.

EMLA®. When lidocaine and prilocaine, in their base forms, are mixed at 2.5 w/w% each, they form a eutectic mixture. This is a mixture where the melting point of the mixture is lower than the melting points of the individual components. In this case the mixture's melting point is 16°C allowing the two local anesthetics to be formulated in high concentration. This preparation's trade name is EMLA®, (eutectic mixture of local anesthetics).

This preparation is available as both a cream and a disk and is used to produce dermal analgesia after topical application to intact skin. The site where the cream is applied has to be covered with an occlusive dressing for maximum absorption into the skin. Both the disk and the cream take up to 20–30 minutes for full effect. EMLA has been used successfully for human neonates and children to facilitate per cutaneous vascular catheterization. EMLA has found sporadic use in veterinary medicine (Erkert and MacAllister 2005), but those uses may be challenged with the advent of lidocaine patches.

COCAINE. Cocaine was the original local anesthetic and has continued as the drug of choice for topical anesthesia of the nasal passage because of the quality and duration of the analgesia plus its innate vasoconstrictor properties. Cocaine has been placed in Schedule II by the DEA (high abuse potential and limited medical use) but is not considered a valid therapeutic option in veterinary practice today. In human medicine, cocaine has been discarded for topical ophthalmic use, and now it is being replaced by the compounded mixture of tetracaine and oxymetazoline (Noorily et al. 1995).

TOPICAL USE: OPTHAMOLOGY

There are only two local anesthetic approved for topical use on the cornea—proparacaine and tetracaine. These are formulated to minimize corneal irritation and often contain no preservatives. For that reason they have to be administered as true drops because contact with the eye or another surface may lead to contamination of the preparations. It is also important to note that their use is to provide topical anesthesia of the cornea and conjunctiva for diagnostic and therapeutic manipulations. They neither prevent blinking nor are intended to provide continuing pain relief for injured or infected corneas as such use exposes the drugs' cytotoxic potential.

PROPARACAINE. Proparacaine is marketed as a 0.5 w/v% sterile solution that is pH adjusted to minimize corneal irritation. Proparacaine has a faster onset and shorter duration than tetracaine. The duration of action varies between species (15 minutes for cats and 45 minutes for dogs) (Bruelle et al. 1996).

TETRACAINE. Tetracaine (Amethocaine BP) is a derivative of procaine but is 100-fold more potent. Its uses today are for spinal anesthesia and topical anesthesia of the cornea. In ophthalmology its potency allows very small amounts to be effective and it lasts longer than proparacaine. It is rapidly metabolized by deesterification but it is not as chemically stable as the amide local anesthetics.

USING LOCAL ANESTHETICS

The modes of use of local anesthetics include the following:

Topical anesthesia. The local anesthetic penetrates through open wounds, skin, or mucous membranes. Penetration of mucous membranes is widely shared by local anesthetics and can result in significant system absorption—especially of the respiratory tract. Penetration of intact skin is much harder. EMLA is a reliable agent for producing dermal analgesia to a maximum depth of about 5 mm.

Infiltration anesthesia. These techniques involve injection of local anesthesia directly into tissue independent of the course of nerves in the area. The method does involve the use of more local anesthetic, with resultant increased risk of toxicity. This risk can be dramatically reduced by mixing vasoconstrictors such as epinephrine with the local anesthetic. This vasoconstriction also increases the duration of action.

Field-block anesthesia. The local anesthetic is injected across the direction of sensory nerve supply so that areas distal to the injection line have sensation blocked. It requires knowledge of the innervation to the region. Examples of this would be infiltrating the bovine foot with a ring block and the inverted L for flank blocks. The use of vasoconstrictors in this type of technique is limited to where there is collateral blood supply to the region distal to the vasoconstriction.

Nerve-block anesthesia. The local anesthetic is injected in immediate proximity to a nerve and prevents passage of action potentials. This is used to block specific nerves or plexus. Toxicity is limited because the drug is specifically placed and limited quantities are used.

IVRA (Bier Block). The distal limb is isolated by a tourniquet and then the local anesthetic is injected intravenously distal to the tourniquet. Two problems are associated with this method. Toxicity occurs when the tourniquet leaks or is released early before the local anesthetic has time to bind to tissue and be gradually released into the systemic circulation. Additionally, prolonged use of the tourniquet produces ischemia with resulting tissue damage. There can be pain associated with the ischemia at quite early stages of the tourniquet's use. The agents most commonly used for IVRA are lidocaine and mepivacaine. There is some evidence that the block produced by mepivacaine is superior (Prieto-Alvarez et al. 2002). Clonidine has also been added to 0.5% lidocaine at 1 mcg/kg with an improvement in postrelease analgesia with minimal side effects (Reuben et al. 1999).

Spinal and epidural anesthesia. With spinal or subarachnoid anesthesia, a local anesthetic is injected into the lumbar dural space immediately surrounding the spinal cord where it mixes with the cerebrospinal fluid (CSF). Besides producing the block of sensory innervation, the most notable physiological effect is the sympathetic blockade produced in the spinal nerve roots. The degree of spinal anesthesia produced relates to the volume of the injectate and its concentration and how far it diffuses along the spinal cord. The sympathetic block is usually one or two segments further rostral since the preganglionic sympathetic fibers are more sensitive to low concentrations of local anesthetic. The movement of anesthetics along the neural axis is determined by volume of injection and by patient position. Drugs commonly used for this technique include bupivacaine, lidocaine, tetracaine, and ropivacaine.

In epidural local anesthetic the drug is injected into the space bounded by the ligamentum flavum dorsally and the dura covering the spinal cord. Although the technique involves a single injection, development of fine catheters has increased the number of clinicians maintaining analgesia for long periods by repeated administration or CRI. The primary site of action in epidural anesthesia is on the spinal nerve roots. A significant absorption of drug takes place in the epidural space compared with spinal administration, but in the former, local toxicity and trauma are always of concern.

FUTURE OUTLOOK

Besides the perpetual search for better and safer drugs, local anesthesia is finding a new niche, with physicians discharging their patients home earlier and earlier. These patients need long-acting analgesia under conditions of minimal monitoring, which local anesthetics with prolonged duration of action and limited toxicity seem prime candidates to provide.

Development of local anesthesia holds promise in a number of directions (White and Durieux 2005). First is reformulation to lengthen the duration; here, work is underway to incorporate the long-acting amides in liposomes and biodegradable polymer microcapsules (Pedersen et al. 2004). Then there is development of drugs that act on specific sodium channels without affecting the other channel subtypes and nonsodium ion channels that are not involved in impulse blockade. As mentioned at the start of this chapter, there are compounds that have been found serendipitously to provide reversible local anesthesia that is novel and unrelated chemically or functionally to the classic drugs discussed in this chapter. Studies of these compounds may lead to new and better mechanisms to provide local anesthesia. Caveats to the prolonged association of local anesthetic in tissues is that, with some prolonged in vitro studies, there have been observations of time related changes in neutrophil function.

REFERENCES

Arthur, G.R. 1987. Pharmacokinetics of local anesthetics. Local Anesthetics (ed. by G. R. Strichartz), pp. 165–186. Springer-Verlag, Berlin.

Aydin, N., Gultekin, B., Ozgun, S., Gurel, A. 2002. Bacterial contamination of propofol: the effects of temperature and lidocaine. Eur J Anaesthesiol, 19, 455–458.

Biehl, D., Shnider, S.M., Levinson, G., Callender, K. 1978. Placental transfer of lidocaine: effects of fetal acidosis. Anesthesiology, 48, 409–412.

Bishop, Y.M. 1996. The Veterinary Formulary, 3rd ed, p. 243.

Bruelle, P., LeFrant, J.Y., de La Coussaye, J.E., Peray, P.A., Desch, G., Sassine, A., Eledjam, J.J. 1996. Comparative electrophysiologic and hemodynamic effects of several amide local anesthetic drugs in anesthetized dogs. Anesth Analg, 82, 648–656.

Burm, A.G., Cohen, I.M., van Kleef, J.W., Vletter, A.A., Olieman, W., Groen, K. 1997. Pharmacokinetics of the enantiomers of mepivacaine after intravenous administration of the racemate in volunteers. Anesth Analg, 84, 85–89.

Burm, A.G., van der Meer, A.D., van Kleef, J.W., Zeijlmans, P.W., Groen, K. 1994. Pharmacokinetics of the enantiomers of bupivacaine following intravenous administration of the racemate. Br J Clin Pharmacol, 38, 125–129.

Carpenter, R.L. 1997. Local anesthetic toxicity: The case for Ropivacaine. Am J Anesthesiol, 24, 4.

Cederholm, I., Evers, H., Lofstrom, J.B. 1992. Skin blood flow after intradermal injection of ropivacaine in various concentrations with and without epinephrine evaluated by laser Doppler flowmetry. Reg Anesth, 17, 322–328.

Chandan, S.S., Faoagali, J., Wainwright, C.E. 2005. Sensitivity of respiratory bacteria to lignocaine. Pathology, 37, 305–307.

Covino, B.G. 1987. Toxicity and systemic effects of local anesthetic agents. Local Anesthetics (ed. by G. R. Strichartz), pp. 187–212. Springer-Verlag, Berlin.

Craigmill, A.L., Rangel-Lugo, M., Damian, P., Riviere, J.E. 1997. Extralabel use of tranquilizers and general anesthetics. J Am Vet Med Assoc, 211, 302–304.

Craigmill, A.L., Riviere, J.E., Webb, A.I. 2006. Tabulation of FARAD Comparative and Veterinary Pharmacokinetic Data, Blackwell Publishing, Ames, IA.

Davis, N.L., de Jong, R.H. 1982. Successful resuscitation following massive bupivacaine overdose. Anesth Analg, 61, 62–64.

Doherty, T.J., Frazier, D.L. 1998. Effect of intravenous lidocaine on halothane minimum alveolar concentration in ponies. Equine Vet J, 30, 300–303.

Erkert, R.S., MacAllister, C.G. 2005. Use of a eutectic mixture of lidocaine 2.5% and prilocaine 2.5% as a local anesthetic in animals. J Am Vet Med Assoc, 226, 1990–1992.

Finster, M., Morishima, H.O., Boyes, R.N., Covino, B.G. 1972. The placental transfer of lidocaine and its uptake by fetal tissues. Anesthesiology, 36, 159–163.

Grimm, K.A. 2002. Dental nerve blocks. Veterinary anesthesia and pain management secrets (ed. by S. A. Greene), pp. 311–314. Hanley Belfus, Philadelphia.

Groban, L., Deal, D.D., Vernon, J.C., James, R.L., Butterworth, J. 2001. Cardiac resuscitation after incremental overdosage with lidocaine, bupivacaine, levobupivacaine, and ropivacaine in anesthetized dogs. Anesth Analg, 92, 37–43.

Harkins, J.D., Stanley, S., Mundy, G.D., Sams, R.A., Woods, W.E., Tobin, T. 1995. A review of the pharmacology, pharmacokinetics, and regulatory control in the US of local anaesthetics in the horse. J Vet Pharmacol Ther, 18, 397–406.

Himes, R.S., Jr., DiFazio, C.A., Burney, R.G. 1977. Effects of lidocaine on the anesthetic requirements for nitrous oxide and halothane. Anesthesiology, 47, 437–440.

Johnson, R.F., Cahana, A., Olenick, M., Herman, N., Paschall, R.L., Minzter, B., Ramasubramanian, R., Gonzalez, H., Downing, J.W. 1999. A comparison of the placental transfer of ropivacaine versus bupivacaine. Anesth Analg, 89, 703–708.

Kalow, W., Genest, K. 1957. A method for the detection of atypical forms of human serum cholinesterase. Determination of dibucaine numbers. Can J Biochem Physiol, 35, 339–346.

Keenaghan, J.B., Boyes, R.N. 1972. The tissue distribution, metabolism and excretion of lidocaine in rats, guinea pigs, dogs and man. J Pharmacol Exp Ther, 180, 454–463.

Koller, C. 1928. Historical notes on the beginning of local anesthesia. J Am Vet Med Assoc, 90, 1742–1743.

Kuhnert, B.R., Zuspan, K.J., Kuhnert, P.M., Syracuse, C.D., Brown, D.E. 1987. Bupivacaine disposition in mother, fetus, and neonate after spinal anesthesia for cesarean section. Anesth Analg, 66, 407–412.

Lamont, L.A. 2002. Local anesthetics. Veterinary anesthesia and pain management secrets (ed. by S. A. Greene), pp. 105–108. Hanley Belfus, Philadelphia.

Leuschner, J., Leblanc, D. 1999. Studies on the toxicological profile of the local anaesthetic articaine. Arzneimittel-Forschung-Drug Research, 49, 126–132.

Liu, P., Feldman, H.S., Covino, B.M., Giasi, R., Covino, B.G. 1982. Acute cardiovascular toxicity of intravenous amide local anesthetics in anesthetized ventilated dogs. Anesth Analg, 61, 317–322.

Liu, P.L., Feldman, H.S., Giasi, R., Patterson, M.K., Covino, B.G. 1983. Comparative CNS toxicity of lidocaine, etidocaine, bupivacaine, and tetracaine in awake dogs following rapid intravenous administration. Anesth Analg, 62, 375–379.

Malone, E., Ensink, J., Turner, T., Wilson, J., Andrews, F., Keegan, K., Lumsden, J. 2006. Intravenous Continuous Infusion of Lidocaine for Treatment of Equine Ileus. Vet Surg, 35, 60–66.

Mao J., Chen L.L. 2000. Systemic lidocaine for neuropathic pain relief. Pain, 87, 17.

McIntyre, J.W. 1999. Regional anesthesia safety. Complications of regional anesthesia (ed. by B. T. Finucane), pp. 1–30. Churchill Livingstone, Edinburgh.

Moore, D.C., Balfour, R.I., Fitzgibbons, D. 1979. Convulsive arterial plasma levels of bupivacaine and the response to diazepam therapy. Anesthesiology, 50, 454–456.

Muir, W.W., III, Wiese, A.J., March, P.A. 2003. Effects of morphine, lidocaine, ketamine, and morphine-lidocaine-ketamine drug combination on minimum alveolar concentration in dogs anesthetized with isoflurane. Am J Vet Res, 64, 1155–1160.

Noorily, A.D., Noorily, S.H., Otto, R.A. 1995. Cocaine, lidocaine, tetracaine: which is best for topical nasal anesthesia? Anesth Analg, 81, 724–727.

Ogata, N., Ohishi, Y. 2002. Molecular diversity of structure and function of the voltage-gated Na+ channels. Jpn J Pharmacol, 88, 365–377.

Olsen, K.M., Peddicord, T.E., Campbell, G.D., Rupp, M.E. 2000. Antimicrobial effects of lidocaine in bronchoalveolar lavage fluid. J Antimicrob Chemother, 45, 217–219.

Parr, A.M., Zoutman, D.E., Davidson, J.S.D. 1999. Antimicrobial activity of lidocaine against bacteria associated with nosocomial wound infection. Ann Plast Surg, 43, 239–245.

Pedersen, J.L., Lilleso, J., Hammer, N.A., Werner, M.U., Holte, K., Lacouture, P.G., Kehlet, H. 2004. Bupivacaine in microcapsules prolongs analgesia after subcutaneous infiltration in humans: a dose-finding study. Anesth Analg, 99, 912–8, table.

Pere, P., Salonen, M., Jokinen, M., Rosenberg, P.H., Neuvonen, P.J., Haasio, J. 2003. Pharmacokinetics of ropivacaine in uremic and nonuremic patients after axillary brachial plexus block. Anesth Analg, 96, 563–9, table.

Phoenix Scientific, I. Freedom of Information Summary: NADA 141–245, Tributame Euthanasia Solution. 1–23. 2005. Ref Type: Report

Picard, J., Meek, T. 2006. Lipid emulsion to treat overdose of local anaesthetic: the gift of the glob. Anaesthesia, 61, 109.

Prieto-Alvarez, P., Calas-Guerra, A., Fuentes-Bellido, J., Martinez-Verdera, E., et-Catala, A., Lorenzo-Foz, J.P. 2002. Comparison of mepivacaine and lidocaine for intravenous regional anaesthesia: pharmacokinetic study and clinical correlation. Br J Anaesth, 88, 516–519.

Pypendop, B.H., Ilkiw, J.E. 2005. The effects of intravenous lidocaine administration on the minimum alveolar concentration of isoflurane in cats. Anesth Analg, 100, 97–101.

Reidenberg, M.M. 1972. The procaine esterase activity of serum from different mammalian species. Proc Soc Exp Biol Med, 140, 1059–1061.

Reuben, S.S., Steinberg, R.B., Klatt, J.L., Klatt, M.L. 1999. Intravenous regional anesthesia using lidocaine and clonidine. Anesthesiology, 91, 654–658.

Rex, M.A.E. 1971. Laryngospasm and respiratory changes in the cat produced by mechanical stimulation of the pharynx and respiratory tract: Problems of intubation in the cat. Br J Anaesth, 43, 54–57.

Rimback, G., Cassuto, J., Tollesson, P.O. 1990. Treatment of postoperative paralytic ileus by intravenous lidocaine infusion. Anesth Analg, 70, 414–419.

Rosenberg, P.H., Kytta, J., Alila, A. 1986. Absorption of bupivacaine, etidocaine, lignocaine and ropivacaine into n-heptane, rat sciatic nerve, and human extradural and subcutaneous fat. Br J Anaesth, 58, 310–314.

Sakuragi, T., Ishino, H., Dan, K. 1996. Bactericidal activity of clinically used local anesthetics on *Staphylococcus aureus*. Reg Anesth, 21, 239–242.

———. 1997. Bactericidal activity of 0.5% bupivacaine with preservatives on microorganisms in the human skin flora. Reg Anesth, 22, 178–184.

Simpson, D., Curran, M.P., Oldfield, V., Keating, G.M. 2005. Ropivacaine: a review of its use in regional anaesthesia and acute pain management. Drugs, 65, 2675–2717.

Sinnott, C.J., Garfield, J.M., Thalhammer, J.G., Strichartz, G.R. 2000. Addition of sodium bicarbonate to lidocaine decreases the duration of peripheral nerve block in the rat. Anesthesiology, 93, 1045–1052.

Skarda, R.T. 1996. Local and regional anesthetic and analgesic techniques: dogs. Lumb and Jones' Veterinary Anesthesia (ed. by J. C. Thurmon W. J. B. J. G. Tranquilli), pp. 426–447. Lippincott, Williams & Wilkins, Baltimore.

Specialized Information Services. ChemIDplus Lite. 2006. Bethesda, National Library of Medicine. Ref Type: Data File.

Stratford, A.F., Zoutman, D.E., Davidson, J.S.D. 2002. Effect of lidocaine and epinephrine on *Staphylococcus aureus* in a guinea pig model of surgical wound infection. Plast Reconstr Surg, 110, 1275–1279.

Strichartz, G.R., Sanchez, V., Arthur, G.R., Chafetz, R., Martin, D. 1990. Fundamental properties of local anesthetics. II. Measured octanol: buffer partition coefficients and pK_a values of clinically used drugs. Anesth Analg, 71, 158–170.

Sundlof, S.F., Duer, W.C., Hill, D.W., Gancarz.T, Dorvil, M.G., Rosen, P. 1983. Procaine in the urine of racing greyhounds: possible sources. Am J Vet Res, 44, 1583–1587.

Tecles, F., Ceron, J.J. 2001. Determination of whole blood cholinesterase in different animal species using specific substrates. Res Vet Sci, 70, 233–238.

Thomas, J., Long, G., Moore, G., Morgan, D. 1976. Plasma protein binding and placental transfer of bupivacaine. Clin Pharmacol Ther, 19, 426–434.

Tranquilli, W.J., Grimm, K.A., Lamont, L.A. 2004. Pain management for the small animal practitioner, 2nd ed, pp. 17–19. Teton NewMedia, Jackson.

USP Expert Committee. 2006. 2006 USP dictionary of USAN and international drug names, 42 ed, United States Pharmacopeia, Rockville.

Viscomi, C.M. 2004. Pharmacology of local anesthetics. Regional Anesthesia: The requisites in anesthesiology (ed. by J. P. Rathmell, J. M. Neal, C. M. Viscomi), pp. 13–31. Elsevier Mosby, Philadelphia.

Weinberg, G., Ripper, R., Feinstein, D.L., Hoffman, W. 2003. Lipid emulsion infusion rescues dogs from bupivacaine-induced cardiac toxicity. Reg Anesth Pain Med, 28, 198–202.

Weinberg, G.L., Ripper, R., Murphy, P., Edelman, L.B., Hoffman, W., Strichartz, G., Feinstein, D.L. 2006. Lipid Infusion Accelerates Removal of Bupivacaine and Recovery From Bupivacaine Toxicity in the Isolated Rat Heart. Reg Anesth Pain Med, 312, 296–303.

Weinberg, G.L., VadeBoncouer, T., Ramaraju, G.A., Garcia-Amaro, M.F., Cwik, M.J. 1998. Pretreatment or resuscitation with a lipid infusion shifts the dose-response to bupivacaine-induced asystole in rats. Anesthesiology, 88, 1071–1075.

White, J.L., Durieux, M.E. 2005. Clinical pharmacology of local anesthetics. Anesthesiol Clin North America, 23, 73–84.

Wilcke, J.K., Davis, L.E., Neff-Davis, C.A. 1983. Determination of lidocaine concentrations producing therapeutic and toxic effects in dogs. J Vet Pharm Therap, 6, 105–112.

Zink, W., Graf, B.M. 2004. Local anesthetic myotoxicity. Reg Anesth Pain Med, 29, 333–340.

CHAPTER 15

EUTHANIZING AGENTS

ALISTAIR I. WEBB

Euthanasia is derived from the Greek ευ (*eu* meaning "good") and θανατοξ (*thanatos*) meaning "death"—combined they imply "good death." In the context of animals cared for by man, euthanasia indicates killing an animal in such a manner that there is minimal pain or suffering involved in the procedure. The charge for this chapter is to explore the role chemicals and drugs can play in meeting the letter and the spirit of the term euthanasia.

Universally accepted requirements for chemically mediated euthanasia include UK recommendations (Close et al. 1996; American Veterinary Medical Association 2001; AHAW Panel 2005; Artwohl et al. 2006):

- The method must produce death with both reliability and consistency.
- Prior to death, animals must be rendered unconscious rapidly and with no element of asphyxia.
- The method should require minimal restraint.
- The delivery method of the lethal chemicals must minimize any pain or stress.
- The delivery method and chemicals used must not expose personnel to unnecessary risk.

There are not many agents that fit these criteria, but those that do are inhaled, swallowed, or injected, or they are immersed.

In considering pharmacological methods of euthanasia the animal's resilience, its size, and the variable degree of experience of the persons performing euthanasia can cause marked uncertainty of efficacy. For this reason, when using a pharmacological method, there are usually legal requirements for either a physical disruption to be performed or visual confirmation of cardiac standstill employed (National Institutes of Health 2002).

INHALED AGENTS

The inhalation route utilizes gases or vapors that either 1) displace oxygen and cause death by hypoxia or 2) induce anesthesia per se and produce death by deliberate overdosage or by permitting the use of other methods to produce death. Carbon dioxide is an example of an agent that can produce both—anesthesia and fatal hypoxia. The use of gases has considerable logistical advantages of allowing multiple animals to be killed simultaneously with minimal restraint. An additional advantage is that often the small laboratory animals can be rendered unconscious in their home cage or box with no handling required at all. These are significant advantages, but there is growing concern regarding how aversive the various gases and administration techniques are (Ewbank 1983; Close et al. 1996, 1997; Hawkins et al. 2006).

CARBON DIOXIDE. Carbon dioxide (CO_2) is a heavier-than-air gas that is available in compressed gas form. Dry ice is the frozen, solid form of CO_2 and was used as a generator of CO_2 gas. However, concerns about the low temperatures engendered and lack of control over gas concentrations has curtailed its use. Today use of solid CO_2 requires use of specialized electrical heaters to ensure the vapors produced are warmed. Compressed gas cylinders require a pressure regulator and a flow meter to control the gas flow. In the cylinder a pressure greater than 31 atmospheres liquefies the CO_2, so the regulator gauge pressure does not indicate how much CO_2 is left in a cylinder and weight loss is the only reliable guide. CO_2 is heavier than air so it settles to the bottom of containers and allows the concentration to gradually build up as the level of the gas rises. This can be a problem where animals are tall and able to breathe at the top of the container where the CO_2 concentration is lowest.

CO_2 has been used successfully in a number of species ranging from small laboratory animals to farm animals (pigs). The advantage of using CO_2 in the larger food-producing animals is that there are no drug residues of concern in animals destined for human consumption. The anesthesia and sedation caused by CO_2 is concentration dependent—5–8% producing sedation, 10–12% stupor, and 25–30% complete anesthesia (Danneman et al. 1997b). Higher concentrations of CO_2 result in death from overwhelming central nervous system (CNS) depression or hypoxia from the displacement of oxygen during alveolar gas exchange. The latter can be illustrated when a concentration of 75% CO_2 in air is used and results in the dilution of oxygen to a concentration of only 5%.

Considerable work has been carried out on the aversiveness of carbon dioxide (CO_2). In humans this has been well established, but studies in animals have been slow to yield definitive answers. Aversive behavior such as preferring to avoid food rather than be exposed to the CO_2 has been demonstrated in several species of farm animals (chickens, turkeys, mink, and pigs) (Raj 1999). Recent evaluations of its use in laboratory animals have raised concerns about nasal and ocular irritation occurring on immediate contact with high concentrations (above 50%). This is largely derived from single-breath human studies (Danneman et al. 1997a) although follow-up studies have demonstrated aversive reactions in rodents. The irritation of mucus membranes probably derives from dissolution of the CO_2 in moist membranes lowering the pH and forming carbonic acid. Despite that, CO_2 remains the most common method of euthanasia in laboratory rodents.

Given the above, there is controversy about the methods of initiating the administration of CO_2 for euthanasia because the objective of producing unconsciousness and subsequent death as quickly as possible uses high CO_2 concentrations which are the most aversive. The high initial concentration technique involves priming equipment with 100% CO_2 even though some studies have shown that these concentrations produce acute discomfort to the animals. Euthanasia methodology researchers consider that even brief periods of pain and stress are unacceptable. Instead these workers propose starting at concentrations of about 2–5% with gradual increases (20% of chamber volume per minute flow rate) (Hawkins et al. 2006) in concentration as sedation overtakes the animal. This gradual increase in CO_2 concentration produces "air hunger" or dyspnea at about 15% CO_2, even when the oxygen concentration is increased. As the CO_2 concentration rises further, the animals become unconscious but death takes 5–6 minutes. Other workers have suggested administering oxygen with the CO_2 so as to minimize the feeling of asphyxia in the initial period. The effect of this maneuver has not been universally accepted as being effective.

When introduced to CO_2, many types of rodents show a sniffing type of action that has been interpreted as curiosity and testing the environment. More recently, workers have proposed that this activity is triggered by chemical stimulation of branches of the glossopharyngeal nerve (Benacka and Tomori 1995).

Thus it can be seen that there seems no ideal way of introducing animals to the CO_2 (American Veterinary Medical Association 2001; AHAW Panel 2005; Artwohl et al. 2006; Hawkins et al. 2006). A lot of the information for the high concentration of adverse effects was based on human experience and workers projecting those experiences onto the animals. However, the Newcastle group (Hawkins et al. 2006) reviewed data on rats submitted to both acute and gradual introduction to lethal concentrations of CO_2 and considered data (ECG and EEG telemetry) that supported both scenarios (prefilling the CO_2 chambers and a 20%/minute chamber filling). The group did not reach consensus on which method was to be preferred.

A major concern with the use of CO_2 is the lack of certainty of animal death. This is especially true with small animals such as rodents and rabbits. There have been reports of animals that are deeply cyanotic, have no palpable pulse and no corneal reflexes, and are considered dead. Yet, some of these animals, after removal from the CO_2 chamber, prove to be alive and capable of self-resuscitation. This risk is considered sufficiently significant that the U.S. National Institutes of Health Office of Laboratory Welfare (OLAW) has mandated that persons euthanizing small animals with CO_2 use a secondary physical method. This is to obtain certainty that death is nonreversible (National Institutes of Health 2002).

Birds, reptiles, burrowing animals, and neonates present a challenge in using CO_2 for euthanasia because of their relative insensitivity to hypoxia. 100% CO_2 is recommended for birds under 72 hours of age (Raj and Gregory 1990). The same concentration has been recommended for non–slaughterhouse killing of large numbers of birds, as might be needed in cases of disease outbreak or end-of-lay house clearing (Anonymous 2007). That recommendation incorporated requirements for a priori official authorization and inspection. The end-of-lay scenario is important as the birds may be in such low calcium status by then that handling and transportation will expose the birds to appreciable risk of bone fractures.

Today, CO_2 is no longer recommended for cats and larger species (Klemm 1964) and, in pigs where later consumption of the body is a concern, it is being replaced by argon.

In summary the advantages of CO_2 as a method for euthanasia are its availability, its relative safety to the operator (in UK handlers must wear dosimeters), the number of species for which it can be used, the ability to perform euthanasia in small laboratory animals in their own cage avoiding any transshipping stress, and its lack of a residue in edible tissues of euthanized animals. Its disadvantages are its slowness when using lower concentrations, uncertainty of death, and concerns about adverse effects on the animals prior to loss of consciousness.

CARBON MONOXIDE. Carbon monoxide (CO) produces hypoxia by displacing oxygen from hemoglobin with such avidity that it takes high partial pressures of oxygen to competitively reverse the association. In humans the initial signs of CO poisoning are headaches and nausea. As the concentration increases unconsciousness intervenes and clonic convulsions take place because of CO's stimulation of the CNS motor centers. Death occurs at concentrations above 4%; concentrations above 2% cause unconsciousness within minutes. CO is produced on site by a combustion engine, but the 100% CO gas produced needs cooling and filtering because otherwise it will cause gross aversive activity. Operators of this type of equipment are advised not to place animals in the chambers before a 1% concentration is present and to keep the animals in the chamber until killed by the CO or a secondary method.

ARGON. Argon may be a future competitor to CO_2 as it is also heavier than air and has anesthetic properties at high concentrations and animals seem to show less aversion to it. It is, however, much more expensive than the other available hypoxia-producing gases. Although it is slower to kill than CO_2, argon has found some use in pigs and other large animals because of the no residue factor.

NITROGEN. With concentrations above 90% nitrogen (N_2) produces hypoxia resulting in sedation and disorientation before finally producing unconsciousness and death. However, because it is lighter than air, N_2 requires special airtight chambers for use in euthanasia. Nitrous oxide (N_2O) could be used as a hypoxic agent but is too weak to be used for anesthetic properties in animals. N_2O has not been used even for producing hypoxia because of expense and the fact that it is actually better at supporting combustion than air.

CO is rarely used today because of improper administration techniques and the appearance of convulsions during the period of unconsciousness. The humane aspects of argon and nitrogen have not been investigated enough for any conclusions about the humaneness of their use, although initial information seems promising for argon in pigs and birds (AHAW Panel 2005).

INHALANT ANESTHETIC OVERDOSE. The major concerns about the inhalant agents are 1) the question of what degree of discomfort they produce before unconsciousness intervenes and 2) effects that workplace and atmospheric pollution have on the health of human operators (Arnold and Nicholau 2005). The aversion animals have with inhalant anesthetics can range from dislike for the odors and breath holding with low concentrations to struggling with sudden introduction to high concentrations.

The anesthetics in use today are halothane, isoflurane, and sevoflurane. These three fluorinated hydrocarbons, which are nonflammable, can be administered easily with a saturated pledget of cotton wool in a container or with a temperature and flow compensated calibrated vaporizer.

Many workers have used inhalation anesthesia to induce unconsciousness because the inhalants can be administered in home cages or with minimal restraint. Then, with the animals unconscious, they can use other methods to kill the animal.

The major differences between the inhalant agents are the speed at which they can induce anesthesia and the concentrations needed to produce unconsciousness.

Speed of Induction (solubility in blood): sevoflurane > isoflurane > halothane

Concentration Needed (potency): halothane ≥ isoflurane > sevoflurane

Cost (drug per se plus amount needed): sevoflurane > isoflurane ≥ halothane

The reader is referred to the chapter on inhalant anesthetics for actual values for these anesthetics. Halothane or sevoflurane seem the most preferred because isoflurane and desflurane have pungent odors.

INJECTED AGENTS

The major disadvantage of using injectable drugs for euthanasia is that individual animals have to be handled and that this can be stressful to the operator. Against that is the speed of the drug delivery and, when administered intravenously (IV), death is very rapid. Again like the inhalation methods there can be failure to produce death when the dose is not sufficient or the injection technique is poor. For that reason most regulators require a secondary physical method of ensuring that the animal is dead for injectable as well as inhaled agents. Another disadvantage with the most popular drug group, the barbiturates, is that they are controlled substances and require special registration, storage, and record keeping. Pentobarbital and the potent mu-agonist opioids incur the most stringent requirements as they are classed as Schedule 2 or C-II under most national drug laws (Drug Enforcement Administration, DEA) in the U.S.A.

BARBITURATE. The short-acting and ultrashort-acting barbiturates are considered by many to be the ideal agents for euthanasia. The only ultrashort-acting barbiturate that is universally available is thiopental. Thiopental crosses the blood brain barrier very rapidly, and a dose of 15–20 mg/kg will produce anesthesia within 15–30 seconds without excitement. A dose of at least three times that given rapidly is needed to produce anesthesia and death. If given too slowly, the thiopental is redistributed away from the brain and death may not occur. It is principally used for induction of anesthesia as a prelude to actual euthanasia. Thiopental, available as a dry powder that is made up freshly for use in induction of anesthesia, has to be dissolved and administered by IV route to be effective. This limit on the route of administration allows a lesser DEA scheduling (C-III). Typically thiopental is constituted as a 2–5% w/v solution; a 10% solution is used in anesthesia of large farm animals, but it starts precipitating within 24 hours. The limited solubility necessitates high volumes for euthanasia and that limits thiopental's utility as a euthanasia method to small mammals or just to anesthetize larger animals before administering other agents to achieve death.

PENTOBARBITAL. Pentobarbital is the most commonly used parenteral euthanasia agent. It is a short-acting barbiturate that takes up to 2 or 3 minutes to have its peak effect. Its status as a C-II controlled substance makes its availability somewhat limited. Some manufacturers add other drugs to the euthanasia formulation to lower its abuse potential and obtain a less stringent scheduling (C-III, which does not require use of special ordering procedures and makes storage a lot more flexible). The drugs used for this include phenytoin, tetracaine, and dibucaine. Evans and colleagues (1993) compared the character of euthanasia in cats using pentobarbital with and without lidocaine. They found the only difference was a shorter time for appearance of an isoelectric (flat waves) EEC. In Europe the closely related barbiturate, secobarbital (quinalbarbital), is used in euthanasia solutions. Secobarbital is not commercially available in the U.S.

Pentobarbital can be administered IV or intraperitoneally (IP). When given IV (anesthetic dose 10–25 mg/kg) it must be administered quickly or the animal may become stimulated and excited. When that happens, the animal struggles against restraint and may void and eliminate spontaneously. This problem can be compounded if venous access is lost. The risk of this happening when the drug is given IP is similar and the animal is subjected to stress and stimulation before anesthesia has occurred. Pentobarbital is conventionally formulated as an anesthetic (45–65 mg/ml) but the euthanasia formulations are of much higher concentration (≥325 mg/ml) and contain a blue or pink dye to clearly define the preparation as nontherapeutic. The high-concentration preparations are very viscous and require minimally a 22 gauge needle for injection.

The minimal dosage of pentobarbital needed for euthanasia is 100 mg/kg, which is over three times the anesthetic dose. Major advantages of pentobarbital compared with other injectable agents are its versatility in route of administration and the fact that it does not sting when injected. Its disadvantages are its controlled drug status and, as with all of the injectables where death occurs quickly, the agonal or gasping-like breathing that can take place. This agonal breathing does not indicate any sort of pain or suffering because it occurs after the animals are deeply anesthetized and there is no cardiac output or heart beat. Rather, it appears to be rooted in some primitive reflex generated by the dying brain (American Veterinary Medical Association 2001).

Pentobarbital can be administered IV or IP. Intrathoracic and intracardiac injections are too difficult and painful in conscious animals and those routes are only used when an animal is already unconscious. The IP route is impractical in larger animals with real risk of ataxia and excitement. When administering pentobarbital IP to small animals, they should be left unhandled in a quiet place until the animal has lost consciousness. Pentobarbital takes 45–90 seconds to cross into the brain after IV injection and 5–15 minutes to have an effect after IP injection. IP injection does not appear to upset rodents, rabbits, cats, and puppies when it is performed with minimal restraint and the injection is done quickly with a needle of at least 20 gauge with a long sharp bevel. Workers (Grier and Schaffer 1990; Grier 1991) have advocated that, in cats, the IP injection be angled cranially to deliver the drug directly into the liver with almost instantaneous loss of consciousness. Seif disagreed (Seif 1991), citing risk of the drug going intrathoracic.

Clients in clinical practice often want to be present during euthanasia of their animal and can become distressed at any movement or vocalization during and immediately after euthanasia. The chances of this can be lessened by prior sedation of the animal although there should not be a reduction in the pentobarbital dose. Use of muscle relaxants after the pentobarbital has been injected has been advocated in the past but is strongly discouraged because there is the very real risk of masking failure of the pentobarbital injection, which would leave an animal conscious and not able to move or even breathe.

The carcasses of animals euthanized with CNS depressants, such as barbiturates, must be buried or incinerated as the drugs will not have had any opportunity to clear from the body and other animals consuming the flesh of such animals as pet food or carrion will themselves be intoxicated (Hall et al. 1972; Polley and Weaver 1977; Fucci 1986). Disposal of large farm animal carcasses will be dictated by local, state, and federal law, and those involved with the euthanasia need to be familiar with these.

Euthanizing conscious large farm animals exposes both the animal and personnel to potential injury. It is recommended that these animals first be anesthetized as in a clinical situation (Thurman 1991) and then killed by injection of a lethal dose of more barbiturate or potassium chloride (KCl).

EMBUTRAMIDE. Embutramide is a derivative of gamma-hydroxybutyrate that produces general anesthesia when injected IV. It has a narrow margin of safety (Phoenix Scientific 2005) and has not been used clinically as an anesthetic agent. Instead it is the principal component of a commercial euthanasia formulation, Tributame™. This formulation is water and alcohol based with embutramide (135 mg/ml), chloroquine (45 mg/ml), and lidocaine (1.9 mg/ml). The chloroquine is used as an antimalarial drug in humans with some degree of myocardial depression. In humans the dose is 5 mg/kg per os once a week, while the euthanasia formulation dosage is 20 mg/kg by bolus IV injection. The lidocaine is cited by the manufacturer (Anonymous 2001) to produce both CVS and CNS depression. This seems to be an exaggeration because the lidocaine dosage would be 0.8 mg/kg, which is on the low side of the dosage traditionally used in treatment of ventricular dysrhythmias. However, the combination of the chloroquine and lidocaine lower the dosage of embutramide needed for euthanasia and facilitate the commercial preparation to have a lesser controlled drug scheduling in the U.S. (C-III). Embutramide dissolved in alcohol by itself caused death when the dose exceeded 61 mg/kg IV but also caused pain at the injection site. It seems this problem has been resolved in the Tributame™ formulation. Tributame™ produces unconsciousness in less than 30 seconds with death taking up to 2 minutes although 60–70% have some agonal breathing.

Embutramide had problems in a past formulation (T61) where it was combined with mebenzonium, tetracaine, and an organic solvent (DMF) (Hellebrekers et al. 1990; Giorgi and Bertini 2000). The mebenzonium was a nondepolarizing muscle relaxant, which caused paralysis and asphyxia before the embutramide produced unconsciousness. T61 was withdrawn from the market because of these concerns but now, with a new formulation devoid of the potential for paralysis, embutramide has won a reprieve. Embutramide in the old T61 formulation was supposed to produce less agonal gasping compared to pentobarbital during the euthanasia procedure. This has not been claimed for Tributame™, which most likely reflects the removal of the muscle relaxant component.

Tributame™ has only been approved for use in dogs with the instruction to administer the product IV at the rate of 1 ml per 5 lb (0.45 mg/kg) within 10–15 seconds.

OTHER INJECTABLE ANESTHETICS AND SEDATIVES

Propofol, etomidate, and other drugs that produce general anesthesia when injected IV can be administered in doses 3–4 times as much to produce death. When injected rapidly, propofol has its greatest lethal potential but it still requires a large volume to be injected. Attempts to make high concentration preparations without the viscosity seen in the pentobarbital euthanasia formulations have been unsuccessful (unpublished observations). Although the costs of these agents have fallen, they are still not generally used for euthanasia. Two other drugs that had been considered for euthanasia were chloral hydrate and ketamine. Although they may be used in sedation in preparation for euthanasia, their use as sole agent for euthanasia is not accepted. Neither drug produces true anesthesia nor does increasing their dosages produce death reliably. Ketamine actually causes seizures as the dosage increases. Both drugs are controlled substances (ketamine C-III and chloral hydrate C-IV).

OPIOIDS AND ALPHA-2 SYMPATHOMIMETICS. A potent mu agonist would generally be considered as part of a preeuthanasia sedative cocktail, but carfentanil and etorphine are potent enough to be administered intramuscularly (IM) and produce anesthesia and potentially death in high doses. They are especially useful in zoological species where IV administrations are impractical. The etorphine and carfentanil require special licensing for their use and a high level of training in correct use to avoid operator tragedy.

Alpha-2 sympathomimetics (xylazine, detomidine, medetomidine and romifidine) have very marked species differences in potencies but could be considered for basal narcosis according to species and drug. Xylazine and medetomidine are very potent in dogs and cats while xylazine is even more potent in the ruminants. Given in high doses (multiples of clinical sedative doses), these could kill a susceptible animal through CVS collapse but have not been generally considered for this role.

ELECTROLYTES. The technique of inducing fatal electrolyte abnormalities has long been an acceptable method of producing death in animals once they are anesthetized. The two electrolyte solutions that have been most widely used were KCl and magnesium sulfate ($MgSO_4$). $MgSO_4$ contributes to death by respiratory arrest and development of fatal hypoxemia and therefore is considered unsuitable for euthanasia. KCl injection into a conscious animal causes firing of the C-nerve fibers, which causes extreme pain before death occurs. In an anesthetized animal that problem is avoided and the use of a saturated solution of KCl, injected IV at the rate 1–2 ml per 5 kg body weight, induces cardiac ventricular fibrillation and death within 1–2 minutes. It may be accompanied by some agonal gasping motion as the cessation of cerebral circulation comes before total CNS quiescence. The use of IV administered KCl in anesthetized animals is both rapid and cheap. However, it must be stressed that the technique needs high concentrations of the KCl administered IV and should be administered only to unconscious animals.

INGESTED AGENTS

The use of drugs in food or drink to produce euthanasia is neither reliable nor humane. Intake can be capricious and free-ranging animals may be incapacitated just enough to permit injury or predation. The real role of ingested CNS depressants is to provide sufficient sedation to allow safe (animal and operator) handling. This role can be subverted when too small a dose is used and there is paradoxical excitement with release of inhibitory behavior. Drugs that can be hidden in feed or water include barbiturates, chloral hydrate, benzodiazepines, and ketamine. Toxic baits that do not produce anesthesia before death are universally condemned.

IMMERSION AGENTS

Immersion is a method used to administer fatal overdoses of anesthetics for euthanasia of fish and amphibians. The drugs used for that are MS-222, benzocaine, etomidate, metomidate (note do not confuse this with medetomidine which is an alpha-2 sympathomimetic CNS depressant), phenoxyethanol, and quinaldine (Close et al. 1997; Hartman 2006). Availability of these can vary as some have no FDA approval in the USA. Standard methods are to use a double-strength anesthetic bath and leave the fish for 10 minutes after all opercular movement has ceased. Death should be confirmed by a secondary physical method (pithing or opening the thorax/heart). Lay texts warn operators to wear gloves during immersion and handling of the fish or amphibians.

MISCELLANEOUS CONSIDERATIONS

When euthanasia is performed as part of a research project or when a postmortem examination may be performed, operators need to be cognizant that euthanasia per se may cause agonal-related pathological lesions. Pentobarbital has not been implicated in any gross or microscopic changes except for the characteristic splenomegaly. CO_2 has been implicated in some pulmonary vasculature changes reflective of local irritation. Embutramide, in its original T61 formulation, caused pulmonary congestion and edema, endothelial swelling of glomerular tuft vessels, and a dose-related hemolysis (Feldman and Gupta 1976; Port et al. 1978; Prien et al. 1988).

Euthanasia using pharmacological agents carries some very important caveats. First, after euthanasia death must be confirmed physically by inspection of the thorax to observe cardiac standstill, CNS destruction, or a terminal procedure such as exsanguination and whole body perfusion. The second caveat is never to use a euthanasia method that produces pain or distress before unconsciousness. Examples of such prohibited drugs or chemicals include paralytic agents (muscle relaxants or nicotine), or concentrated electrolyte solutions used in nonanesthetized animals (KCl or $MgSO_4$).

For the most comprehensive and up-to date discussion of all methods of euthanasia, the reader is referred to the American Veterinary Medical Association website (www.avma.org/) where the most recent Report of the AVMA Panel on Euthanasia can be found.

REFERENCES

AHAW Panel. (2005) Aspects of the biology and welfare of animals used for experimental and other scientific purposes. EFSA J, 292, 1–136.

American Veterinary Medical Association. (2001) 2000 Report of the AVMA panel on euthanasia. J Am Vet Med Assoc, 218, 669–696.

Anonymous. (2001) MS222 (tricaine methane sulphonate), Alpharma Animal Health Limited, Hampshire, U.K.

Anonymous. (2007) The welfare of animals at slaughter: Consultation on the proposed amendment to the Welfare of Animals (Slaughter or Killing) Regulations 1995: Use of gas as a killing method for birds outside of a slaughter house., Department for the Environment, Food and Rural Affairs, London.

Arnold, W.P. and Nicholau, D. (2005) Environmental safety including chemical dependency. In: Miller's Anesthesia (ed. R.D. Miller), pp. 3151–3174. Elsevier/Churchill Livingstone, New York.

Artwohl, J., Brown, P., Corning, B., and Stein, S. (2006) Report of the ACLAM task force on rodent euthanasia. J Am Assoc Lab Anim Sci, 45, 98–105.

Benacka, R. and Tomori, Z. (1995) The sniff-like aspiration reflex evoked by electrical stimulation of the nasopharynx. Resp Physiol, 102, 163–174.

Close, B., Banister, K., Baumans, V., Bernoth, E., Bromage, N., Bunyan, J., Erhardt, W., Flecknell, P., Gregory, N., Hackbarth, H., Morton, D., and Warwick, C. (1997) Recommendations for euthanasia of experimental animals: Part 2. Lab Anim, 31, 1–32.

———. (1996) Recommendations for euthanasia of experimental animals: Part 1. Lab Anim, 30, 293–316.

Danneman, P.J., Stein, S., and Walshaw, S.O. (1997a) Humane and practical implications of using carbon dioxide mixed with oxygen for anaesthesia or euthanasia of rats. Lab Anim Sci, 47, 376–385.

———. (1997b) Humane and practical implications of using carbon dioxide mixed with oxygen for anesthesia or euthanasia of rats. Lab Anim Sci, 47, 376–385.

Evans, A.T., Broadstone, R., Stapleton, J., Hooks, T.M., Johnston, S.M., and McNeil, J.R. (1993) Comparison of pentobarbital alone and pentobarbital in combination with lidocaine for euthanasia of dogs. J Am Vet Med Assoc, 203, 664–666.

Ewbank, R. (1983) Is CO_2 Euthanasia Humane. Nature, 305, 268.

Feldman, D.B. and Gupta, B.N. (1976) Histopathologic changes in laboratory animals resulting from various methods of euthanasia. Lab Anim Sci, 26, 218–221.

Fucci V, Monroe, W.E., Riedesel, D.H., and Jackson, L.L. (1986) Oral pentobarbital intoxication in a bitch. J Am Vet Med Assoc, 188, 191–192.

Giorgi, M. and Bertini, S. (2000) TANAX (T-61): an overview. Pharmacol Res, 41, 379–383.

Grier, R.L. (1991) Administration of euthanasia agents—reply. J Am Vet Med Assoc, 198, 1102–1103.

Grier, R.L. and Schaffer, C.B. (1990) Evaluation of intraperitoneal and intrahepatic administration of a euthanasia agent in animal shelter cats. J Am Vet Med Assoc, 197, 1611–1615.

Hall, L.W., Jeffcott, L.B., and Moss, M.S. (1972) Poisoning of dogs by horse meat containing chloral hydrate. Vet Rec, 91, 480.

Hartman, K.H. (2006) Fish. In: Guidelines for euthanasia of nondomestic animals (ed. C.K. Baer), pp. 28–37. American Association of Zoo Veterinarians.

Hawkins, P., Playle, L., Golledge, H., Leach, M., Banzett, R., Coenan, A., Cooper, J., Danneman, P., Flecknell, P., Kirkden, R., Niel, L., and Raj, M. (2006) Newcastle consensus meeting on carbon dioxide euthanasia of laboratory animals: 27 and 28 February 2006. Anim Tech Welf, 5, 125–142.

Hellebrekers, L.J., Baumans, V., Bertens, A.P., and Hartman, W. (1990) On the use of T61 for euthanasia of domestic and laboratory animals; an ethical evaluation. Lab Anim, 24, 200–204.

Klemm, W.R. (1964) Carbon dioxide anesthesia in cats. Am J Vet Res, 25, 1201–1205.

National Institutes of Health. (2002) PHS policy on humane care and use of laboratory animals clarification regarding use of carbon dioxide for euthanasia of small laboratory animals. NIH NOT-OD-02-062. 7-17-2002.

Phoenix Scientific. (2005) Freedom of Information Summary NADA 141–245: Tributame euthanasia solution.

Polley, L. and Weaver, B.M.Q. (1977) Accidental poisoning of dogs by barbiturates in meat. Vet Rec, 100, 48.

Port, C.D., Garvin, P.J., Ganote, C.E., and Sawyer, D.C. (1978) Pathologic changes induced by an euthanasia agent. Lab Anim Sci, 28, 448.

Prien, T., Traber, D.L., Linares, H.A., and Davenport, S.L. (1988) Haemolysis and artifactual lung damage induced by an euthanasia agent. Lab Anim, 22, 170–172.

Raj, A.B.M. (1999) Behaviour of pigs exposed to mixtures of gases and the time required to stun and kill them: welfare implications. Vet Rec, 144, 165–168.

Raj, A.B.M. and Gregory, N.G. (1990) Investigation Into the Batch Stunning/Killing of Chickens Using Carbon-Dioxide Or Argon-Induced Hypoxia. Res Vet Sci, 49, 364–366.

Seif, D.P. (1991) Administration of euthanasia agents. J Am Vet Med Assoc, 198, 1102–1103.

Thurman, J.C. (1991) Euthanasia. In: Equine Anesthesia: Monitoring and Emergency Therapy (eds. W.Muir and J.Hubbell), pp. 485–495.

SECTION

4

Autacoids and Antiinflammatory Drugs

CHAPTER

16

HISTAMINE, SEROTONIN, AND THEIR ANTAGONISTS

H. RICHARD ADAMS

HISTAMINE

Histamine is a biogenic amine detected in the early 1900s as a common bacterial-source contaminant of ergot extracts (Dale and Laidlaw 1910; Skidgel and Erdös 2006). Because histamine evoked a contractile response in smooth muscles and also lowered blood pressure, attention was drawn to similarities between its actions and allergic and anaphylactic-type reactions. Histamine was discovered in mammalian tissues and found to be released upon cellular trauma, leading to the theory of histamine as an endogenous mediator of cell injury. Subsequent studies have provided a wealth of physiologic and pathophysiologic roles for histamine quite apart from simple cellular trauma (Barnes et al. 1990; Skidgel and Erdös 2006). Mainly through one type of receptor (H_1), histamine is involved in inflammations, anaphylaxis, allergies, and certain types of drug reactions. Using yet a second type of receptor (H_2), it regulates gastric secretion (Obrink 1991; Morris 1992; Mitsuhashi and Payan 1992). The H_3 receptors modulate neurotransmitter release from neurons (Lovenberg et al. 1999), whereas H_4 receptors participate in inflammation involving eosinophils and other inflammatory cell types (Ling et al. 2004). Histamine itself is not used therapeutically, but histamine receptor blocking agents (histamine receptor inverse agonists) are commonly used to inhibit effects of endogenous histamine (Macglashan 2003).

HISTAMINE RECEPTORS. Histamine contracts several types of smooth muscles, including those of the bronchi, gut, and large blood vessels. In contrast, small arterioles are relaxed by histamine to the extent that peripheral vascular resistance and blood pressure fall while capillary permeability is increased. Gastric secretion of hydrochloric acid is stimulated, as are secretory activities of other exocrine glands. In humans, flushing of the facial skin and burning and itching sensations also are evoked. With large doses of histamine, blood pressure progressively falls and is accompanied by hemoconcentration caused by extravasation of plasma. "Histamine shock" may terminate in death (Pearce 1991).

A tissue in which effects of histamine are most recognizable is the skin. Histamine is an important mediator of immediate allergic reactions (MacGlashan 2003; De Mora et al. 2006), and in the skin, mast cells represent its principal source (DeMora et al. 2006). Although H_1 and H_2 receptors are the dominant subtypes in the skin, the affinity of histamine for the H_1 receptors is markedly higher than for the H_2 receptors. Therefore, cutaneous vasodilatation, edema, pruritus, and wheal formation are caused primarily from the interaction between histamine and H_1 receptors (Clough et al. 1998). Moreover, histamine stimulates C-type nerve fibers, and thus induces a perception of pruritus (Johanek et al. 2007). Finally, histamine can also recruit the major effector cells such as eosinophils into the site of inflammation, and it affects their maturation and activation, which leads to chronic skin inflammation (Akdis and Simons 2006).

The other major system affected by histamine is the respiratory tract. Histamine is stored in respiratory tract mast cells and is released in the lungs in response to allergic stimulation. Histamine induces bronchoconstriction and is a chemoattractant and activator of eosinophils and produces airway inflammation. Despite these documented effects, antihistamines alone are only moderately effective for treating inflammatory airway disorders in people and animals, suggesting that other inflammatory mediators play a dominant role.

Responses to histamine can be explained by activation of specific histamine receptors on various target cells (Oda 2000; Rizk et al. 2004). Analysis of histamine-receptor interactions was advanced by Bovet and Staub (1937), who described the first antihistamine. This type of drug competitively inhibits several biologic effects of histamine and protects guinea pigs from the high lethality of anaphylactic shock. Ash and Schild (1966) subsequently pointed out the likelihood for two types of histamine receptors in mammalian tissue. This theory was based on the knowledge that conventional antihistaminic drugs available at that time, such as pyrilamine and diphenhydramine, blocked only certain actions of histamine. Other activities, most notably stimulation of gastric secretion, were not amenable to inhibition by such drugs and were therefore thought to be mediated by a second type of receptor.

The existence of two specific types of histamine receptors was confirmed by Black et al. (1972), who conducted a systematic pharmacologic study of compounds derived from the basic structural components of histamine. Based on this investigation, histamine receptors were designated as histamine type 1 (H_1) and histamine type 2 (H_2). Histamine-induced contraction of bronchial and intestinal smooth muscle is mediated through H_1 receptors and inhibited by pyrilamine and other standard antihistamines (now called H_1 blockers). In contrast, histamine-induced stimulation of gastric acid secretion is mediated by H_2 receptors and inhibited by the newly available H_2 blockers such as burimamide, metamide, famotidine, and cimetidine. (These drugs are discussed in more detail in Chapter 47, "Drugs Affecting Gastrointestinal Function.") Different histamine receptor agonists likewise display preferential action at receptor subtypes. For example, 2-methylhistamine evokes rather selective agonist action at H_1 receptors, whereas 4-methylhistamine acts preferentially at H_2 receptors (Skidgel and Erdös 2006).

Studies have also indicated third and fourth classes of histamine receptors (Hough 2001; Hancock et al. 2003; Hofstra et al. 2003). The H_3 receptors are localized on nerve terminals where they modulate release of neurotransmitters. This action is believed to be linked to inhibition of adenylyl cyclase through an inhibitory G_i protein (Arang et al. 1987; Esbenshade et al. 2003). H_3 receptors are concentrated within the central nervous system (CNS), and their therapeutic relevance to veterinary medicine remains to be clearly defined (Stark et al. 2001). The H_4 receptors are localized on cells of hematopoietic origin where they are believed to participate in allergic and inflammatory reactions (Takeshita et al. 2004; Thurmond et al. 2004). However, there seems to be structural overlap between the H_3 and H_4 receptors, and many questions remain about their pharmacologic applications in clinical medicine (Skidgel and Erdös 2006).

ENDOGENOUS HISTAMINE. Histamine is 2-(4-imidazolyl) ethylamine (Fig. 16.1); it is derived from the decarboxylation of an amino acid, histidine. Conversion of histidine to histamine is catalyzed in mammalian tissues

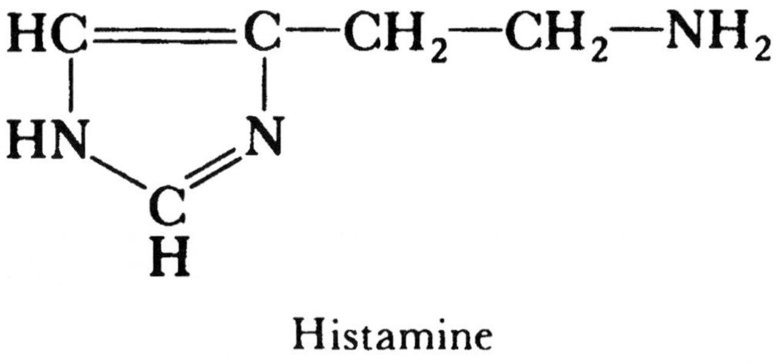

Histamine

FIG. 16.1 Histamine.

by a specific enzyme, histidine decarboxylase; this enzyme is present in all cell types that contain histamine.

Histamine is widely distributed throughout mammalian tissue, but concentrations vary considerably in different species; e.g., quantities of circulating histamine are relatively high in the goat and rabbit but low in the horse, dog, cat, and human. Most of the histamine stored within the body is derived locally from enzymatic decarboxylation of histidine. Two general stores of histamine can be identified in mammalian species: the mast cell pool made up of mast cells and basophils, and the non–mast-cell pool localized in the gastrointestinal (GI) tract, CNS, dermis, and other organs. These two pools differ not only in cellular locale but also in responsiveness to physiologic and pharmacologic stimuli.

The mast cell pool of highly concentrated histamine is distributed in connective tissue throughout the body. Circulating basophils, free counterparts of fixed-tissue mast cells, also contain high concentrations of histamine and are grouped with mast cells because of basic similarities. Within these two cell types, histamine is synthesized rather slowly and stored tenaciously in secretory granules; hence, turnover rate is low. Because of the slow turnover rate, mast cell stores are replenished slowly after exposure to a histamine-releasing agent. The mast cell pool represents the histamine that participates in inflammatory responses, allergic phenomena, shock, some adverse drug reactions, and other forms of cellular insult.

The precise cellular localizations and physiologic functions of the non–mast-cell pool of histamine within the gastric mucosa, brain, and skin are still being identified. Histamine in the stomach mucosa—the source of stimulation of acid secretion on H_2-receptors of the gastric parietal cells—is derived from the enterochromaffin-like cells. Histamine in these regions, in contrast to the mast cell pool, undergoes a rapid turnover rate; it is synthesized and released continuously rather than being stored. Portions of this newly synthesized or nascent histamine are present within neural elements, and neurotransmitter functions have been proposed. In the gastric mucosa, a "local hormone" action of histamine controls acid secretion. Interestingly, non–mast-cell histamine is generally resistant to histamine-releasing drugs such as compound 48/80.

HISTAMINE RELEASE. Histamine is highly concentrated in mast cell granules, where it is stored with a heparin-protein complex, proteolytic enzymes, and other autacoids. Release of histamine basically is a two-step process: sudden exocytotic extrusion of granules from the cell and release of histamine from the granules into the interstitial milieu. The latter occurs as an ionic exchange reaction between extracellular cations and molecules of granular histamine. Release can be initiated by a variety of stressful stimuli, including anaphylaxis-allergy, different drugs and chemicals, and physical injury.

Anaphylaxis and Allergy. Hypersensitivity phenomena associated with antigen-antibody reactions evoke active release of histamine from the mast cell pool. Free histamine then plays an important role in mediating physiologic manifestations of such reactions as vasodilation, itching, smooth muscle contraction, and edema. Other autacoids also participate in tissue responses to hypersensitivity reactions. Signs of histamine involvement in systemic anaphylaxis vary in different species. In carnivores, histamine and anaphylaxis produce pronounced hypotension and hepatomegaly. In rabbits, pulmonary arterioles constrict and the right heart dilates in response to either histamine injection or exposure of a sensitized individual to the appropriate antigen. In guinea pigs, dominant manifestations are bronchial constriction and death by asphyxiation. Humans seem to respond like guinea pigs and dogs in that severe hypotension, bronchial constriction, and laryngeal edema are principal signs of anaphylaxis.

The mast cell pool of histamine represents a major target for acute types of hypersensitivity-allergy reactions. Expulsion of the granular contents of mast cells and basophils is initiated by interaction of specific antigen and cell-bound reaginic (IgE) antibody. This interaction increases permeability of the cell to calcium ions (Ca^{++}). The resulting influx of Ca^{++} from the interstitium evokes release of histamine in a manner basically analogous to the secretory responses of various endocrine and exocrine cells to their respective secretagogues (Douglas 1974). Release is an active process, requiring metabolic energy as well as Ca^{++}, and should be distinguished from simple release secondary to cell destruction and cytolysis.

The ubiquitous cyclic adenosine 3′,5′-monophosphate (cAMP) system is involved in histamine release evoked by antigen-antibody interactions. An increase in cAMP concentration suppresses histamine release (Lichtenstein and Margolis 1968). Agents that activate adenylyl cyclase (e.g., catecholamines), inhibit phosphodiesterase (e.g., methylxanthines), or activate β_2-adrenergic receptors on mast cells can be anticipated to inhibit the release of histamine. The beneficial effects of drugs widely used in treating allergic disorders, such as the catecholamines, β_2-agonists, and theophylline, may therefore involve inhibition of histamine release in addition to their well-known and more important physiologic antagonism of histamine actions on target cells.

Drugs and Chemicals. Many drugs and chemicals produce direct degranulation of mast cells with release of histamine independently from development of allergy. This characteristic action represents an untoward side effect associated either with intravenous (IV) administration of a relatively large dose or direct intradermal injection. Certain chemicals have as their dominant property the ability to release histamine from the mast cell pool.

The curare-alkaloids are used clinically as neuromuscular blocking agents (Chapter 9), but they also are notorious for releasing histamine as an adverse side effect; in some species, IV injection of these agents can be followed by histamine-induced bronchospasm and hypotension. Other clinically used drugs that may release histamine include morphine (Guedes et al. 2007), codeine, doxorubicin, vancomycin, and polypeptide antibiotics (polymyxin). However, other opiates such as oxymorphone and hydromorphone are not associated with as much histamine release (Guedes et al. 2006, 2007).

Certain chemicals have been classified simply as histamine-releasing agents because this particular activity supersedes their other pharmacologic properties. The best known and most active is an organic base called compound 48/80, a condensation product of *p*-methoxyphenylethylmethylamine with formaldehyde (Goth and Johnson 1975). Injection of compound 48/80 or other similar agents evokes classic pharmacologic signs of histamine release that are susceptible to blockade by antihistaminic drugs. Tachyphylaxis to repeated injections is characteristic of these chemicals, presumably because of decreased availability of releasable stores of histamine. Endogenous substances that provoke histamine release and may be involved in physiologic release mechanisms include bradykinin, kallidin, and substance P. Cellular reactions to many venoms and toxins also involve histamine release.

Physical Injury. When the skin is scratched or pricked, the characteristic redness and urtication that result are due to histamine. This response is quite pronounced in humans. Dermal reactions to severe cold or heat stress likewise depend on histamine liberated by local mast cells. Physical injury of virtually any type sufficiently intense to damage the cells will evoke release of histamine.

ROLE IN HEALTH AND DISEASE

Gastric Secretion. Histamine is a potent stimulant of hydrochloric acid secretion by the gastric mucosa. This finding led early investigators to portray endogenous histamine as the final common mediator of gastric secretion, irrespective of whether stimulation arises from chemical, mechanical, or nervous elements. Full acceptance of this theory was delayed for over 50 years because conventional antihistaminic drugs available at the time (i.e., the H_1 blockers) failed to prevent gastric effects of histamine (Leurs et al. 2001). This impediment was surmounted when Black et al. (1972) reported that newly discovered H_2-blocking agents are quite efficacious in inhibiting gastric stimulant activities of histamine and its congeners. H_2-blocking drugs also reduce the gastric secretory response evoked by ingestion of a meal or administration of either the gastric hormone gastrin or its synthetic derivative pentagastrin, further supporting a final H_2-dependent step in gastric acid secretion. (H_2-blocking drugs used to treat stomach disorders are discussed in more detail in Chapter 47.)

Neurons. Locally released or injected histamine stimulates sensory nerve endings, thereby evoking the classic symptoms of itching and pain. Histamine also is present in the brain, where it is concentrated in the hypothalamus; subcellular distribution studies have localized histamine to some nerve endings. These and related studies, in conjunction with the obvious CNS effects of H_1-blockers, have prompted the suggestion that histaminergic neurons are present in the brain and that histamine released from these fibers functions as a neurotransmitter. Peripheral efferent histaminergic nerves are envisioned as active components of reflex vasodilation in conjunction with the passive withdrawal of sympathetic vasoconstrictor tone in this reflex.

Histamine release in the central nervous system is one of the neurotransmitters of the emetic response. Histamine is involved in the emetic response to vestibular stimulation (motion sickness) that may be directed either through the chemorecptor zone (CRTZ) located in the area postrema, or directly to the emetic center of the brain. Histamine-blocking drugs have been used to treat vomiting from these stimuli, although they are less effective in dogs than in people (Yates et al. 1998).

Others. A variety of biologic roles have been proposed for endogenous histamine in addition to those previously addressed, including local regulation of the microcirculatory response to injury and inflammation, some type of anabolic activity in rapidly growing or repairing tissues, systemic signs associated with excessive numbers of mast cells or basophils, and involvement in different types of headaches in humans. In domestic animals, histamine released from damaged tissue has been suggested as a mediator in several pathologic states, including allergic reactions to drugs, venoms, and other antigens; ruminant bloating; overeating and other GI disorders of ruminants; laminitis; azoturia; retained placenta; pneumonia; gut edema of the pig; and various types of anaphylactic shock syndromes (Eyre and Wells 1973). Except for allergic phenomena, however, the role of histamine in these conditions usually is more empirically based than experimentally founded.

PHARMACOLOGIC EFFECTS. Histamine administered orally has essentially no effect because it is destroyed rapidly by the GI tract and liver. Intravenous histamine produces a spectrum of characteristic effects including smooth muscle contraction, hypotension, increased gastric secretion, and dermal reactions.

Difficulties are encountered when attempts are made to designate H_1- or H_2-receptor responsibility for each action of histamine. In some tissues, H_1 and H_2 receptors are complementary and subserve similar tissue responses. In contrast, distinct and even opposing functions of the two receptor types have been identified in some tissues. Species differences are formidable and in most cases await further study for classification. In the following paragraphs, only the more representative examples of H_1- or H_2-receptor involvement, when known, are discussed.

Cardiovascular System. The principal circulatory effects of histamine are dilation of terminal arterioles and other vessels of the microcirculation, edema formation caused by increased capillary permeability, and contraction of large arteries and veins. Relative dominance of the actions varies in different species so that net circulatory response to histamine changes as the zoologic scale is ascended; e.g., arterioles are contracted strongly by histamine in rodents, less so in cats, and actually are dilated in dogs, nonhuman primates, and humans.

In rabbits, histamine is a pressor agent as a result of pronounced constriction of large blood vessels. This constrictor activity is feeble in carnivores where vasodilation of the microcirculation dominates instead. Thus the blood pressure response to histamine in cats, dogs, and primates is hypotension caused by a sharp fall in peripheral vascular resistance. The fall in blood pressure is dose dependent but is usually short-lived because of compensatory reflexes and inactivation of histamine.

The striking effects of histamine on the microcirculation can be demonstrated quite convincingly in the human subject. When this agent is administered intradermally, a characteristic triple response is produced, which includes localized redness at the injection site, developing within a few seconds and attaining maximal hue within a minute; localized edema fluid, forming a wheal in about 90 seconds; and diffuse redness or "flare," extending about 1 cm from the original red spot. The central redness and edema are from the dilation and increased permeability of local microcirculatory vessels (terminal arterioles, capillaries, and venules). The surrounding flush, which is accompanied by itching and perhaps pain, is due to dilation of neighboring arterioles brought about by a poorly understood axonal reflex mechanism. The triple response of human skin may be similar to manifestations of urticaria in animals.

Vascular actions of histamine formerly were believed to be mediated solely by H_1 receptors; however, it now seems that both types of histamine receptors are involved. The vasodilator response to H_1-receptor activation occurs at low doses of histamine and is rapid in onset and of brief duration. The H_2-receptor vasodilator response is evoked with larger doses and is slower in onset and of longer duration. The small-vessel permeability changes evoked by histamine are clearly mediated by H_1 receptors, while the role of H_2 events is uncertain. The precise ratio of H_1- and H_2-receptor involvement in vascular responses to histamine varies in domestic animal species.

Cardiac effects of histamine are minimal when compared to vascular actions. In the intact animal, slight tachycardia is a common finding. This response is mainly secondary to baroreceptor reflexes activated by the depressor effect. In isolated heart muscle, histamine can elicit positive inotropic and chronotropic effects that are produced partly by release of norepinephrine from nerve endings and also to direct activation of H_2 receptors in the heart muscle. There is some evidence that in vivo cardiac responses to histamine injection may partially reflect activation of cardiac H_2 receptors.

Nonvascular Smooth Muscle. Histamine contracts bronchial smooth muscle via H_1 receptors in numerous mammals including the guinea pig, cat, rabbit, dog, goat, calf, pig, horse, and human (Chand and Eyre 1975; Mohammed et al. 1993). Guinea pigs are exceptionally sensitive, and even minute doses of histamine can evoke bronchoconstriction leading to death. Humans with bronchial asthma likewise demonstrate increased sensitivity to bronchial effects of histamine and other bronchial smooth muscle stimulants. In contrast, histamine can mediate relaxation of respiratory smooth muscle in some species. Histamine-induced tracheal relaxation in cats involves both H_1 and H_2 receptors, while bronchial relaxation in sheep seems to be mediated by H_2 receptors (Hirschowitz 1979).

Relaxation of the rat uterus by histamine is mediated by H_2 receptors, but uterine muscle of other species is generally contracted by histamine. Responses of intestinal muscle also vary with species and region, but the classic effect is a contractile response caused by H_1 receptors.

Exocrine Glands. The following exocrine glands are listed in descending order of response to histamine: gastric, salivary, pancreatic, bronchial, and lacrimal. Gastric secretion of hydrochloric acid and, to a lesser degree, pepsinogen is unquestionably the most important; this response is mediated by H_2 receptors.

Mechanism of Action. The H_1 receptors in some cell types are linked to activation of phospholipase C and the resulting increase in inositol triphosphate and intracellular Ca^{++}. This process most likely involves a G protein, as discussed in Chapter 5 (Lambert 1993). The H_2 receptors also utilize G proteins linked to activation of adenylyl cyclase and its increased synthesis of cAMP, culminating in activation of the latter's intracellular receptor, protein kinase A. The vasodilator response elicited by endothelial H_1 receptors involves activation of nitric oxide synthase and release of endothelium-derived nitric oxide, whereas the vasodilatory H_2 receptors directly relax the vascular smooth muscle cells. The H_3 presynaptic receptors are coupled to inhibitory G-proteins and cause a decrease in adenylyl cyclase activity and a corresponding reduction in intracellular cyclic amp concentrations. The H_4 receptors in cells of hematopoietic origin are believed to act through similar G-protein–linked mechanisms as do the H_3 class (Skidgel and Erdös 2006).

BIOTRANSFORMATION. Histamine administered orally is poorly absorbed, but absorption is virtually complete after parenteral injection. Pharmacologic actions are brief because of rapid metabolism and distribution into tissues. Biotransformation of histamine involves methylation and oxidation, as shown in Figure 16.2. Histamine is acted upon by the enzyme histamine-*N*-methyltransferase (imidazole-*N*-methyltransferase) to form methylhistamine; most of this metabolite is oxidized to methylimidazole acetic acid by the enzyme monoamine oxidase (>50%). The second pathway is oxidative deamination catalyzed by the enzyme diamine oxidase (histaminase) to form imidazoleacetic acid, which is conjugated with ribose as riboside (>25%). Only a small percentage of the primary amine can be acetylated in the GI tract, absorbed, and excreted in urine (1%). Some free histamine is also excreted in urine (2–3%).

MEDICAL USE. Clinical applications in humans involve use of histamine as a test agent for achlorhydria, in diagnosis of pheochromocytoma, and for production of the triple response to evaluate the integrity of sensory innervations and circulatory competency. The polypeptide pentagastrin and histamine analogs such as the H_2-selective agonist impromidine have been used as alternative means of evaluating gastric secretory function because of less objectionable H_1-mediated side effects. Repeated injec-

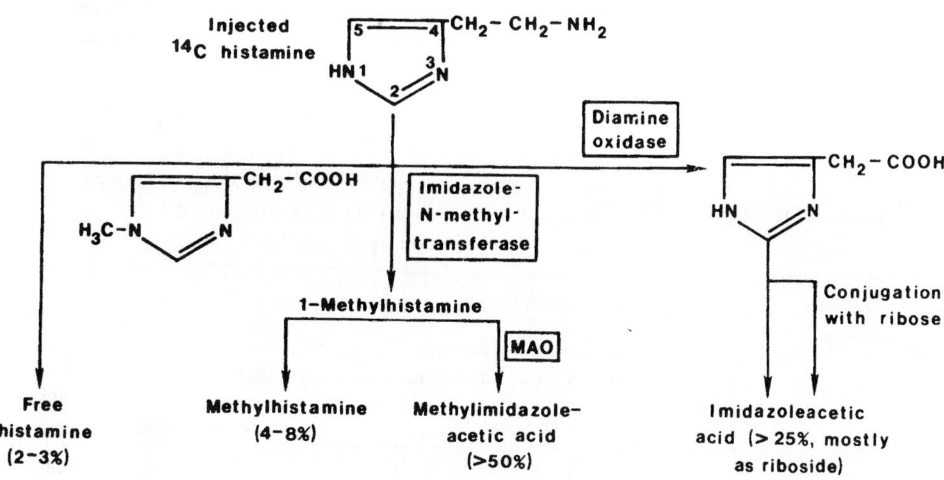

FIG. 16.2 Synthesis, metabolism, and urinary metabolites of histamine recovered in 12 hours following intradermal injection of ^{14}C histamine in a human male (% values from Schayer and Cooper 1956).

tions of histamine, in an attempt to desensitize patients with allergies, has not met with general acceptance.

Cromolyn is an interesting drug used in human medicine, and occasionally in horses, as a prophylactic treatment of bronchial asthma. Cromolyn exerts this activity by inhibiting the release of histamine and other autacoids that participate in the asthmatic syndrome. A more complete discussion of the use of cromolyn in animals will be covered in Chapter 49, "Drugs Affecting the Respiratory System."

ANTIHISTAMINES

Although the pharmacologic effects of histamine can be antagonized by several types of drugs, the term *antihistamine* is restricted to agents that act on histamine receptors. The receptors are not activated by such interaction, but their occupancy by the antihistamine limits accessibility to histamine and thereby prevents the latter from exerting its cellular actions. In recent years, the terminology has changed and H_1-antihistamines are classified as inverse agonists, rather than histamine antagonists (Simons 2004). This new terminology reflects their true mechanism of action, which is to stabilize the H_1 receptor in an inactive state. However, the term *histamine antagonists* is still often used in veterinary literature.

The H_1-antagonists have been divided into the first-generation antihistamines (e.g., chlorpheniramine, diphenhydramine, and hydroxyzine) and the second-generation antihistamines (e.g., cetirizine, desloratadine, fexofenadine, terfenadine, astemizole, and loratadine). The first-generation antihistamines are generally the older, more familiar drugs. The second-generation antihistamines are the newer, nonsedating antihistamines. This group includes most of the newer antihistamines introduced since 1981. Some of these drugs are related: cetirizine is a metabolite of hydroxyzine; diphenhydramine is a metabolite of dimenhydrinate; desloratidine is a metabolite of loratidine.

The primary difference between the first- and second-generation antihistamines is that the second-generation antihistamines lack the antimuscarinic properties and do not cross the blood-brain barrier as easily as first-generation antihistamines. Therefore these drugs lack the central-nervous system side effects, particularly sedation that is common with the first-generation antihistamines. The effects of each group of antihistamines will be discussed in more detail below.

Agents such as catecholamines and xanthines exhibit pharmacologic activities that are, among other things, antagonistic to actions of histamine. However, these opposing actions are mediated by different receptors and cellular pathways; they represent physiologic antagonism.

DEVELOPMENT. Bovet and Staub (1937) of the Pasteur Institute in Paris first demonstrated that two phenolic esters possessed antihistaminic activity. One of these com-

TABLE 16.1 Preparations and doses of some H_1 antihistamines in veterinary use

First Generation Antihistamines (H_1 antagonists)			
Drug Class	Drug Name	Brand Name	Dose in Animals
Alkylamine	Chlorpheniramine	Chlor-Trimeton	Dog: 4–8 mg/dog to a maximum of 0.5 mg/kg q8–12h Cat: 2–4 mg/cat, q12h
Ethanolamine	Diphenhydramine	Benadryl	2–4 mg/kg q8–12h
Ethanolamine	Clemastine	Tavist and generic	0.05–0.1 mg/kg q12h
Piperazine	Hydroxyzine	Atarax	0.5–2 mg/kg q6–8h
Phenothiazine	Trimeprazine	Temaril, Panectyl	0.5 mg/kg q12h
Tricyclic	Doxepin	Sinequan	Dose not established

Second Generation Antihistamines (H_1 antagonists)	
Drug	Brand Name
Terfenadine	Seldane (discontinued)
Fexofenadine	Allegra
Astemizole	Hismanal (discontinued)
Loratadine	Claratin (nonprescription OTC)
Cetirizine	Zyrtec
Desloratidine	Clarinex

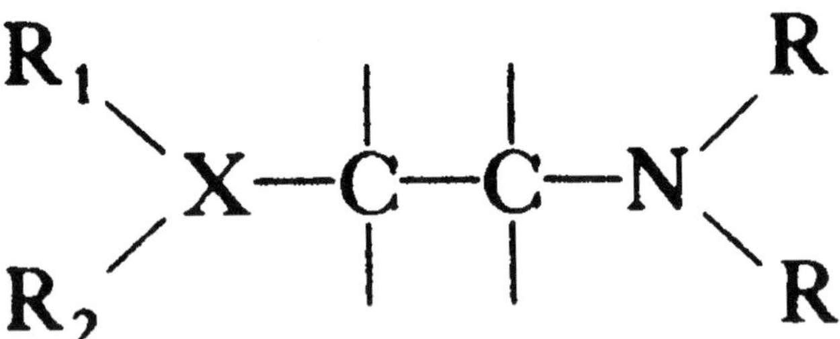

FIG. 16.3 General formula of most H_1 antihistaminic agents.

pounds, 929F (thymoxyethyldiethylamine), protected guinea pigs against several lethal doses of histamine. Although the original drugs were too toxic for therapeutic use, their discovery led to development of many modern antihistamines. Such compounds are now referred to as H_1 and H_2 antihistamines, based on the previously described differentiation of histamine receptors into H_1 and H_2 subtypes (Ash and Schild 1966; Black et al. 1972).

CHEMISTRY. Some of the more frequently used H_1 antihistamines are listed in Table 16.1. The chemical structure of nearly all the H_1 antihistaminic drugs can be depicted by the structural formula shown in Figure 16.3. The nucleus of the structure is ethylamine (CH_2CH_2N), which is also present in histamine. This moiety is thought to be the molecular component necessary for competition with histamine for specific cell receptors.

Three types of H_1 antihistaminics are known in which the element X (as depicted in Fig. 16.3) is nitrogen, oxygen, or carbon. The X represents a nitrogen for the ethylenediamine class (e.g., pyrilamine, Neoantergan), oxygen for the ethanolamine class (e.g., diphenhydramine, Benadryl), and carbon for the alkylamine class (e.g., Teldrin). The fourth class of antihistaminics contains a piperazine in place of the conventional ethylenediamine linkage (e.g., cyclizine, Marezine). The representative of the fifth class (e.g., promethazine, Phenergan) is not related directly to the previous drugs; it is a phenothiazine derivative. The sixth class comprises the peperidines terfenadine and astemizole; these agents have aromatic ring moieties on either end of the ethylamine chain. These different chemical substitutions influence the potency of H_1-antihistaminic action as well as their side effects.

The H_2 antihistamines differ from the H_1 blockers in their chemistry, pharmacokinetics, and pharmacodynamics. The imidazole ring structure of histamine is modified extensively or replaced by other substituents in the H_1 antagonists. In the H_2-blocking agents, however, the side chain is modified extensively, while the imidazole moiety is preserved. In contrast to the H_1 antihistaminics, the H_2 antagonists are somewhat less lipid soluble and do not effectively penetrate the blood-brain barrier. Hence the H_2

antagonists do not cause sedation, a prominent side effect of most of their H_1 counterparts.

Burimamide was the first H_2 antagonist, but it was absorbed too poorly to be effective after oral administration. Metiamide was subsequently synthesized; it was absorbed effectively from the GI tract, but several human patients treated with the drug developed agranulocytosis. A newer H_2 blocker, cimetidine, was then introduced into clinical medicine and so far has not been associated with hematologic toxicity. Ranitidine, famotidine, and nizatidine are some of the newer H_2 blockers. (H_2-blocking drugs used to treat stomach disorders are discussed in more detail in Chapter 47.)

PHARMACOLOGIC EFFECTS. Pharmacokinetic information for the antihistaminics of the H_1 subtype is very sparse. Chlorpheniramine is well absorbed in dogs, with a short time to peak absorption after oral administration and a half-life of 24 hours. Some are absorbed poorly (clemastine) (Hansson et al. 2004), while others appear to be well absorbed, but rapidly converted to a metabolite (hydroxyzine) (Bisikova et al. 2008). There is little data available for horses or ruminants. When clemastine was administered to horses (Törneke et al. 2003), there was a rapid decline in plasma concentrations. Oral absorption was only 3% at a dose of 0.2 mg/kg. Although the pharmacologic response was attributed to the plasma concentrations of cetirizine in horses after the IV administration (0.05 mg/kg, duration 5 hours), there was little, or no response from the oral dose.

In species for which oral absorption occurs, effects are usually expected within 20–45 minutes, and the duration of action ranges from 3 to 12 hours (Table 16.1). IV administration elicits immediate effects, but this route is not used except for treatment of acute anaphylaxis (for which epinephrine is the preferred treatment of choice). Rapid IV injection can produce stimulation of the CNS and other side effects. The intramuscular route rarely gives rise to side effects and is more commonly used than IV administration. Topical application may be suitable in certain skin conditions.

Antihistamines act as reverse agonists to stabilize the histamine H_1-receptors in the tissue cells; their binding to the cell receptors evokes no direct cellular action. This mechanism of action is based on quantitative considerations; therefore, histamine in excess may displace antihistaminics. Generally, antihistaminics are more effective against exogenously administered histamine than against endogenously released histamine. They are also more effective in preventing actions of histamine than in reversing them (Simons 2003).

H_1 antihistaminics are useful in countering action of histamine on bronchial, intestinal, uterine, and vascular smooth muscle (Gelfand et al. 2004). They antagonize both the vasoconstrictor effects of histamine and the more important vasodilator effects as well as the increase in capillary permeability produced by this agent. These antihistaminic effects counteract urticaria, wheal formation, and other types of edema formation in response to injury, antigens, allergens, or histamine-liberating drugs. H_1 antihistaminics also suppress itching and flare in humans and greatly reduce itching associated with allergic reaction. In addition to the traditional effect on histamine response, these drugs may have other antiinflammatory effects, including decrease of the release of inflammatory mediators from inflammatory cells such as mast cells (Simons and Simons 1994; Walsh 2005). The relevance of this activity to clinical response is not known, nor is it known if this occurs at clinically achieved plasma concentrations. The effect of three drugs—terfenadine (a second generation antihistamine that has been discontinued), cetirizine, and loratidine—on histamine release from isolated canine cutaneous mast cells was examined (Garcia et al. 1997). Of these, loratidine and terfenadine produced potent inhibition of histamine release, but at high concentrations terfenadine actually stimulated release. An additional mechanism of action for the antihistamines may also decrease NFκB-mediated inflammatory effects, such as antigen presentation, expression of cell-adhesion molecules, chemotaxis, and proinflammatory cytokines.

H_1 antihistaminics only partially antagonize histamine-induced arterial hypotension because portions of this response are associated with H_2 receptors. The H_1 antagonists do not block the stimulant effect of histamine on gastric secretion, which is an H_2-dependent function. Importantly, neither H_1 nor H_2 antihistamines prevent histamine release; some antihistaminics possess histamine-liberating properties. As mentioned earlier terfenadine stimulate release of histamine from isolated mast cells (Garcia et al. 1997).

H_2 antagonists block the gastric stimulating effects of histamine as well as other actions of histamine that have been defined as H_2-receptor dependent (e.g., stimulation of rat uterus, cardiac excitatory effects, and some vascular effects).

SIDE EFFECTS AND INTERACTIONS. Side effects of clinical importance for the H_1 blockers include sedation or CNS excitement, GI disturbances, parasympatholytic action, local anesthetic properties, allergenic properties, and teratogenic effects. In therapeutic doses, the first generation H_1 antihistaminics elicit a sedative effect expressed by drowsiness or ataxia. As described below, the newer, second-generation antihistamines are more popular in people because they are considered nonsedating. Some dermatologists have acknowledged that the effect on reducing pruritus in dogs after administration of first-generation antihistamines may be partially attributed to the sedation produced (DeBoer and Griffin 2001; Olivry et al. 2003). Despite an assumption that first-generation antihistamines cause sedation in animals, a study of diphenhydramine in dogs indicated that this assumption may be incorrect. When dogs were administered doses of 2, 4, or 8 mg/kg IM compared to acepromazine or saline, the dogs receiving acepromazine showed significant sedation but sedation in dogs receiving diphenhydramine was no different from saline (Hofmeister and Egger 2005).

In much higher doses they produce irritability, convulsions, hyperpyrexia, and even death. Intestinal disorders include anorexia, nausea, vomiting, constipation, or diarrhea when antihistamines are administered orally for a prolonged period. The anticholinergic effects are expressed by dry mouth, pupillary dilation, blurred vision, and tachycardia. Local anesthetic properties are of value when these agents are used as antipruritic drugs in topical application. The teratogenic effects of certain of these agents suggest caution in their use during pregnancy. These drugs possess antiserotonin properties as well as cocainelike effects on catecholamine uptake.

The newer, second-generation H_1 antihistamines—fexofenadine, levocabastine, loratadine, ebastine, mezolastine, and astemizole—are largely excluded from the CNS when given in therapeutic doses because they are better substrates for the P-glycoprotein (P-gp) membrane pump that is an important component of the blood-brain barrier (Sun et al. 2003; Janssens and Howart 1993; Meeves and Appajosyula 2003). Their lack of sedation as a side effect is a distinct advantage in human medicine. Study is needed in veterinary medicine to determine their clinical efficacy and whether lack of sedation is an important attribute in animals (Miller et al. 1989).

TOXICITY. In recommended doses H_1 antihistaminics are relatively nontoxic; however, overdosage can elicit toxic effects expressed by hyperexcitability and even convulsions. At doses of 30–45 mg/kg orally to dogs—much higher than therapeutic doses—diphenhydramine produced stimulation, tremors, and increased reactivity and muscle tone. Anecdotally, excitement has been more common in cats than dogs. Chlorpheniramine has been reported to cause more side effects than other antihistamines (Scott and Buerger 1988). Treatment of acute toxicity is symptomatic; sedative or ultrashort-acting barbiturates may be of value, but caution is indicated because additive effects are possible.

THERAPEUTIC USES. H_1 antihistaminics frequently used in animals and representative doses are given in Table 16.1. Clinically, H_1 antagonists are used to prevent reactions from endogenous histamine as a response to certain allergic disorders and anaphylactic syndromes. However, the clinician must be aware that autacoids other than histamine also play important roles in allergy-anaphylaxis disorders. Eyre and Burka (1978) reviewed this field and listed the following compounds as primary or secondary mediators of hypersensitivity reactions: histamine, serotonin, dopamine, kinins, leukotrienes (slow-reacting substance of anaphylaxis), platelet activating factor, eosinophil chemotactic factor of anaphylaxis, prostaglandins, complement, and lymphokines. Thus it is not surprising that antihistamines alone are often ineffective in treating allergic-type reactions in animals.

Clinical signs of allergy vary among different species. The most frequently observed signs are restlessness, anorexia, yawning, salivation, lacrimation, nasal discharge, coughing, edema, urticaria, pruritus, eczema, necrosis, hemorrhage, inflammation of the mucous membranes and eyes, contraction of smooth muscle (bronchoconstriction), and cardiovascular disturbances. In acute or delayed anaphylaxis, clinical signs occur quickly and, if not treated, are followed by collapse and death in minutes.

Treatment of allergic conditions (e.g., atopic dermatitis) consists of further avoidance of allergens, hyposensitization, corticosteroids, cykclosporine, and occasionally administration of H_1 antihistaminics.

Treatment of Pruritus. The most extensively studied clinical problem in veterinary medicine for which antihistamines have been used is pruritus associated with atopic dermatitis (Papich 2000; DeBoer and Griffin 2001). An evidence-based review was published by Olivry et al. (2003). In some reports the incidence of response is approximately the same as a placebo. Several of the reported studies are uncontrolled, or the studies are not published in reviewed references. Nevertheless, these drugs are used by dermatologists to decrease the reliance on corticosteroids or used in conjunction with other antiinflammatory medications. As reported by Zur and colleagues (2002), dermatologists will often try three to five antihistamines in 2-week trials to find the one that is most effective for a patient. As expected, because of these individual variations, there also are a variety of results reported. Zur and colleagues (2002) evaluated hydroxyzine, diphenhydramine, chlorpheniramine, and clemastine in a retrospective study. Overall, 54% of the dogs had a good to moderate response. In that study, diphenhydramine and hydroxyzine were the most often used, and the most often effective.

Clemastine (Tavist), an ethanolamine antihistamine, is one of the most commonly used in dogs (Paradis et al. 1991) even though there is reliable evidence that it is not absorbed orally (Hansson et al. 2004). Chlorpheniramine, diphenhydramine, and hydroxyzine may be effective in some dogs (Scott and Buerger 1988). Trimeprazine, a phenothiazine derivative with antihistamine effects, has little effect on its own, but is among the most effective drugs when combined with a corticosteroid.

Cetirizine, one of the second-generation drugs, is an active metabolite of hydroxyzine. Some veterinarians have claimed some success, but it was modest at 1 mg/kg/day (18% response). In a study in dogs (Bisikova et al. 2008), it was shown that hydroxyzine (a first generation antihistamine) was rapidly converted to cetirizine (a second generation antihistamine) in dogs. This conversion was rapid regardless of the route (IV or oral at a dose of approximately 2 mg/kg). Moreover, the observed reaction to histamine was attributed to the plasma concentrations of cetirizine, not hydroxyzine. Therefore, hydroxyxine—one of the most popular antihistamines used in dogs—appears to act as a prodrug.

Chlorpheniramine and clemastine also have been reported to reduce pruritus in cats (Miller and Scott 1990). The effects or pharmacokinetics of antihistamines in this species have not been studied as much as in dogs. In one study, cetirizine was well absorbed in cats (approximately 1 mg/kg) and produced plasma concentrations that were above the levels considered therapeutic in humans.

Some studies have shown that combinations of antihistamines with fatty acids or other drugs may improve efficacy. There may be a synergistic effect of antihistamines (e.g., clemastine, chlorpheniramine) in combination with n-3/n-6 fatty acids (Paradis et al. 1991), and evidence for a synergistic effect with fatty acids and corticosteroids. When antihistamines were combined with corticosteroids in one report, the effective dose of prednisone was lowered (30% reduction) (Paradis et al. 1991). In a study in dogs, a combination of a fatty acid product plus clemastine was more effective (43% response) than either drug used alone (Paradis et al. 1991). One unpublished trial showed that a combination of fatty acids and corticosteroids were synergistic when used in combination, allowing for a reduction in the corticosteroid dose by 25–50%. In cats, chlorpheniramine plus fatty acids were more effective than either drug used alone. Despite these positive results, the study by Zur et al. (2002) did not show combinations to be helpful.

Treatment of Anaphylaxis. Anaphylactic syndrome requires emergency treatment because it progresses rapidly to irreversible cardiovascular collapse. The drug of choice is epinephrine; this catecholamine does not directly inhibit mediators of anaphylaxis but reverses their effects. Thus epinephrine acts as a physiologic antagonist (Chapter 6).

Treatment of Respiratory Disorders. The use of antihistamines for treatment of inflammatory airway disease and asthma has been of only minor benefit, suggesting the important contribution of other inflammatory mediators in this disease.

Cetirizine, a second-generation antihistamine (and metabolite of hydroxyzine) produced a protection against bronchoconstriction in humans affected with mild asthma during histamine challenge and may have other antiiflammatory properties (Walsh 2005). However, in sensitized asthmatic cats, cetirizine at a dose that produces plasma concentrations considered effective in people (5 mg per cat every 12 h) was ineffective in attenuating the infiltration of inflammatory eosinophils in airways or in altering other immune variables (Schooley et al. 2007). These authors recommended that cetirizine (and perhaps other antihistamines) should not be considered as sole therapy for asthma in cats. Antihistamines also are considered to be of value in treatment of bovine asthma (pulmonary emphysema). Chapter 49 presents a more detailed discussion of drugs that affect the respiratory system.

Treatment of Other Conditions with Antihistamines. Nonallergic but suspected histamine-related phenomena, which in empirical experience respond to antihistaminic therapy in animals, include many pathologic conditions. Those in which H_1 antihistaminics are reported to be of therapeutic value are urticaria, various types of dermatitis, moist eczema, acute eczematous otitis, insect stings, nutritional types of laminitis, pregnancy laminitis, paroxysmal myoglobinuria or azoturia, periodic ophthalmia, and pulmonary emphysema in horses. In cattle, antihistamines also are considered to be of value in treatment of some types of bloat and acetonemia in ruminants, acute septic and gangrenous mastitis, septic metritis and retained placenta, pregnancy toxemia, and gut edema of pigs. Treatment of vestibular stimulation (motion sickness) in animals has been variable. Although these drugs are sold over-the-counter for this purpose for humans, they appear to be less effective for vestibular vomiting in animals (Yates et al. 1998).

H_2 antagonists are used extensively in treatment of gastric ulceration and other gastric hypersecretory states in humans. H_2 blockers also are utilized commonly in animal patients when suppression of gastric hyperacidity and prevention of gastric mucosal ulceration are indicated. (H_2-blocking drugs used to treat stomach disorders are discussed in more detail in Chapter 47.)

SEROTONIN

Rapport et al. (1948) isolated a vasoconstrictor substance from serum and gave it the name serotonin; it was subsequently identified as 5-hydroxytryptamine (5-HT). Another group of researchers studying histochemical properties of the intestinal mucosa discovered an active agent in enterochromaffin cells and gave it the name enteramine (Erspamer and Asero 1952). After discovery of 5-HT in blood, it was soon confirmed that enteramine and 5-HT were the same chemical structure.

Following discovery of 5-HT and multiple types of 5-HT receptors in the CNS, it was soon discovered that drugs affecting 5-HT in the brain had beneficial CNS actions including modification of behavior, antidepressant actions, and antianxiety effects (Sanders-Bush and Mayer 2006). Drugs that modulate 5-HT action are being used increasingly in veterinary medicine in attempts to control behavioral problems in animals, and modify gastrointestinal motility (for additional information see Chapters 21 and 47) (Crowell-Davis and Murray 2006; Mohammad-Zadeh et al. 2008).

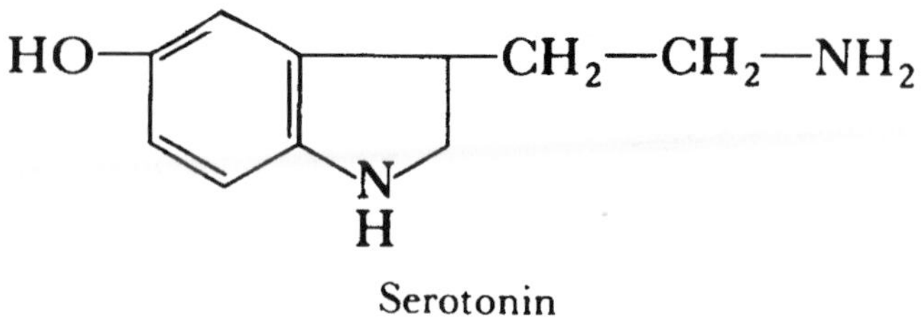

HO—(indole ring, N–H)—CH_2—CH_2—NH_2

Serotonin

FIG. 16.4 Serotonin.

SYNTHESIS. 5-HT is synthesized from dietary tryptophan in a two-stage chemical reaction (Walther et al. 2003). First, tryptophan is hydroxylated by the enzyme tryptophan 5-hydroxylase to give 5-hydroxytryptophan (5-HTP). The latter is then decarboxylated to yield 5-HT (serotonin), as shown in Figure 16.4.

Like histamine, 5-HT is widely distributed in animals and plants (Sanders-Bush and Mayer 2006). It occurs in high concentration in some fruits such as bananas, pineapples, and plums; it also is present in stings (common stinging nettle) and venoms. Endogenous 5-HT is synthesized from about 1% of the dietary tryptophan. It is formed and localized in three essential pools; enterochromaffin cells of the intestine, select neurons in the CNS, and mast cells of rodents (rats, mice, hamsters) along with histamine and heparin. Although 5-HT is concentrated in blood platelets, it is not synthesized there because of lack of decarboxylase. It appears to be bound within cytoplasmic granules and is also continually produced and destroyed in the pool of the intestine and brain. In platelets it appears to be released only upon their destruction.

Most 5-HT is metabolized by oxidative deamination to form 5-hydroxyindoleacetic acid (5-HIAA); the enzyme catalyzing this reaction is monoamine oxidase. The end product of metabolism, 5-HIAA, is excreted in urine. However, in the pineal gland, *N*-acetylation and 5-methylation of 5-HT form the hormone melatonin.

NEURONAL UPTAKE OF 5-HT. After 5-HT is synthesized, it is stored within secretory granules in the axon terminal from which it is released by exocytosis upon arrival of the action potential. The action of intrasynaptic 5-HT is terminated in large part by a neuronal membrane uptake transporter localized in the axon terminals of the 5-HT neurons. This reuptake by the neurons diminishes 5-HT availability at the postsynaptic 5-HT receptors of the effector cells, thereby regulating the duration and intensity of action of 5-HT. Pharmacologic blockade of the 5-HT uptake mechanism thereby prolongs the availability and action of 5-HT at its receptors on the effector cells. The action of 5-HT is subsequently intensified. The 5-HT transporter has been cloned; it is selective for 5-HT and distinctly different from the intraneuronal storage granule uptake mechanism.

The 5-HT neuronal uptake transporter has become important to neuropharmacology in both human and veterinary medicine (Crowell-Davis and Murray 2006). Drugs that inhibit 5-HT uptake, known as selective serotonin reuptake inhibitors (SSRIs or SRIs), are used extensively to treat depression and other neurological disorders, alone or cojointly with drugs that inhibit norepinephrine reuptake into noradrenergic neurons (Sanders-Bush and Mayer 2006). In veterinary medicine SSRIs are used in attempts to control various behavioral disorders in small animals (see Chapter 21). Their clinical use is becoming more common in animals owing to the increased recognition by veterinarians that treatment of behavioral problems in dogs and cats can often be facilitated by drugs that enhance the action of CNS neurotransmitters such as 5-HT, norepinephrine, and dopamine (Crowell-Davis and Murray 2006). The SSRIs include citalopram, sertraline (Zoloft), fluoxetine (Prozac, Reconcile), venlafaxine (effexor), paroxetine, fluvoxamine, and bupropion (Wellbutrin). Of these, only fluoxetine has been registered for dogs, although the others have been used off-label. Clomipramine (Clomicalm) (anafranil) is a tricyclic antidepressant that has been approved for the treatment of separation anxiety in dogs; it inhibits the neuronal reuptake of both 5-HT and norepinphrine (Crowell-Davis and Murray 2006).

SUBTYPES OF 5-HT RECEPTORS. Because of the wide variety of pharmacologic actions produced by 5-HT, multiple types of receptors seemed likely (Bonasera and Tecott 2000). Subsequent investigations including cloning of receptor cDNAs confirmed that there was indeed an impressive variety of 5-HT receptor families comprising at least seven major receptor types and several respective subtypes. Although their full spectrum of physiologic effects and pharmacodynamic actions has only been partially characterized, most of the 5-HT receptors (except 5-HT_3) are believed to be typical G-protein coupled receptor complexes (Sanders-Bush and Mayer 2006).

The seven major 5-HT receptor families are designated as 5-HT_1 through 5-HT_7. The 5-HT_1 family has five members designated 5-HT_{1A}, 5-HT_{1B}, 5-HT_{1D}, 5-HT_{1E}, and 5-HT_{1F}. All five 5-HT_1 receptors inhibit adenylyl cyclase, thereby reducing intracellular concentrations of the cyclic nucleotide cyclic AMP. The 5-HT_{1A} receptor also inhibits a voltage gated Ca^{2+} channel, but activates a receptor-coupled K^+ channel. The 5-HT_1 receptors in the CNS subserve a variety of excitatory and inhibitory neurotransmitter actions in different regions of the brain. 5-HT_{1A}-receptor agonists include buspirone, gepirone, and ipsapirone; these agents comprise a new class of antianxiety drugs in human medicine. The 5-HT_{1D} agonist sumatriptan constricts intracranial blood vessels, an action that helps reduce migraine headaches in humans. The 5-HT_{1B} selective agonists seem to share this action.

Three subtypes of 5-HT_2 receptors (5-HT_{2A-C}) also have been identified; they activate the phospholipase C-diacylglycerol-inositol triphosphate triade, culminating in mobilization of intracellular Ca^{2+} stores (Janssen 1983; Gray and Roth 2001).

Unlike the other 5-HT receptor types, the 5-HT_3 receptor is the only known monoamine receptor believed to serve as a ligand-operated ion channel (Derkach et al. 1989), somewhat analogous to the nicotinic cholinergic receptor (see Chapter 9). The 5-HT_3 receptor promotes a rapidly desensitizing depolarization, presumably due to the efflux of K^+ through its opened channels. The 5-HT_3 receptors are present both in the CNS and peripheral neurons, with one action associated with coordination of the emetic response.

The 5-HT_4 receptors are located in various regions of the CNS and the gastrointestinal tract (Hegde and Eglen 1996), where they are coupled to activation of adenyl cyclase through the excitatory G-protein (G_S). The actions and effects of the 5-HT_5, 5-HT_6, and 5-HT_7 receptor types remain to be clearly defined (Descarries et al. 1990; Skidgel and Erdös 2006).

PHARMACOLOGIC EFFECTS. 5-HT exerts multiple actions with great variation in different species, reflecting its multiple locations and plethora of receptor types. Its essential effects are on smooth muscle and central and peripheral nerves, including afferent nerve endings. Given orally, it is quickly degraded and produces no effect.

Rapid IV injection of 5-HT produces a triphasic response: an initial fall of systemic arterial pressure accompanied by paradoxical bradycardia, caused mainly by reflex chemoreceptor stimulation (Bezod-Jarisch effect); a short period of pressor effect (similar to epinephrine effect); and a prolonged fall in systemic blood pressure attributed to a vasodilator effect in the vascular bed of skeletal muscle. 5-HT also causes a fall in pulmonary arterial pressure (pulmonary depressor reflex). A continuous infusion of 5-HT, which most closely resembles endogenous release of this agent, causes a prolonged fall in arterial pressure as a result of vascular bed dilation. Only in rodents does this agent increase small vessel permeability similar to effects of histamine.

The nonvascular smooth muscle of the bronchi and intestines is stimulated by 5-HT. In the intestine, as a local hormone, 5-HT initiates a peristaltic reflex in response to local stimulation. Among the receptors, 5-HT_3 is inhibitory, and 5-HT_4 is excitatory. Several drugs affect these receptors: cisapride is an agonist for 5-HT_4; metoclopramide is an agonist for 5-HT_4 and antagonist for 5-HT_3. Ondansetron, which is used as an antiemetic agent has modest prokinetic activity via 5-HT_3 antagonism. Tagaserod and Prucalopride, two new drugs not yet used in animals, act as 5-HT_4 agonists with colon-specific effects. The clinical use of these drugs to affect GI motility is discussed in more detail in Chapter 47.

When 5-HT is injected, it has no effect on the brain or spinal cord because it is strongly polar and cannot effectively cross the blood-brain barrier. However, 5-HTP can penetrate into the brain and be decarboxylated to 5-HT; this may produce behavioral changes. 5-HT can also stimulate afferent nerve endings, ganglion cells, and adrenal medullary cells. 5-HT can also stimulate vomiting because the chemoreceptor trigger zone that stimulates vomiting in the area postrema is outside of the blood-brain barrier.

ROLE IN PHYSIOLOGIC AND PATHOLOGIC PROCESSES. The finding that 5-HT is present in the CNS, the hypothalamus, and other areas led to identification of its role as a central neurotransmitter. 5-HT influences sleep, sensory perception, cognition, motor activity, appetite, intestinal motility, temperature regulation, and mood and behavior (Crowell-Davis and Murray 2006). An excess of this agent brings about CNS stimulation and mood elevation, while a deficiency produces mood depression. The addition of SSRIs as a separate class of antidepressant drugs followed the realization that increasing the concentration of 5-HT at its CNS receptor sites could improve mood (see Chapter 21). The role of 5-HT in platelets is related to the mechanism of hemostasis via both vasoconstriction and platelet aggregation.

5-HT AGONISTS AND ANTAGONISTS. Because several classes and subclasses of 5-HT receptors have been identified (Derkach et al. 1989), it is not surprising that 5-HT receptor antagonists and agonists comprise a broad group of chemically unrelated compounds. Neural effects of 5-HT in smooth muscle of the digestive tract are antagonized by morphine, atropine, and cocaine; the direct effects on smooth muscle are antagonized by phenoxybenzamine and two derivatives of ergot alkaloids, LSD and methysergide. An antihistamine, cyproheptadine, is also a clinically important antiserotonin agent. Chlorpromazine and phenoxybenzamine are weak 5-HT receptor blocking agents. Reserpine and compound 48/80 are examples of drugs that deplete serotonin in the brain. Another antagonist frequently used experimentally is *p*-chlorphenylamine, but this agent acts by inhibition of serotonin synthesis. Methysergide blocks both 5-HT_{2A} and 5-HT_{2C} receptors; it has been used in human medicine to prevent migraine headaches and gastrointestinal signs of dumping syndrome and the carcinoid syndrome (Sanders-Bush and Mayer 2006). Cyproheptadine acts on 5-HT_{1A} receptors, but it is also a H_1 antihistamine. Ketanserin is a 5-HT antagonist that acts preferentially at the 5-HT_{2A} receptor subtype without significant action at the 5-HT_1 or 5-HT_3 receptors. It is also an H_1 antihistamine and an α-adrenergic blocker.

The areas in which drugs have been most widely investigated in veterinary medicine are the use of cyproheptadine in animals to treat inflammatory conditions and to stimulate appetite, the use of serotonin antagonists to treat vomiting, the use of serotonin agonists to stimulate gastrointestinal motility, and the use of drugs that modify serotonin CNS receptors or alter the reuptake of serotonin to treat behavioral disorders. The use for treating behavior disorders is discussed in detail in Chapter 21 and by Crowell-Davis and Murray (2006). The gastrointestinal uses of these drugs (agonists and antagonists) are discussed in Chapter 47.

Cyproheptadine. Cyproheptadine (Periactin) is a serotonin antagonist and a modest antagonist for histamine (H_1). It has been used to treat inflammatory conditions of the skin (dermatitis) and the airways. It is also used as an appetite stimulant in cats, presumably by inhibiting serotonergic receptors in the hypothalamus that control satiety. Doses used to stimulate appetite in cats are in the range of 1 mg per cat orally once daily, to as high as 8 mg orally, every 8 hours. In cats the half-life is approximately 8 and 12 hours after IV and oral administration, respectively, suggesting that twice-daily administration would be sufficient in most cats (Norris et al. 1998). It was completely absorbed after oral administration (Norris et al. 1998).

Serotonin is reported to be one of the inflammatory mediators in the airways of animals—particularly the acute phase response of asthma. Serotonin is a mediator released from mast cells in the respiratory tract. Therefore, serotonin antagonists such as cyproheptadine in cats should theoretically produce some benefit against smooth muscle constriction, vasodilation, increased vascular permeability, and inflammatory cell influx. Cyproheptadine attenuated the smooth muscle constriction induced by serotonin in airway smooth muscle from sensitized cats (Padrid et al. 1995). Cyproheptadine also has decreased airway reactivity to serotonin infusion in healthy cats (Reiche and Frey 1983) and at a dose of 2 mg/kg orally q12h it decreased airway reactivity in cats with airway hyperresponsiveness (Reinero et al. 2005). However, in cats with experimentally induced asthma, cyproheptadine at a dose of 8 mg per cat orally it produced limited results (Schooley et al. 2007). It did not decrease eosinophilic infiltration in the airways of treated cats. These authors suggested that perhaps mediators other than histamine and serotonin are responsible for airway responses in asthmatic cats and antihistamines and cetirizine as sole therapy will produce minimal benefit. Adverse effects in cats have not been studied, but side effects of aggression and stimulation have been observed. Additional discussion of drugs that affect the respiratory tract is included in Chapter 49.

REFERENCES

Akdis, C. A., Simons, F. E. 2006. Histamine receptors are hot in immunopharmacology. Eur J Pharmacol 533:69–76.

Arang, J. M., Garbarg, M., Lancelot, J. C., Lecomte, J. M., Pollard, H., Robba, M., Schunack, W., Schwartz, J. C. 1987. Highly potent and selective ligands for histamine H_3-receptors. Nature 327:117–23.

Ash, A. S., Schild, H. O. 1966. Receptors mediating some actions of histamine. Br J Pharmacol 27:427–39.

Barnes, P. J., Belvisi, M. G., Rogers, D. F. 1990. Modulation of neurogenic inflammation: novel approaches to inflammatory disease. TIPS 11:185–89.

Bizikova, P., Papich, M. G., Olivry, T. 2008. Hydroxyzine and cetirizine pharmacokinetics and pharmacodynamics after oral and intravenous administration of hydroxyzine to healthy dogs. (In press)

Black, J. W., Duncan, W. A., Durant, C. J., et al. 1972. Definition and antagonism of histamine H2-receptors. Nature 236:385–90.

Bonasera, S. J., Tecott, L. H. 2000. Mouse models of serotonin receptor function: Toward a genetic dissection of serotonin systems. Pharmacol Ther 88:133–142.

Bovet, D., Staub, A. M. 1937. Action protectrice des ethers phenoliques au cours de l'intoxication histaminique. CR Soc Biol (Paris) 124:547–49.

Chand, N., Eyre, P. 1975. Classification and biological distribution of histamine receptor subtypes. Agents Actions 5:277–95.

Clough, G. F., Bennett, A. R., Church, M. K. 1998. Effects of H1 antagonists on the cutaneous vascular response to histamine and bradykinin: a study using scanning laser Doppler imaging. Br J Dermatol 138:806–14.

Crowell-Davis, S., Murray, T. 2006. Veterinary Psychopharmacology. Iowa: Blackwell Publishing.

Dale, H. H., Laidlaw, P. P. 1910. The physiological action of β-iminazolylethylamine. J Physiol (Lond) 41:318–44.

DeBoer, D. J., Griffin, C. E. 2001. The ACVD task force on canine atopic dermatitis (XXI): antihistamine pharmacotherapy. Vet Immunol Immunopath 81:323–329.

DeMora, F., Puigdemont, A., Torres, R. 2006. The role of mast cells in atopy: what can we learn from canine models? A thorough review of the biology of mast cells in canine and human systems. Br J Dermatol 155:1109–23.

Derkach, V., Surprenant, A., North, R. A. 1989. 5-HT_3 receptors are membrane ion channels. Nature 339:706–9.

Descarries, L., Audet, M. A., Doucet, G., et al. 1990. Morphology of central serotonin neurons. Brief review of quantified aspects of their distribution and ultrastructural relationships. Ann NY Acad Sci 600:81–92.

Douglas, W. W. 1974. Involvement of calcium in exocytosis and the exocytosis-vesiculation sequence. Biochem Soc Symp 39:1–28.

Erspamer, V., Asero, B. 1952. Identification of entermine, a specific hormone of enterochromaffin cell system, as 5-hydroxytryptamine. Nature 169:800–801.

Esbenshade, T. A., Krueger, K. M., Miller, T. R., et al. 2003. Two novel and selective nonimidazole histamine H_3 receptor antagonists A-304121 and A-317920: I. In vitro pharmacological effects. J Pharmacol Exp Ther 305:887–896.

Eyre, P., Burka, J. F. 1978. Hypersensitivity in cattle and sheep: A pharmacological review. J Vet Pharmacol Ther 1:97–109.

Eyre, P., Wells, P. W. 1973. Histamine H2-receptors modulate systemic anaphylaxis: a dual cardiovascular action of histamine in calves. Br J Pharmacol 49:364–67.

Falus, A., Meretey, K. 1992. Histamine: an early messenger in inflammatory and immune reactions. Immunol Today 13:154–56.

Garcia, G., DeMora, F., Ferrer, L., Puigdemont, A. 1997. Effect of H1-antihistamines on histamine release from dispersed canine cutaneous mast cells. Am J Vet Res 58:293–297.

Gelfand, E. W., Appajosyula, S., Meeves, S. 2004. Antiinflammatory activity of H_1-receptor antagonists: Review of recent experimental research. Curr Med Res Opin 20:73–81.

Goth, A., Johnson, A. R. 1975. Current concepts on the secretory function of mast cells. Life Sci 16:1201–13.

Gray, J. A., Roth, B. L. 2001. Paradoxical trafficking and regulation of $5HT_{2A}$ receptors by agonists and antagonists. Brain Res Bull 56:441–451.

Green, T. K., Harvey, J. A. 1974. Enhancement of amphetamine action after interruption of ascending serotonergic pathways. J Pharmacol Exp Ther 190:109–17.

Guedes, A. G., Papich, M. G., Rude, E. P., Rider, M. A. 2007. Comparison of plasma histamine levels after intravenous administration of hydromorphone and morphine in dogs. J Vet Pharmacol Ther 30(6):516–22.

Guedes, A. G., Rudé, E. P., Rider, M. A. 2006. Evaluation of histamine release during constant rate infusion of morphine in dogs. Vet Anaesth Analg 33(1):28–35.

Hancock, A. A., Esbenshade, T. A., Krueger, K. M., Yao, B. B. 2003. Genetic and pharmacological aspects of histamine H_3 receptor heterogeneity. Life Sci 73:3043–3072.

Hansson, H., Bergvall, K., Bondesson, U., Hedeland, M., Törneke, K. 2004. Clinical pharmacology of clemastine in healthy dogs. Vet Derm 15:152–158.

Hegde, S. S., Eglen, R. M. 1996. Peripheral 5-HT_4 receptors. FASEB J 10:1398–1407.

Hirschowitz, B. I. 1979. H-2 histamine receptors. Annu Rev Pharmacol 19:203–44.

Hofmeister E. H., Egger C. M. 2005. Evaluation of diphenhydramine as a sedative for dogs. J Am Vet Med Assoc 226:1092–1094.

Hofstra, C. L., Desai, P. J., Thurmond, R. L., Fung-Leung, W.-P. 2003. Histamine H_4 receptor mediates chemotaxis and calcium mobilization of mast cells. J Pharmacol Exp Ther 305:1212–1221.

Hough, L. B. 2001. Genomics meets histamine receptors: New subtypes, new receptors. Mol Pharmacol 59:415–419.

Janssen, P. A. J. 1983. 5-HT_2 receptor blockade to study serotonin-induced pathology. Trends Pharmacol Sci 4:198–206.

Janssens, M. M. L., Howart, P. H. 1993. The antihistamines of the nineties. Clin Rev Allergy 11:111–53.

Johanek, L. M., Meyer, R. A., Hartke, T., et al. 2007. Psychophysical and physiological evidence for parallel afferent pathways mediating the sensation of itch. J Neurosci 27:7490–7.

Lambert, D. G. 1993. Signal transduction: G proteins and second messengers. Br J Anaesth 71:86–95.

Leurs, R., Church, M. K., Taglialatela, M. 2002. H_1 antihistamines: Inverse agonism, antiinflammatory actions and cardiac effects. Clin Exp Allergy 32:489–498.

Leurs, R., Wantanabe, T., Timmerman, H. 2001. Histamine receptors are finally "coming out." Trends Pharmacol Sci 22:337–339.

Lichtenstein, L. M., Margolis, S. 1968. Histamine release in vitro: Inhibition by catecholamines and methylxanthines. Science 161: 902–3.

Ling, P., Ngo, K., Nguyen, S., et al. 2004. Histamine H_4 receptor mediates eosinophil chemotaxis with cell shape change and adhesion molecule up-regulation. Brit J Pharmacol 142:161–178.

Lovenberg, T. W., Roland, B. L., Wilson, S. J., et al. 1999. Cloning and functional expression of the human histamine H_3 receptor. Mol Pharmacol 55:1101–1105.

MacGlashan, D. 2003. Histamine: A mediator of inflammation. J Allergy Clin Immunol 112:S13–S19.

Meeves, S. G., Appajosyula, S. 2003. Efficacy and safety profile of fexofenadine HCL: A unique therapeutic option in H_1-receptor antagonist treatment. J Allergy Clin Immunol 112:S29–S37.

Merchant S. R., Taboada J. 1989. Antihistaminic drugs: H1-receptor antagonists in dogs and cats. J Am Vet Med Assoc 195:647–649.

Miller, W. H., Jr., Griffin, G. E., Scott, D. W., et al. 1989. Clinical trial of DVM DermCaps in the treatment of allergic disease in dogs: a nonblinded study. J Am Anim Hosp Assoc 25:163.

Miller, W. H., Scott, D. W. 1990. Efficacy of chlorpheniramine maleate for management of pruritus in cats. JAVMA 197(1):67–70.

Mitsuhashi, M., Payan, D. G. 1992. Functional diversity of histamine and histamine receptors. J Invest Dermatol 98:8S–11S.

Mohammed, S. P., Higenbottam, T. W., Adcock, J. J. 1993. Effects of aerosol-applied capsaicin, histamine, and prostaglandin F2 on airway sensory receptors of anesthetized cats. J Physiol 469–451.

Mohammad-Zadeh, L. F., Moses, L., Gwaltney-Brant, S. M. 2008. Serotonin: a review. J Vet Pharmacol Ther (In press)

Morris, A. I. 1992. The success of histamine-2 receptor antagonists. Scand J Gastroenterol 27(Suppl 194):71–75.

Norris, C. R., Boothe, D. M., Esparza, T., Gray, C., Ragsdale, M. 1998. Disposition of cyproheptadine in cats after intravenous or oral administration of a single dose. Am J Vet Res 59:79–81.

Obrink, K. J. 1991. Histamine and gastric acid secretion. Scand J Gastroenterol 26(Suppl 180):4–8.

Oda, T., Morikawa, N., Saito, Y., Masuho, Y., Matsumoto, S.-I. 2000. Molecular cloning and characterization of a novel type of histamine receptor preferentially expressed in leukocytes. J Biol Chem 275:36781–36786.

Olivry, T., Mueller, R. S., et al. 2003. Evidence-based veterinary dermatology: a systemic review of the pharmacotherapy of canine atopic dermatitis. Vet Dermatol 14:121–146.

Padrid, P. A., Mitchell, R. W., Ndukwu, I. M., et al. 1995. Cyproheptadine-induced attenuation of type-1 immediate-hypersensitivity reactions of airway smooth muscle from immune-sensitized cats. Am J Vet Res 56:109–115. *(Erratum published in Am J Vet Res 56:402, 1995).*

Papich, M. G. 2000. Antihistamines: current therapeutic use. In J. D. Bonagura, ed., Kirk's Current Veterinary Therapy 13th Edition. Philadelphia: W.B. Saunders Company. pp. 48–53.

Paradis, M., Lemay, S., Scott, D. W. 1991. The efficacy of clemastine (Tavist), a fatty acid-containing product (Derm Caps) and the combination of both products in the management of canine pruritus. Vet Derm 2:17–20.

Paradis, M., Scott, D. W., Giroux, D. 1991. Further investigations on the use of nonsteroidal and steroidal anti-inflammatory agents in the management of canine pruritus. J Am Anim Hosp Assoc 27:44–48.

Pearce, F. L. 1991. Biological effects of histamine: an overview. Agent Actions 33:4–7.

Rapport, M. M., Green, A. A., Page, I. H. 1948. Serum vasoconstrictor (serotonin); isolation and characterization. J Biol Chem 176:1243–51.

Reiche, R., Frey, H. H. 1983. Antagonist of the 5-HT induced bronchoconstriction in the cat. Arch Int Pharmacodyn 263:139–145.

Reinero, C. R., Decile, K. C., Byerly, J. R., et al. 2005. Effects of drug treatment on inflammation and hyper-reactivity of airways and on immune variables in cats with experimentally induced asthma. Am J Vet Res 66:1121–1127.

Rizk, A., Curley, J., Robertson, J., Raber, J. 2004. Anxiety and cognition in histamine H_3 receptor/mice. Eur J Neurosci 19:1992–1996.

Roudebush, P. 2001. Consumption of essential fatty acids in selected commercial dog foods compared to dietary supplementation: an update. Proceedings of the Annual AAVD/ACVD Meeting.

Sanders-Bush, E., Fentress, H., Hazelwood, L. 2003. Serotonin 5-HT_2 receptors: molecular and genomic diversity. Mol Interv 3:319–330.

Sanders-Bush, E., Mayer, S. E. 2006. 5-Hydroxtryptamine (Serotonin): Receptor Agonists and Antagonist. In L. L. Brunton, J. S. Lazo, K. L. Parker, eds., The Pharmacologic Basis of Therapeutics, 11th ed. New York: McGraw Hill.

Schayer, R. W., Cooper, J. A. D. 1956. Metabolism of C14 histamine in man. J Appl Physiol 9:481–83.

Schooley, E. K., McGee, J. B., McGee Turner, J. B., Jiji, R. D., Spinka, C. M., Reinero, C. R. 2007. Effects of cyproheptadine and cetirizine on eosinophilic airway inflammation in cats with experimentally induced asthma. 68:1265–1271.

Schror, K. 1992. Role of prostaglandins in the cardiovascular effects of bradykinin and angiotensin-converting enzyme inhibitors. J Cardiovasc Pharmacol 20(Suppl 9):S68–S73.

Schwieler, J. H., Hjemdahl, P. 1992. Influence of angiotensin-converting enzyme inhibition on sympathetic neurotransmission: possible roles of bradykinin and prostaglandins. J Cardiovasc Pharmacol 20(Suppl9): S39–S46.

Scott, D. W., Buerger, R. G. 1988. Nonsteroidal antiinflammatory agents in the management of canine pruritus. J Am Animal Hosp Assoc 24:425–428.

Simons, F. E. 2003. H_1-Antihistamines: More relevant than ever in the treatment of allergic disorders. J Allergy Clin Immunol 112: S42–S52.

———. 2004. Advances in H1-antihistamines. N Engl J Med 351:2203–17.

Simons, F. E. R., Simons, K. J. 1994. The pharmacology and use of H_1-receptor-antagonists. New Engl J Med 330:1663–1670.

Skidgel, R. A., Erdös E. G. 2006. Histamine, bradykinin, and their antagonists. In L. L. Brunton, J. S. Lazo, K. L. Parker, eds., The Pharmacologic Basis of Therapeutics, 11th ed. New York: McGraw Hill.

Stark, H., Arrang, J. M., Ligneau, X., et al. 2001. The histamine H_3 receptor and its ligands. Prog Med Chem 38:279–308.

Sun, H., Dai, H., Shaik, N., Elmquist, W. F. 2003. Drug efflux transporters in the CNS. Adv Drug Deliv Rev 55:83–105.

Takeshita, K., Sakai, K., Bacon, K. B., Gantner, F. 2003. Critical role of histamine H_4 receptor in leukotriene B_4 production and mast cell-dependent neutrophil recruitment induced by zymosan in vivo. J Pharmacol Exp Ther 307:1072–1078.

Thurmond, R. L., Deais, P. J., Dunford, P. F., et al. 2004. A potent and selective histamine H_4 receptor antagonist with anti-inflammatory properties. J Pharmacol Exp Ther 309:404–413.

Törneke, K., Ingvast-Larsson, K., Bergvall, K., Hedeland, M., Bondesson, U., Broström, H. 2003. Pharmacokinetics and pharmacodynamics of clemastine in healthy horses. J Vet Pharmacol Therap 26: 151–157.

Walsh, G. M. 2005. Anti-inflammatory properties of antihistamines: an update. Clin Exper Allergy Rev 5:21–25.

Walther, D. J., Peter, J. U., Bashammakh, S., et al. 2003. Synthesis of serotonin by a second tryptophan hydroxylase isoform. Science 299:76.

Yates, B. J., Miller, A. D., Sucot, J. B. 1998. Physiological basis and pharmacology of motion sickness: an update. Brain Res Bull 47:395–406.

Zur, G., Ihrke, P. J., White, S. D., Kass, P. H. 2002. Antihistamines in the management of canine atopic dermatitis: a retrospective study of 171 dogs (1992–1998). Vet Therapeut 3:88–96.

CHAPTER

17

PEPTIDES: ANGIOTENSIN AND KININS

H. RICHARD ADAMS

ANGIOTENSIN

The ischemic kidney releases a pressor agent into the circulation where it provokes a systemic hypertensive response. The pressor substance, identified as renin, is an enzyme that acts on a plasma substrate, resulting in formation of a peptide with exceptional vasoconstrictor potency. The peptide was called "hypertensin" and "angiotonin" until 1958 when the compromise term *angiotensin* was adopted (Braun-Menendez and Page 1958).

Angiotensin is a bloodborne polypeptide that serves as a circulating link between the kidney and systemic hemodynamic control systems (Matsusaka and Ichikawa 1997). This peptide is not manufactured directly by the kidney but is formed within the blood by a complex series of reactions initiated by the renal enzyme renin. Release of renin by the kidney is accelerated when this organ is subjected to physiologic stimuli associated with hypovolemia, hypotension, or hyponatremia (Bernstein 1993; Jackson 2006).

The renin-angiotensin relationship was complicated by the discovery that, after entering the bloodstream, renin and its substrate (angiotensinogen) yielded an inactive precursor, the decapeptide angiotensin I, which was then converted by other enzymes to the active octapeptide angiotensin II. The latter is an exceptionally potent vasoconstrictor agent and a stimulant of aldosterone secretion. Angiotensin II evokes an increase in peripheral vascular resistance and a reduction of urine and salt output, thereby tending to restore blood pressure and blood volume to more normal values. Pharmacologic manipulation of this system has recently gained considerable importance in clinical medicine. The angiotensin-converting enzyme inhibitors are now one of the most commonly used drugs to treat heart failure and hypertension (Dietz et al. 1993; Holtz 1993). Because angiotensin modulates cardiac cellular growth and hypertrophy, angiotensin-converting enzyme inhibitors are also being evaluated in treatment of cardiac hypertrophic states (Matsusaka and Ichikawa 1997; Jackson 2006).

The biologic half-life of angiotensin II was found to be quite brief because of the presence in plasma and tissues of proteolytic enzymes, collectively referred to as *angiotensinases.* A heptapeptide fragment of angiotensin II, originally thought to be an inactive metabolite, was found to possess considerable pharmacologic activity. The active fragment is now referred to as angiotensin III. In the following discussion, the term angiotensin is used to refer to angiotensin II unless otherwise noted.

ENDOGENOUS RENIN-ANGIOTENSIN SYSTEM

Renin Release. Renin is a proteolytic enzyme synthesized and stored within cytoplasmic granules of modified smooth muscle cells that line the afferent arteriole of the glomerulus. Both the afferent and efferent arterioles are associated anatomically and functionally with the macula densa, a group of specialized cells localized at the origin of the distal tubule of the nephron. The entire structure is referred to as the juxtaglomerular apparatus (Oparil and Haber 1974; Johnston 1992).

Renin is released from the juxtaglomerular apparatus in response to several stimuli associated with hypotension, hypovolemia, or hyponatremia (Friis et al. 2002). Factors that reduce blood volume, renal perfusion pressure, or plasma sodium concentration tend to stimulate release of renin, while factors that increase these parameters tend to lower it (Gibbons et al. 1984; Bernstein 1993). Secretion of renin is regulated by an intrarenal baroreceptor mechanism of the afferent arteriole, an intrarenal chemoreceptor mechanism of the macula densa, the renal sympathetic nerves acting through a β_1 adrenoceptor, and several humoral agents. These factors often interact with each other, resulting in considerable complexity. Basic aspects are summarized below and in Figure 17.1.

An intrarenal baroreceptor mechanism detects and responds to changes in wall tension or transmural pressure gradients in the afferent arteriole of the glomerulus. Renin release from the juxtaglomerular apparatus is increased when renal blood flow and, especially, renal blood pressure are decreased. Intrarenal prostaglandins serve as a chemical link between pressure and sodium changes and the resulting increase in renin secretion, at least within the autoregulatory range of renal blood flow (Schror 1992; Schwieler and Hjemdahl 1992). Both COX-1 and COX-2 are found in the kidney (Cheng et al. 2001; Kammerl et al. 2002), but it is the inducible isoform COX-2 that is localized in the macula densa, where it is up-regulated by chronic hyponatremia. The constitutive form of nitric oxide synthase in local neurons is also believed to participate in controlling renin release (Cheng et al. 2000).

The macula densa serves as a Na^+-sensitive and perhaps Cl^--sensitive chemoreceptor that detects these ions in renal tubular fluid. If Na^+ and/or Cl^- concentrations are reduced, renin release is increased.

Activation of the renal sympathetic nerves evokes release of renin. This response is mediated by an intrarenal β-adrenergic receptor. An α-adrenergic receptor that subserves an inhibitory effect on renin release seems to be present within the kidney, but its importance is not known.

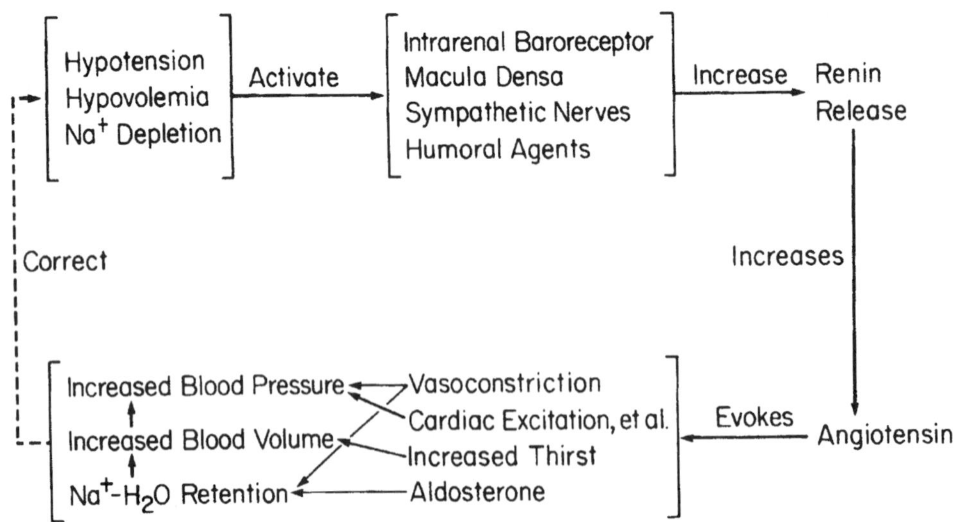

FIG. 17.1 Hemodynamic interrelationships of the renin-angiotensin system.

Several circulating humoral agents and electrolytes influence renin release. Angiotensin itself can feed back to inhibit renin release; vasopressin is also inhibitory. Because angiotensin acts on the brain to increase release of vasopressin, there seems to be a vasopressin-angiotensin feedback loop. Other agents that can influence renin release include catecholamines, prostaglandins, cyclic nucleotides, K^+, Mg^{++}, Ca^{++}, serotonin, adenosine, and others. The importance of all these factors to normal control of renin release has not been fully determined (Jackson 2006), and there may be species differences in which factors are dominant.

Angiotensin Formation. The renin substrate, angiotensinogen, is a large glycoprotein synthesized by the liver. Once in the blood, renin cleaves the bond that joins the *N*-terminal 10 amino acid sequence to the remainder of angiotensinogen. The released decapeptide is angiotensin I; it can be considered as a circulating and essentially inactive prohormone to angiotensin II (Ardaillou 1997). After the decapeptide angiotensin I is formed, two amino acids are removed from its *C*-terminus by angiotensin converting enzyme (ACE) to yield the octapeptide angiotensin II. The sequential formation of angiotensin is summarized in Figure 17.2. Converting enzymes are present in endothelial cells throughout the body, but especially the lungs. Virtually all the circulating angiotensin I can be converted to angiotensin II by a single passage through the pulmonary vascular circuit. The angiotensin-converting enzyme is also known as kininase II, the enzyme responsible for inactivating bradykinin.

In addition to the standard ACE, a novel ACE-related carboxypeptidase termed ACE2 has been identified (Yagil and Yagil 2003). ACE2 cleaves angiotensin I to angiotensin (1–9) and angiotensin II to angiotensin (1–7). The physiologic function of ACE2 is unknown, but it may serve as a counterregulatory mechanism to oppose ACE (Moore et al. 2001; Yagil and Yagil 2003). Interestingly, it seems ACE2 may be a receptor for the SARS virus (Li et al. 2003). ACE2 is not susceptible to the ACE inhibitory drugs used clinically, but it may participate in cardiac function (Crackower 2002). Angiotensin II is metabolized rapidly by plasma and tissue angiotensinases. The best characterized of the plasma enzymes are an aminopeptidase (angiotensinase A) and a less important endopeptidase (angiotensinase B). A heptapeptide fragment of

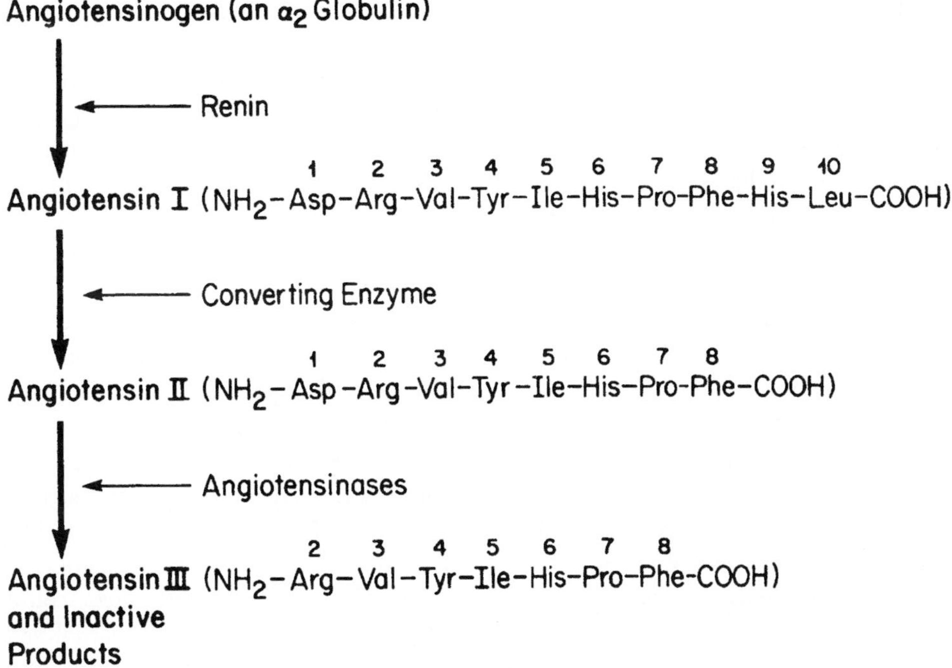

FIG. 17.2 Sequential formation of angiotensins I, II, and III. The structure of angiotensin shown is that found in the rat, pig, horse, and human. Bovine angiotensin contains valine in position 5.

angiotensin II is des-Asp[1] angiotensin II or, as it is now named, angiotensin III. This peptide shares many of the pharmacologic actions of its parent molecule, especially the ability to stimulate aldosterone secretion. However, the physiologic significance of angiotensin III in the intact animal remains debatable.

Cardiovascular Effects. Angiotensin II exerts a wide spectrum of circulatory effects that are directed toward maintenance of blood pressure and volume (Cody 1997; Matsusaka and Ichikawa 1997). First, angiotensin produces a pronounced vasoconstriction as a result of direct stimulation of vascular smooth muscle cells that contain an angiotensin (AT) receptor (Berk and Corson 1997). Both AT_1 and AT_2 receptor subtypes have been identified (Hansen et al. 2000), but the AT_1 receptor is believed to mediate most of the known biological actions of angiotensin II (Carey et al. 2001). Physiologic functions of the AT_2 receptor are incompletely defined (Henrion et al. 2001), but it may participate in effects opposing those subserved by AT_1 receptors (AbdAlla et al. 2001; Bautista et al. 2004).

The vasoconstrictor effect of angiotensin II is most prominent on arteries and, especially, small arterioles, with less influence on veins. The vasoconstrictor action is most pronounced in the kidney, skin, and splanchnic tissues and less pronounced in the brain, heart, and skeletal muscle. The net result is an increase in peripheral vascular resistance and hence in blood pressure (Griendling and Alexander 1990).

Angiotensin also increases cardiac output by direct stimulation of the heart and action on the sympathetic nervous system. By an effect on the brain, angiotensin elicits an increase in sympathetic discharge to the heart and blood vessels. This contributes further to increases in cardiac output and vascular resistance. Angiotensin also provokes release of norepinephrine and epinephrine from the adrenal medulla, facilitates release of norepinephrine from postganglionic sympathetic neurons, stimulates sympathetic ganglia, and decreases uptake of norepinephrine into adrenergic axons. Thus angiotensin produces a state of cardiovascular excitation through several pathways (Peart 1975; Cody 1997; Matsusaka and Ichikawa 1997).

Aside from its direct cardiovascular effects, angiotensin accelerates steroidogenesis in the adrenal cortex. This action results in increased synthesis and release of the mineralocorticoid aldosterone, which acts in turn on the distal tubule of the kidney to increase reabsorption of Na^+ and, subsequently, water (Vecsei et al. 1978). Angiotensin also releases vasopressin (antidiuretic hormone) from the brain and produces a marked dipsogenic effect. All these actions help to expand or restore blood volume and hence assist in maintaining normal blood pressure and circulatory function.

From the above description, it is obvious that the renin-angiotensin system can play an important role in electrolyte-water balance and hemodynamics. Disruptions of this system contribute to certain pathophysiologic states such as renovascular hypertension and aldosteronism. Angiotensin is believed to contribute to maintenance of blood pressure in states of low cardiac output, but may also become part of the pathophysiologic attempt at overcompensation of circulatory adjustments during chronic heart failure syndromes. The physiologic functions of extrarenal renins (the "isorenins" found in blood vessels, the brain, and other tissues) are under considerable study (Ganong 1984; Lee et al. 1993).

PHARMACOLOGY OF THE RENIN-ANGIOTENSIN SYSTEM. Several drugs interact with the renin, angiotensin, and associated enzyme system (Keeton and Campbell 1981; Csajka et al. 1997). The amide of angiotensin II (1-*l*-asparaginyl-5-*l*-valyl angiotensin octapeptide, Hypertensin) activates AT_1 receptors throughout the body. This drug is diluted and administered by slow intravenous infusion for its pressor actions; blood pressure should be monitored continuously.

Saralasin acetate (1-sar-8-ala angiotensin II, Sarenin) was an early prototype for peptide drugs defined as angiotensin receptor blockers. These agents interact with the receptors, thereby preventing angiotensin from eliciting its physiologic-pharmacologic actions. Saralasin and other peptide angiotensin receptor blockers are used experimentally in attempts to define biologic roles of angiotensin. Although these peptide analogs of angiotensin were effective blockers of the angiotensin receptor (Célérier et al. 2002), they were clinically ineffective because they were poorly absorbed after oral administration and they also had partial agonist activity at the receptor sites. Through structural chemistry, a series of non-peptide AT receptor blockers were synthesized; these compounds are orally effective and do not express partial agonist activity. The original non-peptide AT_1 selective blocker was losartan (Cozaar); it was approved for clinical use in humans to counter high blood pressure. Other non-peptide AT blockers include valsartan (Diovan), candesartan cilexetil (Atacand), telmisartan (Micardis), eprosartan (Teveten), olmesartan medoxomil (Benicar), and irbesartan (Avapro). The non-peptide angiotensin receptor blockers are finding considerable use in human medicine as antihypertensive agents, but their extension into veterinary medicine remains unvalidated. In heart failure syndromes, the use of AT receptor blockers after therapy with ACE inhibitors has proven ineffective.

ANGIOTENSIN-CONVERTING ENZYME INHIBITORS. The proline derivative captopril (Capoten) and the related drug enalapril (Vasotec) are inhibitors of angiotensin-converting enzyme. They prevent transformation of angiotensin I to angiotensin II. They also inhibit the inactivation of bradykinin and kallidin. Converting enzyme inhibitors are used to diagnose and treat certain forms of hypertension in humans. Converting enzyme inhibitors also are being used increasingly in human and veterinary medicine to relieve vasoconstriction and lessen fluid retention in patients with congestive heart failure (Knowlen et al. 1983; Dietz et al. 1993; Holtz 1993). An important part of the endogenous compensatory attempt in heart failure syndrome involves increased formation of angiotensin and aldosterone, leading in turn to peripheral vasoconstriction and enhanced urinary reabsorption of salt and water. By preventing the conversion of angiotensin I to angiotensin II, ACE inhibitors lower peripheral vascular resistance, decrease cardiac work load, and diminish the propensity for edema formation by decreasing sodium and water retention (Lage et al. 2002). ACE inhibitors have found therapeutic application in humans with management of hypertension, left ventricular systolic failure, acute myocardial infarction, chronic renal failure during diabetes mellitus, and stroke in high-risk patients. In clinical veterinary medicine, ACE inhibitors are used widely in the management of chronic heart failure (see Chapter 22). ACE inhibitors now available include captopril (Capoten), enalapril (Vasotec), perindopril (Aceon), ramipril (Altace), moexipril (Univasc), lisonopril (Prinivil), trandolapril (Mavik), and quinapril (Accupril).

A large number of drugs used for other therapeutic purposes also influence the renin-angiotensin system; e.g., vasodilators indirectly cause renin release resulting from a reflex increase in sympathetic nervous system discharge to the kidney. General anesthetics also provoke nonspecific increase in renin release. Propranolol inhibits renin secretion by blocking the intrarenal β-adrenergic receptors that subserve release of renin from the juxtaglomerular apparatus (Schwieler and Hjemdahl 1992).

KININS

Discovery of the mammalian kallikrein-kinin system can be traced to the old observation that urine produces a fall in blood pressure when injected intravenously. The urinary principle responsible for the hypotensive activity is an enzyme called kallikrein. However, kallikrein itself does not affect blood pressure directly but converts an inactive α-2 globulin in the plasma, kininogen, into bradykinin, the active depressor substance. Bradykinin and other related polypeptide kinins such as kallidin are exceptionally potent vasodilators. The kinins also increase permeability of the microcirculation, cause contraction of several nonvascular smooth muscles, and evoke pain (Schmaier 2004; Skidgel and Erdös 2006).

Because the kallikrein enzymes are present in various glandular tissues and bodily fluids of mammals, the kinins have been proposed as endogenous mediators of cellular responses to certain types of physiologic and pathophysiologic stimuli. Many aspects remain unresolved, however, and pharmacologic control of the kallikrein-kinin system is still in its infancy (Gainer et al. 1998).

Early studies of kinins were carried out independently by two groups of scientists. The resulting terminology was confusing because of the development of different nomenclatures. One group called their plasma enzyme kallikrein; it formed the active peptide kallidin from the inactive precursor kallidinogen. Other workers reported that trypsin released an active peptide (bradykinin) from a plasma globulin substrate (bradykininogen) (Rocha e Silva et al. 1949).

Similarities between the trypsin-bradykininogen-bradykinin system and the kallikrein-kallidinogen-kallidin system soon became apparent. Schachter and Thain (1954) subsequently introduced the generic term *kinin* to encompass both bradykinin and kallidin, since these two polypeptides exert essentially identical pharmacologic actions. Bradykinin and kallidin are now recognized as members of a group of closely related kinin peptides occurring naturally in wasp, hornet, and other venoms or released from mammalian plasma substrate by kallikreins, trypsin, and certain snake venoms.

Current terminology for the kinin system uses kallikrein-kininogen-kinin as general terms for designating the enzymes, the inactive precursors (substrates), and the active polypeptides, respectively (Skidgel and Erdös 2006).

KININ FORMATION: COMPONENTS AND CHEMISTRY.

A schematic representation of the contributions of kallikrein, kininogen, and other factors to kinin formation is depicted in Figure 17.3.

Kallikreins, Prekallikreins, and Kallikrein Inhibitors

Kallikreins. The term *kallikreins* denotes the endogenous serine protease enzymes that liberate kinins from specific kininogen substrates by limited proteolysis. The term *kininogenase* encompasses the kallikreins and other serine proteases such as trypsin, thrombin, fibrinolysin, and other enzymes that share the common property of releasing kinins from kininogen (Schachter 1980).

Mammals have two basic kallikrein types: plasma and glandular. The latter is localized in exocrine glands and their secretions and has been isolated from porcine pancreas; guinea pig coagulation gland; intestine of the rat, pig, dog, and human; urine from the horse, rat, and human; and saliva from humans. Structurally, the kallikreins are glycoproteins with molecular weights between 24,000 and 43,000 for those of glandular origin and at least 100,000 for the plasma form. In general, the glandular kallikreins yield kallidin, from which bradykinin is formed rapidly by aminopeptidase activity in plasma and tissue (Erdös 1976). Bradykinin is formed directly by plasma kallikrein and also by trypsin, fibrinolysin, and snake venom (Fig. 17.3).

Prekallikreins. Kallikrein is present in some tissues (especially the pancreas, intestines, and plasma) in inactive or prekallikrein forms (referred to formerly as *kallikreinogens*). Prekallikreins are converted to the active mode by various factors that disrupt plasma homeostasis (Fig. 17.3). These include pH changes; organic solvents; trypsin; and contact with glass, collagen, skin, or damaged tissue. The major plasma activators of prekallikreins are the Hageman factor and its fragments, i.e., blood clotting factor XII.

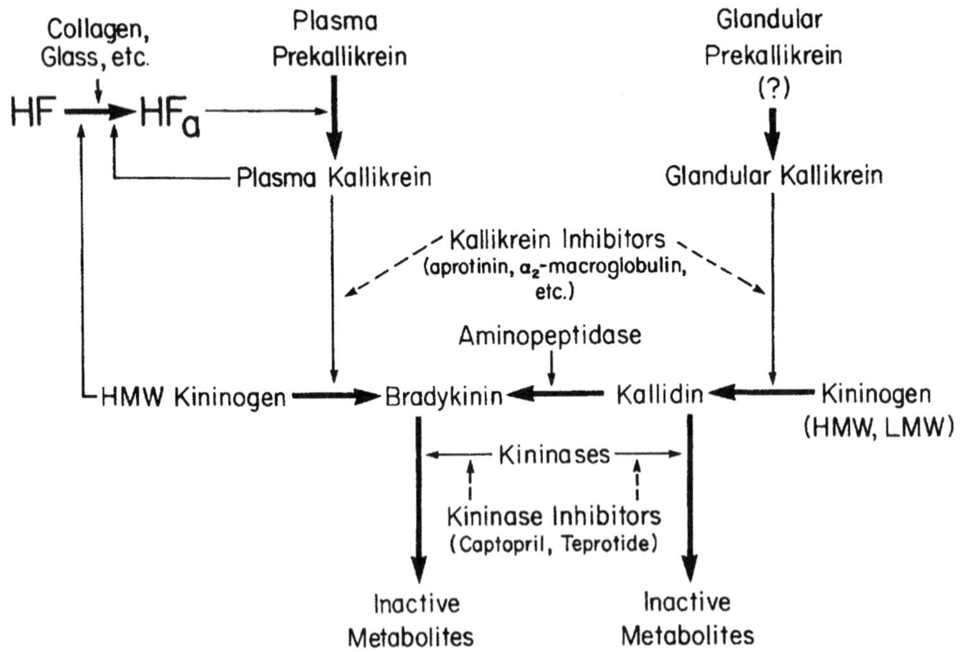

FIG. 17.3 Formation and inactivation of kinins. HF = Hageman factor; HFa = activated HF; HMW and LMW = high and low molecular weight, respectively. Wide solid lines represent conversion of substrate to product. Narrow solid lines represent enzyme acceleration of substrate conversion to product. Dashed lines represent sites of inhibitory actions.

Kallikrein Inhibitors. Once kallikrein is activated, its capability to form kinins is short-lived because of rapid inhibition by several plasma protease inhibitors. These include α_2 macroglobulin, α_1 antitrypsin, antithrombin III, and C,1 esterase inhibitor (Fig. 17.3).

In addition, a polyvalent kallikrein-trypsin inhibitor called aprotinin has been isolated from bovine tissues where it is localized in mast cells (Fritz et al. 1979). This inhibitor is a low-molecular-weight (LMW) protein; it is prepared commercially as Trasylol. Aprotinin has been used outside the USA with varying success in treatment of acute pancreatitis and the carcinoid syndrome in humans.

Kininogens. The kinin precursors, kininogens, are acidic glycoproteins of the α-2 globulin fraction of plasma; they have been isolated from human, bovine, equine, and rabbit blood. At least two plasma kininogens have been identified, the high-molecular-weight (HMW) and the LMW forms. Both types have been isolated from different species, and the HMW and LMW kininogens of bovine origin have molecular weights of 76,000 and 48,000, respectively. The HMW form, also referred to as *substrate 1*, is a good substrate for both plasma and glandular kallikrein. Substrate 2, the LMW type, is a good substrate for glandular kallikrein only (Fig. 17.3).

Kinins and Kinin Inhibitors.

Kinins. The amino acid sequence of the two most important plasma kinins, bradykinin and kallidin, is shown in Figure 17.4. Bradykinin is a nonapeptide, whereas kallidin is a decapeptide identical to the former except for the addition of an *N*-terminal lysine. Thus kallidin also is referred to as lysylbradykinin. Addition of methionine to the *N*-terminal lysine of kallidin yields a third biologically active kinin called methionyl-kallidin or methionyl-lysylbradykinin.

Kinin Inhibitors. Specific inhibitors or antagonists of kinin actions on effector cells have not yet been satisfactorily identified. Accordingly, little is known about kinin-specific receptors, although they have been divided into a series of subtypes (Drouin et al. 1979; Burch et al. 1990; Farmer et al. 1989). Analgesic and antiinflammatory drugs such as aspirin and indomethacin reduce pain and inflammatory responses to kinins. However, these drugs probably act by blocking synthesis of prostaglandins, which mediate or modulate certain activities of kinins (Marceau et al. 1983).

Kallidin

Lys—Arg—Pro—Gly—Phe—Ser—Pro—Phe—Arg

Bradykinin

FIG. 17.4 Amino acid sequence of bradykinin and kallidin.

Kininases and Kininase Inhibitors

Kininases. Plasma and other tissues contain enzymes, collectively called *kininases*, that rapidly inactivate kinins (Fig. 17.3). The most important kininases have been named simply *kininase I* and *II*.

Kininase I is a carboxypeptidase probably synthesized by the liver, but it can be recovered from the lungs and, possibly, the skin. More attention has been directed to kininase II, a peptidyl dipeptide hydrolase. Kininase II also converts angiotensin I to angiotensin II and in this context is referred to more commonly as angiotensin-converting enzyme. It is present in many tissues but is extremely active in the lungs (Erdös 1975).

Kininase Inhibitors. Captopril and enalopril are drugs that inhibit kininase activity, thereby retarding inactivation of bradykinin. As discussed earlier in this chapter, the kininase inhibitors also reduce the conversion of angiotensin I to angiotensin II (Erdös 1976). Although captopril and enalopril are increasingly being used to diagnose and treat forms of hypertension in humans, the importance of the kininases to normal and abnormal circulatory function remains uncertain (Mills 1979; Bhoola et al. 1992; Yousef and Diamandis 2002).

PHARMACOLOGIC EFFECTS OF KININS. At least two separate receptors have been identified that respond to kinins: B_1 and B_2 (Hecquet et al. 2000; Pesquero et al. 2000). The B_2 receptor recognizes as ligands bradykinin and kallidan (Heitsch 2003). The B_2 receptor is constituitively expressed; whereas, the B_1 receptor is induced by inflammation, endotoxin, cytokines, and growth factors. Under basal conditions, the B_1 receptor is expressed at low levels or is absent (Blaukat 2003).

Kinins are extremely potent vasodilators, being about 10 times as active as histamine. They act directly on vascular smooth muscle, but the net effect in different vascular beds varies with species and dose. Smooth muscle of the microcirculation (i.e., of terminal arterioles and small venules) is relaxed by the kinins, yielding a marked decrease in systemic vascular resistance. Blood pressure falls accordingly, but a reflex increase in heart rate and cardiac output may occur. Large arteries and veins, in contrast to the microcirculatory vessels, tend to contract upon exposure to kinins. Permeability of the microcirculation is increased by the kinins, resulting in edema formation similar to the wheal and flare response seen with histamine (Chapter 16). Bradykinin is believed to act in part through receptor-linked activation of the phospholipase C-inositol trisphosphate-Ca^{++} triad (Fasolato et al. 1988).

Intestinal and uterine smooth muscle generally is contracted by kinins, but the duodenum in the rat is relaxed. Bronchoconstriction by kinins is prominent in the guinea pig and in some asthmatic humans but is generally unremarkable in other species. Kinins are potent algesic substances, and they evoke pain when applied topically to exposed blisters or when injected intraarterially. These responses are thought to be associated with stimulation of sensory nerve endings. Since aspirin and other inhibitors of prostaglandin synthesis reduce kinin-induced pain, prostaglandins may mediate or modulate the algesic activities of the kinins (Marceau et al. 1983). Kinins also can stimulate autonomic ganglia and release catecholamines from the adrenal medulla.

ROLE OF ENDOGENOUS KININS. Considerable speculation has centered on the possible roles of kinins in physiologic and pathophysiologic processes. Pathologic conditions in which kinins may participate include acute inflammations, arthritic states, carcinoid syndrome, pancreatitis, migraine headache, allergic reactions, endotoxin shock, and anaphylactic shock. Kinins most likely interact with other autacoids in some of these pathologic states, but their precise involvement remains speculative in most cases (Schror 1992). The physiologic roles of the kallikreins-kinins, even in tissues where they exist in large concentrations (e.g., pancreas, plasma, and parotid gland), also remain uncertain. There is evidence that kallikreins-kinins influence blood flow in exocrine glands and even participate in reproductive activities and cell proliferation (Schachter 1980).

Studies have focused on the roles of plasma kallikrein and HMW kininogen in blood coagulation independently from their involvement in kinin formation. There is considerable evidence that plasma kallikrein activates the Hageman factor (factor XII). Activated Hageman factor and its fragments in turn accelerate conversion of prekallikrein to kallikrein. This establishes a local positive feedback system for sustained activation of clotting factor XII for the coagulation cascade (Fig. 17.3). In addition, the HMW kininogen may participate in the coagulation process by increasing the activation of factor XII, prekallikrein, factor XI, and plasminogen activator. Since plasma kallikrein and plasminogen activator are chemotactic for leukocytes, there seem to be functional interactions between blood coagulation, kallikreins and other kininogenases, and inflammation (Cochrane et al. 1973; Mandle et al. 1976; Ratnoff and Saito 1979).

Studies also have suggested that renal kallikrein may be of significance in regulating fluid and electrolyte balance and, perhaps, renal hemodynamics. In contrast to the renin-angiotensin system, however, kallikrein and bradykinin are diuretic and natriuretic agents; i.e., they increase urine volume and salt excretion. Part of the physiologic actions of the kinins seems to be mediated or modulated by prostaglandins and other autacoids (Busse and Fleming 1996), but the contribution of kinins to the regulation of renal blood flow and nephron function remains speculative (Margolius 1978; Mills 1979). The exact physiologic roles of the kinins probably will not be delineated until specific blockers of kinin receptors are thoroughly identified (Regoli et al. 1996).

OTHER PEPTIDES

Several other vasoactive peptides, of which the actions in pathophysiologic states are less known, are substance P, vasoactive intestinal polypeptide (VIP), eledoisin, physalaemin, coerulein, colostrokinin, urokinin, and the kinins of wasp and hornet venoms. VIP is present in the small intestine and also widely distributed in peripheral nerves and the central nervous system. Although VIP exerts multiple pharmacologic actions in different tissues, its physiologic relevance remains questionable. Substance P was first extracted from horse intestine and brain; it is an endecapeptide structurally similar to eledoisin and physalamin. Substance P has some bradykininlike action and is a potent stimulant of the gut. Eledoisin (from the octopus) and physalamin (from the skin of an amphibian) are endecapeptides with bradykinin-like activity. Coerulein, a related decapeptide, is an extremely potent stimulator of pancreatic and other exocrine secretions.

Atrial natriuretic factor is released from the right atrial musculature of the heart in response to blood volume overload and cardiac stretch. This peptide promotes sodium excretion and diuresis and may have future application in the therapy of congestive heart failure.

Other vasoactive peptides such as oxytocin and vasopressin are discussed in the chapters on hormones, and the cytokines are addressed in Chapter 18 along with the eicosanoids.

REFERENCES

AbdAlla, S., Lother, H., Abdel-tawab, A. M., and Quitterer, U. 2001. The angiotensin II AT_2 receptor is an AT_1 receptor antagonist. J Biol Chem 276:39721–39726.

Ardaillou, R. 1997. Active fragments of angiotensin II: enzymatic pathways of synthesis and biological effects. Current Opinion in Nephrology and Hypertension 6:28–34.

Bautista, R., Manning, R., Martinez, F., et al. 2004. Angiotensin II-dependent increased expression of Na^+-glucose cotransporter in hypertension. Am J Physiol Renal Physiol 286:F127–F133.

Berk, B. C., Corson, M. A. 1997. Angiotensin II signal transduction in vascular smooth muscle. Circ Res 80:607–16.

Bernstein, K. E. 1993. The renin-angiotensin system: a biological machine. Ann Med 24:113–15.

Bhoola, K. D., Figueroa, C. D., Worthy, K. 1992. Bioregulation of kinins: kallikreins, kininogens, and kininases. Pharmacol Rev 44:1–80.

Blaukat, A. 2003. Structure and signaling pathways of kinin receptors. Andrologia 35:17–23.

Braun-Menendez, E., Page, I. H. 1958. Suggested revision of nomenclature—angiotensin. Science 127:242.

Burch, R. M., Farmer, S. G., Steranka, L. R. 1990. Bradykinin receptor antagonists. Med Res Rev 10:143–75.

Busse, R., Fleming, I. 1996. Molecular responses of endothelial tissue to kinins. Diabetes 45:S58–S13.

Carey, R. M., Howell, N. L., Jin, X.-H., and Siragy, H. M. 2001. Angiotensin type 2 receptor-mediated hypotension in angiotensin type 1 receptor-blocked rats. Hypertension 38:1272–1277.

Célérier, J., Cruz, A., Lamandé, N., Gasc, J.-M., and Corvol, P. 2002. Angiotensin and its cleaved derivatives inhibit angiogenesis. Hypertension 39:224–228.

Cheng, H.-F., Wang, J.-L., Zhang, M.-Z., McKanna, J. A., and Harris, R. C. 2000. Nitric oxide regulates renal cortical cyclooxygenase-2 expression. Am J Physiol Renal Physiol 279:F122–F129.

Cheng, H.-F., Wang, J.-L., Zhang, M.-Z., et al. 2001. Genetic deletion of COX-2 prevents increased rennin expression in response to ACE inhibition. Am J Physiol Renal Physiol 280:F449–F456.

Cochrane, C. G., Revak, S. D., Wuepper, K. D. 1973. Activation of Hageman factor in solid and fluid phases: a critical role of kallikrein. J Exp Med 138:1564–83.

Cody, R. J. 1997. The integrated effects of angiotensin II. Amer J Cardiol 79(5A):9–11.

Crackower, M. A., Sarao, R., Oudit, G. Y., et al. 2002. Angiotensin-converting enzyme 2 is an essential regulator of heart function. Nature 417:822–828.

Csajka, C., Buclin, T., Brunner, H. R., Biollaz, J. 1997. Pharmacokinetic-pharmacodynamic profile of angiotensin II receptor antagonists. Clin Pharmacokinet 32(1):1–29.

Dietz, R., Waas, W., Susselbeck, T., Willenbrock, R., Osterziel, K. J. 1993. Improvement of cardiac function by angiotensin converting enzyme inhibition: sites of action. Circulation 87 (Suppl IV):108–16.

Drouin, J. N., St. Pierre, S. A., Regoli, D. 1979. Receptors for bradykinin and kallidin. Can J Physiol Pharmacol 57:375–79.

Erdös, E. G. 1975. Angiotensin I converting enzyme. Circ Res 36:247–55.

———. 1976. The kinins: a status report. Biochem Pharmacol 25:1563–69.

Farmer, S. G., Burch, R. M., Meeker, S. A., Wilkins, D. E. 1989. Evidence for a pulmonary B_3 bradykinin receptor. Mol Pharmacol 36:1–8.

Fasolato, C., Pandiella, A., Meldolesi, J., Pozzan, T. 1988. Generation of inositol phosphates, cytolsolic Ca^{2+}m and ionic fluxes in Pc12 cells treated with bradykinin. J Biol Chem 263:17350–59.

Friis, U. G., Jensen, B. L., Sethi, S., et al. 2002. Control of rennin secretion from rat juxtaglomerular cells by cAMP-specific phosphodiesterases. Circ Res 90:996–1003.

Fritz, H., Kruck, J., Russe, I., et al. 1979. Immunofluorescence studies indicate that the basic trypsin-kallikrein-inhibitor of bovine organs (Trasylol) originates from mast cells. Hoppe Seylers Z Physiol Chem 360:437–44.

Gainer, J. V., Morrow, J. D., Loveland, A., King, D. J., and Brown, N. J. 1998. Effect of bradykinin-receptor blockade on the response to angiotensin-converting-enzyme inhibitor in normotensive and hypertensive subjects. New Engl J Med 339:1285–1292.

Ganong, W. F. 1984. The brain renin-angiotensin system. Annu Rev Physiol 46:17–31.

Gibbons, G. H., Dzau, V. J., Farhi, E. R., et al. 1984. Interaction of signals influencing renin release. Annu Rev Physiol 46:291–308.

Griendling, K. K., Alexander, R. W. 1990. Angiotensin, other pressors, and the transduction of vascular smooth muscle contraction. In J. H. Laragh and B. N. Brenner, eds., Hypertension: Pathophysiology, Diagnosis and Management, Vol. 1, pp. 583–600. New York: Raven Press.

Hansen, J. L., Servant, G., Baranski, T. J., et al. 2000. Functional reconstitution of the angiotensin II type 2 receptor and G_i activation. Circ Res 87:753–759.

Hecquet, C., Tan, F., Marcic, B. M., and Erdös, E. G. 2000. Human bradykinin B(2) receptor is activated by kallikrein and other serine proteases. Mol Pharmacol 58:828–836.

Heitsch, H. 2003. The therapeutic potential of bradykinin B_2 receptor agonists in the treatment of cardiovascular disease. Expert Opin Invest Drugs 12:759–770.

Henrion, D., Kubis, N., and Levy, B. I. 2001. Physiological and pathophysiological functions of the AT_2 subtype receptor of angiotensin II: From large arteries to the microcirculation. Hypertension 38:1150–1157.

Holtz, J. 1993. The cardiac renin-angiotensin system: physiological relevance and pharmacological modulation. Clin Investig 71:S25–S34.

Jackson, E. 2006. In L. L. Brunton, J. S. Lazo, and K. L. Parker, eds., The Pharmacological Basis of Therapeutics, 11th ed. New York: McGraw Hill.

Johnston, C. I. 1992. Renin-angiotensin system: a dual tissue and hormonal system for cardiovascular control. J Hypertens 10(Suppl 7):S13–S26.

Kammerl, M. C., Richthammer, W., Kurtz, A., and Kramer, B. K. 2002. Angiotensin II feedback is a regulator of renocortical rennin, COX-2, and nNOS expression. Am J Physiol Regul Integr Comp Physiol 282: R1613–R1617.

Keeton, T. K., Campbell, W. B. 1981. The pharmacologic alteration of renin release. Pharmacol Rev 32(2):81–227.

Knowlen, G. G., Kittleson, M. D., Nachreiner, R. F., et al. 1983. Comparison of plasma aldosterone concentration among clinical status groups of dogs with chronic heart failure. J Am Vet Med Assoc 183:991–96.

Lage, S. G., Kopel, L., Medeiros, C. C. J., Carvalho, R. T., and Creager, M. A. 2002. Angiotensin II contributes to arterial compliance in congestive heart failure. Am J Physiol Heart Circ Physiol 283: H1424–H1429.

Lee, M. A., Bohm, M., Paul, M., Ganten, D. 1993. Tissue renin-angiotensin systems: their role in cardiovascular disease. Circulation 87 (Suppl IV):7–13.

Li, W., Moore, M. J., Vasilieva, N., et al. 2003. Angiotensin-converting enzyme 2 is a functional receptor for the SARS coronavirus. Nature 426:450–454.

Mandle, R. J., Colman, R. W., Kaplan, A. P. 1976. Identification of prekallikrein and high-molecular-weight kininogen as a complex in human plasma. Proc Natl Acad Sci USA 73:4179–83.

Marceau, F., Lussier, A., Regoli, D., et al. 1983. Pharmacology of kinins: their relevance to tissue injury and inflammation. Gen Pharmacol 14:209–29.

Margolius, H. S. 1978. Kallikrein, kinins, and the kidney: what's going on in there? J Lab Clin Med 91:717–20.

Matsusaka T., Ichikawa I. 1997. Biological functions of angiotensin and its receptors. Annu Rev Physiol 59:395–412.

Mills, I. H. 1979. Kallikrein, kininogen and kinins in control of blood pressure. Nephron 23:61–71.

Moore, A. F., Heiderstadt, N. T., Huang, E., et al. 2001. Selective inhibition of the renal angiotensin type 2 receptor increases blood pressure in conscious rats. Hypertension 37:1285–1291.

Oparil, S., Haber, E. 1974. The renin-angiotensin system (first of two parts). N Engl J Med 291:389–401.

Peart, W. S. 1975. Renin-angiotensin system. N Engl J Med 292:302–6.

Pesquero, J. B., Araujo, R. C., Heppenstall, P. A., et al. 2000. Hypoalgesia and altered inflammatory responses in mice lacking kinin B_1 receptors. Proc Natl Acad Sci USA 97:8140–8145.

Proud, D., Kaplan, A. P. 1988. Kinin formation: mechanisms and role in inflammatory disorders. Annu Rev Immunol 6:49–83.

Ratnoff, O. D., Saito, H. 1979. Interactions among Hageman factor, plasma prekallikrein, high molecular weight kininogen, and plasma thromboplastin antecedent. Proc Natl Acad Sci USA 76:958–61.

Regoli, D., Calo, G., Rizzi, A., Bogoni, G., Gobeil, F., Campobasso, C., Mollica, G., Beani, L. 1996. Bradykinin receptors and receptor ligands (with special emphasis on vascular receptors). Regulatory Peptides 65:83–89.

Rocha e Silva, M., Bernaldo, W. T., Rosenfeld, G. 1949. Bradykinin, hypotensive and smooth muscle stimulating factor released from plasma globulin by snake venom and by trypsin. Am J Physiol 156:261–73.

Schachter, M. 1980. Kallikreins (kininogenases)—a group of serine proteases with bioregulatory actions. Pharmacol Rev 31:1–17.

Schachter, M., Thain, E. M. 1954. Chemical and pharmacological properties of potent, slow contracting substance (kinin) in wasp venom. Br J Pharmacol 9:352–59.

Schmaier, A. H. 2004. The physiologic basis of assembly and activation of the plasma kallikrein/kinin system. Thromb Haemost 91:1–3.

Schror, K. 1992. Role of prostaglandins in the cardiovascular effects of bradykinin and angiotensin-converting enzyme inhibitors. J Cardiovasc Pharmacol 20(Suppl 9):S68–S73.

Schwieler, J. H., Hjemdahl, P. 1992. Influence of angiotensin-converting enzyme inhibition on sympathetic neurotransmission: possible roles of bradykinin and prostaglandins. J Cardiovasc Pharmacol 20(Suppl 9):S39–S46.

Skidgel, R. A., Erdös, E. G. 2006. In L. L. Brunton, J. S. Lazo, and K. L. Parker, eds., The Pharmacological Basis of Therapeutics, 11th ed. New York: McGraw Hill.

Vescei, P., Hackenthal, E., Ganten, D. 1978. The rennin-angiotensin-aldosterone system: past, present and future. Klin Wochenschr 56(Suppl 1):5–21.

Yagil, Y., and Yagil, C. 2003. Hypothesis: ACE2 modulates pressure in the mammalian organism. Hypertension 41:871–873.

Yousef, G. M., and Diamandis, E. P. 2002. Human tissue kallikreins: A new enzymatic cascade pathway? Biol Chem 383:1045–1057.

CHAPTER

18

PROSTAGLANDINS, RELATED FACTORS, AND CYTOKINES

H. RICHARD ADAMS

Prostaglandins, thromboxanes, and leukotrienes are members of a diverse family of endogenous fatty acid derivatives synthesized from cell membrane phospholipids by virtually all types of mammalian cells (Smyth et al. 2006). These compounds and their relatives are referred to collectively as the eicosanoids, because their fatty acid precursors share "eicosa" as the prefix in their chemical nomenclatures. Eicosanoids and other related fatty acid derivatives such as platelet-activating factor (PAF) have a remarkable spectrum of biologic activities involved in homeostatic regulation. Biologic effects of the eicosanoids are believed to encompass practically every bodily function, including various reproductive activities, blood pressure control, renal function, thrombus formation, inflammation, and many more. Details of the biosynthesis, biological effects in physiologic and pathophysiologic states, cellular mechanisms of action, and pharmacologic manipulations of this broad group of lipid-derived autacoids were reviewed by Smyth et al. (2006).

Because of the extraordinarily wide array of biological actions of the eicosanoids in health and disease, it has been difficult to identify drugs that would have beneficial pharmacological effects by acting only on one group of eicosanoids, without concomitantly inducing adverse effects by also affecting another group of related compounds. This dilemma has led to the development of only a relatively few drug groups used clinically to specifically affect the prostaglandins, thromboxanes, prostacyclins, leukotrienes, or platelet-activating factor. By far, the most important class of drugs used to affect the eicosanoids is the nonsteroidal antiinflammatory drugs (NSAIDs) discussed in Chapter 19.

In the current chapter, the biological characteristics of the eicosanoid family and platelet activating factor are briefly reviewed with emphasis on those compounds and affiliated enzymes that have been established as therapeutic targets for the NSAIDs and the limited number of other clinically useful agents that affect the eicosanoids (Masferrer and Kulkarni 1997; de Brum-Fernandes 1997; Donnelly and Hawkey 1997; Smyth et al. 2006).

In addition to eicosanoids and PAF, this chapter briefly addresses another group of endogenous proinflammatory mediators, the cytokines. These agents are not chemically related to the eicosanoids or other fatty acid derivatives; rather, the cytokines are proteins secreted by a variety of cell types in response to inflammation and other stimuli that often concomitantly promote increased synthesis of the eicosanoids.

HISTORY

Recognition of the eicosanoids can be traced to the early 1930s. Two American gynecologists reported that human semen affected the contractile activity of human uterine strips (Kurzrok and Lieb 1930). Extracts of seminal fluid and accessory reproductive glands affected systemic blood pressure and smooth muscle contractile function. The active substance was distinct from the then known autacoids and was identified as a lipid-soluble acid and was named prostaglandin (PG).

Continuing investigations revealed that PG actually comprised a large family of closely related acidic lipids with unique chemical structure. The basic structural unit of the PG compounds proved to be a 20-carbon unsaturated carboxylic acid (Bergström and Samuelsson 1968); the initial PGs were named according to chemical structure and were designated by the letters A–F. $PGF_{2\alpha}$ continues to receive attention relative to animal reproductive problems, which represent a clinical use of PG compounds in veterinary medicine (Schultz 1980; Seguin 1980). Recent advancements have shifted emphasis away from the classic PGs (i.e., PGA–PGF) and toward newer compounds such as the cyclic endoperoxides PGG_2 and PGH_2,

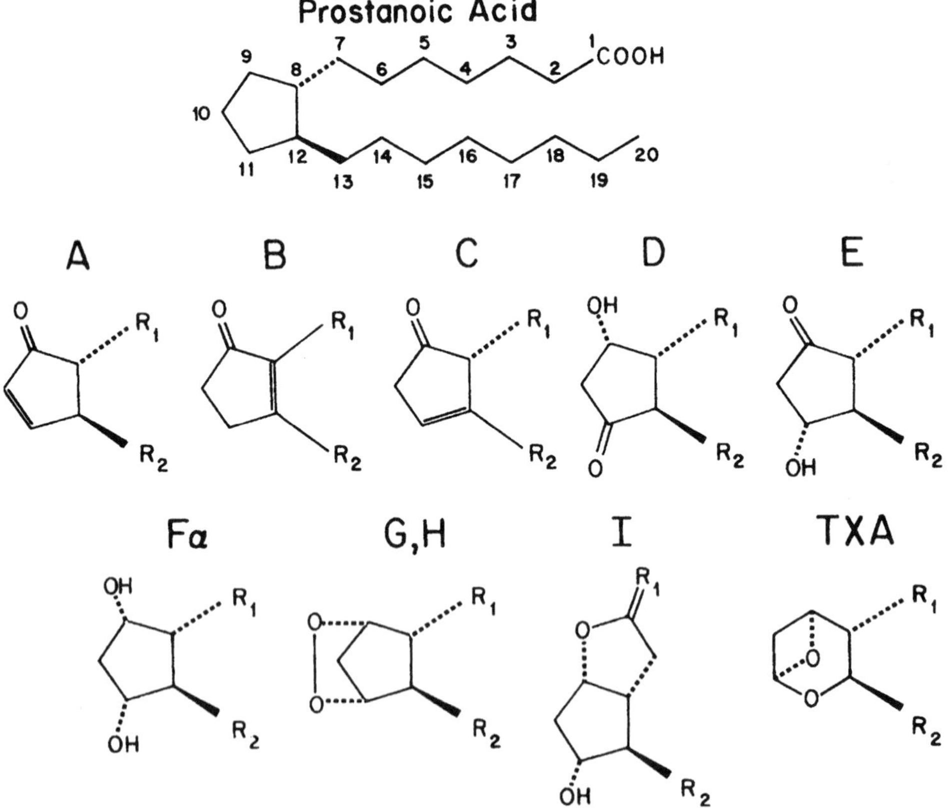

FIG. 18.1 Structures of prostanoic acid and the ring moieties of the six primary PGs (A–F_α), the cyclic endoperoxides (G, H), prostacyclin (I), and thromboxane A (T×A). In the stereochemical convention used in this and subsequent illustrations, the substituents indicated by the triangle lie in front of the plane of the ring structure, whereas those indicated by the dashed line lie behind it.

prostacyclin, thromboxane A_2, leukotrienes, other eicosanoids, and the related PAF (Campbell 1990; Smyth et al. 2006). However, despite the plethora of eicosanoids and related enzymes that have been discovered, the NSAIDs remain the most important class of drug used clinically in veterinary medicine to modulate eicosanoid actions (Chapter 19).

CHEMISTRY AND TERMINOLOGY OF PROSTAGLANDINS

Common to the structure of naturally occurring PGs is the unnatural fatty acid named prostanoic acid; this compound is a 20-carbon carboxylic acid with a cyclopentane ring (Fig. 18.1). The primary or classic PGs are individually named according to substituents on the cyclopentane ring; these are PGA, PGB, PGC, PGD, PGE, and PGF, as shown in Figure 18.1. This figure also pictures the ring moieties of the newer PG-related compounds: PGG, PGH, prostacyclin (PGI), and thromboxane (Fig. 18.1).

The PGs and related substances are further categorized as mono-, di-, or triunsaturated depending on the number of carbon-carbon double bonds in the side chains. This classification appears as a subscript to the letter; e.g., a PG_1 has one double bond between C-13 and C-14, a PG_2 has an additional double bond between C-5 and C-6, and a PG_3 has an additional double bond between C-17 and C-18. As an example, the structural formulas of PGE_1, PGE_2, and PGE_3 are compared in Figure 18.2.

Biosynthetically, the PGs are derived from 20-carbon polyunsaturated fatty acids that contain a total of three, four, or five double bonds. These acids are 8, 11, 14-eicosatrienoic acid (dihomo-γ-linolenic acid); 5, 8, 11, 14-eicosatetraenoic acid (arachidonic acid); and 5, 8, 11, 14, 17-eicosapentaenoic acid (Fig. 18.3). These essential fatty acids yield PGs with one, two, or three double bonds remaining in the side chains, which account for the previ-

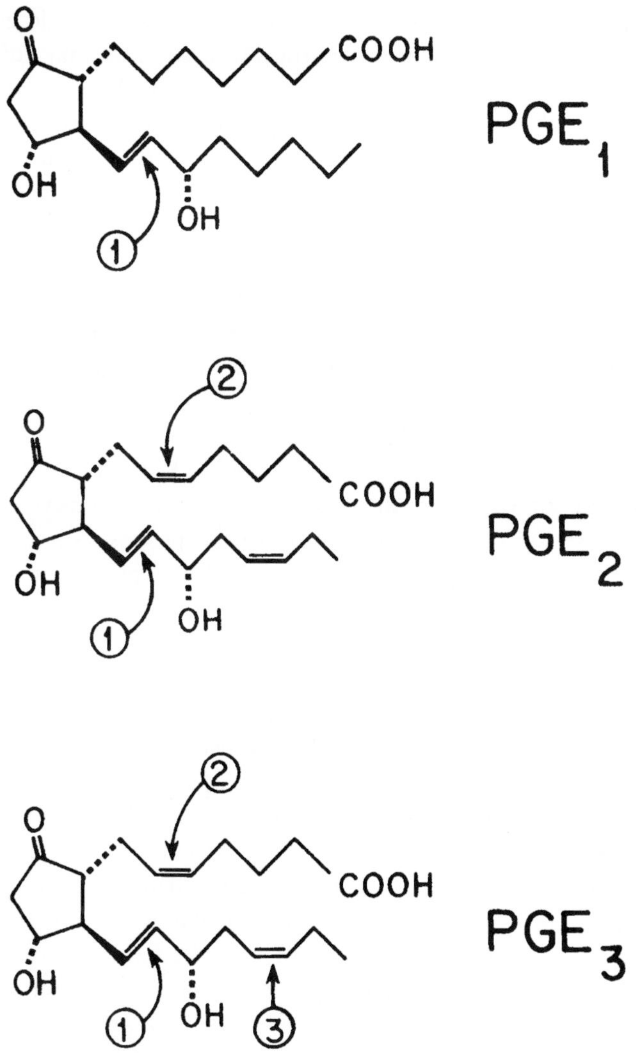

FIG. 18.2 Structures of PG E_1, E_2, and E_3.

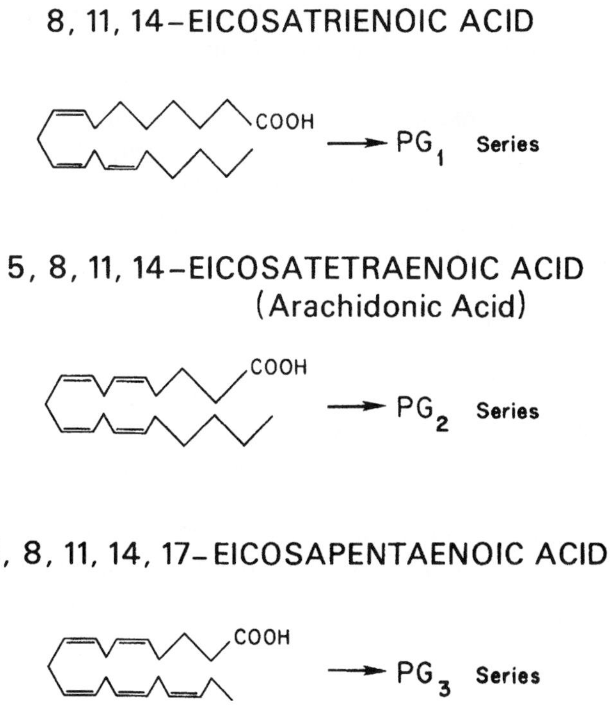

FIG. 18.3 Structures of fatty acid precursors of the 1, 2, and 3 series PGs.

ously described classification as mono- (PG_1), bis- (PG_2), or trienoic (PG_3) PGs (see Fig. 18.3) (Wolfe 1982).

BIOSYNTHESIS OF EICOSANOIDS

The eicosanoids, in contrast to many other autacoids, are not localized or stored in tissue pools. Instead, release of these compounds from cellular components reflects increased rate of their synthesis from available fatty acid precursors (Smyth et al. 2006). Arachidonic acid, the precursor of the bisenoic PGs, is the most important source of the PG compounds found in higher mammalian species. The trienoic PGs are important in marine animals, where the eicosapentaenoic acid seems to be the predominant fatty acid precursor.

Arachidonic acid is an essential fatty acid. It is incorporated by ester linkage into phospholipids of cell membranes and may be contained in other complex lipids such as the triglycerides. Cellular phospholipids release arachidonic acid in response to acyl hydrolases, most notably phospholipase A_2. This is a Ca^{2+}-dependent enzyme activated by a wide array of physiologic, pharmacologic, and pathologic stimuli. Hormones, neurohormones, and other autacoids can participate in initiation of this process; e.g., vasoactive kinins and angiotensin activate tissue phospholipase A_2 and thereby accelerate PG synthesis. This activity in turn results in changes in intensity and range of action of bradykinin and angiotensin, because PG can also modulate the biologic effects of these polypeptides (McGiff 1979; Qi et al. 2002). Thus complex feedback systems exist, which regulate PG synthesis relative to the physiologic status of the animal and the resulting activities of other biologically active autacoids. Even simple mechanical agitation or trauma of tissues can result in phospholipase activation with release of arachidonic acid (Moncada and Vane 1978).

After its liberation from cell membrane phospholipids, arachidonic acid is subject to rapid oxidative catabolism by different enzymatic pathways. Although cytochrome P450 can metabolize arachidonic acid to eicosanoids, the more important enzymes in the PG cascade are a cyclooxygenase and a lipoxygenase. Transformation of arachidonic acid to some of its more important PG derivatives through the cyclooxygenase pathway is illustrated in Figure 18.4 and summarized below.

CYCLOOXYGENASE. The biosynthesis of the PGs from arachidonic acid begins with the action of prostaglandin endoperoxide G/H synthase, which is referred to more commonly as *cyclooxygenase* or *COX*; this enzyme has both cyclooxygenase activity (COX) and hydroperoxidase activity (HOX). COX is widely distributed in mammals, and arachidonic acid can be metabolized to its PG derivatives by virtually all tissue types that have been tested.

The immediate product of cyclooxygenase and arachidonic acid is the cyclic endoperoxide PGG_2, which is formed by the COX-mediated oxygenation and cyclization of unesterified arachidonic acid. PGG_2 is then transformed to the closely related cyclic endoperoxide PGH_2 (Fig. 18.4) through the HOX activity of cyclooxygenase (Boutaud et al. 2002).

Endoperoxides PGG_2 and PGH_2 are quite unstable, with biologic half-lives less than 5 minutes at physiologic pH and body temperature. The endoperoxides undergo enzymatic or nonenzymatic transformation, yielding different PG products (i.e., PGD_2, PGE_2, and $PGF_{2\alpha}$) (Fig. 18.4). PGA, PGB, and PGC compounds are formed from the corresponding PGE during chemical extraction procedures and may not occur biologically. $PGF_{2\alpha}$ can be transformed from PGE_2 in some tissues by a 9-keto-reductase enzyme, but the presence of this enzyme under biologic conditions is debatable. In addition, enzymelike activity called PG endoperoxide $F_{2\alpha}$ reductase, which can form $PGF_{2\alpha}$ from the endoperoxides, has been detected in the bovine uterus (Kindahl 1980).

In addition to yielding PGs of the D, E, and F series, endoperoxide PGH_2 also is metabolized into two other compounds called thromboxane A_2 and prostacyclin. These substances are highly active but possess structures that differ somewhat from those of the primary PGs (Fig. 18.4).

There are two major isoforms of cyclooxygenase: cyclooxygenase-1 (COX-1) and cyclooxygenase-2 (COX-2). The former enzyme is constitutively expressed in most cells under basal conditions, and it serves to synthesize the small amounts of PGs that participate in normal physiologic functions (Cipollone et al. 2004). COX-1 is especially important in producing those eicosanoids that have protective actions on gastrointestinal mucosa. Inhibition of COX-1 activity can be detrimental to the patient because of loss of gastrointestinal protection of mucosal epithelial cells (Masferrer and Kulkarni 1997; Atherton et al. 2004).

The other isoform of cyclooxygenase, COX-2, is not constitutively present; it is nondetectable under basal non-

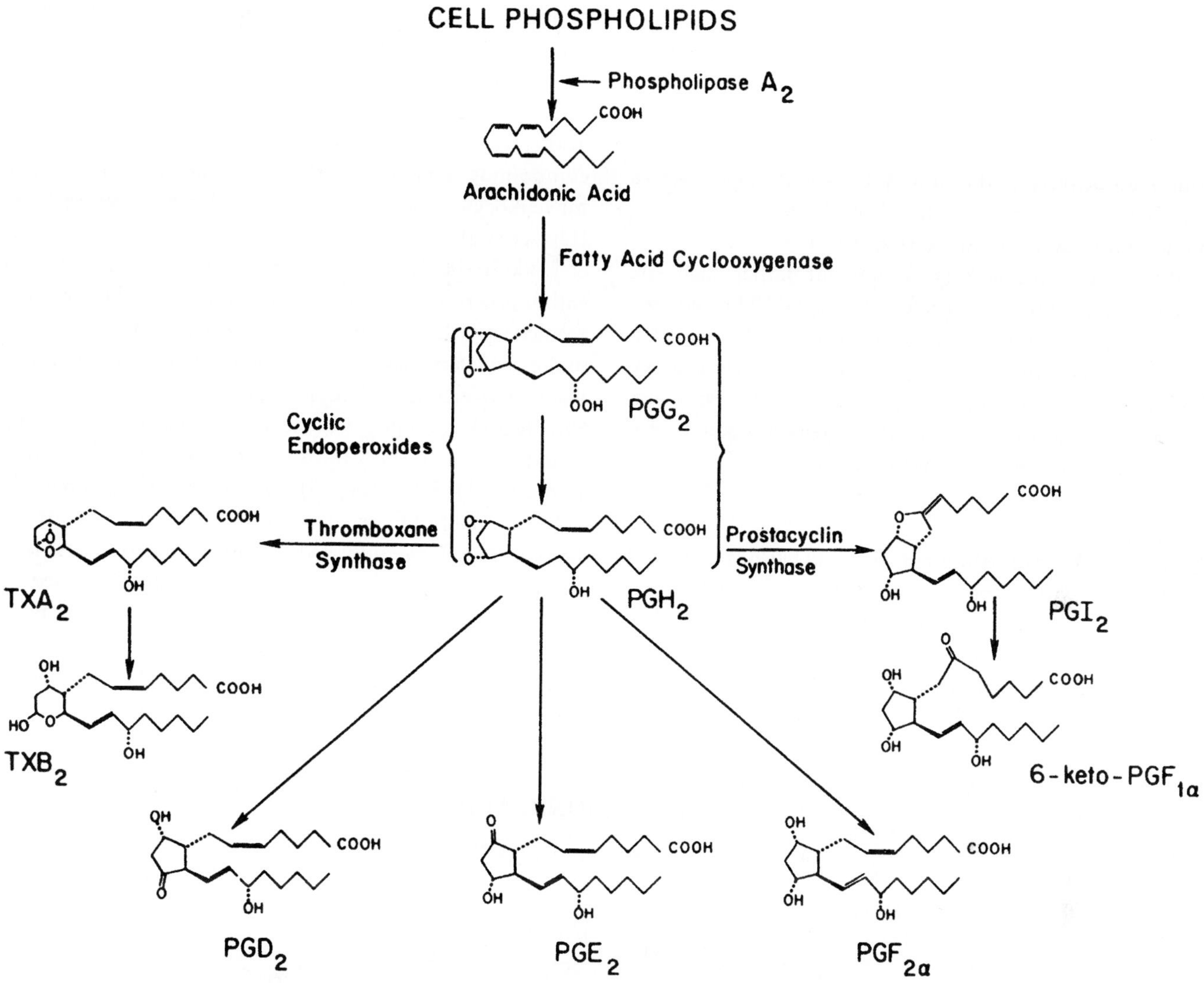

FIG. 18.4 Cyclooxygenase-catalyzed conversion of arachidonic acid to major PG compounds.

stimulated conditions. However, when cells are exposed to bacterial lipopolysaccharide and certain inflammatory cytokines and growth factors, the synthesis of COX-2 is induced. The inducible COX-2 results in increased concentrations of PGs that participate in inflammatory reactions (de Brum-Fernandes 1997; Atherton et al. 2004). The absolute separation of COX-1 and COX-2 into "good" and "bad," respectively, is an oversimplification. Although there are certain physiologic or pathophysiologic functions in which each isoform is predominantly responsible, in other circumstances COX-1 and COX-2 seem to function in a coordinated manner (Smith and Langenbach 2001). Validation of an isoform of COX-1 called COX-3 has been described by Chandrasekharan et al. (2002), but its relevance to eicosanoid metabolism remains unknown.

Thromboxane A_2. An enzyme first isolated from equine and human thrombocytes was found to convert PGH_2 into a compound containing an oxane ring instead of the cyclopentane ring of the PGs. This substance was named thromboxane A_2 (TxA_2), and the responsible enzyme was named thromboxane synthase (Fig. 18.4).

TxA_2 has a brief half-life of about 30 seconds under physiologic conditions, and it degrades into the stable compound thromboxane B_2 (Fig. 18.4). As will be discussed subsequently, TxA_2 plays an important physiologic role as a vasoconstrictor and proaggregate in thrombus formation (see Chapter 26).

Prostacyclin. An enzyme localized in vascular tissue was found to convert PGH_2 into yet another highly active metabolite called prostacyclin or PGI_2; the enzyme was named prostacyclin synthase (Fig. 18.4).

PGI_2 has a double-ring component rather than the single cyclopentane ring (Figs. 18.1, 18.4). The biologic half-life of PGI_2 is quite short, between 2 and 3 minutes; it is converted nonenzymatically into a relatively inactive but stable product, 6-keto-$PGF_{1\alpha}$ (Fig. 18.4). PGI_2 is a potent vasodilator and exerts antiaggregatory activity on blood platelets (see below and Chapter 26).

LIPOXYGENASE. Although fatty acid cyclooxygenase is widely distributed, lipoxygenases have so far been found mainly in lung, platelets, and white blood cells. Metabolism of arachidonic acid via lipoxygenase pathways yields unstable hydroperoxides, which then break down to the stable hydroxyacids or are further transformed into other derivatives such as the leukotrienes (Brink et al. 2003). Selected products of lipoxygenases are shown in Figure 18.5; these include 12-hydroperoxyarachidonic acid (HPETE) and its stable metabolite 12-hydroxyarachidonic acid (HETE). The breadth of physiologic actions of these compounds remains uncertain, but they are chemotactic for leukocytes and participate in inflammatory responses (Dwyer et al. 2004).

Leukotrienes comprise a group of noncyclized, 20-carbon, carboxylic acid products of arachidonic acid formed by 5-lipoxygenase activity (Fig. 18.5). The trivial name *leukotriene* was chosen because these compounds were discovered in leukocytes and shared a common structural feature as conjugated trienes (Samuelsson 1983). The initial reaction of the 5-lipoxygenase pathway is the formation of 5-HPETE (Fig. 18.5); 5-HPETE is converted either to 5-HETE or to leukotriene A_4, a 5,6 epoxide. Leukotriene A_4 is converted in turn either to leukotriene B_4 or C_4. The latter is a glutathionyl derivative, formed by the enzyme glutathione-*S*-transferase (Fig. 18.5). Leukotriene D_4 is formed via the cleavage of the glycine moiety from leukotriene C_4, while E_4 is synthesized by the subsequent removal of glycine. The biologic importance of the

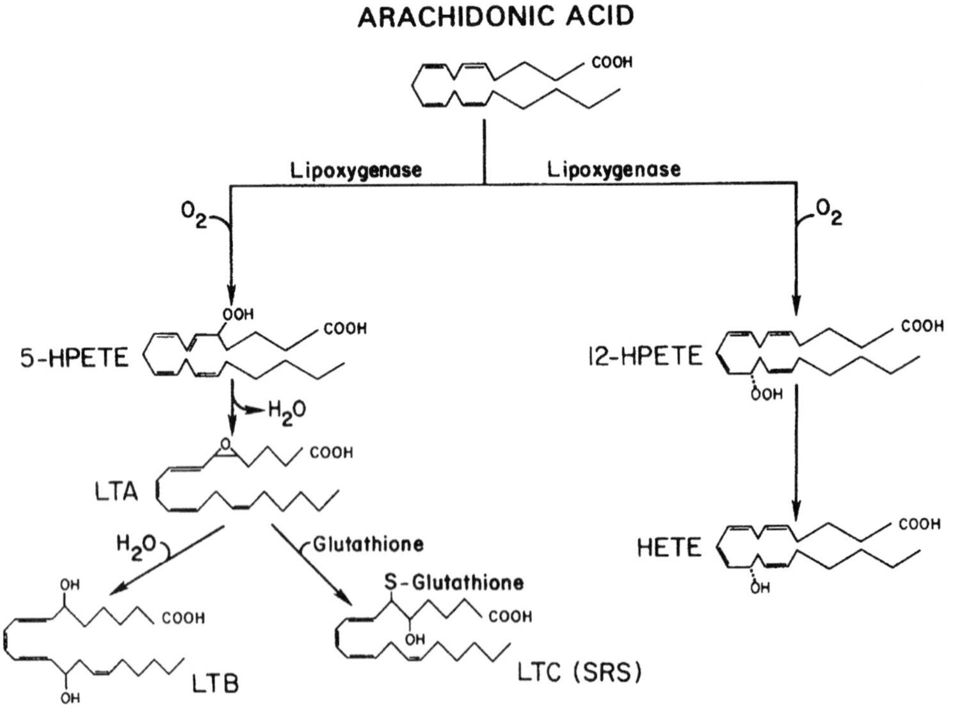

FIG. 18.5 Lipoxygenase-catalyzed conversion of arachidonic acid to hydroperoxyarachidonic acids (HPETE), hydroxyarachidonic acid (HETE), and leukotriene (LT) A_4, B_4, and C_4. SRS = slow-reacting substance of anaphylaxis.

leukotrienes is under intensive investigation; there is considerable evidence that these substances participate in inflammatory reactions, and a combination of the cysteine-containing leukotrienes (i.e., C_4, D_4, and E_4) is now believed to compose the slow-reacting substance of anaphylaxis (Samuelsson 1983; Samuelsson et al. 1980). As a general rule, the dihydroxy acids are chemotactic for leukocytes but have minimal smooth muscle-stimulating properties, whereas the sulfur linkage and amino acid residues at C-6 are required for smooth muscle-stimulating properties (Piper 1983).

INHIBITION OF BIOSYNTHESIS OF EICOSANOIDS

Tissue distribution of the different enzymes involved in PG biosynthesis is important to medicine. These enzymes currently represent the most vulnerable targets for pharmacologic manipulation of the PG system (FitzGerald 2003; Smyth et al. 2006).

Cyclooxygenase seems to be rather ubiquitous, because most tissues are able to convert arachidonic acid to the intermediate endoperoxides PGG_2 and PGH_2. However, the fate of the latter compounds varies considerably in different tissues.

Reproductive organs of several species are able to synthesize PGE_2 and $PGH_{2\alpha}$, whereas the spleen and lung can produce the whole range of PG compounds. The major PG formed by blood vessel endothelial cells is PGI_2; hence, prostacyclin synthase is of major importance in this tissue. On the other hand, thromboxane synthase is dominant in blood platelets; TxA_2 is a primary PG product of this cell type. Various drugs have been studied in attempts to regulate the PG system via individual effects on the participating enzymes.

Starting with Vane's work in 1971, the rather pronounced influence of aspirinlike drugs on the PG system became apparent. Aspirin and other antiinflammatory agents of the nonsteroidal type disrupt the cellular release of PGs by interfering with their biosynthesis. The site of inhibitory action of these drugs is localized high in the PG cascade, at the cyclooxygenase level (Fig. 18.4). By inhibiting cyclooxygenase, aspirin prevents conversion of arachidonic acid to the endoperoxides PGG_2 and PGH_2. Accordingly, the formation of PG products below PGG_2 and PGH_2 in the metabolic pathway is likewise retarded by the action of aspirin (Vane 1971; Szczeklik et al. 2004).

Other nonsteroidal antiinflammatory agents that inhibit cyclooxygenase include other salicylates, indomethacin, phenylbutazone, naproxen, flunixin, and meclofenamic acid (see Chapter 19). The antiinflammatory, antipyretic, and analgesic actions of such drugs all are mediated principally by inhibition of PG biosynthesis at the cyclooxygenase level (Capone et al. 2004). The side effects of this group of drugs also depend on inhibition of PG synthesis (see Chapter 19). Aspirinlike drugs are not inhibitors of the lipoxygenase enzymes that participate in other metabolic pathways of arachidonic acid (Catella-Lawson et al. 2001).

Traditional nonsteroidal antiinflammatory agents are nonselective inhibitors of both the constitutive COX-1 and the inducible COX-2 isoenzymes (Juni et al. 2002). Inhibition of COX-2 results in therapeutically useful reductions in the synthesis of proinflammatory eicosanoids, but inhibition of COX-1 would at the same time result in loss of protective and other physiologic functions of PGs necessary for normal cellular functions (de Brum-Fernandes 1997; Donnelly and Hawkey 1997). Drugs with greater inhibitory action on COX-2 than on COX-1 would be therapeutically beneficial because they would selectively reduce synthesis of inflammatory PGs while sparing cellular protective actions of COX-1 products (Brune and Hinz 2004). Newer nonsteroidal antiinflammatory agents with selective COX-2 inhibitory actions are addressed in Chapter 19 (Tacconelli et al. 2004).

Glucocorticoids interfere with PG formation by inducing the synthesis of a group of proteins called *annexins* (previously *lipocortins*). Annexins inhibit eicosanoid biosynthesis by suppressing phospholipase A_2 activity, thereby retarding release of arachidonic acid from cellular phospholipids (Wolfe 1982). Glucocorticoids also down-regulate expression of the inducible COX-2 enzyme, while apparently not affecting COX-1 (Masferrer and Kulkarni 1997; de Brum-Fernandes 1997; Donnelly and Hawkey 1997).

Considerable interest is directed toward characterization of selective inhibitors of the PG-synthesizing enzymes; e.g., imidazole and certain of its analogs preferentially inhibit thromboxane synthase. Certain analogs of PGG_2 and PGH_2 also exert selective inhibitory actions on this enzyme. Conversely, prostacyclin synthase is inhibited by lipid peroxides such as 15-HPETE. Clinical application of the above enzyme inhibitors is unproven, but potential advantages over the aspirinlike cyclooxygenase inhibitors reside in the possibility of selectively reducing production of one PG derivative without affecting others (Ouellet and Percival 2001; Charlier and Michaux 2003; Patrignani et al. 2003).

PHYSIOLOGIC-PHARMACOLOGIC ASPECTS OF EICOSANOIDS

Although a multitude of biologic activities has been assigned to the different eicosanoids, the physiologic value of all such effects and relative importance of individual derivatives undergo almost continual reappraisal as new discoveries are unfolded. Artifactual conversion of one PG to another during tissue isolation has delayed attempts to designate biologic responsibility. In addition, data obtained from one animal species may not apply to others because there are formidable species differences in responsiveness to many members of the eicosanoid complex. In the following paragraphs, some of the better defined physiologic and pharmacologic aspects of the biologic activities of this system are summarized.

REPRODUCTIVE SYSTEM. The involvement of PGs in reproductive physiology is covered later in this volume. Briefly, PG compounds have been associated with luteolysis, abortion, and parturition. $PGF_{2\alpha}$ is believed to be the long-sought luteolytic hormone produced by the uterus in some nonprimate species (e.g., mare, cow, sow, ewe, and guinea pig). This factor is believed to control the life span of the corpus luteum; e.g., in nonpregnant cows the luteolytic hormone or $PGF_{2\alpha}$ is released about day 14 or 15 of the estrous cycle. The corpus luteum degenerates, which evokes the return of estrus. Pregnancy inhibits release of the luteolytic factor; hence the corpus luteum persists and the fetus develops.

In addition to producing luteolysis, $PGF_{2\alpha}$ also causes contraction of uterine smooth muscle. Because blood concentrations of PG increase during labor, $PGF_{2\alpha}$ is viewed as important for prepartum lysis of the corpus luteum, which removes the progesterone block, and for evoking uterine contractions during parturition. Increased PG production has also been associated with abortion and premature labor. Inhibition of COX-1 prolongs parturition in rodents without affecting closure of the ductus arteriosus (Loftin et al. 2002). In support of these concepts, aspirin was found to delay parturition, reduce uterine contractions during labor, retard premature labor, and delay abortion. The participation of PG in reproductive events has been reviewed by Schultz (1980), Seguin (1980), and Stabenfeldt et al. (1980).

CARDIOVASCULAR SYSTEM. Systemic administration of PGs can evoke pronounced hemodynamic responses, depending upon the individual compound and animal species tested (Camu et al. 1992). Blood pressure effects of all the PG derivatives mainly reflect changes in peripheral vascular resistance; these agents affect smooth muscle contractile activity in large arteries, arterioles, precapillaries, venules, and large veins. Primary PGs of the E and A series, particularly PGE_2, are potent vasodilators in most species. Conversely, vascular smooth muscle is generally contracted by $PGF_{2\alpha}$. Vasodilator effects of the latter and vasoconstrictor effects of PGE_2 have been seen in certain vascular beds (McGiff 1979).

TxA_2 is a potent stimulant of vascular smooth muscle and has produced vasoconstriction in all blood vessel systems yet tested. TxA_2 was originally detected as rabbit aorta-contracting substance released from guinea pig lungs during anaphylaxis (Piper and Vane 1969). As opposed to TxA_2, PGI_2 is an exceptional vasodilator. It is several times more potent than PGE_2. Pronounced vasodilator effects of PGI_2 have been demonstrated in several regions, including the coronary, renal, skeletal muscle, and omental vascular beds.

A systemic depressor response is evoked by the vasodilators PGI_2, PGE_2, and PGE_1, whereas a pressor response is produced by the vasoconstrictors $PGF_{2\alpha}$ and TxA_2. Interestingly, PGI_2 is equipotent as a vasodilator whether administered intravenously or intraarterially. This is an important difference from PGE_1 or PGE_2, which are much less active when given intravenously. These differences were explained when it was discovered that PGE_1 and PGE_2 undergo almost complete metabolism during a single passage through the pulmonary vascular circuit, whereas PGI_2 is not metabolized rapidly by the lungs. In fact, the lungs seem able to release PGI_2 into the circulation. Persistence of PGI_2 in the blood contributed to the suggestion that this agent may be a circulating PG with more hemodynamic responsibility than the rapidly inactivated PGE_2 (Moncada and Vane 1978).

The intermediate endoperoxides PGG_2 and PGH_2 exert variable effects on vascular smooth muscle; both vasoconstriction and vasodilation have been reported. This scope of activity reflects some intrinsic vasoconstrictor actions of the endoperoxides as well as their rapid conversion to other potent agents such as PGI_2. Similarly, injection of arachidonic acid can elicit circulatory effects that are mediated by its metabolites; such effects are inhibited by aspirin.

Cardiac output is increased slightly by PGs of the A, E, and F series, but cardiac responses to PG in intact subjects are mainly a result of reflex adjustment to systemic blood pressure changes. Only weak inotropic effects are seen with isolated heart muscle preparations. The heart can release endogenously produced PGI_2 upon exposure to certain stimuli, but this activity reflects PG synthesis by the coronary vasculature and not by the cardiac muscle cell (Sivakoff et al. 1979).

There is increasing evidence that different eicosanoids participate in the pathogenicity of circulatory depressant effects associated with gram-negative endotoxicosis. Most studies have focused on TxA_2 and PGI_2, and the concentrations of both increase during endotoxin shock in dogs and horses (Moore et al. 1986).

Although leukotrienes C_4 and D_4 exert potent cardiovascular effects, differences exist relative to animal species and to route of administration. Both agents cause an initial hypertensive response followed by long-lasting hypotension when injected intravenously. When given arterially, the pressor phase is reduced, while the depressor response is prolonged. Interestingly, at least a portion of the cardiovascular response to the leukotrienes may be secondary to release of PGs, because cyclooxygenase inhibitors attenuate the prolonged hypotensive response to the leukotrienes. Piper (1983) has reviewed the cardiovascular profile of the leukotrienes.

Since certain fetal and maternal blood vessels can synthesize PGI_2, this agent may participate in circulatory adjustments to pregnancy and parturition (Terragno and Terragno 1979). Locally synthesized PGI_2 has been implicated in maintenance of the patency of the ductus arteriosus. This concept was based in part on the observation that aspirin could produce closure of the ductus in neonates. Indomethacin has proven superior to aspirin in this respect, but mixed results have been seen in clinical trials.

BLOOD. Compared to most cell types, erythrocytes lack the capacity to generate significant amounts of PG. In contrast, blood platelets are prolific producers of the endoperoxides PGG_2 and PGH_2 and of TxA_2. These compounds, especially the more active TxA_2, are potent aggregating agents; their involvement in thrombus formation is contrasted with the antiaggregating action of PGI_2 in Figure 26.1 in Chapter 26.

Briefly, the platelet-aggregating effects of TxA_2 are believed to be important to the thrombus-forming and thus hemostatic mechanisms provoked by damage to blood and blood vessels. Conversely, the antiaggregating action of PGI_2 may serve to modulate thrombus formation. Indeed, PGI_2 is the most potent endogenous inhibitor of platelet aggregation yet discovered. It is 1,000 times more potent than adenosine and 30–40 times more active than PGE_1. Also, PGI_2 disaggregates platelets in vitro, in vivo in the circulatory system, and in extracorporeal circuits where platelet clumping has occurred.

It has been suggested that small amounts of PGI_2 are present in the circulation, circulating PGI_2 is responsible for lack of aggregation of normal platelets, locally produced PGI_2 is involved in providing vascular endothelium with its smooth-surfaced characteristics, and vascular endothelium may even scavenge endoperoxides from platelets for use in production of PGI_2. The latter activity is envisioned to serve as a control mechanism to prevent spread of thrombi onto normal vascular endothelium when adjacent injuries have evoked TxA_2 formation and platelet aggregation. Thus platelet TxA_2 and vascular PGI_2 serve as biologically opposite regulators of interactions between platelets and blood vessels (Cheng et al. 2002; Moncada and Vane 1978).

The antiaggregating action of PGI_2, PGE_1, and PGD_2 has been associated with an increase in the concentration of cyclic adenosine monophosphate (cAMP). Although different PG receptors may be involved, it seems that adenylyl cyclase is activated by each of the antiaggregating PG compounds. Conversely, the endoperoxides and TxA_2 inhibit the stimulatory effect of PGI_2 on adenylyl cyclase, thereby lowering cAMP concentration. Drugs that increase cAMP concentration, such as the phosphodiesterase inhibitor dipyridamole (Persantine), enhance the antiaggregating effects of PGI and antagonize the proaggregating effects of TxA_2.

KIDNEY. Although cyclooxygenase is present in various regions of the kidney, the major products of arachidonic acid metabolism are thought to be tissue-specific in this organ (McGiff and Wong 1979; Cheng and Harris 2004). PGI_2 is synthesized within the kidney primarily by the vascular smooth muscle compartment. Small quantities of this PG cause renal vasodilation and thereby lower vascular resistance and increase blood flow in the kidney. Urinary excretion of sodium, potassium, chloride, and water is increased by PGI_2; these changes may reflect direct effects on tubular transport mechanisms or secondary effects caused by redistribution of blood flow. There is increasing evidence that PGI_2 also regulates release of renin through actions exerted at the vascular pole of the glomerulus, and PG formation may be involved in certain types of hypertension (Oates et al. 1979). Salt handling by the kidneys is affected by prostanoids, and blood pressure can be influenced through this pathway (O'Shaughnessy and Karet 2004).

The major PG derivative of renal medullary interstitial cells seems to be PGE_2. Collecting ducts also are capable of generating PGE_2. This PG can increase salt and water excretion independently of blood flow changes, an effect caused in part by inhibition of the action of antidiuretic hormone on permeability of collecting ducts. There is increasing evidence that effects of PGE_2 and also $PGF_{2\alpha}$ on salt and water excretion involve interaction with the kallikrein-kinin system within the renal urinary compartment (McGiff and Wong 1979; Moncada and Vane 1978).

TxA_2 is believed to be synthesized by the kidney only under pathologic conditions, e.g., after ligation or other obstructions of the ureter. Pathophysiologic stimuli such as hemorrhage or laparotomy can also increase synthesis of renal PG, especially PGE_2, which then contributes to maintenance of renal blood flow. The physiologic value of PG to renal blood flow in normal nonstressed animals remains unclear.

INFLAMMATION AND PAIN. PGs and other eicosanoids are released from soft tissues in response to a variety of noxious stimuli such as infection and mechanical, thermal, and chemical trauma. Once liberated from irritated or damaged cells, PG contributes importantly to different phases of the local inflammatory reaction and its pain. Large concentrations of PG elicit pain by direct stimulation of sensory nerve endings. More typically, PGs in quite small concentrations sensitize sensory nerve endings to other pain-provoking stimuli such as bradykinin, histamine, and other mediators of inflammation (Samad et al. 2002). Edema-inducing and hyperemic effects of kinins and other autacoids are likewise enhanced by certain PGs, e.g., PGE_2 and PGI_2 (Coggins et al. 2002). These PGs do not seem to directly affect vascular permeability but facilitate leukocyte infiltration and edema formation through vasodilation-induced increase in blood flow. Metabolites of the lipoxygenase pathway also contribute to the inflammatory process, and increasing evidence has linked these compounds and certain PG derivatives with immunologic phenomena.

The peptide leukotrienes increase vascular permeability and contribute further to inflammation by their chemotactic effect on leukocytes (Kanaoka and Boyce 2004). Leukotriene B_4 is especially active as a chemoattractant for polymorphonuclear leukocytes. Other lipoxygenase products such as 5-HPETE and 5-HETE may facilitate the release of histamine and other inflammatory autacoids from mast cells.

OTHERS. PGs affect contractile activity of several smooth muscles besides those of the reproductive and vascular systems. Many species differences exist, and the net effect in each tissue is influenced by the age, health, sex, and endocrine status of the test subject. PGs of the F series, especially $PGF_{2\alpha}$, generally contract tracheal and bronchial smooth muscle in several species. Members of the E series generally relax respiratory muscle. In asthmatic humans, $PGF_{2\alpha}$ has induced intense bronchospasm, while PGE_1 and PGE_2 are potent bronchodilators. TxA_2, PGG_2, and PGH_2 contract tracheal muscle and induce bronchospasm.

PGI_2 affects smooth muscle motility and fluid transport mechanisms in the intestine, where it exerts an antidiarrheal effect. In contrast, PGE_2 produces diarrhea, which is an important limitation to therapeutic use of this agent.

PGI_2 is a major product of the gastric mucosa of several species. It is a potent vasodilator in this tissue, where it also inhibits the acid secretion evoked by pentagastrin. Thus PGI_2 may serve as a suppressant modulator of gastric acid secretion and as a participant in functional hyperemia of the stomach. The untoward ability of aspirin-like drugs to induce gastric irritation and ulceration has been attributed to inhibition of PGI_2 synthesis (Ma et al. 2002).

Numerous central nervous system effects have been attributed to PG, but large concentrations are generally needed to demonstrate such actions. Several PG derivatives depress release of norepinephrine from adrenergic neurons of the autonomic nervous system, but physiologic significance remains questionable.

MECHANISM OF ACTION. Membrane receptors for PG have been identified in certain tissues, and smooth muscle-stimulating effects of PG have been associated with alterations in calcium movement induced by cell membrane depolarization. Changes in cellular metabolism of calcium may also be involved in other actions of PG, secondary to changes in various enzyme activities. Certain of the PGs increase cAMP concentrations by stimulating adenylyl cyclase activity, e.g., PGI_2 in platelets. Others are inhibitory to such relationships, e.g., TxA_2 in platelets. In certain tissues, however, cAMP can inhibit PG biosynthesis.

The biological complexity of the eicosanoids is exemplified by the complexity of PG receptors and their associated signal-transduction mechanisms. The G-protein-adenylyl cyclase-cAMP system is linked with some PG receptors (Smith 1992), whereas the phospholipase C-inositol trisphospate-Ca^{++} system is linked with others (Mitchell and Trautman 1993). This area was reviewed by Campbell (1990) and Smyth et al. (2006), and Table 18.1 summarizes some of the PG receptor types and their affiliated receptor mechanisms. Although antagonists for PG receptors and leukotriene receptors are under intense investigation (Toda et al. 2002), inhibition of biosynthetic enzymes in the eicosanoid cascades (Figs. 18.4 and 18.5) is the most viable therapeutic mechanism for currently altering eicosanoid actions (Martel-Pelletier et al. 2003).

CLINICAL ASPECTS. Bell et al. (1980) compiled lengthy lists of possible therapeutic uses of different members of the PG group in veterinary medicine. Disorders that were listed as potentially responsive to PG or to anti-PG treatment varied from such diverse disorders as equine laminitis and feline cardiomyopathies to paralytic ileus and porcine gastric ulceration. Use of PG in treating such pathophysiologic states may well prove to have clinical value in the future. Currently, pharmacologic manipulation of the PG complex involves mainly the cardiovascular system, reproductive functions, and inflammation.

The capability of $PGF_{2\alpha}$ and synthetic analogs to influence reproductive performance represents a common clinical application of PG compounds in veterinary medicine. Use of COX-1 and COX-2 inhibitors for analgesic, anti-inflammatory, and antipyretic effects is discussed elsewhere in this volume (Chapter 19).

Pharmacologic manipulation of the PG system also has application in treating or preventing disorders of the cardiovascular system, but such uses are mainly experimental; e.g., PGI_2 has been used to retard platelet aggregation and thromboembolism in several systems of extracorporeal circulation such as renal dialysis and cardiopulmonary bypass. PGI_2 and its analogs may also become important in controlling thromboembolism in the intact circulation. Intra-arterial infusions of the vasodilators PGE_2 and PGI_2 were reported to increase blood flow, reduce pain, and accelerate healing of ulcers in human patients with peripheral vascular disease (Szczeklik et al. 1979). Considering the breadth of physiologic actions of the eicosanoids, it is not surprising that inhibitors of the cyclooxygenase enzymes can also produce adverse side effects (Sigthorsson et al. 2002; Nussmeier et al. 2005).

Platelet cyclooxygenase is more sensitive to the inhibitory action of aspirin than the cyclooxygenase of blood vessels. Aspirin irreversibly inhibits cyclooxygenase by acetylating its active site. Since platelets cannot synthesize

TABLE 18.1 Classification of some eicosanoid receptors and their affiliated signal-transduction pathways in vascular smooth muscle and platelets

Receptor Type	Endogenous Agonist	Transduction Mechanism	Vascular Effect	Platelet Aggregation
DP	PGD_2	cAMP	—	Inhibit
EP_1	PGE_2; $PGF_{2\alpha}$	IP_3–Ca^{++}	Vasoconstrict	—
EP_2	PGE_2; PGE_1	cAMP	Vasodilate	Inhibit
FP	$PGF_{2\alpha}$	IP_3–Ca^{++}	Vasoconstrict	—
IP	PGI_2; PGE	cAMP	Vasodilate	Inhibit
TP	TxA_2; PGH_2	IP_3–Ca^{++}	Vasoconstrict	Enhance

Source: Campbell 1990; Smith 1992; Mitchell and Trautman 1993.

Note: P = prostaglandin; cAMP = the $G_s$protein-adenylyl cyclase-cAMP-protein kinase A pathway; IP_3–Ca^{++} = the phospholipase C-IP_3-diacylglycerol–protein kinase C–Ca^{++} pathway. The—designates unknown or vasoconstriction and vasodilation depending on tissues. cAMP = cyclic adenosine monophosphate.

new protein during their sojourn in the bloodstream, the inhibitory effect of aspirin persists for several days, i.e., until new platelets are produced by the bone marrow. Thus small doses of aspirin preferentially inhibit platelet production of the proaggregating TxA_2 without marked reduction of vascular production of the antiaggregating PGI_2. The net result is expressed as an antithrombotic effect with increased bleeding time. Aspirin therefore is an antithrombotic agent used for prevention of conditions characterized by excessive platelet aggregation. However, large doses also inhibit vascular cyclooxygenase, resulting in loss of preferential block of TxA_2 synthesis. The clinical application of such interrelationships in animals remains to be clearly defined.

PLATELET-ACTIVATING FACTOR

Platelet-activating factor (PAF) is another autacoid derived from membrane phospholipids rich in arachidonic acid and other precursors of polyunsaturated fatty acids, and is therefore chemically related to the ubiquitous eicosanoid family. Whereas the eicosanoids are formed from a wide variety of cell types, PAF is synthesized principally by platelets, endothelial cells, and circulating leukocytes. The wide distribution of these cells throughout the body ensures PAF the opportunity to affect a host of tissue and cellular functions.

PAF not only provokes platelet aggregation, as its name implies, but it also modulates smooth muscle

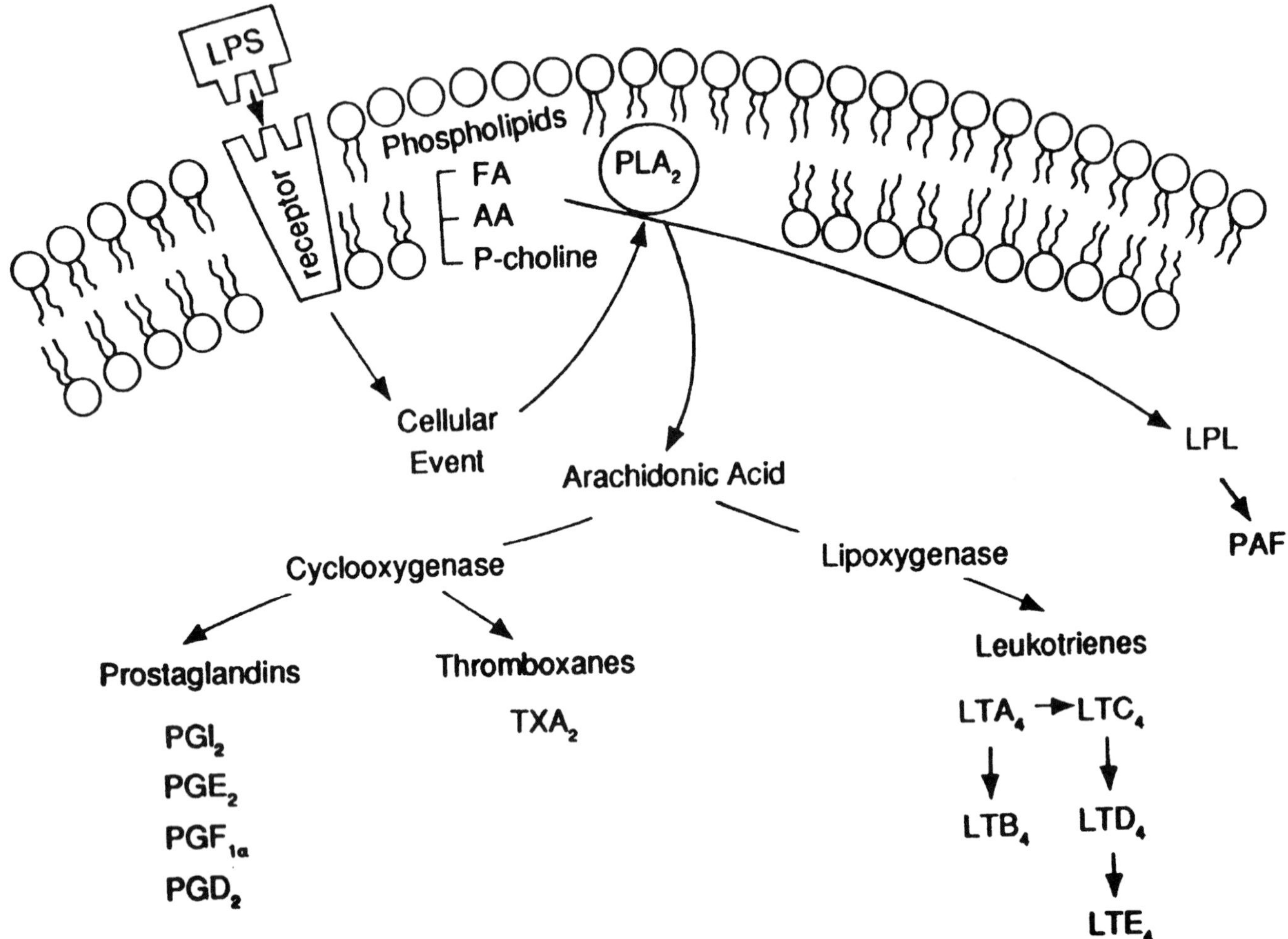

FIG. 18.6 Schematic diagram of endotoxin (lipopolysaccharide, LPS)-induced activation of phospholipase A_2 (PLA_2). Activated PLA_2 results in the release of arachidonic acid from the 2-acyl position of membrane phospholipids, leaving a lysophospholipid (LPL) that can be used to form platelet-activating factor (PAF). Arachidonic acid is metabolized to prostaglandins (PG), thromboxanes (TX), and leukotrienes (LT). FA = fatty acid; AA = arachidonic acid; and P-choline = phosphatidylcholine (Bottoms and Adams 1992.)

activity in blood vessel walls and promotes leakage of vascular fluid across endothelial surfaces. Although PAF lowers blood pressure due to its relaxing effect on vascular smooth muscle, it markedly contracts smooth muscle of the gut, stomach, uterus, and peripheral airways of the lungs. PAF can promote the synthesis and release of thromboxane A_2 and therefore exerts both direct and indirect effects on blood pressure. Since some of the smooth muscle and proinflammatory effects of PAF can be prevented by cyclooxygenase inhibitors, PAF is considered to be one of the most active endogenous activators of prostaglandins and related eicosanoids. In this regard, PAF and cyclooxygenase products are commonly activated concomitantly in response to inflammatory stimuli such as bacterial infection. This type of cohort relationship is exemplified in Figure 18.6, wherein the response of a mammalian cell membrane to bacterial lipopolysaccharide (endotoxin) is schematized. Endotoxin lipopolysaccharide interacts with cellular constituents, culminating in activation of the cell membrane enzyme phospholipase A_2. Not only does the latter release arachidonic acid for eicosanoid biosynthesis through the cyclooxygenase (Fig. 18.4) and lipoxygenase pathways (Fig. 18.5), but this same reaction also yields a lysophospholipid that can be formed into PAF (Fig. 18.6). Thus, biological roles for PAF are often linked to those exhibited by the eicosanoid family. Despite the wealth of physiologic and pathophysiologic activities proposed for PAF (Campbell 1990), pharmacologic manipulation of PAF synthesis and receptors is at a preliminary stage. The clinical significance of PAF antagonists is currently unknown for veterinary medicine.

CYTOKINES

In response to certain inflammatory and immunologic stimuli, many types of mammalian cells produce one or more of a variety of small proteins termed cytokines. Cytokines include tumor necrosis factor-α (TNF-α), gamma interferon, and the interleukins (IL). Currently, monoclonal antibodies raised against these specific proteins represent the primary pharmacotherapeutic intervention relevant to the area of cytokines. However, because of the likely future importance of cytokines to pharmacologic management of bacterial invasion and other inflammatory conditions, the following discussion briefly summarizes key aspects about TNF-α and the interleukins.

TUMOR NECROSIS FACTOR-α. The polypeptide cytokine TNF-α occupies a prominent and perhaps central role as proximal mediator of endotoxic shock (Tracey et al. 1989; Morris et al. 1990). Macrophages exposed to endotoxin and related stimuli release large quantities of TNF-α. On reaching the circulation, TNF-α binds to high-affinity receptors in normal tissues and triggers a wide array of biological effects. The infusion of recombinant TNF-α from human beings can induce lethal shock and tissue injury in animals, closely simulating key elements of the pathophysiologic derangements characteristic of endotoxemia (Tracey et al. 1986; 1987a,b).

The production and release of other cytokines, eicosanoids, and humoral factors are elicited by TNF-α (Fig. 18.7). In addition to induction of IL-1, IL-4, and IL-6 synthesis, other biological activities attributed to TNF-α include T-cell activation, endogenous pyrogen activity, induction of eicosanoid synthesis, activation of osteoclastic bone resorption, inhibition of bone collagen synthesis, induction of acute-phase reactant synthesis and granulocyte/monocyte colony-stimulating factor, and inhibition of lipoprotein lipase and other enzymes of lipid metabolism (Grunfield and Palladino 1990; Beutler and Cerami 1989; Rosonblum and Donato 1989). In neutrophils, TNF-α stimulates activation, respiratory burst, degranulation, and adherence to the vascular endothelium.

At low concentrations, TNF-α exerts its primary effects locally as a paracrine and autocrine regulator of leukocytes and endothelial cells. These actions are critical for the containment of infection. However, when TNF-α gains access to the systemic circulation, signs of septicemia develop and high concentrations of TNF-α can be lethal. Cyclooxygenase inhibitors can block the rapid-onset monophasic fever that is induced by TNF-α. Lethal effects of endotoxin and TNF-α can be reduced under certain conditions by the administration of neutralizing TNF-α antiserum (Tracey et al. 1987a,b; Shimamoto et al. 1988). Long-term exposure to TNF-α results in cachexia, which accounts for its synonym, cachectin.

INTERLEUKIN-1. The polypeptide IL-1 has been termed lymphocyte activating factor, because it enhances T-cell responses during antigen presentation, and endogenous pyrogen, because it induces fever. Production of IL-1, primarily by mononuclear phagocytes (Fig. 18.7), is stimulated by endotoxin, other macrophage-derived cytokines

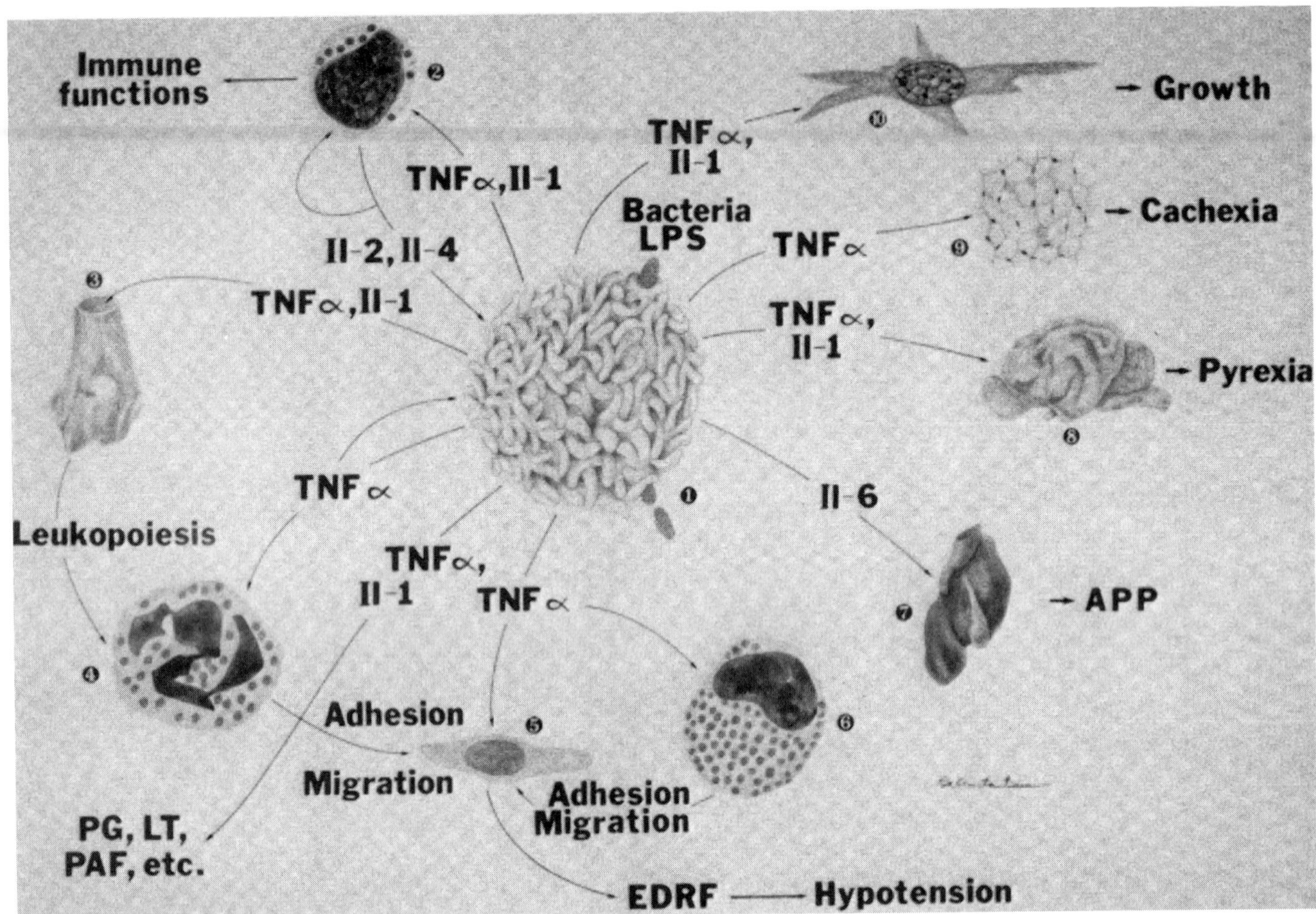

FIG. 18.7 Reaction of macrophage to gram-negative bacteria and endotoxin and representative responses of tissues to liberation of tumor necrosis factor-a (TNF-α) and interleukin (IL) cytokines from macrophages. The following numbered items refer to corresponding numbers in the figure: (1) macrophage: recognizes and assimilates bacteria and endotoxin (lipopolysaccharide, LPS), resulting in macrophage activation and release of cytokine mediators such as TNF-α and IL-1; (2) T and B lymphocytes: TNF-α and IL-1 enhance immunoregulatory functions, and lymphocytes release IL-4 and IL-2, which can affect macrophage function in an autocrine manner; (3) bone marrow: cytokines increase leukopoiesis; (4) neutrophils: activated by TNF-α to enhance migration and adhesion to vascular endothelium; (5) endothelium: TNF-α enhances adhesion and modulates release of hypotensive agents such as endothelium-derived relaxing factor (EDRF); (6) eosinophils: TNF-α promotes migration and adhesion; (7) liver: cytokines promote synthesis of acute-phase proteins (APP); (8) brain: cytokines modulate thermoregulatory functions, resulting in pyrexia; (9) adipocytes: TNF-α modulates metabolic regulatory enzymes, yielding cachexia; and (10) fibroblasts: cytokines enhance proliferation and growth. Cytokines also modulate the release of other mediators, such as prostaglandins (PG), leukotrienes (LT), and platelet-activating factor (PAF). (This figure was modeled after the illustration in Old 1988 and was drawn by Dr. Gheorghe M. Constantinescu, Department of Veterinary Biomedical Sciences, University of Missouri, Columbia (Green and Adams 1992).)

such as TNF-α, other microbial products, and antigens. Although they are structurally distinct, IL-1 performs many of the same biological activities as TNF-α (Dinarello 1985). The principal biological function of IL-1 is believed to be mediation of the host response in natural immunity; IL-1 interacts with antigen-stimulated T cells to induce the release of IL-2 by T cells and synthesis of IL-2 receptors. By direct effect on B cells, IL-1 invokes B-cell activation, proliferation, and antibody synthesis. Natural killer cell activity is enhanced by synergism of IL-1 with other cytokines. Arachidonic acid metabolism, secretion of inflammatory proteins, neutrophil chemoattraction, and fibroblast proliferation are stimulated by IL-1. With TNF-α and IL-6, IL-1 participates in the acute-phase response, which is characterized by fever, hepatic production of acute-phase proteins, neutrophilia, procoagulant activity, and hypoferremia. Endothelial cells are stimulated by IL-1 to synthesize prostacyclin, procoagulant activity, PAF, and neutrophil adherence protein. Evidence suggests that IL-1 and TNF-α interact synergistically to induce many of the tissue reactions associated with endotoxemia.

INTERLEUKIN-6. The phosphoglycoprotein IL-6 is produced and secreted by macrophages, monocytes, fibroblasts, vascular endothelial cells, T lymphocytes, and mast cells (Kishimoto 1989). Cells are stimulated to produce IL-6 by various inflammatory stimuli, including IL-1 and, to a lesser extent, endotoxin, TNF-α, platelet-derived growth factor, and viral infection. The primary inflammatory action of IL-6 is the induction of hepatic production of acute-phase proteins (Fig. 18.7), such as fibrinogen, C-reactive protein, serum amyloid A, haptoglobin, ferroxidase, α-1-antitrypsin, and complement. Growth and differentiation of B cells are enhanced by IL-6, and IL-6 serves as a costimulator of T cells. High concentrations of IL-6 have been measured in serum and body fluids in human beings after the administration of endotoxin, TNF-α, and IL-1, and during acute bacterial infection and sepsis. Whereas the effects of TNF-α and IL-1 may be detrimental, IL-6 appears to be beneficial. Acute-phase reactants protect the host nonspecifically against microorganisms, and IL-6 does not cause tissue injury and vascular thrombosis characteristic of endotoxin and TNF-α.

The wide spectrum of biological actions of TNF-α and IL-1 are illustrated in Figure 18.7. Despite the wealth of physiologic activities ascribed to cytokines, the clinical significance of their pharmacologic manipulation remains unclear (Green and Adams 1992).

REFERENCES

Atherton, C., Jones, J., McKaig, B., et al. 2004. Pharmacology and gastrointestinal safety of lumiracoxib, a novel cyclooxygenase-2 selective inhibitor: an integrated study. Clin Gastroenterol Hepatol 2:113–120.

Bell, T. G., Smith, W. L., Oxender, W. D., Maciejko, J. J. 1980. Biologic interaction of prostaglandins, thromboxane, and prostacyclin: potential nonreproductive veterinary clinical applications. J Am Vet Med Assoc 176(10 Spec No):1195–200.

Bergström, S., Samuelsson, B. 1968. The prostaglandins. Endeavour 27(102):109–13.

Beutler, B., Cerami, A. 1989. The biology of cachectin/tumor necrosis factor-α primary mediator of the host response. Ann Rev Immunol 7:625–55.

Bottoms, G. D., Adams, H. R. 1992. Involvement of prostaglandins and leukotrienes in the pathogenesis of endotoxemia and sepsis. J Am Vet Med Assoc 200:1842–48.

Boutaud, O., Aronoff, D. M., Richardson, J. H., Marnett, L. J., Oates, J. A. 2002. Determinants of the cellular specificity of acetaminophen as an inhibitor of prostaglandin H(2) synthases. Proc Natl Acad Sci USA 99:7130–7135.

Brink, C., Dahlen, S. E., Drazen, J., et al. 2003. International Union of Pharmacology: XXXVII. Nomenclature for leukotriene and lipoxin receptors. Pharmacol Rev 55:195–227.

Brune, K., Hinz, B. 2004. Selective cyclooxygenase-2 inhibitors: similarities and differences. Scand J Rheumatol 33:1–6.

Campbell, W. B. 1990. Lipid-derived autacoids: eicosanoids and platelet-activating factor. In A. G. Gilman, T. W. Rall, A. S. Nies, P. Taylor, eds., Pharmacological Basis of Therapeutics, 8th ed., pp. 600–617. New York: Pergamon Press.

Camu, F., VanLersberghe, C., Lauwers, M. H. 1992. Cardiovascular risks and benefits of perioperative nonsteroidal anti-inflammatory drug treatment. Drugs 44 (Suppl 5):42–51.

Capone, M. L., Tacconelli, S., Sciulli, M. G., et al. 2004. Clinical pharmacology of platelet, monocyte, and vascular cyclooxygenase inhibition by naproxen and low-dose aspirin in healthy subjects. Circulation 109:1468–1471.

Catella-Lawson, F., Reilly, M. P., Kapoor, S. C., et al. 2001. Cyclooxygenase inhibitors and the antiplatelet effects of aspirin. N Eng J Med 345:1809–1817.

Chandrasekharan, N. V., Dai, H., Roos, K. L., et al. 2002. COX-3, a cyclooxygenase-1 variant inhibited by acetaminophen and other analgesic/antipyretic drugs: cloning, structure, and expression. Proc Natl Acad Sci USA 99:13926–13931.

Charlier, C., Michaux, C. 2003. Dual inhibition of cyclooxygenase-2 (COX–2) and 5-lipoxygenase (5-LOX) as a new strategy to provide safer non-steroidal anti-inflammatory drugs. Eur J Med Chem 38:645–659.

Cheng, H. F., Harris, R. C. 2004. Cyclooxygenases, the kidney, and hypertension. Hypertension 43:525–530.

Cheng, Y., Austin, S. C., Rocca, B., et al. 2002. Role of prostacyclin in the cardiovascular response to thromboxane A_2. Science 296: 539–541.

Cipollone, F., Toniato, E., Martinotti, S., et al. 2004. A polymorphism in the cyclooxygenase 2 gene as an inherited protective factor against myocardial infarction and stroke. JAMA 291:2221–2228.

Coggins, K. G., Latour, A., Nguyen, M. S., et al. 2002. Metabolism of PGE_2 by prostaglandin dehydrogenase is essential for remodeling the ductus arteriosus. Nat Med 8:91–92.

de Brum-Fernandes, A. J. 1997. New perspectives for nonsteroidal antiinflammatory therapy. J Rheumatol 24:246–48.

Dempsey, P. W., Doyle, S. E., He, J. Q., Cheng, G. 2003. The signaling adaptors and pathways activated by TNF superfamily. Cytokine Growth Factor Rev 14:193–209.

Dinarello, C. A. 1985. An update on human IL-1: From molecular biology to clinical relevance. J Clin Immunol 5:287–97.

Donnelly, M. T., Hawkey, C. J. 1997. Review article: COX-II inhibitors—a new generation of safer NSAIDs? Aliment Pharmacol Ther 11:227–36.

Dwyer, J. H., Allayee, H., Dwyer, K. M., et al. 2004. Arachidonate 5-lipoxygenase promoter genotype, dietary arachidonic acid, and atherosclerosis. New Engl J Med 350:29–37.

Fam, S. S., Morrow, J. D. 2003. The isoprostanes: Unique products of arachidonic acid oxidation—A review. Curr Med Chem 10:1723–1740.

FitzGerald, G. A. 2003. COX-2 and beyond: Approaches to prostaglandin inhibitors in human disease. Nat Rev Drug Discov 2:879–890.

FitzGerald, G. A., Patrono, C. 2001. The coxibs, selective inhibitors of cyclooxygenase-2. N Engl J Med 345:433–442.

Green, E. M., Adams, H. R. 1992. New perspectives in circulatory shock: pathophysiologic mediators of the mammalian response to endotoxemia and sepsis. J Am Vet Med Assoc 200:1834–41.

Grunfield, C., Palladino, M. A. 1990. Tumor necrosis factor immunologic, antitumor, metabolic, and cardiovascular activities. Adv Intern Med 35:45–72.

Juni, P., Rutges, A. W., Dieppe, P. A. 2002. Are selective COX 2 inhibitors superior to traditional nonsteroidal anti-inflammatory drugs? BMJ 324:1287–1288.

Kanaoka, Y., Boyce, J. A. 2004. Cysteinyl leukotrienes and their receptors: Cellular distribution and function in immune and inflammatory response. J Immunol 173:1503–1510.

Kindahl, H. 1980. Prostaglandin biosynthesis and metabolism. J Am Vet Med Assoc 176(10 Spec No):1173–77.

Kishimoto, T. 1989. The biology of interleukin-6. Blood 74:1–10.

Kurzrok, R., Lieb, C. C. 1930. Proc Soc Exp Biol Med 28:268.

Loftin, C. D., Trivedi, D. B., Langenbach, R. 2002. Cyclooxygenase-1-selective inhibition prolongs gestation in mice without adverse effects on the ductus arteriosus. J Clin Invest 110:549–557.

Ma, L., del Soldato, P., Wallace, J. L. 2002. Divergent effects of new cyclooxygenase inhibitors on gastric ulcer healing: shifting the angiogenic balance. Proc Natl Acad Sci USA 99:13243–13247.

Martel-Pelletier, J., Lajeunesse, D., Reboul, P., Pelletier, J. P. 2003. Therapeutic role of dual inhibitors 5-LOX and COX, selective and non-selective nonsteroidal anti-inflammatory drugs. Ann Rheum Dis 62:501–509.

Masferrer, J. L., Kulkarni, P. S. 1997. Cyclooxygenase-2 inhibitors: a new approach to the therapy of ocular inflammation. Surv Ophthalmol 41: S35–S40.

McGiff, J. C. 1979. Prostaglandins in circulatory disorders. Triangle 18(4):101–7.

McGiff, J. C., Wong, P. Y. 1979. Compartmentalization of prostaglandins and prostacyclin within the kidney: Implications for renal function. Fed Proc 38(1):89–93.

McMahon, B., Godson, C. 2004. Lipoxins: Endogenous regulators of inflammation. Am J Physiol Renal Physiol 286:F189–201.

Mitchell, M. D., Trautman, M. S. 1993. Molecular mechanisms regulating prostaglandin action. Mol Cell Endocrinol 93:C7–C10.

Moncada, S., Vane, J. R. 1978. Pharmacology and endogenous roles of prostaglandin endoperoxides, thromboxane A_2, and prostacyclin. Pharm Rev 30(3):293–331.

Moore, J. N., Hardee, M. M., Hardee, G. E. 1986. Modulation of arachidonic acid metabolism in endotoxic horses: Comparison of flunixin meglumine, phenylbutazone, and a selective thromboxane synthetase inhibitor. Am J Vet Res 47(1):110–13.

Morris, D. D., Crowe, N., Moore, J. N. 1990. Correlation of clinical and laboratory data with serum tumor necrosis factor activity in horses with experimentally induced endotoxemia. Am J Vet Res 51:1935–40.

Nussmeier, N. A., Whelton, A. A., Brown, M. T., et al. 2005. Complications of COX-2 inhibitors parecoxib and valdecoxib after cardiac surgery. N Engl J Med 352:1081–1091.

Oates, J. A., Whorton, A. R., Gerkens, J. F., Branch, R. A., Hollifield, J. W., Frolich, J. C. 1979. The participation of prostaglandins in the control of renin release. Fed Proc 38(1):72–74.

Old, L. J. 1988. Tumor necrosis factor. Sci Am 258:59–75.

O'Shaughnessy, K. M., Karet, F. E. 2004. Salt handling and hypertension. J Clin Invest 113:1075–1081.

Ouellet, M., Percival, M. D. 2001. Mechanism of acetaminophen inhibition of cyclooxygenase isoforms. Arch Biochem Biophys 38:7273–7280.

Patrignani, P., Capone, M. L., and Tacconelli, S. 2003. Clinical pharmacology of etoricoxib: a novel selective COX2 inhibitor. Expert Opin Pharmacother 4:265–284.

Piper, P. J. 1983. Pharmacology of leukotrienes. Br Med Bull 39(3):255–59.

Piper, P. J., Vane, J. R. 1969. Release of additional factors in anaphylaxis and its antagonism by anti-inflammatory drugs. Nature 223(201):29–35.

Prescott, S. M., McIntyre, T. M., Zimmerman, G. A., Stafforini, D. M. 2002. Sol Sherry Lecture in Thrombosis: Molecular events in acute inflammation. Arterioscler Thromb Vasc Biol 22:727–733.

Qi, Z., Hao, C. M., Langenbach, R. I., et al. 2002. Opposite effects of cyclooxygenase-1 and -2 activity on the pressor response to angiotensin II. J Clin Invest 110:61–69.

Rijneveld, A. W., Weijer, S., Florquin, S., et al. 2004. Improved host defense against pneumococcal pneumonia in platelet-activating factor receptor-deficient mice. J Infect Dis 189:711–716.

Rosonblum, M. G., Donato, N. J. 1989. Tumor necrosis factor-alpha: A multifaceted peptide hormone. Crit Rev Immunol 1:21–44.

Samad, T. A., Sapirstein, A., Woolf, C. J. 2002. Prostanoids and pain: Unraveling mechanisms and revealing therapeutic targets. Trends Mol Med 8:390–396.

Samuelsson, B. 1983. Leukotrienes: Mediators of immediate hypersensitivity reactions and inflammation. Science 220(4597):568–75.

Samuelsson, B., Hammarstrom, S., Murphy, R. C., Borgeat, P. 1980. Leukotrienes and slow reacting substance of anaphylaxis (SRS-A). Allergy 35(5):375–81.

Schultz, R. H. 1980. Experiences and problems associated with usage of prostaglandins in countries other than the United States. J Am Vet Med Assoc 176(10 Spec No):1182–86.

Seguin, B. E. 1980. Role of prostaglandins in bovine reproduction. J Am Vet Med Assoc 176 (10 Spec No):1178–81.

Seibert, K., Zhang, Y., Leahy, K., et al. 1997. Distribution of COX-1 and COX-2 in normal and inflamed tissues. Adv Exp Med Biol 400A:167–170.

Shimamoto, Y., Chen, R. L., Bollon, A., et al. 1988. Monoclonal antibodies against human recombinant tumor necrosis factor: Prevention of endotoxic shock. Immunol Lett 17:311–18.

Sigthorsson, G., Simpson, R. J., Walley, M., et al. 2002. COX-1 and -2, intestinal integrity, and pathogenesis of nonsteroidal anti-inflammatory drug enteropathy in mice. Gastroenterology 122:1913–1923.

Sivakoff, M., Pure, E., Hsueh, W., Needleman, P. 1979. Prostaglandins and the heart. Fed Proc 38(1):78–82.

Smith, W. L. 1992. Prostanoid biosynthesis and mechanisms of action. Am J Physiol 263:F181–F191.

Smith, W. L., Langenbach, R. 2001. Why there are two cyclooxygenase isozymes. J Clin Invest 107:1491–1495.

Smyth, E. M., Burke, A., FitzGerald, G. A. 2006. Lipid-derived autocoids: eicosanoids and platelet-activating factor. In L. L. Brunton, J. S. Lazo,

K. L. Parker, eds., The Pharmacological Basis of Therapeutics, 11th ed. New York: McGraw Hill.

Smyth, E. M., FitzGerald, G. A. 2003. Prostaglandin mediators. In R. D. Bradshaw, ed., Handbook of Cell Signaling, pp. 265–273. San Diego: Academic Press.

Soares, A. C., Pinho, V. S., Souza, D. G., et al. 2002. Role of the platelet-activating factor (PAF) receptor during pulmonary infection with gram-negative bacteria. Br J Pharmacol 137:621–628.

Stabenfeldt, G. H., Hughes, J. P., Neely, D. P., Kindahl, H., Edqvist, L. E., Gustafsson, B. 1980. Physiologic and pathophysiologic aspects of prostaglandin F2 alpha during the reproductive cycle. J Am Vet Med Assoc 176(10 Spec No):1187–94.

Szczeklik, A., Nizankowski, R., Skawinski, S., Szczeklik, J., Gluszko, P., Gryglewski, R. J. 1979. Successful therapy of advanced arteriosclerosis obliterans with prostacyclin. Lancet 1(8126):1111–14.

Szczeklik, A., Sanak, M., Nizankowska-Mogilnicka, E., and Kielbasa, B. 2004. Aspirin intolerance and the cyclooxygenase-leukotriene pathways. Curr Opin Pulm Med 10:51–56.

Tacconelli, S., Capone, M. L., Patrignami, P. 2004. Clinical pharmacology of novel selective COX-2 inhibitors. Curr Pharm Des 10:589–601.

Terragno, N. A., Terragno, A. 1979. Prostaglandin metabolism in the fetal and maternal vasculature. Fed Proc 38(1):75–77.

Toda, A., Yokomizo, T., Shimizu, T. 2002. Leukotriene B_4 receptors. Prostaglandins Other Lipid Mediat 68–69:575–585.

Tracey, K. J., Beutler, B., Lowry, S. F., et al. 1986. Shock and tissue injury induced by recombinant human cachectin. Science 234:470–74.

Tracey, K. J., Cerami, A., Morris, D. D., Crowe, N., Moore, J. N. 1989. Cachectin/tumor necrosis factor and other cytokines in infectious disease. Curr Opin Immunol 1:454–64.

Tracey, K. J., Fong, Y., Hesse, D. G., et al. 1987a. Anti-cachectin/TNF monoclonal antibodies prevent septic shock during lethal bacteremia. Nature 330:662–64.

Tracey, K. J., Lowry, S. F., Fahey, T. F., et al. 1987b. Cachectin/tumor factor necrosis factor induces shock and stress hormone responses in the dog. Surg Gynecol Obstet 164:415–22.

Vane, J. R. 1971. Inhibition of prostaglandin synthesis as a mechanism of action for aspirin-like drugs. Nature 231(25):232–35.

Wolfe, L. S. 1982. Eicosanoids: Prostaglandins, thromboxanes, leukotrienes, and other derivatives of carbon-20 unsaturated fatty acids. J Neurochem 38(1):1–14.

CHAPTER

19

ANALGESIC, ANTIINFLAMMATORY, ANTIPYRETIC DRUGS

PETER LEES

THE ROLE OF EICOSANOIDS IN INFLAMMATION AND MECHANISMS OF ACTION OF NSAIDS

The inflammatory process is driven by a diverse range of mediators, synthesized de novo or released from storage sites, in both the early and resolution phases of acute inflammation and in chronic inflammation. Many mediators are formed at each stage and they interact with each other in ways that are not fully understood. These interactions may involve addition, antagonism, or synergism. Acute inflammation is characterized by the four cardinal signs of heat, redness, swelling, and pain, as first characterized by the Roman physician Celsus in the first century A.D., to which Virchow added the fifth sign, loss of function, in the 19th century. Three of the cardinal signs involve the microcirculation, being caused by arteriolar dilation and increased permeability of capillaries and postcapillary venules to protein, leading to formation of an inflammatory exudate rich in leukocytes. The leukocyte infiltrate is first dominated by polymorphonuclear leukocytes and later by mononuclear cells, which transform to macrophages in the interstitial space. Leukocytes are the scavengers of the inflammatory process, engulfing microorganisms, particulate matter and dead and dying cells, and releasing enzymes and chemicals, the mediators of inflammation.

Arachidonic acid (AA), a 20-carbon unsaturated fatty acid, plays a pivotal role in inflammation as the precursor of the eicosanoid group of mediators. AA is an esterified component of cell membrane phospholipid, which is released in tissue damage following activation of phospholipase A_2 (Chapter 18). There are many isoforms of phospholipase A_2 and it is the cytosolic 85 kDa isoform that normally supplies AA. After its release from cell membrane phospholipid, AA serves as a substrate not only for prostaglandin(PG)Hsynthase, more commonly known as *cyclo-oxygenase (COX),* of which there are two isoforms COX-1 and COX-2, but also several lipoxygenases (LO), including 5-LO, 12-LO, and 15-LO. Each enzyme is part of a cascade, in which the action of further enzymes leads to the formation of many inflammatory mediators of the eicosanoid family. The mediators are short-lived, so that continued effect depends on maintained synthesis and release. COX catalyses both the formation of PGG_2 and then PGG_2 conversion to PGH_2 via a peroxidase function.

As described in Chapter 18, at an early stage of acute inflammation several PGs (including PGE_2, PGI_2, and PGD_2) are synthesized from AA, the product profile being determined by differing downstream enzymes. For example, cytosolic PGEsynthase is mainly coupled with COX-1 and an inducible microsomal or membrane-associated perinuclear PGEsynthase, regulated by cytokines and glucocorticoids, is coupled with COX-2 (Murakami et al. 1999). PGI_2 is formed from PGH_2 by the catalytic action of PGIsynthase, a member of the P450 superfamily.

The precise role in inflammation of each PG is not yet determined, and in future studies this will be facilitated by the use of selective receptor site antagonists for individual compounds. Prostanoid receptors are cell membrane spanning G-protein coupled receptors and five subdivisions have been classified pharmacologically, corresponding to each COX metabolite: DP for PGD_2, EP for PGE_2, FP for $PGF_{2\alpha}$, IP for PGI_2 and TP for TxA_2. The actions of PGE_2 are mediated by a range of receptor subtypes (EP1, EP2, EP3, and EP4), activation of which leads to ongoing intracellular signalling pathways. The use of selective antagonists for prostanoid receptors has shown that the EP1 receptor is associated with visceral pain and EP4 antagonists induce colitis and suppress osteoclastogenesis (Sarkar et al. 2003).

As well as the peripheral role of PGs as inflammatory mediators, they are involved in pain perception at the spinal level. PGE_2 is also an endogenous pyrogen, leading to upward resetting of the temperature regulating center in the anterior hypothalamus.

Following intracellular synthesis, PGs must exit the cell of origin. As water-soluble molecules, they are unlikely to cross cell membranes by passive diffusion. ABC genes provide ABC transporters to consume ATP and a wide variety of endogenous and exogenous compounds, including eicosanoids, thereby traverse cell membranes. A subfamily of ABC transporters are the multidrug resistance proteins (MRPs), of which MRP1 is a high affinity LTC_4 transporter, and MRP4, which is widely distributed in tissues, has particular affinity for the transport of PGE_2, TxA_2, and $PGF_{2\alpha}$ (Warner and Mitchell 2003).

Three important examples of synergism between proinflammatory PGs and other inflammatory mediators may be cited. First, both histamine (Chapter 16) and bradykinin (Chapter 17) are primary inflammatory mediators, which stimulate nociceptors (peripheral nerve endings) to increase the discharge in afferent nerves so that pain is sensed in spinal and brain centers. The role of PGs such as PGE_2 is to synergize with these primary mediators; they do not directly stimulate nociceptors but increase both intensity and duration of the afferent discharge caused by histamine and bradykinin (Ferreira 1983). This phenomenon is hyperalgesia and it is linked to a PGE_2-induced increase in the concentration of cyclic AMP in nociceptors. In addition, when tissues are damaged, stimuli (e.g., touch) that are not normally painful, become painful, a phenomenon termed *allodynia*; PGs are again implicated (Nolan 2001). It is by inhibiting PG synthesis that nonsteroidal antiinflammatory drugs (NSAIDs) exert their analgesic actions.

Second, histamine and bradykinin (among other mediators) increase endothelial intercellular gaps in capillary and small postcapillary venules to increase loss of plasma to the interstitial space. This alteration to the Starling balance of forces (hydrostatic pressure exceeding plasma protein oncotic pressure causing loss of fluid to the interstitial space at the arteriolar end of the capillary and oncotic pressure exceeding hydrostatic pressure leading to uptake of fluid at the venular end) causes exudation of plasma. This is the basis of one of the classical signs of acute inflammation, edema. PGs do not alter capillary permeability directly but, by dilating small arterioles, they enhance the edema induced by the primary mediators. They therefore have been described as inflammatory modulators. Inhibition of synthesis of PGs by NSAIDs explains their antiedematous actions.

Third, there is synergy between proinflammatory mediators in the induction of COX-2 protein and in the supply of AA to enhance prostanoid production at inflammatory sites (Hamilton et al. 1999). These authors showed that LPS-induced COX-2 induction alone did not greatly increase prostanoid production, but it was markedly increased by bradykinin administration through an increase in the supply of the substrate AA.

A relatively recent discovery is that COX-2 generates *anti*inflammatory as well as *pro*inflammatory PGs. Studies by Gilroy and co-workers (1998, 1999) demonstrated, in a rat pleurisy model of inflammation, that COX-2 is upregulated not only in the early stage (2 hours) of acute inflammation but also in the resolution phase (around 48 hours). The early peak of COX-2 production was associated with the synthesis of proinflammatory PGE_2 by polymorphonuclear leukocytes, while the later peak was associated with the synthesis of antiinflammatory PGs e.g., 15deoxy$\Delta^{12-14}PGJ_2$ (15dPGJ_2) by mononuclear cells (Gilroy et al. 1999). 15dPGJ_2 is a ligand for the nuclear receptor peroxisome proliferator-activated receptor-γ (PPAR-γ) and some of the actions of 15dPGJ_2 may result from activation of PPAR-γ. For example, 15dPGJ_2 induces apoptosis of synoviocytes from rheumatoid arthritis patients by activating PPAR-γ (Kawahito et al. 2000). 15dPGJ_2 also promotes adipogenesis by activating PPAR-γ (Urade and Eguchi 2002). Inhibition of synthesis of 15dPGJ_2 with COX-2 selective as well as with nonselective NSAIDs potentially might lead to a more protracted resolution/healing phase in acute inflammation.

Proinflammatory PGs and leukotrienes (LTs) are synthesized from AA, which is an ω-6 fatty acid, by the catalytic actions of COX and 5-LO, respectively. ω-3 fatty acids, present in high concentrations in fish oils, include eicosapentanoic acid (EPA) and docosahexanoic acid (DHA). EPA and DHA also serve as substrates for COX and 5-LO. They can thereby suppress the proinflammatory activities of AA both competitively and through the synthesis of products with less inflammatory or even antiinflammatory activity. Thus, resolvin E1, an EPA derivative, is present in inflammatory exudate in the resolution phase of acute inflammation. Resolvin E1 synthesis involves first conversion of EPA to 18R-hydroxyEPA by COX-2 in endothelial cells and its subsequent transformation to resolvin E1 by 5-LO in adjacent leukocytes. Resolvin E1 suppresses both leukocyte infiltration to inflammatory sites and the production of proinflammatory cytokines and chemokines.

12-LO leads to 12-HPETE and 12-HETE formation, while 15-LO forms lipoxins A and B. The lipoxins possess antiinflammatory properties; together with 15dPGJ_2 and resolvin E1 they may subserve roles in the resolution stage of acute inflammation. On the other hand, 5-LO generates the LT family of proinflammatory eicosanoids, such as LTB_4 and the peptidoleukotrienes LTC_4, LTD_4, and LTE_4. LTB_4 is a potent proinflammatory chemoattractant, drawing first neutrophils and later mononuclear cells to inflammatory sites. In addition, it activates leukocytes at these sites so that mediators of other classes are released. LTC_4 constricts arterioles and decreases blood flow. LTs are mediators not only of local vascular and cellular changes at sites of tissue damage and nonimmune inflammation but also in immune-mediated inflammatory conditions. Possible roles of LTs in conditions such as reactive airway obstruction in the horse and skin allergies in the dog have been investigated, and the use of 5-LO inhibitors as well as inhibitors of the actions of released LTs as therapeutic agents in immune-based inflammatory diseases has been researched (Marr et al. 1998a,b,c).

ISOFORMS OF CYCLOOXYGENASE: CHARACTERISTICS, LOCATIONS, AND ROLES

CYCLOOXYGENASE-1 (COX-1). COX-1 is a membrane-bound enzyme present in the endoplasmic reticulum (Table 19.1). It first cyclizes AA to form PGG_2 and then adds a 15-hydroperoxy group to convert PGG_2 to PGH_2. COX-1 is expressed constitutively in many tissues

TABLE 19.1 Characteristics, actions, and roles of COX-1 and its inhibition

A membrane-bound hemo- and glycoprotein of molecular weight 71 kDa, present in the endoplasmic reticulum and comprising approximately 600 amino acids.
Encoded by a 22 Kb gene.
Constitutively expressed by cells in a wide range of tissues involved in housekeeping functions.
Enzyme concentrations are relatively stable, although small (two- to fourfold) increases occur in response to stimulation by hormones and growth factors and by agents causing cell differentiation.
Responsible for generation of TxA_2 and PGs e.g., PGE_2 and PGI_2 with local hormonal (autacoid) functions, such as gastroprotection, renoprotection, and hemostasis.
Inhibited by classical NSAIDs (which generally are nonselective for COX-1 and COX-2).
NSAIDs, which may show some selectivity for inhibition of COX-1 relative to COX-2, include aspirin, ketoprofen, indomethacin, piroxicam, and, from preliminary equine studies, vedaprofen.
Aspirin irreversibly inhibits COX-1 by covalent acetylation of amino acid Ser 530. Other NSAIDs inhibit COX-1 by excluding arachidonic acid from the upper portion of a long, hydrophobic channel.

and in blood platelets. It is involved in "housekeeping" functions, including blood clotting, regulation of vascular homeostasis, renoprotection, gastroprotection, and coordination of the actions of circulating hormones.

CYCLOOXYGENASE-2 (COX-2). COX-2 is both an inducible and constitutive isoform (Table 19.2). It is encoded by a different gene than COX-1. Induction of COX-2 synthesis is stimulated by proinflammatory cytokines, growth factors and lipopolysaccharide (LPS) as well as mitogens. COX-2 produces both pro- and antiinflammatory PGs at sites of inflammation. The cloning, expression, and selective inhibition of canine COX-1 and COX-2 have been reported (Gierse et al. 2002).

While most data support COX-2 as the isoform which generates pro- and antiinflammatory PGs at sites of inflammation, some findings indicate a role for COX-1 (Smith et al. 1998). In a chronic granulomatous model of inflammation, aspirin (preferential for COX-1 inhibition) was more effective than nimesulide and NS-398 (both selective for COX-2) in reducing granuloma weight, vascularity, and COX activity (Gilroy et al. 1998).

TABLE 19.2 Characteristics, actions, and roles of COX-2 and its inhibition

Molecular weight of 70 kD comprising approximately 600 amino acids and having 60% homology with COX-1 at the amino acid level.
Has similar active sites to COX-1 for binding AA and NSAIDs, although the active site of COX-2 is larger and more flexible than that of COX-1 and can accept a wider range of structures as substrates, as a consequence of exchange of Ile in COX-1 for Val in COX-2 at positions 434 and 523.
Encoded by an 8.3 Kb gene descended from a common ancestor with COX-1 but much smaller than COX-1.
One of a family of primary response genes (which also includes iNOS), induced during inflammation and cell growth, with many regulatory sites.
Unlike COX-1 possesses a TATA box and binding sites for transcription factors e.g., NFκB and a cyclic AMP response binding element in the promoter region of the immediate-early gene.
A better competitor than COX-1 for AA released within the cell.
Expression of COX-2 is increased on exposure to LPS, cytokines (e.g., IL-1, TNFα), growth factors, bacterial toxins, and phorbol esters. Induced also by mitogens, immune and inflammatory stimuli. Induction is generally marked but transient.
COX-2 expression regulated at the posttranslational level, for example, by Ras which exerts this influence at least partly through protein kinase B, leading to stabilization of COX-2mRNA.
Present constitutively in monocytes, macrophages, endothelial cells, brain, spinal cord, kidney, ovary, uterus, and ciliary body in the eye.
Produces proinflammatory PGs (e.g., PGE_2) in the early stages of the acute inflammatory response and antiinflammatory PGs (e.g., $15dPGJ_2$) in the resolution phase.
Down-regulated at the mRNA level by corticosteroids (due to transcriptional and posttranscriptional repression of COX-2 mRNA), and also down-regulated by TGFβ.
Exerts significant roles in certain cancers, Alzheimer's disease, and arthritides, and activation inhibits apoptosis (NSAIDs induce apoptosis).
Aspirin preferentially inhibits COX-1 (acetylating Ser 530), although higher concentrations also acetylate irreversibly Ser 516 on COX-2. Other NSAIDs compete reversibly with AA, the substrate for COX-1 and COX-2 for the active sites on the enzymes.
Specific and selective inhibitors of COX-2, the COXIBs, are antiinflammatory and analgesic and have higher gastrointestinal tolerance than nonselective COX inhibitors.

HISTORY OF NSAIDS

The historical antecedents of the modern range of NSAIDs were extracts of various plants, in therapeutic use for more than 3,500 years, and comprising particularly the leaves and bark of the willow tree. These contain saligenin (salicyl alcohol) or salicylic acid either in free form or as glycosides such as salicin. The analgesic and antiinflammatory properties of willow extracts were described in early writings—

for example, by Dioscorides in his pharmacopoeia in the first century A.D, as follows: "the leaves being beaten small and dranke with a little pepper and wine doe help such as are troubled with the Iliaca Passio (colic) . . . the concoction of ye leaves and barke is an excellent fomentation for ye gout." In a classical text, the Rev. Edward Stone of Chipping Norton, U.K., described in his letter to the United Kingdom's Royal Philosophical Society in 1795 the antipyretic properties (cure of agues) of the willow noting, "as this tree delights in a moist or wet soil, where agues (fever) chiefly abounds the general maxim that many natural remedies carry their cures along with them or that remedies lie not far from their causes was so very apposite to this particular case that I could not help applying it." In 1827 an extract of willow bark was shown to contain the glycoside salicin and, on hydrolysis, this yielded salicyl alcohol. From the alcohol, salicylic acid was synthesized in 1838 and reaction with sodium hydroxide converted this to sodium salicylate.

Discovery of salicyl alcohol/salicylic acid as the active principles of plants in the early 19th century led to the use of sodium salicylate as the first synthetic NSAID in 1875 and then to the introduction of the acetyl ester of salicylic acid (aspirin) in 1898 by Felix Hoffman of the Bayer Pharmaceutical Company. In human medicine aspirin has gained the distinction of being the most extensively used drug of all time; the world consumption rate is estimated at 1 million tablets per hour. By the sixth decade of the 20th century, aspirin, cinchophen, phenylbutazone, dipyrone, and isopyrin were, for several years, the most frequently used NSAIDs in veterinary therapy. However, in the 1970s flunixin and meclofenamate and then in the last 20 years a greater number of NSAIDs have received worldwide marketing authorizations for veterinary use. Now, an extensive range of licensed drugs in both oral and parenteral formulations is available for use in animals. Over the last 15 years in particular, there have been intensive searches for novel agents within the NSAID class, stimulated by several factors.

First, there has been the recognition that all species of animal of veterinary interest feel, and almost certainly suffer, pain in a manner similar to the human animal. The debate on the welfare benefits of controlling animal pain has been stimulated and conducted by all members of the veterinary community, including anesthetists, pharmacologists, surgeons, and orthopedic specialists, as well as general practitioners and most particularly colleagues in the pharmaceutical industry. Second, it has been recognized that available drugs of the NSAID class, while commonly very efficacious, do not consistently in all animals or in all circumstances provide adequate levels of analgesia, especially when pain is severe. Third, the need to improve safety margins has been recognized, notably in relation to gastrointestinal (g.i.t.) tolerance of NSAIDs, but also to ensure renal safety and to avoid any possibility of uncontrolled hemorrhage. In other words, a high and consistent level of efficacy combined with a wide safety margin in both short- and long-term use have not been provided by existing drugs in all subjects or all circumstances.

Although much less evidence is available from pharmacovigilance studies in animals, the data on g.i.t. toxicity of NSAIDs in humans is compelling. In the U.S. the ARAMIS (Arthritis, Rheumatism and Aging Medical Information System) study indicated that 117,000 hospitalizations per year arise from NSAID-induced g.i.t. side effects and there are at least 16,500 annual deaths (Singh 1998). For the U.K., the estimated comparable annual human death rate is 2,000 per annum. These absolute numbers are unacceptably high for both morbidity and mortality, but set against the extensive use of NSAIDs in humans the percentage of subjects displaying life-threatening side effects is very low. Clinical veterinary experience suggests a similar situation for NSAID safety in animals, i.e., most of the modern licensed drugs are used in formulations and at dose rates that are efficacious and clinically safe in the great majority of treated animals. There are several qualifications to this statement. First, it is possible to cite equine examples (vide infra) of narrow margins between clinically recommended NSAID doses and doses causing significant toxicity. Second, side effects may be related to age and physiological/pathological status (for example, conditions and circumstances involving hypotension and hypovolemia predispose towards renotoxicity). Third, NSAID toxicity may be idiosyncratic, occurring unpredictably even with manufacturers' recommended dose rates. Therefore, the desire to improve efficacy, but more especially the safety concerns on older drugs, have driven the search for novel agents for human and veterinary use.

THE VETERINARY NSAID MARKET

There are strong geographical distributions in the world veterinary NSAID market, with approximately 60% of the total companion animal market occurring in North

America, 30% in Europe, 3% in Australia, and 2% in Japan. The small animal populations in North America and Europe have been estimated to be 62 and 32 million (dog) and 71 and 34 million (cat), respectively. It is of further interest to note that 40% of the EU market for NSAIDs is in the U.K., where there has been 100% growth since 1998 under the influence of animal welfare concerns, a high percentage of breeds disposed to osteoarthritis, a high percentage of surgical cases, an increasing level of NSAID usage in the cat, and the early introduction and hence availability of new drugs to the U.K. veterinary market. It seems likely that NSAID usage will increase in many countries, as animal welfare aspects of pain control are increasingly recognized. Moreover, there is now extensive veterinary use of NSAIDs for their antiinflammatory (antiedematous) properties in farm animal medicine in conditions such as calf and piglet pneumonias, bovine mastitis, and endotoxemia in several species. Other therapeutic uses, likely to increase in the future, include the therapy of cancers and (in humans) dementias.

CLASSIFICATION OF NSAIDS AND PHYSICOCHEMICAL PROPERTIES

Although useful to chemists, classifications based on chemical structure are of limited value pharmacologically, toxicologically, and clinically because, despite some differences between subgroups, all of the older NSAIDs have similar pharmacological actions (analgesic, antiinflammatory, and antipyretic), similar toxicity profiles (notably potential g.i.t. and renotoxicity) and the same clinical uses. Moreover, physicochemical properties are generally similar; almost all are weak organic acids (pKa of the order of 3.5 to 6.0) of moderate to high lipid solubility (USP Veterinary Pharmaceutical Information Monographs 2004) and these properties impact on their pharmacokinetic profiles.

The older (classical) NSAIDs are divided on the basis of chemical structure into two main groups: carboxylic acids and enolic acids. Each group may be further divided into subgroups on the basis of chemical structure (Table 19.3).

NSAIDs of the 2-arylpropionate group contain a single center of asymmetry; they are therefore chiral compounds. They are produced commercially as racemic (50 : 50) mixtures of the two optical enantiomers (R[−] and S[+]) and thus comprise a mixture of two drugs.

TABLE 19.3 Classification of Classical NSAIDs

Carboxylic Acids (R-COOH)	Enolic Acids (R-COH)
Salicylates	**Oxicams**
Sodium salicylate**	*Meloxicam**
*Acetylsalicylic acid**	Piroxicam
	Tenoxicam
Indoleacetic acids	
*Etodolac****	**Pyrazolones**
	*Phenylbutazone**
Indolines	Oxyphenbutazone***
Indomethacin	*Isopyrin (ramifenazone)**
	*Dipyrone**
Thiopheneacetic acids	
Diclofenac	
*Eltenac**	
2-Arylpropionic acids	
*Carprofen**	
*Ketoprofen**	
*Vedaprofen**	
Flurbiprofen	
Ibuprofen	
Naproxen	
Anthranilic acids	
*Flunixin**	
*Meclofenamic acid**	
*Tolfenamic acid**	
Mefenamic acid	
Quinolines	
*Cinchophen**	

*Drugs licensed for veterinary use.
**Also a metabolite of acetylsalicylic acid.
***Also a metabolite of phenylbutazone.

The COXIBs, a newer group of NSAIDs, include celecoxib, rofecoxib, and etoricoxib. They are preferential or selective inhibitors of the COX-2 isoform and they have differing structures to classical NSAIDs. Most are sulphones or sulphonamides (also described as diarylheterocycles), although lumiracoxib (developed for human use) is exceptional, being a carboxylic acid similar in structure to diclofenac. Their relatively bulky structure limits COX-1 inhibition by steric hindrance. Deracoxib, firocoxib, mavacoxib and robenacoxib have been developed for veterinary use; others are under development. Also relatively new to human and veterinary medicine are the dual COX/5-LO inhibitors, tepoxalin and licofelone.

PHARMACOLOGY OF NSAIDS

As indicated in Chapter 1, *pharmacology* may be defined as a study of drug action on the body (*Pharmacodynamics*) together with a study of drug absorption into, distribution within, and elimination from the body (*Pharmacokinetics*). The application of both components is essential for designing dosage schedules that are effective and safe for therapeutic use (Lees et al. 2004a,b).

NSAID PHARMACOKINETICS

ABSORPTION. As lipid soluble weak organic acids, NSAIDs are generally well absorbed when administered orally to both companion animal and ruminant species (Table 19.4). In monogastric species absorption from the stomach is favored by the Henderson-Hasselbalch ion trapping mechanism, which maintains a diffusion gradient for undissociated acid molecules between acidic gastric juice and plasma of pH 7.4. In ruminants, initial absorption from the four-compartment stomach and subsequent intestinal absorption creates the basis for a biphasic absorption pattern. In young ruminants, early studies reported operation of the esophageal groove reflex as another mechanism to explain double peaks in the plasma concentration-time curve (Marriner and Bogan 1979). Despite dilution in a large volume of rumen liquor (approximately 120 litres in an adult cow), bioavailability of phenylbutazone and meclofenamate was shown to be 50–60% in cattle (Lees et al. 1988a, Marriner and Bogan 1979).

TABLE 19.4 General pharmacokinetic properties of NSAIDs

Generally good bioavailability in monogastric species after oral dosing due to medium to high lipid solubility. Absorption may be (a) delayed by binding to digesta (e.g., in horses and ruminants) or (b) enhanced in the presence of food (e.g., tepoxalin in the dog).
Good bioavailability after parenteral (IM, SC) dosing.
Penetrate blood-brain barrier to act centrally.
High degree of plasma protein binding of most drugs (except salicylate) in all species limits passage from plasma into interstitial and transcellular fluids but *facilitates* passage into inflammatory exudate.
Glomerular ultrafiltration and the renal excretion of parent drug markedly limited by high degree of plasma protein binding—only the free fraction is available for ultrafiltration in glomerular capillaries.
Low volume of central compartment and low volume of distribution (with some exceptions).
Elimination predominantly by metabolism in liver, usually to inactive compounds, but some metabolites are active:
  Phenylbutazone → oxyphenbutazone
  Aspirin → salicylate
For most drugs there are marked species (and possibly breed) differences in the following:
  Clearance
  Terminal half-life
Reduced clearance, increased half-life in neonates.
Enterohepatic recycling occurs for some drugs.

There are exceptions to the high bioavailability of NSAIDs after oral dosing. In one study involving the administration an oil-based formulation of RS-ketoprofen orally to horses, bioavailability was <5% for both enantiomers, both in the presence and absence of feed availability at the time of dosing. However, when the pure drug substance was administered in gelatin capsules, bioavailability was of the order of 50% for each enantiomer (Landoni and Lees 1995a). As well as formulation, a factor affecting the availability of NSAIDs for absorption, of significance in herbivores, and particularly the horse, is binding of drugs to hay (shown in vitro) and to digesta (demonstrated in vivo). This has been studied for phenylbutazone, meclofenamic acid, and flunixin (Lees et al. 1988b). However, the degree of binding to hay in vitro varied with the drug. It was highest (greater than 98%) for phenylbutazone and least (approximately 70%) for flunixin, accounting for differing absorption patterns in vivo. These were characterized by double peaks in plasma concentration-time curves for both drugs but with much greater delay in absorption for phenylbutazone compared to flunixin (Maitho et al. 1986; Welsh et al. 1992). However, for neither drug was bioavailability reduced by the availability of feed.

In monogastric species administration of NSAIDs with food is a common practice, as it may lessen irritant effects on the g.i.t. As in horses, this practice is likely to delay absorption but to reduce absorption only moderately or not at all. For individual drugs, administration with food may *increase* bioavailability. This has been demonstrated for the highly lipid soluble drug, tepoxalin, in the dog; absorption is increased when administered with both low and high fat meals, especially the latter, compared to dosing in fasting dogs (Homer et al. 2005).

Other factors, including product formulation, may influence the rate and/or extent of absorption of NSAIDs. In aspirin for example, plain, water-soluble, film-coated, buffered, enteric-coated, and time-release formulations have been developed and these can influence disintegration and dissolution rates and hence absorption patterns.

DISTRIBUTION. Most NSAIDs are highly bound to plasma protein (95–99% or even greater) (Galbraith and McKellar 1996). Therefore, there is limited passage from plasma into interstitial fluid. The volume of the central compartment and volume of distribution are generally low and values of 0.1–0.3 l/kg or less for the latter are common. There are exceptions, however, and moderate to high volumes of distribution have been reported for flunixin in cattle (but not in other species); for tolfenamic acid in the dog, calf, and pig; and for firocoxib and robenacoxib in the dog (McCann et al. 2004; King et al., in press). The cause of these apparently paradoxical findings is not clear but one possibility is enterohepatic recirculation, as has been established for indomethacin and tolfenamic acid in the dog, or to a high level of extravascular accumulation/tissue binding at unidentified sites.

A potential therapeutic advantage of the high degree of plasma protein binding is accumulation of NSAIDs in inflammatory exudate. Since exudate is rich in plasma protein, which has leaked from the circulation, the binding of NSAIDs to this protein accounts for ready penetration into and persistence at sites of acute inflammation. This is illustrated by studies using tissue cage models of inflammation in which fluid is harvested from inflamed (exudate) or noninflamed (transudate) cages, which allows comparison of area under curve (AUC) values of these fluids with plasma AUC (Table 19.5).

Exudate concentrations often exceed plasma AUC when drug body clearance is high and terminal half-life is short. Accumulation in exudate is a likely explanation for 1) the maintained effectiveness of NSAIDs when plasma concentrations have decreased to low levels and 2) why those NSAIDs with short elimination half-lives in most species (e.g., flunixin, ketoprofen, vedaprofen and tolfenamic acid) may be effective with twice or even once daily dosing. The longer duration of effect than would be predicted from plasma concentrations is associated with the negative hysteresis described in in vivo studies, which indicate that maximal inhibition of PGE_2 synthesis in inflammatory exudate occurs some time after peak drug concentrations in plasma have occurred (Giraudel et al. 2005b).

For the 2-arylpropionate NSAIDs enantioselectivity of extravascular distribution into exudate and transudate (in models of inflammation) (Table 19.5) and also into synovial fluid (Armstrong et al. 1999a) has been demonstrated. These findings illustrate the importance of establishing differences in the extravascular distribution of the enantiomers of chiral NSAIDs, particularly as the enantiomers exhibit significant pharmacodynamic differences as well (vide infra).

The penetration of NSAIDs into milk in the absence of mammary gland infection is poor, milk concentrations being of the order of 1% or less of plasma total (protein-bound plus free) concentration. This results from the high degree of binding to plasma protein. Distribution into milk is also limited by the Henderson-Hasselbalch mechanism, as milk pH is less than that of plasma. In mastitis, however, penetration is likely to be increased from these low levels.

TABLE 19.5 Penetration of NSAIDs administered intravenously into acute inflammatory exudate and transudate relative to plasma

Administered Drug	Species	Dose (mg/kg)	AUC (μg·h/ml)		
			Plasma	Exudate	Transudate
RS-carprofen**[1]	Horse	4.0	558 (R) 138 (S)	451 (R) 133 (S)	336 (R) 93 (S)
Flunixin*[2]	Calf	2.2	11.8	27.6	7.0
Flunixin*[3]	Horse	1.1	19.3	36.0	12.1
RS-ketoprofen*[3]	Horse	2.2	4.2 (R) 5.7 (S)	8.6 (R) 11.9 (S)	2.7 (R) 3.5 (S)
S-ketoprofen*[4]	Horse	1.1	2.7	32.6	3.4
S-ketoprofen*[5]	Calf	1.5	13.2	26.1	20.9
Phenylbutazone*[6]	Horse	4.4	156	128	49
Phenylbutazone*[7]	Donkey	4.4	19.2	8.0	5.0
Phenylbutazone**[8]	Calf	4.4	3604	1117	766
Tolfenamic acid*[9]	Calf	2.0	8.7	16.1	11.3

*Short plasma elimination half-life; **longer half-life.

Data from [1]Armstrong et al. (1999a); [2]Landoni et al. (1995c); [3]Landoni and Lees (1995b); [4]Landoni and Lees (1996); [5]Landoni and Lees (1995c); [6]Lees et al. (1986); [7]Cheng et al. (1996); [8]Arifah et al. (2002); [9]Landoni et al. (1996).

TABLE 19.6 Terminal half-life of NSAIDs (intravenous administration unless stated)

Species	Salicylate	Flunixin	Meloxicam	Carprofen S(+) R(−)	Ketoprofen S(+) R(−)	Naproxen	Tolfenamic Acid
Horse	1.0–3.0	1.6–2.1	3	16, 21	1.0, 0.7	5	7.3
Cow/calf	0.5, 3.7 (p.o.)	8	13	37, 50	0.4, 0.4	—	11.3
Pig	5.9	—	4	—	—	5	3.1
Dog	8.6	3.7	12–36	7, 8	3.5[3]	35–74[2]	5.3
Cat	22–45[1]	—	37	15, 20	1.5, 0.6	—	10.8
Monkey	—	—	—	—	—	1.9	—
Man	3.0 (p.o.)	—	20–50	12[3]	—	14	—

[1]Dose-dependent pharmacokinetics.

[2]Breed-dependent pharmacokinetics (lower value refers to beagles, higher value to mongrels).

[3]Values quoted in the literature for total drug, a concept that is flawed. For the COXIBs half-life values in the dog are 6.31 h (firocoxib) and 0.63 h (robenacoxib). Mavacoxib has a prolonged half-life in the dog.

EXCRETION AND METABOLISM (ELIMINATION). As all classical NSAIDs are weak organic acids, their elimination in urine can be expected to vary with urine pH. Ion trapping of the poorly lipid soluble ionized moiety in alkaline urine will favor excretion in herbivores (e.g., horses and ruminants) but not in omnivores and carnivores (e.g., dogs and cats), as the urine is generally acidic. However, of greater importance for renal excretion in all species is the high degree of plasma protein binding of NSAIDs, which limits passage into glomerular ultrafiltrate to a small amount of the total drug present in plasma. Hence, for most NSAIDs only small fractions of the administered dose are excreted in unchanged form in urine, irrespective of species and urine pH. This is illustrated by phenylbutazone excretion in the alkaline urine of horses; as a percentage of administered dose, the 24-hour excretions of phenylbutazone, and the metabolites oxyphenbutazone and γ-hydroxyphenylbutazone, were 1.9, 11.2 and 12.9, respectively (Lees et al. 1987b).

Although data on pathways of metabolism are limited, most NSAIDs are eliminated primarily by hepatic metabolism to less active (or inactive) metabolites. However, some drugs, such as aspirin and phenylbutazone, are converted to the active metabolites, salicylate and oxyphenbutazone, respectively (Lees et al. 1987a,b). The deacetylation of aspirin is, in part, a spontaneous reaction, so that aspirin only has a half-life of several minutes in plasma. Therefore, salicylate accounts for most of the analgesic and antiinflammatory properties of administered aspirin, although aspirin itself accounts for the platelet-based antithrombotic actions. This is because aspirin is unique among NSAIDs in blocking platelet COX covalently and irreversibly and therefore for the lifespan of the platelet. This permanent inhibition of the platelet enzyme occurs after exposure for only a limited period, so that the short half-life of aspirin (approximately 9 minutes) in the horse is not a limiting factor in platelet COX-1 inhibition (Lees et al. 1987a).

TABLE 19.7 Species differences in phenylbutazone pharmacokinetics

Species	Elimination Half-Life (h)	Clearance (ml/h/kg)
Man	72–96	—
Cow	42–65	1.24–2.90
Sheep	18	—
Goat	16	13.0
Camel	13	4.9–10.0
Horse	4–6	16.3–26.0
Dog	4–6	—
Rat	2.8–5.4	35–86
Donkey	1–2	170

Examples of elimination half-life are presented in Table 19.6. Interpretation of these values must take account of the fact that half-life is a hybrid variable, controlled by body clearance and volume of distribution.

Species differences in some aspects of the pharmacokinetics of NSAIDs are the rule rather than the exception. For example, while plasma protein binding is almost invariably high and volume of distribution is low with most drugs in most species, rate of elimination (clearance) varies markedly, giving rise to differences in terminal half-life. The example of phenylbutazone (administered intravenously) is presented in Table 19.7. Because dosing interval is dependent on terminal half-life, this varies considerably between species and must be separately determined for each species.

Although no longer extensively used in veterinary medicine, aspirin, like phenylbutazone, provides a useful example of the impact of elimination rate on dosing intervals. The terminal half-life ranges from 32 minutes in cattle to 22 to 45 hours in the cat, in which species elimination is zero order (dose-dependent pharmacokinetics).

The pharmacokinetics of the 2-arylpropionate subgroup of NSAIDs (carprofen, ketoprofen, and vedaprofen) is further complicated by the fact that these agents exist in two mirror-image enantiomeric forms, R and S. The licensed products are the racemic (50:50) mixtures. Etodolac, though not a 2-arylpropionate, also possesses a single chiral center. The importance of NSAID chirality derives from the fact that the body is a chiral environment, whose cell membranes, macromolecules, and enzymes are based on D-monosaccharides and L-amino acids. Therefore, while NSAID enantiomers have virtually identical physicochemical properties (melting point, lipid solubility, water solubility); they do *not* have the same pharmacological properties in the body's chiral environment, as manifested by both pharmacokinetic and pharmacodynamic differences. These differences impact on clinical response, because only the S-enantiomer is believed to be pharmacologically active, although a few authors have proposed that the R-enantiomer may contribute to therapeutic effects (Brune et al. 1992). Pharmacokinetic data for 2-arylpropionates based on "the total drug" concept must be viewed with caution; such data may comprise "highly sophisticated scientific nonsense" (Ariens 1985), because racemic mixtures are simply combinations, in equal proportions, of two distinct drugs. Pharmacokinetic differences are reflected in clearance, elimination half-life, and plasma AUC ratios for the two enantiomers. As illustrated by carprofen, these ratios vary between species and may be as high as 4:1, despite the 1:1 ratio in the administered products (Tables 19.5, 19.8).

Differences in pharmacokinetics for each enantiomer of chiral NSAIDs may arise in one or both of two ways (in the case of carprofen the extent of distribution and rate of elimination differ for the two enantiomers, the degrees of difference varying between species). First, a major and possible sole cause of enantiomer differences in elimination is the differing rates of hepatic metabolism (Soraci et al. 1995). Second, for other chiral NSAIDs, including ketoprofen, there is, over and above the inherent differences in elimination rate between R and S enantiomers, an additional factor, namely, chiral inversion. This involves the in vivo conversion of one enantiomer to the other and this, almost invariably, is unilateral, comprising R to S inversion. The extent to which this occurs has been studied and quantified for ketoprofen by administering intravenously each enantiomer separately and then measuring plasma concentration-time profiles for both enantiomers. Species (and possibly breed) differences in the extent of chiral inversion occur (Table 19.9). Thus, when RS-

TABLE 19.8 Species variation in stereoselective pharmacokinetics of carprofen enantiomers*

Species	Dose of Rac-carprofen (mg/kg)	Administration Route (and Dosing Duration)	AUC (% of total)	
			R (−)	S (+)
Dog (beagle)[1]	4.0	Oral	64	36
Dog (various breeds)[2]	2.0	Oral (day 1)	52	48
		Oral (day 7)	52	48
		Oral (day 28)	57	43
Cat[3]	0.7	Intravenous	69	31
	0.7	Subcutaneous	67	33
	4.0	Intravenous	70	30
	4.0	Subcutaneous	72	28
Calf[4]	0.7	Intravenous	58	42
Horse[5,6]	0.7	Intravenous	80–84	16–20
	4.0	Intravenous	80	20
Sheep[7]	4.0	Intravenous	74	26

*Single dose unless stated.
[1]McKellar et al. 1994b.
[2]Lipscomb et al. 2002.
[3]Taylor et al. 1996.
[4]Delatour et al. 1996.
[5]Lees et al. 2002.
[6]Armstrong et al. 1999a.
[7]Cheng et al. 2003.

TABLE 19.9 Species differences in extent of chiral inversion of R(−)- to S(+)-ketoprofen

Species	Inversion (% of Administered Dose)
Horse	48.8
Calf	31.7
Cat	22.4
Goat	15.0
Sheep (female, Dorset Cross)	13.8
Sheep (male, Corriedale)	5.9
Man	8.9

TABLE 19.10 Interanimal variation in S-carprofen pharmacokinetics in the dog*

Day of Dosing	Cmax (μg/ml)		AUC (μg/ml·h)	
	Mean	Range	Mean	Range
1	2.95	1.78–3.86	27.4	21.7–35.0
7	3.94	0.00–5.10	35.3	0.00–51.3
28	3.95	1.80–6.72	37.1	14.6–61.2

*Six dogs, various breeds with osteoarthritis; aged 0.7 to 12 years. 2 mg/kg RS-carprofen administered orally daily for 28 days (Lipscomb et al. 2002).

TABLE 19.11 Interanimal variation in firocoxib pharmacokinetics in the beagle dog*

Parameter	Mean	Range
Cmax (μg/ml)	1.01	0.51–1.37
Tmax (h)	2.63	0.79–4.45
AUC (μg/ml·h)	11.00	8.55–14.27
V/F (l/kg)	4.21	2.78–5.08
T1/2el (h)	6.31	3.31–9.99

*Eight young beagles, both sexes: 5 mg/kg single dose administered orally (Lees et al. unpublished data).

ketoprofen is administered, the measured S-ketoprofen in plasma is due, in part, to chiral inversion from R-ketoprofen.

There is, as with drugs of all classes, inevitable interanimal variation in the pharmacokinetics of NSAIDs. This is illustrated by the range of values for Cmax and AUC for S-carprofen in various canine breeds (Table 19.10) and for firocoxib in beagles (Table 19.11).

As well as interanimal and interbreed differences, a report on celecoxib in a colony of 245 beagle dogs revealed a *within*-breed difference in pharmacokinetics, such that, based on capacity to eliminate the drug, the population was classified into two subpopulations, an extensive metabolizer (EM) phenotype for which mean half-life was 1.72 h and clearance was 18.2 ml/kg/min, and a poor metabolizer (PM) phenotype for which corresponding values were 5.18 h and 7.15 ml/kg/min (Paulson et al. 1999). This example points to the possibility and indeed likelihood of significant genetic differences in clearance and terminal half-life of NSAIDs within as well as between canine breeds. In veterinary medicine the science of pharmacogenetics is in its infancy and there is clearly a need for further studies.

In addition to species, inter- and intrabreed, and interanimal differences in NSAID pharmacokinetics, there are inevitable intraanimal differences, for which pathological or physiological state can be of importance. While there are few studies in this field, two investigations with carprofen may be cited. Lascelles et al. (1998) reported, in dogs undergoing anesthesia, greater values of Cmax (20.6 versus 11.0 μg/ml) and AUC (175 versus 115 μg/ml·h) when carprofen was administered postoperatively compared to preoperatively. Second, in adult cows with an *E. coli* endotoxin-induced mastitis, values of AUC and Cl were 507 mg/l.h and 1.4 ml/kg/h for carprofen (0.7 mg/kg) administered intravenously (Lohuis et al. 1991). Values for healthy control cows were 294 mg/l·h and 2.4 ml/kg/h, respectively. There is an urgent need to conduct population pharmacokinetic studies on NSAIDS on a species by species basis.

Although relatively few data are available, age is another factor that will potentially affect the clearance and terminal half-life of NSAIDs. Clearance is slower and half-life is longer in neonates, as established, for example, for phenylbutazone in goats (Eltom et al. 1993). Slower clearance has also been suggested for carprofen in young calves (Lees et al. 1996; Delatour et al. 1996) and for phenylbutazone in older horses (Lees et al. 1985). There is evidence for biliary secretion of some NSAIDs, creating the basis for possible enterohepatic recirculation (Priymenko et al. 1993).

SITES OF ACTION OF NSAIDS. Of the four principal classes of analgesics, it was assumed for many years that opioid receptor and α-2 receptor agonists act centrally, and that NSAIDs and local anesthetics act peripherally, i.e., at sites of tissue damage. It is now recognized that both opioids and NSAIDs exert central and peripheral actions (Dolan and Nolan 2000). COX-1 and COX-2 are expressed constitutively in dorsal root ganglia, in spinal dorsal and ventral grey matter, and in nonneuronal cells including astrocytes (Svensson and Yaksh 2002). Central

COX-2 up-regulation in response to inflammation at peripheral sites is widespread, leading to release of PGE_2, which lowers spinal depolarization thresholds, thereby increasing action potentials and repetitive spiking. PGE_2-induced neuronal effects involve a central sensitization (comparable to that occurring peripherally) "wind-up" phenomenon (Malmberg and Yaksh 1992). Thermal hyperalgesia induced by injection of carrageenan into the paw was suppressed by both intrathecal and systemically administered COX-2 selective drugs and by a COX-1 selective inhibitor administered systemically (Yaksh et al. 2001). Moreover, intraspinal administration of a COX-2 inhibitor decreased central PGE_2 concentrations and suppressed mechanical hyperalgesia (Samad et al. 2001). Thus, the central actions of nonselective and COX-2 selective NSAIDs contribute to their anti-hyperalgesic actions.

NSAID PHARMACODYNAMICS

INHIBITION OF COX AND 5-LO. In addition to pharmacokinetic differences, a second basis for the variation in clinical response to NSAIDs between species, breeds, and individual animals is differences in their pharmacodynamics. NSAID pharmacodynamics has been studied extensively at several body levels: molecular, cellular, tissue, and whole animal, and can be considered in terms of the action-effect-response relationship (Table 19.12). The principal action is inhibition of COX, an enzyme with a pivotal position in the AA cascade, which leads to inhibition of synthesis of proinflammatory mediators, such as PGE_2 and PGI_2. This inhibitory action has been demonstrated with clinically recommended dose rates of several NSAIDs in several species of veterinary interest (Lees and Higgins 1985; Landoni and Lees 1995a,b,c; Landoni et al. 1995a,b,c; Cheng et al. 2002; Jones et al. 2002). Whole animal responses are the analgesic, antipyretic, antiinflammatory, antithrombotic, and antiendotoxemic responses of NSAIDs (Lees et al. 1986; Welsh and Nolan 1994; Welsh et al. 1997; Nolan 2001; Cheng et al. 2002; Giraudel et al. 2005b). Current evidence suggests that a high level (80 or even 95%) of inhibition of PGs is required to achieve adequate clinical responses (analgesia, etc.).

TABLE 19.12 The principal action-effect-response relationships of NSAIDs

Actions	Inhibition of COX-1, COX-2, and, *for some drugs,* 5-LO
Effects	*COX inhibition*: reduced synthesis of eicosanoids with proaggregatory and vasoconstrictor properties (TxA_2); antiaggregatory and vasodilator properties (PGI_2); proinflammatory properties (PGE_2, PGD_2, PGI_2); and antiinflammatory properties (15deoxyΔ^{12-14} PGJ_2). *5-LO inhibition:* for some NSAIDs only, decreased synthesis of proinflammatory leukotrienes (LTB_4, LTC_4, LTD_4, LTE_4).
Responses	Inhibition of body temperature rise (antipyretic), suppression of pain (analgesic), decreased swelling (antiinflammatory) and *possibly* reduced rate of recovery in the resolution phase of acute inflammation—further research required.

Our understanding of the pharmacodynamics of NSAIDs at the molecular level was transformed when Vane (1971) and Smith and Willis (1971) independently discovered that the principal mechanism of action was inhibition of COX, leading to decreased synthesis of proinflammatory mediators of the prostanoid group. A further step forward occurred 20 years later with the discovery that two COX isoforms, COX-1 and COX-2, exist (Kujubu et al. 1991; Xie et al. 1991). It was immediately recognized that most if not all classical NSAIDs inhibit both isoforms; COX-1 inhibition producing toxic effects and COX-2 inhibition providing therapeutic effects. COX-1 was classified as a constitutive enzyme present in most cells of the body (except erythrocytes) with physiological/housekeeping functions, such as gastro- and reno-protection and blood clotting. COX-2 was initially regarded solely as an inducible enzyme, normally absent from cells or present at low basal levels but markedly up-regulated at sites of inflammation and responsible for producing proinflammatory mediators. Since 1991, much effort has been directed to identifying the following: which tissues express the two isoforms constitutively; the physiological and pathological roles of each isoform; the role of COX-2 induction at sites of inflammation and centrally; and the nature, incidence, and severity of side effects produced by drugs that inhibit one or both isoforms.

The overall roles of COX isoforms and the actions of NSAIDs as perceived in 1991, are still generally accepted, but have been modified significantly in several respects:

1. A third isoform, COX-3, has been isolated from dog brain (Chandrasekharan et al. 2002). Originally it was suggested that it might be involved as a central mediator of pain. It was further suggested that, as COX-3 is a splice variant of COX-1, it might more properly be

described as a COX-1 subtype, e.g., COX-lb (Warner and Mitchell 2004). However, it is not clear that COX-3 exists in all species. For example, humans are unlikely to express COX-3 (Dinchuk et al. 2003) and its actual function in the dog is unknown. There is a one nucleotide difference in intron 1, between humans and rats on the one hand and dogs on the other, that results in a shift in the reading frame and which renders it impossible for a full-length, catalytically active form of COX-3 to exist in humans and rats. Nevertheless, the interesting proposal was made that certain older NSAIDs e.g., acetaminophen, phenacetin, and dipyrone, may be preferential inhibitors of COX-3 and that this hypothesis could account for their central analgesic action with little peripheral effect either as antiinflammatory agents or in producing deleterious effects on the g.i.t. (Chandrasekharam et al. 2002). This hypothesis concerning COX-3 now seems improbable. Warner and Mitchell (2004) have concluded that there are only two genes for COX enzymes, COX-1 and COX-2, but multiple COX isoforms may exist across a range of tissues.

2. It is now recognized that COX-2 is a constitutive enzyme, present in brain, kidney, ovary, uterus, and ciliary body, for example (Kujubu et al. 1991; Xie et al. 1991). Therefore, it has been postulated that complete inhibition of COX-2, especially over long periods, might be associated with such side effects as abortion, fetal abnormalities, delayed bone healing, delayed healing of soft tissue, renotoxicity, and "cardiovascular events." Nevertheless, the widespread clinical use over prolonged periods of COX-2 inhibitors in individual humans has been associated with a generally good safety profile for the g.i.t. and other organs. However, preferential and selective COX-2 inhibitors (vide infra) are not free of adverse effect on the g.i.t. and there remains considerable controversy over the cardiovascular events associated with their clinical use in human medicine. This involved the withdrawal of one drug of this class, rofecoxib. COX-2 is both constitutive and inducible in endothelial cells and its selective inhibition might disturb the endothelial PGI_2 (an antiaggregatory and vasodilator PG synthesized via COX-1 and COX-2) platelet TxA_2 (a proaggregatory and vasoconstrictor eicosanoid synthesized by COX-1) balance in the direction of platelet aggregation and vasoconstriction. The cardiovascular events in humans, which have been the subject of much public discussion, might reflect this imbalance. However, some reports have suggested an increased cardiovascular risk in humans receiving long-term therapy with nonselective as well as COX-2 selective drugs.
3. Some reports indicate that COX-1 may contribute to the synthesis of proinflammatory PGs. In knock-out mice with the COX-1 gene deleted, the inflammatory response was suppressed. Therefore, as well as COX-2 inhibition, inhibition of COX-1, as provided by the older nonselective NSAIDs, might be required for optimal efficacy. However, this concept is controversial and most experimental and clinical data in man and increasing data in animals suggest that selective COX-2 inhibitors are as efficacious as nonselective NSAIDs in relieving inflammatory pain.
4. The introduction of a novel class of NSAIDs, the dual inhibitors, which inhibit two enzymes that use AA as a substrate, COX and 5-LO, has made it necessary to compare the older NSAIDs with this newer drug class.

EFFICACY, POTENCY, AND SENSITIVITY OF INHIBITORY ACTIONS OF NSAIDS ON COX ISOFORMS. As discussed in Chapter 4, the three pharmacodynamic properties of any drug that define and quantify its action on a given tissue, organ, or enzyme are efficacy, potency, and sensitivity. Efficacy (Imax/Emax) is the maximal response a drug is capable of producing. It is important to the clinician because it defines, for example, for a NSAID, the level of pain relief that the drug can provide. Potency is the in vitro drug concentration or in vivo drug dose producing a given level of response. It is usually determined as the concentration or dose producing 50% of maximal response (EC_{50} or ED_{50}) or, for drugs such as NSAIDs acting to inhibit an enzyme, potency is usually expressed as IC_{50}, although IC_{80} or IC_{95} can be more useful. Potency is of less relevance than efficacy to the clinician, but it is important to pharmaceutical companies when selecting a recommended dose rate of a NSAID for clinical use. Usually, NSAID concentration-response data are best described by the sigmoidal Emax (Hill) relationship (Chapter 4) and the steepness of this relationship (slope, denoted as N) determines the third pharmacodynamic parameter, sensitivity. Slope may be shallow (less than 1) or steep (10 or greater) and in the latter circumstance the concentration-effect relationship becomes almost quantal (all-or-none).

TABLE 19.13 COX inhibitor classification****

Classification	Example	Comment
Preferential or selective COX-1 inhibitors	Aspirin, carprofen**, ketoprofen*, vedaprofen*, tepoxalin	COX-1 inhibitory potency at least 5-fold greater than COX-2 inhibition
Nonspecific COX inhibitors	Carprofen**, flunixin, ketoprofen*, meloxicam*, phenylbutazone, tolfenamic acid*, vedaprofen*	No significant biological or clinical differences in concentrations producing COX-1 and COX-2 inhibition
Preferential and moderately selective COX-2 inhibitors***	Carprofen**, celecoxib, deracoxib, etodolac, meloxicam*, nimesulide, tolfenamic acid*, Mavacoxib	COX-2 inhibition potency 5- to 100-fold greater than COX-1 inhibition Some antiinflammatory and analgesic activity may be obtained at concentrations inhibiting COX-2 but not COX-1 At higher concentrations, significant inhibition of COX-1 may occur
Highly selective COX-2 inhibitors***	Etoricoxib, firocoxib, lumiracoxib, robenacoxib	More than 100-fold greater potency for COX-2 inhibition Little or no inhibition of COX-1 in vivo (normally no g.i.t. ulceration or antiplatelet effect) even at maximum therapeutic dose

*Differing findings on selectivity from studies in various laboratories.

**Likely species differences in selectivity.

***Selectivity versus specificity depends on position and slope of COX-1 and COX-2 inhibition curves and therefore on the level of inhibition considered e.g., IC_{50}, IC_{80}, IC_{95}, etc.

*****Ratios of inhibition (COX-1 : COX-2) are markedly affected by experimental conditions.*

Using separate in vitro assays to determine COX-1 and COX-2 inhibition, the Hill relationships for NSAIDs have been used to determine Imax, IC_{50}, IC_{80}, IC_{95} etc. and N for each isoform. Depending on both the position and slope of each curve, it is then possible to determine a fourth pharmacodynamic parameter, selectivity, expressed, for example, as the ratio IC50COX-1 : IC50COX-2. The higher the ratio the greater the selectivity for COX-2. However, a high ratio (of say 50 : 1 or even higher) does not guarantee that at clinical dose rates in vivo a drug will inhibit COX-2 with no inhibition of COX-1 (vide infra).

Based on the degree of selectivity for one or the other COX isoform, NSAIDs are classified as COX-1 selective, nonselective or as preferential or selective (denoting increasing degrees of selectivity) for COX-2 (Table 19.13).

Validating, confirming, and interpreting the data in Table 10.13 is problematic, as the scientific literature reports widely differing potency ratios (COX-1 : COX-2) for individual drugs. The in vitro conditions used to determine COX activity impact markedly on the COX-1 : COX-2 inhibition ratios, with much higher values (i.e., higher selectivity for COX-2) commonly obtained when isolated enzyme, broken cell, or intact cell determinations in buffer are used in comparison with whole blood assays. The latter are accepted as the "gold standard" and most relevant to conditions in the whole animal. Thus, Gierse et al. (2002), using isolated enzyme assays, reported for deracoxib an IC_{50} COX-1 : COX-2 ratio of 380 : 1 in humans and 1295 : 1 in the dog, whereas McCann et al. (2004) for the same drug, in a canine whole blood assay, obtained a ratio of 12 : 1. Ricketts et al. (1998) reported a higher COX-1 : COX-2 ratio for rac-carprofen in isolated cell assays than those obtained in whole blood assays (Table 19.14).

TABLE 19.14 Whole blood assays in four species for RS-, S-, and R-carprofen COX-1 : COX-2 IC_{50} and IC_{80} ratios

Species	Enantiomer	IC_{50}	IC_{80}
Human[1]	RS	0.020	0.253
Canine[2]	RS	16.8	101.2
Canine[3]	RS	7	6
Canine[4]	RS	5.4	—
Canine[5]	RS	6.5	—
Canine[6]	S	25.0	—
Canine[6]	R	2.4	—
Equine[6]	S	1.7	—
Equine[6]	R	2.7	—
Feline[5]	RS	5.5	—
Feline[7]	S	25.6	64.9

[1]Warner et al. 1999.
[2]Streppa et al. 2002.
[3]McCann et al. 2004.
[4]Wilson et al. 2004.
[5]Brideau et al. 2001.
[6]Lees et al. 2004a.
[7]Giraudel et al. 2005a.

An additional complication is the possibility (indeed likelihood) of species differences in NSAID potency for COX-1 and COX-2 inhibition and therefore differences also in COX-1 : COX-2 inhibition ratios. For example, on the basis of published data from whole blood assays, carprofen would be classified as COX-1 selective or preferential in humans, nonselective in the horse and COX-2 preferential or selective in the dog and cat (Table 19.14).

Those compounds with a chiral center have differing potencies and potency ratios for each enantiomer for COX-1 and COX-2 inhibition. Data for carprofen enantiomers are presented in Table 19.15. For this drug and other 2-arylpropionates, each enantiomer should be regarded as a separate drug. Studies using the racemate are based on a mixture of two drugs in equal amounts, and (in light of the information in Table 19.15) data on racemates reported in Table 19.14 must be interpreted with caution.

Thus, in vitro data (Tables 19.14 and 19.15) are complex, as they indicate the likelihood for carprofen of 1) differing ratios for IC_{50} and IC_{80} inhibition in each of the species cat, dog, and human, because of lack of parallelism between the COX-1 and COX-2 curves; 2) species differences in selectivity, with carprofen being apparently preferential or selective for COX-1 in man, preferential or selective for COX-2 in the dog and cat, and nonselective in the horse; and 3) differences in both potency and potency ratios for the two enantiomers, with S-carprofen being significantly more potent than R-carprofen in the horse and dog.

A high level of COX-2 inhibition (80–95% of Imax) seems to be necessary to obtain clinically desirable levels of antiinflammatory and analgesic activity. It is therefore possible to integrate plasma concentration-time data obtained in vivo with pharmacodynamic data such as IC_{80} for COX-2 generated in whole blood assays in vitro. The estimated daily dose of S-carprofen required to produce an average 80% inhibition of COX-2 over 24 hours in the cat was 0.32 mg/kg (Giraudel et al. 2005a). However, the recommended dose of RS-carprofen is 4.0 mg/kg. Assuming that R-carprofen makes no contribution to COX-2 inhibition, the dose of the S-enantiomer, 2.0 mg/kg, is still six and one-quarter times the predicted dose. Giraudel et al. (2005a) calculated that the recommended dose of carprofen in the cat should produce 50, 80, and 95% inhibition of COX-2 for periods of 72, 57, and 42 hours, respectively, after a single intravenous dose. In contrast, corresponding values for the clinically recommended dose of meloxicam (0.3 mg/kg) in the cat were 23, 9, and 0 hours, respectively (Giraudel et al. 2005a).

TABLE 19.15 IC_{50} values and IC_{50} COX-1:COX-2 ratios for S- and R-carprofen enantiomers in the dog and horse (whole blood assays)

Enantiomer	COX-1 IC_{50} (μM)	COX-2 IC_{50} (μM)	COX-1 : COX-2 Ratio
DOG			
S(+) carprofen	176	7	25
R(−) carprofen	380	161	2.4
HORSE			
S(+) carprofen	25	14	1.7
R(−) carprofen	373	137	2.7

Data from Lees et al. (2000, 2004a).

The full implications of COX isomer inhibition studies for clinical efficacy and safety have not been determined but, on the basis of COX-1 : COX-2 inhibition ratios and drug concentrations obtained in plasma in vivo with clinical dose rates, it is likely that (in contrast to the cat) RS-carprofen inhibition of COX-2 is at most moderate in the dog and horse when administered at recommended dose rates, 4.0 and 0.7 mg/kg, respectively. This led to the suggestion that carprofen may act, in part, by one or more non-COX mechanisms. On the other hand, COX-2 inhibition data suggest that optimal efficacy might be achieved with a lower dose than that recommended in the cat. Moreover, with the recommended dose in this species, the potential for a high level of inhibition of COX-2 but with virtually no inhibition of COX-1 is lost (Giraudel et al. 2005a).

To date, based on evidence from whole blood in vitro assays, two drugs highly selective for COX-2 have been introduced into veterinary medicine. Firocoxib was found to have IC_{50} and IC_{80} COX-1 : COX-2 ratios of 384 : 1 and 427 : 1 in the dog, while robenacoxib was shown to have corresponding ratios of 140 : 1 and 150 : 1 in the dog (King et al. in press) and 502 : 1 and 478 : 1 in the cat (Giraudel et al. in press). A third drug of this class, mavacoxib, has been introduced for canine use.

IN VIVO AND EX VIVO DETERMINATION OF COX INHIBITION. An alternative to in vitro assays of inhibition of COX isoforms is to determine pharmacodynamic parameters for NSAIDs in vivo or ex vivo. This has the advantage that in vivo and ex vivo conditions are directly relevant to the whole animal. The problem with in vitro assays is both one of uncertain physiological/pharmacological/clinical relevance and also of variability in potency for COX-1 and COX-2 inhibition, depending on in vitro assay conditions. As a supplement to in vitro assays, a tissue cage model of inflammation (Higgins et al. 1984) has been used to undertake ex vivo and in vivo modeling of pharmacokinetic and pharmacodynamic data on NSAIDs, providing estimates of pharmacodynamic parameters. The model is based on stimulation of the granulation tissue in subcutaneously implanted tissue cages with the mild irritant carrageenan to form inflammatory exudate and measurement of the magnitude and time course of inhibition of exudate PGE_2 in vivo as a tentative indicator of COX-2 inhibition. In the same study ex vivo measurement of the magnitude and time course of inhibition of synthesis of serum TxB_2 in blood allowed to clot under standard conditions is used as an indicator of COX-1 inhibition. Based on this approach it is suggested that tolfenamic acid, S-ketoprofen, and flunixin are essentially nonselective inhibitors of COX isoforms (Table 19.16). However, there are apparent small differences in degree of selectivity between species; tolfenamic acid is a preferential COX-2 inhibitor in the goat (but not in calves), while vedaprofen is preferential for COX-1 in the horse (Lees et al. 1999; Sidhu et al. 2005, 2006).

Using data from these studies and assuming 95% inhibition of COX-2 for clinical efficacy, it has been calculated that a once-daily intravenous dose of tolfenamic acid is 1.76 mg/kg, which is similar to the clinically recommended dose of 2.0 mg/kg. For flunixin the predicted dose is 1.06 mg/kg, while the recommended dose is 2.2 mg/kg (Lees 2003). In vivo studies in the dog have suggested that carprofen, deracoxib, etodolac and meloxicam are COX-1 sparing (for platelet TxA_2 and gastric mucosal PGE_2 production), while suppressing the synthesis of synovial fluid PGE_2 concentrations. However, in the final analysis the dose required in clinical use must be determined using clinical end points.

Toutain and co-workers (1994) have undertaken PK-PD modeling of NSAIDs using clinical indices (or surrogates thereof) together with Monte Carlo simulations to predict dosage schedules for clinical use. In an equine model of inflammatory joint disease flunixin was shown to be more potent (IC_{50} values) and efficacious (Imax) than phenylbutazone based on measurements of stride length, rest angle flexion, and carpal skin temperature. Concentration-response relationships for stride length for these drugs, and also for meloxicam (Toutain and Cester 2004) were steep and almost quantal (slope greater than 10). Simulations predicted, for flunixin for stride length, virtually no response at a dose of 0.5 mg/kg, maximal response persisting up to 10 hours at 1 mg/kg and maximal response up to 16 hours with a dose of 2 mg/kg.

Based on PK-PD modeling and simulations in a model of soft tissue inflammation in the cat, Giraudel et al. (2005b) calculated dosages of meloxicam required to provide 50, 70, and 90% of maximal responses for a range of indices of pain and inflammation (Table 19.17).

An example of species differences in NSAID pharmacodynamics is provided by phenylbutazone. Much higher plasma concentrations (more than tenfold) are achieved in man than in the horse with therapeutic doses. Moreover, Lees et al. (2004b) reported that phenylbutazone plasma concentrations 15 times greater in cattle than in the horse produced *less* inhibition of COX-2 in the former species.

For the 2-arylpropionate subgroup of NSAIDs, the S-enantiomers are generally much more potent COX inhibi-

TABLE 19.16 Generation by PK-PD modeling of pharmacodynamic parameters for NSAIDs

	IC_{50} Ratio Serum TxB_2 : Exudate PGE_2			
DRUG	Horse	Calf	Sheep	Goat
S(+) ketoprofen	0.48	1.12	3.38	1.10
Flunixin	1.84	0.32	—	—
Tolfenamic acid	—	1.37	—	12.0
RS(±) vedaprofen	0.015	—	—	—
S(+) carprofen	—	—	6.30	—

TABLE 19.17 Simulated doses of meloxicam required to provide 50, 70, and 90% of maximal responses in the cat

	Meloxicam Dose (mg/kg)		
Endpoint	ED_{50}*	ED_{70}*	ED_{90}*
Skin temperature difference	0.40	0.50	0.67
Pain score	0.30	0.36	0.45
Body temperature	0.24	0.29	0.39
Lameness score	0.26	0.32	0.42
Overall locomotion variable	0.28	0.33	0.43

*ED (mg/kg) is the meloxicam dose producing 50, 70, or 90% of the maximum possible average drug response that can be obtained with a single subcutaneous administration of meloxicam. The manufacturer's recommended dose is 0.3 mg/kg.

Data from Giraudel et al. (2005b).

tors than the R-enantiomers. However, experimentally both enantiomers have been claimed to be analgesic (Brune et al. 1992). The mechanism of action is unclear but R-flurbiprofen suppresses PG production in the spinal cord.

In summary, for NSAIDs there are distinct species, and likely, between-breed, within-breed, and inter- and intra-animal, differences in some pharmacokinetic parameters, notably clearance and terminal half-life. It also seems likely that species, breed, and animal differences occur in pharmacodynamic parameters, such as IC_{50}, IC_{80}, etc., for inhibition of COX-1 and COX-2 and for clinical responses. Taken together, these two components of each drug's pharmacological profile account for the differences commonly encountered by clinicians and owners in therapeutic responses and tolerance to NSAIDs. A drug that clinically best suits one animal may not suit the next, and an agent with poor efficacy or low tolerance in a particular animal may be efficacious and well tolerated in another. Clinical assessment and judgment on a case-by-case basis are still required with available agents.

TABLE 19.18 Novel classes of NSAIDs

Drug Class	Characteristics
Selective COX-2 inhibitors	Inhibition of COX-2 with absence or only partial inhibition of COX-1 at recommended dose rates Improved g.i.t. safety profiles
COX inhibiting nitric oxide donors (CINODs)	Nitrosoesters of NSAIDs (e.g., aspirin, indomethacin, phenylbutazone), releasing nitric oxide and parent drug in vivo Improved g.i.t. safety profile and possibly greater efficacy and/or potency
Dual COX, 5-LO inhibitors	Inhibition of both COX and 5-LO, thus reducing or abolishing at therapeutic dose rates synthesis of two groups of inflammatory mediators derived from arachidonic acid, PGs, and LTs Improved g.i.t. and possibly renal safety profiles

NOVEL NSAID CLASSES

Veterinary medicine has benefited indirectly from the drive to develop safer NSAIDs for human use, driven in turn by the estimated morbidity rate, of 117,000 hospitalizations per year relating to g.i.t. complications in the U.S. alone (Table 19.18).

COX-2 INHIBITORS. Drugs with preferential, selective, or specific activity against COX-2 have provided a major advance in pain therapy (Wilson et al. 2004). COX-2 specific inhibitors are of particular interest in view of the introduction of several COXIBs into human medicine. The introduction of firocoxib into canine medicine for the therapy of canine osteoarthritis constituted the first truly COX-2 selective drug for veterinary use (McCann et al. 2004), and others including deracoxib, mavacoxib and robenacoxib have followed. In the dog the oral bioavailability of firocoxib is high and systemic clearance (7.7 ml/kg/min) is relatively low. In contrast to classical NSAIDs, the volume of distribution (2.9l/kg) is high, despite a high degree (96%) of binding to plasma protein. Steady-state concentrations are achieved after 3 days of dosing. In clinical trials at the recommended dose rates, analgesia was equal to or greater than that of carprofen or etodolac. Robenacoxib has a relatively rapid clearance and short terminal half-life in both dog and cat. Binding to plasma protein is high.

Although not universally accepted, the improved g.i.t. tolerance of selective COX-2 inhibitors over nonselective inhibitors is well established (Warner et al. 1999). However, when g.i.t. ulceration has occurred from any cause, COX-2 is rapidly induced; the enzyme then generates cytoprotective prostaglandins. Furthermore, COX-2 inhibitors have been shown in experimental rodent studies to inhibit the healing of preexisting ulcers. Selective COX-2 inhibitors are therefore unlikely to cause ulcers at recommended dose rates but they might delay the healing of preexisting ulcers. Further evaluation of this possibility is required.

CINODS. CINODs are nitrosoesters of the older nonselective COX inhibitors (e.g., aspirin, indomethacin, phenylbutazone). The ester linkage is hydrolyzed in vivo to yield parent NSAID and the vasodilator NO. The latter may (by an unknown mechanism) enhance potency and it also increases gastric tolerance (Wallace et al. 2004). Again, the mechanism is unknown but the vasodilator action of NO, to inhibit the ischemia, which arises when NSAIDs block synthesis of the endogenous local dilator prostacyclin (PGI_2), is a possibility. NO has also been shown to prevent neutrophil adherence to g.i.t. endothelial cells, which precedes the ischemic, ulcerogenic effects of NSAIDs, and this is another possible mechanism to explain reduced toxicity. No drug of this class has to date been introduced into veterinary therapeutics.

DUAL COX/5-LO INHIBITORS. A third field of advance is dual inhibition of both COX and 5-LO. Compounds of this class first became available in the early 1980s, when they were investigated experimentally in the horse (Higgins et al. 1987a,b). However, the drugs evaluated (BW540C, BW755C) proved to be of low potency, and clinical development was prevented by hepatotoxic properties. More recently, second-generation dual inhibitors have been introduced. Tepoxalin is used in canine medicine and licofelone has been developed for human use and possible veterinary use (Argentiere et al. 1994; Fiorucci et al. 2001; Kay-Mugford et al. 2004; Moreau et al. 2005). These compounds should be distinguished from older NSAIDs, such as tolfenamic acid and ketoprofen, which have been shown to inhibit 5-LO as well as COX in vitro, but which fail to do so when administered at recommended dose rates as licensed products in in vivo models of inflammation (Landoni et al. 1995a,b; 1996). This in vivo, in vitro difference is likely due to the use of high drug concentrations in protein free media in vitro. In vivo lower total concentrations are achieved in plasma and inflammatory exudate and the biologically active free concentrations may be less than 1% of total concentration.

Tepoxalin is converted rapidly in vivo to an acid metabolite, which is a potent COX inhibitor and is cleared more slowly than the parent compound. Tepoxalin produces most of its COX inhibitory effect via the metabolite. However, the parent compound (but not the metabolite) also inhibits 5-LO. In whole blood ex vivo assays, COX inhibition was more persistent than inhibition of 5-LO. *Potentially,* dual inhibitors have a broader spectrum of antiinflammatory activity than that of pure COX inhibitors (Agnello et al. 2005). Indeed, licofelone has been shown to inhibit immune inflammation in a sheep model of asthma (Laufer 2001; Triese and Laufer 2001). This is not surprising as such models are LT-dependent.

In vitro studies indicate that the potency of both tepoxalin and its metabolite for inhibition of COX-1 is approximately thirtyfold greater than for COX-2 so that they are preferential COX-1 inhibitors when assessed using enzymes isolated from ram seminal vesicle (COX-1) and ovine uterus (COX-2). However, the COX-1 : COX-2 potency ratio in canine whole blood in vitro assays or in ex vivo and in vivo studies is not known.

As well as inhibiting COX and 5-LO, tepoxalin has been shown experimentally to inhibit another lipoxygenase, 12-LO, and to block release of the proinflammatory cytokines IL-1, IL-6, and TNF-α. Whether these actions occur with clinical dose rates in the target species (dog) is not known, but potentially they provide additional bases for a broad antiinflammatory spectrum.

The pharmacokinetics of tepoxalin is of interest not only because of the formation of an active metabolite but also because absorption of orally administered parent drug from the g.i.t. is affected by food. Tepoxalin bioavailability is increased when administered with both a high-fat and a low-fat meal in comparison with dosing on an empty stomach (Homer et al. 2005). Therefore, to achieve optimal efficacy, consideration should be given to dosing in feed or at the time of feeding. Both tepoxalin and its active metabolite are highly protein-bound and both are excreted almost entirely (≥99%) in feces. The very low urinary excretion rates may have positive benefits in terms of renal safety.

ADDITIONAL MECHANISMS OF ACTION OF NSAIDS

As well as inhibition of one or both COX isoforms and, for the newer dual inhibitors, inhibition of 5-LO, NSAIDs possess many other actions at the molecular level (Table 19.19).

Other actions claimed for NSAIDs include interference of protein-protein interactions in cell membranes and inhibitory effects on signal transduction pathways (Weissmann 1991). Several NSAIDs, including phenylbutazone and flunixin, inhibit leukocyte migration in in vitro assays (Dawson et al. 1987) but not in vivo. Likewise, actions such as inhibition of NFκB demonstrated in vitro (Bryant et al. 2003) may or may not occur with therapeutic concentrations in vivo.

What is not known is the extent (if any) to which these additional actions contribute to the therapeutic effects of NSAIDs, when administered at clinical dose rates and by recommended routes of administration, since many literature reports describe in vitro studies in which drug concentrations used may be classed as heroic. Nevertheless, some in vitro data do correlate with in vivo findings. For

TABLE 19.19 Possible mechanisms of action of NSAIDs

INHIBITION OF CYCLOOXYGENASE IN THE ARACHIDONIC ACID CASCADE LEADING TO BLOCKADE OF SYNTHESIS OF PROINFLAMMATORY MEDIATORS IS THE PRINCIPAL MECHANISM OF ACTION	
Additional Actions of Some Drugs	Examples
Inhibit 5-LO	Licofelone, tepoxalin
Inhibit prostanoid release from cells, e.g., by blockade of MRP4	2-arylpropionic acids, indomethacin
Inhibit IκB kinases or NFκB to inhibit COX expression	Aspirin, carprofen, flunixin, indomethacin, diarylheterocycles (COXIBs)
Inhibit the actions of eicosanoids on their receptors	Fenamate subgroup, e.g., tolfenamic acid
Inhibit the actions of bradykinin	Flunixin, ketoprofen, tolfenamic acid
Modulate the release of proinflammatory cytokines, e.g., IL-1,IL-6,TNF-α	Carprofen (IL-6), tepoxalin (IL-1, IL-6, TNF-α)
Stimulate nuclear receptors, e.g., PPAR-γ	Salicylates, 2-arylpropionic acids, arthranilic acids, indene acetic acids
Increase intracellular breakdown of ATP to adenosine	Salicylates
Modulate the synthesis of nitric oxide	Several drugs
Inhibit neutrophil chemotaxis and/or chemokinesis*	Vedaprofen, salicylates
Inhibit neutrophil activation, thereby preventing: Release of oxygen radicals e.g., superoxide, hydroxyl Release of both lysosomal and nonlysosomal enzymes	Flunixin, ketoprofen, piroxicam, tolfenamic acid
Increased synthesis and reduced breakdown of cartilage matrix (proteoglycans)	Carprofen, licofelone
Increased apoptosis and inhibition of carcinogenesis by a non-COX mechanism	Sulphone metabolite of sulindac

*Most NSAIDs inhibit leukocyte movement in a concentration-dependent manner in in vitro assays (Dawson et al. 1987) but clinically recommended doses in vivo usually do not inhibit leukocyte chemotaxis or chemokinesis.

example, rac-carprofen (dog) and rac-carprofen and individual R- and S-carprofen enantiomers (horse) have been shown in vitro to stimulate the synthesis and retard the breakdown of cartilage matrix molecules, proteoglycans, by both chondrocytes and cartilage explants in culture (Benton et al. 1997; Armstrong and Lees 1999b; Frean et al. 1999). This may provide a biochemical explanation for the beneficial effects of carprofen in an experimental model of osteoarthritis in the dog (Pelletier et al. 2000). However, the effects of carprofen enantiomers on cartilage proteoglycan synthesis are concentration-dependent, higher concentrations inhibiting synthesis. In similar studies the dual COX/5-LO inhibitor licofelone has been shown to improve the integrity of cartilage structure, both macro- and microscopically, while also reducing synovial fluid concentrations of the inflammatory mediators, PGE_2 and LTB_4 (Lajeunesse et al. 2004). On the other hand, Brandt (1991) reported that some NSAIDs, including salicylate, inhibit cartilage proteoglycan synthesis in vitro.

TOXICITY OF NSAIDS

The capacity for synthesis of PGs is common to almost all cell types; they are therefore ubiquitous compounds, associated with a range of physiological-autacoid and pathophysiological functions. Inhibition of these functions is the main basis for their toxicity as well as their therapeutic effects. The most frequent and clinically significant side effects of NSAIDs are the irritant, ulcerogenic, erosive effects on the gastrointestinal tract (g.i.t.). The principal target organs for *potential* toxicity are as follows:

- Gastrointestinal irritation associated with vomiting (possibly blood-stained), ulceration, erosions, leading to plasma protein losing enteropathy and melena
- Renotoxicity including occasional acute renal failure
- Hepatotoxicity (cholestastic or parenchymal)
- Inhibition of hemostatic mechanisms leading to hemorrhage
- Blood dyscrasias
- Delayed parturition
- Delayed soft tissue healing
- Delayed fracture healing

It must be emphasized that clinical manifestations of toxicity do not occur in the great majority of animals receiving recommended dose rates of NSAIDs. For example, after use for more than 2 years pharmacovigilance data on tepoxalin indicated an estimated incidence of side effects in 0.1–

0.3% of treated dogs (Pappas, personal communication). The majority of cases involved g.i.t.-related effects e.g., emesis (33%), diarrhea (34%), melena (4%), and gastroenteritis (3%). It is in the nature of pharmacovigilance data that a proportion of the 0.1–0.3% reports will be incidental and not drug-related, and some are due to overdosing or reflect drug interactions. On the other hand, a proportion of reactions to NSAIDs will not be reported. Therefore, it is important to 1) consider the incidence and severity of side effects (usually mild and/or transient) and 2) distinguish between side effects actually reported in clinical use and those postulated on the basis of the molecular actions of NSAIDs or predicted from experimental animal studies.

An important aspect of NSAID toxicity in animals is the ready (over-the-counter) availability of certain drugs to animal owners. A possible consequence is severe toxicity, if an uninformed owner has little or no knowledge of pharmacokinetic, pharmacodynamic, and toxicity profiles of a given agent. For example, in the cat the metabolite of aspirin (salicylate) is cleared slowly and has a long elimination half-life (Table 19.6), so that approximately *one-tenth* of a 300 mg tablet represents a *maximum* dose, which should not be administered more frequently than at 48-hour intervals.

GASTROINTESTINAL TOXICITY. Serious g.i.t.-related side effects of NSAIDs in clinical use are rare, but mortality can and does occur. This normally involves marked g.i.t. ulceration and erosion and loss of blood or plasma into the peritoneal cavity. There may be sufficient fluid loss to cause hypovolemic shock. Moreover, through disruption of the mucosal g.i.t. barrier, normally harmless organisms within the g.i.t. may gain access to the circulation, leading to endotoxic shock. Alternatively, NSAID-induced irritation in the stomach can lead to persistent emesis, with associated fluid losses, requiring therapy with proton pump inhibitors or selective H_2-receptor antagonists. Another means of suppressing NSAID-induced mucosal injury is to coadminister a cytoprotective E-type prostaglandin, as a form of replacement therapy. Thus, misoprostol, a stable derivative of PGE_1, has been used in combination with diclofenac in man. Misoprostol significantly inhibits the gastric ulceration in dogs produced by aspirin and flunixin, although no products for veterinary use containing misoprostol have received a Marketing Authorization.

In early studies the g.i.t. toxicity of NSAIDs was ascribed to their "local actions" on the stomach. However, as pointed out by Rainsford (1977) many factors may be involved. For example, the irritant actions of NSAIDs can occur 1) throughout the tract and 2) after parenteral as well as oral administration. Therefore, it is now recognized that toxicity is *not* a sole consequence of high local concentrations in the stomach. Many studies have demonstrated that ulcerogenic doses of NSAIDs reduce PG concentrations in the gastric mucosa, in turn leading to reduced production in the stomach of bicarbonate-rich mucus secretion, which provides a protective, viscous, alkaline lining fluid. Thus, the g.i.t. damaging effects of NSAIDs have been linked to inhibition of the cytoprotective effects of COX-1. However, knock-out mice in which the COX-1 gene has been deleted fail to develop mucosal ulcers. Moreover, in the rat neither SC-540 (a selective COX-1 inhibitor) nor celecoxib (selective for COX-2) alone caused ulcers, but erosions were induced when they were given in combination (Wallace et al. 2000).

COX-2 expression is increased on the edges of gastric ulcers; it leads to the synthesis compounds, which accelerate ulcer healing, possibly by increasing angiogenesis via inhibition of cellular kinase activity and up-regulation of vascular endothelial growth factor in the gastric mucosa. There may be roles for both PGE_2 and $15dPGJ_2$ in ulcer healing. COX-2 inhibitors have been shown experimentally to delay ulcer healing (Bataar et al. 2002).

A role for neutrophils in NSAID-induced g.i.t. toxicity has been proposed, on the evidence that NSAID administration increases neutrophil adherence to the mucosal vascular endothelium. In addition, monoclonal antibodies, which block leukocyte adhesion reduce the severity of NSAID-induced gastropathic effects. The gastropathy is also reduced in animals that are neutropenic. NSAID-induced neutrophil adherence to endothelium may contribute to mucosal injury by releasing oxygen derived free radicals, proteases, and other compounds from activated neutrophils. Moreover, neutrophil adherence might cause capillary obstruction, resulting in reduced gastric mucosal blood flow and hypoxia. However, not all data support the proposed role of neutrophils in NSAID-induced g.i.t. ulceration.

Another theory of NSAID-induced gastropathy implicates reduced formation of the free radical gas NO. This is supported by the observed reduction or abolition of gastric damage induced experimentally by NSAIDs when they are used as nitrosoesters (CINODs). The nitroso group acts as a NO donor in vivo. The increased leukocyte adherence to the mucosal vascular endothelium caused by NSAIDs does not occur with the nitroso derivatives. Additionally, released NO may, through its vasodilator action, increase gastric and intestinal mucosal blood flows directly, thereby inhibiting NSAID-induced ischemia and hypoxia.

An approach commonly employed to minimize g.i.t. irritation is to administer NSAIDs in feed or with water, to reduce drug concentration in contact with the g.i.t. mucosa. In addition, NSAID-induced g.i.t. ulceration in the horse involves a specific interaction with feed. When administered with hay or horse nuts, phenylbutazone, meclofenamate, and flunixin bind to the feed (Lees et al. 1988b). This initially limits absorption of a high proportion of the administered drug, most markedly for phenylbutazone and least for flunixin, as binding to feed is of the order of 98 and 70%, respectively. It has been postulated that, when the fibrous component of the feed is partially digested in the large intestine, bound drug is released and this mechanism may account for the two distinct peaks recorded in the plasma concentration-time profile. The availability of released drug, not only for absorption but also to exert a local irritant action, accounts for the high incidence of lesions in the distal parts of the g.i.t., when high doses of phenylbutazone are administered to horses (Snow et al. 1979).

Several reports in the late 1970s/early 1980s described extensive erosions throughout the g.i.t., as well as oral ulceration, associated with a protein losing enteropathy (with plasma total protein and albumin decreasing by 20% or more) and high mortality in ponies receiving oral phenylbutazone doses only moderately in excess of those then recommended for clinical use (Snow et al. 1979; Lees et al. 2003). Similar findings were reported in horses receiving ketoprofen (MacAllister et al. 1993). Another group reported, on the basis of clinical, hematological, and biochemical analyses, that the 20% decrease in plasma protein in the horse, caused by a phenylbutazone dosage regimen of 8.8 mg/kg for 4 days, followed by 4.4 mg/kg for 4 days, and then 2.2 mg/kg for 7 days, could be avoided by restricting the 8.8 mg/kg dosage to a loading dose on day 1 only (Lees et al. 1983; Taylor et al. 1983). This and other studies indicated a steep dose-effect relationship for the toxicity of phenylbutazone. Reports that ponies are more susceptible than larger equine breeds to the toxic effects of phenylbutazone have not been confirmed. Other manifestations of phenylbutazone toxicity in the horse include neutropenia, bone marrow suppression, and necrotizing phlebitis of the portal vein (Murray 1985). Oral dosing of flunixin and meclofenamate for 5 successive days at the recommended dose rate (1.1 mg/kg) also reduced plasma total protein and albumin significantly, and these agents may have a similar narrow margin between therapeutic and safe doses in the horse (Lees and Higgins 1985; Lees et al. 1983; Taylor et al. 1983). Carprofen, on the other hand, has a wider safety margin in this species. In a recent comparative study in the dog, using clinically recommended dose rates, the greatest incidence and severity of g.i.t.-related side effects were reported for flunixin and ketoprofen, while carprofen was best tolerated (Luna et al. 2007).

Carprofen has been described as a "PG sparing" NSAID in the dog and horse and available evidence suggests that it is less likely than many other available agents to cause g.i.t. irritation in these species (Lees et al. 2004a). An alternative explanation for its g.i.t. safety profile (in the dog, but not in the horse) is its selectivity for COX-2 over COX-1. It is likely that improved g.i.t. tolerance is also a property of 1) nimesulide, etodolac, and meloxicam, as these compounds have been classified as having some (though variable between studies) selectivity for inhibition of COX-2; 2) the newer COXIBs such as firocoxib, mavacoxib and robenacoxib; and 3) the dual COX/5-LO inhibitors such as tepoxalin.

COX-2 is expressed throughout the human g.i.t. but COX-1 probably has the greater role in protecting its integrity; hence the ulcerative/erosive actions of nonselective NSAIDs. However, as indicated above, COX-2 is likely to have an important role in resolving tissue damage and COX-2 inhibition delays ulcer healing (Bataar et al. 2002). COX-2 products promote g.i.t. healing (Wallace et al. 2000; Wallace and Devchand 2005).

While all reports are not unanimous, the human literature strongly indicates a better g.i.t. safety profile for selective and specific COX-2 inhibitors in comparison with nonselective inhibitors (Lanza et al. 1999; Hawkey et al. 2000). Thus, the balance of evidence from the CLASS, VIGOR, and other human studies indicates a better safety profile of rofecoxib and celecoxib in comparison with naproxen, ibuprofen, and diclofenac (Bombardier et al. 2000; Silverstein et al. 2000). In other human studies valdecoxib and lumiracoxib were found to provide similar levels of gastroduodenal tolerability to placebo treatments (Goldstein et al. 2003; Rordorf et al. 2003). However, in both humans and animals COX-2 selective and specific drugs at high dose rates are not free of g.i.t.-related side effects. For example, for firocoxib in the dog at five times the recommended daily dose for 3 months, toxic signs included inappetence, emesis, duodenal ulcers, lipid accumulation in the liver, and vacuolization in the brain. However, emesis and duodenal ulcers did not occur with three times the recommended dose, administered daily for 6 months. Puppies aged 10–13 weeks were more susceptible than dogs aged 6–12 months.

The g.i.t. tolerance of dual inhibitors differs from that of the older nonselective COX inhibitors. In preclinical toxicity studies, beagle dogs receiving up to 10 times the therapeutic dose of tepoxalin over periods of many months did not display major g.i.t. side effects either in life or at postmortem. The explanation for this may reside in the dual inhibition phenomenon. When classical NSAIDs inhibit COX-1 there may be "shunting" of the substrate AA toward 5-LO. It is postulated that this leads to increased synthesis of LTs 1) with vasoconstrictor properties (e.g., LTC_4) and 2) that cause neutrophils to adhere to gastric mucosal blood vessels (e.g., LTB_4). The potential consequence is mucosal ischemia and the release of tissue damaging mediators from neutrophils (Rainsford 1993). In this way LTs may contribute to the g.i.t. side effects of NSAIDs. Tepoxalin and licofelone avoid this mechanism of g.i.t. toxicity by blocking the LT synthetic pathway (Wallace et al. 1993). In the dog, licofelone was shown to possess a good safety profile with no gastroduodenal ulceration at a dose rate of 2.5 mg/kg twice daily (Moreau et al. 2005).

LOCAL IRRITANCY. As well as irritancy to the g.i.t. after oral or parenteral dosing, some NSAIDs are irritants and may cause tissue necrosis after injection by nonvascular routes. This is particularly true for phenylbutazone, which is formulated as a high-strength alkaline solution (as the sodium salt), whereas other NSAIDs such as carprofen and meloxicam have been specifically formulated for parenteral, nonvascular administration.

RENOTOXICITY. *Renotoxic effects of NSAIDs at recommended dose rates do not generally occur in healthy animals with free access to drinking water.* However, PGs do play subtle (even key) roles in renal physiology. PGs regulate glomerular filtration, renin release, and tubular sodium reabsorption. Potential side effects of COX inhibitors include sodium retention (with accompanying edema), reduced glomerular filtration rate (GFR), and systemic hypertension. Both isoforms of COX are likely to be involved. In the dog COX-2 is expressed constitutively in the macula densa, thick ascending limb of the Loop of Henle, and interstitial cells and also in humans in glomerular podocytes and the afferent arteriole. The activation of renin release is a property of COX-2.

Thus, both isoforms of COX are present at several intrarenal sites, with some apparent differences between species. COX products (possibly both COX-1 and COX-2 derived) are involved in maintaining renal blood flow and GFR in the face of reduced arterial pressure and/or fluid and sodium depletion. General anesthesia is a particular circumstance in which hypotension may arise from the cardiovascular actions of premedicant, induction, and maintenance agents, and reduction in blood pressure may be compounded by losses of blood and insensible water losses during surgery. Under these conditions, enhanced sympathetic nervous activity and stimulation of the renin-angiotensin system occur. Angiotensin II, formed from angiotensin I, is a potent vasoconstrictor, which decreases renal blood flow, notably to the renal medulla. Increased production of the prostanoid vasodilators, PGI_2 in the glomerulus and PGE_2 in the medulla, offsets the vasoconstrictor actions of both angiotensin II and noradrenaline and glomerular and tubular functions are thereby protected from ischemic damage. The release of COX-2–derived PGE_2 from the macula densa dilates the afferent arteriole to maintain GFR.

Blockade of the renoprotective actions of intrarenally released PGs explains renal pharmacological effects of NSAIDs, and there have been several reports of acute renal failure with clinical doses of some drugs such as flunixin in the dog. Some licensing authorities recommend restriction for some NSAIDs to postoperative administration, when blood pressure has been restored to normal and fluid losses have been replaced. Despite these considerations, an experimental study in eight healthy beagle dogs revealed no adverse effects on renal function of oral meloxicam as a single dose, when the animals had been rendered hypotensive by anesthesia with acepromazine, thiopentone, and isoflurane (Bostrom et al. 2006). On the other hand, several reports of renal papillary necrosis in horses receiving clinical dose rates of phenylbutazone or flunixin appeared in the 1980s, but this occurred only when horses on NSAID therapy also had restricted access to water.

Ko et al. (2000) found that carprofen did not alter renal function in healthy dogs anesthetized with propofol and isoflurane. However, Forsyth et al. (2000) reported reductions in GFR in dogs premedicated with carprofen and then anesthetized with isoflurane. Markers of renal and hepatic function were unaffected by tepoxalin administered preoperatively in adult dogs anesthetized for 30 minutes with propofol/isoflurane (Kay-Mugford et al. 2004). Based on known mechanisms of action, there is potential for adverse interactions between NSAIDs and angiotensin converting enzyme (ACE) inhibitors. However, Fusellier et al. (2005) reported no significant effects on GFR from the combined effects of tepoxalin and benazepril administered daily for 7 or 28 days.

Murine knock-out studies suggest that COX-2 is crucially involved in kidney maturation. In COX-2 null mice renal cortical development (involving tubular atrophy, nephron hypoplasia, and reduced glomerulogenesis) was impaired and neonatal death rates increased (Dinchuk et al. 1995). There is therefore concern on the use of NSAIDs (both selective and nonselective) in pregnancy as well as in neonates. This may have implications for the use of both nonselective and selective COX-2 inhibitors in young animals, especially neonates since, in addition to a role for COX-2 in renal maturation, very young animals are likely to have immature mechanisms of elimination of drugs, including NSAIDs.

In summary, in physiological or pathological conditions of hyponatremia, fluid depletion, and hypotension, and in disease states such as diabetes mellitus and diminished adrenocortical function, COX isoforms maintain renal perfusion, GFR, and tubular function. Both nonselective and COX-2 selective NSAIDs have the potential, in these conditions, to cause edema, reduced GFR, hyperkalemia, and hypertension. Moreover, in man rofecoxib has been found to interfere with antihypertensive drugs, such as ACE inhibitors and β-adrenoceptor blockers, which exert their actions, in part, through the renal vasodilator actions of PGs. Similarly, NSAIDs can interfere with the actions of loop diuretics, such as frusemide. Manufacturers' product literature on NSAIDs often contains warnings of potential toxicity arising from their combined use with agents of other classes with known nephrotoxic properties, such as aminoglycoside and polymixin antimicrobial drugs and loop diuretics such as frusemide.

BONE, TENDON, AND LIGAMENT HEALING. A physiological role for COX-2 is indicated by studies in COX-2 null mice, which develop to normal skeletal maturity but in which fracture healing may be impaired. The genes cbfa and osterix, which are required for bone formation, are regulated by COX-2 (Zhang et al. 2002). However, the roles of PGs in bone metabolism are complex; they stimulate both new bone formation by osteoblasts and resorption by osteoclasts through EP_2 and EP_4 receptors (Kawagachi et al. 1995). Moreover, in response to particulate wear debris, COX-2 increased the concentration of several proinflammatory cytokines (TNF-α, IL-1β, IL-6) and other osteotrophic factors. PGs are thus involved in inflammatory bone conditions. They are released in high concentrations by osteoblasts in the 2 weeks following injury (Gajraj 2003; Gerstenfeld et al. 2003). PGE_2 (and also PGI_2 and TxA_2) first stimulate bone reabsorption via osteoclast activity, which is then followed by bone remodeling.

COX-1 is present constitutively in osteocytes, osteoblasts, and osteoclasts, whereas COX-2mRNA levels are raised and PGE_2 synthesis is increased in the early stages of bone healing. Experimental studies in mice and rats have demonstrated reduced fracture healing in response to nonselective COX inhibitors and to COX-2 selective drugs (Simon et al. 2002; Goodman et al. 2003). These effects are reversed if dosing is not prolonged.

In reviewing the experimental literature in this field Radi and Khan (2005) noted that COX-2 is up-regulated only during the initial stages of bone healing and various orthopedic inflammatory and neoplastic conditions, such as canine and human osteosarcoma and canine pulmonary osteosarcoma. Reports of impairment of bone, tendon and ligament healing by NSAIDs are conflicting, with some studies failing to show any deleterious effects from either nonselective or COX-2 selective inhibitors. Radi and Khan (2005) concluded that, in animal models, NSAIDs do retard bone and also ligament and tendon healing, but that the effects are confined to the early stages of healing, with no significant impact on long-term outcome. Indeed in one study, both COX-2 selective and nonselective inhibitors improved mechanical strength in the later phase of healing (Riley et al. 2001). Unfortunately, there is little published clinical data in human and veterinary medicine in this field.

SOFT TISSUE HEALING AND REPAIR. As with hard tissues, there is potential for nonselective and COX-2 selective inhibitors to affect the healing of soft tissues, given the postulated role of COX-2 products in the resolution phase of acute inflammation. Experimental data in mice both for (Laudederkind et al. 2002) and against

(Blomme et al. 2003) a role for COX-2 in dermal wound healing have been presented. Wilgus et al. (2003) reported that, in mice, celecoxib suppresses the early inflammatory phase of epidermal wound healing and reduces scar tissue formation but without disrupting reepithelialization or decreasing tensile strength. Data on wound healing relevant to species of veterinary interest is lacking, although one conference report suggested a negative effect of phenylbutazone on wound healing in the horse.

CARDIOVASCULAR SYSTEM AND BLOOD CELLS.

The principal eicosanoids with local hormonal roles on blood vessels and blood cells are TXA_2 (a vasoconstrictor, proaggregatory agent with smooth muscle proliferation properties, which is released from platelets and involved in blood clotting) and PGI_2 (a vasodilator, antiaggregatory, antiplatelet adhesive, antiproliferative agent released from endothelial cells, which prevents clotting in normal circulatory function). Platelet COX-1 is constitutive and endothelial cell COX comprises both isoforms. For example, the sheer stress associated with each arterial pulse probably maintains COX-2 levels in vivo. The TXA_2/PGI_2 system maintains a homeostatic balance, which can be disrupted by selective COX-2 inhibitors, potentially causing increases in blood pressure (through removal of the vasodilator influence) and a tendency toward clotting (through loss of the antiaggregatory effect). In humans, celecoxib and rofecoxib reduce PGI_2 synthesis, as assessed by measurement of urinary metabolites (Fitzgerald and Patrono 2001).

The potential for COX-2 inhibition to cause "cardiovascular events," including thrombus formation and myocardial infarction, which may be life threatening, has been the subject of considerable debate and concern in human medicine, leading to the withdrawal from use of rofecoxib. Even in man, however, for whom very large-scale clinical trials have been undertaken, the situation is unclear. This is partly because there is an incidence level of cardiovascular events in untreated or placebo-treated subjects as well as those receiving nonselective NSAIDs. While several studies indicate an increase in relative cardiovascular risk in patients receiving selective or specific COX-2 inhibitors, adverse cardiovascular effects are generally not apparent until continuous treatment has been given for periods of 18 months or longer. Furthermore, in the VIGOR study the greater relative risk with rofecoxib compared to naproxen was ascribed to a possible protective action of naproxen (which may be a preferential COX-1 inhibitor) rather than deleterious effects of the COX-2 inhibitor, a suggestion that has caused vigorous debate.

Even at supratherapeutic dose rates, rofecoxib (in contrast to naproxen) does not inhibit ex vivo TxB_2 formation in whole blood assays (Warner and Mitchell 2004). Moreover, the adverse cardiovascular effects of selective COX-2 inhibitors in humans are dose related and rofecoxib did not significantly increase relative risk at low dose rates (Ray et al. 2002). Some studies have shown an increase in relative risk for cardiovascular effects for nonselective NSAIDs, as well as selective and specific COX-2 inhibitors, in placebo controlled studies. Others have failed to demonstrate any increase in risk; a meta-analysis of eight osteoarthritis trials indicated similar rates of thrombotic cardiovascular events with placebo, nabumetone, rofecoxib, and comparator nonselective NSAIDs, which included ibuprofen and diclofenac (Reicin et al. 2002). However, the median treatment duration was short, 3.5 months. Finally, some studies have been criticized on the grounds of insufficient or incorrect statistical analyses. Warner and Mitchell (2004) concluded, from a review of the then available literature, that COX-2 inhibitors in humans do not increase the risk of thrombotic events.

The relevance of these human pharmacovigilance studies for major veterinary species is unclear. The dog (but not the cat) is relatively resistant to thromboembolic diseases. In humans, increased risk is not associated with all drugs at all dose rates. When it has been found to be significant, it has been revealed only because of the large numbers of patients treated, usually over long periods. Therefore, while the potential for adverse cardiovascular effects in veterinary patients must be borne in mind, veterinary experiences to date indicate a risk/benefit relationship clearly in favor of benefits.

Among NSAIDs in veterinary use, aspirin is a special case, because of its irreversible action and the inability of platelets, being anuclear, to synthesize new COX-1. The potential for inhibition of hemostasis and prolonged bleeding time must therefore be borne in mind when aspirin is used therapeutically, even at low dose rates, and when other NSAIDs are used at high dose rates. In the horse aspirin's antiplatelet action is manifested by virtually complete inhibition of TXA_2 synthesis for up to 1 week after a single dose, yet the terminal half-life after intravenous dosing is only 9 minutes (Lees et al. 1987a). The latter authors suggested this might be due to inhibition of COX-1 in bone marrow megakaryocytes as well as circulating platelets. In humans, there is concern that concomitant administration of aspirin (for its antithrombotic effects) and other NSAIDs (for their analgesic, antiinflammatory effects) may result in interference with aspirin's antiplatelet actions (MacDonald and Wei 2003). This might occur as a consequence of the very short half-life of aspirin, combined with NSAID prevention of aspirin entry to the COX-1 active site. In fact, concomitant administration of ibuprofen, but not celecoxib, rofecoxib, acetaminophen, or diclofenac, antagonized the irreversible action of aspirin on platelets (Catella-Lawson et al. 2001).

In the dog, phenylbutazone usage was linked in early studies to blood dyscrasias (Tandy and Thorpe 1967; Watson et al. 1980). It is not known whether this is a dose-related phenomenon or an idiosyncratic response, but blood dyscrasias are also associated with high doses of phenylbutazone (and possibly other NSAIDs) in the horse. Early studies indicated marked depression of the bone marrow in cats receiving aspirin or phenylbutazone; in retrospect it seems likely that the doses used were much greater than those required for clinical efficacy and thus may represent the effects of gross overdosage (Larson 1963; Carlise et al. 1968).

Acetaminophen (paracetamol) has been extensively used as an analgesic in human medicine for many years, with a generally wide safety margin. Its antiinflammatory properties are weak, it has good g.i.t. tolerance, and it is assumed to be a centrally acting analgesic. However, acetaminophen is toxic to the cat, in which species it is metabolized to oxidative compounds with cytotoxic properties. The metabolites overwhelm the glutathione scavenging system, resulting in methemoglobinemia and, less commonly, centrolobular hepatic necrosis. Recommended antidotes are antioxidants such as vitamin C or n-acetylcysteine (St Omer and McKnight 1980). In addition, the H_2-receptor antagonist, cimetidine, a hepatic microsomal enzyme inhibitor, has been recommended to inhibit formation of the toxic metabolites; it should be administered within 48 hours (Jackson 1982). Similar signs of toxicity may occur with high dose rates of acetaminophen in the dog (Hjelle and Grasser 1986).

RESPIRATION. A subset of human asthmatic patients display signs of respiratory distress when administered aspirin (and in some subjects other NSAIDs also). This may be due to diversion of the substrate, AA, towards 5-LO and the increased synthesis of LTs, which have been implicated as mediators of asthma. COX-2 selective drugs seem not to share this untoward effect of nonselective NSAIDs.

SKIN. Occasional skin reactions to NSAIDs, including urticaria, rashes, and angioedema have been reported. The mechanisms are unclear but, in some instances, a hypersensitivity reaction may be involved. This is not surprising in view of the high degree of binding to plasma proteins.

REPRODUCTIVE SYSTEM. Prostanoids are involved in ovulation, fertilization, and blastocyte implantation (Kniss 1999). COX-2 null mice do not ovulate, and fertilization, implantation, and decidualization do not proceed normally. In early pregnancy COX-2 is present in the uterine epithelium and is likely to be involved in ova implantation, angiogenesis, and labor. It has been suggested that COX-1 mediates the early stages of labor onset, involving uterine contractions and early stages of cervix dilation, whereas COX-2, induced by cytokines from the decidua, trophoblast, or fetal membranes, generates prostanoids to sustain myometrial contractions and cervical ripening leading to fetal expulsion. In humans, COX-2 but not COX-1 is induced during labor. Experimental studies have also indicated a role for PGE_2 in maintaining in utero the patency of the ductus arteriosus, and treatment with COXIBs postpartum leads to premature closure. Based on these roles of COX, various effects might be predicted from dosing with NSAIDs; in fact, rofecoxib produces delayed follicular rupture and nimesulide reduces preterm labor. In the testes COX-2 is the main isoform and PGs formed include $PGF_{2\alpha}$, PGE_2, and PGD_2. The effects of NSAIDs on testicular function have not been extensively studied.

NERVOUS SYSTEM. COX-2 is present constitutively, particularly in neonates, in neuron cell bodies and dendrites at several brain sites. Centrally, PGs are involved in body temperature regulation, hyperalgesia and neuron development. PGs are not neurotransmitters but they do modulate nerve transmission. In view of these roles of COX in CNS functions, it is perhaps surprising that so few significant central side effects are associated with NSAID use.

HEPATOTOXICITY. Liver toxicity is rare in animals treated with clinical dose rates of NSAIDs. However, parenchymal hepatotoxicity has been described for phenylbutazone in the aged horse (Lees et al. 1983), possibly as a consequence of increased blood levels in older subjects receiving the same dose rates as younger animals (Lees et al. 1985). Cholestatic toxicity has also been described in the horse treated with phenylbutazone. Acute hepatic necrosis is a rare complication of carprofen in the dog, with a likely predisposition of the Labrador breed (MacPhail et al. 1998). When therapy was discontinued in the dog, resolution of biochemical associated liver changes and clinical signs occurred.

TABLE 19.20 Conditions that may cause severe pain for which NSAID usage should be considered

Surgical Conditions	Medical Conditions
Orthopedic surgery	Bone tumors
Aural surgery	Disc lesions
Oral surgery	Otitis externa
Anal surgery	Various ophthalmic conditions
Upper abdominal surgery	Pancreatitis
Onychectomy	Acute moist dermatitis
	Equine colic

THERAPEUTIC USES OF NSAIDS

Over the last decade, the number of NSAIDs approved by registration bodies has increased significantly. This has been matched by a considerable increase in the extent of usage, driven by recognition of the wide range of circumstances in which the control of inflammation and pain is desirable for medical, welfare, and economic reasons.

ACUTE PAIN AND INFLAMMATION. Pain in animals is often difficult to recognize and assessment of its intensity can be particularly difficult. Nevertheless, it has been increasingly recognized that animals "feel" pain and we must assume that they also "suffer" pain as do humans. Therefore, both subjective (e.g., semiquantitative scoring systems and visual analogue scales) and more objective (e.g., force plate) indices of pain/lameness have increasingly been used (Flecknell and Waterman-Pearson 2000; Holton et al. 1998; Lipscomb et al. 2002). In consequence, there is now widespread use of NSAIDs in all major veterinary species: 1) perioperatively, 2) to treat acute trauma (e.g., lameness, road accident cases, and equine/canine sports injuries), 3) for a range of musculoskeletal conditions, and 4) to treat the severe pain associated with colic in the horse (Balmer et al. 1998; Lascelles et al. 1995, 1998; Welsh et al. 1997; Robertson 2005). In the latter condition, however, drugs such as flunixin can mask the signs of colic, so that diagnosis of the underlying cause should be made prior to dosing. NSAIDs are used extensively to control acute pain associated with surgical and medical conditions as shown in Table 19.20.

Some reports suggest that, for the control of postoperative pain in companion animals, NSAIDs may be as effective as opioids (Lascelles et al. 2007). However, NSAIDs are generally longer acting, do not possess the central nervous depressant side effects of opioids, and are subject to fewer legal restrictions. They are, therefore, commonly used as alternatives to opioids or to extend the duration of analgesia initiated by opioids. Preemptive analgesia with both drug classes has been widely advocated in human and veterinary medicine (Welsh et al. 1997). It involves the administration of analgesics as premedicants or very early in general anesthesia prior to surgical intervention, i.e., pre- or early intraoperatively, not only to enhance surgical conditions but also to control pain in the postoperative period. It is based on the observation that postoperative analgesic dose requirements are reduced when preemptive analgesia has been provided. Lascelles et al. (1998) demonstrated greater postoperative analgesia in dogs undergoing ovariohysterectomy when the drug was administered preoperatively than when given in the early postoperative phase. The use of NSAIDs perioperatively can have the additional advantage of reducing edematous swelling and thus preventing wound breakdown. However, antiedematous doses, at least for some drugs, may be higher than those required to provide analgesia.

There is concern that the administration of NSAIDs before recovery from anesthesia may be associated with low incidence but life-threatening acute renal failure (vide supra). Of the agents in veterinary use, carprofen and tepoxalin may be the drugs of choice for pre- and perioperative use. Carprofen has been described as "PG sparing" because clinical dose rates in the dog and horse do not markedly inhibit either COX-1 or COX-2, although this "sparing action" does *not* apply to sheep or the cat, because of the high dose rate recommended for the latter species.

CHRONIC PAIN. The main nonsurgical use of NSAIDs in companion animals is the treatment of chronic pain, associated, for example, with cancer. However, the chronic pain conditions of primary significance in veterinary medicine are those associated with the arthritides and of these, in the horse and dog, osteoarthritis is by far the most common. NSAIDs are the only class of analgesic suitable for medium- to long-term oral treatment of the pain associated with osteoarthritis. As with other forms of inflammation, many mediators are involved in joint conditions, leading to inflammation and increased angiogenesis of the synovial lining. The inflammation is particularly acute in canine rheumatoid arthritis compared to osteoarthritis and in osteoarthritis acute inflammation is a more prominent component in the dog than in the horse. Some authors therefore prefer the term degenerative joint disease (DJD) in the horse.

The defining characteristics of osteoarthritis and DJD are pain, stiffness, restriction of movement, catabolism of cartilage, and, in advanced cases, erosion of subchondral bone. Cartilage catabolism involves loss of the matrix proteoglycans molecules as breakdown exceeds neosynthesis. The roles of COX-2 in osteoarthritis have not been fully elucidated, but the enzyme is up-regulated and PGE_2 concentrations in synovial fluid are increased in inflammatory joint diseases but not in DJD in the horse (May et al. 1994). Nevertheless, it is likely that PGE_2 is involved in the pain of osteoarthritis and it also suppresses chondrocyte proliferation, increases IL1-β release (which is catabolic for cartilage), and inhibits chondrocyte aggrecan synthesis. It may therefore contribute to the loss of cartilage matrix, as well as to the pain of osteoarthritis.

Carprofen enhances SO_4 incorporation to stimulate the synthesis of proteoglycans by equine chondrocytes in culture and, to a lesser degree, it exerts similar actions on equine cartilage explants (Armstrong and Lees 1999b; Frean et al. 1999). Carprofen exerts a similar action on canine chondrocytes (Benton et al. 1997). Moreover, carprofen in vitro reverses IL-1–induced suppression of proteoglycan synthesis by equine chondrocytes (Armstrong and Lees 1999b). Whether such actions demonstrated in vitro have significance for clinical subjects is not clear. *Nevertheless,* it is of interest to note that a disease-modifying action of carprofen has been demonstrated in the dog in the Pond-Nuki model of osteoarthritis (Pelletier et al. 2000), when the drug was administered at the recommended dose rate. An action on subchondral bone was postulated, since carprofen delayed or prevented the abnormal metabolism of subchondral osteoblasts. Licofelone, also in a canine osteoarthritis model, retarded degradative changes in cartilage, both macroscopically and histologically. These effects were accompanied by significant suppression of synthesis of PGE_2 and LTB_4 (Boileau et al. 2002; Lajeunesse et al. 2004).

Preclinical assessment of doses providing analgesic efficacy of NSAIDs for joint pain is often obtained using models providing intense but transient pain, for example, urate crystal–induced synovitis (Millis et al. 2002; Toutain et al. 2001b). While such models differ significantly from clinical osteoarthritis, it can be argued that they provide a major challenge to analgesic efficacy and are therefore justified for dosage selection for osteoarthritic treatment. Toutain et al. (2001a,b) have carefully validated these models, comparing them 1) with data for COX inhibition in whole blood assays and 2) against a Freund's adjuvant arthritis model in the dog.

Clinical trials comparing tepoxalin with either carprofen or meloxicam in canine osteoarthritis have revealed similar efficacy at clinically recommended dose rates for signs indicating analgesia and suppression of lameness. This may reflect a relative insensitivity of the subjective pain indexes used to assess and discriminate between drugs. Alternatively, it may be that mediators generated by COX alone cause the pain associated with osteoarthritis with no contribution from products of 5-LO metabolism. On available evidence the benefit provided by tepoxalin seems to be principally the greater g.i.t. (and possibly renal) tolerance in comparison with nonselective COX inhibitors.

ANTIHEMOSTATIC ACTIONS OF ASPIRIN. At high dose rates all NSAIDs inhibit blood clotting by blocking platelet production of TxA_2 by COX-1. At clinically recommended dose rates NSAIDs do not, as far as is known, markedly prolong bleeding times, although there are anecdotal reports that some prolongation occurs with some drugs. Among available NSAIDs, the action of aspirin on hemostatic mechanisms is unique. By covalently acetylating COX-1, the enzyme is inhibited irreversibly and hence for the life span of the platelet, as platelets contain no nuclei and cannot synthesize new enzyme. Therefore, aspirin is the NSAID of choice as an antithrombotic drug, for example, in prophylaxis of aortic embolism in cats. For the same reason, however, aspirin is more likely than all other NSAIDs (which act reversibly) to exacerbate hemorrhage at high dose rates. The antithrombotic action of aspirin may also be of value in equine conditions such as laminitis, navicular disease, and disseminated intravascular coagulation, although definitive studies are lacking.

ATHEROSCLEROSIS. Atherosclerosis, which involves the deposition of fatty plaques (atheromas) in the intima of medium and large arteries, is now recognized as a chronic inflammatory condition of the circulation. The plaques obstruct blood flow and cause ischemia. In addition, plaque disruption can act as a focus for thrombus formation, leading to myocardial or cerebral infarction. Many inflammatory mediators are involved, including COX derivatives. In humans, there may be a therapeutic role for NSAIDs in atherosclerosis, but more data are required to establish this.

CANCER. Epidemiological studies on human patients receiving long-term treatment with NSAIDs (for example, elderly subjects with osteoarthritis) have indicated a potential beneficial effect against colonic cancers. Overexpression of COX-2 in epithelial colon cells causes resistance to apoptosis and promotion of tumor growth by stimulating the production of growth factors and by angiogenesis. In humans and rats cancerous colonic tissue has increased PGE_2 concentrations. A possible mechanism of the procancerous action of PGE_2 is transactivation of epidermal growth factor receptor, promoting growth of colonic polyps and cancers (Pai et al. 2002). Colon tumor cells (adenomas and adenocarcinomas) show increased COX-2 (two- to fiftyfold) and decreased COX-1 expression at mRNA and protein levels compared with normal colon epithelial cells, and a therapeutic role for COX-2 inhibitors has been established in the prevention, treatment, and palliation of certain cancers. In dogs, PGE_2 concentrations were increased in osteosarcoma tissue compared to normal bone (Mohammed et al. 2001). Moreover, colorectal tumors and polyps in the dog, canine transitional cell bladder carcinomas and canine osteosarcomas (Mullins et al. 2004) involve COX-2 up-regulation. High COX-2 expression levels have also been reported in humans in lung, breast, gastric, hepatic, pancreatic, and head and neck tumors.

Antineoplastic actions of NSAIDs have been demonstrated in many experimental studies. For example, in a rat model celecoxib was effective in the prevention and treatment of azoxymethane-induced carcinogenesis. Moreover, the incidence of adenomas is reduced and possibly even tumor regression has been described in response to celecoxib and rofecoxib (Steinbach et al. 2000; Hallak et al. 2003). Thus, NSAIDs reduce cell numbers in various cancers, and studies demonstrating that NSAIDs can directly induce apoptosis in neoplastic cells and inhibit angiogenesis may provide an explanation for this finding.

Clinically, in canine prostatic carcinomas carprofen and meloxicam increased median survival time and piroxicam has been used in the treatment of transitional cell tumors in dogs; Knapp et al. (1992) reported a reduction in tumor sizes. In the dog piroxicam has a long terminal half-life of 40–45 hours (Galbraith and McKellar 1991). In dogs with rectal polyps piroxicam reduced polyp size and suppressed clinical signs (Knottenbelt et al. 2000). Wolfsberger et al. (2006) reported that meloxicam at low concentrations (1–10 μM) *increased* numbers of D-17 canine osteosarcoma cells in vitro after exposure for 3 days, whereas high concentrations (100 and 200 μM) exerted a marked antiproliferative effect. It should be noted that the maximum serum concentrations of meloxicam in the dog after therapeutic doses are 1.3 μM (oral dosing) and 2.1 μM (subcutaneous injection), and most of the drug is bound to protein (Busch et al. 1998).

In a human study low-dose aspirin (81 mg daily), but not a higher dose (325 mg daily), reduced the adenomas occurring in colon cancer (Baron et al. 2003), but in another study the 325 mg dose of aspirin did suppress adenomas (Sandler et al. 2003). Neither the low nor the high dose is likely to produce significant and persistent COX-2 inhibition, whereas the antiplatelet COX-1 inhibitory actions are exerted at both the low and higher doses. Furthermore, much evidence correlates platelets to cancer spread. Nevertheless, low-dose aspirin (82 mg) does reduce colonic prostanoid synthesis by more than 50% and (surprisingly) a higher daily dose (650 mg) produced no greater inhibition (Krishnan et al. 2001; Sample et al. 2002). The effects of NSAIDs on cancer are clearly complex and in some, but not all, instances are concentration or dose related. Moreover, antiproliferative effects of COX inhibitors have been described in COX negative cell lines, so that non-COX mechanisms of action are possible and even likely (Waskewich et al. 2002). In human lung cancer cells in culture the effects of sulindac seem to be independent of COX and possibly involve the PPAR-γ pathway (Wick et al. 2002).

NEURODEGENERATIVE DISEASES. COX-2 is present constitutively in the brain. It is up-regulated in the hippocampus and cortex in human subjects with dementia. PGs decrease neuronal function in patients with Alzheimer's disease, a condition characterized by the accumulation of extracellular deposits of β-amyloid in regions concerned with memory and cognition (Hwang et al. 2002). COX-2–derived PGs accelerate neurodegeneration, possibly by enhancing glutamate excitotoxicity. A key event in dementia is the transformation by Aβ peptides of resting microglia and astrocytes into activated cells, which then release a wide range of inflammatory mediators.

Human epidemiological studies have indicated a lower incidence of Alzheimer's disease in subjects on long-term NSAID therapy (Launer 2003). This may be linked to their antiinflammatory properties; COX-2 containing inflammatory cells are present in the vicinity of amyloid-β plaques. This action of NSAIDs is not shared by acetaminophen. Although there is unlikely to be a beneficial effect of NSAIDs on disease progression, disease incidence was lower when subjects were receiving a NSAID prior to the onset of neurological symptoms. A trial in humans showed no slowing of cognitive decline in patients with mild to moderate Alzheimer's disease receiving rofecoxib and naproxen over 12 months (Aisen et al. 2003).

One human trial revealed positive clinical effects in Alzheimer's disease from a COX-1 inhibitor but not from celecoxib. Stewart et al. (1997) reported relative risks of 0.4 and 0.65 for patients receiving NSAIDs for more than, and less than 2 years, respectively. However, for acetaminophen the relative risk was 1.35. The mechanism of action of NSAIDs is unclear and does not necessarily involve COX-1 or COX-2 inhibition. For example, ibuprofen confers protection by modulating γ-secretase cleavage to reduce Aβ42 production by a non-COX pathway. The antiplatelet properties of NSAIDs may be beneficial through reducing ischemia and blockade of brain capillaries. Maintaining low density lipoprotein levels is beneficial in dementias, and this suggests a role for statins, as these drugs possess both cholesterol lowering and antiinflammatory properties.

MASTITIS, METRITIS, AND ENDOTOXEMIA. When gram-negative bacteria gain access to the circulation, the associated endotoxemia produces many systemic effects. For example, acute and peracute *E. coli* mastitis is a major welfare concern and source of economic loss in the dairy industry, involving reduced milk production, treatment costs, discarded milk, and mortality. As well as inflammation in the affected quarter, systemic signs include depression, fever, tachycardia, neutropenia, and inhibition of reticulorumen motility. Endotoxin causes the release or de novo synthesis of many inflammatory mediators and endotoxemia may be regarded as an acute inflammatory condition of the circulatory system. Endotoxic shock may be associated with a range of diseases in addition to mastitis, including equine colic, metritis, and septic peritonitis. Several reports in the 1980s indicated a therapeutic role for phenylbutazone and flunixin in equine endotoxemia (Moore 1986; Moore et al. 1986) and for septic shock in dogs (Hardie et al. 1983).

For the treatment of acute mastitis and endotoxemia, systemically administered NSAIDs are used frequently as adjuncts to antimicrobial drugs. For example, responses to carprofen therapy included lowering of rectal temperature, restoration of reticulorumen motility, and more rapid normalization of the clinical severity score in an *E. coli* model of mastitis (Vangroenweghe et al. 2005). In this study carprofen did not significantly affect either plasma or milk concentrations of PGE_2 or TxB_2, indicating the possibility of clinical benefit through a mechanism of action other than COX inhibition. The beneficial effects of carprofen confirm the findings of many previous workers for flunixin (Anderson et al. 1986a,b; Lohuis et al. 1989; Ziv and Long 1991), flurbiprofen (Lohuis et al. 1989; Vandeputte-Van Messom et al. 1987), indomethacin (Burvenich and Peeters 1982), ketoprofen (Shpigel et al. 1994), phenylbutazone (Shpigel et al. 1996), dipyrone (Shpigel et al. 1996) and meloxicam (Banting et al. 2000). In addition to beneficial clinical responses, Anderson et al. (1986b) reported reduced PGE_2 and TxA_2 concentrations in the udder in response to flunixin; increased whey IgG1 and IgM concentrations were also obtained. Insofar as the effects of endotoxin are COX-mediated, it is likely that both isoforms are implicated. Therefore, a nonselective COX inhibitor may be a more rational therapeutic choice than a selective COX-2 inhibitor.

Systemically administered NSAIDs may be of less benefit in cases of mild or chronic mastitis. Pyorala et al. (1988) examined the influence of phenylbutazone and flunixin administered intravenously in cases of chronic subclinical mastitis. Neither drug influenced bacterial growth; somatic cell count; or concentrations of inflammatory markers, N-acetyl-β-D-glucosaminidase activity, and trypsin-inhibitory capacity. However, Fitzpatrick

(1998) reported that allodynia was abrogated by a single intravenous dose of flunixin, an effect that lasted for 24 hours, after which the allodynic state recurred. This indicates the potential value of NSAIDs to provide analgesia in inflammatory conditions in cattle, although further work is required to establish optimal dosage regimens. There have been few investigations of NSAIDs administered locally by intramammary infusion to determine whether analgesic and antiinflammatory effects provide symptomatic relief of mastitis. Such use has probably been precluded by the irritant properties of many NSAIDs.

Some studies have shown no beneficial effect of NSAIDs in reproductive disorders such as retained placenta and postpartum endometritis (Konigsson et al. 2001). However, flunixin reduced the incidence of pyrexia in cows with either acute or subacute metritis compared to nontreated controls (Amiridis et al. 2001). Uterine involution and onset of estrus occurred earlier in cows that received flunixin.

RESPIRATORY DISEASES. Acute and potentially life-threatening inflammatory lung infections occur in such conditions as calf and piglet pneumonias of viral, bacterial, or mixed etiology. Disease models and/or clinical trials have indicated positive responses to NSAID treatment, although findings have been conflicting. Selman et al. (1984) showed that flunixin reduced lung consolidation scores in calves infected with P13 virus. The effects of flunixin on lung lesions, postmortem lung weights (reflecting an antiedematous action) and clinical signs in an experimental bovine pasteurellosis model based upon challenge with *Mannheimia haemolytica* A1 were investigated. The benefits of flunixin therapy were apparent not when the drug was administered alone but when used in combination with oxytetracycline (Selman 1988). The author claimed benefits on the basis of several indices, but the findings were equivocal. Anderson (1988) investigated a flunixin/oxytetracycline product in comparison with oxytetracycline alone in field cases of pneumonia, with treatment daily for 3 days. Reduction in coughing, return to normal food intake, and weight gain were said to be better improved with the combination product compared to oxytetracycline alone and there were fewer relapses.

Other NSAIDs, including ketoprofen, meloxicam, carprofen, and tolfenamic acid, have been used in combination with antibiotics in the therapy of calf pneumonias. Not all studies have demonstrated clear benefits of NSAID therapy, and the mechanism of any beneficial actions is not established. One may speculate that the antiinflammatory action reducing pulmonary edema improves lung function and respiratory gas exchange, while the antipyretic action may improve the clinical status so that animals begin to eat and drink. As cattle rely principally on respiration for temperature regulation, they may be stressed from infections causing pyrexia and hence benefit from the antipyretic actions of NSAIDs. The analgesic action of NSAIDs might also contribute to any improvement in clinical status.

Ingestion of 3-methylindole in cattle causes a chemical toxicosis characterized by signs of respiratory distress, congestion, edema, and interstitial emphysema. It is termed fog fever. Selman (1988) reported that flunixin reduced respiratory rate and the extent of lung lesions, assessed by pathological and histopathological examinations, reducing the degree and severity of alveolar epithelial hyperplasia. Further evaluation of NSAIDs in acute life-threatening respiratory infections is needed. Nevertheless, carprofen, flunixin, ketoprofen, tolfenamic acid, and meloxicam all possess marketing authorizations for use in the therapy of pneumonia in calves.

CALF AND PIGLET SCOURS. Infections of the gastrointestinal tract in young calves and piglets are associated with high morbidity and, in the absence of effective treatments, possible mortality. Early studies suggested possible benefits from aspirin treatment. Jones et al. (1977) described the benefit of flunixin therapy in suppressing inflammation, reducing fluid losses in feces, and lowering morbidity and mortality in calf scours. Meloxicam is licensed for use in calf scours in combination with antimicrobial drugs.

REFERENCES

Agnello, K.A., Reynolds, L.R. and Budsberg, S.C. 2005. In vivo effects of tepoxalin, an inhibitor of cyclooxygenase and lipoxygenase, on prostanoid and leukotriene production in dogs with chronic osteoarthritis. Am J Vet Res 66:966–972.

Aisen, P.S., Schafer, K.A. Grundman, M. et al. 2003. Effects of rofecoxib or naproxen vs placebo on Alzheimer disease progression: a randomised controlled trial. Alzheimer's Disease Cooperative Study. J Am Med Assoc 289:2819–2826.

Amiridis, G.S., Leontides, L., Tassos, E. et al. 2001. Flunixin meglumine accelerates uterine involution and shortens the calving-to-first-oestrus interval in cows with puerperal metritis. J Vet Pharmacol Therap 24:365–367.

Anderson, D. 1988. Clinical use of flunixin. Br Vet J Suppl 1:7–8.

Anderson, K.L., Smith, A.R., Shanks, R.D. et al. 1986a. Efficacy of flunixin meglumine for the treatment of endotoxin-induced bovine mastitis. Am J Vet Res 47:1366–1372.

———. 1986b. Endotoxin-induced bovine mastitis: immunoglobulins, phagocytosis and effect of flunixin meglumine. Am J Vet Res 47:2405–2410.

Argentieri, D.C., Ritchie, D.M., Ferro, M.P. et al. 1994. Tepoxalin: A dual cyclooxygenase/5-lipoxygenase inhibitor of arachidonic acid metabolism with potent anti-inflammatory activity and a favourable gastrointestinal profile. J Pharmacol Exp Therap 271:1399–1408.

Ariens, E.J. 1985. Stereochemistry, a basis for sophisticated nonsense in pharmacokinetics and clinical pharmacology. Eur J Clin Pharmacol 26:663–668.

Arifah, K.A. and Lees, P. 2002. Pharmacodynamics and pharmacokinetics of phenylbutazone in calves. J Vet Pharmacol Therap 25:299–309.

Armstrong, S., Tricklebank, P., Lake, A. et al. 1999a. Pharmacokinetics of carprofen enantiomers in equine plasma and synovial fluid—A comparison with ketoprofen. J Vet Pharmacol Therap 22:196–201.

Armstrong, S. and Lees, P. 1999b. Effects of R and S enantiomers and a racemic mixture of carprofen on the production and release of proteoglycan and prostaglandin E_2 from equine chondrocytes and cartilage explants. Am J Vet Res 60:98–104.

Armstrong, S. and Lees, P. 2002. Effects of carprofen (R and S enantiomers and racemate) on the production of IL-1, IL-6 and TNF-α by equine chondrocytes and synoviocytes. J Vet Pharmacol Therap 25: 145–153.

Balmer, T.V., Irvine, D., Jones, R.S. et al. 1998. Comparison of carprofen and pethidine as postoperative analgesics in the cat. J Small Anim Pract 39:158–164.

Banting, A., Schmidt, H. and Banting, S. 2000. Efficacy of meloxicam in lactating cows with E coli endotoxin induced acute mastitis. Abstract no. E4. in Proc 8th Int Congr EAVPT, Jerusalem, Israel. Blackwell Scientific Publications, Oxford, U.K.

Baron, J.A., Cole, B.F., Sandler, R.S. et al. 2003. A randomised trial of aspirin to prevent colorectal adenomas. N Engl J Med 348:891–899.

Bataar, D., Jones, M.K., Pai, R. et al. 2002. Selective cyclooxygenase-2 blocker delays healing of esophageal ulcers in rats and inhibits ulceration-triggered c-Met/hepatocyte growth factor receptor induction and extracellular signal-regulated kinase 2 activation. Am J Pathol 160:963–972.

Benton, H.P., Vasseur, P.B., Broderick-Villa, G.A. et al. 1997. Effect of carprofen on sulphated glycosaminoglycan metabolism, protein synthesis and prostaglandin release by cultured osteoarthritic canine chondrocytes. Am J Vet Res 58:286–292.

Blomme, E.A., Chinn, K.S., Hardy, M.M. et al. 2003. Selective cyclooxygenase-2 inhibition does not affect the healing of cutaneous full-thickness incisional wounds in SKH-1 mice. Br J Dermatol 148:211–223.

Boileau, C., Martel-Pelletier, J., Jouzeau, J.Y. et al. 2002. Licofelone (ML-3000), a dual inhibitor of 5-lipoxygenase and cyclooxygenase, reduces the level of cartilage chondrocyte death in vivo in experimental dog osteoarthritis: Inhibition of pro-apoptotic factors. J Rheumatol 29:1446–1452.

Bombardier, C., Lain, L., Reicin, A. et al. 2000. Comparison of upper gastrointestinal toxicity of rofecoxib and naproxen in patients with rheumatoid arthritis. N Engl J Med 343:1520–1528.

Bostrom, I.M., Nyman, G., Hoppe, A. et al. 2006. Effects of meloxicam on renal function in dogs with hypotension during anaesthesia. Vet Anaesth Analg 33:62–69.

Brandt, K.D. 1991. The mechanism of action of nonsteroidal anti-inflammatory drugs. J Clin Pharmacol 28:512–517.

Brideau, C., Van Staden, C. and Chung, C. 2001. In vitro effects of cyclooxygenase inhibitors in whole blood of horses, dogs and cats. Am J Vet Res 62:1755–1760.

Brune, K., Geisslinger, G. and Menzel-Soglowek, S. 1992. Pure Enantiomers of 2-arylpropionic acids: Tools in pain research and improved drugs in rheumatology. J Clin Pharmacol 32:944–952.

Bryant, C.E., Farnfield, B.A. and Janicke, H.J. 2003. Evaluation of the ability of carprofen and flunixin meglumine to inhibit activation of nuclear factor kappa B. Am J Vet Res 64:211–215.

Burvenich, C. and Peeters, G. 1982. Effect of prostaglandin synthetase inhibitors on mammary blood flow during experimentally induced mastitis in lactating goats. Arch Int Pharmacodyn Therap 258:128–137.

Busch, U., Schmid, J., Heinzel, G. et al. 1998. Pharmacokinetics of meloxicam in animals and the relevance to humans. Drug Metab Dispos 26:576–584.

Carlisle, C.H., Penny, R.H.C., Prescott, C.W. et al. 1968. Toxic effects of phenylbutazone on the cat. Brit Vet J 124:560–568.

Catella-Lawson, F., Reilly, M.P., Kapoor, S.C. et al. 2001. Cyclooxygenase inhibitors and the antiplatelet effects of aspirin. N Engl J Med 345:1809–1817.

Chandrasekharan, N.V., Hu Dai, K., Roos, L.T. et al. 2002. COX-3, a cyclooxygenase-1 variant inhibited by acetaminophen and analgesic/antipyretic drugs: cloning, structure and expression. Proc Nat Acad Sci 99:13926–13931.

Cheng, Z., McKellar, Q.A., Nolan, A. et al. 1996. Pharmacokinetics and pharmacodynamics of phenylbutazone and oxyphenbutazone in the donkey. J Vet Pharmacol Therap 19:149–151.

Cheng, Z., Nolan, A. and McKellar, Q. 2002. Anti-inflammatory effects of carprofen, its enantiomers and Ng-nitro-L-arginine methyl ester in vivo using sheep as a model. Am J Vet Res 63:782–788.

Cheng, Z., Nolan, A., Moneiro, A. et al. 2003. Enantioselective pharmacokinetic and cyclooxygenase inhibition of carprofen and carprofen enantiomers in sheep. J Vet Pharmacol Therap 26:391–394.

Dawson, J., Lees, P. and Sedgwick, A.D. 1987. Actions of non-steroidal anti-inflammatory drugs on equine leucocyte movement in vitro. J Vet Pharmacol Therap 10:150–159.

Delatour, P., Foot, R., Foster, A.P. et al. 1996. Pharmacodynamics and chiral pharmacokinetics of carprofen in calves. Brit Vet J 152:183–198.

Dinchuk, J.E., Car, B.D., Focht, R.J. et al. 1995. Renal abnormalities and an altered inflammatory response in mice lacking cyclooxygenase II. Nature 378:406–409.

Dinchuk, J.E., Liu, R.Q. and Trzaskos, J.M. 2003. COX-3 in the wrong frame in mind. Immunol Lett 86:121.

Dolan, S. and Nolan, A.M. 2000. Behavioural evidence supporting a differential role for group I and II metabotropic glutamate receptors in spinal nociceptive transmission. Neuropharmacology 39:1132–1138.

Eltom, S.E., Guard, C.H. and Schwark, W. 1993. The effect of age on phenylbutazone pharmacokinetics, metabolism and protein binding in goats. J Vet Pharmacol Therap 16:141–151.

Ferreira, S.H. 1983. Prostaglandins: peripheral and central analgesia. In Advances in Pain Research and Therapapy, Raven Press, New York, U.S.

Fiorucci, S., Meli, R., Bucci, M. et al. 2001. Dual inhibitors of cyclooxygenase and 5-lipoxygenase. A new avenue in anti-inflammatory Therapy? Biochem Pharmacol 62:1433–1438.

FitzGerald, G.A. and Patrono, C. 2001. The coxibs, selective inhibitors of cyclooxygenase-2. N Engl J Med 345:433–442.

Fitzpatrick, J. 1998. Personal communication.

Flecknell, P.A. and Waterman-Pearson, A. 2000. Pain management in animals. W B Saunders, London.

Forsyth, S.F., Guilford, W.G. and Pfeiffer, D.U. 2000. Effect of NSAID administration on creatinine clearance in healthy dogs undergoing anaesthesia and surgery. J Small Anim Prac 41:547–550.

Frean, S.P., Abraham, L.A. and Lees, P. 1999. In vitro stimulation of equine articular cartilage proteoglycan synthesis by hyaluronan and carprofen. Res Vet Sci 67:181–188.

Fusellier, M., Desfontis, J.C., Madec, S. et al. 2005. Effect of tepoxalin on renal function in healthy dogs receiving an angiotensin-converting enzyme inhibitor. J Vet Pharmacol Therap 28:581–586.

Gajraj, N.M. 2003. The effect of cyclooxygenase-2 inhibitors on bone healing. Reg Anesth Pain Med 28:456–65.

Galbraith, E.A. and McKellar, Q.A. 1991. Pharmacokinetics and pharmacodynamics of piroxicam in dogs. Vet Rec 128:561–565.

———. 1996. Protein binding and in vitro serum thromboxane B2 inhibition by flunixin meglumine and meclofenamic acid in dog, goat and horse blood. Res Vet Sci 61:78–81.

Gerstenfeld, L.C., Cullinane, D.M., Barnes, G.L. et al. 2003. Fracture healing as a post-natal developmental process: molecular, spatial, and temporal aspects of its regulation. J Cell Biochem 88:873–84.

Gierse, M.S., State, N.R., Casperson, G.F. et al. 2002. Cloning, expression and selective inhibition of canine cyclooxygenase-1 and cyclooxygenase-2. Vet Therap 3:270–280

Gilroy, D.W., Tomlinson, A. and Willoughby, D.A. 1998. Differential effects of inhibition of isoforms of cyclooxygenase (COX-1, COX-2) in chronic inflammation. Inflamm Res 47:79–85.

Gilroy, D.W., Colville-Nash, P.R., Willis, D. et al. 1999. Inducible cyclooxygenase may have anti-inflammatory properties. Nat Med 6:698–701.

Giraudel, J.M., Toutain, P.L. and Lees, P. 2005a. Development of in vitro assays for the evaluation of cyclooxygenase inhibitors and application for predicting the selectivity of NSAIDs in the cat. Am J Vet Res 66:700–709.

Giraudel, J.M., Diquelou, A., Laroute, V. et al. 2005b. Pharmacokinetic/pharmacodynamic modelling of NSAIDs in a model of reversible inflammation in the cat. Brit J Pharmacol 146:642–653.

Goldstein, J.L., Kivitz, A.J., Verburg, K.M. et al. 2003. A comparison of the upper gastrointestinal mucosal effects of valdecoxib, naproxen and placebo in healthy elderly subjects. Aliment Pharmacol Therap 18:125–132.

Goodman, S.B., Ma, T., Genovese, M. et al. 2003. COX-2 selective inhibitors and bone. Int J Immunopathol Pharmacol 16:201–205.

Hallak, A., Alon-Baron, L., Shamir, R. et al. 2003. Rofecoxib reduces polyp recurrence in familial polyposis. Dig Dis Sci 48:1998–2002.

Hamilton, L.C., Mitchell, J.A., Tomlinson, A.M. et al. 1999. Synergy between cyclo-oxygenase-2 induction and arachidonic acid supply in vivo: consequences for nonsteroidal anti-inflammatory drug efficacy. FASEB J 13:245–251.

Hardie, E.M., Kolata, R.J. and Rawlings, C.A. 1983. Canine septic peritonitis: treatment with flunixin meglumine. Circ Shock 11:159–173.

Hawkey, C., Laine, L., Simon, T. et al. 2000. Comparison of the effect of rofecoxib (a cyclooxygenase 2 inhibitor), ibuprofen and placebo on the gastroduodenal mucosa of patients with osteoarthritis: a randomised, double-blind, placebo-controlled trial. The Rofecoxib Osteoarthritis Endoscopy Multinational Study Group. Arthritis Rheum 43:370–377.

Higgins, A.J., Lees, P. and Wright, J.A. 1984. Tissue-cage model for the collection of inflammatory exudate in ponies. Res Vet Sci 36:284–289.

Higgins, A.J., Lees, P., Sedgwick, A.D. et al. 1987a. Studies on the use of a novel non-steroidal anti-inflammatory drug in the horse. Equine Vet J 19:60–66.

Higgins, A.J., Lees, P. and Sedgwick, A.D. 1987b. Actions of BW 540C in an equine model of acute inflammation: A preliminary study. Vet Quarterly 9:103–110.

Hjelle, J.J. and Grasser, C.F. 1986. Acetaminophen induced toxicosis in dogs and cats. J Am Vet Med Assoc 188:742–746.

Holton, L.L., Scott, E.M. and Nolan, A.M. 1998. Comparison of three methods used for assessment of pain in dogs. J Am Vet Med Assoc 212:61–66.

Homer, L.M., Clarke, C.R. and Weingarten, A.J. 2005. Effect of dietary fat on oral bioavailability of tepoxalin in dogs. J Vet Pharmacol Therap 28:287–291.

Hwang, D.Y., Chae, K.R. Kang, T.S. et al. 2002. Alterations in behavior, amyloid beta-42, caspase-3, and Cox-2 in mutant PS2 transgenic mouse model of Alzheimer's disease. FASEB J 16: 805–813.

Jackson, J.E. 1982. Cimetidine protects against acetaminophen toxicity. Life Sci 31:31–35.

Jones, E.O., Hamm, D., Cooley, L. et al. 1977. Diarrhoeal diseases of the calf: observations on treatment and prevention. New Z Vet J 25:312–16.

Jones, C.J., Streppa, H.K., Harmon, B.G. et al. 2002. In vivo effects of meloxicam and aspirin on blood, gastric mucosal and synovial fluid prostanoid synthesis in dogs. Am J Vet Res 63:1527–1531.

Kawaguchi, H., Pilbeam, C.C., Harrison, J.R. et al. 1995. The role of prostaglandins in the regulation of bone metabolism. Clin Orthop 313:36–46.

Kawahito, Y., Kondo, M., Tsubouchi, Y. et al. 2000. 15-deoxy-$\Delta^{12,14}$-PGJ_2 induces synoviocyte apoptosis and suppresses adjuvant-induced arthritis in rats. J Clin Invest 106:189–197.

Kay-Mugford, P., Grimm, K.A., Weingarten, A.J. et al. 2004. Effect of preoperative administration of tepoxalin on hemostasis and hepatic and renal function in dogs. Vet Therap 5:120–127.

Knapp, D.W., Richardson, R.C., Bottoms, G.D. et al. 1992. Phase I. Trial of piroxicam in 62 dogs bearing naturally occurring tumors. Cancer Chem Pharmacol 29:214–218.

Kniss, D.A. 1999. Cyclooxygenases in reproductive medicine and biology. J Soc Gynecol Invest 6:285–292.

Knottenbelt, C.M., Simpson, J.W., Tasker, S. et al. 2000. Preliminary clinical observations on the use of piroxicam in the management of rectal tubulopapillary polyps. J Small Anim Prac 41:393–397.

Ko, J.C.H., Miyabiyashi, T., Mandsager, R.E. et al. 2000. Renal effects of carprofen administered to healthy dogs anesthetized with propofol and isoflurane. J Amer Vet Med Assoc 217:346–349.

Konigsson, K., Gustafsson, H., Gunnarsson, A. et al. 2001. Clinical and bacteriological aspects on the use of oxytetracycline and flunixin in primiparous cows with induced retained placenta and post-partal endometritis. Reprod Domest Anim 36:247–256.

Krishnan, K., Ruffin, M.T., Normolle, D. et al. 2001. Colonic mucosal prostaglandin E_2 and cyclooxygenase expression before and after low aspirin doses in subjects at high risk or at normal risk for colorectal cancer. Cancer Epidemiol Biomarkers Prev 10:447–453.

Kujubu, D.A., Fletcher, B.S., Varnum, B.C. et al. 1991. TIS10, a phorbol ester tumor promoter-inducible mRNA from Swiss 3T3 cells, encodes a novel prostaglandin synthase/cyclooxygenase homologue. J Biol Chem 266:12866–12872.

Lajeunesse, D., Martel-Pelletier, J., Fernandes, J.C. et al. 2004. Treatment with licofelone prevents abnormal subchondral bone cell metabolism in experimental dog osteoarthritis. Annals Rheum Dis 63:78–83.

Landoni, M.F., Comas, W., Mucci, N. et al. 1999. Enantiospecific pharmacokinetics and pharmacodynamics of ketoprofen in sheep. J Vet Pharmacol Therap 22:349–359.

Landoni, M.F., Cunningham, F.M. and Lees, P. 1995a. Comparative pharmacodynamics of flunixin, ketoprofen and tolfenamic acid in calves. Vet Rec 137:428–431.

Landoni, M.F., Cunningham, F.M. and Lees, P. 1995b. Pharmacokinetics and pharmacodynamics of ketoprofen in calves applying PK-PD modelling. J Vet Pharmacol Therap 18:315–324.

Landoni, M.F., Cunningham, F.M. and Lees, P. 1995c. Determination of pharmacokinetics and pharmacodynamics of flunixin in calves by use of pharmacokinetic/pharmacodynamic modelling. Am J Vet Res 56:786–793.

Landoni, M.F., Cunningham, F.M. and Lees, P. 1996. Pharmacokinetics and pharmacodynamics of tolfenamic acid in calves. Res Vet Sci 61:26–32.

Landoni, M.F. and Lees, P. 1995a. Influence of formulation on the pharmacokinetics and bioavailability of racemic ketoprofen in horses. J Vet Pharmacol Therap 18:446–450.

Landoni, M.F. and Lees, P. 1995b. Comparison of the anti-inflammatory actions of flunixin and ketoprofen in horses applying PK/PD modelling. Equine Vet J 27:247–256.

Landoni, M.F. and Lees, P. 1995c. Pharmacokinetics and pharmacodynamics of ketoprofen enantiomers in calves. Chirality 7:586–597.

Landoni, M.F. and Lees, P. 1996. Pharmacokinetics and pharmacodynamics of ketoprofen enantiomers in the horse. J Vet Pharmacol Therap 19:466–474.

Lanza, F.L., Rack, M.F., Simon, T.J. et al. 1999. Specific inhibition of cyclooxygenase-2 with MK-0966 is associated with less gastroduodenal damage than either aspirin or ibuprofen. Aliment Pharmacol Therap 13:761–767.

Larson, E.J. 1963. Toxicity of low doses of aspirin in the cat. J Am Vet Med Assoc 143:837–840.

Lascelles, B.D., Cripps, P., Mirchandani, S. et al. 1995. Carprofen as an analgesic for postoperative pain in cats: dose titration and assessment of efficacy in comparison to pethidine hydrochloride. J Small Anim Pract 36:535–541.

Lascelles, B.D., Cripps, P.J., Jones, A. et al. 1998. Efficacy and kinetics of carprofen, administered preoperatively or postoperatively, for the prevention of pain in dogs undergoing ovariohysterectomy. Vet Surg 27:568–582.

Lascelles, B.D., Court, M.H., Hardie, M. et al. 2007. Nonsteroidal anti-inflammatory drugs in cats: a review. Vet Anaes Analg 34: 2228–2250.

Laudederkind, S.J., Thompson-Jaeger, S., Goorha, S. et al. 2002. Both constitutive and inducible prostaglandin H synthase affect dermal wound healing in mice. Lab Invest 82:919–927.

Laufer, S. 2001. Discovery and development of ML3000. Inflammopharm 9:101–112.

Launer, L. 2003. Nonsteroidal anti-inflammatory drug use and the risk for Alzheimer's disease: dissecting the epidemiological evidence. Drugs 63:731–739.

Lees, P., Creed, R.F.S., Gerring, E.L. et al. 1983. Biochemical and haematological effects of recommended dosage with phenylbutazone in horses. Equine Vet J 15:158–167.

Lees, P. and Higgins, A.J. 1985. Clinical pharmacology and therapeutic uses of non-steroidal anti-inflammatory drugs in the horse. Equine Vet J 17:83–96.

Lees, P., Maitho, T.E. and Taylor, J.B. 1985. Pharmacokinetics of phenylbutazone in young and old ponies. Vet Rec 116:229–32.

Lees, P, Taylor, J.B.O., Higgins, A.J. et al. 1986. Phenylbutazone and oxyphenbutazone distribution into tissue fluids in the horse. J Vet Pharm Therap 9:204–212.

Lees, P., Ewins, C.P., Taylor, J.B.O. et al. 1987a. Serum thromboxane in the horse and its inhibition by aspirin, phenylbutazone and flunixin. Brit Vet J 143:462–476.

Lees, P., Taylor, J.B.O., Maitho, T.E. et al. 1987b. Metabolism, excretion, pharmacokinetics and tissue residues of phenylbutazone in the horse. Cornell Vet 77:192–211.

Lees, P., Ayliffe, T., Maitho, T.E. et al. 1988a. Pharmacokinetics, metabolism and excretion of phenylbutazone in cattle following intravenous, intramuscular and oral administration. Res Vet Sci 44:57–67.

Lees, P., Taylor, J.B.O., Higgins, A.J. et al. 1988b. In vitro and in vivo studies on the binding of phenylbutazone and related drugs to equine feeds and digesta. Res Vet Sci 44:50–56.

Lees, P., Taylor, P.M., Landoni, M.F. et al. 2003. Ketoprofen in the cat: pharmacodynamics and chiral pharmacokinetics. The Vet J 165:21–35.

Lees, P., Delatour, P., Foster, A.P. et al. 1996. Evaluation of carprofen in calves using a tissue cage model of inflammation. Brit Vet J 152:199–211.

Lees, P., May, S.A., Hoeijmakers, M. et al. 1999. A pharmacodynamic and pharmacokinetic study with vedaprofen in an equine model of acute nonimmune inflammation. J Vet Pharmacol Therap 22: 96–106.

Lees, P., Landoni, M.F., Armstrong, S. et al. 2000. New insights into inflammation with particular reference to the role of COX enzymes. 8th EAVPT International congress Proceedings. J Vet Pharm Therap Supplement.

Lees, P., AliAbadi, F.S. and Landoni, M.F. 2002. Pharmacodynamics and enantioselective pharmacokinetics of racemic carprofen in the horse. J Vet Pharmacol Therap 25:433–448.

Lees, P. 2003. Pharmacology of drugs used to treat osteoarthritis in veterinary practice. Inflammopharmacology 11:385–399.

Lees, P., Landoni, M.F., Giraudel, J. et al. 2004a. Pharmacodynamics and pharmacokinetics of nonsteroidal anti-inflammatory drugs in species of veterinary interest. J Vet Pharmacol Therap 27:479–490.

Lees, P., Giraudel, J., Landoni, M.F. et al. 2004b. PK-PD integration and PK-PD modelling of nonsteroidal anti-inflammatory drugs: principles and applications in veterinary pharmacology. J Vet Pharmacol Therap 27:491–502.

Leese, P.T., Hubbard, R.C., Karim, A. et al. 2000. Effects of celecoxib, a novel cyclooxygenase-2 inhibitor, on platelet function in healthy adults: a randomised, controlled trial. J Clin Pharmacol 40:124–132.

Lipscomb, V.J., AliAbadi, F.S., Lees, P. et al. 2002. Clinical efficacy and pharmacokinetics of carprofen in the treatment of dogs with osteoarthritis. Vet Rec 150:684–689.

Lohuis, J.A.C.M., Van Leeuwen, W., Verheijden, J.H.M. et al. 1989. Flunixin meglumine and flurbiprofen in cows with experimental Escherichia coli mastitis. Vet Rec 124:305–308.

Lohuis, J.A., van Werven, T., Brand, A. et al. 1991. Pharmacodynamics and pharmacokinetics of carprofen, a non-steroidal anti-inflammatory drug, in healthy cows and cows with Escherichia coli endotoxin-induced mastitis. J Vet Pharmacol Therap 14:219–229.

Luna, S.P.L., Basilio, A.C., Steagall, D.V.M. et al. 2007. Evaluation of adverse effects of long-term oral administration of carprofen, etodolac, flunixin, meglumine, ketoprofen and meloxicam in dog. Am J Vet Res 68:258–264.

MacAllister, C.G., Morgan, S.J., Borne, A.T. et al. 1993. Comparison of adverse effects of phenylbutazone, flunixin meglumine and ketoprofen in horses. J Am Vet Med Assoc 202:71–77.

MacDonald, T.M. and Wei, L. 2003. Effect of ibuprofen on cardioprotective effect of aspirin. Lancet 361:573–574.

MacPhail, C.M., Lappin, M.R., Meyer, D.J. et al. 1998. Hepatocellular toxicosis associated with administration of carprofen in 21 dogs. J Am Vet Med Assoc 212:1895–1901.

Maitho, T.D., Lees, P. and Taylor, J.B. 1986. Absorption and pharmacokinetics of phenylbutazone in Welsh Mountain ponies. J Vet Pharmacol Therap 9:26–39.

Malmberg, A.B. and Yaksh, T.L. 1992. Antinociceptive actions of spinal nonsteroidal anti-inflammatory agents on the formalin test in the rat. J Pharmacol Exp Therap 263:136–146.

Marr, K., Marsh, K., Hernandez, L. et al. 1998a. Pharmacokinetics and pharmacodynamics of fenleuton, a 5-lipoxygenase inhibitor in ponies. Res Vet Sci 64:111–117.

Marr, K.A., Lees, P., Page, C.P. et al. 1998b. Effect of the 5-lipoxygenase inhibitor, fenleuton, on antigen-induced neutrophil accumulation and lung function changes in horses with chronic obstructive pulmonary disease. J Vet Pharmacol Therap 21:241–246.

———. 1998c. Inhaled leukotrienes cause bronchoconstriction and neutrophil accumulation in horses. Res Vet Sci 64:219–224.

Marriner, S. and Bogan, J.A. 1979. The influence of the rumen on the absorption of drugs; study using meclofenamic acid administered by various routes to sheep and cattle. J Vet Pharmacol Therap 2:109–15.

May, S.A., Hooke, R.E., Peremans, K.Y. et al. 1994. Prostaglandin E2 in equine joint disease. Vlaams Diergeneeskd. Tijdschr. 63:187–191.

McCann, M., Andersen, D.R., Zhang, D. et al. 2004. In vitro effects and in vivo efficacy of a novel cyclooxygenase-2 inhibitor in dogs with experimentally induced synotitis. Am J Vet Res 65:503–512.

McKellar, Q.A., Lees, P. and Gettinby, G. 1994a. Pharmacodynamics of tolfenamic acid in dogs. Evaluation of dose response relationships. Eur J Pharmacol 253:191–200.

McKellar, Q.A., Delatour, P. and Lees, P. 1994b. Stereospecific pharmacodynamics and pharmacokinetics of carprofen in the dog. J Vet Pharmacol Therap 17:447–454.

Millis, D.L., Weigel, J.P., Moyers, T. et al. 2002. Effect of deracoxib, a new COX-2 inhibitor, on the prevention of lameness induced by chemical synovitis in dogs. Vet Therap 3:453–464.

Mohammed, S.I., Coffman, K., Glickman, N.W. et al. 2001. Prostaglandin E_2 concentrations in naturally occurring canine cells. Prostaglandins, Leukotrienes, Essent Fatty Acids 70:479–483.

Moore, J.N. 1986. Treatment of equine colic and endotoxemia. In International Symposium on Nonseteroidal Anti-inflammatory Agents pp 11–14, Trenton, NJ: Vet Learning Systems Co.

Moore, J.N., Hardee, M.M. and Hardee, G.E. 1986. Modulation of arachidonic acid metabolism in endotoxic horses: comparison of flunixin meglumine, phenylbutazone and a selective thromboxane synthetase inhibitor. Am J Vet Res 47:110–113.

Moreau, M., Daminet, S., Martel-Pelletier, J. et al. 2005. Superiority of the gastroduodenal safety profile of licofelone over rofecoxib, a COX-2 selective inhibitor, in dogs. J Vet Pharmacol Therap 28:81–86.

Mullins, M.N., Lana, S.E., Dernell, W.S. et al. 2004. Cyclooxygenase-2 expression in canine appendicular osteosarcomas. J Vet Int Med 18:859–865.

Murakami, M., Kambe, T., Shimbara, S. et al. 1999. Functional coupling between various phospholipase A_2s and cyclooxygenase in immediate and delayed prostanoid biosynthetic pathways. J Biol Chem 274: 3103–3115.

Murray, M.J. 1985. Phenylbutazone toxicity in a horse. Compendium on Continuing Education 7:S389–S394.

Nolan, A.M. 2001. Patterns and its management of pain in animals. In Pain: its nature and management in man and animals. International Congress and Symposium Series 246:93–100. Eds. Lord Soulsby of Swaffham Prior, Professor David Morton. Royal Soc. of Med. Press, U.K.

Pai, R., Soreghan, B., Szabo, I.L. et al. 2002. Prostaglandin E_2 transactivates EGF receptor: a novel mechanism for promoting colon cancer growth and gastrointestinal hypertrophy. Nat Med 8:289–293.

Paulson, S.K., Engel, L., Reitz, B. et al. 1999. Evidence for polymorphism in the canine metabolism of the cyclooxygenase 2 inhibitor, celecoxib. Drug Metab Dispos 27:1133–1142.

Pelletier, J.P., Lajeunesse, D., Jovanovic, D.V. et al. 2000. Carprofen simultaneously reduces progression of morphological changes in cartilage and subchondral bone in experimental dog osteoarthritis. J Rheumatol 27:2893–2902.

Priymenko, N., Ferre, J.P., Rascol, A. et al. 1993. Migrating motor complex of the intestine and absorption of a biliary excreted drug in the dog. J Pharmacol Exp Therap 267:1161–1167.

Pyorala, S., Patila, J. and Sandholm, M. 1988. Phenylbutazone and flunixin meglumine fail to show beneficial effects on bovine subclinical mastitis. Acta Vet Scand 29:501–503.

Radi, Z.A. and Khan, N.K. 2005. Effects of cyclooxygenase inhibition on bone, tendon, and ligament healing. Inflamm Res 54:358–366.

Rainsford, K.D. 1977. The comparative gastric ulcerogenic activities of non-steroid anti-inflammatory drugs. Agents and Actions 7:573–7.

———. 1993. Leukotrienes in the pathogenesis of NSAID-induced gastric and intestinal mucosal damage. Agents and Actions 39:C24–C26.

Ray, W.A., Stein, C.M., Daugherty, J.R. et al. 2002. COX-2 selective nonsteroidal anti-inflammatory drugs and risk of serious coronary heart disease. Lancet 360:1071–1073.

Reicin, A.S., Shapiro, D., Sperling, R.S. et al. 2002. Comparison of cardiovascular thrombotic events in patients with osteoarthritis treated with rofecoxib versus non-selective nonsteroidal anti-inflammatory drugs (ibuprofen, diclofenac and nabumetone). Am J Cardiol 89:204–209.

Ricketts, A.P., Lundy, K.M. and Seibel, S.B. 1998. Evaluation of selective inhibition of canine cyclooxygenase 1 and 2 by carprofen and other nonsteroidal anti-inflammatory drugs. Am J Vet Res 59:1441–1446.

Riley, G.P., Cox, M., Harrall, R.L. et al. 2001. Inhibition of tendon cell proliferation and matrix glycosaminoglycan synthesis by non-steroidal anti-inflammatory drugs in vitro. J Hand Surg [Br] 26:224–228.

Robertson, S.A. 2005. Managing pain in feline patients. Vet Clin Small Anim 35:129–146.

Rordorf, C., Kellett, N., Mair, S. et al. 2003. Gastroduodenal tolerability of lumiracoxib vs placebo and naproxen: a pilot endoscopic study in healthy male subjects. Aliment Pharmacol Therap 18:533–541.

Samad, T.A., Moore, K.A., Sapirstein, A. et al. 2001. Interleukin-1β-mediated induction of Cox-2 in the CNS contributes to inflammatory pain hypersensitivity. Nature 410:471–475.

Sample, D., Wargovich, M., Fischer, S.M. et al. 2002. A dose-finding study of aspirin for chemoprevention utilizing rectal mucosal prostaglandin E_2 levels as a biomarker. Cancer Epidemiol Biomarkers Prev 11:275–279.

Sandler, R.S., Halabi, S., Baron, J.A. et al. 2003. A randomised trial of aspirin to prevent colorectal adenomas in patients with previous colorectal cancer. N Engl J Med 348:883–890.

Sarkar, S., Hobson, A.R., Hughes, A. et al. 2003. The prostaglandin E_2 receptor-1 (EP-1) mediates acid-induced visceral pain hypersensitivity in humans. Gastroenterology 124:18–25.

Selman, I.E., Allan, E.M., Gibbs, M.A. et al. 1984. Effect of anti-prostaglandin therapy in experimental parainfluenza type 3 pneumonia in weaned conventional calves. Vet Rec 115:101–105.

Selman, I.E. 1988. The veterinary uses of a non-steroidal anti-inflammatory agent: flunixin meglumine. Brit Vet J Suppl. No.1:4–6.

Shpigel, N.Y., Chen, R., Winkler, M. et al. 1994. Anti-inflammatory ketoprofen in the treatment of field cases of bovine mastitis. Res Vet Sci 56:62–68.

Shpigel, N.Y., Winkler, M., Saran, A. et al. 1996. The anti-inflammatory drugs phenylbutazone and dipyrone in the treatment of field cases of bovine mastitis. Am J Vet Med Assoc 43:331–336.

Sidhu, P.K., Landoni, M.F. and Lees, P. 2005. Influence of marbofloxacin on the pharmacokinetics and pharmacodynamics of tolfenamic acid in calves. J Vet Pharmacol Therap 28:109–119.

———. 2006. Pharmacokinetic and pharmacodynamic interactions of tolfenamic acid and marbofloxacin in goats. Res Vet Sci 80:79–90.

Silverstein, F.E., Faich, G., Goldstein, J.L. et al. 2000. Gastrointestinal toxicity with celecoxib vs nonsteroidal anti-inflammatory drugs for osteoarthritis and rheumatoid arthritis: the CLASS study: A randomised controlled trial. Celecoxib Long-term Arthritis Safety Study. J Am Med Assoc 284:1247–1255.

Simon, A.M., Manigrasso, M.B. and O'Connor, J.P. 2002. Cyclooxygenase 2 function is essential for bone fracture healing. J Bone Miner Res 17:963–976.

Singh, G. 1998. Recent considerations in nonsteroidal anti-inflammatory drug gastropathy. Am J Med 105:315–385.

Smith, C.J., Zhang, Y., Koboldt, C.M. et al. 1998. Pharmacological analysis of cyclooxygenase-1 in inflammation. Proc Nat Acad Sci 95:13313–13318.

Smith, J.B. and Willis, A.I. 1971. Aspirin selectively inhibits prostaglandin production in human platelets. Nature 231:235–237.

Snow, D.H., Bogan, J.A., Douglas, T.A. et al. 1979. Phenylbutazone toxicity in ponies. Vet Rec 105:26–30.

Solomon, D.H., Karlson, E.W., Rimm, E.B. et al. 2003. Cardiovascular morbidity and mortality in women diagnosed with rheumatoid arthritis. Circulation 107:1303–1307.

Soraci, A., Benoit, E., Jaussaud, E. et al. 1995. Enantioselective glucuronidation and subsequent biliary excretion of carprofen in horses. Am J Vet Res 56:358–361.

St Omer, V.V. and McKnight, E.D. 1980. Acetylcysteine for treatment of acetaminophen toxicosis in the cat. J Am Vet Med Assoc 176:911–913.

Steinbach, G., Lynch, P.M., Phillips, R.K. et al. 2000. The effect of celecoxib, a cyclooxygenase-2 inhibitor, in familial adenomatous polyposis. N Engl J Med 342:1946–1952.

Stewart, W.F., Kawas, M.D., Corrada, M. et al. 1997. Risk of Alzheimer's disease and duration of NSAID use. Neurology 48:626–631.

Streppa, H.K., Jones, C.J. and Budsberg, S.C. 2002. Cyclooxygenase selectivity of non-steroidal anti-inflammatory drugs in canine blood. Am J Vet Res 63:91–94.

Svensson, C.I. and Yaksh, T.L. 2002. The spinal phospholipase-cyclooxygenase-prostanoid cascade in nociceptive processing. Ann Rev Pharmacol Toxicol 42:553–583.

Tandy, J. and Thorpe, E. 1967. A fatal syndrome in a dog following administration of phenylbutazone. Vet Rec 81:398–399.

Taylor, J.B., Walland, A., Lees, P. et al. 1983. Biochemical and haematological effects of a revised dosage schedule of phenylbutazone in horses. Vet Rec 112:599–602.

Taylor, P.M., Delatour, P., Landoni, F.M. et al. 1996. Pharmacodynamics and enantioselective pharmacokinetics of carprofen in the cat. Res Vet Sci 60:144–151.

Toutain, P.L., Autefage, A., Legrand, C. et al. 1994. Plasma concentrations and therapapeutic efficacy of phenylbutazone and flunixin meglumine in the horse: pharmacokinetic/pharmacodynamic modelling. J Vet Pharmacol Therap 17:459–469.

Toutain, P.L. and Cester, C.C. 2004. Dose titration responses to meloxicam in an equine carpitis model and pharmacokinetic/pharmacodynamic relationships. Am J Vet Res. In press.

Toutain, P.L., Cester, C.C., Haak, T. et al. 2001a. Pharmacokinetic profile and in vitro selective cyclooxygenase-2 inhibition by nimesulide in the dog. J Vet Pharmacol and Therap 24:35–42.

———. 2001b. A pharmacokinetic/pharmacodynamic approach vs. a dose titration for the determination of a dosage regimen: the case of nimesulide, a Cox-2 selective nonsteroidal anti-inflammatory drug in the dog. J Vet Pharmacol Therap 24:43–55.

Tries, S. and Laufer, S. 2001. The pharmacological profile of ML3000: A new pyrrolizine derivative inhibiting the enzymes cyclooxygenase and 5-lipoxygenase. Inflammopharmacol 9:113–124.

Urade, Y. and Eguchi, N. 2002. Lipocalin-type and hematopoietic prostaglandin D synthases as a novel example of functional convergence. Prostaglandins and other Lipid Mediators 68–69:375–382.

USP Veterinary Pharmaceutical Information Monographs, Anti-inflammatories. 2004. J Vet Pharmacol Therap 27:Suppl 1, 1–110.

Vandeputte-Van Messom, G., Reynaert, R., Burvenich, C. et al. 1987. Effects of flurbiprofen on endotoxin-induced changes of plasma tyrosine in lactating goats. Arch Int Pharmacodyn Therap 290:159–160.

Vane, J.R. 1971. Inhibition of prostaglandin synthesis as a mechanism of action for aspirin-like drugs. Nat New Biol 231:232–235.

Vangroenweghe, F., Duchateau, L., Boutet, P. et al. 2005. Effect of carprofen treatment following experimentally induced Escherichia coli mastitis in primiparous cows. J Dairy Sci 88:2361–2376.

Wallace, J.L. and Devchand, P.R. 2005. Emerging roles for cyclooxygenase-2 in gastrointestinal mucosal defense. Brit J Pharmacol 145:275–282.

Wallace, J.L., McCafferty, D.D. and Carter, L. 1993. Tissue-selective inhibition of prostaglandin synthesis in rat by tepoxalin: anti-inflammatory without gastropathy. Gastroenterology 105:1630–1636.

Wallace, J.L., McKnight, W., Reuter, B.K. et al. 2000. NSAID-induced gastric damage in rats: requirement for inhibition of both cyclooxygenase 1 and 2. Gastroenterology 119:706–714.

Wallace, J.L., Muscara, M.N., de Nucci, G. et al. 2004. Gastric tolerability and prolonged prostaglandin inhibition in the brain with a nitric oxide-releasing flurbiprofen derivative, NCX-2216 [3-[4-(2-fluoro-alpha-methyl-[1,1′-biphenyl]-4-acetyloxy)-3-methoxyphenyl]-2-propenoic acid 4-nitrooxy butyl ester]. J Pharmacol Exp Therap 309:626–633.

Warner, T.D., Giuliano, F., Vojnovic, I. et al. 1999. Nonsteroid drug selectivities for cyclooxygenase-1 rather than cyclooxygenase-2 are associated with human gastrointestinal toxicity: a full in vitro analysis. Proc Nat Acad Sci 96:7563–7568.

Warner, T.D. and Mitchell, J.A. 2003. Nonsteroidal anti-inflammatory drugs inhibiting prostanoid efflux: As easy as ABC? Proc Nat Acad Sci 100:9108–9110.

———. 2004. Cyclooxygenases: new forms, new inhibitors, and lessons from the clinic. The FASEB J 18:790–804.

Waskewich, C., Blumenthal, R.D. Li, H. et al. 2002. Celecoxib exhibits the greatest potency amongst cyclooxygenase (COX) inhibitors for growth inhibition of COX-2-negative hematopoietic and epithelial cell lines. Cancer Res 62:2029–2033.

Watson, A.D.J., Wilson, J.T., Turner, D.M. et al. 1980. Phenylbutazone-induced blood dyscrasias suspected in three dogs. Vet Rec 107:239–241.

Weissmann, G. 1991. The actions of NSAIDs. Hosp Pract 15:60–76.

Welsh, E.M. and Nolan, A.M. 1994. Repeated intradermal injection of low dose carrageenan induces tachyphylaxis to evoked hyperalgesia. Pain 59:415–421.

Welsh, E.M., Nolan, A.M. and Reid, J. 1997. Beneficial effects of administering carprofen before surgery in dogs. Vet Rec 14:251–253.

Welsh, J.C.M., Lees, P., Stodulski, G. et al. 1992. Influence of feeding schedule on the absorption of orally administered flunixin in the horse. Equine Vet J Suppl 11:62–65.

Wick, M., Hurteau, G., Dessey, C. et al. 2002. Peroxisome proliferator-activated receptor-γ is a target of nonsteroidal anti-inflammatory drugs mediating cyclooxygenase-independent inhibition of lung cancer cell growth. Mol Pharmacol 62:1207–1214.

Wilgus, T.A., Vodovotz, Y., Vittadini, E. et al. 2003. Reduction of scar formation in full-thickness wounds with topical celecoxib treatment. Wound Repair Regen 11:25–34.

Wilson, J.E., Chandrasekharan, N.V., Westover, K.D., et al. 2004. Determination of expression of cyclooxygease-1 and -2 isozymes in canine tissues and their differential sensitivity to nonsteroidal anti-inflammatory drugs. Am J Vet Res 65:810–818.

Wolfsberger, B., Hoelzl, C., Walter, I. et al. 2006. In vitro effects of meloxicam with or without doxorubicin on canine osteosarcoma cells. J Vet Pharmacol Therap 29:15–23.

Xie, W.L. Chipman, J.G., Robertson, D.L. et al. 1991. Expression of a mitogen-responsive gene encoding prostaglandin synthase is regulated by mRNA splicing. Proc Nat Acad Sci 88:2692–2696.

Yaksh, T.L., Dirig, D.M., Conway, C.M. et al. 2001. The acute antihyperalgesic action of nonsteroidal, anti-inflammatory drugs and release of spinal prostaglandin E_2 is mediated by the inhibition of constitutive spinal cyclooxygenase-2 (COX-2) but not COX-1. J Neurosci 21:5847–5853.

Zhang, X., Schwarz, E.M., Young, D.A. et al. 2002. Cyclooxygenase-2 regulates mesenchymal cell differentiation into the osteoblast lineage and is critically involved in bone repair. J Clin Invest 109:1405–1415.

Ziv, G. and Longo, F. 1991. Comparative clinical efficacy of ketoprofen and flunixin in the treatment of induced E coli endotoxin mastitis in lactating dairy cows. In Mammites des Vaches Laitières, Société Française de Buiatrie, Paris, France, pp. 207–208.

CHAPTER

20

ANTICONVULSANT DRUGS

Mark G. Papich

INTRODUCTION

Treatment of seizure disorders first requires that an accurate diagnosis is made and underlying problems ruled out, such as metabolic disorders, neoplasia, congenital disorders, and intoxication. If a diagnosis of idiopathic epilepsy is made, treatment is usually initiated with one of the maintenance anticonvulsants described in this chapter. Occasionally, animals are presented to veterinary hospitals with continuous seizures—status epilepticus. These animals require prompt treatment with one of the rapidly acting anticonvulsants.

The methods used to classify and diagnosis seizure disorders will not be discussed in this chapter. One should rely on a reputable internal medicine textbook, review paper (Olby 2006), or reference that specifically addresses seizure disorders in animals (Podell 2004).

Anticonvulsant drugs act to limit either the initialization or spread of the seizure focus in the central nervous system. These drugs act to suppress nerve conduction, stabilize neurons, or enhance and potentiate the action of the inhibitory neurotransmitter gamma-aminobutyric acid (GABA). For a few drugs, the exact mechanism of action is unknown. Some drugs, such as the barbiturates, are used for other indications as well. Some barbiturates are better at providing an anticonvulsant effect, and others are better at producing anesthesia. An anticonvulsant is distinguished from an anesthetic by an action that suppresses seizure activity, without producing unconsciousness. Table 20.1 lists anticonvulsant drugs used in veterinary medicine.

The application of pharmacokinetic principles to treatment of epilepsy in animals has been a major contribution to veterinary neurology. Therefore, the focus of many research publications has been on the pharmacokinetics of the anticonvulsant medications. The pharmacokinetics of several anticonvulsants in dogs, with comparison to humans, was reported by Frey and Löscher (1985), and other relevant papers will be discussed in this chapter among individual drugs. In the paper by Frey and Löscher (1985), they reported significant differences for some drugs, with generally much more rapid clearance in dogs than humans. Protein binding was generally similar for drugs in dogs and people, with the exception of valproate and phenytoin.

PHENOBARBITAL

Phenobarbital is the most widely used anticonvulsant drug in small animals. Although it is classified as a barbiturate and shares properties with barbiturates discussed in Chapter 11, phenobarbital is unique in its ability to produce an anticonvulsant effect at doses below those that produce anesthesia.

MECHANISM OF ACTION. Phenobarbital increases the seizure threshold and decreases the electrical activity of the seizure focus by potentiating the action of the neurotransmitter gamma-aminobutyric acid (GABA). Potentiating GABA increases chloride conductance in neurons, stabilizes electrical activity, and raises the potential necessary for depolarization. Barbiturates also decrease the influx of calcium into nerve cells and thereby decrease release of neurotransmitters. This property may be more important at high phenobarbital levels than at the concentrations that produce an anticonvulsant effect.

PHARMACOKINETICS. The pharmacokinetics of phenobarbital have been studied in a variety of animals (Frey and Löscher 1985). Protein binding in serum is 24–30% in sheep, 34–52% in goats, 31% in horses, 19–28% in rabbits, 10–25% in pigs, and 4–23% in cows (Bailey 1998). This compares with a value of 30–38% in humans.

TABLE 20.1 Anticonvulsants used in veterinary medicine

Barbiturates	Succinimides	Oxazoldinediones	Others
Phenobarbital	Ethosuximide	Trimethadione	Valproate
Mephobarbital		Paramethadione	Carbamazepine
Primidone	*Benzodiazepines*		Potassium Bromide
	Diazepam	*Dicarbamates*	Lamotrigine
Hydantoins	Clonazepam	Felbamate	Gabapentin
Phenytoin	Oxazepam	Meprobamate	Lorazepam

Phenobarbital is well absorbed with systemic availability that is almost complete in monogastric animals (Pedersoli et al. 1987). The volume of distribution is large and is similar to total body water at 600 to 700 ml/kg. The high lipophilicity produces penetration across lipid membranes, including the blood-brain barrier (BBB) of the central nervous system (CNS). Phenobarbital clearance is low in dogs (0.09–0.1 ml/kg/min) (Pedersoli et al. 1987), but it is highly metabolized and relies on hepatic cytochrome P450 enzymes for biotransformation. In people the half-life is in the range of 70–100 hours. In dogs the range has been from 37 to 75 hours (average 53 h) (Ravis et al. 1984), 89 ± 20 hours (Ravis et al. 1989), and 92.6 (±24) hours (Pedersoli et al. 1987). In a study that examined variations during the dosing interval in epileptics, the range in half-life among dogs was 20 to 140 hours, with a mean of 65 hours, (Levitski and Trepanier 2000). As demonstrated from these studies, the half-lives can vary considerably among animals, which may explain a range of plasma concentrations despite similar doses among dogs and which supports individualized dosing based on therapeutic drug monitoring (discussed below and in Chapter 51). Changes in half-life and clearance that occur during multiple dosing is caused by autoinduction of hepatic metabolism (Ravis et al. 1989), and may also be influenced by diet (Maguire et al. 2000). With multiple-dosing, the half-life decreased from 89 hours (±19.6) on day 1 to 47 hours (±11) at day 90. Clearance almost doubled during that time (Ravis et al. 1989).

In cats the half-life ranges from 35–56 hours, (average 43 hr); and 59–76 hours, depending on the study (Cochrane et al. 1990). In horses the half-life is approximately 18–19 hours, but one study showed a half-life of 24 hours after a single dose, but 11.2 hours after multiple doses (Knox et al. 1992; Duran et al. 1987; Ravis et al. 1987). In foals the mean half-life was 13 hours (Spehar et al. 1984). These values for horses indicate a more rapid clearance in horses than in other species.

DRUG INTERACTIONS. Phenobarbital is a well-known inducer of microsomal cytochrome P450 (CYP450) enzymes (microsomal enzymes) that metabolize drugs (Hojo et al. 2002). Increased levels of CYP450 enzymes have been documented and are found in the endoplasmic reticulum of hepatocytes. Induction of microsomal enzymes may cause enhanced biotransformation of other drugs, which can diminish the pharmacologic effect for a drug that is administered concurrently (e.g., digoxin, corticosteroids, phenylbutazone, some anesthetics, and antipyrine). Enzyme induction will also increase phenobarbital's own metabolism. In one study (Maguire et al. 2000), the half-life at the beginning of the study was 47–49 hours in dogs. But, after chronic treatment for 2 months, the phenobarbital $T^1/_2$ decreased to 24–33 hours.

Other drugs that are microsomal enzyme inhibitors (CYP450 inhibitors) may inhibit the metabolism of phenobarbital and cause toxicity if the two drugs are administered concurrently. Chloramphenicol and ketoconazole are examples of CYP450 enzyme inhibitors.

SIDE EFFECTS, ADVERSE EFFECTS, AND TOLERANCE. Side effects that one may expect include sedation, polyphagia, polyuria/polydipsia (PU/PD), and mild behavior changes. These may subside somewhat after the first few weeks of treatment because both pharmacokinetic and pharmacodynamic tolerance develops with chronic therapy. Pharmacokinetic tolerance is caused by enhanced metabolism owing to induction of the hepatic enzymes (i.e., phenobarbital increases its own metabolism) with chronic dosing. Pharmacodynamic tolerance is determined by the sensitivity of receptors.

Liver. Elevated hepatic enzymes have been observed after chronic therapy in healthy animals (alanine aminotransferase—ALT, alkaline phosphatase—ALP) without an association with hepatic injury (Aitken et al. 2003; Gieger et al. 2000; Müller et al. 2000; Chauvet et al. 1995). The highest elevations occur with serum ALP. Elevations in hepatic enzymes that are not associated with liver pathology are reported to be caused by induction of the enzymes by the drug and are expected to return to normal 3–5 weeks after discontinuation of the drug (Gieger et al. 2000). In one study of 95 epileptic dogs controlled with phenobarbital, the increases in liver enzymes were related to the phenobarbital plasma concentration (Aitken et al. 2003). Dogs with the highest levels of phenobarbital also had the highest ALT increases.

Hepatotoxicosis also is possible from phenobarbital. It has been described as both an intrinsic and idiosyncratic hepatic injury. In clinical reports, most affected dogs had high serum phenobarbital concentrations (>40 μg/ml) (Dayrell-Hart et al. 1991). Animals with phenobarbital-induced hepatotoxicosis had bilirubin increases that are disproportionately elevated in comparison to the ALP. There also may be elevations in bile acids or other signs of hepatic disease. Liver lesions include chronic fibrosis with nodular regeneration, biliary hyperplasia, necrosis, and cirrhosis (March et al. 2004). Animals receiving high doses of phenobarbital to control seizures should be examined periodically because they may be at a higher risk of developing liver disease.

Hepatocutaneous Disease. As a consequence of phenobarbital-induced liver disease, the skin also may be affected. This has been described as *superficial necrolytic dermatitis,* more commonly known as *hepatocutaneous syndrome.* The hepatocutaneous syndrome has been associated with phenobarbital administration in some dogs (March et al. 2004). Prolonged phenobarbital exposure and high plasma drug levels may contribute to this disease in dogs.

Blood Disorders. Anemia, thrombocytopenia, and neutropenia have been described as a result of phenobarbital administration (Jacobs et al. 1998). It is rare, and probably idosyncratic, but should be considered in a patient that shows signs of a blood disorder in association with phenobarbital treatment.

Effect on Hormones. Phenobarbital administration may alter thyroid hormone levels (Gieger et al. 2000; Kantrowitz et al. 1999). After multiple doses, it may decrease thyroxine (T-4) and free T-4 in dogs, but not T-3 (Kantrowitz et al. 1999). In one study, T-3 was increased slightly (Müller et al. 2000). Thyroid stimulating hormone (TSH) has been mildly elevated in some studies, but not others (Müller et al. 2000; Gieger et al. 2000). Thyroid hormones and TSH return to normal within 4 weeks after discontinuing phenobarbital treatment. The mechanism for the effect on thyroid hormone is probably via an increase in T-4 metabolism induced by phenobarbital (Kantrowitz et al. 1999; Gieger et al. 2000).

Corticosteroid Metabolism. In experimental animals and humans phenobarbital accelerates steroid metabolism. This may decrease the therapeutic effects of corticosteroid administration. However, there is no evidence that phenobarbital treatment induces adrenal disease in dogs.

The effect of phenobarbital administration to dogs on adrenal cortex diagnostic tests has been examined (Dyer et al. 1994; Chauvet et al. 1995). Phenobarbital administration to dogs did not affect response to exogenous ACTH or the levels of endogenous ACTH.

CLINICAL USE. Phenobarbital is considered the first drug of choice for long-term treatment of seizure disorders in dogs and cats. Its efficacy has been estimated to be approximately 60% to 90%. It also has been used to treat some behavior disorders in dogs and cats. Daily dosages of 4 to 16 mg/kg/day have been used, but dogs are usually started on 2.5–3 mg/kg q12h and adjusted up to 6–8 mg/kg q12h, gradually—if necessary. Even though the half-life is long in dogs, most animals are initially treated with phenobarbital on an every-12-hour schedule to decrease side effects and ensure minimal peak-trough fluctuations. In some patients, however, once-a-day dosing may be effective.

The typical starting dose for cats is 1.5 to 2.5 mg/kg q12h, PO (Quesnel et al. 1997; Platt 2001). In some cats, doses are increased to 2 to 4 mg/kg, q12h, PO. A common dose in cats is 7.5 mg per cat, q12h (1/2 of a 15 mg tablet), and the dose may be adjusted by 7.5 mg increments.

In horses, the initial doses are 11 mg/kg q24h. When chronic therapy has been needed the dose may be increased to 25 mg/kg every 24 hr.

CLINICAL MONITORING. To adjust dose, monitor compliance, and assess toxicity, it is the usual practice to monitor plasma or serum phenobarbital concentrations regularly during therapy. (Therapeutic drug monitoring is discussed in more detail in Chapter 51.) Assays are available at most diagnostic laboratories. This can be done initially after the first 2 weeks of starting treatment and then every 6–12 months, or as needed to assess treatment. The recommended plasma/serum therapeutic concentration for dogs is 15–40 μg/ml (65–180 mmol/l). Some textbooks list this range as 20–45 μg/ml and 15–45 μg/ml. If dogs are also receiving bromide (bromide therapy discussed below), phenobarbital concentrations in the range of 10 to 36 μg/ml have been reported as therapeutic (Trepanier et al. 1998). For cats, the plasma concentrations can be variable, but the optimum range has been cited as 23–30 μg/ml (Quesnel, et al. 1997). In the cited study by Quesnel et al. (1997), cats were more unstable than dogs, possibly because of more serious CNS disease and required more frequent monitoring.

Because phenobarbital has such a long half-life, fluctuations between plasma peaks and troughs are minimized when it is administered on an every-12-hour schedule. Therefore, the timing of sample makes no difference when a sample is collected during a 12-hour schedule for the assessment of plasma phenobarbital concentrations (Levitski and Trepanier 2000).

PRIMIDONE

Primidone (Mylepsin, Mysoline) is a barbiturate derivative metabolized to phenobarbital and phenylethylmalonamide (PEMA). Primidone and its two major metabolites have anticonvulsant activity, but, at least 85% of the pharmacologic activity is derived from phenobarbital.

PHARMACOKINETICS. In addition to the differences in potency, PEMA and primidone do not persist in the plasma for as long as phenobarbital, which raises questions regarding the activity of PEMA and primidone throughout a long dosing interval (Frey et al. 1979). When primidone was administered to dogs, the half-life (mean value) of PEMA was 7.1 hours, the half-life of primidone was 1.85 hours, and the half-life of phenobarbital, was 41 hours (Yeary 1980). After multiple dosing in this study, the primidone concentrations decreased, probably caused by accelerated metabolism.

CLINICAL EFFICACY. Although seizures can be controlled with primidone in dogs (Schwartz-Porsche et al. 1982), primidone has little advantage over phenobarbital in dogs. Control of seizures in dogs is correlated with the plasma concentrations of phenobarbital, rather than primidone (Cunningham et al. 1983). In a comparison between primidone and phenobarbital in epileptic dogs (Schwartz-Porsche et al. 1982), there was no significant difference between phenobarbital and primidone with respect to seizure control, and primidone appeared more likely to induce liver injury than phenobarbital. The authors concluded that phenobarbital, rather than primidone, should be the drug of first choice for treatment of canine epilepsy.

However, there may be rare cases that respond to primidone when phenobarbital alone has not been effective (1 out of 15 according to Farnbach 1984). Primidone is more expensive than phenobarbital, but it is not classified as a controlled drug in the U.S.; therefore it does not require the same degree of record keeping.

ADVERSE EFFECTS. Most adverse effects and side effects are the same as those listed for phenobarbital; however, primidone administration may be associated with a higher incidence of hepatotoxicity. Hepatic necrosis, fibrosis, and cirrhosis have been associated with chronic use of primidone (Bunch 1989). Intrahepatic cholestasis has occurred in dogs in which primidone was combined with phenytoin.

Manufacturers do not recommend its use in cats; in fact it is stated on the package insert that its use should be cautioned in cats. However, studies in cats have demonstrated that primidone is probably safe.

CLINICAL USE. Initial dosages in dogs are 3–5 mg/kg q 8–12 hours, but have been increased up to 12 mg/kg q8h. If one is converting a patient from primidone to phenobarbital or vice versa, the conversion is the following: 65 mg phenobarbital = 250 mg primidone.

THERAPEUTIC MONITORING. Because the clinical effects are associated with the concentrations of the metabolite, phenobarbital, and these levels can be monitored in patients. Measurements of PEMA or primidone are not available in most laboratories. (See Chapter 51 for more details on therapeutic drug monitoring.)

PHENYTOIN

Phenytoin (Dilantin, formerly diphenylhydantoin) is one of the most commonly prescribed anticonvulsants in human medicine. In veterinary medicine, its use is rare because of pharmacokinetic differences and susceptibility to adverse effects. It is *not* a recommended anticonvulsant for dogs or cats. It is used occasionally in horses for muscle disorders or as an antiarrhythmic agent.

MECHANISM OF ACTION. Phenytoin stabilizes neuronal membranes and limits the spread of neuronal or seizure activity from the focus. It blocks inward movement of Na^+, and stabilizes excitable tissue (this drug is also used as a Class I antiarrhythmic agent, see Chapter 23). Phenytoin also decreases Ca^{++} inward flow during depolarization, thus, inhibiting Ca^{++}-dependent release of neurotransmitters (presynaptic).

PHARMACOKINETICS. There are important interspecies differences among animals and between animals and humans that cause difficulty in maintaining effective concentrations. Phenytoin is eliminated much more rapidly in dogs than in people (Frey and Löscher 1985). Because of its rapid elimination, phenytoin is not recommended as an anticonvulsant in small animals. In cats, the elimination is very slow, and toxicity has been a concern. In horses the pharmacokinetics have been described (Soma et al. 2001), but are highly variable among horses. The half-life was approximately 12–13 hours, depending on the route of administration, but the oral absorption ranged from 14–85% among horses.

CLINICAL USE. Phenytoin is available in 25 mg/ml oral suspension; 30 and 100 mg capsules (sodium salt); and 50 mg/ml injection (sodium salt). For dogs, these formulation sizes result in an impractical dose (several capsules per day) for a large-size dog. Nevertheless, a dose recommended for dogs is 20–35 mg/kg q8h and the antiarrhythmic dose is 30 mg/kg q8h PO or 10 mg/kg IV over 5 minutes. It should not be used in cats.

Horses. Phenytoin has been used in horses for tying-up syndrome. This is a use primarily employed on the racetrack in athletic horses. The use is not related to the anticonvulsant property. In horses, at high doses recumbency and excitement have been observed. Sedation in horses may be an initial sign of high plasma phenytoin concentrations. Pharmacokinetic studies have shown that phenytoin pharmacokinetics are highly variable in horses, particularly the extent of absorption (Soma et al. 2001). Because of this variability it is difficult to maintain consistent plasma concentrations. Monitoring plasma concentrations may be necessary to adjust the dose to maintain an optimum level and prevent adverse effects. Suggested doses for horses are to administer an initial bolus of 20 mg/kg q12h PO, for 4 doses, followed by 10–15 mg/kg q12h PO. A single IV dose in horses of 7.5–8.8 mg/kg can be used, followed by oral maintenance doses.

THERAPEUTIC MONITORING. Therapeutic drug monitoring can be performed; however, therapeutic concentrations have not been established for dogs and cats. Effective plasma concentrations listed for people are between 5 and 20 μg/ml. In the absence of other data, an average peak concentration of 15 μg/ml has been used as a target for animals. In horses, effective plasma concentrations are 5–20 μg/ml (average 8.8 μg/ml ± 2 μg/ml) (Soma et al. 2001). Therapy should be aimed at producing concentrations above 5 μg/ml in horses, or a peak concentration of 15 μg/ml.

VALPROIC ACID (VALPROATE)

Valproic acid (Depakene®) has been used in dogs primarily when they are refractory to other medications. The use has declined after other drugs became available (see gabapentin and levetiracetam, below), but it has been used in some dogs successfully. The mechanism of action is unknown. It may interfere with GABA metabolism.

PHARMACOKINETICS. Absorption from oral valproate is high in dogs, with values for the immediate release tablets of 100% (Bialer et al. 1984) and sustained release preparations of approximately 80%. The half-life in dogs is 1.0 to 2.8 hours (15–20 hrs in people), or approximately 1.4 hrs in another study in dogs (Bialer et al. 1984). This short half-life severely limits its therapeutic effectiveness unless frequent dosing schedules are used or sustained-release products are employed. But, some evidence suggests that the anticonvulsant effects of valproate persist long after the drug is eliminated from the plasma.

CLINICAL USE. According to some studies in dogs (Bialer et al. 1984; Bialer 1992), the sustained-release tablets provide a more sustained plasma concentration than the plain tablets. However, half-life and extent of absorption may be different between valproate pharmacokinetics in dogs and humans; therefore, the human extended-release dosage forms may be applied to dogs, but should be administered more frequently than in humans (Bialer 1992; Bialer et al. 1986).

Divalproex sodium is composed of equal parts of valproic acid and valproate. It is pharmacologically equivalent to valproic acid and is available in delayed-release tablets of 125 and 500 mg (Depakote®, Epival®).

Although valproate is not commonly used, some neurologists have reported it to be "reasonably effective" and well tolerated. Combining this drug with another anticonvulsant such as phenobarbital may increase its efficacy. Dosages that have been used in dogs range from 75–200 mg/kg q8h when used alone, or 30–40 mg/kg/day with phenobarbital (phenobarbital dose is usually decreased). Drug assays exist for therapeutic monitoring, but this is not commonly performed for animals. The therapeutic concentrations are reported to be 350–830 μmol/ml (50–120 μg/ml), but the true "therapeutic range" for valproate in animals is not known.

DIAZEPAM

Diazepam belongs to the class of benzodiazepines. Diazepam (Valium) is an important drug for treating acute seizures and status epilepticus, but is not practical for long-term therapy. Diazepam, like other benzodiazepines, was discussed in Chapters 11, 13, and 21.

MECHANISM OF ACTION. The mechanism of action as an anticonvulsant is similar to phenobarbital, in that it hyperpolarizes neurons and suppresses neuronal activity. Benzodiazepines accomplish this action by binding to a specific GABA-binding site. It may modify the GABA-binding sites and increase the action of GABA on nerve cells.

PHARMACOKINETICS. In people the half-life is 43 hours (mean) but may range from 24–48 hours, and as high as 60 hours. It has a low hepatic extraction rate compared to dogs. In dogs, the half-life is much shorter (Frey and Löscher 1985), with a high hepatic extraction rate, which makes this drug unsuitable for most dogs for chronic anticonvulsant therapy. The half-life from IV administration has been reported to be as rapid as 15 minutes and as long as 3.2 hours, depending on the study (Papich and Alcorn 1995). Diazepam is rapidly converted to two metabolites. It is first demethylated to N-desmethyldiazepam (also called nordiazepam), then to oxazepam. The metabolites are eliminated more slowly than diazepam and have equal to one-third the potency of diazepam, depending on the study used to determine potency. The half-life of the desmethyldiazepam metabolite is 2.2 to 3.6 hours. and of oxazepam is 3.83 to 5.7 hours. In cats, the half-life of diazepam is reported to be 5.5 hours, with the half-life of the metabolite 21 hours. Diazepam is highly lipophilic, more so than other drugs in this class. Its high lipophilicity produces high concentrations in the CNS rapidly after IV injection.

CLINICAL USE. Diazepam is usually the first drug of choice for treating status epilepticus because it is distributed rapidly to the CNS after IV administration. But, it is unsuitable for chronic treatment in dogs because frequent administration is required. There are also other disadvantages: tolerance develops with repeated administration, animals may develop dependence, and there is abuse potential (by animal owners). In cats it has a longer half-life than dogs and has been used as a drug to control seizures, treat behavioral problems, and stimulate appetite. In cats, dosages of 0.25 to 0.5 mg/kg q8h, PO are used. This dose may be increased to 1–2 mg/kg, q8h for seizure control. Adverse hepatic effects (discussed below) have caused a decline in the long-term administration to cats.

ADVERSE REACTIONS AND TOLERANCE. Some neurologists have observed that patients may become refractory to chronic treatment (tachyphylaxis) because there may be a feedback decrease in benzodiazepine receptor synthesis or a decreased synthesis of GABA. Tolerance in dogs may be seen after 1 week of dosing. After long-term administration, withdrawal should be done gradually and carefully because some dependence occurs. Signs of withdrawal may include increased anxiety and tremors.

Hepatic Toxicosis in Cats. Hepatic necrosis in cats has been reported from oral administration of diazepam (Center et al. 1996). This reaction appears to be idiosyncratic (that is, unpredictable) and reactions can be severe and fatal. The liver injury usually appears after the initial 5 days of treatment. Because of this reaction, diazepam therapy in cats should be monitored closely.

OTHER USES

Skeletal Muscle Relaxant. Benzodiazepines may act as muscle relaxants by inhibiting certain spinal pathways, or by directly depressing motor nerve and muscle function. Examples of their use have been relaxation of urethral skeletal muscle in cats following obstruction and relaxation of skeletal muscle associated with spinal disk disease. Their clinical efficacy as muscle relaxants has been questioned.

Treatment of Anxiety, Aggression, and Behavioral Disorders in Small Animals. Because benzodiazepines are common drugs in human medicine for emotional disorders—anxiety, stress, phobias, aggression, insomnia, etc.—they have also been administered to dogs and cats for a large variety of disorders with varied success. (See Chapter 21 for more detailed description of these uses.) Other benzodiazepines also are used for treatment of anxiety disorders in animals, such as alprazolam. A discussion of the use of alprazolam and other benzodiazepines for behavior problems can be found in a review paper (Simpson and Papich 2003) and in Chapter 21.

Diazepam-Induced Eating in Anorexic Cats. Benzodiazepines stimulate the appetite in anorexic cats (less effective in dogs). Diazepam has been administered for this purpose at dosages of 0.04–0.05 mg/kg, IV. Oral oxazepam also has been used for this indication.

CLONAZEPAM

Clonazepam (Klonopin) is another benzodiazepine with a mechanism of action similar to diazepam, but it is more potent. There is anecdotal evidence that it is a good anticonvulsant in dogs that are refractory to phenobarbital therapy, but this should be considered only as a last resort. Clonazepam undergoes saturable (zero order) elimination. As the dose is increased, or if animals are dosed for longer than 1 week, the half-life increases (e.g., from 1.5 hours to 3 hr). As for other antiepileptic drugs, the half-life is much longer in humans compared to dogs. The starting dose recommended for dogs is 0.5 mg/kg, 2–3 times a day (Frey and Löscher 1985). In cats, clonazepam has been used as an alternative to diazepam to avoid the risk of hepatotoxicity. Because of a difference in metabolism, there have been no cases of hepatotoxicity reported from use of clonazepam in cats. The starting dose is 0.5 mg/kg once or twice daily in cats.

Withdrawal syndrome is possible from chronic therapy with clonazepam. If dogs are receiving clonazepam and there is abrupt cessation of therapy, signs of acute withdrawal can be seen, which include listlessness, weight loss, pyrexia, and recumbency. Cessation of this drug should be tapered over a period of 1 month to minimize these effects.

CLORAZEPATE

Clorazepate (Traxene) is another benzodiazepine also used occasionally for treating seizures in animals. There is no published information regarding its efficacy in dogs, but anecdotal evidence indicates that it may be effective in some refractory cases.

Clorazepate is hydrolyzed to desmethyldiazepam (nordiazepam), an active metabolite of diazepam. The half-life of desmethyldiazepam is 3.6 to 6 hours in dogs (30 to 100 hr in man) (Frey and Löscher 1985). Dosages of 2 mg/kg every 12 hours may provide therapeutic concentrations in dogs. Therapeutic plasma concentrations of desmethyldiazepam are usually greater than 1 μg/ml.

As mentioned for clonazepam, clorazepate is also used in cats as an alternative to diazepam. There has not been much experience in cats, but doses in the range of 3.75 to 7.5 mg per cat once daily have been used.

FELBAMATE

Felbamate (Felbatol) has been used in dogs that are refractory to other anticonvulsant drugs. Since it is more expensive than older therapies, it is usually considered as a last resort. The action is not completely understood, but it is an antagonist at the N-methyl-D-aspartate (NMDA) receptor-ionophore complex. Antagonism of NMDA may block effects of excitatory amino acids and suppress seizure activity (increase seizure threshold and decrease seizure spread). It addition there may be some neuroprotective effects from antagonizing excitatory amino acids. Because this mechanism is unique, this drug may be considered in patients refractory to other anticonvulsant drugs.

PHARMACOKINETICS. In dogs the half-life has been reported to be approximately 5–6 hours (Adusumalli et al. 1992). The pharmacokinetics have not been examined in other animals.

CLINICAL USE. The initial dose in dogs is approximately 15–20 mg/kg q8h, orally. In practice, the starting dose is 200 mg/dog orally q8h (small dogs) and increases by 200 mg per week until seizures are controlled to a maximum of 600 mg/dog q8h. For large dogs, start with

400 mg/dog q8h and increase gradually to a maximum of 1,200 mg/dog q8h. (This dose range is approximately 15–65 mg/kg q8h.) Felbamate has induced its own metabolism in dogs; therefore, there may be a need to increase doses as therapy progresses. Felbamate is registered for people as Felbatol® in 120/ml oral liquid and 400 and 600 mg tablets.

ADVERSE EFFECTS. Adverse reactions have not yet been documented with clinical use in dogs, but it has not been used frequently. It does not seem to produce the sedation and behavior changes that other drugs have been known to cause. Toxic signs have not been seen in dogs unless the dose exceeded 300 mg/kg/day. In people the most severe reactions have been aplastic anemia, and severe hepatic toxicity. In people it has been shown to increase phenobarbital concentrations by 20–30% so careful monitoring of phenobarbital concentrations is suggested.

GABAPENTIN

Gabapentin (Neurontin, and generic brands) has been used successfully in dogs and cats to control seizures when other anticonvulsant drugs have not been effective, or when others have been too toxic. It is not used as commonly as the others because of its high cost of therapy compared to bromide or phenobarbital. However, the availability of a generic brand has decreased the cost of therapy to animals.

Gabapentin is a structural analog of gamma-aminobutyric acid (GABA). The mechanism of action as an anticonvulsant is not entirely known. However, it does not interact with GABA receptors and is not a GABA agonist, and does not affect GABA uptake or degradation. It also does not interfere with sodium-dependent channels or exhibit affinity for other neurotransmitter receptors such as those affected by benzodiazepines, glutamate, dopamine, or N-methyl-D-aspartate (NMDA).

The same action that is responsible for its use for treating neuropathic pain may also explain the anticonvulsant activity. The mechanism of action appears to be via blocking calcium-dependent channels. Gabapentin inhibits the alpha-2-delta ($\alpha_2\ \delta$) subunit of the N-type voltage-dependent calcium channel on neurons. After binding to the $\alpha_2\ \delta$ subunit it reduces calcium influx that is needed for release of neurotransmitters—specifically excitatory amino acids—from presynaptic neurons. This channel becomes up-regulated when nerves are stimulated, such as in epileptic conditions or associated with neuropathology. Blocking the channels has little effect on normal neurons, but appears to suppress stimulated neurons. Therefore, there are few adverse effects associated with use of gabapentin.

PHARMACOKINETICS. Gabapentin is absorbed in dogs with systemic oral availability that is practically complete (80% or greater) and is not affected by food. Compared to the elimination in people, gabapentin has a short half-life of 2–4 hours (Radulovic et al. 1995). The systemic clearance resembles renal clearance values in dogs of 2–3 ml/kg/min (Radulovic et al. 1995), which has led to the conclusion that gabapentin is excreted by renal mechanisms and does not rely on hepatic biotransformation, except for small biotransformation in dogs to N-methyl-gabapentin. Therefore, it has been used in animals when hepatic disease or impaired metabolism is a concern. Protein binding in dogs is negligible (Radulovic et al. 1995).

Lipophilicity and Penetration. The volume of distribution is small for an anticonvulsant (0.158 l/kg) (Radulovic et al. 1995), an octanol/water partition coefficient (Log P) of only −1.10 and a partition coefficient at pH 6–8.5 (Log D) of only −1.44. These values indicate that lipophilicity is lower than what is needed to penetrate the blood-brain barrier. Therefore, gabapentin must rely on a carrier for penetration to the CNS. Gabapentin mimics an alpha-amino acid and utilizes the large amino acid transporter (LAT) to penetrate the brain (Jolliet-Riant and Tillement 1999).

CLINICAL USE. Gabapentin is available in 100, 300, and 400 mg capsules; 100, 300, 400, 600, and 800 mg scored tablets; and 50 mg/ml oral solution. The oral solutions contains xylitol, which is known to be toxic to dogs. The dose of oral solution administered to dogs must consider the amount of xylitol delivered.

Anticonvulsant Use. Gabapentin is used primarily for refractory seizures that have not responded to other drugs. It is rarely used alone as an anticonvulsant in animals. In people the dose varies from 900 to 1,800 mg per person per day, and up to 3,600 mg per day. In dogs it has been

TABLE 20.2 Drugs for treatment of neuropathic pain*

Drug	Action	Discussed In
Gabapentin and Pregabalin	Blocks alpha-2-delta calcium channels	Chapter 20
Amantadine	NMDA receptor antagonist	Chapter 39
Tricyclic antidepressants (Clomipramine, Amitryptyline)	Serotonin reuptake inhibitor	Chapter 21
Local Anesthetics	Blocks sodium channels	Chapter 14
Opioids	Blocks opiate receptors (mu- and kappa-)	Chapter 12
Tramadol	Multiple effects (opiate receptor blocker, serotonin reuptake inhibitor, and norepinephrine reuptake inhibitor)	Chapter 12

**Neuropathic pain* is defined as dysfunction of peripheral or central nerves. It is caused by nerve injury characterized by an exaggerated response to painful stimuli (hyperalgesia) and pain response to normally innocuous stimuli (allodynia). The syndrome can also include central sensitization changes in expression and changes in ion channel expression.

administered at an initial dose of 2–10 mg/kg and as high as 30–60 mg/kg q8–12h, PO (start low and titrate up). In cats, it has been administered at a dose of 5–10 mg/kg per day orally, increasing the frequency to twice daily. Sedation can be an adverse effect in cats.

Use for Treatment of Pain. Another use of gabapentin in animals is for treatment of pain syndromes—particulary those identified with neuropathic pain (Table 20.2). The mechanism responsible for this effect is via blockade of the calcium channels that may be up-regulated in painful neuropathic conditions, as discussed previously. Neuropathic pain is difficult to diagnose in animals, but may result from nerve pathology linked to another underlying disease. In people, gabapentin (Neurontin) is one of the few drugs registered for use in treating neuropathic pain. Another related drug is pregabalin (Lyrica), used in people for neuropathic pain. However, there is no information on pregabalin for treatment in animals. For neuropathic pain the dose used is 10–15 mg/kg q8h PO, and increase as necessary to levels similar to the anticonvulsant dose.

Gabapentin also was used to treat neuropathic pain in horses. After a dose of 2.5 mg/kg orally every 12 hours gabapentin appeared subjectively to relieve pain in a horse that was secondary to surgery (Davis et al. 2007).

ADVERSE EFFECTS. There have been no reported serious safety problems with gabapentin in animals during routine use. Sedation and ataxia are reported as the only significant adverse effects. In people a withdrawal syndrome from abrupt discontinuation has been described, but it is not reported in animals.

LEVETIRACETAM

Levetiracetam (Keppra) is a relatively new anticonvulsant that is used in people. Levetiracetam is structurally and mechanistically different from other anticonvulsant drug classes. The mechanism of action of levetiracetam is not completely understood, but it has significant anticonvulsant activity for several types of seizures. It does not appear to affect membrane channels, GABA, membrane receptor activity, or glutamate receptor neurotransmission. Levetiracetam is capable of suppressing seizure activity without affecting normal neuronal excitability. One proposed mechanism of action is via modulation of calcium-dependent neurotransmitter release from vesicles in neurons. The site of binding is exclusively in the CNS, without any known peripheral effects.

Because of favorable pharmacokinetics (Isoherranen et al. 2001; Dewey et al. 2007; Patterson et al. 2007; Moore et al. 2008) in dogs and few reported adverse effects, it has been preferred in dogs for treatment of refractory epilepsy or as an add-on to phenobarbital and bromide.

According to Isoherranen et al. (2001) levetiracetam is the ethyl analogue of piracetam, which has been used, among other things, for cognition enhancement in elderly people. Levetiracetam is a the S-isomer of a chiral drug that exists in two enantiomers. Only the S-form, levetiracetam, has anticonvulsant activity and is administered in the available formulations. It has high solubility (>1 grams/ml), and octanol/water partition coefficient (Log D at 7.4) of −0.64.

PHARMACOKINETICS. In pharmacokinetic studies performed in dogs with IV, IM, and oral doses (Isoherranen et al. 2001; Dewey et al. 2007; Patterson et al. 2007), levetiracetam had 100% absorption from both routes of administration. Protein binding of levetiracetam is small (<10%); therefore, drugs or conditions that affect plasma protein will not alter levetiracetam pharmacokinetics. The volume of distribution ranged from 0.45 to 0.89 l/kg, depending on the study. With a half-life that ranged from 3 to 4.5 hours, it can be administered three times daily and maintain plasma concentrations that are within the range cited for humans as effective (Moore et al. 2008). After multiple doses for 6 days, there was no change in pharmacokinetic parameters. In cats, the half-life was 5.3 hours in a limited study (Dewey et al. 2005).

Levetiracetam does not undergo significant hepatic metabolism, and it is mostly excreted unchanged in the urine. Therefore, the pharmacokinetics are unaffected by other drugs that may alter cytochrome P450 (CYP450) enzymes (drug-drug interactions), and liver disease is not expected to affect the pharmacokinetics. This drug has been one of the preferred drugs when it is anticipated that liver function may be altered by other drugs or diseases.

CLINICAL USE. Levetiracetam is used clinically in dogs for refractory epilepsy when other drugs have not been sufficient, often as an add-on to phenobarbital and/or bromide therapy. Levetiracetam (Keppra) is available in 250, 500, and 750 mg tablets. The usual human dose is 500 mg q12h. In dogs, the typical dose is 20 mg/kg orally, every 8 hours. With repeated doses in dogs, it was shown that this dose will maintain plasma concentrations within a range that is reported to produce anticonvulsant activity in people. At this dose it has been used successfully as an add-on drug for refractory epileptic dogs.

There has been only limited evaluation of levetiracetam in a small number of cats (Dewey et al. 2005). At 20 mg/kg q8h, orally, it was well tolerated and effective in some cats.

ADVERSE EFFECTS AND INTERACTIONS. No adverse effects have been reported in dogs at the currently recommended dosages. Intravenous levetiracetam has been administered to dogs at doses of 60 mg/kg without reported adverse effects (Dewey et al. 2007; Patterson et al. 2007). At high doses in excess of 600 mg/kg/day, nausea and vomiting in dogs has been observed, but no deaths. At this time, the clinical use is not common; therefore, adverse effects in a larger population of treated animals have not been evaluated. In people, adverse effects are uncommon and may be idiosyncratic because there has been no relationship between plasma drug concentrations and adverse events (Contin et al. 2004).

Because it does not rely on extensive hepatic metabolism by cytochrome P450 enzymes, drug interactions are expected to be uncommon. However, studies in people have shown that elderly people may have lower clearance, and some anticonvulsant drugs have induced a more rapid clearance (Hirsch et al. 2007; Contin et al. 2004; May et al. 2003). Lower clearance in the elderly was associated with decreased creatinine clearance.

ZONISAMIDE

Zonisamide (Zonebran) is a human anticonvulsant that has been used in some canine epileptics that are refractory to other drugs. Zonisamide is chemically classified as a sulfonamide, but unrelated to other anticonvulsants. It has a high pKa of 10.2, a low molecular weight of 212.23, and solubility in water that is close to 1 mg/ml. It can suppress seizures induced by a variety of stimuli. Mechanism of action is unclear. It does not affect GABA-mediated mechanisms, but may block sodium and calcium channels (T-type calcium channels). The result of these actions is to stabilize neuronal membranes and suppress neuronal hyperactivity.

PHARMACOKINETICS. There is not much known about the pharmacokinetics in animals. In people, it has low (40%) protein binding, a high volume of distribution, low clearance (0.3 ml/kg/min), and half-life of 63 hours in plasma and 105 hours in red blood cells. Levels are much higher in RBCs (eightfold 8-fold higher higher), which are sometimes used for drug assays. It is excreted primarily in urine as the parent drug or as a glucuronide metabolite. It also undergoes N-acetylation. Because these two mechanisms—N-acetylation and glucuronidation—are deficient in dogs and cats, respectively, this may contribute to important pharmacokinetic differences in dogs and cats compared to people. Dogs are known to have adverse reactions to sulfonamide antimicrobial drugs, which may be related to their deficiency in N-acetylation metabolism (discussed in more detail in Chapter 33, Sulfonamides).

The disposition of zonisamide has been studied in a limited number of dogs (Matsumoto et al. 1983). The half-life in dogs was 15 hours and the desired plasma concentration is 10–20 μg/ml.

CLINICAL USE. In dogs, a recommended dose of zonisamide is 6–10 mg/kg twice daily orally. It is available in 100 mg capsules. It has been used in a few instances for treating epilepsy in animals as an add-on to other drugs. There have been two studies of efficacy reported in animals (Dewey et al. 2004; von Klopmann et al. 2007). In the study by Dewey et al. (2004) 12 dogs with refractory epilepsy were treated with an average dose of 8.9 mg/kg every 12 hours orally. 58% of dogs responded favorably, but 5 of 12 dogs actually had an increase in seizure frequency. In the study by von Klopmann et al. (2007) dogs were administered 10 mg/kg twice daily for treatment of refractory epilepsy. Of 11 dogs, 9 were responders. In 3 of the dogs there was a decrease in response over time, which may reflect tolerance that develops with long-term treatment.

Zonisamide is typically not monitored clinically, but effective concentrations in dogs were reported to be above 12.6 μg/ml (Masuda et al. 1979). Neurotoxic effects in dogs were seen at concentrations above 96 μg/ml. In the study by Dewey et al. (2004) cited above, the effective concentrations were 10–40 μg/ml and similarly in the report by von Klopmann et al. (2007) were 15–38 μg/ml.

ADVERSE EFFECTS. The administration of zonisamide to animals has been infrequent; therefore, there is not a full appreciation for the incidence of adverse effects. In clinical studies, the adverse effects reported were sedation (transient), ataxia, and vomiting (Dewey et al. 2004). There were also some adverse effects that occurred that are similar to those caused by sulfonamides. Because of structural similarity between zonisamide and sulfonamides, this may be of concern.

In safety studies, dogs tolerated doses of 10–175 mg/kg for 52 weeks (pharmaceutical company data). At doses of 1,000 mg/kg to dogs, there was a decrease of locomotor movement, ataxia, and vomiting (pharmaceutical company data).

POTASSIUM BROMIDE

Bromide is the oldest, yet most chemically simple, of the anticonvulsants. It was used in people as early as the mid 1800s and its use was first described in dogs as early as 1907. Because it is toxic in people, it was replaced by other anticonvulsants after the introduction of phenobarbital in 1918. It is now used commonly in dogs, and sometimes in cats (Podell and Fenner 1994; Trepanier 1995).

The exact mechanism of action is unknown, but it appears to stabilize neuronal cell membranes by interfering with chloride transport across cell membranes.

PHARMACOKINETICS. The half-life in humans is 12 days. The half-life in dogs is approximately 25 days, but can be variable. Elimination rate can vary depending on the patient's diet. Because the half-life is long, chronic daily administration will be necessary for this drug to accumulate to steady-state plasma concentrations. However, during the accumulation phase (loading dose period) the half-life is shorter (15 days, March et al. 2002) which results in faster accumulation. The half-life in cats appears to be a bit less than dogs; about 14 days, and perhaps as short as 10 days (Boothe et al. 2002).

CLINICAL USE IN DOGS. Bromide has been used in combination with phenobarbital to treat refractory seizures, and also has been used as monotherapy (single drug). When bromide is administered as a single drug, bromide doses may need to be higher than compared to administering bromide with phenobarbital. When used with phenobarbital, phenobarbital doses can be decreased by as much as one-half. One study reported that, in 19% of dogs receiving phenobarbital and bromide, eventually the phenobarbital was discontinued while still maintaining seizure control (Trepanier et al. 1998).

When potassium bromide (KBr) has been used to treat canine epileptics that have not responded to phenobarbital alone, success rates have been 60% and higher. One author reported as high as 72% improvement in seizure control (Trepanier et al. 1998).

Maintenance Doses. Usually the potassium salt of bromide is used, but sodium bromide also can be substituted. Most veterinary compounding pharmacies have recipes for preparing an oral solution and it is reasonably inexpensive. Compounded forms have been tested and shown to be stable for several months. The typical dosage of potassium bromide for dogs is 30 to 40 mg/kg, orally, once per day. (This translates to 20–27 mg/kg of bromide once per day.) The lower doses are more common when used with phenobarbital, while the higher doses are given when monotherapy is used.

There is high variability among animals with respect to absorption and excretion. Therefore, it is suggested that each patient be monitored for signs of toxicity (ataxia, CNS depression), as well as plasma concentration monitoring, and the dose adjusted if necessary.

Loading Doses. Loading doses of 600 mg/kg orally over 3–4 days have been administered in patients that need therapeutic concentrations quickly in the range of 1.0 to 1.5 mg/ml. If dogs are receiving bromide alone (without phenobarbital), use a starting dose of 40–50 mg/kg/day. In one study, March and colleagues (2002) administered loading doses of 30 mg/kg twice daily for 115 days to achieve steady-state concentrations in the range of 200–300 mg/dl.

In some cases it has been necessary to administer sodium bromide IV as a loading dose. This has been accomplished by mixing sodium bromide (potassium bromide may be too toxic if given IV), in a solution to deliver an initial dose of 600–1,200 mg/kg over approximately 8 hours. If the plasma concentration is still in the low range, an additional IV loading dose can be administered.

EFFECT OF DIET. Diets high in chloride will cause bromide to be excreted more rapidly (as much as 50% decrease in half-life with high chloride diets); therefore, the diet should be kept constant throughout therapy, or monitor serum bromide concentrations each time the diet is changed. Some prescription diets have either high, or restricted chloride content and patients receiving these diets may need dose adjustments.

CLINICAL USE IN CATS. The most common dose for cats is 30 mg/kg per day. A report and accompanying review evaluated use of bromide in cats (Boothe et al. 2002). In that report, the authors identified a half-life in cats of only 11.2 days. An evaluation of the clinical use showed that there was inadequate seizure control in approximately half of the cats, despite serum concentrations that are reported to be effective in dogs. More importantly, approximately half of the cats developed adverse reactions. The most common adverse effect was coughing.

THERAPEUTIC MONITORING. Plasma concentrations can be measured at most veterinary diagnostic laboratories (see Chapter 51 for more information on Therapeutic Drug Monitoring). Ordinarily, effective concentrations are reported as between 1 and 2 mg/ml (100–200 mg/dl). If concentrations are less than 1.0 mg/ml, one should increase the dose. If bromide is used as the sole anticonvulsant (without phenobarbital) concentrations as high as 2–3 mg/ml (200–300 mg/dl) may be necessary.

SIDE EFFECTS AND ADVERSE EFFECTS. Side effects of polyphagia and behavior changes have been reported in some dogs. Bromide toxicosis (bromism) has been reported with high serum concentrations. The signs of toxicosis are largely related to CNS depression and include depression, weakness, ataxia, and decreased proprioception. A unique sign of high bromide concentrations is joint stiffness in the rear limbs. Some animals may show signs of sedation for the first 3 weeks of therapy, but develop tolerance with chronic treatment. In cats, respiratory signs resembling feline asthma (coughing) have been reported (Boothe et al. 2002). The mechanism is not known, but it is not believed to be an allergic reaction, but rather a result of airway inflammation.

DRUG INTERACTIONS. When an animal is receiving potassium bromide therapy, it may cause an falsely elevated chloride serum measurement with some assays.

TREATMENT OF STATUS EPILEPTICUS

DIAZEPAM (VALIUM). Diazepam, IV at a dose of 5–20 mg/animal (diazepam concentration is 5 mg/ml) has been the drug used most commonly in small animals. The equivalent dose is approximately 0.5 mg/kg. Diazepam is the most rapidly acting of the anticonvulsants, but it has a short duration of action. However, the metabolites (desmethyldiazepam and oxazepam) are active and have longer half-lives. Repeated doses may be administered to patients that continue to seize, but some veterinarians have utilized constant rate infusions. Infusion doses are in the range of 0.5 mg/kg per hour, IV (Bateman et al. 2000). One must be aware of the potential for diazepam to adsorb and absorb to plastic IV infusion sets when administered as an IV infusion.

Rectal Administration of Diazepam. Rectal administration is a convenient alternative to IV dosing in an animal with status epilepticus when intravenous or oral administration is not practical. Diazepam is rapidly absorbed by this route (Papich and Alcorn 1995) and has been effective in dogs for at-home treatment of cluster seizures (Podell 1995). Diazepam is readily metabolized to metabolites, which are active. The 5 mg/ml injectable solution has been instilled in the rectum with a syringe starting at a dose of 0.5–1 mg/kg, and as high as 2 mg/kg. A small plastic teat cannula attached to the end of the syringe has been used to facilitate administration. A formulation in gel has been made available for this use (Dreifuss et al. 1998), but it is more expensive.

Other Routes. Other routes have been used, such as intranasal and mucosal (gingival). However, these routes are not as convenient as rectal for emergency treatment to a patient with seizures.

BARBITURATES. Phenobarbital also has been administered to animals for the treatment of status epilepticus, IV in increments of 10–20 mg/kg, or approximately 15–200 mg/animal (to effect). Phenobarbital infusions have been given at the rate of 3–6 mg/dog per hour, IV (Bateman et al. 2000). If the patient has already been receiving maintenance doses of phenobarbital, this dose should be lower. Phenobarbital does not cross the blood-brain barrier as fast as diazepam; therefore, it may take several minutes for an anticonvulsant effect to treat status epilepticus. In severe cases pentobarbital, IV, to effect (4–20 mg/kg) has been administered. Pentobarbital is not a good anticonvulsant; its use in this instance is simply to anesthetize the patient until additional therapy can be provided.

OTHER DRUGS. Other drugs that have been used for treatment of status epilepticus include: other benzodiazepines (midazolam, lorazepam), inhalent anesthetics, and lidocaine.

REFERENCES AND ADDITIONAL READING

Abramson FP. Autoinduction of phenobarbital elimination in the dog. J Pharm Sci Sep;77(9):768–70, 1988.

Adusumalli VE, Gilchrist JR, Wichmann JK, Kucharczyk N, Sofia RD. Pharmacokinetics of felbamate in pediatric and adult beagle dogs. Epilepsia Sep–Oct;33(5):955–60, 1992.

Aitken MM, Hall E, Scott L, Davot JL, and Allen WM. Liver-related biochemical changes in the serum of dogs being treated with phenobarbitone. Vet Rec 153:13–16, 2003.

Bailey DN. Relative binding of therapeutic drugs by sera of seven mammalian species. J Anal Toxicol Nov–Dec;22(7):587–90, 1992.

Bateman SW, Parent JM. Clinical findings, treatment, and outcome of dogs with status epilepticus or cluster seizures: 156 cases (1990–1995). J Am Vet Med Assoc 215:1463–1468, 2000.

Bialer M. Pharmacokinetic evaluation of sustained release formulations of antiepileptic drugs: clinical implications. Clin Pharmacokin 22:11–21, 1992.

Bialer M, Friedman M, Dubrovsky J. Comparative pharmacokinetic analysis of a novel sustained release dosage form of valproic acid in dogs. Biopharmaceut & Drug Dispos 5:1–10, 1984.

———. Relation between absorption half-life values of four novel sustained-release dosage forms of valproic acid in dogs and humans. Biopharmaceut Drug Dispos 7:495–500, 1986.

Boothe DM, George KL, Couch P. Disposition and clinical use of bromide in cats. J Am Vet Med Assoc 221:1131–1135, 2002.

Brockmöller J, Thomsen T, Wittstock M, Coupez R, Lochs H, Roots I. Pharmacokinetics of levetiracetam in patients with moderate to severe liver cirrhosis (Child-Pugh classes A, B, and C): Characterization by dynamic liver function tests. Clin Pharmacol Ther 77:529–541, 2005.

Bunch SE. Drug-induced hepatic diseases of dogs and cats. In Kirk RW (ed). Curr Vet Ther X, pp. 879–883, 1989.

Center SA, Elston TH, Rowland PH, et al. Fulminant hepatic failure associated with oral administration of diazepam in 11 cats. J Am Vet Med Assoc 209:618–625, 1996.

Chauvet AE, Feldman EC, Kass PH. Effects of phenobarbital administration on results of serum biochemical analyses and adrenocortical function tests in epileptic dogs. J Am Vet Med Assoc 207:1305–1307, 1995.

Cochrane SM, Black WD, Parent JM, et al. Pharmacokinetics of phenobarbital in the cat following intravenous and oral administration. Can J Vet Res 54:132–138, 1990.

Cochrane SM, Parent JM, Black WD, Allen DG, Lumsden JH. Pharmacokinetics of phenobarbital in the cat following multiple oral administration. Can J Vet Res 54:309–312, 1990.

Contin M, Albani F, Riva R, Baruzzi A. Levetiracetam therapeutic monitoring in patients with epilepsy. Therapeut Drug Monit 26:375–379, 2004.

Cunningham JG, Haidukewych D, Jensen HA. Therapeutic plasma concentrations of primidone and its metabolites, phenobarbital and phenylethylmalonamide in epileptic dogs. J Am Vet Med Assoc 182(10):1091–1094, 1983.

Davis JL, Posner LP, Elce Y. Gabapentin for the treatment of neuropathic pain in a pregnant horse. J Am Vet Med Assoc 231:755–758, 2007.

Dayrell-Hart B, Steinberg SA, VanWinkle TJ, et al. Hepatotoxicity of phenobarbital in dogs: 18 cases (1985–1989). J Am Vet Med Assoc 199:1060–1066, 1991.

Dewey CW, Bailey KS, Badgley BL, Boothe DM. Pharmacokinetics of single-dose intravenous levetiracetam administration in normal dogs. [Abstract 70] ACVIM Forum 2007.

Dewey CW, Barone G, Boother DM, Smith K, O'Connor JH. The use of oral levetiracetam as an add-on anticonvulsant drug in cats receiving phenobarbital. [Abstract 211] ACVIM Forum, 2005.

Dewey CW, Guiliano R, Boothe DM, Berg JM, Kortz GD, Joseph RJ, Budsberg SC. Zonisamide therapy for refractory idiopathic epilepsy in dogs. J Am Anim Hosp Assoc Jul–Aug;40(4):285–91, 2004. PMID: 15238558.

Dreifuss FE, Rosman NP, Cloyd JC, et al. A comparison of rectal diazepam gel and placebo for acute repetitive seizures. New Engl J Med 338:1869–1875, 1998.

Duran SH, Ravis WR, Pedersoli WM, Schumacher J. Pharmacokinetics of phenobarbital in the horse. Am J Vet Res May;48(5):807–10, 1987.

Dyer KR, Monroe WE, Forrester SD. Effects of short- and long-term administration of phenobarbital on endogenous ACTH concentration and results of ACTH stimulation tests in dogs. J Am Vet Med Assoc 205:315–318, 1994.

Farnbach GC. Serum concentrations and efficacy of phenytoin, phenobarbital, and primidone in canine epilepsy. J Am Vet Med Assoc 184:1117–1120, 1984.

Foster SF, Church DB, Watson AD. Effect of phenobarbitone on the low-dose dexamethasone suppression test and the urinary corticoid: creatinine ratio in dogs. Aust Vet J Jan;78(1):19–23, 2000.

Frey H-H, Löscher W. Pharmacokinetics of anti-epileptic drugs in the dog: a review. J Vet Pharmacol Therapeut 8:219–233, 1985.

Frey HH, Göbel W, Löscher W. Pharmacokinetics of primidone and its active metabolites in the dog. Arch Int Pharmacodyn Ther Nov;242(1):14–30, 1979.

Gieger TL, Hosgood G, Taboada J, et al. Thyroid function and serum hepatic enzyme activity in dogs after phenobarbital administration. J Vet Intern Med 14:277–281, 2000.

Hirsch LJ, Arif H, Buschsbaum R, Weintraub D, Lee J, Chang JT, Resor SR, Bazil CW. Effect of age and comedication on levetiracetam pharmacokinetics and tolerabilitiy. Epilepsia 48:1351–1359, 2007.

Hojo T, Ohno R, Shimoda M, Kokue E. Enzyme and plasma protein induction by multiple oral administration of phenobarbital at a therapeutic dosage regimen in dogs. J Vet Pharmacol Therapeut 25:121–127, 2002.

Isoherranen N, Yagen B, Soback S, Roeder M, Schurig V, Bialer M. Pharmacokinetics of levetiracetam and its enantiomer (R)-alpha-ethyl-2-oxo-pyrrolidine acetamide in dogs. Epilepsia 42:825–830, 2001.

Jacobs G, Calvert C, Kaufman A. Neutropenia and thrombocytopenia in three dogs treated with anticonvulsants. J Am Vet Med Assoc 212:681–684, 1998.

Jolliet-Riant P, Tillement J-P. Drug transfer across the blood-brain barrier and improvement of brain delivery. Fundam Clin Pharmacol 13:16–26, 1999.

Kantrowitz LB, Peterson ME, Trepanier LA, Melian C, et al: Serum total thyroxine, total triiodothyronine, free thyroxine, and thyrotropin concentrations in epileptic dogs treated with anticonvulsants. J Am Vet Med Assoc 214:1804–1808, 1999.

Knox DA, Ravis WR, Pedersoli WM, Spano JS, Nostrandt AC, Krista LM, Schumacher J. Pharmacokinetics of phenobarbital in horses after single and repeated oral administration of the drug. Am J Vet Res May;53(5):706–10, 1992.

Levitski RE, Trepanier LA. Effect of timing of blood collection on serum phenobarbital concentrations in dogs with epilepsy. J Am Vet Med Assoc Jul 15;217(2):200–4, 2000. Erratum in: J Am Vet Med Assoc Aug 15;217(4):468, 2000.

Maguire PJ, Fettman MJ, Smith MO, Greco DS, Turner AS, Walton JA, Ogilvie GK. Effects of diet on pharmacokinetics of phenobarbital in healthy dogs. J Am Vet Med Assoc Sep 15;217(6):847–52, 2000.

March PA, Hillier A, Weisbrode SE, Mattoon JS, Johnson SE, DiBartola SP, Brofman PJ. Superficial necrolytic dermatitis in 11 dogs with a history of phenobarbital administration (1995–2002). J Vet Intern Med 18:65–74, 2004.

March PA, Podell M, Sams RA. Pharmacokinetics and toxicity of bromide following high-dose oral potassium bromide administration in healthy Beagles. J Vet Pharmacol Therapeut 25:425–432, 2002.

Masuda Y, Utsui Y, Shiraishi Y, Karasawa T, Yoshida K, Shimizu M. Relationships between plasma concentrations of diphenylhydantoin, phenobarbital, carbamazepine, and 3-sulfamoylmethyl-1,2-benzisoxazole (AD-810), a new anticonvulsant agent, and their anticonvulsant or neurotoxic effects in experimental animals. Epilepsia Dec;20(6):623–33, 1979. PMID: 115675.

Matsumoto K, Miyazaki H, Fujii T, Kagemoto A, Maeda T, Hashimoto M. Absorption, distribution and excretion of 3-(Sulfamoyl [C] methyl)-1,2-bnzisoxazole (AD-810) (zonisamide) in rats, dogs, and monkeys and of AD-810 in men. Arzeimittel Forschung 33:961–968, 1983.

May TW, Rambeck B, Jürgens U. Serum concentrations of levetiracetam in epileptic patients: the influence of dose and co-administration. Therapeut Drug Monit 25:690–699, 2003.

Moore S, Papich MG, Munana K, Osborne JN. Pharmacokinetics of levetiracetam (Keppra) in dogs after single and multiple oral doses. [Abstract] ACVIM Forum, 2008.

Müller PB, Taboada J, Hosgood G, et al. Effects of long-term phenobarbital treatment on the liver in dogs. J Vet Intern Med 14:165–171, 2000.

Müller PB, Wolfsheimer KJ, Taboada J, Hosgood G, et al. Effects of long-term phenobarbital treatment on the thyroid and adrenal axis and adrenal function tests in dogs. J Vet Intern Med 14:157–164, 2000.

Olby N. Seizure management in dogs. NAVC Clinicians Brief June; 7–13, 2006.

Papich MG, Alcorn J. Absorption of diazepam after its rectal administration in dogs. Am J Vet Res 56:1629–1636, 1995.

Patterson EE, Leppik IE, O'Brien TD, Goel V, Fisher JE, Dunn AW, Cloyd JC. Safety and pharmacokinetics of intramuscular and intravenous levetiracetam in dogs. [Abstract 73]. ACVIM Forum, 2007.

Pedersoli WM, Wike JS, Ravis WR. Pharmacokinetics of single doses of phenobarbital given intravenously and orally to dogs. Am J Vet Res Apr;48(4):679–83, 1987.

Platt SR. Feline seizure control. J Am An Hosp Assoc 37:515–517, 2001.

Podell M. The use of diazepam per rectum at home for the acute management of cluster seizures in dogs. J Vet Intern Med 9:68–74, 1995.

———. Seizures. Chapter 7. In Platt SR, Olby N (eds): BSAVA Manual of Canine and Feline Neurology, Third Edition. British Small Animal Veterinary Association, pp 97–112, 2004.

Podell M, Fenner WR. Bromide therapy in refractory canine idiopathic epilepsy. J Vet Intern Med 7:318–327, 1993.

———. Use of bromide as an antiepileptic drug in dogs. Compendium of Continuing Education for the Practicing Veterinarian, June 1994;767–774.

Quesnel AD, Parent JM, McDonell W. Clinical management and outcome of cats with seizure disorders: 30 cases (1991–1993). J Am Vet Med Assoc 210:72–77, 1997.

Radulovic LL, Türck D, Von Hodenberg A, Vollmer KO, McNally WP, DeHart PD, Hanson BJ, Brockbrader HN, Chang T. Disposition of gabapentin (Neurontin) in mice, rats, dogs, and monkeys. Drug Metabol Dispos 23:441–448, 1995.

Ravis WR, Duran SH, Pedersoli WM, Schumacher J. A pharmacokinetic study of phenobarbital in mature horses after oral dosing. J Vet Pharmacol Ther Dec;10(4):283–9, 1987.

Ravis WR, Nachreiner RF, Pedersoli WM, Houghton NS. Pharmacokinetics of phenobarbital in dogs after multiple oral administration. Amer J Vet Res 45(7):1283–1286, 1984.

Ravis WR, Pedersoli WM, Wike JS. Pharmacokinetics of phenobarbital in dogs given multiple doses. Amer J Vet Res Aug;50(8):1343–7, 1989.

Reimer JM, Sweeney RW. Pharmacokinetics of phenobarbital after repeated oral administration in normal horses. J Vet Pharmacol Ther Sep;15(3):301–4, 1992.

Schwartz-Porsche D, Löscher W, Frey H-H. Treatment of canine epilepsy with primidone. J Am Vet Med Assoc 181:592–595, 1982.

———. Therapeutic efficacy of phenobarbital and primidone in canine epilepsy: a comparison. J Vet Pharmacol Therap 8:113–119, 1985.

Simpson BS, Papich MG. Pharmacologic management in veterinary behavioral medicine. Vet Clin N Am (Sm An) 33:365–404, 2003.

Soma LR, Uboh CE, Guan F, Birks EK, Teleis DC, Rudy JA, Tsang DS, Watson AO. Disposition, elimination, and bioavailability of phenytoin and its major metabolite in horses. Am J Vet Res 62:483–489, 2001.

Spehar AM, Hill MR, Mayhew IG, et al. Preliminary study on the pharmacokinetics of phenobarbital in the neonatal foal. Equine Vet J 16:368–371, 1984.

Suzuki R, Rahman W, Rygh LJ, Webber M, Hunt SP, Dickenson AH. Spinal-supraspinal serotonergic circuits regulating neuropathic pain and its treatment with gabapentin. Pain 117:292–303, 2005.

Trepanier L. Optimal bromide therapy and monitoring. ACVIM Proceedings. 15th ACVIM Forum, pp 100–101, 1997.

Trepanier LA. Use of bromide as an anticonvulsant for dogs with epilepsy. J Am Vet Med Assoc Jul 15;207(2):163–166, 1995.

Trepanier LA, Babish JG. Pharmacokinetic properties of bromide in dogs after the intravenous and oral administration of single doses. Res Vet Sci 58:248–251, 1995.

Trepanier LA, Van Schoick A, Schwark WS, Carrillo J. Therapeutic serum drug concentrations in epileptic dogs treated with potassium bromide alone or in combination with other anticonvulsants: 122 cases (1992–1996). J Am Vet Med Assoc 213:1449–1453, 1998.

von Klopmann T, Rambeck B, Tipold A. Prospective study of zonisamide therapy for refractory idiopathic epilepsy in dogs. J Sm An Pract Mar;48(3):134–8, 2007. PMID: 17355603.

Watson AD, Church DB, Emslie DR, Tsoukalas G, Griffin DL, Baggot JD. Effects of ingesta on systemic availability of phenobarbitone in dogs. Aust Vet J Mar;73(3):108–9, 1996.

Yeary RA. Serum concentrations of primidone and its metabolites, phenylethylmalonamide and phenobarbital, in the dog. Am J Vet Res 41:1643–1645, 1980.

CHAPTER

21

DRUGS AFFECTING ANIMAL BEHAVIOR

BARBARA L. SHERMAN AND MARK G. PAPICH

INTRODUCTION

In recent years, the use of drugs to influence animal behavior has expanded commensurate with that of human behavioral medicine (Crowell-Davis and Murray 2006; Simpson and Papich 2003). Drugs, in combination with behavior modification, have been used to manage difficult animal behavior problems. Often these problems are those insufficiently responsive to nonpharmacologic approaches alone. In a general way, drugs may decrease arousal, excitability, and impulsivity and promote behavioral calming. More specifically, behavioral drugs may be used to attenuate repetitive compulsive behaviors, modulate aggression, and help manage organic states (Stein et al. 1994). Psychotropic drugs may be used to decrease the latency to response to behavioral treatment.

The use of behavioral drugs to reduce fears and anxieties may enhance animal welfare and promote safe and humane handling. Extrapolating from the reports of humans who suffer from anxiety disorders and from our direct observations, highly anxious or fearful animals suffer as well and should be treated, behaviorally and pharmacologically, consistent with our mission as veterinarians to reduce animal suffering. We suggest that, particularly for anxiety-related disorders, pharmacologic treatment should be considered as a first, rather than last, resort.

This chapter focuses on commonly used behavioral drugs, their presumed mechanism of action, their side effects and their application to clinical veterinary practice. In addition, some new agents, with potential for use in veterinary behavior, are introduced. Although the activities of behavioral drugs have been elucidated in vitro, our knowledge of their activity in the brain of humans or nonhuman animals remains imperfect. Radioactive labeling, advanced imaging and other techniques have revealed the remarkable complexity of the brain and the interrelationships of systems previously considered distinct. For example, there is increasing evidence that affective disorders are modulated by neuroactive steroids that, in turn, modulate specific neurotransmitters, including those described in this chapter (Eser et al. 2006). In spite of recent expansion in our understanding and application of behavioral drugs, behavioral pharmacology is in its infancy.

With few exceptions, the drugs discussed herein are approved for use in humans for the treatment of behavioral disorders; their use in animals is extralabel (Simpson and Voith 1997). Without an approved claim, it has fallen upon veterinary behaviorists, pharmacologists, and other specialists to examine the relevant data and conduct studies to examine the published record on these medications to predict clinical use and response. One of the greatest challenges in evaluating the studies published in human medicine or from laboratory animal studies is to interpret the data in light of the various species differences that exist in drug metabolism, receptor sensitivity, and susceptibility to toxicosis.

PHARMACOKINETIC ISSUES FOR BEHAVIOR DRUGS

Pharmacokinetics is covered in more detail in this book in earlier chapters (Chapters 2 and 3). In this section are some comments regarding the importance of pharmacokinetic issues to behavior drug therapy. When there is a relationship of the plasma or serum drug concentrations to clinical effect, pharmacokinetics can be helpful to predict pharmacological response. This becomes particularly important when we have few controlled clinical trials of drugs in animals, but comparative pharmacokinetic data. Pharmacokinetics is the science that describes the effect of the body on a drug and a description of the absorption, distribution, metabolism, and elimination (Janicek et al. 1997).

ABSORPTION, METABOLISM, CLEARANCE, AND DISTRIBUTION. Bioavailability of a drug depends on both the extent and rate of drug absorption. Since most behavior drugs discussed in this paper are administered orally, absorption becomes a critical pharmacokinetic parameter. Drug absorption is determined by examining the relative concentrations in plasma or serum, because the availability of a drug to the central nervous system cannot be easily measured.

Drugs given orally can be absorbed quickly and avoid significant metabolism, be poorly absorbed because of unfavorable dissolution or solubility, or be absorbed from the gastrointestinal tract (GIT) and then undergo first-pass metabolism, which is the process of intestinal or hepatic metabolism prior to reaching systemic circulation.

Many of the behavior drugs to be discussed in this article are weak bases, for example, the substituted amines that are the tricyclic antidepressants and other centrally acting drugs. These weak bases generally have good lipophilicity, but poor water solubility. However, most are formulated as water-soluble salts (hydrochloride salts of clomipramine, fluoxetine, buspirone). This allows for more rapid dissolution in the gastrointestinal tract, followed by good permeability in the intestine. Subsequently, the oral absorption of most of these drugs is good. However, these drugs—being lipophilic—are also subject to enzyme metabolism in the intestine and liver. For some drugs, extensive intestinal and hepatic metabolism may render these drugs susceptible to the first-pass metabolic effects, which reduces the overall systemic availability.

Drug metabolism is the process whereby drugs are metabolized to active and inactive metabolites or an inactive drug can be metabolized to an inactive drug (if administered as a prodrug). For the drugs discussed in this chapter, the metabolic fate is determined primarily by hepatic and intestinal metabolism. To our knowledge, there are few drugs used in behavior therapy that are affected much by renal clearance. Although, the kidneys may be the ultimate route of elimination for conjugated water-soluble metabolites.

Many behavioral drugs are substrates for, or affect cytochrome P450 (CYP) enzymes, which are microsomal drug-metabolizing enzymes (DeVane 1997; Janicak et al. 1997) located primarily in the liver and GIT. These enzymes have potential for important pharmacokinetic drug-drug interactions. They are designated by family, subfamily, and isoforms by a number and letter sequence (Tables 21.1, 21.2). In humans the important CYP enzymes include CYP1A2, CYP2C9-10, CYP2C19, CYP2D6, and CYP3A3/4. The enzymes CYP3A3/4 and CYP2D6 are responsible in humans for 50% and 30%,

TABLE 21.1 Psychotropic agents used in dogs

Drug Class	Drug Name	Dose in Dogs	References
Benzodiazepine (BZD)	Diazepam	0.55–2.2 mg/kg PRN	Plumb 2008
BZD	Alprazolam	0.02–0.1 mg/kg q8–12h	Landsberg et al. 2003
		0.02 mg/kg PRN (w/clomipramine)	Crowell-Davis et al. 2003
BZD	Clorazepate	2 mg/kg q12h	Papich 2007
			Forrester et al. 1990
BZD	Lorazepam	0.02–0.1 mg/kg q8–24h	Mills and Simpson 2002
BZD	Oxazepam	0.2–1.0 mg/kg q12–24h	Landsberg et al. 2003
Azapirone	Buspirone	2.5–10 mg/dog q12–24h or 1.0–2.0 mg/kg q12h	Papich 2007
Tricyclic antidepressant (TCA)	Amitriptyline	2.2–4.4 mg/kg q12–24h	Juarbe-Diaz 1997a,b
		2 mg/kg q24h	Takeuchi et al. 2000
		0.74–2.5 mg/kg q12h	Reich et al. 2000
		1–2 mg/kg q12–24h	Papich 2007
TCA	Clomipramine	1–3 mg/kg q12h	Papich 2007
		1–2 mg/kg q12h	King et al. 2000b
		1–2 mg/kg q12h	Moon-Fanelli and Dodman 1998
		1–2 mg/kg q12h	Seksel and Lindeman 2001
		3 mg/kg q12h	Hewson and Luescher 1998a,b
		3 mg/kg q24h	Rapoport et al. 1992
TCA	Imipramine	2–4 mg/kg q12–24h	Papich 2007
Selective serotonin reuptake inhibitor (SSRI)	Fluoxetine	Start 0.5 mg/kg q24h, increase to 1.0 mg/kg q24h	Papich 2007
			Dodman et al. 1996a
		1 mg/kg q24h	Rapoport et al. 1992
		0.96 mg/kg q24h	Wynchank and Berk 1998
		20 mg/dog q24h	
SSRI	Paroxetine	0.5–1 mg/kg q24h	Papich 2007
SSRI	Sertraline	3.42 mg/kg q24h	Rapoport et al. 1992
		2.5 mg/kg q24h	N. Dodman, Pers. Comm. 2000
			Larson and Summers 2001
Monoamine oxidase inhibitor (MAOI)	Selegiline	0.5–1.0 mg/kg q am	Calves 2000
Atypical antidepressant	Trazodone	2–5 mg/kg q12h and/or bolus 1+ hour prior to an anxiety-inducing event	Gruen and Sherman (2008), Simpson and Papich 2003
	Mirtazapine	Small dogs 3.75 mg q24h	Mandelker 2006
		20–35 pounds dogs: 7.5 mg q24h	
		40–50 pounds dogs: 15 q24h	
		>75 pounds: 22.5 mg q24h	
		>100 pounds: 30 mg q24h	
Anticonvulsant	Phenobarbital	0.45 mg/kg q24h	Crowell-Davis et al. 1989
		1.5–2.0 mg/kg q12h	Dodman et al. 1992
		5 mg/kg q12h (with clorazepate)	Forrester et al. 1993
		2–8 mg/kg q12h	Papich 2007
	Carbamazepine	4–8 mg/kg q12h	Holland 1988
Beta antagonist	Propranolol	2–3 mg/kg q12hrs (w/phenobarbital)	Walker et al. 1997
Narcotic antagonist	Naltrexone	2.2 mg/kg q12–24h	White 1990
		2.2 mg/kg q12h	Papich 2007
Progestogen hormones	Megoestrol acetate (see text)	Males: 2 mg/kg q 24h × 7d, then if improved 1 mg/kg × 14d	Joby et al. 1984
		2.2 mg/kg q24h × 14d, then 1.1 mg/kg q24h × 14d, then 0.5 mg/kg q24h × 14d	Borchelt and Voith 1986
		2–4 mg/kg q24h × 8 days, reduce for maintenance	Papich 2007
Hormone	Melatonin	0.1 mg/kg q8–24h (w/amitriptyline)	Aronson 1999

Note: See text for special considerations and side effects.
All doses are *per os*.

TABLE 21.2 Psychotropic Agents Used in Cats

Drug Class	Drug Name	Dose in Cats	References
Benzodiazepine (BZD)	Diazepam	1–4 mg/cat q12–24h	Papich 2007
		0.2–0.4 mg/kg q12–24h	Cooper and Hart 1992
		1–2 mg/cat q12h	
BZD	Alprazolam	0.125–0.25 mg/cat q12h	Marder 1991
BZD	Clorazepate	2 mg/kg q12h	Papich 2007
BZD	Oxazepam	2.5 mg/cat PRN appetite stimulation	Papich 2007
Azapirone	Buspirone	2.5–5 mg/cat q12–24h	Hart et al. 1993
		5.0 mg/cat q12h	Sawyer et al. 1999
		2.5–5.0 mg/cat q8–12h	Marder 1991
Tricyclic antidepressant (TCA)	Amitriptyline	5–10 mg/cat q24h	Papich 2007
		2.5–5.0 mg/cat q12–24h	Sawyer et al. 1999
		0.5–1.0 mg/kg q12h	Halip et al. 1998
		10 mg/cat qHS	Chew et al. 1998
TCA	Clomipramine	0.5 mg/kg q24h	DeHasse 1997
		1.25–2.5 mg/cat q24h	Sawyer et al. 1999
		1–5 mg/cat q12–24h	Papich 2007
TCA	Imipramine	2–4 mg/kg q12–24h	Papich 2007
Selective serotonin reuptake inhibitor (SSRI)	Fluoxetine	0.5–4.0 mg/cat q24h	Papich 2007
		1 mg/kg q24h	Pryor et al. 2001
		1–1.5 mg/cat q24h	Hartmann 1995
		2 mg/cat q24–72h	Romatowski 1998
SSRI	Paroxetine	1.25–2.5 mg/cat q24h	Papich 2007
Monoamine Oxidase Inhibitor (MAOI)	Selegiline	0.5 mg/kg q24h	
Atypical Antidepressant	Mirtazapine	Cats: 1/8–1/4 × 15 mg tablet (1.87–3.75 mg)/cat q72h	Mandelker 2006
Anticonvulsant	Carbamazepine	25 mg q12hrs	Schwartz 1994
	Megestrol acetate (see text)	2.5–5 mg/cat q24h × 7d, then 5 mg 1–24 × 4/wk	Papich 2007
		5 mg/cat q 24h × 7–10d, then 5 mg eod × 14d, then 5 mg 2 ×/wk;	Hart 1980
		2 mg/kg q24h × 5d, then 1 mg/kg q24h × 5d, then 0.5 mg/kg q24h × 5d	Romatowski 1989

Note: See text for special considerations and side effects. All doses are *per os*.
qHS = at bedtime.

respectively, of known oxidative drug metabolism. Because these enzymes can be both induced and inhibited by certain drugs, such as those classified as antidepressants, concentrations of other drugs, metabolized by the same CYP enzymes, will increase. For example, in humans fluoxetine and paroxetine inhibit CYP2D6, important in the oxidative metabolism of the tricyclic antidepressants (TCAs). When fluoxetine or paroxetine is used in combination with a TCA, a significant increase of the TCA plasma concentration occurs, potentially causing toxicity unless the TCA dose is reduced (Janicak et al. 1997).

One of the problems in veterinary medicine is that the enzymes, and subsequently their substrates and inhibitors, are not as well characterized as in human medicine (Chauret et al. 1997). The enzyme responsible for the greatest proportion of metabolism in humans is CYP3A4 oxidase. There are only low levels of CYP3A4 in dogs and cats, but other enzymes play a larger role (for example, CYP3A12) (Kuroha et al. 2002). Other enzymes present in dogs are the 1A, 2C, 3A, and 2D families and subfamilies (Chauret et al. 1997; Kuroha et al. 2002). There are large interspecies differences in the P450-mediated metabolism in dog and cat microsomes compared to human. The variation is in the metabolic activity, as well as the effect of specific inhibitors on P450 enzyme activity (Chauret et al. 1997). Information on the inhibitory activity of drugs on various enzyme systems in humans should not be broadly extrapolated to dogs and cats (Kuroha et al. 2002).

The other step in drug metabolism is a biosynthetic reaction called conjugation. Drug metabolic conjugation is the process whereby the drug or metabolite is linked with endogenous compounds such as amino acids, glucuronic acid, sulfate, glutathione, or acetyl (acetate). These polar conjugates are more water-soluble and more easily excreted than the parent compound. The conjugated products are usually inactive, but there are exceptions.

Just as with the other metabolic reactions, there are tremendous species differences in the conjugation reactions. Dogs lack the ability to acetylate drugs such as sulfonamides; cats have a deficient ability to form glucuronide metabolites with drugs such as salicylate and phenols (such as with acetaminophen metabolites).

The rate of hepatic metabolism is measured by hepatic clearance. Clearance is one of the determinants of elimination half-life ($T^1/_2$) the time needed for plasma drug concentrations to decrease by 50% (Janicek 1997). Drugs with short elimination half-lives must be given more frequently to maintain a consistent plasma concentration. With repeated dosing, these drugs also achieve steady-state more quickly. Usually after five half-lives, a drug reaches steady-state, the plasma concentration achieved as long as the dosing schedule or other metabolic processes remain constant. Once plasma steady-state is achieved, drug concentration in other tissues, such as the brain, is at equilibrium. The time to reach steady-state is relevant to the use of behavior drugs. Some drugs, such as diazepam in the dog have short half-lives [$T^1/_2$ less than 1 hour; (Papich and Alcorn 1995)]. Unless administered more frequently than once every five half-lives, these drugs will never reach a steady-state. On the other hand, drugs with long half-lives will accumulate with chronic dosing and attain steady-state in approximately five half-lives. But, if the half-life is 24 hours or longer, several days may be necessary before the drug accumulates to a level high enough to produce a consistent clinical response. This may be one reason that some antidepressant drugs do not have immediate effects when administered chronically in animals.

The pharmacokinetic term that describes drug distribution is the *volume of distribution*, often called the *apparent volume of distribution (VD)* because its physiological relevance is only apparent. The term does not attempt to describe a physiological process; it is only a proportionality constant relating drug concentration in the plasma or serum to drug dose, as in the following formula:

$$VD = [\text{dose}]/[\text{plasma concentration}]$$

The physiological distribution of drugs is determined by their lipid solubility and protein binding. The higher the lipophilicity, the greater is the ability to distribute across biological lipid membranes, as long as plasma protein binding is not so high as to limit the diffusion. Because most behavior drugs are weak bases, protein binding is expected to be low for these drugs. However, this is only assumed, because there is little or no published data documenting the true plasma protein binding for these drugs in dogs and cats. Tissue protein binding, or intracellular trapping of drugs, can increase the distribution of drugs from the plasma to tissue compartment. Most of the behavior drugs are weak bases and unionized and lipophilic at physiological pH. Some may be trapped in the brain or CSF owing to pH partitioning because these spaces are relatively more acidic than the plasma. Because the tissue concentrations may be high relative to plasma concentrations of these drugs, the apparent volume of distribution for this group of drugs is usually greater than 1.0 l/kg.

Relevant to the behavior drugs is the distribution across the blood-brain barrier (BBB). The BBB consists of unfenestrated capillaries, with tight junctions that prevent large or poorly lipophilic molecules from passing from the blood to the brain (Pardridge 1999; Jolliet-Riant and Tillement 1999). There is also a blood-CSF barrier, but it makes up a relatively smaller component to the distribution of drugs to the central nervous system. The BBB also is comprised of transmembrane pumps that effectively transport drugs (and probably other compounds) from the brain back to the blood stream. One of the best known of these transporters is p-glycoprotein. Some drugs are good substrates for p-glycoprotein and other drugs serve as inhibitors of these pumps (Jolliet-Riant and Tillement 1999).

NEUROTRANSMITTERS

Many of the autononomic nerve function and transmission are covered in more detail in Chapters 5 and 6. Presented here are some of the neurotransmitters that are most affected by behavior-modifying drugs. Behavioral drugs act either as stimulators (agonists) or blockers (antagonists) of neurotransmitter receptors, or as inhibitors of associated regulatory enzymes (Baldessarini 1995; Stahl 2008). Drugs that modulate naturally occurring neurosignals affect the monoamine neurotransmitters serotonin (5-hydroxytryptamine or 5-HT), norepinephrine (NE), and dopamine (DA), as well as acetylcholine (ACh), glutamate, and γ-aminobutyric acid (GABA) receptors, among others. Neurotransmitters have multiple receptor subtypes distributed in specific areas of the body with which they interact. The most selective drugs mimic the natural neurotransmitter's action at only one receptor subtype. Other substances, such as circulating hormones, pituitary peptides, opioid peptides, and neurokinins can also affect behavior (Stahl 2008).

At the cellular level, neurotransmission alters the function of postsynaptic target neurons. This process, in turn, affects gene expression (Stahl 2008). The neurotransmitter released from the presynaptic neuron is considered the first messenger. It binds to its postsynaptic receptor and the bound neurotransmitter regulates a second messenger inside the cell of the postsynaptic neuron. This second messenger, in turn, forms transcription factors that, when activated, bind to regulatory regions of genes. This process activates RNA polymerase and the gene transcribes itself into its mRNA, leading to translation of the corresponding protein. The protein can influence cellular processes that modulate behavior. Because multiple neurotransmitters are involved in CNS function, each working through multiple receptors, chemical signaling provides the features of both selectivity and amplification.

Discussed below are neurotransmitters or regulatory enzymes known to influence behavior and be affected by commonly used behavioral drugs. The monoamine neurotransmitters include norepinephrine, dopamine, and serotonin. It is now known that many neurons respond to more than one neurotransmitter, a process called *cotransmission* (Stahl 2008). This may explain why multiple drugs in combination may be particularly effective and why some beneficial drugs act on more than one neurotransmitter. At this time, there is no rational treatment approach based on cotransmission. However, a strategic multiple drug program may enhance treatment success in the future.

NOREPINEPHRINE. Norepinephrine (NE) is derived from the amino acid tyrosine, which is transported from the blood and into each noradrenergic neuron by means of an active transport pump (Stahl 2008). There, tyrosine is acted upon by three enzymes, eventually converting it to dopamine, and then to NE, which is stored in vesicles. NE can be destroyed by monoamine oxidase (MAO), located in mitochondria, and catechol-O-methyl transferase (COMT), located outside the presynaptic nerve terminal. There are three postsynaptic receptors for NE: β 1, α 1, and α 2. Norepinephrine has little activity on β-2 receptors. α-2 receptors are also found presynaptically. Called autoreceptors, they regulate NE release via a negative feedback system.

Most cell bodies for noradrenergic neurons are located in the locus coeruleus area of the brainstem. This region determines whether attention is focused on the external environment (as in response to a threat) or to internal signals (such as pain). There are many specific noradrenergic pathways in the brain, controlling both psychological and physiological activities. For example, projections from the locus coeruleus to the limbic cortex regulate emotions; projections in cardiovascular centers may control blood pressure.

DOPAMINE. Like norepinephrine, dopamine is synthesized intraneuronally from the amino acid tyrosine. Dopamine (DA) neurons lack the third enzyme that leads to conversion to norepinephrine. The same enzymes that destroy norepinephrine (MAO and COMT) destroy DA. There are at least 5 DA receptor subtypes. Best known is the DA2 receptor, which is stimulated by dopaminergic agonists for the treatment of Parkinson's disease in humans and blocked by DA antagonist antipsychotics. Although DA1, 3, and 4 receptors respond to antipsychotics, it is not clear to what extent they contribute to the behavioral effects of these drugs. When dopamine receptors are blocked, as with an antipsychotic drug, acetylcholine activity increases. This is because dopamine normally suppresses acetylcholine activity. An increase in acetylcholine activity can lead to extrapyramidal symptoms, discussed below.

SEROTONIN. Serotonin, is also called 5-hydroxytryptomine or 5-HT. The chemistry and pharmacology of serotonin and other transmitters were covered in more detail in Chapter 16. Abnormalities in central serotonin function have been hypothesized to underlie disturbances in mood, anxiety, satiety, cognition, aggression, and sexual drives (Tollefson and Rosenbaum 1998). Drugs that enhance serotonin are among the most effective modulators of behavior (Simpson and Simpson 1996a). Abnormalities in serotonin production or metabolism may underlie some behavior problems in companion animals. For example, dogs that exhibit affective (dominance type) aggression have significantly lower levels of serotonin-metabolites in their cerebrospinal fluid than nonaggressive control dogs (Reisner et al. 1996). Canine compulsive disorder may be linked to 5HT dysfunction, based on the responsiveness of dogs that exhibit repetitive spinning, object-licking, or light-chasing to treatment with drugs that inhibit serotonin reuptake (Hewson et al. 1998a; Luescher 2003).

For synthesis of serotonin, the amino acid tryptophan is transported into the brain from plasma. Two enzymes are involved in the conversion of tryptophan to 5-HT. Analogous enzymes, transport pumps, and receptors exist in the 5HT neuron. Classification of 5HT receptors was reviewed thoroughly by Hoyer and colleagues (1994). There are two key presynaptic receptors, 5HT1A and 5HT1D, and at least six postsynaptic receptors, 5HT1A, 5HT1D, 5HT2A, 5HT2C, 5HT3, and 5HT4 (Hoyer et al. 1994). As with NE and DA, presynaptic receptors act as autoreceptors that detect high concentrations of 5HT, inhibit further 5HT release, and slow 5HT neuronal impulse flow. Postsynaptic 5HT receptors regulate 5HT release from the presynaptic nerve ending. The 5HT2A, 5HT2C, and 5HT3 receptors are implicated in several serotonin pathways in the CNS (Hoyer et al. 1994). Although some 5HT4 receptors are in the CNS, their action is primarily localized to the gastrointestinal tract. Additional roles of this receptor on gastrointestinal function is discussed with specific drugs in Chapter 47. Serotonergic nuclei are localized to the raphe nucleus of the brainstem (Tollefson and Rosenbaum 1998). This area has projections to the frontal cortex, which may regulate mood; the basal ganglia, which may control movement and compulsive behaviors; and the limbic area, which may be involved in anxiety and panic.

There is evidence that the serotonin system may exert "tonic inhibition" on the central dopaminergic system (Tollefson and Rosenbaum 1998). This may explain the occasional unexpected occurrence of extrapyramidal side effects during therapy with a selective serotonin reuptake inhibitor (Tollefson and Rosenbaum 1998).

ACETYLCHOLINE. Acetylcholine (ACh) is formed in cholinergic neurons from two precursors: choline, derived from dietary sources, and acetyl coenzyme A, which is synthesized in the neuron. There are two major types of cholinergic receptors: nicotinic and muscarinic. Each of these is further divided into numerous receptors subtypes. There are five muscarinic receptor subtypes, M_1 through M_5. M_1 receptors are found on ganglia. M_3 and M_4 are found on smooth muscle and secretory organs, such as those of the GIT and all five subtypes are found in the central nervous system. A nonspecific blocker of muscarinic receptors is atropine. One of the side effects of some behavior-modifying drugs (e.g., tricyclic antidepressants) is to block of muscarinic receptors producing cardiovascular, gastrointestinal, and other side effects. Additional discussion of the cholinergic nervous system is provided in Chapter 7.

GAMMA AMINO BUTYRIC ACID. Gamma amino butyric acid (GABA) is the major inhibitory neurotransmitter in the CNS, localized particularly in the cortex and thalamus (Ballenger 1998). GABA is synthesized from the amino acid precursor glutamate. Glutamate participates in multiple metabolic functions. The GABA neuron has a presynaptic transporter similar to those of NE, DA, and 5HT. There are two subtypes of GABA: $GABA_A$ and $GABA_B$. $GABA_A$ subtype receptors are allosterically modulated by benzodiazepine receptors and others. Some of the anticonvulsant drugs that affect the GABA receptor are discussed in Chapter 20.

MAJOR DRUG CLASSES

Historically, behavioral drugs are classified according to their first human clinical application (for example, the antidepressant category), although such categorical descriptions have become functionally obsolete. Most behavioral drugs used in human and veterinary medicine have expanded their use well beyond their original clinical application. Traditionally, drugs are further classified according to their chemical structure and neurochemical activity. Tricyclic antidepressants (referring to a common chemical structure), and selective serotonin reuptake inhibitors (referring to neurochemical activity) are examples of drugs classified by their chemical structure, and mechanism of action, respectively. The historic and functional drug classifications are retained here, since they provide a useful framework for our understanding of action and side effects of behavioral drugs. Drugs in the same category share many characteristics, including mechanism of action and common side effects. In addition, many reference sources utilize this traditional and logical categorization.

ANTIPSYCHOTICS. The antipsychotics include a number of structurally dissimilar drugs used in humans to treat psychosis, typified by conditions such as schizophrenia, affective disorder, and psychoses associated with organic mental disorders (Marder 1998). Most veterinarians are familiar with acepromazine, one of the drugs in this class that is registered for veterinary medicine (e.g., Atravet, PromAce, or "ACE"). Acepromazine and other sedatives in this class are discussed in more detail in the anesthetic section (Chapter 13). Since the conventional antipsychotics produce neurological side effects, they are sometimes called *neuroleptics*. This term is generally not applied to newer, atypical antipsychotics for which neurological side effects are less likely. Antipsychotics block central dopamine (DA) receptors, particularly of the subtype D_2. Antipsychotics produce ataraxia, a state of relative indifference to external stimuli (Baldessarini 1995). Most antipsychotics are metabolized by the CYP-450 enzymes belonging to family 2 and 3; therefore it is possible that drug-drug interactions described for people also would be a concern for animals (Simpson and Papich 2003).

Except for acepromazine (and prolixin for horses), antipsychotics are not commonly used in modern veterinary behavioral medicine for a number of reasons. First, small animals are rarely diagnosed with "psychosis"; and the anxiolytic properties of antipsychotics in animals are minimal. Second, side effects limit their usefulness. When animals are given traditional antipsychotics at relatively high or repeated doses, they often develop catalepsy, a syndrome with immobility, increased muscle tone, and abnormal postures, although reflexes (including the bite reflex) are preserved. Most veterinarians are familiar with the effects of acepromazine on dogs and cats. Third, spontaneous motor activity, caused by dopamine-receptor blockade in the striatum and inactivation of dopamine neurons in the substantia nigra may result from the administration of phenothiazines to animals (Marder 1998). Finally, other important side effects of antipsychotic drugs, summarized below, can be unacceptable.

Antipsychotics can cause extrapyramidal signs (EPS) because of their effect of inhibiting the action of dopamine. EPS are most likely in older, high-potency antipsychotics such as haloperidol. EPS documented in humans include pseudoparkinsonism (stiffness, tremor, shuffling gait), akathesia (motor restlessness), acute dystonic reactions (tightening of facial and neck muscles). The involuntary muscle movements of EPS have been confused with seizures. Antipsychotic drugs may also reduce blood pressure and elevate prolactin levels. One subclass of antipsychotics, the phenothiazines, may disinhibit learned responses (Aronson 1999) and may inhibit the learning processes necessary for behavior modification techniques. It has been reported in several textbooks that this group of drugs, particularly acepromazine, increases the risk of seizures in animals and may actually be contraindicated in animals at risk of seizures. However, recent clinical studies have shown that acepromazine does not increase the risk of seizures in dogs (Tobias et al. 2006; Garner et al. 2004; McConnell et al. 2007).

These EPS should not be confused with another adverse effect of long-term antipsychotic medication called *tardive dyskinesia*. Tardive dyskinesia is characterized by oral-facial, limb, or trunchal dyskinesia or twisting postures. The differentiation is that EPS usually occur soon after administration of the drugs. Tardive dyskinesia occurs after prolonged chronic treatment. The other important differentiation is that EPS are believed to be caused by a deficiency of dopamine and tardive dyskinesia is caused by an excess of dopamine, or increased dopamine receptor sensitivity caused by chronic administration. Decreasing the dose or withdrawal of the antipsychotic drug will worsen tardive dyskinesia. To our knowledge, tardive dyskinesia has not been described in veterinary patients.

Historically, one phenothiazine antipsychotic, acepromazine (PromAce, ACE, Atravet), has been used in the management of veterinary behavior problems, such as noise phobia, by reducing animals' general attendance to environmental stimuli, and producing sedation. The effectiveness of acepromazine as an oral anxiolytic is often disappointing and causes undesirable side effects (Overall 1998a). However, its intramuscular use may decrease presurgical patient apprehension and reduce the dose of other drugs used as general anesthetics (Light et al. 1993). It also may reduce the dose of other coadministered anesthetics. Owing to the sedative and extrapyramidal effects, acepromazine is not satisfactory for chronic administration. Other agents, such as the benzodiazepines or antidepressants, are preferred because they are more specific for their antianxiety effects and have fewer side effects. A small proportion of companion animals—especially cats—that are administered acepromazine orally will experience spontaneous motor activity, possibly akathesia.

Phenothiazines have been used to treat compulsive behaviors not satisfactorily responsive to serotonergic drugs or in combination with serotonergic agents (Goodman et al. 1990). Dopamine has been implicated in some forms of stereotypic behaviors, perhaps because of the effect of serotonin (Kennes et al. 1988). Dopaminergic agents such as apomorphine and amphetamine and the dopamine precursor L-dopa can induce stereotypies in animals (Goodman et al. 1990). Thioridazine has been used in one case of aberrant motor behavior in a dog (Jones 1987). In 2000, proprietary thioridazine (Mellaril) added a label warning that the drug has been shown to prolong the QTc interval and been associated with arrhythmias and sudden death in humans. It was recommended that thioridazine not be used concurrently with fluvoxamine, fluoxetine, paroxetine, propranolol, pindolol, or any drug that affects the QTc interval of the EKG or the CYP P450 2D6 enzymes.

Some newer atypical antipsychotics, such as risperidone (Risperdal), may prove to be useful in cases of environmental-specific anxiety (including veterinary visits) or impulsive, explosive behaviors in dogs and cats (Chouinard and Arnott 1993). However, at this time, there is not sufficient information available to recommend safe dosage regimens. The side effects associated with the traditional antipsychotics may not apply to the newer drugs, although immobility and transient loss of conditioned responses may be observed. At present their high cost and lack of published data make them impractical for animal use.

ANXIOLYTICS. The anxiolytic drugs include benzodiazepines, azapirones, barbiturates, and antihistamines. Antidepressants (discussed separately, below) also have anxiolytic properties. Discussed here are the benzodiazepine and azapirone classes, as well as a special class, nonbenzodiazepine hypnotics.

Benzodiazepines (BZD). The benzodiazepines (BZDs) constitute a large class of drugs with a long history of safe and efficacious use in humans. Examples used in veterinary medicine are shown in Figure 21.1. All drugs in the class act on BZD receptors in the CNS to facilitate $GABA_A$, an inhibitory neurotransmitter. After binding to the $GABA_A$ receptor, these drugs enhance the GABA-mediated conductance through ionic channels and stabilize excitable membranes. The effects of BZD on behavior may be attributed to potentiation of GABA pathways that act to regulate release of monoamine neurotransmitters in the CNS. Examples of drugs in this class with veterinary application

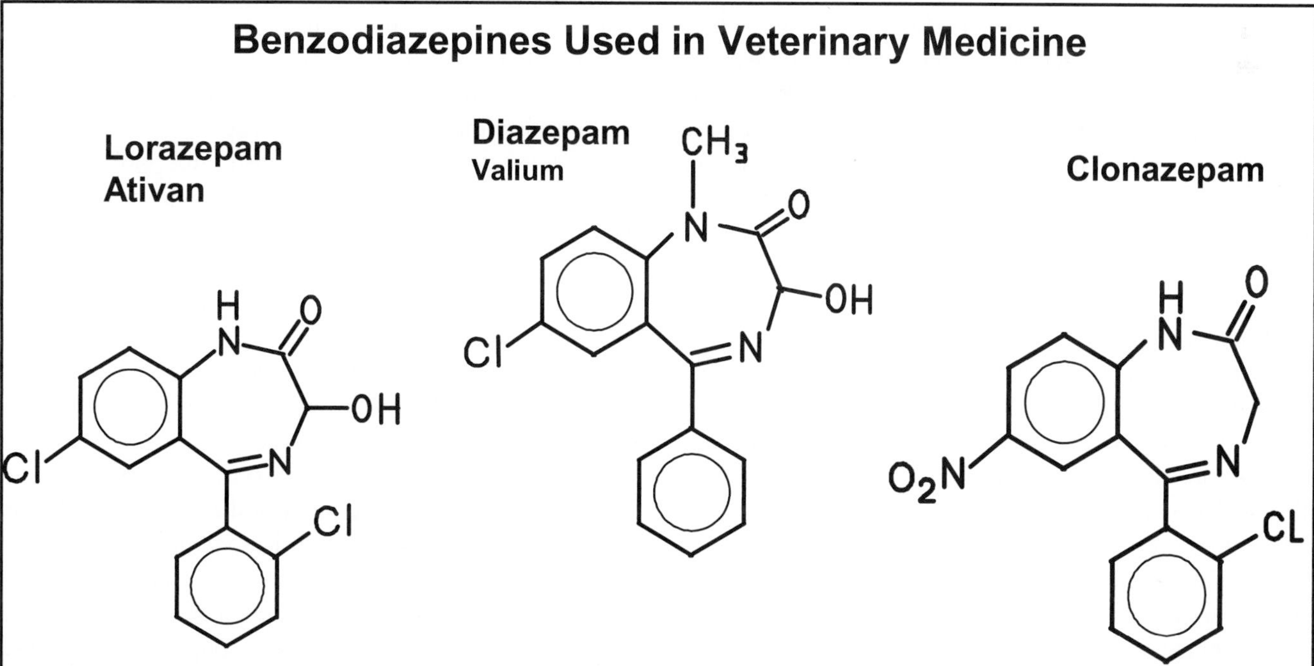

FIG. 21.1 Benzodiazepines used in veterinary medicine. Lorazepam (left), diazepam (center), and clonazepam (right).

are diazepam, clorazepate, alprazolam, oxazepam, orazepam, and temazepam. Anesthetic uses of benzodiazepines are discussed in more detail with anesthetic agents in Chapter 13. The use of benzodiazepines for treating seizures is discussed in Chapter 20 on anticonvulsant drugs.

There are more differences in the pharmacokinetic properties among these drugs than differences that affect the receptor (pharmacodynamic effect). BZDs are used in humans primarily for generalized anxiety disorder or panic disorder (Ballenger 1998); they are used similarly in small animals (Simpson and Simpson 1996b). Dosing schedule can affect pharmacokinetics. For example, diazepam given one time for anxiety will have a lower maximal nordiazepam concentration compared to the same BZD given twice daily for anxiety (Ballenger 1998; Forrester et al. 1990).

After oral administration, behavioral responses to BZDs generally occur within 1 hour, although conflicting studies in animals suggest that the anxiolytic effects are greater after they have been administered for several days (File 1985). Sedation, ataxia, muscle relaxation, increased appetite, paradoxical excitation, and memory deficits may be observed (Roy-Byrne and Cowley 1991). Tolerance to sedation, ataxia, and muscle relaxation may develop over the first few days of therapy (Löscher and Frey 1981). Animals may become ataxic and unstable; therefore, pet owners should be cautioned to assist older animals to avoid falls. Animals should be observed for hyperphagia when given BZDs on a regular basis. Agitation and restlessness may occur as an idiosyncratic response to BZDs. Paradoxic reactions of excitement have been observed in dogs, particularly with administration of alprazolam. If these are observed, the drug should be discontinued and another drug from another class should be selected. Amnesia from BZD has been observed in humans for many years (King 1992). Also, in animals, memory deficits and diminished conditioned responses may be observed, i.e., the animal may seem to "forget" what it has been previously taught. Difficulty in learning new behaviors, such as desensitization protocols, may be affected by the memory deficits.

At routine doses, BZDs have little, if any, effect on cardiovascular and respiratory systems (Ballenger 1998). BZDs may disinhibit behavior. In humans, manifestations of disinhibition include hostility, aggressiveness, rage reactions, paroxysmal excitement, irritability, and behavioral dyscontrol (Dietch and Jennings 1988). These effects are also reported in animals (Dodman 2000), thus benzodiazepines should be used with caution in aggressive animals, particularly dogs, since bite inhibition may be lessened. The potential for behavioral disinhibition serves as a contraindication for the use of benzodiazepines in fearful, but aggressive dogs. Bite inhibition may be diminished and the net effect may be an increased, rather than decreased, tendency to bite. Benzodiazepines are controlled substances with the potential for human substance abuse. Pet owners should be screened prior to prescribing and refill requests should be carefully scrutinized.

Although BZDs have a high safety margin, occasionally animals may be exposed to overdoses (accidental ingestion, for example) or have a paradoxical, unexpected reaction. In these instances it may be necessary to reverse the effects. Flumazenil (Romazicon) is a benzodiazepine-receptor antagonist and will inhibit the effects of BZDs. Flumazenil has been used to counteract the adverse effects of large overdoses of BZDs.

After daily administration for more than 1 week, a benzodiazepine should be withdrawn gradually to avoid discontinuation syndrome. Discontinuation syndrome, especially common in high-potency benzodiazepines such as alprazolam, includes nervousness, tremors, or even seizures (Roy-Byrne and Cowley 1991; Roy-Byrne et al. 1993). The longer a BZD is administered and the higher the dose used, the greater the likelihood of withdrawal reactions when it is discontinued, especially abruptly (Janicek 1997). Signs may be reversed by administration of the BZD. Discontinuation syndrome may be avoided by tapering the BZD dose 25% per week for 1 month. If a discontinuation reaction is observed, signs can be relieved by administering the implicated drug.

BZDs are used in dogs to treat fears and phobias as well as generalized anxiety. Benzodiazepines may be combined with a tricyclic antidepressant such as clomipramine to decrease latency to effect and reduce the paniclike states of thunderstorm phobia (Crowell-Davis et al. 2003) and separation anxiety (Sherman, pers. comm.). Among cats, BZDs are used for management of urine spraying, travel, and generalized anxiety, such as anxiety associated with changes in a new home environment.

Diazepam (Valium) is the best-known of the BZD (Fig. 21.1). It has been used for behavior disorders as a sedative, muscle relaxant, anxiolytic, anticonvulsant, and adjunct for anesthesia. It is a weak base with a low pK_a, has a benign taste, and is relatively easy to administer directly or by mixing in moist food. Its high lipophilicity and rapid distribution make it suitable for the emergency treatment of seizures because it crosses the blood-brain barrier quickly.

Its high lipophilicity allows it to be absorbed across membranes quickly and is even rapidly and almost completely absorbed from a rectal administration (Papich and Alcorn 1995). However, the vehicle carrier is not suitable for intramuscular administration. As an oral anxiolytic in dogs, particularly for paniclike states of thunderstorm phobia and separation anxiety, clinicians anecdotally report the anxiolytic performance of diazepam to be disappointing. Because hepatic clearance is high in dogs, oral doses are likely to be less effective than IV doses. If used orally in dogs, high doses may be sufficient to produce ataxia but insufficient to reduce anxiety. Other agents, such as alprazolam, may be more satisfactory, or a regime of daily, rather than PRN dosing, may be more effective.

In cats, diazepam has been used for treatment of urine spraying (Cooper and Hart 1992; Hart et al. 1993). In open trials, efficacy was approximately 55%, although relapse was common on discontinuation (Marder 1991; Cooper and Hart 1992).

The pharmacokinetics of diazepam are complex, but have been examined in both dogs and cats (Ballenger 1998; Löscher and Frey 1981; Papich and Alcorn 1995; Cotler et al. 1984). Diazepam undergoes metabolism first to a demethylated metabolite, desmethyldiazepam (also called nordiazepam), and then to oxazepam. Both of these metabolites are active, but not as active, or as lipid soluble as diazepam. Desmethyldiazepam is believed to have anticonvulsant properties that are equal to, (Randall et al. 1965), or about one-third of (Frey and Löscher 1982), the potency of diazepam. The pharmacokinetics of diazepam illustrate the tremendous species differences in clearance and elimination. In people, diazepam is considered a drug with low hepatic clearance and a long half-life. The half-life in people is 43 hours, (but may range from 24–48 hours) and systemic clearance is 0.38 ml/min/kg. In dogs, the half-life is less than 1 hour, and clearance is in excess of liver blood flow at 57–60 ml/min/kg (Papich and Alcorn 1985). Cats are intermediate between dogs and humans; the half-life in cats is 5.5 hours and the systemic clearance is 4.7 ml/min/kg (Cotler et al. 1984). In all species, the metabolites of diazepam have longer elimination half-lives than diazepam. For example, the half-life of desmethyldiazepam is 51–120 hr, 21.3 hours, and 2.2–2.8 hours for humans, cats, and dogs, respectively (Papich and Alcorn 1995; Cotler et al. 1984). These differences show that for long-term treatment, diazepam is not suitable for dogs because frequent administration is necessary to avoid high peaks and low troughs. However, its short half-life and ability to attain therapeutic concentrations makes it suitable for short-term use. This large difference in pharmacokinetics among species for diazepam means that information published for diazepam in humans will not apply to dogs. For example, P450 enzyme inhibition and other drug interactions cited for people are not likely in dogs because of the already-high systemic clearance. But, because liver clearance is dependent primarily on hepatic blood flow, changes in hepatic perfusion will drastically affect diazepam clearance. Clearance is expected to be altered in dogs with congenital or acquired hepatic vascular shunts.

The most serious adverse reaction associated with diazepam in companion animals is that of idiopathic hepatic necrosis in cats. Idiopathic hepatic necrosis is a rare but often-fatal condition, and has been documented in cats given oral diazepam. The specific etiology is not known (Center et al. 1996; House et al. 1996; Hughes et al. 1996). Diazepam undergoes complex metabolism to intermediate compounds. It is possible that in susceptible cats, an aberrant metabolite is produced that is responsible for the hepatic toxicosis. In the cats reported, the reaction occurred within 7 days of oral administration of generic or proprietary diazepam (House et al. 1996; Hughes et al. 1996). It is possible that in susceptible individuals, metabolites responsible for the toxicosis are more likely to be produced from oral administration because of first-pass metabolism, compared to parenteral administration. Idiopathic hepatic necrosis has not been reported after administration of other oral benzodiazepines, although that negative finding does not eliminate the possibility. However, the adverse event may be less likely with lorazepam and oxazepam, which are conjugated directly without undergoing intermediate metabolism. Alprazolam and temazepam appear to have only one intermediate (alpha-hydroxy) metabolite before undergoing conjugation. Compared to diazepam, these alternative drugs may be less likely to induce hepatic toxicosis in cats but safety studies are needed to confirm this theory.

The BZD clorazepate (Tranxene) is metabolized in the acidity of the stomach to its active metabolite before absorption (Ballenger 1998; Forrester et al. 1993). Clorazepate is used in dogs for treatment of anxiety disorders, particularly thunderstorm/noise phobia. Mean peak nordiazepam levels were detected approximately 98 minutes after a single oral dose of clorazepate, and 153 minutes after multiple oral doses (Forrester et al. 1990). The elimination half-life after a single dose (284 minutes) was not significantly different than after multiple doses (355 minutes) (Forrester et al. 1990). An oral dose of 2 mg/kg q12h maintains concentrations of the active metabolite, nordiazepam, in the range considered therapeutic in humans (Forrester et al. 1990). Excessive ataxia and sedation are uncommon (Forrester et al. 1990). Although available in a sustained-delivery formulation, one pharmacokinetic study in dogs found no difference in the serum disposition compared to immediate-release clorazepate (Brown and Forrester 1991).

Alprazolam (Xanax) is a high-potency benzodiazepine shown in humans to be an effective treatment for panic disorder (Fig. 21.1). It is used in dogs to treat the paniclike states of separation anxiety, thunderstorm phobia, and other phobias, as well as generalized anxiety. In people, it has a more rapid onset of action and shorter elimination half-life than diazepam, but these comparisons have not been reported for animals. In humans (Ballenger 1998; Brandwein 1993), plasma concentrations vary greatly among patients administered identical doses of alprazolam. As in humans, higher doses of alprazolam may be required for paniclike states in dogs, such as thunderstorm phobia and separation anxiety, compared to general anxiety. Thus, individualized dosing may be required to achieve treatment success with the fewest side effects (Ballenger 1998). Paradoxical excitement occurs in some canine patients given alprazolam. In such cases, the drug should be discontinued and a drug in another class should be selected. The mechanism of this paradoxical reaction is not known. Canine patients receiving alprazolam at a moderately high dose once a day, as may occur with separation anxiety or thunderstorm phobia, are at risk for withdrawal-induced anxiety or tremors prior to the next day's dose, due to its short elimination half-life (Moore 2000). This may be avoided by administering the drug twice a day and not skipping doses. To terminate the drug, alprazolam should be withdrawn slowly, decreasing the dose over weeks.

As mentioned previously, oxazepam (Serex) and lorazepam (Arivan) are metabolized directly via Phase II conjugation to inactive compounds (Ballenger 1998). Both oxazepam and lorazepam have been used by veterinarians as sedatives, anxiolytics, and anticonvulsants, but they are not as well-known as diazepam. There are no active metabolites. Because conjugation reactions are usually preserved, even when there is hepatic disease, these drugs are recommended for individuals with compromised liver function, for aged canine subjects in which metabolism may be slowed (Ballenger 1998), and in cats, in which Phase II metabolism may be less likely to trigger idiopathic hepatic necrosis.

In cats, oxazepam has been used as an appetite stimulant. Lorazepam has the advantage of a greater and more prolonged distribution to the CNS than other BZDs. Lorazepam in healthy dogs has a half-life of 0.88 hrs, a systemic clearance less than half that of diazepam at 19.3 ml/min/kg, and oral availability of 60% (Papich, unpublished research). Therefore, as an oral drug it may be a suitable alternative to diazepam.

In dogs, tricyclic antidepressants may be used with benzodiazepines for treatment of thunderstorm phobia (Crowell-Davis et al. 2003) and separation anxiety (Takeuchi et al. 2000). When alprazolam is given concomitantly with fluoxetine in humans, the result is a 30% increase in alprazolam levels (but no significant increases in fluoxetine or norfluoxetine plasma concentrations) due to cytochrome P450 CYP 3A inhibition (Lasher et al. 1991). Therefore, coadministration may permit a lower dose of alprazolam to be effective. Fluvoxamine inhibits the CYP450 3A4 enzyme and can be associated with increased levels of alprazolam (Ballenger 1998). In fact, the use of a BZD and an SSRI is a useful strategy with panic disorder in humans refractory to single drug therapy (Stahl 2008). Similar strategies may be helpful in animals, particularly dogs. Oxazepam has been shown in humans to decrease turnover of serotonin and norepinephrine (Ballinger 1998). In one pharmacokinetic study in dogs, clorazepate was used concurrently with phenobarbital (Forrester et al. 1993). The amount of the active metabolite nordiazepam in circulation during each dose interval was significantly reduced compared to administration of clorazepate alone (Forrester et al. 1990).

Azapirones. This class of anxiolytics is represented clinically by one drug, buspirone (Buspar). Buspirone was the first nonsedating, nonbenzodiazepine anxiolytic drug to be developed and marketed (Ninan et al. 1998). Buspirone acts as a full agonist at presynaptic $5HT_{1A}$ receptors, with resulting decrease in serotonin synthesis and inhibition of neuronal firing. It also acts as a partial agonist at postsynaptic $5HT_{1A}$ receptors. In serotonin deficit states, buspirone acts as an agonist (Ninan et al. 1998). Buspirone also has dopaminergic effects.

Buspirone is not a substrate for CYP450 enzymes, nor does it inhibit them (Ninan et al. 1998). It has no interactions with benzodiazepines and there are no withdrawal concerns after long-term use (Stahl 2008). In humans, buspirone has been effective for treatment of generalized anxiety disorder, but not for the control of panic disorder. Buspirone has demonstrated efficacy in certain animal models of anxiety, such as the conditioned avoidance response. In dogs, buspirone does not appear to be particularly therapeutic for the paniclike condition of thunderstorm phobia or separation anxiety, but it has been used for generalized anxiety.

Because it has a short elimination half-life, buspirone must be administered two or three times per day. Buspirone has a benign taste and may be given with food. In contrast to benzodiazepines, buspirone produces no sedation, no memory or psychomotor impairment, and no disinhibition phenomenon. Unlike the benzodiazepines, buspirone produces no immediate behavioral effects. Its beneficial effects are not observed until administration for several weeks. Side effects are uncommon and mild, but may be noted immediately. They include gastrointestinal signs and alterations in social behavior (often reported as increased "friendliness"). Buspirone has no potential for abuse.

In cats, buspirone is used to modulate states of high arousal, including feline urine spraying. In an open trial, improvement was observed in 55% of cats, with a 50% relapse rate following the cessation of treatment (Hart et al. 1993). It has also been used to reduce anxiety in the "pariah" cat in cases of intercat aggression within a household (Overall 1994a, 1999a).

Buspirone can be used to augment certain antidepressants. If used with an SSRI, increased efficacy is possible if intraneuronal serotonin has been depleted. Buspirone also may act directly on autoreceptors to inhibit neuronal impulse flow, possibly allowing repletion of 5HT stores. Also, buspirone may act at $5HT_{1A}$ receptors to aid in the targeted desensitization of $5HT_{1A}$ autoreceptors (Stahl 2008). In humans, buspirone may be used to augment SSRI treatment for OCD with success in some studies (Janicak et al. 1997) but not others (Grady et al. 1993). In dogs, buspirone has been used with tricyclic antidepressants to treat separation anxiety (Takeuchi et al. 2000) and with an SSRI (fluoxetine) to treat a complex case involving anxiety, aggression, and stereotypic behavior (Overall 1995).

NONBENZODIAZEPINE HYPNOTICS. In cases of acute-onset and severe phobic states, such as thunderstorm phobia and separation anxiety, there is a need for safe and rapid reduction in responsiveness to environmental stimuli and initiation of sleep, with relatively short duration of action and rapid recovery. The unpredictable and often disappointing effect of benzodiazepines and phenothiazines, and the long latency to effect of buspirone, leave a void with regard to such application. Nonbenzodiazepine hypnotics hold promise, since they are used to facilitate and maintain sleep for 3–7 hours in humans, although no published reports on their clinical use in dogs are available to date. Drugs in this class include zaleplon (Sonata), eszopiclone (Lunesta), and zolpidem (Ambien). Zaleplon has an ultrashort elimination half-life in humans, suggesting it unlikely to be useful in dogs. The newest agent, eszopiclone, is registered for the long-term treatment of insomnia in humans (Brielmaier 2006), but there are no reports of its clinical use in animals.

Zolpidem is a sedative of the imidazopyridine class. The usual human dose is 5–10 mg (also available as *CR*, controlled release formulation), used to promote and maintain sleep. Paradoxical excitation has been noted in some cases of administration to dogs (B. Sherman, pers. obs. 2000–2006). In a report of 33 cases of accidental ingestion of zolpidem by dogs presented to a poison control center, 40% exhibited signs of depression/sedation and 40% demonstrated signs of hyperactivity (Richardson et al. 2002). Although doses were extreme (up to 21 mg/kg), all dogs recovered. Clinical experience suggests at doses of 5–10 mg/dog, responses range from mild sedation (Juarbe-Diaz, pers. comm. 2006) to paradoxical CNS stimulation (B. Sherman, pers. obs. 2000–2006). These antecdotal reports suggest that, with appropriate case screening, zolpidem may be used to initiate sedation and diminish severe anxiety responses in dogs.

ANTIDEPRESSANTS. The general category of antidepressants includes a number of classes of drugs. Depending on the reference consulted, various classification systems have been used to group these drugs. Following convention, here, the structurally similar tricyclic antidepressants (TCAs) are discussed together. Drugs in this class include amitriptyline, imipramine, doxepin, and clomipramine. The functionally similar selective serotonin reuptake inhibitors (SSRIs) are discussed as a class. Drugs that act to inhibit the enzyme monoamine oxidase (MAOIs) are discussed as a class. Grouped as a separate "atypical" class are those antidepressants that fall outside the aforementioned three groups. This group includes the newer, heterocyclic drugs, such amoxapine, maprotiline, venlafaxine, and mirtazapine, which resemble TCAs, and older drugs, such as trazodone and bupropion, which have distinct chemical structures. The classes described above differ in their mode of action, their side effect profile, and their relative efficacy in certain behavioral disorders.

All antidepressants have important antianxiety properties, and at routine doses are generally well tolerated by animals. To some extent, all share a similar action, which is to alter neurotransmitter concentration (primarily norepinephrine and serotonin) at the receptor sites. The unifying theory that explains their efficacy is the *monoamine theory of depression* described by Schildkraut in 1965 (Maes and Meltazer 1995), which stated that depression in people is caused by a deficiency of monoamine neurotransmitters. Initially this theory focused on norepinephrine, but it became clear later that serotonin (5HT) also was an important neurotransmitter. The relationship of the mechanism to the neuronal effects and clinical response is complex. The action affecting reuptake of neurotransmitters occurs rapidly, but the clinical response may take days to weeks for maximum effect. This implies that the increased presence of neurotransmitters norepinephrine and 5HT also may affect the sensitivity of receptors, either presynaptically or postsynaptically.

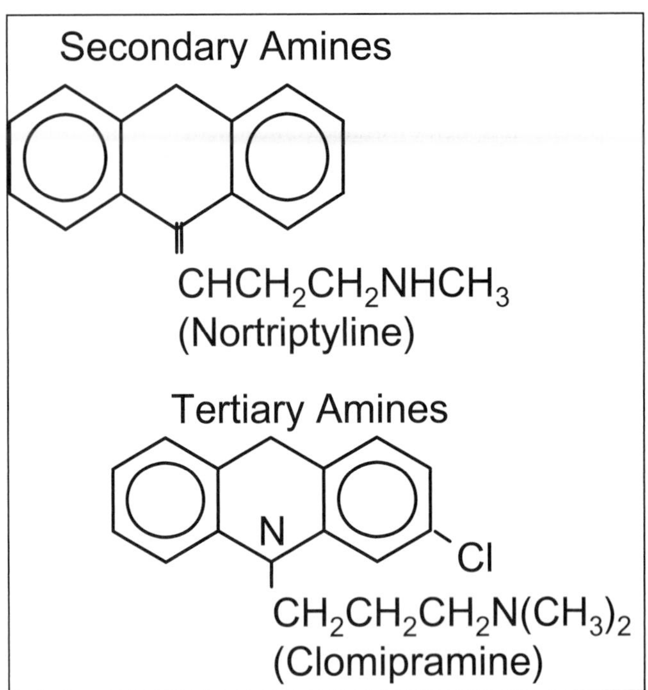

FIG. 21.2 Tricyclic antidepressants (TCAs) used to treat behavior disorders in veterinary medicine. Nortriptyline is a secondary amine and clomipramine is a tertiary amine. Most of the other TCAs used in veterinary medicine—amitriptyline (Elavil), doxepin (Sinequan), and imipramine (Tofranil)—are also tertiary amines.

Tricyclic Antidepressants. The tricyclic antidepressants (TCAs) are so-called because they have a three-ring nucleus (Fig. 21.2). Chemically they resemble phenothiazines, but their actions differ considerably. The TCAs inhibit the reuptake of serotonin and norepinephrine. Specific drugs vary in the extent to which they inhibit one transmitter more than the other. Some of these drugs familiar to veterinarians are human-label drugs that are used off-label. These include amitriptyline (Elavil), doxepin (Sinequan), and imipramine (Tofranil). All are tertiary amines (Fig. 21.2) and block the reuptake of both 5HT, and norepinephrine (Fig. 21.3). The secondary amines, such as nortriptyline (Pamelor) and desipramine (Norpramin), are not as well known to veterinarians. Secondary amines (Fig. 21.2) are relatively selective inhibitors of norepinephrine, but the tertiary amines inhibit both serotonin and norepinephrine (Fig. 21.3). Clomipramine (Clomicalm, veterinary label; and Anafranil human label), another tertiary amine, is most selective among the TCAs for blocking the reuptake of 5HT. TCAs also have antagonist activity for the α-adrenergic (alpha-1) receptor, and can produce antihistaminic and anticholinergic effects. The antagonist activity on these receptors is responsible for some of the side effects reported with TCAs, but most likely plays little role in their efficacy. As with other drugs in this article, there are species-specific differences in metabolism, elimination, and susceptibility to side effects that will be discussed in more detail with specific drugs.

TCAs have a long history of efficacious use in humans, but in recent years, they have been largely replaced by the more specific selective serotonin reuptake inhibitors. The low cost, efficacy, and tolerance of the TCAs make them particularly useful in small animal behavioral therapy. In general, the TCAs moderate excessive arousal and reduce anxiety. TCAs may enhance learning in specific circumstances (Mills and Ledger 2001). Unlike the benzodiazepines, the TCAs do not disinhibit behavior. TCAs are used in dogs to manage mild aggression, canine compulsive disorders, and various anxiety states (Juarbe-Diaz 1997a,b). TCAs may be used in cats to control certain forms of

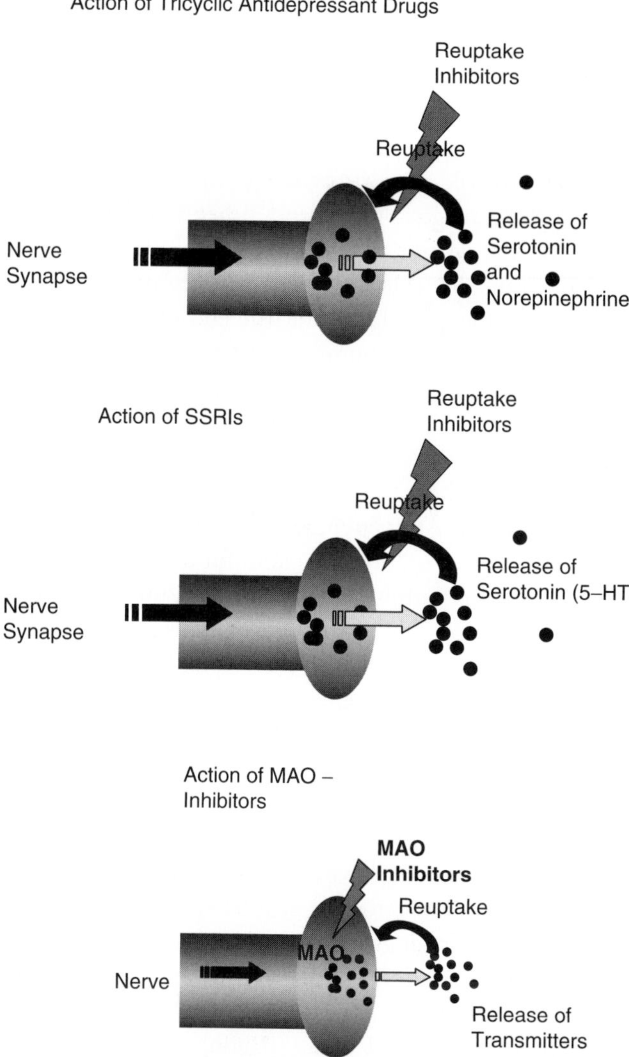

FIG. 21.3 Action of drugs used to treat behavior disorders in animals. Tricyclic antidepressants (top panel) inhibit the reuptake of serotonin and norepinephrine. Selective serotonin reuptake inhibitors (SSRI) (middle panel) selectively inhibit reuptake of serotonin without much effect on other receptors. Monoamine oxidase inhibitors (MAO-inhibitors) (bottom panel) inhibit the enzymatic breakdown of monoamines in the presynaptic nerve terminal. Specific types of MAO exist in the nervous system, such as MAO-type A and MAO-type B, depending on location.

aggression, inappropriate urination and spraying, excessive grooming, anxiety states, and excessive vocalization.

Because of the time to reach pharmacokinetic steady-state, and the time for modulation of the receptors affected by TCAs, therapeutic effects may not be seen for 2–4 weeks. Slow discontinuation of any TCA is recommended to avoid withdrawal responses, although these are generally not problematic and withdrawal reactions in animals have not been described.

In horses the TCAs have had limited use and there is little known about pharmacokinetics. Tricylic antidepressants, such as amitriptyline or imipramine, via their serotonin and norepinephrine reuptake inhibitor effects, may enhance behavioral calming; side effects can include mild sedation and anticholinergic effects in horses. Imipramine has been used to reduce anxiety in breeding males and is associated with masturbation and erection in males in sexual context. At high doses, imipramine (2–4 mg/kg q 24h, PO) can cause muscle fasciculations, tachycardia, and hyperresponsiveness to sound, likely due to norepinephrine effects.

TCAs are extensively metabolized and are CYP450 enzyme substrates. In people, coadministration of drugs that inhibit the CYP450 enzyme that is important for their metabolism can cause a fourfold increase in serum levels of TCAs. Drugs of the selective serotonin reuptake inhibitor class, described below, are potent inhibitors of CYP450 enzymes (Mealey 2002). Despite these potential risks, specific reports in the veterinary literature of drug interactions caused by coadministration of other drugs with TCAs are lacking. One reason for the lack of reported problems may be the high systemic clearance compared to humans, which indicates that there is less influence on changes in enzyme activity (discussed in more detail in the clomipramine section) and the high therapeutic index in animals. Nevertheless, because of the potential for drug-drug interactions in humans, caution is advised when prescribing a TCA with other drugs known to affect drug metabolism.

Adverse Effects. Adverse effects may occur soon after administration of the drug, or after chronic use. Side effects include mild sedation, gastrointestinal side effects—especially vomiting—antihistamine effects, and anticholinergic effects (Potter et al. 1998). Anticholinergic effects may include dry mouth (and consequent increased water consumption), constipation, and urinary retention. The use of TCAs is contraindicated in cases of glaucoma or keratoconjunctivitis sicca.

A particularly serious adverse effect is possible when TCAs are administered at high doses, as in an accidental ingestion by a pet, for example. High concentrations of TCAs can cause a quinidinelike membrane-stabilizing effect that can lead to fatal cardiac arrhythmias if patients are not treated promptly (Potter et al. 1998; Johnson 1990; Wismer 2000). If animals receive a high dose (a toxic dose may be over 15 mg/kg), an ECG should be monitored immediately for conduction disturbances. If available, blood pressure should be monitored as well. Treatment of overdoses should be initiated at once, because deaths have occurred within 2 hours. Contact an animal poison control center for specific therapy. Treatment consists of gastric lavage, activated charcoal, a suitable cathartic (*not* containing magnesium), and sodium bicarbonate therapy. Antiarrhythmics that do not affect conduction may be indicated, such as lidocaine, but other Class I antiarrhythmics such as procainamide and quinidine are contraindicated (antiarrhythmic drugs are discussed in more detail in Chapter 23).

The cardiotoxic effect described above should not be confused with the effect on the heart produced as an anticholinergic side effect or adrenergic-blockade by TCAs. These drugs may elevate heart rate in some individuals caused by the anticholinergic effects, or lower the heart rate in others as a reflex response to the alpha-1 adrenergic effects. Before administering a TCA to animals, it is suggested to conduct a cardiac assessment (evaluate history, auscultate, ECG if indicated) prior to administration (Pacher et al. 1999). In a study in which effects on the cardiac ECG were evaluated in otherwise healthy dogs administered either clomipramine or amitriptyline, there was no evidence of ECG abnormalities (Reich et al. 2000). In this study, the drugs were administered at doses recommended for treatment of behavior problems.

Tricyclic antidepressants may also lower seizure threshold and potentiate seizures in predisposed animals (Juarbe-Diaz 1997a). Agranulocytosis has been associated with TCA administration, but it is rare (Alderman et al. 1993).

TCAs may be difficult to administer directly or disguised in food since they have a lingering bitter taste. Biting the tablet can induce taste aversion, future dosing avoidance, and hypersalivation.

The TCAs have also been used to treat pain syndromes. As reviewed by Micó et al. (2006), there is good evidence that TCAs are effective in people for treating pain, especially neuropathic pain and may be used in combination with other drugs. Some veterinarians have also used these drugs for treatment of pain, although there are no published reports. The mechanism for analgesia is not entirely understood. It is probably not via the same mechanism that affects anxiety and depression because the analgesic effects have been documented to occur at lower doses and the onset of pain relief occurs faster than relief from depression and anxiety. The proposed mechanism of action for analgesia is via increased availability of norepinephrine and serotonin at the synapse, but other neurotransmitters also could be involved. Amitriptyline seems to be the gold standard for analgesic uses, and other antidepressants, such as SSRIs, do not appear to be as effective. Of note, the drug tramadol (Ultram) used for treatment of pain (discussed in Chapter 12 and at the end of this chapter) has some opioid effects, but in addition, has similar effects as TCAs—inhibition of serotonin and norepinephrine reuptake.

Amitriptyline. Amitriptyline is used in humans for depression, anxiety disorders, and for certain types of chronic or neuropathic pain (Anderson 2001). It exerts active reuptake inhibition on serotonin receptors relative to norepinephrine receptors. It has strong anticholinergic, antihistamine, alpha-1 adrenergic, and analgesic properties (Anderson 2001; Potter et al. 1998). Nortriptyline, also commercially available (Pamelor), is the active metabolite (Anderson 2001; Boothe 2001).

Amitriptyline (Elavil) has been a useful drug in animals to enhance behavioral calming and augment a behavioral treatment program (Anderson 2001; Hart and Cooper 1996). In dogs, amitriptyline has been used for treatment of separation anxiety (Takeuchhi et al. 2000), aggression (Anderson 2001; Reich 1999), and repetitive self-trauma (Overall 1997a, 1998b). The time for maximum effect is 2–4 weeks (Anderson 2001). In cats, amitriptyline has been used for psychogenic alopecia (Sawyer et al. 1999).

Reported side effects in cats include weight gain, somnolence, and decreased grooming (Chew et al. 1998). Once-a-day, nighttime dosing is recommended to avoid excessive daytime sedation (Chew et al. 1998). Because there is a generic formulation, it has been popular among veterinarians desiring inexpensive treatments for patients.

Among the most common use in cats is administration for urinary disorders. It has been used for urine marking and inappropriate urination secondary to idiopathic interstitial cystitis (Chew et al. 1998). Amitriptyline stimulates β-adrenergic receptors in smooth muscle, including the urinary bladder, to cause a decrease in smooth muscle excitability and an increase in bladder capacity (Anderson 2001;

Chew et al. 1998). It also has been one of the more effective drugs for treating pain syndromes (Micó et al. 2006). For these reasons, it has been used to treat feline interstitial cystitis at an initial dose of 10 mg/cat once in the evening (Chew et al. 1998; Buffington et al. 1999). It is not known if an analgesic effect or behavior-modifying effect plays a role in the efficacy for treatment of this disease.

Imipramine. Imipramine (Tofranil) is a TCA with properties similar to amitriptyline except that imipramine has similar affinity for norepinephrine and serotonin receptors. Imipramine has only moderate affinity for H_1, or muscarinic (anticholinergic) receptors. Imipramine has more serotonergic activity, fewer anticholinergic effects, and modest alpha-agonist properties. In humans, imipramine has an elimination half-life of approximately 12 hours. Pharmacokinetics have not been reported for dogs, but empirically it has been administered twice daily to dogs.

Imipramine has been successfully used in humans to treat panic disorder in adults and nocturnal enuresis (bed-wetting) in children. It is a modestly priced treatment for narcolepsy in dogs and horses (Coleman 1999). Imipramine may be used to treat separation anxiety (Marder 1991; Overall et al. 2001), particularly in those cases in which urine house-soiling is problematic (Sherman, pers. obs.). Imipramine may also be used in cases of estrogen-dependent urinary incontinence in dogs intolerant to phenylpropanolamine. In one study of laboratory beagles, after 14 days treatment at a high dose (10 mg/kg q24h), imipramine improved abnormal "withdrawn and depressed" behavior (Iorio et al. 1983).

Clomipramine. Clomipramine (Clomicalm, veterinary label; Anafranil, human label) has the most serotonergic activity of all the TCAs. It is approved in humans for the treatment of obsessive-compulsive disorder (OCD) and was the first veterinary drug registered to treat separation anxiety in dogs.

Dogs metabolize clomipramine more rapidly than humans, which affects clinical use. The average half-life in dogs is 5 hours (King et al. 2000a), 7.2 hours (Hewson et al. 1998a) after single dose administration, and 2.1–4 hours after repeated doses (King et al. 2000b) The half-life of, desmethylclomipramine, an active metabolite, is 2.9 hours (King et al. 2000a), 1.9 hours (Hewson et al. 1998a) and 2.2–3.8 hours after multiple doses (King et al. 2000b). By comparison, the half-life in humans is 24 hours (Potter et al. 1998) to 33 hours, and has been reported to be as high as 36–50 hours (Evans et al. 1980). The systemic clearance in dogs is rapid (23.3 ml/kg/min). The evidence indicates therefore, that in dogs, clomipramine is a high clearance drug for which hepatic blood flow is the most important factor in clearance. Changes in enzyme activity (cytochrome P450 alterations) or protein binding are not expected to affect clomipramine pharmacokinetics as it does in humans.

Oral absorption is only 16–20% in dogs (King et al. 2000a); the low systemic availability is probably reduced because of first-pass hepatic clearance. There are also differences between humans and dogs regarding metabolite profile. In dogs, the ratio of clomipramine to the desmethylclomipramine metabolite is 3 : 1, whereas in people this ratio is only 1 : 2.5. Clomipramine is believed to act primarily as a serotonin reuptake inhibitor, but the desmethyl metabolite is probably most responsible for the anticholinergic side effects. This may explain why there appears to be fewer anticholinergic side effects in dogs compared to people from this drug.

Despite the relatively short half-life in dogs, it has been effective when administered every 12 or 24 hours (King et al. 2000b). Clomipramine has been effective for treatment of canine compulsive disorder (Hewson et al. 1998b; Seksel and Lindeman 2001) such as tail chasing (Moon-Fanelli and Dodman 1998), or acral lick granuloma (Goldberger and Rapoport 1991; Rapoport et al. 1992). Clomipramine (Clomicalm) is approved in the U.S. for the treatment of separation anxiety in dogs (King et al. 2000; Simpson 2000), although there is debate concerning the relative merits of behavioral versus pharmacological components to treatment (Podberscek et al. 1999). In one study, clomipramine was no more effective than controls for the treatment of dominance-related aggression in dogs (White et al. 1999). Clomipramine may be helpful in some cases of noise phobia (Seksel and Lindeman 2001), but additional treatment with a benzodiazepine, such as alprazolam, may be necessary (Crowell-Davis et al. 2003).

Clomipramine has been used in cats to manage urine spraying (DeHasse 1997; King et al. 2004), hyperesthesia (Sherman, pers. obs. 2000–2002), and some feline compulsive behavior, including psychogenic alopecia (Sawyer et al. 1999).

Selective Serotonin Reuptake Inhibitors. As the name implies, selective serotonin reuptake inhibitors (SSRIs), are more specific than the TCAs. SSRIs block the reuptake of serotonin, making more available in the synapse, with little effect on the reuptake of norepinephrine (Fig. 21.3).

The SSRIs include fluoxetine (Reconcile, veterinary label; Prozac, human label), paroxetine (Paxil), sertraline (Zoloft), fluvoxamine (Luvox), citalopram (Celexa), and escitalopram (Lexapro). All are approved by the FDA for treatment of depression in humans. SSRIs are efficacious for the treatment of panic disorder in humans (Tollefson and Rosenbaum 1998). Only fluoxetine (Reconcile) is registered for use in dogs (Simpson et al. 2007). Often a low dose is used to initiate therapy, then it is titrated upward as necessary (Tollefson and Rosenbaum 1998). Most SSRIs have been shown to be effective in treatment of human obsessive-compulsive disorder (Tollefson and Rosenbaum 1998). Higher doses and longer treatments may be required to obtain satisfactory response for this problem (Tollefson and Rosenbaum 1998). In humans, eating disorders, impulsivity, aggression, pain syndromes, and premenstrual dysphoria also have been successfully treated with SSRIs, compared to controls (Tollefson and Rosenbaum 1998).

In dogs, SSRIs have been used clinically for management of separation anxiety (Simpson et al. 2007), compulsive behaviors, and dominance-type (Dodman et al. 2001) or impulsive aggression (Peremans et al. 2005). Fluoxetine is the first drug of this class to be registered by the FDA for use in dogs (Simpson et al. 2007). In cats, SSRIs are used to treat urine spraying, aggression, and compulsive behavior such as psychogenic alopecia and fabric chewing. Due to concerns about GIT side effects, cats medicated with SSRIs should be closely monitored for food and water consumption, and fecal and urinary elimination, as well as body weight.

There is evidence that individuals who exhibit violent behavior have low CNS serotonin activity, as measured by the CSF concentrations of serotonin metabolites (rhesus macaques, Mehlman et al. 1994; dogs, Reisner 1996). Therefore, serotonin enhancing agents have been used to treat certain forms of aggression, particularly dominance-related aggression (Dodman et al. 1996a; Peremans et al. 2005).

In horses, there is little known about the metabolism and effects of SSRIs. Fluoxetine, a selective serotonin reuptake inhibitor with anxiolyic and anticompulsive effects, may require 1–4 weeks to effect. Fluoxetine may decrease libido in breeding animals; higher doses of fluoxetine may cause serotonin effects in the intestine.

Adverse Effects. In general, SSRIs have an excellent safety record. Side effects vary from agent to agent, but include gastrointestinal effects and nervous system alterations ranging from sedation to agitation, irritability, and insomnia. In a study of fluoxetine in dogs (Sherman et al. 2007) in which 122 dogs were treated with fluoxetine and 120 with placebo, the most common side effect was lethargy/depression/calming (45%). The second most common effect reported was anorexia/decreased appetite (29%). Sexual dysfunction is reported in humans under treatment with SSRIs. Fluoxetine and fluvoxamine shorten REM sleep in animal models (Tollefson and Rosenbaum 1998). Gastrointestinal effects (up to 25% of humans) are likely due to the concentration of serotonin receptors in the GIT. SSRIs are considered to cause less effect on cardiac impulse conduction than TCAs (Pacher et al. 1999). Starting a patient at a low dose and then increasing after 1 week may reduce the likelihood of problematic side effects (Sherman, pers. obs.). Onset to action may be 1–4 weeks (Simpson et al. 2007).

In people, there is great variation in the effect of SSRIs on cytochrome P450 enzymes. These differences have not been reported in animals. In people, fluoxetine, fluvoxamine, and paroxetine all inhibit one or more CYP enzymes; sertraline, citalopram, and escitalopram do not. Phenobarbital and other anticonvulsants induce specific CYP enzymes, principally CYP1A2 and CYP3A3/4. Drug interactions have been infrequently reported from administration of an SSRI to animals. Because the type and extent to which the CYP450 enzymes are responsible for metabolism of SSRIs in animals, it is difficult to predict potential drug interactions.

Fluoxetine. Fluoxetine (Reconcile, veterinary ↓ Fever label, Prozac, human label) is widely used to treat a range of human behavioral disorders, including depression, generalized anxiety, panic disorder, obsessive-compulsive disorder, eating disorders, and premenstrual dysphoria (Figure 21.4).

Among dogs, fluoxetine has been used for treatment of dominance-related aggression (Overall 1999a; Dodman et al. 1996a), interdog aggression (Dodman 2000) and acral lick dermatitis (Rapoport et al. 1992; Wynchank and Berk 1998a) as well as other compulsive disorders (Irimajiri and Luescher 2005). It is licensed by the FDA for canine separation anxiety (Simpson et al. 2007). Fluoxetine has also been used to successfully treat stereotypical

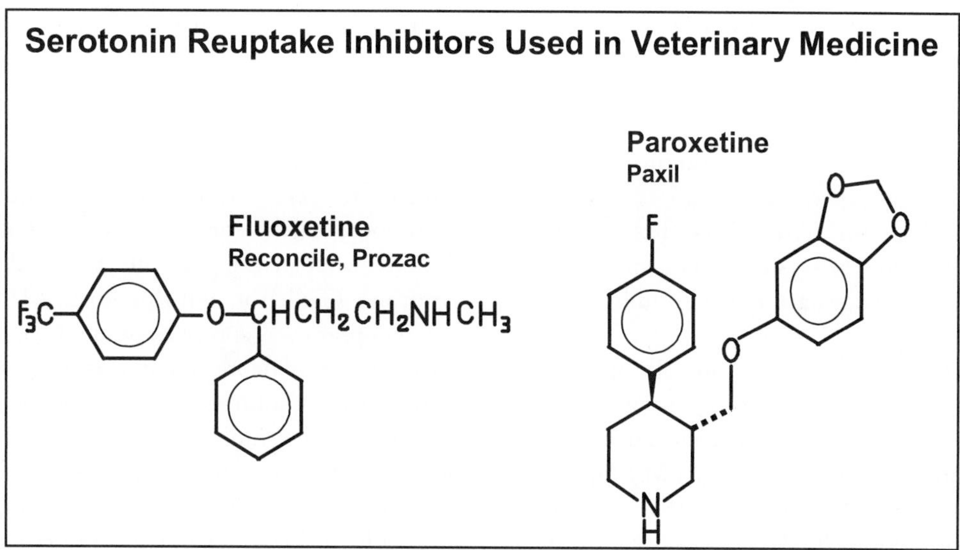

FIG. 21.4 Selective serotonin reuptake inhibitors (SSRIs) used in veterinary medicine. Fluoxetine (left) and paroxetine (right). Only fluoxetine (Reconcile) is licensed for veterinary use.

pacing of 22 years' duration in a captive polar bear; relapse occurred after discontinuation of treatment (Poulsen et al. 1996).

Among cats, fluoxetine has been used for treatment of refractory urine spraying (Pryor et al. 2001), inappropriate urination (Romatowski 1998), psychogenic alopecia (Hartman 1995; Romatowski 1998), and aggression (Overall 1999b; Romatowski 1998).

The approved canine form is available as 8, 16, 32, and 64 mg chewable flavored tablets. The human form is available in solid dose form as 10 and 20 mg capsules that must be divided or compounded for smaller animals, or 10 or 20 mg tablets that can be broken. There is a 4 mg/ml oral liquid solution, but it has 0.23% alcohol, which some animals (especially cats) may find unpalatable. The usual dose for dogs is 1–2 mg/kg oral per day (Simpson et al. 2007); the dose for cats is 0.5–1.0 mg/kg oral per day (Landsberg et al. 2003; Pryor et al. 2001).

Fluoxetine is metabolized to norfluoxetine, its active metabolite. Norfluoxetine has an elimination half-life of 4–16 days in humans (Tollefson and Rosenbaum 1998). After a single dose in dogs, fluoxetine has an elimination half-life of 3–13 hours; norfluoxetine has an elimination half life of 33–64 hours (Reconcile package insert, Lilly 2007). This long half-life offers protection from the discontinuation syndromes associated with abrupt interruption or termination of treatment. It also necessitates a washout period after discontinuation of fluoxetine and initiation of a monoamine oxidase inhibitor such as selegiline (Tollefson and Rosenbaum 1998; Reconcile package insert, Lilly 2007).

In people, extrapyramidal side effects are a rare consequence of therapy with fluoxetine. These are likely due to inhibition of dopaminergic transmission (Tollefson and Rosenbaum 1998). Inappetence is a common side effect (Pryor et al. 2001; Simpson et al. 2007); lethargy has been reported (Simpson et al. 2007; Hartman 1995; Pryor et al. 2001); vomiting is rare (Pryor et al. 2001).

In dogs the most common effect in clinical trials was sedation and calming effects, followed by anorexia and weight loss. Less common effects observed were vomiting, shaking, diarrhea, restlessness, vocalization, aggression, and, in rare cases, seizures. Treatment with fluoxetine in dogs for acral lick dermatitis was well-tolerated (Wynchank and Berk 1998b).

Paroxetine. Like fluoxetine, paroxetine is used in humans to treat a range of psychiatric complaints, including depression, social anxiety, and panic disorder (Fig. 21.4). It has shown efficacy for the management of episodic aggressive rages in Tourette's patients (Bruun and Budman 1998). Paroxetine is considered by some to be the first choice for treatment of generalized anxiety (Moore 2000).

In dogs, paroxetine may be helpful for the treatment of canine aggression and canine compulsive disorders but efficacy has not been documented as well as for fluoxetine. In cats, paroxetine has been used for compulsive behaviors, redirected aggression, and generalized anxiety. Paroxetine is available in 10, 20, 30, and 40 mg tablets that can be more easily divided than capsules and administered orally to cats.

Compared to fluoxetine, paroxetine has a shorter elimination half-life and reaches steady-state more rapidly. However, pharmacokinetics have not been fully reported for animals.

Unlike fluoxetine, anticholinergic side effects, such as dry mouth and constipation, are more common with paroxetine. Paroxetine can cause an idiosyncratic, dose-dependent increase in arousal, wakening, and REM suppression in humans (Tollefson and Rosenbaum 1998) and dogs (Sherman, pers. obs. 2000–2002). After chronic administration, paroxetine should be gradually withdrawn over several weeks to avoid a discontinuation reaction, typified by increased anxiety (Michelson et al. 2000).

Constipation is a common anticholinergic side effect of paroxetine use in cats. Cats should be carefully monitored for food and water consumption and urine and feces production during the first week of therapy. Reducing the target dose by half for the first week can avoid such side effects (Sherman, pers. obs. 2000–2006). Weight gain is a common side effect in cats with paroxetine treatment (Sherman, pers. obs. 2000–2006). To avoid negative metabolic consequences of weight gain, the body weight of cats receiving paroxetine treatment should be monitored closely.

Other SSRIs. Sertraline is an SSRI with pharmacokinetic properties in humans similar to paroxetine. Like other SSRIs, in humans, it is used for a range of behavioral disorders including panic disorder, chronic depression, compulsive disorders, and anxiety (Sheikh et al. 2000). It is considered by some to be the first choice for treatment of panic disorder in humans (Moore 2000) and may provide some cognitive benefits to elderly patients, compared to other SSRIs. Like other SSRIs, sertraline has been used as a treatment for eating disorders. In one report, sertraline was used to successfully treat chronic regurgitation, deemed to be a compulsive behavior in a chimpanzee (Howell et al. 1997). In a study of male anoles (*Anolis carolinensis*), sertraline reversed dominant social status (Larson and Summers 2001).

In dogs, sertraline can be helpful for compulsive behaviors (Rapoport et al. 1992), aggression (Larson and Summers 2001) and anxiety disorders. In dogs, diarrhea is a common side effect. This may be circumvented by starting the drug at a low dose and increasing over 2 weeks.

Fluvoxamine is distinguished by its lack of activity in humans at CYP2D6 isozyme. Therefore in people it has been more safely combined with TCAs. Fluvoxamine should be taped off gradually to avoid discontinuation syndrome (Tollefson and Rosenbaum 1998).

Citalopram was approved by the U.S. FDA in 1998 for the treatment of depression in humans, after a long history of safe human administration in Europe (Pollock 2001). Although early studies of citalopram administration to dogs at high doses (20 mg/kg, Boeck et al. 1982) revealed no cardiac effects, one toxicity study of 10 beagle dogs given a high dose of citalopram (8 mg/kg/day) for 17–31 weeks suffered 50% mortality due to cardiac effects (Forest Pharmaceuticals, Inc. *Celexa Product Information.* p. 16. St. Louis: Warner-Lambert Company, 1998). Citalopram has been used to treat acral lick dermatitis in dogs at a dose of 0.5–1.0 mg/kg/day (Stein et al. 1998). Citalopram may modulate aggressive behavior in humans (Reiste et al. 2003) and dogs. One study of impulsive aggressive dogs (N = 9) treated for 6 weeks with citalopram demonstrated behavioral improvement (Peremans et al. 2005). Based on the suggestion of increased cardiac sensitivity to citalopram particularly in beagle dogs, cardiac screening (Pacher at al. 1999) and conservative dosing, or alternative drug selection are recommended. To date, there are no published reports of the use of citalopram in cats.

The S-isomer of racemic citalopram, escitalopram (Lexapro, Forest Pharmaceuticals), may be promising for the treatment of behavioral disorders in dogs, but at this time, there is limited information. It is a potent and highly selective inhibitor of CNS neuronal reuptake of serotonin. No published studies are currently available for its use in companion animals. At present, the relatively high price of escitalopram limits its veterinary use.

It has recently been recognized that SSRIs may have effects other than those on the central nervous system. The SSRIs have been shown to have antimicrobial activity, primarily against gram-positive bacteria (Munoz-Bellido et al. 2000). They have little activity on gram-negative bacteria. They also have activity against fungi such as *Candida* spp. and *Aspergillus* spp. (Lass-Florl et al. 2001). Despite the attractiveness of this feature of the SSRIs, they have not been employed as antiinfective drugs at this time. It is not known if the antimicrobial effects are relevant at clinical dosages.

As discussed for the TCAs, antidepressants have been used for treatment of pain (Micó et al. 2006). However, the strongest evidence has been for TCA drugs, which have effects on neurotransmitters (norepinephrine, histamine, dopamine) other than serotonin. Although there is some evidence for an analgesic effect from SSRI drugs, it is not as convincing as for TCA drugs.

Atypical Antidepressants. The atypical antidepressants are a diverse category of heterocyclic drugs. These include trazodone (Desyrel), nefazodone (Serzone), bupropion (Welbutrin, Welbutrin XL, Zyban), and mirtazapine (Remeron). Because of its rare association in humans with life-threatening liver failure, nefazodone is now rarely prescribed. Because of its stimulating effect, buproprion does not sufficiently enhance behavioral calming in animals to be clinically useful. Discussed below are the atypical antidepressants trazodone and mirtazapine.

Most notable in this group for clinical use in small animals is trazodone. Trazodone is a mixed serotonergic agonist/antagonist. It has no anticholinergic effects, moderate antihistaminergic activity, and is an antagonist of postsynaptic α_1-adrenergic receptors. Trazodone is well absorbed after oral administration, with peak blood levels in humans approximately 1 hour after administration on an empty stomach, 2 hours after dosing when given with food (Golden et al. 1998). Empirically, rapid absorption also occurs in dogs (Sherman, pers. obs. 1997–2007).

In humans, the cytochrome isozyme CYP2D6 is involved in the metabolism of trazodone and caution is advised when prescribing trazodone with SSRIs that inhibit CYP2D6 (Golden et al. 1998). However, the wide safe dose range for trazodone makes this less problematic than other drugs, such as the TCAs. Trazodone is used in humans for treatment of major depression and to counter the sleep disturbances caused by SSRIs. When given over weeks, it produces anxiolytic properties similar to diazepam (Golden et al. 1998).

Trazodone has been used in dogs for mild thunderstorm phobia and as an adjunct to TCA or SSRI treatment (Sherman, pers. obs. 1997–2002; Gruen and Sherman 2008). However, trazodone may have some limitations. In one study of four "depressed" laboratory beagles, no effect was noted after administration of trazodone at a high dose (10 mg/kg; Iorio et al. 1983); its effects appear insufficient in severe cases of thunderstorm phobia (Sherman, pers. obs. 1997–2002). Side effects in dogs include sedation and GIT issues, including vomiting and diarrhea (Sherman, pers. obs. 1997–2002), particularly during the first few days of dosing. Starting at a low dose and titrating the dose up over the initial days and subsequent weeks may be helpful (Gruen and Sherman 2008). Priapism, noted as a rare side effect in human males, has not been observed in neutered male dogs (Sherman, pers. obs. 1997–2007).

Trazodone may be used in combination with antidepressants, particularly SSRIs, to enhance behavioral calming, decrease agitation, and to aid with sleep. This can be helpful in humans with depression, obsessive-compulsive disorder, and other anxiety disorders (Stahl 2008). It may be similarly effective in dogs (Sherman, pers. obs. 1997–2002).

Mirtazapine exhibits noradrenergic and serotonergic activity through its activity as an α-2 antagonist. In humans, it is used to manage depression and anxiety. Mirtazapine is a potent antagonist of histamine H1 receptors, which may account for its sedative effects. The antagonism of $5HT_3$ receptors by mirtazapine results in an antiemetic effect, suggesting that mirtazapine could be considered a successful antiemetic agent in patients suffering from nausea and vomiting. Although uncommonly used for the treatment of primary behavior problems in animals, it has recently found safe and useful application in the management of anorexia in dogs and cats. Elimination half-life in dogs ranges from 20–40 hours and reaches a steady-state in 4–6 days (Mandelker 2006). The elimination half-life in cats is approximately three times that of dogs; cats are effectively dosed every 3 days (Mandelker 2006).

Monoamine Oxidase Inhibitors. Monoamine oxidase inhibitors (MAOIs) are drugs that inhibit the intracellular enzyme monoamine oxidase (MAO). Since MAO catabolizes intracellular monoamine neurotransmitters, such as serotonin, dopamine, norepinephrine, and tyramine, MAOIs inhibit this process, causing an increase in monoamines. There are two MAO subtypes, A, which affect serotonin, dopamine, norepinephrine, and tyramine, and B, which affect the metabolism of phenylethylamine as well as dopamine. Location of the enzymes also characterizes the differences between Type A and B. Type A is located in the intestine as well as the CNS. If MAO-Type A is inhibited, it can produce a decrease in the metabolism of compounds from foods that can produce systemic effects. However, this effect has not been well characterized in animals, perhaps because of the rare clinical use of these drugs.

The nonselective (Type A and B) MAO-inhibitors are not used to any extent in veterinary medicine. Only one MAO-B inhibitor, selegiline (L-deprenyl, Anipryl), is clinically important as a behavioral treatment in animals. Selegiline is approved by the FDA for treatment of canine cognitive dysfunction, a disorder of elderly dogs characterized by decreased social interactions, loss of housetraining, confusion, and changes in sleep cycle (Milgram et al. 1993; Ruehl et al. 1995). Selegiline has been known by many names. Selegiline hydrochloride is the official USP drug name, but most clinicians know it by the older name L-deprenyl. (L-deprenyl is distinguished from its steroisomer D-deprenyl.) It was used in humans for treatment of Parkinson's disease and occasionally for Alzheimer's disease with the trade name *Eldepryl.* (Efficacy for Alzheimer's disease has not been established.) It has recently become available as a patch used for treatment of cognitive impairment and depression in humans. The veterinary formulation is *Anipryl.*

There is evidence that these behavioral changes have a histolopathologic (Cummings et al. 1996) and metabolic (Milgram et al. 1993) basis and selegiline may affect these changes. However, at currently registered doses for dogs, it has not produced beneficial effects on anxiety or depression and is generally not used for this purpose by veterinary behavior experts in the United States.

The action of selegiline is to inhibit MAO type B (and other MAOs at higher doses). Studies in dogs showed that MAO inhibition was specific at doses of 1 mg/kg (Milgram et al. 1993, 1995). The proposed mechanism of action of this drug is to inhibit the metabolism of dopamine in the central nervous system (Bruyette et al. 1995). The theory to explain the beneficial response is that dopamine depletion in the brain and loss of dopaminergic neurons leads to cognitive dysfunction (dementia) in old dogs. Treatment with selegiline inhibits MAO type B and increases dopamine concentrations in the brain, which restores neurotransmitter balance and improves cognitive ability. It also inhibits the metabolism of phenylethylamine (Milgram et al. 1993, 1995). (Phenylethylamine in laboratory animals produces amphetaminelike effects.) There are two active metabolites, L-amphetamine and L-methamphetamine. In dogs, even though there were increases in amphetamine concentrations, (Milgram et al. 1993) they were not high enough to produce adverse effects. However, at high doses (>3 mg/kg) the authors proposed that increased amphetamine concentrations could explain the observed behavioral changes. The L-isomer metabolites are not as active as their D-forms and studies have not supported a potential for amphetamine-like abuse or dependency from selegiline, compared to other amphetaminelike drugs.

In clinical trials, selegiline significantly improved clinical signs of cognitive dysfunction in treated dogs compared to controls. Selegiline may also improve learning (Mills and Ledger 2001). In general, selegiline is given daily for a month. Any improvement in clinical signs dictates continuation of treatment: additional improvement is often seen in subsequent months (Calves 2000). Treatment failure should prompt an increase in daily dose and an additional trial of medication. As an extralabel application, selegiline has also been used in geriatric cats diagnosed with cognitive dysfunction.

Side effects are uncommon, but high doses can cause hyperactivity and stereotypic behavior in dogs. In studies in dogs in which selegiline was administered a doses of 1, 4, or 16 mg/kg for 1 year, adverse effects were rare. At high doses salivation, panting, repetitive movements, decreased weight, and changes in activity level were noted. In one report (Milgram et al. 1993), changes in behavior were not seen until doses exceeded 3 mg/kg, which the authors attributed to amphetaminelike effects.

Selegiline is also FDA-approved for treating canine pituitary-dependent hyperadrenocorticism (PDH). The mechanism of action to explain selegiline's effect for treating PDH is potentiation of dopamine. Increased dopamine levels in the brain decreases ACTH release, resulting in lower cortisol levels (Bruyette et al. 1995, 1996). (Blockade of dopamine enhances CRH-mediated ACTH release in normal dogs.) In 52 dogs with PDH, administered selegiline at 1.0 mg/kg once daily, there was significant improvement in polyuria-polydipsia, appetite, activity, thinning of skin and alopecia, body weight, and body conformation (Bruyette et al. 1996). There was also a significantly lower mean response in the low-dose dexamethasone suppression test (LDDS). Overall, selegiline was evaluated as effective in 71% of dogs and not effective in 21%. Side effects of therapy were rare. However, other studies released after the drug's FDA registration have not been as convincing. In one study, the authors found a much smaller percentage of PDH dogs that responded to selegiline and they did not recommend this drug for treatment (Reusch et al. 1999). Perhaps only dogs with pars intermedia lesions of the pituitary will respond to selegiline, which represents 30% or less of canine PDH cases (Peterson 1999).

Tricyclic antidepressants and selective serotonin reuptake inhibitors should not be used concurrently with monoamine oxidase inhibitors such as selegiline (L-deprenyl) or amitraz, a topical product used for control of ticks and mites.

MAOIs can sufficiently inhibit catabolism of monoamines that their concentration, particularly serotonin, becomes toxic. This may occur when other antidepressants that inhibit reuptake of serotonin or inhibit MAO are used concurrently. This can lead to serotonin syndrome, a potentially fatal condition, characterized by hypertension, hyperthermia, restlessness, tremor, seizures, and altered mental status (Calves 2000; Tollefson and Rosenbaum 1998; Wismer 2000). Thus, an MAOI should not be used with an antidepressant, including TCAs (Anderson 2001). Drugs from one class should be discontinued 14 days before agents from the other class are initiated (Anderson 2001).

Because selegiline may affect other monoamine synthesis, there has been concern about its administration with sympathetic amines used to treat urinary incontinence in dogs, such as phenylpropanolamine (PPA). However, when this was studied, selegiline had no effect on pulse rate, ECG, or behavior compared to administration of phenylpropanolamine alone in dogs (Cohn et al. 2002).

Concurrent use of α-2 agonists, phenothiazines, and opiate analgesics is discouraged with selegiline. A standard recommendation is to wait at least five times the elimination half-life of the SSRI or its active metabolite (whichever is longer), before administering the next serotonergic agent (Tollefson and Rosenbaum 1998). A washout period of 1–3 weeks is recommended after discontinuation of an MAOI and initiation of another drug that affects monoamines.

MISCELLANEOUS DRUGS

Anticonvulsant Drugs. Anticonvulsants are covered in more detail in Chapter 20. However, they are mentioned briefly here because some anticonvulsants have been used to manage veterinary behavior problems. Some maladaptive behaviors, such as tail chasing and unprovoked rage aggression in Bull Terriers, have been postulated to be partial complex seizures at least in part due to their positive response to phenobarbital (Crowell-Davis et al. 1989; Dodman et al. 1992, 1996b). In other cases with similar presentations, phenobarbital treatment is ineffective (Brown et al. 1987). Response may be obtained with narcotic antagonists (Brown et al. 1987) or anticompulsive agents (Hewson 1998b).

Other applications exist for the behavioral use of anticonvulsants. Carbamazepine (Tegretol) has been used for the treatment of aggression in two cats (Schwartz 1994) and for treatment of psychomotor seizures in a dog (Holland 1988). Since blood dyscrasias may result (at least in humans), regular evaluation of the CBC is recommended for patients given carbamazepine. New anticonvulsants, such as gabapentin (Neurontin), topiramate (Topamax), lamotrigine (Lamictal), and tiagabine (Gabitril), show promise for management of anxiety disorders and other behavioral disturbances, but their current high cost limits their practical use.

Opiates. Opiates are presented in more detail in Chapter 12. Stereotypic, compulsive behaviors, such as self-traumatic licking, tail chasing, and pacing are seen in animals confined to zoos and laboratory settings (Kenny 1994). It has been postulated that such behaviors are "coping strategies" that lead to release of endogenous opiates (endorphins). Some cases of dogs and other animals have been successfully treated with the oral narcotic antagonist naltrexone (Brown et al. 1987; Dodman et al. 1988; Kenny 1994; White 1990) or other opiate antagonists (Dodman et al. 1988). Horses with "crib biting" have also been treated with opiate antagonists.

There is evidence that there may be a developmental component to the expression of stereotypies (Kennes et al. 1988). Other cases of client-owned dogs develop acral lick dermatitis associated with repetitive licking for unknown reasons (Dodman et al. 1988; White 1990). Since the etiology of stereotypic behavior (based on response to treatment) is uncertain, treatment with anticompulsive (Hewson et al. 1998b) or anticonvulsant (Dodman et al. 1992) agents should also be considered in such cases.

Hormonal Therapy. Reproductive hormones are discussed in more detail in Chapter 28. Historically, synthetic progestins have been used to treat a wide range of behavioral disorders. Most likely the response to these drugs is caused by their mild sedating effects on steroid receptors in the CNS (McEwan et al. 1979). This nonspecific use has declined with the advent of more specific agents, described above. The use of progestin hormones for behavioral therapy is now considered a "last resort" therapy to avoid abandonment or euthanasia of the offending animal.

In castrated and entire male dogs, megestrol acetate (Ovaban) has been used for the treatment of dominance (Borchelt and Voith 1986) and intermale aggression, mounting, urine marking, and tendency to roam (Joby et al. 1984). In one study of 123 males, 75% improved with hormone treatment (Joby et al. 1984). Side effects included increased appetite and lethargy. Relapse within 3 months was most common in dogs that had signs of dominance aggression and marking (Joby et al. 1984). However, such treatment significantly impairs adrenocortical function as measured by ACTH stimulation during treatment (van den Broek and O'Farrell 1994).

In cats, megestrol acetate may reduce the incidence of aggression (Henick et al. 1985; Marder 1993) and urine spraying, particularly among neutered male cats (Hart 1980). Side effects of progestins in cats include hyperphagia, obesity, hyperglycemia leading to diabetes, lethargy, mammary gland hyperplasia and adenocarcinoma, pyometra, and bone marrow suppression (Romatowski 1989; Henick et al. 1985).

Another class of drugs that has been used in male animals for behavior treatment are long-acting progestins. Medroxyprogesterone acetate (DepoProvera) is the most common of this group. It has a long-acting depot effect after a single injection that may last several days up to 3–4 weeks. A dose that has been used is 10–20 mg/kg, injected SC or IM. This drug may be as effective as megestrol acetate for some indications. Medroxyprogesterone acetate (Depo-Provera) has been used in cats for urine spraying in a manner similar to that of megestrol acetate (Hart 1980).

Reproductive hormones have been used in postmenopausal women in combination with a first-line SSRI to enhance therapeutic effects (Stahl 2008). Although controlled clinical trials are not available, clinicians anecdotally report benefits. Such a strategy may be helpful in spayed female dogs with refractory behavioral problems, although no published reports are currently available.

Thyroid hormone has been used to accelerate (Altshuler et al. 2001) or augment (Stahl 2008) TCA response, particularly in women. Thyroid supplementation may increase cortical 5HT concentrations and desensitize autoinhibitory $5HT_{1A}$ receptors in the raphe area, resulting in disinhibition of cortical and hippocampal 5HT release (Altshuler et al. 2001).

Melatonin is produced by the pineal gland according to the light/dark cycle, with light acting as a production suppressant. The nocturnal secretion of melatonin is primarily induced by increased noradrenergic neurotransmission, resulting in increased activity of the rate-limiting enzyme that converts serotonin to melatonin. In recent years, melatonin has become a popular over-the-counter remedy for insomnia in humans and behavioral calming in dogs, although data on safely, efficacy, or appropriate doses are not available (Stahl 2008). Melatonin given with amitriptyline was used in one dog to improve signs of generalized anxiety disorder (Aronson 1999).

Melatonin is an endogenous hormone, produced from serotonin in the pineal gland. At high doses in dogs (1–1.3 mg/kg q12h), melatonin affects endogenous sex hormones, but does not affect prolactin or thyroid concentrations in adult dogs (Ashley et al. 1999). Melatonin has been used with amitriptyline to manage thunderstorm phobia (Aronson 1999), since it impairs psychomotor vigilance (Graw et al. 2001). No controlled studies on the behavioral effects of melatonin on dogs have been conducted.

Beta Blockers. The beta adrenergic antagonist propranolol (Inderal) has been used to ameliorate the sympathetic symptoms of anxiety in humans, including trembling, sweaty palms, and tachycardia (McNaughton 1989) and to treat organically based aggression (Williams et al. 1982). No controlled studies have investigated the efficacy of beta blockers for treatment of anxiety disorders in small animals (Shull-Selcer and Stagg 1991).

Pindolol is a beta adrenergic blocker that is also an antagonist and partial agonist at $5HT_{1A}$ receptors. Pindolol may disinihbit serotonin neurons and may serve as a useful adjuvant therapy (Stahl 2008).

In Great Britain, propranolol is used in combination with phenobarbital to manage phobic behavior (Walker et al. 1997). When propranolol is used in combination with the antipsychotic thioridazine, thioridazine plasma levels increase.

A beta blocker with $5HT_{1A}$ autoreceptor antagonist properties, pindolol, may disinihbit serotonin neurons and may serve as a useful adjuvant therapy to TCAs (Altshuler et al. 2001; Stahl 2008). However, in one study, pindolol was not superior to placebo for augmenting the effects of paroxetine of social anxiety symptoms (Stein et al. 2001).

Tramadol. Of perhaps equal or greater importance with respect to efficacy of tramadol for some conditions—including behavior problems—is the effect on serotonin and norepinephrine reuptake. Tramadol has three effects that may act synergistically: opiate agonist, inhibition of synaptic reuptake of norepinephrine, and inhibition of synaptic reuptake of serotonin. The latter two effects resemble the action of tricyclic antidepressants discussed earlier in this chapter. One of the stereo isomers is more prominent at inhibiting serotonin reuptake and the other isomer has more of an effect on norepinephrine reuptake. Some studies in experimental animals and people with tramadol have elicited significant behavior-modifying effects. However, veterinary clinical studies for this use are lacking.

Analgesia may also play a role in the action of this drug for some behavior problems. Veterinary behaviorists are often faced with uncertainty about the role of pain in the presentation of a behavior problem. Older animals or those with chronic degenerative orthopedic diseases may be irritable, leading to anxiety or irritable aggression. Although a thorough physical examination and appropriate diagnostic tests are indicated, the role of pain may remain uncertain. Often, a trial of analgesics may be initiated as a way to determine if pain management improves behavior. In addition to the many new nonsteroidal agents discussed in Chapter 19, tramadol also may be useful, alone or in combination with other behavioral drugs. See Chapter 12 for a more complete discussion of tramadol.

DRUG COMBINATIONS

COMBINED USE OF BEHAVIORAL DRUGS. When the effect of one drug is inadequate, a second drug may be added. In fact, this strategy is utilized in commercially available combination products, such as the combination of olanzapine (an antipsychotic) and fluoxetine (an SSRI) marketed by Lilly under the trade name Symbyax approved by the FDA for treatment of bipolar depression in humans (www.symbyax.com). One strategy is to start with an antidepressant, such as a TCA or SSRI. Then, if needed, a benzodiazepine, buspirone, or other agent may be added. A cautious approach is to add the second agent at a low dose, and then titrate the dose to a therapeutic level as response is monitored. Failure to sufficiently manage severe behavior problems, such as separation anxiety, can lead to animal relinquishment and even euthanasia, so aggressive treatment, in combination with behavior modification, may be necessary.

TREATMENT SUCCESS

In each case to which psychotropic medication is administered, there must be a means of documenting treatment response. The first step is to determine target signs that can be documented by the client with regard to frequency, intensity and duration. The second step is to document the occurrence of these signs over time. Treatment response is often defined as 50% or greater improvement in symptoms.

Clients must also be educated as to probable side effects and duration to effect. Many behavioral drugs will produce side effects within hours or days of first administration, but may require weeks to onset of desired behavioral effects.

The duration of treatment has not been systematically investigated. One strategy is to continue treatment for 2 months after satisfactory treatment response, and then gradually decrease the dose over weeks. If the status quo is maintained, the drug can be discontinued. If treatment success wanes, the previous dose should be reinstated for an additional 6 months and the process repeated.

With the exception of clomipramine (Clomicalm), fluoxetine (Reconcile), and selegiline (Anipryl), the behavioral drugs discussed here are not approved by the FDA for animal use. The limitations and risks of extralabel prescribing should be explained to the pet owner (Simpson and Voith 1997; Papich and Davidson 1995). An evaluation of the medical and behavioral history, a physical and neurological examination, and appropriate laboratory tests should precede prescribing any psychotropic agent, and should be repeated at reasonable intervals during treatment. The risk associated with treating animals aggressive to people, especially children, should be carefully considered (Baumgardner 1997). Patients should be monitored at regular intervals.

SUMMARY

As our knowledge expands, behavioral pharmacology plays an increasingly important role in behavioral medicine. Drugs traditionally categorized as anxiolytics, antidepressants, anticonvulsants, and hormones may be used to help manage a range of animal behavior problems. Knowledge of how these agents act in the body and interact with other agents is imperative for safe, efficacious use.

REFERENCES

Alderman CP, Atchison MM, McNeece JI. Concurrent agranulocytosis and hepatitis secondary to clomipramine therapy. Brit J Psychiatry 162:688–689, 1993.

Altshuler LL, Bauer M, Frye MA, et al. Does thyroid supplementation accelerate tricyclic antidepressant response? A review and meta-analysis of the literature. Am J Psychiatry 158(10):1617–1622, 2001.

Anderson P. Pharm Profile: Amitriptyline. Compend Contin Educ Pract Vet 23:433–437, 2001.

Aronson L. Animal Behavior Case of the Month: Extreme fear in a dog. J Am Vet Med Assoc 215:22–24, 1999.

Ashley PF, Frank LA, Schmeitzel LP, et al. Effect of oral melatonin administration on sex hormone, prolactin, and thyroid hormone concentrations in dogs. J Am Vet Med Assoc 215:1111–1115, 1999.

Baldessarini RJ. Drugs and the treatment of psychiatric disorders: psychosis and anxiety. *In* Hardman JG, Limbird LE (eds): Goodman and Gilman's The Pharmacological Basis of Therapeutics, 9th ed. New York, McGraw-Hill, pp 431–446, 1995.

Ballenger JC. Benzodiazepines. *In* Schatzberg AF, Nemeroff CB (eds): The American Psychiatric Press Textbook of Psychopharmacology, 2nd ed. Washington D.C., American Psychiatric Press, pp 271–286, 1998.

Baumgardner K. Aggressive dogs cause problems for owners, insurance companies. DVM Mag 29:1 & 28, 1997.

Boeck V, Overo KF, Svendsen O. Studies on acute toxicity and drug levels of citalopram in the dog. Acta Pharmacol Toxicol (Copenh) 50(3):169–74, 1982.

Boothe DM. Drugs that modify animal behavior. *In* Small Animal Clinical Pharmacology and Therapeutics. Philadelphia, WB Saunders, pp 457–472, 2001.

Boothe DM, George KL, Couch P. Disposition and clinical use of bromide in cats. J Am Vet Med Assoc 221:1131–1135, 2002.

Borchelt PL, Voith VL. Dominance aggression in dogs. Compend Contin Educ Pract Vet 8(1):36–44, 1986.

Bowen J, Heath S. Behaviour Problems in Small Animals: Practical advice for the veterinary team, Elsevier Saunders, pp 49–58, 2005.

Brandwein J. Benzodiazepines for the treatment of panic disorder and generalized anxiety disorder: clinical issues and future directions. Can J Psychiatry 38:S109–S113, 1993.

Brielmaier B. Eszopiclone (Lunesta): a new nonbenzodiazepine hypnotic agent. Proc Baylor University Medical Center, 19(1):54–59, 2006.

Brown SA, Crowell-Davis S, Malcolm T, et al. Naloxone-responsive compulsive tail chasing in a dog. J Am Vet Med Assoc 190:884–886, 1987.

Brown SA, Forrester SD. Serum disposition of oral clorazepate from regular-release and sustained-delivery tablets in dogs. J Vet Pharmacol Therap 14:426–429, 1991.

Bruun R, Budman C. Paroxetine treatment of episodic rages associated with Tourette's disorder. J Clin Psychiatry 59:581–584, 1998.

Bruyette DS, Darling LA, Griffen D, Ruehl WW. L-deprenyl for canine pituitary dependent hyperadrenocorticism: Pivotal efficacy trial. J Vet Int Med 10:182, 1996.

Bruyette DS, Ruehl WW, Smidberg TL. Canine pituitary-dependent hyperadrenocorticism: a spontaneous animal model for neurodegenerative disorders and their treatment with L-deprenyl. Prog Brain Res 106:207–215, 1995.

Buffington CAT, Chew DJ, Woodworth BE. Feline interstitial cystitis. J Am Vet Med Assoc 215(5):682–687, 1999.

Calves S. Pharm Profile: Selegeline. Compend Contin Educ Pract Vet 22:204–205 214, 2000.

Catalano G, Catalano MC, Epstein MA, et al. QTc interval prolongation associated with citalopram overdose: A case report and literature review. Clin Neuropharmacol 24(3):158–162, 2001.

Center SA, Elston TH, Rowland PH, et al. Fulminant hepatic failure associated with oral administration of diazepam in 11 cats. J Vet Emerg Crit Care 6:618–625, 1996.

Chauret N, Gauthier A, Martin J, and Nicoll-Griffith DA. In Vitro comparison of cytochrome P450-mediated metabolic activities in human, dog, cat, and horse. Drug Metab Dispos 25:1130–1136, 1997.

Chew DJ, Buffington CA, Kendall MS, et al. Amitriptyline treatment for severe recurrent idiopathic cystitis in cats: 15 cases (1994–1996). J Am Vet Med Assoc 213:1282–1286, 1998.

Chouinard G, Arnott W. Clinical review of risperidone. Can J Psychiatry 38:S89–S95, 1993.

Ciribassi J, Luescher A, Pasloske KS, Robertson-Plouch C, Zimmerman A, Kaloostian-Whittymore L. Comparative bioavailability of fluoxetine after transdermal and oral administration to healthy cats. Am J Vet Res 64:949–1068, 2003.

Clayton AH. Antidepressant-induced tardive dyskinesia—Review and case report. Psychopharmacol Bull 31:259–264, 1995.

Cohn LA, Dodam JR, Szladovits B. Effects of selegiline, phenylpropanolamine, or a combination of both on physiologic and behavioral variables in healthy dogs. Am J Vet Res 63:827–832, 2002.

Coleman ES. Canine narcolepsy and the role of the nervous system. Compend Contin Educ Pract Vet 21:641–650, 1999.

Cooper L, Hart BL. Comparison of diazepam with progestin for effectiveness in suppression of urine spraying behavior in cats. J Am Vet Med Assoc 200:797–801, 1992.

Cotler S, Gustafson JH, Colburn WA. Pharmacokinetics of diazepam and nordiazepam in the cat. J Pharmaceutical Sci 73:348–351, 1984.

Crowell-Davis SL, Lappin M, Oliver JE, et al. Stimulus-responsive psychomotor epilepsy in a Doberman pinscher. J Am Anim Hosp Assoc 25:57–60, 1989.

Crowell-Davis SL, Murray T. Veterinary Psychopharmacology. Blackwell Publishing, 2006.

Crowell-Davis SL, Seibert LM, Sung W, et al. Use of clomipramine, alprazolam, and behavior modification for treatment of storm phobia in dogs. J Am Vet Med Assoc 222:744–748, 2003.

Cummings BJ, Head E, Afagh AJ, et al. B-amyloid accumulation correlates with cognitive dysfunction in the aged canine. Neurobiol Learn Mem 66:11–23, 1996.

Davidson G. Evaluating transdermal medication forms for veterinary patients, part 1. Inter J Pharmaceut Compound 5:214–215, 2001.

Davidson G. Update on transdermals for animal patients. Inter J Pharmaceut Compound 9(3):178–182, 2005.

DeHasse J. Feline urine spraying. Appl An Behav Sci 52:365–371, 1997.

DeVane CL. Principles of pharmacokinetics and pharmacodynamics. *In* Schatzberg AF, Nemeroff CB (eds): The American Psychiatric Press Textbook of Psychopharmacology, 2nd ed. Washington D.C., American Psychiatric Press, pp 155–169, 1998.

Dietch JF, Jennings RK. Aggressive dyscontrol in patients treated with benzodiazepines. J Clin Psychiatry 49:184–188, 1988.

Dodman NH. Animal behavior case of the month: Interdog intrahousehold aggression. J Am Vet Med Assoc 217:1468–1472, 2000.

Dodman NH, Donnelly R, Shuster L, et al. Use of fluoxetine to treat dominance aggression in dogs. J Am Vet Med Assoc 209:1585–1587, 1996a.

Dodman NH, Knowles KE, Shuster L, et al. Behavioral changes associated with suspected complex partial seizures in Bull Terriers. J Am Vet Med Assoc 208:688–691, 1996b.

Dodman NH, Miczed KA, Knowles K, et al. Phenobarbital-responsive episodic dyscontrol (rage) in dogs. J Am Vet Med Assoc 201:1580–1583, 1992.

Dodman NH, Shuster L, White SD, et al. Use of narcotic antagonists to modify stereotypic self-licking, self-chewing, and scratching behavior in dogs. J Am Vet Med Assoc 193:815–819, 1988.

Eser D, Schule C, Baghai TC, Romeo E, Uzunov DP, Rupprecht R. Neuroactive steroids and affective disorders. Pharmacol Biochem Behav 84(4):656–555, 2006.

Evans LE, Bett JH, Cox JR, Dubois JP, Van Hees T. The bioavailability of oral and parenteral chlorimipramine (Anafranil). Prog Neuropsychopharmacol 1980;4(3):293–302.

File SE. Animal models for predicting clinical efficacy of anxiolytic drugs: social behavior Neuropsychobiology 13:55–62, 1985.

Forrester SD, Brown SA, Lees GE, et al. Disposition of clorazepate in dogs after single- and multiple-dose oral administration. Am J Vet Res 51:2001–2005, 1990.

Forrester SD, Wilcke JR, Jacobson JD, et al. Effects of a 44-day administration of phenobarbital on disposition of clorazepate in dogs. Am J Vet Res 54:1136–1138, 1993.

Frey H-H, Löscher W. Anticonvulsant potency of unmetabolized diazepam. Pharmacology 25:154–159, 1982.

Garner JL, Kirby R, Rudloff E. The use of acepromazine in dogs with a history of seizures. J Vet Emerg Crit Care 14:S1, 2004.

Goldberger E, Rapoport JL. Canine acral lick dermatitis: response to the antiobsessional drug clomipramine. J Am Anim Hosp Assoc 27:179–182, 1991.

Golden RN, Dawkins K, Nicholas L, et al. Trazodone, nefazodone, bupropion, and mirtazapine. *In* Schatzberg AF, Nemeroff CB (eds): The American Psychiatric Press Textbook of Psychopharmacology, 2nd ed. Washington D.C., American Psychiatric Press, pp 251–269, 1998.

Goodman WK, McDougle CJ, Price LH, et al. Beyond the serotonin hypothesis: a role for dopamine in some forms of obsessive compulsive disorder? J Clin Psychiatry 51:36–43, 1990.

Grady TA, Pigott TA, L'Heureux F, Hill JL, Bernstein SE, Murphy DL. Double-blind study of adjuvant buspirone for fluoxetine-treated patients with obsessive-compulsive behavior. Am J Psychiatry May;150(5):819–821, 1993.

Graw P, Werth E, Krauchi K, et al. Early morning melatonin administration impairs psychomotor vigilance. Behav Brain Res 121:167–172, 2001.

Gruen ME, Sherman BL. Use of trazodone as an adjunctive agent in the treatment of canine anxiety disorders: 56 cases (1995–2007) J Am Vet Med Assoc, in press, 2008.

Halip JW, Vaillancourt JP, Luescher UA. A descriptive study of 189 cats engaging in inappropriate elimination behaviors. Fel Pract 26:18–21, 1998.

Hart BL. Objectionable urine spraying and urine marking in the cat: evaluation of progestin treatment in gonadectomized males and females. J Am Vet Med Assoc 177:529–533, 1980.

Hart BL, Cliff KD. Interpreting published results of extra-label drug use with special reference to reports of drugs used to correct problem behavior in animals. J Am Vet Med Assoc 209:1382–1385, 1996.

Hart BL, Cliff KD, Tynes VV, Bergman L. Control of urine marking by use of long-term treatment with fluoxetine or clomipramine in cats. J Am Vet Med Assoc 226:378–382, 2005.

Hart BL, Cooper LL. Integrating use of psychotropic drugs with environmental management and behavioral modification for treatment of problem behavior in animals. J Am Vet Med Assoc 209:1549–1551, 1996.

Hart BL, Eckstein RA, Powell KL, et al. Effectiveness of buspirone on urine spraying and inappropriate urination in cats. J Am Vet Med Assoc 203:254–258, 1993.

Hart BL, Hart LA, Bain MJ. Canine and Feline Behavior Therapy, 2nd ed., Blackwell Publishing, pp 763–90, 2006.

Hartmann L. Cats as possible obsessive-compulsive disorder and medication models. Am J Psychiatry 152:8, 1995.

Harvey A, Preskorn SH. Cytochrome P450 enzymes: interpretation of their interaction with selective serotonin reuptake inhibitors. J Clin Psychopharmacol 16:273–285, 1996.

Henik RA, Olson PN, Rosychuk RAW. Progestogen therapy in cats. Compend Contin Educ Pract Vet 7(2):132–140, 1985.

Hewson CJ, Conlon PD, Luescher UA, et al. The pharmacokinetics of clomipramine and desmethylclomipramine in dogs: parameter estimates following a single oral dose and 28 consecutive daily oral doses of clomipramine. J Vet Pharmacol Ther 21:214–222, 1998a.

Hewson CJ, Luescher A, Parent JM, et al. Efficacy of clomipramine in the treatment of canine compulsive disorder. J Am Vet Med Assoc 213:1760–1766, 1998b.

Holland CT. Successful long term treatment of a dog with psychomotor seizures with carbamezepine. Aust Vet J 65:389–392, 1988.

House J, Banks S, Lynch L, et al. Fulminant hepatic failure associated with oral administration of diazepam in 12 cats. J Am Vet Med Assoc 209:618–625, 1996.

Howell SM, Fritz J, Downing S, et al. Treating chronic regurgitation behavior: a case study. Lab An 26:30–33, 1997.

Hoyer D, Clarke DE, Fozard JR, et al.. International union of pharmacology classification of receptors for 5-hydroxytryptamine (serotonin). Pharm Rev 46:157–194, 1994.

Hughes D, Moreau RE, Overall KL, et al. Acute hepatic necrosis and liver failure associated with benzodiazepine therapy in six cats, 1986–1995. J Vet Emerg Crit Care 6,13–20, 1996.

Iorio LC, Eisenstein N, Brody PE, et al. Effects of selected drugs on spontaneously occurring abnormal behavior in beagles. Pharmacol Biochem Behav 18:379–382, 1983.

Irimajiri M, Luescher AU. Effect of fluoxetine hydrochloride in treating canine compulsive disorder. Proc International Veterinary Behavior Meeting, Minneapolis MN, 5:198–200, 2005.

Janicak PG, Davis JM, Preskorn SH, et al. Pharmacokinetics. *In* Principles and Practice of Psychopharmacotherapy, 2nd ed. Baltimore, Williams and Wilkins, pp 61–84, 1997.

Joby R, Jemmett JE, Miller ASH. The control of undesirable behaviour in male dogs using megestrol acetate. J Sm An Pract 25:567–572, 1984.

Johnson LR. Tricyclic antidepressant toxicosis. Vet Clin North Am Sm An Pract 20:393–403, 1990.

Jolliet-Riant P, Tillement J-P. Drug transfer across the blood-brain barrier and improvement in brain delivery. Fundam Clin Pharmacol 13:16–26, 1999.

Jones RD. Use of thioridazine in the treatment of aberrant motor behavior in a dog. J Am Vet Med Assoc 191:89–90, 1987.

Juarbe-Diaz SV. Social dynamics and behavior problems in multiple dog households. Vet Clin North Am Small Anim Pract 27:497–514, 1997a.

———. Assessment and treatment of excessive barking in the domestic dog. Vet Clin North Am Small Anim Pract 27:515–532, 1997b.

Kennes D, Odberg FO, Bouquet Y, et al. Changes in naloxone and haloperidol effects during the development of captivity-induced jumping stereotypy in bank voles. Eur J Pharmacol 153:19–24, 1988.

Kenny DE. Use of naltrexone for the treatment of psychogenically induced dermatoses in five zoo animals. J Am Vet Med Assoc 205:1021–1023, 1994.

King DJ. Benzodiazepines, amnesia and sedation: theoretical and clinical issues and controversies. Hum Psychopharmacol 7:79–87, 1992.

King JN, Maurer MP, Altmann BO, et al. Pharmacokinetics of clomipramine in dogs following single-dose and repeated-dose oral administration. Am J Vet Res 61:80–85, 2000a.

King JN, Simpson BS, Overall KL, et al. Treatment of separation anxiety in dogs with clomipramine: results from a prospective, randomized, double-blind, placebo-controlled, parallel-group, multicenter clinical trial. Appl An Behav Sci 67:255–275, 2000b.

King JN, Steffan J, Heath SE, Simpson BS, Crowell-Davis SL, Harrington LJM, Weiss A-B, Seewald W. Determination of the dosage of clomipramine for the treatment of urine spraying in cats. J Am Vet Med Assoc 225:881–887, 2004.

Kuroha M, Kuze Y, Shimoda M, Kokue E. In vitro characterization of the inhibitory effects of ketoconazole on metabolic activities of cytochrome P450 in canine hepatic microsomes. Am J Vet Res 63:900–905, 2002.

Landsberg G, Hunthausen W, Ackerman L. Handbook of Behaviour Problems of the Dog and Cat, 2nd ed. New York, WB Saunders, 2003.

Larson ET, Summers CH. Serotonin reverses dominant social status. Behav Brain Res 121:195–102, 2001.

Lasher TA, Fleishaker JC, Steenwyk RC, et al. Pharmacokinetic pharmacodynamic evaluation of the combined administration of alprazolam and fluoxetine. Psychopharmacology 104:323–327, 1991.

Lass-Flörl C, Dierich MP, Fuchs D, et al. Antifungal properties of selective serotonin reuptake inhibitors against Aspergillus species in vitro. J Antimicrob Chemother 48:775–779, 2001.

Levitski RE, Trepanier LA. Effect of timing of blood collection on serum phenobarbital concentrations in dogs with epilepsy. J Am Vet Med Assoc Jul 15;217(2):200–4, 2000. Erratum in: J Am Vet Med Assoc Aug 15;217(4):468, 2000.

Light GS, Hardie EM, Young MS, et al. Pain and anxiety behaviors of dogs during intravenous catheterization after premedication with placebo, acepromazine, or oxymorphone. Appl An Behav Sci 37:331–343, 1993.

Lindell EM. Diagnosis and treatment of destructive behavior in dogs. Vet Clin N Am Sm An Pract 27:533–547, 1997.

Löscher W, Frey H-H. Pharmacokinetics of diazepam in the dog. Arch Int Pharmacodyn Ther 254:180–195, 1981.

Luescher AU. Diagnosis and management of compulsive disorders in dogs and cats. Vet Clin N Am Sm An Pract 33(2):253–267, 2003.

Maes M, and Meltzer HY. The serotonin hypothesis of major depression. *In* Psychopharmacology: The 4th Generation of Progress. New York, Raven Press, 1995.

Mandelker L. Mirtazepine dose for appetite stimulation. Posting Veterinary Information Network, Clinical Pharmacology Board, 10/11/2006, 11/12/2006.

Marder AR. Psychotropic drugs and behavioral therapy. Vet Clin N Am Sm An Pract 21:329–342, 1991.

———. Diagnosing and treating aggression problems in cats. Vet Med 88:736–742, 1993.

Marder SR. Antipsychotic medications. *In* Schatzberg AF, Nemeroff CB (eds): The American Psychiatric Press Textbook of Psychopharmacology, 2nd ed. Washington D.C., American Psychiatric Press, pp 309–321, 1998.

McConnell J, Kirby R, Rudloff E. Administration of acepromazine maleate to 31 dogs with a history of seizures. J Vet Emerg Crit Care 17:262–267, 2007.

McEwan BS, Davis PG, Parsons B, et al. The brain as a target for steroid hormone action. Ann Rev Neurosci 2:65–112, 1979.

Mealey KL. Clinically significant drug interactions. Compend Contin Educ Pract Vet 24(1):10–22, 2002.

Mealey KL, Peck KE, Bennett BS, Sellon RK, Swinney GR, Melzer K, Gokhale SA, Drone TM. Systemic absorption of amitriptyline and buspirone after oral and transdermal administration to healthy cats. J Vet Intern Med 18:43–46, 2004.

Mehlman PT, Higley JD, Faucher BA, et al. Low CSF 5-HIAA concentrations and severe aggression and impaired impulse control in nonhuman primates. Am J Psychiatry 151(10):1485–1491, 1994.

Michelson D, Fava M, Amsterdam J, et al. Interruption of selective serotonin reuptake inhibitor treatment. Brit J Psychiatry 176:363–368, 2000.

Micó JA, Ardid D, Berrocoso E, Eschaller A. Antidepressants and pain. Trends Pharmacol Sci 27:348–354, 2006.

Milgram NW, Ivy GO, Head E, et al. Effect of L-Deprenyl on behavior, cognitive function, and biogenic amines in the dog. Neurochem Res 18:1211–1219, 1993.

Milgram NW, Ivy GO, Murphy MP, et al.. Effects of chronic oral administration of L-deprenyl in the dog. Pharmacol Biochem Behav 51:421–428, 1995.

Mills DS. Medical paradigms for the study of problem behaviour: A critical review. Appl An Behav Sci 81:265–277, 2003.

Mills DS, Ledger R. The effect of oral selegiline hydrochloride on learning and training in the dog: a psychobiological interpretation. Prog Neuropsychopharmacol Biol Psychiatry 25:1597–1613, 2001.

Mills D, Simpson BS. Psychotropic agents. *In* Horwitz D, Mills D, Heath S (eds): British Small Animal Veterinary Association Manual of Canine and Feline Behavioural Medicine, pp. 237–248, 2002.

Mohr N, Vythilingum B, Emsley R, et al. Quetiapine augmentation of serotonin reuptake inhibitors in obsessive-compulsive disorder. Inter Clin Psychopharmacol 17:37–40, 2002.

Moon-Fanelli AA, Dodman NH. Description and development of compulsive tail chasing in terriers and response to clomipramine treatment. J Am Vet Med Assoc 212:1252–1257, 1998.

Munoz-Bellido JL, Munoz-Criado S, Garcia-Rodriguez JA. Antimicrobial activity of psychotropic drugs selective serotonin reuptake inhibitors. Inter J Antimicrobial Agents 14:177–180, 2000.

Ninan PT, Cole JO, Yonkers KA. Nonbenzodiazepine anxiolytics. *In* Schatzberg AF, Nemeroff CB (eds): The American Psychiatric Press Textbook of Psychopharmacology, 2nd ed. Washington D.C., American Psychiatric Press, pp 287–300, 1998.

Ostroff RB, Nelson JC. Risperidone augmentation of selective serotonin reuptake inhibitors in major depression. J Clin Psychiatry 60(4):256–259, 1999.

Overall KL. Animal behavior case of the month: use of buspirone to treat spraying associated with intercat aggression. J Am Vet Med Assoc 205:694–696, 1994a.

———. Use of clomipramine to treat ritualistic stereotypic motor behavior in three dogs. J Am Vet Med Assoc 205:1733–1741, 1994b.

———. Animal behavior case of the month: Treatment of a dog with interdog aggression, stereotypic circling, and fearful avoidance of strangers. J Am Vet Med Assoc 206:629–632, 1995.

———. Pharmacologic treatments for behavior problems. Vet Clin N Am Sm An Pract 27:637–665, 1997a.

———. Clinical Behavioral Medicine for Small Animals. Mosby, New York, 1997b.

———. Animal Behavior Case of the Month: separation anxiety in a dog. J Am Vet Med Assoc 212:1702–1704, 1998a.

———. Correct diagnosis, correct dose of amitriptyline (letter). Vet Forum 15:10–11, 1998b.

———. The role of pharmacotherapy in treating dogs with dominance aggression. Vet Med 94:1049–1055, 1999a.

———. Intercat aggression: why can't they all just get along? Vet Med 94:688–693, 1999b.

———. Dealing with dogs affected by separation anxiety. Vet Forum 18:4053, 2001.

Overall KL, Dunham AE, Frank D. Frequency of nonspecific clinical signs in dogs with separation anxiety, thunderstorm phobia, and noise phobia, alone or in combination. J Am Vet Med Assoc 219:467–473, 2001.

Pacher P, Ungvari Z, Nanasi PP, Furst S, Kecskemeti V. Speculations on difference between tricyclic and selective serotonin reuptake inhibitor antidepressants on their cardiac effects. Is there any? Curr Medicinal Chem 6(6):469–480, 1999.

Papich MG. Saunders Handbook of Veterinary Drugs, 2nd ed. Philadelphia, WB Saunders, 2007.

Papich MG, Alcorn J. Absorption of diazepam after its rectal administration in dogs. Am J Vet Res 56:1629–1635, 1995.

Papich MG, Davidson G. Unapproved use of drugs in small animals. *In* Bonagura JD (ed): Kirk's Current Veterinary Therapy XII: Small Animal Practice. Philadelphia, WB Saunders, pp 48–53, 1995.

Pardridge WM. Blood-brain barrier biology and methodology. J Neurovirol 5:556–569, 1999.

Peremans K, Audenaert K, Hoybergs Y, Otte A, Goethals I, Gielen I, Blankaert P, Vervaet M, van Heeringen C, Dierckx R. The effect of citalopram hydrobromide on 5-HT2A receptors in the impulsive-aggressive dog, as measured with I-123-5-I-R91150 SPECT. Eur J Nucl Med Molec Imaging 32(6):708–716, 2005.

Peterson ME. Medical treatment of pituitary-dependent hyperadrenocorticism in dogs: should L-Deprenyl (Anipryl) ever be used? J Vet Intern Med 13:289–290, 1999.

Plumb DC. Veterinary Drug Handbook, 6th ed. Ames, IA, Blackwell Publishing, 2008.

Podberscek AL, Hsu Y, Serpell JA. Evaluation of clomipramine as an adjunct to behavioural therapy in the treatment of separation-related problems in dogs. Vet Rec 145:365–369, 1999.

Podell M, Fenner WR. Use of bromide as an antiepileptic drug in dogs. Compendium of Continuing Education for the Practicing Veterinarian, June; 767–774, 1994.

———. Bromide therapy in refractory canine idiopathic epilepsy. J Vet Intern Med 7:318–327, 1993.

Pollock BG. Citalopram: a comprehensive review. Exp Omin Pharmacother 2:681–698, 2001.

Potter WZ, Manji HK, Rudorfer MV. Tricyclics and tetracyclics. *In* Schatzberg AF, Nemeroff CB (eds): The American Psychiatric Press Textbook of Psychopharmacology, 2nd ed. Washington, D.C., American Psychiatric Press, pp 199–218, 1998.

Poulsen EMB, Honeyman V, Valentine PA, et al. Use of fluoxetine for the treatment of stereotypical pacing behavior in a captive polar bear. J Am Vet Med Assoc 209:1470–1474, 1996.

Pryor PA, Hart BL, Cliff KD, Main MJ. Effects of a selective serotonin reuptake inhibitor on urine spraying behavior in cats. J Am Vet Med Assoc 219:1557–1713, 2001.

Randall LO, Scheckel CL, Banziger RF. Pharmacology of the metabolites of chlordiazepoxide and diazepam. Curr Ther Res 149:423–435, 1965.

Rapoport JL, Ryland DH, Kriete M. Drug treatment of canine acral lick dermatitis: an animal model of obsessive-compulsive disorder. Arch Gen Psychiatry 49:517–521, 1992.

Reich MR. Animal Behavior Case of the Month: Food aggression in a Cocker Spaniel puppy. J Am Vet Med Assoc 215:1780–1782, 1999.

Reich MR, Ohad DG, Overall KL, Dunham AE. Electrocardiographic assessment of antianxiety medication in dogs and correlation with serum drug concentration. J Am Vet Med Assoc 216:1571–1575, 2000.

Reisner I, Houpt K. Behavioral disorders: *In* Ettinger S, Feldman E (eds). Textbook of Veterinary Internal Medicine: Diseases of the Dog and Cat. Philadelphia, WB Saunders, pp 156–162, 2000.

Reisner IR, Mann JJ, Stanley M, Huang Y, Houpt KA. Comparison of cerebrospinal fluid monoamine metabolite levels in dominant-aggressive and non-aggressive dogs. Brain Res 714:57–64, 1996.

Reist C, Nakamura K, Sagart E, Sokolski KN, Fujimoto KA. Impulsive aggressive behavior: Open-label treatment with citalopram. J Clin Psychiatry 64:81–85, 2003.

Reusch CE, Steffen T, Hoerauf A. The efficacy of L-deprenyl in dogs with pituitary-dependent hyperadrenocorticism. J Vet Intern Med 13:291–301, 1999.

Richardson JA, Gwaltney-Brant SM, Albretsen JC, Khan SA, Porter JA. Clinical syndrome associated with zolpidem ingestion in dogs: 33 cases (January 1998–July 2000). J Vet Intern Med 16:208–210, 2002.

Romatowski J. Use of megestrol acetate in cats. J Am Vet Med Assoc 194:700–702, 1989.

Romatowski J. Two cases of fluoxetine-responsive behavior disorders in cats. Fel Pract 26:14–15, 1998.

Roy-Byrne PP, Cowley DS. Benzodiazepines in clinical practice: risks and benefits. American Psychiatric Press, Washington D.C., 1991.

Roy-Byrne PP, Sullivan MD, Cowley DS, Ries RK. Adjunctive treatment of benzodiazepine discontinuation syndromes: a review. J Psychiatric Res 27S1:143–153, 1993.

Ruehl WW, Bruyette DS, DePaoli A, et al. Canine cognitive dysfunction as a model for human age-related cognitive decline, dementia, and Alzheimer's disease: clinical presentation, cognitive testing, pathology, and response to L-deprenyl therapy. Prog Brain Res 106:217–225, 1995.

Sawyer LS, Moon-Fanelli AA, Dodman NH. Psychogenic alopecia in cats: 11 cases (1993–1996). J Am Vet Med Assoc 214:71–74, 1999.

Seksel K, Lindeman MJ. Use of clomipramine in treatment of obsessive-compulsive disorder, separation anxiety and noise phobia in dogs: a preliminary, clinical study. Aust Vet J 79:252–256, 2001.

Schwartz S. Carbamazepine in the control of aggressive behavior in cats. J Am Animal Hosp Assoc 30:515–519, 1994.

Sheikh JI, Longbord P, Clary CM, et al. The efficacy of sertraline in panic disorder: combined results from two fixed dose studies. Inter Clin Psychopharmacol 15:235–242, 2000.

Shull-Selcer E, Stagg W. Advances in the understanding and treatment of noise phobias. Vet Clin North Am Small Anim Pract 21:353–367, 1991.

Simpson BS. Canine separation anxiety. Compend Contin Educ Pract Vet 22:328–339, 2000.

Simpson BS, Davidson G. Letter to the editor: Concerns about concurrent use of a tricyclic antidepressant and an amitraz tick collar. J Am Vet Med Assoc 209 (8):1380–1381, 1996.

Simpson BS, Landsberg GM, Reisner IR, Ciribassi JJ, et al. (10 other authors). Effects of Reconcile (Fluoxetine) chewable tablets plus behavior management for canine separation anxiety. Vet Therapeut 8:18–31, 2007.

Simpson BS, Papich MG. Pharmacologic Management in Veterinary Behavioral Medicine. Vet Clin N Am Sm An Pract 33:365–404, 2003.

Simpson BS, Simpson DM. Behavioral Pharmacotherapy. Part 1. Antipsychotics and Antidepressants. Compend Contin Educ Pract Vet 18:1067–1081, 1996a.

———. Behavioral Pharmacotherapy. Part II. Anxiolytics and Mood Stabilizers. Compend Contin Educ Pract Vet 18:1203–1213, 1996b.

Simpson BS, Voith VL. Extralabel Drug Use in Veterinary Behavioral Medicine. Compend Contin Educ Pract Vet 19:329–331, 1997.

Stahl SM. Essential Psychopharmacology: Neuroscientific Basis and Practical Applications, 3rd ed. Cambridge University Press, 2008.

Stein DJ, Dodman NH, Borchelt P, Hollander E. Behavioral disorders in veterinary practice. Comp Psychiatry 35:25–285, 1994.

Stein DJ, Mendelsohn I, Potocnik MB, Van Kradenberg J, Wessels C. Use of the selective serotonin reuptake inhibitor citalopram in a possible animal analogue of obsessive-compulsive disorder. Depress Anx 8:39–42, 1998.

Stein MB, Sareen J, Hami S, et al. Pindolol potentiation of paroxetine for generalized social phobia: a double-blind, placebo-controlled, crossover study. Am J Psychiatry 158:1725–1727, 2001.

Takeuchhi Y, Houpt KA, Scarlett JM. Evaluation of treatments for separation anxiety in dogs. J Am Vet Med Assoc 217:342–345, 2000.

Tobias KM, Marioni-Henry K, Wagner R. A retrospective study on the use of acepromazine maleate in dogs with seizures. J Am Anim Hosp Assoc 42:283–289, 2006.

Tollefson GD, Rosenbaum JF. Selective serotonin reuptake inhibitors. *In* Schatzberg AF, Nemeroff CB (eds): The American Psychiatric Press Textbook of Psychopharmacology, 2nd ed. Washington, D.C., American Psychiatric Press, pp 219–235, 1998.

Trepanier LA. Use of bromide as an anticonvulsant for dogs with epilepsy. J Am Vet Med Assoc Jul 15;207(2):163–6, 1995.

Vail J, Davidson G. Compounding for behavior problems in companion animals. Inter J Pharmaceut Compound 9(3):185–192, 2005.

van den Broek AHM, O'Farrell V. Suppression of adrenocortical function in dogs receiving therapeutic doses of megestrol acetate. J Sm An Pract 35:285–288, 1994.

Walker R, Fisher J, Neville P. The treatment of phobias in the dog. Appl An Behav Sci 52:275–289, 1997.

White MM, Neilson JC, Hart BL, Cliff KD. Effects of clomipramine hydrochloride on dominance-related aggression in dogs. J Am Vet Med Assoc 215:1288–1291,1999.

White SD. Naltrexone for treatment of acral lick dermatitis in dogs. J Am Vet Med Assoc 196:1073–1076, 1990.

Williams DT, Mehl R, Yudofsky S, et al. The effect of propranolol on uncontrolled rage outbursts in children and adolescents with organic brain dysfunction. J Am Acad Child Psychiatry 21(2):129–135, 1982.

Wismer TA. Antidepressant drug overdoses in dogs. Vet Med 95:520–525, 2000.

Wynchank D, Berk M. Fluoxetine treatment of acral lick dermatitis in dogs: a placebo-controlled randomized double blind trial. Depress Anx 8:21–23, 1998a.

———. Behavioural changes in dogs with acral lick dermatitis during a 2-month extension phase of fluoxetine treatment. Hum Psychopharmacol Clin Exp 13:435–437, 1998b.

Yen HCY, Krop S, Mendez HC, et al. Effects of some psychoactive drugs on experimental "neurotic" (conflict induced) behavior in cats. Pharmacol 3:32–40, 1970.

SECTION 5

Drugs Acting on the Cardiovascular System

CHAPTER

22

DIGITALIS, POSITIVE INOTROPES, AND VASODILATORS

MATTHEW W. MILLER AND H. RICHARD ADAMS

Understanding of the clinical pharmacodynamics of cardiac drugs is essential to veterinary medicine for two important reasons. First, the indispensable pumping function of the heart in maintaining circulation rules that life-threatening events are often present when pharmacologic agents are needed to control the heart. Second, cardiac dysfunctional states amenable to drug therapy are common in many species. This chapter considers the more important drugs used in therapeutic management of cardiac disorders, with focus on basic aspects of cardiac function, positive inotropes, inodilators, and vasodilators. Antiarrhythmic drugs are covered in Chapter 23. Other classes of drugs that elicit prominent cardiac responses (e.g., adrenergic and cholinergic agents and diuretics) are addressed specifically in appropriate chapters.

BASIC ASPECTS OF CARDIAC FUNCTION

The heart, blood, lungs, and blood vessels comprise an integrated physiologic system that supplies oxygen and other nutrients to tissues and removes carbon dioxide and other waste products in return. This exchange necessitates a series of sensitive and dynamic control mechanisms to ensure that cardiac output is sufficient to supply cellular demands.

The three primary pathways by which the heart can increase cardiac output in response to body needs for increased blood flow are an intrinsic response of the muscle to changes in muscle length, changes in heart rate, and adjustments in contractility. These physiologic control systems are of considerable importance to pharmacology because the net response of the heart to drugs is controlled by these mechanisms.

INTRINSIC REGULATION. Contractile response of cardiac muscle to a change in its own length is the primary mechanism whereby the heart adjusts its pumping activity under normal physiologic conditions (Fozzard 1976). Individual myofibers are stretched as the intraventricular diastolic volume expands to accommodate increased venous return. The stretched muscle responds in turn with enhanced contractile strength, thereby pumping the increased volume of blood into the arterial circuits.

The fundamental capability of the heart to autoregulate its pumping capacity in response to end-diastolic filling is referred to as the *Frank-Starling Law of the Heart* (Frank 1895; Starling 1918). This length-force relationship is the result of stretching the sarcomere to a more optimal interdigitating arrangement of the actin and myosin elements. The relationship between end-diastolic filling and cardiac output under basal conditions and under dominance by the sympathetic and parasympathetic nervous systems is shown in Figure 22.1.

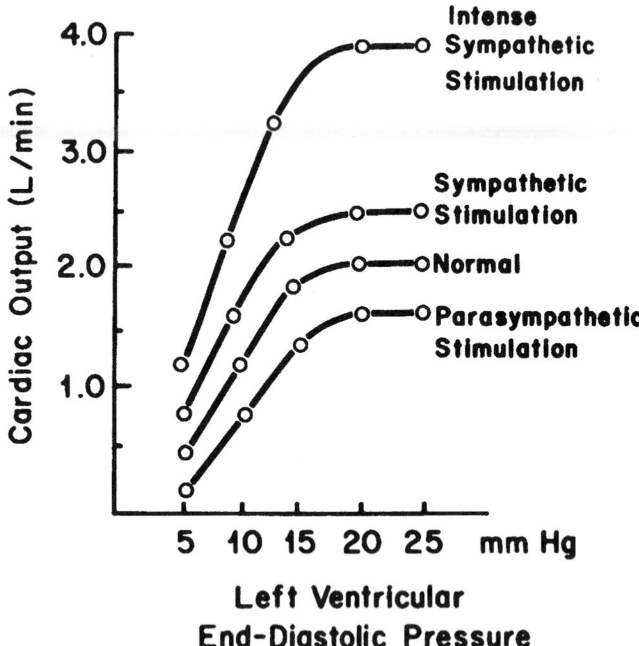

FIG. 22.1 Frank-Starling Law of the Heart. As end-diastolic ventricular volume increases, the myofiber is stretched, enhancing the contractile state of the muscle; cardiac output is thus increased. The cardiac output curve can be influenced by different degrees of sympathetic and parasympathetic stimulation.

REGULATION BY THE NERVOUS SYSTEM. The autonomic nervous system regulates the heart mainly by adjusting cardiac rate and myocardial contractility. Details concerning cardiac effects and mechanisms of action of the sympathetic neurotransmitter norepinephrine and the parasympathetic neurotransmitter acetylcholine (ACh) are presented in Chapters 5–7.

Sympathetic stimulation of cardiac muscle markedly increases the force of contraction irrespective of end-diastolic muscle length. A change in contractile strength that is independent of muscle length is referred to as a change in contractility (inotropy). In the presence of inotropic stimulation by the sympathetic system, cardiac output at each level of ventricular filling is enhanced considerably over the basal state (Fig. 22.1). Conversely, parasympathetic nerves exert their primary influences on cardiac output, not by changing the inotropic state, but by adjusting heart rate. Vagal discharge produces bradycardia; with fewer heartbeats per unit of time, less blood is pumped and cardiac output is decreased at all levels of venous return (Fig. 22.1). In contrast, sympathetic stimulation produces marked tachycardia and, within physiologic limits, cardiac output is increased proportionately. Coronary blood flow increases in response to sympathetic stimulation, but much of this change is secondary to increased metabolic-oxygen demands of the heart muscle.

Myocardial oxygen demand varies directly with three main factors: heart rate, myocardial wall tension, and inotropic state. Myocardial wall tension is directly proportional to ventricular radius (cardiac size) and intraventricular pressure, i.e., the law of Laplace. Primary determinants of ventricular wall tension are preload (i.e., end-diastolic volume and stretch) and afterload (aortic blood pressure). By reducing preload or afterload, certain drugs can elicit marked reduction in cardiac work without direct inotropic action on a heart muscle cell.

CELLULAR CONCEPTS. The basic contractile unit of a heart muscle cell is the sarcomere, composed of the interdigitating protein filaments actin (thin filament) and myosin (thick filament). Activation of the filaments is regulated by a protein assembly unit composed of tropomyosin and troponin and associated with actin molecules. Availability of ionized calcium (Ca^{++}) in the vicinity of troponin is the obligate modulator of the relaxation-contraction cycle.

Binding of Ca^{++} to a high-affinity subunit of the troponin molecule evokes the movement of tropomyosin from its diastolic blocking position on actin. Cross-linkages or "cross-bridges" are formed between projections of the myosin molecules and exposed sites on actin. As cross-bridges are formed, the thick and thin filaments move laterally in relation to one another, and contraction occurs. Calcium delivery to the myofibrils is initiated by bioelectric events at the cell membrane, represented by the cardiac action potential.

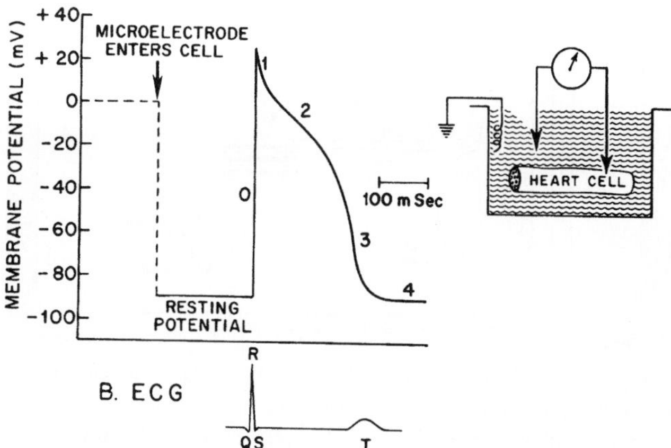

FIG. 22.2 (A) Cardiac action potential recorded from a single myocardial cell. The following phases are listed: 0 = rapid depolarization upstroke, 1 = rapid repolarization, 2 = plateau, 3 = delayed repolarization, and 4 = diastolic potential. The plateau phase is due partly to a slow current representing entry of Ca^{++} into the cell during excitation-contraction coupling. (B) Electrocardiogram (ECG) of the ventricle correlating with the respective phases above (Parker and Adams 1977).

Cardiac Action Potential. The diastolic (resting) membrane potential in heart cells is maintained at about −90 mV (negative intracellular relative to extracellular), primarily as a result of uneven distribution of potassium ions (K^+) inside, $(K^+)_i$, and outside, $(K^+)_o$, the cell. The cell membrane (sarcolemma) is selectively permeable to K^+ during diastole compared to other electrolytes like sodium ions (Na^+), and yet an active ion transport system maintains high $(K^+)_i$ relative to $(K^+)_o$, and low $(Na^+)_i$ relative to $(Na^+)_o$. The high permeability of the cell membrane to K^+ allows a net outward leakage of this positively charged ion. This outward current, in combination with impermeate organic anions within the cell, yields a negatively charged intracellular space. When the cell is stimulated, selective permeability characteristics of the sarcolemma to K^+ are lost. The resulting change in ion distribution can be recorded as an action potential by using a microelectrode capable of penetrating a single myocardial cell (Fozzard and Gibbons 1973).

The action potential of a ventricular muscle cell contains two basic components, depolarization and repolarization, which can be differentiated into five phases (Fig. 22.2). The rapid upstroke, phase 0, is similar to the depolarization spike seen in skeletal muscle and neurons; it represents a rapid flux of Na^+ into the cell. As the permeability characteristics of the cell membrane are reestablished, rapid (phase 1) and delayed (phase 3) repolarization occur, restoring the membrane potential to its diastolic level (phase 4).

The plateau (phase 2) is due partly to a slow inward current that is carried by Ca^{++} through membrane passageways (channels or pores) that are distinct from those participating in the rapid Na^+ upstroke phase of the action potential. The plateau phase is critically important because the slow inward Ca^{++} current is believed to be the link in heart muscle that couples membrane excitation with activation of the contractile apparatus (Reuter 1979, 1985; see Chapter 23).

Excitation-Contraction Coupling. The amount of Ca^{++} that enters by the slow-current pathway is insufficient by itself for optimal activation of the contractile apparatus (Solaro et al. 1974). Instead, the small amount of Ca^{++} entering the cell during the plateau of the action potential fills sarcoplasmic reticulum stores of Ca^{++} and also acts as a trigger to cause a regenerative release of additional amounts of this cation previously sequestered within the sarcoplasmic reticulum (Fabiato and Fabiato 1979).

Two separate pathways of movement of superficial Ca^{++} are believed to be involved (Langer 1976, 1980; Parker and Adams 1977). The primary electrogenic route is associated with the previously discussed plateau phase of the action potential. An additional influx of Ca^{++} is linked with a Ca^{++}-Na^+ exchange across the sarcolemma. A schematic representation of excitation-contraction

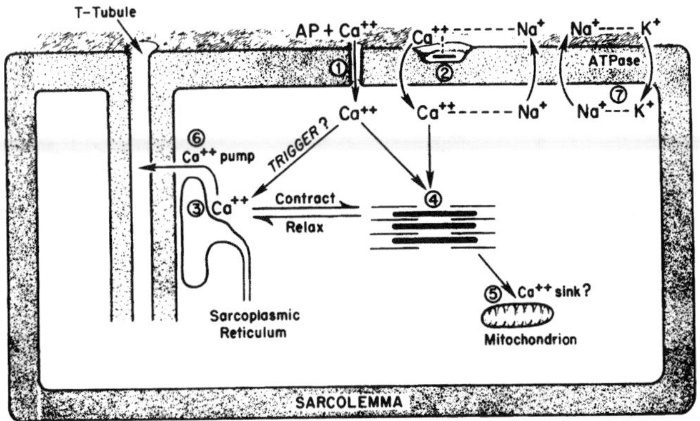

FIG. 22.3 Schematic representation of cellular ion movements controlling excitation-contraction coupling in heart muscle. An action potential (AP) instigates the inward movement of Ca^{++} through slow Ca^{++} channels of the sarcolemma (1). Inward-moving calcium fills sarcoplasmic reticulum stores of the cation and also serves as a trigger to release additional Ca^{++} from storage sites of the sarcoplasmic reticulum (3). These Ca^{++} sources and that resulting from Na^+–Ca^{++} exchanges across the sarcolemma (2) activate the contractile proteins (4). Relaxation occurs as calcium is sequestered at storage sites of sarcoplasmic reticulum (3). Mitochondrion (5). Ca^{++} is pumped out of the cell (6). Altered sodium pump activity (7) may also affect sodium concentrations available from Na^+–Ca^{++} exchange (Parker and Adams 1977).

coupling in mammalian heart muscle is shown in Figure 22.3.

Relaxation. During repolarization, Ca^{++} is actively sequestered by the sarcoplasmic reticulum, which avidly binds and stores myoplasmic Ca^{++} with affinity greater than troponin. Relaxation occurs as Ca^{++} moves to the sarcoplasmic reticulum from troponin binding sites on the myofibrils, and the cytoplasmic Ca^{++} concentration decreases below the threshold required to trigger actin-myosin cross-bridge formation (Fig. 22.3).

Maintenance of Electrolyte Gradients. There is a net influx of Na^+ and Ca^{++} and efflux of K^+ with each action potential. Membrane-bound enzymes act as pumps to relocate ions and prevent their improper accumulation (Gadsby 1984). Sodium-potassium–activated adenosine triphosphatase (Na^+,K^+-ATPase) localized in the cell membrane propels Na^+ out of and K^+ into the cell, against their respective concentration gradients. Excess intracellular Ca^{++} is pumped out of the cell by systems localized in regions of the sarcoplasmic reticulum in close approximation to the sarcolemma (Fig. 22.3). A sarcolemmal Ca^{++}-ATPase also contributes to extrusion of Ca^{++}.

POSITIVE INOTROPES AND INODILATORS

DIGITALIS AND RELATED CARDIAC GLYCOSIDES.

Digitalis and several closely allied chemicals are derived from the purple foxglove plant (*Digitalis purpurea*), other related species of the figwort family, and some plant species unrelated to digitalis. Medicinal use of plant extracts containing cardioactive principles has a long and colorful history, dating to ancient times of the Greeks and Romans.

Application of digitalis to modern medicine can be traced to 1785, when William Withering, a physician of Birmingham, England, reported his account of the therapeutic use of foxglove. This remarkable story starts with an old woman from Shropshire who for many years had concocted an herbal folk remedy purported to be efficacious in treating dropsy (edema). Although the remedy was a family secret and included at least 20 different herbs, Withering correctly ascribed beneficial therapeutic results to the foxglove ingredient. After 10 years of study, Withering was convinced of the therapeutic value of the plant and published his now classic monograph, "An Account of the Foxglove and Some of Its Medical Uses: With Practical Remarks on Dropsy and Other Diseases."

Because of the often pronounced diuretic response, the kidney was thought to be the primary target organ of foxglove; however, Withering stated, "It has the power over the motion of the heart, to a degree yet unobserved in any other medicine, and this power may be converted to salutary ends."

Subsequent studies by numerous investigators identified the heart as the focus of digitalis action in congestive failure patients and designated a positive inotropic effect on the myocardium as the relevant mechanism of action. These agents also exert important antiarrhythmic action that has therapeutic application whether or not congestive failure is present.

Chemistry and Sources. Chemical and structure-activity relationships of the digitalis glycosides are quite complex, but several basic similarities are retained in the different compounds. The nomenclature is interesting, since it is not derived from specific chemical structures but is based instead on botanical origins.

Official digitalis is the dried leaf of the purple foxglove plant. Digitoxin, digoxin (another glycoside used therapeutically), and gitoxin also can be extracted from the leaf of a related plant, *D. lanta,* the woolly foxglove. Strophanthidin and ouabain are glycosides contained in the seeds of *Strophanthus* sp.; *S. gratus,* the source of ouabain, is an African tree. Ouabain is not used clinically because of a high risk of toxicity. Digitoxin is not used clinically any longer and dosage forms are unavailable. Of toxicologic interest, several cardioactive glycosides are found in the skin of some toads (*Bufo vulgaris, B. maritimus*), in certain oleander plants, and in a large number of other unrelated botanical species.

Only digoxin is currently relevant to veterinary therapeutics; the focus of discussion in this chapter will be on digoxin. With respect to terminology, because of considerable pharmacologic similarities between the different glycosides, the collective term *digitalis* has been used to designate the entire group of drugs, including digoxin. The term "*glycoside*" in general refers to a compound linked by an oxygen atom to a sugar molecule(s). The basic steroid-type nucleus is a cyclopentanoperhydrophenanthrene to which is attached an unsaturated lactone ring at carbon atom 17 (C-17). The sugar molecules usually are attached at C-3; they influence water solubility, cell penetrability, duration of action, and other pharmacokinetic characteristics. Cardioactivity of the molecule resides principally in the aglycone moiety, but the positive myocardial actions of these entities are somewhat less potent and of briefer duration than the parent glycoside.

The structures of digitoxin, digoxin, and the aglycones digitoxigenin and digoxigenin are shown for comparative purposes in Figure 22.4; some chemical aspects of several important compounds are summarized in Table 22.1.

Cardiovascular Effects. The therapeutic response to digitalis in congestive heart failure patients entails a broad scope of hemodynamic adjustments: augmented myocardial contractility; increased cardiac output; diuresis and diminution of edema; control of cardiac arrhythmias; and reductions in blood volume, venous pressures, heart size, and heart rate. Improved myocardial contractility is the most important; it is the primary action on which other effects depend.

Myocardial Contractility. The ability of cardiac glycosides to increase contractility has been demonstrated in

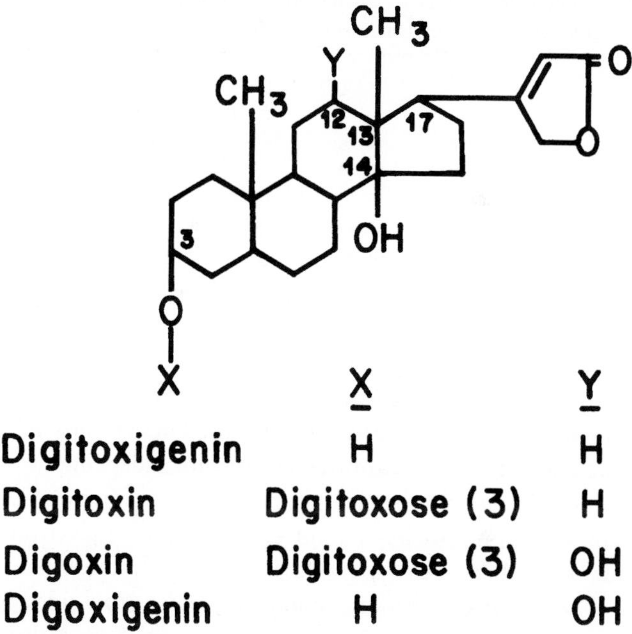

FIG. 22.4 Structural arrangements of digoxin and digitoxin and the aglycones digoxigenin and digitoxigenin.

TABLE 22.1 Plant sources and chemical composition of selected digitalis glycosides

Plant	Glycoside	Sugar	Aglycone
Digitalis purpurea (leaf)	Digitoxin*	Digitoxose (3)	Digitoxigenin
	Gitoxin	Digitoxose (3)	Gitoxigenin
	Gitalin	Digitoxose (3)	Gitoxigenin hydrate
D. lanta (leaf)	Digitoxin*	Digitoxose (3)	Digitoxigenin
	Digoxin*	Digitoxose (3)	Digoxigenin
	Gitoxin	Digitoxose (3)	Gitoxigenin
Strophanthus kombé (seed)	Strophanthin	Glucose and cymarose	Strophanthidin
S. gratus (seed)	Ouabain* (G-Strophanthin)	Rhamnose	Ouabagenin (G-Strophanthidin)

Source: Moe and Farah 1975.

*Clinically important to veterinary medicine.

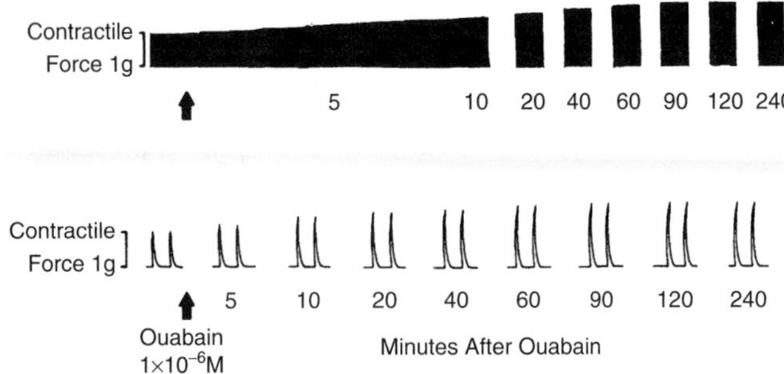

FIG. 22.5 Myographic recordings from a heart muscle before and after exposure to the cardiac glycoside ouabain. Top tracings were taken at a slow recording speed; bottom tracings show individual muscle contractions at designated intervals after addition of ouabain. Notice that contractile force increased by almost 100% and that this effect lasted for the 4-hour measurement period.

a multitude of experimental preparations. Heart muscle suspended at constant external length responds to digitalis with an increase in isometric systolic force; studied under isotonic conditions, muscle shortening is enhanced. Intravenous (IV) infusion of the drug augments intraventricular pressure development in intact subjects even when heart rate, venous return, and blood pressure are maintained constant by experimental means. These results validate a direct effect on contractile strength independent of changes in resting fiber length, heart rate, or afterload. A typical response of heart muscle to the cardiac glycoside ouabain is shown in Figure 22.5.

The positive inotropic action of cardiac glycosides is particularly pronounced in the hypodynamic or failing heart. However, this should not be construed as evidence that digitalis selectively corrects the specific biochemical defect in the chronically failing heart. This defect has yet to be identified in a satisfactory manner. Digitalis, by increasing Ca^{++} availability in the myocardial fiber, increases contractility of the normal as well as the failing heart. Thus cardiac glycosides may increase contractile strength by way of a cellular pathway that bypasses or only partially involves the spontaneous defect (Aranow 1992).

Cellular Mechanisms of Inotropic Action. The mechanism of digitalis action that is helpful in congestive failure is a positive inotropic effect on the heart muscle, but only portions of this mechanism can be answered without controversy (Feldman 1993; Ezrailson et al. 1977).

Inhibition of Na^+,K^+-ATPase. The Mg^{++}-dependent Na^+,K^+-ATPase of the cell membrane supplies energy for the active pumping of Na^+ outward and K^+ inward against their large concentration gradients (Fig. 22.3). The Na^+,K^+-ATPase is believed to be the cellular receptor for digitalis glycosides (Schwartz 1977; Akera and Ng 1991; Schatzmann 1953). Inhibition of Na^+,K^+-ATPase by digitalis results in progressive reduction of $(K^+)_i$ as the ability of the pump to transport K^+ inward and Na^+ outward progressively fails (Fozzard and Sheets 1985; Katz 1985). A decrease in $(K^+)_i$ and/or an increase in $(K^+)_o$ reduces resting membrane potential to a less negative value, which can lead to increased automaticity and eventually impaired conduction and excitability. Inhibition of ATPase and resulting depletion of $(K^+)_i$ are responsible for many toxic arrhythmogenic activities of digitalis.

The inotropic effect involves activation of a Na^+-Ca^{++} exchange mechanism through accumulation of $(Na^+)_i$. Baker et al. (1969) demonstrated with the giant squid axon that an increase in $(Na^+)_i$ enhanced the uptake of Ca^{++} by a Na^+-Ca^{++} exchange process. This mechanism seems to be operative in other excitable tissues and has been evoked as the link between inhibition of Na^+,Ka^+-ATPase and digitalis inotropy in the heart (Langer 1977). The sequence of events can be visualized to include the following progression: digitalis interacts with and inhibits cell membrane Na^+,K^+-ATPase, outward pumping of Na^+ is slowed, $(Na^+)_i$ accumulates, increased $(Na^+)_i$ augments transmembrane exchange of intracellular Na^+ for extracellular Ca^{++}, $(Ca^{++})_i$ is increased, and Ca^{++} delivery to the contractile proteins is increased; thus the positive inotropic effect is gained. A schematic that illustrates the dominance of Na^+-K^+ exchange in the normal state and the augmentation of Na^+-Ca^{++} exchange after inhibition of ATPase by digitalis is shown in Figure 22.6.

Cardiac Output. Digitalis glycosides exert a fundamentally similar action on the normal and failing myocardium, an increase in contractility. However, changes in cardiac output are influenced by the functional status of the cardiovascular system at the time of digitalis administration.

Normal Heart. Output of the normal heart increases minimally and may even decrease slightly after treatment with digitalis (Braunwald 1985). Total peripheral resistance is increased by digitalis in the normal subject as a result of a centrally mediated increase in sympathetic vaso-

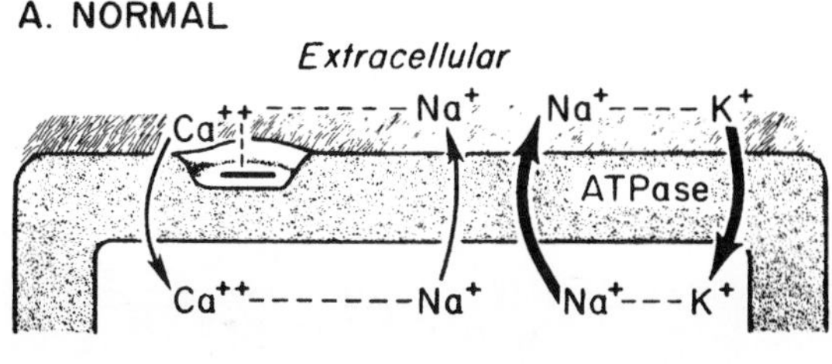

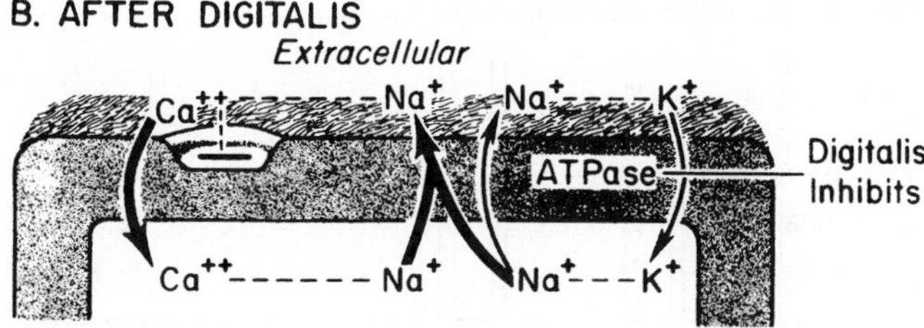

FIG. 22.6 Schematic representation of a proposed mechanism for the positive inotropic action of cardiac glycosides. Inhibition of Na^+,K^+–ATPase (sodium pump) by digitalis results in increased intracellular concentrations of sodium available for exchange with calcium. Heavy arrows designate the dominant pathway of ion exchange during normal conditions (A) and after inhibition by digitalis of Na^+,K^+–ATPase (B). (After Langer 1976; from Parker and Adams 1977.)

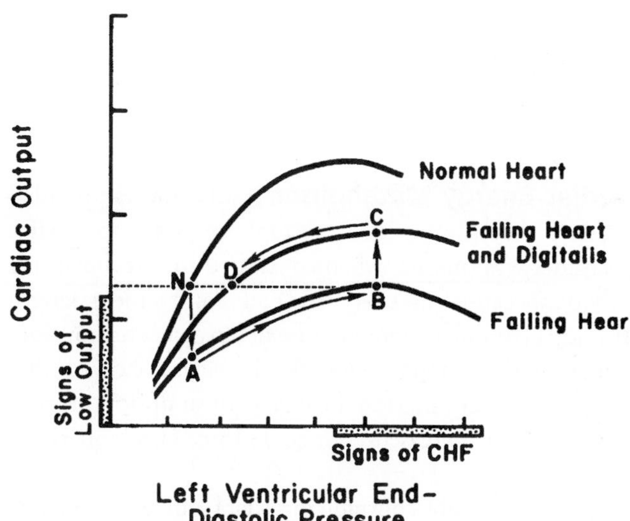

FIG. 22.7 Diagrammatic representation of how changes in left ventricular filling influence cardiac output by the Frank-Starling mechanism in a normal heart and in a failing heart before and after digitalis. The points N to D represent in sequence: N–A, normal cardiac output falls to A because of initial contractile depression from congestive heart failure (CHF); A–B, shift to higher end-diastolic filling and thus higher cardiac output in accord with the Frank-Starling law; B–C, increase in contractility after digitalization; C–D, reduction in use of Frank-Starling compensation, which digitalis allows. N, B, and D: identical cardiac output on the vertical axis but achieved at different end-diastolic filling pressure on the horizontal axis. Levels of cardiac output and end-diastolic filling associated with signs of low output (e.g., fatigue) or CHF (e.g., dyspnea, edema) are represented by the dotted areas. (Modeled after Mason 1973.)

motor tone and direct vasoconstrictor effect. Impedance of the arterial circuit to ventricular ejection is thereby increased, which opposes the trend toward increased output produced by positive inotropic response to the drug. Increased outflow impedance and increased cardiac contractility tend to counteract each other, yielding little net change in cardiac output in normal populations.

Failing Heart. The work capacity of the failing ventricle at any given end-diastolic volume or pressure is inadequate to generate a normal stroke volume (Fig. 22.7). The ejection fraction is diminished accordingly, which increases residual blood in the ventricle after systole (Moalic et al. 1993). If diastolic filling continues at a near normal rate, the ventricle will dilate to accommodate increased end-diastolic volume. After digitalization, the above processes are reversed. Digitalis-increased contractile vigor of the heart muscle augments work capacity of the ventricle at any given end-diastolic filling pressure, as illustrated in Figure 22.7, where ventricular function curves derived in the prefailure state (normal) are compared with curves derived from congestive failure patients prior to and after digitalis therapy. Digitalis shifts the complete ventricular function curve upward in the direction of improved contractility (Mason 1973; Braunwald 1985). Systolic emptying is now more complete, and residual ventricular volume is diminished. Cardiac output increases and size of the heart is reduced as ventricular filling volume is lowered.

Subsequent hemodynamic adjustments evoke other responses that contribute to maintenance of improved cardiac output in the congestive heart failure patient; e.g., sympathetically mediated vasoconstriction and its attending increase in peripheral vascular resistance are already in progress in these individuals as part of the compensatory response to their pathophysiologic condition; increased impedance to ventricular ejection is in force. After digitalis, the pronounced augmentation of myocardial contractility and stroke volume set into motion a reflex withdrawal of vasomotor tone. This in turn evokes peripheral vasodilation, reduced peripheral resistance, and diminished outflow impedance. This sequence of events continues to dominate as peripheral perfusion and tissue oxygenation improve, and it compensates for the direct vasoconstrictor effect of digitalis. The increase in cardiac output persists as long as the state of myocardial compensation prevails.

Cardiac Energy Metabolism. Early studies provided evidence that the positive inotropic response to cardiac glycosides was unique, when contrasted to catecholamine activity, because digitalis increased contractile strength without a commensurate increase in oxygen consumption. Studies with nonfailing muscle, however, showed that cardiac glycosides increased oxygen consumption proportionately with increased contractile force (Lee and Klaus 1971).

These seemingly contradictory data can be reconciled by comparing the cardiodynamics of digitalis in normal and failing hearts. The heart with a normal ventricular volume responds to digitalis with increase in oxygen consumption commensurate with increase in contractility. Increased oxygen consumption is the direct result of increased contractility, in accordance with the concept that myocardial oxygen demand (MVO_2) is influenced directly by the inotropic state, heart rate, and wall tension. Ventricular wall tension is directly proportional to ventricular pressure and radius (tension < pressure × radius; Laplace relation); tension will decrease if either pressure or radius is reduced. In the failing and dilated heart, reduction in cardiac size secondary to the inotropic action of digitalis therapy leads to a significant reduction in wall tension, which in turn leads to decreased MVO_2.

Blood Pressure. Adjustments in blood pressure after cardiac glycoside therapy are secondary to cardiodynamic improvement in the congestive failure patient, and systemic pressure tends to normalize (Fig. 22.8).

Neuroendocrine Effects. In heart failure patients, a lowering of heart rate accompanies the positive inotropic effect. This effect is apparently the result of a *neuroendocrine effect* and has been recognized as perhaps more important than the positive inotropic effects at therapeutic doses. It also appears that the neuroendocrine effects are independent from the positive inotropic action.

Neuroendocrine effects are achieved because digitalis increases the baroreceptor reflex sensitivity that has been lost during heart failure. The desensitization is thought to cause the high catecholamine levels in patients with heart failure. Digitalis restores the sensitivity and decreases sympathetic tone in patients with heart failure. The neuroendocrine effects also are attributed to vagal stimulation (parasympathomimetic effect). The neuroendocrine effects are responsible for a decrease in sinus rate and a slowing of atrioventricular (AV) impulse conduction.

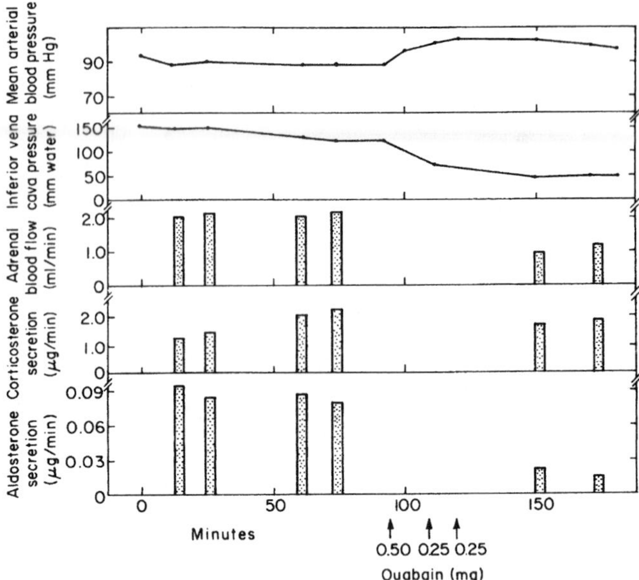

FIG. 22.8 The effects of IV ouabain injection (total dose 0.05 mg/kg) in an 8-year-old, 20 kg male Pointer with naturally occurring congestive heart failure. Following injection, mean arterial blood pressure increased from 88 mm Hg to a maximum of 110 mm Hg, and inferior vena cava pressure fell from a control value of 150–140 mm water to a minimum of 38 mm water; these changes started within 5 minutes after beginning the ouabain injection and reached a maximum 40–50 minutes postinjection. Following drug administration, there was also a marked fall in adrenal corticosterone and aldosterone secretion (Carpenter et al. 1962).

Excitability. Direct and indirect electrophysiologic effects of digitalis can be demonstrated throughout the heart (Gillis and Quest 1980). The reduced intracellular K^+ and increased intracellular Na^+ resulting from inhibition of Na^+,K^+-ATPase yield a partial depolarization of the cell; i.e., negativity of the cell interior is diminished. The resulting decrease in diastolic potential brings this value closer to threshold, thus tending to enhance excitability. Increased excitability can be observed in atria and ventricles with a small dose of digitalis; however, excitability becomes depressed with progressively larger amounts of the drug as diastolic depolarization progresses beyond a critical limit.

Automaticity. Pacemaker cells are characterized by phase 4 spontaneous depolarization, which moves diastolic potential to the threshold required for activation of phase 0, thereby firing automatically (see Chapter 23). Therapeutic doses of cardiac glycosides produce a decrease in the slope of spontaneous depolarization of the sinoatrial pacemaker, which yields a reduced firing rate. This effect, however, is secondary to increased vagal tone and decreased sympathetic tone. After pretreatment with atropine, or with relatively high doses of digitalis, the nonvagal effects dominate, and an increase in automaticity is observed; this response is prevalent in the specialized conducting systems of atria and, especially, ventricles. A typical transmembrane potential recording of a subsidiary pacemaker cell prior to and after digitalis is shown in Figure 22.9.

Increased automaticity evoked by cardiac glycosides is due to an accelerated rate of spontaneous diastolic depolarization (Fig. 22.9). The normally latent pacemaker activities of cells within the ventricular conducting system are thereby magnified, leading to ectopic ventricular beats as an important early sign of digitalis toxicity. In contrast, muscle fibers in atria and ventricles can be depolarized to the extent of inexcitability without demonstrating spontaneous impulse generation. If excitability of ventricular muscle falls below normal concomitantly with increased frequency of ectopic impulses from specialized conduction fibers, the tendency for ventricular fibrillation is promoted.

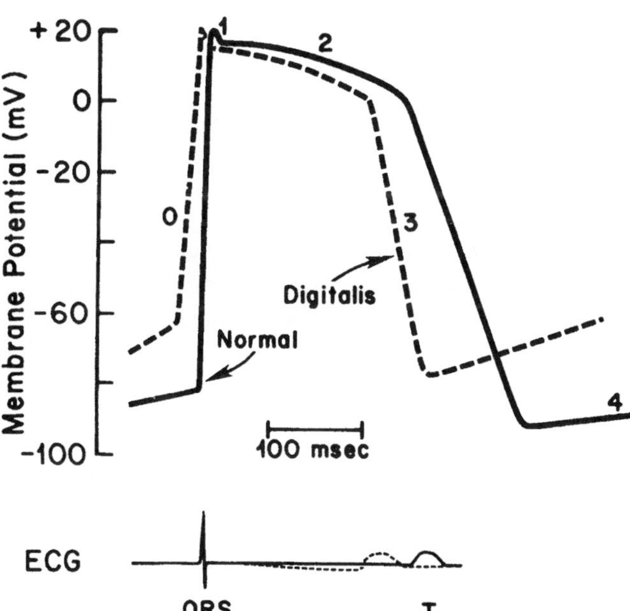

FIG. 22.9 Electrophysiologic effects of digitalis on transmembrane potential of a subsidiary pacemaker cell. Digitalis (*a*) decreases (less negative) the maximal diastolic potential, (*b*) decreases the maximal rate of depolarization of phase 0, *V*max, and (*c*) enhances automaticity by increasing the slope of phase 4 spontaneous depolarization. (*a*) and (*b*) lead to decreased conduction velocity and, in conjunction with (*c*), can lead to arrhythmias of both impulse formation and impulse conduction. (Modeled after Mason et al. 1971.)

The clinical significance of the unusual "delayed afterdepolarizations" that can be seen with digitalis toxicity is not completely resolved. These secondary depolarizations of the transmembrane potential initially are subthreshold and appear spontaneously during diastole after a usual action potential. The afterdepolarizations can reach threshold as toxicity worsens; the resulting extrasystoles contribute to ectopic arrhythmias associated with digitalis intoxication.

Impulse Conduction and Refractory Periods. The dominant effect of digitalis on impulse conduction is to slow conduction velocity by both vagal and nonvagal mechanisms. This response is particularly prevalent in the AV transmission system and contributes importantly to the beneficial effects of digitalis in controlling ventricular rate during atrial fibrillation and flutter.

Vagal-dependent actions in the intact animal shorten the refractory period of atrial fibers, which tends to exacerbate atrial fibrillatory rhythms. In contrast, the refractory period of the AV conduction system is prolonged markedly by vagal mechanisms. Digitalis shortens the refractory period in the ventricle, which contributes to reentry arrhythmias (Table 22.2).

Combined Effects During Atrial Fibrillation and Flutter. During atrial fibrillation, the ventricular rate is rapid and dysrhythmic as a result of rapid but irregular transmission of impulses through the AV node. This contributes further to heart failure syndrome by promoting incomplete ventricular filling and ejection. Because digitalis prolongs the refractory period and delays impulse conduction through the AV junction, the ventricle will be bombarded by fewer impulses effectively traversing the junction. Thus ventricular rate is adjusted to a slower, more physiologic level (Meijler 1985).

Similar benefits are gained during atrial flutter. Digitalis can convert this rhythm to atrial fibrillation (or increase the frequency of the latter) by vagal-dependent mechanisms, evoking a reduction in the atrial refractory period. Ventricular rate is still decreased, however, through pro-

TABLE 22.2 Characteristic effects of digitalis on electrophysiologic properties of the heart

Electrophysiologic	Cardiac Property Region	Effects	Response
Automaticity	SA node	Decreases as a result of vagal-dependent actions and sympathic withdrawal (may increase after atrophine)	Decreases sinus rate
	Atrial specialized conducting fibers	Little change; increases with toxicity	Increases ectopic pacemakers
	AV junctional tissues	Variable; increases with larger doses	Increases AV junctional rhythms
	Purkinje fibers	Variable; increases with larger doses	Increases ectopic pacemakers
	Atrial and ventricular muscle	Usually little change; rarely increases with toxic doses	
Excitability	Atrial and ventricular muscle	Variable; progressively decreases with larger doses; severe decrease with toxicity	
	Purkinje fibers	Variable; progressively decreases with larger doses	
Conduction	Atrial and ventricular muscle	Increases slightly; decreases with larger doses	Promotes atrial fibrillation
	AV junctional tissues	Decreases as a result of vagal-dependent actions; progressively decreases with toxicity	Decreases ventricular rate in atrial fibrillation; AV block
	Purkinje fibers	Decreases; further decrease with toxicity	Promotes ventricular reentry forms of arrhythmias
Refractoriness	Atrium	Decreases as a result of vagal-dependent actions; (increase after atropine)	Promotes atrial fibrillation
	Ventricle	Decreases	Favors reentry forms of arrhythmias
	AV junctional tissues	Increases as a result of vagal-dependent actions	Contributes to ventricular rate decreases in atrial fibrillation; AV block with toxicity
	Purkinje fibers	Increases; progressively decreases with larger doses	Favors reentry forms of arrhythmias

Note: SA = sinoatrial; AV = atrioventricular.

longed AV refractoriness and slowed impulse conduction. Conversion of atrial flutter to fibrillation by digitalis is viewed optimistically because ventricular rate is controlled more easily during fibrillation than during flutter.

Effects on the Electrocardiogram. The multiplicity of electrophysiologic effects of cardiac glycosides in myocardial tissues can be expressed as equally complex changes in the electrocardiogram (ECG). Most types of conduction disturbances and dysrhythmias detected in diseased animals can be reproduced in normal individuals by the cardiac glycosides. Most of these changes are more important to diagnosis of digitalis toxicosis than to therapy.

Congestive failure patients with sinus tachycardia or other supraventricular tachyarrhythmias usually demonstrate return toward more normal ECG patterns after digitalization. Rapid ventricular rates associated with atrial fibrillation or flutter should be reduced as the AV depressing action of digitalis is manifested. Prolonged PR intervals, reflecting delayed AV conduction, are relatively common ECG features of digitalized dogs. Conversely, a lengthened PR interval is not necessarily a prerequisite for the therapeutic response. Some cardiologists believe that prolongation of the PR interval can be a borderline sign of digitalis toxicity (Tilley 1979).

Different types of ECG abnormalities can appear if therapeutic response to digitalis degenerates into intoxication. The following progression of ECG signs has been recognized as evidence of digoxin action (Detweiler 1977): 1) signs occasionally observed in normal dogs but also characteristic of digoxin effects (first degree AV block or AV block with dropped beats), 2) signs unlikely to occur spontaneously in normal resting dogs (sinus bradycardia less than 50 beats/min or sinus tachycardia exceeding 200 beats/min), and 3) signs not occurring in normal dogs (AV dissociation, paroxysmal atrial tachycardia with or without block, ectopic atrial beats, fusion beats, intraventricular block, or ventricular ectopic beats).

Kidneys and Diuresis. Compensatory mechanisms that participate in an attempt to restore blood flow in congestive failure include reflex increases in sympathetic vasoconstrictor tone. Arteriolar constriction in the kidney is particularly crucial because diminished renal blood flow reduces glomerular filtration rate, resulting in sodium and water retention. Renal underperfusion also activates a kidney-dependent humoral mechanism that further promotes salt and water reabsorption. This sequence involves the following progressive pathway: diminished cardiac output, hypotension, baroreceptor reflexes, increased sympathetic activity, renal arteriolar constriction, reduced renal flow, release of renin, increased formation of angiotensin, increased release of aldosterone, sodium retention, water retention, and blood volume expansion.

Increased blood volume tends to increase cardiac output; however, a detrimental consequence is increased interstitial fluid volume, which promotes edema formation. As blood volume expands and intravascular pressures increase, likelihood for edema increases proportionately. Edema forms in the lungs and more peripheral tissue, respectively, if left and right ventricular failure progressively worsens.

After digitalization, the above processes are reversed. Reflex vasoconstriction withdraws as cardiac output and hemodynamics are improved; renal blood flow and glomerular filtration rate increase and stimuli for increased release of aldosterone are diminished. A remarkable fall in aldosterone secretion can be measured after digitalization in the dog with naturally occurring congestive failure (Fig. 22.8). Profuse diuresis results as salt and water retention by the kidneys is decreased. Diuresis and a lowering of capillary hydrostatic pressure move tissue water from the interstitial compartment into the vascular space, providing relief from edema. Diuresis is not a prominent feature of digitalis therapy if edema does not accompany the congestive failure syndrome. Similarly, digitalis does not evoke diuresis if edema is not cardiogenic. Thus the diuretic response to digitalis is secondary to circulatory improvement and is not from a direct effect on the kidney (Robinson 1972).

Extracirculatory Effects. Cardiac glycosides can affect cellular functions throughout the body, apparently by inhibiting the ubiquitous Na^+,K^+-ATPase; e.g., these agents can affect skeletal muscle function, thyroid gland activity, hematologic parameters, and numerous other functions. Such activities are believed to have little therapeutic importance except for overt toxicosis and generally require quantities of the drug in excess of those that should be administered.

Vomiting reactions after digitalis are due mainly to a central action and occur even after parenteral administration in the eviscerated animal. Both the chemoreceptor trigger zone and the medullary emetic center seem to be involved; local irritation of the gastric mucosa also may participate in the emetic response after oral administration.

Pharmacokinetics. The small intestine is the principal site of digitalis absorption after oral administration, but the rate and extent of this process vary with different compounds and their formulations. Absorption of digoxin after oral administration of an elixir usually is uniform, up to 75–90%, with peak serum concentrations attained in 45–60 minutes (Krasula et al. 1976). The peak serum value is smaller and occurs somewhat later (90 minutes) when the tablet form is used. Depending on the pharmaceutical methods used in formulating tablets, absorption of digitalis glycosides can be erratic and inefficient to the extent that therapeutically useful serum concentrations are not gained.

After IV administration, the maximal positive inotropic responses to digoxin were obtained within 60 minutes after injection (Hamlin et al. 1971). There is an initial fall in serum concentration as the drug mixes in the vascular compartment and distributes through the tissues; a slower exponential decline follows. Biologic half-life values for digitalis glycosides in dogs remain uncertain because of variable results obtained from laboratory to laboratory and even within the same one. Breznock (1973, 1975) reported that the plasma half-life value for digoxin was 38.9 and 55.9 hours in different studies. Other approximate values for digoxin include 27 hours (Barr et al. 1972), 30 hours (Hahn 1977), 24 hours (Doherty 1973), and 31 hours (De Rick et al. 1978). Differences are probably caused by interpatient variability; e.g., the half-life for digoxin in dogs after therapy for 13 days varied from 14.4 to 46.5 hours (De Rick et al. 1978). These variables strengthen the need for adoption of individual dosage regimens depending on the patient's response.

Digoxin is 25% protein bound (Breznock 1973) and urinary excretion seems to be the more important route of elimination. Digitalis glycosides and their biotransformation products can follow an enterohepatic cycle in which compounds are excreted by the liver into bile and some parent glycoside and metabolites are subsequently reabsorbed.

Digitalis Toxicity

Plasma Concentrations. Development of an accurate radioimmunoassay for measuring quantities of digoxin and digitoxin in biologic fluids was an important advancement in the field of pharmacology. The clinical application of this method permits correlation of serum concentrations of the drugs with therapeutic or toxic effects (Haber 1985).

In humans, therapeutic and toxic plasma concentrations of digoxin usually are set at 0.8–1.6 ng/ml and greater than 2.4 ng/ml, respectively (Moe and Farah 1975). Similar numbers have been derived from studies with animals; e.g., digoxin plasma concentrations of 0.5–2 ng/ml were nontoxic in horses (Button et al. 1980c); 2.3 ng/ml were not toxic in cats (Ericksen et al. 1980). Plasma digoxin concentrations up to 2.5 ng/ml were reported to be essentially nontoxic in healthy dogs and in dogs with spontaneous cardiac failure; importantly, values from 0.8 to 1.9 ng/ml may have been therapeutically effective in the latter group. Concentrations of digoxin greater than 2.5–3 ng/ml were associated with increased probability of toxicosis in these animals (De Rick et al. 1978).

The acute toxic IV dose of digoxin in dogs was determined in one study as approximately 0.177 mg/kg (Beck 1969). Subacute digoxin toxicosis could be induced and maintained in healthy Beagle dogs by an IV loading dose of 0.125–0.150 mg/kg given in increments at 0, 1, 4, and 24 hours, followed by a daily IV maintenance dose of 0.015–0.025 mg/kg (Fillmore and Detweiler 1973; Teske et al. 1976). Signs of toxicity were generally mild or absent when serum digoxin concentrations were less than 2.5 ng/ml. Moderate signs of intoxication were associated with concentrations of 2.5–6 ng/ml, whereas severe toxicosis and some deaths occurred when levels exceeded 6 ng/ml. The highest digoxin concentrations were associated with mild hypothermia (0.6–1.7°C reduction), increased blood urea nitrogen (BUN), and increased serum creatinine. The unexpected increase in serum creatinine and BUN concentrations was interpreted as evidence that digoxin toxicity compromised renal function.

Clinical Signs. Digitalis intoxication is characterized by several clinical signs varying from mild GI upset to chronic weight loss and life-threatening arrhythmias (Detweiler 1977; Tilley 1979). Initial anorexia and loose stools are common side effects; if they do not progressively worsen, a reduction in dose may not be necessary. Vomiting after IV administration of cardiac glycosides is a relatively common reaction and usually not cause for alarm. Vomiting in dogs receiving oral digitalis preparations is viewed more seriously, especially if protracted diarrhea is an accompaniment; these individuals should be examined for additional evidence of toxicity. GI disturbances are certainly troublesome and may debilitate the patient; however, the lethal outcome of digitalis intoxication is due to cardiac arrhythmias.

A variety of abnormalities can appear in the ECG as digitalis toxicity develops. The reduced sinus rate and slowed AV conduction attained with digitalis therapy can progress to incomplete or complete heart block with dropped beats and ST segment changes as intoxication supervenes. AV block, in turn, may progress to junctional escape rhythms and ventricular premature systoles. If an extra QRS complex recurs after each regular systole, digitalis has evoked ventricular bigeminy (coupled ventricular systoles). Ventricular bigeminal rhythm can appear prior to, with, or after development of other arrhythmias that may be associated with digitalis intoxication. Paroxysmal ventricular or atrial tachycardia with block and multifocal premature ventricular systoles are further evidence of serious cardiac disturbances. Occurrence of these or any other important ECG abnormalities necessitates complete withdrawal of digitalis therapy; treatment with smaller doses should not be instituted until the ECG is free of such arrhythmias.

Species differences in sensitivity to acute toxic effects of digitalis glycosides were reviewed by Detweiler (1967). The relative median lethal dose in several species, taking the cat as unity, are: cat, 1; rabbit, 2; various frogs, 28; various toads, >400; and rat, 671. Resistance to digitalis toxicity seems to reside in the heart and may be a reflection of the relative sensitivity of the Na^+,K^+-ATPase to glycoside inhibition.

Electrolyte Involvement. Cardiac toxicity of digitalis is affected by availability of electrolytes, especially K^+ and Ca^{++}. In essence, reduced K^+ potentiates digitalis arrhythmogenicity, whereas excess K^+ antagonizes arrhythmogenic activity. The antiarrhythmic activity of K^+ in digitalis intoxication is probably related to inhibition by the cation of glycoside binding to the Na^+,K^+-ATPase. The intracellular-extracellular ratio of K^+ seems to be a primary determinant of the interaction between this ion and digitalis rather than interstitial concentrations of K^+ alone. Digitalis-induced dysrhythmia can occur in the presence of normal K^+ plasma concentration because of the intracellular depletion of this cation that accompanies Na^+,K^+-ATPase inhibition (Rosen 1985).

Treatment. Although radioimmunoassay techniques can distinguish obviously subtherapeutic and toxic plasma concentrations of digitalis, considerable overlap occurs; a therapeutic concentration in one patient may be toxic to another. Clinical experience and judgment must still be exercised when digitalis intoxication is differentiated from exacerbation of cardiac failure with its attending dysrhythmias.

When digitalis intoxication is diagnosed, the first procedure is to withdraw glycoside therapy; the patient's progress should then be followed closely with frequent ECG monitoring. These conservative measures in conjunction with cage rest often are effective in controlling cardiac arrhythmias and other signs of intoxication; however, appropriate therapy should be instituted if arrhythmias worsen or fail to revert spontaneously.

Potassium chloride (KCl) has been administered in an attempt to increase plasma K^+ concentrations to upper limits of the normal range and thereby suppress glycoside arrhythmias. Conversely, if plasma K^+ is already high in the digitalis-intoxicated dog, administration of exogenous K^+ can actually cause further deterioration of ECG patterns. Obviously, considerable care should be exerted when K^+ therapy is employed in managing digitalis toxicity. In dogs, the dosage schedule for KCl has included 0.6–1 g orally as the initial dose, followed by 0.3–0.5 g every 1–2 hours for 2 doses, and continued at 4-hour intervals as necessary to control arrhythmias (Detweiler 1977). Slow IV infusion of KCl with frequent monitoring of the ECG and serum K^+ concentrations may be attempted (Ettinger and Suter 1970). However, too rapid an infusion of potassium salts may precipitate other arrhythmias, including ventricular fibrillation.

Cholestyramine Resin, USP, is an exchange resin that binds glycoside within the digestive tract; it has been used experimentally in attempts to interrupt the enterohepatic cycle and thereby hasten elimination of the digitalis compound.

The use of specific antiglycoside antibodies is another therapy (Haber 1985; Kurowski et al. 1992). Digoxin Immune FAB (Digibind®) is an ovine source of antidigoxin antibodies. This treatment has been used in animals but is expensive. One vial contains 38 mg digoxin immune FAB and will neutralize 500 mcg of digoxin. Animals will improve quickly after administration. If this is used in animals, a clinical assay for digoxin serum concentrations will be misleading due to interference and should not be used to monitor toxicity.

Agents such as Mg^{++}, procainamide, quinidine, EDTA, sodium citrate, saturated lactones, and salts of canrenoate have received little clinical use in animals. Of the antiarrhythmic agents, lidocaine, propranolol, and, especially, phenytoin are the most useful in controlling digitalis-induced arrhythmias (see Chapter 23). Atropine may be helpful in cases with severe sinus bradycardia. In the presence of AV block, antiarrhythmic agents and K^+ therapy should be avoided. Use of antiarrhythmic interventions so that the dose of digitalis can be increased in the hope of attaining a larger inotropic response is dangerous and unwarranted. Quinidine may actually cause an increase in plasma concentrations of digoxin, probably by blocking efflux transporters, p-glycoprotein.

Therapeutic Indications for Digitalis

Congestive Heart Failure. Controversy exists relative to the actual survival benefits of digitalis glycosides in the long-term therapeutic management of cardiac disease in animal patients (Hamlin et al. 1973; Patterson et al. 1973; Braunwald 1985; Kittleson et al. 1985a).

Cardiac glycosides are indicated in congestive heart failure resulting from an absolute or relative chronic overload in which the supply of energy to the heart is uncompromised is an indication for digitalis therapy. These types of problems include hypertension, passive outflow impedance (e.g., dirofilariasis), and idiopathic dilated cardiomyopathy. New inodilator drugs have largely taken the place of digitalis in managing heart failure in animals.

Atrial Arrhythmias. Digitalis is sometimes used in treatment of atrial fibrillation or flutter, whether or not congestive heart disease is present. However, the drug is not employed for ablation of the arrhythmic pattern. The goal of digitalis therapy in either of these states is to reduce ventricular rate by slowing AV conduction, eliminate the pulse deficit if present, and improve cardiac efficiency (Meijler 1985). The potential involvement of latent or hidden congestive heart failure in pathogenesis of atrial fibrillation in some animals should not be discounted; the beneficial results from digitalis in treating what seems to be uncomplicated atrial fibrillation may well involve such complexities.

Precautions. Digitalis is not indicated in cases of circulatory shock, renal failure, hepatic failure, ventricular premature contractions, ventricular tachycardia, or heart block unless the abnormality is associated with congestive heart failure (Braunwald and Kahler 1964). Digitalis therapy in congestive failure patients with heart block or ventricular tachycardia should be supervised in a particularly intensive manner, and digitalization should be monitored closely with an ECG. Digitalis can accentuate AV block and a serious decrease in ventricular rate may result. Digitalis treatment can also transform ventricular tachyarrhythmias to fibrillation.

Although digitalis slows sinus rate in congestive heart disease, this activity is complex and has no application in attempts to reduce heart rate when sinus tachycardia is present without evidence of congestive failure. Tachycardia associated with other conditions such as fever, thyrotoxicosis, constrictive pericarditis, or cardiac tamponade is not amenable to digitalis therapy. Hypertrophic cardiomyopathies and ruptured chorda tendinae constitute other nonindications for digitalis therapy.

Digitalis toxicosis can simulate certain aspects of cardiac disease, especially serious arrhythmias. Clinicians should always ascertain that any patient scheduled for cardiac glycoside treatment has not recently received any digitalis preparation; otherwise, an attempt to produce therapeutic digitalization in a patient actually suffering from unrecognized digitalis intoxication can have negative results.

Clinical Procedures. When initiating treatment with digoxin, the precise dosage schedule can be less important than the care taken in monitoring patient response during implementation. In all cases, a predetermined dose should not be administered indiscriminately until toxic effects are seen. If signs of intoxication supervene early in the digitalization schedule before salutary effects are attained, treatment must be halted and resumed at a lower dose after signs of toxicosis are absent. Similarly, if toxicity develops during maintenance therapy, the dose must be readjusted to a lower level. Conversely, the dose may have to be increased or administered at shorter intervals if therapeutic effects are not achieved with the predetermined schedule. Thus semantics about rigid time schedules should be interpreted in the clinic in accordance with needs of the individual patient. A listing of average dose levels of digitalis glycosides is provided in Table 22.3.

Data published by De Rick et al. (1978) indicated that administration of 0.025 mg/kg digoxin every 12 hours for 36 hours (i.e., a total digitalization dose of 0.1 mg/kg), followed by a maintenance dose of 0.01 mg/kg every 12 hours, was associated with less toxicity than larger loading dose techniques. The digoxin data presented in Figure 22.10 show that this schedule leads to therapeutic blood levels, whereas a larger loading dose results in initial plasma concentrations associated with toxicosis.

Harris (1974) and Hahn (1977) advocated that a loading dose of digoxin is not necessary in dogs and that daily maintenance doses of 0.022 mg/kg given in two equal amounts at 12-hour intervals should be implemented as the original procedure. Using complex pharmacokinetic

TABLE 22.3 Guidelines for approximating doses and dosage schedules for digitalis glycosides in dogs

	Loading Dose Technique		
Drug	Total Dose	Administration Schedule	Daily Maintenance Dose and Schedule
Oral			
Digitoxin*	0.11–0.22 mg/kg	0.022–0.044 mg/kg q12 h for 48 hr	0.011 mg/kg q12 h
Digoxin[†]	0.066 mg/kg	Three divided doses on day 1 of therapy	0.022 mg/kg daily
Digoxin[§]	0.1 mg/kg	0.025 mg/kg q12 h for 36 hr	0.011 mg/kg q12 h
Digoxin[‖]	. . .	. . .	0.011 mg/kg q12 h
Digitoxin*	0.022–0.044 mg/kg	0.0044–0.0088 mg/kg q12 h	0.0022–0.0044 mg/kg q12 h
Digitoxin[#]	0.44 mg/kg	Divided doses over 48 hr	0.11 mg/kg daily
Parental			
Ouabain	0.022–0.033 mg/kg	Three divided doses over 24 hr	Oral digoxin 0.011 mg/kg q12 h
Digoxin	0.022–0.044 mg/kg	Three divided doses over 24 hr	Oral digoxin 0.011 mg/kg q12 h

Sources: *Drug companies and others, [†]Detweiler and Knight 1977; [§]De Rick et al. 1978; [‖]Harris 1974; [#]Hahn 1977.
Note: q12 h = every 12 hours.

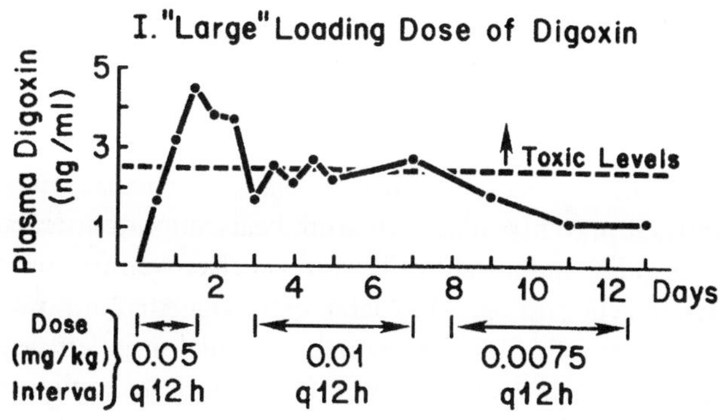

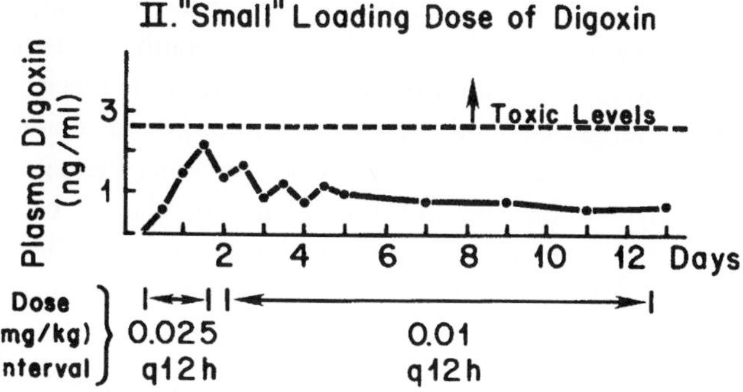

FIG. 22.10 Dosage schedules and plasma concentrations of digoxin after oral digitalization with a "large" (I) or "small" (II) loading dose. Notice in the top graph that with a large loading dose technique (0.05 mg/kg every 12 hr), plasma concentrations initially were in the toxic range (>2.5 ng/ml), whereas in the bottom graph with the smaller loading dose technique (0.025 mg/kg/12 hr), plasma concentrations did not exceed toxic levels and remained within presumed therapeutically effective concentrations. (Modeled after De Rick et al. 1978.)

calculations based on individual animals, Button et al. (1980a,b) found that the standard 0.022 mg/kg was a likely daily maintenance dose of digoxin in dogs.

Kittleson (1983) pointed out that because of its high toxic/therapeutic dose ratio, digitalis should be administered according to body surface area rather than body weight. Thus, since the body surface area/body weight ratio generally decreases as the size of the dog increases, larger canine breeds would require less digitalis per kilogram of body weight than the small breeds. According to a recommended twice-a-day digoxin dose of 0.22 mg/m^2 body surface area (Kittleson 1983), dogs weighing 10, 20, 30, 40, and 50 kg would receive 0.011, 0.009, 0.008, 0.007, and 0.006 mg digoxin/kg, respectively, twice daily. Clinical trials support the merit of this approach (Kittleson et al. 1985a).

Parenteral Schedules. IV administration increases the likelihood for toxic arrhythmias, and this limitation should be considered. Intramuscular injection reduces the danger, but pain and swelling at the injection site limits patient acceptance of this method. Oral maintenance doses should be substituted if feasible.

The positive inotropic response to digoxin can be detected within 15–30 minutes after IV administration in dogs (Hamlin et al. 1971). The rapid hemodynamic effects of ouabain in a dog with congestive failure are illustrated in Figure 22.8. When an emergency is presented, the total IV loading dose for digoxin is approximately 0.044 mg/kg (Ettinger and Suter 1970), with 25–50% of the total dose administered initially by slow IV injection; an additional 25% is given every 30–60 minutes (ouabain) or 60–120 minutes. Patients treated with these techniques should be closely examined for signs of intoxication and monitored continuously for ECG abnormalities.

Preparations

Digoxin, USP—cardiotonic glycoside from *D. lanata.*
Digoxin Injection, USP—digoxin in 10% alcohol; injections, 0.5 mg/2 ml.
Digoxin Tablets, USP—tablets, 0.25 and 0.5 mg.
Digoxin Elixir—digoxin, 0.05 or 0.15 mg/ml in 30% alcohol.

INODILATORS: PIMOBENDAN. Agents that have both vasodilator and positive inotropic properties have been labeled *inodilators* (Opie 2001). Historically, short-term management of acute or decompensated heart failure characterized by systolic dysfunction benefited from a combination of dobutamine (positive inotrope) and nitroprusside (vasodilator). Agents in this class combine these properties and agents such as pimobendan, which is available in an oral formulation, make chronic therapy a possibility. Levosimendan is another drug from this class investigated in animals but it is not available for clinical use at this time.

Clinical Application. Pimobendan is a novel agent with properties useful in the clinical management of canine heart failure secondary to either dilated cardiomyopathy (DCM) or chronic degenerative valvular disease (CVD).

The efficacy of pimobendan in the treatment of heart failure (HF) arising from DCM and CVD has been evaluated more thoroughly in dogs than has other cardioactive medications to date, including angiotensin converting enzyme inhibitors (ACEI). In a prospective blinded placebo controlled study, O'Grady et al. (2003a) demonstrated a doubling of overall survival in Doberman pinschers with HF secondary to DCM, from a median of 63 ± 14 days with furosemide, an ACEI and placebo, versus 128 ± 29 days with furosemide, an ACEI and pimobendan (0.25 mg/kg by mouth twice daily). Additional studies suggest a survival benefit with the combination of pimobendan and furosemide when compared to an ACEI and furosemide (with or without digoxin) in dogs with HF secondary to DCM or CVD. Other studies offer conflicting evidence with respect to the superiority of pimobendan for the treatment of HF secondary to CVD.

Preliminary analysis of an ongoing study by O'Grady et al. (2003b) showed no survival advantage using pimobendan and furosemide compared to an ACEI and furosemide in dogs with HF due to CVD. Conversely, Smith et al. (2005) and Lombard et al. (2006) (VetScope study) demonstrated superiority of a combination of pimobendan and furosemide over an ACEI (ramipril or benazepril, respectively) and furosemide for the treatment of HF due to CVD. Smith et al. (2005) reported a significant reduction of overall adverse outcomes, including death (euthanized or died) and treatment failure when furosemide and ramipril (48%) were compared to furosemide and pimobendan (18%) over 6 months of treatment. Lombard et al. (2006) reported the median survival (i.e., death or treatment failure) for dogs receiving pimobendan and furosemide was 415 days versus 128 days for those receiving benazepril and furosemide. In these studies no substantial side effects were observed, suggesting that the combination of pimobendan and furosemide may be superior to furosemide and an ACE inhibitor for the treatment of HF caused by atrioventricular valvular disease.

Pimobendan appears to be safe and well tolerated in dogs with HF associated with CVD. Unreported studies by Miller et al. (2007) in over 300 dogs with HF due to DCM or CVD showed overall beneficial effects of pimobendan when added to standard HF therapies. In addition to pimobendan these dogs received furosemide and an ACEI and one or more of the following drugs: spironolactone (>75%), a beta-blocker (20%), digoxin (11%), and hydrochlorothiazide (3%). Hemodynamic effects were evaluated prior to initiation of pimobendan and again approximately 45 days later. No significant changes were detected in indirect systemic blood pressures, body weight, hematocrit, total solids, serum creatinine, or electrolytes. Blood urea nitrogen concentration increased in some dogs. Heart rate and respiratory rate were reduced and no changes occurred in the combined frequency of arrhythmias (i.e., ventricular premature beats, ventricular tachycardia, supraventricular premature beats, supraventricular tachycardia, and atrial fibrillation) on electrocardiograms. Certain echocardiographic parameters suggested improvement in systolic function, namely a reduction in left ventricular (LV) internal dimension in systole, reduction of LV end-systolic area, and an increase in the percentage of LV area shortening. Reduction in the regurgitant fraction was suggested by a decrease in the radiographic vertebral heart score, a reduction in systolic left atrial diameter on echocardiography, and a decrease in the M-mode derived ratio of left atrial to aortic size. Taken together these findings suggest that the addition of pimobendan to background HF therapy had no detectable adverse side effects, while it enhanced systolic function and also reduced diastolic filling pressures. Although these beneficial effects were observed (on average) 45 days after initiating pimobendan, more recent experience suggests that these effects may be apparent as soon as 24 hours, which indicates potential application in the treatment of acute, decompensated HF. The median survival of the dogs in this 6-year study was 17 months (range 2 to 50 months) (Miller et al. 2007).

This clinical experience is in agreement with currently available prospective data supporting the efficacy of adjunctive pimobendan therapy in improving the quality and length of life in dogs with HF arising from both CVD and DCM (Smith et al. 2005; Lombard et al. 2006; O'Grady et al. 2003a). Pimobendan is easy to use clinically, requires no additional monitoring, and enjoys client compliance. Pimobendan works rapidly and can be used during the initial, acute phase of HF treatment. Peak hemodynamic effects following oral administration on an empty stomach are achieved in 1 hour and last 8 to 12 hours. The rapid onset of action, low incidence of side effects, and decreased time of hospitalization with the use of pimobendan have had a positive impact on the willingness of clients to pursue the treatment of HF. Ongoing studies (QUEST) will further test survival benefits associated with the use of pimobendan in dogs with HF due to CVD.

Pimobendan has been licensed for use in dogs with CHF since 2000 in many countries around the world, including the United States, Great Britain, Australia, Canada, and Mexico.

Mechanism of Action

Inotropy. Pimobendan is a benzimidazole pyridazinone derivative and is classified as an inodilator (i.e., positive inotrope and balanced arteriovenous dilator). In failing hearts it exerts its positive inotropic effects primarily through sensitization of the cardiac contractile apparatus to intracellular calcium. As a phosphodiesterase (PDE) III inhibitor it can potentially increase intracellular calcium concentration and increase myocardial oxygen consumption. However, the cardiac PDE effects of pimobendan are reportedly minimal at pharmacologic doses in dogs with heart disease, which is a major advantage relative to other inotropic PDE inhibitors such as milrinone. Pimobendan's calcium sensitization of the contractile apparatus is achieved by enhancement of the interaction between calcium and troponin C complex resulting in a positive inotropic effect that enhances systolic function, but does not increase myocardial oxygen consumption. Another advantage of pimobendan is its relative lack of arrhythmogenicity associated with positive inotropes whose sole mechanism of action is to increase myocardial intracellular calcium or cyclic AMP concentrations.

Vasodilation. Phosphodiesterase III and V are found in vascular smooth muscle. Inhibitors of PDE III such as pimobendan result in balanced vasodilation (combination of venous and arterial dilation) leading to a reduction of both cardiac preload and afterload, a cornerstone of therapy in HF. In addition, pimobendan may have some PDE V inhibitory effects. PDE V concentrations are relatively high in the vascular smooth muscle of pulmonary arteries, so PDE V inhibition may help ameliorate elevations in pulmonary artery pressure (pulmonary hypertension) that tend to parallel long-standing elevations in left atrial pressure, a clinically important complication of CVD.

Cytokine Modulation. The significance of alterations in proinflammatory cytokines such as tumor necrosis factor-α and interleukins 1-β and 6 on the progression of heart failure has been documented in several forms of heart disease. Maladaptive alterations in these cytokine concentrations are associated with increased morbidity and mortality; pimobendan has demonstrated beneficial modulation of several such cytokines in models of HF.

Antiplatelet Effects. Pimobendan reportedly has antithrombotic effects on platelets in the dog. The clinical significance of this property is not clear at this time.

Positive Lusiotropic Effects. Via PDE III inhibition in cardiomyocytes, pimobendan increased intracellular cAMP, facilitating phosphorolation of receptors on the sarcoplasmic recticulum. Diastolic reuptake of calcium is thus enhanced, and the speed of relaxation increased, indicating a positive lusiotropic property.

Formulations and Dose Rates. Pimobendan is supplied as hard gelatin capsules (most countries) containing 1.25, 2.5, or 5 mg pimobendan. In the United States it is approved as a chewable formulation in three sizes: *Vetmedin* 1.25, 2.5, and 5 mg. It is not stable in suspension and should not be reformulated in this manner. The labeled dose recommendation is 0.25–0.3 mg/kg q 12 hours (twice daily). Initial efficacy may be enhanced by administration on an empty stomach but once steady state is reached (a few days) it can be administered with food.

Levosimendan has been investigated as another veterinary drug for treating heart failure in dogs. At this time, it is still investigational and not available for clinical use.

Pharmacokinetics. Bioavailability is reduced by food until steady state is reached after a few days of administration. Consequently, the drug should be administered on an empty stomach at least 1 hour before feeding for maximal effects when starting therapy. Peak hemodynamic effects following oral administration on an empty stomach are achieved in 1 hour and last 8 to 12 hours. Thus although pimobendan is an oral preparation it can provide rapid short-term support to dogs with acute or decompensated heart failure.

Adverse Effects. Pimobendan is well tolerated clinically in dogs with HF. A case report documented chordal rupture in two dogs treated with pimobendan for an off-label indication. One additional case study reported ventricular hypertrophy, but the dogs in this study did not have HF and thus do not represent the patient population pimobendan was intended to treat. No prospective randomized controlled blinded study in either human or veterinary medicine has reported an increase in the frequency of arrhythmias, and veterinary studies report improved quality and quantity of life, arguing against clinically important side effects when pimobendan is used for treatment of canine HF. However, according to the Canadian package insert, suspected adverse effects that have been reported following clinical use include cardiovascular (systemic hypotension, tachycardia, usually dose dependent and avoided by reducing the dose), gastrointestinal (inappetence, anorexia, vomiting), nervous system/behavior (uneasiness, incoordination, convulsions), and renal (polyuria, polydyspnea). In addition, as for all positive inotropic agents, pimobendan should not be administered to patients with hypertrophic cardiomyopathy or patients with any type of outflow tract obstruction (e.g., subaortic stenosis, pulmonic stenosis). There are no data on the safety of pimobendan in pregnant or lactating dogs.

The inotropic effect may have a negative effect in dogs with early valvular lesions. In a study in asymptomatic dogs with mitral valve disease (Chetboul et al. 2007), pimobendan worsened mitral valve lesions and other indices of cardiac function in dogs treated with pimobendan compared to the group treated with the ACE inhibitor benazepril. The authors of the study proposed that the cardiotoxic effects were caused by an exaggerated pharmacodynamic effect rather than from intrinsic toxicity.

INAMRINONE AND MILRINONE. Inamrinone (formerly amrinone) and milrinone are bipyridine derivatives commonly referred to as nonglycoside, noncatecholamine inotropic drugs. These compounds were discovered during an investigative search for cardiac stimulant agents that could be used to replace digitalis in the therapy of heart failure (Alousi et al. 1979). Numerous studies confirmed that inamrinone and milrinone evoke both a positive inotropic action in the heart and a peripheral vasodilator effect. The mechanism of action of the bipyridines is dissimilar from that of digitalis and does not involve adrenergic nor other cell surface receptors. Rather, the cardiac inotropic and peripheral vasodilator actions of inamrinone and milrinone involve inhibition of the type III cyclic nucleotide phosphodiesterase enzyme. This enzyme is responsible for the selective metabolism of cAMP; hence, inhibition of type III phosphodiesterase by inamrinone or milrinone results in the accumulation of intracellular cAMP in cardiac and vascular tissues. Cyclic AMP subserves a positive inotropic response in myocardium and a vasodilator response in blood vessels. Because of concurrent inotropic and vasodilator actions, considerable attention has been focused first on inamrinone and later on milrinone as alternatives to digitalis in managing congestive heart failure patients (Mancini et al. 1985; Colucci et al. 1986a,b).

Inamrinone. IV administration of inamrinone (1–10 mg/kg) to anesthetized and unanesthetized dogs increased cardiac contractile force and left ventricular pressure with relatively small changes in heart rate and blood pressure. Administered orally to dogs, inamrinone (2–10 mg/kg) produced a positive inotropic effect with rapid onset (within 15 minutes) and long duration of action (approximately 5 hours). Acute hemodynamic response to inamrinone also has been studied in human patients with refractory heart failure. Inamrinone by oral or IV administration consistently enhanced cardiac contractile indexes while decreasing ventricular filling pressure/volume (preload) and systemic vascular resistance (afterload). Heart rate and blood pressure were affected slightly by therapeutic doses.

Despite some beneficial actions of inamrinone in managing acute exacerbation of heart failure, studies in humans have questioned whether long-term oral administration of inamrinone is clinically effective in therapy of chronic congestive heart failure (Massie et al. 1985). These results illustrate the potential pitfalls of trying to extrapolate results from acute studies to the exceedingly more complex situation of chronic therapy of heart failure. Moreover, adverse side effects occurred in 83% of these inamrinone-treated patients after long-term therapy, necessitating drug withdrawal in 34%. Thrombocytopenia is a serious side effect of inamrinone in about 15% of human patients chronically treated. This untoward reaction does not seem to be a problem in dogs. Inamrinone is used rarely in dogs except for treatment of acute HF when other more conventional therapy fails.

Milrinone. Milrinone is a structural congener of inamrinone, and the former is 20–30 times more potent than the latter. Initial studies suggested that milrinone might be relatively free of adverse side effects in reasonable doses and could be helpful in the management of heart failure patients in human medicine (Colucci et al. 1986a,b). However, studies with human patients with moderately severe heart failure indicated that milrinone was less effective than digoxin, and the combination of milrinone and digoxin was no more effective than digoxin alone. Moreover, milrinone administration was associated with an increased incidence of both ventricular and supraventricular tachyarrhythmias as adverse side effects (DiBianco et al. 1989).

Tachyarrhythmias could have been predicted as an adverse side effect of milrinone and other type III phosphodiesterase inhibitors inasmuch as their mechanism of action depends upon accumulation of cAMP. The latter not only subserves positive inotropic actions in the heart but also increases cardiac automaticity in sinoatrial pacemaker cells and other cardiac tissues that carry spontaneous automaticity. Emergence of latent pacemakers and associated ectopic beats and tachyarrhythmias can be expected as limiting side effects of drugs that affect the heart through the cAMP system. Hence, the initial enthusiasm for cardiac uses of milrinone and other type III phosphodiesterase inhibitors has decreased (Massie et al. 1985; DiBianco et al. 1989).

A collaborative investigation involving three veterinary medical teaching hospitals provided evidence that milrinone may be effective in dogs with spontaneous heart failure (Kittleson et al. 1985b). This study included a randomized blinded evaluation of milrinone (0.5–1.0 mg/kg) versus placebo for a 4-week period in a total of 14 dogs, 11 with left ventricular failure and 3 with right ventricular failure. Dogs in this study with echocardiographic evidence of mild-to-severe myocardial failure and clinical evidence of poor-to-good compensation for their heart failure responded favorably to treatment with milrinone as the sole therapeutic agent, as determined by echocardiography. This salutary effect was sustained for the 4 weeks of the study; it was not due to spontaneous remission of the disease because heart failure worsened when milrinone was withdrawn and improved when the drug was reinstituted. The only apparent adverse reactions were asymptomatic ventricular dysrhythmias in two dogs. The improved ventricular performance observed in this study was attributed to a direct increase in myocardial contractility owing to milrinone's positive inotropic action, to a decrease in cardiac work load owing to milrinone's vasodilator effects or, more likely, to a combination of both. These investigators concluded that milrinone may be an effective drug for treating myocardial failure in the dog when administered orally twice daily in 0.5–1 mg/kg doses.

The biologic half-life of milrinone is about 2 hours in dogs; the onset of action occurs within 30 minutes of oral administration and the duration of effect has been reported to be about 6 hours. The maximal response to milrinone in dogs with spontaneous heart failure develops about 1.5–2 hours after administration and dissipates rather quickly thereafter. Kittleson et al. (1985b) suggested, therefore, that dogs with severe decompensation of their heart failure may benefit from 3–4 daily doses of milrinone to take advantage of the maximal effects of the drug.

Milrinone was advanced as either a primary drug of choice in congestive heart failure or as an alternative in congestive failure patients who become refractory to digitalis. Additional controlled clinical trials with milrinone are needed to determine whether the beneficial results observed by Kittleson et al. (1985b) during their 4-week study are sustained over longer intervals without limiting side effects. It is unclear if arrhythmogenic side effects will be a limiting factor for milrinone in dogs, as it is in humans (DiBianco et al. 1989).

Indeed, clinicians should remember that effects of drugs on cardiovascular function may not be causally linked to effects on long-term survival. As examples, clinical studies in humans have shown that despite some apparent improvement in hemodynamic parameters, all the following drugs have actually been associated with increased mortality: the type III PDE inhibitors inamrinone, milrinone, and vesnarinone; the dopamine agonist ibopamine; and the benzimedazoline PDE inhibitor with calcium-sensitizing properties pimobendan (Cohn et al. 1998; Hampton et al. 1997; Packer et al. 1991; Rocco and Fang 2006). Such results have prompted some to caution that chronic inotropic therapy may even hasten death. But, as referenced previously, studies have documented prolonged survival of HF dogs treated with pimobendan when it was used in conjunction with other drugs that act by noncardiac actions (Smith et al. 2005; Lombard et al. 2006; Miller et al. 2007). Synergism between mechanistically different pharmacodynamic agents should be carefully appraised by the clinician in attempts to treat animals with chronic heart failure.

Despite experience with oral milrinone in dogs, there is currently no approved oral formulation available. Milronone lactate (Primacor) is available as an injectable solution in a strength of 1 mg/ml.

ANGIOTENSIN-CONVERTING ENZYME INHIBITORS

CAPTOPRIL AND ENALAPRIL MALEATE. Recognition of the contribution of the renin-angiotensin-aldosterone axis to the pathophysiology of congestive heart failure led to development of a new group of vasodilator agents. These compounds are the angiotensin-converting enzyme (ACE) inhibitors such as captopril, enalapril maleate, and benazepril (Holtz 1993; Dietz et al. 1993; Jackson 2006). Subsequent studies in experimental animals and humans have led to the identification of almost a dozen different ACE inhibitors (Jackson 2006). Although each ACE inhibitor has its own pharmacologic characteristics, all share the central and primary action of inhibiting the conversion of angiotensin I to angiotensin II (Jackson 2006; see Chapter 17).

Reduced perfusion of the kidneys during heart failure evokes release into the circulation of the renal enzyme renin. As detailed in Chapter 17, renin synthesizes the formation of angiotensin I. The latter is relatively inactive; however, it is metabolized by ACE into the potent vasoconstrictor angiotensin II. Thus, by inhibiting ACE, captopril and enalapril decrease the formation of angiotensin II and through this mechanism evoke peripheral vasodilation in the heart failure patient. Angiotensin II-mediated release of aldosterone also is decreased by ACE inhibitors, thus facilitating sodium excretion and diuresis. Captopril improves hemodynamics in dogs with experimental heart failure (Kittleson et al. 1993), and reduces blood concentrations of aldosterone and improves clinical status in dogs with naturally occurring heart failure (Knowlen et al. 1983); 1–2 mg/kg orally three times daily has been suggested as a successful dose for captopril in congestive failure in dogs (Kittleson 1983).

Studies with ACE inhibitors in human medicine have indicated that these agents exert substantial beneficial effects in heart failure patients (Dietz et al. 1993; Swedberg 1993; Jackson 2006). Enalapril and other ACE inhibitors improve exercise tolerance, decrease signs and symptoms of heart failure, and prolong life. Partly because of the rapidly expanding role of ACE inhibitors in cardiovascular therapeutics in human medicine, these drugs also are being used in animals with spontaneous cardiac disease.

In studies with cats presenting with hypertrophic cardiomyopathy, enalapril therapy improved hemodynamic status (Rush et al. 1998). The therapeutic efficacy of enalapril was also examined in a carefully controlled study involving over 400 dogs with naturally occurring dilated cardiomyopathy or chronic valvular heart disease (Ettinger et al. 1994). Some of the dogs were subjected to invasive monitoring of cardiodynamic functions, while other dogs were observed for signs of clinical improvement or mortality. Nearly all of the dogs continued to receive conventional therapy for heart failure involving diuretics (usually furosemide) without or with digoxin. Thus, this multicenter trial actually examined the ability of ACE inhibition to augment digitalis and diuretic therapy of heart failure, rather than therapeutic benefits from enalapril alone. Nevertheless, this study yielded convincing evidence that inhibition of ACE with enalapril can improve quality of life and delay mortality in dogs with heart failure.

Enalapril reduced the following variables in dogs with heart failure: pulmonary capillary wedge pressure, heart rate, mean blood pressure, and pulmonary arterial pressure (Sisson 1992). Similar results were also seen in experimental studies with captopril (Kittleson et al. 1993). Improvements in cardiovascular functions were evident over the first 24 hours of treatment with enalapril. After 3–4 weeks of enalapril plus conventional therapy, improvement was detected in several clinical markers of hemodynamic function. These included increased exercise capacity and resulting reduction in class of heart failure, reduced signs of pulmonary edema, and overall improvement in well being. Mortality was lower in the dogs treated with enalapril, and fewer of these patients exhibited progressive worsening of heart failure (Ettinger et al. 1994).

In a subset of 148 dogs, the long-term efficacy of enalapril was evaluated by measuring when the patients died or when they had to be removed from the study because of clinical deterioration. Dogs treated with enalapril (plus standard heart failure therapy) remained in the trial for 169 ± 14 days, compared to 90 ± 17 days for dogs receiving placebo (plus standard heart failure therapy). A group of 17 Doberman Pinschers treated with enalapril and standard therapy remained in the study for 80 ± 11 days, compared to only 38 ± 8 days in the placebo cohort group of 19 Dobermans. All other breeds of dogs treated with enalapril remained in the trial 189 ± 15 days, compared to 110 ± 14 days for the placebo group. When the dogs that died from congestive heart failure or died suddenly were analyzed separately, dogs treated with enalapril lived approximately 50% longer than placebo-treated dogs. Although these studies did not evaluate enalapril alone, they clearly indicate that enalapril is beneficial in the management of heart failure when added to conventional therapy with diuretics and digoxin (Ettinger et al. 1994).

1. Dogs with Class I heart disease do not have clinical evidence of heart disease except in response to exceptionally powerful exercise or other severe cardiovascular challenges. In general, these patients do not require drugs. High-salt diets should be avoided to prevent water retention and hypervolemia. Both chronic valvu-

lar disease and idiopathic dilated cardiomyopathy are progressive and usually irreversible conditions. Their rate of progression may be abated by therapeutic intervention; however, currently there are no reliable drugs that will cease progressive deterioration of the heart in these pathologic entities.

2. Dogs with Class II heart disease exhibit signs of insufficient cardiac function upon mild or moderate exercise. Enalapril at a dosage of 0.5 mg/kg once daily should be considered along with a restricted-salt diet. Renal function should be monitored regularly as signs of clinical improvement are followed.
3. Dogs with Class III heart disease have overt signs of heart failure during mild exercise; signs include dyspnea, orthopnea, cardiac cough, and episodes of pulmonary edema. Exercise tolerance is markedly diminished. Ascites and other evidence of right side heart failure commonly appear. Aggressive drug therapy should be implemented along with restriction of physical activity and dietary salt. A diuretic such as furosemide is usually started first for 2–4 days, followed by institution of enalapril at 0.5 mg/kg once daily. The dose of enalapril may be increased to a total of 1 mg/kg per day in two divided doses, depending upon clinical response. Digoxin may also be prescribed at a standard dosage and concomitantly with the diuretic, depending on signs of heart failure and cardiac tachyarrhythmias.
4. Dogs with Class IV heart failure are in acute decompensation and usually require aggressive emergency therapy with oxygen, morphine, cardiac inotropes, IV diuretics, and preload reducers. ACE inhibitors should be reserved until the patient is out of danger from acute pulmonary edema and cardiac decompensation.

ACE inhibitors such as enalapril truly represent a major addition to drug therapy of heart failure. However, renal function should be monitored to ensure adequate perfusion of the kidneys. Furthermore, despite the impressive results of the multicenter trial with enalapril (Ettinger et al. 1994), it should be remembered that enalapril was studied as an adjunct to conventional therapy with digoxin and diuretics. The results with these combined therapies will most likely be improved upon as additional studies examine the full therapeutic spectrum for ACE inhibitors such as enalapril, benzapril, and the several newer ACE inhibitors now available for therapeutic use in humans (Jackson 2006; see Chapter 17).

ADVERSE EFFECTS. Because of the importance of angiotensin in maintaining renal perfusion in heart failure and other low cardiac output conditions, renal function should be monitored during therapy with ACE inhibitors. However, results from the multicenter trial with enalapril in dogs indicated that sporadic episodes of azotemia (elevated BUN and/or serum creatinine) were seen with approximately the same frequency in the enalapril and placebo groups (Atkins et al. 2002). Furthermore, regression analysis indicated that BUN was correlated with the dose of furosemide but not with the dose of either digoxin or enalapril. Based on these data, Ettinger et al. (1994) supported the position that the dose of furosemide should be decreased first should azotemia occur in a dog with heart failure receiving furosemide and enalapril with or without digoxin. Nevertheless, the potential for renal failure should be closely followed whenever ACE inhibitors are used. Because of this potential, concurrent use of diuretics should be limited and renal parameters should be monitored in treated animals periodically. Preexisting renal disease and dehydration will increase this risk. Nonsteroidal antiinflammatory drugs (NSAIDs) also have been suggested to increase the risk. For example, in humans, there is concern that, in some patients, the combination of an ACE inhibitor and an NSAID may increase the risk of renal injury (Loboz and Shenfield 2005). Only one study examining this combination has been published for dogs (Fusellier et al. 2005). It was concluded in that study that tepoxalin did not alter renal function in healthy Beagle dogs receiving an ACE inhibitor. Such an effect of other NSAID combinations has not been adequately studied in veterinary medicine to make adequate conclusions.

Based on results from the multicenter study with enalapril, Ettinger et al. (1994) proposed the following guidelines for pharmacologic treatment of dogs with chronic valvular heart disease or dilated cardiomyopathy. Treatment programs should be customized to the severity of the patient's disease.

An unusual side effect is coughing and angioedema. This has been well-documented in people, but not in animals. The cause for coughing is unclear but it may be caused by increased levels of bradykinin or prostaglandins in the respiratory tract.

DRUG INTERACTIONS. A complete list of pharmacokinetic drug interactions is listed in the article by Shionoiri

(1993). Interactions that affect renal function are listed by Loboz and Shenfield (2005).

Captopril and enalapril have been used with other cardiovascular drugs (including diuretics) safely. However, ACE inhibitors will potentiate the effect of diuretics and these drugs should be used together cautiously.

When ACE inhibitors are administered concurrently with NSAIDs, it may diminish the effect. Some of the antihypertensive effect of ACE inhibitors is caused by generation of prostaglandins (Guazzi, et al. 1998; Davie et al. 2000).

USE OF ACE INHIBITORS IN CHRONIC RENAL FAILURE. A comprehensive review of the use of ACE inhibitors in patients with renal disease was published by Lefebvre and Toutain (2004). As reviewed by these authors, ACE inhibitors can be beneficial in chronic renal failure because they relieve glomerular pressure, slow progression of lesions, and decrease proteinuria. In the same article, and in other papers (Lefebvre et al. 2006), the authors have documented the changes in disposition of ACE inhibitors in animals with renal impairment. In dogs and cats enalaprilat (metabolite of enalapril) is predominantly cleared by the kidneys. In dogs, ramiprilat, and benazeprilat (metabolites of ramipril and benazepril) are cleared by both liver and kidney. Subsequently, these authors have demonstrated ACE inhibitor changes (both pharmacokinetic and pharmacodynamic) caused by renal impairment for enalaprilat in dogs but not ramiprilat and benazeprilat. In cats with reduction in GFR, there was no difference in disposition measured for benazeprilat.

OTHER ACE INHIBITORS. Benazapril has been approved for use in dogs in Europe (Fortekor®) and has been investigated in the U.S. for use in cats in dogs. Clinical doses of benazepril have been 0.25–0.5 mg/kg q12–24h, PO. Lisinopril (Prinivil, Zestril) also has been investigated in animals, but is not in common use. The clinical doses used in animals are in the range of 0.5 mg/kg, q12–24h, PO.

VASODILATOR DRUGS

Careful use of peripheral vasodilator drugs has been developed extensively as treatment in congestive failure to "unload" the failing heart (Hamlin 1977; Zelis et al. 1979; Remme 1993). The rationale for this treatment is the idea that decreasing the work load of the heart is better for the patient than administering a positive inotropic agent with considerable toxic potential (i.e., digitalis). If systemic arterial pressure (i.e., left ventricular afterload) is reduced by a vasodilator drug, the left ventricle will be ejecting blood into a circuit with lowered resistance. Further, peripheral venodilation will divert blood volume from the pulmonary to the systemic vasculature. This response is antagonistic to the formation of pulmonary edema and also tends to restrict venous return to the heart (i.e., ventricular preload). Left ventricular size and wall tension decrease in response to reduction in ventricular preload and afterload. Myocardial oxygen demands decrease accordingly as the workload of the heart is reduced; cardiac output and hemodynamics should improve (Packer 1984; Abrams 1985).

Before initiating vasodilator therapy in treating congestive failure in animals, the clinician should be aware of potential problems; e.g., it has been assumed that drug-induced vasodilation would automatically increase peripheral perfusion and thereby increase oxygen availability to all tissues. However, vasodilator agents of the nitroglycerin type exert a predominant reduction in peripheral venous resistance as compared to arteriolar resistance. Pooling of blood in the venous capacitance beds in no way ensures increased perfusion of all tissues. Vasodilators are beneficial to the failing heart because they decrease cardiac workload, not by directly improving peripheral perfusion but because of vascular dilation. Furthermore, if arterial pressure is critically decreased, blood flow through the coronary and renal vascular beds may be compromised further. Reflex tachycardia accompanied by increased myocardial oxygen demand is another potential problem associated with fall in systemic blood pressure.

PRAZOSIN. Atwell (1979) indicated that peripheral vasodilation induced by prazosin hydrochloride (Minipress), an α_1-adrenergic selective blocking agent (Chapter 6), was effective in four dogs with congestive failure that were refractory to digoxin. However, digoxin was actually continued in three of the four dogs at reduced dosage levels. Thus the beneficial response may well have resulted from a combination of mechanisms involving both a positive inotropic action on the heart (digoxin) and peripheral vasodilation (prazosin).

HYDRALAZINE HYDROCHLORIDE. *Hydralazine Hydrochloride*, USP (Apresoline), is an arteriolar dilator that has undergone limited clinical trial in dogs with volume-overload heart failure (Kittleson et al. 1983). Because of its vasodilator action in systemic arterial beds, hydralazine reduces peripheral vascular resistance and lowers impedance to left ventricular ejection. Stroke volume and cardiac output increase proportionately, thereby initiating hemodynamic improvement.

Beneficial effects of hydralazine are manifested mainly in congestive heart failure that is secondary to mitral valve insufficiency. In this pathophysiologic state, forward left ventricular stroke volume is reduced owing to a regurgitant fraction being pumped backward through the incompetent AV valve into the left atrium. By lowering systemic impedance to left ventricular ejection, hydralazine increases forward stroke volume and thereby reduces the regurgitant fraction. End-systolic volume and cardiac size are reduced because more blood is pumped out of the cardiac chambers per beat. Reduction in cardiac size leads to commensurate decreases in wall tension and myocardial oxygen consumption and, also importantly, to reduction of the orifice of the incompetent mitral valve. The latter contributes in turn to further diminution of the regurgitant fraction. This cycle leads to hemodynamic improvement and, it is hoped, pharmacologically supported compensation of the heart failure patient. Indeed, clinical studies indicate that hydralazine therapy is effective in dogs with volume-overload congestive failure caused by mitral valve insufficiency (Kittleson et al. 1983). Hydralazine may be similarly effective in aortic valvular insufficiency.

Hydralazine is absorbed rapidly after oral administration in dogs; its onset of action develops within 1 hour, and peak response occurs at 3–5 hours. The drug undergoes extensive hepatic metabolism during its initial passage through the liver in the portal blood. There is evidence that uremia in some way affects biotransformation of hydralazine, so that blood concentrations may increase in uremic patients. A recommended dose schedule for hydralazine in dogs involves the initial oral administration of 1 mg/kg; this dose can be adjusted upward, depending upon evidence of clinical improvement, but should not exceed 3 mg/kg. Average-size adult cats may require an initial oral dose of 2.5 mg, which may be adjusted upward to 10 mg. The therapeutic response generally lasts 11–13 hours; thus twice daily administration is suggested as the standard (Kittleson 1983).

Important side effects of hydralazine therapy in humans are tachycardia and hypotension. It was reported that hypotension was not a problem in dogs when hydralazine dosage was titrated carefully against signs of clinical improvement; however, tachycardia does seem to be a common untoward development in congestive-failure dogs treated with hydralazine (Kittleson et al. 1983). Because tachycardia increases myocardial oxygen consumption and may therefore lead to cardiac decompensation, heart rate should be monitored during therapeutic implementation with hydralazine or any other vasodilating drug.

Concomitant administration of a β-blocking drug might reduce the reflex tachycardia produced by hypotensive reactions to hydralazine. On the other hand, the potential negative inotropic response to β-receptor blockade in the heart may exacerbate heart failure (see Chapter 6).

CALCIUM CHANNEL BLOCKING DRUGS. These agents suppress calcium ion (Ca^{++}) influx through plasma membrane channels in cardiac tissues, vascular smooth muscle, and other excitable cell types (Katz 1985; Allert and Adams 1987; Opie 1984). The resulting decrease in intracellular Ca^{++} concentration leads to characteristic changes in physiologic activity of affected tissues, including reduction in myocardial contractility, vasodilation in coronary and peripheral arterial beds, lowered impedance to left ventricular ejection, reduced myocardial oxygen demand, and slowed AV impulse conduction. Because of this diverse pharmacologic profile, Ca^{++} channel blockers have been studied extensively for therapeutic application in a wide spectrum of cardiovascular disorders. Drugs of this group have been approved for the management of ischemic heart disease, hypertension, and some forms of cardiac dysrhythmias in human medicine. Other indications in people include obstructive cardiomyopathies, asthma, and cerebral ischemia (Stone and Antmann 1983; Conti et al. 1985).

Although Ca^{++} channel blockade is an important therapeutic modality in human medicine (Katz 1985), less is known about the clinical application of this concept in veterinary medicine (Adams 1986a; Novotny and Adams 1986; Johnson 1985; Bright 1992). Most of the experience has been with amlodipine, primarily in cats. The present discussion is an overview of this topic and addresses the pharmacodynamic rationale for Ca^{++} channel blocking drugs in cardiovascular therapeutics in animals, as summarized by Allert and Adams (1987). The use of verapamil and diltiazem as Class IV antiarrhythmics in treating supraventricular tachyarrhythmias is addressed in Chapter 23.

History and Terminology. Discovery of Ca^{++} channel blocking drugs can be traced to 1964, when the German cardiologist Fleckenstein reported that the newly synthesized drug verapamil mimicked the cardiac effects of Ca^{++} withdrawal (Fleckenstein 1983). Verapamil was being developed as a coronary vasodilator, but it also inhibited myocardial contractile strength while leaving the cardiac action potential essentially intact. Importantly, the cardiodepressant effects of verapamil could be antagonized promptly and completely by excess Ca^{++}. Fleckenstein coined the term *Ca^{++} antagonists* to describe verapamil and other drugs that exerted this basic Ca^{++}-dependent inhibitory effect as their predominant pharmacologic property (Fleckenstein 1983). Dozens of drugs that share this action subsequently have been identified, and several have been approved for clinical use in human medicine, including nifedipine, verapamil, and diltiazem.

These agents interfere with the function of plasma membrane channels that mediate Ca^{++} entry into excitable cells (Katz 1985). The pharmacologic rationale for their therapeutic use resides in the fundamental importance of Ca^{++} influx as an intracellular messenger system in cardiovascular tissues (Schramm and Towart 1985; Janis and Triggle 1984).

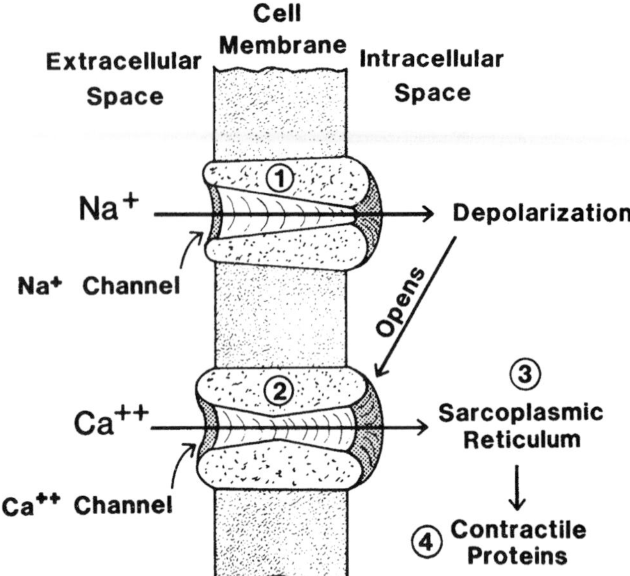

FIG. 22.11 Schematic representation of cell membrane Ca^{++} channel involvement in excitation-contraction coupling in mammalian heart. Na^{+} channels (1) open during cell excitation, and the inward Na^{+} current depolarizes the cell membrane. Depolarization opens Ca^{++} channels (2), and Ca^{++} influx triggers shift of additional Ca^{++} from sarcoplasmic reticulum (3) to contractile proteins (4). Calcium channel blocking drugs reduce Ca^{++} influx through the Ca^{++} channels (2) (Allert and Adams 1987).

Fundamentals of Ca^{++} Channel Blockade

Pharmacologic Concepts. The essential roles of Ca^{++} in coupling cell membrane excitation to intracellular functions in cardiac and vascular muscle have been reviewed in detail (Janis and Triggle 1984; Reuter 1985). In essence, Ca^{++} influxing through specific plasma membrane channels gains access to intracellular organelles and through this pathway leads to activation of Ca^{++}-dependent cellular functions.

The molecular architecture and biophysical operation of the cell membrane Ca^{++} channels are incompletely understood. The channel structures are protein moieties embedded within and spanning the permeability barrier of the phospholipid plasma membrane biolayer, as illustrated in Figure 22.11. Some of the Ca^{++} channel blocking drugs interact with specific ligand binding sites of channel elements, others seem to "plug" the outer orifice of the channel pore, whereas others may have to gain access to the cytosolic face of the cell membrane to interfere with channel operation (Schramm and Towart 1985; Janis and Triggle 1984). Despite dissimilar molecular mechanisms, the Ca^{++} channel blockers share a common pharmacodynamic property: they all inhibit Ca^{++} influx and the associated Ca^{++}-dependent physiologic responses of affected cells.

Physiologic Concepts. A schematic representation of excitation-contraction coupling in heart muscle cells and the importance of Ca^{++} channels in this physiologic process are presented in Figure 22.11. Cardiac excitation initially involves a rapid influx of sodium ions (Na^{+}) through plasma membrane passageways referred to as *fast Na^{+} channels*. Rapid Na^{+} influx depolarizes the cell membrane. Depolarization then leads to a voltage-dependent opening of another type of plasma membrane channel, referred to as *slow Ca^{++} channels* or simply as *Ca^{++} channels* (Reuter 1985). Calcium moves inward through these open channels and serves two critical interconnected functions on a beat-to-beat basis. It replenishes sarcoplasmic reticulum stores of Ca^{++} and triggers the release of additional amounts of Ca^{++} from sarcoplasmic reticulum storage sites into the cytosol. The resulting increase in intracellular Ca^{++} concentration ($[Ca^{++}]_i$) proportionately activates the contractile proteins of the cardiac myocyte (Figure 22.11), and the heart contracts. Diastolic relaxation develops as the sarcoplasmic reticulum avidly resequesters Ca^{++} away from the contractile apparatus. Thus, Ca^{++} channel blocking drugs induce negative inotropic effects in the heart by reducing trans-sarcolemmal influx of activator Ca^{++} (Fig. 22.11).

Contraction of vascular smooth muscle is mediated by Ca^{++} and depends on the influx of Ca^{++} through cell membrane channels (Somlyo 1985). Therefore, Ca^{++} channel blockade in vascular smooth muscle evokes vascular smooth muscle relaxation and vasodilatory responses in different vascular beds. The resultant peripheral vasodilation and accompanying decrease in peripheral vascular resistance lower impedance to left ventricular ejection, thereby reducing ventricular wall tension during stroke volume ejection. Diminution of ventricular wall tension during systole (i.e., reduced cardiac afterload), coupled to direct negative inotropic actions of Ca^{++} channel blockade in the heart muscle, proportionately lowers myocardial oxygen demand. Hence, and this is an important aspect, Ca^{++} channel blocking drugs can preserve cardiac integrity by hemodynamically lowering myocardial oxygen demand. Certain Ca^{++} channel blocking drugs also have pronounced coronary vasodilator effects, which further improve tissue perfusion-metabolic demand relationships in the heart. This complex pharmacologic spectrum probably explains the salutary effects of Ca^{++} channel blockade in managing coronary artery–ischemic heart disease and the resulting anginal pain in people (Katz 1985; Nayler 1980; Opie 1984; Stone and Antmann 1983; Conti et al. 1985).

Electrophysiologic Concepts. The importance of slow inward Ca^{++} currents to normal and abnormal rhythmicity mechanisms in the heart is reviewed in Chapter 23 (Adams 1986b; Novotny and Adams 1986). Briefly, usual electrophysiologic mechanisms of the sinoatrial (SA) and AV nodes involve Ca^{++} influx through the plasma membrane Ca^{++} channels in these tissues. Calcium channel blockade can suppress these normal mechanisms, reduce sinus rate, and slow AV conduction velocity. There also is evidence that aberrant Ca^{++} currents can arise from injured cardiac tissue and lead to reentry and automaticity forms of arrhythmias that are responsive to Ca^{++} channel blockade. Because of their unique Ca^{++}-dependent antiarrhythmic mechanism, the Ca^{++} channel blockers are considered Class IV antiarrhythmic agents (Adams 1986b; Novotny and Adams 1986; Vaughn Williams 1984) (see Chapter 23).

Pathophysiologic Concepts. Cellular Ca^{++} influx-efflux control mechanisms are set awry during ischemia and perhaps in many other fundamental forms of cellular injury (Trump et al. 1982; White et al. 1984). During ischemic and hypoxemic conditions the ability of the cell to maintain energy-dependent ionic gradients is impaired, leading to intracellular potassium ion (K^+) depletion and concomitant intracellular Na^+ and Ca^{++} overloads. One consequence of increased $[Ca^{++}]_i$ is activation of Ca^{++}-regulated catabolic and lysosomal enzyme systems (Trump et al. 1982; White et al. 1984). These degradative enzymes disrupt cellular regulatory functions with further compromise of cell membrane integrity and further loss of ion permeability barriers. The $[Ca^{++}]_i$ progressively overloads the cell via this putative pathway and sequentially inhibits mitochondrial oxidative phosphorylation, impairs Ca^{++} uptake-release functions of sarcoplasmic reticulum, and eventually culminates in cell death and necrosis (Trump et al. 1982; White et al. 1984). Calcium channel blocking drugs reduce the increase in $[Ca^{++}]_i$ by lowering the quantity of Ca^{++} influx, at least that component occurring through Ca^{++} channels. Decreased $[Ca^{++}]_i$ and then should reduce activation of Ca^{++}-dependent degradative enzymes, thereby preserving cell viability after ischemic-related injuries (Trump et al. 1982; White et al. 1984).

Clinical Precautions. On the basis of the foregoing schema of physiologic and pathophysiologic roles for Ca^{++}, it is now possible to discuss three basic types of pharmacodynamic pathways incorporating Ca^{++} channel blocking drugs into cardiovascular therapeutics in veterinary medicine. First, by evoking arteriolar dilatation and lowering total peripheral vascular resistance, these drugs should improve blood flow–oxygen demand relationships during hypodynamic circulatory conditions such as heart failure or arterial hypotension. Second, these drugs should be able to restore hemodynamic stability in patients with cardiac arrhythmias caused by abnormal Ca^{++} influx patterns. Third, these drugs should directly prolong cell viability in various tissues during ischemic-related syndromes by modulating the cellular Ca^{++} overload cascade. Some essential issues remain unresolved, however, and these drugs have found minimal therapeutic use.

Pharmacologic Heterogeneity. The Ca^{++} channel blockers comprise chemically unrelated subgroups with disparate tissue and systemic pharmacologic profiles (Spedding 1985; Defeudis 1985). Nifedipine, e.g., directly reduces myocardial contractile strength and slows AV conduction in isolated cardiac tissues. However, these direct cardiodepressant effects of nifedipine may not be manifested in patients with normal myocardial contractile reserves, owing to more potent vasodilator actions and the resulting baroreflex-induced cardiac stimulation. In contrast, verapamil can induce direct myocardial contractile depression and antiarrhythmic responses at dosages that induce peripheral vasodilatation. Diltiazem is a potent vasodilator that also directly decreases sinus firing rate in dosages that usually spare cardiac contractile mechanisms. Dissimilarities in systemic pharmacologic profiles rule that the various Ca^{++} channel blockers should not be construed as being therapeutically interchangeable.

Cardiovascular Side Effects. Because of the essential physiologic roles for Ca^{++} influx in activation of cardiovascular tissues, the Ca^{++} channel blocking agents can be likened to a "double-edged sword" relative to benefit-risk relationships. On the one hand, the negative inotropic effects and vasodilator actions of Ca^{++} channel blockade can benefit hemodynamics by reducing cardiac workload. On the other hand, if unexpected or unabated, these same cardiovascular depressant responses obviously carry the risk of exacerbating underlying abnormalities of the circulatory system.

Adverse circulatory side effects of Ca^{++} channel blockade include contractile depression of the heart, with reduced cardiac output and hypotension. This combination of effects can result in decompensation of preclinical or compensated heart failure, precipitation of pulmonary edema, and worsening of the primary ailment. Other potential side effects are sinus bradycardia and heart block attributable to direct depression of SA firing rate and AV conduction, respectively. The propensity for cardiovascular depression should be considered whenever Ca^{++} channel blocking drugs are used. This precaution is especially valid in patients with preexisting or suspected myocardial contractile failure.

Clinical Applications. The clinical antiarrhythmic applications are discussed in Chapter 23.

Heart Failure Syndromes. Initial studies with nifedipine, verapamil, and diltiazem indicated favorable results in human beings with chronic myocardial contractile failure, valvular insufficiencies, or obstructive cardiomyopathies (Katz 1985; Conti et al. 1985; Lorell 1985; Rosing et al. 1979). The therapeutic use of Ca^{++} channel blockade in congestive cardiomyopathies with severe cardiac contractile failure is controversial (Colucci et al. 1985; Josephson and Singh 1985; Brooks et al. 1980; Packer 1985). Josephson and Singh (1985) suggested caution in the use of these agents in patients with impaired ventricular performance and stated that available data do not support the use of calcium antagonists as afterload-reducing agents in chronic heart failure. Packer (1985) cautioned that both verapamil and nifedipine may exert notable depressant effects on right ventricular performance in patients with impaired right ventricular function. Colucci et al. (1985) similarly warned that Ca^{++} channel blockade in the setting of severe left ventricular dysfunction can result in abrupt decompensation and development of overt pulmonary edema. In contrast, treatment with verapamil or nifedipine seemed particularly effective in human patients with hypertrophic cardiomyopathy (Lorell 1985; Rosing et al. 1979).

Hypertrophic Cardiomyopathy. In contrast to the lack of clinical interest for Ca^{++} channel blockers in dilated cardiomyopathy, verapamil and diltiazem have been used in dogs and cats with hypertrophic cardiomyopathy (Bright 1992). Because of reduced propensity for side effects associated with cardiac contractile depression, diltiazem is commonly the preferred drug for this condition. Recommended doses range from 1.75 to 2.5 mg/kg orally BID to TID. As with any highly active cardiovascular drug, therapy with diltiazem or other Ca^{++} channel blocker should be implemented with careful patient monitoring.

Hypertension in Cats. Amlodipine (Norvasc® and generic) is one of the calcium-channel blockers of the dihydropyridine group and is the most common one of this group used in veterinary medicine. It is primarily effective for arterial dilation. In people, this drug is longer-acting than other dihydropyridines, which may be an advantage over other drugs.

Amlodipine has become the drug of choice to treat hypertension in cats. Hypertension in cats may be secondary to other diseases such as renal failure, hyperthyroidism, or diabetes mellitus. According to one study, cats responded to 0.625 mg/cat once daily (0.18 mg/kg).

Circulatory Shock and Trauma. Calcium channel blocking drugs have been tested for salutary pharmacologic effects in experimental models of hemorrhagic shock, traumatic shock, cerebral ischemia, cardiopulmonary resuscitation, and endotoxemic shock. Studies have involved various representatives of this drug group, including verapamil, diltiazem, lidoflazine, nimodipine, nisoldipine, nivadipine, and nitrendipine (Adams 1986a). Initial data favored the general conclusion that Ca^{++} channel blocking drugs can improve the short-or long-term outcome of various induced forms of shock and trauma. Other studies, however, have indicated that Ca^{++} channel blocking effects were not helpful in some forms of induced shock and ischemia (Denis et al. 1985; Lanza et al. 1984) and could result in further reductions in blood pressure and cardiac output. Ca^{++} channel blocking drugs are not used in emergency medicine dealing with circulatory shock and trauma (Adams 1986a).

NITROVASODILATORS (NITROGLYCERINE). The organic nitrates are nitrogen esters that exert their effect by acting as an exogenous source for nitric oxide. Nitric oxide is the endothelium-derived relaxing factor (EDRF) discussed in other scientific papers. The nitrate vasodilators are esters of nitrous acid. They are metabolized to inorganic nitrite and denitrated metabolites. Nitrites, organic nitrates, and nitroso compounds all act to activate the enzyme *guanylate cyclase*.

Increased intracellular cyclic-GMP (3′,5′-guanosine monophosphate) acts to inhibit contraction of vascular smooth muscle. This mechanism may involve a decrease in the availability of intracellular Ca^{++} in vascular smooth muscle cells, or may interfere with the myosin-actin interaction. Nitrates may also stimulate synthesis of the vasodilator prostaglandins: PGI_2 and PGE, but this may not have clinical relevance.

Action on Smooth Muscle. Nitrates relax smooth muscle in both arteries and veins, but they are often used clinically as *preload* reducers. When used as preload reducers, they decrease myocardial O_2 requirements (decrease workload of heart). Because of this effect, they have been commonly used to manage human patients with angina pectoris (chest pain caused by cardiovascular disease).

Pharmacokinetics. Nitroglycerin is metabolized quickly with a half-life of only a few minutes. Nitrates have significant *first-pass* effects, and metabolites are at least 10× less potent. Owing to the first-pass effects it is administered either topically, sublingually, or intravenously to avoid first-pass metabolism by the liver.

Examples Used Clinically. Nitroglycerin (NitroBid®, Nitrol®) is applied topically as a cream or ointment, sublingual tablet, lingual spray, or buccal tablet. Half-life is 1–3 minutes. In dogs it has been used as 3 to 5 inches of ointment every 6 hr (1 inch equals 15 mg). In cats it has been used at 1 to 3 inches every 4–6 hr. It is usually applied to an area on the patient that lacks hair and where the patient will not lick it off (such as pinnae of ears). In horses, patches or ointment are applied to the legs, usually for treatment of laminitis.

Isosorbide dinitrate (Isordil®) is available as oral tablets (even though it has poor systemic availability), topical ointments, and lingual spray (dose: 2.5–5.0 mg/dog). Isosorbide mononitrate has better absorption and longer half-life.

Sodium nitroprusside (Nipride) is a potent vasodilator administered as a constant rate infusion. Tolerance does not develop to nitroprusside, compared to the other nitrate compounds, because it provides intracellular nitric oxide. It is administered at an infusion rate of 1–10 mcg/kg/min to veterinary patients, to maintain the blood pressure at a stable level. It is mixed in 5% dextrose in an infused IV. Cyanide toxicity can develop in patients in which renal elimination is compromised.

Amyl nitrite has been used occasionally in people to treat angina, but its medical use is not as popular as it once was. Amyl nitrite has been a popular recreational drug and its use in veterinary medicine has not been reported.

Clinical Uses. In people, the organic nitrates are primarily used for the relief of anginal pain (angina pectoris) (Parker and Adams 1987). Their use in veterinary medicine is limited because the dosage forms available can be inconvenient to use and the duration of action is brief (15 to 30 min). They may be helpful for vasodilation and the acute treatment of pulmonary edema associated with congestive heart failure.

In horses, nitroglycerin is used to treat disease of the feet, such as laminitis. Nitroglycerin is applied to the skin of the leg in an attempt to improve distal blood flow.

Tolerance. Tolerance to nitrovasodilators develops with repeated administration. The exact mechanism is not known, but one of the proposed causes is a progressive depletion of sulfhydral groups necessary for the formation of nitric oxide. Efficacy is improved if the drug is used intermittently instead of continuously because intermittent use allows time for regeneration of sulfhydral groups. Optimum intermittent use is to provide a nitrate free interval of 8 hours or more during the day.

Adverse Effects. The most common and limiting side effect of these drugs is hypotension. (People can inadvertently become exposed when they apply ointment it to their animals.) Methemoglobinemia can occur with accumulation of nitrites but is not a common clinical problem.

PHOSPHODIESTERASE V INHIBITORS: SILDENAFIL. Sildenafil (Viagra®) is an orally active phosphodiesterase V inhibitor (PDEVI). Phosphodiesterase V is found in relatively high concentration in lung and erectile penile tissue and is elevated in humans with pulmonary hypertension. Pulmonary hypertension is a clinically important disease associated with high morbidity and mortality in dogs. Canine pulmonary hypertension is most often a sequelae of other disease processes and thus requires a balanced therapeutic approach, which targets the underlying etiology and palliation of clinical signs. An important goal of therapy is to reduce pulmonary artery pressures. However, historically, vasodilators have had no preferential effect on pulmonary vasculature and thus have had no benefit and often worsen the clinical signs of pulmonary hypertension. Type V phosphodiesterase inhibitors prevent degradation of cGMP resulting in relaxation of smooth muscle in pulmonary vasculature and, to a lesser degree, systemic vessels, i.e., preferential pulmonary vasodilation.

Sildenafil is currently the most extensively researched of the PDE V inhibitors, and has been shown to improve both exercise tolerance and quality of life in humans with pulmonary hypertension, resulting in FDA approval for its use in this condition. Sildenafil (Viagra®) is also used in humans to treat erectile dysfunction of the penis. Subsequently Viagra® was recently re-released as Revatio® (which is even more expensive). Sildenafil is now available as a generic preparation in some countries further reducing its cost, although efficacy of the generic preparations has not been reported. Clinical improvement in erectile function in humans has been documented at multiple dosages ranging from 20 mg to 80 mg three times a day.

Well-controlled dose-studies of vasodilator effects of sildenafil are lacking in the veterinary literature. In dogs, some clinicians start at a dose of approximately 0.25 mg/kg every 12 hours and increase the dosage until circulatory status improved. Until further studies are conducted, it is recommended that the dosage should not exceed 1–2 mg/kg every 8–24 hours, unless cardiovascular parameters can be closely monitored. Using a liquid form of sildenafil for oral dosage has been reported in people and thus suspension formulations may facilitate cost effective accurate dosing.

One retrospective study reported few adverse side effects with clinical improvements in 10 dogs with pulmonary hypertension treated with a median dose of approximately 2 mg/kg sildenafil every 8–24 h (Bach et al. 2006).

Because of the complexity of the systemic response to pulmonary hypertension, sildenafil has been used in combination with other medications including conventional heart failure therapeutics such as diuretics, ACEI, and pimobendan (Hoskins 2006). Adverse side effects have been minimal or nonrecognizable. Additional study is needed with this new class of vasodilators.

CARVEDILOL. This compound has been approved for use in humans to treat hypertension and heart failure. It is both a nonselective β_1–β_2-receptor antagonist and an α_1-receptor antagonist (see Chapter 6). The ratio of β_{1-2}- to α_1-receptor antagonist potency for carvedilol is 10:1; thus, this agent should reduce myocardial workload by lowering heart rate and peripheral vascular resistance. It is used mostly in conjunction with other agents used in treating heart failure. Studies in dogs show promise with this agent (Arsenault et al. 2005; Gordon et al. 2005, 2006). Carvedilol is also discussed with the antiarrhythmic drugs in Chapter 23.

OTHER VASODILATORS. Several other vasodilator drugs have been studied and employed therapeutically in humans with heart failure, including nitroprusside, nitroglycerin, isosorbide dinitrate, and Ca^{++} entry-blocking drugs. Clinical trials with these compounds are lacking in veterinary medicine. Indeed, with the notable exception of a few outstanding studies (Kittleson et al. 1983, 1985a,b; Knowlen et al. 1983; Ettinger et al. 1994; Smith et al. 2005; Lombard et al. 2006; Roland et al. 2006), clinical drug trials in spontaneous heart failure in animal patients are almost nonexistent. This is in sharp contrast to human medicine, where literally dozens of double-blind, placebo-controlled drug trials appear almost annually in the cardiovascular literature. Until such studies are done in animals with spontaneous cardiac disease, cardiovascular drug therapy in veterinary internal medicine will involve a somewhat empiric approach and should be implemented carefully, with close supervision of each patient.

ANCILLARY THERAPY IN CONGESTIVE HEART FAILURE

The basic goal of therapeutic management of patients with congestive heart failure is to adjust cardiac output to meet bodily needs and, importantly, vice versa. In addition to improving mechanical performance of the heart with digitalis, other procedures helpful in attaining this goal include reducing oxygen demand by the tissues, improving oxygen uptake into the pulmonary capillary bed, decreasing pulmonary capillary pressure, reducing respiratory froth, and reducing salt intake. Except for dietary changes, all these goals theoretically can be achieved by effective drug therapy and its attendant hemodynamic improvement; however, other interventions may be necessary. This is particularly relevant in emergency situations when time may not be available for the full effects of digitalis to become manifested. Several clinical aspects concerning emergency management of congestive failure patients have been reviewed by Adams (1981).

OXYGEN DEMAND AND DELIVERY. In animals with mild stages of congestive failure to be treated as outpatients, severe restriction of physical exertion may be adequate to decrease oxygen needs. The owner of the animal should be advised that reduced physical activity will in all likelihood be necessary throughout the remainder of the animal's life. Initial therapy of severe cases of congestive failure includes complete inactivity in a well-oxygenated cage, especially if acute cardiac decompensation is presented. An oxygen mask, nasal catheter, or even endotracheal tube may be necessary in severe episodes of cardiogenic pulmonary edema; intermittent positive pressure ventilation is sometimes required if fluid accumulation in the lungs is overwhelming.

DIURETICS. Diuretics are covered in more detail in Chapter 25. The use of potent loop-acting diuretics usually is indicated in congestive failure, and some clinicians believe these agents are drugs of choice in this condition (Hamlin et al. 1973). However, therapy with diuretics alone should be carefully monitored. Pronounced diuresis could reduce blood volume to the extent that ventricular filling would be inadequate. A reduced ventricular filling pressure is good on the one hand because it reduces wall tension and myocardial oxygen demand and propensity for edema. Conversely, excessive loss of venous return without concurrent positive inotropic effects may well lead to reduced cardiac output. Most cardiologists routinely advocate the use of diuretics as a standard addition to therapy with positive inotropic drugs. Pharmacodynamic details addressing the use of diuretics are discussed in Chapter 25.

MORPHINE. Morphine has been advocated as an agent of choice, second only to effective delivery of oxygen, in managing pulmonary edema (Davis 1979). Morphine purportedly exerts beneficial effects by three actions: sedation and relief of anxiety; conversion of rapid, violent ventilatory patterns to slow, deep respirations by depressing the respiratory centers; and dilation of splanchnic vasculature, thereby diverting blood volume from the pulmonary to the systemic circuit. IV administration of small quantities of morphine (0.05–0.1 mg/kg) can be made every 3–6 minutes while the patient's progress is monitored closely.

OTHER PROCEDURES. Bronchodilating drugs (e.g., aminophylline) have been advocated in treatment of congestive failure (Bolton 1977). Aminophylline and other xanthines are potent bronchodilators, but they also have direct stimulatory activity on the heart, some diuretic activity, and vasodilator effects. The pharmacology of this class of drugs will be discussed more thoroughly in Chapter

49. A usual dose of aminophylline is 10 mg/kg given orally or parenterally 2 to three times a day. IV administrations should be infused slowly, preferably in dilute solution. A large number of bronchodilatory antitussive-expectorant preparations have been used in congestive failure, but the potential for unexpected drug interactions should be considered. Nebulization of a 20% solution of ethanol into the respiratory tract may be of some help in reducing foaming of respiratory fluids in acute cases. Sodium intake should be restricted on a long-term basis to reduce the potential for edema formation. Low-salt dog foods are available commercially.

NEW/EXPERIMENTAL HEART FAILURE DRUGS

Because there is no cure for most cardiovascular diseases that result in heart failure, new drugs are sought to treat cardiac disease and heart failure. Some drugs eventually make it to the marketplace while others fall by the wayside during drug development. This section presents a few drugs that may become useful for treating heart failure in the future.

AQUARETICS. Aquaretics are vasopressin-receptor antagonists, e.g., tolvaptan (OPC-41061). Tolvaptan is a selective V_2-receptor antagonist, which is showing promise in the acute and chronic treatment of human CHF. In contrast to loop diuretics like furosemide, V_2-receptor antagonism has demonstrated free water excretion with little to no sodium loss. In addition, the water loss associated with V_2 antagonism has not been associated with activation of the renin-angiotensin-aldosterone system in contrast to the loop diuretics. Thus, this novel class of agents may prove to be a useful addition to our pharmacologic arsenal against HF.

PROSTACYCLIN ANALOGUES. Prostacyclin analogues have been shown to improve symptoms and short-term survival in human patients with pulmonary hypertension (PH). Epoprostenol (Flolan, GlaxoSmithKline) was the first available prostacyclin used to treat PH in humans. It is administered via continuous rate intravenous infusion and due to a very short half-life, abrupt withdrawal is associated with increased morbidity and mortality. Adverse effects related to the drug are mild and dose related while sepsis and thrombosis are important adverse effects related to chronic central venous access. Treprostinil (Remodulin, United Therapeutics Corp.) has similar hemodynamic effects as epoprostenol but is administered as a constant rate subcutaneous infusion, which lowers the risk of sepsis associated with direct venous access. Intravenous Iloprost (Berlex Labs) has similar hemodynamic effects as epoprostenol with a longer half-life diminishing the adverse effects associated with abrupt withdrawal. Inhaled iloprost is also available and has a short half-life of 20–25 minutes requiring administration every 2–3 hours. Beraprost (United Therapeutics Corp), the first orally stable prostacyclin analogue, requires administration four times a day to maintain adequate blood levels.

ENDOTHELIN (ET)-RECEPTOR ANTAGONISTS. ET-1 is converted to functional ET by endothelin converting enzyme. ET is a potent vasoconstrictor and smooth-muscle mitogen resulting in vascular hypertrophy. ET levels are elevated in humans with PH and dogs with experimentally induced dirofilariasis. Two types of ET receptors have been identified, ET_A and ET_B. ET_A receptors are located on vascular smooth muscle cells and mediate vasoconstriction and vascular smooth muscle proliferation, while ET_B receptors are located on both endothelial and vascular smooth muscle cells and mediate vasodilation and vasoconstriction. ET_B receptors are up regulated in pulmonary hypertension (PH). The ET-receptor antagonist bosentan (Tracleer, Actelion Pharmaceuticals US) competitively antagonizes the ET receptor types ET_A and ET_B, with slightly more affinity for ET_A receptors. Optimal dosage in humans is 125 mg every 12 hours. In human studies, bosentan resulted in significant increases in exercise capacity. A potentially important adverse effect of bosentan therapy is elevations in hepatic enzyme activity that typically resolve with discontinuation of the drug but require monthly monitoring of serum biochemistries. Bosentan was developed initially for the treatment of HF but failed to be proven useful in clinical trials for this indication. The selective ET_A-receptor antagonists, sitaxsentan and ambrisentan, are currently being evaluated in human clinical trials.

REFERENCES

Abrams, J. 1985. Vasodilator therapy for chronic congestive heart failure. J Am Med Assoc 254:3070–74.

Adams, H. R. 1981. Cardiovascular emergencies: drug and resuscitative principles. Vet Clin North Am 11:77–102.

———. 1986a. Ca^{++} channel blocking drugs in shock and trauma: new approaches to old problems? Am J Emerg Med 15:1457–60.

———. 1986b. New perspectives in cardiology: pharmacodynamic classification of antiarrhythmic drugs. J Am Vet Med Assoc 189:525–32.

Akera, T., Ng, Y. C. 1991. Digitalis sensitivity of Na^+,K^+-ATPase, myocytes and the heart. Life Sci 48:97–106.

Allert, J. A., Adams, H. R. 1987. New perspectives in cardiovascular medicine: the calcium channel blocking drugs. J Am Vet Med Assoc 190:573–78.

Alousi, A. A., Farah, A. E., Lesher, G. Y., et al. 1979. Cardiotonic activity of amrinone—Win 40680 [5-amino-3,4′-bipyridine-6(1H)-one]. Circ Res 45:666–77.

Aranow, W. S. 1992. Clinical use of digitalis. Comp Ther 18:38–41.

Arsenault, W. G., Boothe, D. M., Gordon, S. G., et al. 2005. Pharmacokinetics of carvedilol in healthy conscious dogs. Am J Vet Res 66(12):2172–2176.

Atkins, C. E., Brown, W. A., Coats, J. R., et al. 2002. Effects of long-term administration of enalapril on clinical indicators of renal function in dogs with compensated mitral regurgitation. J Am Vet Med Assoc 221(5):654–658.

Atwell, R. B. 1979. The use of alpha blockade in the treatment of congestive heart failure associated with dirofilariasis and mitral valvular incompetence. Vet Rec 104:114–16.

Bach, F. J., Rozanski, E. A., MacGregor, J., et al. 2006. Retrospective evaluation of sildenafil citrate as a therapy for pulmonary hypertension in dogs. J Vet Intern Med 20:1132–1135.

Baker, P. F., Blaustein, M. P., Hodgkin, A. L., et al. 1969. The influence of calcium on sodium efflux in squid axons. J Physiol (Lond) 200:431–58.

Barr, I., Smith, T. W., Klein, M. D., et al. 1972. Correlation of the electrophysiologic action of digoxin with serum digoxin concentration. J Pharmacol Exp Ther 180:710–22.

Beck, A. M. 1969. M.S. thesis, Univ. of Pennsylvania.

Bolton, G. R. 1977. In R. W. Kirk, ed., Veterinary Therapy, VI: Small Animal Practice, p. 340. Philadelphia: W. B. Saunders.

Braunwald, E. 1985. Effects of digitalis on the normal and the failing heart. J Am Coll Cardiol 5:51A–59A.

Braunwald, E., Kahler, R. L. 1964. The mechanism of action of cardiac drugs. Physiol Physicians 2:1–5.

Breznock, E. M. 1973. Application of canine plasma kinetics of digoxin and digitoxin to therapeutic digitalization in the dog. Am J Vet Res 34:993–99.

———. 1975. Effects of phenobarbital on digitoxin and digoxin elimination in the dog. Am J Vet Res 36:371–73.

Bright, J. M. 1992. Update: diltiazem therapy of feline hypertrophic cardiomyopathy. In Kirk's Current Veterinary Therapy XI, Ed. R. W. Kirk, J. D. Bonagura, p. 766–73. Philadelphia: W.B. Saunders.

Brooks, N., Cattell, M., Pidgeon, J., et al. 1980. Unpredictable response to nifedipine in severe cardiac failure. Br Med J 281:1324.

Button, C., Gross, D. R., Allert, J. A. 1980b. Application of individualized digoxin dosage regimens to canine therapeutic digitalization. Am J Vet Res 41:1238–42.

Button, C., Gross, D. R., Johnston, J. T., et al. 1980a. Pharmacokinetics, bioavailability, and dosage regimens of digoxin in dogs. Am J Vet Res 41:1230–37.

———. 1980c. Digoxin pharmacokinetics, bioavailability, efficacy, and dosage regimens in the horse. Am J Vet Res 41:1388–95.

Carpenter, C. C., Davis, J. O., Wallace, C. R., et al. 1962. Acute effects of cardiac glycosides on aldosterone secretion in dogs with hyperaldosteronism secondary to chronic right heart failure. Circ Res 10:178–87.

Chetboul, V., Lefebvre, H. P., Sampedrano, C., et al. 2007. Comparative adverse cardiac effects of pimobendan and benazepril monotherapy in dogs with mild degenerative mitral valve disease: a prospective, controlled, blinded, and randomized study. J Vet Intern Med 21:742–753.

Cohn, J. N., Goldstein, S. O., Greenberg, B. H., et al. 1998. A dose-dependent increase in mortality with vesnarinone among patients with severe heart failure. Vesnarinone Trial Investigators. N Engl J Med 339:1810–1816.

Colucci, W. S., Fifer, M. A., Lorell, B. H., et al. 1985. Calcium channel blockers in congestive heart failure: theoretic considerations and clinical experience. Am J Med 78(Suppl 2B):9–17.

Colucci, W. S., Wright, R. F., Braunwald, E. 1986a. New positive inotropic agents in the treatment of congestive heart failure: mechanisms of action and recent clinical developments, 1. N Engl J Med 314:290–99.

———. 1986b. New positive inotropic agents in the treatment of congestive heart failure: mechanisms of action and recent clinical developments, 2. N Engl J Med 314:349–58.

Conti, C. R., Pepine, C., Feldman, R. L., et al. 1985. Calcium antagonists. Cardiology 72:297–321.

Davie, A. P., Love, M. P., McMurray, J. J. V. 2000. Even low-dose aspirin inhibits arachidonic acid-induced vasodilation in heart failure. Clin Pharm Therap 67:530–537.

Davis, L. E. 1979. Management of acute pulmonary edema. J Am Vet Med Assoc 175:97–98.

Defeudis, F. V. 1985. Calcium antagonist subgroups. Trends Pharmacol Sci 6:237–38.

Denis, R., Lucas, C. E., Ledgerwood, A. M., et al. 1985. The beneficial role of calcium supplementation during resuscitation from shock. J Trauma 25:594–600.

De Rick, A., Belpaire, F. M., Bogaert, M. G., et al. 1978. Pharmacokinetics of digoxin. Am J Vet Res 39:811–18.

Detweiler, D. K. 1967. Comparative pharmacology of cardiac glycosides. Fed Proc 26:1119–24.

———. 1977. In L. M. Jones, N. H. Booth, and L. E. McDonald, eds., Veterinary Pharmacology and Therapeutics, 4th ed. Ames: Iowa State Univ Press.

Detweiler, D. K., Knight, D. H. 1977. Congestive heart failure in dogs: therapeutic concepts. J Am Vet Med Assoc 171:106–14.

Detweiler, D. K., Patterson, D. F. 1963. In J. F. Bone, ed., Equine Medicine and Surgery. Wheaton, Ill.: American Veterinary Publications.

DiBianco, R., Shabetai, R., Kostuk, W., Moran, J., Schlaut, R. C., Wright, R. 1989. A comparison of oral milrinone, digoxin, and their combination in the treatment of patients with congestive heart failure. N Eng J Med 320:677–83.

Dietz, R., Waas, W., Susselbeck, T., Willenbrock, R., Osterziel, K. J. 1993. Improvement of cardiac function by angiotensin converting enzyme inhibition: sites of action. Circulation 87 (Suppl IV): 108–16.

Doherty, J. E. 1973. Digitalis glycosides: pharmacokinetics and their clinical implications. Ann Int Med 79:229–38.

Erichsen, D. F., Harris, S. G., Upson, D. W. 1980. Therapeutic and toxic plasma concentrations of digoxin in the cat. Am J Vet Res 41:2049–58.

Ettinger, S. J., Benitz, A. M., Ericsson, G. F. 1994. Relationships of enalapril with other CHF treatment modalities. In Proc 12th Amer Col Vet Int Med Forum, pp. 251–53.

Ettinger, S. J., Suter, P. F. 1970. Canine Cardiology, p. 237. Philadelphia: W. B. Saunders.

Ezrailson, E. G., Potter, J. D., Michael, L., et al. 1977. Positive inotropy induced by ouabain, by increased frequency, by X537A (RO2–2985), by calcium and by isoproterenol: the lack of correlation with phosphorylation of TnI. J Mol Cell Cardiol 9:693–98.

Fabiato, A., Fabiato, F. 1979. Calcium and cardiac excitation-contraction coupling. Ann Rev Physiol 41:473–84.

Feldman, A. M. 1993. Modulation of adrenergic receptors and G-transduction proteins in failing human ventricular myocardium. Circulation 87(Suppl IV):27–34.

Fillmore, G. E., Detweiler, D. K. 1973. Maintenance of subacute digoxin toxicosis in normal beagles. Toxicol Appl Pharmacol 25:418–29.

Fleckenstein, A. 1983. History of calcium antagonists. Circ Res 52(Suppl 1):3–16.

Fozzard, H. A. 1976. In M. Vassale, ed., Cardiac Physiology for the Clinician, p. 61. New York: Academic Press.

Fozzard, H. A., Gibbons, W. R. 1973. Action potential and contraction of heart muscle. Am J Cardiol 31:182–92.

Fozzard, H. A., Sheets, M. F. 1985. Cellular mechanism of action of cardiac glycosides. J Am Coll Cardiol 5:10A–15A.

Frank, O. 1895. Z Biol 32:370.

Fusellier, M., Desfontis, J. C., Madec, S., Gautier, F., Marescaux, L., Debailleul, M., Gogny, M. 2005. Effect of tepoxalin on renal function in healthy dogs receiving an angiotensin-converting enzyme inhibitor. J Vet Pharmacol Ther 28(6):581–586.

Gadsby, D. C. 1984. The Na/K pump of cardiac cells. Ann Rev Biophys Bioeng 13:373–98.

Gillis, R. A., Quest, J. A. 1980. The role of the nervous system in the cardiovascular effects of digitalis. Pharmacol Rev 31:19–97.

Gordon, S. G., Arsenault, W. G., Longnecker, M., et al. 2006. Pharmacodynamics of carvedilol in healthy conscious dogs. J Vet Int Med 20(2):297–304.

Gordon, S. G., Bahr, A., Miller, M. W., et al. 2005. Short-term hemodynamic effects of chronic oral carvedilol in Cavalier King Charles Spaniels with asymptomatic degenerative valve disease. Abstract. J Vet Int Med 19(3) Abstract Number 69:417–418.

Guazzi, M. D., Campodonico, J., Celeste, F., et al. 1998. Antihypertensive efficacy of angiotensin converting enzyme inhibition and aspirin counteraction. Clin Pharmacol & Therap 63:79–86.

Haber, E. 1985. Antibodies and digitalis: the modern revolution in the use of an ancient drug. J Am Coll Cardiol 5:111A–117A.

Hahn, A. W. 1977. In R. W. Kirk, ed., Veterinary Therapy, VI: Small Animal Practice, p. 329. Philadelphia: W. B. Saunders.

Hamlin, R. L. 1977. New ideas in the management of heart failure in dogs. J Am Vet Med Assoc 171:114–18.

———. 1986. Clinical and experimental studies with verapamil in the dog. In Proc 5th Symp Am Acad Vet Pharm Therap, pp. 89–96.

Hamlin, R. L., Dutta, S., Smith, C. R. 1971. Effects of digoxin and digitoxin on ventricular function in normal dogs and dogs with heart failure. Am J Vet Res 32:1391–98.

Hamlin, R. L., Pipers, F. S., Carter, K. L., et al. 1973. Treatment of heart failure in dogs without use of digitalis glycosides. Vet Med Small Anim Clin 68:349–50.

Hampton, J. R., van Velduisen, D. J., Kleber, F. X., et al. 1997. Randomised study of effect of ibopamine on survival in patients with advanced severe heart failure. Second Prospective Randomised Study of Ibopamine on Mortality and Efficacy (PRIME II) Investigators. Lancet 349:971–977.

Harris, S. G. 1974. In R. W. Kirk, ed., Veterinary Therapy, V: Small Animal Practice, p. 320. Philadelphia: W. B. Saunders.

Holtz, J. 1993. The cardiac renin-angiotensin system: physiological relevance and pharmacological modulation. Clin Investig 71: S25–S34.

Hoskins, J. D. 2006. Cardiac Therapy: New Treatments Emerge. DVM Magazine. May 1, 2007.

Jackson, E. K. 2006. In L. L. Brunton, J. S. Lazo, and K. L. Parker, eds., Goodman & Gilman's The Pharmacological Basis of Therapeutics, 11th ed., p. 789–821. New York: McGraw-Hill.

Jacobs, A. S., Nielsen, D. H., Gianelly, R. E. 1985. Fatal ventricular fibrillation following verapamil in Wolff-Parkinson-White syndrome with atrial fibrillation. Ann Emerg Med 14:159–60.

Janis, R. A., Triggle, D. J. 1984. 1,4-Dihydropyridine Ca^{++} channel antagonists and activators: a comparison of binding characteristics with pharmacology. Drug Dev Res 4:257–74.

Johnson, J. T. 1985. Conversion of atrial fibrillation in two dogs using verapamil and supportive therapy. J Am Anim Hosp Assoc 21:429–34.

Josephson, M. A., Singh, B. N. 1985. Use of calcium antagonists in ventricular dysfunction. Am J Cardiol 55:81B–88B.

Kae, A. M., Hager, W. D., Messineo, F. C., et al. 1985. Cellular actions and pharmacology of the calcium channel blocking drugs. Am J Med 77(Suppl 2B):2–10.

Katz, A. M. 1985. Effects of digitalis on cell biochemistry: sodium pump inhibition. J Am Coll Cardiol 5:16A–21A.

Kittleson, M. D. 1983. In R. W. Kirk, ed., Veterinary Therapy, VIII: Small Animal Practice, p. 285. Philadelphia: W. B. Saunders.

Kittleson, M. D., Eyster, G. E., Knowlen, G. G., et al. 1985a. Efficacy of digoxin administration in dogs with idiopathic congestive cardiomyopathy. J Am Vet Med Assoc 186:162–65.

Kittleson, M. D., Eyster, G. E., Olivier, M. B., et al. 1983. Oral hydralazine therapy for chronic mitral regurgitation in the dog. J Am Vet Med Assoc 182:1205–9.

Kittleson, M. D., Johnson, L. E., Pion, P. D., Mekhamer, Y. E. 1993. The acute hemodynamic effects of captopril in dogs with heart failure. J Vet Pharmacol Therap 16:1–7.

Kittleson, M. D., Keene, B., Woodfield, J. A. 1986. The acute therapy of supraventricular tachycardia with verapamil. In Proc 5th Symp Am Acad Vet Pharm Therap., p. 97–102.

Kittleson, M. D., Pipers, F. S., Knauer, K. W., et al. 1985b. Echocardiographic and clinical effects of milrinone in dogs with myocardial failure. Am J Vet Res 46:1659–64.

Knowlen, G. G., Kittleson, M. D., Nachreiner, R. F. 1983. Comparison of plasma aldosterone concentration among clinical status groups of dogs with chronic heart failure. J Am Vet Med Assoc 183:991–96.

Krasula, R. W., Gardella, L. A., Zaroslinsk, J. F., et al. 1976. Comparative bioavailability of four dosage forms of digoxin in dogs. Fed Proc 35:327(abst.).

Kurowski, V., Iven, H., Djonlagic, H. 1992. Treatment of a patient with severe digitoxin intoxication by Fab fragments of anti-digitalis antibodies. Intensive Care Med 18:439–42.

Langer, G. A. 1976. Events at the cardiac sarcolemma: localization and movement of contractile-dependent calcium. Fed Proc 35:1274–78.

———. 1977. Relationship between myocardial contractility and the effects of digitalis on ionic exchange. Fed Proc 36:2231–34.

———. 1980. The role of calcium in the control of myocardial contractility: an update. J Mol Cell Cardiol 12:231–39.

Lanza, R. P., Cooper, D. K. C., Barnard, C. N. 1984. Lack of efficacy of high-dose verapamil in preventing brain damage in baboons and pigs after prolonged partial cerebral ischemia. Am J Emerg Med 2:481–85.

Lee, K. S., Klaus, W. 1971. The subcellular basis for the mechanism of inotropic action of cardiac glycosides. Pharmacol Rev 23:193–261.

Lefebvre, H. P., Jeunesse, E., Laroute, V., Toutain, P. L. 2006. Pharmacokinetic and pharmacodynamic parameters of ramipril and ramiprilat in healthy dogs and dogs with reduced glomerular filtration rate. J Vet Intern Med 20(3):499–507.

Lefebvre, H. P., Toutain, P. L. 2004. Angiotensin-converting enzyme inhibitors in the therapy of renal diseases. J Vet Pharmacol Ther 27(5):265–281.

Loboz, K. K., Shenfield, G. M. 2005. Drug combinations and impaired renal function—The triple whammy. British J Clin Pharmacol 59:239–243.

Lombard, C. W., Jons, O., Bussadori, C. M. 2006. Clinical efficacy of pimobendan versus benazepril for the treatment of acquired atrioventricular valvular disease in dogs. J Am Anim Hosp Assoc 42:249–261.

Lorell, B. H. 1985. Use of calcium channel blockers in hypertrophic cardiomyopathy. Am J Med 78(Suppl 2B):43–54.

Lown, B., Black, H., Moore, F. D. 1960. Digitalis, electrolytes and the surgical patient. Am J Cardiol 6:309–37.

Mancini, D. M., Keren, G., Aogaichi, K., et al. 1985. Inotropic drugs for the treatment of heart failure. J Clin Pharmacol 25:540–54.

Mason, D. T. 1973. Regulation of cardiac performance in clinical heart disease: interactions between contractile state mechanical abnormalities and ventricular compensatory mechanisms. Am J Cardiol 32:437–48.

Mason, D. T., Zelis, R., Lee, G., et al. 1971. Current concepts and treatment of digitalis toxicity. Am J Cardiol 27:546–59.

Massie, B., Bourassa, M., DiBianco, R., et al. 1985. Long-term oral administration of amrinone for congestive heart failure: lack of efficacy in a multicenter controlled trial. Circulation 71:963–71.

Meijler, F. L. 1985. An "account" of digitalis and atrial fibrillation. J Am Coll Cardiol 5:60A–68A.

Mendez, C., Aceves, J., Mendez, R. 1961a. The anti-adrenergic action of digitalis on the refractory period of the A-V transmission system. J Pharmacol Exp Ther 131:199–204.

———. 1961b. Inhibition of adrenergic cardiac acceleration by cardiac glycosides. J Pharmacol Exp Ther 131:191–98.

Miller, M. W. et al. 2007. (unpublished data)

Moalic, J. M., Charlemagne, D., Mansier, P., Chevalier, B., Swynghedauw, B. 1993. Cardiac hypertrophy and failure—a disease of adaptation. Circulation 87(Suppl IV):21–26.

Moe, G. K, Farah, A. E. 1975. In L. S. Goodman and A. Gilman, eds., The Pharmacological Basis of Therapeutics, 5th ed., p. 653. New York: Macmillan.

Nayler, W. G. 1980. Calcium antagonists. Eur Heart 1:225–37.

Novotny, M. J., Adams, H. R. 1986. New perspectives in cardiology: recent advances in antiarrhythmic drug therapy. J Am Vet Med Assoc 189:533–39.

O'Grady, M. R., Minors, S. L., O'Sullivan, L., et al. 2003a. Evaluation of the efficacy of pimobendan to reduce mortality and morbidity in Doberman Pinschers with congestive heart failure due to dilated cardiomyopathy. J Vet Int Med 17, Abstract 248.

———. 2003b. Evaluation of the efficacy of pimobendan to reduce mortality and morbidity in dogs with congestive heart failure due to chronic mitral valve insufficiency. J Vet Int Med 17:410, Abstract 12.3.

Opie, L. E. 2001. Mechanisms of cardiac contraction and relaxation. In E. Braumwald, D. Zipes, and P. Libby, eds., Heart Disease: A Textbook of Cardiovascular Medicine, 6th ed. New York: W. B. Saunders.

Opie, L. H., ed. 1984. Calcium antagonists and cardiovascular disease. New York: Raven Press.

Packer, M. 1984. Conceptual dilemmas in the classification of vasodilator drugs for severe chronic heart failure: advocacy of a pragmatic approach to the selection of a therapeutic agent. Am J Med 76:3–13.

———. 1985. Therapeutic application of calcium channel antagonists for pulmonary hypertension. Am J Cardiol 55:81B–88B.

Packer, M., Carver, J. R., Rodeheffer, R. J., et al. 1991. Effect of oral milrinone on mortality in severe chronic heart failure. PROMISE Study Research Group. N Engl J Med 325:1468–1475.

Parker, J. L., Adams, H. R. 1977. Drugs and the heart muscle. J Am Vet Med Assoc 171:78–84.

Patterson, D. F., Abt, D. A., Detweiler, D. K., et al. 1973. On digitalis glycosides in treatment of heart failure: Criticism and reply. Vet Med Small Anim Clin 68:708.

Pion, P. D., Batish, J., Schwark, W., et al. 1986. Pharmacokinetics and electrocardiographic effects of verapamil in the cat. In Proc 5th Symp Am Acad Vet Pharm Therap., pp. 141–53.

Remme, W. J. 1993. Vasodilator therapy for heart failure: early, late, or not at all? Circulation 87(Suppl IV):97–107.

Reuter, H. 1979. Properties of two inward membrane currents in the heart. Ann Rev Physiol 41:413–24.

———. 1985. Calcium movements through cardiac cell membranes. Med Res Rev 5:427–40.

Rick, A. D., Belpaire, F. M., Bogaert, M. G., et al. 1978. Plasma concentrations of digoxin and digitoxin during digitalization of healthy dogs and dogs with cardiac failure. Am J Vet Res 39:811–15.

Robinson, J. W. 1972. The inhibition of glycine and beta-methyl glucoside transport in dog kidney cortex slices by ouabain and ethacrynic acid: contribution to the understanding of sodium-pumping mechanisms. Com Gen Pharmacol 3:145–59.

Rocco, T. P. and Fang, J. C. 2006. In L. L. Brunton, J. S. Lazo, and K. L. Parker, eds., Goodman & Gilman's The Pharmacological Basis of Therapeutics, 11th ed., p. 869–897. New York: McGraw-Hill.

Roland, R., Gordon, S. G., Bahr. A., et al. 2006. Acute cardiovascular effects of oral pimobendan in dogs with heart failure due to chronic valve disease. J Vet Int Med 20(3):731, Abstract Number 75.

Rosen, M. R. 1985. Cellular electrophysiology of digitalis toxicity. J Am Coll Cardiol 5:22A–34A.

Rosing, D. R., Kent, K. M., Borer, J. S., et al. 1979. Verapamil therapy: a new approach to the pharmacologic treatment of hypertrophic cardiomyopathy, 1. Hemodynamic effects. Circulation 60:1201–7.

Rush, J. E., Freeman, L. M., Brown, D. J., et al. 1998. The use of enalapril in the treatment of feline Hypertrophic cardiomyopathy. J Am Anim Hosp Assoc 34:38–41.

Schatzmann, H. J. 1953. Herzglykoside als Hemmstoffe für den aktiven kalium—und natriumtransport durch die erythrocytenmembran. Helv Physiol Pharmacol Acta 11:346–54.

Schramm, M., Towart, R. 1985. Modulation of calcium channel function by drugs. Life Sci 37:1843–60.

Schwartz, A. 1977. New aspects of cardiac glycoside action: introduction. Fed Proc 36:2207–8.

Shionoiri, H. 1993. Pharmacokinetic drug interactions with ACE inhibitors. Clin Pharmacokin 25:20–58.

Sisson, D. D. 1992. Hemodynamic, echocardiographic, radiographic, and clinical effects of enalapril in dogs with chronic heart failure. In Proc 10th Amer Col Vet Int Med Forum, pp. 589–91.

Smith, P. J., French, A. T., Van Israel, N., et al. 2005. Efficacy and safety of pimobendan in canine heart failure caused by myxomatous mitral valve disease. J Small Anim Pract 46:121–130.

Smith, W. J., Wenger, T. L., Grant, A. O., et al. 1981. The antiarrhythmic spectrum of verapamil. Drug Ther (Hosp) 6:63–75.

Solaro, R. J., Wise, R. M., Shiner, J. S., et al. 1974. Calcium requirements for cardiac myofibrillar activation. Circ Res 34:525–30.

Somlyo, A. P. 1985. Excitation-contraction coupling and the ultrastructure of smooth muscle. Circ Res 57:497–507.

Spedding, M. 1985. Calcium antagonists subgroups. Trends Pharmacol Sci 6:109–14.

Starling, E. H. 1918. The Linacre Lecture on the Law of the Heart. London: Longmans, Green.

Stone, P. H., Antmann, E. M, eds. 1983. Calcium channel blocking agents in the treatment of cardiovascular disorders. New York: Fritina Publishing Co.

Swedberg, K. 1993. Reduction in mortality by pharmacological therapy in congestive heart failure. Circulation 87(Suppl IV):126–29.

Teske, R. H., Bishop, S. P., Righter, H. F., et al. 1976. Subacute digoxin toxicosis in the beagle dog. Toxicol Appl Pharmacol 35:283–301.

Tilley, L. P. 1979. Essentials of Canine and Feline Electrocardiography. St. Louis: C. V. Mosby.

Tilley, L. P., Liusk, Gilbertson, S. R., et al. 1977. Primary myocardial disease in the cat: a model for human cardiomyopathy. Am J Pathol 86:493–513.

Tilley, L. P., Weitz, J. 1977. Pharmacologic and other forms of medical therapy in feline cardiac disease. Vet Clin North Am 7:415–28.

Trump, B. F., Berezesky, I. K., Cowley, R. A. 1982. The cellular and subcellular characteristics of acute and chronic injury with emphasis on the role of calcium. In R. A. Cowley, B. F. Trump, eds., Pathophysiology of Shock, Anoxia, and Ischemia, p. 646. Baltimore: Williams & Wilkins.

Vaughn Williams, E. M. 1984. Classification of antiarrhythmic actions reassessed after a decade of new drugs. J Clin Pharmacol 24:129–47.

Wasman, H. L., Myerburg, R. J., Appel, R., et al. 1981. Verapamil for control of ventricular rates in paroxysmal supraventricular tachycardia and atrial fibrillation or flutter. Ann Intern Med 94:1–6.

Watanabe, A. M. 1985. Digitalis and the autonomic nervous system. J Am Coll Cardiol 5:35A–42A.

White, B. C., Aust, S. D., Arfors, K. E., et al. 1984. Brain injury by ischemic anoxia: hypothesis extension—a tale of two ions? Ann Emerg Med 13:862–67.

Withering, W. 1785. Reprinted 1937. Account of foxglove, and some of its medical uses; with practical remarks on dropsy, and other diseases. Med Classics 2:305–443.

Zelis, R., Flaim, S. F., Moskowitz, R. M., et al. 1979. How much can we expect from vasodilator therapy in congestive heart failure? Circulation 59:1092–97.

CHAPTER 23

ANTIARRHYTHMIC AGENTS

MATTHEW W. MILLER AND H. RICHARD ADAMS

An arrhythmia is an abnormality in the rate, regularity, or site of origin of the cardiac impulse or a disruption in impulse conduction such that the normal sequence of atrial and ventricular activation is changed. Although numerous drugs have been identified that suppress cardiac rhythm disturbances, relatively few antiarrhythmic drugs have found strong clinical use in veterinary medicine. This chapter focuses on the more common antiarrhythmic agents along with their principal pharmacodynamic actions on cardiac rate and rhythm.

RHYTHMICITY OF THE HEART

Normal cardiac rhythmicity is maintained by 1) dominance of a single pacemaker discharging regularly with the highest frequency, 2) rapid and uniform conduction through normal routes of impulse conduction, and 3) long and uniform duration of the action potential and refractory period of cardiac myofibers. In addition, duration of the Purkinje fiber action potential normally outlasts that of the ventricular muscle, thus providing a safety factor preventing reentry and reexcitation of the Purkinje system by the muscle action potential. A disturbance in any of the preceding factors can be arrhythmogenic, e.g., an inappropriate increase in automaticity of normally latent pacemaker cells, abbreviation of the refractory period, slowing of conduction velocity, or disparate refractory periods of adjacent fibers.

Arrhythmias often are associated with imbalance of the parasympathetic and sympathetic branches of the autonomic nervous system; changes in serum electrolyte concentrations, especially potassium and calcium ions (K^+ and Ca^{++}); hypoxemia; acidosis; changes in concentration of carbon dioxide; excessive stretch of cardiac tissue; mechanical trauma; myocardial disease states such as congestive heart failure and viral myocarditis; numerous drugs; and ischemia and infarction of the heart muscle.

Hemodynamic instability occurring during cardiac arrhythmias results from alterations in heart rate, changing the regularity of heartbeats, and losing atrial assistance in ventricular filling. Electromechanical synchrony of the cardiac chambers is thereby lost, culminating in ineffectual filling and ejection of the ventricles and hemodynamic deterioration of the patient. Antiarrhythmic drugs suppress arrhythmias and help restore hemodynamic stability by altering basic electrophysiologic processes in the heart.

ELECTROPHYSIOLOGIC PROPERTIES OF CARDIAC CELLS. The classification system for clinically useful antiarrhythmic drugs is based mainly on the predominant pharmacologic effects of a drug on the action potential of cardiac cells (Vaughn Williams 1984; Adams 1986). Accordingly, a useful understanding of antiarrhythmic drug actions and affiliated nomenclature depends first on a good comprehension of basic bioelectric properties of the heart. An overview of salient features of this topic is outlined below relative to action potentials of cardiac cells and types of cardiac arrhythmogenesis.

Action Potentials of Cardiac Cells. The electrical activity of individual heart muscle cells can be recorded with a microelectrode capable of entering the intracellular space of a single cell, as shown schematically in Figure 23.1. Some of the common terms used to describe the configuration and ionic determinants of cardiac action potential components are defined below (Adams 1986):

1. Membrane potential is the voltage difference across the cell membrane, i.e., the difference in electrical voltage between the intracellular and extracellular spaces. By convention, the resting membrane potential is defined as the charge inside the cell relative to the

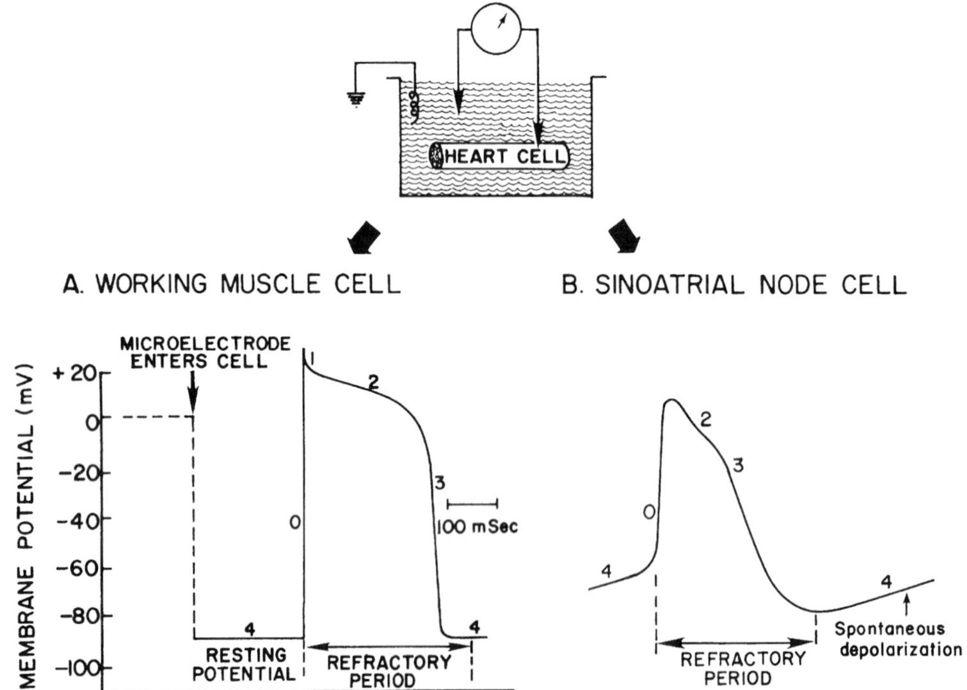

FIG. 23.1 Cardiac action potentials recorded from a working myocardial cell (A) and a sinoatrial pacemaker cell (B). The nonautomatic working muscle cell (A) exhibits a constant phase 4 resting potential during diastole, whereas the automatic cell (B) undergoes spontaneous depolarization during phase 4, leading to threshold and spontaneous excitation. The cell is inexcitable or poorly responsive to additional stimuli during much of the action potential, and this refractory period helps prevent premature excitation. See text for further details. (Source: Adams 1986.)

extracellular side, in which case the resting potential is a negative charge. An increase in resting membrane potential would therefore designate a more negative intracellular charge (e.g., an increase from −70 to −90 mV), while a decrease in resting membrane potential would designate a less negative intracellular charge (e.g., a decrease from −70 to −50 mV).

2. Depolarization is the loss or decrease in electronegativity of the intracellular space, e.g., a decrease in membrane potential from −90 to −50 mV (partial depolarization) or from −90 to 0 mV (complete depolarization).
3. Hyperpolarization is an increase in electronegativity of the intracellular space.
4. Inward current is the change in electrical charge across the cell membrane that results from influx of positively charged ions or, alternatively, from efflux of negatively charged ions.
5. Spontaneous depolarization of automatic cells is a physiologic and progressive decrease in resting potential during diastole, leading spontaneously to threshold and automatic firing.
6. Threshold potential is the membrane potential required for excitation of the cell, initiating the action potential and affiliated cellular responses.
7. Phase 0 is the rapid depolarization phase of the action potential of the excited cell, mediated by a rapid inward current carried by Na^+ through fast sodium channels of the cell membrane.
8. Phase 1 is the initial early repolarization phase of the action potential.
9. Phase 2 is the plateau phase of the action potential, mediated in part by a slow inward current carried by Ca^{++} through slow calcium channels of the cell membrane.
10. Phase 3 is the rapid repolarization phase of the action potential, returning membrane potential to the diastolic level.
11. Phase 4 is the membrane potential during diastole; it is constant in working muscle cells but undergoes spontaneous depolarization in cells with automaticity.
12. Refractory period is that early and late interval of the action potential during which excitability of the cell is essentially absent (functional refractory period) or depressed (relative refractory period), respectively.
13. Depressed fast sodium ion (Na^+) responses are slowly rising phase 0 depolarizations due either to premature excitation during the relative refractory period of normal cells or excitation of sick cells with low diastolic potentials; depressed fast Na^+ response action potentials develop cardiac impulses that propagate poorly with reduced conduction velocity.
14. Slow Ca^{++} responses are analogous to the slow inward Ca^{++} current during phase 2; this term is used to describe the very slowly rising phase 0 depolarizations mediated by Ca^{++} when the fast Na^+ channels are inoperative. Slow Ca^{++} action potentials develop cardiac impulses that propagate poorly with extremely slow conduction.

When a cardiac cell is stimulated, the electrical potential measured across the cell membrane undergoes a depolarization and repolarization cycle that can be differentiated into five interconnected components. These components are referred to as phases 0, 1, 2, 3, and 4 (Fig. 23.1). The precise morphology of the 5 phases of the cardiac action potential varies with the anatomic region of the heart. A schematic diagram illustrating the configuration of action potentials derived from sinoatrial (SA) tissue, atrial muscle (AM), Purkinje fibers (PF), and ventricular muscle (VM) is depicted in Figure 23.2 along with corresponding waveforms of the electrocardiogram (ECG). Action potentials of a sinoatrial pacemaker cell (Fig. 23.1B) and a typical working heart muscle cell (Fig. 23.1A) will be addressed as examples of cardiac tissue with and without normal automaticity, respectively.

Working Heart Muscle Cells. Electrical diastole is designated by phase 4 of the cardiac action potential (Fig. 23.1A); this resting membrane potential is steady at about −90 mV. Polarization across the cell membrane is maintained primarily because of the unequal distribution of K^+ inside and outside the cell. The Na^+,K^+-adenosine triphosphatase transport system maintains high intracellular K^+ relative to extracellular K^+, and the cell membrane is selectively permeable to K^+ during phase 4 diastole when compared to other ions such as Na^+ or Ca^{++}. When the cell is stimulated to its particular threshold level, however, the selective permeability characteristics of the cell membrane to K^+ are momentarily lost. Other ions now cross the sarcolemma and produce the typical depolarization-repolarization cycle that comprises the action potential (Fig. 23.1).

Phase 0 of the action potential reflects the extremely rapid depolarization spike produced by Na^+ rushing into

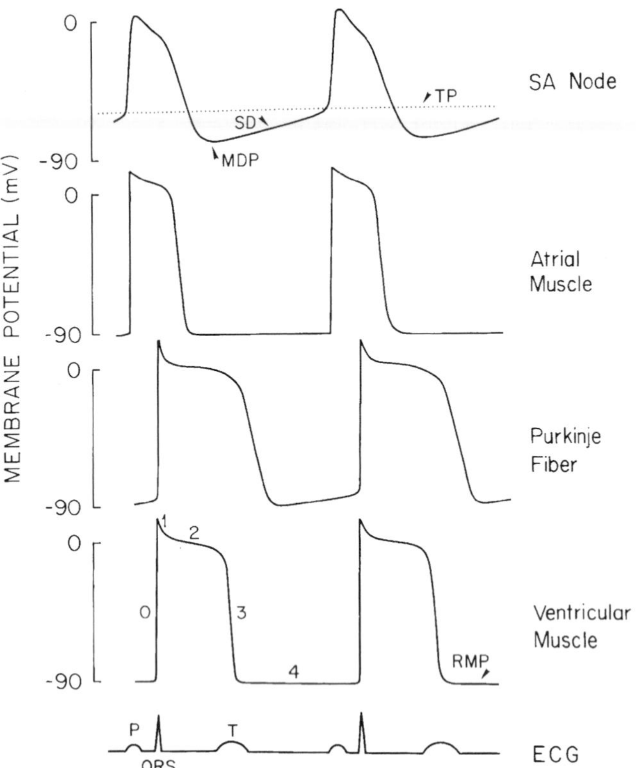

FIG. 23.2 Schematic diagrams demonstrating the temporal relationships between transmembrane action potentials recorded from cells of the sinoatrial node (SA), atrial muscle, Purkinje fibers, and ventricular muscle (see text for discussion). (Modeled after Trautwein 1963. Source: Adams 1986.)

the cell through specific "fast Na^+ channels" or passageways of the sarcolemma. Phase 0 is terminated as early (phase 1) and delayed (phase 3) repolarization occur, restoring the membrane potential to its resting diastolic level of phase 4 (Fig. 23.1). The cell is inexcitable or refractory to additional stimuli during the early and intermediate phase of the action potential cycle; it is only partially responsive if stimulated prior to complete repolarization and return to normal phase 4 diastolic potential.

The phase 2 plateau of the action potential partially represents a brief anomalous delay in restoration of K^+ permeability (Fig. 23.1). A critically important component of phase 2 comprises an influx of Ca^{++} through specific "slow Ca^{++} channels" or "slow cation channels" of the cell membrane. This slow inward Ca^{++} current is the mechanism whereby membrane excitation is coupled to activation of the contractile elements of heart muscle cells (Parker and Adams 1977). The influx of Ca^{++} during phase 2 triggers a release of greater amounts of Ca^{++} from intracellular storage sites, and the increased cytosolic Ca^{++} proportionately activates the contractile machinery of the myocardial cells.

Sinoatrial Pacemaker Cells. Unlike working myocardial cells, automatic cells do not exhibit a clearly definable resting membrane potential during phase 4. Instead, phase 4 is characterized by a slow spontaneous depolarization to threshold potential (Fig. 23.1B), thereby discharging automatically and leading into the more rapid depolarization of phase 0. However, the slope of phase 0 depolarization of SA pacemaker cells is much less than that of working muscle cells (Figs. 23.1, 23.2). This distinction may be explained by a component of slow Ca^{++} influx in the genesis of phase 0 depolarization in these types of automatic cells (Adams 1986). Cells with normal automaticity (i.e., spontaneous phase 4 depolarization) also are found in specialized atrial conduction tracts, the distal region of the AV node, AV valves, and PF.

CLASSIFICATION OF ARRHYTHMOGENIC MECHANISMS. The basic mechanisms involved in genesis of cardiac arrhythmias involve abnormalities of impulse formation (i.e., arrhythmias caused by changes in automaticity), impulse conduction (i.e., arrhythmias caused by reentry phenomena), and a combination of automaticity and reentry (Singh et al. 1980; Binah and Rosen 1984; Boyden and Wit 1985).

Disturbances in Automaticity. The action potential from the SA node, AM, PF, and VM are shown in Fig. 23.2. The five phases of the action potential (0, 1, 2, 3, 4) are numbered in the first complex of VM. Notice spontaneous depolarization (SD), maximal diastolic potential (MDP), and threshold potential (TP) in the automatic cells of SA and PF. The resting membrane potential (RMP) is shown in the nonautomatic cells of the AM and VM. The P wave of the ECG corresponds to depolarization of SA and AM, while the QRS complex and T wave correspond to depolarization and repolarization, respectively, of ventricular cells (Fig. 23.2).

Automatic cells of the SA node normally are the dominant pacemaker, reaching threshold first with the resultant propagating impulse exciting all other potential pacemaker cells before they spontaneously attain threshold values (Fig. 23.2). If automaticity of the SA node is depressed or the spontaneous firing rate in some other tissue (latent pacemaker) is accelerated, regions of the heart other than the SA node may serve as the pacemaker and initiate ectopic impulses. Examples are shown in Figure 23.3.

Automaticity is enhanced when the slope of phase 4 SD is increased (e.g., from a to b in I of Fig. 23.3); this decreases the time required to reach TP, thereby increasing the frequency of spontaneous discharge. The result is an increase in heart rate when the SA pacemaker is involved or emergence of ectopic beats if a normally latent pacemaker is involved. By decreasing the slope of spontaneous depolarization (e.g., from b to a or from a to c in I of Fig. 23.3), drugs can depress ectopic foci and restore normal sinus rhythm without affecting MDP or TP. If a drug raises TP to less negative values (e.g., from TP-a to TP-b in II of Fig. 23.3), additional time will be required to reach TP, thereby depressing automaticity. By increasing the MDP (e.g., from MDP-a to MDP-b in III of Fig. 23.3), a drug can suppress automaticity because additional time would be required before TP is attained.

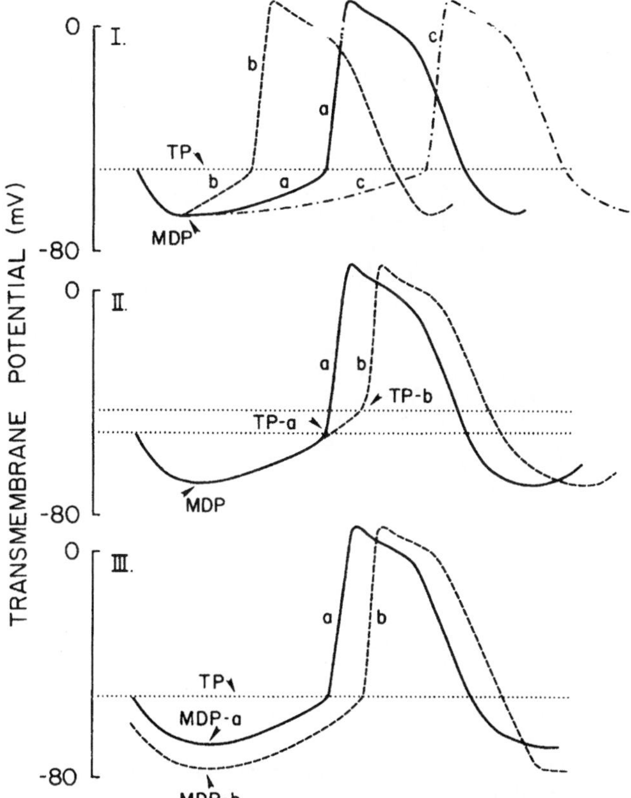

FIG. 23.3 Schematic representations of transmembrane action potentials of cardiac cells with the property of automaticity and potential mechanisms whereby antiarrhythmic drugs can influence automaticity (see text for discussion). (Modeled after Hoffman and Cranefield 1960; Mason et al. 1973.)

Disturbances in Impulse Conduction. Arrhythmias caused by disturbances in impulse conduction are thought to be associated with a phenomenon of reentry or circus movement. The concept of reentry is based on very slow conduction velocity, an area of the heart demonstrating unidirectional block of impulse conduction and perhaps an abnormally brief refractory period (Schmidt and Erlanger 1929; Wit et al. 1972, 1974). This theory holds that a cardiac impulse can travel circuitously around an anatomic loop of fibers in which slowed conduction velocity and brief refractoriness permit the impulse to arrive at cells that are no longer refractory, thereby permitting perpetual reexcitation.

A schematic demonstration of impulse reentry at a junctional region between PF and ventricular muscle is shown in Figure 23.4 (Adams 1986). Acceptance of this theory was delayed by difficulty in visualizing a decrease in conduction velocity adequate to comply with the value deemed necessary for establishing reentry phenomena. After all, the normal conduction velocity in PF can be as high as 2–4 m/sec, thus displaying a high safety factor for impulse propagation. However, the velocity of impulse conduction can be diminished to as low as 0.01–0.1 m/sec by pathologic emergence of action potentials that demonstrate activation-deactivation kinetics that are remarkably slower than the normal fast responses.

Reentry theoretically could be controlled by a drug that either creates bidirectional block or bidirectional conduction through the region of cells causing the unidirectional block; accelerates speed of impulse conduction, thus returning the impulse to the site of reentry when cells are still inexcitable; prolongs action potential duration of normal cells, thereby extending their refractory period; or exhibits a combination of the above actions.

Other forms of cardiac electrophysiologic disturbances, in addition to primary abnormalities of impulse conduction and automaticity, may be important. Examples include abnormal excitability, early/late afterdepolarizations, triggered electrical activities, and perhaps others. However, these types of abnormalities overlap mechanistically with disturbances of automaticity and impulse conduction. Arrhythmias arising from primary automaticity and conduction abnormalities are adequate for modeling the classes of antiarrhythmic drugs relative to their

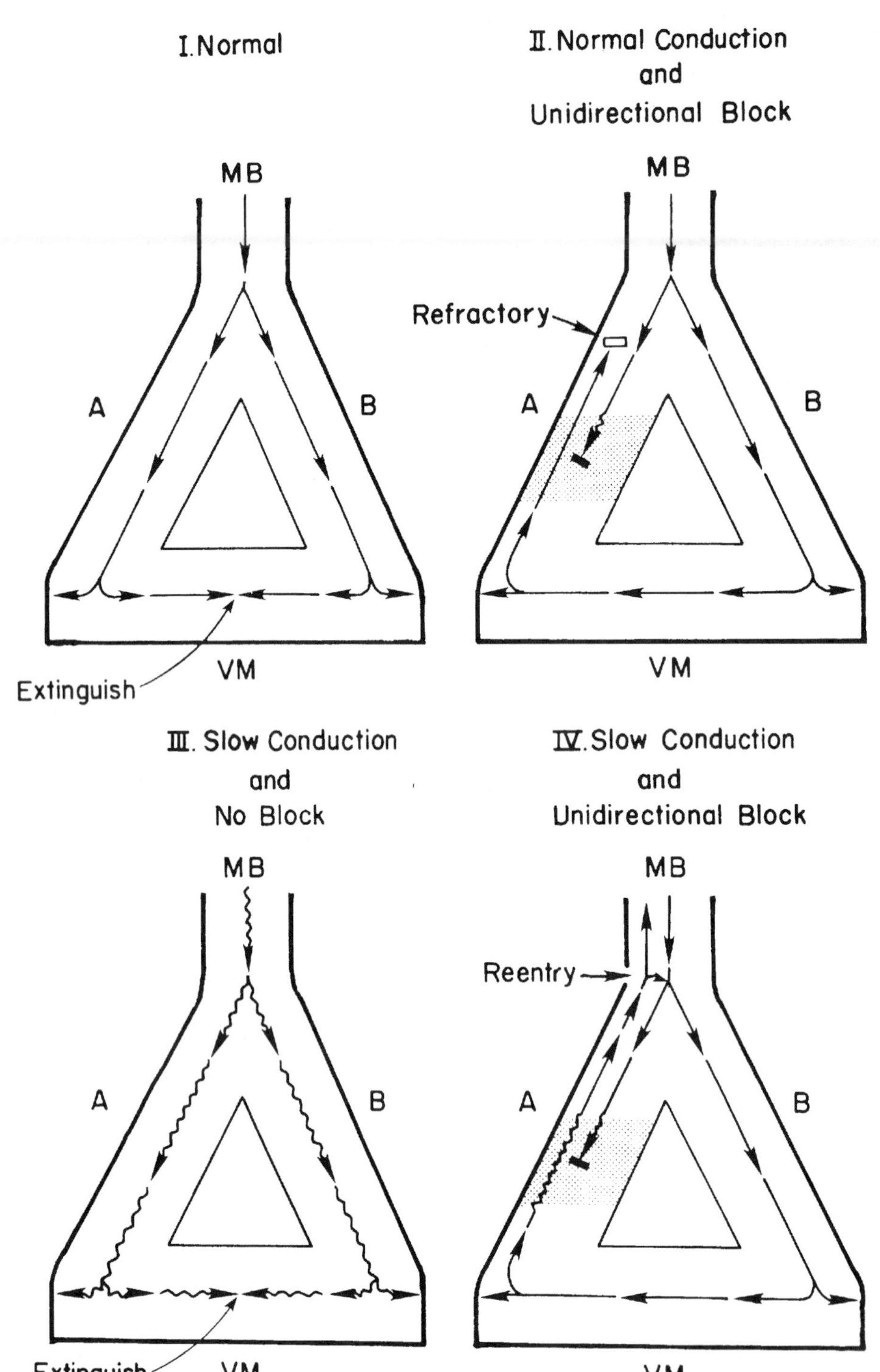

FIG. 23.4 Schematic representations of potential mechanisms involved in cardiac arrhythmias caused by reentry phenomena.

I. Normal. The cardiac impulse (arrows) exits a main bundle branch (MB) of the Purkinje system and enters terminal Purkinje branches A and B. The impulse uniformly and rapidly excites a segment of ventricular muscle (VM) and would be extinguished within the VM due to refractoriness of the cells just excited.

II. Normal conduction and unidirectional block. Because of an area of damaged tissue (shaded area) that blocks antegrade conduction in branch A, the impulse traversing branch B and the VM will excite branch A. The impulse will traverse branch A and the area of unidirectional block through a retrograde pathway; however, since it is conducted at a normally fast speed, it will encounter refractory cells (open square) and be extinguished.

III. Slow conduction velocity and no block. Although the cardiac impulse may be conducted at an abnormally slow velocity (wavy arrows), the lack of unidirectional conduction block causes the impulse to arrive at refractory cells and extinguish.

IV. Slow conduction and unidirectional block. Same as II but the speed of impulse conduction through the area of unidirectional block (wavy arrows), and perhaps through B and VM as well, is so slow that the impulse encounters cells after their refractory period. Thus the impulse can reenter the conduction pathway, thereby establishing perpetual reexcitation. (Modeled after Cranefield 1973; Mason et al. 1973. Source: Adams 1986.)

effects on cardiac action potential characteristics and arrhythmogenesis.

ANTIARRHYTHMIC DRUGS

CLASSIFICATION. Disagreements have arisen owing to lack of consensus over which drug-induced changes in the cardiac transmembrane potential are responsible for antiarrhythmic activity. The classification system advocated by Vaughn Williams (1984) and co-workers is rather straightforward; it is based on the observation that most antiarrhythmic drugs have one dominant electrophysiologic action on the myocardial cell, which may be influenced by the drug's subsidiary myocardial effects as well as its extracardiac activities (Adams 1986). Antiarrhythmic drugs are divided into Class I to IV in this system, as summarized in Table 23.1.

Class I drugs are potent local anesthetics for nerves as well as the myocardial cell membrane, but this activity is generally more pronounced in the heart than in nerve fibers. By inhibiting spontaneous diastolic depolarization, Class I drugs can control arrhythmias caused by enhanced automaticity. Class I drugs that also prolong the refractory period are likely to be effective in abolishing reentrant tachyarrhythmias. Quinidine was the original and prototypical Class I drug.

Clinically useful Class II drugs are β-adrenergic blocking agents (Chapter 6). Propranolol is the prototype of Class II; newer agents include oxyprenolol, alprenolol, metoprolol, timolol, and pindolol. By reducing sympathetic input, β-blocking drugs are effective in controlling arrhythmias associated with increased sympathetic activity (Singh et al. 1980).

Class III drugs produce a prominent prolongation of the action potential, thereby extending the refractory period. An antianginal drug, amiodarone, was found to exert antiarrhythmic activity associated with a prolonged action potential duration without effect on resting membrane potential. Bretylium, an adrenergic neuronal-blocking agent (Chapter 6), has Class III activity.

Ca^{++} channel blockers exert little local anesthetic activity on fast Na^+ responses, but have relatively specific inhibitory effects on Ca^{++}-dependent slow responses. Because of slow Ca^{++} current participation in AV nodal conduction, Ca^{++} blockers slow AV conduction and thereby have application for controlling supraventricular arrhythmias that

TABLE 23.1 Classification and mechanisms of action of antiarrhythmic drugs

Class	Drug	Depression of Fast $Na^+ \dot{V}_{max}$	Action Potential Duration	β-Blockade	Depression of slow responses	Extracardiac Effects
I	*Local anesthetic agents—membrane stabilizers*					
	Quinidine	4+	Lengthen +	Slight	0	Anticholinergic
	Procainamide	4+	Lengthen +	0	0	Anticholinergic
	Lidocaine	4+[a]	Shorten +	0	0	Local anesthetic
	Phenytoin	4+[a]	Shorten +	0	0	Anticonvulsant
	Disopyramide	4+	Lengthen	0	0	Anticholinergic
	Aprindine	4+	0	0	0	Anticonvulsant
	Tocainide	4+	0	0	0	Local anesthetic
II	*β blockers*					
	Propranolol	+	Shorten +	4+	0[b]	Slight
	Oxyprenolol	+	Shorten +	4+	0[b]	Slight
	Alprenolol	+	Shorten +	4+	0[b]	Slight
III	*Agents that prolong action potential duration*					
	Bretylium	0	Lengthen 4+	Neuron blockade	0	Hypotension
	Amiodarone	0	Lengthen 4+	0	0	Coronary vasodilator
IV	*Ca^{++} channel blockers*					
	Verapamil	0	Lengthen phase 1 and 2+	0	4+	Coronary vasodilator

Source: Singh et al. 1980; Vaughn Williams 1984.
Note: 4+ = principal electrophysiologic action; + = subsidiary action; 0 = little or no effect in presumed therapeutic plasma concentrations.
[a]May decrease Na^+ conductance in injured, rather than normal, cells (see text for subclassification of IA, IB, and IC).
[b]May indirectly inhibit slow responses that are initiated by catecholamines.

involve AV reentry pathways (Allert and Adams 1987). Verapamil and diltiazem were the original prototype drugs of Class IV, but many newer agents are now available.

The drugs used to treat supraventricular and ventricular tachyarrhythmias can be divided into separate classes based on their generalized mechanisms of cellular action. Antiarrhythmic drugs exert their effects primarily by blocking sodium, potassium, or calcium channels, or β-adrenergic receptors. This classification scheme is somewhat helpful clinically when deciding to use particular drugs for specific arrhythmias. However, clinical experience with these drugs is the more important means of determining efficacy of various drugs to suppress different tachyarrhythmias.

Class I. Class I drugs are most frequently used to treat ventricular tachyarrhythmias, although they may also be used to treat supraventricular tachyarrhythmias. They are the so-called "membrane stabilizers." Their common mechanism of action is the blockade of fast sodium channels in the myocardial cell membrane. Sodium-channel blockade results in a decrease in the upstroke (phase 0) velocity of the action potential in atrial and ventricular myocardium and Purkinje cells. The upstroke velocity is a major determinant of conduction velocity. Consequently, class I drugs slow conduction velocity in normal cardiac tissue, abnormal cardiac tissue, or both.

Class I agents have variable effects on repolarization. Some of them prolong repolarization while others shorten it or have no effect. Primarily on the basis of differences in repolarization characteristics, class I agents are subdivided into classes IA, IB, and IC (Keefe et al. 1981):

1. Class IA agents include quinidine, procainamide, and disopyramide. These agents depress conduction in normal and abnormal cardiac tissue and prolong repolarization.
2. Class IB agents include lidocaine and its derivatives, tocainide and mexiletine, along with phenytoin. Class IB agents do not prolong conduction velocity in normal cardiac tissue as much as class IA drugs. They do, however, have profound effects on conduction velocity in abnormal cardiac tissue. They also shorten the action potential duration by accelerating repolarization. A greater degree of shortening occurs in fibers that have a longer action-potential duration. Consequently, this effect is most profound in Purkinje fibers and does not significantly alter the effective refractory period of normal atrial and ventricular muscle. In contrast, class IB agents may prolong the effective refractory period of damaged myocardium.
3. Class IC antiarrhythmic drugs include encainide and flecainide. These drugs slow conduction and have little effect on action potential duration; they are rarely used in veterinary medicine.

Class II. Class II drugs are the β-adrenergic blocking drugs. Class II drugs are useful for treating both supraventricular and ventricular tachyarrhythmias. Although few tachyarrhythmias are the direct result of catecholamine stimulation, β-adrenergic receptor stimulation by catecholamines commonly exacerbates abnormal cellular electrophysiology. This can result in initiation or enhancement of a tachyarrhythmia. For example, drugs that block β-adrenergic receptors decrease heart rate and myocardial contractility, and thereby reduce myocardial oxygen consumption. The resultant improvement in myocardial oxygenation may improve cellular electrophysiology and reduce arrhythmia formation.

Class II drugs are most commonly used to alter the electrophysiological properties of the AV junction in patients with supraventricular tachyarrhythmias. β-receptor blockade at the AV junction slows impulse conduction time through the AV junction and therefore prolongs the time that the AV junction is refractory to further stimulation. Both changes effectively disrupt reentrant circuits that use the AV node as part of the circuit.

Class III. Class III drugs act primarily by prolonging the action potential duration and, hence, the refractory period. By such action, they increase the fibrillation threshold and are used commonly to prevent sudden death due to ventricular tachyarrhythmias. They also can be effective in suppressing ventricular arrhythmias. Examples of class III drugs are amiodarone, bretylium, and sotalol. The clinical use of these drugs is evolving in veterinary medicine.

Class IV. Class IV drugs are the calcium channel blocking drugs. They are also known as calcium entry blockers, calcium-channel antagonists and slow-channel inhibitory blockers. They act by inhibiting the function of the slow L-type calcium channels on cardiac cell membranes. Slow calcium channels participate in depolarization of sinus node and AV junctional tissues. Calcium channel blocking drugs slow the upstroke velocity of sinus node and AV junctional cell action potentials, resulting in slowing of sinoatrial and AV junctional conduction times. They also slow the depolarization rate of the sinoatrial node. Calcium channel blocking drugs prolong the time for recovery from inactivation of the slow calcium channel and, as a result, markedly prolong the refractory period of the AV junctional tissue. Calcium channel blocking drugs are also negative inotropic agents because of their effects on L-type slow calcium channels during phase 2 of the action potential in myocardial cells.

Because the primary effects of the calcium channel blocking drugs are on the sinus node and the AV junction, these drugs are most effective for treating supraventricular tachyarrhythmias.

AUTONOMIC DRUGS. With the exception of the β-adrenoceptor blocking agents, autonomic drugs usually are not included in classic groupings of antiarrhythmics. However, the clinician should not overlook the fact that during the actual practice of medicine, drugs other than the classic antiarrhythmic agents generally are preferred in controlling arrhythmias associated with uncomplicated autonomic imbalance. Atropine, e.g., would be an obvious choice when severe sinus bradycardia or sinus arrest is presented secondary to vagal discharge and accumulation of acetylcholine (ACh). Epinephrine is indicated in attempts to restart the heart after cardiac arrest; isoproterenol is useful in reversing AV block; and both can be effective in increasing heart rate if sinus bradycardia associated with impaired sympathetic drive is diagnosed (Adams 1981; Tilley 1985). Pharmacologic actions of the autonomic drugs are covered in Chapters 5–7.

DIGITALIS. The pharmacologic action of digitalis, a quite useful antiarrhythmic agent for controlling ventricular rate in atrial tachyarrhythmias such as atrial fibrillation, is discussed in Chapter 22.

CLASS I AGENTS

QUINIDINE SULFATE. *Quinidine Sulfate,* USP (Quinidex, Quinicardine), is the dextrorotatory isomer of quinine. Both compounds are present in cinchona bark, and their use as antiarrhythmic drugs can be traced to Wenckebach in 1914. This Viennese cardiologist learned that quinine, used to treat malaria, could also control irregular pulse rates in patients with atrial fibrillation. Subsequent investigation indicated that quinidine was more effective than quinine, and the former became a drug of choice in controlling atrial fibrillation.

Quinidine has both direct and indirect effects on cardiac rhythmicity. Similar to other Class I agents (Table 23.1), quinidine decreases the maximal rate of phase 0 depolarization of cardiac cells. This activity is demonstrable in atrial, ventricular, and Purkinje fibers; it reflects a direct depressant effect on Na^+ permeability or the relationship between resting membrane potential and Na^+ conductance (see Fig. 23.5). Quinidine also decreases the slope of spontaneous depolarization of Purkinje fibers but usually spares automaticity of the SA node except when excessive amounts are administered. Thus careful use of quinidine can control ectopic automaticity with less effect on firing frequency of normal pacemaker cells.

Clinically useful doses of quinidine prolong the effective refractory period of atrial and ventricular muscle with relatively less effect on the refractory period of normal pacemaker cells. Quinidine is subtyped as a Class IA drug owing to its characteristic prolongation of the refractory period. The capability of quinidine to directly prolong the refractory period of atrial fibers is thought to

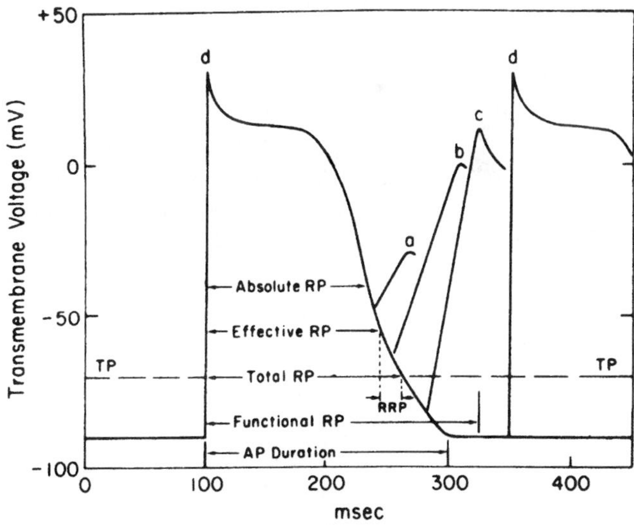

FIG. 23.5 Schematic diagram of transmembrane potentials (TMP) of a working ventricular muscle cell. The maximal rate of rise of phase 0 depolarization of the action potentials labeled a, b, c, and d depends on the magnitude of the TMP at the time of excitation. Thus the rate of depolarization is least at low levels of membrane potential (a), becomes progressively greater as TMP increases (b, c), and finally reaches a maximum at the resting potential (d). RP = refractory period, RRP = relative refractory period, AP = action potential, TP = threshold potential (Mason et al. 1973).

account for its ability to convert atrial fibrillation to sinus rhythm.

As a subsidiary action, quinidine exerts an atropinelike vagolytic effect and therefore antagonizes the cardiac actions of vagally released ACh. This activity contributes to the effectiveness of quinidine in controlling atrial tachyarrhythmias because the action of ACh to shorten the atrial refractory period would be antagonized. Thus quinidine not only directly lengthens the refractory period, it also acts indirectly to lengthen this parameter by its anticholinergic action (Moss and Patton 1973). An adverse result of the atropinelike activity of quinidine, however, is improved AV conduction. Accordingly, an untoward effect of quinidine in treating supraventricular tachyarrhythmias is a sometimes pronounced increase in ventricular rate before the atrial dysrhythmia itself is controlled. This characteristic seems to be particularly prevalent when quinidine is administered by the intravenous (IV) route.

To avoid the potentially dangerous acceleration of ventricular rate by quinidine, it is traditional to first pretreat with a digitalis glycoside. The latter slows AV conduction and can thereby provide control of ventricular rate in atrial fibrillation and flutter. However, care should be exercised in the concomitant use of digoxin and quinidine, since the latter may substantially increase the plasma concentration of the former (Leahey et al. 1978).

Acute quinidine toxicoses is characterized by hemodynamic changes due largely to nonselective depression of various electromechanical functions of the heart. Impulse conduction through the AV node can be depressed to the extent that AV block develops. SA block and even ventricular fibrillation may also occur. Hypotension, decreased cardiac output, decreased myocardial contractility, and prolongation of the PR, QRS, and QT intervals of the ECG can result if large amounts of quinidine are administered intravenously. IV administration is not advocated because of potential dangers. Quinidine and other Class I agents usually are considered to be contraindicated in AV block or intraventricular block.

Quinidine is absorbed efficiently and rapidly when administered by the oral or intramuscular (IM) route. After IV administration, quinidine rapidly passes from the blood and distributes in tissues; distribution equilibrium is complete within 30 minutes (Neff et al. 1972). Approximate plasma half-life values in hours are: dogs (5.5), swine (5.5), ponies (4.4), cats (1.9), and goats (0.9). Protein binding varies from 82 to 92%. A large portion of quinidine undergoes metabolic degradation in the liver, and less than 40% is excreted in urine. Dissimilar rates of biotransformation and elimination probably account for species differences with this drug.

Clinical Aspects. Quinidine has become less available commercially in recent years because the use has declined so much in human medicine. Consequently, veterinarians have found that quinidine formulations are difficult to obtain. This has limited the use of quinidine clinically in animals, and has caused veterinarians to seek alternatives (for example, other drugs to treat atrial fibrillation in horses).

Quinidine has generally been less successful in treatment of atrial fibrillation in small breeds of dogs (Detweiler 1957) than in large breeds such as the Great Dane, St. Bernard, and Newfoundland (Pyle 1967; Bohn et al. 1971). This may be because atrial fibrillation can occur in large or giant breed dogs with minimal cardiac pathology, so-called "lone" atrial fibrillation. Quinidine is rarely used clinically in dogs for management of atrial fibrillation.

Quinidine has been used in the treatment of atrial fibrillation in horses (Detweiler and Patterson 1963; Reef et al. 1995); however, because of decreased availability discussed above, alternatives have been sought (Young van Loon 2005). When used in horses, quinidine is administered at 22 mg/kg quinidine sulfate via nasogastric tube every 2 hours until conversion to sinus rhythm, a cumulative dose of 88 to 132 mg/kg had been administered in 2-hour increments, or the horse has adverse or toxic effects from the drug. Treatment intervals are typically prolonged to every 6 hours if conversion had not occurred. Digoxin should be administered before treatment if the horse has evidence of systolic dysfunction, was prone to tachycardia (resting heart rate ≥60 beats/min) or had a previous history of sustained tachycardia of over 100 beats/min during prior conversion. Digoxin should be administered during day 1 of quinidine sulfate treatment if the horse developed a sustained tachycardia of over 100 beats/min during treatment or on day 2 if conversion had not occurred. Adverse effects of quinidine in horses include urticarial wheals, digestive disturbances, inflammation of the nasal mucosa with respiratory difficulty, laminitis, cardiovascular dysfunction, and even sudden death (Detweiler 1977). IV administration of quinidine has been employed by some clinicians, but this route is more hazardous than oral therapy (Muir and McGuirrk 1984). An IV preparation is available (*Quinidine Gluconate,* USP), but none of the quinidine products have been approved by the U.S. Food and Drug Administration for use in animals.

PROCAINAMIDE HYDROCHLORIDE. *Procainamide Hydrochloride,* USP (Pronestyl), is a derivative of procaine containing an amide linkage in place of the ester linkage in the procaine molecule. This structural modification prolongs the biologic half-life of procainamide to 3–4 hours, making it more useful than the shorter-lasting procaine.

The pharmacologic actions of procainamide, a Class IA agent, are qualitatively similar to those of quinidine (Table 23.1). In general, procainamide is considered more effective in controlling ventricular arrhythmias than atrial arrhythmias.

In dogs the half-life is 2.5 to 3 hours with oral absorption 85% (Papich et al. 1986b). In horses the half-life is 6 hours. A significant feature of procainamide metabolism in animals is differences in conversion to the active metabolite. In people, and other animals, when procainamide is metabolized, an active metabolite is formed, N-acetylprocainamide (NAPA), which has moderate antiarrhythmic effects (Class-III antiarrhythmic effects). Canines are the only mammals that do not produce this metabolite (Papich et al. 1986a). Acetylator status (rapid acetylator versus slow acetylator) determines to what degree people produce this metabolite. Slow acetylators are the most prone to lupuslike adverse effects. The lack of metabolism to an active form may explain the higher doses and plasma concentrations of procainamide in dogs compared to people. It also may explain the safety in dogs, because some adverse effects in people (QT prolongation) may be caused by the Class III antiarrhythmic effects of NAPA.

Huisman and Teunissen (1963) recommended IV infusion of procainamide at the rate of 100 mg/min when used in controlling dangerous ventricular tachycardias in dogs. Ettinger and Suter (1970) employed doses of 250 mg injected intramuscularly as frequently as every 2 hours in dogs weighing 11–16 kg (i.e., about 15–20 mg/kg). Hilwig (1976) listed the dose of procainamide as 4–8 mg/kg when given by IV injection or 25–50 mg/min by constant rate infusion (CRI). Tilley (1979) listed an oral dose of procainamide as 125–500 mg every 6–8 hours (not to exceed 33 mg/kg/day), an IM dose as 8–16 mg/kg every 3–6 hours, and an IV dose as 1–2 mg/kg every 5 minutes to effect or to signs of intoxication (not to exceed 1 g). In a pharmacokinetic study, the dose to suppress experimental arrhythmias in dogs was 8–20 mg/kg and as high as 20–40 mg/kg q6 hr. To produce similar plasma concentrations a CRI of 20–50 mcg/kg/min would be needed. This is in the range of doses found in a clinical study. In a comparison of lidocaine and procainamide for treating ventricular arrhythmias in dogs (Chandler et al. 2006), procainamide was safe and effective at a dose of 10 mg/kg given in 5 minutes, followed by 20 mcg/kg/min CRI.

When used clinically in dogs, it is recommended that one should start at the lowest dose and increase if needed in refractory patients. It is available in 250, 375, and 500 mg tablets or capsules (Pronestyl®). It is also available in 100 mg/ml injection. To prepare IV infusion, remove 5 ml fluid from a 500 ml bag of fluids. To this, add 5 ml of 10% solution (100 mg/ml) to deliver 1,000 μg/ml. At a rate of 70 ml/kg/hr for dogs, this delivers 50 μg/kg/min.

Signs of procainamide toxicosis include greater than 50% widening of the QRS complex of the ECG, additional arrhythmias, bradycardia, tachycardia, hypotension and proarrhythmia (Meurs et al. 2002). Ideally, the ECG and blood pressure should be monitored during administration of procainamide, especially if given by a parenteral route.

In people there is a high incidence (as much as 20%) of immune-mediated drug reactions associated with chronic therapy. A high percentage of people that receive procainamide develop antinuclear antibodies (ANA) and systemic lupuslike syndromes (manifest as arthritis, arthralgia, skin rash, etc). However, similar reactions have not been identified in animals, even though dogs are poor acetylators.

PHENYTOIN SODIUM. *Phenytoin Sodium,* USP (Dilantin, Diphenytoin), originally referred to as diphenylhydantoin, is a primary anticonvulsant drug used in humans and animals for control of epileptic seizures (see Chapter 20). Phenytoin also exerts antiarrhythmic activity in the heart, but this characteristic has a narrow spectrum of therapeutic application. Studies in isolated cardiac tissues have shown that phenytoin exerts direct antiarrhythmic actions similar in some respects to those of quinidine. Because it minimally shortens the refractory period, phenytoin is subtyped as a Class IB drug. Under some circumstances, phenytoin actually may enhance membrane responsiveness and increase conduction velocity, thereby improving impulse conduction through damaged tissue; however, the clinical significance of these activities is uncertain (Singh et al. 1980).

In general, phenytoin is considered to be effective in controlling digitalis-induced arrhythmias of all types; it also is useful in treating ventricular arrhythmias from other causes but is relatively ineffective in abolishing atrial dysrhythmias unless they are related to digitalis toxicosis (Hayes 1972). When administered slowly by the IV route, the usual dose of phenytoin for dogs is approximately 5–10 mg/kg at an infusion rate of about 25–50 mg/min. This appears to be effective in treatment of digitalis-induced arrhythmias without depressant effect on myocardial contractile function (Helfant et al. 1967; Scherlag et al. 1968; Damato 1969). Tilley (1979) and Hilwig (1976) have used 4 mg/kg phenytoin for slow IV administration in dogs. Data pertaining to phenytoin use in cats are lacking; in view of the remarkably long plasma half-life of phenytoin in this species (Roye et al. 1973), much smaller doses than those used in dogs should be considered.

The complete pharmacokinetic disposition of phenytoin has not been determined, but studies in dogs indicate that the drug is absorbed somewhat poorly from the gastrointestinal (GI) tract (approximately 40%) and has a short serum half-life (approximately 3 hours) Sanders and Yeary (1978) proposed that 35 mg/kg of phenytoin administered three times daily (i.e., a total daily dose of 105 mg/kg) may be necessary to achieve plasma concentrations likely to be therapeutically effective in controlling convulsions or cardiac arrhythmias in dogs.

Phenytoin is metabolized in dogs by the microsomal enzymes of the liver, and pharmacokinetic-based drug interactions are likely. Dogs receiving phenytoin were reported to develop signs of phenytoxin toxicosis (postural ataxia and hypermetric gait) when chloramphenicol was added to the therapeutic regimen; this adverse drug interaction was attributed to the inhibitory effect of chloramphenicol on phenytoin metabolism (Adams 1975; Sanders et al. 1979).

LIDOCAINE HYDROCHLORIDE. *Lidocaine Hydrochloride,* USP (Xylocaine), is a local anesthetic drug found to exert antidysrhythmic action that has therapeutic application in treating ventricular tachyarrhythmias. Lidocaine is classified as a Class IB agent. Lidocaine is not recommended for controlling supraventricular arrhythmias but is considered to be useful primarily in reverting ventricular dysrhythmias that develop during general anesthesia, surgery, ischemia, and other forms of trauma. In humans it also is used following myocardial infarction. Lidocaine has been advocated in cardiac emergencies to antagonize the profibrillatory activity of epinephrine (Clark 1977).

The pharmacokinetics have been studied in most veterinary species. Lidocaine undergoes extensive presystemic metabolism (first-pass metabolism in the liver) and therefore lidocaine is not effective if administered orally. In dogs the half-life is less than 1 hour (Wilcke et al. 1983b). In cats, the half-life is approximately 5 hours (cats are also more susceptible to adverse effects and therefore require lower doses). In horses, the half-life is 80 minutes in conscious animals.

Therapeutic assets of lidocaine in emergency situations are its rapid onset and short duration of action after IV injection. However, it is not useful for maintenance therapy because of ineffective absorption after oral administration and short duration of action. In large doses, lidocaine can produce hypotension and exert negative chronotropic and inotropic actions on the heart.

In animals, lidocaine is used as a short-term treatment for acute arrhythmias. It is administered as a bolus, 2–4 mg/kg IV in dogs or 0.5–2 mg/kg every 20–60 minutes by slow injection. If necessary, this may be followed by a constant rate infusion. Rapid IV administration of more than approximately 4 mg/kg lidocaine is likely to cause CNS seizures.

Cats and horses have been given doses of 0.25 to 0.75 mg/kg IV. Cats are particularly susceptible to adverse effects and should be dosed carefully. Continuous rate infusions in dogs have been calculated to deliver 50 μg/kg/min then adjusted as needed within a range of 25 to 75 μg/kg/min (Wilcke et al. 1983a,b; Tilley 1979), or 0.025–0.060 mg/kg/min by constant infusion with ECG monitoring. To prepare this, 25 ml of fluid is removed from a 500 ml bag of fluids. To this, replace with 25 ml of 2% lidocaine (20 mg/ml). This provides 1,000 μg/ml and can be administered as per standard maintenance fluids (e.g., 70 ml/kg/24 hrs for a dog).

Other Clinical Uses of Lidocaine. IV infusions of lidocaine are used in horses to treat postoperative ileus. It has been reported to decrease the duration of ileus after abdominal surgery by returning the intestine to normal motility. The mechanism of action for this effect on GI motility in horses is not known, but may be via suppression of pain receptors, or inhibition of sympathetic inhibitory reflexes in the gastrointestinal tract and peritoneum. In one study (Malone et al. 2006) lidocaine had less reflux and shorter time of hospitalization. Doses in horses are 1.3 mg/kg loading dose (bolus), followed by 0.05 mg/kg/min IV infusion. Adverse effects in horses include muscle fasciculations, ataxia, and seizures.

DISOPYRAMIDE. Disopyramide is a Class IA agent. The spectrum of electrophysiologic actions and the range of therapeutic effectiveness of disopyramide basically resemble respective characteristics of the other two Class IA drugs, procainamide and quinidine (Novotny and Adams 1986). Most data indicate that disopyramide is therapeutically effective mainly against tachyarrhythmias of ventricular origin. In this respect, clinical applications for disopyramide more closely resemble those for procainamide than for quinidine. However, Because of pharmacokinetic disadvantages and limiting side effects, Bonagura and Muir (1985) indicated that disopyramide may prove to have limited application in veterinary medicine.

TOCAINIDE. Tocainide is a Class IB antiarrhythmic drug; it was discovered as a structural congener of lidocaine that shared basic electrophysiologic and antiarrhythmic actions with the parent compound. Tocainide has distinct pharmacokinetic advantages because it is effective after oral administration and has a long duration of action. Like lidocaine, tocainide is a narrow spectrum antiarrhythmic drug with clinical efficacy against ventricular arrhythmias.

Patients that respond to parenterally administered lidocaine usually respond to oral tocainide. Reports in the human literature often concern patients whose arrhythmias were refractory to other antiarrhythmic agents before tocainide was tried, so the actual efficacy of tocainide as an initial antiarrhythmic drug may be higher than some studies would indicate.

There currently are no indications for the use of tocainide in dogs or cats. Doses that are adequate to suppress arrhythmias result in unacceptable toxicity. Tocainide is structurally similar to lidocaine (lignocaine). The major difference is that it is not metabolized extensively on its first pass through the liver after absorption (first-pass effect). Its actions on the normal action potential are almost identical to lidocaine. Although its effects on abnormal action potentials have not been well studied, they are likely to be similar to lidocaine's effects. The depression of the sodium current is more pronounced in abnormal than in normal myocardial tissue. Tocainide does increase the fibrillation threshold. Tocainide is supplied as tablets. Clinical experience with the use of tocainide in small-animal veterinary medicine is limited. Doses required to adequately suppress ventricular arrhythmias in Doberman pinschers range between 15 and 25 mg/kg every 8 hours orally. These doses produce a serum tocainide concentration between 6.2 and 19.1 μg/ml 2 hours after dosing and between 2.3 and 11.1 μg/ml 8 hours after dosing. Apparently, smaller doses are not effective.

The half-life of the drug after oral administration is dose-dependent. After oral doses of 50 and 100 mg/kg the half-life is 8.5 and 12 hours, respectively. These doses are much higher than those used clinically, so the half-life of the drug at clinical doses is unknown but probably shorter. Tocainide is metabolized by the liver and excreted in the urine. About 30% of an intravenous dose is excreted unchanged in the urine. Therapeutic plasma concentration is thought to be in the range 4–10 μg/ml.

At doses adequate to suppress arrhythmias, tocainide causes about 25% of dogs to acutely develop anorexia, and about 10–15% develop central nervous signs of ataxia or head tremor. Chronically, these doses produce intolerable side effects of corneal dystrophy in 10–15% of dogs, and renal failure in about 25% of dogs within 4 months. Consequently, it does not appear that tocainide is a drug that should be used in dogs for the suppression of ventricular arrhythmias and the prevention of sudden death.

MEXILETINE. Mexiletine is a Class IB drug that exerts electrophysiologic and antiarrhythmic actions similar to those of lidocaine and tocainide (Novotny and Adams 1986). As with tocainide, mexiletine was developed for its lidocainelike effectiveness in treating serious ventricular arrhythmias in a formulation suitable for oral administration. Mexiletine undergoes minimal first-pass metabolism by the liver after nearly complete absorption from the GI tract. As with tocainide, mexiletine may find its greatest clinical utility in controlling ventricular arrhythmias that are found to be lidocaine-sensitive and when continued outpatient therapy by the oral route is desirable. In one clinical study involving a small group of dogs (Bonagura and Muir 1985), success was limited when mexiletine was administered orally 2 or 3 times daily at doses of 1–2 mg/kg, but as with tocainide, more extensive clinical trials are necessary.

Mexiletine is indicated for chronic treatment of ventricular tachyarrhythmias in dogs. One group of investigators reported limited success in suppressing ventricular arrhythmias with mexiletine in canine patients. Another group reported good efficacy. However, in the latter report, many dogs had what appeared to be benign and self-limiting ventricular tachyarrhythmias, so determining whether the drug was effective is difficult. One investigator reported that mexiletine appears to be effective at controlling ventricular tachyarrhythmias and preventing sudden death in Doberman pinschers with dilated cardiomyopathy. Although this has not been tested in clinical trials, this report is encouraging and is consistent with the reported increase in the fibrillation threshold.

Mexiletine can interrupt reentry circuits by slowing conduction and depressing membrane responsiveness. Abnormal automaticity is suppressed by mexiletine. Most important, mexiletine can increase the ventricular fibrillation threshold in the dog. In one study of experimental dogs with myocardial infarction, ventricular fibrillation or a rapid ventricular tachycardia could be induced in 6 of 10 dogs at baseline by stimulating the heart with two premature beats. These arrhythmias were prevented by mexiletine administration. Combination therapy is sometimes more effective than administration of one drug alone. A combination of mexiletine and quinidine was more effective at preventing induced ventricular arrhythmias in experimental dogs with myocardial infarction than was either drug alone in one study.

Mexiletine is supplied as capsules. The dose in dogs is 5–10 mg/kg every 8 hours orally. An effective serum concentration may be achieved after three doses. Mexiletine is well absorbed from the gastrointestinal tract in dogs, with a bioavailability of approximately 85%. Approximately 80% is excreted in the urine in dogs and 10% is metabolized by the liver and excreted in the feces. It has a plasma half-life of 3–4 hours in the dog. Therapeutic serum concentration is thought to be between 0.5 and 2 μg/ml.

Toxic effects of mexiletine include vomiting and disorientation/ataxia but are uncommon at the suggested dosage range. A dose of 25 mg/kg orally to dogs can induce seizure activity while 40 mg/kg orally consistently produces ataxia, tremor, and salivation within 10 minutes after administration. These signs last for up to 2.5 hours. Tonic–clonic spasms often begin within 15–40 minutes after administration and last for up to 1 hour. Vomiting and diarrhea can be seen at doses of 15–30 mg/kg. In humans, mexiletine has no effect on sinus rate, PR interval and QRS duration in patients without preexisting conduction system disease. In human patients with sinus node or conduction system disease, bradycardia and AV block can be produced. Mexiletine has been studied in normal dogs at doses ranging from 3 mg/kg to 15 mg/kg for 13 weeks. No effects on heart rate, PR interval, QRS complex duration, or QT interval were noted. No clinical signs of toxicity were seen.

APRINDINE. Aprindine is a Class I agent that shares basic electrophysiologic actions with lidocaine, except that aprindine seems to have a somewhat broader spectrum of antiarrhythmic efficacy. Aprindine is effective against premature ventricular beats and ventricular tachycardias but also has potential for suppressing supraventricular premature beats. Aprindine is less effective and is not used in the settings of atrial fibrillation, atrial flutter, or supraventricular paroxysmal tachycardia. Aprindine may accelerate AV conduction and precipitate increased ventricular rate responses. Aprindine's usefulness in humans has been somewhat limited, owing to a rather narrow toxic-therapeutic ratio; leukopenia, agranulocytosis, and hepatotoxicosis are potential side effects. Dose-related and reversible untoward reactions include hypotension, ataxia, nausea, seizures, transient depression of myocardial contractile function, and prolongation of the PR, QRS, and QT intervals (Novotny and Adams 1986).

Aprindine underwent clinical trial in 20 dogs with spontaneous ventricular arrhythmias (Muir and Bonagura 1982); 17 of the dogs had failed to respond to treatment with quinidine, procainamide, lidocaine, propranolol, or a combination of these drugs. Aprindine was administered by IV infusion at a dose of 0.1 mg/kg/min for 5 minutes and repeated at 10-minute intervals until the arrhythmia was controlled or signs of intoxication intervened. The subsequent oral dose was 1–2 mg/kg, 3 times daily. Aprindine was effective with this schedule in converting ventricular tachycardia to sinus rhythm in 15 of the dogs and in slowing ventricular rate in 4 others; one dog had an increased ventricular rate. Aprindine likewise was effective in controlling ventricular tachycardia in another clinical trial involving Doberman pinschers with congestive cardiomyopathy (Calvert et al. 1982).

ENCAINIDE, FLECAINIDE, AND LORCAINIDE. Encainide, flecainide, and lorcainide are Class IC members discovered and characterized during a search for drugs with efficacy against arrhythmias resistant to standard treatment regimens. They share basic Na^+ conductance-blocking properties with quinidine; however, they are distinct from other quinidinelike drugs because they do not prolong the refractory period. Because of this spectrum of electrophysiologic actions, encainide, flecainide, and lorcainide are subgrouped as Class IC antiarrhythmic drugs (Novotny and Adams 1986). These drugs have found no application in veterinary cardiology.

CLASS II AGENTS

PROPRANOLOL HYDROCHLORIDE. Drugs that exhibit β-adrenoceptor blocking properties have an established place in treating and preventing cardiac dysrhythmias in humans but have received less clinical use in animals. In view of the effectiveness of β-blocking agents in controlling a wide variety of dysrhythmias, it seems likely that these drugs will be used increasingly in animals with spontaneous cardiac arrhythmias.

Propranolol Hydrochloride, USP (Inderal), is the prototype; newer agents include oxprenolol, metoprolol, timolol, alprenolol, pindolol, and practolol. Experimental evidence in animals and clinical studies in humans support the view that β blockade is the primary determinant of the antiarrhythmic activity of this group of drugs. Their local anesthetic or quinidinelike activities currently are considered to be less important (perhaps unimportant) in most clinical situations (Table 23.1). The efficacy of β-blocking agents in preventing various cardiac dysrhythmias emphasizes the importance of autonomic imbalance, particularly sympathetic overactivity, in the genesis of different rhythm disturbances in the heart.

Propranolol slows the rate of spontaneous discharge of the SA and ectopic pacemakers and slows both antegrade and retrograde conduction through anomalous pathways of the heart. Thus propranolol can provide relief from arrhythmias associated with disturbances of automaticity, reentry phenomena, or both. Propranolol increases the refractory period of the AV node, which has therapeutic application in slowing ventricular rate during atrial fibrillation or flutter. During the latter conditions, propranolol usually does not slow the fibrillatory or flutter frequency of the atria and only rarely does it restore sinus rhythm. However, the slowing of ventricular rate by propranolol often is effective and is reported to be useful in some cases that are refractory to other antiarrhythmic agents.

Propranolol and other β blockers are effective in reducing frequency of paroxysmal supraventricular tachycardia, especially in the Wolff-Parkinson-White syndrome (Singh and Jewitt 1974). Tachyarrhythmias associated with digitalis intoxication and physical exertion respond well to β-blocking agents. Arrhythmias evoked during inhalation anesthesia with halogenated hydrocarbon anesthetics often can be prevented or reversed by propranolol administration prior to or during anesthesia, respectively.

Propranolol is well absorbed from the gut and is eliminated largely from portal blood by the liver before it reaches the systemic circulation. Because of this large first-pass effect, six to ten times larger doses are necessary when propranolol is administered by mouth as compared to the IV route (Weidler et al. 1979). The order of plasma clearance for propranolol in different species is: rat > dog > cat > human > monkey.

In a study in cats, a two-step IV infusion technique was found to be more effective in attaining and maintaining steady-state plasma concentrations of propranolol than IV bolus injection. The two-step technique involved the following schedule: continuous IV infusion first at a rapid rate of approximately 8–11 μg/kg/min for 15 minutes, than a slow rate of approximately 1–4 μg/kg/min for 4 hours (Weidler et al. 1979). Steady-state plasma concentrations of propranolol achieved with this schedule were 60–80 ng/ml. Application of such techniques to clinical management of arrhythmias probably would be useful depending upon severity of the dysrhythmia and whether the animal is ill enough or tractable enough to allow prolonged IV infusions.

In the dog, suppression of catecholamine-induced arrhythmias by propranolol requires smaller IV doses (0.1–1 mg/kg) than abolition of ouabain-induced arrhythmias (3–5 mg/kg). Relatively large IV doses of propranolol (3 and 5 mg/kg) are toxic in dogs subjected to myocardial infarction after ligation of the anterior descending branch of the left coronary artery (Shanks and Dunlop 1967). Care must be exercised when β-blocking agents are administered to animals with reduced cardiac reserve.

Importantly, rapid bolus injections of large amounts of propranolol can produce nonspecific cardiovascular depressant effects. Ideally, blood pressure and the ECG should be monitored closely when β blockers are administered intravenously. Oral doses of propranolol in animals vary from approximately 2 mg/kg to as high as 40 mg/kg 2 or 3 times daily (Hilwig 1976; Tilley 1979).

ATENOLOL. Atenolol is a specific β_1-adrenergic blocking drug. It has the same potency as propranolol but different pharmacokinetics. In dogs, atenolol is most commonly used in conjunction with digoxin to slow the heart rate in patients with atrial fibrillation. It is also used in dogs to treat supraventricular tachycardia and ventricular tachyarrhythmias and is used in attempts to prevent sudden death in dogs with severe subaortic stenosis. It is used in cats most commonly to decrease systolic anterior motion of the mitral valve in feline hypertrophic cardiomyopathy and to treat ventricular tachyarrhythmias.

Atenolol is supplied as tablets and as a solution for IV injection. The IV dosage for dogs and cats is not known, but the oral dose in dogs is 6.25–50 mg every 12 hours orally. Because of its shorter half-life in the dog, it is recommended that atenolol be administered every 12 hours to dogs. In large dogs with atrial fibrillation, the starting dose is 12.5 mg every 12 hours orally. The dose is titrated upward until the heart rate is above 160 beats/min. In small dogs, the starting dose is 6.25 mg every 12 hours orally. If used to treat ventricular arrhythmias in dogs without underlying myocardial failure or in an attempt to prevent sudden death in dogs with subaortic stenosis, the dose should be at the upper end of the dosage range.

In cats with hypertrophic cardiomyopathy, atenolol can be used to decrease the subaortic pressure gradient that occurs secondary to systolic anterior motion of the mitral valve. The starting dose is 6.25 mg every 12 hours orally. It is then titrated upwards to as high as 25 mg every 12 hours orally.

Atenolol is more water-soluble than propranolol. In the dog, bioavailability appears to be approximately 80%. Atenolol is eliminated unchanged in the urine. There is little hepatic metabolism. The half-life of atenolol is longer than the half-life of propranolol, being 5–6 hours in the dog. This is somewhat shorter than the half-life in humans, which is 6–9 hours. In the cat, atenolol has a half-life of 3.5 hours. Its bioavailability is high at 90% and the pharmacokinetic variability from cat to cat is small. When administered to cats at a dose of 3 mg/kg, atenolol attenuates the increase in heart rate produced by isoprenaline for 12 but not for 24 hours.

ESMOLOL. Esmolol is a β_1-blocker used in several clinical situations, including acute termination of supraventricular tachycardia. It can also be used, at low doses, acutely to decrease the heart rate in dogs with severe ventricular tachycardia (heart rate > 250 beats/min) due to atrial fibrillation. In cats with hypertrophic cardiomyopathy, it has been used as an agent to determine if β-blockade will reduce the dynamic left ventricular outflow tract obstruction due to systolic anterior motion of the mitral valve.

Esmolol is ultrashort-acting (half-life <10 minutes) used commonly for intravenous administration. Steady state β-blockade is produced within 10–20 minutes after starting intravenous administration of esmolol in dogs. After discontinuation of drug administration, no detectable β-blockade is apparent at 20 minutes postinfusion, regardless of the dose administered. Esmolol decreases the sinus node rate. At an infusion rate of 25 μg/kg/min, approximately 30% of the effect of isoprenaline-induced tachycardia is inhibited. This value increases to approximately 60% with a 50 μg/kg/min dose and to approximately 70% with a 100 μg/kg/min infusion rate. Myocardial contractility is depressed with esmolol. In normal conscious dogs, an infusion rate of 10 μg/kg/min does not change ventricular dP/dt. An infusion rate of 40 μg/kg/min decreases dP/dt by approximately 30% and an infusion rate of 160 μg/kg/min decreases it by 50%. Because esmolol predominantly blocks β_1-adrenergic receptors, it produces no increase in peripheral vascular resistance associated with block of β_2-vascular receptors.

Formulations and Dose Rates. Esmolol hydrochloride is supplied as a solution for intramuscular injection and a concentrated solution for dilution in intravenous infusions. Esmolol can be administered in two different ways to dogs. An initial loading dose of 0.25–0.5 mg/kg (250–500 μg/kg) can be administered intravenously as a slow bolus over 1–2 minutes followed by a constant rate infusion of 50–200 μg/kg/min. Alternatively, a constant rate infusion of 10–200 μg/kg/min can be started without a loading dose. In this manner, maximal effect should be apparent within 10–20 minutes. With the loading dose, an effect should be apparent more rapidly.

An initial loading dose and the high end of the dosage range should be used only in dogs with normal cardiac function. In dogs with severe dilated cardiomyopathy or severe mitral regurgitation and atrial fibrillation with a high ventricular rate, esmolol should be infused without a loading dose. The infusion should start at 10–20 μg/kg/min and titrated upward every 10 minutes to an effective endpoint.

Esmolol has the basic structure of a β-adrenergic blocking drug but it contains an ester on the phenoxypropanolamine nucleus that is rapidly hydrolyzed by red-blood-cell esterases. The major metabolite of esmolol is ASL-8123. It has a half-life in dogs of 2.1 hours. This metabolite has 1/1500 the beta-blocking activity of esmolol, which is clinically insignificant.

METOPROLOL TARTRATE. Metoprolol tartrate, USP (Lopressor), is considered to be a cardioselective β-blocking agent; i.e., it is relatively more effective in blocking β_1 receptors of the heart than β_2 receptors of vascular and bronchiolar smooth muscles (see Chapter 6). This selectivity is important, because a limiting side effect of propranolol and other nonselective β-blockers is airway obstruction owing to a block of adrenergically regulated dilation of bronchioles. Thus metoprolol or other β_1 selective blockers may well be the β-blocking agents of choice in patients with a history of chronic obstructive airway disease.

Precautions. Beta-blocking agents should be administered with caution in patients with reduced cardiac reserve (e.g., congestive heart failure). Under such pathophysiologic conditions, cardiac function is characterized by increased dominance of the sympathetic nervous system as part of the compensatory attempt to maintain cardiac output (see Chapter 22). Blockade of sympathetic input to the heart by propranolol, particularly if sudden, can precipitate cardiac decompensation and all the associated problems that entails (Kittleson and Hamlin 1981). This warming is valid despite the increasing realization that β-blockade, by reducing myocardial oxygen consumption, is a useful adjunct to treating chronic heart failure.

CARVEDILOL. Carvedilol (Coreg) is considered a *3rd generation beta blocker*. This is a unique drug administered as a racemic mixture (R+ and S– forms). The S isomer is a beta blocker, but the R and S isomer also have α1-adrenergic blocking activity. The α-blocking effects contribute to vasodilation. It is a nonselective (β_1 and β_2) blocker. However, it may be beneficial in patients with heart failure because there is evidence that β_2-mediated effects are important in heart failure as well as the β_1 effects. Also, the α-blocking effects counter the vasoconstrictive action of the β_2-blocking action.

Although oral doses for dogs have been cited as 1.5 mg/kg every 12 hours, studies in dogs have demonstrated poor and variable oral systemic absorption. Oral absorption is less than 10% and is highly variable (Arsenault et al. 2005). Response in dogs is also highly variable and inconsistent (Gordon et al. 2006). Therefore, the oral use of carvedilol in dogs may have limitations caused by inconsistent systemic absorption. In the future, newer agents such as bisoprolol may be preferred because of better and more consistent oral absorption in dogs.

CLASS III AGENTS

AMIODARONE. Amiodarone hydrochloride (Cordarone) has been suggested for use in dogs with dilated cardiomyopathy at risk of sudden death. There have been no controlled studies examining amiodarone's effectiveness in this situation, although anecdotal evidence supports its effectiveness. More recently amiodarone has been reported to offer good ventricular rate control in atrial fibrillation and may result in conversion to sinus rhythm in as many as 25% of dogs. Amiodarone is potentially useful and may become more popular in small-animal medicine as veterinarians gain more experience with the drug (Oyama and Prosek 2006; Saunders et al. 2006).

Amiodarone is a benzofurane derivative. It is structurally related to levothyroxine (thyroxine) and has a high iodine content. It is metabolized to desethylamiodarone in the dog. Desethylamiodarone has important antiarrhythmic effects because of its ability to block fast sodium channels. It is more effective in suppressing ventricular arrhythmias 24 hours after myocardial infarction in experimental dogs than is amiodarone.

Amiodarone is supplied as tablets. The effective dose of amiodarone in the dog is unknown. Because of its bizarre and variable pharmacokinetics, predicting the ultimate serum concentration is difficult and predicting the myocardial concentration is untenable. For years, amiodarone was administered to humans at higher doses than are currently used. More recently, clinical use showed lower doses to be more efficacious.

Because amiodarone has not been used extensively in clinical veterinary medicine, it is unknown whether lower doses than those used in experimental studies are effective.

It is known that an oral dose of approximately 10 mg/kg/day to experimental dogs increases the defibrillation threshold after 9 days.

No established relationship between plasma concentration and efficacy in humans exists. However, a plasma concentration below 1 mg/l is often not effective and a plasma concentration above 2.5 mg/l is usually associated with a higher incidence of side effects in humans.

It is known that the plasma concentration was 1.9 ± 1.1 mg/l within 3 weeks in experimental dogs administered 40 mg/kg/day orally for 10 days followed by 30 mg/kg/day orally for 4 days followed by 20 mg/kg orally day for 6 weeks. It is also known that this dose was effective at preventing inducible ventricular tachycardia/fibrillation in these dogs with experimentally induced myocardial infarction. From these data, it would appear that this dose might be effective in clinical canine patients. However, lower doses were not tested in this study so it is unknown whether a lower dose might have been equally effective.

The dose outlined above resulted in a plasma concentration above 2.5 mg/l in some dogs. This may suggest that a lower dose might be safer. One veterinary clinician has reported that a dose of 10–15 mg/kg every 12 hours (20–30 mg/kg/day) orally for 7 days followed by 5–7.5 mg/kg every 12 hours (10–15 mg/kg/day) orally produced an improvement in ventricular arrhythmias in a few dogs treated in this manner.

Amiodarone has unusual pharmacokinetics. After repeated administration, the drug has a long half-life of 3.2 days in the dog. It is very lipophilic and accumulates in adipose tissue up to 300 times the plasma concentration. Once drug administration is discontinued, amiodarone is cleared rapidly from all tissues except adipose tissue.

Myocardial concentration of the drug is approximately 15 times that of plasma. The long half-life of the drug means that it takes a long time to produce a significant effect once administration starts. It also takes a long time for the drug effect to dissipate once administration is discontinued. For example, the time to reach one-half of the peak value ultimately achieved for the increase in left ventricular refractory period in dogs is 2.5 days. The time to fall to one-half the peak value after drug administration is discontinued is 21 days in dogs. Because of the long time to onset, loading doses of amiodarone are commonly administered in human medicine. In humans it may take 1–3 weeks to observe onset of action, even with loading doses. Antiarrhythmic effects are present for weeks to months after discontinuing the drug in humans.

Numerous side effects of amiodarone have been reported in the human literature. In humans who receive more than 400 mg/day of amiodarone (i.e., approximately 6 mg/kg/day), 75% patients experience adverse reactions and 7–18% discontinue the drug because of side effects. Most of the adverse sequelae occur after 6 months of drug use.

Adverse reactions in humans consist of neurological problems (20–40%), gastrointestinal disturbances (25%), visual disturbances including corneal microdeposits (4–9%), dermatological reactions including photosensitivity and blue discoloration of the skin (5%), cardiovascular reactions including congestive heart failure and bradycardia (3%), abnormal liver function tests (4–9%), pulmonary inflammation and fibrosis (4–9%), and hypothyroidism and hyperthyroidism.

Pulmonary fibrosis is a common severe sequela of amiodarone administration in humans. Pulmonary fibrosis, heart failure, and elevation of liver enzymes necessitate discontinuing the drug in humans. Pulmonary toxicity appears to be multifaceted but inhibition of phospholipase A with resultant phospholipidosis is one mechanism responsible for producing pulmonary lesions.

Amiodarone's side-effect profile in dogs is poorly documented. In two studies elevated liver enzymes and neutropenia were reported in some dogs. The liver enzymes returned to normal following discontinuation of the medication in most dogs. Gastrointestinal disturbances have also been reported. Comparable lung changes to those seen in humans are induced in rats and mice. Dyslipidic lesions can be produced in dogs in the gastrointestinal tract by amiodarone administration but only at high doses (>50 mg/kg/day for 30 days). It is also known that amiodarone increases the phospholipid content of feline myocardium. Consequently, it is suspected that chronic amiodarone toxicity could occur in dogs and cats.

Amiodarone can result in either hypothyroidism or hyperthyroidism in humans. Amiodarone inhibits T_4 and T_3 secretion from canine thyroid glands. Consequently, thyroid function should be monitored when amiodarone is chronically administered in veterinary patients. Amiodarone alters the pharmacokinetics and increases the serum concentrations or the effects of several drugs in humans, including digoxin, quinidine, procainamide, phenytoin, and warfarin. Amiodarone administration increases the bioavailability of diltiazem and decreases total body clearance and volume of distribution of the drug in the dog. This results in an increased serum diltiazem concentration and could produce a toxic concentration. This combination should be used cautiously and the dose of diltiazem reduced.

SOTALOL. Sotalol is a class III antiarrhythmic with subsidiary β-adrenergic blocking properties. The information provided on this drug in this chapter is based on studies reported from experimental use in animals, on reports of its use in human medicine, on limited clinical experience, and on anecdotal reports from individuals who have used the drug. Sotalol is potentially a useful drug in small-animal veterinary medicine but this potential has not yet been fully explored.

In human medicine, sotalol is effective for treating various arrhythmias. It is not as successful as quinidine at converting primary atrial fibrillation to sinus rhythm. However, it is as effective as quinidine at preventing recurrence of atrial fibrillation after electrical cardioversion. Sotalol is effective at terminating supraventricular tachycardia due to AV nodal reentry or preexcitation in humans. In human patients with ventricular tachycardia, sotalol may be one of the more effective agents for terminating or slowing tachycardia. It also appears to be efficacious for preventing sudden death. These effects, however, are not profound and have required large clinical trials to reach statistical significance.

A major indication in veterinary medicine is boxer dogs with severe ventricular tachyarrhythmias and syncope. Sotalol is very effective at suppressing the arrhythmias and stopping the syncopal events in this breed (Meurs et al. 2002).

Mechanism of Action. Sotalol is marketed as the racemic mixture of its stereo isomers, D- and L-sotalol. The D-isomer has less than 1/50 the β-blocking activity of the L-isomer. The L-isomer's potency is similar to that of propranolol. The D- and L-isomers both prolong action potential duration and refractoriness. The increase in action potential duration is caused by blockade of potassium channels.

Sotalol, when administered intravenously or at high doses orally, increases the QT interval on the ECG in experimental dogs. As for any β-blocker, the heart rate is decreased with sotalol administration. It also prolongs the AV nodal refractory period and the PR interval because of its β-blocking effect. Sotalol increases the atrial and the ventricular fibrillation threshold in experimental dogs. The effect on atrial refractoriness should make it a good drug for preventing atrial fibrillation in dogs, especially those with primary atrial fibrillation after cardioversion. The effect on the ventricular fibrillation threshold should make it an effective agent for preventing sudden death in dogs. Its effects on defibrillation are less well understood. In one study, sotalol decreased the success rate for defibrillation, while in another study, it decreased the energy required for defibrillation.

The hemodynamic effects of sotalol are mixed. Because it is a β-blocker, a decrease in myocardial contractility is expected and has been identified in anesthetized, experimental dogs with normal hearts and in experimental dogs after myocardial infarction. However, in isolated cardiac tissues, sotalol does not have a negative inotropic effect and may induce a modest (20–40%) positive inotropic effect in catecholamine-depleted experimental cats. This effect may be caused by the prolongation of the action potential allowing more time for calcium influx in systole.

In experimental dogs, sotalol has less of a negative inotropic effect than does propranolol. In humans with compromised myocardial function, sotalol can induce or exacerbate heart failure but the incidence is much lower than one might expect. In one study, heart failure was aggravated by sotalol in only 3% of human patients. The potential negative inotropic effects of sotalol could theoretically produce myocardial depression and produce or aggravate heart failure in small-animal patients. As in human patients, if one uses this drug, the dose must be carefully titrated and canine or feline patients with moderate to severe cardiac disease must be monitored carefully.

Formulations and Dose Rates. Both the D- and L-isomers prolong action potential duration, while the L-isomer is responsible for the β-blocking properties of the drug. In one study in experimental dogs, sotalol successfully converted atrial flutter to sinus rhythm in 14 of 15 dogs at a dose of 2 mg/kg IV administered over 15 minutes. Quinidine converted only 9 of the 15 dogs at a dose of 10 mg/kg IV over 15 minutes. In another study to examine sotalol's ability to terminate and to prevent atrial fibrillation, sotalol was administered intravenously to dogs with induced atrial fibrillation. At a dose of 2 mg/kg IV, sotalol did not terminate or prevent atrial fibrillation. At a cumulative dose of 8 mg/kg, however, it terminated the arrhythmia in 7 of 8 dogs and prevented its reinduction in all 8 dogs. This effect was due to a prolongation of atrial refractory period.

It takes a high dose of D-sotalol to suppress the formation of ventricular arrhythmias in experimental dogs. This compound has no β-blocking activity and one would expect that a lower dose of the racemic mixture would be effective. In one study of conscious experimental dogs 3–5 days after myocardial infarction, four doses of 8 mg/kg D-sotalol administered intravenously successfully prevented the induction of ventricular tachycardia by programmed electrical stimulation in 6 of 9 dogs and slowed the rate of the tachycardia in 2 of the 3 remaining dogs.

D-sotalol is also effective in increasing the ventricular fibrillation threshold in experimental dogs with myocardial infarction. Again, the dose required to produce this beneficial effect appears to be quite high, although the data are conflicting and lower doses were not used in most studies. In one study that examined conscious dogs, four doses of 8 mg/kg of D-sotalol orally were administered over 24 hours. This dose prevented ventricular fibrillation secondary to ischemia produced distal to a previous myocardial infarction. The use of lower doses was not reported. In another study using conscious dogs subjected to distal myocardial ischemia and infarction, sotalol was administered at 2 mg/kg and at 8 mg/kg intravenously. Although the two groups were not reported separately, it appears that both doses prevented ventricular fibrillation and sudden death. In the group of dogs given sotalol, 13 of 20 dogs survived while only 1 of 15 dogs given a placebo lived.

Boxers with severe ventricular arrhythmias and syncope without severe myocardial failure often respond favorably to the administration of sotalol; syncopal episodes cease and a marked reduction in ventricular arrhythmias occurs. The dose ranges from 40 mg to 120 mg every 12 hours (approximately 1–4 mg/kg every 12 hours) orally. This dose is comparable to the human pediatric dose of 50 mg/m^2 of body surface area every 12 hours orally. The dose is generally titrated, starting at 40 mg every 12 hours. If that dose is ineffective the dose is increased to 80 mg in the morning and 40 mg in the evening, followed by 80 mg every 12 hours.

Sotalol may, in some circumstances, be used cautiously in dogs with moderate to severe myocardial failure; they should be monitored very carefully during the initial stages of sotalol administration. If this cannot be done, sotalol should not be used. In dogs with myocardial failure, the most common response to a relative overdose is weakness, presumably secondary to a low cardiac output. In patients in heart failure, exacerbation of edema can occur. In most cases, withdrawal of the drug should be the only action required if evidence of low cardiac output or exacerbation of the edema becomes apparent. If this does not suffice or if the clinical abnormalities are severe, the administration of a bipyridine compound, calcium, or glucagon may be beneficial. Administration of a catecholamine, such as dobutamine or dopamine, will not produce the desired response, because β receptors are blocked by sotalol.

Pharmacokinetics. In experimental dogs, sotalol is rapidly absorbed from the gastrointestinal tract and has a bioavailability in the 85–90% range. Less than 1% of the drug is metabolized. Elimination is via renal clearance and is linearly related to the glomerular filtration rate. Consequently, the drug dose must be reduced in patients with compromised renal function due to any cause. Sotalol is not protein-bound in plasma of dogs. The elimination half-life is 4.8 ± 1.0 hour. The apparent volume of distribution is in the 1.5–2.5 L/kg range.

Following oral administration of sotalol at 5 mg/kg every 12 hours for 3 days (when steady-state is reached in experimental dogs), the plasma concentration is in the 1.1–1.6 mg/l range. In humans given the same dose, the plasma concentration is in the 2–3 mg/l range. This discrepancy probably occurs because the elimination half-life in humans is longer (7–18 hours). This suggests that the dose in dogs should be roughly double that used in humans. The human dosage recommendation is to administer 40–80 mg every 12 hours as an initial dose. This dose then can be increased as necessary every 3–4 days. The maximum dose is 320 mg every 12 hours. Assuming an average weight of 70 kg for humans means the dose starts at approximately 0.5–1.0 mg/kg every 12 hours and can achieve a maximum dose of approximately 5 mg/kg every 12 hours.

A plasma concentration of 0.8 mg/l is needed to produce half-maximal β-adrenergic blockade in experimental dogs. This suggests that a dose of 5 mg/kg every 12 hours orally to a dog should result in near maximal blockade. The plasma concentration required to prolong cardiac refractoriness is higher. In humans, a plasma concentration of 2.6 mg/l is necessary to increase the QT interval. Doses between 2 and 5 mg/kg every 12 hours orally in humans prolong the QT interval by 40–100 ms. In experimental dogs, a dose of 5 mg/kg every 12 hours orally also prolongs the QT interval.

Adverse Effects. Adverse effects of sotalol in humans are related to its negative inotropic effects and to its ability to prolong the QT interval. As stated earlier, the negative inotropic effects appear to be minor and few human patients experience exacerbation of heart failure. The most dangerous adverse effect of sotalol in humans is aggravation of existing arrhythmias or provocation of new arrhythmias. Excessive QT-interval prolongation can provoke *torsades de pointes* in humans. *Torsades de pointes* has also been produced in experimental dogs. One canine model requires that the dog be bradycardic from experimentally induced third-degree AV block and hypokalemic (serum potassium concentration in the 2.5 mEq/l range) before sotalol can produce this serious arrhythmia. The arrhythmia in this model can be terminated with intravenous magnesium administration (1–2 mg/kg/min for 20–30 minutes). Sotalol apparently can also induce other forms of ventricular tachyarrhythmia because of the prolongation of the QT interval.

As for any other β-blocker, withdrawal of sotalol should be performed gradually over 1–2 weeks because of upregulation of β-receptors. Sudden cessation of use can produce fatal ventricular arrhythmias. The drug should not be used in patients with conduction system disease such as sick sinus syndrome, AV block, or bundle branch block.

BRETYLIUM. Bretylium tosylate (Bretylol) is a bromobenzyl quaternary ammonium compound originally introduced as an antihypertensive agent in humans. This drug is broadly classified as an adrenergic neuronal-blocking agent because it inhibits release of norepinephrine from adrenergic nerve endings (see Chapter 6). Although bretylium is no longer considered useful as an antihypertensive agent, subsequent studies have shown that it exerts direct antiarrhythmic actions in the heart. This characteristic is thought to reside with a relatively "pure" prolongation of action potential duration. Thus bretylium is designated a Class III agent (Table 23.1).

Bretylium lengthens the action potential duration as well as the refractory period in ventricular muscle cells and PF in a homogeneous manner; however, this characteristic effect is not manifested in the atria. Accordingly, bretylium is particularly effective in controlling ventricular arrhythmias, but supraventricular tachycardias are poorly responsive to the drug. Bretylium has received little clinical application in animals, but it has been approved for management of refractory and recurrent ventricular tachycardia or fibrillation in humans (Koch-Weser 1979; Singh et al. 1980).

Bretylium has been reported to bring about defibrillation in clinical episodes of ventricular fibrillation in humans and in experimental episodes in dogs (Koch-Weser 1979). Conflicting data have been presented, however, as Breznock et al. (1977) reported that bretylium (6–24 mg/kg) did not induce chemical defibrillation in dogs when administered by the IV or intracardiac route. Furthermore, bretylium did not seem to stabilize ventricular irritability or facilitate resuscitation by electrical defibrillation. Additional work is needed in both the clinic and laboratory before therapeutic applications of bretylium are identified in animals with spontaneous cardiac dysrhythmias.

Administration of bretylium to animals anesthetized with halogenated hydrocarbon anesthetics may be contraindicated, since a study demonstrated severe and long-lasting ventricular arrhythmias under such circumstances in cats (Condouris et al. 1979). These anesthetics are known to sensitize the heart to the arrhythmogenic activities of the catecholamines. Because bretylium initially causes a release of catecholamines from adrenergic nerves prior to neuronal blockade, the ventricular arrhythmias evoked by the drug may have been secondary to release of norepinephrine.

The pharmacokinetics of bretylium are not fully elucidated, but it is effective after parenteral (IM, IV) or oral administration. Absorption from the GI tract is somewhat poor and erratic; bretylium is not biotransformed to a significant extent and is excreted essentially unchanged in urine, accounting for its long elimination half-life (Hurley et al. 1960).

CLASS IV AGENTS

VERAPAMIL AND DILTIAZEM. Verapamil (Isoptin) is a systemic and coronary vasodilator that also exerts important antiarrhythmic action (Allert and Adams 1987). Verapamil has a unique cellular action in selectively inhibiting transmembrane influx of Ca^{++} (and perhaps Na^{+}) through the aforementioned slow cation channels of the cardiac sarcolemma. Since this action seems crucial to the antiarrhythmic effects of these drugs, verapamil and diltiazem

TABLE 23.2 Comparison of properties of fast Na^+ and slow Ca^{++} inward currents in cardiac muscle

Electrophysiologic Property	Fast Current (Fast Response)	Slow Current (Slow Response)
Activation-inactivation kinetics	Rapid	Slow
Dependent on extracellular concentration of:	Na^+	Ca^{++}
Blocked by:	Tetrodotoxin	Verapamil, D600
Threshold	−60 to −70 mV	−30 to −40 mV
Diastolic membrane potential	*−80 to −90 mV*	*−40 to −70 mV*
Conduction velocity	*0.5 to 3.0 m/sec*	*0.01 to 0.1 m/sec*
Overshoot	+20 to +35 mV	0 to +15 mV
V_{max}	*100 to 1000 V/sec*	*1 to 10 V/sec*
Safety factor for conduction	*High*	*Low*
Relationship to nodal tissues	Probably none	May mediate pacemaker potentials
Catecholamines	Little effect	Significant enhancement

Source: Singh et al. 1980.
Note: Particularly important differences are italicized.

are placed in a separate category (i.e., the calcium antagonists or Ca^{++} channel blockers of Class IV) (Table 23.1).

Arrhythmias caused by disturbances in either impulse formation (automaticity) or impulse conduction (reentry) are theoretically amenable to Ca^{++}-channel blockade by verapamil if their origin is associated with the emergence of slow response depolarizations (see Table 23.2). In addition, verapamil depresses SA and AV nodal discharge rates and conduction velocity, because slow Ca^{++}-dependent events are normal characteristics of automaticity in these tissues (Spedding 1985). Thus verapamil has application in certain types of atrial arrhythmias and in aborting supraventricular tachycardias that depend on continuous reentry of impulses utilizing the AV node as part of the reentrant pathway (Singh et al. 1980).

In veterinary medicine the clinical antiarrhythmic applications for Ca^+ channel blockade mainly involve use of verapamil and diltiazem for treatment of supraventricular tachyarrhythmias (Allert and Adams 1987; Kittleson et al. 1988). Verapamil is used in human medicine for short-term conversion of paroxysmal atrial tachycardia to sinus rhythm. Atrial fibrillation and flutter constitute other important indications. Verapamil and diltiazem usually do not convert these high-frequency atrial patterns to sinus rhythm but effectively reduce AV conduction and thereby lower the ventricular rate response. Primary ventricular arrhythmias generally are unresponsive to Ca^{++} channel blockade, unless they are secondary to myocardial ischemia. Nifedipine has little clinical antiarrhythmic utility because reflex cardiac stimulation evoked by this drug's systemic vasodilator effects usually nullifies any direct Ca^{++}-dependent antiarrhythmic properties.

Few clinical trials have examined the antiarrhythmic efficacy of Ca^{++} channel blockade in animals with cardiac disease. Verapamil was reported to be effective in converting paroxysmal or chronic atrial fibrillation to sinus rhythm in 3 of 7 dogs (Johnson 1985). Further, one of the 3 responding dogs developed ventricular tachycardia within 1 day after verapamil treatment was started. Verapamil was discontinued and replaced effectively by combination therapy with quinidine and propranolol. Clinical details were presented for only 2 dogs in the study, and apparently other cardioactive agents (e.g., digoxin, milrinone) were routinely administered along with verapamil. Thus it is difficult to determine whether improvement or lack of improvement in cardiac rhythmicity could be ascribed solely to verapamil.

In one study, verapamil was successful in terminating supraventricular tachycardia in 12 of 14 dogs when administered intravenously in 1 to 3 doses at the rate of 0.05 mg/kg (Kittleson et al. 1988). One nonresponding dog developed a transient hypotensive crisis after a total verapamil dose of 0.15 mg/kg. A second study involved 27 dogs with either atrial tachycardia (17 dogs) or atrial fibrillation with rapid ventricular rate responses (10 dogs) (Hamlin 1986). A qualification for subjects in that study was the absence of overt heart failure, as evidenced by lack of dyspnea and severe cardiomegaly. Verapamil was administered orally at a dose of 0.5 mg/kg every 6 hours, but greater doses were used for some dogs at the beginning of the study. Seven dogs retained their arrhythmia after verapamil, 5 dogs with atrial fibrillation had a reduction in ventricular rate of more than 50 beats/min, and 9 dogs with supraventricular tachycardia converted to sinus rhythm (Hamlin 1986).

Thus about 50% of the dogs with supraventricular tachyarrhythmia responded favorably to verapamil. Importantly, however, 6 dogs died within 2–3 hours after the initial dosing of verapamil. Five of these dogs were treated at the rate of 1.5–2.5 mg/kg. Because the deaths occurred so rapidly, they probably were attributable to verapamil rather than to natural progression of the disease. Cardiovascular depressant effects resulting from these relatively large doses of verapamil may have exacerbated underlying cardiac dysfunction, thus evoking acute decompensation of preexisting subclinical heart failure.

A combination of Wolff-Parkinson-White syndrome and atrial fibrillation may constitute a serious precaution or even a contraindication to verapamil treatment. Clinical reports in human medicine have indicated that when these conditions exist simultaneously, verapamil may paradoxically evoke an increase in ventricular rate and lead to fatal ventricular fibrillation (Jacobs et al. 1985). Perhaps episodes of ventricular tachycardia or mortality associated with verapamil therapy in dogs with atrial fibrillation (Johnson 1985; Hamlin 1986) might have involved occult Wolff-Parkinson-White or analogous syndromes.

Adverse circulatory side effects of Ca^{++} channel blockade include contractile depression of the heart, with reduced cardiac output and hypotension. This combination of effects can result in decompensation of preclinical or compensated heart failure, precipitation of pulmonary edema, and worsening of the primary ailment. Other potential side effects are sinus bradycardia and heart block attributable to direct depression of SA firing rate and AV conduction, respectively. The propensity for cardiovascular depression should be considered whenever Ca^{++} channel blocking drugs are used. This precaution is especially valid in patients with preexisting or suspected myocardial contractile failure (Allert and Adams 1987).

In summary, important clinical uses of antiarrhythmic drugs were discussed when appropriate in the preceding sections on individual drugs. Data shown in Table 23.3 provide a listing of drugs of choice for several common arrhythmias and also point out relevant contraindications of some of the older agents (Tilley 1979, 1985). Tables 23.4 and 23.5 provide schedules for approximating doses of several drugs in dogs and cats, respectively. The fact remains, however, that although several antiarrhythmic drugs routinely are advocated for control of spontaneous arrhythmias in animals, well-controlled clinical data on the subject generally are lacking. Dosage recommendations by different investigators often vary widely in the same species, necessitating careful judgment in the clinical setting.

The clinician should integrate basic knowledge about the pharmacologic control of arrhythmias into a rational

TABLE 23.3 Suggested antiarrhythmic drugs of choice in treating canine arrhythmias

	Supraventricular				Ventricular			Symptomatic Second- and Third-Degree AVBlock
Treatment	Sinus Bradycardia	Atrial Tachycardia	Atrial Flutter	Atrial Fibrillation	Ventricular Premature Complexes	Ventricular Tachycardia	Ventricular Fibrillation	
Drugs								
Atropine	+++	0	0	0	0	0	0	+++
Digoxin	0	+++	+++	+++	0	0	0	0
Isoproterenol	++	0	0	0	0	0	0	++
Lidocaine	0	0	0	0	+++	+++	0	0
Phenytoin	0	+	0	0	++	++	0	0
Procainamide	0	++	++	+	+++	+++	0	0
Propranolol	0	++	++	++	+	+	0	0
Quinidine	0	+	++	+	+++	++	0	0
Electrical methods								
Cardioversion	0	+	+++	++	0	+++	+++	0
Pacing	+	+	+	0	0	+	0	+++

Source: Tilley 1979, 1985.

Note: For each arrhythmia the drug or procedure of first choice (response excellent) is indicated by + + +; of second choice (response good) by + +; of third choice (response fair and rarely indicated) by +; and contraindicated by 0. Combination antiarrhythmic therapy is often based on this table, with first- and second-choice therapies used concurrently.

TABLE 23.4 Dose recommendations for drugs used to treat cardiac arrhythmias in dogs

Drug	Dose and route of administration	Indications
Atropine sulfate, 1/200 g tablets; 0.4 mg/ml injectable	Oral: 0.04 mg/kg every 6–8 hours SC, IM, IV: 0.04 mg/kg every 4–6 hours	Sinus bradycardia, AV block, SA arrest
Calcium chloride	IV, IC: 0.05–0.10 ml/kg of 10% solution	Ventricular asystole (to increase cardiac irritability), electrical-mechnical dissociation
Digoxin (Lanoxin), 0.125, 0.25, and 0.50 mg tablets; 0.05 mg/ml oral elixir; 0.25 mg/ml IV	Oral: 0.1–0.2 mg/kg in 4 divided doses over 48 hours or to effect (rapid method); 0.02 mg/kg average daily maintenance divided into 2 doses IV: 0.02–0.03 mg/kg in 4 divided doses over 4 hours or to effect	Congestive heart failure, APCs, atrial tachycardia, atrial fibrillation, atrial flutter, sick sinus syndrome (after pacemaker insertion)
Epinephrine hydrochloride* (Adrenalin), 1 : 1000 solution; 1 mg/ml injectable	IC: 6–10 μg/kg IV: 0.1–0.3 mg of 1 : 10,000 dilution	Ventricular asystole, changing fine ventricular fibrillation to coarse fibrillation
Isoproterenol (Proternol), 15 and 30 mg tablets; (Isuprel), 0.2 mg/ml injectable	Oral: 15–30 mg 4–6 times daily SC, IM: 0.1–0.2 mg every 4 hours IV:1 mg/500 ml 5% dextrose/water and titrate to effect	Sinus bradycardia, complete AV block, to initiate heartbeat
Lidocaine (2% without epinephrine) (Xylocaine), 20 and 40 mg/ml injectable	IV:2–4 mg/kg as bolus over 1–2 min, 0.5–2.0 mg/kg every 20–60 min (slow injection), 25–60 μg/kg/min with monitoring (constant infusion)	Ventricular tachycardia, ventricular premature complexes (especially multiform)
Phenytoin (diphenylhydantoin) (Dilantin), 30 and 100 mg capsules; 125 mg/5 ml syrup; 50 mg/ml injectable	Oral: 4–8 mg/kg divided 3–4 times daily IV: 4 mg/kg slowly once	Ventricular arrhythmias, digitalis-induced arrhythmias
Procainamide (Pronestyl), 250, 375, and 500 mg capsules or tablets; 100 mg/ml injectable	Oral: 125–500 mg every 6–8 hr (not to exceed 33 mg/kg day) IM: 8–16 mg/kg every 3–6 hr IV: 1–2 mg/kg/5 min to effect or toxicity (>50% widening of QRS), not to exceed 1 g	Ventricular premature complexes, ventricular tachycardia
Propranolol (Inderal), 10, 20, and 40 mg tablets; 1 mg/ml injectable	Oral: 2.5–40 mg 2–3 times daily unless desired effect at lower dose or toxicity IV: 0.05 to 0.15 mg/kg slowly to effect or toxicity	Sinus tachycardia, digitalis-induced atrial arrhythmias, supraventricular tachycardias and ventricular arrhythmias, preexcitation arrhythmias, and with digoxin for atrial fibrillation
Quinidine sulfate (short-acting form) 3 g tablets; quinidine sulfate (Quinidex Extentabs) (long-acting form), 300 mg tablets; quinidine gluconate injectable (IM), 80 mg/ml; quinidine gluconate (Quinaglute Duratabs) (long-acting form), 5 g tablets; quinidine polygalacturonate (Cardioquin) (long-acting form), 3 g tablets	Oral: 6–20 mg/kg every 6–8 hours (short-acting form), 8–12 hours (long-acting form) IM: 2.0–6.0 mg/kg every 6–8 hours	Ventricular premature complexes, ventricular tachycardia, maintenance therapy after electroconversion of atrial fibrillation and/or flutter, Wolff-Parkinson-White syndrome

Source: Tilley 1979, 1985. See text for other recommendations.

Note: IV = intravenous, IM = intramuscular, SC = subcutaneous, IC = intracardiac, AV = atrioventricular, SA = sinoatrial, APC = atrial premature contraction.

*Drugs for cardiac arrest.

TABLE 23.5 Dose recommendations for drugs used to treat cardiac arrhythmias in cats

Drug	Dose and Route of Administration	Indications
Atropine sulfate, 0.4 mg/ml injectable	SC, IM, IV: 0.04 mg/kg every 4–6 hours	Sinus bradycardia, AV block
Calcium chloride	IC, IV: 0.05–0.10 ml of 10% solution/kg	Ventricular asystole (to increase cardiac irritability), electrical-mechanical dissociation
Digoxin (Lanoxin), 0.125 mg tablets; 0.25 mg/ml IV	Oral: 0.008–0.01 mg/kg, average daily maintenance divided into 2 doses (e.g., 1/4 of a 0.125 mg tablet twice daily for 6 kg cat) IV: 0.02–0.03 mg/kg in 4 divided doses over 4 hours or to effect	Congestive heart failure, APC, atrial tachycardia, atrial fibrillation, atrial flutter
Epinephrine hydrochloride (Adrenalin), 1 : 1000 solution; 1 mg/ml injectable	IC: 6–10 μg/kg IV: 0.05–0.1 mg of 1 : 10,000 dilution	Ventricular asystole, changing fine ventricular fibrillation to coarse fibrillation
Isoproterenol (Isuprel), 0.2 mg/ml injectable	IV: 0.5 mg/250 ml 5% dextrose/water and titrate to effect	Sinus bradycardia, complete AV block
Propranolol (Inderal), 10 mg tablets; 1 mg/ml injectable	Oral: 2.5 mg every 8–12 hours for average 5 kg cat; higher doses to effect IV: 0.25 mg diluted in 1 ml of saline, given as 0.2 ml boluses to effect	Sinus tachycardia, supraventricular tachycardia and ventricular arrhythmias, preexcitation arrhythmias, and with digoxin for atrial fibrillation

clinical approach to managing cardiac dysfunction in patients. A precise classification of individual drugs is of less importance to the clinician than a basic understanding of their pharmacodynamic and therapeutic applications. Initial therapy should be directed at correcting specific etiologies; e.g., if serum electrolyte abnormalities are responsible, obviously these should be corrected before a potent antiarrhythmic drug is introduced into the animal. Arrhythmias secondary to congestive heart failure may respond to restitution of cardiac compensation, and initial treatment with a primary antiarrhythmic drug may worsen rather than lessen the severity of the arrhythmia. Use of physical maneuvers such as ocular pressure, massage of the carotid sinus region, or a blow to the chest should not be disregarded (Ettinger and Suter 1970; Hilwig 1976; Tilley 1979, 1985).

REFERENCES

Adams, H. R. 1975. Acute adverse effects of antibiotics. J Am Vet Med Assoc 166:983–87.

———. 1981. Cardiovascular emergencies: drug and resuscitative principles. Vet Clin North Am 11:77–102.

———. 1986. New perspectives in cardiology: pharmacodynamic classification of antiarrhythmic drugs. J Am Vet Med Assoc 189:525–32.

Allert, J. A., Adams, H. R. 1986. New perspectives in cardiovascular medicine: the calcium channel blocking drugs. J Am Vet Med Assoc 190:573–78.

Arsenault, W. G., Boothe, D. M., Gordon, S. G., Miller, M. W., Chalkley, J. R., Petrikovics, I. 2005. Pharmacokinetics of carvedilol after intravenous and oral administration in conscious healthy dogs. Am J Vet Res 66:2172–2176.

Binah, O., Rosen, M. R. 1984. The cellular mechanisms of cardiac antiarrhythmic drug action. Ann NY Acad Sci 432:31–44.

Bohn, F. K., Patterson, D. F., Pyle, R. L. 1971. Atrial fibrillation in dogs. Br Vet J 127:485–96.

Bonagura, J. D., Muir, W. W. 1985. In L. D. Tiley, ed., Essentials of Canine and Feline Electrocardiography, 2nd ed., p. 266. Philadelphia: Lea & Febiger.

Boyden, P. A., Wit, A. L. 1985. In L. D. Tiley, ed., Essentials of Canine and Feline Electrocardiography, 2nd ed., p. 266. Philadelphia: Lea & Febiger.

Breznock, E. M., Kagan, K., Hibser, N. K. 1977. Effects of bretylium tosylate on the in vivo fibrillating canine ventricle. Am J Vet Res 38:89–94.

Calvert, C. A., Chapman, W. L., Jr., Toal, R. L. 1982. Congestive cardiomyopathy in Doberman pinscher dogs. J Am Vet Med Assoc 181:598–602.

Chandler, J. C., Monnet, E., Staatz, A. J. 2006. Comparison of acute hemodynamic effects of lidocaine and procainamide for postoperative ventricular arrhythmias in dogs. J Am Anim Hosp Assoc 42:262–268.

Clark, D. R. 1977. Recognition and treatment of cardiac emergencies. J Am Med Assoc 171:98–106.

Clark, D. R., Knauer, K. 1980. Personal communication.

Condouris, G. A., Ortiz, J., Lyness, W. 1979. Cardiac arrhythmias produced by bretylium in cats anesthetized with halothane. Eur J Pharmacol 55:93–97.

Cranefield, P. F. 1973. Ventricular fibrillation. N Engl J Med 289:732–36.

———. 1975. The Conduction of the Cardiac Impulse, p. 1. Mt. Kisco, N.Y.: Futura.

Damato, A. N. 1969. Diphenylhydantoin: pharmacological and clinical use. Prog Cardiovasc Dis 12:1–15.

Detweiler, D. K. 1957. Electrocardiographic and clinical features of spontaneous auricular fibrillation and flutter (tachycardia) in dogs. Zntralbl Veterinaermed 4:509–56.

———. 1977. In L. M. Jones, N. H. Booth, and L. E. McDonald, eds., Veterinary Pharmacology and Therapeutics, 4th ed., p. 496. Ames: Iowa State Univ. Press.

Detweiler, D. K., Patterson, D. F. 1963. In J. F. Bone, ed., Equine Medicine and Surgery. Wheaton, Ill.: American Veterinary Publications.

Ettinger, S. J., Suter, P. F. 1970. Canine Cardiology, p. 237. Philadelphia: W. B. Saunders.

Gordon, S. G., Arsenault, W. G., Longnecker, M., Boothe, D. M., Miller, M. W., Chalkley, J. 2006. Pharmacodynamics of carvedilol in conscious, healthy dogs. J Vet Intern Med 20:297–304.

Hamlin, R. L. 1977. New ideas in the management of heart failure in dogs. J Am Vet Med Assoc 171:114–18.

———. 1986. Clinical and experimental studies with verapamil in the dog. In Proc 5th Symp Am Acad Vet Pharm Therap, pp. 89–96.

Hayes, A. H., Jr. 1972. The actions and clinical use of the newer antiarrhythmic drugs. Ration Drug Ther 6:1–6.

Helfant, R. H., Scherlag, B. J., Damato, A. N. 1967. Protection from digitalis toxicity with the prophylactic use of diphenylhydantoin sodium: an arrhythmic-inotropic dissociation. Circulation 36: 119–24.

Hilwig, R. W. 1976. Cardiac arrhythmias in the dog: detection and treatment. J Am Vet Med Assoc 169:789–98.

Hoffman, B. F., Cranefield, P. F. 1960. Electrophysiology of the Heart. New York: McGraw-Hill.

Huisman, G. H., Teunissen, G. H. B. 1963. Paroxysmal ventricular tachycardia in the dog. Zentralbl Veterinaermed 10:273–85.

Hurley, R. E., Page, I. H., Dustan, H. R. 1960. Bretylium tosylate as an antihypertensive drug. J Am Med Assoc 172:2081–83.

Jacobs, A. S., Nielsen, D. H., Gianelly, R. E. 1985. Fatal ventricular fibrillation following verapamil in Wolff-Parkinson-White syndrome with atrial fibrillation. Ann Emerg Med 14:159–60.

Johnson, J. T. 1985. Conversion of atrial fibrillation in two dogs using verapamil and supportive therapy. J Am Anim Hosp Assoc 21:429–34.

Keefe, D. L., Kates, R. E., Harrison, D. C. 1981. New antiarrhythmic drugs: their place in therapy. Drugs 22:363–400.

Kittleson, M. D., Hamlin, R. L. 1981. Hydralazine therapy for severe mitral regurgitation in a dog. J Am Vet Med Assoc 179:903–5.

Kittleson, M. D., Keene, B. W., Pion, P. 1988. Verapamil administration for acute termination of supraventricular tachycardia in dogs. J Am Vet Med Assoc 193:1525–30.

Koch-Weser, J. 1979. Drug therapy: bretylium. N Engl J Med 300:473–77.

Leahey, E. B., Jr., Reiffel, J. A., Drusin, R. E., et al. 1978. Interaction between quinidine and digoxin. J Am Med Assoc 240:533–34.

Malone, E., Ensink, J., Turner, T., Wilson, J., Andrews, F., Keegan, K., Lumsden, J. 2006. Intravenous continuous infusion of lidocaine for treatment of equine ileus. Veterinary Surgery 35:60–66.

Mason, D. T., Demaria, A. N., Amsterdam, E. A., et al. 1973. Antiarrhythmic agents. I. Mechanisms of action and clinical pharmacology. Drugs 5:261–91.

Meurs, K. M., Spier, A. W., Wright, N. A., et al. 2002. Comparison of the effects of four antiarrhythmic treatments for familial ventricular arrhythmias in Boxers. J Am Vet Med Assoc 221:522–527.

Moss, A. J., Patton, R. D. 1973. Antiarrhythmic Agents. Springfield, Ill.: Charles C. Thomas.

Muir, W. W., Bonagura, J. D. 1982. Aprindine for treatment of ventricular arrhythmias in the dog. Am J Vet Res 43:1815–19.

Muir, W. W., McGuirrk, S. M. 1984. J Am Vet Med Assoc 184(8):965–970.

Neff, C. A., Davis, L. E., Baggot, J. D. 1972. A comparative study of the pharmacokinetics of quinidine. Am J Vet Res 33:1521–25.

Novotny, M. J., Adams, H. R. 1986. New perspectives in cardiology: recent advances in antiarrhythmic drug therapy. J Am Vet Med Assoc 189:533–39.

Oyama, M. A. and Prosek, R. 2006. Acute conversion of atrial fibrillation in two dogs by intravenous amiodarone administration. J Vet Intern Med 20:1224–1227.

Papich, M. G., Neff-Davis, C. A., Davis, L. E. 1986a. Procainamide in the dog: antiarrhythmic plasma concentrations after intravenous administration. J Vet Pharmacol Therap 9:359–369.

Papich, M. G., Neff-Davis, C. A., Davis, L. E., McKiernan, B. C., Brown, S. 1986b. Pharmacokinetics of procainamide in dogs. Am J Vet Res 47:2351–2358.

Parker, J. L., Adams, H. R. 1977. Drugs and the heart muscle. J Am Vet Med Assoc 171:78–84.

Pyle, R. L. 1967. Conversion of atrial fibrillation with quinidine sulfate in a dog. J Am Vet Med Assoc 151:582–89.

Reef, V. B., Reimer, J. M., and Spencer, P. A. 1995. Treatment of atrial fibrillation in horses: new perspectives. J Vet Intern Med 9(2):57–67.

Roye, D. B., Serrano, E. E., Hammer, R. H., et al. 1973. Plasma kinetics of dephenylhydantoin in dogs and cats. Am J Vet Res 34:947–50.

Sanders, J. E., Yeary, R. A. 1978. Serum concentrations of orally administered diphenylhydantoin in dogs. J Am Vet Med Assoc 172:153–56.

Sanders, J. E., Yeary, R. A., Fenner, W. R., et al. 1979. Interaction of phenytoin with chloramphenicol or pentobarbital in the dog. J Am Vet Med Assoc 175:177–80.

Saunders, A. B., Miller, M. W., Gordon, S. G., et al. 2006. Oral amiodarone therapy in dogs with atrial fibrillation. J Vet Intern Med 20:921–926.

Scherlag, B. J., Helfant, R. H., Ricciutti, M. A., et al. 1968. Dissociation of the effects of digitalis on myocardial potassium flux and contractility. Am J Physiol 215:1288–91.

Schmitt, F. O., Erlanger, J. 1929. Directional differences in conduction of impulse through heart muscle and their possible relation to extrasystolic and fibrillary contractions. Am J Physiol 87:326–47.

Shanks, R. G., Dunlop, D. 1967. Effect of propranolol on arrhythmias following coronary artery occlusion. Cardiovasc Res 1:34–41.

Singh, B. N., Collett, J. T., Chew, C. Y. 1980. New perspectives in the pharmacologic therapy of cardiac arrhythmias. Prog Cardiovasc Dis 22:243–301.

Singh, B. N., Jewitt, D. E. 1974. Beta-adrenergic receptor blocking drugs in cardiac arrhythmias. Drugs 7:426–61.

Spedding, M. 1985. Calcium antagonist subgroups. Trends Pharmacol Sci 6:109–14.

Tilley, L. P., ed. 1979. Essentials of Canine and Feline Electrocardiography. St. Louis: C. V. Mosby.

———. 1985. Essentials of Canine and Feline Electrocardiography, 2nd ed. Philadelphia: Lea & Febiger.

Trautwein, W. 1963. Generation and conduction of impulses in the heart as affected by drugs. Pharmacol Rev 15:277–332.

Vaughn Williams, E. M. 1984. A classification of antiarrhythmic actions reassessed after a decade of new drugs. J Clin Pharmacol 24:129–47.

Weidler, D. J., Jallad, N. S., Garg, D. C., et al. 1979. Pharmacokinetics of propranolol in the cat and comparisons with humans and three other species. Res Commun Chem Pathol Pharmacol 26:105–14.

Wilcke, J. R., Davis L. E., Neff-Davis, C. A. 1983a. Determination of lidocaine concentrations producing therapeutic and toxic effects in dogs. J Vet Pharmacol Therap 6:105–112.

Wilcke, J. R., Davis, L. E., Neff-Davis, C. A., Koritz, G. D. 1983b. Pharmacokinetics of lidocaine and its active metabolites in dogs. J Vet Pharmacol Therap 6:49–58.

Wit, A. L., Hoffman, B. F., Cranefield, P. F. 1972. Slow conduction and reentry in the ventricular conducting system. I. Return of extrasystole in canine Purkinje fibers. Circ Res 30:1–10.

Wit, A. L., Rosen, M. R., Hoffman, B. F. 1974. Electrophysiology and pharmacology of cardiac arrhythmias. II. Relationship of normal and abnormal electrical activity of cardiac fibers to the genesis of arrhythmias B. Re-entry. Section I. Am Heart J 88:664–70.

Young, L., van Loon, G. 2005. Atrial fibrillation in horses: new treatment choices for the new millennium? J Vet Intern Med 19:631–632.

SECTION 6

Drugs Affecting Renal Function and Fluid-Electrolyte Balance

CHAPTER

24

PRINCIPLES OF ACID-BASE BALANCE: FLUID AND ELECTROLYTE THERAPY

DEBORAH T. KOCHEVAR AND MAYA M. SCOTT

COMPOSITION AND DISTRIBUTION OF BODY FLUIDS

UNITS OF MEASURE. The units of measure commonly utilized in discussion of fluid balance are presented in Table 24.1. Ions or electrolytes combine according to valence (charge) rather than molecular weight. Hence in the case of univalent ions, 1 mM = 1 mEq. One mM of a divalent ion provides 2 mEq. By expressing most electrolyte concentrations in milliequivalents per liter (mEq/l), and comparing the concentration of cations to anions in the body, it becomes clear that electroneutrality exists. Although extracellular cations are often more completely documented in the course of clinical investigations, anions, particularly chloride and bicarbonate, are the electrical counterbalance. Some electrolytes are measured in millimoles per liter (mM/l) because they exist in variable states of protein binding or valence. An example is total calcium, because protein binding confounds any simple assessment of ionized fraction. Phosphorus exists in variable

TABLE 24.1 Units of measure and conversions commonly used in fluid therapy

Term	Abbreviation	Description and Conversion
Molecular (formula) weight	MW	Sum of atomic weights of all elements in a chemical formula
Millimole	mmol (mM)	Molecular (formula) weight of a substance in mg, equals 1 mM
Milliequivalent	mEq	Weight, in mg, of an element that combines or replaces 1 mg (1 mmol) of hydrogen (H^+)
Milliosmole	mOsm	Always contains 6.0×10^{23} molecules and equals 1 mmol of a nondissociable substance
Milliequivalent per liter	mEq/l	= mmol/l × valence = [(mg/dl × 10)/MW] × valence

proportions of phosphate and monohydrogen and dihydrogen phosphate, so no valence can be assigned and calculation of milliequivalence is therefore inaccurate. Since mEq/l are the most common and informative unit of comparison for most electrolytes, conversion formulas are also provided in Table 24.1.

Solutes exert an osmotic effect in solution that is dependent only on the number of particles in solution, not on molecular weight or valence. Hence for nondissociable substances, 1 osmole contains 1 mole of substance. If a substance dissociates in solution, the number of osmoles is increased according to the number of particles generated per mole of dissociated substance. For example, each mmol of a completely dissociated NaCl solution yields 2 mOsm. Osmolarity refers to the number of osmoles per liter, and osmolality indicates the number of osmoles per kilogram of solvent (Rose 1989). In physiological systems the difference between these two is usually small. The concept of osmolality explains why solutions of diverse chemical and electrical composition (e.g., 5% dextrose, 0.9% NaCl, and 1.3% sodium bicarbonate) can all be considered isotonic. For mammals, isotonic solutions equal approximately 300 mOsm.

BODY FLUID COMPARTMENTS. Semipermeable membranes separate most body compartments, allowing the free passage of water and selected solutes. The effective osmolality, or tonicity, of a solution is related to the ability of a solute to attract water and to sustain an increase in osmotic pressure as a result of water movement. For example, two substances with equal ability to attract water down a concentration gradient and across a semipermeable membrane may have very different effects on osmotic pressure, depending upon the movement of the substance itself through the semipermeable membrane. While the measured osmolality of a solution includes all osmoles, whether effective or ineffective, tonicity of a solution relates only to effective osmolality. For example, a solution containing 300 mOsm of nonpenetrating NaCl and 100 mOsm of urea, which can cross plasma membranes, would have a total osmolarity of 400 mOsm and would be hyperosmotic. However, if one put red blood cells in this solution, they would not shrink or swell, because the urea would diffuse into the cells and reach equilibrium inside and outside the cells. Thus, both extracellular and intracellular solutions would have the same osmolarity. There would be no difference in the water concentration across the membrane and no change in cell volume. The solution is therefore considered isotonic.

Ultimately all fluids within the body are in dynamic equilibrium, but it is helpful during fluid therapy to consider body water as existing in several compartments since critical fluid shifts can and do occur. Determination of the volumes of these compartments is problematic, as can be deduced from the large number of different methods that have been used to estimate these volumes (Kohn and DiBartola 1992). The most common method for assessment of volume in body fluid compartments depends upon intravenous administration of a known amount of a dye or radioisotope-tagged substance that distributes only in the compartment of interest. This is followed by assessment of dye or radioisotope concentration in the compartment. Ideally, the indicator substance must distribute rapidly and homogeneously, remain in the space to be measured, not be metabolized or bound, and be nontoxic. The volume of distribution (Vd) of a drug, or in this case a volume marker, may be derived according to the same principles of pharmacokinetics described elsewhere in this text.

Total body water (TBW) is approximated at 60% of body weight, but this figure varies from 50 to 75% depending upon age, lean body mass, and individual animal variations. Since fat is lower in water content than lean tissue, obesity is associated with decreased TBW (approximately 50%). To avoid overhydration of obese patients, fluid

TABLE 24.2 Approximate volumes of selected fluid compartments in the dog

Compartment	% Body Weight (BW)	Method
Total body water (TBW)	60	Indicator substance
ECF	20–27	Indicator substance
Red blood cells (RBC)	3	Counted + calculations
Plasma volume (PV)	5	Indicator substance
Total blood volume (BV)	5.7–10	Calculated: RBC volume + PV
Interstitial lymph fluid	15	Calculated: ECF – BV
Transcellular fluid	1–6	Estimated
Bone and dense connective tissue	5	Estimated
ICF	33–40	TBW – ECF

Source: Estimated from data collected in multiple studies as detailed in Kohn and DiBartola 1992, 5–7.

TABLE 24.3 Approximate values for blood volumes of various animals expressed as percentages of body weight

Species	Total Blood Volume	Plasma Volume	RBC Volume
Dogs	8.5	4.5	4.0
Cats	6.7	4.7	2.0
Chickens	6.5	4.5	2.0
Cattle	5.7	3.8	1.9
Goats	7.0	5.4	1.6
Horses			
Draft	7.0	4.0	3.0
Thoroughbred	10.0	6.0	4.0
Saddle	7.7	5.2	2.5
Pigs	7.5	4.8	2.7
Sheep	6.5	4.5	2.0

Source: Smith 1970. Values represent averages from approximately 30 references.

requirements are best estimated based on lean body mass. Very young animals are about 70–75% water, with TBW declining with advancing age. Table 24.2 provides estimates of selected volumes in dogs. TBW is broadly divided into two types: intracellular (ICF) and extracellular fluid (ECF). The ECF is further divided into four subcompartments: plasma volume, interstitial lymph fluid, transcellular fluid, and fluid present in dense connective tissue and bone. Table 24.3 provides experimentally derived blood volumes as percentages of body weight for various species.

Transcellular fluid is found in diverse locations, including cerebrospinal fluid, pleural cavity, gastrointestinal tract, bladder, synovia, aqueous humor, and peritoneal cavity. Transcellular volumes vary greatly from monogastrics (1–6%) to horses and ruminants (10–15%), dependent largely upon the amount of fluid sequestered in the gastrointestinal tract. Transcellular volumes are not readily mobilized during volume deficits but are of importance in terms of drug disposition and equilibrium. In certain disease processes, transcellular fluids may accumulate, causing ascites, hydropericardium, hydrothorax, synovitis, or other conditions, depending on the location of fluid accumulation.

FLUID AND ELECTROLYTE DISTRIBUTION. Body solutes are not distributed homogeneously throughout TBW. Like drugs, every solute has a defined space or volume of distribution that can be assessed experimentally. As with estimation of body compartment volumes, determination of solute distribution is limited by the features of the labeled solute used. Because normal vascular endothelium is largely impermeable to formed blood elements and plasma protein, these cells and solutes are usually limited to the plasma. Vascular endothelium is freely permeable to ionic solutes, and the concentration of these ions is almost the same in interstitial as in plasma fluid. Table 24.4 provides estimations of ion composition in plasma of normal mammals.

The volume of ICF and ECF compartments is determined by the number of osmotically active particles in each space. ECF osmolality can be estimated from the following formula (Rose 1989):

$$\text{ECF osmolality (mOsm/kg)} = 2([\text{Na}^+]+[\text{K}^+]) + \text{glucose}/18 + \text{blood urea nitrogen (BUN)}/2.8$$

Because cell membranes are permeable to urea and K^+, these substances contribute only ineffective osmoles, as

TABLE 24.4 Approximate average concentrations of cations and anions in plasma in normal mammals

Cations	mEq/l	Anions	mEq/l
Sodium	135–160	Chloride	110–125
Potassium	3–5	Bicarbonate	18–22
Calcium (total calcium 5–10 mM/l)	4–6	Phosphate	1–3*
Magnesium	1–3	Sulfate	1–2
Trace elements	1	Lactate	1–2
		Other organic acids	3–5
		Protein	10–16
Total	144–175		144–175

Source: Gross 1994.

*Phosphate exists in variable proportions of phosphate and monohydrogen and dihydrogen phosphate, so no valance can be identified and the number of mEq/l is therefore an estimate (Gross 1994).

described earlier. At normal blood glucose concentrations, Na^+ is the primary determinant of effective ECF osmolality. Because Na^+ is the most abundant and osmotically active ECF cation, maintenance of an extracellular-to-intracellular sodium gradient is critical and is accomplished by the cell membrane Na^+,K^+-adenosine triphosphatase (ATPase) pump. This pump is also responsible for maintaining appropriate concentrations of intracellular K^+. Because K^+ is the most abundant intracellular cation, the ratio of intracellular-to-extracellular K^+ concentration is the major determinant of the resting cell membrane potential (−70 to −90 mV). Because all body fluid spaces are isotonic with one another, the effective osmolality of the ICF, and indeed TBW, must be equal to that of the ECF. Acute addition or loss of fluid and/or solutes from the body inevitably results in alterations in compartment volumes and tonicity. Homeostatic shifts of fluid between compartments must then occur to return the system to isotonicity.

The critical distribution of water between the plasma and the interstitium is maintained by the colloidal osmotic pressure of plasma protein (oncotic pressure). This is the force that draws water into the capillaries and balances the hydrostatic pressure driving water out. These so-called "Starling forces" describe the capillary balance between forces that favor filtration of water from plasma and those that retain vascular volume:

$$\text{Net filtration (NF)} = K_f[(P_{cap} - P_{if}) - (\pi_p - \pi_{if})]$$

where K_f represents permeability of the capillary wall, P represents hydrostatic pressure in the capillaries (P_{cap}) (blood) or tissues (P_{if}) (interstitial fluid), and π represents oncotic pressure generated by plasma protein (π_p) or filtered proteins and glycosaminoglycans in the interstitium (π_{if}). Applying Starling's relationships yields the prediction that hypoproteinemia (decreased π_p) will increase loss of vascular fluid and that water depletion (with a relative increase in π_p and a decrease in P_{cap}) will promote reabsorption of interstitial fluid into the vasculature (Kohn and DiBartola 1992). The volume of intracellular water in a given tissue is maintained by intracellular protein. As plasma water decreases, plasma protein competes with intracellular protein for water, resulting in cellular dehydration. Clinical alterations in plasma osmolality may be assessed by comparing measured osmolality in a patient to calculated serum osmolality as determined using Na^+, K^+, glucose, and BUN measurements (see the ECF osmolality equation provided above). Observed changes in the osmolal gap (difference between measured osmolality and the osmolality calculated from normal concentrations) may be useful in determining the presence of unmeasured osmoles associated with toxic substances such as ethylene glycol. The osmolal gap may also be useful in assessing shifts in plasma sodium concentration (Kohn and DiBartola 1992).

The number of cations in the ECF must equal the number of anions in order to maintain electroneutrality. In practice, only selected cations and anions are routinely measured in a clinical setting. Calculation of the difference between the commonly measured cations and anions in ECF yields the unmeasured anions, or anion gap (Oh and Carrol 1977; Emmett and Narins 1977). The anion gap calculation can be useful in assessing the etiology of metabolic acidosis and will be discussed in this context subsequently.

WATER, SODIUM, AND CHLORIDE

HOMEOSTASIS. Daily intake of water, nutrients, and minerals is normally balanced by daily excretion of these substances. Water turnover is the term used to describe input and output of body water over a given period of time. Values for water turnover, per 24 hours, in various domestic animals resting in cages or stalls range from about 40 to 132 ml/kg/day. The range is influenced by species, age, and physiologic state (Adolph 1939; Smith 1970). Extremes of temperature, psychologic state, disease, and other variables may change water demands markedly. Water turnover in mature dogs is approximated as 40–

60 ml/kg/day, while immature and lactating animals may turn over approximately twice this amount (Muir and DiBartola 1983). Maintenance fluid needs are defined as the volume of fluid required daily to maintain an animal in zero fluid balance, that is, no net gain or loss of water.

Normal water intake occurs in response to thirst, which is stimulated by plasma hypertonicity and/or contracted ECF volume. Plasma hypertonicity, the primary stimulus, prompts osmoreceptors in the supraoptic and paraventricular nuclei of the hypothalamus to release vasopressin, also called antidiuretic hormone (ADH), which is released into the circulation at the level of the pituitary neurohypophysis. Binding of vasopressin to receptors in the distal nephron and renal collecting duct cells activates adenylyl cyclase and increases intracellular cyclic AMP. A protein kinase cascade initiated by activation of protein kinase A results in opening of luminal water pores in the tubule cell. Permeability of the collecting duct to water and reabsorption of water increase. Sustained release of vasopressin depends additionally upon calcium cycling across the plasma membrane and activation of protein kinase C–dependent pathways. Prostaglandins inhibit the renal response to vasopressin. Drugs with anticyclooxygenase activity that inhibit prostaglandin synthesis thereby enhance the action of endogenous vasopressin. Figure 24.1 summarizes the effects of selected drugs and electrolytes on vasopressin release and action.

If ECF volume and renal perfusion decrease, volume receptors in the renal juxtaglomerular apparatus respond, causing the secretion (or release) of renin, which converts angiotensinogen to angiotensin I. This is the rate-limiting step in the renin-angiotensin system. Angiotensin I is activated to the potent vasoconstrictor angiotensin II in the lung and in endothelial cells throughout the body by angiotensin-converting enzyme (ACE). Angiotensin II stimulates the zona glomerulosa of the adrenal cortex to secrete aldosterone, which, in turn, causes increased reabsorption of sodium from the distal nephron with excretion of K^+ and H^+. Due to the increased concentration of sodium, plasma becomes hypertonic, causing vasopressin release and water retention.

Water intake occurs in response not only to thirst but also to hunger. Water content of food may be as low as 10% (dry food) or as high as 90% (succulent green pasture). Canned pet foods generally contain more than 70% water, and semimoist foods are intermediate (20–40% water) (Lewis and Morris 1987). Intake of dietary water is governed centrally by appetite control mechanisms rather than by fluid and electrolyte homeostasis. In addition to water intake related to eating and drinking, metabolic water is produced endogenously by catabolism of proteins, fats, and carbohydrates (approximately 5 ml/kg/day) and represents about 10–15% of total water intake in dogs and cats (Anderson 1983).

Normal water loss occurs via urine, fecal water, and saliva (sensible loss), with insensible losses occurring via evaporation from cutaneous and respiratory epithelia. Insensible losses account for TBW elimination of about 15–30 ml/kg/day in healthy, sedentary animals in a thermoneutral environment (Kohn and DiBartola 1992).

Metabolic rate, and therefore a portion of daily water turnover, are directly proportional to the ratio of body surface area to total volume. For example, the surface area to volume ratio in a puppy is much larger than in an adult dog and the puppy has a higher basal metabolic rate. Both lead to a much greater evaporative loss of water from the skin per unit volume. Hence, daily water turnover per unit body weight may be nearly twice that of the adult animal. Small, immature animals are therefore at greater risk for insensible water loss than large, mature animals.

The most important and predictable loss of water in healthy, sedentary animals, in a thermoneutral environment, occurs via the urine. Urinary losses can vary from 2 to 20 ml/kg/day. Daily urinary water losses may be divided into obligatory water loss and free water loss (Kohn and DiBartola 1992). Obligatory water loss represents water eliminated in order to excrete the daily renal solute load. The renal solute load is derived from dietary sources of protein and minerals and consists of urea, Na^+, K^+, Ca^{++}, Mg^{++}, NH_4^+, and other cations, and PO_4^{3-}, Cl^-, SO_4^{2-}, and other anions. Hence, daily renal solute load is a function of the quantity and composition of food ingested. Urea accounts for two-thirds of the urinary solute load in dogs (O'Connor and Potts 1969).

In normal animals increased urine solute load is eliminated by an increase in urine volume (obligatory water loss) rather than a marked increase in urine osmolality. Hence, urine osmolality is not generally maximized in order to accomplish steady-state elimination of solutes. Obligatory renal water loss is clinically important for removal of renal solutes but also because this type of water loss will continue even in states of relative water deficit. Free water loss represents water excreted unaccompanied by solute. Excretion of free water is controlled by

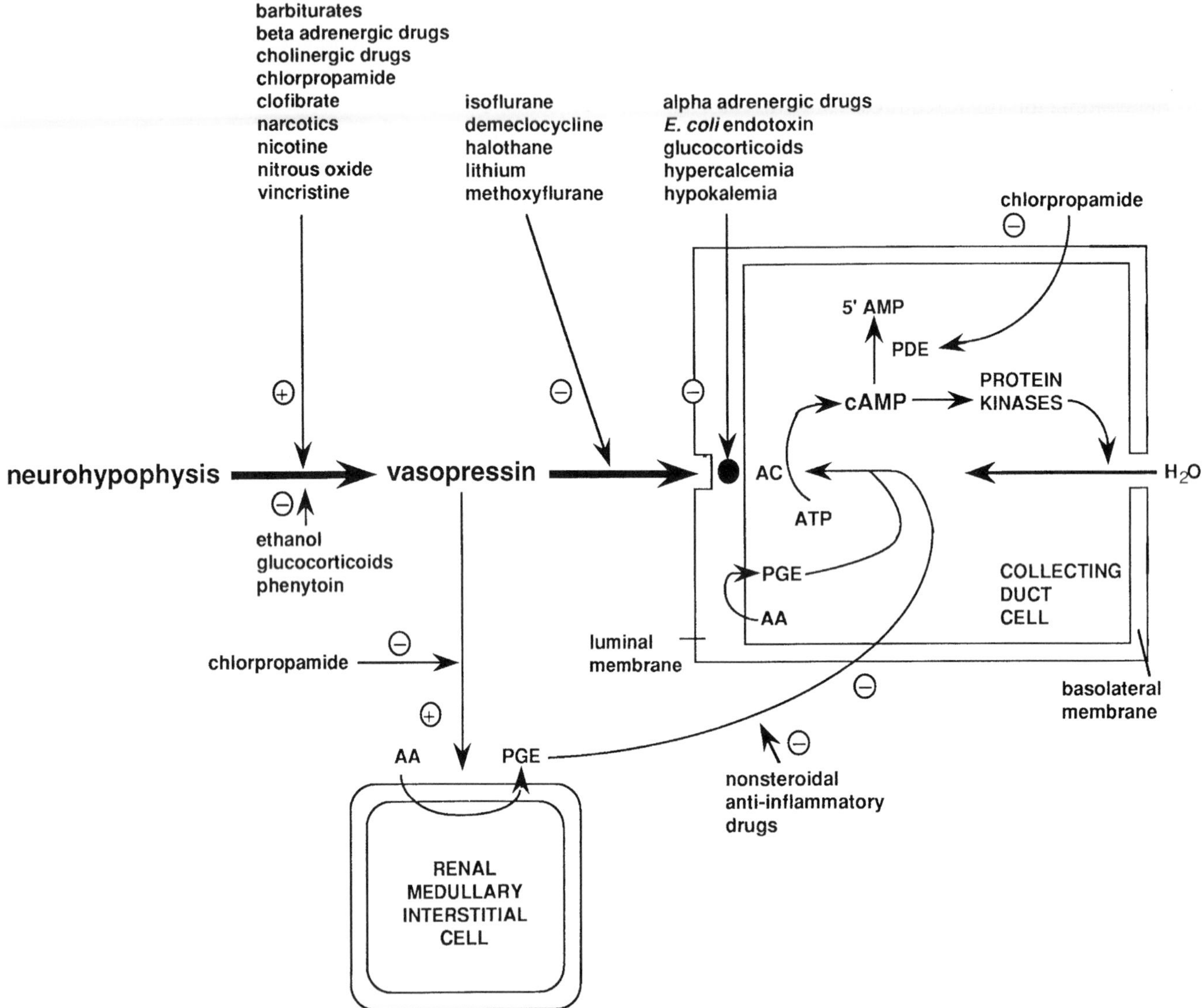

FIG. 24.1 Effects of drugs and electrolytes on vasopressin release and mechanisms of cellular action. AA = arachidonic acid; AC = adenylyl cyclase; ATP = adenosine triphosphate; cAMP = cyclic adenosine monophosphate; PDE = phosphodiesterase; PGE = prostaglandin E. (Adapted from DiBartola 1992c, Fig. 3-3.)

vasopressin and increases during relative water excess or hypotonicity and decreases during water deficit or hypertonicity. Obligatory fecal water loss occurs in order to excrete fecal solutes. Fecal losses ordinarily account for 2–5% of TBW losses and vary with the species. Feces typically contain 50–80% water (Kohn and DiBartola 1992).

RENAL REGULATION OF SODIUM, CHLORIDE, AND WATER EXCRETION. Elimination or conservation of body water and solutes via the kidneys depends upon the processes of glomerular filtration and renal tubular reabsorption and secretion. A major mechanism for conservation of water is urine concentration. The canine kidney can concentrate urine to as much as 2400 mOsm, compared to 1200–1400 mOsm achieved in human urine. Elimination of substances via the urine depends upon renal clearance of each substance from the plasma. The volume of plasma that must be filtered each minute to account for the amount of substance appearing in the urine each minute under steady-state conditions defines renal clearance of that substance.

As much as 20% of cardiac output is directed to the kidneys, with blood entering a renal glomerulus through an afferent arteriole and leaving through an efferent arteriole. Resistance changes in afferent and efferent capillaries regulate glomerular filtration rate (GFR). For discussions of normal and abnormal renal physiologic function the reader is referred to any standard physiology text. An understanding of the complexities of renal function is crucial to the understanding of water, acid-base, and electrolyte balances.

As glomerular filtrate flows through the tubules, most of the water (greater than 90%) and varying amounts of solute are reabsorbed into the peritubular capillaries. The composition of the tubular reabsorbate closely approximates that of ECF. Reabsorption is largely achieved by transport of electrolytes and other solutes in two steps: 1) absorption of solutes from tubular fluid into tubular cells and 2) movement of solutes from tubular cells into the ECF. Several types of transport account for tubular reabsorption of solutes, including passive transport (simple diffusion), facilitated diffusion, active transport, and cotransport. These mechanisms are discussed in more detail in the context of diuretic drugs (Chapter 25) and are summarized in Figure 24.2, which depicts some of the functional processes for regulation of salt and water transport in different segments of the nephron.

As much as 60–65% of filtered solute is reabsorbed in the proximal tubule accompanied by osmotically proportional amounts of water. The tubular fluid at the distal portion of the proximal tubule becomes slightly hypo-osmotic. Passive reabsorption of substances, especially sodium and chloride, continues in the thin segment of the

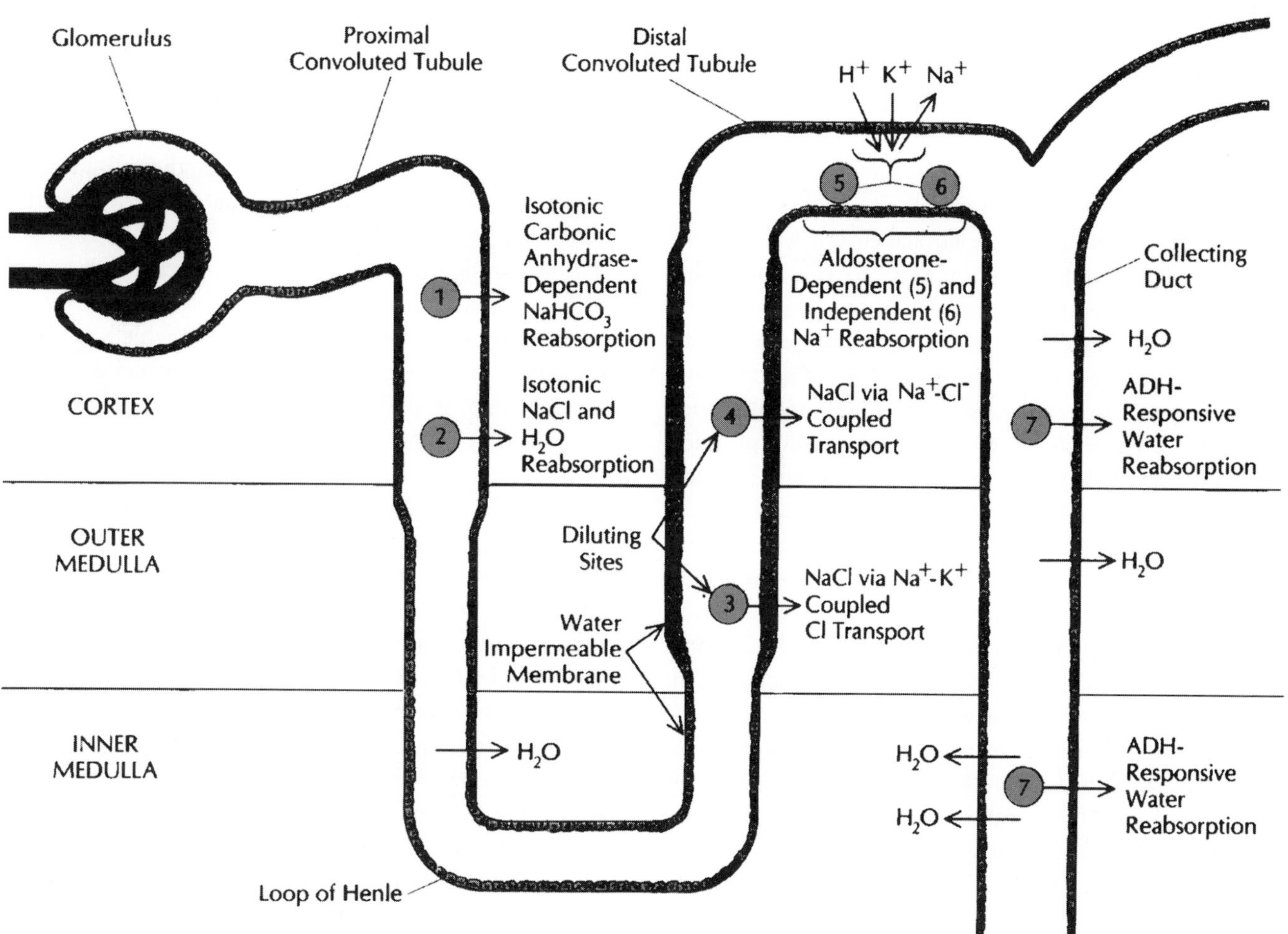

FIG. 24.2 Functional processes for regulation of salt and water transport in a nephron. (Reprinted from Thier 1987, 83, Fig. 1.)

loop of Henle. The thick ascending limb of the loop of Henle and the distal convoluted tubule are relatively impermeable to water but actively reabsorb solute. Sodium and chloride enter tubular cells in the thick ascending limb of Henle's loop by crossing the luminal membrane coupled to potassium in a proportion of 1 Na^+:1 K^+:2 Cl^-. Sodium is then actively extruded across the basolateral membrane to maintain intracellular sodium at low levels. Potassium and chloride leave the tubular cell passively. Two consequences of this are decreased concentration of sodium and chloride in the tubular lumen and increased concentration of each in interstitial fluid. A concentration gradient across the tubular epithelium is established, and this becomes multiplied in a longitudinal direction by the countercurrent mechanism. The collecting ducts are responsive to vasopressin, and in its presence the ducts become highly permeable to water. Tubular fluid equilibrates with hyperosmotic interstitium, and hypertonic (concentrated) urine results. In the absence of vasopressin, the ducts are relatively impermeable to water. In this case, sodium and chloride have been reabsorbed proximally to the collecting ducts, tubular fluid is hypoosmotic, and voided urine is dilute (Thier 1987).

Renal reabsorption of sodium in the distal nephron is increased by aldosterone, a mineralocorticoid synthesized in the zona glomerulosa of the adrenal cortex. Aldosterone is produced and released in response to stimulation by angiotensin II, hyperkalemia, and by a decrease in dietary sodium intake. Adrenocorticotropic hormone (ACTH) and hyponatremia play permissive roles in promoting aldosterone secretion. Increased dietary sodium and atrial natriuretic peptide (ANP) decrease aldosterone production. ANP is a polypeptide released from atrial and ventricular myocytes in response to atrial distention associated with volume expansion. ANP causes vascular smooth muscle relaxation, inhibits production of aldosterone in the adrenal glands, and blocks the production of angiotensin II. Study results suggest that parathyroid hormone (PTH) is required for augmented ANP secretion in response to acute volume loading in rats. PTH may play an important role in the regulation of fluid homeostasis via control of ANP (Geiger et al. 1992).

In general, chloride is reabsorbed with sodium throughout the nephron. As previously noted, chloride is exchanged in a ratio of 1 Na^+:1 K^+:2 Cl^- in the thick ascending limb of Henle's loop during sodium reabsorption. Because the cotransporter in this exchange has a very high affinity for both Na^+ and K^+, luminal Cl^- concentration is normally the rate-limiting step in NaCl entry into the cell (Gregor and Velazquez 1987). Additional active and passive processes contribute to proximal Cl^- reabsorption in the renal tubules. Chloride exchange for formate appears to occur via an anion exchanger in the luminal membrane. Low concentrations of filtered formate combine with H^+ to form formic acid (HF) in the tubular lumen. Because HF is uncharged, it moves freely into the tubular cell. Two additional mechanisms set the stage for conversion of HF back to formate and H^+. First, basolateral Na^+,K^+-ATPase pumps maintain a low intracellular sodium concentration, and this, in turn, allows for the continued exchange of Na^+-H^+ across the luminal membrane. As Na^+ is reabsorbed and H^+ is secreted, the interior of the cell is left with a lower $[H^+]$ than the tubular lumen. Under these conditions HF is converted back to H^+ and formate, providing for continued chloride-formate exchange. Reabsorbed chloride is returned to the ECF across the basolateral membrane by selective Cl^- channels and a K^+-Cl^- cotransporter (Rose 1994). Additional transport mechanisms in type B intercalated cells in the cortical collecting tubule may exchange bicarbonate for chloride. The favorable inward concentration gradient for chloride (lumen concentration greater than inside the cell) presumably provides the energy for bicarbonate secretion via this mechanism (Bastani et al. 1991).

Understanding the mechanisms for renal regulation of acid-base balance and electrolyte transport is increasingly dependent upon use of transgenic mice in which the function and regulation of key transporter proteins can be assessed (Cantone et al. 2006).

DISORDERS OF WATER, SODIUM, AND CHLORIDE BALANCE

Types of Dehydration. Dehydration may be considered in three general categories: hypertonic, isotonic, and hypotonic. Pure water loss and loss of hypotonic fluid lead to hypertonic dehydration. As pure water is lost from the ECF, fluid shifts from the intra- to the extracellular compartment in response to increased osmolality. The resulting proportionate distribution of volume loss results in fewer clinically detectable signs of volume depletion in the patient. Causes of dehydration associated with pure water deficit include hypodypsia due to neurologic disease, diabetes insipidus, respiratory losses during exposure to elevated temperatures, fever, and inadequate access to water.

Loss of hypotonic fluid, as compared to pure water, results in a greater depletion of ECF volume since there is less osmotic drive to pull volume from the intracellular space. Hypotonic fluid losses are common and have been subclassified as extrarenal and renal. Extrarenal losses could include gastrointestinal (e.g., vomiting or diarrhea) or third-space loss (e.g., pancreatitis, peritonitis, as a result of surgery or cutaneous injury). Third spacing is a term used to describe extravasation of fluid from the vascular compartment into extravascular spaces. As tonicity of lost fluid approaches or exceeds normal plasma osmolality (about 300 mOsm/kg), disproportionate depletion of ECF causes more evident clinical signs of dehydration. Volume depletion would likely be the most clinically apparent in cases of hypertonic fluid loss.

Estimations of percent dehydration based on clinical signs are given in Table 24.5. Skin elasticity is a useful indicator of hydration status. However, age of the animal, body condition, and the technique used for evaluating elasticity may affect hydration assessment. With advancing age or cachexia, loss of fat and protein may account for decreased skin elasticity unrelated to hydration. Conversely, obese animals are likely to retain skin elasticity longer in the face of dehydration. Possibly as a result of variations in elastin content of skin, some species display smaller changes in elasticity for a given degree of dehydration. This may be clinically important in the horse. While dry mucous membranes can indicate dehydration, open-mouthed breathing associated with respiratory disease may cause misleading mucous membrane dryness. Degree of enopthalmos is considered a very useful parameter in assessment of dehydration in large animals. For example, the measured gap between the eyeball and orbit has been included as a guideline for assessment of dehydration in neonatal calves. A gap less than 0.5 cm is correlated with 9–10% dehydration, and a gap greater than 0.5 cm suggests 11–12% loss of hydration (Naylor 1996). A recent study evaluated several clinical and laboratory parameters to determine which were most useful in assessment of dehydration in diarrheic calves. Factors assessed included extent of enophthalmos, skin-tent duration on neck, thorax, and upper and lower eyelids, heart rate, mean central venous pressure, peripheral (extremities) and core temperatures, packed-cell volume, and hemoglobin and plasma protein concentration. The best predictors of degree of dehydration were extent of enophthalmos, skin elasticity on neck and thorax, and plasma protein concentration (Constable et al. 1998). Laboratory parameters such as hematocrit, plasma protein, and osmolality are often useful, but assessment should include consideration of possible preexisting derangements, such as anemia or hypoproteinemia, that could confound interpretation. If an accurate previous body weight is known, serial changes in weight are considered a very useful and accurate measurement in determining degree of dehydration.

Hypernatremia. As the most important and abundant ECF cation, sodium is essential for proper maintenance of membrane potentials, initiation of action potentials, and, according to strong ion difference theory, maintenance of acid-base balance. Plasma sodium concentration and plasma osmolality generally vary in parallel since sodium and its associated anions account for greater than 95% of plasma osmolality. Plasma sodium concentration reflects the ratio of body sodium ion concentration to TBW. Total body sodium content, however, is independent of plasma sodium concentration and may be increased, decreased, or unchanged in the presence of hyper- or hyponatremia.

Clinical signs associated with alterations in serum sodium are more related to the rapidity of change rather than to the magnitude of sodium increase or decrease. Hypernatremia (e.g., >155 mEq sodium/l in dogs) and

TABLE 24.5 Physical findings in dehydration

Percent Dehydration	Clinical Signs
4 or less	History of fluid loss, mucous membranes still moist, evidence of thirst
5–6	Subtle loss of skin elasticity, slight delay in return of skin to normal position, hair coat dull, mucous membranes slightly dry but tongue still moist
7–8	Definite delay in return of skin to normal position, both mucous membranes and tongue may be dry, eyeballs may be soft and sunken, slight prolongation of capillary refill time
9–11	Tented skin does not return to normal position, definite prolongation of capillary refill time, eyes definitely sunken in orbits, all mucous membranes dry, may be signs of shock such as tachycardia, cool extremities, rapid and weak pulses
12–15	Definite signs of shock and circulatory collapse, death is imminent.

ECF hypertonicity can be caused by a loss of pure water, a loss of hypotonic fluid (extrarenal or renal), or a gain of impermeable sodium-containing solute (see Fig. 24.3). Clinical signs of hypernatremia are usually observed in dogs and cats as sodium concentration approaches and exceeds 170 mEq/ml. The signs seen are related to the osmotic movement of water out of cells. Negative effects of cellular dehydration are most pronounced in the brain and lead to the characteristic neurologic deficits associated with hypernatremia. These deficits include abnormal behavior and mentation, ataxia, seizures, and coma. The more rapidly water shifts out of brain cells, the greater the chance that decreased brain volume will lead to rupture of cerebral vessels and focal hemorrhage (Arieff and Guisado 1976). If sodium concentration or concentration of sodium-containing impermeable solute increases slowly, the brain attempts to adapt to the hypertonic state by production of intracellular solutes (e.g., sugars, amino acids) known as "idiogenic" osmoles. Production of these osmotically active substances protects the cell by retaining intracellular volume and preventing cellular dehydration. In addition to neurologic deficits, other clinical signs of hypernatremia include thirst, anorexia, lethargy, vomiting, and muscle weakness. If hypernatremia is related to hypotonic fluid loss, then clinical signs of dehydration (as previously described) may be present. If a gain of sodium has caused the hypernatremia, volume overload may be a problem, especially in patients with cardiac disease.

Restoration of ECF volume and tonicity is of primary importance in treatment of hypernatremia. Volume replacement must be accomplished slowly to avoid rapid shifts in plasma osmolality. In general, the rate of fluid administration is determined by the rate of onset of the hypernatremia. When treating chronic hypernatremia, the serum sodium concentration should drop at a rate that does not exceed 0.7 mEq/l/hr (O'Brien 1995). If plasma

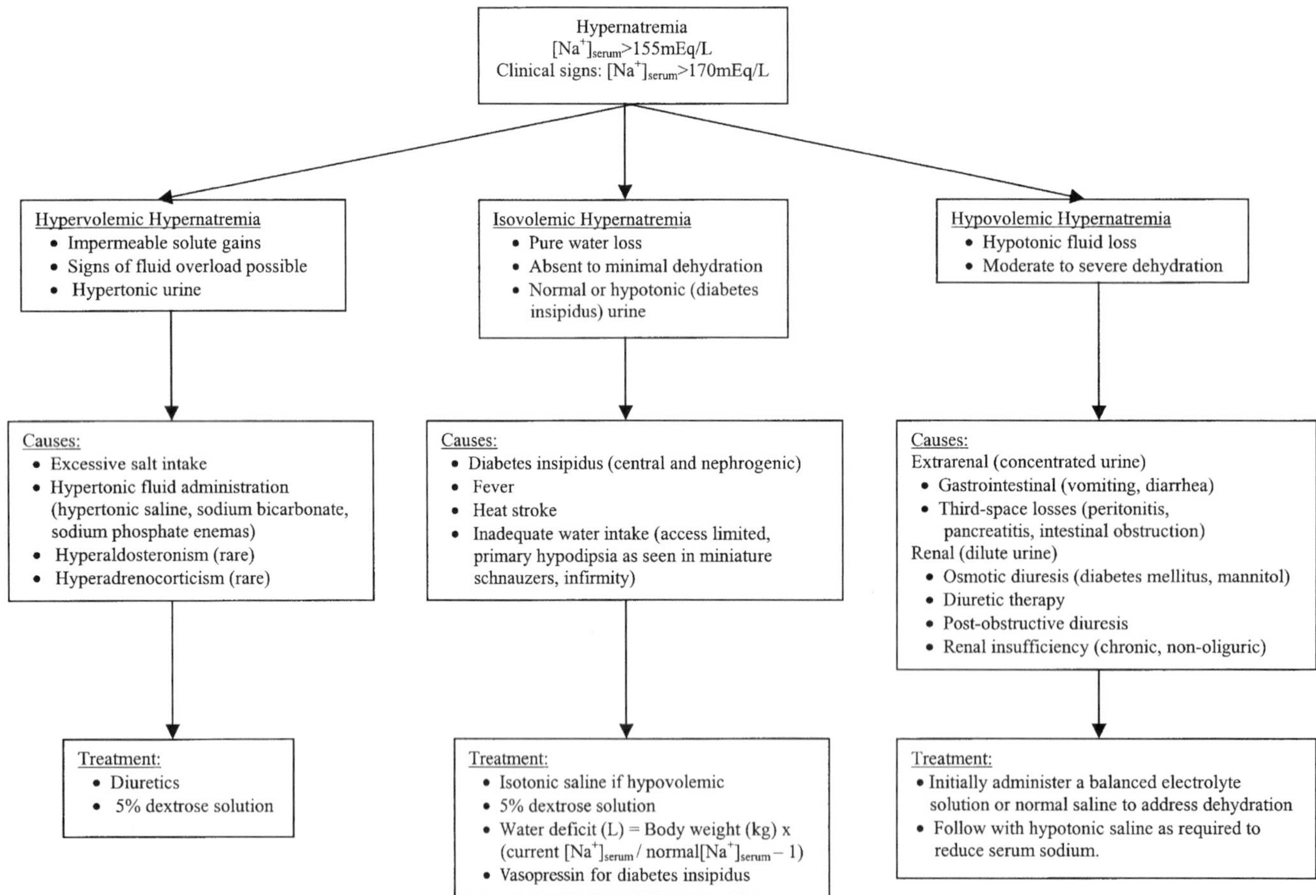

FIG. 24.3 Summary of classification, causes, and treatment of hypernatremia. See text for additional details of treatment.

osmolality drops quickly, water may be attracted intracellularly by idiogenic osmoles, resulting in development of cerebral edema. In the case of pure-water loss, volume can be replaced with 5% dextrose in water over a 48- to 72-hour period. Since the dextrose ultimately enters cells and is metabolized, 5% dextrose administration is essentially replacement with pure water. Use of a 1:1 mixture of normal saline with 5% dextrose solution yields an isotonic solution of 2.5% dextrose, 0.45% saline that has also been utilized. This solution decreases plasma tonicity more slowly and decreases the chance for cerebral edema. Hypotonic fluid losses should generally be replaced with an isotonic crystalloid solution. If hypernatremia has resulted from addition of sodium or sodium-containing impermeable solute, then administration of 5% dextrose and water should be accomplished cautiously to avoid pulmonary edema. Diuretics may be useful in promoting saluresis (sodium excretion) as ECF volume is restored (Marks 1998).

Evaluation and treatment of hypernatremia in critically ill cats was reviewed with emphasis on the importance of careful monitoring and early recognition of signs for positive therapeutic outcomes (Temol et al. 2004).

Hyponatremia. Causes of hyponatremia (<135–140 mEq sodium/l) are best categorized if two additional variables, osmolality and hydration, are also considered. As indicated in Figure 24.4, the more common causes of

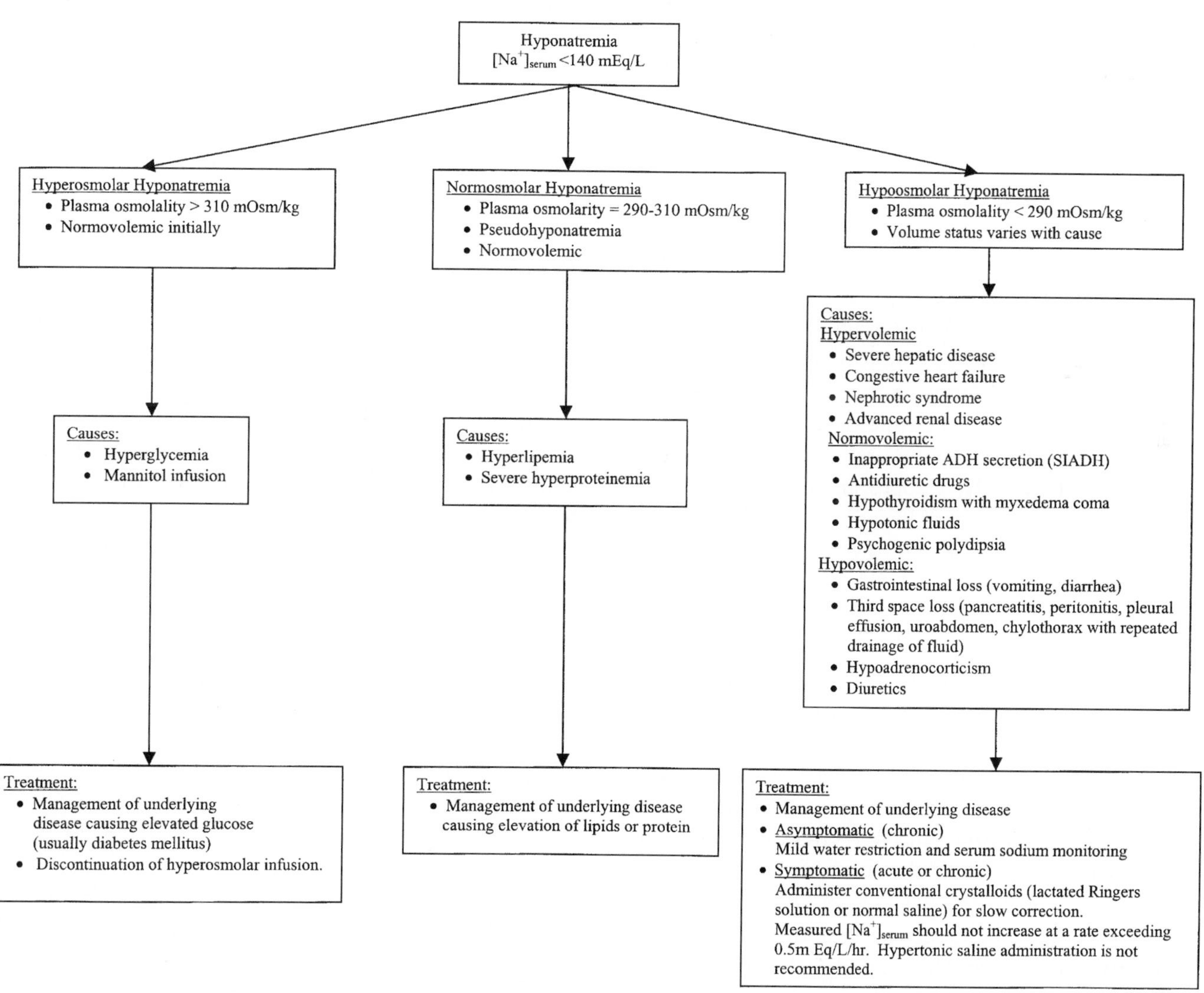

FIG. 24.4 Summary of classification, causes, and treatment of hyponatremia. See text for additional details of treatment.

hyponatremia are accompanied by decreased plasma osmolality (<290 mOsm/kg) with or without volume depletion. If volume depletion exists with hyponatremia, then loss of body sodium has exceeded water loss. Physiologic responses to hypovolemia lead to impaired water excretion and a relative dilution of the sodium remaining in body fluids. Hypovolemia causes decreased renal perfusion and GFR, leading to a decline in water excretion. Slower movement of filtrate through renal tubules enhances isosmotic reabsorption of salt and water in the proximal tubules and decreases presentation of tubular fluid at distal diluting sites. Additionally, hypovolemia prompts vasopressin release, further impairing water elimination. Finally, thirst related to hypovolemia results in consumption of low-sodium fluids that also dilute existing plasma sodium (DiBartola 1992c).

Hyponatremia accompanied by hypervolemia and low plasma osmolality occurs in clinical disorders where there is a physiological perception of volume depletion by in vivo volume detectors. The physiological response is volume expansion. For example, in congestive heart failure, decreased cardiac output is sensed as volume depletion by baroreceptors. Release of vasopressin impairs water excretion, leading to expanded vascular volume. Decreased effective circulating volume and decreased renal perfusion also lead to activation of the renin-angiotensin-aldosterone system. Enhanced renal retention of sodium contributes to expanded vascular volume. In cirrhosis and the nephrotic syndrome, hypoalbuminemia and decreased oncotic pressure may contribute to decreased effective circulating volume and, ultimately, vasopressin release and volume expansion. Other features of hepatic and renal disease also contribute to decreased circulating volume and/or impaired water excretion (DiBartola 1992c).

Hyponatremia is relatively less common when associated with increased plasma osmolality. The most frequent cause of sodium decreases in the presence of increased plasma osmolality is the increased circulating glucose levels associated with diabetes mellitus. Each 100 mg/dl increase in glucose results in a measured decrease of serum sodium by 1.6 mEq/l (Katz 1973). In response to the increased concentration of serum glucose, water shifts from the intracellular to the extracellular compartment, resulting in dilution of measured sodium. Serum osmolality remains high due to elevated glucose concentrations.

Hyponatremia associated with normal plasma osmolality is referred to as pseudohyponatremia. The decreased sodium concentrations are spurious and are almost universally related to technical difficulties in sodium measurement when plasma lipid or protein concentrations are high.

As with hypernatremia, clinical signs of hyponatremia are more severe if sodium concentration changes rapidly than if it changes over a more prolonged period of time. If sodium concentrations and plasma osmolality decrease quickly, water shifts out of the ECF and into cells. The central nervous system (CNS) is most affected by a rapid fluid shift, which, in hyponatremia, results in development of cerebral edema. If onset of hyponatremia is slow, the brain can adjust cell volume by decreasing intracellular osmolality and preventing influx of water from the ECF. Patients with chronic hyponatremia will also adjust intracellular osmolality to an extent that clinical signs may not be obvious even though sodium concentrations are quite low.

Treatment of hyponatremia varies with etiology of the disorder. The goals of therapy are to manage the underlying disease and, if necessary, to increase serum sodium and osmolality. Infusion with conventional crystalloid solutions (e.g., normal saline or lactated Ringer's solution) is reported to accomplish sodium and volume replacement in hyponatremic, hypovolemic patients (DiBartola 1992c). Use of hypertonic saline solutions is not recommended since overly rapid correction of hyponatremia may do more harm than good. Chronic hyponatremia, in which the brain has adjusted to the decrease in osmolality and sodium, must be handled cautiously to avoid brain dehydration and injury, including osmotic demyelination syndrome. This syndrome, often occurring several days after correction of hyponatremia, results from areas of demyelination caused by treatment-induced increases in serum sodium concentration. Dogs with asymptomatic chronic hyponatremia are best treated by mild water restriction and monitoring of serum sodium. Chronic, symptomatic dogs should be treated such that the rate of increase of serum sodium does not exceed 10–12 mEq/l/day (0.5 mEq/l/hr) (DiBartola 1998). Again, the most important therapeutic goal in management of hyponatremia should be treatment of the underlying disease.

Hyperchloremia. Fluid loss associated with small bowel diarrhea often results in greater loss of HCO_3^- than chloride due to loss of alkaline pancreatic secretions and bile and HCO_3^- secretion in exchange for Cl^- in the ileum. The resulting hyperchloremic metabolic acidosis is characterized by a normal anion gap. Additional causes and treatment for hyperchloremic metabolic acidosis will be considered subsequently under the heading of metabolic acidosis. Please refer to the discussion of hypernatremia for treatment of hyperchloremia associated with loss of free water.

Hypochloremia. Hypochloremia may be seen in patients with fluid losses due to vomiting or excessive diuretic administration. Hypochloremic metabolic alkalosis may develop in these cases because an excess of chloride is lost, leading to decreased filtered Cl^- in the renal tubules. As previously noted, activity of the Na^+-K^+-$2Cl^-$ cotransporter in the luminal membrane of the macula densa cell is primarily determined by the availability of Cl^-. In hypochloremia, less Cl^- is delivered, resulting in less NaCl reabsorption, promotion of renin release leading to secondary hyperaldosteronism, and increased distal H^+ secretion. If further Na^+ reabsorption does occur, then Na^+ must be accompanied by an anion other than chloride, usually bicarbonate, or must be exchanged for a secreted cation, either H^+ or K^+. In addition, bicarbonate secretion in exchange for chloride, which is thought to occur in intercalated cells of the cortical collecting tubule, will decrease since this process is presumably driven by a favorable inward gradient for Cl^-. As luminal $[Cl^-]$ decreases, the gradient is dissipated and bicarbonate is retained in the system. All of the foregoing mechanisms promote retention of base and excretion of H^+, leading to a hypochloremic metabolic alkalosis (Rose 1994). Treatment with chloride-replete fluid such as normal saline is usually adequate to resolve chloride-responsive alkalosis. As will be discussed below, potassium depletion may also promote a metabolic alkalosis and should be addressed as needed by addition of potassium chloride to fluids.

POTASSIUM

HOMEOSTASIS. As the major intracellular cation, potassium concentrations inside (145 mEq/l) and outside (3.5–5.5 mEq/l) the cell are maintained by the Na^+,K^+-ATPase pump. Under normal circumstances each pump actively transports three sodium ions out of and two potassium ions into the cell, but the ratio can change depending upon the circumstances. The ratio of intra- to extracellular concentration of potassium ($[K^+]i/[K^+]o$) is the major determinant of resting membrane potential. Resting membrane potential is crucial to normal membrane excitability associated with cardiac conduction, muscle contraction, and nerve impulse transmission.

The normal dietary intake of potassium is much more than the body requires. About 90% of this intake is excreted in the urine, with the remainder of what is not required eliminated in the stool. Plasma potassium concentration is determined by the movement of potassium into or out of cells. Two important factors stimulating the transport of potassium into cells are insulin and beta-adrenergic stimulation (Clausen and Flatman 1987). Aldosterone is the primary determinant of potassium secretion across renal tubular epithelial surfaces.

RENAL REGULATION OF POTASSIUM EXCRETION. Most filtered potassium (60–80%) is reabsorbed in the proximal tubule. In the early proximal tubule, potassium enters the tubular cell at the luminal surface by active transport. The intracellular concentration of potassium is high, and the lumen of the tubule is negatively charged relative to the interior of the early proximal tubular cell. Potassium passively exits the basolateral membrane of the tubular cell down a favorable chemical concentration gradient. In the mid-to-late proximal tubule, the tubular lumen is relatively more positively charged than the tubular cell interior. This favors the passive reabsorption of potassium. Potassium again exits on the basolateral side of the tubular cell down a concentration gradient. Potassium reabsorption by intercalated cells in the distal nephron is similar to the process in the early proximal tubule and involves active transport at the luminal cell membrane followed by passive diffusion from the cell at the basolateral membrane.

Tubular secretion of potassium is aldosterone mediated and occurs in the distal nephron (late distal tubule or connecting tubule of the collecting duct system) primarily in the "principal" cells of the collecting tubules. Additional information on mechanisms of collecting duct system reabsorption and secretion is given in Chapter 25 (Fig. 25.2). Principal cells are rich in Na^+,K^+-ATPase and respond to aldosterone by increasing the number and activity of Na^+,K^+-ATPase pumps in the basolateral membrane. The increasing luminal membrane permeability to sodium causes greater lumen negativity relative to the tubular cell interior and increases luminal permeability to potassium. This facilitates potassium secretion into the tubule lumen. Aldosterone-stimulated Na^+,K^+-ATPase actively pumps potassium out of the peritubular fluid through the basolateral tubular cell membrane. Movement of potassium from the tubular cell through the luminal membrane and into the tubule lumen is favored by relative negativity of the lumen compared to the interior of the distal tubule cell (Black 1993).

When plasma potassium concentration is low, secretion of potassium by the principal cells is reduced while hydrogen ion secretion may be increased. Active potassium reabsorption by intercalated cells in the distal nephron is also stimulated by a potassium deficit. An additional factor affecting the movement of potassium across tubular cells is related to tubular flow rate. A rapid flow of filtrate through the tubules maximizes the potassium concentration gradient between the tubular cell interior and the lumen of the tubule and enhances potassium excretion. A reduction of tubular flow slows secretion by allowing a relatively greater concentration of potassium to be maintained in the lumen of the distal tubule (DiBartola and Autran de Morais 1992).

DISORDERS OF POTASSIUM BALANCE. Disorders of potassium balance have marked effects on excitable membranes. The difference between the resting membrane potential and the membrane potential required for depolarization (threshold potential) determines the excitability of a cell. Hypokalemia makes the resting membrane potential more negative, thereby hyperpolarizing the cell and increasing the difference between resting and threshold potentials. Hyperkalemia causes the resting membrane potential to become more positive, hypopolarizing the cell and causing hyperexcitability. In hyperkalemia, if the resting potential decreases to less than the threshold potential, the cell depolarizes but is incapable of repolarizing, resulting in loss of cell excitability (DiBartola and Autran de Morais 1992). In cardiac muscle this results in diastolic arrest; in vascular smooth muscle hyperkalemia causes vasoconstriction.

Changes in pH affect the distribution of potassium between the ICF and the ECF. When acidosis is present, potassium moves out of cells in exchange for hydrogen, which moves intracellularly. In the distal tubule more hydrogen, and relatively less potassium, may be exchanged for sodium at the luminal membrane, leading to decreased potassium excretion. Based on these general principles, a clinical rule of thumb predicts that each 0.1 unit decrease in pH will be accompanied by a 0.6 mEq/l increase in serum potassium concentration.

Conversely, in alkalosis potassium tends to move into cells in exchange for extracellular movement of hydrogen. Hypokalemia has been thought to promote alkalosis because less potassium is available to be exchanged for sodium in the distal tubule. Instead, sodium exchanges for hydrogen at the luminal membrane, leading ultimately to reclamation of bicarbonate and increased systemic pH. At the same time that systemic pH is increasing, secreted hydrogen ions exchanged for sodium cause the urine pH to decline.

Although the principles outlined above are commonly stated and widely applied clinically, it is not clear that these explanations are adequate. In acidosis, the effect of pH changes on potassium translocation varies with the nature of the acid anion, blood pH and HCO_3^- concentration, osmolality, hormonal activity, and liver and renal function (DiBartola and Autran de Morais 1992). Although changes in serum potassium have been documented during acute mineral acidosis caused by HCl or NH_4Cl (Adrogue and Madias 1981), acute metabolic acidosis caused by organic acids did not increase serum potassium as predicted (Oster et al. 1980; Adrogue and Madias 1981). In certain conditions (e.g., diabetic ketoacidosis), hyperkalemia may be more directly associated with hyperosmolality and insulin deficiency than with the acidosis itself. In lactic acidosis, increased serum potassium concentration may be the result of release of intracellular potassium caused by cell breakdown associated with decreased peripheral perfusion (Black 1993). Metabolic acidosis associated with both mineral and organic acids may directly or indirectly stimulate aldosterone secretion. The effects of aldosterone facilitate excretion of the acid load and, presumably, potassium, although one study failed to show any changes in serum potassium concentration (Perez et al. 1980).

Early studies of the effects of hypokalemia on acid-base balance may have overlooked the key role of chloride depletion in causing metabolic alkalosis (DiBartola and Autran de Morais 1992). When pure potassium depletion is created iatrogenically in rats, metabolic alkalosis results. However, in dogs, potassium deficit with normal chloride levels leads to metabolic acidosis due, presumably, to a distal renal tubular acidification defect (Garella et al. 1979).

Hyperkalemia. Total body potassium may be normal, decreased, or increased with hyperkalemia. Clinical signs of hyperkalemia (>7.5 mEq/l) are generally associated with changes in membrane excitability and are more severe if the increase in potassium has been rapid. Muscle weakness, twitching, and irritability may occur. Electrocardiographically determined cardiac effects may include extrasystoles, intraventricular conduction blocks, high-peaked T waves, altered QT interval, widened QRS interval, decreased amplitude or disappearance of P waves, depressed ST segment, ventricular asystole, or fibrillation.

Causes of hyperkalemia are summarized in Table 24.6. The more common causes are related to decreased urinary potassium excretion. Pseudohyperkalemia related to hemolysis can occur in species that have high red cell potassium concentrations similar to humans. Dogs, sheep, and cattle can be divided into two groups based on Na^+,K^+-ATPase activity in red cell membranes. Those animals with high activity and high intracellular potassium concentrations are at risk for hyperkalemia caused by hemolysis. Animals with genetically determined low activity and low intracellular concentrations of potassium are unlikely to suffer from pseudohyperkalemia since the concentration of potassium in red cells resembles the concentration in the ECF (DiBartola and Autran de Morais 1992).

TABLE 24.6 Causes of hyperkalemia

Decreased Excretion
- Urethral obstruction
- Ruptured bladder
- Anuric or oliguric renal failure
- Hypoadrenocorticism
- Gastrointestinal diseases (e.g., trichuriasis, salmonellosis, perforated duodenal ulcers)
- Chylothorax with repeated drainage of the pleural effusion
- Drugs
  - ACE inhibitors (e.g., captopril, enalapril)
  - Potassium-containing drugs (e.g., potassium chloride)
  - Potassium-sparing diuretics (e.g., spironolactone, amiloride, triamterene)
  - Nonsteroidal antiinflammatory agents
  - Heparin

Translocation from the ICF to ECF
- Acute mineral acidosis (e.g., HCl or NH_4Cl administration)
- Insulin deficiency (e.g., diabetic ketoacidosis)
- Ischemia reperfusion
- Drugs (e.g., propranolol)
- Acute tumor lysis syndrome
- Hyperkalemic periodic paralysis (rare)

Increased Intake (rare)

Pseudohyperkalemia
- Thrombocytosis
- Hemolysis

Source: Adapted from DiBartola and Autran de Morais 1992, 108, Table 4.6.

The effects of several different drugs may impact serum potassium concentration. Since potassium uptake by cells is mediated in part by catecholamines at beta receptors, beta blockers decrease intracellular potassium movement and increase ECF potassium concentrations. Angiotensin-converting enzyme (ACE) inhibitors may cause hyperkalemia by interfering with angiotensin II–mediated aldosterone secretion. Prostaglandin inhibitors, heparin, and selected potassium-sparing diuretics (e.g., spironolactone) increase serum potassium by decreasing the secretion of aldosterone or by blocking its activity. In many cases drugs alone may not have a marked effect on serum potassium concentration but if combined with a potassium load or decreased renal function may cause clinically significant hyperkalemia.

Treatment of hyperkalemia varies with the severity of the condition in terms of magnitude and rapidity of onset. Emergency treatment is indicated if potassium rises quickly and exceeds 6.0–8.0 mEq/l (Phillips and Polzin 1998). Serum potassium concentrations less than these do not typically induce life-threatening cardiotoxicity and can usually be managed with administration of potassium-free fluids. More aggressive treatment is necessary if electrocardiographic signs suggest toxicity. Additional measures that may be taken in treatment of severe hyperkalemia are summarized in Table 24.7. Some are directed toward increasing movement of potassium from the extracellular to the intracellular compartment (i.e., glucose, insulin, and sodium bicarbonate), while others are intended to decrease potassium from the ECF by enhanced renal excretion (e.g., diuretics) or decreased gastrointestinal absorption (i.e.,

TABLE 24.7 Therapeutic considerations in the management of severe hyperkalemia

- Establish venous access and administer potassium-deficient fluids
- Discontinue potassium intake, including drugs that may promote hyperkalemia
- Administer the following as needed:
  - $NaHCO_3$ (0.5–1 mEq/kg, slowly IV) if animal is acidotic
  - Calcium gluconate (10% solution; 0.5–1 ml/kg slowly IV up to 10 ml maximum)
  - Glucose (20% solution; 0.5–1.0 g/kg IV)
  - Insulin (0.5 IU/kg) and glucose (20% solution; l g/kg; half given IV bolus and the remainder infused over 2 hours)
- Potassium-wasting diuretics (furosemide, chlorothiazide, hydrochlorothiazide)
- Sodium polystyrene (20 g with 100 ml 20% sorbitol) per os or 50 g in 100–200 ml tap water (retention enema)
- Peritoneal dialysis (last resort)

orally administered potassium-binding resins such as sodium polystyrene sulfonate).

Therapy with calcium gluconate is included as part of the emergency treatment of hyperkalemia because changes in membrane excitability associated with alterations in potassium may be exacerbated by abnormalities in ionized calcium. Ionized calcium affects the threshold potential of a membrane and, when calcium is decreased, brings threshold closer to resting membrane potential, resulting in greater membrane excitability. An increase in ionized calcium has an opposing effect on membrane excitability by increasing the threshold potential and making depolarization more difficult. Hence, hypocalcemia exacerbates hyperkalemia while hypercalcemia counteracts hyperkalemia.

Hypokalemia. Since 97% of total body potassium is intracellular, depletion can occur with no change in plasma potassium concentration or even with an increase if acidosis is present. Clinical signs of hypokalemia (<2.5–3.0 mEq/l) can include weakness of skeletal and respiratory muscles and intestinal smooth muscle loss of tone. As in hyperkalemia, cardiac changes occur as potassium concentration changes. Supraventricular and ventricular arrhythmias are most commonly observed in animals. ECG hallmarks of hypokalemia in humans are flattened or inverted T waves, depressed S-T segment, and the appearance of U waves. Prolongation of the QT interval and U waves have been reported in dogs but are not as consistently seen as they are in humans. Hypokalemia is increasingly recognized as an important clinical problem in cats, especially in association with chronic renal failure and geriatric animals (Phillips and Polzin 1998). Feline hypokalemic polymyopathy syndrome, characterized by generalized muscle weakness associated with hypokalemia, is often manifest in cats as ventroflexion of the head and a stiff, stilted gait.

Increased loss associated with the gastrointestinal or the urinary system is a common cause of hypokalemia, as indicated in Table 24.8. Differentiating gastrointestinal from urinary causes of hypokalemia is largely accomplished by clinical signs and physical exam, but fractional potassium excretion rates (FE_K) may also be useful. Fractional potassium excretion can be calculated using the following formula:

$$FE_K = (U_K/S_K)/(U_{CR}/S_{CR}) \times 100$$

TABLE 24.8 Causes of hypokalemia

Increased Loss
- Gastrointestinal (FE_K <4–6%)
  - Persistent vomiting of stomach contents
  - Diarrhea
- Urinary (FE_K >4–6%)
  - Chronic renal failure in cats
  - Diet-induced hypokalemic nephropathy in cats
  - Renal tubular acidosis
  - Postobstructive diuresis
- Excess circulating mineralocorticoid
  - Hyperadrenocorticism
  - Primary hyperaldosteronism (hyperplastic or neoplastic)
- Iatrogenic (drug induced)
  - Diuretics (loop acting, thiazides and osmotic)
  - Antibiotics (penicillins, amphotericin B, aminoglycosides)

Translocation from ECF to ICF
- Alkalemia
- Overadministration of insulin and glucose-containing fluids
- Hyperthyroidism
- Hypokalemic periodic paralysis
- Possible complication of hypothermia

Decreased intake
- Unlikely as sole cause

Source: Adapted from DiBartola and Autran de Morais 1992, 99, Table 4.3.

where *U* indicates the urine concentration of potassium (K^+) or creatinine (CR), and *S* indicates the serum concentration.

Treatment of hypokalemia is indicated if significant potassium loss is expected based on history and clinical signs (e.g., vomiting, diarrhea, overzealous use of diuretics) or if clinical signs of hypokalemia are present. Appropriate potassium administration is often required with prolonged fluid therapy. If feasible, oral potassium supplementation is most desirable since this is the safest route of administration. If intravenous potassium supplementation is warranted, the amount administered should be based on clinical status of the animal and measured serum potassium values. Oral and parenteral products for potassium supplementation are discussed later in this chapter. Table 24.9 provides approximate potassium dosages for treatment of hypokalemia in small animals. Alternatively, a rule of thumb may be applied in which 20 mEq/l of potassium is supplemented with careful monitoring of changes in serum potassium. An important admonition in the administration of intravenous potassium is not to exceed a rate of 0.5 mEq/kg/hr. Parenteral potassium administration should always be monitored to ensure that rate of potas-

TABLE 24.9 Potassium supplementation in treatment of hypokalemia

Serum potassium concentration (mEq/l)	Supplement fluids (mEq/l)*
3.5 to 4.5	20
3.0 to 3.5	30
2.5 to 3.0	40
2.0 to 2.5	60
<2.0	80

*Quantity of potassium to add per liter of fluid. Do not exceed administration rate of 0.5 mEq K^+/kg/hr.

sium addition does not exceed rate of potassium movement into cells.

PRINCIPLES OF ACID-BASE METABOLISM

HOMEOSTASIS. Blood pH is highly regulated and is normally maintained between 7.38 and 7.42. Pulmonary and renal functions are necessary for precise regulation of pH of all body fluids, blood, and extravascular tissues. An acid is defined by Bronsted and Lowry as a substance that can supply H^+ (protons), and a base is defined as a substance that can accept H^+. In aqueous solutions, H^+ are hydrated; therefore, H_3O^+ is considered an acid and is implied by the symbol H^+. Blood pH is the negative logarithm of the hydrogen ion concentration. Although hydrogen ion concentration cannot be measured directly, hydrogen ion activity is measured chemically using a pH electrode. In body fluids, the difference between activity of hydrogen ions and concentration of hydrogen ions is negligible; hence hydrogen ion concentration and pH are commonly referred to in acid-base discussions. The hydrogen ion concentration of blood at pH 7.4 is 40 nmol/l (nanoequivalents per L) and is therefore approximately a millionfold lower than the blood concentration of electrolytes such as sodium and potassium. Appropriate hydrogen ion concentration is critical in order to maintain body proteins in configurations required for enzymatic and structural function. An increase in hydrogen ion concentration with a decrease in blood pH is termed acidemia and can be caused by pathophysiologic processes that cause accumulation of acids in the body. As the concentration of hydrogen ions decreases, and blood pH increases, alkalemia occurs and can be associated with pathophysiologic processes that cause accumulation of alkali in the body. The disordered processes leading to acidemia and alkalemia are termed acidosis and alkalosis, respectively.

On a daily basis, an excess of acid (70–100 mEq) is generated in the body as a result of dietary intake and intermediary metabolism. Catabolism of carbohydrate, fat, and protein account for most of this as a result of oxidation of sulfur-containing amino acids to sulfuric acid; oxidation of phosphoproteins to phosphoric acid; incomplete oxidation of fats and carbohydrates to organic acid; production of lactate/lactic acid during anaerobic glycolysis; and conversion of carbon dioxide and water produced in the tricarboxylic acid cycle to carbonic acid. Buffers throughout the body minimize changes in blood pH associated with alterations of acid-base balance. The most effective physiological buffers have pK_a values between 6.1 and 8.4, with buffering capacity being maximal within one pH unit of the pK_a. Important extracellular buffers include bicarbonate, inorganic phosphates, and plasma proteins.

Most extracellular buffering occurs as a result of the bicarbonate-carbonic acid buffer pair (pKa = 6.1). Equilibrium of this buffer pair is indicated with the following:

$$CO_2 + H_2O \leftrightarrow H_2CO_3 \leftrightarrow H^+ + HCO_3^-$$

The hydration of CO_2 is a rapid reaction in the presence of the enzyme carbonic anhydrase (CA), which is found primarily in red blood cells and renal tubular cells. The dissociation of any acid, in this case carbonic acid, can be described utilizing the concept that the velocity of a reaction is proportional to the product of the concentration of the reactants. In the case of the bicarbonate buffer system, the carbonic anhydrase–catalyzed hydration of CO_2 to form H_2CO_3 reaches equilibrium almost instantaneously, with the number of dissolved CO_2 molecules far exceeding the number of carbonic acid molecules. By defining dissociation constants and rearranging, the useful Henderson-Hasselbalch form of the dissociation equilibrium equation can be derived:

$$pH = pK_a + \log[HCO_3^-]/[H_2CO_3]$$

Gaseous CO_2 produced in the tissues, primarily via the tricarboxylic acid cycle, is soluble in water; the concentration of dissolved CO_2 in body fluids can be related to the partial pressure of CO_2 in the gas phase, PCO_2, by the following expression:

$$[\text{dissolved } CO_2] = 0.03 \times PCO_2$$

Hence the clinically useful form of this equation for the bicarbonate–carbonic acid buffer system becomes

$$pH = 6.1 + \log[HCO_3^-]/(0.03 \times PCO_2)$$

The bicarbonate–carbonic acid system is the most physiologically important extracellular buffer system because it is present in relatively high concentrations in the blood and because it can effectively buffer by rapid regulation of PCO_2 through alveolar ventilation. As carbonic acid is formed from the buffering of excess H^+ by HCO_3^-, this drives the dissociation equation of carbonic acid to the left, causing an increase in PCO_2. An increase in ventilation enhances CO_2 excretion and lowers the PCO_2.

Intracellular buffers also contribute to maintenance of body pH. The primary intracellular buffers are proteins, organic and inorganic phosphates, and, in the red cell, hemoglobin. Hemoglobin is an especially important buffer for carbonic acid since the primary extracellular buffer, the bicarbonate system, cannot buffer this acid. Bone also acts as a tissue-based buffer by exchanging surface Na^+ and K^+ for H^+ under conditions of acid load. Additionally, dissolution of bone mineral results in release of buffer compounds into the ECF.

REGULATION OF HYDROGEN ION, CARBON DIOXIDE, AND BICARBONATE. Pulmonary and renal control of dissolved CO_2 and bicarbonate concentrations, respectively, is responsible for maintenance of body pH. The "tail" of the Henderson-Hasselbalch equation for the bicarbonate system (i.e., HCO_3^-/dissolved CO_2) provides a simplistic but useful means to consider pulmonary and renal adjustments during simple acid-base disturbances. Under normal physiological conditions, the ratio of HCO_3^- to dissolved CO_2 is 20:1. This ratio can be disturbed by addition or loss of CO_2 or bicarbonate to the system. Table 24.10 depicts changes in the tail of the bicarbonate–carbonic acid dissociation equation that might occur during simple acid-base disturbances. The respiratory component of acid-base regulation (the denominator of the tail, or dissolved CO_2) involves changes in respiratory rate and volume prompted by changes in PCO_2. Initiation of these processes requires only minutes.

The renal component of acid-base regulation (the numerator of the tail, or HCO_3^-) involves selective absorption of bicarbonate and secretion of H^+. During periods of acidosis, relatively more H^+ are secreted, while relatively

TABLE 24.10 Examples of changes in the "tail" of the Henderson-Hasselbalch equation occurring during simple acid-base disturbances

Respiratory acidosis (↓ CO_2 elimination) associated with inadequate ventilation:								
$\frac{20HCO_3^-}{1CO_2}$	$+\ 2CO_2$	→	$\frac{20HCO_3^-}{3CO_2}$	$+\ 40HCO_3^-$	→	$\frac{60HCO_3^-}{3CO_2}$	=	$\frac{20}{1}$
(Normal)	(↓ Ventilation)		(Uncompensated)	(Renal production)		(Compensated)		
Respiratory alkalosis (↑ CO_2 elimination) associated with hyperventilation:								
$\frac{20HCO_3^-}{1CO_2}$	$-\ 0.5CO_2$	→	$\frac{20HCO_3^-}{0.5CO_2}$	$-\ 10HCO_3^-$	→	$\frac{10HCO_3^-}{0.5CO_2}$	=	$\frac{20}{1}$
(Normal)	(↑ Ventilation)		(Uncompensated)	(Renal excretion)		(Compensated)		
Metabolic acidosis (bicarbonate deficit) associated with diarrhea:								
$\frac{20HCO_3^-}{1CO_2}$	$-\ 10HCO_3^-$	→	$\frac{10HCO_3^-}{2CO_2}$	$-\ 0.5CO_2$	→	$\frac{10HCO_3^-}{0.5CO_2}$	=	$\frac{20}{1}$
(Normal)	(Loss in feces)		(Uncompensated)	(Eliminated by ↑ ventilation)		(Compensated)		
Metabolic alkalosis (bicarbonate excess) associated with administration of alkali:								
$\frac{20HCO_3^-}{1CO_2}$	$+\ 20HCO_3^-$	→	$\frac{40HCO_3^-}{1CO_2}$	$-\ 1CO_2$	→	$\frac{40HCO_3^-}{2CO_2}$	=	$\frac{20}{1}$
(Normal)	(Alkali) administration)		(Uncompensated)	(Eliminated by ↓ ventilation)		(Compensated)		

more K^+, Na^+, and HCO_3^- are retained. During alkalosis, K^+ is secreted, while relatively more H^+ and less Na^+ and HCO_3^- are retained. This process requires hours to days to produce an effect. The kidney regulates acid-base balance by maintaining the appropriate HCO_3^- in the plasma. The kidney accomplishes this by reclaiming virtually all filtered HCO_3^- and excreting an amount of acid that equals the amount of ingested or endogenously generated nonvolatile acid. In the proximal tubule of the kidney, cytoplasmic carbonic anhydrase catalyzes the formation of H^+ and bicarbonate from cellular carbon dioxide and water, controlling the rate of hydrogen secretion and bicarbonate reabsorption. In the luminal membrane, carbonic anhydrase converts carbonic acid to carbon dioxide and water, increasing net bicarbonate reabsorption (Fig. 24.5, panel A). In the distal nephron, intercalated cells specialized for hydrogen secretion contain large quantities of carbonic anhydrase, again yielding hydrogen and bicarbonate. In this case, secreted H^+ serves to titrate buffers in the urine (phosphate buffering is shown in Figure 24.5, panel B) and lower urinary pH. As titratable acidity of the urine reaches a maximum, another adaptation, increased ammonia (NH_3) production by tubular cells, contributes to excretion of acid loads. Figure 24.5, panel C, shows production of freely diffusable NH_3 from glutamine moving into the tubular lumen, where it combines with H^+ to form ammonium (NH_4^+). Ammonium, in turn, combines with chloride for excretion as ammonium chloride. While this is an oversimplification of the physiological events, it is acceptable to consider ammonium chloride as a flexible mechanism for H^+ secretion based on the ability of the kidney to generate ammonia.

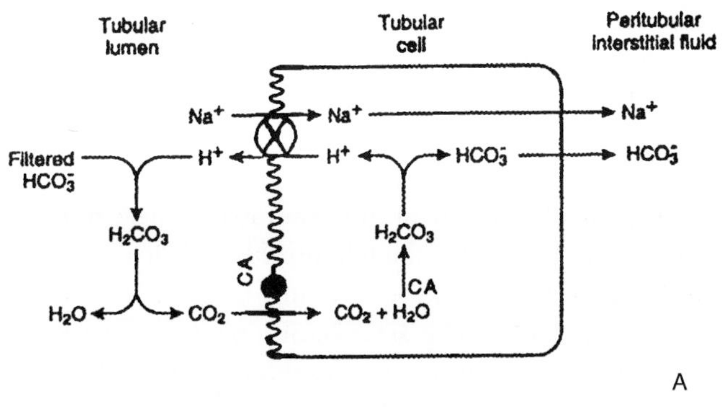

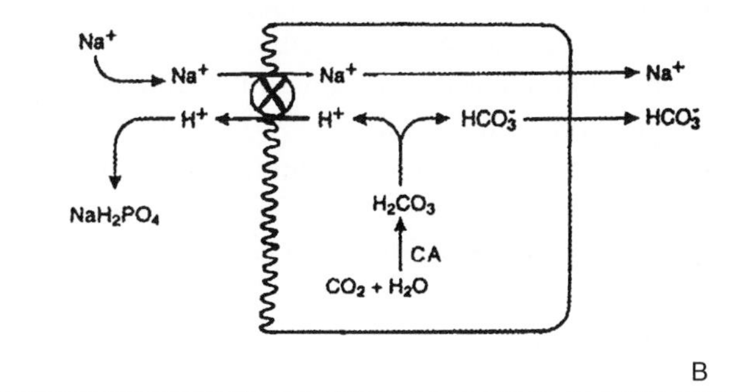

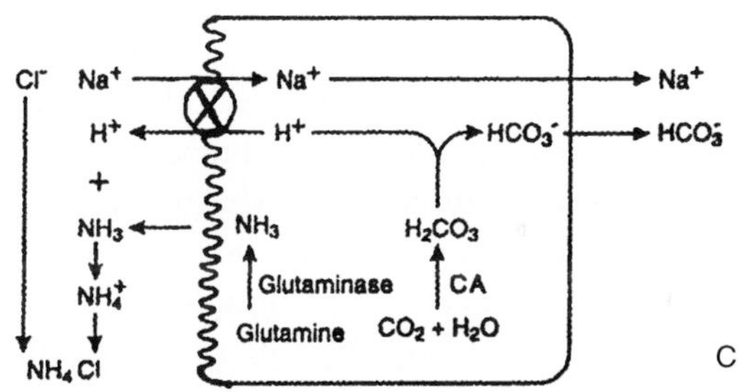

FIG. 24.5 Renal mechanisms for H^+ excretion. See text for explanation of each panel.

ASSESSMENT OF ACID-BASE DISTURBANCES. Disorders of acid-base equilibrium can result from a primary disturbance in pulmonary regulation of the concentration of H_2CO_3 in body fluids via changes in alveolar ventilation and PCO_2 levels, from metabolic changes in concentration of bicarbonate, or from a combination of these mechanisms.

The partial pressure of CO_2 (PCO_2) is generally accepted as the best measure of respiratory disturbances. Assessment of PCO_2 depends upon availability of a blood gas analyzer and proper arterial sample collection. A blood gas analysis provides three measured parameters (pH, PCO_2, PO_2) and typically two calculated values (actual bicarbonate and base excess). Acidemia and alkalemia (using pH), eucapnia, hypercapnia or hypocapnia (using PCO_2), and hypoxemia (using PO_2 if the sample is arterial) may be directly assessed. In-house blood gas and electrolyte analyzers have become much more common in practice, making assessment of these parameters practical and economical. Results obtained with one handheld analyzer appropriate for in-house testing were similar to those obtained from a standard chemistry analyzer with the exception of sodium concentration in canine samples and hematocrit in equine samples (Looney et al. 1998).

Actual bicarbonate values are useful in assessment of nonrespiratory disorders, but these values will vary with compensatory changes in alveolar ventilation and PCO_2. Bicarbonate values are derived using the Henderson-Hasselbalch equation and measured values for pH and PCO_2. Plasma bicarbonate values may also be estimated by measurement of total CO_2. Total CO_2 combines measurement of both the numerator and the denominator of the tail of the Henderson-Hasselbalch equation ($[HCO_3^-]/[H_2CO_3]$) by converting both to measurable CO_2. Total CO_2 and plasma bicarbonate are used interchangeably in reporting plasma bicarbonate concentrations even though total CO_2 is actually plasma bicarbonate plus 1.1–1.3 mEq of H_2CO_3. As compared to actual plasma bicarbonate, standard bicarbonate is defined as the concentration of bicarbonate after fully oxygenated whole blood has been equilibrated with CO_2 at a PCO_2 of 40 mm Hg at 38°C; this measurement eliminates the influence of respiration on plasma HCO_3^-.

Standard base excess (BE) is the concentration of titratable base of ECF; this value may be calculated using a Siggaard-Anderson alignment nomogram that interrelates BE and total CO_2 and HCO_3^- when pH and PCO_2 are measured. Because this calculation is based on a constant oxygen saturation, error may be introduced by inclusion of air bubbles in a poorly handled blood sample. In veterinary medicine, error may also be inherent because the nomogram is based on human blood and excludes the effects of plasma protein and electrolytes on acid-base equilibrium. BE is useful because it accounts for the effects of CO_2 on carbonic acid equilibrium and identifies nonrespiratory causes of acid-base derangement. Base deficit is defined as the negative of base excess (Bailey and Pablo 1998).

ANION GAP. Further analysis, beyond pH, PCO_2, HCO_3^-, and BE, may be useful in assessment of complex acid-base disturbances. The anion gap (AG) is defined as the difference between the quantity of unmeasured cations (UCs) and unmeasured anions (UAs) in the blood. Major UAs include phosphates, sulfates, and organic acids (e.g., lactate, citrate, ketones), with chloride and bicarbonate being the measured anions. Major UCs include calcium and magnesium, with sodium and potassium being the measured cations. Calculation of the AG according to the following equations reflects the law of electroneutrality, according to which total cations must equal total anions (DiBartola 1992d).

$$[Na^+]+[K^+]+[UC]=[Cl^-]+[HCO_3^-]+[UA]$$

$$\text{Anion gap} = UC - UA = ([Na^+]+[K^+]) - ([Cl^-]+[HCO_3^-])$$

The normal AG varies with the species but is approximately 13–24 mEq/l in dogs and cats. AG is most often used to identify causes of metabolic acidosis. In organic acidoses, HCO_3^- buffers hydrogen ions that are generated from dissociation of organic acid (e.g., lactic acid). In theory, the measured $[HCO_3^-]$ should decrease as the concentration of the UA (the organic acid) increases. As long as $[Cl^-]$ remains unchanged (normochloremic metabolic acidosis), the gap will increase proportionately with the increase in acid. Several factors that may confound this simple relationship include the following: 1) other buffers besides HCO_3^- also respond to the influx of organic acid; 2) the volume of distribution of HCO_3^- may be different from that of the acid; and (3) the patient's AG baseline (prior to the presenting illness) is often not known. Hence the AG is useful but not fully predictable.

Increased AG often occurs in lactic acidosis, diabetic ketoacidosis, azotemic renal failure (due to increased phosphates and sulfates), and poisoning (ethylene glycol, salicylate). Constable and Morin (1997) demonstrated a useful correlation between AG and serum creatinine concentration in calves with experimentally induced diarrhea and adult cattle with abomasal volvulus. Although the AG was not a useful predictor of all anion-associated changes (e.g., no correlation was found between AG and blood lactate levels), the AG could alert clinicians to the potential presence of uremic acidosis.

A normal AG usually occurs in metabolic acidosis related to diarrhea, renal tubular acidosis, excessive use of carbonic anhydrase inhibitors, or ammonium chloride administration and in iatrogenic expansion acidosis caused by excessive normal saline administration. The two most common causes of a decreased AG are hypoalbuminemia or dilution of plasma proteins caused by infusion of crystalloid solutions. In both cases the gap decreases as a result of a decreased concentration of net negative charges associated with plasma proteins. Each 1.0 g/dl decrease in albumin is associated with an approximately 2.4 mEq/l decrease in the AG (Gabow 1985).

NONTRADITIONAL (STEWART'S) ACID-BASE ANALYSIS. An understanding of the traditional interrelationships between H^+, CO_2, and HCO_3^- is adequate to explain the behavior of aqueous solutions; however, it does not account for the effects of plasma proteins and electrolytes, particularly sodium and chloride, on acid-base status in biological systems. Stewart described a new approach to understanding acid-base physiology based on three fundamental concepts of electrolyte chemistry (Stewart 1978, 1983). First, electroneutrality must always be maintained. Hence, as with the concept of the AG, the sum of all positive charges must equal the sum of all negative charges. Second, mass must be conserved even though it may change in form within a solution. Finally, the dissociation or ionization of a substance in water is determined by its dissociation constant. Weak electrolytes relevant to acid-base physiology include proteins, water, and CO_2. In contrast, sodium and chloride are considered strong electrolytes because they are fully dissociated in water. Evaluation of acid-base status using the Stewart approach requires assessment of independent, or primary, variables; dependent, or unknown, variables; and dissociation constants of all variables. Values of independent variables are controlled externally and cannot be changed by processes occurring within the solution. Independent variables dictate the acid-base status of a solution.

The independent variables controlling acid-base status in biological solutions are strong ion difference (SID), PCO_2, and total weak acid concentration (A_{TOT}). The first variable, SID, is the sum of the strong cation concentrations minus the sum of the strong anion concentrations:

$$SID = ([Na^+]+[K^+])-([Cl^-]+[lactate^-]+[ketoacid])$$

Unless lactic acidosis or ketoacidosis is suspected in a given case, these terms may be eliminated from the equation since their values would be quite small. Likewise, $[K^+]$ is often dropped from the equation since it contributes a relatively small number to the total cation population. If PCO_2 and A_{TOT} remain constant, increases in SID suggest nonrespiratory alkalosis and decreases suggest nonrespiratory acidosis. Mean normal SID values are derived by each laboratory based on their reference population, and these values vary across species. The second independent variable, PCO_2, is an indication of the amount of CO_2 dissolved in plasma. As in traditional acid-base theory, an increase in PCO_2 shifts the dissociation equation for carbonic acid to the right, increasing the $[H^+]$ and making the solution more acidic. The final independent variable, $[A_{TOT}]$, is accounted for by plasma proteins (95%), primarily albumin, and inorganic phosphates (5%). A_{TOT} has been calculated for horses (Constable 1997) using the formula

$$[A_{TOT}](mEq/l) = 2.25[albumin](g/dl) + 1.4[globulin](g/dl) + 0.59[phosphate](mg/dl)$$

These three independent variables influence several dependent, or unknown, variables. Dependent variables are affected by processes occurring within the solution and do not change unless independent variables change. Values for dependent variables are thus the result, not the cause, of events in solution. Dependent variables include $[H^+]$, $[HCO_3^-]$, carbonate ion concentration ($[CO_3^{2-}]$), $[OH^-]$, concentration of dissociated weak acids ($[A^-]$), and concentration of nondissociated weak acids ([AH]). Values of dependent variables are not affected by the values of other dependent variables. Because the values for $[CO_3^{2-}]$ and $[OH^-]$ are so small, they are not measured or evaluated in a clinical setting. The variables for dissociated and nondissociated weak acids reflect the dynamic relationship between acid-base balance and protein ionization. The ability of proteins to function as enzymes, cell membrane pumps, ion channels, receptors, etc., depends upon their state of ionization, and this is directly affected by changes in independent variables (PCO_2, SID, and A_{TOT}). Likewise, the ratio of ionized to unionized calcium depends upon protein binding, which changes with alterations of A_{TOT} and pH.

Independent variables are controlled via respiration (PCO_2) and renal function (SID). As in traditional acid-base theory, rate and depth of respiration control retention or elimination of CO_2, which may lead to respiratory acidosis or alkalosis, respectively. Control of SID is primarily accomplished by the kidney with a smaller contribution from the gastrointestinal tract. Changes in SID via the kidneys are achieved much more slowly than respiratory changes and are on the order of hours to days. The kidney regulates SID by differential reabsorption of Na^+ and Cl^-. Since Na^+ reabsorption is strongly related to renal regulation of ECF volume, net Cl^- excretion relative to net Na^+ excretion is the primary mechanism for renal regulation of acid-base balance. Control of PCO_2 and SID is the primary determinant of acid-base balance because there is no evidence that the body alters the third independent variable, protein concentration $[A_{TOT}]$, in order to regulate acid-base balance.

In summary, the most important premise of Stewart's approach is that concentrations of HCO_3^- and H^+ are dependent on concentrations of primary, or independent, variables, notably CO_2, Na^+, and Cl^-. The complex equations derived by Stewart address the changes induced by independent variables and quantitate each potential influence by solving for the dependent variables. Much simplified versions of Stewart's formula have been adopted on a limited basis by clinicians who value Stewart's theories and believe that they provide a more complete picture of acid-base derangements. Table 24.11 summarizes the equations being applied for nontraditional analysis of nonrespiratory acid-base status (Russell et al. 1996). In brief, increases in SID suggest nonrespiratory alkalosis, whereas decreases suggest nonrespiratory acidosis. Negative values for Δ albumin suggest hyperproteinemic acidosis, whereas positive values reflect hypoproteinemic alkalosis. Negative values for Δ phosphorus suggest hyperphosphatemic acidosis. Negative changes in free water point to dilutional acidosis, and positive values suggest concentration alkalosis. Positive values for Δ chloride suggest hypochloremic alkalosis, and negative values suggest hyperchloremic acidosis.

While most clinicians still favor the traditional approach to evaluation of acid-base balance, modified applications of Stewart's theories broaden this scope and lend useful quantitative insights into the complexities of acid-base disturbances (Constable 1999).

DISORDERS OF ACID-BASE METABOLISM

Disorders of acid-base equilibrium can result from a primary disturbance in pulmonary regulation of the concentration of CO_2, from metabolic changes in strong ions and, dependently, bicarbonate, or from a combination of these mechanisms. An acid-base disturbance is considered simple if it is limited to a primary disturbance and an appropriate secondary or compensatory response. Primary disturbances and expected compensatory responses are modeled using the tail of the Henderson-Hasselbalch equation in Table 24.10 and summarized in Table 24.12. Mixed acid-base disturbances are suspected when the compensatory response to a primary disorder is not as expected

TABLE 24.11 Formulas for quantitative analysis of nonrespiratory acid-base status

I. Estimation of [SID]. (All values expressed as mEq/l.)
  $[\text{SID approx.}] = [Na^+_{\text{mean normal}}] - [Cl^-_{\text{corrected}}]$
  $[Cl^-_{\text{corrected}}] = [Cl^-_{\text{patient}}] \times ([Na^+_{\text{mean normal}}] / [Na^+_{\text{patient}}])$
II. Alterations in acid-base balance
  A. Changes in acid-base balance due to weak acids
    Δ albumin (mEq/l) $= 3.7 \times ([alb_{\text{mean normal}}] \text{ (mg/dl)} - [alb_{\text{patient}}] \text{ (mg/dl)})$
    Δ phosphorus:
      $[phos_{\text{adjusted}}] \text{ (mg/dl)} = [phos_{\text{mean normal}}] \text{ (mg/dl)} - [phos_{\text{patient}}] \text{ (mg/dl)}$
      $phos_{adj} \text{ (mg/dl)} \times 0.3229 = \text{phos (mmol/l)}$
      effective phos (mEq/l) $= 1.8 \times$ phos (mmol/l)
  B. Changes in acid-base balance due to alterations in [SID]. (All values expressed in mEq/l.)
    $\Delta \text{ free water} = z([Na^+_{\text{patient}}] - [Na^+_{\text{mean normal}}])$
      where $z = [\text{SID}] / [Na^+_{\text{mean normal}}]$
    $\Delta \text{ chloride} = [Cl^-_{\text{mean normal}}] - [Cl^-_{\text{corrected}}]$
    Δ unmeasured anions (UA) $= \text{BE} - (\Delta \text{ free water} + \Delta Cl^- + \Delta \text{ phos} + \Delta \text{ albumin})$

TABLE 24.12 Characteristics of primary acid-base disturbances

Disorder	pH	$[H^+]$	Primary disturbance	Compensatory response
Metabolic acidosis	↓	↑	↓ $[HCO_3^-]$, ↓ [SID]	↓ PCO_2
Metabolic alkalosis	↑	↓	↑ $[HCO_3^-]$, ↑ [SID]	↑ PCO_2
Respiratory acidosis	↓	↑	↑ PCO_2	↑ $[HCO_3^-]$, ↑ [SID]
Respiratory alkalosis	↑	↓	↓ PCO_2	↓ $[HCO_3^-]$, ↓ [SID]

Source: Adapted from Rose 1994, 506.

or when the pH is changing in a direction opposite that predicted by the primary disorder. Mixed acid-base disturbances are characterized by two or more primary disturbances in the same patient.

METABOLIC (NONRESPIRATORY) ACIDOSIS. Metabolic acidosis may be characterized by a decrease in plasma HCO_3^- concentration, decreased pH, increased concentration of strong anions (such as chloride, lactic acid, or ketoacids), and decreased plasma sodium concentration associated with renal disease or diarrhea. The clinical signs most commonly associated with metabolic acidosis are hyperpnea and CNS depression. Laboratory analysis of blood and urine reveals a lowered urine and blood pH, decreased serum HCO_3^- (<20 mEq/l), decreased [SID], and a variable serum PCO_2 depending upon the degree of respiratory compensation. Figure 24.6 summarizes causes of metabolic acidosis and provides general principles of treatment. Metabolic acidosis is the most common acid-base disorder in dogs, cats, and horses, and causes may be usefully subdivided into those conditions that increase the AG and those that do not.

Loss of Na^+ and HCO_3^- associated with diarrhea is the most common cause of normal AG (hyperchloremic) metabolic acidosis. Intestinal secretions replete in Na^+ and HCO_3^- may also be sequestered in lower obstructive bowel disease and paralytic ileus. Hypoadrenocorticism may also present with a nongap metabolic acidosis, but these patients usually have hypochloremia as a result of impaired water excretion, lack of aldosterone, and poor renal function.

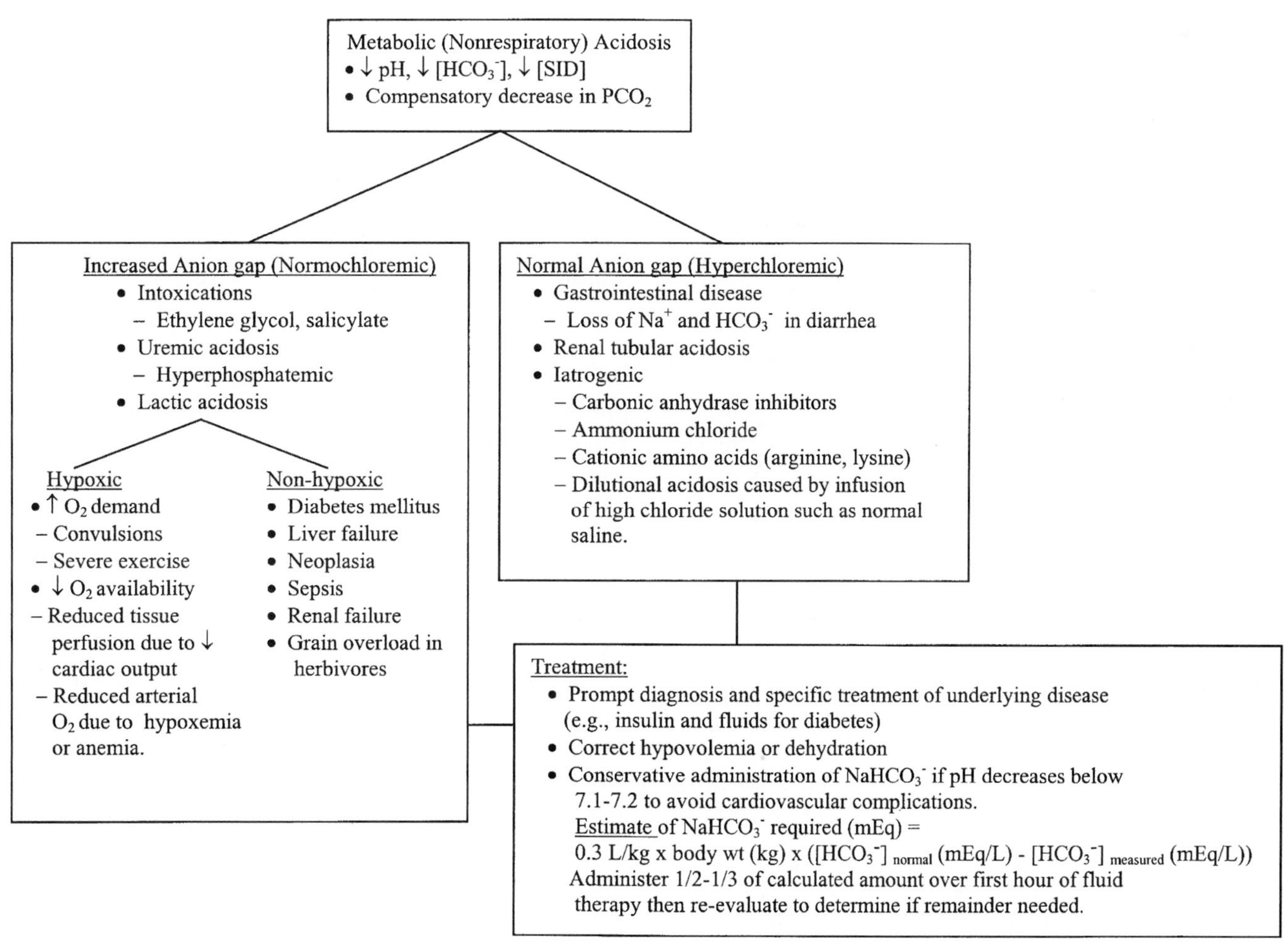

FIG 24.6 Causes of metabolic acidosis and general treatment principles.

Lactic Acidosis. Production of lactic acid and accumulation of lactate, an unmeasured anion, decrease the [SID], resulting in a high AG metabolic acidosis. Lactic acid is the final product of anaerobic glycolysis in eukaryotic cells and is formed by the action of lactate dehydrogenase (LDH) on pyruvic acid with NADH as a cofactor.

$$CH_3COO^- + NADH + H^+ \leftrightarrow CH_3CHOHCOO^- + NAD^+ \text{ (pyruvate) LDH (lactate)}$$

The direction of the LDH reaction depends upon the relative intracellular concentrations of pyruvate and lactate and on the ratio of reduced (NADH) to oxidized (NAD^+) nicotinamide adenine dinucleotide cofactor. Newly produced lactic acid is partially buffered by HCO_3^-, resulting in rapid generation of sodium lactate, which dissociates to lactate and sodium ions. Under aerobic conditions in the liver and the kidney, lactate is converted back to pyruvate, and pyruvate is metabolized through the tricarboxylic acid (TCA) cycle to yield HCO_3^-, CO_2, and H_2O. Alternatively, hepatic uptake of lactate and conversion to pyruvate can feed gluconeogenesis, a process that also regenerates HCO_3^-. In either case, the net result of aerobic lactate metabolism is production of alkalinizing equivalents in the form of HCO_3^-:

Conversion via the TCA cycle:

$$\text{lactate}^- + 3O_2 \rightarrow HCO_3^- + 2CO_2 + 2H_2O$$

Conversion via gluconeogenesis:

$$2\text{ lactate}^- + 2H_2O + 2CO_2 \rightarrow 2HCO_3^- + \text{glucose}$$

If the ratio of NADH/NAD^+ in the cell shifts toward accumulation of NADH (e.g., in exercising muscle or poorly oxygenated tissues), more lactic acid accumulates, decreasing cellular pH. In the case of poorly oxygenated tissues, inability to oxidize NADH via the respiratory chain blocks oxidative phosphorylation and production of ATP. ATP depletion in lactic acidosis causes leaky ATP-dependent K^+ channels, leading to hyperpolarized membranes and decreased Ca^{++} influx via voltage-dependent Ca^{++} channels. Decreased intracellular Ca^{++} produces smooth muscle relaxation, vasodilation, and a potential decline in systemic blood pressure (Landry and Oliver 1992).

Causes of the two types of lactic acidosis, hypoxic (type A) and nonhypoxic (type B), are listed in Figure 24.6. (Only L-lactate is metabolized by animals; hence the discussion that follows refers only to L-lactic acidosis and not D-lactic acidosis, a condition described in humans and associated with small bowel resection or short bowel syndrome.) Reduced tissue perfusion and hypoxia caused by cardiac arrest/cardiopulmonary resuscitation, shock, hypovolemia, left ventricular failure, low cardiac output, and acute pulmonary edema limit oxygen availability and force cells into anaerobic glycolysis. As NADH accumulates, the LDH reaction is pushed to the right, resulting in lactic acid accumulation. Successful management of most of these conditions involves returning tissue perfusion and oxygenation to normal, often with the aid of parenteral fluid administration. Reversal of circulatory failure decreases further lactate accumulation and, if the liver is well perfused, will result in conversion of accumulated lactate to HCO_3^-.

Administration of $NaHCO_3^-$ to animals suffering from lactic acidosis is controversial. Benefits could include improved tissue perfusion related to reversal of acidemia-induced vasodilation and an increase in [SID] (associated with Na^+ administration). Potential risks include overshoot metabolic alkalosis caused by the cumulative effect of $NaHCO_3^-$ administration and metabolism of the accumulated lactate into HCO_3^-. A study in rats (Halperin et al. 1996) concluded that $NaHCO_3^-$ therapy extended the period of survival during acute, hypoxic L-lactic acidosis. Hypoxia was induced in anesthetized, paralyzed rats ventilated with a lowered (5.5%) oxygen concentration, which was sufficient to cause a severe degree of L-lactic acidosis. Survival in rats receiving $NaHCO_3^-$ was close to twofold longer than in rats receiving no sodium bicarbonate or NaCl only. The rate of $NaHCO_3^-$ infusion was titrated to equal the rate of L-lactic acid appearance in the ECF of control hypoxic rats. Part of the benefit of alkali treatment was hypothesized to be increased anaerobic glycolysis, causing enhanced ATP and L-lactic acid production and a decreased oxygen consumption. Despite continued accumulation of L-lactic acid and a decrease in cardiac output that was greater than in control rats, availability of ATP for vital organs was considered critical to prolonged survival in alkali-treated animals. While results using this controlled model are not directly clinically applicable, they suggest that continued consideration of the advantages and disadvantages of alkali supplementation in L-lactic acidosis may be merited. Many clinicians favor a conservative therapeutic approach in which small amounts of $NaHCO_3^-$ are administered to keep the arterial pH above 7.1–7.2 and to avoid progressive decline in cardiovascular function (Rose 1994). In the absence of severely elevated concentrations of lactate, and in the presence of a well-perfused liver, the use of lactate-containing alkalinizing solutions is effective for volume restoration.

Alternatives to lactate-containing solutions include $NaHCO_3^-$, sodium gluconate, sodium acetate, and an equimolar mixture of sodium carbonate and sodium bicarbonate. The latter product, referred to as "Carbicarb" (Cohen 1995), has been promoted as a method of preventing the increased CO_2 production and paradoxical intracellular acidosis that has been reported as a complication of $NaHCO_3^-$ treatment. It has been found, using a canine model of severe hemorrhagic shock, that Carbicarb, $NaHCO_3^-$, and hypertonic saline all possess similar abilities to improve hemodynamics, despite the buffering properties of $NaHCO_3^-$ and Carbicarb. However, correction of arterial pH did not appear to improve the responses to blood retransfusion in this model (Benjamin et al. 1994).

Ketoacidosis and Other Causes. Metabolic acidosis associated with ketonemia and ketonuria occurs when the rate of formation of ketone bodies is greater than the rate of their use. This occurs most often in two conditions, diabetes mellitus and starvation. Excess acetyl coenzyme A (CoA) derived from fatty acid or pyruvate oxidation is diverted, primarily in the liver, to production of ketone bodies (acetoacetate, beta-hydroxybutyrate, acetone). Ketones can be transported in the blood and utilized as an energy source by peripheral tissues. In diabetes the lack of insulin increases lipolysis, and an excess of glucagon indirectly increases fatty acetyl CoA entry into hepatic mitochondria for conversion to ketones. An elevation of ketones in the blood results in acidemia because the carboxyl group of the ketone body has a pK_a of about 4. At physiological pH the ketoacid is fully dissociated, losing a proton (H^+), which lowers blood pH. Addition of an unmeasured anion, the ketoacid, decreases the [SID] driving an acidosis. Ketoacidosis is often complicated by dehydration associated with osmotic (glucose-driven) diuresis. The use of alkali to treat diabetic ketoacidosis is controversial and not generally recommended. Rehydration (usually with normal saline) and administration of insulin is the treatment of choice since circulating ketoacids will subsequently be metabolized to HCO_3^- and move plasma pH toward normal.

Renal failure typically produces a normochloremic, high-AG metabolic acidosis due to accumulation of phosphates, sulfates, and other organic anions, altered handling of chloride, and an inability to excrete the daily dietary acid load. Enhanced generation of ammonia by the renal tubular cells allows the kidney to respond, up to a point, to the chronic retention of fixed acid. Use of alkali to treat metabolic acidosis associated with renal failure is controversial. Three reasons cited in support of treatment are that treatment 1) spares depletion of bone serving as a H^+ buffer, 2) prevents the potentially catabolic effects of acidosis on muscle protein, and 3) limits complement-mediated tubulointerstitial damage that may occur in concert with increased ammoniagenesis. Oral administration of $NaHCO_3^-$ (0.5–1.0 mEq/kg/day) with the goal of maintaining plasma HCO_3^- at 15 mEq/l may be effective if the associated sodium load does not encourage fluid retention.

METABOLIC (NONRESPIRATORY) ALKALOSIS. Metabolic alkalosis is characterized by an excess of HCO_3^- caused by a deficit of H^+ in the ECF. This state may be caused by excessive vomiting (especially from gastrointestinal obstruction), excessive alkaline therapy or use of diuretics that can create iatrogenic metabolic alkalosis, or excessive loss of potassium caused by hyperadrenocorticism or administration of large quantities of K^+-free solutions. Clinical signs of metabolic alkalosis are depressed breathing (slow and shallow), nervous excitement, including tetany, and even convulsions and muscular hypertonicity. Respiratory compensation is not as effective as respiratory compensation for metabolic acidosis.

Values for serum electrolytes usually reveal elevated [HCO_3^-], lowered [Cl^-], and variable [Na^+]. There is usually a low serum [K^+] in this condition. A relationship exists between K^+ loss and metabolic alkalosis in that each can result in the other (positive feedback). In ruminants the situation is much more complex, and unlike in small animals, metabolic alkalosis is much more common. Compensation for metabolic alkalosis requires the kidneys to excrete HCO_3^- and retain H^+. Therapy for metabolic alkalosis involves treatment of the underlying disease and, potentially, use of acidifying solutions such as NaCl (0.9%), NH_4Cl (1.9%) (NH_3^+ is conjugated to urea in the liver, which frees H^+ and Cl^-), and Ringer's solution, which supplies Na^+, K^+, Ca^{++}, and Cl^-.

RESPIRATORY ACIDOSIS. Respiratory acidosis (Table 24.13) involves retention of CO_2 as a consequence of

TABLE 24.13 Causes of respiratory acidosis

- Inadequate mechanical ventilation
- Airway obstruction
- Respiratory center depression
  Neurologic disease
  Drugs (e.g., anesthetic agents, narcotics, sedatives)
- Cardiopulmonary arrest
- Neuromuscular defects
  Myasthenia gravis
  Tetanus
  Botulism
  Polyradiculoneuritis
  Polymyositis
  Tick paralysis
  Hypokalemic periodic paralysis in Burmese cats
  Hypokalemic myopathy in cats
  Drugs (e.g., succinylcholine, pancuronium, aminoglycosides with anesthetics, organophosphates)
- Restrictive defects
  Diaphragmatic hernia
  Pneumothorax
  Pleural effusion
  Hemothorax
  Chest wall trauma
  Pulmonary fibrosis
  Pyothorax
  Chylothorax
- Pulmonary disease
  Respiratory distress syndrome
  Pneumonia
  Severe pulmonary edema
  Diffuse metastatic disease
  Smoke inhalation
  Pulmonary thromboembolism
  Chronic obstructive pulmonary disease
  Pulmonary fibrosis

Source: Adapted from DiBartola 1992a, 267, Table 10.3.

alveolar hypoventilation. The fall in pH is predictable from the Henderson-Hasselbalch equation. Impaired respiration can be caused by pneumonia, pulmonary edema, emphysema, pneumothorax, respiratory muscle paralysis, morphine, barbiturate, or anesthetic poisoning, airway occlusion, or, most commonly, hypoventilation during positive pressure ventilation (iatrogenic). Clinical signs include respiratory distress and CNS depression with progressive disorientation, weakness, and finally coma (CO_2 narcosis). Cyanosis is often present in the advanced stages. Laboratory analysis of blood and urine will show a decreased urine pH, decreased blood pH, increased serum HCO_3^- (from tissue buffers and renal reabsorption of HCO_3^-), and a decrease in serum Cl^- because of renal excretion. Hypoventilation results in CO_2 retention, an excess of H_2CO_3, and thereby an excess of H^+. The compensatory mechanism is for the kidneys to conserve HCO_3^- and excrete H^+. The most important treatment for this condition is proper ventilation of the animal. Use of alkalinizing solutions may aid in cases of lung disease when ventilation alone will not correct the condition. Whenever possible, therapy should be directed at removal of the causative factor.

TABLE 24.14 Causes of respiratory alkalosis

- Overzealous mechanical ventilation
- Hypoxemia (stimulation of peripheral chemoreceptors by decreased oxygen delivery):
  Right-to-left shunts
  Decreased PO_2 (e.g., high altitude)
  Congestive heart failure
  Severe anemia
  Hypotension
  Pulmonary diseases resulting in ventilation-perfusion mismatching:
  Pneumonia
  Pulmonary embolism
  Pulmonary fibrosis
  Pulmonary edema
  Pulmonary disease resulting in stimulation of nociceptive receptors independent of hypoxemia:
  Pneumonia
  Pulmonary embolism
  Interstitial lung disease
  Pulmonary edema
- CNS-mediated hypocapnia with direct stimulation of medullary respiratory center:
  Liver disease
  Gram-negative sepsis
  Drugs (e.g., salicylate intoxication, progesterone, xanthines)
  Recovery from metabolic acidosis
  Central neurologic disease
  Heat stroke

Source: Adapted from DiBartola 1992a, 269, Table 10.4.

RESPIRATORY ALKALOSIS. Causes of respiratory alkalosis are indicated in Table 24.14. The most common cause of this disease in animals is overactive positive pressure ventilation during anesthesia (iatrogenic). Other causes include fever, stimulation of respiratory centers by encephalitis, salicylate intoxication, a deficiency of O_2 (hypoxia), heat prostration, hysteria, or conditions causing chronic hyperventilation (excessive blowing off of CO_2). Clinical signs include hyperpnea (with or without panting), hyperactive tendon reflexes, and CNS stimulation with or without convulsions. Laboratory analysis reveals increased urine pH, increased blood pH, and decreased serum HCO_3^-. Serum Cl^- is usually normal to slightly increased, and pathogenesis of the condition relates to excessive blowing off of CO_2. Compensation occurs by renal excretion of HCO_3^- and retention of H^+. Treatment for this condition should involve correcting the hyperventilation, when feasible, and use of the same acidifying solutions used for metabolic alkalosis. Underlying etiologic factor(s) must be eliminated.

TABLE 24.15 Examples of potential causes of mixed respiratory and metabolic disorders

- Respiratory acidosis and metabolic acidosis
  - Hypoadrenocorticism-like syndrome in dogs with gastrointestinal disease
  - Cardiopulmonary arrest
  - Severe pulmonary edema
  - Thoracic trauma with hypovolemic shock
  - Low-cardiac-output heart failure with pulmonary edema
  - Advanced septic shock
  - Gastric dilatation volvulus
  - Acute tumor lysis syndrome
- Respiratory acidosis and metabolic alkalosis
  - Pulmonary edema and diuretics
  - Gastric dilatation volvulus
- Respiratory alkalosis and metabolic acidosis
  - Hypoadrenocorticism-like syndrome in dogs with gastrointestinal disease
  - Septic shock
  - Salicylate toxicity
  - Heat stroke
  - Gastric dilatation volvulus
  - Liver disease (renal tubular acidosis and impaired metabolism of lactate)
  - Lactic acidosis with excessive hyperventilation
  - Pulmonary edema
  - Parvovirus gastroenteritis and septicemia
  - Severe exercise
  - Acute tumor lysis syndrome
  - Cardiopulmonary resuscitation
- Respiratory alkalosis and metabolic alkalosis
  - Gastric dilatation volvulus
  - Hyperadrenocorticism with pulmonary thromboembolism
  - Ventilator-induced mixed alkalosis (too rapid correction of abnormal arterial PCO_2)
  - Congestive heart failure and diuretics
  - Hepatic disease and diuretics
  - Vomiting or hypoproteinemia
  - Parvovirus gastroenteritis and septicemia

Source: Adapted from DiBartola 1992a, 287, Table 11.9.

MIXED ACID-BASE DISTURBANCES. The preceding discussion of acidosis and alkalosis has purposely dealt with idealized, single etiologic processes in the genesis of acid-base abnormalities. Such states rarely exist in real life. Mixed disturbances usually occur, and treatment will often convert one type of acid-base disturbance into another. Proper therapy must include careful appraisal of repeated laboratory determinations and close observation of the clinical situation. Using these techniques, mixed disturbances can be identified, evaluated, and managed successfully. Examples of potential causes of mixed respiratory and metabolic disorders are noted in Table 24.15.

PRACTICAL ASPECTS OF FLUID THERAPY

DIAGNOSIS AND MONITORING. When fluid therapy is under consideration, the practitioner must ask the following six questions: 1) When should fluid therapy be instituted? 2) What kind(s) of solution(s) should be used? 3) How much fluid should be administered? 4) How fast should the solution be given? 5) What route of administration should be used? 6) How will the success of the therapy be evaluated? The answers to these questions are individual in nature and are critically dependent on a knowledge and understanding of normal homeostatic mechanisms. They are also dependent on the history of the patient, a basic understanding of how a particular disease affects water and electrolyte balance, and a correct diagnosis.

The purpose of fluid and electrolyte therapy is to correct dehydration or overhydration and electrolyte imbalance and/or acid-base imbalance. It may also be indicated to correct a condition of acidosis or alkalosis, treat shock, give parenteral nourishment, or even stimulate organ function (i.e., the kidneys). Causes of fluid, electrolyte, and/or protein loss include situations wherein substances are not available because of lack of supply or condition of the animal; for example, an animal with a fractured mandible may be unable to take in food or liquid, or an animal with a CNS disturbance may be unable to eat or drink because of the primary disease state. Other causes of fluid, electrolyte, and/or protein imbalances may involve excessive elimination.

The following information must be provided by questioning the owner, observation of the patient, and/or clinical examination: duration and frequency of vomiting and/or diarrhea, consistency of stools, frequency of urination, color of urine, presence and character of thirst, fluid and dietary intake, dryness or elasticity (turgor) of the skin, nature and color of the mucous membranes and sclera, presence of excessive salivation or panting, odor of the breath, and weight loss or gain.

In combination with clinical signs, laboratory examination of the blood provides a rational basis for estimating patient fluid and electrolyte needs and monitoring treatment success. Measurements should include hematocrit, plasma protein, blood gases (PO_2, PCO_2, base excess, HCO_3^-, or total CO_2) and electrolytes (Na^+, K^+, Cl^-), blood urea nitrogen, and creatinine. Because red blood cells and plasma protein are largely limited to the vascular space, the concentration of both tends to increase with dehydration. It is best to assess both hematocrit and plasma protein since results of one or the other test alone can be misleading if pre-illness values are out of the normal range. For example, preexisting anemia, hypoproteinemia, or physiologic events such as splenic contraction can confound interpretation of either parameter if considered alone.

Collection, measurement, and analysis of urine are important for proper care of the critically ill patient. Urinalysis should include tests for specific gravity, glucose, acetone, pH, and albumin and microscopic sediment examination. During a state of dehydration, if the kidneys are functioning normally, specific gravity will increase and urine volume will decrease. If the specific gravity of urine is unchanged or lowered and the animal shows clinical signs of dehydration, the kidneys are probably not functioning properly, and more sophisticated renal function tests must be employed. Specific gravity of urine should be monitored during the treatment period. A decrease in this parameter indicates that hydration is taking place. If the animal has not yet received treatment with a solution containing glucose and it is found in the urine, diabetic acidosis is possibly the cause of dehydration. The urine glucose should also be monitored during treatment. If the animal is receiving glucose and the urine glucose reaches $^+3$ or $^+4$, the dosage must be lowered. Acetone in the urine is a frequent finding during dehydration and/or carbohydrate starvation. If the pH of the urine in species with normally acid urine tests alkaline, a diagnosis of alkalosis may be indicated if no kidney or urinary tract disease is present. The presence of urinary albumin and sediment may be an indication of renal disease. If the kidneys are functioning properly, they can adjust markedly to insult. However, in the presence of renal impairment, therapy must be specific or the treatment may be fatal.

TABLE 24.16 Parameters to be monitored during fluid therapy

- Normal bronchovesicular lung sounds on auscultation
- Packed-cell volume
- Total protein
- Electrolytes: Na^+, Cl^-, Ca^{2+}, HCO_3^-
- Arterial pH
- Arterial PCO_2
- Urine output
- Hemodynamics
  Central venous pressure
  Pulmonary capillary wedge pressures
  Mean arterial pressure
  Mean pulmonary arterial pressure

Source: Adapted from DiBartola 1992a, 503, Table 20.9.

Diligent assessment of clinical signs and laboratory parameters is essential to successful diagnosis and monitoring of fluid and electrolyte imbalances. Useful parameters are summarized in Table 24.16.

FLUID VOLUME AND TYPE. A standard approach to estimating fluid volume needs should be used. Replacement of adequate volume is often the single most important key to improved clinical status of animals with multiple fluid and electrolyte disturbances. Volume replacement should have three specific aims: correct existing deficits, satisfy maintenance needs, and replace continuing loss. Initial volume deficits are addressed by administration of replacement fluids. Calculation of the amount of fluid needed is based on clinical and laboratory assessment of percent of dehydration. See Table 24.5 for a summary of signs correlated to degree of dehydration. The volume needed to address the initial deficit is estimated according to the following equation:

$$\text{Replacement volume (l)} = \text{body weight (kg)} \times \%\ \text{dehydration}$$

Clinicians working with both small and large animals should become comfortable with the large differences in volume that will be required to address deficits in different animals. For example, the replacement volume needed to address an 8% fluid deficit in a dehydrated mare weighing 500 kg is 100 times greater than that needed for a similarly dehydrated cat weighing 5 kg. Forty liters of fluid would initially be administered to the mare versus 400 ml to the cat. In general, the composition of replacement fluids should reflect the composition of the volume of fluid lost. For example, if the volume deficit is related to loss of electrolyte-rich gastrointestinal fluid, then a balanced replacement solution containing Na^+, K^+, Cl^-, and bicarbonate equivalents would likely be selected. Table 24.17 details the compositions of commonly utilized replacement fluids.

In addition to replacing existing deficits, maintenance fluid needs must be calculated. Maintenance fluids are needed when a patient does not voluntarily ingest sufficient food and water to replace normal losses occurring via urine, feces, respiratory tract, and skin. The average resting animal at standard conditions of humidity and temperature has a rather constant rate of water turnover. For practical purposes, 40–65 ml/kg/24 hr (30 ml/lb/day is often used as a rule of thumb) for mature animals and 130 ml/kg/24 hr for immature animals serve as average water turnovers for all mammalian species. Based on these assumptions, an average mature dog weighing 20 kg requires about 1.3 l for a daily maintenance supply of water, while a horse weighing 450 kg would require about 29 l/day. Maintenance needs may be modified under conditions of severe stress or fever, extreme environmental conditions, or in the presence of various disease processes. Older animals may need more or less maintenance volume depending upon the presence of polyuria or compromised cardiovascular function, respectively. Administration of various drugs (e.g., glucocorticoids, diuretics) will also affect maintenance needs. The electrolyte composition of fluids used for maintenance differs from that of replacement fluids used to address initial deficits. Because of the composition of fluid lost daily in urine and as insensible loss from the skin and respiratory tract, maintenance fluids are typically lower in sodium (approximately 40 mEq/l) and higher in potassium (approximately 10–16 mEq/l) than replacement fluids. Table 24.17 details the composition of both commercial maintenance fluids and maintenance fluids that can be prepared using other commonly available fluid components.

TABLE 24.17 Composition of selected fluid therapy solutions

		Characteristics		Ion Composition (mEq/l)						
Type	Solution	pH	Osmolarity (mOsm/l)	Na^+	K^+	Cl^-	Ca^{++}	Mg^{++}	Glucose (g/l)	Alkalinizing Equivalents (mEq/l)
Replacement										
Acidifying BES	Ringer's	5.4	309	147	4	155	4	0	0	0
Acidifying BES	Normal saline (0.9%)	5.0	308	154	0	154	0	0	0	0
Alkalinizing BES	Lactated Ringer's	6.6	273	130	4	109	3	0	0	28 (lactate)
Alkalinizing BES	Normosol-R	6.6	294	140	5	98	0	3	0	27 (acetate) 23 (gluconate)
Alkalinizing BES	Plasma-Lyte A	7.4	294	140	5	98	0	3	0	27 (acetate) 23 (gluconate)
Maintenance										
Acidifying	2.5% dextrose/water in 0.45% saline plus potassium addition (16 mEq/l)	4.5	280	77	16	77	0	0	25	0
	Equal volumes 5% dextrose/water and lactated Ringer's plus potassium addition (16 mEq/l)	5.0	309	65.5	18	55	1.5	0	25	14 (lactate)
	Normosol-M with 5% dextrose	5.0	363	40	13	40	0	3	50	16 (acetate)
	Plasma-Lyte M with 5% dextrose	5.5	377	40	16	40	5	3	50	12 (lactate) 12 (acetate)
Other Solutions	5% dextrose/water	4.0	252	0	0	0	0	0	5	0
	50% dextrose/water	4.2	2780	0	0	0	0	0	50	0
	7.5% saline	—	2566	1283	0	1283	0	0	0	0
	8.4% $NaHCO_3$	—	2000	1000	0	0	0	0	0	1000
	14.9% KCl	—	4000	0	2000	2000	0	0	0	0

Note: BES = balanced electrolyte solution.

If the animal being treated continues to lose water during the treatment period (e.g., due to continued vomiting, diarrhea, polyuria) this additional amount must be estimated and added to the replacement and maintenance volumes. The volume required to replace continued loss is based on clinical observation (e.g., frequency of defecation, character and volume of feces in the case of diarrhea). Like the volume used to address the initial deficit, the type of fluid selected to replace continuing loss should, in general, resemble the fluid lost. More often than not, balanced electrolyte solutions such as lactated Ringer's are chosen.

Application of the principles outlined above may be appreciated using the following case example. A 2-year-old, 20 kg mixed-breed dog presents with a chief complaint of diarrhea of 2 days' duration. A physical exam reveals a loss of skin elasticity and a definite delay in return of skin to normal position when tented. Both mucous membranes and tongue are dry and the eyeballs feel soft and slightly sunken. Capillary refill time is slightly prolonged. Based on these clinical signs, dehydration is assessed at 8%. The dog is continuing to pass semifluid stools every 2–3 hours, resulting in an estimated ongoing loss of 150 ml/day. The owner reports that the dog is not eating or drinking. Calculation of the volume of fluid to be administered to this dog over the next 24 hours would include

Replacement of initial deficit:	20 kg × 0.08 =	1.6 l
Maintenance needs:	65 ml/kg/day × 20 kg =	1.3 l
Continued loss:		0.15 l
Total estimated fluid needs:		3.05 l

This volume is considered an estimate because it is based on clinical signs and average maintenance losses. Despite the importance of good data collection and appropriate application of fluid therapy principles, at some level adjusting volume is dependent upon a "guess and reassess" process driven by diligent and thorough patient observation (Roussel 1990).

RATES AND ROUTES OF ADMINISTRATION. The rate of fluid and/or electrolyte replacement should parallel the severity of dehydration and electrolyte or acid-base imbalance. Fluids should be administered rapidly at first and then at decreasing rates until the condition is corrected. Most investigators report that rates of about 15 ml/kg/hr are reasonable. Cornelius et al. (1978) have shown that rates of 90 ml/kg/hr are well tolerated in moderately dehydrated, unanesthetized normal dogs. No deaths occurred, but clinical signs of severe overhydration were evident in dogs given fluids at 360 ml/kg/hr. At 90 ml/kg/hr, pulmonary artery wedge pressures and central venous pressures were increased in dogs with normally functioning hearts. It can be presumed that a seriously ill dog, with compromised cardiac muscle contractility, could be injured by infusion rates that result in acute volume overload. If central venous pressures are being monitored, the infusion rate can be individually adjusted for each patient. This technique is simple and inexpensive. The attending veterinarian should monitor this parameter in the critically ill patient and adjust the rate of fluid administration according to individual needs.

Conservative and reasonable practice would dictate infusion rates of about 50 ml/kg/hr in severely dehydrated cases. Less severe cases should tolerate rates of 15–30 ml/kg/hr. In all cases the rate of infusion should be slowed after the first hour of administration and should be slowed considerably if no urine flow is established. After 4 or more hours of fluid administration without urine flow, the rate of administration should be 2 ml/kg/hr or less. Every attempt must be made to establish renal function if no urine flow is detected after 2 hours of fluid administration. To accurately monitor urine flow, all critically ill animals should have a urinary bladder catheter in place.

Common sense and clinical judgment must be exercised. If an animal is severely dehydrated and in shock, it is difficult to administer fluids too fast during the initial stages of treatment. If, however, an animal is almost normally hydrated and the aim is only to maintain hydration, the rate should be slowed considerably. The importance of renal function has been repeatedly emphasized. A commonly used method of determining if the kidneys are capable of functioning is to inject a small bolus (1–24 ml, depending on size of the animal) of 50% glucose. Urine from the catheterized bladder is then checked every 5 minutes for the presence of glucose, which indicates glomerular filtration is occurring.

The route of fluid administration depends on the type of illness being dealt with and the severity of the condition, degree of dehydration, condition of the patient, type of electrolyte imbalance, organic functions of the patient, and time and equipment available. Probably the easiest, most physiologic, and most overlooked route of administration of fluid and electrolytes is oral or nasogastric. The oral route is the least dangerous, since the solution can be administered without strict attention to tonicity, volume, and asepsis. Oral replacement of electrolytes by using combinations of electrolyte salts, glycine, and dextrose has been especially successful (Hamm and Hicks 1975). Proper technique for oral fluid administration should preclude complications associated with fluid aspiration or administration of excessive amounts of air.

A relatively unused route of administration that might be considered, especially in very young animals, is per rectum. Warm water, K^+, Na^+, and Cl^- are well absorbed via this route. It may be difficult, however, to get the animal to retain material given in this manner, especially in the presence of gastrointestinal disease. Rectal infusion of fluids in birds has been suggested as an effective alternative route to intravenous, intraosseous, oral, or subcutaneous (Ephrati and Lemeij 1997).

The most commonly used and perhaps most practical routes of fluid and electrolyte administration are the parenteral routes: intravenous (IV), subcutaneous (SC), or intraperitoneal (IP). The IV route is the most versatile. Severe disturbances of fluid and electrolyte balance demand it. Nearly all the toxicity of solutions administered in this manner is more related to rate than volume or composition. No indications for hypotonic solutions have been found, but indications for isotonic and hypertonic solutions exist, and some of these have been discussed previously. Some of the problems associated with IV administration include those associated with maintenance and asepsis of indwelling catheters, clotting, and hematomas, as well as the location of a vein on very small or very ill animals. Obviously, the fluids administered and equipment used must be sterile. Large volumes of fluid administered too rapidly may overload the circulatory system, causing pulmonary edema and even death, especially in severely ill or toxic cases. This is the preferred route for blood, blood plasma, and plasma volume expanders.

Subcutaneous administration of fluid is referred to as hypodermoclysis. This technique is convenient for correction of mild to moderate deficits in small animals. Fluids are absorbed more slowly than by the IV route, but if the animal is not in critical condition, this is of no real consequence. Only isotonic solutions should be used in this manner. Dextrose of any tonicity or any solutions lacking electrolytes in isotonic levels are contraindicated because they may produce an initial rapid diffusion of major extracellular electrolytes to the area. This can result in severe reactions, including death, especially if the animal is already in shock. Hypodermoclysis is extremely valuable in very young or very small animals. If the animal is difficult to restrain long enough for a prolonged IV infusion, this is a useful technique. When edema is present, absorption will not occur, and this route of administration is contraindicated. If the animal is chilled by a cold environment or a cold fluid is injected, absorption by this route will be delayed, and it is recommended that fluids be prewarmed to body temperature when feasible. Administration of fluids in one anatomical location should be limited to amounts that are readily absorbed (approximately 10–12 ml/kg) (Greco 1998). Fluid should be deposited dorsally along the area bordered by the scapulae anteriorly and the iliac crests posteriorly. Hypodermoclysis is not commonly used as a route of administration in large animals.

IP infusion of fluids has the same restrictions as those for hypodermoclysis. The technique may predispose to peritonitis, so aseptic procedures must be used. The fluids are mobilized faster than in SC administration, but this route is potentially more hazardous (puncture of abdominal organs). Nevertheless, this is a good route for electrolyte and water absorption. Plasma and a large percentage of red blood cells administered using this technique are rapidly absorbed. In large animals it can be a very practical method of treatment, since a large quantity of fluid can be administered rapidly with few adverse effects. Perhaps the greatest application of this technique is with peritoneal lavage.

PRODUCTS FOR FLUID THERAPY

Major categories of parenteral fluids include crystalloids, colloids, blood replacements, and nutritional solutions. Blood replacement products (whole blood, blood components, and red blood cell substitutes) and nutritional solutions (amino acids and fat emulsions) are considered elsewhere. The composition and characteristics of selected crystalloid solutions and additives used to spike parenteral solutions are listed in Table 24.17. Types and recommended dosages of synthetic colloids are listed in Table 24.18.

CRYSTALLOIDS. As detailed in Table 24.17, crystalloid solutions are polyionic but differ in the amount of each ion and in tonicity. As discussed previously, the tonicity of parenteral fluids partially dictates distribution of volume

TABLE 24.18 Indications, dosages, administration, and side effects associated with use of selected colloids in dogs

Type of Colloid	Indications	Dosage and Administration	Side Effects and Contraindications
Plasma	Coagulopathies; disseminated intravascular coagulation; low antithrombin; acute hypoalbuminemia.	20–30 ml/kg/day administered: (a) continuously over 24 hr, (b) as a 2–4 hr infusion, (c) 6–10 ml/kg in 1 hr infusions every 8 hr, or (d) until plasma albumin is over 2.0 g/dl. Approximately 22.5 ml/kg of plasma needed to increase patient albumin by 5 g/l.	Rapid volume expansion may be detrimental to patients with oliguric or anuric renal failure or congestive heart failure.
Dextran 40	Rapid, short-term intravascular volume resuscitation from hypovolemic shock; rapid improvement of microcirculatory flow by lowering blood viscosity; prophylaxis of deep vein thrombosis and pulmonary emboli.	10–20 ml/kg/day IV bolus to effect; with distributive shock due to SIRS dextran can be followed by a CRI of hetastarch to maintain MAP of at least 80 mm Hg.	*See* plasma. Dilutional effect on serum coagulation factors in addition to possible direct effects on these factors. May be of limited clinical relevance except in patients with preexisting coagulopathies. Contraindicated in patients with severe coagulopathies. Sludging of RBCs in microcirculation in dehydrated patients may occur if sufficient crystalloids are not administered. Anaphylaxis reported in humans. ARF has been reported.
Dextran 70	Rapid, intravascular volume resuscitation from hypovolemic, traumatic, or hemorrhagic shock.	*See* dextran 40.	*See* dextran 40. Dextran 70 is thought to impair coagulation more than dextran 40. No ARF reported.
Hetastarch (hydroxyethyl starch or HES)	Rapid, intravascular volume resuscitation from all forms of shock; small-volume resuscitation; volume replacement and maintenance in SIRS patients.	10–40 ml/kg/day IV bolus to effect; with cardiogenic shock, pulmonary contusions, or head injury, 5 ml/kg boluses are administered to effect, using the smallest volume possible to maintain MAP of 80 mm Hg.	*See* dextran 40. Anaphylaxis has not been reported with hetastarch, but pruritus possibly associated with deposits of HES in cutaneous nerves has been reported in up to 33% of patients treated with long-term infusions. No ARF reported.
Pentastarch (PEN)	Rapid, intravascular volume resuscitation from hypovolemic, traumatic, or hemorrhagic shock.	10–25 ml/kg/day; terminal half-life shorter than HES.	*See* dextran 40. Anaphylaxis and ARF have not been reported with pentastarch.
Oxypolygelatin	Rapid, short-term intravascular volume resuscitation from hypovolemic shock.	5 ml/kg over 15 min; titrate to effect; do not exceed 15 ml/kg total dose. If more volume required, follow with another synthetic colloid.	*See* dextran 40. No ARF reported.

Source: Modified from Rudloff and Kirby 1998. Other sources for information in table include Mathews 1998 and Hughes 2000.
Note: ARF = acute renal failure; CRI = constant-rate infusion; MAP = mean arterial pressure; SIRS = systemic inflammatory response syndrome.

into interstitial and intracellular spaces. Fluids that most closely resemble the ECF are isotonic, high in sodium, and low in potassium and may be acidifying or alkalinizing. These replacement fluids, also referred to as balanced electrolyte solutions (BES), may be given in large volumes at a rapid rate to patients in shock in an attempt to reestablish effective perfusion without severely altering electrolyte concentrations. Alkalinizing solutions depend upon metabolism of various substrates (e.g., lactate, acetate, gluconate) to alkalinizing equivalents in order to reduce acidemia. Lactate and acetate are metabolized in the liver and muscle, respectively, while gluconate is metabolized widely in the body. Perfusion and function of the liver are required for generation of alkalinizing equivalents from the most commonly used replacement fluid, lactated Ringer's solution. A large percentage of veterinary patients that require fluid therapy suffer from nonrespiratory acidosis and are treated with alkalinizing balanced electrolyte solutions. These fluids are generally indicated for animals suffering from diarrhea, vomiting (assuming vomitus contains bile), renal disease, trauma, and shock and those requiring pre- and postsurgical support. To avoid calcium precipitation, calcium-containing balanced electrolyte solutions, such as lactated Ringer's solution, should not be coadministered through the same port with whole blood or sodium bicarbonate.

Normal saline and Ringer's solution are considered acidifying solutions and are used to treat the relatively small percentage of small-animal patients that present with metabolic alkalosis. Both solutions are high in chloride and promote renal excretion of bicarbonate. Normal saline is also commonly used in treatment of patients with electrolyte disorders such as hyperkalemia or hypercalcemia in which absence of electrolytes in parenteral fluids is desirable. Assuming appropriate insulin therapy is instituted, normal saline is also considered the fluid of choice for treatment of diabetic ketoacidosis.

COLLOIDS. The critical distribution of water between plasma and interstitial fluid is maintained in part by the colloid osmotic pressure (COP) of plasma protein. COP includes the osmotic pressure exerted by plasma proteins and their associated electrolyte molecules. This force draws water into capillaries and balances the hydrostatic pressure driving water out (see Starling relationships described earlier in this chapter). Although the basic concept of Starling relationships is straightforward, in vivo application of these concepts is complicated by the heterogeneity of Starling forces within different tissues and the complexity of transvascular fluid dynamics. Despite these caveats, it is practical to say that the balance between intravascular COP and capillary hydrostatic pressure drives net fluid extravasation and forms the basis for intravenous colloid therapy.

Therapeutic colloids may be of two types: natural and synthetic. Natural colloids include whole blood, plasma, and albumin. Synthetic colloids, the focus of this discussion, include dextran 40, dextran 70, hetastarch, pentastarch, and oxypolygelatin. Therapeutic colloid solutions contain large particles and are retained within the vascular space more readily than crystalloids. As a result, smaller volumes of colloids cause greater volume expansion than crystalloids do. Initial tissue perfusion has been found to be better after volume expansion with colloids or combinations of colloids and crystalloids than with crystalloids alone (Funk and Baldinger 1995). The duration of this effect varies and is dependent upon many variables, including the species of animal, dose, specific colloid formulation, preinfusion intravascular volume status, and microvascular permeability (Hughes 2000).

The osmotic effect of colloid solutions is related to the number of particles rather than the size of particles in a solution. However, heterogeneity of particle size causes considerable complexity in the pharmacokinetics of these solutions. Synthetic colloids contain molecules that vary in molecular weight more than the molecules in a solution of a natural colloid such as albumin. After synthetic colloids are administered, the smaller molecules pass rapidly into the urine and are eliminated or move to the interstitium, negating their ability to attract water into the vasculature. Larger molecules remain in the circulation to exert COP until they are hydrolyzed by amylase or removed by the monocyte phagocytic system. Because of differences in particle behavior and in pharmacokinetic study design (e.g., duration of study, volume status of study subjects, volumes and rates of colloid administration), specific half-lives reported for colloids may vary considerably (Mathews 1998). Such variation may pose therapeutic problems since actual duration of action of colloids may not coincide with manufacturer estimates of the same.

Indications for colloid use include perfusion deficits, hypooncotic states, deficiency of blood components, and diseases that lead to systemic inflammatory response syndrome (SIRS). SIRS is a generalized inflammatory process with evidence of decreased organ perfusion. Sepsis may be the source of SIRS but other conditions may also result in generalized systemic pathophysiology (e.g., heat stroke, acute pancreatitis, neoplasia). Hallmarks of SIRS include alterations in temperature, heart rate, respiratory rate, PCO_2, and white blood cell count. Peripheral vasculature dilates, capillary permeability increases, and plasma proteins leak from affected vessels. The resulting hypoalbuminemia leads to a reduction in COP, loss of vascular volume, and hypoperfusion of tissues. High molecular weight colloids administered to SIRS patients are retained more effectively in leaky vessels and force retention of volume. Approximately 20–24% of crystalloid remains within the vasculature 1 hour after infusion into normal animals compared with 100% of the volume of infused colloid. Hence, colloids may initially expand the volume of the intravascular space approximately fourfold more than crystalloids (Hughes 2000).

Colloids are often included in fluid regimens for small-volume resuscitation (e.g., during traumatic, hypovolemic, or cardiogenic shock), improvement of microcirculatory flow and capillary integrity (e.g., SIRS), and management of ongoing hemorrhage. While colloids are useful in reestablishing vascular integrity, replenishment of interstitial and intracellular fluid deficits depends upon appropriate use of colloids and crystalloids in combination. Colloid administration typically reduces the required amount of crystalloid fluid by as much as 40–60% (Rudloff 1998). Care must be taken to adjust amounts and rates of all fluids administered to prevent intravascular volume overload and subsequent interstitial edema. Monitoring of colloid therapy ideally includes direct measurement of COP with a membrane osmometer in addition to measurement of traditional indices of perfusion and hydration.

Problems associated with colloid therapy may include dilutional effects caused by expansion of the intravascular space. Packed-cell volume, albumin concentration, serum potassium concentration, and amount of circulating coagulation factors typically decline following administration of synthetic colloids. Rapid volume expansion may be of greatest concern in patients with oliguric or anuric renal failure or congestive heart failure. Precipitation of acute renal failure has been reported in humans with dextran 40 (Ferraboli et al. 1997). Impairment of coagulation as a result of dilution of coagulation factors is thought to be of limited clinical relevance in veterinary medicine except in patients with preexisting coagulopathies. Anaphylactic or anaphylactoid reactions associated with colloids have been reported in humans. Concern has also been raised over the effects of selected colloids on reticuloendothelial function (Hughes 2000). Because cats are more likely to show signs of allergic reactions, especially when synthetic colloids are administered quickly, only small volumes infused at slow rates (5 ml/kg increments given over 5–10 minutes, repeated to effect up to 20 ml/kg) are recommended for use in this species.

Table 24.18 lists indications, dosages, and administration details for colloids commonly used to treat dogs. Albumin (66,000–69,000 daltons) accounts for 80% of the COP of the only natural colloid listed, plasma. Each gram of albumin can retain as much as 18 ml of fluid in the intravascular space, assuming infused albumin does not leak from damaged vessels. The intravascular half-life of albumin in plasma is approximately 16 hours (Mathews 1998). The three major categories of synthetic colloids are dextrans, hydroxyethyl starches, and gelatins. Dextrans are prepared from a macromolecular polysaccharide produced by bacterial fermentation of sucrose. Because these products represent a range of molecules with different molecular weights, they are described by a weight average molecular weight (MWw). MWw is defined as the sum of the number of molecules at each molecular weight times their mass divided by the total weight of the molecules. Dextran 70 (MWw = 70,000 daltons) is more commonly used and is available as a 6% solution in either 0.9% saline or 5.0% dextrose. Hydroxyethyl starches are derived from plant amylopectin and are modified by hydroxyethylation to reduce hydrolysis by amylase. The most commonly used product in this category, hetastarch (Hespan®), has a MWw of 100,000–300,000 daltons and is available as a 6% (6 g/dl) solution in 0.9% saline. Pentastarch has a narrower range of molecular weights, a shorter duration of action than hetastarch, and is only approved in this country for leukapheresis. Only one gelatin product, oxypolygelatin (Vetaplasma®) derived from bovine bone gelatin, is approved in this country as a plasma substitute for fluid resuscitation.

HYPERTONIC SOLUTIONS. For several decades, resuscitation of experimental and clinical animals suffering from shock has been attempted using hypertonic saline (HSS). Throughout the 1900s, studies have generally supported the benefits of HSS for transient restoration of cardiovascular function. Although a full understanding of the mechanism of action has been elusive, there is agreement that the primary benefits of HSS infusion result from plasma volume expansion. High circulating concentrations of sodium attract water into the vasculature from the interstitial and intracellular spaces and help to restore capillary flow and tissue perfusion. Cardiac output has been reported to increase as a result of increased preload, decreased afterload related to systemic and pulmonary vasodilation (Constable et al. 1995), increased adrenergic activity through release of catecholamines, and improved oxygen delivery to the heart (Tobias et al. 1993). Positive inotropy has also been reported but this remains a controversial point (Cambier et al. 1997). In vitro studies have shown that, at least during the initial treatment period, negative inotropy may predominate (Constable et al.

1994). All of the above effects are short-lived (peak occurs within approximately 1 hour) but resuscitative benefits may be prolonged by combination of HSS with colloids such as dextran 70. Ideally, rapid recovery of cardiovascular parameters occurs with administration of smaller volumes of HSS or HSS plus dextran (HSD) compared to crystalloids, thus decreasing the risk of edema related to volume overload. In addition to primary volume expansion, HSS is thought to invoke a lung vagal reflex important to circulatory control during hypovolemia. How much this reflex contributes to the cardiovascular effects of HSS infusion remains controversial. HSS may also have immunomodulatory effects that protect organs from oxidative injury and enhance cell-mediated immunity (Coimbra et al. 1996).

HSS use is indicated in the treatment of shock associated with hemorrhage (Bauer et al. 1993), trauma (Schertel et al. 1996), gastric-dilatation volvulus (Schertel et al. 1997), acute pancreatitis (Horton et al. 1989), burns (Horton et al. 1990), and sepsis (Fantoni et al. 1999; Maciel et al. 1998). The evidence for use of HSS in the first three of these is most compelling, with fewer studies unequivocally demonstrating advantage under specific study conditions associated with the other disorders. HSS has also been utilized in treatment of head injury since, like mannitol, HSS draws interstitial and intracellular water away from edematous tissues and into the vasculature (Prough and Zornow 1998). Regardless of the indication, HSS effects are transient, necessitating combination with crystalloids or colloids to achieve long-term resuscitative goals. Effects of HSS should be monitored by improvement in cardiovascular parameters correlated with increased perfusion as well as by assessment of mean arterial blood pressure, electrocardiogram, and electrolytes. Monitoring is aimed at preventing volume overload and electrolyte imbalances that may occur as a result of therapy.

HSS use is contraindicated in hypernatremic patients or those with increased plasma osmolality. Use in dehydrated animals is controversial since these patients frequently suffer from increases in both parameters. Studies that support HSS use in the presence of dehydration include those in which resuscitation with HSD of hypovolemic, diarrheic calves found this method to be at least as effective as others (Constable et al. 1996; Walker et al. 1998). In animals suffering from shock related to trauma and hemorrhage, two additional problems, hypokalemia and increased risk of rehemorrhaging, may be of concern. Rehemorrhage—bleeding caused by breakdown of clots in areas where hemorrhage has previously occurred—may be related to the sudden increase in cardiac output and arterial blood pressure associated with HSS resuscitation (Schertel and Tobias 2000). HSS may also dilute circulating coagulation factors and affect platelet function. As with colloids, these concerns may only be of practical significance if the patient suffers from preexisting coagulopathies or thrombocytopenia. Using a swine model of hemorrhagic shock, Dubick et al. (1993) demonstrated that the combination of 7.5% NaCl/6% dextran 70 did not significantly affect various measures of coagulation and platelet aggregation in their model. Studies continue to address the pros and cons of HSS use in various animal models and in clinical patients (Krausz 1995). Variation across species lines, differences in physiological circumstances of each study, and different views of cost versus benefit ratios may account for differing conclusions on the overall value of HSS treatment.

HSS is administered most effectively in combination with colloids or crystalloids in order to optimize resuscitative effects. 5% HSS, at a dose of 6–10 ml/kg, and 7–7.5% HSS, at a dose of 4–8 ml/kg, are administered at a rate of 1 ml/kg/min. Similar dosages may be used for HSD. More rapid administration rates may invoke a vagal-mediated hypotension, decreased heart rate, bronchoconstriction, and rapid, shallow breathing. To prepare 7% saline in 6% dextran 70, 33.0 g of anhydrous sodium chloride is added to a 500 ml bag of 6% dextran 70 in 0.9% saline. Half of the sodium chloride crystals are placed into the barrel of a 35 ml syringe and an adequate volume of dextran 70 solution is drawn into the syringe to dissolve the crystals. This solution is filtered through a 0.22 μm filter and is injected back into the bag of dextran 70. The procedure is repeated a second time to dissolve the remaining half of the sodium chloride (Schertel and Tobias 2000). Although a reported advantage of HSS is presumed sterility due to hypertonicity, St. Jean et al. (1997) have demonstrated the ability of bacteria to adapt and survive in the hypertonic environment of HSS. Hence, aseptic technique consistent with handling of all intravenous fluids should be followed.

BLOOD SUBSTITUTES. The term *oxygen carrier* (or *oxygen therapeutic*) has replaced the terms *blood substitute* and *red blood cell substitute* because it more appropriately describes the common oxygen-carrying role of these agents, which have some but not all of the functions of blood

(Wohl and Cotter 1995; Awasthi 2005). Two types of products have been developed for use as oxygen carriers—perfluorocarbons (PFCs) and hemoglobin-based oxygen carriers (HBOCs).

Perfluorochemicals. Perfluorochemicals are comprised of carbon and fluoride, are chemically inert, and are insoluble in water. They were originally developed as hydraulic fluids and transformer coolants but are used as oxygen carriers because of their ability to dissolve oxygen and carbon dioxide. PFCs have a high oxygen solubility and are emulsified with a surfactant for intravenous administration. Unemulsified PFCs can dissolve 40 to 56 ml of oxygen per 100 ml of liquid while emulsified PFC dissolves 5 to 8 ml O_2/100 ml. The oxygen content of PFC has a linear dependence on PO_2 and in order to transport physiologic quantities of oxygen a very high oxygen tension is needed. This factor limits the use of PFCs as oxygen carriers to situations where high oxygen tension can be maintained (e.g., surgery). PFCs have a short intravascular half-life, can activate the complement cascade, and have a slow elimination (Rentko 1992; Wohl and Cotter 1995).

Fluosal-DA is a 20% (by weight) emulsion licensed by the FDA for use in humans during coronary angioplasty surgery. PFC can also be potentially used during tumor radiation therapy, vascular surgery, extracorporeal organ perfusion, peritoneal lavage, and carbon monoxide poisoning (Rentko 1992; Wohl and Cotter 1995).

The half-life of perfluorochemicals depends upon the molecular size and structure of the agent. PFCs are expired in the lungs after phagocytosis by fixed macrophages, primarily in the liver and spleen (Wohl and Cotter 1995).

Hemoglobin-based Oxygen Carriers (HBOCs). HBOCs are useful for replacing red blood cells in anemic humans and animals. These products contain purified hemoglobin, removed from red blood cells and suspended in solution, and are especially useful when compatible red blood cells are not available. These solutions can pass through microcirculation more readily than red blood cells making them ideal for treating severe anemia or hypovolemia due to acute hemorrhage or poor blood flow distribution (Callan and Rentko 2003; Lichtenberger 2004).

HBOCs are developed from animal or human hemoglobin. Hemoglobin is an iron-containing protein composed of a tetramer of two α-chains and two β-chains with a heme molecule within the folds of each chain. When hemoglobin is administered, it breaks down into its constituent chains and has toxic effects (Awasthi 2005). The dissociation is also associated with a short circulation half-life (Rentko 1992). Small-sized, modified hemoglobin chains tend to extravasate, sequester nitric oxide and cause vasoconstriction (Awasthi 2005).

Cross-linking, glutaraldehyde-polymerization, or polyethylene glycolation of hemoglobin prevents dissociation, improves the circulation half-life, and increases the size of the molecule to reduce extravasation (Rentko 1992; Awasthi 2005). The amount of cross-linking, polymerization, or polymer-linking also affects the viscosity of HBOC solutions. HBOCs cause an increase in plasma hemoglobin concentration and act as colloids to cause volume expansion (Wohl and Cotter 1995; Awasthi 2005).

Encapsulation is another technique used to stabilize hemoglobin. Hemoglobin can be encapsulated in nonantigenic phospholipids (liposomes), which prevents glomerular filtration and increases the half-life compared to free hemoglobin. Initial problems associated with encapsulated hemoglobin are related to reticuloendothelial stimulation, contamination with endotoxins, and rapid clearance (Rentko 1992; Awasthi 2005).

The only commercially available HBOC approved by the FDA for use in veterinary species is Oxyglobin® (Biopure Corporation, Cambridge, MA). Oxyglobin® (hemoglobin glutamer-200 [bovine]), approved for use in the United States for treatment of anemia in dogs, is given as a single dose (10–30 ml/kg, 1.3–3.9 g/kg) administered at a rate no greater than 10 ml/kg/hour (Hamilton et al. 2001; Callan and Rentko 2003). This product is a purified and chemically modified bovine hemoglobin, which is stable at room temperature, has a shelf-life of 3 years, and has a similar oxygen-carrying capacity as endogenous hemoglobin (Senior 1998; Callan and Rentko 2003; Awasthi 2005). The hemoglobin is polymerized to glutaraldehyde and is reconstituted in a modified lactated Ringer's solution (Hamilton et al. 2001; Lichtenberger 2004). Oxyglobin® does not need to be cross-matched and does not have the potential to transmit disease (Lichtenberger 2004); therefore, it may be useful in emergencies when there is not time to cross-match or prepare blood products (Lanevschi and Wardrop 2001).

The product has an osmolality of 300 mOsm/kg, lower viscosity than whole blood, hemoglobin concentration of 13 g/dl, colloidal oncotic pressure of 20–25 mm Hg, and a half-life of around 36 hours (30 to 40 hours) (Rentko 1992; Senior 1998; Callan and Rentko 2003;

Lichtenberger 2004). It has a pH of 7.8 and expands the intravascular space by at least its own volume (Lichtenberger 2004). Oxyglobin® is not associated with renal toxicity, and there is no clinical evidence of allergic reaction with repeated doses (Rentko 1992). Hamilton et al. (2001) demonstrated that multiple administrations of Oxyglobin® (nine administrations over 50 weeks) in eight splenectomized dogs produced neither adverse physiologic effects nor adverse pathologic effects. Although most dogs produced Oxyglobin®-specific IgG antibodies, no anaphylactic or anaphylactoid reactions were noted and the development of IgG antibodies did not affect the oxygen-carrying capacity (Senior 1998; Hamilton et al. 2001).

The oxygen affinity of Oxyglobin® is dependent on chloride ion concentration rather than the concentration of 2,3-diphosphoglycerate (2,3-DPG) (Lichtenberger 2004). In humans and dogs the oxygen affinity of hemoglobin is determined by the interaction of hemoglobin and 2,3-DPG in red blood cells (Rentko 1992). The levels of 2,3-DPG decrease in blood stored over 1 week, which leads to increased oxygen binding and decreased delivery of oxygen to the tissues. Compared to canine blood, Oxyglobin® has a lower oxygen affinity enhancing oxygen delivery to tissues (Lichtenberger 2004). One gram of hemoglobin from Oxyglobin® can deliver the same amount of oxygen to tissues as 3 to 4 grams of red blood cell hemoglobin (Callan and Rentko 2003).

Twenty-four hours after being opened, the product must be discarded due to the production of methemoglobin and to avoid bacterial contamination (Callan and Rentko 2003; Lichtenberger 2004). Oxyglobin® is stored in its deoxygenated state and becomes oxygenated when it passes through the lungs (Senior 1998). The primary effects of Oxyglobin® last about 24 hours, and 90–95% percent of Oxyglobin® is eliminated in 5 to 9 days (Senior 1998; Callan and Rentko 2003; Lichtenberger 2004).

The volume of distribution, plasma clearance, and terminal elimination half-life of Oxyglobin® are dose dependent, and administration of this product increases plasma hemoglobin concentrations. Medications should not be added to the bag, and fluids and drugs should not be administered through the same infusion set as Oxyglobin® (Callan and Rentko 2003).

Hemopure® (hemoglobin glutamer-250 [bovine]) (Biopure Corporation, Cambridge, MA) is a glutaraldehyde-polymerized bovine hemoglobin similar to Oxyglobin® approved in South Africa for use in humans (Callan and Rentko 2003; Awasthi 2005). Hemopure® can transport oxygen, needs no refrigeration, is compatible with all blood types, has a long shelf life, and has a minimized risk of disease transmission (Fitzpatrick et al. 2005). Fitzpatrick et al. (2005) demonstrated in laboratory studies that Hemopure® reversed anaerobic metabolism in the treatment of hemorrhagic shock without end-organ damage. The decreased urine output noted in animals given Hemopure® in laboratory studies has been attributed to the smaller volumes needed to resuscitate the animals and has not been associated with long-term decreased renal function (Fitzpatrick et al. 2005). Animal studies with Hemopure® have demonstrated that it can carry oxygen more efficiently than red blood cells on a per-gram basis (Hamilton et al. 2001).

PolyHeme® (Northfield Laboratories, Evanston, IL) is a glutaraldehyde-polymerized human hemoglobin-based product in development (Awasthi 2005).

Hemospan® (MP4 or MPEG-Hb) (Sangart, San Diego, CA) is a polyethylene glycolated hemoglobin in clinical trials (Awasthi 2005; Björkholm et al. 2005). MP4 is very viscous, made from stroma-free human hemoglobin, has a high oxygen affinity, and is reported to not cause vasoconstriction (Awasthi 2005; Björkholm et al. 2005). Based on in vitro and animal studies, the lack of vasoconstriction (i.e., avoidance of engaging autoregulatory vasoconstriction) is thought to be related to increased molecular size and oxygen affinity, which lead to a decreased diffusive oxygen transfer in the plasma space (Björkholm et al. 2005).

Cross-linking or polymerization stabilizes the structure of HBOCs so that there is almost no urinary excretion. Some modified hemoglobin may still be deposited in renal tubules. Other sites of deposition for HBOCs are lymph, liver, and spleen. HBOCs use fixed macrophages in their metabolism, which may impair macrophage phagocytic ability (Wohl and Cotter 1995).

Adverse Effects. One of the shortcomings of early HBOCs was nephrotoxicity associated with contamination with red blood cell stromal elements. Current HBOCs are ultrapurified to prevent contamination (Callan and Rentko 2003).

HBOCs should be used cautiously in euvolemic or hypervolemic patients to avoid volume overload related to the colloidal effects of HBOCs. Cats and small mammals appear to be more predisposed to pulmonary edema following volume overload (Lichtenberger 2004).

Circulatory overload is dependent on rate of infusion and is most marked in dogs receiving greater than 10 ml/kg/hour and cats receiving more than 5 ml/kg/hour (Wohl and Cotter 1995; Callan and Rentko 2003). Because HBOCs are colloids, they should be used cautiously in patients with preexisting cardiopulmonary disease (Callan and Rentko 2003).

Ischemia-reperfusion injury is common to all HBOCs and occurs due to production of free radicals by hemoglobin and its oxidation products (Awasthi 2005). HBOCs can provide oxygen and iron as electron donors leading to oxygen radical production and tissue damage (Wohl and Cotter 1995).

Anaphylactic reactions are a possibility (though not documented in clinical or research cases) with repeated administration of heterologous HBOCs (Wohl and Cotter 1995; Callan and Rentko 2003; Awasthi 2005). If hypersensitivity occurs, infusion of the HBOC should be discontinued, and appropriate resuscitation measures should be implemented (e.g., crystalloids, epinephrine).

Adverse effects of HBOCs in dogs, cats, and small mammals are discoloration of mucous membranes, sclera, and urine (Wohl and Cotter 1995; Callan and Rentko 2003; Lichtenberger 2004). In bird species no discoloration of urine or mucous membranes is noted. Measurements of colorimetric lab tests are affected for 24–72 hours after Oxyglobin® administration (Lichtenberger 2004).

Hypertension can also be an adverse effect of hemoglobin solutions. HBOCs have a pressor effect that is attributed to sequestration, or scavenging, of nitric oxide following extravasation, but other mechanisms may be involved including endothelin release and sensitization of peripheral α-adrenergic receptors (Callan and Rentko 2003; Fitzpatrick et al. 2005). Polymerization or polyethylene glycolation of hemoglobin decreases extravasation but does not completely eliminate its pressor effect (Awasthi 2005; Fitzpatrick et al. 2005).

It is beyond the scope of this chapter to compare treatments for hemorrhagic shock, but much has been written on the topic, including therapy with blood substitutes. In a recent study comparing autologous/shed blood, hemoglobin-based oxygen carrier/Oxyglobin, crystalloid/saline, colloid/Hespan (6% hetastarch), and vasopressin in a canine hemorrhagic shock model (50–55% total blood loss with a mean arterial pressure of 45–50 mmHg as a clinical criterion), all resuscitation modalities except vasopressin restored microvascular and systemic function changes close to prehemorrhagic values. Autologous blood was the only treatment that restored oxygenation changes to prehemorrhagic levels (Cheung et al. 2007).

SPECIAL TOPICS

HORSES. Horses present some special problems in acid-base management. In cases of severe diarrhea, shock, and intestinal obstruction, the horse seems predisposed to severe metabolic acidosis (Waterman 1977). Electrolyte disorders common in horses with acute abdominal disease have recently been reviewed (Borer and Corley 2006 a,b). Respiratory acidosis is a very common sequel to closed-circuit inhalation anesthesia in the horse. An abnormally low concentration of Na^+ is a common problem in dehydrated horses. Severe hypokalemia, with blood K^+ values less than 2.5–3 mEq/l, may require treatment with solutions high in K^+. Dangerous hyperkalemia, with blood levels greater than approximately 7 mEq/l, may be associated with acidosis in foals. Prompt correction of the acidosis will usually correct the hyperkalemia.

CATTLE. Ruminants also present special fluid and electrolyte management problems. When a diagnosis of abomasal disease is coupled with an obvious fluid balance disorder, hypochloremia, hypokalemia, and alkalosis are usually present. These should be confirmed by appropriate laboratory tests. Grain overloading will result in severe dehydration and metabolic acidosis.

Calf diarrhea also results in severe dehydration and metabolic acidosis, with dangerous hyperkalemia in some cases. If hyperkalemia exists, one must guard against administration of even more K^+. When dealing with herbivores, it is important to remember that normal feed contains high levels of K^+. When these animals are anorexic, they frequently become K^+ depleted. The best way to replace K^+ deficits is by consumption of hay or grass, but K^+ must be added parenterally when the situation dictates. A wide variety of electrolyte mixtures containing K^+ are available for oral administration.

Intravenous administration of 5% dextrose alone or with isotonic sodium bicarbonate to hypernatremic, diarrheic calves has been preliminarily observed to provide benefit (Abutarbush and Petrie 2007). Despite the fact that the average reduction rate of serum sodium concentration in these calves (n=5) was about four times that recommended, no complications were reported in this small cohort. Further studies are needed to determine how this approach compares with other therapies.

ANESTHETIC AND SURGICAL EFFECTS. General anesthesia may exert several effects on water, electrolyte, and acid-base balance. Almost all general anesthetics induce some degree of Ca^{++} channel blockade, resulting in some degree of vasodilation and myocardial depression. The end effect can be a reduction in cardiac output and/or alterations in organ blood flow. Arterial pressures are frequently lowered in a dose-dependent manner, and GFR may be affected. The commonly used inhalation anesthetic agents (halothane, enflurane, and isoflurane) all cause direct systemic vasodilation. Narcotics and some muscle relaxants also can cause vasodilation. As a result of the vasodilation, fluid requirements may be increased during the course of the surgical procedure to maintain adequate blood pressure and cardiac output. After recovery from the general anesthetic, when vascular tone is normalized, the patient may be volume overloaded and hypertensive. Fluid loss may also increase during general anesthesia as a result of tracheal intubation and/or artificial ventilation. Normal mechanisms for the humidification of inspired air are bypassed, and the cold, dry gases from the anesthesia machine can cause a considerable amount of fluid loss. Open body cavities allow for evaporative losses. Third spacing may occur with extravasation of fluid from the vascular to the extravascular, extracellular spaces. If extravasated fluid is replaced to maintain adequate circulatory volumes, the patient with inadequate cardiac reserve or poor renal function may suffer fluid overload and congestive heart failure when postoperative redistribution of the fluid back into the circulation occurs (Gold 1992).

Surgical injury can result in significant reductions in serum albumin, total proteins, and total lymphocyte counts. These decreases are typically greater following abdominal surgery. The decreases have been found to be primarily caused by the volume of IV fluids frequently required for resuscitation and to compensate for blood loss.

REFERENCES

Abutarbush, S. M., and Petrie, L. 2007. Treatment of hypernatremia in neonatal calves with diarrhea. Can Vet J 48:184–187.

Adolph, E. F. 1939. Measurements of water drinking in dogs. Am J Physiol 124:75–86.

Adrogue, H. J., and Madias, N. E. 1981. Changes in plasma potassium concentration during acute acid-base disturbances. Am J Med 71:456–467.

Anderson, R. S. 1983. Fluid balance and diet. In Proceedings of the Seventh Kal Kan Symposium, pp. 19–24. Kal Kan Foods, Inc.

Arieff, A. I., and Guisado, R. 1976. Effects on the central nervous system of hypernatremic and hyponatremic states. Kidney Int 10:104–116.

Astrup, P., Jorgensen, K., Andersen, O. S., and Engel, K. 1960. The acid-base metabolism. Lancet 1:1035–1039.

Awasthi V. 2005. Pharmaceutical aspects of hemoglobin-based oxygen carriers. Curr Drug Deliv 2(2):133–142.

Bailey, J. E., and Pablo, L. S. 1998. Practical approach to acid-base disorders. Vet Clin N Am, Sm An Pract 28:645–662.

Bastani, B., Purcell, H., Hemken, P., et al. 1991. Expression and distribution of renal vacuolar proton-translocating adenosine triphosphatases in response to chronic acid and alkali loads in the rat. J Clin Invest 88:126.

Bauer, M., Marzi, I., Ziegenfuss, T., et al. 1993. Comparative effects of crystalloid and small volume hypertonic hyperoncotic fluid resuscitation on hepatic microcirculation after hemorrhagic shock. Circ Shock 40:187–193.

Benjamin, E., Oropello, J. M., Abalos, A. M., et al. 1994. Effects of acid-base correction on hemodynamics, oxygen dynamics, and resuscitability in severe canine hemorrhagic shock. Crit Care Med 22:1616–1623.

Björkholm, M., Fagrell, B., Przybelski, R., Winslow, N., Young, M., and Winslow, RM. 2005. A phase I single blind clinical trial of a new oxygen transport agent (MP4), human hemoglobin modified with maleimide-activated polyethylene glycol. Haematologica 90(4): 505–515.

Black, R. M. 1993. Disorders of acid-base and potassium balance. In E. Rubenstein and D. D. Federman, eds., Scientific American Medicine, pp. 1–24. New York: Scientific American.

Borer, K., and Corley, K. T. T. 2006a. Electrolyte disorders in horses with colic. Part 1: potassium and magnesium. Equine Veterinary Education. Eq Vet J 18:266–271.

———. 2006b. Electrolyte disorders in horses with colic. Part 2: calcium, sodium, chloride and phosphate. Equine Veterinary Education. Eq Vet J 18:320–325.

Brown, L. W., and Feigin, R. D. 1994. Bacterial meningitis: fluid balance and therapy. Ped Ann 23:93–98.

Button, C. 1979. Metabolic and electrolyte disturbances in acute canine babesiosis. JAVMA 175:475–479.

Callan, M. B., and Rentko, V. T. 2003. Clinical application of a hemoglobin-based oxygen-carrying solution. Vet Clin N Am, Sm An Pract 33(6):1277–1293.

Cambier, C., Ratz, V., Rollin, F., Frans, A., Clerbaux, T., and Gustin, P. 1997. The effects of hypertonic saline in healthy and diseased animals. Vet Res Commun 21:303–316.

Cantone, A., Wang, T., Pica, A., Simeoni, M., and Capasso, G. 2006. Use of transgenic mice in acid-base balance studies. J Nephrol 19:121–127.

Cheung, A. T. W, To, P. L. D., Chan, D. M, Ramanujam, S., Barbosa, M. A., Chen, P. C. Y., Driessen, B., Jahr, J. S., and Gunther, R. A. 2007. Comparison of treatment modalities for hemorrhagic shock. Artif Cells Blood Substit Immob Biotechnol 35:173–190.

Clausen, T., and Flatman, J. A. 1987. Effect of insulin and epinephrine on Na^+-K^+ and glucose transport in soleus muscle. Am J Physiol 242: E492–499.

Cohen, R. D. 1995. New evidence in the bicarbonate controversy. Appl Cardiopul Pathophysiol 5:135–138.

Coimbra, R., Junger, W. G., and Hoyt, D. B. 1996. Hypertonic saline resuscitation restores hemorrhage induced immunosuppression by decreasing prostaglandin E2 and interleukin 4 production. J Surg Res 64:203–209.

Constable, P. D. 1997. A simplified strong ion model for acid-base equilibria: application to horse plasma. J Appl Physiol 83:297–311.

———. 1999. Clinical assessment of acid-base status: strong ion difference theory. Vet Clin N Am, Food An Pract 15:447–471.

Constable, P. D., Gohar, H. M., Morin, D. E., and Thurmon, J. C. 1996. Use of hypertonic saline-dextran solution to resuscitate hypovolemic calves with diarrhea. Am J Vet Res 57:97–104.

Constable, P. D., Muir, W. W., III, and Binkley, P. F. 1994. Hypertonic saline is a negative inotropic agent in normovolemic dogs. Am J Physiol 267:H667–H677.

———. 1995. Effect of hypertonic saline solution on left ventricular afterload in normovolemic dogs. Am J Vet Res 56:1513–1521.

Constable, P. D., Streeter, R. N., Koenig, G., Perkins, N. R., Gohar, H. M., and Morin, D. E. 1997. Determinants and utility of the anion gap in predicting hyperlactatemia in cattle. J Vet Int Med 11:71–79.

Constable, P. D., Walker, P. G., Morin, D. E., and Foreman, J. H. 1998. Clinical and laboratory assessment of hydration status of neonatal calves with diarrhea. JAVMA 212:991–996.

Cornelius, L. M., Finco, D. R., and Culver, D. H. 1978. Physiologic effects of rapid infusion of Ringer's lactate solution into dogs. Am J Vet Res 39:1185–1190.

DiBartola, S. P., ed. 1992a. Fluid Therapy in Small Animal Practice. Philadelphia: W. B. Saunders.

———. 1992b. Renal physiology. In S. P. DiBartola, ed., Fluid Therapy in Small Animal Practice, pp. 35–56. Philadelphia: W. B. Saunders.

———. 1992c. Disorders of sodium and water: hypernatremia and hyponatremia. In S. P DiBartola, ed., Fluid Therapy in Small Animal Practice, pp. 57–88. Philadelphia: W. B. Saunders.

———. 1992d. Introduction to acid-base disorders. In S. P. DiBartola, ed., Fluid Therapy in Small Animal Practice, pp. 207–209. Philadelphia: W. B. Saunders.

———. 1998. Hyponatremia. Vet Clin N Am, Sm An Pract 28:515–532.

DiBartola, S. P., and Autran de Morais, H. S. 1992. Disorders of potassium: hypokalemia and hyperkalemia. In S. P. DiBartola, ed., Fluid Therapy in Small Animal Practice, pp. 89–115. Philadelphia: W. B. Saunders.

Dubick, M. A., Kilani, A. F., Summary, J. J., et al. 1993. Further evaluation of the effects of 7.5% sodium chloride/6% Dextran-70 (HSD) administration on coagulation and platelet aggregation in hemorrhaged and euvolemic swine. Circ Shock 40:200–205.

Emmett, M., and Narins, R. G. 1977. Clinical use of the anion gap. Medicine 56:38–54.

Ephrati, C., and Lemeij, T. 1997. Rectal fluid therapy in birds: an experimental study. J Avian Med Surg 11:4–6.

Fantoni, D., Auler, J., Futema, F., Cortopassi, S., Migliati, E., Faustino, M., deOliveira, C. 1999. Intravenous administration of hypertonic sodium chloride solution with dextran or isotonic sodium chloride solution for treatment of septic shock secondary to pyometra in dogs. JAVMA 215:1283–1287.

Ferraboli, R., Malheiro, P. S., and Abdukader, R. C. 1997. Anuric acute renal failure caused by dextran 40 administration. Ren Fail 19: 303–306.

Fitzpatrick, C. M., Biggs, K. L., Atkins, B. Z., Quance-Fitch, F. J., Dixon, P. S., Savage, S. A., Jenkins, D. H., and Kerby, J. D. 2005. Prolonged low-volume resuscitation with HBOC-201 in a large-animal survival model of controlled hemorrhage. J Trauma 59(2):273–283.

Funk, W., and Baldinger, V. 1995. Microcirculatory perfusion during volume therapy: a comparative study using crystalloid or colloid in awake animals. Anesthesiology 82:975–982.

Gabow, P. A. 1985. Disorders associated with an altered anion gap. Kidney Int 27:472–483.

Garella, S., Chang, B., and Kahn, S. I. 1979. Alterations of hydrogen ion homeostasis in pure potassium depletion: studies in rats and dogs during the recovery phase. J Lab Clin Med 93:321–331.

Geiger, H., Hahner, U., Meissner, M., et al. 1992. Parathyroid hormone modulates the release of atrial natriuretic peptide during acute volume expansion. Am J Nephrol 12:249–264.

Gold, M. S. 1992. Perioperative fluid management. Crit Care Clin 8:409–421.

Greco, D. S. 1998. The distribution of body water and general approach to the patient. Vet Clin N Am, Sm An Pract 28:473–482.

Gregor, R., and Velazquez, H. 1987. The cortical thick ascending limb and early distal convoluted tubule in the urine concentrating mechanism. Kidney Int 31:590.

Gross, D. R. 1994. Animal models in cardiovascular research. Dordrecht: Kluwer.

Halperin, F. A., Cheema-Dhadli, S., Chen, C. B., and Halperin, M. L. 1996. Alkali therapy extends the period of survival during hypoxia: studies in rats. Am J Physiol 271 (Regulatory Integrative Comp Physiol 40):R381–R387.

Hamilton, R. G., Kelly, N., Gawryl, M. S., and Rentko, V. T. 2001. Absence of immunopathology associated with repeated IV administration of bovine HB-hased oxygen carrier in dogs. Transfusion 41(2):219–225.

Hamm, D., and Hicks, W. J. 1975. A new oral electrolyte in calf scours therapy. Vet Med Small Anim Clin 70:279–282.

Hardy, R. M. 1989. Hypernatremia. Vet Clin N Am, Sm An Pract 19:231–240.

Horton, J. W., Dunn, C. W., Burnweit, C. S., and Wlaker, P. B. 1989. Hypertonic saline-dextran resuscitation of acute canine bile-induced pancreatitis. Am J Surg 158:48–56.

Horton, J. W., White, J., and Baxter, C. R. 1990. Hypertonic saline dextran resuscitation of thermal injury. Ann Surg 211:301–311.

Hughes, D. 2000. Fluid therapy with macromolecular plasma volume expanders. In S. P. DiBartola, ed., Fluid Therapy in Small Animal Practice, 2nd ed., pp. 483–495. Philadelphia: W. B. Saunders.

Jenkins, D. H., and Kerby, J. D. 2005. Prolonged low-volume resuscitation with HBOC-201 in a large-animal survival model of controlled hemorrhage. J Trauma 59(2):273–283.

Katz, M. A. 1973. Hyperglycemia-induced hyponatremia: calculation of expected serum sodium depression. N Engl J Med 289:843–844.

Kohn, C. W., and DiBartola, S. P. 1992. Composition and distribution of body fluids in dogs and cats. In S. P. DiBartola, ed., Fluid Therapy in Small Animal Practice, pp. 1–34. Philadelphia: W. B. Saunders.

Krausz, M. M. 1995. Controversies in shock research: hypertonic resuscitation, pros and cons. Shock 3:69–72.

Landry D. W., and Oliver, J. A. 1992.The ATP-sensitive K^+ channel mediates hypotension in endotoxemia and hypoxic lactic acidosis in the dog. J Clin Invest 89:2071.

Lanevschi, A., and Wardrop, K. J. 2001. Principles of transfusion medicine in small animals. Can Vet J 42(6):447–454.

Lewis, L. D., and Morris, M. L. 1987. Small Animal Clinical Nutrition, 3rd ed., pp. 2–22. Topeka: Mark Morris Assoc.

Lichtenberger, M. 2004. Transfusion medicine in exotic pets. Clin Tech Sm An Pract 19(2):88–95.

Looney, A. L., Ludders, J., Erb, H. N., Gleed, R., and Moon, P. 1998. Use of a handheld device for analysis of blood electrolyte concentrations and blood gas partial pressures in dogs and horses. JAVMA 213:526–530.

Maciel, F., Mook, M., Zhang, H., and Vincent, J.-L. 1998. Comparison of hypertonic with isotonic saline hydroxyethyl starch solution on oxygen extraction capabilities during endotoxic shock. Shock 9:33–39.

Marks, S. L. 1998. Hypernatremia and hypertonic syndromes. Vet Clin N Am, Sm An Pract 28:533–543.

Mathews, K. A. 1998. The various types of parenteral fluids and their indications. Vet Clin N Am, Sm An Pract 28:483–513.

McEvoy, G. K. 1997. Electrolyte solutions. In G. K. McEvoy, ed., American Hospital Formulary Service Drug Information, pp. 1991–1994. Bethesda: American Society of Health-System Pharmacists.

Monafo, W. W. 1993. The second quinquennium: 1974–1978. J Burn Care Rehabil 14:236–237.

Muir, W. W., and DiBartola, S. P. 1983. Fluid therapy. In R. W. Kirk, ed., Current Veterinary Therapy VIII, pp. 28–40. Philadelphia: W. B. Saunders.

Naylor, J. M. 1996. Neonatal ruminant diarrhea. In B. P. Smith, ed., Large Animal Internal Medicine, 2nd ed., p. 403. St. Louis: Mosby Yearbook.

O'Brien, D. 1995. Metabolic dysfunction and the CNS. In Proc 13th Ann Vet Med Forum, American College of Veterinary Internal Medicine, Lake Buena Vista, FL, p. 447.

O'Connor, W. J., and Potts, D. J. 1969. The external water exchanges of normal laboratory dogs. Q J Exp Physiol 54:244–265.

Oh, M. S., and Carrol, J. H. 1977. The anion gap. N Engl J Med 297:814–817.

Oster, J. R., Perez, G. O., Castro, A., et al. 1980. Plasma potassium response to acute metabolic acidosis induced by mineral and nonmineral acids. Miner Electrolyte Metab 4:28–36.

Perez, G. O., Kem, D. C., Oster, J. R., et al. 1980. Effect of acute metabolic acidosis on the renin-aldosterone system. J Lab Clin Med 96: 371–378.

Phillips, S. L., and Polzin, D. J. 1998. Clinical disorders of potassium homeostasis. Vet Clin N Am, Sm An Pract 28:545–564.

Prough, D. S., and Zornow, M. H. 1998. Mannitol: an old friend on the skids? Crit Care Med 26:997–998.

Rentko, V.T. 1992. Red blood cell substitutes. Transfus Med 4(4):647–651.

Rose, B. D. 1989. Clinical Physiology of Acid-Base and Electrolytes, 3rd ed., pp. 248–260. New York: McGraw-Hill.

———. 1994. Clinical Physiology of Acid-Base and Electrolytes, 4th ed., pp. 73–75, 500–560, 651–694. New York: McGraw-Hill.

———. In press. Clinical Physiology of Acid-Base and Electrolytes. 5th ed. New York: McGraw-Hill.

Roussel, A. J. 1990. Fluid therapy in mature cattle. Vet Clin N Am, Food An Pract 6:111–123.

Rudloff, E., and Kirby, R. 1998. The critical need for colloids: administering colloids effectively. Compend Contin Educ Pract Vet 20:27–43.

Russell, K. E., Hansen, B. D., and Stevens, J. B. 1996. Strong ion difference approach to acid-base imbalances with clinical applications in dogs and cats. Vet Clin N Am, Sm An Pract 26:1185–1201.

Schertel, R. R., Allen, D. A., Muir, W. W, Bourman, J. D., and DeHoff, W. D. 1997. Evaluation of a hypertonic saline-dextran solution for treatment of dogs with shock induced by gastric dilatation-volvulus. JAVMA 210:226–230.

Schertel, R. R., Allen, D. A., Muir, W. W., and Hansen, B. D. 1996. Evaluation of a hypertonic sodium chloride/dextran solution for treatment of traumatic shock in dogs. JAVMA 208:366–370.

Schertel, E. R., and Tobias, T. A. 2000. Hypertonic fluid therapy. In S. P. DiBartola, ed., Fluid Therapy in Small Animal Practice, 2nd ed., pp. 496–506. Philadelphia: W. B. Saunders.

Senior, K. 1998. Blood substitute receives FDA approval for veterinary use. Molec Med Today 4(4):139.

Smith, C. R. 1970. Unpublished data.

Stewart, P. A. 1978. Independent and dependent variables of acid-base control. Respir Physiol 33:9–26.

———. 1983. Modern quantitative acid-base chemistry. Can J Physiol Pharmacol 61:1444–1461.

St. Jean, G., Chengappa, M. M., and Staats, J. 1997. Survival of selected bacteria and fungi in hypertonic (7.2%) saline. Aust Vet J 75: 137–138.

Sun, X., Iles, M., and Weissman, C. 1993. Physiologic variables and fluid resuscitation in the post-operative intensive care unit patient. Crit Care Med 21:555–561.

Thier, S. O. 1987. Diuretic mechanisms as a guide to therapy. Hosp Pract 22:81–100.

Temol, K., Rudloff, E., Lichtenberger, M., Kirby, R. 2004. Hypernatremia in critically ill cats: evaluation and treatment. Compend Contin Educ Pract Vet. 26:434–445.

Tobias, T. A., Schertel, E. R., Schmall, L. M., et al. 1993. Comparative effects of 7.5% NaCl in 6% Dextran 70 and 0.9% NaCl on cardiorespiratory parameters after cardiac output-controlled resuscitation from canine hemorrhagic shock. Circ Shock 398:139–146.

Vander, A. J., Sherman, J. H., and Luciano, D. S. 1994. Human Physiology: The Mechanisms of Body Function. 6th ed. New York: McGraw-Hill.

Wachtel, T. L., McCahan, G. R., and Monafo, W. W. 1977. Fluid resuscitation in a porcine burn shock model. J Surg Res 23:405–414.

Walker, P. G., Constable, P. D., Morin, D. E., Foreman, J. H., Drackley, J. K., and Thurmon, J. C. 1998. Comparison of hypertonic saline-dextran solution and lactated Ringer's solution for resuscitating severely dehydrated calves with diarrhea. JAVMA 213:113–121.

Waterman, A. 1977. A review of the diagnosis and treatment of fluid and electrolyte disorders in the horse. Equine Vet J 9:43–48.

Wohl, J. S. and Cotter, S. M. 1995. Blood substitutes: oxygen-carrying acellular fluids. Vet Clin N Am, Sm An Pract 25(6):1417–1440.

CHAPTER

25

DIURETICS

DEBORAH T. KOCHEVAR

This chapter presents the physiological basis for fluid and electrolyte balance, including discussion of selected renal mechanisms for regulation of water, sodium, chloride, potassium, hydrogen, and bicarbonate. In this chapter these concepts will be extended in order to understand the mechanism of action, therapeutic uses, and side effects of diuretic agents. Diuretic agents are used to mobilize tissue fluid, most often in the treatment of edema of cardiac, renal, or hepatic origin. The history of diuretics dates back to consumption by Paleolithic humans of caffeine-containing plants. Besides xanthine derivatives such as caffeine, osmotic diuretics were clinically important prior to the 20th century. The use of mercurial diuretics, now therapeutically obsolete, began in the early 1900s and was followed by introduction of the first modern diuretic, acetazolamide, in the mid-1950s. By the late 1950s and early 1960s the formulary of modern diuretics included chlorothiazide, furosemide, and potassium-sparing diuretics (Morrison 1997). These drugs and their relatives constitute the mainstays of diuretic treatment.

RENAL PHYSIOLOGY

NEPHRON FUNCTION. Knowledge of renal anatomy and physiology is essential to understanding the mechanism of action of diuretic drugs. Although a thorough review of these topics is beyond the scope of this text, a brief overview of nephron function is provided. The basic functional unit of the kidney is the nephron, which consists of a filtering apparatus, the glomerulus, connected to an extended tubular structure that reabsorbs and conditions the glomerular ultrafiltrate to produce urine. Each kidney is composed of thousands of nephron units. Figure 25.1 is a schematic drawing of a single nephron unit, indicating the broad subdivisions of nephron segments and the sites of action of diuretic agents. This diagram provides the simplest nomenclature for nephron segments. As knowledge of the function and epithelial morphology of each segment has increased, the tubular portion of the nephron has been subdivided into approximately 14 shorter segments referred to by a standardized nomenclature (Kriz and Kaissling 1992).

Formation of urine starts in the glomerulus, where a portion of plasma water is filtered through fenestrated glomerular capillary endothelial cells, a basement membrane, and, finally, filtration slit diaphragms formed by the visceral epithelial cells that cover the basement membrane on its urinary space side. The filtrate collects in Bowman's space, a double-walled invagination that forms a cup around the glomerular capillaries. From Bowman's capsule the filtered fluid passes into the proximal tubule and begins its passage through the renal tubular system. Small solutes are actively filtered with plasma water while larger elements, such as protein and macromolecules, are retained by the glomerular filter. The rate of filtration in each nephron (referred to as the single-nephron glomerular

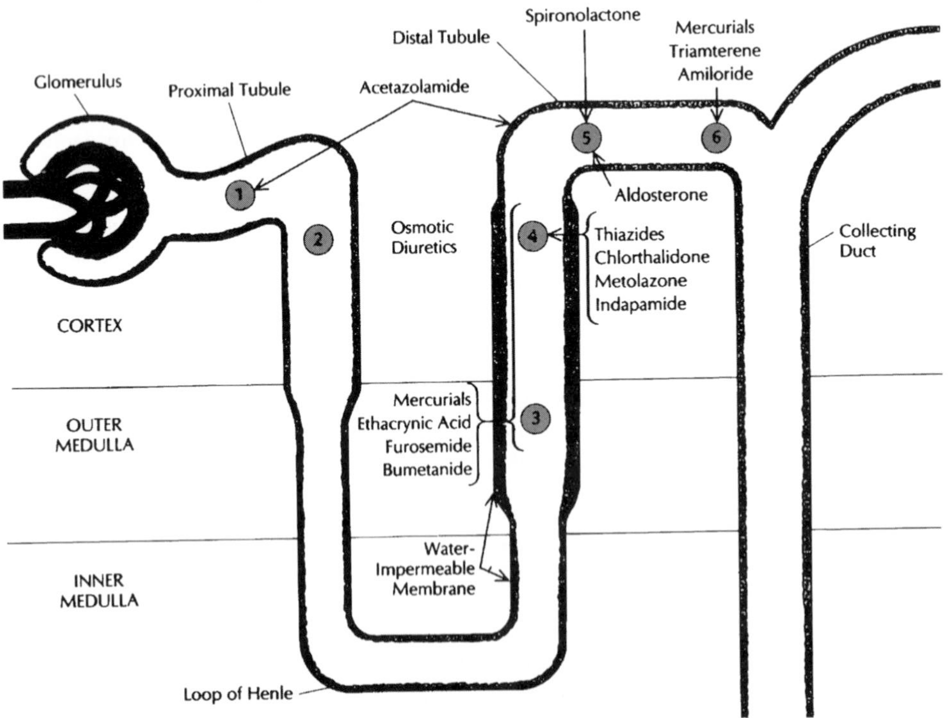

FIG. 25.1 Locations within the nephron where diuretic agents exert their effects.

filtration rate, SNGFR) is a function of hydrostatic pressure in the glomerular capillaries (P_{GC}), hydrostatic pressure in Bowman's space or the proximal tubule (P_T), mean colloid osmotic pressure in the glomerular capillaries (Π_{GC}), colloid osmotic pressure in the proximal tubule (Π_T), and the ultrafiltration coefficient (K_f). The relationship between these forces is summarized by the following equation:

$$SNGFR = K_f[(P_{GC} - P_T) - (\Pi_{GC} - \Pi_T)]$$

This equation is usually simplified by defining $P_{GC} - P_T$ as the transcapillary hydraulic pressure difference (ΔP) and eliminating Π_T since little protein is filtered. Hence the equation below becomes the most useful expression:

$$SNGFR = K_f(\Delta P - \Pi_{GC})$$

Whereas K_f is determined by the properties of the filtering membrane, ΔP is primarily determined by the proportion of arterial pressure conveyed to the glomerular capillaries. As resistance changes in pre- and postglomerular vessels, ΔP varies. The pressure Π_{GC} depends upon the concentration of protein in arterial blood as well as the actual flow of blood to the nephron. SNGFR is an important parameter that may affect, or be affected by, the action of diuretic drugs.

Ultrafiltrate from the glomerulus enters the proximal tubule from Bowman's capsule. By the time urine exits the distal tubule and collecting duct, better than 99% of ultrafiltrate volume will be reabsorbed. Figure 25.2 summarizes the characteristics of reabsorption in broad sections of the

Nephron Segment	Transport Systems
Proximal tubule • Isotonic reabsorption • Reabsorbs the bulk (approximately 65%) of filtered water and solute.	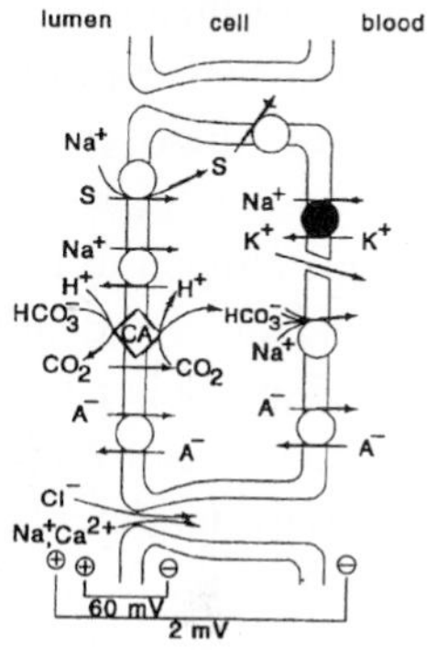
Thick ascending limb of Henle's loop • Actively transports sodium but effectively impermeable to water. • Location of macula densa that senses NaCl concentration in filtrate.	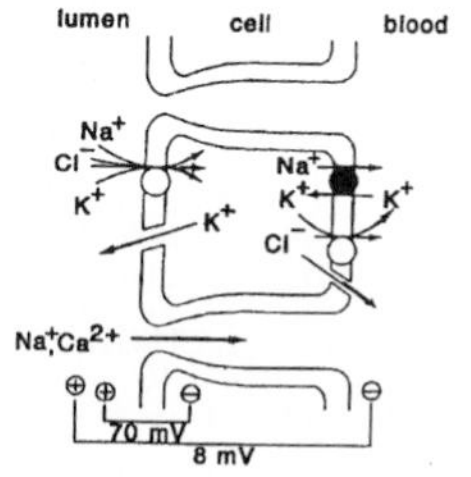
Distaltubule cell • Actively transports sodium but effectively impermeable to water.	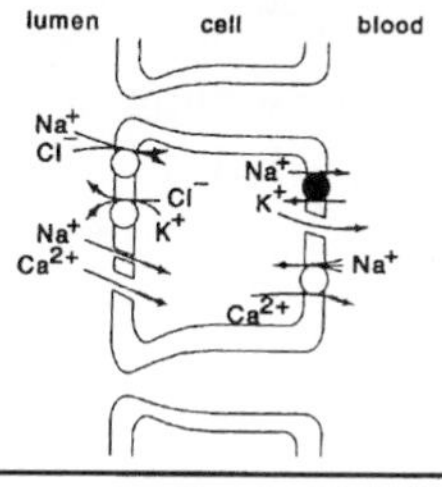
Collecting duct system (includes connecting tubule and collecting duct) • Principal cell (top) • Intercalated cells Type A (middle) Type B (bottom) • Principal cells of connecting tubule are responsive to aldosterone. • Collecting ducts are responsive to vasopressin.	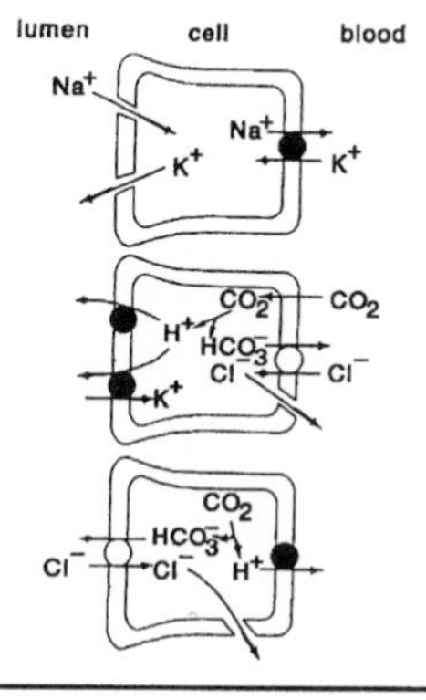

FIG. 25.2 Reabsorption in the nephron. General characteristics of segmental tubular reabsorption *(left)* and details of transport mechanisms in each segment *(right).* Six of seven basic mechanisms for transport of solutes across renal epithelial membranes are shown. Channel-mediated diffusion (shown as an *interrupted cell membrane)* allows solutes to move passively through the membrane. Carrier-mediated, or facilitated, transport *(unfilled circle, single arrow)* (also referred to as a uniport) allows a single substance to move with, but not against, an electrochemical gradient. ATP-driven primary active transport *(filled circles),* usually in the form of Na^+,K^+-ATPase, mediates the bulk of renal transport and can move solutes against an electrochemical gradient. Secondary active transport utilizes the potential energy stored in electrochemical gradients to move solutes across membranes against their gradients. Two types of secondary active transport are shown. Cotransport of solutes (S), such as glucose, inorganic phosphate, and amino acids, with sodium in the same direction occurs through symports *(unfilled circles, two arrows, each pointing in the same direction across the cell membrane).* Countertransport of solutes in the opposite direction occurs through antiports *(unfilled circles, two arrows, each pointing in a different direction across the cell membrane).* Simple diffusion down a concentration gradient can occur through cell membranes if the solute is lipid soluble. Simple diffusion that occurs between cells (paracellular) is shown *(arrows directed between cells).* A final transport mechanism, solvent drag, can occur across membranes through aqueous pores or between cells *(not shown).* A^- = organic acid (anion).

renal tubules. The thick ascending limb of the loop of Henle is of particular importance since this is the site of action of the most potent diuretic drugs. Approximately 25% of filtered solutes are reabsorbed in the loop of Henle, and most of this reabsorption occurs in the thick ascending limb. The thick ascending limb also makes a critical contact with the afferent arteriole through a cluster of specialized epithelial cells referred to as the macula densa. The macula densa monitors the NaCl concentration in filtrate leaving the loop of Henle. Together with extraglomerular mesangial cells and renin-producing cells of the glomerular arterioles, these components form the juxtaglomerular apparatus. A high concentration of salt in tubular fluid prompts a signal to the afferent arteriole causing constriction and decreased SNGFR. This, in combination with other responses, constitutes the tubuloglomerular feedback mechanism that protects the animal from salt and water wasting. Alternatively, excessive volume expansion causes the macula densa to inhibit renin release from the juxtaglomerular cells, leading to dilatation of the afferent arteriole. Because the ascending loop of Henle is poorly water permeable, tubular fluid at the end of this segment is dilute despite the presence of renal interstitial tissues with increasing osmolality toward the medulla. The renal interstitial concentration gradient, amplified by the countercurrent mechanism, provides the driving force for passive water reabsorption later in the nephron. The collecting duct system described in Figure 25.2 includes the connecting tubule (also referred to as the late distal tubule), which is responsive to aldosterone. If extracellular fluid (ECF) sodium concentrations are too low, aldosterone is secreted, causing increased sodium reabsorption in the connecting tubule. Vasopressin, also referred to as arginine vasopressin (AVP) and antidiuretic hormone, is secreted when plasma osmolality is elevated or ECF volume contracts. Stimulation by vasopressin leads to receptor-mediated opening of water channels in the collecting ducts with subsequent retention of water and expansion of ECF volume. In general, modification of filtrate as it passes through the nephron is controlled at two different levels. Systemic regulatory mechanisms and effector hormones such as renin-angiotensin-aldosterone, natriuretic peptides, and vasopressin ensure the balance of salt and water metabolism. Cellular feedback loops and glomerulotubular balance modify tubular function and influence single-cell homeostasis. Diuretics may interfere at either or both levels to cause increases in salt and water excretion.

RENAL EPITHELIAL TRANSPORT AND SECRETION. Just as knowledge of functional renal anatomy has increased, so has understanding of cellular mechanisms for transport of solutes across renal epithelium. Since the early 1990s, many ion transporters and cotransporters that serve as targets for diuretic drugs have been cloned and characterized at the molecular level (Xu et al. 1994; Gamba et al. 1993, 1994). Figure 25.2 (right column) summarizes the general mechanisms for renal epithelial transport in different segments of the renal tubules. Table 25.1 provides approximations of percent renal tubular reabsorption of selected substances by nephron segment.

In addition to ion transport mechanisms, the kidney also has effective and separate transport systems for movement of organic acids and bases. Energy from ATP-driven active transport is used to establish gradients for secondary

TABLE 25.1 Approximate renal tubular reabsorption (%) of filtered substances

	Proximal Tubule	Thick Ascending Limb of Henle's Loop	Distal Tubule	Total Reabsorption (All Segments)
H_2O	60	20	19	99
Na^+	60	34	6	100
Cl^-	55	38	6	99
K^+	60	25	−5	80
HCO_3^-	90	0	10	100
Ca^{++}	60	30	9	99
HPO_4^-	70	10	0	80
Mg^{++}	30	60	0	90
Urea	Reabsorbed	Secreted	Reabsorbed	—

active transport of both anions and cations. Families of proteins representing both anion and cation transporters move a wide variety of related substances (Dresser 2001). While these transporters have flexible stereospecificity, structural features of anions and cations that are efficiently transported have been identified (Jackson 1996). The presence of anion and cation transporters is essential for most highly protein-bound diuretic drugs to gain access to their site of action, the lumen of the renal tubule. Loop and thiazide diuretics and acetazolamide are secreted through the organic acid pathway, and amiloride and triamterene via an organic base transporter (Brater 1998). Renal insufficiency accompanied by reduced creatinine clearance decreases delivery of diuretic drugs to their secretory site and hence to their site of action. Accumulation of endogenous organic acids during chronic renal failure may result in competition with diuretics for transport at proximal tubule secretion sites (Brater 1993). There is also evidence that nonsteroidal antiinflammatory drugs (NSAIDs) compete for tubular secretion of loop diuretics, thus decreasing their efficacy.

PRINCIPLES OF DIURETIC USE

OVERVIEW. The current therapeutic goal of diuretic use is increased excretion of sodium followed by water. The degree of sodium loss in the urine (referred to as natriuresis or, in combination with chloride, saluresis) varies with the mechanism of action of the drug. All except osmotic diuretics inhibit specific enzymes, transport proteins, hormone receptors, or ion channels that function, directly or indirectly, in renal tubular sodium reabsorption. Although saluresis is the primary clinical goal, diuretics also alter elimination of other ions to varying degrees (e.g., K^+, H^+, Ca^{2+}, Mg^{2+}, Cl^-, HCO_3^-, phosphates) and may affect renal hemodynamics. Diuretic-induced depletion of circulating blood volume may lead to adverse effects if therapy is not well monitored. For example, in patients with chronic hepatic disease hypoalbuminemia leads to a decrease in plasma colloidal osmotic pressure and shifts in fluid to other spaces. Even a small diuretic-induced decrease in arterial perfusion under these circumstances may lead to severe exacerbation of disease. Older animals and those with cardiac or renal disease are also at increased risk for adverse effects if diuretic-induced hypovolemia goes untreated. Because these groups are also the primary target groups for diuretic use, rational use of diuretic drugs is essential. Table 25.2 summarizes selected features of diuretic drugs most commonly used in veterinary medicine.

EDEMA FORMATION. The most common indication for diuretic use is mobilization of tissue edema. Understanding the physiological principles underlying edema formation depends upon an understanding of net capillary filtration (see Chapter 24 and the equation above for SNGFR). Net capillary filtration (NF), or fluid flux out of a capillary, is dependent upon Starling forces inside and outside the vessel. NF is determined by the difference between ΔP, which represents the hydrostatic pressure inside the capillary lumen minus the hydrostatic pressure in the interstitial fluid, and $\Delta\Pi$, representing the oncotic pressure inside the capillary minus the oncotic pressure in the interstitial fluid. This value multiplied by a filtration coefficient (K_f), representing the permeability of the capillary wall, predicts the movement of fluid into and out of the vascular compartment.

Normally the flux of fluid out of capillaries is equaled by the lymph flow away from the site. If flux exceeds flow, edema results. A simplistic explanation of edema formation starts with a decrease in plasma oncotic pressure that leads to loss of intravascular volume to the interstitial space. The loss of intravascular fluid leads to decreased plasma volume, which leads to renal salt and water retention. Eventually salt and water retention causes increased plasma volume, increased plasma hydrostatic pressure, and increased flux of fluid out of the capillary, resulting in accumulation of edema in the interstitium. In veterinary medicine the most common causes of edema are cardiac (usually congestive heart failure; CHF), hepatic and renal disease.

CHF causes decreased cardiac output and decreased renal blood flow, leading to activation of the renin-angiotensin-aldosterone system followed by renal retention of salt and water. High baroreceptor activity causes increased peripheral vascular resistance and increased vasopressin, which lead to further salt and water retention by the kidneys. Increased central venous pressure caused by increased left ventricular end-diastolic pressures cause increased capillary hydrostatic pressure. All of these factors lead to greater fluid flux out of vessels, resulting in edema related to cardiac disease.

TABLE 25.2 Summary of diuretic drugs commonly used in veterinary medicine

Drug	Indications, Dosages, Route of Administration	Mechanism of Action, Route of Elimination	Adverse Effects
Mannitol	*Oliguric renal failure:* 0.25–0.5 gm/kg IV over 15–20 min. If diuresis occurs, may repeat every 4–6 hr up to a dose of 1.5 gm/kg in 12–24 hr. Monitor for urine production and dehydration. *Acute glaucoma:* 1–2 gm/kg IV over 15–20 min; withhold water for 30–60 min after dosing.	Osmotic diuretic Renal elimination	Hyper- or hypo-osmolality Hypokalemia Acute hypotension associated with hyponatremia
Furosemide	*Increased intracranial pressure:* 1.5 gm/kg IV once *Edema of cardiac, hepatic or renal origin:* SMALL ANIMALS: 1–3 mg/kg every 8–24 hr PO for chronic use; 2–5 mg/kg every 4–6 hr IV, IM, SC (dogs); 1–2 mg/kg every 12 hr up to 4 mg/kg every 8–12 hr IV, I.M, SC, PO (cats). LARGE ANIMALS: 0.5–1.0 mg/kg twice daily or to effect. *Other uses:* Decrease bleeding in horses with EIPH (controversial). Establish diuresis in renal failure. Promote excretion of other substances (e.g., other drugs, elevated electrolytes).	Inhibits Na^+-K^+-$2Cl^-$ symport. Referred to as loop or high ceiling diuretic. Primarily renal excretion of unchanged drug with remainder biotransformed by glucuronidation and renally excreted.	Hypokalemia Hypochloremic alkalosis Ototoxicity Hyperglycemia GI irritation Enhances aminoglycoside nephrotoxicity
Acetazolamide	Primarily ophthalmic use. *Adjunctive therapy of glaucoma in dogs and cats:* 10–30 mg/kg divided and administered 2–3 times daily orally. 50 mg/kg IV once.	Carbonic anhydrase inhibitor. Renal elimination.	Hypokalemia Acidosis Urinary tract calculi Hepatic encephalopathy

INHIBITORS OF CARBONIC ANHYDRASE

CHEMISTRY/FORMULATIONS. This class of drugs was discovered as a result of the observation that sulfanilamide chemotherapeutic agents were capable of causing metabolic acidosis by inhibition of carbonic anhydrase (CA). Screening of sulfanilamides resulted in identification of compounds whose predominant mechanism of action was CA inhibition. These drugs have been used sparingly in veterinary medicine as diuretics and are more commonly used for ophthalmic purposes. The prototype drug in this class, acetazolamide (Diamox®, Dazamide®), is available in tablets (125 and 250 mg), extended-release capsules (500 mg), and injectable (500 mg per vial). Other CA inhibitors include preparations for oral use, dichlorphenamide (Daranide®) and methazolamide (Neptazane®), and a topical drug, dorzolamide (Trusopt®), for ophthalmic use.

MECHANISMS AND SITES OF ACTION

Renal Mechanisms. Drugs in this class are active in the CA-rich segments of the nephron, in particular the proximal tubule. Noncompetitive, reversible inhibition of CA located in the luminal and basolateral membranes (type IV CA) as well as in the cytoplasm (type II CA) results in decreased formation of carbonic acid from CO_2 and H_2O (see Fig. 25.2 and equation below):

$$HCO_3^- + H^+ \leftrightarrow H_2CO_3 \leftrightarrow H_2O + CO_2$$

Reduction in the amount of carbonic acid yields fewer H^+ within proximal tubular cells. Because H^+ is normally exchanged for Na^+ from the tubular lumen by the Na^+-H^+ antiporter (also referred to as a Na^+-H^+ exchanger or NHE), less Na^+ is reabsorbed and more is available to combine with urinary HCO_3^-. The NHE maintains a low proton concentration in the cell so that $H_2CO_3^-$ ionizes spontaneously to form H^+ and HCO_3^-. This, in turn, creates an electrochemical gradient for HCO_3^- across the basolateral membrane that drives movement of HCO_3^- into the interstitial space. Diuresis is established when water is excreted with sodium bicarbonate. As sodium bicarbonate is trapped in the urine and eliminated, less HCO_3^- is returned to plasma, and a systemic acidosis eventually develops. As a result of the systemic acidosis, H^+ becomes available, Na^+ reabsorption is reestablished, and diuresis decreases. Continual use of CA inhibitors is therefore self-limiting in terms of diuretic action. Diuresis induced by CA inhibitors is mild due to incomplete inhibition of CA, redundancy of Na^+ transporting systems in the proximal tubule, and rescue of Na^+ by reabsorption later in the distal tubule. Because intracellular K^+ can, to some extent, substitute for H^+ in the Na^+ reabsorption step, CA inhibitors cause enhanced K^+ excretion. As more Na^+ is presented to the distal tubule, the potential for K^+ wasting increases. CA inhibitors also decrease secretion of titratable acids and ammonia in the collecting duct (Jackson 1996). For this reason, and due to the increased excretion of sodium bicarbonate, urine pH increases despite the decreasing systemic pH associated with CA-inhibitor–induced acidosis. This class of drugs has little, if any, effect on excretion of Ca^{2+} and Mg^{2+} but does enhance phosphate elimination.

Extrarenal Actions. Other actions of CA inhibitors are related to the wide distribution of CA in body tissues including the eye, gastric mucosa, pancreas, central nervous system (CNS), and red blood cells. The most important therapeutic consequence is associated with CA inhibition in the eye. The ciliary processes of the eye mediate the formation of aqueous humor, which contains an abundance of HCO_3^-. This process is CA dependent and, when inhibited, leads to a decreased rate of formation of aqueous humor and subsequent reduction in intraocular pressure. Although not therapeutically relevant in veterinary medicine, CA inhibition in the CNS has been associated with anticonvulsant actions attributed to this class of drugs.

ABSORPTION AND ELIMINATION. Limited information is available regarding pharmacokinetics of CA inhibitors in animals. Acetazolamide gains access to the renal tubules via the organic acid secretion pathway. A dose of 22 mg/kg is reported to have an onset of action of 30 minutes, maximal effects in 2–4 hours, and a duration of action of 4–6 hours in small animals (Roberts 1985). Oral absorption of drugs in this class is good. Acetazolamide is eliminated primarily through the kidneys.

TOXICITY, ADVERSE EFFECTS, CONTRAINDICATIONS, AND DRUG INTERACTIONS. Because CA inhibitors are sulfonamide derivatives, side effects commonly associated with sulfonamides can occur. CNS drowsiness and disorientation may occur as a result of inhibition of CA in the CNS. In particular, some dogs are sensitive to adverse reactions from sulfonamide drugs (hypersensitivity reactions). Because CA inhibitors decrease ammonia excretion, the severity of preexisting hepatic disease may be worsened and hepatic encephalopathy can be induced. Use is also contraindicated in patients with electrolyte disturbances (due to K^+ and Na^+ wasting) and those with metabolic or respiratory acidosis. Use in patients with severe pulmonary disease who cannot respond to drug-induced metabolic acidosis with respiratory compensation is also contraindicated. Because CA inhibitors alkalinize the urine, calcium phosphate calculi formation is enhanced, and excretion of weak organic bases is reduced. Rare blood dyscrasias associated with CA inhibitors have also been reported in the human, but not in the veterinary, literature.

THERAPEUTIC USES. The primary indication for use of CA inhibitors is to inhibit production of aqueous humor and reduce intraocular pressure. In veterinary medicine, acetazolamide (10–30 mg/kg divided and given three times daily) and methazolamide (2–10 mg/kg given 2–3 times daily) are used in dogs for management of glaucoma. A one-time IV dose of acetazolamide (50 mg/kg) has been reported for management of acute glaucoma. Methazolamide is often preferred over acetazolamide for long-term glaucoma therapy due to fewer side effects. CA inhibitors are also used preoperatively to lower ocular pressure.

In human medicine, CA inhibitors have been used as an adjunctive therapy for epilepsy and in management of acute mountain (high-altitude) sickness. In both human and veterinary medicine, the use of CA inhibitors as diuretics has limited effectiveness due to the rapid development of tolerance. Theoretically, acetazolamide could be used to manage metabolic alkalosis, but this is not a typical clinical practice in veterinary medicine.

OSMOTIC DIURETICS

CHEMISTRY/FORMULATIONS. Solutions used as osmotic diuretics contain simple solutes of low molecular weight that have an increased osmolarity relative to plasma. These substances are typically freely filtered by the glomerulus, undergo limited tubular reabsorption, and are pharmacologically inert. The most common osmotic diuretic is mannitol, a six-carbon nonmetabolizable polyalcohol with a molecular weight of 182. Other agents include glycerin, isosorbide, urea, and hypertonic saline solutions. Because mannitol is the most commonly used osmotic diuretic in both human and veterinary medicine, subsequent discussion will focus primarily on this drug. Concentrated mannitol (15–25%) may crystallize at cooler temperatures, in which case the drug can often be resolubilized by warming the solution. Prior to administration, the solution should be cooled and any remaining crystals removed using an in-line intravenous (IV) filter. There are no veterinary-approved mannitol formulations available. For IV use in animals, the human formulations are used. Human products (Osmitrol®, Resectisol®) range from 5% (275 mOsm/l) to 25% (1375 mOsm/l) and are available for IV administration.

MECHANISMS AND SITES OF ACTION. Hyperosmolar solutions exert part of their effects by establishing an osmotic gradient between plasma and tissue water compartments. Acute effects of this gradient include decreases in hematocrit, blood viscosity, plasma sodium, plasma pH, and, to some degree, the volume of solid organs. Hence, parenchymal dehydration and acute hemodilution are theoretically related as long as the osmotically active particles are effectively separated by a relatively solute-impermeable barrier.

Renal Mechanisms. Initially osmotic diuretics were thought to act primarily at the level of the proximal tubule by limiting the movement of water from the lumen into the interstitial space. Water retained in the tubular lumen diluted concentrations of sodium and other ions, reduced ion reabsorption, and promoted diuresis. It is now held that osmotic diuretics, in particular mannitol, have effects throughout the length of the tubule, with the most prominent action occurring in the loop of Henle. Sodium reabsorption is markedly reduced in the descending and thin limbs of the loop of Henle, as determined by studies in dogs and rats. Sodium load to the thick ascending limb of the loop of Henle and to the distal tubule is consequently increased, but the nephron fails to recapture the increased loads of salt and water. As demonstrated in the dog, sodium reabsorption is also thought to be directly inhibited in medullary collecting ducts (Better et al. 1997).

Other reported renal effects of mannitol include increases in cortical and medullary blood flow due to a decrease in renal vascular resistance, impairment of urinary concentration, dilution by dissipation of medullary hypertonicity, an increase in GFR during renal hypoperfusion (may vary according to species), and an increase in urinary excretion of other electrolytes (e.g., K^+, Ca^{2+}, Mg^{2+}, phosphate, bicarbonate) (Better et al. 1997). Mannitol may also prompt the release of atrial natriuretic factor (ANF) and vasodilatory prostaglandins. Inhibition of renin release by mannitol has also been described.

Extrarenal Mechanisms. The actions of mannitol extend beyond the renal effects and include changes in blood rheology, direct transient effects on vascular tone, and increases in cardiac output. In addition to decreasing the hematocrit by hemodilution, mannitol decreases the volume, rigidity, and cohesiveness of red blood cell membranes. The combination of reduced viscosity and reduced mechanical resistance presumably leads to enhanced blood flow. Mannitol-induced increases in cardiac output are thought to be related to reduced peripheral resistance and reduced afterload, a transient increase in preload, and mild positive inotropy. Mannitol may also exert a cytoprotective effect by acting as an oxygen-free radical scavenger (Paczynski 1997).

ABSORPTION AND ELIMINATION. Mannitol is not metabolized and is handled as an inert substance by the body. Studies in dogs and humans indicate that mannitol distribution and elimination follow a two-compartment model (Cloyd et al. 1986; Rudehill et al. 1993). The distribution half-life of intravenously administered mannitol is measured in minutes. Elimination half-life is dose dependent and ranges from 0.5 to 1.5 hours for doses between 0.25 and 1.5 g/kg. Mannitol is eliminated rapidly by the kidneys unless renal function is impaired. As a result, penetration of mannitol into tissues is limited by rapidly falling plasma concentrations. Mannitol and urea are administered intravenously in a slow bolus over 15–30 minutes. Glycerin and isosorbide are administered orally. Of the available osmotic diuretics, only glycerin is eliminated by biotransformation.

ADVERSE EFFECTS AND DRUG INTERACTIONS

Acute Adverse Effects. Pulse pressure and mean arterial blood pressure usually increase transiently with mannitol administration. However, acute hypotensive, hyponatremic effects of mannitol administration have been reported, especially subsequent to rapid infusion in dehydrated individuals. The mechanism for this acute vasodilatory effect is not well understood, but the problem can largely be prevented by appropriate rates of administration (0.25–1.5 g/kg over 15–30 min). Acute hyponatremia may account for the nausea and vomiting that are sometimes observed with mannitol infusion. Rapid expansion of plasma volume related to attraction of fluid into the vascular compartment may precipitate CHF or pulmonary edema in certain patient populations. However, because the drug is cleared rapidly this problem is not common unless renal function is impaired.

Dehydration and Electrolyte Disturbances. Because the ratio of the volume of fluid eliminated in urine to the volume of mannitol administered is high, care should be taken to avoid hypertonic dehydration. Circulating plasma volume tends to be preserved as hypertonic dehydration develops, making it harder to clinically detect that a problem exists. The presence of dehydration and significant hypernatremia should be closely monitored using body weight, urine output, and other clinical parameters. In addition to hypertonic dehydration, loss of other electrolytes, including potassium, phosphate, and magnesium, can lead to clinically significant cardiac arrhythmias and neuromuscular complications.

Hyperosmolar State and Osmotic Compensation. The phenomenon of osmotic compensation occurs when cells respond to prolonged treatment with a hyperosmolar agent by increasing the presence of intracellular, idiogenic osmoles. Compensation is thought to occur rapidly when the osmolality of plasma is increased by 25 mOsm/kg or more above normal. Newly generated, osmotically active intracellular particles counteract the dehydrating effect of hyperosmolar plasma. Osmotic compensation can limit therapeutic effectiveness by decreasing the osmotic gradient from tissue to plasma. Increased intracellular osmolarity may also promote conditions, especially in the brain, where iatrogenic edema may occur. The risk of edema formation is increased if a hyperosmolar state is reversed rapidly, leaving the intracellular osmoles as the most osmotically active site. To prevent this complication, the duration of return of plasma to normal osmolality should be approximately equal to the duration of the hyperosmolar state.

CONTRAINDICATIONS. The use of mannitol in patients with ongoing intracranial hemorrhage, anuric renal failure, severe dehydration, or pulmonary congestion or edema is contraindicated.

Adequate fluid therapy should be administered to dehydrated animals prior to administration of mannitol. Mannitol should not be added to whole-blood products unless at least 20 mEq/l of sodium chloride is added to the solution; otherwise, pseudoagglutination may occur.

THERAPEUTIC USES. Mannitol is used in the prophylaxis and treatment of renal failure, for the reduction of intracranial and intraocular pressure, and with other diuretics to mobilize edema. For reasons already discussed, short-term use of mannitol is most effective to prevent adverse effects and decreased therapeutic efficacy.

Prophylaxis of Acute Renal Failure. Anuric patients should not be routinely treated with mannitol, although a small (0.25–0.5 g/kg), single test dose may be used to try and induce diuresis. Administration of mannitol to patients with renal dysfunction must be done cautiously to prevent problems associated with decreased elimination and prolonged hyperosmolarity. Acute renal failure (ARF) may be caused extrinsically (pre- and postrenal failure) or intrinsically, often associated with acute renal tubular necrosis (ATN). Mannitol has been found to be effective in limiting the decrease in GFR caused by ATN if administered before the ischemic insult or exposure to nephrotoxins. Protection of tubules from necrosis may be due to dilution of nephrotoxic substances, reduction of swelling of tubular elements, or removal of tubular casts that are obstructing urine flow. In human medicine, mannitol has been shown to be clearly beneficial in the preservation of kidneys for transplant and for decreasing the incidence of posttransplant ARF. Fewer data are available to support the general value of mannitol for treatment of ARF outside the area of transplantation (Better et al. 1997). In vascular and open-heart surgery, prophylactic mannitol maintains urine flow but not GFR. Some evidence suggests that mannitol administration in patients with established ATN may increase the conversion of oliguric to nonoliguric patients (Levinsky and Bernard 1988).

Reduction of Intracranial Pressure. Osmotherapy has been used for decades to decrease intracranial pressure (ICP). Reduction in ICP is rapid and usually appears within minutes of completion of administration, with maximum effects within the hour. Several theories have been formulated to account for the effectiveness of mannitol in reducing ICP. The osmotic theory holds that brain shrinkage occurs as a result of osmotically driven movement of fluid from tissue and into the vascular compartment. Sensitive, high-resolution imaging methods seem to support the significance of osmotically induced changes in brain water content (Betz et al. 1989). The hemodynamic theory of ICP reduction states that cerebral blood volume is decreased as a result of decreased blood viscosity and increased cerebral perfusion pressure, both of which act to enhance oxygen delivery to the brain. Increased oxygen delivery to the brain is thought to trigger a compensatory reduction in vascular caliber and secondarily a reduction in cerebral blood volume. Detractors of this idea suggest that mannitol is just as likely to decrease blood viscosity as a result of hemoconcentration secondary to hypertonic dehydration. While attention to fluid replacement should prevent dehydration, it has recently been suggested that alternative agents, such as hypertonic saline, are safer and equally effective at reducing ICP. Hypertonic saline has been shown to establish a strong transendothelial osmotic gradient but without the tendency to reduce intravascular volume (Prough and Zornow 1998). Finally, the diuretic theory of ICP reduction suggests that mannitol-induced decreases in central venous pressure translate directly to decreases in ICP due to the valveless communication between the central venous system and the jugular drainage system. This effect may be more important in sustaining, rather than inducing, a decrease in ICP (Paczynski 1997). Regardless of the theory, mannitol has been used for temporary reduction of ICP in patients with a variety of intracranial lesions as well as those with spinal cord trauma and edema. Evidence of ongoing intracranial hemorrhage is considered a contraindication for mannitol administration.

Other Uses. Osmotic diuretics have also been used successfully to control intraocular pressure during acute glaucoma attacks and to reduce intraocular pressure before or after ophthalmic surgery. Decreases in intraocular pressure occur by loss of intraocular water to hyperosmolar plasma. As the vitreous shrinks, the lens moves posteriorly and the iridocorneal angle opens, improving drainage from the eye. The duration of action depends upon the degree to which the osmotic diuretic is excluded from ocular fluids. Mannitol is reported to increase retinal oxygen tension and is used at a dose of 1–2 g/kg at a rate of 1 ml/kg/min to reduce intraocular pressure in dogs.

INHIBITORS OF NA^+-K^+-$2CL^-$ SYMPORT (LOOP, OR HIGH-CEILING, DIURETICS)

Drugs belonging to this class are among the most potent and the most commonly prescribed diuretics, and all share a common mechanism of action. By blocking a key sodium transport mechanism in the thick ascending limb of the loop of Henle (hence the name loop diuretic), these drugs inhibit reabsorption of approximately 25% of the filtered sodium load. Nephron segments distal to the thick ascending limb (TAL) are incapable of reabsorbing the additional solute, leading to a marked (or high-ceiling) natriuresis and diuresis. Because furosemide (Lasix®) is by far the most commonly used diuretic in veterinary medicine, the remaining discussion will focus primarily on this drug (also referred to as *frusemide*). Other drugs in this class include ethacrynic acid (Edecrin®), bumetanide (Bumex®), and the most recent addition approved in the United States, torsemide (Demadex®).

CHEMISTRY/FORMULATIONS. Except for ethacrynic acid, the structurally diverse drugs in this class are sulfonamide derivatives. Furosemide is light sensitive and stable under alkaline conditions; the veterinary injectable preparations (Lasix®, Diuride®, or generic; 50 mg/ml) have a light yellow color, whereas the human injectable (Lasix®; 10 mg/ml) should not be used if it appears yellow. A wide range of veterinary preparations of furosemide are available, including oral tablets approved for use in dogs and cats (12.5 mg, 50 mg), oral solution approved for use in dogs (10 mg/ml), large-animal boluses approved for use in cattle (2 g/bolus), and injectable (5%) approved for use in dogs, cats, horses not intended for food, and cattle.

Milk and slaughter withdrawal time for both oral and injectable formulations for cattle is 48 hours. Bumetanide (Bumex® is supplied in 0.5, 1, and 2 mg tablets and as a 0.25 mg/ml parenteral injection. Bumetanide is approximately 40 to 50 times as potent as furosemide in the dog. Torsemide (also torasemide) (Demadex®) is supplied as 5, 10, 20, and 100 mg tablets and in 2 or 5 ml ampules containing 10 mg/ml for intravenous administration. Torsemide dosage in the dog has been estimated at approximately 1/10 the human dose but the drug has not been well studied in dogs and cats (Kittleson and Kienle 2007).

MECHANISMS AND SITES OF ACTION

Renal Effects. Drugs in this class block the Na^+-K^+-$2Cl^-$ symporter in the TAL by binding to the Cl^- binding site of the transporter protein. All of these drugs must be actively secreted into the tubular lumen by an organic acid pathway in order to reach and inhibit the luminal symporter. A high degree of protein binding (>95%) limits glomerular filtration of furosemide and other loop diuretics, making tubular secretion essential. The mechanism involved in Na^+ reabsorption in the TAL depends upon Na^+,K^+-ATPase activity in the basal membrane of tubular cells (see Table 25.1). The transmembrane Na^+ gradient generated by ATPase drives the Na^+-K^+-$2Cl^-$ symporter in the luminal membrane. Basolateral Cl^- conductance and luminal K^+ conductance determine membrane voltage. The polarity of K^+ and Cl^- conductances results in a lumen-positive transepithelial voltage. This voltage drives cations between tubular cells via the paracellular shunt pathway. When loop diuretics block the Na^+-K^+-$2Cl^-$ symporter, Cl^- concentrations in the cell fall, the cell becomes hyperpolarized, transepithelial voltage is disrupted, and paracellular cation reabsorption is blocked (Bleich and Gregor 1997). Because renin-producing cells in the area of the macula densa generate part of their membrane voltage via Cl^- channels, the new Cl^- equilibrium also depolarizes these cells and enhances the secretion of renin. Loop diuretics interfere with establishment of a hypertonic medullary interstitium and disrupt the countercurrent mechanism. Hence, these drugs block the kidney's ability to concentrate and dilute urine appropriately. Inhibitors of the Na^+-K^+-$2Cl^-$ symporter also inhibit Ca^{2+} and Mg^{2+} reabsorption in the TAL by disruption of the transepithelial potential difference. Some loop diuretics, notably furosemide, also have weak carbonic anhydrase-inhibiting activity that leads to enhanced urinary excretion of HCO_3^- and phosphate. All Na^+-K^+-$2Cl^-$ symporter inhibitors increase the urinary excretion of K^+ and H^+ by presenting a greater load of Na^+ to the distal tubule. Sodium is reabsorbed while K^+ and H^+ are excreted.

Nonsteroidal antiinflammatory drugs (NSAIDs) inhibit the diuretic, natriuretic, and chloruretic responses to furosemide. Furosemide enhances production of prostaglandin E2 (PGE2), which in turn inhibits chloride and sodium reabsorption in the TAL. In the presence of NSAIDs, PGE2 production is blocked, and furosemide-induced diuresis is prevented (Kirchner 1987). In the absence of volume depletion, loop diuretics generally increase and redistribute total renal blood flow. The mechanism for this effect is thought to be related to prostaglandins, and the effect is diminished or blocked in the presence of NSAIDs (Data et al. 1978). Furosemide-induced hemodynamic changes correlate with an increase in urinary excretion of PGE2.

Another mechanism that has been used to explain the inhibition of efficacy of furosemide with NSAIDs is that both drugs compete for the organic acid transporter (OAT) in the renal tubular cell. By competing for transport, an NSAID may decrease transport of furosemide into the lumen of the renal tubule, thus decreasing its efficacy.

Extrarenal Effects. Furosemide causes extrarenal hemodynamic effects that include increased venous compliance and decreased right atrial pressure, pulmonary artery pressure, pulmonary artery wedge pressure, and pulmonary blood volume (Hinchcliff and Muir 1991). Prostaglandins are thought to account for the acute increase in systemic venous capacitance and subsequent decrease in left ventricular filling pressure. All of these effects are dependent upon the presence of a functional kidney and the uninhibited production of prostaglandins. In the isolated rabbit heart, furosemide has also been reported to exert a mild negative inotropic effect that is prostaglandin dependent (Feldman et al. 1987). Inhaled furosemide in humans has been shown to protect against the early response to inhaled allergens and to prevent exercise-induced bronchoconstriction (Bianco et al. 1988, 1989). Furosemide may prevent bronchoconstriction in part by inhibiting release of inflammatory mediators from lung cells (Anderson et al. 1991). Pulmonary gas exchange is reportedly improved by furosemide in experimental pulmonary edema. Furosemide also reduces the rate of pulmonary transvascular fluid filtration through a reduction in pulmonary vein pressure (Demling and Will 1978).

ABSORPTION AND ELIMINATION. Furosemide is approximately 77% bioavailable in dogs and has an elimination half-life of about 1 hour following an IV dose of 5 mg/kg (Hirai et al. 1992). The absorption of orally administered furosemide takes place mainly in the upper parts of the canine alimentary tract, decreasing rapidly across the jejunum. Due to variable oral bioavailability and rapid elimination in the dog, a prolonged-release furosemide formulated in hydroxypropyl methylcellulose matrix tablets has been investigated (Smal et al. 1996). Peak effects of an IV dosage of furosemide in the dog are reported at approximately 30 minutes and following oral dosing at about 1–2 hours. The rate of urinary furosemide excretion, more so even than the concentration of plasma furosemide, has been found to closely correlate with diuretic response in dogs. As in humans, the relation between the natriuretic response and the concentration of diuretic in the urine (at the site of action) is represented by a sigmoidal curve (Fig. 25.3). The shape of the curve suggests that a threshold quantity of drug must be achieved at the site of action in order to elicit a response and that a maximal dose can be identified that yields a maximal response. Beyond that maximal dose, the curve plateaus, and limited additional benefits are derived from dose increases (Brater 1998; Hirai et al. 1992). Because intermittent doses produce a brief effect in dogs and higher doses do not produce a greater effect, the use of a constant-rate infusion (CRI) has been explored. In dogs, a loading dose of 0.66 mg/kg is followed by a constant rate infusion (CRI) of 0.66 mg/kg/hr × 8 hours. This results in greater natriuresis, calciuresis, and diuresis than with intermittent treatment (Adin et al. 2003).

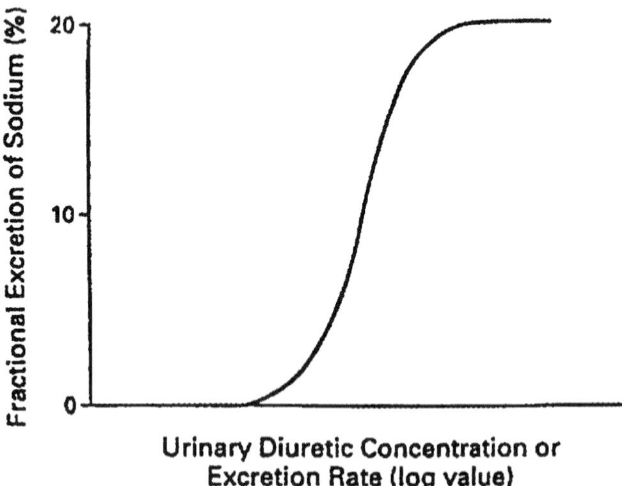

FIG. 25.3 Pharmacodynamics of a loop diuretic. The relation between the natriuretic response and the amount of diuretic reaching the site of action is represented by a sigmoidal curve.

Elimination half-life of IV furosemide in the horse is similar to that in the dog and, in the absence of renal impairment, is slightly less than 1 hour. Preventing renal elimination of the drug in horses by bilateral ureteral ligation increases elimination half-life by approximately threefold to an average of 164 minutes. This result demonstrates that furosemide elimination in the horse is primarily, but not exclusively, renal (Dyke et al. 1998). The hemodynamic effects of furosemide in this model are prevented by ureteral ligation, suggesting that these effects are diuresis dependent (Hinchcliff et al. 1996). Furosemide is typically administered IV or IM 3–4 times daily to horses. A study comparing oral and IV administration of the drug determined that systemic availability of furosemide given orally is poor, erratic, and variable among horses. Median systemic bioavailability was low and, at a dose of 1 mg/kg PO, diuresis was not induced (Johansson 2004). In a study comparing continuous rate infusion (CRI) to intermittent administration (IA) of furosemide in the horse, CRI of the drug produced more uniform urine flow, decreased fluctuations in plasma volume and suppressed renal concentrating ability throughout the study. Although potassium, calcium, and chloride excretion were higher with CRI than IA, CRI was preferred if profound diuresis was required in the horse (Johansson et al. 2003).

In humans and other animals, including the dog and horse, approximately 50–60% of a furosemide dose is excreted unchanged in the urine, and the remaining drug is conjugated to glucuronic acid in either the kidney, the liver, or other extrahepatic site (Brater 1998; Dyke et al. 1998).

Plasma half-life in patients with renal insufficiency is prolonged, and dosage adjustments should be made. Binding of furosemide to excessive amounts of albumin (>4 g/l) in the urine decreases the amount of unbound, active drug and diminishes the diuretic response. In human patients with nephrotic syndrome, doses of two to three times normal are recommended to provide sufficient amounts of active drug to block the Na^+-K^+-$2Cl^-$ symporter.

In humans bumetanide and torsemide are metabolized in large part by the liver, and so dosage generally does not need to be adjusted for renal disease. Bumetanide's potency in the dog is, in part, explained by limited biotransformation. In addition, renal uptake of bumetanide is greater than furosemide and the drug has a more marked effect on sodium transport in the ascending limb of the Loop of Henle. Approximately 67% of bumetanide in dogs is eliminated unchanged in the urine and feces (Schwarz 1981). Oral bioavailability of these drugs is much more predictable than that of furosemide and in humans ranges from 80 to 100% (Brater 1998).

TOXICITY, ADVERSE EFFECTS, CONTRAINDICATIONS, AND DRUG INTERACTIONS. Most adverse effects of furosemide administration are related to abnormalities of fluid and electrolyte balance. Extracellular volume depletion and hyponatremia may lead to reduced blood pressure and diminished organ perfusion. Most at risk for adverse effects related to volume depletion are patients with renal disease (may decrease GFR, increase prerenal azotemia, and, possibly, cause tubular necrosis), cardiac disease (stroke volume and cardiac output may decrease), and hepatic disease (precipitation of hepatic encephalopathy). As noted previously, Na^+-K^+-$2Cl^-$ symporter inhibitors deliver an increased load of Na^+ to the distal tubules, resulting in a renin-angiotensin-aldosterone-driven increase in excretion of K^+ and H^+ in exchange for Na^+. Hypochloremic alkalosis and hypokalemia may result. Risk factors for cardiac dysrhythmias related to diuretic-induced hypokalemia include inadequate dietary intake of K^+, concurrent administration of cardiac glycosides, and additional electrolyte imbalances. A common cause of anorexia in CHF patients is digitalis toxicity, and risk of arrhythmias is increased in these patients if hypokalemia is present. Deficiencies in Mg^{2+} and Ca^{2+} may also be caused by diuretic-enhanced excretion of these substances. Serum electrolyte levels should be monitored in patients receiving ongoing diuretic therapy, especially if risk factors exist related to appetite, diuretic dosage, or severity of disease.

Ototoxicity that is usually transient has been described primarily with ethacrynic acid and less often with all other loop diuretics. In veterinary medicine, ototoxicity may be of greatest concern in treatment of cats with high-dose IV regimens. Other adverse effects reported with use of loop diuretics include gastrointestinal disturbances, bone marrow depression, and hyperglycemia. Hyperglycemia may be related to impairment of proinsulin-to-insulin conversion associated with diuretic-induced decreases in K^+ levels. Patients hypersensitive to sulfonamides may also be hypersensitive to furosemide since this drug contains a sulfonamide moiety. Diuretic-induced depletion of water-soluble vitamins may occur, and supplementation of B-complex vitamins has been recommended for animals receiving continuous diuretic therapy (Keene and Rush 1995).

Loop diuretics are contraindicated in animals with severe fluid and electrolyte disturbances or anuria that does not respond to test doses of diuretics.

Drug interactions may occur when furosemide is administered with theophylline (enhanced effects), aminoglycosides or cisplatin (enhanced ototoxicity and, if volume depleted, nephrotoxicity), digitalis glycosides (diuretic-induced hypokalemia may increase risk of arrhythmias), aspirin or other anticoagulants (anticoagulant activity increased), neuromuscular blockers (alteration in extent of muscle relaxation), corticosteroids (enhanced potassium wasting), insulin (alteration of insulin requirements associated with hyperglycemic effects), lithium and propranolol (increased plasma levels), probenecid (competition for secretion of diuretic into tubular lumen leading to decreased diuretic effect), NSAIDs (as previously described, decreased diuretic effects), and thiazides (synergistic diuretic activity).

THERAPEUTIC USES. Furosemide is used in small animals for treatment of edema of cardiac, hepatic, or renal origin. In general, the dose of drug in dogs (1–3 mg/kg every 8–24 hours PO for chronic use; 2–5 mg/kg every 4–6 hours IV, IM, SC) is higher than that used in cats (1–2 mg/kg every 12 hours up to 4 mg/kg every 8–12 hours IV, IM, SC, PO) (Ware 1998). Furosemide is also used to establish diuresis in renal failure and to promote excretion of other substances, including elevated electrolytes such as Ca^{2+} and K^+. In large animals, furosemide has been used to treat edema in cattle and edema and exercise-induced pulmonary hemorrhage (EIPH) in horses. A general dose of 0.5–1 mg/kg twice daily or as needed to control edema has been recommended in large animals (Reef and McGuirk 1996). Benefits of furosemide use for treatment of EIPH remain controversial (see below).

Specific state guidelines should be consulted for details of furosemide use (dose, frequency, allowable levels) in racing animals.

Diuretic effects of orally administered torsemide (0.3 mg/kg) and furosemide (3 mg/kg) were compared in dogs and cats (Uechi 2003). Both furosemide and torsemide increased urine volume but the effects of furosemide peaked at 2–3 hours and dissipated by 6 hours while the effects of torsemide peaked at 2–4 hours but persisted for 12 hours in normal dogs, dogs with mitral regurgitation, and cats with experimentally induced left ventricular concentric hypertrophy. It was noted that torsemide decreased urine potassium excretion in study dogs with mitral regurgitation. In a previous study, the ratio of sodium to potassium excretion was found to be 20 : 1 for torsemide and 10 : 1 for furosemide (Ghys et al. 1985).

Renal Insufficiency. Decreased GFR and decreased delivery of drug to the tubular site of action and site of elimination in renal insufficiency results in decreased efficacy and increased half-life of furosemide. A sufficiently high dose of drug must be administered to attain an effective amount of drug at the site of action. For the dog, furosemide doses starting at 2 mg/kg IV and increasing in 2 mg/kg increments every hour for 3 hours may be used to try and induce diuresis in severe renal insufficiency. Once a maximal dosage is reached (approximately 6–8 mg/kg), exceeding this amount is not advantageous based on the sigmoidal shape of the fractional sodium excretion curve (Fig. 25.3). In all cases, fluid deficits should be addressed prior to furosemide therapy.

Cardiogenic or Pulmonary Edema. Furosemide has been widely used to reduce extracellular volume and minimize venous and pulmonary congestion in chronic and acute CHF. Human patients with CHF do not require large dosages since furosemide is adequately delivered to the tubular fluid. However, because renal responsiveness to loop diuretics appears to be decreased in these patients, increased frequency of administration has been recommended (Brater 1998). Diuretics have traditionally been considered front-line therapy for the treatment of chronic CHF in small animals, and furosemide is reported to be the most frequently used drug for this purpose (Goodwin and Hamlin 1993; Watson and Church 1995). Despite the popularity of furosemide, human studies have revealed that CHF patients controlled on loop diuretics alone deteriorate more quickly than those treated with either angiotensin-converting enzyme (ACE) inhibitors or digoxin. Use of furosemide alone is thought to enhance early activation of the renin-angiotensin-aldosterone system, with detrimental effects on long-term prognosis (Svedberg et al. 1990). Current recommendations include furosemide for treatment of more advanced stages of heart failure in patients already receiving ACE inhibitors, digoxin, or both. Furosemide remains a drug of choice for treatment of acute cardiogenic pulmonary edema. Within the context of severity and chronicity of disease, the lowest effective dosage and frequency of furosemide administration should be determined by observation of clinical signs and consideration of owner observations.

Exercise-Induced Pulmonary Hemorrhage (EIPH). EIPH, or bleeding from the lungs as a consequence of exercise, occurs in horses engaged in a variety of athletic activities. The problem has been best studied in racing horses, particularly Thoroughbreds.

In most studies, furosemide has been found to reduce right atrial, pulmonary arterial, and pulmonary wedge pressures in exercising horses. Some studies suggest that changes in pulmonary pressures caused by furosemide are due to reduction in plasma and blood volume and not to direct effects of the drug on the pulmonary vasculature. Furosemide produces a rapid reduction in blood and plasma volume, which has been shown in the horse to be essential for subsequent reduction in pulmonary pressures (Hinchcliff et al. 1996). Furthermore, administration of polyionic fluids in an amount equal to the volume lost in urine restores furosemide-induced decreases in right atrial pressure and blood volume in the horse (Rivas and Hinchcliff 1997). Furosemide administration 4 hours prior to exercise has been found to significantly decrease pulmonary capillary hypertension, which is thought to correlate with decreased risk of EIPH. Administration of the drug at shorter intervals prior to exercise did not result in more effective attenuation of exercise-induced pulmonary capillary hypertension (Magid et al. 2000). Combination of furosemide with either clenbuterol (Manohar et al. 2000) or pentoxifylline (Manohar 2001) have not been found to enhance the pulmonary hemodynamic efficacy of furosemide in EIPH.

Data from additional studies leave open the question of direct effects of furosemide on pulmonary pressures and mechanics in EIPH. In one study horses treated with NSAIDs (phenylbutazone and flunixin) prior to administration of furosemide followed by exercise did not show reductions in pulmonary and right atrial pressures (Olsen et al. 1992). In a subsequent study these effects could not be reproduced (Manohar 1994). Differences in the studies may be related to drug dosages, time of administration, amount of diuresis, and degree of cyclooxygenase inhibition. While it is accepted that NSAIDs decrease the diuretic response to furosemide, it is as yet unresolved whether these drugs mitigate furosemide-induced reductions in pulmonary and right atrial pressures. It is also not clear whether the magnitude of reduction of pulmonary capillary transmural pressure with furosemide is sufficient to prevent capillary rupture in exercising horses (Soma and Uboh 1998). This is consistent with clinical observations that furosemide reduces, but does not completely eliminate, pulmonary hemorrhage in exercising horses.

Administration of furosemide to racing animals is thought to enhance their performance, although this conclusion remains somewhat controversial. Use of furosemide in racing Thoroughbreds, Quarter Horses, and Standardbreds is estimated at 74.3, 19, and 22.5%, respectively (Hinchcliff 1999). A recent cross-sectional study concluded that Thoroughbreds receiving furosemide raced faster, earned more money, and were more likely to win or finish in the top three positions than unmedicated horses (Gross et al. 1999). Early studies showed increases in racing times when EIPH was diagnosed and a subsequent improvement of racing times upon administration of furosemide (Soma et al. 1985). Treadmill studies have not consistently shown furosemide-induced changes in maximal O_2 consumption, time to fatigue, or the speed at which fatigue occurred in exercising horses (Hinchcliff et al. 1993). However, in these and later studies, the loss of weight associated with furosemide administration did reduce carbon dioxide production, the respiratory exchange ratio, and plasma lactate. Furosemide-induced gains in performance were reversed by addition of a weight equal to the weight of the volume lost. These results suggest that performance benefits associated with furosemide administration to EIPH horses may be unrelated to reduction in hemorrhage and more related to changes in body weight (Soma and Uboh 1998). Based on human studies, this interpretation should not be extended to circumstances in which the race distance is long and exertion prolonged. In these cases, the detrimental effects of dehydration would rapidly offset the advantage of running under reduced weight.

A final issue related to use of furosemide in racing animals involves the regulation of administration of furosemide and other drugs to equine athletes. The control of drugs in racing animal is discussed in more detail in Chapter 57. Doses of 250–500 mg furosemide per horse (0.5–1.0 mg/kg) administered IV no later than 4 hours prior to post time are permitted for medication of horses with EIPH in most jurisdictions in the United States. Specific regulations at a given track should be consulted. The regulation of furosemide administration according to track rules has been approached in a variety of ways. Some jurisdictions use a combination of urine specific gravity of 1.015 or 1.010 and a plasma concentration of greater than 60 or 100 ng/ml as an indication of a violation of the rules. The combination of these two parameters, low specific gravity and high plasma concentration, will suggest that an irregularity related to dose, time, or route of furosemide administration occurred (Soma and Uboh 1998). By considering both urine specific gravity and plasma furosemide concentration, the probability of misclassifying horses as being in violation of regulatory concentrations is reduced (Chu et al. 2001).

Widespread use of furosemide in racing animals also presents problems related to screening of urine for presence of regulated substances. The urinary concentration of coadministered drugs may be diluted as a function of furosemide-enhanced diuresis. Urinary excretion rates of some drugs, especially those that are water-soluble acids, may be altered as a result of furosemide competition for the organic anion tubular secretion pathway. Furosemide has been shown to decrease the urinary concentration of phenylbutazone through both of these mechanisms. In comparison, the excretion rate of other agents, notably fentanyl, procaine, and methylphenidate, is increased by furosemide. Faster clearance of these substances may make it more difficult to detect illegal use prior to a race (Hinchcliff and Muir 1991).

Other Uses. Furosemide has been shown to decrease pulmonary resistance and increase dynamic compliance in ponies with chronic obstructive pulmonary disease. In this case, the rapidity of the response and the finding that the response could be blocked by NSAIDs suggested a cyclooxygenase-mediated event rather than an effect dependent upon loss of body fluid (Broadstone et al. 1991). Immediate changes in pulmonary pressures in other species (e.g., dogs with pulmonary edema) are thought to be related to direct effects of furosemide on the pulmonary vasculature. Similar to use in small animals, furosemide is indicated for treatment of CHF and associated pulmonary edema by decreasing cardiac preload and plasma volume. Furosemide is also recommended to increase urine flow in acute renal failure in horses.

INHIBITORS OF NA^+-CL^- SYMPORT (THIAZIDE AND THIAZIDELIKE DIURETICS)

CHEMISTRY/FORMULATIONS. Thiazide diuretics are benzothiadiazines or analogs and are derivatives of CA-inhibiting sulfonamides. Compared to loop diuretics, thiazides promote renal excretion of chloride, rather than bicarbonate, with sodium, producing a true saluretic effect. Two of the first thiazides synthesized, and the two drugs most commonly used in veterinary medicine, are chlorothiazide (Diuril®, human-approved 250 and 500 mg tablets, 50 mg/ml suspension, and 500 mg/vial injectable available) and hydrochlorothiazide (Hydrozide®, veterinary-approved 25 mg/ml injectable; HydroDiuril®, human-approved 25, 50, and 100 mg tablets and 10 mg/ml oral suspension). Both drugs are derivatives of benzothiadiazine and are water soluble. Hydrozide® is the only veterinary-approved product for use in cattle and has a 72-hour milk withholding time for lactating dairy cattle; no meat withholding time has been reported. Newer generation, more lipid-soluble benzothiadiazine derivatives include cyclothiazide and methychlothiazide.

Nonbenzothiadiazine derivatives have thiazidelike effects, and these drugs also promote excretion of sodium with chloride. Quinazolinone derivatives are in this class and include metolazone and chlorthalidone. These drugs are not commonly used in veterinary medicine but are examples of thiazidelike diuretics.

MECHANISMS AND SITES OF ACTION. The primary site of action of thiazides is the distal convoluted tubule, with some secondary activity, possibly CA-related, in the proximal tubule. In the distal tubule, NaCl reabsorption is mediated by an electroneutral cotransport (symport) system (see Fig. 25.2). The driving force for Cl^- entry is the transmembrane Na^+ gradient established by the activity of basolateral Na^+,K^+-ATPase. The apical NaCl cotransporter is reversibly inhibited by thiazides. Basolateral movement of Cl^- out of the cell is possibly mediated by a KCl cotransport system. The lumen-negative transepithelial potential generated by the polarity of K^+ and Cl^- exit may drive anion reabsorption via a paracellular shunt pathway. Ca^+ reabsorption is enhanced by thiazides, perhaps by increasing distal tubule Ca^{2+}-binding proteins. Because 90% of filtered Na^+ is reabsorbed prior to the distal tubule, the peak diuresis caused by thiazides is moderate compared to loop diuretics. Like loop diuretics, thiazides enhance excretion of K^+ by increasing the delivery of Na^+ to the distal tubule.

ABSORPTION AND ELIMINATION. Thiazide and thiazidelike diuretics are absorbed slowly and incompletely from the gastrointestinal tract. Most drugs in this class are highly protein bound and are excreted renally (chlorothiazide and hydrochlorothiazide) or by a combination of renal and biliary routes (thiazidelike drugs). Hydrochlorothiazide is less protein bound (40%) than others in the class and partitions and accumulates in red blood cells (Velazquez et al. 1995). All drugs in this class gain access to the lumen of the renal tubule via an organic acid secretory pathway. Hence effectiveness of these drugs is decreased if renal blood flow diminishes.

TOXICITY, ADVERSE EFFECTS, CONTRAINDICATIONS, AND DRUG INTERACTIONS. Similar to loop diuretics, most problems associated with administration of thiazides are related to fluid and electrolyte disturbances. Potassium wasting, especially with concurrent use of digitalis, increases the risk of cardiac arrhythmias. Low K^+ may secondarily affect conversion of proinsulin to insulin, leading to hyperglycemia. Enhanced calcium reabsorption can lead to hypercalcemia, and mild magnesuria may cause magnesium deficiency. Depletion of extracellular volume, hyponatremia, hypochloremia, and hypochloremic metabolic alkalosis may occur as adverse effects with prolonged or aggressive thiazide use. Because thiazides block solute reabsorption at nephron sites involved in dilution of urine, these agents increase the risk of hyponatremia under conditions of increased consumption of hypotonic fluids. CNS and gastrointestinal effects may occur but are not common.

Sensitivity to sulfonamides limits use of thiazide diuretics because of the structural similarity between these two classes of drugs. Patients with severe renal disease, hypovolemia, or electrolyte disturbances are poor candidates for thiazide therapy. Impaired hepatic function that may be worsened by volume contraction (leading to hepatic encephalopathy) is a contraindication for thiazide use. Diabetic patients are at risk for thiazide-induced derangements of glucose and insulin.

Drug interactions include decreased effects of anticoagulants and insulin and increased effects of some anesthetics, diazoxide, digitalis glycosides, lithium, loop diuretics, and vitamin D. Combination therapy using low-dose thiazides with front-line antihypertensives (e.g., ACE inhibitors) is currently considered to be an effective alternative strategy for management of human hypertension (Neutel et al. 1996). At low doses, side effects of thiazides are decreased, making their use in combination regimens particularly appealing.

Thiazides are reported to prolong the half-life of quinidine. In the face of thiazide-induced hypokalemia, an elevated plasma quinidine level increases the risk of polymorphic ventricular tachycardia (torsades de pointes), a condition that can deteriorate into ventricular fibrillation (Jackson 1996). NSAIDs may reduce the effectiveness of thiazides and loop diuretics by increasing solute reabsorption at the TAL of the loop of Henle (Brater 1998).

THERAPEUTIC USES. Thiazides may be used to treat edema of cardiac, hepatic, or renal origin. Typical oral dosages in the dog and cat are 20–40 mg/kg every 12 hours (chlorothiazide) and 2–4 mg/kg every 12 hours (hydrochlorothiazide). Effects of both chlorothiazide and hydrochlorothiazide peak at 4 hours and last up to 12 hours, with hydrochlorothiazide typically having a longer duration (12 hr) than chlorothiazide (6–12 hr). Cattle may be treated for udder edema with hydrochlorothiazide (125–250 mg IV or IM once or twice daily). Oral chlorothiazide (not a veterinary-approved product) at a dose of 4–8 mg/kg once or twice daily has been substituted for injectable hydrochlorothiazide following the first or second day of parenteral treatment.

Thiazides have previously been used in veterinary medicine in management of the early stages of CHF. As mentioned previously, early use of loop and thiazide diuretics in CHF activates aldosterone-mediated mechanisms that eventually lead to cardiac deterioration. For this and other reasons, the use of thiazides in treatment of CHF is not common in veterinary medicine. In general, furosemide is more commonly used in veterinary medicine to treat edema, whether it be cardiac, hepatic, or renal in origin. In human medicine, thiazides are commonly used in the management of hypertension. Because thiazides increase reabsorption of calcium, they may also be beneficial in treatment of calcium nephrolithiasis in humans and animals.

Thiazides are used effectively to reduce the volume of urine in patients with nephrogenic diabetes insipidus. Diuretic-induced volume contraction leads to increased proximal tubule reabsorption and a decrease in urine volume of 30–50%. Although dosages are individualized in these patients, starting ranges of 10–20 mg/kg twice daily (chlorothiazide) or 2.75–5.5 mg/kg (hydrochlorothiazide) twice daily have been suggested (Nichols and Thompson 1995).

INHIBITORS OF RENAL EPITHELIAL SODIUM CHANNELS (K^+-SPARING DIURETICS)

CHEMISTRY/FORMULATIONS. The two relevant drugs in this class, triamterene (Dyrenium®) and amiloride (Midamor®), both belong to the class of cyclic amidine diuretics. Triamterene is a pteridine ring with amino groups at the 2, 4, and 7 positions. It was originally synthesized as a folic acid antagonist. Amiloride consists of a substituted pyrazine ring with a carbonylguanidinium side chain. A number of analogs of this basic structure have been synthesized and have been useful tools in elucidating mechanisms of sodium transport. Both triamterene and amiloride are organic bases and are secreted into the proximal tubule by an organic base transport system. Although neither of these drugs is used with frequency in veterinary medicine, triamterene is the more commonly used and hence will be the focus of these discussions. No parenteral forms of the drug are available; oral preparations are available in 50 and 100 mg capsules.

MECHANISMS AND SITES OF ACTION. Triamterene and amiloride cause a mild increase in excretion of NaCl and a retention of K^+. Both drugs slightly augment diuresis and are used in combination with loop diuretics or thiazides to decrease K^+ excretion (hence the term K^+-sparing). Both drugs act at the late distal tubule (or connecting tubule) and collecting duct to block the electrogenic transport of Na^+ (see Fig. 25.2). As with other diuretics, the basolateral Na^+,K^+-ATPase creates an electrochemical gradient that drives events at the luminal surface of the tubular cell. In this case, the principal cells of the connecting tubule contain a Na^+ channel in their luminal membrane that provides a pathway for entry of Na^+ and sets up a lumen-negative transepithelial potential. The transepithelial voltage is the key force involved in driving K^+ out of the principal cell and into the tubular lumen. Blockade of Na^+ channels by triamterene or amiloride hyperpolarizes the luminal membrane, reduces the lumen–negative potential difference, and decreases the excretion of K^+, H^+, Ca^{2+}, and Mg^{2+}. It has been speculated that effects of both of these drugs may also be mediated by inhibition of a Na^+-H^+ antiport located in the late distal tubule and collecting duct. Additional, direct effects on Mg^{2+} excretion may also occur.

Triamterene has been shown to exert cardiac effects that are not secondary to alterations in renal function. Early studies documented a prolongation of the cardiac action potential duration and functional refractory period and an increase in myocardial contractile force. Triamterene has also been shown to decrease digitalis-induced K^+ loss from the heart and increase the dose of digitalis necessary to induce toxic effects in dogs (Palmer and Kleyman 1995; Netzer et al. 1995). Neither triamterene nor amiloride has been shown to affect renal hemodynamics, and neither acts as an aldosterone antagonist.

ABSORPTION AND ELIMINATION. Both amiloride and triamterene are administered orally; triamterene is up to 70% bioavailable. Amiloride is renally excreted. The pharmacokinetics of triamterene are complex. The parent drug is converted in the liver to an active metabolite, 4-hydroxytriamterene sulfate, which is actively secreted into the renal tubules. Hence renal or hepatic disease could impair elimination of triamterene. The peak onset of action of triamterene is 6–8 hours, with effects persisting up to 12–16 hours.

TOXICITY, ADVERSE EFFECTS, CONTRAINDICATIONS, AND DRUG INTERACTIONS. The most important potential side effect of these drugs is hyperkalemia. The presence of diseases or circumstances that may increase the risk of hyperkalemia (e.g., renal failure, coadministration of other drugs with K^+-sparing properties, including ACE inhibitors and K^+ supplements) should be noted and these patients treated with other diuretic combinations. Triamterene may decrease GFR and, in combination with NSAIDs, has been shown to increase the likelihood of hyperkalemia and renal dysfunction. Triamterene-induced renal casts may be responsible for increased risk of interstitial nephritis and renal stones. Both triamterene and amiloride may induce hypersensitivity reactions that include rash and photosensitivity in humans. CNS, gastrointestinal, and hematological side effects have also been reported. As with most other diuretics, use in patients with severe hepatic disease or renal disease is contraindicated. In human patients with hepatic disease, the mild folic acid antagonism inherent in triamterene may increase the risk of megaloblastosis.

THERAPEUTIC USE. Because these drugs have relatively weak diuretic properties, they are clinically important primarily because of their K^+-sparing properties in combination with loop and thiazide diuretics. Both have been used in this capacity for treatment of edema associated with CHF, liver cirrhosis, nephrotic syndrome, steroid-induced edema, and idiopathic edema. Triamterene is administered at a dose of 2–4 mg/kg/day orally to dogs with food to avoid gastrointestinal side effects.

ANTAGONISTS OF MINERALOCORTICOID RECEPTORS (ALDOSTERONE ANTAGONISTS AND K^+-SPARING DIURETICS)

CHEMISTRY/FORMULATIONS. Spironolactone is a 17-spirolactone and is the only aldosterone antagonist approved in the United States. Canrenone, an active metabolite of spironolactone, and potassium canrenoate are closely related structurally and are available in other countries. All of these drugs share a four-ring, steroid structure similar to the mineralocorticoid aldosterone. Spironolactone is available as a human-approved oral preparation (Aldactone®) in 25, 50, and 100 mg tablets.

MECHANISMS AND SITES OF ACTION. Aldosterone is a steroid hormone that binds to mineralocorticoid receptors (MRs) located in the cytoplasm of target cells. The inactive MR complex is bound to heat shock protein 90 (HSP90), a protective chaperon protein, and is incapable of binding to target DNA sequences. Upon binding of aldosterone, HSP90 dissociates from the receptor-hormone complex, allowing movement of the activated receptor into the nucleus. The complex binds to target sequences of DNA referred to as mineralocorticoid-response elements (also termed hormone-responsive elements) that regulate transcription of downstream, mineralocorticoid-responsive genes. Protein products of these responsive genes, aldosterone-induced proteins (AIPs), cause Na^+ reabsorption and increase excretion of K^+ and H^+ in the late distal tubule and collecting duct. AIPs are thought to have multiple effects, including activation, redistribution, and de novo synthesis of Na^+ channels and Na^+,K^+-ATPase, changes in permeability of tight junctions, and increased mitochondrial production of ATP. These effects combine to cause an increase in Na^+ conductance of the luminal membrane and increased Na^+ pump activity in the basolateral membrane. As a result, NaCl transport is increased across tubular epithelial cells, and the lumen-negative transepithelial voltage is increased. Secretion of K^+ and H^+ into the tubular lumen increases with increasing voltages.

Aldosterone antagonists act by binding to the MR and facilitating the release of HSP90 from the steroid-binding subunit of the receptor. The unprotected MR complex is thought to be inactivated by proteases. In the absence of activated MRs, gene transcription is not induced, AIPs are not produced, and the physiological effects of aldosterone are blocked.

In addition to antagonism of aldosterone, spironolactone is thought to act in a manner similar to calcium channel blockers to cause direct vasodilation. By binding to plasma membrane sites, spironolactone may inhibit inward slow calcium channels and depress contractions dependent on release of calcium from the sarcoplasmic reticulum. Aldosterone antagonists have also been shown to increase circulating levels of atrial natriuretic peptide as evaluated in the dog. Hence direct and aldosterone-mediated effects of the drug may contribute to its usefulness in treatment of cardiac disease (Endou and Hosoyamada 1995).

ABSORPTION AND ELIMINATION. In humans, spironolactone is absorbed moderately well (60–90%), is highly protein-bound, and is extensively biotransformed in the liver, exhibiting a first-pass effect. An active metabolite, canrenone, has a longer half-life than the parent drug and extends the biological effects of spironolactone to about 16 hours in humans. Peak diuresis occurs as late as 2–3 days after initiation of therapy. Aldosterone antagonists do not require secretion into the renal tubule to induce diuresis.

TOXICITY, ADVERSE EFFECTS, CONTRAINDICATIONS, AND DRUG INTERACTIONS. Hyperkalemia, dehydration, and hyponatremia are the most common side effects of aldosterone antagonists. When used alone, these drugs can also cause hyperchloremic metabolic acidosis. In humans, sexual side effects limit the use of spironolactone in some patients. The most likely explanation for these effects relates to the binding of drug not only to renal aldosterone receptors but also to progesterone and dihydrotestosterone receptors. This lack of receptor specificity drives continued efforts to identify a more MR-specific antagonist for use in human medicine.

As previously noted, combination of any K^+-sparing diuretic with ACE inhibitors must be accomplished cautiously to avoid hyperkalemia. This is a clinically significant scenario that merits patient monitoring of plasma K^+ concentrations. Because both spironolactone and digoxin have steroidlike structures, the former is thought to compete with digoxin for renal clearance, thus prolonging the half-life of digoxin (Hedman et al. 1992). The presence of spironolactone in plasma may also confound therapeutic drug monitoring of digoxin if a cross-reactive antidigoxin antibody is used in the assay. Aspirin apparently blocks spironolactone-induced natriuresis (Endou and Hosoyamada 1995).

THERAPEUTIC USES. The effectiveness of aldosterone antagonists in promoting diuresis is largely dependent upon elevated concentrations of endogenous aldosterone. Aldosterone secretion increases upon activation of the renin-angiotensin-aldosterone system, which, in turn, responds to reductions in serum sodium, effective blood volume, and cardiac output, and decreases in serum K^+. Secondary hyperaldosteronism and edema are associated with cardiac failure, hepatic cirrhosis, nephrotic syndrome, and severe ascites. Spironolactone is used in veterinary medicine at a dose of 2–4 mg/kg/day orally in management of refractory edema associated with these conditions and has been used in the management of hepatic cirrhosis. In both human and veterinary medicine, aldosterone antagonists are commonly administered with a thiazide or loop diuretic to increase peak diuresis and to spare K^+.

Elevated aldosterone levels have been shown to be a useful prognostic indicator in heart failure, with higher levels correlated with a poorer prognosis. Activation of the renin-angiotensin-aldosterone system in arterial hypertension is thought to lead to remodeling of the myocardial collagen network with progressive cardiac interstitial fibrosis. As fibrosis increases, diastolic function deteriorates and pathologic cardiac hypertrophy occurs. When aldosterone-mediated effects are blocked by spironolactone, progression of myocardial failure is presumably slowed. A clinical study in humans supported this contention by showing significant delays in progression of CHF in patients treated with spironolactone (Pitt et al. 1999). No comprehensive study has been published to verify this effect in veterinary patients. Diuretic efficacy of spironolactone was not demonstrated in a study combining the drug with furosemide in greyhound dogs (Rioordan and Estrada 2005).

A newer drug, eplerenone, reduced mortality in a human study of heart failure due to myocardial infarction (Weir and McMurray 2005), and the drug has also been shown to have cardioprotective effects in animal models of myocardial failure (McMahon 2003). Despite the potential side effect of hyperkalemia associated with coadministration of aldosterone-antagnonists and ACE inhibitors, this combination with appropriate dosages has been deemed effective in management of CHF. Patient monitoring for K^+ derangements is critical to safe implementation of this approach. In veterinary medicine, spironolactone may be useful in patients with CHF secondary to chronic valvular heart disease or dilated cardiomyopathy that become unresponsive to therapy with ACE inhibitors, digoxin, and furosemide.

NEW AND EXPERIMENTAL AGENTS

AQUARETICS. Vasopressin (or arginine vasopressin, AVP) regulates water and solute excretion in the kidney by binding to V2 receptors in the principal cells of the renal collecting duct system. As one of three G-protein-coupled AVP receptor subtypes (V1a, V1b, V2), V2 receptors mediate the antidiuretic effects of AVP. V2 receptor antagonists, so-called aquaretic agents, promote solute-free water excretion These antagonists hold considerable promise for treatment of edematous states associated with heart failure, liver cirrhosis, nephrotic syndrome, and syndrome of inappropriate secretion of antidiuretic hormone (Verbalis 2006). While peptide derivatives of AVP have been found to have intrinsic antidiuretic properties, several nonpeptide antagonists are in development. These include VPA-985 (lixivaptan), OPC-41061 (tolvaptan), SR-121463, and YM-087 (conivaptan). These drugs typically increase urine volume and decrease urine osmolality and body weight without affecting urinary sodium excretion (Orita and Nakahama 1998; Serradeil-Le Gal 1998; Palm et al. 2006). Conivaptan was shown to improve impaired cardiovascular parameters induced by intravenous infusion of AVP in a dog model, suggesting possible clinical usefulness (Yatsu et al. 2002).

Although vasopressin antagonists represent the most promising area of drug development for induction of aquaresis, drugs that interfere with secretion of AVP from the neurohypophysis and drugs that directly inhibit water channels in the collecting ducts are also of interest. Aquaporin-CD, the water channel of the principal cell of the cortical and medullary collecting duct, has been cloned and provides an attractive site for drugs intended to inhibit diuresis.

NEUTRAL ENDOPEPTIDASE INHIBITORS. Neutral endopeptidase (NEP) is an enzyme that rapidly degrades atrial natriuretic factor (ANF), the cardiac peptide hormone that increases sodium and water excretion, inhibits the renin-angiotensin-aldosterone system and produces vasodilation. NEP inhibitors have been investigated for their possible usefulness in increasing circulating concentrations of ANF and therefore increasing the fractional excretion of sodium. An experimental NEP inhibitor, ecadotril, has been investigated in induced heart failure in dogs (Solter et al. 2000; Mishima et al. 2002) and been shown to attenuate progression of disease. NEP inhibitors have been shown in dogs to enhance the actions of furosemide and prevent the furosemide-induced activation of the renin-angiotensin-aldosterone system (Kittleson and Kienle 2007).

DOPAMINE RECEPTOR AGONISTS. Dopaminergic receptor 1 (DA-1) and dopaminergic receptor 2 (DA-2) have both been considered targets for low-dose dopamine therapy of low output renal failure in dogs and humans. Efficacy of low dose dopamine has been questioned and concerns have been raised over renal morbidity and gastrointestinal side effects. It has been noted that although dopamine increases renal perfusion and urine output, increases in creatinine clearance are not sufficient to achieve therapeutic efficacy in management of renal failure. In comparison, DA-1 selective agonists may be more effective at increasing renal blood flow, inducing diuresis and natriuresis, and increasing glomerular filtration rate. This is particularly true in cats, a species that does not respond well to the renal effects of dopamine. Fenoldopam, a selective DA-1 agonist, has been investigated in both dogs and cats. In cats, fenoldopam at a dose of 0.5 μg/kg/min induced diuresis in a delayed manner, by 6 hours postadministration, increased urine output, sodium excretion, fractional clearance of sodium, and elimination of creatinine (Simmons et al. 2006).

REFERENCES AND ADDITIONAL READING

Adin, D. B., Taylor, A. W., Hill, R. C., Scott, K. C., Martin, F. G. 2003. Intermittent bolus injection versus continuous infusion of furosemide in normal adult greyhound dogs. J Vet Int Med 17:632–636.

Anderson, S., He, W., and Temple, D. 1991. Inhibition by furosemide of inflammatory mediators from lung fragments. N Engl J Med 324:131.

Better, O. S., Rubinstein, I., Winaver, J. M., and Knochel, J. P. 1997. Mannitol therapy revisited (1940–1997). Kidney Int 51:886–894.

Betz, A. L., Ianotti, F., and Hoff, J. T. 1989. Brain edema: a classification based on blood-brain barrier integrity. Cerebrovasc Brain Metab Rev 1:133–154.

Bianco, S., Robuschi, M., and Vaghi, A. 1988. Prevention of exercise-induced bronchoconstriction by inhaled furosemide. Lancet 2:252–255.

Bianco, S., Pieroni, M., and Refini, R. 1989. Protective effect of inhaled furosemide on allergen-induced early and late asthmatic reactions. N Engl J Med 321:1069–1073.

Bleich, M., and Greger, R. 1997. Mechanism of action of diuretics. Kidney Int 51 (Suppl 59):S11–S15.

Brater, D. C. 1993. Resistance to diuretics: mechanisms and clinical implications. Adv Nephrol 22:349–369.

———. 1998. Diuretic therapy. New Engl J Med 339:387–395.

Broadstone, R. V., Robinson, N. E., and Gray, P. R. 1991. Effects of furosemide on ponies with recurrent airway obstruction. Pulm Pharmacol 44:203–208.

Chu, K., Cohen, N., Stanley, S., Wang, N. 2001. Estimation of the probability for exceeding thresholds of urine specific gravity and plasma concentration of furosemide at various intervals after intravenous administration of furosemide in horses. Amer J Vet Res 62:1349–1353.

Cloyd, J. C., Snyder, B. D., and Cleermans, B. 1986. Mannitol pharmacokinetics and serum osmolality in dogs and humans. J Pharmacol Exp Ther 236:301–306.

Data, J., Rane, A., and Gerkens, J. 1978. The influence of indomethacin on the pharmacokinetics, diuretic response, and hemodynamics of furosemide in the dog. J Pharmacol Exp Ther 206:431–438.

Demling, R., and Will, J. 1978. The effect of furosemide on the pulmonary transvascular fluid filtration rate. Crit Care Med 6:317–319.

Dormans, T. P. J, Pickkers, P., Russel, F. G. M. and Smits, P. 1996. Vascular effects of loop diuretics. Cardiovasc Res 32:988–997.

Dresser, M. J., Leabman, M. K., and Giacomini, K. M. 2001. Transporters involved in the elimination of drugs in the kidney: Organic anion transporters and organic cation transporters. J Pharm Sci 90:397–421.

Dyke, T., Hubel, J., Grosenbaugh, D., Beard, W., Mitten, L., Sams, R., and Hinchcliff, K. 1998. The pharmacokinetics of furosemide in anaesthetized horses after bilateral ureteral ligation. J Vet Pharmacol Therap 21:298–303.

Endou, H., and Hosoyamada, M. 1995. Potassium-retaining diuretics: aldosterone antagonists. In R. F. Greger, H. Knauf, and E. Mutschler, eds., Handbook of Experimental Pharmacology, vol. 117, Diuretics, pp. 335–355. Berlin: Springer-Verlag.

Feldman, A., Levine, M., and Gerstenblith, G. 1987. Negative inotropic effects of furosemide in the isolated rabbit heart: a prostaglandin-mediated event. J Cardiovasc Pharmacol 9:493–499.

Gamba, G., Slatzberg, S. N., Lombardi, M., et al. 1993. Primary structure and functional expression of a cDNA encoding the thiazide-sensitive, electroneutral sodium-chloride cotransporter. Proc Natl Acad Sci USA 90:2749–2753.

Gamba, G., Miyanoshita, A., Lombardi, M., et al. 1994. Molecular cloning, primary structure, and characterization of two members of the mammalian electroneutral sodium- (potassium-) chloride cotransporter family expressed in kidney. J Biol Chem 269:17713–17722.

Ghys, A., Denef, J., Delarge, J., Georges, A. 1985. Renal effects of the high ceiling diuretic torasemide in rats and dogs, Arzneimittelforschung 35:1527.

Goodwin, J., and Hamlin, R. 1993. Preferences of veterinarians for drugs used to treat heart disease in dogs and cats: a 20-year follow-up study. J Vet Int Med 7:118.

Gross, D. K., Morley, P. S., Hinchcliff, K. W., and Wittum, T. E. 1999. Effect of furosemide on performance of Thoroughbreds racing in the United States and Canada. JAVMA 215:670–675.

Hedman, A., Angelin, B., Arvidsson, A., and Dahogvist, R. 1992. Digoxin interactions in man: spironolactone reduces renal but not biliary digoxin clearance. Eur J Clin Pharmacol 42:481–485.

Hinchcliff, K. W. 1999. Effects of furosemide on athletic performance and exercise-induced pulmonary hemorrhage in horses. JAVMA 215:630–635.

Hinchcliff, K. W., and Muir, W. 1991. Pharmacology of furosemide in the horse: a review. J Vet Int Med 5:211–218.

Hinchcliff, K. W., McKeever, K. H., and Muir, W. W. 1993. Effect of furosemide and weight carriage on energetic responses of horses to incremental exertion. Amer J Vet Res 54:1500–1504.

Hinchcliff, K. W., Hubbell, J., Grosenbaugh, D., Mitten, L., and Beard, W. 1996. Hemodynamic effects of furosemide are dependent on diuresis. Proc Am Assoc Equine Practitioners, 42:229–230.

Hirai, J., Miyazaki, H., and Taneike, T. 1992. The pharmacokinetics and pharmacodynamics of furosemide in the anaesthetized dog. J Vet Pharmacol Therap 15:231–239.

Jackson, E. K. 1996. Diuretics. In J. G. Hardman and L. E. Limbird, eds., Goodman and Gilman's The Pharmacological Basis of Therapeutics, 9th ed., pp. 685–713. New York: McGraw-Hill.

Johansson, A., Gardner, S., Levine, J. et al. 2003. Furosemide continuous rate infusion in the horse: evaluation of enhanced efficacy and reduced side effects. J Vet Int Med 17:887–895.

Johansson, A., Gardner, S., Levine, J. et al. 2004. Pharmacokinetics and pharmacodynamics of furosemide after oral administration to horses. J Vet Int Med 18:739–743.

Keene, B., and Rush, J. 1995. Therapy of heart failure. In S. Ettinger and E. Feldman, eds., Textbook of Veterinary Internal Medicine, 4th ed., pp. 878–881. Philadelphia: W. B. Saunders.

Kirchner, K. 1987. Indomethacin antagonizes furosemide's intratubular effects during loop segment microperfusion. J. Pharmacol Exp Ther 243:881–886.

Kittleson, M. D., and Kienle R. D. 2007. Chapter 10: Management of heart failure—New or experimental heart failure drugs in the United States. In M.D. Kittleson and R.D. Kienle eds., Small Animal Cardiovascular Medicine, 2nd edition, on-line version, Elsevier Health.

Kriz, W., and Bankir, L. 1988. A standard nomenclature for structures of the kidney. Am J Physiol 254:F1–F8.

Kriz, W., and Kaissling, B. 1992 In D. W. Seldin and G. Giebisch, eds., The Kidney: Physiology and Pathophysiology, 2d ed., pp. 707–777. New York: Raven Press.

Lang, F., and Busch, A. 1995. Basic concepts of renal physiology. In R. F. Greger, H. Knauf, and E. Mutschler, eds., Handbook of Experimental Pharmacology, vol. 117, Diuretics, pp. 67–114. Berlin: Springer-Verlag.

Lester, G., Clark, C., Rice, B., Steible-Hartless, C., and Vetro-Widenhouse, T. 1999. Effect of timing and route of administration of furosemide on pulmonary hemorrhage and pulmonary arterial pressure in exercising Thoroughbred racehorses. Am J Vet Res 60:22–28.

Levinsky, N. G., and Bernard, D. B. 1988. Mannitol and loop diuretics in acute renal failure. In B. M. Brenner and J. M. Lazarus, eds., Acute Renal Failure, 2nd ed., pp. 841–856. New York: Churchill Livingstone.

Magid, J,, Manohar, M., Goetz, T. E. et al. 2000. Pulmonary vascular pressures of Thoroughbred horses exercised 1, 2, 3 and 4 h after furosemide administration. J Vet Pharmacol Ther 23:81–89.

Manohar, M. 1994. Pulmonary vascular pressures of strenuously exercising Thoroughbreds after administration of flunixin meglumine and furosemide. Am J Vet Res 55:1308–1312.

Manohar, M., Goetz, T. E., Rothenbaum, P., Humphrey, S. 2000. Clenbuterol administration does not enhance the efficacy of furosemide in attenuating the exercise-induced pulmonary capillary hypertension in Thoroughbred horses. J Vet Pharmacol Ther 23:389–95.

Manohar, M., Goetz, T. E., Rothenbaum, P, Humphrey, S. 2001. Intravenous pentoxifylline does not enhance the pulmonary haemodynamic efficacy of frusemide in strenuously exercising Thoroughbred horses. Equine Vet J 33:354–9.

McMahon, E. G. 2003. Eplerenone, a new selective aldosterone blocker. Curr Pharm Des 9:1065.

Mindel, J. S. 1997. Dorzolamide: development and clinical application of a topical carbonic anhydrase inhibitor. Surv Ophthalmol 42: 137–151.

Mishima, T., Tanimura, M., Suzuki, A. et al. 2002. Effects of chronic neutral endopeptidase inhibition on the progression of left ventricular dysfunction and remodeling in dogs with moderate heart failure. Cardiovasc Drugs Ther 16:209–14.

Morrison, R. T. 1997. Edema and principles of diuretic use. Med Clin N Am 81:689–704.

Netzer, T., Ullrich, R., Knauf, H., and Mutschler, E. 1995. Potassium-retaining diuretics: triamterene. In R. F. Greger, H. Knauf, and E. Mutschler, eds., Handbook of Experimental Pharmacology, vol. 117, Diuretics, pp. 396–421. Berlin: Springer-Verlag.

Neutel, J., Black, H., and Weber, M. 1996. Combination therapy with diuretics: an evolution of understanding. Am J Med 101 (Suppl 3A): 61S–70S.

Nichols, R., and Thompson, L. 1995. Pituitary-hypothalamic disease. In S. Ettinger, and E. Feldman, eds., Textbook of Veterinary Internal Medicine, 4th ed., p. 1432. Philadelphia: W. B. Saunders.

Olsen, S. C., Coyne, C. P., and Lowe, B. S. 1992. Influence of cyclooxygenase inhibitors on furosemide-induced hemodynamic effects during exercise in horses. Am J Vet Res 53:1562–1567.

Orita, Y., and Nakahama, H. 1998. Vasopressin receptor antagonists. Intern Med 37:219–221.

Paczynski, R. 1997. Osmotherapy: basic concepts and controversies. Crit Care Clin 13:105–129.

Palm, C., Pistrosch, F., Herbrig, K., and Gross, P. 2006. Vasopressin antagonists as aquaretic agents for the treatment of hyponatremia. Am J Med 119(7 Suppl 1):S87–92.

Palmer, L. G., and Kleyman, T. R. 1995. Potassium-retaining diuretics: amiloride. In R. F. Greger, H. Knauf, and E. Mutschler, eds., Handbook of Experimental Pharmacology, vol. 117, Diuretics, pp. 363–388. Berlin: Springer-Verlag.

Pfeiffer, N. 1997. Dorzolamide: development and clinical application of a topical carbonic anhydrase inhibitor. Surv Ophthalmol 42:137–151.

Pitt, B., Zannad, F., Remme, W. J., et al. 1999. The effect of spironolactone on morbidity and mortality in patients with severe heart failure. New Engl J Med 341:709–717.

Prough, D. S., and Zornow, M. H. 1998. Mannitol: an old friend on the skids? Crit Care Med 26:997–998.

Reef, V., and McGuirk, S. 1996. Diseases of the cardiovascular system. In B. Smith, ed., Large Animal Internal Medicine, 2nd ed., p. 531. St. Louis: Mosby Year Book.

Riordan, L., and Estrada, A. 2005. Diuretic efficacy of oral spironolactone when used in conjunction with furosemide in healthy adult greyhounds. J Vet Int Med 19:451.

Rivas, L. J., and Hinchcliff, K. W. 1997. Effect of furosemide and subsequent intravenous fluid administration on right atrial pressure of splenectomized horses. Am J Vet Res 58:632–635.

Roberts, S. E. 1985. Assessment and management of the ophthalmic emergency. Compend Cont Ed 7:739–752.

Rudehill, A., Gordon, E., and Ohman, G. 1993. Pharmacokinetics and effects of mannitol on hemodynamics, blood, and cerebrospinal fluid electrolytes, and osmolality during intracranial surgery. J Neurosurg Anesthesiol 5:4–12.

Schwartz, M. A. 1981. Metabolism of bumetanide, J Clin Pharmacol 21:555.

Serradeil-Le Gal, C. 1998. Nonpeptide antagonists for vasopressin receptors. In Zingg et al., eds., Vasopressin and Oxytocin, pp. 427–438. New York: Plenum Press.

Simmons, J., Wohl, J., Schwartz, D., et al. 2006. Diuretic effects of fenoldopam in healthy cats. J Vet Emerg Crit Care 16: 96–103.

Smal, J., Marvola, M., Liljequist, C., and Happonen, I. 1996. Prolonged-release hydroxypropyl methylcellulose matrix tablets of furosemide for administration to dogs. J Vet Pharmacol Therap 19:482–487.

Solter, P., Sisson, D., Thomas, W., Goetze, L. 2000. Intrarenal effects of ecadotril during acute volume expansion in dogs with congestive heart failure, J Pharmacol Exp Ther 293:989.

Soma, L. R., and Uboh, C. E. 1998. Review of furosemide in horse racing: its effects and regulation. J Vet Pharmacol Therap 21:228–240.

Soma, L. R., Laster, L., and Oppenlander, F. 1985. Effects of furosemide on the racing times of horses with exercise-induced pulmonary hemorrhage. Am J Vet Res 46:763–768.

Svedberg, K., et al. 1990. Hormones regulating cardiovascular function in patients with severe congestive heart failure and their relation to mortality: Consensus Trial Study Group. Circulation 82:1730.

Uechi, M., Matsuoka, M., Kuwajima, E., Kaneko, T., Yamashita, K., Fukushima, U., Ishikawa, Y. 2003. The effects of the loop diuretics furosemide and torasemide on diuresis in dogs and cats. J Vet Med Sci 65:1057-61.

Velazquez, H., Knauf, H., and Mutschler, E. 1995. Thiazide diuretics. In R. F. Greger, H. Knauf, and E. Mutschler, eds., Handbook of Experimental Pharmacology, vol. 117, Diuretics, pp. 275–321. Berlin: Springer-Verlag.

Verbalis, J. G. 2006. AVP receptor antagonists as aquaretics: a review and assessment of clinical data. Cleve Clin J Med 73 Suppl 3:S24–33.

Ware, W. 1998. Disorders of the cardiovascular system. In R. Nelson and C. G. Couto, eds., Small Animal Internal Medicine, 2nd ed., pp. 58–59. St. Louis: Mosby.

Watson, A., and Church, D. 1995. Preferences of veterinarians for drugs to treat heart disease in dogs and cats. Aus Vet J 72:401–403.

Weir, R., McMurray, J. J. 2005. Treatments that improve outcome in the patient with heart failure, left ventricular systolic dysfunction, or both after acute myocardial infarction. Heart 91(Suppl)2:ii17–ii20.

Yatsu, T., Kusayama, T., Tomura, Y. et al. 2002. Effect of conivaptan, a combined vasopressin V(1a) and V(2) receptor antagonist, on vasopressin-induced cardiac and haemodynamic changes in anaesthetized dogs. Pharmacol Res 46:375–81.

Xu, J. C., Lytle, C., Zhu, T. T., Payne, J. A., Benz, E., Jr., and Forbush, B., III. 1994. Molecular cloning and functional expression of the bumetanide-sensitive Na-K-Cl cotransporter. Proc Natl Acad Sci USA 91:2201–2205.

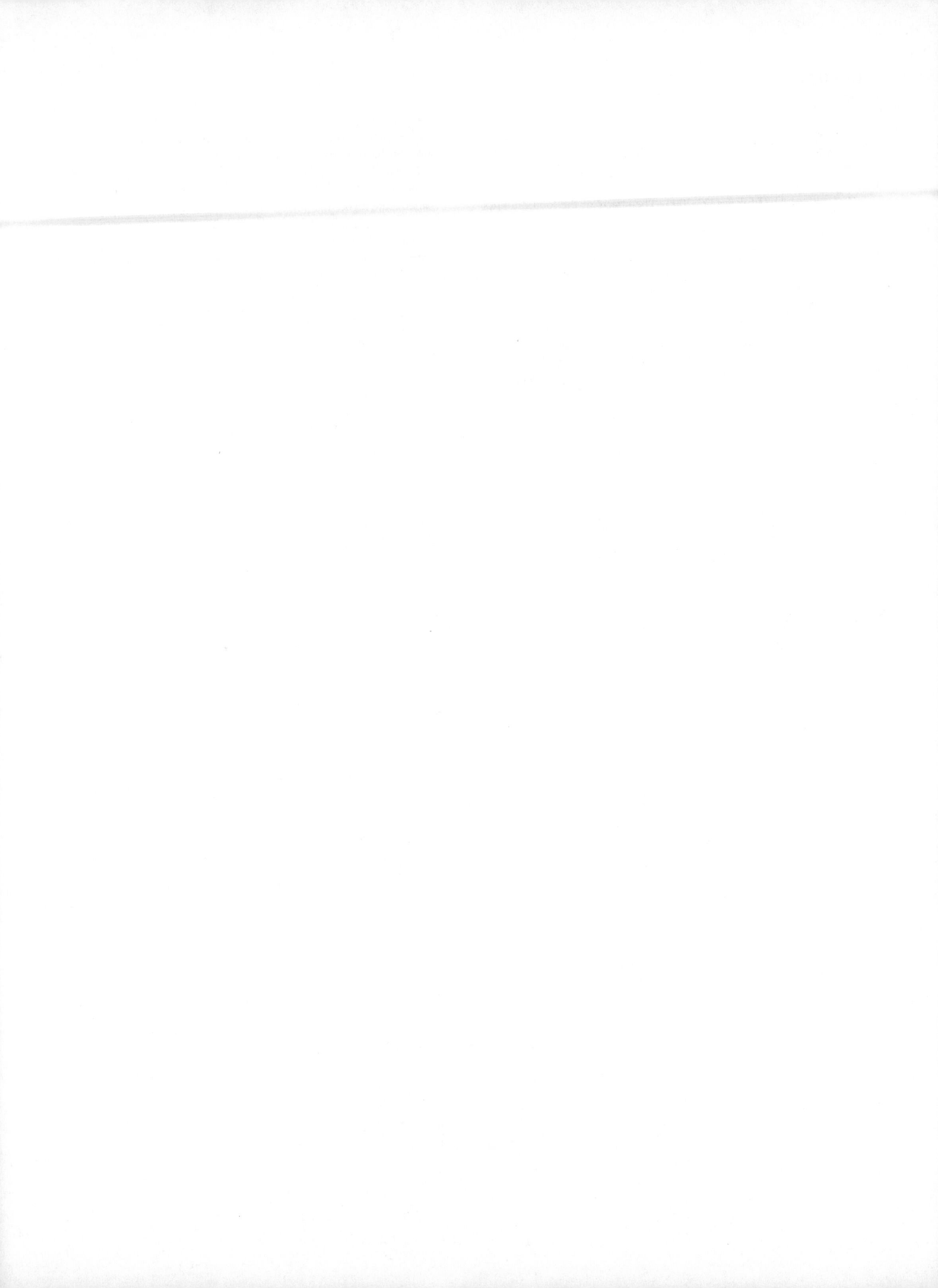

SECTION 7

Drugs Acting on Blood and Blood Elements

CHAPTER

26

HEMOSTATIC AND ANTICOAGULANT DRUGS

H. RICHARD ADAMS

Several drugs and animal tissue extracts have pronounced effects on hemostatic and blood coagulation mechanisms. Some of these substances promote hemostasis and have clinical value in control of blood oozing from small vessels. Hemostatic agents include thrombin, thromboplastin, fibrin, and fibrinogen. In contrast, drugs such as heparin and coumarin retard hemostasis by impeding clot formation. Heparin is used in vivo, as are the coumarin-derivative anticoagulants, in treatment and prevention of thromboembolic disorders. Additional approaches involve the enzyme streptokinase and tissue plasminogen activator, which accelerate fibrinolytic breakdown of formed clots and clotting factors. Thrombus formation also is reduced by inhibitors of platelet aggregation such as aspirin and ticlopidine. A wide variety of new compounds has led to new approaches to anticoagulant and thrombolytic therapy in humans (Majerus and Tollefsen 2006), although their clinical use in animals remains to be validated.

An overview of local factors involved in control of bleeding will first be presented as an aid to understanding how hemostatic and anticoagulant drugs affect hemostasis-related mechanisms.

HEMOSTASIS

Hemostasis refers to prevention or control of hemorrhage. Physiologic control systems operate to ensure fluidity of blood under normal conditions, yet opposing systems promote coagulation when the circulatory system is invaded (Edelberg et al. 2001). Hemostasis is achieved through a series of interdependent mechanisms, including vascular spasm of the injured artery or vein, local aggregation of platelets into a plug, coagulation of the blood into a clot, and subsequent dissolution of the formed clot by fibrinolysis. The basic process of hemostasis can be separated into the vascular, platelet, coagulation, and fibrinolysis phases. The phases overlap considerably, and events in one step promote and even cause development of subsequent phases (Chart and Sanderson 1979).

VASCULAR AND PLATELET PHASES. The vascular and platelet phases are closely allied, with the vascular endothelium having a multitude of both anticoagulant and procoagulant functions (Nawroth et al. 1986). Immediately after a blood vessel is cut or otherwise traumatized, the vascular wall contracts and platelets start adhering to the injured site. The local vasoconstrictor response, or vascular spasm, mechanically retards the flow of blood escaping from the vessel. Vascular spasm may be partly a local reflex or myogenic response and partly humoral owing to vasoactive agents released from platelets and nearby endothelial cells. Local vasoconstriction lasts as long as 20–30 minutes, during which the ensuing phases of platelet aggregation and blood coagulation take place (Moncada and Vane 1979).

Damage to a blood vessel results in exposed subendothelial collagen. Collagen and other proteins localized to the subendothelium are strong stimuli for platelet adherence. For platelets to properly attach to a traumatized area, von Willebrand factor (vWf) must be present because the platelets express a vWf integrin receptor that facilitates adherence. Once adhesion has occurred, the platelets undergo a change in shape and release diverse substances that recruit further platelets to the clot and promote the coagulation cascade. This process is termed platelet aggregation. The substances released include adenosine diphosphate (ADP), adenosine triphosphate (ATP), serotonin (5-HT), platelet factor 3 and 4, thromboxane A_2, and platelet-derived growth factor. This aggregation yields a rather loosely formed plug or platelet thrombus at the injury site.

Involvement of Prostaglandins. Adenosine diphosphate is a potent chemical activator of platelet aggregation, which in turn activates a phospholipase that acts on membrane phospholipid to yield arachidonic acid. The latter is transformed by a platelet cyclooxygenase into short-lived but potent aggregating compounds called cyclic endoperoxides (prostaglandins [PGs] G_2 and H_2). These endoperoxides are converted by platelet thromboxane synthase to a potent aggregating compound called thromboxane A_2. Thus platelet clumping initiates formation of chemical agents that promote further platelet aggregation. In contrast, prostacyclin (PGI_2) is a PG that inhibits platelet aggregation and acts as a counterbalance to thromboxane. PGI_2 is formed from arachidonic acid and intermediate cyclic endoperoxides. Prostacyclin synthase, the enzyme responsible for transformation of PGI_2 from the cyclic endoperoxides, is localized in the vascular endothelium rather than in platelets. The platelet activation sequence is shown in Figure 26.1.

Vascular spasm and platelet adhesion, aggregation, and release of chemical agents are initiated within seconds after vascular trauma. During subsequent events, the platelet plug becomes more tightly bound and organized by incorporation of fibrin strands formed during coagulation.

COAGULATION PHASE. Blood clotting results from a complex series of interdependent events. Clotting ingredients normally exist as inactive factors in blood vessels, perivascular tissue, and the blood itself. Upon injury to the circulatory system, the inactive or procoagulant substances are transformed to active clotting factors. Activation of all factors does not occur simultaneously (Broze 2001). Rather, the activated form of one factor activates a subsequent factor in a sequential series of reactions, yielding a cascade or "waterfall" effect. Biochemically, the activation process is accomplished for most of the clotting factors by the proteolytic splitting off of a small moiety of the inactive procoagulant factor (Majerus and Tollefson 2006).

Blood clotting factors generally are designated by Roman numerals I–V and VII–XIII, as listed in Table 26.1. Nomenclature of the factors has undergone considerable revision over the years (Jain 1993). Factors V and VII–XIII usually are designated by their numbers, whereas factors I and II are referred to commonly as *fibrinogen* and *prothrombin,* respectively. Tissue thromboplastin is factor III and should not be confused with platelet factor 3. There is no factor VI. Important synonyms for the major clotting factors are included in Table 26.1.

Although clotting factors participate in coagulation through different pathways, the overall coagulation process can be divided into three major events: (1) a substance called *prothrombin activator* or *complete thromboplastin* is

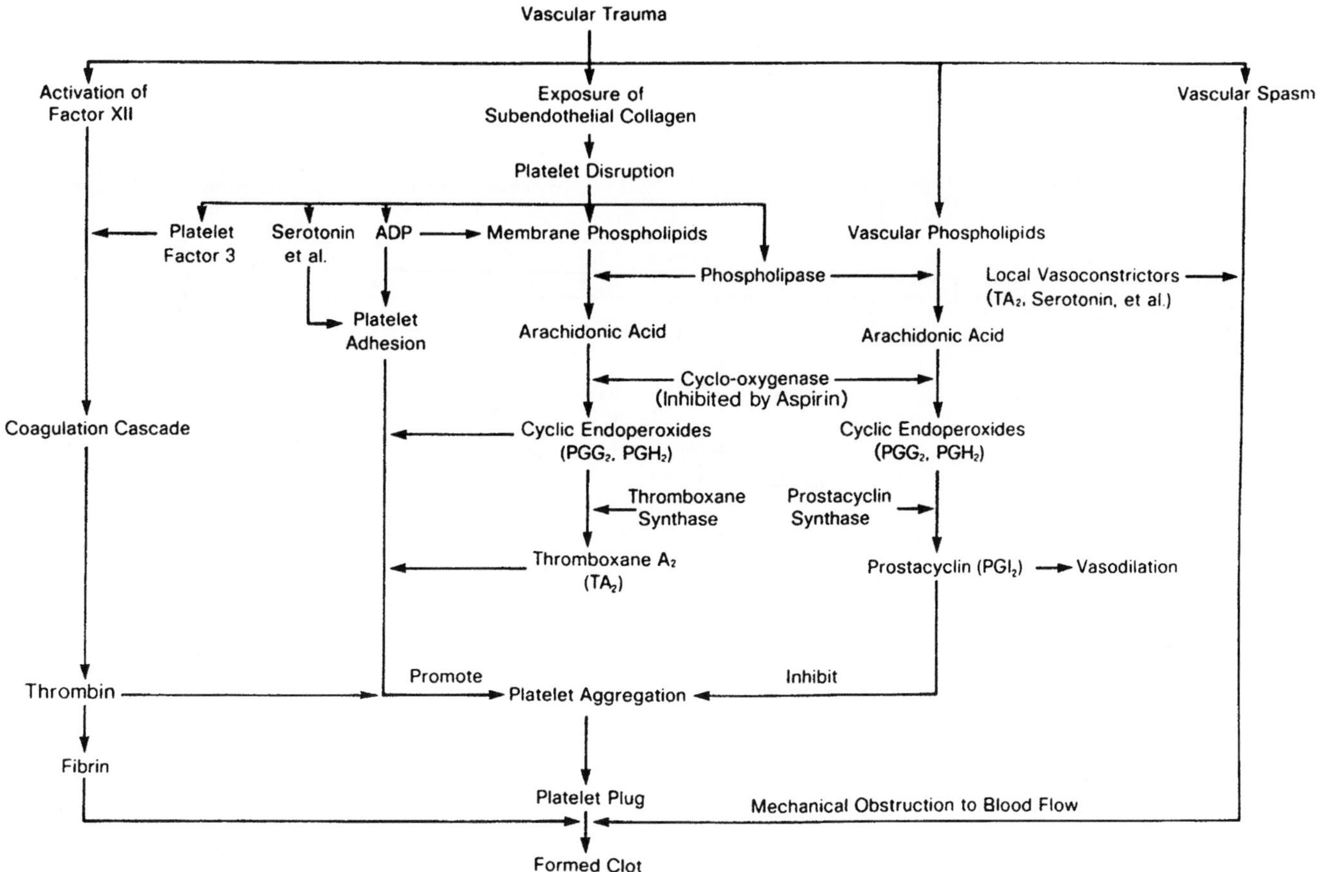

FIG. 26.1 Vascular and platelet phases of hemostasis. PG = prostaglandin; ADP = adenosine diphosphate.

TABLE 26.1 Blood coagulation factors and their synonyms

Factor	Synonym
Factor I	Fibrinogen
Factor II	Prothrombin
Factor III	Tissue thromboplastin
Factor IV	Calcium
Factor V	Proaccelerin
Factor VII	Proconvertin; serum prothrombin conversion accelerator
Factor VIII	Antihemophilic factor
Factor IX	Plasma thromboplastin component; Christmas factor
Factor X	Stuart-Prower factor
Factor XI	Plasma thromboplastin antecedent
Factor XII	Hageman factor
Factor XIII	Fibrin stabilizing factor

formed in response to trauma to blood vessels, extravascular tissues, or the blood itself; 2) prothrombin activator catalyzes the transformation of prothrombin to thrombin; and 3) thrombin rapidly catalyzes conversion of fibrinogen into threads of fibrin, which in turn enmesh platelets, plasma, and erythrocytes to form a clot.

The initial step, formation of prothrombin activator, is the most complex and least understood. This substance can be produced by two basic routes: the intrinsic pathway instigated by trauma to the blood itself and the extrinsic pathway that begins with damage to the vessel wall and extravascular tissues. In vivo the coagulation factors involved in the intrinsic and extrinsic coagulation pathways overlap and interact with each other. The strict separation of the intrinsic and extrinsic coagulation pathways is based upon the in vitro coagulation assays.

Intrinsic Pathway. Blood taken by venipuncture and placed in a glass container clots normally within 5–10 minutes because all factors required for coagulation are present within the blood (Fig. 26.2). This pathway is initiated because trauma to the blood directly affects two important coagulation factors within the blood itself, the

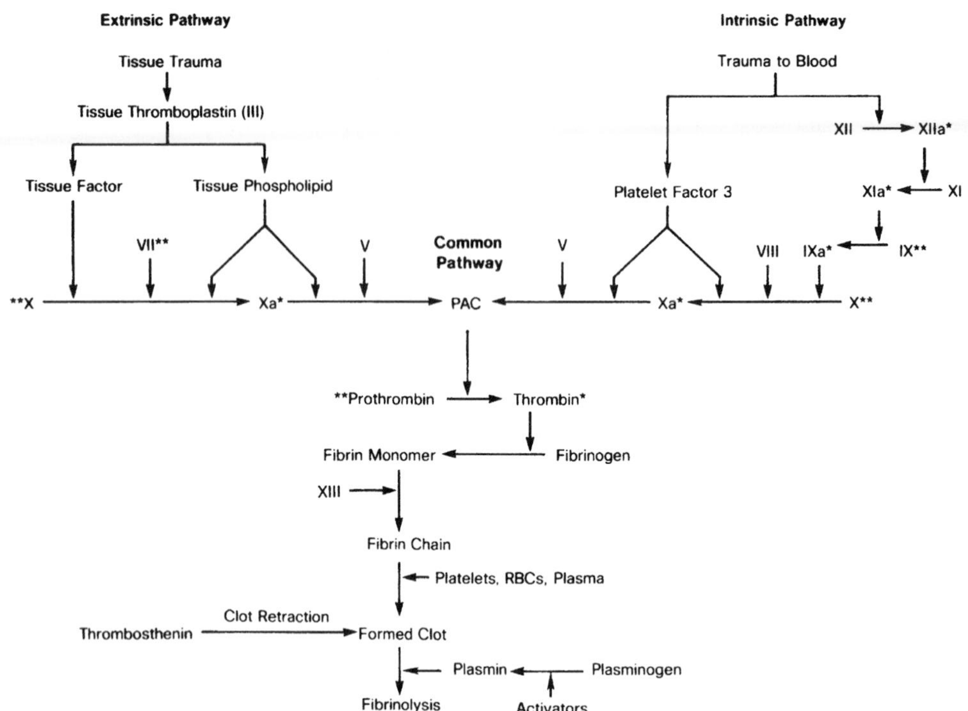

FIG. 26.2 Blood coagulation, clot formation, and fibrinolysis. PAC = prothrombin activator complex (also referred to as complete thromboplastin, prothrombinase, prothrombinase complex, and intrinsic or extrinsic thromboplastin); a = activated forms of clotting factors; * = factors inhibited by heparin; ** = factors inhibited by coumarin derivatives. Calcium is required in most reactions.

platelets and factor XII. Platelets damaged by contact with a wettable surface like glass (or collagen in vivo) release the phospholipid commonly referred to as platelet factor 3. In addition, factor XII is transformed into activated factor XII when disturbed by trauma to the blood. The activated form of factor XII in turn activates factor XI and forms kallikrein. Factor XI converts factor IX to an activated form. The activated factor IX interacts with factor VIII in conjunction with the platelet phospholipid to convert factor X to activated factor X (Xa). Finally, activated factor X interacts with factor V and platelet phospholipids to yield the complex called prothrombin activator (intrinsic thromboplastin system). Prothrombin activator immediately catalyzes the cleavage of prothrombin to thrombin, which converts fibrinogen into fibrin (Fig. 26.2).

Extrinsic Pathway. When tissue extract is added to whole blood, clotting occurs rapidly in about 10–15 seconds. The extrinsic factor that sets the coagulation cascade into motion is released from traumatized tissues (Fig. 26.2). Referred to as tissue thromboplastin, the extrinsic factor includes a combination of a proteolytic enzymes simply called tissue factor and tissue phospholipids that are probably derived from cell membrane components. First, the tissue factor interacts with clotting factor VII; this complex converts factor X to activated factor X in the presence of the tissue phospholipids. In addition, factor IX is activated, which can also lead to further factor X activation. The subsequent step is essentially the same as the last step in the intrinsic pathway; i.e., activated factor X interacts with factor V and tissue phospholipid to form prothrombin activator (extrinsic thromboplastin system). The difference is that tissue phospholipids are used in the extrinsic system while platelet phospholipids are used in the intrinsic system (Fig. 26.2).

Fibrin Formation. Prothrombin activator, whether derived from the intrinsic or extrinsic pathway, converts the α_2-globulin prothrombin into thrombin. Thrombin in turn acts as a proteolytic enzyme and cleaves two low molecular weight peptides from each molecule of fibrinogen, forming a molecule of fibrin monomer (Mann et al. 2003). Thrombin also promotes platelet aggregation and activates factors XIII, XII, VIII, and V. Fibrin monomers immediately polymerize with each other, forming long fibrin threads that act as the reticulum network for the clot. The fibrin chains initially are somewhat loosely bound. However, clotting factor XIII (fibrin-stabilizing factor) quickly acts as an enzyme to cause covalent bonding between fibrin monomers and between adjacent fibrin threads. This process stabilizes and strengthens the meshwork of the clot. The clot comprises the interlocking fibrin chains and the entrapped blood cells, platelets, and plasma. Final clot retraction and serum extrusion are caused by a contractile protein thrombosthenin that is released from platelets (Fig. 26.2).

Involvement of Calcium. Calcium ions (Ca^{++}), referred to as clotting factor IV (Table 26.1), are required for all coagulation reactions except the first two steps in the intrinsic pathway. This dependency is exploited in the laboratory; Ca^{++}-complexing agents such as citrate are used as in vitro anticoagulants. Availability of calcium generally is not a limiting factor in the body except rarely after massive transfusion of citrated blood. Usually, death from tetany and respiratory failure would result from hypocalcemia before the calcium concentration was low enough to significantly affect coagulation.

Involvement of Kallikrein-Kinin System. A deficiency of prekallikrein or high molecular weight kininogen prolongs the partial thromboplastin time of blood in vitro and thus slows the intrinsic clotting pathway. Kallikrein amplifies activation of factor XII, which in turn further increases conversion of prekallikrein to kallikrein (Donaldson et al. 1976).

FIBRINOLYSIS PHASE. A plasma β globulin called plasminogen is bound to fibrin and incorporated into the clot along with other plasma constituents. Fibrinolysis is initiated when plasminogen is activated by local agents to plasmin. Tissue-type plasminogen activator is produced by endothelial cells and fibroblasts and utilizes fibrin as a cofactor in the conversion of plasminogen to plasmin. Plasmin is a proteolytic enzyme that digests the fibrin chains into soluble polypeptides, thereby preventing further fibrin polymerization. Plasmin also digests other substances in the clot and surrounding blood, e.g., prothrombin; fibrinogen; and clotting factors V, VIII, and XII. Formation of plasmin results in dissolution of the clot and also in hypocoagulability of the blood because of loss of clotting factors. Thus fibrinolysis represents the physiologic converse of the coagulation process. It serves as a defense mechanism against overactivity of the coagulation mechanism. The long-term patency of the vascular tree no doubt depends on a balanced equilibrium between coagulation and fibrinolysis.

NATURAL ANTICOAGULANTS. The sensitivity of the coagulation cascade to hematologic disruptions necessitates equally sensitive control systems to prevent indiscriminate clotting. As stated so colorfully by Erslev and Gabuzda (1979), the clotting factors "stand poised as the parts of a loaded gun with trigger cocked, aimed at fibrinogen." Physiologic systems are available that either "clean up" the clotted target after the thrombin bullet is shot or act as "safeties" to prevent the gun from discharging needlessly.

First, the vascular endothelium is exceptionally smooth surfaced, thereby preventing contact activation of platelets and factor XII. Prompt removal of activated factors from the circulation is attained physically by rapid blood flow that washes local concentrations away from the site of thrombus formation. The liver rapidly clears the activated factors with a half-life of only a few minutes.

Humoral inhibitors of intermediate products of coagulation play a vital role in limiting coagulatory processes. Substances with inhibitory effects include heparin, plasmin, antithrombin III, and tissue factor inhibitor (extrinsic pathway inhibitor, lipoprotein-associated coagulation inhibitor). Antithrombin III (AT III) is the most vital of these factors. It is a globulin with a molecular weight of 65,000 and has the ability to inactivate factors Xa, IXa, XIa, and XIIa and thrombin. Binding to heparin markedly increases the rate of inactivation of factor Xa and thrombin. In addition, the surface of the vascular endothelium serves as the site of the thrombomodulin/protein C/protein S anticoagulant system (Esmon 2003). Thrombomodulin is an integral membrane protein, and protein C and protein S are circulating vitamin K–dependent proteins. Thrombomodulin has a receptor site for thrombin. Once thrombin has been bound, its ability to form fibrin and aggregate platelets is nullified. Additionally, it becomes a powerful activator of protein C. Protein C has anticoagulation effects through inactivation of factors Va and VIIIa (Marlar et al. 1982) and promotes fibrinolysis (Roemisch et al. 1991). Protein S increases the rate of inactivation of factor V.

Humoral inhibitors of intermediate products of coagulation include heparin, antithromboplastin, plasmin, and antithrombin III (not to be confused with clotting factor III or platelet factor 3). Antithrombin III also is called the heparin cofactor. This enzyme is a thrombin antagonist, but it additionally inhibits activated forms of factors IX, X, XI, and XII. Antithrombin III combines in a stable manner with the enzymatically active binding sites of these factors, thereby preventing their accessibility to subsequent substrates in the clotting cascade. The combination of heparin with antithrombin III increases approximately hundredfold the affinity of the latter for the activated clotting factors. The anticoagulant activity of heparin is due to its interaction with antithrombin III.

Fibrin itself is an effective antithrombin factor, because it removes from the circulation approximately 90% of the thrombin formed during the clotting process. This action assists in localizing the clot to the target site and retarding its spread to other regions of the vasculature.

COAGULOPATHIES AND DRUGS. Clinically, a large number of pathophysiologic states influence hemostatic events in animals. Abnormalities of one or more of the vascular, platelet, coagulation, and fibrinolytic phases are not uncommon; some of these disorders are summarized in Table 26.2. Drugs can be helpful in managing certain types of coagulopathies, but identification of etiologic factors is important. Some of the more commonly used hemostatic, anticoagulant, fibrinolytic, and antiplatelet drugs are discussed below. Commonly used tests of hemostatic function are listed in Table 26.3.

TABLE 26.3 Hemostatic assays and their clinical relevance

1. **One-step prothrombin time (OSPT):** Screening test of the extrinsic and common pathway. It is most sensitive to factor VII deficiency. First assay to be prolonged with vitamin K deficiency.
2. **Activated partial thromboplastin time (APTT):** Screening test of the intrinsic and common pathway. Will be prolonged with hemophilia and with prolonged vitamin K deficiency.
3. **Activated coagulation test (ACT):** Screening test for the intrinsic pathway, with less sensitivity than APTT.
4. **Buccal mucosal bleeding time:** Screening test for primary hemostasis. Will be prolonged with platelet dysfunction, thrombocytopenia, vWf deficiency, or vasculitis.

TABLE 26.2 Selected hemostatic diseases in animals

- I. Vascular defects (vasculitis)
- II. Platelet defects
  - A. Thrombocytopenia
    1. Idiopathic immune-mediated destruction
    2. Immune-mediated destruction secondary to drug administration, vaccination, and various diseases
    3. Bone marrow suppression (chemotherapeutics, estrogens)
    4. Increased consumption (disseminated intravascular coagulation, microangiopathy associated with neoplasia)
  - B. Thrombocytopathy
    1. Inherited (Otterhounds, Basset Hounds, cattle)
    2. Acquired (drug administration [e.g., aspirin, antibiotics, lidocaine] gammopathy associated, uremia)
- III. Von Willebrand disease (inherited deficiency of von Willebrand factor leading to defective platelet adhesion; found in humans, swine, dogs, and rabbits)
- IV. Coagulation defects
  - A. Inherited
    1. Hemophilia A (lack of functional factor VIII; found in humans, horses, cats, and dogs)
    2. Hemophilia B (lack of factor IX; found in humans, dogs, and cats)
    3. Hagemann factor deficiency (lack of factor XII; will produce significant prolongation of APTT and ACT results but is rarely related to a clinical bleeding disorder)
  - B. Acquired
    1. Deficiency of vitamin K activity (vitamin K-antagonist rodenticide poisoning, malabsorption)
    2. Decreased hepatic synthesis (neoplasia, cirrhosis, infection)
    3. Increased consumption (disseminated intravascular coagulation)
- V. Thrombotic diseases
  - A. Disseminated intravascular coagulation (neoplasia, severe generalized inflammation, pancreatitis, hemolysis)
  - B. Deficiency of AT III (nephrotic syndrome, heartworm adulticide treatment)
  - C. Circulatory abnormalities (cardiomyopathy in cats)

HEMOSTATIC DRUGS

TOPICAL HEMOSTATICS. Several locally applied substances can provide assistance in control of persistent capillary bleeding if blood coagulation mechanisms are otherwise intact. The ideal topical hemostatic substance should provide good hemostasis, have minimal tissue reactivity, and be easy to sterilize and handle. If hemostatic or fibrinolytic defects are present, however, topical agents are of little or no value; replacement therapy is indicated. Although lyophilized concentrates of several clotting factors are available for investigational use, most clinically useful topical hemostatic preparations contain thrombin or collagen. These compounds control bleeding by providing artificial clotting material or forming a structural matrix for coagulation events and clot formation. Because most topical hemostatics are absorbed gradually over varying intervals, they commonly are referred to as the absorbable hemostatics.

The clinician must recognize that locally applied hemostatics are indicated only in the combat of capillary oozing from minute vessels of denuded or superficially bleeding surfaces. These compounds will not effectively prevent loss of blood from arteries or veins where there is appreciable pressure.

Thromboplastin. Thromboplastin (thrombokinase) is produced naturally by platelets and tissues in response to trauma. The commercial preparation is a powder extracted from bovine brains or from acetone-extracted lung and/or brain of rabbits. *Thromboplastin*, USP, aids hemostasis by promoting conversion of prothrombin to thrombin, thereby accelerating the coagulation process. It is employed as a local hemostatic in surgery when applied by spray or direct application in a sponge. Thromboplastin is used in measurement of prothrombin time and activity of blood in vitro, an important guide in anticoagulant drug therapy.

Thrombin. *Thrombin*, USP, is a white sterile powder prepared by interaction of thromboplastin and calcium with prothrombin of bovine origin. It is standardized on the basis of National Institutes of Health (NIH) units; one NIH unit is the amount of thrombin required to clot 1 ml standard fibrinogen solution in 15 seconds. In control of bleeding, thrombin converts endogenous fibrinogen to fibrin for clot formation. It is useful where there is bleeding from parenchymatous tissues, cancellous bone, dental sockets, laryngeal and nasal surgery, and reconstructive surgery. Thrombin is particularly valuable as an adhesive agent for fixation of skin grafts. It can be applied topically as a powder or as a solution in sterile distilled water or isotonic saline (approximately 1000 units/ml); it can also be used in conjunction with absorbable gelatin sponge or fibrin foam. After neutralization of stomach acid, thrombin may be of some value in bleeding of the upper gastrointestinal (GI) tract.

Thrombin must not be injected or otherwise allowed to enter large blood vessels. Extensive intravascular clotting and even death may result. Local ischemia can result from subcutaneous or intramuscular (IM) injection. Thrombin is antigenic, but allergic reactions are encountered rarely when it is applied topically.

Fibrinogen. *Human Fibrinogen*, USP (Fibrogen, Parenogen), is a concentrated fraction of normal human plasma and is available as sterile white powder. It is readily soluble in normal saline and is used principally on denuded mucous membranes and as an adhesive in skin grafts (as a 2% solution). Fibrinogen also is used for restoring normal plasma fibrinogen concentrations in the treatment of hemorrhagic complications arising from massive blood loss or acute hypofibrinogenemia. Adequate amounts of endogenous thrombin are required for conversion of fibrinogen into fibrin.

Fibrin Foam. Fibrin foam is a spongelike material prepared by action of thrombin on human fibrinogen. It is an insoluble substance marketed as strips of fine white sponge. Fibrin foam may be applied directly, with pressure, to the hemorrhagic area or after presoaking it in thrombin solution. This preparation acts as a preformed network to trap blood oozing from the surface area.

Absorbable Gelatin Sponge. *Absorbable Gelatin Sponge*, USP (Gelfoam), is a sterile, water-insoluble, gelatin-base sponge. It is nonantigenic and will absorb several times its weight of whole blood. This denaturized gelatin usually is soaked in bovine thrombin and left in the bleeding area following closure of operative wounds. When applied to the surface of the body or mucosal membranes, it liquefies within 3–5 days. Gelatin sponge is completely absorbed in 4–6 weeks, usually without inducing a reaction or excessive scar tissue formation. It is used primarily for capillary or venous bleeding.

Oxidized Cellulose. *Oxidized Cellulose*, USP (Surgicel, Oxycel, Hemo-Pak), is a specially treated form of surgical gauze or sponge that aids coagulation by reaction between hemoglobin and cellulosic acid. Upon interaction with blood and tissue fluids, oxidized cellulose facilitates formation of a gummy matrix for clot formation. It should be used only as temporary packing because its permanent implantation in tissues and fractures interferes with bone regeneration and may result in cyst formation. Oxidized cellulose also interferes with epithelialization and hence should not be used as a topical dressing except for short-term control of bleeding. Complete absorption of large amounts may require weeks. Also, oxidized cellulose should not be used in conjunction with thrombin since the latter is inactivated by the former's acidity. Oxidized cellulose is available as sterile cotton pledgets and gauze pads and strips.

Microcrystalline Collagen. Microcrystalline collagen is a surface hemostatic agent. A valuable property of this substance is its affinity for wet surfaces, to which it quickly adheres. Microcrystalline collagen is absorbed in about 6 weeks with minimal tissue reaction. It may be effective in the presence of clotting factor deficiencies but is less effective in thrombocytopenia. It has also been shown to be effective in systemically heparinized patients (Abbott 1975). Surface hemostasis obtained with this agent appears to be most effective and reliable in such cases as venoarterial anastomoses or surgery of the spleen and liver.

Epinephrine and Norepinephrine. Topically applied, *Epinephrine*, USP, and *Norepinephrine Bitartrate*, USP, produce an immediate but transitory vasoconstriction, which may be of some value in local control of bleeding from small vessels. See Chapter 6 for indications and limitations.

Miscellaneous Topical Hemostatics. The locally acting hemostatics known as styptics are the oldest blood-clotting drugs. Styptics include such agents as ferric chloride, ferric sulfate, ferric subsulfate, alum, tannic acid, chromium trioxide, silver nitrate, zinc chloride, cotarnine chloride, and a variety of other astringent substances. Some of these drugs are used locally in full strength as powders dusted onto a bleeding area; in solution they are used in concentrations from 1 to 20%. Action of these drugs depends upon precipitation of the protein of blood and soft tissue, and they supposedly seal off the ruptured vessel. However, many of these agents, especially if used in high concentration, may damage tissues, resulting in sloughing and even recurrence of hemorrhage. Thus they should be used carefully and only on superficial lesions.

SYSTEMIC HEMOSTATICS

Blood. Fresh whole blood or blood components are indicated for emergency treatment of acute hemorrhagic syndromes associated with deficiency of clotting factors or platelets.

Vitamin K. Vitamin K is a fat-soluble vitamin that is found in a variety of plants and is produced by microorganisms. Its main therapeutic usage is in the treatment of vitamin K antagonist rodenticide intoxication.

Chemistry and Mechanism of Action. Vitamin K exists in three main forms. Vitamin K-1 (phytonadione) is present in plants, vitamin K-2 (menaquinone) is produced by microorganisms, and vitamin K-3 (menadione) is a synthetic derivative (Fig. 26.3). All of these compounds are naphthoquinone derivatives. Vitamin K aids in the production of clotting factors II, VII, IX, and X by postribosomal carboxylation of glutamyl residues. It also is vital for the production of active protein C and protein S, both of which have anticoagulant effects.

Vitamin K-1 is actively absorbed in the small intestine. Vitamins K-2 and K-3 are passively absorbed in the ileum and colon. Solubilization by bile acids is required for absorption of vitamins K-1 and K-2. Biotransformation in

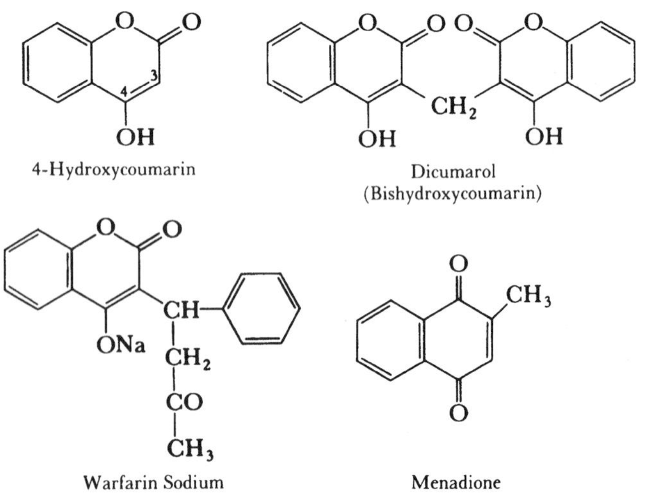

FIG. 26.3 Structures of 4-hydroxycoumarin, dicumarol (bishydroxycoumarin), warfarin, and synthetic vitamin K (menadione).

the organism is required for vitamin K-3 to become active (Mount 1982).

Clinical Use. Deficiency of vitamin K activity will lead to a hypocoagulable state. The major cause of this syndrome in veterinary medicine is the ingestion of vitamin K antagonists. Antagonists can occur naturally (dicumarol, sweet clover poisoning) or as commercial rodenticides (coumarin, warfarin, indandiones, brodifacoum). Occasionally disorders in fat absorption can lead to decreased vitamin K absorption. Coagulopathies have been documented with lymphocytic-plasmacytic enteritis, exocrine pancreatic insufficiency, and bile duct obstruction (Perry et al. 1991; Edwards and Russell 1987; Neer and Hedlund 1987; Li et al. 2004). In birds, prolonged administration of sulfonamides for the treatment of coccidiosis can lead to vitamin K deficiency by destroying the intestinal microorganisms. In swine porcine hemorrhagic syndrome in weaned pigs is believed to be related to low vitamin K levels in feed (Liggett 1989). A heritable multifactor vitamin K–dependent coagulopathy has been documented in Devon Rex cats (Soute et al. 1992).

Hypocoagulability is documented clinically by prolongation of the coagulation times (activated coagulation test [ACT], prothrombine time [PT], activated partial thromboplastin time [APTT]). Factor VII is the vitamin K–dependent clotting factor with the shortest half-life and is also the factor predominantly measured by PT. As a result, PT values will change before APTT or ACT values. This makes PT a good test to detect and monitor the therapy of a vitamin K–deficient state.

The therapeutic agent of choice is vitamin K-1. Vitamin K-3 has demonstrated poor efficacy in veterinary patients as well as toxic side effects (Alstad et al. 1985; Fernandez et al. 1984). Subcutaneous injection or oral administration are the preferred modes of administration. Intramuscular injections in an animal with a coagulopathy may lead to extensive life-threatening hemorrhage. Intravenous administration has been associated with anaphylactoid reactions. Most protocols recommend giving the initial dose of vitamin K by subcutaneous injection to ensure that therapeutic levels are reached. Thereafter, the drug can be given orally. A fatty meal will enhance oral absorption. Duration of treatment and dosage used will vary depending upon the clinical indication. Poisoning from first-generation vitamin K–antagonist rodenticides (coumarin, warfarin) should be treated for 4–6 days with 0.25–2.5 mg/kg divided BID in small animals, 300–500 mg TID in horses (Byars et al. 1986), and 1.1–3.3 mg/kg in cattle (Alstad et al. 1985). For second-generation vitamin K–antagonist rodenticides (diphacinone, brodifacoum), the treatment period should be extended to 14 days and a loading dose of 5 mg/kg should be given initially, followed by 2.5 mg/kg daily (Woody et al. 1992). Determination of PT 48 hours after cessation of therapy is recommended to detect residual toxicity. Substitution of vitamin K will begin to normalize PT values in 12–24 hours.

Desmopressin Acetate (DDAVP). Desmopressin is a synthetic analog of vasopressin, and is used in the treatment of central diabetes insipidus and to transiently elevate levels of vWf. Its actions are via the V_2 receptor rather than the V_1 receptor (Majerus and Tollefson 2006). The elevation in vWf allows surgical procedures to be performed and aids in the control of capillary bleeding from wounds in humans and animals with certain forms of von Willebrand disease. In comparison to vasopressin, DDAVP has minimal pressor effects. Administration of this drug leads to the release of stored vWf from endothelial cells and macrophages. When DDAVP is given, a rapid rise in vWf levels occurs, with larger, more-active multimeres predominating (Kraus et al. 1989; Johnstone and Crane 1986). This effect is reduced if the drug is given repeatedly, because the storage pools will be depleted. The duration of elevation is approximately 2 hours (Mansell and Parry 1991). Though the elevation in vWf levels found in dogs is considerably lower than in humans, clinically a decrease in buccal mucosal bleeding time was seen (Kraus et al. 1989). In some dogs only a minimal response was noted. The recommended dosages for dogs is 0.4 μg/kg given subcutaneously.

Protamine Sulfate. Protamine Sulfate, USP, is a low molecular weight protein found in the sperm of certain fish. It is strongly basic and combines with acidic heparin to form a stable salt that prevents further anticoagulant activity of heparin. Protamine is used as an antagonist only against heparin-evoked hemorrhages. It also arrests action of heparin in vitro. Protamine itself has anticoagulant properties probably caused by interference with the reaction of thrombin and fibrinogen. This would imply that the clinician must take care not to overneutralize the action of heparin.

Protamine is available as a 1–2% solution. It is administered slowly by the IV route at a rate no greater than 50 mg over a 10-minute period. The average dose is 1–1.5 mg to antagonize each 1 mg heparin. The dose is related to the lapse of time from administration; e.g., 30 minutes after heparin injection only 0.5 mg protamine may be required to antagonize each 1 mg heparin.

ANTICOAGULANTS

The principal uses of anticoagulant agents are in vitro to prevent clotting of blood for transfusion or diagnostic use and in vivo to prevent development and enlargement of thrombi.

IN VITRO ANTICOAGULANTS. Essentially two categories of chemicals are used to prevent coagulation of shed blood: those employed in samples of blood intended for physical or chemical examination and those employed to preserve blood for transfusion. Certain of these agents can be used to prevent clotting both in vitro and in vivo (heparin), while others are best used only in vitro because of their toxicity (oxalates).

Anticoagulant agents used in laboratory examination of blood include 1) sodium oxalate in a concentration of 20% at the level of 0.01 ml/ml (2 mg/ml) blood; 2) *Sodium Citrate,* USP, in a concentration of 25% at the rate of 0.01 ml/ml (2.5 mg/ml) blood; 3) *Edetate Disodium,* USP (Endrate, Sodium Versenate), to prevent coagulation when used in a concentration of 1 mg/5 ml blood, the anticoagulant property being related to its ability to chelate calcium; and 4) heparin sodium to prevent coagulation (75 units to each 10 ml whole blood).

Anticoagulants used for blood and blood component transfusions ideally should maintain the function of the individual components and have preservative effects. Anticoagulant agents used for blood and blood plasma transfusion include 1) *Acid Citrate Dextrose,* USP (ACD solution), consisting of sodium citrate 25 g, citric acid 8 g, dextrose 24.5 g, and distilled water to make a total volume of 1000 ml, given at the level of 15 ml/100 ml blood. The toxicity of citrated blood injected intravenously varies with rate of injection and total dose. The lethal dose of sodium citrate for the dog is estimated to be about 132 mg/kg after extensive hemorrhage; in the normal intact dog the lethal dose is about 286 mg/kg. 2) Citrate-phosphate-dextrose-adenine (CPDA-1) is one of the most commonly used anticoagulants in human and veterinary transfusion medicine. It can maintain a high level of erythrocyte posttransfusion viability for up to 20 days in dogs (Price et al. 1988).

Other means also may prevent or retard coagulation. These are cold, at 2–5° C, and collection of blood into a receptacle having smooth and unwettable walls, e.g., paraffin or silicone coated. Silicone coating is the most effective method for many types of mechanical devices used for implantation, transfusion, and dialysis.

PARENTERAL ANTICOAGULANTS. Heparin used parenterally has a direct and almost instantaneous action on the coagulation process, whereas the coumarin derivatives (for oral administration) have an indirect anticoagulant effect by acting as vitamin K antagonists in the hepatic synthesis of select coagulation factors. Therefore, action by the coumarin derivatives is delayed for several hours. For emergency treatment, heparin is used first and then may be followed by the coumarin derivatives.

Heparin. Heparin (Heparin sodium, USP; Heparin calcium, Calciparine) can be used in vivo and in vitro. Heparin has both antithrombotic and anticoagulatory effects, which are not necessarily dependent on each other. Heparin is prepared from bovine lung tissue or porcine intestinal mucosa. Both calcium and sodium salts of heparin are available for therapeutic use and occur as a white hygroscopic powder that is easily soluble in water.

Research has focused on synthetic heparinoids and the clinical applicability of heparin fractions of various molecular weights, referred to collectively as the low-molecular-weight heparin preparations (Vairel et al. 1983). These compounds include: reviparin (Clivarine), enoxaparin (Lovenox), dalteparin (Fragmin), tinzaparin (Innohep), nadroparin (Fraxiparine), and ardeparin (Normiflo). These agents share similar antifactor Xa activity, and have more predictable pharmacokinetic properties than the parent molecule. Their clinical application in veterinary medicine has yet to be defined. Heparin derivatives such as fondaparinux (Arixtra) and idraparinux have been synthesized and are undergoing study for clinical application.

Chemistry and Mechanism of Action. Pharmaceutical-grade heparin is a heterogeneous mixture of anionic sulfated mucopolysaccharides with molecular weights ranging from 1200 to 40,000 daltons (Sugahara and Kitagawa 2002). Relative antithrombotic and anticoagulatory activity is related to molecular size. The variability in both molecular composition and biologic activity necessitates standardization of drug concentration by bioassay of anticoagulant activity (expressed as units).

The reversible binding of heparin to antithrombin III (AT III), a protease inhibitor, is responsible for much of the anticoagulatory effect of heparin. Affinity for AT III is dependent upon molecular size (Fareed et al. 1985). Binding to AT III causes a conformational change in the AT III molecule that significantly enhances its inhibitory effect on various activated coagulation factors, especially thrombin and activated factor X (Xa). The rate of inactivation can increase 2000- to 10,000-fold. After inactivation has occurred, the heparin molecule dissociates from the complex and is available for further interactions. In a pharmaceutical heparin preparation, only 30–50% of the heparin molecules present will bind to AT III. Heparin acts as a template to which thrombin and AT III can bind and thereby interact to form an inactive compound. Simultaneous binding of factor Xa to AT III and heparin is not required for inactivation. Low-molecular-weight (LMW) fractions of heparin inactivate only factor Xa because they are not large enough to bind thrombin and AT III concurrently. The additional inactivation of thrombin by high-molecular-weight (HMW) fractions of heparin increases their anticoagulatory ability. At higher dosages heparin can also bind to heparin cofactor II, which inhibits only thrombin. Heparin also binds to endothelial cell walls, imparting a negative charge, affecting platelet aggregation and adhesion, and increasing levels of plasminogen activator (Hirsh et al. 1992a). In addition, heparin administration leads to an increase in the levels of tissue factor inhibitor (Ostergaard et al. 1993). These effects all contribute to the anticoagulatory and antithrombotic action of heparin and vary with the individual heparin fractions. Heparin-induced thrombocytopenia has been reported in humans (Warkentin 2003).

The pharmacokinetics and pharmacodynamics of heparin are complex. Most of an administered dose of heparin is bound extensively to endothelial cells, macrophages, and plasma proteins, which act as storage pools. Once these pools have been saturated, free heparin appears in the plasma and is excreted slowly by the kidney. Heparin is metabolized by the liver and also by the reticuloendothelial system (RES). Clearance of LMW fractions is slower than that of HMW fractions, which leads to their cumulation in the organism. All of these factors cause the kinetics of heparin to be highly variable between individuals and within the individual. A fixed dose cannot be expected to produce a uniform level of anticoagulation or antithrombotic effect. In addition, since most of heparin's efficacy is dependent on AT III, low levels of this protein will result in reduced anticoagulant activity. Biologic half-life is variable and depends upon the dosage administered and the route of administration. Subcutaneous administration leads to slow release of heparin and has been found to have an effect equivalent to intravenous heparin for the prophylaxis of thrombosis. Intravenous administration leads to high initial levels with a short half-life.

Clinical Use. Heparin is used widely in humans, especially in the prevention of venous thrombosis and pulmonary embolism. Its use in the treatment of established thrombi is also advocated. Uses of heparin in veterinary medicine include the management of disseminated intravascular coagulation (DIC), arterial thrombi in cats, and other potentially hypercoagulable states (Cushing's disease, nephrotic syndrome, cardiomyopathy). Low-dose heparin has been reported to decrease the complications associated with heartworm adulticide treatment (Vezzoni and Genchi 1989).

The major adverse side effect in animals is excessive anticoagulation leading to hemorrhage. Intramuscular administration is contraindicated, as it may lead to extensive hematoma formation. In horses, treatment for several days with doses of heparin that were believed to produce therapeutically desired levels of anticoagulation led to a significant (50%) drop in red blood cell (RBC) mass. This may have been associated with increased RBC removal by the RES (Duncan et al. 1983). Erythrocyte agglutination has also been associated with heparin therapy in horses (Mahaffey and Moore 1986).

Guidelines for heparin dosage vary widely. Both high-dose and low-dose regimens have been developed; their applicability will depend upon the clinical indication. High-dose heparin therapy aims to increase APTT 1.5–2.5 times baseline or ACT 1.2–1.4 times baseline. Its main clinical indication is the treatment of established thromboemboli. The amount of heparin required to achieve this goal will vary with each individual and, since the pharmacokinetics are nonlinear, will vary with each dose administered. In dogs 150–250 U/kg TID and in cats 250–375 U/kg TID will usually suffice to achieve this goal. A higher loading dose may be of benefit. Regular and frequent monitoring of clotting times is essential. Severe anemia was detected in horses administered dosages that led to the desired prolongation of clotting times after several days of treatment. Low-dose regimens are generally 75 U/kg TID in small animals and 25–100 U/kg TID in horses. This regimen is especially useful in the management of DIC. The effect on APTT should be minimal with low-dose heparin therapy, yet antithrombotic efficacy should be maintained. Bleeding tendencies also are reduced.

OTHER INJECTABLE ANTICOAGULANTS. These agents include argatroban, lepirudin (Refludan), bivalirudin (angiomax), danaparoid (Orgaron), and drotrecogin alfa (Xigris). Lepirudin is an interesting compound; it is a recombinant derivative of hirudin, which is a direct thrombin inhibitor present in the salivary glands of the medicinal leach. It is approved for treatment of humans with heparin-induced thrombocytopenia. Bivalirudin is a synthetic peptide that also acts by inhibiting thrombin, as does argotroban. Danaparoid is a mixture of nonheparin gylocosamines isolated from swine intestine; it acts mainly by enhancing the inhibition of factor Xa by antithrombine. Drotrecogin alfa is a recombinant form of protein C that exerts anticoagulant effects through proteolytic inactivation of factors Va and VIIIa. The application of these synthetic compounds to clinical veterinary medicine remains to be defined.

VITAMIN K ANTAGONISTS

Coumarin Derivatives. Coumarin, normally present in some species of sweet clover, has little anticoagulant action. However, bishydroxycoumarin, a derivative of moldy or spoiled sweet clover, is responsible for a hemorrhagic disease in cattle. This compound was synthesized by Link (1943–44). Other drugs have been synthesized with the 4-hydroxycoumarin structure. Of the several coumarin derivatives, bishydroxycoumarin (Dicumarol, USP) was the first oral anticoagulant and 3-(α-acetonylbenzyl)-4-hydroxycoumarin (Warfarin Sodium, USP; Panwarfin, Coumodin) was the second compound used.

Chemistry. Dicumarol is a colorless, crystalline solid; it is relatively insoluble in water but forms soluble salts with strong alkalies. The chemical structures of coumarin, dicumarol, warfarin, and menadione are shown in Figure 26.3. The structure of vitamin K suggests the competitive relation between the vitamin and these inhibitors. Bioavailability of warfarin is much greater than dicumarol because it is approximately 75,000 times more soluble in aqueous media. Warfarin is extensively used as a rodenticide because it produces fatal internal bleeding. Domestic animals also may be poisoned accidentally.

Action. Coumarin derivatives share one major pharmacologic action: in vivo inhibition of blood coagulation mechanisms. This activity is achieved not by direct depression of preformed components of the coagulation cascade, but by inhibition of hepatic synthesis of vitamin K–dependent clotting factors, i.e., prothrombin and factors VII, IX, and X (Fig. 26.2). Unlike heparin, therefore, coumarin compounds are inactive in vitro. Their in vivo anticoagulant activity is apparent only after a latent period of at least several hours, which accounts for the time required for natural breakdown of circulating factors already present in the blood (Wajih et al. 2004). After cessation of administration, anticoagulant effects can last for several days. This reflects the time necessary for reappearance of newly synthesized clotting factors.

The formation of functional clotting factors II, VII, IX, and X is dependent upon the presence of vitamin K. After the precursor proteins of these clotting factors have been synthesized in the liver, they must undergo carboxylation of terminal glutamic acid residues. The carboxylation results in the oxidative inactivation of vitamin K. The resulting vitamin K epoxide is then recycled by epoxide reductase so that it can again participate in the conversion of precursor proteins to functional clotting factors. Vitamin K antagonists exert their effect by inhibiting epoxide reductase. This results in a rapid depletion of vitamin K stores. The coagulation factors are still produced but are not functional. Vitamin K and dicumarol are mutually antagonistic, and administration of vitamin K can reverse hypoprothrombinemia produced by coumarin compounds. This action is clinically important where there is an unusual response to dicumarol, as in overdosage or accidental ingestion. The antidotal effect of vitamin K and its clinical use have been discussed. The characteristics of coumarin derivatives and those of heparin are shown in Table 26.4.

Absorption and Metabolism. Dicumarol, as other coumarin derivatives, is absorbed from the GI tract; over 90% is bound to plasma protein and some is stored in the liver. This binding is reversible and is in part responsible for the long plasma half-life of these drugs. Despite this property, the drug displays great variability in action. This

TABLE 26.4 Pharmacologic characteristics of heparin and coumarin derivative anticoagulants

Characteristic	Heparin	Coumarin Derivatives
Mechanism of action	Antagonist to thrombin and activated factors IX, X, XI, and XII	Inhibit hepatic synthesis of vitamin K-dependent clotting factors (II, VII, IX, and X)
Onset of action	Immediate	Delayed 12–24 hr
Duration of action	4 hr	2–5 days
Route of administration	Parenteral	Oral
Laboratory control test	Clotting time, partial thromboplastin time	Prothrombin time
Antidotal therapy	Protamine, fresh blood	Vitamin K, fresh blood or plasma
In vitro activity	Yes	No

may be due to variable metabolic transformation, GI absorption, a possible influence of diet (amount of vitamin K), and interaction with other drugs. Dicumarol is hydroxylated by hepatic enzymes to inactive compounds that are excreted in urine; the metabolites have no anticoagulant effect. Variations in rate of metabolism are due in part to genetic factors. A small quantity, if any, appears unchanged in urine. However, coumarins cross the placenta and are probably secreted in milk.

Laboratory Control. Because of variability in individual and species response to dicumarol, laboratory monitoring of prothrombin activity is essential in its clinical use. The most widely used method for regulating dosage of the drug is the Quick test, or the one-stage prothrombin time. The prothrombin time for a patient on oral anticoagulant therapy should be two to two and one-half times the control value for that individual.

Clinical Use. Clinical use of dicumarol in humans has been rated as effective for prophylaxis and treatment of venous thrombosis (Hirsh et al. 2003). All coumarin derivatives can cause one principal side reaction, hemorrhage. However, bleeding rarely occurs if the dose is regulated in relation to prothrombin test results. Contraindications include bleeding from any cause, purpura of any type, or a severe state of malnutrition. The coumarin drugs have received relatively little clinical use in animals.

Drug Interaction. A large number of pharmacokinetic interactions may potentiate or inhibit the anticoagulant action of the coumarin group of drugs (Daly and King 2003). The most important prescribed drugs that may increase their response are phenylbutazone, heparin, salicylates, quinine, broad-spectrum antibiotics, and anabolic steroids. Among those that may decrease response are barbiturates (by induction of liver microsomal enzymes), chloral hydrate, and griseofulvin. Experimentally, it has been shown that the hypoprothrombinemic activity of orally administered dicumarol is nullified in sheep pretreated with phenobarbital (Shetty et al. 1972). Coumarins may inhibit metabolism of phenytoin. Some physiologic factors may increase the action of coumarins, e.g., hepatic dysfunction, hypermetabolism, and vitamin K deficiency resulting from poor absorption. Other physiologic factors may decrease response to anticoagulants, e.g., pregnancy and diuresis.

Administration. The dosage of oral anticoagulants in dogs is based on the schedule used in humans. Dicumarol is given on the first day at 5 mg/kg; the average daily maintenance is one-third to two-thirds the first day's dose and is dependent on daily prothrombin time determinations. When prothrombin activity is reduced to less than 25%, the drug must be discontinued.

Other Oral Anticoagulants. In addition to dicumarol and warfarin, other oral anticoagulants have been developed, including ximelagatran, anisindione (Miradon), phenindione (Dindevan), phenprocoumon (Marcumar), and acenocoumarol (Sinthrome). Several of these compounds have been used in human medicine in other countries (Schulman et al. 2003), but they have found little application in clinical veterinary medicine.

FIBRINOLYTIC AGENTS

The basic event of fibrinolysis is abstracted in Figure 26.2. Pharmacologic acceleration of this process involves drugs that enhance the conversion of the inactive precursor plasminogen to the active fibrinolytic enzyme plasmin (Sherry and Gustafson 1985; Armstrong et al. 2003). Plasminogen exists in two phases, the plasma or soluble phase found in the circulating blood and the gel phase bound to fibrin in the formed clot. Thus when a plasminogen-activating agent comes in contact with the clot, fibrin-bound gel-phase plasminogen is activated to plasmin locally with selective fibrinolysis. There is increased tendency for systemic bleeding if, instead, soluble-phase plasminogen circulating in systemic blood is also activated. Plasmin formation would then occur throughout the circulation rather than being localized to the formed clot. Indeed, the presence of plasmin in peripheral blood indicates a pathologic fibrinolytic state. Such a condition reflects overactivation of plasminogen, which overcomes the neutralizing capacity of an endogenous antagonist to plasmin called α_2-antiplasmin.

STREPTOKINASE. Streptokinase is a stable, vacuum-dried powder containing enzymes produced by β-hemolytic streptococcus. Streptokinase complexes with plasminogen, yielding plasmin. The conversion of animal plasminogens to plasmins by streptokinase is variable. Local use is indicated when removal of fibrin or a viscous exudate is desired and drainage can be achieved. Clinical trials have demonstrated its usefulness in treatment of wounds not responding to antibacterial therapy, such as burns, ulcers, chronic eczema, ear hematoma, otitis externa, sinusitis, cysts, fractures with fistulous tracts, and osteomyelitis. Locally, it can be administered as a powder or wet pack by infusion or irrigation. Liquefaction of blood clots and fibrinous exudates may occur in 30 minutes to 12 hours.

Parenteral administration has been used in treatment of eczema, dermatitis, edema, cellulitis, hematoma, trauma, and pneumonia. For parenteral use, the solution may be administered intramuscularly or intravenously. The daily dose for large animals is 5,000–10,000 units/45 kg. The recommended total daily dose for small animals is 5,000–10,000 units. Therapy may be given 1 or 2 times daily for up to 5 days. Streptokinase is used infrequently because of its tendency to cause systemic fibrinolysis.

TISSUE PLASMINOGEN ACTIVATOR. Tissue-type plasminogen activator (t-PA) predominantly exerts its effect in association with fibrin clots. Its selectivity for plasminogen in clots is therapeutically attractive. Unlike other plasminogen activators, t-PA does not readily induce a systemic fibrinolytic state. Though the commercial product is recombinant DNA produced human-type tissue plasminogen activator, its efficacy has been demonstrated in cats (Pion 1988). In addition, the local application of t-PA was efficacious in reducing intraocular fibrin deposition (Gerding et al. 1992). The major clinical use to date has been the lysis of aortic thromboemboli in cats. Intravenous administration of t-PA resulted in a rapid return of function. However, 50% of the animals treated died acutely after treatment. This was attributed to the rapid reperfusion of the rear extremities, which resulted in reperfusion-induced hyperkalemia and heart failure. A factor that may limit the use of t-PA is the expense of the drug.

PLASMINOGEN AND α_2-ANTIPLASMIN. Commercial plasminogen is a glycoprotein activated by cleavage of amino acid residues, with the active metabolite binding to partially degraded fibrin. The latter promotes fibrinolysis. α_2-antiplasmin is a glycoprotein that forms a stable complex with plasmin, thereby preventing its fibrinolytic action. Two drugs are available for treatment of hyperfibrinolytic conditions: *Aminocaproic Acid,* USP (Amicar, Caprocid), and a biologic inhibitor, aprotinin (Transylol). Aprotinin is a kallikrein or protease enzyme inhibitor. In humans, underactive fibrinolysis is postulated to play a role in occlusive vascular disease, as in myocardial infarction, pulmonary thromboembolic disease, massive postsurgical adhesions, and such unrelated processes as inflammation and malignancy.

ANTIPLATELET DRUGS

Platelets have a central role in the initiation and propagation of thrombus formation. They release a variety of substances that promote coagulation, and they also form the initial platelet plug. Platelets adhere and aggregate in response to a myriad of stimuli. A central mechanism in aggregation is alteration of cAMP concentrations in the platelet itself. Increased cAMP is inhibitory to aggregation, while decreased cAMP is proaggregatory. Although a variety of stimuli influence platelet function in vivo, many of the in vitro methods used to assess platelet reactivity suffer from the inability to truly recreate the in vivo environment. Another factor that leads to difficulties in assessing clinical efficacy based on experimental work is that platelet reactivity varies between individuals and with health status.

A variety of drugs can be used to reduce platelet function. Clinically this should be beneficial in the prevention of thrombotic disease, especially if affecting arteries. The efficacy of certain of these drugs in the prevention of myocardial infarction and stroke in humans has been well established. The most common indications in veterinary medicine are to prevent thrombi associated with feline cardiomyopathy and to reduce the severity of pulmonary endarteritis associated with heartworm disease. The efficacy of antiplatelet drugs in alleviating the proliferative changes in arteries associated with heartworm infestation remains controversial (Boudreaux et al. 1991a; Keith et al. 1983; Schaub et al. 1983). Platelet inhibition may also be beneficial in membranous glomerulonephritis, mild DIC, and pulmonary thromboembolism. In horses platelet inhibition may be of benefit in the treatment of thrombotic disorders such as laminitis and navicular disease.

ASPIRIN. A commonly used antiplatelet drug in veterinary medicine is aspirin (acetylsalicylic acid, ASA). Aspirin is a nonsteroidal antiinflammatory drug (NSAID) that inhibits the activity of cyclooxygenase (Chapter 19). Other NSAIDs, such as phenylbutazone and flunixin meglumine, share the same mechanism of action, yet aspirin is unique in that even at low doses it causes irreversible inhibition of platelet cyclooxygenase. Aspirin acetylates this enzyme, which leads to decreased production of eicosanoids by the platelet. The most pivotal eicosanoids for hemostasis are prostacyclin (PGI_2) and thromboxane A_2 (TA_2). PGI_2 is a potent vasodilator and inhibitor of aggregation, while TA_2 is a vasoconstrictor and a strong aggregatory stimulus.

Once ASA has been administered, rapid and irreversible inhibition of platelet cyclooxygenase occurs. Because platelets do not produce appreciable amounts of new enzymes, this results in decreased platelet aggregation response because of lower TA_2 levels throughout the life span of the platelet. Aggregation response will return to normal as new platelets enter the bloodstream. Endothelial cell cyclooxygenase activity is also inhibited but recovers more rapidly. This inhibition is considered deleterious because endothelial cells produce PGI_2, which is antithrombotic. Proposed explanations for the more rapid recovery of endothelial cell cyclooxygenase activity include reduced sensitivity to ASA of the endothelial cell cyclooxygenase, ability to synthesize new cyclooxygenase, and the pharmacologic distribution of ASA (Hirsh et al. 1992b). The last theory postulates that platelets are exposed to ASA in the enterohepatic circulation before ASA is hydrolyzed. At low doses endothelium will primarily be exposed to circulating salicylate rather than ASA. Higher doses will result in circulating ASA leading to endothelial cell cyclooxygenase inhibition. The differential inhibition of platelet and endothelial cell cyclooxygenase has resulted in research efforts to find an ideal dose of ASA that will maximally limit proaggregatory platelet TA_2 and minimally decrease levels of antithrombotic PGI_2. In addition, low dosages should minimize the gastrointestinal side effects seen with ASA. The goal of finding an optimum low ASA dose has proven elusive. In healthy dogs individual variation in the amount of ASA required to inhibit aggregation in vitro is marked. Experimental infestation and embolization with heartworms lead to a pronounced increase in the amount of ASA needed to maintain this level of inhibition (Boudreaux et al. 1991a).

Dosage recommendations for platelet inhibition vary widely. In healthy dogs a dose of 0.5 mg/kg BID aspirin was found to be more effective than higher doses (Rackear et al. 1988). A dose of 10 mg/kg has been recommended to reduce the sequelae of heartworm infestation and adulticide treatment (Keith et al. 1983). In cats 25 mg/kg twice weekly has been found to inhibit platelet aggregation without evidence of toxicity (Greene 1985). Experimental studies in horses showed that oral ASA (12 mg/kg) significantly increased bleeding times for 48 hours posttreatment (Trujillo et al. 1981). A lower dose (4 mg/kg) prolonged bleeding times for 4 hours posttreatment (Cambridge et al. 1991).

TICLOPIDINE. Ticlopidine is an antiplatelet drug used for prevention of thrombotic diseases. In humans it has been proven to be as effective as ASA in the prevention of stroke (Hass et al. 1984). The mechanism of action of ticlopidine is connected to purinergic receptors of the platelet, which presents two types: $P2Y_1$ and $P2Y_{12}$. Both receptors are typical G-protein coupled complexes that recognize ADP as their principal ligand (Hollopeter et al. 2001). The $P2Y_{12}$ receptor is coupled with G_I, leading to inhibition of adenylyl cyclase in response to ADP. Thus, platelet concentrations of the antiaggregating compound cyclic AMP are reduced, leading in turn to platelet aggregation. Ticlopidine is a $P2Y_{12}$ receptor inhibitor, thereby preventing ADP from exerting its strong cyclic AMP-dependent aggregating action. It seems both purinergic receptors are needed for full expression of ADP-induced platelet aggregation, and selective block of $P2Y_{12}$ by ticlopidine is adequate to express efficacious antiaggregating effects. The drug limits platelet aggregation response to a variety of stimuli, illustrating the role of ADP in the aggregating action of various other agents and factors. Cyclooxygenase is not inhibited by ticlopidine, so endothelial PGI_2 levels are not affected.

Inhibition of aggregation persists for the life span of the platelet after treatment with ticlopidine. Onset of antiplatelet effect is approximately 2–5 days after treatment is initiated, indicating that an intermediate breakdown product is the agent actually responsible for the clinical response. Experience with ticlopidine in veterinary medicine is limited. In healthy animals 62 mg/kg daily inhibited platelet aggregation responses. In heartworm-infected and heartworm-embolized dogs, higher dosages were necessary (Boudreaux et al. 1991b). Ticlopidine administration was associated with a reduction of pulmonary lesions caused by the heartworms.

CLOPIDOGREL. This compound is structurally related to ticlopidine, and is believed to exert a similar antiaggregation mechanism. Clopidogrel (Plavix) is a prodrug that undergoes biotransformation into its active metabolite. Its onset of action is therefore slow, but it seems to have fewer objectionable side effects than does ticlopidine. Clopidogrel is commonly used in conjunction with aspirin, and it has been approved for use in humans to prevent recurrence of stroke and myocardial infarction secondary to thrombus formation.

INTEGRIN INHIBITORS. Platelets and endothelial cells express adhesion molecules and integrins on their surfaces in response to various stimuli. An important integrin of platelets is named $\alpha_{11b}\beta_3$; it is a receptor for von Willebrand factor and fibrinogen, which anchor platelets to each other and other surfaces. Platelet stimulants such as collagen, thromboxane A_2, and thrombin activate $\alpha_{11b}\beta_3$ receptors, thereby promoting platelet adhesion and clumping into aggregates. The integrin inhibitors thereby prevent aggregation promoted by almost any pro–aggregation factor. Three integrin inhibitors have been approved for use in human medicine: abcixinab (Reopro), eptifibatide (Integrilin), and tirofiban (Aggrastat).

Eptifibatide is a cyclic peptide that inhibits the fibrinogen binding loci of the $\alpha_{11b}\beta_3$ integrin. Concurrent administration with aspirin is its most common use in the prevention of myocardial infarction after acute coronary syndrome. Triofiban is a nonpeptide molecule, but it is thought to have similar antiplatelet actions as eptifibalide. Abciximab has a different mechanism of action in that it is a Fab fragment of human-source monoclonal antibody raised against the $\alpha_{11b}\beta_3$ integrin receptor itself. Abciximab was effective in preventing restenosis and recurrent myocardial infarction in humans. However, the clinical application of integrin inhibitors remains undetermined in veterinary medicine.

DIPYRIMADOLE. Originally marketed as a vasodilator, dipyrimadole has been shown to have a synergistic effect with ASA. It inhibits cAMP phosphodiesterase, which leads to increased cAMP levels in the platelet. If used alone, its effect on platelets is minimal (Boudreaux et al. 1991a).

REFERENCES

Abbot, W. M., Austen, W. G. 1975. The effectiveness and mechanism of collagen-induced topical hemostasis. Surgery 78:723–29.

Alstad, A. D., Casper, H. H., Johnson, L. J. 1985. Vitamin K treatment of sweet clover poisoning in calves. J Am Vet Med Assoc 187:729–31.

Armstrong, P. W., Collen, D., and Antman, E. 2003. Fibrinolysis for acute myocardial infarction: the future is here and now. Circulation 107:2533–2537.

Boudreaux, M. K., Dillon, A. R., Ravis, W. R., Sartin, E. A., Spano, J. S. 1991a. Effects of treatment with aspirin or aspirin/dipyrimadole combination in heartworm-negative, heartworm-infected, and embolized heartworm-infected dogs. Am J Vet Res 52:1992–99.

Boudreaux, M. K., Dillon, A. R., Sartin, E. A., Ravis, A. R., Spano, J. S. 1991b. Effects of treatment with ticlopidine in heartworm-negative, heartworm-infected, and embolized heartworm-infected dogs. Am J Vet Res 52:2000–2006.

Broze, G., Jr. 2001. Protein Z-dependent regulation of coagulation. Thromb Haemost 86:1–13.

Byars, T. D, Greene, C. E., Kemp, D. T. 1986. Antidotal effect of vitamin K_1 against warfarin induced anticoagulation in horses. Am J Vet Res 47:2309–12.

Cambridge, H., Lees, P., Hooke, R. E., Russell, C. S. 1991. Antithrombotic actions of aspirin in the horse. Equine Vet J 23:123–27.

Chart, I. S., Sanderson, J. H. 1979. General aspects of the blood coagulation system. Pharmacol Ther 5:229–33.

Daly, A. K., and King, B. P. 2003. Pharmacogenetics of oral anticoagulants. Pharmacogenetics 13:247–252.

Donaldson, V. H., Glueck, H. I., Miller, M. A., Movat, H. Z., Habul, F. 1976. Kininogen deficiency in Fitzgerald trait: role of high molecular weight kininogen in clotting and fibrinolysis. J Lab Clin Med 87:327–37.

Duncan, S. G., Meyers, K. M., Reed, S. M. 1983. Reduction of the red blood cell mass of horses: toxic effect of heparin anticoagulant therapy. Am J Vet Res 44:2271–76.

Edelberg, J. M., Christie, P. D., and Rosenberg, R. D. 2001. Regulation of vascular bed-specific prothrombotic potential. Circ Res 89:117–124.

Edwards, D. F., Russell, R. G. 1987. Probable vitamin K–deficient bleeding in two cats with malabsorption syndrome secondary to lymphocytic-plasmacytic enteritis. J Vet Intern Med 1:97–101.

Erslev, A. J., Gabuzda, T. G. 1979. Pathophysiology of Blood, 2nd ed. Philadelphia: W. B. Saunders.

Esmon, C. T. 2003. The protein C pathway. Chest 124(Suppl):26S–32S.

Fareed, J., Walenga, J. M., Williamson, K., Emanuele, R. A., Kumar, A., Hoppensteadt, D. A. 1985. Studies on the antithrombotic effects and pharmacokinetics of heparin fractions and fragments. Sem in Thromb and Hemostasis 11:56–74.

Fernandez, F. R., Davies, A. P., Teachout, D. J., Krake, A., Christopher, M. M., Perman, V. 1984. Vitamin K–induced heinz body formation in dogs. J Am Anim Hosp Assoc 20:711–20.

Gerding, P. A., Essex-Sorlie, D., Yack, R., Vasaune, S. 1992. Effects of intracameral injection of tissue plasminogen activator on corneal endothelium and intraocular pressure in dogs. Am J Vet Res 53:890–93.

Greene, C. E. 1985. Effects of aspirin and propranolol on feline platelet aggregation. Am J Vet Res 46:1820–23.

Hass, W. K., Easton, J. D., Adams, H. P., Pryse-Phillips, W., Molony, B. A., Anderson, S., Kamm, B. 1984. A randomized trial comparing ticlopidine hydrochloride with aspirin for the prevention of stroke in high-risk patients. N Engl J Med 321:501–7.

Hirsh, J., Dalen, J. E., Deykin, D., Poller, L. 1992a. Heparin: mechanism of action, pharmacokinetics, dosing considerations, monitoring, efficacy and safety. Chest 102:337S–351S.

Hirsh, J., Dalen, J. E., Fuster, V., Harker, L. B., Salzman, E. W. 1992b. Aspirin and other platelet-active drugs: the relationship between dose, effectiveness, and side effects. Chest 102:327S–336S.

Hirsh, J., Fuster, V., Ansell, J., and Halperin, J. L. 2003. American Heart Association/American College of Cardiology Foundation guide to warfarin therapy. Circulation 107:1692–1711.

Hollopeter, G., Jantzen, H. M., Vincent, D., et al. 2001. Identification of the platelet ADP receptor targeted by antithrombotic drugs. Nature 409:202–207.

Jain, N. C. 1993. Essentials of Veterinary Hematology. Philadelphia: Lea & Febiger.

Johnstone, I. B., Crane, S. 1986. The effects of desmopressin on hemostatic parameters in the normal dog. Can J Vet Res 50:265–71.

Keith, J. C., Rawlings, C. A., Schaub, R. G. 1983. Pulmonary thromboembolism during therapy of dirofilariasis with thiacetarsamide: modification with aspirin or prednisolone. Am J Vet Res 44:1278–83.

Kraus, K. H., Turrentine, M. A., Jergens, A. E., Johnson, G. S. 1989. Effect of desmopressin acetate on bleeding times and plasma von Willebrand factor in Doberman Pinscher dogs with von Willebrand's disease. Vet Surg 18:103–9.

Kraus, K. H., Turrentine, M. A., Johnson, G. S. 1987. Multimeric analysis of von Willebrand factor before and after desmopressin acetate (DDAVP) administration intravenously and subcutaneously in male Beagle dogs. Am J Vet Res 48:1376–79.

Li, T., Chang, C. Y., Jin, D. Y., et al. 2004. Identification of the gene for vitamin K epoxide reductase. Nature 427:541–544.

Liggett, A. D. 1989. Porcine hemorrhagic syndrome in recently weaned pigs. Comp Cont Ed 11:1409–11.

Link, K. P. 1943–44. The anticoagulant from spoiled sweet clover hay. Harvey Lect 39:162–216.

Mahaffey, E. A., and Moore, J. N. 1986. Erythrocyte agglutination associated with heparin treatment in three horses. J Am Vet Med Assoc 189:1478–80.

Majerus, P. W., and Tollefson, D. M. 2006. Blood coagulation and anticoagulant, thrombolytic, and antiplatelet drugs. In L. L. Brunton, J. S. Lazo, and K. L. Parker, eds., The Pharmacological Basis of Therapeutics, 11th ed., pp. 1467–1488. New York: McGraw Hill.

Mann, K. G., Butenas, S., and Brummel, K. 2003. The dynamics of thrombin formation. Arterioscler Thromb Vasc Biol 23:17–25.

Mansell, P. D., and Parry, B. W. 1991. Changes in factor VII: coagulant activity and von Willebrand factor antigen concentration after subcutaneous injection of desmopressin in dogs with mild hemophilia A. J Vet Intern Med 6:191–94.

Marlar, R. A., Kleiss, A. J., Griffin, J. H. 1982. Mechanism of action of human activated protein C, a thrombin-dependent anticoagulant enzyme. Blood 59:1067–72.

Moncada, S., Vane, J. R. 1979. Arachidonic acid metabolites and the interactions between platelets and blood-vessel walls. N Engl J Med 300:1142–47.

Mount, M. E. 1982. Vitamin K and its therapeutic importance. J Am Vet Med Assoc 180:1354–56.

Nawroth, P. P., Handley, D., Stern, D. M. 1986. The multiple levels of endothelial cell-coagulation factor interactions. Clinics in Haematology 15:293–321.

Neer, T. M., Hedlund, C. S. 1987. Vitamin K–dependent coagulopathy in a dog with bile and cystic duct obstructions. J Am Anim Hosp Assoc 25:461–64.

Ostergaard, P., Nordfang, O., Petersen, L. C., Valentin, S., Kristensen, H. 1993. Is tissue factor pathway inhibitor involved in the antithrombotic effect of heparins. Haemostasis 23:107–11.

Perry, L. A., Williams, D. A., Pidgeon, G. L., Boosinger, T. R. 1991. Exocrine pancreatic insufficiency with associated coagulopathy in a cat. J Am Anim Hosp Assoc 27:109–14.

Pion, P. D. 1988. Feline aortic thromboemboli and the potential utility of thrombolytic therapy with tissue plasminogen activator. Vet Clin North Am: Sm Anim Pract 18:79–86.

Platt, W. R. 1979. Color Atlas and Textbook of Hematology, 2nd ed. Philadelphia: J. B. Lippincott.

Price, G. S., Armstrong, P. J., McLeod, D. A., Babineau, C. A., Metcalf, M. R., Sellett, L. C. 1988. Evaluation of citrate-phosphate-dextrose-adenine as a storage medium for packed canine erythrocytes. J Vet Int Med 2:126–32.

Rackear, D., Feldman, B., Farver, T., Lelong, L. 1988. The effect of three different dosages of acetylsalicylic acid on canine platelet aggregation. J Am Anim Hosp Assoc 24:23–26.

Roemisch, J., Diehl, K. H., Reiner, G., Paques, E. P. 1991. Activated protein C: antithrombotic properties and influence on fibrinolysis in an animal model. Fibrinolysis 5:191–96.

Schaub, R. G., Keith, J. C., Rawlings, C. A. 1983. Effect of acetylsalicylic acid on vascular damage and myointimal proliferation in canine pulmonary arteries subjected to chronic injury by *Dirofilaria immitis.* Am J Vet Res 44:449–54.

Schulman, S., Wahlander, K., Lundstrom, T., et al. 2003. THRIVE III Investigators. Secondary prevention of venous thromboembolism with the oral direct thrombin inhibitor ximelagatran. N Engl J Med 349:1713–1721.

Sherry, S., Gustafson, E. 1985. The current and future use of thrombolytic therapy. Ann Rev Pharmacol Toxicol 25:413–31.

Shetty, S. N., Himes, J. A., Edds, G. T. 1972. Effect of phenobarbital on bishydroxycoumarin plasma concentration and hypoprothrombinemia responses in sheep. Am J Vet Res 33:825–34.

Soute, B. A., Ulrich, M. M., Watson, A. D., Maddison, J. E., Ebberink, R. H., Vermeer, C. 1992. Congenital deficiency of all vitamin K–dependent blood coagulation factors due to a defective vitamin K–dependent carboxylase in Devon Rex cats. Thrombosis and Hemostasis 68:521–25.

Sugahara, K., and Kitagawa, H. 2002. Heparin and heparin sulfate biosynthesis. IUBMB Life 54:163–175.

Szabuniewicz, M., McCrady, J. D. 1977. Hemostasis, hemostatic, anticoagulant and fibrinolytic agents. In L. M. Jones, N. H. Booth, L. E. McDonald, eds., Veterinary Pharmacology and Therapeutics, 4th ed. Ames: Iowa State Univ Press.

Trujillo, O., Rios, A., Maldonado, R., Rudolph, W. 1981. Effect of oral administration of acetylsalicylic acid on haemostasis in the horse. Equine Vet J 13:205–6.

Vairel, E. G., Bouty-Boye, H., Toulemonde, F., Doutremepuich, C., Marsh, N. A., Gaffney, P. J. 1983. Heparin and a low molecular weight fraction enhances thrombolysis and by this pathway exercises a protective effect against thrombosis. Thrombosis Research 30:219–24.

Vezzoni, A., Genchi, C. 1989. Reduction of post-adulticide thromboembolic complications with low dose heparin therapy. Proc Heartworm Symposium 1989:73–83.

Wajih, N., Sane, D. C., Hutson, S. M., and Wallin, R. 2004. The inhibitory effect of calumenin on the vitamin K–dependent γ-carboxylation system. Characterization of the system in normal and warfarin-resistant rats. J Biol Chem 279:25276–25283.

Warkentin, T. E. 2003. Heparin-induced thrombocytopenia: pathogenesis and management. Br J Haematol 121:535–555.

Woody, B. J., Murphy, M. J., Ray, A. C., Green, R. A. 1992. Coagulopathic effects and therapy of brodifacoum toxicosis in dogs. J Vet Intern Med 6:23–28.

SECTION 8

Endocrine Pharmacology

CHAPTER 27

HYPOTHALAMIC AND PITUITARY HORMONES

SRUJANA RAYALAM, MARGARETHE HOENIG, AND DUNCAN FERGUSON

INTRODUCTION

The hypothalamus and pituitary control the function of the thyroid, adrenal glands, and gonads. Neurons and endocrine gland cells share the characteristic of being able to secrete chemical mediators and being electrically excitable. Chemical messengers can be secreted as a neurotransmitter or as a hormone. The neuroendocrine systems consist of clusters of peptide- and monoamine-secreting cells in the anterior and middle portions of the ventral hypothalamus. Their fibers project via nerve fibers to terminals in the outer layer of the median eminence. The capillary plexus of the median eminence is proximate to the nerve terminals of the periventricular nucleus (PVN) hypothalamic neurons, which make corticotropin-releasing hormone (CRH), thyrotropin-releasing hormone (TRH), and somatostatin (growth hormone inhibitory hormone, GHIH); arcuate hypothalamic nucleus neurons make gonadotropic hormone–releasing hormone (GnRH), growth hormone–releasing hormone (GHRH), and the prolactin-inhibiting neurotransmitter dopamine. The concentrations of the releasing and inhibitory hormones in the median eminence are 10 to 100 times as great as in other parts of the hypothalamus because they are stored in the nerve terminals (Cone et al. 2003; Rijnberk 1996). The process of neurosecretion is characteristic of the hypothalamic nuclei, which release hormones into the portal vessels mediating the release of the anterior pituitary

TABLE 27.1 Location of hypothalamic and pituitary peptides

Substance	Neurotransmitter in Nerve Endings	Hormone Secreted by Neurons	Hormones Secreted by Endocrine Cells
GnRH	+	+	+
TRH	+	+	
CRH	+	+	+
GHRH	+	+	+
Somatostatin	+	+	+
POMC Derivatives	+		+
TSH	+		+
FSH	+		+
LH	+		+
GH	+		+
PRL	+		+
Oxytocin	+	+	+
Vasopressin	+	+	+

hormones such as growth hormone (GH), prolactin (PRL), thyrotropin (TSH), follicle-stimulating hormone (FSH), luteinizing hormone (LH), and the pro-opiomelanocortin (POMC)-derived peptides adrenocorticotropic hormone (ACTH), β-lipotropin (β-LPH), α-melanotropin (α-MSH) and the opioid β-endorphin (β-END). For each of the anterior lobe hormone systems (ACTH, LH, FSH, TSH, GH, and PRL), there is a closed-loop feedback system. Anterior lobe hormone and hypophysiotropic hormone secretions are suppressed by hormonal products of the respective end-organs, i.e., the thyroid, gonadal, and adrenal glands. Some hormones like PRL regulate their own secretion by inhibition via short-loop feedback on the hypothalamus. The somatotropes account for 50% or more of the anterior pituitary lobe cells, while other types of anterior lobe cells account for between 5–15% of the gland (Rijnberk 1996). Table 27.1 outlines the location of

TABLE 27.2A Hypothalamic regulatory hormones

Hormone	Action	Structure	Precursor	Target Organ
TRH	Elevates TSH, PRL	Blocked tripeptide (pGlu-His-Pro-NH2)	29-kDa precursor containing five copies of TRH	Pituitary thyrotrope
GnRH	Elevates LH, FSH	Blocked decapeptide (pGlu . . . Gly-NH2)	Amino terminus of 90 amino acid precursor	Pituitary gonadotrope
Somatostatin	Decreases GH	14 amino acid peptide with disulfide bond between residues 3 and 14	Carboxy-terminus of 92 amino-acid precursor	Pituitary somatrotroph
CRH	Elevates ACTH	41 amino acid peptide with amidated carbo xy-terminus	Carboxy-terminus of 190 amino-acid precursor	Pituitary corticotroph
GHRH	Elevates GH	44 amino-acid peptide with amidated carboxy-terminus	Residues 32–75 from a 107 amino-acid precursor	Pituitary somatotroph
Dopamine	Decreases PRL Increases GHRH or GH Decreases CRH or ACTH	Catechol		Pituitary lactotroph, somatotroph, corticotroph

TABLE 27.2B Anterior pituitary hormones

Hormone	Molecular Weight	Amino Acids	Other
I. ACTH-LPH			Derived from POMC
ACTH	4,500	39	
β-LPH	11,200	91	
	4,000	31	
II. GLYCOPROTEIN			
LH	29,000	α subunit: 89 β subunit: 115	α subunits are identical within a species; β subunits contribute biologic specificity
FSH	29,000	α subunit: 89 β subunit: 115	
TSH	28,000	α subunit: 89 β subunit: 112	
III. SOMATOMAMMOTROPINS			
GH	21,500	191	Common ancestral hormone
PRL	22,000	198	

Adapted from Tyrell et al. (1994), p. 74. See text for explanation of abbreviations.

TABLE 27.3 Hormones of the hypothalamus and the pituitary gland

Hormone	Site of Action (Target Organ)	Biologic Activity
Hypothalamus		
Gonadotropin-releasing hormone	Anterior pituitary (AP)	Releases LH and FSH
Thyrotropin-releasing hormone	AP	Releases TSH
Corticotrophin-releasing hormone	AP	Releases ACTH
Somatotropin-releasing hormone	AP	Releases somatotropin
Somatotropin-inhibitory hormone	AP	Inhibits somatotropin output
Prolactin-inhibitory hormone	AP	Inhibits prolactin output
Prolactin-releasing hormone	AP	Releases prolactin
Adenohypophysis		
Par distalis (anterior lobe)		
Somatotropin (growth hormone)	General soma	Body growth (bone, muscle, organs), protein synthesis, carbohydrate metabolism, regulation of renal functions (glomerular filtration rate) and water metabolism; increases cell permeability to amino acids; favors lactation
Adenocorticotropin hormone (ACTH, corticotropin)	Adrenal cortex	Maintenance of structural integrity of adrenal cortex; regulation of glucocorticoid secretion by zona fasciculate
Thyroid-stimulating hormone (TSH, thyrotropin)	Thyroid	Maintenance of normal structure and function of the thyroid gland; production of thyroxin and analogs
Prolactin (lactogenic hormone)	Mammary gland	Possibly favors lactation
Gonadotropins		
Follicle-stimulating hormone (FSH)	Ovary	Growth and maturation of ovarian follicles
		Germ-cell production (spermatogenesis)
	Testis seminiferous tubule	Synergistically with FSH causes estrogen secretion, follicle maturation, and ovulation; corpus luteum development in some species
Interstitial cell–stimulating, luteinizing hormone (LH)	Ovary	
	Testis Leydig cells	Stimulation of interstitial tissue; androgen secretion
Pars intermedia	Melanophore cells of amphibia and reptiles	Melanophore-expanding activity with resultant maintenance of skin color (negligible importance in mammals)
Intermedin (melanocyte-stimulating hormone)		
Neurohypophysis		
Antidiuretic hormone (vasopressin)	Renal tubules (distal convoluted)	Regulation of water excretion by resorption of water, pressor effect only in high doses
Oxytocin	Mammary myoepithelium	Letdown of milk by contraction of myoepithelium
	Uterine myoepithelium	Contraction of uterine musculature to aid parturition and sperm transport

neuroendocrine substances in the nervous system and endocrine organs. Tables 27.2A, 27.2B, and 27.3 show the key features of the structure and function of the hypothalamic regulatory and pituitary hormones. Many of these peptides find their clinical use as agents used for diagnostic tests of pituitary or endocrine end-organ function. Therefore, the related hypothalamic and anterior pituitary hormones will be discussed concomitantly.

The magnocellular neurons in the supraoptic nucleus (SON) and PVN of the hypothalamus terminate in the posterior pituitary lobe and secrete vasopressin (antidiuretic hormone; ADH) and oxytocin into the circulation.

ANTERIOR PITUITARY AND ASSOCIATED REGULATORY HORMONES

The pituitary hormones can be classified into three general categories: ACTH-LPH, glycoproteins (LH, FSH, and

TSH), and somatomammotropins (GH, PRL) (see Table 27.2B).

CORTICOTROPIN AND RELATED PEPTIDES

CORTICOTROPIN-RELEASING HORMONE (CRH).

CRH-secreting neurons are found in the paraventricular nuclei, and their nerve endings terminate in external layers of the median eminence. CRH is synthesized as part of a prohormone of 196 amino acids in length and undergoes enzymatic modification to an amidated form of 41-amino-acid peptide, which is identical in man, dog, rat, and horse (Mol et al. 1994). CRH stimulates synthesis and secretion of pro-opiomelanocortin (POMC) and ACTH by pituitary corticotrophs. Two major CRH receptor subtypes, CRH-R1 and CRH-R2, and a nonmembrane-associated CRH binding protein, have been identified (Hauger et al. 2003). Both the receptors belong to the G protein–coupled receptor superfamily, and are linked to adenylate cyclase. The CRH-R1 is the major subtype in the pituitary corticotroph, and it mediates the stimulatory actions of CRH on ACTH secretion through both the adenylate cyclase and calcium-calmodulin signal transduction systems (Klonoff and Karam 1992; Tyrell et al. 1994). In addition, CRH and its receptors act outside the HPA axis and maintain both acute and chronic synaptic stability to deal with daily or lifelong stressors (Orozco-Cabal et al. 2006). CRH neurons integrate inputs from physiological stressors such as osmotic challenge, hypoxia and blood volume loss, and neurogenic stress such as fear and restraint. Chemical inputs to these neurons include inhibitory effects of GABA and, of course, negative feedback from glucocorticoids. Stimulatory effects are provided by glutamate, serotonin, and cytokines such as IL-1, IL-2, IL-6, and TNFα. Intravenous CRH, acting via CRH-R2β receptors on the cardiac atria and ventricles, results in hypotension and bradycardia (Cone et al. 2003). CRH has also been identified as an anxiogenic and anorexogenic factor, prompting research into CRH antagonists as both mood altering and appetite-stimulating drugs (Cone et al. 2003). A CRH inhibitory factor has been postulated, and atrial natriuretic peptide, activins, and inhibins are considered as candidate peptides (Engler et al. 1999).

ADRENOCORTICOTROPIN (ACTH)

Biosynthesis. ACTH is a 39-amino-acid peptide hormone (MW 4500), which is one of several products from the metabolism of the 267-amino-acid precursor molecule pro-opiomelanocortin (POMC; MW 28,500; see Fig. 27.1). Between species, there is significant sequence homology in the ACTH amino acid structure. Canine ACTH differs by only 1 C-terminal amino acid from ACTH of other species (Mol et al. 1991). The other fragments of POMC with biological activity include β-lipotropin (β-LPH), α-melanocyte–stimulating hormone (α-MSH), β-MSH, and the opioid β–endorphin, as well as the N-terminal fragment (see Fig. 27.1). ACTH is metabolized to $ACTH_{1-13}$, which is identical to α-MSH and CLIP, which represents $ACTH_{18-39}$. These fragments are observed in species with developed intermediate lobes, such as the rat and horse, as well as fish, reptiles, and amphibians. β-LPH is secreted in equimolar amounts to ACTH. The 91 amino acids of β-LPH include the amino acid structure for β-MSH (41–58), γ-LPH (1–58), and β-endorphin (61–91). The first (N-terminal) 23 amino acids of ACTH, which are identical in humans, cattle, pigs, and sheep, produce all of its biological effects (Klonoff and Karam 1992; Tyrell et al. 1994). The sequence of the remaining amino acids varies among species (Chastain and Ganjam 1996). MSH causes pigment granules in melanocytes to disperse so that skin will darken. Although genetic factors associated with skin color are more important in the higher vertebrates, in mammals, MSH may cause transiently increased pigment synthesis. In addition to the pigmentary action, α-MSH exhibits cytoprotective activity against UV-induced apoptosis and DNA damage in cutaneous tissue (Bohml et al. 2006).

Structure. ACTH is a peptide that contains 39 amino acids in a straight chain molecule in sheep, pig, cow, and human. The first 24 and last 7 amino acids are identical and there are minor differences in amino acids 25 through 32 (see Fig. 27.2). The amino acid sequence of canine β-endorphin (β-END) differs from the human sequence by 4 amino acids (Young and Kemppainen 1994). The distribution of molecular forms of β-END in the canine intermediate lobe and anterior pituitary resembles most closely that in rats. In other species, such as sheep or horse, acetylated and shortened forms exist in substantial amounts. In all species studied to date, ACTH and related peptides are synthesized and cleaved from a common precursor molecule POMC. Posttranslational processing of POMC differs in the pars distalis and pars intermedia of the pituitary gland. In the pars distalis, POMC is processed to form ACTH, β-LPH, and some γ-LPH and

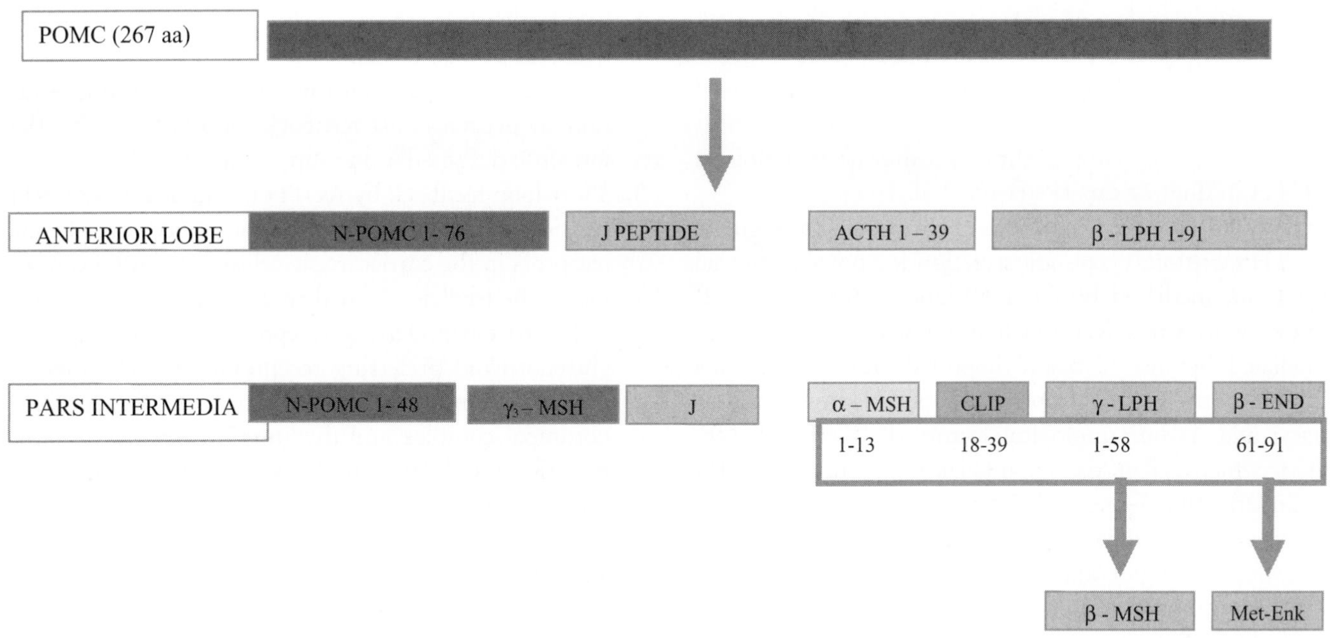

FIG. 27.1 Relationships of pro-opiomelanocortin (POMC)-derived peptides. Following synthesis in the anterior or intermediate lobe of the pituitary, POMC is cleaved to form adrenocorticotropin (ACTH) and β-lipotropin (β-LPH). ACTH further degrades, particularly in the intermediate lobe, to α-melanocyte-stimulating factor (α-MSH) and corticotropin-like intermediate lobe peptide (CLIP). β-LPH is cleaved to produce gamma-LPH and the endogenous opiate β-endorphin (β-END). Gamma-LPH is cleaved to produce β-MSH, and β-endorphin is further processed to produce another opioid met-enkephalin (Met-Enk).

1 2 3 4 5 6 7 8 9 10 11 12 13 -------- 25 26 27 28 29 30 31 32 33 34 35 36 37 38 39
Ser Tyr Ser Met Glu His Phe Arg Trp Gly Lys Pro Val (human) Asp Ala Gly Glu Asp Gln Ser Ala Glu Ala Phe Pro Leu Glu Phe
Ser Tyr Ser Met Glu His Phe Arg Trp Gly Lys Pro Val (pig) Asp Gly Ala Glu Asp Gln Leu Ala Glu
Ser Tyr Ser Met Glu His Phe Arg TRp Gly Lys Pro Val (beef) Asp Gly Glu Ala Glu Asp Ser Ala Gln
Ser Tyr Ser Met Glu His Phe Arg TRp Gly Lys Pro Val (sheep) Ala Gly Glu Asp Asp Glu Ala Ser Glu

FIG. 27.2 Amino acid sequences of human, pig, cattle, and sheep ACTH. Amino acids 1–13 are also present in α-MSH. Note areas of species homology in shaded boxes. (Reprinted from Klonoff and Karam (1992), Fig. 36.2.)

β-endorphin. In the pars intermedia, however, POMC is processed to ACTH and β-LPH; ACTH is then further processed to α-MSH and corticotropin-like intermediate lobe peptide (CLIP), and β-LPH is further processed to β-MSH, β-END, and β-END metabolites. As a result, ACTH and β-LPH are intermediates to α-MSH and the opiate β-END. The pattern of POMC-derived peptide secretion from the pars intermedia has been characterized in rats, horses, pigs, sheep, dogs, and cats. The plasma POMC peptide concentrations found in cats is similar to that in rats, but is markedly different from that in dogs in which the secretion of POMC peptides in the pars intermedia is normally low (Peterson et al. 1994b). The role of N-POMC (1–77) is known to promote adrenocortical cell replication, and the growth-promoting actions may be a result of either direct action of N-POMC (1–77) at the fetal adrenal or a consequence of proteolytic cleavage of N-POMC (1–77) at the adrenal (Coulter et al. 2002).

Regulation of Secretion. β-LPH and β-endorphin are secreted in a pattern similar to ACTH, increasing in response to stress and paralleling ACTH in a variety of disease conditions. The regulation of ACTH is most directly influenced by the hypothalamic hormone corticotropin-releasing hormone (CRH), which stimulates ACTH in a pulsatile fashion. Arginine-vasopressin (ADH) is also a potent stimulus for ACTH secretion (van Wijk et al. 1994). The pulsatility of ACTH release appears to occur in most species. Although a diurnal variation of cortisol exists in man, studies with sampling at 30-minute intervals for 48 hours have not confirmed a diurnal variation in ACTH in dogs or cats (Peterson et al. 1994c).

Four mechanisms have been identified to regulate ACTH secretion: 1) episodic secretion and possible diurnal variation, mediated by the CNS and hypothalamus; 2) response to stress (cat much more sensitive than dog) mediated by the CNS and hypothalamus; 3) feedback inhibition by cortisol at both the hypothalamus and pituitary; and 4) immunological factors (IL-1, IL-6, TNF, etc.), which act at the hypothalamus to increase CRH (Rijnberk 1996, Cone et al. 2003). Facilitatory and inhibitory pathways involving GABAergic, cholinergic, adrenergic, dopaminergic, and serotoninergic systems are all involved in hypothalamic regulation of ACTH and cortisol secretion. Drugs manipulating these systems have been utilized to manage pituitary-dependent hyperadrenocorticism in the dog and horse. Ergot alkaloids (dopamine agonists) and serotonin antagonists (cyproheptadine) have been utilized to manipulate ACTH release without much clinical success. The monoamine oxidase B inhibitor L-deprenyl was developed and approved by the FDA for use in dogs with pituitary-dependent hyperadrenocorticism (Bruyette et al. 1997a,b). In theory, reduction of the rate of dopamine degradation by this class of drugs should increase dopamine and suppress ACTH secretion (Klonoff and Karam 1992). Subsequent studies have been less enthusiastic about this drug as the sole treatment for canine pituitary-dependent hyperadrenocorticism (Reusch CE et al. 1999; Braddock et al. 2004).

Many factors stimulate ACTH secretion: pain, trauma, hypoxia, hypoglycemia, surgery, cold, pyrogens, and vasopressin (at least in man). CRH is often used pharmacologically to release ACTH from the pars distalis, and the drug haloperidol can be used to stimulate pars intermedia secretion with pars distalis effects being removed by dexamethasone. In cultured canine anterior pituitary cells, it appears that CRH stimulates ACTH secretion, but arginine vasopressin, oxytocin, and angiotensin II do not (Kemppainen et al. 1992).

Negative-Feedback Systems. Exogenous corticosteroids suppress the ACTH response to stress. Negative feedback of cortisol occurs via both the hypothalamic and pituitary. Feedback occurs in three ways:

1. Fast feedback is sensitive to the rate of change in cortisol and probably occurs via a nonnuclear receptor.
2. Slow feedback that is sensitive to the cortisol concentration in plasma. This feedback loop is tested by the low-dose dexamethasone suppression test.
3. Short-loop feedback by ACTH on the release of CRH by neurons in the hypothalamus and corticotrope receptors in the corticotropic cells of the anterior pituitary. The feedback is mediated through a type I mineralocorticoid preferring receptor (MR) and a type II glucocorticoid preferring receptor (GR). The highest level of GR in the dog brain is found in the septohippocampal complex and the anterior lobe of the pituitary (Reul et al. 1990; Keller-Wood 1990; Klonoff and Karam 1992; Tyrell et al. 1994).

Function. ACTH stimulates the secretion of glucocorticoids, mineralocorticoids, and adrenal androgens by increasing the activity of cholesterol desmolase, the enzyme that is rate limiting for steroid production and converts cholesterol to pregnenolone. ACTH also stimulates adrenal hypertrophy and hyperplasia. Steroids are not stored in the adrenal cortex, but they are immediately released upon stimulation of the zona fasciculata. ACTH causes growth of both the zona fasciculata and glomerulosa. The biological activity is conveyed by the amino terminal end of the molecule. ACTH stimulates adrenocortical growth and steroidogenesis by increasing cellular cAMP (Tyrell et al. 1994).

LPH induces lipolysis in adipocytes of some species, but its function is largely unknown other than serving as a precursor peptide for β-endorphin, which is an endogenous opiate (Klonoff and Karam 1992; Kuret and Murad 1990). However, a recent comparative study of the central effects of specific POMC-derived melanocortin peptides on food intake and body weight indicated that most of the POMC-derived melanopeptides, including γ-LPH, reduced food intake in POMC null mice (Tung et al. 2006).

DIAGNOSTIC USES OF CRH AND ACTH. The most important applications of CRH and ACTH are as a diagnostic agent to test adrenocorticotroph and adrenal functional reserve.

CRH Stimulation Test. CRH stimulation test is used mainly as a research tool to assess pituitary ACTH secretory capacity. In animals administered exogenous gluco-

TABLE 27.4 Dosage protocols for CRH stimulation test

Preparation	Horses/Cattle	Dogs	Cats
Ovine CRH (μg/kg IV)	NA	1	1
Sampling times (hrs)	NA	0, 0.5	0, 0.5

Sources: Crager et al. (1994); Moore and Hoenig (1992); Peterson et al. (1994b,c).
NA = protocol not available.

corticoids, the ACTH and cortisol response to CRH is diminished. In dogs and cats, ovine CRH is administered at 1 μg/kg intravenously and plasma is sampled for ACTH measurement at 0 and 0.5 hr for peak effect (see Table 27.4). Other sampling times have been employed in research reports (Crager et al. 1994; Moore and Hoenig 1992; Peterson et al. 1994b,c; Scott-Moncrieff et al. 2003). Dogs with primary adrenal insufficiency have high basal plasma immunoreactive-ACTH concentrations and show exaggerated responses to CRH, whereas dogs with secondary adrenal insufficiency showed undetectable basal plasma concentrations of immunoreactive-ACTH that did not increase after stimulation with CRH (Peterson et al. 1992). On the other hand, studies of normal dogs and dogs with pituitary-dependent hyperadrenocorticism have shown that ACTH secretion is less sensitive to CRH than with lysine vasopressin (LVP). It was found also that adrenocortical tumors develop an aberrant sensitivity to LVP, with adrenal tissue appearing to directly respond to LVP (van Wijk et al. 1994).

PREPARATIONS OF ACTH. Synthetic human $ACTH_{1-24}$ is called *cosyntropin.* Repositol ACTH gel from animal (porcine) sources is no longer available commercially. However, when comparing dosage protocols, 1 unit of porcine ACTH is approximately equal to 10 μg of cosyntropin. Synthetic ACTH is well absorbed by the IM route. The biological half-life of all forms of ACTH is 10 to 20 minutes and has an effect on the adrenal cortex for 12 to 48 hours.

ACTH STIMULATION TEST. The main use of ACTH is the differential diagnosis of adrenocortical hyperplasia from adrenocortical neoplasia (primary) in dogs, cats, and horses (see Table 27.5), and in the definitive diagnosis of primary adrenal hypofunction. ACTH is well absorbed following IM injection. Following injection of aqueous synthetic ACTH, largely because of the short half-life of ACTH, plasma cortisol concentrations peak at 30 to 90 minutes. Therefore, most sampling protocols with aqueous ACTH in dogs recommend sampling times at 1 hour after administration for a peak effect. The administration of 250 μg synthetic ACTH to dogs resulted in similar cortisol patterns, whether the dose was given IV or IM, despite the fact that there were much higher peak ACTH concentrations with the intravenous dose. A recent study further confirms that in healthy dogs and dogs with hyperadrenocorticism, administration of cosyntropin, a synthetic derivative of ACTH at a dose of 5 μg/kg, IV or IM, results in equivalent adrenal gland stimulation (Behrend et al. 2006). The peak cortisol concentration was at 60–90 minutes (Hansen et al. 1994). However, in cats, the intravenous dose of synthetic ACTH appeared to provide a greater response compared to the IM dosage but the peak cortisol response is somewhat variable and post-ACTH samples at 45 and 60 minutes are recommended (Peterson et al. 1994b, c).

TABLE 27.5 Dosage protocols for ACTH stimulation test

Preparation	Horses	Dogs	Cats
ACTH, USP (IU/kg IV, IM, SC)	1	2.2	2.2
Sampling times (hrs)	0, 8	0, 2	0,1,2
Synthetic (IV preferred)			
Cosyntropin (μg IV, IM)	100 (foals)	250 or 5 μg/kg	125
Sampling times (hrs)	0,1.5	0,1	0,0.75,1

Sources: Hansen et al. (1994); Moore and Hoenig (1992); Peterson et al. (1994b,c); Behrend et al. (2006). Hart et al. (2007).

Evaluation of Partial or Relative Adrenal Insufficiency in Foals. Recent studies have sought to evaluate the dose-dependency of the cortisol response to ACTH as an index of adrenal insufficiency in systemically ill foals. A randomized crossover study of intravenous ACTH (Cosyntropin®) in healthy foals at 3–4 days of age demonstrated that while 1 μg of ACTH had not yet reached a threshold dose, 10 μ resulted in a peak cortisol at 30 minutes returning to baseline by 90 minutes, while 100 and 250 μ both peaked at 90 minutes with a cortisol response that was indistinguishable (Hart et al. 2007).

MELATONIN

The pineal gland consists of photoreceptive cells, which have functional significance in fish and amphibians, but the pinealocytes function mainly as secretory cells in higher vertebrates. In vertebrates, light-dark cycle information is related to the pineal via indirect multisynaptic input crucial to the control of biologic rhythmicity. The retina provides light information to the suprachiasmatic nucleus (SCN) of the hypothalamus via the retinohypothalamic tract. The SCN provides input to the PVN via intrahypothalamic projections. The PVH then innervates sympathetic preganglionic neurons in the intermediolateral neurons in the cranial cervical ganglion, which then provides noradrenergic input to the pineal gland.

In mammals, the pinealocytes are the source of melatonin. Melatonin is synthesized from the amino acid tryptophan, through serotonin. Melatonin synthesis is tightly controlled in a circadian manner and is entrained to the light-dark cycle with highest melatonin concentrations during dark periods. The signal transduction associated with these changes in melatonin secretion is as follows: the absence of light leads to norepinephrine release from sympathetic nerve terminals that act upon G-protein coupled beta-adrenergic receptors, which increase adenylate cyclase activity. Cyclic AMP–response element in the promoter region for N-acetyltransferase (NAT) is the rate-limiting step for melatonin synthesis. Melatonin then acts on a family of G-protein coupled receptors (Mel1a, Mel1b, and Mel1c), depending upon the species of animal. Melatonin thereby inhibits the activity of neurons in the suprachiasmatic nucleus (SCN), considered the circadian pacemaker of the mammalian brain. This regulation is key to entraining reproductive patterns in species such as the sheep and horse.

Melatonin can be used as therapy for alopecia X in dogs. Alopecia X is a controversially defined condition (or conditions) associated with hair loss in dogs, which cannot be attributed to known endocrinopathies such as hypothyroidism and hyperadrenocorticism. One proposed treatment is melatonin at a dose of 3–6 mg/dog once or twice a day (Frank et al. 2004). Response rate may vary greatly depending on the severity and chronicity of the problem, and recurrence is not uncommon despite therapy.

GLYCOPROTEIN HORMONES AND ASSOCIATED RELEASING HORMONES

Only the thyroid-related peptides TRH and TSH will be discussed in this chapter. Gonadotropin-releasing hormone (GnRH), luteinizing hormone (LH), placental chorionic gonadotropin (HCG), and pregnant mare serum gonatropin (PMSG) are discussed in Chapter 28 on reproductive drugs.

THYROTROPIN-RELEASING HORMONE (TRH). TRH is a tripeptide: PyroGlu-His-Pro-NH_2. Neurons secreting TRH are located in the medial portion of the paraventricular nuclei and their axons terminate in medial portions of the external lamina of medial eminence. TRH is present extensively in the brain outside of the classic "thyrotropic area" of the hypothalamus. An intact amide and the cyclized glutamic acid terminus are essential for activity. TRH is synthesized as a large 242-amino-acid precursor, which contains five repeating sequences in the rat and six in the human called *preprothyrotropin-releasing hormone (preproTRH)* (Jackson 1982; Johnannson et al. 1981; Lechan et al. 1994; Yamada et al. 1990). The prohormone undergoes extensive posttranslational processing, including enzymatic cleavage, cyclization of NH_2-terminal glutamic acid, and exchange of an amide for the COOH-terminal glycine. TRH binds to specific receptors on the plasma membrane of the pituitary cell (Halpern and Hinkle 1981). TRH activates membrane adenylate cyclase with the formation of cAMP and increase in cAMP stimulates TSH secretion. However, cAMP may not increase under all conditions of TRH-induced TSH release, and increased intracellular cAMP is not always associated with an increase in TSH secretion. There is growing evidence that TRH-induced increase in cAMP concentrations may be a secondary event. It is now widely accepted that TRH action is mediated mainly through activation of Phospholipase C. It causes hydrolysis of phosphatidyl-inositol-4,5-biphosphate (PIP_2) into Inositol-1,4,5-triphosphate (IP_3) and 1,2-diacylglycerol (DAG). DAG then activates protein kinase C. Continuous exposure of TRH receptors to TRH causes an increase in IP_3 concentration that peaks within 10 seconds and falls within 1 minute indicating the rapid desensitization of the TRH response (Yu and Hinkle 1997). The binding of β-arrestins is shown to be critical for desensitization (Jones and Hinkle 2005). TRH induces an immediate and rapid increase in intracellular free calcium, which decays rapidly, followed by an extended plateau of elevated calcium. The first phase reflects increased release of intracellular calcium stores, whereas the second phase represents calcium influx. This biphasic action correlates with electrical charges, induction of Ca^{++} fluxes, and secretory activity in pituitary cells (Geras and Gershengorn 1981; Gershengorn et al. 1980; Tashjian et al. 1987; Vale et al. 1977; Winiger and Schlegel 1988).

TRH Stimulation Test

Diagnosing Hypothyroidism in the Dog. The TRH stimulation test, as it is used in the diagnosis of human pituitary and thyroid disease, is designed to evaluate the pituitary's responsiveness to TRH as manifested by the change in serum TSH concentration. In primary thyroid gland failure, the pituitary response to TRH is increased, and, in hyperthyroidism, it is decreased.

TRH has been most commonly applied instead of exogenous TSH to evaluate thyroid functional reserve by the increment in serum T_4 concentrations. Figure 27.3 shows the theoretical response of serum thyroxine (T4) to TRH and TSH administration. In theory, the administration of TRH should lead to an increase in T_4 only if the pituitary-thyroid axis is intact (see Figure 27.3). Therefore, responsiveness to TRH should be observed only in tertiary (hypothalamic) thyroid insufficiency, a condition not yet documented in the dog (Ferguson 1984, 1994, 2007). Since the availability of the canine TSH assay in 1997, more has been learned about regulation of TSH secretion. In human patients, an increased response of TSH to TRH generally demonstrated an enhanced response in early or mild primary hypothyroidism. However, evaluation of TRH-stimulated TSH responsiveness has not proved to be of much more diagnostic value than baseline canine TSH concentrations (Scott-Moncrieff et al. 1998; Hoenig and Ferguson 1997; Ferguson 2007).

A variety of TRH dosages have been proposed for use in the dog. In general, regardless of the species, increasing the TRH or TSH dose increases the duration of the serum T_4 response. In the dog, side effects were more significant at dosages greater than 100 μg/kg; salivation, urination, defecation, vomition, miosis, tachycardia, and tachypnea were observed (see Table 27.6). The recommended protocol for the TRH stimulation test is the administration of 100 μg/kg TRH (Relefact TRH, Rhone-Poulenc Rorer; Thypinone, Abbott Diagnostic) intravenously with the collection of serum for T_4 measurement at 0 and 6 hours post-TRH if serum T_4 is measured, and at 0 and 30

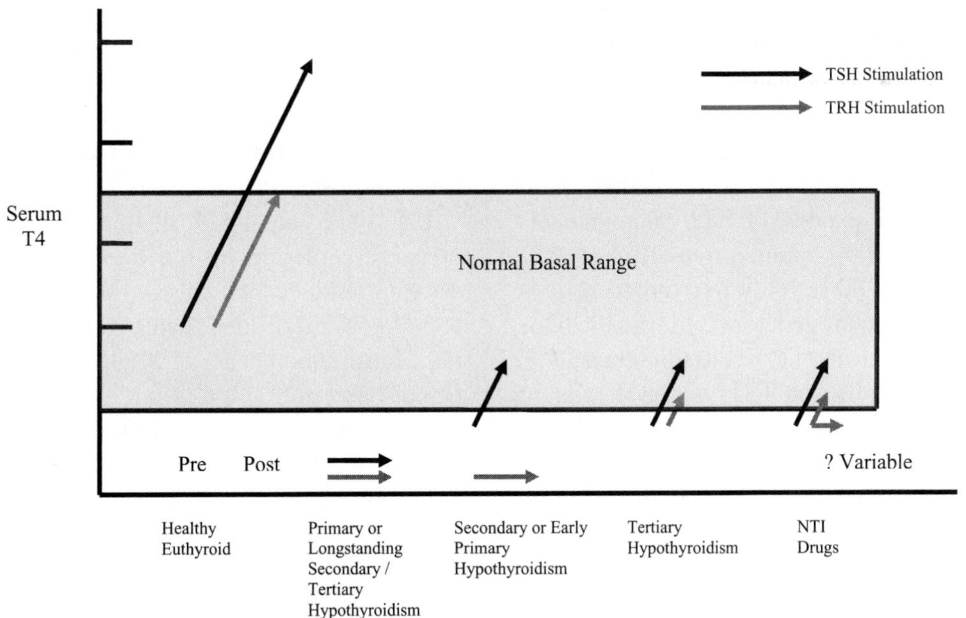

FIG. 27.3 Diagnostic classifications based upon TRH and TSH stimulation tests. The arrows represent in a stylized fashion the classical response of serum T4 concentrations to optimal doses of TRH and TSH. The actual magnitude of response will, in part, be determined by the dosage of TRH and TSH and the time of serum sampling post-TRH or post-TSH. The shaded area represents the normal baseline serum T_4 concentrations. Note the lower relative response to even maximal dosages of TRH compared to TSH. The left arrow (dark-filled) represents the response to TSH and the right arrow (lighter) represents the response to TRH. NTI = nonthyroidal illness. (Reprinted from Peterson and Ferguson (1989), Fig. 95–5.)

TABLE 27.6 Protocols for TRH stimulation test

	Dose	Route	Sampling Times (hr)
Dogs	100 μg/kg or 200 μg total	IV	0,4 (0,0.5 if TSH measured)
Cats	100 μg/kg	IV	0,4
Horse	1000 μg	IV	0,4

Preparations used are Relefact TRH® (Rhone-Poulenc Rorer), Thypinone® (Abbott Diagnostic), TRH (Peninsula Laboratories).

Sources: Ferguson (1984, 1994); Lothrop and Nolan (1986); Lothrop et al. (1984); Peterson and Ferguson (1989); Peterson et al. (1994a,c).

minutes if serum TSH is measured. Using this protocol in normal dogs, at least a 50% increase in serum T_4 was observed in 90% of dogs and all dogs had an increase of at least 0.5 μg/dl (6.4 nmol/l) above baseline (see Figure 27.3). With the lower dose of 200 μg TRH per dog, serum T_4 was shown to be maximal 4 hours after TRH administration. Because of the small increments following TRH, the successful application of the TRH stimulation test requires the use of a T_4 assay with extremely good internal reproducibility or preferentially, measurement of canine TSH.

Diagnosing Hypothyroidism in the Horse. TRH has been evaluated in horses as an alternative for establishing the pituitary thyrotrope and thyroid functional reserve. Intravenous administration of 1000 μg of TRH increases serum concentrations of T_4 and T_3 peaking at 4 hours post-TRH (see Table 27.6) (Lothrop and Nolan 1986). TRH has also been used at a dose of 2000 micrograms IV with samples at 0,30 and 90 minutes, to evaluate possible pituitary disease in the horse. However, no increase in progesterone, 17-hydroxyprogesterone, androstenedione, cortisol, aldosterone, testosterone, or estradiol, raising the question about the validity of TRH for evaluation of adrenal dysfunction in the horse (Fecteau et al. 2005).

Diagnosing Mild Hyperthyroidism in the Cat. In some instances, thyroid hormone concentrations (T_4 and T_3) are normal, are borderline, or even fluctuate into and out of the normal range in cats with mild hyperthyroidism. The TRH stimulation has been studied as a test of thyroid autonomy. In euthyroidism, the thyroid gland of the cat responds significantly to intravenous TRH, but the response in the hyperthyroid cat is considerably less, implying that thyroid function is not under the influence of endogenous TSH. The dosage of 100 μg/kg TRH administered intravenously is followed by serum sampling at 4 hours after injection. Serum T_4 concentrations increased by >50% in all normal cats and cats with nonthyroidal disease, whereas only 11% of hyperthyroid cats showed a 50% increase in serum T_4 concentration after TRH administration. Although case-controlled studies have established relative specificity, others have questioned the specificity the TRH stimulation test results in the presence of nonthyroidal illness (Peterson et al. 1994a, 2001). Adverse side effects in the cat associated with administration of TRH were common and included transient vomiting, salivation, tachypnea, and defecation. As a diagnostic test, the TRH stimulation test compares favorably with the T_3 suppression test while requiring less time, and it is more convenient to perform (Peterson et al. 1994a,c). The biological activity of freshly reconstituted TRH is maintained when frozen at −20°C for 1 to 5 weeks (Rosychuk et al. 1988).

THYROTROPIN (TSH)

Chemistry. Thyroid stimulating hormone (TSH) is a glycoprotein of MW 28,000 that is synthesized by thyrotrope cells of the anterior pituitary (see Table 27.2B). It is chemically related to the family of glycoproteins, including the pituitary gonadotropins luteinizing hormone (LH), follicle-stimulating hormone (FSH) and placental chorionic gonadotropin (CG). Each of these hormones contains two noncovalently linked dissimilar polypeptide chains, alpha and beta.

LH, FSH, and TSH all share similarities in tertiary structure conferred by the evolutionary preservation of cysteine residues, particularly those involved in the "cysteine knot" motif identified by crystallographic information. Furthermore, sites of N-glycosylation also appear to be preserved during evolution. As described below, glycoproteins contribute to the tertiary structure as well as the functional and immunogenic characteristics of the dimers (Zerfaoui and Ronin 1996).

Alpha and Beta Subunits. TSH is a heterodimer composed of two noncovalently bound subunits, alpha and beta. The subunits are synthesized as separate peptides from distinct mRNAs (Vamvakopooulos and Lourides 1979). The alpha subunit is common to all three hormones, but the beta subunit is unique for each hormone and confers biological specificity. For all four glycoproteins within each species, the amino acid sequence of the alpha subunit is common. However, the carbohydrate structure may vary. Microheterogeneity of the carbohydrate constituents of the individual hormones causes heterogeneity in receptor affinity, biological potency, and metabolic clearance (Pierce and Parson 1981; Wondisford et al. 1988).

The alpha subunits are approximately 20 to 22 kD, have 92 to 96 amino acid residues, and contain two N-linked carbohydrate groups. The human, cow, mouse, dog, cat, and rat alpha subunit genes are similar (Yang et al. 2000b, Rayalam et al. 2006a, b). All species have a single mRNA species that is between 730 and 800 bases long. The mRNA encodes the precursor of the alpha subunit and a leader sequence of an average of 24 amino acids.

The TSH beta subunit is approximately 18 kD, consists of approximately 110–113 amino acids and contains one N-linked complex carbohydrate (Green and Baenziger 1988). TSH, like LH, contains sulfate groups that terminate certain chains; such sulfation is found only to a small extent in FSH and not at all in CG. The genes for beta subunit of TSH of mouse, cow, human, dog, and horse have been cloned, and recombinant canine TSH (Yang et al. 2000a, b) and feline TSH (Rayalam et al. 2006a, b) have been expressed in vitro. Each mRNA is approximately 700 bases in length with minor variations. The TSH beta mRNA encodes the precursor TSH beta subunit with a 20–amino-acid leader sequence and a 117– or 118–amino-acid coding region.

The alpha subunit peptide is more abundant than the unique beta subunit of peptides. Free serum alpha subunits are secreted and are present in equivalent concentrations to combined concentration of TSH, LH, and FSH. Free serum beta subunit concentrations are lower, usually below the level of detectability. Overabundance of alpha subunit suggests that regulation of beta subunit synthesis is the rate-limiting step in modulating the levels of TSH, LH, and FSH.

Action. TSH binds to specific receptors on the thyroid plasma membrane. TSH receptors (TSHR) from dog, cat, pig, human, and rat have been completely cloned. The extracellular domain of the receptor contains 398 amino acids with five sites for N-linked glycosylation. The intracellular domain has 346 amino acids with seven putative transmembrane segments. The stimulatory guanine nucleotide regulatory protein binds to the third intracellular loop. The receptor has a glycoprotein component and a ganglioside, which may be involved in TSH activation of adenylate cyclase. TSHR is unique among glycoprotein hormone receptors in that some mature receptors on the cell surface are cleaved into two subunits (Rapoport et al. 1998). Only intact TSH binds to the receptor and the beta subunit does not possess biological activity (Chan et al. 1987; Field 1975). Binding of TSH to its receptor activates adenylate cyclase and subsequent accumulation of cAMP, but is not dependent on the interaction of the TSH from that species with the receptor. This results in the stimulation and dissociation of the regulatory and catalytic subunits of cAMP-dependent protein kinase (protein kinase A) with subsequent phosphorylation of various cellular proteins resulting in an increase in thyrocyte iodide uptake, thyroid hormone organification, and thyroid hormone secretion. This cyclic AMP–mediated pathway appears to be important in both thyroid hormone secretion and thyroid glandular growth (Chayoth et al. 1985).

The binding of TSH is also known to activate the phospholipase C signaling system. Activation of phospholipase C results in hydrolysis of phosphotidylinositol 4,5-biphosphate (PIP_2) with formation of diacylglycerol (DAG) and inositol-1,4, 5-triphosphate (IP_3). The former activates a Ca^{2+}-phospholipid–dependent protein kinase (protein kinase C) and the latter increases intracellular Ca^{2+} concentrations. The effect of TSH on phospholipase C is slower and requires larger amounts of the hormone than its activation of adenylate cyclase, suggesting a high capacity and low affinity TSH binding site. The physiological significance of activation of PIP_2 hydrolysis by TSH is not known, but is suspected to be involved in thyroid glandular proliferation (Chayoth et al. 1985; Taguchi and Field 1988).

Preparations. Two bovine thyrotropin products have been available in the past. Availability of biochemically purified native TSH purified from bovine pituitary glands as a pharmaceutical has been drastically reduced following the introduction of human recombinant TSH and following the emergence of bovine spongiform encephalopathy (BSE). Nonetheless, investigators occasionally still use cell culture grade product for animal use. Regardless of the source, it is stored in a lyophilized form for reconstitution and parenteral administration. A study evaluated the effects of freezing reconstituted bovine TSH and demonstrated that bioactivity remained intact for at least 3 weeks at 4°C (Bruyette et al. 1987; Ferguson 1994). Furthermore, the effect of storage conditions on the use of recombinant human thyrotropin (rhTSH) for thyroid-stimulating hormone (TSH) stimulation testing in dogs indicated that reconstituted rhTSH can be stored at 4°C for 4 weeks and at −20°C for 8 weeks without loss of biological activity (De Roover et al. 2006).

Thyrotropin (TSH) Stimulation Test. The administration of exogenous bovine or human TSH followed by the measurement of serum T_4 and/or T_3 provides important information in the diagnosis of hypothyroidism, used primarily in the dog, cat, and horse, because it tests thyroid secretory reserve. The availability of immunoassays measuring endogenous canine TSH have reduced the practicality and need for this test. However, the TSH stimulation test continues to be considered a noninvasive test for confirming the reduced thyroid functional reserve associated with hypothyroidism.

Protocols for this test vary widely in the dog and are summarized in Table 27.7. Although the TSH dose and serum sampling times are often dictated by practical and economic considerations, increasing the TSH dose administered generally delays the time of the T_4 peak, and, up to a limit, results in a higher serum T_4 response and a plateau that is maintained for a longer period of time. The route of administration may be intravenous, intramuscular, or subcutaneous; however, the most consistent and rapid response is seen after intravenous dosing. For the dog, the suggested protocol is to draw a baseline blood sample for serum T_4 determination, and then administer 0.1 IU/kg TSH intravenously (maximum dose 5 units), followed by a blood sample at 4 or 6 hours post-TSH (Ferguson DC 1984, 1994, 2007). Recent studies using 1 unit of bovine TSH (bTSH) per dog have indicated that the mean increase in serum T_4 and T_3 above baseline at 6 hours post-TSH was significantly lower following TSH at 1 IU than TSH at 5 IU but was not significantly different at 4 hours post TSH for the 2 doses of TSH evaluated. Based on the criteria for adequate response to TSH, TSH at 1 IU led to classification of 35% of the dogs as having a decreased response to TSH at 4 hours and 35% at 6 hours. TSH at 5 IU resulted in no dogs having a decreased response at 4 hours and 1 dog in 20 (5%) at 6 hours (Beale et al. 1990).

TABLE 27.7 Protocols for TSH stimulation test

	Dose or Dosage	Route	Sampling Times (hr)
Dog	0.1 unit/kg(max. 5 units)	IV	0,4
	1 unit/dog	IV	0,4
	50 or 75 mg/dog*	IV	0,4,6
Cat	1 unit/kg	IV	0,6
	1 unit/cat	IV	0,4
	25–200 μg/cat*	IV	0,6
Horse	5–10 units	IV	0,4,6

Preparation used was bovine TSH (Thytropar®; Rhone-Poulenc Rorer).

*Preparation used is recombinant hTSH (Thyrogen®, Genzyme Corporation).

For older protocols in the dog, see Ferguson (1984) for a review.

Sources: Hoenig and Ferguson (1983); Beale et al. (1990); Chen and Li (1987); Ferguson (1984,1994); Peterson and Ferguson (1989); Sauvé and Paradis (2000); Stegeman et al. (2003); DeRoover et al. (2006).

Pituitary-source preparations of TSH have been standardized according to bioactivity, which is reported as International Units (IU). Highly purified TSH approaches a biological specific activity of 12.5 IU activity/mg protein. A recent study compared the biological activity of recombinant human TSH (rhTSH) with bTSH in dogs, where bTSH was administered (1 unit corresponding to 500 μg in 0.5 ml of sterile water) intramuscularly and rhTSH was administered (75 μg in 0.5 ml sterile water) both intramuscularly and intravenously. Blood samples were collected immediately before and 6 hours after TSH administration. There were no significant differences in post-TSH stimulation T_4 concentrations among the three groups (Boretti et al. 2006). Another study suggested that 50 μg rhTSH was the optimal dose in euthyroid dogs to get a significant increase in serum TT4 concentrations (Sauvé and Paradis 2000). Similarly, IV administration of 25–200 micrograms significantly increased serum TT4 concentrations 6–8 hours later in euthyroid cats (Stegeman et al. 2003). A previous study with bovine TSH in cats had shown that the peak of serum T_4 was simply extended to later time points with higher dosages (Hoenig and Ferguson 1983).

Assuming a pharmacological dosage of TSH is used, the diagnosis of hypothyroidism in the dog is usually confirmed when the post-TSH serum T_4 concentration is below the normal range for basal T_4 (usually <1.0 μg/dl or <13 nmol/l in the dog) and rarely increases greater than 0.2 μg/dl (2.6 nmol/l) above the baseline. In pituitary forms of hypothyroidism, the thyroid gland should remain responsive to TSH. The rare cases of long-standing secondary (pituitary) or tertiary (hypothalamic) hypothyroidism with subsequent thyroid atrophy may require 2 or 3 consecutive daily doses of TSH to eventually demonstrate thyroid responsiveness (Ferguson 1984, 1994, 2007).

A study of normal dogs evaluated the predictive value of blood sampling times after 5 units of intravenous TSH:

in 80% of the animals, a doubling of the serum T_4 concentration was not achieved by 4 hours but was achieved in all cases by 6 hours post-TSH. Animals that responded favorably to thyroid replacement therapy have, on average, virtually no increase in serum T_4 concentration following TSH. An advantage of the TSH stimulation test is that post-TSH T_4 concentrations tend to be less variable because the thyroid is maximally stimulated.

Thyrotropin: Structural Homology Among Species. The TSH beta subunit is approximately 18 kD in molecular weight, consists of approximately 110–113 amino acids, and contains one N-linked complex carbohydrate. TSH, like LH, contains sulfate groups that terminate certain chains; such sulfation is found only to a small extent in FSH and not at all in CG. The genes for the beta subunit of TSH of mouse, rat, human, cattle, sheep, dog, cat, horse, opossum, teleost fish, chicken, quail, and horse have been cloned and sequenced. For most mammalian species, the mRNA is approximately 700 bases in length with minor variations. The TSH beta mRNA encodes the precursor TSH beta subunit with a 20-amino-acid leader sequence and a 117– or 118–amino-acid coding region. There is 80 to 90% homology at the amino-acid level among the sequences of most of the mammalian TSH beta molecules. As an example of avian species, the amino acid sequence of the quail TSH beta subunit shows homologies of about 70% to that of mammalian species, about 60% to that of amphibian, and about 50% to that of teleost fish. There is evidence that the functional domains of the TSH beta subunit and the TSH receptor have diverged cooperatively during evolution. Many regions of identical sequences are apparent in various beta subunits of glycoprotein hormones and the regions around residues 51 through 57 and 75 through 80 in the beta-structures are suggested to be involved in interaction with the common alpha subunit (Szkudlinski et al. 2002).

Glycosylation Patterns: Relevance to Bioactivity and Immunoreactivity. The pituitary glycoproteins LH, FSH, and TSH are produced and secreted in multiple molecular forms. In vivo, microheterogeneity of the carbohydrate constituents of the individual hormones causes heterogeneity in affinity for the receptor and in metabolic clearance of the hormone. In vitro, immunoreactivity is affected by this heterogeneity. Much has been learned from studies of human and equine chorionic gonadotropin because of the use of these agents as pharmaceuticals. For example, highly sialylated human FSH variants exhibit lower receptor binding, bioactivity, and immunoactivity compared to less sialylated counterparts. Each isoform appears to have a different affinity for the receptor. For example, FSH glycosylation variants appear to induce or stabilize distinct receptor conformations, resulting in different degrees of activation or inhibition of a given signal transduction pathway. Moreover, the FSH microheterogeneity depends on not only the variations in the sialic acid content but also on the differences in the internal structure of the carbohydrate chains, which determine the full biological expression of FSH glycosylation variants (Creus et al. 2001).

The oligosaccharide chains of pituitary glycoprotein hormones such as human thyroid-stimulating hormone (hTSH) have been shown to be important in biosynthesis, subunit association, secretion, and bioactivity. However, the exact biological significance of these glycosylation isoforms remains controversial. Human TSH glycosylation variants more basic in isoelectric point were found to be significantly more active than acidic ones in stimulating cAMP formation; however, there were no differences in stimulation of inositol phosphate release. In support of efforts to develop recombinant pituitary glycoproteins as pharmaceuticals, the bioactivity of glycoproteins produced in vitro appears to be as great or, in some cases, greater than, that of the pituitary derived form (Thotakura et al. 1991). Deglycosylation of recombinant feline TSH appears not to have reduced the in vitro bioactivity of this product (Rayalam 2006c). No studies have evaluated the rate of clearance of recombinant TSH in domestic species.

Effects of Drugs on TSH Concentrations. This subject was reviewed recently (Daminet and Ferguson 2003, Ferguson 2007). Drugs with significant effects on the thyroid axis include glucocorticoids and barbiturates. However, suppression of TSH concentrations by glucocorticoids have not been observed probably due to the lack of sensitivity of the TSH assay.

Two recent studies (Daminet et al. 1999; Gaskill et al. 1999) have examined the effects of phenobarbital on thyroid function tests. Daminet and co-workers prospectively examined the effect of a 3-week course of phenobarbital on TT4, FT4D, and TSH, and observed no significant alteration of these values over this time frame. Gaskill and co-workers, in an effort to dissect out the effects of phenobarbital, documented TT4 and TSH in 78 dogs receiving phenobarbital and compared them with 48 untreated epileptic dogs. Of the dogs on phenobarbital, 40% had low TT4 and 7% had elevated TSH, while only 8% of untreated dogs had low TT4 and none had elevated TSH. Of the latter group, only dogs with recent seizure activity had low TT4 values. The investigators found no effect of phenobarbital on serum binding of T4. The mean serum TT4 was significantly lower, and mean serum TSH significantly higher in the phenobarbital-treated group. As with the subacute study (Daminet et al. 1999), there did not appear to be a correlation between phenobarbital dosage or duration of treatment and the serum TT4 and TSH concentrations.

SOMATOMAMMOTROPINS AND REGULATORY HORMONES. Growth hormone (GH) and prolactin have similarities in amino acid structure and also share some biological activities. As a result they are called somatomammotropic or somatolactotropic hormones.

Growth Hormone–Releasing Hormone (GHRH). GHRH is secreted by neurons located in the arcuate nuclei with their axons terminating in external lamina of median eminence. GHRH is synthesized from a precursor of 108 amino acids. Initially, two peptides of 44 and 40 amino acids with GH-releasing activity were isolated. Synthetic peptides that contain only the first 29-amino-acid residues of GHRH are shown to be as potent as natural GHRH. GHRH stimulates synthesis and secretion of growth hormone by somatotrophs. GHRH binds to specific cell-surface receptors that are coupled to adenylyl cyclase though G proteins. Cyclic AMP mediates the GHRH effect on GH gene transcription and regulation GH secretion. GHRH also has a mitogenic effect on somatotrophs (Brazeau et al. 1982; Guillemin et al. 1981; Mayo et al. 1983; Michel et al. 1983; Reul et al. 1990).

Ghrelin. Ghrelin is a 28-amino-acid peptide with O-n-octanoylation at the serine in the third position, a modification essential for biological activity. This posttranslational modification is unique among known neuropeptides. Ghrelin is produced by the stomach in anticipation of a meal, but has stimulatory effects on GHRH neurons and GH secretion by the pituitary (Kojima et al. 1999; Cone et al. 2003).

Somatostatin: Growth Hormone Release Inhibiting Hormone (GHRIH). Somatostatin-producing neurons within the CNS are concentrated mainly in the anterior periventricular region of the hypothalamus with nerve terminals in external lamina of the median eminence. However, somatostatin-producing neurons are distributed also in other regions of CNS and outside CNS in epithelial cells (D cells) of the gastric mucosa, small intestine, kidney, islets of Langerhans of the pancreas, and parafollicular cells of thyroid. Somatostatin is synthesized as a precursor of 116 amino acids that is processed proteolytically to peptides with 14 or 28 amino acids. Somatostatin exerts its effects by binding to specific receptors on surface of target cells, which interact with G proteins. G proteins mediate a number of intracellular events, namely inhibition of adenyl cyclase activity leading to suppression of cAMP accumulation and inhibition of calcium fluxes leading to enhanced K^+ conductance and hyperpolarization. The fall in intracellular calcium reduces hormone secretion. GHRH also exerts a direct antiproliferative effect; inhibiting DNA synthesis and cell replication, by blocking epidermal growth factor induced centrosomal separation. This action might occur by interfering with movement of microfilaments and by preventing microtubule disassembly by inhibiting calcium influx. Table 27.8 summarizes the wide biological effects of somatostatin (Brazeau et al. 1973; Lamberts 1986; Montminy et al 1984; Reichlin 1983; Schmeitzel and Lothrop 1990).

Octreotide. Somatostatin has a limited clinical utility because of its short half-life (2–3 minutes) and its multiple effects. The somatostatin analogue octreotide has been used to help manage pituitary disorders (Klonoff and Karam 1992). Octreotide (Sandostatin®; Novartis) has been employed in the management of acromegaly, gastrinoma, pancreatic beta cell tumors, and glucagonoma in the dog.

Somatotropin: Growth Hormone (GH)

Structure and Secretion. Somatotropin (growth hormone) is a polypeptide hormone with a molecular weight of approximately 22 kD. The principal form of human somatotropin is a single chain, 191-amino-acid hormone, and was published in 1969 by Li (Li 1969). There is considerable species specificity for somatotropin (Kyosto and Reagan 1976; Wallis 1975), and human, bovine, and porcine somatotropin used clinically are now commercially produced by recombinant techniques. The sequence of canine growth hormone was first identified in

TABLE 27.8 Actions of somatostatin

Inhibits Hormone Secretion By
Pituitary gland—TSH, GH
PRL, ACTH
Gastrointestinal tract
Gastrin
Secretin
GIP
Motilin
Enteroglucagon
VIP
Pancreas
Insulin
Glucagon
Somatostatin
Genitourinary tract
Renin

Inhibits Other Gastrointestinal Actions By
Gastric acid secretion
Gastric emptying
Pancreatic enzyme and bicarbonate secretion
Intestinal absorption
Gastrointestinal blood flow
AVP stimulated water transport
Bile flow

TABLE 27.9 Factors influencing growth hormone secretion

Stimulate	Inhibit
Hypoglycemia	Hyperglycemia
Exercise	Free fatty acids
Sleep	Somatostatin
Amino acids	Growth hormone (negative feedback)
Hypoglycemia	ADH
GHRH	
Ghrelin	
ACTH	
α2-adrenergic agonists (clonidine)	α-adrenergic antagonists
M1 cholinergic agonists	M1 cholinergic antagonists
β-adrenergic antagonists	β2-adrenergic agonists
Dopamine or agonists	Dopamine antagonists (phenothiazines)
GABA or agonists	
Histamine 1 agonists	H1-histamine antagonists
Serotonin agonists	Serotonin antagonists
m opioids	Neuropeptide Y (NPY)
Testosterone	Progesterone
Estrogen	
Stress glucocorticoids (acute)	Glucocorticoids (chronic)

1994 and that of the cat was identified in 1995 (Asacio-Martinez and Barrera-Saldana 1994; Castro-Peralta and Barrera-Saldana 1995).

Somatotropin is synthesized and released under the influence of growth hormone releasing hormone (GHRH), a 44-amino-acid peptide. The secretion of somatotropin occurs in a pulsatile fashion, which results from the asynchronous release of GHRH and somatostatin (Growth Hormone Inhibition Hormone (GHIH), a potent inhibitor of somatotropin release (Müller 1987). Pulsatile release of GH appears to be the effect of GHRH pulsatile secretion, whereas between-pulse concentrations are largely determined by somatostatin (somatotropin-release inhibiting hormone; SRIH) (Rijnberk 1996). Many physiologic, pharmacologic, and pathologic factors influence the secretion of somatotropin, including exercise and hypoglycemia, which increase somatotropin secretion as do alpha adrenergic agonists, beta adrenergic antagonists, and dopamine agonists. Glucocorticoids, alpha adrenoceptor blockers, and beta adrenergic agonists decrease somatotropin secretion, as do hyperglycemia and obesity. See Table 27.9 for a review of regulatory factors for growth hormone release (Cone et al. 2003).

Function. Growth hormone's effects can be divided into two main categories: rapid or metabolic actions, and slow or hypertrophic actions (Rijnberk 1996). Acute catabolic effects are mediated by GH by decreasing carbohydrate utilization and impairing glucose uptake into cells, which results in glucose intolerance and secondary hyperinsulinism (Lean et al. 1992). The slower anabolic effects are mediated via insulinlike growth factors (IGFs). These hormones are produced in many tissues, particularly liver, in response to somatotropin. Growth hormone, via IGF-1, increases protein synthesis and decreases protein catabolism by mobilizing fat. This protein-sparing effect is important for linear growth and development.

Therapeutic Use. *Small animal applications.* In young dogs, growth hormone deficiency can occur as a primary endocrine abnormality resulting in pituitary dwarfism. It may be treated with bovine, porcine, or human somatotropin. Porcine somatotropin (pGH) is structurally identical to canine somatotropin and may be preferred for treatment in the dog (Asacio-Martinez et al. 1994). The pharmacological and toxicological effects of exogenous porcine somatotropin administration in normal adult dogs was evaluated. The results indicated that pGH caused a dose-dependent increase in body weight and the weights of liver, kidney, thyroid, and pituitary gland; increased skin thickness; and increased serum IGF-1 levels. However, minimal or no biologically significant effect of pGH on serum T3, T4, and cortisol levels in dogs was noticed (Prahalada et al. 1998).

Preparations and dosage protocols. It has been recommended to administer somatotropin at 0.1 IU/kg to dogs subcutaneously three times weekly for 4–6 weeks (Eigenmann 1982). If ACTH and TSH secretion are also abnormal, the animals need to be treated with replacement doses of glucocorticoids and thyroid hormone. Growth hormone–responsive dermatosis has been treated successfully with 0.15 IU/kg two times weekly for 6 weeks (Schmeitzel and Lothrop 1990).

Large animal applications. Bovine somatotropin (bST) has been used in cattle for several reasons. Somatotropin improves feed efficiency and leads to an effective increase in protein and reduction of fat, thus providing a desirable carcass in terms of degree of fatness and meat quality (Groenwegen et al. 1990; Schwarz et al. 1993). This has also been seen when bST was administered in finishing lambs (McLaughlin et al. 1993). In the pig, porcine somatotropin also leads to increased growth rates, and improved meat quality (Campbell et al. 1988; Etherton et al. 1987). A recent study indicated that use of bST was effective in reducing carcass fat and increasing edible lean of Holstein steers, but administering bST to young lightweight steers decreased carcass quality (Schlegel et al. 2006).

In addition to improvements in meat quality, bST has been used to increase milk production in the cow, and in the U.S., this application has been approved since 1994. Somatotropin also has an effect on milk composition, resulting in less short- and medium-chain fatty acids and more long-chain fatty acids (Bauman 1992, 1999; Lean et al. 1992).

Bovine milk naturally contains less than 1 ng/ml of GH whereas humans secrete 500 to 875 micrograms of GH per day. GH does not significantly increase in milk when cows are treated with bGH. Bovine growth hormone itself is degraded by the gastric acid when ingested orally and it is reported that the human growth hormone receptor does not respond to bovine GH.

Administration of bST increases IGF-1 concentrations in bovine milk, and some researchers have postulated that dairy products may increase the risk of breast cancer due to their content of fat, insulin like growth factor-1, estrogens, or growth hormone. However, a meta-analysis review concluded that the available evidence does not support this association. Although IGF-1 concentrations are not affected by pasteurization, the average milk content of IGF-1 has been estimated at 4 ng/ml. Based upon a 1.5 l/day milk intake, this would contribute 6 micrograms of IGF-1 to the gastrointestinal tract About 380 micrograms are contributed by gastrointestinal secretions. These amounts compare to the 10,000 micrograms produced daily in the liver and extrahepatic tissues. Thus, milk-derived IGF-1 is estimated to contribute less than 0.06% of the total IGF-1, and that would likely be an overestimate as it assumes that all IGF-1 survives proteolysis in the gastrointestinal tract (Parodi 2005).

It is important to note, however, that the European Union (EU) currently has a moratorium banning the use of bST in order to increase milk yield. An immunoassay for IGF-1 concentrations in milk has been developed and proposed as a regulatory test in milk samples.

Preparations and dosage protocols. Several formulations of bovine somatotropin (bST) are on the market. These include a daily dose, and 7, 14, and 28-day prolonged release preparations. The 14- and 28-day preparations are methionyl BST preparations. Exogenous bST must be present every day in order to continue an augmented milk response. The reason is that the bST peptide is rapidly cleared from the body. When given to cattle daily, maximum milk response is achieved with bST doses of 30–40 mg/day, and no further increase is observed with higher doses. Most production trials have employed doses between 10 to 50 mg/day. POSILAC® (Monsanto) is 500 mg of met^{-1} . . . leu^{126} bovine somatotropin (Sometribove, USAN), a 14-day prolonged release preparation of bST (Sometribove, USAN), which is administered every 14 days. Milk yield generally increases the first few days of bST treatment, reaching the maximum about the 6th day. In swine, prolonged release (4–6 weeks) injectables or ear tags are also available (Bauman 1992, 1999; Lean et al. 1992).

Adverse Effects. In dogs, diabetes mellitus is the major potential side effect of growth hormone administration; therefore, fasting blood glucose concentrations should be determined before and at weekly intervals while on growth hormone therapy. Hypersensitivity reactions might also occur after treatment with growth hormone (Schmeitzel and Lothrop 1990).

In cattle, treatment with growth hormone has been reported to cause an initial decrease in food intake; however, after a few weeks an increase is seen. It has also been suggested that growth hormone treatment increases the incidence of mastitis, which may be a function of the increase in milk production (Bauman 1992, 1999; Lean et al. 1992). However, in a multinational study involving over 900 cows no effect on incidence of clinical mastitis was seen (White et al. 1994). There are no indications that growth hormone administration leads to an increase in metabolic diseases in this species (Bauman 1992, 1999; Lean et al. 1992).

Prolactin

Structure and Biosynthesis. Prolactin (PRL) is a 198-amino-acid polypeptide hormone with a molecular weight of 22,000, which is synthesized and secreted by the lactotrophs of the anterior pituitary. It is classified as a somatomammotropic hormone and about 10–15% of the molecule represents glycosylation. Although glycosylated PRL is less potent, the glycosylation appears to stabilize the molecule to degradation in the body. In the species for which its structure has been identified, PRL has 3 intrachain disulfide bridges. The amino acid sequences of canine and feline prolactin have been recently identified (Gomez-Ochoa et al. 2004; Warren et al. 1996).

There are no pharmaceutical preparations of this hormone and few, if any therapeutic applications. Prolactin regulation is of relevance to the reproductively cycling animal in a variety of species. PRL evolved from a hormone common to GH and human placental lactogen (hPL), but it now shares only a minority of residues (13 and 16%, respectively) with these hormones. The precursor molecule for PRL is a 227 amino-acid with a molecular weight of 40,000 to 50,000 and contributes to some of the plasma PRL immunoreactivity (Klonoff and Karam 1992; Tyrell et al. 1994).

Function. PRL stimulates lactation in the postpartum period. It appears to have functions related to reproduction, particularly related to the care, feeding, and protection of offspring, even in fish and birds. Prolactin seems to have effects on salt and water metabolism, and is important in the ability of the salmon, for example, in changing from a saltwater to a freshwater environment. In mammals, the increasing concentrations of prolactin during pregnancy, combined with the hormonal effects of estrogens and progestins, induce the development of mammary tissue. In rodents, prolactin prolongs the life of the corpus luteum, but does not perform this function in humans or domestic mammals. The secretion of prolactin with suckling in certain species, most notably humans, is also likely to inhibit ovarian function and prevent ovulation and fertility (Klonoff and Karam 1992; Tyrell et al. 1994).

Regulation of Secretion. Secretion of prolactin by the pituitary is normally under inhibitory control by the hypothalamus, specifically by the neurotransmitter dopamine. Therefore, dopamine agonists inhibit prolactin secretion. Factors influencing secretion of growth hormone often have similar effects on PRL: sleep, stress, hypoglycemia, and exercise all increase PRL and GH. Other PRL-releasing hormones include TRH, which may explain galactorrhea in some hypothyroid bitches. Also the dopamine antagonists phenothiazines and metoclopramide, as well as butyrophenones, increase prolactin secretion. The half-life of prolactin in plasma is only 15–20 minutes. A prolactin inhibiting hormone (PRIH) of peptide nature has been investigated in rats. In humans, heavy athletic training, likely through opioid release, may inhibit PRL production and result in reproductive alterations, specifically amenorrhea in women (Kuret and Murad 1990).

Therapeutic Uses. There are no applications of clinical relevance. Milk production in cattle does not seem to be limited by the usual concentrations of circulating prolactin. However, research has focused upon the ability of GH to be galactopoietic.

POSTERIOR PITUITARY HORMONES

There are two known pituitary hormones: vasopressin (antidiuretic hormone or ADH) and oxytocin. Both hormones differ from vasotocin found in nonmammalian vertebrates by only 1 amino acid. Posterior pituitary hormones are synthesized in the hypothalamus and transported to the posterior pituitary where they are released into the circulation.

ANTIDIURETIC HORMONE (ADH)

Two 9-amino-acid peptides are secreted by the neurohypophyseal system: antidiuretic hormone (ADH or arginine vasopressin) and oxytocin. They are synthesized by the magnocellular neurons of the supraoptic nuclei and the lateral and superior parts of the paraventricular nuclei. ADH regulates the water permeability of the distal tubules and collecting duct of the nephron. It also is a vasoconstrictor and influences cardiovascular function.

STRUCTURE. ADH has a molecular weight of 1084 and is characterized by a 6-amino-acid ring and a 3-amino-acid side chain with a disulfide linkage. The prohormone for ADH includes the ADH sequence and neurophysin II, which binds to ADH. Following synthesis of the peptide, secretory granules containing the prohormone move down the axon to the nerve terminal in the posterior lobe of the pituitary. Upon exocytosis, equimolar amounts of the neurophysin and ADH are released. The neurons also project to the choroid plexus where they also release ADH into the cerebrospinal fluid.

STIMULI FOR RELEASE. The primary physiological stimulus for ADH release is an increase in plasma osmolality. However, hypovolemia, pain, exercise, and some drugs may stimulate ADH release.

MECHANISM OF ACTION. Three receptor subtypes that mediate the actions of AVP have been identified (V1A, V2, and V1B). V1A receptors are located in vascular smooth muscle cells and the heart and mediate vasopressin-induced vasoconstriction and increased afterload. The V1B receptor is located in the anterior pituitary and mediates ACTH release. V2 receptors are found on the renal tubule cells and are involved in the mediation of antidiuresis through increased water permeability and water reabsorption in the collecting ducts. ADH increases cyclic AMP in the tubule, which increases water permeability by stimulating the insertion of aquaporin 2 proteins at the luminal surface resulting in increased water permeability and reabsorption, urine osmolality, and decreased urine volume. V2 receptors outside of the kidney also mediate the release of the coagulation factor VIII and von Willebrand's factor. Aside from its value in treating conditions like central diabetes insipidus where vasopressin is deficient, irreversible shock has also been postulated to be exacerbated by a vasopressin deficiency, leading to its use in shock therapy.

Desmopressin acetate (DDAVP, 1-desamino-8-D-arginine vasopressin), is a long-acting synthetic analogue of predominately V2 or antidiuretic activity. Several nonpeptide AVP antagonists (vaptans) have been developed and are being evaluated for treating hyponatremia and fluid overload (Ali et al. 2007).

Table 27.10 summarizes the actions of vasopressin and the respective ADH receptors (V1A, V1B, and V2) mediating the actions.

ABSORPTION, METABOLISM, AND EXCRETION. Vasopressin must be administered parenterally and has a very short half-life of about 20 minutes.

PREPARATIONS. Natural and synthetic ADH is available commercially for the diagnosis and treatment of diabetes insipidus. Natural ADH (Pitressin) from cows and pigs is available as a water-soluble product. Dogs, cats, horses, and humans produce arginine-ADH and pigs produce lysine ADH. Desmopressin or deamino-D-arginine vasopressin (DDAVP) is available for parenteral (sub-

TABLE 27.10 Actions of vasopressin

Target Organ	Receptor Type	Action
Renal glomerulus	V_{1A}	Mesangial cell contraction
Vasa recta	V_{1A}	Decreases medullary blood flow
Juxtaglomerular cells	V_{1A}	Suppresses renin release
Arterioles	V_{1A}	Constriction
Liver	V_{1A}	Increases glycogenolysis
Anterior pituitary	V_{1B}	Increases ACTH release
Baroreceptors	?	Desensitization of baroreflex
Cortical/medullary collecting tubules	V_2	Increases H_2O permeability
Papillary collecting ducts	V_2	Increase H_2O permeability
Thick ascending loop of Henle	V_2	Increases Na^+, K^+, Cl^- reabsorption
Baroreceptors	?	Sensitization of baroreflex

cutaneous) injection and the acetate form is available for nasal administration and as 0.1 and 0.2 mg tablets.

DIAGNOSIS OF DIABETES INSIPIDUS. Diabetes insipidus (DI) is caused by the deficiency of antidiuretic hormone (central DI) or by absence of a renal response to this anterior pituitary hormone (nephrogenic DI). The main presenting signs, in the absence of other conditions, are polyuria and polydipsia.

Central diabetes insipidus is due to the absolute deficiency of antidiuretic hormone (vasopressin; ADH). In partial central diabetes insipidus, some endogenous ADH secretion remains. These conditions are the result of the destruction of the supraoptic and paraventricular nuclei of the hypothalamus, which have axons terminating in the posterior pituitary. The damage may be due to head trauma from surgical transection of the pituitary stalk (usually only transient DI) or primary or metastatic tumors, or—most commonly in veterinary medicine—the cause is not known (idiopathic DI).

Nephrogenic diabetes insipidus results when the renal tubule is insensitive to antidiuretic hormone. In this condition, ADH does not increase intratubular cAMP concentrations, a necessary prerequisite to the increased water permeability normally induced by ADH. This abnormality of ADH responsiveness may also be partial or total. Primary causes of nephrogenic diabetes are rare. However, secondary nephrogenic DI may result from pyometra, liver disease, hyperadrenocorticism, hyperthyroidism, hypercalcemic disorders, renal failure, and pyelonephritis.

Diabetes insipidus is diagnosed if the urine specific gravity is dilute (less than 1.008) in the face of dehydration and/or an elevated plasma osmolality. However, it is not infrequent for the animal to present in a hydrated state and to have a normal or only slightly elevated plasma osmolality. A modified water deprivation test is recommended to confirm that endogenous ADH and urine osmolality will not rise in the face of moderate dehydration. Following carefully monitored gradual water withdrawal over 3 days, water is completely withdrawn on the 4th day and the urine osmolality and plasma osmolality are monitored. If greater than 5% dehydration is achieved and no urine concentration is observed, exogenous ADH is administered to test the ability to respond to exogenous hormone.

Vasopressin can be administered in two ways in this test:

1. 0.55 units per kg intramuscular aqueous ADH (Pitressin Synthetic, Parke-Davis; Vasopressin USP, Quad) up to a maximum of 5 units. Urine volume and osmolality (or specific gravity) should be measured at 30, 60, and 120 minutes after administration.
2. The administration of 1 milliunit/ml of aqueous ADH (Pitressin Synthetic, Monarch; Vasopressin USP) in Lactated Ringer's or 5% dextrose. This solution is then administered over 1 hour at the rate of 10 ml per kg body weight. Urine samples should be obtained at 15-minute intervals for 90 minutes following ADH administration.

In an animal with complete central diabetes insipidus, the urine osmolality will not have risen above isoosmolality (300 mOsm per kg) with dehydration, and subsequent ADH administration will increase urine osmolality at least 50%. In an animal with partial central DI, the urine osmolality will increase above isoosmolality, but it will increase an additional 10–50% following exogenous ADH. Animals with nephrogenic DI do not concentrate their urine upon dehydration above isoosmolality, and also do not respond to exogenous ADH.

THERAPEUTIC USES. Aqueous ADH or ADH analogues are currently the only formulations available for the treatment of total and partial central DI. Synthetic ADH analogues DDAVP (DDAVP®, Stimate®, Minirin®, Ferring Pharmaceuticals) and LVP (Lysine-8-vasopressin, Lypressin®, Diapid Nasal Spray®, Novartis) are the most commonly used. Both of these preparations can be administered intranasally or into the conjunctival sac. The latter route appears to be better tolerated by the animals. Ocular or conjunctival irritation is a rare problem.

DDAVP is a drug with greater potency and slower metabolism than the natural ADH molecule. Administration of 5 to 20 μg of DDAVP (2–4 drops) in single or divided doses controls polyuria in most animals. The peak drug action is seen at 2–6 hours and its duration may last from 10 to 27 hours. The clear advantage of this medication is that it does not require parenteral administration. However, the conjunctival route results in variable amounts of drug reaching the blood stream and variable duration of effect even in the same patient. DDAVP is also quite expensive and therefore it might be prudent to use the drug only when polyuria is observed or to avoid excessive nocturnal urine production.

LVP is another product that is available for managing DI via nasal or conjunctival administration. However, its duration of action is shorter and expense greater than the other products. As a result, it has not found much application in veterinary medicine (Chastain and Ganjam 1986; Ferguson et al. 1992).

DDAVP has also been used for bleeding disorders (von Willebrand's disease and hemophilia A). In pharmacologic doses, it increases plasma levels of factor VIII:C and von Willebrand factor, via preferentially increasing levels of larger vWF multimers and by increasing platelet adhesion. Controlled studies on the use of DDAVP in dogs are lacking, but the clinical impression is that DDAVP is beneficial in some, but not all, von Willebrand's dogs. The initial parenteral dose of DDAVP (with either preparation) is 0.5–2 micrograms SQ once or twice daily. In animals, administration as eye drops is often more convenient. For chronic therapy of central diabetes insipidus, the DDAVP tablets are dosed initially at 0.1 mg given three times a day. The dose is gradually increased to effect if there still is unacceptable polyuria and polydipsia persisting a week after starting therapy. Most dogs require 0.1–0.2 mg of DDAVP two to three times a day for chronic therapy.

TOXICITY. Immediately following a dose, in order to avoid water intoxication, dogs should not be given unlimited quantities of water. The transiently high levels of ADH will prevent the excretion of a free water load by the kidney and result in overhydration and possible neurological sequela such as cerebral edema. Cerebral edema may be manifested by depression, vomiting, salivation, ataxia, muscle tremors, and convulsions. Animals with central or nephrogenic DI disease may also be successfully managed by providing free access to water at all times and by housing the animals outdoors. Another inexpensive maneuver that reduces the urine output is the restriction of dietary sodium using homemade diets or the commercial diets designed for use in congestive heart failure (e.g., Hill's H/D). Such products generally contain less than 0.1% sodium on a dry weight basis (Ferguson et al. 1992).

OTHER DRUGS FOR TREATMENT OF CENTRAL DIABETES INSIPIDUS. Oral agents have also been used primarily as adjuncts to ADH therapy of central DI. Chlorpropamide (Diabinese®, Pfizer), a sulfonylurea hypoglycemic agent used to treat noninsulin-dependent diabetes in humans, has produced inconsistent antidiuretic effects in the dog and cat. Chlorpropamide's effect is to enhance the effect of ADH on the renal tubules and collecting duct by increasing intracellular cyclic AMP. It may also stimulate pituitary ADH release. As a result, it is only effective in the presence of sufficient endogenous (partial central DI) or exogenously administered ADH. Careful dosage studies for chlorpropamide have not been performed in the dog. Reported doses include 250 mg every 12 hours and 10–40 mg/kg/day. Reduction in urinary volumes ranging from 18–50% has been reported. Maximal antidiuretic effects take 1–2 weeks to develop. Side effects of hypoglycemia can be minimized by frequent feedings and periodic monitoring of blood glucose concentrations.

Carbamazepine (Tegretol®, Novartis), an antiepileptic, is also effective in some cases of central DI. In contrast to the other drugs, these agents may increase the secretion of ADH and therefore would be rational therapy only in partial central DI. However, there have been no reports in the veterinary literature of the use of these drugs for the successful treatment of DI.

Thiazide diuretics when used together with salt restriction may serve to potentiate the effect of exogenous or endogenous ADH (see below) (Ferguson et al. 1992; Klonoff and Karam 1992; Tyrell et al. 1994).

TREATMENT OF NEPHROGENIC DIABETES INSIPIDUS. Treatment for nephrogenic DI should, if possible, start with correction of the underlying cause of the nephrogenic DI (hypercalcemia, renal infection, hyperadrenocorticism without a compressive pituitary tumor). Except for institution of a low-sodium diet, the thiazide diuretics are the only agents that have been shown to be effective in the treatment of nephrogenic DI.

Thiazide diuretics have a paradoxical antidiuretic effect in central and nephrogenic DI. These agents may reduce the reabsorption of sodium in the ascending loop of Henle, resulting in enhanced urinary sodium loss, mild reduction in plasma osmolality and, therefore, diminished thirst. The reduction in water intake causes contraction of the extracellular volume, and proximal tubular sodium reabsorption is increased and the glomerular filtration rate decreased. The urine volume is thereby reduced without overt concentration of the urine osmolality. Hydrochlorothiazide (Hydrodiuril®, Merck) at a dosage of 2.5–5 mg per kg has succeeded in reducing water intake by 50–85% in cases of ADH-resistant polyuria. Due to the kaliuretic effect of the thiazides, serum potassium should be monitored and oral potassium gluconate administered if the animal becomes anorexic (Ferguson et al. 1992). However, in human patients, combined use of thiazide diuretics and selective serotonin reuptake inhibitors synergistically impaired renal free water clearance resulting in severe hyponatremia (Rosner 2004).

OXYTOCIN

Oxytocin induces contraction of smooth muscle, most importantly of the myoepithelial cells of the mammary gland, which results in milk ejection. Furthermore, it also results in uterine smooth muscle contraction, an effect that increases during pregnancy. Its clinical use in the management of milk letdown and uterine contraction (induction of parturition and treatment of pyometra) is described in detail in the chapter on reproductive pharmacology. Oxytocin is also involved in endocrine and neuroendocrine regulation through receptor-mediated actions exerted on the heart, vasculature, and kidneys (Gutkowska et al. 1997; Jankowski et al. 2000; Conrad et al. 1993).

MECHANISM OF ACTION. Oxytocin affects the transmembrane ionic currents in uterine smooth muscle cells resulting in sustained uterine contraction. Oxytocin-induced myometrial contractions can be inhibited by tocolytic agents such as beta-adrenergic agonists, magnesium sulfate and inhalation anesthetics (Klonoff and Karam 1992; Tyrell et al. 1994).

REFERENCES

Ali F, Guglin M, Vaitkevicius P, Ghali JK. 2007. Therapeutic potential of vasopressin receptor antagonists. Drugs 67(6):847–858.

Ascacio-Martinez JA, Barrera-Saldana HA. 1994. A dog growth hormone cDNA codes for a mature protein identical to pig growth hormone. Gene 143:277–280.

Bauman DE. 1992. Bovine somatotropin: review of an emerging animal technology. J Dairy Sci 75:3432–3451.

Bauman DE. 1999. Bovine somatotropin and lactation: from basic science to commercial application. Domest An Endocrinol 17:101–116.

Beale KM, Helm LJ, Keisling K. 1990. Comparison of two doses of aqueous bovine thyrotropin for thyroid function testing in dogs. J Am Vet Med Assoc 197:865.

Behrend EN, Kemppainen RJ, Bruyette DS, Busch KA, Lee HP. 2006. Intramuscular administration of a low dose of ACTH for ACTH stimulation testing in dogs. J Am Vet Med Assoc 229(4): 528–530.

Böhm M, Luger TA, Tobin DJ, Garcia-Borron JC. 2006. Melanocortin receptor ligands: New horizons for skin biology and clinical dermatology. J Invest Dermatol 126:1966–1975.

Boretti FS, Sieber-Ruckstuhl NS, Willi B, Lutz H, Hofmann-Lehmann R, Reusch CE. 2006. Comparison of the biological activity of recombinant human thyroid-stimulating hormone with bovine thyroid-stimulating hormone and evaluation of recombinant human thyroid-stimulating hormone in healthy dogs of different breeds. Am J Vet Res 67(7):1169–1172.

Braddock JA, Church DB, Robertson ID, Watson AD. 2004. Inefficacy of selegiline in treatment of canine pituitary-dependent hyperadrenocorticism. Aust Vet J 82(5):272–277.

Brazeau P, Ling N, Esch F, et al. 1982. Somatocrinin (growth hormone-releasing factor) in vitro bioactivity: Ca^{++} involvement, cAMP mediated action and additivity of effect with PGE_2. Biochem Biophys Res Commun 109:588–594.

Brazeau P, Vale W, Burgus R, et al. 1973. Hypothalamic polypeptide that inhibits the secretion of immunoreactive pituitary growth hormone. Science 179:77–79.

Bruyette DS, Nelson RW, Bottoms GD. 1987. Effect of thyrotropin storage on thyroid-stimulating hormone response testing in normal dogs. J Vet Intern Med 1(2):91–94.

Bruyette DS, Ruehl WW, Entriken TL, Darling LA, Griffin DW. 1997a. Treating canine pituitary-dependent hyperadrenocorticism with L-deprenyl. Vet Med 92(8):711–727.

Bruyette DS, Ruehl WW, Entriken TL, Griffin DW Darling LA. 1997b. Management of canine pituitary-dependent hyperadrenocorticism with L-deprenyl (Anipryl). Vet Clin North Am Small Anim Pract 27(2):273–286.

Campbell RG, Steele NC, Caperna TJ, McMurtry JP, Solomon MB, Mitchell AD. 1988. Interrelationships between energy intake and endogenous porcine growth hormone administration on the performance, body composition and protein and energy metabolism of growing pigs weighing 25–55 kilograms live weight. J Anim Sci 66:1643.

Castro-Peralta F, Barrera-Saldana HA. 1995. Cloning and sequencing of cDNA encoding the cat growth hormone. Gene 160(2):311–312.

Chan J, Sandisteban P, De luca M, Isozedi E, Grollman E, Kohn L. 1987. TSH receptor structure. Acta Endocrinol (Copenh) 281(suppl):166.

Chastain CB, Ganjam VK. 1986. The endocrine brain and clinical tests of its function. In: Clinical Endocrinology of Companion Animals. Philadelphia: Lea and Febiger, pp. 37–68.

Chayoth R, Arem R, Yoshimura Y, Field JB. 1985. The role of calcium in the induction of refractoriness to cyclic AMP stimulation by TSH. Metabolism 34:1128.

Chen DCL, Li OW. 1987. Hypothyroidism. In: Robinson, NE (ed). Current Therapy in Equine Medicine 2. Philadelphia: W.B. Saunders, pp. 185–187.

Cone RD, Low Malcolm JL, Elmquist JK, Cameron JL. 2003. Neuroendocrinology. In: Larsen PR, Kronenberg HM, Melmed R, Polonsky KS (eds). Williams Textbook of Endocrinology, 10th ed. Philadelphia: Elsevier-Saunders, pp. 81–176.

Conrad KP, Gellai M, North WG. 1993. Valtin H. Influence of oxytocin on renal hemodynamics and sodium excretion. Ann N Y Acad Sci 689:346–362.

Coulter CL, Ross JT, Owens JA, Bennett, HP, McMillen IC. 2002. Role of pituitary POMC-peptides and insulin-like growth factor II in the developmental biology of the adrenal gland. Arch Physiol Biochem 110(1–2):99–105.

Crager CS, Dillon AR, Kemppainen RJ, Brewer WG, Angarano DW. 1994. Adrenocorticotropic hormone and cortisol concentrations after corticotropin-releasing hormone stimulation tests in cats administered methylprednisolone. Am J Vet Res 44(5):704–709.

Creus S, Chaia Z, Pellizzari EH, Cigorraga SB, Ulloa-Aguirre A, Campo S. 2001. Human FSH isoforms: carbohydrate complexity as determinant of in-vitro bioactivity. Mol Cell Endocrinol 174(1–2):41–49.

Daminet S, Ferguson DC. 2003. Influence of drugs on thyroid function in dogs. J Vet Int Med 17:463–472.

Daminet S, Paradis M, Refsal KR, Price C. 1999. Short-term influence of prednisone and phenobarbital on thyroid function in euthyroid dogs. Can Vet J 40(6):411–415.

De Roover K, Duchateau L, Carmichael N, van Geffen C, Daminet S. 2006. Effect of storage of reconstituted recombinant human thyroid-stimulating hormone (rhTSH) on thyroid-stimulating hormone (TSH) response testing in euthyroid dogs. J Vet Intern Med 20(4):812–817.

Eigenmann JE. 1982. Diagnosis and treatment of pituitary dwarfism in dogs. Proc 6th KalKan Symposium. Columbus, Ohio 81.

Engler D, Redei E, Kola I. 1999. The corticotropin-release inhibitory factor hypothesis: a review of the evidence for the existence of inhibitory as well as stimulatory hypophysiotropic regulation of adrenocorticotropin secretion and biosynthesis. Endocr Rev 20(4):460–500.

Etherton TD, Wiggins JP, Chung CS, Evock CM, Rebhun JF, Walton PE, Steele, NC. 1987. Stimulation of pig growth performance by porcine growth hormone: Determination of the dose-response relationship. J Anim Sci 64:433.

Fecteau KA, Haffner JC, Eiler H, Andrews FM, Oliver JW. 2005. Equine pars intermedia pituitary adenoma (Cushing's Disease): Steroid hormone profiles in healthy horses undergoing dexamethasone suppression, thyrotropin releasing hormone (TRH), and adrenocorticotropic hormone (ACTH) stimulation. ACVIM Forum Proceedings, abstract.

Ferguson DC. 1984. Thyroid function tests in the dog. Vet Clin N Amer 14:783–808.

Ferguson DC. 1994. Update on the Diagnosis of Canine Hypothyroidism. Vet. Clin. No. Am. 24(3):515–540.

Ferguson DC. 2007. Testing for hypothyroidism in dogs. Veterinary Clinics of North America Small Animal 37:647–669.

Ferguson DC, Hoenig M, Cornelius LM. 1992. Endocrinologic Disorders. In: Lorenz MD, Cornelius LM, Ferguson DC (eds). Small Animal Medical Therapeutics. Philadelphia: JB Lippincott, pp. 85–148.

Field JB. 1975. Thyroid stimulating hormone and cyclic adenosine 3′,5′-monophosphate in the regulation of thyroid gland function. Metabolism 24:381.

Frank LA, Hnilica KA, Oliver JW. 2004. Adrenal steroid hormone concentrations in dogs with hair cycle arrest (Alopecia X) before and during treatment with melatonin and mitotane. Vet Dermatol 15(5): 278–284.

Gaskill CL, Burton SA, Gelens HC, Ihle SL, Miller JB, Shaw DH, Brimacombe MB, Cribb AE. 1999. Effects of phenobarbital treatment on serum thyroxine and thyroid-stimulating hormone concentrations in epileptic dogs. J Am Vet Med Assoc. 215(4):489–496.

Geras EJ, Gershengorn MD. 1981. Evidence that TRH stimulates secretion of TSH by two calcium-mediated mechanisms. Am J Physiol 242:109.

Gershengorn MC, Rebecchi MJ, Geras E, Arelvalo CO. 1980. Thyrotropin releasing hormone (TRH) action in mouse thyrotropic tumor cells in culture; evidence against a role for adenosine, 3′,5′-monophosphate as a mediator of TRH-stimulated thyrotropin release. Endocrinology 207:665.

Gomez-Ochoa P, Fernandez-Juan M, Cebrian JA, Gascon M, Lucientes J, Larraga V, Castillo JA. 2004. GenBank Direct Submission. Canis familiaris prolactin mRNA, complete cds. ACCESSION # AY741405.

Green ED, Baenzinger JU. 1988. Asparagine-linked oligosaccharides on lutropin, follitropin, and thyrotropin. I. Structural elucidation of the sulfated oligosaccharides on bovine, ovine, and human pituitary glycoprotein hormones. J Biol Chem 263(1):25–35.

Groenwegen PP, McBride BW, Burton JJ, Elsasser TH. 1990. Effect of bovine somatotropin on the growth rate, hormone profiles and carcass composition in Holstein bulls. Domest Anim Endocrinol 7:43.

Guillemin R, Barazeau P, Bohlen P, et al. 1981. Growth hormone-releasing factor from a human pancreatic tumor that caused acromegaly. Science 218:585–587.

Gutkowska J, Jankowski M, Lambert C, Mukaddam-Daher S, Zingg HH, McCaan SM. 1997. Oxytocin releases atrial natriuretic peptide: evidence for oxytocin receptors in the heart. Proc Nat Acad Sci USA 94:11704–11709.

Halpern J, Hinkle PM. 1981. Direct visualization of receptors for thyrotropin releasing hormone with a fluorescein-labeled analog. Proc Natl Acad Sci USA 78:587–591.

Hansen BL, Kemppainen RJ, MacDonald JM. 1994. Synthetic ACTH (Cosyntropin) stimulation tests in normal dogs: comparison of intravenous and intramuscular administration. J Am An Hosp Assoc 30:38–41.

Hart KA, Ferguson DC, Heusner GL, Barton MH. 2007. Synthetic adrenocorticotropic hormone stimulation tests in healthy neonatal foals. J Vet Intern Med 21(2):314–321.

Hauger RL, Grigoriadis DE, Dallman MF, Plotsky PM, Vale WW, Dautzenberg FM. 2003. International Union of pharmacology. XXXVI. Current status of the nomenclature for receptors for corticotrophin-releasing factor and their ligands. Pharmacol Rev 5:21–26.

Hoenig M, Ferguson DC. 1983. Assessment of thyroid functional reserve in the cat by the thyrotopin stimulation test. Amer J Vet Res 44:1229–1232.

Hoenig M, Ferguson DC. 1997. Comparison of TRH-stimulated thyrotropin (cTSH) to TRH- and TSH-stimulated T4 in euthyroid, hypothyroid, and sick dogs. Proc ACVIM.

Jackson IMD. 1982. Thyrotropin releasing hormone. N Engl J Med 306:145–155.

Jankowski M, Wang D, Hajjar F, Mukaddam-Daher S, McCaan SM, Gutkowska J. 2000. Oxytocin and its receptors are synthesized and present in the vasculature of rats. Proc Natl Acad Sci U S A 97: 6207–6211.

Jones BW, Hinkle PM. 2005. Beta-arrestin mediates desensitization and internalization but does not affect dephosphorylation of the thyrotropin-releasing hormone receptor. J Biol Chem 280(46):38346–38354.

Keller-Wood, M. 1990. Fast feedback control of canine corticotropin by cortisol. Endocrinology 126 (4):1959–1966.

Kemppainen RJ, Clark TP, Sartin JL, Zerbe CA. 1992. Regulation of adrenocorticotropin secretion from cultured anterior pituitary cells. Am J Vet Res 53(12):2355–2358.

Klonoff DC, Karam JH. 1992. Hypothalamic and pituitary hormones. In: Katzung BC (ed). Basic and Clinical Pharmacology, 5th ed. East Norwalk: Appleton and Lange, pp. 513–528.

Kojima M, Hosoda H, Date Y, et al. 1999. Ghrelin is a growth hormone–releasing acylated peptide from stomach. Nature 402:656–660.

Kuret JA, Murad F. 1990. Adenohypophyseal hormones and related substances. In: The Pharmacological Basis of Therapeutics. New York: Pergamon Press, pp. 1334–1360.

Lamberts SWJ. 1986. Non-pituitary actions of somatostatin: a review on the therapeutic role of SM 201–995. (Sandostatin). Acta Endocrinol 276 (suppl):41–55.

Lean IJ, Troutt HF, Bruss ML, Baldwin RL. 1992. Bovine somatotropin. Vet Clinics North Amer 8:147–163.

Lechan RM, Adelman LS, Forte S, et al. 1984. organization of thyrotropin releasing hormone immunoreactivity in the human spinal cord. Proc Soc Neurosci 431.

Lewin MJ, Reyl-Desmars F, Ling N. 1983. Somatocrinin receptor coupled with cAMP-dependent protein kinase on anterior pituitary granules. Proc Natl Acad Sci USA 80:6538–6541.

Li CH. 1969. Recent studies on the chemistry of human growth hormone. In: Fontaine, M (ed). La specificite zoologique des hormones hypophysaires et de leurs activites. Paris: Centre National de la Recherche Scientifique.

Lothrop CD, Nolan HL. 1986. Equine thyroid function assessment with the thyrotropin-releasing hormone response test. Am J Vet Res 47(4):942–4.

Lothrop CD, Tamas PM, Fadok VA. 1984. Canine and feline thyroid function assessment with the thyrotropin-releasing hormone response test. Am J Vet Res 45:2310–2313.

Mayo KE, Vale W, Rivier J, et al. 1983. Expression-cloning and sequence of a cDNA encoding human growth hormone-releasing factor. Nature 306:86–88.

McLaughlin CL, Byatt JC, Hedrick HB, Veenhuizen JJ, Curran DF, Hintz RL, Hartnell GF, Kasser TR, Collier RJ, Baile CA. 1993. Performance, clinical chemistry, and carcass responses of finishing lambs to recombinant bovine somatotropin and bovine placental lactogen. J Anim Sci 71:3307–3318.

Michel D, Lefevre G, Labrie F. 1983. Interactions between growth hormone-releasing factor, prostaglandin E_2 and somatostatin on cyclic AMP accumulation in rat adenohypophysial cells in culture. Mol Cell Endocrinol 33:255–264.

Mol JA, Van Mansfeld DM, Kwant MM, Van Wolferen M, Rothuizen J. 1991. The gene encoding proopiomelanocortin in the dog. Acta Endocrinol 125(Suppl 1):77–83.

Mol JA, Van Wolferen M, Kwant M, Meloen R. 1994. Predicted primary and antigenic structure of canine corticotropin releasing hormone. Neuropeptides 27:7–13.

Montminy MR, Goodman RH, Horovitch SJ, et al. 1984. Primary structure of the gene encoding rat pre-prosomatostatin. Proc Natl Acad Sci USA 81:3337–3340.

Moore GE, Hoenig M. 1992. Duration of pituitary and adrenocortical suppression after long-term administration of anti-inflammatory doses of prednisone in dogs. Am J Vet Res 53(5):716–720.

Müller EE. 1987. Neural control of somatotropic function. Physiol Rev 67:962–1053.

Murakami K, Hashimoto K, Ota Z. 1985. Calmodulin inhibitors decrease the CRF and AVP-induced ACTH release in vitro: Interaction of calcium-calmodulin and cyclic AMP system. Neuroendocrinology 41:7–12.

Orozco-Cabal L, Pollandt S, Liu J, Shinnick-Gallagher P, Gallagher JP. 2006. Regulation of synaptic transmission by CRF receptors. Rev Neurosci 17(3):279–307.

Parodi PW. 2005. Dairy product consumption and the risk of breast cancer. J Am Coll Nutr 24(6):556–568.

Peterson ME, Broussard JD, Gamble DA. 1994a. Use of the thyrotropin releasing hormone stimulation test to diagnose mild hyperthyroidism in cats. J Vet Int Med 8(4):279–286.

Peterson ME, Ferguson DC. 1989. Thyroid Diseases. In: Ettinger SJ (ed). Textbook of Veterinary Internal Medicine, Vol. 2, Philadelphia: W.B. Saunders and Co, pp. 1632–1675.

Peterson ME, Kemppainen RJ, Orth DN. 1992. Effects of synthetic ovine corticotropin-releasing hormone on plasma concentrations of immunoreactive adrenocorticotropin, alpha-melanocyte-stimulating hormone, and cortisol in dogs with naturally acquired adrenocortical insufficiency. Am J Vet Res 53(3):421–425.

Peterson ME, Kemppainen RJ, Orth DN. 1994b. Plasma concentrations of immunoreactive proopiomelanocortin peptides and cortisol in clinically normal cats. Am J Vet Res 55 (2):295–300.

Peterson ME, Melian C, Nichols R. 2001. Measurement of serum concentrations of free thyroxine, total thyroxine, and total triiodothyronine in cats with hyperthyroidism and cats with nonthyroidal disease. J Am Vet Med Assoc 218 (4):529–536.

Peterson ME, Randolph JF, Mooney CT. 1994c. Endocrine diseases. In: Sherding RG (ed). The Cat:Diseases and Clinical Management, 2nd ed, Volume 2. New York: Churchill Livingstone, pp. 1403–1506.

Pierce JG, Parson TF. 1981. Glycoprotein hormones: structure and function. Ann Rev Biochem 50:465–495.

Prahalada S, Stabinski LG, Chen HY, Morrissey RE, De Burlet G, Holder D, Patrick DH, Peter CP, van Zwieten MJ. 1998. Pharmacological and toxicological effects of chronic porcine growth hormone administration in dogs. Toxicol Pathol 26(2):185–200.

Rapoport B, Chazenbalk GD, Jaume JC, McLachlan SM. 1998. The thyrotropin (TSH) receptor: interaction with TSH and autoantibodies. Endocr Rev 19:673–716.

Rayalam S, Eizenstat LD, Davis RR, Hoenig M, Ferguson DC. 2006b. Expression and purification of feline thyrotropin (fTSH): immunological detection and bioactivity of heterodimeric and yoked glycoproteins. Domest An Endocrinol 30:185–202.

Rayalam S, Eizenstat LD, Hoenig M, Ferguson DC. 2006a. Cloning and sequencing of feline thyrotropin (fTSH): heterodimeric and yoked constructs. Domestic Animal Endocrinology 30:203–217.

Reichlin S. 1983. Somatostatin. N Engl J Med 309:1495–1501, 1556–1563.

Reul JMHM, DeKloet ER, Van Sluijs FJ, Rijberk A, Rothuizen J. 1990. Binding characteristics of mineralocorticoid and glucocorticoid receptors in dog brain and pituitary. Endocrinology 127:907–915.

Reusch CE, Steffen T, Hoerauf A. 1999. The efficacy of L-deprenyl in dogs with pituitary-dependent hyperadrenocorticism. J Vet Intern Med 13(4):291–301.

Rijnberk A. 1996. Hypothalamus-pituitary system. In: Rijnberk, A (ed). Clinical Endocrinology of Dogs and Cats : An Illustrated Text. Netherlands: Kluwer Academic Publishers.

Rosner MH. 2004. Severe hyponatremia associated with the combined use of thiazide diuretics and selective serotonin reuptake inhibitors. Am J Med Sci. 327(2):109–11.

Sauvé F, Paradis M. 2000. Use of recombinant human thyroid-stimulating hormone for thyrotropin stimulation test in euthyroid dogs. Can Vet J. 41(3):215–219.

Schlegel ML, Bergen WG, Schroeder AL, VandeHaar MJ, Rust SR. 2006. Use of bovine somatotropin for increased skeletal and lean tissue growth of Holstein steers. J Anim Sci 84(5):1176–1187.

Schmeitzel LP, Lothrop CD. 1990. Hormonal abnormalities in Pomeranians with normal coat and in Pomeranians with growth hormone-responsive dermatosis. J Amer Vet Med Assoc 197:1333–1341.

Schonbrunn A. 1990. Somatostatin action in pituitary cells involve two independent transduction mechanisms. Metabolism 39(suppl2): 96–100.

Schwarz FJ, Schams D, Röpke R, Kirchgessner M, Kögel J, Matzke P. 1993. Effects of somatotropin treatment on growth performance, carcass traits, and the endocrine system in finishing beef heifers. J Anim Sci 71:2721–2731.

Scott-Moncrieff JC, Koshko MA, Brown JA, Hill K, Refsal KR. 2003. Validation of a chemiluminescent enzyme immunometric assay for plasma adrenocorticotropic hormone in the dog. Vet Clin Pathol 32(4):180–7.

Scott-Moncrieff JCR, Nelson RW, Bruner JM, Williams DA. 1998. Comparison of serum concentrations of thyroid stimulating hormone in healthy dogs, hypothyroid dogs, and euthyroid dogs with concurrent disease. J Am Vet Med Assoc 212(3):387–391.

Stegeman JR, Graham PA, Hauptman JG. 2003. Use of recombinant human thyroid-stimulating hormone for thyrotropin-stimulation testing of euthyroid cats. Am J Vet Res 64(2):149–152.

Szkudlinski MW, Fremont V, Ronin C, Weintraub BD. 2002. Thyroid-stimulating hormone and thyroid-stimulating hormone receptor structure-function relationships. Physiol Rev 82(2):473–502.

Taguchi M, Field JB. 1988. Effect of thyroid stimulating hormone, carbachol, norepinephrine and cAMP on polyphosphatidylinositol phosphate hydrolysis in dog thyroid slices. Endocrinology 123:2019.

Tashjian AH, Jr, Heslop JP, Berridge MJ. 1987. Subsecond and second changes in inositol polyphosphates in GH4C1 cells induced by thyrotropin releasing hormone. Biochem J 243:305–308.

Thotakura NR, Desai RK, Bates LG, Cole ES, Pratt BM, Weintraub BD. 1991. Biological activity and metabolic clearance of a recombinant human thyrotropin produced in Chinese hamster ovary cells. Endocrinology 28:341–348.

Tung YC, Piper SJ, Yeung D, O'Rahilly S, Coll AP. 2006. A comparative study of the central effects of specific proopiomelancortin (POMC)-derived melanocortin peptides on food intake and body weight in *Pomc* null mice. Endocrinology 147(12):5940–5947.

Tyrell JB, Findling JW, Aron DC. 1994. Hypothalamus and pituitary. In: Greenspan FS, Baxter JD (eds). East Norwalk: Appleton and Lange, 64–127.

Vale W, Rivier C, Brown M. 1977. Pharmacology of thyrotropin releasing factor (TRF) and somatostatin. In: Porter JC (ed). Hypothalamic Peptide Hormones and Pituitary Regulation. New York: Plenum, pp. 123–156.

Vamvakopoulos NC, Kourides IA. 1979. Identification of separate mRNAs coding for the alpha and beta subunits of thyrotropin. Proc Natl Acad Sci USA 76:3809–3813.

van Wijk, PA, Rijnberk A, Croughs RJM, Wolfswinkel J, Selman PJ, Mol JA. 1994. Responsiveness to corticotropin-releasing hormone and vasopressin in canine Cushing's syndrome. Eur J Endocrinol 130: 410–416.

Wallis M. 1975. The molecular evolution of pituitary hormones. Biol Rev 50:35.

Warren WC, Bentle KA, Bogosian G. 1996. Cloning of the cDNAs coding for cat growth hormone and prolactin. Gene 168(2):247–249.

White TC, Madsen KS, Hintz RL, et al. 1994. Clinical mastitis in cows treated with sometribove (recombinant bovine somatotropin) and its relationship to milk yield. J Dairy Sci 77:2249–2260.

Winiger BP, Schlegel W. 1988. Rapid transient elevations of cytosolic calcium triggered thyrotropin releasing hormone in individual cells of pituitary line GH3B6. Biochem J 255:161–167.

Wondisford FE, Radovic S, Moates JM, et al. 1988. Isolation and characterization of the human thyrotropin beta-subunit gene. Differences in gene structure and promoter function from murine species. J Biol Chem 263:12538–12542.

Yamada M, Radovic S, Wondisford FE, et al. 1990. Cloning and structure of human genomic DNA and hypothalamic cDNA encoding human preprothyrotropin-releasing hormone. Mol Endocrinol 4: 551–556.

Yang X, McGraw RA, Ferguson DC. 2000b. cDNA cloning of canine common α gene and its co-expression with canine β gene in baculovirus expression system. Domest An Endocrinol 18:379–393.

Yang X, McGraw RA, Su X, Katakam P, Grosse WM, Li OW, Ferguson DC. 2000a. Canine thyrotropin β-subunit gene: cloning and expression in *Escheria coli*, generation of monoclonal antibodies and transient expression in the Chinese ovary cells. Domestic Animal Endocrinology 18:363–378.

Young DW, Kemppainen RJ. 1994. Molecular forms of β-endorphin in the canine pituitary gland. Am J Vet Res 55(4):567–571.

Yu R, Hinkle PM. 1997. Desensitization of thyrotropin-releasing hormone receptor-mediated responses involves multiple steps. J Biol Chem 272:28301–28307.

Zerfaoui M, Ronin C. 1996. Glycosylation is the structural basis for changes in polymorphism and immunoreactivity of pituitary glycoprotein hormones. Eur J Clin Chem Clin Biochem 34(9):749–753.

CHAPTER

28

HORMONES AFFECTING REPRODUCTION

DOODIPLA S. REDDY AND JOHN E. GADSBY

INTRODUCTION

The brain (hypothalamus) regulates overall reproduction in animals via the synthesis and release of several peptide hormones. Hypothalamic hormones are released from hypothalamic neurons in the region of the median eminence, and they reach the anterior pituitary through the hypothalamic-adenohypophyseal portal system. The two main hypothalamic hormones relevant to reproduction are gonadotropin-releasing hormone (GnRH) and the prolactin-inhibitory hormone known as *dopamine*. The primary function of these hormones is to stimulate or inhibit the release of a specific anterior pituitary hormone.

The pituitary gland is essential for the regulation of reproduction, as well as growth, stress, and intermediary metabolism. The pituitary gland consists of three separate lobes in vertebrates: the anterior (adenohypophysis), posterior (neurohypophysis), and intermediate. The anterior pituitary lobe releases two distinct types of reproductive "trophic" hormones; the gonadotropins, (follicle-stimulating hormone, FSH, and luteinizing hormone, LH), and prolactin. Based on evolutionary and structural considerations, FSH and LH are grouped together and are glycoprotein hormones, while prolactin is related to growth hormone and is known as a *somatomammotropin*. A large number of reproductive states as well as a diverse group of drugs also affects their secretion and function (Wright and Malmo 1992).

Steroid hormones play vital roles in reproduction. The ovary (females) and testis (males) are the primary sources

TABLE 28.1 Reproductive hormones and related agents

Hormone	Indications
GnRH and GONADOTROPINS	
GnRH	Ovulation induction, infertility therapy
Gonadorelin (synthetic GnRH)	Ovulation induction, infertility therapy
Follicle-stimulating hormone (FSH)	Follicle development for embryo transfer
Human chorionic gonadotropin (hCG)	Ovulation induction, infertility therapy
Equine chorionic gonadotropin (eCG)	Ovulation induction, infertility therapy
OXYTOCICS (Ecbolics = uterotonics)	
Oxytocin	Labor induction
PROGESTINS	
Altrenogest	Synchronization of estrus in mare and pig
Melengestrol acetate (MGA)	Synchronization of estrus in cattle
Progesterone (injectable or intravaginal delivery—CIDR)	Synchronization of estrus in cattle, sheep, goats, and mares
ANDROGENS	
Nandrolone	Catabolic disease states in horses and dogs
Stanazolol	Catabolic disease states in horses and dogs
ANTIANDROGENS	
Finasteride	Benign prostatic hypertrophy in dogs
PROSTAGLANDINS	
Lutalyse®	Regulation of the estrous cycle in ruminants (e.g., cows)
	Induction of abortion (various species)
Estrumate® (Cloprostenol)	Induction of parturition in sows
	Induction of abortion (various species)

of reproductive steroid hormones in animals. The gonadotropins, FSH and LH, which are secreted in response to hypothalamic GnRH, stimulate the secretion of gonadal steroids (estrogens and progesterone in the female, and testosterone in the male). A list of hormones and drugs affecting reproduction is summarized in Table 28.1.

ESTROUS CYCLE

In females, GnRH from the hypothalamus and the gonadotropins, FSH and LH, from the pituitary regulate the estrous cycle (Fig. 28.1). GnRH secreted from the hypothalamus is transported by the hypophyseal portal blood vessels to the pituitary gland, where it increases secretion of the gonadotropins, FSH and LH. Gonadotropins stimulate the secretion of gonadal steroids (estrogens and progesterone). Estrogens and progesterone have prominent stimulatory effects upon the endometrium and the mammary gland, while increased circulating levels of these steroids decrease gonadotropin secretion (via negative feedback). Each estrous cycle consists of the following phases:

1. *Follicular phase (= proestrus and estrus).* During the follicular phase ovarian follicles (one or more depending on the species) develop and mature, secreting increasing amounts of estrogen. Estrogen triggers a surge release of LH from the pituitary gland, causing ovulation of follicles and the release of ova into the oviduct.
2. *Luteal phase (= metestrus and diestrus).* Following ovulation the remnants of each follicle develop into a corpus luteum, whose primary function is secretion of progesterone, which is required to act on the uterus to create an environment compatible with attachment/implantation of the embryo. If the ova are not fertilized, or if embryos fail to develop or attach/implant, the corpus luteum regresses (degenerates) leading to the cessation of progesterone secretion. However, during pregnancy, the life span of the corpus luteum is lengthened (except in the bitch), resulting in continued progesterone secretion, which is necessary for pregnancy maintenance.

In nonpregnant animals, during the late stages of the luteal phase of the estrous cycle, the uterus (endometrium)

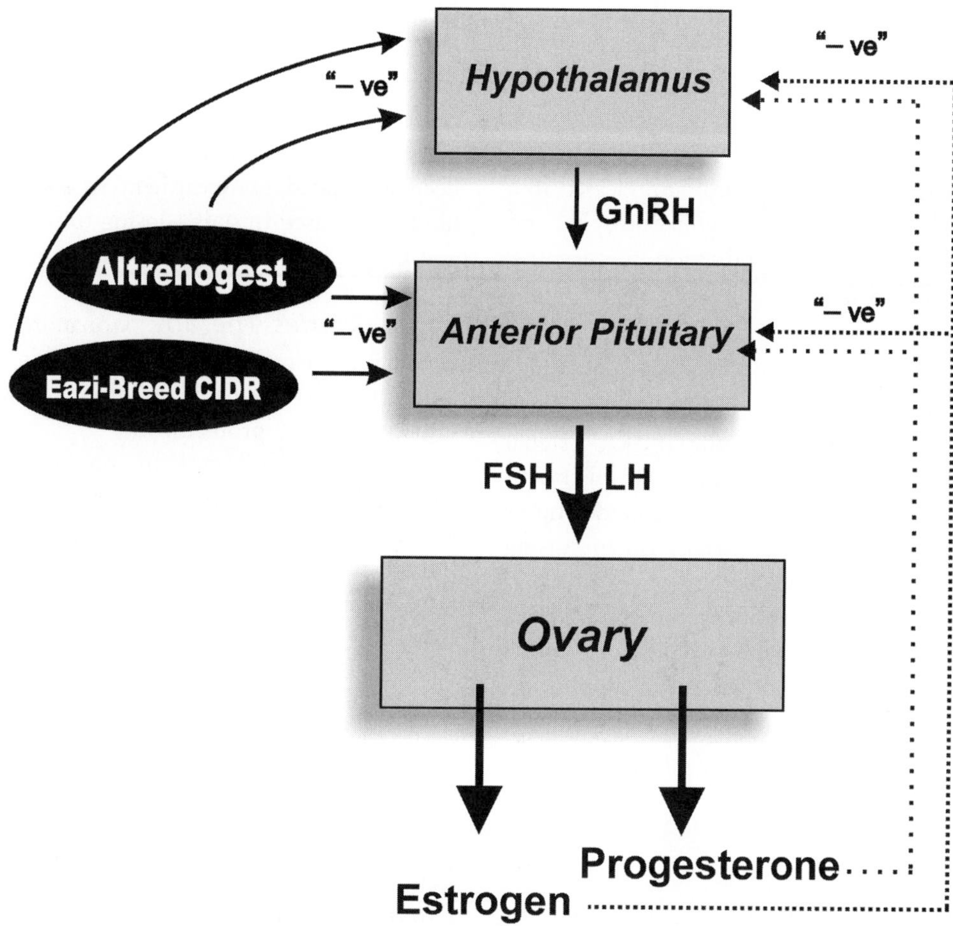

FIG 28.1 Regulation of estrous cycle and gonadal hormone secretion. Gonadotropin-releasing hormone (GnRH) stimulates gonadotropin (FSH, LH) release, which subsequently increases ovarian steroid hormone production during the estrous cycle. Like natural estrogen and progesterone, synthetic agents such as Altrenogest and Melengestrol Acetate (MGA) control the estrous cycle by *negative feedback* mechanisms.

releases the hormone prostaglandin $F_{2\alpha}$ ($PGF_{2\alpha}$). (Additional discussion on prostaglandin pharmacology is listed in Chapter 18). This hormone causes corpus luteum regression, which is then followed by another estrous cycle (follicular phase followed by luteal phase). Estrus (female reproductive behavior induced by follicular estrogen) follows corpus luteum regression within a few days. Because ovarian steroids generally decrease gonadotropin secretion through negative feedback mechanisms, administration of exogenous gonadal steroids, or their analogs, inhibits gonadotropin secretion and consequently inhibits gonadal function (see Fig. 28.1). Progesterone, estrogen, and $PGF_{2\alpha}$ (or analogs) have all been used in the control and synchronization of estrous cycles for breeding purposes. Progesterone like hormones (progestins; e.g., melengestrol acetate [MGA] or altrenogest) are the most commonly used hormones in theriogenology (Wright and Malmo 1992).

GNRH, GONADORELIN, AND GONADOTROPINS

The neurohormones, such as GnRH (and analogs), gonadotropins (FSH and LH), prolactin, and oxytocin, that are important in veterinary medicine are discussed below.

GONADOTROPIN-RELEASING HORMONE (GNRH)

Structure and Function. GnRH is the decapeptide hypothalamic-releasing hormone responsible for stimulating the release of gonadotropins, FSH and LH, by the anterior pituitary gonadotropes. It has a very short half-life (2–4 min). GnRH release is intermittent and controlled by a neural pulse generator in the hypothalamus. Such intermittent release is crucial for the proper synthesis and release of the gonadotropins, which also are released in a pulsatile fashion (Peters 2005). Both gonadotropins and gonadal steroids regulate GnRH production in a negative feedback manner (Peters 2005).

Mechanism. GnRH stimulates the synthesis and release of gonadotropins by binding to the GnRH receptor, a G protein-coupled receptor linked to the IP_3-Ca^{2+} signal transduction pathway. Pulsatile or episodic administration of GnRH stimulates the secretion of gonadotropins and forms the basis of infertility therapy by increasing gonadal stimulation (see use 1 in the next section). Alternatively, continuous administration of GnRH leads to desensitization and down-regulation of GnRH receptors on pituitary gonadotropes. This leads to the suppression of gonadotropin secretion and forms the basis for the clinical use of long-acting GnRH analogs (*e.g., leuprolide, gonadorelin*) to cause medical castration (see use 2 in the next section) (Yoshimoto et al. 2005; Stout and Colenbrander 2004).

Clinical Use. The two principal uses of GnRH are 1) management of infertility and 2) suppression of gonadotropin secretion (medical castration). A number of clinical GnRH analogs have been synthesized. These include synthetic GnRH (gonadorelin) and other potent, long-acting GnRH analogs (e.g., leuprolide).

GONADORELIN. Gonadorelin (Cystorelin® or Factrel®) is a synthetic preparation of GnRH used to treat animals with infertility disorders secondary to GnRH deficiency or dysfunction in GnRH secretion. It stimulates the synthesis and secretion of FSH and LH by interacting with GnRH receptors on the pituitary gonadotropes. Since GnRH is released in a pulsatile manner, gonadorelin therapy should be used in an "*intermittent* or *pulse-dosing*" schedule. The continuous administration of gonadorelin leads to desensitization and down-regulation of GnRH receptors on pituitary gonadotropes, which may be the basis for its clinical use to limit estrus in some animals (Thatcher et al. 2001).

Clinical Use

Infertility Therapy. Gonadorelin has been used empirically to induce ovulation at the time of breeding in both cattle and horses, and is a component of the "Ovsynch" protocol (see discussion later in this chapter). It has also been advocated for treatment of stallions with lowered libido. It is used in pulse-dosing to induce estrus in dogs, and in cats with prolonged anestrus.

Cystic Ovaries Therapy. Gonadorelin is the drug of choice for *ovarian follicular cysts* ("cystic ovaries") in cattle (and camelids) in clinical conditions in which incomplete luteinization is a problem.

Ovarian follicular cysts in cows are defined as follicle-like structures that persist rather than ovulate. These are more than 25 mm in diameter and have been present for 10 days or more in the absence of a corpus luteum (CL). Their occurrence is frequent in the postpartum dairy cow but rare in beef cows (Farin and Estill 1993). The first choice for treatment is 100 mcg GnRH, which generally produces luteinization of the cystic structure, with estrus occurring in 18–23 days. The administration of $PGF_{2\alpha}$ 9 days after GnRH will often shorten the interval to estrus. (Refer to additional discussion later in the chapter.)

Estrus Synchronization in Conjunction with $PGF_{2\alpha}$. "Ovsynch" or "Timed AI" protocol is used in cows (Lucy et al. 2004): Day 0–100 mcg GnRH, Day 7–25 mg $PGF_{2\alpha}$, Day 9–100 mcg GnRH, breed cattle by AI 20–24 h after 2nd GnRH. This allows synchronization of estrous cycles for AI without estrus detection.

Timed Embryo Transfer (ET) Protocol. This protocol is used for recipient cows (Al-Katanani et al. 2002) using the Ovsynch treatment protocol as above, but instead of AI, using transfer of embryos (ET) into recipients on Day 16–17. This enables preparation of recipients and ET without the need for estrus detection.

Terminating Estrus. Gonadorelin is used in ferrets and induced ovulators (cats and camelids) to terminate estrus.

Diagnostic Purposes. Gonadorelin can be used experimentally for diagnostic purposes to differentiate between pituitary and hypothalamic defects in dogs with hypogonadotropic hypogonadism.

Identifying Intact Animals. Gonadorelin is also used to identify intact animals from spayed or neutered animals by estimating gonadorelin-stimulated release of FSH and LH.

Dosage. Veterinary products are listed in Table 28.2.

GONADOTROPINS

Secretion and Function. The pituitary hormones, FSH and LH, as well as the related placental *human chorionic gonadotropin* (hCG), are referred to as the "gonadotropic" hormones. Each hormone is a glycosylated heterodimer containing a common α-subunit and a distinct β-subunit that confers specificity of action. A single hypothalamic-releasing factor, GnRH, controls the synthesis and release of gonadotropins, LH and FSH, in males and females. LH and FSH are synthesized and secreted by gonadotropes, which make up ~20% of anterior pituitary cells. hCG is produced only in primates and horses (equine chorionic gonadotropin, eCG—see below)—and is made by syncytiotrophoblast cells of the placenta. Gonadal

TABLE 28.2 Drugs affecting reproduction in animals

Class	Drug Name	Preparation	Dosage
Gonadotropins			
Follicle-stimulating hormone	Follitropin®-V		
Equine chorionic gonadotropin (eCG)	Ovagen® PG600®	Combination of 400 IU eCG, 200 IU hCG	Pig: 1 ml PG600 IM
Human chorionic gonadotropin (hCG)	Follutein® Chrorulon®	Injection 5,000 U and 10,000 U	Dog: 50–100 μg, SC, IV Cat: 25 μg, IM Horse:1,000 U, IV Cattle: 1,000–2,500 U, IV Sheep: 400–800 U, IV, IM Goat: 3,000 U, IV
Gonadorelin (synthetic GnRH)	Cystorelin® Factrel®	Injection 50, 100 μg/ml	Dog: 50–100 μg, SC, IV Cat: 25 μg, IM Horse: 50 mg, SC Cattle: 100 mg, IM (100 mcg)
Oxytocics			
Oxytocin	Pitocin® Syntocinon®	Synthetic oxytocin injection 20 U/ml	Dog: 5–20 U, IM or IV once Cat: 2.5–5 U, IM once Pig: 10–20 U, IM Horse: 50–100 U, IV, IM, SC Cattle: 50–100 U, IV, IM, SC Sheep: 30–50 U, IV, IM, SC
Progestins			
Altrenogest	Regumate®	Solution: 2.2 mg/ml	Horse: 0.044 mg/kg/day for 15 days
Syncro-Mate B	SMB™	Ear implant + Inj.	(Not available in U.S.)
Progesterone	Eazi-Breed CIDR™	Vaginal drug delivery devices	Cattle: 1.38 g for 7 days
Androgens			
Stanazolol	Vinstrol-V®	Tabs: 2 mg Inj. 50 mg/ml	Horse: 0.55 mg/kg, IM up to 4 doses once weekly
Antiandrogens			
Finasteride	Proscar®	Tablets	Dog: 0.1–0.5 mg/kg, once daily for up to 16 weeks
Prostaglandins			
(PGF2α agents) Dinoprost	Lutalyse®	Vials: 5 mg/ml	Cattle: 25 mg, IM inj. Pig: 10 mg, IM inj. *(= 2 ml!)* Horse: 1 mg/100 lb body weight, IM inj.
Cloprostenol	Estrumate®	Vials: 0.25 mg/ml	Cattle: 0.5 mg, IM inj.

steroid hormones (androgens, estrogens, and progesterone) cause feedback inhibition at the level of the pituitary and the hypothalamus. The preovulatory surge of estrogen also can exert a stimulatory effect at the level of the pituitary and the hypothalamus (Day 2004):

- *In males,* LH acts on testicular Leydig cells to stimulate the synthesis of androgens, primarily testosterone. FSH acts on the Sertoli cells to stimulate the production of proteins and nutrients required for sperm maturation.
- *In females,* FSH and LH stimulate the growth and development of ovarian follicles, induce ovulation, and thereby stimulate the follicle to produce estrogen, while LH stimulates the developing corpus luteum (after ovulation) to secrete progesterone.

Mechanism. The actions of LH and hCG are mediated by the LH receptor, and those of FSH are mediated by the FSH receptor. Both of these G protein-coupled receptors are linked to adenylate cyclase and raise the intracellular levels of cAMP.

Therapeutic Uses. Apart from diagnostic application in pregnancy detection kits, gonadotropins are used in 1) female and male fertility and 2) cryptorchidism (see Table 28.2).

Three distinct gonadotropins—hCG, human menopausal gonadotropin (hMG), and equine chorionic gonadotropin (eCG)—are available for clinical use in animals. (See Table 28.2 for a list of available products.)

HUMAN CHORIONIC GONADOTROPIN. Human chorionic gonadotropin (hCG) is a gonadal-stimulating hormone obtained from the urine of pregnant women. It is synthesized by syncytiotrophoblast cells of the placenta. It possesses primarily LH-like activity; therefore, it serves as a substitute for LH to promote follicle maturation, ovulation, and formation of corpus luteum. hCG is a glycoprotein and nonpituitary gonadotropin with long-lasting biological effects (>24 hr). A single injection is adequate for reproductive therapy. For example, because of its predominant LH-like activity, hCG is used to induce ovulation in the mare after an appropriate follicular size has been achieved (Wathes et al. 2003).

Clinical Use

Infertility Therapy. hCG is widely used for infertility therapy. It is used in female horses for hypogonadism due to pituitary hypofunction, and to hasten or induce ovulation (Samper 2001).

Cystic Ovaries. hCG is used for the treatment of cystic ovaries in cows. Treatment recommendations are either hCG 5,000 IU IV or 10,000 IU IM. Most cows respond with the establishment of an estrous cycle within 3–4 weeks.

Inducing Estrous Cycles. eCG (400 IU) and hCG (200 IU) together make up PG600®, which is used in pigs for inducing estrous cycles in prepubertal gilts.

Impotence. hCG is useful for treating male infertility due to *impotence*, particularly in the mare. In the male, hCG stimulates the interstitial cells to produce testosterone.

Cryptorchidism. hCG is the preferred drug for the correction of *cryptorchidism*, a genetically influenced condition in which one or both testes fail to descend into the scrotum. Cryptorchidism can be treated with early injections of hCG. Cryptorchid testes have defective spermatogenesis.

Inducing Pseudopregnancy. hCG may be used in sequence with eCG for the induction of pseudopregnancy in cats.

Toxicity. Immunological reactions such as anaphylaxis due to antihormone antibody production have been reported. Prolonged usage may produce loss of efficacy because of circulating antibody.

Dose Veterinary preparations and dosage are listed in Table 28.2.

EQUINE CHORIONIC GONADOTROPIN (ECG). Equine chorionic gonadotropin (eCG; formerly known as *Pregnant Mare Serum Gonadotropin,* or PMSG) is secreted from the endometrial cups of pregnant mares in early pregnancy in order to induce secondary corpora lutea—by developing and ovulating accessory follicles—and to maintain the primary corpora lutea (and thus progesterone secretion) in the mare. Its gonadotropic activity is primarily FSH-like and increases ovarian follicular growth, but it has sufficient LH-like activity to induce ovulation and luteinization. Like hCG, eCG is a glycoprotein and nonpituitary gonadotropin with long-lasting biological effects (>24 hr). A single injection is generally sufficient for marked growth of ovarian follicles (Shelton 1990).

Clinical Use

Ovarian Follicular Growth. eCG is frequently used to stimulate ovarian follicular growth in the anestrous sheep or goat. It is used in combination with hCG for induction of ovulation and corpus luteum formation.

Inducing Estrous Cycle. eCG (400 IU) and hCG (200 IU) together make up PG600®, which is used in pigs for inducing estrous cycle in prepubertal gilts.

HUMAN MENOPAUSAL GONADOTROPIN (HMG). Human menopausal gonadotropin (hMG), also known as *menotropin,* is extracted from the urine of postmenopausal women. hMG contains approximately equal amounts of FSH and LH activity. This preparation is not widely used in veterinary medicine.

FOLLICLE STIMULATING HORMONE (FSH). Two preparations are available: Folltropin V® (porcine FSH), Vetrepharm, Canada; and Ovagen® (ovine FSH), ICP Bio, New Zealand.

FSH is used to develop multiple follicles of donor cattle for ovulation (superovulation) and oocyte collection, and for production of embryos used in embryo transfer procedures (Hasler 2002).

PROLACTIN

Structure and Function. Prolactin is synthesized in lactotropes of the anterior pituitary and is classified as a somatomammotropic hormone. It is a 198-amino acid polypeptide with 3-intra-chain disulfide bridges. Prolactin stimulates lactation in the postpartum period. During pregnancy, prolactin secretion increases and, in concert with other hormones (e.g., estrogen, progesterone), promotes additional mammary development in preparation for milk production (Kooistra and Okkens 2001). The secretion of prolactin during suckling maintains milk secretion by the mammary gland, and also inhibits ovarian function by suppression of the hypothalamic-pituitary-gonadal axis, and thus prevents ovulation. Prolactin is secreted in a pulsatile manner (half-life, 15–20 min).

Mechanism. Prolactin, acting via the prolactin receptor, plays an important role in inducing growth and differentiation of the ductal and lobuloalveolar epithelium; lactation does not occur in the absence of this hormone.

Regulation. Prolactin is unique among the anterior pituitary hormones in that hypothalamic regulation inhibits its secretion. The major regulator of prolactin secretion is *dopamine* (also known as *prolactin inhibiting hormone, PIH*), which is released by tuberoinfundibular neurons and activates the D_2 receptors on lactotropes to inhibit secretion of prolactin. Hence, dopamine agonists or antagonists can affect prolactin release. Prolactin is the only anterior pituitary hormone for which a unique stimulatory releasing factor has not been identified. Thyroptopin-releasing hormone (TRH) can stimulate prolactin release, but its physiological role is unclear. Prolactin is not under feedback control by peripheral hormones.

Therapeutic Uses. Prolactin has no therapeutic uses. Milk production in cattle does not appear to be limited by the circulating prolactin. It may be useful for treatment of unwanted lactation associated with pseudopregnancy in the bitch and to treat atypical or idiopathic lactation in the mare.

Other Drugs that Affect Prolactin. Metoclopramide (Reglan) is used as an antiemetic in small animals and to stimulate stomach emptying and small intestinal motility in small and large animals. The mechanism of acting is via dopamine antagonism. This drug also transiently increases prolactin secretion. Women at risk for developing mammary gland carcinoma are advised to avoid use of metoclopramide, but such a risk factor has not been identified for animals. There has been interest in using this drug for treating agalactia in animals, but efficacy has not been determined. Use in horses is cautioned because of reported undesirable behavioral effects. (Gastrointestinal drugs are discussed in more detail in Chapter 47.)

Domperidone (Motilium, Equidone) has been available as a tablet for people outside the U.S. to stimulate gastrointestinal motility. Its mechanism of action and GI effect are similar to metoclopramide. A difference between metoclopramide and domperidone is that the latter does not cross the blood brain barrier. Therefore, adverse CNS effects are not as much of a problem in horses compared to metoclopramaide. There have been studies to investigate the use of domperidone for use in horses to treat fescue toxicity and agalactia. Fescue toxicosis is caused by a fungus that produces a toxin that induces reproductive problems in horses. The action of domperidone to increase lactation is through the stimulation of prolactin. Although not currently registered for use by the FDA, the equine formulation of domperidone is called *Equidone oral gel* (11%) for prevention and treatment of fescue toxicosis and related agalactia in periparturient mares. It is to be administered for 10 days prior to foaling. The dose administered to horses is 1.1 mg/kg, daily PO, starting 10 days before the scheduled foaling date. (This dose is equivalent to 5 ml per 500 kg [5 ml per horse], daily, PO of the 11% oral gel). Administration should continue until foaling. If there is not adequate milk production after foaling, continue for 5 additional days. Because of drug interactions, do not administer with stomach antacids such as omeprazole, cimetidine, or antacids.

OXYTOCIN

Structure. Oxytocin is a cyclic nonapeptide that is structurally similar to vasopressin. It is synthesized as a large precursor molecule in cell bodies of the paraventricular nucleus (PVN) in the hypothalamus. It is packaged as an oxytocin-neurophysin complex and secreted from nerve endings that terminate primarily in the posterior pituitary gland. Stimuli for oxytocin secretion include sensory stimuli arising from the cervix and vagina and from suckling of the mammary gland. Oxytocin is under tonic inhibition by GABAergic inhibitory transmission in the magnocellular neurons in the hypothalamus. Disinhibition of such control results in rapid firing of oxytocin-containing neurons, leading to oxytocin release.

Functions. The two principal targets of oxytocin are uterus and mammary gland:

- *Uterus.* Oxytocin stimulates both the frequency and force of uterine (myometrial smooth muscle) contraction. These effects are highly dependent on estrogen, and the immature uterus is quite resistant to the effects of oxytocin. Progesterone antagonizes the stimulant effect of oxytocin, and the decline in progesterone seen in late pregnancy may play an important role in the normal initiation of parturition. Oxytocin is also found in birds, fish, and reptiles and in these species, its effects are mostly osmoregulatory (antidiuretic hormone or vasopressinlike).
- *Mammary gland.* Oxytocin plays an important physiological role in milk ejection. It induces contraction of smooth muscle, most importantly of the myoepithelial cells of the mammary gland, which results in milk ejection. Suckling is the main stimulus that causes oxytocin secretion (Goodman and Grosvenor 1983).

Mechanism of Action. Oxytocin acts via specific G protein-coupled membrane receptors, which upon activation lead to generation of inositol triphosphate (IP_3) from phosphoinositide hydrolysis. IP_3 mobilizes intracellular Ca^{2+} and consequently causes depolarization-contraction of smooth muscle tissues containing oxytocin receptors.

Clinical Uses. Oxytocin (Pitocin®, Syntocinon®, or generic ceterinary formulations—e.g., Oxoject, Vetus Pharmaceuticals) is primarily used in 1) labor induction, 2) milk letdown (Jeffcott and Rossdale 1977), and 3) to aid in the treatment of mastitis in dairy cows caused by *Escherichia coli.* Oxytocin, originally extracted from animal posterior pituitaries, is now chemically synthesized. The dosage of oxytocin is listed in Table 28.2.

Induction of Labor. Oxytocin is widely used in small, large, and exotic animal practice to assist parturition (uterine inertia), to induce early or timed parturition, and to encourage postpartum uterine involution and emptying. To induce labor, it is administered intramuscularly or intravenously. Oxytocin is used for uterine prolapse in dogs and cats.

Milk Letdown. Oxytocin is used to stimulate milk letdown in bitches. Oxytocin spray is used intranasally to stimulate milk letdown, 5–10 min before nursing. In dairy cattle, treatment of *E. coli* mastitis involves supportive therapy, including stripping of the affected quarters. Administration of oxytocin may aid in the treatment by producing contraction of the affected quarter to facilitate stripping.

Persistent Endometritis. Oxytocin is a treatment for mating-induced persistent endometritis in the mare; it aids myometrial contractions to clear the uterus of debris following mating.

Side Effects. Toxicity is uncommon with oxytocin. Overdose or repeated dosing can lead to painful contractions and even uterine rupture and fetal death.

PROSTAGLANDIN ANALOGS

Dinoprost, Prostaglandin $F_{2\alpha}$ ($PGF_{2\alpha}$). $PGF_{2\alpha}$ is a luteolytic agent produced by the endometrium in farm animals, where it is released in late diestrus in the cycling animal and near term in the pregnant animal (Kindahl et al. 1981). Dinoprost is the accepted name for the commercial form of this compound known by several brand names (e.g., ProstaMate, Lutalyse, In-Sync), but many veterinarians and reference sources refer to it as $PGF_{2\alpha}$. The two names are interchangeable when referring to the commercial compounds. $PGF_{2\alpha}$ mediates a decrease in circulating progesterone via luteolysis (corpus luteum regression) and decreased placental progesterone production. $PGF_{2\alpha}$ acts via activation of G protein-coupled receptor linked to IP_3-Ca^{2+}–protein kinase C pathway, which leads to decreased steroidogenesis and luteolysis. There are several prostaglandin analogs (see Tables 28.1 and 28.2) that are widely used to regulate estrous cycles, to induce abortion, and to induce parturition in animals (Schultz and Copeland 1981).

Clinical Uses

Estrus Synchronization. Dinoprost ($PGF_{2\alpha}$) and its analogs are used for estrus synchronization. It will decrease estrous cycle length and thereby hasten the onset of estrus. Used strategically, in most large animal species except the pig, $PGF_{2\alpha}$, alone or in conjunction with progesterone/progestin treatment withdrawal (refer to section on Progestins) can be used. It can also be used in conjunction with GnRH for timed AI or ET (see Gonadorelin).

Abortion and Parturition. Dinoprost ($PGF_{2\alpha}$) is used to induce abortion and parturition in the bitch (Romagnoli et al. 1991). $PGF_{2\alpha}$ administered at a dose of at least 250 micrograms/kg twice daily subcutaneously for at least 4 days starting no earlier than day 5 of cytologic diestrus induces luteolysis and pregnancy termination in the mated bitch. The resulting shortening of the luteal phase is associated with a shortening of the interestrous interval by 1 to 4 months. Bitches treated with PGF show emesis, diarrhea, and panting within 5 minutes and transient hypothermia, which lasts 2 to 3 hours, but generally have no further reaction. Bitches with cardiac or respiratory dysfunctions are not considered safe patients for early pregnancy termination with PGF because of the cardiovascular effects of this drug.

Uterine Contractions. In the cow, dinoprost ($PGF_{2\alpha}$) is used to stimulate uterine contractions to facilitate placental delivery at birth. It is also used to induce abortion in first 100 days of gestation.

Mating-Induced Persistent Endometritis. In the mare, dinoprost ($PGF_{2\alpha}$) can be used to treat mating-induced persistent endometritis (but *not* after 2 days following ovulation, since it may interfere with normal corpus luteum development/function)—also see "Oxytocin," above.

Uterine Infections. In the bitch, dinoprost ($PGF_{2\alpha}$) is used to treat uterine infections via luteolytic and ecbolic effects. It has been administered to dogs for treatment of open pyometra. Extreme care must be used. If the cervix is not open at the time of administration, there is a risk of uterine rupture.

Inducing Parturition. In pigs, dinoprost is used to induce parturition when given within 3 days of farrowing.

Adverse Reactions. $PGF_{2\alpha}$ causes increased smooth muscle tone, resulting in diarrhea, abdominal discomfort, bronchoconstriction, and increase in blood pressure. In small animals, other side effects include vomiting. Induction of abortion may cause retained placenta.

Dinoprost should not be administered intravenously. It should never be administered to pregnant animals, unless abortion is a desired outcome.

Veterinarians and their assistants should use caution when handling this drug. It should not be handled by pregnant women. Absorption through the skin is possible. People with respiratory problems also should not handle dinoprost.

Available Sources and Doses. Dinoprost is available in 5 mg/ml solution for injection (e.g., ProstaMate, Lutalyse, In-Sync). It has been administered at the following dose rates: dogs with pyometra, 0.1–0.2 mg/kg once daily for 5 days SQ; for inducing abortion in dogs, 0.025–0.05 mg (25–50 mcg)/kg q12h IM; in cats for treating pyometra, 0.1–0.25 mg/kg once daily for 5 days

SQ; to induce abortion in cats, 0.5–1 mg/kg IM for 2 injections.

In cattle, it is used to induce abortion at a dose of 25 mg total dosage, administered once IM; to produce estrous synchronization, 25 mg once IM or twice at 10–12 day intervals; to treat pyometra in cattle, 25 mg IM administered once. In pigs, induction of parturition is accomplished by 10 mg administered once IM. Parturition occurs within 30 hours.

In horses for estrous synchronization, dosage is 1 mg/100 pounds (1 mg/45 kg) IM or 1–2 ml administered once IM. Mares should return to estrous within 2–4 days and ovulate 8–12 days after treatment.

ESTROGENS AND PROGESTERONE

A wide range of steroid hormonal treatment programs have been developed to regulate or induce estrous cycles in small and large animals for breeding purposes. Programs structured to provide increased levels of progesterone, estradiol, and related steroids at the appropriate times leading to ovulation and pregnancy have been commonly used in theriogenology (Day 2004). The three distinct classes of reproductive steroid hormones (estrogens, progesterone, and androgens) are discussed below, including their general mechanism of action, pharmaceutical preparations, and therapeutic applications in veterinary medicine.

MECHANISM OF STEROID ACTION. The mechanism of action of steroid hormones (estrogens, progestins, and androgens) involves binding to intracellular steroid receptors, which mediate most biological actions of steroids. These steroid receptors are located *inside* the cell, in the nucleus or cytoplasm. Steroid hormones diffuse readily across the cell membrane and bind to intracellular receptors in the cytoplasm. The hormone-receptor complex interacts directly and specifically to sites on the DNA (in the nucleus) called *hormone response elements (HRE),* and act as transcription factors to activate or inhibit "gene expression" (*transcription*) of the nearby gene. The resulting mRNA is translated into a specific protein and brings about a change in the metabolism or other function of the cell. In contrast to hormones acting via membrane receptors that produce effects rapidly within few minutes or less, the biological effects of steroid hormones generally take longer to occur (hours to days) because of the complex signaling cascade.

A brief description of some important pharmacological steroidal agents used in veterinary practice is given in Table 28.2.

ESTROGENS. The major ovarian estrogen in females is estradiol. Other estrogens include estrone, and estriol, which are produced in other tissues. Estrogens are transported in the blood by binding to sex hormone–binding globulin (SHBG). Estradiol is active by the oral route for pharmacotherapy, but has low bioavailability because of high first-pass hepatic metabolism. Therefore, for some treatments injectable preparations are used. For oral administration, semisynthetic derivatives (ethinyl estradiol), synthetic estrogens (mestranol), or nonsteroidal derivatives (diethyl stilbosterol, DES) have been developed for clinical use.

Therapeutic Uses. Estrogen is essential for normal development of secondary sexual phenotype and reproductive behavior in females. Estrogen modifies serum protein levels and reduces bone resorption. It is also an effective feedback suppressor of pituitary LH and FSH secretion. Estrogens are useful in the treatment of the following conditions: hypogonadism, postmenopausal symptoms (humans), oral contraceptives (humans), and carcinoma of prostate. DES was used in the 1940s and 1950s to treat pregnant women with a history of spontaneous abortion. Because of a link to cancer in the offspring of treated women, its use was discontinued.

Toxicity. The most common adverse effects in humans associated with chronic estrogen usage include breast cancer, endometrial hyperplasia, breakthrough bleeding, and uterine carcinoma.

Veterinary Uses. Estrogens are not widely used in veterinary medicine, especially in food animals, due to the concerns about drug residues in meat for human consumption. The following sections describe clinical uses and estrogen preparations that have been used in veterinary medicine.

Uterine Infection and Uterine Involution. *Estradiol benzoate* or other derivatives have been suggested for the treatment of the postpartum cow to decrease uterine infection and to hasten uterine involution.

Estrus Synchronization. *Estradiol valerate* is a component of *Syncro-Mate B*, which is a treatment for estrus synchronization in heifers and postpartum cows (SMB is not available in the U.S., see below).

Metritis in Cattle, Parturition Induction in Horses. *Estradiol cypionate* (ECP) is a semisynthetic form of esterified estradiol. It has been used to treat metritis in cattle to enhance epithelial cornification and defense mechanisms. In horses, it was used to facilitate induction of parturition.

In dogs, it was given within 48 hours of mating (mismating) to terminate pregnancy (0.02 mg/kg IM as a single dose). However, the frequent adverse effects of ECP injection in dogs have decreased this use. A single dose, even within the recommended dose range, has caused severe bone marrow depression in dogs. There is also a risk of pyometra developing in dogs. Commercial forms of ECP have been withdrawn from the market.

Urinary Incontinence and Perianal Gland Adenoma in Dogs. *Diethylstilbestrol* (DES, Stilboestrol®) is a nonsteroidal estrogenic agent used in the management of estrogen-responsive urinary incontinence and perianal gland adenoma in dogs. Commercial forms have been withdrawn from the market. Compounded formulations are still available from some pharmacies. It was once used as an anabolic agent in cattle. It improved growth rate and efficiency in feedlot cattle. However, because it has been identified as a potential carcinogen, it is prohibited from use in food-producing animals by federal regulation. (See Chapter 57 for a discussion on federal regulations that govern use of drugs in food-producing animals.)

PROGESTINS. Progesterone is the major progestin in humans and animals. Progesterone is rapidly metabolized in the liver and therefore has a very low bioavailability and a short half-life. Synthetic progestins (allyl-trenbolone—Altrenogest = Regumate®; melengestrol acetate, MGA) are widely used in veterinary practice to induce long-lasting ovarian suppression and synchronization of the estrous cycle following progestin withdrawal in small and large animals. Progestins act on progesterone receptors in the hypothalamus/pituitary, increasing the negative feedback and decreasing FSH and LH output. The withdrawal of progestin therapy initiates a new estrous cycle and ovulation.

The following sections discuss preparations of natural progesterone or synthetic progestins that are widely used in veterinary medicine.

Altrenogest. Altrenogest (Regumate®), also known as *allyl-trenbolone*, is a synthetic, orally active progestin indicated for controlling the estrous cycle of the mare and pig (see Fig. 28.1).

Altrenogest is indicated to suppress estrus in mares to allow a more predictable occurrence of estrus following withdrawal of the drug (Davis et al. 1985; Shimatsu et al. 2004). Altrenogest (0.044 mg/kg, PO) is recommended for 15 days to suppress estrus and allow for a predictable occurrence of estrus. Suppression of estrus will encourage regular cycles following winter anestrus, facilitate scheduled breeding, and help manage mares exhibiting prolonged estrus. Ovulation occurs 9–11 days after altrenogest therapy. Use of $PGF_{2\alpha}$ immediately following altrenogest withdrawal will induce estrus. Low-dose altrenogest can be used in pregnancy to minimize the abortion in mares, but high doses may cause fetal abnormalities. Generally, altrenogest may be helpful to control the equine estrous cycle, but it has not always been able to exert predictable control over the estrous cycle of the mare (Lofstedt and Patel 1989).

Altrenogest can also be used in synchronizing estrus in the gilt (Davis et al 1985). Swine producers are interested in synchronizing estrus in gilts to reduce the number of replacement gilts and for optimizing breeding by AI. Altrenogest is given to gilts at 15–20 mg daily for 18 days, which results in 95% expression of estrus 4–7 days after Altrenogest withdrawal.

Contraindications. Altrenogest is contraindicated in pregnant mares because higher doses may cause fetal abnormalities.

Syncro-Mate B. Syncro-Mate B (SMB) is a progesterone-estrogen combination product for estrous synchronization in cattle (Gary et al. 1998; Williams 2002). However, SMB is not available in the U.S. but may still be available in other countries. The objective of a SMB-based synchronization program is to breed a high percentage of the females in a given group of heifers or cows in a short period, using either artificial insemination or natural service (bulls). SMB treatment is composed of an ear implant containing

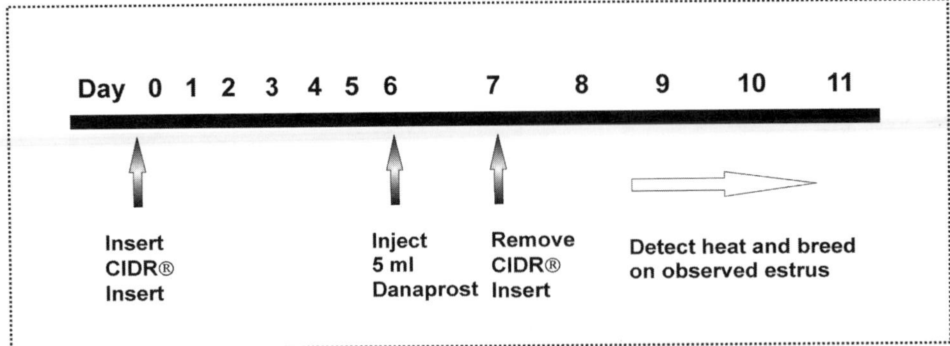

FIG 28.2 Eazi-Breed™ CIDR protocol for synchronization of estrus in cattle. The Eazi-Breed CIDR for cattle consists of 1.38 g progesterone releasing device for vaginal insertion in breeding programs.

the progestin norgestomet (6 mg) and an injectable solution of norgestomet (3 mg) and estradiol valerate (5 mg). The initial norgestomet/progestogen implant has an inhibitory effect on the release of LH and FSH necessary for estrous cycles to continue. Norgestomet inhibits LH secretion and thereby inhibits corpus luteum function. The estradiol valerate causes a breakdown of the corpus luteum by stimulating $PGF_{2\alpha}$ release. This treatment synchronizes estrus in heifers and postpartum cows. Animals are given an ear implant for 9 days, and norgestomet and estradiol valerate are injected intramuscularly at the time of implantation. An SMB program can also be used in cattle and goats.

Melengestrol Acetate (MGA). Melengestrol acetate is a progestin-based, feed-additive system to synchronize estrous in cattle. This product is indicated for use in heat suppression in feedlot steers and has been used with increased frequency to synchronize breeding females. MGA can be fed at a rate of 0.5 mg per head per day to suppress estrus. Once MGA is removed from the feed, females can be expected to begin cycling within a few days, normally two to three. Briefly, the MGA program consists of feeding MGA at the prescribed level in a feed product the cattle will consume, once daily for 11 to 14 days. Then, after removal of the MGA from the feed, estrus follows after 48 to 72 hours. At this point, breeding can begin with bulls or artificial insemination. MGA is a simple treatment, but is generally less efficient than other estrous synchronization products.

CIDR®—Progesterone-Containing Controlled Internal Drug Release Intravaginal Device. Several CIDR (Controlled Internal Drug Release) intravaginal progesterone-releasing devices are marketed for cattle (Eazi-Breed™), sheep (CIDR-S™), and goats (CIDR-G™). The main objective of these products is synchronization of estrus to improve the timing and efficiency of breeding programs (Yavas and Walton 2000). The Eazi-Breed CIDR contains 1.38 g progesterone in silicon molded over a nylon spine. These inserts are to be administered intravaginally, one per animal, in dairy heifers for breeding. It releases progesterone during the 7-day treatment period (see Fig. 28.2). To induce definitive synchronization, an injection of a prostaglandin dinoprost tromethamine (Lutalyse®) is given to all heifers 1 day before insert removal. Removal of the insert on treatment day 7 results in a decline in plasma progesterone, triggering estrus within 3 days.

SPECIFIC REPRODUCTIVE CONDITIONS

SUPEROVULATION. Some cattle may be induced to ovulate multiple follicles (superovulation) so that embryos can be transferred to recipient animals to increase the number of progeny. In cattle, superovulation results in about 10 ovulations, compared to the normal, single ovulation. Superovulation, on the average, results in about 6 usable embryos. The ideal response is 5–12 embryos from one-third of the donors. The donor superovulation injection program is begun between day 9 and 14 of the estrous cycle, with FSH given over 4 days and $PGF_{2\alpha}$ given on days 3 and 4. In case of goats and sheep, the drug regime for superovulation depends upon the reproductive status. During the breeding season, $PGF_{2\alpha}$ is used to mediate luteolysis, and gonadotropins are given to increase the ovulatory rate. The anestrous animal is given a progestin followed by gonadotropin treatment. Dairy goats were superovulated successfully during the breeding season by placement of an intravaginal sponge (medroxyprogesterone; MAP, 60 mg) for 11 days, 125 μg cloprostenol IM on days 1 and 9 of sponge treatment, and twice-daily injections of FSH-P (2.5 mg) IM for 3 days beginning on day 9 of sponge treatment (Thompson 2001).

PSEUDOPREGNANCY. For treatment of a queen (female cat) in heat, animals may be treated with GnRH or hCG. These animals are induced ovulators and in the absence of the mating stimulus, ovulation and corpus luteum formation must be induced with GnRH or hCG, as described above, to prevent repeated estrus periods every 3–5 days. In some rodents (rats and mice), a state of pseudopregnancy associated with prolonged high serum progesterone levels can be induced by sequential administration of eCG and hCG elevated progesterone (Reddy et al. 2001). This sequential regimen may be useful in transgenic mice breeding programs.

PARTURITION. Parturition may be induced in cattle by glucocorticoids and $PGF_{2\alpha}$. The reasons for induced parturition include 1) allowing more time postpartum before the next breeding, 2) attempting to reduce calf size and therefore dystocia, 3) preventing excessive udder edema in dairy cattle, and 4) taking advantage of available forage for milk production. Dexamethasone (20–30 mg) or flumethasone (8–10 mg) IM is 80–90% effective in parturition induction, with calving occurring 24–72 hours posttreatment. Calving may be induced with $PGF_{2\alpha}$ (25–30 mg) or cloprostenol (500 μg) IM, with results similar to that found with short-acting glucocorticoids. The interval from injection to calving is 24–72 hours. A combination of treatments with dexamethasone and cloprostenol has resulted in a shorter interval from treatment to delivery and a greater percentage induced compared to either drug alone or two injections of cloprostenol. Induced farrowing in the pig is a practical management aid to allow for increased supervision of the event and to improve utilization of labor. The optimal farrowing response to $PGF_{2\alpha}$ is achieved by administration within 2 days of normal delivery for a herd. Oxytocin is the most widely used drug for induction of parturition in the mare. Delivery is usually complete within 90 minutes of administering oxytocin but may occur as soon as 10 minutes. Oxytocin may be delivered via several schemes. One method involves the administration of 60–100 U oxytocin IM. Second-stage labor is generally experienced within 30–60 minutes, with delivery complete within 45–90 minutes.

TERMINATION OF PREGNANCY (ABORTION). Pregnancy termination is one of the most common "reproductive" requests from dog and cat owners because of mismating or other reasons. Pharmacological agents are available that can prevent or terminate pregnancy (Eilts 2002). Drugs that can be given during estrus to prevent pregnancy include estrogens and tamoxifen. A pregnancy examination should be performed before any drug is given to terminate pregnancy. If a dog is known to be pregnant, multiple doses of natural or synthetic prostaglandins can be used throughout pregnancy, whereas multiple doses of inhibitors of prolactin secretion (cabergoline, bromocriptine, metergoline) or dexamethasone can be used in the second half of pregnancy. Combined protocols of prostaglandin and prolactin inhibitors are also effective at terminating pregnancy. Progesterone blockers such as mifepristone and aglepristone are effective, but very expensive. Other drugs, such as the isoquinolones and progesterone synthesis inhibitor epostane are available outside of the United States and appear to be very effective at terminating pregnancy. A discussion of the approaches to terminating pregnancy in dogs and cats was discussed in the review by Concannon and Meyers-Wallen (1991).

CRYPTORCHIDISM. Cryptorchidism (dog) is the failure of one or both testes to be present in the scrotum by 6–8 weeks of age. The testes migrate from the caudal pole of the kidney to the scrotum via guidance from the gubernaculum testis. At birth, the testes in the dog are usually within the abdomen near the internal inguinal ring. The testes move through the inguinal canal and are in the scrotum by 10–14 days of age. Because this condition has a genetic basis, dogs with this condition should not be used for breeding purposes. The most common method of treatment is serial injections of hCG. Dogs younger than 16 weeks of age are the best candidates. The IM injection of 100–1,000 IU hCG 4 times in a 2-week period is expected to result in descent in the majority of dogs. However, cryptorchidism in cattle, sheep, and goats is typically not treated and they are not encouraged to enter the genetic pool.

ANDROGENS

TESTOSTERONE. Testosterone is the principal circulating androgen in males. It is secreted by the Leydig cells of the testes in response to LH from the pituitary gland. Testosterone regulates the male reproductive system by binding to the androgen receptors present especially in reproductive tissue, muscle, and fat. It is particularly responsible for normal male sexual differentiation. Some physiological effects of testosterone are mediated by conversion to dihydrotestosterone, a more potent androgen than testosterone (see Fig. 28.3). Testosterone also is converted to estradiol. Several analogs of testosterone that possess greater *anabolic* (protein building) than *androgenic* (male sexual) effects have been synthesized. They are called *anabolic steroids*. These include *nandrolone, stanazolol, oxymethalone,* and others. The major indication for anabolic steroids is in equine medicine to increase athletic performance. Anabolic steroids increase muscle size and strength, and increase RBC production. Excretion of urea nitrogen is reduced ("positive nitrogen balance").

ANABOLIC STEROIDS. Anabolic steroids are controlled substances that predominantly produce greater anabolic than androgenic effects, and, as described below, are used in equine practice to increase athletic performance. In addition, these agents have been used in the treatment of aplastic anemia (dogs and cats), myeloproliferative disease, and lymphoma accompanied by nonregenerative anemia. They increase myelopoiesis, stimulate the production of erythropoietin, and increase production of erythrocytes. They stimulate appetite, promote a positive nitrogen balance and muscle calcium levels (Brower 1993). Several weeks to months may be required for a positive response to be seen, and even with this prolonged therapy only one-third of dogs and cats show a positive erythropoietic response to anabolic steroids. Anabolic steroids bind to androgen receptors present especially in reproductive tissue, muscle, and fat. The ratio of anabolic ("bodybuilding") effects to androgenic ("virilizing") effects may differ among the members of the class, but in practice all agents possess both properties to some degree (see Fig. 28.3).

Anabolic steroid drugs can be classified into two groups:

1. Alkylated agents: Stanazolol
    - Fluoxymesterone
    - Oxymethalone
    - Norethandrolone
2. Nonalkylated agents: Nandrolone
    - Methenolone

Stanozolol. Stanozolol (Winstrol-V®) is an anabolic steroid with strong anabolic and weak androgenic activity. It is potentially useful as an adjunct to the management of catabolic disease states (Cowan 1997). It has been recommended to stimulate erythropoiesis, arouse appetite, and promote weight gain, and increase strength and vitality. However, the efficacy of stanozolol is conflicting and requires 3–6-month treatment before a positive change can be seen. Stanozolol is most commonly used in horses to enhance athletic performance.

Adverse Effects. Stanozolol may produce weight gain, sodium and water retention, and exacerbate azotemia. It may promote hypercalcemia, hyperphosphatemia, and hyperkalemia. Stanozolol is potentially hepatotoxic and has been associated with hepatopathy in cats. When cats

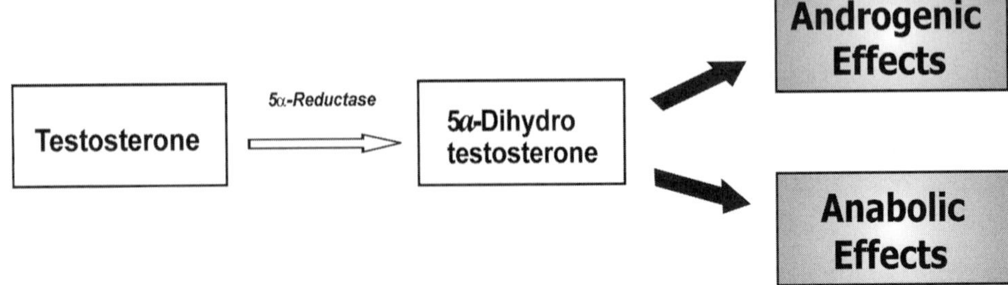

FIG 28.3 Metabolism and major effects of testosterone. Testosterone is converted in several organs to dihydrotestosterone (DHT), which is the active hormone in those tissues. Testosterone and DHT produce both androgenic and anabolic actions.

were treated with 25 mg IM on the first day, and then 2 mg orally every 12 hours for 4 weeks, most developed clinical adverse reactions and elevated liver enzymes (Harkin et al 2000).

Contraindication. Stanozolol and all other anabolic steroids are contraindicated in dogs with benign prostatic hypertrophy. Anabolic steroids may produce carcinogenicity and teratogenicity.

Nandrolone. Nandrolone laurate (Nandrabolin, also referred to as *19-nortestosterone*) is a potent synthetic anabolic androgenic steroid. Nandrolone is useful in the treatment of certain rare forms of aplastic anemia, which are or may be responsive to anabolic androgens. It has been used in some cases to counteract catabolic states, for example, after major trauma or strenuous physical exercise (Hyyppa 2001). Side effects and other properties are similar to stanozolol.

Boldenone Undecylenate. Boldenone (Equipoise) is a steroid ester anabolic agent. It is used, primarily in horses, to improve nitrogen balance, reduce overexertion associated with exercise, and improve training. It may also improve appetite and improve weight gain when used with a well-balanced diet. Boldenone is a long-lasting agent and effects may persist for 6 weeks after an intramuscular injection.

BENIGN PROSTATIC HYPERTROPHY. Benign prostatic hypertrophy (BPH) is a spontaneous and age-related disorder of intact male dogs. It occurs in more than 80% of male dogs over 5 years of age. BPH is associated with clinical signs of sanguineous prostatic fluid, constipation, and dysuria. BPH is linked to the testosterone's androgenic activity (enlargement of prostate gland). BPH can be identified by signs such as increased frequency of urination, constipation or blood in urine. BPH often occurs concurrently with prostatic infection, abscessation, cysts and neoplasia in the intact dog. The treatment of choice is castration or antiandrogenic agents such as finasteride, a 5α-reductase inhibitor, or flutamide, an androgen receptor antagonist (Fig. 28.4) (Iguer-Ouada and Verstegen 1997; Johnston 2000).

FINASTERIDE. Finasteride (Proscar®) is an irreversible 5α-reductase inhibitor that blocks the conversion of testosterone to 5α-dihydrotestosterone, a potent androgen receptor agonist (see Fig. 28.4). Testosterone itself interacts weakly with androgen receptors. Therefore, most of the

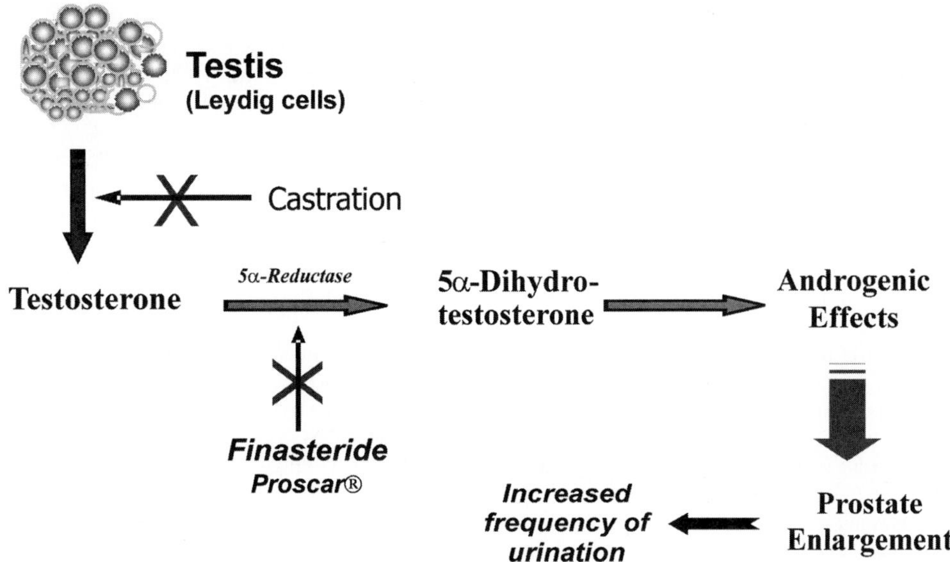

FIG 28.4 Treatment options for benign prostatic hypertrophy. Reduction of androgen effects is an important therapeutic goal for benign prostatic hypertrophy (BPH). Inhibition of dihydrotestosterone produced by finasteride is a key pharmacotherapy in dogs affected by BPH.

biological effects of testosterone have been attributed to the synthesis of endogenous 5α-dihydrotestosterone. In the prostate gland, 5α-dihydrotestosterone has been implicated to cause benign prostatic hypertrophy.

Uses. Finasteride is the drug of choice for benign prostatic hypertrophy in dogs. Finasteride induces prostatic involution by apoptosis in dogs with spontaneous benign prostatic hypertrophy (Sirinarumitr et al. 2002). Finasteride has been highly effective in benign prostatic hypertrophy cases. Finasteride has not proven valuable in prostatic carcinoma.

Dose. Finasteride (0.1 to 0.5 mg/kg, PO once daily) therapy for 16 weeks may reduce prostate size in canine prostatic hypertrophy.

Toxicity. The major potential side effect is impotence. Finasteride, however, did not affect semen quality or serum testosterone concentrations in experimental studies in dogs.

REFERENCES

Al-Katanani YM, Drost M, Monson RL. Pregnancy rates following timed embryo transfer with fresh or vitrified in vitro produced embryos in lactating dairy cows under heat stress conditions. Theriogenology. 2002;58:171–182.

Brower KJ. Anabolic steroids. Psychiatr Clin North Am. 1993;16(1): 97–103.

Concannon PW, Meyers-Wallen VN. Current and proposed methods for contraception and termination of pregnancy in dogs and cats. J Am Vet Med Assoc. 1991;198:1214–1225.

Cowan LA, McLaughlin R, Toll PW, Brown SA, Moore TI, Butine MD, Milliken G. Effect of stanozolol on body composition, nitrogen balance, and food consumption in castrated dogs with chronic renal failure. J Am Vet Med Assoc. 1997;211(6):719–722.

Davis DL, Stevenson JS, Schmidt WE. Scheduled breeding of gilts after estrous synchronization with altrenogest. J Anim Sci. 1985;60(3): 599–602.

Day ML. Hormonal induction of estrous cycles in anestrous Bos taurus beef cows. Anim Reprod Sci. 2004;82–83:487–494.

Eilts BE. Pregnancy termination in the bitch and queen. Clin Tech Small Anim Pract. 2002;17(3):116–123.

Farin PW, Estill CT. Infertility due to abnormalities of the ovaries in cattle. Vet Clin North Am Food Anim Pract. 1993;9(2):291–308.

Geary TW, Whittier JC, Downing ER, LeFever DG, Silcox RW, Holland MD, Nett TM, Niswender GD. Pregnancy rates of postpartum beef cows that were synchronized using Syncro-Mate-B or the Ovsynch protocol. J Anim Sci. 1998;76(6):1523–1527.

Goodman GT, Grosvenor CE. Neuroendocrine control of the milk ejection reflex. J Dairy Sci. 1983;66(10):2226–2235.

Harkin KR, Cowan LA, Andrews GA, Basaraba RJ, Fischer JR, DeBowes LJ, Roush JK, Guglielmino JL, Kirk CA. Hepatotoxicity of stanozolol in cats. J Am Vet Med Assoc. 2000;217:681–684.

Hasler JF. The current status and future of commercial embryo transfer in cattle. Anim Reprod Sci. 2002;79:245–264.

Hyyppa S. Effects of nandrolone treatment on recovery in horses after strenuous physical exercise. Vet Med A Physiol Pathol Clin Med. 2001;48(6):343–352.

Iguer-Ouada M, Verstegen JP. Effect of finasteride (Proscar MSD) on seminal composition, prostate function and fertility in male dogs. J Reprod Fertil Suppl. 1997;51:139–149.

Jeffcott LB, Rossdale PD. A critical review of current methods for induction of parturition in the mare. Equine Vet J. 1977;9(4):208–215.

Johnston SD, Kamolpatana K, Root-Kustritz MV, Johnston GR. Prostatic disorders in the dog. Anim Reprod Sci. 2000;60:405–415.

Kindahl H, Lindell JO, Edqvist LE. Release of prostaglandin F2 alpha during the oestrous cycle. Acta Vet Scand Suppl. 1981;77:143–158.

Kooistra HS, Okkens AC. Secretion of prolactin and growth hormone in relation to ovarian activity in the dog. Reprod Domest Anim. 2001;36(3–4):115–119.

Lofstedt RM, Patel JH. Evaluation of the ability of altrenogest to control the equine estrous cycle. J Am Vet Med Assoc. 1989;194(3): 361–364.

Lucy MC, McDougall S, Nation DP. The use of hormonal treatments to improve the reproductive performance of lactating dairy cows in feedlot or pasture-based management systems. Anim Reprod Sci. 2004;82–83:495–512.

Peters AR. Veterinary clinical application of GnRH-questions of efficacy. Anim Reprod Sci. 2005;88(1–2):155–167.

Reddy DS, Kim H-Y, Rogawski MA. Neurosteroid withdrawal model of perimenstrual catamenial epilepsy. Epilepsia. 2001;42(3):328–336.

Romagnoli SE, Cela M, Camillo F. Use of prostaglandin F2 alpha for early pregnancy termination in the mismated bitch. Vet Clin North Am Small Anim Pract. 1991;21(3):487–499.

Samper JC. Management and fertility of mares bred with frozen semen. Anim Reprod Sci. 2001;68(3–4):219–228.

Schultz RH, Copeland DD. Induction of abortion using prostaglandins. Acta Vet Scand Suppl. 1981;77:353–361.

Shelton JN. Reproductive technology in animal production. Rev Sci Tech. 1990;9(3):825–845.

Shimatsu Y, Uchida M, Niki R, Imai H. Effects of a synthetic progestogen, altrenogest, on oestrus synchronisation and fertility in miniature pigs. Vet Rec. 2004;155(20):633–635.

Sirinarumitr K, Sirinarumitr T, Johnston SD, Sarkar DK, Root Kustritz MV. Finasteride-induced prostatic involution by apoptosis in dogs with benign prostatic hypertrophy. Am J Vet Res. 2002;63(4): 495–498.

Stout TA, Colenbrander B. Suppressing reproductive activity in horses using GnRH vaccines, antagonists or agonists. Anim Reprod Sci. 2004;82–83:633–643.

Thatcher WW, Moreira F, Santos JE, Mattos RC, Lopes FL, Pancarci SM, Risco CA. Effects of hormonal treatments on reproductive performance and embryo production. Theriogenology. 2001;55(1):75–89.

Thompson FN. Hormones affecting reproduction. In: H.R. Adams, ed. Veterinary Pharmacology and Therapeutics, 8th edition, Ames: Iowa State University Press, 2001; 612–625.

Wathes DC, Taylor VJ, Cheng Z, Mann GE. Follicle growth, corpus luteum function and their effects on embryo development in postpartum dairy cows. Reprod Suppl. 2003;61:219–237.

Williams SW, Stanko RL, Amstalden M, Williams GL. Comparison of three approaches for synchronization of ovulation for timed artificial insemination in Bos indicus-influenced cattle managed on the Texas gulf coast. J Anim Sci. 2002;80(5):1173–1178.

Wright PJ, Malmo J. Pharmacologic manipulation of fertility. Vet Clin North Am Food Anim Pract. 1992;8(1):57–89.

Yavas Y, Walton JS. Induction of ovulation in postpartum suckled beef cows: a review. Theriogenology. 2000;54(1):1–23.

Yoshimoto N, Shimoda K, Mori Y, Honda R, Okamura H, Ide Y, Nakashima T, Nakagata N, Torii R, Yoshikawa Y, Hayasaka I. Ovarian follicular development stimulated by leuprorelin acetate plus human menopausal gonadotropin in chimpanzees. J Med Primatol. 2005;34(2): 73–85.

CHAPTER 29

THYROID HORMONES AND ANTITHYROID DRUGS

DUNCAN C. FERGUSON

INTRODUCTION

HYPOTHYROIDISM. Hypothyroidism is the most common endocrinopathy of the dog, and is diagnosed with some frequency in the horse, but spontaneous hypothyroidism is rare in the cat and other domestic species. Less commonly, hypothyroidism can be caused by iodine deficiency or by the ingestion of goitrogenic substances in the environment or food; goitrogenic substances are compounds that interfere with thyroid hormone synthesis by the thyroid gland.

Clinical signs of hypothyroidism common to most species generally reflect the reduction in basal metabolic rate of the body and include lethargy, mental depression, weakness, inability to train and/or nonpruritic hair loss (Ferguson 1989a, 1993; Ferguson and Hoenig 1991b; Ferguson et al. 1992; Peterson and Ferguson 1990; Feldman and Nelson 2004a).

HYPERTHYROIDISM. Hyperthyroidism is now the most common endocrine disorder in the cat, and is only occasionally seen in other domestic species. Hyperthyroidism or thyrotoxicosis is caused by excessive concentrations of the circulating thyroid hormones, thyroxine (T_4) and triiodothyronine (T_3), most commonly the result of hyperplastic or benign adenomatous malignant thyroid glands in cats and adenocarcinomas in dogs. Hyperthyroidism occurs most frequently in middle-aged to geriatric cats and discussion of therapeutic agents will focus on those used in this species. The most common clinical signs associated with hyperthyroidism, which can be directly related to thyroid hormone excess are weight loss in spite of ravenous appetite, hyperactivity, polydipsia, polyuria, diarrhea, intermittent fever, vomiting and symptoms of cardiovascular disease such as tachycardia and dyspnea. Often the cats shed excessive amounts of hair or the coat may be matted. Rarely, hyperthyroid cats present in a way similar to what has been called "apathetic hyperthyroidism"; the cats are lethargic and often anorectic, perhaps representing an end-stage form of the disease (Feldman and Nelson 2004b; Ferguson and Hoenig 1991a; Peterson and Ferguson 1990).

THYROID PHYSIOLOGY

IODINE METABOLISM. Thyroid hormones are the only iodinated organic compounds in the body with the 2 major secretory products of the thyroid gland, thyroxine (L-T_4) and 3,5,3′-triiodothyronine (L-T_3) containing 65% and 59% iodine, respectively. The minimum iodine requirement of most animals is unknown, but the daily amount needed in the ration to prevent goiter in all animals is generally accepted to be 1 μg/kg body weight. The daily recommended amount of iodine in the dog is 15 μg/kg and while it has not been carefully studied in the cat, it is believed to be about 100 μg/cat/day. Commercial cat foods have been shown to be quite variable in the amount of iodide provided, probably a result of the variable amount of seafood used to create the diet. Indeed, dietary iodide has been shown to be inversely related to free T_4 concentrations (Tartellin and Ford 1994). Although true nutrient requirements for this micronutrient are not well established, most commercial dog and cat food preparations include at least three to five times this minimum requirement for iodine when fed in recommended amounts. As a result, iodine deficiency has become a rare condition in domestic animals. During pregnancy, the recommended minimum daily requirement for iodine is increased fourfold. Areas of iodine deficiency in North America include the Great Lakes region and eastern British Columbia (Belshaw et al. 1974; Kaptein et al. 1994; Peterson and Ferguson 1990).

Ingested iodine is converted to iodide in the gastrointestinal tract and absorbed into the circulation. The dog has plasma iodide concentrations of 5 to 10 μg/dl, which are 10 to 20 times the levels in human plasma. In the thyroid gland, iodide is concentrated or "trapped" by the sodium-iodide symporter (NIS), which utilizes the sodium gradient developed by the Na^+,K^+-ATPase to move iodide through the basolateral plasma membrane of the thyroid follicular cell. This results in intracellular iodide concentrations, which are 10 to 200 times that of serum. This process is stimulated by the interaction of thyrotropin (TSH) with G-protein coupled TSH receptors on the surface of the follicular cell leading to the stimulation of cAMP (see Fig. 29.1). The transcription of NIS is stimulated by TSH or cyclic AMP. NIS is also up-regulated directly by thyroidal mechanisms reacting to iodide insufficiency or blockade of iodide transport by compounds such as perchlorate. Other tissues, including the salivary glands, gastric mucosal cells, renal proximal tubule cells, placenta, ciliary body, choroid plexus, and mammary glands, can take up considerable amounts of radioiodide in a TSH-independent fashion.

Diagnostically, radioactive iodide or pertechnetate (TcO_4^-), which, unlike iodine, cannot be organified, can be used to assess the anion transport function (uptake) by the thyroid gland. Iodide trapping can be inhibited by other anions such as thiocyanate (SCN^-), NO_3^- and ClO_4^-. Thiocyanate is a metabolic product of some naturally occurring compounds in plants and may result in goitrogenic (antithyroid) activity of the plant. Domestic animals may also be exposed to thiocyanate produced as a by-product of cigarette smoke in a household environment. Oral administration of perchlorate following the administration of a tracer dose of radioiodine can be used to diagnose congenital defects in the thyroidal organification of iodide (perchlorate discharge test) (Greenspan 1994; Taurog 1971).

THYROID HORMONE SYNTHESIS. Thyroglobulin (Tg), an iodinated glycoprotein with a molecular weight of 660,000 daltons, serves as a synthesis and storage site

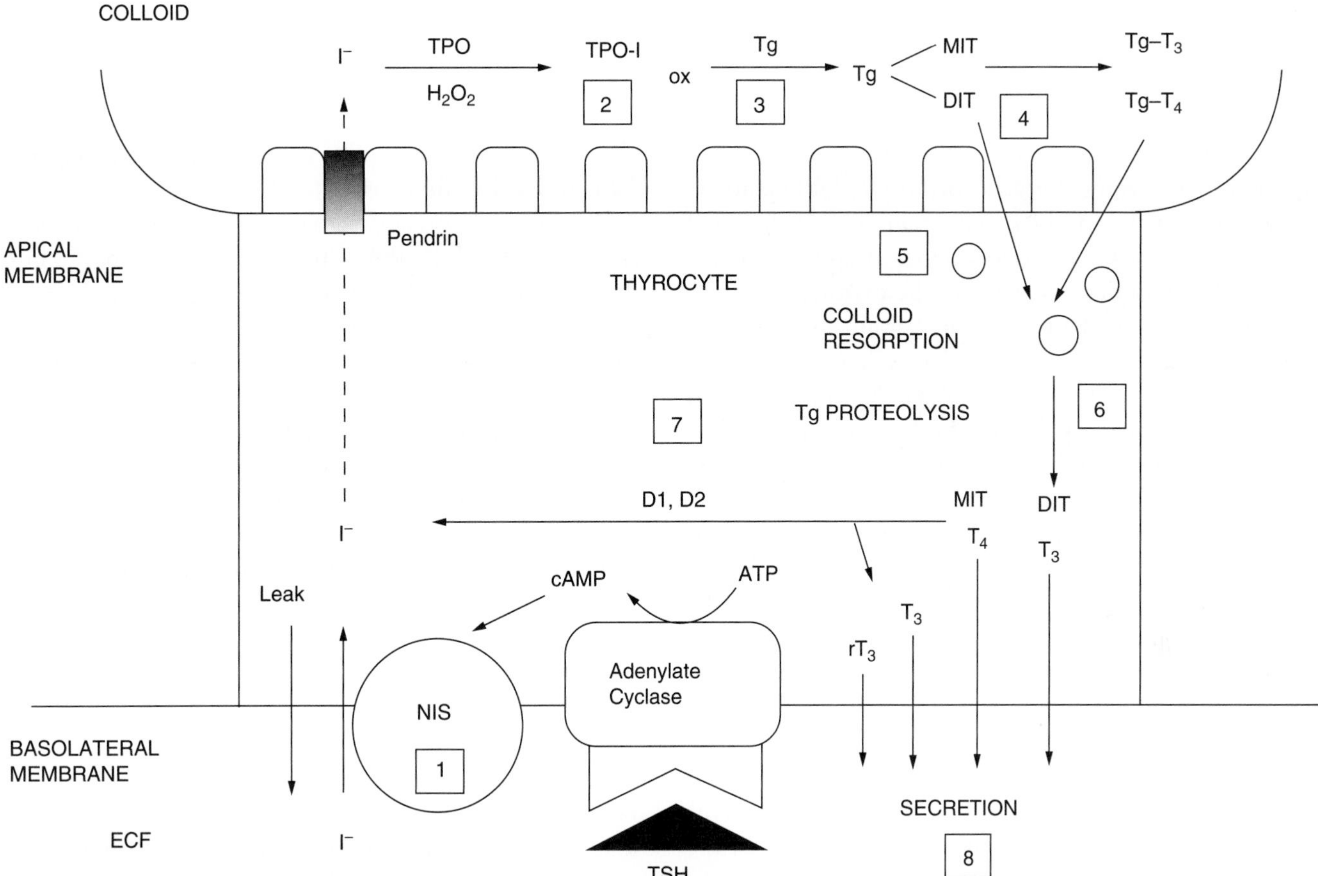

FIG 29.1 TSH-stimulated iodide uptake and organification by the thyrocyte. **Step 1:** Inorganic iodide (I^-) is actively translocated by the sodium-iodide symporter (NIS), using the Na+ gradient established by the Na+K+-ATPase. NIS is stimulated directly by the G protein-coupled TSH receptor, and is influenced by availability of iodide, being stimulated by iodide insufficiency and suppressed by excess iodide. After diffusing to the apical or brush border membrane, the pendrin protein carries it into the lumen of the colloid. **Steps 2 and 3—Oxidation and organification:** Iodide is oxidized by the thyroid peroxidase enzyme (TPO) (step 2) and added to a tyrosine residue of preformed thyroglobulin (Tg) (step 3) to form monoiodotyrosine (MIT) and diiodotyrosin (DIT). **Step 4—Coupling:** The MIT and DIT residues on Tg couple to form T_3, and two DIT residues couple to form T_4. Steps 2–4 are sensitive to thionamide antithyroid drugs like PTU or MMI. **Step 5—Colloid resorption:** Under the influence of TSH, follicular colloid–containing Tg is resorbed by the thyrocyte by pinocytosis. **Step 6—Tg proteolysis:** Thyroid hormones, MIT and DIT are released from Tg under the influence of TSH. **Step 7—Deiodination:** Also stimulated by TSH at the time of secretion, deiodinase enzymes (D1,D2) are stimulated, resulting in the removal of iodide and increasing the T_3/T_4 ratio in the secreted pool. **Step 8—Secretion:** T_4, T_3, and rT_3 are released into the bloodstream. (Figure modified from Peterson and Ferguson, 1990, Fig. 95-1.)

for thyroid hormone and its precursors in the thyroid follicle. After synthesis within the endoplasmic reticulum of the thyroid follicular cell, membrane vesicles containing noniodinated Tg fuse with the apical membrane and are released (by exocytosis) into the follicullar cell lumen where thyroglobulin is stored as colloid. Once inside the thyroid cell, iodide is transported to the follicular lumen by the protein pendrin, then oxidized by the enzyme thyroid peroxidase (TPO) to iodine (Fig. 29.1). Pendrin is an apical transmembrane protein that transports sulfate, chloride, iodide, and bicarbonate (Larsen et al. 2003). Iodide is then incorporated by the heme protein enzyme thyroid peroxidase (TPO), which, in the presence of hydrogen peroxide, adds iodide onto tyrosine residues of Tg in a process called *organification,* forming monoiodotyrosine (MIT) and diiodotyrosine (DIT). TPO also forms thyroxine (T_4) by coupling two DIT molecules, and 3,5,3′-triiodothyronine (T_3) by coupling one MIT molecule with one DIT molecule (Burrow et al. 1989; Greenspan 1994; Peterson and Ferguson 1990; Taurog 1991).

The reaction catalyzed by TPO is inhibited by the thionamide drugs propylthiouracil (PTU) and methimazole (MMI) and by high concentrations of iodide (*the Wolff-Chaikoff effect*). The intermediate product of peroxidation of iodide is either hypoiodous acid (HIO_2^-) or iodinium (I^+). The H_2O_2 required is generated by NADPH oxidase. In normal humans and rats, more than 90% of thyroidal radioiodine is organified to iodotyrosines and iodothyronines within minutes of entry into the thyroid.

When iodine intake is adequate, production of T_4 is favored. However, in iodine-deficient states and impending thyroid failure, the intrathyroidal synthesis of T_3 is preferred over that of T_4. By this autoregulation, the thyroid gland produces the most active thyroid hormone (T_3 is 3 to 10 times more potent than T_4) while using less iodide. Conversely, chronic iodine excess may lead to excessive storage of thyroidal hormone.

The Wolff-Chaikoff effect, another intrathyroidal regulatory mechanism, is key to understanding the potential acute antithyroid effect of large amounts of ingested iodide. Mediated via inhibition of the thyroid peroxidase (TPO) enzyme, iodide decreases the rate of its own relative and absolute organification. In humans, this effect is transient and "escape" is seen within several weeks. This inhibitory effect may be a mechanism through which the organism is protected from massive thyroid hormone release following a large dietary iodine load (Taurog 1991; Wolff 1989). Iodine has been shown to inhibit Ca^{++}- and NADPH-dependent H_2O_2-generating activity associated with NADPH oxidase, a mechanism characterized in dog, pig, and human thyroid glands. NADPH oxidase seems to be inhibited by iodinated compounds in vivo and probably is an enzyme involved in the Wolff-Chaikoff effect.

THYROID HORMONE SECRETION. Thyroid hormone secretion is initiated as the epithelial follicular cells take up thyroglobulin in colloid droplets by a process called *pinocytosis.* Simultaneously, lysosomes (containing proteases and hydrolytic enzymes) migrate from the basal region of the cell and fuse with the colloid droplets (see Fig 29.1). Degradation of thyroglobulin by the lysosomal proteolytic enzymes produces both the iodotyrosines (MIT and DIT) and iodothyronines (T_4 and T_3). Little of the released MIT and DIT enters the circulation because the iodine is removed from these compounds by a deiodinase enzyme (see Fig. 29.1). Some of this iodine is recycled internally for iodination of new tyrosine residues in thyroglobulin, but in carnivores, much iodine is released to the circulation (Belshaw et al. 1974; Kaptein et al. 1994). This inefficient thyroidal reutilization of iodine may help explain the high daily iodine requirements of the dog and cat compared to humans.

Proteolysis of Tg, as described above, liberates relatively large amounts of T_4, but only small quantities of T_3, into the cytosol. Enzymes present within the thyroid gland, however, can deiodinate T_4 to either T_3 or 3′,5′,3-T_3 (reverse T_3). As a result, although the T_4:T_3 ratio stored in the gland is 12:1 in the canine thyroid, the ratio of secreted products is 4:1. Production rates of the thyroid hormones in the dog have been estimated to be 8 μg/kg/day for T_4 and 0.8 to 1.5 μg/kg/day for T_3. In cats, T_4 production rates have been estimated to be 5.6 μg/kg/day, and 0.4 μg/kg/day for T_3. These production rates are greater than twice those for T_4 and greater than three times the rate for T_3 in humans (Kaptein et al. 1993, 1994).

HYPOTHALAMIC-PITUITARY-THYROID EXTRATHYROID AXIS. Thyrotropin (thyroid-stimulating hormone; TSH), a glycoprotein produced in the thyrotropes of the pituitary pars distalis, has a stimulatory effect on thyroid hormone synthesis and secretion. In addition, TSH stimulates thyroid growth, probably in conjunction with actions of the insulinlike growth factors (IGF I and II). Thyrotropin has a molecular weight of about 30,000 consisting of an α subunit (identical to the a subunit of the other glycoprotein pituitary hormones LH and FSH), and a β subunit, which is specific to the TSH molecule (see Chapter 27). TSH binds to a specific TSH receptor on the thyroid follicular cell membrane and stimulates adenylate cyclase, the production of cyclic AMP and the active uptake of inorganic iodide (see Fig. 29.1). The TSH receptors in dog, cat, and humans have been cloned and expressed. TSH also stimulates the synthesis of thyroglobulin, its release into the colloid, and its iodination by TPO (i.e., organification). As a final step in the delivery of hormone into plasma, TSH stimulates thyroglobulin resorption and proteolysis to release T_3 and T_4. The thyroidal enzymes deiodinating T_4 to T_3 and reverse T_3 are also stimulated by TSH (Magner 1990; Rapaport and Nagayama 1992; Shupnick et al. 1989).

A detailed study of the hypothalamic-pituitary-thyroid-extrathyroid axis is only possible with the availability of a valid TSH radioimmunoassays (RIA) for each species. Availability of this assay has helped to demonstrate that most of the replacement dosages of L-thyroxine recommended for the dog are well in excess of those needed for suppression of endogenous TSH into the normal range. The currently available assays do not reliably distinguish between normal and low TSH concentrations making it more difficult to confirm an overdosage (Braverman and Utiger 1991; Ferguson 1984; Greenspan 1994; Williams et al. 1996; Bruner et al. 1998).

The tripeptide TRH is produced in the paraventricular nucleus of the hypothalamus and transported to the pituitary pars distalis by the hypophyseal portal system in the pituitary stalk. In the pituitary gland, TRH binds to specific receptors on the thyrotrope cell and stimulates TSH secretion (see Fig. 29.2A). In the dog, as in other species, TRH also stimulates the secretion of prolactin. The hypothalamic hormone somatostatin acts to inhibit TSH secretion and may function as a thyrotropin inhibitory factor (Reichlin 1986).

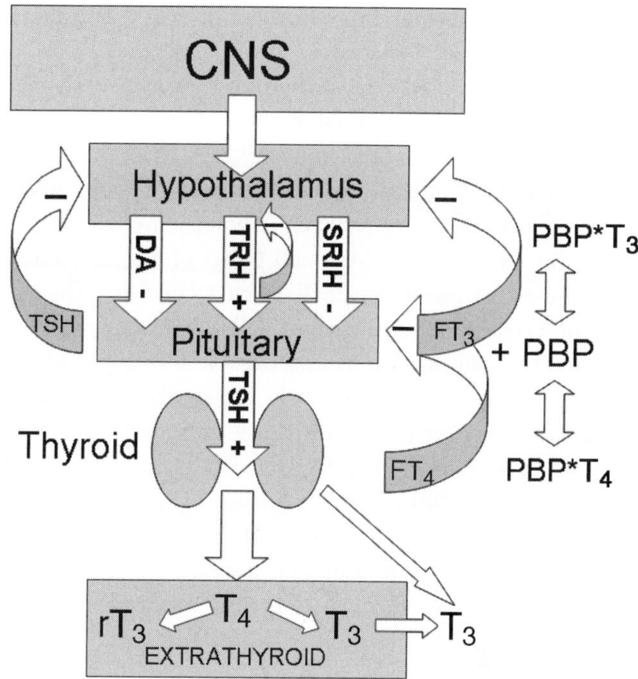

FIG. 29.2A Hypothalamic-pituitary-thyroid-extrathyroid axis. Please see text for details.
Abbreviations: TSH = thyrotropin; CNS = central nervous system; DA = dopamine; TRH = thyrotropin releasing hormone; SRIH = somatostatin; TSH = thyrotropin; FT_3 = free T_3; FT_4 = free T_4; PBP = plasma binding proteins; + = stimulation; − = inhibition.

Negative Feedback Regulation. The negative feedback effect of thyroid hormones (in the free or unbound form) is the principal mechanism regulating TSH secretion. Tonic stimulation by TRH has a permissive role in TSH secretion. The pituitary thyrotope cell completely deiodinates T_4 (derived from the plasma) to T_3 which subsequently inhibits TSH synthesis and secretion through alteration of nuclear receptor binding, mRNA transcription, and protein synthesis. The Type II 5′-deiodinase (D2) mediates the intrapituitary conversion of T_4 to T_3, but at the same time, T_4 inhibits D2 activity at a post-translational level by shortening the enzymes cellular half-life through ubiquitination and subsequent proteasomal degradation (Fig. 29.2B). D2 and TSH are co-expressed in thyrotrophs and hypothyroidism increases D2 expression in the thyrotroph. Through these mechanisms, intrapituitary T_3 concentration is maintained even when free T_4 concentrations are several-fold above the physiological level. As a result FT_4 concentration and D2-mediated T_3 production correlate negatively with expression of mRNA for TSH (Christoffelete et al. 2006).

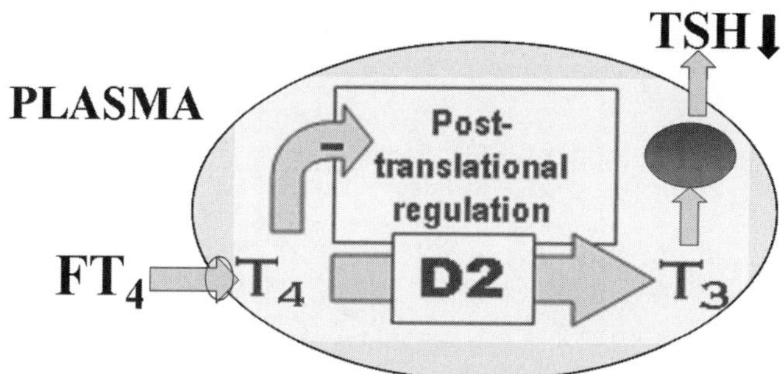

FIG. 29.2B Postranslational regulation of the D2 enzyme by T_4 in the thyrotroph cell. Free T_4 (FT_4) in the circulation is available to enter the thyrotroph, and the quantity of T_4 in the pituitary cell directly and rapidly inhibits the D2 enzyme, which converts T_4 to T_3. Posttranslational modification of the D2 enzyme by ubiquitination shortens the half-life of the enzyme and ultimately reduces the amount of T_3 produced from T_4. Most of the T_3 binding to the nuclear receptor in the thyrotroph is derived from T_4 deiodination. Occupancy of the TR results in down-regulation TSH mRNA and TSH secretion completing the negative feedback loop between FT_4 and TSH.

Circulating T_4 taken up by the pituitary is the preferred source of T_3 in the pituitary, at least in the rat (Larsen et al. 1981). In human patients with hypothyroidism, thyroid replacement therapy with L-T_4 normalizes serum TSH concentrations only when the serum T_4 value is high-normal to slightly high; serum T_3 concentration usually remain within normal range in these patients (Fish et al. 1987; Larsen et al. 1981).

There is also evidence that thyroid hormones may have a direct negative-feedback effect on the hypothalamus to inhibit the release of TRH (Fig. 29.2A). Also, TSH and TRH may have "short-loop" and "ultrashort-loop" negative-feedback effects, respectively, upon the hypothalamus to inhibit TRH release. Although pulses of TSH secretion and an evening rise in serum TSH have been described in humans (possibly resulting from a fall in circadian circulating cortisol concentrations), studies in the dog and cat have failed to demonstrate such a circadian rhythm in circulating thyroid hormone concentrations (Fish et al. 1987; Larsen et al. 1981; Magner 1990; Reichlin 1986; Bruner et al. 1998). Pulsatile release of TSH has been confirmed in hypothyroid but not euthyroid dogs, but there was no overlap in values. However, TSH may not be elevated in a large percentage of confirmed cases (Kooistra et al. 2000).

METABOLISM OF THYROID HORMONE. The metabolically active thyroid hormones are the iodothyronines L-thyroxine (L-T_4) and 3,5,3′- L-triiodothyronine (L-T_3) (see Fig. 29.3). Thyroxine is the main secretory product of the normal thyroid gland. However, T_3, which is about 3 to 10 times more potent than T_4, as well as smaller amounts of 3,3′,5′- L-triiodothyronine (reverse T_3), a thyromimetically inactive product, and other deiodinated metabolites, are also secreted by the thyroid gland of most mammals (see Figs. 29.2A, 29.3) (Belshaw et al. 1974; Ferguson 1984; Inada et al. 1975; Kaptein et al. 1993, 1994; Laurberg 1980).

Although all T_4 is secreted by the thyroid, a considerable amount (40 to 60% in the dog) of T_3 is derived from extrathyroidal enzymatic 5′-deiodination of T_4. Therefore, although it also has intrinsic metabolic activity, T_4 has been called a "prohormone," and its "activation" to the more potent T_3 is a step regulated individually by peripheral tissues (see Figs. 29.3, 29.4). The vast majority (approximately 90%) of reverse T_3 (rT_3) is derived from extrathyroidal sources in the dog (Belshaw et al. 1974; Kaptein et al. 1993, 1994; Larsen et al. 1981).

Types and Regulation of Deiodinase Enzymes. The identification of three distinct types of deiodinase

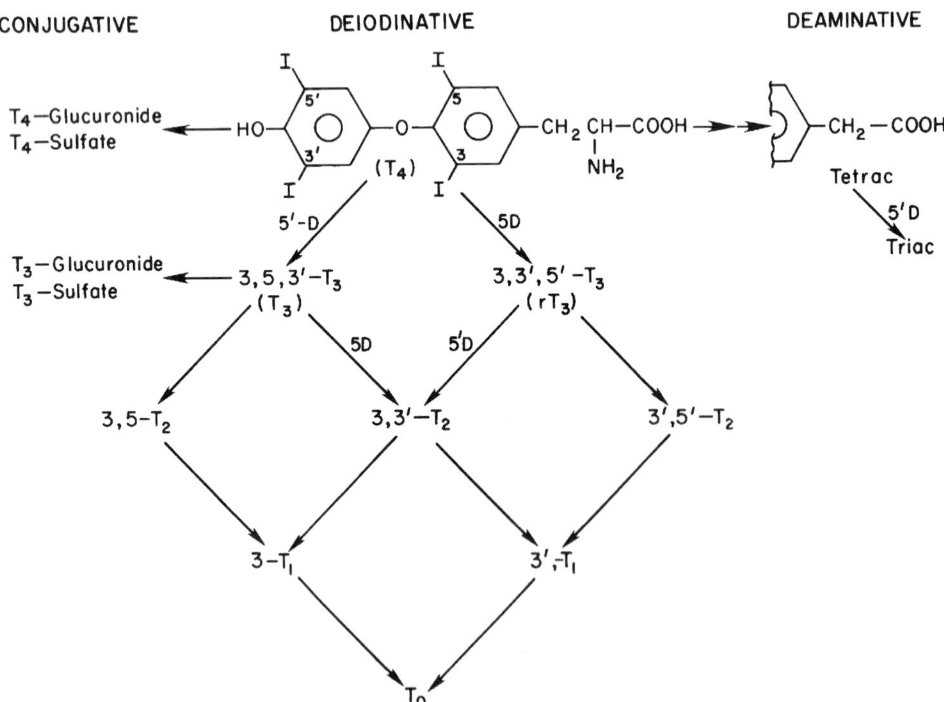

FIG. 29.3 Pathways of metabolism of thyroid hormones. 5′-D = 5′-deiodinase. 5-D = 5-deiodinase. (Reprinted from Ferguson 1984).

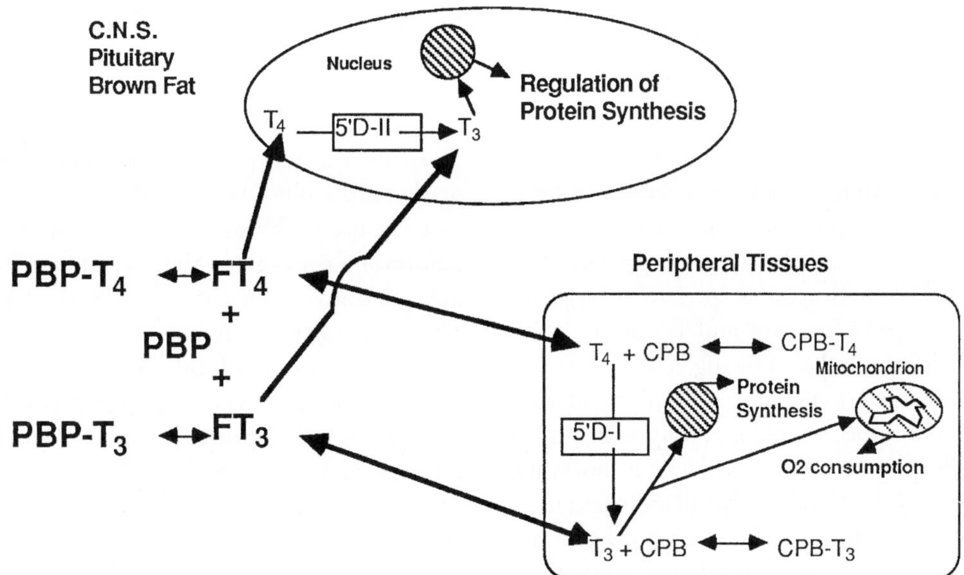

FIG. 29.4 Peripheral action of thyroid hormones. T_4 and T_3, in amounts proportional to their free forms (FT_4 and FT_3) in plasma at equilibrium with plasma binding proteins (PBP), are taken up by peripheral tissues such as liver and kidney, which have the type I 5′-deiodinase enzyme (5′-D-I). T_3 from the plasma (or that derived from T_4) interacts with mitochondrial receptors to rapidly increase oxygen consumption and with nuclear receptors to initiate protein synthesis. Cytosolic binding proteins (CBP) buffer the effects of intracellular hormones and provide a relatively unsaturable hormone reservoir. In the brain, pituitary, and brown fat, another isoenzyme of the 5′-deiodinase enzyme (5′-D-II) converts T_4 to T_3. This enzyme is regulated very differently from the type I enzyme. (Reprinted from Peterson and Ferguson 1990.)

enzymes has underscored the importance of the regulation of T_3 production in individual tissues from T_4. Type I 5′-D (D1) is found in most tissues, but has its highest activity in liver, kidney, muscle and thyroid gland. This enzyme is now known to be a selenoenzyme requiring trace quantities of selenium for optimal activity. Muscle, although it has low enzyme activity, may produce a significant amount (approximately 60% in the rat) of the body's T_3 solely because of its large mass. The physiological role of D1 is the provision of *circulating* T_3 during conditions of euthyroidism. This enzyme is capable of "outer-ring" and "inner-ring" deiodination and can deiodinate T_4 with a high capacity and is sensitive to the thionamide antithyroid agent, propylthiouracil (PTU). Type II 5′-D (D2) is found in the CNS, pituitary, brown fat, and placenta and its physiological role is provision of *intracellular* T_3. Its role in contributing circulating T_3 may increase with primary hypothyroidism. This enzyme acts upon T_4 and other compounds with outer ring iodine at concentrations within the physiological range and is resistant to PTU. Type III deiodinase (D3), which is a 5-deiodinase, removes only inner ring iodines. D3 is present in placenta, CNS, skin, and fetal brain and liver and has as its physiologic role *inactivation* of T_4 and T_3 through inner-ring (ring with amino acid moiety) deiodination, with preference for T_3 as a substrate. Relevant to understanding the rationale for L-thyroxine therapy in hypothyroidism, hypothyroidism dramatically reduces the activity of D1 and D3 while increasing the activity of D2. Through this type of regulation, the brain may continue to obtain adequate cellular T_3 levels necessary to prevent or delay neurologic dysfunction resulting from T_4 deficiency, while the liver reduces its production of T_3, thereby leading to decreased systemic metabolism (see Fig. 29.4). It is interesting to note that in rodents, D1 and D3 are increased in hyperthyroidism resulting in both increased production and degradation rates for T_3. The characteristics of D1 and D2 have been examined in dogs, cats, and cattle. In cats, renal and hepatic D1 has been shown to metabolize T_4 with similar Vmax and Km of the rat enzyme, but the ability of the enzyme to degrade rT_3 was only about 0.2% of that of rat D1 with a Km 500-fold higher. The D1 enzyme was not identified in the cat's thyroid gland, unlike in rat, dog, and humans. These differences would imply that D1 does not metabolize rT_3 under physiological conditions. However, muscle D1 mRNA is stimulated by T_3 treatment of lean cats, as seen in most species. D2 has been identified in human keratinocytes as well as in dog skin. Previous studies have indicated important differences in catalytic specificity between dog and human D1, in particular with respect to the 5′-deiodination of rT_3. While D1 and D2 are found in the microsomal fraction of cells, D3 seems to be a plasma membrane protein, positioning it well to inactivate both excess T_4 and T_3 in tissues such as the placenta and brain (Baqui et al. 2003; Burrow et al. 1989; Ferguson 1988; Larsen et al. 1981; Peterson and Ferguson 1990; Foster et al. 2000; Bianco 2002; Hoenig et al. 2008).

The process of deiodination continues until the thyroid hormone nucleus is stripped of its remaining iodine molecules thereby allowing iodine to recycle for hormone resynthesis (see Fig. 29.3). These further deiodinated metabolic products (other than T_3 and T_4) do not have thyromimetic activity. Evidence is accumulating that reverse T_3 may have an important role in regulating thyroid T_4 and T_3's activity in the central nervous system. A number of nonthyroidal illnesses and drugs may affect the local tissue regulation of thyroid hormone deiodination. Other pathways of thyroid hormone metabolism include conjugation to form soluble glucuronides and sulfates for biliary or urinary excretion as well as cleavage of the ether linkage of the iodothyronine molecule (Braverman and Utiger 1991; Burrow et al. 1989; Ferguson 1984, 1988; Kaptein et al. 1994).

With oral administration of thyroid hormone preparations, the first-pass effect must be considered, as a large quantity of hormone can be conjugated and secreted into the bile where the hormone may either be deconjugated and reabsorbed by bacteria in the large intestine, or eliminated in the feces. The intestinal pool of thyroid hormone is known to be very large. In the dog, over 50% of the T_4 and about 30% of the T_3 produced each day are lost into the feces. In both the dog and cat, the extrathyroidal body stores of T_4 are eliminated and replaced in about one day, whereas stores of T_3 are lost and replaced twice daily (Kaptein et al. 1993, 1994). Such fecal wastage is responsible, in part, for the higher daily replacement doses of thyroid hormone required on a per body weight basis in dogs and cats. Nonetheless, upon administration of a physiological dosage of L-T_4 to a dog, serum TSH appears to be suppressed for at least 24 hours. However, it is the clinical impression of some specialists that dividing the daily oral replacement dose may serve to reduce the loss of hormone due to the hepatic first-pass effect resulting in a more consistent clinical response.

PLASMA HORMONE BINDING OF THYROID HORMONE. Thyroid hormones are water-insoluble lipophilic compounds. Their ability to circulate in plasma is dependent upon binding by specific binding proteins, thyroxine-binding protein (TBG) and transthyretin (TTR) or thyroxine-binding prealbumin (TBPA), as well as by albumin itself. Thyroid hormone–binding proteins provide a hormone reservoir in the plasma and "buffer" hormone delivery into tissue (see Fig. 29.4). TTR and possibly albumin, also may serve as intermediary carriers for specific tissue uptake of the hormone by tissues (Mendel 1989; Pardridge 1981). The dog has a high affinity thyroid hormone–binding protein comparable to TBG in humans, but plasma concentrations of TBG in the dog are only 25% of those in humans. In addition to TBG, TBPA, and albumin, circulating T_4 in canine plasma appears to bind to certain plasma lipoproteins. These include a high-density lipoprotein (HDL_2), which migrates in the $alpha_1$ region on the electrophoretic pattern and a very low-density lipoprotein (VLDL), which migrates in the beta region. At normal serum T_4 concentrations in the dog, about 60% of T_4 is bound to TBG, 17% to TBPA, 12% to albumin and 11% to the HDL_2. Thyroxine-binding globulin in the dog is not saturated until the total T_4 concentration is six times the normal serum T_4 values, while the other serum proteins are virtually unsaturable (Inada et al. 1975). The cat does not appear to have a high affinity thyroid binding protein (such as TBG) but has only TTR and albumin as serum thyroid hormone–binding proteins. Partly as a result of weaker serum protein binding, total T_4 concentrations are lower, the unbound or free fraction of circulating T_4 is higher, and hormone metabolism is more rapid in most domestic animals than in humans (Bigler 1976; Kaptein et al. 1994; Larsson 1987; Larsson et al. 1985).

TISSUE THYROID HORMONE UPTAKE: THE "FREE HORMONE" HYPOTHESIS. The free hormone hypothesis, proposed by Robbins and Rall 5 decades ago (1960) and restated by Mendel (1989) states that it is the unbound fraction of hormone that is available to tissues and therefore proportional to the action, metabolism, and elimination of that hormone. This hypothesis has stood the clinical test of time; direct or indirect measurements of free T_4 have been a mainstay in the diagnosis of thyroid disease in human medicine. There is also strong evidence that certain cell types actively transport or exchange thyroid hormone from the plasma into the cytosol. The presence of a plasma membrane protein specific for thyroid hormone transport certainly reflects the premium the cell is willing to pay to facilitate entry and possibly concentration of thyroid hormone. However, some investigators would argue that the serum binding proteins, particularly albumin and TTR may serve to distribute hormones to specific tissues. TTR serves to carry both thyroid hormones and retinoic acid in the circulation. Most theories of thyroid hormone exchange have assigned a passive "reservoir" role to cytosolic thyroid hormone-binding proteins (CTBP; CBP in Fig. 29.4), the proteins that retain thyroid hormone in a predominantly bound state inside the cell. Little is known about the regulation of these proteins, which are often called "intracellular albumin" for their low specificity, low affinity, and high capacity. However, in renal cytosol, the affinity of CTBP may be acutely regulated by cellular redox potential, increasing when NADPH levels are high. CTBP has just recently been shown to be identical to the protein μ-crystallin (Burrow et al. 1989; Hashizume et al. 1987; Kaptein et al. 1994; Mendel 1989; Pardridge 1981; Suzuki et al. 2007).

Irrespective of the mechanisms, the following observations in the clinical patient must be recognized:

1. The linear correlation between the serum free T_4 concentration, rate of hormonal degradation, and basal metabolic rate in humans.
2. The inverse correlation between the serum free T_4 concentration and the cellular distribution volume of T_4, which exists in all subjects regardless of thyroid state.
3. The positive correlation between the in vitro perfused organ free T_4 concentration and tissue T_4 uptake and T_3 production in vivo and in vitro. Most researchers agree that it is the steady-state tissue concentrations of hormone that are the driving force for thyroid hormone metabolism and action (Mendel 1989).

In the healthy euthyroid dog or cat, about 0.1% of total concentration of serum T_4 is free (i.e., not bound to thyroid hormone-binding proteins), whereas about 1% of circulating T_3 is free (Ferguson and Peterson 1992; Kaptein et al. 1994). The proportion of free hormone may change in response to drug administration or illness. For example, in obese cats, increased nonesterified free fatty acids compete for hormone binding resulting in an increase in free serum thyroid hormone concentrations and may have a similar effect to compete with cellular binding, leading to a form of thyroid hormone resistance to negative feedback manifested by an increase in total and/or free T_4 concentrations. However, it appears that thyroid status of the animal does not change, since the absolute level of the free hormone concentrations tends to soon return to within normal range or remains relatively constant (Ferguson 1988, 1989b, 1994; Ferguson et al. 2007).

Most evidence suggests that the thyroid hormone uptake by tissues is proportional to, but not limited to, the free or unbound fraction of circulating hormone. Approximately 50 to 60% of the body's T_4 and 90 to 95% of the body's T_3 is located in the intracellular compartment (Fish et al. 1997). Certain organs, particularly the liver and kidney, can concentrate thyroid hormones and exchange hormone rapidly with the plasma. In humans, about 60% of the intracellular T_4 is in these *rapidly equilibrating* tissues (liver and kidney), whereas only 6% of the intracellular T_3 is in these tissues. About 80% of all extrathyroidal T_3 is located in the *slowly equilibrating* tissues (e.g., muscle, skin), while only 20% of intracellular T_4 is in this compartment. As a result, most of the body's T_4 is located in plasma, interstitial fluid, liver, and kidney. The majority of the body's extrathyroidal T_3 is in the cells of the muscle and skin and in a conjugated form in the intestinal tract. Kaptein et al. (1994) have used a three-pool model to describe the distribution and metabolism of thyroid hormone metabolites and iodide (see Fig. 29.5). Table 29.1 compares the model parameters for T_4, T_3, rT_3, and iodide in dogs, cats, and humans.

As a principle impacting the diagnosis and treatment of thyroidal diseases, the tissue-specific regulation of deiodinases and TR receptor subtypes (vide infra) suggests that the determination of thyroid status really must be established on a tissue-by-tissue basis.

METABOLIC CLEARANCE RATES. The plasma half-life of T_4 in the dog has been estimated to be 8 hours (Kaptein et al. 1993, 1994) or 10–16 hours (Fox and Nachreiner 1981) and 11 hours in the cat (Kaptein et al. 1994) compared to a plasma half-life of about 7 days in humans. Similarly, the plasma half-life of T_3 in the dog has been estimated to be 5–6 hours, compared to 24–36 hours in humans (see Table 29.2). Studies in the normal cat indicate that the plasma half-lives of T_4 and T_3 are similar to that of the dog (Fox and Nachreiner 1981; Kaptein et al. 1994). Despite these rates of plasma clearance, the suppressive effect on pituitary TSH secretion

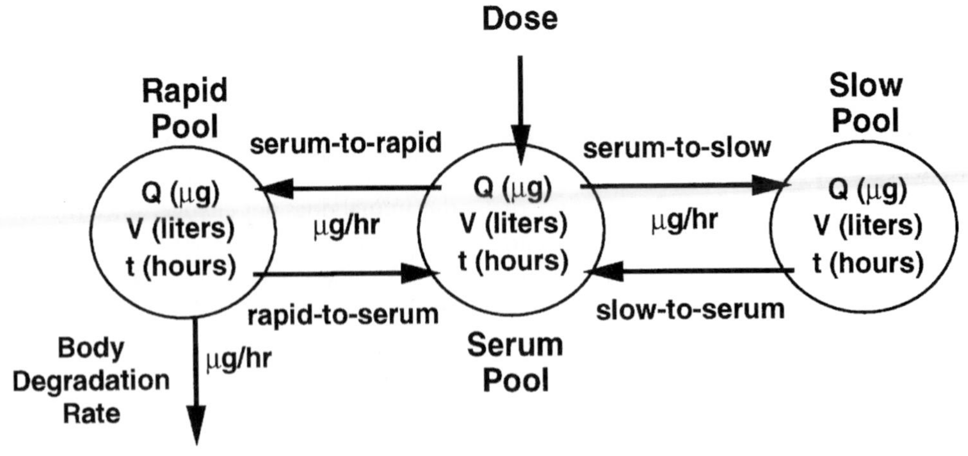

FIG. 29.5 Compartmental model of thyroid hormone metabolism.

TABLE 29.1 Thyroid hormone and iodide kinetics in normal dogs, cats, and humans using a three-pool model

	Dogs	Cats	Humans
T_4			
Plasma concentration (ng/dL)	2.8	1.68	6.8
Free fraction (%)	0.102	0.056	0.030
Total mean residence time (d)	0.54	0.69	6.8
Clearance rate (L/[kg·d])	0.24	0.38	0.017
Degradation rate (μg/[kg·d])	6.81	6.2	1.14
Total pool size (μg/kg)	3.7	4.3	7.8
Distribution (%)			
Plasma pool	46	13	32
Rapidly equilibrating pool	23	19	26
Slowly equilibrating pool	31	68	42
T_3			
Plasma concentration (ng/dL)	43	32	140
Free fraction (%)	1.426	0.48	0.299
Total mean residence time (d)	0.40	0.62	1.50
Clearance rate (L/[kg·d])	1.99	1.77	0.32
Degradation rate (μg/[kg·d])	0.84–0.89	0.52–2.2	0.43–0.46
Total pool size (μg/kg)	0.34	0.30	0.66
Distribution (%)			
Plasma pool	7	3.6	9
Rapidly equilibrating pool	29	18	19
Slowly equilibrating pool	64	79	73
Reverse T_3			
Plasma concentration (ng/dL)	22	—	13
Free fraction (%)	0.560	—	0.111
Total mean residence time (d)	0.12	—	0.16
Clearance rate (L/[kg·d])	1.44	—	1.78
Degradation rate (μg/[kg·d])	0.32–0.42	—	0.23–0.33
Total pool size (μg/kg)	0.039	—	0.036
Distribution (%)			
Plasma pool	31	—	15
Rapidly equilibrating pool	29	—	29
Slowly equilibrating pool	40	—	55
Inorganic iodide[a]			
Plasma mass (μg/kg)[b]	21	—	1.67
Total mean residence time (d)	1.07	0.82	0.35–0.36[c]
Clearance rate (L/[kg·d])	0.43	0.63	1.00–1.01
Total distribution volume (L/kg)	0.46	0.44	0.35–0.36
Distribution (%)			
Plasma pool	19	11	13[c]
Rapidly equilibrating pool	9	32	38
Slowly equilibrating pool	72	57	50

Source: Kaptein et al. 1994. Dog and human data from Kaptein et al. 1990; Kaptein et al. 1993. Cat data from Hays et al. 1988.

Note: Parameter values were estimated using a three-pool model. Only mean values are presented. Conversion to SI units: Total T_4 in μg/dL × 12.87 = nmol/L; total T_3 and reverse T_3 in ng/dL × 0.01536 = nmol/L.

[a]Thyroid gland unblocked for all species.

[b]Dog data from Belshaw et al. 1974.

[c]Data from Hays and Solomon 1965 (reanalyzed in three-pool model); Belshaw et al. 1974.

TABLE 29.2 Thyroxine kinetics in dogs, cats, and humans following intravenous, subcutaneous, and oral L-thyroxine administration

	Dogs	Cats	Humans
T_4 degradation rate (μg/[kg·day])	6.81	6.2	1.14
Intravenous			
Time to peak (hr)	0.02–0.03	0.02–0.03[a]	0.02–0.03
Total mean residence time (hr)	13.0	16.6[a]	164
Terminal half-life (hr)	7.6	10.7[b]	168
Subcutaneous			
Dosage (μg/[kg·day])	5–7	—	—
Absorption (%)	100[c]	—	81
Time to peak (hr)	1.5–1.8	—	72
Terminal half-life (hr)	14.7	—	120
Oral			
Dosage (μg/[kg·day])	20–40[c]	20–30[c]	2.11
Absorption (%)	10–50[c]	10.5[c]	50–80
Time to peak (hr)	—	3–4[c]	2–4
Terminal half-life (hr)	7.6	10.7[c]	168

Source: Kaptein et al. 1994. Data on dogs and humans from Kaptein et al. 1993.
Note: Conversion to SI units: Total T_4 in μg × 1.287 = nmol.
[a]Data from Hays et al. 1988.
[b]Data from Hays et al. 1992.
[c]Data from Hulter et al. 1984.

appears to persist at least 24 hours after a dose, suggesting that intrapituitary T_3 persists longer than the serum half-life (Ferguson 2007). Therefore, as with many lipophilic nuclear receptor–mediated hormones, the plasma disappearance rates may underestimate the extent or duration of biological action.

EXTRATHYROIDAL FACTORS ALTERING THYROID HORMONE METABOLISM

EFFECT OF ILLNESS AND MALNUTRITION IN HUMANS. In humans, a wide range of clinical conditions such as chronic starvation or malnutrition, surgery, diabetes mellitus, hepatic and renal disease, and chronic systemic illness may result in decreased serum T_3 concentrations together with elevated serum rT_3 values. This "low T_3" syndrome results from inhibition of 5′-deiodinase, the enzyme necessary for conversion of T_4 to T_3 and the conversion of rT_3 to 3,3′-T_2 (Braverman and Utiger 1991; Burrow et al. 1989; Kaptein et al. 1994; Kaptein 1986; Daminet and Ferguson 2003.)

The reduction in the production of T_3, the most potent thyroid hormone, appears to be a beneficial adaptive mechanism by which the body serves to limit the loss of protein and perhaps blunt the metabolic rate during illness. Maintenance of serum T_3 concentrations (with triiodothyronine replacement therapy) in euthyroid fasting humans leads to excessive nitrogen excretion and blunting of the pituitary's TSH response to TRH, as if there was a state of hyperthyroidism. The body of evidence does not support the contention that lowering of serum T_3 during malnutrition and illness is associated with "tissue" hypothyroidism. Also, outside of these regulatory mechanisms, there is, as yet, no evidence that an isolated 5′-deiodinase deficiency exists in animals or in specific tissues (Braverman and Utiger 1991; Ferguson 1984, 1988; Kaptein et al. 1993, 1994; Kaptein 1986).

In acute and severe illnesses in humans, serum T_4 and T_3 concentrations may also fall, in what is called the "low T_4 state of medical illness." Impaired serum protein binding of T_4 caused by inhibitors of binding (such as free fatty acids) or a reduction in binding protein concentration results in reduced total serum T_4 concentrations and increased free fractions of T_4. In most cases, however, the absolute free T_4 concentrations remain normal. A fall in serum TSH concentrations may also contribute to the subnormal serum T_4 concentrations, especially in human patients treated with dopamine or glucocorticoids, drugs inhibiting TSH release. No studies have examined systematically the benefit or detriment of thyroid hormone therapy in domestic animals; however, studies of critically ill patients with low serum T_4 and T_3 concentrations have revealed that thyroxine therapy is not beneficial and fails to improve survival (Kaptein 1986; Kaptein et al. 1993, 1994).

The effects of nonthyroidal illness on thyroid hormone metabolism in the dog are less well characterized than in humans. In the dog, depressed serum T_4 concentrations have been reported in various nonthyroidal illnesses such as hyperadrenocorticism (e.g., Cushing's syndrome), diabetes mellitus, hypoadrenocorticism (e.g., Addison's disease), chronic renal failure, hepatic disease, as well as a variety of other critical medical illnesses requiring intensive care (Ferguson 1984, 1988, 1994, 2007; Ferguson and Peterson 1992).

EFFECT OF DRUGS ON THYROID FUNCTION. This topic was reviewed by Daminet and Ferguson in 2003. A variety of drugs may impair plasma or tissue binding of the thyroid hormones or alter thyroid hormone metabolism. Drugs used in veterinary medicine that are most likely to alter circulating thyroid hormone concentrations include the glucocorticoids, anticonvulsants, quinidine, salicylates, phenylbutazone, and radiocontrast agents. The mechanisms by which these drugs exert their effect vary. Quinidine and other membrane stabilizing drugs may inhibit 5′-deiodinase. Salicylates, furosemide and oleic acid may directly displace thyroid hormone from plasma binding sites (Daminet and Ferguson 2003; Ferguson 2007; Ferguson et al. 2007). Phenylbutazone appears also to have a direct antithyroid (goitrogenic) effect in some species, having been shown to decrease total and free T_4 in the horse (Ramirez et al. 1997). In vitro, it appears to decrease serum hormone binding. Radiocontrast agents (e.g, diatrizoate, iopanoic acid, ipodate, tyropanoate and metrizamide) may act by preventing the uptake of T_4 by tissue, by directly inhibiting 5′-deiodinase, or by releasing the iodine they contain to exert an antithyroid effect on the thyroid gland. No studies have been reported in domestic animals to evaluate the influence of these iodine containing drugs on thyroid function tests or on subsequent radioiodine uptake (Ferguson 1984, 1989b, 1994).

Exogenous glucocorticoids have also been shown to have a profound effect on thyroid function tests in the dog, but similar studies have had little effect on serum T_4 levels in the cat and horse. A single high immunosuppressive dosage of glucocorticoid (2.2 mg/kg prednisone, 0.6 mg/kg dexamethasone) will lower serum T_3, but not serum T_4 concentrations in the dog (Kemppainen et al. 1983; Laurberg and Boye 1984). Serum T_3 concentrations may be decreased because of glucocorticoid inhibition of 5′-deiodinase or simply because of a reduced availability of plasma T_4, the substrate for the enzyme. Most dogs on chronic, high dose, daily glucocorticoid therapy will have very low or undetectable serum T_4 concentrations, as well as subnormal serum T_3 values (Ferguson and Peterson 1992; Kaptein et al. 1992; Kemppainen et al. 1983; Moore et al. 1993; Torres et al. 1992). Based upon electron microscopic examination of thyroid tissue, it was postulated that glucocorticoids may interfere with thyroid hormone secretion by inhibiting lysosomal hydrolysis of colloid in the follicular cell (Woltz et al. 1983). *Immunosuppressive* dosages (1.1–2 mg/kg q 12h) of prednisolone in dogs for 3 to 4 weeks significantly decreased serum total T_4 and to a lesser extent, free T_4 (FT_4) concentrations. These changes were observed as soon as 1 day after initiation of treatment (Torres et al. 1991; Daminet et al. 1999). Endogenous TSH was not affected by 3 weeks of an immunosuppressive dosage of prednisone, but the assay may not allow detection of a mild decrease. No changes in serum total T_4 levels were seen after a month of prednisone administration at an *antiinflammatory* dosage (0.5 mg/kg q 12h) (Moore et al. 1993). However, a decrease in total T_3 concentrations, with a supranormal T_4 increase after TSH administration was observed. Another study also showed that prednisone at an antiinflammatory dosage of 1 mg/kg/day had no effect on TSH concentration of dogs with experimental hypothyroidism, but higher dosages have not been studied. In summary, glucocorticoids can markedly decrease total T_3 and T_4 concentrations and to a lesser extent FT_4 concentrations in dogs. Therefore, thyroid function test results should be interpreted carefully in any dog receiving glucocorticoids if prescribed an immunosuppressive dosage or for a period greater than 1 month (Ferguson 1984, 1994; Moore et al. 1993; Daminet and Ferguson 2003).

Other drugs have been well documented to alter thyroid hormone metabolism or serum or tissue binding of the thyroid hormones in the dog. The anticonvulsants diphenylhydantoin and phenobarbital, which are mixed function oxidase inducers, consistently decrease serum T_4 concentrations. Phenobarbital increases the rate of clearance of T_4. Increased hepatic deiodination of thyroid hormones, biliary clearance, and fecal excretion result in decreased concentrations of circulating thyroid hormones.

The *short-term* administration (3 weeks) of phenobarbital to dogs did not affect total or free T_4 nor TSH serum concentrations in beagle dogs. However, several studies have looked at the *long-term* effects of phenobarbital administration. Total and free T_4 can be decreased to a range consistent with hypothyroidism. Endogenous TSH concentrations can remain within reference range or be slightly increased. Serum phenobarbital concentrations did correlate with the decrease in total and free T_4 concentrations in one study, but not in another. The reduction of free T_4 concentration particularly supports the idea that phenobarbital influences the steady-state clearance of T_4. Difficulty of interpretation of drug effects is compounded by the observation in dogs that seizure activity reduces serum total T_4 concentrations in proportion to the frequency of seizure episodes (von Klopmann et al. 2006). In one study, thyroid function normalized 1 to 4 weeks after discontinuation of phenobarbital. It is therefore recommended, when this is an option clinically, to evaluate thyroid function at least 4–6 weeks after discontinuation of phenobarbital (Kantrowitz et al. 1999; Gaskill et al. 1999; Müeller et al. 2000; Gieger et al. 2000; Daminet et al. 1999; McClain et al. 1989; Curran and DeGroot 1991; Johnson et al. 1993; Barter and Klaassen 1994; Theodoropoulos and Zolman 1989; Liu et al. 1995; DeSandro et al. 1991; Attia and Aref 1991).

The antiepileptic potassium bromide is a halide chemically related to iodide and could potentially interact with iodine in the thyroid gland. In rats, bromide produces a relative iodine deficiency, thereby interfering with iodine uptake, iodine transport, and iodination of tyrosine and tyrosyl residues on thyroglobulin. In one study of epileptic dogs and another of healthy dogs receiving KBr at therapeutic dosages up to 6 months, no abnormal thyroid function test results were seen (Kantrowitz et al. 1999, Paull et al. 2000).

A study evaluated the effect of a standard dosage of trimethoprim/sulfamethoxazole on thyroid function tests in dogs with pyoderma and normal baseline serum thyroxine concentrations. The average serum T_4, but not T_3 concentration, fell significantly during the treatment period of 6 weeks. The TSH response also fell in several dogs and radionuclide imaging suggested that the preparation (likely the sulfa component) interfered with iodine metabolism by the thyroid gland. The thyroid carcinogenic potential of sulfonamides, which has resulted in restriction of some forms in food animals, is likely due to its goitrogenic potential, chronic elevation of serum TSH, and subsequent stimulation of thyroid growth (Hall et al. 1993). Sulfonamides are known goitrogens in domestic species because they can markedly interfere with thyroid hormone synthesis through reversible inhibition of TPO activity and reduction of serum concentrations of thyroid hormones. With reduced negative feedback, there is an increase in pituitary secretion of TSH, which induces proliferative changes in the thyroid gland. Long-term administration of sulfonamides and prolonged stimulation of the thyroid gland by TSH have been associated with thyroid neoplasia in rats. There is considerable interspecies variation with respect to TPO inhibition by sulfonamides. For example, only mild effects of sulfonamides are observed on human thyroid function. Several prospective studies have evaluated the effects of sulfonamide administration on canine thyroid function. Trimethoprim-sulfadiazine administered at a dosage of 15 mg/kg q12h to healthy dogs for 4 weeks had no effect on serum total T_4 or T_3 or free T_4 concentrations or upon the results of TSH stimulation tests. When trimethoprim-sulfadimethoxazole was administered to dogs with pyoderma for 6 weeks at a higher dosage of 30 mg/kg q 12h, serum total T_4 and T_3, and FT_4 concentrations decreased. Half of the dogs in this experiment had TT_4 levels below the reference range at the end of the treatment, which could easily have resulted in the inappropriate diagnosis of primary thyroid failure. In another study, the same dosage of trimethoprim-sulfadimethoxazole was given to healthy dogs for 6 weeks, and thyroid hormones were markedly decreased and endogenous TSH increased as soon as 7 days after initiation of the treatment. Thyroid imaging showed increased uptake of pertechnetate, and thyroid gland biopsies revealed hyperplasia of thyroid follicles and absence of colloid production. These findings further support the concept that sulfonamides act as goitrogens, resulting in primary hypothyroidism with secondary changes associated with the proliferative effects of TSH. The effects of sulfonamides on thyroid function are species-specific, and dosage- and duration-dependent. Normalization of thyroid function test results in dogs after cessation of sulfonamide administration can take up to 8 or 12 weeks. Sulfa drugs can lead to clinical hypothyroidism in some dogs (Cohen et al. 1980, 1981; Lagler et al. 1976; Panciera and Post 1992; Post et al. 1993; Hall et al. 1993; Campbell et al. 1996; Gookin et al. 1999).

Many nonsteroidal antiinflammatory drugs (NSAIDs) have been shown to alter thyroid function tests in humans, since circulating thyroid hormones are highly protein-bound, and various NSAIDs can displace thyroid hormones from serum protein-binding sites. Short-term administration of therapeutic dosages of salicylates leads to a transient increase in unbound hormone levels and suppression of TSH concentrations. After long-term treatment with salicylates, a new steady-state is reached, reflecting an increased T_4 turnover rate, and serum total T_4 concentrations have been reported to be reduced 20–40%. Free T_4 concentrations can be unchanged or decreased, and TSH concentrations return to the reference range within a few weeks of treatment. Carprofen is a commonly used NSAID in dogs and is highly protein-bound. One abstract reports a mild decrease in serum total T_4 and TSH measurements after administration of carprofen to dogs (2.2–3.3 mg/kg q 12 h for 5 weeks). Free T_4 also decreased mildly, but this was not statistically significant. The proposed mechanism includes displacement of T_4 from serum-binding sites and displacement of pituitary intracellular binding of thyroid hormone (Daminet et al. 2003; Ferguson et al. 1999).

MECHANISMS OF THYROID HORMONE ACTION

CORRELATION OF CLINICAL EFFECTS WITH CELLULAR ACTIONS. Thyroid hormone (T_4 and/or T_3) acts on many different cellular processes via specific ligand-receptor interactions with the nucleus, the mitochondria, and the plasma membrane (see Fig. 29.4). The effects of thyroid hormone are seen in most tissues throughout the body. Although both L-T_4 and L-T_3 have intrinsic metabolic activity, L-T_3 is 3 to 10 times more potent in binding to the nuclear receptors and similarly more potent in stimulating oxygen consumption (see Table 29.3). Except for the deaminated form of T_4 and T_3 (tetraiodothyroacetic acid (Tetrac) and triiodothyroacetic acid (Triac), respectively), most thyroid hormone metabolites have little thyromimetic activity. Reverse T_3 (3,3′,5′-T_3) has recently been linked to some potential developmental effects in the central nervous system.

The effects of thyroid hormone can generally be divided into those that are rapid and evident within minutes to hours of administration, such as stimulation of amino acid transport and mitochondrial oxygen consumption, and those that require protein synthesis and a longer period of time (usually no sooner than 6 hours) to be manifested. Of course, the clinical manifestations may require weeks to months to clearly appreciate. About one-half of the increment in oxygen consumption produced by thyroid hormone has been related to activation of the plasma membrane-bound Na^+,K^+-ATPase, which, at least in the kidney and liver, is secondary to increases in passive K^+ fluxes caused directly and primarily by thyroid hormone via as yet undetermined mechanisms. These changes have been linked directly to the calorigenic effect of thyroid hormone. The rapid hormone effects can be observed clinically in the hypothyroid patient starting on thyroid replacement therapy by signs such as increased physical and mental activity (Braverman and Utiger 1991; Burrow et al. 1989; Greenspan 1994).

TABLE 29.3 Relative nuclear binding affinity of thyroid hormone analogs to T_3

Analog	Relative binding affinity (T_3 = 1) In vitro	In vivo
L-T_3	1.0	1.0
D-T_3	0.6	0.7
Triiodothyroacetic acid (triac)	1.6	1.0
Isopropyl T_2	1.0	1.0
L-T-$_4$	0.1	0.1
Tetraiodothyroacetic acid (tetrac)	0.16	0.05
3,3′,5′-T_3 (reverse T_3)	0.001	0
Monoiodotyrosine	0	0
Diiodotyrosine	0	0

Source: Oppenheimer 1983.

Chronic effects of thyroid hormone invariably are related to the cellular actions of the hormone requiring interaction with nuclear thyroid hormone receptors (TRs) followed by an increase in protein synthesis. Clinically, these are effects such as growth, differentiation, proliferation, and maturation. A common clinical presentation of thyroid insufficiency is bilateral symmetrical alopecia, the result of diminished turnover of shafts of hair within the hair follicle, resulting in greater amounts of telogen hairs. Such changes are slow in onset and, upon treatment, slow to resolve.

PLASMA MEMBRANE TRANSPORTERS AND CYTOSOLIC BINDING PROTEINS. The details of the following processes will vary depending upon the specific cell type. Free thyroid hormone, translocated by passive diffusion or specific plasma membrane transporters into the cell, binds to cytosolic thyroid binding protein (CTBP, now known as μ-crystallin) to maintain intracellular solubility and buffering and as act as a form of intracellular hormone storage. There is evidence that the affinity of μ-crystallin for TH may be increased by NADPH resulting in another possible mechanism for an impact on cellular action. Cytosolic TH presumably exchanges with specific nuclear thyroid hormone receptors (see Fig. 29.6A).

NUCLEAR THYROID HORMONE RECEPTORS (TRS). Most, but not all, of the cellular actions of thyroid hormone can be linked to binding to nuclear receptors. Thyroid hormones act by binding to a specific nuclear thyroid hormone receptor (TR), which is a heterodimer with the retinoid X receptor (RXR). TRs are members of a family of nuclear receptors similar to the v-erb A receptor, which is a receptor for the avian erythroblastosis virus, including the glucocorticoid, mineralocorticoid, estrogen, progestin, vitamin D_3 and retinoic acid receptors. There are three major functional domains of this receptor, one binding DNA, one binding the ligand, and two major transcriptional activation domains (Fig. 29.6B). T_3 has a higher binding affinity for TRs than does T_4, leading to its function as the most potent thyroid hormone analogue. There are two TR genes (TR α and TR β). Alternatively spliced gene products from each of these genes produce active (TRα-1 and TRs β1, β2, and β3) and inactive (α-2 and α-3) gene products, which are expressed in a tissue-specific manner. TRβ-2 is the subtype of the receptor in the cochlea, hypothalamus, and pituitary gland, and it mediates negative feedback and is down-regulated by T_3. TRβ-1 is expressed in all tissues, with the highest levels in kidney, liver, brain, and heart. TRα-1 mRNA is expressed most highly in the brain, with lower levels in skeletal muscle, heart, and lungs. TRβ-3 mRNA is not very abundant but is found in highest levels in the liver, kidneys, and lungs. TRα-2 is found only in the heart, and in human, dog, and guinea pig, but not rodents. While not binding T_3, TRα-2 does bind the TRE and may antagonize TRα-1's action. In addition, there are truncated proteins, with unclear physiological roles, which do not bind either T_3 or the TRE (Blange et al. 1997; Larsen et al. 2003; Bernal 2003).

For a function directly regulated by a TR, the binding affinity of thyroid analogues directly predicts the biological activity of that analogue (see Table 29.3). The binding of T_3 to the TR-TRE complex leads to stimulation or inhibition of the mRNA and protein synthesis (Figs. 6A, B). Upon binding TH, a conformational change in the TR results in dissociation of repressors of transcription, which are replaced by coactivators, including those stimulating DNA acetylation or histone acetyltransferase activity. The latter enzyme causes dissociation of thyroid hormone–regulated genes, which then bind the transcriptional initiation complex. The action of T_3 is terminated by its dissociation from the receptor or by ubiquitination and proteasomal degradation of the hormone-bound complex.

L-T_4 is the preferred choice of thyroid hormone for therapy of hypothyroidism; although T_3 activates cellular thyroid hormone–dependent genes with highest potency, T_4 negatively regulates its own activation to T_3 by post-translationally down-regulating D2 in the pituitary and other tissues, reducing TSH, and therefore, indirectly as well as directly, inactivating D1 (Larsen et al. 2003). Topological studies suggest that D1 is a plasma membrane protein with its catalytic site on the cytosolic surface, therefore facilitating access of the enzyme to circulating rT_3 and T_4 as well as the entry of produced T_3 into the plasma. D2 is localized to endoplasmic reticulum. These subcellular distribution patterns of the 5′-deiodinases may explain why T_3 produced by D2 is most likely to impact nuclear receptor occupancy and T_3 produced by D1 is most likely to be released to the circulation (Bianco et al. 2002; Larsen et al. 2003).

EXTRANUCLEAR ACTIONS OF THYROID HORMONE. Some of the actions of thyroid hormone occur in the absence of new protein synthesis. Nongenomic actions, which include stimulation of cardiac plasma membrane Na^+ channel, the inward-rectifying and voltage-activated K^+ channels, Na^+/H^+ exchange, and the calcium pump (Ca^{2+}-ATPase), have been shown in intact cells and isolated plasma membranes. Actions on channels or pumps may contribute to setting of basal activity of these transport functions perhaps by influencing protein kinases that modulate channel activity. A mitochondrial T_3 receptor has also been identified and has been postulated to mediate the activity of the mitochondrial ATP/ADP translocase indirectly stimulating oxygen consumption. The density of β-adrenergic receptors on cardiomyocytes is increased by T_3 within 2 hours even when protein synthesis is inhibited. Another nongenomic effect already described is the posttranslational inhibition by ubiquitination of pituitary D2. (Greenspan et al. 1994; Davis and Davis 2002).

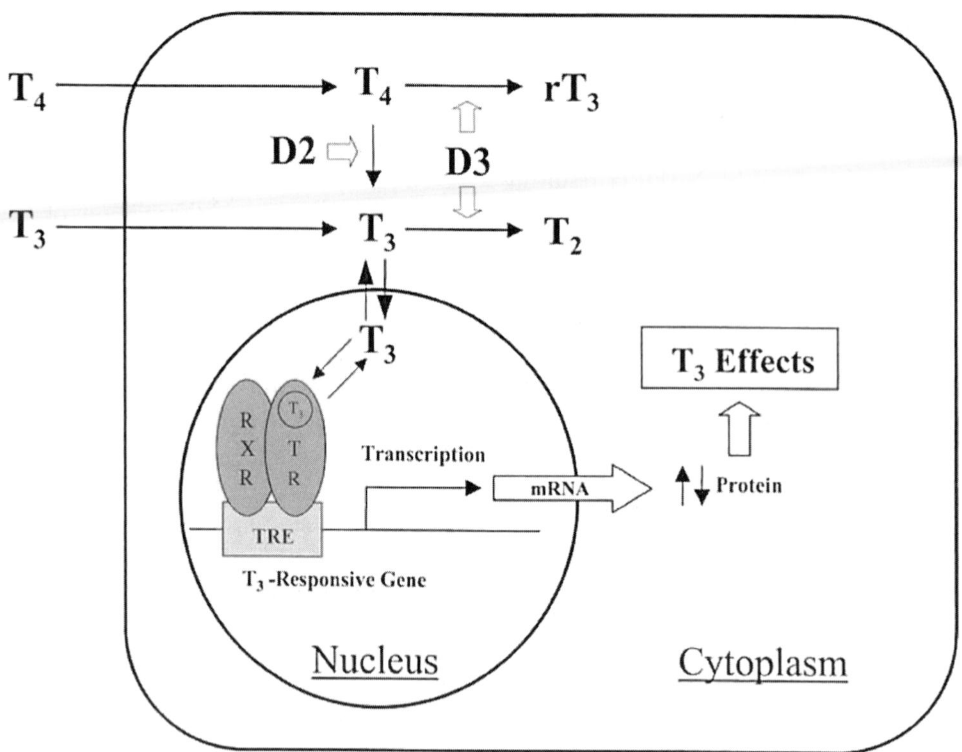

FIG. 29.6A Cellular deiodinative metabolism and nuclear action of thyroid hormone in a cell in the central nervous system. Thyroid hormone enters the cell by diffusion or active transport. T_4 may be activated by the D2 enzyme to T_3, which can enter the nucleus and interact with the thyroid hormone receptor (TR) as a heterodimer with the retinoic X receptor (RXR), which binds to the thyroid-response element (TRE) leading to a change in mRNA transcription (increase or decrease) and effects secondary to altered protein synthesis. The D3 enzyme can remove the 5-position iodines to produce inactive products (rT_3 from T_4) and 3,3′-T2 from T_3 (Larsen et al. 2003; Fig. 10-8, p. 345).

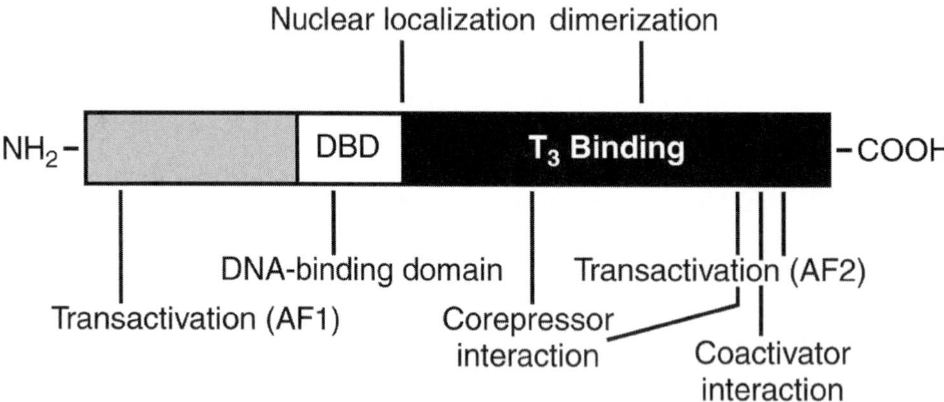

FIG. 29.6B Functional domains of a nuclear thyroid hormone receptor. The functional domains of the thyroid hormone receptor are similar among the four active isoforms (α1, β1, β2, and β3), with the only difference being in the amino-terminal section. Coactivators and corepressors interact with the T_3 binding domain, which dimerizes with the retinoic acid receptor (RXR). DBD = DNA binding domain; AF = activating factor (from Larsen et al. 2003; Figure 10-9, p. 345).

PHYSIOLOGIC AND PHARMACOLOGIC EFFECTS OF THYROID HORMONE. Thyroid hormones, in physiological quantities, are anabolic. Working in conjunction with growth hormone and insulin, protein synthesis is stimulated and nitrogen excretion is reduced. However, in excess (i.e., hyperthyroidism), they can be catabolic, with an increase in gluconeogenesis, protein breakdown, and nitrogen wasting. Table 29.4 summarizes the multiple organ effects of thyroid hormone and the clinical manifestations of hormone deficit (hypothyroidism).

Calorigenesis and Thermoregulation. Thyroid hormones increase oxygen consumption and heat production to a large extent by stimulating Na^+,K^+-ATPase in all tissues except the brain, spleen and, testis. As such, thyroid hormones determine the basal (resting) metabolic rate (BMR) of the animal. This results in the development of mental dullness, lethargy, and an unwillingness to exercise. The reduced basal metabolic rate results in hypothermia and the tendency for the animal to seek heat (Greco et al. 1998). Once-daily administration of 0.022 mg/kg was sufficient to normalize basal metabolic rate in dogs when measured by indirect calorimetry. Clinical signs improved in 93% of dogs with either improvement or complete resolution. This dosage was also shown to suppress TSH values to undetectable levels in most thyroidectomized dogs (Ferguson and Hoenig 1997).

Effects on Growth and Maturation. The fetus obtains thyroid hormone from maternal sources during the first half of gestation in most mammals, after which the fetal thyroid function matures. Thyroid hormones are crucial for growth and development of the skeleton and central nervous system. Therefore, in addition to the well-recognized signs of adult-onset hypothyroidism, disproportionate dwarfism and impaired mental development (cretinism) are prominent signs of congenital and juvenile-onset hypothyroidism. With primary congenital hypothyroidism, enlargement of the thyroid gland (goiter) is also often observed. Puppies, kittens, and foals with this condition are behaviorally dull and less active, may have a shuffling gait, and have a poor appetite. On neurological examination, the animal is often weak, hyporeflexic, or hyperreflexic (if there is muscle tremor or spasticity), and it may lack conscious proprioception. Angular deformities have been observed in foals. Radiographic signs of

TABLE 29.4 Physiological effects of thyroid hormone

Site of action	Effect of hormone	Effects of deficit
Calorigenesis	Increase in BMR	Lethargy, weakness
Thermoregulation	O_2 consumption	Distal extremity hypothermia, heat-seeking
Growth and maturation	Normal CNS development	Mental retardation of cretin and dullness in adults; neuropathies
Carbohydrate metabolism	Increase in glycogenolysis and glycolysis, anti-insulin effects	Obesity despite normal or decreased appetite
Protein metabolism	Increased synthesis and degradation	Muscle weakness, poor hair coat and regrowth
Dermatologic	Normal maintenance of anagen hairs, maintenance of fatty acid turnover in skin, normal keratin turnover rates	Bilateral symmetrical alopecia, hyperkeratosis, myxedema
Cardiovascular	Stimulation of myosin ATPase, stimulation of Na^+,K^+-ATPase, increased β-receptor numbers	Decreased heart rate, pulse, pressure, and cardiac output
Neuromuscular	Normal myelin production, maintenance of balance between slow-twitch and fast-twitch fibers	Polyneuropathy, muscle atrophy, weakness, stiffness, myotonia
Gastrointestinal	Maintenance of normal electrical activity of GI smooth muscle, normal segmentation	Diarrhea or constipation
Reproductive	Maintenance of normal protein synthetic rates	*Female:* anestrus, irregular cycles, galactorrhea, stillbirth *Male:* azospermia, lack of libido
Immunologic	Stimulus of humoral and cell-mediated immunity	Recurrent infections (especially pyodermas)
Hematologic	Bone marrow stimulation, factor VIII and VIIIAg production, normal platelet synthesis and function	Nonresponsive anemia, possible bleeding tendency
Endocrine	Normal secretion of growth hormone, gonadotropins, cortisol; inhibition of secretion of prolactin	Secondary growth hormone deficiency, galactorrhea

Source: Modified from Ferguson 1989a.
Note: BMR = basal metabolic rate; CNS = central nervous system; GI = gastrointestinal.

underdeveloped epiphyses, shortened vertebral bodies, and delayed epiphyseal closure are common.

Effects on Lipid and Carbohydrate Metabolism. Thyroid hormone increases gluconeogenesis and glycogenolysis, contributing to its insulin antagonistic properties. Cholesterol synthesis and degradation are both increased by thyroid hormones and mediated by an increase in hepatic low density lipoprotein (LDL) receptors. Therefore, hypercholesterolemia is a common finding in hypothyroidism. Thyroid hormones stimulate lipolysis releasing nonesterified fatty acids (NEFAs) and glycerol. Obesity may develop in some hypothyroid animals despite a normal appetite and caloric intake. In a study of lean and obese cats, T_3 administration increased thermogenesis and NEFA concentrations, as well as mRNA for adipose tissue peroxisome proliferator-activating receptor γ (PPARγ) and D1 for lean cats (Hoenig et al. 2008).

Dermatologic Effects. Thyroid hormones in physiological quantities are necessary for normal hair and skin turnover. Thyroid insufficiency results in an increased percentage of telogen (inactive) hair follicles and an increase in keratin and sebum production. Dryness of the hair coat, excessive shedding, and retarded regrowth of hair are early signs of hypothyroidism in dogs. Alopecia, present in about two-thirds of affected dogs, is usually bilateral and symmetrical in distribution, and is most obvious over points of friction, such as the ventral trunk and neck, and axilla, and tail ("rattail" appearance) but also is common in the perineal area, and the dorsum of the tail and nose. The alopecia is classically nonpruritic unless secondary seborrhea or dermatitis has developed. Thickening of the skin and/or the development of myxedema (subcutaneous accumulation of glycosaminoglycans), develops in some cases. Myxedema is most prominent in the facial features, which may take on a puffy or "tragic" appearance. The type and distribution of dermal fatty acids can even be stimulated by replacement dosages of thyroid hormone in euthyroid animals. It is possible that this effect is truly a pharmacological effect of thyroid hormones and might explain the improvement in hair coat some dogs experience following thyroid hormone administration even when diagnostic tests fail to confirm hypothyroidism (Campbell and Davis 1990).

Cardiovascular Effects. The major physiologic effects of thyroid hormone on the myocardium are 1) a direct positive inotropic effect, 2) stimulation of myocardial hypertrophy, and 3) increased responsiveness to adrenergic stimulation. Thyroid hormones increase the sarcolemmal Na^+,K^+-ATPase activity and favor the transcription of the α or "fast-twitch" form of the cardiac myosin ATPase improving cardiac contractility. In addition, myocardial contractility is improved by increasing the number of L-type calcium channels and enhancing sarcoplasmic reticulum calcium uptake and release. Thyroid hormones increased the number of beta-adrenergic receptors in the heart, skeletal muscle, adipose tissue, and lymphocytes. In hyperthyroidism, tachycardia often results from this mechanism. Thyroid hormones also decrease alpha-adrenergic receptors in cardiac and vascular tissue. In hypothyroidism, the sensitivity to catecholamines in the peripheral vasculature is increased and may lead to peripheral hypothermia.

In dogs with hypothyroidism examined by an ECG, there is evidence of left ventricular dysfunction based upon cardiac echocardiography and electrocardiography. Following treatment with a replacement dosage of L-T_4 (0.5 mg/m^2 q12h) for 2 months, a significant decrease in shortening fraction and velocity of circumferential fiber shortening, as well as an increase in left ventricular end-systolic diameter, and prolongation of preejection period were noted when comparing measurements before and after levothyroxine supplementation. On electrocardiography, P and R wave amplitudes were significantly higher after treatment than before. Therefore, changes in cardiac function during hypothyroidism can be reversed (Panciera 1994). Despite this, administration of the same dosage of L-T_4 to euthyroid dogs did not lead to any alteration of echocardiographic or electrocardiographic measurements (Panciera and Post 1992).

Neuromuscular Effects. Thyroid hormones stimulate the synthesis of many proteins associated with normal nerve and muscle activity. For example, nerve Na^+,K^+-ATPase and fast forms of the myosin ATPase in muscle are stimulated by thyroid hormone. Myopathies have also been associated with hypothyroidism in domestic animals. Severe muscle weakness and delayed reflexes may be the clinical manifestation, or the signs may be vague such as stiffness, reluctance to move, and muscle wasting. Facial muscle and eyelid weakness (lip and lid droop) attributable to cranial nerve VII paralysis or paresis have been observed in dogs. Also, head tilt may be observed consistent with vestibular nerve disruption. These changes are likely due to the swelling of and around the dural sheath of the facial, vestibular, and cochlear nerves as they pass through bony foramina in the facial bones. Bilateral laryngeal paralysis has been associated with hypothyroidism in dogs as well. The pathophysiology of polyneuropathies associated with hypothyroidism is poorly understood but may be due to altered neuronal metabolism. Segmental demyelination and axonopathy has also been shown. Alternatively, compressive neurologic abnormalities may be the result of tissue swelling (myxedema) surrounding the spinal cord or peripheral nerve. Clinically and electrodiagnostically, the polyneuropathy is indistinguishable from those caused by other diseases with hyporeflexia, slow nerve conduction velocities, fibrillation potentials, and positive sharp waves on electromyography. Although extremely rare, central nervous system (CNS) signs of seizures, disorientation, and circling also have been reported in hypothyroid dogs with cerebrovascular atherosclerosis caused by the hyperlipidemia associated hypothyroidism. Severe mental obtundation can be also observed in the syndromes of cretinism and myxedema coma.

Gastrointestinal Effects. Studies in hypothyroid dogs have demonstrated a decrease in the intestinal and gastric electrical and motor activity. Although hypothyroid dogs usually have normal bowel movements, constipation and diarrhea have been also observed.

Reproductive Effects. Normal thyroid hormone concentrations appear to be important for normal reproductive cycling of mammals. Hypothyroidism has been associated with a variety of reproductive disturbances in dogs and horses. In breeding bitches, persistent or sporadic anestrus, infertility, abortion, and high puppy mortality have been observed. Galactorrhea is a rare sign of hypothyroidism that develops in some intact female dogs whose mammae have been primed for lactation. Hyperprolactinemia, perhaps resulting from the excessive stimulation of prolactin-secreting pituitary cells by TRH, appears to be the cause of galactorrhea in susceptible bitches and may be at least partially responsible for the infertility associated with canine hypothyroidism. Lack of libido, testicular atrophy, hypospermia, or infertility have been suspected in the male with hypothyroidism, but studies of thyroidectomized dogs showed no changes in sperm count or motility. It is possible that there are components of autoimmune orchitis coexisting with autoimmune thyroiditis in the spontaneously developing form of hypothyroidism.

Immunologic Effects. Any dog with a recurrent infection, particularly of the skin, should be evaluated for hypothyroidism. Pyoderma, which is unresponsive or only temporarily responsive to appropriate antibacterial agents, may be exacerbated by the reduced phagocytic function of white blood cells in hypothyroidism.

Hematologic Effects. The increased cellular demand for oxygen stimulated by thyroid hormone leads to increased production of erythropoietin and increased red blood cell production by the bone marrow. Thyroid hormones also increase the 2,3-diphosphoglycerate content of erythrocytes, allowing increased oxygen dissociation from hemoglobin and increased availability to tissues.

A cause-and-effect relationship between canine hypothyroidism and the development of an acquired coagulation defect (von Willebrand's disease) has been postulated, but controlled studies in hypothyroid dogs have not confirmed a relationship. Similarly, in dogs with von Willebrand's disease treated with thyroid hormone, a rise in factor VIII antigen has been described even when little evidence of primary hypothyroidism exists. The mechanism of action of thyroxine in these circumstances is uncertain, but may reflect the nonspecific action of thyroid hormone on protein synthesis. Since the breed incidence of von Willebrand's disease and hypothyroidism overlap (e.g., Doberman Pinscher, Golden Retriever, Miniature Schnauzer), it is critical to rule out the coexistence of these conditions in individual dogs where hypothyroidism may unmask a subclinical bleeding tendency. Platelet number and function can be decreased in hypothyroidism.

Endocrine Effects. Thyroid hormones influence the normal secretion and metabolism of a variety of hormones and xenobiotics. Secretion of growth hormone, gonadotropins, and cortisol are stimulated by thyroid hormones and prolactin secretion is inhibited. Hypothyroidism may cause galactorrhea due to the subsequent increase in prolactin secretion in this condition (Braverman and Utiger 1991; Burrow et al. 1989; Ferguson 1989a, 1990, 1993; Ferguson and Hoenig 1991b; Greenspan 1994; Panciera and Johnson 1994, 1996; Johnson et al. 1999).

THYROID HORMONE PREPARATIONS

Thyroid hormone preparations can be classified into the following groups: 1) crude hormones prepared from animal thyroid gland; 2) synthetic L-thyroxine (L-T_4), and 3)

TABLE 29.5 Thyroid hormone replacement products

Drug	Product Names	Dosage Range and Routes		
		Dog	Cat	Horse
L-Thyroxine	**Veterinary Products** Soloxine (Virbac) Nutrived Chewable Tablets (Vedco) Thyro-Tabs (Vet-A-Mix, Lloyd) Thyro-Form (Vet-A-Mix) Thyro-L powder (Vet-A-Mix) ThyroSyn (Vedco) LevoTabs and Levo-Powder (Vetus) Thyroxine-L Tablets and Powder (Butler) Thyrozine (Phoenix, Vedco) Amtech Levothyroxine Sodium (Phoenix) Leventa (Intervet) Liquid 1 mg/ml Canine Thyroid Chewable Tablets (Pala-Tech) Chewable Thyroid Supplement Equine Thyroid Supplement (Pala-Tech) Am-Vet T_4 Powder (Neogen) **Human Products:** Levothroid (Forest) Levoxyl (Jones Pharma) Synthroid (Abbott) Levo-T (Lederle) Eltroxin (Roberts) Levothyroxine Sodium (several) Unithroid (Watson)	0.02–0.04 mg/kg q24h or divided q12h PO or 0.5 mg/m^2 B.S.A. q24h or divided q12h PO **Rarely Necessary to Exceed:** 1 mg/day	0.02–0.04 mg/kg q24h or divided q12h PO 0.2 mg/day	0.01–0.1 mg/kg q24h or divided q12h PO 100 mg/day
L-Thyroxine Sodium for Injection:	Synthroid (Boots-Flint) Levothroid (Rorer)	100–200 μg IV or SC once	NA	NA
L-Triiodothyronine	Cytomel (Monarch)-human	4–6 μg/kg q8h po 4.4 μg/kg q8–12 h po	NA	
L-Triiodothyronine Sodium for Injection	Triostat Injection (Monarch)-human	NA	NA	NA
Combination T_4/T_3 products	Thyrolar (Forest)-human 4 : 1 T_4/T_3 ratio	Based upon T_4 dosage: see above	NA	NA
Dessicated Thyroglobulin-human	Thyroid USP (various generics) Armour Thyroid (Pfizer Canada) Thyroid Strong (Jones Medical)	NA	NA	15 grains/day/horse

NA = not appropriate, applicable, or available.
Products listed in Plumb (2005).

synthetic L-triiodothyronine (L-T_3), and combinations of T_4 and T_3. The available products and dosage ranges are listed in Table 29.5.

CRUDE THYROID PRODUCTS. Thyroid hormone products derived from thyroid tissue from hog, sheep, or cattle are available in the forms of desiccated thyroid (thyroglobulin). There are no good reasons to continue to use these products for replacement therapy in small animals; however, due to decreased cost, these products still have some utility in large animals. Problems with dessicated thyroid products include a highly variable content of T_4 and T_3, unphysiologically low ratios of T_4/T_3 (2 : 1 to 4 : 1), and short shelf life; these drawbacks outweigh the lower cost of these products. Standards set by the U.S. Pharmacopoeia for control of hormone content may have improved the reproducibility of these products but are unlikely to eliminate the other disadvantages.

SYNTHETIC L-THYROXINE. Thyroxine (L-T_4) is the thyroid hormone replacement compound of choice in all species. It is generally formulated and used as levothyroxine sodium for oral administration. Injectable forms are also available (for the rare indication of myxedema coma). Thyroxine is recommended for the following reasons:

1. L-T_4 is the main secretory product of the thyroid gland.
2. L-T_4 is the physiological "prohormone"; administration of L-T_4 does not bypass the cellular regulatory processes controlling the production of the more potent T_3 from T_4 (5′-deiodination)
3. In human patients with untreated hypothyroidism, serum TSH concentrations correlate inversely with serum free T_4 concentrations but to a lesser extent with serum T_3 concentrations. However, as mentioned previously, there is some recent evidence that there might be some clinical benefits associated with administration of a small amount of T_3 in humans, and studies in rodents have long shown that normalization of TSH values with T_4 monotherapy often results in T_4 values, which are in the high normal or high range.
4. The therapeutic goal should be to normalize both tissue and serum T_4 and T_3 concentrations, and this is accomplished only in tissues with exogenous T_4 administration.
5. The central nervous system and pituitary derive a large proportion of intracellular T_3 from local 5′-deiodination of T_4 by D2. With administration of T_3, the serum T_3 concentrations must be higher than normal to normalize serum TSH (see Fig. 29.7).

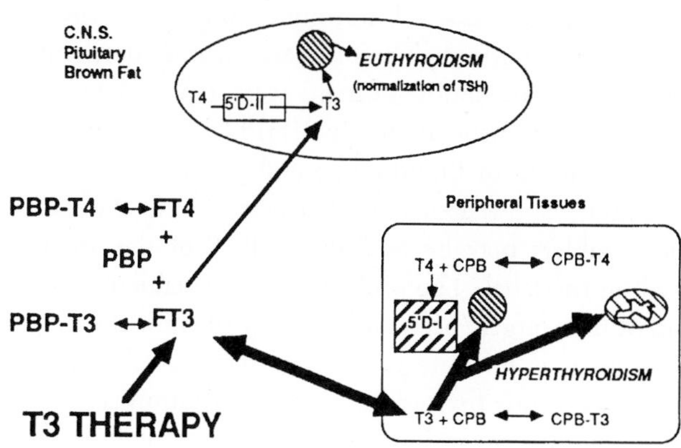

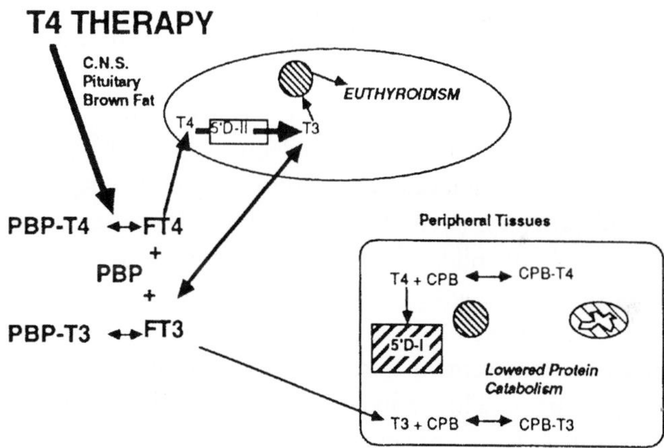

FIG. 29.7 Thyroid replacement therapy of hypothyroidism with L-T_3 (*top*) or L-T_4 in supervening nonthyroidal illness. *Top*, L-T_3 therapy during nonthyroidal illness bypasses the individual tissue regulation of the 5′-deiodinase enzymes. Shown is the scenario when the amount of T_3 administered is sufficient to re-create euthyroidism in the pituitary, brown fat, or CNS. In the pituitary, TSH secretion would be reduced to normal. This amount of T_3 would be excessive for tissues such as the liver and kidney, which are trying to limit protein catabolism during illness. A state of tissue hyperthyroidism results. *Bottom,* In contrast to therapy with L-T_3, L-T_4 therapy allows individual tissues to regulate T_3 production. Therefore, the brain, pituitary, and brown fat continue to produce adequate amounts of T_3 derived from plasma T_4, but the liver, kidney, and other tissues reduce local T_3 production, allowing a lowering of protein catabolism in illness. PBP = plasma binding protein, CBP = cytosolic binding protein, FT_3 = free triiodothyronine, FT_4 = free thyroxine. (Reprinted from Peterson and Ferguson 1990, Fig. 95-7.)

6. In general, variability in the bioavailability of synthetic T_4 preparations is less than for the crude products.
7. L-T_4 is less expensive than other synthetic preparations.

Quality Control of Thyroid Hormone Products. In 1982, the U.S. Pharmacopoeia (USP) adopted a new method for the assay of hormone content in thyroid hormone preparations. The old, less accurate determinations based upon iodine content were replaced by high pressure liquid chromatographic (HPLC) determination. Initially, studies of brand-name and generic L-thyroxine preparations showed that the hormonal content of some generic tablets may be as little as 30% of the amount stated on the label. The problems with variable hormone content have largely been addressed by the new standards. However, it is not safe to assume that the relative bioavailability of one thyroid hormone preparation is equivalent to another. Therefore, when starting an animal on a thyroid replacement product, it is recommended to start with a brand-name product (or proven generic product) with which broad experience has been obtained and use this product until a distinct clinical response has been seen. If no response is seen at a reasonable dose after a period of at least 4–6 weeks, and normal serum T_4 concentrations are achieved after administration, the diagnosis should be reevaluated. Except for financial reasons, the concern about mild overreplacement is minimal in most cases since the dog (as well as the cat) is very resistant to the development of thyrotoxic signs, requiring 10 to 20 times the replacement dose chronically in order to demonstrate signs. This is likely the result of the dog's and cat's capacity to efficiently clear thyroid hormone via biliary and fecal excretion (Ferguson 1986; Kaptein et al. 1994).

Dosage Considerations for L-Thyroxine. Thyroid hormone replacement therapy is almost always indicated for the remainder of the dog's life. Therefore, careful initial diagnosis and tailoring of treatment is essential. A variety of dosage regimens for T_4 therapy have been recommended. This probably reflects the variation between animals in hormone absorption and metabolism, the variable degree of remaining endogenous hormone secretion by the failing thyroid, the possible effect of circulating anti-T_4 antibodies in a subgroup of animals, the resistance to the development of thyrotoxicosis with overdoses in the dog, and the vague and variable criteria by which clinical improvement is judged. With the advent of the canine TSH assay, objective analysis of the body's response (at least the pituitary's) to exogenous hormone replacement is now possible and is routinely used in the monitoring of human patients with hypothyroidism. In one study, serum TSH concentration was suppressed to undetectable concentrations by a 0.02 mg/kg or less of L-T_4 given only once daily (Ferguson 2007).

In addition to the aforementioned effects of concomitant drug therapy on thyroid hormone metabolism, increased doses of T_4 appear to be necessary in hypothyroid humans during the colder months of winter. While similar studies of L-T_4 dosage have not been performed in animals, seasonal variations have been seen in dogs exposed to significant seasonal changes in light, as in racing dogs in Alaska. It is possible that an animal housed outdoors might require a higher dose of T_4 than an animal predominantly in the house, particularly during the colder months. In the dog, as in humans, basal serum concentrations of T_4 decrease with age. It has been observed in humans that older hypothyroid patients require lower doses of T_4 for adequate replacement, and are more apt to develop the adverse effects of slight thyroid hormone overdoses (Ferguson 1986; Rosychuk 1982).

Levothyroxine Dosages for the Dog. Based upon isotopic kinetic studies, L-thyroxine is produced and degraded at the rate of 7 μg/kg/day in dogs (see Table 29.2) (Kaptein et al. 1993, 1994). In general, reported oral replacement doses for T_4 in the dog range from a total dose of 0.02–0.04 mg/kg daily. Based upon this indirect evidence and unpublished studies by the author of the oral bioavailability of common brand names of levothyroxine, the fraction of oral absorption of L-T_4 products may range from 10 to 50%, averaging 35% (Ferguson and Hoenig 1997), in part explaining the variation of necessary oral dosage to attain clinical euthyroidism. Therefore, if the daily production rate of T_4 is 7 μg/kg/day, and average bioavailability is 35%, a total daily dosage of 20 μg/kg or 0.02 mg/kg is predicted. The relevance of this calculation was confirmed by observations that serum TSH was consistently suppressed to undetectable levels by once-daily dosing with a similar dosage (see Fig. 29.8) (Ferguson and Hoenig 1997; Ferguson 2007). It has also been proposed that the dosage might be calculated according to body surface area (0.5 mg/M^2) with the reasoning that it is proportional to the metabolic rate. When the L-T_4 dosage is determined on a body weight basis, large breed dogs

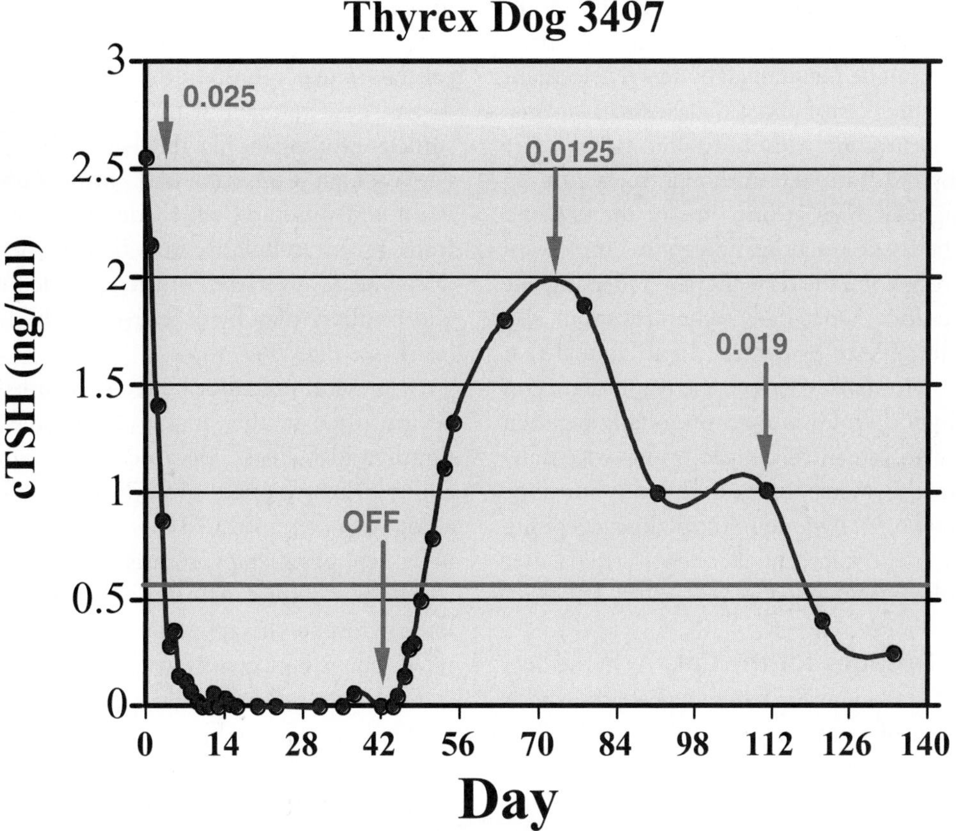

FIG. 29.8 Effect of L-T4 administration to a thyroidectomized dog on serum TSH concentrations. The numbers next to the arrows represent the dosage of L-T4 administered once daily in mg/kg. Serum samples were taken 24 hours after the last dosing. On day 42, L-T4 administration was terminated until day 70. The horizontal line represents the upper limit of the normal range for serum TSH concentration. Note the manner in which the varied L-T4 dosage titrates the serum TSH concentration demonstrating the negative feedback system on the hypothalamus and pituitary.

have a greater tendency to develop thyrotoxicosis or, at least elevated serum T_4 concentrations. For example, according to body surface area, a 5 kg (0.29 M^2 BSA) dog would start on a dose of 0.15 mg L-T_4 daily, or 0.03 mg/kg. A 50 kg dog (1.36 M^2 BSA) would start on 0.70 mg/day, or less than half the dose according to body weight, 0.014 mg/kg. There are no published experimental studies, however, to confirm the validity of this dosing method. It is rarely necessary to exceed 1 mg of levothyroxine per day in dogs, but some experts place the upper dosage at 1.6 mg per day (Ferguson 1986; Ferguson and Hoenig 1991b; Ferguson et al. 1992; Rosychuk 1982).

As thyroid replacement therapy is initiated, a common practice is to divide the total daily dosage into two separate doses given at 12-hour intervals. Because of the significant intracellular capacity for storage of T_4, particularly in rapidly exchanging pools like liver and kidney, the initial oral doses of thyroid hormone may be substantially distributed into tissue stores. As previously outlined, hypothyroidism reduces the deiodinative and conjugative rate of thyroid hormone metabolism. Division of the daily dose reduces the metabolic effect of a bolus of thyroid hormone on hypothyroid tissues and decreases the "one-pass" effect (i.e., hepatic metabolism and excretion of a portion of a bolus dose of hormone before ever reaching the systemic circulation). In the rat, the largest compartment for thyroid hormone has been shown to be the gastrointestinal tract. During the initial days to weeks of replacement therapy in a hypothyroid animal, the hormone stores of the liver and kidney are repleted to euthyroid levels, and then can serve to "buffer" serum concentrations when the circulating hormone "store" bound to binding proteins begins to be depleted. The clinical result is that many hypothyroid animals can be maintained on once-daily T_4 therapy despite the fact that the serum half-life is much shorter. In humans, it seems that clinical improvement and suppression of serum TSH can be maintained by any replacement regimen that, over the course of a day, leads to a normal average serum concentration without leading to the acute toxic effects of thyroid hormone. Although the serum T_4 concentration might be high at one time of the day and low at another, the tissue response "integrates" the serum concentration throughout the day, thereby reflecting the average concentration. Once-daily administration also leads to greater compliance by owners. In an animal that has responded to twice-daily therapy, the reappearance of clinical signs of hypothyroidism on a once-daily regimen should be a signal to return to the successful twice-daily regimen. Because the metabolism of thyroid hormone changes with correction of hypothyroidism, dosage regimes should be reassessed by clinical and laboratory criteria after at least 4 weeks of initial therapy.

Levothyroxine Dosages for the Cat. As in the dog, the recommended treatment for feline hypothyroidism is daily administration of L-thyroxine, using an initial dose of 0.1 to 0.2 mg/day. This dosage should subsequently be adjusted on the basis of the cat's clinical response and postpill serum T_4 evaluation (as described below under "Monitoring Therapy"). Complete resolution of clinical signs can usually be expected in cats with adult-onset iatrogenic hypothyroidism. However, the mental dullness and dwarfism that develops in kittens with hypothyroidism usually persist because of delayed period of time from onset to diagnosis in these cats (Peterson and Ferguson 1990; Rosychuk 1982).

Levothyroxine Dosages for the Horse. There is little published information establishing therapeutic criteria for levothyroxine dosing in the horse. The oral L-T_4 dosage required clinically appears to depend largely on the form of hormone (crude versus synthetic) used for replacement therapy.

SYNTHETIC L-TRIIODOTHYRONINE. Although T_3 is the active intracellular hormone, there are few valid reasons to use this product for replacement therapy and some good reasons not to use it. Triiodothyronine therapy is not physiological as it bypasses the final cellular regulatory step of 5′-deiodination of T_4 (see Fig. 29.7). Thyroxine does have intrinsic thyromimetic activity. Its role is particularly important in the central nervous system and pituitary, tissues in which normalization of the intracellular T_3 concentration depends upon the normalization of both serum T_4 and T_3. Treatment with T_3 alone may provide amounts sufficient for organs like the liver, kidney, and heart, which derive a high proportion of T_3 from plasma. However, the brain and pituitary, which derive a majority of their T_3 from T_4 intracellularly, may then be deficient in thyroid hormone. Conversely, T_3 therapy adequate for the brain and pituitary may be excessive for the liver, kidney, and heart (see Fig. 29.7, top).

At present, it cannot be recommended that T_3 therapy be instituted in the "low T_3 syndrome" associated with nonthyroidal illness. Because of its higher oral bioavailability, it may be used to improve the clinical response in a dog with demonstrated or suspected poor T_4 absorption in which posttherapy serum T_4 and T_3 concentrations remain low despite increases in the oral daily T_4 dose. Triiodothyronine therapy may be indicated when thyroid replacement is necessary with the simultaneous administration of drugs, such as glucocorticoids, which inhibit the conversion of T_4 to T_3.

Anecdotal reports suggest that a small fraction of hypothyroid dogs convert T_4 to T_3 poorly in the absence of obvious nonthyroidal illness, and therefore, do not respond to L-T_4 therapy. Triiodothyronine therapy has been recommended in these cases as an adjunct to T_4 or as sole therapy. The most likely cause of apparently low serum T_3 concentrations and normal or high T_4 concentrations following T_4 therapy is the presence of anti-T_3 antibodies that, in certain T_3 radioimmunoassays, will result an extremely low reading for the T_3 concentration. This observation is an in vitro artifact, which has no relevance to the choice of replacement therapy products. Because the binding capacity of antithyroid hormone antibodies is easily overcome in most cases, it is recommended that usual dosages of L-T_4 be administered and the dose increased (if needed) until a clinical response is seen. The posttreatment serum T_3 concentration should be ignored in these dogs with T_3 autoantibodies (Ferguson 1986; Rosychuk 1982).

Combination T_4/T_3 Therapy. A study in humans compared the administration of solely T_4, with replacing 50 μg of the normal T_4 dose with 12.5 μg of T_3. Using neuropsychological methods for evaluation, the T_3-treated individuals showed improved cognitive performance (Bunevicius et al. 1999). This approach is controversial because other studies have not confirmed the finding. Similar studies have not been conducted in domestic animals.

Triiodothyronine (T_3) Suppression Test in the Cat. As part of a workup for hyperthyroidism in cats, the administration of L-T_3 is utilized to evaluate the autonomy of thyroid secretion from the influence of pituitary TSH. L-triiodothyronine is administered at a dose of 25 μg every 8 hours for 2 days giving a seventh dose on the morning of the 3rd day. A blood sample for serum T_4 measurement is taken before T_3 administration and again at 4 hours after the last dose. Presumably mediated via a fall in pituitary TSH, serum T_4 is depressed by at least 50% in normal cats, whereas little suppression is seen in cats with hyperthyroidism because TSH is already depressed. The advantages of this test are that the doses of T_3 can be given at home on an outpatient basis with an office visit 4 hours after the last dose (Graves and Peterson 1994; Peterson and Ferguson 1990). The disadvantage is that there may be less than full compliance with successful administration of the seven doses of L-T_3 by the owner.

EFFECTS OF THYROID HORMONE OVERDOSE (IATROGENIC THYROTOXICOSIS). Except for financial reasons, the concern about mild overreplacement is minimal in most cases as the dog is very resistant to the development of thyrotoxic signs. This resistance to iatrogenic thyrotoxicosis is the result of the dog's capacity to efficiently clear thyroid hormone via biliary and fecal excretion. Animals on replacement therapy, particularly with a T_3-containing product, can develop signs of thyrotoxicosis, particularly in large breed dogs dosed on a body weight basis; however, the incidence at recommended doses is rare. Animals should be monitored for signs suggesting an overdose including polyuria, polydipsia, nervousness, weight loss, increase in appetite, panting, and fever. Diagnosis is confirmed by elevated serum T_4 and/or T_3 concentrations and the amelioration of signs by temporary discontinuation of therapy. Following accidental ingestion of massive amounts of levothyroxine, dogs should be treated with activated charcoal within several hours of ingestion, possibly managed with beta-adrenergic blockers if tachycardic, and heart rate and body temperature should be carefully monitored. Clinical experience has generally shown that dogs survive intoxication with few side effects despite considerable elevations in serum T_4 and T_3 concentrations.

THERAPEUTIC TRIAL FOR DIAGNOSIS OF HYPOTHYROIDISM. Thyroid replacement therapy, without confirmatory laboratory evidence of hypothyroidism, has been suggested as a valid diagnostic step in a dog suspected to be hypothyroid. Although the major factor cited in defense of this practice is the cost of the diagnostic testing for the owner, it should be emphasized to an owner that replacement therapy is generally necessary for the remainder of the animal's life. Therefore, an incorrect diagnosis (and unnecessary long-term thyroid hormone treatment) can also be quite expensive. In one study of normal dogs given L-T_4 at the dosage of 0.5 mg/m^2 twice daily, the mean serum T_4 response to exogenous TSH had suppressed to 56% and 46% of the pretreatment value when retested at 4 and 8 weeks on treatment, respectively. Four weeks after cessation of L-T_4 therapy, the serum T_4 response to TSH was still slightly suppressed, indicative of residual thyroid atrophy (Panciera et al. 1990). Therefore, if TSH stimulation testing is used to confirm the diagnosis of hypothyroidism in a dog that has recently been receiving thyroid hormone, TSH testing should not be performed for at least 4 weeks following discontinuation of thyroid hormone replacement therapy.

MONITORING THERAPY. The most important indicator of the success of thyroid replacement therapy is the progress made toward ameliorating clinical signs. Before therapy is begun, the clinician and owner should have a clear idea of the goals of therapy and the time frame in which these goals can reasonably be achieved. The reversal of changes in haircoat and body weight should be assessed no sooner than after 2 months of therapy. In cases in which clinical improvement is marginal or signs of thyrotoxicosis are seen, the clinical observations can be supported by therapeutic monitoring of serum thyroid hormone concentrations (postpill testing). Clearly, the documentation of distinctly elevated serum T_4 concentrations following T_4 administration and elevated serum T_3 concentrations following T_3 administration, concomitant with signs of thyrotoxicosis, confirm an overdose. The interpretation of postpill serum thyroid hormone concentrations in cases of suspected underdosing can be more complicated because the timing of sampling may be critical to the proper interpretation. Ideally, therapeutic monitoring should not be attempted until steady-state conditions are reached, minimally 1 week after the initiation of therapy from a pharmacokinetic standpoint, but probably 1 month after initiation of therapy from a pharmacodynamic and clinical standpoint. With once-daily T_4 administration, the peak serum concentrations of T_4 generally should be in the high-normal to slightly high range 4–8 hours after dosing and should be low normal to normal 24 hours after dosing. Given the dog's resistance to signs of thyrotoxicosis, it may be reasonable and adequate to check the serum T_4 concentration 24 hours after the previous day's dose. This is the method of choice of the author. In this situation, serum T_4 concentrations should still be in the normal range. Some endocrinologists prefer to measure "peak" T_4 concentrations at 4 or 6 hours after once-daily dosing, and some measure at "peak" and "trough" times. Animals on twice-daily administration probably can be checked at any time, but peak concentrations can be expected at the middle of the dosing interval (4–8 hours) and the nadir just prior to the next dose. Once the dog's dose is stabilized, once- or twice-yearly checks of serum T_4 (with or without T_3) concentrations are recommended

Monitoring L-T_4 therapy may also be accomplished by documenting suppression of serum TSH. Although with the current generation of TSH, concentrations are elevated only in about 75% of cases, detectable TSH concentrations within the normal range still appear sensitive to titration of T_4 dosage (Fig. 29.8). In a study of treatment of thyroidectomized dogs, it was shown that dosages as little as 0.02 mg/kg once a day will almost always suppress endogenous TSH concentrations into the normal or undetectable range. This observation establishes that the biological half-life of thyroid hormone exceeds by far the serum half-life (Ferguson and Hoenig 1997). However, although titration of L-T_4 dosage by monitoring endogenous TSH concentrations is standard practice in hypothyroid human patients, no study has yet evaluated whether TSH suppression correlates consistently with a satisfactory clinical response in dogs. Therefore, it appears clear that dosing protocols recommending the dosage of 0.02 mg/kg twice daily probably reflect the dosage necessary for dogs with the lowest T_4 bioavailability. Unfortunately, the assay sensitivity does not allow the distinction of normal values from low values, so establishment of overtreatment and hyperthyroidism is not yet possible.

Although not recommended routinely, serum T_3 measurements following L-thyroxine administration should be interpreted together with the serum T_4 results and, most importantly, the clinical response. Low serum T_3 and T_4 concentrations, together with a poor clinical response, suggest an underdose or inadequate bioavailability (absorption). With T_3 administration, serum concentrations are reported to peak 2–3 hours after administration. Serum T_4 concentrations are routinely low or undetectable in dogs receiving T_3 therapy. Any remaining endogenous thyroidal T_4 secretion will be inhibited because of the suppression of pituitary TSH secretion by T_3 (Ferguson 1986; Peterson and Ferguson 1990; Rosychuk 1982).

THERAPEUTIC FAILURE. If clinical signs of hypothyroidism remain despite the use of reasonable doses of thyroid hormone, the following possibilities must be considered: 1) the dose or frequency of administration is improper; 2) the owner is not complying with instructions or is not successfully administrating the product; 3) the animal may not be absorbing the product well, or is metabolizing and/or excreting it too rapidly; 4) the product is outdated; or 5) the diagnosis is incorrect. A syndrome of tissue resistance to thyroid hormone, while described in humans, has not yet been documented in the dog or cat.

TREATMENT OF MYXEDEMA COMA. Myxedema coma is a rare condition in domestic animals, only described in dogs, and is caused by severe untreated hypothyroidism. Often induced by an anesthetic episode or concurrent infectious disease, it results in severe mental obtundation or coma, and hypothermia. Common physical examination abnormalities include obesity and nonpitting edema (myxedema), and anemia and hypercholesterolemia are clinicopathological findings (Pullen and Hess 2006). Because of the extremely high mortality associated with this condition, it is essential that treatment be instituted promptly and vigorously as soon as the diagnosis is made. Treatment should include an intravenous dose of L-T_4 prepared for injection (100–200 μg total dose or 4–5 μg/kg), passive rewarming (wrapping in blankets, etc.), and mechanical respiratory support as needed. Therapy for shock must include glucocorticoids and fluid and electrolyte replacement. Oral thyroxine therapy can be instituted when the animal stabilizes. A recent study (Pullen and Hess 2006) of seven severely hypothyroid dogs treated with 4–5 μg/kg of L-T_4 IV observed improvement in mentation or ambulation and systolic hypotension within 30 hours of IV levothyroxine administration. Prognosis is good in most treated dogs.

ANTITHYROID DRUGS

GOITROGENS. With the isolation and purification of thyroid peroxidase (TPO) enzyme of the thyroid gland, it became apparent that most compounds with antithyroid (goitrogenic) activity are inhibitors of TPO-catalyzed iodination. Plants of the genus *Brassica,* such as rutabaga, cabbage, and turnip contain a compound called *goitrin* (see structure in Fig. 29.9), which has antithyroid activity. In addition, plants such as broccoli and rapeseed include glucosinolates, which are metabolized to thiocyanate, an inhibitor of thyroid iodide uptake and organification. The so-called "cyanogenic glucosides," found in foods such as cassava, lima beans, and sweet potatoes can be a source of cyanide, which then is detoxified to thiocyanate. Substituted phenols, such as resorcinol, phloroglucinol and 2,4, dihydroxybenzoic acid, which may be found as contaminants in the water supply near coal conversion plants and may arise from degradation of flavonoids in plant material, also have goitrogenic activity (Taurog 1991; Brucker-Davis 1998).

Studies have raised questions about the goitrogenic potential of environmental polyhalogenated aryl hydrocarbons (PHAHs), polychlorinated biphenyls (PCBs), polybrominated diphenyl ethers (PBDEs), plasticizer bisphenol A (BPA), and perchlorate on thyroid function. PHAHs have the particular potential to be retained by cats who have low glucuronyltransferase activity, and very high serum concentrations of PBDEs; dietary concentrations of BPA in cat food have been linked epidemiologically if not mechanistically to the development of feline hyperthyroidism. Confirmation of the link and the possible mechanisms still awaits further research (Edinboro et al. 2004; Dye et al. 2007; Mensching et al. 2007).

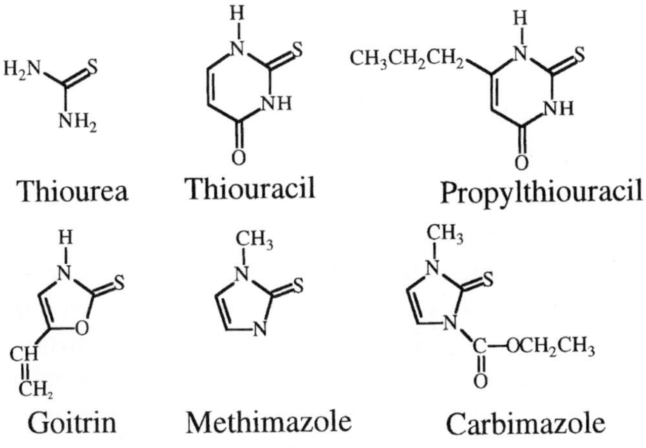

Thiourea Thiouracil Propylthiouracil

Goitrin Methimazole Carbimazole

FIG. 29.9 Thioureylene antithyroid drugs.

THIOUREYLENES OR THIONAMIDES. Antithyroid thioureylene or thionamide drugs act by being direct inhibitors of the thyroid peroxidase (TPO) leading to a reduction in the organification and coupling steps of thyroid hormone synthesis. Figure 29.9 shows the structure of thiourea, goitrin, and the antithyroid drugs thiouracil, propylthiouracil, methimazole, and carbimazole. After administration, these drugs are actively concentrated by the thyroid gland, where they act to inhibit the synthesis of thyroid hormones through the following mechanisms: 1) blocking the incorporation of iodine into the tyrosyl groups in thyroglobulin, 2) preventing the coupling of iodotyrosyl groups (mono- and diiodotyrosines) to form the ether linkage of T_4 and T_3, and 3) direct interactions with the thyroglobulin molecule (see Fig. 29.1). Processes 1 and 2 are mediated via inhibition of the enzyme thyroid peroxidase (TPO). Thionamide antithyroid drugs do not interfere with the thyroid gland's ability to concentrate, or "trap," inorganic iodine, do not block the release of stored thyroid hormone into the circulation, and do not damage the thyroid glandular tissue.

The thionamide drugs propylthiouracil (PTU) and methimazole (MMI) are the most commonly used antithyroid drugs in veterinary clinical practice (see Table 29.6 for products and dosages). Following initiation of treatment with MMI or PTU there is usually a slight delay in the fall of serum thyroid hormone concentrations as glandular hormone stores are becoming depleted. PTU has the additional beneficial effect of blocking the conversion of T_4 to the more active T_3 in peripheral tissues like the liver and kidney. Therefore, serum T_4 may fall following both PTU and MMI therapy, but with MMI, due to autoregulatory mechanisms in the peripheral tissues (most likely up-regulation of D2 activity), serum T_3 is usually maintained within the normal range even when T_4 is quite low. As a result of this mechanism, it is rare to see a cat on MMI develop clinical signs of hypothyroidism. In some elderly hyperthyroid cats, elevations in serum creatinine with occasional overt renal failure develops. In cases where pretreatment renal function is in question, the use of MMI has gained favor because it provides a reversible and more gradual mode of therapy for returning the animal to euthy-

TABLE 29.6 Antithyroid drugs

Drug	Product Name	Dosage Range and Route (Cats Only)
Methimazole	Tapazole™ (Jones Pharma)	Initial: 2.5–5 mg q8–12 h PO mg q24h or divided q12h PO Maintenance: 2.55–20 mg daily
Carbimazole	Neomercazole™ (Available in Europe, Canada)	Same as Methimazole
Propylthiouracil	Propylthiouracil USP	50 mg q8–12 h PO (generic)
Iopanoic Acid	Telepaque™ (Amersham Health)	50 mg q12h PO (Note: dosage lowers serum T_3 only)
Potassium Iodine (Lugol's)		50 mg q12–24 h PO

roidism. It is not yet known whether the changes in renal function parameters are associated with the correction of hyperthyroidism to euthyroidism or rather to the transient development of hypothyroidism.

Propylthiouracil. Propylthiouracil (PTU) is the prototype D1 inhibitor as well as being a TPO inhibitor. Despite its apparent additional therapeutic effects, the use of PTU has fallen out of favor because of its potential for serious side effects. Like MMI, it can cause anorexia, vomiting, lethargy, and the development of positive antinuclear antibody titers, but has been associated with the development of autoimmune hemolytic anemia and immune-mediated thrombocytopenia. Because of the latter two complications, which are a particular problem in the animal being prepared for surgery, PTU can no longer be recommended for routine use in the hyperthyroid cat (Ferguson and Hoenig 1991a; Ferguson et al. 1992; Kintzer 1994; Peterson and Ferguson 1990).

Methimazole. Methimazole is now the antithyroid medication of choice in the cat. The use of this drug in the cat has been well-documented by a 20-year-old study of a 3-year experience with the drug in almost 300 cats. In this study, doses as high as 5 mg q8h were applied, which reduced the serum T_4 into the normal range by 2–3 weeks. Since that time, most cats are diagnosed at an earlier phase of disease and MMI doses most commonly begin at 2.5 mg once or twice daily and are titrated upward in 2.5 mg (1/2 tablet) intervals until the serum T_4 concentration falls within the normal range. As mentioned, even cats with low serum T_4 may not become hypothyroid because the serum T_3 concentration generally remains normal. Once a satisfactory therapeutic effect is seen, many cats can be maintained on once-daily therapy, a major advantage for owner compliance. However, if a daily dose is missed, the serum T_4 concentration may rise rapidly. Cats on chronic MMI therapy should be checked every 3 to 6 months to draw blood for serum T_4 measurement and to monitor for signs of drug toxicity (see below) (Peterson et al. 1988; Trepanier 2007).

Pharmacokinetics and Pharmacodynamics of Methimazole. In euthyroid cats, the serum half-life has ranged from 4–6 hours following an IV dose. Following 2 weeks of oral methimazole, an average half-life of 3.4 ± 0.2 hours was measured with less variability. In hyperthyroid cats, while the half-life was no different from euthyroid cats (2.3 ± 0.4 hours), the mean residence time was shorter. Several studies in euthyroid and normal cats show bioavailability as averaging about 80%, with significant variability in bioavailability between animals. Studies in human hyperthyroid patients have shown that the drug has an intrathyroidal residence time of approximately 20 hours, which is fourfold longer than the serum half-life. Since antithyroid drugs act to inhibit thyroid hormone synthesis only after they are concentrated within the thyroid gland, serum half-life of these drugs may be of lesser importance than the intrathyroidal drug concentration for adequate control of the hyperthyroid state. There is usually a 1–3-week lag time between starting the drug and significant reductions in serum T_4 (Trepanier et al. 1989, 1991a,b).

Adverse Effects of Methimazole. Methimazole has been associated with the following adverse effects: anorexia (11.1%), vomiting (10.7%), lethargy (8.8%), excoriations (2.3%), bleeding (2.3%), hepatopathy (1.5%), thrombocytopenia (2.7%), agranulocytosis (1.5%), leukopenia (4.7%), eosinophilia (11.3%), lymphocytosis (7.2%), positive ANA (21.8%), and positive direct antiglobulin test (1.9%). The gastrointestinal adverse effects generally developed within the first month of treatment and usually resolved even with continued therapy.

Mild clinical side effects associated with methimazole treatment are relatively common (approximately 15% of cats) and include anorexia, vomiting, and lethargy. In most cats, these adverse signs are transient and resolve despite continued administration of the drug. Severe gastrointestinal signs persist in some cats, however, necessitating discontinuation of the drug. Self-induced excoriations of the face and neck also may develop in a few cats within the first 6 weeks of therapy. Although these cutaneous lesions tend to be partially responsive to treatment with systemic glucocorticoids, cessation of methimazole administration is usually required for complete resolution of these excoriations. Finally, hepatic toxicity is an uncommon but serious reaction that can develop during drug treatment. Methimazole-induced hepatopathy is characterized by the development of marked increases in serum concentrations of ALT, AST, SAP, and total bilirubin. Clinical improvement, with resolution of anorexia, vomiting, and lethargy, usually occurs within a few days after cessation of methimazole, but jaundice and abnormal serum biochemical tests indicative of liver disease may not resolve for several weeks. Rechallenge with the drug will again induce clinical signs and serum biochemical abnormalities indicative of hepatic disease within a few days. A variety of hematologic abnormalities may develop in cats during treatment with methimazole. Those abnormalities that do not appear to be associated with any adverse effects include eosinophilia, lymphocytosis, and transient leukopenia with a normal differential count. As with PTU treatment, more serious hematologic reactions that develop in a few cats treated with methimazole include severe thrombocytopenia (platelet count <75,000 cells/mm^3) and agranulocytosis (severe leukopenia with a total granulocyte count <250 cells/mm^3). Most cats that develop severe thrombocytopenia also show concomitant overt bleeding (i.e., epistaxis, oral hemorrhage). Development of agranulocytosis during methimazole treatment predisposes to severe bacterial infections, systemic toxicity, and fever. If serious hematologic reactions develop during methimazole therapy, the drug should be stopped and supportive care given; these adverse reactions should resolve within 5 days after the methimazole is withdrawn. Since most life-threatening side effects (e.g., hepatopathy, thrombocytopenia, agranulocytosis) caused by methimazole treatment usually again develop quickly after rechallenge with the drug, alternative therapy with either surgery or radioiodine should be considered in these cases.

During methimazole therapy, serum antinuclear antibodies (ANA) develop in a high percentage of cats after treatment with methimazole. The risk of developing ANA appears to increase with the duration of methimazole treatment, with ANA developing in approximately half of cats treated for greater than 6 months. The risk of developing serum ANA also appears to be greater for cats treated with higher daily methimazole doses, since most cats that develop ANA are receiving doses ≥15 mg/day and ANA will disappear in most cats after the dosage is decreased. Despite the high prevalence of ANA development during long-term treatment with methimazole, clinical signs associated with a lupuslike syndrome (i.e., dermatitis, polyarthritis, glomerulonephritis, hemolytic anemia, or fever) have not been observed in any of these cats. The daily drug dosage should therefore be decreased to as low as possible (while still maintaining serum T_4 values within the low-normal range), since ANA tests will become negative in many cats when the methimazole dosage is decreased.

Transdermal Methimazole. Methimazole compounded in a pluronic lecithin organogel (PLO) dosage form has begun to be offered by compounding pharmacists. Transdermal pluronic gels have been shown to modulate permeation of a variety of drugs from small organics to peptides. Lecithin is an emulsifying agent that increases fluidity of stratum corneum, and can result in exfoliation and low-grade inflammation, resulting in greater absorption when given chronically. Transdermal administration may be considered when oral therapy of MMI is impractical in a cat. Although a pharmacokinetic study initially showed poor to no bioavailability for methimazole formulated in PLO and administered as a single dose inside the pinna of healthy cats, studies of daily administration to hyperthyroid cats for 4 weeks have reported clinical response and reduction of serum T_4 concentrations. The time to optimal reduction of serum T_4 response to treatment tends to be slower than with oral therapy. Furthermore, the response is more variable, possibly because of greater variability in factors determining transdermal bioavailability. Despite questionable absorption in euthyroid cats following a single dose, a study by Sartor et al. (2004) evaluated the efficacy and safety of transdermal MMI in 47 hyperthyroid cats. A randomized clinical trial compared transdermal with oral MMI at 2.5 mg q12h for both routes. While 88% of cats treated by oral route had serum T_4 concentrations within the reference range after 2 weeks, 56% of transdermally treated cats reached this goal. This efficacy gap reduced to 80% with oral administration and 67% by transdermal administration (not significant). Oral MMI cats had a higher incidence of gastrointestinal (GI) adverse effects (24%) compared to the cats treated with transdermal methimazole (4%), but no differences were found between groups in the incidence of other side effects. In this study, the absolute bioavailability (compared to IV route) was 40% for the oral and transdermal routes. Another study of 13 hyperthyroid cats given 5 mg/0.1 ml of MMI q12h showed that total T_4 concentrations fell to 28% of baseline at 14 days and 15% of baseline (low normal range) at 28 days. The gastrointestinal side effects also appeared reduced with the transdermal route (Lecuyer et al. 2006).

Methimazole and Thyroid Scintigraphy. Based on a study in hyperthyroid cats, concurrent methimazole treatment does not affect results of diagnostic pertechnetate [$^{99m}TcO_4$] thyroid scans. However, some hyperthyroid cats were diagnosed by thyroid scan as having unilateral disease before MMI treatment, and then, once euthyroid, appeared to have bilateral disease when scanned again. Enhanced uptake of pertechnetate occurred for 2 to 3 weeks after the end of methimazole treatment of normal cats. These scintigraphic findings are likely an artifact of seeing intense pertechnetate uptake in large hyperfunctional thyroid nodules, and then, upon reduction of T_4, the increase of TSH would stimulate the normal tissue or less active tissue to take up [$^{99m}TcO_4$.]

Monitoring Patients on Methimazole. In addition to serum total T_4 or possibly even TSH concentrations, the following liver function tests are recommended: alanine aminotransferase (ALT), alkaline phosphatase (SAP) and/or aspartate aminotransferase (AST), and total bilirubin. Alkaline phosphatase is likely high in hyperthyroidism because of an elevation of the bone isoenzyme associated with increased calcium turnover. Renal function tests including blood urea nitrogen (BUN) and creatinine concentrations are important in the first month of treatment to monitor the effect of correction of hyperthyroidism on reduction of GFR. Complete blood count (CBC) and platelet count should be periodically monitored as peak chance of autoimmune phenomena is at about 3 months of therapy (Peterson et al. 1988; Trepanier 2007).

Carbimazole. The antithyroid drug carbimazole is a carbethoxy derivative of methimazole that is rapidly and completely metabolized to the parent compound, which is reponsible for its antithyroid activity. It is commonly used in treatment of feline hyperthyroidism outside of North America. Carbimazole is a larger molecule than methimazole; 10 mg of carbimazole is equimolar to 6 mg methimazole. To achieve the same effect with carbimazole as with methimazole, approximately twice the dosage of carbimazole would be required. Clinical experience in Europe describes fewer gastrointestinal side effects for this medication likely because this prodrug reduces direct contact of methimazole on gastrointestinal mucosa. Transdermal administration of MMI has also been associated with lower gastrointestinal side effects (Peterson and Becker 1984; Trepanier 2007).

MEDICAL OPTIONS TO THIONAMIDE DRUGS. When cats have adverse reactions to the thionamides, if the reaction is gastrointestinal, often a reduction of the dosage or conversion to carbimazole or transdermal therapy will reduce side effects (see above). However, if the reaction is an allergic one, the antithyroid drug class must be changed if medical therapy is still going to be pursued. PTU and carbimazole as thionamides with similar structure would not then be an option; transdermal therapy with methimazole would also not be an option.

Iodinated Radiocontrast Agents. In human medicine, iodinated radiocontrast agents have been employed as adjunctive antithyroid drugs. These agents have several potential mechanisms of action:

1. *Release of iodide, which can transiently suppress thyroid secretion through the Wolff-Chaikoff effect.* This effect seems insignificant in cats as serum T_4 concentrations rarely fall with these agents; however, the effect should be considered if therapy is to precede ^{131}I treatment.
2. *Direct inhibition of both D1 and D2 enzymes reducing the production of more bioactive T_3.* This effect appears to be the most dramatic effect in cats, and efficacy is best monitored by documenting the reduction of serum T_3 into the normal range despite an elevated serum T_4 concentration
3. *Inhibition of uptake and/or nuclear receptor binding of T_3.* This mechanism has not been documented in cat tissues.

The first such agent used in managing feline hyperthyroidism was the biliary contrast agent, ipodate, which was shown in both experimental hyperthyroidism and in spontaneously hyperthyroid cats to be an alternative medical treatment for patients not tolerating MMI or PTU. In a study of cats in which hyperthyroidism was experimentally induced by the administration of T_4, ipodate significantly reduced the serum T_3 concentrations and was well-tolerated by otherwise healthy cats (Chopra et al. 1984; Ferguson et al. 1988; Murray and Peterson 1997). Ipodate was removed from the market several years ago and has largely been replaced in veterinary use by iopanoic acid. Iopanoic acid contains three iodines and is 67% iodine by weight (Figure 29.10). The recommended dose of 50 mg q12h has apparently been borrowed directly from pharmacodynamic studies in experimental cats with ipodate, and reports of clinical efficacy of iopanoic acid have largely been anecdotal to date. Other drugs in this class include diatrizoic acid.

Radioactive Iodine (^{131}I) Therapy. Although only available in specialty referral centers, radioiodine treatment is the most effective and selective cure for toxic goiter in the cat because it selectively destroys the functioning thyroid tissue after being taken up and incorporated into thyroid hormone precursors in the thyroid gland. There is rarely, if ever, damage to the nearby tissue responsible for regulating serum calcium by the secretion of parathyroid hormone and calcitonin. Iodine-131 has a half-life of 8 days and produces both gamma and beta radiation. The beta particles, with a short pathlength, serve to produce most of the local tissue destruction. Radioiodine is also used in much higher doses in an attempt to ablate thyroid adenocarcinomas in cats and dogs. Following a therapeutic dose (generally 1–5 mCi) of ^{131}I, the serum T_4 and T_3 concentrations will commonly normalize within 1 to 2 weeks. The major disadvantage of radioiodine therapy is that certain radiation safety precautions must be taken. Radioiodine is secreted in saliva, and excreted in urine and feces. As such, handling of the cat's haircoat or waste may result in contamination. Unlike human patients who may receive therapeutic doses on a outpatient basis, radioiodine-treated cats must be hospitalized for periods of time (3 days to 4 weeks), which depend upon the dose administered and the state's radiation safety regulations. Despite these drawbacks, radioiodine therapy is the least invasive cure for bilateral adenomatous goiter, has no hypoparathyroidism or toxicity associated with it, and can be implemented without anesthesia or sedation, an important consideration in the elderly cat with other medical complications (Kintzer and Peterson 1991, 1994; Meric et al. 1986).

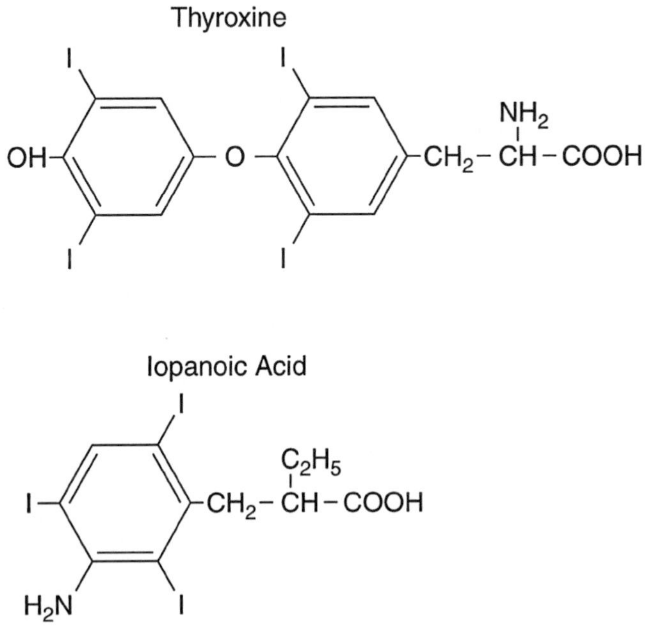

Regarding the efficacy and prognosis for survival following radiiodide therapy, a study of 231 cats being treated with ^{131}I was performed (Slater et al. 2001). With a mean age at diagnosis of 13 years, the treated cats had a median survival time of 25 months. Hypothyroidism was present in five cats (2.2%), and hyperthyroidism was present in one (0.4%). While there was a 33% incidence of renal disease after treatment, it was not clear how many cats might have had this problem at diagnosis.

Thyroxine

Iopanoic Acid

FIG. 29.10 Comparison of structure of radiocontrast agent iopanoic acid to L-thyroxine. (Modified from Larsen et al., 2003; Williams Textbook of Endocrinology, 10th edition, Fig. 10-7, p. 344.)

THYROID IMAGING

Thyroid imaging is performed using radioactive iodine or $^{99m}TcO_4^-$ (pertechnetate), which is taken up by mechanisms similar to iodide, but is not incorporated into iodothyronines on thyroglobulin. Because of its rapid uptake and increased safety, technetium can be given in higher diagnostic doses and provides a better image than radioiodine. In cats with palpable goiter but normal serum total T_4 and/or free T_4 concentrations, a semiquantitative thyroid scintigraphy would seem to be a more sensitive method for confirmation of disease. With this assumption, Daniel and co-workers (2002) used this approach to quantify pertechnetate uptake in 43 cats with hyperthyroidism and 8 normal control cats. The 20-minute thyroid:salivary ratio of the most intense lobe correlated best with serum T_4 concentrations, and the authors concluded that this ratio was a valuable predictor of the thyroid status. However, another study (Tomsa et al. 2001) found increased thyroid : salivary (T : S) ratios in cats with no demonstrable histopathology, suggesting that either the cats were true false positives, false positives associated with iodine depletion, or true positives with false negative histopathology. These results do raise the important issue of controlling for iodine repletion when establishing normal T : S pertechnetate ratios. Thyroid imaging also aids the diagnosis when an obvious enlargement of one thyroid lobe exists. Imaging is particularly useful in the diagnosis of the 30% of cases that are unilateral as the function of the contralateral lobe is suppressed and not apparent on the scan. Thyroid imaging is also useful in cats with adenomas that have slipped into the mediastinum or the 1–2% of cats with adenocarcinomas that have a tendency to metastasize by extension into the mediastinum (Kintzer and Peterson 1991, 1994).

REFERENCES

Attia MA, Aref H. 1991. Hepatic microsomal enzyme induction and thyroid function in rats treated with high doses of phenobarbital or chlorpromazine. Deutsch Tierarzt Wschr 98:205–244.

Baqui M, Botero D, Gereben B, Curcio C, Harney JW, Salvatore D, Sorimachi K, Larsen PR, Bianco AC. 2003. Human type 3 iodothyronine selenodeiodinase is located in the plasma membrane and undergoes rapid internalization to endosomes. J Biol Chem 278(2):1206–1211.

Barter RA, Klaassen CD. 1994. Reduction of thyroid hormone levels and alteration on thyroid function by four representative UDP-glucuronosyltransferase inducers in rats. Toxicol Appl Pharmacol 128:9–17.

Becker TJ, Graves TK, Kruger JM, et al. 2000. Effects of methimazole on renal function in cats with hyperthyroidism. J Am Anim Hosp Assoc 36(3):215–23.

Belshaw BE, Barandes M, Becker DV. 1974. A model of iodine kinetics in the dog. Endocrinology 95:1078–1093.

Bernal J, Guadano-Ferraz A, Morte B. 2003. Perspectives in the study of thyroid hormone action on brain development and function. Thyroid 13(11):1005–12.

Bianco AC, Salvatore D, Gereben B, Berry MJ, Larsen PR. 2002. Biochemistry, cellular and molecular biology, and physiological roles of the iodothyronine selenodeiodinases. Endocr Rev 23(1): 38–89.

Bigler B. 1976. Thyroxine-binding serum proteins in the cat: A comparison with dog and man. Schweiz Archiv Tierheilkd 118(12):559–662.

Blange I, Drvota V, Yen PM, Sylven C. 1997. Species differences in cardiac thyroid hormone receptor isoforms protein abundance. Biol Pharm Bull 20(11):1123–6.

Braverman LE, Utiger RD (eds). 1991. Werner and Ingbar's The Thyroid: A Fundamental and Clinical Text, 6th ed. Philadelphia: Lippincott.

Brent GA, Moore DD, Larsen PR. 1991. Thyroid hormone regulation of gene expression. Ann Rev Physiol 53:17–35.

Brucker-Davis, F. 1998. Effects of environmental synthetic chemicals on thyroid function. Thyroid 8:827–856.

Bruner JM, Scott-Moncrieff CR, Williams DA. 1998. Effect of time of sample collection on serum thyroid-stimulating hormone concentrations in euthyroid and hypothyroid dogs. J Am Vet Med Assoc 212:1572–1575.

Bunevicius R, Kazanavicius G, Zalinkevicius R, Prange AJ, Jr. 1999. Effects of thyroxine as compared with thyroxine plus triiodothyronine in patients with hypothyroidism. N Engl J Med 340(6): 424–9.

Burrow GN, Oppenheimer JH, Volpé R. 1989. Thyroid Function and Disease. Philadelphia: WB Saunders.

Campbell KL, Davis CA. 1990. Effects of thyroid hormones on serum and cutaneous fatty acid concentrations in dogs. Am J Vet Res 51(5):752–6.

Campbell KL, Nachreiner R, Schaeffer DJ, et al. 1996. Effects of trimethoprim/sulfamethoxazole on endogenous thyroid stimulating hormone concentration in dogs. 3rd World Congress of Veterinary Dermatology, Edinburgh Scotland, 29.

Cardoso LC, Martins DC, Figueiredo MD, Rosenthal D, Vaisman M, Violante AH, Carvalho DP. 2001. Ca(2+)/nicotinamide adenine dinucleotide phosphate-dependent H(2)O(2) generation is inhibited by iodide in human thyroids. J Clin Endocrinol Metab 86(9): 4339–43.

Chopra IJ, Huang TS, Hurd RE, Solomon DH. 1984. A study of the cardiac effects of thyroid hormone: Evidence of amelioration of the effects of thyroxine by sodium ipodate. Endocrinology 114:2039–2045.

Christoffolete MA, Ribeiro R, Singru P, Fekete C, da Silva WS, Gordon DF, Huang SA, Crescenzi A, Harney JW, Ridgway EC, Larsen PR, Lechan RM, Bianco AC. 2006. Atypical expression of type 2 iodothyronine deiodinase in thyrotrophs explains the thyroxine-mediated pituitary thyrotropin feedback mechanism. Endocrinology 147:1735–1743.

Cohen HN, Beastall GH, Ratcliffe WA, et al. 1980. Effects on human thyroid function of sulfonamide and trimethoprim combination drugs. British Medic J 81:646–647.

Cohen HN, Fyffe JA, Ratcliffe WA, et al. 1981. Effects of trimethoprim and sulfonamide preparations on the pituitary-thyroid axis of rodents. J Endocrinol 91:299–303.

Corvilain B, Van Sande J, Laurent E, Dumont JE. 1991. The H2O2-generating system modulates protein iodination and the activity of the pentose phosphate pathway in dog thyroid. Endocrinology 128:779–785.

Curran PG, DeGroot LJ. 1991. The effect of hepatic enzyme-inducing drugs on thyroid hormones and the thyroid gland. 1991. Endocr Rev 12:135–150.

Daminet S, Ferguson DC. 2003. Influence of drugs on thyroid function in dogs. J Vet Int Med 17:463–472.

Daminet S, Paradis M, Refsal KR, et al. 1999. Short term influence of prednisone and phenobarbital on thyroid function in euthyroid dogs. Can Vet J 40:411–415.

Daniel GB, Sharp DS, Nieckarz JA, et al. 2002. Quantitative thyroid scintigraphy as a predictor of serum thyroxin concentration in normal and hyperthyroid cats. Vet Radiol Ultrasound 43(4):374–82.

Davis PJ, Davis FB. 2002. Nongenomic actions of thyroid hormone on the heart. Thyroid 12(6):459–466.

Deda G, Akinci A, Teziç, et al. 1992. Effects of anticonvulsivant drugs on thyroid hormones in epileptic children. Turk J Pediatr 34:239–244.

DeSandro V, Chevrier M, Boddaert A, et al. 1991. Comparison of the effects of propylthiouracil, amiodarone, diphenylhydantoin, Phenobarbital, and 3-methylcholanthrene on hepatic and renal T4 metabolism and thyroid gland function in rats. Toxicol Appl Pharmacol 111:263–278.

Dong BJ, Hauck WW, Gambertoglio JG, Gee L, White JR, Bubp JL, Greenspan FS. 1997. Bioequivalence of generic and brand-name levothyroxine products in the treatment of hypothyroidism. J Am Med Assoc 227:1205–1213.

Dye JA, Venier M, Zhu L, Ward CR, Hites RA, Birnbaum LS. 2007. Elevated PBDE levels in pet cats: sentinels for humans? Environ Sci Technol 41(18):6350–6.

Edinboro CH, Scott-Moncrieff JC; Janovitz E, et al. 2004. Epidemiologic study of relationships between consumption of commercial canned food and risk of hyperthyroidism in cats. J Am Vet Med Assoc 224(6):879–86.

Feldman EC, Nelson RW (eds). 2004a. Hypothyroidism. In Canine and Feline Endocrinology and Reproduction, 3rd ed. St. Louis: Saunders Elsevier, 86–151.

———. 2004b. Feline hyperthyroidism and thyrotoxicosis. In Canine and Feline Endocrinology and Reproduction, 3rd ed. St. Louis: Saunders Elsevier, 152–218.

Ferguson DC. 1984. Thyroid function tests in the dog. Vet Clin N Amer 14:783–808.

———. 1986. Thyroid hormone replacement therapy. In Kirk RW (ed): Current Veterinary Therapy IX. Philadelphia: WB Saunders, 1018–1025.

———. 1988. Effect of nonthyroidal factors on thyroid function tests in the dog. Comp Cont Ed (Sm An) 10(12):1365–1377.

———. 1989a. Hypothyroidism: Many presentations, one treatment. Small animal geriatrics: Viewpoints in veterinary medicine. Proc Alpo Symposium on Geriatrics, 30–36.

———. 1989b. Influence of common drugs on the free thyroxine fraction in canine serum. Proc Annual Forum of the ACVIM, San Diego, 5:1032 (abstract).

———. 1993. An Internal Medical Perspective of Hypothyroidism. Daniels Pharmaceuticals, Inc. monograph, 3–9.

———. 1994. Update on the diagnosis of canine hypothyroidism. Vet Clin N Am 24(3):515–540.

———. 2007. Testing for hypothyroidism in dogs. Vet Clin N Am Sm An 37:647–669.

Ferguson DC, Hoenig ME. 1991a. Feline hyperthyroidism. In Allen, D.G. (ed.): Small Animal Medicine. Philadelphia: JB Lippincott Co, 831–843.

———. 1991b. Canine hypothyroidism. In Allen DG (ed): Small Animal Medicine. Philadelphia: JB Lippincott Co, 845–865.

———. 1997. Re-examination of dosage regimens for L-thyroxine (T4) in the dog: Bioavailability and persistence of TSH suppression. Proc 15th ACVIM Forum, abstract 72, 668.

Ferguson DC, Hoenig M, Cornelius L. 1992. Endocrinologic disorders. In Lorenz MD, Cornelius LM, Ferguson DC (eds): Small Animal Medical Therapeutics. Philadelphia: JB Lippincott, 85–148.

Ferguson DC, Jacobs GJ, Hoenig M, 1988. Ipodate as an alternative medical treatment for hyperthyroidism: preliminary results in experimentally induced disease. Proc Am Coll Vet Med Annual Forum, Washington, D.C., abstract 3, 718.

Ferguson DC, Moore GE, Hoenig M. 1999. Carprofen lowers total T4 and TSH, but not free T4 concentrations in dogs. Proc 17th Annual Vet Med Forum of the ACVIM, Chicago, 709.

Ferguson DC, Peterson M.E. 1992. Serum free and total iodothyronine concentrations in dogs with spontaneous hyperadrenocorticism. Am J Vet Res 53:1636–1640.

Fish LH, Schwartz HL, Cavanagh J, Steffens MW, Bantle JP. 1987. Replacement dose, metabolism and bioavailability of levothyroxine in the treatment of hypothyroidism: Role of triiodothyronine in pituitary feedback in humans. N Engl J Med 316: 764–770.

Foster DJ, Thoday KL, Beckett GJ. 2000. Thyroid hormone deiodination in the domestic cat. J Mol Endocrinol 24(1):119–26.

Fox LE, Nachreiner RF. 1981. The pharmacokinetics of T_3 and T_4 in the dog. Proc 62nd Conference of Research Workers in Animal Disease, 13.

Gaskill CL, Burton SA, Gelens HC, et al. 1999. Effects of phenobarbital treatment on serum thyroxine and thyroid-stimulating hormone concentrations in epileptic dogs. J Am Vet Med Assoc 215:489–496.

Gieger TL, Hosgood G, Taboada J, et al. 2000. Thyroid function and serum hepatic enzyme activity in dogs after phenobarbital administration. J Vet Int Med 14:277–281.

Gookin JL, Trepanier LA, Bunch SE. 1999. Clinical hypothyroidism associated with trimethoprim-sulfadiazine administration in a dog. J Am Vet Med Assoc 214:1028–1031.

Graham PA, Refsal KR, Nachreiner RF. 1998. Oral prednisone did not suppress serum thyrotropin in radiothyroidectomized beagles. Proc 16th Annual Vet Med Forum of the ACVIM, San Diego, 732.

Graves TK, Peterson ME. 1994. Diagnostic tests for feline hyperthyroidism. Vet Clin N Am 24(3):567–576.

Greco DS, Rosychuk RAW, Ogilvie GK, Harpold LM, Van Liew H. 1998. The effect of levothyroxine treatment on resting energy expenditure of hypothyroid dogs. J Vet Intern Med 12:7–10.

Greenspan FS. 1994. The thyroid gland. In Greenspan FS, Baxter JD (eds): Basic and Clinical Endocrinology, 4th ed. Norwalk: Appleton and Lange, 160–226.

Hall IA, Campbell KL, Chambers MD, et al. 1993. Effect of trimethoprim/sulfamethoxazole on thyroid function in dogs with pyoderma. J Am Vet Med Assoc 202:1959–1962.

Hashizume K, Takahide M, Nishiano Y, Kobayashi M. 1987. Evidence for the presence of active and inactive forms of cytosolic triiodothyronine (T_3) binding protein in the rat kidney: cooperative action of Ca^{++} in NADPH activation. Endocrinol Jpn 34:379.

Hoenig M, Caffall Z, Ferguson DC. 2008. Triiodothyronine differentially regulates key metabolic factors in lean and obese cats. Domest An Endocrinol, in press.

Hoenig M, Ferguson DC. 1983. Assessment of thyroid functional reserve in the cat by the thyrotropin-stimulation test. Am J Vet Res 44:1229–1232.

Hoffman SB, Yoder AR, Trepanier LA. 2002. Bioavailability of transdermal methimazole in a pluronic lecithin organogel (PLO) in healthy cats. J Vet Pharmacol Ther 25:189–93.

Hoffmann G, Marks SL, Taboada J, et al. 2003. Transdermal methimazole treatment in cats with hyperthyroidism. J Feline Med Surg 5(2):77–82.

Inada M, Kasagi K, Kurata S, Kazama Y, Takayama H, Torizuka K, Fukase M, Soma T. 1975. Estimation of thyroxine and triiodothyronine distribution and of the conversion rate of thyroxine to triiodothyronine in man. J Clin Invest 55:1337–1348.

Johnson C, Olivier B, Nachreiner R, Mullaney T. 1999. Effect of 131I-induced hypothyroidism on indices of reproductive function in adult male dogs. J Vet Intern Med 13:104–110.

Johnson S, McKillop D, Miller J, et al. 1993. The effects on rat thyroid function of an hepatic microsomal enzyme inducer. Hum Experiment Toxicol 12:153–158.

Kantrowitz LB, Peterson ME, Trepanier LA, et al. 1999. Serum total thyroxine, total triiodothyronine, free thyroxine, and thyrotropin concentrations in epileptic dogs treated with anticonvulsants. J Am Vet Med Assoc 214:1804–1808.

Kaptein EM. 1986. Thyroid hormone metabolism in illness. In Henneman G (ed): Thyroid Hormone Metabolism. New York: Marcel Dekker, 297.

Kaptein EM, Hays MT, Ferguson DC. 1994. Thyroid hormone metabolism: A comparative evaluation. Vet Clin N Am 24(3):431–466.

Kaptein, EM, Moore GM, Ferguson DC, Hoenig M. 1992. Effects of prednisone on thyroxine and 3,5,3′-triiodothyronine metabolism in normal dogs. Endocrinology 130(3):1669–1679.

———. 1993. Thyroxine and triiodothyronine distribution and metabolism in thyroxine-replaced athyreotic dogs and normal humans. Am J Physiol 264:E90–E100.

Kemppainen RJ, Thompson FN, Lorenz MD, et al. 1983. Effects of prednisone on thyroid and gonadal endocrine function in dogs. J Endocrinol 96:293–302.

Kintzer PP. 1994. Considerations in the treatment of feline hyperthyroidism. Vet Clin N Am 24(3):577–585.

Kintzer PP, Peterson ME. 1991. Thyroid scintigraphy in small animals. Semin Vet Med Surg (Sm An) 6:131.

———. 1994. Nuclear medicine of the thyroid gland. Vet Clin N Am 24(3):587–605.

Kooistra HS, Diaz-Espineira M, Mol JA., van den Brom WE, Rijnberk A. 2000. Secretion pattern of thyroid-stimulating hormone in dogs during euthyroidism and hypothyroidism Dom Anim Endocrinol 18(1):19–29.

Lagler F, Kretzschmar R, Leuschner F, et al. 1976. Toxikologische untersucchungen der kombination sulfamoxoll/trimethoprim (CN 3123) eines neuen briet-brandchemotherapeutikums. Arzheimmittelforsch 26:634–643.

Larrson M. 1987. Diagnostic methods in canine hypothyroidism and influence of nonthyroidal illness on thyroid hormones and thyroxine-binding proteins. PhD thesis, Uppsala, Sweden.

Larsen PR, et al. 1981. Relationships between circulating and intracellular thyroid hormones: Physiological and clinical implications. Endocr Rev 2:87.

Larsen PR, Davies TF, Schlumberger M-J, Hay ID. 2003. Thyroid physiology and diagnostic evaluation of patients with thyroid disorders. In Larsen PR, Kronenberg HM, Melmed S, Polonsky KS.(eds): Williams Textbook of Endocrinology, 10th ed. St. Louis: Saunders Elsevier, 331–352.

Larsson M, Pettersson T, Carlstrom A. 1985. Thyroid hormone binding in serum of 15 vertebrate species: isolation of thyroxine-binding globulin and prealbumin analogs. Gen Comp Endocrinol 58:360.

Laurberg P. 1980. Iodothyronine release from the perfused canine thyroid. Acta Endocrinol (Suppl)236:1.

Laurberg P, Boye N. 1984. Propylthiouracil, ipodate, dexamethasone, and periods of fasting induce different variations in serum rT_3 in dogs. Metabolism 33:323.

Lazar MA, Chin WW. 1990. Nuclear thyroid hormone receptors. J Clin Invest 86:1777.

Lecuyer M, Prini S, Dunn ME, et al. 2006. Clinical efficacy and safety of transdermal methimazole in the treatment of feline hyperthyroidism. Can Vet J 47:131–5.

Liu J, Liu Y, Barter RA, et al. 1995. Alteration of thyroid homeostasis by UDP-glucuronosyltransferase inducers in rats: a dose-response study. J Pharmacol Exp Ther 273:977–985.

Magner JA. 1990. Thyroid-stimulating hormone: Biosynthesis, cell biology and bioactivity. Endocr Rev 11:354.

McClain M, Levin AA, Posch R, et al. 1989. The effect of phenobarbital on the metabolism and excretion of thyroxine in cats. Toxicol Appl Pharmacol 99:216–228.

Mendel, C M. 1989. The free hormone hypothesis: a physiologically based mathematical model. Endocrine Rev 10:232.

Mensching DA, Ferguson DC, Bordson G, Scott J, Piwoni M, Beasley V. 2007. The feline thyroid gland: a model for endocrine disruption by PBDEs? Program, Annual Meeting of the American Thyroid Association, New York, NY, 2007; abstract 3786.

Meric SM , Hawkins EC, Washabau RJ, Turrel JM, Feldman EC. 1986. Radioactive iodine therapy in cats with hyperthyroidism. J AVMA 188:1038–1040.

Moore GE, Ferguson DC, Hoenig M. 1993. Effects of oral administration of antiinflammatory doses of prednisone on thyroid hormone response to thyrotropin-releasing hormone and thyrotropin in clinically normal dogs. Am J Vet Res 54:130–135.

Müller PB, Wolfsheimer KJ, Tabaoda J, et al. 2000. Effects of long-term phenobarbital treatment on the thyroid and adrenal axis and adrenal function tests in dogs. J Vet Intern Med 14:157–164.

Munira B, Diego B, Gereben B, Curcio C, Harney JW, Salvatore D, Sorimachi K, Larsen PR, Bianco AC. 2003. Human type 3 iodothyronine selenodeiodinase is located in the plasma membrane and undergoes rapid internalization to endosomes. J Biol Chem 278(2): 1206–11.

Murray LAS, Peterson ME. 1997. Ipodate treatment of hyperthyroidism in cats. JAVMA 211:63–67.

Ohnhaus EE, Bürgi H, Burger A, et al. 1981. The effects of antipyrine; phenobarbitol and rifampicin on thyroid hormone metabolism in man. Eur J Clin Invest 11:381–387.

Oppenheimer JH. 1983. The nuclear receptor-triiodothyronine complex: relationship to thyroid hormone distribution, metabolism and biological action. In Oppenheimer JH, Samuels HH (eds): Molecular Basis of Thyroid Hormone Action. New York: Academic Press, 1–35.

Panciera DL. 1994. An echocardiographic and electrocardiographic study of cardiovascular function in hypothyroid dogs. J Am Vet Med Assoc 205(7):996–1000.

Panciera DL, Johnson GS. 1996. Plasma von Willebrand factor antigen concentration and buccal mucosal bleeding time in dogs with experimental hypothyroidism. J Vet Intern Med 10(2):60–4.

Panciera DL, Keene BW, Mier HC. 1992. Administration of levothyroxine to euthyroid dogs does not affect echocardiographic and electrocardiographic measurements. Res Vet Sci 53(1):130–2.

Panciera DL, MacEwen EG, Atkins CE, Bosu WTK, Refsal KR, Nachreiner RF. 1990. Thyroid function tests in euthyroid dogs treated with L-thyroxine. Am J Vet Res 51:22–26.

Panciera DL, Post K. 1992. Effect of oral administration of sulfadiazine and trimethoprim in combination on thyroid function in dogs. Can J Vet Res 56:349–352.

Papich MG. 2007. Saunders Handbook of Veterinary Drugs, 2nd ed. St. Louis: Saunders Elsevier.

Pardridge WM. 1981. Transport of protein-bound hormones into tissues in vivo. Endocrine Rev 2:103.

Paull LC, Scott-Moncrieff JC, DeNicola DB, et al. 2000. Effect of potassium bromide (KBr) at anticonvulsant dosages on thyroid function and morphology in dogs. Proc 18th Annual Vet Med Forum of the ACVIM, Seattle, 753.

Peterson ME, Aucoin DP. 1993. Comparison of the disposition of carbimazole and methimazole in clinically normal cats. Res Vet Sci 54:351–355.

Peterson ME, Becker DV. 1984. Radionuclide thyroid imaging in 135 cats with hyperthyroidism. Vet Radiol 25:23–27.

Peterson ME, et al. 1984. Effects of spontaneous hyperadrenocorticism on serum thyroid hormone concentrations in the dog. Am J Vet Res 45:2034–2038.

Peterson ME, Ferguson DC. 1990. Thyroid Diseases, In Ettinger SJ, Textbook of Veterinary Internal Medicine, Vol. 2, Philadelphia: WB Saunders and Co, 1632–1675.

Peterson ME, Kintzer PP, Hurvitz AI. 1988. Methimazole treatment of 262 cats with hyperthyroidism. J Vet Intern Med 2:150–7.

Plumb DC. 2005. Veterinary Drug Handbook, 5th ed. Ames, Iowa: Blackwell Publishing.

Post K, Panciera DL, Clark EG. 1993. Lack of effect of trimethoprim and sulfadiazine in combination in mid- to late gestation on thyroid function in neonatal dogs. J Reprod Fertil Suppl 47:477–482.

Pullen WH, Hess RS. 2006. Hypothyroid dogs treated with intravenous levothyroxine. J Vet Intern Med 20(1):32–7.

Ramirez S, Wolfsheimer KJ, Moore RM, Mora F, Bueno AC, Mirza T. 1997. Duration of effects of phenylbutazone on serum total thyroxine and free thyroxine concentrations in horses. J Vet Intern Med 11:371–374.

Rapaport B, Nagayama Y 1992. The thyrotropin receptor 25 years after its discovery: New insights after molecular cloning. Mol Endocrinol 6:145.

Reichlin S. 1986. Neuroendocrine control of thyrotropin secretion. In Ingbar SH and Braverman LE (eds): The Thyroid, 5th ed. Philadelphia: JB Lippincott, 241.

Robbins JR, Rall JE. 1960. Proteins associated with the thyroid hormones. Physiol Rev 40:415.

Rosychuk RAW. 1982. Thyroid hormones and antithyroid drugs. Vet Clin N Am 12(1):111–148.

Sartor LL, Trepanier LA, Kroll MM, et al. 2004. Efficacy and safety of transdermal methimazole in the treatment of cats with hyperthyroidism. J Vet Intern Med 18:651–5.

Sartor LL, Trepanier LA, Kroll MM, Rodan I, Challoner L. 2004. Efficacy and safety of transdermal methimazole in the treatment of cats with hyperthyroidism. J Vet Intern Med 18:651–655.

Shupnick MA, Ridgeway EC, Chin WW. 1989. Molecular biology of thyrotropin. Endocr Rev 4:459.

Slater MR, Geller S, Rogers K. 2001. Long-term health and predictors of survival for hyperthyroid cats treated with iodine 131. J Vet Intern Med 15(1):47–51.

Toyoda N, Kaptein E, Berry MJ, et al. 1997. Structure-activity relationships for thyroid hormone deiodination by mammalian type I iodothyronine deiodinases. Endocrinology 138(1):213–9.

Su X, Katakam P, Yang X, Grosse WM, Li OW, McGraw RA, Ferguson DC. 1995. Cloning, expression, and development of monoclonal antibodies against the beta subunit of canine thyrotropin. J Vet Int Med 9(3):185, (abstract).

Suzuki S, Mori J, Hashizume K. 2007. μ-crystallin, a NADPH-dependent T3-binding protein in cytosol. Trends Endocrinol Metab 18(7):286–9.

Suzuki S, Suzuki N, Mori J, Oshima A, Usami S, Hashizume K. 2007. μ-crystallin as an intracellular 3,5,3′-triiodothyronine holder in vivo. Molec Endocrinol 21(4):885–894.

Tarttelin MF, Ford HC. 1994. Dietary iodine level and thyroid function in the cat. J Nutr 124(12Suppl):2577S–2578S.

Taurog A. 1991. Hormone synthesis: Thyroid iodine metabolism. In Braverman LE, Utiger RD (eds): Werner and Ingbars The Thyroid: A Fundamental and Clinical Text, 6th ed. Philadelphia: Lippincott, 1991.

Theodoropoulos TJ, Zolman JC. 1989. Effects of phenobarbital on hypothalamic-pituitary-thyroid axis in the rat. Am J Med Sci 297:224–227.

Tomsa K, Hardegger R, Glaus T, Reusch C. 2001. 99mTc-pertechnetate scintigraphy in hyperthyroid cats with normal serum thyroxine concentrations. J Vet Int Med 15(3):299, abst 109.

Torres S, McKeever P, Johnston S. 1996. Hypothyroidism in a dog associated with trimethoprim-sulfadiazine therapy. Vet Dermatol 7:105–108.

Torres S, McKeever PJ, Johnston SD. 1991. Effects of oral administration of prednisolone on thyroid function in dogs. Am J Vet Res 52:416–421.

Toyoda N, Kaptein E, Berry MJ, Harney JW, Larsen PR, Visser TJ. 1997. Structure-activity relationships for thyroid hormone deiodination by mammalian type I iodothyronine deiodinases. Endocrinology 138(1): 213–9.

Trepanier LA. 2007. Pharmacologic management of feline hyperthyroidism. Vet Clin Sm An 37:775–88.

Trepanier LA, Hoffman SB, Kroll M, et al. 2003. Efficacy and safety of once versus twice daily administration of methimazole in cats with hyperthyroidism. J Am Vet Med Assoc 222(7):954–8.

Trepanier LA, Peterson ME, Aucoin DP. 1991. Pharmacokinetics of intravenous and oral methimazole following single- and multiple-dose administration in normal cats. J Vet Pharmacol Ther 14(4):367–73.

———. 1991. Pharmacokinetics of methimazole in normal cats and in cats with hyperthyroidism. Res Vet Sci 50(1):69–74.

Verma NP, Haidukewych D. 1994. Differential but infrequent alterations of hepatic enzyme levels and thyroid hormone levels by anticonvulsivant drugs. Arch Neurol 51:381–384.

von Klopmann T, Boettcher IC, Rotermund A, Rohn K, Tipold A. 2006. Euthyroid sick syndrome in dogs with idiopathic epilepsy before treatment with anticonvulsant drugs. J Vet Intern Med 20(3): 516–22.

Williams DA, Scott-Moncrieff C, Bruner J, Sustarsic D, Panosian-Sahakian N, el Shami AS. 1996. Validation of an immunoassay for canine thyroid-stimulating hormone and changes in serum concentration following induction of hypothyroidism in dogs. J Am Vet Med Assoc 209(10):1730–2.

Wolff J. 1989. Excess iodide inhibits the thyroid gland by multiple mechanisms. In Eckholm R, Kohn LD, Wollman SH (eds): Control of the Thyroid Gland. New York: Plenum.

Woltz HH, et al. 1983. Effect of prednisone on thyroid gland: Morphology and plasma thyroxine and triiodothyronine concentrations in the dog. Am J Vet Res 44:2000–2003.

CHAPTER

30

GLUCOCORTICOIDS, MINERALOCORTICOIDS, AND ADRENOLYTIC DRUGS

DUNCAN C. FERGUSON, LEVENT DIRIKOLU, AND MARGARETHE HOENIG

GLUCOCORTICOIDS

Glucocorticoids (GCs) are among the most widely used (and misused) class of drugs in veterinary medicine. Despite this, scientific information on glucocorticoid therapy in most domestic species is scarce, particularly with respect to optimal dosages and dosage intervals, physical and endocrine side effects, and efficacy in clinical applications. Therefore, therapeutic protocols are often the product of clinical experience, common sense, and information from human medicine. Though the following discussion emphasizes systemic use of glucocorticoids, it should be recognized that local application (ophthalmic, otic, intraarticular, topical, intralesional) also has similar systemic effects.

MANAGEMENT OF HYPOADRENOCORTICISM.

Spontaneous glucocorticoid deficiency without concomitant mineralocorticoid deficiency is a relatively rare occurrence in dogs, the species that most commonly suffers from Addison's disease (gluco- and mineralocorticoid deficiency). The underlying cause is suspected to be an immune-mediated destruction of the adrenal cortex, making replacement of the physiological hormones aldosterone and cortisol (in most domestic animals) to be the primary clinical goal. Spontaneous selective glucocorticoid deficiency is rare; however, exogenous glucocorticoids may themselves induce selective atrophy of the glucocorticoid-producing part of the adrenal cortex (zonae fasciculata and reticularis) (Addison 1855; Feldman and Nelson

1987; Ferguson 1985a; Ferguson et al. 1978; Hoenig and Ferguson 1991b).

MANAGEMENT OF NONADRENAL DISORDERS: INFLAMMATORY, ALLERGIC, AND AUTOIMMUNE DISORDERS. Glucocorticoids are potent antiinflammatory and immunosuppressant agents. The majority of therapeutic applications for these agents fall into these classifications. However, the adverse metabolic effects, as described below, are difficult to separate pharmacologically from the therapeutic benefits, making glucocorticoids potent, yet potentially dangerous, compounds.

REVIEW OF PHYSIOLOGY

Biosynthesis of Steroids. The adrenal cortex synthesizes a variety of steroids from cholesterol and releases them into the circulation. Those steroids with effects on intermediary metabolism are termed "glucocorticoids" and are produced mainly in the layers of the adrenal gland called the *zonae fasciculata* and *reticularis*. The steroids with primarily salt-retaining activity are called *mineralocorticoids* and are synthesized in the zona glomerulosa. The adrenal gland is also capable of synthesizing steroids with androgenic and estrogenic activity. The major glucocorticoid in most domestic animals is cortisol, and in most mammals, the most important mineralocorticoid is aldosterone. In some species (e.g., the rat), corticosterone is the major glucocorticoid. It is less firmly bound to protein and therefore metabolized more rapidly. Quantitatively, dehydroepiandrosterone (DHEA) is the major androgen, with part of it being sulfated to DHEA-sulfate. Both DHEA and androstenedione are very weak androgens. A small amount of testosterone is secreted by the adrenal gland and may be of greater importance as an androgen. Little is known about the estrogens secreted by the adrenal gland. However, the adrenal androgens such as testosterone and androstenedione can be converted to estrone in small amounts by nonendocrine tissues (Aron and Tyrrell 1994; Tyrrell et al. 1994).

The biochemical pathways involved in adrenal steroidogenesis are shown in Figure 30.1. The initial ACTH-dependent rate-limiting step is the transport of intracellular

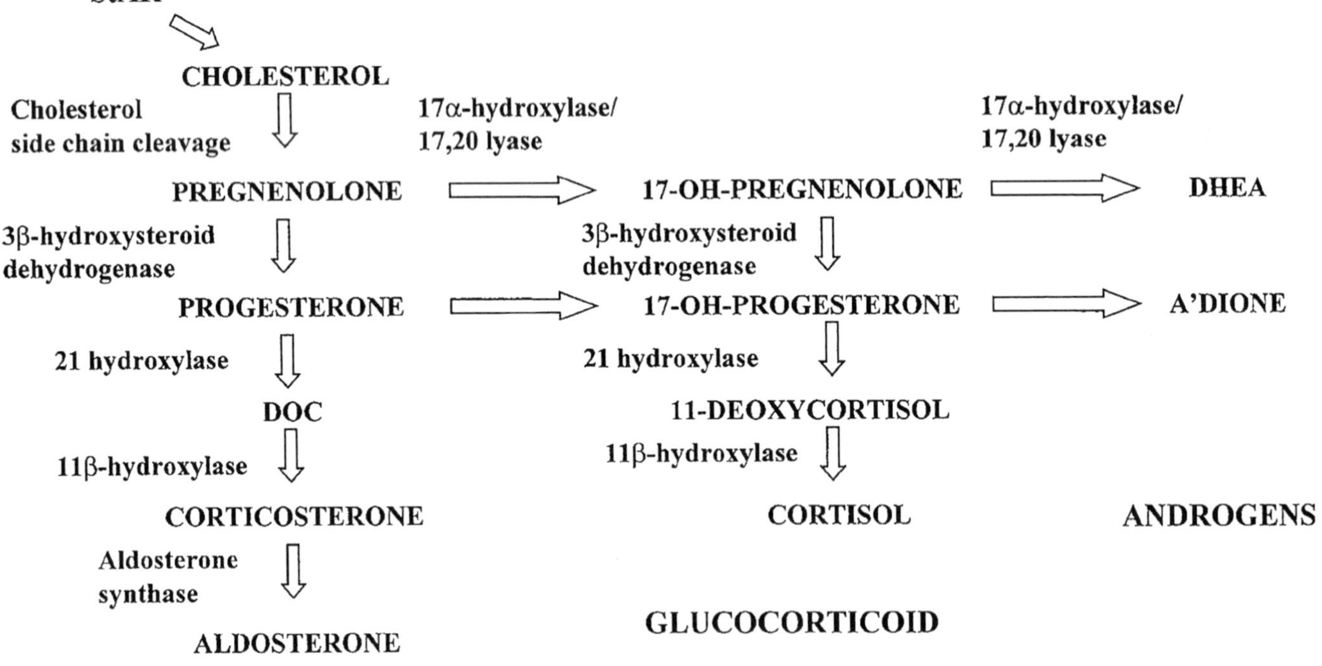

FIG. 30.1 Adrenal steroidogenesis. Steroidogenic acute regulatory (StAR) protein mediates uptake of cholesterol into mitochondria within adrenocortical cells. Then aldosterone, cortisol, and adrenal androgens are synthesized through a series of steroidogenic enzymes. A'dione = androstenedione; DHEA = dehydroepiandrosterone; DOC = deoxycorticosterone (from Stewart 2003; Fig. 14.3, p. 495).

TABLE 30.1 Nomenclature for adrenal steroidogenic enzymes and their genes

Enzyme Name	Gene
Cholesterol side-chain cleavage (SCC) (desmolase)	*CYP11A1*
3β-hydroxysteroid dehydrogenase (3β-HSD) (type II isozyme)	*HSD3B2*
17α-hydroxylase/17,20 lyase	*CYP17*
21-Hydroxylase	*CYP21A2*
11β-hydroxylase	*CYP11B1*
Aldosterone synthase	*CYP11B2*

Modified from Stewart (2003), Table 14.3, p. 495.

cholesterol from the outer to the inner mitochondrial membrane by Steroidogenic Acute Regulatory (StAR) protein, where it is then converted to pregnenolone by cytochrome P450scc (SCC; side-chain cleavage enzyme). The synthesis of the various adrenal steroids then involves a series of cytochrome P450 enzymes (Table 30.1). SCC and the CYP11B enzymes are localized to the mitochondria and utilize a specific electron shuttle system to hydroxylate steroids. 17α-hydroxylase and 21-hydroxylase are localized in the endoplasmic reticulum. In the cytoplasm, pregnenolone is converted to progesterone by 3β-hydroxysteroid dehydrogenase (3β-HSD), which is the target of the antiadrenal drug trilostane. Progesterone is hydroxylated to 17-OHP by 17α-hydroxylase, and this step is necessary for glucocorticoid synthesis. 21-hydroxylation of either progesterone in the zona glomerulosa or 17-OHP in the zona fasciculata is accomplished by 21-hydroxylase yielding deoxycorticosterone (DOC) or 11-deoxycortisol, respectively. Cortisol is then synthesized in the mitochondria by the conversion of 11-deoxycortisol to cortisol by the enzyme 11-β-hydroxylase. In the zona glomerulosa, 11β-hydroxylase also converts DOC to corticosterone. Aldosterone synthase also accomplishes this reaction and converts corticosterone to aldosterone through the intermediate 18-OH corticosterone.

Adrenal steroids are metabolized in extradrenal tissues as well. Cortisol is interconverted with biologically inactive cortisone by the 11-β hydroxysteroid dehydrogenase system (11-β HSD). 11-β HSD1 uses NADPH to convert cortisone to active cortisol. Conversely, 11-β HSD2 uses NAD^+ to convert cortisol to cortisone, essentially inactivating it. Likewise, the synthetic glucocorticoid prednisone must be converted by 11-β-HSD1 in the liver for bioactivity (Stewart 2003).

Hypothalamic-Pituitary-Adrenal Axis (Fig. 30.2). Production of ACTH is stimulated by corticotropin-releasing hormone (CRH), which is a hypothalamic hormone (see also Chapter 27); production of ACTH is also influenced by vasopressin (antidiuretic hormone; ADH), particularly during stress. There is also central nervous system (CNS) input into hypothalamic hormone secretion. A "short-loop" feedback system of ACTH on the corticotrophs (ACTH-producing cells) in the pituitary has also been described. In humans, cortisol is secreted in response to pulsatile ACTH release with diurnal variation.

Negative feedback of glucocorticoids on ACTH secretion occurs at both the hypothalamic and pituitary levels via two mechanisms:

1. "Fast-feedback" is sensitive to the rate of change of cortisol levels and likely occurs without interaction with nuclear steroid receptors (see cellular mechanisms below).
2. "Slow-feedback" is sensitive to the absolute cortisol concentration and is a nuclear receptor–mediated effect, which results in a decrease in ACTH synthesis. The clinical test for spontaneous hyperadrenocorticism, called the dexamethasone suppression test, is mediated by this mechanism of feedback (Keller-Wood 1990; Tyrrell et al. 1994).

Pharmacologic doses of glucocorticoids have a profound effect on endogenous glucocorticoid regulation, suppressing both hypothalamic and pituitary hormone production (Fig. 30.2). Cortisol inhibits ACTH secretion and CRH secretion through negative feedback at both hypothalamic and pituitary levels, a point that is important when considering recovery of the hypothalamic-pituitary-adrenal axis (HPAA) from exogenous glucocorticoid administration. Glucocorticoids with antiinflammatory effects but no effects on the HPAA have not been identified to date. As a result, long-term use of supraphysiologic doses may lead to adrenocortical atrophy and decreased adrenal secretory reserve (Chastain et al. 1981; Chastain and Graham 1979; Hench 1952; Kemppainen et al. 1982; Moore and Hoenig 1992).

Cellular Mechanisms of Negative Feedback. Glucocorticoids inhibit POMC gene transcription (and therefore, ACTH synthesis and secretion) in the anterior pituitary and CRH and vasopressin (AVP) mRNA synthesis and secretion in the hypothalamus. This negative

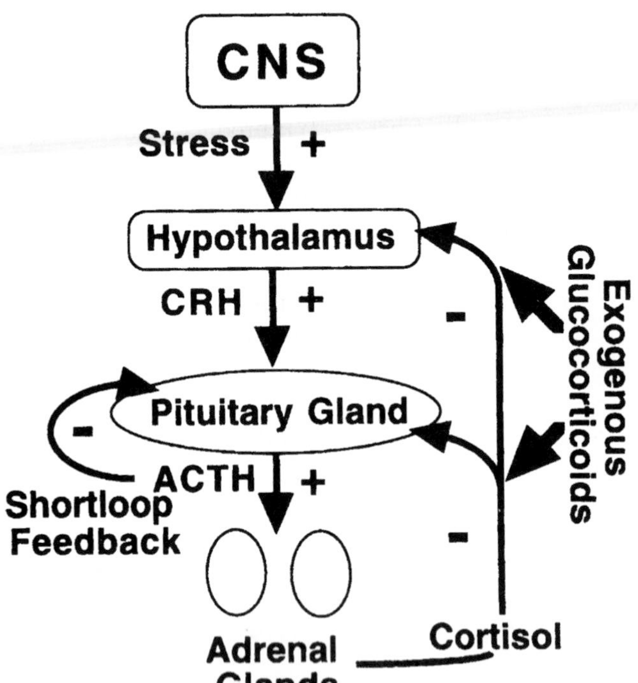

FIG. 30.2 Hypothalamic-pituitary-adrenal axis. Exogenous glucocorticoids inhibit the hypothalamic and pituitary function in a negative-feedback fashion. ACTH, through "shortloop" feedback, inhibits its own production. Therefore, recovery of the entire hypothalamic-pituitary-adrenal axis requires withdrawal of glucocorticoid and is not enhanced by the administration of exogenous ACTH. CNS = central nervous system; CRH = corticotropin-releasing hormone; ACTH = adrenocorticotropic hormone; + represents stimulation; − represents inhibition.

feedback is dependent upon the dose, potency, half-life, and duration of administration of the glucocorticoid administered. Although feedback inhibition is principally mediated by the glucocorticoid receptor (GR), there is evidence of fast-loop feedback, which can account for as much as 50% of the negative feedback effect. Glucocorticoids have shown negative effects on spiking of periventricular nucleus (PVN) neurons in hypothalamus by an effect blocked by a glucocorticoid receptor antagonist. However, GCs also acutely suppress voltage-activated K^+ currents of PVN neurons, and inhibit glutamatergic excitatory postsynaptic currents by PVN neurons within minutes. This effect appears to be due to the release of endocannabinoids, which suppress in a retrograde fashion the presynaptic release of glutamate and GABA. Furthermore, GCs induce a rapid facilitatory effect on GABA release by these hypothalamic neurons. There is some evidence that the membrane-bound GCRs mediating these rapid effects engage directly or indirectly the Gs-adenylate cyclase-PKA signaling pathway. The combined effect of suppression of excitatory synaptic input with facilitation of inhibition of PVN neurons results in rapid inhibition of PVN output controlling the HPA axis (Di et al. 2003; Tasker et al. 2006).

Therapeutic Significance. In humans, single daily doses of exogenous glucocorticoids are most commonly recommended to be given in the morning to mimic the adrenal gland's secretory pattern (Tyrrell et al. 1994). Although older reports claimed the existence of a diurnal cortisol variation in dogs and cats, with plasma cortisol level peaking in the morning in dogs and in the evening in cats, carefully designed studies have not confirmed these observations (Kemppainen 1986). Under basal (nonstressful) conditions, the adrenal gland produces cortisol (hydrocortisone) at about 1 mg/kg body weight daily in most species.

Plasma Binding, Metabolism, and Excretion. In plasma, cortisol is over 90% bound to plasma proteins. The remaining 10% free hormone is the active moiety according to the free-hormone hypothesis. Corticosteroid-binding globulin (CBG), an α_2 globulin synthesized by the liver, binds the majority of circulating hormone under normal circumstances. The remainder is free or loosely bound to albumin and is available to exert its effect on target cells. Cortisol is removed from the circulation by the liver, where it is reduced and conjugated to form water-soluble glucuronides and sulfates, which are excreted into the urine (Aron and Tyrrell 1994; Grote et al. 1993; Hammond 1990; Tyrrell et al. 1994).

Molecular Mechanisms of Action. Glucocorticoids have four cellular mechanisms of action: 1) the classical genomic mechanism of action caused by the cytosolic glucocorticoid receptor (cGCR); 2) secondary nongenomic effects also initiated by the cGCR; 3) membrane-bound glucocorticoid receptor (mGCR)-mediated nongenomic effects; and 4) nonspecific, nongenomic effects caused by interactions with cellular membranes (see Fig. 30.3; Loewenberg et al. 2007). Which of these effects is seen will depend upon the tissue and the dose of glucocorticoids (see Table 30.2) (Stahn et al. 2007; Buttgereit 2004).

Genomic Mechanisms of Action. Genomic mechanisms mediate most effects associated with eventual protein

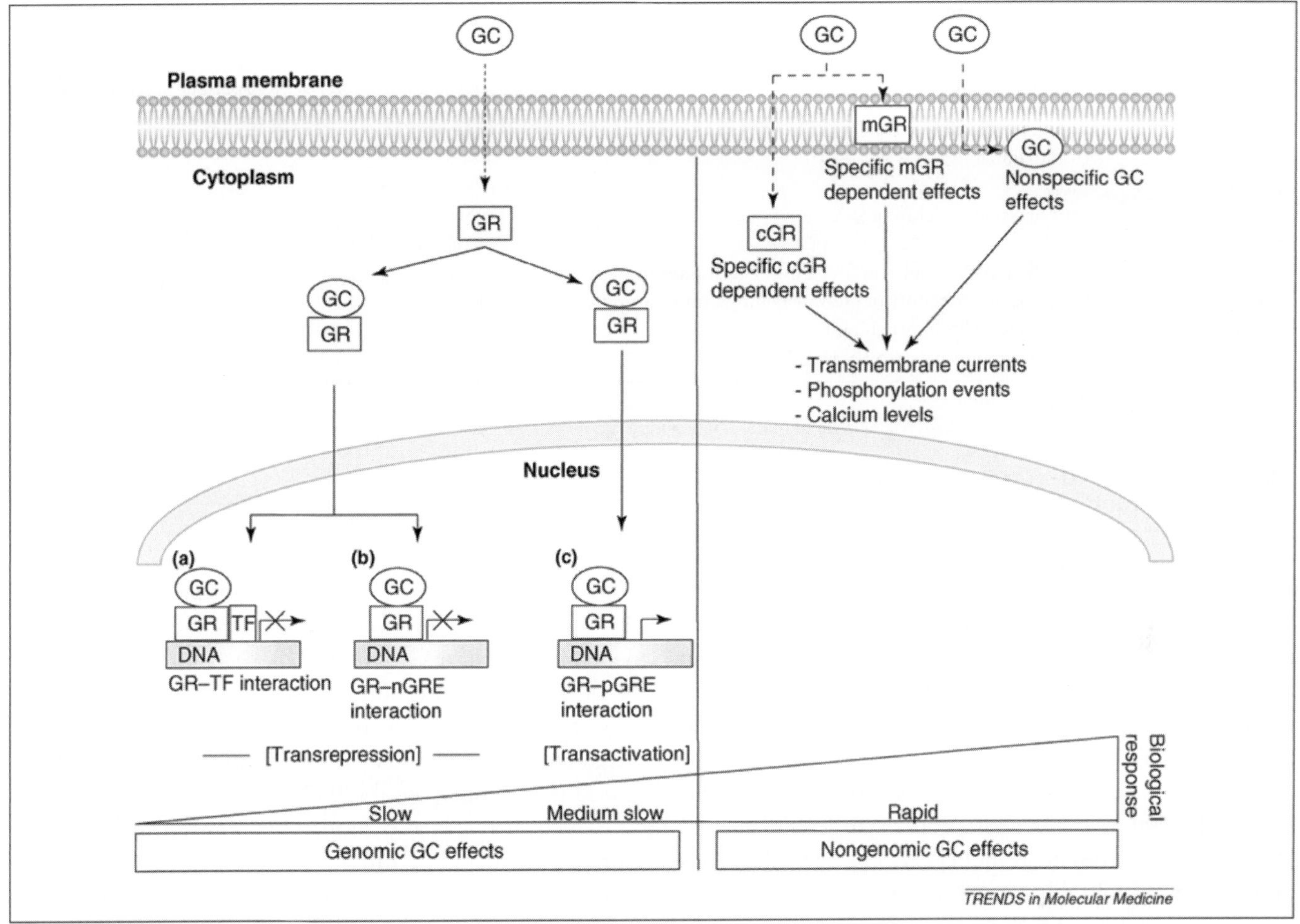

FIG. 30.3 Genomic and nongenomic cellular mechanisms of glucocorticoid (GC) action (from Loewenberg et al. 2007). GCs diffuse into cells and bind to the cytoplasmic GR, after which the GC–GR complex translocates into the nucleus.

Left side of figure: (a) Ligated GR directly inhibits proinflammatory transcription factors such as AP-1,NF-κB and STAT (b) Ligated GR actively suppresses transcription (transrepression) of inflammatory genes (such as IL-1 and IL-2) through binding to negative GREs (nGREs). GC-induced transrepression is slow because time is required before RNA and protein levels of target genes are fully degraded. (c) Activated GR induces transcription (transactivation) of immunosuppressive genes (e.g., lipocortin-1) via positive GREs (pGREs). Transactivation of genes that encode regulator proteins is less slow (medium slow) compared to transrepression.

Right side of figure: GCs induce rapid effects (occurring within minutes) on transmembrane currents, signal transduction (such as MAPK signaling pathways), second-messenger cascades, or intracellular Ca^{2+} mobilization. Nongenomic GC effects are mediated by cytosolic or membrane-bound GRs, or via nonspecific interactions with cell membranes.

In this simplified scheme, no GR–chaperones are depicted.

Abbreviations: cGR, cytosolic glucocorticoid receptor; GC, glucocorticoid; GRE, glucocorticoid receptor responsive element; MAPK, mitogen activated protein kinase; mGR, membrane-bound glucocorticoid receptor; TCR, T-cell receptor; TF, transcription factor.
(Legend modified from Loewenberg et al. [2007], Elsevier.)

synthesis, such as low-dose physiological replacement therapy and antiinflammatory and immunomodulatory effects; however, it is now clear that some effects, particularly the more rapid ones seen at high glucocorticoid doses, cannot be explained through this mechanism (see "Nongenomic Effects of Glucocortoids" below). The genomic mechanisms of glucocorticoid action are cGCR-mediated by the cytoplasmic glucocorticoid receptor. The unliganded cGCR is a 94-kD protein that exists in the cytoplasm as a multiprotein complex including heat-shock proteins (Hsp), such as Hsp90, Hsp70, Hsp56 and Hsp40. There is also an interaction with immunophilins, (chaperones

TABLE 30.2 Current knowledge on the relationship between clinical dosing and cellular actions of glucocorticoids

Daily Prednisolone Dosage (mg/kg)	Therapeutic Application	Genomic Actions (% Receptor Saturation)	Nongenomic Nonspecific	Nongenomic cGR-mediated
Low (≤0.2)	Replacement or low maintenance	+ (<50%)	–	?
Medium (0.2–0.5)	Antiinflammatory Initial	++ (50–100%)	(+)	(+)
High (0.5–1)	Antinflammatory (chronic disease) Initial	+++ (almost 100%)	+	+
Very high (1–3)	Antiinflammatory (subacute) or chronic immunosuppressive Acute antiinflammatory or life-threatening immunosuppressive	+++ (almost 100%)	+++	++
Pulse or shock therapy (≥3)	Very severe or life-threatening Immunosuppressive or initial lymphocytolytic	++++ (100%)	++++	+++

cGCR = cytosolic glucocorticoid receptor.

? = unknown; – = not relevant; (+) = perhaps relevant, but of minor importance; + = relevant; ++ = relevant to very relevant; +++ = very relevant; ++++ = most relevant.

Modified from Buttgereit et al. (2004) for small animal veterinary applications).

such as p23 and Src) and several kinases in the mitogen-activated protein kinase (MAPK) signaling system. The glucocorticoid receptor itself consists of three domains: an N-terminal domain containing transactivation functions, a DNA-binding domain with a "zinc-finger" motif and a glucocorticoid-binding domain. Binding to the cGCR ultimately induces (also known as *transactivation*) or inhibits (also known as *transrepression*) the synthesis of regulatory proteins. The genomic effects are generally not observed prior to 30 minutes because of the time necessary for cGCR activation/translocation, transcription, and translation. It is estimated that glucocorticoids influence the transcription of ~1% of the entire genome either directly or indirectly through interaction with transcription factors and coactivators (Stahn et al. 2007).

Genomic Effects Via the Cytosolic Glucocorticoid Receptor (cGCR). The cholesterol-like structure and low molecular weight (~300 daltons) allow GCs to pass easily through the cell membrane and bind to the inactive cGCR. Conformational changes in the GC/cGCR complex result in dissociation from heat shock proteins (HSPs) 70 and 90 followed by migration within 20 minutes to the nucleus. Binding occurs as a homodimer to the glucocorticoid response element (GRE) in association with the activator protein-1 (AP-1) comprised of *c-fos* and *c-jun*. Binding of the GC/cGPR to a positive GRE (pGRE) results, for example, in induced synthesis of antiinflammatory proteins (e.g., lipocortin 1, IκB, annexin-1, MAP kinase phosphatase 1, and IL-10), as well as metabolic proteins (e.g., those key to gluconeogenesis) often associated with common side effects. Transcription of genes can be inhibited by GCs via direct interaction between the GCR and negative GREs (nGRE), such as those associated with pituitary expression and secretion of pro-opiomelanocortin, the precursor to ACTH, which constitutes the negative feedback system in the pituitary (see Figs. 30.2, 30.3) (Loewenberg et al. 2007).

Glucocorticoids also suppress expression of inflammatory genes, including interleukin 1 and 2 (IL-1 and IL-2) via the same mechanism (Loewenberg et al. 2007; Stahn et al. 2007). The repressive effect of GR on NF-κB regulation is balanced by the fact that since NF-κB negatively regulates GCR α–mediated transcription even though the mechanism underlying such antagonism is as yet unclear (Duma et al. 2006). Transcription factors may also be displaced from a positive GRE through direct interaction of the factor and the GCR. In addition, GR-mediated transcriptional modulation can be achieved through direct protein-protein interaction with proinflammatory transcription factors, such as activator protein-1 (AP-1), nuclear factor-κB (NF-κB), or signal transducers and activator of transcription (STAT), leading to inhibition of target gene expression (van der Velden 1998; Loewenberg et al. 2007).

Induction of Lipocortin and Inhibition of Phospholipase A_2. An important mechanism for antiinflammatory and immunosuppressive effects of glucocorticoids is the inhibition of phospholipase A_2 (PLA_2), the enzyme responsible for the release of arachidonic acid from membranes prior to its further metabolism by the cyclooxygen-

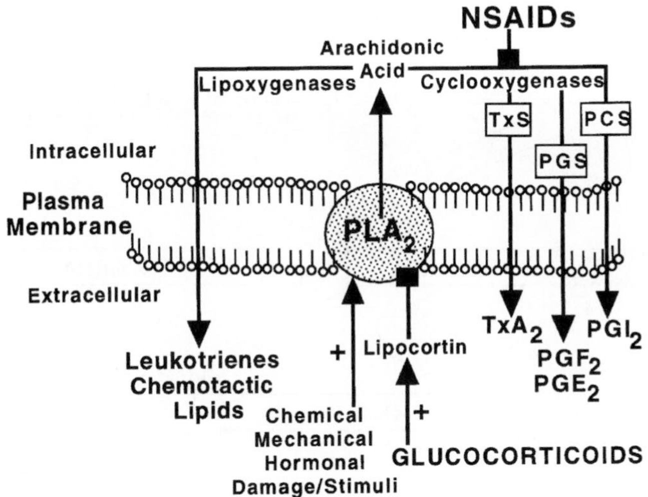

FIG. 30.4 Comparison of the effects of glucocorticoids and nonsteroidal anti-inflammatory drugs (NSAIDs) on arachidonic acid–derived mediators of inflammation. Glucocorticoids stimulate the production of lipocortin, which inhibits the activity of plasma phospholipase A_2 (PLA_2) and thereby inhibits the release of arachidonic acid and indirectly the production of newly formed inflammatory mediators of the cyclooxygenase pathway as well as the lipoxygenase pathway. The net result is a reduction in production of leukotrienes and chemotactic compounds, as well as less formation of thromboxane A_2 (TxA_2) by thromboxane synthase (TxS), of prostaglandins E_2 and $F_{2\alpha}$ by prostaglandin synthase (PGS), and of prostacyclin (PGI_2) by prostacyclin synthase (PCS).

ase (COX) and lipoxygenase (LOX) pathways (Fig. 30.4). Glucocorticoids enhance the production of a protein called *lipocortin,* which inhibits the enzyme phospholipase A_2 in the cell membrane, thereby inhibiting the formation of prostaglandins, leukotrienes, and PAF (see Fig. 30.4). Glucocorticoids also may inhibit other phospholipases, such as phospholipase C (Barragry 1994; Goldfien 1992; Sorenson et al. 1988). Lipocortin-1, a 37 kDa member of the annexin superfamily of proteins, plays a major regulatory role in systems as diverse as cell growth regulation and differentiation, neutrophil migration, CNS responses to cytokines, neuroendocrine secretion, and neurodegeneration (Flower and Rothwell 1994).

Steroid Receptor Isoforms. Glucocorticoid and mineralocorticoid receptors form a class of proteins within the nuclear receptor superfamily of receptors including glucocorticoids, mineralocorticoids, estrogens, progesterone, androgen, Vitamin D, and retinoic acid. They are widely conserved throughout the species. Glucocorticoid receptors are critical for normal development and differentiation and are essential for life (Duma et al. 2006). For the human glucocorticoid receptor, there exists a steroid-binding isoform of 777 amino acids, termed α and a nonsteroid binding β isoform of 742 amino acids, which is identical to the α isoform through the first 727 amino acids (Fig. 30.5). Initially, it was thought that GCR β was not physiologically significant. However, it is now known to convey a dominant negative effect. GCR α is considered the classical GCR responsible for most genomic actions, whereas the β isoform has been implicated in the conveyance of glucocorticoid resistance, and possibly a role in autoimmune and inflammatory disorders. It has been suggested that GCR β inhibits GCR α transcriptional activity by interference with formation of the coactivator complex. Much remains to be clarified mechanistically, but it has been suggested that GCR β overexpression may either be neutral, or might lead to anti or proinflammatory states. There would be pharmacological relevance of GCR β overexpression as an antiinflammatory or to suppress metabolic side effects of glucocorticoids. To date, most studies report higher expression of GCR β in autoimmune, inflammatory, or glucocorticoid-resistant states. Neutrophils have a normally high β:α GCR ratio, and this may account for their relative glucocorticoid-resistance. However, no study has yet evaluated the effect of acute or chronic glucocorticoid administration on GCR β expression. Nonetheless, proinflammatory cytokines induce an overexpression of GCR β and expression of this GCR isoform has been postulated as a possible predictor of therapeutic failure with glucocorticoid therapy (Duma et al. 2006).

Posttranslational Modifications. The function of GCR can be subsequently altered by posttranslational modifications, such as phosphorylation, ubiquitination, and SUMOylation. Ultimately, such changes may alter subcellular distribution, transcriptional activity, and protein-protein interactions. Ubiquitination is believed to be a major mechanism by which the degradation rates of GCRs are regulated, regulating targeting to proteasome degradation. This is a highly conserved mechanism among eukaryotes. Addition of a small ubiquitin-related modifier-1 (SUMO-1) is called *SUMOylation* and may also impact protein stability and localization. For example, of significance to immunosuppressive or anticancer therapy, the phosphorylation state of the GCR may impact glucocorticoid-sensitivity during the cell cycle. Glucocorticoid treatment increases phosphorylation during the S phase,

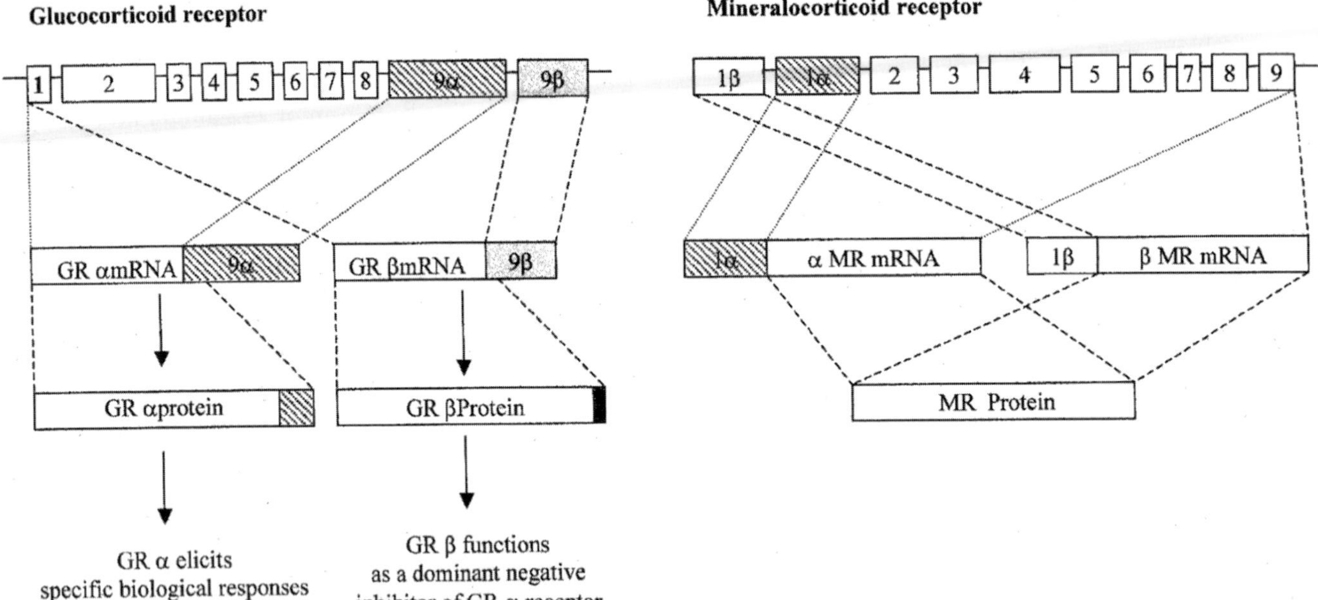

FIG. 30.5 Schematic structure of the human genes encoding the glucocorticoid receptor (GR) and mineralocorticoid receptor (MR). Splice variants have been described for both receptors; in the case of the glucocorticoid receptor, there is evidence that the GR β isoform can act as a dominant negative inhibitor of GR α action. mRNA = messenger ribonucleic acid (from Stewart 2003; Fig. 14-9; p. 500).

but not during the G2 or M phases. As a result, cells synchronized to the S phase were responsive to glucocorticoids, whereas those in G2/M phase were not (Duma et al. 2006).

Nongenomic Effects of Glucocorticoids. In shock and pulse immunosuppressive therapy, very high doses of glucocorticoids are administered. At such doses, cGCRs are believed to be saturated (see Table 30.2) and effects are unlikely to be limited to receptor-mediated phenomena. At high GC concentrations, nonspecific effects due to direct interaction with the cell membrane lipid may occur (Fig. 30.3). These effects are too rapid to be regulated transcriptionally and are termed *nongenomic* but represent several possible mechanisms. Rapid GC effects might occur by interaction of GCs with specific membrane receptors. For example, a plasma-membrane form of GCR has been shown in B cells and peripheral blood mononuclear cells. GCs may also act on the plasma membrane by nonspecific physicochemical mechanisms, particularly when at high concentrations. Through such mechanisms, they may inhibit Na^+ and Ca^{++} plasma membrane transport or increase H^+ leak of the mitochondria. The former mechanism in lymphocytes has been implicated as part of the rapid immunosuppression induced by glucocorticoids. The effects of GCs on ion fluxes and vascular permeability are independent of protein synthesis (Muller and Rankawitz 1991; Reull et al. 1990). Nongenomic effects of glucocorticoids have been described on different cellular processes, such as actin polymerization, neuronal membrane conductance, intracellular calcium release, and other signal transduction mechanisms. For example, short-term glucocorticoid treatment reduced antigen-induced phosphorylation of mitogen-activated protein (MAP)–extracellular signal-regulated kinase (ERK, MEK) as well as reduced phospholipase A_2 (PLA_2) (Song and Buttgereit 2006).

Specific membrane-associated receptors for glucocorticoids may be involved in the rapid effects of these agents in shock conditions (Gametchu et al. 1991; Grote et al. 1993; Liposits and Bohn 1993). Glucocorticoids as cholesterol-like compounds, may change membrane fluidity, thereby regulating plasma membrane $GABA_A$, EGF, insulinlike growth factor-I (IGF-I), and dopamine receptors. Receptor-mediated insertion of steroid hormones into DNA may also take place, with the steroid acting as a transcription factor. These diverse modes of action provide for integrated rapid and/or prolonged effects to address the physiological needs of the individual (Brann et al. 1995).

Glucocorticoids can induce the rapid phosphorylation and membrane translocation of annexin-1, an important antiinflammatory protein. They also have been shown to activate endothelial nitric oxide synthase (eNOS) via actions on phosphatidylinositol 3-kinase and protein kinase B, resulting in vasodilatation associated with cardioprotective effects of glucocorticoids. Neuroprotection following high dose glucocorticoids may also be associated with a nongenomic effect, again possibly by eNOS activation and increased cerebral blood flow (Song and Buttgereit 2006).

Membrane-bound states of the cytosolic glucocorticoid and mineralocorticoid receptors have also been described. Aldosterone receptors on plasma membranes of lymphocytes and smooth muscle cells appear to trigger changes in Ca^{++}, IP3, cAMP, and protein kinase C. Supporting clinical significance, the number of plasma membrane-bound GCRs correlates with the ability of GCs to induce lymphocyte death. Further work is necessary to clarify the functional role and cellular mechanisms associated with membrane-bound GR. Current thinking is that there is only one cytosolic GCR, which may be either unliganded and membrane-associated, or liganded and act as a "classical" nuclear transcription factor. In future pharmaceutical development, glucocorticoids with preference for membrane-bound GCRs may have enhanced immunosuppressive activity with fewer side effects (Buttgereit 2004; Song and Buttgereit 2006; Loewenberg et al. 2007).

PHYSIOLOGICAL EFFECTS OF GLUCOCORTICOIDS. A principal role of glucocorticoids is the maintenance of fluid homeostasis by regulation of volume and composition of body fluids and by being permissive for essential cellular metabolism. Without glucocorticoids, an animal cannot survive a stressful incident. The glucocorticoids have widespread effects because they influence the function of most cells in the body. Glucocorticoids in physiological quantities are essential for the dilution of the renal filtrate into the hyposthenuric range. Other physiological roles of glucocorticoids are to increase gluconeogenesis, decrease protein synthesis, and increase lipolysis with the release of glycerol and free fatty acids (an insulin-antagonistic effect). Although many of the effects are dose-related, glucocorticoids may also act in a permissive manner to optimize certain cellular reactions such as the gluconeogenesis stimulated by glucagon and catecholamines. The physiological effects of glucocorticoids in the fed state are not very significant; however, during fasting, glucocorticoids contribute to the maintenance of glucose concentrations by increasing the release of glucose by the liver and increasing gluconeogenesis and glycogen deposition by stimulating glycogen synthase. The effect on muscle is catabolic because glucose uptake decreases and amino acid release (gluconeogenesis) increases.

Glucocorticoids stimulate adipocyte differentiation, promoting adipogenesis through activation of key adipocyte differentiation genes such as lipoprotein lipase, glycerol-3-phosphate dehydrogenase, and leptin. Glucocorticoids also are permissive for activity of the hormone-sensitive lipase (HSL), which is responsible for mobilization of free fatty acids from adipose stores. Lipolysis is stimulated; therefore, when insulin is lacking or being greatly antagonized, ketogenesis may result (Aron and Tyrrell 1994; Feldman and Nelson 1987; Ferguson 1985a; Goldfien 1992; Haynes 1990; Melby 1974; Wilcke and Davis 1982).

Glucocorticoids also maintain microcirculation, normal vascular permeability, and stability of lysosomal membranes, and suppress inflammatory reactions, although these functions are more commonly associated with the pharmacologic effects of glucocorticoids (Aron and Tyrrell 1994; Tyrrell et al. 1994).

PHARMALOGIC EFFECTS

Growth and Development. Glucocorticoids play a physiological role in the development of pulmonary surfactant in the near-term fetus, allowing an adaptation to air breathing. GCs stimulate lung maturation through the synthesis of surfactant proteins. GCR knockout mice do not survive because of lung atelectasis. Prematurity with delayed development of the adrenal axis in foals has been suspected as a cause of neonatal respiratory distress syndrome. Although glucocorticoids stimulate growth hormone (GH) gene transcription in physiological quantities, glucocorticoids in excess inhibit linear skeletal growth, via catabolic effects on connective tissue and muscle and inhibition of IFG-1 effects. GCs also stimulate the adrenal medullary enzyme converting norepinephrine to epinephrine (Aron and Tyrrell 1994; Tyrrell et al. 1994; Stewart 2003).

Energy Metabolism. Glucocorticoids have an antagonistic effect to that of insulin, leading to increased glucose production from amino acids (gluconeogenesis) and reduced incorporation of amino acids into protein. As stated above, glucocorticoids enhance lipolysis; however, glucocorticoid excess (pharmacologic amounts) or spontaneous hyperadrenocorticism may result in redistribution of fat because glucocorticoids stimulate appetite, thereby stimulating hyperinsulinemia, which results in lipogenesis. As a result, diabetes mellitus may result from prolonged glucocorticoid use at high dosages in animals with diminished insulin secretory capacity (prediabetics). Muscle wasting and weakness are not uncommon with glucocorticoid excess; although glucocorticoids stimulate protein and RNA synthesis in the liver, they have catabolic effects in lymphoid and connective tissue, muscle, fat, and skin. While not usually a recognizable clinical problem in domestic animals, osteoporosis may result in people with Cushing's syndrome or on chronic glucocorticoid administration. The problem likely is most significant in areas of healing bone; glucocorticoids directly inhibit bone formation by inhibiting osteoblast proliferation and the synthesis of bone matrix while stimulating osteoclast activity. In addition, glucocorticoids potentiate the action of parathyroid hormone (PTH) and 1,24-dihydroxycholecalciferol ($1,25(OH)_2$-D_3) and inhibit the gut absorption of calcium, an effect that can be used to advantage in hypercalcemic states. In the young animal, the catabolic effects of excessive amounts of glucocorticoid reduce growth. In children, this reduced growth is not prevented by growth hormone (Aron and Tyrrell 1994; Tyrrell et al. 1994).

Water and Electrolyte Balance. Glucocorticoid use invariably leads to polyuria and polydipsia via inhibition of ADH release and action, as well as alteration of the animal's psyche, resulting in increased water intake. No glucocorticoid given in large doses is completely devoid of mineralocorticoid (salt-retaining and K^+-losing) activity; therefore, excessive use may precipitate or exacerbate hypertension and induce hypokalemia. In part by increasing extracellular fluid volume, glucocorticoids increase the glomerular filtration rate and are required in physiologic amounts for maximal dilution of urine (Ferguson 1985a; Melby 1974; Nakamoto et al. 1992).

Immune and Hematologic Effects. Often the desired result of a therapeutic application, antiinflammatory effects of glucocorticoids are primarily seen at pharmacologic doses. Glucocorticoids result in alterations in the concentration, distribution, and function of peripheral leukocytes and in inhibition of phospholipase A_2 activity in the plasma membranes of these cells. Glucocorticoids act indirectly by inducing lipocortin synthesis, which in turn inhibits arachidonic acid release from membrane-bound stores, and also by inducing TGF-β expression, which subsequently blocks cytokine synthesis and T-cell activation. In addition to contributing to maintenance of the microcirculation and cell membrane integrity, glucocorticoids interfere with progressive dissolution and disruption of connective tissue and cells, possibly by stabilizing lysosomal membranes (Aron and Tyrrell 1994; Aucoin 1982; Barragry 1994). Although lysosomal stabilization by glucocorticoids has been demonstrated experimentally, it is hard to know what benefit these effects have in clinical situations. Glucocorticoids also decrease formation of induced histamine (histamine produced locally by cells during injury), the action of which is not effectively blocked by standard doses of antihistamines. They also antagonize toxins and kinins, reducing the resultant inflammation. It is important to realize, however, that most of their effects are *nonspecific;* that is, they have profound metabolic effects regardless of the initial insult.

Glucocorticoids are used to advantage to suppress both the number of cells and the actions of the immune system. The suppressive effects on cell-mediated immunity predominate over those on humoral immunity. Antibody production is generally unaffected by moderate dosages of glucocorticoids and is inhibited only at high dosages and with long-term therapy. They cause lymphopenia and eosmopenia, an effect secondary to cell redistribution and/or lysis, and lead to increased vascular demargination of neutrophils from the vascular bed to lymphoid tissue. Glucocorticoids inhibit virus-induced interferon synthesis and diminish the functional capacity of monocytes, macrophages, and eosinophils through inhibition of the formation of ILs such as IL1 (macrophages), IL2 (lymphocytes), IL3, and IL6 and other chemotactic factors. Glucocorticoids can induce apoptosis on normal lymphoid cells and play a key role in the physiology of thymic selection. They inhibit monocyte differentiation into macrophages and macrophage phagocytosis and cytotoxic activity (Barragry 1994; Ehrich et al. 1992; McDonald and Langston 1994; Melby 1974; Tyrrell et al. 1994; Buttgereit et al. 2004).

In the clinical setting, GCs are used for their ability to induce apoptosis of malignant lymphoid cells. The mechanisms of apoptosis induced by glucocorticoids fall roughly in two categories, depending on the type of lymphocytes: induction of "death genes" such as IκB and *c-jun* or repression of survival factors such as AP-1 and *c-myc*. By inhibiting the production of Th1 cytokines, glucocorticoids may enhance Th2 cell activity and generate a long-lasting state of tolerance. Although the ultimate apoptotic mechanisms of GCs on lymphocytes are still unclear, the roles of chromatin degradation, endonucleases, and several oncogenes has been suspected. However, GCs appear to up-regulate repair-phase cytokines like TGF-β and PDGF, possibly explaining the suppressive effect on healing and fibrosis (Pallardy and Biola 1998; Buttgereit et al. 2004).

Cardiorespiratory Effects. In addition to indirect effects on electrolyte metabolism, glucocorticoids have direct positive chronotropic and inotropic actions on the heart. They appear to block the increased permeability of capillaries induced by acute inflammation, reducing transport of protein into damaged areas and maintaining microcirculation. Because glucocorticoids are necessary for maximal catecholamine sensitivity, they contribute to maintenance of vascular tone (Ferguson et al. 1978; Nakamoto et al. 1992). In shock, production of vasoactive products of lipid peroxidation (arachidonic acid cascade), such as the vasoconstrictor thromboxane A_2, may be decreased by glucocorticoids, but probably only in the early stage of cell disruption. Glucocorticoids cause vasoconstriction when applied directly to vessels. They decrease capillary permeability by inhibiting the activity of kinins and bacterial endotoxins and by reducing the amount of histamine released by basophils.

Glucocorticoids may induce hypertension in animals and humans through the following mechanisms: 1) activation of the renin-angiotensin (R-A) system due to an increase in plasma renin substrate (PRS); 2) reduced activity of the hypotensive kallikrein-kinin (K-K) system, prostaglandins (PGs), and the endothelium-derived relaxing factor (EDRF), nitric oxide (NO); and (3) increased pressor responses to angiotensin II (Ang II) and norepinephrine. Furthermore, the number of Ang II type 1 receptors of vascular smooth muscle cells is significantly increased by glucocorticoids (Saruta 1996).

Glucocorticoids increase the number and affinity of β-adrenergic receptors. Glucocorticoids prevent receptor down-regulation and therefore tachyphylaxis, resulting in potentiation of the effects of β-adrenergic agonists on bronchial smooth muscle, an important effect in the asthmatic patient (Sprung et al. 1984; Tyrrell et al. 1994; Wilcke and Davis 1982).

CNS Effects. Although rarely described in domestic animals, glucocorticoids (or lack of them) have marked effects on the psyche, resulting in a form of mental, as well as physical, dependence (Ferguson 1985a; Metz et al. 1982).

It is known that pretreatment of neonatal rats with dexamethasone provides protection against hypoxic-ischemic brain damage. This effect is likely mediated via glucocorticoid receptors, because glucocorticoid receptor antagonist RU38486 reverses the benefit. The neuroprotection also appears to be related to alterations in cerebral metabolism. Glucose utilization is reduced prior to hypoxia-ischemia by dexamethasone and is better maintained during hypoxia-ischemia. High-energy phosphates in the brain are higher in dexamethasone-treated animals. Thus, glucocorticoids may provide their protection against hypoxic-ischemic damage by decreasing basal metabolic energy requirements and/or increasing the availability or efficiency of use of energy substrates (Tuor 1997).

Endocrine Effects. Glucocorticoids, in addition to being diabetogenic, also have marked effects on hypothalamic and pituitary function. ACTH, β-lipotropin, thyroid-stimulating hormone (TSH), follicle-stimulating hormone (FSH), and growth hormone (GH) synthesis and secretion are all suppressed; however, β-endorphin levels are unaffected. Glucocorticoids, even at "physiological" dosages (0.22 mg/kg prednisolone once daily orally in the dog), result in HPAA suppression, as indicated by reduction in the ACTH-stimulated cortisol concentration increment and by reduction of the ratio of the zona fasciculata and reticularis to zona glomerulosa in the adrenal gland. Antiinflammatory dosages of prednisolone (0.5 mg/kg q12h orally) resulted in adrenal suppression within 2 weeks of therapy (Chastain and Graham 1979). In another study in dogs, 1 month of the same dosage of prednisolone orally resulted in profound suppression of endogenous plasma ACTH and cortisol concentrations, CRH-stimulated ACTH release, and ACTH-stimulated cortisol release. However, following withdrawal of the prednisolone, the HPAA returned to normal within 2 weeks (Moore and Hoenig 1992). A similar ability to recover from exogenous glucocorticoids was seen in the cat. A dosage of 2 mg/kg q12h of methylprednisolone given orally for 7 days resulted in suppression of ACTH-stimulated cortisol and CRH-stimulated ACTH, but these changes completely reversed by 7 days after withdrawal of the exogenous glucocorticoid (Crager et al. 1994). Higher dosages and long-acting preparations (dexamethasone, triamcinolone, depot products) may result in more pronounced HPAA suppression (Kemppainen and Sartin 1984; Kemppainen 1986; Kemppainen et al. 1982).

The effect of glucocorticoids on glucose metabolism is time- and dose-dependent: insulin and glucose concentrations, or glucose tolerance, were not significantly altered by the administration for 28 days of an antiinflammatory dosage of oral prednisone (Moore and Hoenig 1993). However, daily administration of high dosages of dexamethasone and growth hormone is a reliable model for induction of diabetes mellitus in the cat (Hoenig et al. 2000). There also have been case reports of diabetes mellitus induced in dogs after administration of corticosteroids and methylprednisolone pulse therapy (Jeffers et al. 1991).

Pharmacologic doses of glucocorticoids generally reduce serum thyroid hormone concentrations, presumably through suppression of pituitary TSH. These effects have been well documented in the dog, are not as significant in the cat, and are not well studied in other domestic species (Ferguson and Peterson 1992; Kaptein et al. 1992; Moore et al. 1993). The metabolic consequences of these lowered concentrations of thyroid hormones are not known in the dog; however, a state of hypothyroidism is not believed to be the result (Jennings and Ferguson 1984).

Gastrointestinal Effects. In human patients, large doses of glucocorticoids stimulate excessive production of acid and pepsin in the stomach and may cause peptic ulcer. Despite reasonable clinical concern in animals, similar controlled clinical studies of the propensity for glucocorticoids to induce gastric ulcers have not been conducted. However, in an experimental canine fundic pouch model of acid secretion, the effect of prednisolone (2 mg/kg per day given parenterally for 3 doses, 2 weeks or 12 weeks) on gastric mucosal H^+ permeability was studied. Acute administration (<2 weeks) had no effect. Chronic administration (12 weeks) increased slightly the basal H^+ secretion rate, and increased mucosal permeability by 50% when simultaneously administered with aspirin (Chung et al. 1978). In rats, dexamethasone-induced ulceration has led to alterations in the phospholipid fatty acid profile (increased linoleic acid and decrease in other polyunsaturated fatty acids [PUFAs]). PUFA supplementation or the administration of an H2 receptor antagonist reduced ulcerization with near normalization of changes in the phospholipid fatty acid profile (Manjari and Das 2000). Similar studies have not been conducted in domestic animals.

Prednisolone and dexamethasone, studied in canine colon cell culture, had no effect on the intestinal cell tight junction barrier function, but did prevent the increase in permeability induced by TNF-α. Specifically, glucocorticoids, acting through nuclear receptors, inhibited the TNF-α–induced increase in myosin light chain kinase (MLCK) protein expression, which was shown to mediate increased intestinal tight junction permeability (Boivin et al. 2007).

Glucocorticoids facilitate fat absorption and appear to antagonize the effect of vitamin D on calcium absorption. Therefore, glucocorticoids are employed in chronic hypercalcemic states in an attempt to inhibit gastrointestinal calcium absorption (Aron and Tyrrell 1994; Tyrrell et al. 1994).

CHEMISTRY

Source. Although the natural corticosteroids can be obtained from animal adrenal glands, they are usually synthesized from cholic acid or steroid sapogenins found in plants of the Liliaceae and Dioscoreaceae families. Further modifications of these steroids have led to the marketing of a large group of synthetic steroids with special characteristics that are pharmacologically and therapeutically important (see Table 30.3 and Figs. 30.6 and 30.7).

Structure-Activity Relationships. The actions of the synthetic steroids are similar to those of cortisol (see above). They bind to the specific intracellular receptor proteins and produce the same effects but have different ratios of glucocorticoid-to-mineralocorticoid potency (see Table 30.3).

Steroid Base. Figures 30.6 and 30.7 show the steroid base, or carbon skeleton, of glucocorticoids. The structure of the base determines the *antiinflammatory (glucocorticoid) potency, mineralocorticoid potency,* and the *duration of action once at the site of action.*

Alterations in the steroid base structure influence its affinity for glucocorticoid and mineralocorticoid receptors, as well as its protein-binding avidity, side-chain

TABLE 30.3 Characteristics of various glucocorticoid bases

Drug	Potency			Alternate-day therapy possible?
	Glucocorticoid[a]	Mineralocorticoid	HPAA suppression[b]	
Short-acting (duration of action: <24 hr)				
Hydrocortisone	1	++	+	No (too short)
Cortisone	0.8	++	+	Yes (not ideal)
Prednisone	4	+	+	Yes
Prednisolone	4	+	+	Yes
Methylprednisolone	5	+	+	Yes
Intermediate-acting (duration of action: 24–48 hr)				
Triamcinolone	5	0	++	No
Long-acting (duration of action: <48 hr)				
Flumethasone	15	0	+++	No
Dexamethasone	30	0	+++	No
Betamethasone	30	0	+++	No

Note: Effective anti-inflammatory time equals the HPAA suppression time in most cases. However, the therapeutic success and fewer side effects with alternate-day therapy stem from the fact that some preparations have slightly longer anti-inflammatory or immunosuppressive action than their action to suppress the HPAA.

[a]Compared with hydrocortisone on a mg-for-mg basis.

[b]HPAA = hypothalamic-pituitary-adrenal axis.

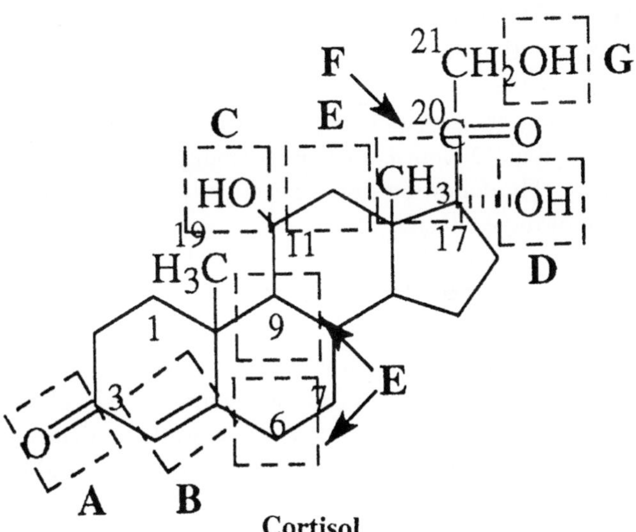

FIG. 30.6 Structure-activity relationships of glucocorticoids. Shown on the structure of the compound cortisol are the important structural sites determining the activity of a glucocorticoid base. *A:* 3 keto group essential for glucocorticoid activity; *B:* 4,5 double bond essential for glucocorticoid activity; *C:* 11 hydroxyl essential for optimal glucocorticoid activity; *D:* 17 α hydroxyl is important for glucocorticoid activity; *E:* 16 methylation or fluorination reduces mineralocorticoid activity considerably and increases glucocorticoid activity; *F:* 20 keto group is important for glucocorticoid activity; *G:* 21 hydroxyl is essential for mineralocorticoid activity and is the site of esterification.

stability, rate of reduction, and metabolic products. Certain structures on the steroid base are essential for glucocorticoid activity (Figs. 30.6, 30.7). An 11-ketol is essential for glucocorticoid activity, and compounds like cortisone and prednisone must first be reduced in the liver from the 11-carbon ketone to the ketol before full activity is seen. The 1,2 double bond provides a fourfold increase in glucocorticoid activity. The C-3 and C-20 ketone groups are also essential for glucocorticoid activity. The addition of 16-α-methyl 9-α-fluoro groups results in compounds with enhanced antiinflammatory activity. Further substitution at the 17 ester position results in a new group of extremely potent steroids (e.g., beclomethasone and betamethasone) that are effective when applied topically for skin diseases and by inhalation for treating asthma. Modifications of the glucocorticoid molecular structure also alter the tendency for the molecule to bind with CBG in the plasma. An increase in binding to CBG results in a lower tendency for the hormone to be metabolized. Halogenation at the 9 position, unsaturation of the 1,2 bond, and methylation at the 2 or 16 position will prolong the half-life by more than 50–70%. The 11-hydroxyl group also appears to inhibit destruction, since the half-life of 11-deoxycortisol is half that of cortisol. In some cases, the agent administered is a prodrug: prednisone is rapidly reduced to prednisolone, and cortisone is rapidly converted to cortisol by

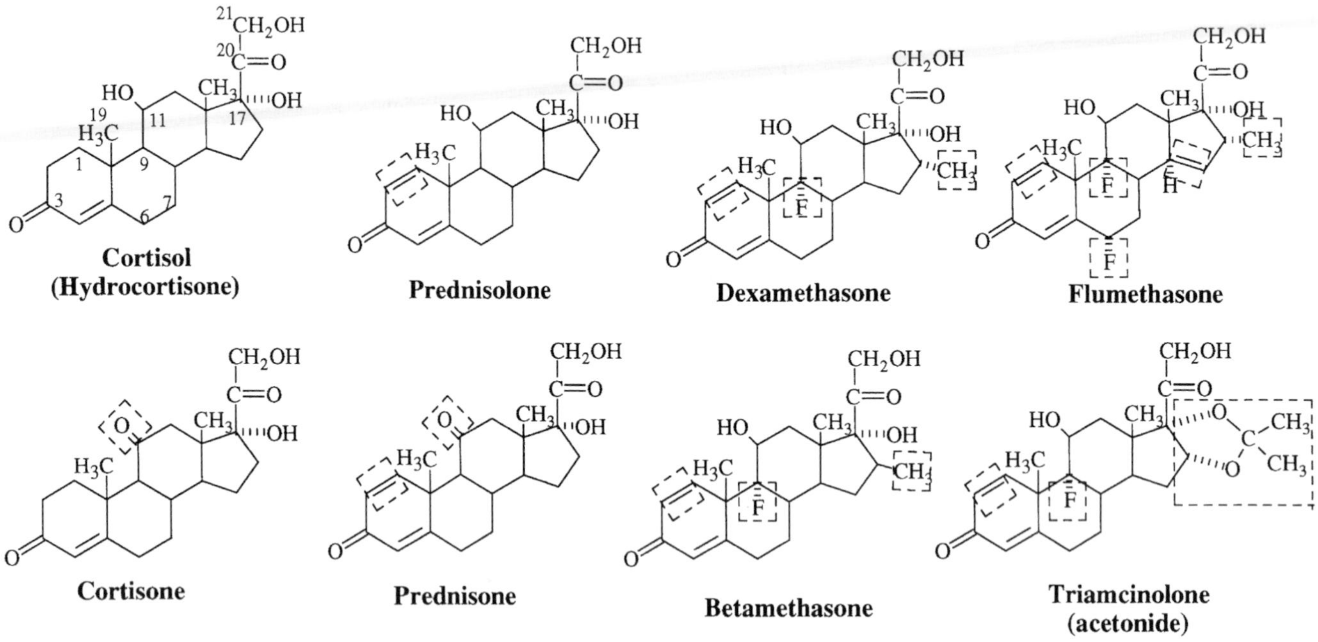

FIG. 30.7 Structures of common glucocorticoids used in veterinary medicine. The key elements of structure differing from cortisol are identified by the outlined areas.

the liver. The synthetic corticosteroids for oral use are in most cases rapidly and completely absorbed when given by mouth.

Ester. Esterification of the alcohol at C-21 serves a number of potential purposes. The ester moiety determines to a significant extent the water/lipid solubility ratio and also influences the duration of action of the base compound's release from subcutaneous or intramuscular sites. Tissue esterases cleave the ester, resulting in free base, which then is distributed via the circulation to tissue sites of action. Routes of administration and duration of release are given for the following esters:

1. Phosphate and hemisuccinate: IV or IM, rapid action and metabolism
2. Acetate, diacetate, tebutate: subcutaneous or IM depots, 2–14 days
3. Acetonide: subcutaneous or IM depots, poorly H_2O soluble
4. Pivalate: subcutaneous or IM depots; weeks to months

The ability of a formulation to suppress the HPAA is determined by the *dosage,* the *potency of the base,* and the *duration of action of the formulation* (base + ester).

TOXICITY. The main limiting factors for glucocorticoid administration are the global toxic effects of these agents. Table 30.4 lists most of the reported side effects as described in the dog, the species in which glucocorticoids are most widely used. Of course, there is variability from species to species. The following discussion highlights the basis for some of these effects.

Metabolic/Endocrine Effects. The endocrine manifestations of glucocorticoid administration can be severe. Iatrogenic Cushing's syndrome may develop with adrenal insufficiency on withdrawal of the medication. The gluconeogenic effects may unmask or exacerbate diabetes, and polyuric and polydipsic states and may induce hypertension.

CNS Effects. In animals, the effects on mental status are difficult to assess or compare with those in humans; however, glucocorticoids likely induce a state of well-being. Neurologically, there is also evidence that glucocorticoids may decrease the threshold for seizures. Lethargy and panting occasionally develop in dogs and cats. Rapid withdrawal of glucocorticoids can induce depression and irritability (Ferguson 1985a,b; McDonald and Langston 1994).

TABLE 30.4 Reported side effects of glucocorticoid treatment (with emphasis on dogs)

Blood and blood chemistry	**Gastrointestinal**
Increases in:	Polyphagia
Neutrophils	Anorexia (rare)
Erythrocytes	Diarrhea (may be bloody)
Monocytes	Increased gastric acid secretion
Platelets	Hepatomegaly
Alkaline phosphatase*	Hepatopathy
Cholesterol	Pancreatitis
Glucose	Colonic perforation
Alanine aminotransferase	**Renal**
Decreases in:	Polyuria with secondary polydipsia*
Eosinophils*	Increased urinary calcium excretion
Lymphocytes	**Musculoskeletal**
Blood urea nitrogen	Muscle atrophy
Central nervous system	Weakness, exercise intolerance
Behavioral and mood changes (depression, increased irritability)	Myotonia (rare)
Lethargy	Osteoporosis
Panting	**Skin**
Endocrine	Calcinosis cutis
Iatrogenic Cushing's disease, HPAA suppression*, secondary adrenocortical insufficiency	Thin skin
Reduced thyroid hormone (T_4 and T_3) levels	Bilateral hair loss
Reduced gonadotropin and sex steroid levels	Increased bruising
Anestrus, testicular atrophy, reduced libido	**Other**
Elevated insulin levels, carbohydrate intolerance	Increased risk of infection
Reduced vitamin D levels	Enhanced spread of infection
Elevated parathyroid hormone levels	Poor wound healing
	Redistribution of body fat
	Reduced growth

Source: Summarized from Kemppainen 1986.
*Relatively common finding in dogs.

Lending to the understanding of their potential protective effects at high doses in central nervous system injury, glucocorticoids have been shown to protect neurons from apoptosis by a mechanism involving the cyclin-dependent kinase inhibitor $p21_{Waf1/cip1}$, an effect reversed by receptor antagonists as well as inhibitors of PI3- and Akt-kinase (Harms et al. 2007).

Gastrointestinal and Hepatic Effects. The gastrointestinal and hepatic effects of glucocorticoids are among the most limiting regarding chronic administration. Glucocorticoids clearly induce a form of micronodular cirrhosis and stimulate the steroid-specific isozyme of alkaline phosphatase. In addition to hepatopathy and hepatomegaly, glucocorticoid excess may result in increased gastric acid and gastric ulceration, but more commonly high doses of potent glucocorticoids cause colonic perforation in dogs. Of course, glucocorticoids may stimulate appetite, an effect occasionally used to advantage in some therapeutic situations. Rarely, the animal will respond with anorexia. It has been postulated that glucocorticoids may also cause pancreatitis.

Musculoskeletal Effects. Chronic glucocorticoid administration induces excessive catabolism and muscle atrophy. Animals may become clinically weak and be unable to exercise optimally. Bone growth may be inhibited and antagonism of vitamin D activity may result in osteoporosis with chronic administration of glucocorticoids.

Dermatologic Effects. Glucocorticoids reduce collagen synthesis and thereby reduce the rate of wound healing. The skin becomes thin and more easily stretched and bruised due to increased capillary fragility. Dogs on large dosages of glucocorticoids often develop bilateral symmetrical alopecia, known as a "Cushingoid" appearance. Cats tend to be less susceptible to these effects. Occasionally, exogenous glucocorticoid administration will induce calcium deposition in the dystrophic epidermis; however, the incidence in dogs appears to be less than with spontaneous hyperadrenocorticism (Scott 1982).

Immunologic Effects. Although immune suppression is often the desired therapeutic effect of glucocorticoids, these agents are notorious for exacerbation of clinical or latent infectious disease processes. Animals on chronic glucocorticoid therapy have a higher incidence of bacterial infections; in one study, 75% of dogs on glucocorticoids for allergic skin disease had clinical or subclinical urinary tract infections. Of course, by inhibiting the cell-mediated immune response to an infection, glucocorticoids slow the function of immune cells that help contain an infection (Aucoin 1982; Fauci 1976; Feldman and Nelson 1987; Ferguson 1985a,b; Siegel 1985).

Reproductive Effects. High doses of glucocorticoids induce parturition during the latter part of pregnancy in ruminants and horses (Barragry 1994). There is also now evidence that dexamethasone can cause abortion in the dog. Glucocorticoids generally have teratogenic effects during early pregnancy and should be avoided in the breeding animal if possible.

Fatal Sequela in the Dog. As an example of the severe consequences of glucocorticoid excess in the dog, the following clinical case, reported in the veterinary literature (Bellah et al. 1989), is provided:

A dog was given multiple doses of glucocorticoids for treatment of intervertebral disk disease over a 25-day period: methylprednisolone acetate (Depo-Medrol)—20 mg IM; dexamethasone sodium phosphate—2 mg IM; flumethasone—0.5 mg and 1 mg IM; dexamethasone—0.25 mg q8h orally as needed; triamcinolone diacetate—40 mg IM (60 times the manufacturer's recommended dose).

The dog presented to the examining clinician with historical and physical findings of polyuria/polydipsia, fever, murmur, pendulous abdomen, marked hepatomegaly, hindlimb paraparesis, midlumbar hyperpathia, and normal pain perception in the hindlimbs. Initial laboratory findings included anemia; leukocytosis; neutrophilia; hyperalbuminemia; increased serum alkaline phosphatase (SAP), alanine aminotransferase (ALT), and glucose; increased bromsulfophthalein (BSP) retention; isosthenuria; bacteriuria (staphylococci); and low baseline and post-ACTH stimulation plasma cortisol levels.

Subsequently, laboratory findings demonstrated a deteriorating state of anemia, hypoproteinemia, leukocytosis, neutrophilia, thrombocytopenia, hyperglycemia, hyperbilirubinemia, and increased SAP and ALT. Radiographic findings included cardiomegaly, hepatomegaly, and a herniated intervertebral disk at L5–L6. Needle biopsy of the liver revealed a micronodular cirrhosis, changes consistent with glucocorticoid hepatopathy. Despite extensive supportive treatment, the dog succumbed following the development of *Haemobartonella*-induced hemolytic anemia, more vomiting, depression, anorexia, melena, and multiple cutaneous abscesses. The dog was euthanized and necropsy revealed generalized atrophy, icterus, and thinning of the skin; hepatomegaly; severe adrenocortical atrophy; hepatic vacuolization; and pancreatic fibrosis with foci of necrosis and inflammation. Although this case represents an extreme overdosage, it illustrates the severe and potentially fatal toxicity that can result from excessive dosage or duration of glucocorticoid administration (Bellah et al. 1989).

Laminitis in the Horse. High-dose glucocorticoids can induce or exacerbate laminitis in the horse. Glucocorticoids appear to potentiate the action of catecholamines in the equine digit. Because this constriction is more pronounced on venous beds than on arteriolar beds, the net result is often digital congestion and edema (Barragry 1994). The enzyme 11-β steroid dehydrogenase Type 1 (11-β HSD1) is occasionally elevated in hoof lamellar tissues during conditions of glucocorticoid excess resulting in a greater tendency toward metabolically active glucocorticoids. Glucocorticoids have been postulated to reduce digit perfusion by a direct action on smooth muscle as well as by inducing insulin-resistance. Endothelial damage associated with elevated glucose leads to increased production of endothelin-1 and a reduction in nitric oxide (NO) production tending to promote vasoconstriction (Johnson et al. 2004).

PRINCIPLES OF RATIONAL GLUCOCORTICOID THERAPY. Because of their wide-ranging and nonspecific effects, reports of the clinical use of glucocorticoids are replete with pragmatic recommendations regarding dosage, duration of therapy, and severity of side effects. Much has been adopted from clinical use in humans, and much more is known about the fine points of glucocorticoid therapy in dogs and cats than in other species. In the following discussion, most of the specific comments will apply to the use of glucocorticoids in the dog; however, when available, appropriate information for other species will be mentioned. It is important to recognize that glucocorticoids rarely cure disease. With the possible exception of spontaneous glucocorticoid deficiency, they are used to try to suppress clinical signs long enough for a condition to run its natural course (Fauci 1976; Ferguson 1985a,b; Melby 1974; Wilcke and Davis 1982).

A well-known endocrinologist named Thorn proposed in 1966 that physicians ask themselves the following questions *before using* glucocorticoid therapy (Hench 1952). A similar approach is proposed for use in animals:

1. How serious is the underlying disorder?
2. How long will therapy be required?
3. Is the patient predisposed to any complications of glucocorticoid therapy?
4. What is the anticipated glucocorticoid dosage?
5. Which glucocorticoid preparation should be used?
6. Have other types of treatment been used to minimize glucocorticoid dosage and side effects?
7. Is an alternate-day regimen indicated?

These questions may help develop guidelines for practical and rational glucocorticoid therapy.

How Serious Is the Underlying Disorder? How Long Will Therapy Be Required? The following general principles should be considered when glucocorticoid therapy is employed:

Diagnose the disease first, if possible. Glucocorticoids are generally only palliative and do not provide a true cure for any disease. In addition, if used before all reasonable diagnostic tests have been completed, they may mask signs of underlying disease and complicate specific diagnosis and therapy. Though a definitive diagnosis is not always possible, a presumptive diagnosis should be proposed (Ferguson 1985a,b).

Classify the disorder into one of the following categories of glucocorticoid therapy, according to a definitive or presumptive diagnosis: physiologic replacement, intensive short-term, antiinflammatory and antiallergic, immunosuppressive, and chronic palliative. Each of these usage classifications will be discussed in more detail. By using these classifications, the clinician clearly defines the goal of therapy and can choose a starting dose and formulation appropriate for the disorder.

Use glucocorticoids to accomplish specific objectives. It is important to decide on the therapeutic endpoint *before* therapy is started in order to objectively assess efficacy and determine the smallest effective dose. For example, in treatment of a dog with autoimmune hemolytic anemia, the goal for initial glucocorticoid therapy might be to raise the hematocrit from 10% to 25%. In a horse with chronic obstructive pulmonary disease ("heaves"), the goal might be to suppress the allergic reaction for 1–2 weeks in order to allow the owners to change the feeding regimen to eliminate the offending allergen. By defining a therapeutic objective, the clinician can then judge the efficacy of a treatment protocol and decide when the glucocorticoid dose should be altered or alternative therapy chosen.

The length of therapy should also be anticipated. For example, immunosuppressive therapy generally requires several months of glucocorticoid use. Accordingly, a plan for instituting and later decreasing the dose should be considered from the outset. In such a case, intermittent or alternate-day therapy would not be appropriate, and an intermediate- or long-acting glucocorticoid could be used.

Is the Patient Predisposed to Any Complications of Glucocorticoid Therapy? Because many of the therapeutic effects of glucocorticoids are nonspecific, clinicians should anticipate the impact on the patient of the previously outlined complications of glucocorticoid use. In doing so, the risk/benefit ratio of using these potent agents is considered.

What Is the Anticipated Glucocorticoid Dosage? Which Glucocorticoid Preparation Should Be Used? It is important to understand the relative potency and, perhaps more important, the relative *duration of action* of a glucocorticoid preparation, because the duration of antiinflammatory effects usually parallels the duration of effects on the HPAA. Success with alternate-day therapy, more commonly applied in small-animal practice, depends on selecting a glucocorticoid preparation with slightly longer antiinflammatory or immunosuppressive (beneficial) actions than HPAA-suppressive effects. *Dosages of glucocorticoids are derived by trial and error and should* *be constantly reevaluated.* Due to the aforementioned hazards of long-term daily glucocorticoid use, intermittent or alternate-day therapy is preferred when long-term use is necessary. As shown in Table 30.3, short- or intermediate-acting formulations, generally given orally, are most appropriate and safe for long-term use and alternate-day therapy. The goal of rational therapy is to maintain a condition in remission at the lowest effective glucocorticoid dosage (Fauci 1976; Feldman and Nelson 2004; Ferguson 1985a,b; Wilcke and Davis 1982).

CLASSES OF GLUCOCORTICOID USAGE

Physiological Replacement Therapy. Replacement therapy involves use of glucocorticoids in amounts similar to those of the naturally occurring glucocorticoids (cortisol in virtually all domestic species) from the adrenal gland. Ideal replacement therapy should mimic the adrenal gland's hormonal output under basal conditions, with doses increasing if the animal is stressed by illness or surgery. Practically, this ideal is never achieved; however, the following regimens have been used successfully in adrenalectomized and Addisonian dogs and cats. As a general rule, animals produce approximately 1 mg/kg of cortisol (hydrocortisone) every day. It is not rational to employ alternate-day or intermittent glucocorticoid replacement therapy in a glucocorticoid-deficient animal, because the animal's metabolic well-being depends upon the presence of glucocorticoids *every day.* Therefore, physiological replacement therapy is aimed at providing a small daily amount of glucocorticoid. Physiological replacement therapy is rarely indicated or applied in large animals. In small animals, hydrocortisone or cortisone at 0.2–1 mg/kg/day or, more commonly, equipotent amounts of prednisolone or prednisone at 0.1–0.2 mg/kg/day once daily orally are indicated. There have been reports that the diurnal variation of cortisol results in a peak in the morning in dogs and in the evening in cats; however, more-recent studies have not confirmed this pattern (Kemppainen 1986; Scott 1982). Therefore, the timing of the single daily dosage would not appear to be critical, other than that it be provided approximately the same time each day. Because stress results in higher adrenal output of glucocorticoids, this pattern should be mimicked; in general, in moderate stress, give 2–5 times the physiologic dosage, and in severe stress (e.g., surgery), administer 5–20 times this dosage until the stressful experience has ended (Ferguson 1985a,b).

Intensive Short-Term and Shock Therapy. The effects of glucocorticoids in all forms of shock are still controversial; however, some evidence suggests that early treatment (probably about 4 hours postinduction in dogs) may lead to increased survival, particularly in hemorrhagic and septic shock. The nature of the formulation (particularly the ester) may affect the speed of cellular entry of glucocorticoids during shock; however, other conclusions have also been reached (Ferguson 1985a,b; Ferguson et al. 1978; Sprung et al. 1984; Wilcke and Davis 1982; Wilson 1979).

Glucocorticoids improve hemodynamics and enhance survival in canine models of endotoxic and hemorrhagic shock. However, therapy for shock should also include aggressive fluid therapy. Septic (endotoxic) shock is the most responsive form to glucocorticoid therapy; however, although human trials have shown improved short-term survival, most patients succumbed to chronic septicemia later (Sprung et al. 1984). Suspected endotoxic shock should be treated with fluid therapy and a broad-spectrum antimicrobial, with or without glucocorticoids. Glucocorticoids and antibiotics were synergistic when given within 2 hours of induction of septic shock in baboons.

The potential detrimental effects of massive doses of glucocorticoids should always be considered. However, proponents of glucocorticoid therapy for shock point out that short-term (~48 hr) glucocorticoid therapy has few negative effects, and the positive effects far outweigh the risks. Most human patients with sepsis survive beyond the acute stages of endotoxemia but succumb later to chronic septicemia (Sprung et al. 1984). Certainly, the immunosuppressive effects of glucocorticoids make their use contraindicated during chronic sepsis, and those supporting glucocorticoid use in septic shock do not generally advocate use other than during the early acute hypotensive state. Opponents to glucocorticoid use generally are not convinced that experimental studies in anesthetized animals adequately duplicate clinical situations and do not believe even short-term treatment to be innocuous, because of immunosuppressive effects (Wilcke and Davis 1982).

Antiinflammatory and Antiallergic Therapy. A large proportion of glucocorticoid use in veterinary practice is designed to combat inflammation or allergy. Unfortunately, many such diseases are difficult to definitively diagnose. Therefore, misuse of glucocorticoids is not uncommon in this category. Examples of antiinflammatory and antiallergic use of glucocorticoids include symptomatic treatment of pruritic dermatoses, allergic pulmonary disease, and allergic gastroenteritis. Guidelines for antiinflammatory and antiallergic dosages vary from species to species. Prednisolone or prednisone is most commonly used in small animals at 0.55 mg/kg q12h given orally for induction, and then at 0.55–2.2 mg/kg every other day for maintenance. Although all dosages should be adjusted according to effect, a general, but undocumented, observation has been that cats require approximately twice the glucocorticoid dosage that dogs require to manage a similar condition. Methylprednisolone acetate may also be administered subcutaneously or intramuscularly at 1.1 mg/kg every 1–3 weeks; however, use of depot products brings the distinct disadvantage that the drug dosage cannot be stopped or reduced. Other long-acting injectable products and their duration include prednisolone acetate, 1–2 days; dexamethasone in propylene glycol, 1–7 days; triamcinolone acetonide, 3–7 days; and betamethasone valerate, 7–60 days. For practical reasons of cost and potency, dexamethasone is the most commonly used glucocorticoid in large animals.

Immunosuppressive Therapy. Protracted glucocorticoid use generally is required for immunosuppression. Therefore, use of a glucocorticoid with well-documented side effects and efficacy is recommended. It is important to use the highest recommended dosage until clinical signs abate. After that point, the dosage may be decreased in increments. In general, in small animals, the dosage may be decreased until the equivalent prednisolone dosage of 1.1 mg/kg is being given on alternate days (Aucoin 1982; Ferguson 1985a,b). Long-term side effects of alternate-day therapy are few, and the dosage rarely must be decreased further. Therapy should not be discontinued until the autoimmune disease is in remission for 2–3 months; otherwise, signs are likely to recur (Aucoin 1982; Fauci 1978; Ferguson 1985a,b).

Glucocorticoids provide very nonspecific protective benefits: "The hormone appears not to extinguish the fire or to act like a carpenter to repair the damage of the fire. Instead, it appears to 'dampen the fire,' or to provide, as it were, an asbestos suit behind which the patient, like some Biblical Shadrach, Meshach or Abednego, protects his tissues from the fire. If this protection is removed prematurely, before the fire has spent itself, the patient and his tissues will react again to the burning. But, if the protection is not discarded until the natural duration of the fire is over, the patient remains largely free of symptoms and apparently 'well'" (Hench 1952). Unlike other immunosuppressants, glucocorticoids do not significantly inhibit antibody production by B lymphocytes until possibly very high dosages. If glucocorticoids provide incomplete remission of an immune-mediated disorder, other immunosuppressant agents such as the alkylating agent cyclophosphamide may be added to complement the effects of glucocorticoids. Furthermore, if side effects of the glucocorticoids are too great, other immunosuppressants may be added to the regimen. If no clinical response is obtained with glucocorticoid therapy alone, addition of other immunosuppressants is less likely to succeed. Immune-mediated thrombocytopenia and autoimmmune hemolytic anemia are examples of diseases treated with immunosuppressive doses of glucocorticoids.

In small animals, immunosuppression is generally accomplished with prednisolone at 2.2–6.6 mg/kg or the equipotent dosage of dexamethasone at 0.33–1.1 mg/kg q12h for induction, and prednisolone at 1.0–2.2 mg/kg every other day for maintenance. Note that, because its duration of action exceeds 24 hours, dexamethasone is acceptable for induction but not for alternate-day maintenance therapy (Ferguson 1985a,b).

The adverse effects of chronic immunosuppressive doses of glucocorticoid use can be serious. Therefore, clinicians should eventually attempt to maintain a satisfactory therapeutic result with the smallest possible dose of glucocorticoids on alternate days if possible. Nonsteroidal drugs (e.g., cyclophosphamide or cyclosporine for immunosuppression) may be used as adjunctive therapy if necessary.

Chronic Palliative Therapy. Historically, glucocorticoids were commonly used when nonsteroidal antiinflammatory therapy no longer succeeded at managing chronic conditions, such as arthritis in most species or hip dysplasia in dogs. If nonsteroidal analgesics are not satisfactory, glucocorticoids may be used on an intermittent or alternate-day basis. It is important not to administer glucocorticoids erratically, as rapid withdrawal may precipitate signs of lameness or stiffness ("pseudorheumatism") (Fauci 1976 1978; Ferguson 1985a,b).

Although no controlled clinical studies of simultaneous administration have been conducted in domestic animals, it would seem prudent to heed evidence in human studies suggesting that simultaneous use of glucocorticoids with nonsteroidal antiinflammatory drugs be used cautiously out of concern over the synergistic adverse gastrointestinal ulcerative effects. It is worth noting that in a large case control study of over 1,400 human patients, there was no significant increased peptic ulcerative risk (1.1 times) with oral glucocorticoid therapy alone. However, concomitant NSAID and oral glucocorticoid administration increased the relative risk of fatal ulcers to 21.8 and nonfatal ulcers 4.4-fold. The highest risk was for upper gastrointestinal bleeding (Piper et al. 1991).

Alternate-Day Therapy. Side effects of long-term glucocorticoid use can be dramatically reduced by alternate-day therapy. Allowing the HPAA to recover on "off" days provides greater safety if therapy should suddenly be discontinued. Successful use of alternate-day therapy depends upon the therapeutic effects lasting longer than HPAA-suppressive effects. As a result, this approach is not successful for all diseases. Also, true alternate-day therapy is rarely applied to large-animal cases because it is less practical to give large animals agents with low or intermediate potency like prednisolone. Weaning of more-potent agents such as dexamethasone often is accomplished by extending the between-dose interval to as long as 3–4 days in large animals; however, this is technically not considered alternate-day therapy, because full recovery of the HPAA is not allowed on alternate days (Barragry 1994; Ferguson 1985a,b).

Several common pitfalls of alternate-day therapy should be avoided. Alternate-day therapy is rarely, if ever, effective as primary therapy. It is usually first necessary to use daily therapy to achieve the desired clinical effect. Alternate-day therapy with long-acting glucocorticoids is not rational. The change to alternate-day glucocorticoid use ideally should be gradual, particularly after prolonged high-dosage therapy. Rapid change to alternate-day use may result in signs of glucocorticoid withdrawal. Finally, alternate-day glucocorticoid therapy may fail if used exclusively; supplemental use of alternative therapy should be considered, particularly on "off" days (Fauci 1978; Ferguson 1985a,b).

In inflammatory joint disease caused by infectious or immune-mediated conditions, early aggressive therapy is usually necessary to limit subsequent joint dysfunction. Of course, the primary therapy for immune-mediated arthritis, immunosuppression, can jeopardize the health of patients with infectious arthropathies. So before initiating immunosuppressive therapy, follow a thorough diagnostic plan to exclude infectious causes (Michels and Carr 1997).

Changing to Alternate-Day Therapy. Because glucocorticoid administration to dogs for longer than 2 weeks generally results in significant loss of adrenal functional reserve, for the sake of this discussion, administration of greater than 0.5 mg/kg/day of prednisolone or an equipotent dosage of a more potent drug for longer than 2 weeks should be considered chronic therapy (Chastain and Graham 1979). However, when 0.5 mg/kg q12h (an anti-inflammatory dosage) was administered to dogs for 35 days and stopped abruptly, it took less than 2 weeks for the HPAA to totally recover (Moore and Hoenig 1992). This contrasts drastically with the experience in humans, where normalization of cortisol secretion and pituitary function may take as long as 6–9 months (Fauci 1976 1978). Similar studies have not been performed in large-animal species.

There is no "correct" way to taper an animal from glucocorticoids. The following guidelines are suggested. If the glucocorticoid dosage is large (>1 mg/kg/day prednisolone or an equivalent) or therapy prolonged (>2 weeks in duration), some process of gradually reducing the steroid dosage (i.e., weaning) is indicated. One highly conservative approach is to double the glucocorticoid dose for "on" days and taper the dose for "off" days by 25% per cycle (a cycle may vary from 1 day to several weeks). Another conservative method includes increasing the dose for "on" days by the same amount as the dose for "off" days is decreased. Practical experience indicates that, in many canine patients, rapid tapering has few recognizable side effects unless the animal is severely stressed. Subtle adverse effects may be missed unless the owners and clinician are vigilant. Patient tolerance defines the success of any change. If therapy is for less than 2 weeks, it is probably safe to rapidly taper the dog and have no therapy on "off" days. If clinical signs are observed on "off" days, supplement with a replacement dose of glucocorticoids on those days, or add nonsteroidal therapy. If alternate-day therapy is ineffective, use of a single dose each morning (to mimic diurnal variation) may also minimize adverse effects. Examples of two conservative approaches to weaning a dog from prednisolone and application of alternate-day therapy are shown in Table 30.4.

Withdrawal from Glucocorticoids. The identification of clinical signs of glucocorticoid deficiency may be very difficult. Animals cannot complain of minor aches and pains or of mood swings as do people being withdrawn from glucocorticoids. Signs of glucocorticoid withdrawal may include dullness, depression, decreased exercise tolerance, incoordination, unthriftiness and weight loss, loose stools, and behavioral changes. Significant adrenocortical suppression occurs in dogs within 2 weeks of initiating daily glucocorticoid therapy. Therefore, it is reasonable to assume that dogs and cats may require supplementation of glucocorticoids during episodes of stress, such as illness or surgery, particularly if signs of glucocorticoid withdrawal are present. It should be emphasized that short-term use of glucocorticoids in physiological amounts has few risks despite the evidence that these "physiological" quantities significantly suppress the HPAA, resulting in adrenal atrophy (Byyny 1976; Chastain and Graham 1979).

Test of Adrenal Reserve. Laboratory tests usually are not necessary to diagnose most cases of iatrogenic adrenal insufficiency; a good history usually indicates the cause of the problem. Occasionally, in the absence of an accurate history or when surgery is considered for a dog with suspected adrenal insufficiency, an ACTH stimulation test is performed to test adrenal functional reserve.

ACTH Stimulation Test Protocol. A venous blood sample is collected in heparin tubes and centrifuged within 15 minutes, with the plasma immediately frozen for later plasma cortisol determination. A dose of 0.25 mg (25 units or an entire vial, though less will work, regardless of the animal's size) of synthetic ACTH (Cortrosyn, Organon) is given intravenously or intramuscularly. For the dog or horse, a postinjection venous blood sample, handled as for the preinjection sample, is collected 1 hour after IV Cortrosyn injection. If cost is a concern, valuable information on adrenal secretory reserve can be obtained by giving ACTH and collecting a blood sample only at the appropriate time after injection. Blood samples are then assayed by a clinical pathology laboratory for plasma cortisol levels. In cats, peak cortisol concentrations should be measured 30 minutes after intravenous ACTH administration (Feldman and Nelson 1987).

Interpretation of Test Results. Healthy unstressed animals have basal plasma cortisol levels in the normal range that increase by 50–100% after ACTH stimulation. Some dogs, after chronic glucocorticoid treatment, may have normal basal cortisol levels but a post-ACTH increase of less than 50%. Such dogs do well until stressed and then require glucocorticoid supplementation (see below). Other dogs may have low basal levels as well as low post-ACTH cortisol levels, indicating a need for continued regular glucocorticoid supplementation as well as additional glucocorticoids during periods of stress (Ferguson 1985a,b).

Glucocorticoid Supplementation During Stress. Animals with marginally adequate or deficient adrenal function require supplementation of glucocorticoids during periods of stress. In situations of minor stress such as minor surgery, general anesthesia, a minor illness, or even a visit to the veterinarian, glucocorticoid can be given to avoid collapse and other complications. For example, hydrocortisone or cortisone can be given at 2–5 mg/kg or prednisolone or prednisone at 0.4–1.0 mg/kg. In severely stressful situations, such as in severe illness or major surgery, higher dosages may be necessary. In preparing an animal for major surgery (including adrenalectomy), prednisolone acetate can be given intramuscularly at 0.4–2 mg/kg the night before and the morning of surgery. Alternatively, or in addition, 100–300 mg hydrocortisone can be given by IV drip. These large doses should be gradually reduced within 3–5 days to maintenance levels unless there are complications (Ferguson 1985a,b).

Miscellaneous or Special Usages

Topical and Intralesional Usage. Topical and intralesional glucocorticoid administration is occasionally used to manage localized lesions of the skin. Despite the route of administration, systemic effects, including suppression of the HPAA, should be expected. Acute inflammatory conditions such as pyotraumatic dermatitis and urticaria are usually managed with nonocclusive, nonheating glucocorticoid preparations. However, chronic conditions are most commonly managed with penetrating glucocorticoid creams and ointments. The potent fluorinated bases such as betamethasone, dexamethasone, triamcinolone, and fluocinolone are the most commonly preferred. The topical, intralesional, or intraarticular use of compounds (e.g., prednisone, cortisone) requiring hepatic activation is of questionable value (Coppoc 1984; Glaze et al. 1988; Kemppainen 1986; McDonald and Langston 1994; Scott 1982; Scott and Greene 1974; Wilcke and Davis 1982).

Intraarticular Administration. Intraarticular glucocorticoids have been utilized to manage the orthopedic conditions of traumatic arthritis, myositis, bursitis, and tendinitis. Used primarily in equine medicine to manage joint inflammation and pain, the practice of intraarticular glucocorticoid therapy is controversial and potentially dangerous. Glucocorticoids tend to reduce the pain for a working animal but also diminish chondrocyte collagen and synovial fluid production. The benefits cited for this practice include the reduction of proteolytic enzymes in joint fluid and reduction of joint swelling and discomfort. The hazards include encouragement of further mechanical damage, loss of joint proteoglycan, development of septic arthritis, and inhibition of chondrocyte and osteoblast activity, with the end result being joint or bone breakdown. Intraarticular administration of glucocorticoids leads to systemic absorption and HPAA suppression (Barragry 1994).

Special Considerations for Intraarticular Glucocorticoid Usage in Horses. The rationale for intraarticular administration in the horse includes the following: 1) the size of the animal, which requires a large systemic dose of drug to be administered, 2) the higher incidence of acute arthritis conditions in these animals, and 3) the adverse systemic effects of corticosteroids. This route is effective for the treatment of synovitis and capsulitis; however, imaging techniques should confirm that there is no prior structural damage, and strict aseptic technique is mandatory. Chronic degenerative joint conditions tend to respond less well than acute ones. Surgery following glucocorticoid therapy can be problematic as corticosteroids slow the rate of healing as described above. Additional forced exercise may compound the joint damage; therefore, at least 3 months should be given to allow damaged cartilage and subchondral bone to heal (Gabel 1977). In some cases, complete breakdown of the affected joint has occurred during the race following intraarticular glucocorticoid treatment (Tobin 1979; Upson 1978). It has been suggested that the rational usage of corticosteroids are effective in prolonging the performance career of carefully selected equine patients, particularly those in which surgical intervention and/or rest will not be of benefit (McKay and Milne 1976). Furthermore, as previously discussed, glucocorticoid administration has been considered a risk factor for laminitis. In summary, the intraarticular route of administration must be used judiciously (Barragry 1994).

Ophthalmic Applications. Glucocorticoids are used topically and subconjunctivally to manage inflammatory conditions of the eye, including retinitis, choroiditis, optic neuritis, and orbital cellulitis. These agents stabilize the blood-aqueous and blood-retinal barriers, reducing the leakage of protein into the aqueous that accompanies edema and inflammation. Topical ophthalmic administration of glucocorticoid preparations is also employed to minimize neovascularity and, by inhibiting fibroblast activity, to inhibit corneal scarring, pigmentation, and the formation of synechia.

Topical glucocorticoids are available in solutions, ointments, and suspensions. Penetration, therefore, is determined by two factors: the chemical composition of the base and the vehicle. Except for prednisolone acetate, the alcoholic forms of cortisone, hydrocortisone, and prednisone penetrate the cornea more readily than the acetate ester forms.

Subconjunctival administration of glucocorticoids is used to manage conjunctivitis, keratitis, scleritis, and anterior uveitis. However, it is not the route of choice for diseases of the posterior segment. High concentrations of glucocorticoids can be achieved with subconjunctival administration because the sclera is very permeable to steroids.

Glucocorticoids are contraindicated in corneal ulcers because they slow the process of reepithelialization of the cornea. Furthermore, glucocorticoids enhance the activity of collagenase, which is produced by bacteria like *Pseudomonas* and by leukocytes, and may contribute to the development of "melting" corneal ulcers (Brightman 1982; Glaze et al. 1988; McDonald and Langston 1994). Iatrogenic Cushing's syndrome has resulted from topical ophthalmic preparations (Murphy et al. 1990).

Neurological Applications. Neurological applications of glucocorticoid therapy are numerous. Potent anti-inflammatory action is often necessary to manage acute spinal or CNS trauma, acute cervical or lumbar pain, vestibular disease, acute traumatic and some chronic peripheral neuropathies, polymyositis, and CNS neoplasia (Ferguson 1985a,b; McDonald and Langston 1994; Metz et al. 1982; Wilcke and Davis 1982; Meintjes et al. 1996).

Newer Preparations

Selective Glucocorticoid Receptor Agonists. Given the previously discussed existence of cGCR isoforms, future drug development is likely to include qualitatively new drugs, such as selective glucocorticoid receptor agonists (SEGRAs). Several such compounds are under development and are showing promising results. The advantage would be to allow selective therapeutic antiinflammatory benefits associated with transrepression of AP-1 and NF-κ B-stimulated synthesis of inflammatory mediators, while adverse effects were associated with the transactivation of genes involved in metabolic processes (Buttgereit 2004; Stahn et al. 2007).

21-Aminosteroids (Lazaroids). Neuroprotective effects of GCs at high dosages are independent of GCR interaction. 21-aminosteroids have been developed as highly lipophilic drugs, which retain neuroprotective (antilipid peroxidase) effects, in part by reducing fluidity of membranes. They may also appear to scavenge hydroxyl radicals and reduce eicosanoid mediators and tumor necrosis factor, without metabolic effects such as alterations in hematology, glucose, ACTH, or cortisol. Although still largely in development as human pharmaceuticals, their projected use is in acute nervous system trauma, membrane protectants in most forms of shock, and in chronic neurodegenerative diseases (Buttgereit et al. 2004).

Nitrosteroids. This class of glucocorticoids releases low levels of nitric oxide (NO) and it is believed that post-translational modification of GCR by tyrosine nitration is responsible for its enhanced antiinflammatory activity and reduced side effects. Further studies are required in the clinical setting and none have been performed to date in domestic animals (Buttgereit et al. 2004).

"Soft" Steroids. Budesonide, ciclesonide, and loteprednol etabonate are examples of "soft" steroids that are designed for delivery near to their site of action to exert their effect, and then undergo metabolism to inactive metabolites. This retrometabolic drug design has the goal of reducing systemic side effects. Budesonide has been used as an orally administered product in dogs and cats primarily for the treatment of inflammatory bowel disease. It is absorbed in the intestine and undergoes first-pass metabolism to an inactive metabolite. Approximately 15 times more potent than prednisolone, it still has shown systemic glucocorticoid side effects. Ciclesonide (CIC) is a new-generation inhaled corticosteroid, which is hydrolyzed by esterases in the upper and lower airways to its pharmacologically active metabolite desisobutyrl-CIC. In human patients, it is used for treating asthma and allergic rhinitis.

Limited studies in dogs have shown long-lasting antiallergic (antiasthmatic) effects without influencing the hypothalamic-pituitary axis (HPA). Loteprednol is an inactive metabolite soft steroid that has been used in human medicine as an ophthalmic or inhaled product (Belvisi and Hele 2003; Bodor and Buchwald 2006).

MINERALOCORTICOIDS

HISTORY. In 1855, Thomas Addison first described the clinical manifestations of primary adrenal insufficiency (Addison 1855); however, it was not until 1929 that crude extracts of adrenal cortex were used in clinical treatment trials of patients with Addison's disease (glucocorticoid and mineralocorticoid deficiency) (Rogoff and Stewart 1969). In 1937, the adrenocortical steroid 11-desoxycorticosterone was finally produced and made available for treatment of Addison's disease (Thorn et al. 1942). It was able to prevent the urinary sodium loss and was the major therapy for the treatment of Addison's for several years. It was not until the early 1950s that aldosterone was discovered, and it was established that this hormone was involved in water and electrolyte balance (Luetscher 1956; Simpson et al. 1954). Aldosterone was isolated and synthesized in the mid-1950s (Ham et al. 1955; Simpson et al. 1954). It is by far the most potent of the naturally occurring corticosteroids with regard to water and electrolyte balance.

SECRETION AND MECHANISM OF ACTION. Almost all naturally occurring and synthetically derived corticoids have both mineralocorticoid and glucocorticoid activity but are usually designated on the basis of their predominant activity. Mineralocorticoid hormones are secreted by both the zona glomerulosa and zona fasciculata. The zona glomerulosa produces aldosterone and 18-hydroxycorticosterone under the major control of angiotensin II, while the zona fasciculata produces mainly desoxycorticosterone, 18-hydroxydeoxycorticosterone, and corticosterone under ACTH regulation (Mantero et al. 1990). Most of our knowledge of mineralocorticoid action is derived from studies on the classical target organ for mineralocorticoids, the kidney. Mineralocorticoids bind to a specific receptor, the mineralocorticoid receptor

(MR). The MR is a member of the steroid/thyroid/retinoid superfamily of intracellular receptors that are ligand-dependent transcription factors. In the absence of hormone the MR resides predominantly in the cytoplasm (Fejes-Toth et al. 1998) complexed with heat-shock proteins (HSPs) (Couette et al. 1998). Upon hormone binding, there is a conformational change in the receptor's structure; the HSPs dissociate and the receptor migrates to the nucleus where it binds to the promoter region of target genes and regulates transcription from these genes (Rogerson and Fuller 2000). The human MR was cloned in 1987 by Arriza (Arriza et al. 1987), and its mRNA was demonstrated in various tissues such as kidney, hippocampus, pituitary, heart, and spleen. The naturally occurring MR ligands are predominantly aldosterone and deoxycorticosterone, although other steroids such as progesterone show a high-affinity binding to MR. Aldosterone is the most potent regulator of electrolyte excretion and is essential for life (Sutanto and deKloet 1991). It is believed to exist in at least five isoforms, which may have different biological activity. Deoxycorticosterone is also a naturally occurring mineralocorticoid with similar binding patterns to MR as aldosterone. Mineralocorticoids exert their effect in target tissues through interaction with the MR receptor. Hormone-receptor complex binds to chromatin and induces transcription of mRNA, which is subsequently translated to generate proteins. All physiological actions of mineralocorticoids depend on gene activation and new protein synthesis (Johnson 1992). A two-step model for mineralocorticoid action has been proposed. Changes in membrane electrolyte transport in the kidney are fast (within minutes) and involve the stimulation of Na+,K+-ATPase and activation of the Na+/H+ exchanger, which leads to Na+ influx into the cell at the expense of H+ and K+, while de novo synthesis of Na+,K+-ATPase is a late response (within hours or days). Aldosterone also affects the epithelial Na-channel and aldosterone rapidly induces the transcription of gene(s) encoding regulatory protein(s) that increase ENaC activity in the renal collecting duct and distal colon (Snyder 2002; Pearce and Kleyman 2007). The net effect of mineralocorticoid action is, therefore, Na+ retention, proton excretion, and K+ excretion (Wehling et al. 1991, 1992). The Addisonian patient typically has hypernatremia, hyperkalemia, and metabolic acidosis.

PREPARATIONS AND PROPERTIES. The following preparations are currently available for the treatment of mineralocorticoid deficiency:

1. Desoxycorticosterone pivalate (DOCP), a long-acting ester of desoxycorticosterone acetate (DOCA), is available as a sterile suspension for intramuscular injection (Percorten™-V, Novartis). It has been approved for use in the dog.
2. Fludrocortisone acetate is available for oral use in generic form only. It is manufactured as 0.1 mg tablets (Barr Laboratories, Global Pharmaceuticals). It has a half-life of approximately 8 hours in humans. Fludrocortisone also has substantial glucocorticoid activity.

Note: Aldosterone is available only for research, not for therapeutic applications. The structures of the available mineralocorticoid preparations used in veterinary medicine are shown in Figure 30.8.

THERAPEUTIC USE. Historically, DOCA was the treatment of choice for the mineralocorticoid deficiency in acute primary adrenal failure but the drug has been discontinued for many years. For the acute crisis situation or maintenance therapy, either DOCP or fludrocortisone

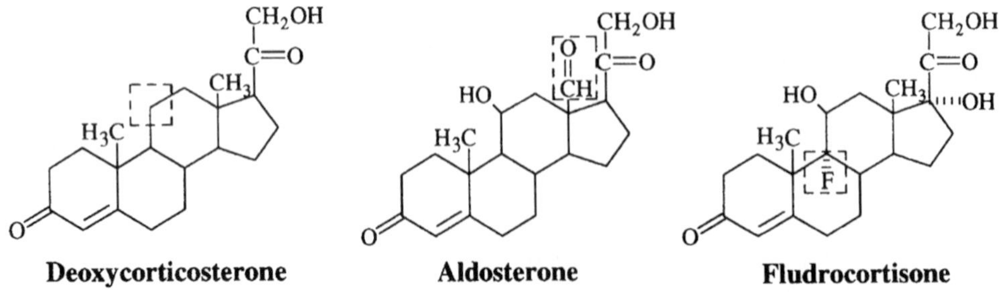

Deoxycorticosterone **Aldosterone** **Fludrocortisone**

FIG. 30.8 Structures of common mineralocorticoid drugs used in veterinary medicine. The key elements of structure differing from cortisol are identified by the outlined areas.

acetate may be used. An initial starting dose of 2.2 mg DOCP/kg of body weight every 25 days has been recommended (Lynn et al. 1993). In the cat a dose of 12.5 mg every 3–4 weeks has been recommended (Greco and Peterson 1989). These doses and the time intervals of injections may be adjusted depending on the response to therapy as measured by serum Na+ and K+ concentrations.

Fludrocortisone acetate must be administered daily for the treatment of hypoadrenocorticism. In the dog the dose is 0.1–0.5 mg orally twice daily or 0.01 mg/kg divided every 12 hours orally. In the cat the dose is 0.1–0.2 mg divided every 12 hours orally. The dose may have to be adjusted based on weekly electrolyte measurements. Once the animal is stable, rechecks including serum Na+ and K+ measurement should be made on a monthly basis. Dogs metabolize this drug rapidly and high doses may be necessary even for less-than-optimal results (Hoenig and Ferguson 1991b).

SIDE EFFECTS. Adverse effects of mineralocorticoid replacement therapy are rare but may include hypokalemia, hypernatremia, muscle weakness, and hypertension, particularly in patients with borderline renal disease (Hoenig and Ferguson 1991b). Because fludrocortisone also has glucocorticoid activity, animals on large doses may show signs of glucocorticoid excess (Lynn et al. 1993). It is important that any fluid deficits be corrected prior to treatment with mineralocorticoids.

ADRENOLYTIC DRUGS AND STEROID SYNTHESIS INHIBITORS

THERAPY FOR HYPERADRENOCORTICISM. Spontaneous hyperadrenocorticism is characterized by excess secretion of the glucocorticoid cortisol. In 85–90% of cases in the dog and the majority of cases in the horse, the primary species suffering from this condition, the cause is excess ACTH production by the pituitary. The term *Cushing's disease* is used when the adrenal glands are bilaterally hypertrophied and producing excess cortisol in response to overproduction of ACTH by the pituitary corticotrophs. In the horse, an intermediate lobe pituitary tumor is the most common cause. Accordingly, in the dog and horse, there have been attempts to reduce ACTH production with dopaminergic compounds (like bromocryptine mesylate or pergolide mesylate) or the antiserotoninergic agent cyproheptadine. The experience with these agents has largely been unsatisfactory in the dog due to toxicity and lack of efficacy. In the horse, pergolide seems to be a more effective treatment than cyproheptadine or bromocryptine (Schott 2002).

Low hypothalamic dopamine concentrations have been observed in dogs with pituitary-dependent hyperadrenocorticism. As such, dopamine deficiency has been proposed as an underlying etiology for this condition. L-Deprenyl (Anypril®, Pfizer Animal Health), a monoamine oxidase B enzyme inhibitor that inhibits the breakdown of dopamine, has been approved for the treatment of pituitary-dependent hyperadrenocorticism in the dog.

Medical therapy for hyperadrenocorticism in the dog has been primarily aimed at reducing glucocorticoid production by the adrenal cortex. The two most frequently used drugs are mitotane and trilostane (Feldman and Nelson 1987; Hoenig and Ferguson 1991a; Neiger et al. 2002). Both drugs are used for hyperadrenocorticism regardless of etiology. This is not true for l-deprenyl. Because it influences dopamine concentrations, it is approved only for pituitary-dependent hyperadrenocorticism. Trilostane has also been used in horses (McGowan and Neiger 2003). Hyperadrenocorticism rarely occurs in cats and the response to medical therapy is inconsistent.

MITOTANE (*o,p′*-DDD)

Chemistry and Mechanism of Action. Mitotane (1-(*o*-chlorophenyl)-1-(*p*-chlorophenyl)-2,2-dichlorethane; *o,p′*/4-DDD) (Fig. 30.9) is a compound that is chemically similar to the insecticides DDD and DDT and leads to a relatively selective destruction of the zonae fasciculata and reticularis by an unknown mechanism.

Metabolism. Clinical studies in human patients indicate that approximately 40% of orally administered mitotane is absorbed, while the remainder is recovered in the feces. Similar studies are not available for the dog or cat.

Preparations and Properties. Mitotane (Lysodren, Bristol-Myers Oncology Division) is available in 500 mg scored tablets.

Therapeutic Uses. The cytotoxic effect of mitotane to the dog adrenal cortex was first described in 1959 (Vilar and Tullner 1959); however, it was not until 1973 that

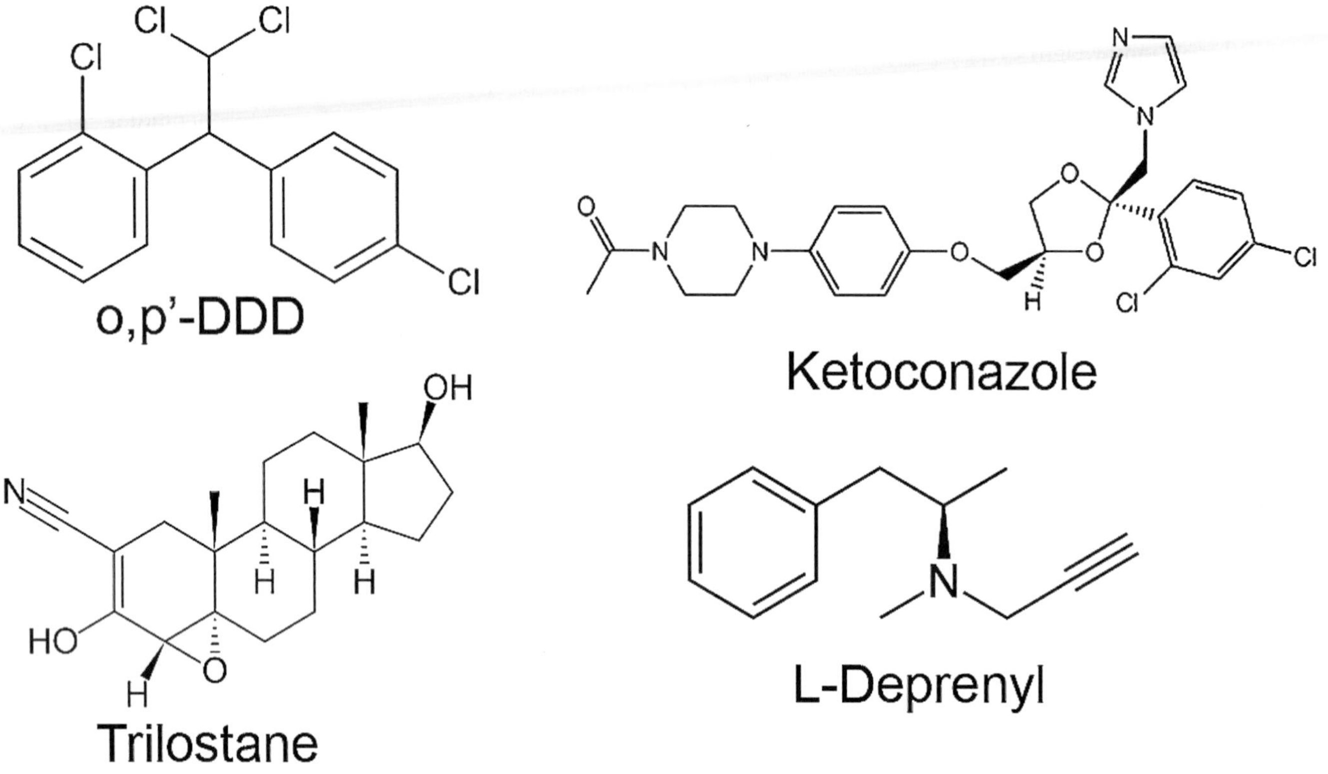

o,p'-DDD

Ketoconazole

Trilostane

L-Deprenyl

FIG. 30.9 Structures of antiadrenal drugs.

mitotane was used therapeutically in veterinary medicine (Lorenz et al. 1973; Schechter et al. 1973). It is now the most commonly used form of treatment for pituitary-dependent hyperadrenocorticism (Peterson 1983) but has also proven to be efficacious in cases with adrenal neoplasia (Kintzer and Peterson 1989). Usually 50 mg/kg are given daily or divided twice daily for 7–10 days. The goal of this so-called "loading period" is to decrease the capacity of the adrenal cortex to the point that cortisol secretion becomes minimal and the animal is unable to respond to exogenous ACTH with an increase in cortisol secretion. If, after the loading period, the ACTH stimulation test indicates little or no response of the adrenal glands to ACTH and cortisol concentrations are low, the dog is kept on the same dose of mitotane, and a maintenance dose is given once weekly. To reduce side effects, it is advisable to divide the dose and give it over a 2-day period. If the ACTH stimulation test indicates a normal or even exaggerated response, the treatment with mitotane is continued and the dog retested at 5- to 10-day intervals until the desired response is obtained. In some cases, the mitotane dose needs to be increased to 75 mg/kg or 100 mg/kg to obtain the desired response. Higher doses are generally necessary to decrease cortisol concentrations in dogs with adrenal neoplasia. Cortisol-secreting tumors seem to be more resistant and sometimes even unresponsive to the adrenolytic effect of mitotane.

Diabetic animals need to be monitored carefully while on mitotane treatment because the decrease in cortisol concentrations makes the animal more sensitive to insulin. For that reason, some clinicians prefer to use 25–35 mg/kg of mitotane instead of 50 mg/kg in the diabetic. Dogs on maintenance treatment need to be reevaluated regularly. An ACTH stimulation test is the most accurate assessment of adrenal functional reserve. If the ACTH test shows normal or exaggerated cortisol response, the animal should undergo "loading" again for several days, with an increase in the maintenance dosage. Mitotane has not proven to have any therapeutic value in the Cushingoid cat (Hoenig and Ferguson 1991a; Kintzer and Peterson 1989; Schechter et al. 1973).

Side Effects. The side effects of mitotane at routine therapeutic doses are usually mild and may consist of gastrointestinal problems such as vomiting and anorexia, mild hypoglycemia, CNS depression, and mild liver damage with increases in alkaline phosphatase. However, in some cases the rapid fall in cortisol levels may lead to weakness, diarrhea, and lethargy. In rare cases, the zona glomerulosa is affected by mitotane, and electrolyte abnormalities compatible with Addison's disease are seen (Kintzer and Peterson 1989; Schechter et al. 1973).

TRILOSTANE

Chemistry and Mechanism of Action. Trilostane ($4\alpha,5\alpha$-Epoxy-17β-hydroxy-3-oxoandrostane-2α-carbonitrile; Fig. 30.9) produces suppression of the adrenal cortex by reversibly inhibiting enzymatic conversion of steroids by 3-beta-hydroxysteroid dehydrogenase/delta 5,4 ketosteroid isomerase, thus blocking synthesis of adrenal steroids, including cortisol and aldosterone. The effect on aldosterone is less than that on cortisol (Wenger et al. 2004).

Metabolism. Trilostane is metabolized by the liver in people. There are no reports to date that describe the metabolism in dogs, cats, or horses.

Preparation and Properties. Trilostane (Vetoryl®, Arnold Veterinary Products, U.K.) is available in 30, 60, and 120 mg capsules. It should be stored at room temperature in airtight, light-resistant containers. Pregnant women should wear gloves when handling the drug (trilostane has been shown to cause abortion in pregnant monkeys) and all users should wash their hands after handling the capsules.

Therapeutic Uses. Trilostane has been used for treatment of hyperadrenocorticism (pituitary-dependent and adrenal-dependent) in dogs (Neiger et al. 2002; Ruckstuhl et al. 2002, Wenger et al. 2004), cats (Neiger et al. 2004), and horses (McGowan and Neiger 2003). In dogs, trilostane has been effective in reducing polydipsia/polyuria in over 90%, and polyphagia in over 80%. Trilostane causes a significant reduction in pre- and post-ACTH cortisol concentrations. It also leads to a significant decrease in alanine aminotransferase and alkaline phosphatase. Potassium concentrations increase but not usually to a level that requires medical intervention. Similarly, in horses, trilostane caused a reduction in polyuria/polydipsia and recurrent or chronic laminitis.

Trilostane is administered once daily at 2–10 mg per kg in dogs. Because accurate dosing with capsules is difficult, miniature dogs (<5 kg) usually receive 30 mg, small dogs (<20 kg) receive 60 mg; medium-size dogs (<40 kg) 120 mg, and large dogs 240 mg. This needs to be adjusted according to clinical signs and cortisol values. The goal of therapy is to decrease post-ACTH cortisol concentrations measured 4–6 hours after administration of trilostane to 27–55 nmol/l (1–2 μg/dl). Some dogs may need twice-daily administration for control (Bell et al. 2006).

The dose in horses is 0.4–1.0 mg/kg once daily. The initial dose for cats is 30 mg once daily.

Side Effects. Trilostane seems to be generally well tolerated. Diarrhea, vomiting, and lethargy have been described, which are usually mild and self-limiting. However, acute deaths have also been seen in a small number of dogs (Neiger et al. 2002), and necrosis of the adrenal cortex (Chapman et al. 2004) has been described. Interestingly, ultrasonographically, adrenal glands increase in size in dogs on trilostane (Mantis et al. 2003). This increase may be caused by the increase in ACTH.

Trilostane is not licensed for use in the U.S. It can be obtained from England with a prescription and new drug waiver permit from the FDA.

KETOCONAZOLE

Chemistry and Mechanism of Action. Ketoconazole (*cis*-1-acetyl-4-[4-[[2-(2,44-dichlorophenyl)-2-(1H-imidazol-1-ylmethyl)-1,3-dioxolan-4-yl] methoxyl] phenyl]piperazine; Fig. 30.9) is an imidazole derivative whose major effect is to inhibit sterol synthesis in fungi (Schechter et al. 1973). In mammalian cells, it inhibits the conversion of lanosterol to cholesterol by inhibition of cytochrome P450–dependent enzyme systems (Loose et al. 1983). Ketoconazole also inhibits the synthesis of hormones from cholesterol such as cortisol, estradiol, and testosterone (Pont et al. 1940; Pont et al. 1982; Willard et al. 1986). In male dogs it greatly increases serum progesterone concentrations (Willard 1989).

Preparations and Properties. Ketoconazole (Nizoral®, Janssen) is available in tablet form, each containing 200 mg ketoconazole base, for oral administration. It is soluble in acids.

Metabolism. Ketoconazole requires an acidic environment for the dissolution of the drug. Its bioavailability is therefore decreased in patients on antacids. After oral ketoconazole administration, maximal blood concentrations occur 1–2 hours later. There is considerable variation in the bioavailability of the drug in dogs (Baxter et al. 1986). Approximately 50% of ketoconazole is excreted unchanged in the feces, and the rest is metabolized mainly by the liver. Inactive metabolites are excreted primarily in the feces; a small amount is excreted in the urine.

Therapeutic Uses. Ketoconazole is used to decrease cortisol concentrations in dogs with pituitary-dependent hyperadrenocorticism and cortisol-secreting adrenal neoplasms. The drug is expensive but is a valuable alternative in those cases where mitotane is ineffective or as initial therapy prior to adrenalectomy in order to control the hyperadrenocorticism and reduce the risk of anesthesia and surgery. However, about 25% of dogs will not respond to this therapy. The recommended dose is 15 mg/kg twice daily. As ketoconazole inhibits cortisol synthesis only reversibly, it should be given on a daily basis.

No consistent therapeutic effect of ketoconazole has been demonstrated in the Cushingoid cat. The dose in the cat is 10 mg/kg twice daily.

Side Effects. The main side effects are vomiting and anorexia. Hepatic enzymes can transiently increase. In rare cases, a reversible hepatopathy with icterus may be seen (Willard 1989). Gynecomastia and azoospermia have been reported in human patients (DeFelice et al. 1981). Ketoconazole is teratogenic and should not be used in pregnant animals.

L-DEPRENYL

Chemistry and Mechanism of Action. L-Deprenyl hydrochloride (selegiline hydrochloride) is phenylisopropyl-*N*-methylpropinylamine (Fig. 30.9) and is an irreversible inhibitor of monoamine oxidase B. L-Deprenyl is thought to decrease the metabolism of dopamine and also other catecholamines, to inhibit the reuptake of dopamine, and to increase its synthesis. It is hypothesized that the increase in dopamine concentrations decreases ACTH secretion from the pituitary and in turn cortisol secretion from the adrenal gland. In a study by Milgram and coworkers (1995), however, brain levels of dopamine were unaffected when dogs were given l-deprenyl for 3 weeks at different doses. The authors concluded that although dopamine was not increased, l-deprenyl could still affect dopaminergic transmission through one of its metabolites, phenylethylamine, whose levels were increased in dogs on l-deprenyl.

Preparations and Properties. L-Deprenyl (Anipryl®, Pfizer Animal Health) is available for oral administration as white, convex tablets containing 2, 5, 10, 15, or 30 mg.

Metabolism. The metabolism of l-deprenyl in the dog is unknown. In humans, l-deprenyl is metabolized to amphetamine and metamphetamine; amphetamine concentrations also were increased in dogs on l-deprenyl (Reynolds et al. 1978). Pharmacokinetic analysis in four dogs indicated that the drug had a short half-life, which was attributed to high clearance and large volume of distribution of the drug. After oral administration, the bioavailability of the drug was less than 10% (Mahmood et al. 1994).

Therapeutic Uses. L-Deprenyl is used for the treatment of uncomplicated Cushing's disease. In 125 cases with naturally occurring pituitary-dependent hyperadrenocorticism, l-deprenyl was shown to be effective in controlling clinical signs associated with the disease such as panting, polyuria, polydipsia, obesity, reduced activity, abdominal distention, and others. The initial dose is 1 mg/kg body weight once daily; this dose might have to be increased if a response is not seen after 4 weeks. The maximum dose is 2 mg/kg body weight per day. It is recommended that the drug be administered for a 2- to 3-month period to allow sufficient time to assess its clinical usefulness. Should the dog's condition deteriorate during that time or should the dog show complications due to high cortisol levels, l-deprenyl should be discontinued and treatment with mitotane initiated. Although the company claims that 80% of dogs with hyperadrenocorticism respond favorably to l-deprenyl treatment, a recent study in a very small group of dogs suggests that only about 20% show an improvement of the clinical signs associated with the disease (Reusch et al. 1999). It has been argued that only Cushingoid dogs with pituitary pars intermedia tumors might respond to this treatment. Pars intermedia tumors account for approximately 30% of pituitary tumors in dogs with Cushing's disease (Peterson 1999). More clinical studies are needed to evaluate the efficacy of this drug.

Side Effects. L-Deprenyl is a very safe drug. The following adverse effects were noted infrequently in dogs on long-term treatment: vomiting, diarrhea, hyperactivity, anorexia, diminished hearing, weight loss, anemia, polydipsia, and weakness.

REFERENCES

Addison, T. 1855. On the Constitutional and Local Effects of Disease of the Suprarenal Capsules. London: Highley.

Almawi, W. Y., Beyhum, H. N., Rahme, A. A., and Rieder M. J. 1996. Multiplicity of glucocorticoid action in inhibiting allograft rejection. J Leukoc Biol 60(5):563–572.

Almawi, W. Y., Hess, D. A., and Rieder, M. J. 1998. Regulation of cytokine and cytokine receptor expression by glucocorticoids. Cell Transpl 7(6):511–523.

Aron, D. C., and Tyrrell, J. B. 1994. Glucocorticoids and adrenal androgens. In F. S. Greenspan, and J. D. Baxter, eds., Basic and Clinical Endocrinology, pp. 307–346. Norwalk: Appleton & Lange.

Arriza, J. L., Weinberger, C., Cerelli, G., Glaser, T. M., Handelin, B. L., Housman, D. E., and Evans, R. M. 1987. Cloning of human mineralocorticoid receptor complementary DNA: structural and functional kinship with the glucocorticoid receptor. Science 237:268–275.

Aucoin, D. P. 1982. Treatment of immune-mediated disease. Vet Clin No Am 12(l):61–66.

Barragry, T. B. 1994. Veterinary Drug Therapy, pp. 530–545. Philadelphia: Lea & Febiger.

Baxter, J. G., Brass, C., Schentag, J. J., and Slaughter, R. L. 1986. Pharmacokinetics of ketoconazole administered intravenously to dogs and orally as tablet and solution to humans and dogs. J Pharmaceut Sci 75:443–447.

Bell, R., Neiger, R., McGrotty, Y., and Ramsey, I.K. 2006. Study of the effects of once daily doses of trilostane on cortisol concentrations and responsiveness to adrenocorticotrophic hormone in hyperadrenocorticoid dogs. Vet Rec 26:277–81.

Bellah, J. R., Lothrop, C. D., and Helman, R. G. 1989. Fatal iatrogenic Cushing's syndrome in a dog. J Am Anim Hosp Assoc 25(6):673–676.

Belvisi, M.G., and Hele, D.J. 2003. Soft steroids: a new approach to the treatment of inflammatory airways diseases. Pulm Pharmacol Ther 16(6):321–5.

Bodor, N., and Buchwald, P. 2006. Corticosteroid design for the treatment of asthma: structural insights and the therapeutic potential of soft corticosteroids. Curr Pharm Des 12(25):3241–3260.

Boivin, M. A., Ye, D., Kennedy, J. C., Al-Sadi, R., Shepela, C., and Ma, T. Y. 2007. Mechanism of glucocorticoid regulation of the intestinal tight junction barrier. Am J Physiol Gastrointest Liver Physiol 292: G590–G598.

Brann, D. W., Hendry, L. B., and Mahesh, V. B. 1995. Emerging diversities in the mechanism of action of steroid hormones. J Steroid Biochem Mol Biol 52(2):113–133.

Bratts, R., and Linden, M. 1996. Cytokine modulation by glucocorticoids: mechanisms and actions in cellular studies. Aliment Pharmacol Ther 10(Suppl2):81–90.

Brightman, A. H. 1982. Ophthalmic use of glucocorticoids. Vet Clin No Am 12(l):33–40.

Buttgereit, F., Straub, R.H., Wehling, M., and Burmester, G.R. 2004. Glucocorticoids in the treatment of rheumatic diseases: an update on the mechanisms of action. Arthritis Rheum 50:3408–3417.

Byyny, R. L. 1976. Withdrawal from glucocorticoid therapy. New Engl J Med 295:30–32.

Chapman, P. S., Kelly, D. F., Archer, A., et al. 2004. Adrenal necrosis in a dog receiving trilostane for the treatment of hyperadrenocorticism. J Sm An Pract 45(6):307–310.

Chastain, C. B., and Graham, C. L. 1979. Adrenocortical suppression in dogs on daily and alternate-day prednisone administration. Am J Vet Res 40:936–941.

Chastain, C. B., Graham, C. L., and Nichols, C. E. 1981. Adrenocortical suppression in cats given megestrol acetate. Am J Vet Res 42:2029–2035.

Chung, R. S. K., Field, M., and Silen, W. 1978. Effects of methylprednisolone on hydrogen ion absorption in the canine stomach. J Clin Invest 62(2):262–270.

Coppoc, G. L. 1984. Relationship of dosage form of a corticosteroid to its therapeutic efficacy. J Am Vet Med Assoc 186(10):1098.

Couette, B., Jalaguier, S., Hellal-Levy, C., Lupo, B., Fagart, J., Auzou, G., and Rafestin-Oblin, M. E. 1998. Folding requirements of the ligand-binding domain of the human mineralocorticoid receptor. Mol Endocrinol 12:855–863.

Crager, C. S., Dillon, A. R., Kemppainen, R. J., Brewer, W. G., and Angarano, D. W. 1994. Adrenocorticotropic hormone and cortisol concentrations after corticotropin-releasing hormone stimulation testing in cats administered methylprednisolone. Am J Vet Res 55:704–709.

Dallman, M. F. 2005. Fast glucocorticoid actions on brain: Back to the future. Front Neuroendocrinol 26:103–108.

DeFelice, R., Johnson, D. G., and Galgiani, J. N. 1981. Gynecomastia with ketoconazole. Antimicrob Agents Chemother 19:1073–1074.

Di, S., Malcher-Lopes, R., Halmos, K. C., and Tasker, J. G. 2003. Nongenomic glucocorticoid inhibition via endocannabinoid release in the hypothalamus: a fast feedback mechanism. J Neurosci 23:4850–4857.

Duma, D., Jewell, C.M., and Cidlowski, J.A. 2006. Multiple glucocorticoid receptor isoforms and mechanisms of post-translational modification. J Ster Biochem Molec Biol 102:11–21.

Ehrich, E., Lambert, E. R., and McGuire, J. L. 1992. Rheumatic disorders. In K. L. Melmon, H. F. Morrelli, B. B. Hoffman, and D. W. Nierenberg, eds., Clinical Pharmacology: Basic Principles in Therapeutics, 3rd ed., pp. 469–485. New York: McGraw-Hill.

Eyre, P., and Elmes, P, J. 1980. Corticosteroid-induced laminitis? Further observations on the isolated, perfused hoof. Vet Res Commun 4:139–43.

Fauci, A. S. 1976. Glucocorticosteroid therapy: mechanisms of action and clinical considerations. Annals Int Med 84:304–315.

———. 1978. Alternate-day corticosteroid therapy. Am J Med 64:729–731.

Fejes-Tóth, G., Pearce, D., and Náray-Fejes-Tóth, A. 1998. Subcellular localization of mineralocorticoid receptors in living cells: Effects of receptor agonists and antagonists. Proc Natl Acad Sci USA 95:2973–2978.

Feldman, E. C., and Nelson, R. W. 2004. Glucocorticoid therapy, in Feldman, E. C., Nelson, R. W., eds., Canine and Feline Endocrinology and Reproduction, 3rd ed. St. Louis: Saunders Elsevier.

Ferguson, D. C. 1985a. Rational steroid therapy. 1. Principles. Mod Vet Prac (Feb):101–105.

———. 1985b. Rational steroid therapy. 2. Therapeutic protocols. Mod Vet Prac (Mar):175–179.

Ferguson, D. C., and Peterson, M. E. 1992. Serum free and total iodothyronine concentrations in dogs with spontaneous hyperadrenocorticism. Am J Vet Res 53(9):1636–1640.

Ferguson, D. C., Hoenig, M., and Cornelius, L. 1991. Endocrinologic disorders. In M. D. Lorenz, L. M. Cornelius, and D. C. Ferguson, eds., Small Animal Medical Therapeutics, pp. 85–157. Philadelphia: J. B. Lippincott.

Ferguson, J. L., Roesel, O. F., and Bottoms, G. D. 1978. Dexamethasone treatment during hemorrhagic shock: blood pressure, tissue perfusion, and plasma enzymes. Am J Vet Res 39:817–824.

Flower, R. J., and Rothwell, N. J. 1994. Lipocortin-1: cellular mechanisms and clinical relevance. Trends Pharmacol Sci 15(3):71–76.

Gabel, A. A. 1977. Corticosteroids-side effects and toxicity. Proc Am Assoc Equine Pract 23:393.

Gametchu, B., Watson, C. S., Shih, C. C., and Dashew, B. 1991. Studies on the arrangement of glucocorticoid receptors in the plasma membrane of S-49 lymphoma cells. Steroids 56(8):411–419.

Glaze, M. B., Crawford, M. A., Nachreiner, R. F., Casey, H. W., Nafe, L. A., and Kearney, M. T. 1988. Ophthalmic corticosteroid therapy: systemic effects in the dog. J Am Vet Med Assoc 192(l):73–75.

Goecke, A., and Guerrero, J. 2006. Glucocorticoid receptor β in acute and chronic inflammatory conditions: Clinical implications. Immunobiology 211:85–96.

Goldfien, A. 1992. Adrenocorticosteroids and adrenocortical antagonists. In B. G. Katzung, ed., Basic and Clinical Pharmacology, 5th ed., pp. 543–558. Norwalk: Appleton & Lange.

Greco, D. S., and Peterson, M. E. 1989. Feline hypoadrenocorticism. In R. W. Kirk, ed., Current Veterinary Therapy X, pp. 1042–1045. Philadelphia: W. B. Saunders.

Grote, H., Ioannou, I., Voigt, J., and Sekeris, C. E. 1993. Localization of the glucocorticoid receptor in rat liver cells: evidence for plasma membrane bound receptor. Int J Biochem 25(11):1593–1599.

Ham, E. A., Harman, R. E., Brink, N. G., and Sarett, L. H. 1955. Studies on the chemistry of aldosterone. J Am Chem Soc 77:1637.

Hammond, G. L. 1990. Molecular properties of corticosteroid binding globulin and the sex-steroid binding proteins. Endocr Rev 11:65.

Harms, C., Albrecht, K., Harms, U., Seidel, K., Hauck, L., Baldinger, T., Huebner, D., Kronenberg, G., An, J., Ruscher, K., Meisel, M., Dirnagl, U., von Harsdorf, R., Endres, M., and Hoertnag, H. 2007. Phosphatidylinositol 3-Akt-kinase-dependent phosphorylation of $p21_{Waf1/cip1}$ as a novel mechanism of neuroprotection by glucocorticoids. J Neurosci 27(17):4562–4571.

Haynes, R. C. 1990. Adrenocorticotropic hormone; adrenocortical steroids and their synthetic analogs; inhibitors of the synthesis and actions of adrenocortical hormones. In A. G. Gilman, T. W. Rall, A. S. Nies, and P. Taylor, The Pharmacological Basis of Therapeutics, pp. 1431–1462. New York: Pergamon Press.

Hench, P. S. 1952. Quoted in J. C. Krantz and C. J. Carr, Pharmacological Principles of Medical Practice, 5th ed., p. 1287. Baltimore: Williams & Wilkins, 1961.

Hoenig, M., and Ferguson, D. C. 1991a. Hyperadrenocorticism. In D. G. Allen, ed., Small Animal Medicine, pp. 807–820. Philadelphia: J. B. Lippincott.

Hoenig, M., and Ferguson, D. C. 1991b. Hypoadrenocorticism. In D. G. Allen, ed., Small Animal Medicine, pp. 821–830. Philadelphia: J. B. Lippincott.

Hoenig, M., Hall, G., Ferguson, D., Jordan K, Henson, M., Johnson, K., and O'Brien, T. 2000. A feline model of experimentally induced islet amyloidosis. Am J Pathology 157(6):2143–2150.

Jeffers, J. G., Shanley, K. J., and Schick, R. O. 1991. Iatrogenic Cushing's syndrome in a dog caused by topical ophthalmic medications. J Am Vet Med Assoc 199:77–80.

Jennings, A. S., and Ferguson, D. C. 1984. Effect of clexamethasone on triiodothyronine production in perfused rat liver and kidney. Endocrinology 114:3136.

Johnson, P. J., Messer, N. T., Slight, S. H., Wiedmeyer, C., Buff, P., Ganjam, V. K. 2004. Endocrinopathic laminitis in the horse. Clin Tech Equine Pract 3:45–56.

Johnson, J. P. 1992. Cellular mechanisms of action of mineralocorticoid hormones. Pharm Ther 53:1–29.

Kaptein, E. M., Moore, G. E., Ferguson, D. C., and Hoenig, M. 1992. Effects of prednisone on thyroxine and 3,5,3'-triiodothyronine metabolism in normal dogs. Endocrinology 130(3):1669–1679.

Keller-Wood, M. 1990. Fast feedback control of canine corticotropin by cortisol. Endocrinology 126(4):1959–1966.

Kemppainen, R. J. 1986. Principles of glucocorticoid therapy in nonendocrine disease. In R. W. Kirk, ed., Current Veterinary Therapy IX, pp. 954–962. Philadelphia: W. B. Saunders.

Kemppainen, R. J., and Sartin, J. L. 1984. Effects of single intravenous doses of dexamethasone on base-line plasma cortisol concentrations and responses to synthetic ACTH in healthy dogs. Am J Vet Res 45:742.

Kemppainen, R. J., Lorenz, M. D., and Thompson, F. N. 1982. Adrenocortical suppression in the dog given a single intramuscular dose of prednisone or triamcinolone acetonide. Am J Vet Res 42:204.

Kintzer, P. P., and Peterson, M. E. 1989. Mitotane (*o,p'*-DDD) treatment of cortisol-secreting adrenocortical neoplasia. In R. W. Kirk, ed., Current Veterinary Therapy X, pp. 1034–1037. Philadelphia: W. B. Saunders.

Kuhlenschmidt, M. S., Hoffmann, W. E., and Rippy, M. K. 1991. Glucocorticoid hepatopathy: effect on receptor mediated endocytosis of asialoglycoproteins. Biochem Med Metab Biol 46(2):152–168.

Liposits, Z., and Bohn, M. C. 1993. Association of glucocorticoid receptor immunoreactivity with cell membrane and transport vesicles in hippocampal and hypothalamic neurons of the rat. J Neurosci Res 35(l):14–19.

Loewenberg, M., Verhaar, A. P., van den Brink, G. R., and Hommes, D. W. 2007. Glucocorticoid signaling: a nongenomic mechanism for T-cell immunosuppression. Trends in Molec Med 13(4):158–163.

Loose, D. S., Kan, P. B., Hirst, M. A., Marcus, R. A., and Feldman, D. 1983. Ketoconazole blocks adrenal steroidogenesis by inhibiting cytochrome P450-dependent enzymes. J Clin Invest 7:1495–1499.

Lorenz, M. D., Scott, D. W., and Pulley, L. T. 1973. Medical treatment of canine hyperadrenocorticoidism with *o,p'*-DDD. Cornell Vet 63:646.

Luetscher, J. A. 1956. Studies of aldosterone in relation to water and electrolyte balance in man. Recent Prog Horm Res 12:175–184.

Lynn, R. C., Feldman, E. C., and Nelson, R. W. 1993. Efficacy of microcrystalline desoxycorticosterone pivalate for treatment of hypoadrenocorticism in dogs. J Am Vet Med Assoc 202:392–396.

Mahmood, I., Peters, D. K., and Mason, W. D. 1994. The pharmacokinetics and absolute bioavailability of selegiline in the dog. Biopharm Drug Disp 15:653–664.

Manjari, V., Das, U. N. 2000. Effect of polyunsaturated fatty acids on dexamethasone–induced gastric mucosal damage. Prostaglandins Leukot Essent Fatty Acids 62(2):85–96.

Mantero, F., Armanini, D., Biason, A., Boscaro, M., Carpene, G., Fallo, F., Cipocher, G., Rocco, S., Scarom, C., and Sonino, N. 1990. New aspects of mineralocorticoid hypertension. Horm Res 34:175–180.

Mantis, P. Lamb, C. R., Witt, L., Neiger, R. 2003. Changes in ultrasonic appearance of adrenal glands in dogs with pituitary-dependent hyperadrenocorticism treated with trilostane. Vet Radiol Ulstrasound 44:682–5

McDonald, R. K., and Langston, V. C. 1994. Use of corticosteroids and nonsteroidal antiinflammatory agents. In S. Ettinger and E. C. Feldman, eds., Textbook of Veterinary Internal Medicine, pp. 284–293. Philadelphia: W. B. Saunders.

McGowan, C., and R. Neiger. 2003. Efficacy of trilostane for the management of equine Cushing's syndrome. Equine Vet J 35:414–8.

McKay, A. G., and Milne, F. J. 1976. Observations of the intra-articular use of corticosteroids in the racing Thoroughbred. Am J Vet Res 168:1039.

Meintjes, E., Hosgood, G., and Daniloff, J. 1996. Pharmaceutic treatment of acute spinal cord trauma. Compend Contin Educ Pract Vet 18(6):625–635.

Melby, J. C. 1974. Systemic corticosteroid therapy: pharmacology and endocrinology considerations. Annals Int Med 81:505–512.

Metz, S. R., Taylor, S. R., and Kay, W. J. 1982. The use of glucocorticoids for neurological disease. Vet Clin No Am 12(l):41–60.

Michels, G. M., and Carr, A. P. 1997. Treating immune-mediated arthritis in dogs and cats. Vet Med 92(9):811–814.

Milgram, N. W., Ivy, G. O., Murphy, M. P., Head, E., Wu, P. H., Ruehl, W. W., Yu, P. H., Durden, D. A., Davis, B. A., and Boulton, A. A. 1995. Effects of chronic oral administration of l-deprenyl in the dog. Pharm Biochem Behav 51:421–428.

Moore, G. E., Ferguson, D. C., and Hoenig, M. 1993. Effects of oral administration of anti-inflammatory doses of prednisone on thyroid hormone response to thyrotropin-releasing hormone and thyrotropin in clinically normal dogs. Am J Vet Res 54(1):130–135.

Moore, G. E., and Hoenig, M. 1992. Duration of ACTH and adrenocortical suppression following long-term anti-inflammatory doses of prednisone in the dog. Am J Vet Res 53:716–720.

———. 1993. Effects of orally administered prednisone on glucose tolerance and insulin secretion in clinically normal dogs. Am J Vet Res 54(l):126–129.

Moore, G. E., Mahaffey, E. A., and Hoenig, M. 1992. Hematologic and biochemical effects of long-term anti-inflammatory doses of prednisone in the dog. Am J Vet Res 53:1033–1037.

Muller, M., and Rankawitz, R. 1991. The glucocorticoid receptor. Biochem Biophys Acta 1088:171.

Murphy, C. J., Feldman, E., and Bellhorn, R. 1990. Iatrogenic Cushing's syndrome in a dog caused by topical ophthalmic medications. J Am Anim Hosp Assoc 26(6):640–642.

Nakamoto, H., Suzuki, H., Kageyama, Y., Murakami, M., Ohishi, A., Naitoh, M., Ichihara, A., and Saruta, T. 1992. Depressor systems contribute to hypertension induced by glucocorticoid excess in dogs. J Hypertens 10(6):561–569.

Neiger, R., Ramsey, I., O'Connor, J., et al. 2002. Trilostane treatment of 78 dogs with pituitary-dependent hyperadrenocorticism. Vet Rec 150(26):799–804.

Neiger, R., Witt, A. I., Noble, A., German, A. J. 2004. Trilostane therapy for treatment of pituitary-dependent hyperadrenocorticism in 5 cats. JIVM 18:160–4.

Pallardy, M., and Biola, A. 1998. Induction de l'apoptose par les glucocorticoides dans les lymphocytes: entre physiologie et pharmacologie. C R Seances Soc Biol 192(6):1051–1063.

Pearce, D., Kleyman, T. R. 2007. Salt, sodium channels, and SGK1. J Clin Invest 117:592–595.

Peterson, M. E. 1983. *o,p'*-DDD (Mitotane) treatment of canine pituitary dependent hyperadrenocorticism. J Am Vet Med Assoc 182:527.

———. 1999. Medical treatment of pituitary-dependent hyperadrenocorticism in dogs: should l-deprenyl (Anipryl) ever be used? J Vet Int Med 13:289–290.

Peterson, M. E., Ferguson, D. C., Kintzer, P. P., and Drucker, W. D. 1984. Effects of spontaneous hyperadrenocorticism on serum thyroid hormone concentrations in the dog. Am J Vet Res 45(10):2034–2038.

Piper, J. M., Ray, W. A., Daugherty, J. R., Griffin, M. R. 1991. Corticosteroid use and peptic ulcer disease: role of nonsteroidal anti-inflammatory drugs. Ann Inter Med 114:735–740.

Plumb, D. C. 2005. Veterinary Drug Handbook, 5th ed. Ames, Iowa: Blackwell Publishing.

Pont, A., Williams, P. L., Azhar, S., Reitz, R. E., Bochra, C., Smith, E. R., and Stevens, D. A. 1940. Ketoconazole blocks testosterone synthesis. Arch Intern Med 142:2137–2140.

Pont, A., Williams, P. L., Loose, D. S., Feldman, D., Reitz, R. E., Bochra, C., and Stevens, D. A. 1982. Ketoconazole blocks adrenal steroid synthesis. Ann Intern Med 97:370–372.

Restrepo, A., Stevens, D. A., and Utz, J. P., eds. 1980. First International Symposium on Ketoconazole. Rev Infect Dis 2:519–699.

Reull, J. M., de Kloet, E. R., van Sluijs, F. J., Rijnberk, A., and Rothuizen, J. 1990. Binding characteristics of mineralocorticoid and glucocorticoid receptors in dog brain and pituitary. Endocrinology 127(2):907–915.

Reusch, C. E., Steffen, T., and Hoerauf, A. 1999. The efficacy of l-deprenyl in dogs with pituitary-dependent hyperadrenocorticism. J Vet Int Med 13:291–301.

Reynolds, G. P., Elsworth, J. D., Blau, K., Sandler, M., Lees, A. J., and Stern, G. M. 1978. Deprenyl is metabolized to metamphetamine and amphetamine in man. Br J Clin Pharm 6:542–544.

Rogerson, F. M., and Fuller, P. J. 2000. Mineralocorticoid action. Steroids 65:61–73.

Rogoff, J. M., and Stewart, G. N. 1969. Suprarenal cortical extracts in suprarenal insufficiency (Addison's disease). J Am Med Assoc 92:1569.

Ruckstuhl, N. S., Nett, C. S., Reusch, C. E. 2002. Results of clinical examinations, laboratory tests, and ultrasonography in dogs with pituitary-dependent hyperadrenocorticism treated with trilostane. Am J Vet Res 63:506–512.

Saruta, T. 1996. Mechanism of glucocorticoid-induced hypertension. Hypertens Res 19(1):1–8.

Schechter, R. D., Stabenfeldt, G. H., Gribble, D. H., and Ling, G. 1973. Treatment of Cushing's syndrome in the dog with an adrenocorticolytic agent, *o,p'*DDD. J Am Vet Med Assoc 162:629.

Schott, H. C. 2002. Pituitary pars intermedia dysfunction: equine Cushing's disease. Vet Clin N Am Pract 18:237–270.

Schwartzman, R. A., and Cidlowski, J. A. 1994. Glucocorticoid-induced apoptosis of lymphoid cells. Int Arch Allergy Immunol 105(4):347–354.

Scott, D. W. 1982. Dermatologic use of glucocorticoids: systemic and topical. Vet Clin No Am 12(l):19–32.

Scott, D. W., and Greene, C. E. 1974. Iatrogenic secondary adrenocortical insufficiency in dogs. JAAHA 10:555–564.

Siegel, S. C. 1985. Corticosteroid agents: overview of corticosteroid therapy. J Allergy Clin Immunol 76:312.

Simpson, S. A., Tait, J. F., and Bush, I. E. 1952. Secretion of a salt-retaining hormone by the mammalian adrenal gland. Lancet 263:226–227.

Simpson, S. A., Tait, J. F., Wettstein, A., Neher, R., von Euw, J., Schindler, O., and Reichstein, T. 1954. Constitution of aldosterone, a new mineralocorticoid. Experientia 10:132.

Snyder, P. M. 2002. The epithelial Na+ channel: cell surface insertion and retrieval in Na+ homeostasis and hypertension. Endocr Rev 23:258–75.

Solter, P. F., Hoffmann, W. E., Hungerford, L. L., Peterson, M. E., and Dorner, J. L. 1993. Assessment of corticosteroid-induced alkaline phosphatase isoenzyme as a screening test for hyperadrenocorticism in dogs. J Am Vet Med Assoc 203(4):534–538.

Song, I.-H., Buttgereit, F. 2006. Non-genomic glucocorticoid effects to provide the basis for new drug developments. Molec Cell Endocrinol 246:142–146.

Sorenson, D. K., et al. 1988. Corticosteroids stimulate an increase in phospholipase A_2 inhibitor in human serum. J Steroid Biochem 2:271.

Sprung, C. L., Caralis, P. V., Marcial, E. H., Pierce, M., Gelbard, M. A., Long, W. M., Duncan, R. C., Tendler, M. D., and Karpf, M. 1984. The effects of high-dose corticosteroids in patients with septic shock. N Engl J Med 311:1137–43.

Stahn, C., Loewenberg, M., Hommes, D. W., Buttgereit, F. 2007. Molecular mechanisms of glucocorticoid action and selective glucocorticoid receptor agonists. Molec Cell Endocrinol 275:71–78.

Stewart, P. M. 2003. The adrenal cortex, in Larsen, P. R., Kronenberg, H. M., Melmed, S., and Polonsky K. S., eds. Williams Textbook of Endocrinology, 10th ed., pp. 491–550. St. Louis: Saunders Elsevier.

Streeten, D. H. P. 1975. Corticosteroid therapy. 1. Pharmacological properties and principles of corticosteroid use. JAMA 232:1046–1049.

Sutanto, W., and deKloet, E. R. 1991. Mineralocorticoid receptor ligands: biochemical, pharmacological, and clinical aspects. Med Res Rev 11:617–639.

Tasker, J.G., Di, S., Malcher-Lopes, R. 2006. Minireview: Rapid glucocorticoid signaling via membrane-associated receptors. Endocrinology 147:5549–5556.

Thorn, G. W., Dorrance, S. S., and Day, E. 1942. Addison's disease: evaluation of synthetic desoxycorticosterone acetate therapy in 158 patients. Ann Intern Med 16:1053.

Tobin, T. 1979. Pharmacology review, the corticosteroids. J Equine Med Surg 3:10.

Tuor, U. I. 1997. Glucocorticoids and the prevention of hypoxic-ischemic brain damage. Neurosci Biobehav Rev 21(2):175–179.

Tyrrell, J. B., Aron, D. C., and Forsham, P. H. 1994. Glucocorticoids and adrenal androgens. In F. S. Greenspan and J. D. Baxter, eds., Basic and Clinical Endocrinology, pp. 307–346. Norwalk: Appleton & Lange.

Upson, D. W. 1978. Clinical pharmacology of corticosteroids. Equine pharmacology. Powers, J.D., Powers, T.E., eds.: Proc 2nd Equine Pharmacol symp. Am Assoc Equine Pract, p 233.

van der Velden, V. H. 1998. Glucocorticoids: mechanisms of action and anti-inflammatory potential in asthma. Mediators Inflamm 7(4):229–237.

Vilar, O., and Tullner, W. W. 1959. Effects of *o,p'*-DDD on the histology and 17-hydroxy corticosteroid output in the dog adrenal cortex. Endocrinology 65:80.

Ward, D. A., Ferguson, D. C., Ward, S. L., Green, K., and Kaswan, R. L. 1992. Comparison of the blood-aqueous barrier stabilizing effects of steroidal and non-steroidal anti-inflammatory agents in the dog. Prog in Vet and Comp Ophthalmol 2(3):117–124.

Wehling, M., Eisen, C., and Christ, M. 1992. Aldosterone-specific membrane receptors and rapid non-genomic actions of mineralocorticoids. Mol Cell Endocrinol 90:C5–C9.

Wehling, M., Kaesmayr, J., and Theisen, K. 1991. Rapid effects of mineralocorticoids on sodium-proton exchanger: genomic or non-genomic pathway? Am J Physiol 260:E719–E726.

Wenger, M., Sieber-Ruckstuhl, N. S., Müller, C. et al. 2004. Effect of trilostane on serum concentrations of aldosterone, cortisol, and potassium in dogs with pituitary-dependent hyperadrenocorticism. Am J Vet Res 265:1245–1250.

Wilcke, J. R., and Davis, L. E. 1982. Review of glucocorticoid pharmacology. Vet Clin No Am 12(1):3–18.

Willard, M. D. 1989. Treatment of fungal and endocrine disorders with imidazole derivatives. In R. W. Kirk, ed., Current Veterinary Therapy X, pp. 82–84. Philadelphia: W. B. Saunders.

Willard, M. D., Nachreiner, R., and Roudebush, P. 1986. Hormonal and clinical pathologic changes with long-term ketoconazole therapy in the dog and cat. Washington, DC: ACVIM Scient Proc.

Wilson, J. W. 1979. Cellular localization of ^{3}H-labeled corticosteroids by electron microscopic autoradiography after hemorrhagic shock. In Upjohn Proc Symp on Steroids and Shock, pp. 275–299.

CHAPTER

31

DRUGS INFLUENCING GLUCOSE METABOLISM

MARGARETHE HOENIG

INSULIN

HISTORY. Diabetes mellitus has been recognized for centuries as a debilitating disease, characterized by the excretion of "sweet urine" (mellituria), polydipsia, wasting of tissue, and the development of ketoacidosis, hyperosmolar coma, and death. The role of the pancreas in the development of diabetes was first recognized in 1886 when Minkowski and von Mering produced diabetes by total pancreatectomy in the dog. In 1921 Banting and Best extracted the active compound from pancreas and showed that was able to control hyperglycemia in diabetic dogs and humans. Insulin was prepared for the first time in crystalline form in 1926 by Abel, and it took 34 more years until its amino acid sequence was demonstrated by Sanger. Finally, in 1963 insulin was synthesized by Meyenhofer and co-workers, and in 1964 by Katsoyannis and co-workers. In 1967, Steiner discovered that insulin was synthesized as a larger precursor, proinsulin. An even larger molecule, named preproinsulin, was identified as a precursor for proinsulin in 1976 by Chan and co-workers (for a detailed review, see Bliss 1983). These research efforts have culminated in the biosynthesis of human insulin by recombinant DNA techniques, allowing large-scale production of the hormone in 1983 (Frank and Chance 1983; Johnson 1983).

Spontaneous diabetes has been reported in many species. Diabetes is a major health problem and one of the leading causes of death in humans. In animals, it occurs most frequently in the dog and cat, with an incidence of approximately 0.2–0.5%. Diabetes is rare in horses, cattle, and sheep. Isolated cases have been reported in mules, ferrets, pigs, newts, buffalos, monkeys, and fish (Stogdale 1986). Diabetes also has been reported in several breeds of birds (Stogdale 1986). Diabetes in humans has been classified into two major categories that are of interest to veterinary medicine: type 1 diabetes, previously called insulin-dependent diabetes mellitus or juvenile onset diabetes, and type 2 diabetes, previously called non–insulin–dependent diabetes mellitus or maturity onset diabetes. Based on glucose-tolerance testing (Kaneko et al. 1977; O'Brien et al. 1985), it has been determined that most diabetic dogs and cats are insulin deficient.

CHEMISTRY AND BIOSYNTHESIS. Insulin is produced in the beta cells of the islets of Langerhans in the endocrine pancreas. The islet also contains glucagon-secreting, somatostatin-secreting delta cells and PP or F cells, which secrete pancreatic polypeptide. The beta cells compose about 60–80% of the islet. The endocrine cells are arranged in a nonrandom distribution, with beta cells forming a central core surrounded by a mantle of the other three cell types in some animals and humans (Bonner-Weir and Orci 1982). In the cat, the beta cells are located in the periphery (O'Brien et al. 1986), while in the horse, the alpha cells form a central core (Helmstaedter et al. 1976).

Insulin exists initially as preproinsulin, which is cleaved to proinsulin in the endoplasmic reticulum. Proinsulin is a large polypeptide consisting of an A and B chain and a connecting peptide (Fig. 31.1). By proteolytic cleavage, four basic amino acids and the connecting peptide are removed, and proinsulin is converted to insulin (Steiner et al. 1969). This reduces the molecular weight from 9000 (proinsulin) to one of 6000 (insulin) and one of 3000

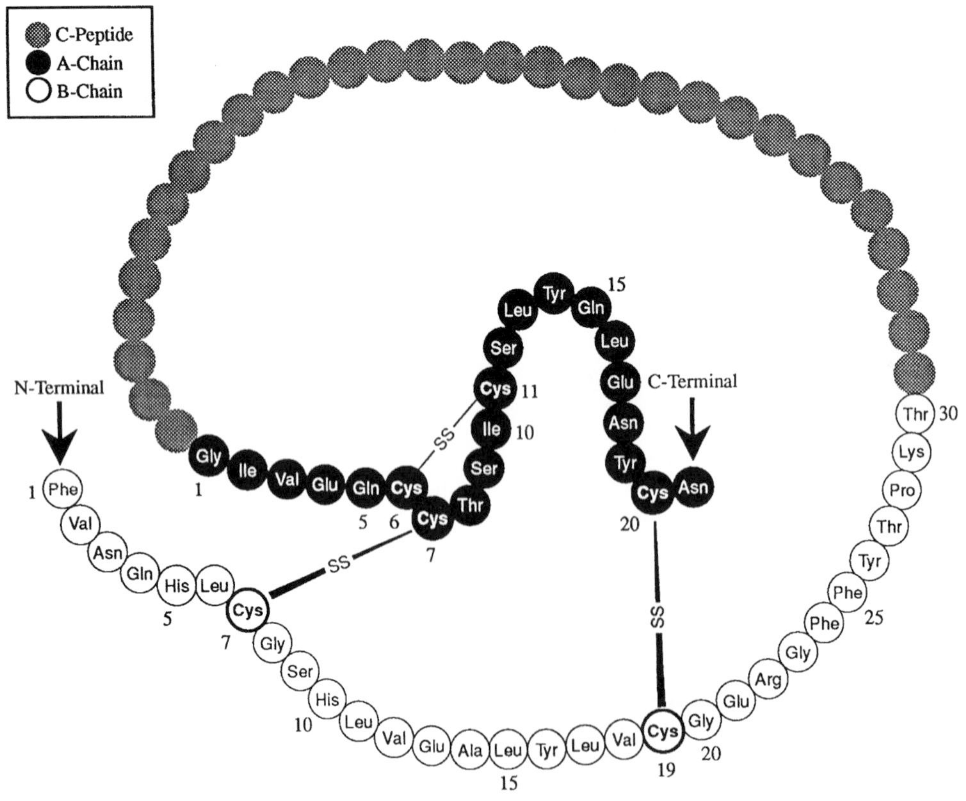

FIG. 31.1 Proinsulin.

(C-peptide). This conversion occurs soon after proinsulin is transported to the Golgi complex, where it is packaged into secretory granules. These granules therefore contain an equimolar amount of insulin and C-peptide. In the secretory granules, insulin is complexed with zinc and stored.

The amino acid sequence of insulin shows little species variation. Human insulin differs from porcine and rabbit insulin by a single amino acid, whereas dog insulin is identical to porcine insulin. Bovine insulin differs from human insulin by three amino acids and from feline insulin by one amino acid (Neubauer and Schoene 1978; Porte and Halter 1981; Hoenig et al. 2006). Antiserum directed against insulin of one species usually cross-reacts with insulin of other species. Antiinsulin serum generally also cross-reacts with heterologous proinsulin, while C-peptides have no immunoreactivity against insulin antiserum. The biological activity of proinsulin, however, is much less than that of insulin. Feline proinsulin has been cloned and expressed (Hoenig et al. 2006).

SECRETION. The secretion of insulin from the beta cell occurs through the process of exocytosis in which there is fusion of the secretory granule with the plasma membrane. Insulin secretion is highly regulated primarily by glucose, but also by other fuels, hormones, and neurotransmitters (Porte and Halter 1981). On a cellular level, insulin release stimulated by glucose and other fuels is thought to be initiated by closure of ATP (adenosine triphosphate)–dependent K channels, which leads to depolarization of the beta cell and influx of calcium into the cytosol through voltage-gated calcium channels (Arkhammar et al. 1987; Cook et al. 1988). The increase in cytosolic free calcium triggers insulin secretion. In addition, insulin is also secreted in a pathway that is Ca-dependent but independent of ATP-K channels. This pathway is called the amplification pathway. The exact mechanism is not understood (for a review, see Straub and Sharp 2002). Insulin is released from the beta cell in a pulsatile fashion. It is currently thought that these rapid oscillations are generated through intra-islet mechanisms, because they can be seen even in isolated islets and beta cells (Berman et al. 1993). Pulsatile secretion becomes abnormal in diabetes; however, pulsatility can be restored by beta-cell rest (Laedtke et al. 2000).

In both type 1 and type 2 diabetes, islet function and insulin secretion are abnormal. It is now clear that in both types a loss of beta-cell mass has occurred and that the fundamental difference between the two major types of diabetes lies in the etiology of the beta-cell dysfunction and its severity but not its presence or absence (Porte 1991). Insulin resistance, frequently caused by obesity (Hoenig et al. 2006) or other factors, is an important concomitant factor in type 2 diabetes and puts an additional stress on the beta cell. The beta cell tries to overcome the resistance by increasing the insulin output. Islet dysfunction in type 2 diabetes is therefore an essential element in the development of hyperglycemia. In fact, it has been shown that defects in pulsatile insulin secretion are an early marker of beta cell dysfunction and are seen even in glucose-tolerant first-degree relatives of type 2 diabetics (Pørksen 2002). An early marker is also a change in the proinsulin/insulin secretion ratio (Haffner et al. 1997). In some of the dogs and cats that are obese, the hyperglycemia, as in the human counterpart, can be alleviated, at least in part, by dietary manipulations resulting in weight loss. In rats, cats, and humans, the increase in insulin release from a reduced beta-cell mass in type 2 diabetes is associated with release and deposition of islet amyloid polypeptide, leading to further loss of beta cells (Porte and Kahn 1989; Hoenig et al. 2000a). In type 1 the loss of beta cells is caused by immune-mediated destruction (MacLaren et al. 1989). About 50% of dogs have beta-cell antibodies, and the pathogenesis of the disease may therefore be similar to that in humans (Hoenig and Dawe 1992). Beta-cell antibodies have not been demonstrated in diabetic cats (Hoenig et al. 2000b).

Insulin secretion can also become autonomous, resulting in hyperinsulinemia associated with hypoglycemia. Insulin-secreting tumors (adenomas or carcinomas; also called insulinomas) occur infrequently and have been described in the dog, cat, ferret, cattle, and a pony (Capen 1990). The diagnosis of an insulinoma can be difficult, but frequently it can be made on the basis of an inappropriately high serum insulin concentration. In humans, the diagnosis is often made based on high proinsulin and/or C-peptide concentrations (Chammas et al. 2003).

MECHANISM OF ACTION. Insulin is the most potent physiological anabolic agent. In insulin-responsive tissues, it facilitates cellular uptake and metabolism of glucose. Insulin promotes the synthesis of glycogen, protein, and fat and is involved in the uptake of ions such as K into the cell. Insulin exerts its effect by binding to specific receptors on the plasma membrane of cells. The insulin receptor is a tetrameric structure consisting of two subunits: an alpha and a beta subunit. Two of each of these subunits are joined together via disulfide bonds. Both subunits are glycosylated and exposed to the extracellular milieu; only the beta subunit is exposed to the intracellular environment. The insulin receptor has tyrosine kinase activity, which is enhanced by the binding of insulin. Not only does binding of insulin lead to receptor autophosphorylation, but the insulin receptor will also phosphorylate other cellular proteins (Schinner et al. 2005). Once the insulin receptor kinase is activated, the presence of insulin is not necessary for its continued activity. The receptor is inactivated by dephosphorylation.

Despite our knowledge of insulin-receptor interaction, our understanding of molecular events that link the insulin-receptor interactions to the regulation of cellular metabolism is poor. Some, but not all, of the actions are due to the phosphorylation or dephosphorylation of target proteins on serine and threonine residues. Recently, diabetes has been linked to alterations in the function of both endoplasmic reticulum (Kaneto et al. 2005) as well as mitochondria (Lowell and Shulman 2005).

METABOLISM. The existence of a relatively specific insulin-degrading enzyme (IDE, insulinase, insulin-specific protease) has been reported by several investigators (for a review, see Duckworth 1990). Insulin-degrading activity has been found in essentially all tissues examined, and high activity has been seen in liver, kidney, muscle, brain, fibroblasts, and red blood cells. The enzyme seems to be located predominantly in the cytoplasm but can be found in other subcellular compartments. Plasma membrane preparations also contain this enzyme. Some receptor-bound insulin is degraded on the membrane, while some insulin is released intact from the receptor, and some is internalized with the receptor, and insulin degradation is then initiated in endosomes. The degradation of insulin via this process is rapid. Other enzymes may also be involved in the degradation of insulin, and further studies are needed to assess their role and to examine factors controlling insulin-degrading activity in various tissues and disease states.

PREPARATIONS AND PROPERTIES. The biological activity of insulin preparations is documented using a bioassay that is based on the capacity of insulin to lower blood glucose concentrations. All but one insulin preparation have been standardized at 100 U/ml several years ago; a U 500 (500 U/ml) regular insulin preparation is available from Eli Lilly. Vetsulin (Intervet), a solution of beef insulin, and protamine zinc insulin (PZIVet®, Idexx Laboratories), a beef-pork insulin mixture, contains 40 U/ml. Vetsulin is the only insulin preparation that has been approved by the Federal Drug Administration (FDA) for use in animals. PZI insulin has recently been discontinued. For correct dosage, insulin preparations are administered with syringes that are calibrated for the appropriate standardization (e.g., U 100 syringes, U 40 syringes). All commercially available insulins in the United States contain no more than 25 parts per million of proinsulin. The insulin preparations currently available are summarized in Table 31.1.

In general, based on action profiles, insulin preparations can be divided into fast, intermediate, and long-acting. Generally, lispro and aspart, as well as the regular insulin preparations have a quick onset of action (15–30 min) and short duration, whereas the NPH, glargine, detemir, and the animal source insulin preparations have a longer onset and duration of action. There is, however, considerable species and individual variation in the insulin action profiles. It is important for the practitioner to realize that the time course of action of any insulin preparation may not only vary considerably between different individuals, but also in the same individual from day to day (Hoenig and Ferguson 1991; Church 1981). It is also important to realize that the pharmacokinetics change with different doses. The time periods listed by manufacturers should only be considered as initial guidelines for the treatment of a diabetic. Individual responses to insulin and the "fine-tuning" of insulin therapy have to be assessed by measuring blood glucose concentrations at frequent intervals, yielding what is often called a "glucose curve." In order to decrease stress effects, glucose monitoring also can be performed by measuring interstitial glucose concentrations using a continuous glucose monitoring system (Medtronic). There are currently no reports of the use of lispro, aspart, and detemir in pets.

Insulin thus far needs to be injected for the effective treatment of diabetes. The short-acting regular insulin preparations can be injected intravenously, intramuscularly, and subcutaneously, the intermediate and long-acting insulin preparations are for subcutaneous injection. The preferred injection site is the flank for those injec-

TABLE 31.1 Insulin preparations

Trademark	Common Name	Strength	pH	Administration	Company
HUMALOG®	LISPRO	U100	Neutral	Subcutaneous	Eli Lilly
NOVOLOG®	ASPART			External pump, subcutaneous	Novo Nordisk
APIDRA®	GLULISINE				Aventis
HUMULIN® R	REGULAR HUMAN INSULIN, RECOMBINANT DNA ORIGIN	U100		External pump, Intravenous Intramuscular Subcutaneous	Eli Lilly
HUMULIN® R		U 500		Subcutaneous	
NOVOLIN® R		U100		Intravenous	Novo Nordisk
VELOSULIN® R	HUMAN INSULIN (semisynthetic)			Intramuscular Subcutaneous	
HUMULIN® N	NPH HUMAN INSULIN,			Subcutaneous	Eli Lilly
NOVOLIN® N	RECOMBINANT DNA ORIGIN				Novo Nordisk
VETSULIN®	PORK INSULIN	U40			Intervet
LANTUS® (GLARGINE)	GLARGINE	U100	Acidic (pH4)		Idexx
LEVEMIR® (DETEMIR)	DETEMIR		Neutral		Aventis
					Novo Nordisk

tions. Intermediate and long-acting insulin preparations are suspensions and need to be gently mixed before administration. The shelf life of most insulin preparations is 28 days when stored at room temperature. If refrigerated, unopened bottles last until the expiration date of the vial.

Exubera®, produced by Pfizer, Sanofi-Aventis, and Nektar Therapeutics, was a rapid-acting, dry-powder type of insulin that was delivered to the lungs via a special bong-shaped inhaler device, and received FDA approval in 2006. It was withdrawn from the market in 2007 because of weak sales. Oral-lyn® has been developed by Generex. It is a novel oral (buccal) insulin spray product, which is delivered into the human mouth by way of the company's proprietary RapidMist drug delivery system. It is currently available in Ecuador, India, and the United Arab Emirates, and is in clinical trials in the U.S. It remains to be seen whether these applications could ever be used in the cat and dog.

THERAPEUTIC USES

Treatment of Diabetes Mellitus in Dogs and Cats. Insulin deficiency is characterized by increased catabolism. The breakdown of glycogen and the decreased utilization of glucose in peripheral tissues lead to hyperglycemia. There is increased protein breakdown, and the increased release of amino acids fuels gluconeogenesis. Finally, lipolysis leads to an increase in free fatty acids, which are transferred to the liver, where they are either reesterified or oxidized, resulting in fatty liver and ketoacidosis.

Treatment of diabetes must be adjusted to the clinical presentation of the animal. Usually two forms can be differentiated: uncomplicated and complicated diabetes mellitus. For practical purposes, complicated diabetics are those that cannot take food orally, such as the vomiting ketoacidotic patient or the comatose hyperosmolar patient (Hoenig and Ferguson 1991).

The goal of treatment of any diabetic animal is to maintain blood glucose concentrations in a mild hyperglycemic state; i.e., the blood glucose should stay between 150 and 200 mg/dl for most of the day and should not drop into the low-normal range. Ideally, the glucose curve after the injection of insulin should look like a shallow bowl. The practical therapeutic goal in diabetic animals is more conservative than the goal in a human diabetic, where tight control of normoglycemia has been demonstrated to prevent diabetic complications such as retinopathy, neuropathy, nephropathy, and other chronic sequelae. In the diabetic animal, one has to be more concerned with avoiding the dangers of hypoglycemia in a patient that cannot convey the more subtle signs of low blood glucose. In addition, the complications of persistent hyperglycemia play a lesser role in animals due in part to the shorter life span of the animal.

The fast-acting insulin preparations are used for the complicated diabetic patient. These animals can be treated with low-dose insulin infusions or several intramuscular insulin injections during the day while their blood glucose concentration is maintained with a 2.5 or 5% dextrose infusion (see Tables 31.2 and 31.3 for treatment protocols).

The intermediate and long-acting insulin preparations are used in the diabetic that is able to eat and drink without vomiting. Food is given before the insulin peak, which is characterized by the glucose nadir, and should not be given after insulin action has waned. As stated above, it is important to realize that each animal reacts differently to a given insulin preparation. As an example, in some animals NPH insulin has to be given twice daily to achieve adequate control; in others, it can be given once daily. However, most animals need twice daily insulin administrations for good control. Treatment protocols are shown in Tables 31.4 and 31.5 and can serve as guidelines. It is prudent to maintain a treatment regimen for several days before trying to regulate the time and dose of insulin or the time of feeding, unless, of course, insulin leads to hypoglycemia. It may take several weeks before an animal shows a consistent response to a given preparation.

Treatment of Ketosis in Cattle. Insulin is a powerful antiketogenic agent and has been used as adjunct treatment in ketosis therapy. It has been suggested that insulin therapy is particularly beneficial in those cases of ketosis

TABLE 31.2 Low-dose, continuous IV infusion protocol for the treatment of diabetic ketoacidosis

1. Place intravenous catheter.
2. Start fluid therapy (0.9% NaCl; consider replacement and maintenance fluid requirements).
3. Insert urinary catheter and attach to a closed monitoring system.
4. Add regular insulin to the saline solution (0.5 units/kg/day). Use pediatric infusion set or infusion pump for accurate administration.
5. Monitor blood glucose concentrations every 2 hr. If no change after 4 hr, increase insulin by 25%. Repeat if necessary.
6. Monitor urinary output.
7. Monitor electrolytes. Adjust if necessary.
8. Change saline solution to 2.5% dextrose in either 0.45% saline or in a balanced electrolyte solution when blood glucose reaches 250 mg/dl (13.8 mmol/l). Continue to administer regular insulin. Supplement K. Adjust glucose or insulin (glucose may have to be increased to 5%).
9. Keep animals on this regimen until they are able to eat without vomiting.
10. Stop insulin infusion in the evening. Start treatment of the uncomplicated diabetic the next morning.

TABLE 31.3 Alternative treatment of the complicated diabetic: intramuscular low-dose method

Initial dose of regular insulin: 0.25 units/kg
Followed by injections of 0.1 units/kg as needed (i.e., when blood glucose >250 mg/dl).

TABLE 31.4 Suggested initial protocol for the uncomplicated diabetic animal assuming BID insulin administration

7:50	Check blood glucose.
7:55	Feed one-half of caloric needs.
8:00	Administer insulin, 0.5 units/kg subcutaneously[a].
10:00–4:00	Check blood glucose every 2–4 hr.
5:50	Check blood glucose.
5:55	Feed one-half of caloric needs.
6:00	Administer insulin, 0.5 units/kg subcutaneously[b].
8:00	Check blood glucose.
10:00	Check blood glucose.

Note: The animal may not show a consistent response for several days. The owner should monitor and record blood or urine glucose and ketones at home. In addition, weekly blood glucose checks by the veterinarian should be performed initially at the time of insulin peak, or perform continuous glucose monitoring (Medtronic system).

Insulin dose can be increased 10–25% per day if necessary. Feeding time can be adjusted to optimize response if needed.

[a]Insulin is not administered if the blood glucose is <200 mg/dl.

[b]The second insulin injection can be administered after 10 hr to allow the owner to observe the animal's reaction to insulin at a reasonable time. Usually, if insulin is metabolized fast enough to warrant a BID administration, the peak insulin action is approximately 4 hr after the injection.

TABLE 31.5 Suggested initial protocol for the uncomplicated diabetic animal assuming SID insulin administration

7:50	Check blood glucose.
7:55	Feed one-half of caloric needs.
8:00	Administer insulin, 0.5 units/kg subcutaneously.
10:00	Check blood glucose.
Noon	Check blood glucose.
2:00	Feed one-half of caloric needs.
4:00–24:00	Check blood glucose every 2–4 hr.

Note: Blood glucose concentrations need to be monitored only until glucose concentrations start rising after the insulin peak action has been seen.

The owner should monitor and record urine glucose and ketones at home. Ketonuria indicates insulin deficiency. In addition, weekly blood glucose checks by the veterinarian should be performed initially at the time of insulin peak.

Insulin dose can be increased by 10–25%. Feeding time can be adjusted to optimize response if needed.

that occur within the first week of lactation and are nonresponsive to glucose or glucocorticoid therapy alone (Herdt and Emery 1992). A dose of 200–300 IU of protamine zinc insulin per animal repeated as necessary at 24- to 48-hour intervals was administered.

ADVERSE EFFECTS. Acute hypoglycemia may result from excessive insulin dose or inadequate food intake. The brain is particularly sensitive to glucose deficiency, and nervous system dysfunction is seen. Initially, confusion, nervousness, trembling, or hyperexcitability may be seen, which progress to convulsions if the hypoglycemia is not treated. Karo® syrup or other glucose-containing solutions can be used orally; however, the intravenous administration of dextrose solutions may be necessary to alleviate the hypoglycemic symptoms. Glucagon may also be used intramuscularly (see below).

The body itself combats hypoglycemia through the release of insulin-antagonistic hormones, primarily catecholamines, glucagon, glucocorticoids, and growth hormone. This frequently leads to hypoglycemia-induced hyperglycemia, also called Somogyi rebound (Cryer and Gerich 1990).

Antibody formation has been documented in diabetic dogs (Davison 2003) and diabetic cats (Hoenig et al. 2000). While this has not been examined in dogs, in cats the insulin dose was not different in the presence or absence of antibodies, and the clinical significance therefore seems to be minor.

ORAL HYPOGLYCEMIC AGENTS

SULFONYLUREAS

History. During World War II, Janbon and colleagues (1942) found that certain sulfonamide derivatives being used to treat typhoid fever caused hypoglycemia. After the end of the war, derivatives of these antibiotics were first used to treat patients with diabetes. Studies by Loubatieres (1946) showed that sulfonylureas did not alter blood glucose concentrations in pancreatectomized dogs and juvenile diabetics (i.e., type I), which suggested that sulfonylureas stimulated the pancreas to secrete insulin. Indeed, sulfonylureas have become the major therapeutic agent used to treat type 2 diabetes in humans until recently. In type 2 diabetics insulin secretion is still present although insufficient to control blood glucose concentrations. In most diabetic animals the insulin-secretory capacity of the beta cells is lost, and they require insulin for treatment.

Chemistry. The chemical structure of the most commonly used sulfonylurea in veterinary medicine, glipizide, is shown in Figure 31.2. Oral sulfonylurea agents available in the United States are listed in Table 31.6. Sulfonylureas differ in potency, duration of action, metabolism, and side effects.

Mechanism of Action. In the pancreatic beta cells, sulfonylureas inhibit ATP-dependent potassium (K+) channels in the plasma membrane. This results in depolarization and release of insulin (Antomarchi et al. 1987). Because ATP-sensitive K+ channels also exist in other tissues, sulfonylureas exert tissue-specific responses through the activation of the channels. The extrapancreatic effects of sulfonylureas have been described in detail by Gerich (1989). Sulfonylurea therapy augments the ability of insulin to inhibit hepatic glucose production and to stimulate glucose utilization. It is unclear whether these effects are direct effects of the drugs or secondary to the reduced hyperglycemia caused by improved insulin secretion.

metabolism. In people, sulfonylureas are readily absorbed from the gastrointestinal tract and are highly protein-bound. Glipizide has a half-life in plasma of approximately 2–4 hours, but its hypoglycemic effects may persist for up to 24 hours. It is metabolized in the liver, and its inactive

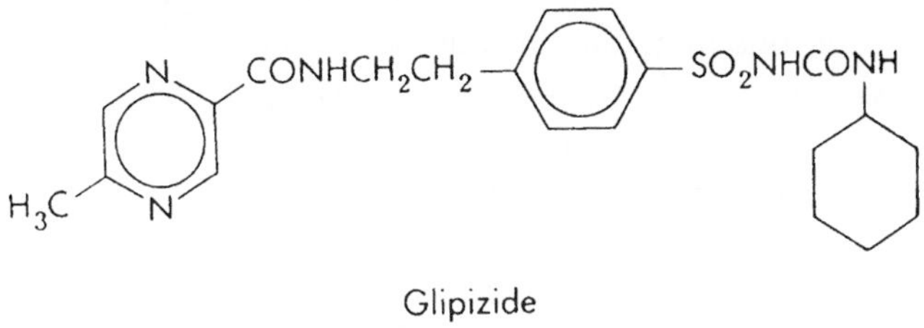

Glipizide

FIG. 31.2 Chemical structure of the sulfonylurea glipizide.

TABLE 31.6 Oral sulfonylurea agents available in the United States

Tolbutamide: Orinase (Upjohn) and generics
Tolazamide: Tolinase (Upjohn) and generics
Chlorpropamide: Diabinese (Pfizer) and generics
Acetohexamide: Dymelor (Lilly) and generics
Glyburide: Micronase (Upjohn) and DiaBeta (Hoechst-Roussel)
Glipizide: Glucotrol (Pfizer)
Glimepiride: Amaryl (Hoechst Marion Roussel)

metabolites are excreted in the urine (Gerich 1989). Sulfonylureas should not be administered in patients with renal or hepatic insufficiency.

No studies on the pharmacokinetics of glipizide have been done in the cat or dog. Studies in healthy cats showed an immediate release of insulin after oral administration. Peak insulin concentrations were achieved 15 minutes later, and baseline concentrations were reached again after 60 minutes (Miller et al. 1992). In our own studies, the insulin concentration peaked 30 minutes after glipizide administration and did not return to baseline levels until several hours later (Hoenig, unpublished). Glipizide is usually administered orally. A recent study has evaluated transdermal administration of glipizide. The absorption was low and inconsistent and it was concluded that a transdermal preparation cannot be recommended at this time (Bennet et al. 2005).

Preparations and Properties. The preparation used in veterinary medicine is glipizide (Glucotrol®; Pfizer). It is marketed as 5 and 10 mg tablets.

Therapeutic Uses. Glipizide has been advocated as an antidiabetic agent for the cat (Miller et al. 1992). The drug seemed to be effective in some cats; however, these cats were also on a high-fiber diet, which might have influenced the therapeutic response. A dose of 5 mg BID was given to each cat.

For glipizide to be effective, it is necessary for beta cells to still have the capacity to release insulin. Therefore, in theory, this drug should only be administered in those cases in which insulin secretion has been documented (with glucose/glucagon stimulation tests, etc.). However, it has recently been shown that glipizide accelerates amyloid deposition in cat islets (Hoenig et al. 2000), which confirmed evidence in rats that these drugs may actually be harmful (Kahn et al. 1993). It is therefore prudent to treat all diabetic cats with insulin at this time until other oral antihypoglycemic agents have been evaluated and shown to be effective: the insulin-deficient patient whose beta cells no longer can secrete insulin and the patient who still has insulin but whose secretion rate is insufficient to control blood glucose concentrations. In the latter, the use of insulin will alleviate the overstimulation of the beta cells and amyloid formation.

Adverse Effects. Hypoglycemia is the most frequently observed side effect of sulfonylureas in humans; however, severe life-threatening hypoglycemic reactions are rare. The hypoglycemic reactions may be potentiated by drugs that are highly protein-bound. Hepatotoxicity has been reported in dogs after tolbutamide administration. In cats, vomiting, hypoglycemia, and an increase in alanine aminotransferase (ALT) has been reported. Other side effects seen in humans include increased cardiovascular mortality, gastrointestinal disturbances, allergic skin reactions, and hematologic changes (Gerich 1989).

METFORMIN. Metformin (N,N-dimethylbiguanide; Glucophage®, Bristol-Myers Squibb) is an oral antihyperglycemic agent used primarily in the management of type 2 diabetes in people. Metformin reduces blood glucose concentrations primarily by reducing hepatic glucose output and by improving peripheral sensitivity to insulin without affecting insulin secretion. It does not cause hypoglycemia at therapeutic doses. Although the pharmacokinetics of metformin have been established in the cat (Michels et al. 1999) and are similar to those in people, data on the efficacy of the drug in clinical diabetes cases are not available. Since the drug is eliminated primarily by renal clearance in the cat (Michels et al.1999), it should not be used in cats with significant renal dysfunction.

THIAZOLIDINEDIONES. Thiazolidinedione compounds have been developed to counteract the insulin resistance that is seen in type 2 diabetes. Thiazolidinediones are high-affinity ligands of PPAR γ (peroxisome-proliferator-activated receptor γ), a subtype of the nuclear receptor superfamily of ligand-activated transcription factors that is involved in the differentiation of adipose tissue. They regulate the transcription of insulin-responsive genes involved in the control of glucose production, transport, and utilization and lead to lower fasting and postprandial glucose concentrations, and improved insulin sensitivity (for review, see Yki-Järvinen 2004).

Among the thiazolidinedione compounds, troglitazone (Rezulin®, Parke Davis) was the first to become widely available (Nolan et al. 1994). The serious liver side effects have forced the discontinuation of the use of this drug. Pioglitazone (Actos®, Takeda) and Rosiglitazone (Avandia®, GlaxoSmithKline) were approved by the FDA in 1999 for the treatment of type 2 diabetics. There are no reports about the efficacy of this drug in the diabetic dog or cat. The pharmokinetics of troglitazone in the cat is similar to that in people (Michels et al. 2000). Recently, darglitazone (Pfizer) was evaluated in lean and obese cats. It was found to markedly improve indices of insulin resistance (Hoenig and Ferguson 2003). However, this drug was not made available for veterinary use.

ACARBOSE. Acarbose (Precose®, Bayer) is an alpha glucosidase inhibitor, a term applied to inhibitors of alpha amylase, which digests starch, and of brush border oligo- and disaccharidases, which cleave off glucose. Acarbose delays and reduces postprandial hyperglycemia after a carbohydrate meal. It has been used in human diabetic patients in combination with insulin and oral antihyperglycemic agents but also as monotherapy. Gastrointestinal disturbances such as diarrhea, flatulence, and abdominal pain are the major side effects (Scheen and Lefebvre 1998). The pharmacokinetics of acarbose has been established in the dog (Ahr et al. 1989), and a small number of diabetic dogs needed less insulin when treated with acarbose (Robertson et al. 1998). It has also been used in diabetic cats in combination with a low carbohydrate diet (Mazzaferro et al. 2003). Because of the high cost of this drug, it remains to be seen whether the clinical effect justifies its use.

GLUCAGON

HISTORY. Although the existence of a pancreatic hyperglycemic hormone was postulated in 1923 by Kimball and Murlin (1923), it was not until 1955 that Staub and co-workers succeeded in purifying glucagon (1955). In 1957, Bromer and co-workers identified its amino acid sequence.

CHEMISTRY AND BIOSYNTHESIS. Glucagon is a polypeptide hormone containing 29 amino acids. Its structure is highly preserved in different species, and the various glucagons differ usually only by 1 or 2 amino acids. Glucagon is synthesized in the alpha cells of the islets of Langerhans as a prohormone with a molecular mass of 18 kilodaltons. The exact mechanism of glucagon secretion into the blood is still controversial (Unger and Orci 1989). However, it seems that glucagon is co-released with two major proglucagon fragments. Glucagon-like immunoreactive peptides are also synthesized in the gastrointestinal tract. Glucagon bears striking structural similarity to secretin, gastric inhibitory peptide, and vasoactive intestinal peptide.

SECRETION. Glucagon is a hyperglycemic hormone and as such is antagonistic to the action of insulin. The special arrangement of beta and alpha cells in the islet makes a close interaction of both hormones possible, and both, glucagon and insulin, exert a major regulatory function on metabolism. It seems that for many metabolic effects, the ratio of insulin to glucagon is important for the regulation of cellular responses (Smith 1989). In general, glucagon secretion is stimulated by low glucose concentrations, by protein intake, and by lowered fatty acid concentrations. Glucagon secretion is also under control of intestinal hormones and neurotransmitters (Unger and Orci 1989).

MECHANISM OF ACTION. Glucagon is a major antagonist of insulin action. Glucagon stimulates glycogenolysis, gluconeogenesis, and lipolysis. Administration of glucagon leads to a rapid increase in intracellular cyclic adenosine monophosphate (cAMP) concentrations, which is followed by activation of cAMP-dependent protein kinase and subsequent substrate phosphorylation (Smith 1989).

METABOLISM. Glucagon is degraded in liver, kidney, plasma, and at its receptor on the plasma membrane. Its half-life in plasma is approximately 3–6 minutes (Unger and Orci 1989).

PREPARATIONS AND DOSAGE. Glucagon is extracted from beef and pork pancreases. Glucagon for injection (Eli Lilly) contains glucagon as the hydrochloride and is dispensed in 1 or 10 mg vials. It is packaged with diluent containing glycerin and phenol. One mg is usually administered to dogs for insulin-induced hypoglycemia.

THERAPEUTIC USES. Glucagon can be used for the treatment of insulin-induced hypoglycemia when dextrose is unavailable. It is only useful as a hyperglycemic agent in those patients that have sufficient hepatic glycogen. Glucagon should not be used in hypoglycemia due to insulinoma or in patients with pheochromocytoma, because it can induce hormone release from the tumors. In humans it is also used for radiographic and endoscopic examination of the gastrointestinal tract, because it acts as a smooth muscle relaxant. Glucagon has been used in small animals for double-contrast gastroscopy (Evans and Biery 1983); however, a recent study could not confirm a beneficial effect for endoscopic examinations in the dog (Matz et al. 1991).

ADVERSE EFFECTS. Glucagon is relatively free of adverse effects. Generalized allergic reactions have been reported in human patients after glucagon administration.

GLUCAGON-LIKE PEPTIDE 1 RECEPTOR AGONIST

Glucagon-like peptide 1 (GLP-1) is an incretin that augments insulin secretion after food intake. It also inhibits glucagon release and gastric emptying. Because of its poor stability, it cannot be used therapeutically. However, exendin-4 (Extendine; Byetta®, Eli Lilly/Amylin), a synthetic version of a peptide isolated from the saliva of the gila monster, has been shown to bind and activate the known human GLP-1 receptor and is now used therapeutically for the treatment of type 2 diabetics. In people, it is injected subcutaneously twice daily within 60 minutes before the morning and evening meal. There are no reports yet of the use of this drug in animals. Because the half-life of GLP-1 is very short, a new class of drugs has been developed, the dipeptidyl peptidase 4 (DPP-4) inhibitors. Their mechanism of action is thought to result from increased incretin levels (GLP-1 and glucose-dependent insulinotropic polypeptide, GIP) leading to increased insulin concentrations (Valk 2007). Sitagliptine (Januvia®, Merck) and Vildagliptine (Galvus®, Novartis) have been approved for use in human type 2 diabetics. There are no reports of their use in pets.

SOMATOSTATIN

HISTORY. Somatostatin was isolated from ovine hypothalamus in 1973 by Brazeau and co-workers (1973). Soon it became evident that somatostatin was not only present in hypothalamus but also in other tissues, including the pancreas (Hökfeldt et al. 1975; Arimura et al. 1975). It became apparent that the islet D cells, first described by Bloom (1931), secreted this hormone, which inhibited insulin and glucagon secretion (Koerker et al. 1974).

CHEMISTRY AND BIOSYNTHESIS. Somatostatin is synthesized as a high-molecular weight precursor, which is differently processed in a tissue-specific manner. In the pancreas and hypothalamus it is cleaved mainly to a 14-residue peptide containing an internal disulfide bridge, whereas in the gastrointestinal tract the predominant form is a 28-residue peptide. Very little is yet known about the regulation of its biosynthesis.

SECRETION. Much still needs to be learned about the regulation of somatostatin secretion. In the pancreas, somatostatin may act in a paracrine or endocrine manner when released from the delta cells.

MECHANISM OF ACTION. The mechanism of action by which somatostatin inhibits insulin and glucagon release from the islet cells is not well understood. It has recently been shown that somatostatin inhibits insulin gene expression through a posttranslational mechanism, however, at concentrations well above those measured in the peripheral blood. Somatostatin release is stimulated by most nutrients, including glucose, amino acids, and a fat-protein meal. Somatostatin also inhibits growth hormone release and a variety of gastrointestinal hormones (for a review, see Long 1987).

METABOLISM. It is unknown how somatostatin is metabolized. It has an apparent half-life of 3–5 minutes.

PREPARATIONS AND DOSAGE. The only preparation available with pharmacologic actions similar to somatostatin is the synthetic agent octreotide acetate (L-cysteinamide; Sandostatin® Injection, Sandoz Pharmaceuticals), a cyclic octapeptide prepared as a clear solution of octreotide acetate in buffered saline for deep subcutaneous injection. In humans, peak concentrations are reached within 0.4 hours; the half-life is approximately 1.5 hours in humans and approximately 75 minutes in dogs (for a review, see Long 1987). The duration of action of octreotide is variable but can extend up to 12 hours.

THERAPEUTIC USES. In humans, octreotide acetate is used most frequently in patients with VIP(vasoactive intestinal polypeptide)oma and carcinoid.

In dogs, the use of octreotide has been used for the treatment of some insulinomas and for gastrinomas. Not all of the tumors treated responded to octreotide, likely because of the absence of specific receptors. Octreotide has not proven to be useful in the treatment of acromegaly. The dose for the treatment of insulinomas is 10–20 μg BID to TID; in gastrinomas 20–60 μg TID has been recommended (Lothrop 1991).

ADVERSE EFFECTS. In humans, gastrointestinal problems are most frequently encountered after octreotide administration. Side effects in dogs have not been described.

MISCELLANEOUS

DIAZOXIDE. Diazoxide (Proglycem®; Schering) is 7-chloro-3-methyl-2*H*-1,2,4-benzothiadiazine 1,1-diazoxide. It is a white powder practically insoluble in water. This nondiuretic benzothiadiazine inhibits insulin release from the beta cell by increasing the permeability to potassium, thereby hyperpolarizing the cell membrane (Trube et al. 1986). It also has extrapancreatic effects and promotes hepatic glycogenolysis and decreases glucose uptake in the liver (Altzuler et al. 1977). It is used in the treatment of insulin-secreting tumors. The initial dose of diazoxide is 10 mg/kg body weight divided into two daily doses. This dose can be increased gradually but should not exceed 40 mg/kg daily. Diazoxide is available as 50 mg capsules or as a suspension containing 50 mg/ml diazoxide.

REFERENCES

Ahr, H. J, Boberg, M., Krause, H. P., Maul, W., Muller, F. O., Ploschke, H. J., Weber, H., and Wunsche, C. 1989. Pharmacokinetics of acarbose. Part I: Absorption, concentration in plasma, metabolism and excretion after single administration of [^{14}C]acarbose to rats, dogs and man. Arzneimittelforschung 39:1254–1260.

Altzuler, N., Hampshire, J., and Moraru, E. 1977. On the mechanism of diazoxide-induced hyperglycemia. Diabetes 26:931–935.

Antomarchi, S. H., Weille, J. D., Fosset, M., and Lazdunski, M. 1987. The receptor for antidiabetic sulfonylureas controls the activity of the ATP-modulated K channel in insulin-secreting cells. J Biol Chem 262:15840–15844.

Arimura, A., Sata, H., and Dupont, A. 1975. Abundance of immunoreactive hormone in rat stomach and pancreas. Science 189:1007.

Arkhammar, P., Nilsson, T., Rorsman, P., and Berggren, P.-O. 1987. Inhibition of ATP-regulated K channels precedes depolarization-induced increase in cytoplasmic free Ca concentration in pancreatic beta cells. J Biol Chem 262:5448–5454.

Bennett, N., Papich, M. G., Hoenig, M., Fettman, M. J., and Lappin M. R. 2005. Evaluation of transdermal application of glipizide in a pluronic lecithin gel to healthy cats. Am J Vet Res 66:581–8.

Berman, N., Chou, H.-F., Berman, A., et al. 1993. A mathematical model of oscillatory insulin secretion. Am J Physiol 264:R839–851.

Bliss, M. 1983. The Discovery of Insulin. Chicago: Univ Chicago Press.

Bloom, W. 1931. A new type of granular cell in the islets of Langerhans of man. Anat Rec 49:363.

Bonner-Weir, S., and Orci, L. 1982. New perspectives on the microvasculature of the islets of Langerhans in the rat. Diabetes 31:883–889.

Brazeau, P., Vale, W., Burgus, R., et al. 1973. Hypothalamic peptide that inhibits the secretion of immunoreactive pituitary growth hormone. Science 179:77–79.

Bromer, W. W., Sinn, L. G., and Behrens, O. K. 1957. Amino acid sequence of glucagon. V. Location of amide groups, acid-degradation studies, and summary of sequential evidence. J Am Chem Soc 79:2807.

Capen, C. C. 1990. Tumors of the pancreatic islets. In J. E. Moulton, ed., Tumors in Domestic Animals, pp. 616–622. Berkeley: Univ California Press.

Chammas, N. K., Teale, J. D., and Quin, J. D. 2003. Insulinoma: how reliable is the biochemical evidence? Ann Clin Biochem 40:689–693.

Church, D. B. 1981. The blood glucose response to three prolonged duration insulins in canine diabetes mellitus. J Small Anim Pract 22:301–310.

Cook, D. L., Satin, L. S., Ashford, L. J., et al. 1988. ATP-sensitive K channels in pancreatic beta cells: spare channel hypothesis. Diabetes 37:495–498.

Cryer, P. E., and Gerich, J. E. 1990. Hypoglycemia in insulin dependent diabetes mellitus: insulin excess and defective glucose counterregulation. In H. Rifkin and D. Porte, eds., Ellenberg and Rifkin's Diabetes Mellitus: Theory and Practice, 4th ed., pp. 526–546. New York: Elsevier.

Davison, L. J., Ristic, J. M., Herrtage, M. E., Ramsey, I. K., and Catchpole, B. 2003. Anti-insulin antibodies in dogs with naturally occurring diabetes mellitus. Vet Immunol Immunopathol 91:53–60.

Diem, P., and Robertson, R. P. 1991. Preventive effects of octreotide (SMS 201-995) on diabetic ketogenesis during insulin withdrawal. J Clin Pharm 32:563–567.

Duckworth, W. C. 1990. Insulin-degrading enzyme. In P. Cuatrecasas and S. Jacobs, eds., Insulin, pp. 143–165. New York: Springer Verlag.

Evans, S. M., and Biery, D. N. 1983. Double contrast gastroscopy in the cat. Vet Rad 4:3–5.

Frank, B. H., and Chance, R. E. 1983. Two routes for producing human insulin utilizing recombinant DNA technology. Münch Med Wochenschr 125(Suppl 1):14–20.

Gerich, J. 1989. Oral hypoglycemic agents. N Engl J Med 321:1231–1245.

Haffner, S. M., Gonzalez, C., Mykkänen, L., and Stern, M. 1997. Total immunoreactive proinsulin, immunoreactive insulin and specific insulin in relation to conversion to NIDDM: the Mexico City Diabetes Study, Diabetologia 40:830–837.

Helmstaedter, V., Feurle, G. E., and Forssmann, W. G. 1976. Insulin-, glucagon-, and somatostatin-immunoreactive endocrine cells in the equine pancreas. Cell Tiss Res 172:447–454.

Herdt, T. H., and Emery, R. S. 1992. Therapy of diseases of ruminant intermediary metabolism. Vet Clin North Am 8(Appl Pharm Therap II):91–106.

Hoenig, M., and Dawe, D. L. 1992. A qualitative assay for beta cell antibodies: preliminary results in dogs with diabetes mellitus. Vet Immunol Immunopathol 32:195–203.

Hoenig, M., and Ferguson, D. C. 1991. Diabetes mellitus. In D. G. Allen, ed., Small Animal Medicine, pp. 795–805. Philadelphia: Lippincott.

———. 2003. Effect of darglitazone on glucose clearance and lipid metabolism in obese cats. Am J Vet Res 64:1409–13.

Hoenig, M., Caffall, Z. F., McGraw, R. A., Ferguson, D. C. 2006. Cloning, expression and purification of feline proinsulin. Domest Anim Endocrinol 30:28–37.

Hoenig, M., Hall G., Ferguson, D., Jordan, J., Henson, M., Johnson, K., and O'Brien, T. D. 2000a. A feline model of experimentally induced islet amyloidosis. Am J Pathol 157:2143–2150.

Hoenig, M., Reusch, C., and Peterson, M. E. 2000b. Beta cell and insulin antibodies in treated and untreated diabetic cats. Vet Immunol Immunopathol 77:93–102.

Hoenig, M., Thomaseth, K., Brandao, J., Waldron, M., Ferguson, D. C. In press. Assessment and mathematical modeling of glucose turnover and insulin sensitivity in lean and obese cats. Dom Anim Endocrinol.

Hökfeldt, T., Efendic, S., and Hellerström, C. 1975. Cellular localization of somatostatin in endocrine-like cells and neurons of the rat with special reference to the A_1-cells of the pancreatic islets and to the hypothalamus. Acat Endocrinol 80(Suppl 200):5.

Johnson, I. S. 1983. Human insulin from recombinant DNA technology. Science 219:632–637.

Kahn, S. E., Verchere, C. B., D'Alessio, D. A., Cook, D. L., and Fujimoto, W. Y. 1993. Evidence for selective release of rodent islet amyloid polypeptide through the constitutive secretory pathway. Diabetologia 36:570–573.

Kaneko, J. J., Mattheeuws, D., Rottiers, R. P., and Vermeulen, A. 1977. Glucose tolerance and insulin response in diabetes mellitus of dogs. J Small Anim Pract 18:85.

Kaneto, H., Nakatani, Y., and Kawamori, D. 2005. Role of oxidative stress, endoplasmic reticulum stress, and c-Jun N-terminal kinase in pancreatic beta-cell dysfunction and insulin resistance. Int J Biochem Cell Biol 37:1595–1608.

Kimball, C. B., and Murlin, J. R. 1923. Aqueous extracts of pancreas: some precipitation reactions of insulin. J Biol Chem 58:337.

Koerker, D. J., Ruch, W., Chideckel, E., et al. 1974. Somatostatin: hypothalamic inhibitor of the endocrine pancreas. Science 184:482.

Laedtke, T., Kjems, L., Pørksen, N., Schmitz, O., Veldhuis, J., Kao, P. C., and Butler, P. C. 2000. Overnight inhibition of insulin secretion restores pulsatility and proinsulin/insulin ratio in type 2 diabetes. Am J Physiol Endocrinol Metab 279:E520–E528.

Long, R. G. 1987. Review: long-acting somatostatin analogues. Aliment Pharmacol Therap 1:191–200.

Lothrop, C. D. 1991. Octreotide treatment in canine and feline endocrine tumors. Proc 9th ACVIM Forum, pp. 755–757.

Loubatieres, A. 1946. Etude physiologique et pharmacodynamique de certains derives sulfamides hypoglycemiants. Arch Int Physiol 54:174–177.

Lowell, B. B., and Shulman, G. I. 2005. Mitochondrial dysfunction and type 2 diabetes. Science 307:384–387.

MacLaren, N., Schatz, D., Drash, A., et al. 1989. Initial pathogenic events in IDDM. Diabetes 38:534–538.

Matz, M. E., Leib, M. S., Monroe, W. E., Davenport, D. J., Nelson, L. P., and Kenny, J. E. 1991. Evaluation of atropine, glucagon, and metoclopramide for facilitation of endoscopic intubation of the duodenum in dogs. Amer J Vet Res 52:1948–1950.

Mazzaferro, E. M., Greco, D. S., Turner, A. S., and Fettman, M. J. 2003. Treatment of feline diabetes mellitus using an alpha-glucosidase inhibitor and a low-carbohydrate diet. J Feline Med Surg 5:183–9.

Michels, G. M., Boudinot, F. D., Ferguson, D. C., and Hoenig, M. 1999. Pharmacokinetics of the antihyperglycemic agent, metformin, in cats. Am J Vet Res 60:738–742.

———. 2000. Pharmacokinetics of the insulin-sensitizing agent, troglitazone, in cats. Am J Vet Res 61:775–778.

Miller, A. B., Nelson, R. W., Kirk, C. A., Neal, L., and Feldman, E. C. 1992. Effect of glipizide on serum insulin and glucose concentrations in healthy cats. Res Vet Sci 52:177–181.

Neubauer, H. P., and Schoene, H. H. 1978. The immunogenicity of different insulins in several animal species. Diabetes 27:8–15.

Nolan, J. J., Ludvik, B., Beerdsen, P., Joyce, M., and Olefsky, J. 1994. Improvement in glucose tolerance and insulin resistance in obese subjects treated with troglitazone. N Engl J Med 331:1188–1193.

O'Brien, T. D., Hayden, D. W., Johnson, K. H., and Stevens, J. B. 1985. High-dose intravenous glucose-tolerance test and serum insulin and glucagon levels in diabetic and non-diabetic cats: relationship to insular amyloidosis. Vet Path 22:250.

O'Brien, T. D., Hayden, D. W., Johnson, K. H., et al. 1986. Immunohistochemical morphometry of pancreatic endocrine cells in diabetic, normoglycaemic glucose-intolerant and normal cats. J Comp Path 96:357–369.

Pørksen, N. 2002. Early changes in beta-cell function and insulin pulsatility as predictors for type 2 diabetes. Diabetes Nutr Metab 15Suppl:9–14.

Porte, D., Jr. 1991. Beta cells in type 2 diabetes mellitus. Diabetes 40:1660–1680.

Porte, D., Jr., and Halter, J. B. 1981. The endocrine pancreas and diabetes mellitus. In R. H. Williams, ed., Textbook of Endocrinology, 6th ed., p. 716. Philadelphia: W. B. Saunders.

Porte, D., Jr., and Kahn, S. E. 1989. Hyperproinsulinemia and amyloid in NIDDM: clues to etiology of islet beta cell dysfunction? Diabetes 38:1333–1336.

Robertson, J., Nelson, R., Feldman, E., and Neal, L. 1998. Effect of α-glucosidase inhibitor acarbose in healthy and diabetic dogs. Proc 16th ACVIM Forum, A54.

Scheen, A. J., and Lefebvre, P. J. 1998. Oral antidiabetic agents: a guide to selection. Drugs 55(2):P225–236.

Schinner, S., Scherbaum, W. A., Bornstein, S. R., and Barthel, A. 2005. Molecular mechanisms of insulin resistance. Diabet Med 22:674–82.

Smith, R. J. 1989. Biological actions and interactions of insulin and glucagon. In L. J. DeGroot, ed., Endocrinology, vol. 2, pp. 1333–1345. Philadelphia: W. B. Saunders.

Staub, A., Sinn, L., and Behrens, O. K. 1955. Purification and crystallization of glucagon. J Biol Chem 214:619.

Steiner, D. F., Clark, J. L., and Nolan, D., et al. 1969. Proinsulin and the biosynthesis of insulin. Recent Prog Horm Res 25:207.

Stogdale, L. 1986. Definition of diabetes. Cornell Vet 76:156–174.

Straub S. G., and Sharp G. W. 2002. Glucose-stimulated signaling pathways in biphasic insulin secretion. Diabetes Metab Res Rev 18:451–63.

Trube, G., Rorsman, P., and Ohno-Sahosaku, T. 1986. Opposite effects of tolbutamide and diazoxide on the ATP-dependent K-channel in mouse pancreatic beta cells. Pflügers Arch 407:493–499.

Unger, R. H., and Orci, L. 1989. Glucagon secretion and metabolism in man. In L. J. DeGroot, ed., Endocrinology, vol. 2, pp. 1318–1332. Philadelphia: W. B. Saunders.

Valk, H. W. 2007. DPP-4 inhibitors and combined treatment in type 2 diabetes: Re-evaluation of clinical success and safety. Rev Diabet Stud 4:126–133.

Yki-Järvinen, H. 2004. Thiazolidinediones. NEJM 351:1106–1118.

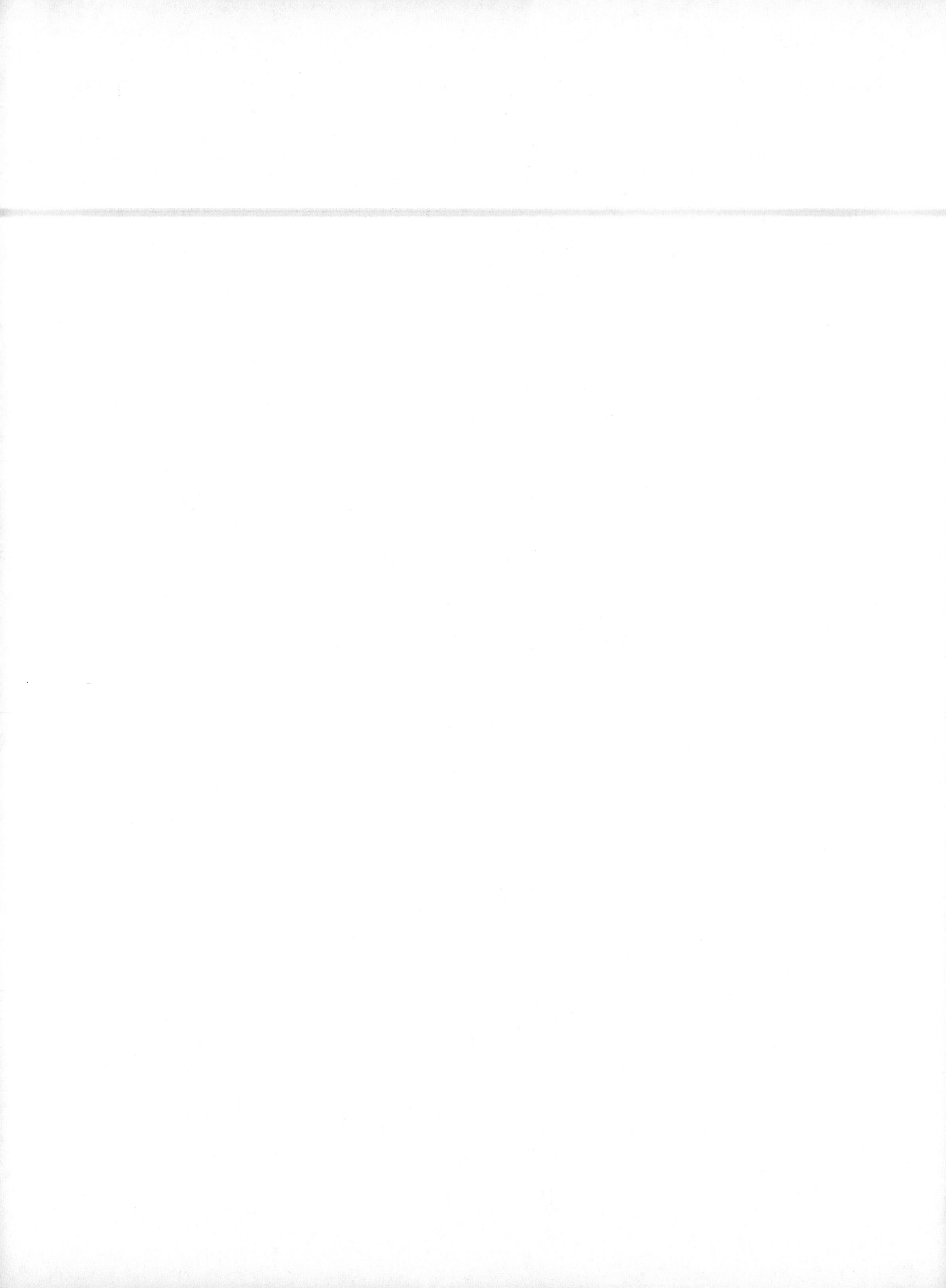

SECTION 9

Chemotherapy of Microbial Diseases

CHAPTER

32

ANTISEPTICS AND DISINFECTANTS

MARK C. HEIT AND JIM E. RIVIERE

Long before the ability to view microorganisms with a microscope and three centuries before Koch and Pasteur, Fracastoro postulated that germs caused infections. In the 1840s, Ignaz Semmelweis, a Hungarian obstetrician, demonstrated the beneficial effects of hand washing between patients as well as the antiseptic effect of chlorine in the form of chlorinated lime. Following Pasteur's identification of infective agents as the cause of disease, Joseph Lister suggested the use of antiseptics in the field of surgery. His treatment of the hands with 1:20 carbolic lotion and his initiation of methods for chemical sterilization of bandages, dressings, and surgical instruments and for antisepsis of wounds began aseptic surgery. Although originally targeted toward the surgeon, general cleanliness and the use of antiseptics and disinfectants have spread to all fields of the medical, dental, and veterinary professions.

Cleansers, antiseptics, and disinfectants are differentiated by their intended use and characteristic properties and not by their chemical content. A cleanser aids in physical removal of foreign material and is not a germicide. An antiseptic is a biocide applied to living tissue, and a disinfectant is a biocide applied to inanimate objects. Because certain antiseptics may be inactivated on inanimate surfaces and because certain disinfectants are hazardous to living tissue, the two should not be used interchangeably. Even products with the identical active chemical moiety may be formulated in such a way as to prevent their interchangeable use. Products to be used on inanimate surfaces, objects, or instruments are regulated by the Environmental Protection Agency (EPA), whereas chemicals in antiseptics for use on the human body must be registered with the Food and Drug Administration (FDA).

CLEANSERS

Cleansers (surfactants, detergents) remove dirt and contaminating organisms by solubilization and physical means. Cleaning an area to remove gross contamination prior to disinfection or antisepsis treatment maximizes their efficacy. Cleansers can be classified into three types based on the presence and sign of the charge of the hydrophilic portion of the molecule: anionic, cationic, and nonionic.

Soaps are anionic surfactants of the general structure R-COO^-Na^+. Dissociation in water to R-COO^- liberates a molecule with both a hydrophilic and a hydrophobic portion which can emulsify and solubilize hydrophobic dirt, fat, and protoplasmic membranes. Once solubilized, this contamination can be rinsed away with water. The ability to solubilize membranes renders soaps antibacterial against gram-positive and acid-fast bacteria. The anionic nature of soaps, however, causes them to be inactivated in the presence of certain positive ions such as free Ca^+ in hard water and in the presence of cationic detergents. The mixture of soaps and quaternary ammonium compounds forms a precipitate, which terminates the activity of both compounds. Inclusion of antiseptic compounds in soap preparations has given them a wider antibacterial spectrum.

The quaternary ammonium compounds are examples of cationic surfactants with germicidal activity. These compounds have been widely used as disinfectants. Cationic surfactants combine readily with proteins, fats, and phosphates and are thus of limited value in the presence of serum, blood, and other tissue debris (Huber 1988). In addition, use with materials such as gauze pads and cotton balls makes them less microbicidal owing to absorption of the active ingredients. For these reasons, and because several outbreaks of infections have been associated with use of contaminated solutions, the Center for Disease Control (CDC) no longer recommends cationic surfactants for antisepsis.

Second- and third-generation quaternary ammonium compounds are less affected by hard water and other anions. These quaternaries are fungicidal, bactericidal, and virucidal against lipophilic viruses but are not sporicidal, tuberculocidal, or active against hydrophilic viruses. Benzalkonium chloride, the first commercially available quaternary compound, has been shown to cause chemical burns when used undiluted (Bilbrey et al. 1989).

ANTISEPTICS AND DISINFECTANTS

An antiseptic is a chemical agent that reduces the microbial population on skin and other living tissues. Because, in most cases, its mechanism of action involves nonspecific disruption of cellular membranes or enzymes, caution must be taken not to harm host tissue. An ideal antiseptic would have a broad spectrum of activity, low toxicity, high penetrability, would maintain activity in the presence of pus and necrotic tissue, and would cause little skin irritation or interference with the normal healing process.

The use of antiseptics has been suggested in situations which require maximal reduction of bacterial contamination (Larson 1987) such as when defense mechanisms are compromised after surgery, during catheterization or insertion of other invasive implants, and in immunocompromised states due to immune defects, cytotoxic drug therapy, extreme old or young age, or extensive skin damage (burns and wounds).

Disinfection is the elimination of many or all pathogenic organisms, excluding spore forms, from an inanimate object. The treatment of objects that are too large to soak in disinfectant, such as cabinets, exam tables, chairs, lights, and cages, is considered surface disinfection. Immersion disinfection, sometimes wrongly referred to as cold sterilization, is the immersion of smaller objects in disinfectant for sufficient time to kill the majority of contaminating organisms. True chemical sterilization necessitates the use of an EPA-registered agent capable of killing all infective organisms, including fungal and bacterial spores, usually within 10 hours. Chemical sterilization should not replace heat-pressure sterilization.

The ideal characteristics of a disinfectant include a broad spectrum, fast action, activity in the presence of organic material (including blood, sputum, and feces), compatibility with detergents, low toxicity, and residual surface activity. They should not corrode instruments or metallic surfaces or disintegrate rubber, plastic, or other materials, and should be odorless and economical (Molinari et al. 1982).

Microorganisms can be ranked from least to most resistant to disinfectant killing as follows: vegetative bacteria, medium-size lipid-coated viruses, fungi, small nonlipid enveloped viruses, *Mycobacterium tuberculosis*, and bacterial endospores. Using these different resistances, disinfection can be further divided into three levels. Low-level disinfection kills most bacteria, some viruses, and some fungi, but not tubercle bacilli or bacterial spores. Intermediate-level disinfection inactivates *M. tuberculosis*, most viruses and fungi, but not necessarily bacterial spores. High-level disinfection destroys all microorganisms except high numbers of bacterial spores.

A second classification system divides instruments and patient-care items into three categories based on risk of infection involved in their use (Spaulding 1968). In this system, items are classified as 1) critical—those that enter or penetrate skin or mucous membranes (e.g., needles, scalpels), 2) semicritical—those that touch intact mucous membranes (e.g., anesthesia equipment, endoscopes), and, 3) noncritical—those that do not touch mucous membranes but may contact intact skin (e.g., cages, tables, food bowls). In general, items classified as critical should be sterilized, semicritical items require high-level disinfection, and noncritical items require low- to intermediate-level disinfection.

The following is a discussion of biocidal agents categorized by the active chemical entity. Where appropriate, considerations and recommendations for their use as cleansers, disinfectants, or antiseptics are noted.

ALCOHOL. Although many alcohols are germicidal, the two most commonly used are ethyl and isopropyl alcohol. These compounds are both lipid solvents and protein denaturants. They kill organisms by solubilizing the lipid cell membrane and by denaturing membrane cellular proteins. Alcohols are most effective when diluted with water to a final concentration of 70% ethyl or 50% isopropyl alcohol by weight. It is thought that at greater concentrations, initial dehydration of cellular proteins makes them resistant to the denaturing effect (Molinari and Runnel 1991). The alcohols have excellent antibacterial activity against most vegetative gram-positive, gram-negative, and tubercle bacillus organisms but do not inactivate bacterial spores. They are active against many fungi and viruses, principally enveloped viruses due to alcohol's lipid-solubilizing action. They are active against cytomegalovirus and herpes simplex and human immunodeficiency viruses.

Both isopropyl and ethyl alcohol are commonly used, effective antiseptics, with only subtle differences in their action. Because their effectiveness is drastically reduced by organic matter such as excreta, mucus, and blood, they are most effective on "clean" skin. Of all agents, they produce the most rapid and largest reduction in bacterial counts (Lowbury et al. 1974), with contact times of 1–3 minutes resulting in elimination of almost 80% of organisms. Rapid evaporation limits contact time; however, residual decreases in bacterial counts are seen to occur after the alcohol has evaporated from the skin. Although alcohols are among the safest antiseptics, toxic reactions have been reported in children. Alcohol is very drying to the skin and can cause local irritation. In efforts to minimize this drying effect, emollients such as glycerine have been added with good results (Larson et al. 1986).

The alcohols are not recommended for high-level disinfection or chemical sterilization due to their inactivity against bacterial spores and reduced efficacy in the presence of protein or other bioburden. Blood proteins are denatured by alcohol and will adhere to instruments being disinfected. Fatal *Clostridium* spp. infections have occurred postoperatively that were the result of contaminated surgical instruments that had been disinfected with alcohol containing bacterial spores (Nye and Mallory 1923). After repeated and prolonged use, alcohols can damage the shellac mounting of lensed instruments, can swell or harden rubber and certain plastic tubing (Rutala 1990), and can be corrosive to metal surfaces. Alcohols are flammable; thus caution must be taken in their storage and when used prior to electrocautery or laser surgery. In deciding between ethyl and isopropyl alcohol, it is important to consider isopropyl's inactivity against hydrophilic viruses, its less corrosive nature, and the abuse potential for ethyl alcohol (grain alcohol).

HALOGENS. Elemental iodine has activity against gram-positive and gram-negative bacteria, bacterial spores, fungi, and most viruses. It exerts these lethal effects by diffusing into the cell and interfering with metabolic reactions and by disrupting protein and nucleic acid structure and synthesis. Iodine has a characteristic odor and is corrosive to metals. It is insoluble in water and thus is prepared in alcohol (tincture) or with solubilizing surfactants ("tamed" iodines). Tincture of iodine, used as early as 1839, in the French Civil War, is most effectively formulated as a 1–2% iodine solution in 70% ethyl alcohol. In this form, most (−90%) bacteria are killed within 3 minutes of application. The antibacterial activity of this combination is greater than that of the alcohol alone. Tincture of iodine, however, is irritating and allergenic, corrodes metals, and stains skin and clothing. It is also painful when applied to open wounds and is harmful to host tissue; therefore, it can delay healing and thereby increase the chance of infection. For these reasons, this preparation has fallen out of favor as an antiseptic or disinfectant. Strong tinctures of iodine have been used as blistering agents in the equine industry.

Efforts to reduce the undesirable aspects of tinctures while retaining the powerful killing action of iodine have led to the introduction of tamed iodines known as iodophors. In this preparation, iodine is solubilized by surfactants, which allow it to remain in a dissociable form. Application of this product allows for slow continual release of free iodine to exert its germicidal effects. The iodophors have a similar spectrum of activity to aqueous solution; are less irritating, allergenic, corrosive, and staining; and have prolonged activity after application (4–6 h). Common solubilizing carriers include polyvinylpyrrolidone (called PVP-iodine or povidone-iodine [PI]) as well as other nonionic surfactants, making iodophors excellent cleansing agents as well as antiseptics and disinfectants. Iodophor solutions retain their activity in the presence of organic matter at pH <4 (Huber 1988). The water-soluble carriers have been postulated to interact with epithelial surfaces to increase tissue permeability, thereby enhancing iodine's killing efficacy.

Free iodine released by the iodophor complex is apparently responsible for its germicidal activity. Proper dilution to 1% iodine is necessary for maximum killing effect and minimal toxicity. More-concentrated solutions are actually less efficacious, presumably due to stronger complexation preventing free iodine release. It takes approximately 2 minutes of contact time for release of free iodine (Lavelle et al. 1975). Literature reports indicate that iodophors are quickly bactericidal, virucidal, and mycobactericidal but may require prolonged contact times to kill certain fungi and bacterial spores. Iodophors formulated as antiseptics are not suitable as hard-surface disinfectants, due to insufficient concentrations of iodine.

Consideration must be taken of iodine's ability to be systemically absorbed through the skin and mucous membranes. The extent of absorption is related to the concentration used, frequency of application, and status of renal function (the principal excretory route) (Swaim and Lee 1987). Complications of iodophor absorption include increased serum enzyme levels, renal failure, metabolic acidosis (Pretsch and Meakins 1976), and increased serum free iodide. If renal function is normal, serum iodine concentrations quickly return to normal. Clinical hyperthyroidism and thyroid hyperplasia have been reported after treatment with PI (Scheider et al. 1976; Altemeier 1976).

Chlorine-containing solutions were first introduced by Dakin in the early 1900s in the chemical form of sodium hypochlorite. They are effective antibacterial, fungicidal, virucidal, and protozoacidal agents. The chemical forms most commonly used today include the hypochlorites (sodium and calcium) and organic chlorides (chloramine-T). In either form, the germicidal activity is due to release of free chlorine and formation of hypochlorous acid (HOCl) from water. The mechanisms of action of these compounds include inhibition of cellular enzymatic reactions, protein denaturation, and inactivation of nucleic acids (Dychdala 1983). Dissociation of HOCl to the less microbicidal hypochlorite ion (OCl^-) increases as pH increases, and thus the solution may be rendered ineffective above pH 8.0 (Weber 1950). Mixing NaOCl with acid liberates toxic chlorine gas, and NaOCl decomposes when exposed to light.

Low concentrations of free chlorine are active against *M. tuberculosis* (50 ppm) and vegetative bacteria (<1 ppm) within seconds. Concentrations of 100 ppm destroy fungi in less than 1 hour, and many viruses are inactivated in 10 minutes at 200 ppm. Household bleach is 5.25% (52,500 ppm); thus dilutions of 1:100–1:250 should result in effective germicidal concentrations although more-concentrated solutions are often recommended (1:10–1:100).

The use of the hypochlorites as disinfectants is limited by several characteristics. Chlorine solutions are corrosive to metals and destroy many fabrics. Because chlorine solutions are unstable to light, they must be prepared fresh daily. Hypochlorites are inactivated by the presence of blood more so than are the organic chlorides (Bloomfield and Miller 1989). They have a strong odor and are not suitable for enclosed spaces. Despite these shortcomings, chlorine solutions are commonly used as low-level disinfectants to sanitize dairy equipment, animal housing quarters, hospital floors, and other noncritical items. Of 12 disinfectant solutions evaluated for their ability to kill the dermatophyte *Microsporum canis*, those containing hypochlorite were most effective. Also found effective were benzalkonium chloride- and glutaraldehyde-based products; phenolics and anionic detergents were considered inadequate (Rycroft and McLay 1991). The hypochlorites are not recommended for use as antiseptics because they are very irritating to skin and other tissues and they delay healing.

Several compounds from a class called N-halamines (oxazolidinones or imidazolidinones) have been developed which are water-soluble solids that have been shown to be bactericidal, fungicidal, virucidal, and protozoacidal in water disinfection at low total halogen concentrations (1–10 mg/l). They are noncorrosive and tasteless and odorless in water. They are extremely stable in water even in the presence of organic loads. Their potential use in poultry processing to control *Salmonella* has been evaluated (Smith et al. 1990).

BIGUANIDES. Chlorhexidine (Chx) is a synthetic cationic compound (1-1'-hexamethylenebis[5-(p-chlorophenyl)biguanide]) with better activity against gram-positive organisms than against gram-negative ones. It was found to be superior to PI against *Staphylococcus aureus* infection in dogs (Amber et al. 1983), but some gram-negative bacteria were found to be resistant (Russell 1986). Chlorhexidine kills bacteria by disrupting the cell membrane and precipitating cell contents. It has also been suggested that membrane bound adenosine triphosphatases, specifically inhibition of the F1 ATPase, may be a primary target for Chx (Gale et al. 1981). It is active against fungi, fairly active against *M. tuberculosis*, but poorly active against viruses. The antibacterial activity of Chx is not as rapid as that of the alcohols; however, as a 0.1% aqueous solution, significant killing action is evident after only 15 seconds. Additionally, Chx solutions have the longest residual activity, remaining chemically active for 5–6 hours and retaining their activity in the presence of blood and other organic material. Being cationic, it is inactivated by hard water, nonionic surfactants, inorganic anions, and soaps. Dilution with saline causes precipitation and its activity is pH dependent. It has extremely low toxicity even when used on intact skin of newborns (O'Neill et al. 1982).

Chlorhexidine is available in a detergent base as a 4% solution or as a 2% liquid foam. It is widely used as a presurgical antiseptic, wound flush, and teat dip. Its use as a disinfectant has not been described.

Polyhexamethylene biguanide (PHMB) is a polymeric biguanide with activity against gram-positive and gram-negative bacteria, including methicillin-resistant *Staphylococcus aureus*, *Pseudomonas aeruginosa*, and *Streptococcus equi*. PHMB rapidly kills bacteria by disrupting the cytoplasmic membrane resulting in leakage and precipitation of cellular contents (Broxton et al. 1983). PHMB has been used to treat infections in the eye, mouth and vagina and has been formulated in contact lens disinfectants and mouth rinses. It was shown to be nontoxic as a component of an ear flush for dogs (Mills et al. 2005) and when impregnated in a gauze wound dressing, reduced growth of underlying gram-positive and gram-negative bacteria in vitro (Lee et al. 2004).

ALDEHYDES. Two related aldehyde disinfectants are formaldehyde and glutaraldehyde (GLT). Formaldehyde has antimicrobial activity both as a gas (see later) and in liquid form. Formalin, the aqueous form, is 37% formaldehyde by weight. It inactivates microorganisms by alkylating the amino and sulfhydryl groups of proteins and ring nitrogen atoms of purine bases (Favero 1983). Formaldehyde is an effective but slow bactericide, virucide, and fungicide, requiring 6–12 hours contact time. It is effective against *M. tuberculosis*, bacterial spores, and most animal viruses, including foot-and-mouth disease virus. Its action is not affected by organic matter and it is relatively noncorrosive to metals, paint, and fabric. Formaldehyde alone is considered a high-level disinfectant and in combination with alcohol can be used as a chemical sterilant for surgical instruments. However, due to irritating fumes and pungent odor at low concentrations (−1 ppm), and because the National Institute for Occupational Safety and Health requires it to be handled as a potential carcinogen, thereby limiting worker exposure time, formaldehyde's use as a disinfectant has been limited to certain veterinary applications (see later).

Glutaraldehyde, a saturated dialdehyde, is similar to formaldehyde but without some of its shortcomings. GLT has better bactericidal, virucidal, and sporicidal activity than formaldehyde. Its biocidal activity is related to its ability to alkylate sulfhydryl, hydroxyl, carboxyl, and amino groups affecting RNA, DNA, and protein synthesis (Scott and Gorman 1983). Acidic GLT solutions are not sporicidal; thus, they must be "activated" by alkalinizing agents to a pH between 7.5 and 8.5. Once activated, these solutions have a limited shelf life (14 days) due to polymerization of the GLT molecules (Rutala 1990). Newer formulations (stabilized alkaline GLT, potentiated acid GLT, GLT-phenate) have increased shelf life (28–30 days) and excellent germicidal activity (Pepper 1980).

GLT has gained wide acceptance in high-level disinfection and chemical sterilization due to several favorable properties, including wide spectrum of activity. Low surface tension allows GLT to penetrate blood and exudate without coagulating proteins. It retains its biocidal activity in the presence of organic matter. It is noncorrosive to metal, rubber, and plastic and does not damage lensed instruments. GLT solutions must be used in well-ventilated areas, since air concentrations of 0.2 ppm are irritating to the eyes and nasal passages (CDC 1987).

Contact times of less than 2 minutes for vegetative bacteria, 10 minutes for fungi, and 3 hours for bacterial spores were necessary using a 2% aqueous alkaline GLT solution (Stonehill et al. 1963). Activity against the tubercle bacillus was found to be somewhat variable; at least 20 minutes at room temperature is needed to reliably kill these organisms with 2% GLT. When used as a high-level disinfectant, a minimum of 1% GLT should be used. GLT-phenate formulations should be used with caution since they were shown to be less effective than other aldehyde solutions in decreasing bacterial counts from some medical instruments (Ayliffe et al. 1986). GLT disinfectants were found to more effectively reduce duck hepatitis B virus infectivity when they contained additives such as alcohol, an ammonium chloride derivative, and a surfactant (Murray et al. 1991).

The caustic nature of both formaldehyde and GLT makes them inappropriate as antiseptics, and in fact, protective gloves should be worn when using the aldehyde disinfectants.

OXIDIZING COMPOUNDS. Conflicting reports concerning hydrogen peroxide's efficacy as a germicide make evaluating its utility in disinfection and antisepsis difficult. Although it has been reported to have bactericidal (Schaeffer et al. 1980), virucidal (Mentel and Schmidt 1973), and fungicidal (Turner 1983) activity, others believe it to be more effective against bacterial spores (Reybrouk 1985; Baldry 1983) than against vegetative bacteria. For this reason, one author suggests that hydrogen peroxide antiseptic use be restricted to initial treatment of recently contaminated wounds suspected of containing clostridial spores (Reybrouk 1985). Because 3% hydrogen peroxide has been shown to be damaging to tissues including fibroblasts (Lineweaver et al. 1982), it is not considered suitable for routine wound care. It is, however, considered a stable and effective disinfectant and is used in the disinfection of soft contact lenses.

Potassium peroxymonosulfate (PPMS) is an oxidizing agent used in disinfection systems of pools and hot tubs. Recently, it has been formulated with potassium chloride and organic acids and salts (i.e., sulphamic acid, malic acid, sodium hexametaphosphate, and sodium dodecyl benzene sulphonate) resulting in a disinfectant effective against over 580 infectious agents including viruses, gram-positive and gram-negative bacteria, fungi (molds and yeasts), and mycoplasma (EPA Master Label). Its mechanism of action is not well characterized but is thought to be the result of the synergistic activity of its components to attack the key structures within microbial organisms (Antec International website). It is marketed as a powder because it is stable in solution for approximately 1 week. It is not inactivated by organic challenge and has been found to be user friendly to both humans and animals. It is widely used as a high-level disinfectant for surfaces in laboratories, dental care facilities, and hospitals; for decontaminating laundry; for air disinfection; and in food processing and transport.

PHENOLS. Carbolic acid, a phenol, is the oldest example of an antiseptic compound. However, due to severe toxicity, it is no longer appropriate for use as an antiseptic. These agents act as cytoplasmic poisons by penetrating and disrupting microbial cell walls. Most commercially available phenolic products contain two or more compounds that act synergistically, resulting in a wider spectrum of activity, including against *M. tuberculosis.* Sodium o-phenylphenol is effective against staphylococci, pseudomonads, mycobacteria, fungi, and lipophilic viruses and against ascarids, strongyles, and tichurids. Cresols are substituted phenols and are more bactericidal and less toxic and caustic than phenols. Phenolics are not recommended for disinfection of anything other than noncritical items, because of residual disinfectant on porous materials causing tissue irritation even when the items have been thoroughly rinsed, because of strong odors and because of absorption into feed.

Triclosan (Irgasan DP 300; 2,4,4′ trichloro-2′-hydroxydiphenyl ether) is a chlorinated diphenyl ether or bisphenol that possesses high antibacterial activity particularly against many gram-positive (e.g., *B. subtilis, M. smegmatis, S. aureus*) and gram-negative bacteria (*E. coli, S. typhinmurium, S. flexneri*) as well as fungi and yeasts (Stewart et al. 1999). Triclosan has been used for over 30 years and was first introduced in the health care industry in a surgical scrub in 1972. However, recently there has been a rapid increase in the use of triclosan-containing products including soaps, disinfectants, deodorants, shampoos, and medical supplies. In addition, it can be incorporated into plastics (e.g., children's toys) and fibers to retard decomposition.

The mechanisms of action of triclosan have been debated, but it is likely that they are concentration-dependent. At low concentrations, triclosan acts as a competitive inhibitor of bacterial enoyl-acyl carrier protein reductase, which is involved in the bacterial fatty acid elongation cycle. At higher concentrations, because of its lipophilicity, triclosan has been shown to incorporate into bacterial membranes to alter the physicochemical properties of the lipid bilayer including perturbation of the packing and interaction between membrane phospholipids (Guillen et al. 2004). Resistance due to specific mutations (Heath et al. 1999) of the bacterial carrier protein has been demonstrated in *S. aureus* and *E. coli* (Fan et al. 2002). The clinical significance of this decreased sensitivity remains questionable since concentrations achieved during triclosan use are likely high enough for the generalized bactericidal activity to prevail. Decreased sensitivity has been demonstrated in bacteria that overexpress the AcrAB efflux pump (Wang et al. 2001). The possibility and data suggesting that these resistance mechanisms may not only confer resistance to triclosan but also to other antibiotics has led to concern about the ubiquitous use of this compound in detergents, toothpaste, and other household items.

GASES. Gases are used primarily as disinfectants for large spaces and for sterilization of sensitive surgical equipment. Ethylene oxide (C_2H_4O) is a water soluble flammable gas used for gas sterilization. Mixing ethylene oxide with carbon dioxide or fluorocarbons reduce its flammability. Ethylene oxide kills bacteria, fungi, yeasts, viruses, and spores. Bacterial spores are only 2–10 times more resistant to the cidal activity than are vegetative cells. It has been shown that the relative humidity of the microenvironment is critical to microbial susceptibility to ethylene oxide. Activity is decreased in the presence of organic matter due to interaction with proteins and nucleic acids. Care must be used to contain the gas as it has an irritant effect on the skin and eyes and may cause headaches and nausea.

Formaldehyde gas inactivates viruses, fungi, bacteria, and bacterial spores. Its activity is dependent on relative humidity and its efficacy is thought to peak at less than 50 % relative humidity. Formaldehyde has been used for disinfection of hospital linen and for terminal disinfection in certain food producing industries (see later). Propriolactone, methyl bromide, and propylene oxide have also been used as gas disinfectants.

FACTORS AFFECTING EFFICACY OF ANTISEPTICS

Several factors influence the efficacy of antiseptics and disinfectants, including concentration and contact time, temperature, pH, presence of organic or other material, type and concentration of offending organism.

CONCENTRATION. The time to effectively kill an organism is inversely dependent upon antimicrobial concentration (Figure 32.1). For certain compounds (compound A), small decreases in concentration may result in large increases required for killing whereas other compounds (compound B) are less sensitive to changes in concentration. In this example it would be much more critical to achieve the appropriate concentration of compound A to ensure adequate antisepsis/disinfection. Alcohols are very concentration-dependent as are phenolics, whereas QACs, aldehydes, and chlorhexidine are less sensitive.

TEMPERATURE. Increased temperature results in increased antimicrobial activity. This relationship can be described by $Q_{(T2-T1)}$ = (time to kill at T_1) / (time to kill at T_2), where T_2 and T_1 are two different temperatures in centigrade degrees. This equation is commonly referred to as the Q_{10} coefficient and describes the change in activity caused by a 10 C rise in temperature. Table 32.1 lists the Q_{10} coefficient for certain disinfectant compounds.

pH. The pH at the site of action may affect a compound's activity by influencing the compound itself or the microbial cell. Certain molecules such as phenols, and certain acids, including hypochlorous acid (bleach), are effective only in the unionized form thus as pH increases they become less efficacious. Glutaraldehyde is more potent at alkaline pH but is more stable at acid pH. Increased pH results in higher numbers of negative charges on cell sur-

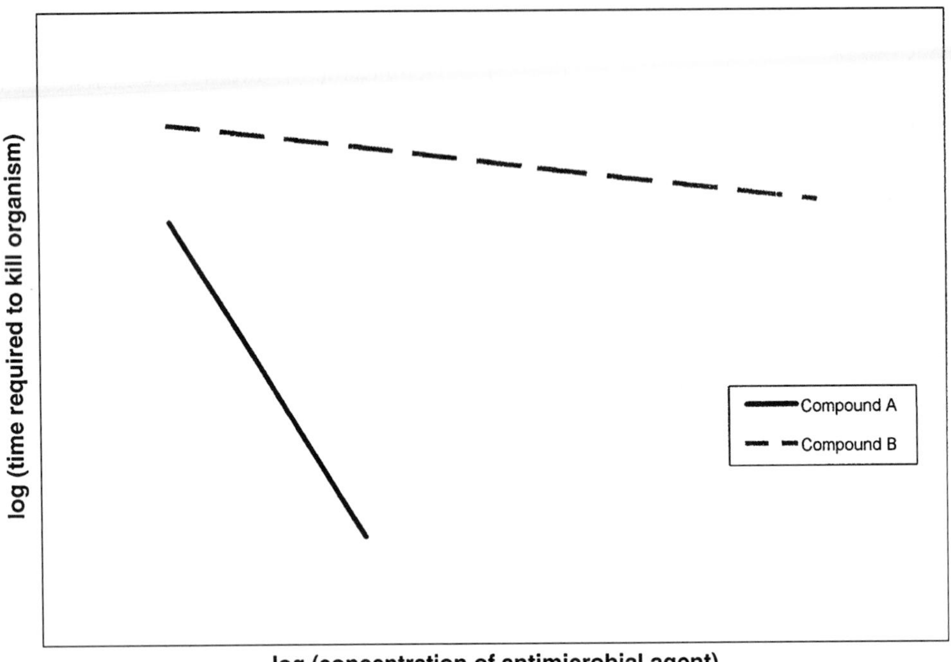

FIG. 32.1 The relationship of the concentration of two theoretical antimicrobial agents to the time required to kill a theoretical organism. The efficacy of compound A is more sensitive to change in concentration than that of compound B.

TABLE 32.1 Q_{10} coefficients for selected disinfectant/antiseptic compounds

Compound	Q_{10} Coefficient
Formaldehyde	1.5
β-propriolactone	2–3
Ethylene oxide	2.7
Phenol and cresol	3–5
Aliphatic alcohols	30–40

faces with which positively charged molecules, such as QACs and chlorhexidine can interact, thereby increasing their activity. Lastly, in a process similar to absorption through any cell membrane, pH can effect partitioning from the bathing solution into the cell's interior.

CONTAMINATION. The most important step in attempting to maximize the efficacy of antisepsis and disinfection is thorough cleansing of the site. Organic matter such as blood, pus, feces, soil, food, and milk, are believed to directly reduce the activity of antimicrobial compounds via a chemical reaction which results in a smaller amount of compound available for killing microorganisms or by spatial nonreaction (the inability of the disinfectant molecule to get to the organism). Certain compounds (hypochlorites and iodines) are more susceptible to this type of interference than others. Glutaraldehyde is less affected by organic contamination than other compounds and is therefore useful for instruments whose surface or design make it impossible to thoroughly clean. Soil contamination can make disinfection of large animal facilities difficult and may require removal of surface layers of soil and bedding for complete treatment. The presence of inorganic ions, Ca^{+2}, Mg^{+2}, Na^{+}, and Cl^{-} may be physically incompatible with certain antiseptics/disinfectants and therefore dilution with either hard water or saline solutions may render these formulations ineffective.

ORGANISM TYPE. The sensitivity of different classes (bacteria, fungus, virus, etc.) of organisms has been previously discussed. Within each group, however, differences in sensitivities exist to the various chemical compounds, which may render a particular disinfection process ineffective against certain microbes yet effective against others. Gram-positive bacteria are in general less resistant to disinfectant/antiseptic compounds than are gram-negative organisms due to a less complex and less lipid-rich outer membrane. Staphylococci are less susceptible to alcohols, glycols and ethylene oxide than are other cocci. Of the gram-negative bacteria, *Pseudomonas aeruginosa*, *Escherichia coli*, and spp. seem to be more resistant to antimicrobial agents, especially QACs and chlorhexidine, than other species. Mycobacteria, due to the hydrophobic nature of their cell wall, are highly resistant to many compounds. *M. tuberculosis* is resistant to chlorhexidine, acids, and alkalis while QACs are tuberculostatic. The tuberculosis organism is killed by alcohols, formaldehyde (glutaraldehyde), and ethylene oxide. Bacterial sporicides include the aldehydes, hydrogen peroxide, hypochlorites, iodine, acid alcohol and ethylene oxide. By inhibiting germination or spore outgrowth, phenols, QACs, biguanides, and alcohols are sporostatic. The efficacy of most germicides against bacterial spores increases with temperature; however, the most effective method against bacterial spores is moist heat (115°C autoclaving). Fungi are sensitive to chlorine, phenols, iodine compounds, ethylene oxide, and the aldehydes, whereas QAC are fungistatic. Fungal spores are resistant to most disinfectants. The sensitivity of viruses to disinfectant compounds relates to the composition of the viral envelope. The lipid-enveloped viruses are readily inactivated by lipophilic agents such as ether, chloroform, phenols, QACs, and even detergents. The nonenveloped viruses are resistant to these agents but are sensitive to chlorine and the aldehydes. Formaldehyde and β-propriolactone are used to inactivate viruses in the production of viral vaccines utilized in veterinary medicine.

FORMATION OF BIOFILMS. Bacteria present on metal or other surfaces may form a biofilm (Mafu et al. 1990) that is an adherent slimy layer of organic polymer matrix in which microbes are embedded. In addition, the intercellular matrix contains products of cellular metabolism including ions, nutrients, and enzymes such as polysaccharases, proteases, and β-lactamases. Differing cellular densities and extracellular concentrations of factors results in diverse cellular phenotypes with regard to growth rate, nutrient deprivation, etc. Bacteria in biofilm are less sensitive to disinfectant inactivation than are those grown in culture broth (i.e., planktonic). Proposed reasons for this increased resistance include decreased diffusion of disinfectant solution through polymer matrix preventing centrally located cells from being exposed to lethal concentrations of the compound. Chemical or enzymatic modification by extracellular components or decreased inherent microbe susceptibility due to slow growth rate or starvation responses may also contribute to increased bacterial survival in biofilms (Gilbert et al. 2002).

MICROBIAL RESISTANCE TO DISINFECTANTS AND ANTISEPTICS

Bacterial resistance to antibiotics is a well-documented and well-researched phenomenon. Concern regarding the development of resistance to antiseptics and disinfectants is not new (Lowbury 1951). Recent evidence confirming resistance to these compounds has been reported in the literature.

Staph. aureus has been shown to be resistant to triclosan, quaternary ammonia compounds, and chlorhexidine (Heath and Rock 2000; Suller and Russell, 1999, 2000). There are also reports of low-level resistance to QACs and chlorhexidine in Pseudomonas species (Mechin et al. 1999; Bamber and Neal, 1999; Tattawasart et al. 1999). However, this resistance has been considered unstable and not clinically significant (Russell 2000). The possibility that the mechanisms of resistance developed against a disinfectant or antiseptic could confer resistance to an antibiotic, however, is considered quite possible and potentially clinically disastrous.

The mechanisms of action of antibiotics are well known and in most cases, take advantage of a single specific target (e.g., inhibitors of peptidoglycan, protein, and nucleic acid synthesis, inhibitors of RNA polymerase, DNA gyrase) in their ability to kill or suppress the growth of bacteria. This is in contrast to mechanisms of action of disinfectants and antiseptics, which are less well understood and often involve more general and multiple cellular targets (Denyer and Stewart 1998). These include interactions with the cell wall or the envelope, disruption of membrane integrity, interruption of the proton-motive force, and inhibition of membrane enzymes, or as alkylating, cross-linking, and intercalating agents. Similarly, the mechanisms of resistance to antibiotics have been better characterized than those to biocides. Changes in the drug's target (e.g., methylation of the ribosome, penicillin-binding protein alterations), impermeability to the drug (e.g., intrinsic gram-negative resistance, biofilm formation), enzymatic modification or destruction of the drug (e.g., β-lactamases), and increased efflux of the drug can confer resistance to antibiotics.

As mentioned previously, there is evidence of resistance to disinfectants developing or being measured in vitro; however, because of redundancy in the number of targets for activity and the ability to achieve very high concentrations of biocide chemicals at the site of contamination, in vivo or clinical resistance to these compounds is not thought to be prevalent. However, because several of the mechanisms that allow for this resistance are common to those that provide resistance to antibiotics (efflux, impermeability, modification of target sites), the possibility for decreased efficacy to antibiotics is real.

β-lactam resistance in association with resistance to quaternary ammonia compounds has been demonstrated in *S. aureus* (Akimitsu et al. 1999). Triclosan-resistant mycobacteria were also resistant to isoniazid (McMurry et al. 1999), and there are many reports of biocide-antibiotic cross resistance in gram-negative bacteria. For example, *E. coli* that are resistant to triclosan (McMurry et al. 1998) or pine oil (Moken et al. 1997) have been shown to display the multiple antibiotic resistance (mar) phenotype. It is generally believed that in E. coli the mar phenotype is attributable to increased efflux due to up-regulation of the efflux pump (e.g., AcrAB-ToIC) (Okusu et al. 1996), which can cause resistance to β-lactams, chloramphenicol, fluoroquinolones, and tetracyclines.

The discovery of ciprofloxacin-resistant *E. coli* on farms with no previously reported quinolone exposure suggests that a disinfectant caused antibiotic resistance (Randall et al. 2005). Based on laboratory investigations designed to induce antibiotic resistance by repeated exposure to three different disinfectants, these authors conclude that, although bacteria became less sensitive to fluoroquinolones, this mechanism could not produce clinically resistant strains from fully susceptible ones. They further conclude that the risk of disinfectant exposure giving rise to multiple antibiotic resistant bacteria is outweighed by the value of sanitation provided by these compounds.

ANTISEPTIC USAGE IN VETERINARY MEDICINE

The role of antiseptics in veterinary medicine includes use in skin cleansers, wound scrubs, and teat dips.

SKIN CLEANSERS. Skin cleansers are important in the presurgical antisepsis of both the surgeon and the patient. The recommendations of the Association of Practitioners of Infection Control for presurgical antisepsis of the surgeon include two alternatives. The first involves an initial water-and-soap cleansing followed by use of an alcohol emollient scrub for at least 5 minutes. The second and more traditional method consists of a 5-minute chlorhexidine or iodophor hand scrub. This latter technique has the advantage that the active agents have residual bactericidal activity under surgical gloves. The presence of organic material and dirt can decrease the effectiveness of most antiseptics; thus removal of gross contamination should precede any antiseptic scrub. Additionally, an important reservoir of dirt and bacteria that needs to be specifically addressed is the subungual space (McHinley et al. 1988).

Preoperative preparation of the veterinary patient varies depending on the surgical environment, yet attempts to achieve the optimal antiseptic cleansing can aid in limiting postsurgical infections. Contrary to human surgery, hair removal from the operative site is almost always a necessity with animal patients. Clipping hair is superior to shaving since it causes less damage and less favorable conditions for bacterial colonization of the surgical skin site (Alexander et al. 1983). Removal of gross contamination and dirt should precede use of antiseptics for previously mentioned reasons. Gentle antiseptic scrubbing should begin at the incision site and move outward over the entire surgical area. Consideration of proper antiseptic contact times should be made. A final antiseptic spray is often applied and left to dry on the surgical site. Despite even the most careful presurgical preparation, up to 20% of skin-resident bacteria may be unaffected by skin antiseptic cleansing (Smeak and Olmstead 1984). Characteristics of an ideal skin antiseptic include broad spectrum, rapid killing, persistent lethal effect, cleansing effect, lack of skin irritation, noninhibition of healing, and activity in the presence of organic material.

Three antiseptic combinations were evaluated for surgical preparation of canine paws (Swaim et al. 1991): 7.5% PI scrub/10% PI solution, 2% Chx acetate scrub/2% Chx diacetate solution, and tincture of green soap/70% isopropyl alcohol combinations were each shown to effectively reduce bacterial colony counts. The first two combinations were also effective in residual killing when applied under a sterile bandage for 24 hours. However, no significant advantage of applying the antiseptics 24 hours prior to surgery was shown. This is in contrast to results in human patients, where antiseptic cleaning the night prior to surgery has resulted in fewer wound infections (Garibaldi et al. 1988). A similar technique involving prophylactic antiseptic cleansing and wrapping of a limb overnight has been shown to reduce contamination of equine orthopedic surgical sites (Stewart 1984). For surgery of the foot, additional reduction in bacteria load was achieved by removal of the superficial layer of the hoof; however, counts remained above a level that might predispose the surgical site to infection (Hennig et al. 2001). Antibacterial agents found in shampoos were shown to prevent infections caused by *S. intermedius* in a skin infection model in beagles. Shampoo containing 3% benzoyl peroxide was most effective, followed by shampoos containing 0.5% Chx acetate and iodine (1.0% polyalkyleneglycol-iodine) (Kwochka and Kowalski 1991).

A recent study compared the presurgical efficacy of chlorhexidine to a stabilized glutaraldehyde compound. Glutaraldehyde is most commonly associated with disinfection of inanimate objects; however, in its stabilized form it was noncorrosive, nonvolatile, nontoxic, biodegradable, stable, and highly microbiocidal at neutral pH. Stabilized glutaraldehyde (SG), with and without alcohol, and chlorhexidine with alcohol had similar and significant ability to reduce and maintain surface bacteria levels and therefore were recommended for presurgical antiseptic prophylaxis in elective (noncontaminated) procedures (Lambrechts et al. 2004).

TREATMENT OF OPEN WOUNDS. The treatment of open wounds is an important procedure in veterinary medicine. The important processes involved in wound healing and proper wound care have been reviewed (Swaim and Wihalf 1985; Berk et al. 1992). Issues involved in the decision of how to properly treat a wound include host age and general health status, and the age, cause, size, and extent of contamination of the wound. Treatment options include surgical closure, bandaging (of different types), and irrigation or application of a varied group of topical agents, including saline, antiseptics, antibiotics, and local anesthetics. It is important to recognize that each wound has different characteristics and thus treatment must be individualized. For all wounds, however, a basic principle to which all caregivers should adhere is "above all, do no harm"; that is, any agent chosen should not impede the healing process. When treating a wound topically, a general guideline would be not to apply anything that should not be placed in the patient's conjunctival sac (Peacock 1984).

The literature is divided concerning the utility of antiseptics in routine wound care. Some authors contend that this practice reduces the incidence of infections as a complication (Zukin and Simon 1987), while others believe that any benefit is outweighed by the potential for these agents to cause tissue damage (Oberg and Lindsey 1987). It is the opinion of these authors that in the initial care of grossly contaminated wounds, antiseptic application may be beneficial. Once the healing process has begun, however, the use of more-benign agents may be indicated. Saline has been shown to be an effective means of eliminating debris and lowering bacterial counts (Stevenson et al. 1976). Hypertonic saline has also been proposed as a wound dressing (Lowthian and Oke 1993). Archer et al. (1990) report that surface colonization of wounds does not impede healing and thus recommend a move away from potentially damaging antiseptics.

Many reports in the literature discuss potential toxic and harmful effects of antiseptics on fragile healing tissues, making their use controversial. A 5% PI solution inhibited local leukocyte migration, fibroblast activity, and wound cellularity (Viljanto 1980). In vitro, neutrophil migration was inhibited at concentrations greater than 0.05% (Tvedten and Till 1985), whereas 1% PI killed fibroblasts and resulted in weaker wound breaking strength (Lineweaver et al. 1985). Detergent scrubs containing PI and other surfactants were found to damage wound tissue and therefore are not recommended for wound care (Rodheaver et al. 1982). A maximum of 1% PI solution has been recommended as the most effective and least tissue-toxic dilution for wound irrigation (Swaim and Lee 1987). Because antibacterial activity lasts 4–6 hours, repeated treatment is necessary for optimal results.

Chlorhexidine's residual activity (possibly by binding to proteins of the stratum corneum) and its activity against many organisms, make it a useful wound treatment. In an experimental wound infection model, wounds irrigated with 0.05–1% Chx diacetate solution had fewer infections than those treated with 0.1–0.5% PI. Concentrations of Chx gluconate 0.5% or greater were effective against *S. aureus* in vitro; however, concentrations above 0.05% were lethal to equine fibroblasts (Redding and Booth 1991) and in a wound model in pigs. Unfortunately, it also delayed healing to a greater extent than other solutions tested, including PI (Archer et al. 1990).

Chlorine solution, such as sodium hypochlorite, was used as an effective wound flush in World War I. Full strength Dakin's solution (0.5% NaOCl) kills bacteria and fibroblasts, as well as retarding epithelialization in vivo in rats (Lineweaver et al. 1985). Other studies have shown low concentrations (0.025–0.0025%) to be toxic to neutrophils, fibroblasts, and endothelial cells, prompting one author to recommend abandoning the use of NaOCl as an irrigant (Kozol et al. 1988). In contrast, a concentration of 0.025% NaOCl was shown to be bactericidal while having no in vitro or in vivo tissue toxicity, suggesting a modified Dakin's solution may be a safe and effective fluid dressing (Heggers et al. 1991. Chloramine-T (Chlorazene), was shown to reduce in vitro *Pseudomonas aeruginosa* growth and the ability of the bacteria to colonize experimentally created wounds in guinea pigs. Additionally, Chlorazene was seen not to delay the healing of these wounds at a concentration of 0.03% (Henderson et al. 1989). Thus, it was concluded that this preparation should have no effect on healing of wounds when used to sanitize hydrotherapy units.

TEAT ANTISEPSIS. Postmilking teat antisepsis is one of the most effective procedures for reducing clinical and subclinical mastitis during lactation (Bramley and Dodd 1984). An ideal teat dip kills bacteria left on the skin after milking, prevents colonization of the teat orifice by pathogens, and cleans teat lesions without irritating the skin (Pankey et al. 1984). Many products exist with proven efficacy against intramammary infections (IMI) caused by *Streptococcus agalactiae* and *S. aureus*. Mastitis caused by environmental pathogens such as coliforms and non-*S. agalactiae Streptococcus* spp. is more difficult to combat. Since the environment is the reservoir for these organisms, residual activity of an antibacterial is necessary for infection control. In a natural-exposure trial (Oliver et al. 1990), a 0.35% Chx/glycerine emollient was shown to lower new infections caused by non-*S. agalactiae Streptococcus* spp. This combination was also effective against coagulase-negative *Staphylococcus* spp. and *Corynebacterium bovis*. No irritation or chapping of the quarters resulted.

The in vitro germicidal activity of nine commercial teat dips was tested (Larocque et al. 1992). All products tested were found to be effective against *E. coli*, *S. aureus*, and *S. agalactiae*. Chx acetate was found to be only bacteriostatic against *Nocardia*; thus, dips containing this compound should not be used if this organism is present on a farm. The automatic application of an iodine-containing teat dip through the milking machine cluster appeared to be as effective as manual teat dipping in preventing IMI under conditions of artificially high levels of bacterial exposure (Grindal and Priest 1989).

Chlorous acid and chlorine dioxide were seen to reduce IMI caused by *Streptococcus uberis* and *S. aureus* significantly better when used for premilk and postmilk dipping than when used as a postmilking teat dip alone. There were no treatment differences against gram-negative bacteria, coagulase-negative *Staphylococcus* spp., and *C. bovis* (Oliver et al. 1993). These authors warn against assuming all teat dips to be safe and effective as premilking dips. Correct use of a premilk dip requires careful drying of the udder since studies have shown that cleaning-liquid containing bacteria can drain into the teat cups after milk machine attachment (Galton et al. 1986). These bacteria can both increase milk bacterial counts and cause mastitis. In addition, premilk dip liquid runoff may leave chemical residues in milk. In an attempt to avoid these pitfalls, a 0.5% iodophor-containing gel was developed and compared to routine udder preparation and to premilk dipping with a 0.5% iodophor solution. Gel treatment resulted in low bacterial contamination of milk and teat ends, low somatic cell counts, low milk iodine content, and reduced mastitis. In addition, parlor throughput was higher than with standard predip therapy (Ingawa et al. 1992).

DISINFECTANT USAGE IN VETERINARY MEDICINE

Disinfectants are widely used in veterinary medicine as hospital disinfectants on floors, tables, walls, on surgical equipment and other instruments before storage, and for disinfection of animal housing facilities. For effective germicidal activity, manufacturer recommendations regarding contact time, dilution, and useful life of a disinfectant solution should be followed. The best disinfectant for a particular situation will depend on the surface's shape, structure, chemical reactivity, and use as well as on the type of contaminating organisms anticipated. The previous edition of this text chapter discussed disinfection principles in varying veterinary applications (e.g., dairy parlors, stockyards). Although detailed descriptions of guidelines for disinfectant use in all circumstances is beyond the scope of this chapter, it is justified to provide a short discussion of their use in situations involving microbes that cause significant health concerns or that can be easily transmitted.

SALMONELLA. Salmonella species have been estimated to be the most frequent cause of foodborne related hospitalizations and cause illness in an estimated 1.4 million people in the U.S. each year (Mead et al. 1999). These numbers have increased in the recent past, and outbreaks have been linked to contaminated ground beef, dairy products, poultry, and fresh produce fertilized with cattle manure. The origin or mechanism of transfer of the organism is often unknown, but in many cases it is the contaminated carcass, transport container, or cattle manure fertilizer. There is evidence that *Salmonella* can persist despite thorough cleaning and disinfecting procedures (Gradel and Rattenberg, 2003) possibly due to rodents, insects, or lack of hygiene barriers (Gradel et al. 2004).

Glutaraldehyde was found to be the most effective compound in reducing *Salmonella enteritidis* and *S. senftenberg* bacterial load in a study designed to mimic worst-case conditions in disinfecting poultry houses (Gradel et al. 2004). Four types of materials (e.g., concrete, wood) were contaminated with bacteria mixed with several types of organic matter (e.g., feed, egg yolk) and disinfection was attempted at high and low temperatures. Formaldehyde was considered effective even at low temperatures despite reports that a minimum temperature of 16°C is required for activity, whereas a peroxygen compound was found to be least effective except for one material/organic matter combination. This lack of efficacy was attributed to peroxygen compounds inactivation in the presence of organic matter.

In a similar study that investigated disinfection of poultry transport containers, real-world conditions were created by testing five compounds against bacteria growing isolated and in a biofilm. Although halogen compounds and QAC were effective against artificially contaminated surfaces, after the biofilm had matured, only sodium hypochlorite or an iodine-containing disinfectant was able to achieve 100% reduction. In the ultimate test of disinfectant activity in the face of organic matter, sodium carbonate, ammonia, and sodium hydroxide were shown to reduce foodborne pathogen load in cattle manure (Park and Diez-Gonzalez 2003).

Salmonella outbreaks have caused interruptions in services at several veterinary teaching hospitals prompting the search for effective methods of detection, prevention, and disinfection. Environmental contamination (Patterson et al. 2005) or affected individuals (Schott et al. 2001) may have been the initiating events; however, housing of sick and immunocompromised patients as well as incomplete disinfection likely contributed to routine shedding developing into epidemics. Sites and methods of sampling for monitoring for *Salmonella* contamination have been proposed and a high frequency of positive results have been recorded (~50%). However, this high percentage may reflect the fact that the polymerase chain reaction assay used may be measuring only DNA remnants rather than pathogenic bacteria; therefore bacterial culture should remain the definitive test (Alinovi et al. 2003). The ability to decontaminate a veterinary hospital quickly, efficiently, and effectively is paramount to preventing loss of income and public confidence and to ensuring high quality treatment of the veterinary population. Following one outbreak, the hospital was at least partially closed for 3 months (Colorado State, 1996) to allow manual decontamination/disinfection. Recently, mist application of a 4% peroxymonosulfate compound was shown to be an effective method of eliminating artificially induced contamination of an animal holding facility (Patterson et al. 2005).

Disinfectant footbaths have been used as a hygiene barrier to prevent spread of microbes in veterinary hospital environments. Footbath efficacy has been shown to be dependent upon the disinfectant used and the compliance with which it is utilized. In one study, a peroxygen compound was shown to be more effective than a QAC; however, a maximal reduction in contamination of only 75% was observed (Morley et al. 2005). These results suggest that footwear hygiene can be improved through appropriate use of disinfectant footbaths, but it should not be relied on as the only method of controlling the spread of infectious agents.

AVIAN INFLUENZA. The spread of the avian influenza virus (Orthomyxoviridae) among poultry populations and its ability to cause morbidity and mortality in man have become a recently publicized concern. Strain H5N1 is of particular concern because of its ability to mutate rapidly and to acquire genes from viruses infecting other animal species. Studies have demonstrated that isolates from this virus are highly pathogenic and can cause severe disease in humans. Birds that survive infection excrete virus for at least 10 days, orally and in feces, thus facilitating further spread.

As an enveloped virus, the Orthomyxoviridae, including influenza viruses, are very sensitive to most detergents and disinfectants. They are readily inactivated by pH, heating, and drying. Treatment with either 70% alcohol or a commercial disinfectant containing formaldehyde/ QAC for at least 15 minutes resulted in complete loss of viral infectivity of the H7N2 strain (Lu et al. 2003). Other classes of disinfectants considered effective at destroying avian influenza virus include phenolics, oxidizing agents, and dilute acids. However, flu viruses are well-protected from inactivation by organic material, and infectious virus can be recovered from manure for up to 105 days. It is therefore suggested that complete removal of all organic material is part of any effective disinfection procedure. Contaminated litter and manure should be composted or buried to ensure that it does not spread infectious virus.

REFERENCES

Akimitsu N, Hamamoto H, Inoue R, Shoji M, Akamine A, Takemori K, Hamasaki N, and Sekimizu K. 1999. Increase in resistance of methicillin-resistant *Staphylococcus aureus* to b-lactams caused by mutations conferring resistance to benzalkonium chloride, a disinfectant widely used in hospitals. Antimicrob Agents Chemother 43:3042–3043.

Alexander JW, Fisher J, Boyajiani M, Palmquist J, and Morris MJ. 1983. The influence of hair removal methods on wound infections. Arch Surg 118:347–349.

Alinovi CA, Ward MP, Couetil LL, and Wu CC. 2003. Detection of Salmonella organisms and assessment of a protocol for removal of contamination in horse stalls at a veterinary teaching hospital. J Am Vet Med Assoc. 223(1):1640–1644.

Altemeier WA (ed.). 1976. Manual on Control of Infection in Surgical Patients, p. 212. Philadelphia: JP Lippincott.

Amber EI, Henderson RA, Swaim SF, and Gray BW. 1983. A comparison of antimicrobial efficacy and tissue reaction of four antiseptics on canine wounds. Vet Surg 12:63–68.

Antec International website: http://www.antecint.co.uk/, accessed 26 Mar 2006.

Archer HG, Barrett S, Irving S, Middleton KR, and Seal DV. 1990. A controlled model of moist wound healing: comparison between semi-permeable film, antiseptics and sugar paste. J Exp Path 71:155–170.

Ayliffe GAJ, Babb JR, and Bradley CR. 1986. Disinfection of endoscopes. J Hosp Infect 7:296–299.

Baldry MGC. 1983. The bactericidal, fungicidal, and sporicidal properties of hydrogen peroxide and peracetic acid. J Appl Bacteriol 54:417–423.

Bamber A, and Neal TJ. 1999. An assessment of triclosan susceptibility in methicillin-resistant and methicillin-sensitive *Staphylococcus aureus*. J Hosp Infect 41:107–109.

Berk WA, Welch RD, and Brooks BF. 1992. Controversial issues in clinical management of the simple wound. Annal Emerg Med 21:72–80.

Bilbrey SA, Dulisch JL, and Stallings B. 1989. Chemical burns caused by benzalkonium chloride in eight surgical cases. J Am Anim Hosp Assoc 25:31–34.

Bloomfield SF, and Miller EA. 1989. A comparison of hypochlorite and phenolic disinfectants for disinfection of clean and soiled surfaces and blood spillages. J Hosp Infect 13:231–239.

Bramley AJ, and Dodd FH. 1984. Reviews of the progress of dairy science: mastitis control progress and prospects. J Dairy Res 51:481–512.

Broxton P, Woodcock PM, and Gilbert P. 1983. A study of the antibacterial activity of some polyhexamethylene biguanides towards Escherichia coli ATCC 8739. J Appl Bacteriol 54:345–353.

Center for Disease Control (CDC). 1987. Symptoms of irritation associated with exposure to glutaraldehyde. Colorado MMWR 36: 190–191.

Denyer SP, and Stewart GSAB. 1998. Mechanisms of action of disinfectants. Int Biodet Bideg 41:261–268.

Dychdala GR. 1983. Chlorine and chlorine compounds. In Block SS (ed.), Disinfection, Sterilization, and Preservation, 3rd ed, pp. 157–182. Philadelphia: Lea & Febiger.

Fan F, Yan K, Wallis NG, Reed S, Moore TD, Rittenhouse SF, DeWolf WE Jr, Huang J, McDevitt D, Miller WH, Seefeld MA, Newlander KA, Jakas DR, Head MS, and Payne DJ. 2002. Defining and combating the mechanisms of triclosan resistance in clinical isolates of *Staphylococcus aureus*. Antimicrob Agents Chemother 46(11):3343–3347.

Favero MS. 1983. Chemical disinfection of medical and surgical materials. In Block SS (ed.), Disinfection, Sterilization, and Preservation, pp. 469–492. 3rd ed. Philadelphia: Lea & Febiger.

Gale EF, Cundliffe E, Reynolds PE, Richmond MH, and Waring MJ. 1981. Molecular Basis of Antibiotic Action. London: John Wiley & Sons.

Galton DM, Petersson LG, and Merril WG. 1986. Effects of premilking udder preparation practices on bacterial counts in milk and on teats. J Dairy Sci 69:260–266.

Garibaldi RA, Skolnick D, and Lerer T. 1988. The impact of preoperative skin disinfection on preventing intra-operative wound contamination. Infect Control Hosp Epidemiol 9:109–113.

Gilbert P, Allison DB, and McBain AJ. 2002. Biofilms in vitro and in vivo: do singular mechanisms imply cross-resistance? J Appl Mic Sym Suppl 92:98S–110S.

Gradel KO, and Rattenberg E. 2003. A questionnaire-based, retrospective field study of persistence of *Salmonella Enteritidis* and *Salmonella Typhimurium* in Danish broiler houses. Prev Vet Med 56:267–284.

Gradel KO, Sayers AR, and Davies RH. 2004. Surface disinfection tests with *Salmonella* and a putative indicator bacterium, mimicking worst-case scenarios in poultry houses. Poultry Sci 83:1636–1643.

Grindal RJ, and Priest DJ. 1989. Automatic application of teat disinfectant through the milking machine cluster. J Dairy Res 56:579–585.

Guillen J, Bernabeu A, Schapir S, and Villalain J. 2004. Location and orientation of triclosan in phospholipid model membranes. Eur Biophys J 33:448–453.

Heath RJ, and Rock CO. 2000. A triclosan-resistant bacterial enzyme. Nature 406:145–146.

Heath RJ, Rubin JR, Holland DR, Zhang E, Snow ME, and Rock CO. 1999. Mechanism of triclosan inhibition of bacterial fatty acid synthesis. J Bio Chem 274:11110–11114.

Heggers JP, Sazy JA, Stenberg BD, Strock LL, McCauley RL, Herndon DN, and Robson MC. 1991. Bactericidal and wound healing properties of sodium hypochlorite solutions: the 1991 Lindberg Award. J Burn Care Rehabil 12:420–424.

Henderson JD, Leming JT, and Melon-Niksa DB. 1989. Chloramine-T solutions: effect on wound healing in guinea pigs. Arch Phys Med Rehabil 70:628–631.

Hennig GE, Kraus BH, Fister R, King VL, Steckel RR, and Kirker-Head CA. 2001. Comparison of two methods for presurgical disinfection of the equine hoof. Vet Surg 320:336–373.

Huber WG. 1988. Antiseptics and disinfectants. In Booth NH, McDonald LE (eds.), Veterinary Pharmacology and Therapeutics, pp. 765–784. 6th ed. Ames: Iowa State University Press.

Ingawa KH, Adkinson RW, and Hough RH. 1992. Evaluation of a gel teat cleaning and sanitizing compound for premilking hygiene. J Dairy Sci 75:1224–1232.

Kozol RA, Gillies C, and Elgebaly SA. 1988. Effects of sodium hypochlorite (Dakin's solution) on cells of the wound module. Arch Surg 123:420–423.

Kwochka KW, and Kowalski JJ. 1991. Prophylactic efficacy of four antibacterial shampoos against *Staphylococcus intermedius* in dogs. Am J Vet Res 52(1):115–118.

Lambrechts NE, Hurter K, Picard JA, Goldin JP, and Thompson PN. 2004. A prospective comparison between stabilized glutaraldehyde and chlorhexidine gluconate for preoperative skin antisepsis in dogs. Vet Surg 33:636–643.

Larocque L, Malik SS, Landry DA, Presseault S, Sved S, and Matula T. 1992. In vitro germicidal activity of teat dips against *Nocardia asteroides* and other udder pathogens. J Dairy Sci 75:1233–1240.

Larson E. 1987. Draft guidelines for the use of topical antimicrobial agents. (Abstr.) Am J Infec Control 15:25–30.

Larson EL, Eke PI, and Laughon BE. 1986. Efficacy of alcohol based hand rinses under frequent use conditions. Antimicrob Agents Chemother 30:542–544.

Lavelle KJ, Doedus DJ, Kleit SA, and Forney RB. 1975. Iodine absorption in burn patients treated topically with povidone iodine. Clin Pharmacol Ther 17:355–356.

Lee WR, Tobias KM, Bemis DA, and Rohrbach BW. 2004. In vitro efficacy of a polyhexamethylene biguanide-impregnated gauze dressing against bacteria found in veterinary patients. Vet Surg 33:404–411.

Lineweaver W, Howard R, Soucy D, McMorris S, Freeman J, Crain C, Robertson J, and Rumley T. 1985. Topical antimicrobial toxicity. Arch Surg 120:267–270.

Lineweaver W, McMorris S, and Howard R. 1982. Effects of topical disinfectants and antibiotics on human fibroblasts. Surg Forum 33:37–39.

Lowbury EJL. 1951. Contamination of cetrimide and other fluids with *Pseudomonas pyocyanea*. Br J Ind Med 8:22–25.

Lowbury EJL, Lilly HA, and Ayliffe GAJ. 1974. Preoperative disinfection of surgeon's hands: use of alcoholic solutions and effects of gloves on skin flora. Br Med J 4:369–372.

Lowthian P, and Oke S. 1993. Hypertonic saline solution as a disinfectant. Lancet 341:182.

Lu H, Castro AE, Pennick K, Liu J, Yang Q, Dunn P, Weinstock D, and Henzler D. 2003. Survival of avian influenza virus H7N2 in SPF chickens and their environments. Av Dis 47:1015–1021.

Mafu AA, Roy D, Goulet J, Magney P. 1990. Attachment of Listeria monocytogenes to stainless steel, glass, polypropylene, and rubber surfaces after short contact times. J Food Protect 53:742–746.

McHinley KJ, Larson EL, and Leyden JJ. 1988. Composition and density of microflora in the subungual space of the hand. J Clin Microbiol 26:950–953.

McMurry LM, McDermott PF, and Levy SB. 1999. Genetic evidence that InhA of *Mycobacterium smegmatis* is a target for triclosan. Antimicrob Agents Chemother 43:711–713.

McMurry LM, Oethinger M, and Levy SB. 1998. Overexpression of marA, soxS, or acrAB produces resistance to triclosan in laboratory and clinical strains of *Escherichia coli*. FEMS Microbiology Letters 166:305–309.

Mead PS, Slutsker L, Dietz V, McCaig LF, Bresee JS, Shapiro C, Griffin PM, Tauxe RV. 1999. Food-related illness and death in the United States. Emerg Infect Dis 5:607–625.

Mechin L, Dubois-Brissonnet F, Heyd B, and Leveau JY. 1999. Adaptation *Pseudomonas aeruginosa* ATCC 15442 to didecyldimethylammonium bromide induces changes in membrane fatty acid composition and in resistance of cells. J Appl Microbiol 86:859–866.

Mentel R, and Schmidt J. 1973. Investigations on rhinovirus inactivation by hydrogen peroxide. Acta Virol 17:351–354.

Mills PC, Ahlstrom L, Wilson WJ. 2005. Ototoxicity and tolerance assessment of a TrisEDTA and polyhexamethylene biguanide ear flush formulation in dogs. J Vet Pharmacol Therap 28:391–397.

Moken MC, McMurry LM, and Levy SB. 1997. Selection of multiple-antibiotic-resistant (mar) mutants of *Escherichia coli* by using the disinfectant pine oil: roles of the mar and acrAB loci. Antimicrob Agents Chemother 41:2770–2772.

Molinari JA, Campbell MD, and York JJ. 1982. Minimizing potential infections in dental practice. Mich Dent Assoc 64:411–416.

Molinari JA, and Runnel RR. 1991. Role of disinfectants in infection control. Dental Clin North Am 35(2):323–337.

Morley PS, Morris SN, Hyatt DR, Van Metre DC. 2005. Evaluation of the efficacy of disinfectant footbaths as used in veterinary hospitals. J Am Vet Med Assoc 226:2053–2058.

Murray SM, Freiman JS, Vickery K, Lim D, Cossart TE, and Whiteley RK. 1991. Duck hepatitis B virus: a model to assess efficacy of disinfectants against hepadnavirus infectivity. Epidemiol Infect 106:434–443.

Nye RN, and Mallory TB. 1923. A note on the fallacy of using alcohol for the sterilization of surgical instruments. Boston Med Surg J 189:561–563.

Oberg MS, and Lindsey D. 1987. Do not put hydrogen peroxide or povidone-iodine into wounds. Am J Dis Child 141:27–28.

Okusu H, Ma D, and Nikaido H. 1996. AcrAB efflux pump plays a major role in the antibiotic resistance phenotype of *Escherichia coli* multiple-antibiotic-resistance (Mar) mutants. J Bacteriol 178:306–308.

Oliver SP, King SH, Lewis MJ, Torre PM, Matthews KR, and Dowlen HH. 1990. Efficacy of chlorhexidine as a postmilking teat disinfectant for the prevention of bovine mastitis during lactation. J Dairy Sci 73:2230–2235.

Oliver SP, Lewis MJ, Ingle TL, Gillespie BE, and Matthews KR. 1993. Prevention of bovine mastitis by a premilking teat disinfectant containing chlorous acid and chlorine dioxide. J Dairy Sci 76:287–292.

O'Neill J, Hosmer M, Challup RM, Driscoll J, Speck W, and Sprunt K. 1982. Percutaneous absorption potential of chlorhexidine in neonates. Curr Ther Res 31:485–487.

Pankey JW, Eberhart RJ, Cuming AL, Dagget RD, Farnsworth RJ, and McDuff CK. 1984. Update on postmilking antisepsis. J Dairy Sci 67:1336–1353.

Park GW, and Diez-Gonzalez F. 2003. Utilization of carbonate and ammonia-based treatments to eliminate *Exherichia coli* O157:H7 and

Salmonella typhimurium DT104 from cattle manure. J Appl Micr 94:675–685.

Patterson G, Morley PS, Blehm KD, Lee DE, and Dunowska M. 2005. Efficacy of directed misting application of a peroxygen disinfectant for environmental decontamination of a veterinary hospital. J Am Vet Med Assoc 227(4):597–602.

Peacock EE Jr. 1984. Wound Repair, pp. 141–186. 3rd ed. Philadelphia: WB Saunders Co.

Pepper RE. 1980. Comparison of the activities and stabilities of alkaline glutaraldehyde sterilizing solutions. Infect Contr 1:90–92.

Pretsch J, and Meakins JL. 1976. Complications of povidone-iodine absorption in topically treated burn patients. Lancet 1:280–282.

Randall LP, Clouting CS, Gradel KO, Clifton-Hadley FA, Davies RD, Woodward MJ. 2005. Farm disinfectants select for cyclohaxane resistance, a marker of multiple antibiotic resistance, in *Escherichia coli*. J Appl Microbiol 98:556–563.

Redding WR, and Booth LC. 1991. Effects of chlorhexidine gluconate and chlorous acid-chlorine dioxide on equine fibroblasts and *Staphylococcus aureus*. Vet Surg 20(5):306–310.

Reybrouk G. 1985. The bactericidal activity of aqueous disinfectants applied on living tissues. Pharm Weekbl (Sci) 7:100–103.

Rodheaver G, Bellamy W, Kody M, Spatafora G, Fitton L, Leyden K, and Edlich R. 1982. Bacterial activity and toxicity of iodine-containing solutions in wounds. Arch Surg 117:181–186.

Russell AD. 1986. Chlorhexidine: antibacterial action and bacterial resistance. Infection 14:212–215.

———. 2000. Do biocides select for antibiotic resistance? J Pharm Pharmacol 52:227–233.

Rutala WA. 1990. APIC guideline for selection and use of disinfectants. Am J Inf Control 18(2):99–117.

Rycroft AN, and McLay C. 1991. Disinfectants in the control of small animal ringworm due to *Microsporum canis*. Vet Rec 129:239–241.

Schaeffer AJ, Jones JM, and Amundsen SK. 1980. Bactericidal effect of hydrogen peroxide on urinary tract pathogens. Appl Environ Microbiol 40:337–340.

Scheider W, Ahuja S, and Klebe I. 1976. Clinical and bacteriological studies of the polyvinylpyrrolidone-iodine complex. In World Congress on Antisepsis, pp. 79–81. New York: PH Publishing Co.

Schott HC 2nd, Ewart SL, Walker RD, Dwyer RM, Dietrich S, Eberhart SW, Kusey J, Stick JA, and Derksen FJ. 2001. An outbreak of salmonellosis among horses at a veterinary teaching hospital. J Am Vet Med Assoc 218(7):1152–9.

Scott EM, and Gorman SP. 1983. Sterilization with glutaraldehyde. In Block SS (ed.), Disinfection, Sterilization, and Preservation, pp. 65–68. 3rd ed. Philadelphia: Lea & Febiger.

Smeak DO, and Olmstead ML. 1984. Infections in clean wounds: the roles of the surgeon, environment, and the host. Comp Contin Educ Pract Vet 6:629–634.

Smith MS, Williams DE, and Worley SD. 1990. Potential uses of combined halogen disinfectants in poultry processing. Poultry Sci 69:1590–1594.

Spaulding EH. 1968. Chemical disinfection of medical and surgical materials. In Lawrence CA, Block SS (eds.), Disinfection, Sterilization, and Preservation, pp. 517–531. Philadelphia: Lea & Febiger.

Stevenson TR, Thacker JG, and Rodheaver GT. 1976. Cleansing the traumatic wound by high pressure irrigation. J Am Col Emer Phys 141:357–362.

Stewart K. 1984. Equine intensive care: preoperative, intraoperative, and postoperative procedures. Vet Tech 5:177–180.

Stewart MJ, Parikh S, Xiao G, Tonge PJ, and Kisker C. 1999. Structural bases and mechanism of enoyl reductase inhibition by triclosan. J Mol Biol 290:859–865.

Stonehill AA, Krop S, and Borick PM. 1963. Buffered glutaraldehyde: a new chemical sterilizing solution. Am J Hosp Pharm 20:458–465.

Suller MT, and Russell AD. 1999. Antibiotic and biocide resistance in methicillin-resistant *Staphylococcus aureus* and vancomycin-resistant enterococcus. J Hosp Infect 43:281–291.

———. 2000. Triclosan and antibiotic resistance in *Staphylococcus aureus*. J Antimicrob Chemother 46:11–18.

Swaim SF, and Lee AH. 1987. Topical wound medications: a review. JAVMA 190(12):1588–1592.

Swaim SF, Riddell KP, Geiger MS, Hathcock TL, and McHuire JA. 1991. Evaluation of surgical scrub and antiseptic solutions for surgical preparation of canine paws. JAVMA 198(11):1941–1945.

Swaim SF, and Wihalf D. 1985. The physics, physiology, and chemistry of bandaging open wounds. Comp Cont Educ Pract Vet 7(2):146–156.

Tattawasart U, Maillard J-Y, Furr JR, and Russell AD. 1999. Development of resistance to chlorhexidine diacetate and cetylpyridinium chloride in *Pseudomonas stutzeri* and changes in antibiotic susceptibility. J Hosp Infect 42:219–229.

Turner FJ. 1983. Hydrogen peroxide and other oxidant disinfectants. In Block SS (ed.), Disinfection, Sterilization, and Preservation, pp. 240–250. 3rd ed. Philadelphia: Lea & Febiger.

Tvedten HW, and Till GO. 1985. Effect of povidone, povidone-iodine and iodide on locomotion (in vitro) of neutrophils from people, rats, dogs and rabbits. Am J Vet Res 46:1797–1800.

Viljanto J. 1980. Disinfection of surgical wounds without inhibition of normal healing. Arch Surg 115:253–256.

Wang H, Dzink-Fox JL, Chen M, and Levy SB. 2001. Genetic characterization of high-level fluoroquinolone resistant clinical *Escherichia coli* strains from China: role for acrR mutations. Antimicrob Agents Chemother 45:1515–1521.

Weber GR. 1950. Effect of concentration and reaction (pH) on germicidal activity of chloramine T. Public Health Rep 65:503–512.

Zukin DD, and Simon RR. 1987. Emergency Wound Care: Principles and Practice, pp. 30–31. Rockville, Md.: Aspen Publishers.

CHAPTER

33

SULFONAMIDES AND POTENTIATED SULFONAMIDES

MARK G. PAPICH AND JIM E. RIVIERE

The sulfonamides are one of the oldest groups of antimicrobial compounds still in use today. Sulfanilamide, an amide of sulfanilic acid, was the first sulfonamide used clinically. It was derived from the azo dye Prontosil. Other sulfonamides also share the same structure. Sulfonamides have been in clinical use for 50 years, but resistance is common when these drugs are used alone (without addition of trimethoprim or ormetoprim). Most of the use of sulfonamides in dogs, cats, horses, and some exotic and zoo animals rely on the addition of trimethoprim (trimethoprim-sulfonamide) or ormetoprim (e.g., ormetoprim-sulfadimethoxine) to broaden the spectrum and increase antibacterial activity against bacteria that would have been resistant to either drug used alone. Technically, trimethoprim and ormetoprim are chemically called *diaminopyrimidines,* but they will be referred to by their respective names in this chapter. In companion animals, trimethoprim-sulfonamide combinations have all but replaced single or combination sulfonamide (triple-sulfas) treatment regimens. Sulfonamide administration is restricted in food animals, particularly dairy cattle, because of a concern for drug residues. Previous editions of this text should be consulted for a review of this extensive historical database.

PHARMACOLOGY OF SULFONAMIDES

All sulfonamides are derivatives of sulfanilamide (structurally similar to para-aminobenzoic acid), which was, in the 1940s, the first sulfonamide discovered to have antimicrobial activity (see Fig. 33.1) . Note that in some countries and certain formularies outside the United States, different spellings have been used for sulfonamides (e.g., *sulphamethoxazole* for sulfamethoxazole; *sulphadiazine* for sulfadiazine; *sulphadimethoxine* for sulfadimethoxine, and so forth). This textbook uses the United States Adopted Names (USAN) and United States Pharmacopeia (USP) official names throughout.

Many structural derivatives of sulfanilamide with differing pharmacokinetic and antimicrobial spectrums have been used in veterinary medicine to treat microbial infections of the respiratory, urinary, gastrointestinal, and central nervous systems. Susceptible organisms include many bacteria, coccidia, chlamydia, and protozoal organisms, including *Toxoplasma* spp. Treatment of protozoa infections is discussed in more detail in Chapter 43 of this book.

Name	Chemical name (Empirical formula) [Molecular weight]	Chemical structure
Sulfadiazine	4-amino-*N*-2-pyrimidinylbenzenesulfonamide ($C_{10}H_{10}N_4O_2S$) [250.28]	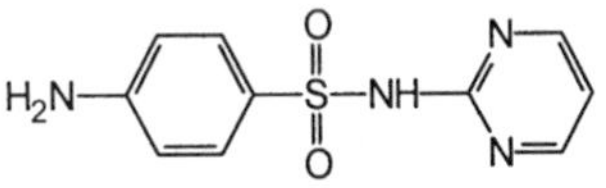
Sulfadimethoxine	4-amino-*N*-(2,6-dimethoxy-4-pyrimidinyl)-benzenesulfonamide ($C_{12}H_{14}N_4O_4S$) [310.33]	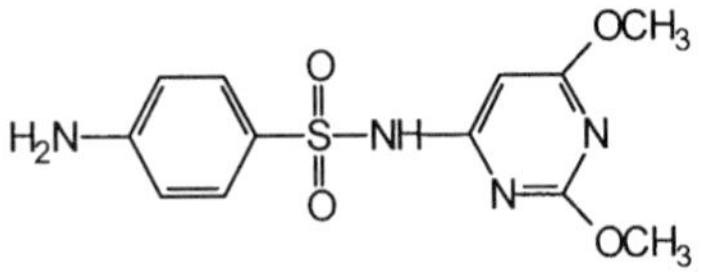
Sulfadoxine	4-amino-*N*-(5,6-dimethoxy-4-pyrimidinyl)-benzenesulfonamide ($C_{12}H_{14}N_4O_4S$) [310.34]	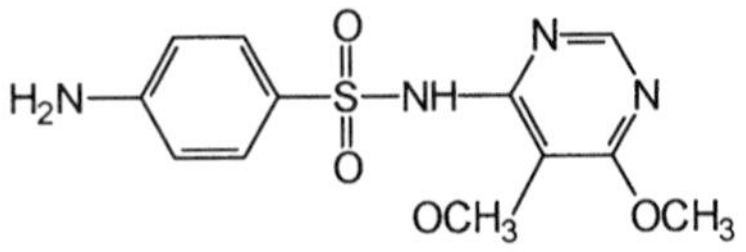
Sulfaguanidine	4-amino-*N*-(aminoiminomethyl)-benzenesulfonamide ($C_7H_{10}N_4O_2S$) [214.24]	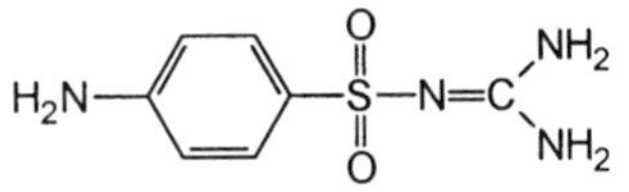
Sulfamethazine	4-amino-*N*-(4,6-dimethyl-2-pyrimidinyl)-benzenesulfonamide ($C_{12}H_{14}N_4O_2S$) [278.32]	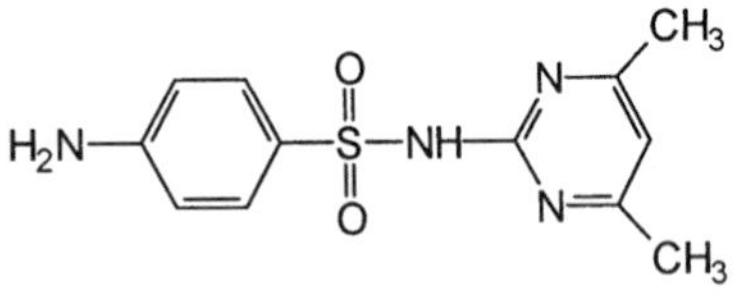
Sulfamethoxazole	4-amino-*N*-(5-methyl-3-isoxazolyl)-benzenesulfonamide ($C_{10}H_{11}N_3O_3S$) [253.31]	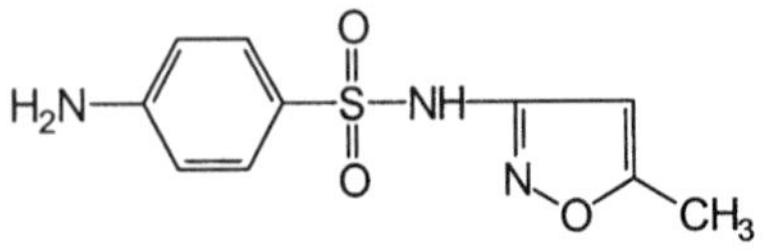
Sulfaquinoxaline	4-amino-*N*-2-quinoxalinyl-benzenesulfonamide ($C_{14}H_{12}N_4O_2S$) [300.33]	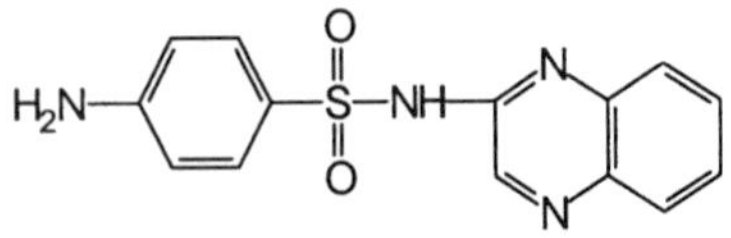
Sulfanitran	4′-[(*p*-nitrophenyl)sulfamoyl]acetanilide ($C_{14}H_{13}N_3O_5S$) [335.34]	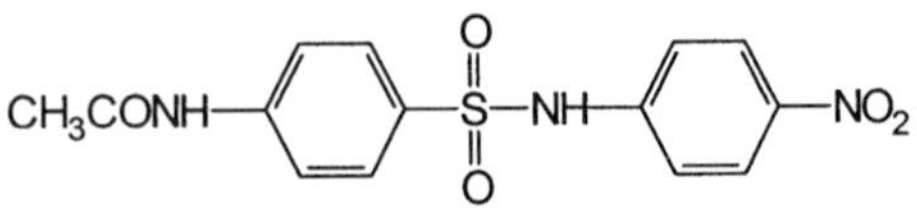

FIG. 33.1 Sulfonamides.

Sulfonamides are white crystalline powders that are weak organic acids, with solubility in water that varies among the specific drugs (ranging from slightly soluble to practically insoluble), and have a wide range of pK_a values, as shown in Table 33.1. The pK_a values of these compounds and their ionization are important because—among other properties—the antibacterial activity, solubility, and protein binding has been associated with the pK_a value (Mengelers et al. 1997). Drugs with high pK_a are less soluble and exhibit lower protein binding; drugs with low pK_a tend to have higher protein binding. The sulfonamides all share a similar structure, which contains a $-SO_2$ group linked to a benzene ring, and a para NH_2- group on N-4. An attached pyrimidine ring may contain zero, one, or two methyl groups (sulfamethazine, sulfamerazine, and sulfadiazine, respectively), which may undergo hydroxylation during metabolism. The other major site of metabolism is acetylation of the para-NH_2, which can vary among species. Acetylated forms of the drug tend to be less soluble.

The sulfonamides exhibit large variation in the extent to which they bind to plasma proteins. In general, the plasma protein binding is higher than other antimicrobials (>70% in many animals), and ranges from 90% (sulfadimethoxine in some species) to as low as 50% (sulfamethazine in some species). Sulfonamides are more soluble in alkaline than in neutral or acidic pHs; solubility is enhanced when the sulfonamides are formulated as sodium salts or when in solution in more alkaline environments. Some sulfonamide solutions have pHs between 9 and 10, prohibiting extravascular use. Sulfonamides in general are relatively insoluble in water and may become particularly insoluble and crystallize in renal tubules when urine pH is low, especially when high doses are administered, or animals are dehydrated or acidemic. To minimize crystalluria and obtain high blood or urine levels of the sulfonamides, they are often given in combination with other sulfonamides. Each sulfonamide in a mixture of sulfonamides exhibits its own solubility in solution (law of independent solubility); i.e., sulfonamides do not significantly affect the solubility of each other, which has important clinical considerations in the excretion of parent compound and any metabolites. However, the antimicrobial effect is additive; thus the use of "triple-sulfas" (three sulfonamides formulated in solution together) allows increased efficacy without a significant increased risk of adverse effects (Bevill 1988).

TABLE 33.1 Physical chemistry properties of sulfonamides, trimethoprim, and ormetoprim

Drug	pK_a	Log P
Sulfanilamide	10.1	−0.072
Sulfadimidine	7.7	0.691
Sulfamerazine	7.0	0.812
Sulfadiazine	6.4, 6.5, 6.6	0.631
Sulfadimethoxine	6.3, 6.2	1.648
Sulfachlorpyridazine	6.1, 6.0	1.305
Sulfamethoxazole	5.9, 6.0	1.396
Sulfisoxazole	5.0, 4.9	2.259
Sulfadoxine	6.1	1.271
Trimethoprim	7.12, 7.6	0.91
Ormetoprim	na	1.23

The pK_a is the dissociation rate constant. For some drugs, more than one pK_a value is listed because of variation among sources. For pK_a values, all sulfonamides are weak acids; trimethoprim and ormetoprim are weak bases. Log P is the logarithm of the partition coefficient between an organic solvent (oil) and water. The higher the Log P, the more lipophilic is the drug. Some values are from Mengelers et al. (1997) and van Duijkeren et al. (1994a).

MECHANISM OF ACTION. Sulfonamides rely on the requirement of susceptible organisms to synthesize folic acid as a precursor of other important molecular molecules in the cell. Sulfonamides act as false substrates in the synthesis of folic acid. Trimethoprim and ormetoprim (diaminopyrimidines, discussed later in this chapter) produce a synergistic effect when used together by inhibiting the enzyme dihydrofolate reductase.

Folic acid metabolism is presented in Figure 33.2. Para-aminobenzoic acid (PABA), pteridines, glutamic acid, and the enzyme dihydropterate synthase interact to form dihydropteroic acid, the immediate precursor to dihydrofolic acid. Dihydropteroic acid is enzymatically converted to dihydrofolic acid by dihydrofolate synthase, followed by another enzymatic conversion of dihydrofolic acid to tetrahydrofolic acid (THFA) via dihydrofolate reductase (DHFR). The combination of sulfonamides and trimethoprim inhibits formation of tetrahydrofolic acid at two steps. This action is synergistic. Tetrahydrofolate is a coenzyme in a number of complex enzymatic reactions and also is a coenzyme in the synthesis of thymidylic acid (a nucleotide), which is a building block of DNA. Trimethoprim and sulfonamides are bacteriostatic by themselves; together, they can be bactericidal. Bacteria are more susceptible to this combination than to either drug when tested alone (White et al. 1981).

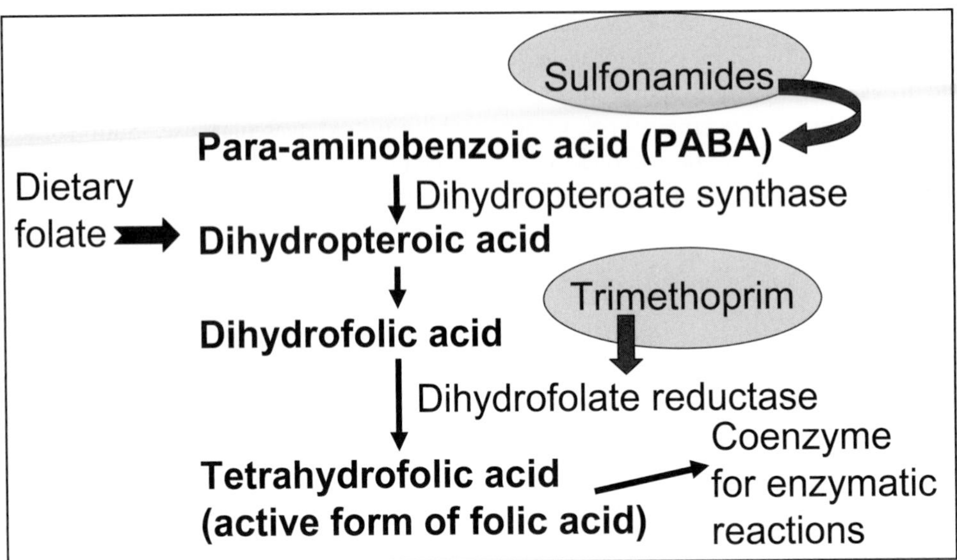

FIG. 33.2 Simplified pathway for the action of trimethoprim-sulfonamide combinations. Sulfonamides provide a false substrate for para-aminobenzoic acid (PABA) inhibiting the synthesis to dihydropteroic acid, a precursor for synthesis to dihydro- and tetrahydrofolic acid. Trimethoprim inhibits the enzyme dihydrofolate reductase, an enzyme critical to the synthesis of tetrahydrofolic acid.

Trimethoprim-sulfonamides are formulated in a ratio of 1:5 (trimethoprim:sulfonamide). In the animal, it is usually cited that the optimum ratio to produce antibacterial activity is 1:20 (Bushby 1980; van Duijkeren et al. 1994b). However, this ratio is often much lower in animals because the trimethoprim component is excreted faster in animals than the sulfonamide. Nevertheless, most reviews on this subject suggest that the optimum ratio may actually be much wider than the value of 1:20 cited in human medical references.

Sulfonamide action is dependent on the chemical similarity with PABA. Therefore, sulfonamides act as a false substrate in this reaction and synthesis of THFA is inhibited. Folic acid synthesis microorganisms are more selectively inhibited than animal cells. The sulfonamides are relatively safe to mammalian cells because mammals utilize dietary folate for the synthesis of dihydrofolic acid, and they do not require PABA. The enzyme dihydrofolate reductase of bacteria has a much higher affinity (50,000- to 60,000-fold, and in some references as high as 100,000-fold) for trimethoprim than mammalian dihydrofolate reductase.

The mechanism of action of sulfonamides does not entirely explain the activity against protozoa. Sulfonamides may inhibit protozoal dihydrofolate synthetase. Protozoal dihydrofolate reductase also is susceptible to the action of trimethoprim, which may explain some of the effect to support the use of these drugs for protozoal infections.

CLINICAL USES AND MICROBIAL SUSCEPTIBILITY. The spectrum of activity for the sulfonamides is broad, affecting gram-positive, gram-negative, and many protozoal organisms. The action is bacteriostatic rather than bactericidal. Sulfonamides have been used clinically for approximately 50 years and many organisms once susceptible to the sulfonamides are now resistant. To increase the activity, most of the sulfonamides used in clinical practice are combinations with either trimethoprim or ormetoprim (diaminopyrimidines). These combinations (referred to in this chapter as *trimethoprim-sulfonamides,* but also referred to in clinical practice as *trimethoprim-sulfa* or simply abbreviated as *TMP/SU*) have increased the activity.

However, in livestock, single or combination sulfonamide therapy is common in food-animal medicine. In the United States, there are no approved formulations of trimethoprim-sulfonamides available for food animals, but trimethoprim-sulfadoxine is available in some countries.

Table 33.2 illustrates the general susceptibility/resistance patterns of most sulfonamides, trimethoprim, and

TABLE 33.2 Comparative activity of sulfonamides, trimethoprim, and trimethoprim-sulfamethoxazole against selected microorganisms

Organism	Sulfonamide[a]	Trimethoprim	Trimethoprim-sulfamethoxazole[b]
A. pyogenes	30	10	0.15
C. pseudotuberculosis	NA	NA	≤0.5
C. renale	>50	NA	NA
E. rhusiopathiae	10	0.15	0.05
L. monocytogenes	10	0.06	0.01
N. asteroides	128	128	8/160
R. equi	>100	50	32/608
S. aureus	30	1.5	0.2
S. agalactia	30	0.5	0.05
S. dysgalactia	>250	3.1	0.05
S. uberis	>100	3	0.5
β-hemolytic streptococci	>100	10	1.5
C. perfringens	16	50	NA
Actinobacillus spp.	64	NA	≤0.05
A. pleuropneumonia	≥100	2	8
B. bronchiseptica	400	NA	≤0.05
B. abortus	15	3	0.05
B. canis	1.6	NA	NA
C. jejuni	≥256	≥512	≥512
E. coli	≥128	1	≤0.5
H. somnus	≥100	NA	NA
K. pneumoniae	>100	3.1	≤0.5
M. bovis	>60	>75	<0.15
P. multocida	>128	3.1	NA
Proteus spp.	>1000	6.3	≤0.5
P. aeruginosa	>1000	1000	100
Salmonella spp.	128	1000	100
T. equigenitalis	>100	3	0.5
Y. enterocolitica	>128	1	8

Source: Adapted from Prescott and Baggot 1993.

[a]The sulfonamide in most instances was sulfadimethoxine.

[b]Single values refer to trimethoprim concentration; second figure refers to sulfamethoxazole. Trimethoprim:sulfamethoxazole ratio is usually 1 : 20.

Note: Concentrations are MIC_{90}s in μg/mL. MIC_{90} = the minimum inhibitory concentration that inhibits 90% of the microbes.

trimethoprim-sulfamethoxazole combinations against the most commonly encountered veterinary pathogens. The in vitro susceptibility patterns of many pathogens (van Duijkeren et al. 1994b) and more specifically *Salmonella* spp. (van Duijkeren et al. 1994a), which affect the horse, have also been recently reported.

The use of sulfonamides alone has been restricted to respiratory infections, urinary tract and soft tissue infections, and intestinal infections (intestinal protozoa). Susceptible organisms include *Arcanobacterium, Bacillus* spp., *E. rhusiopathiae, L. monocytogenes, Streptococcus* spp., *Chlamydia* spp., and protozoa (coccidia and *Pneumocystis carinii*).

When less sensitive organisms are encountered, the activity can be increased with the addition of trimethoprim (or ormetoprim). The following organisms are usually susceptible: *Pasteurella* spp., *Proteus* spp., *Salmonella* spp, *Histophilus* (formerly *Hemophilus*), the protozoa *Toxoplasma,* and coccidia. Other bacteria that may be susceptible, but for which resistance can develop include *Staphylococcus* spp., *Corynebacterium,* anaerobes (see below), *Nocardia* asteroides, *Klebsiella* indole-positive *Proteus, Enterobacter, E. coli,* and *Streptococcus* spp.

The organisms that are consistently resistant to trimethoprim-sulfonamide combinations include: *Pseudomonas* spp., *Enterococcus* sp., and *Bacteriodes.*

The activity of trimethoprim-sulfonamides against anaerobic bacteria can be variable. When measured in vitro, trimethoprim-sulfonamides have good activity against anaerobic bacteria (Indiveri and Hirsh 1986), but clinical results are not as good (Dow 1988) because thymidine and PABA (inhibitors of trimethoprim-sulfonamide activity) may be present in anaerobic infections.

Trimethoprim-sulfonamides have been used to treat infections caused by protozoa (including *Toxoplasma gondii*) and intestinal coccidia. Trimethoprim-sulfonamide combinations have also been used to treat Equine Protozoal Myeloencephalitis (EPM) caused by *Sarcocystis neurona*. (See also pyrimethamine for treating EPM in a later section.)

INTERACTIONS AFFECTING ANTIMICROBIAL ACTIVITY. As mentioned above, the study by Indiveri and Hirsh (1986), suggested that in some tissue environments, inhibitors of trimethoprim-sulfonamide activity—thymidine and PABA present in infected tissue—may interfere with activity. This has been demonstrated in tissue cages in horses. Ensink et al. (2005) showed an inability to eliminate the infection in an infected environment, despite in vitro sensitivity. They cited inhibitors—such as PABA and thymidine—present in abscessed and infected tissues that may inhibit the effects of these drugs. In another study in which trimethoprim-sulfadoxine was administered to cattle with infected tissue cages (Greko et al. 2002) it was shown that high levels of thymidine in the tissue cage fluid inhibited trimethoprim and compromised the ability to eradicate the infection.

SUSCEPTIBILITY TESTING. For susceptibility testing, trimethoprim-sulfamethoxazole may be used, even when trimethoprim-sulfadiazine is used for therapy (CLSI, 2007). In addition to in vivo interactions caused by PABA and thymidine present in tissues, this also is an issue when performing susceptibility tests. The CLSI susceptibility testing standards state that Mueller-Hinton agar containing excessive amounts of thymidine or thymine can reverse the inhibitory effect of sulfonamides and of trimethoprim, which may result in false-resistant reports (CLSI 2007). Susceptibility testing agar that is as thymidine-free as possible should be obtained.

DRUG RESISTANCE. Resistance by many bacterial and protozoal organisms has become widespread due to the extensive use of sulfonamides over many years. Resistance occurs via chromosomal and plasmid-mediated mechanisms. Chromosomal resistance tends to occur slowly and confers resistance via impaired drug penetration into the microbial cell, producing an insensitive dihydropteroate enzyme and an increased production of PABA. Plasmid-mediated resistance, the most commonly encountered form of sulfonamide resistance, occurs quickly and manifests itself via the impaired drug penetration mechanism in addition to producing sulfonamide-resistant dihydropteroate synthase enzymes. If an organism becomes resistant to one sulfonamide, it is generally resistant to all other sulfonamides.

Resistance to trimethoprim occurs via overproduction of the dihydrofolate reductase enzyme or synthesis of an enzyme that resists binding of the drug.

PHARMACOKINETICS OF SULFONAMIDES

Pharmacokinetics of sulfonamides that are used in veterinary medicine are listed in Tables 33.3, 33.4, 33.5, and 33.6.

ORAL ABSORPTION. Sulfonamides can be rapidly absorbed from the gastrointestinal tract when administered orally. In dogs, absorption is excellent and not affected by feeding (Sigel et al. 1981). There has been considerable interest in the oral absorption of trimethoprim-sulfonamide combinations in horses and the effect of feeding. The observation has been made that when administered to a horse that has not been fed, rapid absorption occurs. Oral absorption in horses is not as complete as for dogs or people, but is high enough for oral administration to be effective in horses. The fraction absorbed for trimethoprim was reported to be 67%, and for sulfadiazine 58%, but for both components the variability was high (van Duijkeren et al. 1994c). When administered to horses that have been fed or when it is added to the horses' concentrate, a delayed and biphasic absorption is observed (van Duijkeren et al. 2002, 1995). For example, when trimethoprim sulfachlorpyridazine was administered to horses, oral absorption appeared to be delayed, with the first peak appearing 1 hour after dosing and the second appearing 8–10 hours postdosing. Dual absorption peaks were not found after nasogastric

TABLE 33.3 Some pharmacokinetic parameters of sulfamethazine (sulfadimidine) in animals

Species	Dose (mg/kg)	Route	V_d (L/kg)	$t_{1/2}$ (hr)	Clearance (mL/hr/kg)	Reference
Cattle	107	IV	0.346	NR	NR	Bevill et al. 1977a
Cattle (male)	200	IV	0.37	5.82	45	Witcamp et al. 1992
Cattle (female)	200	IV	0.24	3.64	54	Witcamp et al. 1992
Calves (62–70 days old)	10	IV	NR	5.2	NR	Nouws et al. 1988c
Calves (68–76 days old)	100	IV	NR	5.7	NR	Nouws et al. 1988c
Cows (4–5 yr old)	10	IV	NR	4	NR	Nouws et al. 1988c
Cows (3–5 yr old)	100	IV	NR	5.9	NR	Nouws et al. 1988c
Cows (5–6 yr old)	200	IV	NR	5.5	NR	Nouws et al. 1988c
Pigs (9 wk old)	50	IV	0.51	16	21	Sweeney et al. 1993
Pigs (10 wk old)	20	IV	0.604	10	42	Nouws et al. 1989a
Pigs (10 wk old, given in drench)	20	PO	NR	11.9	NR	Nouws et al. 1989a
Pigs (10 wk old, given in medicated feed)	20	PO	NR	16.6	NR	Nouws et al. 1989a
Pigs (male, 18–32 kg)	20	IV	0.55	12.4	25	Nouws et al. 1989a
Gilts (12–13 wk old)	107.5	IA	0.493	15.61	NR	Duffee et al. 1984
Barrows (12–13 wk old)	107.5	IA	0.614	17.7	NR	Duffee et al. 1984
Boars (12–13 wk old)	107.5	IA	0.542	16.63	NR	Duffee et al. 1984
Pigs (normal castrated males and intact females)	50	IV	0.50	15	23	Yuan et al. 1997
Pigs (castrated males and intact females infected with *S. suum*)	50	IV	0.52	20	17	Yuan et al. 1997
Goat	100	IV	0.316	2.77	81	Elsheikh et al. 1991
Goats (adult and fed)	100	IV	0.9	4.75	135.6	Abdullah and Baggot 1988
Goats (adult and fasted)	100	IV	0.897	7.03	69.6	Abdullah and Baggot 1988
Goats (adult male)	20	IV	0.28	8.7	20	Witcamp et al. 1992
Goats (adult female)	20	IV	0.18	2.13	70	Witcamp et al. 1992
Goats (12 wk old)	100	IV	0.43	1.97	134	Nouws et al. 1989b
Goats (18 wk old)	100	IV	0.507	2.56	106	Nouws et al. 1989b
Sheep	100	IV	0.297	4.72	44.6	Elsheikh et al. 1991
Sheep (male)	100	IV	0.4	4.5	90	Srivastava and Rampal 1990
Ewes	100	IV	0.474	9.51	35.07	Youssef et al. 1981
Ewes (dosed in summer months)	100	IV	0.37	3.64	63	Nawaz and Nawaz 1983
Ewes (dosed in winter months)	100	IV	0.49	3.92	85	Nawaz and Nawaz 1983
Sheep (ewes and rams)	100	IV	0.41	10.8	41	Bulgin et al. 1991
Sheep (ewes and rams)	100	PO	NR	4.3	NR	Bulgin et al. 1991
Sheep (ewes and rams)	391	PO	NR	14.3	NR	Bulgin et al. 1991
Sheep (ewes and rams)	100	IV	0.37	3.64	NR	Bulgin et al. 1991
Sheep (ewes and rams)	107.5	IV	0.293	5.87	NR	Bulgin et al. 1991
Sheep (ewes and rams)	107.5	IV	0.327	7.09	NR	Bulgin et al. 1991
Ponies (breed unknown)	160	IV	0.63	11.4	42.1	Wilson et al. 1989
Ponies (Shetland)	20	IV	0.33	5.4	55.2	Nouws et al. 1987
Mare (2 yr old)	20	IV	0.47	5	65	Nouws et al. 1985a
Mare (2 yr old)	200	IV	0.56	6	67	Nouws et al. 1985a
Mare (22 yr old)	20	IV	0.38	9.5	28	Nouws et al. 1985a
Mare (22 yr old)	200	IV	0.36	14.6	27	Nouws et al. 1985a
Stallion (1.5 yr old)	20	IV	0.44	9.5	32	Nouws et al. 1985a
Stallion (1.5 yr old)	200	IV	0.65	11	41	Nouws et al. 1985a
Dogs (normal)	100	IV	0.628	16.2	22.4	Riffat et al. 1982
Dogs (febrile)	100	IV	0.495	16.7	20.2	Riffat et al. 1982
Rabbits (male)	35	IV	0.42	0.4	73.6	Witcamp et al. 1992
Rabbits (female)	35	IV	0.23	0.39	40.8	Witcamp et al. 1992
Carp (10°C)	100	IV	1.15	50.3	16.14	van Ginneken et al. 1991
Carp (20°C)	100	IV	0.9	25.6	24.66	van Ginneken et al. 1991
Rainbow trout (10°C)	100	IV	1.2	20.6	41.1	van Ginneken et al. 1991
Rainbow trout (20°C)	100	IV	0.83	14.7	39.9	van Ginneken et al. 1991
Camel	50	IV	0.73	13.2	40	Younan et al. 1989
Camel	100	IV	0.394	7.36	40.9	Elsheikh et al. 1991
Buffalo (female)	200	IV	1.23	12.36	193.2	Singh et al. 1988

Note: NR = not reported; IV = intravenously; IA = intra-arterially; PO = orally.

TABLE 33.4 Some pharmacokinetic parameters of sulfadiazine in animals

Species	Dose (mg/kg)	Route	V_d (L/kg)	$t_{1/2}$ (hr)	Clearance (mL/hr/kg)	Reference
Pigs	25/5[a]	PO	NR	3.1–4.31	NR	Soli et al. 1990
Pigs	20	IV	0.54	4.0[b]	140	Nielsen and Gyrd-Hansen 1994
Pigs (fed)	40	PO	NR	11.5[b]	NR	Nielsen and Gyrd-Hansen 1994
Pigs (fasted)	40	PO	NR	8.1[b]	NR	Nielsen and Gyrd-Hansen 1994
Carp (10°C)	100/20[a]	IV	0.53	47.1	7.9	Nouws et al. 1993
Carp (20°C)	100/20[a]	IV	0.60	33	12.2	Nouws et al. 1993
Ewes	100	IV	0.39	37.15	38.75	Youssef et al. 1981
Dogs	100/20[a]	PO	NR	9.84	NR	Sigel et al. 1981
Calves (milk diet, 7 wk)	25/5[a]	SC	NR	3.4	NR	Shoaf et al. 1987
Calves (milk diet, 13 wk)	25/5[a]	SC	SC	3.4	NR	Shoaf et al. 1987
Calves (grain diet, 7 wk)	25/5[a]	SC	NR	4.4	NR	Shoaf et al. 1987
Calves (grain diet, 13 wk)	25/5[a]	SC	NR	3.6	NR	Shoaf et al. 1987
Calves (8–20 days)	20	IV	NR	6.2	NR	Nouws et al. 1988c
Calves (0.5 yr)	100	IV	NR	7	NR	Nouws et al. 1988c
Cattle (5 yr)	10	IV	NR	4.1	NR	Nouws et al. 1988c
Calves (male, 1 day)	25/5[a]	IV	0.72	5.78	5.8	Shoaf et al. 1989
Calves (male, 7 days)	25/5[a]	IV	0.67	4.4	102	Shoaf et al. 1989
Calves (male, 42 days)	25/5[a]	IV	0.59	3.6	112.8	Shoaf et al. 1989
Calves (7 days, with synovitis)	25/5[a]	IV	28.7	24.44	102	Shoaf et al. 1986

Note: NR = not reported; IV = intravenously; PO = orally; SC = subcutaneously.
[a]Sulfadiazine-trimethoprim dose.
[b]Reported as mean residence time (MRT).

TABLE 33.5 Some pharmacokinetic parameters of trimethoprim in animals

Species	Dose[a] (mg/kg)	Route	V_d (L/kg)	$t_{1/2}$ (hr)	Clearance (mL/hr/kg)	Reference
Cows	8/40	IV	NR	1.18	NR	Davitiyananda and Rasmussen 1974
Pigs	4	IV	1.8	3.3[b]	0.55	Nielsen and Gyrd-Hansen 1994
Pigs (fed)	8	PO	NR	10.6[b]	NR	Nielsen and Gyrd-Hansen 1994
Pigs (fasted)	8	PO	NR	6.5[b]	NR	Nielsen and Gyrd-Hansen 1994
Calves (male, 1 day old)	5/25	IV	1.67	8.4	2.8	Shoaf et al. 1989
Calves (male, 7 days old)	5/25	IV	2.23	2.11	2.0	Shoaf et al. 1989
Calves (male, 42 days old)	5/25	IV	2.36	0.9	28.9	Shoaf et al. 1989
Calves (7 wk old, milk diet)	5/25	SC	NR	3.4	126.0	Shoaf et al. 1987
Calves (13 wk old, milk diet)	5/25	SC	NR	3.4	124.8	Shoaf et al. 1987
Calves (7 wk old, grain diet)	5/25	SC	SC	4.4	105.6	Shoaf et al. 1987
Calves (13 wk old, grain diet)	5/25	SC	NR	3.6	112.2	Shoaf et al. 1987
Calves (7 days old)	5/25	IV	28.72	4.44	102.0	Shoaf et al. 1986
Carp (10°C)	20/100	IV	3.1	40.7	47.0	Nouws et al. 1993
Carp (20°C)	20/100	IV	4.0	20.0	141.0	Nouws et al. 1993
Broilers	4/2[c]	PO	NR	0.63	NR	Dagorn et al. 1991
Quail (*Coturnix coturnix japonica;* male and female)	10	PO	NR	2.98	NR	Lashev and Mihailov 1994
Quail (*Coturnix coturnix japonica;* male and female)	4	IV	2.99	2.38	1.129	Lashev and Mihailov 1994
Pigs	5/25 (Tribrissen 12%)	PO	NR	3.35	NR	Soli et al. 1990
Pigs	5/25 (Trimazin 12%)	PO	NR	4.86	4.86	Soli et al. 1990
Pigs	5/25 (Trimazin Forte 24%)	PO	NR	5.92	NR	Soli et al. 1990

Note: NR = not reported; IV = intravenously; SC = subcutaneously; PO = orally.
[a]First dose is trimethoprim; second dose is sulfadiazine (except for Davitiyananda and Rasmussen 1974 reference, in which the sulfonamide is sulfadoxine).
[b]Reported as mean residence time (MRT).
[c]Dose reported in mg/kg/24 hr.

TABLE 33.6 Some pharmacokinetic parameters of aditoprim, ormetoprim, tetroxoprim, and metioprim in animals

Species	Dose (mg/kg)	Route	V_d (L/kg)	$t_{1/2}$ (hr)	Clearance (mL/hr/kg)	Reference
Aditoprim:						
Calves (80 kg, milk fed)	5.0	IV	10.44	13.0	11.03	Sutter et al. 1993
Calves (80 kg, conventionally fed)	5.0	IV	9.72	14.8	8.20	Sutter et al. 1993
Calves (160 kg, milk fed)	5.0	IV	9.64	10.7	12.17	Sutter et al. 1993
Calves (160 kg, conventionally fed)	5.0	IV	6.29	8.8	10.29	Sutter et al. 1993
Calves (210 kg, conventionally fed)	5.0	IV	7.16	7.2	13.75	Sutter et al. 1993
Calves (80 kg, milk fed)	5.0	PO	NR	11.6	NR	Sutter et al. 1993
Calves (80 kg, conventionally fed)	5.0	PO	NR	11.60	NR	Sutter et al. 1993
Calves (160 kg, milk fed)	5.0	PO	NR	10.2	NR	Sutter et al. 1993
Calves (160 kg, conventionally fed)	5.0	PO	NR	NR	NR	Sutter et al. 1993
Calves (210 kg, conventionally fed)	10.0	PO	NR	16.6	NR	Sutter et al. 1993
Dairy cows (3–7 yr old)	5.0	IV	6.28	7.26	820.0	Lohuis et al. 1992
Dairy cows (3–7 yr old, mammary endotoxin)	5.0	IV	12.25	about 7 hr	1000.0	Lohuis et al. 1992
Ormetoprim:						
Calves (6–8 months old)	5.5/27.5[a]	IV	1.450	1.37	13.71	Wilson et al. 1987
Mare[b]	9.2/45.8[a]	IV	1.66	1.19	671.0	Brown et al. 1989
Tetroxoprim:						
Dogs	5.0	IV	NR	5.45	NR	Vergin et al. 1984
Metioprim:						
Dogs	5.0	IV	NR	3.07	NR	Vergin et al. 1984

Note: NR = not reported; IV = intravenously; PO = orally.
[a]First dose is trimethoprim; second dose is sulfadimethoxine.
[b]One mare studied.

administration (van Duijkernen et al. 1995). The best explanation for this phenomenon is that that there is an initial peak of absorption in the small intestine where much of drug absorption is known to occur. However, the drug that is bound to feed (adsorption) is unavailable for absorption until it travels to the cecum, and after digestion of the carbohydrates, the drug is released, producing a delayed and biphasic peak in absorption. Trimethoprim-sulfachlorpyridazine bound equine cecal contents 60–90%, which was responsible for the "double peak" produced after oral administration to horses and reduced systemic availability from 70% (fasted) to 45% when fed (van Duijkernen et al. 1996).

In ruminants, age and diet can markedly affect trimethoprim and oral sulfadiazine disposition in calves (Guard et al. 1986; Shoaf et al. 1987). Orally administered sulfadiazine (30 mg/kg) was absorbed very slowly in those calves fed milk diets, with absorption slightly higher in ruminating calves. Trimethoprim was absorbed in preruminant calves, but not absorbed in mature ruminants after oral administration (Shoaf et al. 1987), probably because of inactivation in the rumen.

Sulfasalazine is not absorbed as a whole molecule to any extent but rather is cleaved into two more active compounds by native resident colonic bacteria. (Discussed in more detail in Chapter 47 on gastrointestinal drugs.)

DISTRIBUTION. Sulfonamides are widely distributed throughout the body and into many soft tissues, including the CNS (cerebrospinal fluid) and joints (synovial fluid). Binding to plasma proteins, usually to albumin, varies from sulfonamide to sulfonamide and from species to species and ranges from 15 to 90%. High protein binding affects the distribution and markedly increases the half-life of sulfonamides.

Sulfonamides are weak acids (Table 33.1) and trimethoprim is a weak base. The ionization affects distribution, which favors the distribution and ion trapping of trimethoprim in tissues (intracellular environment is typically more negative than plasma). Therefore trimethoprim has a higher volume of distribution than sulfonamides. Also, because sulfonamides are weak acids, the pH-partition hypothesis shows that these drugs do not attain therapeutic concentrations in milk; however, enough passive diffusion occurs to limit their use in dairy cattle.

The prostate is another example in which pH-dependent distribution is known to occur (Robb et al. 1971). Sulfadiazine (a weak acid) penetrated the prostate to approximately 11% that of the mean plasma concentration. Because trimethoprim is a weak base (pK_a of 7.3) the concentrations in the prostate are higher owing to ion trapping. The concentration in the prostatic fluid has been measured to be 380% higher than that of plasma.

In horses, studies have been conducted to examine tissue concentrations in urine, peritoneal fluid, endometrium, and synovial fluid (Brown et al. 1983, 1988, 1989) of trimethoprim or ormetoprim-sulfonamide combinations. In each tissue, drug concentrations were adequate for treating infections in these sites. Urine concentrations—as expected because of the route of elimination—were much higher than plasma, but otherwise, the plasma concentration and tissue concentration curves were parallel. The only tissue for which drug concentrations are low is the central nervous system (Brown et al. 1988). Although trimethoprim-sulfonamides can be used to treat CNS infections, higher doses may be required in order to reach effective concentrations (Brown et al. 1988), and administration of dimethylsulfoxide (DMSO) concurrently does not increase the penetration across the blood-brain barrier (Green et al. 1990).

METABOLISM. Metabolism and elimination have been examined in several of the veterinary species. One phenomenon that is apparent from these studies is that herbivores metabolize sulfonamides and trimethoprim at a faster rate and more extensively than carnivores or omnivores. This may be caused by a higher metabolic capacity among herbivores—because of the nature of their diet and compounds to which they are exposed—compared to carnivores. Metabolic pathways are discussed in more detail by Nouws et al. (1988c) and (1987). Acetylation of the NH_2 group on N-4 is a major mechanism of metabolism. Hydroxylation of the methyl group on the pyrimidine ring, in addition to carboxylation also occur. The extent to which these metabolites are produced is drug- and species-dependent. In general, acetylation and hydroxylation increases the polarity of the sulfonamides, which increases excretion (Nouws et al. 1988c). Acetylation (mainly occurring in the liver and lung) is the major pathway by which sulfonamides are metabolized in most species. Ruminants metabolize sulfonamides by acetylation pathways, and acetylated metabolites are the major urinary metabolites in cattle, sheep, and swine. The canine (dogs and other canine species) lacks the ability to acetylate aromatic amines, relying on alternative metabolic pathways to convert sulfonamides to less active forms. Acetylated metabolites are less soluble than the parent compounds and increase the risks of renal tubular injury caused by precipitation and crystal formation. Glucuronide conjugation and aromatic hydroxylation are two additional metabolic pathways by which sulfonamides are metabolized in animals. Glucuronide metabolites are water-soluble and are excreted in urine, decreasing the risk of precipitation in renal tubules. Deacetylation, oxidation, deamination, conjugation with sulfate, and cleavage of heterocyclic rings of sulfonamide molecules have also been reported (Bevill 1988). Regardless of the metabolic pathway taken, metabolites have either reduced therapeutic activity (hydroxy metabolite) or are therapeutically inactive (N4-acetyl metabolite).

EXCRETION. Sulfonamides that are capable of obtaining therapeutic blood concentrations are excreted by the kidneys, either as the parent compound or as metabolites via glomerular filtration (unbound to plasma proteins). There also is some active carrier-mediated proximal tubular excretion and passive absorption of the nonionized drug from the distal tubular fluid. Small concentrations of sulfonamides are also excreted in the tears, feces, bile, milk, and sweat. Low urine pHs favor tubular reabsorption and hence longer half-lives of the sulfonamides, whereas alkalinization of the urine increases urinary excretion by slowing this pH-dependent passive reabsorption in the tubules. Many of the long-acting sulfonamides, with long half-lives in the body, undergo extensive tubular reabsorption. Nonabsorbed sulfonamides intended for intestinal activity are primarily eliminated via the feces, with little of the active or metabolized drug being absorbed systemically to be excreted by these renal mechanisms.

ADVERSE EFFECTS CAUSED BY SULFONAMIDES

Sulfonamides can produce a variety of adverse effects in animals. Likewise, when trimethoprim- or ormetoprim-sulfonamide combinations are administered, the adverse effects are primarily attributed to the sulfonamide component.

CRYSTALLURIA. Crystalluria, hematuria, and renal tubule blockage can occur owing to precipitation of the sulfonamide in the glomerular filtrate of the kidney. Subsequently, crystals of sulfonamides can form in the renal tubules. This problem is not as important as it once was because it was caused primarily from older insoluble preparations. Sulfadiazine is the least soluble and can precipitate in renal tubules at acidic pH. Even though this complication is rare with the current use of sulfonamides, one should ensure that patients are well hydrated when receiving sulfonamides because renal failure caused by sulfonamide crystals has been reported in human patients that are dehydrated. (Note that this effect is more likely with acetylated-metabolites of sulfonamides, which are not formed in dogs.)

KERATOCONJUNCTIVITIS SICCA (KCS). Keratoconjunctivitis sicca (KCS), also known as dry eye is a lack of adequate tear production resulting in ocular inflammation, irritation, and susceptibility to infection. Several cases of sulfonamide-induced KCS have been reported in dogs treated with sulfasalazine, sulfadiazine, and sulfamethoxazole (Morgan and Bachrach 1982; Slatter and Blogg 1978; Collins et al. 1986). The reaction apparently is caused by a lacrimotoxic effect of the sulfonamide component (toxic to the lacrimal acinar cells). The reaction is seen most commonly after chronic treatment, but cases have been reported that received only short-term administration. Berger et al. (1995) observed 33 dogs of various breeds for the occurrence of KCS after trimethoprim-sulfadiazine treatment, as characterized by changes in the Schirmer tear test (STT) values. There has been disagreement as to whether this effect is caused by an intrinsic dose-related effect, or is idiosyncratic. The prognosis appears to depend on the animal's age and duration of exposure (Morgan and Bachrach 1982). Dogs treated with sulfonamides should have tear production checked periodically.

The lacrimotoxic effect may be caused by the nitrogen-containing pyridine ring on the lacrimal acinar cells (Collins et al. 1986; Slatter and Blogg 1978). Reversal of KCS may or may not occur once sulfonamide therapy has been discontinued.

HYPERSENSITIVITY. A delayed hypersensitivity reaction has been described primarily in dogs (Trepanier 1999; Trepanier et al. 2003). The reaction may be caused by either sulfadiazine, sulfadimethoxine, or sulfamethoxazole. Doberman Pinschers may be more susceptible than other breeds (Giger et al. 1985; Cribb 1989; Cribb and Spielberg 1990). This may be a serum sickness reaction (Type III hypersensitivity) or involve another mechanism of cytotoxicity and hypersensitivity, or may be idiosyncratic (Trepanier 2004). The lesions include, but are not limited to, glomerulopathy, polymyositis, polyarthritis, skin rash, skin eruptions, fever, hepatotoxicity, thrombocytopenia, neutropenia, and anemia (Giger et al. 1985; Cribb 1989; Rowland et al. 1992). The most important of these reactions are described in more detail below. The reaction is caused by the sulfonamide component rather than trimethoprim (Giger et al. 1985). In affected dogs, the clinical signs quickly resolved after the sulfonamide was discontinued. However, some problems such as hepatopathy did not resolve in dogs after the initial drug-induced injury (Trepanier et al. 2003). There is some evidence that a reaction to a metabolite of the sulfonamide, rather than an immunologic reaction to the parent drug is responsible for these signs (see "Effect of Acetylator Status on Adverse Reactions," below).

HEPATIC NECROSIS. A component of the hypersensitivity reaction described above is hepatic necrosis. Trimethoprim-sulfadiazine and trimethoprim-sulfamethoxazole combination therapy in dogs has resulted in hepatic necrosis (Twedt et al. 1997; Dodds 1997). Hepatotoxicity may be caused by a hypersensitivity reaction or a result of an abnormal metabolic pathway, which allows the production or accumulation of hepatotoxic metabolites.

HYPOPROTHROMBINEMIA. Hypoprothrombinemia has been reported in dogs (Neer and Savant 1992; Patterson and Grenn 1975), in coyote pups (Brown et al. 1982), and in Leghorn chickens (Daft et al. 1989) given sulfaquinoxaline. Sulfaquinoxaline is unique among the sulfonamides in that it can induce hypoprothrombinemia in animals within 24 hours after dosing by lengthening prothrombin times. It is thought that this adverse effect is unrelated to the individual sulfonamide or to the quinoxaline portion of the sulfaquinoxaline molecule but occurs when the two entities are combined into a single molecule.

Sulfaquinoxaline is not an anticoagulant in vitro, nor does it destroy or otherwise inactivate prothrombin. Nevertheless, recent studies have reported that sulfaquinoxaline is a potent inhibitor of vitamin K epoxide reductase, and this inhibition is the most likely reason for the hypothrombinemic reaction seen in the reported cases of sulfaquinoxaline toxicosis. Treatment is by vitamin K1 administration for 4–7 days, and recovery is usually uneventful.

BLOOD DYSCRASIAS. Anemia and thrombocytopenia from sulfonamides has been reported (Weiss and Adams 1987; Weiss and Klausner 1990; Stockner 1993). Mammals derive their folic acid preformed either in the diet or from bacteria that produce the vitamin in the intestinal tract. The anemia induced by trimethoprim-sulfonamide combinations may be caused by decreased serum folate reductions, presumably by inhibiting the folate production by intestinal bacteria or by blocking its reduction to tetra- and dihydrofolate, resulting in lowered serum folate concentrations in the animal's serum that eventually induce an anemia. Folate deficiency anemia is rare but should be monitored with long-term use. Some veterinarians administer folic acid or folinic acid (vitamin B supplements) to patients receiving trimethoprim-sulfonamides. Whether this is routinely necessary, or whether this is effective, is controversial.

Thrombocytopenia has been reported in animals and in humans (Sullivan et al. 1992; Dodds 1993). The thrombocytopenia in animals, as in humans, is probably associated with an immune-mediated or hypersensitivity reaction. The thrombocytopenia usually resolves after the drug is discontinued.

THYROID METABOLISM DISORDERS. Both sulfamethoxazole and sulfadiazine have been associated with hypothyroidism in dogs. The effect is probably caused by the ability of sulfonamides to inhibit thyroid peroxidase activity. Studies have demonstrated that, administration of trimethoprim-sulfamethoxazole at a dose of 30 mg/kg, q12 h for 6 weeks, or 15 mg/kg q12 h for as short as 3 weeks decreased T_4 levels in dogs and decreased TSH response (Frank et al. 2005; Hall et al. 1993; Williamson et al. 2002; Hall et al. 1993). The hypothyroidism is reversible, and can return to normal in as short as 1 week, or in most dogs by 3 weeks after discontinuing the drug (Hall et al. 1993; Williamson et al. 2002). Only one study (Panciera and Post 1992) has produced conflicting evidence in which administration of trimethoprim-sulfadiazine at a dose of 15 mg/kg, q12 h × 4 weeks had no effect on total T_4, free-T_4, or TSH tests. Sulfadimethoxine has also been implicated as being goitrogenic to swine fetuses in late gestation (Blackwell et al. 1989).

SKIN REACTIONS. Sulfonamides are among the most common drugs to cause skin eruptions in people, especially the drug-induced Stevens-Johnson syndrome and toxic epidermal necrolysis (Roujeau et al. 1995). These skin reactions are believed to be a manifestation of the immune reaction described above (Trepanier 1999). In dogs, skin reactions (drug eruptions) also are commonly reported adverse reactions (Medleau et al. 1990).

EFFECT OF ACETYLATOR STATUS ON ADVERSE REACTIONS. Adverse effects in people have been associated with acetylator status. In slow acetylators a greater proportion of the drug may be directed to conversion of a more toxic metabolite, sulfonamide-hydroxylamine or nitroso compounds, which are more toxic to cells. Ordinarily, these metabolites are detoxified by glutathione conjugation, but some patients may lack this ability. Dogs lack ability to acetylate drugs; therefore, they may be more susceptible to adverse effects than other animals. There is evidence that some dogs are more susceptible to the adverse effects of the hydroxylamine-sulfonamide metabolite than mixed-breed dogs because of decreased ability to handle the metabolite, which may explain the higher incidence of adverse effects reported in Dobermans (Cribb and Spielberg 1990). (Other drugs that are acetylated in people include dapsone and isoniazid and these also may present a higher risk of toxicity in dogs.)

DIARRHEA. Diarrhea has been associated with trimethoprim-sulfonamide therapy in horses. However, this effect may not be any more common from trimethoprim-sulfonamides than from other orally administered antimicrobials in horses. When healthy horses were administered doses of 25 to 100 mg of sulfadiazine in combination with 5 to 20 mg/kg of trimethoprim there was no evidence of increased *Clostridium perfringens*–associated colitis (White and Prior 1982). In another study, Gustafsson et al. (1999) administered trimethoprim-sulfadiazine twice daily for 5 days to horses and measured the effect on intestinal flora. There was an initial decline in bacterial numbers, but these rebounded and the authors concluded that this treatment did not produce a disturbance of the intestinal bacterial flora.

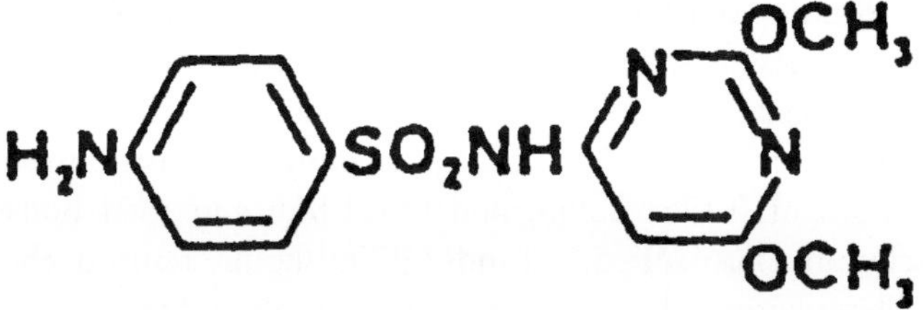

FIG. 33.3 Sulfadimethoxine.

CARCINOGENESIS. Sulfamethazine (discussed later in this chapter) has been demonstrated to induce thyroid hyperplasia in rats (Astwood et al. 1943; MacKenzie and MacKenzie 1943; Swarm et al. 1973) but has more recently been shown to induce specific types of thyroid cancer in both mice and rats. Fullerton et al. (1987) found that male and female Fischer 344 rats fed diets containing 1200 or 2400 ppm of sulfamethazine had thyroid weights that were increased significantly more than controls and that these increased weights were most likely due to thyroid hyperplasia related to increased thyroid-stimulating hormone levels. Littlefield et al. (1989) fed sulfamethazine to mice and induced follicular cell adenomas of the thyroid gland after 24 months of continuous feeding at the 4800 ppm dose with focal follicular cell hyperplasia and other organ aberrations being noted at some of the lower doses of sulfamethazine. In a similar study, there was a statistically significant increase in the incidence of thyroid follicular cell adenocarcinomas in rats sacrificed after 24 months of continuous feeding of sulfamethazine, with other nonneoplastic lesions of the thyroid also being reported in other treatment groups.

SULFONAMIDES IN VETERINARY MEDICINE

SULFADIMETHOXINE. Sulfadimethoxine (Fig. 33.3) is a long-acting sulfonamide that has been used alone or in combination with ormetoprim (ormetoprim-sulfadimethoxine) for the treatment of susceptible microbial infections of cattle, swine, horses, poultry, fish, and dogs, in addition to other vertebrate and invertebrate animals. The combination is discussed later in this chapter.

Sulfadimethoxine pharmacokinetics have been reported for many species. In dogs, the oral absorption is 49%, with a half-life of 13.1 hours (Baggot et al. 1976). Peak serum concentrations in dogs at a dose of 55 mg/kg oral was 67 μg/ml (mean). Systemic clearance in dogs was 0.36 ml/kg/min, with most clearance occurring via the kidneys.

Sulfadimethoxine pharmacokinetics in cattle has been described by many investigators. Bourne et al. (1981) dosed adult cattle with 107 mg/kg either intravenously (IV) or orally. In the IV study, sulfadimethoxine plasma concentrations peaked at 0.5 hours after administration and slowly declined over time, with the parent compound, acetylsulfadimethoxine, and a "polar" metabolite being found in the urine for at least 48 hours after the IV dose. The volume of distribution (Vd) was 0.315 l/kg in those cattle. In the oral study, plasma concentrations of sulfadimethoxine started low at 0.5 hours and gradually peaked at 10 hours after dose and then began to drop, with detectable levels of parent compound and all metabolites being found in the urine for at least 84 hours after dosing. Bioavailability of sulfadimethoxine was calculated to be 59.1%. Boxenbaum et al. (1977) administered 55 mg/kg IV sulfadimethoxine (40% solution) or 55 mg/kg orally to cattle, followed by 27.5 mg/kg sulfadimethoxine administered orally at 24, 48, and 72 hours after the initial loading dose. After IV injection, the half-life of sulfadimethoxine was determined to be 12.5 hours, with a volume of distribution of 0.31 l/kg. This study also confirmed that adequate plasma concentrations (>50 μg/ml) were maintained throughout the oral-dosing study, and this method could be used when IV administration was not possible. By comparison, a study by Wilson et al. (1987) demonstrated that sulfadimethoxine (27.5 mg/kg) in combination with ormetoprim (5.5 mg/kg) administered IV to cattle had a shorter half-life, 7.91 hours, and volume of distribution of 0.185 l/kg. When given the same dose orally, bioavailability of sulfadimethoxine was 56.6%.

Studies by Righter et al. (1979) examined the pharmacokinetics of sulfadimethoxine in mature, growing, and suckling pigs. Mature pigs dosed with 20, 50, or 100 mg/kg of sulfadimethoxine IV had volume of distribution values of 0.178, 0.258, and 0.331 l/kg and total body clearance of 4.21, 5.54, and 7.37 ml/kg/hr, respectively. The pharmacokinetic parameters of 55 mg/kg sulfadimethoxine given IV to growing and suckling pigs have also been reported. Suckling pigs (1–2 weeks old) had sulfadimethoxine half-lives of 16.16 hours, volume of distribution of 0.483 l/kg, and total body clearance of 20.9 ml/kg/hr. In contrast, growing pigs (11–12 weeks old) had sulfadimethoxine half-lives of 9.35 hours, volume of distribution of 0.347 l/kg, and total body clearance of 26.1 ml/kg/hr, indicating an age-related effect of sulfadimethoxine pharmacokinetics in young pigs. Weanling pigs consuming water dosed with 0.05 g sulfadimethoxine/100 ml showed mean plasma concentrations of 80 ppm 12 hours after introduction of the medicated water, with plasma concentrations declining to approximately 50 ppm thereafter. Total water consumption was not affected, which indicated that sulfadimethoxine may be of therapeutic use in swine provided that water consumption is maintained throughout the medication period. Mengelers et al. (1995) dosed 34–40 kg healthy and febrile (inoculated endobronchially with *A. pleuropneumoniae* toxins) pigs with 25 mg/kg sulfadimethoxine and 5 mg/kg trimethoprim intravenously. Sulfadimethoxine plasma half-lives for both healthy and pneumonic pigs were not significantly different (approximately 13 hr). Trimethoprim half-lives were not significantly different between healthy and pneumonic pigs (approximately 2.7 hr); however, the half-lives were significantly shorter than the half-life of sulfadimethoxine. In addition, the volume of distribution values of healthy and pneumonic pigs receiving sulfadimethoxine were not significantly different (approximately 0.25 l/kg), but trimethoprim did show significant differences between healthy (1.21 l/kg) and pneumonic (1.49 l/kg) pigs. The mean area under the curve (AUC) of trimethoprim was decreased and the total body clearance was increased in the febrile pigs, but with no significant changes in these sulfadimethoxine pharmacokinetic parameters.

Sulfadimethoxine is available in a concentrated solution (e.g., Albon 12.5%) for cattle or poultry; oral suspension (e.g., 5% Albon Suspension) and tablets and boluses for dogs, cats, and cattle; extended release tablets (Albon SR); 40% injection used in dogs, cats, and cattle; and soluble powder that can be added to drinking water for cattle and poultry. The clinical use for this formulation is described on product labels for treatment of intestinal coccidiosis, bacterial enteritis, fowl cholera, bacterial pneumonia, pododermatitis in cattle, skin and soft tissue infections in dogs and cats, and bacterial cystitis in dogs. On the product labels for treating bacterial infections, it states "for treatment of susceptible bacteria causing these infections." Because resistance can be common, some of the conditions listed above may not respond appropriately to treatment.

The clinical use of sulfadimethoxine has been described for turkeys (Epstein and Ashworth 1989), dogs (Yagi et al. 1981; Fish et al. 1965; Dunbar and Foreyt 1985; Imamura et al. 1986, 1989), primates (Adamson et al. 1970; Bridges et al. 1968), lobsters (James and Barron 1988), channel catfish (Squibb et al. 1988), and rainbow trout (Kleinow and Lech 1988). Detection of violative levels of sulfadimethoxine residues in channel catfish has also been reported (Walker and Barker 1993).

SULFAMETHAZINE (SULFADIMIDINE). Sulfamethazine (sulfadimidine), (Fig. 33.4) like many sulfonamides, has been utilized for decades in veterinary medicine; hence, the veterinary literature contains many reports on its usage in a wide variety of animals, including cattle, horses, swine, poultry, small ruminants, and rabbits (among others). Table 33.3 summarizes some of the pharmacokinetic parameters of sulfamethazine in animals.

Sulfamethazine has been administered to cattle and swine, and is formulated for use in drinking water (Church et al. 1979), as a feed additive, an extended-release bolus, and an IV preparation. Sulfamethazine has been marketed by itself and in combination with other antimicrobials, such as other sulfonamides, tylosin, chlortetracycline, and procaine penicillin G.

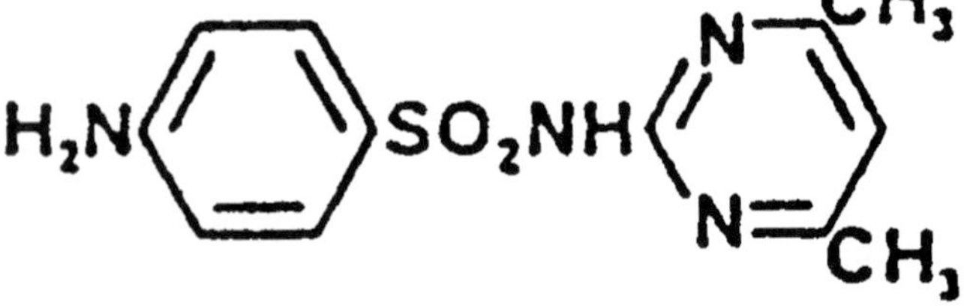

FIG. 33.4 Sulfamethazine (sulfadimidine).

The product labels for sulfamethazine products include uses for treating intestinal coccidiosis, bacterial enteritis, pneumonia, and pododermatitis in cattle. Sulfamethazine is available as an oral solution for calves, poultry, pigs, and cattle. It is available as a 12.5% solution to be added to drinking water. It is also available as a powder for oral solution to be added to the drinking water of these species. Tablets (Sulmet 2.5 and 5 gram tablets) are also available for large animals, as well as extended-release tablets (e.g., Sulfa-Max) in a range of sizes for calves and adult cattle. Triple-sulfa products containing sulfamethazine (sulfamethazine, sulfanilamide, and sulfathiazole) as well as sulfamethazine-sulfathiozole combination oral powder are no longer available in the United States, but may still be available in other countries.

The basic pharmacokinetic parameters of sulfamethazine in cattle have been reported by Bevill et al. (1977a) and Nouws et al. (1988c), among many others. Of particular interest are the oral forms of sulfamethazine that have been formulated in extended-release (sustained-release) form for cattle. Several reports on the efficacy and clinical uses of the extended-release form of sulfamethazine in cattle are available (Clark et al. 1966; Ellison et al. 1967; Miller et al. 1969; Carlson et al. 1976). This sustained-release formulation has been reported to achieve therapeutic blood concentrations within 6–12 hours after oral administration and to maintain or exceed that level for 2–5 days after dosing. The sustained-release formulation of sulfamethazine has been reported to be effective for treating Bovine Respiratory Disease, diphtheria, and pneumonia in cattle (Carlson et al. 1976; Clark et al. 1966). Clearance of sulfamethazine and its metabolites in cattle are age- and dose-dependent (Nouws et al. 1986a, 1985, 1983; Lapka et al. 1980). Several metabolites of sulfamethazine have been identified and described in both adult cattle and calves (Nouws et al. 1988c).

The pharmacokinetics of sulfamethazine and its metabolites are of particular interest in swine. Sulfonamides had been one of the most common causes of food-residue violations reported by the U.S. Food Safety Inspection Service, with swine being the food-animal species with the greatest number of residue violations (Sweeney et al. 1993). Sulfamethazine and its metabolites are most often associated with violative levels in pork products because of sulfamethazine's widespread use as a swine feed additive. Sulfamethazine has been used extensively to treat a host of susceptible microbial infections in swine, including *Salmonella typhisuis* (Fenwick and Olander 1987) and *Bordetella bronchiseptica* (Kobland et al. 1984).

Pharmacokinetic parameters for swine have been described by Sweeney et al. (1993) and others (see Table 33.3), including pharmacokinetics of metabolites (Nouws et al. 1989a, 1986b). Several studies have used radiolabeled (Mitchell et al. 1986; Mitchell and Paulson 1986) and nonradiolabeled (Biehl et al. 1981; Ashworth et al. 1986) sulfamethazine to determine the elimination patterns of sulfamethazine and its metabolites from the tissues in swine. Other studies have shown that the major metabolites produced from sulfamethazine metabolism in swine are N_4-acetylsulfamethazine, N_4-glucose conjugate of sulfamethazine, and desaminosulfamethazine (Mitchell et al. 1986). Studies using pigs fed 110 ppm of ^{14}C-sulfamethazine in the feed for 3–7 days, euthanized, and their tissues examined for total radioactivity and metabolite content found the highest concentration of radioactivity in the gut (undigested feed). Blood, kidney, urine, and liver all had high concentrations of radioactivity (i.e., parent compound and metabolite). Adipose tissue contained the least amount of radioactivity of all tissues assayed (Mitchell et al. 1986). Specific metabolites found in these and other tissues of swine given ^{14}C-labeled sulfamethazine in the feed have been reported by Mitchell and Paulson (1986). Other studies have also reported on sulfamethazine residues in swine (Ashworth et al. 1986; Biehl et al. 1981).

Cattle and swine are the two major species in which sulfamethazine is approved for use, with fewer reports in other species. Pharmacokinetic parameters and/or tissue-depletion kinetics of sulfamethazine and metabolites have been established in ponies (Wilson et al. 1989; Nouws et al. 1987) and horses (Nouws et al. 1985a). Studies on pharmacokinetics of sulfamethazine in goats (Abdullah and Baggot 1988; Witcamp et al. 1992; Nouws et al. 1988b, 1989b; Elsheikh et al. 1991; Youssef et al. 1981; van Gogh et al. 1984; Witcamp et al. 1993), sheep (Srivastava and Rampal 1990; Bourne et al. 1977; Bevill et al. 1977c; Bulgin et al. 1991; Nawaz and Nawaz 1983), dogs (Riffat et al. 1982), chickens (Righter et al. 1971; Nouws et al. 1988a; Goren et al. 1987), rabbits (Yuan and Fung 1990), mice (Littlefield et al. 1989), buffalo (Singh et al. 1988), camels (Younan et al. 1989), and carp and rainbow trout (van Ginneken et al. 1991), also have been published.

Lashev et al. (1995) described altered pharmacokinetics in roosters treated with a single 50 mg/kg IV dose of sulfadimidine only or IV sulfadimidine after 2 weeks of four 3.5 mg/kg subcutaneous (SC) testosterone treatments. Normal and castrated roosters provided no significant differences in half-life values, which ranged from 7.62 hours (castrated) to 9.38 hours (intact). Roosters pretreated with testosterone and then dosed with sulfadimidine had half-lives of 23.85 hours, as well as significantly decreased clearance and volume of distribution. Chickens metabolize sulfamethazine in relatively equal parts through hydroxylation and acetylation. It was hypothesized in this study that the acetylation pathway of sulfamethazine metabolism was retarded by the testosterone treatments and resulted in the prolonged half-lives.

SULFAQUINOXALINE. Sulfaquinoxaline (Fig. 33.5) has been used primarily for control of coccidia and some susceptible bacterial diseases in poultry. The veterinary literature also contains a few reports of sulfaquinoxaline use in rabbits (Eppel and Thiessen 1984; Joyner et al. 1983) and dogs (Brown et al. 1982; Patterson and Grenn 1975), but clinical use in these species is rare today.

Sulfaquinoxaline is available as an oral solution in a range of concentrations (20–32%). These solutions are intended to be mixed with drinking water. In some countries (but not the U.S.) there are combinations of pyrimethamine and sulfaquinoxaline solution for administration to drinking water.

For the use in poultry, sulfaquinoxaline has been administered to control coccidiosis. Mathis and McDougald (1984) described the therapeutic effectiveness of sulfaquinoxaline and sulfaquinoxaline-pyrimethamine against several coccidia species of *Eimeria*. It was determined from that study that both sulfaquinoxaline and sulfaquinoxaline-pyrimethamine were highly effective against *E. acervulina* but less effective against *E. tenella*. In addition, the potentiated mixture was determined to be more effective

H_2N–C₆H₄–SO_2NH–quinoxaline

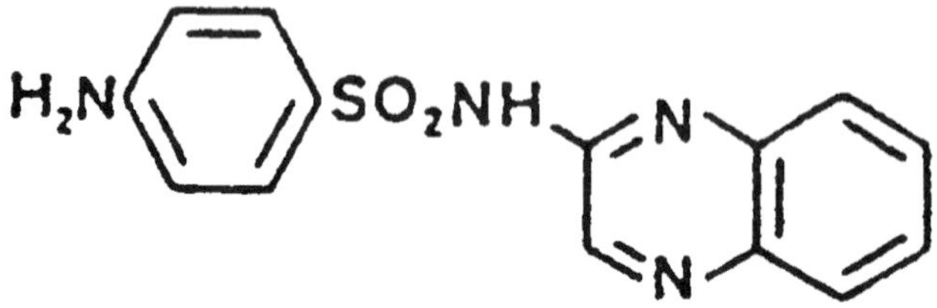

FIG. 33.5 Sulfaquinoxaline.

against *E. tenella* than sulfaquinoxaline alone, although neither mixture was found to be particularly effective against any cecal coccidia. Amprolium was found to be efficacious against cecal-dwelling forms of coccidia; hence amprolium has been combined with sulfaquinoxaline or sulfaquinoxaline-pyrimethamine to enhance the spectrum of activity. Ineffectiveness of sulfaquinoxaline-pyrimethamine against *E. tenella* has also been documented in another study (Chapman 1989), underlining the importance of correct coccidia species identification before instituting anticoccidial therapy with sulfaquinoxaline or any other sulfonamide.

Banerjee et al. (1974) reported on the blood concentrations after administration of sulfaquinoxaline, which were in the therapeutic range. In that same study, sulfaquinoxaline was found in high concentrations in the liver, kidney, and cecum, with the lowest concentrations found in the yolk sac and brain. A single oral dose of ^{35}S-labeled sulfaquinoxaline in 1-week-old chicks showed rapid uptake from the gastrointestinal tract and wide distribution throughout the body, including crossing of the blood-brain barrier. At 0.5 hours after dosing, autoradiography showed that all tissues (brain, lung, liver, kidney, fat, and muscle), except the lens of the eye had measurable concentrations of sulfaquinoxaline. Similar findings resulted from IV administration of ^{35}S-labeled sulfaquinoxaline, and it was also found that excretion of sulfaquinoxaline by the bile and secretion by the cecal mucosa, crop, and gizzard probably occur. Oral absorption was higher (3.5 times) in birds infected with *E. acervulina* and *E. tenella* compared to uninfected birds (Williams et al. 1995). A study by Qiao et al. (1995) found that in 7- to 8-week-old male and female broilers given a single 200 mg/kg oral dose of sulfaquinoxaline, peak concentration times in plasma and liver were similar (4 hr) but were longer in the heart, kidney, and muscle (6 hr). The half-life of sulfaquinoxaline was the shortest in the muscle (4.5 hr), with significantly longer half-lives in the heart (10 hr), plasma (11 hr), liver (13 hr), and kidney (18 hr).

The safety and efficacy of sulfaquinoxaline alone or in combination with trimethoprim (trimethoprim:sulfaquinoxaline ratio is 1:3) have been reported in poultry (White and Williams 1983; Piercy et al. 1984; Sainsbury 1988). A total dose of 30 mg/kg/day PO satisfactorily controlled experimentally induced colisepticemia and pasteurellosis in addition to five species of coccidia (White and Williams 1983). A wide margin of safety has been shown for the 1:3

combination of trimethoprim:sulfaquinoxaline in poultry, although decreased appetite and water consumption and lowered egg production, egg weight, and hatchability were noted when these antimicrobials were incorporated in the feed or water in higher than recommended concentrations (Piercy et al. 1984).

Toxicosis from sulfaquinoxaline use in animals is rare. Toxicity from sulfaquinoxaline has occurred in Leghorn chickens (Daft et al. 1989), where a mortality of 47% was reported in a commercial flock given a 0.05% concentration of sulfaquinoxaline in the feed. Lesions included mildly enlarged livers; swollen and pale livers; hemorrhages on the epicardium, kidney, oviduct, small intestine, and cecum; pale bone marrow; gangrenous dermatitis; and some lung involvement was present. Patterson and Grenn (1975) reported a situation where 12 adult Miniature Poodles that received 3.16 g/l of sulfaquinoxaline in the drinking water as treatment for coccidiosis suffered similar lesions as described above in poultry, in addition to depressed body temperature, pale mucous membranes, microscopic hemorrhages of the jejunum and ileum, and prolonged prothrombin times. Although the exact mechanism has not been reported, sulfaquinoxaline possesses an ability to produce a marked hypothrombinemia, even in animals receiving balanced diets containing adequate amounts of vitamin K. These animals also responded to vitamin K treatment. It is thought that this adverse effect is not related to the individual sulfonamide or quinoxaline portion of the sulfaquinoxaline molecule but occurs only when the two entities are combined. A similar toxicosis has also been reported in coyote pups treated with sulfaquinoxaline (Brown et al. 1982).

SULFAMERAZINE. Sulfamerazine (Fig. 33.6) has primarily been utilized in adult sheep and lambs to treat susceptible microbial infections. In these ruminants, sulfamerazine has been used alone or in combination with other antibiotics (tylosin) and other sulfonamides (sulfamethazine, sulfadiazine).

The pharmacokinetics of sulfamerazine has been described for ewes and lambs. Hayashi et al. (1979) described the pharmacokinetics of sulfamerazine in ewes after either IV or oral administration of 107 mg/kg (see Table 33.3). After oral administration of the oral solution systemic availability was 81 ± 19%. Urinary concentrations of parent compound and metabolites were

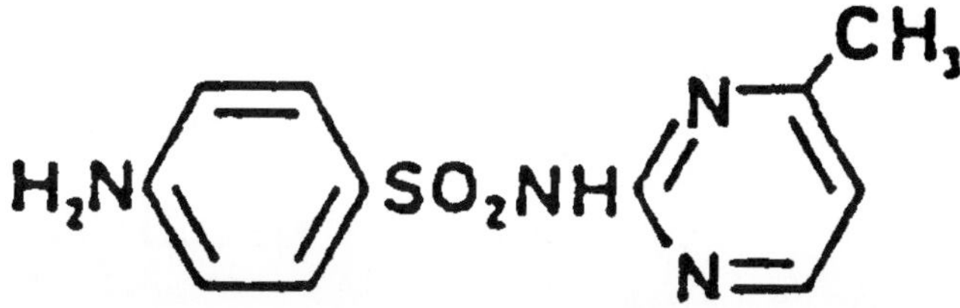

FIG. 33.6 Sulfamerazine.

also reported for both IV- and PO-dosing studies. Both routes produced appreciable concentrations of sulfamerazine and three metabolites in the urine (described as a polar metabolite acetylsulfamerazine). Intravenous sulfamerazine produced more parent compound and fewer metabolites were found in the urine, which is attributed to lack of rumen metabolism, while more metabolite than parent compound was found in the PO study due to rumen metabolism. In a similar pharmacokinetic study, Garwacki et al. (1991) administered 60 mg/kg sulfamerazine IV in fasted sheep and in sheep fed ad libitum. That study determined that sheep fed ad libitum had a sulfamerazine half-life of 5.72 hours and a volume of distribution of 0.40 l/kg, while those sheep that were fasted had a half-life of 6.91 hours and similar volume of distribution.

The pharmacokinetics of sulfamerazine has also been reported in neonatal and young lambs (Debacker et al. 1982). Lambs from birth to 16 weeks of age were administered either IV or PO, 100 mg/kg of sulfamerazine. In the IV study, it was found that the sulfamerazine half-life was longest in the first week of life (9–14 hours) and decreased to 4–7 hours by 9–16 weeks of age. The volume of distribution was highest during the first week of life and steadily decreased with age, while clearance of sulfamerazine was lowest in the first week of life (20–40 ml/kg/hr) and steadily increased with age up to 9–16 weeks of age (50–80 ml/kg/hr). In the oral study, plasma concentrations of sulfamerazine tended to decrease more slowly after dosing in the early weeks of life (<4 weeks of age), with plasma clearance of the drug steadily increasing after 4 weeks of age until 16 weeks, when it approached the adult values.

SULFATHIAZOLE. Sulfathiazole (Fig. 33.7) use in veterinary medicine has declined. It has been formulated in

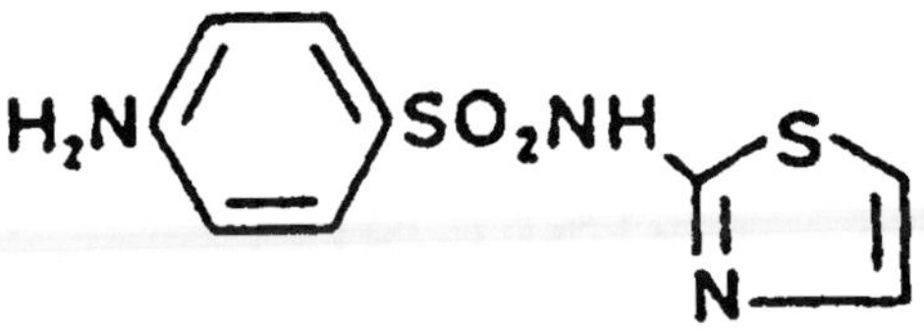

FIG. 33.7 Sulfathiazole.

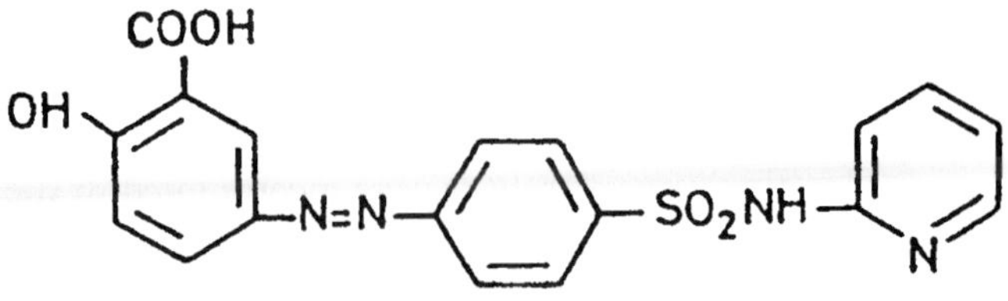

FIG. 33.8 Sulfasalazine.

combination with chlortetracycline HCl and procaine penicillin G. Recent reports of its use are rare and earlier editions of this text should be consulted for more details. A few reports have described the pharmacokinetics of sulfathiazole in sheep and swine.

Sulfathiazole pharmacokinetics in sheep has been outlined by Koritz et al. (1977), and sulfathiazole tissue residues in sheep have been described by Bevill et al. (1977b). When 36 or 72 mg/kg of 5% aqueous solution of sulfathiazole sodium IV was given to ewe lambs, it cleared quickly from the plasma, with a low volume of distribution of 0.34 and 0.59 l/kg and half-lives of 1.2 and 1.4 hours, respectively. Ewes given 214 mg/kg orally of a 12.5% aqueous solution of sulfathiazole sodium cleared the drug from plasma much more slowly than by the IV route, with the systemic bioavailability being approximately 73%, with a half-life of approximately 18 hours. Both oral and IV routes produce parent compound, acetylsulfathiazole, and a third "polar" metabolite in the urine of these sheep. Sulfathiazole residues in sheep are highest in the kidney (308 ppm), followed by the liver (40 ppm), heart (34 ppm), shoulder muscle (23 ppm), leg and loin muscle (22 ppm), body fat (11 ppm), and omental fat (6.7 ppm). Residues quickly dropped to very low (<0.13 ppm) or to nondetectable levels by 24 hours after dosing in all tissues tested.

Pharmacokinetic parameters have also been reported for swine. Pigs given 72 mg/kg of sulfathiazole sodium IV had quick plasma elimination of the drug, with mean Vd of 0.54 l/kg and a biological half-life of 1.39 hours, similar to those for sheep. Given 214 mg/kg orally, sulfathiazole had a Vd of 0.32 l/kg and a systemic bioavailability of 73%, identical to that of sheep.

SULFASALAZINE (SALICYLAZOSULFAPYRIDINE). Sulfasalazine (Fig. 33.8) was originally developed as a possible treatment for rheumatoid arthritis in humans. It was found, however, to be more effective in the treatment of inflammatory bowel disease. The most frequent use is to treat various forms of colitis (Aronson and Kirk 1983). The gastrointestinal use is discussed in more detail in Chapter 47 of this book. Inflammatory bowel diseases (most commonly ulcerative colitis and Crohn's disease) have been treated with sulfasalazine in humans.

Sulfasalazine consists of two components, 5-aminosalicylic acid and sulfapyridine, which are linked by an azo bond. This bond is broken by the bacterial enzymes in the colon. After oral administration, the sulfonamide component is absorbed systemically, but the 5-aminosalicylic acid component has a local effect in the bowel. Therefore, this drug produces a local inflammatory effect in the colon. 5-aminosalicylic acid is also known as *mesalamine* and there are now other forms of mesalamine (e.g., olsalazine) or enteric-coated (pH-sensitive) tablets that release mesalamine in the colon, while avoiding the systemic effects of the sulfonamide component.

The intestinal antiinflammatory effects may be due to prostaglandin inhibition (Hoult and Moore 1978), inhibition of leukotrienes, decreased intestinal oxygen free radicals (Del Soldato et al. 1985) or sulfhydryls (Garg et al. 1991). For further discussion of sulfasalazine, refer to Chapter 47.

SULFADIAZINE. The most commonly used formulation containing sulfadiazine is a trimethoprim-sulfadiazine combination (e.g., Tribrissen). This combination will be discussed in more detail in the section about potentiated sulfonamides because of its common use.

Sulfadiazine (Fig. 33.9) use alone has been reported in some studies. Sulfadiazine has been used to control plaque and gingivitis in Beagles (Howell et al. 1989) and has attained concentrations in the cerebrospinal fluid (when administered IV) above the reported MIC values for many of the Enterobacteriaceae family (Vergin et al. 1984). In pigs, sulfadiazine administration was reported from various studies (Soli et al. 1990; Guise et al. 1986).

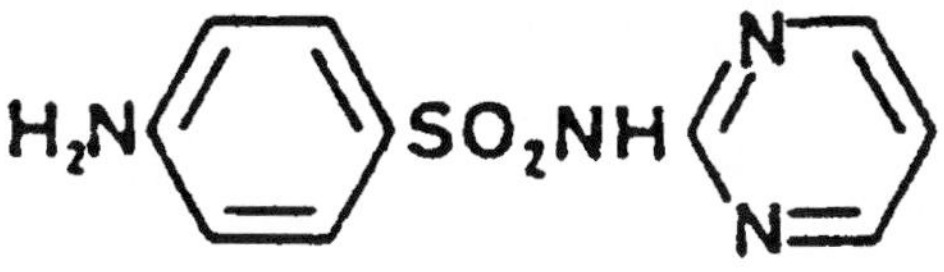

FIG. 33.9 Sulfadiazine.

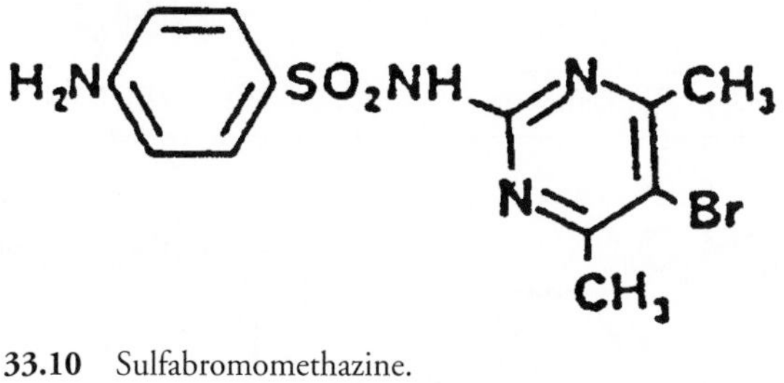

FIG. 33.10 Sulfabromomethazine.

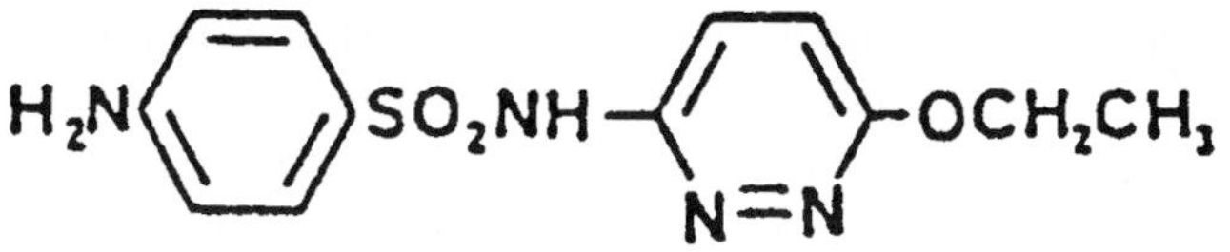

FIG. 33.11 Sulfaethoxypyridazine.

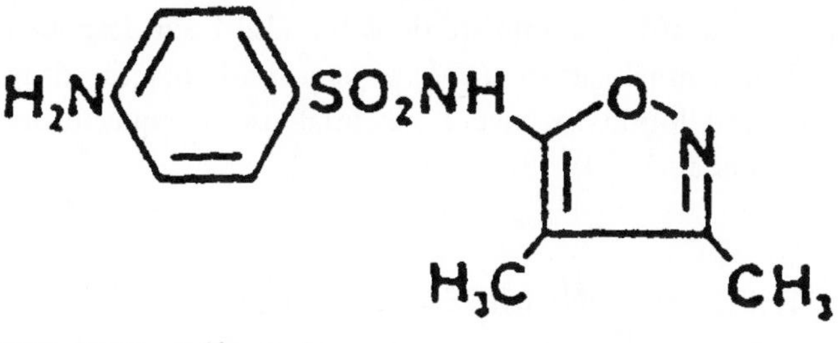

FIG. 33.12 Sulfisoxazole.

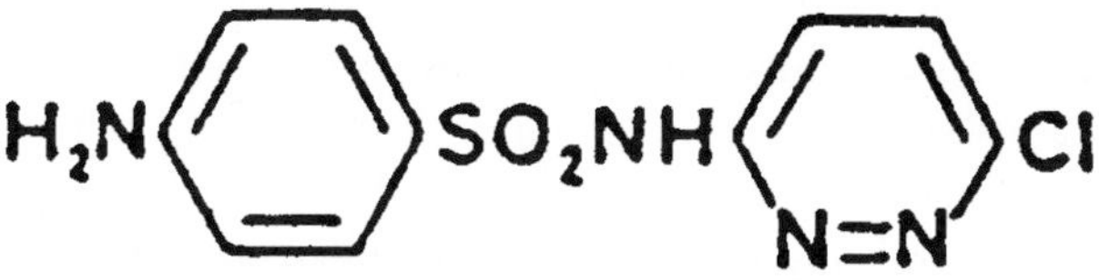

FIG. 33.13 Sulfachlorpyridazine.

SULFABROMOMETHAZINE. Sulfabromomethazine (Fig. 33.10) is the brominated derivative of sulfamethazine and is considered a long-acting sulfonamide that is now rarely used. Sulfabromomethazine has a lower solubility than sulfamethazine, and single oral doses of the drug have been used to treat calf diphtheria and pneumonia, metritis, foot rot, and septic mastitis in cattle, with a repeated dose 48 hours later sometimes required. Use of sulfabromomethazine during the last 3 months of pregnancy should be avoided (Bevill 1988).

SULFAETHOXYPYRIDAZINE. Sulfaethoxypyridazine (Fig. 33.11) also is rarely used today. It is rapidly absorbed after oral administration to swine, sheep, and cattle and is extensively bound to plasma proteins. The parent compound and the N4-acetylated metabolite and another unidentified glucuronide conjugate seem to be the major urinary excretion products (Bevill 1988). Sulfaethoxypyridazine has also been reported to induce cataracts at some doses when fed to dogs and rats over a period of 27 and 118 weeks, respectively (Ribelin et al. 1967).

SULFISOXAZOLE. Sulfisoxazole (Fig. 33.12) has limited use today but has found some application in the treatment of urinary tract infections in the dog and cat, especially infections caused by susceptible bacteria (Bevill 1988). The pharmacokinetics of sulfisoxazole has been studied in dogs, swine, and humans (Suber et al. 1981), as well as its delivery across the skin using iontophoresis (Inada et al. 1989). A formulation of combined trimethoprim-sulfisoxazole is available in some countries for injection of cattle.

SULFACHLORPYRIDAZINE. When used alone, sulfachlorpyridazine (Fig. 33.13) is administered most often to calves and pigs. Sulfachlorpyridazine powder, to be mixed into an oral solution (Vetisulid powder) or tablets (Vetisulid 2 gram tablets), has been administered to calves and pigs for treatment of enteritis at a dose of 33–49.5 mg/kg for calves and 44–77 mg/kg per day to pigs. There is also an injectable solution available (Vetisulid injection 200 mg/ml) for intravenous use in calves. Sulfachlorpyridazine has also been used in combination with trimethoprim and this combination is discussed in more detail in the section on potentiated sulfonamides.

Sulfachlorpyridazine is rapidly eliminated from the plasma following IV administration. Intramuscular injections in swine result in maximum blood concentrations within 30 minutes after injection, which are maintained for up to 3 hours (Bevill 1988). A single 50 mg/kg IV dose of sulfachlorpyridazine demonstrated significantly different volume of distribution in cocks (0.34 l/kg) versus hens (0.36 l/kg), with the sulfonamide being more slowly excreted in hens (Lashev et al. 1995).

The pharmacokinetics of sulfachlorpyridazine after oral and intracardiac administrations has also been described in the channel catfish (*Ictalurus punctatus*), and the drug has been found to have a potential use in aquaculture (Alavi et al. 1993).

OTHER SULFONAMIDES. This chapter has discussed the major sulfonamides in use in veterinary medicine today. However, other sulfonamides exist that are not currently, or are no longer, used in the U.S. markets. Other sulfonamides that may be of interest, either historically or because of use in other countries include sulfadimethoxypyrimidine (Walker and Williams 1972), sulfasomidine and sulfamethomidine (Bridges et al. 1969), sulfamethoxypyridazine (Garg and Uppal 1997), sulfamethoxydiazine (Weijkamp et al. 1994), and sulfamethylphenazole (Austin and Kelly 1966).

The combination of sulfadimethoxine-sulfamethoxazole use in healthy and pneumonic pigs (Mengelers et al. 1995), trimethoprim-sulfamethoxazole in goats (kids) (Koudela and Bokova 1997), and trimethoprim-sulfamethoxazole combinations in Japanese quails (Lashev and Mihailov 1994) have also been reported. Previous editions of this textbook or the individual references listed above may be consulted for more in-depth information on the older and less commonly used sulfonamides not discussed in this chapter.

POTENTIATED SULFONAMIDES

The combination of sulfonamides with trimethoprim (Fig. 33.14) or ormetoprim (Fig. 33.15) produces greater antibacterial activity than either drug used alone. Consequently in humans, dogs, cats, horses, and occasionally other animals, these formulations are used more commonly than sulfonamides alone.

Sulfonamide and trimethoprim combinations have been reviewed in some depth by Bushby (1980) and van Miert (1994). An extensive review of trimethoprim-sulfonamide combinations in the horse is also available (van Duijkeren et al. 1994b).

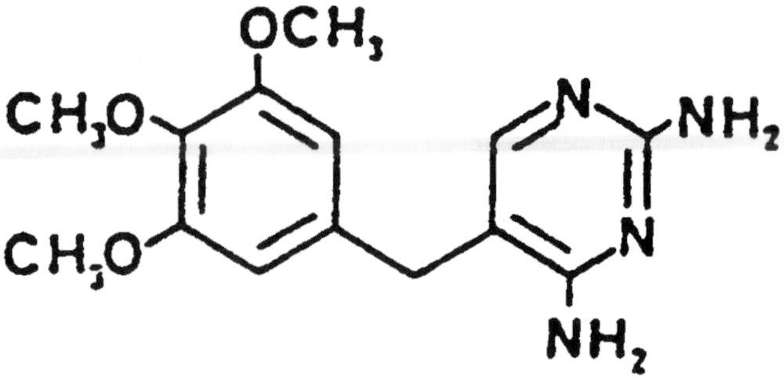

OCH_3 CH_3O CH_3O N NH_2 N NH_2

FIG. 33.14 Trimethoprim.

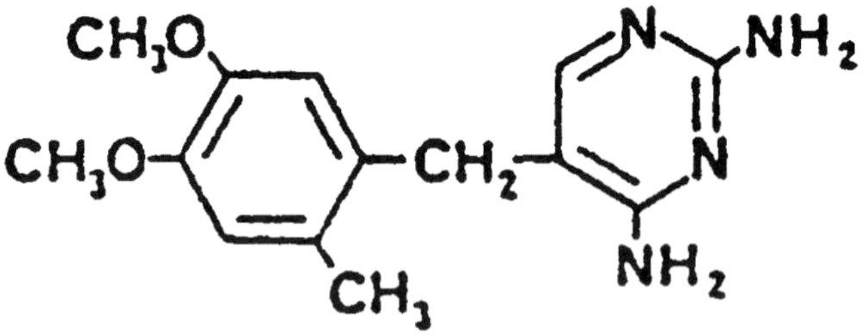

CH_3O CH_3O CH_2 CH_3 N NH_2 N NH_2

FIG. 33.15 Ormetoprim.

The pharmacokinetic parameters of diaminopyrimidines (trimethoprim, ormetoprim, and others) have been established for some species and are listed in Tables 33.5 and 33.6. Specific properties of these diaminopyrimidines are also discussed by Ascalone et al. 1986, Mengelers et al. 1990, Lohuis et al. 1992, Sutter et al. 1993, Wilson et al. 1987, Brown et al. 1989, Iversen et al. 1984, Vergin et al. 1984, and Aschhoff 1979.

The full range of combinations possible include a sulfonamide with trimethoprim (2,4-diamino-5-(3,4,5-trimethoxybenzyl) pyrimidine), aditoprim (2,4-diamino-5-[4-(dimethylamino)-3,5-dimethoxybenzyl] pyrimidine), ormetoprim (2,4-diamino-5-[4,5-dimethoxy-2-methylbenzyl] pyrimidine), or tetroxoprim (2,4-diamino-5-[3,5-dimethoxy-4(2-methoxy ethoxy)benzyl] pyrimidine). These are commonly referred to as *potentiated sulfonamides*.

TRIMETHOPRIM-SULFADIAZINE. Sulfadiazine is most often administered in combination with trimethoprim (e.g., Tribrissen). Pharmacokinetic values are presented in Table 33.4. This combination has been used for respiratory infections, urinary tract infections, urogenital infections, protozoal infections, bone and joint infections, and skin and soft-tissue infections. It is available as an oral paste for horses (400 mg per gram, e.g., Tribrissen). It also is available as a powder (e.g., Tucoprim, Uniprim) to be added to feed for horses. Feeding does not affect absorption of sulfadiazine in horses, but it may delay the absorption of the trimethoprim component. Tablets of sulfadiazine and trimethoprim (5:1 ratio) have been available in a range of sizes for small animals, but the availability of the small animal products has diminished in recent years. Injectable formulations have become less available, but 24% and 48% injections (e.g., Tribrissen) have been used in a range of species.

Trimethoprim-sulfadiazine combination in a 1:5 ratio has been one of the most popular antimicrobials in dogs, cats, and horses as a general "first-line" antimicrobial that can be useful for treating a wide variety of pathogens, in particular *Staphylococcus* spp., *Streptococcus* spp., and some gram-negative organisms, such as *Proteus mirabilis* spp., *Pasteurella* spp., and *Klebsiella* spp. However, resistance among the gram-negative bacilli *Enterobacteriacea* can be common.

Dosing Recommendations. It is difficult to correlate plasma drug levels (and plasma elimination rates) with clinical efficacy and dosing intervals because trimethoprim is excreted faster (shorter half-life) than the sulfadiazine component, but trimethoprim persists longer in some tissues than in the plasma. Among the various species, doses range from 15 mg/kg twice daily, to 30 mg/kg twice daily. (See specific species recommendations below.) Doses are generally listed as the combined product; that is, 30 mg/kg is equivalent to 5 mg/kg trimethoprim + 25 mg/kg of the sulfonamide.

The safety is generally acceptable for use in dogs, except for general concerns discussed for sulfonamides previously in this chapter. Specific toxicologic studies have been conducted in both dogs and cats (Craig and White 1976). In the Craig and White study, dogs were administered up to 300 mg/kg/day orally (10 times the recommended dose) of trimethoprim-sulfadiazine for as long as 20 days with no abnormal clinical signs or blood or serum chemistry abnormalities reported. Cats were more sensitive to adverse effects. When cats were administered 30 to 300 mg/kg/day orally for 10 to 30 days, the high dose (300 mg/kg) produced signs of lethargy, anorexia, anemia, leukopenia, and altered blood urea nitrogen (BUN).

Equine Use. Trimethoprim-sulfadiazine use in horses is common. Pharmacokinetics have been reported for horses and dosing protocols have been established (White and Prior 1982; Divers et al. 1981; Bertone et al. 1988). A common use in horses includes treatment of *Streptococcus zooepidemicus* (McCandlish and Thompson 1979). However, in tissue cages placed in horses, trimethoprim-sulfadiazine did not eliminate infection of *Streptococcus zooepidemicus* (Ensink et al. 2005). The inability to eliminate the infection in an infected environment may be caused by inhibitors—such as PABA and thymidine—present in abscessed and infected tissues that may inhibit the effects of these drugs.

For horses, the proper dosing regimen was reviewed by van Duijkeren et al., (1994c). The conclusion reached from most studies in horses is that twice daily administration is needed because of the rapid elimination in horses—particularly of the trimethoprim component—and the need to maintain concentrations above the MIC throughout most of the dosing interval. For example, in horses with joint infections the optimum dosage is 30 mg/kg q12 h (Bertone et al. 1988). van Duijkeren et al. (2002) also concluded from an analysis of plasma concentrations that twice-daily administration to horses at 30 mg/kg (25 sulfadiazine; 5 trimethoprim) was necessary.

Small Animal Use. Trimethoprim-sulfadiazine has been used to treat urinary tract infections in dogs and cats (Ling et al. 1984). The combination was effective for treating urinary tract infections caused by *Staphylococcus intermedius* (Turnwald et al. 1986) as well as the more common pathogens such as *E. coli, Proteus mirabilis, Klebsiella pneumoniae,* and *Streptococcus* spp. (Ling and Ruby 1979; Ling et al. 1984). Beagle dogs treated with trimethoprim-sulfadiazine (240 mg total of a 1:5 combination) once a day or the same daily dose divided into twice daily had high concentrations of both sulfadiazine and trimethoprim in their urine that greatly exceeded the MIC values for most susceptible pathogens (Sigel et al. 1981).

An overall success rate of 85% was reported in dogs and cats treated with a trimethoprim-sulfadiazine combination for microbial diseases involving the alimentary, respiratory, urogenital, skin, and other systems (Craig 1972). A common use of trimethoprim-sulfadiazine is for the treatment of bacterial skin infections. Success rates of 90% (skin diseases either cured or improved) in bacterial skin infections; foot infections; interdigital abscesses; anal abscesses; and infections of the eye, ear, and mouth in dogs have been reported. A similar success rate was reported in cats (89%) with infections caused from bite wounds and other infections.

In dogs, pharmacokinetic studies have reported that 30 mg/kg (25 sulfadiazine + 5 trimethoprim) administered once daily, should be adequate for most infections caused by susceptible organisms (Sigel et al. 1981). In a specific study in which response for treating skin infections was examined (Messinger and Beale 1993), there was no difference in response between once- or twice-daily administration. However, the authors acknowledged that the sample size may have been too small to detect a significant difference. Supporting a once daily schedule, a study in dogs with skin infections showed that 30 mg/kg once daily is adequate (Pohlenz-Zertuche et al. 1992). These authors reported that 30 mg/kg of trimethoprim-sulfadiazine orally at 12- or 24-hour intervals were found to attain therapeutically useful concentrations of both trimethoprim and sulfadiazine in the skin (Pohlenz-Zertuche et al. 1992).

In dogs, it also has been used for *Bordetella bronchiseptica* (Powers et al. 1980), ocular infections (Sigel et al. 1981), and prostate infections. The distribution into the prostate was discussed earlier in the chapter (see the section "Distribution"). The use for treatment of protozoan infections is discussed in more detail in Chapter 43 of this book.

Cattle Use. Trimethoprim-sulfadiazine has been used to treat infections in cattle (Slaughter 1972), but because there are no longer any licensed formulations of trimethoprim-sulfadiazine for cattle, the use has diminished. Nevertheless, the pharmacokinetics have been described in calves with values reported for tissue fluids (Shoaf et al. 1986). The pharmacokinetics of sulfadiazine and trimethoprim are reported for calves and in cattle in Tables 33.4 and Table 33.5. Calves given sulfadiazine subcutaneously (30 mg/kg) had a rapid absorption of the drug; age and diet had no effect on sulfadiazine or trimethoprim disposition in those calves (Shoaf et al. 1987). In another study by Guard et al. (1986), calves 1 day of age showed higher serum and synovial fluid concentrations of trimethoprim and sulfadiazine than did calves of 1 week or 6 weeks of age. Sulfadiazine is acetylated in calves and cows, with no glucuronide or 5-hydroxy derivatives detected in this species (Nouws et al. 1988c). Trimethoprim-sulfadiazine concentrations also have been documented in the cerebrospinal fluid of neonatal calves (Shoaf et al. 1989). A pharmacokinetic model has been developed for determining the metabolic depletion of sulfadiazine (Woolly and Sigel 1982).

Pig Use. Trimethoprim (8 mg/kg)-sulfadiazine (40 mg/kg) was administered orally to pigs to determine bioavailability and other pharmacokinetic parameters. Bioavailability of sulfadiazine was 89% and 85% in fasted and fed pigs, respectively, while the trimethoprim resulted in bioavailability values of 90% and 92%. After IV administration of trimethoprim (4 mg/kg)-sulfadiazine (20 mg/kg), sulfadiazine was detectable in plasma up to 30 hours after administration, while the trimethoprim was found in the plasma only during the first 12 hours after dosing (Nielsen and Gyrd-Hansen 1994).

Other species in which trimethoprim-sulfadiazine was investigated include carp (Nouws et al. 1993), and ewes (Youssef et al. 1981).

TRIMETHOPRIM-SULFAMETHOXAZOLE. The most common human formulation is trimethoprim-sulfamethoxazole (Bactrim and Septra) and it is referred to as *cotrimoxazole*. Although there are no registered veterinary formulations, the generic human formulation is inexpensive and has been used commonly in dogs and horses for oral administration.

Trimethoprim-sulfamethoxazole combinations (human formulations, e.g. Septra, Bactrim) are available as liquid suspensions (48 mg/ml) or oral tablets (480 or 960 mg). The injectable formulation is 96 mg/ml (80 mg sulfamethoxazole + 16 mg trimethoprim). The injectable form should be given slowly IV. It has been used at a dose of 43.5 mg/kg (combined drugs) to treat CNS infections in foals.

Because of the availability of the human generic formulation of trimethoprim-sulfamethoxazole, it is often used in horses, dogs, and other species for oral administration. Many veterinarians consider trimethoprim-sulfamethoxazole to be interchangeable with trimethoprim-sulfadiazine. The pharmacokinetics have been examined in horses (Brown et al. 1988) and the pharmacokinetics are favorable for clinical use and dosage regimens that essentially mirror that of the use of trimethoprim-sulfadiazine.

TRIMETHOPRIM-SULFACHLORPYRIDAZINE. The studies of trimethoprim-sulfachlorpyridazine have been primarily in horses. Horses given 5 mg/kg trimethoprim and 25 mg/kg sulfachlorpyridazine IV revealed an elimination half-life of 2.57 hours (trimethoprim) and 3.78 hours (sulfachlorpyridazine) and a volume of distribution of 1.51 l/kg (trimethoprim) and 0.26 l/kg (sulfachlorpyridazine) (van Duijkeren et al. 1995). Bioavailability of the same dose of sulfachlorpyridazine in a powder formulation administered in the feed was about 46%. The dose of trimethoprim-sulfachlorpyridazine of 30 mg/kg (combined drug) twice daily is recommended for most indications in horses (Van Duijkeren et al. 1995).

SULFADIMETHOXINE-ORMETOPRIM. Sulfadimethoxine has been formulated with ormetoprim to enhance the spectrum of antimicrobial activity in a similar manner that trimethoprim enhances the activity of other sulfonamides. Commercial preparations of ormetoprim-sulfadimethoxine are available for dogs (Primor tablets), poultry (Rofenaid premix for feed) and for fish (Romet). These combinations offer the same advantages as trimethoprim-sulfonamide combinations because the ormetoprim component produces the same synergistic effect as trimethoprim.

Sulfadimethoxine-ormetoprim is available as a premix for medicated feed (Rofenaid). In this form, sulfadimethoxine-ormetoprim is used for prevention of coccidioisis in chickens and turkeys caused by susceptible *Eimeria* species and for prevention of fowl cholera. A similar formulation (Romet) also is available for treating furunculosis in salmon and trout. Sulfadimethoxine-ormetoprim oral tablets for dogs (Primor) have been used for skin and soft tissue infections, urinary tract infections, and intestinal coccidia infections. It has been administered once-daily for these indications.

There are no commercially available cattle formulations of sulfadimethoxine-ormetoprim in the U.S. However, this combination has been shown to be highly effective in treating calves with experimentally induced *Pasteurella (Mannheimia) hemolytica* pneumonia. Wilson et al. (1987) investigated the potential efficacy of a sulfadimethoxine-ormetoprim combination administered orally and IV to treat *Moraxella bovis* infections in cattle. In cattle, sulfadimethoxine-ormetoprim administered IV was effective in maintaining sufficiently high concentrations of both drugs in the tears to exceed the known MICs of 13 *Moraxella bovis* isolates and in maintaining those concentrations for approximately 6 hours. However, when the same concentration of sulfadimethoxine-ormetoprim was administered orally, sulfadimethoxine appeared in low concentrations and ormetoprim in very low or trace concentrations in the tears, indicating this combination of drugs when administered orally is not suitable for treating *Moraxella bovis* infections in cattle.

In horses, sulfadimethoxine pharmacokinetics were described by Brown et al. (1989). That study administered sulfadimethoxine-ormetoprim (45.8 mg/kg:9.2 mg/kg) orally, followed by lower oral doses (22.9 mg/kg:4.6 mg/kg) at 24-hour intervals, to healthy adult mares. Sulfadimethoxine produced peak plasma concentrations 8 hours after the initial dose, and plasma concentrations above 50 μg/mL were maintained for the entire dosing schedule. Significant concentrations were also found in the synovial fluid, peritoneal fluid, endometrium, and urine, with a small amount (2.1 mg/ml) appearing in the cerebrospinal fluid approximately 100 hours after the initial dose.

The pharmacokinetic parameters of sulfadimethoxine-ormetoprim were determined in 1- to 3-day-old foals given a sulfadimethoxine-ormetoprim dose (17.5 mg/kg:3.5 mg/kg) orally (Brown et al. 1993). In the foals, sulfadimethoxine concentrations peaked at 8 hours (55 μg/mL) after the oral dose and declined to 37.6 μg/mL 24 hours after the dose.

RESIDUES IN FOOD ANIMALS

Tissue residues from sulfonamide use in food-producing animals are a concern of both U.S. government agencies and the end consumers (Bevill 1989). FARAD (Food Animal Residue Avoidance Databank), a computerized databank of scientific and regulatory data, has specific information on the withdrawal times for sulfonamides used extralabel (www.farad.org) in food-producing animals (Riviere et al. 1986). Detection methods for sulfonamides and metabolites have also been described (Sharma et al. 1976; Agarwal 1992).

Sulfonamide residues were a problem in the United States for at least 25 years, having produced more drug-residue violations than any other drug, with the highest incidence occurring in pork, followed by veal and poultry. Residues in animal tissues consumed by humans are considered to be potential health hazards to humans. Toxic or allergic reactions to the sulfonamide class of antimicrobials have been reported in humans receiving therapeutic doses of sulfonamides. However, we are aware of no reports in the open literature about toxicity or other adverse reactions in humans consuming animal products containing trace amounts of sulfonamides or its metabolites. Evidence indicating that sulfonamides (in particular, sulfamethazine) may be carcinogenic in humans consuming small amounts over long periods of time (based on in vivo rat and mouse data) has heightened the Food Safety Inspection Service's (FSIS's) concern for controlling sulfonamide residues in food animals (USDA 1988).

The highest rate of sulfonamide-residue violations has historically occurred in swine. Sulfamethazine and sulfathiazole are the two most commonly used sulfonamides in swine feeds today. However, sulfamethazine is responsible for most of the sulfonamide-residue violations (97%) due to its mass incorporation in swine feeds and its longer half-life when compared to that of sulfathiazole (12.7 versus 1.2 hr). The primary reasons for the occurrence of violative levels of sulfonamides in pork were failure to observe drug withdrawal time, improper feed mixing, and improper cleaning of feed-mixing equipment, causing a cross-contamination of feed (Bevill 1984, 1989). During the late 1970s, 13% of swine livers were found to be in violation of federal sulfonamide tissue concentrations. At that time the maximum amount of sulfonamide (parent compound) permitted in animal tissues was 0.1 ppm, with a 7-day withdrawal period. Drug manufacturers at this time increased the withdrawal time for sulfonamides used in animal feed from 7 to 15 days, and by 1980, the violation rate in liver tissue had fallen to 4%. In 1987, the rate was reported to be 3.8% (Augsburg 1989), with the rate decreasing significantly by the end of the 1990s.

In veal calves presented for slaughter, similar problems with sulfamethazine residues have been reported. The prevalence rate of sulfamethazine violations in veal calves was 1.9% in 1979 and 2.9% in 1981. Reasons for violations in this species include administering the drug to calves by individuals unaware of the drug withdrawal time constraints, unknowingly selling calves treated with sulfonamides, not following drug label directions, not seeking professional advice regarding drug use, and failing to maintain drug use records (Bevill 1989).

Legal control of veterinary drugs is discussed in Chapter 54 of this book, and more information about residues in food-producing animals is presented in Chapter 61 of this textbook and also in previous editions. Several references are also available on this subject (Kaneene and Miller 1992; Bevill 1984; Dalvi 1988; Rosenberg 1985).

REFERENCES AND ADDITIONAL READING

Abdullah, A.S., and Baggot, J.D. 1988. The effect of food deprivation on the rate of sulfamethazine elimination in goats. Vet Res Commun 12:441–446.

Adamson, R.H., Bridges, J.W., Kibby, M.R., Walker, S.R., and Williams, R.T. 1970. The fate of sulfphdimethoxine in primates compared with other species. Biochem J 118:41–45.

Agarwal, V.K. 1992. High-performance liquid chromatographic methods for the determination of sulfonamides in tissue, milk, and eggs. J Chromatography 624:411–423.

Alavi, F.K., Rolf, L.L., and Clarke, C.R. 1993. The pharmacokinetics of sulfachlorpyridazine in channel catfish, *Icthlurus punctatus*. J Vet Pharmacol Therap 16:232–236.

Ames, T.R., Casagranda, C.L., Werdin, R.E., and Hanson, L.J. 1987. Effect of sulfadimethoxine-ormetroprim in the treatment of calves with induced Pasteurella pneumonia. AJVR 48(1):17–20.

Aronson, A.L., and Kirk, R.W. 1983. Antimicrobial drugs. In S.J. Ettinger, ed., Textbook of Veterinary Internal Medicine: Diseases of the Dog and Cat. Philadelphia: WB Saunders Co. pp. 338–366.

Ascalone, V., Jordan, J.C., and Ludwig, B.M. 1986. Determination of aditoprim, a new dihydrofolate reductase inhibitor, in the plasma of cows and pigs. J Chromatography 383:111–118.

Aschhoff, H.S. 1979. Tetroxoprim: A new inhibitor of bacterial dihydrofolate reductase. J Antimicrob Chemotherapy 5(Suppl B):19–25.

Ashworth, R.B., Epstein, R.L., Thomas, M.H., and Frobish, L.T. 1986. Sulfamethazine blood/tissue correlation study in swine. AJVR 47(12):2596–2603.

Astwood, E.B., Sullivan J., Bissell, A., and Tyslowitz, R. 1943. Action of certain sulfonamides and thiourea upon the thyroid gland of the rat. Endocrinology 32:210–225.

Augsberg, J.K. 1989. Sulfa residues in pork: An update. J Anim Sci 67:2817–2821.

Austin, F.H., and Kelly, W.R. 1966. Sulphamethylphenazole: A new long-acting sulphonamide. II. Some pharmacodynamic aspects in dogs, pigs and horses. Vet Rec 78(6):192–195.

Azad Kahn, A.K., Guthrie, G., Johnston, H.H., Truelove, S.C., and Williamson, D.H. 1983. Tissue and bacterial splitting of sulphasalazine. Clin Sci 64(3):349–354.

Baggot, J.D., Ludden, T.M., and Powers, T.E. 1976. The bioavailability, disposition kinetics and dosage of sulfadimethoxine in dogs. Can J Comp Med 40:310–317. (Correction in 1977; 41: 479–480.)

Banerjee, N.C., Yadava, K.P., and Jha, H.N. 1974. Distribution of sulphaquinoxaline in tissues of poultry. Ind J Physiol Pharmacol 18(4):361–363.

Berger, S.L., Scagliotti, R.H., Lund, E.M. 1995. A quantitative study of the effects of tribrissen on canine tear production. JAAHA 31:236–241.

Bertone, A.L., Jones, R.L., and McIlwraith, C.W. 1988. Serum and synovial fluid steady-state concentrations of trimethoprim and sulfadiazine in horses with experimentally induced infectious arthritis. AJVR 49(10):1681–1687.

Bevill, R.F. 1984. Factors influencing the occurrence of drug residues in animal tissues after the use of antimicrobial agents in animal feeds. JAVMA 185(10):1124–1126.

———. 1988. Sulfonamides. In N.H. Booth and L.E. McDonald, eds., Veterinary Pharmacology and Therapeutics, 6th ed., pp. 785–795. Ames: Iowa State Univ Press.

———. 1989. Sulfonamide residues in domestic animals. J Vet Pharmacol Therap 12:241–252.

Bevill, R.F., Dittert, L.W., and Bourne, D.W.A. 1977a. Disposition of sulfonamides in food-producing animals IV: Pharmacokinetics of sulfamethazine in cattle following administration of an intravenous dose and three oral dosage forms. J Pharm Sci 66(5):619–623.

Bevill, R.F., Koritz, G.D., Dittert, L.W., and Bourne, W.A. 1977b. Disposition of sulfonamides in food-producing animals. V. Disposition of sulfathiazole in tissue, urine, and plasma of sheep following intravenous administration. J Pharm Sci 66(9):1297–1300.

Bevill, R.F., Sharma, R.M., Meachum, S.H., Wozniak, S.C., Bourne, D. W.A., and Dittert, L.W. 1977c. Disposition of sulfonamides in food-producing animals: Concentrations of sulfamethazine and its metabolites in plasma, urine, and tissues of lambs following intravenous administration. AJVR 38:973–977.

Biehl, L.G., Bevill, R.F., Limpoka, and Koritz, G.D. 1981. Sulfamethazine residues in swine. J Vet Pharmacol Therap 4:285–290.

Blackwell, T.E., Werdin, R.E., Eisenmenger, M.C., and FitzSimmons, M.A. 1989. Goitrogenic effects in offspring of swine fed sulfadimethoxine and ormetoprim in late gestation. JAVMA 194(4):519–523.

Bourne, D.W.A., Bevill, R.F., Sharma, R.M., Gural, R.P., and Dittert, L.W. 1977. Disposition of sulfonamides in food-producing animals: pharmacokinetics of sulfamethazine in lambs. AJVR 38:967–972.

Bourne, D.W.A., Bialer, M., Kittert, L.W., Hayashi, M., Rudawsky, G., Koritz, G.D., and Bevill, R.F. 1981. Disposition of sulfadimethoxine in cattle: inclusion of protein binding factors in a pharmacokinetic model. J Pharm Sci 70(9):1068–1074.

Boxenbaum, H.G., Fellig, J., Hanson, L.J., Snyder, W.E., and Kaplan, S.A. 1977. Pharmacokinetics of sulphadimethoxine in cattle. Res Vet Sci 23:24–28.

Bridges, J.W., Kibby, M.R., Walker, S.R., and Williams, R.T. 1968. Species differences in the metabolism of sulfadimethoxine. Biochem J 109:851–856.

Bridges, J.W., Walker, S.R., and Williams, R.T. 1969. Species differences in the metabolism and excretion of sulphasomidine and sulphamethomidine. Biochem J 111:173–179.

Brown, M.J., Wojcik, B., Burgess, E.D., and Smith, G.J. 1982. Adverse reactions to sulfaquinoxaline in coyote pups. JAVMA 181(11): 1419–1420.

Brown, M.P., Gronwall, R., and Castro, L. 1988. Pharmacokinetics and body fluid and endometrial concentrations of trimethoprim-sulfamethoxazole in mares. Am J Vet Res 49:918–922.

Brown, M.P., Gronwall, R.R., Cook, L.K., and Houston, A.E. 1993. Serum concentrations of ormetoprim/sulfadimethoxine in 1–3-day-old foals after a single dose of oral paste combination. Eq Vet J 25(1):73–74.

Brown, M.P., Gronwall, R.R., and Houston, A.E. 1989. Pharmacokinetics and body fluid and endometrial concentrations of ormetoprim-sulfadimethoxine in mares. Can J Vet Res 53:12–16.

Brown, P., Kelly, R.H., Stover, S.M., and Gronwall, R. 1983. Trimethoprim-sulfadiazine in the horse: serum, synovial, peritoneal, and urine concentrations after single-dose administration. Am J Vet Res 44:540–543.

Bulgin, M.S., Lane, V.M., Archer, T.E., Baggot, and Craigmill, A.L. 1991. Pharmacokinetics, safety and tissue residues of sustained-release sulfamethazine in sheep. J Vet Pharmacol Therap 14:36–45.

Bushby, S.R.M. 1980. Sulfonamide and trimethoprim combinations. JAVMA 176(10):1049–1053.

Campbell, K.L. 1999. Sulphonamides: updates on use in veterinary medicine. Vet Derm 10:205–215.

Cannon, R.W. 1976. Clinical evaluation of tribrissen: New antibacterial agent for dogs and cats. VMSAC 71(8):1090–1095.

Carlson, A., Rupe, B.D., Buss, D., Homman, C., and Leaton, J. 1976. Evaluation of a new prolonged-release sulfamethazine bolus for use in cattle. VMSAC 71(5):693–696.

Chapman, H.D. 1989. Chemotherapy of caecal coccidiosis: efficacy of toltrazuril, sulphaquinoxalin/pyrimethamine and amprolium/ethopabate, given in drinking water, against field isolated *Eimeria tenella*. Res Vet Sci 46:419–420.

Church, T.L., Janzen, E.D., Sisodia, C.S., and Radostits, O.M. 1979. Blood levels of sulfamethazine achieved in beef calves on medicated drinking water. Can Vet J 20:41–44.

Clark, J.G., Mackey, D.R., and Scheel, E.H. 1966. Evaluation of sustained-release sulfamethazine in infectious diseases of cattle. VMSAC 11:1103–1104.

Clarke, C.R., Short, C.R., Corstvet, R.E., and Nobles, D. 1989. Effect of *Pasteurella haemolytica* infection on the distribution of sulfadiazine and trimethoprim into tissue chambers implanted subcutaneously in cattle. Am J Vet Res 50: 1551–1556.

CLSI. 2007. Performance Standards for Antimicrobial Disk and Dilution Susceptibility Tests for Bacteria Isolated From Animals; Approved Standard—Third Edition. CLSI document, M31-A3. Wayne, PA: Clinical and Laboratory Standards Institute.

Collins, B.K., Moore, C.P., and Hagee, J.H. 1986. Sulfonamide-associated keratoconjunctivitis sicca and corneal ulceration in a dysuric dog. JAVMA 189(8):924–926.

Cordle, M.K. 1989. Sulfonamide residues in pork: past, present, and future. J Anim Sci 67(10):2810–2816.

Craig, G.R. 1972. The place for potentiated trimethoprim in the therapy of diseases of the skin in dogs and cats. J Small Animal Pract 13:65–70.

Craig, G.R., and White, G. 1976. Studies in dogs and cats dosed wtih trimethoprim and sulphadiazine. Vet Rec 98(5):82–86.

Cribb, A.E. 1989. Idiosyncratic reactions to sulfonamides in dogs. JAVMA 195(11):1612–1614.

Cribb, A.E., Spielberg, S.P. 1990. An in vitro investigation of predisposition to sulphonamide idiosyncratic toxicity in dogs. Vet Res Comm 14:241–252.

Daft, B.M., Bickford, A.A., and Hammarlund, M.A. 1989. Experimental and field sulfaquinoxaline toxicosis in Leghorn chickens. Avian Dis 33:30–34.

Dagorn, M., Moulin, G., Laurentie, M., and Delmas, J.M. 1991. Plasma and lung pharmacokinetics of trimethoprim and sulphadiazine combinations administered to broilers. Acta Veterinaria Scandinavica 87:273–277.

Dalvi, R.F. 1988. Comparative in vitro and in vivo drug metabolism in major and minor food-producing species. Vet Human Toxicol 30(Suppl 1):22–25.

Das, K.M., Chowdhury, J.R., Zapp, B., and Fara, J.W. 1979. Small bowel absorption of sulfasalazine and its hepatic metabolism in human beings, cats, and rats. Gastroenterology 77:280–284.

Das, K.M., and Dubin, R. 1976. Clinical pharmacokinetics of sulphasalazine. Clin Pharmacokinetics 1:406–425.

Davis, R.E., and Jackson, J.M. 1973. Trimethoprim/sulphmethoxazole and folate metabolism. Pathology 5:23–29.

Davitiyananda, D., and Rasmussen F. 1974. Half-lives of sulfadoxine and trimethoprim after a single intravenous infusion in cows. Acta Vet Scand 15:356–365.

Debacker, P., Belpaire, F.M., Bogaert, M.G., and Debackere, M. 1982. Pharmacokinetics of sulfamerazine and antipyrine in neonatal and young lambs. AJVR 43(10):1744–1751.

Del Soldato, P., Campieri, M., Brignola, C., Bazzocchi, G., Gionchetti, P., Lanfranchi, G.A., and Tamba, M. 1985. A possible mechanism of action of sulfasalazine and 5-aminosalicylic acid in inflammatory bowel disease: interaction with oxygen free radicals. Gastroenterology 89(5):1215–1216.

Divers, J., Byars, T.D., Murch, O., and Sigel, C.W. 1981. Experimental induction of *Proteus mirabilis* cystitis in the pony and evaluation of therapy with trimethoprim-sulfadiazine. AJVR 42:1203–1205.

Dodds, W.J. 1993. Hemorrhagic complications attributable to certain drugs. JAVMA 202(5):702–703.

———. 1997. Letter to the Editor. J Vet Internal Med 11:267–268.

Dow, S.W. 1988. Management of anaerobic infections. Vet Clin N Am Sm An Pract 18(6):1167–1182.

Duffee, E., Bevill, R.F., Thurmon, J.C., Luther, H.G., Nelson, D.E., and Hacker, F.E. 1984. Pharmacokinetics of sulfamethazine in male, female, and castrated male swine. J Vet Pharmacol Therap 7:203–211.

Dunbar, R., and Foreyt, W.J. 1985. Prevention of coccidiosis in domestic dogs and captive coyotes (*Canis latrans*) with sulfadimethoxine-ormetoprim combination. AJVR 46(9):1899–1902.

Eastwood, M.A. 1980. Pharmacokinetic patterns of sulfasalazine. Therapeutic Drug Monitoring 2:149–152.

Ellison, T., Scheidy, S.F., Tucker, S., Scott, G.C., and Bucy, C.B. 1967. Blood concentration studies in cattle of a sustained-release form of sulfamethazine. JAVMA 150(6):629–633.

Elsheikh, H.A., Ali, B.H., Homeida, A.M., Hassan, T., and Hapke, H.J. 1991. Pharmacokinetics of antipyrine and sulphadimidine (sulfamethazine) in camels, sheep, and goats. J Vet Pharmacol Therap 14:269–275.

Ensink, J.M., Bosch, G., and van Duikjeren, E. 2005. Clinical efficacy of prophylactic administration of trimethoprim-sulfadiazine in a *Streptococcus equi subsp. zooepidemicus* infection model in ponies. J Vet Pharmacol Therap 28:45–49.

Eppel, J.G., and Thiessen, J.J. 1984. Liquid chromatographic analysis of sulfaquinoxaline and its application to pharmacokinetic studies in rabbits. J Pharm Sci 73(11):1635–1638.

Epstein, R.L., and Ashworth, R.B. 1989. Tissue sulfonamide concentration and correlation in turkeys. AJVR 50(6):926–928.

Fenwick, B.W., and Olander, H.J. 1987. Experimental infection of weanling pigs with *Salmonella typhisuis:* effect of feeding low concentrations of chlortetracycline, penicillin, and sulfamethazine. AJVR 48(11): 1568–1573.

Fish, J.G., Morgan, D.W., and Horton, C.R. 1965. Clinical experiences with sulfadimethoxine in small animal practice. VMSAC 60(12): 1201–1203.

Frank, L.A., Hnilica, K.A., May, E.R., Sargent, S.J., and Davis, J.A. 2005. Effects of sulfamethoxazole-trimethoprim on thyroid function in dogs. Am J Vet Res 66:256–259.

Fullerton, F.R., Kushmaul, R.J., Suber, R.L., and Littlefield, N.A. 1987. Influence of oral administration of sulfamethazine on thyroid hormone levels in Fischer 344 rats. J Toxicol Environ Health 22:175–185.

Garg, G.P., Cho, C.H., and Ogle, C.W. 1991. The role of the gastric mucosal sulphydryls in the ulcer-protecting effects of sulfasalazine. J Pharm Pharmacol 43:733–734.

Garg, S.K., and Uppal, R.P. 1997. Bioavailability of sulfamethoxypyridazine following intramuscular or subcutaneous administration in goats. Vet Res 28:101–104.

Garwacki, S., Hornik, H., Karlik, W., and Dabrowski, J. 1991. Pharmacokinetics of sulfamerazine in sheep fed ad libitum and fasted. Acta Veterinaria Scandinavica 87:145–146.

Giger, U., Werner, L.L., Millichamp, N.J., and Gorman, N.T. 1985. Sulfadiazine-induced allergy in six Doberman Pinschers. JAVMA 186(5):479–484.

Giwercman, A., and Skakkebaek, N.E. 1986. The effect of salicylazosulphapyridine (sulfasalazine) on male fertility. A review. Inter J Andrology 9:38–52.

Gomez-Bautista, M., and Rojo-Vazauez, F.A. 1986. Chemotherapy and chemoprophylaxis of hepatic coccidiosis with sulphadimethoxine and pyrimethamine. Res Vet Sci 41:28–32.

Goren, E., de Jong, W.A., and Doornenbal, P. 1987. Additional studies on the therapeutic efficacy of sulphadimidine sodium in experimental *Eschericha coli* infection of broilers. Vet Quarterly 9(1):86–87.

Green, S.L., Mahew, I.G., Brown, M.P., et al. 1990. Concentrations of trimethoprim and sulfamethoxazole in cerebrospinal fluid and serum in mares with and without a dimethyl sulfoxide pretreatment. Can J Vet Res 54(2):215–222.

Greko, C., Bengtsson, B., Franklin, A., Jacobsson, S.-O., Wiese, B., and Luthman, J. 2002. Efficacy of trimethoprim-sulfadoxine against *Escherichia coli* in a tissue cage model in calves. J Vet Pharmacol Therap 25:413–423.

Guard, C.L., Schwark, W.S., Friedman, D.S., Blackshear, P., and Haluska, M. 1986. Age-related alterations in trimethoprim-sulfadiazine disposition following oral or parenteral administration in calves. Can J Vet Res 50:342–346.

Guise, H.J., Penny, H.C., and Petherick, D.J. 1986. Streptococcal meningitis in pigs: field trial to study the prophylactic effect of trimethoprim/sulphadiazine medication in feed. Vet Rec 119(16):395–400.

Gustafsson, A., Båverud, V., Franklin, A., Gunnarsson, A., Ögren, G., Ingvast-Larsson, C. 1999. Repeated administration of trimethoprim-sulfadiazine in the horse—pharmacokinetics, plasma protein binding, and influence on the intestinal flora. J Vet Pharmacol Therap 22:20–26.

Hall, I.A., Campbell, K.L., Chambers, M.D., and Davis, C.N. 1993. Effect of trimethoprim/sulfamethoxazole on thyroid function in dogs with pyoderma. JAVMA 202:1959–1962.

Hayashi, M., Bourne, D.W.A., Bevill, R.F., and Koritz, G.D. 1979. Disposition of sulfonamides in food-producing animals: pharmacokinetics of sulfamerazine in ewe lambs. AJVR 49(11):1578–1582.

Hoult, J.R.S., and Moore, P.K. 1978. Sulphasalazine is a potent inhibitor of prostaglandin 15-hydroxydehydrogenase: possible basis for therapeutic action in ulcerative colitis. Br J Pharmacol 64:6–8.

Howell, T.H., Reddy, M.S., Weber, H.P., Li, K.L., Alfano, M.C., Vogel, R, Tanner, ACR, and Williams, RC. 1989. Sulfadiazines prevent plaque formation and gingivitis in beagles. J Periodont Res 25:197–200.

Imamura, Y., Nakamura, H., and Otagiri, M. 1986. Effect of phenylbutazone on serum protein binding of sulfadimethoxine in different animal species. J Pharmacobio-Dyn 9:694–696.

———. 1989. Effect of phenylbutazone on serum protein binding and pharmacokinetic behavior of sulfadimethoxine in rabbits, dogs and rats. J Pharmacobio-Dyn 12:208–215.

Inada, H., Endoh, M., Katayama, K., Kakemi, M., and Koizumi, T. 1989. Factors affecting sulfisoxizole transport through excised rat skin during iontophoresis. Chem Pharm Bull 37(7):1870–1873.

Indiveri, M.C., and Hirsh, D.C. 1986. Susceptibility of obligate anaerobes to trimethoprim-sulfamethoxazole. J Am Vet Med Assoc 188(1): 46–48.

———. 1992. Tissues and exudates contain sufficient thymidine for growth of anaerobic bacteria in the presence of inhibitory levels of trimethoprim-sulfamethoxazole. Vet Microbiol 31(2–3):235–242.

Iverson, P., Vergin, H., and Madsen, P.O. 1984. Renal handling and lymph concentration of tetroxoprim and metioprim: An experimental study in dogs. J Urology 132:362–362.

James, M.O., and Barron, M.G. 1988. Disposition of sulfadimethoxine in the lobster (*Homarus americanus*). Vet Human Toxicol 30(Suppl 1): 36–40.

Joyner, L.P., Catchpole, J., and Berrett, S. 1983. *Eimeria stiedai* in rabbits: The demonstration of responses to chemotherapy. Res Vet Sci 34:64–67.

Kajinuma, H., Kuzuya, T., and Ide, T. 1974. Effects of hypoglycemic sulfonamides on glucagon and insulin secretion in ducks and dogs. Diabetes 23(5):412–417.

Kaneene, J.B., and Miller, R. 1992. Description and evaluation of the influence of veterinary presence on the use of antibiotics and sulfonamides in dairy herds. JAVMA 201(1):68–76.

Khan, A.K.A., Guthrie, G., Johnston, H.H., Truelove, S.C., and Williamson, D.H. 1983. Tissue and bacterial splitting of sulphasalazine. Clin Sci 64:349–354.

Kleinow, K.M., and Lech, J.J. 1988. A review of the pharmacokinetics and metabolism of sulfadimethoxine in the rainbow trout. Vet Human Toxicol 30(Suppl 1):26–30.

Kobland, J.D., Gale, G.O., Maddock, H.M., Garces, T.R., and Simkins, K.L. 1984. Comparative efficacy of sulfamethazine and sulfathiazole in feed for control of *Bordetella bronchiseptica* infection in swine. AJVR 45(4):720–723.

Koritz, G.D., Bevill, R.F., Bourne, D.W.A., and Dittert, L.W. 1978. Disposition of sulfonamides in food-producing animals: pharmacokinetics of sulfathiazole in swine. AJVR 39(3):481–484.

Koritz, G.D., Bourne, D.W.A., Dittert, L.W., and Bevill, R.F. 1977. Disposition of sulfonamides in food-producing animals: pharmacokinetics of sulfathiazole in sheep. AJVR 38:979–982.

Koudela, B., and Bokova, A. 1997. The effect of cotrimoxazole on experimental *Cryptosporidium parvum* infection in kids. Vet Res 28:405–412.

Lapka, R., Urbanova, Z., Raskova, H., Cerny, J., Sykora, Z., Vanecek, J., Ploak, L., and Kubicek, A. 1980. Acetylation of sulphadimidine in calves. Gen Pharmacol 11:147–148.

Lashev, L.D., Bochukov, A.K., and Penchev, G. 1995. Effect of testosterone on the pharmacokinetics of sulphadimidine and sulphachloropyrazine in roosters: a preliminary report. Br Vet J 151:331–336.

Lashev, L.D., and Mihailov, R. 1994. Pharmacokinetics of sulphamethoxazole and trimethoprim administered intravenously and orally to Japanese quails. J Vet Pharmacol Therap 17:327–330.

Li, T., Qiao, G.L., Hu, G.Z., Meng, F.D., Qiu, U.S., Zhang, X.Y., Guo, W.X., Yie, H.L., Li, S.F., and Li, S.Y. 1995. Comparative plasma and tissue pharmacokinetics and drug residue profiles of different chemotherapeutants in fowls and rabbits. J Vet Pharmacol Therap 18:260–273.

Ling, G.V., Rohrich, P.J., Ruby, A.L., Johnson, D.L., and Jang, S.S. 1984. Canine urinary tract infections: a comparison of in vitro antimicrobial susceptibility test results and response to oral therapy with ampicillin or with trimethoprim-sulfa. JAVMA 185(3):277–281.

Ling, G.V., and Ruby, A.L. 1979. Trimethoprim in combination with a sulfonamide for oral treatment of canine urinary tract infections. JAVMA 174(9):1003–1005.

Littlefield, N.A., Gaylor, D.W., Blackwell, B.N., and Allen, R.R. 1989. Chronic toxicity/carcinogenicity studies of sulphamethazine in B6C3F1 mice. Fd Chem Toxicol 27(7):455–463.

Littlefield, N.A., Sheldon, W.G., Allen, R., and Gaylor, D.W. 1990. Chronic toxicity/carcinogenicity studies of sulphamethazine in Fischer 344/N rats: Two-generation exposure. Food Chem Toxicol 28(3):157–167.

Lohuis, J.A.C.M., Sutter, H.M., Graser, T., Ludwig, B., van Miert, A. S.J.P.A.M., Rehm, W.F., Rohde, E., Schneider, B., Wanner, and van Werven, T. 1992. Effects of endotoxin-induced mastitis on the pharmacokinetic properties of aditoprim in dairy cows. AJVR 53(12):2311–2314.

MacKenzie, C.G., and MacKenzie, J.B. 1943. Effect of sulfonamides and thiourea on thyroid gland and basal metabolism. Endocrinology 32:185–209.

Mathis, G.F., and McDougald, L.R. 1984. Effectiveness of therapeutic anticoccidial drugs against recently isolated coccidia. Poultry Sci 63:1149–1153.

McCaig, J. 1970. A clinical trial using trimethoprim-sulphadiazine in dogs and cats. Vet Rec 87(9):265–266.

McCandlish, I.A.P., and Thompson, H. 1979. Canine bordetellosis: chemotherapy using a sulphadiazine-trimethoprim combination. Vet Rec 105(3):51–54.

Medleau, L., Shanley, K.J., Rakich, P.M., et al. 1990. Trimethoprim-sulfonamide-associated drug eruptions in dogs. J Am Anim Hosp Assoc 26:305–311.

Mengelers, M.J.B., Hougee, P.E., Janssen, L.H.M., and van Miert, A.S.J.P.A.M. 1997. Structure activy relatinoshops between antibacterial activities and physiochemical properties of sulfonamides. J Vet Pharmacol Ther 20:276–283.

Mengelers, M.J.B., van Klingeren, B., and van Miert, A.S.J.P.A.M. 1990. In vitro susceptibility of some porcine respiratory tract pathogens to aditoprim, trimethoprim, sulfadimethoxine, sulfamethoxazole, and combinations of these agents. AJVR 51(11):1860–1864.

Mengelers, M.J.B., van Gogh, E.R., Kuiper, H.A., Pijpers, A., Verheijden, J.H.M., and van Miert, A.S.J.P.A.M. 1995. Pharmacokinetics of sulfadimethoxine and sulfamethoxazole in combination with trimethoprim after intravenous administration to healthy and pneumonic pigs. J Vet Pharmacol Therap 18:243–253.

Messinger, L.M., Beale, K.M. 1993. A blinded comparison of the efficacy of daily and twice daily trimethoprim-sulfadiazine and daily sulfadimethoxine-ormetoprim therapy in the treatment of canine pyoderma. Vet Derm 4:13–18.

Miller, G.E., Stowe, C.M., Jegers, A., and Bucy, C.B. 1969. Blood concentration studies of a sustained release form of sulfamethazine in cattle. JAVMA 154(7):733–779.

Mitchell, AD, and Paulson, GD. 1986. Depletion kinetics of 14C-sulfamethazine {4-amino-N-(4,6-dimethyl-2-pyr}midinyl)benzene[U-14C]sulfonamide metabolism in swine. Drug Metabol Disposition 14(2):161–165.

Mitchell, A.D., Paulson, G.D., and Zaylskie, R.G. 1986. Steady state kinetics of 14C-sulfamethazine {4-amino-N-(4,6-dimethyl-2-pyr}midinyl)benzene[U-14C]sulfonamide metabolism in swine. Drug Metabol Disposition 14(2):155–160.

Morgan, R.V., and Bachrach, A. 1982. Keratoconjunctivitis sicca associated with sulfonamide therapy in dogs. JAVMA 180(4):432–434.

Nawaz, M., and Nawaz, R. 1983. Pharmacokinetics and urinary excretion of sulphadimidine in sheep during summer and winter. Vet Rec 112(16):379–381.

Neer, T.M., and Savant, R.L. 1992. Hypoprothrombinemia secondary to administration of sulfaquinoxaline to dogs in a kennel setting. JAVMA 200(9):1344–1345.

Nielsen, P., and Gyrd-Hansen, N. 1994. Oral bioavailability of sulphadiazine and trimethoprim in fed and fasted pigs. Res Vet Sci 56:48–52.

Noli, C., Koeman, J.P., and Willemse, T. 1995. A retrospective evaluation of adverse reactions to trimethoprim-sulphonamide combinations in dogs and cats. Vet Quarterly 17:123–128.

Nouws, J.F.M., Firth, E.C., Vree, T.B., and Baakman, M. 1987. Pharmacokinetics and renal clearance of sulfamethazine, sulfamerazine, and sulfadiazine and their N_4-acetyl and hydroxy metabolites in horses. AJVR 48(3):392–402.

Nouws, J.F.M., Geertsma, M.F., Grondel, J.L., Aerts, M.M.L., Vree, T.B., and Kan, C.A. 1988a. Plasma disposition and renal clearance of sulphadimidine and its metabolites in laying hens. Res Vet Sci 44:202–207.

Nouws, J.F.M., Meesen, B.P.W., van Gogh, H., Korstanje, C., van Miert, A.S.J.P.A.M., Vree, T.B., and Degen, M. 1988b. The effect of testosterone and rutting on the metabolism and pharmacokinetics of sulphadimidine in goats. J Vet Pharmacol Therap 11:145–154.

Nouws, J.F.M., Mevius, D., Vree, T.B., Baakman, M., and Degen, M. 1988c. Pharmacokinetics, metabolism, and renal clearance of sulfadiazine, sulfamerazine, and sulfamethazine and of their N4-acetyl and hydroxy metabolites in calves and cows. AJVR 49(7):1059–1065.

Nouws, J.F.M., Mevius, D., Vree, T.B., and Degen, M. 1989a. Pharmacokinetics and renal clearance of sulphadimidine, sulphamerazine, and sulphadiazine and their N4-acetyl and hydroxy metabolites in pigs. Vet Quarterly 11(2):78–86.

Nouws, J.F.M., van Ginneken, J.T., Grondel, J.L., and Degen, M. 1993. Pharmacokinetics of sulphadiazine and trimethoprim in carp (*Cyprinus carpio* L.) acclimated at two different temperatures. J Vet Pharmacol Therap 16:110–113.

Nouws, J.F.M., Vree, T.B., Baakman, M., Driessens, F., Breukink, H.J., and Mevius, D. 1986a. Age and dosage dependency in the plasma disposition and the renal clearance of sulfamethazine and its N4-acetyl and hydroxy metabolites in calves and cows. AJVR 47(3):642–649.

Nouws, J.F.M., Vree, T.B., Baakman, M., Driessens, F., Smulders, A., and Holtkamp, J. 1985a. Disposition of sulfadimidine and its N4-acetyl and hydroxy metabolites in horse plasma. J Vet Pharmacol Therap 8:303–311.

Nouws, J.F.M., Vree, T.B., Baakman, M., Driessens, F., Vellenga, L., and Mevius, D.J. 1986b. Pharmacokinetics, renal clearance, tissue distribution, and residue aspects of sulphadimidine and its N4-acetyl metabolite in pigs. Vet Quarterly 8(2):123–135.

Nouws, J.F.M., Vree, T.B., Baakman, M., and Tijhuis, M. 1983. Effect of age on the acetylation and deacetylation reactions of sulphadimidine and N4-acetylsulphadimidine in calves. J Vet Pharmacol Therap 6:13–22.

Nouws, J.F.M., Vree, T.B., Breukink, H.J., Baakman, M., Driessens, F., and Smulders, A. 1985b. Dose dependent disposition of sulphadimidine and of its N4-acetyl and hydroxy metabolites in plasma and milk of dairy cows. Vet Quarterly 7(3):177–186.

Nouws, J.F.M., Watson, A.D.J., van Miert, A.S.J.P.A.M., Degen, M., van Gogh, H., and Vree, T.B. 1989b. Pharmacokinetics and metabolism of sulphadimidine in kids at 12 and 18 weeks of age. J Vet Pharmacol Therap 12:19–24.

Panciera, D.L., and Post, K. 1992. Effect of oral administration of sulfadiazine and trimethoprim in combination on thyroid function in dogs. Can J Vet Res 56:349–352.

Patterson, J.M., and Grenn, H.H. 1975. Hemorrhage and death in dogs following the administration of sulfaquinoxaline. Can Vet J 16(9):265–268.

Piercy, D.W.T., Williams, R.B., and White, G. 1984. Evaluation of a mixture of trimethoprim and sulphaquinoxaline for the treatment of poultry: safety and palatability studies. Vet Rec 114(3):60–62.

Pohlenz-Zertuche, H.O., Brown, M.P., Gronwall, R., Kunkle, G.A., and Merritt, K. 1992. Serum and skin concentrations after multiple-dose oral administration of trimethoprim-sulfadiazine in dogs. American Journal of Veterinary Research 53(7):1273–1276.

Powers, T.E., Powers, J.D., Garg, R.C., Scialli, V.T., and Hajian, G.H. 1980. Trimethoprim and sulfadiazine: Experimental infection of beagles. AJVR 41(7):1117–1122.

Prescott, J.F., and Baggot, J.D., eds. 1993. Sulfonamides, trimethoprim, ormetoprim, and their combinations. In Antimicrobial Therapy in Veterinary Medicine, 2d ed., pp. 229–251. Ames: Iowa State Univ Press.

Ribelin, W.E., Owen, G., Rubin, L.F., Levinskas, G.J., and Agersborg, H. P.K. 1967. Development of cataracts in dogs and rats from prolonged feeding of sulfaethoxypyridazine. Toxicol Appl Pharmacol 10:557–564.

Riffat, S., Nawaz, M., and Rehman, Z.U. 1982. Pharmacokinetics of suphadimidine in normal and febrile dogs. J Vet Pharmacol Therap 5:131–135.

Righter, H.F., Worthington, J.M., and Mercer, H.D. 1971. Tissue-residue depletion of sulfamethazine in calves and chickens. AJVR 32(7):1003–1006.

Righter, H.R., Showalter, D.H., and Teske, R.H. 1979. Pharmacokinetic study of sulfadimethoxine depletion in suckling and growing pigs. AJVR 49(5):713–715.

Riviere, J.E., Craigmill, A.L., and Sundlof, S.F. 1986. Food animal residue avoidance databank (FARAD): an automated pharmacologic databank for drug and chemical residue avoidance. J Food Protection 49(10):826–830.

Robb, C.A., Carroll, P.T., Tippett, L.O., and Langston, J.B. 1971. The diffusion of selected sulfonamides, trimethoprim, and diaveridine into prostatic fluid of dogs. Invest Urology 8(6):679–685.

Rosenberg, M.C. 1985. Update on the sulfonamide residue problem. JAVMA 187(7):704–705.

Roujeau, J.-C., Kelly, J.P., Naldi, L., et al. 1995. Medication use and the risk of Stevens-Johnson syndrome or toxic epidermal necrolysis. New Engl J Med 333:1600–1607.

Rowland, P.H., Center, S.A., and Dougherty, S.A. 1992. Presumptive trimethoprim-sulfadiazine-related hepatotoxicosis in a dog. JAVMA 200(3):348–350.

Sainsbury, D.W.B. 1988. Potentiated sulphaquinoxaline used as "strategic medication" for broiler poultry. Vet Rec 122(16):395.

Scheidy, S.F., and Bucy, C.B. 1967. Evaluation of a prolonged-acting oral dose form of sulfamethazine in cattle. VMSAC 62(12):1161–1164.

Shafii, A., Chowdhury, J.R., and Das, K.M. 1982. Absorption, enterohepatic circulation, and excretion of 5-aminosalicylic acid in rats. Am J Gastroenterology 77(5):297–299.

Sharma, J.P., Perkins, E.G., and Bevill, R.F. 1976. High-pressure liquid chromatographic separation, identification, and determination of sulfa drugs and their metabolites in urine. J Pharm Sci 1606–1608.

Shimoda, M., Kokue, E., Itani, M., Hayama, T., and Vree, T.B. 1989. Nonlinear pharmacokinetics of intravenous sulphadimethoxine and its dosage regimen in pigs. Vet Quarterly 11(4):242–250.

Shoaf, S.E., Schwark, W.S., and Guard, C.L. 1987. The effect of age and diet on sulfadiazine/trimethoprim disposition following oral and subcutaneous administration to calves. J Vet Pharmacol Therap 10:331–345.

———. 1989. Pharmacokinetics of sulfadiazine/trimethoprim in neonatal male calves: effect of age and penetration into cerebrospinal fluid. AJVR 50(3):396–403.

Shoaf, S.E., Schwark, W.S., Guard, C.L., and Schwartsman, R.V. 1986. Pharmacokinetics of trimethoprim/sulfadiazine in neonatal calves: influence of synovitis. J Vet Pharmacol Therap 9:446–454.

Sigel, C.W., Ling, G.V., Bushby, R.M., Woolley, J.L., DeAngelis, D., and Eure, S. 1981. Pharmacokinetics of trimethoprim and sulfadiazine in the dog: urine concentrations after oral administration. AJVR 42(6): 996–1001.

Sigel, C.W., Macklin, A.W., Grace, M.E., and Tracy, C.H. 1981. Trimethoprim and sulfadiazine concentrations in aqueous and vitreous humors of the dog. VMSAC 76(7):991–993.

Singh, M.K., Jayachandran, C., Roy, G.P., and Banerjee, N.C. 1988. Pharmacokinetics and distribution of sulphadimidine in plasma, milk and uterine fluid of female buffaloes. Vet Res Commun 12:41–46.

Slatter, D.H., and Blogg, J.R. 1978. Keratoconjunctivitis sicca in dogs associated with sulphonamide administration. Aust Vet J 54:444–446.

Slaughter, R.E. 1972. Potentiated trimethoprim for the therapy of calf scours. New Zealand Vet J 20:221–223.

Slavik, D., Oehme, F.W., and Schoneweis, D.A. 1980. Plasma levels of sulfadimethoxine in swine given the medication in their water. VMSAC 75(6):1035–1038.

Soli, N.E., Framstad, T., Skjerve, E., Sohlberg, S., and Odegaard, S.A. 1990. A comparison of some of the pharmacokinetic parameters of three commercial sulfphadiazine/trimethoprim combined preparations given orally to pigs. Vet Res Commun 14:403–410.

Squibb, K.S., Michel, C.M.F., Zelikoff, J.T, and O'Conner, J.M. 1988. Sulfadimethoxine pharmacokinetics and metabolism in the channel catfish (*Ictalurus punctatus*). Vet Human Toxicol 30(Suppl 1):31–35.

Srivastava, A.K., and Rampal, S. 1990. Disposition kinetics and dosage regimen of sulphamethazine in sheep (*Ovis aries*). Br Vet J 146:239–242.

Stampa, S. 1986. A field trial comparing the efficacy of sulphamonomethoxine, penicillin, and tarantula poison in the treatment of pododermatitis circumspecta of cattle. J So African Vet Assn 57(2):91–93.

Stockner, P.K. 1993. More on hemorrhagic complications attributable to certain drugs. JAVMA 202:1547.

Suber, R.L., Lee, C., Torosian, G., and Edds, G.T. 1981. Pharmacokinetics of sulfisoxazole compared to humans and two monogastric species. J Pharm Sci 70(9):981–984.

Sullivan, P.S., Arrington, K., West, R., and McDonald, T.P. 1992. Thrombocytopenia associated with administration of trimethoprim/sulfadiazine in a dog. JAVMA 201(11):1741–1744.

Sutter, H.M., Riond, J.L., and Wanner, M. 1993. Comparative pharmacokinetics of aditoprim in milk-fed and conventionally fed calves of different ages. Res Vet Sci 54:86–93.

Swarm, R.L., Robers, G.K.S., Levy, A.C., and Hines, L.R. 1973. Observations on the thyroid gland in rats following the administration of sulfamethoxazole and trimethoprim. Toxicol Appl Pharmacol 24:351–363.

Sweeney, R.W., Bardalaye, P.C., Smith, C.M., Soma, L.R., and Uboh, C.E. 1993. Pharmacokinetic model for predicting sulfamethazine disposition in pigs. AJVR 54(5):750–754.

Trepanier, L.A. 1999. Delayed hypersensitivity reactions to sulphonamides: syndromes, pathogenesis, and management. Vet Derm 10:241–248.

———. 2004. Idiosyncratic toxicity associated with potentiated sulfonamides in the dog. J Vet Pharmacol Ther 27(3):129–38.

Trepanier, L.A., Danhof, R., Toll, J., Watrous, D. 2003. Clinical findings in 40 dogs with hypersensitivity associated with administration of potentiated sulfonamides. J Vet Intern Med 17:647–652.

Turnwald, G.H., Gossett, K.A., Cox, H.U., Kearney, M.T., Roy, A.F., Thomas, D.E., and Troy, G.C. 1986. Comparison of single-dose and conventional trimethoprim-sulfadiazine therapy in experimental *Staphylococcus intermedius* cystitis in the female dog. AJVR 47(12):2621–2623.

Twedt, D.C., Kiehl, K.J., Lappin, M.R., and Getzy, D.M. 1997. Association of hepatic necrosis with trimethoprim sulfonamide administration in 4 dogs. J Vet Internal Med 11:20–23.

Ueda, M., Tsurui, Y., and Koizumi, T. 1972. Studies on metabolism of drugs. XII. Quantitative separation of metabolites in human and rabbit urine after oral administration of sulfamonomethoxine and sulfamethomidine. Chem Pharm Bull 20:2042–2046.

Uno, T., Kushima, T., and Hiraoka, T. 1967. Studies on the metabolism of sulfadimethoxine. II. Determinations of metabolites in human and rabbit urine after oral administration of sulfadimethoxine. Chem Pharm Bull 15:1272–1276.

USDA Food Safety Inspection Service, Residue Evaluation and Planning Division. 1988. Program Report: Sulfamethazine (SMZ) Control Program, part 1: Mar 7–June 13, 1988.

USPDI. 1998. Potentiated Sulfonamides. In USPDI Vols. I and II Update, pp. 1503–1518. Sept. US Pharmacopeial Convention, Rockville, MD.

van Duijkeren, E., Ensink, J.M., and Meijer, L.A. 2002. Distribution of orally administered trimethoprim and sulfadiazine into noninfected subcutaneous tissue chambers in adult ponies. J Vet Pharmacol Therap 25:273–277.

van Duijkeren, E., Kessels, B.G.F., Sloet van Oldruitenborgh-Oosterbaan, M. M., Breukink, J.H., Vulto, A.G., and van Miert, AS.J.P.A.M. 1996. In vitro and in vivo binding of trimethoprim and sulfachlorpyridazine to equine food and digesta and their stability in caecal contents. J Vet Pharmacol Therap 19:281–287.

van Duijkeren, E., van Klingeren, B., Vulto, A.G., Sloet van Oldruitenborgh-Oosterbann, M.M., Breukink, H.J., van Miert, A.S.J.P.A.M. 1994a. In vitro susceptibility of equine *Salmonella* strains to trimethoprim and sulfonamide alone or in combination. Am J Vet Res 55:1386–1390.

van Duijkeren, E., Vulto, A.G., and van Miert, A.S.J.P.A.M. 1994b. Trimethoprim/sulfonamide combination in the horse: a review. J Vet Pharmacol Therap 17:64–73.

van Duijkeren, E., Vulto, A.G., Sloet van Oldruitenborgh-Oosterbaan, M. M., Mevius, D.J., Kessels, B.G.F., Breukink, J.H., and van Miert, A.S.J.P.A.M. 1994c. A comparative study of the pharmacokinetics of intravenous and oral trimethoprim—sulfadiazine formulations in the horse. J Vet Pharmacol Therap 17: 440–446, 1994c.

van Duijkeren, E., Vulto, A.G., Sloet van Oldruitenborgh-Oosterbann, M.M., Kessels, B.G.F., van Miert, A.S.J.P.A.M., and Breukink, H.J. 1995. Pharmacokinetics of trimethoprim/sulphachlorpyridazine in horses after oral, nasogastric and intravenous administration. J Vet Pharmacol Therap 18:47–53.

van Ginneken, V.J.T., Nouws, J.F.M., Grondel, J.L., Driessens, F., and Degen, M. 1991. Pharmacokinetics of sulphadimidine in carp (*Cyprinus carpio* L.) and rainbow trout (*Salmo gairdneri* Richardson) acclimated at two different temperature levels. Vet Quarterly 13(2):88–96.

van Gogh, R., van Deurzen, E.J.M., van Duin, C.T.M., and van Miert, A.S.J.P.A.M. 1984. Effect of staphylococcal enterotoxin B–induced diarrhoea on the pharmacokinetics of sulphadimidine in the goat. J Vet Pharmacol Therap 7:303–305.

van Miert, A.S.J.P.A.M. 1994. The sulfonamide-diaminopyrimidine story. J Vet Pharmacol Therap 17:309–316.

van Miert, A.S.J.P.A.M., Peters, R.H.M., Basudde, C.D.K., Nijmeijer, S. N., van Duin, C.T.M., van Gogh, H., and Korstanje, C. 1988. Effect of trenbolone and testosterone on the plasma elimination rates of SMZ, trimethoprim, and antipyrine in female dwarf goats. AJVR 49(12):2060–2064.

Vergin, H., Bishop-Freudling, G.B., Foing, N., Szelenyi, I., Armengaud, H., and van Tho, T. 1984. Diffusion of metioprim, tetroxoprim and sulphadiazine in the cerebrospinal fluid of dogs with healthy meninges and dogs with experimental meningitis. Chemotherapy 30:297–304.

Walker, C.C., and Barker, S.A. 1994. Extraction and enzyme immunoassay of sulfadimethoxine residues in channel catfish (*Ictalurus punctatus*) muscle. JAOAC Internat 77:908–916.

Walker, S.R., and Williams, R.T. 1972. The metabolism of sulphadimethoxypyrimidine. Xenobiotica 2(1):69–75.

Weijkamp, K., Faghihi, S.M., Nijmeijer, S.M., Witkamp, R.F., and van Miert, A.S.J.P.A.M. 1994. Oral bioavailability of sulphamethoxydiazine, sulphathiazole and sulphamoxazole in dwarf goats. Vet Quarterly 16:33–37.

Weiss, D.J., and Adams, L.G. 1987. Aplastic anemia associated with trimethoprim-sulfadiazine and fenbendazole administration in a dog. JAVMA 191(9):1119–1120.

Weiss, D.J., and Klausner, J.S. 1990. Drug-associated aplastic anemia in dogs: Eight cases. 1984–1988. JAVMA 196(3):472–475.

White, G., Piercy, D.W., Gibbs, H.A. 1981. Use of a calf salmonellosis model to evaluate the therapeutic properties of trimethoprim and sulphadiazine and their mutual potentiation in vivo. Res Vet Sci 31(1):27–31.

White, G., and Prior, S.D. 1982. Comparative effects of oral administration of trimethoprim/sulphadiazine or oxytetracycline on the faecal flora of horses. Vet Rec 111(14):316–318.

White, G., and Williams, R.B. 1983. Evaluation of a mixture of trimethoprim and sulphaquinoxaline for the treatment of bacterial and coccidial diseases of poultry. Vet Rec 113(26–27):608–612.

Williams, R.B., Farebrother, D.A., and Latter, V.S. 1995. Coccidiosis: a radiological study of sulphaquinoxaline distribution in infected and uninfected chickens. J Vet Pharmacol Therap 18:172–179.

Williamson, N.L., Frank, L.A., Hnilica, K.A. 2002. Effects of short-term trimethoprim-sulfamethoxazole administration on thyroid function in dogs. J Am Vet Med Assoc 221:802–806.

Wilson, R.C., Hammond, L.S., Clark, C.H., and Ravis, W.R. 1989. Bioavailability and pharmacokinetics of sulfamethazine in the pony. J Vet Pharmacol Therap 12:99–102.

Wilson, W.D., George, L.W., Baggot, J.D., Adamson, P.J.W., Hietala, S.K., and Mihalyi, J.E. 1987. Ormethoprim-sulfadimethoxine in cattle: pharmacokinetics, bioavailability, distribution to the tears, and in vitro activity against Moraxella bovis. AJVR 48(3):407–414.

Witcamp, R.F., van't Klooster, G.A.E., Nijmeijer, S.M., Kolker, H.J., Noordhoek, J., and van Miert, A.S.J.P.A.M. 1993. Hormonal regulation of oxidative drug metabolism in the dwarf goat: the effect of sex hormonal treatment on plasma disposition and metabolite formation of sulphadimidine. J Vet Pharmacol Therap 16:55–62.

Witcamp, R.F., Yun, H.-I., van't Klooster, G.A.E., van Mosel, J.F., van Mosel, M., Ensink, J.M., Noordhoek, J., and van Miert, A.S.J.P.A.M. 1992. Comparative aspects and sex differentiation of plasma sulfamethazine elimination and metabolite formation in rats, rabbits, dwarf goats, and cattle. AJVR 53(10):1830–1835.

Woolly, J.L., and Sigel, C.W. 1982. Development of pharmacokinetic models for sulfonamides in food animals: metabolic depletion profile of sulfadiazine in the calf. AJVR 43(5):768–774.

Yagi, N., Agata, I., Kawamura, T., Tanaka, Y., Sakamoto, M., Itoh, M., Sekikawa, H., and Takada, M. 1981. Fundamental pharmacokinetic behavior of sulfadimethoxine, sulfamethazole and their biotransformed products in dogs. Chem Pharm Bull 29(12):3741–3747.

Younan, W., Nouws, J.F.M., Homeid, A.M., Vree, T.B., and Degen, M. 1989. Pharmacokinetics and metabolism of suphadimidine in the camel. J Vet Pharmacol Therap 12:327–329.

Youssef, S.A.H., el-Gendi, A.Y.I., el-Sayed, M.G.A., Atef, M., and Abdel, S.A. 1981. Some pharmacokinetic and biochemical aspects of sulphadiazine and sulphadimidine in ewes. J Vet Pharmacol Therap 4:173–182.

Yuan, Z.-H., and Fung, K.-F. 1990. Pharmacokinetics of sulfadimidine and its N4-acetyl metabolite in healthy and diseased rabbits infected with *Pasteurella multocida*. J Vet Pharmacol Therap 13:192–197.

Yuan, Z.-H., Miao, X.-Q., and Yin, Y.-H. 1997. Pharmacokinetics of ampicillin and sulfadimidine in pigs infected experimentally with *Streptococcus suum*. J Vet Pharmacol Therap 20:318–322.

CHAPTER

34

β-LACTAM ANTIBIOTICS: PENICILLINS, CEPHALOSPORINS, AND RELATED DRUGS

MARK G. PAPICH AND JIM E. RIVIERE

In 1928, Alexander Fleming observed that a *Penicillium* mold contaminating a Petri dish culture of staphylococci colonies was surrounded by a clear zone free of growth. Fleming cultured the contaminating mold on a special medium and demonstrated that the culture broth contained a potent antibacterial substance that was relatively nontoxic to animals, but was active against a variety of gram-positive organisms. He named the substance *penicillin*. In 1940, penicillin was isolated in the form of a brown, impure powder and was the most powerful chemotherapeutic agent known at that time. Since then, more than 40 penicillins have been identified. Some occur naturally; others are biosynthesized (semisynthetic penicillins).

In 1945, *Cephalosporium acremonium* was isolated from raw sewage. The first cephalosporin, cephalosporin C, was derived from this fungus. All other cephalosporins are semisynthetic antibiotic derivatives of cephalosporin C. The first cephalosporin was available for clinical use in 1964. The reader may notice differences in spelling. The older cephalosporins, derived from the fungus are spelled *ceph*, whereas the newer semisynthetic derivatives are spelled *cef.*

Although penicillins, penicillin derivatives, and cephalosporins are still the most commonly used β-lactam antibiotics, much progress has been made in the development of new β-lactams during recent years. Most notably, these include the β-lactamase inhibitors (e.g., clavulanic acid), the carbapenems, also known as *penems* (e.g., imipenem, meropenem, ertapenem, doripenem), and the monobactams (e.g., aztreonam) (Abraham 1987).

MECHANISM OF ACTION OF β-LACTAM ANTIBIOTICS

β-lactam antibiotics exert their effects by preventing bacterial cell wall synthesis and disrupting bacterial cell wall integrity. These drugs are considered *bactericidal* in a time-dependent manner. They kill bacteria by inhibiting or weakening the cell wall. The cell wall of bacteria consists of alternating units of *N-acetylglucosamine* and *N-acetylmuramic acid,* which are cross-linked by short strands of peptides. A transpeptidation reaction is responsible for cross-linking the strands to form a strong, netlike structure. Inhibition of this transpeptidation reaction is one of the sites of action for β-lactam antibiotics. When they interfere with transpeptidation it results in a weak cell wall and rupture of the bacteria.

The binding sites for β-lactam antibiotics are called penicillin-binding proteins (PBPs), which are the enzymes that form the cell wall. There can be anywhere from 2–8 distinct PBPs in bacteria, which are numbered according to their molecular weight. The most common PBPs affected by β-lactams are PBP-1, -2, or -3. Some of the variation in spectrum of action and bactericidal action of β-lactam antibiotics can be related to their relative affinity for different PBPs. For example, inhibition of PBP-1a and -1b generally cause lysis, PBP-2 results in rounded cells called *spheroblasts,* and PBP-3 produces long filamentous forms. The drugs that cause rapid lysis (for example, carbapenems) are the most bactericidal and have highest affinity for PBP-1. On the other hand, mutations in the enzyme, produced by the resistance gene *mecA*, produces PBP-2a, a penicillin-binding protein that resists binding of the β-lactam drugs and renders bacteria with this gene resistant. The PBP-2a target is the basis for resistance to methicillin and oxacillin, known as *methicillin-resistant staphylococci (MRS)* (Weese 2005).

In order to reach the site of action, these drugs first must penetrate the outer layer of the bacteria. They penetrate the outer layer of bacteria through a pore (a porin protein) that is ordinarily present in bacteria to allow nutrients to enter the cell. It is generally easier to reach the target site in gram-positive bacteria and they usually are more susceptible to the effects of β-lactam antibiotics than gram-negative bacteria. Gram-negative bacteria may have a thick outer membrane and have pores more difficult to penetrate. The drugs most effective against gram-negative bacteria are those that can rapidly penetrate the outer membrane of the cell wall.

PHARMACOKINETIC-PHARMACODYNAMIC (PK-PD) PROPERTIES. The β-lactam antibiotics are time-dependent in their activity (Turnidge et al. 1998). β-lactam antibiotics are slowly bactericidal and the time of drug concentration above the MIC (T > MIC) is important to clinical success. In some cases, drug concentrations can fall below the MIC for treating staphylococcal infections and still attain a cure because of a post-antibiotic effect (PAE), but not against gram-negative bacilli (Zhanel et al. 1991). Additionally, since the MICs are lower for gram-positive bacteria, longer dose intervals may be possible for infections caused by gram-positive as compared to gram-negative bacteria because it is easier to keep the plasma concentration above the MIC.

The optimum duration of plasma concentrations above the MIC has varied among studies, but a general assumption is that the drug concentration should be above the MIC for 50%—and perhaps less—of the dosing interval (Turnidge 1998). This may vary depending on the immune competence of the animal and specific drug class. The carbapenem group of drugs (for example, imipenem and meropenem) are used with increasing popularity in small animal practice. These drugs are more bactericidal than penicillins and cephalosporins and the T > MIC for successful therapy may be less for these drugs than other β-lactams (for example, 30% of the dose interval).

Dosage regimens for the β-lactam antibiotics should consider these pharmacodynamic relationships. Therefore, for treating a gram-negative infection, especially a serious one, it is necessary to administer many of the penicillin derivatives and cephalosporins three to four times per day if they have short half-lives. Some of the third-generation cephalosporins have long half-lives and less frequent regimens have been used for some of these drugs (e.g., ceftiofur—Naxcel, cefovecin—Convenia, and cefpodoxime proxetil—Simplicef).

MICROBIAL RESISTANCE TO β-LACTAM ANTIBIOTICS

Three independent factors determine the bacterial susceptibility to β-lactam antibiotics: 1) production of β-lactamases, 2) decreased penetration through the outer cell membrane to access the cell wall enzymes, and 3) the resistance of the target (PBP) to binding by β-lactam agents (Gold and Moellering 1996; Frere et al. 1991). An example of an altered target (PBP) is the one found in methicillin-resistant isolates, mentioned earlier.

β-LACTAMASE ENZYMES. The elaboration of β-lactamases, enzymes that inactivate the drugs by hydrolyzing the β-lactam ring, is the major mechanism of drug resistance (Jacoby and Munoz-Price 2005). Different bacteria produce β-lactamases that possess a range of physical, chemical, and functional properties. Some β-lactamases are specific for penicillins (penicillinases), some are specific for cephalosporins (cephalosporinases), and others have affinity for both groups.

The genes that code for β-lactamases can occur via mutations in chromosomes, or they may be transferred by genetic elements. The genetic elements carrying these genes—which may be transferred among bacteria—include plasmids, which may be organized into integrons or carried on tranposons. A transposon may move (transpose) from DNA to plasmids, and vice versa. Integrons may be part of a transposon. The integrons may also contain genes that code for resistance to other drugs—thus producing multidrug resistance.

There are many β-lactamase enzymes that are capable of hydrolyzing the cyclic amide bond of the β-lactam structure and inactivating the drug. Investigators have described over 190 unique β-lactamase proteins that have this ability. Classification schemes may vary, and β-lactamase enzymes have been categorized according to molecular structure and substrate, bacterial type (gram-negative versus gram-positive), transmission (plasmid coded versus chromosomal coded), and whether they are inducible or constitutive. The Ambler Class (Class A, B, C, and D), which uses amino acid sequencing, is now widely accepted (Rice and Bonomo 2000). Class A enzymes are the most important in veterinary medicine. These include those listed in the following sections.

Staphylococcal β-Lactamase. These are produced by coagulase-positive *Staphylococcus* sp. and some coagulase-negative strains. The synthesis of these enzymes is determined by specific resistance genes and the enzymes are exocelluar. These enzymes typically do not inactivate cephalosporins and antistaphylococcal penicillins (e.g., isoxazolyl penicillins such as oxacillin or dicloxacillin). These β-lactamases can be inactivated by β-lactamase inhibitors (e.g., clavulanate acid, and sulbactam).

Gram-Negative β-Lactamases. This is a very diverse group that can arise through mutation or via transferable genetic elements. These enzymes are more wide-spectrum and can hydrolyze penicillins (penicillinases), cephalosporins (cephalosporinases), or both. β-lactamase produced by *E. coli,* (TEM is the most common enzyme) are coded by resistance genes and hydrolyze both cephalosporins and penicillins (broad spectrum). Some, but not all, of these enzymes are inhibited by β-lactamase inhibitors (e.g., clavulanate, sulbactam). Gram-negative bacteria secrete small amounts of β-lactamases into their periplasmic space, allowing for optimal location of the enzyme to degrade the β-lactam upon entry into the organism. The advantage of newer drugs such as third-generation cephalosporins (also called *oxyimino-β-lactams*) and penems is their ability to remain stable to gram-negative β-lactamases.

Among the most serious of the gram-negative β-lactamases are the ESBLs—extended-spectrum β-lactamases. These β-lactamases can be induced and will cause resistance to even the most active (extended-spectrum) cephalosporins. Bacteria positive for ESBL can be difficult to treat because of limited drug options.

RESISTANCE TO DRUG ACCESS TO BINDING SITES. Gram-negative bacteria can produce a cell wall with a modified outer membrane that is no longer permeable to β-lactam antibiotics. These impenetrable porin proteins can resist entry by β-lactam drugs. They can also delay or slow the rate of entry, thus making the drugs more susceptible to attack by β-lactamase enzymes. Therefore, this mechanism can enhance resistance produced by the elaboration of β-lactamases.

PENICILLINS

GENERAL PHARMACOLOGY. Penicillin G is historically important because it was the first antibiotic introduced in medicine. Alexander Fleming discovered penicillin in 1928, but it was not used clinically until the early 1940s. Much of the early supply was designated for military use during WW II. It remains a popular antibiotic and is still the drug of choice for initial treatment of many infections in horses and cattle. It has little usefulness in small animals because of the high incidence of resistance.

Unitage. Penicillin is one of the few antibiotics that is still measured in terms of units rather than weight in mg or μg. One unit of penicillin represents the specific activity in 0.6 μg of sodium penicillin. Thus, one mg of penicillin sodium represents 1,667 units of penicillin. Doses of other β-lactams are expressed in weight (mg) rather than units.

Structure. Penicillin contains a fused ring system, the β-lactam thiazolidine (Fig. 34.1). The physical and chemical properties, especially solubilities, of penicillins are determined by the acyl side chain and the cations used to form salts.

Hydrolysis is the main cause of penicillin degradation, which can occur via bacterial enzymes (β-lactamases). This reaction also can occur from drug interactions (for example, in the syringe when penicillin is mixed with another drug). Some penicillins are poorly orally absorbed because they are unstable in the stomach and hydrolyzed by gastric acid. Penicillin is incompatible with heavy metal ions, oxidizing agents, and strong concentrations of alcohol.

1. *Natural penicillins* are produced by mold cultures and then extracted and purified. Penicillin G is the only one of the natural penicillins of any clinical relevance today.
2. *Aminopenicillins* (e.g., amoxicillin, ampicillin) are semisynthetic derivatives that have a free amino group at position R on the penicillin nucleus. Amoxicillin and ampicillin are identical, except for a parahydroxy group on amoxicillin that changes the pharmacokinetics.
3. *Antistaphylococcal penicillis.* This group of antibiotics includes the isoxazolylpenicillins (e.g., oxacillin, cloxacillin, and dicloxacillin) and synthetic derivatives of penicillin (e.g., methicillin and nafcillin). This group has a ring structure attached to the carbonyl carbon of the amide side chain and are stable against the β-lactamase produced by *Staphylococcus*.
4. *Extended-spectrum penicillins*, which are active against *Pseudomonas* and other gram-negative bacilli (e.g., piperacillin, ticarcillin, carbenicillin) have either a carboxylic acid group or a basic group at position R. These drugs have anti-*Pseudomonas* activity, but also have better activity against some of the other gram-negative fermenting bacilli. However, they are susceptible to β-lactamase, which led to combinations such as ticarcillin-clavulanate, and piperacillin-tazobactam (β-lactamase inhibitors will be discussed in more detail later in the chapter).

MICROBIAL SUSCEPTIBILITY. The natural penicillins are active against many *Streptococci* spp. and nonpenicillinase-producing *Staphylococci* spp. They are active against some gram-positive, but only selected gram-negative bacteria that include *Arcanobacterium* (formerly *Actinomyces*), *Listeria monocytogenes*, and *Pasteurella multocida*. Therefore, these drugs are narrow-spectrum drugs that are active against non–β-lactamase–producing gram-positive bacteria but few gram-negative bacteria. Many anaerobic bacteria are susceptible, including *Fusobacterium*, *Peptococcus*, *Peptostreptococcus*, and some strains of *Bacteroides* (except *Bacteriodes fragilis* group) and *Clostridium*. These drugs are also active against most spirochetes, including *Leptospira* and *Borrelia burgdorferi*. Natural penicillins are consistently inactive against *Pseudomonas*, most Enterobacteriaceae, and penicillinase-producing *Staphylococcus* spp.

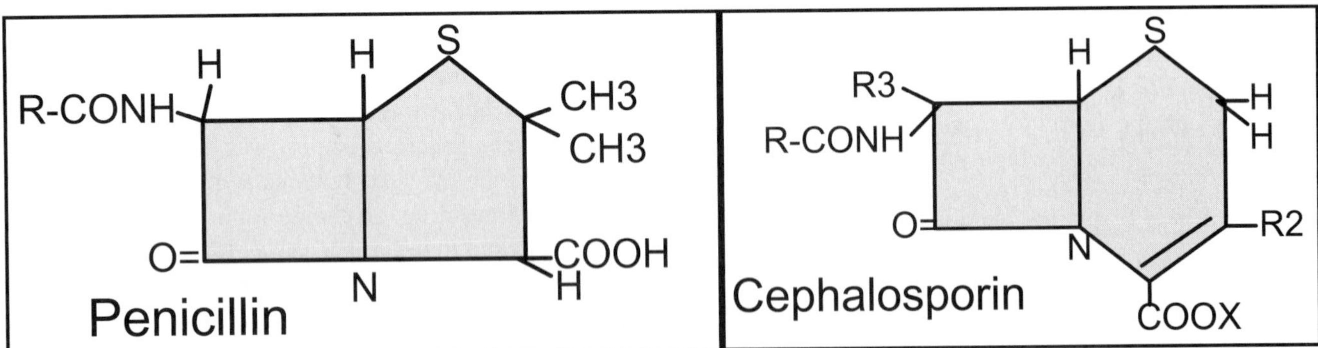

FIG. 34.1 Structure of penicillins and cephalosporins. Penicillins are composed of a five-member thiazolidine ring; cephalosporins are composed of a six-member dihydrothiazine ring. The most critical feature of the structure to exert its antibacterial action is the β-lactam ring. If the β-lactam ring is broken (hydrolyzed), the drug is inactive.

Aminopenicillins are active against the bacteria that are susceptible to penicillin G. They can penetrate through the outer membrane of gram-negative bacilli better than penicillin, which increases the spectrum to include some Enterobacteriaceae, including strains of *E. coli, Proteus mirabilis,* and *Salmonella.* Aminopenicillins are inactive against *Pseudomonas, Bacteroides fragilis,* and penicillinase-producing *Staphylococcus* spp. There are only subtle differences in antimicrobial activity between amoxicillin and ampicillin, and for susceptibility testing purposes, they are considered equivalent (CLSI 2007).

The antistaphylocccal penicillins include methicillin and nafcillin as well as the isoxazolylpenicillins (oxacillin, cloxacillin, and dicloxacillin). The isoxazolylpenicillins are considered as a group because of their structural similarity. These semisynthetic penicillins are active against many penicillinase-producing *Staphylococcus* spp. that would ordinarily be resistant to penicillin G and the aminopenicillins. They also have some activity against other gram-positive and gram-negative bacteria and spirochetes.

The antipseudomonas penicillins have the most activity against gram-negative aerobic and anaerobic bacteria of all of the penicillin groups. The drugs are active against many strains of Enterobacteriaceae and some strains of *Pseudomonas.* Carbenicillin and ticarcillin are active against some strains of *E. coli, Morganella morganii, Proteus* spp., and *Salmonella.* In addition to these organisms, mezlocillin and piperacillin are active against some strains of *Enterobacter, Citrobacter, Klebsiella,* and *Serratia.* These extended-spectrum penicillins have some activity against gram-positive aerobic and anaerobic bacteria but have no advantages against these organisms compared to penicillin G and aminopenicillins. Extended-spectrum penicillins are generally more active against *Bacteroides fragilis* than are other available penicillins.

PHARMACOKINETICS. Ampicillin and amoxicillin have been the most studied of the penicillin group and Table 34.1 lists the pharmacokinetic parameters in several domestic species. Penicillin G pharmacokinetics are presented in Table 34.2. Most penicillins are rapidly absorbed when injected in aqueous suspension, usually the sodium salt, by the IM or SC route. The trihydrate formulations of ampicillin or amoxicillin are chemically more stable, and available as aqueous suspensions. These formulations may be injected IM or SC and produce slow absorption profiles to prolong the action. When sodium salts of these drugs are injected, maximum blood concentrations occur usually within an hour.

Absorption. For the penicillin G formulations, distinct absorption patterns are observed, depending on which form is administered, the formulation, and the site of injection. The long-acting formulations (procaine- or benzathine-penicillin) are given IM or SC (never IV). The slow absorption from the injection site prolongs the plasma concentration. Injections of penicillin G IM to horses produced prolonged plasma concentrations, even when the sodium salt of penicillin was administered (Uboh et al. 2000). The half-life was longer from the procaine formulation, but at 24 hours, concentrations were similar in horses, regardless of whether the procaine- or potassium formulation of penicillin G was administered. Benzathine formulations produce lower, but much longer, plasma concentrations because of insolubility and extremely slow absorption from the injection site (Papich et al. 1994).

For all the penicillins, as expected, the maximum plasma concentration will be lower, and the time to reach maximum concentration delayed, from an IM route versus IV route. More rapid absorption occurs from IM injection than SC. Also, there are differences depending on the location in large animals, with an injection in the neck muscle being absorbed faster than an injection in gluteal muscle (Papich et al. 1993). This pattern of absorption has been shown for other penicillins in cattle and horses (Firth 1986), in which injections in the neck muscle are absorbed more rapidly and completely than injections in the rear leg.

For ampicillin and amoxicillin, these can be administered IM or IV as sodium salts, or they may be formulated as the trihydrate form that is more stable in aqueous solutions and may be administered SC or IM to produce a more prolonged absorption phase and a longer duration of activity (Traver and Riviere 1982). Sodium salts of the other penicillin derivatives also are available for IM or IV administration (e.g., ticarcillin sodium, piperacillin sodium, etc.).

Penicillin is easily inactivated in the acidic pH of the stomach (a pH of 6–6.5 is optimum for chemical stability), and therefore is not absorbed orally (except the acid-stable penicillin V, which is discussed under the specific formulations below). Because oral absorption of penicillin G is not sufficient to be of therapeutic value in animals this route is not used.

TABLE 34.1 Ampicillin and amoxicillin pharmacokinetics (mean values)

Species	Dose (mg/kg)	Half-Life (hr)	VD (l/kg)	CL (ml/kg/hr)	C_{max} (μg/ml)	T_{max} (hr)	F (%)	Reference
Ampicillin Trihydrate IM Administration								
Calves	11				2.62			Martinez et al. 2001
Pigs	6.6				3.25			Martinez et al. 2001
Horse	11				1.48	1		Beech et al. 1979
Horse	22				2.9	6		Beech et al. 1979
Horse	20				2.49	6		Brown et al. 1982
Cattle	17 studies	6.66	4.49	467.8				Gehring et al. 2005
Ampicillin Sodium IV								
Horses		0.62	0.18	210	6.7–9.7			Sarasola and McKellar 1993
Horses	10	0.725	0.303	268	59.9			Sarasola and McKellar 1992
Horses		1.55						Durr et al. 1976
Horses		1.41	0.17					Bowman et al. 1986
Horses		0.75	0.21					Horspool et al. 1992
Horses	15	1.72	0.705	285				Ensink et al. 1992
Horses	10	0.7	0.2628	365.4				Sarasola and McKellar 1995
Cats		1.22						Mercer et al. 1977
Pigs		0.55						Galtier and Charpenteau 1979
Dogs	15	1.35	0.679	387				ten Voorde et al. 1990
Sheep	10	0.78	0.156	372.6				Oukessou and Toutain 1992
Ampicillin Sodium IM								
Cows	10	2.3			6.18	1.5		Nelis et al. 1992
Horses	15	2.3	0.71	209.8	31.1	0.32		Van Den Hoven et al. 2003
Horses	11				10	0.5		Beech et al. 1979
Horses	22	2			12.88	0.5		Traver and Riviere 1982
Dogs	15	5.2–5.5			7.76–12.18	.92–1.03		ten Voorde et al. 1990
Ampicillin Oral								
Dogs	14.5	0.9			4.6			Nelis et al. 1992
Dogs	10	0.96			3.9	1.6		Watson et al. 1986
Foal	20				5.0	1		Brown et al. 1984
Cat							42	Mercer et al. 1977
Horse	15				0.84	0.69	2	Ensink et al. 1996
Amoxicillin								
Foals (30 d) IM	22	0.991	0.986	691	23.21			Carter et al. 1986
Foals (6–7 d) IV	20	0.74	0.369	343.2				Baggot et al. 1988
Foals (6–7d) Oral	20	1.09			6.23	2	36.2	Baggot et al. 1988
Horses IV	10	0.657	0.325	340.8				Wilson et al. 1988
Horses IM					3.9–11.9			Evans et al. 1971
Horses Oral	20	0.85			11.05	0.3	10.4	Wilson et al. 1988
Horses Oral	20	0.75			2.03		5	Ensink et al. 1992
Horses IV	10	1.43	0.556	273				Ensink et al. 1992
Dogs IV	20	1.3	0.312	204				Kung and Wanner 1994
Dogs IV	15	1.18	0.449	270				ten Voorde et al. 1990
Dogs IM	15	6.98–9.02			7.64–8.13	1.61–1.89		ten Voorde et al. 1990
Pigs IV	8.6	1.8	0.55, 0.63	370, 520				Agerso and Friis 1998
Pigs IM	14.7	15.5			5.1	2	83	Agerso and Friis 1999
Sheep IV	10	0.77	0.22	606				Craigmill et al. 1992
Sheep IV	20	1.43	0.18	90				Carceles et al. 1995
Goats IV	10	1.15	0.47	684.6				Craigmill et al. 1993
Goats IV	20	1.13	0.18	110				Carceles et al. 1995
Dogs oral		1.06	0.284	182				Marier et al. 2001
Dogs oral	16.9	1.52	0.71	460	11.4	1.38		Vree et al. 2003
Dogs oral	21	1.5			18–21	1.4–2	64–77	Kung and Wanner 1994
Dogs oral	10	1.4		8.1	1.6			Watson et al. 1986
Pigs oral	10	9, 9.9	2.25		0.8, 1.6	1.9, 3.6	28, 33	Agerso et al. 1998
Pigs oral	20	4.2			7.5	1.5		Jensen et al. 2004

VD = volume of distribution; CL = systemic clearance; C_{max} = peak concentration; T_{max} = time of peak concentration after absorption; F = fraction of dose absorbed.

TABLE 34.2 Pharmacokinetic parameters for penicillin

Species	Form	Dose (Units/kg)	Route/Site	C_{max} (μg/ml)	T_{max} (hrs)	Half-Life (hrs)	Reference
Calves (6–9 mo)	Potassium	10,000	IM/Neck	4.71 ± 3.86	1 to 1.5	—	Bengtsson et al. 1989
	Procaine	30,000	IM/Neck	1.55 ± 0.33	1.5 to 6	—	Bengtsson et al. 1989
Cattle	Procaine	66,000	IM/Neck	4.24 ± 1.08	6.00 ± 0.00	8.9	Papich et al. 1993
		66,000	SC/Neck	1.85 ± 0.27	5.33 ± 0.67	17	
After 5-day administration	Procaine	24,000	IM/Gluteal	0.99 ± 0.04	5.33 ± 0.67	17	Papich et al. 1993
		66,000	IM/Gluteal	2.63 ± 0.27	6.00 ± 0.00	17	
Horses	Sodium	10,000	IV/Jugular				Love, et al. 1983
		20,000	IV/Jugular				
		40,000	IV/Jugular				
	Procaine	10,000	IM/Gluteal				Sullins et al.
		20,000	IM/Gluteal				
		40,000	IM/Gluteal				
	Procaine	22,000	IM/Gluteal	1.42 ± 0.22	3		Stover et al. 1981
	Procaine	22,000	IM/Neck	1.8	3.5	24.7	Uboh et al. 2000
	Potassium	22,000	IM/Neck	5.8	1.0	12.9	Uboh et al. 2000
Foals (0–7 d)	Procaine	22,000	IM/Semimembranous	2.17 ± 0.27	2		Brown et al. 1984

IM = intramuscular; IV = intravenous; SC = subcutaneous; C_{MAX} = peak concentration; T_{MAX} = time of peak concentration after absorption.

Amoxicillin, ampicillin, and the antistaphylococcal penicillins can be administered to small animals. Amoxicillin differs from ampicillin only by the addition of a hydroxyl group. This decreases the lipophilicity of amoxicillin, but increases the oral absorption, whereby systemic availability of amoxicillin administered orally is higher than a similar dose of ampicillin (Watson et al. 1986). For example, absorption of ampicillin in dogs and cats has been reported to range from 30–40%, and for amoxicillin 64–68% (Kung and Wanner 1994). Ampicillin had wide variation of oral absorption in cats (18% for suspension; 42% for capsule), depending on the dosage form (Mercer et al. 1977). Amoxicillin also has twice the systemic bioavailability of ampicillin when administered orally in pigs and preruminant calves.

Other penicillin derivatives may have low oral absorption, which limits their clinical usefulness. Cloxacillin, is absorbed poorly in dogs (Watson et al. 1986; Dimitrova et al. 1998) and with its short half-life is unsuitable for therapy in dogs.

The effect of feeding on oral absorption of these drugs has been debated, and results have varied, depending on the species of dogs studied. The most complete study on this subject was reported by Watson et al. (1986). They found that feeding dogs inhibited oral absorption of amoxicillin, ampicillin, penicillin V, and cloxacillin. The effect was modest for ampicillin and amoxicillin (feeding decreased ampicillin tablets by 38%, but only 20–25% for amoxicillin). Feeding had a large effect for cloxacillin, decreasing oral absorption by 74%.

Aminopenicillins are absorbed poorly in horses and ruminants following oral administration. They can be absorbed in preruminant calves, but not ruminating (6 weeks of age) calves (Soback et al. 1987a). Oral absorption of ampicillin in adult horses has been reported to be only 2–3.5% (Ensink et al. 1996; Sarasola and McKellar 1994). Systemic availability of oral amoxicillin is higher than ampicillin in adult horses but is only 2–10% (Wilson et al. 1988; Ensink et al. 1992, 1996; Baggot 1988; Sarasola and McKellar 1994); still too low to be practical for dosing. In foals, oral absorption of amoxicillin has been higher at 36.2–42.7% (Baggot et al. 1988), but this is a seldom-used route of administration.

Absorption of some oral drugs has been improved by administering them as prodrugs. The ester prodrugs of ampicillin such as bacampicillin and pivampicillin produce systemic availability in horses of 35 to 45% after oral administration (Sarasola and McKellar 1994). However, these prodrugs are no longer available as commercial products in the U.S.

Elimination. The elimination half-life for IV penicillin is short (0.5 to 1.2 hour). Slow-release formulations are designed to lengthen this half-life. For example, because of slow release from the injection site, procaine penicillin may produce a terminal half-life of 20 hours or more and can maintain concentrations against susceptible bacteria for 24 hours after a single injection. The prolonged terminal half-life is caused by slow absorption (see the section "Absorption," above), rather than slow elimination, which is referred to as the "flip-flop effect" determining the plasma profile. All penicillins rely on renal elimination (primarily tubular secretion) and reach high drug concentrations in the urine.

Distribution. Penicillins diffuse into extracellular fluid easily unless protein binding is high. Protein binding is low to moderate in most species, ranging from approximately 30–60%. Penicillin is a weak acid with a pK_a of 2.7, therefore it is mostly ionized in the plasma and the volume of distribution is moderate. For example, volume of distribution (V_D) listed in some studies is 0.2 to 0.3 l/kg. In some studies, and in some species, however, it may be as high as 0.6 to 0.7 l/kg. These values represent a distribution to extracellular fluid, and possibly reaching intracellular concentrations. Sufficient concentrations are attained for susceptible bacteria in kidneys, synovial fluid, liver, lung, skin, and soft tissues (Stover et al. 1981; Brown et al. 1982; Beech et al. 1979). Penicillins do not penetrate the blood brain barrier to reach concentrations in the central nervous system (CNS) to a large extent, but they have been used to treat infections of the CNS when administered at high doses.

Metabolism. Penicillin G, penicillin V, nafcillin, ticarcillin, and the aminopenicillins are metabolized to some extent by hydrolysis of the β-lactam ring. The metabolites are microbiologically inactive. Penicillins and their metabolites are excreted in the urine by tubular secretion. Most of the drug is excreted in the urine within 1 hour of IM injection of sodium or potassium penicillin in aqueous solution. Probenecid competitively inhibits renal tubular secretion of penicillins and can prolong the half-life of penicillin. However, probenecid is rarely used for this purpose.

SUMMARY OF PENICILLINS AND DERIVATIVES

Natural Penicillins. The only natural penicillins still in use are penicillin G and penicillin V. Penicillin V has a phenoxymethyl group that provides more acid stability in the stomach, allowing for oral administration. It has been used orally in people, but it is of limited value in calves because of low oral absorption and limited spectrum (Soback et al. 1987b). In dogs, oral administration of penicillin V tablets produces maximum plasma concentrations of 3.5–4.8 μg/ml, but the concentrations decline quickly and were above 0.5 μg/ml for only approximately 3 hours (Watson et al. 1987a, b).

Penicillin Formulations. There are three injectable formulations. Pharmacokinetics of these formulations are provided in Table 34.2:

1. *Na^+ and K^+ salts of penicillin, also called crystalline penicillin:* These are water soluble and may be injected intravenously (IV), intramuscularly (IM), or subcutaneously (SC). They achieve rapid, but short-lived, plasma concentrations.
2. *Procaine penicillin G (Crysticillin, Pen-Aqueous):* This compound is a poorly soluble salt in an aqueous vehicle suspension that is slowly absorbed following intramuscular (IM) or subcutaneous (SC) injection. *Do not administer IV.*
3. *Benzathine penicillin G (Benza-pen, Durapen, Flo-cillin):* This preparation is the so-called "long-acting penicillin". It is absorbed more slowly than the procaine salt because of its insolubility. It produces persistent, but low, plasma concentrations. Most formulations of long-acting penicillin contain 50% procaine penicillin G, and 50% benzathine penicillin G. *Do not administer IV.*

Additional formulations and route of administration are the formulations of penicillin G administered via intramammary routes to treat bovine mastitis.

The doses of penicillin G vary greatly depending on the formulation, the species of animal, and the disease treated. It is best to consult references related to the specific disease being treated. In general, Na^+ or K^+ penicillin G are administered IM, or IV at doses of 20,000 to 50,000 U/kg every 4 to 6 hours. Procaine penicillin G is administered IM or SC at dosages of 22,000 to 70,000 U/kg, every 12 to 24 hours. Treatment of streptococcal infections may use a lower dose, but for some infections such as those caused by *Arcanobacterium Actinomyces* (formerly called) doses as high as 100,000 U/kg have been recommended.

The United States FDA–approved label dose for cattle is 7,500 U/kg, but the approved withdrawal time for food animals—10 days—applies only to an approved food animal dose. Since the doses used in food animals are extralabel, extended withdrawal times must be applied.

Aminopenicillins. Ampicillin and amoxicillin have been used in the treatment of a variety of diseases in domestic animals. The half-life of all aminopenicillins is short (Table 34.1), requiring frequent administration for some infections, particularly gram-negative pathogens that may have high MIC values.

Aminopenicillins are popular because they have a broader spectrum of activity compared to penicillin G, can be administered orally, and are relatively inexpensive and safe. The aminopenicillins differ from penicillin by the addition of an amino group, and amoxicillin has a para-hydroxy group that ampicillin lacks. Compared to penicillin G, these compounds have two ionization points (pK_a 2.7 and 7.3). Ampicillin is more soluble than amoxicillin, and is also more lipophilic (Log P ampicillin 1.35; Log P amoxicillin 0.87), but amoxicillin is better absorbed by a factor of approximately two in most animals.

Compared to penicillin G, the aminopenicillins can penetrate the outer layer of gram-negative bacteria better than penicillin G; therefore, they have a spectrum of activity that includes those listed for penicillin but is extended to include some of the gram-negative bacteria (e.g., susceptible Enterobacteriaceae). However, acquired resistance can be common and this group is still quite susceptible to β-lactamase. To overcome resistance the β-lactamase inhibitors clavulanic acid and sulbactam have been added to amoxicillin (Clavamox) and ampicillin (Unasyn), respectively, to increase the spectrum. β-lactamase inhibitors are discussed later in the chapter.

Aminopenicillin Formulations. The formulations of aminopenicillins used in veterinary medicine (examples of brand names in parentheses) that are available include

1. *Sodium ampicillin:* This formulation is used for injection IM, IV, SC (Omnipen®).
2. *Ampicillin trihydrate (Polyflex®):* This is a poorly soluble, slow-release aqueous suspension. Absorption of this formulation is erratic, and it produces prolonged, but low, blood concentrations.
3. *Amoxicillin trihydrate:* (Amoxi-inject®).
4. *Ampicillin:* These are oral products such as tablets, capsules, and liquid suspensions (for example, Omnipen®).
5. *Amoxicillin:* These are oral products, such as tablets and liquids (Amoxi-Tabs®, Amoxi-Drops®, and others).
6. *Intramammary preparations:* These include Amoxi-Mast, which is used for treating mastitis.

TABLE 34.3 Common dosages for ampicillin and amoxicillin

Amoxicillin oral: dogs, cats 10–22 mg/kg q8, 12, or 24 h
Ampicillin trihydrate injection: cattle 6.6–22 mg/kg q8, 12, or 24 h (24 h most common); the approved label dose in cattle is 4.4–11 mg/kg IM, q24 h
Ampicillin sodium: horses IV 10–20 mg/kg q6–8 h
Ampicillin sodium: horses IM 10–22 mg/kg q12 h

The elimination of the aminopenicillins is slightly longer that what is reported for sodium salts of penicillin, but this difference does not appear to relate to a difference in clinical efficacy (Table 34.1). Common doses are listed in Table 34.3. A common formulation used in animals is ampicillin trihydrate (Polyflex), a poorly soluble preparation. After IM injection, the half-life is 6.7 hours in cattle, which is adequate for once-daily administration (Gehring et al. 2005). The IM injection in horses also prolongs the plasma concentration (Table 34.1).

An important difference between the aminopenicillins and penicillin G is that the aminopenicillins are not inactivated by gastric acid and may be administered orally. There appears to be a saturable transport process for absorption of aminopenicillin in the intestine. Oral absorption of the penicillins in various species and effect of feeding and age is discussed in the section "Absorption."

In addition to the formulations listed above there are ester derivatives of ampicillin, but these are not currently available. The advantage of these esters is that they are stable in the gastrointestinal tract and are absorbed intact, but esterases release the active drug after absorption across the intestinal mucosa. They are absorbed much better than the parent drugs. Examples of these drugs are *pivampicillin* and *bacampicillin* (Sarasola and McKellar 1994; Ensink et al. 1996).

Antistaphylococcal Penicillins. Also called the β-lactamase stable penicillins, this group of antibiotics includes the isoxazolylpenicillins (e.g., oxacillin, cloxacillin, and dicloxacillin) and synthetic derivatives of penicillin (e.g., methicillin and nafcillin). The value of this group lies in their resistance to the β-lactamase of *Staphylococcus* spp. They have minimal activity against gram-negative bacteria because they do not exhibit good penetration of the outer layer of these bacteria.

One of the drugs in this group is methicillin. If *Staphylococcus* shows phenotypic resistance to methicillin, it is a marker for resistance mediated by the *mecA*-gene, which codes for a resistant PBP protein. When it occurs in *S. aureus,* this type of resistance is called *methicillin-resistant Staphylococcus aureus*—MRSA. Today, oxacillin is used to test for this resistance, even though the resistant strains are still referred to as "methicillin-resistant" (CLSI 2007).

Preparations Available. The antistaphylococcal penicillins are available in oral and parenteral forms, but decreased availability has limited their use. Many human preparations of oxacillin are not currently available. Cloxacillin, which is used to treat staphylococcal and streptococcal mastitis, is also available as an intramammary infusion for dry cows (cloxacillin benzathine).

In the species studied (dogs, horses) the pharmacokinetics of oxacillin, dicloxacillin, and cloxacillin are similar. The elimination half-life ranges from 30 to 40 minutes and volume of distribution from 0.2 to 0.3 l/kg. Methicillin and nafcillin are not administered orally because they are not acid stable and produce erratic oral absorption. Oral preparations exist for oxacillin, cloxacillin, and dicloxacillin, but oral absorption is low for these drugs in small animals. Cloxacillin is so poorly and variably absorbed and produces such low plasma concentrations that it is not suitable for oral administration to treat most infections (Watson et al. 1986). Oral absorption is greatly reduced for cloxacillin when it is administered with food. Dicloxacillin is absorbed only 23% in dogs after oral administration and the half-life is so short (2.6 hours) that frequent administration is necessary (Dimitrova et al. 1998). Likewise, dicloxacillin half-life is rapid in cats, and absorption was low even with IM administration (Dimitrova 1996).

Clinical Use. Intramammary infusions are used for treating mastitis (cloxacillin). Drugs in this class are ordinarily not used systemically in large animals. In small animals, these drugs have been used to treat staphylococcal infections such as pyoderma. The following doses are used but not evaluated for efficacy: cloxacillin at 20 to 40 mg/kg, q6–8h, (oral, IM); dicloxacillin at 11–25 mg/kg, orally, every 8 hours; or oxacillin at 20 to 40 mg/kg, orally, q8h. Cloxacillin is best administered on an empty stomach.

Extended-Spectrum Penicillins. The extended-spectrum penicillins have also been called the *antipseudomonas penicillins* because they are among the few drugs active against *Pseudomonas*. This group includes the carboxypenicillins—carbenicillin and ticarcillin—because of a substitution of a carboxy group for the amino group on ampicillin, and the ureidopenicillins, which include piperacillin, and azlocillin. The carboxy group decreased activity against *Streptococcus*, but improved penetration through the outer cell membrane of gram-negative bacteria. Substitution of a ureido for the carboxy group produced ureido penicillins, which maintained ampicillin's activity against *Streptococcus* and also produced good penetration through the outer membrane of gram-negative bacteria.

The value of this group of penicillins is that they are able to penetrate the outer wall of *Pseudomonas* and some other gram-negative bacteria (e.g., *Proteus*, *Providencia,* and *Enterobacter*) better than other penicillins. Like the other penicillins, they are susceptible to β-lactamase inactivation. This group has good synergistic activity when administered with the aminoglycosides (e.g., gentamicin, amikacin). The ureido penicillins also have good activity against anaerobic bacteria, and piperacillin may have some activity against enterococci.

Pharmacokinetic Features. The disadvantage of this group of penicillins is the short half-life, which necessitates frequent administration. The half-life for carbenicillin in dogs and horses is 75 and 90 minutes, respectively. The half-life for ticarcillin ranges from 50 minutes to 73 minutes in dogs and horses (VanCamp et al. 2000; Garg et al. 1987; Tilmant et al. 1985). The apparent volume of distribution is between 0.2 and 0.4 l/kg for most drugs in this class. The pharmacokinetics of ticarcillin have been studied in horses more than other animals. One of the more recent studies provides a thorough review of the studies and details on the pharmacokinetic features (VanCamp et al. 2000).

Clinical Use. Ticarcillin is probably the most common of this group used in veterinary medicine. (However, there are no longer any veterinary preparations marketed.) Ticarcillin is more active than carbenicillin against gram-negative bacteria, but whether this relates to clinical differences is not clear. Ticarcillin is available in a formulation for people in combination with the β-lactamase inhibitor clavulanic acid (Timentin®) and clinical use of ticarcillin in veterinary medicine usually is with this formulation, rather than ticarcillin alone. More detail about this combination is presented in the section "β-Lactamase Inhibitors," later in this chapter. These drugs are available as sodium salts for injection; there are *no* orally effective formulations in this class, except indanyl carbenicillin (Geocillin®, Geopen®), which is poorly absorbed and not useful for systemic infections. These drugs can be more expensive than other penicillins.

These drugs are primarily used in small animals for resistant gram-negative infections. Their use is rare in cattle. There has been a preparation of ticarcillin (Ticillin®) approved for intrauterine treatment for endometritis in horses, but it is currently unavailable. When used in animals, the doses are wide, because no clinical trials have been conducted to establish efficacy. The following doses have been used: carbenicillin at 15–50 mg/kg (dog, cats, horses) IM, IV, q6h; ticarcillin at 40 mg/kg IM, IV, q4–6h (dogs, cats) and at 44 mg/kg IM, IV, q6–8h (horses). Ticarcillin also is used intrauterine in mares at a dose of 12.4 mg/kg diluted in saline (VanCamp et al. 2000).

ADVERSE EFFECTS. Penicillins are very safe drugs, with relatively few adverse effects reported. Like most β-lactams, adverse effects are rare. The most common, and often most serious, adverse effects are attributed to allergy—immune-mediated reactions or allergic reactions. These are common in people from penicillins (approximately 15% of the human population) and are seen in veterinary species. Treatment may require administration of medications to attenuate the allergic response and avoidance of future use. Coomb's-positive hemolytic anemia has been reported in horses following penicillin administration (Blue et al. 1987; Step et al. 1991).

After oral administration, there can be disruption of intestinal bacteria. *Clostridium* bacterial intestinal overgrowth from oral administration is a risk in guinea pigs, hamsters, gerbils, and rabbits.

Central nervous system reaction can be produced by penicillins (and other β-lactam antibiotics). At high concentrations these drugs can inhibit GABA (an inhibitory neurotransmitter) and cause excitement and seizures. Procaine, which is in some preparations, also causes excitement in some animals (horses) (Neilsen et al. 1988). There may be free procaine in some formulations of aqueous procaine penicillin G. When injected IM, (or inadvertently IV) it can elicit an excitatory response. Because procaine can mask pain, and produce excitation in horses, its use is regulated in racing horses (see Chapter 57 on control of drugs in racing animals for additional information). Injections of procaine-penicillin in a horse may cause a positive procaine test reaction at the race track for as long as 2 weeks. In severe cases it can cause bacterial overgrowth with *Clostridium* species and enteritis. Oral administration of ampicillin, amoxicillin, and similar formulations may also cause vomiting at high doses.

SPECIAL SPECIES CONSIDERATIONS. The penicillins are excreted similarly in all mammalian animals. In general, doses and intervals are similar among mammals, except that in larger species, dose intervals may be longer because of slower renal clearance. Renal clearance can be scaled allometrically to show that the larger body weight is associated with slower renal clearance.

In reptile species, clearance of all penicillin drugs is slow. The half-lives are much longer in reptiles, which allows for infrequent dosing intervals of once every 3–5 days. In birds, renal clearance and metabolic rate is high. This difference results in high doses and frequent intervals. Because of the need for frequent dosing, and because injectable drugs of this group may cause intramuscular pain, these drugs may be impractical in many clinical situations involving birds.

β-LACTAMASE INHIBITORS. The β-lactamase inhibitors are a specific class of drugs with little antibacterial effects of their own, but they act to inhibit the β-lactamase enzyme. They are always combined with another active drug of the β-lactam class. The veterinary use of this group was reviewed by Mealey (2001). The primary drugs of this group are clavulanic acid (also called *potassium clavulanate*) and sulbactam. Tazobactam is a newer addition to this group, but veterinary use has not been reported.

Mechanism of Action. The β-lactamase inhibitors bind to the β-lactamase enzyme that is produced by gram-negative or gram-positive bacteria. This usually is an irreversible, noncompetitive binding. Clavulanate is considered an irreversible, suicide inhibitor. A wide range of β-lactamases are inhibited by clavulanate, including Class B β-lactamases, TEM and SHV enzymes found in Enterobacteriaceae, many of the extended-spectrum β-lactamases, and various chromosomally mediated enzymes (Finlay et al. 2003). An inactive enzyme complex is formed and the coadministered antibiotic (e.g., amoxicillin or ampicillin) can exert its antibacterial effect. All β-lactamase inhibitors are not equal with respect to potency and ability to bind β-lactamase enzymes. For example, compared to clavulanate, sulbactam is less active against β-lactamase of *Staphylococcus, Bacteroides,* and some *E. coli.* However, whether these differences are important clinically is not known.

Pharmacokinetics. The pharmacokinetics of clavulanate in animals has been studied more than the other inhibitors (Bywater et al. 1985; Vree et al. 2003). Clavulanate is notoriously unstable and should be protected from moisture. Tablets are packaged in foil-protective packaging. Although clavulanate is absorbed orally (the only one of the β-lactamases absorbed orally), the absorption is variable and can vary highly among animals administered similar doses (Vree et al. 2003). There is evidence that high doses of amoxicillin inhibit the absorption of clavulanate in dogs and people (Vree et al. 2003). Clavulanate is susceptible to enzymatic degradation and is excreted by glomerular filtration, whereas amoxicillin is eliminated by renal tubular excretion.

Examples and Clinical Use

Amoxicillin-Clavulanic Acid (Clavamox®, Synulox). This is one of the most popular oral antibiotics used in small animals. Amoxicillin-clavulanate extends the spectrum of amoxicillin to include many of the β-lactamase–producing bacteria. There is an equivalent drug used in people (Augmentin), which is one of the most popular drugs in human medicine. The human drug Augmentin is not entirely equivalent because the proportion of amoxicillin : clavulanate may be different. Clavamox has a 4 : 1 ratio, whereas Augmentin is either in a 4 : 1 ratio or a 7 : 1 ratio. The dose administered to animals is a fixed ratio of 4 : 1 (amoxicillin : clavulanate), but because of lower absorption of clavulanate and more rapid excretion, the ratio in the body can be highly variable and as low as 20 : 1.

In small animals Clavamox® has been used to treat infections in almost all tissues (except CNS). It has been successful for skin infections and urinary tract infections (Bywater et al. 1985; Senior et al. 1985). It is particularly useful to treat infections caused by β-lactamase–producing staphylococci. Amoxicillin-clavulanate also is useful for treating anaerobic infections in dogs and cats, such as those of the oral cavity (Indiveri and Hirsh 1985).

In large animals, amoxicillin-clavulanate has not been an important drug. As reported previously, the oral absorption of amoxicillin in horses is small and unlikely to reach therapeutic concentrations. The oral administration has also been examined in calves (Soback et al. 1987a). There is sufficient absorption of amoxicillin-clavulanate in preruminant calves, but three-times-daily administration was recommended (Soback et al. 1987a), which is impractical. Oral absorption was not high enough in ruminant calves—because of degradation in the rumen—to produce therapeutic concentrations.

Sulbactam-Ampicillin (Unasyn®). This is a human drug, but veterinary preparations exist in other countries. This drug has been administered IM, IV, and SC to dogs, horses, and cattle. (Sulbactam is not absorbed orally.) In some countries (e.g., Canada) this combination is used as an intramuscular drug (ampicillin trihydrate + sulbactam, Synergistin) in cattle for the treatment of diseases such as pneumonic pasteurellosis (Risk and Bentley 1987; Risk and Cummins 1987; Girard et al. 1987).

Ticarcillin-Clavulanic Acid (Timentin®). This is available as a human drug, but also has been used in veterinary medicine. Because ticarcillin is susceptible to β-lactamase inactivation, clavulanate increases the spectrum of ticarcillin to include *Staphylococcus*, and many Enterobacteriaceae. Ticarcillin-clavulanate has been examined in dogs and horses (Garg et al. 1987; VanCamp et al. 2000). Ticarcillin-clavulanate is a fixed combination (Timentin) in a 30 : 1 ratio. It has been administered at a dose of 50 mg/kg and 1.67 mg/kg for the ticarcillin and clavulanate portion, respectively. This dose was derived from pharmacokinetic studies in dogs and horses (VanCamp et al. 2000; Garg et al. 1987). The short half-life requires frequent administration (every 6 hours).

There are several reports that investigated the administration of ticarcillin-clavulanate (30 : 1 ratio) as an intrauterine infusion in mares. These studies were summarized in the most recent report (VanCamp et al. 2000). The conclusion from this study was that it was possible to attain effective concentrations of ticarcillin in the uterine tissue of mares from either IV administration (50 and 1.67 mg/kg of ticarcillin and clavulanate, respectively) or intrauterine administration (12.4 and 0.4 mg/kg of ticarcillin and clavulanate, respectively), but that clavulanate concentrations either declined too rapidly to be effective or were undetectable.

Piperacillin-Tazobactam (Zosyn®). This is a relatively newer combination that has not been used in veterinary medicine. Tazobactam has essentially the same activity as clavulanate. Piperacillin has good extended-spectrum activity against streptococci and gram-negative bacilli.

CEPHALOSPORINS

Cephalosporins that are veterinary-labeled, as well as drugs registered for humans (e.g., cephalexin, cefazolin) have commonly been used in veterinary medicine for many infections, including pyoderma, urinary tract infection, pneumonia, soft-tissue infection, osteomyelitis, and pre- and postsurgical use. They are considered first-line treatments, often employed empirically for routine outpatient and in-hospital use. One of the advantages of the use of the generic formulations intended for humans (cefazolin and cephalexin) is their low cost. For more resistant infections caused by *Pseudomonas aeruginosa* or the Enterobacteriaceae such as *E. coli,* extended-spectrum drugs of the second- and third-generation have been used.

GENERAL PHARMACOLOGY. The spectrum is similar to amoxicillin and ampicillin, but also includes some β-lactamase–producing bacteria, depending on the specific generation of cephalosporin. Many in this class have greater activity against gram-negative bacteria than amoxicillin or ampicillin. In general (exceptions noted below in the section "Classification"), the cephalosporins owe their usefulness to activity against the following: *Staphylococcus* (β-lactamase–positive), streptococci (but not enterococci), gram-negative bacteria, except *Pseudomonas* (exceptions noted below), and anaerobic bacteria (except *Bacteroides fragilis*). Although cephalosporin antibiotics show activity against some anaerobic bacteria, they are ordinarily *not* considered a drug of choice for the gram-negative anaerobes. The cephamycins (a subclass of cephalosporins), however, have good anaerobic activity.

Cephalosporins contain a 7-aminocephalosporanic acid nucleus, which is composed of a β-lactam ring fused with a 6-membered dihydrothiazine ring (see Fig. 34.1). Additions of various groups at the R positions form derivatives with differences in antimicrobial activity, stability against β-lactamases, protein binding, intestinal absorption, metabolism, and toxicity.

The cephalosporin antibiotics are extremely important in veterinary medicine. They were first produced by a fungus isolated from raw sewage from the sea in Sardinia. Although the antibiotic was first isolated from *Cephalosporium acremonium* in 1948, it was not available commercially until 1962. There are now over 30 cephalosporin antibiotics on the market (most on the human pharmaceutical market), but new recent ones have been introduced to the veterinary market.

CLASSIFICATION. The cephalosporins are broadly classified into first-, second-, third-, and fourth-generation cephalosporins. This classification system is somewhat arbitrary, depending on when they were synthesized. Rather than by their structure, the cephalosporins are classified on the basis of activity. Against gram-negative bacteria, these drugs are grouped according to their susceptibility to β-lactamase. Various other classifications of cephalosporins have been proposed (Williams et al. 2001). For this chapter, we retain the classification categories listed in the United States Pharmacopeia (USP-DI 2004), provided in Table 34.4.

First Generation. The first-generation drugs are effective against almost all gram-positive bacteria, except enterococcus, and their activity includes β-lactamase–positive staphylococcus. They also have greater activity against members of the Enterobacteriaceae than penicillin G. Compared to others in this group, cefazolin has the greatest gram-negative activity (Petersen and Rosin 1995), and it has been grouped with the second-generation drugs in some references based on this activity (Williams et al. 2001). Gram-negative bacteria may develop resistance by inhibiting penetration and by producing β-lactamase enzymes.

Second Generation. In general, these drugs have greater activity against many gram-negative bacteria that are resistant to the first-generation drugs (e.g., resistant *E. coli, Klebsiella, Proteus, Enterobacter*), but are no more active against the gram-positive bacteria. Improved activity against gram-negative bacteria compared to first-generation drugs is attributed to an increased resistance to β-lactamases. Cefoxitin and cefotetan belong to the cephamycin group and are often used clinically because of good activity against anaerobic bacteria (e.g., *Bacteroides fragilis,* and the *Bacteroides fragilis* group). Cefaclor (Ceclor®), cefprozil (Cefzil®), and cefuroxime axetil (Cefetin®) can be administered orally, but their use has not been reported for small animals.

TABLE 34.4 Classification of cephalosporins

First Generation		Second Generation		Third Generation	
Drug Name	Brand Name	Drug Name	Brand Name	Drug Name	Brand Name
cephalexin	generic, Keflex*	cefamandole	Mandol	cefoperazone	Cefobid
cephalothin	Keflin	cefmetazole	Zefazone	cefotaxime	Claforan
cefadroxil	Cefa-Tabs*	cefonicid	Monocid	ceftazidime	Fortaz
cephapirin	Cefadyl	cefprozil	Cefzil*	ceftizoxime	Cefizox
cefazolin	Kefzol	cefotetan	Cefotan	ceftriaxone	Rochephin
cephradine	Velosef*	cefoxitin	Mefoxin	moxalactam	Moxam
cefaparin	Cefa-Lak and Cefa-Dri	cefuroxime	Kefurox	cefixime	Suprax*
		cefuroxime axetil	Ceftin*	cefdinir	Omnicef*
		cefaclor	Ceclor*	ceftiofur	Naxcel
				cefpodoxime proxetil	Vantin* Simplicef*
				Cefovecin	Convenia

*Oral drugs.

Third Generation. This group of antibiotics has more activity against gram-negative bacteria than the earlier generations of cephalosporins. Only ceftazidime and cefoperazone have good activity against *Pseudomonas aeruginosa*, with ceftazidime having the greatest activity. For this reason, ceftazidime has been an important drug for some infections in small animals.

The third-generation drugs, in general, are less active against gram-positive cocci, but there is considerable variability in the activity against staphylococci and streptococci among this group. For example, cefotaxime has the highest activity against streptococci, but others have less activity. There are only three that can be administered orally. Of these, two have been used in veterinary medicine, cefixime (Suprax®) (Lavy et al. 1995), and cefpodoxime proxetil (Simplicef veterinary formulation and Vantin human formulation).

Most of the human-labeled injectable third-generation drugs are expensive and used in veterinary medicine only when resistance has been shown to other drugs. An exception is ceftiofur (Naxcel®), which has been used extensively in cattle and is also registered for use in horses and dogs. The activity of the major metabolite, desfuroylceftiofur is similar to cefotaxime, which is listed as a typical third-generation cephalosporin. A new addition to the veterinary drugs is cefovecin (Convenia) which is an injectable formulation that has an extremely long half-life compared to other cephalosporins.

Fourth Generation. Recently, there has been designation of a fourth-generation of cephalosporins. The use of these has not been reported in veterinary medicine except for some experimental studies. The first fourth-generation cephalosporin is cefepime (Maxipime®). It is unique among cephalosporins because of its broad spectrum of activity that includes gram-positive cocci, enteric gram-negative bacilli, and *Pseudomonas aeruginosa*. It is active against β-lactamase–producing strains of *E. coli* that are resistant to other β-lactam antibiotics. Doses for dogs and foals have been developed from pharmacokinetic studies (Gardner and Papich 2001), but its clinical use has not been evaluated in veterinary medicine. The other fourth-generation cephalosporin is cefquinome, which has been licensed for use in cattle in Europe since 1994 and also has not undergone FDA review in the United States for use in cattle.

MECHANISM OF ACTION. Similar to other β-lactam antibiotics, the cephalosporins bind to PBPs and disrupt the cell wall. They are usually bactericidal and most often bind the PBP-2 and -3.

PHARMACOKINETICS. The pharmacokinetic features of specific drugs are provided in Table 34.5 and are also listed in the article by Caprile (1988) (see Table 34.5).

Pharmacokinetics-Pharmacodynamics. Pharmacokinetic-pharmacodynamic (PK-PD) relationships for cephalosporins are the same as for other β-lactam antibiotics discussed earlier in this chapter. Like other β-lactam

TABLE 34.5 Pharmacokinetic parameters of selected cephalosporins in domestic species

Drug	Species	V_d[a] (L/kg)	Clearance (mL/kg/min)	Elimination half-life (hr)	Reference
Cephapirin	Foals[b]	1.06	18.4	0.70	Brown et al. 1987
	Horses	0.17	10.0		Brown et al. 1986a
	Cows[c]		12.7		Prades et al. 1988
	Dogs	0.32	8.9	0.42	Cabana et al. 1976
Cephalothin	Horses	0.15	13.6	0.25	Ruoff and Sams 1985
Cefadroxil	Horses	0.46	7.0	0.77	Wilson et al. 1985
Cefazolin	Foals	0.45	0.4	1.37	Duffee et al. 1989
	Horses	0.19	5.5	0.67	Sams and Ruoff 1985
	Calves	0.17	5.8	0.62	Soback et al. 1987
	Dogs	0.70	10.4	0.80	
Cephalexin	Calves	0.32	1.9	2.00	Garg et al. 1992
	Cows	0.39	10.5	0.58	Soback et al. 1988
	Sheep	0.17	5.0	1.20	Villa et al. 1991
Cefoxitin	Calves			1.12	Soback 1988
	Horses	0.12	4.3	0.82	Brown 1986b
Cepfaronide	Sheep	0.39	2.7		Guerrini et al. 1985
Ceftriaxone	Dogs			0.85	Matsui et al. 1984
	Sheep	0.30	3.7		Guerrini et al. 1985
	Calves			1.40	Soback and Ziv 1988
Ceftazidime	Dogs			0.82	Matusi et al. 1984
	Sheep	0.36		1.60	Rule et al. 1991
Cefoperazone	Calves			0.89	Carli et al. 1986
	Sheep	0.16	2.7		Guerrini et al. 1985
Moxalactam	Calves			2.40	Soback 1989

[a]V_d = volume of distribution.
[b]Neonatal.
[c]Lactating.

antibiotics, cephalosporins are considered to be bactericidal in action; they kill bacteria if the drug concentrations are maintained above the MIC for a critical period during the dosing interval (Nishida et al. 1978). Thus the important parameter is considered time above MIC (T > MIC). It is the duration of exposure, rather than the magnitude of the concentration above the MIC that determines efficacy of cephalosporins. Dosage regimens for the cephalosporins have been formulated to consider these PK-PD relationships (Craig 1995, 2001; MacGowan 2001; Turnidge 1998). Among the β-lactams, penicillins are not as bactericidal as carbapenems, and cephalosporins are not as bactericidal as penicillins. Therefore, among the β-lactams, cephalosporins should be maintained above the MIC longer than others in this class. Although the optimum time above the MIC has not been determined for most cephalosporins used in companion animals, in humans and laboratory animals, the optimum time above the MIC is regarded as 50% of the dosing interval. However, for treating gram-negative infections, maximum bactericidal effect occurs at 60–70% of the dosing interval, and as the duration of the T > MIC increases, improved clinical outcomes are possible. In some experimental studies the T > MIC may be less than 50%. For example, when four cephalosporins were examined to determine the T > MIC necessary for optimum dosing, the T > MIC was 30–40% of the dosing interval for Enterobacteriaceae and streptococcus, but less than 30% for staphylococcus.

Because the half-lives of most cephalosporins in mammals are short, many regimens for cephalosporins use require an administration frequency of three to four times per day. Alternatively, some of the third-generation cephalosporins have long half-lives, and less frequent regimens have been used for some of these drugs (for example cefpodoxime, cefovecin, cefotaxime, and ceftiofur). However, the long half-life for ceftriaxone in people does not occur in animals because of differences in drug protein binding (Popick et al. 1987).

The dosing regimen that produces the greatest T > MIC is the constant rate intravenous infusion (CRI), and superior efficacy has been reported from CRI regimens rather than intermittent dosing (Zeisler et al. 1992). Constant rate intravenous infusions have also been calculated for some third-generation cephalosporins for dogs (Moore et al. 2000).

Gram-positive organisms are more susceptible to the bactericidal effect of cephalosporins than are gram-negative bacteria. Additionally, since the MICs are lower for gram-positive bacteria, and antibacterial effects occur at concentrations below the MIC for *Staphylococcus* (post-antibiotic effect, PAE), longer dose intervals may be possible for infections caused by gram-positive as compared to gram-negative bacteria. For example, cephalexin or cefadroxil have been used successfully to treat staphylococcal infections when administered twice daily (discussed further in the later section "Clinical Features and Specific Drugs Used in Veterinary Medicine"). Some studies have reported efficacy for cephalexin treating staphylococcal pyoderma in dogs with administration of only once daily (although twice-daily administration is recommended to obtain maximum response).

In neutropenic patients, Turnidge (1998) proposes that the T > MIC should be greater than 50%, and he presents compelling evidence in his review to support this view. In neutropenic animals, the T > MIC for cephalosporins should be 90–100% of the dosing interval against gram-negative bacilli and streptococci, but can be lowered to only 50–60% of the dosing interval because of the post-antibiotic effect when treating *Staphylococcus*.

Tissue Concentrations and Protein Binding. Cephalosporins are relatively polar antibiotics. They are minimally lipid soluble and have poor intracellular penetration. The volume of distribution is generally in the range of 0.2 to 0.3 l/kg and rarely exceeds 0.5 l/kg. However, they have good distribution into the extracellular fluid of most tissues, except prostate and the CNS. Some of the third-generation cephalosporins are an exception because they have an improved ability to penetrate the CNS. Specific features of each drug will be discussed in more detail later in this chapter.

Pharmacokinetic-pharmacodynamic–based dosing regimens use plasma concentrations as the surrogate marker for determining the optimum dose and interval (Hyatt et al. 1995). This presumes that the plasma drug concentration and tissue fluid concentration are similar. Because cephalosporins do not penetrate cells, the intracellular drug concentrations are low. Tissue homogenates will underestimate the drug concentration at the site of infection, which is in the extracellular fluid (Craig 1995; Nix et al. 1991; Liu et al. 2002).

In general, plasma drug concentrations for cephalosporins will predict the interstitial tissue fluid concentrations. There is an exception to this assumption if there is high protein binding that prevents drug diffusion from the plasma through capillaries into the tissue (Nix et al. 1991; Liu et al. 2002). When protein binding is high, it decreases drug diffusion from the plasma and reduces the concentration of active drug at the site of infection. (Only protein-unbound drug is microbiologically active.) Protein binding for most cephalosporins is low in companion animals compared to humans. However, this has been examined and reported for only a few drugs, and there are many drugs for which we do not have enough information to make extrapolations. Ceftriaxone has high protein binding of 90–95% in people, which restricts clearance and causes a long half-life (Popick et al. 1987). But the same drug in dogs has protein binding of only 25% at low concentrations to 2% at high concentrations. Cefazolin has high protein binding in people (85%), but low protein binding in dogs (19%), which favors rapid distribution from plasma to interstitial fluid. The most highly protein-bound cephalosporin in animals is cefovecin, which is greater than 99% bound in dogs and cats. This property prolongs the plasma concentrations, although because of lower protein binding in tissue fluids does not decrease antibacterial effectiveness in infected tissues.

The effect of protein binding on drug distribution was demonstrated for cephalexin and cefpodoxime, two orally administered cephalosporins used in dogs (Papich et al. 2007). Protein binding is higher for cefpodoxime in dogs (>80%), which prolongs the half-life compared to cephalexin. The free drug concentration for cefpodoxime in tissue fluid represented the unbound drug fraction in plasma, reflecting the effect of protein binding to restrict drug diffusion from capillaries into tissues. This phenomenon has also been observed in humans (Liu et al. 2002).

Oral Absorption. Many of the cephalosporins are absorbed orally. Cefadroxil and cephalexin of the first-generation group are well-absorbed in small animals, but not in large animals. Oral absorption of the ester formulations, (cefpodoxime proxetil) is enhanced. This feature will be discussed in more detail later for individual drugs. For cefadroxil, but not cephalexin, absorption was enhanced somewhat with food (Campbell and Rosin 1998).

In horses cefadroxil is absorbed better in the foal than in adult horses (Wilson et al. 1985; Duffee et al. 1989). Oral absorption of cephalexin is low in horses (5%) (Davis et al. 2005) but at 30 mg/kg orally q8h, concentrations can be maintained above the MIC of susceptible bacteria.

Metabolism. Cephalosporins are minimally metabolized by the liver, but degree of metabolism can vary widely among the various drugs. Ceftiofur is transformed almost completely to the metabolite desfuroylceftiofur, which is responsible for its antibacterial efficacy. Most cephalosporins rely on renal elimination.

Elimination. The cephalosporins are eliminated rapidly after systemic administration. The route of elimination is primarily renal, and concentrations in the urine are usually high. This feature makes cephalosporins good choices for treatment of urinary tract infections.

In general, the cephalosporins have half-lives of 1 to 2 hours, but some (particularly the third-generation cephalosporins) may have longer half-lives, which may allow for infrequent dosing. For example, ceftiofur is metabolized to an active metabolite and has a half-life of approximately 3–6 hr in cattle, 4 hr in dogs, and 2.5 hr in horses. The longer half-life of ceftiofur and its metabolites is probably caused by their high protein binding.

CLINICAL FEATURES AND SPECIFIC DRUGS USED IN VETERINARY MEDICINE. The drugs in the first-generation group have a spectrum of activity that includes staphylococci, streptococci, and many of the enteric gram-negative bacilli. However, resistance among gram-negative bacteria develops easily, primarily from synthesis of β-lactamase enzymes that can hydrolyze these drugs. Resistance was demonstrated in two clinical studies in which samples were collected from dogs and cats (Oluoch et al. 2001; Walker et al. 2000; Cooke et al. 2002). These studies reported that more than half of the gram-negative isolates were resistant to first-generation cephalosporins.

Extended-spectrum cephalosporins include cephalosporins from the second, third, and fourth generation. The situations in veterinary medicine in which extended-spectrum cephalosporins are most often used are for treatment of bacterial infections that are resistant to other drugs. The bacteria often identified in these resistance problems have been *Escherichia coli, Klebsiella pneumoniae, Enterobacter* species, *Proteus* species (especially indole-positive), and *Pseudomonas aeruginosa.*

First-Generation Cephalosporins. Veterinarians are familiar with the cephalosporins commonly referred to as the *first-generation cephalosporins* represented by the oral drugs cephalexin (Keflex) and cefadroxil (Cefa-Tabs, Cefa-Drops), and the injectable drug cefazolin (generic). Cefadroxil and cephalexin have been the most extensively used of the oral first-generation cephalosporins in dogs. (Older drugs such as cephradine are no longer available.) Cefadroxil is more lipophilic than cephalexin and has the advantage of being better absorbed orally. The differences between cephalexin and cefadroxil were illustrated in the study by Campbell and Rosin (1998) in which they examined the oral absorption of each drug and the influence of food in dogs after 30 mg/kg every 12 hours. Being more lipophilic, cefadroxil was absorbed better when administered with food and attained higher concentrations in plasma. Cephalexin was less influenced by the presence of food. Because cefadroxil was also more active, with lower MIC values for *E. coli*, the time above MIC was longer for cefadroxil than for cephalexin. These differences were not observed for *Staphylococcus*. Every 12-hour dosing was determined to be adequate for both drugs against *Staphylococcus* because it is more sensitive to both drugs than is *E. coli*.

Cefadroxil. Cefadroxil is available as oral suspension (50 mg/ml) and oral tablets (although the availability of some formulations has diminished in recent years). In cats, cefadroxil pharmacokinetics are similar to that in dogs (Chatfield et al. 1984) and it has a half-life of 2.5 to 2.7 hours. Clinical trials in cats showed that cefadroxil was effective for dermal infections with cure rates of 88% at 10–20 mg/kg and 100% cure rate at 20 mg/kg twice daily. Cefadroxil also is recommended for urinary tract infections in cats at a dose of 20 mg/kg once daily.

In dogs, cefadroxil has been effective for treatment of urinary tract infections, skin infections, and respiratory infections (Chatfield et al. 1984, Angarano and

MacDonald 1989; Barsanti et al. 1985). The dose for which efficacy has been demonstrated for pyoderma has been 22 mg/kg every 12 hours orally for 21 to 30 days, but efficacy at a once-daily dose of 20 mg/kg once daily also has been reported (Scarampella et al. 2000). Cefadroxil at a dose of 22 mg/kg every 12 hours for 21 days was effective in an experimental model of canine cystitis (Barsanti et al. 1985) and has been registered for dogs for the treatment of urinary tract infections.

Cephalexin. Cephalexin is perhaps the most common oral cephalosporin administered to dogs. The generic formulation is inexpensive, and studies have been performed to establish its efficacy for some conditions, even though it is not registered for veterinary use in the United States. Cephalexin has a half-life of 2.2 to 2.5 hours after oral administration. (It is not available in other formulations in the U.S.) Its oral absorption ranges from 57% to 73–79% (Lavy et al. 1997; Carli et al. 1999). Another study reported higher values for half-life of 6.5 hours after oral administration (Wackowiez et al. 1997), and oral absorption of 91% in dogs.

Practitioners sometimes make the mistake of administering cephalexin doses used for staphylococcal pyoderma when they are treating infections caused by gram-negative bacteria. At the doses typically administered to dogs, cephalexin concentrations can be maintained above the MIC for staphylococci for at least 12 hours, which is sufficient for clinical cure. However, the ability of cephalexin to reach effective levels against many gram-negative bacteria (e.g., *E. coli*) at 20–30 mg/kg every 12 hours is doubtful. The conclusion from an analysis of published pharmacokinetic studies is that cephalexin must be administered at least every 8 hours (and perhaps as often as every 6 hours) to maintain the T > MIC values for susceptible gram-negative bacteria such as *E. coli* (Wackowiez et al. 1997; Carli et al. 1999).

Oral absorption of cephalexin in cats is about 56%, with a half-life of 2.25 hours (Wackowiez et al. 1997). At usual recommended doses, this will maintain concentrations for pathogens in cats that may cause dermal or urinary tract infections with 12-hour dosing.

One of the most common uses of first generation cephalosporins is for skin infections. Patterns of in vitro susceptibility of *Staphylococcus* have been reported for over 15 years (Lloyd et al. 1996; Medleau et al. 1986; Noble and Kent 1992; Petersen et al. 2002; Prescott et al. 2002). These published surveys have confirmed that a high proportion of organisms have retained susceptibility to cephalosporins, including cephalexin and cefadroxil. Cephalexin has been evaluated for superficial and deep pyoderma. It has been equally effective as cefadroxil in dogs (Frank and Kunkle 1993) when each was administered at 22 to 35 mg/kg twice daily for at least 3 weeks. Deep pyoderma required longer treatment than superficial pyoderma. In this study generic cephalexin was as effective as proprietary cephalexin (Keflex). Cephalexin also has been effective administered at either 15 mg/kg twice a day or 30 mg/kg once a day orally (Guaguère et al. 2000; Maynard et al. 2002a).

Cephalexin oral absorption in horses is only 5% (Davis et al. 2005), but can be administered at 30 mg/kg q8h orally to achieve effective plasma concentrations above 0.5 μg/ml.

Cefazolin. Cefazolin is the injectable cephalosporin most often used in small animals. It is inexpensive, has a broad spectrum of activity, and is stable after reconstitution for 1 week if refrigerated (Bornstein et al. 1974). It has been administered IV, IM, and SC to dogs. There are several papers that have examined its activity and pharmacokinetics in animals (Petersen and Rosin 1995; Rosin et al. 1989, 1993; Dickson et al. 1987; Marcellin-Little et al. 1996). It is more active against *E. coli* than cephalothin (Petersen and Rosin 1995), and after standard doses of 20–22 mg/kg IV, concentrations can be maintained during surgical procedures. Cefazolin, like many other cephalosporins has low plasma protein binding (19%, in dogs, which is much lower than in humans) and diffuses into tissue fluid to reach concentrations that parallel those in plasma (Rosin et al. 1989, 1993). Cefazolin also penetrated normal and osteomyletic bone in concentrations similar to plasma concentrations (Daly et al. 1982). Distribution was not impaired in osteomyletic bone. This advantage of good penetration has allowed it to be used for prevention and treatment of bone infections (Daly et al. 1982) and as a common antibiotic to use prophylactically prior to orthopedic surgery (Rosin et al. 1993). Richardson et al. (1992) showed that at a dose of 22 mg/kg IV every hour, cefazolin concentrations in bone were above the MIC_{90} for pathogens causing common postoperative infections. The optimum dose was further evaluated in a follow-up study by Marcellin-Little et al. (1996). As in previously reported studies, cefazolin concentrations in bone of dogs paralleled the plasma concentrations. To maintain cefazolin concentrations above 20 μg/ml (10× the MIC_{90} for organisms in the author's laboratory), a dose of 22 mg/kg administered IV every 2 hours or 8 mg/kg administered IV every hour was determined. During surgery, disease, anesthesia, and blood loss may affect distribution and clearance of some drugs. However, when cefazolin was administered to dogs with hemorrhagic shock, the clearance was slower, but it was offset by an increased volume of distribution (Dickson et al. 1987). Consequently, the plasma concentrations were not different in dogs when compared before and after shock. Some cephalosporins affect blood clotting and platelet function in animals and may be risky to use prior to surgery. However, when cefazolin was compared to cephalothin and cefmetazole in dogs, the investigators showed that cephalothin decreased platelet aggregation, and cefmetazole prolonged bleeding time (Wilkens et al. 1994), but cefazolin caused no adverse effects on platelet aggregation, bleeding time, platelet count, platelet size, or bleeding times.

Cefazolin also is used in large animals. Cefazolin is used occasionally in horses as an injectable preoperatively or perioperatively. Pharmacokinetic studies are available to guide dosing (Sams and Ruoff 1985; Donecker et al. 1986). Cefazolin has a slower terminal half-life from IM than from IV administration. The IM injection is thought to have a longer half-life because of slower absorption (caused by the flip-flop effect discussed earlier). Subsequent doses of 10 to 20 mg/kg can be administered q8h IM or q6h IV.

Cephapirin. Cephapirin is not used very often for systemic use in animals, but there are dry cow and lactating cow preparations (Cefa-Dri®, Cefa-Lak®, respectively) of cephapirin for intramammary infusion. Cephapirin is used for treatment of mastitis caused by *Streptococcus* or *Staphylococcus*.

Cephapirin benzathine is used for dry cow treatment 300 mg/10 ml, administered in each quarter at the time of drying. Cephapirin sodium 200 mg/10 ml is infused 200 mg to each affected quarter every 12 hours.

Second-Generation Cephalosporins. Of the second-generation cephalosporins, the ones used most often in veterinary medicine are cefoxitin and cefotetan (Petersen and Rosin 1993). Their use has been valuable for treating organisms resistant to the first-generation cephalosporins or in cases in which there are anaerobic bacteria present. Anaerobic bacteria such as those of the *Bacteroides fragilis* group can become resistant by synthesizing a cephalosporinase enzyme, but cefoxitin and cefotetan, which are in the cephamycin group, are resistant to this enzyme. Therefore, these drugs may be valuable for some cases such as septic peritonitis that may have a mixed population of anaerobic bacteria and gram-negative bacilli.

Both drugs were evaluated for activity and pharmacokinetics in dogs (Petersen and Rosin 1993). Cefotetan was much more active against *E. coli*. Even though both drugs had similar pharmacokinetics and were absorbed after SC administration, the T > MIC was greater for cefotetan resulting in a longer dose interval compared to cefoxitin. The recommended dose for cefotetan was 30 mg/kg every 8 hours IV, or every 12 hours SC.

There are no reports of clinical use of oral second-generation cephalosporins in small animals, but doses have been extrapolated from human studies. Cefaclor was shown to have 75% oral bioavailability in dogs (Waterman and Scharfenberger 1978). Interstitial drug levels were lower than serum, but urine concentrations were high for 4 hours after dosing.

Third-Generation Cephalosporins. The third-generation cephalosporins are the most active of the cephalosporins against gram-negative bacteria, especially enteric organisms that are resistant to other cephalosporins. The injectable drugs are administered IV, SC, IM. The SC route is often used for convenience (Moore et al. 2000; Guerrini et al. 1986). Veterinarians have observed that the IM or SC administration of some of these drugs can be irritating and painful. One of the most frequently administered of the human-labeled drugs in this group is cefotaxime (Claforan) because of its potency and activity against most enteric gram-negative bacteria and some streptococci. Except for a few pharmacokinetic studies (Guerrini et al. 1986; McElroy et al. 1986), there are no published studies in which cefotaxime has been evaluated in veterinary patients. However, the pharmacokinetics between dogs and humans are similar enough that doses, as well as clinical uses, have been extrapolated from human medicine. Generally, cefotaxime is administered IV, IM, or SC to dogs and cats at a dose of 30 mg/kg every 8 hours. When administered SC to dogs, and IM to cats, the absorption was high (McElroy et al. 1986; Guerrini et al. 1986), but IM and SC injections can cause pain.

Ceftiofur. Ceftiofur (Naxcel) is registered for use in small animals. It is registered for use only for treating urinary tract infections caused by gram-negative bacilli of the Enterobacteriaceae. It is registered for a dose of 2.2 mg/kg SC once a day. It is converted to an active metabolite, desfuroylceftiofur, which is similar in activity to cefotaxime, and therefore this drug has a spectrum of action representative of other third-generation cephalosporins. According to a published study (Brown et al. 1995), the dose of 2.2 mg/kg once daily will be sufficient for treatment of bacteria with low MIC values; higher MIC values of 2.0 μg/ml or greater may require a higher dose of 4.4 mg/kg. The CLSI (CLSI 2007) breakpoint for ceftiofur use in cattle is ≤2.0 μg/ml, but the breakpoint for cephalosporins used in people is usually ≤8.0 μg/ml. Therefore, susceptibility to other cephalosporins does not necessarily mean susceptibility to ceftiofur. The use of ceftiofur for treating systemic infections in small animals has not been reported. But, on the basis of the pharmacokinetic profile of plasma concentrations (Brown et al. 1995), it appears that the frequency of administration should be greater than once a day to maintain the drug concentrations above the MIC for a sufficient duration. In dogs, anemia and thrombocytopenia are possible if ceftiofur is administered at doses of 3 times and 5 times the registered dose of 2.2 mg/kg.

Ceftiofur is perhaps the most frequently used cephalosporin in horses. Ceftiofur was approved for use in horses for treatment of respiratory tract infections caused by *Streptococcus equi* subsp. *zooepidemicus* at a dose of 2.2 to 4.4 mg/kg q24h IM. Higher doses or more frequent intervals have been recommended for treating gram-negative organisms (e.g., *Klebsiella, Enterobacter, Salmonella*). Because these organisms are inherently more resistant, higher plasma concentrations are needed for efficacy. The susceptibility breakpoint for ceftiofur use in horses is low ≤0.25 μg/ml (CLSI 2007), and organisms other than streptococci may be classified in vitro as resistant. Studies in foals indicated that a dose of 2.2 to 6.6 mg/kg could be given to foals IM or IV q12h for treatment of neonatal sepsis. Based on pharmacokinetic studies (Jaglan et al. 1994) a dose of 4.4 mg/kg injected q12h will produce plasma concentrations above the MIC to meet the criteria for effective therapy. Toxicity studies have shown that horses tolerate ceftiofur doses up to 11 mg/kg/day IM, with pain at the injection site and decreased feed consumption as the most common adverse effects at the highest dose.

The other major use of ceftiofur is for cattle and pigs. Ceftiofur is available in three formulations: 1) ceftiofur sodium—Excenel, 2) ceftiofur hydrochloride suspension (Naxcel), and 3) ceftiofur crystalline-free acid (Excede). The crystalline-free acid is a slow-releasing drug that is injected at the base of the ear in cattle and in the neck of pigs. It has been used for treating respiratory infections (BRD) in cattle (1–2 mg/kg q24h) caused by *Mannheimia haemolytica* (formerly called *Pasteurella haemolytica*), *Histophilus somni* (formerly *Haemohilus somnus*), and *Pasteurella multocida*. It is also used for treating respiratory disease in pigs. Ceftiofur hydrochloride and ceftiofur crystalline-free acid have also been administered intramammary to dairy cattle.

Ceftazidime. Compared to other cephalosporins, ceftazidime is the most active against *Pseudomonas*, against which all the other cephalosporins, except cefoperazone, have little or no activity. Ceftazidime has been studied in dogs (Moore et al. 2000; Matsui et al. 1984; Acred 1983) and it has a short half-life (less than 1 hour) and volume of distribution similar to that in humans. Dosages have ranged from 20–30 mg/kg every 12 hours for Enterobacteriaceae, to 30 mg/kg administered every 4 hours for *Pseudomonas* (Moore et al. 2000).

In vitro activity of ceftazidime is good against most gram-negative bacilli (Martin Barrasa et al. 2000). Isolates of *Pseudomonas aeruginosa* from otitis media showed that 97% were susceptible to ceftazidime (Colombini et al. 2000). In a study that isolated *Pseudomonas aeruginosa* from the skin and ears of dogs, a similar pattern of resistance was reported (Petersen et al. 2002). In a study that examined 183 isolates of *Pseudomonas aeruginosa* from various sites in dogs (1993–2000), with the ADD test (Seol et al. 2002), percent sensitivity to ceftazidime was 77%.

Because of the good activity against Enterobacteriaceae and *Pseudomonas aeruginosa*, ceftazidime has been used in exotic and zoo animals. In a killer whale, the half-life was greater than 6 hours after IM administration and therapeutic concentrations were maintained after doses of 20 mg/kg every 24 hours, IM (unpublished observations by one of the authors [MGP]). In reptiles, cephalosporins are excreted slowly. Ceftazidime pharmacokinetics in sea turtles determined that a half-life of 20 hours allowed for dosing of 20 mg/kg as infrequently as every 72 hours (Stamper et al. 1999).

Cefovecin. In December 2006 cefovecin (Convenia) was introduced to small animal medicine in Europe. The same drug and formulation were available in Canada in October 2007 and in the United States in 2008. There have also been pharmacokinetic studies (Stegemann et al. 2006a,b) published for dogs and cats, pharmacodynamic studies published (Stegemann et al. 2006c), and clinical efficacy studies in dogs and cats (Stegemann et al. 2007a,b; Passmore et al. 2007). In the clinical studies, cefovecin was compared to another active antimicrobial (cefadroxil, cephalexin, or amoxicillin-clavulanate) and was found noninferior to these other drugs.

In dogs and cats, cefovecin is registered for treatment of skin infections. In some countries it is also registered for urinary tract infections. The approved label dose in the United States allows for a repeat injection at seven days at a dose of 8 mg/kg SC. However, concentrations are maintained against some bacteria for 14 days, and the approved dose interval in Canada and Europe lists a 14-day dose interval. The studies published show efficacy with a 14-day interval for administration. The injection may be repeated for infections that require longer than 14 days for a cure (e.g., canine pyoderma).

The long duration of cefovecin is attributed to the long half-life in dogs and cats. Cefovecin is >99% protein bound in cats and >98% in dogs. With such a small fraction unbound (fu) there is little drug available for excretion and some tubular reabsorption may also occur. Subsequently, the terminal half-life is approximately 7 days in cats and 5 days in dogs. Effective concentrations can be maintained in the tissue fluid for a 14-day interval or longer (Stegemann et al. 2006a,b). Cefovecin is a third-generation cephalosporin. Therefore, against many bacteria, it is more active with lower MIC values than first-generation cephalosporins. This was demonstrated for pathogens from Europe and the United States (Stegemann et al. 2006c). Cefovecin MIC_{90} values were 0.25 μg/ml for *Staphylococcus intermedius* compared to 2 μg/ml for cephalexin and cefadroxil. As a third-generation cephalosporin, it is expected to have even greater activity against gram-negative bacteria, as was demonstrated by the MIC_{90} values of 1 μg/ml compared to 16 μg/ml for cephalexin and cefadroxil. Many other MIC comparisons are provided in the tables in the paper by Stegemann et al. (2006c). Susceptibility breakpoints based on the distribution of organisms reported (Stegemann et al. 2006c) ≤2.0 μg/ml should be considered.

Oral Third-Generation Cephalosporins. Since the drugs mentioned above are all injectable, there has been a need for an oral extended-spectrum cephalosporin. Cefixime (Suprax) has been used in small animals because of the data on the pharmacokinetics to support a clinical dose (Lavy et al. 1995; Bialer et al. 1987). Oral tablets or liquid suspension formulated for adults and children provided convenient dosage forms (200, 400 mg tablets and 20 mg/ml oral suspension). According to investigators, cefixime has adequate oral absorption (52–58% oral absorption) and a long enough half-life for once or twice daily administration at 5 mg/kg orally. One investigator reported a half-life of 7.3–7.8 hours (Bialer et al. 1987) and another reported two phases for the half-life at 8 to 8.5 hours, and a later phase with a half-life of 12 to 14.5 hours (Lavy et al. 1995). Irrespective of which half-life is considered, the longer duration should be considered an advantage for a drug with time-dependent pharmacodynamics. The long half-life in dogs may be attributed to the high protein binding in dogs which is 82–92% (Bialer et al. 1987; Tonelli et al. 1985). However, this high degree of protein binding may limit the usefulness of this drug for systemic infections, as mentioned earlier. (See the section "Tissue Concentrations and Protein Binding," above.)

Cefpodoxime Proxetil. Cefpodoxime proxetil is the oral third-generation cephalosporin used most often in veterinary medicine. It is a prodrug ester (Borin et al. 1991) that is designed to remain stable in the stomach, but the prodrug is converted to the active cefpodoxime after intestinal absorption. As a lipophilic ester, it is anticipated that oral absorption will be enhanced if the drug is administered with food, which has been confirmed in people, but not specifically reported for dogs. Cefpodoxime has similar gram-negative in vitro activity as cefixime, but greater activity against *Staphylococcus.*

In dogs pharmacokinetics have been studied to show good oral absorption and a long half-life (4.7 and 5.6 hours) compared to other cephalosporins that allow for once-daily administration at 5–10 mg/kg (Brown et al. 2007; Klesel et al. 1992; Papich et al. 2007). Cherni and colleagues (2006) reported that cefpodoxime proxetil administered once a day (5 mg/kg) to dogs with pyoderma was as effective as twice-daily (26 mg/kg) administration of cephalexin (Cherni et al. 2006).

In horses, cefpodoxime proxetil oral absorption was good enough that a dose of 10 mg/kg q6–12h produced plasma concentrations that would potentially treat infections in horses (Carrillo et al. 2005).

Fourth-Generation Cephalosporins. The most recent development is the fourth generation cephalosporins. The first fourth generation cephalosporin is *cefepime* (Maxipime). It is unique because of its broad spectrum of activity that includes gram-positive cocci, enteric gram-negative bacilli, and *Pseudomonas*. It has the advantage of activity against some extended-spectrum β-lactamase (ESBL)–producing strains of *Klebsiella* and *E. coli* that have become resistant to many other β-lactam drugs and fluoroquinolones. Except for investigations in dogs, adult horses, and foals, the use of cefepime has been limited in veterinary medicine (Gardner and Papich 2001). In the study in dogs, there was a short half-life of 1 hour, and to maintain drug concentrations above an MIC value of 8 μg/ml for 67% of the dosing interval, a dose of 40 mg/kg IV every 6 hours would be necessary. However, this dose would maintain the concentration above an MIC of 2 μg/ml for 100% of the dosing interval so that for the more sensitive bacteria (MIC ≤2 μg/ml) dose intervals of every 8 to 12 hours could be considered. In foals and mares this drug possibly could be used for infections resistant to other drugs. A cefepime dose for foals of 11 mg/kg IV q8h (Gardner and Papich,. 2001) and for adults of 2.2 mg/kg IV q8h (Gardner and Papich 2001; Guglick et al. 1998) is recommended. When cefepime was administered to horses orally, signs of colic were observed (Guglick et al. 1998).

ADVERSE REACTIONS. Cephalosporins have a high therapeutic index and have been administered to small animals safely. Some of the adverse reactions are listed in the following sections.

Hypersensitivity Reactions. Hypersensitivity allergic reactions (Type I, II, or III) have been observed in small animals after administration, but they are infrequently reported. There appears to be some cross-sensitivity with penicillins, but the incidence has not been reported. One should not assume that if animals are sensitive to penicillin drugs, they will have adverse effects from cephalosporins. Sensitivity to penicillins may increase the risk of sensitivity to cephalosporins by a factor of 4 (Kelkar and Li 2001), but many patients who are sensitive to penicillins can receive cephalosporins safely. Cephalexin has a side chain identical to that of amoxicillin, so animals with sensitivity to ampicillin should be administered cephalexin cautiously. Likewise, cefadroxil has the same identical side chain as amoxicillin.

Gastrointestinal. Some dogs vomit after receiving oral cephalosporins (e.g., cefadroxil, Cefa-Tab®; cephalexin), particularly at high doses. Dogs also may vomit after rapid injections of intravenous cephalosporins (Petersen and Rosin 1993). In clinical studies with oral cephalosporins, vomiting and diarrhea are the most common adverse reaction (Frank and Kunkle 1993). Cephalexin and cefadroxil were the third and fifth most common oral drugs to cause adverse events in dogs according to one survey (Kunkle et al. 1995). In this survey, the most common adverse effects associated with oral cephalospsorins were gastrointestinal (vomiting, diarrhea, and loss of appetite). It is believed to be caused by irritation to the stomach mucosa, but the exact mechanism has not been investigated.

Blood Disorders. Cephalosporin-induced hemolysis has been reported in people (Ehmann 1992). Such a disorder has not been reported from use of cephalosporins in small animals. A positive Coombs test reaction can occur with patients receiving cephalosporins, but it is not associated with hemolytic anemia. High doses of ceftiofur in dogs can cause anemia and thrombocytopenia.

Bleeding Disorders. Bleeding disorders have been reported with some cephalosporins in humans because they may produce a prolongation of the prothrombin bleeding time. Even though this effect can be demonstrated in experimental dogs, it has not been reported to be a clinical problem in veterinary medicine, probably because it is associated only with a few of the cephalosporins that are rarely used in animals. Cephalothin was shown to prolong mucosal bleeding times and ADP-induced platelet aggregation in dogs, but did not affect platelet numbers or platelet aggregation from collagen (Schermerhorn et al. 1994). This is a moot point for cephalothin because it is no longer used clinically in dogs. The most commonly injected cephalosporin in dogs is cefazolin. When cefazolin was compared to cephalothin and cefmetazole in dogs, the investigators showed that cephalothin decreased platelet aggregation, and cefmetazole prolonged bleeding time (Wilkens et al. 1994). However, cefazolin caused no adverse effects on platelet aggregation, bleeding time, platelet count, platelet size, or bleeding times.

In people, only the cephalosporins with NMTT (N-methylthiotetrazole) side chains are prone to producing bleeding problems. *(The NMTT drugs include cefoperazone, cefotetan, and cefamandole.)* Bleeding problems appear to be related to vitamin K antagonism and/or platelet dysfunction.

Glycosuria. Cephalosporins may cause a false-positive glucose test on a urine sample test, but this occurs only if the test employs the copper-reduction test. Others such as the glucose enzymatic tests are not affected. This is of little clinical significance.

SPECIAL SPECIES CONSIDERATIONS. In zoo hoofstock, ceftiofur and other cephalosporins are important injectable drugs. Pharmacokinetics are similar as in other large animals, and doses for the cephalosporins are similar among the large zoo species.

In reptiles, cephalosporins are excreted slowly. Ceftazidime pharmacokinetics in sea turtles determined that a half-life of 20 hours allowed for dosing of 20 mg/kg as infrequently as every 72 hours (Stamper et al. 1999). Regimens for cephalosporins in other reptiles have been published that also allow for long dosing intervals (Jacobson 1999).

In birds, rapid elimination and poor oral absorption are a problem. This requires high doses and frequent administration for cephalosporins (Flammer 1998). Doses for cephalexin and cefotaxime in birds has been listed as high as 100 mg/kg, q8h.

CARBAPENEMS (PENEMS)

Carbapenems (also called *penems*) include imipenem, doripenem, ertapenem, and meropenem. They have the broadest antibacterial action in comparison to other β-lactams, even surpassing many third-generation cephalosporins. The penems have become valuable antibiotics because of a broad spectrum that includes many bacteria resistant to other drugs (Edwards and Betts 2000). Penems are not active against methicillin-resistant staphylococci or resistant strains of *Enterococcus faecium*. The high activity of the carbapenem group of β-lactams is attributed to its stability against most of the β-lactamases (including ESBL) and ability to penetrate porin channels that usually exclude other drugs (Livermore 2001). Resistance to carbapenems has been extremely rare in veterinary medicine.

The penems have been used primarily for serious, resistant infections that would otherwise require multiple drugs, including aminoglycosides. They are more bactericidal than other β-lactam antibiotics against gram-negative bacteria because they affect PBP-1 and -2 and produce postantibiotic effects (PAE) that are not seen with other β-lactams. The rapid bactericidal activity is less likely to induce release of endotoxin in patients from gram-negative sepsis during treatment. In veterinary medicine, their use has been limited to serious infections caused by bacteria resistant to other antibiotics. Imipenem and meropenem are the most commonly used of this group.

IMIPENEM (PRIMAXIN®). Imipenem has been used occasionally for treating serious infections in veterinary medicine. Imipenem is ordinarily metabolized extensively by the renal tubules (a brush border enzyme) to a potentially toxic compound. The drug cilastatin inhibits the renal enzymes and imipenem is combined with cilastatin in the product Primaxin® 1) to avoid renal toxicity, and 2) to achieve high urine concentrations of active drug.

Some disadvantages of imipenem are the inconvenience of administration, short shelf-life after reconstitution, and high cost. It must be diluted in fluids prior to administration. A common dose for small animals is 10 mg/kg q8h or 5 mg/kg q6h. This dose must be given by constant rate infusion over 30–60 minutes, but it has been administered subcutaneously. One of the adverse effects caused from imipenem therapy is seizures. Another problem is the risk of renal injury, which should be minimized by the addition of cilastatin (Barker et al. 2003).

MEROPENEM (MERREM®). Meropenem is one of the newest of the carbapenem class. It has antibacterial activity approximately equal to, or greater than, imipenem. Other characteristics are similar to imipenem. Its advantage over imipenem is that it is more soluble and can be administered in less fluid volume and more rapidly. For example, small volumes can be administered subcutaneously with almost complete absorption. There also is a lower incidence of adverse effects to the central nervous system, such as seizures (Edwards and Betts 2000). Based on pharmacokinetic experiments (Bidgood and Papich 2002), the recommended dose for Enterobactericeae and other sensitive organisms is 8.5 mg/kg SC every 12 hours, or 24 mg/kg IV every 12 hours. For infections caused by *Pseudomonas aeruginosa*, or other similar organisms that may have MIC values as high as 1.0 μg/ml, the dose is 12 mg/kg q8h, SC, or 25 mg/kg q8h, IV. For sensitive organisms in the urinary tract, 8 mg/kg, SC, every 12 hours can be used. In the experience of the authors, these doses have been well-tolerated except for slight hair loss over some of the SC dosing sites.

ERTAPENEM (INVANZ). Ertapenem is one of the newest of the carbapenems. Ertapenem has good activity against most gram-negative organisms, except *Pseudomonas aeruginosa.*

It has a longer half-life in people allowing for once-daily administration. However, in dogs the protein binding is not as high and the half-life is not prolonged.

REFERENCES AND ADDITIONAL READING

Abraham EP. 1987. Cephalosporins, 1945–1986. Drugs 34:1–14.

Acred P. 1983. Therapeutic and kinetic properties of ceftazidime in animals. Infection 11(Suppl1):S44–S48.

Agersø H, Friis, C. 1998. Bioavailability of amoxycillin in pigs. J Vet Pharmacol Ther 21:41–46.

Agersø H, Friis C, Haugegaard J. 1998. Water medication of a swine herd with amoxicillin. J Vet Pharmacol Ther 21:199–202.

AHFS Drug Information. 1994a. Cephalosporins. 95–101.

———. 1994b. Penicillins. 213–308.

Ambrose PG, Owens RC, Garvey MJ, Jones RN. 2002. Pharmacodynamic considerations in the treatment of moderate to severe pseudomonal infections with cefepime. J Antimicrob Chemo 49:445–453.

Ampicillin package insert (Polyflex, Fort Dodge Laboratories, Inc.—US). Downloaded 2/11/03 from www.wyeth.com.

Andes D, Craig WA. 2002. Animal model pharmacokinetics and pharmacodynamics: a critical review. Inter J Antimicrob Agents 19:261–268.

Angarano DW, MacDonald JM. 1989. Efficacy of cefadroxil in the treatment of bacterial dermatitis in dogs. J Am Vet Med Assoc 194:57–59.

Baggot JD. 1988. Bioavailability and disposition kinetics of amoxicillin in neonatal foals. Equine Vet J 20:125–127.

Baggot JD, Love D, Love RJ, Raus J, Rose RJ. 1990. Oral dosage of penicillin V in adult horses and foals. Equine Vet J 22:290–291.

Barker CW, Zhang W, Sanchez S, et al. 2003. Pharmacokinetics of imipenem in dogs. Am J Vet Res 64:694–699.

Barsanti JA, Chatfield RC, Shotts EB, Crowell WA, Hardin JA. 1985. Efficacy of cefadroxil in experimental canine cystitis. J Am An Hosp Assoc 21:89–93.

Beech J, Leitch M, Kohn CW, et al. 1979. Serum and synovial fluid levels of sodium ampicillin and ampicillin trihydrate in horses. J Equine Med Surg 3:350–4.

Bennett K, editor. 1993. Polyflex. In Compendium of Veterinary Products. 3rd ed., p. 47. Hensall, ON: North American Compendiums Inc.

Bialer M, Wu WH, Look AM, Silber BM, Yacobi A. 1987. Pharmacokinetics of cefixime after oral and intravenous doses in dogs: Bioavailability assessment for a drug showing nonlinear serum protein binding. Res Commun Chem Pathol Pharmacol 56:21–32.

Bidgood T, Papich MG. 2002. Plasma pharmacokinetics and tissue fluid concentrations of meropenem after intravenous and subcutaneous administration in dogs. Am J Vet Res 63(12):1622–1628.

Blue, JT, Dinsmore RP, Anderson KL. 1987. Immune-mediated hemolytic anemia induced by penicillin in horses. Cornell Vet 77:263–276.

Borin MT. 1991. A review of the pharmacokinetics of cefpodoxime proxetil. Drugs 42(Suppl 3):13–21.

Bornstein M, Thomas PN, Coleman DL, Boylan JC. 1974. Stability of parenteral solutions of cefazolin sodium. Am J Hosp Pharm 31:296–298.

Bowman KF, Dix LP, Riond JL, Riviere JE. 1986. Prediction of pharmacokinetic profiles of ampicillin sodium, gentamicin sulfate, and combination ampicillin sodium-gentamicin sulfate in serum and synovia of healthy horses. Am J Vet Res 47(7):1590–6.

Brown SA, Arnold TS, Hamlow PJ, et al. 1995. Plasma and urine disposition and dose proportionality of ceftiofur and metabolites in dogs after subcutaneous administration of ceftiofur sodium. J Vet Pharmacol Ther 18:363–269.

Brown MP, Bronwall R, Kroll WR, Beal C. 1984. Ampicillin trihydrate in foals: serum concentrations and clearance after a single oral dose. Equine Vet J 16(4):371–373.

Brown SA, Boucher JF, Hubbard VL, Prough MJ, Flook TF. 2007. The comparative plasma pharmacokinetics of intravenous cefpodoxime sodium and oral cefpodoxime proxetil in beagle dogs. J Vet Pharmacol Ther 30(4):320–326.

Brown MP, Gronwall RR, Gossman TB, Houston AE. 1987. Pharmacokinetics and serum concentrations of cephapirin in neonatal foals. Am J Vet Res 48:805–806.

Brown MP, Gronwall RR, Houston AE. 1986a. Pharmacokinetics and body fluid and endometrial concentrations of cephapirin in mares. Am J Vet Res 47:784–788.

———. 1986b. Pharmacokinetics and body fluid and endometrial concentrations of cefoxitin in mares. Am J Vet Res 47:1734–1737.

Brown MP, Stover SM, Kelly RH, Farver TB. 1982. Body fluid concentrations of ampicillin trihydrate in 6 hours after a single intramuscular dose. Equine Vet J 14:83–85.

Bywater RJ, Palmer GH, Buswell JF, Stanton A. 1985. Clavulanate-potentiated amoxycillin: activity in vitro and bioavailability in the dog. Vet Rec 116:33–36.

Cabana BC, VanHarken DR, Hottendorf GH. 1976. Comparative pharmacokinetics and metabolism of cephapirin in laboratory animals and humans. Antimicrob Agents Chemo 10:307–317.

Campbell BG, Rosin E. 1998. Effect of food on absorption of cefadroxil and cephalexin in dogs. J Vet Pharmacol Ther 21:418–420.

Caprile KA. 1988. The cephalosporin antimicrobial agents: a comprehensive review. J Vet Pharmacol Ther 11:1–32.

Carceles CM, Escudero E, Baggot JD. 1995. Comparative pharmacokinetics of amoxicillin/clavulanic acid combination after intravenous administration in sheep and goats. J Vet Pharmacol Ther 18:132–136.

Carli S, Anfossi P, Villa R, Castellani G, Mengozzi G, Montesissa C. 1999. Absorption kinetics and bioavailability of cephalexin in the dog after oral and intramuscular administration. J Vet Pharmacol Ther 22:308–313.

Carli S, Montesissa C, Sonzogni O, Madonna M. 1986. Pharmacokinetics of sodium cefoperazone in calves. Pharmacol Res Commun 18:481–490.

Carrillo NA, Giguère S, Gronwall, RR, et al. 2005. Disposition of orally administered cefpodoxime proxetil in foals and adult horses and minimum inhibitory concentration of the drug against common bacterial pathogens of horses Am J Vet Res 66:30–35.

Carter GK, Martens RJ, Brown SA, Martin MT. 1986. Pharmacokinetics of sodium amoxicillin in foals after intramuscular administration. Am J Vet Res 47:2126–2128.

Chatfield RC, Gingerich DA, Rourke JE, Strom PW. 1984. Cefadroxil: a new orally effective cephalosporin antibiotic. Vet Med 79:339–346.

Cherni JA, Boucher JF, Skogerboe TL, Tarnacki S, Gajewski KD, Lindeman CJ. 2006. Comparison of the efficacy of cefpodoxime proxetil and cephalexin in treating bacterial pyoderma in dogs. Inter J Appl Res Vet Med 4(2):85–93.

CLSI. 2007. Performance Standards for Antimicrobial Disk and Dilution Susceptibility Tests for Bacteria Isolated from Animals; Approved Standard—Third Edition. CLSI document M31-A3. Wayne, PA: Clinical and Laboratory Standards Institute.

Cole LK, Kwochka KW, Kowalaski JJ, Hillier A. 1998. Microbial flora and antimicrobial susceptibility patterns of isolated pathogens from the horizontal ear canal and middle ear in dogs with otitis media. J Am Vet Med Assoc 212:534–538.

Colombini S, Merchant RS, Hosgood G. 2000. Microbial flora and antimicrobial susceptibility patterns from dogs with otitis media. Vet Dermatol 11:235–239.

Cooke CL, Singer RS, Jang SS, Hirsh DC. 2002. Enrofloxacin resistance in *Escherichia coli* isolated from dogs with urinary tract infections. J Am Vet Med Assoc 220(2):190–192.

Craig WA. 1995. Interrelationship between pharmacokinetics and pharmacodynamics in determining dosage regimens for broad-spectrum cephalosporins. Diagn Microbiol Infect Dis 22:89–96.

———. 2001. Does the dose matter? Clin Infect Dis 33(Suppl3): S233–237.

Craigmill AL, Pass MA, Wetzlich S. 1992. Comparative pharmacokinetics of amoxicillin administered intravenously to sheep and goats. J Vet Pharmacol Ther 15:72–77.

Crosse R, Burt DG. 1984. Antibiotic concentrations in the serum of dogs and cats following a single dose of cephalexin. Vet Rec 115:106–107.

Daly RC, Fitzgerald RH, Washington JA. 1982. Penetration of cefazolin into normal and osteomyletic canine cortical bone. Antimicrob Agents Chemo 22:461–469.

Davis JL, Salmon JH, Papich MG. 2005. Pharmacokinetics and tissue fluid distribution of cephalexin in the horse after oral and i.v. administration. J Vet Pharmacol Ther 28(5):425–431.

Dickson PL, DiPiro JT, Michael KA, Cheung RPF, Hall EM. 1987. Effect of hemorrhagic shock on cefazolin and gentamicin pharmacokinetics in dogs. Antimicrob Agents Chemo 31:389–392.

Dimitrova DJ, Pashov DA, Dimitrov DS. 1998. Dicloxacillin pharmacokinetics in dogs after intravenous, intramuscular and oral administration. J Vet Pharmacol Ther 21:414–417.

Dimitrova DJ. 1996. Pharmacokinetics of dicloxacillin sodium following intravenous and intramuscular administration to domestic cats. J Vet Pharmacol Ther 19:405–407.

Donecker JM, Sams RA, Ashcraft SM. 1986. Pharmacokinetics of probenecid and the effect of oral probenecid administration on the pharmacokinetics of cefazolin in mares, Am J Vet Res 47(1):89–95.

Dorrestein GM, van Gogh H, Rinzema JD. 1984. Pharmacokinetic aspects of penicillins, aminoglycosides and chloramphenicol in birds compared to mammals: a review. Vet Quarterly 6(4):216–224.

Duffee NE, Christensen JM, Craig AM. 1989. The pharmacokinetics of cefadroxil in the foal. J Vet Pharmacol Ther 12:322–326.

Durr A. 1976. Comparison of the pharmacokinetics of penicillin G and ampicillin in the horse. Res Vet Sci 20:24–9.

Edwards JR, Betts MJ. 2000. Carbapenems: the pinnacle of the Beta-lactam antibiotics or room for improvement? J Antimicrob Chemo 45:1–4.

Ehmann WC. 1992. Cephalosporin-induced hemolysis: a case report and review of the literature. Am J Hematol 40:121–125.

Ensink JM, Klein WR, Mevius DJ, et al. 1992. Bioavailability of oral penicillins in the horse: a comparison of pivampicillin and amoxicillin. J Vet Pharmacol Ther 15:221–230.

Ensink JM, Vulto AG, van Miert ASJPAM, et al. 1996. Oral bioavailability and in vitro stability of pivampicillin, bacampicillin, talampicillin, and ampicillin in horses. Am J Vet Res 57:1021–1024.

Finlay J, Miller L, Pooupard JA. 2003. A review of the antimicrobial activity of clavulanate. J Antimicrob Chemo 52:18–23.

Firth EC, Klein WR, Nouws JFM, et al. 1988. Effect of induced synovial inflammation on pharmacokinetics and synovial concentration of sodium ampicillin and kanamycin sulfate after systemic administration in ponies. J Vet Pharmacol Ther 11:56–62.

Firth EC, Nouws JFM, Driessens F, et al. 1986. Effect of the injection site on the pharmacokinetics of procaine penicillin G in horses, Am J Vet Res 47:2380–2383.

Flammer, K. 1998. Common bacterial infections and antibiotic use in companion birds. Compendium on Continuing Education for the Practicing Veterinarian 20(Suppl3A):34–48.

Francis ME, Marshall AB, Turner WT. 1978. Amoxycillin: clinical trials in dogs and cats. Vet Rec 102:377–80.

Frank LA, Kunkle GA. 1993. Comparison of the efficacy of cefadroxil and generic and proprietary cephalexin in the treatment of pyoderma in dogs. J Am Vet Med Assoc 203(4):530–533.

Frere JM, Joris B, Granier B, Matagne A, Jacob F, Bourguignon-Bellefroid C. 1991. Diversity of the mechanisms of resistance to beta-lactam antibiotics. Res Microbiol 142:705–710.

Galtier P, Charpenteau JL. 1979. Pharmacokinetics of ampicillin in pigs. J Vet Pharmacol Ther 2:173–80.

Gardner SY, Papich MG. 2001. Comparison of cefepime pharmacokinetics in neonatal foals and adult dogs. J Vet Pharmacol Ther 24:187–192.

Garg RC, Keefe TJ, Vig MM. 1987. Serum levels and pharmacokinetics of ticarcillin and clavulanic acid in dog following parenteral administration of Timentin. J Vet Pharmacol Ther 10:324–330.

Garg SK, Chaudhary RK, Srivastava AK. 1992. Disposition kinetics and dosage of cephalexin in cow calves following intramuscular administration. Annales de Recherches Veterinaires 23:399–402.

Gehring R, van der Merwe D, Pierce AN, Baynes RE, Craigmill AL, Riviere JE. 2005. Multivariate meta-analysis of pharmacokinetic studies of ampicillin trihydrate in cattle. Am J Vet Res 66:108–112.

Girard AE, Schelkly WU, Murphy KT, Sawyer PS. 1987. Activity of beta-lactamase inhibitor subactam plus ampicillin against animal isolates of *Pasterurella, Haemophilus,* and *Staphylococcus.* Am J Vet Res 48: 1678–1683.

Gold HS, Moellering RC, Jr. 1996. Antimicrobial resistance mechanisms. N E J Med 335(19):1445–1453.

Goldberg DM. 1987. The cephalosporins. Med Clin North Am 71:1113–1133.

Gortel K, Campbell KL, Kakoma I, Whittem T, Schaeffer DJ, Weisiger RM. 1999. Methicillin resistance among staphylococci isolated from dogs. Am J Vet Res 60:1526–1530.

Graham JM, Oshiro BT, Blanco JD. 1992. Limited-spectrum (first-generation) cephalosporins. Obstet Gynecol Clin North Am 19:449–459.

Guaguère E, Maynard L, Salomon C. 1996. Cephalexin in the treatment of canine pyoderma: comparison of two dose rates. Eur Coll Vet Dermatol Proceedings, page 82, [abstract].

Guaguère E, Salomon C, Cadot P. 2000. Comparison of two protocols of administration of cephalexin in the treatment of deep pyoderma in dogs. Vet Dermatol 11(Suppl1):20.

Guerrini VH, English PB, Filippich LJ, Schneider J, Bourne DWA. 1986. Pharmacokinetic evaluation of a slow-release cefotaxime suspension in the dog and in sheep. Am J Vet Res 47:2057–2061.

Guerrini VH, Filippich LJ, Cao GR, English, PB, Bourne DW. 1985. Pharmacokinetics of cefaronide, ceftriaxone, and cefoperazone in sheep. J Vet Pharmacol Ther 8:120–127.

Guglick MA, MacAllister CG, Clarke CR, et al. 1998. Pharmacokinetics of cefepime and comparison with those of ceftiofur in horses, Am J Vet Res 59(4):458–463.

Holmgren N, Haggmar B, Tolling S. 1985. A field trial evaluating the use of cefoperazone in the treatment of bovine clinical mastitis. Nord Vet Med 37:228–233.

Horspool LJ, Sarasola P, McKellar QA. 1992. Disposition of ampicillin sodium in horses, ponies and donkeys after intravenous administration. Equine Vet J (Suppl)11:59–61.

Huber WG. 1988. Penicillins. In LE McDonald, NH Booth, eds., Veterinary Pharmacology and Therapeutics, 6th ed., pp. 796–812. Ames: Iowa State Univ Press.

Hyatt JM, McKinnon PS, Zimmer GS, Schentag JJ. 1995. The importance of pharmacokinetic/pharmacodynamic surrogate markers to outcome. Clin Pharmacokinet 28:143–160.

Indiveri MC, Hirsh DC. 1985. Clavulanic acid potentiated activity of amoxicillin against *Bacteriodes fragilis.* Am J Vet Res 46:2207–2209.

Jacobson ER. 1999. Antimicrobial therapy in reptiles. Compendium on Continuing Education for the Practicing Veterinarian 21(Suppl3E): 33–48.

Jacoby GA, Archer GL. 1991. New mechanisms of bacterial resistance to antimicrobial agents. N E J Med 324(9):601–612.

Jacoby GA, Munoz-Price LS. 2005. The new beta-lactamases. N E J Med 352:380–391.

Jaglan PS, Roof RD, Yein FS, et al. 1994. Concentration of ceftiofur metabolites in the plasma and lungs of horses following intramuscular treatment, J Vet Pharmacol Ther 17:24–30.

Jayachandran C, Singh MK, Banerjee NC. 1990. Pharmacokinetics and distribution of ampicillin in plasma, milk and uterine fluid of female buffaloes. Vet Res Commun 14:47–51.

Jensen GM, Kykkesfeldt J, Frydendahl K, Møller K, Svendsen O. 2004. Pharmacokinetics of amoxicillin after oral administration in recently weaned piglets with experimentally induced *Escherichia coli* subtype 0149:F4 diarrhea. Am J Vet Res 65:992–995.

Kelkar PS, Li JT-C. 2001. Cephalosporin allergy. N E J Med 345: 804–809.

Klesel N, Adam F, Isert D, Limbert M, Markus A, Schrinner E, Seibert G. 1992. RU 29 246, the active compound of the cephalosporin prodrug-ester HR 916.III. Pharmacokinetic properties and antibacterial activity in vivo. J Antibiot 45:922–931.

Koch H, Peters S. 1996. Antimicrobial treatment in German Shepherd dog pyoderma (GSP). Vet Dermatol 7:171–181.

Konig C, Simmen HP, Blaser J. 1998. Bacterial concentrations in pus and infected peritoneal fluid—implication of bactericidal activity of antibiotics. J Antimicrob Chemo 42:227–232.

Kruse H, Hofshagen M, Thoresen SI, et al. 1996. The antimicrobial susceptibility of *Staphylococcus* species isolated from canine dermatitis. Vet Res Commun 20:205–14.

Küng K, Wanner M. 1994. Bioavailability of different forms of amoxicillin administered orally to dogs. Vet Rec 135:552–554.

Kunkle GA, Sundlof S, Keisling K. 1995. Adverse side effects of oral antibacterial therapy in dogs and cats: an epidemiologic study of pet owners' observations. J Am An Hosp Assoc 31(1):46–55.

Lavy E, Shem-Tov M, Or-Bach A, Ziv G, Glickman A, Saran A. 1997. Oral availability and bioequivalence studies in dogs for two cephalexin tablets and a cephalexin capsule. J Vet Pharmacol Ther 20(Suppl 1):63–64.

Lavy E, Ziv G, Aroch I, Glickman A. 1995. Clinical pharmacologic aspects of cefixime in dogs. Am J Vet Res 56:633–638.

Lee FH, Pfeffer M, VanHarken DR, Smyth RD, Hottendorf GH. 1980. Comparative pharmacokinetics of ceforanide (BL-S786R) and cefazolin in laboratory animals and humans. Antimicrob Agents Chemo 17:188–192.

Ling GV, Conzelman GM, Franti CE, Ruby AL. 1980. Urine concentrations of five penicillins following oral administration to normal adult dogs. Am J Vet Res 41:1123–1125.

Liu P, Müller M, Derendorf H. 2002. Rational dosing of antibiotics: the use of plasma concentrations versus tissue concentrations. Inter J Antimicrob Agents 19:285–290.

Livermore DM. 2001. Of *Pseudomonas,* porins, pumps, and carbapenems. J Antimicrob Chemo 47:247–250.

Lloyd DH, Lamport AI, Feeney C. 1996. Sensitivity to antibiotics amongst cutaneous and mucosal isolates of canine pathogenic staphylococci in the UK, 1980–96. Vet Dermatol 7:171–175.

Lloyd DH, Noble WC. 1999. Use and abuse of antibiotics in veterinary dermatology. Vet Dermatol 10:161.

MacGowan AP. 2001. Role of pharmacokinetics and pharmacodynamics: Does the dose matter? Clin Infect Dis 33(Suppl3):S238–S239.

Marcellin-Little DJ, Papich MG, Richardson DC, DeYoung DJ. 1996. Pharmacokinetic model for cefazolin distribution during total hip arthroplasty in dogs. Am J Vet Res 57:720–723.

Marier J-F, Beaudry F, Ducharme MP, Fortin D, Moreau J-P, Masse R, Vachon P. 2001. Pharmacokinetic study of amoxicillin in febrile beagle dogs following repeated administrations of endotoxin. J Vet Pharmacol and Ther 24:379–383.

Martin Barrasa JL, Lupiola Gomez P, Gonzalez Lama Z, et al. 2000. Antibacterial susceptibility patterns of *Pseudomonas* strains isolated from chronic canine otitis externa. J Vet Med B Infect Dis Vet Pub Health 47:191–196.

Martinez MN, Pedersoli WM, Ravis WR, Jackson JD, Cullison R. 2001. Feasibility of interspecies extrapolation in determining the bioequivalence of animal products intended for intramuscular administration. J Vet Pharmacol Ther 24:125–135.

Matsui H, Komiya M, Ikeda C, Tachibana A. 1984. Comparative pharmacokinetics of YM-13115, ceftriaxone, and ceftazidime in rats, dogs, and rhesus monkeys. Antimicrob Agents Chemo 26:204–207.

Maynard L, Guaguère E, Medaille C. Clinical efficacy of cefalexin administered once or twice daily by oral route in the treatment of superficial pyoderma in dogs. 18th ESVD-ECVD Annual Congress, page 198.

———. Clinical efficacy of cefalexin administered by oral route at two dosages in the treatment of deep pyoderma in dogs. 18th ESVD-ECVD Annual Congress, page 197.

McElroy D, Ravis WR, Clark CH. 1986. Pharmacokinetics of cefotaxime in the domestic cat. Am J Vet Res 47:86–88.

McKellar QA, Sanchez Bruni SF, Jones DG. 2004. Pharmacokinetic/pharmacodynamic relationships of antimicrobial drugs used in veterinary medicine. J Vet Pharmacol Ther 27:503–514.

Mealey KL. 2001. Penicillins and beta-lactamase inhibitor combinations. J Am Vet Med Assoc 218:1893–1896.

Medleau L, Long RE, Brown J, Miller WH. 1986. Frequency and antimicrobial susceptibility of *Staphylococcus* species isolated from canine pyoderma. Am J Vet Res 47:229–231.

Mercer HD, et al. 1977. Bioavailability and pharmacokinetics of several dosage forms of ampicillin in the cat. Am J Vet Res 1977 38(9): 1353–1359.

Montesissa C, et al. 1988. Pharmacokinetics of sodium amoxicillin in horses. Res Vet Sci 44:233–6.

Moore KW, Trepanier LA, Lautzenhiser SJ, et al. 2000. Pharmacokinetics of ceftazidime in dogs following subcutaneous administration and continuous infusion and the association with in vitro susceptibility of *Pseudomonas aeruginosa*. Am J Vet Res 61:1204–1208.

Nawaz, M., Kahn, H. 1991. Bioavailability, elimination kinetics, renal clearance and excretion of ampicillin following intravenous and oral administration in sheep and goats. Acta Veterinaria Scandinavica 8:131–132.

Nawaz M, Tabassum R, Iqbal T, Perveen Z. 1990. Disposition kinetics, renal clearance and excretion of ampicillin after oral administration in goats. Zentralblatt für Veterinarmedizin 37:247–252.

Neilsen IL, Jacobs KA, Huntington PJ, Chapman CB, Lloyd KC. 1988. Adverse reaction to procaine penicillin G in horses. Austral Vet J 65:181–185.

Nelis HJ, Vandenbranden J, Verhaeghe B, De Kruif A, Mattheeuws D, De Leenheer AP. 1992. Liquid chromatographic determination of ampicillin in bovine and dog plasma by using a tandem solid-phase extraction method. Antimicrob Agents Chemo 36:1606–1610.

Nicolau DP, Quintiliani R, Nightingale CH. 1995. Antibiotic kinetics and dynamics for the clinician. Med Clin N Am 79:477–495.

Nishida M, Murakawa T, Kaminura T. 1978. Bactericidal activity of cephalosporins in an in vitro model of simulating serum levels. Antimicrob Agents Chemo 14:6–12.

Nix DE, Goodwin SD, Peloquin CA, et al. 1991. Antibiotic tissue penetration and its relevance: Impact of tissue penetration on infection response. Antimicrob Agents Chemo 35:1953–1959.

Noble WC, Kent LE. 1992. Antibiotic resistance in *Staphylococcus intermedius* isolated from cases of pyoderma in the dog. Vet Dermatol 3:71–74.

Normand EH, Gibson NR, Taylor DJ, et al. 2000. Trends of antimicrobial resistance in bacterial isolates from a small animal referral hospital. Vet Record 146:151–155.

Oluoch AO, Kim CH, Weisiger RM, Koo HY, Siegel AM, Campbell KL, Burke TJ, McKiernan BC, Kakoma I. 2001. Nonenteric *Escherichia coli* isolates from dogs: 674 cases (1990–1998). J Am Vet Med Assoc 218(3):381–384. (Erratum in: J Am Vet Med Assoc 2001 Mar 1;218(5):732.)

Oukessou M, Toutain PL. 1992. Effect of water deprivation on absorption (oral, intramuscular) and disposition of ampicillin in sheep. J Vet Pharmacol Ther 15:421–432.

Oukessou M, Benlamlih S, Toutain PL. 1990a. Benylpenicillin kinetics in the ewe: influence of pregnancy and lactation. Res Vet Sci 49(2): 190–193.

Oukessou M, Hossaini J, Zine-Filali R, Toutain PL. 1990b. Comparative benzylpenicillin pharmacokinetics in the dromedary *Camelus dromedarius* and in sheep. J Vet Pharmacol Ther 13:298–303.

Palmer GH, Bywater RJ, Stanton A. 1983. Absorption in calves of amoxicillin, ampicillin, and oxytetracycline given in milk replacer, water or an oral rehydration formulation. Am J Vet Res 44(1):68–71.

Papich MG, Korsrud GO, Boison J, et al. 1994. Disposition of penicillin G after administration of benzathine penicillin G, or a combination of benzathine G and procaine penicillin G in cattle. Am J Vet Res 55:825–830.

Papich MG, Korsrud GO, Boison J, et al. 1993. A study of the disposition of procaine penicillin G in feedlot steers following intramuscular and subcutaneous injection. J Vet Pharmacol Ther 16: 317–327.

Papich MG, Davis JL, Floerchinger AM. 2007. Cefpodoxime and cephalexin plasma pharmacokinetics, protein binding, and tissue distribution after oral administration to dogs. [abstract # 161] American College of Veterinary Internal Medicine Annual Forum, Seattle, Washington.

Passmore CA, Sherington J, Stegemann MR. 2007. Efficacy and safety of cefovecin (Convenia) for the treatment of urinary tract infections in dogs. J Sm An Pract 48(3):139–44.

Pellerin JL, Bourdeau P, Sebbag H, et al. 1998. Epidemiosurveillance of antimicrobial compound resistance of *Staphylococcus intermedius* clinical isolates from canine pyodermas. Comp Immunol Microbiol Infect Dis 21:115–33.

Periti P, Mazzei T. 1999. New criteria for selecting the proper antimicrobial chemotherapy for severe sepsis and septic shock. Int J Antimicrob Agents 12:97–105.

Petersen AD, Walker RD, Bowman MM, Schott HC, Rosser EJ. 2002. Frequency of isolation and antimicrobial susceptibility patterns of *Staphylococcus intermedius* and *Pseudomonas aeruginosa* isolates from canine skin and ear samples over a 6 year period (1992–1997). J Am An Hosp Assoc 38:407–413.

Petersen SW, Rosin E. 1992. In vitro antibacterial activity of cefoxitin and cefotetan and pharmacokinetics in dogs. Am J Vet Res 54:1496–1499.

———. 1993. In vitro antibacterial activity of cefoxitin and cefotetan and pharmacokinetics in dogs. Am J Vet Res 54(9):1496–1499.

———. 1995. Cephalothin and cefazolin in vitro antibacterial activity and pharmacokinetics in dogs. Vet Surg 24(4):347–351.

Popick AC, Crouthamel WG, Bekersky I. 1987. Plasma protein binding of ceftriaxone. Xenobiotica 17:1139–1145.

Prades M, Brown MP, Gronwall R, Miles NS. 1988. Pharmacokinetics of sodium cephapirin in lactating dairy cows. Am J Vet Res 49:1888–1890.

Prescott JF, Hanna WJB, Reid-Smith R, Drost K. 2002. Antimicrobial drug use and resistance in dogs. Can Vet J 43:107–116.

Rice LB, Bonomo RA. 2000. Beta-lactamases: which ones are clinically important? Drug Resistance Updates 3:178–189.

Richardson DC, Aucoin DP, DeYoung DJ, Tyczkowska KL, DeYoung BA. 1992. Pharmacokinetic disposition of cefazolin in serum and tissue during canine total hip replacement. Vet Surg 21:1–4.

Risk JE, Bentley OE. 1997. Efficacy of sulbactam, a beta-lactamase inhibitor, combined with ampicillin in the therapy of ampicillin-resistant pneumonic pasteurellosis in veal calves. Can Vet J 28:595–599.

Risk JE, Cummins JM. 1987. Efficacy of sulbactam, a beta-lactamase inhibitor, combined with ampicillin in the therapy of ampicillin-resistant pneumonic pasteurellosis in feedlot calves. Can Vet J 28:591–594.

Rolinson GN. 1991. Evolution of beta-lactamase inhibitors. Surg Gyn Obstet 172:11–16.

Rosin E, Ebert S, Uphoff TS, Evans MH, Schultz-Darken NJ. 1989. Penetration of antibiotics into the surgical wound in a canine model. Antimicrob Agents Chemo 33:700–704.

Rosin E, Uphoff TS, Schultz-Darken NJ, Collins MT. 1993. Cefazolin antibacterial activity and concentrations in serum and the surgical wound in dogs. Am J Vet Res 54:1317–1321.

Rule R, Rubio M, Perelli MC. 1991. Pharmacokinetics of ceftazidime in sheep and its penetration into tissue and peritoneal fluids. Res Vet Sci 51:233–238.

Ruoff WW, Sams RA. 1985. Pharmacokinetics and bioavailability of cephalothin in horse mares. Am J Vet Res 46:2085–2090.

Sams RA, Ruoff WW. 1985. Pharmacokinetics and bioavailability of cefazolin in horses. Am J Vet Res 46:348–352.

Sanders WE Sanders CC. 1988. Inducible beta-lactamases: clinical and epidemiologic implications for use of newer cephalosporins. Rev Infect Dis 10:830–838.

Sarasola P, McKellar QA. 1992. Effect of probenecid on disposition kinetics of ampicillin in horses. Vet Rec 131:173–5.

———. 1993. Pharmacokinetics and applications of ampicillin sodium as an intravenous infusion in the horse. J Vet Pharmacol Ther 16:63–69.

———. 1994. Ampicillin and its congener prodrugs in the horse (review). Br Vet J 150(2):173–87.

———. 1995. Pharmacokinetics of bacampicillin in equids. Am J Vet Res 56(11):1486–92.

Saxon, A. 1989. Aztreonam in the management of gram-negative infections in penicillin-allergic patients: a review. Pediatr Infect Dis J 8:S124–S127.

Scarampella F, Noli C, and Horspool LJI. 2000. Cefadroxil in the treatment of canine pyoderma. Vet Dermatol 11(Suppl1):19.

Schermerhorn T, Barr SC, Stoffregen DA, Koren-Roth Y, Erb HN. 1994. Whole-blood platelet aggregation, buccal mucosa bleeding time, and serum cephalothin concentration in dogs receiving a presurgical antibiotic protocol. Am J Vet Res 55:1602–1607.

Senior DF, Gaskin JM, Buergelt CD, Franks PP Keefe TJ. 1985. Amoxycillin and clavulanic acid combination in the treatment of experimentally induced bacterial cystitis in cats. Res Vet Sci 39:42–46.

Seol B, Naglić T, Madić J, Bedeković M. 2002. In vitro antimicrobial susceptibility of 183 *Pseudomonas aeruginosa* strains isolated from dogs to selected antipseudomonal agents. J Vet Med B 49:188–192.

Soback, S. 1988. Pharmacokinetics of single doses of cefoxitin given by the intravenous and intramuscular routes to unweaned calves. J Vet Pharmacol Ther 11:155–162.

———. 1989. Pharmacokinetics of single-dose administration of moxolactam in unweaned calves. Am J Vet Res 50:498–501.

Soback S, Bor A, Kurtz B, Paz R, Ziv G. 1987a. Clavulanate-potentiated amoxycillin: in vitro antibacterial activity and oral bioavailability in calves. J Vet Pharmacol Ther 10:105–113.

Soback S, Bor A, Ziv G. 1987. Clinical pharmacology of cefazolin in calves. J Vet Med Assoc 34:25–32.

Soback S, Kurtz B, Ziv G. 1987b. Pharmacokinetics of phenoxymethyl penicillin (penicillin V) in calves. J Vet Pharmacol Ther 10:17–22.

Soback S, Ziv G. 1988. Pharmacokinetics and bioavailability of ceftriaxone administered intravenously and intramuscularly to calves. Am J Vet Res 49:535–538.

Soback S, Ziv G, Bor A, Shapira M. 1988. Pharmacokinetics of cephalexin glycinate in lactating cows and ewes. J Vet Med Assoc 35:755–760.

Stamper MA, Papich, MG, Lewbart GA, May SB, Plummer D, Stoskopf MK. 1999. Pharmacokinetics of ceftazidime in loggerhead sea turtles (*Caretta caretta*) after single intravenous and intramuscular injections. J Zoo Wildlife Med 30(1):32–35.

Stegemann MR, Coati N, Passmore CA, Sherington J. 2007a. Clinical efficacy and safety of cefovecin in the treatment of canine pyoderma and wound infections. J Sm An Pract 48(7):378–86.

Stegemann MR, Sherington J, Passmore C. 2007b. The efficacy and safety of cefovecin in the treatment of feline abscesses and infected wounds. J Sm An Pract 48(12):683–9.

Stegemann MR, Sherington J, Blanchflower S. 2006a. Pharmacokinetics and pharmacodynamics of cefovecin in dogs. J Vet Pharmacol Ther 29(6):501–11.

Stegemann MR, Sherington J, Coati N, Brown SA, Blanchflower S. 2006b. Pharmacokinetics of cefovecin in cats. J Vet Pharmacol Ther 29(6): 513–24.

Stegemann MR, Passmore CA, Sherington J, Lindeman CJ, Papp G, Weigel DJ, Skogerboe TL. 2008c. Antimicrobial activity and spectrum of cefovecin, a new extended- spectrum cephalosporin, against pathogens collected from dogs and cats in Europe and North America. Antimicrob Agents Chemo 50(7):2286–92.

Step DL, Blue FT, Dill SG. 1991. Penicillin-induced hemolytic anemia and acute hepatic failure following treatment of tetanus in a horse. Cornell Vet 81:13–18.

Stover SM, Brown MP, Kelly RH, Farver TB, Knight HD. 1981. Aqueous procaine penicllin G in the horse: serum, synovial, peritoneal, and urine concentrations after single-dose intramuscular administration. Am J Vet Res 42:629–631.

ten Voorde G, Broeze J, Hartmen EG, van Gogh H. 1990. The influence of the injection site on the bioavailability of ampicillin and amoxicillin in beagles. Vet Quarterly 12:73–79.

Thompson RL. 1987. Cephalosporin, carbapenem, and monobactam antibiotics. Mayo Clin Proc 62:821–834.

Tilmant L, Brown MP, Gronwall RR. 1985. Pharmacokinetics of ticarcillin in the dog. Am J Vet Res 46:479–481.

Tomlin J, Pead MJ, Lloyd DH, Howell S, et al. 1999. Methicillin-resistant *Staphylococcus aureus* infections in 11 dogs. Vet Rec 144:60–64.

Tonelli AP, Bialer M, Yacobi A. 1985. Relationship between protein binding and renal clearance of a new oral cephalosporin in the dog. J Pharm Sci 74:1242–1244.

Traver DS, Riviere JE. 1982. Ampicillin in mares: a comparison of intramuscular sodium ampicillin or sodium ampicillin-ampicillin trihydrate injection. Am J Vet Res 43(3):402–4.

Traver DS, Riviere JE. 1981. Penicillin and ampicillin therapy in horses. J Am Vet Med Assoc 178(11):1186–9.

Turnidge JD. 1998. The pharmacodynamics of β-lactams. Clinical Infectious Diseases. 27:10–22.

Uboh CE, Soma LR, Luo Y, McNamara E, Fennel MA, May L, Teleis DC, Rudy JA, Watson AO. 2000. Pharmacokinetics of penicillin G procaine versus penicillin G potassium and procaine hydrochloride in horses. Am J Vet Res 61:811–815.

USP monograph. Aminopenicillins. 2003. J Vet Pharmacol Ther 26(Suppl2): 36–45.

USP-DI, United States Pharmacopeia. 2004. Drug monographs. Rockville, MD (www.usp.org).

VanCamp SD, Papich MG, Whitacre MD. 2000. Administration of ticarcillin in combination with clavulanic acid intravenously and intrauterinely to clinically normal oestrous mares. J Vet Pharmacol Ther 23:373–378.

Van Den Hoven R, Hierweck B, Bobretsberger M, Ensink JM, Meijer LA. 2003. Intramuscular dosing strategy for ampicillin sodium in horses, based on distribution into tissue chambers before and after induction of inflammation. J Vet Pharmacol Ther 26:405–411.

Villa R, Carli S, Montesissa C, Sonzogni U. 1991. Influence of probenecid on cephalexin pharmacokinetics in sheep. Acta Veterinaria Scandinavica 8:124–126.

Vree TB, Dammers E, Van Duuren E. 2003. Variable absorption of clavulanic acid after an oral dose of 25 mg/kg of Clavubactin® and Synulox® in healthy dogs. J Vet Pharmacol Ther 26:165–171.

Wackowiez G, Richard JJ, Fabreguettes G. 1997. Pharmacokinetics of cephalexin in plasma and urine after single intravenous and oral (tablets) administration in dogs. J Vet Pharmacol Ther 20(Suppl1):63–64.

Walker AL, Jang S, Hirsh DC. 2000. Bacteria associated with pyothorax of dogs and cats: 98 cases (1989–1998). J Am Vet Med Assoc 216:359–363.

Waterman NG, Scharfenberger LF. 1978. Concentration relationships of cefaclor in serum, interstitial fluid, bile, and urine of dogs. Antimicrob Agents Chemo 14:614–616.

Watson ADJ, Emslie DR, Martin ICA, Egerton JR. 1986. Effect of ingesta on systemic availability of penicillins administered orally in dogs. J Vet Pharmacol Ther 9:140–149.

Watson ADJ, Emslie DR, Martin ICA. 1987a. Systemic availability of penicillin V from six oral preparations in dogs. J Vet Pharmacol Ther 10:180–183.

———. 1987b. Effect of different intervals between dosing and feeding on systemic availability of penicillin V in dogs. J Vet Pharmacol Ther 10:90–95.

Weese JS. 2005. Methicillin-resistant *Staphylococcus aureus*: An emerging pathogen in small animals. J Am An Hosp Assoc 41:150–157.

Wilkens BE, Sullivan PS, McDonald TP, Krahwinkel DJ. 1994. Effects of cephalothin, cefazolin and cefmetazole on the hemostatic mechanism in normal dogs: Implications for the surgical patient. 1994 ACVS Symposium, October 16–19, Washington, D.C.

Williams JD, Naber KG, Bryskier A, Høiby N, Gouild IM, Periti P, Giamarellou H, Rouveix B. 2001. Classification of oral cephalosporins. A matter of debate. Inter J Antimicrob Agents 17:443–450.

Wilson WD, Baggot JD, Adamson PJW, et al. 1985. Cefadroxil in the horse: pharmacokinetics and in vitro antibacterial activity. J Vet Pharmacol Ther 8:246–253.

Wilson WD, Spensley MS, Baggot JD, Hietala SK. 1988. Pharmacokinetics and estimated bioavailability of amoxicillin in mares, after intravenous, intramuscular, and oral administration. Am J Vet Res 49:1688–1693.

Yeoman GH. 1997. Microbiology and bioavailability of amoxicillin. Vet Med Sm An Clin 4(Suppl):720–38.

Zeisler JA, McCarthy JD, Richelieu WA, Nichol MB. 1992. Cefuroxime by continuous infusion: a new standard of care? Infect Med 9:54–60.

Zhanel GG. 1990. Cephalosporin-induced nephrotoxicity: does it exist? DICP 24:262–265.

Zhanel GG, Hoban DJ, Harding GK. 1991. The postantibiotic effect: a review of in vitro and in vivo data. DICP 25:153–163.

Ziv G, Horsey J. 1979. Elevation and prolongation of serum ampicillin and amoxycillin concentrations in calves by the concomitant administration of probenecid. J Vet Pharmacol Ther 2:187–94.

CHAPTER

35

TETRACYCLINE ANTIBIOTICS

MARK G. PAPICH AND JIM E. RIVIERE

GENERAL PHARMACOLOGY OF TETRACYCLINES

The tetracycline antibiotics were isolated from various species of *Streptomyces* in the late 1940s and early 1950s. Since that time, many semisynthetic structural modifications have been made on the tetracycline molecule to yield other tetracyclines with differing pharmacokinetic properties and antimicrobial activities. Chlortetracycline and oxytetracycline were discovered in 1948, tetracycline in 1953, doxycycline in 1967, and minocycline in 1972. Chlortetracycline and oxytetracycline are natural products; the others are semisynthetic. The newest development is the glycylcyclines, which are derivatives of minocycline. Tigecycline is the only available representative of this group, which possesses better antimicrobial activity than older drugs (Agwuh and MacGowan 2006). Tigecycline use in veterinary medicine has not been reported.

The tetracyclines are a group of four-ringed amphoteric compounds (Fig. 35.1) that differ by specific chemical substitutions at different points on the rings. As a group, the tetracyclines are acidic, hygroscopic compounds in aqueous solutions and easily form salts with acids and bases, with which they are commonly formulated. The most common salt form is the hydrochloride formulation, as is the case with oxytetracycline. However, some tetracyclines, especially oxytetracycline, are formulated with vehicles (excipients) to prolong absorption from the injection site. Some of the chemical and physical properties of the tetracyclines used in veterinary medicine today are listed in Table 35.1.

Tetracyclines are broad-spectrum and used for a wide variety of diseases. Accepted indications include abscesses, enteritis, Leptospirosis, pneumonia, bovine and swine respiratory disease, pododermatitis, treatment of tick-borne pathogen skin and soft tissue infections, and uterine infections.

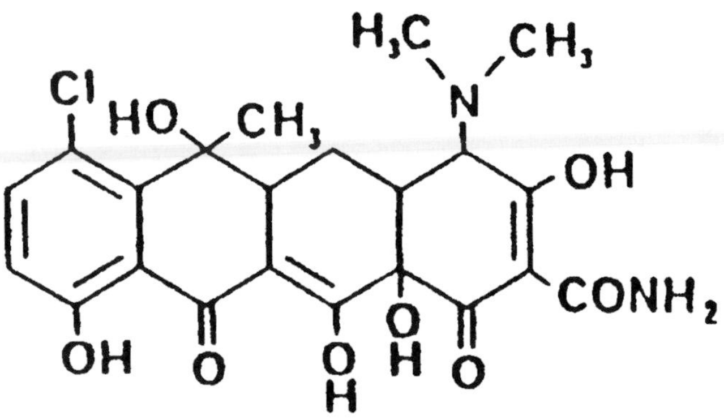

FIG. 35.1 Chemical structure of chlortetracycline.

TABLE 35.1 Chemical and physical properties of tetracyclines

Drug	Molecular weight	pK_a
Chlortetracycline	478.88	3.3, 7.4, 9.3
Doxycycline	462.46	NA
Minocycline	457.48	2.8, 5.0, 7.8, 9.3
Oxytetracycline	460.44	NA
Tetracycline	444.43	8.3, 10.2

Note: NA = information not available.

Many formulations are intended for medication in water and for feed (growth promotion). These products will not be considered here because the levels administered are considered subtherapeutic for production use, and the pharmacokinetics of these formulations in the target species is incomplete. Formulations listed that are added to feed and water also have incomplete pharmacokinetic information.

MECHANISM OF ACTION. Tetracyclines possess antimicrobial activity by binding to the 30S ribosomal subunit of susceptible organisms. After binding to the ribosome, the tetracyclines interfere with the binding of aminoacyl-tRNA to the messenger RNA molecule/ribosome complex, thereby interfering with bacterial protein synthesis in growing or multiplying organisms (Gale and Folkes 1953; Suzuka et al. 1966). Tetracyclines have much less affinity for mammalian ribosomes. Tetracyclines are bacteriostatic, with the pharmacokinetic-pharmacodynamic properties described in a later section.

Resistance. Resistance occurs among many bacteria. The mechanisms of acquired resistance include 1) energy dependent efflux of antibiotic (membrane efflux proteins), or 2) altered target whereby the ribosome is protected from binding of tetracyclines (Chopra et al. 1992). A third mechanism whereby the drug is attacked by enzymes liberated by the bacteria is possible, but has not yet been fully characterized. The genes mediating resistance may be carried on plasmids or transposons. Resistance to one tetracycline will produce cross-resistance to the others in the group. However, the newest tetracycline, tigecycline, is active against many organisms (e.g., methicillin-resistant staphylococci) that are resistant to older tetracyclines (Agwuh and MacGowan 2006).

Susceptibility Testing. For susceptibility testing, tetracycline is used to test all others in the class (CLSI 2007). For veterinary isolates, the susceptible breakpoint is ≤2 μg/ml for bovine respiratory pathogens and ≤0.5 μg/ml for swine pathogens. For other isolates, the breakpoint for sensitive organisms in humans is used, which is ≤4 μg/ml for all organisms, except streptococci, which is ≤2 μg/ml.

PHARMACOKINETIC-PHARMACODYNAMIC (PK-PD) PROPERTIES. Based on an evaluation of tetracycline PK-PD, the effectiveness is best expressed as a ratio of the area-under-the-curve for a 24-hour interval to the MIC (AUC_{24}/MIC) (Agwuh and MacGowan 2006). The optimal AUC/MIC ratio is in the range of 30–40. In veterinary studies this has been explored insufficiently. One study (Prats et al. 2005) examined PK-PD parameters after administration of doxycycline to swine in drinking water at 10 mg/kg. They reported high AUC/MIC ratios ranging from 60 for *Pasteurella,* 155 for *Mycoplasma,* and 585 for *Bordetella.* For *Actinobacillus,* which exhibits a higher MIC, the AUC/MIC was only 13. However, these ratios did not factor the protein binding, which is at least 90% (Table 35.2). Using a fraction unbound (fu) value of 0.1, reduces these ratios substantially. Ideal AUC/MIC ratios would be achieved only for *Bordetella bronchiseptica.*

ABSORPTION. Tetracyclines can be administered intravenously (most tetracyclines) or intramuscularly (oxytetracycline). The oral route has been used, but oral absorption is low for all the drugs, except doxycycline (Table 35.3). Although some formulations (e.g., chlortetracycline and tetracycline) are commonly administered to feed and water for pigs, cattle, and poultry, the systemic effects of this route of administration may be much less than antici-

TABLE 35.2 Protein binding of tetracyclines in various species

Drug	Species	% Protein Binding
Chlortetracycline	Cows	47–51
	Sheep	46–50
Doxycycline	Calves	92
	Cats	98
	Horses	81
	Dogs	91
	Pigs	93
	Sheep	84–90
	Turkeys	70–85
Oxytetracycline	Buffalo	42
	Cows	18–22
	Horses	50
	Pigs	75.5
	Sheep	21–25
	Trout	55
Tetracycline	Cows	31–41
	Sheep	28–32

TABLE 35.3 Comparison of oral absorption of tetracyclines in animals (mean values of studies reported)

Drug	Species	Systemic Absorption (F%)
Chlortetracycline	Chickens	1
	Turkeys	6
	Pigs	6, 11, 19 (depending on the study and fasting conditions)
Oxytetracycline	Pigs	3–5
	Fish	6
	Turkeys	9–48
Tetracycline	Pigs	5, 8, 18, 23 (depending on the study and fasting conditions)
	Dogs	40
	Cats	50
Doxycycline	Pigs	21.2
	Chickens	41.3
	Turkeys	25, 37, 41, 63.5 (depending on age)
	Horses	2.7% (estimated)
	Dogs	53% (hyclate), 33.5% (monohydrate)

pated. In a study in which oxytetracycline was fed to pigs (Hall et al. 1989) the authors concluded that feeding this medication at a rate of 0.55 g/kg of feed resulted in plasma concentrations so low that only highly susceptible bacteria would be inhibited, with plasma concentrations reaching only one-tenth of the MIC for most pathogens. If fed for growth promotion purposes, the effect is likely a local one—influencing the intestinal bacteria. Several studies have examined use of tetracyclines added in subtherapeutic concentrations to feed rations (in particular, chlortetracycline) (Zinn 1993; Jones et al. 1983; Dawson et al. 1983; Williams et al. 1978; Quarles et al. 1977; Richey et al. 1977; Nivas et al. 1976). The explanation for low oral absorption is not clear, but may be multifactorial. Tetracyclines are zwitterions and ionized at physiological pH values (see Table 35.1). Although the tetracyclines are relatively lipophilic drugs, they are ionized in the gastrointestinal tract and may not cross membranes easily. The oral absorption of tetracycline can be drastically reduced in the presence of food (Nielsen and Gyrd-Hansen 1996). Tetracyclines can easily chelate to polyvalent cations, which decreases the absorption several-fold. Thus, tetracycline oral absorption can be decreased with the coadministration of food, dairy products, polyvalent cations (i.e., Ca^{++}, Mg^{++}, Fe^{++}, Al^{3+}), kaolin/pectin preparations, iron-containing supplements, and antacids (Weinberg 1957; Waisbren and Hueckel 1950; Harcourt and Hamburger 1957; Neuvonen et al. 1970; Hagermark and Hoglund 1974; Gothoni et al. 1972). Doxycycline is much less effected by chelation to food and has higher oral absorption in most animals than other tetracyclines (Table 35.3).

DISTRIBUTION. Once absorbed, tetracyclines bind to plasma proteins to varying degrees in each species (Table 35.2). The high protein binding for some drugs may limit the microbiologically active fraction in the plasma. Tetracyclines are widely distributed throughout most tissues of the body after oral and intravenous administration. Tables 35.4–35.8 show the pharmacokinetic variables for some of these drugs. In most species, the tetracyclines have volumes of distribution that are equal to or larger than cellular water, and in most studies higher than 1.0 l/kg. A volume of distribution in excess of 1.0 l/kg indicates concentration outside the extracellular water (e.g., intracellular or binding to tissue sites). In one study in loggerhead sea turtles, (Harms et al. 2004) the volume of distribution after IV administration of oxytetracycline was in excess of 18 l/kg (mean value), suggesting high binding to the large bony mass in this species.

Tetracyclines are more lipophilic than some other classes of antibiotics (e.g., β-lactams, and aminoglycosides); therefore at physiological pH they are capable of crossing lipid membranes. Some tetracyclines penetrate tissues better than others do. For example, minocycline and

TABLE 35.4 Pharmacokinetic parameters of chlortetracycline in some food-animal species

Species	Dose (mg/kg)	Route	V_d (L/kg)	$t_{1/2}$ (hr)	Clearance (mL/min/kg)	Reference
Turkey	0.9	IV	0.2284	0.877	3.77	Dyer 1989
Pigs	11.0	IV	1.3883	NR	0.3071	Kilroy et al. 1990
Pigs	10	IV	0.7	3.6 (MRT)	3.33	Nielsen & Gyrd-Hansen, 1996
Pigs	39.9	Oral	—	8.7 (MRT)	—	Nielsen & Gyrd-Hansen, 1996
Calves (milk fed)	11.0	IV	3.34	8.89	260.52 L/hr/kg	Bradley et al. 1982
Calves (conventionally fed)	11.0	IV	1.93	8.25	162.12 L/hr/kg	Bradley et al. 1982

Note: NR = information not reported; IV = intravenous.

TABLE 35.5 Pharmacokinetic parameters of tetracycline in some species

Species	Dose (mg/kg)	Route	V_d (L/kg)	$t_{1/2}$ (hr)	Clearance (mL/min/kg)	Reference
Gilts	11	IA	1.06	NR	0.4	Kniffen et al. 1989
Chickens	65	IV	0.174	2.772	1.632	Anadon et al. 1985
Rabbits (male and female)	10	IV	1.047	2	6.1	Percy and Black 1988
Channel catfish (*Ictalurus punctatus*) (27°C)	4	IV	0.513	16.5	0.365	Plakas et al. 1988
Pigs	11	IV	4.5	16	3.1	Kniffen et al. 1989
Pigs	9.6	IV	1.2	5.6 (MRT)	3.5	Nielsen & Gyrd-Hansen, 1996
Pigs	46.4	Oral	—	9.0 (MRT)	—	Nielsen & Gyrd-Hansen, 1996

Note: NR = information not reported; IV = intravenous; IA = intra-arterial.

doxycycline penetrate brain, ocular tissues, spinal fluid, and prostate better than other tetracyclines, such as oxytetracycline or chlortetracycline. Tetracyclines are commonly reported to concentrate intracellularly, and doxycycline has a higher affinity for intracellular accumulation than other tetracyclines (Gabler 1991; Forsgren and Ballahsene 1985; Davis et al. 2006). In vitro analysis of the penetration of radiolabeled doxycycline into isolated human PMNLs revealed a cellular-to-extracellular concentration ratio of 13 (Forsgren and Ballahsene 1985). In horses the ratio was 17 at peak concentrations (Davis et al. 2006). These high leukocyte concentrations may explain the reported antiinflammatory effects. Minocycline is found in high concentrations in the bronchial secretions (Kelly and Kanegis 1967a; MacCulloch et al. 1974); prostate (Fair 1974); brain (Barza et al. 1975); thyroid, saliva, and tears (Hoeprich and Warshauer 1974).

METABOLISM, EXCRETION, AND ELIMINATION.

The elimination rates and half-lives are presented in the pharmacokinetic tables for each drug and various species (Tables 35.4–35.8). Although it varies considerably from species to species, the half-life is long enough for once-, or twice-daily administration in most animals. The intramuscular administration of formulations that contain viscosity excipients (e.g., 2-pyrrolidone) (Table 35.9) may prolong the terminal half-life because of a "flip-flop" effect. This is discussed in more detail in the section on oxytetracycline below.

Approximately 60% of the dose is eliminated in the urine via glomerular filtration, with the other 40% eliminated in the feces. An examination of Tables 35.4–35.8 indicates that systemic clearance is similar to, or somewhat higher than GFR. The glomerular filtration pathway does not appear to be of importance with doxycycline, as most of the dose is excreted in the large intestine. Doxycycline was shown to be metabolically inert in calves (with mature or immature rumen function) and pigs (Riond et al. 1989b; Riond and Riviere 1990a). Tetracyclines are also excreted in the bile, with up to 20 times the plasma concentration of tetracyclines being present in the bile (Kunin and Finland 1961; Schach von Wittenau and Twomey 1971).

TABLE 35.6 Pharmacokinetic parameters of oxytetracycline in some species

Species	Dose (mg/kg)	Route	V_d (L/kg)	$t_{1/2}$ (hr)	Clearance (mL/min/kg)	Reference
Horses	10	IV	0.6728	12.953	0.6583	Horspool and McKellar 1990
Ponies	10	IV	1.0482	14.949	1.013	Horspool and McKellar 1990
Donkeys	10	IV	0.7765	6.464	1.523	Horspool and McKellar 1990
Horses (adult)	2.5	IV	1.35	10.5	NR	Pilloud 1973
Pigs	10	IV	1.49	5.99	2.88	Pijpers et al. 1991
Pigs (normal)	50	PO	1.44	5.92		Pijpers et al. 1991
Pigs (pneumonia)	50	PO	1.9	14.1		Pijpers et al. 1991
Pigs	20	IV	5.18	3.68	4.15	Mevius et al. 1986b
Cows (adult)	2.5	IV	1.04	9.12	NR	Pilloud 1973
Dairy cows	5	IV	0.917	2.63	1.24	Nouws et al. 1985a,b
Dairy cows[a]	5.23	IV	1.01	2.58	1.45	Nouws et al. 1985a,b
Veal calves	40	IV	18.144	7.34	2.246	Meijer et al. 1993a
Veal calves	20	IV	18.541		2.167	Meijer et al. 1993a
Calves (3 wk old)	7.54	IV	2.48	13.5		Nouws et al. 1983
Calves (12 wk old)	6.88	IV	1.52	8.8		Nouws et al. 1983
Calves (14 wk old)	17	IV	1.83	10.8		Nouws et al. 1983
Buffalo calves (female)	22	IV	0.32	3.6	1.02	Varma and Paul 1983
Dogs	5	IV	2.096	6.02	4.23	Baggot et al. 1977
Rabbits	10	IV	0.668	1.32	14.6	McElroy et al. 1987
Turkeys	1	IV	3.622	0.7298	3.6579	Dyer 1989
Rainbow trout	5	IV	2.988	81.5	0.423	Black et al. 1991
African catfish	60	IV	1.33	80.3	0.19	Grondel et al. 1989
Red-necked wallaby	40	IV	2.041	11.4	NR	Kirkwood et al. 1988
Foal	59	IV	1.95–2.2	6.7–7.3	3.3	Papich et al. 1995
Cattle	20	IM	3.34 (Vd/F)	21.6	—	Craigmill et al. 2004 (meta-analysis)
Cattle (young)	20	IV	0.94	5.67	—	Toutain & Raynaud 1983
Calves	40	IM	—	23.9	—	TerHune et al. 1989
Calves (healthy)	11	IV	2.32	11.8	3.35	Ames et al. 1983
Calves (disease)	11	IV	3.6	14.8	4.01	Ames et al. 1983
Pigs	9.5	IV	1.4	6.5 (MRT)	3.67	Nielsen & Gyrd-Hansen. 1996
Pigs	45.5	Oral	—	10.3 (MRT)	—	Nielsen & Gyrd-Hansen. 1996
Sea Turtles	25	IV	18.4	66.1	4.8	Harms et al. 2004
Sea Turtles	25	IM	28.5 (Vd/F)	61.9	5.3 (CL/F)	Harms et al. 2004
Alligator	10	IV	0.77	74.1	0.12	Helmick et al. 2004

Note: NR = information not reported; IV = intravenous; PO = per os. All formulations were reported to be or are assumed to be HCl unless otherwise noted.
[a]Oxytetracycline dihydrate formulation tested.

TABLE 35.7 Some pharamcokinetic parameters of doxycycline in some species

Species	Dose (mg/kg)	Route	V_d (L/kg)	$t_{1/2}$ (hr)	Clearance (mL/min/kg)	Reference
Pigs (9 wk old)	20	IV	0.53	4.04	1.67	Riond and Riviere 1989
Pigs	12	Oral	—	7.2	—	Prats et al. 2005
Pigs	10.5	IV	0.89	4.2	2.8	Baert et al. 2000
Pigs	10.5	Oral	0.97	2.9	2.9	Baert et al. 2000
Horses	20	Oral	—	11.8	—	Davis et al. 2006
Dogs	0.1 mg/kg/hr	IV	0.65	4.56	1.66	Bidgood & Papich 2003
Calves	5	IV	NR	9.5	1.2 (mg/L)	Meijer et al. 1993
Calves (functional rumen)	20	IV	1.31	14.9	1.07	Riond et al. 1989
Calves (nonfunctional rumen)	20	IV	1.81	9.9	2.2	Riond et al. 1989
Cats	5	IV	0.34	4.56	1.09	Riond et al. 1990
Dogs	5	IV	0.93	6.99	1.72	Riond et al. 1990
Dogs	5	IV	1.468	10.36	1.68	Wilson et al. 1988
Goats (lactating)	5	IV	9.78	16.63	6.91	Jha et al. 1989

Note: IV = intravenous; NR = information not reported.

TABLE 35.8 Some pharmacokinetic parameters of minocycline HCl in some species

Species	Dose (mg/kg)	Route	V_d (L/kg)	$t_{1/2}$ (hr)	Clearance (mL/min/kg)	Reference
Dogs (2-compartment model)	5	IV	1.952	6.93	3.347	Wilson et al. 1985
Dogs (3-compartment model)	5	IV	2.001	7.24	3.424	Wilson et al. 1985
Sheep (normal)	2.2	IV	1.32	2.58	5.94	Wilson and Green 1986
Sheep (hypoproteinemic)	2.2	IV	1.67	2.91	5.60	Wilson and Green 1986

Note: IV = intravenous.

TABLE 35.9 Formulations of tetracyclines used in animals

Formulations Registered by U.S. FDA for Animals

Oxytetracycline hydrochloride soluble powder: added to drinking water for poultry, cattle, pigs

Oxytetracycline for medicated feed: added to feed for cattle, poultry, fish, pigs

Oxytetracycline tablets: oral treatment for calves.

Oxytetracycline injection: IM injection for cattle and pigs. These products are occasionally used in horses and other species. There is both a conventional and long-acting formulation. The long-acting formulation contains a viscosity excipient used to prolong the absorption from the injection site.

Tetracycline bolus: oral treatment for cattle.

Tetracycline hydrochloride soluble powder: added to drinking water for cattle, pigs and poultry

Tetracycline oral suspension: Oral treatment for cats and dogs

Chlortetracycline hydrochloride soluble powder: added to drinking water for poultry, calves, and pigs

Chlortetracycline for medicated feed: premix added to feed for pigs, cattle, poultry

Formulations Registered for Humans, but Used Off-Label in Animals

Doxycycline capsules and tablets: used in dogs, cats, birds, horses, and some exotic animals

CLINICAL USES. The use and dosages of specific agents in this group will be discussed later in this chapter for each drug. The tetracyclines are broad-spectrum antibiotics and, as a class, inhibit the growth of a wide variety of bacteria, protozoa, and many intracellular organisms such as mycoplasma, chlamydia, and rickettsia. Differences in antimicrobial spectrum of the tetracyclines in vivo result mainly from differences in lipid solubility, which influences the absorption, distribution, metabolism/excretion, and concentration of a specific tetracycline within the cell. Higher concentrations of the tetracycline within the organism or cell (as is the case with the more lipid soluble doxycycline and minocycline) usually result in an increase in antimicrobial activity.

Tetracyclines in general have good or moderate activity against the following organisms: *Bacillus* spp., *Corynebacterium* spp., *Erysipelothrix rhusiopathiae, Listeria monocytogenes,* streptococci, *Actinobacillus* spp., *Bordetella* spp., *Brucella* spp., *Francisella tularensis, Haemophilus* spp., *Pasteurella multocida, Yersinia* spp., *Campylobacter fetus, Borrelia* spp., *Leptospira* spp., *Actinomyces* spp., and *Fusobacterium* spp. The family Rickettsiaceae includes *Rickettsia* and *Ehrlichia,* and tetracyclines, particularly doxycycline, are considered the first drug of choice for these infections. In birds, doxycycline is the drug of choice for treatment of *Chlamydophila psittaci* (formerly called *Chlamydia psittaci*). Tetracyclines are also useful against organisms that lack a cell wall, which would ordinarily be resistant to β-lactam antibiotics, for example, *Mycoplasma,* as well as other Mycoplasma organisms such as *Mycoplasma haemofelis* (formerly called *Haemobartonella felis*).

Resistance is common among staphylococcus and enterococcus species and members of the family Enterobacteriaceae (*Enterobacter* spp., *E. coli, Klebsiella* spp., *Proteus* spp., *Salmonella* spp.). Anaerobes (such as *Bacteroides* spp. and *Clostridium* spp.) have shown variable susceptibility. Commonly resistant to the tetracyclines are those infections involving *Mycobacterium* spp., *Proteus vulgaris, Pseudomonas aeruginosa,* and *Serratia* spp. Increased activity against staphylococcus has been reported when doxycycline or minocycline has been used, presumably due to their increased ability to permeate the cell wall of this organism, which results in higher intracellular concentrations of drug.

ADVERSE EFFECTS AND INTERACTIONS

Interactions. Calcium-containing products or other di- or trivalent cations (Mg^{++}, Fe^{++}, Al^{+3}) will chelate with tetracyclines and interfere with GI absorption. Doxycycline is less susceptible to this interaction and has been shown that it can be administered to people (children) even when mixed with milk before oral administration. It is stable for 6 days when refrigerated.

Gastrointestinal Microflora Changes. In horses the oral administration of oxytetracycline has been associated with proliferation of *Clostridium perfringens*, or *Salmonella* in the colon, which has led to enteritis. This syndrome has been called *AColitis-X.* A more detailed discussion of the effects of tetracyclines in horses is reviewed by Papich (2003a,b).

Esophageal Lesions. Doxycycline entrapped in the esophagus from a broken tablet or incompletely dissolved capsule can cause injury to the esophagus and stricture. It has been demonstrated that, in cats, administration of a capsule or broken tablet can be lodged in the esophagus unless followed by some water. Therefore, one should be cautious about giving oral doxycycline medications to cats. This problem has been primarily associated with doxycycline hyclate (the form most common in the U.S.), rather than doxycycline monohydrate.

Problems in Young Animals. Tetracyclines bind to bone and teeth. They may produce teeth discoloration and inhibit growth of long bones in young animals or the offspring of pregnant animals treated with tetracyclines. The true incidence of this problem is not known in veterinary medicine, but in human medicine, tetracyclines are avoided in children less than 7 years of age (before tooth eruption). Tooth discoloration is related more to the duration of treatment than the dose. The discoloration is related to the chelation of tetracyclines to the calcium deposits in the developing teeth in the dentin (where it is mostly visible) and to a lesser extent in the enamel (Hamp 1967; Hennon 1965; Finerman and Milch 1963; Moffit et al. 1974).

It is prudent to avoid tetracyclines in animals during time of teeth development. The effects on bones are probably only important with high doses. Doxycycline has less potential to stain dental enamel than other tetracyclines.

Renal Tubular Necrosis. Renal tubular necrosis has been associated with high doses and prolonged administration of oxytetracycline to ruminants (Riond and Riviere 1989a), and dogs (Stevenson 1980). When high doses are administered, the drug vehicle (such as propylene glycol) has been suspected to contribute to renal effects.

Although the combination of tetracyclines and the inhalent anesthetic methoxyflurane has been implicated in renal injury, this was not confirmed in a study in dogs (Fleming and Pedersoli 1980). Methoxyflurane is not in common use any longer.

Using Outdated Formulations. It often is stated in publications that renal injury may occur when outdated tetracyclines are administered. The degradation products of the tetracyclines have been found to be nephrotoxic and are formed in the presence of heat, low pH, and moisture (Cleveland et al. 1965; Teuscher et al. 1982; Lowe and Tapp 1966; Riond and Riviere 1989a). Although we do not advocate administering outdated products, this problem does not occur with currently available formulations because the citric acid excipient is no longer used.

Hepatic Disease. Idiosyncratic toxic hepatitis is possible (Bocker et al. 1982; Hopf et al. 1985). Drug-induced hepatitis has been described in people, and pregnant women appear to be at the greatest risk. The significance of hepatic reactions in veterinary medicine is unknown, but may be important at high doses.

Allergy. Hypersensitivity and drug fever have been reported. Cats appear to be more prone to drug fever from tetracyclines than other animals.

Photosensitivity. This is a direct toxic effect that damages cutaneous membranes when exposed to light. This reaction is rare in animals, but rather common in people. The incidence appears to be highest with doxycycline and demeclocycline.

Risks from IV Administration. Tetracyclines administered intravenously rapidly can cause hypotension and collapse (McPherson et al. 1974; Wivagg et al. 1976; Gyrd-Hansen et al. 1981). In one study, a fast IV administration (60 sec or less) to cattle caused collapse in 50% of the animals. Affected animals had low blood pressure, low heart rate, and ECG abnormalities. Collapse from IV injection has been prevented when the cattle were premedicated with calcium borogluconate, indicating that tetracycline may decrease the amount of calcium available to the heart for its role in contraction to the point of producing collapse of the animals.

Rather than decreased calcium, it may instead be the vehicle that is responsible for the problems. In calves, Gross et al. (1981) studied the cardiovascular effects of both oxytetracycline and the different vehicles used for injection (propylene glycol, saline, polyvinylpyrrolidine). They determined that the cardiovascular adverse effects were caused by the vehicles used and not the oxytetracycline. The propylene glycol vehicle studied resulted in increased pulmonary arterial pressures and a decrease in cardiac output and stroke volume. Aortic pressure and heart rates were also depressed in association with the vehicle. They concluded that the cardiovascular effects observed were due to the endogenous release of histamine after propylene glycol injection, and this histamine release was not dependent on the animal being sensitized prior to exposure. No discernible cardiovascular effects were observed after injection with the oxytetracycline-saline combination, while the polyvinylpyrrolidine preparation and vehicle resulted in higher aortic pressure, heart rate, and overall systemic resistance.

Tetracycline has been reported to induce anaphylactic shock in dogs after intravenous injection (Ward et al. 1982) as well as possibly increasing alanine transaminase activity in the cat (Kaufman and Greene 1993).

The most serious concern is intravenous injection in horses, which can be fatal (Riond et al. 1989a, 1992). IV administration of doxycycline to horses has caused sudden death, most likely caused by a cardiac arrhythmia. Oral administration of doxycycline to horses has not produced this problem (Davis et al. 2006).

COMMONLY USED TETRACYCLINES

CHLORTETRACYCLINE. Chlortetracycline was the first tetracycline discovered and was first introduced for clinical use in 1948 (see Fig. 35.1). Chlortetracycline has historically been used to treat several of the susceptible organisms listed above. Chlortetracycline is not utilized to any significant degree in small-animal medicine for treatment of disease, but it is still in use today in some feed and water additives for food-producing animals. Systemic absorption is low, as reported previously (Table 35.3). Some of the pharmacokinetic parameters of chlortetracycline in food-producing animals are listed in Table 35.4. (Doses for drugs are listed in Table 35.10.)

In a study by Kelly and Kanegis (1967b), ^{14}C-labeled chlortetracycline was administered intravenously (10 mg/kg) to dogs, which were then sacrificed to determine the extent of penetration of the radiolabeled chlortetracycline in the tissues. Significant amounts of drug accumulated in most tissues of the body except for the cerebrospinal fluid (CSF), vitreous and aqueous humors, and fat deposits. In cattle, chlortetracycline given intravenously at 2.27 mg/kg showed blood levels of 1.0–4.4 μg/ml for at least 12 hours after injection and low levels present in serum in some animals for 48 hours after administration. Chlortetracycline appeared in milk at 1–3 μg/ml for 4–12 hours following intravenous injection of 2.5 g/cow. At the 2.27 mg/kg dose, milk concentration of chlortetracycline was between 2.5 and 5 μg/ml between 2 and 8 hours postadministration, with levels slowly falling off to 0.25 μg/ml at 48 hours after dose (Schipper 1965).

Chlortetracycline has been fed orally at varying concentrations to food animals such as pigs, calves, cattle, chickens, and turkeys. As a feed additive, 350 mg of chlortetracycline per animal daily resulted in significant increases in daily weight gain (Perry et al. 1971; Brown et al. 1975). Tylosin and chlortetracycline have been compared with respect to their ability to prevent liver abscesses in feedlot cattle (Brown et al. 1975). In that study, chlor-

TABLE 35.10 Clinical dosages used for tetracyclines in animals—Most frequently cited on product labels, or in reputable references based on a consensus of the literature (USP 2003).

Drug	Species	Dose
Doxycycline	Dogs and cats	5 mg/kg q12 h oral
Doxycycline	Horses	10–20 mg/kg q12 h oral (never administer IV)
Oxytetracycline	Calves, cattle, and pigs	22 mg/kg q24 h added to drinking water or in feed
Oxytetracycline	Calves, cattle	6.6 to 11 mg/kg q24 h, IM
Oxytetracycline	Calves, cattle	20 mg/kg q24 h, IM or SC. Off label doses have been as high as 40 mg/k
Oxytetracycline	Pigs	6.6–11 mg/kg q24 h IM. Doses as high as 20 mg/kg IM, q24 h are also used
Oxytetracycline	Sea turtles	40 mg/kg IM, followed by 20 mg/kg q72 h, IM
Tetracycline HCL	Calves	11 mg/kg q12 h PO

tetracycline reduced the number of liver abscesses by about 12% compared to controls, but tylosin was better than chlortetracycline at preventing these abscesses. Low levels of chlortetracycline have been fed to cattle at a dose of 1.1 mg/kg for 120 days to eliminate latent infections of anaplasmosis as determined using complement-fixation testing (Richey et al. 1977). In contrast, Royal et al. (1970) reported that chlortetracycline fed at levels of 50 mg or 100 mg daily did not alter the excretion patterns of *Salmonella typhimurium* in calves.

Chlortetracycline has been used in pigs as a feed additive for promotion of growth as well as being used orally for the treatment of *Salmonella typhimurium* (Jones et al. 1983; Williams et al. 1978), coccidiosis (Onawunmi and Todd 1976), and many other porcine diseases. Similar infections have been treated with chlortetracycline in poultry (Fagerberg et al. 1978; Nivas et al. 1976; Quarles et al. 1977; Landgraf et al. 1981; Dawson et al. 1983). Chlortetracycline has been reported to decrease the breeding rate of sows, although it did increase conception and farrowing rates. Birth weights, overall litter weights of pigs born alive, and weights of pigs at weaning were also significantly higher than unmedicated controls (Soma and Speer 1975).

TETRACYCLINE. The chemical structure of tetracycline is shown in Figure 35.2. The drug was first introduced for clinical use in 1952 and is still used today, primarily in small animals and some exotic species, although some use occurs in food-producing animals. Relatively little has been published in recent years on the pharmacokinetics of tetracycline. Pharmacokinetic information on tetracycline is presented in Table 35.5; older information on tetracycline pharmacokinetics in other species can be obtained from previous editions of this text.

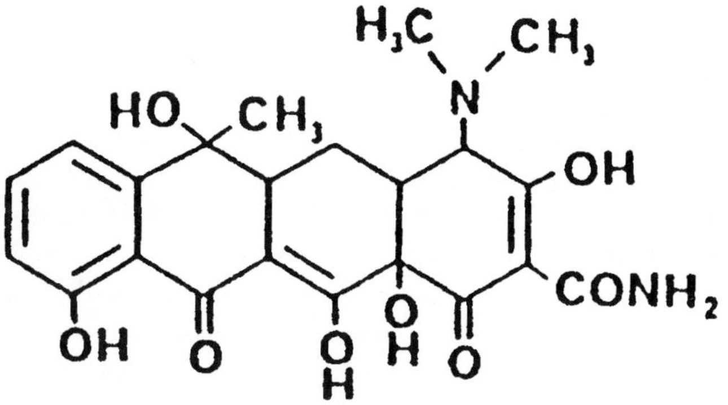

FIG. 35.2 Chemical structure of tetracycline.

In a study by Kelly and Kanegis (1967b), ^{3}H-labeled tetracycline was administered intravenously (10 mg/kg) to dogs, which were then sacrificed to determine the extent of penetration of the radiolabeled tetracycline in the tissues. Significant amounts of drug accumulated in most tissues of the body except for the CSF, vitreous and aqueous humors, and fat deposits. Tissue penetration of tetracycline was found to be somewhat less than that of chlortetracycline in the dog. Jun and Lee (1980) studied the distribution of tetracycline in the red blood cells of dogs and humans and determined that tetracycline enters red blood cells quickly, forming a steady-state equilibrium with the extracellular fluid within 10 minutes. Hypoalbuminemia in the dog seemed to accelerate the uptake of tetracycline into the red blood cell. Tetracycline has also been explored for use in parakeets (Schachter et al. 1984). These and other studies have shown that tetracycline is absorbed and distributed well to many tissues.

Tetracycline has been used in small animals to treat various diseases such as *Rickettsia rickettsii* (Rocky Mountain spotted fever). A study by Breitschwerdt et al. (1991) determined that tetracycline, chloramphenicol, and enrofloxacin were all equally effective in treating this disease in experimentally infected dogs. However, doxycycline is now used more frequently for this disease (see section on doxycycline later in this chapter.) Tetracycline was also found to be efficacious in the treatment of canine ehrlichiosis (*E. canis*). Amyx et al. (1971) found that oral administrations of tetracycline at 30 mg/lb (13.6 mg/kg) resulted in the remission of the clinical signs associated with the disease. In addition, tetracycline administered at the dose of 3 mg/lb (1.36 mg/kg) was adequate as a prophylactic agent for the prevention of the disease. In a later study by Davidson et al. (1978), oral treatments of dogs with canine ehrlichiosis in Thailand at a dose of 66 mg/kg for 14 days caused remission of the clinical signs of this disease. However, another report (Price and Dolan 1980) found that tetracycline was less effective at clearing ehrlichiosis in dogs compared to imidocarb dipropionate. Tetracycline (10 mg/kg every 8 hr) has also been reported to be efficacious in other intracellular infections, such as *Brucella canis* (Lewis et al. 1973). Tetracycline and the other tetracyclines can be useful in treating borreliosis, chlamydiosis (especially in cats and poultry), *Mycoplasma* spp., *Leptospira* spp., and *Listeria* spp.

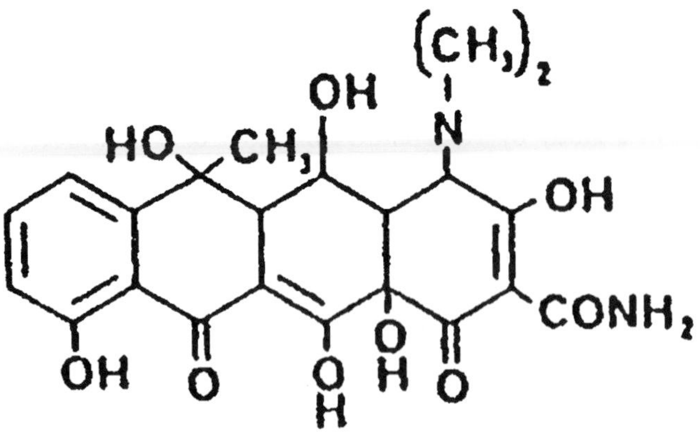

FIG. 35.3 Chemical structure of oxytetracycline.

OXYTETRACYCLINE. By far the most commonly used tetracycline in veterinary practice today is oxytetracycline. Numerous reports are available in the literature on the uses of oxytetracycline in veterinary medicine. Its chemical structure is shown in Figure 35.3.

The most complete pharmacokinetic analysis was performed by the Food Animal Residue Avoidance Databank (Craigmill et al. 2004) for oxytetracycline in cattle. This analysis was derived from 41 data sets and 25 published papers (489 data points) for oxytetracycline. A meta-analysis of this data from a dose of 20 mg/kg IM of long-acting tetracycline yielded the following population data: half-life 21.6 hours, peak concentration (C_{MAX}) 5.61 µg/ml, clearance 0.115 l/kg/hr, and volume of distribution per fraction absorbed (VD/F) 3.34 l/kg.

Oxytetracycline solution in propylene glycol is 50–100 mg/ml (Oxy-Mycin®, Terramycin, Oxy-Tet®), and is available as a solution in povidone (IM use only). A "long acting" preparation is available with the viscosity excipient 2-pyrrolidone (200 mg/ml) in formulations such as Liquamycin® LA-200. The clinical usefulness of oxytetracycline has been documented in most domestic species of animals, and previous editions of this textbook should be consulted for historic work on oxytetracycline. Oxytetracycline has been a common treatment for lung infections associated with Bovine Respiratory Disease (BRD). Although the in vitro susceptibility may not always be favorable, oxytetracycline appears to accumulate in pneumonic lung preferentially over normal lung, and an increased volume of distribution has been shown in diseased animals (Ames et al, 1983). Tissue levels are maintained for 24 hours after dosing. Other uses for cattle have included treating cases of mastitis and anaplasmosis. Although oxytetracycline has been used as an intrauterine infusion for cows with retained fetal membranes (RFM), this practice has been discouraged (Dinsmore et al. 1996). Intrauterine use in cows may not improve reproductive performance in cows with RFM and may cause illegal residues in milk of dairy cows (Dinsmore et al. 1996; Stevens et al. 1995).

Oxytetracycline has been used to treat ehrlichiosis in dogs (Adawa et al. 1992), although doxycycline is more frequently used for this disease. Oxytetracycline has also been used for treating Potomac Fever (*Neorickettsia risticii*, formerly called *Ehrlichia risticii*) in horses (Palmer et al. 1992). Oxytetracycline has also been studied in normal and diseased ovine lung tissue (Baxter and McKellar 1990) and in calves with pneumonic pasteurellosis (Burrows et al. 1986). Long-acting oxytetracycline has also found clinical usefulness in the treatment of *Moraxella bovis*/infectious bovine keratoconjunctivitis infections in calves (Smith and George 1985; George and Smith 1985; George et al. 1985, 1988). The distribution of oxytetracycline in the genital tracts of cows has also been reported (Bretzlaff et al. 1982, 1983a,b). Absorption of oxytetracycline is known to vary with injection site in calves. A report by Nouws and Vree (1983) found that site-to-site intramuscular injection bioavailability varied widely at 52 hours postinjection, with bioavailability being 79% in the buttock, 86% in the neck, and 98% in the shoulder.

Larson and Stowe (1981) reported high serum concentrations obtained in clinically normal horses given 10 mg/kg oxytetracycline intravenously, with serum concentrations peaking at 30 minutes postinjection (16.85 µg/ml) and high concentrations persisting through at least 240 minutes (4.67 µg/ml). In addition to the high serum concentrations, oxytetracycline was demonstrated to penetrate well into pulmonary and renal tissue, as well as into bronchial fluid. In another study of oxytetracycline in horses, Brown et al. (1981) used a dose of 5 mg/kg intravenously and found a peak concentration of oxytetracycline in the serum at 0.5 hours after dose, with a steady decline in serum levels through 36 hours. Similar fluid-concentration versus time profiles were also demonstrated for oxytetracycline detected in the synovial fluid, peritoneal fluid, and urine after intravenous injection, suggesting that oxytetracycline crosses those membranes easily and that the concentrations obtained would be adequate for combating such infections as *Corynebacterium equi, Streptococcus zooepidemicus,* and *Actinobacillus* spp., with limited efficacy in treating some *Staphylococcus aureus, Escherichia coli,* and *Salmonella* spp., and no efficacy in treating common *Pseudomonas aeruginosa* pathogens.

The pharmacokinetic parameters of oxytetracycline for some species are shown in Table 35.6. More information on the pharmacokinetics of oxytetracycline is available for dogs (Baggot et al. 1977; Cooke et al. 1981), calves (Burrows et al. 1987; Banting et al. 1985; Banting and Baggot 1996; Schifferli et al. 1982; Meijer et al. 1993a,c; TerHune and Upson 1989; Toutain and Raynaud 1983), ponies and donkeys (Horspool and McKellar 1990), horses (Larson and Stowe 1981; Brown et al. 1981; Teske et al. 1973), foals (Papich, et al. 1995), chickens (Black 1977), swine (Nielsen and Gyrd-Hansen 1996; Hall et al. 1989; Pijpers et al. 1990), sheep (Immelman and Dreyer 1986), elephants (Bush et al. 2000), and other species (Teare et al. 1985; Martinsen et al. 1992).

Oxytetracycline is the tetracycline of choice for reptiles. Studies were conducted in reptiles (Harms et al. 2004; Helmick et al. 2004) and demonstrated that the elimination of oxytetracycline from reptiles is slow. Harms et al. (2004) showed that the half-life in sea turtles was over 60 hours, which would allow for extended-interval dosing (41 mg/kg once IM, followed by 21 mg/kg every 72 hours IM). In another study, Helmick et al. (2004), showed that in alligators the half-life of oxytetracycline was 74 hours, which allows for long intervals between doses (for example every 5 days).

Oxytetracycline is exceptional among the tetracyclines for having a conventional as well as long-acting formulations, the differences in formulation being in the different vehicles (viscosity excipient) for injection. Several solvent systems are available around the world that produce a long-acting effect for oxytetracycline, but only one long-acting formulation, oxytetracycline and 2-pyrrolidone, is approved for veterinary use in the United States (e.g., LA-200). These solvent systems induce varying degrees of local irritation at the site of injection in calves, pigs, and sheep and, coupled with the high dose used, are responsible for the long-acting pharmacokinetic behavior of the long-acting oxytetracycline formulations (Nouws et al. 1990; Nouws 1984).

Use of a long-acting formulation, particularly in food animals, has the main advantage of obtaining clinically useful sustained serum and tissue concentrations for long periods of time—usually every 48 hours, but may be up to 3–5 days for some pathogens. Several studies have described the differing pharmacokinetic patterns of the conventional and long-acting formulations in dogs, sheep, cattle, and pigs. Toutain and Raynaud (1983) examined the pharmacokinetic parameters of oxytetracycline with the 2-pyrrolidone carrier (long-acting formulation) injected intramuscularly in young beef cattle. This intramuscular formulation resulted in rapid development of serum concentrations of 4 μg/ml within 60–90 minutes, followed by persistence of these levels for approximately 12 hours. Serum half-life was calculated to be 21.8 hours, and bioavailability was 51.5%. Extended serum concentrations exceeding 0.5 μg/ml were found to persist for approximately 87 hours, in contrast to approximately 52 hours for the conventional formulation in another study using cattle (Mevius et al. 1986a). Davey et al. (1985) injected cattle with the conventional oxytetracycline hydrochloride or the long-acting formulation, both at a standard 20 mg/kg dose, and found that although the long-acting formulation had lower peak serum concentrations when compared to the conventional formulation, the long-acting formulation had a longer serum half-life (36.9 hr) than the conventional formulation (11.1 hr). In addition, the time it took for serum concentrations to drop below 0.5 μg/ml was 86.8 hours for the long-acting formulation and 51.5 hours for the conventional formulation. Similar findings have been reported for dairy cows (Nouws et al. 1985b), calves (Nouws and Vree 1983), pigs (Nouws et al. 1990; Xia et al. 1983; Nouws 1984; Banting and Baggot 1996), dogs (Immelman and Dreyer 1981), and sheep (Nouws et al. 1990).

Despite the advantages of the long-acting oxytetracycline formulation cited above, there are also studies that cast doubt on the value of a long-acting formulation. In one such study, the long-acting oxytetracycline (in 2-pyrrolidone) was compared to a conventional formulation in pigs at a dose of 20 mg/kg of each formulation (Hall et al. 1989). There was no difference in area-under-the-curve (AUC) or disappearance rate constant from either formulation. The authors concluded that the long-acting formulation did not provide an advantage for pigs.

DOXYCYCLINE. Doxycycline is available in two forms, doxycycline hyclate and doxycycline monohydrate. Doxycycline hyclate (hydrochloride) has been used more commonly but the monohydrate also is available. There are no reported differences between these two formulations with respect to oral absorption, but the hyclate form is associated with more injury to the esophagus (see the previous section "Adverse Effects and Interactions").

Doxycycline is commonly used in small animals and is available in tablets (50, 75, 100 mg) and oral suspension (5 mg/ml suspension and 10 mg/ml syrup). Doxycycline hyclate (Vibramycin IV) also can be administered IV to patients (except horses) that cannot tolerate oral medications. The IV formulation is reconstituted before use and is stable for only 12 hours following reconstitution (72 hr in refrigerator, 8 wk in the freezer).

Doxycycline, like all other derivatives of tetracycline, is a structural isomer of the parent molecule and is synthesized from oxytetracycline or methacycline. Doxycycline and minocycline (discussed later in this chapter) differ from tetracycline, oxytetracycline, and chlortetracycline in that they are more lipophilic (five- to tenfold increase), resulting in higher tissue penetration, higher intracellular penetration, larger volumes of distribution, and better overall antimicrobial properties. Doxycycline is unique from other tetracyclines in that more is excreted in the intestine, compared to renal clearance. Doxycycline also has greater plasma protein binding than the other tetracyclines (Table 35.2), which produces a prolonged half-life of the drug in humans and animals. The chemical structure of doxycycline is shown in Figure 35.4.

The pharmacokinetics of doxycycline has been studied in dogs and cats (Wilson et al. 1988; Riond et al. 1990; Bidgood and Papich 2003), pigs (Riond and Riviere 1990a,b; Prats et al. 2005), calves (Meijer et al. 1993b; Riond et al. 1989b), goats (Jha et al. 1989), rhesus monkeys (Kelly et al. 1992), horses (Davis et al. 2006), and birds (Flammer et al. 2001 2003; Powers et al. 2000; Prus et al. 1992; Greth et al. 1993). Some of the pharmacokinetic data for doxycycline for commonly encountered species of animals are listed in Table 35.7.

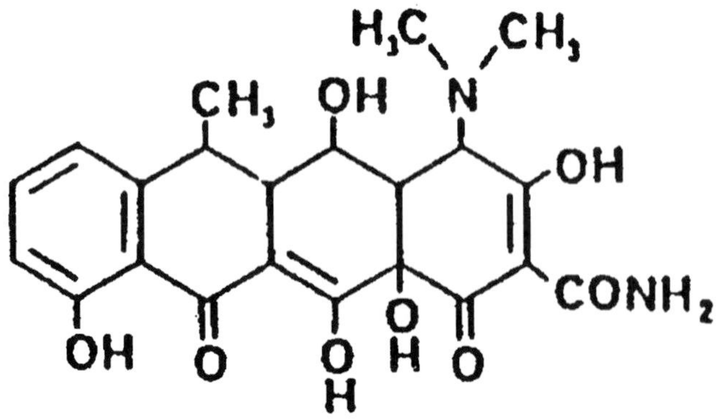

FIG. 35.4 Chemical structure of doxycycline.

Doxycycline pharmacokinetics has been extensively studied in humans and to a lesser degree in animals. An excellent review of doxycycline's use in humans is available (Cunha et al. 1982). Riond et al. (1990) compared the pharmacokinetics of doxycycline in dogs and cats given 5 mg/kg intravenously. In dogs, a peak serum concentration of 11.56 μg/ml was detected in serum 0.17 minutes after injection, steadily falling to 0.33 μg/ml 32 hours after injection and to nondetectable serum levels at 44 hours and beyond. Similar serum pharmacokinetics have been reported in dogs by others (Wilson et al. 1988). In cats, the peak serum concentration was 22.89 μg/ml and fell to 0.89 μg/ml 20 hours after injection, falling to nondetectable levels at 32 hours and beyond. Doxycycline was more extensively bound to serum proteins in cats than in dogs (Table 35.2) . Protein binding was reported to be 98.35% in cats and 91–92% in dogs, with albumin binding being 76.46% in cats and 53.87% in dogs (Riond et al. 1990; Bidgood & Papich 2003). Doxycycline pharmacokinetics has also been reported in pigs (Riond and Riviere 1990a). The half-life for doxycycline in this species was significantly shorter than that in other food-producing animals. Also, no doxycycline biotransformation was detected in those pigs, and no metabolites were detected in calves (Riond et al. 1989b).

Oral absorption was reported for various species (Table 35.3) and shown to be higher than for other tetracyclines. Systemic absorption in calves of doxycycline fed orally with milk replacer was approximately 70%, with an elimination half-life of 9.5 (±3.0) hours (Meijer et al. 1993b). Doxycycline use in the goat has also been reported (Jha et al. 1989).

The pharmacokinetics of doxycycline can be extrapolated across species using allometric procedures (Riond and Riviere 1990b). Riond and Riviere (1989b) reported on the binding of doxycycline to plasma albumin in dogs, sheep, cats, cows, pigs, and humans by measuring the association constants (Ka, l/mol).

High intracellular drug concentrations produce good activity against intracellular pathogens. Doxycycline is the first drug of choice for treatment of tickborne infections caused by *Ehrlichia canis* and *Rickettsia,* as well as *Mycoplasma haemofelis* (formerly called *Haemobartonella felis).* Efficacy of doxycycline for rickettsial disease in animals was demonstrated by Breitschwerdt et al. (1997, 1999). The most common dose for dogs and cats is 5 mg/kg q12 h orally (25 mg/cat q12 h). It also has been considered one of the treatments of choice, in addition to azithromycin, for treatment of infections caused by *Bartonella* (Kordick et al. 1997; Brunt et al. 2006), although the most appropriate drug for *Bartonella* is still unknown (Brunt et al. 2006).

Doxycycline has also been used for infections in other species, including respiratory tract disease and systemic colibacillosis in poultry (Migaki and Babcock 1977; George et al. 1977) and anaplasmosis in splenectomized calves (Kutter and Simpson 1978).

An important use of doxycycline is in birds. Doxycycline has become a treatment of choice for psittacosis caused by *Chlamydophila psittaci* (formerly called *Chlamydia psittaci*) in birds because of its good oral absorption, tolerance and efficacy (Flammer et al. 2001, 2003; Powers et al. 2000). The oral route is preferred for doxycycline because IM injections cause pain and tissue irritation and did not maintain concentrations in a range thought to be therapeutic. Oral doxycycline can be administered to pet birds by simply adding doxycycline hyclate to drinking water. When doxycycline hyclate was added to drinking water at concentrations of 0.28 mg/ml and 0.83 mg/ml (280 and 830 mg/l), plasma concentrations in treated birds were maintained high enough for susceptible organisms during a 45-day treatment (Powers et al. 2000). Another study confirmed that when added to drinking water at a concentration of 0.8 mg/ml (800 mg/l) it produced effective concentrations in Psittacine birds for a treatment duration of 42 days (Flammer et al. 2001). Lower water concentrations of 400 mg/l also may produce effective concentrations in some birds.

Because of the unique way doxycycline is eliminated (fecal), concentrations of doxycycline do not tend to accumulate in the blood of human patients with renal failure. Doxycycline is thus ideal for treating susceptible infections when renal failure or renal insufficiency is a complicating factor in antimicrobial therapy (Shaw and Rubin 1986). Doxycycline accumulation in normal and diseased kidneys in dogs and humans has been studied (Whelton et al. 1975).

MINOCYCLINE. Like doxycycline, minocycline is a product of chemical manipulations of the tetracycline base molecule that enhance antimicrobial action by improving gastrointestinal tract absorption, prolonging the half-life, and increasing the tissue penetration of the drug. The chemical structure of minocycline is shown in Figure 35.5. Increased penetration of minocycline into bacterial cells results in more activity against penicillinase-resistant strains of *Staphylococcus aureus* and a variety of other gram-positive and gram-negative organisms (Jonas and Cunha 1982). The increased concentration of the drug within the cell, which results in an overall increase in pharmacologic activity, is the primary advantage of minocycline.

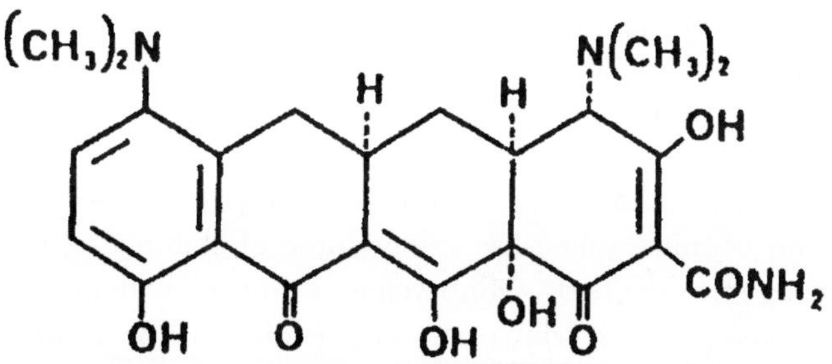

$(CH_3)_2N$ … $N(CH_3)_2$ … H H … OH … $CONH_2$ … OH O OH OH O

FIG. 35.5 Chemical structure of minocycline.

Minocycline has been studied less in veterinary medicine than the other tetracyclines. In humans, minocycline is rapidly and completely absorbed from the gastrointestinal tract, which results in high bioavailability by this route and produces less disturbance of the normal bacterial flora of the gastrointestinal tract. As with other tetracyclines, food, milk, and iron decrease the absorption of minocycline, but not to as great an extent (Leyden 1985). A high degree of protein binding occurs with minocycline in the plasma, with 80% protein binding reported for sheep serum (Wilson and Green 1986).

Some studies have been performed with minocycline in dogs. A toxicologic study performed by Noble et al. (1967) examined the use of minocycline in Beagles administered a daily dose of 5, 10, 20, or 40 mg/kg intravenously for 1 month. Adverse effects occurred only in the high dose groups. Minocycline produced erythema of the skin and mucous membranes, characterized by papules around the eyes, muzzle, ears, and abdomen; the intensity of these lesions was directly proportional to the dose administered. Decreases in red blood cell packed cell volumes, hemoglobin concentrations, and red cell counts were noted in dogs receiving 10 mg/kg or more of minocycline intravenously. Similar adverse effects were noted by Wilson et al. (1985). Other toxicologic studies with minocycline have been performed in dogs, rats, mice, and monkeys (Benitz et al. 1967).

Tissue distribution studies in dogs given a 10 mg/kg intravenous dose of minocycline showed that the drug penetrated most tissues very well, much like the other tetracyclines (Kelly and Kanegis 1967a). Metabolism may not play a major role in the elimination of minocycline in the rat or dog (Wilson and Green 1986). The major route of elimination for minocycline appears to be through the feces. Like doxycycline, minocycline excretion seems to be independent of renal function, indicating that renal excretion of minocycline is a minor route of eliminating the drug from the body. Minocycline is extensively bound to plasma proteins, which may in part account for its prolonged biological half-life.

The pharmacokinetics of minocycline in some species is summarized in Table 35.8. Pharmacokinetic parameters of other tetracycline analogs (including minocycline) have also been reported in dairy cows and ewes (Ziv and Sulman 1974) and in rabbits (Nicolau et al. 1993).

NEW DRUGS. The newest development in tetracyclines has been the modification of the minocycline structure to produce glycylcyclines (Agwuh and MacGowan 2006). Tigecycline is unique compared to the older tetracyclines (Agwuh and MacGowan 2006). It has a broader spectrum of activity that includes methicillin-resistant staphylococci (MRSA), Enterococcus, and multiresistant Enterobacteriaceae. It can be administered only IV. It has only been used in people; its use in animals has not been reported.

OTHER NON-ANTIMICROBIAL USES OF TETRACYCLINES

Tetracyclines also have been used as immunomodulating drugs and antiinflammatory drugs. This use of tetracyclines has focused on treatment of osteoarthritis, vasculitis, and dermatitis.

DERMATOLOGY. A review of the uses of tetracyclines in dermatology is available by Tsankov et al. (2003). The action of tetracyclines appears to be via inhibition of inflammatory cell infiltration. Tetracyclines also may affect COX-2 mediated PGE-2 synthesis during inflammation. The antiinflammatory activity was reviewed by Suomalainen et al. (1992). The combination of tetracycline and niacinamide has been used in dogs for the treatment of discoid lupus erythematosus (DLE), pemphigus foliaceus (PF), ulcerative dermatosis of Collies and Shetland Sheepdogs (vesicular cutaneous lupus erythematosus), lupoid onychodystrophy, and sterile pyogranulomatous disease (including sterile nodular panniculitis) (Auxilia et al. 2001; Rothstein et al. 1997; White et al. 1992). The exact mechanism to explain the efficacy of this combination is uncertain, but some inflammatory mechanisms are probably important. However, as an antipruritic treatment, this combination is not impressive (Beningo et al. 1999).

Alone, tetracyclines have been used for conditions in which an antiinflammatory mechanism may play a role (Suomalainen et al. 1992). Doxycycline was used in one study of plasmacytic pododermatitis in cats (Bettenay et al. 2001). Remission of signs occurred in 26% of cats.

ANGULAR LIMB DEFORMITIES IN FOALS. Another use of oxytetracycline has been the administration of high doses to newborn foals for the purpose of correcting angular limb deformities (Madison et al. 1994). The doses have been as high as 50–70 mg/kg, IV, q48 h. There is no known explanation for the effect of oxytetracycline on tendon or ligament laxity in horses. The pharmacokinetics in foals at this dose and adverse effects were explored by Papich et al. (1995) and no adverse effects were reported.

ARTHRITIS. Both in vivo and in vitro studies have documented antiinflammatory, chondroprotective, and antiarthritic effects of tetracyclines, particularly doxycycline and minocycline. These studies were summarized in other studies (Schanbel et al. 2007; Haerdi-Landerer, et al. 2007). The effects on arthritis may be caused by decreased inflammatory mediators, such as prostaglandins, and the reduced matrix metalloproteinases (MMP). In calves, the predominant effect was lower activity of MMP.

Yu et al. (1992) indicated that doxycycline administered prophylactically markedly reduced the severity of osteoarthritis in dogs with surgically induced transactions of the anterior cruciate ligament. Inhibition of classical lesions in that model was felt to be due to doxycycline's ability to inhibit (chelate) metalloproteases (collagenase, gelatinase, stromelysin) in the degenerating cartilage of the canine knee.

REFERENCES CITED AND ADDITIONAL READING

Adawa, D. A. Y., Hassan, A. Z., Abdullah, S. U., Ogunkoya, A. B., Adeyanju, J. B., and Okoro, J. E. 1992. Clinical trial of long-acting oxytetracycline and piroxicam in the treatment of canine ehrlichiosis. Vet Quarterly 14(3):118–120.

Agwuh, K. N., and MacGowan, A. 2006. Pharmacokinetics and pharmacodynamics of the tetracyclines including glycylcyclines. J Antimicrob Chemo 58:256–265.

Amyx, H. L., Huxsoll, D. L., Zeiler, D. C., and Hildebrandt, P. K. 1971. Therapeutic and prophylactic value of tetracycline in dogs infected with the agent of tropical canine pancytopenia. JAVMA 159(11):1428–1432.

Anadon, A., Martinez-Larranaga, M. R., and Diaz, M. J. 1985. Pharmacokinetics of tetracycline in chickens after intravenous administration. Poultry Sci 64:2273–79.

Aronson, A. L. 1980. Pharmacotherapeutics of the newer tetracyclines. JAVMA 176(10):1061–68.

Auxilia, S. T., Hill, P. B., Thoday, and K. L. 2001. Canine symmetrical lupoid onychodystrophy: a retrospective study with particular reference to management. J Sm An Pract 42:82–7.

Baert, K., Croubels, S., Gasthuys, F., DeBusser, J, and DeBacker. 2000. Pharmacokinetics and oral bioavailability of a doxycycline formulation (Doxycycline 75%) in nonfasted young pigs. J Vet Pharmacol Ther 23:45–48.

Baggot, J. D., Powers, T. E., Powers, J. D., Kowalski, J. J., and Kerr, K. M. 1977. Pharmacokinetics and dosage of oxytetracycline in dogs. Res Vet Sci 24:77–81.

Banting, A. de L., Baggot, J. D. 1996. Comparison of the pharmacokinetics and local tolerance of three injectable oxytetracycline formulations in pigs. J Vet Pharmacol Ther 19:50–55.

Banting, A. de L., Duval, M., and Gregoire, S. 1985. A comparative study of serum kinetics of oxytetracycline in pigs and calves following intramuscular administration. J Vet Pharmacol Ther 8:418–20.

Barza, M., Brown, R. B., Shanks, C., Gamble, C., and Weinstein, L. 1975. Relation between lipophilicity and pharmacological behavior of minocycline, doxycycline, tetracycline, and oxytetracycline in dogs. Antimicrob Agents Chemo 8(6):713–20.

Baxter, P., and McKellar, Q. A. 1990. Distribution of oxytetracycline in normal and diseased ovine lung tissue. J Vet Pharmacol Ther 13:428–31.

Beningo, K.E., Scott, D.W., Miller, W.H., Jr, and Rothstein, E. 1999. Observations on the use of tetracycline and niacinamide as antipruritic agents in atopic dogs. Can Vet J 40(4):268–270.

Benitz, K.-F., Roberts, G. K. S., and Yusa, A. 1967. Morphologic effects of minocycline in laboratory animals. Toxicol Appl Pharmacol 11:150–70.

Bettenay, S. V., Mueller, R. S., Dow, K., Friend, S. 2001. Feline plasmacytic pododermatitis—a prospective study of a novel treatment using systemic doxycycline. Proceedings of 16th Annual AAVD and ACVD Meeting.

Bidgood, T., Papich, M. G. 2003. Comparison of plasma and interstitial fluid concentrations of doxycycline and meropenem following constant rate intravenous infusion in dogs. Am J Vet Res 64:1040–1046.

Black, W. D. 1977. A study of the pharmacokinetics of oxytetracycline in the chicken. Poultry Sci 56:1430–34.

Black, W. D., Ferguson, H. W., Byrne, P., and Claxton, M. J. 1991. Pharmacokinetic and tissue distribution study of oxytetracycline in rainbow trout following bolus intravenous administration. J Vet Pharmacol Ther 14:351–58.

Bocker, R., Estler, C. J., Muller, S., Pfandzelter, C., and Spachmuller, B. 1982. Comparative evaluation of the effects of tetracycline, rolitetracycline and doxycycline on some blood parameters related to liver function. Arzneim Forsch 32(1):237–41.

Bradley, B. D., Allen, E. H., Showalter, D. H., and Colaianne, J. J. 1982. Comparative pharmacokinetics of chlortetracycline in milk-fed versus conventionally fed calves. J Vet Pharmacol Ther 5:267–78.

Breitschwerdt, E. B., Davidson, M. G., Aucoin, D. P., Levy, M. G., Szabados, N. S., Hegarty, B. C., Kuehne, A. L., and James, R. L. 1991. Efficacy of chloramphenicol, enrofloxacin, tetracycline for treatment of experimental rocky mountain spotted fever in dogs. Antimicrob Agents Chemo 35(11):2375–81.

Breitschwerdt, E. B., Davidson, M. G., Hegarty, B. C., Papich, M. G., and Grindem, C. B. 1997. Prednisolone at anti-inflammatory or immunosuppressive dosages in conjunction with doxycycline does not potentiate the severity of *Rickettsia rickettsii* infection in dogs. Antimicrob Agents Chemo 41:141–147.

Breitschwerdt, E. B., Papich, M. G., Hegarty, B. C., Gilger, B., Hancock, S. I., and Davidson, M. G. 1999. Efficacy of doxycycline, azithromycin, or trovafloxacin for treatment of experimental Rocky Mountain Spotted Fever in dogs. Antimicrob Agents Chemo 43:813–821.

Bretzlaff, K. N., Ott, R. S., Koritz, G. D., Bevill, R. F., Gustafsson, B. K., and Davis, L. E. 1983a. Distribution of oxytetracycline in the genital tract tissues of postpartum cows given the drug by intravenous and intrauterine routes. AJVR 44(5):764–69.

———. 1983b. Distribution of oxytetracycline in the healthy and diseased postpartum genital tract of cows. AJVR 44:760–63.

Bretzlaff, K. N., Ott, R. S., Koritz, G. D., Lock, T. F., Bevill, R. F., Shawley, R. V., Gustafsson, B. K., and Davis, L. E. 1982. Distribution of oxytetracycline in the genital tract of cows. AJVR 43:12–16.

Brown, H., Bing, R. F., Grueter, H. P., McAskill, J. W., Cooley, C. O., and Rathmacher, R. P. 1975. Tylosin and chlortetracycline for the prevention of liver abscesses, improved weight gains and feed efficiency in feedlot cattle. J Anim Sci 40(2):207–13.

Brown, M. P., Stover, S. M., Kelly, R. H., Farber, T. B., and Knight, H. D. 1981. Oxytetracycline hydrochloride in the horse: serum, synovial, peritoneal and urine concentrations after single dose intravenous administration. J Vet Pharmacol Ther 4:7–10.

Brunt, J., Guptill, L., Kordick, D. L., Kudrak, S., and Lappin, M. R. 2006. American Association of Feline Practitioners 2006 Panel report on diagnosis, treatment, and prevention of *Bartonella spp.* infections. J Feline Med Surg 8:213–226.

Burrows, G. E., Barto, P. B., and Martin, B. 1987. Comparative pharmacokinetics of gentamicin, neomycin and oxytetracycline in newborn calves. J Vet Pharmacol Ther 10:54–63.

Burrows, G. E., Barto, P. B., and Weeks, B. R. 1986. Chloramphenicol, lincomycin and oxytetracycline disposition in calves with experimental pneumonic pasteurellosis. J Vet Pharmacol Ther 9:213–22.

Bush, M., Stoskopf, M. K., Raath, J. P., and Papich, M. G. 2000. Serum oxytetracycline concentrations in African elephant (*Loxodonta africana*) calves after long-acting formulation injection. J Zoo Wildlife Med 31:41–46.

Chopra, I., Hawkey, P. M., Hinton, M. 1992. Tetracyclines, molecular and clinical aspects. J Antimicrob Chemo 29:245–277.

Cleveland, W. W., Adams, W. C., Mann, J. B. 1965. Acquired fanconi syndrome following degraded tetracycline. J Pediatr 66:333–42.

CLSI. 2007. Performance Standards for Antimicrobial Disk and Dilution Susceptibility Tests for Bacteria Isolated From Animals; Approved Standard—Third Edition. CLSI document M31-A3. Wayne, PA: Clinical and Laboratory Standards Institute.

Cooke, R. G., Knifton, A., Murdoch, D. B., and Yacoub, I. S. 1981. Bioavailability of oxytetracycline dihydrate tables in dogs. J Vet Pharmacol Ther 4:11–13.

Craigmill, A. L., Miller, G. R., Gehring, R., Pierce, A. N., and Riviere, J. E. 2004. Meta-analysis of pharmacokinetic data of veterinary drugs using the Food Animal Residue Avoidance Databank: oxytetracycline and procaine penicillin G. J Vet Pharmacol Ther 27:343–353.

Cunha, B. A., Sibley, C. M., and Ristuccia, A. M. 1982. Doxycycline. Ther Drug Monit 4:115–35.

Davey, L. A., Ferber, M. T., and Kaye, B. 1985. Comparison of the serum pharmacokinetics of a long acting and a conventional oxytetracycline injection. Vet Rec 117:426–29.

Davidson, D. E., Jr., Dill, G. S., Jr., Tingpalapong, M., Premabutra, S., Nguen, P. L., Stephenson, E. H., and Ristic, M. 1978. Prophylactic and therapeutic use of tetracycline during an epizootic of ehrlichiosis among military dogs. J Am Vet Med Assoc 172(6):697–700.

Davis, J. L., Salmon, J. H., Papich, M. G. 2006. Pharmacokinetics and tissue distribution of doxycycline after oral administration of single and multiple doses in horses. Am J Vet Res 67(2):310–6.

Dawson, K. A., Langlois, B. E., Stahly, T. S., and Cromwell, G. L. 1983. Multiple antibiotic resistance in fecal, cecal and colonic coliforms from pigs fed therapeutic and subtherapeutic concentrations of chlortetracycline. J Anim Sci 57(5):1225–34.

Dietz, D. D., Abdo, K. M., Haseman, J. K., Eustis, S. L., and Huff, J. E. 1991. Comparative toxicity and carcinogenicity studies of tetracycline and oxytetracycline in rats and mice. Fund Appl Toxicol 17:335–46.

Dinsmore, R. P., Stevens, R. D., Cattell, M. B., Salman, M. D., Sundlof, S. F. 1996. Oxytetracycline residues in milk after intrauterine treatment of cows with retained fetal membranes. J Am Vet Med Assoc 209(10):1753–5.

Dyer, D. C. 1989. Pharmacokinetics of oxytetracycline in the turkey: evaluation of biliary and urinary excretion. AJVR 50(4):522–24.

Fagerberg, D. J., Quarles, C. L., George, B. A., Fenton, J. M., Rollins, L. D., Williams, L. P., and Hancock, C. B. 1978. Effect of low level chlortetracycline feeding on subsequent therapy of *Escherichia coli* infection in chickens. J Anim Sci 46(5):1397–1412.

Fair, W. R. 1974. Diffusion of minocycline into prostatic secretions in dogs. Urology 3:339–44.

Finerman, G. A. M., and Milch, R. A. 1963. In vitro binding of tetracyclines to calcium. Nature 198:486–87.

Flammer, K., Trogdon, M. M., and Papich, M. G. 2003. Assessment of plasma concentrations of doxycycline in budgerigars fed medicated seed or water. J Am Vet Med Assoc 223:993–998.

Flammer, K., Whitt-Smith, D., Papich, M. G. 2001. Plasma concentrations of doxycycline in selected Psittacine birds when administered in water for potential treatment of *Chlamydophila psittaci* infection. J Avian Med Surg 15:276–282.

Fleming, J. T., and Pedersoli, W. M. 1980. Serum inorganic fluoride and renal function in dogs after methoxyflurane anesthesia, tetracycline treatment, and surgical manipulation. AJVR 41:2025–29.

Forsgren, A., and Bellahsene, A. 1985. Antibiotic accumulation in human polymorphonuclear leucocytes and lymphocytes. Scand J Infect Dis Suppl 44:16–23.

Gabler, W. L. 1991. Fluxes and accumulation of tetracyclines by human blood cells. Res Commun Chem Pathol Pharmacol 72(1):39–51.

Gale, E. F., and Folkes, J. P. 1953. The assimilation of amino acids by bacteria: actions of antibiotics on nucleic acid and protein synthesis in *Staphylococcus aureus*. Biochem J 53:493–98.

George, B. A., Fagerberg, D. J., and Quarles, C. L. 1977. Comparison of therapeutic efficacy of doxycycline, chlortetracycline and lincomycin-spectinomycin on *E. coli* infection of young chickens. Poultry Sci 56:452–58.

George, L., Mihalyi, J., Edmondson, A., Daigneault, J., Kagonyera, G., Willits, N., and Lucas, M. 1988. Topically applied furazolidone or parenterally administered oxytetracycline for the treatment of infectious bovine keratoconjunctivitis. JAVMA 192(10):1415–22.

George, L. W., and Smith, J. A. 1985. Treatment of *Moraxella bovis* infections in calves using a long-term oxytetracycline formulation. J Vet Pharmacol Ther 8:55–61.

George, L. W., Smith, J. A., and Kaswan, R. 1985. Distribution of oxytetracycline into ocular tissues and tears of calves. J Vet Pharmacol Ther 8:47–54.

Gothoni, G., Neuvonen, P. J., Mattila, M. 1972. Iron-tetracycline interaction: effect of time interval between the drugs. Acta Med Scand 191:409–11.

Greth, A., Gerlach, H., Gerbermann, H., Vassart, M., and Richez, P. 1993. Pharmacokinetics of doxycycline after parenteral administration in the Houbara Bustard (*Chlamydotis undulata*). Avian Dis 37:31–36.

Grondel, J. L., Nouws, J. F. M., Schutte, A. R., and Driessens, F. 1989. Comparative pharmacokinetics of oxytetracycline in rainbow trout (*Salmo gairdneri*) and African catfish (*Clarias gariepinus*). J Vet Pharmacol Ther 12:157–62.

Gross, D. R., Dodd, K. T., Williams, J. D., and Adams, H. R. 1981. Adverse cardiovascular effects of oxytetracycline preparations and vehicles in intact awake calves. AJVR 42(8):1371–77.

Gyrd-Hansen, N., Rasmussen, F., and Smith, M. 1981. Cardiovascular effects of intravenous administration of tetracycline in cattle. J Vet Pharmacol Ther 4:15–25.

Haerdi-Landerer, M. C., Suter, M. M., and Steiner, A. 2007. Intra-articular administration of doxycycline in calves. Am J Vet Res 68:1324–1331.

Hagermark, O., and Hoglund, S. 1974. Iron metabolism in tetracycline-treated acne patients. Acta Derm Venereol 54:45–48.

Hall, W. F., Kniffen, T. S., Bane, D. P., Bevill, R. F., and Koritz, G. D. 1989. Plasma concentrations of oxytetracycline in swine after administration of the drug intramuscularly and orally in feed. JAVMA 194(9):1265–68.

Hamp, S. E. 1967. The tetracyclines and their effect on teeth: a clinical study. Odontologisk Tidskrift 75:33–49.

Harber, L. C., Tromovitch, T. A., and Baer, R. L. 1961. Studies on photosensitivity due to demethylchlortetracycline. J Invest Dermatol 37:189–93.

Harcourt, R. S., and Hamburger, M. 1957. The effect of magnesium sulfate in lowering tetracycline blood levels. J Lab Clin Med 50:464–68.

Harms, C. A., Papich, M. G., Stamper, M. A., Ross, P. M., Rodriguez, M. X., and Hohn, A. A. 2004. Pharmacokinetics of oxytetracycline in loggerhead sea turtles (*Caretta caretta*) after single intravenous and intramuscular injections. J Zoo Wildlife Med 35(4):477–488.

Helmick, K., Papich, M. G., Vliet, K. A., Bennett, R. A., Jacobson, E. R. 2004. Pharmacokinetic disposition of a long-acting oxytetracycline formulation after single-dose oral and intravenous administrations in the American alligator (*Alligator mississippiensis*). J Zoo Wildlife Med 35(3):341–346.

Hennon, D. K. 1965. Dental aspects of tetracycline therapy: literature review and results of a prevalence survey. J Indiana Dent Assoc 44:484–92.

Hoeprich, P. D., and Warshauer, D. M. 1974. Entry of four tetracyclines into saliva and tears. Antimicrob Agents Chemo 5:330–36.

Hopf, G., Bocker, R., and Estler, C. J. 1985. Comparative effects of tetracycline and doxycycline on liver function of young adult and old mice. Arch Int Pharmacodyn 278:157–68.

Horspool, L. J. I., and McKellar, Q. A. 1990. Disposition of oxytetracycline in horses, ponies and donkeys after intravenous administration. Eq Vet J 22(4):284–85.

Immelman, A., and Dreyer, G. 1981. Oxytetracycline plasma levels in dogs after intramuscular administration of two formulations. J S African Vet Assoc 52(3):191–93.

———. 1986. Oxytetracycline concentration in plasma and semen of rams. J S African Vet Assoc 57(2):103–104.

Jha, V. K., Jayachandran, C., Singh, M. K., and Singh, S. D. 1989. Pharmacokinetic data on doxycycline and its distribution in different biological fluids in female goats. Vet Res Commun 13:11–16.

Jonas, M., and Cunha, B. A. 1982. Minocycline. Ther Drug Monitoring 4(2):137–45.

Jones, F. T., Langlois, B. E., Cromwell, G. L., and Hays, V. W. 1983. Effect of feeding chlortetracycline or virginiamycin on shedding of salmonellae from experimentally infected swine. J Anim Sci 57(2):279–85.

Jun, H. W., and Lee, B. H. 1980. Distribution of tetracycline in red blood cells. J Pharm Sci 69(4):455–57.

Kasper, C. A., Clayton, H. M., Wright, A. K., Skuba, E. V., and Petrie, L. 1995. Effects of high doses of oxytetracycline on metacarpophalangeal joint kinematics in neonatal foals. J Am Vet Med Assoc 207:71–73.

Kaufman, A. C., and Greene, C. E. 1993. Increased alanine transaminase activity associated with tetracycline administration in a cat. JAVMA 202(4):628–30.

Kelly, D. J., Chulay, J. D., Mikesell, P., and Friedlander, A. M. 1992. Serum concentrations of penicillin, doxycycline, and ciprofloxacin during prolonged therapy in rhesus monkeys. J Infect Dis 166:1184–87.

Kelly, R. G., and Kanegis, L. A. 1967a. Metabolism and tissue distribution of radioisotopically labeled minocycline. Toxicol Appl Pharmacol 11:171–83.

———. 1967b. Tissue distribution of tetracycline and chlortetracycline in the dog. Toxicol Appl Pharmacol 11:114–20.

Kilroy, C. R., Hall, W. F., Bane, D. P., Bevill, R. F., and Koritz, G. D. 1990. Chlortetracycline in swine: bioavailability and pharmacokinetics in fasted and fed pigs. J Vet Pharmacol Ther 13:49–58.

Kirkwood, J. K., Gulland, F. M. D., Needham, J. R., and Vogler, M. G. 1988. Pharmacokinetics of oxytetracycline in clinical cases in the red-necked wallaby (*Macropus rufogriseus*). Res Vet Sci 44:335–37.

Kniffen, T. S., Bane, D. P., Hall, W. F., Koritz, G. D., and Bevill, R. F. 1989. Bioavailability, pharmacokinetics, and plasma concentration of tetracycline hydrochloride fed to swine. AJVR 50(4):518–21.

Kordick, D.L., Papich, M.G., and Breitschwerdt, E.B. 1997. Efficacy of enrofloxacin or doxycycline for treatment of *Bartonella henselae* or *Bartonella clarridgeiae* infection in cats. Antimicrob Agents Chemother 41(11):2448–2455.

Kunin, C. M., and Finland, M. 1961. Clinical pharmacology of the tetracycline antibiotics. Clin Pharmacol Ther 2:51–69.

Kutter, K. L., and Simpson, J. E. 1978. Relative efficacy of two oxytetracycline formulations and doxycycline in the treatment of acute anaplasmosis in splenectomized calves. AJVR 39:347–49.

Landgraf, W. W., Ross, P. F., Cassidy, D. R., and Clubb, S. L. 1981. Concentration of chlortetracycline in the blood of yellow-crowned Amazon parrots fed medicated pelleted feeds. Avian Dis 26(1):14–17.

Larson, V. L., and Stowe, C. M. 1981. Plasma and tissue concentrations of oxytetracycline in the horse after intravenous administration. AJVR 42(12):2165–66.

Lewis, G. E., Crumrine, M. H., Jennings, P. B., and Fariss, B. L. 1973. Therapeutic value of tetracycline and ampicillin in dogs infected with *Brucella canis*. JAVMA 163:239–41.

Leyden, J. J. 1985. Absorption of minocycline hydrochloride and tetracycline hydrochloride. J Am Acad Dermatol 12:308–12.

Ling, G. V., Conzelman, G. M., Franti, C. E., and Ruby, A. L. 1980. Urine concentrations of chloramphenicol, tetracycline, and sulfisoxazole after oral administration to healthy adult dogs. AJVR 41(6):950–52.

Ling, G. V., Creighton, S. R., and Ruby, A. L. 1981. Tetracycline for oral treatment of canine urinary tract infection caused by *Pseudomonas aeruginosa*. JAVMA 179(6):578–79.

Lowe, M. B., and Tapp, E. 1966. Renal damage caused by anhydro-4-epitetracycline. Arch Pathol 81:362–64.

MacCulloch, D., Richardson, R. A., and Allwood, G. K. 1974. The penetration of doxycycline, oxytetracycline and minocycline into sputum. NZ Med J 80:300–302.

Madison, J. B., Garber, J. L., Rice, B., et al. 1994. Effect of oxytetracycline on metacarpophalangeal and distal interphalangeal joint angles in newborn foals. J Am Vet Med Assoc 204:246–249.

Martinsen, B., Oppegaard, H., Wichstrom, R., and Myhr, E. 1992. Temperature-dependent in vitro antimicrobial activity of four 4-quinolones and oxytetracycline against bacteria pathogenic to fish. Antimicrob Agents Chemother 36(8):1738–43.

McElroy, D. E., Ravis, W. R., and Clark, C. H. 1987. Pharmacokinetics of oxytetracycline hydrochloride in rabbits. AJVR 48(8):1261–63.

McPherson, J. C., Ellison, R. G., Davis, H. N., Hawkridge, F. M., Ellison, L. T., and Hall, W. K. 1974. The metabolic acidosis resulting from intravenous tetracycline administration (37829). Proc Soc Exper Biol Med 145:450–55.

Meijer, L. A., Ceyssens, G. F., deJong, W. T., and de Greve, B. I. J. A. C. 1993a. Correlation between tissue and plasma concentrations of oxytetracycline in veal calves. J Toxicol Environ Health 40:35–45.

Meijer, L. A., Ceyssens, K. G. F., de Greve, B. I. J. A. C., and de Bruijn, W. 1993b. Pharmacokinetics and bioavailability of doxycycline hyclate after oral administration in calves. Vet Quarterly 15(1):1–5.

Meijer, L. A., Ceyssens, K. G. F., deJong, W. T., and deGreve, B. I. J. A. C. 1993c. Three phase elimination of oxytetracycline in veal calves: the presence of an extended terminal elimination phase. J Vet Pharmacol Ther 16:214–22.

Mevius, D. J., Nouws, J. F. M., Breukink, H. J., Vree, T. B., Driessens, F., and Verkaik, R. 1986a. Comparative pharmacokinetics, bioavailability and renal clearance of five parenteral oxytetracycline-20% formulations in dairy cows. Vet Quarterly 8(4):285–94.

Mevius, D. J., Vellenga, L., Breukink, H. J., Nouws, J. F. M., Vree, T. B., and Driessens, F. 1986b. Pharmacokinetics and renal clearance of oxytetracycline in piglets following intravenous and oral administration. Vet Quarterly 8(4):274–84.

Migaki, T. T., and Babcock, W. E. 1977. Efficacy of doxycycline against experimental complicated chronic respiratory disease compared with commercially available water medicants in broilers. Poultry Sci 56:1739.

Moffit, J. M., Cooley, R. O., and Olsen, N. H. 1974. Prediction of tetracycline-induced tooth discoloration. J Am Dental Assoc 88:547–52.

Neuvonen, P. J., Gothoni, G., Hackman, R., and Bjorksten, K. 1970. Interference of iron with the absorption of tetracyclines in man. Brit Med J 4:532–34.

Nicolau, D. P., Freeman, C. D., Nightingale, C. H., and Quintiliani, R. 1993. Pharmacokinetics of minocycline and vancomycin in rabbits. Lab An Sci 43(3):222–25.

Nielsen, P., and Gyrd-Hansen, N. 1996. Bioavailability of oxytetracycline, tetracycline and chlortetracycline after oral administration to fed and fasted pigs. J Vet Pharmacol Ther 19:305–311.

Nivas, S. C., York, M. D., and Pomeroy, B. S. 1976. Effects of different levels of chlortetracycline in the diet of turkey poults artificially infected with *Salmonella typhimurium*. Poultry Sci 55:2176–89.

Noble, J. F., Kanegis, L. A., and Hallesy, D. W. 1967. Short-term toxicity and observations on certain aspects of the pharmacology of a unique tetracycline—minocycline. Toxicol Appl Pharmacol 11:128–49.

Nouws, J. F. M. 1984. Irritation, bioavailability, and residue aspects of ten oxytetracycline formulations administered intramuscularly to pigs. Vet Quarterly 6(2):80–84.

Nouws, J. F. M., Breukink, H. J., Binkhorst, G. J., Lohuis, J., van Lith, P., Mevius, D. J., and Vree, T. B. 1985a. Comparative pharmacokinetics and bioavailability of eight parenteral oxytetracycline-10% formulations in dairy cows. Vet Quarterly 7(4):306–14.

Nouws, J. F. M., Smulders, A., and Rappalini, M. 1990. A comparative study on irritation and residue aspects of five oxytetracycline formulations administered intramuscularly to calves, pigs and sheep. Vet Quarterly 12(3):129–38.

Nouws, J. F. M., van Ginneken, C. A. M., and Ziv, G. 1983. Age-dependent pharmacokinetics of oxytetracycline in ruminants. J Vet Pharmacol Ther 6:59–66.

Nouws, J. F. M., and Vree, T. B. 1983. Effect of injection site on the bioavailability of an oxytetracycline formulation in ruminant calves. Vet Quarterly 5(4):165–70.

Nouws, J. F. M., Vree, T. B., Termond, E., Lohuis, J., van Lith, P., Binkhorse, G. J., and Breukink, H. J. 1985b. Pharmacokinetics and renal clearance of oxytetracycline after intravenous and intramuscular administration to dairy cows. Vet Quarterly 7(4):296–305.

Onawunmi, O. A., and Todd, A. C. 1976. Suppression and control of experimentally induced porcine coccidiosis with chlortetracycline combination, buquinolate, and lincomycin hydrochloride. AJVR 37:657–60.

Palmer, J. E., Benson, C. E., and Whitlock, R. H. 1992. Effect of treatment with oxytetracycline during the acute stages of experimentally induced equine ehrlichial colitis in ponies. AJVR 53(12):2300–2304.

Papich, M. G. 2003a. Antimicrobial Therapy for Horses. Chapter 1.2. In Robinson NE (Editor). Current Theory in Equine Medicine, 5th Edition, pp. 6–10.

Papich, M. G. 2003b. Antimicrobial therapy for gastrointestinal diseases. Vet Clin N Am: Equine Pract 19(3):645–63.

Papich, M. G., Wright, A. K., Petrie, L., and Korsrud, G. O. 1995. Pharmacokinetics of oxytetracycline administered intravenously to 4- to 5-day-old foals. J Vet Pharmacol Ther 18:375–378.

Percy, D. H., and Black, W. D. 1988. Pharmacokinetics of tetracycline in the domestic rabbit following intravenous or oral administration. Can J Vet Res 52:5–11.

Perry, T. W., Beeson, W. M., Mohler, M. T., and Harrington, R. B. 1971. Value of chlortetracycline and sulfamethazine for conditioning feeder cattle after transit. J Anim Sci 32(1):137–40.

Pijpers, A., Schoevers, E. J., van Gogh, H., van Leengoed, L. A. M. G., Visser, I. J. R., van Miert, A. S. J. P. A. M., and Verheijden, J. H. M. 1990. The pharmacokinetics of oxytetracycline following intravenous administration in healthy and diseased pigs. J Vet Pharmacol Ther 13:320–26.

———. 1991. The influence of disease on feed and water consumption and on pharmacokinetics of orally administered oxytetracycline in pigs. J Anim Sci 69:2947–54.

Pilloud, M. 1973. Pharmacokinetics, plasma protein binding and dosage of oxytetracycline in cattle and horses. Res Vet Sci 15:224–30.

Plakas, S. M., McPhearson, R. M., and Guarino, A. M. 1988. Disposition and bioavailability of 3H-tetracycline in the channel catfish (*Ictalurus punctatus*). Xenobiotica 18(1):83–93.

Powers, L. V., Flammer, K., Papich, M. 2000. Preliminary investigation of doxycycline plasma concentrations in cockatiels (*Nymphicus hollandicus*) after administration by injection or in water or feed. J Avian Med Surg 14:23–30.

Prats, C., ElKorchi, G., Giralt, M., Cristòfol, C., Pea, J., Zorrilla, I., Saborit, J., and Peréz, B. 2005. PK and PK/PD of doxycycline in drinking water after therapeutic use in pigs. J Vet Pharmacol Ther 28:525–530.

Prescott, J. F., and Baggot, J. D. (eds.) 1993. Tetracyclines. In Antimicrobial Therapy in Veterinary Medicine, 2nd ed., pp. 215–228. Ames: Iowa State Univ Press.

Price, J. E., and Dolan, T. T. 1980. A comparison of the efficacy of imidocarb dipropionate and tetracycline hydrochloride in the treatment of canine ehrlichiosis. Vet Rec 107:275–77.

Prus, S. E., Clubb, S. L., Flammer, K. 1992. Doxycycline plasma concentrations in macaws fed a medicated corn diet. Avian Dis 36:480–83.

Quarles, C. L., Fagerberg, D. J., and Greathouse, G. A. 1977. Effect of low level feeding chlortetracycline on subsequent therapy of chicks infected with *Salmonella typhimurium*. Poultry Sci 56:1674–75.

Richey, E. J., Brock, W. E., Kliewer, I. O., and Jones, E. W. 1977. Low levels of chlortetracycline for anaplasmosis. AJVR 38(2):171–72.

Riond, J.-L., Duckett, W. M., Riviere, J. E., Jernigan, A. D., and Spurlock, S. L. 1989a. Concerned about intravenous use of doxycycline in horses. JAVMA 195(7):846–47.

Riond, J.-L., and Riviere, J. E. 1988. Pharmacology and toxicology of doxycycline. Vet Human Toxicol 30(5):431–43.

———. 1989a. Effects of tetracyclines on the kidney in cattle and dogs. JAVMA 195(7):995–97.

———. 1989b. Doxycycline binding to plasma albumin of several species. J Vet Pharmacol Ther 12:253–60.

———. 1990a. Pharmacokinetics and metabolic inertness of doxycycline in young pigs. AJVR 51(8):1271–75.

———. 1990b. Allometric analysis of doxycycline pharmacokinetic parameters. J Vet Pharmacol Ther 13:404–07.

Riond, J.-L., Riviere, J. E., Duckett, W. M., Atkins, C. E., Jernigan, A. D., Rikihisa, Y., and Spurlock, S. L. 1992. Cardiovascular effects and fatalities associated with intravenous administration of doxycycline to horses and ponies. Eq Vet J 24(1):41–45.

Riond, J.-L., Tyczkowska, K., and Riviere, J. E. 1989b. Pharmacokinetics and metabolic inertness of doxycycline in calves with mature or immature rumen function. AJVR 50(8):1329–33.

Riond, J.-L., Vaden, S. L., and Riviere, J. E. 1990. Comparative pharmacokinetics of doxycycline in cats and dogs. J Vet Pharmacol Ther 13:415–24.

Rothstein, E., Scott, D. W., Riis, R. C. 1997. Tetracycline and niacinamide for the treatment of sterile pyogranuloma/granuloma syndrome in a dog. J Am Anim Hosp Assoc 33:540–3.

Royal, W. A., Robinson, R. A., and Loken, K. I. 1970. The influence of chlortetracycline feeding on *Salmonella typhimurium* excretion in young calves. Vet Rec 86:67–69.

Schach von Wittenau, M., and Delahunt, C. S. 1966. The distribution of tetracycline in tissues of dogs after repeated oral administration. J Pharmacol Exp Ther 152:164–69.

Schach von Wittenau, M., and Twomey, T. M. 1971. The disposition of doxycycline by man and dog. Chemotherapy 16:217–28.

Schachter, J., Bankowski, R. A., Sung, M. L., Miers, L., and Strassburger, M. 1984. Measurement of tetracycline levels in parakeets. Avian Dis 28(1):295–302.

Schanbel, L. V., Watts, A. E., Papich, M. G., Torre, C. H., Mohammed, H. O., Fortier, L. A. 2007. Orally administered subantimicrobial concentrations of doxycycline attains synovial fluid levels capable of inhibiting matrix metalloproteinases 3 and 13. [abstract] Presented at the Orthopaedic Research Society Annual Meeting 2007, and the American Association of Equine Practitioners Annual Meeting.

Schifferli, D., Galeazzi, R. L., Nicolet, J., and Wanner, M. 1982. Pharmacokinetics of oxytetracycline and therapeutic implications in veal calves. J Vet Pharmacol Ther 5:247–57.

Schipper, I. A. 1965. Milk and blood levels of chemotherapeutic agents in cattle. JAVMA 147(12):1403–7.

Segal, B. M. 1963. Photosensitivity, nail discoloration, and onycholysis: side effect of tetracycline therapy. Arch Int Med 112:165–67.

Shaw, D. H., and Rubin, S. I. 1986. Pharmacologic activity of doxycycline. JAVMA 189(7):808–10.

Smith, J. A., and George, L. W. 1985. Treatment of acute ocular *Moraxella bovis* infections in calves with a parenterally administered long-acting oxytetracycline formulation. AJVR 46(4):804–7.

Soma, J. A., and Speer, V. C. 1975. Effects of pregnant mare serum and chlortetracycline on the reproductive efficiency of sows. J Anim Sci 41(1):100–105.

Stevens, R. D., Dinsmore, R. P., Cattell, M. B. 1995. Evaluation of the use of intrauterine infusions of oxytetracycline, subcutaneous injections of fenprostalene, or a combination of both, for the treatment of retained fetal membranes in dairy cows. J Am Vet Med Assoc 15;207(12): 1612–5.

Stevenson, S. 1980. Oxytetracycline nephrotoxicosis in two dogs. JAVMA 176(6):530–31.

Suomalainen, K., Sorsa, T., Golub, L. M., et al. 1992. Specificity of the anticollagenase action of tetracycline: relevance to the anti-inflammatory potential. Antimicrob Agents Chemother 36:227–229, 1992.

Suzuka, I., Kaji, H., and Kaji, A. 1966. Binding of specific sRNA to 30S ribosomal subunits: effect of 50S ribosomal subunits. Proc Natl Acad Sci 55:1483–86.

Teare, A., Schwark, W. S., Shin, S. J., and Graham, D. L. 1985. Pharmacokinetics of a long-acting oxytetracycline preparation in ring-necked pheasants, great horned owls, and Amazon parrots. AJVR 46(12): 2639–43.

TerHune, T. N., and Upson, D. W. 1989. Oxytetracycline pharmacokinetics, tissue depletion, and toxicity after administration of a long-acting preparation at double the label dosage. J Am Vet Med Assoc 194: 911–916.

Teske, R. H., Rollins, L. D., Condon, R. J., Carter, G. G. 1973. Serum oxytetracycline concentrations after intravenous and intramuscular administration in horses. J Am Vet Med Assoc 162:119–120.

Teuscher, E., Lamothe, P., Tellier, P., and Lavallee, J.-C. 1982. A toxic nephrosis in calves treated with a medication containing tetracycline degradation products. Can Vet J 23:327–31.

Toutain, P. L., and Raynaud, J. P. 1983. Pharmacokinetics of oxytetracycline in young cattle: comparison of conventional vs. long-acting formulations. AJVR 44:1203–9.

Tsankov, N., Broshtilova, V., and Kazandjieva, J. 2003. Tetracyclines in dermatology. Clin Dermatol 21:33–39.

USP. (United States Pharmacopeia.) 2003. Veterinary Pharmaceutical Information Monographs—Antibiotics. Tetracyclines. J Vet Pharmacol Ther 26(Suppl 2):225–252.

Varma, K. J., and Paul, B. S. 1983. Pharmacokinetics and plasma protein binding (in vitro) of oxytetracycline in buffalo (*Bubalus bubalis*). AJVR 44(3):497–99.

Waisbren, B. A., and Hueckel, J. S. 1950. Reduced absorption of Aureomycin caused by aluminum hydroxide gel (Amphojel). Proc Soc Exp Biol Med 73:73–74.

Ward, G. S., Guiry, C. C., and Alexander, L. L. 1982. Tetracycline-induced anaphylactic shock in a dog. JAVMA 180(7):770–71.

Weinberg, E. D. 1957. The mutual effects of antimicrobial compounds and metallic cations. Bacteriol Rev 21:4–68.

Whelton, A., Nightingale, S. D., Carter, G. G., Gordon, L. S., Bryant, H. H., and Walker, W. G. 1975. Pharmacokinetic characteristics of doxycycline accumulation in normal and severely diseased kidneys. J Infect Dis 132(4):467–71.

White, S. D., Rosychuk, A. W., Reinke, S. I., and Paradis, M. 1992. Use of tetracycline and niacinamide for treatment of autoimmune skin disease in 31 dogs. JAVMA 200(10):1497–1500.

Williams, R. D., Rollins, L. D., Pocurull, D. W., Selwyn, M., and Mercer, H. D. 1978. Effect of feeding chlortetracycline on the reservoir of *Salmonella typhimurium* in experimentally infected swine. Antimicrob Agents Chemother 14(5):710–19.

Wilson, R. C., and Green, N. K. 1986. Pharmacokinetics of minocycline hydrochloride in clinically normal and hypoproteinemic sheep. AJVR 47(3):650–52.

Wilson, R. C., Kemp, D. T., Kitzman, J. V., and Goetsch, D. D. 1988. Pharmacokinetics of doxycycline in dogs. Can J Vet Res 52:12–14.

Wilson, R. C., Kitzman, J. V., Kemp, D. T., and Goetsch, D. D. 1985. Compartmental and noncompartmental pharmacokinetic analyses of minocycline hydrochloride in the dog. AJVR 46(6):1316–18.

Wivagg, R. T., Jaffe, J. M., and Colaizzi, J. L. 1976. Influence of pH and route of injection on acute toxicity of tetracycline in mice. J Pharm Sci 65(6):916–18.

Xia, W., Gyrd-Hanson, N., and Nielsen, P. 1983. Comparison of pharmacokinetic parameters for two oxytetracycline preparations in pigs. J Vet Pharmacol Ther 6:113–20.

Yu, L. P., Smith, G. N., Brandt, K. D., Myers, S. L., O'Connor, B. L., and Brandt, D. A. 1992. Reduction of the severity of canine osteoarthritis by prophylactic treatment with oral doxycycline. Arthritis and Rheum 35(10):1150–59.

Zinn, R. A. 1993. Influence of oral antibiotics on digestive function in Holstein steers fed a 71% concentrate diet. J Anim Sci 71(1):213–17.

Ziv, G., and Sulman, F. G. 1974. Analysis of pharmacokinetic properties of nine tetracycline analogues in dairy cows and ewes. AJVR 35:1197–1201.

CHAPTER

36

AMINOGLYCOSIDE ANTIBIOTICS

MARK G. PAPICH AND JIM E. RIVIERE

Aminoglycoside antibiotics are important treatments against gram-negative infections. Aminoglycosides are a therapeutically essential class of antibiotics whose usefulness is often restricted by their toxic potential and residues in food animals. This chapter reviews the pharmacokinetics, toxicity, and tissue disposition of aminoglycoside antibiotics in various species.

PHARMACOLOGY OF AMINOGLYCOSIDES

GENERAL. Aminoglycosides include the familiar drugs gentamicin, amikacin, kanamycin, and tobramycin. They also include less familiar drugs such as neomycin, dihydrostreptomycin, and paromomycin. Spectinomycin has been included with aminoglycosides in some textbooks, but we have instead included it with the miscellaneous antibiotics in Chapter 37. Aminoglycosides are a class of antimicrobial compounds produced from strains of *Streptomyces* spp., *Micromonospora* spp., and *Bacillus* spp. Chemically, they are aminocyclitols: hydroxyl and amino or guanidine substituted cyclohexane with amino sugars joined by glycosidic linkages to one or more of the hydroxyl groups. These molecules have excellent solubility in water, but poor lipid solubility, are thermodynamically stable over a wide range of pH values and temperatures (Lancini and Parenti 1982; Leitner and Price 1982; Nagabhusban et al. 1982; Pechere and Dugal 1979), and have molecular weights ranging from 400 to 500 g/mol. The aminoglycosides are basic polycations with pK_a values that range from 7.2 to 8.8 (Ziv and Sulman 1974; Katzung 1984; Prescott and Baggot 1988).

The chemical structures of some of the commonly used aminoglycosides are shown in Figure 36.1. The chemical structure determines the antimicrobial activity, resistance

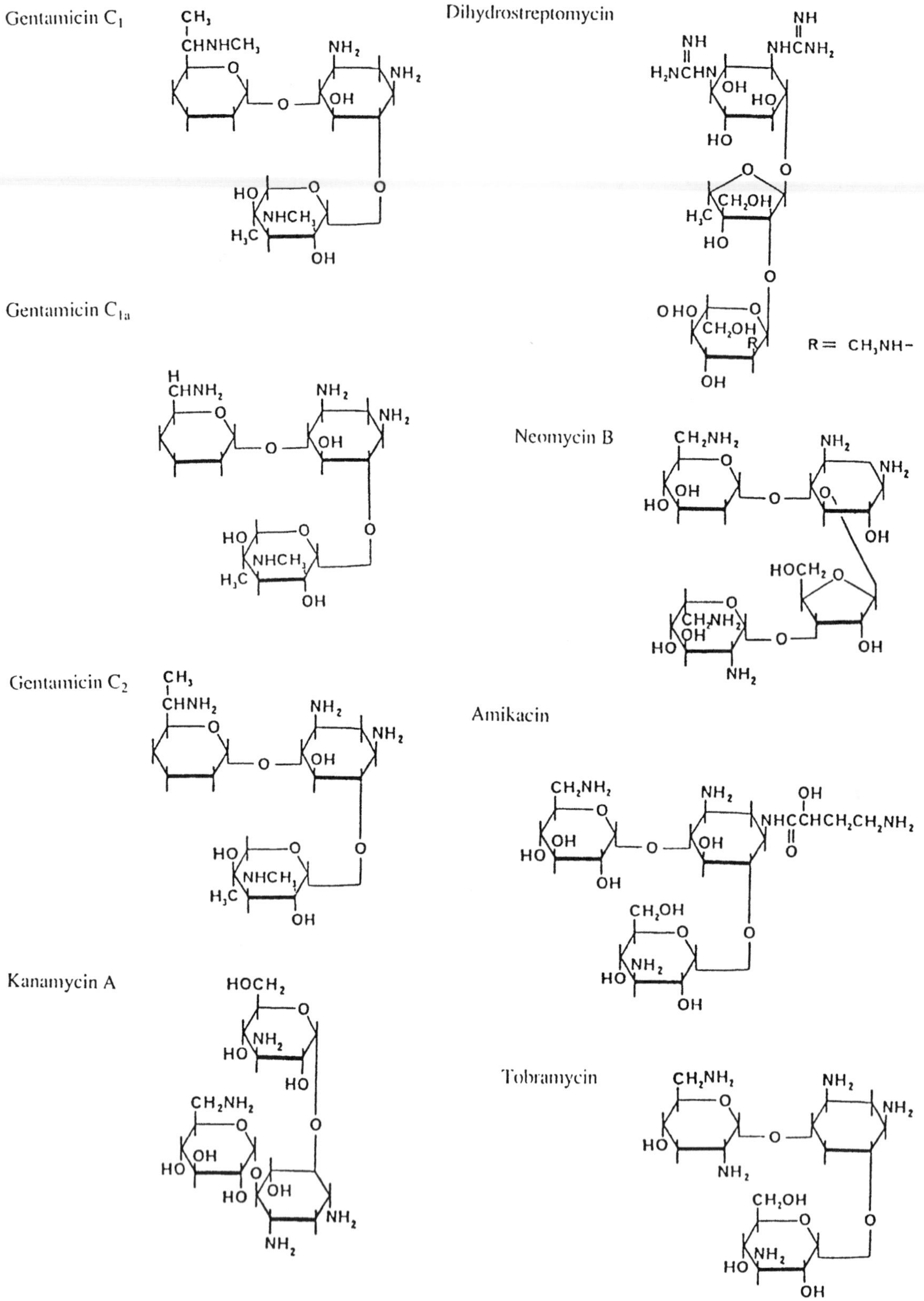

Gentamicin C_1

Dihydrostreptomycin

$R = CH_3NH-$

Gentamicin C_{1a}

Neomycin B

Gentamicin C_2

Amikacin

Kanamycin A

Tobramycin

FIG. 36.1 Chemical structures of the commonly used aminoglycosides.

patterns, and inherent propensity to cause toxicosis. The various mechanisms of nephrotoxicity (binding to proximal tubule brush-border vesicles and phospholipids, inhibition of mitochondrial function, etc.) may be associated with the number of free amino groups on the aminoglycoside molecule. In general, the most ionized aminoglycosides (i.e., neomycin, with six groups) are more toxic and show greater binding affinity than the least ionized aminoglycosides of the class (i.e., streptomycin, with three groups) (Bendirdjian et al. 1982; Cronin 1979; Feldman et al. 1981; Humes et al. 1982; Just and Habermann 1977; Kunin 1970; Lipsky and Lietman 1982; Luft and Evan 1980a,b; Weinberg et al. 1980). Other structural characteristics may account for differences in toxicity within groups of drugs with similar total ionization potentials (i.e., netilmicin, tobramycin, amikacin, and gentamicin, all with five ionizable groups).

MECHANISM OF ACTION. Aminoglycosides exert their antibacterial action by irreversibly binding to one or more receptor proteins on the 30S subunit of the bacterial ribosome and thereby interfering with several mechanisms in the mRNA translation process. These include disrupting an initiation complex between the mRNA and the 30S subunit, blocking further translation and thereby causing premature chain termination, or causing incorporation of an incorrect amino acid in the protein product. Although most antimicrobials that interfere with ribosomal protein synthesis are bacteriostatic, aminoglycosides are bactericidal.

The mechanism of bacterial penetration by the aminoglycoside through the cell membrane is biphasic. Drug diffuses through the outer membrane of gram-negative bacteria through aqueous channels formed by the porin proteins. Once in the periplasmic space, an oxygen-requiring transport process transports the drug into the cell, where it interacts with the ribosome. Anaerobic bacteria are therefore resistant to the antibacterial effects of aminoglycosides. The oxygen-dependent transport is linked to an electron transport system, which causes the bacterial cytoplasm to be negatively charged with respect to the periplasm and external environment. The positively charged aminoglycosides are attracted electrostatically into the bacterial cytoplasm. Some divalent cations (such as calcium and magnesium) are competitive inhibitors of this transport system. This proton-motive force also functions in the lysosomes and mitochondria in which aminoglycosides accumulate and may also be a factor in the intralysosomal accumulation of the aminoglycosides.

A characteristic of aminoglycoside activity is that bacterial killing is concentration-dependent, and a postantibiotic effect (PAE) is evident. By definition, the PAE is a persistent suppression of bacterial growth following the removal of an antimicrobial agent. Bactericidal action persists after serum concentrations fall below minimum inhibitory concentrations (MICs). This has ramifications for the design of clinical dosage regimens.

CLINICAL USES. The drugs used most often to any extent in veterinary medicine are amikacin, gentamicin, kanamycin, and neomycin (topically only). Netilmicin, sisomicin, and dibekacin are newer compounds that may be used clinically in the future. Many streptomycin products have either been removed from the human market or are used only for certain infections (e.g., tuberculosis). Penicillin-dihydrostreptomycin combinations have been discontinued in the United States for use in animals.

Aminoglycosides are still considered to be important drugs of choice for treating serious aerobic gram-negative infections in veterinary medicine, although newer and less toxic antimicrobials (i.e., third-generation cephalosporins and fluoroquinolones) have replaced the use of aminoglycosides for some bacterial infections.

Neomycin is too toxic to be used systemically but is still used topically. Kanamycin, first introduced in the late 1950s, has a primarily gram-negative spectrum of antimicrobial activity. However, many organisms are now resistant to this aminoglycoside and its use has subsequently declined. Gentamicin, introduced in the 1960s, has a broader spectrum and is associated with less resistance than kanamycin. Amikacin, a semisynthetic derivative of kanamycin, was introduced clinically in the 1970s, has the broadest spectrum of activity of all the aminoglycoside antibiotics used clinically to date, and is the preferred antibiotic in severe gram-negative infections that are resistant to gentamicin or tobramycin.

Table 36.1 lists the dosage regimens for gentamicin, kanamycin, apramycin, and amikacin that have been used for several years in which administration is given more than once per day. Although these regimens are still used occasionally, it is more common currently to use a once-daily dosing regimen for mammals. Table 36.2 includes the once-daily dosing recommendations. It is important to note that these are recommended doses that should be

TABLE 36.1 Recommended dosage regimens based on target maximum concentrations of 10–12 μg/mL for gentamicin and 30–40 μg/mL for kanamycin, apramycin, and amikacin and target minimum concentrations of 1–2 μg/mL for gentamicin and 2.5–5 μg/mL for kanamycin, apramycin, and amikacin

Species	Dosage regimen	Reference
Gentamicin		
Dogs (juvenile)	2–4 mg/kg q6h IV	Riviere and Coppoc 1981a
Cats	3 mg/kg q8h IV	Jernigan et al. 1988a–e
	3 mg/kg q6h IM/SC	Jernigan et al. 1988a–e
Ponies	4 mg/kg q8h IV/IM	Haddad et al. 1985a,b
	5 mg/kg q8h IM	
Horses	4.2 mg/kg q8-12h IV/IM	Pedersoli et al. 1980
Horses (adult)	2 mg/kg q8h IV/IM	Sojka and Brown 1986
Horses (foals)	3 mg/kg q12h IV/IM	Sojka and Brown 1986
Cows	5 mg/kg q8h IV/IM	Haddad et al. 1987
Cows (lactating)	3.5 mg/kg q8h IM	Haddad et al. 1986
Birds of prey	2.5 mg/kg q8h IM	Bird et al. 1983
Catfish	3.5 mg/kg q33h IM	Setzer 1985
	1.6 mg/kg q33h	Setzer 1985
Roosters	2 mg/kg q12h IM	Pedersoli et al. 1990
Kanamycin		
Dogs	10 mg/kg q6-8h IM/IV	Baggot 1978
Apramycin		
Calves	20 mg/kg q12h IM	Ziv et al. 1985
Amikacin		
Cats	10 mg/kg q8h IV/IM/SC	Jernigan et al. 1988a
Dogs	10 mg/kg q8h IM/SC	Baggot et al. 1985
Dogs[a]	10 mg/kg q12h IM/SC	Baggot et al. 1985

Source: Adapted from Brown and Riviere 1991.
[a]Urinary tract infections; based on IV infusion of 0.35 mg/kg/hr and a half-life of 2.5 hr.

modified proportionately to correct for age, clinical or subclinical disease processes, renal insufficiency, or any of the other factors that may predispose the patient to aminoglycoside toxicosis (see the section "Aminoglycoside Toxicity," below). Alterations in the dose can be best determined by monitoring serum creatinine concentrations or optimally by monitoring aminoglycoside serum concentrations at predetermined time points after dosing (See Chapter 52).

Single Daily Dose Administration. Recent studies in humans, laboratory animals, and veterinary species suggest that single daily dosing (SID) of aminoglycosides may be as efficacious as administering the same dose divided over 24 hours. The concept of single daily dosing of aminoglycosides has been utilized and generally accepted within the human medical community (Bass et al. 1998; Christensen et al. 1997; Freeman et al. 1997; Karachalios

TABLE 36.2 Once-daily dosages for selected aminoglycosides

Species	Dosage (In Most cases the Dose Can Be Administered IV, IM, or SC)
Gentamicin	
Dog	9–14 mg/kg q24h
Cat	5–8 mg/kg q24h
Horse	Adult: 4–6.8 mg/kg q24h
	Foal (<2 weeks): 12–14 mg/kg q24h
Cattle	Adult: 5–6 mg/kg q24h
	Calf (<2 weeks): 12–15 mg/kg q24h
Sheep	Same as cattle
Amikacin	
Dog	15–30 mg/kg q24h
Cat	10–15 mg/kg, q24h
Horse	Adult: 20 mg/kg q24h
	Foal (<weeks): 20–25 mg/kg q24h

et al. 1998; Rodvold et al. 1997). A report from a guinea pig infection model indicates that the recommended total daily dose of gentamicin given once daily (6–12 mg/kg/day) has the same antibacterial efficacy as two or three times daily therapy (Campbell et al. 1996). The efficacy of single dose administration is rooted in the PAE. Because of the PAE phenomenon, the aminoglycoside can be given less frequently and will continue to inhibit bacterial growth after levels fall below the MIC for the organism. Fortuitously, as will be discussed later relative to nephrotoxicity, aminoglycoside dosage regimens that produce high peak and low trough concentrations also have less propensity to induce renal toxicity than multiple-dose regimens, which produce lower peak but higher trough concentrations. For example, in a classic study rats given gentamicin at a dose of 40 mg/kg once daily had significantly lower serum creatinine concentrations than rats given the same dose of gentamicin divided twice daily or three times a day indicating that once daily induced less renal damage than the lower, divided dosing scheme (Bennett et al. 1979).

The concept of once-daily dosing has been adopted for dogs and cats (doses listed in Table 36.2). In one study, once-daily dosing to dogs at 6 mg/kg produced adequate serum drug concentrations with minimal risk of nephrotoxicity (Albarellos et al. 2004). The PAE and efficacy of once-daily therapy have also been suggested for the horse (Geor & Papich 2003; Godber et al. 1995; Tudor et al. 1999; Martin et al. 1998; Magdesian et al. 1998). Once-daily therapy for adults should be administered at a dose of 4.4 mg/kg (Tudor et al. 1999) for highly susceptible bacteria, or at a dose of 6.6 mg/kg for other organisms. These doses produce adequate plasma concentrations of gentamicin to meet pharmacokinetic-pharmacodynamic (PK-PD) criteria.

PHARMACOKINETICS OF AMINOGLYCOSIDES

GENERAL. A comprehensive review of aminoglycoside pharmacokinetics has been reported by Brown and Riviere (1991) and serves as the basis for this review. The pharmacokinetics of the aminoglycosides is similar across species lines, but the variability within each animal population is large, indicating a significant amount of heterogeneity in aminoglycoside disposition in both diseased and normal animals (Sojka and Brown 1986; Frazier et al. 1988). In addition, the inherent variability caused by many different disease states necessitates close monitoring of serum or plasma concentrations to optimize efficacy and minimize toxicosis (see Chapter 52). A similarly large variability in aminoglycoside pharmacokinetics has also been reported in humans (Kaye et al. 1974; Sawchuk et al. 1977; Zaske et al. 1982; Blaser et al. 1983).

Although there is variability in aminoglycoside pharmacokinetic parameters, the therapeutic range for all of the aminoglycosides is relatively narrow, and the potential for toxicosis is greater than for most other classes of antimicrobials. Altered physiologic or pathologic states such as pregnancy (Lelievre-Pegorier et al. 1985), obesity (Sketris et al. 1981), subnormal body weight (Tointon et al. 1987), renal disease (Frazier and Riviere 1987), dehydration (LeCompte et al. 1981; Brown et al. 1985), immaturity (Sojka and Brown 1986), sepsis (Mann et al. 1987), dietary protein (Grauer et al. 1994; Behrend et al. 1994), endotoxemia (Wilson et al. 1984; Jernigan et al. 1988c), and intraindividual variability (Mann et al. 1987), among many others, may alter the distribution, clearance, and half-life of aminoglycosides by as much as 1000-fold between individuals in a single study (Zaske et al. 1982). In order to achieve target therapeutic concentrations, dosage adjustment seems to be required in 80–90% of both human and equine patient populations receiving aminoglycosides therapeutically (Bauer and Blouin 1981; Sojka and Brown 1986), with therapeutic drug monitoring highly recommended for any patient receiving multiple doses of parenteral aminoglycosides (Sveska et al. 1985; Sojka and Brown 1986; Frazier et al. 1988). The variability among horses expressed in terms of underlying physiological parameters was recently incorporated into a population pharmacokinetic model for gentamicin in horses (Martin et al. 1998) where pharmacokinetic parameters could be expressed with significantly less variability if the individual animal's creatinine and body weight were known. In a follow-up study using population pharmacokinetic methods, the performance of the model improved when certain covariates were entered into the model (Martin-Jimenez & Riviere 2001). The authors concluded that the pharmacokinetics of aminoglycosides can be predicted across species using population pharmacokinetic modeling, and the predictions are enhances by incorporating clinical features that affect animals. This approach holds much promise for increasing the ability to tailor aminoglycoside dosage regimens to specific clinical scenarios (Martin and Riviere 1998).

ABSORPTION. Aminoglycosides are not appreciably absorbed from the gastrointestinal tract because of their highly polar and cationic nature. However, if there is significant disruption of the intestinal mucosa from enteritis (i.e., parvovirus infections) (Gemer et al. 1983; Miranda et al. 1984; Gookin et al. 1999), some absorption may occur. The low absorption in the normal gastrointestinal tract is relevant to achieving therapeutically effective plasma concentrations of drug but may not be accurate if tissue residues are the relevant endpoint (for example, neomycin oral administration to calves). The aminoglycosides are not inactivated in the intestine and are eliminated in the feces unchanged after oral administration to normal animals. This lack of significant absorption through the gastrointestinal tract requires that all aminoglycosides be given by parenteral routes if therapeutic plasma concentrations are desired. Aminoglycoside absorption is practically complete after IM or subcutaneous (SC) injection. The peak serum concentrations after extravascular injection occur 14–120 minutes after the dose (Blaser et al. 1983; Ristuccia 1984). Absorption is extremely rapid and complete if aminoglycosides are instilled into body cavities that contain serosal surfaces; administration by this route closely mimics IV administration (Jawetz 1984; Sande and Mandell 1985). Absorption from topical administration in open wounds also is possible and may increase the risk of nephrotoxicosis if high doses are used (Mealey and Boothe 1994).

DISTRIBUTION. The distribution of aminoglycoside antibiotics after an IV bolus dose is virtually complete within 1 hour. Because of the polycationic nature of these antibiotics, the penetration of aminoglycosides across membranous barriers by simple diffusion is very limited; therefore, very low concentrations of aminoglycosides are found in cerebrospinal fluid or in respiratory secretions (Riviere and Coppoc 1981b; Strausbaugh and Brinker 1983). Aerosol or intratracheal administration of gentamicin produces negligible serum concentrations in both dogs and sheep, although substantial bronchial and pulmonary concentrations can be achieved (Riviere et al. 1981b; Wilson et al. 1981). Plasma protein binding is generally less than 20% in all species studied (Riond et al. 1986) and has a minimal effect on distribution from the vascular compartment. Binding to erythrocytes has been suggested to be approximately 10%, which is considered insignificant for aminoglycoside disposition (Lee et al. 1981). The molecular weight of aminoglycosides is small enough to allow unhindered passage through the capillary fenestrae and gap junctions of the vasculature (Huber 1982; Ristuccia 1984; Sande and Mandell 1985). Aminoglycoside distribution increases in lean and/or cachectic humans (Tointon et al. 1987) because of decreased plasma protein production leading to extravasation of fluid and resultant edema. A similar phenomenon probably occurs in animals, which may also require a concurrent dose adjustment.

Distribution is altered in young animals. In studies performed in calves, foals, and puppies, the high body water—particularly extracellular water—produces a high volume of distribution for aminoglycosides. Because the plasma concentration is proportional to the volume of distribution: the larger the volume of distribution, the higher the dose that is needed to attain a targeted peak plasma concentration (C_{MAX}). These properties are discussed in more detail in the gentamicin section titled "Effect of Age on Disposition of Gentamicin," and in the amikacin section under the heading of "Horses."

METABOLISM AND EXCRETION. Whole animal and human renal clearance (Black et al. 1963; Chiu et al. 1976; Chung et al. 1980; Gyselynck et al. 1971; Schentag and Jusko 1977; Silverman and Mahon 1979), isolated perfused rat kidney (Collier et al. 1979; Mitchell et al. 1977), and micropuncture studies (Pastoriza-Munoz et al. 1979; Senckjian et al. 1981; Sheth et al. 1981) have clearly demonstrated that aminoglycosides are eliminated nonmetabolized from the body in all animal species studied so far, primarily by renal glomerular filtration. The sole route of excretion for all aminoglycosides is the kidney. Some degree of proximal tubular reabsorption does occur and results in an intracellular sequestration or storage in the tubule cells without a significant transepithelial flux from the intraluminal to peritubular space. Net aminoglycoside secretion along more distal nephron segments may also occur. Proximal tubule luminal absorption of aminoglycoside appears quantitatively to be the primary mechanism of intracellular uptake; however, selective peritubular or basolateral reabsorption, evident in isolated tissue slice studies, does occur and may be of toxicologic significance in specific situations. Reabsorption requires metabolic energy and occurs along the midconvoluted and straight portions of the proximal tubule (Barza et al. 1980; Bennett et al. 1982; Hsu et al. 1977; Kaloyanides and Pastoriza-

Munoz 1980; Kluwe and Hook 1978a,b; Kuhar et al. 1979; Pastoriza-Munoz et al. 1979; Senckjian et al. 1981; Silverblatt 1982; Silverblatt and Kuehn 1979; Silverman and Mahon 1979; Tulkens and Trouet 1978; Vandewalle et al. 1981; Williams et al. 1981a,b; Zaske 1980). Several laboratories have demonstrated that renal cortical uptake of the aminoglycosides is dose-dependent up to a threshold concentration; then, cortical accumulation increases at a progressively slower rate as the dose is increased. Cumulative uptake of aminoglycosides in tissues indicates that the kidney is the major site of drug sequestration, although other organs with larger volumes (e.g., liver) may also contain substantial total drug (Brown et al. 1985).

Aminoglycoside disposition generally follows a three-compartment pharmacokinetic model with a three-phase plasma concentration–time profile curve (α, β, γ) as shown in Figure 36.2 Using those parameters, the half-life of α (alpha) represents the distribution half-life, the half-life of β (beta) reflects the classic elimination phase governed largely by renal elimination, and the half-life of γ (gamma) reflects the slow release of drug sequestered in tissues (i.e., renal cortex and liver). Typically, the α phase occurs within the first hour after IV dosing, the β phase occurs between 1 and 24 hours after IV dosing (and probably the most useful in determining dose adjustments in clinical situations), and the γ phase occurs 24 hours after dosing and is the most important part of the elimination curve of aminoglycosides when considering drug residues in food-producing animals. The primary determinant of aminoglycoside disposition is reflected in the phase that correlates to renal glomerular filtration. The primary difference in pharmacokinetics among species is related to the glomerular filtration rate (GFR), which decreases on a weight basis in larger animals. Larger animals tend to have prolonged half-lives and require smaller doses on a mg/kg basis. In contrast, doses are similar across all species if based on a body surface area or a measure of basal metabolic rate (0.75 mg/kg) (Riviere 1985; Riviere et al. 1997).

The prolonged terminal elimination phase of aminoglycosides has major implication for veterinary therapeutics in food-producing animals. As discussed above, aminoglycosides accumulate in the renal cortex for prolonged periods of time, resulting in violative tissue residues even after short periods of administration. In some cases, aminoglycosides such as gentamicin may be detected for a year after parenteral administration! The veterinary profession had originally recommended a withdrawal time of 18 months for cattle treated with gentamicin but now suggests that the drug not be used in adult food-producing animals. Piglets may be treated up to 3 days of age, but even in this case the withdrawal time is 40 days.

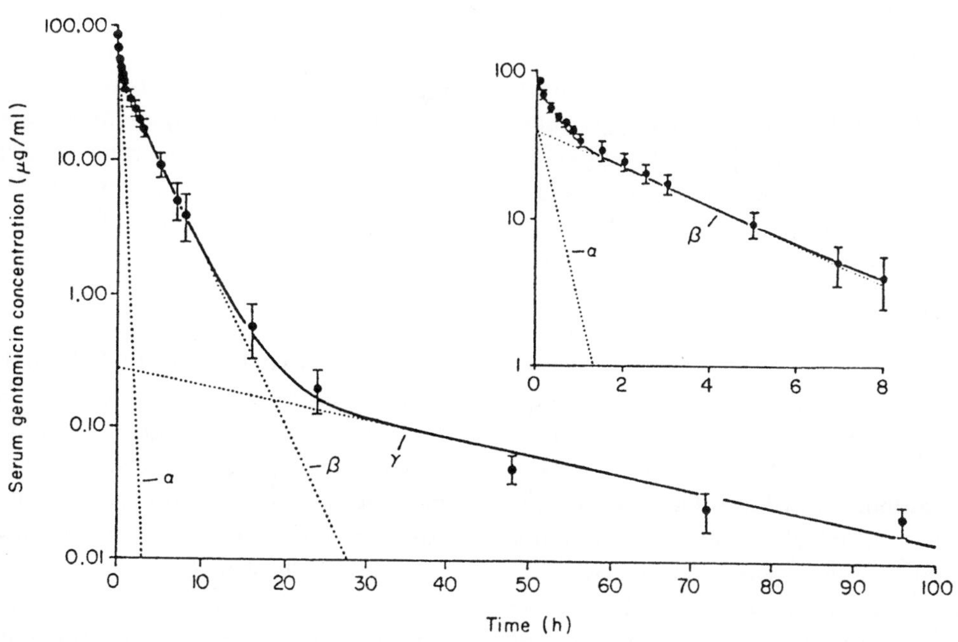

FIG. 36.2 Graphic representation of the three elimination curves associated with aminoglycoside excretion. (From Brown et al. 1991, reproduced by permission.)

.3 Selected risk factors that predispose to aminoglycoside toxicosis

Age	Peak and trough serum concentrations
Volume contraction (shock)	
Acidosis	Hepatic disease
Sodium or potassium depletion	Total dose of drug administered
Sepsis	Duration of treatment
Renal transplantation	Concurrent administration of loop diuretics
Prior renal insufficiency	
Prior aminoglycoside exposure	Methoxyflurane anesthesia
Cumulative dose of aminoglycoside	Cephalosporin antibiotics
	Nephrotoxic drugs

AMINOGLYCOSIDE TOXICITY

Aminoglycoside toxicity in domestic and laboratory animals has been reviewed by Riviere (1985). The possible risk factors that may predispose a patient to aminoglycoside toxicity are shown in Table 36.3.

Aminoglycosides can induce ototoxicity and nephrotoxicity because both organs have higher-than-normal concentrations of phospholipid (in particular, phosphatidylinositol) (Sastrasinh et al. 1982a,b) in their cellular matrixes. Cationic aminoglycosides are chemically attracted to anionic membrane phospholipids, the so-called *aminoglycoside receptors.* The two tissues into which gentamicin preferentially accumulates (renal cortex and cochlear tissue) have disproportionately high amounts of phosphatidylinositol in their membranes compared with other tissues of the body (Hauser and Eichberg 1973). Basolateral membranes of the renal proximal tubular epithelium also have a higher capacity for binding aminoglycosides than brush-border membranes because of their higher phosphatidylinositol content (Josepovitz et al. 1985). This nearly twofold lower uptake in brush-border membranes is even lower in female rats than in male rats (Williams and Hottendorf 1985, 1986). Ototoxicity studies in a variety of species have shown a progressive accumulation of the aminoglycoside in the perilymph and endolymph of the inner ear that may affect both auditory and vestibular function due to destruction of the sensory hair cells in the cochlea and vestibular labyrinth. The likelihood of inducing ototoxicity is mainly dependent on the duration of treatment, cumulative dose, average daily dose, peak and trough serum concentration, concurrent diuretic use, underlying disease status, and previous exposure to aminoglycoside therapy. Ototoxicity may be irreversible in some cases (Johnson and Hardin 1992). Of pertinence to veterinary medicine, dogs tend to present with auditory toxicity, and cats tend to present with vestibular toxicity, although both usually occur after nephrotoxicity has ensued.

More complete information is available on the toxicosis of the aminoglycosides in the kidney (Ali et al. 1992; Beauchamp et al. 1992; Riviere 1985). The interaction between the cationic aminoglycosides and the kidney anionic phospholipids appears to be electrostatic and proportional to the cationic charge of the drug. This interaction is saturable and is competitively inhibited by divalent cations (magnesium and calcium), spermine, poly-l-lysine, and other aminoglycosides. For example, diets high in calcium may decrease the risk of aminoglycoside nephrotoxicity (Schumacher et al. 1991). Intravenous administration of calcium also decreases the risk of aminoglycoside-induced nephrotoxicosis (Brashier et al. 1998). After binding, the aminoglycoside is internalized into the cell by pinocytosis (Bennett et al. 1982; Elliott et al. 1982; Feldman et al. 1981; Humes et al. 1982; Lipsky et al. 1980; Lipsky and Lietman 1982; Pastoriza-Munoz et al. 1979; Schacht 1978), where concentrations of the aminoglycoside can reach as high as 50 times the concentrations achieved in serum or plasma. Cytosegresomes are formed and are the primary locus of intracellular aminoglycoside storage. This intralysosomal binding within the proximal tubules results in drug sequestration and is primarily responsible for the prolonged half-life and extended withdrawal times of aminoglycosides, which are pertinent to food-animal tissue residues. The uptake of aminoglycosides into lysosomes is competitive and is dependent in part upon the charge density of the aminoglycoside molecule, which is a function of the number of amino groups. For example, neomycin (valence + 4.37 at pH 7.40) accumulates in the renal cortex more than gentamicin (valence + 3.46 at pH 7.40) due to a higher cationic charge.

Because the renal proximal tubules and inner-ear tissues actively take up aminoglycosides, concentrations in the renal cortex and cochlear tissues are far greater than those observed concurrently in the serum and other tissues. In emergency-slaughtered ruminants, renal cortical concentrations of dihydrostreptomycin or neomycin ranged from 4.1 to 237 μg/g of renal cortex (Nouws and Ziv 1978). Studies have also demonstrated a substantially higher renal cortical concentration of other aminoglycosides compared with other tissues in humans (Schentag et al. 1977b; Schentag and Jusko 1977), rats (Luft and Kleit 1974;

Fabre et al. 1976; Luft et al. 1978), dogs (Cowan et al. 1980), cats (Jernigan et al. 1988c), sheep (Brown et al. 1985, 1986b; Brown and Garry 1988), lambs (Weisman et al. 982), cattle (Haddad et al. 1987), pigs (Riond and Riviere 1988), and birds (Bush et al. 1981). Endotoxemia increases the renal concentrations of aminoglycosides above normal (Bergeron and Bergeron 1986). Substantial concentrations are also found in the renal medulla, liver, spleen, and lungs in sheep (Brown et al. 1985, 1986b), cattle (Haddad et al. 1987), birds (Bush et al. 1981), and rats (Cowan et al. 1980).

Diabetic animals do not accumulate aminoglycosides in their renal cortex to the same extent as normal animals (Teixeira et al. 1982; Vaamonde et al. 1984; Pastoriza-Munoz et al. 1987; Ramsammy et al. 1987). Streptozotocin-induced diabetes mellitus in laboratory rats substantially decreases the renal uptake of aminoglycosides by depressing the uptake and accumulation process of renal proximal tubular cells (Vaamonde et al. 1984; Ramsammy et al. 1987). As an apparent result, single-dose gentamicin disposition in diabetic dogs does not show a γ phase at all, whereas normal dogs do exhibit that terminal elimination phase, with a terminal half-life of the γ phase of several days (Brown et al. 1991). This abolition of the γ phase, noted in alloxan-induced diabetic dogs and in dogs with naturally occurring diabetes mellitus, was observed in spite of exogenous insulin therapy to control hyperglycemia. Other endocrine disorders such as familial hypothyroidism also affect the terminal elimination phase (and perhaps renal accumulation) of certain aminoglycosides in certain species (Riond et al. 1986; Riviere and Carver 1984).

Controvery exists over the precise mechanism by which aminoglycosides initially damage the proximal renal tubule cells (Swann et al. 1990; Schumacher et al. 1991; Beauchamp et al. 1992). Abundant evidence suggests that lysosomal dysfunction is a component of the early phase of renal injury (Carbon et al. 1978; Feldman et al. 1982; Hull et al. 1981; Kaloyanides and Pastoriza-Munoz 1980; Laurent et al. 1982; Lipsky and Lietman 1982; Mazze 1981; Meisner 1981; Morin et al. 1980, 1981; Tulkens and Trouet 1978). This view is consistent with the idea that lysosomes are the primary locus of aminoglycoside sequestration in proximal tubule cells. Lysosomes are also the first organelle to demonstrate morphologic changes (myeloid body or cytosegresome formation) after exposure to the drugs (Riviere et al. 1981a). Studies have demonstrated that lysosomal enzyme activities (i.e., sphingomyelinase, cathepsin B, α-d-galactosidase) are decreased and that the structural latency of lysosomes, reflected by leakage of *N*-acetyl-β-d-glucosaminadase in the cytosol is increased. Inhibition of lysosomal enzymes may cause an intralysosomal accumulation of membrane-associated lipids, which would be reflected morphologically as myeloid body formation. However, this process by itself should not be acutely lethal to the cell. Decreased lysosomal function may also result in a decreased ability to degrade endogenous intracellular proteins and exogenous low-molecular weight proteins reabsorbed from the tubular filtrate, events that would perturb nephron function (Cojocel et al. 1983; Cojocel and Hook, 1983). The increase in lysosomal permeability could result in proximal tubule cell dysfunction, although this event is probably a late change in aminoglycoside-induced toxic nephropathy occurring after cell necrosis has been initiated by another factor (Humes et al. 1982). Myeloid body formation is most likely a marker of aminoglycoside exposure rather than toxicosis. The appearance of lysosomal enzymes (for example, urinary GGT) in the urine of aminoglycoside-induced toxic nephropathy patients is secondary to proximal tubule cell necrosis, apical plasma membrane damage, or lysosome exocytosis.

Mitochondria are a second possible target of aminoglycosides because, both in vitro and in vivo, aminoglycosides decrease mitochondrial respiration, thereby impairing the tubule cell's bioenergetic profile (Appel and Neu 1977; Cuppage et al. 1977; Kaloyanides and Pastoriza-Munoz 1980; Kluwe and Hook 1978a; Sastrasinh et al. 1982b; Simmons et al. 1980; Weinberg et al. 1980, 1990; Weinberg and Humes 1980). This could selectively produce tubule dysfunction, which would initially be detectable biochemically but not morphologically. The mechanism of this toxicity may be secondary to a direct aminoglycoside interaction with mitochondrial membrane phospholipids, to a competitive interaction with the divalent cations magnesium or calcium, or to an alteration in the intracellular milieu that would indirectly affect mitochondrial function. The magnitude of aminoglycoside effects on mitochondrial respiration is roughly correlated to the net positive charge of the specific drug.

The third possible site of initial intracellular aminoglycoside interaction is the proximal tubule cell plasma membrane's phospholipids and enzymes (Feldman et al. 1981; Humes et al. 1982; Knauss et al. 1983; Lullmann and Vollmer 1982; Sastrasinh et al. 1982a,b; Schacht 1979; Silverman and Mahon 1979; Williams et al. 1981a,b). Binding of aminoglycosides to membrane polyphosphoinositides could perturb the regulation of membrane permeability, thereby promoting cellular dysfunction. Aminoglycosides induce a phospholipidosis that may be secondary to inhibition of cytoplasmic phospholipase activity. This event affecting multiple membrane systems may affect other cellular metabolic processes. Aminoglycosides also inhibit basolateral membrane Na^+,K^+-ATPase activity in vitro and in vivo when used at high doses or incubating concentrations (Appel 1982; Chahwala and Harpur 1982; Cronin et al. 1982). Aminoglycosides have also been found to inhibit adenylate cyclase activity in proximal tubule basolateral membranes and in toad bladder epithelium in vitro (Humes and Weinberg 1980; Ross et al. 1980; Souliere et al. 1978). The enzyme interactions at the basolateral membrane could result in significant cellular dysfunction by altering intracellular electrolyte balance or osmolality.

A final possible site of aminoglycoside interaction with the nephron is at the level of the glomerulus, where gentamicin has been demonstrated to reduce the glomerular ultrafiltration coefficient and to reduce the number and size of glomerular endothelial fenestrae (Avasthi et al. 1981; Huang et al. 1979; Luft and Evan 1980a,b; Luft et al. 1978). These effects may be mediated by a charge interaction between the cationic aminoglycosides and the anionic endothelial cell surfaces or could be a feedback response to a primary tubular injury. The mediator of this mechanism is not known.

The relative contributions of the lysosomal, mitochondrial, and membrane tubular mechanisms and glomerular injury to clinical aminoglycoside-induced toxic nephropathy is not known. The relative importance of each as a primary insult is largely a function of the pattern of intracellular distribution of toxicologically active aminoglycosides. In all probability, cellular dysfunction is a result of a combination of the above processes. Whatever the mechanism, dysfunction of the proximal tubule cell ultimately results in a decrease in nephron function, the sum of which determines whole kidney function.

Aminoglycoside-induced nephropathy has been studied in many species of animals. In general, the syndrome is similar across species lines, with any peculiarities being a result of pharmacokinetic factors or inherent differences in underlying renal morphology or physiology.

DOGS. Aminoglycosides are used in the dog to treat a variety of susceptible bacteria populations. Toxicosis may occur at the recommended therapeutic doses if given to dogs for protracted lengths of time. Canine clinical doses are provided in Tables 36.1 and 36.2.

In a controlled study, 8 mg/kg/day, divided every 12 hours, produced a statistically significant decrease in urine osmolarity by day 7, an increase in fractional sodium excretion by day 8, an increase in serum urea nitrogen concentration by day 17, and an increase in serum creatinine concentration by day 18 (McNeil et al. 1983). This study documents a bimodal course of aminoglycoside-induced toxic nephropathy in the dog administered low-dose gentamicin therapy: an initial subclinical (subazotemic) phase marked by a urinary concentrating defect followed by a clinical (azotemic) phase. It also serves as the basis for simple noninvasive clinical monitoring (for example, monitoring urine specific gravity and proteinuria) for toxicosis since urinary changes preceded the more irreversible systemic changes.

Urine GGT (γ-glutamyl transferase):creatinine and NAG (*N*-acetyl-β-d-glucosaminidase):creatinine ratios and 24-hour urinary excretions of NAG and GGT were calculated on days 2, 4, 6, and 8 of gentamicin administration. Urinary excretion of GGT increased through day 6 of administration. Urinary excretion of NAG increased through day 8 of treatment, while creatinine clearance tended to decrease during the study period. Similarly, Rivers et al. (1996) found that in dogs dosed with gentamicin at 3 mg/kg and 30 mg/kg for 10 days, urine GGT: creatinine ratios in the 30 mg/kg dose group were approximately 3 times that of baseline values. The elevated GGT: creatinine ratio indicator preceded clinically significant elevations in serum creatinine, urine specific gravity, and urine protein:creatinine ratios. The authors concluded that urine GGT:creatinine ratios were a much earlier indicator of aminoglycoside-induced renal toxicity and may have potential applications in detecting early gentamicin-induced nephrotoxicity in dogs.

High-dose studies of 30 mg/kg/day, divided every 8 hours, administered for 10–12 days, produced clinically significant increases in serum creatinine and serum urea nitrogen 9–12 days after the start of drug administration (Adelman et al. 1979; Cronin et al. 1980). Almost complete recovery occurred in dogs after discontinuation of gentamicin for 28 days, with only focal, tubulointerstitial nephritis being present on histopathologic examination (Cronin et al. 1980). In other studies conducted in dogs either high doses, prolonged administration, or both were used, (Black et al. 1963; Powell et al. 1983).

These studies suggest that prolonged low-dose or very high-dose therapy may produce deleterious results. In a clinical study (Brown et al. 1985), the risk factors were identified that contributed to nephrotoxicosis in ten dogs. Risk factors included dehydration, fever, old age, and preexisting renal disease. In addition, low protein and electrolyte abnormalities were documented in these dogs.

Ototoxicity in dogs, manifested as either vestibulotoxic and/or ototoxic effects, can occur after systemic aminoglycoside therapy, but toxicity after topical use of aminoglycosides is apparently rare (Strain et al., 1995). Although it is sometimes recommended among dermatologists to avoid topical gentamicin in animals with a ruptured tympanum (ear drum) this apparently is not a risk. In a study designed to detect ototoxicity in dogs treated with topically administered gentamicin using brain stem auditory evoked potential (BAEP), dogs underwent a unilateral myringotomy, followed by instillation of 7 drops of the 3 mg/ml buffered aqueous solution of gentamicin instilled into one ear twice a day for 3 weeks. There was no evidence in any treated dogs of drug-induced detectable changes in cochlear or vestibular function.

CATS. Doses for cats are presented in Tables 36.1 and 36.2. Cats appear to have a relatively more concentrated urine and retain the ability to produce concentrated urine even when the GFR is significantly reduced (Ross and Finco 1981), making urine monitoring less successful than in dogs.

Consistent with the studies cited in dogs, studies in cats have shown that high doses, prolonged administration, or both, can produce renal injury, with histologic changes and increases in serum urea nitrogen and creatinine (Welles et al. 1973; Waitz et al. 1971).

Nephrotoxicosis associated with the topical use of gentamicin has been reported in cats (Mealey and Boothe 1994). A cat was administered 10 ml of an undiluted gentamicin injectable solution (50 mg/ml) to lavage an open wound twice. The cat eventually progressed to an azotemic state and was euthanized. Histologically, the kidneys showed severe acute proximal tubular necrosis compatible with aminoglycoside toxicosis. Elevated serum levels of gentamicin were noted as late as 96 hours after administration. Although a number of factors may have contributed to the death of this cat, the topical administration of such large quantities of gentamicin was most likely the major determinant.

HORSES. Aminoglycoside toxic nephropathy as well as ototoxicity (Nostrandt et al. 1991) has been studied in horses. Clinically, aminoglycoside-induced toxic nephropathy is more common in young animals, with toxicity rarely reported in adults (Riviere et al. 1982; Tobin 1979). The effect of neomycin on the kidneys of adult horses has been studied (Fuentes et al. 1997). Horses (4–7 years old) dosed with 10 mg/kg IM twice daily for 15 days failed to demonstrate liver or renal histopathology by the end of the dosing period. There was no significant change in serum and urinary values of creatinine. There was, however, a significant increase in urinary GGT beginning on or about the third day of treatment, peaking between 12 and 15 days, and decreasing through the end of the study, indicative of damage to the brush border of the proximal tubular cells of the nephron. The use of GGT as a biomarker for nephrotoxicity in horses has been debated. Rossier et al. (1995) studied three groups of horses: normal horses, normal horses treated with 2.2 mg/kg gentamicin IV four times daily for 10 days, and sick horses (pleuropneumonia) treated with 2.2 mg/kg gentamicin IV four times daily for 10 days. All groups had urinary GGT, urinary creatinine, and plasma creatinine measured at days 1, 3, and 10 of treatment. Sick horses had significantly higher mean urinary GGT:urinary creatinine ratios than either of the other groups. There was no significant difference between the urinary GGT:urinary creatinine ratios in normal (untreated) horses and normal horses treated with gentamicin. The study further concluded that, at least with horses, the urinary GGT:urinary creatinine ratio could, but does not necessarily, correspond to clinically significant changes in renal function due to aminoglycoside toxicity, mainly due to assay methodology and variability in normal baseline values.

Daily doses of 8.8 mg/kg/day for 5–14 days induced toxic nephropathy marked by elevations in serum creatinine and serum urea nitrogen (Tobin 1979; Riviere 1982). In an experimental study of aminoglycoside-induced toxic nephropathy in young horses, 1 of 3 horses given 8.8 mg/kg/day and 1 of 3 given 17.6 mg/kg/day for 14 days developed elevated serum urea nitrogen and creatinine concentrations and decreased urine osmolarity (Riviere et al. 1983). Three foals given 4.4 mg/kg/day for 14 days did not develop functional evidence of aminoglycoside-induced toxic nephropathy, but there was dose-related histopathologic evidence of proximal tubular nephrosis, including tubular necrosis and regeneration. Ultrastructurally, cytosegresomes were present in gentamicin-treated animals. The severity of the aminoglycoside-induced toxic nephropathy seen at the low dose above is expected since the human-equivalent equine dose predicted using allometry (0.75 mg/kg) would be only 2–3 mg/kg/day. Once per day dosing (6.6 mg/kg/day IV for 10 days) did not produce signs of nephrotoxicosis (elevated blood urea nitrogen, serum creatinine, urine GGT, etc.) in adult animals (Godber et al. 1995), suggesting again that a once daily regimen may be preferred both for efficacy and for reduced toxicity.

RUMINANTS. Calves given 5 or 9 mg/kg/day neomycin IM for 12–13 days developed aminoglycoside-induced toxic nephropathy marked by increased serum creatinine and urea nitrogen concentrations, decreased creatinine clearance, decreased urine specific gravity, cylindruria, proteinuria, and enzymuria (γ-glutamyltranspeptidase and alanine aminopeptidase) (Crowell et al. 1981). On histopathologic examination, tubular hyaline droplet change, degeneration, and necrosis were present. This apparent sensitivity is again primarily caused by the large body size of cows, for which 5–9 mg/kg/day is an overdosage on a 0.75 mg/kg basis. Gentamicin-induced toxic nephropathy was not detected in adult sheep given 9 mg/kg/day for 7 days when serum creatinine and urea nitrogen concentrations were monitored and tissues were examined at necropsy by light microscopy (Brown et al. 1985). Sheep have recently been advocated as a stable animal model for human renal diseases (Eschbach et al. 1980). They may be a useful animal model of gentamicin toxic nephropathy because body weight is essentially identical to that seen in humans and the pharmacokinetic parameters describing gentamicin disposition are also similar. The use of urinary enzyme indices as a function of aminoglycoside nephrotoxicosis has been reported (Garry et al. 1990a,b).

EXAMPLES OF DRUGS

GENTAMICIN. Gentamicin is available in solutions of 5, 50, and 100 mg/ml (Garasol, Gentocin, and generic), as well as oral solution for pigs (4.35 or 5 mg/ml) and powder for oral solution (66.7 or 333.3 mg per gram of powder) Gentamicin has been the most widely studied aminoglycoside antibiotic to date. Gentamicin is a combination of four components produced by *Micromonospora purpurea,* which all cross-react in common immunoassay procedures and are usually considered a single antimicrobial entity.

The plasma elimination phase (β phase) is correlated well with GFR in dogs and horses (Sojka and Brown 1986; Frazier et al. 1988). Selected pharmacokinetic data for gentamicin in animals are shown in Tables 36.4 and 36.5.

The parenteral absorption patterns of gentamicin have been studied in several species of animals. Bioavailability (F) of gentamicin from IM sites is reported to be 68 ± 13% in cats (Jernigan et al. 1988e), 92 ± 15% in cows (Haddad et al. 1986), 87 ± 14% in horses (Haddad et al. 1985b), 95 ± 20% in dogs (Wilson et al. 1989), 95 ± 18% in roosters (Pedersoli et al. 1990), 21% in turkeys (Pedersoli et al. 1989), ≥95% in hawks and owls (Bird et al. 1983), ≥70% in eagles (Bird et al. 1983), and 60% in catfish (Setzer 1985). Bioavailability from different IM sites is considered identical (Wilson et al. 1989) and bioavailability from SC sites is similar to IM bioavailability (Gilman et al. 1987; Jernigan et al. 1988e; Wilson et al. 1989). The maximum concentration after SC administration is usually lower and occurs later after injection than that observed after an equivalent IM dose (Jernigan et al. 1988a; Wilson et al. 1989), which is most likely due to less blood flow to the SC injection sites than to the IM injection sites, resulting in a slower rate of absorption but not altering the extent of absorption. Systemic availability from intrauterine (IU) administration is 30% in normal cows, with maximum plasma concentrations of 3.70 μg/mL and 17.5 μg/mL being observed 30 minutes after IU doses of 2 and 4 mg/kg, respectively (al-Guedawy et al. 1983). Oral availability is near 0% in normal animals with intact intestinal mucosa, although necrotizing enteritis and/or diarrhea have been reported to increase availability in humans (Gemer et al. 1983; Miranda et al. 1984). Concentrations in renal tissue are observed after oral doses of 1 mg/kg/day for 7 days, for 10 days (>0.1 μg/g of renal tissue), and for 30 days (>0.02 μg/g of renal tissue) after the last dose in calves (Takahashi et al. 1985). Serum concentrations after IU dosing were minimal in normal horses; however, in horses treated with progesterone, systemic availability was 8–10 times higher, with greater penetration into endometrial tissue (Pedersoli et al. 1985). Estradiol also increased the systemic availability and endometrial penetration after IU infusion, but not to the same extent as that observed after progesterone.

TABLE 36.4 Single-dose intravenous serum or plasma pharmacokinetics of gentamicin in various species

Species	Dose (mg/kg)	$V_{d(area)}$ (L/kg)	$V_{d(ss)}$ (L/kg)	Cl_B (mL/min/kg)	$t_{1/2(\beta)}$ (hr)	$t_{1/2(\gamma)}$ (hr)	Reference
Dogs (juvenile)	10	0.354	ND	4.08	1.01	N/A	Riviere and Coppoc 1981a
		(0.036)		(0.62)	(0.12)		
Dogs	10	0.38	ND	4.20	1.05	N/A	Riviere et al. 1981a; Riviere et al. 1981b
		(0.029)		(0.70)	(0.13)		
Dogs	10	0.30	ND	3.44	1.01	N/A	Rivierie et al. 1981a; Riviere et al. 1981b
		(0.06)		(0.38)	(0.08)		
Dogs	10	0.335	ND	2.94	1.36	N/A	Baggot 1977
		(0.094)		(0.67)	(0.09)		
Dogs	4.4	0.227	0.175	2.27	1.09[a]	N/A	Brown et al. 1991
		(0.076)	(0.033)	(0.41)			
Dogs	4	0.255	ND	3.33	1.06	N/A	Batra et al. 1983
Dogs	3	NR	0.172	2.29	0.91	N/A	Wilson et al. 1989
			(0.025)	(0.48)	(0.25)		
Cats	4.4	0.190	0.180	1.61	1.36	N/A	Short et al. 1986
Cats	5	ND	0.14	1.38	1.25	86[a]	Jernigan et al. 1988e
			(0.20)	(0.35)	(0.30)		
Cows	5	0.19	0.16	1.32	1.83	N/A	Haddad et al. 1986
		(0.04)	(0.032)	(0.17)	(0.18)		
Cattle (1 day old)	4.4	0.393	0.376	1.92	2.49	N/A	Clarke et al. 1985
		(0.040)	(0.041)	(0.43)	(0.73)		
Cattle (5 days old)	4.4	0.413	0.385	2.44	1.99	N/A	Clarke et al. 1985
		(0.050)	(0.044)	(0.34)	(0.33)		
Cattle (10 days old)	4.4	0.341	0.323	2.02	1.97	N/A	Clarke et al. 1985
		(0.021)	(0.020)	(0.27)	(0.21)		
Cattle (15 days old)	4.4	0.334	0.311	2.10	1.85	N/A	Clarke et al. 1985
		(0.039)	(0.029)	(0.32)	(0.13)		
Cattle (4–5 weeks old)	3	1.95	0.75	4.9	3.96	N/A	Ziv et al. 1982
		(1.24)	(0.20)	(1.9)	(1.67)		
Cattle (adult)	4.4	0.140	0.140	1.29	1.26	N/A	Clarke et al. 1985
		(0.020)	(0.020)	(0.26)	(0.19)		
Horse (mare)	6.6	0.21	0.16	1.1	2.2	ND	Santschi et al. 2000.
Horse (clinical)	4.4	0.17	ND	1.2	1.61	ND	Tudor et al. 1999
Horse (clinical)	6.6	0.17	ND	1.3	1.47	ND	Tudor et al. 1999
Horse	2.2	0.46	ND	ND	0.83	ND	Godber et al. 1995
Horse	6.6	0.115	ND	ND	0.78	ND	Godber et al. 1995
Horse (foal)	4.0	0.32–0.38	0.28–0.35	1.7–3.7	1–2.1	ND	Cummings et al. 1990
Horse (adult)	4.0	0.17	0.15	1.7	1.1	ND	Cummings et al. 1990
Horse	2.2	0.18	0.15	1.1	1.82–1.96	ND	Jones et al. 1998
Horse	2.2	0.48	0.24	1.2	4.4	ND	Whittem et al. 1996
Horse	6.6	0.19	0.14	0.95	2.3	ND	Magdesian et al. 1998
Horses	5	0.254	0.24	2.54	2.54	N/A	Pedersoli et al. 1980
		(0.031)	(0.03)	(0.33)	(0.33)		
Horses (2–3 months old)	4.5	ND	0.306	1.65	3.23	N/A	Riviere et al. 1983
			(0.094)	(0.79)	(0.62)		
Horses	2.2	ND	0.15	0.87	3.85	N/A	Bowman et al. 1986
			(0.001)	(0.05)	(0.40)		
Horses	2.2	ND	1.74	0.68	3.51	142	Bowman et al. 1986
			(0.59)	(0.17)	(0.59)	(31)	
Horses	3	0.202	0.173	1.41	1.66	N/A	Wilson et al. 1983
		(0.028)	(0.012)	(0.19)	(0.06)		
Ponies	5	0.20	0.19	1.27	1.82	N/A	Haddad et al. 1985b
		(0.01)	(0.01)	(0.18)	(0.22)		
Mammoth asses[d]	2.2	0.12	ND	1.22	2.07	ND	Miller et al. 1994
		(0.025)		(0.18)			

TABLE 36.4—*continued*

Species	Dose (mg/kg)	$V_{d(area)}$ (L/kg)	$V_{d(ss)}$ (L/kg)	Cl_B (mL/min/kg)	$t_{1/2(\beta)}$ (hr)	$t_{1/2(\gamma)}$ (hr)	Reference
Mammoth asses[e]	2.2	0.088 (0.028)	ND	1.29 (0.07)	0.84	5.12	Miller et al. 1994
Sheep	2.2	0.194 (0.059)	ND	1.56 (0.40)	1.44 (0.085)	N/A	Wilson et al. 1981
Sheep	3	ND	0.408 (0.196)	0.660 (0.256)	1.33[a]	41.9 (18.5)	Brown et al. 1986b
Sheep	10	ND	0.243 (0.026)	1.03 (0.015)	2.4 (0.5)	30.4 (18.9)	Brown et al. 1985
Sheep	10	ND	0.384 (0.195)	0.805 (0.317)	1.72[a]	88.9 (19.8)	Brown et al. 1986b
Sheep	20	ND	0.709 (0.751)	0.882 (0.342)	1.77[a]	167.2 (42.7)	Brown et al. 1986b
Sheep (Desert)	3	0.27	ND	0.07	4.20	ND	Elsheikh et al. 1997
Goat	3	0.22	ND	0.08	1.041	ND	Elsheikh et al. 1997
Pigs	2	0.32 (0.032)	0.24 (0.03)	1.66 (0.12)	1.9 (1.47–4.89)	20.2 (13.9–34.6)	Riond and Riviere 1988
Pigs (newborn)	5	ND	0.80	ND	5.19	ND	Giroux et al. 1995
Pigs (42 days)	5	ND	0.50	ND	3.50	ND	Giroux et al. 1995
Rabbits	20	ND	0.52–0.95[b]	2.90–4.0	0.98–1.15	11.4–15.1	Huang et al. 1979
Rabbits	3.5	ND	0.114 (0.020)	2.82 (0.97)	0.74	ND	Ogden et al. 1995
Hawks[c]	10	0.24 (0.03)	N/A	2.09 (0.16)	1.35 (0.18)	N/A	Bird et al. 1983
Owls[c]	10	0.23 (0.02)	N/A	1.41 (0.10)	1.93 (0.24)	N/A	Bird et al. 1983
Eagles[c]	10	0.21 (0.01)	N/A	1.01 (0.06)	2.46 (0.32)	N/A	Bird et al. 1983
Catfish	1	0.156	NR	0.126	12.2	N/A	Setzer 1985
Catfish	10	0.176	ND	0.215	11.87	N/A	Rolf et al. 1986
Guinea pigs	40	ND	ND	3.4	1.01	1.01	Chung et al. 1982
Buffalo calves	5	0.43	ND	54.61	5.69	ND	Garg et al. 1991a,b
Turkeys	5	0.190	0.172	49.8	2.570	ND	Pedersoli et al. 1989
Roosters	5	0.228 (0.019)	0.209 (0.013)	0.775 (0.132)	3.38 (0.62)	N/A	Pedersoli et al. 1990
Turtles	3	ND	ND	ND	40–44	ND	Beck et al. 1995

Source: Adapted from Brown and Riviere 1991.

Note: Values reported as arithmetic mean followed by SD or SEM in parentheses. N/A = not applicable (inappropriate term for the model used); ND = not determined; NR = not reported.

[a]Harmonic mean; data are IV and IM data pooled together.

[b]Range.

[c]One-compartment model used.

[d]Best described using a two-compartment open model.

[e]Best described using a three-compartment open model.

Effect of Age on Disposition of Gentamicin. Age appreciably affects gentamicin disposition. Because neonatal animals have a larger proportion of their body weight as extracellular fluid, gentamicin volume of distribution (Vd) is larger in immature animals than in adults. For example, Vd(area) of gentamicin in juvenile dogs is 0.35 l/kg (Riviere and Coppoc 1981a), whereas Vd(area) in normal dogs is 0.227 l/kg (Brown et al. 1991). Foals less than 3 months of age exhibited a Vd of 0.344 l/kg, whereas adult horses in the same study had Vd of 0.184 l/kg (Sojka and Brown 1986). Another study, in young horses 2–3 months old, demonstrated Vd(ss) of 0.306 l/kg

TABLE 36.5 Terminal (γ) elimination half-lives of gentamicin from different species (mean ± SD unless otherwise specified)

Species	Dose (mg/kg)	Route	Interval (hr)	No. of doses	$t_{1/2\gamma}$ (hr)	Reference
Cattle	3.5	IM	8	30	44.9 ± 9.4	Haddad et al. 1987
Sheep	10	IV	NA	1	30.4 ± 18.9	Brown et al. 1985
Sheep	3	IM	8	21	82.1 ± 17.8	Brown et al. 1985
Sheep	3	IV	8	21	129.5[a]	Brown et al. 1986a
Sheep	3	IV	NA	1	42.6[a]	Brown et al. 1986a
Sheep	10	IV	NA	1	107.6[a]	Brown et al. 1986a
Sheep	20	IV	NA	1	164.2[a]	Brown et al. 1986a
Dogs	4.4	IV	NA	1	154.3[a]	Brown et al. 1991
Dogs (diabetic)	4.4	IV	NA	1	NF	Brown et al. 1991
Pigs	6	IV	NA	1	10.6 ± 1.8	Riond et al. 1986
Pigs	2	IV	8	21	13.9 ± 34.6	Riond and Riviere 1988
Rabbits	20	IV	NA	1	11.4 ± 15.1	Huang et al. 1979
Cats	5	IV	NA	1	86.6[a]	Jernigan et al. 1988e
Horses	2.2	IV	NA	1	142 ± 31	Bowman et al. 1986
Dogs	10	IV	NA	1	31 ± 10	Riviere and Carver 1984
Dogs (hypothyroid)	10	IV	NA	1	5.6 ± 4.1	Riviere and Carver 1984
Pigs	6	IV	NA	1	11.0 ± 0.4	Riond et al. 1986

929

Source: Adapted from Brown and Riviere 1991.
Note: NF = not found in diabetic dogs (only 1 out of 7 dogs had a detectable $t_{1/2\gamma}$ = 46.8 hr); NA = not applicable.
[a]Harmonic mean; range.

(Riviere et al. 1983). A similar pattern was observed in foals 1 to 30 days of age compared to adult mares (Cummings et al. 1990), with Vd higher in foals, and clearance lower in younger foals. Clarke et al. (1992) reported that the half-life, Vd(area), and Cl_B (clearance) of gentamicin (3 mg/kg IV, once) did not change appreciably as the horses aged, even up to the highest age group at 20–30 years. The authors concluded that there was no pharmacologic reason to adjust the dose in older animals.

Clearance of gentamicin is notably dependent on renal function and has been shown to be so in (among others) horses (Sojka and Brown 1986; Sweeney et al. 1992, Martin et al., 1998), dogs (Frazier et al. 1988), and pigs (Riond et al. 1986). When horses were being treated for bacterial infections (pleuropneumonia, peritonitis, pericarditis, abscess, etc.) with gentamicin, clearance was correlated with the plasma creatinine concentration in both healthy and clinically ill horses (Sweeney et al. 1992), allowing serum creatinine concentrations to be used to individualize gentamicin doses in horses (Martin et al. 1998). As predicted by allometric principles, on a ml/min/kg basis, gentamicin clearance decreases as body weight increases (Martin-Jimenez and Riviere 2001).

Recovery of gentamicin in the urine has been reported to be 91 ± 28% within the first 24 hours in sheep (Brown et al. 1985, 1986a,b), 96% in the first 5 hours in dogs (Chisholm et al. 1968), 83 ± 8% in the first 8 hours in adult cattle (Haddad et al. 1986), and 90% recovered in the first 24 hours in 4- to 5-week-old calves (Ziv et al. 1982). Urinary recovery data of gentamicin appears to indicate that the β phase of elimination accounts for the majority of gentamicin elimination from the body.

Effect of Body Condition and Disease on Gentamicin Disposition. Because gentamicin and other drugs from this class are water-soluble, dehydration reduces the apparent volume of distribution (Hunter et al. 1991; LeCompte et al. 1981). Gentamicin pharmacokinetics changes appreciably between lean and obese cats (Wright et al. 1991). Obese cats given a 3 mg/kg IV dose of gentamicin had significantly lower Vd(ss) and Cl values compared to lean cats. Bioavailability and half-life values for obese cats were unchanged when compared to the values obtained in lean cats. These changes were attributed to the chemical characteristics of gentamicin, in that the poorly lipid soluble gentamicin fails to distribute adequately into the excess adipose tissue, resulting in reduced Vd values and necessitating a dose adjustment based on the cat's estimated lean body mass and not its overall body mass. In a related study, obese rats were found to sustain more nephrotoxicity due to increased renal uptake and retention of gentamicin in the kidneys than did their lean counterparts (Salazar et al. 1992).

Gentamicin disposition has been extensively studied in animals given IV endotoxin. Endotoxemia decreased plasma gentamicin concentrations in dogs and cats by approximately 20–30% (Pennington et al. 1975; Jernigan et al. 1988c). However, differences in healthy and febrile goats were not significant (Ahmad et al 1994). In a population pharmacokinetic model across species, the covariate of fever seemed to influence gentamicin volume of distribution (Martin-Jimenez and Riviere 2001). Other conditions that have been shown to alter gentamicin disposition include endocrinopathies, pregnancy, and other concurrent drug administrations.

In dogs, familial hypothyroidism effectively abolishes the γ phase of serum disposition (Riviere and Carver 1984), as does experimentally induced and naturally occurring diabetes mellitus (Brown et al. 1991). In rats, hypoparathyroidism (Holohan et al. 1987) and streptozotocin-induced diabetes mellitus (Ramsammy et al. 1987) reduce the renal accumulation of gentamicin without affecting the number or affinity of the gentamicin binding sites (Holohan et al. 1987). In pigs, hypothyroidism reduced mean (±SEM) gentamicin systemic clearance from 2.51 ± 0.17 (normal pigs) to 1.52 ± 0.12 ml/min/kg (Riond et al. 1986), an effect caused by reduction in the GFR. Finally, horses under halothane anesthesia showed longer gentamicin half-life than when in the awake state (4.03 hours versus 2.01 hours), as a result of reduced GFR during anesthesia.

Regional Limb Perfusion. Gentamicin has been used to treat infections in horses using regional limb perfusion, particularly for lower limb and joint infections (Whitehair et al. 1992a,b). The disposition of gentamicin in equine plasma, synovial fluid, and lymph has also been reported (Anderson et al. 1995). The half-life of gentamicin in the plasma was 2.17 hours (range = 1.92–2.5), and the half-life in the lymph was 3.03 hours (range = 2.63–3.57). It was concluded that the plasma concentration of gentamicin was a reliable predictor of concentration in lymph fluid and that plasma-based pharmacokinetics could be used with a good degree of confidence to predict the concentrations that would be obtained in the lymph in horses.

Renal Effects of Gentamicin. Gentamicin is accumulated in renal proximal tubules to concentrations several-fold higher than in serum or any other tissue in every species investigated (Schentag and Jusko 1977; Riviere et al. 1981a; Aronoff et al. 1983; Trnovec et al. 1984; Brown et al. 1985, 1986b; Haddad et al. 1987; Jernigan et al. 1988c; Ziv et al. 1982).

Urine concentrations are reported to be as high as 107 ± 33 μg/mL after 2.2 mg/kg every 8 hours in dogs (Ling et al. 1981), and 362 ± 163 μg/mL 3 hours after 3 mg/kg in cats (Jernigan et al. 1988b). Urine concentrations in animals with pyelonephritis (Bergeron et al. 1982) and endotoxemia (Jernigan et al. 1988b) are lower than in control animals given gentamicin, perhaps in part due to retention in the renal medulla (Jernigan et al. 1988b).

Renal uptake is inhibited by urinary alkalinization with sodium bicarbonate, theoretically because gentamicin is less ionized and therefore is less able to bind to the acidic phospholipids of the proximal tubular membranes (Chiu et al. 1979). High proteinuria due to high-protein diet or diabetes mellitus and proteinuria induced primarily by renal disorders reduce gentamicin uptake into renal proximal tubules (Pattyn et al. 1988), although factors other than proteinuria may also play a role (Ramsammy et al. 1987). In sheep, diet may also play a significant role in gentamicin pharmacokinetics. A study by Oukessou and Toutain (1992) reported that sheep fed a low-protein diet (25 g/day) had significantly lower Vd(ss) and Cl values for gentamicin (4 mg/kg IV) than did sheep fed a high-protein diet (120 g/day), while AUC values were higher in the sheep fed the low-protein diet, indicating higher overall serum concentrations of gentamicin in this treatment group. Coupled with IV inulin clearance data, it was surmised that the protein content of the diet can appreciably modify the distribution of body water and also modulate kidney function, resulting in altered gentamicin kinetics. A similar study in horses found that horses fed a diet of oats (low in calcium and potassium) had a higher incidence of gentamicin-induced nephrotoxicosis than horses fed an all-alfalfa hay diet high in vitamins and minerals (Schumacher et al. 1991). Intravenous administration of calcium also decreased the risk of gentamicin-induced nephrotoxicosis (Brashier et al. 1998). Based on these results, anorectic horses or horses consuming diets low in mineral content are seemingly predisposed to aminoglycoside nephrotoxicosis. Diet composition in dogs also can affect gentamicin toxicosis. Diets fed to dogs that varied in protein content from high to low produced renal changes that corresponded to the diet protein content (Grauer et al. 1994). The highest protein content diet produced the least degree of renal toxicity after gentamicin administration. In a similar study (Behrend et al. 1994), protein diet content was varied from high to low. The dogs with the highest protein diet content induced faster gentamicin clearance, a larger volume of distribution, and greater preservation of renal function.

Tissue Uptake of Gentamicin. Skeletal muscle concentrations are either very low or nondetectable (Bush et al. 1981; LeCompte et al. 1981). Although gentamicin does not partition into and sequester in skeletal muscle (Brown et al. 1986b; Haddad et al. 1987; Riond and Riviere 1988), substantial retention of gentamicin did occur at the site of IM injections (Haddad et al. 1987; Brown et al. 1986b).

Gentamicin does not accumulate in the central nervous system after systemic administration. Gentamicin residues can be found in milk after IV, IM, or intramammary (IMM) administration. Pedersoli et al. (1995) administered a single IV or IM dose of gentamicin (5 mg/kg) or a single 500 mg dose of gentamicin to the udder of lactating cows and followed the elimination of the drug via the milk over several days. After a single IMM infusion, the gentamicin levels did not fall below a safe level (≤30 ng/ml) until the seventh milking, 84 hours after treatment. Single IV or IM doses of gentamicin yielding safe milk levels of gentamicin occurred at the third milking, 36 hours after dosing. In another experiment, the cows were given two IV or IM doses of gentamicin (5 mg/kg) or two 500 mg doses of gentamicin to the udders of lactating cows for 5 days. Gentamicin levels did not fall below a safe level (≤30 ng/ml) until the eleventh milking, 132 hours after treatment. Single IV doses again produced safe milk levels of gentamicin at 36 hours after dosing.

AMIKACIN. Amikacin is available as a 50 mg/ml injectable solution (e.g., Amikin, Amiglyde) as well as an intrauterine infusion (250 mg/ml intrauterine solution) for horses. Tables 36.6 and 36.7 list some selected pharmacokinetic parameters for amikacin in various species of animals. The parenteral absorption patterns of amikacin have been studied in several species of animals, including birds (Gronwall et al., 1989; Bloomfield et al. 1997).

Bioavailability of amikacin ranges from 90% after IM and 100% after SC doses in cats (Jernigan et al. 1988d). Mean absorption time is 55 ± 36 minutes after IM doses and 53 ± 19 minutes after SC doses in cats (Jernigan et al. 1988d).

In dogs and calves, amikacin concentrations peak at approximately 0.5–0.85 hours (Cabana and Taggart 1973; Ziv 1977), with plasma depletion half-lives slightly longer after IM dosing and particularly after SC dosing than after an IV dose (Baggot et al. 1985; Carli et al. 1990). The urine amikacin concentration in dogs after 15 mg/kg divided into three daily doses was 342 ± 153 μg/mL when obtained as a 6- to 9-hour collection after dosing (Ling et al. 1981).

In reptiles the absorption half-life is 5.7 ± 2.8 hours after IM dosing in snakes and is independent of the ambient temperature (Mader et al. 1985). In tortoises (Caligiuri et al. 1990), the Vd of amikacin at 20°C (0.221 l/kg) was not appreciably different from that when the body temperature was at 30°C (0.241 l/kg); however, clearance in the 30°C tortoises was markedly higher (10.65 ml/min/kg) than in the 20°C animals (5.27 ml/min/kg). Similar differences were also noted for mean residence time and AUC values, indicating that clearance of amikacin (like many other drugs in cold-blooded animals) is temperature dependent.

Horses. Pharmacokinetic parameters for amikacin in normal, premature, uremic, and hypoxic foals have been reported (Wichtel et al. 1992; Adland-Davenport et al. 1990; Green et al. 1992). In one report, the half-life, Vd, and Cl for amikacin in premature foals (3.5 hr, 0.48 l/kg, and 98.2 ml/hr/kg, respectively) were not very different from the values for full-term nonuremic foals (3.3 hours, 0.40 l/kg, and 85.8 ml/hr/kg, respectively). However, full-term uremic foals less than 4 days old had higher values for two out of three of these parameters (20.1 hr, 0.80 l/kg, and 38.4 ml/hr/kg, respectively) when given 7 mg/kg (IV or IM) either twice or three times daily. Septic foals (less than 1 week old) have increased amikacin AUC and mean residence times and lower values for clearance when compared to clinically normal foals of similar age.

The pharmacokinetics of IV versus intraosseous (IO) administration of amikacin was studied in 3- and 5-day-old foals (Golenz et al. 1994). Foals were given 7 mg/kg amikacin IV or IO (tibia) and blood samples taken at predetermined times. The pharmacokinetics of amikacin administered IV and IO were almost identical in these foals with nearly complete absorption from the site of administration. No significant differences were noted between the major pharmacokinetic parameters of IV and

TABLE 36.6 Single-dose intravenous pharmacokinetics of amikacin in various species

Species	Dose (mg/kg)	$V_{d(area)}$ (L/kg)	$V_{d(ss)}$ (L/kg)	Cl_B (mL/min/kg)	$t_{1/2\beta}$ (hr)	Reference
Cats	5	0.134 (0.008)	NR	110 (15)	NR	Shille et al. 1985
Cats	10	0.14 (0.008)	NR	121 (22)	NR	Shille et al. 1985
Cats	20	0.18 (0.022)	NR	138 (2.6)	NR	Shille et al. 1985
Cats	5	NR	0.17 (0.02)	1.46 (0.26)	79[b] (19)	Jernigan et al. 1988c
Horses	4.4	0.20 (0.05)	NR	89.3 (23.4)	1.44[b]	Orsini et al. 1985
Horses	6.6	0.17 (0.03)	NR	76.6 (11.3)	1.57[b]	Orsini et al. 1985
Horses	11	0.14 (0.02)	NR	84.7 (13.4)	1.14	Orsini et al. 1985
Horses	6	0.214	0.207	0.75	2.8	Horspool et al. 1994
Ponies	6	0.191	0.162	1.37	1.6	Horspool et al. 1994
Donkeys	6	0.156	0.150	0.97	1.9	Horspool et al. 1994
Dogs[a]	5	0.26 (0.23–0.29)	NR	2.82 (2.29–3.22)	1.07 (0.95–1.22)	Baggot et al. 1985
Dogs[a]	10	0.239 (0.18–0.27)	NR	2.66 (2.32–2.89)	0.98 (0.90–1.07)	Baggot et al. 1985
Dogs[a]	20	0.36 (0.32–0.38)	NR	3.57 (3.31–4.73)	1.03 (0.90–1.33)	Baggot et al. 1985
Calves	7.5	350	NR	1.5	150.5	Carli et al. 1990
Sheep	7.5	200	NR	0.7	115.5	Carli et al. 1990
African grey parrots	5	289	233	188	1.06	Gronwall et al. 1989
African grey parrots	10	184	122	142	0.90	Gronwall et al. 1989
African grey parrots	20	444	308	229	1.34	Gronwall et al. 1989
Dogs	25	0.25	NR	34	0.85	Cabana and Taggart 1973
Humans	125	16.26 (1.7)	NR	81 (6)	2.8 (0.26)	Yates et al. 1978

Source: Adapted from Brown and Riviere 1991.
Note: NR = not reported.
[a]Median (range); total dose (mg); mL/min.
[b]Harmonic mean (±SD).

IO amikacin in this study. Five-day-old foals did have statistically significant higher ClB values than the 3-day-old foals. The study concluded by stating that the IO infusion methodology in neonatal foals is a safe and effective technique for drug delivery when the IV route cannot be used, particularly in cases of circulatory collapse. Amikacin, like other aminoglycosides, is poorly absorbed from the gastrointestinal tract of the horse. Horspool et al. (1994) administered a single dose of amikacin IV and two PO doses to horses, ponies, and donkeys. Detectable blood levels of amikacin were not found in any of the animals dosed orally with amikacin; likewise, no amikacin was found in the fecal material of animals dosed with amikacin by the IV route. Amikacin had little, if any, effect on the numbers of viable bacteria of the normal gastrointestinal flora of these study animals.

Serum concentrations of amikacin have also been studied in mares in estrus. After induction of estrus, mares were dosed with 1.0 or 2.0 g amikacin by intrauterine (IU) infusion every 24 hours for 3 days, or given an IM injection of either 9.7 or 14.5 mg/kg every 24 hours for 3 days. Amikacin blood concentrations were detected after IU administration, indicating low systemic absorption from this route.

TABLE 36.7 Nonintravenous disposition values for amikacin in various species (means with standard deviations in parentheses)

Species	Dose (mg/kg)	Route	V_d/F (L/kg)	Cl_B/F (mL/min/kg)	$t_{1/2}$ (hr)	F (%)	Reference
Horses	4.4	IM	NR	NR	NR	100	Orsini et al. 1985
Horses	6.6	IM	NR	NR	NR	100	Orsini et al. 1985
Horses	11	IM	NR	NR	NR	100	Orsini et al. 1985
Cats	5	IM	0.16 (0.004)	132[a] (13)	NR	NR	Shille et al. 1985
Cats	10	IM	0.2 (0.02)	150[a] (10)	NR	NR	Shille et al. 1985
Cats	20	IM	0.19 (0.02)	121[a] (21)	NR	NR	Shille et al. 1985
Cats	5	SC	0.19 (0.01)	138[a] (13)	NR	NR	Shille et al. 1985
Cats	10	SC	0.21 (0.01)	117[a] (6)	NR	NR	Shille et al. 1985
Cats	20	SC	0.19 (0.01)	141[a] (21)	NR	NR	Shille et al. 1985
Cats	5	IM	ND	ND	119	90 (36)	Jernigan et al. 1988d
Cats	5	SC	ND	ND	118	100 (19)	Jernigan et al. 1988d
Sheep	7.5	IM	ND	ND	1.96	87	Carli et al. 1990
Calves	7.5	IM	ND	ND	1.94	99	Carli et al. 1990
African grey parrot	5	IM	ND	ND	1.08	98	Gronwall et al. 1989
African grey parrot	10	IM	ND	ND	1.04	61	Gronwall et al. 1989
African grey parrot	15	IM	ND	ND	0.97	106	Gronwall et al. 1989
Gopher snake (25° C)	5	IM	0.29 (0.04)	2.8 (0.29)	1.2 (0.17)	ND	Mader et al. 1985
Gopher snake (37° C)	5	IM	0.63 (0.31)	5.83 (1.6)	1.25 (0.5)	ND	Mader et al. 1985

Source: Adapted from Brown and Riviere 1991.
ND = not determined; NR = not reported.
[a]mL/min.

KANAMYCIN. Because of the structural similarities between kanamycin and amikacin (amikacin is synthesized from kanamycin), the pharmacokinetics of kanamycin and amikacin are very similar. However, kanamycin is among the least active aminoglycosides in comparison to gentamicin and amikacin. Subsequently, the clinical use of kanamycin has fallen out of popularity in veterinary medicine in recent years For example, against clinical isolates of *Pseudomonas aeruginosa* the highest rate of resistance was for kanamycin (90% resistant) compared to gentamicin (7%) and amikacin (3%) (Rubin et al. 2008).

Lashev et al. (1992) studied species differences in the pharmacokinetics of kanamycin in sheep, goats, rabbits, adult chickens, and pigeons given a 10 mg/ml IV dose of kanamycin. The differences in the Vd in these animals were small, all being between 0.254 and 0.292 l/kg. Eighteen-day-old chicks had the largest Vd (0.671 l/kg). In calves, IM doses of 10, 25, and 50 mg/kg produced peak concentrations at 30 minutes of 31 ± 3.1 μg/mL, 57.3 ± 4.9 μg/mL, and 64 ± 14 μg/mL, respectively. The kanamycin elimination half-lives of 2 hours in all three instances were identical to amikacin (Ziv 1977). Similar half-lives of 1.80 ± 0.17 hours were observed in horses (Baggot et al. 1981) and sheep (Andreini and Pignatelli 1972). IM availability (F) of kanamycin in horses has been reported to be approximately 100% (Baggot et al. 1981). After a dose of 25 mg/kg of either kanamycin or amikacin IV in dogs, Vd was 0.23–0.25 l/kg, and after IM dosing in that same study, absorption half-life was 0.4–0.75 hours, with apparent elimination half-life of 0.9–1.2 hours for both amikacin and kanamycin (Cabana and Taggart 1973). The kanamycin half-life in dogs after a 10 mg/kg IV dose was 0.97 ± 0.31 hours; after IM dosing, the fraction absorbed was 89 ± 16%, with an absorption half-life of 0.15 ± 0.003 hours (Baggot 1978). Synovial fluid kanamycin concentrations in horses were equivalent to serum concentrations 4 hours after a 5 mg/kg dose IM, whereas peritoneal kanamycin concentrations were equal to or higher than serum kanamycin concentrations at 3 hours postadministration. Firth et al. (1993) gave adult ponies a single 10 mg/kg kanamycin dose IM. At 2 and 5 hours after dosing, the metacarpophalangeal, intercarpal, radiocarpal, tibiotarsal, and metatarsophalangeal joints underwent arthrocentesis to determine kanamycin concentrations in the synovial fluid. There was considerable variation between joints sampled at each time point, and the authors reported that the variations were not consistent between animals and that these variations were not statistically significant. At 2 hours after dosing, synovial fluid concentrations fluctuated between joints but averaged 50% that of serum concentration. At 5 hours, synovial fluid concentrations were approximately 145% of plasma concentrations. Urine concentrations of kanamycin in dogs given 5.5 μg/mL twice a day were 473 ± 306 μg/ml urine when obtained as a 6-hour collection after dosing (Ling et al. 1981).

APRAMYCIN. Apramycin, an aminoglycoside derived from *Streptomyces tenebrarius* (Ryden and Moore 1977), is the newest aminoglycoside introduced for veterinary use. The only formulations currently registered in the U.S. of this drug are powder (Apralan) to be added to feed (Type A medicated feed article) at 150 grams per ton of feed, and the soluble powder to be added to water (100 mg per liter) to deliver 12.5 mg/kg for 12 days of treatment in medicated water. For each formulation, the indication is to treat porcine colibacillosis (pig scours) caused by *Escherichi coli.*

Administration of 10 mg/kg apramycin IV to preruminant dairy calves resulted in a Vd(ss) of 0.71 ± 0.042 l/kg, and systemic clearance of 3.22 ± 0.44 ml/min/kg, and a half-life of 4.4 ± 1.2 hours (Ziv et al. 1985). Urine recovery of apramycin accounted for approximately 85% of the dose after 24 hours. Apramycin peak concentrations after IM doses of 10 and 20 mg/kg were 19 and 40 μg/mL, respectively, although peak concentrations occurred somewhat later after the larger dose. There was no plasma accumulation when IM doses of 10 or 20 mg/kg were given daily. Bioavailability of apramycin from IM sites was quite variable, ranging from 50 to 100% (Ziv et al. 1985).

Although apramycin is primarily used only in pigs, the pharmacokinetics were described in lactating cows, ewes, and goats (Ziv et al. 1995). The IV pharmacokinetics of 20 mg/kg apramycin was very similar in the lactating cow, ewe, and goat, with an elimination half-life of approximately 2 hours, a Vd between 1.26 and 1.5 l/kg, and an IM absorption bioavailability between 60% and 70%. All species had higher penetration of apramycin in the milk from inflamed udders than from clinically normal (nonmastitic) udders. The pharmacokinetics of apramycin in Japanese quails has also been described (Lashev and Mihailov 1994).

Pharmacokinetic data for apramycin in selected species are presented in Table 36.8

TOBRAMYCIN. Tobramycin is produced by *Streptomyces tenebrarius* and is structurally similar to kanamycin.

TABLE 36.8 Selected pharmacokinetic parameters of apramycin

Species	$V_{d(ss)}$ (L/kg)	Cl_B (L/kg/hr)	$t_{1/2}$ (hr)	Reference
Sheep	0.167	0.078	90.96	Lashev et al. 1992
Cow (lactating)	1.263	12.164[a]	2.10	Ziv et al. 1995
Ewe (lactating)	1.446	14.142[a]	1.85	Ziv et al. 1995
Goat (lactating)	1.357	11.68[a]	2.14	Ziv et al. 1995
Rabbits	0.284	0.258	48.06	Lashev et al. 1992
Adult chickens	0.182	0.078	100.54	Lashev et al. 1992
18-day-old chicks	0.254	0.218	48.0	Lashev et al. 1992
Japanese quail	0.133[b]	0.186	0.50	Lashev and Mihailov 1994
Pigeons	0.077	0.210	15.24	Lashev et al. 1992

[a]Value in mL/kg/min.
[b]V_α is area, not steady state.

Tobramycin is not extensively used in veterinary medicine, although it is used occasionally in dogs and cats because of its good activity against most *Pseudomonas aeruginosa* organisms. In cats, tobramycin systemic clearance was 2.21 ± 0.59 and 1.69 ± 0.36 ml/min/kg after doses of 5 mg/kg and 3 mg/kg IV, respectively, and a Vd(ss) of 0.19 ± 0.03 and 0.18 ± 0.03 l/kg, respectively (Jernigan et al. 1988b). In that same study, IV doses of 3 mg/kg and 5 mg/kg resulted in mean residence time (MRT) of 90 ± 16 and 108 ± 21 minutes, respectively. Bioavailability after IM and SC tobramycin administration in cats was complete (Jernigan et al. 1988d). The mean absorption times were 35 and 60 minutes, respectively. Urine tobramycin concentrations following 2.2 mg/kg 3 times a day were 66 ± 39 μg/mL when urine was obtained as a 6-hour collection in dogs (Ling et al. 1981).

After IV administration to camels (Hadi et al. 1994), tobramycin (1.3 mg/kg) elimination half-life was 189 minutes. The apparent Vd (area method) was 245 ml/kg and Vd(ss) was 228 ml/kg. Clearance was measured at 0.9 ml/min/kg. After a 1.0 mg/kg IM dose of tobramycin, bioavailability was almost 91%, with an elimination half-life of 201 minutes.

NEOMYCIN. Most neomycin is used topically or administered orally (e.g., Biosol used for enteritis caused by *E. coli*) to achieve a local effect in the intestine. Registered formulations are powder for addition to feed at 715 grams per kg of feed (Neomix), or neomycin oral solution (200 mg/ml) to be added to drinking water, both the oral solution and feed additive are designed to deliver 22 mg/kg up to 14 days. The oral solution also may be administered directly to individual animals.

Pharmacokinetic information about neomycin's use in human and veterinary medicine is very limited. In calves administered 12 mg/kg IV, Vd was 0.39 ± 0.13 l/kg, and half-life was reported as 167 ± 48 minutes (Black et al. 1983) although half-lives of approximately 1 hour have been observed (Drury 1952). Bioavailability after IM dosing of neomycin was 56 ± 5.4% in calves (Black et al. 1983) and 74 ± 27% in horses (Baggot et al. 1981). The pharmacokinetics of IV, IM, single PO, and repeated PO neomycin in ruminating Holstein calves has been described (Pedersoli et al. 1994). Variable absorption rates were also observed. In horses, terminal half-life of 2.1 ± 1.0 hours has been reported, in addition to a Vd(area) of 0.232 ± 0.061 l/kg and systemic clearance of 1.3 ± 0.4 ml/min/kg (Baggot et al. 1981). Neomycin did not accumulate in inner-ear tissue as did other aminoglycosides (Desrochers and Schacht 1982) but was more potent than any other clinically used aminoglycoside at displacing gentamicin from renal binding sites (Josepovitz et al. 1982). Concentrations in guinea pig tissues other than the kidney continued to increase during 3 weeks of treatment with a dosing regimen of 100 mg/kg/day administered SC (Desrochers and Schacht 1982). Terminal half-lives have been estimated in cattle to be between 55 and 65 hours after single parenteral doses (Siddique et al. 1965).

DIHYDROSTREPTOMYCIN AND STREPTOMYCIN. The clinical use of dihydrostreptomycin and streptomycin has declined substantially in veterinary medicine. An old formulation of penicillin-dihydrostreptomycin (Pen-Strep) is off the market in North America. There is still a formulation containing dihydrostreptomycin sulfate (500 mg/ml) registered for treatment of *Leptospira* in dogs, horses, pigs, and ruminants. Although dihydrostreptomycin has been used in the treatment of cows infected with *Leptospira interrogans* serovar *hardjo* subtype *hardjobovis* (Gerritsen et al. 1994), this use is not common and the product is not marketed.

There is an oral formulation of streptomycin (250 mg/ml) still registered for oral treatment of bacterial enteritis in pigs, cattle, and poultry. It has been administered directly to the patient or added to drinking water. Because the use of these products is uncommon, previous editions of this book will contain more detailed information on their use.

After IM doses of 5.5 mg/kg dihydrostreptomycin, maximum concentrations ranged from 5.1 to 17.0 μg/mL, with peak concentrations occurring earlier and more variable from the commercial preparation containing procaine penicillin G, dihydrostreptomycin, dexamethasone, and chlorpheniramine than from the commercial product containing only dihydrostreptomycin and procaine penicillin G (Rollins et al. 1972). Half-lives range from 2.35–4.50. Because streptomycin and dihydrostreptomycin are chemically very similar, their dispositions also may be nearly identical.

PAROMOMYCIN. Paromomycin is a wide-spectrum aminoglycoside antibiotic produced by *Streptomyces rimosus* var. *paromomycinus* and, unlike others in this class, has

TABLE 36.9 Pharmacokinetic parameters of paromomycin in the dog

Parameter	IV	IM	SC
$t_{1/2\alpha}$	21.54	15.31	12.43
$t_{1/2\beta}$	91.03	114.22	120.86
V_d (L/kg)	0.51	ND	ND
V_{ss} (L/kg)	0.33	ND	ND
Cl_B (L/min/kg)	0.0037	ND	ND
C_{max} (μg/mL)	ND	32.1	36.3
F	ND	>0.99	>0.99
MRT (min)	98.7	204.8	203.8
K_{el} (min^{-1})	0.0186	0.0061	0.0057

Source: Belloli et al. 1996.
Note: ND = not determined.

both gram-positive and gram-negative activity. Paromomycin is poorly absorbed from the gastrointestinal tract, which is clearly an advantage if used to treat certain bacterial or protozoal gastrointestinal infections. The pharmacokinetics of paromomycin in the dog has been described by Belloli et al. (1996); see Table 36.9.

Giardia, Leishmania, Entamoeba histolytica, and *Balantidium coli* are susceptible to paromomycin (Barr et al. 1994; Belloli et al. 1996). Paromomycin has been used to treat cryptosporidiosis in a cat (Barr et al. 1994) and leishmaniasis (*Leishmania infantum*) in dogs (Poli et al. 1997). However, a retrospective case study in cats treated with high-dose oral paromomycin (165 mg/kg) suggested that 4 of 31 individuals developed acute nephrotoxicity, deafness, and/or possible cataract formation (Gookin et al. 1999), implying that enough oral absorption occurred for this large and highly charged aminoglycoside to exert an adverse effect. Therefore, use of this drug at these high doses should be approached with caution until further data are available.

REFERENCES

Adelman, R.D., Spangler, W.L., Beasom, F., Ishizaki, G., and Conzelman, G. 1979. Furosemide enhancement of experimental gentamicin nephrotoxicity, comparison of functional-morphological changes with activities of urinary enzymes. J Infect Dis 140:342–352.

Adland-Davenport, P., Brown, M.P., Robinson, J.D., and Derendorf, H.C. 1990. Pharmacokinetics of amikacin in critically ill neonatal foals treated for presumed or confirmed sepsis. Equine Vet J 22(1):18–22.

Ahmad, A.H., Bahga, H.S., and Sharma, L.D. 1994. Pharmacokinetics of gentamicin following single dose intravenous administration in normal and febrile goats. J Vet Pharmacol Therap 17:369–373.

Albarellos, G., Montoya, L., Ambros, L., Kreil, V., Hallu, R., and Rebuelto, M. 2004. Multiple once-daily dose pharmacokinetics and renal safety of gentamicin in dogs. J Vet Pharmacol Therap 27:21–25.

al-Guedawy, S.S., Neff-Davis, C.A., Davis, L.E., Whitmore, H.L., and Gustafusson, B.K. 1983. Disposition of gentamicin in the genital tract of cows. J Vet Pharmacol Therap 6:85–92.

Ali, B.H., Abdel Gayoum, A.A., and Bashir, A.A. 1992. Gentamicin nephrotoxicity in rats: some biochemical correlates. Pharmacol Toxicol 70:419–423.

Anderson, B.H., Firth, E.C., and Whittem, T. 1995. The disposition of gentamicin in equine plasma, synovial fluid and lymph. J Vet Pharmacol Therap 18:124–131.

Andreini, G., and Pignatelli, P. 1972. Kanamycin blood levels and residues in domestic animals. Veterinaria 21:51–72.

Appel, G.B. 1982. Aminoglycoside nephrotoxicity: physiologic studies of the sites of nephron damage. In A. Whelton and H.C. Neu, eds., The Aminoglycosides: Microbiology, Clinical Use and Toxicology, pp. 269–382. New York: Marcel Dekker.

Appel, G.B., and Neu, H.C. 1977. The nephrotoxicity of antimicrobial agents. N Engl J Med 296:722–728.

Aronoff, G.R., Pottratz, S.T., Brier, M.E., et al. 1983. Aminoglycoside accumulation kinetics in rat renal parenchyma. Antimicrob Agents Chemother 23:74–78.

Avasthi, P.S., Evan, A.P., Huser, J.W., and Luft, F.C. 1981. Effect of gentamicin on glomerular ultrastructure. J Lab Clin Med 98:444–454.

Baggot, J.D. 1977. Principles of Drug Disposition in Domestic Animals. Philadelphia: W.B. Saunders.

———. 1978. Pharmacokinetics of kanamycin in dogs. J Vet Pharmacol and Therap 1:163–170.

Baggot, J.D., Ling, G.V., Chatfield, R.C., and Raus, J. 1985. Clinical pharmacokinetics of amikacin in dogs. Am J Vet Res 46:1793–1796.

Baggot, J.D., Love, D.N., Rose, R.J., and Raus, J. 1981. The pharmacokinetics of some aminoglycoside antibiotics in the horse. J Vet Pharmacol and Therap 4:277–284.

Barr, S.C., Jamrosz, G.F., Hornbuckle, W.E., Bowman, D.D., and Fayer, R. 1994. Use of paromomycin for treatment of cryptosporidiosis in a cat. JAVMA 205(12):1742–1743.

Barza, M., Murray, T., and Hamburger, R.J. 1980. Uptake of gentamicin by separated, viable renal tubules from rabbits. J Infect Dis 141:510–517.

Bass, K.D., Larkin, S.E., Paap, C., and Haase, G.M. 1998. Pharmacokinetics of once-daily gentamicin dosing in pediatric patients. J Ped Surg 33(7):1104–1107.

Batra, V.K., Morrison, J.A., and Hoffman, T.R. 1983. Pharmacokinetics of piperacillin and gentamicin following intravenous administration to dogs. J Pharmaceut Sci 72:894–898.

Bauer, L.A., and Blouin, R.A. 1981. Influence of age on tobramycin pharmacokinetics in patients with normal renal function. Antimicrob Agents Chemother 20:587–589.

Beauchamp, D., Gourde, P., Theriault, G., and Bergeron, M.G. 1992. Age-dependent gentamicin experimental nephrotoxicity. J Pharmacol Exp Therap 260(2):444–449.

Beck, K., Loomis, M., Lewbart, G., Spellman, L., and Papich, M.G. 1995. Preliminary comparison of plasma concentrations of gentamicin injected into the cranial and caudal limb musculature of the eastern box turtle (*Terrapene carolina carolina*). Journal of Zoo and Wildlife Medicine 26:265–268.

Behrend, E.N., Grauer, G.F., Greco, D.S., Fettman, M.J., and Allen, T.A. 1994. Effects of dietary protein conditioning on gentamicin pharmacokinetics. J Vet Pharmacol Therap 17:259–264.

Belloli, C., Crescenzo, G., Carli, S., Villa, R., Sonzogni, O., Carelli, G., and Ormas, P. 1996. Pharmacokinetics and dosing regimen of aminosidine in the dog. Vet Res Commun 20:533–541.

Bendirdjian, J.P., Fillastre, J.P., and Foucher, B. 1982. Mitochondria modifications with the aminoglycosides. In A. Whelton and H.C. Neu, eds., The Aminoglycosides: Microbiology, Clinical Use and Toxicology, pp. 325–354. New York: Marcel Dekker.

Bennett, W.M., Plamp, C.E., Gilbert, D.N., Parker, R.A., and Porter, G. A. 1979. The influence of dosage regimen on experimental gentamicin nephrotoxicity: dissociation of peak serum levels from renal failure. J Infect Dis 140(4):576–580.

Bennett, W.M., Plamp, C.E., Elliott, W.C., Parker, R.A., and Porter, G.A. 1982. Effect of basic amino acids and aminoglycosides on 3H gentamicin uptake in cortical slices of rat and human kidney. J Lab Clin Med 99:156–162.

Bergeron, M.G., Bastille, A., Lessard, C., and Gagnon, P.M. 1982. Significance of intrarenal concentrations of gentamicin for the outcome of experimental pyelonephritis in rats. J Infect Dis 146: 91–96.

Bergeron, M.G., and Bergeron, Y. 1986. Influence of endotoxin on the intrarenal distribution of gentamicin, netilmicin, tobramycin, amikacin, and cephalothin. Antimicrob Agents Chemother 29:7–12.

Bird, J.E., Miller, K.W., Larson, A.A., and Duke, G.E. 1983. Pharmacokinetics of gentamicin in birds of prey. Am J Vet Res 44:1245–1247.

Black, J., Calesnick, B., Williams, D., and Weinstein, M. 1963. Pharmacology of gentamicin, a new broad spectrum antibiotic. Antimicrob Agents Chemother 3:138–147.

Black, W.D., Holt, J.D., and Gentry, R.D. 1983. Pharmacokinetic study of neomycin in calves following intravenous and intramuscular administration. Canad J Comparative Med 47:433–435.

Blantz, R.C. 1980. The glomerulus, passive filter or regulatory organ? Klin Wochenschr 58:957–964.

Blaser, J., Rieder, H., Niederer, P., and Lüthy, R. 1983. Biological variability of multiple dose pharmacokinetics of netilmicin in man. Europ J Clin Pharmacol 24:359–406.

Blaser, J., Simmon, H.P., Gonzenbach, H.R., Sonnabend, W., and Lüthy, R. 1985. Aminoglycoside monitoring: timing of peak levels is critical. Therap Drug Monitor 7:303–307.

Bloomfield, R.B., Brooks, D., and Vulliet, R. 1997. The pharmacokinetics of a single intramuscular dose of amikacin in red-tailed hawks (*Buteo jamaicensis*). J Zoo Wildlife Med 28(1):55–61.

Bowman, K.F., Dix, L.P., Riond, J.-L., and Riviere, J.E. 1986. Prediction of pharmacokinetic profiles of ampicillin sodium, gentamicin sulfate, and combination ampicillin sodium-gentamicin sulfate in serum and synovia of healthy horses. Am J Vet Res 47:1590–1596.

Brashier, M.K., Geor, R.J., Ames, T.R., and O'Leary, T.P. 1998. Effect of intravenous calcium administration on gentamicin-induced nephrotoxicosis in ponies. Am J Vet Res 59:1055–1062.

Brown, M.P., Stover, S.M., Kelly, R.H., and Farver, T.B. 1981. Kanamycin sulfate in the horse: serum, synovial fluid, peritoneal fluid, and urine concentrations after single-dose intramuscular administration. Am J Vet Res 42:1823–1825.

Brown, S.A., Coppoc, G.L., and Riviere, J.E. 1986a. Effects of dose and duration of therapy on gentamicin tissue residues in sheep. Am J Vet Res 47:2373–2379.

Brown, S.A., Coppoc, G.L., Riviere, J.E., and Anderson, V.L. 1986b. Dose-dependent pharmacokinetics of gentamicin in sheep. Am J Vet Res 47:789–794.

Brown, S.A., and Garry, F.B. 1988. Comparison of serum and renal gentamicin concentrations and fractional urinary excretion tests as indicators of nephrotoxicity. J Vet Pharmacol Therap 11:330–337.

Brown, S.A., Nelson, R.W., and Scott-Moncrieff, C. 1991. Pharmacokinetics of gentamicin in diabetic dogs. J Vet Pharmacol Therap 14:90–95.

Brown, S.A., and Riviere, J.E. 1991. Comparative pharmacokinetics of aminoglycoside antibiotics. J Vet Pharmacol Therap 14:1–35.

Brown, S.A., Riviere, J.E., Coppoc, G.L., Hinsman, E.J., Carlton, W.W., and Steckel, R.R. 1985. Single intravenous and multiple intramuscular dose pharmacokinetics and tissue residue profile of gentamicin in sheep. Am J Vet Res 47:69–74.

Brown, S.A., Barsanti, J.A., and Crowell, W.A. 1985. Gentamicin-associated acute renal failure in the dog. J Am Vet Med Assoc 186:686–690.

Burrows, G.E. 1979. Gentamicin. JAVMA 175:301–302.

Bush, M., Locke, D., Neal, L.A., and Carpenter, J.W. 1981. Gentamicin tissue concentrations in various avian species following recommended dosage therapy. Am J Vet Res 46:2114–2116.

Busse, H.J., Wostmann, C., and Bakker, E.P. 1992. The bacterial action of streptomycin: Membrane permeabilization caused by the insertion of mistranslated proteins into the cytoplasmic membrane of *Escherichia coli* and subsequent caging of the antibiotic inside the cells due to degradation of these proteins. J Gen Microbiol 138(Pt3):551–561.

Cabana, B.E., and Taggart, J.G. 1973. Comparative pharmacokinetics of BB-K8 and kanamycin in dogs and humans. Antimicrob Agents Chemotherapy 3:478–483.

Caligiuri, R., Kollias, G.V., Jacobson, E., McNab, B., Clark, C.H., and Wilson, R.C. 1990. The effects of ambient temperature on amikacin pharmacokinetics in gopher tortoises. J Vet Pharmacol Therap 13:287–291.

Campbell, B.G., Bartholow, S., and Rosin, E. 1996. Bacterial killing by use of once daily gentamicin dosage in guinea pigs with *Escherichia coli* infection. AJVR 57(11):1627–1630.

Campbell, B.G., and Rosin, E. 1992. Optimal gentamicin dosage regimen in dogs (Abstr). Vet Surg 21(5):385.

Carbon, C., Contrepois, A., and Lamotte-Barrillon, S. 1978. Comparative distribution of gentamicin, tobramycin, sisomicin, netilmicin, and amikacin in interstitial fluid in rabbits. Antimicrob Agents Chemother 13:368–372.

Carli, S., Montesissa, C., Sonzogni, O., Madonna, M., and Said-Faqi, A. 1990. Comparative pharmacokinetics of amikacin sulphate in calves and sheep. Res Vet Sci 48:231–234.

Chahwala, S.B., and Harpur, E.S. 1982. An investigation of the effects of aminoglycoside antibiotics on Na-K ATPase as a possible mechanism of toxicity. Res Commun Chem Pathol Pharmacol 35:63–78.

Chisholm, G.D., Calnan, J.S., Waterworth, P.M., and Reis, N.D. 1968. Distribution of gentamicin in body fluids. Brit Med J 2:22–24.

Chiu, P.T.S., Brown, A., Miller, G., et al. 1976. Renal extraction gentamicin in anesthetized dogs. Antimicrob Agents Chemother 10:227–282.

Chiu, P.T.S., Miller, G.H., Long, J.F., and Waitz, J.A. 1979. Renal uptake and nephrotoxicity of gentamicin during urinary alkalinization in rats. Clin and Experim Pharmacol and Physiol 6:317–326.

Christensen, S., Ladefoged, K., and Frimodt-Moller, N. 1997. Experience with once daily dosing of gentamicin: considerations regarding dosing and monitoring. Chemotherapy 43:442–450.

Chung, M., Costello, R., and Symchowicz, S. 1980. Comparison of netilmicin and gentamicin pharmacokinetics in humans. Antimicrob Agents Chemother 17:184–187.

Chung, M., Parravicini, L., Assael, B.M., Cavanna, G., Radwanski, E., and Symchowicz, S. 1982. Comparative pharmacokinetics of aminoglycoside antibiotics in guinea pigs. Antimicrob Agents Chemother 10:1017–1021.

Clarke, C.R., Lochner, F.K., and Bellamy, J. 1992. Pharmacokinetics of gentamicin and antipyrine in the horse-effect of advancing age. J Vet Pharmacol Therap 15:309–313.

Clarke, C.R., Short, C.R., Hsu, R.-C., and Baggot, J.D. 1985. Pharmacokinetics of gentamicin in the calf: developmental changes. Am J Vet Res 46:2461–2466.

Cojocel, C., Dociu, N., Malta, K., Sleight, S.D., and Hook, J.B. 1983. Effects of aminoglycosides on glomerular permeability, tubular reabsorption, and intracellular catabolism of the cationic low-molecular weight protein lysozyme. Toxicol Appl Pharmacol 68:96–109.

Cojocel, C., and Hook, J.B. 1983. Aminoglycoside nephrotoxicity. Trends Pharmacol Sci 4:174–179.

Collier, V.U., Lictman, P.S., and Mitch, W.E. 1979. Evidence for luminal uptake of gentamicin in the perfused rat kidney. J Pharmacol Exp Ther 210:247–251.

Conzelman, G.M. 1980. Pharmacotherapeutics of aminoglycoside antibiotics. JAVMA 176:1078–1084.

Cowan, R.H., Jukkola, A.F., and Arant, B.S. 1980. Pathophysiologic evidence of gentamicin nephrotoxicity in neonatal puppies. Pediatric Res 14:1204–1211.

Cronin, R.E. 1979. Aminoglycoside nephrotoxicity, pathogenesis and nephotoxicity. Clin Nephrol 11:251–256.

Cronin, R.E., Bulger, R.E., Southeru, P., and Henrich, W.L. 1980. Natural history of aminoglycoside nephotoxicity in the dog. J Lab Clin Med 95:463–474.

Cronin, R., Nix, K., and Ferguson, E. 1982. Renal cortex ion composition and Na-K ATPase activity in early gentamicin nephrotoxicity. Am J Physiol 242:F477–F483.

Crowell, N.A., Divers, T.J., Byars, T.D., Marshall, A.E., Nusbaum, K.E., and Larsen, L. 1981. Neomycin toxicosis in calves. Am J Vet Res 42:29–34.

Cummings, L.E., Guthrie, A.J., Harkins, J.D., and Short, C.R. 1990. Pharmacokinetics of gentamicin in newborn to 30 day-old foals. Am J Vet Res 51:1988–1992.

Cuppage, F.E., Setter, K., Sullivan, L.P., Reitzes, E.J., and Meinykovych, A.D. 1977. Gentamicin nephrotoxicity 11: Physiological, biochemical and morphological effects of prolonged administration to rats. Virchows Arch B 24:121–138.

Desrochers, C.S., and Schacht, J. 1982. Neomycin concentrations in inner ear tissues and other organs of the guinea pig after chronic drug administration. Acta Otalarnygologica 93:233–236.

Drury, A.R. 1952. Evaluation of neomycin sulfate in treatment of bovine mastitis. Vet Med 47:407–411.

Easter, J.L., Hague, B.A., Brumbaugh, G.W., Nguyen, J., Chaffin, M.K., Honnas, C.M., and Kemper, D.L. 1997. Effects of postoperative peritoneal lavage on pharmacokinetics of gentamicin in horses after celiotomy. AJVR 58(10):1166–1170.

Elliott, W.C., Gilbert, D.N., DeFehr, J., Bennett, W.M., and McCarron, D.A. 1982. Protection from experimental gentamicin toxicity by dietary calcium loading. Kidney Int 21:216.

Elsheikh, H.A., Osman, L.A., and Ali, B.H. 1997. Comparative pharmacokinetics of ampicillin trihydrate, gentamicin sulphate and oxytetracycline hydrochloride in Nubian goats and desert sheep. J Vet Pharmacol Therap 20:262–266.

Errecalde, J.O., and Marino, E.L. 1990. A discriminatory study of pharmacokinetic models for intramuscular gentamicin in sheep. Vet Res Commun 14:53–58.

Erskine, J., Wilson, R.C., Riddell, M.G., Tyler, W., and Spears, H.J. 1992. Intramammary administration of gentamicin as treatment for experimentally induced *Escherichia coli* mastitis in cows. Am J Vet Res 53(3):375–381.

Eschbach, J.W., Adamson, J.W., and Dennis, M.B. 1980. Physiologic studies in normal and uremic sheep 1: the experimental model. Kidney Int 18:725–731.

Fabre, J., Rudhardt, M., Blanchard, P., and Regamey, C. 1976. Persistence of sisomicin and gentamicin in renal cortex and medulla compared with other organs and serum of rats. Kidney Int 10:444–449.

Feldman, S., Josepovitz, C., Scott, M., Pastoriza, E., and Kaloyanides, G.J. 1981. Inhibition of gentamicin uptake in rat kidney by polycations. Kidney Int 19:222.

Feldman, S., Wang, M.Y., and Kaloyanides, G.J. 1982. Aminoglycosides induce a phosphaolipidosis in the renal cortex of the rat: an early manifestation of nephrotoxicity. J Pharmacol Exp Ther 220:514–520.

Firth, E.C., Whittem, T., and Nouws, J.F.M. 1993. Kanamycin concentrations in synovial fluid after intramuscular administration in the horse. Aust Vet J 70(9):324–325.

Forsyth, S.F., Ilkiw, J.E., and Hildebrand, S.V. 1990. Effect of gentamicin administration on the neuromuscular blockade induced by atracurium in cats. Am J Vet Res 51(10):1675–1678.

Frazier, D.L., Aucoin, D.P., and Riviere, J.E. 1988. Gentamicin pharmacokinetics and nephrotoxicity in naturally acquired and experimentally induced disease in dogs. JAVMA 192:57–63.

Frazier, D.L., and Riviere, J.E. 1987. Gentamicin dosing strategies for dogs with subclinical renal dysfunction. Antimicrob Agents Chemother 31:1929–1934.

Freeman, C.D., Nicolau, D.P., Belliveau, P.P., and Nightingale, C.H. 1997. Once-daily dosing of aminoglycosides: review and recommendation for clinical practice. J Antimicrob Chemother 39:677–686.

Fuentes, V.O., Gonzalez, H., Sanchez, V., Fuentes, P., and Rosiles, R. 1997. The effect of neomycin on the kidney function of the horse. J Vet Med 44:201–205.

Garg, S.K., and Garg, B.D. 1989. Disposition kinetics and urinary excretion of gentamicin in buffalo bulls (*Bubalus bubalis*). Vet Res Commun 13:331–337.

Garg, S.K., Verma, S.P., and Garg, B.D. 1991a. Disposition kinetics of gentamicin in buffalo calves (*Bubalus bubalis*) following single intravenous administration. J Vet Pharmacol Therap 14:335–340.

———. 1991b. Pharmacokinetics and urinary excretion of gentamicin in *Bubalus bubalis* calves following intramuscular administration. Res Vet Sci 50:102–105.

Garg, S.K., Verma, S.P., and Uppal, R.P. 1995. Pharmacokinetics of gentamicin following single-dose parenteral administration to goats. Br Vet J 151:453–458.

Garry, F., Chew, D.J., Hoffsis, G.F. 1990a. Urinary indices of renal function in sheep with induced aminoglycoside nephrotoxicosis. Am J Vet Res 51(3):420–427.

———. 1990b. Enzymuria as an index of renal damage in sheep with induced aminoglycoside nephrotoxicosis. Am J Vet Res 51(3): 428–432.

Gemer, O., Zaltztein, E., and Gorodischer, R. 1983. Absorption of orally administered gentamicin in infants with diarrhea. Pediatric Pharmacol 3:119–123.

Geor, R.J., and Papich, M.G. 2003. In Robinson NE (Editor). Once-daily Aminoglycoside Dosing Regimens. Chapter 17.11 Current Therapy in Equine Medicine, 5th Edition, page 850–853.

Gerber, A.U., Craig, W.A., Brugger, H.-P., Feller, C., Vastola, A.P., and Brandel, J. 1983. Impact of dosing intervals on activity of gentamicin and ticarcillin against *Pseudomonas aeruginosa* in granulocytopenic mice. J Infect Dis 147:910–917.

Gerritsen, M.J., Koopmans, M.J., Dekker, T.C.E.M., De Jong, M.C.M., Moerman, A., and Olyboek, T. 1994. Effective treatment with dihydrostreptomycin of naturally infected cows shedding *Leptospira interrogans* serovar hardjo subtype hardjobovis. Am J Vet Res 55(3):339–343.

Gilman, J.M., Davis, L.E., Neff-Davis, C.A., Koritz, G.D., and Baker, G. J. 1987. Plasma concentrations of gentamicin after intramuscular or subcutaneous administration to horses. J Vet Pharmacol Therap 10:101–103.

Giroux, D., Sirois, G., and Martineau, G.P. 1995. Gentamicin pharmacokinetics in newborn and 42-day-old male piglets. J Vet Pharmacol Therap 18:407–412.

Godber, L.M., Walker, R.D., Stein, G.E., Hauptman, J.G., and Derksen, F.J. 1995. Pharmacokinetics, nephrotoxicosis, and in vitro antibacterial activity associated with single versus multiple (three times) daily gentamicin treatments in horses. Am J Vet Res 56(5):613–220.

Golenz, M.R., Wilson, W.D., Carlson, G.P., Craychee, T.J., Mihaly, J.E., and Knox, L. 1994. Effect of route of administration and age on the pharmacokinetics of amikacin administered by the intravenous and intraosseous routes to 3- and 5-day-old foals. Equine Vet J 26:367–373.

Gookin, J.L., Riviere, J.E., Gilger, B.C., and Papich, M.G. 1999. Acute renal failure in four cats treated with paromomycin. JAVMA 215:1821–1823.

Grauer, G.F., Greco, D.S., Behrend, E.N., Mani, I., Fettman, M.J., and Allen, T.A. 1995. Estimation of quantitative enzymuria in dogs with gentamicin-induced nephrotoxicosis using urine enzyme/creatinine ratios from spot urine samples. J Vet Int Med 9(5):324–327.

Grauer, G.F., Green, D.S., Behrend, E.N., Fettman, M.J., Jaenke, R.S., and Allen, T.A. 1994. Effects of dietary protein conditioning on gentamicin-induced nephrotoxicosis in healthy male dogs. Am J Vet Res 55:90–97.

Green, S.L., Conlon, P.D., Mama, K., and Baird, J.D. 1992. Effects of hypoxia and azotaemia on the pharmacokinetics of amikacin in neonatal foals. Equine Vet J 24(6):475–479.

Gronwall, R., Brown, M.P., and Clubb, S. 1989. Pharmacokinetics of amikacin in African grey parrots. Am J Vet Res 50(2):250–252.

Gyselynck, A.M., Forrey, A., and Cutler, R. 1971. Pharmacokinetics of gentamicin distribution and plasma and renal clearance. J Infect Dis 124S:70–76.

Haddad, N.S., Pedersoli, W.M., Ravis, W.R., Fazeli, M.H., and Carson, R.L., Jr. 1985a. Pharmacokinetics of gentamicin at steady-state in ponies: serum, urine, and endometrial concentrations. Am J Vet Res 46:1268–1271.

———. 1985b. Combined pharmacokinetics of gentamicin in pony mares after a single intravenous and intramuscular administration. Am J Vet Res 46:2004–2007.

Haddad, N.S., Ravis, W.R., Pedersoli, W.M., and Carson, R.L., Jr. 1986. Pharmacokinetics of single doses of gentamicin given by intravenous and intramuscular routes to lactating cows. Am J Vet Res 47:808–813.

———. 1987. Pharmacokinetics and residues of gentamicin in lactating cows after multiple intramuscular doses are administered. Am J Vet Res 48:21–27.

Hadi, A.A., Wasfi, I.A., Gadir, F.A., Amir, M.H., Bashir, A.K., and Baggot, J.D. 1994. Pharmacokinetics of tobramycin in the camel. J Vet Pharmacol Therap 17:48–51.

Hammond, P.B. 1953. Dihydrostreptomycin dose-serum level relationships in cattle. JAVMA 122:203–206.

Hauser, G., and Eichberg, J. 1973. Improved conditions for the preservation and extraction of polyphosphoinositides. Biochemica et Biophysiologica Acta 326:201–209.

Holohan, P.D., Elliot, W.C., Grace, E., and Ross, C.R. 1987. Effect of parathyroid hormone on gentamicin plasma membrane binding and tissue accumulation. J Pharmacol Exp Therap 243:893–986.

Horspool, L.J.I., Taylor, D.J., and Mckellar, Q.A. 1994. Plasma disposition of amikacin and interactions with gastrointestinal microflora in Equidae following intravenous and oral administration. J Vet Pharmacol Therap 17:291–298.

Hottendorf, G.H., and Gordon, L.L. 1980. Comparative low-dose nephrotoxicities of gentamicin, tobramycin, and amikacin. Antimicrob Agents Chemother 18:176–181.

Hsu, C.H., Kurtz, T.W., and Weller, J.M. 1977. In vitro uptake of gentamicin by rat renal cortical tissue. Antimicrob Agents Chemother 19:192–194.

Huang, S.M., Huang, Y.C., and Chiou, W.L. 1979. Triexponential disposition pharmacokinetics of gentamicin in rabbits. Res Commun Chem Pathol Pharmacol 26:115–127.

Huber, W.G. 1982. Aminoglycosides, macrolides, lincosamides, polymyxins, chloramphenicol, and antibacterial drugs. In N.H. Booth and L. E. McDonald, eds., Veterinary Pharmacology and Therapeutics, 5th ed., pp. 748–756. Ames: Iowa State Univ Press.

Hull, J.H., Hak, L.J., Koch, G.G., Wargin, W.A., Chi, S.L., and Mattocks, A.M. 1981. Influence of range of renal function and liver disease on the predictability of creatinine clearance. Clin Pharmacol Ther 29:516–521.

Humes, H.D., and Weinberg, J.M. 1980. Importance of membrane bound calcium on the hydroosmotic water flow response of ADH in toad urinary bladder. Clin Res 28:449.

Humes, H.D., Weinberg, J.M., and Knauss, T.C. 1982. Clinical and pathophysiologic aspects of aminoglycoside nephrotoxicity. Am J Kidney Dis 2:5–29.

Hunter, R.P., Brown, S.A., Rollins, J.K., and Nelligan, D.F. 1991. The effects of experimentally induced bronchopneumonia on the pharmacokinetics and tissue depletion of gentamicin in healthy and pneumonic calves. J Vet Pharmacol and Therap 14:276–292.

Itoh, N., and Okada, H. 1993. Pharmacokinetics and potential use of gentamicin in budgerigars (*Melopsittacus undulatus*). J Vet Med 40:194–199.

Jawetz, E. 1984. Aminoglycosides and polymyxins. In B.G. Katzung, ed., Basic and Clinical Pharmacology, 2nd ed., pp. 538–545. Los Altos, CA: Lange Medical Publications.

Jernigan, A.D., Hatch, R.C., Brown, J., and Crowell, W.A. 1988a. Pharmacokinetic and pathological evaluation of gentamicin in cats given a small intravenous dose repeatedly for 5 days. Can J Vet Res 52:177–180.

Jernigan, A.D., Hatch, R.C., and Wilson, R.C. 1988b. Pharmacokinetics of tobramycin in cats. Am J Vet Res 49:608–612.

Jernigan, A.D., Hatch, R.C., Wilson, R.C., Brown, J., and Tulelr, S.M. 1988c. Pharmacokinetics of gentamicin in cats given *Escherichia coli* endotoxin. Am J Vet Res 49:603–607.

Jernigan, A.D., Wilson, R.C., and Hatch, R.C. 1988d. Pharmacokinetics of amikacin in cats. Am J Vet Res 49:355–358.

Jernigan, A.D., Wilson, R.C., Hatch, R.C., and Kemp, D.T. 1988e. Pharmacokinetics of gentamicin after intravenous, intramuscular, and subcutaneous administration in cats. Am J Vet Res 49:32–35.

Johnson, J.G., and Hardin, T.C. 1992. Aminoglycosides, imipenem, and aztreonam. Clin Podiat Med Surg 9(2):443–464.

Johnson, J.H., Wolf, A.M., Johnson, T.L., and Jensen, J. 1993. Gentamicin toxicosis in a North American cougar. JAVMA 203(6):854–856.

Jones, G.F., and Ward, G.E. 1990. Evaluation of systemic administration of gentamicin for treatment of coliform mastitis in cows. JAVMA 197(6):731–735.

Jones, S.L., Wilson, W.D., and Milhalyi, J.E. 1998. Pharmacokinetics of gentamicin in healthy adult horses during intravenous fluid administration. J Vet Pharmacol Therap 21:247–249.

Josepovitz, C., Levine, R., Farraggulla, T., Lane, B., and Kaloyanides, G.J. 1985. [3H]netilmicin binding constants and phospholipid composition of renal plasma membranes of normal and diabetic rats. J Pharmacol Exp Therap 233:298–303.

Josepovitz, C., Pastoriza-Munoz, E., Timmerman, D., Scott, M., Feldman, S., and Kaloyanides, G.J. 1982. Inhibition of gentamicin uptake in rat renal cortex in vivo by aminoglycosides and organic polycations. J Pharmacol Exp Therap 223:314–321.

Just, M., and Habermann, E. 1977. The renal handling of polybasic drugs II: in vitro studies with brush border and lysosomal preparations. Naunyn Schmiedebergs Arch Pharmacol 300:67–76.

Kaloyanides, G.J., and Pastoriza-Munoz, E. 1980. Aminoglycoside nephrotoxicity. Kidney Int 18:571–582.

Karachalios, G.N., Houpas, P., Tziviskou, E., Papalimneou, V., Georgiou, A., Karachaliou, I., and Halkiadake, D. 1998. Prospective randomized study of once-daily versus twice-daily amikacin regimens in patients with systemic infections. Internat J Clin Pharmacol Therap 36(10):561–564.

Katzung, B.G. 1984. Introduction. In B.G. Katzung, ed., Basic and Clinical Pharmacology, 2d ed., p. 2. Los Altos, CA: Lange Medical Publications.

Kaye, D., Levison, M.E., and Labovitz, E.D. 1974. The unpredictability of serum concentrations of gentamicin: pharmacokinetics of gentamicin in patients with nomal and abnormal renal function. J Infect Dis 130:150–154.

Kluwe, W.M., and Hook, J.B. 1978a. Analysis of gentamicin uptake by rat renal cortical slices. Toxicol Appl Pharmacol 45:531–539.

———. 1978b. Functional nephrotoxicity of gentamicin in the rat. Toxicol Appl Pharmacol 45:163–175.

Knauss, T.C., Weinberg, J.M., and Humes, U.D. 1983. Alterations in renal cortical phospholipid content induced by gentamicin, time course, specificity, and subcellular localization. Am J Physiol 244F:535–536.

Kuhar, M.J., Mak, L.I., and Lietman, P.S. 1979. Autoradiographic localization of 3H gentamicin in the proximal renal tubules of mice. Antimicrob Agents Chemother 15:131–133.

Kunin, C.M. 1970. Binding of antibiotics to tissue homogenates. J Infect Dis 121:55–64.

Lancini, G., and Parenti, F., eds. 1982. Antibiotics: An Integrated View, pp. 169–196. New York: Marcel Dekker.

Lashev, L.D., and Mihailov, R. 1994. Pharmacokinetics of apramycin in Japanese quails. J Vet Pharmacol Therap 17:394–395.

Lashev, L.D., Pashov, D.A., and Marinkov, T.N. 1992. Interspecies differences in the pharmacokinetics of kanamycin and apramycin. Vet Res Commun 16:293–300.

Laurent, G., Carlier, M.B., Rollman, B., Van Hoof, F., and Tulkens, P. 1982. Mechanisms of aminoglycoside-induced lysosomal phospholipidosis, in vitro and in vivo studies with gentamicin and amikacin. Biochem Pharmacol 31:3861–3870.

LeCompte, J., Dumont, L., DuSouich, P., and LeLorier, J. 1981. Effect of water deprivation and rehydration on gentamicin disposition in the rat. J Pharmacol Exp Therap 218:231–236.

Lee, M.G., Chen, M.-L., Huang, S.-M., and Chiou, W.L. 1981. Pharmacokinetics of drugs in blood I: unusual distribution of gentamicin. Biopharm Drug Dispos 2:89–97.

Leitner, F., and Price, K.E. 1982. Aminoglycosides under development. In A. Whelton and H.C. Neu, eds., The Aminoglycosides: Microbiology, Clinical Use and Toxicology, pp. 29–64. New York: Marcel Dekker.

Lelievre-Pegorier, M., Sagly, R., Meulemans, A., and Merlet-Benichou, C. 1985. Kinetics of gentamicin in plasma of nonpregnant, pregnant, and fetal guinea pigs and its distribution in fetal tissues. Antimicrob Agents Chemother 28:565–569.

Ling, G.V., Conzelman, G.M., Franti, C.E., and Ruby, A.L. 1981. Urine concentrations of gentamicin, tobramycin, amikacin, and kanamycin after subcutaneous administration to healthy dogs. Am J Vet Res 42:1792–1974.

Ling, G.V., and Ruby, A.L. 1979. Gentamicin for treatment of resistant urinary tract infections in dogs. JAVMA 175:480–481.

Lipsky, J.J., Cheng, L., Sacktor, B., and Lietman, P.S. 1980. Gentamicin uptake by renal tubule brush border membrane vesicles. J Pharmacol Exp Ther 215:390–393.

Lipsky, J.J., and Lietman, P.S. 1980. Neomycin inhibition of adenosine triphosphatase, evidence for a neomycin-phospholipid interaction. Antimicrob Agents Chemother 18:532–535.

———. 1982. Aminoglycoside inhibition of a renal phosphatidylinositol phospholipase C. J Pharmacol Exp Ther 220:287–292.

Luft, F.C., Bloch, R., Sloan, R.S., Yum, M.N., Costello, R., and Maxwell, D.R. 1978. Comparative nephrotoxicity of aminoglycoside antibiotics in rats. J Infect Dis 138:541–545.

Luft, F.C., and Evan, A.P. 1980a. Comparative effects of tobramycin and gentamicin on glomerular ultrastructure. J Infect Dis 142:910–914.

———. 1980b. Glomerular filtration barrier in aminoglycoside induced nephrotoxic acute renal failure. Renal Physiol 3:265–271.

Luft, F.C., and Kleit, S.A. 1974. Renal parenchymal accumulation of aminoglycoside antibiotics in rats. J Infect Dis 130:656–659.

Luft, F.C., Patel, V., Yum, M.N., Patel, B., and Kleit, S.A. 1975. Experimental aminoglycoside nephrotoxicity. J Lab Clin Med 86: 213–220.

Lullmann, H., and Vollmer, B. 1982. An interaction of aminoglycoside antibiotics with Ca binding to lipid monolayers and to biomembranes. Biochem Pharmacol 31:3769–3773.

Mader, D.R., Conzelman, G.M., Jr, and Baggot, J.D. 1985. Effects of ambient temperature on the half-life and dosage regimen of amikacin in the gopher snake. JAVMA 187:1134–1136.

Magdesian, K.G., Hogan, P.M., Cohen, N.D., Brumbaugh, G.W., and Bernard, W.V. 1998. Pharmacokinetics of a high dose of gentamicin administered intravenously or intramuscularly to horses. J Am Vet Med Assoc 213(7):1007–1011.

Mann, H.J., Fuhs, D.W., Awang, R., Ndemo, F.A., and Cerra, F.B. 1987. Altered aminoglycoside pharmacokinetics in critically ill patients with sepsis. Clin Pharmacol 6:148–153.

Martin, T., Papich, M., and Riviere, J.E. 1998. Population pharmacokinetics of gentamicin in horses. Am J Vet Res 59:1589–1598.

Martin-Jimenez, T., and Riviere, J.E. 2001. Mixed effects modeling of the disposition of gentamicin across domestic animal species. J Vet Pharmacol Therap 24:321–332.

Martin, T., and Riviere, J.E. 1998. Population pharmacokinetics in veterinary medicine: potential uses for therapeutic drug monitoring and prediction of tissue residues. J Vet Pharmacol Therap 21:167–189.

Mazze, R.I. 1981. Methoxyflurane nephropathy. In J.B. Hook, ed., Toxicology of the Kidney, pp. 135–149. New York: Raven Press.

McNeil, J.S., Jackson, B., Nelson, L., and Butkas, D.E. 1983. The role of prostaglandins in gentamicin induced nephrotoxicity in the dog. Nephron 33:202–207.

Mealey, K.L., and Boothe, D.M. 1994. Nephrotoxicosis associated with topical administration of gentamicin in a cat. JAVMA 204(12):1919–1921.

Meisner, H. 1981. Effect of gentamicin on the subcellular distribution of renal beta-N-acetylglucosaminidase activity. Biochem Pharmacol 30:2949–2952.

Mercer, H.D., Rollins, K.D., Garth, M.A., and Carter, G.C. 1971. A residue study and comparison of penicillin and dihydrostreptomycin concentration in cattle. JAVMA 158:776–779.

Miller, S.M., Matthews, N.S., Mealey, K.L., Taylor, T.S., and Brumbaugh, G.W. 1994. Pharmacokinetics of gentamicin in mammoth asses. J Vet Pharmacol Therap 17:403–406.

Miranda, J.C., Schimmel, M.S., Mimms, G.M., et al. 1984. Gentamicin absorption during prophylactic use for necrotizing enterocolitis. Devel Pharmacol Therap 7:303–306.

Mitchell, C.J., Bullock, S., and Ross, B.D. 1977. Renal handling of gentamicin and other antibiotics by the isolated perfused rat kidney, mechanisms of nephrotoxicity. J Antimicrob Chemother 3:593–600.

Morin, J.P., Viotte, G., Vandewalle, A., Van Hoof, F., Tulkens, P., and Fillastre, J.P. 1980. Gentamicin-induced nephrotoxicity, a cell biology approach. Kidney Int 18:583–590.

Morin, J.P., Viotte, G., Van Hoof, F., Tulkens, P., Godin, M., and Fillastre, J.P. 1981. Functional, biochemical and morphological events related to gentamicin therapy in rats. Drugs Exp Clin Res 7:345–348.

Nagabhusban, T.L., Miller, G.H., and Weinstein, M.J. 1982. Structure-activity relationships in aminoglycoside-aminocyclitol antibiotics. In A. Whelton and H.C. Neu, eds., The Aminoglycosides: Microbiology, Clinical Use and Toxicology, pp. 3–27. New York: Marcel Dekker.

Nostrandt, A.C., Pedersoli, W.M., Marshall, A.E., Ravis, W.R., and Robertson, B.T. 1991. Ototoxic potential of gentamicin in ponies. Am J Vet Res 52(3):494–498.

Nouws, J.F.M., and Ziv, G. 1978. Tissue distribution and residues of benzylpenicillin and aminoglycoside antibiotics in emergency-slaughtered ruminants. Tijdschrift voor Diergeneeskunde 102:140–151.

Ogden, L., Wilson, R.C., Clark, C.H., and Colby, E.D. 1995. Pharmacokinetics of gentamicin in rabbits. J Vet Pharmacol Therap 18:156–159.

Orsini, J.A., Park, M.I., and Spencer, P.A. 1996. Tissue and serum concentrations of amikacin after intramuscular and intrauterine administration to mares in estrus. Can Vet J (37):157–160.

Orsini, J.A., Soma, L.R., Rourke, J.E., and Park, M. 1985. Pharmacokinetics of amikacin in the horse following intravenous and intramuscular administration. J Vet Pharmacol Therap 8:194–201.

Oukessou, M., and Toutain, P.L. 1992. Effect of dietary nitrogen intake on gentamicin disposition in sheep. J Vet Pharmacol Therap 15: 416–420.

Pastoriza-Munoz, E., Bowman, R.L., and Kaloyanides, G.J. 1979. Renal tubular transport of gentamicin in the rat. Kidney Int 16:440–450.

Pastoriza-Munoz, E., Josepovitz, C., Ramsammy L., and Kaloyanides, G.J. 1987. Renal handling of netilmicin in the rat with streptozotocin-induced diabetes mellitus. J Pharmacol Exp Therap 241:166–173.

Pattyn, V.M., Verpooten, G.A., Guiliano, R.A., Aheng, F., and DeBroe, M.E. 1988. Effect of hyperfiltration, proteinuria and diabetes mellitus on the uptake kinetics of gentamicin in the kidney cortex of rats. J Pharmacol Exp Therap 244:694–698.

Pechere, J.C., and Dugal, R.D. 1979. Clinical pharmacokinetics of aminoglycoside antibiotics. Clin Pharmacokinet 4:170–199.

Pedersoli, W.M., Belmonte, A.A., Purohit, R.C., and Ravis, W.R. 1980. Pharmacokinetics of gentamicin in the horse. Am J Vet Res 41:351–354.

Pedersoli, W.M., Fazeli, M.H., Haddad, N.S., Ravis, W.R., and Carson, R.L., Jr. 1985. Endometrial and serum gentamicin concentrations in pony mares given repeated intrauterine infusions. Am J Vet Res 46:1025–1028.

Pedersoli, W.M., Jackson, J., and Frobish, R.A. 1995. Depletion of gentamicin in the milk of Holstein cows after single and repeated intramammary and parenteral treatments. J Vet Pharmacol Therap 18: 457–463.

Pedersoli, W.M., Ravis, W.R., Askins, D.R., et al. 1990. Pharmacokinetics of single-dose intravenous and intramuscular administration of gentamicin in roosters. Am J Vet Res 51:286–289.

Pedersoli, W.M., Ravis, W.R., Askins, D.R., Krista, L.M., Spano, J.S., Whitesides, J.F., and Tolbert, D.S. 1989. Pharmacokinetics of single doses of gentamicin given intravenously and intramuscularly to turkeys. J Vet Pharmacol Therap 12:124–132.

Pedersoli, W.M., Ravis, W.R., Jackson, J., and Shaikh, B. 1994. Disposition and bioavailability of neomycin in Holstein calves. J Vet Pharmacol Therap 17:5–11.

Pennington, J.E., Dale, D.C., Reynolds, H.Y., and MacLowry, J.D. 1975. Gentamicin sulfate pharmacokinetics: lower levels of gentamicin in blood during fever. J Infect Dis 132:270–275.

Pickerell, J.A., Oehme, F.W., and Cash, W.C. 1993. Ototoxicity in dogs and cats. Sem Vet Med Surg (Sm An) 8(1):42–49.

Poli, A., Sozzi, S., Guidi, G., Bandinelli, and Mancianti, F. 1997. Comparison of aminosidine (paromomycin) and sodium stibogluconate for treatment of canine leishmaniasis. Vet Parasitol 71:263–271.

Powell, S., Thompson, W.L., Luthe, M.A., Stern, R.C., Grossniklaus, D.A., Bloxham, D.D., Groden, D.L., et al. 1983. Once-daily vs. continuous aminoglycoside dosing, efficacy, and toxicity in animal and clinical studies of gentamicin, netilmicin and tobramycin. J Infect Dis 147:918–932.

Prescott, J.F., and Baggot, J.D. 1988. Antimicrobial Therapy in Veterinary Medicine. Boston: Blackwell Scientific Publications.

Ramsammy, L.S., Josepovitz, C., Jones, D., Ling, K.-Y., Lane, B.P., and Kaloyanides, G.J. 1987. Induction of nephrotoxicity by high doses of gentamicin in diabetic rats. Proc Soc Exper and Biol Med 186:306–312.

Ramsay, E.C., and Vulliet, R. 1993. Pharmacokinetic properties of gentamicin and amikacin in the cockatiel. Avian Dis 37:628–634.

Riond, J.-L., Dix, L.P., and Riviere, J.E. 1986. Influence of thyroid function on the pharmacokinetics of gentamicin in pigs. Am J Vet Res 47: 2142–2146.

Riond, J.-L., and Riviere, J.E. 1988. Multiple intravenous dose pharmacokinetics and residue depletion profile of gentamicin in pigs. J Vet Pharmacol Therap 11:210–214.

Ristuccia, A.M. 1984. Aminoglycosides. In A.M. Ristuccia and B.A. Cunha, eds., Antimicrobial Therapy, pp. 305–328. New York: Raven Press.

Rivers, B.J., Walter, P.A., O'Brien, T.D., King, V.L., and Polzin, D.J. 1996. Evaluation of urine gamma-glutamyl transpeptidase-to-creatinine ratio as a diagnostic tool in an experimental model of aminoglycoside-induced acute renal failure in the dog. J Am Animal Hosp Assoc 32:323–336.

Riviere, J.E. 1982. The aminoglycosides. In D.E. Johnston, ed., The Bristol Veterinary Handbook of Antimicrobial Therapy, pp. 186–189. Syracuse: Veterinary Learning Systems.

———. 1985. Aminoglycoside-induced toxic nephropathy. In S.R. Ash and S.A. Thornhill, eds., CRC Handbook of Animal Models of Renal Failure, pp. 145–182. Boca Raton, FL: CRC Press.

Riviere, J.E., and Carver, M.P. 1984. Effects of familial hypothyroidism and subtotal nephrectomy on gentamicin pharmacokinetics in Beagle dogs. Chemotherapy 30:216–220.

Riviere, J.E., and Coppoc, G.L. 1981a. Pharmacokinetics of gentamicin in the juvenile dog. Am J Vet Res 42:1621–1623.

———. 1981b. Determination of cerebrospinal fluid gentamicin in the Beagle using an indwelling cerebral ventricular cannula. Chemotherapy 27:309–312.

Riviere, J.E., Coppoc, G.L., Hinsman, E.J., Carlton, W.W., and Traver, D.S. 1983. Species-dependent gentamicin pharmacokinetics and nephrotoxicity in the young horse. Fund Appl Toxicol 3:448–457.

Riviere, J.E., Craigmill, A.L., and Sundlof, S.F. 1990. Handbook of Comparative Pharmacokinetics and Tissue Residues of Veterinary Antimicrobial Drugs. Boca Raton, FL: CRC Press.

Riviere, J.E., Hinsman, E.J., Coppoc, G.L., and Carlton, W.W. 1981a. Single dose gentamicin nephrotoxicity in the dog: Early functional and ultrastructural changes. Res Commun Chem Pathol Pharmacol 33:403–418.

Riviere, J.E., Martin, T., Sundlof, S., and Craigmill, A.L. 1997. Interspecies allometric analysis of the comparative pharmacokinetics of 44 drugs across veterinary and laboratory species. J Vet Pharmacol Therap 20:453–463.

Riviere, J.E., Silver, G.R., Coppoc, G.L., and Richardson, R.C. 1981b. Gentamicin aerosol therapy in 18 dogs: failure to induce detectable serum concentrations of the drug. JAVMA 179:166–168.

Riviere, J.E., Traver, D.S., and Coppoc, G.L. 1982. Gentamicin toxic nephropathy in horses with disseminated bacterial infection. JAVMA 180:648–651.

Rodvold, K.A., Danziger, L.H., and Quinn, J.P. 1997. Single daily doses of aminoglycosides. Lancet 350:1412.

Rolf, L.L., Setzer, M.D., and Walker, J.L. 1986. Pharmacokinetics and tissue residues in channel catfish, *Ictalurus pluctatus*, given intracardiac and intramuscular injections of gentamicin sulfate. Vet Human Toxicol 28(Suppl 1):25–30.

Rollins, L.D., Teske, R.H., Condon, R.J., and Carter, G.G. 1972. Serum penicillin and dihydrostreptomycin concentrations in horses after intramuscular administration of selected preparations containing those antibiotics. JAVMA 161:490–493.

Ross, L.A., and Finco, D.R. 1981. Relationship of selected clinical renal function tests to glomerular filtration rate and renal blood flow in cats. Am J Vet Res 42:1704–1710.

Ross, M., Parker, R.A., and Elliot, W.C. 1980. Gentamicin induced resistance to ADH stimulated water flow in the toad bladder explained by drug induced pH changes. Clin Res 28:46–64.

Rossier, Y., Divers, T.J., and Sweeney, R.W.W. 1995. Variations in urinary gamma glutamyl transferase/urinary creatinine ratio in horses with or without pleuropneumonia treated with gentamicin. Equine Vet J 27(3):217–220.

Rubin, J., Walker, R.D., Blickenstaff, K., Bodeis-Jones, S., and Zhao, S. 2008. Antimicrobial resistance and genetic characterization of fluoroquinolone resistance of *Pseudomonas aeruginosa* isolated from canine infections. Vet Microbiol 131:164–172.

Ryden, R., and Moore, B.J. 1977. The in vitro activity of apramycin, a new aminocyclitol antibiotic. J Antimicrob Chemother 3:609–613.

Salazar, D.E., Schentag, J.J., and Corcoran, G.B. 1992. Obesity as a risk factor in drug-induced organ injury: toxicokinetics of gentamicin in the obese overfed rat. Drug Metabol Dispos 20(3):402–406.

Sande, M.A., and Mandell, G.L. 1985. Antimicrobial agents: the aminoglycosides. In A.G. Gilman, L.S. Goodman, T.W. Rall, and F. Murad, eds., The Pharmacological Basis of Therapeutics, 7th ed., pp. 1157–1169. New York: Macmillan.

Santschi, E.M., and Papich, M.G. 2000. Pharmacokinetics of gentamicin in mares in late pregnancy and early lactation. Journal of Veterinary Pharmacology and Therapeutics 23:359–363.

Sastrasinh, M., Knauss, T.C., Weinberg, J.M., and Humes, H.D. 1982a. Identification of the aminoglycoside binding site in rat renal brush border membranes. J Pharmacol Exp Therap 222:350–355.

Sastrasinh, M., Weinberg, J.M., and Humes, H.D. 1982b. Effect of gentamicin on calcium uptake by renal mitochondria. Life Sci 26: 2309–2315.

Sawchuk, R.J., Zaske, D.E., Cipolle, R.J., Wargin, W.A., and Strate, R.G. 1977. Kinetic model for gentamicin dosing with the use of the individual patient parameters. Clin Pharmacol Therap 21:362–369.

Schacht, J. 1978. Purification of polyphosphoinositides by chromatography on immobilized neomycin. J Lipid Res 19:1063–1067.

———. 1979. Isolation of an aminoglycoside receptor from guinea pig inner ear tissues and kidney. Arch Otorhinolaryngol 224:129–134.

Schentag, J.J., and Jusko, W.J. 1977. Renal clearance and tissue accumulation of gentamicin. Clin Pharmacol Therap 22:364–370.

Schentag, J.J., Jusko, W.J., Plaut, M.E., Cumbo, T.J., Vance, J.W., and Abrutyn, E. 1977a. Tissue persistence of gentamicin in man. JAVMA 238:327–329.

Schentag, J.J., Jusko, W.J., Vance, J.W., et al. 1977b. Gentamicin disposition and tissue accumulation on multiple dosing. J Pharmacokin Biopharma 5:559–579.

Schentag, J.J., Lasezkay, G., Cumbo, T.J., Plaut, M.E., and Jusko, W.J. 1978. Accumulation pharmacokinetics of tobramicin. Antimicrob Agents Chemother 13:649–656.

Schumacher, J., Wilson, R.C., Spano, J.S., Hammond, L.S., McGuire, J., Duran, S.H., Kemppainene, R.J., and Hughes, F.E. 1991. Effect of diet on gentamicin-induced nephrotoxicosis in horses. Am J Vet Res 52(8):1274–1278.

Senckjian, H.O., Knight, T.F., and Weinman, E.J. 1981. Micropuncture study of the handling of gentamicin by the rat kidney. Kidney Int 19:416–423.

Setzer, M.D. 1985. Pharmacokinetics of gentamicin in channel fish (*Ictalurus punctatus*). Am J Vet Res 46:2558–2561.

Sheth, A.V., Senckjian, H.O., Babino, H., Knight, T.F., and Weinman, E. J. 1981. Renal handling of gentamicin by the Munich-Wistar rat. Am J Physiol 241F:645–648.

Shille, V.M., Brown, M.P., Gronwall, R., and Hock, H. 1985. Amikacin sulfate in the cat: serum, urine, and uterine tissue concentrations. Theriogenology 23:829–839.

Short, C.R., Hardy, M.L., Clarke, C.R., Taylor, W., and Baggot, J.D. 1986. The nephrotoxic potential of gentamicin in the cat: a pharmacokinetic and histopathologic investigation. J Vet Pharmacol Therap 9: 325–329.

Siddique, I.H., Loken, K.I., and Hoyt, H.H. 1965. Concentrations of neomycin, dihydrostreptomycin and polymyxin in milk after intramuscular or intramammary administration. JAVMA 146:594–599.

Silverblatt, F.J. 1982. Autoradiographic studies of intracellular aminoglycoside disposition in the kidney. In A. Whelton and H.C. Neu, eds., The Aminoglycosides: Microbiology, Clinical Use, and Toxicology, pp. 223–233. New York: Marcel Dekker.

Silverblatt, F.J., and Kuehn, C. 1979. Autoradiography of gentamicin uptake by the rat proximal tubule cell. Kidney Int 15:335–345.

Silverman, M., and Mahon, W. 1979. Gentamicin interaction in vivo with luminal and antiluminal nephron surfaces of dog kidney. Abstracts—Am Soc Nephrol 12:89A.

Simmons, C.F., Jr, Bogusky, R.T., and Humes, H.D. 1980. Inhibitory effects of gentamicin on renal mitochondria oxidative phosphorylation. J Pharmacol Exp Ther 214:709–715.

Sketris, I., Lesar, T., Zaske, D.E., and Cipolle, R.J. 1981. Effect of obesity on gentamicin pharmacokinetics. J Clin Pharmacol 21:288–293.

Smeltzer, B.D., Schwartzman, M.S., and Bertino, J.S., Jr. 1988. Amikacin pharmacokinetics during continuous peritoneal dialysis. Antimicrob Agents Chemother 32:236–240.

Sojka, J.E., and Brown, S.A. 1986. Pharmacokinetic adjustment of gentamicin dosing in horses with sepsis. JAVMA 189:784–789.

Souliere, C.R., Goodman, D.B.P., and Appel, G.B. 1978. Gentamicin selectively inhibits antidiuretic hormone induced water flow in the toad urinary bladder. Kidney Int 14:733.

Strain, G.M., Merchant, S.R., Neer, T.M., and Tedford, B.L. 1995. Ototoxicity assessment of a gentamicin sulfate otic preparation in dogs. Am J Vet Res 56(4):532–538.

Strausbaugh, L.J., and Brinker, G.S. 1983. Effect of osmotic blood-brain disruption on gentamicin penetration into the cerebrospinal fluid and brain of normal rats. Antimicrob Agents Chemother 24:147–150.

Sveska, K.J., Roffe, B.D., Solomon, D.K., and Hoffmann, R.P. 1985. Outcome of patients treated by an aminoglycoside pharmacokinetic dosing service. Am J Hosp Pharm 42:2472–2478.

Swann, J.D., Ulrich, R., and Acosta, D. 1990. Lack of changes in cytosolic ionized calcium in primary cultures of rat kidney cortical cells exposed to cytotoxic concentrations of gentamicin. Toxicol Appl Pharmacol 106:38–47.

Sweeney, R.W., Divers, T.J., and Rossier, Y. 1992. Disposition of gentamicin administered intravenously to horses with sepsis. JAVMA 200(4): 503–506.

Takahashi, Y., Kido, Y., Naoi, M., and Kokue, E.-I. 1985. The serial biopsy technique for estimation of drug residue in calf kidney using gentamicin as a model drug. Japn J Vet Sci 47:179–183.

Teixeira, R.B., Kelley, J., Alpert, H., Pardo, V., and Vaamonde, C.A. 1982. Complete protection from gentamicin-induced acute renal failure in the diabetes mellitus rat. Kidney Int 21:600–612.

Tobin, T. 1979. Pharmacology review: streptomycin, gentamicin and the aminoglycoside antibiotics. J Equine Med Surg 4:206–212.

Tointon, M.M., Job, M.L., Pletier, T.T., Murphy, J.E., and Ward, E.S. 1987. Alterations in aminoglycoside volume of distribution in patients below ideal body weight. Clin Pharmacy 6:160–162.

Trnovec, T., Bezek, S., Kállay, Z., Durisová, M., and Navarová, J. 1984. Non-linear accumulation of gentamicin in guinea-pig kidney. J Antimicrob Ther 14:543–548.

Tudor, R.A., Papich, M.G., and Redding, W.R. 1999. Gentamicin disposition and dosage determination of once daily administration of gentamicin sulfate in horses after abdominal surgery. J Am Vet Med Assoc 215(4):503–506.

Tulkens, P., and Trouet, A. 1978. The uptake and intracellular accumulation of aminoglycoside antibiotics in lysosomes of cultured rat fibroblasts. Biochem Pharmacol 27:415–424.

Vaamonde, C.A., Bier, R.T., Guovea, W., Alpert, H., Kelley, J., and Pardo, V. 1984. Effect of duration of diabetes on the protection observed in the diabetic rat against gentamicin-induced acute renal failure. Mineral Electrolyte Metab 10:209–216.

Vandewalle, A., Farman, N., Morin, J.P., Fillastre, J.P., Liatt, P.Y., and Bonvalet, J.P. 1981. Gentamicin incorporation along the nephron, autoradiographic study on isolated tubules. Kidney Int 19:529–539.

Waitz, J.A., Moss, E.L., and Weinstein, M.J. 1971. Aspects of the chronic toxicity of gentamicin sulfate in cats. J Infect Dis 124S:125–129.

Weinberg, J.M., Harding, P.G., and Humes, H.D. 1980. Mechanisms of gentamicin induced dysfunction of renal cortical mitochrondria II: effects on mitochondrial monovalent cation transport. Arch Biochem Biophys 205:232–239.

Weinberg, J.M., and Humes, B.D. 1980. Mechanisms of gentamicin induced dysfunction of renal cortical mitochondria I: effects on mitochondrial respiration. Arch Biochem Biophys 205:222–231.

Weinberg, J.M., Simmons, C.F., Jr, and Humes, H.D. 1990. Alterations of mitochondrial respiration induced by aminoglycoside antibiotics. Res Commun Chem Pathol Pharmacol 27:521–531.

Weisman, D., Herrig, J., and McWeeny, O. 1982. Tissue distribution of gentamicin in lambs: effect of postnatal age and acute hypoxemia. Devel Pharmacol Therap 5:194–206.

Welles, J.S., Emmerson, J.L., Gibson, W.R., Nickander, R., Owen, N.V., and Anderson, R.C. 1973. Preclinical toxicology studies with tobramycin. Toxicol Appl Pharmacol 25:398–409.

Whitehair, K.J., Blevins, T.L., Fessler, J.F., Van Sickle, D.C., White, M.R., and Bill, R.P. 1992a. Regional perfusion of the equine carpus for antibiotic delivery. Vet Surg 21(4):279–285.

Whitehair, K.J., Bowersock, T.L., Blevins, W.E., Fessler, J.F., White, M.R., and Van Sickle, D.C. 1992b. Regional limb perfusion for antibiotic treatment of experimentally induced septic arthritis. Vet Surg 21(5):367–373.

Whittem, T., Firth, E.C., Hodge, H., and Turner, K. 1996. Pharmacokinetic interactions between repeated dose phenylbutazone and gentamicin in the horse. Journal of Veterinary Pharmacology and Therapeutics 19:454–459.

Wichtel, M.G., Breuhaus, B.A., and Aucoin, D. 1992. Relation between pharmacokinetics of amikacin sulfate and sepsis score in clinically normal and hospitalized neonatal foals. JAVMA 200(9):1339–1343.

Williams, P.D., Holohan, P.D., and Ross, C.R. 1981a. Gentamicin nephrotoxicity I: acute biochemical correlates in rats. Toxicol Appl Pharmacol 61:234–242.

———. 1981b. Gentamicin nephrotoxicity II: plasma membrane changes. Toxicol Appl Pharmacol 61:243–251.

Williams, P.D., and Hottendorf, G.H. 1985. Inhibition of renal membrane binding and nephrotoxicity of gentamicin by polysaparagine and polyaspartic acid in the rat. Res Commun Chem Pathol Pharmacol 47:317–320.

———. 1986. [3H]Gentamicin uptake in brush border and basolateral membrane vesicles from rat kidney cortex. Biochem Pharmacol 35:2253–2256.

Wilson, R.C., Duran, S.H., Horton, C.R., Jr, and Wright, L.C. 1989. Bioavailability of gentamicin in dogs after intramuscular or subcutaneous injections. Am J Vet Res 50:1748–1750.

Wilson, R.C., Goetsch, D.D., and Huber, T.L. 1984. Influence of endotoxin-induced fever on the pharmacokinetics of gentamicin in ewes. Am J Vet Res 45:2495–2497.

Wilson, R.C., Moore, J.N., and Eakle, N. 1983. Gentamicin pharmacokinetics in horses given small doses of *Escherichia coli* endotoxin. Am J Vet Res 44:1746–1749.

Wilson, R.C., Whelan, S.C., Coulter, D.B., Mahaffey, E.A., Mahaffey, M.B., and Huber, T.L. 1981. Kinetics of gentamicin after intravenous, intramuscular, and intratracheal administration in sheep. Am J Vet Res 42:1901–1904.

Wright, L.C., Horton, C.R., Jernigan, A.D., Wilson, R.C., and Clark, C. H. 1991. Pharmacokinetics of gentamicin after intravenous and subcutaneous injection in obese cats. J Vet Pharmacol Therap 14:96–100.

Yates, R.A., Mitchard, M., and Wise, R. 1978. Disposition studies with amikacin after rapid intravenous and intramuscular administration to human volunteers. J Antimicrob Chemother 4:335–341.

Zaske, D.E. 1980. Aminoglycosides. In W.E. Evans, J.J. Schentag, and W.J. Jusko, eds., Applied Pharmacokinetics and Therapeutics, pp. 210–239. San Francisco.

Zaske, D.E., Cipolle, R.J., Rotschafer, J.C., Solem, L.D., Mosier, N.R., and Strate, R.G. 1982. Gentamicin pharmacokinetics in 1,640 patients: method for control of serum concentrations. Antimicrob Agents Chemother 21:407–411.

Ziv, G. 1977. Comparative clinical pharmacology of amikacin and kanamycin in dairy calves. Am J Vet Res 38:337–340.

Ziv, G., Bor, A., Soback, S., Elad, D., and Nouws, J.F.M. 1985. Clinical pharmacology of apramycin in calves. J Vet Pharmacol Therap 8:95–104.

Ziv, G., Kurtz, B., Risenberg, R., and Glickman, A. 1995. Serum and milk concentrations of apramycin in lactating cows, ewes and goats. J Vet Pharmacol Therap 18:346–351.

Ziv, G., Nouws, J.F.M., and Van Ginneken, C.A.M. 1982. The pharmacokinetics and tissue levels of polymyxin B, colistin, and gentamicin in calves. J Vet Pharmacol Therap 5:45–58.

Ziv, G., and Sulman, F.G. 1974. Distribution of aminoglycoside antibiotics in blood and milk. Res in Vet Sci 17:68–71.

CHAPTER 37

CHLORAMPHENICOL AND DERIVATIVES, MACROLIDES, LINCOSAMIDES, AND MISCELLANEOUS ANTIMICROBIALS

MARK G. PAPICH AND JIM E. RIVIERE

Several of the drugs discussed in this chapter do not fit into other categories or are not important enough for a separate chapter. They are grouped together here because they have certain features in common: they inhibit protein synthesis in bacteria (with macrolides, lincosamides, and chloramphenicol acting at a similar site), are relatively broad-spectrum, and have a large volume of distribution (i.e., they achieve effective concentrations in most tissues).

Some of these drugs are not as common or as available as in previous years. Some older drugs have given way to newer derivatives. For example, newer macrolides such as azithromycin have replaced erythromycin for some uses in small-animal medicine, and florfenicol has replaced chloramphenicol for use in cattle. Earlier editions of this text should be consulted for more in-depth discussion of these older agents.

CHLORAMPHENICOL

CHEMICAL FEATURES. Chloramphenicol chemically is d-(-)-threo-1-*p*-nitrolphenyl-2-dichloroacetamido 1,3-propanediol (Fig. 37.1), has a pK_a of 5.5, and was first isolated from the soil organism *Streptomyces venezuelae* in 1947. The chloramphenicol used today is manufactured synthetically. Chloramphenicol is slightly soluble in water and freely soluble in propylene glycol and organic solvents. Chloramphenicol is a broad-spectrum antibiotic, affecting gram-positive and gram-negative organisms, aerobic and anaerobic bacteria, and many intracellular organisms. Chloramphenicol has three functional groups that largely determine its biological activity: the *p*-nitrophenol group, the dichloroacetyl group, and the alcoholic group at the third carbon of the propanediol chain (Yunis 1988). Replacement of the *p*-NO_2 group by a methylsulfonyl (HC_3-SO_2) moiety produces thiamphenicol and a substantial change in biological activity, while modification of the propanediol group by the addition of a fluorine atom results in the synthesis of florfenicol. Both thiamphenicol and florfenicol will be discussed in more detail later in this chapter. Loss of the dichloroacetyl group altogether results in loss of biological activity (Yunis 1988; Hird and Knifton 1986).

DRUG FORMULATIONS. Three formulations of chloramphenicol have been administered for systemic therapy in animals. Chloramphenicol base is the unconjugated form of chloramphenicol and is available only in an oral formulation. Chloramphenicol base has a bitter taste, so to increase the palatability, the ester chloramphenicol palmitate was manufactured as an alternative oral formulation. Chloramphenicol palmitate is insoluble in water but soluble in acetone and ether. Before systemic absorption, chloramphenicol palmitate is hydrolyzed in the small intestine by esterases, which release the free base form of chloramphenicol to systemic circulation. Similarly, chloramphenicol succinate is a formulation for parenteral use that requires hydrolysis reactions in the plasma to produce the active drug (Ambrose 1984). The succinate form of the drug is freely soluble in water and can be administered intravenously (IV) or intramuscularly (IM). Topical formulations of chloramphenicol have been used for otic and ophthalmic use. Because of the decreased use of chloramphenicol in human medicine, some of the formulations mentioned above are not as readily available today, if at all.

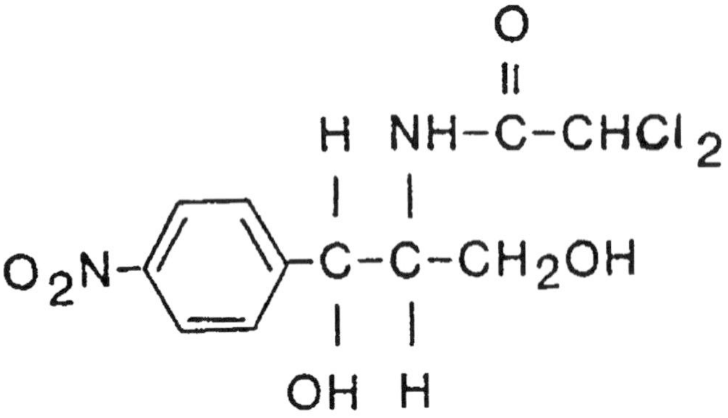

FIG. 37.1 The chemical structure of chloramphenicol.

MECHANISM OF ACTION. Chloramphenicol inhibits protein synthesis. Its biologic activity is due to interference with peptidyltransferase activity at the 50S ribosomal subunit, which is near the site of action of macrolide antibiotics and for which there can be competition (Yunis 1988). Because of the interaction with peptidyltransferase, binding with the amino acid substrate cannot occur, and peptide bond formation is inhibited. Chloramphenicol affects mammalian protein synthesis to some degree, especially mitochondrial protein synthesis. Mammalian mitochondrial ribosomes have a strong resemblance to bacterial ribosomes (both are 70S), with the mitochondria of the bone marrow especially susceptible. Prolonged administration to animals has been associated with a dose-related bone marrow suppression, especially in cats (Watson 1980).

SPECTRUM OF ACTIVITY. Chloramphenicol has a broad spectrum of activity. It is active against *Staphylococcus pseudintermedius* (*Staphylococcus intermedius* has been renamed *Staph. pseudintermedius* by most laboratories), *S. aureus*, streptococci, and some gram-negative bacteria, such as *Pasteurella multocida*, *Mannheimia haemolyticia* (previously called *Pasteurella haemolytica*), and *Histophilus somni* (previously named *Haemophilus somnus*) *Escherichia coli*, *Proteus vulgaris*, and *Salmonella* spp. may be susceptible, but resistance can occur with many gram-negative bacteria, especially the Enterobacteraceae. Resistance by staphylococci may occur with increased use. Anaerobic bacteria, *Mycoplasma* spp., and many rickettsiae also are susceptible. The Clinical Laboratory Standards Institute (CLSI, 2007; formerly called NCCLS) approved break point for susceptibility is ≤4 μg/ml for streptococci and ≤8 μg/ml for other organisms (Watts et al. 1999).

BACTERIAL RESISTANCE. Four mechanisms of resistance to chloramphenicol have been described (Yunis 1988). The most important is plasmid mediated due to the presence of the chloramphenicol acetyltransferase enzyme, which catalyzes a reaction that modifies the hydroxyl groups. Chloramphenicol acetyltransferase was reviewed by Shaw and Leslie (1991). Other mechanisms of resistance include decreased bacterial cell wall permeability, altered binding capabilities at the 50S ribosomal subunit, and inactivation by nitroreductases.

PHARMACOKINETICS

Absorption and Distribution. The pharmacokinetic parameters of chloramphenicol have been studied in several animal species and are summarized in Table 37.1. Chloramphenicol in animals is well absorbed via both oral and parenteral routes, with a few notable species exceptions. Plasma half-lives vary, ranging from 0.9 hours in ponies to 5.1 hours in the cat (Davis et al. 1972). Watson (1992) reports that fasted cats showed differences in absorption between the chloramphenicol tablets and the chloramphenicol palmitate suspension. The liquid formulation showed a lower systemic drug availability, indicating that hydrolysis of the palmitate form is necessary and that there is a higher risk of drug failure when the palmitate suspension is used to treat sick cats that are also not eating. In ruminants, microflora present in the ruminant forestomach tend to metabolize chloramphenicol faster than it can be absorbed, making chloramphenicol administered orally of little systemic therapeutic use in ruminant animals. This point is rather moot since administration of chloramphenicol to food animals in the United States is currently illegal (discussed in more detail in Chapter 54). In most animals, 30–46% of chloramphenicol is bound to plasma proteins, leaving much of the drug in the free and active form. Chloramphenicol is widely distributed to many tissues of the body due to its nonionized state and high lipophilicity, enabling it to cross lipid bilayers quite easily. The volume of distribution (Vd) is typically greater than 1.0 l/kg and has been measured at 1–2.5 l/kg (Table 37.1). Chloramphenicol reaches sufficient concentrations in most tissues of the body, including the eye, central nervous system (CNS), heart, lung, prostate, saliva, liver, and spleen, among others (Ambrose 1984; Hird and Knifton 1986). Chloramphenicol concentrations in cerebrospinal fluid (CSF) are approximately 50% of corresponding plasma concentrations. Chloramphenicol can also cross the placental barrier in pregnant animals and can diffuse into the milk of nursing animals.

Metabolism and Excretion. Chloramphenicol is metabolized by the liver after absorption into the systemic circulation. One of the largest drawbacks to chloramphenicol administration is the rapid metabolic clearance, producing short half-lives in many species and necessity for frequent administration. In dogs, it should be administered three times daily. In horses, because of rapid elimination rates, tissue fluid concentrations persisted for only 3 hours after IV administration of chloramphenicol sodium succinate (Brown et al. 1984). Phase II glucuronidation is the principal pathway for the hepatic biotransformation of chloramphenicol, with the principal metabolite being chloramphenicol glucuronide. A few hydrolysis products have also been identified. Cats excrete chloramphenicol more slowly than other animals, perhaps owing to the cat's deficiency in some glucuronidase enzymes. One report notes that 25% of the total dose of chloramphenicol is excreted in the urine in the active form in cats compared to 6% in normal dogs (Hird and Knifton 1986). Most of the absorbed chloramphenicol (approximately 80%) is excreted into the urine as inactive metabolites via tubular secretion.

When chloramphenicol is administered to young animals, there may initially be reduced excretion. Calves showed decreased hepatic glucuronidation of chloramphenicol soon after birth, but this metabolic pathway matured quickly. Calves also showed higher oral availability than older animals because of immaturity of the rumen, with a marked decrease in oral absorption as the calves age (Burrows et al. 1984). Brumbaugh et al. (1983) found that in neonatal horses, elimination and Vd did not differ from adults. Bioavailability in foals was 83%, with an oral half-life of 2.54 hours. A dose of 50 mg/kg orally every 6 hours should be adequate for treating most susceptible bacteria in foals.

ADVERSE EFFECTS AND PRECAUTIONS. Bone marrow suppression has been the most important adverse

TABLE 37.1 Selected serum pharmacokinetic parameters of chloramphenicol in animals

Species	Dose (mg/kg)	Route	Formulation	Half-life ($t_{1/2\beta}$) (hr)	V_d (l/kg)	Comments	Reference
Dogs	22	IV	Base	4.2	1.77	Dissolved in 50% aqueous solution of N,N,di-methylacetamide	Davis et al. 1972
Felines	22	IV	Base	5.1	2.36	Dissolved in 50% aqueous solution of N,N,di-methylacetamide	Davis et al. 1972
Sheep	30	IV	Base	1.702	0.691		Dagorn et al. 1990
	30	SC	Base	17.93	NA		Dagorn et al. 1990
	30	IM	Base	2.71	NA		Dagorn et al. 1990
Adult swine	22	IV	Base	1.3	1.05	Dissolved in 50% aqueous solution of N,N,di-methylacetamide	Davis et al. 1972
Piglets	25	IV	Base	12.7	0.9411	Normal piglets	Martin and Weise 1988
	25	IV	Base	17.2	0.9549	Colostrum-deprived piglets	Martin and Weise 1988
Goats	25	IV	Succinate	1.22	1.683	Nonfebrile animals	Kume and Garg 1986
	25	IV	Succinate	1.29	1.962	Febrile animals	Kume and Garg 1986
	25	IM	Succinate	1.46	3.019	Nonfebrile animals	Kume and Garg 1986
	25	IM	Succinate	1.45	2.769	Febrile animals	Kume and Garg 1986
Goats	22	IV	Base	2.0	1.33	Dissolved in 50% aqueous solution of N,N,di-methylacetamide	Davis et al. 1972
Goats	10	IV	Succinate	1.47	0.312	Normal animals	Abdullah and Baggot 1986
	10	IV	Succinate	3.97	0.287	Starved animals	Abdullah and Baggot 1986
Goats	22	IV	Base	2.0	1.33	Dissolved in 50% aqueous solution of N,N,di-methylacetamide	Davis et al. 1972
Goats	10	IV	Succinate	1.47	0.312	Normal animals	Abdullah and Baggot 1986
	10	IV	Succinate	3.97	0.287	Starved animals	Abdullah and Baggot 1986
Cattle	40	IV	Base	2.81	0.351		Sanders et al. 1988
	90	IM	Base	1.345	NA	2 doses 48 hr apart	Sanders et al. 1988
	90	SC	Base	1.153	NA	2 doses 48 hr apart	Sanders et al. 1988
Calves	30	IV	Base	3.98	1.208	Age not reported; average weight = 73 kg	Guillot and Sanders 1991
Calves							
(1 day old)	25	IV	Base in PG vehicle	7.56	1.031		Burrows et al. 1983
(7 days old)	25	IV	Base in PG vehicle	5.96	0.808		Burrows et al. 1983
(14 days old)	25	IV	Base in PG vehicle	4.0	0.903		Burrows et al. 1983
(28 days old)	25	IV	Base in PG vehicle	3.69	0.69		Burrows et al. 1983
(9 months old)	25	IV	Base in PG vehicle	2.47	1.38		Burrows et al. 1983
Horses	22	IV	Base in PG vehicle	0.51–0.78	0.86–1.26		Varma et al. 1987
Ponies	22	IV	Base	0.9	1.02	Dissolved in 50% aqueous solution of N,N,di-methylacetamide	Davis et al. 1972
Foals							
(1 day old)	25	IV	Succinate	5.29	1.1		Adamson et al. 1991
(3 days old)	25	IV	Succinate	1.35	0.759		Adamson et al. 1991
(7 days old)	25	IV	Succinate	0.61	0.491		Adamson et al. 1991
(14 days old)	25	IV	Succinate	0.51	0.426		Adamson et al. 1991
(42 days old)	25	IV	Succinate	0.34	0.362		Adamson et al. 1991
(1–9 days old)	50	IV	Succinate	0.95	1.6	After oral suspension administered oral, availability was 83% and half-life of 2.54 hr	Brumbaugh et al. 1983
Rabbits	100	IV	Succinate	1.1575	NA		Mayers et al. 1991
Chickens	20	IV	Succinate	8.32	0.24	Normal animals	Atef et al. 1991a
	20	IV	Succinate	26.21	0.3	*E. coli*-infected animals	Atef et al. 1991a
	20	IM	Succinate	7.84	0.44		Atef et al. 1991a
	20	PO	Succinate	8.26	0.41		Atef et al. 1991a

Note: NA = data not available; PG = propylene glycol.

effect associated with chloramphenicol administration to people. Bone marrow injury from chloramphenicol takes two forms (Yunis 1988). The first type is the most common and involves a dose-related suppression of the bone marrow precursor erythroid series. This toxicosis is reversible. The evidence suggests that this bone marrow suppression is the result of mitochondrial injury and the suppression of mitochondrial protein synthesis in bone marrow cells. Studies in animal species have described the pathology of bone marrow cell toxicity as a decreased entry into S phase in dividing bone marrow cells, vacuolation of the myeloid and erythroid series precursor cells, and inhibition of erythroid and granulocytic colony forming units (IARC 1976, 1990). In both the dog and the cat, dose-related bone marrow suppression is possible. However, signs of toxicity reverse when chloramphenicol therapy is discontinued.

The second type of bone marrow toxicity, aplastic anemia, has been described in people but not in animals. In people, it is rare and independent of dose and treatment duration, and it causes bone marrow aplasia, chiefly characterized by a profound and persistent pancytopenia. This aplastic anemia occurs in approximately 1:10,000 to 1:45,000 humans who receive chloramphenicol. There may be a genetic predisposition to this form of toxicity. It appears that the para-nitro group of the chloramphenicol molecule is responsible for this more serious form of bone marrow toxicity. The para-nitro group undergoes nitroreduction, leading to the production of nitrosochloramphenicol and other toxic intermediates, which trigger the stem cell damage in humans (IARC 1976, 1990; Yunis 1988). Modification of the molecule to eliminate the para-nitro group to produce either thiamfenicol or florfenicol reduces the risk of chloramphenicol-associated aplastic anemia.

Chloramphenicol-induced aplastic anemia in humans is important from a food-animal residue standpoint. If chloramphenicol is used to treat infections in food animals, it is possible that low concentrations of chloramphenicol in milk, meat, and other edible tissues from the animals will be consumed by people and cause aplastic anemia in susceptible individuals. Chloramphenicol residues have been known to persist for prolonged periods in food animals (Korsrud et al. 1987). Even though the amount consumed may be small, the reaction is not concentration-dependent. Thus, there is a public health risk for individuals consuming these products. For this and other reasons, the use of chloramphenicol in food-producing animals has been banned in the United States. The hazards of using chloramphenicol in food animals have also been reviewed (Settepani 1984; Lacey 1984).

Other adverse effects caused by chloramphenicol in animals are uncommon. However, young animals and cats are the most sensitive to intoxication due to impaired glucuronidation pathways. Cats given 60 and 120 mg/kg/day PO every 8 hours for 21 and 14 days (respectively) showed clinical signs of depression, dehydration, reduced fluid intake, weight loss, emesis, and diarrhea. Bone marrow hypoplasia was also documented in addition to pancytopenia (Watson 1980). Other investigators (Penny et al. 1967, 1970) administered to cats 50 mg/kg/day IM, with the cats showing marked depression and inappetence by day 7 of administration, severe bone marrow changes by day 14, and becoming extremely ill by day 21. Dogs showed milder signs of toxicity, mainly gastrointestinal (GI), but doses required to produce these effects were higher than what was administered to cats (225 mg/kg for 2 weeks).

DRUG INTERACTIONS. Chloramphenicol is an inhibitor of the cytochrome P450 drug-metabolizing enzymes. It is not known which specific family of enzymes is inhibited in animals. However, chloramphenicol administration to dogs has been shown to inhibit drug metabolism, and in dogs and cats, it prolongs pentobarbital anesthesia (Adams and Dixit 1970). Sleeping times may be prolonged by 120% in dogs and 260% in cats due to impaired metabolism of pentobarbital. Chloramphenicol also may inhibit the metabolism of digoxin, phenobarbital, propofol, primidone, and perhaps other drugs metabolized by the same enzymes. Erythromycin and chloramphenicol compete for the same site of action on bacteria, and both drugs used together may produce antibacterial antagonism.

CLINICAL USE. Chloramphenicol has been used for treatment of a wide range of susceptible microbial infections, including those caused by salmonellae, intracellular and extracellular bacteria, rickettsiae, and mycoplasmata; infections of the eyes and CNS; and infections due to anaerobic organisms (IARC 1976, 1990). One of the reasons for its popularity has been the high lipophilicity. Chloramphenicol readily penetrates cells, making it active against intracellular bacteria, and it penetrates tissues that otherwise are difficult to treat, such as the CNS. Chloramphenicol was shown in one study to be equally effective for treatment of Rocky Mountain spotted fever in dogs as enrofloxacin and tetracyclines (Breitschwerdt et al. 1990). Although less popular than it once was, chloramphenicol has been used to treat infections caused by *Staphylococcus* spp., streptococci, *Brucella* spp., *Pasteurella* spp., *E. coli, Proteus* spp., *Salmonella* spp., *Bacillus anthracis, Arcanobacterium pyogenes, Erysipelothrix rhusiopathiae,* and *Klebsiella pneumoniae*. It is consistently active against anaerobic bacteria.

Chloramphenicol has been popular for treatment of infections of the CNS (encephalitis, meningitis) because it is able to cross the inflamed or uninflamed blood-brain barrier and attain therapeutic concentrations in the CSF and the brain. Despite the popularity for this use, some experts have suggested that since chloramphenicol is merely bacteriostatic against gram-negative pathogens, and there is a lack of phagocytes or immunoglobulins in CSF, chloramphenicol is not well suited to treat serious infections of the CNS (Rahal and Simberkoff 1979).

Chloramphenicol attains high concentrations in the eye when given systemically or after topical application on the cornea and is useful in treating susceptible bacterial conjunctivitis, panophthalmitis, endophthalmitis, and bacterial diseases of the cornea (Conner and Gupta 1973). Topical formulations are not as readily available owing to the risk of aplastic anemia (discussed previously), which can be caused by topical exposure. Florfenicol has been administered systemically for treating eye infections in cattle (see below.)

Chloramphenicol has been used to treat bacterial infections of the respiratory tract because it may have better penetration across the blood-bronchus barrier into respiratory secretions and respiratory lining fluid than more polar or less lipophilic antibiotics. Respiratory infections are among the infections in horses treated with oral chloramphenicol.

Chloramphenicol is one of the few drugs that can be administered orally to horses with safety. It achieves moderate systemic absorption of 21–40% (Gronwall et al. 1986) and has no serious adverse effects on the equine digestive system. However, oral administration resulted in intestinal mucosal damage and diarrhea in calves and reduced glucose absorption (Rollin et al. 1986). For treatment in horses, tablets or capsules are mixed with substances like molasses or corn syrup to facilitate oral administration. Chloramphenicol has been administered to horses for respiratory infections, pleuritis, CNS infections, and joint infections. Despite this widespread use, because of rapid elimination and poor-to-moderate absorption, one author has discouraged its use (Gronwall et al. 1986), but for foals oral doses of 50 mg/kg every 4–12 hours (frequency of administration was dependent on the minimum inhibitory concentration (MIC) of the pathogen) have been recommended (Brumbaugh et al. 1983).

Chloramphenicol has been administered to exotic animals, especially reptiles and amphibians, to treat a variety of infections (Clark et al. 1985). Chloramphenicol administration in 15 species of birds was examined, and the investigators concluded that after IM injections of 50 mg/kg, chloramphenicol would produce adequate concentrations to treat susceptible bacteria for 8–12 hours, except in pigeons, macaws, and conures because effective concentrations could not be achieved in these birds (Clark et al. 1982). However, oral absorption was poor, and this route of administration was discouraged for all birds.

CHLORAMPHENICOL DERIVATIVES

The ban on the use chloramphenicol in food-producing animals in the mid-1980s left a gap in the veterinarian's armamentarium of effective antimicrobial drugs. Because the idiosyncratic aplastic anemia is associated with the presence of the para-nitro group on the chloramphenicol molecule, attempts were made to modify the chloramphenicol structure to simultaneously retain chloramphenicol's broad spectrum of antimicrobial activity and eliminate the induction of aplastic anemia in people. Compounds synthesized in attempts to accomplish this goal are thiamphenicol and florfenicol. Thiamfenicol is not approved in the United States and will be discussed here only briefly. However, florfenicol has been approved for use in pigs, cattle and fish (in some countries) and has been effective for treatment of various infections, especially bovine respiratory disease in cattle and swine respiratory disease in pigs intended for human consumption.

THIAMPHENICOL. Thiamphenicol is a semisynthetic structural analog of chloramphenicol (Fig. 37.2). The major structural difference between chloramphenicol and thiamphenicol is that the para-nitrophenol group has been replaced by the methyl sulfonyl moiety. Thiamphenicol inhibits bacterial protein synthesis at the 50S ribosomal

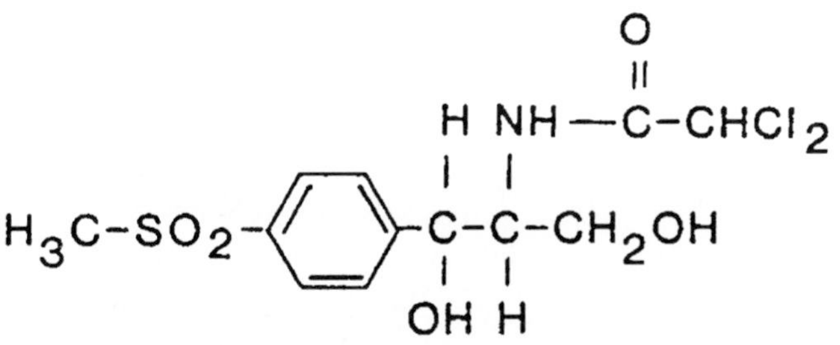

FIG. 37.2 The chemical structure of thiamphenicol.

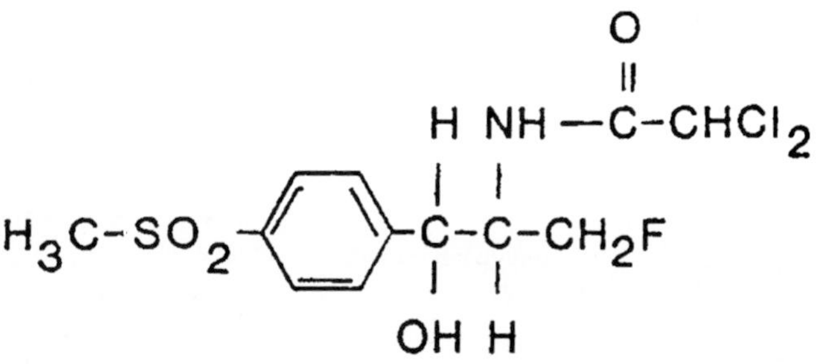

FIG. 37.3 The chemical structure of florfenicol.

subunit at the same location as does chloramphenicol. Thiamphenicol has an antimicrobial spectrum similar to that of chloramphenicol. However, its structural differences result in different pharmacokinetic properties and decreased potency. Thiamphenicol is more water soluble and less lipid soluble and therefore diffuses more slowly through lipid membranes. It is not metabolized to a significant extent in the liver (Ferrari and Bella 1974) and most of the dose is excreted in the urine as the unchanged active compound (Yunis 1988; Lavy et al. 1991a; Gamez et al. 1992). Resistance to thiamphenicol is also similar to that of chloramphenicol, with bacterial acetylation of the thiamphenicol molecule, but at a rate approximately 50% less than that of chloramphenicol.

Few pharmacokinetic studies have been performed on food-producing animals, but thiamphenicol pharmacokinetics has been studied in veal calves (Gamez et al. 1992) and lactating goats (Lavy et al. 1991a). Both studies found thiamphenicol to have a large Vd and to be rapidly eliminated in the urine. In dogs, thiamfenicol had a half-life of 1.7 hours and a Vd of 0.66 l/kg (Castells et al. 1998). In dogs the injection of thiamfenicol was well absorbed, with availability of 97%, but the terminal half-life was longer (5.6 hr), suggesting slow release from the injection site.

Thiamphenicol is considered to be less toxic than chloramphenicol, yet a reversible bone marrow suppression has been reported in humans. However, millions of people have been treated with thiamphenicol in countries in which it is approved, with no reports linking its use to aplastic anemia (Adams et al. 1987). In a thiamphenicol toxicity study in rabbits (Kaltwasser et al. 1974), no changes attributed to thiamphenicol in erythrocyte, reticulocyte, or plasma iron parameters were noted after long-term treatments of up to 90 mg/kg/day. Despite some of the advantages cited here, thiamfenicol is not presently available in North America.

FLORFENICOL. Florfenicol is structurally related to thiamphenicol; however, florfenicol contains fluorine at the 3' carbon position (Fig. 37.3). The fluorine molecule substitution at this position also reduces the number of sites available for bacterial acetylation reactions to occur, possibly making the antibiotic more resistant to bacterial inactivation. Florfenicol is as potent or more potent than either chloramphenicol or thiamphenicol against many organisms in vitro. The list of susceptible bacteria for florfenicol is the same as listed previously for chloramphenicol, except that some bacteria resistant to chloramphenicol due to acetylation may be sensitive to florfenicol. The CLSI (formerly called NCCLS) (CLSI 2007) quality control ranges of MIC for florfenicol are 2–8 μg/ml (Marshall et al. 1996). However, *Mannheimia haemolytica, Pasteurella multocida,* and *Histophilus somni* (previously named *Haemophilus somnus*) are several-fold more sensitive in vitro than bacteria of the Enterobacteriaceae, with MIC_{90} for *Pasteurella* and *Histophilus somni* in the range of 0.5–1.0 μg/ml. Against these bacteria, florfenicol may actually be bactericidal.

The advantage of florfenicol for administration to food animals is that it lacks the para-nitro group (Figures 37.1 and 37.3) that could contribute to the induction of aplastic anemia associated with chloramphenicol use in humans. Therefore, if residues were to occur in animals treated with florfenicol, no dangerous public health risk would ensue. However, it is possible that florfenicol can still produce a dose-related form of reversible bone marrow suppression with prolonged use or high doses, although such reactions have not been reported from routine use of florfenicol in animals. However, in one clinical account in a zoo animal, high doses induced bone marrow suppression (Tuttle et al. 2006).

Pharmacokinetics. The pharmacokinetics of florfenicol are summarized in Table 37.2.

TABLE 37.2 Selected pharmacokinetic parameters of florfenicol in animals

Species	Dose mg/kg	Half-life (hr)	Absorption (%)	V_d (L/kg)	C_{MAX} (µg/mL)	Reference
Cats	22 (all routes)	4 (IV)		0.61	57 (IV)	Papich 1999
		7.8 (oral)	>100 (oral)		28 (oral)	
		5.6 (IM)	>100 (IM)		20 (IM)	
Dogs	20 mg/kg (all routes)	2 (IV)	28 (SC)	1.2	44 (IV)	Papich 1999
		18 (SC)	16 (IM)		0.93 (SC)	
		9 (IM)			1.64 (IM)	
		3 (oral)	>100 (oral)		17 (oral)	
Sea turtles	20 (IM, IV)	2–7.8 hr (IM)	67 (IM)	10–60	0.5–0.8 (IM)	Stamper et al. 1999
Sharks	40 (IM)	269	ND	2.9	10.5	Zimmerman et al. 2006
Fish (red pacu)	10 (IM)	4.25	ND	5.69	1.09	Lewbart et al. 2005
Horses	22 (IV)	1.83	81 (IM)	0.72	4 (IM)	McKellar et al. 1996
			83 (oral)		13 (oral)	
Cattle	50 (IV)	3.2	ND	0.67	157.7	Bretzlaff et al. 1987
Feeder calves	20 (IV)	2.65	ND	0.88	73	Lobell et al. 1994
Feeder calves	20 (IM)	18.3	78.5	ND	3.07	Lobell et al. 1994
Veal calves	22 (oral)	ND	88	ND	11.3	Varma et al. 1986
Veal calves	22 (IV)	2.87	ND	0.78	66	Varma et al. 1986
Veal calves	11 (IV)	3.71	ND	0.91	26.35	Adams et al. 1987
Veal calves	11 (oral)	3.7	89	ND	5.7	Adams et al. 1987

Note: Route of administration used is listed in parentheses. V_d is volume of distribution, C_{MAX} is the maximal concentration after administration with route listed in parentheses. ND = not determined.

Absorption. Studies in calves (Varma et al. 1986; Adams et al. 1987; Lobell et al. 1994) showed high bioavailability after oral and parenteral administrations, but there was decreased oral absorption when florfenicol was administered with milk. After IM injection in cattle, the absorption is almost complete, with systemic availability of 78%, but absorption is slow, which is demonstrated in cattle by an IV half-life of 2.65 hours but an average of 18 hours after IM injection (Lobell et al. 1994). This suggests that it is more slowly released from an IM injection site, thus prolonging the duration of effective levels. This slow elimination after IM injection in cattle prolongs the effective plasma concentration (above 1 µg/ml for respiratory pathogens) for 23 hours in calves. In horses, florfenicol is absorbed well after oral and IM administration (81% IM and 83% oral) (McKellar and Varma 1996). Oral absorption in Atlantic salmon was 96%.

Distribution. Like chloramphenicol, florfenicol has a wide distribution in most tissues of the body (Adams et al. 1987), including high concentrations in the kidney, urine, bile, and small intestine, but less penetration in the CSF, brain, and aqueous humor of the eye than that attained with chloramphenicol. Concentrations in brain and CSF are 1/4 to 1/2, respectively, the corresponding concentrations in plasma. Although in one study the distribution into CSF was only 46% relative to plasma, these levels were high enough to produce concentrations in CSF of cattle to inhibit *Histophilus somni* for over 20 hours (DeCraene et al. 1997). Florfenicol also penetrated well into the milk of lactating goats after IV and IM administration, making it of possible use in the treatment of microbial infections in the udder of lactating animals (Lavy et al. 1991b). The Vd is 0.7–0.9 l/kg in most studies in cattle. Protein binding is low in cattle (13–19%) (Bretzlaff et al. 1987; Lobell et al. 1994) but has not been reported for other species.

Elimination. The elimination half-life is 2–4 hours in cattle (Table 37.2). The half-life of less than 2 hours in horses is shorter than that in cattle. The half-life is dependent on the route of administration, which can be seen in Table 37.2 for studies in calves and dogs. The injection IM or SC can prolong the terminal half-life because of slow absorption ("flip-flop" effect).

Metabolism. Most of the dose administered to cattle is excreted as the parent drug (64%) in the urine. The rest of the drug is excreted as urinary metabolites. This possibly indicates its use in the treatment of organisms infecting the genitourinary tract of animals. Florfenicol amine is the metabolite that persists longest in tissues of cattle and is used as the marker residue for withdrawal determination.

Pharmacokinetic Studies in Other Species. In small animals, florfenicol has limited application, but disposition was studied after oral, IM, and subcutaneous (SC) administration (Papich 1999). After IV administration in dogs, the half-life was less than 1 hour for three out of four dogs and clearance was rapid. After oral administration, inhibitory concentrations were maintained for only 4 hours. In dogs after IM injection, florfenicol mean peak plasma concentrations were 1.64 μg/ml and mean elimination half-life was 9.2 hours. Concentrations were above a MIC of 1.0 μg/ml for only 2 hours. After SC administration, florfenicol was absorbed poorly and inconsistently, with peak concentrations less than 1.0 μg/ml. By contrast, florfenicol solution in cats was absorbed well from both routes, with peak concentrations of 20 μg/ml and 27 μg/ml after IM and oral dose, respectively. Absorption was high from both routes (greater than 100% from IM and oral). IV elimination half-life was 4 hours, and Vd was 0.6 l/kg. The half-life was 5.6 hours and 7.8 hours for IM and oral dose, respectively. In cats, florfenicol produced inhibitory concentrations for 12 hours.

Florfenicol has been administered orally for treatment of infections in captive fish and is approved in some countries for this use (Aqua-Flor®). In rainbow trout at a water temperature of 10°C and given an oral dose of 10 mg/kg, florfenicol has a mean residence time of 21 hours and a peak (C_{max}) of 3.23 μg/ml and is well distributed to tissues (Pinault 1997). In salmon, florfenicol has a half-life of 12.2 hours at 10.8°C (Martinsen et al. 1993) and is also well distributed (Horsberg et al. 1994), with a Vd of 1.12 l/kg (Martinsen et al. 1993). In salmon the systemic availability of an oral dose is 96.5%. In red pacu, after a florfenicol dose of 10 mg/kg IM, the half-life was 4.25 hours, and the maximum concentration was only 1 μg/ml (Lewbart et al. 2005). To maintain concentrations effective for fish pathogens, a dose of 20–30 mg/kg every 24 hours was recommended by the authors. In sharks at a dose of 40 mg/kg IM, florfenicol produced effective levels for 120 hours (Zimmerman et al. 2006). Dosing every 3–5 days will produce concentrations in a therapeutic range.

Pharmacokinetic studies in horses show that florfenicol has longer half-life than chloramphenicol, good distribution, and good absorption. However, in experimental horses there were consistent loose stools and elevated bilirubin (McKellar and Varma 1996). Until additional studies establish safe doses, florfenicol cannot be recommended for horses.

In snakes (Boas), the half-life was 28 hours from IM injection. It was estimated that 50 mg/kg once daily for Boas is the best dose to produce therapeutic plasma concentrations, even though efficacy studies are not available. In sea turtles the clearance was rapid (60–100 ml/kg/hr) and the half-life was short (Stamper et al. 2003). It was concluded that florfenicol was not a practical drug for treatment of infections in sea turtles.

Clinical Use. Florfenicol is available in a 300 mg/ml solution for injection (Nuflor), a solution to be added to drinking water for swine and powder to be added to feed for swine. For fish there is a 500 gram per kilogram premix for fish (Aqua-Flor).

Cattle and Pigs. Several studies in cattle have been conducted to support the use of florfenicol for treating bovine respiratory disease caused by *Mannheimia haemolytica, Pasteurella multocida,* and *Histophilus somni* (previously named *Haemophilus somnus*). Florfenicol has been effective for treating undifferentiated bovine respiratory disease in cattle with doses of 20 mg/kg IM, given every 48 hours and injected in the neck (Hoar et al. 1998; Jim et al. 1999). It is also approved as a single dose for cattle at 40 mg/kg SC in the neck (withdrawal times listed below). Florfenicol is also approved for treatment of bovine interdigital phlegmon (foot rot, acute interdigital necrobacillosis, infectious pododermatitis) associated with *Fusobacterium necrophorum* and *Bacteroides melaninogenicus*.

Florfenicol has been effective in calves for treating experimentally induced infections and naturally occurring infectious bovine keratoconjunctivitis (Dueger et al. 1999; Angelos et al. 2000). In the naturally occurring case, florfenicol was administered one dose SC at 40 mg/kg or IM two doses 48 hours apart at 20 mg/kg. Concentrations persist in CSF for a long enough period after administration of 20 mg/kg in cattle that concentrations are above MIC of susceptible pathogens for at least 20 hours. When florfenicol was administered by intramammary infusion (750 mg/cow) to cattle (Wilson et al. 1996) with subclinical mastitis, there was poor efficacy, which could, perhaps, be attributed to an interval between treatments that was too long or to a duration of treatment that was too short.

For pigs, florfenicol is added to the feed (182 g per ton of feed), or drinking water (400 mg per gallon) for 5 days for the control of swine respiratory disease (SRD) associated with *Actinobacillus pleuropneumoniae, Pasteurella multocida, Streptococcus suis,* and *Bordetella bronchiseptica.*

Small Animals. Although some pharmacokinetic studies have been conducted in small animals and exotic animals, there are no reports of efficacy. Pharmacokinetic studies in reptiles and dogs suggest that frequent dosing with high doses would be necessary to maintain plasma concentrations above the MIC for susceptible organisms throughout the dosing interval. In cats, the pharmacokinetic evidence (discussed earlier) indicates that a dose of 22 mg/kg administered every 12 hours orally or parenterally would be adequate to produce sustained plasma concentrations for treatment of susceptible bacteria.

Use in Fish. Florfenicol has been demonstrated to be efficacious against bacteria of fish, especially trout and salmon (Fukui et al. 1987). Florfenicol premix is approved in some countries for treatment of furunculosis in salmon caused by *Aeromonas salmonicida.* Florfenicol has been administered orally for treatment of furunculosis caused by susceptible strains of *Aeromonas salmonicida* in captive fish and is approved in other countries. The premix (Aqua-Flor®) is approved for use in catfish and salmonids at a dose of 10 mg/kg for 10 days to treat susceptible fish pathogens.

Adverse Effects. Effect of florfenicol on bovine pregnancy, reproduction, and lactation have not been determined. Mild diarrhea and elevated bilirubin have been reported from administration to horses (McKellar and Varma 1996). Reversible, dose-related bone marrow suppression is possible but not reported, except for a reaction reported in a zoo animal that was mentioned previously (Tuttle et al. 2006). In cattle, diarrhea and decreased feed consumption have been observed, which are transient. A local tissue reaction from IM or SC injection is possible. When toxic overdoses were administered to calves (200 mg/kg) there was marked anorexia, decrease in body weight, ketosis, and elevated liver enzymes. In dogs administered high doses for prolonged periods there was CNS vacuolation, hematopoietic toxicity, and renal tubule dilation.

Regulatory Information. The tolerance for florfenicol is 3.7 ppm for florfenicol amine (the marker residue) in liver and 0.3 ppm in muscle. Withdrawal time for use in salmon is 12 days. Withdrawal time for oral administration to pigs in feed is 13 days and for administration in water 16 days. After injection to cattle, the withdrawal time for slaughter is 28 days if injected at a dose of 20 mg/kg IM (36 days in Canada). If injected at a dose of 40 mg/kg SC, the withdrawal time for slaughter is 38 days. A formulation with different excipients (Nuflor Gold) has a withdrawal time of 44 days in cattle when injected at 40 mg/kg SC, once. Do not inject more than 10 ml in one site. Give injections in the neck only (both SC and IM). Do not administer to dairy cows older than 20 months, to calves under 1 month of age, or to calves on an all-milk diet.

MACROLIDE ANTIBIOTICS

SOURCE AND CHEMISTRY. The macrolide antibiotics are a group of structurally similar compounds, most of which are derived from various species of *Streptomyces* soilborne bacteria. Chemically, all the drugs in this group are classified as macrocyclic lactones, with members containing 12–20 atoms of carbon in the lactone ring structure. Attached to this lactone ring are various combinations of deoxy sugars held to the lactone ring by glycosidic linkages. Since erythromycin's discovery in the early 1950s from the soil organism *Streptomyces erythreus,* numerous other macrolides have been isolated or synthesized from the parent molecule erythromycin, including tylosin, roxithromycin, erythromycylamine, tilmicosin, dirithromycin, azithromycin, tulathromycin, clarithromycin, spiramycin, and flurithromycin (Kirst and Sides 1989).

Erythromycin, tylosin (see Fig. 37.4), and tilmicosin have found the most clinical applications of the macrolide class in veterinary medicine. The newest introduced drug in this group is tulathromycin (Draxxin), approved for use in cattle for treatment of respiratory disease. New human-label derivatives such as azithromycin are increasing in popularity. Other macrolides such as oleandomycin and carbomycin have been used as feed additives for growth promotion in food animals.

Erythromycin is a large molecule consisting of a 14-atom polyhydroxylactone erythronolide ring and the two sugars clandinose and desosamine. Similarly, tylosin is composed of a 16-atom lactone ring (a tylonolide) to

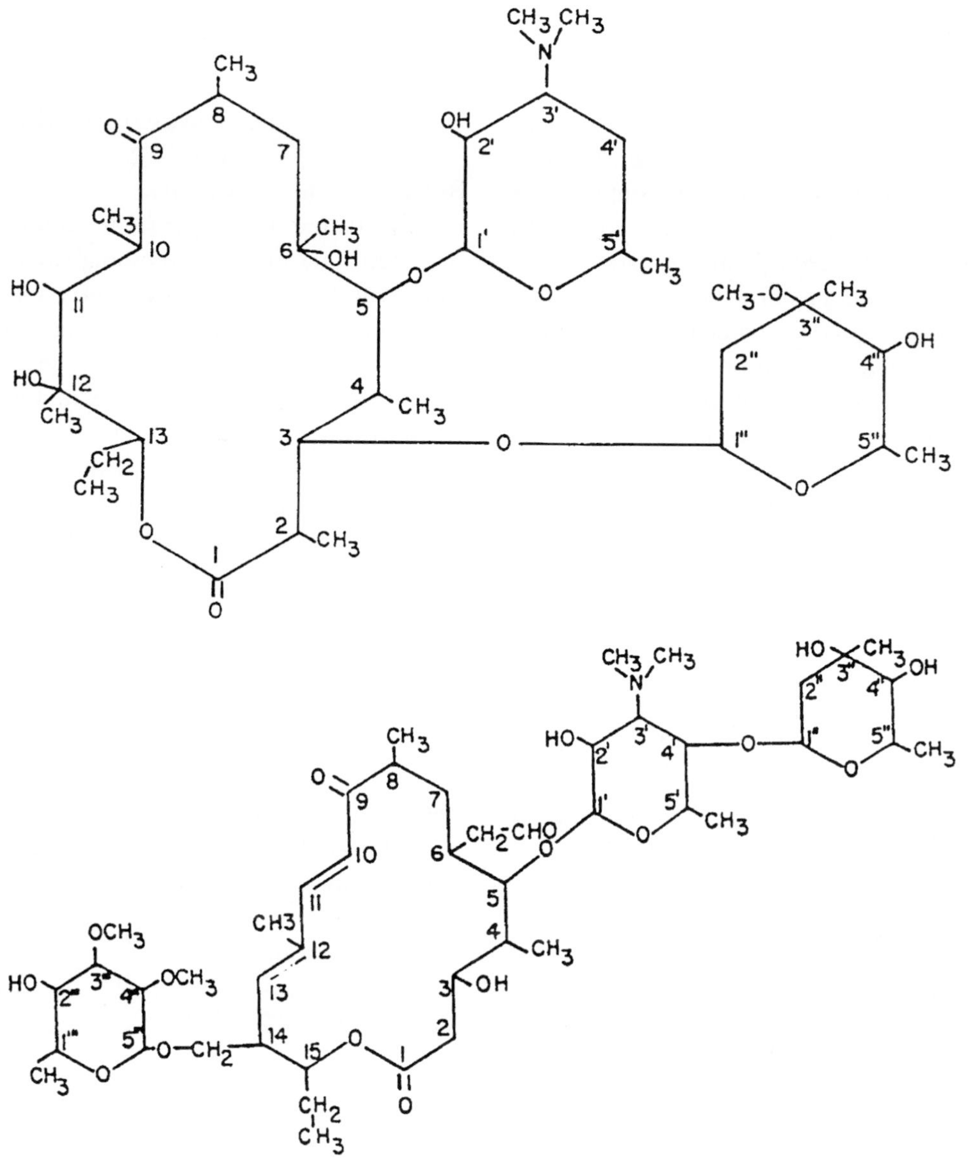

FIG. 37.4 The chemical structures of erythromycin (top) and tylosin.

which three sugars—mycinose, mycaminose, and mycarose—are attached (Wilson 1984; Kirst et al. 1982). Other macrolides with 16-member rings include josamycin and spiramycin. Azithromycin is the first drug in the group of azalides, which are semisynthetic derivatives of erythromycin (Lode et al. 1996). Azithromycin has a 15-member ring structure. Tulathromycin, the newest drug for cattle, is also a 15-member ring structure derived from the azalides. Tulathromycin has three basic nitrogen groups (tribasic) that produce a higher positive charge and increased affinity for intracellular sites compared to other drugs.

DRUG FORMULATIONS. All macrolides are weak bases, with pK_a ranges from 6 to 9; erythromycin has a pK_a of 8.7–8.8 and tylosin has a pK_a of 7.1. Erythromycin base is poorly absorbed, and oral formulations are modified to increase absorption and improve oral tolerability. Oral formulations are estolate or ethylsuccinate esters of erythromycin. The esters are absorbed systemically, then hydrolyzed to the erythromycin base by enzymes in the body before they are active. Alternatively, other oral forms of erythromycin are formulated as a salt of stearate or phosphate. After oral administration of the salt, erythromycin dissociates from the salt in the intestine and is absorbed as free drug. There are also oral formulations intended to be added to the feed or drinking water to treat infections for poultry. Examples of these preparations are erythromycin thiocynate premix and erythromycin phosphate powder (Ery-Mycin). In addition, there are formulations of other macrolides to be added to the feed or water of cattle, pigs, or poultry for control of respiratory and other infections. Examples of these formulations are tilmicosin premix (Pulmotil) to be added to feed for pigs, tylosin phosphate premix to be added to feed for cattle, pigs, or poultry, and tylosin tartrate (Tylan soluble) for the drinking water of poultry. Veterinary forms of erythromycin injectable (e.g., Erythro-100 and Gallimycin-100) are 100 mg/ml formulations intended for IM injection only; they should not be administered SC or IV. The injectable formulation of tulathromycin (Draxxin) is 100 mg/ml for use as a single SC injection at 2.5 mg/kg, and tilmicosin (Micotil) 300 mg/ml for SC injection (10 mg/kg) to cattle and sheep.

MECHANISM OF ACTION. The antibacterial action of macrolides is produced by an inhibition of protein synthesis by binding to the 50S ribosomal subunit of prokaryote organisms. The binding site on the ribosome is near but not identical to that of chloramphenicol, and antagonism of effect is possible if macrolides are administered with chloramphenicol. Macrolides inhibit translocation of tRNA from the amino acid acceptor site, which disrupts addition of new peptide bonds and thus prevents synthesis of new proteins within the microbial cell. Macrolides can bind to mitochondrial ribosomes but are unable to cross the mitochondrial membrane (in contrast to chloramphenicol) and therefore do not produce bone marrow suppression in mammals. Macrolides in general do not bind to mammalian ribosomes, making them a relatively safe group of drugs for veterinary use.

Although most authors have listed macrolides as bacteriostatic at therapeutic concentrations (Wilson 1984), they can be slowly bactericidal, especially against streptococci. Their bactericidal action is time dependent (Carbon 1998). The antimicrobial action of erythromycin is enhanced by a high pH (Sabath et al. 1968), with the optimum antibacterial effect at a pH of 8. Therefore, in an acidic environment, such as in an abscess, necrotic tissue, or urine, the antibacterial activity is suppressed.

Resistance Mechanisms. Resistance to macrolides is usually plasmid-mediated, but modification of ribosomes may occur through chromosomal mutation. Resistance can occur from 1) decreased entry into bacteria (most common with the gram-negative organisms), 2) synthesis of bacterial enzymes that hydrolyze the drug, and 3) modification of target (the ribosome in this instance). The ribosomal attenuation involves methylation of the 50S drug receptor site. This resistance may also lead to cross-resistance with other antibiotics that preferentially bind to these sites, such as other macrolides and lincosamides (Wilson 1984). Resistance to erythromycin in animals in several microorganisms has been discussed in more detail elsewhere (Maguire et al. 1989; Dutta and Devriese 1981, 1982a,b; Leclercq and Courvalin 1991; Devriese and Dutta 1984). In small animals with staphylococcal infections, resistance was more likely if antibiotics had previously been prescribed, especially in cases of recurrent pyoderma (Lloyd et al. 1996; Medleau et al. 1986; Noble and Kent 1992). As summarized by Noli and Boothe (1999), an increasing trend toward resistance to macrolides by staphylocci has been demonstrated when treating pyoderma (increasing from 7 to 22%), whereas in some countries, the incidence of resistance has remained relatively stable at around 22–24%.

SPECTRUM OF ACTIVITY. Erythromycin is mainly effective against gram-positive organisms such as streptococci, staphylococci, including staphylococci that may be resistant to β-lactams because of β-lactamase synthesis or modification of the penicillin-binding protein target. Other organisms that show in vitro susceptibility include *Mycoplasma, Arcanobacterium, Erysipelothrix, Bordetella,* and *Bartonella*. Although the spectrum favors the gram-positive group, a few gram-negatives are susceptible, especially *Pasteurella* spp. Activity against anaerobic bacteria is only moderate. Gram-negative anaerobic bacteria often are resistant. Most other gram-negative bacteria, such as those of the Enterobacteriaceae or *Pseudomonas* spp., are resistant. The activity of tilmicosin is similar to that of erythromycin, but most of the in vitro data concern its activity against *Pasteurella, Mannheimia* *haemolytica,* and *Histophilus somni,* for which it maintains good activity. Other gram-negative bacteria are resistant to tilmicosin. Tulathromycin also has activity against these organisms, as well as *Mycoplasma bovis,* with lower MIC_{90} values compared to tilmicosin.

The CLSI (CLSI 2007) guidelines for susceptibility (Watts et al. 1999) list the erythromycin breakpoint for sensitivity as ≤0.25 μg/ml for streptococci and ≤0.5 μg/ml for organisms other than streptococci.

PHARMACOKINETICS

Absorption and Distribution. Erythromycin pharmacokinetics has been studied in most animals and in humans; some of these parameters are shown in Table 37.3. Oral erythromycin is absorbed well, but inactivation of erythromycin due to gastric acidity is common for the base form of erythromycin, which is the reason that other formulations, such as erythromycin estolate or stearate forms or enteric-coated formulations, are used. They have better bioavailability owing to decreased destruction of erythromycin in the acidic environment of the stomach. The presence of food in the stomach also tends to decrease absorption of erythromycin in most species, including the dog (Wilson 1984; Eriksson et al. 1990). Erythromycin salts (erythromycin-stearate and erythromycin-phosphate) dissociate in the intestine and are absorbed as the active drug. Erythromycin esters (erythromycin-ethylsuccinate and erythromycin-estolate) are absorbed as the esters and hydrolyzed in the body to release active drug. There is no proven difference among these formulations as to which is the most favorable in most animals. However, in horses,

TABLE 37.3 Selected serum pharmacokinetic parameters of erythromycin in animals

Species	Dose (mg/kg)	Route	Formulation	Half-life ($t_{1/2\beta}$) (hr)	V_d (L/kg)	Reference
Cows	12.5	IV	Base	3.16	0.789	Baggot and Gingerich 1976
Calves	15	IV	Base in PG vehicle	2.91	0.835	Burrows et al. 1989
	15	IM	Base in PG vehicle	5.81	NA	Burrows et al. 1989
	15	SC	Base in PG vehicle	26.87	NA	Burrows et al. 1989
Calves	30	IV	Base in PG vehicle	4.09	1.596	Burrows et al. 1989
	30	IM	Base in PG vehicle	11.85	NA	Burrows et al. 1989
	30	SC	Base in PG vehicle	18.3	NA	Burrows et al. 1989
Mice	10	IV	Base	0.65	3.6	Duthu 1985
Rats	25	IV	Base	1.27	9.3	Duthu 1985
Rabbits	10	IV	Base	1.4	6.8	Duthu 1985
Dogs	10	IV	Base	1.72	2.7	Duthu 1985
Pigs (1 day)	10	IV	Base	3.0	0.68	Kinoshita et al. 1995
Pigs (3 day)	10	IV	Base	1.43	3.28	Kinoshita et al. 1995
Foal	25	Oral	Ethylsuccinate	1.52	ND	Lakritz et al. 2002
Foal	25	Oral	Base	1.8, 1.3	ND	Lakritz et al. 2000
Foal	25	Oral	Estolate	0.52	ND	Lakritz et al. 2000
Foal	25	Oral	Phosphate	0.81	ND	Lakritz et al. 2000
Foal	10	IV	Lactiobionate	1.18	0.91	Lakritz et al. 2000
Foal	10	IV	Lactiobionate	0.97	3.52	Lakritz et al. 1999
Foal	25	Oral	Base	17.6 (MRT)	ND	Lakritz et al. 1999
Foal	5	IV	Gluceptate	1.0	3.7	Prescott et al. 1983
Foal	20	IV	Gluceptate	1.1	7.2	Prescott et al. 1983
Horse (Mares)	5	IV	Gluceptate	1.0	2.3	Prescott et al. 1983
Horse	25	Oral	Estolate	2.42	ND	Ewing et al. 1994
Horse	37.5	Oral	Estolate	6.2	ND	Ewing et al. 1994
Horse	25	Oral	Phosphate	2.49	ND	Ewing et al. 1994
Horse	37.5	Oral	Phosphate	1.68	ND	Ewing et al. 1994
Horse	25	Oral	Stearate	1.84	ND	Ewing et al. 1994
Horse	25	Oral	Ethylsuccinate	4.76	ND	Ewing et al. 1994
Cats	25	PO	Base	2.83	2.6	Jernigan et al. 1990

Note: NA = data not available; PG = propylene glycol.

it was shown that the salt forms (erythromycin-phosphate or erythromycin-stearate) are preferred for oral administration (Ewing et al. 1994) because they provided the most favorable blood concentrations. A series of studies by Lakritz et al (1999, 2000a, 2000b, 2002) examined the absorption of various oral formulations in foals. The ethylsuccinate form was poorly absorbed, but the phosphate, estolate, and microencapsulated forms were better absorbed (16%, 14.7%, and 26%, respectively). Absorption is better in foals when food was withheld. Crushed tablets of enteric-coated preparations are substantially degraded in the stomach or are metabolized in the intestine wall and are not recommended for oral administration to animals.

SC or IM injections of erythromycin can be painful and irritating; therefore, the PO route is preferred whenever possible. The only formulations that can be given IV are the glucoptate and lactobionate forms, because these are the only forms soluble in aqueous solution.

Macrolides tend to concentrate in some cells because the basic drug is trapped in cells that are more acidic than plasma. Tissue concentrations for erythromycin, tylosin, and tilmicosin are higher than serum concentrations, especially in the lungs, which is relevant because these drugs are often used to treat respiratory infections. The lung concentrations are so high for tilmicosin that they persist for at least 72 hours after a single dose. Tulathromycin levels in lung tissue persist much longer than in plasma (184 hr half-life in lungs versus 58–99 hrs for plasma). In addition to the lungs, erythromycin concentrations are equal to or higher than plasma concentrations in several body fluids such as bile and prostatic, seminal, pleural, and peritoneal fluids, as well as in many tissues, such as the liver, spleen, heart, and kidneys, among others. Erythromycin does not penetrate the blood-brain barrier in high enough concentrations to be therapeutic; however, it can cross the placenta and attain therapeutic concentrations in the fetus. High concentrations are also obtained in the feces of animals due to biliary excretion (Wilson 1984). These high tissue concentrations are reflected in a relatively large Vd of 3–6 l/kg (Riviere et al. 1991). The tylosin Vd is 1–2.5 l/kg for most species of animals. The new macrolide azithromycin is discussed in more detail later in this section. Its distribution to tissues is higher than other macrolides discussed so far, and its Vd has been measured at over 20 l/kg in animals. For tulathromycin, the Vd is over 11 l/kg. Protein binding for macrolides is low, with values of 18–30% for most species. Protein binding in some species may be predominantly to the alpha-1-acid glycoprotein, rather than albumin (Kinoshita et al. 1995).

Tylosin has good absorption from the GI tract, and no enteric coating is required to maintain the stability of the compound in the stomach. It is widely distributed to basically the same tissues as described for erythromycin, metabolized by the liver, and excreted via the bile and feces.

Tilmicosin has slow absorption, 22% bioavailability, a half-life in plasma of 4 hours, and extensive penetration in milk (Ziv et al. 1995). However, because of the high and persistent distribution to tissues, especially lungs, the plasma pharmacokinetics seem to have little correlation to the observed clinical effects (Gourlay et al. 1989).

Metabolism and Excretion. Metabolism of erythromycin is via hepatic microsomal enzymes, which cause a demethylation of one of the methyl groups on the desosamine sugar moiety of the erythromycin molecule. Little of the antimicrobial action is retained after demethylation by these enzymes. These metabolic enzymes can be induced with phenobarbital (and possibly other enzyme inducers); therefore, patients given phenobarbital and erythromycin simultaneously may experience more antimicrobial treatment failures due to increased metabolism. Most (90%) of the drug in the bile is in the metabolized form. Some active erythromycin (2–5%) is found excreted into the urine, with higher levels found in the urine after IV dosing. Renal dysfunction seemingly does not have an appreciable effect on its elimination half-life in the body (Wilson 1984). Although macrolides are not a popular choice for treating urinary tract infections because of their limited spectrum of activity, high urine pH tends to favor antimicrobial activity in the urine environment (Sabath et al. 1968).

Half-lives for erythromycin are listed in Table 37.3 and range from less than 1.0 hour in rodents and rabbits to 3–4 hours in cattle. Tylosin follows a similar pattern, with half-lives of 1–2 hours in most animals.

ADVERSE EFFECTS AND PRECAUTIONS. Side effects are reported more frequently in humans than in animals. Humans dosed with macrolides (in particular, erythromycin) have experienced nausea and vomiting (oral forms), fever, skin eruptions, cholestatic hepatitis, elevated serum aspartate aminotransferase, epigastric distress, and transient auditory impairment, among many other side effects. Cholestatic hepatitis, most commonly associated with the estolate ester, is the most common of these adverse reactions, with the symptoms starting 10–20 days after beginning therapy and ending a few days after the cessation of therapy. Cholestasis associated with erythromycin use in humans is considered to be a hypersensitivity reaction (Sande and Mandell 1990a). In animals, however, few of these side effects are observed, and hepatitis has not been a reported association. However, regurgitation and/or vomiting has been commonly reported in small animals, especially dogs after oral administration of erythromycin. In one report, erythromycin was the drug that most frequently caused side effects after oral dosing in dogs (Kunkle et al. 1995). Stimulation of GI motility may play a role in small-animal vomiting (discussed below under clinical uses). In horses, erythromycin may induce diarrhea, which stops after therapy is discontinued and is generally not fatal. The effect of erythromycin on producing diarrhea in horses was discussed more extensively in a review (Papich 2003). Although these reactions in the horse may limit its use by some clinicians, erythromycin is still commonly used in horses to treat a variety of infections, especially in the foal. Hyperthermia (febrile syndrome) has also been observed in foals associated with erythromycin treatment (Stratton-Phelps et al. 2000), which was accompanied in some foals by diarrhea and respiratory distress.

DRUG INTERACTIONS. Erythromycin is a well-known hepatic microsomal enzyme inhibitor. Erythromycin is both a substrate and an inhibitor for the cytochrome P450 enzyme, which is the enzyme system that is most often involved in drug metabolism. As an inhibitor of the cytochrome P450 enzyme, it may inhibit metabolism of drugs such as theophylline, cyclosporine, digoxin, and warfarin. Concentrations of these drugs may increase when animals receive erythromycin, resulting in a potentiation of the pharmacologic effect or toxicity.

CLINICAL USE OF ERYTHROMYCIN. Doses of erythromycin are listed in Table 37.3. Erythromycin is primarily used for treating infections caused by gram-positive organisms. Because of the high distribution into tissues and long persistence in some cells, macrolides are particularly useful for treating some infections caused by bacteria that more polar or less lipid-soluble drugs may have difficulty reaching. Erythromycin and other macrolide antibiotics are sometimes used as a penicillin alternative when penicillins have either failed or when there is allergy to penicillins. Infections treated by erythromycin include those caused by *Staphylococcus* spp., *Streptococcus* spp., *Arcanobacterium* spp., *Clostridium* spp., *Listeria* spp., *Bacillus* spp., *Erysipelothrix* spp., *Histophilus*, *Brucella* spp., *Fusobacterium* spp., *Pasteurella* spp., *Borrelia* spp., and *Mycoplasma* spp. (Wilson 1984).

In small animals, erythromycin is used to treat pyoderma caused by staphylococci (Noli and Boothe 1999), respiratory infections caused by *Mycoplasma,* and diarrhea caused by *Campylobacter* organisms. When treating *Campylobacter,* erythromycin stopped the shedding but did not eliminate the organism. Respiratory infections are sometimes treated with erythromycin, even when a causative organism has not been identified because erythromycin crosses the blood-bronchus barrier and achieves favorable concentrations in respiratory tract secretions. Erythromycin has also been used as a treatment for undifferentiated bovine respiratory disease and for pig infections caused by *Erysipelothrix* and for pig respiratory infections caused by *Streptococcus* and *Pasteurella.* In poultry, erythromycin is used for treatment of respiratory infections caused by *Mycoplasma.* In foals, erythromycin is used, in combination with rifampin, for treatment of pneumonia caused by *Rhodococcus equi.* However, there is some evidence that erythromycin administered alone may be equally efficacious.

Clinical Use of Erythromycin to Modify Gastrointestinal Motility. Erythromycin is a common cause of vomiting and regurgitation in small animals. In one study erythromycin oral administration produced the most common adverse effects in comparison to other drugs (Kunkle et al. 1995). Although some nausea from the oral preparations is possible, most of this effect is believed to be related to a drug-induced increase in GI motility. This mechanism appears to be related to an increase in activation of motilin receptors, via release of endogenous motilin, or via cholinergic mechanisms in the upper GI tract (Hall and Washabau 1997; Lester et al. 1998). At small doses (1 mg/kg) erythromycin has been considered for use as a motility-stimulating drug in animals. In calves, administration of erythromycin, tylosin, or tilmicosin increased the rate of abomasal emptying, with erythromycin (8.8 mg/kg IM) producing the most significant effect (Nouri and Constable 2007; Nouri et al. 2008; Wittek and Constable 2005). These properties of erythromycin are discussed in more detail in Chapter 47. In calves, these drugs increase the abomasal emptying rate and erythromycin (10 mg/kg IM) has been used to improve postoperative abomasal rate in dairy cows undergoing surgical correction of left abomasal displacement (Wittek et al. 2008). The clinical benefits for treating GI motility disorders has also been explored. Although 14-membered macrolides appear to have the most profound effect on the gastrointestinal tract, there is also an effect from 16-membered macrolides such as tylosin and tilmicosin (Nouri and Constable 2007).

Regulatory Considerations. Erythromycin has a 6-day withdrawal time when used according to label in cattle in the United States. Erythromycin added to feed or water for poultry has a withdrawal time of 1–2 days; the specific product label should be consulted for the exact withdrawal time. In the United States erythromycin should not be administered to lactating dairy cattle because macrolides concentrate in the milk for a long time after treatment. However, Canadian labeling lists a milk withholding time of 72 hours after a dose of 2.2–4.4 mg/kg.

TYLOSIN. Pharmacokinetic data for tylosin are listed in Table 37.4. Tylosin has been used therapeutically to treat "pinkeye" (*Moraxella bovis*) in cattle; respiratory tract infections; swine dysentery; pleuropneumonia due to *Haemophilus parahemolyticus;* and other infections in cats, chickens (Ose and Tonkinson 1985), quail (Jones et al. 1976), and turkeys (Wilson 1984). Tylosin has been used more extensively as a feed additive to promote growth in food-producing animals, such as swine, cattle, and chickens, among others (Wilson 1984). Residues from tylosin have been discussed in other papers (Knothe 1977a,b; Anderson et al. 1966). After administration to cattle there is a 21- and 14-day withdrawal time for slaughter for cattle and pigs, respectively. Tylosin concentrates in milk for a long time after administration and should not be administered to lactating dairy cattle. Specific product information should be consulted for withholding times when tylosin is administered in feed or water to pigs or poultry because withdrawal times can vary from 0 to 5 days, depending on the use.

Tylosin has also been used to treat diarrhea in dogs, which is discussed in Chapter 47 in more detail. This type of diarrhea has been characterized as "Tylosin-Responsive Chronic Diarrhea in Dogs" (Westermarck et al. 2005). In these animals, tylosin has been effective at improving clinical signs that occur with or without organisms being identified.

TILMICOSIN. Tilmicosin is 20-deoxo-20-(3,5-dimethylpiperidin-1-yl)desmycosin, a newer macrolide antibiotic that is closely related to erythromycin. Tilmicosin phosphate (Micotil 300) has been effective for treating bovine respiratory disease (Musser et al. 1996; Hoar et al. 1998;

TABLE 37.4 Selected serum pharmacokinetic parameters of tylosin in animals

Species	Dose (mg/kg)	Route	Half-life ($t_{1/2\beta}$) (hr)	V_d (L/kg)	Reference
Dogs (Beagle)	10	IV	0.9	1.7	Weisel et al. 1977
Ewes	20	IV	2.05	NA	Ziv and Sulman 1973b
Goats	15	IV	3.04	1.7	Atef et al. 1991b
Cows	12.5	IV	1.62	1.1	Gingerich et al. 1977
Cows	20	IV	2.14	NA	Gingerich et al. 1977
Calves					
(2 days old)	10	IV	2.32	7	Burrows et al. 1983
(1 wk old)	10	IV	1.26	7.2	Burrows et al. 1983
(2 wk old)	10	IV	0.95	11.1	Burrows et al. 1983
(4 wk old)	10	IV	1.53	9	Burrows et al. 1983
(>6 wk old)	10	IV	1.07	11.1	Burrows et al. 1983
Avians (emus)	15	IV	4.7	NA	Locke et al. 1982
Avians (quail, pigeons, cranes)	15	IM	1.2	NA	Locke et al. 1982

Note: NA = data not available.

Jim et al. 1999). One study (Ose and Tonkinson 1988) reports that 90% of the *Mannheimia haemolytica* and *Pasteurella multocida* isolates tested were sensitive to tilmicosin at concentrations of ≤6.25 μg/ml, and the drug was also active against *Mycoplasma,* including those from bovine isolates. Other organisms with in vitro susceptibility to tilmicosin include staphylococci and streptococci. Most gram-negative organisms other than those causing bovine respiratory disease are frequently resistant.

Tilmicosin administered to calves with pneumonia were found to respond better when treated with 10 mg/kg SC tilmicosin than with a 20 mg/kg IM dose of oxytetracycline (Laven and Andrews 1991). In a study by Gourlay et al. (1989) using calves treated with 20 mg/kg SC tilmicosin, the high success rate in treating bovine pneumonia was believed to be due in part to the prolonged presence of therapeutic concentrations of tilmicosin in the lung tissues. Due to high affinity for certain tissues, tilmicosin concentrations remain above the MIC of susceptible organisms for at least 72 hours. Resistance among cattle respiratory pathogens has been recognized (Musser et al. 1996). However, because tilmicosin has such a high concentration in some tissues (e.g., the lung), in vitro measurements of resistance may have little relationship to whether or not the drug produces a cure in cattle with respiratory disease (Musser et al. 1996).

Tilmicosin also has been used as a prophylactic antibiotic (metaphylaxis) for administration to calves entering a feedlot situation. Tilmicosin reduced the incidence of pneumonia in susceptible calves when administered prophylactically as a single 10 mg/kg SC injection (Morck et al. 1993; Schumann et al. 1990). Tilmicosin used as a metaphylactic treatment in newly arrived feedlot calves reduced prevalence of bovine respiratory disease and improved growth of calves (Vogel et al. 1998).

The CLSI break point for tilmicosin susceptibility is ≤8 μg/ml for cattle respiratory pathogens (*Mannheimia haemolytica*) and ≤16 μg/ml for swine respiratory disease pathogens (CLSI 2007). The currently approved dose is 10 mg/kg SC as a single treatment. After treatment with tilmicosin phosphate in cattle, there is a 28-day withdrawal time. Tilmicosin should not be administered to lactating dairy cattle because residues may persist in milk for more than 30 days.

Tilmicosin phosphate is approved for treatment of swine respiratory disease caused by *Actinobacillus pleuropneumoniae* and *Pasteurella multocida*. This form (Pulmotil) is administered as a feed additive and has been shown to be effective for controlling pneumonia in swine (Moore et al. 1996). There is a 7-day withdrawal time for slaughter when administered to swine.

Tilmicosin has also been used for treatment of pasteurellosis in rabbits (McKay et al. 1996). Single doses of 25 mg/kg SC were an effective treatment for pasteurellosis in rabbits.

Adverse Reactions to Tilmicosin. Injections of tilmicosin to horses, goats, swine, or nonhuman primates can be fatal. The heart is the target of toxicity in animals, perhaps mediated via depletion of cardiac intracellular calcium, resulting in a negative inotropic effect (Main et al. 1996). Epinephrine worsens the cardiac toxicity in pigs, but dobutamine has alleviated the cardiac depression in dogs (Main et al. 1996). The effects of toxicity are increased heart rate, arrhythmia, and depressed contractility. Injected doses of 20 and 30 mg/kg to pigs caused death, but oral tilmicosin in pigs produces no toxic effects. In cattle, injected SC doses of 50 mg/kg caused myocardial toxicity; 150 mg/kg was lethal. Doses as low as 10 mg/kg IV have caused cardiac toxicity as well (Ziv et al. 1995). The risk of toxicity is particularly important for humans.

There are warnings on the tilmicosin label that accidental injection into humans has caused death. Published reports (Veenhuizen et al. 2006) indicate that more than 12 people have died as a result of tilmicosin administration—some have been accidental. The deaths are caused by cardiovascular toxicity.

TULATHROMYCIN. Tulathromycin (Draxxin) is the most recent addition to this group of drugs. Tulathromycin is an azalide derivative of erythromycin, with three charged nitrogen groups; therefore it has been called a *triamilide* (Evans 2005). These charged groups may be important to increase the intracellular concentrations compared to older macrolides with fewer charges. It is registered for use in cattle and pigs; it has not been used in other species. In cattle and pigs it is registered for treating respiratory infections (Bovine Respiratory Disease—BRD, and Swine Respiratory Disease—SRD), for which the pathogens have been discussed earlier in this chapter. In addition to these pathogens the label includes *Mycoplasma bovis* in this drug's indications. It also is used to prevent BRD when administered to cattle (metaphylaxis) that are at risk for developing respiratory disease (Booker et al. 2007).

Tulathromycin has improved gram-negative activity compared to other drugs in this group, which translates to lower MIC values for cattle and swine respiratory pathogens (e.g., *Pasteurella, Mannheimia, Histophilus,* etc.) and bactericidal activity for many pathogens. Another important feature is the long half-life in tissues. The serum half-life was 90 hours, but the half-life in lung tissues was 184 hours and 142 hours in cattle and swine, respectively (Evans 2005). Because of this long half-life, it can be administered only once (e.g., 2.5 mg/kg SC in cattle and IM in swine) and produces high drug concentrations for several days. Withdrawal times are 18 days for cattle, and 5 days for swine.

There is some limited evidence that tulathromycin may be useful for treating pulmonary infections in foals (Venner et al. 2007). At 2.5 mg/kg IM once per week, it resolved pulmonary lesions and, except for diarrhea in some foals, was well tolerated.

The susceptible break point for tulathromycin for cattle respiratory disease pathogens is ≤16 μg/ml (CLSI 2007).

CLARITHROMYCIN. Clarithromycin (Biaxin®) is one of the newer macrolides that is semisynthetically derived from erythromycin. It is primarily used in people because it is tolerated better than erythromycin, has a broader spectrum, and concentrates in leukocytes. Clarithromycin in combination with ranitidine and bismuth (Tritec®) is currently used to treat *Helicobacter pylori* infections in people. In dogs, clarithromycin does not have pharmacokinetic features that are as favorable as those of azithromycin (the half-life is not as long), and except for pharmacokinetic studies, its use in veterinary medicine has not been reported (Vilmànyi et al. 1996).

Most veterinary experience has been in foals, where clarithromycin has been investigated as a potential treatment for respiratory infections. It has more activity against *Rhodococcus equii* isolated from foals (Jacks et al. 2003). In foals, clarithromycin is absorbed orally and has a half-life of 4.8 and 5.4 hours, depending on the study (Jacks et al. 2002), but it does not persist in tissues for as long as azithromycin (Suarez-Mier et al. 2007). Oral absorption was 57% (Womble et al. 2006), compared to 70–75% in dogs. In foals, oral clarithromycin at a dose of 7.5 mg/kg every 12 hours produces concentrations sufficient for treatment of *Rhodococcus equi* infections (Jacks et al. 2002). It has been more successful at this dose than azithromycin (Giguère et al. 2004).

AZITHROMYCIN. Azithromycin (Zithromax®) is the first drug in the class of azalides approved for people, and it is used frequently in small animals, exotic species, and horses off-label. Azalides are derived from erythromycin and their mechanisms of action are similar. (Erythromycin has a 14-member ring structure, and azithromycin has a 15-member ring structure.) Azithromycin has better oral absorption, is better tolerated, has a much longer half-life (especially in tissues), and has a broader spectrum of activity than erythromycin.

Azithromycin is active against gram-positive aerobic bacteria (staphylococci and streptococci) and anaerobes. However, the activity against staphylococci is not as good as erythromycin. It has some activity against gram-negative bacteria such as *Haemophilus* but not against enteric gram-negative bacteria or *Pseudomonas.* It has activity against many intracellular organisms, including *Chlamydophilia* (formerly called *Chlamydia*) and *Toxoplasma.* It is also active against mycobacteria and *Mycoplasma* (Lode et al. 1996)

The primary pharmacokinetic difference between azithromycin and erythromycin is the long half-life and high concentration in tissues. Azithromycin has an extraordinary ability to concentrate in tissues, particularly leukocytes, macrophages, and fibroblasts. The tissue concentration can be as much as 100 times serum concentrations. Concentrations in leukocytes can be at least 200–300 times the concentrations in serum (Panteix et al. 1993). In cats, the serum half-life is 35 hours, tissue half-lives vary from 13 to 72 hours, and the Vd is 23 l/kg (Hunter et al. 1995). In dogs, it also exhibits rapid uptake and persistent concentrations in tissues; the Vd is 12 l/kg, and plasma and tissue half-lives are 29 and 90 hours, respectively (Shepard and Falkner 1990). Oral absorption is high, with bioavailability values of 58% in cats (Hunter et al. 1995) and 97% in dogs (Shepard and Falkner 1990). In people, azithromycin is absorbed much better on an empty stomach (Lode et al. 1996).

In horses, azithromycin also demonstrates favorable pharmacokinetic and pharmacodynamic properties (Davis et al. 2002; Jacks et al. 2002, 2003; Suarez-Mier et al. 2007). For example, Davis et al. (2002) showed that oral absorption was 39% and had a plasma half-life of 18 hours in foals. More importantly, the drug persisted in leukocytes and alveolar macrophages for at least 120 hours after a single dose at concentrations greater than 5.0 μg/ml, with a half-life in leukocytes of over 49 hours. Concentrations in PMNs were over 200 times the plasma concentrations. These results were similar to those reported by Suarez-Mier et al. (2007). It had a volume of distribution of 12 l/kg, which probably accounts for the long persistence in inflammatory cells.

Of particular interest is the fact that the intracellular reservoir of azithromycin can apparently produce effective drug concentrations in the interstitial fluids, even after the plasma concentrations have declined below detectable levels (Girard et al. 1990). In fact, plasma pharmacokinetic parameters have little correlation to the in vivo efficacy of azithromycin. Intracellular stores of azithromycin in leukocytes also can serve as a mode of delivery of azithromycin to infected tissues, especially early abscesses, since the leukocytes are attracted to these sites via chemotaxis (Girard et al. 1993). The slow release of azithromycin from leukocytes distinguishes azithromycin from other macrolides and fluoroquinolones, which, despite achieving high concentrations in leukocytes, are released rapidly from cells in a drug-free environment (Panteix et al. 1993).

Clinical Use of Azithromycin. The therapeutic uses for azithromycin are similar to those of other macrolides such as erythromycin (Lode et al. 1996). The MIC for susceptible organisms is 2 μg/ml. It has become popular for treating infections in dogs, cats, exotic animals, and birds. Results of treatment of intracellular infections caused by *Toxoplasma* spp. and *Mycobacterium* spp. have been conflicting in people and are not yet reported for animals. Because of the long half-life and persistence of drug in tissues, the regimen employed in people is to administer a dose once daily for 3–5 days. Thereafter, effective drug concentrations are expected in tissues for up to 10 days. In dogs, doses of 5–10 mg/kg once daily orally for 1–5 days have been suggested. In cats, doses of 5 mg/kg once daily or every other day or one dose two to three times a week orally have been used.

There are several reports of azithromycin clinical use in foals with pulmonary infections, such as those caused by *Rhodococcus equii.* Because of favorable pharmacokinetics, cited above, plasma, leukocyte, and alveolar macrophage concentrations persist long enough to allow for every-other-day administration. Based on this work the dose for foals is 10 mg/kg every 24 hours initially, followed by treatment every 48 hours orally.

Safety of Azithromycin. Azithromycin is generally well tolerated. In people, gastrointestinal disturbances are the most common side effects (nausea, vomiting, diarrhea, abdominal pain). In dogs, high doses may cause vomiting. From the clinical reports, it appears to have been well tolerated in foals. Some transient diarrhea is possible. Adult horses may be more prone to developing diarrhea and more caution is urged with clinical use in these animals.

Erythromycin is well known to decrease the activity of drug-metabolizing enzymes in the liver. This can increase the toxicity of some drugs administered concurrently. Although azithromycin is reported to have less effect on the hepatic enzymes, some caution is needed when combining azithromycin with other drugs.

LINCOSAMIDES

Lincosamides are a group of monoglycoside antibiotics containing an amino-acidlike side chain. There are two antibiotics within this group: lincomycin and clindamycin. Lincomycin and clindamycin are structurally similar. Lincomycin has a hydroxyl moiety at the 7 position of the molecule, and clindamycin contains a chlorine at this position, making clindamycin a more active molecule against bacteria than its parent molecule, lincomycin, and better absorbed orally. The lincosamides, like the macrolides, are used primarily to treat gram-positive infections in cases where there is resistance or intolerance to penicillins. Clindamycin also is a common drug for treatment of anaerobic infections. Common infections treated with lincosamides include infections involving *Staphylococcus* spp. and *Streptococcus* spp. (Burrows 1980).

LINCOMYCIN

Source and Chemistry. Lincomycin is the antibiotic produced by *Streptococcus lincolnensis* var. *lincolnensis,* discovered in the 1950s; its name comes from cultures of soil that originated in Lincoln, Nebraska (Fig. 37.5). Lincomycin was first marketed for human clinical use in 1964 and for veterinary use in dogs and cats in 1967. Lincomycin was added to feed premixes for chickens in 1970 and to swine premixes in 1976 for growth promotion. An injectable form was ready for clinical use in swine in 1979 (Ford and Aronson 1985; Kleckner 1984). Lincomycin is a weak base with a pK_a of 7.6 (Riviere et al. 1991).

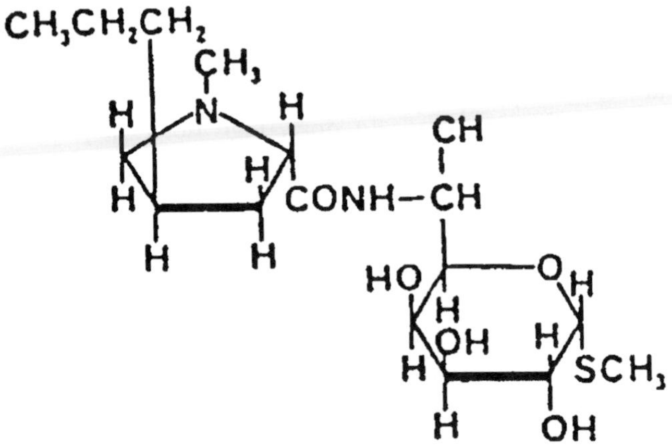

FIG. 37.5 The chemical structure of lincomycin.

Formulations. Lincomycin is available as an oral premix for pigs and chickens (Lincomix) and a soluble powder for drinking water (Lincomix). Lincomycin hydrochloride oral syrup and tablets have been used for dogs and cats (Lincocin), as well as lincomycin hydrochloride injection, but use in small animals is not as common as it once was. Ruminants and horses should not be exposed to lincomycin-supplemented feed. The toxicity is described in more detail below.

Mechanism of Action. Lincomycin inhibits protein synthesis in the microbial cell by binding to the 50S ribosomal subunit in much the same way described for macrolides. Other antibiotics, such as erythromycin and clindamycin, function similarly by binding at different sites to the same ribosomal subunit. Concurrent use of these antibiotics typically results in a decrease in the overall efficacy against the microbe due to one bound antibiotic physically overlapping the binding site of another (Burrows 1980).

Spectrum of Activity. Lincomycin is active against essentially the same bacteria as listed for macrolides.

Absorption and Distribution. Lincomycin is rapidly but incompletely absorbed when administered orally to animals, with one report stating that lincomycin oral absorption in swine given 10 mg/kg is in the range 20–50% (Hornish et al. 1987). Peak serum levels in most animals are reached within 60 minutes after an oral dose and within 2–4 hours after IM injection. Lincomycin is well distributed in the body, with highest tissue concentrations in the liver and kidneys, while very low levels are obtained in the CSF (Burrows 1980; Ford and Aronson 1985; Kleckner 1984). The Vd in animals ranges from 1 to 1.3 l/kg.

Metabolism and Excretion. The half-life after oral, IM, or IV administration is approximately 2–4 hours. Most of the oral dose, measured as ^{14}C-labeled lincomycin, was recovered in the feces and 14% in the urine after a single oral administration to the dog (Kleckner 1984); thus, biliary secretion of lincomycin appears to be an important route of elimination. After a single IM injection, 38% of the dose was found in the feces and 49% in the urine of the dog. Urine excretion of the radiolabeled drug was complete in 24 hours and fecal excretion was complete within 48 hours for both dosing routes. It is not known whether this radioactivity was associated with an unchanged/unmetabolized lincomycin or with the metabolites of this compound. An unpublished report cited by Hornish et al. (1987) stated the parent drug was the primary form present in the urine of dogs and humans.

Because of the potential for residues in meat, from a food-animal residue viewpoint, the metabolism and excretion of lincomycin have been studied more extensively in swine and chickens (Hornish et al. 1987). When administered to animals, lincomycin concentrations are highest in the liver and kidney, with low, albeit detectable, levels in muscle and skin. Lincomycin can pass unchanged from the body via the bile and feces or urine or can be metabolized to the glucuronide, *N*-demethyl lincomycin, or lincomycin sulfoxide forms by the liver. Swine given oral doses of lincomycin showed that 11–21% was excreted into the urine: 50% unchanged lincomycin, trace amounts of *N*-demethyl lincomycin, no lincomycin sulfoxide or glucuronide forms, and the rest labeled "unidentified substances." The feces contained the remainder of the excreted lincomycin: 17% unchanged lincomycin, possible trace amounts of lincomycin sulfoxide, and 83% uncharacterized metabolites (Hornish et al. 1987). Similarly conducted studies in chickens treated orally for 7 days with lincomycin showed that the excreta contained ≈80% lincomycin, ≤10% lincomycin sulfoxide, ≤5% *N*-demethyl lincomycin.

Adverse Effects and Precautions. Dogs and cats have few adverse reactions to lincomycin. Loose stools in the dog and vomiting in the cat have been the major side effects reported (Kleckner 1984). Pigs may occasionally develop diarrhea and/or swelling of the anus within the first 2 days of treatment and will self-correct within a week after withdrawal from the antibiotic.

The most serious adverse effect from lincomycin reported in people is that of pseudomembranous colitis. This is a serious disease in people caused by an overgrowth and production of toxin from *Clostridium difficile,* which may be fatal. In animals with fermenting GI tracts (horses, ruminants, rabbits, hamsters, chinchillas, and guinea pigs) there also is a high risk of GI bacterial overgrowth with *Clostridium* from lincomycin treatment. Severe enteritis, enterocolitis, may lead to diarrhea and death. Other bacteria also have been implicated in this reaction, such as *Salmonella* spp. or *E. coli* (Burrows 1980; Plenderleith 1988). Rehg and Pakes (1982) have implicated *Clostridium difficile* and *Clostridium perfringens* toxins in lincomycin toxicity in rabbits. Lincomycin-induced enterocolitis has been reported for rabbits (Maiers and Mason 1984; Thilsted et al. 1981), horses (Raisbeck et al. 1981; Plenderleith 1988), sheep (Bulgin 1988), and large ruminants (Plenderleith 1988). Lincomycin has been reported to produce ketosis in dairy cows (Rice and McMurray 1983).

Clinical Use. Lincomycin is used to treat gram-positive aerobic and anaerobic infections in patients for many of the same indications for which one would use erythromycin or other macrolide. In dogs and cats, lincomycin has been used to treat penicillin-resistant or suspected penicillin-resistant strains of *Staphylococcus* spp. and *Streptococcus* spp. bacteria found in bone, the upper respiratory tract, and the skin. Although it has been used for skin infections, it is not as popular as it once was (Noli and Boothe 1999). Doses in dogs and cats generally are 22 mg/kg every 12 hours orally. The use of lincomycin to treat bacterial infections in dogs and cats has been largely replaced by clindamycin therapy.

Lincomycin has been utilized to treat bacterial arthritis in swine caused by *Staphylococcus* spp., *Streptococcus* spp., *Erysipelothrix* spp., and *Mycoplasma* spp. and pneumonia caused by *Mycoplasma* spp. Doses in pigs are 11 mg/kg every 24 hours IM. It has also been used as a feed additive (Rainier et al. 1980), drinking-water supplement (Hamdy 1978), and parenteral product (Hamdy and Kratzer 1981) to control or treat swine dysentery.

In broiler chickens, lincomycin has been used as a feed additive to increase the rate of weight gain and improve feed efficiency, in addition to treating necrotic enteritis in this species. The addition of 2 g/ton of lincomycin to the feed of broilers resulted in a significant decrease in the incidence of necrotic enteritis (Maxey and Page 1977). Lincomycin has also been used with success in psittacines (Mandel 1977). Lincomycin use in the eyes of rabbits has also been reported (Kleinberg et al. 1979). Topical corneal administration of 1% lincomycin in water to rabbits showed local therapeutic levels could be maintained from 30–45 minutes to 2 hours postdose in the cornea, aqueous humor, and iris-ciliary body and that de-epithelialization of the corneal epithelium served to enhance the ocular topical absorption of this antibiotic.

Sheep, goats, and calves have been treated with parenteral lincomycin-spectinomycin antibiotic combinations for gram-positive and gram-negative respiratory tract infections. The lincomycin-spectinomycin combination (50 mg lincomycin with 100 mg spectinomycin [Linco-Spectam] per ml) at a dose of 1 ml/10 kg body weight IM has been used to treat foot rot in sheep caused by *Bacteroides nodosus* with better success than systemic penicillin-streptomycin therapy (Venning et al. 1990).

Regulatory Considerations. When added to feed for poultry and pigs, the slaughter withdrawal time ranges from 0 to 6 days, depending on the preparation and dose. Consult the package insert for specific recommendations. When injected in pigs, the withdrawal time for slaughter is 2 days.

CLINDAMYCIN

Source and Chemistry. Clindamycin chemically is 7-chlorolincomycin, a derivative of lincomycin and an antibiotic produced by *Streptococcus lincolnensis* var. *lincolnensis.* The replacement of the hydroxyl group at the C7 position of the lincomycin molecule by a chloride results in a more active antibacterial effect when compared to lincomycin. The chemical structure of clindamycin is shown in Figure 37.6. It is a weak base with a pK_a of 7.6. Both clindamycin hydrochloride (HCl) and clindamycin palmitate are for oral administration. Clindamycin HCl is directly active when administered, whereas the palmitate form must be converted to clindamycin in the small intestine. Clindamycin palmitate is more palatable than clindamycin HCl. Clindamycin phosphate is the parenteral form of clindamycin and must undergo hydrolysis in the plasma for it to become active.

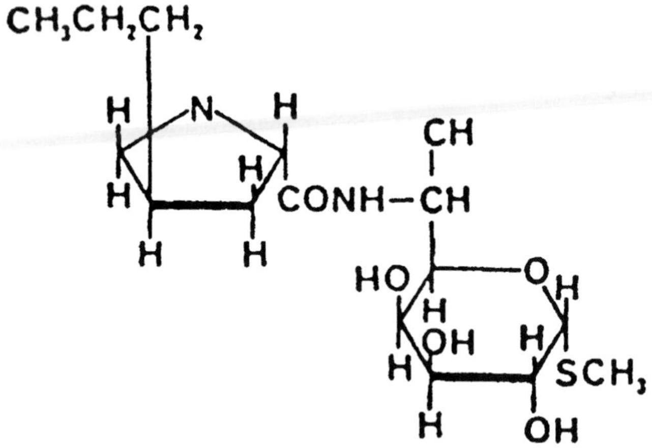

$CH_3CH_2CH_2$ ... CONH–CH ... SCH_3

FIG. 37.6 The chemical structure of clindamycin.

Mechanism of Action. Clindamycin exerts its antibiotic activity by inhibiting protein synthesis at the 50S ribosomal subunit (Hedstrom 1984) in a manner identical to that described for lincomycin. Plasmid-mediated resistance to clindamycin has been reported in *Bacteroides fragilis* (Tally et al. 1979) and cross-resistance to lincomycin can occur (Harari and Lincoln 1989).

Spectrum of Activity. Clindamycin is distinguished from the macrolide antibiotics and lincomycin by its high activity against anaerobic bacteria, including gram-negative anaerobes such as *Bacteroides* spp. In small animals, anaerobic infections are one of the major uses of clindamycin. However, one report (Jang et al. 1997) indicated that only 83% of *Bacteroides* from small animals were sensitive to clindamycin and only 80% of the *Clostridium.* Other than anaerobes, clindamycin is active against the same bacteria previously listed for macrolides and lincomycin. An additional organism for which there is activity is *Toxoplasma,* but the clinical use of clindamycin for treating toxoplasmosis in cats is controversial (described in more detail below).

Absorption and Distribution. Clindamycin is better absorbed from the GI tract in humans and animals than lincomycin, yielding higher serum concentrations, and is more active than lincomycin due to the chlorine substitution (Nichols and Keys 1984). Brown and co-workers (1989, 1990) have described the pharmacokinetics of oral clindamycin HCl disposition in the cat. Groups of cats were given oral doses of either 5.5, 11.0, or 22.0 mg/kg once daily of clindamycin (Antirobe), with physical, histologic, and hematologic changes recorded during therapy. Mean residence time ranged from 4.5 to 6.5 hours. It was also found that the 5.5 and 11.0 mg/kg oral doses maintained a serum MIC above that necessary for most *Staphylococcus aureus* infections and that the 11.0 and 22.0 mg/kg doses gave serum concentrations above the MIC for many susceptible anaerobes. Clindamycin is distributed well to tissues and attains high intracellular concentrations as exhibited by the high Vd. The apparent Vd in cats ranged from 1.6 to 3.1 L/kg. The highest concentrations of clindamycin were found in the lung, followed by liver, spleen, jejunum, and colon. Although the CSF had very low but detectable levels of clindamycin, the brain had higher than anticipated concentrations. This was most likely due to clindamycin's lipophilic nature, having a greater affinity for the lipid matrix of the brain than for the aqueous CSF. Bone marrow also had appreciable levels of clindamycin accumulation, due to sequestration of clindamycin in the fat, the concentration of clindamycin in the white blood cell precursors, or a combination of both factors.

In the dog (Budsberg et al. 1992; Lavy et al. 1999), clindamycin phosphate was administered IV, IM, and SC at 10 and 11 mg/kg. The elimination half-life was 2–3.2 hours IV but longer (5–7 hr) from IM and SC injection. The Vd was 0.9–1.4 l/kg. The bioavailability of clindamycin in one study after IM injection was 87% (Budsberg et al. 1992), but in another study bioavailability was greater than 100% from an IM dose and over 300% from the SC dose (Lavy et al. 1999). It appears that the prolonged elimination half-life from the SC administration ("flip-flop" effect) resulted in a falsely high estimate of the true availability following IM and SC administration in these studies. In one study, it was reported that clindamycin is too painful for IM administration (Budsberg et al. 1992), but in another study, IM administration of a buffered, more concentrated 20% solution was better tolerated. However, the SC dose was much better tolerated (Lavy et al. 1999) and produced more prolonged concentrations. When clindamycin was administered to dogs at a dose of 11 mg/kg oral and IV, the half-life was identical from each route (4.37 hr), and the volume of distribution was 2.48 L/kg (Batzias et al. 2005). Oral absorption was 73%.

In sea turtles (unpublished data from the author), clindamycin had extremely rapid clearance and a short half-life. There was very little oral absorption. These results in sea turtles suggest that it would be impractical to use in these animals.

Unlike lincomycin, the presence of food does not appear to affect oral absorption of clindamycin. There is good penetration into respiratory secretions, pleural fluid, the prostate, bones, and joints, but with low concentrations appearing in the CSF. The concentrations of clindamycin in phagocytes are ten- to twentyfold (and as high as 40) times the plasma concentrations (Harari and Lincoln 1989). Despite the high intracellular concentrations of clindamycin in phagocytes, intracellular killing is poor (Yancy et al. 1991), perhaps because the drug is sequestered in subcellular sites. Macrophages take up clindamycin by an active transport mechanism and concentrate clindamycin up to 50 times the extracellular concentration (Dhawan and Thadepalli 1982). Because phagocytes are the cells most likely to enter infected tissues, such as abscesses, it is possible for clindamycin to be transported to an abscess and eradicate the bacteria (Yancy et al. 1991). Clindamycin also crosses the placental barrier, but its safety during pregnancy has not been determined.

Metabolism and Excretion. Clindamycin HCl requires no metabolism to be active once administered orally. Clindamycin phosphate requires hydrolysis to occur in the plasma to be active; similarly, clindamycin palmitate requires the removal of the palmitate moiety in the small intestine to be active. The commercial form for small animals (Antirobe) is clindamycin HCl.

Clindamycin metabolites are much like those described for lincomycin. In dogs, 36% of the administered dose of clindamycin is excreted unchanged by the bile and urine. The balance of the dose appears to be active or inactive metabolites, 28% excreted by the liver in the glucuronide form (no antimicrobial activity), 28% as clindamycin sulfoxide (25% of the antimicrobial activity of the parent antibiotic), and 9% as *N*-demethyl clindamycin, which has 4–8 times the antimicrobial activity of the parent compound (Dhawan and Thadepalli 1982). The bile is the major excretion route. The colonic contents of humans administered clindamycin were found to suppress microbial activity for as long as 2 weeks after the discontinuation of therapy.

Adverse Effects and Precautions. Like lincomycin, the most serious adverse effect in humans is pseudomembranous colitis, from overgrowth of *Clostridium difficile*. This has not been a reported problem in animals. In dogs and cats, vomiting and diarrhea are possible but they are transient and not serious. However, GI problems such as those discussed above for lincomycin in ruminants, horses, rabbits, and rodents are possible, and the same precautions apply that were discussed for lincomycin. Greene et al. (1992) orally administered to cats 25 and 50 mg/kg clindamycin HCl divided in 2 doses and found that diarrhea and vomiting are two clinical signs most often associated with oral therapy. The highest frequency for both of these clinical signs occurred in the 50 mg/kg treatment group and was thought to be related to either a direct irritant effect on the GI tract or some effect on intestinal water absorption. Cats are also reluctant to accept the oral liquid form of clindamycin because of poor palatability. As reported for other oral drugs in cats (eg, doxycycline hyclate) oral administration of clincamycin hydrochloride has been associated with esophageal injury (Beatty et al. 2006).

A study was performed in cats to ascertain the effect of prolonged clindamycin therapy on vitamin K–dependent blood clotting times (Jacobs et al. 1989). The study showed that factor VII levels did not significantly change in cats treated with a total daily dose of 25 mg/kg orally once daily for 6 weeks compared to controls.

Clinical Use. Clindamycin possesses an antimicrobial spectrum similar to that of lincomycin, but it is much more extensively used clinically than lincomycin because of higher activity against anaerobes, increased potency, and more complete oral absorption. Clindamycin has been reported to be as much as 20 times more potent than lincomycin in the treatment of *Staphylococcus* and *Streptococcus* infections in humans (Harvey 1985). Clindamycin is active against aerobic species of organisms, including *Staphylococcus, Streptococcus, Actinomyces, Nocardia, Mycoplasma,* and *Toxoplasma*. The anaerobic bacterial spectrum of activity includes *Bacteroides fragilis, Fusobacterium* spp., *Peptostreptococcus* spp., and *Clostridium perfringens* (Harari and Lincoln 1989). Clindamycin has been used to treat wounds, abscesses, osteomyelitis, and periodontal diseases caused by these organisms. Clindamycin is found in high concentrations in the prostate, making it an acceptable choice for treating bacterial prostatitis when caused by gram-positive organisms.

The use of clindamycin for treating toxoplasmosis is controversial. Lappin et al. (1989) performed a retrospective study of cats diagnosed with *Toxoplasma gondii* infections and found that those cats treated with clindamycin resolved all clinical signs of the disease except those lesions involving the eyes. Clindamycin alone or in combination with a corticosteroid helped to resolve the active retinochoroiditis and the anterior uveitis associated with this disease. Even though clindamycin may help clinical signs associated with toxoplasmosis, it may not help to clear organisms from the CNS or the eye. In experimentally infected cats, there was a paradoxical effect in that cats with toxoplasmosis treated with clindamycin had a worsening of clinical signs. As discussed in more detail by Davidson et al. (1996), this paradoxical effect may be due to an inhibition of intracellular killing of organisms by clindamycin.

Clindamycin can be used to treat *Staphylococcus* spp. infections in dogs with experimentally induced posttraumatic osteomyelitis (Braden et al. 1987, 1988). An oral dose of 11 mg/kg twice daily for 28 days was found to be efficacious in treatment of these infected dogs, resulting in a 94% recovery rate in the clindamycin-treated dogs. Clindamycin also has been shown to be effective for treatment of superficial and deep pyoderma in dogs and is a common choice as an alternative to β-lactam antibiotics (Harvey et al. 1993; Noli and Boothe 1999; Scott et al. 1998). Although 11 mg/kg every 24 hours has been used to treat staphylococcal infections (pyoderma) in dogs, for most infections dosing 11 mg/kg every 12 hours is used by many veterinarians for treating most *Staphylococcus* spp. infections.

MISCELLANEOUS ANTIBIOTICS

BACITRACIN. Bacitracin is a complex labile polypeptide consisting of 5–10 separate chemical components first isolated from a *Bacillus subtillus*–contaminated wound in 1943 (Teske 1984). Bacitracin A ($C_{66}H_{103}N_{17}O_{16}S$) is the major component of this mixture and accounts for most of the antibiotic activities. Bacitracin inhibits peptidoglycan synthesis in bacteria by nonspecifically blocking phosphorylase reactions, some of which occur during cell wall synthesis (Lancini and Parenti 1982). Development of resistance to bacitracin is rare.

Bacitracin is active against gram-positive organisms. Bacitracin is not absorbed from the GI tract when given orally. Systemic administration has resulted in a high incidence of nephrotoxicity (albuminuria, cylindruria, azotemia), in addition to pain, induration, and petechiae at the site of injection. In contrast, bacitracin is nonirritating and rarely induces allergic reactions when used topically. Bacitracin (bacitracin, bacitracin methylenedisalicylate, bacitracin manganese, zinc bacitracin) has been used as a feed additive to promote growth in many species of animals, but its most common use today is in topical applications to treat susceptible skin, ear, and eye infections. Bacitracin inhibits many organisms found on skin, such as hemolytic and nonhemolytic *Streptococcus* spp., coagulase-positive *Staphylococcus* spp., and some *Clostridium* spp., and it is often combined with other antibiotics that have a gram-negative spectrum of activity (polymyxin B, neomycin). Zinc bacitracin administered topically may increase the activity of bacitracin due to zinc's astringent properties, which decrease inflammation (Harvey 1985).

NOVOBIOCIN. Novobiocin is a dibasic acid ($pK_a = 4.3$ and 9.1) derived from coumarin and is utilized clinically as a mono- (Na^+) or dibasic- (Ca^{++}) salt form. Novobiocin possesses activity against both gram-positive and gram-negative bacteria but is more active against the gram–positive bacteria, in particular *Staphylococcus* species. Other susceptible organisms include *Neisseria* spp., *Haemophilus* spp., *Brucella* spp., and some strains of *Proteus* spp. It may be used as an alternative to penicillins in cases involving penicillin-resistant *Staphylococcus* spp., although other penicillin substitutes (cephalosporins, macrolides, clindamycin) are better clinical choices.

Novobiocin has several toxic effects on bacteria, but its exact mechanism and site of action are unknown. Novobiocin has been shown to cause nonspecific inhibition of cell wall synthesis by inhibiting formation of alternating *N*-acetylmuramic acid pentapeptide and *N*-acetylglucosamine residues; it also inhibits teichuronic acid in some species of bacteria. The concentrations needed to inhibit these cell wall components are greater than the minimal concentration needed to inhibit growth, suggesting these effects on bacteria are secondary effects. DNA and RNA synthesis, protein synthesis (β-galactosidase), respiration, and oxidative phosphorylation are also inhibited in some species of bacteria and in rat liver homogenates (Morris and Russell 1971), with none seemingly being the primary antibiotic effect. Novobiocin is also known to induce an intracellular magnesium deficiency, but there is no direct convincing evidence that this is the mechanism responsible for novobiocin's antimicrobial activity.

Novobiocin is initially highly effective against *Staphylococcus* spp. infections, but resistance to this antibiotic develops quickly (Morris and Russell 1971; Harvey 1985).

Synergism occurs when novobiocin is combined with tetracycline. Novobiocin has been combined with tetracycline to broaden the spectrum of activity and to decrease the resistance to novobiocin, but these older combinations are used infrequently today. Novobiocin and tetracycline have been reported to be efficacious in cases of canine upper respiratory diseases such as "kennel cough" and tonsillitis (Maxey 1980), but the use for this problem in dogs has declined substantially. Toxic side effects in animals and humans given novobiocin systemically have been reported and include skin rashes, leucopenia, pancytopenia, anemia, agranulocytosis, thrombocytopenia, nausea, vomiting, and diarrhea. Few side effects have been reported for this antibiotic used in its topical form in domestic animals.

THIOSTREPTON. Thiostrepton is a polypeptide antibiotic produced by *Streptomyces aureus* and has a predominately gram-positive spectrum, although some gram-negative organisms are also affected. Thiostrepton is not absorbed from the GI tract and is used primarily for topical local therapy, usually combined with other antibiotics and/or glucocorticosteroids for dermatologic therapy (Huber 1982).

RIFAMPIN. Rifampin is a complex macrocyclic high-molecular-weight semisynthetic antibiotic derived from rifamycin B, produced by *Nocardia mediterrea.* Rifamycin B is chemically modified to produce rifampin (U.S. and Canadian name), also known as *rifampicin* in Europe. The chemical structure of rifampin is shown in Figure 37.7. Rifampin has a high activity against gram-positive bacteria (*Staphylococcus* spp.), *Mycobacterium* spp., *Haemophilus* spp., *Neisseria* spp., and *Chlamydia* spp., but more limited activity against the gram-negative bacteria.

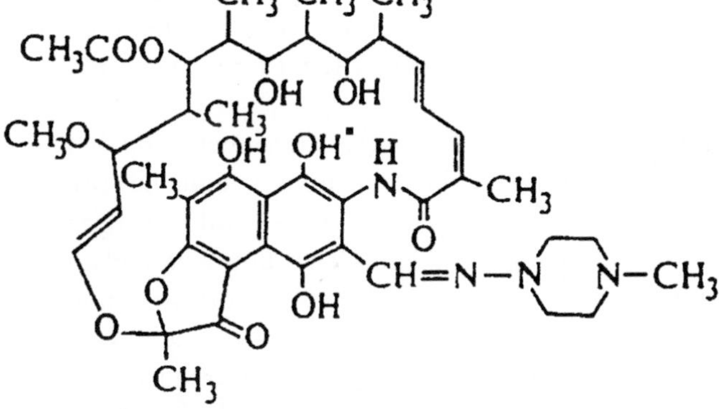

FIG. 37.7 The chemical structure of rifampin.

Rifampin is highly lipid soluble, is stable in acidic environments, and can concentrate in neutrophils and macrophages, which is therapeutically advantageous in diseases involving intracellular organisms (*Brucella, Mycobacterium, Rhodococcus, Chlamydophilia,* etc.) and chronic granulomatous diseases. Rifampin enters the microbial cell and forms stable complexes with the β subunit of DNA-dependent RNA polymerases of microorganisms. This binding results in inactive enzymes and inhibition of RNA synthesis by preventing chain initiation. This inhibition can also occur in mammalian cells, but much higher concentrations are needed. MICs for gram-positive organisms generally occur at 0.1 μg/ml, while gram negative bacteria have MIC values ranging from 8 to 32 μg/ml. This large disparity in MIC values is attributed to rifampin's ability to more easily permeate the gram-positive organism cell wall than the gram-negative organism cell wall rather than differences in bacterial RNA polymerases.

Pharmacokinetics. Rifampin is rapidly absorbed from the GI tract after oral administration in humans, dogs, calves, horses, and foals. Rifampin absorption is highest in an acidic environment. Rifampin is approximately 80% bound to plasma proteins, with the remainder being widely distributed to all tissues of the body, with particularly high concentrations of the drug found in the lungs, liver, bile, and urine. After oral absorption or parenteral administration, rifampin is primarily metabolized to the bioactive metabolite 25-desacetylrifampin, with some minor glucuronidation products formed in the liver. Both parent and metabolite compounds are excreted in the bile. Both forms are passively filtered through the kidneys, with renal clearance being approximately 12% of total glomerular filtration rate.

Multiple dosing of rifampin often results in decreased, rather than increased, peak serum concentrations. This phenomenon is due to autoinduction of liver enzymes and is known to occur in humans, swine, dogs, calves, and rodents (Frank 1990). Hepatic enzyme induction by rifampin will also alter the disposition of other drugs. Plasma ketoconazole levels decrease and the metabolism of progestin, digitalis, warfarin, ciprofloxacin, glucocorticosteroids, and several other drugs increases when they are concurrently administered with rifampin (Kenny and Strates 1981; Frank 1990; Barriere et al. 1989). In addition to being a potent inducer of hepatic cytochrome P450 enzymes, rifampin also can induce the MRD membrane efflux pump (P-glycoprotein), which may have the consequence of decreasing oral absorption of other drugs.

The pharmacokinetics of rifampin has been studied in humans (Acocella 1983; Kenny and Strates 1981), in the adult horse (Burrows et al. 1985), and in the foal (Castro et al. 1986). Adult horses given 10 mg/kg of rifampin IV, IM, or PO showed a rapid absorption of rifampin by the oral route versus the IM route, but the IM route provided longer detectable plasma concentrations in 50% of the horses than did the oral route. Adult horses given 10 mg/kg IV showed a serum half-life of 6.05 hours and an apparent Vd of 0.7 l/kg. Doses of 10 mg/kg administered IM and PO had half-lives of 7.32 and 5.84 hours, respectively. Oral doses of 25 mg/kg in adult horses had a serum half-life of 4.78 hours. It was determined that the 10 mg/kg PO dose was adequate for susceptible gram-positive infections in the adult horse, whereas the 10 mg/kg IV or the 25 mg/kg PO dose was necessary to treat susceptible gram-negative infections. The rate of excretion in the foal is lower than in the adult horse, mainly due to biliary excretion mechanisms being less developed in the foal. Foals given 10 mg/kg of rifampin orally had a mean serum half-life of 17.5 hours, significantly longer than that found in the adult horse. The authors of that study indicated that 5 mg/kg orally was sufficient in the foal to combat susceptible gram-positive infections and that higher or more-frequent doses were needed to treat susceptible gram-negative infections.

The pharmacokinetics of rifampin has also been studied in sheep (Jernigan et al. 1986), with the recommended dose from that study being 20 mg/kg orally once a day. In sheep administered a 50 mg/kg dose of rifampin IV, the serum half-life was 4.56 hours and the apparent Vd was 0.5 l/kg.

Clinical Use. Rifampin has been used to treat a wide variety of microbial infections. Susceptible organisms of interest to veterinarians include *Staphylococcus* species (including methicillin-resistant strains), *Streptococcus* spp., *Rhodococcus equi*, *Corynebacterium pseudotuberculosis*, and most strains of *Bacteroides* spp., *Clostridium* spp., *Neisseria* spp., and *Listeria* spp. Organisms known to be resistant to rifampin are *Pseudomonas aeruginosa, E. coli, Enterobacter* spp., *Klebsiella pneumoniae, Proteus* spp., *and Salmonella* spp. Wilson et al. (1988) obtained samples from clinically ill horses and tested the isolated bacteria for susceptibility to rifampin. It was found that all strains of coagulase-positive *Staphylococcus* spp., *Streptococcus zooepidemicus, Streptococcus equi, Streptococcus equisimilus, Rhodococcus equi*, and *Corynebacterium pseudotuberculosis* were highly susceptible to rifampin at MICs of 0.25 μg/ml. Gram-negative organisms isolated in that study were *Actinobacillus suis, Actinobacillus equuli*, and *Bordetella bronchiseptica*, and MIC values ranged from <0.008 to >16 μg/ml. Other isolates, such as *Pseudomonas aeruginosa, Enterobacter cloacae, Klebsiella pneumoniae, Proteus* spp., and *Salmonella* spp., were found to be resistant, having MICs greater than 4 μg/ml.

Most of rifampin use has been in horses. Rifampin is used to treat equine diseases of a gram-positive bacterial origin (e.g., *Rhodococcus equi, Streptococcus equi*). However, resistance to rifampin is quickly acquired when administered alone to combat these infections. Resistance is readily accomplished by a single mutation of the amino acid sequence of the β subunit of the DNA-dependent RNA polymerase enzyme. Mutations result in rifampin having less affinity for the RNA polymerase enzyme. Higher concentrations of rifampin are necessary to overcome this resistance in vitro. Resistance can be minimized if other antibiotics are used concurrently with rifampin that will kill the mutant strains of bacteria produced in response to rifampin. Antibiotics that can be so used are erythromycin, most of the β-lactam antibiotics, vancomycin, and gentamicin, depending on the bacterial sensitivity to these drugs (Frank 1990).

Synergism may occur between amphotericin B and rifampin against some fungi, particularly *Saccharomyces cerevisiae, Histoplasma capsulatum*, several species of *Aspergillus*, and *Blastomyces dermatitidis* (Medoff 1983). Increased permeability of rifampin across the fungal cell wall (and hence increased inhibition of RNA polymerases) due to amphotericin B–induced cell wall damage is probably the mechanism responsible for this synergism.

Adverse Effects. Rifampin is teratogenic in laboratory animals, so its use in pregnant animals should be restricted. Rifampin will color the urine, saliva, and tears of treated animals an orange-red. This effect should be explained to animal owners when prescribing so that this reaction does not cause alarm. Dogs given the human dose of 10 mg/kg orally developed increases in hepatic enzyme activity, some of which eventually progressed to clinical cases of hepatitis. Hepatitis is the most common reason to discontinue rifampin treatment in dogs. However, lowering the total daily dose of rifampin will decrease the chances of inducing toxic side effects, especially in dogs. Although rare, rifampin can induce thrombocytopenia, hemolytic anemia, anorexia, vomiting, and diarrhea. Preexisting renal disease does not normally require a dose modification of rifampin.

NITROFURANS. Nitrofurans comprise several synthetic compounds derived from 5-nitrofuran and possess antimicrobial activity, the 5-nitro group being required for this activity. Over 3,500 nitrofurans have been synthesized to date, with only a handful being useful in animal chemotherapy. Nitrofurans and furazolidone are banned from use in food-producing animals.

Nitrofurans as a group are bacteriostatic and function by blocking oxidative decarboxylation of pyruvate to acetyl coenzyme A, depriving susceptible organisms of vital energy production pathways. Their spectrum of activity includes gram-positive and gram-negative bacteria and some protozoans, but they are most effective against the gram-negative bacteria. Nitrofurans can be administered orally or topically. Oral absorption is enhanced when administered with feed; it is widely distributed throughout the body but in low concentrations. Approximately 50% of the total dose of nitrofurans are excreted in the active form. Acidification of the urine promotes tubular reabsorption, which also decreases the overall urine concentration of the drug. An acid environment is required for the nitrofurans to diffuse across the cell membranes. Nitrofurantoin has a broad gram-positive and gram-negative spectrum and also high concentrations in the urine, making it useful as a urinary antiseptic in small animals. Nitrofuran use today is mainly in topical preparations for the eye, ear, mucous membranes, and skin; it finds limited use in treating bacterial GI tract and urinary tract disorders (Ali 1989; Ford and Aronson 1985).

The major disadvantage of nitrofurans to treat systemic infections is that the concentrations needed to reach the MIC also induce systemic toxicity. There are many reports in the veterinary literature on the toxicities induced when the nitrofurans are used systemically (Ali 1983). The toxicology of furazolidone (*N*-5-nitro-2-furfurylidene amino-2-oxazolidinone) has been investigated extensively in laboratory, food, and companion animals as well as in humans and has been reviewed by Ali (1989). The effects of feeding furazolidone to poultry have been reported (Ali 1989; Mustafa et al. 1975; Czarnecki et al. 1974a; Jankus et al. 1972; Czarnecki et al. 1974b).

Furazolidone has also been demonstrated to be carcinogenic when used at a 0.15% w/w concentration in feed for 1 year, inducing mammary tumors in a dose-related manner. Mice fed a 0.03% w/w concentration in feed for life developed bronchial adenocarcinomas in both sexes (Ali 1983). DNA is the principal target of furazolidone in some cells in vivo, causing cuts and mutations in DNA and binding to DNA, hence blocking the replication and transcription processes. Mutagenesis by nitrofurans in general also occurs and has been extensively reviewed by McCalla (1983), who notes several possible metabolic pathways by which nitrofurans can cause mutagenesis in mammalian cells. This potential for mutagenesis and carcinogenesis has caused the ban from use in food-producing animals.

VIRGINIAMYCIN. Virginiamycin is a combination of two chemicals produced by *Streptomyces virginiae,* isolated from soil samples in Belgium in the early 1960s. Virginiamycin is classified as a peptolide antibiotic composed of the predominate M fraction ($C_{28}H_{35}N_3O_7$) and the lesser S fraction ($C_{43}H_{49}NO_{10}$) (Crawford 1984). The optimum ratio of M:S is 4:1 (Gottschall et al. 1988). Administered separately, both M- and S- fractions have a reversible bacteriostatic action on susceptible bacterial populations; used together, their activity is synergistic, bactericidal, and approximately 100 times that found when used separately. Virginiamycin is not known to be synergistic with other classes of antibiotics. Virginiamycin is primarily active against gram-positive organisms, *Haemophilus* spp., and *Neisseria* spp. and has mild activity against the protozoan *Toxoplasma* spp. It works by inhibiting protein synthesis at the 23S ribosomal subunit, blocking translation but not transcription in susceptible bacteria. Virginiamycin is rapidly absorbed when administered orally, is excreted by the bile with no enterohepatic circulation, and has an affinity for dermal tissues (Crawford 1984). Gottschall et al. (1988) reported that ^{14}C-virginiamycin, specifically the M fraction, was extensively metabolized in the rumen. The S fraction underwent no detectable metabolism in the rumen, and the M fraction metabolites had considerably less antimicrobial activity than the parent compound.

All virginiamycin-like antibiotics fall into one of two groups. Group A consists of polyunsaturated cyclic peptolides that have a molecular weight of approximately 500 and that contain substituted aminodecanoic acid and an oxanzole system. Group B consists of cyclic hexadepsipeptides with an approximate molecular weight of 800, and most members contain one molecule of pipecolic acid or its derivative. Both groups have low solubilities in aqueous solvents and are more soluble in organic solvents. All strongly absorb ultraviolet radiation and are therefore degraded in its presence. Virginiamycin-like antibiotics tend to affect gram-positive bacteria more than the gram-negative, with *Mycobacteria* spp. being relatively resistant and *Haemophilus* spp. and *Neisseria* spp. being very sensitive. Differences in bacterial sensitivity to different virginiamycin-like antibiotics are caused by each antibiotic's particular ability to permeate that bacteria's cell wall to gain access to the ribosomes (Cocito 1979).

Virginiamycin and virginiamycin-like antibiotics are not commonly used to treat clinical bacterial disease in domestic animals, despite their rather broad spectrum of activity. They have been used to treat swine dysentery (*Treponema hyodysenteriae*) (Olsen and Rodabaugh 1977), but other antibiotics have proven to be more efficacious. Its main use has been as a feed additive for growth promotion in food animals such as swine (Ravindran and Kornegay 1984; Moser et al. 1985), being approved for this use since 1975. Virginiamycin has also been studied in turkeys (Salmon and Stevens 1990), broilers (Miles et al. 1984), and laying hens (Miles et al. 1985) as a growth promotant, all of which experienced either increased weight gain or increased egg production.

CARBADOX. Carbadox (methyl 3-(2-quinoxalinylmethylene) carbazate N_1,N_4 dioxide) is a synthetic antibacterial agent primarily active against the gram-positive bacteria, although some gram-negative bacteria are affected as well. Available in 1973, carbadox was marketed as a growth promotant in swine and also for the control of swine dysentery (*Treponema hyodysenteriae*), bacterial enteritis (in particular, *Salmonella cholerasuis*), and nasal infections of *Bordetella bronchiseptica* in swine (Farrington and Shively 1979; Huber 1982). Carbadox was shown to be better than lincomycin for the treatment of swine dysentery (Anonymous 1980; Rainier et al. 1980). Resistance to carbadox has been reported in *E. coli* via R-plasmids (Ohmae et al. 1981).

The daily feeding of carbadox in feed concentrations of more than 100 ppm for growth promotion in pigs has resulted in toxicities in some weaned pigs, which include growth retardation, dry feces, wasting, dehydration, urine drinking, and a strong interest in salt-containing products (van der Molen et al. 1989a). It is now known that carbadox suppresses aldosterone production, leading to hypoaldosteronism, which then leads to decreased plasma sodium and increased plasma potassium concentrations. These ion alterations are due to stimulation of the renin-angiotensin system with subsequent morphological changes in the zona glomerulosa of the adrenal cortex (van der Molen et al. 1989a,b,c).

VANCOMYCIN. Of the glycopeptides, vancomycin is the only one used in veterinary medicine. Teicoplanin has been used in Europe but is not available in the United States. Vancomycin was discovered in the 1950s. In the 1960s and 1970s it was not used much because the penicillins and cephalosporins were active against most gram-positive bacteria. But in the last 10–15 years resistant enterococcal and staphylococcal infections have generated more reliance on vancomycin in human medicine. Vancomycin is a tricyclic glycopeptide having an approximate molecular weight of 1500. It is produced by the soilborne actinomycete *Streptomyces orientalis*. It is freely soluble in water, odorless, and slightly bitter to the taste. Vancomycin is highly active against gram-positive cocci (in particular, *Staphylococcus* spp. and streptococci), enterococci (*Enterococcus faecium* and *E. faecalis*), as well as *Neisseria* spp. Because it has activity against methicillin-resistant *Staphylococcus* species, including *S. aureus* (MRSA) and *Staphylococcus pseudintermedius* and β-lactam resistant *Enterococcus* species, it has become extremely valuable for the treatment of these infections. It also is active against gram-positive anaerobic cocci (but not anaerobic gram-negative bacteria) and has been administered to people for diarrhea caused by *Clostridium* spp.

Vancomycin functions as a bactericidal antibiotic by inhibiting the synthesis of the linear peptidoglycan in the bacterial cell wall during replication, resulting in the bacterium's rapid death. Its action is time-dependent, but the pharmacokinetic-pharmacodynamic (PK-PD) that best predicts clinical results is the area-under-the-curve (AUC) to MIC ratio (AUC:MIC). Over 80 *n*-alkyl vancomycins have been synthesized by reductive alkylation of vancomycin, with some forms being five times more active than vancomycin and with some having longer elimination half-lives (Nagarajan et al. 1989).

Adverse Effects. The most common adverse effect is kidney injury. Early formulations of vancomycin were associated with a high incidence of adverse effects. Most of these effects were associated with rapid IV administration, which induced flushing of the skin, pruritus, tachycardia, and other signs attributed to histamine release. Ototoxicity also was reported. The incidence of nephrotoxicity and ototoxicity may be partially caused by the common practice of simultaneously administering vancomycin with aminoglycosides. Newer formulations are safer, but histamine release still is possible from IV administration. Toxicity studies on vancomycin have been performed in many species of laboratory animals (Wold and Turnipseed 1981). The LD_{50} for the canine was 292 mg/kg, but death did not occur until several days after dosing. Dogs that died typically had blood urea nitrogen (BUN) values between 250 and 300 mg/dl, death presumably being due to acute nephrotoxic renal failure.

Clinical Use and Administration Guidelines. Clinical use of vancomycin has been limited in veterinary medicine and most of our clinical recommendations for use are derived from pharmacokinetic studies performed in dogs and horses and recommendations of effective blood concentrations for people. Vancomycin must be administered via IV infusion, although in rare instances intraperitoneal administration has been used. Vancomycin is poorly absorbed orally and this route is not used except to treat intestinal infections. IM administration is painful and irritating.

In dogs the half-life is somewhat shorter and the Vd smaller than in humans (Zaghlol and Brown 1988). In order to keep the plasma concentration within a suggested window of 10–30 μg/ml, the dose rate of 15 mg/kg q6-8h IV is recommended. (This dose actually produces peaks and troughs of approximately 40 and 5 μg/ml, respectively, but it is the most convenient dose that can be used because of the short half-life in dogs.) This dose should be infused slowly over 30–60 minutes, or at a rate of approximately 10 mg/min. The total dose to be administered can be diluted in 0.9% saline or 5% dextrose solution, but not alkalinizing solutions. Vancomycin is available in vials of 500 mg to 5 g (Vancocin, other brands, and generic). If vancomycin is used to treat enterococcal infections, it is strongly recommended to coadminister an aminoglycoside (e.g., amikacin or gentamicin) because when used alone, vancomycin is not bactericidal.

Vancomycin is used much less frequently in horses, but has been necessary occasionally for treatment of methicillin-resistant *Staphylococcus* infections and drug-resistant infections caused by *Enterococcus*. The guidelines for treatment were developed by Orsini et al. (2005) from their pharmacokinetic studies. A dose of 7.5 mg/kg is infused over at least 30 minutes every 8 hours in horses. Adverse reactions with this protocol have been minimal. To treat distal limb infections in horses regional limb perfusion or interosseous regional infusions have been used according to a protocol developed by Rubio-Martinez et al. (2005, 2006), in which 300 mg total dose is diluted in 60 ml saline solution and infused in the distal limb.

If vancomycin is administered according to the recommended dosing rates, adverse reactions described earlier are rare. A slow infusion is recommended to minimize histamine release. To avoid other toxic reactions, dose recommendations are designed to avoid high plasma concentrations. In people, therapeutic drug monitoring is often performed to ensure that peak concentrations are below 50 μg/ml and the trough concentrations are above 5 μg/ml. If animals have renal disease or unique physiologic changes (e.g., pregnant or a neonatal animal), drug disposition may change, and peak and trough plasma concentrations should be monitored to adjust the dose appropriately.

Regulatory Considerations. In August 20, 1997, the US FDA prohibited the extralabel use of glycopeptides in food-producing animals for fear of glycopeptide-resistant bacteria being transmitted to humans from treated animals (Bates et al. 1994). Feeding glycopeptides to animals is not legal in the United States.

METHENAMINE. Methenamine (hexamethylenetetramine) is a urinary antiseptic most commonly used to treat urinary tract infections in small animals. It may be used in conjunction with an antibiotic or occasionally by itself in some cases of bacterial urinary tract infections that have become refractory to conventional antibiotic therapies. Methenamine is activated by a hydrolysis reaction to form formaldehyde and ammonia in acidic urine. It has been proven to be effective against a wide variety of gram-positive and gram-negative organisms but will not affect the growth of *Candida albicans*. It can be either bacteriostatic or bactericidal depending on the pH of the urine (Huber 1982; Harvey 1985).

Methenamine is quickly absorbed when given orally, but absorption is not complete because some is hydrolyzed in the stomach. It is excreted via the urine, and is associated with a low systemic toxicity. For this drug to be efficacious, the urine must be at an acidic pH in order to liberate free formaldehyde. Methenamine has been administered with a urinary acidifier to lower the urine pH. Acid urine also exerts some independent weak antibacterial activity. Concurrent use of other urinary acidifiers, such as ascorbic acid, arginine HCl, methionine, cranberry juice (hippurate), and ammonium chloride, will enhance the antibacterial action of methenamine. Methenamine is most effective when the urine pH is 6 or below. One of the forms of methenamine used is methenamine hippurate, which is available in human tablet form and is administered to dogs. Sulfonamides should not be administered with methenamine due to the formation of insoluble formaldehyde-sulfonamide precipitates. Since methenamine is largely eliminated via the kidney, its use should be restricted or closely monitored in cases of renal insufficiency (Huber 1982; Harvey 1985). Methenamine is less effective for treating infections caused by urea-splitting organisms which increase the urine pH (e.g., *Proteus mirabilis*).

Methenamine mandelate has been used experimentally in the treatment of burn wounds in rats. Topical doses of 5% and 10% were highly efficacious against experimentally induced burns infected with a virulent strain of *Pseudomonas* spp. (Taylor et al. 1970).

POLYMYXINS. Polymyxins are a group of *N*-monoacetylated decapeptides discovered in 1947 and are produced by *Bacillus polymyxa*. They contain seven amino acids in a cyclic configuration and have a molecular weight of approximately 1000. Several polymyxins have been isolated and have been named A, B, C, D, E, and M. Of these six antibiotics, B and E in their sulfate salt forms are the only ones used clinically. The largest use of polymyxin has been in topical ointment preparations. Polymyxin B sulfate is a mixture of polymyxin B1 ($C_{56}H_{98}N_{16}O_{3}$) and polymyxin B2 ($C_{55}H_{96}N_{16}O_{13}$); polymyxin E is more commonly known as colistin (Harvey 1985). Polymyxin B1 has a pK_a ranging from 8 to 9.

Polymyxins are basic surface-active cationic detergents that interact with the phospholipid within the cell membrane, penetrate that membrane, and then disrupt its structure. This action subsequently induces permeability changes within the cell that result in cell death, giving polymyxins bactericidal properties.

Polymyxins are not absorbed to any extent from the GI tract when administered orally but are rapidly absorbed when given parenterally, with 70–90% plasma protein binding. Polymyxin B is rapidly distributed to the heart, lungs, liver, kidney, and skeletal muscle, with excretion mainly via the urine (Sande and Mandell 1990a). The pharmacokinetics of some of the polymyxins in calves, ewes, rabbits, and dogs is reviewed in greater detail elsewhere (Ziv and Sulman 1973a; Ziv et al. 1982; Craig and Kunin 1973; al-Khayyat and Aronson 1973a,b). Ziv and Sulman (1973a) reported that an IV administration of 5 mg/kg polymyxin B in ewes resulted in a serum half-life of 2.7–4.3 hours and a Vd of 1.29 l/kg.

Polymyxins have a gram-negative antibacterial spectrum, which includes *Aerobacter, Escherichia, Histophilus, Klebsiella, Pasteurella, Pseudomonas, Salmonella,* and *Shigella. Proteus* spp. and most strains of *Serratia* spp. are not affected by polymyxins, and all gram-positive bacteria are resistant. If bacteria are sensitive to the polymyxins, they rarely acquire resistance. The ability of each antibiotic in this group to kill these bacteria varies (Harvey 1985). The antimicrobial actions of polymyxin B are inhibited by divalent cations, unsaturated fatty acids, debris, purulent exudate, and quaternary ammonium compounds.

Since the polymyxins are not absorbed into the body when given orally, polymyxin B has been used for "bowel sterilization" prior to abdominal surgeries and in irrigation solutions to flush the peritoneal cavities during those procedures. Polymyxins used to be the major drugs for treatment of *Pseudomonas* infections in humans, but since the advent of better penicillins, aminoglycosides, and cephalosporins, their use has declined over time. Nephrotoxicity occurs due to glomerulus and tubular epithelium damage. In addition, respiratory paralysis (usually due to a rapid IV injection, too much peritoneal lavage, or a preexisting renal condition); and CNS dysfunction, including depression, pyrexia, and anorexia, also occurs. Polymyxins are mainly used in topical skin, mucous membrane, eye, and ear preparations. No adverse systemic effects have been reported when they are applied to intact or denuded skin surfaces. Polymyxin antibacterial activity is markedly decreased in the presence of pus, in tissues containing acidic phospholipids, and in the presence of anionic detergents or other chemicals that antagonize cationic detergents (Harvey 1985).

In addition to its narrow-spectrum antimicrobial properties, polymyxin B has demonstrated a protective effect against the adverse effects of endotoxin produced by gram-negative bacteria. This property has been studied more in horses than in other species and has been part of an anti-endotoxin protocol in equine medicine (Morresey and Mackay 2006). Infusions ranging from 1,000 to 10,000 units per kg (a common dose is 6,000 units/kg, equivalent to 1 mg/kg) administered every 8 hours have been shown to be safe and effective for treating endotoxemia in horses. Mechanistically, the cationic portion of polymyxin B binds to the anionic lipid A portion of this endotoxin. This effectively renders the endotoxin inactive, thereby preventing most of the adverse effects that gram-negative endotoxin has on the mammalian body.

SPECTINOMYCIN. Spectinomycin (Spectam) resembles aminoglycosides in some properties. It is highly water soluble and is easily mixed in aqueous solutions. Compared to aminoglycosides, it does not contain amino sugars or glycosidic bonds, but it has an aminocyclitol nucleus like the aminoglycosides. An important difference between spectinomycin and the aminoglycosides is in the adverse effects and spectrum of activity. Spectinomycin lacks the toxic effects of aminoglycoside antibiotics and can be used without the concern about renal injury.

Antimicrobial Activity. Spectinomycin, like aminoglycosides inhibits protein synthesis via a 30S ribosomal target. It is a broad-spectrum drug with activity against gram-positive and some gram-negative bacteria, but little anaerobic activity. It also has good activity against *Mycoplasma.* It is used in cattle because it has activity against *Mannheimia (Pasteurella) haemolytica, Pasteurella multocida,* and *Histophilus somni* (formerly *Haemohilus somnus).*

Pharmacokinetics. Like the aminoglycosides, spectinomycin has a small volume of distribution. It is poorly absorbed after oral administration (10% or less), but some systemic levels are achieved after oral administration in monogastric animals. Most of an oral dose is eliminated in the feces, but after an injection the primary route of elimination is the kidneys. Oral administration has been used for a local effect for treatment of diarrhea.

The half-life of spectinomycin is approximately 2 hours in cattle at a dose of 10 mg/kg IM or IV, and 1.2 hours after a dose of 20 mg/kg IV. After oral dosing in dogs of 100 or 500 mg/kg, the plasma concentrations (peak) were 22 and 80 μg/ml, respectively. The half-life in dogs is 2.72 hours at the 100 mg/kg dose. After IM injection in dogs, the half-life was 1.1 hours. In pigs, the half-life was 1 hour after IM administration.

Clinical Use. Older formulations have been used that contain both lincomycin and spectinomycin (linco-spectin). Formulations containing only spectinomycin (Spectam) include spectinomycin oral solution, spectinomycin powder for drinking water, and spectinomycin hydrochloride injection for poultry. Spectinomycin sulfate is used for injection in cattle (Adspec®), which is more highly absorbed than the hydrochloride salt. Spectinomycin tablets for dogs are an old formulation that is not currently used. (The sponsor of Adspec® [Pfizer Animal Health] has announced discontinuation of the manufacture of this drug.)

Clinical use is primarily confined to food animals. There are no small animal formulations currently available. Administration to horses has not been reported. In pigs, spectinomycin has been used orally as spectinomycin hydrochloride oral solution. It has in vitro activity against some gram-negative bacteria and has been used as a feed additive for pigs because of its activity against *Mycoplasma.* It has also been administered orally to pigs for treatment of bacterial enteritis caused by *E. coli* (50–100 mg/animal oral) and as an injection for treatment of respiratory infections. In poultry, spectinomycin has been used as injection and added to drinking water for prevention and treatment of respiratory disease and other infections.

In cattle, spectinomycin has been used as an IM injection for treatment of respiratory infections (10–15 mg/kg SC in the neck, q24 h × 3–5 days). Poultry formulations were used in cattle off-label prior to approval of Adspec®, when it was a past practice to mix the water soluble powder intended for drinking water as an IV solution for administration to cattle. Studies have shown that this practice may result in severe pulmonary edema and death.

REFERENCES AND ADDITIONAL READING

Abdullah, A.S., and Baggot, J.D. 1986. Effect of short term starvation on disposition kinetics of chloramphenicol in goats. Res Vet Sci 40: 382–385.

Acocella, G. 1983. Pharmacokinetics and metabolism of rifampin in humans. Rev Infect Diseases 5(Suppl 3):S428–S432.

Adams, H.R., and Dixit, B.N. 1970. Prolongation of pentobarbital anesthesia by chloramphenicol in dogs and cats. JAVMA 156:902–905.

Adams, P.E., Varma, K.J., Powers, T.E., and Lamendola, J.F. 1987. Tissue concentrations and pharmacokinetics of florfenicol in male veal calves given repeated doses. Am J Vet Res 48(12):1715–1732.

Adamson, P.J.W., Wilson, W.D., Baggot, J.D., Hietala, S.K., and Mihalyi, J.E. 1991. Influence of age on the disposition kinetics of chloramphenicol in equine neonates. Am J Vet Res 52(3):426–431.

Ali, B.H. 1983. Some pharmacologic and toxicologic properties of furazolidone. Vet Res Commun 6:1–11.

———. 1989. Pharmacology and toxicity of furazolidone in man and animals: some recent research. Gen Pharmac 5:557–563.

Ali, B.H., Hassan, T., Wasfi, I.A., and Mustafa, A. 1984. Toxicity of furazolidone to Nubian goats. Vet Hum Toxicol 26(3):197–200.

al-Khayyat, A.A., and Aronson, A.L. 1973a. Pharmacologic and toxicologic studies with the polymyxins. II. Comparative pharmacologic studies of the sulfate and methanesulfonate salts of polymyxin B and colistin in dogs. Chemotherapy 19:82–97.

———. 1973b. Pharmacologic and toxicologic studies with the polymyxins. III. Considerations regarding clinical use in dogs. Chemotherapy 19:98–107.

Ambrose, P.J. 1984. Clinical pharmacokinetics of chloramphenicol and chloramphenicol succinate. Clin Pharmacokin 9:222–238.

Anderson, R.C., Worth, H.M., Small, R.M., and Harris, P.N. 1966. Toxicologic studies on tylosin: its safety as a food additive. Fd Cosmet Toxicol 4:1–15.

Angelos, J.A., Dueger, E.L., George, L.W. et al. 2000. Efficacy of florfenicol for treatment of naturally occurring infectious bovine keratoconjunctivitis. J Am Vet Med Assoc 216:62–64.

Anonymous. 1980. Carbadox vs. lincomycin in swine dysentery control. Mod Vet Pract 61:152–153.

———. 1990. Chloramphenicol. IARC Monographs 50:169–193.

Atef, M., Atta, A.H., and Amer, A.M. 1991a. Pharmacokinetics of chloramphenicol in normal and *Escherichia coli* infected chickens. Br Poultry Sci 32:589–596.

Atef, M., Youssef, H., Atta, A.H., and el-Maaz, A.A. 1991b. Disposition of tylosin in goats. Br Vet J 147:207–215.

Baggot, J.D., and Gingerich, D.A. 1976. Pharmacokinetic interpretation of erythromycin and tylosin activity in serum after intravenous administration of a single dose to cows. Res Vet Sci 21:318–323.

Baquero, F. 1990. Resistance to quinolones in gram-negative microorganisms: mechanisms and prevention. Eur Urol 17(Suppl 1):3–12.

Barriere, S.L., Kaatz, G.W., and Seo, S.M. 1989. Enhanced elimination of ciprofloxacin after multiple-dose administration of rifampin to rabbits. Antimicrob Agents Chemother 33(4):589–590.

Bates, J., Jordens, J.Z., and Griffiths, D.T. 1994. Farm animals as a putative reservoir for vancomycin-resistant enterococcal infection in man. J Antimicrob Chemother 34:507–516.

Batzias, G.C., Delis, G.A., and Athanasiou, L.V. 2005. Clindamycin bioavailability and pharmacokinetics following oral administration of clindamycin hydrochloride capsules in dogs. The Veterinary Journal 170:339–345.

Beatty, J.A., Swift, N., Foster, D.J., and Barrs, V.R.D. 2006. Suspected clindamycin-associated oesophageal injury in cats: five cases. J Feline Med & Surg 8:412–419.

Booker, C.W., Abutarbush, S.M., Schunicht, O.C., Jim, G.K., Perrett, T., Wildman, B.K., Guichon, P.T., Pittman, T.J., Jones, C., and Pollock, C.M. 2007. Evaluation of the efficacy of tulathromycin as a metaphylactic antimicrobial in feedlot calves. Vet Therap 8(3):183–200.

Braden, T.D., Johnson, C.A., Gabel, C.L., Lott, G.A., and Caywood, D.D. 1987. Posologic evaluation of clindamycin, using a canine model of posttraumatic osteomyelitis. Am J Vet Res 48(7):1101–1105.

Braden, T.D., Johnson, C.A., Wakenell, P., Tvedten, H.W., and Mostosky, U.V. 1988. Efficacy of clindamycin in the treatment of *Staphylococcus aureus* osteomyelitis in dogs. JAVMA 192(12):1721–1725.

Breitschwerdt, E.B., Davidson, M.G., Aucoin, D.P., Levy, M.G., Szabados, N.S., Hegarty, B.C., Kuehne, A.L., and James, R.L. 1990. Efficacy of chloramphenicol, enrofloxacin, and tetracycline, for treatment of experimental Rocky Mountain spotted fever in dogs. Antimicrob Agents Chemother 35:2375–2381.

Bretzlaff, K.N., Neff-Davis, C.A., Ott, R.S., Koritz, G.D., Gustafsson, B. K., and Davis, L.E. 1987. Florfenicol in non-lactating dairy cows: pharmacokinetics, binding to plasma proteins, and effects on phagocytosis by blood neutrophils. J Vet Pharmacol Therap 10:233–240.

Brown, M.P., Kelly, R.H., Gronwall, R.R., and Stover, S.M. 1984. Chloramphenicol sodium succinate in the horse: serum, synovial, peritoneal, and urine concentrations after single-dose intravenous administration. Am J Vet Res 45:578–580.

Brown, S.A., Dieringer, T.M, Hunter, R.P., and Zaya, M.J. 1989. Oral clindamycin disposition after single and multiple doses in normal cats. J Vet Pharmacol Therap 12:209–216.

Brown, S.A., Zaya, M.J., Dieringer, T.M, Hunter, R.P., Nappier, J.L., Hoffman, G.A., Hornish, R.E., and Yein, F.S. 1990. Tissue concentrations of clindamycin after multiple oral doses in normal cats. J Vet Pharmacol Therap 13:270–277.

Brumbaugh, G.W., Martens, R.J., Knight, H.D., and Martin, M.T. 1983. Pharmacokinetics of chloramphenicol in the neonatal horse. J Vet Pharmacol Ther 6(3):219–227.

Budsberg, S.C., Kemp, D.T., and Wolski, N. 1992. Pharmacokinetics of clindamycin phosphate in dogs after single intravenous and intramuscular administrations. Am J Vet Res 53(12):2333–2336.

Bulgin, M.S. 1988. Losses related to the ingestion of lincomycin-medicated feed in a range sheep flock. JAVMA 192(8):1083–1086.

Burrows, G.E. 1980. Pharmacotherapeutics of macrolides, lincomycins, and spectinomycin. JAVMA 176(10):1072–1077.

Burrows, G.E., Barto, P.B., Martin, B., and Tripp, M.L. 1983. Comparative pharmacokinetics of antibiotics in newborn calves: chloramphenical, lincomycin, and tylosin. Am J Vet Res 44(6):1053–1057.

Burrows, G.E., Griffin, D.D., Pippin, A., and Harris, K. 1989. A comparison of the various routes of administration of erythromycin in cattle. J Vet Pharmacol Therap 12:289–296.

Burrows, G.E., MacAllister, C.G., Beckstrom, D.A., and Nick, J.T. 1985. Rifampin in the horse: comparison of intravenous, intramuscular, and oral administrations. Am J Vet Res 46(2):442–446.

Burrows, G.E., Tyler, R.D., Craigmill, A.L., and Barto, P.B. 1984. Chloramphenicol and the neonatal calf. Am J Vet Res 45(8):1586–1591.

Buss, W.C., Morgan, R., Guttmann, J.G., Barela, T., and Stalter, K. 1978. Rifampin inhibition of protein synthesis in mammalian cells. Science 200(28):432–434.

Carbon, C. 1998. Pharmacodynamics of macrolides, azalides, and streptogramins: effect on extracellular pathogens. Clin Infect Dis 27:28–32.

Castells G, Intorre, L., Franquelo, C., et al. 1998. Pharmacokinetics of thiamfenicol in dogs. Am J Vet Res 59:1473–1475.

Castro, L.A., Brown, M.P., Gronwall, R., Houston, A.E., and Miles, N. 1986. Pharmacokinetics of rifampin given as a single oral dose in foals. Am J Vet Res 47(12):2584–2586.

Christie, P.J., Davidson, J.N., Novick, R.P., and Dunny, G.M. 1983. Effects of tylosin feeding on the antibiotic resistance of selected gram-positive bacteria in pigs. Am J Vet Res 44:126–128.

Clark, C.H., Roger, E.D., and Milton, J.L. 1985. Plasma concentrations of chloramphenicol in snakes. Am J Vet Res 46(12):2654–2657.

Clark, C.H., Thomas, J.E., Milton, J.L., and Goolsby, W.D. 1982. Plasma concentrations of chloramphenicol in birds. Am J Vet Res 43:1249–1253.

CLSI (Clinical Laboratory Standards Institute). 2007. Performance Standards for Antimicrobial Disk and Dilution Susceptibility Tests for Bacteria Isolated From Animals; Approved Standard—Third Edition. CLSI document M31-A3. Wayne, PA: Clinical and Laboratory Standards Institute.

Cocito, C. 1979. Antibiotics of the virginiamycin family, inhibitors which contain synergistic components. Microbiologic Rev 43(2):145–198.

Conner, G.H., and Gupta, B.N. 1973. Bone marrow, blood and assay levels following medication of cats with chloramphenicol ophthalmic ointment. VMSAC, Aug:895–899.

Craig, W.A., and Kunin, C.M. 1973. Dynamics of binding and release of the polymyxin antibiotics by tissues. J Pharmacol Exper Therap 184(3):757–765.

Cravedi, J.P., Heuillet, G., Peleran, J.C., and Wal, J.M. 1985. Disposition and metabolism of chloramphenicol in trout. Xenobiotica 15(2):115–121.

Crawford, L.M. 1984. Virginiamycin. In J.H. Steele and G.W. Beran, eds.-in-chief, Handbook Series in Zoonoses, Section D: Antibiotics, Sulfonamides, and Public Health, vol. I, pp. 345–349. Boca Rotan, FL: CRC Press.

Czarnecki, C.M., Jankus, E.R., and Hultgren, B.D. 1974a. Effects of furazolidone on the development of cardiomyopathies in turkey poults. Avian Dis 18(1):125–133.

Czarnecki, C.M., Reneau, J.K., and Jankus, E.F. 1974b. Effect of furazolidone on glycogen deposition in the left ventricle of turkey hearts. Avian Dis 18(4):551–558.

Dagorn, M., Guillot, P., and Sanders, P. 1990. Pharmacokinetics of chloramphenicol in sheep after intravenous, intramuscular and subcutaneous administration. Vet Quart 12(3):166–174.

Davidson, M.G., Lappin, M.R., Rottman, J.R., et al. 1996. Paradoxical effect of clindamycin in experimental, acute toxoplasmosis in cats. Antimicrob Agents Chemother 40:1352–1359.

Davis, J.L., Gardner, S.Y., Jones, S.L., Schwabenton, B.A., and Papich, M.G. 2002. Pharmacokinetics of azithromycin in foals after i.v. and oral dose and disposition into phagocytes. J Vet Pharmacol Ther 25(2):99–104.

Davis, L.E., Baggot, J.D., and Powers, T.E. 1972. Pharmacokinetics of chloramphenicol in domesticated animals. Am J Vet Res 33(11):2259–2266.

DeCraene, B.A., Deprez, P., D'Haese, E., et al. 1997. Pharmacokinetics of florfenicol in cerebrospinal fluid and plasma of calves. Antimicrob Agents Chemother 41:1991–1995.

Devriese, L.A., and Dutta, G.N. 1984. Effects of erythromycin-inactivating *Lactobacillus* crop flora on blood levels of erythromycin given orally to chicks. J Vet Pharmacol Therap 7:49–53.

Dhawan, V.K., and Thadepalli, H. 1982. Clindamycin: a review of fifteen years of experience. Rev Infect Dis 4(6):1133–1153.

Dorrestein, G.M., van Gogh, H., and Rinzema, J.D. 1984. Pharmacokinetic aspects of penicillins, aminoglycosides and chloramphenicol in birds compared to mammals: a review. 6(4):216–224.

Dueger, E.L., Angelos, J.A., Cosgrove, S., Johnson, J., and George, L. 1999. Efficacy of florfenicol in the treatment of experimentally induced infectious bovine keratoconjunctivitis. Am J Vet Res 60:960–964.

Duthu, G.S. 1985. Interspecies correlation of the pharmacokinetics of erythromycin, oleandomycin, and tylosin. J Pharm Sci 74(9): 943–946.

Dutta, G.N., and Devriese, L.A. 1981. Macrolide-lincosamide-streptogramin resistance patterns in *Clostridium perfringens* from animals. Antimicrob Agents Chemother 19(2):274–278.

———. 1982a. Resistance to macrolide-lincosamide-streptogramin antibiotics in enterococci from the intestine of animals. Res Vet Sci 33:70–72.

———. 1982b. Resistance to macrolide, lincosamide and streptogramin antibiotics and degradation of lincosamide antibiotics in streptococci from bovine mastitis. J Antimicrob Chemother 10:403–408.

Eriksson, A., Rauramaa, V., Happonen, I., and Mero, M. 1990. Feeding reduced the absorption of erythromycin in the dog. Acta Vet Scand 31:497–499.

Evans, N.A. 2005. Tulathromycin: an overview of a new triamilide antimicrobial for livestock respiratory disease. Vet Therap 6(2):83–95.

Ewing, P.J., Burrows, G., Macallister, C., and Clarke, C. 1994. Comparison of oral erythromycin formulations in the horse using pharmacokinetic profiles. J Vet Pharmacol Therap 17:17–23.

Farrington, D.O., and Shively, J.E. 1979. Effect of carbadox on growth, feed utilization, and development of nasal turbinate lesions in swine infected with *Bordetella bronchiseptica*. JAVMA 174(6):597–600.

Ferrari, V., and Bella, D.D. 1974. Comparison of chloramphenicol and thiamphenicol metabolism. Postgrad Med J 50(Suppl 5):17–22.

Finnie, J.W. 1992. Two clinical manifestations of furazolidone toxicity in calves. Aust Vet J 69(1):21.

Fisher, A.A. 1983. Adverse reactions to topical clindamycin, erythromycin and tetracycline. Cutis 32:415–428.

Ford, R.B., and Aronson, A.L. 1985. Antimicrobial drugs and infectious diseases. In L. Davis, ed., Handbook of Small Animal Therapeutics, pp. 45–88. New York: Churchill Livingstone.

Frank, L.A. 1990. Clinical pharmacology of rifampin. JAVMA 197(1):114–117.

Fukui, H., Fujihara, Y., and Kano, T. 1987. In vitro and in vivo antibacterial activities of florfenicol, a new fluorinated analog of thiamfenicol, against fish pathogens. Fish Pathol 22:201–207.

Gamez, A., Perez, Y., Marti, G., Cristofol, C., and Arboix, M. 1992. Pharmacokinetics of thiamphenicol in veal calves. Br Vet J 148:535–539.

George, L., Mihalyi, J., Edmondson, A., Daigneault, J., Kagonyera, G., Willits, N., and Lucas, M. 1988. Topically applied furazolidone or parenterally administered oxytetracycline for the treatment of infectious bovine keratoconjunctivitis. JAVMA 192(10):1415–142[illegible].

Gerken, D.F., and Sams, R.A. 1985. Inhibitory effects of intravenous chloramphenicol sodium succinate on the disposition of phenylbutazone in horses. J Pharmacokin and Biopharmaceutics [illegible](5):467–476.

Giguère, S., Jacks, S., Roberts, G.D., Hernandez, J., Long, M.T., Ellis, C. 2004. Retrospective comparison of azithromycin, clarithromycin, and erythromycin for the treatment of foals with *Rhodococcus equi* pneumonia. J Vet Intern Med 18(4):568–73.

Gingerich, D.A., Baggot, J.D., and Kowalski, J.J. 1977. Tylosin antimicrobial activity and pharmacokinetics in cows. Can Vet J 18(4):96–100.

Girard, A.E., Girard, D., and Retsema, J.A. 1990. Correlation of the extravascular pharmacokinetics of azithromycin with in-vivo efficacy in models of localized infection. J Antimicrob Chemother 25(Suppl A):61–71.

Girard, D., Bergeron, J.M., Milisen, W.B., and Retsema, J.A. 1993. Comparison of azithromycin, roxithromycin, and cephalexin penetration kinetics in early and mature abscesses. J Antimicrob Chemother 31(Suppl E):17–28.

Gottschall, D.W., Wang, R., and Kingston, G.I. 1988. Virginiamycin metabolism in cattle rumen fluid. Drug Metab and Dispos 16(6):804–812.

Gourlay, R.N., Thomas, L.H., and Wyld, S.G. 1989. Effect of a new macrolide antibiotic (tilmicosin) on pneumonia experimentally induced in calves by *Mycoplasma bovis* and *Pasteurella haemolytica*. Res Vet Sci 47:84–89.

Greene, C.E., Cook, J.R., and Mahaffey, E.A. 1985. Clindamycin for treatment of *Toxoplasma* polymyositis in a dog. JAVMA 187(6):631–634.

Greene, C.E., Lappin, M.R., and Marks, A. 1992. Effect of clindamycin on clinical, hematological, and biochemical parameters in clinically healthy cats. JAAHA 29:323–326.

Gronwall, R., Brown, M.P., Merritt, A.M., and Stone, H.W. 1986. Body fluid concentrations and pharmacokinetics of chloramphenicol given to mares intravenously or by repeated gavage. Am J Vet Res 47(12):2591–2595.

Guillot, P., and Sanders, P. 1991. Pharmacokinetics of chloramphenicol and oxytetracycline in calves after intravenous and intramuscular administrations. Acta Veterinaria Scandinavica 87:136–138.

Hall, J.A., and Washabau, R.J. 1997. Gastrointestinal prokinetic therapy: motilin-like drugs. Compend Cont Educ Pract 19:281–288.

Hamdy, A.H. 1975. Efficacy of lincomycin and spectinomycin on canine pathogens. Lab An Sci 25(5):570–574.

———. 1978. Therapeutic effects of various concentrations of lincomycin in drinking water on experimentally transmitted swine dysentery. Am J Vet Res 39(7):1175–1180.

Hamdy, A.H., and Kratzer, D.D. 1981. Therapeutic effects of parenteral administration of lincomycin on experimentally transmitted swine dysentery. Am J Vet Res 42(2):178–182.

Harari, J., and Lincoln, J. 1989. Pharmacologic features of clindamycin in dogs and cats. J Am Vet Med Assoc 195(1):124–125.

Harvey, R.G., Noble, W.C., and Ferguson, E.A. 1993. A comparison of lincomycin hydrochloride and clindamycin hydrochloride in the treatment of superficial pyoderma in dogs. Vet Rec 132:351–353.

Harvey, S. 1985. Antimicrobial drugs. In A. R. Gennaro, ed., Remington's Pharmaceutical Sciences, 17th ed., pp. 1158–1233. Easton, PA: Mack Publishing Co.

Hedstrom, S.A. 1984. Clindamycin as an anti-staphylococcal agent: indications and limitations. Scand J Infect Dis Suppl 43:62–66.

Hird, J.F.R., and Knifton, A. 1986. Chloramphenicol in veterinary practice. Vet Rec 119:248–250.

H[illegible] B.R., Jelinski, M.D., Ribble, C.S., et al. 1998. A comparison of the clinical field efficacy and safety of florfenicol and tilmicosin for the treatment of undifferentiated bovine respiratory disease in cattle in western Canada. Can Vet J 39:161–166.

Hornish, R.E., Gosline, R.E., and Nappier, J.M. 1987. Comparative metabolism of lincomycin in the swine, chicken and rat. Drug Metab Rev 18(2–3):177–214.

Horsberg, T.E., Martinsen, B., and Varma, K.J. 1994. The disposition of 14C-florfenicol in Atlantic salmon (*Salmo salar*). Aquaculture 122:97–106.

Huber, W.G. 1982. Aminoglycosides, macrolides, lincomycin, polymyxins, chloramphenicol, and other antibacterial drugs. In N.H. Booth and L.E. McDonald, eds., Veterinary Pharmacology and Therapeutics, 5th ed., pp. 748–771. Ames: Iowa State Univ Press.

Hunter, R.P., Lynch, M.J., Ericson, J.F., et al. 1995. Pharmacokinetics, oral bioavailability and tissue distribution of azithromycin in cats. J Vet Pharmacol Therap 18:38–46.

IARC Monographs on the Evaluation of Carcinogenic Risk of Chemicals to Man. 1976. Chloramphenicol, vol. 10:85–98.

———. 1990. Chloramphenicol, vol. 50:169–193.

Jacks, S., Giguère, S., Gronwall, R.R., Brown, M.P., and Merritt, K.A. 2001. Pharmacokinetics of azithromycin and concentration in body fluids and bronchoalveolar cells in foals. Am J Vet Res 62(12): 1870–5.

———. 2002. Disposition of oral clarithromycin in foals. J Vet Pharmacol Therap 25:359–362.

Jacks, S.S., Giguère, S., and Nguyen, A. 2003. 2003. In vitro susceptibilities of *Rhodococcus equi* and other common equine pathogens to azithromycin, clarithromycin, and 20 other antimicrobials. Antimicrob Agents Chemother 47(5):1742–5.

Jacobs, G.J., Lappin, M., Marks, A., and Greene, C.E. 1989. Effect of clindamycin on factor-VII activity in healthy cats. Am J Vet Res 50(3):393–395.

Jang, S.S., Breher, J.E., Dabaco, L.A., and Hirsh, D.C. 1997. Organisms isolated from dogs and cats with anaerobic infections and susceptibility to selected antimicrobial agents. J Am Vet Med Assoc 210: 1610–1614.

Jankus, E.F., Noren G.R., and Staley, N.A. 1972. Furazolidone-induced cardiac dilatation in turkeys. Avian Dis 16(4):958–961.

Jernigan, A.D., St. Jean, G.D., Rings, D.M., and Sams, R.A. 1986. Pharmacokinetics of rifampin in adult sheep. Am J Vet Res 52(10):1626–1629.

Jim, G.K., Booker, C.W., Guichon, P.T., et al. 1999. A comparison of florfenicol and tilmicosin for the treatment of undifferentiated fever in feedlot calves in western Canada. Can Vet J 40:179–184.

Jones, J.E., Hughes, B.L., and Mulliken, W.E. 1976. Use of tylosin to prevent early mortality in bobwhite quail. Poultry Sci 55: 1122–1123.

Jones, P.W. 1974. Treatment of calf pneumonia with tylosin. Vet Rec 94:200.

Kaltwasser, J.P., Werner, E., Simon, B., Bellenberg, U., and Becker, H.J. 1974. The effect of thiamphenicol on normal and activated erythropoiesis in the rabbit. Postgrad Med J 50(Suppl 5):118–122.

Kelly, D.J., Chulay, J.D., Mikesell, P., and Friedlander, A.M. 1992. Serum concentrations of penicillin, doxycycline, and ciprofloxacin during prolonged therapy in rhesus monkeys. J Infect Dis 166:1184–1187.

Kenny, M.T., and Strates, B. 1981. Metabolism and pharmacokinetics of the antibiotic rifampin. Drug Metab Rev 12(1):159–218.

Kinoshita, T., Son, D.-S., Shimoda, M., and Kokue, E. 1995. Impact of age-related alteration of plasma alpha-1-acid glycoprotein concentration on erythromycin pharmacokinetics in pigs. Am J Vet Res 56:362–365.

Kirst, H.A., and Sides, G.D. 1989. New directions for macrolide antibiotics: structural modifications and in vitro activity. Antimicrob Agents Chemother 33(9):1413–1418.

Kirst, H.A., Wild, G.M., Baltz, R.H., Hamill, R.L., Ott, J.L., Counter, F.T., and Ose, E.E. 1982. Structure-activity studies among 16-membered macrolide antibiotics related to tylosin. J Antibiotics 35(12):1675–1682.

Kleckner, M.D. 1984. Lincomycin. In J.H. Steele and G.W. Beran, eds.-in-chief, Handbook Series in Zoonoses, Section D: Antibiotics, Sulfonamides, and Public Health, vol. I, pp. 337–345. Boca Rotan, FL: CRC Press.

Kleinberg, J., Dea, F.J., Anderson, J.A., and Leopold, I.H. 1979. Intraocular penetration of topically applied lincomycin hydrochloride in rabbits. Arch Ophthamol 97:933–936.

Knothe, H. 1977a. Medical implications of macrolide resistance and its relationship to the use of tylosin in animal feeds. Infection 5: 137–139.

———. 1977b. A review of the medical considerations of the use of tylosin and other macrolide antibiotics as additives in animal feeds. Infection 5:183–187.

Korsrud, G.O., Naylor, J.M., MacNeil, J.D., and Yates, W.D.G. 1987. Persistence of chloramphenicol residues in calf tissues. Can J Vet Res 51:316–318.

Kume, B.B., and Garg, R.C. 1986. Pharmacokinetics and bioavailability of chloramphenicol in normal and febrile goats. J Vet Pharmacol Therap 9:254–263.

Kunkle, G.A., Sundlof, S., and Keisling, K. 1995. Adverse side effects of oral antibacterial therapy in dogs and cats: an epidemiologic study of pet owners' observations. JAAHA 31:46–55.

Lacey, R.W. 1984. Does the use of chloramphenicol in animals jeopardise the treatment of human infections? Vet Rec Jan; 7:6–8.

Lakritz, J., Wilson, W.D., Marsh, A.E., and Mihalyi, J.E. 2000a. Effects of prior feeding on pharmacokinetics and estimated bioavailability after oral administration of a single dose of microencapsulated erythromycin base in healthy foals. Am J Vet Res 61(9):1011–1015.

Lakritz, J., Wilson, W.D., Marsh, A.E., and Mihalyi, J.E. 2000b. Pharmacokinetics of erythromycin estolate and erythromycin phosphate after intragastric administration to healthy foals. Am J Vet Res 61(8):914–919.

Lakritz, J., Wilson, W.D., and Mihalyi, J.E. 1999. Comparison of microbiologic and high-performance liquid chromatography assays to determine plasma concentrations, pharmacokinetics, and bioavailability of erythromycin base in plasma of foals after intravenous or intragastric administration. Am J Vet Res 60(4):414–419.

Lakritz, J., Wilson, W.D., Marsh, A.E., and Mihalyi, J.E. 2002. Pharmacokinetics of erythromycin ethylsuccinate after intragastric administration to healthy foals. Veterinary Therapeutics 3(2):189–195.

Lancini, G., and Parenti. 1982. Antibiotics: An Integrated View. New York: Springer-Verlag.

Lappin, M.R., Greene, C.E., Winston, S., Toll, S.L., and Epstein, M.E. 1989. Clinical feline toxoplasmosis: serologic diagnosis and therapeutic management of 15 cases. J Vet Int Med 3:139–143.

Laven, R., and Andrews, A.H. 1991. Long-acting antibiotic formulations in the treatment of calf pneumonia: a comparative study of tilmicosin and oxytetracycline. Vet Rec 129(6):109–111.

Lavy, E., Ziv, G., Lkikman, A., and Ben-Zvi, Z. 1991a. Single-dose pharmacokinetics of thiamphenicol in lactating goats. Acta Veterinaria Scandinavica Suppl 87:99–102.

Lavy, E., Ziv, G., Shem-Tov, M., Glickman, A., and Dey, A. 1999. Pharmacokinetics of clindamycin HCl administered intravenously, intramuscularly, and subcutaneously to dogs. J Vet Pharmacol Therap 22:261–265.

Lavy, E., Ziv, G., Soback, S., Glickman, A., and Winkler, M. 1991b. Clinical pharmacology of florfenicol in lactating goats. Acta Veterinaria Scandinavica Suppl 87:133–136.

Leclercq, R., and Courvalin, P. 1991. Intrinsic and unusual resistance to macrolide, lincosamide, and streptogramin antibiotics in bacteria. Antimicrob Agents Chemother 35(7):1273–1276.

Lester, G.D., Merritt, A.M., and Neuwirth, L. 1998. Effect of erythromycin lactobionate on myoelectric activity of ileum, and cecal emptying of radiolabeled markers in clinically normal ponies. Am J Vet Res 59:328–334.

Lewbart, G.A., Papich, M.G., and Whitt-Smith, D. 2005. Pharmacokinetics of florfenicol in the red pacu (*Piaractus brachypomus*) after single dose intramuscular administration. J Vet Pharmacol Therap 28(3):317–319.

Lloyd, D.H., Lamport, A.I., and Feeney, C. 1996. Sensitivity of antibiotics amongst cutaneous and mucosal isolates of canine pathogenic staphylococci in the UK, 1980–1996. Vet Derm 7:171–175.

Lobell, R.D., Varma, K.J., Johnson, J.C., et al. 1994. Pharmacokinetics of florfenicol following intravenous and intramuscular doses to cattle. J Vet Pharmacol Therap 17:253–258.

Locke, D., Bush, M., and Carpenter, J.W. 1982. Pharmacokinetics and tissue concentrations of tylosin in selected avian species. 43(10):1807–1810.

Lode, H., Borner, K., Koeppe, P., and Schaberg, T. 1996. Azithromycin: review of key chemical, pharmacokinetic, and microbiological features. J Antimicrob Chemother 37(Suppl C):1–8.

Maguire, B.A., Deaves, J.K., and Wild, D.G. 1989. Some properties of 2 erythromycin-dependent strains of *Escherichia coli*. J Gen Micro 135:575–581.

Maiers, J.D., and Mason, S.J. 1984. Lincomycin-associated enterocolitis in rabbits. JAVMA 185(6):670–671.

Main, B.W., Means, J.R., and Rinkema, L.E. 1996. Cardiovascular effects of the macrolide antibiotic tilmicosin, administered alone or in combination with popranolol or dobutamine, in conscious unrestrained dogs. J Vet Pharmacol Therap 19:225–232.

Mandel, M. 1977. Lincomycin in treatment of out-patient psittacines. VMSAC 72:473–474.

Marshall, S.A., Jones, R.N., Wanger, A., et al. 1996. Proposed MIC quality control guidelines for National Committee for Clinical Laboratory Standards susceptibility tests using seven veterinary antimicrobial agents: ceftiofur, enrofloxacin, florfenicol, penicillin G–Novobiocin, pirlimycin, premafloxacin, and spectinomycin. J Clin Microbiol 34:2027–2029.

Martin, K., Wiese, B. 1988. The disposition of chloramphenicol in colostrum-fed and colostrum-deprived newborn pigs. Pharmacol Toxicol 63:16–19.

Martinsen, B., Horsberg, T.E., Varma, K.J., et al. 1993. Single dose pharmacokinetic study of florfenicol in Atlantic salmon (*Salmo salar*) in seawater at 11°C. Aquaculture 112:1–11.

Matsuoka, T., Muenster, O.A., Ose, E.E., and Tonkinson, L. 1980. Orally administered tylosin for the control of pneumonia in neonatal calves. Vet Rec 106:149–151.

Maxey, B.W. 1980. Efficacy of tetracycline/novobiocin combination against canine upper respiratory infections. VMSAC 75:89–92.

Maxey, B.W., and Page, R.K. 1977. Efficacy of lincomycin feed medication for the control of necrotic enteritis in broiler-type chickens. Poultry Sci 56:1909–1913.

Mayers, M., Rush, D., Madu, A., Motyl, M., and Miller, M.H. 1991. Pharmacokinetics of amikacin and chloramphenicol in the aqueous humor of rabbits. Antimicrob Agents Chemother 35(9):1791–1798.

McCalla, D.R. 1983. Mutagenicity of nitrofuran derivative: review. Environmental Mutagenesis 5:745–765.

McKay, S.G., Morck, D.W., Merrill, J.K., et al. 1996. Use of tilmicosin for treatment of pasteurellosis in rabbits. Am J Vet Res 57:1180–1184.

McKellar, Q.A., and Varma, K.J. 1996. Pharmacokinetics and tolerance of florfenicol in Equidae. Equine Vet J 28:209–213.

Medleau L., Long R.E., Brown J., and Miller, W.H. 1986. Frequency and antimicrobial susceptibility of staphylococcus species isolated from canine pyoderma. Am J Vet Res 47:229–231.

Medoff, G. 1983. Antifungal action of rifampin. Rev Infect Dis 5(Suppl 3):S614–S619.

Miles, R.D., Janky, D.M., and Harms, R.H. 1984. Virginiamycin and broiler performance. Poultry Sci 63:1218–1221.

———. 1985. Virginiamycin and laying hen performance. Poultry Sci 64:139–143.

Moore, G.M., Mowrey, D.H., Tonkinson, L.V., et al. 1996. Efficacy dose determination study of tilmicosin phosphate in feed for control of pneumonia caused by *Actinobacillus pleuropneumoniae* in swine. Am J Vet Res 57:220–223.

Morck, D.W., Merrill, J.K., Thorlakson, B.E., Olson, M.E., Tonkinson, L.V., and Costerton, J.W. 1993. Prophylactic efficacy of tilmicosin for bovine respiratory tract disease. JAVMA 202(2):273–277.

Morresey, P.R., Mackay, R.J. 2006. Endotoxin-neutralizing activity of polymyxin B in blood after IV administration in horses. Am J Vet Res 67(4):642–647.

Morris, A., and Russell, A.D. 1971. The mode of action of novobiocin. Progress Med Chem 8(1):39–59.

Moser, R.L. Cornelius, S.G. Pettigrew, J.E. Jr., Hanke, H.E., and Hagen, CD. 1985. Response of growing-finishing pigs to decreasing floor space allowance and(or) virginiamycin in diet. J Anim Sci 61(2):337–342.

Musser, J., Mechor, G.D., Grohn, Y.T., et al. 1996. Comparison of tilmicosin with long-acting oxytetracycline for treatment of respiratory tract disease in calves. J Am Vet Med Assoc 208:102–106.

Mustafa, A.I., Ali, B.H., Hassan, T., and Satti, A.M. 1985. Furazolidone concentrations in plasma, milk and some tissues of Nubian goats. J Vet Pharmacol Therap 8:190–193.

Mustafa, A.I., Idris, S.O., Ali, B.H., Mahdi, M., and Elgasim, A.I.A. 1975. Furazolidone poisoning associated with cardiomyopathy in chickens. Avian Dis 19:596.

Nagarajan, R., Schabel, A.A., Occolowitz, J.L., Counter, F.T., Ott, J.T., and Felty-Duckworth, A.M. 1989. Synthesis and antibacterial evaluation of *N*-alkyl vancomycins. J Antibiotics 42(1):63–72.

Nakata, K., Maeda, H., Fujii, A., Arakawa, S., Umezu, K., and Kamidono, S. 1992. In vitro and in vivo activities of sparfloxacin, other quinolones, and tetracyclines against *Chlamydia trachomatis*. Antimicrob Agents Chemother 36(1):188–190.

Neu, H.C. 1992. The crisis in antibiotic resistance. Science 257:1064–1073.

Nichols, D.R., and Keys, T.F. 1984. An historical overview of antibiotics and sulfonamides in society. In J.H. Steele and G.W. Beran, eds.-in-chief, Handbook Series in Zoonoses, Section D: Antibiotics, Sulfonamides, and Public Health, vol. I, pp. 35–43. Boca Rotan, FL: CRC Press.

Noble, W.C., and Kent, L.E. 1992. Antibiotic resistance in *Staphylococcus intermedius* isolated from cases of pyoderma in the dog. Vet Derm 3:71–74.

Noli, C., and Boothe, D.M. 1999. Macrolides and lincosamides. Vet Dermatology 10:217–223.

Nouri, M., and Constable, P.D. 2007. Effect of parenteral administration of erythromycin, tilmicosin, and tylosin on abomasal emptying rate in suckling calves. Am J Vet Res 68(12):1392–8.

Nouri, M., Hajikolaee, M.R., Constable, P.D., and Omidi, A. 2008. Effect of erythromycin and gentamicin on abomasal emptying rate in suckling calves. J Vet Intern Med 22(1):196–201.

Ohmae, K., Yonezaw, S., and Terakadok, N. 1981. R plasmid with carbadox resistance from *Escherichia coli* of porcine origin. Antimicrob Agents Chemother 19:86–90.

Olsen, D., and Rodabaugh, D.E. 1977. Evaluation of virginiamycin in feed for treatment and retreatment of swine dysentery. Am J Vet Res 38(10):1485–1490.

Orsini, J.A., Snooks-Parsons, C., Stine, L., Haddock, M., Ramberg, C.F., Benson, C.E., and Nunamaker, D.M. 2005. Vancomycin for the treatment of methicillin-resistant staphylococcal and enterococcal infections in 15 horses. Can J Vet Res 69(4):278–286.

Ose, E.E. 1976. Synergistic action of tylosin and oxytetracycline against bovine pasteurella isolates. VM/SAC. 71:92–95.

Ose, E.E., and Tonkinson, L.V. 1985. Comparison of the antimycoplasma activity of two commercially available tylosin premixes. Poultry Sci 64:287–293.

———. 1988. Single-dose treatment of neonatal calf pneumonia with the new macrolide antibiotic tilmicosin. Vet Rec 123(14):367–369.

Panteix, G., Guillaumond, B., Harf, R., et al. 1993. In-vitro concentration of azithromycin in human phagocytic cells. J Antimicrob Chemother 31(Suppl E):1–4.

Papich, M.G. 1999. Florfenicol pharmacokinetics in dogs and cats. Proc 1999 ACVIM Annual Forum.

———. 2003. Antimicrobial therapy for gastrointestinal diseases. Vet Clin N Am: Equine Pract 19(3):645–63,

Penny, R.H.C., Carlisle, C.H., Prescott, C.W., and Davidson, H.A. 1967. Effects of chloramphenicol on the haemopoietic system of the cat. Br Vet J 123(4):145–153.

———. 1970. Further observations on the effect of chloramphenicol on the haemopoietic system of the cat. Br Vet J 126:453–457.

Pinault, L.P., Millot, L.K., Sanders, P.J. 1997. Absolute oral bioavailability and residues of florfenicol in the rainbow trout (*Onchorynchus mykiss*). J Vet Pharmacol Therap 20:297–298.

Plenderleith, R. 1988. Treatment of cattle, sheep and horses with lincomycin: case studies. Vet Rec 122:112–113.

Prescott, J.F., Hoover, D.J., and Dohoo, J.R. 1983. Pharmacokinetics of erythromycin in foals and in adult horses. J Vet Pharmacol Therap 6:67–74.

Rahal, J.J., and Simberkoff, M.S. 1979. Bactericidal and bacteriostatic action of chloramphenicol against meningeal pathogens. Antimicrob Agents Chemother 16:13–18.

Rainier, R.H., Harris, D.L., Glock, R.D., Kinyon, J.M., and Brauer, M.A. 1980. Carbadox and lincomycin in the treatment and carrier state of swine dysentery. Am J Vet Res 41(9):1349–1356.

Raisbeck, M.F., Holt, G.R., and Osweiler, G.D. 1981. Lincomycin-associated colitis in horses. JAVMA 179:362–363.

Ravindran, V., and Kornegay, E.T. 1984. Effects of fiber and virginiamycin on nutrient absorption, nutrient retention and rate of passage in growing swine. J Anim Sci 59(2):400–408.

Rehg, J.E., and Pakes, S.P. 1982. Implication of *Clostridium difficile* and *Clostridium perfringens* iota toxins in experimental lincomycin-associated colitis in rabbits. Lab Anim Sci 32(3):253–256.

Renneberg, J., and Walder, M. 1989. Postantibiotic effects of imipenum, norfloxacin, and amikacin in vitro and in vivo. Antimicrob Agents Chemother 33(10):1714–1720.

Rice, D.A., and McMurray, C.H. 1983. Ketosis in dairy cows caused by low levels of lincomycin in concentrate feed. Vet Rec 113:495–496.

Riviere, J.E., Craigmill, A.L., and Sundlof, S.F. 1991. Handbook of Comparative Pharmacokinetics and Residues of Veterinary Antimicrobials. Boca Raton, FL: CRC Press.

Rollin, R.E., Mero, K.N., Kozisek, P.B., Phillips, R.W. 1986. Diarrhea and malabsorption in calves associated with therapeutic doses of antibiotics: absorptive and clinical changes. Am J Vet Res 47:987–991.

Rootman, D.S., Savage, P., Hasany, S.M., Chisholm, L., and Basu, P.K. 1992. Toxicity and pharmacokinetics of intravitreally injected ciprofloxacin in rabbit eyes. Can J Ophthalmol 27(6):277–282.

Rubio-Martinez, L.M., López-Sanromán, J., Cruz, A.M., Santos, M., Andrés, M.S., Román, F.S. 2005. Evaluation of safety and pharmacokinetics of vancomycin after intravenous regional limb perfusion in horses. Am J Vet Res 66(12):2107–2113.

Rubio-Martinez, L.M., López-Sanromán, J., Cruz, A.M., Tendillo, F., Rioja, E., and San Román, F. 2006. Evaluation of safety and pharmacokinetics of vancomycin after intraosseous regional limb perfusion and comparison of results with those obtained after intravenous regional limb perfusion in horses. Am J Vet Res 67(10):1701–1707.

Sabath, L.D., Gerstein, D.A., Loder, P.B., and Finland, M. 1968. Excretion of erythromycin and its enhanced activity in urine against gram-negative bacilli with alkalinization. J Lab Clin Med 72(6):916–923.

Salmon, R.E., and Stevens, V.I. 1990. Response of large white turkeys to virginiamycin from day-old to slaughter. Poultry Sci 69:1383–1387.

Sande, M.A., and Mandell, G.L. 1990a. Antimicrobial agents: tetracyclines, chloramphenicol, erythromycin, and miscellaneous antibacterial agents. In A.G. Goodman, T.W. Rall, A.S. Nies, and P. Taylor, eds., Goodman and Gilman's The Pharmacologic Basis of Therapeutics, 8th ed., pp. 1117–1145. New York: Pergamon Press.

Sanders, P., Guillot, P., and Mourot, D. 1988. Pharmacokinetics of a long-acting chloramphenicol formulation administered by intramuscular and subcutaneous routes in cattle. J Vet Pharmacol Therap 11:183–190.

Schumann, F.J., Janzen, E.D., and McKinnon, J.J. 1990. Prophylactic tilmicosin medication of feedlot calves at arrival. Can Vet J 31:285–288.

Scott, D.W., Beningo, K.E., Miller, W.H., and Rothstein, E. 1998. Efficacy of clindamycin hydrochloride capsules for the treatment of deep pyoderma due to *Staphylococcus intermedius* infection in dogs. Can Vet J 39:753–756.

Settepani, J.A. 1984. The hazard of using chloramphenicol in food animals. JAVMA 184:930–931.

Shaw, W.V., and Leslie, A.G.W. 1991. Chloramphenicol acetyltransferase. Annu Rev Biophys Chem 20:363–386.

Shepard, R.M., and Falkner, F.C. 1990. Pharmacokinetics of azithromycin in rats and dogs. J Antimicrob Chemother 25(Suppl A):49–60.

Shukla, V.K., Garg, S.K., and Mathur, V.S. 1984. Influence of prednisolone on antipyrine and chloramphenicol disposition in rabbits. Pharmacol 29:117–120.

Smith, M.J. 1966. Efficacy of furazolidone in the treatment of topical bacterial infections in dogs. VM/SAC 61:459–462.

Stamper, M.A., Papich, M.G., Lewbart, G.A., May, S.B., Plummer, D.D., and Stoskopf, M. K. 2003. Pharmacokinetics of florfenicol in loggerhead sea turtles (*Caretta caretta*) after single intravenous and intramuscular injections. J Zoo Wildl Med 34(1):3–8.

Stern, I.J., Hollifield, R.D., Wilk, S., and Buzard, J.A. 1967. The antimonoamine oxidase effects of furazolidone. J Pharmacol Exp Therap 156(3):492–499.

Stratton-Phelps, M., Wilson, W.D., and Gardner, I.A. 2000. Risk of adverse effects in pneumonic foals treated with erythromycin versus other antibiotics: 143 cases (1986–1996). J Am Vet Med Assoc 217:68–73.

Suarez-Mier, G., Giguère, S., Lee, E.A. 2007. Pulmonary disposition of erythromycin, azithromycin, and clarithromycin in foals. J Vet Pharmacol Ther 30(2):109–15.

Tally, F.P., Snydman, D.R., Gorbach, S.L., and Malamy, M.H. 1979. Plasmid-mediated transferable resistance to clindamycin and erythromycin in *Bacteroides fragilis*. J Infect Dis 139:83–88.

———. 1981. Plasmid-mediated transferable resistance to clindamycin and erythromycin in *Bacteroides fragilis*. Am J Med 139:83–88.

Taylor, J.D., Gibson, J.A., and Yeates, C.E.F. 1991. Furazolidone toxicity in dairy calves. Aust Vet J 68(5):182–183.

Taylor, P.H., Gulupo, P., Naille, R., Heydinger, D.K., and Bowers, J.D. 1970. Experimental use of methanamine mandelate in treatment of burn wounds in rats. J Trauma 10(4):331–333.

Tennent, D.M., and Ray, W.H. 1971. Metabolism of furazolidone in swine. Proc Soc Exper Biology and Med 138(3):808–810.

Teske, R.H. 1984. The polypeptide antibiotics. In J.H. Steele and G.W. Beran, eds.-in-chief, Handbook Series in Zoonoses, Section D: Antibiotics, Sulfonamides, and Public Health, vol. I, pp. 333–335. Boca Raton, FL: CRC Press.

Thilsted, J.P., Newton, W.M, Crandel, R.A., and Bevill, R.F. 1981. Fatal diarrhea in rabbits resulting from the feeding of antibiotic-contaminated feed. JAVMA 179:360–361.

Tuttle, A.D., Papich, M.G., and Wolfe, B.A. 2006. Bone marrow hypoplasia secondary to florfenicol toxicity in a Thomson's gazelle (*Gazella thomsonii*). J Vet Pharmacol Therap 29(4):317–9.

van der Molen, E.J., Baars, A.J., deGraaf, G.J., and Jager, L.P. 1989a. Comparative study of the effect of carbadox, olaquindox and cyadox on aldosterone, sodium and potassium plasma levels in weaned pigs. Res Vet Sci 47:11–16.

van der Molen, E.J., deGraaf, G.J., and Baars, A.J. 1989b. Persistence of carbadox-induced adrenal lesions in pigs following drug withdrawal and recovery of aldosterone plasma concentrations. J Comp Path 100:295–304.

van der Molen, E.J., van Lieshout, J.H.L.M., Nabuurs, M.J.A., Derkx, F., Michelakis, A. 1989c. Changes in plasma renin activity and renal immunohistochemically demonstrated renin in carbadox treated pigs. Res Vet Sci 46:401–405.

Varma, K.J., Adams, P.E., Powers, T.E., Powers, J.D., and Lamendola, J.F. 1986. Pharmacokinetics of florfenicol in veal calves. J Vet Pharmacol Therap 9:412–425.

Varma, K.J., Powers, T.E., and Powers, J.D. 1987. Single and repeat-dose pharmacokinetic studies of chloramphenicol in horses: values and limitations of pharmacokinetic studies in predicting dosage regimens. Am J Vet Res 48(3):403–406.

Veenhuizen, M.F., Wright, T.J., McManus, R.F., and Owens, J.G. 2006. Analysis of reports of human exposure to Micotil 300 (tilmicosin injection). J Am Vet Med Assoc 1;229(11):1737–42.

Venner, M., Kerth, R., and Klug, E. 2007. Evaluation of tulathromycin in the treatment of pulmonary abscesses in foals. Vet J 174(2):418–21.

Venning, C.M, Curtis, M.A., and Egerton, J.R. 1990. Treatment of virulent footrot with lincomycin and spectinomycin. Aust Vet J 67(6):258–260.

Vernimb, G.D. 1969. A furazolidone aerosol powder in the prevention and treatment of keratoconjunctivitis in cattle and sheep. VM/SAC 64:708–710.

Vilmànyi, E., Küng, K., Riond, J.-L., et al. 1996. Clarithromycin pharmacokinetics after oral administration with or without fasting in crossbred Beagles. J Sm Anim Pract 37:535–539.

Vogel, G.J., Laudert, S.B., Zimmerman, A., et al. 1998. Effects of tilmicosin on acute undifferentiated respiratory tract disease in newly arrived feedlot cattle. J Am Vet Med Assoc 212:1919–1924.

Watson, A.D.J. 1980. Further observations on chloramphenicol toxicosis in cats. Am J Vet Res 41:293–294.

———. 1992. Bioavailability and bioinequivalence of drug formulations in small animals. J Vet Pharmacol Therap 15:151–159.

Watts, J.L., et al. 1999. Performance standards for antimicrobial disk and dilution susceptibility tests for bacteria isolated from animals: approved standard (M31-A). NCCLS 19, no. 11.

Weisel, M.K., Powers, J.D., Powers, T.E., and Baggot, J.D. 1977. A pharmacokinetic analysis of tylosin in the normal dog. Am J Vet Res 38(2):273–275.

Westermarck, E., Skrzypczak, T., Harmoinen, J., Steiner, J.M., Ruaux, C. G., Williams, D.A., Eerola, E., Sundbäck, P., and Rinkinen, M. 2005. Tylosin-responsive chronic diarrhea in dogs. J Vet Intern Med 19(2):177–86.

Wilson, D.J., Sears, P.M., Gonzalez, R.N., et al. 1996. Efficacy of florfenicol for treatment of clinical and subclinical bovine mastitis. Am J Vet Res 57:526–528.

Wilson, R.C. 1984. The Macrolides. In J.H. Steele, ed.-in-chief, Handbook Series in Zoonoses, Section D: Antibiotics, Sulfonamides, and Public Health, vol. I. Boca Raton, FL: CRC Press.

Wilson, W.D., Spensley, M.S., Baggot, J.D., and Hietala, S.K. 1988. Pharmacokinetics, bioavailability, and in vitro antibacterial activity of rifampin in the horse. Am J Vet Res 49(12):2041–2046.

Wittek, T., and Constable, P.D. 2005. Assessment of the effects of erythromycin, neostigmine, and metoclopramide on abomasal motility and emptying rate in calves. Am J Vet Res 66(3):545–52.

Wittek T., Tischer, K., Gieseler, T., Fürll, M., and Constable, P.D. 2008. Effect of preoperative administration of erythromycin or flunixin meglumine on postoperative abomasal emptying rate in dairy cows undergoing surgical correction of left displacement of the abomasum. J Am Vet Med Assoc 1;232(3):418–23.

Wold, J.S., and Turnipseed, S.A. 1981. Toxicology of vancomycin in laboratory animals. Rev Infect Dis 3:S224–229.

Wolfensohn, S.E. 1991. Clindamycin treatment of mandibular osteomyelitis in a cynomolgus monkey. Vet Rec 129:265–266.

Womble, A.Y., Giguère, S., Lee, E.A., and Vickroy, T.W. 2006. Pharmacokinetics of clarithromycin and concentrations in body fluids and bronchoalveolar cells of foals. Am J Vet Res 67:1681–1686.

Yancy, R.J., Sanchez, M.S., and Ford, C.W. 1991. Activity of antibiotics against *Staphylococcus aureus* within polymorphonuclear neutrophils. Eur J Clin Microbiol Infect Dis 10:107–113.

Yunis, A.A. 1988. Chloramphenicol: relation of structure to activity and toxicity. Ann Rev Pharmacol Toxicol 28:83–100.

Zaghlol, H.A., and Brown, S.A. 1988. Single- and multiple-dose pharmacokinetics of intravenously administered vancomycin in dogs. Am J Vet Res 49:1637–1640.

Zimmerman, D.M., Armstrong, D.L., Curro, T.G., Dankoff, S.M., Vires, K.W., Cook, K.K., Jaros, N.D., and Papich, M.G. 2006. Pharmacokinetics of florfenicol after a single intramuscular dose in white-spotted bamboo sharks (*Chiloscyllium plagiosum*). J Zoo Wildl Med 37(2):165–73.

Ziv, G., Nouws, J.F.M., and Ginneken, C.A.M. 1982. The pharmacokinetic and tissue levels of polymyxin B, colistin and gentamicin in calves. J Vet Pharmacol Therap 5:45–58.

Ziv, G., Shem-Tov, M., Glickman, A., et al. 1995. Tilmicosin antibacterial activity and pharmacokinetics in cows. J Vet Pharmacol Therap 18:340–345.

Ziv, G., and Sulman, F.G. 1973a. Passage of polymyxins from serum into milk in ewes. Am J Vet Res 34(3):317–322.

———. 1973b. Serum and milk concentrations of spectinomycin and tylosin in cows and ewes. Am J Vet Res 34:329–333.

CHAPTER

38

FLUOROQUINOLONE ANTIMICROBIAL DRUGS

MARK G. PAPICH AND JIM E. RIVIERE

The use of the fluoroquinolone antibacterial agents in veterinary medicine has increased tremendously in the last 15 years. The fluoroquinolones are synthetic antibacterial agents introduced in veterinary medicine first as enrofloxacin. Since then, there has been a great deal of research on this class of drugs to better understand their mechanism of action, antimicrobial spectrum, pharmacokinetics in a wide variety of animal species, and clinical use. In addition, pharmaceutical companies have developed new compounds to increase the number of these drugs available to veterinarians. The advantages of the fluoroquinolones are that they are rapidly bactericidal against a wide variety of clinically important bacterial organisms, are potent, are well tolerated by animals, and have been administered via a variety of routes (orally via tablets and drinking water, subcutaneously, intravenously, intramuscularly and topically).

Fluoroquinolones approved for use in veterinary medicine for small animals include enrofloxacin, difloxacin, orbifloxacin, and marbofloxacin. Danofloxacin and enrofloxacin were approved for cattle, and enrofloxacin for pigs. Enrofloxacin and sarafloxacin were once approved for poultry but have been withdrawn because of *Campylobacter* resistance concerns. Fluoroquinolones that are labeled for humans and are of potential interest for veterinary medicine include ciprofloxacin. The newest generation of fluoroquinolones with increased activity against gram-positive cocci and anaerobic bacteria includes grepafloxacin, trovafloxacin, levofloxacin, moxifloxacin, gatifloxacin, and pradofloxacin. Grepafloxacin and trovafloxacin already have been discontinued because of adverse effects in people.

CHEMICAL FEATURES

The currently available fluoroquinolones have the same quinolone structure (Fig. 38.1); various chemical substitutions and side groups account for the different physical characteristics of each drug. These differences may account for variations in lipophilicity, volume of distribution (Vd), oral absorption, and elimination rate, but they do not change the antibacterial spectrum appreciably. For example, enrofloxacin has one fluorine substitution, difloxacin has two fluorine substitutions, and orbifloxacin has a three-fluorine substitution, but the presence of more than one fluorine does not increase antibacterial effects (Asuquo and Piddock 1993). When lipid solubility is expressed as the octanyl:water partition coefficient, enrofloxacin and difloxacin have high lipophilicity. Ciprofloxacin has a partition coefficient that is approximately 100-fold less than that of enrofloxacin; the corresponding partition coefficients of orbifloxacin and marbofloxacin are slightly higher than that of ciprofloxacin (Asuquo and Piddock 1993; Takács-Novák et al. 1992). (Some of these octanyl:water partition coefficients were determined in the laboratory of one of the authors and are unpublished.)

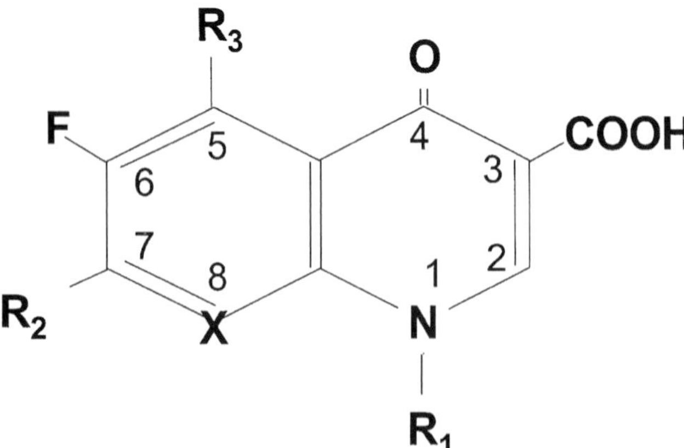

FIG. 38.1 Structure of fluoroquinolone. Features necessary for antibacterial activity are fluorine at position 6, ketone at position 4, and carboxyl at position 3. Addition of cyclopropyl, ethyl, or fluorophenyl at position 1 and of piperazine at position 7 increases the spectrum of antibacterial activity.

No studies are available to show that these chemical differences among the drugs can account for differences in clinical response. However, the differences may account for some variation in absorption and distribution. For example, ciprofloxacin oral absorption is approximately one-half that of enrofloxacin in dogs; ciprofloxacin absorption in horses is less than 10%, compared to 60% for enrofloxacin. The less lipid-soluble fluoroquinolones (marbofloxacin, orbifloxacin) have a lower Vd than the ones with higher lipid solubility (enrofloxacin, difloxacin) (Table 38.1). One explanation for this observation is that the more lipid-soluble drugs have higher intracellular concentrations, but higher tissue binding also could explain the differences in Vd.

Quinolones are amphoteric molecules that can be protonated at the carboxyl and the tertiary amine portion of the molecule. The pK_a varies among the drugs slightly, but generally the pK_a for the carboxyl group is 6.0–6.5 (5.5–6.3 in some references) and the pK_a for the nitrogen of the piperazine group is 7.5–8 (Nikaido and Thanassi 1993) (as high as 7.6–9.3 in some references). For two common drugs, enrofloxacin and ciprofloxacin, the pK_a for the carboxyl group is 6.0 and 6.1, respectively, and 8.8 and 7.8 for the amine, respectively. The isoelectric point is midway between the pK_a for each ionizable group. Therefore, at physiologic pH fluoroquinolones exist as zwitterions, in which both of the respective anionic and cationic groups are charged. It is at the isoelectric point (near the physiologic pH) that fluoroquinolones are the most lipophilic (Takács-Novák et al. 1992).

STRUCTURE-ACTIVITY RELATIONSHIPS. Figure 38.1 shows the basic quinolone structure. The carboxyl group at position 3 and the ketone at position 4 are necessary for the antibacterial activity. The fluorine at position 6 differentiates the quinolones from the fluoroquinolones and accounts for the improved gram-negative and gram-positive activity over the nonfluorinated quinolones, increased potency, and increased entry into bacteria. At position 1, addition of a cyclopropyl (as for enrofloxacin and ciprofloxacin in Fig. 38.2), an ethyl, or a fluorophenyl improve the spectrum of activity against gram-positive and gram-negative bacteria. Addition of a piperazine at position 7, as demonstrated for ciprofloxacin and enrofloxacin (Fig. 38.2), improves the spectrum of activity to include

TABLE 38.1 Pharmacokinetic comparison of fluoroquinolones

Drug	Dose studied (mg/kg)	Recommended daily dose (mg/kg)	$t_{1/2}$[a] (hr)	Vd (area)[a] (L/kg)	C_{max} (μg/mL)	AUC[a] (μg · hr/mL)	%*F*	Assay[b]	Reference
Dogs									
Enrofloxacin	5	5	4.61	ND	1.75	11.65	Nd	HPLC	Frazier et al. 2000
Enrofloxacin	5	5	2.23	3.64	1.24	4.46	63.22	HPLC	Bidgood & Papich 2005
Marbofloxacin	5	5	7.63	1.54	3.63	42.08	104.6	HPLC	Bidgood & Papich 2005
Marbofloxacin	5	5	4.07	Nd	1.41	8.74	Nd	Bioassay	Heinen 2002
Marbofloxacin	2	2	9.07	Nd	1.47	13.07	Nd	Bioassay	Heinen 2002
Marbofloxacin	2.75	2.75	10.9	Nd	2.53	35.44	Nd	HPLC	Frazier et al. 2000
Orbifloxacin	2.5	2.5	2.42	Nd	1.37	12.72	Nd	Bioassay	Heinen 2002
Difloxacin	5	5	6.9	Nd	1.1	9.34	Nd	Bioassay	Heinen 2002
Cats									
Levofloxacin	10	10	8.37	1.57	4.38	57.5	71.2	Bioassay	Albarellos et al. 2005
Enrofloxacin	5	5	6.7	2.5	1.0	20.3	107	HPLC	Seguin et al. 2004
Enrofloxacin (kitten)	5	5	3.7–6.3	1.8–3.9	0.5–1.1	5–12.7	33.7–72.8	HPLC	Sequin et al. 2004
Horses									
Moxifloxacin	5.8	NR	34	5.3	3.12	50.9	Nd	HPLC	Gardner et al. 2004
Ciprofloxacin	5	NR	5.8	4.9 (VDss)	0.6 (PO)	8.1	10.5	HPLC	Wilson et al. 2009
Enrofloxacin	7.5	7.5 (oral)	5.9 (IV)	4.2	2.22	14.37	65.6	HPLC	Boeckh et al. 2001
Enrofloxacin	7.5	7.5 (oral)	5.3 (IV)	2.9	1.85	21.0	78.3	Bioassay	Haines et al. 2000
Enrofloxacin	5	5 (IV)	6.7	1.9	12.4 (IV)	25.3	Nd	HPLC	Papich et al. 2002
Enrofloxacin	5	Nd	6.15 (IV)	2.32 (VDss)	1.0 (approx)	13.8	55	HPLC	Peyrou et al. 2006
Marbofloxacin	2	Nd	7.42 (IV)	1.6 (VDss)	0.8 (approx)	7.36	59	HPLC	Peyrou et al. 2006
Marbofloxacin	2	2	4.74 (IV)	1.17 (VDss)	1.42 (IM)	11.27	87.9 (IM)	HPLC	Carretero et al. 2002
Marbofloxacin	2	2	7.56 (IV)	2.83	0.89 (PO)	8.26	62 (PO), 98 (IM)	HPLC	Bousquet-Melou et al. 2002
Dogs									
Enrofloxacin	5.0 IV	5.0	2.7–3	5.0–5.6	—	4.05–4.34	—	HPLC	Intorre et al. 1995
Enrofloxacin	5.0	5.0	2.52	2.5	1.12 (oral)	7.27	72.3	HPLC	Cester et al. 1996
Enrofloxacin	5.8	5.0	4.4 (IV) 2.7 (oral)	4.5	1.44 (oral)	8.2	83.0	HPLC	Monlouis et al. 1997
Enrofloxacin	5.5	2.75–11.0	4.0 (oral)	nd	2.45 (oral)	16.32	Nd	Bioassay	Walker et al. 1992
Enrofloxacin	5.0	5.0	2.4	4.5	1.16 (oral)	3.9	100	HPLC	Küng et al. 1993a
Enrofloxacin	5.0	5.0–20.0[c]	4.8	4.2	1.6	8.15	—	HPLC	Stegemann et al. 1996
Ciprofloxacin	5.0	nd	3.17	2.23	0.35	4.18	43.0	HPLC	Cester et al. 1996
Ciprofloxacin	5.8[f]	nd	5.2	nd	0.34	7.2	Nd	HPLC	Monlouis et al. 1997
Ciprofloxacin	10.0	10.0–20.0	2.4	3.0	—	12.93	—	HPLC	Abadia et al. 1994
Ciprofloxacin	10.0	10.0–20.0	7.5	—	1.18 (oral)[d]	9.58 (oral)[d]	46[e]	Bioassay	Walker et al. 1990
Difloxacin	5.0	5.0–10.0[c]	9.3	4.63	1.8 (oral)	12.93	96.0	nd	Manufacturer's data
Orbifloxacin	2.5	2.5–7.5[c]	5.6	1.5	2.33 (oral)	14.3	97–100	HPLC	Manufacturer's data
Marbofloxacin	2.0	2.0	12.4–14.0	1.9–2.25	1.38 (oral) 1.52 (SC)	18.6–20.95 99 (SC)	100 (oral)	HPLC	Schneider et al. 1996

TABLE 38.1—*continued*

Drug	Dose studied (mg/kg)	Recommended daily dose (mg/kg)	$t_{1/2}$[a] (hr)	Vd (area)[a] (L/kg)	C_{max} (μg/mL)	AUC[a] (μg · hr/mL)	%F	Assay[b]	Reference
Marbofloxacin	2.0	2.0	9.8	1.4	1.35 (oral)	23.31	99.8	HPLC	Cester et al. 1996
Marbofloxacin	5.55 and 2.8 mg/kg	2.75–5.55[c]	9.5 (IV) 11 (oral)	1.27	2.0 at 2.8 mg/kg oral; 4.2 at 5.55 mg/kg oral	59.0	94.0	HPLC	Manufacturer's data
Cats									
Enrofloxacin	4.7	5[c]	6.7	6.3	1.66 (oral)	7.2	100	HPLC	Richez et al. 1997b
Orbifloxacin	2.5	2.5–7.5[c]	5.5	1.4	2.06	10.82	100	HPLC	Manufacturer's data
Horses									
Ciprofloxacin	3.0	Not recommended	4.9 (IV) 10.7 (IM)	0.147	0.77 (IM)	6.97	96.0 (IM)	HPLC	Yun et al. 1994
Ciprofloxacin	5.0	Not recommended	2.6 (IV)	3.88	na	4.83	6.8	Bioassay	Dowling et al. 1995
Enrofloxacin	2.5 and 5.0	5.0 (IV, IM) 5.0–7.5 (oral)	5.9–6.1	0.78 (5 mg/kg)	5.44	58.3	62.5	Bioassay	Giguere et al. 1996
Orbifloxacin	2.5	2.5–5.0 (oral)	5.1	2.4	1.25 (oral)	9.06	68.3 (oral)	HPLC	Davis et al. 2006
Enrofloxacin	5.0 (IV, IM)	5.0 (IV or IM)	4.4 (IV) 9.9 (IM)	2.4	1.28 (IM)	13.2	>100% (IM)	HPLC	Pyorala et al. 1994
Enrofloxacin (foals)	5.0	2.5–5.0	16.5	2.31	2.12 (10 mg/kg oral)	48.54	42.0	HPLC	Bermingham et al. 2000
Cattle									
Enrofloxacin	12.5	12.5	6.79	ND	0.96	14.95	ND	HPLC	Davis et al. 2007
Enrofloxacin	8	8	7.28	NS	0.81	7.51	ND	HPLC	TerHune et al. 2005
Danofloxacin	6	6	4.21	ND	1.7	9.72	ND	HPLC	TerHune et al. 2005
Danofloxacin	1.25	Nd	2.25	2.04	0.28	132.85	289	Bioassay	Shem-Tov et al. 1998
Danofloxacin	5	Nd	2.9	ND	0.82	4.7	78 (IM)	HPLC	Mann & Frame 1992
Danofloxacin	1.25	Nd	6.26	4.0	0.18	2.9	91	HPLC	Apley & Upson 1993
Rabbits									
Moxifloxacin	5	Nd	1.84	2.12	1.3 (PO)	6.28	75.5 (PO)	HPLC	Fernandex-Varon et al. 2005
Pigs									
Danofloxacin	5	Nd	8.0	ND	0.8	6.0	76 (IM)	HPLC	Mann & Frame 1992
Goats									
Danofloxacin	1.25	Nd	4.67	3.8	0.33	2.29	110 (SC)	HPLC	Aliabadi & Lees 2001
Enrofloxacin	5	5	1.1	1.3	6.7	6.7	ND	HPLC	Rao et al. 2000
Marbofloxacin	2	2	7.2	1.3 (VDss)	1.9	8.44	100.7 (IM)	HPLC	Waxman et al. 2001
Sheep									
Enrofloxacin	5	10	4.8	1.15	2.69	57.5	98.07	HPLC	Bermingham & Papich 2002
Alpacas									
Enrofloxacin	5 & 10	5–10	13.0	1.6	7.8 (SC), 15.3 (PO)	58.4	90 (SC), 29 (PO)	HPLC	Gandolf et al. 2005

Elephants									
Enrofloxacin	2.5 (PO)	2.5 (PO)	18.4	Nd	1.31	34.93	Nd	HPLC	Sanchez et al. 2005
Mice									
Enrofloxacin	10.0	nd	1.48	10.5	nd	2.45	na	HPLC	Bregante et al. 1999
Rats									
Enrofloxacin	7.5	nd	1.8	4.78	nd	5.65	nc	HPLC	Bregante et al. 1999
Rabbits									
Enrofloxacin	7.5	nd	2.2	4.94	nd	5.52	nd	HPLC	Bregante et al. 1999
Enrofloxacin	7.5 (IV)	nd	1.87	3.97	na	5.38	na	HPLC	Aramayona et al. 1996
Enrofloxacin	5.0 (IV)	5.0	2.18 (IV)	4.4	na	3.89	na	HPLC	Cabanes et al. 1992
Enrofloxacin	5.0 (IM)	5.0	1.8	na	3.04	3.84	92.0	HPLC	Cabanes et al. 1992
Enrofloxacin	5.0 (IV)	5.0	2.5	2.12	na	8.6	na	HPLC	Broome et al. 1991
Enrofloxacin	5.0 (oral)	5.0	2.4	na	0.45	5.4	61.0	HPLC	Broome et al. 1991
Cattle									
Enrofloxacin (1-day-old calves)	2.5	2.5–5 per day or 7.5–12.5 SC once	6.61	1.70	nd	13.94	nd	HPLC	Kaartinen et al. 1997
Enrofloxacin (1-week-old calves)	2.5	2.5–5 per day or 7.5–12.5 SC once	4.87	2.61	nd	6.73	nd	HPLC	Kaartinen et al. 1997
Enrofloxacin (lactating cows)	5.0	nd	1.68 (IV) 5.9 (IM) 5.55 (SC)	1.63	0.73 (IM) 0.98 (SC)	7.42	82.0 (IM) 137.0 (SC)	HPLC	Kaartinen et al. 1995
Enrofloxacin (cows)	2.5	nd	2.82	2.98	nd	5.28	nd	HPLC	Bregante et al. 1999
Enrofloxacin (adult cattle)	5.0	2.5–5 per day or 7.5–12.5 SC once[c]	2.3	1.65	0.73 (SC)	10.08	88.0 (SC)	HPLC	Richez et al. 1997
Enrofloxacin (calves)	5.0	2.5–5 per day or 7.5–12.5 SC once[c]	2.2	1.98	0.87 (SC)	7.99	97.0 (SC)	HPLC	Richez et al. 1997
Ciprofloxacin (calves)	2.8	nd	2.4	2.5	0.27	nd	53.0 (oral)	HPLC	Nouws et al. 1988
Sheep									
Enrofloxacin	2.5	5.0 mg/kg/day SC	3.73	2.18	0.78 (IM)	5.47	85.0 (IM)	HPLC	Mengozzi et al. 1996
Enrofloxacin	2.5	5.0 mg/kg/day SC	3.8	1.3	0.6 (oral)	10.4	60.6 (oral)	Bioassay	Pozzin et al. 1997
Enrofloxacin	2.5	nd	2.5	1.53	nd	8.98	nd	HPLC	Bregante et al. 1999
Chickens									
Ciprofloxacin	5.0	5.0–15.0 IM, SC, oral	9.01	2.02	4.67	78.04	70.0	Bioassay	Atta and Sharif 1997
Enrofloxacin	10.0	10.0	5.6 (IV)	5.0	1.88 (oral)	16.17	89.2	HPLC	Knoll et al. 1999
Enrofloxacin	10.0	10.0	10.3 (IV)	4.3	2.44 (oral)	34.51	64.0	HPLC	Anadón et al. 1995
Ciprofloxacin	5.0	5.0	9.0	2.0	4.67	78.04	70.0 (oral)	Bioassay	Atta and Sharif 1997
Camels									
Enrofloxacin	2.5	2.5 IM, SC	3.58	1.4	1.44 (IM)	18.95	85.0 (IM)	Bioassay	Gavrielli et al. 1995

TABLE 38.1—*continued*

Drug	Dose studied (mg/kg)	Recommended daily dose (mg/kg)	$t_{1/2}$[a] (hr)	Vd (area)[a] (L/kg)	C_{max} (μg/mL)	AUC[a] (μg · hr/mL)	%F	Assay[b]	Reference
Chickens									
Enrofloxacin	10 (PO)	NR	14	Nd	1.5	35	Nd	HPLC	Da Silva et al. 2006
Harbor Seals									
Enrofloxacin	5	5	5	1.4	3	30	Nd	HPLC	KuKanich et al. 2007
Cuttlefish									
Enrofloxacin	10	10	1.0	Nd	10.95	26.71	Nd	HPLC	Gore et al. 2005
Pigs									
Enrofloxacin	2.5		345	3.34	1.17	5.97	150	HPLC	Zeng and Fung 1997
Enrofloxacin	2.5		7.73	3.5	0.61 (IM)	9.94	95.0 (IM)	HPLC	Richez et al. 1997a
Enrofloxacin	2.5		5.5	3.95	0.75 (IM)	5.03	101 (IM)	Bioassay	Pijpers et al. 1997.
Enrofloxacin	10.0 oral		nd	nd	nd	27.0	73.0–80.0	HPLC	Gyrd-Hansen and Nielsen 1994
Ciprofloxacin	3.06	nd	2.57	3.83	0.17	2.88	37.0	HPLC	Nouws et al. 1988
Dolphins									
Enrofloxacin	5.0	5.0 q24h oral	6.4	nd	1.4	15.4	Nd	Bioassay	Linnehan et al. 1999
Fish									
Enrofloxacin trout	5.0 and 10.0	5.0 mg/kg q24h	24.0 and 30.0	3.22 and 2.56	0.945 and 1.28 (15E)	109.2 and 171.3	(oral at 15°) 42 and 49	Bioassay	Bowser et al. 1992
Enrofloxacin (red pacu)	5.0	5.0 mg/kg q48h IM	29.0	nd	1.64 (IM) 0.8 (oral)	46.3 (IM)	57.0 (relative)	HPLC	Lewbart et al. 1997
Enrofloxacin (Atlantic salmon)	10.0	5.0 mg/kg q24h oral	131.0	22.4	0.29 (oral) 0.54 (oral)	84.3 1.3 (IP)	89.0 (IP) 46 (oral)	Bioassay 66 (IM)	Stoffregen et al. 1997

Na = Data not available or not applicable.

Nd = Not determined, NR = not recommended.

$t_{1/2}$ = Half-life of the terminal portion of the plasma concentration vs. time curve.

Vd = Apparent volume of distribution (area method).

AUC = Area under the curve of the plasma concentration vs. time curve.

C_{max} = Maximum plasma concentration after administration of oral or IM dose.

%F = Percentage of oral or IM administered dose absorbed (determined from comparison of IV dose).

[a]Half-life, Vd, and AUC are from an IV dose unless otherwise noted.

[b]Assay type = Assay using HPLC is able to distinguish between enrofloxacin and ciprofloxacin, and values shown in table represent enrofloxacin. Assays performed by bioassay represent the parent drug and active metabolites. Bioassay may include concentrations of ciprofloxacin.

[c]Registered dose with the FDA in the United States. In some European countries doses may vary or may not include the flexible range. In most cases, when treating non-*Pseudomonas* infections, the lowest dose in the range listed is used.

[d]After multiple dosing with ciprofloxacin, the C_{max} was 1.18 mg/mL and the 12 hr AUC was 9.58 mg/hr/mL.

[e]Oral absorption of ciprofloxacin estimated from a comparison of independent oral and IV studies.

[f]These parameters determined after administration of 5.8 mg/kg of enrofloxacin.

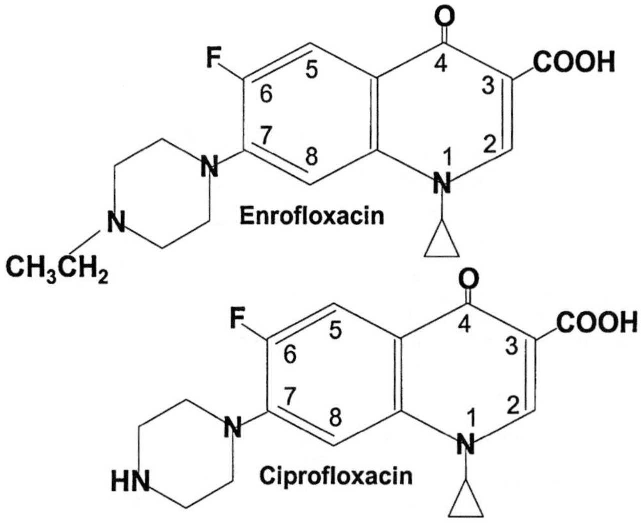

FIG. 38.2 Structure of enrofloxacin and ciprofloxacin.

pseudomonads, among other gram-negative bacteria. The change to a carbon from a nitrogen at position 8 decreased some of the adverse central nervous system effects and increased activity against staphylococci.

The newer generation of quinolones have a bicyclic substitution at position 7, instead of a piperazine. This increased the activity to include a wider range of bacteria. In addition, a substitution at the 8 position on the ring enhances the bactericidal effects and improves the spectrum of activity to include more gram-positive and anaerobic bacteria. For example, the 8-methoxy substitution produces the drug moxifloxacin, a human quinolone with improved activity against gram-positive bacteria (Behra-Miellet et al. 2002; Aktaç et al. 2002; Pestova et al. 2000). Pradofloxacin, a new veterinary quinolone with similar activity has a cyano substitution at position 8, and this drug has improved gram-positive and anaerobic activity compared to enrofloxacin and ciprofloxacin (Silley et al. 2007). This drug is discussed in more detail at the end of this chapter in the section "New Developments."

MECHANISM OF ACTION

Quinolones are bactericidal by inhibiting bacterial DNA replication and transcription. Two-stranded DNA is tightly coiled in the cell and must be separated for transcription and translation. To facilitate coiling, winding, and unwinding, the enzyme DNA gyrase allows the strands to be cut and reconnected. This allows coiling because negative supercoils can be introduced. DNA gyrase, a topoisomerase, consists of A and B subunits. The most common target site for quinolones is the A subunit of DNA gyrase coded by the gene *gyrA*. Mammals are resistant to the killing effects of quinolone antimicrobials because Topoisomerase II in mammalian cells is not inhibited until the drug concentration reaches 100–1000 μg/ml. Bacteria are inhibited by concentrations of 0.1–10 μg/ml or less. The Clinical Laboratory Standards Institute (CLSI, formerly called *NCCLS*) break point for ciprofloxacin, the prototypical fluoroquinolone, for susceptible bacteria is 1.0 μg/ml (CLSI 2007). Another target is the Topoisomerase IV enzyme composed of subunits *parC* and *parE*. This site of action is less important for gram-negative bacteria but is a target of fluoroquinolones in some gram-positive bacteria such as streptococci and staphylococci (Ferrero et al. 1995). Among the newer fluoroquinolones (e.g., moxifloxacin, gatifloxacin) the primary target for gram-positive bacteria may be the DNA-gyrase rather than Topoisomerase IV, or these drugs also may be dual inhibitors against both targets (Intorre et al. 2007). The action of quinolones on DNA gyrase and Topoisomerase IV has been reviewed in more detail in other papers (Drlica and Zhao1997; Blondeau et al. 2004).

ANTIBACTERIAL SPECTRUM

Fluoroquinolones in general exhibit good activity against most gram-negative bacteria, especially those of the Enterobacteriaceae. Representative minimum inhibitory concentration (MIC) values are shown in Table 38.2. *Escherichia coli, Klebsiella* spp., *Proteus* spp., *Salmonella* spp., and *Enterobacter* spp. are usually susceptible. *Pseudomonas aeruginosa* is variably susceptible and, when it is susceptible, usually has a higher MIC than other susceptible organisms. Against *P. aeruginosa,* ciprofloxacin is the most active (Rubin et al. 2008).

Gram-positive bacteria are variably susceptible. *Staphylococcus aureus, Staphylococcus pseudintermedius* and other *Staphylococcus* species usually are susceptible. However, the MIC values for staphylococci typically are higher than for gram-negative bacteria, and staphylococcal resistance to fluoroquinolones has been a problem in human patients. Methicillin-resistant strains of staphylococci (MRSA) are often resistant to fluoroquinolones.

The use of the newest generation of fluoroquinolones has not yet been reported in veterinary medicine, except in experimental studies. These drugs, such as moxifloxa-

TABLE 38.2 Comparative microbiological data for common pathogens

Drug	MIC of bacteria (μg/mL)			
	Pasteurella multocida	*Escherichia coli*	*Staphylococcus intermedius*	*Pseudomonas aeruginosa*
Ciprofloxacin	0.015	0.03	0.25	0.5
Difloxacin	<0.05	0.11–0.23	0.25–0.91	0.92
Enrofloxacin	0.03	0.03–0.06	0.125	2.0
Marbofloxacin	0.04	0.125–0.25	0.23–0.25	0.94
Orbifloxacin	0.05	0.125–0.39	0.25–0.39	6.25–12.5

Sources: Pirro et al. 1997, 1999; Asuquo and Piddock 1993; Stegemann et al. 1996; Spreng et al. 1995; and manufacturer data.
Note: MIC values listed are MIC_{90} and represent an average from available published literature or manufacturer technical information.

TABLE 38.3 Interpretive criteria for susceptibility break points (CLSI 2007)

Drug	Sensitive (μg/ml)	Intermediate (μg/ml)	Resistant (μg/ml)
Danofloxacin (cattle BRD)	≤0.25	—	—
Enrofloxacin (dogs and cats)	≤0.5	1–2	≥4
Enrofloxacin (cattle BRD)	≤0.25	0.5–1	≥2
Difloxacin (dogs)	≤0.5	1–2	≥4
Marbofloxacin (dogs and cats)	≤1	2	≥4
Orbifloxacin (dogs and cats)	≤1	2–4	≥8
Ciprofloxacin (human)*	≤1	2	≥4

*The break point listed for ciprofloxacin is based on human use, not veterinary use.

cin, gatifloxacin, and the veterinary drug pradofloxacin have increased activity against gram-positive cocci and anaerobic bacteria and may have advantages for certain infections (Behra-Miellet et al. 2002; Aktaç et al. 2002; Pestova et al. 2000; Silley 2007). Against gram-negative bacteria, such as the Enterobacteriaceae, they have equal or similar activity. Against *Pseudomonas aeruginosa,* these drugs are not as active as ciprofloxacin. Whether these newer fluoroquinolones will replace standard treatment with β-lactam antibiotics for treatment of streptococci remains a question (Legg and Bint 1999).

Factors that may affect activity are cations at the site of infection and low pH. Cations such as Al^{+3}, Mg^{+3}, Fe^{+2}, and Ca^{+2} can bind a carboxyl group on the drug and significantly decrease activity. Low pH at the site of action also can affect the MIC (Ross and Riley 1994), especially for drugs that have a piperazine at position 7 (Fig. 38.1). For example, in urine, the MIC for fluoroquinolones may increase due to the presence of cations in the urine and low pH (Fernandes 1988). This activity in urine may increase the MIC from 4- to 64-fold. Fluoroquinolone activity in an abscess is not diminished despite the observation that in pus there is cellular material that can bind drugs, a low pH, and slow-growing bacteria (Bryant and Mazza 1989). The activity of fluoroquinolones in this milieu may explain its efficacy for treating infections associated with abscessation.

SUSCEPTIBILITY TESTING. Susceptibility testing is performed either by the agar-disk-diffusion (ADD) method or broth dilutions (MIC test). The CLSI (formerly NCCLS) (CLSI 2007) has published interpretive criteria to set break points for most fluoroquinolones (Table 38.3). For isolates in the "Intermediate" range , the organism "could be considered as susceptible if appropriate dosing modifications, explained in the package insert, are applied. The MIC quality-control ranges for wild-type organisms are also available from CLSI.

RESISTANCE

Resistance most frequently develops via the *gyrA* mutation that codes for the A subunit of the DNA gyrase enzyme. A mutation at the serine-83 residue has been one of the most common, but at least 10 additional mutations at the *gyrA* gene have been identified to confer resistance (Ferrero et al. 1995). Mutations in the *parC* gene that codes for Topoisomerase IV enzyme also are important (e.g., GrlA mutation). A mutation in *parC* coding for resistant Topoisomerase IV may be more important in gram-positive bacteria than in gram-negative isolates, but may also produce high-level resistance. The *parC* mutation causes a high-level resistance when detected with mutations of *GyrA*. The multidrug resistance membrane efflux mechanisms reduce the accumulation of antibiotics in the bacteria. These efflux mechanisms are known to produce a high-level resistance to fluoroquinolones when they are present with other target site mutations (Zhanel et al. 2004). Efflux mechanisms may play an important role in *Pseudomonas aeruginosa* fluoroquinolone resistance and could explain why resistance is high among these bacteria (Zhanel et al. 2004). Because the efflux membrane pumps may affect other drugs, this may produce cross-resistance to other antimicrobials.

Resistance can occur through a multistep process (Everett et al. 1996). A single mutation can increase the MIC slightly (perhaps one dilution), and each subsequent mutation produces a progressively higher level resistance in a stepwise fashion. For example, resistant strains of *E. coli* with MIC >8 μg/ml may possess multiple mutations for the target genes and may also show enhanced drug efflux. Unlike plasmid-mediated bacterial resistance, in which resistance may disappear after selective antibiotic pressure is removed, chromosomal (mutational) resistance exhibited by fluoroquinolone-resistant bacteria can be maintained in bacteria after drug administration is discontinued. Plasmid-mediated resistance has been found in *E. coli* and *Klebsiella* organisms, but the clinical significance of plasmid-mediated resistance has not been identified (Martinez-Martinez et al. 1998). Chromosomal mutations, rather than plasmid-mediated resistance, is overwhelmingly the most important source of clinical resistance.

CLINICAL RESISTANCE PROBLEMS. Resistance to fluoroquinolones has become a problem in human medicine that some investigators have attributed to increased prescribing of these drugs. Resistance to fluoroquinolones by *E. coli, Staphylococcus aureus,* and *Streptococcus pneumoniae* has been documented (Chen et al. 1999; Murphy et al. 1997; Sanders et al. 1995; Neu 1992; Peña et al. 1995; Perea et al. 1999; Everett et al. 1996). Clinical resistance in human hospitals among staphylococci appeared relatively quickly after introduction of ciprofloxacin (Neu 1992; Sanders et al. 1995; Hedin and Hambreus 1991). Resistant bacteria also have been identified in companion animals. Resistance in small animals has been documented for *E. coli, P. aeruginosa, Enterobacter, Proteus,* and other gram-negative bacteria. Resistance among staphylococci isolated from small animals has also been documented (Lloyd et al. 1999), but the prevalence remains low (Pinchbeck et al. 2007; Petersen et al. 2002; Ganière et al. 2001; Intorre et al. 2007). Frequent use may increase this prevalence. In a study of bacteria causing chronic otitis in dogs, 14% of *Staphylococcus intermedius* from the middle ear were resistant to enrofloxacin (Cole et al. 1998). If methicillin-resistant strains of *Staphylococcus* are identified, many are multidrug resistant and often exhibit fluoroquinolone resistance in addition to resistance to other drugs (Jones et al. 2007). The newer generation of fluoroquinolones, discussed previously, such as moxifloxacin and gatifloxacin may have better activity against these resistant strains (Intorre et al. 2007).

Pseudomonas organisms have been particularly troublesome because single-step mutations are common for this bacteria, which can easily lead to high-level resistance after exposure. This is an important problem in companion animal medicine because; except for the fluoroquinolones, there are no other oral drugs with which to treat infections caused by *Pseudomonas aeruginosa.* Resistance is primarily caused by a *GyrA* mutation, but an additional mutation in *parC* could cause a high-level resistance (Jalal and Wretlind 1998). Strains with both mutations were significantly more resistant than strains with one mutation. As discussed earlier, efflux mechanisms may also contribute to resistance among *Pseudomonas* (Zhanel et al. 2004). Factors leading to resistant *P. aeruginosa* are an inadequate dosage and extended treatment at low doses. From the horizontal and middle ear of dogs with chronic otitis, 87 and 65%, respectively, of the pseudomonads cultured were resistant to enrofloxacin (Cole et al. 1998). Other studies have confirmed increased frequency of resistance among *Pseudomonas aeruginosa* isolated from chronic infections in dogs (Petersen et al. 2002; Martin Barrasa et al. 2000).

HUMAN HEALTH RISKS. Infectious disease experts have warned that frequent usage of fluoroquinolones may lead to increased resistance in animals (WHO 1997). Transfer of fluoroquinolone resistance from animals to people has been suggested to occur for *Campylobacter* species (Endtz et al. 1991) and *Salmonella typhimurium* type DT-104 (Threlfall et al. 1995; Threlfall et al. 1997; Griggs et al. 1994). An increase in the incidence of resistant *Campylobacter jejuni* infecting people was linked to consumption of *Campylobacter*-contaminated chicken. The increased resistance occurred primarily after 1995, which coincides with the time that fluoroquinolones were approved for use in poultry as an additive to drinking water (Smith et al. 1999). Investigators have also associated resistance in salmonellae with veterinary use of fluoroquinolones in livestock (Piddock et al. 1998). However, resistant strains of *Salmonella typhimurium* may have occurred spontaneously because some of the resistant salmonellae have come from farms in which fluoroquinolones were not administered to animals (Griggs et al. 1994). Nevertheless, some scientists have warned that continued use of fluoroquinolones in livestock is a public health risk because it can potentially lead to resistant mutants of salmonellae being passed on to humans through the food chain. Because of these concerns, there have been limited approvals of fluoroquinolones for food-producing animals, and the extralabel use of fluoroquinolones is prohibited in food-producing animals in the United States. Because of the risk of *Campylobacter* resistance, all fluoroquinolone formulations for poultry have been removed from the market.

PHARMACOKINETICS

Mammals are relatively consistent in elimination half-life and Vd. Reptiles with lower renal clearance generally demonstrate longer half-lives—as long as 55 and 36 hours for enrofloxacin in alligators and Monitor lizards, respectively (Papich 1999). There may be an allometric relationship in pharmacokinetic parameters among mammals ranging in size from mice to cattle (Bregante et al. 1999; Cox et al. 2004). The allometric relationship was improved considerably when the pharmacokinetic parameters were corrected for the percentage of protein-unbound enrofloxacin in the plasma. In particular, for enrofloxacin the Vd was the most directly proportional to animal body weight, with the animals with largest body weight having the largest Vd.

Among the drugs, there are differences in the pharmacokinetic parameters, which in animals are listed in Table 38.1. Whether these differences translate to clinical differences, however, has not been shown, because there are no comparative studies. For example, it does not appear that differences in half-life can account for different clinical results for skin infection treatment in dogs because enrofloxacin, which has the shortest half-life (Table 38.1), and marbofloxacin, which has the longest half-life, have both been reported to be effective when administered once daily (Paradis et al. 1990; Carlotti et al. 1995; Carlotti 1996; Gruet et al. 1997; Koch and Peters 1996; Lloyd 1992; Kwochka 1993; Ihrke 1996, 1998; Cester et al. 1996). Likewise, even though there is a range of values for Vd among the drugs, this has not translated into a superior clinical efficacy. Marbofloxacin and orbifloxacin, which have a Vd in the range of 1–2 l/kg, achieve effective skin concentrations and appear as clinically effective as drugs such as enrofloxacin with a Vd of 2.5–5 l/kg. The data published (Walker et al. 1990, 1992) or available from manufacturer technical information show that all the fluoroquinolones, regardless of their Vd and lipophilicity, achieve concentrations in tissues, except for the central nervous system and eye, that are at least as high as plasma. Differences in Vd, however, account for a range of maximum plasma concentrations (Cmax) among the drugs (Table 38.1). Drugs with the lowest Vd are diluted less in body fluid and produce higher plasma concentrations than drugs with a higher Vd. The consequence of this difference is reflected in the dose administered (dose = Vd × Cmax).

ORAL ABSORPTION. Oral absorption of fluoroquinolones is high for most animals studied (Table 38.1). Whether fluoroquinolones are administered with or without food has little effect on oral absorption. Fluoroquinolones administered with food may exhibit a slow or a prolonged absorption, but the extent of absorption, determined by the total AUC (area under the curve of the plasma concentration versus time curve) is not affected significantly. Administration with food has prolonged the terminal half-life when enrofloxacin was administered orally to reptiles (Papich 1999), sheep, pigs (Gyrd-Hansen and Nielsen 1994), and chickens (Anadón et al. 1995).

In clinical situations involving animals difficult to dose, fluoroquinolones may be added to a patient's food in order to provide a more convenient dosing form. For example, enrofloxacin tablets were placed in whole fish, which were fed to dolphins to produce good absorption (Linnehan et al. 1999), and enrofloxacin was injected into mice and fed to Monitor lizards also producing good absorption (Hungerford et al. 1997). Chewable tablets of enrofloxacin (Taste-Tabs) do not affect oral absorption (manufacturer's data).

In dogs, cats, and pigs, oral absorption of fluoroquinolones approaches 100% (Table 38.1), but in large animals, extent of absorption has been less. Oral absorption of fluoroquinolones is variable in horses. Ciprofloxacin showed an oral absorption of only 6.8% in ponies (Dowling et al. 1995) and only 10% (mean) in adults (Torill et al. 2009). But enrofloxacin absorption is 63% (Giguère et al. 1996) in adult horses and 42% in foals (Bermingham et al. 2000). The value reported for adult horses is probably artificially high because the study used a bioassay that overestimates the concentration of enrofloxacin in plasma. With the exception of ciprofloxacin, other studies listed in Table 38.1 indicate relatively good oral absorption of these drugs in horses. Studies in ruminants produce conflicting results on oral absorption. In sheep, oral absorption was reported to be 61% (Pozzin et al. 1997), but absorption in ruminant calves was listed as less than 10% (Vancutsem et al. 1990). In sheep, absorption from oral administration was high (Bermingham et al. 2002). In addition, this study showed that when enrofloxacin was mixed with food and administered orally to sheep, absorption was high and half-life longer than after the IV dose. The long oral half-life was the result of slow release from the feed (possible adsorption) or slow emptying from the rumen ("flip-flop" effect). Absorption is also good in nondomestic ruminants such as the hoofstock kept in zoological parks (Gandolf et al. 2003, 2006). In camels (although not a true ruminant), oral absorption was reported to be negligible (Gavrielli et al. 1995), but our laboratory found that absorption was 29% (mean) in alpacas and was capable of producing high enough concentrations to treat susceptible gram-negative pathogens at 10 mg/kg (Gandolf et al. 2005).

In birds, oral absorption of enrofloxacin has been reported to be good, with effective levels being achieved by adding the drug to the bird's drinking water. This method of administration has been employed to treat sick pet birds (Flammer 1998) and chickens (Knoll et al. 1999). However, as mentioned previously, administration to food-producing poultry is prohibited in the United States. After continuous medication in the drinking water, steady-state plasma concentrations of enrofloxacin are 0.53 μg/ml (Knoll et al. 1999). In fish enrofloxacin absorption has been estimated to be 40–50% (Lewbart 1998).

INTRAMUSCULAR AND SUBCUTANEOUS INJECTION. Absorption is virtually complete from intramuscular (IM) injection. There have not been many studies that examined subcutaneous (SC) injection, but in the studies that are available, absorption was nearly complete. Delayed absorption from injection is possibly due to a slow release from the injection site caused by tissue binding or tissue injury that disrupts blood flow.

In cattle, e.g. (Kaartinen et al. 1995), half-life was 1.68 hours from IV injection of enrofloxacin (5 mg/kg), but 5.9 and 5.55 hours from IM and SC injection, respectively, even though the extent of absorption was high. In the study by Davis et al., (2007) the half-life of enrofloxacin after a SC injection to calves at 12.5 mg/kg was 6.79 hr (mean), and 7.25 hr for the metabolite ciprofloxacin. For danofloxacin, the IV half-life in cattle was 0.9 hours and the IM half-life was 2.26 hours. In some animals there was delayed absorption from IM or SC injections, which produced longer half-lives from these routes compared to IV administration (this is known as "flip-flop" absorption kinetics).

METABOLISM. Metabolism of enrofloxacin to ciprofloxacin occurs via deethylation of the ethyl group on the piperazine ring. Other metabolites are produced from further metabolism of ciprofloxacin, but these are minor and do not contribute to the antibacterial effects. There are also minor insignificant metabolites of some of the other drugs. Examination of the extent of metabolism of enrofloxacin to ciprofloxacin in dogs and cats was reported in several studies (Küng et al. 1993a; Monlouis et al. 1997; Cester et al. 1996; Richez et al. 1997b; Kordick et al. 1997; Heinen 1999; Seguin et al. 2004) in which high-pressure liquid chromatography (HPLC) was used to determine the specific concentrations of enrofloxacin and ciprofloxacin after enrofloxacin administration. An analysis of the data shows that at Cmax 20% and 10% in dogs and cats, respectively, of the total fluoroquinolone concentration is contributed by ciprofloxacin. (That is, ciprofloxacin accounts for 20 and 10% of enrofloxacin plus ciprofloxacin concentrations.) In cats, the proportion of ciprofloxacin to total quinolone concentration was 17% and was not affected by age (Seguin et al. 2004). In cattle, the proportion of ciprofloxacin in plasma has been measured as 25% (Richez et al. 1994) and as high as 41% (Davis et al. 2007). Also, in the latter study, the proportion of ciprofloxacin in tissues of calves was higher than that of enrofloxacin. But in pigs, foals, and some reptiles there were only small traces of ciprofloxacin metabolized from enrofloxacin (Zeng and Fung 1997; Bermingham et al. 2000; Richez et al. 1997a). Studies in fish show that after administration of enrofloxacin, about 2% of the maximal concentration is made up of ciprofloxacin (Lewbart et al. 1997). Difloxacin is metabolized to the active metabolite sarafloxacin by demethylation, but the amount of sarafloxacin from difloxacin in dogs has been small (Heinen 1999).

In chickens, the concentrations of ciprofloxacin in plasma and tissues after administration of enrofloxacin are minimal (Knoll et al. 1999; Anadón et al. 1995). However, similar to studies in cattle (Davis et al. 2007), one of these studies reported that the ratio of ciprofloxacin:enrofloxacin tissue concentrations was greater than 1.0 after administration of enrofloxacin despite the low plasma concentrations of ciprofloxacin (Anadón et al. 1995). The ciprofloxacin concentration residues were still present in tissues of chickens 12 days after dosing.

If there are active metabolites produced, such as ciprofloxacin from enrofloxacin, this can cause errors in the interpretation of drug assays when a bioassay (microbiological assay) is used because a bioassay does not distinguish parent drug from active metabolite. Pharmacokinetic studies performed using bioassay techniques and compared with HPLC methods have demonstrated that bioassay can overestimate the combined enrofloxacin and ciprofloxacin concentrations in animals by as much as 70% for the AUC and 29% for the Cmax (Cester et al. 1996). This finding agrees with another study in dogs: a microbiological assay overestimated the total enrofloxacin + ciprofloxacin AUC determined by HPLC by as much as 30–70% (Küng et al. 1993b).

EXCRETION. The fluoroquinolones are primarily excreted via the kidneys by glomerular filtration and tubular excretion (Bregante et al. 1999). The role of tubular excretion has been demonstrated by showing that probenecid can decrease the clearance for some fluoroquinolones. For most of the drugs a major portion of the parent drug or metabolites can be recovered in the urine, with a smaller amount recovered in the feces. An exception is difloxacin, for which 80% of a dose was recovered in the feces and renal clearance accounted for less than 5% of the total systemic clearance.

PROTEIN BINDING. No studies have shown that fluoroquinolones are so highly protein bound that this limits distribution to tissues or causes a protein-binding interaction if displaced by another drug. Table 38.4 shows some of the protein-binding data generated. In most instances protein binding is low, but for animals for which multiple studies are available, as shown in Table 38.4, there is a lack of consistency among studies, which is probably related to differences in technique used to measure protein binding.

TISSUE DISTRIBUTION. Distribution to most tissues is listed for each drug in the manufacturer's package insert or Freedom of Information (FOI) summary. Specific

TABLE 38.4 Plasma/serum protein binding of fluoroquinolones in animals (% bound)

Animal	Enrofloxacin	Ciprofloxacin	Marbofloxacin	Orbifloxacin
Camel	17–24			
Cattle	56, 36–45, 60, 46	31, 70, 19		
Sheep	69			
Horse	22	37		21 (at 1 μg/mL)
Pig	27	23.6, 35		
Dog	15–25, 27, 35, 72	44, 18.5	9.1, 22	13.24 (at 1 μg/mL)
Rabbit	53, 50, 35, 6.0	33, 28		
Chicken	21	30		
Mouse	42			
Rat	50			

Sources: Villa et al. 1997; Gavrielli et al. 1995; Nouws et al. 1988; Aramayona et al. 1994; Davis et al. 2007; Bidgood & Papich 2005 and author Papich's unpublished data.

Note: When two or more values are listed, they represent results from independent studies.

studies for enrofloxacin have been conducted to show that it distributes to bone (Duval and Budsberg 1995), prostate (Dorfman et al. 1995), and skin (DeManuelle et al. 1998). In tissues in which high intracellular distribution does not occur, total tissue concentrations will generally be in equilibrium with drug concentrations in the extracellular fluid (Nix et al. 1991). For example, concentrations of enrofloxacin in canine cortical bone were approximately 30% of the corresponding plasma concentration (determined by bioassay), which approximates the concentration in the extracellular fluid space (Duval and Budsberg 1995).

Definitive studies that examined fluoroquinolone concentrations in tissue extracellular fluids (the site of action for these antibiotics) showed that the protein binding (discussed above) does not appreciably affect distribution to tissues. The protein unbound fraction in plasma (active drug) can be used to predict free drug concentrations of fluoroquinolone in tissue fluids (Bidgood and Papich 2005; Davis et al. 2007). In tissues in which the fluoroquinolones accumulate intracellularly, high tissue concentrations are reported because measurement of tissue concentrations is typically performed by homogenizing the tissue, which disrupts cells and releases intracellular concentrations. Tissue concentrations measured in this manner represent both intracellular and extracellular concentrations and can overestimate active drug concentrations. Some tissues, such as liver and kidney, may have fluoroquinolone concentrations several-fold higher than corresponding plasma concentrations.

Fluoroquinolones attain particularly high intracellular concentrations in macrophages and neutrophils: intracellular concentrations of 4–10 times plasma concentrations can be expected (Pascual et al. 1990; Tulkens 1990; Garaffo et al. 1991; Easmon and Crane 1985). In canine alveolar macrophages, the accumulation of enrofloxacin was 10 times the plasma concentration (Hawkins et al. 1998). The intracellular concentrations occur because fluoroquinolones are sufficiently lipid soluble to cross the cell membrane, or there may be active mechanisms to transport these drugs into cells. Fluoroquinolones also have a slower efflux from these cells. In humans, ciprofloxacin has an intracellular half-life of 6.7 hours in neutrophils versus 3.7 hours in serum (Easmon et al. 1986).

The high intracellular distribution in leukocytes may account for higher drug concentrations of fluoroquinolones in infected tissue compared to healthy tissue. Leukocytes, attracted via chemotaxis, may transport active drug to the site of infection. Dogs with superficial and deep pyoderma had significantly higher enrofloxacin concentrations in affected skin compared to healthy skin from control dogs (DeManuelle et al. 1998). Skin from dogs with deep pyoderma had higher enrofloxacin concentrations than skin from dogs with superficial pyoderma and there was significant correlation between dermal inflammation (dermal inflammatory cell count) and drug concentration.

Concentrations in urine may be several times higher than plasma concentrations. Concentrations of enrofloxacin, marbofloxacin, and orbifloxacin in urine of dogs are listed by the manufacturer to be 43, 40, and 84.5 μg/ml, respectively. One exception to the high urine excretion is difloxacin, of which, according to the manufacturer, less than 5% of the dose is cleared in the urine. Fluoroquinolones are among the few drugs that adequately penetrate the prostate gland in sufficient concentrations to treat infection. Enrofloxacin concentration (determined by bioassay) in the prostatic fluid and prostate tissue exceeded serum concentration at all times after administration (Dorfman et al. 1995). There were no differences in tissue concentrations when infected prostate was compared to healthy tissue. Concentrations of other fluoroquinolones in prostate tissue have been reported by the manufacturers to be 3.36, 5.6, and 1.35 μg/gram for difloxacin, marbofloxacin, and orbifloxacin, respectively.

PHARMACODYNAMICS (PK-PD)

MIC values for bacteria are listed in Table 38.2. Even though there are differences in potency among the currently available fluoroquinolones, a pattern is apparent: *Pasteurella,* such as the strains found in skin wounds, are the most susceptible; the gram-negative enteric bacilli (e.g., *E. coli* and *Klebsiella*) also have low MIC values. The gram-positive cocci such as the common skin pathogen *Staphylococcus pseudintermedius* have MIC values at a somewhat higher range, and *P. aeruginosa,* if sensitive at all, has MIC values that are among the highest for susceptible bacteria. Although not listed in Table 38.2, streptococci, enterococci, and anaerobic bacteria typically have MIC values high enough that they are usually in the resistant category.

Fluoroquinolones are bactericidal and that they act in a concentration-dependent manner rather than a time-dependent manner. The exposure to the bacteria has been measured by using the maximum peak concentration

(Cmax) in relation to the bacteria MIC and expressed as the Cmax:MIC ratio. A Cmax:MIC ratio that is at least 8–10 times (i.e., a peak concentration that is 8–10 times the MIC) is desirable. In the last 5–8 years, the favored parameter for predicting efficacy has been the area under the curve (AUC) for a 24-hour dose interval in relation to the MIC, expressed as the AUC_{24}:MIC ratio. An AUC: MIC ratio of 125–250 has been associated with the optimum antibacterial effect (Lode et al. 1998; Hyatt et al. 1995; Dudley 1991; Nicolau et al. 1995; Wright et al. (2000).

These targeted Cmax:MIC and AUC:MIC ratios were based on in vitro or in vivo studies performed with immunosuppressed laboratory animals or on clinical studies involving people with serious illness (Forrest et al. 1993; Blaser et al. 1987; Sullivan et al. 1993). A study in neutropenic mice showed that the optimum therapeutic effect was attained when the Cmax:MIC ratio was greater than 10, but at lower drug doses when the Cmax:MIC ratio was less than 10, the AUC:MIC was better linked to outcome (Drusano et al. 1993). A Cmax:MIC ratio of at least 8–10 has been associated with less resistance (Blaser et al. 1987). When lower ratios were achieved, the mutant strains that occur spontaneously were not suppressed, and resistance was allowed to emerge because these mutant strains have MIC values that are at least 4–8 times that of the parent (wild-type) strain (Drusano et al. 1993).

As reviewed by Wright et al. (2000), there is evidence that for some clinical situations, AUC:MIC ratios as low as 30–55 are necessary for a clinical cure, since the study in which 125 was cited involved critically ill human patients. AUC:MIC ratios for clinical success may be lower for gram-positive bacteria than for gram-negative bacteria. This was also shown in the paper by Ambrose and Grasela (2000), in which they presented data and reviewed the relevant publications. Because some of the studies above that cited ratios for target attainment used laboratory animals (usually immunosuppressed) or people with severe illness, the ratios needed for a cure may have been higher than needed in many veterinary patients. For example, if one compares the AUC in Table 38.1 to representative MIC values from Table 38.2, an AUC:MIC ratio of 50–60 in some patients appears adequate (Cester et al. 1996). In one model of skin infection in dogs caused by *Staphylococcus intermedius* (MIC 0.5 μg/ml), infections were prevented with Cmax:MIC ratios of only 3–5.5 μg/ml of marbofloxacin (Gruet et al. 1997). Perhaps a more competent immune system or less serious infection accounts for this discrepancy between laboratory studies and clinical observations in veterinary medicine. Other veterinary studies also reveal that the ratios necessary for clinical results may not be as high as reported from studies in laboratory rodents or people (Lees and Aliabadi 2002).

DOSE GUIDELINES

Doses listed in Tables 38.1 and 38.5 cover a wide MIC range among susceptible bacteria, from as low as 0.03 μg/ml, to as high as 1.0 μg/ml. The upper end of the dose is limited by safety (such as gastrointestinal effects); the lower dose is determined by efficacy. There is no advantage to frequent dosing (multiple times/day) as long

TABLE 38.5 Dose recommendations for enrofloxacin in exotic animals

Animal	Dose	Route	Interval	Reference
Alligator	5 mg/kg	IV, oral	Every 96 hr	Helmick et al. 1997
Savanna monitor	5 mg/kg (10 mg/kg for *Pseudomonas* spp.)	IM, oral	Every 96 hr	Hungerford et al. 1997
Burmese python	5 mg/kg (higher doses for *Pseudomonas* spp.)	IM	Every 48 hr	Young et al. 1997
Indian star tortoise	5 mg/kg	IM	Every 24 hr	Raphael et al. 1994
Red-eared slider	5 mg/kg	oral, IM	Every 72 hr (oral), every 48 hr (IM)	James et al. forthcoming
Gopher tortoise	5 mg/kg	IM	Every 24–48 hr	Prezant et al. 1994
Bottlenose dolphin	5 mg/kg	oral	Every 24 hr	Linnehan et al. 1999
Parrot and cockatoo	7.5–15 mg/kg	oral	Every 12 hr	Flammer 1998
Fish (ornamental)	5 mg/kg	IM, oral, or IP	Every 48 hr	Lewbart 1998

Note: These recommendations are based on an analysis of pharmacokinetic data and limited clinical experience. There have been no well-controlled efficacy studies or safety studies in these animals.

as a sufficiently high Cmax:MIC or the same AUC:MIC is achieved; therefore, the doses discussed for mammals and listed in Table 38.1 are intended for once-daily administration.

A range of doses allows relatively low doses of fluoroquinolones to be administered to treat the most susceptible organisms. That is, for susceptible *E. coli* or *Pasteurella* organisms, the lowest approved dose can be administered. To achieve the necessary concentration for some *Staphylococcus* or gram-positive bacteria that have higher MIC values, a higher dose may be needed, e.g., a dose in the middle of the dose range in Table 38.1. When the MIC values are high for organisms such as *P. aeruginosa,* the highest safe dose should be considered (Walker et al. 1992; Meinen et al. 1995).

CLINICAL USE

DOGS AND CATS. The administration of fluoroquinolones to dogs and cats constitutes one of the largest applications of these drugs for veterinary medicine. They have been used extensively during the past 20 years for infections of the skin, soft tissue, oral cavity, urinary tract, prostate, external and middle ear, wounds, respiratory tract, and bone (Paradis et al. 1990; Ihrke and DeManuelle 1999; Ihrke 1996; Ihrke et al. 1999; Carlotti et al. 1999; Griffin 1993; Hawkins et al. 1998; Dorfman et al. 1995; Cotard et al. 1995). The first veterinary quinolone was enrofloxacin, and veterinarians now have experience with marbofloxacin, orbifloxacin, and difloxacin. The efficacy of the fluoroquinolones is established for indications listed on the labels approved by the U.S. Food and Drug Administration (FDA). In the United States, enrofloxacin, marbofloxacin, and orbifloxacin are approved for dogs and cats; difloxacin is registered for dogs only. In Europe, ibafloxacin also is available.

The efficacy of enrofloxacin and marbofloxacin has been demonstrated specifically for canine pyoderma through published reports (Ihrke and DeManuelle 1999; Ihrke 1996; Paradis et al. 1990; Carlotti et al. 1999; Ihrke et al. 1999). One disease in particular for which enrofloxacin's efficacy has been demonstrated is German Shepherd dog pyoderma when the drug is administered orally once daily at a dose rate of 5–10 mg/kg (Ihrke and DeManuelle 1999; Koch and Peters 1996).

In addition to treatment of infections in these common sites, fluoroquinolones also have been used to treat rickettsial infections (Breitschwerdt et al. 1990, 1999) and have been examined for treating *Bartonella* infections in cats (Kordick et al. 1997). Against *Rickettsia rickettsii,* enrofloxacin is equally as effective as doxycycline or chloramphenicol (Breitschwerdt et al. 1990), but the success for eliminating *Bartonella* in cats has been equivocal (Kordick et al. 1997). Enrofloxacin has been used successfully to treat acute ehrlichiosis in dogs caused by *E. canis* and *E. platys* at a dosage of 5 mg/kg once daily for 15 days (Kontos and Athanasiou 1998). However, success in treating chronic ehrlichiosis has not been demonstrated. Fluoroquinolones also have been used to treat infections caused by *Mycoplasma* and *Mycobacteria*. Although the activity against *Mycoplasma* can be variable (Hannan et al. 1997), it has been effective for some opportunistic mycobacterial infections in cats (Studdert and Hughes 1992). Enrofloxacin and danofloxacin were consistently more active against veterinary *Mycoplasma* isolates than flumequine (Hannan et al. 1997).

SMALL MAMMALS. Enrofloxacin and other fluoroquinolone antibiotics are used frequently in small mammals such as rabbits, mice, rats, and exotic species for skin and visceral infections (Göbel 1999; Cabanes et al. 1992; Broome and Brooks 1991). One of the reasons fluoroquinolones are popular for treatment in small mammals is the potent activity against gram-negative pathogens affecting these animals and the excellent oral absorption. Another important advantage is the good safety record of the fluoroquinolones in small mammals. Oral tablets of fluoroquinolones have been administered directly or crushed to make a suspension that can be conveniently administered orally to the small mammals mixed with water, fruit, or some other palatable flavoring. Small mammals such as rodents and rabbits are prone to gastrointestinal disturbances and enteritis caused by overgrowth of bacteria, especially *Clostridium* organisms after administration of β-lactam and macrolide antibiotics. Because fluoroquinolones are not active against the anaerobic bacteria that compete with *Clostridium* organisms, bacterial overgrowth of pathogenic opportunistic bacteria has not been a problem as it has with other drugs, such as penicillins or macrolides.

Of the available drugs, enrofloxacin has been the most extensively studied. The doses listed in textbooks and review articles for mice, gerbils, hamsters, rats, and guinea pigs are 2.5–5.0 mg/kg up to 10–20 mg/kg IM, SC, or orally administered twice daily. The pharmacokinetics has been reported (Table 38.1), and there is some experience with the drug's efficacy. In rabbits oral enrofloxacin has been effective for improving clinical signs associated with pasteurellosis. The recommended dose of enrofloxacin for rabbits is 5 mg/kg IM, SC, or oral. Although it does not completely eradicate the bacteria in pasteurellosis in rabbits, it is considered the drug of choice (Göbel 1999; Broome and Brooks 1991).

REPTILES. The use of fluoroquinolones in reptiles has become popular because of their activity, safety, and convenience of administration (Papich 1999; Jacobson 1999; Rosenthal 1999). The only fluoroquinolone studied extensively is enrofloxacin. It is active against gram-negative organisms often implicated in serious infection of reptiles, including *Salmonella* spp., *Aeromonas hydrophilia, Klebsiella* spp., and *P. aeruginosa,* and its pharmacokinetics has been summarized in a review (Papich 1999). It shows remarkable differences among the reptiles, but generally the elimination is longer than in mammals or birds, which allows long dose intervals—as long as every 96 hours in some species. The elimination rate of drugs in reptiles varies with the animal's body temperature, because body temperature affects metabolic rate. When enrofloxacin is administered, there is variable metabolism to the active metabolite ciprofloxacin among the reptiles. Elimination half-life ranged from 55 hours in alligators to 5.1 hours in tortoises (Young et al. 1997; Raphael et al. 1994; Helmick et al. 1997; Hungerford et al. 1997; Prezant et al. 1994). Monitor lizards, pythons, and turtles had half-lives of 36, 17.6, and 6.4 hours, respectively. Analysis of pharmacokinetic data and appraisal of clinical experience (Jacobson 1999; Papich 1999) suggest a range of doses (Table 38.5), but safety and efficacy studies have not been performed.

Pharmacokinetic studies have shown good absorption of enrofloxacin from IM administration, and this route may prolong the half-life, probably because of delayed absorption from the injection site. Although some authors have suggested that oral administration should be avoided in reptiles because of unreliable absorption, absorption was good after oral administration to alligators, lizards, and turtles (Helmick et al. 1997; Hungerford et al. 1997; James et al. forthcoming). Because of slow gastrointestinal transit time, oral absorption may prolong the half-life (flip-flop effect).

BIRDS. The fluoroquinolones are an important group of antibiotics for pet birds and exotics kept in zoo collections. Despite pharmacokinetic studies in poultry, these drugs are prohibited in poultry in the United States. Administration is via drinking water oral gavage, or by injection. Fluoroquinolones have the advantage of good activity against bacterial pathogens important to birds, including *E. coli, Klebsiella* spp., *Pseudomonas* spp., *Staphylococcus* spp., and for treatment of *Chlamydophila psittaci* (formerly called *Chlamydia psittaci*). Resistance is possible for *E. coli* and *Pseudomonas* spp., however, and activity against gram-positive cocci (e.g., streptococci and enterococci) is low. Although there is in vitro susceptibility of *Chlamydophila* to fluoroquinolones, experience suggests that enrofloxacin can decrease clinical signs but not eliminate the infections (Flammer 1998). Therefore, fluoroquinolones are not recommended for mass medication of pet birds, and doxycycline is still the choice for this indication.

For pet birds, the dose is higher than for mammals because the clearance is faster and metabolic rate is higher. Pharmacokinetic studies of enrofloxacin in birds (see Table 38.1) indicate a dose of 15 mg/kg IM or orally every 12 hours (Flammer 1998; Flammer et al. 1991). One advantage of enrofloxacin for treating birds is that it has been possible to add it to the drinking water of pet birds so they can be conveniently medicated. Enrofloxacin added to drinking water at a concentration of 0.3–0.5 mg/ml has been used to treat highly susceptible bacteria (Flammer et al. 1990). Enrofloxacin is well absorbed via this route, and as long as the bird is drinking, effective plasma concentrations can be attained. One concern with the IM injection is that it can produce irritation at the site of injection, which is problematic because birds have a limited muscle mass into which one can inject.

Enrofloxacin has been administered to ducks at a dose of 10 mg/kg every 24 hours IM or orally.

FISH. Fluoroquinolones have been considered for treatment of infections in ornamental fish and for use in aquaculture. These drugs are active against important gram-negative bacterial pathogens of fish, and they appear to be well tolerated. Enrofloxacin has been administered orally to Rainbow trout kept in water maintained at 10° and 15°C. Although oral absorption is less than in mammals, it was good enough to produce effective plasma concentrations (Bowser et al. 1992). MIC values for pathogens infecting fish range from 0.0064–0.032 μg/ml for the most sensitive organisms to 0.25–0.45 μg/ml for *Streptococcus* spp. Thus the dose of 5 mg/kg should produce effective plasma concentrations for most susceptible pathogens (Bowser et al. 1992). In Atlantic salmon, enrofloxacin administered at 10 mg/kg intraperitoneally, intramuscularly, and orally was well absorbed from these routes, with no advantage of one route over another, but it produced a wide range of half-lives and Vd. Oral absorption in salmon was 46%, but the authors concluded that at 5 mg/kg this route would be suitable for therapeutic treatment (Stoffregen et al. 1997). Tissue concentrations were high, with concentrations detected at 120 hours after dosing.

Enrofloxacin has also been studied in red pacu as a model for other ornamental fish (Lewbart et al. 1997). For treatment of bacterial infections in ornamental fish, Lewbart (1998) recommends enrofloxacin at a dose of 5 mg/kg. This can be administered IM, IP, or orally with a recommended interval of every 48 hours, but the IM route produces the most predictable plasma concentrations. The oral dose can be prepared as a mixture of 0.1% in fish food (10 mg per 10 g of food). Enrofloxacin also has been added to water and used as a bath for fish in which the drug is absorbed across the surface area of the gill to produce systemic levels. In this treatment 2.5–5.0 mg enrofloxacin per liter is used as a 5-hour treatment bath repeated every 24 hours (Lewbart et al. 1997). The resulting peak plasma concentration after such a treatment was 0.17 μg/ml. Studies of the stability of enrofloxacin in water at various degrees of salinity and pH showed enrofloxacin to be stable when added to a water bath (unpublished results from the laboratory of one of the authors, MGP). However, the effect of the drug on nitrifying bacteria in the water should be considered. Studies in cuttlefish showed that clearance was surprisingly rapid, and doses of 5 mg/kg every 12 hours would be necessary to maintain effective concentrations (Gore et al. 2005). However, the same study indicated that systemic absorption from immersion of cuttlefish in an enrofloxacin medicated bath was possible.

LARGE ANIMALS. In horses, there is no fluoroquinolone approved for use, but increasing interest in use in these animals. Although none is registered for use in horses in the U.S., several pharmacokinetic studies have generated data for these drugs. These data, as well as clinical experience, have shown that this class of drugs can be valuable for treating infections in horses. Their valuable properties include the following: 1) ability to administer by oral, IV, and IM routes, although only enrofloxacin is available in an injectable formulation in the United States; 2) spectrum of activity that includes staphylococci and gram-negative bacilli such as *Klebsiella pneumoniae, Escherichia coli,* and *Proteus* spp.; 3) spectrum of activity that does *not* include anaerobic bacteria, therefore posing little risk of disrupting bacteria in the GI tract; and 4) good safety profile in adult horses.

The oral absorption of enrofloxacin in horses has generally been in the range of 50–70% (Table 38.1). Most bacteria that infect horses are susceptible, but resistance is expected for streptococci and anaerobes. Strains of *P. aeruginosa* may be resistant or only moderately susceptible. *Rhodococcus equi* can be resistant, and success in treating *Rhodococcus* infections in horses with enrofloxacin has not been encouraging. Based on the studies cited in this section, as well as clinical experience to date, an injectable dose of enrofloxacin at 2.5 to 5 mg/kg once daily or an oral dose of 7.5 to 10 mg/kg once daily is recommended (Giguère et al. 1996). The higher oral dose is used to accommodate the decreased systemic availability from an oral dose. For orbifloxacin (Orbax), an oral dose of 5 mg/kg once daily is recommended (Davis et al. 2006). These doses meet PK-PD criteria for susceptible bacteria discussed earlier in this chapter. For marbofloxacin (Zeniquin), IV doses of 2 mg/kg q24h may be adequate for treatment of most gram-negative infections caused by Enterobacteriaceae (Bousquet-Mélou et al. 2002; Peyrou et al. 2004; Carretero et al. 2002). However, this dose would not be adequate for many gram-positive bacteria, such as *Staphylococcus* spp., with MIC values of 0.25 μg/ml or higher. The injectable formulation is not available in the United States; therefore, oral tablets of marbofloxacin would be required for administration. Marbofloxacin has systemic availability of approximately 62% in horses. (Bousquet-Mélou et al. 2002). Oral dosing at 2 mg/kg may be adequate for susceptible Enterobacteriaceae with MIC values less than 0.2 μg/ml, but not for other bacteria. Doses higher than 2 mg/kg have not been studied in horses. As mentioned earlier, ciprofloxacin is not recommended because the oral absorption was poor in ponies and adult horses. Enteritis may occur in horses owing to the poor absorption and disruption of intestinal bacteria.

The method of administration for horses has been to 1) crush up tablets used in small animals, 2) administer the injectable solution (2.27% or 10%) IM (neck muscle) or

IV, or 3) administer the concentrated 10% solution orally (Baytril-100 cattle formulation). All these methods appear to produce adequate plasma concentrations, except for the administration of the concentrated 10% solution (Baytril-100) orally. This solution has produced inconsistent and incomplete absorption in horses, possibly because of its insolubility in solutions of low pH (Haines et al. 2000). In other studies, absorption of this solution was better when horses were fed (Boeckh et al. 2001). This solution also has been associated with oral mucosal lesions in horses. Some clinicians have produced more consistent oral absorption and reduced mucosal irritation when the 100 mg/ml solution was compounded into a gel (Epstein et al. 2004).

Moxifloxacin (Avelox) is a human drug of this group and has been used on a limited basis for treatment of infections in dogs and cats caused by bacteria that have been refractory to other drugs. When administered to horses, moxifloxacin had favorable pharmacokinetics that could make it suitable for oral use in horses (Gardner et al. 2004). However, oral administration also produced diarrhea in the experimental horses studied, and one of these horses tested positive for *Clostridium difficile* toxins A and B. The spectrum of activity of this drug may be broad enough to disrupt the normal flora.

In cattle and sheep, the pharmacokinetics of enrofloxacin and danofloxacin has been reported (Table 38.1) and doses have been derived from these studies or clinical trials. Enrofloxacin and danofloxacin are approved for use in cattle in the United States and some European countries. These fluoroquinolones have been highly active against important pathogens causing Bovine Respiratory Disease (BRD) in cattle. The MIC_{90} values listed for *Histophilus somni, Mannheimia haemolytica,* and *P. multocida* are 0.03, 0.06, and 0.03 μg/ml, respectively. Extralabel use is not allowed in food-producing animals (see Chapter 54). The dose ranges from a single SC dose of 7.5–12.5 mg/kg, or treatment for 3 days at 2.5–5.0 mg/kg, once daily, SC. The withdrawal time is 28 days. It is not approved for lactating cattle or dairy calves, but disposition into milk of lactating cows has been studied. Enrofloxacin is highly excreted in milk. (See the section on administration of fluoroquinolones to nursing animals below.)

Danofloxacin (A-180). Danofloxacin (A-180) is also approved in the U.S. for treatment of BRD in cattle. In Europe, this drug has been approved for several years, as the name Advocin®. It has a broad spectrum of activity, similar to enrofloxacin, including bovine isolates of *Pasteurella, Mannheimia haemolytica, Haemophilus somnus,* and *Mycobacterium bovis.* The manufacturer reported a half-life values of 4.35, and volume of distribution of 3.6 l/kg at the label dose of 6 mg/kg. Some earlier work at lower doses (Giles et al. 1991) reported similar results (half-life 4 hrs and Vd of 2.76 l/kg). Lung tissue concentrations were higher than the corresponding serum concentration and persist above the MIC for 12–24 hrs after injection (Giles et al. 1991; Apley and Upson 1993). In a comparison between enrofloxacin and danofloxacin (Terhune et al. 2005) danofloxacin produced plasma concentrations that were 56 times the MIC of 0.03 μg/ml, which is the MIC reported for North American BRD isolates. Although it is not legal to use fluroquinolones in the U.S. in an off-label manner, studies have also shown danofloxacin to be effective for bacterial enteritis in calves.

ADMINISTRATION TO NURSING, PREGNANT, OR YOUNG ANIMALS

Nursing Animals. Distribution also has been measured for milk in rabbits and cattle. Enrofloxacin is excreted rapidly in the milk after administration. In cattle after administration of enrofloxacin at 5 mg/kg, enrofloxacin concentrations in milk parallel the concentrations in serum, with a Cmax of 1.3–2.5 μg/ml, but concentrations of the active metabolite ciprofloxacin exceed those of enrofloxacin (Kaartinen et al. 1995; Tyczkowska et al. 1994). Danofloxacin distribution into milk of cows exceeded serum concentrations (Shem-Tov et al. 1998). In rabbits the milk-to-plasma ratios were 3.6 and 2.6 for enrofloxacin and ciprofloxacin, respectively, after administration of 7.5 mg/kg IV (Aramayona et al. 1996). The reason for the high distribution of fluoroquinolones into milk is not known, because these concentrations do not match what is predicted from simple diffusion into milk, even after considering ion trapping. Protein binding is higher in milk, and the milk proteins may act as a reservoir for enrofloxacin and ciprofloxacin (Aramayona et al. 1996). Despite these concentrations of fluoroquinolones in milk, the activity of enrofloxacin in mastitic milk is decreased, possibly owing to lower pH, chelation with cations, or other factors in milk that inhibit fluoroquinolone activity (Kaartinen et al. 1995), and it has not been shown that fluoroquinolones are effective drugs for treating clinical mastitis. In the United States, this would be considered extralabel use and is prohibited.

When administering fluoroquinolones to nursing animals, the amount in the milk should be considered because fluoroquinolones may cause arthropathy in some species of young animals (discussed further in the section on safety below). Disposition into milk was studied in two mares after administration, and it was shown that although both ciprofloxacin and enrofloxacin were present in milk at levels that were as high or higher than the mares' plasma concentrations, the total doses administered to the foals via suckling were small, and the plasma concentrations in the foals were negligible (author's observations). Young nursing animals may have decreased oral absorption caused by interference from calcium in milk (see information below on kittens in the section on young animals).

Pregnant Animals. When administering fluoroquinolones to pregnant animals, there will be some drug transfer across the placenta because these drugs are lipophilic and have low protein binding, and drug transfer is not limited by tissue barriers. Placental transfer has been specifically examined in rabbits, in which it was shown that the more lipophilic drug, enrofloxacin, crossed the placenta to a greater degree (80%) than ciprofloxacin (5% placental transfer), which is less lipophilic (Aramayona et al. 1994). Despite the rather high transfer of enrofloxacin across the placenta, there have been no reports of adverse effects when fluoroquinolones were administered to pregnant animals. Manufacturer studies have not shown any adverse effects on pregnancy or reproduction.

Young Animals. There is a risk that fluoroquinolones may cause damage to the developing cartilage of young animals. This is discussed more thoroughly in the section on safety. There have been few pharmacokinetic comparisons of young animals versus older animals, but the studies available demonstrate that young animals were exposed to more drug than adults because of slower clearance. After administration of enrofloxacin, calves at 1 day of age had smaller Vd, longer half-life, and decreased clearance than at 1 week of age (Kaartinen et al. 1997). There also was a smaller amount of metabolism of enrofloxacin to ciprofloxacin in 1-week-old calves than in older ones. Rabbit pups exhibited lower clearance and longer half-life for enrofloxacin than adult rabbits (Aramayona et al. 1996). This pattern was also seen in horses: foals at 1–2 weeks of age showed little metabolism of enrofloxacin to ciprofloxacin after administration of IV and oral doses. Foals also exhibited slower clearance and longer half-life than adults (Bermingham et al. 2000).

In kittens, enrofloxacin was administered at 5 mg/kg via various routes (oral, IV, SC) (Seguin et al. 2004). There was no evidence of adverse effects or impaired excretion of enrofloxacin in kittens. The half-life in young cats (2, 6, and 8 weeks old) was shorter, and clearance more rapid, than in adult cats, Volume of distribution in 6–8-week-old cats was larger, and combined with the shorter half-life, produced lower plasma concentrations than in adults. Oral administration to kittens produced low plasma concentrations and it was hypothesized that interference with milk in nursing kittens may lower oral absorption (see section "Drug Interactions," below).

SAFETY

The fluoroquinolones have had a remarkably good safety record. For enrofloxacin, the LD_{50} in laboratory rats is 5000 mg/kg. When high doses were administered to animals during safety testing, one of the most common problems was gastrointestinal disturbances (nausea, vomiting, diarrhea), but these were usually produced at high doses and were not serious. Because these drugs currently registered for animals do not alter the anaerobic flora of the gastrointestinal tract, there usually is minimal disruption of the intestinal bacterial population, even when these drugs are administered orally to small rodents. There have been no reports of cutaneous drug reactions resulting from fluoroquinolone usage in the veterinary literature, but some of the FOI summaries from manufacturers report an occasional reddening of the skin of dogs when high doses were administered.

There have been no reports of adverse effects on reproduction or pregnancy from administration of fluoroquinolones. Although the use in pregnant animals has been discouraged because of toxicity to developing cartilage, there have been no clinical reports where this effect has been described in offspring of treated animals.

With very high concentrations, adverse central nervous system (CNS) effects have been observed. The mechanism responsible for the CNS effects is believed to be inhibition of the inhibitory neurotransmitter GABA. Fluoroquinolones injected rapidly IV or administered at high doses can induce CNS excitement. Fluoroquinolones can precipitate convulsions in some animals and should not be administered to animals that are prone to seizures.

BLINDNESS IN CATS. In cats high doses of fluoroquinolones have caused ocular problems from drug-induced changes in the retina (Corrado et al. 1987). This concern was precipitated by a report by Gelatt and colleagues (Gelatt et al. 2001) in which retinal degeneration was associated with enrofloxacin administration. This was followed by studies by the manufacturer in which toxicosis from enrofloxacin was described and new dose labeling was announced. The most common ophthalmologic abnormalities were mydriasis, lack of menace reflex, and poor papillary light reflexes. Acute blindness may occur and retinal lesions may be observed, which include increased tapetal reflectivity and attenuation of retinal blood vessels. In one review of safety studies (Corrado et al. 1987) nalidixic acid (one of the earlier quinolones) at 100 mg/kg/day, but not norfloxacin at 200 mg/kg/day produced both electrical and histopathologic changes in feline retinas. In another review (Schluter 1987), the author states that feline retinas are particularly sensitive to fluoroquinolones. When cats received 100 mg/kg of nalidixic acid there was suppression of electroretinographic waves and histologic changes in the cones and rods, but ciprofloxacin treatment at the same dose to cats had no effect on the electroretinographic findings or on the fundus.

In studies performed by the manufacturer, enrofloxacin was administered to cats at doses of 0, 5, 20, and 50 mg/kg for 21 days (8 cats per group). There were no adverse effects observed in cats treated with 5 mg/kg/day of enrofloxacin. However, the administration of enrofloxacin at 20 mg/kg or greater caused salivation, vomiting, and depression. At doses of 20 mg/kg or greater, there were mild to severe fundic lesions on ophthalmologic examination, including changes in the fundus and retinal degeneration. There was also abnormal electroretinograms, including blindness. Ford et al. (2007) reported on a study in 24 cats that received 3, 5, or 7 days of enrofloxacin at a high dose of 50 mg/kg (10 times the label dose). Ocular changes were observed by day 3 of the study. At this dose, both retinal degeneration and systemic toxic effects were observed. Because the blindness has been associated with high doses, the manufacturer has limited the dose to 5 mg/kg/day in cats.

Besides enrofloxacin, the other fluoroquinolones registered for use in cats are orbifloxacin (Orbax) and marbofloxacin (Zeniquin). The current approved dose of orbifloxacin for cats is 2.5–7.5 mg/kg/day. In a published abstract (Kay-Mugford et al. 2001), orbifloxacin oral liquid was administered to cats at 0, 15, 45, and 75 mg/kg for at least 30 days (8 cats/group). This represents 6, 18, and 30 times the lowest label dosage. No ocular lesions were observed in any cats treated with 15 mg/kg. At the higher doses, (18 and 30 times dose) there was tapetal hyperreflectivity in the area centralis and minimal photoreceptor degeneration. When marbofloxacin was administered to cats at 5.55, 16.7, and 28 mg/kg, representing 2, 6, and 10 times the lowest label dose, for 6 weeks there were no ocular lesions in cats (manufacturer's data). At 55.5 mg/kg (10 times the lowest label dose) for 14 days there were also no lesions from marbofloxacin.

PROBLEMS IN YOUNG ANIMALS. In young, rapidly growing animals it is well known that fluoroquinolones can produce an arthropathy (Gough et al. 1992; Burkhardt et al. 1997). Fluoroquinolones also have caused tendinitis and tendon rupture in people, but this effect has not been reported for animals. The species most susceptible to developmental arthropathy are rats and dogs. Dogs between the ages of 4 and 28 weeks are the most susceptible. Affected dogs may show signs of lameness and joint swelling, but if the drug is discontinued, the lesions may be reversible. Kittens, calves, and pigs are much more resistant to this effect. For example, feeder calves and 23-day-old calves were administered 25 mg/kg for 15 days without evidence of articular cartilage lesions. Young foals are susceptible to the joint arthropathy from enrofloxacin at 10 mg/kg orally (Bermingham et al. 2000). However, studies in adult horses treated with enrofloxacin have not demonstrated articular toxicity (Bertone et al. 2000; Giguère et al. 1999).

The risk increases with higher doses and in most instances has been more clinically obvious only when the highest maximum dose was exceeded (e.g., at 25 mg/kg of enrofloxacin); however, even enrofloxacin dosages of 10 mg/kg/day have induced cartilage damage in young dogs. Lesions have been observed in as few as 2 days after initiation of treatment (Yabe et al. 2001). The use of fluoroquinolones has been discouraged in children, but thousands of children have been treated with these drugs under a compassionate protocol with no reports of joint arthropathy.

Joint arthropathy is best described as a toxicity to the chondrocyte that causes vesicles to form on the articular surface. The mechanism for damage to cartilage apparently is via chelation of magnesium by the drug (Egerbacher et al. 2001). Magnesium is necessary for proper development of the cartilage matrix, especially in young, growing animals. Chelation of the magnesium results in a local magnesium deficiency leading to loss of proteoglycan in the articular cartilage. Studies in which magnesium was supplemented to decrease cartilage damage had equivocal results. (Magnesium added to the diet while oral drugs are administered would cause a chelation and significantly decrease oral absorption.)

DISEASES OR CONDITIONS. There has been limited study of the disposition of fluoroquinolones in animals that have other conditions. In most of these instances, there were no changes in the drug's pharmacokinetics that would necessitate a change in dosage. Since the fluoroquinolones rely on both the kidneys and liver for clearance, insufficiency in one organ may result in compensation by the other clearance route. For example, renal failure may result in more reliance on hepatic clearance. In dogs with renal impairment, clearance of marbofloxacin was only slightly decreased and there was no significant effect on Vd or mean residence time (Lefebvre et al. 1998). In camels that were deprived of water for 14 days and lost 12.5% of their body weight, there was little effect on the distribution, clearance, or half-life of enrofloxacin. However, water deprivation resulted in a slower and less complete absorption from a SC injection compared to normal camels or camels injected IM (Gavrielli et al. 1995).

DRUG INTERACTIONS

Combinations with other antibiotics neither antagonize nor enhance the microbiologic effects of fluoroquinolones. The currently used fluoroquinolones will kill bacteria whether or not they are dividing (Lode et al. 1998). Therefore, use of a bacteriostatic agent should not interfere with the action of a fluoroquinolone. Although there is no evidence that other antibiotics produce a synergistic effect when administered with fluoroquinolones, they may produce an additive effect and broaden the spectrum of activity.

Fluoroquinolones are involved in some drug interactions, but few of these are serious. Drugs containing di- and trivalent cations (e.g., Ca^{++}, Mg^{++}, Al^{+3}, Fe^{+3}), such as antacids, sucralfate, and nutritional supplements can inhibit oral absorption (Nix et al. 1989). These cations, when mixed with fluoroquinolones in extemporaneously compounded preparations can chelate the drug and decrease oral absorption. Fluoroquinolones may inhibit metabolism of some drugs through an interaction with hepatic metabolism. One such example is the inhibition of theophylline metabolism by enrofloxacin (Intorre et al. 1995), in which enrofloxacin significantly increased the Cmax and decreased systemic clearance of theophylline in dogs.

FORMULATIONS AVAILABLE

Fluoroquinolones licensed for small-animal use are available as oral preparations as tablets or chewable tablets. There are no oral liquid preparations currently available in the United States, but veterinarians have used compounding pharmacists to create oral liquid preparations from tablets dissolved in an aqueous vehicle. There are two formulations of enrofloxacin, an IM injectable preparation for dogs (2.27% solution, 22.7 mg/ml), and an injectable for cattle (100 mg/ml). It is registered for IM administration, but veterinarians have administered this preparation IV. The IV administration has not produced serious problems, but one should avoid rapid IV injection; otherwise, CNS reactions are possible. In addition, mixing a solution with some intravenous solutions may cause chelation and precipitation in the IV line. Fluids of particular concern are those that contain calcium or magnesium. The formulation approved for SC injection in cattle in the United States is 100 mg/ml in an l-arginine base. This preparation may cause tissue irritation if injected in small animals. It is very alkaline and has also produced oral mucosal lesions when used for oral administration to horses (Boeckh et al. 2001).

There is an otic preparation available (Baytril otic) containing 5 mg/ml enrofloxacin and 10 mg/ml silver sulfadiazine. Some veterinarians have also used topical administration of enrofloxacin for otitis externa caused by pseudomonads (Griffin 1993, 1999; Rosychuk 1994). Other otic preparations have been mixed extemporaneously by veterinarians, even though these are not licensed or evaluated for efficacy. For example, veterinarians have mixed the 2.27% injectable solution of enrofloxacin with saline, water, or other topical ear solutions in a 1:1 to 4:1 ratio (e.g., 4 parts saline, 1 part enrofloxacin). Stability studies by one of the authors (M.G.P.) with HPLC analysis confirmed these solutions to be stable for 2 weeks at room temperature. When the infection is believed to extend to the middle ear, topical treatment alone is not sufficient, and systemic treatment for pseudomonads should be administered.

Difloxacin (Dicural) is available in tablet form for administration to dogs, but safety has not been evaluated for cats. Danofloxacin mesylate (A-180) is used for administration to cattle, SC in the neck area. It has a 2-pyrrolidone and polyvinyl alcohol vehicle. Marbofloxacin (Zeniquin) is available in tablets for dogs and cats. There is an injectable formulation available in other countries for small animals and horses (Marbocyl), but not in the United States. Orbifloxacin is available in tablet form for dogs and cats.

NEW DEVELOPMENTS

Pradofloxacin (Veraflox) is one of the newest generation of fluoroquinolones (sometimes referred to as fourth-generation *quinolones*, or third-generation *fluoroquinolones*), which is related to the human drugs trovafloxacin, grepafloxacin, gatifloxacin, gemifloxacin, and moxifloxacin (discussed earlier in this chapter). Because the older, more familiar, fluroroquinolones, (e.g., enrofloxacin, marbofloxacin, orbifloxacin, difloxacin) have less activity against gram-positive cocci and anaerobic bacteria, and have been associated with development of resistance, these new drugs have been explored for use in veterinary medicine, as they have in human medicine (Blondeau et al. 2004).

Pradofloxacin has been evaluated in dogs and cats for skin, soft-tissue, oral, and urinary tract infections (deJong et al. 2004; Stephan et al. 2008; Spindel et al. 2008; Hartmann et al. 2008; Litster et al. 2007; Mueller and Stephan 2007). Pharmacokinetic studies are also available (Hartmann et al. 2008). Susceptibility data indicate that it is more active than other fluoroquinolones against bacterial isolates from dogs and cats (deJong et al. 2004; Ganière et al. 2005; Silley et al. 2007; Stephan et al. 2007). Because it is active against two targets of fluoroquinolones (Topoisomerase IV and DNA gyrase) development of resistant mutants may be less likely (Wetzstein 2005; Stephan et al. 2007).

Pradofloxacin has been safe in cats with respect to ocular lesions (Messias et al. 2008). At a dose of 3 mg/kg orally it was effective for treatment of urinary tract infections in dogs (Stephan et al. 2008) and at 5 mg/kg was effective for canine pyoderma (Mueller and Stephan 2007). At a dose of 5 mg/kg in a 2.5% oral suspension it was effective for urinary tract infections in cats (Litster et al. 2007).

At the time of this writing (July 2008) pradofloxacin was not registered for use. However, a closely related human drug, moxifloxacin (Avelox) of this group has been used on a limited basis for treatment of infections in dogs and cats caused by bacteria that have been refractory to other drugs.

REFERENCES AND ADDITIONAL READING

Abadia, A. R., Aramayona, J. J., Munoz, M. J., Pla Delfina, J. M., Saez, M. P., and Bregante, M. A. 1994. Disposition of ciprofloxacin following intravenous administration in dogs. Journal of Veterinary Pharmacology and Therapeutics 17:384–388.

Aktaç, Z., Gönüllü, N., Salcioğlu, M., Bal, C., and Anğ, O. 2002. Moxifloxacin activity against clinical isolates compared with the activity of ciprofloxacin. International Journal of Antimicrobial Agents 20(3):196–200.

Ambrose, P. G., and Grasela, D. M. 2000. The use of Monte Carlo simulation to examine pharmacodynamic variance of drugs: fluoroquinolone pharmacodynamics against *Streptococcus pneumoniae*. Diagnostic Microbiology and Infectious Disease 38:151–157.

Anadón, A., Martinez-Larranaga, M. R., Diaz, J., Bringas, P., Martinez, M. A., Fernandez-Cruz, M. L., and Fernandez, R. 1995. Pharmacokinetics and residues of enrofloxacin in chickens. American Journal of Veterinary Research 56:501–506.

Apley, M.D., and Upson, D.W. 1993. Lung tissue concentrations and plasma pharmacokinetics of danofloxacin in calves with acute pneumonia. American Journal of Veterinary Research 54:1122–1127.

Aramayona, J. J., Garcia, M. A., Fraile, L., Abadia, A. R., and Bregante, M. A. 1994. Placental transfer of enrofloxacin and ciprofloxacin in rabbits. American Journal of Veterinary Research 55:1313–1318.

Aramayona, J. J., Mora, J., Fraile, L., Garcia, M. A., Abadia, A. R., and Bregante, M. A. 1996. Penetration of enrofloxacin and ciprofloxacin into breast milk, and pharmacokinetics of the drugs in lactating rabbits and neonatal offspring. American Journal of Veterinary Research 57:547–553.

Asuquo, A. E., and Piddock, L. J. V. 1993. Accumulation and killing kinetics of fifteen quinolones for *Escherichia coli, Staphylococcus aureus,* and *Pseudomonas aeruginosa*. Journal of Antimicrobial Chemotherapy 31:865–880.

Atta, A. H., and Sharif, L. 1997. Pharmacokinetics of ciprofloxacin following intravenous and oral administration in broiler chickens. Journal of Veterinary Pharmacology and Therapeutics 20:326–329.

Bailly, S., Fay, M., Roche, Y., and Gougerot-Pocidalo, M. A. 1990. Effect of quinolones on tumor necrosis factor production by human monocytes. International Journal of Immunopharmacology 12:31–36.

Barsanti, J. A. 1995. Diseases of the prostate gland. In C. A. Osborne and D. R. Finco, eds., Canine and Feline Nephrology and Urology, pp. 726–755. Baltimore: Lea & Febiger.

Behra-Miellet, J., Dubreuil, L., and Jumas-Bilak, E. Antianaerobic activity of moxifloxacin compared with that of ofloxacin, ciprofloxacin, clindamycin, metronidazole and beta-lactams. International Journal of Antimicrobial Agents 20(5):366–374.

Bermingham, E.C., and Papich, M.G.. 2002. Pharmacokinetics after intravenous and oral administration of enrofloxacin in sheep. American Journal of Veterinary Research 63:1012–1017.

Bermingham, E. C., Papich, M. G., and Vivrette, S. 2000. Pharmacokinetics of enrofloxacin after oral and IV administration to foals. American Journal of Veterinary Research 61:706–709.

Bertone, A.L., Tremaine, W.H., Macoris, D.G., Simmons, E.J., Ewert, K.M., Herr, L.G., and Weisbrode, S.E. 2000. Effect of long-term administration of an injectable enrofloxacin solution on physical and musculoskeletal variables in adult horses. Journal of American Veterinary Medical Association 15;217(10):1514–1521.

Bidgood, T.L., and Papich, M.G. 2005. Plasma and interstitial fluid pharmacokinetics of enrofloxacin, its metabolite ciprofloxacin, and marbofloxacin after oral administration and a constant rate intravenous infusion in dogs. Journal of Veterinary Pharmacology and Therapeutics 28(4):329–341.

Blaser, J., Stone, B. J., Groner, M. C., and Zinner, S. H. 1987. Comparative study with enoxacin and netilmicin in a pharmacodynamic model to determine importance of ratio of antibiotic peak concentration to MIC for bactericidal activity and emergence of resistance. Antimicrobial Agents and Chemotherapy 31:1054–1060.

Blondeau, J.M., Hansen, G., Metzler, K., and Hedlin, P. 2004. The role of PK/PD parameters to avoid selection and increase of resistance: mutant prevention concentration. Journal of Chemotherapy 16 (Suppl3):1–19.

Boeckh, C., Buchanan, C., Boeckh, A., et al. 2001. Pharmacokinetics of the bovine formulation of enrofloxacin (Baytril 100) in horses, Veterinary Therapeutics 2:129–134.

Bousquet-Mélou, A., Bernard, S., Schneider, M., and Toutain, P.L. 2002. Pharmacokinetics of marbofloxacin in horses, Equine Veterinary Journal 34:366–372.

Bowser, P. R., Wooster, G. A., St. Leger, J., and Babish, J. G. 1992. Pharmacokinetics of enrofloxacin in fingerling rainbow trout (*Oncorhynchus mykiss*). Journal of Veterinary Pharmacology and Therapeutics 15:62–71.

Bregante, M. A., Saez, P., Aramayona, J. J., Fraile, L., Garcia, M. A., and Solans, C. 1999. Comparative pharmacokinetics of enrofloxacin in mice, rats, rabbits, sheep, and cows. American Journal of Veterinary Research 60:1111–1116.

Breitschwerdt, E. B., Davidson, M. G., Aucoin, D. P., Levy, M. G., Szabados, N. S., Hegarty, B. C., Kuehne, A. L., and James, R. L. 1990. Efficacy of chloramphenicol, enrofloxacin, and tetracycline, for treatment of experimental Rocky Mountain Spotted Fever in dogs. Antimicrobial Agents and Chemotherapy 35:2375–2381.

Breitschwerdt, E. B., Papich, M. G., Hegarty, B. C., Gilger, B., Hancock, S. I., and Davidson, M. G. 1999. Efficacy of doxycycline, azithromycin, or trovafloxacin for treatment of experimental Rocky Mountain Spotted Fever in dogs. Antimicrobial Agents and Chemotherapy. 43:813–821.

Broome, R. L, and Brooks, D. L. 1991. Efficacy of enrofloxacin in the treatment of respiratory pasteurellosis in rabbits. Laboratory Animal Science 41:572–576.

Broome, R. L., Brooks, D. L., Babish, J. G., Copeland, D. D., and Conzelman, G. M. 1991. Pharmacokinetic properties of enrofloxacin in rabbits. American Journal of Veterinary Research 52:1835–1841.

Bryant, E. E., and Mazza, J. A. 1989. Effect of the abscess environment on the antimicrobial activity of ciprofloxacin. American Journal of Medicine 87(Suppl5A):23S–27S.

Burkhardt, J.E., Hill, M.A., Turek, J.J., and Carlton, W.W. 1992. Ultrastructural changes in articular cartilages of immature Beagle dogs dosed with difloxacin, a fluoroquinolone. Veterinary Pathology 29:230–238.

Burkhardt, J.E., Walterspiel, J.N., and Schaad, U.B. 1997. Quinolone arthropathy in animals versus children. Clinical Infectious Diseases 25:1196–1204.

Cabanes, A., Arboix, M., Anton, J. M. A., and Reig, F. 1992. Pharmacokinetics of enrofloxacin after intravenous and intramuscular injection in rabbits. American Journal of Veterinary Research 53:2090–2093.

Carlotti, D. N. 1996. New trends in systemic antibiotic therapy of bacterial skin disease in dogs. Compendium on Continuing Education for the Practicing Veterinarian 18(Suppl.):40–47.

Carlotti, D. N., Guaguere, E., Pin, D., et al. 1999. Therapy of difficult cases of canine pyoderma with marbofloxacin: a report of 39 cases. Journal of Small Animal Practice 40:265–270.

Carlotti, D. N., Jasmin, P., Guaguere, E., et al. 1995. Utilisation de la marbofloxacine dans le traitement des pyodermites du chien. Pratique Medicale et Chirurgicale de l'Animal de Compagnie 30:281–293.

Carretero, M., Rodriguez, C., San Andres, M.I., et al. 2002. Pharmacokinetics of marbofloxacin in mature horses after single intravenous and intramuscular administration, Equine Veterinary Journal 34:360–365.

Cester, C. C., Schneider, M., and Toutain, P.-L. 1996. Comparative kinetics of two orally administered fluoroquinolones in dog: enrofloxacin versus marbofloxacin. Revue Med Vet 147:703–716.

Chen, D. K., McGeer, A., de Azavedo, J. C., and Low, D. E. 1999. Decreased susceptibility of *Streptococcus pneumoniae* to fluoroquinolones in Canada. New England Journal of Medicine 341:233–239.

Chew, D. J. 1997. An overview of prostatic disease. Compendium of Continuing Education for the Practicing Veterinarian 19:80–85.

CLSI (Clinical Laboratory Standards Institute). 2007. Performance Standards for Antimicrobial Disk and Dilution Susceptibility Tests for Bacteria Isolated From Animals; Approved Standard—Third Edition. CLSI document M31-A3. Wayne, PA: Clinical and Laboratory Standards Institute.

Cole, L. K., Kwochka, K. W., Kowalski, J. J., and Hillier, A. 1998. Microbial flora and antimicrobial susceptibility patterns of isolated pathogens from the horizontal ear canal and middle ear in dogs with otitis media. Journal of the American Veterinary Medical Association 212:534–538.

Collins, B. 1994. Antimicrobial drug use in rabbits, rodents, and other small mammals. Proceedings of an International Symposium on Antimicrobial Selection, Orlando: The North American Veterinary Conference, pp. 12–17.

Corrado, M. L., Struble, W. E., Peter, C., et al. 1987. Norfloxacin: review of safety studies. American Journal of Medicine 82(Suppl6B):22–26.

Cotard, J. P., Gruet, P., Pechereau, D., Moreau, P., Pages, J. P., Thomas, E. and Deleforge, J. 1995. Comparative study of marbofloxacin and amoxicillin-clavulanic acid in the treatment of urinary tract infections in dogs. Journal of Small Animal Practice 36:349–353.

Cox, S.K., Cottrell, M.B., Smith, L., Papich, M.G., Frazier, D.L., and Bartges, J. 2004. Allometric analysis of ciprofloxacin and enrofloxacin pharmacokinetics across species. Journal of Veterinary Pharmacology and Therapeutics 27(3):139–146.

da Silva, R.G., Reyes, F.G., Sartori, J.R., and Rath, S. 2006. Enrofloxacin assay validation and pharmacokinetics following a single oral dose in chickens. J Vet Pharmacol Ther Oct;29(5):365–372.

Davis, J.L., Foster, D.M., and Papich, M.G. 2002. Pharmacokinetics and tissue distribution of enrofloxacin and its active metabolite ciprofloxacin in calves. Journal of Veterinary Pharmacology and Therapeutics 30(6):564–71.

Davis, J.L., Papich, M.G., and Weingarten, A. 2006. The pharmacokinetics of orbifloxacin in the horse following oral and intravenous administration, Journal of Veterinary Pharmacology and Therapeutics 29:191–197.

DeBoer, D. J. 1995. Management of chronic and recurrent pyoderma in the dog. In J. D. Bonagura, ed., Kirk's Current Veterinary Therapy XII, pp. 611–617. Philadelphia: W. B. Saunders.

deJong, A., Stephan, B., and Friederichs, S.. 2004. Antibacterial activity of pradofloxacin against canine and feline pathogens isolated from clinical cases, [abstract] AAVM, Ottawa, Canada, June 2004.

DeManuelle, T. C., Ihrke, P. J., Brandt, C. M., Kass, P. H., and Vuilliet, P. R. 1998. Determination of skin concentrations of enrofloxacin in dogs with pyoderma. American Journal of Veterinary Research 59:1599–1604.

Dorfman, M., Barsanti, J., and Budsberg, S. C. 1995. Enrofloxacin concentrations in dogs with normal prostate and dogs with chronic bacterial prostatitis. American Journal of Veterinary Research 56:386–390.

Dowling, P. M., Wilson, R. C., Tyler, J. W., and Duran, S. H. 1995. Pharmacokinetics of ciprofloxacin in ponies. Journal of Veterinary Pharmacology and Therapeutics 18:7–12.

Drlica, K., and Zhao, X. 1997. DNA gyrase, Topoisomerase IV, and the 4-quinolones. Microbiology and Molecular Biology Reviews 61:377–392.

Drusano, G. L., Johnson, D. E., Rosen, M., and Stadiford, H. C. 1993. Pharmacodynamics of a fluoroquinolone antimicrobial agent in a neutropenic rat model of *Pseudomonas* sepsis. Antimicrobial Agents and Chemotherapy 37:483–490.

Dudley, M. N. 1991. Pharmacodynamics and pharmacokinetics of antibiotics with special reference to the fluoroquinolones. American Journal of Medicine 91(Suppl6A):45S–50S.

Duval, J. M., and Budsberg S. C. 1995. Cortical bone concentrations of enrofloxacin in dogs. American Journal of Veterinary Research 56:188–192.

Easmon, C. S. F., and Crane, J. P. 1985. Uptake of ciprofloxacin by macrophages. Journal of Clinical Pathology 38:442–444.

Egerbacher, M., Wolfesberger, B., and Gabler, C. 2001. In vitro evidence for effects of magnesium supplementation on quinolone-treated horse and dog chondrocytes. Veterinary Pathology 38(2):143–148.

Endtz, H. P., Ruijs, G. J., van Klingeren, B., et al. 1991. Quinolone resistance in *Campylobacter* isolated from man and poultry following the introduction of fluoroquinolones in veterinary medicine. Journal of Antimicrobial Chemotherapy 27:199–208.

Epstein, K., Cohen, N., Boothe, D., et al. 2004. Pharmacokinetics, stability, and retrospective analysis of use of an oral gel formulation of the bovine injectable enrofloxacin in horses, Veterinary Therapeutics 5(2):155–167.

Everett, M. J., Jin, Y. F., Ricci, V., and Piddock, L. J. V. 1996. Contributions of individual mechanisms to fluoroquinolone resistance in 36 *Escherichia coli* strains isolated from humans and animals. Antimicrobial Agents and Chemotherapy 40:2380–2386.

Fernandes, P. B. 1988. Mode of action and in vitro and in vivo activities of the fluoroquinolones. Journal of Clinical Pharmacology 28:156–168.

Ferrero, L., Cameron, B., and Crouzet, J. 1995. Analysis of gyrA and grlA mutations in stepwise-selected ciprofloxacin-resistant mutants of *Staphylococcus aureus*. Antimicrobial Agents and Chemotherapy 39:1554–1558.

Flammer, K. 1998. Common bacterial infections and antibiotic use in companion birds. Compendium on Continuing Education for the Practicing Veterinarian 20(Suppl3A):34–48.

Flammer, K., Aucoin, D. P., and Whitt, D. A. 1991. Intramuscular and oral disposition of enrofloxacin in African grey parrots following single and multiple doses. Journal of Veterinary Pharmacology and Therapeutics 14:359–366.

Flammer, K., Aucoin, D. P., Whitt, D. A., and Prus, S. A. 1990. Plasma concentrations of enrofloxacin in African grey parrots treated with medicated water. Avian Disease 34:1017–1022.

Ford, M.M., Dubielzig, R.R., Giuliano, E.A., Moore, C.P., and Narfström, K.L. 2007. Ocular and systemic manifestations after oral administration of a high dose of enrofloxacin in cats. American Journal of Veterinary Research 68:190–202.

Forrest, A., Nix, D. E., Ballow, C. H., Goss, T. F., Birmingham, M. C., and Schentag, J. J. 1993. Pharmacodynamics of intravenous ciprofloxacin in seriously ill patients. Antimicrobial Agents and Chemotherapy 37:1073–1081.

Gandolf, A.R., Atkinson, M.W., Papich, M.G., and Shurter, S.S. 2003. Oral enrofloxacin as a promising antibiotic therapy for non-domestic ruminants. American Association of Zoo Veterinarians Annual Meeting, Proceedings.

Gandolf, A.R., Papich, M.G., Bringardner, A.B., and Atkinson, M.W. 2005. Pharmacokinetics after intravenous, subcutaneous, and oral administration of enrofloxacin to alpacas. American Journal of Veterinary Research. 66(5):767–771. (Erratum in: American Journal of Veterinary Research 66(7):1291.)

———. 2006. Single-dose intravenous and oral pharmacokinetics of enrofloxacin in goral (*Nemorrhaedus goral arnouxianus*). Journal of Zoo Wildlife Medicine 37(2):145–150.

Ganière, J.P., Medaille, C., Limet, A., et al. 2001. Antimicrobial activity of enrofloxacin against *Staphylococcus intermedius* strains isolated from canine pyodermas. Veterinary Dermatology 12:171–5.

Garaffo, R., Jambou, D., Chichmanian, R. M., et al. 1991. In vitro and in vivo ciprofloxacin pharmacokinetics in human neutrophils. Antimicrobial Agents and Chemotherapeutics 35:2215–2218.

Gardner, S.Y., Davis, J.L., Jones, S.L., et al. 2004. Moxifloxacin pharmacokinetics in horses and disposition into phagocytes after oral dosing. Journal of Veterinary Pharmacology and Therapeutics 27(1):57–60.

Gavrielli, R., Yagil, R., Ziv, G., Creveld, C. V., and Glickman, A. 1995. Effect of water deprivation on the disposition kinetics of enrofloxacin in camels. Journal of Veterinary Pharmacology and Therapeutics 18:333–339.

Gelatt, K.N., van der Woerdt, A., Ketring, K.L., et al. 2001. Enrofloxacin-associated retinal degeneration in cats. Veterinary Ophthalmology 4:99–106. (Erratum in: Veterinary Ophthalmology 2001 Sep;4(3):231.)

Giguère, S., Sweeney, R. W., and Belanger, M. 1996. Pharmacokinetics of enrofloxacin in adult horses and concentration of the drug in serum, body fluids, and endometrial tissues after repeated intragastrically administered doses. American Journal of Veterinary Research 57:1025–1030.

Giguère, S., Sweeney, R.W., Habecker, P.L., Lucas, J., and Richardson, D.W. 1999. Tolerability of orally administered enrofloxacin in adult horses: a pilot study. Journal of Veterinary Pharmacology and Therapeutics 22(5):343–347.

Giles, C.J., Magonigle, R.A., Grimshaw, W.T.R., et al. 1991. Clinical pharmacokinetics of parenterally administered danofloxacin in cattle. Journal of Veterinary Pharmacology and Therapeutics 14:400–410.

Giuliano, E.A., and van der Woerdt, A. 1999. Feline retinal degeneration: clinical experience and new findings(1994–1997). Journal of the American Animal Hospital Association 35:511–514

Göbel, T. 1999. Bacterial diseases and antimicrobial therapy in small mammals. Compendium on Continuing Education for the Practicing Veterinarian 21(Suppl3E):5–20.

Gore, S.R., Harms, C.A., Kukanich, B., Forsythe, J., Lewbart, G.A., and Papich, M.G. 2005. Enrofloxacin pharmacokinetics in the European cuttlefish, *Sepia officinalis*, after a single i.v. injection and bath administration. Journal of Veterinary Pharmacology and Therapeutics 28(5):433–439.

Gough, A. W., Kasali, O. B., Sigler, R. E., and Baragi, V. 1992. Quinolone arthropathy: acute toxicity to immature articular cartilage. Toxicological Pathology 20:436–447.

Griffin, C. E. 1993. Otitis externa and otitis media. In C. E. Griffin, K. W. Kwochka, and J. M. MacDonald, eds., Current Veterinary Dermatology: The Science and Art of Therapeutics, pp. 245–262. Philadelphia: W. B. Saunders.

———. 1999. Pseudomonas otitis therapy. In J. D. Bonagura, ed., Current Veterinary Therapy XIII. Philadelphia: W. B. Saunders.

Griggs, D. J., Hall, M. C., Jin, Y. F., and Piddock, J. V. 1994. Quinolone resistance in veterinary isolates of *Salmonella*. Journal of Antimicrobial Chemotherapy 33:1173–1189.

Gruet, P., Richard, P., Thomas, E., and Autefage, A. 1997. Prevention of surgical infections in dogs with a single intravenous injection of marbofloxacin: an experimental model. Veterinary Record 140:199–202.

Gyrd-Hansen, N., and Nielsen, P. 1994. The influence of feed on the oral bioavailability of enrofloxacin, oxytetracycline, penicillin V, and spiramycin in pigs. Proceedings of the 6th EAVPT Congress, pp. 242–243.

Haines, G.R., Brown, M.P., Gronwall, R.R., and Merritt, K.A. 2000. Serum concentrations and pharmacokinetics of enrofloxacin after intravenous and intragastric administration to mares, Canadian Journal of Veterinary Research 64:171–177.

Hannan, P. C. T., Windsor, G. D., De Jong, A., Schmeer, N., and Stegemann, M. 1997. Comparative susceptibilities of various animal-pathogenic mycoplasmas to fluoroquinolones. Antimicrobial Agents and Chemotherapy 41:2037–2040.

Hartmann, A., Krebber, R., Daube, G., and Hartmann, K. 2008. Pharmacokinetics of pradofloxacin and doxycycline in serum, saliva, and tear fluid of cats after oral administration. Journal of Veterinary Pharmacology and Therapeutics 31(2):87–94.

Hartmann, A.D., Helps, C.R., Lappin, M.R., Werckenthin, C., and Hartmann, K. 2008. Efficacy of pradofloxacin in cats with feline upper respiratory tract disease due to *Chlamydophila felis* or *Mycoplasma* infections. Journal of Veterinary Internal Medicine 22(1):44–52.

Hawkins, E. C., Boothe, D. M., Guin, A., et al. 1998. Concentration of enrofloxacin and its active metabolite in alveolar macrophages and pulmonary epithelial lining fluid of dogs. Journal of Veterinary Pharmacology and Therapeutics 21:18–23.

Hedin, G., and Hambreus, A. 1991. Multiply antibiotic-resistant *Staphylococcus* epidermidis in patients, staff, and environment—a one-week survey in a bone marrow transplant unit. Journal of Hospital Infection 17:95–106.

Heinen, E. 1999. Comparative pharmacokinetics of enrofloxacin and difloxacin as well as their main metabolites in dogs. Compendium for Continuing Education for the Practicing Veterinarian 21(Suppl10) 12–18.

Helmick, K. E., Papich, M. G., Vliet, K. A., et al. 1997. Preliminary kinetics of single dose intravenously administered enrofloxacin and oxytetracycline in the American alligator (*Alligator mississippiensis*). Proceedings of the American Association of Zoo Veterinarians pp. 27–28.

Hungerford, C., Spelman, L., and Papich, M. G. 1997. Pharmacokinetics of enrofloxacin after oral and intramuscular administration in Savanna monitors (*Varanus exanthematicus*). Proceedings of the American Association of Zoo Veterinarians, pp. 89–92.

Hyatt, J. M., McKinnon, P. S., Zimmer, G. S., and Schentag, J. J. 1995. The importance of pharmacokinetic/pharmacodynamic surrogate markers to outcome. Clinical Pharmacokinetics 28:143–160.

Ihrke, P. J. 1996. Experiences with enrofloxacin in small animal dermatology. Compendium of Continuing Education for the Practicing Veterinarian 18(2):35–39.

———. 1998. Bacterial infections of the skin. In C. E. Greene, ed., Infectious Diseases of the Dog and Cat, 2nd ed., pp. 541–547. Philadelphia: W. B. Saunders.

Ihrke, P. J., and DeManuelle, T. C. 1999. German Shepherd dog pyoderma: an overview and antimicrobial management. Compendium of Continuing Education for the Small Animal Practitioner 21(Suppl10).

Ihrke, P. J., Papich, M. G., and DeManuelle, T. C. 1999. The use of fluoroquinolones in veterinary dermatology. Veterinary Dermatology 10:193–204.

Intorre, L., Mengozzi, G., Maccheroni, M., Bertini, S., and Soldani, G. 1995. Enrofloxacin-theophylline interaction: influence of enrofloxacin on theophylline steady-state pharmacokinetics in the Beagle dog. Journal of Veterinary Pharmacology and Therapeutics 18:352–356.

Intorre, L., Vanni, M., Di Bello, D., Pretti, C., Meucci, V., Tognetti, R., Soldani, G., Cardini, G., and Jousson, O. 2007. Antimicrobial susceptibility and mechanism of resistance to fluoroquinolones in *Staphylococcus intermedius* and *Staphylococcus schleiferi*. Journal of Veterinary Pharmacology and Therapeutics 30(5):464–469.

Jacobson, E. R. 1999. Antimicrobial therapy in reptiles. Compendium on Continuing Education for the Practicing Veterinarian 21(Suppl3E):33–48.

Jalal, S., and Wretlind, B. 1998. Mechanisms of quinolone resistance in clinical strains of *Pseudomonas aeruginosa*. Microbial Drug Resistance 4:257–261.

James, S., Papich, M. G., and Raphael, B. (Unpublished) Forthcoming. Pharmacokinetics of enrofloxacin after oral and intramuscular administration in red-eared sliders (*Chrysemys scripts elegans*). (Unpublished data; manuscript in preparation).

Janbon, F., Jonquet, O., Reynes, J., and Bertrand, A. 1989. Use of pefloxacin in the treatment of rickettsiosis and coxiellosis. Review of Infectious Diseases 11(Suppl.5):990–991.

Jones, R.D., Kania, S.A., Rohrbach, B.W., Frank, L.A., and Bemis, D.A. 2007. Prevalence of oxacillin- and multidrug-resistant staphylococci in clinical samples from dogs: 1,772 samples (2001–2005). Journal of American Veterinary Medical Association 230(2):221–7.

Jordan, F. T. W., Horrocks, B. K., Jones, S. K., Cooper, A. C., and Giles, C. J. 1993. A comparison of the efficacy of danofloxacin and tylosin in the control of *Mycoplasma gallisepticum* infection in broiler chicks. Journal of Veterinary Pharmacology and Therapeutics 16:79–86.

Kaartinen, L., Pyörälä, S., Moilanen, M., and Räisänen, S. 1997. Pharmacokinetics of enrofloxacin in newborn and one-week-old calves. Journal of Veterinary Pharmacology and Therapeutics 20:479–482.

Kaartinen, L., Salonen, M., Älli, L., and Pyörälä, S. 1995. Pharmacokinetics of enrofloxacin after single intravenous, intramuscular, and subcutaneous injections in cows. Journal of Veterinary Pharmacology and Therapeutics 18:357–362.

Kay-Mugford, P.A., Ramsey, D.T., Dubielzig, R.R., et al. 2001. Ocular effects of orally administered orbifloxacin in cats. American College of Veterinary Ophthalmologists 32nd Annual Meeting, (abstract) October 9–13, 2001.

Knoll, U., Glunder, G., and Kietzmann, M. 1999. Comparative study of the plasma pharmacokinetics and tissue concentrations of danofloxacin and enrofloxacin in broiler chickens. Journal of Veterinary Pharmacology and Therapeutics 22:239–246.

Knöller, J., Brom, J., Schönfeld, W., and König 1989. Influence of ciprofloxacin on leukotriene generation from various cells in vitro. Journal of Antimicrobial Chemotherapy 25:605–612.

Koch, H.-J., and Peters, S. 1996. Antimicrobial therapy in German Shepherd dog pyoderma (GSP). An open clinical study. Veterinary Dermatology 7:177–181.

Kontos, V. I., and Athanasiou, L. V. 1998. Use of enrofloxacin in the treatment of acute ehrlichiosis. Canine Practice 23:10–14.

Kordick, D., Papich, M. G., and Breitschwerdt, E. B. 1997. Efficacy of enrofloxacin or doxycycline for treatment of *Bartonella henselae* or *Bartonella clarridgeiae* infection in cats. Antimicrobial Agents and Chemotherapy 41:2448–2455.

Kukanich, B., Huff, D., Riviere, J.E., and Papich, M.G. 2007. Naive averaged, naive pooled, and population pharmacokinetics of orally administered marbofloxacin in juvenile harbor seals. J Am Vet Med Assoc Feb 1;230(3):390–5.

Küng, K., Riond, J.-L., and Wanner, M. 1993a. Pharmacokinetics of enrofloxacin and its metabolite ciprofloxacin after intravenous and oral administration of enrofloxacin in dogs. Journal of Veterinary Pharmacology and Therapeutics 16:462–468.

Küng, K., Riond, J.-L., Wolfram, S., and Wanner, M. 1993b. Comparison of an HPLC and bioassay method to determine antimicrobial concentrations after intravenous and oral administration of enrofloxacin in four dogs. Research in Veterinary Science 54:247–248.

Kwochka, K. W. 1993. Recurrent pyoderma. In C. E. Griffin, K. W. Kwochka, J. M. MacDonald, eds., Current Veterinary Dermatology, pp. 3–21. St. Louis: Mosby Yearbook.

Langston, V. C., Sedrish, S., and Boothe, D. M. 1996. Disposition of single-dose oral enrofloxacin in the horse. Journal of Veterinary Pharmacology and Therapeutics 19:316–319.

Lees, P., and Aliabadi, F.S. 2002. Rational dosing of antimicrobial drugs: animal versus humans. International Journal of Antimicrobial Agents 19:269–284.

Lefebvre, H. P., Schneider, M., Dupouy, V., Laroute, V., Costes, G., Delesalle, L., and Toutain, P. L. 1998. Effect of experimental renal impairment on disposition of marbofloxacin and its metabolites in the dog. Journal of Veterinary Pharmacology and Therapeutics 21:453–461.

Legg, J. M., and Bint, A. J. 1999. Will pneumococci put quinolones in their place? Journal of Antimicrobial Chemotherapy 44:425–427.

Lewbart, G. A. 1998. Koi medicine and management. Compendium on Continuing Education for the Practicing Veterinarian 20(Suppl3A):5–12.

Lewbart, G. A., Vaden, S., Deen, J., et al. 1997. Pharmacokinetics of enrofloxacin in the red pacu (*Colossoma brachypomum*) after intramuscular, oral and bath administration. Journal of Veterinary Pharmacology and Therapeutics 20:124–128.

Ling, G. V. 1995. Lower Urinary Tract Diseases of Dogs and Cats: Diagnosis, Medical Management, Prevention, pp. 116–128. St. Louis: Mosby Yearbook.

Linnehan, R. M., Ulrich, R. W., and Ridgway, S. 1999. Enrofloxacin serum bioactivity in bottlenose dolphins, *Tursiops truncatus,* following oral administration of 5 mg/kg in whole fish. Journal of Veterinary Pharmacology and Therapeutics 22:170–173.

Litster, A., Moss, S., Honnery, M., Rees, B., Edingloh, M., and Trott, D. 2007. Clinical efficacy and palatability of pradofloxacin 2. 5% oral suspension for the treatment of bacterial lower urinary tract infections in cats. Journal of Veterinary Internal Medicine 21(5):990–5.

Lloyd, D. H. 1992. Therapy for canine pyoderma. In R. W. Kirk and J. D. Bonagura, eds., Kirk's Current Veterinary Therapy XI, pp. 539–544. Philadelphia: W. B. Saunders.

Lloyd, D. H., Lamport, A. I., Noble, W. C., and Howell, S. A. 1999. Fluoroquinolone resistance in *Staphylococcus intermedius*. Veterinary Dermatology 10:249–251.

Lode, H., Borner, K., and Koeppe, P. 1998. Pharmacodynamics of fluoroquinolones. Clinical Infectious Diseases 27:33–39.

Martin Barrasa, J.L., Lupiola Gomez, P., Gonzalez Lama, Z., et al. 2000. Antibacterial susceptibility patterns of Pseudomonas strains isolated from chronic canine otitis externa. Journal of Veterinary Med B Infectious Disease Vet Public Health 47:191–6.

Martinez-Martinez, L., Pascual, A., and Jacoby, G. A. 1998. Quinolone resistance from a transferable plasmid. Lancet 351:797–799.

Meinen, J. B., Rosin, E., and McClure, J. T. 1995. Pharmacokinetics of enrofloxacin in clinically normal dogs and mice and drug pharmacodynamics in neutropenic mice with *Escherichia coli* and staphylococcal infections. American Journal of Veterinary Research 56:1219–1224.

Mengozzi, G., Intorre, L., Bertini S., and Soldani, G. 1996. Pharmacokinetics of enrofloxacin and its metabolite ciprofloxacin after intravenous and intramuscular administration in sheep. American Journal of Veterinary Research 57:1040–1043.

Messias, A., Gekeler, F., Wegener, A., Dietz, K., Kohler, K., and Zrenner, E. 2008. Retinal safety of a new fluoroquinolone, pradofloxacin, in cats: assessment with electroretinography. Doc Ophthalmol May;116(3):177–191.

Monlouis, J.-D., DeJong, A., Limet, A., and Richez, P. 1997. Plasma pharmacokinetics and urine concentrations after oral administration of enrofloxacin to dogs. Journal of Veterinary Pharmacology and Therapeutics 20(Suppl1):61–63.

Mueller, R.S., and Stephan, B. 2007. Pradofloxacin in the treatment of canine deep pyoderma: a multicentered, blinded, randomized parallel trial. Veterinarian Dermatology 18(3):144–51.

Murphy, O. M., Marshall, C., Stewart, D., and Freeman, R. 1997. Ciprofloxacin-resistant Enterobacteriaceae. Lancet 349:1028–1029.

Neu, H. C. 1992. The crisis in antibiotic resistance. Science 257:1064–1073.

Nicolau, D. P., Quintiliani, R., and Nightingale, C. H. 1995. Antibiotic kinetics and dynamics for the clinician. Medical Clinics of North America 79:477–495.

Nikaido, H., and Thanassi, D. G. 1993. Penetration of lipophilic agents with multiple protonation sites into bacterial cells: tetracyclines and fluoroquinolones as examples. Antimicrobial Agents and Chemotherapy 37:1393–1399.

Nix, D. E., Goodwin, S. D., Peloquin, C. A., Rotella, D. L., and Schentag, J. J. 1991. Antibiotic tissue penetration and its relevance: impact of tissue penetration on infection response. Antimicrobial Agents and Chemotherapeutics 35:1953–1959.

Nix, D. E., Watson, W. A., Lener, M. E., et al. 1989. Effects of aluminum and magnesium antacids and ranitidine on the absorption of ciprofloxacin. Clinical Pharmacology and Therapeutics 46:700–705.

Nouws, J. F. M., Mevius, D. J., Vree, T. B., Baars, A. M., and Laurensen, J. 1988. Pharmacokinetics, renal clearance, and metabolism of ciprofloxacin following intravenous and oral administration to calves and pigs. Veterinary Quarterly 10:156–163.

Papich, M. G. 1999. Pharmacokinetics of enrofloxacin in reptiles. Compendium for Continuing Education for the Practicing Veterinarian 21(Suppl10).

Papich, M.G.,VanCamp, S.D., Cole, J., and Whitacre, M.D. 2002. Pharmacokinetics and endometrial tissue concentrations of enrofloxacin and the metabolite ciprofloxacin after IV administration of enrofloxacin to mares. Journal of Veterinary Pharmacology and Therapeutics 25:343–350.

Paradis, M., Lemay, S., Scott D. W., et al. 1990. Efficacy of enrofloxacin in the treatment of canine bacterial pyoderma. Veterinary Dermatology 1:123–127.

Pascual, A., Garcia, I., and Perea, E. J. 1990. Uptake and intracellular activity of an optically active ofloxacin isomer in human neutrophils and tissue culture cells. Antimicrobial Agents and Chemotherapy 34:277–280.

Peña, C., Albareda, J. M., Pallares, R., Pujol, M., Tubau, F., and Ariza, J. 1995. Relationship between quinolone use and emergence of ciprofloxacin-resistant *Escherichia coli* in bloodstream infections. Antimicrobial Agents and Chemotherapy 39:520–524.

Perea, S., Hidalgo, M., Arcediano, A., et al. 1999. Incidence and clinical impact of fluoroquinolone-resistant *Escherichia coli* in the faecal flora of cancer patients treated with high dose chemotherapy and ciprofloxacin prophylaxis. Journal of Antimicrobial Chemotherapy 44:117–120.

Pestova, E., Millichap, J.J., Noskin, G.A., and Peterson, L.R. 2000. Intracellular targets of moxifloxacin: a comparison with other fluoroquinolones. Journal of Antimicrobial Chemotherapy 45:583–590.

Petersen, A.D., Walker, R.D., Bowman, M.M., Schott, H.C., and Rosser, E.J. 2002. Frequency of isolation and antimicrobial susceptibility patterns of *Staphylococcus intermedius* and *Pseudomonas aeruginosa* isolates from canine skin and ear samples over a 6 year period (1992–1997). Journal of the American Animal Hospital Association 38:407–413.

Peyrou, M., Ducet, M.Y., Vrins, A., et al. 2004. Population pharmacokinetics of marbofloxacin in horses: preliminary analysis, Journal of Veterinary Pharmacology and Therapeutics 27:283–288.

Peyrou, M., Bousquet-Melou, A., Laroute, V., Vrins, A., and Doucet, M.Y. 2006. Enrofloxacin and marbofloxacin in horses: comparison of pharmacokinetic parameters, use of urinary and metabolite data to estimate first-pass effect and absorbed fraction. J Vet Pharmacol Ther Oct;29(5):337–344.

Piddock, L. J. V., Ricci, V., McLaren, I., and Griggs, D. J. 1998. Role of mutation in the *gyrA* and *parC* genes of nalidixic-acid-resistant salmonella serotypes isolated from animals in the United Kingdom. Journal of Antimicrobial Chemotherapy 41:635–641.

Pijpers, A., Heinen, E., DeJong A., and Verheijden, J. H. M. 1997. Enrofloxacin pharmacokinetics after intravenous and intramuscular administration in pigs. Journal of Veterinary Pharmacology and Therapeutics 20(Suppl1):42–43.

Pinchbeck, L.R., Cole, L.K., Hillier, A., Kowalski, J.J., Rajala-Schultz, P.J., Bannerman, T.L., and York, S. 2007. Pulsed-field gel electrophoresis patterns and antimicrobial susceptibility phenotypes for coagulase-positive staphylococcal isolates from pustules and carriage sites in dogs with superficial bacterial folliculitis. American Journal of Veterinary Research. 68(5):535–42.

Pirro, F., Edingloh, M., and Schmeer, N. 1999. Bactericidal and inhibitory activity of enrofloxacin and other fluoroquinolones in small animal pathogens. Compendium on Continuing Education for the Practicing Veterinarian 21(Suppl12):19–25.

Pirro, F., Scheer, M., and de Jong, A. 1997. Additive in vitro activity of enrofloxacin and its main metabolite ciprofloxacin. 14th Annual Congress of the ESVD-ECVD, p. 199.

Pozzin, O., Harron, D. W. G., Nation, G., Tinson, A. H., Sheen, R., and Dhanasekharan, S. 1997. Pharmacokinetics of enrofloxacin following intravenous/intramuscular/oral administration in Nedji sheep. Journal of Veterinary Pharmacology and Therapeutics 20(Suppl1):60.

Prezant, R. M., Isaza, R., and Jacobson, E. R. 1994. Plasma concentrations and disposition kinetics of enrofloxacin in gopher tortoises (*Gopherus polyphemus*). Journal of Zoo and Wildlife Medicine 25:82–87.

Pyörälä, S., Panu, S., and Kaartinen, L. 1994. Single dose pharmacokinetics of ciprofloxacin in horses. Proceedings of EAVPT, pp. 45–46.

Raoult, D., and Drancourt, M. 1991. Antimicrobial therapy of rickettsial diseases. Antimicrobial Agents of Chemotherapy 35:2457–2462.

Raphael, B. L., Papich, M. G., and Cook, R. A. 1994. Pharmacokinetics of enrofloxacin after a single intramuscular injection in Indian star tortoises (*Geochelone elegans*). Journal of Zoo Wildlife Medicine 25:88–94.

Richez, P., Dellac, B., Froyman, R., and DeJong, A. 1994.Pharmacokinetics of enrofloxacin in calves and adult cattle after single and repeated subcutaneous injections. Proceedings of European Association for Veterinary Pharmacology and Toxicology, Proceedings of the 6th International Congress, Deinburgh, UK, pp. 232–233.

Richez, P., Pedersen Morner, A., DeJong, A., and Monlouis, J. D. 1997a. Plasma pharmacokinetics of parenterally administered danofloxacin and enrofloxacin in pigs. Journal of Veterinary Pharmacology and Therapeutics 20(Suppl1):41–42.

Richez, P., Monlouis, J. D., Dellac, B., and Daube, B. 1997b. Validation of a therapeutic regimen for enrofloxacin in cats on the basis of pharmacokinetic data. Journal of Veterinary Pharmacology and Therapeutics 20(Suppl1):152–153.

Riddle, C., Lemons, C., Papich, M.G., and Altier, C. 2000. Evaluation of ciprofloxacin as a representative of veterinary fluoroquinolones in susceptibility testing. Journal of Clinical Microbiology 38: 1636–1637.

Rosenthal, K. L. 1999. Avian bacterial infections and their treatment. Compendium on Continuing Education for the Practicing Veterinarian 21(Suppl3E):21–32.

Ross, D. L., and Riley, C. M. 1994. Dissociation and complexation of the fluoroquinolone antimicrobials—an update. Journal of Pharmaceutical and Biomedical Analysis 12:1325–1331.

Rosychuk, R. A. W. 1994. Management of otitis externa. In R. A. W. Rosychuk and S. R. Merchant, eds., Veterinary Clinics of North America: Small Animal Practice 24(5):921–952.

Rubin, J,. Walker, R.D., Blickenstaff, K., Bodeis-Jones, S., and Zhao, S. 2008. Antimicrobial resistance and genetic characterization of fluoroquinolone resistance of *Pseudomonas aeruginosa* isolated from canine infections. Veterinary Microbiology 131:164–172.

Sanchez, C.R., Murray, S.Z., Isaza, R., and Papich, M.G. 2005. Pharmacokinetics of a single dose of enrofloxacin administered orally to captive Asian elephants (*Elephas maximus*). American Journal of Veterinary Research Nov;66(11):1948–1953.

Sanders, C. C., Sanders, W. E., and Thomson, K. S. 1995. Fluoroquinolone resistance in staphylococci: new challenges. European Journal of Clinical Microbiology and Infectious Disease 14(Suppl1):S6–S11.

Schluter, G., 1987. Ciprofloxacin: Review of potential toxicologic effects. American Journal of Medicine 82(Suppl4A):91–93.

Schneider, M., Thomas, V., Boisrame, B., and Deleforge, J. 1996. Pharmacokinetics of marbofloxacin in dogs after oral and parenteral administration. Journal of Veterinary Pharmacology and Therapeutics 19:56–61.

Seguin, M.A., Papich, M.G., Sigle, K.J., Gibson, N.M., and Levy, J.K. 2004. Pharmacokinetics of enrofloxacin in neonatal kittens. American Journal of Veterinary Research 65:350–356.

Shem-Tov, M., Rav-Hon, O., Ziv, G., Lavi, E., Glickman, A., and Saran, A. 1998. Pharmacokinetics and penetration of danofloxacin from the blood into the milk of cows. Journal of Veterinary Pharmacology and Therapeutics 21:209–213.

Silley, P., Stephan, B., Greife, H.A., and Pridmore, A. 2007. Comparative activity of pradofloxacin against anaerobic bacteria isolated from dogs and cats. Journal of Antimicrobial Chemotherapy 60(5):999–1003.

Smith, K. E., Besser, J. M., Hedberg, C. W., et al. 1999. Quinolone-resistant *Campylobacter jejuni* infections in Minnesota, 1992–1998. New England Journal of Medicine 340:1525–1532.

Spindel, M.E., Veir, J.K., Radecki, S.V., and Lappin, M.R. 2008. Evaluation of pradofloxacin for the treatment of feline rhinitis. Journal of Feline Medical Surgery 10(5):472–79.

Spreng, M., Deleforge, J., Thomas, V., Boisrame, B., and Drugeon, H. 1995. Antibacterial activity of marbofloxacin: a new fluoroquinolone for veterinary use against canine and feline isolates. Journal of Veterinary Pharmacology and Therapeutics 18:284–289.

Stegemann, M., Heukamp, U., Scheer, M., and Krebber, R. 1996. Kinetics of antibacterial activity after administration of enrofloxacin in dog serum and skin: in vitro susceptibility of field isolates. Compendium on Continuing Education for the Practicing Veterinarian 18(Suppl.):30–34.

Stegemann, M., Wollen, T. S., Ewert, K. M., Terhune, T. N., and Copeland, D. D. 1997. Plasma pharmacokinetics of enrofloxacin administered to cattle at a dose of 7.5 mg/kg. Journal of Veterinary Pharmacology and Therapeutics 20(Suppl1):22.

Stephan, B., Greife, H.A., Pridmore, A., and Silley, P. 2007. Mutant prevention concentration of pradofloxacin against *Porphyromonas gingivalis*. Veterinary Microbiolpgy 31;121(1–2):194–5.

———. Activity of pradofloxacin against *Porphyromonas* and *Prevotella* spp. Implicated in periodontal disease in dogs: susceptibility test data from a European multicenter study. Antimicrobial Agents and Chemotherapy 52(6):2149–55.

Stoffregen, D. A., Wooster, G. A., Bustos, P. S., Bowser, P. R., and Babish, J. G. 1997. Multiple route and dose pharmacokinetics of enrofloxacin in juvenile Atlantic salmon. Journal of Veterinary Pharmacology and Therapeutics 20:111–123.

Studdert, V. P., and Hughes, K. L. 1992. Treatment of opportunistic mycobacterial infections with enrofloxacin in cats. Journal of the American Veterinary Medical Association 201:1388–1390.

Sullivan, M. C., Cooper, B. W., Nightingale, C. H., Quintiliani, R., and Lawlor, M. T. 1993. Evaluation of the efficacy of ciprofloxacin against *Streptococcus pneumoniae* by using a mouse protection model. Antimicrobial Agents and Chemotherapy 37:234–239.

Takács-Novák, K., Jozan, M., Hermecz, I., and Szasz, G. 1992. Lipophilicity of antibacterial fluoroquinolones. International Journal of Pharmaceutics 79:89–96.

TerHune, T.N., Skogerboe, T.L., Shostrom, V.K., and Weigel, D.J. 2005. Comparison of pharmacokinetics of danofloxacin and enrofloxacin in calves challenged with Mannheimia haemolytica. American Journal of Veterinary Research 66:342–349.

Threlfall, E. J., Cheasty, T., Graham, A. and Rowe, B. 1997. High-level resistance to ciprofloxacin in *Escherichia coli*. Lancet 349:403 (Letter).

Threlfall, E. J., Frost, J. A., Ward, L. R., and Rowe, R. 1995. Epidemic in cattle of *S. typhimurium* DT 104 with chromosomally integrated multiple drug resistance. Veterinary Record 134:577.

Torill, A., Yamarick, T.A., Papich, M.G., Wiebe, V.J., Edman, J., and Wilson, W.D. Pharmacokinetics and toxicity of ciprofloxacin in adult horses (unpublished data, submitted for publication).

Tulkens, P. M. 1990. Accumulation and subcellular distribution of antibiotics in macrophages in relation to activity against intracellular bacteria. In R. J. Fass, ed., Ciprofloxacin in Pulmonology, pp. 12–20. Bern: W. Zuckschwerdt Verlag Munchen.

Tyczkowska, K. L., Voyksner, R. D., Anderson, K. L., and Papich, M. G. 1994. Simultaneous determination of enrofloxacin and its primary metabolite ciprofloxacin in bovine milk and plasma by ion-pairing liquid chromatography. Journal of Chromatography B: Biomedical Applications 658:341–348.

Vancutsem, P. M., Babish, J. G., and Schwark, W. S. 1990. The fluoroquinolone antimicrobials: structure, antimicrobial activity, pharmacokinetics, clinical use in domestic animals, and toxicity. Cornell Veterinarian 80:173–186.

Villa, R., Prandini, E., Caloni, F., and Carli, S. 1997. Serum protein binding of some sulfonamides, quinolones, and fluoroquinolones in farm animals and domestic animals. Journal of Veterinary Pharmacology and Therapeutics 20(Suppl1):60.34–35.

Walker, R. D., Stein, G. E., Hauptman, J. G., and MacDonald, K. H. 1992. Pharmacokinetics evaluation of enrofloxacin administered orally to healthy dogs. American Journal of Veterinary Research 53:2315–2319.

Walker, R. D., Stein, G. E., Hauptman, J. G., MacDonald, K. H., Budsberg, S. C., and Rosser, E. J. 1990. Serum and tissue cage fluid concentrations of ciprofloxacin after oral administration of the drug to healthy dogs. American Journal of Veterinary Research 51:896–900.

Waxman, S., Rodríguez, C., González, F., De Vicente, M.L., San Andrés, M.I., and San Andrés, M.D. 2001. Pharmacokinetic behavior of marbofloxacin after intravenous and intramuscular administrations in adult goats. J Vet Pharmacol Ther Dec;24(6):375–378.

Wetzstein, H.G. 2005. Comparative mutant prevention concentrations of pradofloxacin and other veterinary fluoroquinolones indicate differing potentials in preventing selection of resistance. Antimicrobial Agents and Chemotherapy 49(10):4166–73.

WHO (World Health Organization). 1997. Reduction in use of antimicrobials decreases resistance. WHO Drug Information 11(4):241–243.

Wright, D.H., Brown, G.H., Peterson, M.L., and Rotschafer, J.C. 2000. Application of fluoroquinolone pharmacodynamics. Journal of Antimicrobial Chemotherapy 46:669–683.

Yabe, K., Murakami, Y., Nishida, S., Sekiguchi, M., Furuham, K., Goryo, M., and Okada, K. 2001. Journal of Veterinary Medical Science 63(8):867–872.

Young, L. A., Schumacher, J., Papich, M. G., et al. 1997. Disposition of enrofloxacin and its metabolite ciprofloxacin after intramuscular injection in juvenile Burmese pythons (*Python molurus bivittatus*). Journal of Zoological and Wildlife Medicine 28:71–79.

Yun, H. I., Park, S. C., Jun, M. H., Hur, W., and Oh, T. K. 1994. Ciprofloxacin in horses: antimicrobial activity, protein binding, and pharmacokinetics. Proceedings of the 6th EAVPT Congress, pp. 28–29.

Zeng, Z., and Fung, K. 1997. Effects of experimentally induced *Escherichia coli* infection on the pharmacokinetics of enrofloxacin in pigs. Journal of Veterinary Pharmacology and Therapeutics 20(Suppl1):39–40.

Zhanel, G.G., Hoban, D.J., Schurek, K., and Karlowsky, J.A. 2004. Role of efflux mechanisms on fluoroquinolone resistance in *Streptococcus pneumoniae* and *Pseudomonas aeruginosa*. International Journal of Antimicrobial Agents 24:529–535.

CHAPTER

39

ANTIFUNGAL AND ANTIVIRAL DRUGS

JENNIFER L. DAVIS, MARK G. PAPICH, AND MARK C. HEIT

ANTIFUNGAL DRUGS

The need for safe and effective antifungal drugs has become important, particularly in small-animal medicine, with the recognition of serious systemic fungal diseases as well as the need for effective drugs to treat skin infections caused by dermatophytes and yeasts. Some animals are at a greater risk of fungal infections because they are immunosuppressed, receiving cancer drugs, radiation therapy, or prolonged courses of corticosteroids. Fortunately, there have

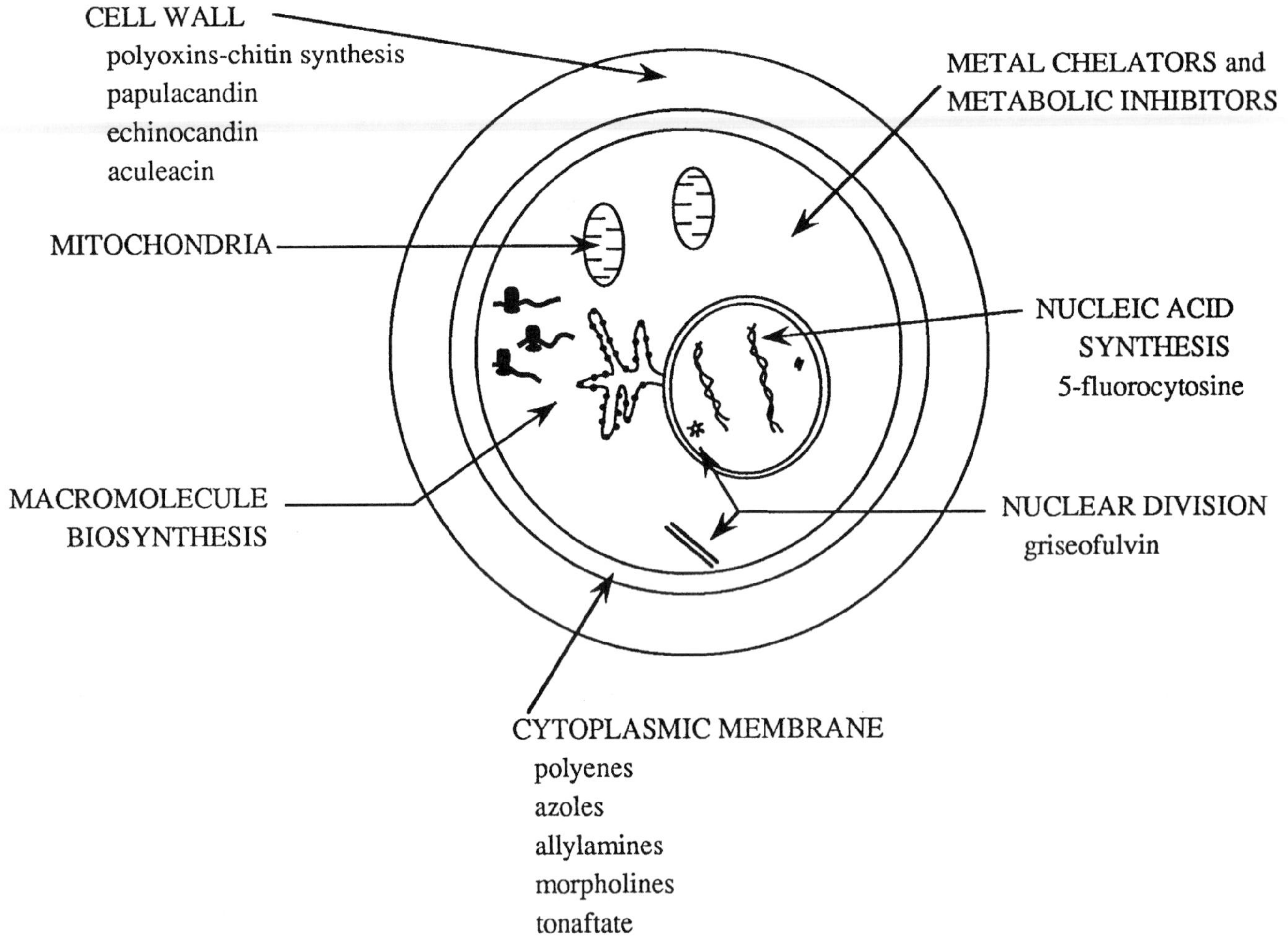

FIG. 39.1 Schematic anatomy of a fungal cell and potential sites where antifungal drugs act.

been many advances in the development of antifungal drugs in the last 10 years. Effective oral drugs are more widely used and there are newer, safer formulations of injectable agents. Figure 39.1 illustrates the sites of drug action for common antifungal drugs used in veterinary medicine.

GRISEOFULVIN

Griseofulvin (Fulvicin U/F®, Fulvicin P/G®, Grifulvin V®, Grisactin®, Grisactin ultra®), is a fungistatic antibiotic produced by *Penicillium griseofulvin dierckx*. It is colorless, slightly bitter, and virtually insoluble in water. There are two types of preparations, the microsized and the ultramicrosized. Due to increased surface area, the ultramicrosized formulations have almost 100% bioavailability, whereas oral absorption of microsized formulations is lower and more variable (25–70%). The ultramicrosized preparations are not used often in veterinary medicine due to the higher cost. If the ultramicrosized form is used, the dose must be decreased to account for differences in absorption.

MECHANISM OF ACTION. Griseofulvin's selective toxicity is based on an energy-dependent uptake into susceptible fungi that occurs preferentially in fungal cells rather than mammalian cells. Once inside the cell, griseofulvin disrupts the mitotic spindle by interacting with polymerized microtubules, thus causing mitotic arrest in metaphase. Grossly this may appear as shortened fungal hyphae that have fewer branching points. This is known as the *curling* phenomenon. Griseofulvin may also interfere with cytoplasmic tubule formation, thereby inhibiting normal cellular trafficking.

SPECTRUM OF ACTIVITY. Griseofulvin's activity is limited to organisms causing dermatophytosis, *Microsporum* spp., *Trichophyton* spp., and *Epidermophyton*. Fungal resistance to griseofulvin, caused by decreased energy-dependent uptake into the fungal cell, has not been reported to be a clinically important problem in veterinary medicine.

PHARMACOKINETICS. Pharmacokinetic properties were reviewed by Hill et al. (1995). Within hours of oral administration, griseofulvin can be detected in the stratum corneum. Because of low water solubility, griseofulvin absorption is enhanced when given with a meal with high fat content. Griseofulvin distributes to the keratin of skin, hair, and nails. Only a small fraction of the dose is present in other body fluids or tissues. The plasma half-life in the dog is 47 minutes (Harris and Riegelman 1969); however, the half-life at the site of action—the stratum corneum—is prolonged because the drug is bound tightly to keratinocytes and remains in the skin until these cells are shed. Thus, new hair or nail growth is first to become free of disease as keratin infected by fungus is replaced by new cells.

Griseofulvin is metabolized primarily by the liver to demethylgriseofulvin and the glucuronide. It is metabolized approximately six times faster in animals than in people, which is the reason animal doses are higher than human doses (half-life in dogs is less than 1 hour, compared to 20 hours in people) (Shah et al. 1972).

CLINICAL USE

Small Animals. Griseofulvin is still used for treating dermatophytosis, but is being gradually replaced by azole drugs (see below). The recommended doses have varied, depending on the author. The label dose in dogs and cats for Fulvicin U/F® tablets is 11 to 22 mg/kg per day, but recommendations by specialists in dermatology have ranged from 44 mg/kg/day (Sousa and Ihrke 1983) to 110 to 132 mg/kg per day in divided treatments (Scott 1980). One review suggested a dose of 50 mg/kg once a day of the microsize formulation (Hill et al. 1995), and another review listed 25 mg/kg every 12 hours (deJaham et al. 2000), but the dose can be doubled for refractory cases. The most common dose is in the range of 50 mg/kg/day, which was confirmed in a report in which it was used in cats and was as effective as itraconazole for treatment of dermatophytosis (Moriello and DeBoer 1995).

Griseofulvin is available in 125 and 250 mg capsules; 125, 250, and 500 mg tablets; and 125 mg/ml oral syrup. Often, at least 4 weeks are needed for successful therapy, and some patients require 3 months (or more) of continuous therapy. As long as 4 months may be necessary to treat infections of the nail bed (onychomycosis).

Large Animals. Griseofulvin is labeled for use in horses at a dose of 2.5 gm/day orally in adult horses for a minimum of 10 days. This translates to one packet of the powder formulation or one bolus per day, administered on feed. The dose for foals is 1/2 packet or 1/2 bolus. Its use is limited to cases of dermatophytosis. There are currently no alternative registered products for use in food animals in the United States. Nevertheless, when used off-label, griseofulvin has been effective in the prevention and treatment of dermatophytes in cattle (Reuss 1978). Doses used are approximately 7.5–10 mg/kg for 7 to 35 days. A dose rate of 1 g/100 kg has been recommended for pigs for a duration of 30–40 days (Kielstein and Gottschalk 1970). Because this drug is not approved, veterinarians must determine proper food animal withdrawal times for this drug prior to administration.

ADVERSE EFFECTS. The most serious adverse effects associated with griseofulvin occur in cats and include leukopenia, anemia, increased hepatic enzyme activity, and neurotoxicosis (Helton et al. 1986). Ataxia in a kitten (Levy 1991) and bone marrow hypoplasia in an 8-year-old cat (Rottman et al. 1991) have been reported.

Prolonged treatment of eight cats with griseofulvin at the high end of the dosage range resulted in no untoward clinical, hematologic, or hepatic side effects, suggesting that griseofulvin toxicity may be idiosyncratic (Kunkle and Meyer 1987). Cats with the feline immunodeficiency virus (FIV) appear to be at increased risk for griseofulvin-associated neutropenia (Shelton et al. 1990); however, toxicity has also been reported in FIV-negative cats (Rottman et al. 1991). The mechanism of this increased risk is unknown but may involve griseofulvin-enhanced binding of immune complexes to granulocytic cells in infected cats (Shelton et al. 1991).

Griseofulvin should never be administered to pregnant cats. Its teratogenicity has been well-documented (Scott et al. 1975; Gruffydd-Jones and Wright 1977). The teratogenic effects include cranial and skeletal malformations as well as ocular, intestinal, and cardiac problems (Scott et al. 1975). It has been given to pregnant horses with no apparent ill effect (Hiddleston 1970); however, this may be dependent on the stage of pregnancy in which the drug was given. One report documented bilateral microphthalmia, brachygnathia superior, and palatocheiloschisis of the drug when given to a mare in the second month of pregnancy (Schutte and Van den Ingh 1997).

AMPHOTERICIN B

Amphotericin B (Fungizone®, ABELCET®, Amphotec®, AmBisome®) is a polyene antibiotic with a large macrolide ring with a hydrophobic conjugated double-bond chain and a hydrophilic hydroxylated carbon chain and attached sugar (Figure 39.2) (Mechlinsk et al. 1970). It is a yellowish powder that is insoluble in water and somewhat unstable (Bennett 1990). There are several formulations of amphotericin B available, including the conventional formulation which is a micellar complex with the bile salt deoxycholate, and several new formulations which are lipid based complexes that are less toxic, but also more expensive (reviewed by Plotnick 2000).

Amphotericin B lipid complex (ABELCET) is a suspension of amphotericin B complexed with two phospholipids. Amphotericin B cholesteryl sulfate complex (Amphotec, ABCD) is a colloidal dispersion of amphotericin B. The liposomal complex of amphotericin B (AmBisome) is a unilamellar liposomal formulation which, when reconstituted, produces small vesicles of encapsulated amphotericin B. Some investigators have attempted to achieve the benefits of lipid formulations without the added cost by mixing the deoxycholate salt in a 10 or 20% lipid solution (Intralipid). This formulation is stable for up to 3 weeks after mixing (Walker and Whitaker 1998); however, the reports of the benefit of this emulsion versus the conventional formulation are inconsistent.

In comparison to the conventional formulation of amphotericin B, lipid formulations can be administered at higher doses to produce greater efficacy with less toxicity (Hiemenz and Walsh 1996). Decreased toxicity is attributed to a selective transfer of the lipid complex amphotericin B, releasing the drug directly to the fungal cell membrane and sparing the mammalian cell membranes. Reduced drug concentrations in the kidneys and diminished release of inflammatory cytokines from amphotericin lipid complex compared to the conventional formulation also may prevent adverse reactions.

MECHANISM OF ACTION. The major action of amphotericin B is to bind ergosterol in the fungal plasma cell membrane, making the membrane more permeable and resulting in leakage of cell electrolytes and cell death

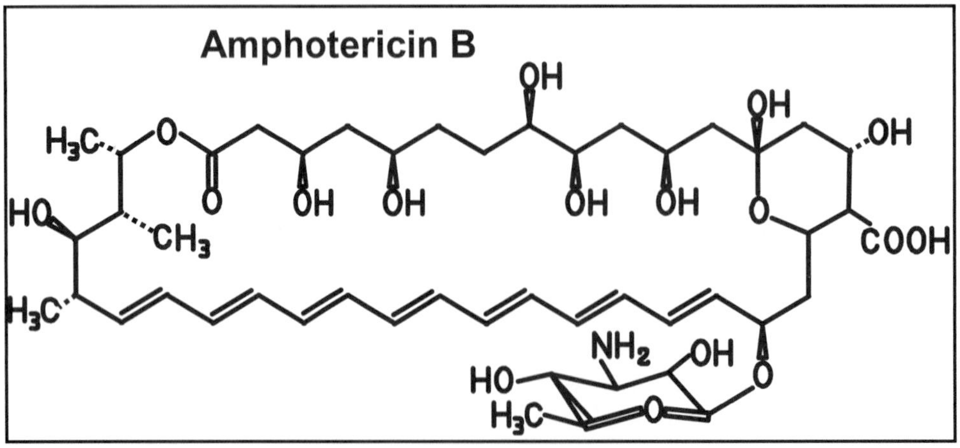

FIG. 39.2 Amphotericin B.

(Brajtburg et al. 1990). At high concentrations, amphotericin B is thought to cause oxidative damage to the fungal cell (Warnock 1991) or disruption of fungal cell enzymes. The selective toxicity of amphotericin B is based on its decreased binding to the major cell membrane sterol of mammalian cells (cholesterol) as compared to that of fungal cells (ergosterol).

Amphotericin B demonstrates concentration-dependent fungicidal activity. There is also a postfungal effect whereby a persistent antifungal effect persists after drug concentrations have declined. This property allows for intermittent therapy (e.g., every other day in dogs).

SPECTRUM OF ACTIVITY. The growth of strains of most veterinary fungal pathogens is inhibited in vitro at amphotericin B concentrations between 0.05 and 1.0 μg/ml and there is good correlation between the MIC values and clinical response (O'Day et al. 1987). Because of concentration-dependent killing, peak (C_{MAX}) concentrations should be 2–4 times above the MIC (C_{MAX}/MIC ratio of 2:4) (Goodwin and Drew 2008).

Sensitive fungi include *H. capsulatum, C. neoformans, C. immitis, B. dermatitidis, Candida* spp., and many strains of *Aspergillus*. Amphotericin B has been indicated for treatment of mucormycosis, sporotrichosis, and phycomycosis (Drouhet and Dupont 1987). Most strains of *Pseudallescheria boydii,* as well as some agents causing chromoblastomycosis and phaeohyphomycosis, are resistant to amphotericin. Clinical fungal resistance to amphotericin B, either primary or acquired, does not appear to occur commonly, although resistant strains occur in vitro. In most cases, these resistant strains contain decreased levels of membrane ergosterol (Pierce et al. 1978) and increased catalase levels may allow these fungi to be resistant to oxidative-dependent damage (Sokol-Anderson et al. 1988). The MIC concentrations were increased in some human patient populations, such as neutropenic patients (Dick et al. 1980), transplant patients (Powderly et al. 1988), and patients undergoing cytotoxic therapy.

PHARMACOKINETICS. Despite its long history of use, much is still unknown concerning the pharmacokinetics of amphotericin B, especially in the veterinary-treated animals. It is poorly absorbed from the GI tract and therefore must be given locally, intravenously, or intrathecally. Amphotericin B binds extensively (~95%) to serum proteins, mainly β-lipoprotein (Bennett 1977). Much of the drug is thought to leave the vascular space and bind to cholesterol-containing membranes. The highest concentrations are found in liver, spleen, kidney, and lungs, with little accumulation in either muscle or adipose tissue. Concentrations of amphotericin B in fluids from inflamed pleura, peritoneum, synovium, and aqueous humor are about two-thirds of those in serum. Amphotericin B readily crosses the human placenta. Penetration into normal or inflamed meninges, vitreous humor, and normal amniotic fluid is poor. This differential distribution may explain treatment failures for infections in some tissues. Although amphotericin B binds ergosterol with higher affinity than cholesterol, it was suggested that because there are more binding sites for cholesterol in the body than for ergosterol, this may sequester amphotericin B from its site of action (Bennett 1977).

CLINICAL USE. A variety of dosage protocols for amphotericin B have been described in the veterinary literature. These are summarized in Table 39.1. One such protocol for small animals was published by Rubin (1986) that is still used today. During infusion, it should be mixed with 5% dextrose solution because if it is added to an electrolyte solution the drug will precipitate, although a solution of amphotericin B with 0.45% saline and 2.5% dextrose has been used successfully subcutaneously without any visible precipitation (Malik et al. 1996). Amphotericin B is used only sporadically in equine medicine and there are no pharmacokinetic data available on amphotericin in the horse. There are no reports of use of this drug in food animals, and there are no approved formulations for use in these species.

Combination therapy using amphotericin B and flucytosine has been shown to be synergistic against cryptococcal infections (see section on flucytosine). Combinations of amphotericin B and azole antifungals have been less successful. Azole-induced depletion of fungal cell membrane ergosterol results in fewer binding sites on which polyene antifungals can exert their effect. Antagonism and synergism between these two classes of antifungal agents have been reported experimentally (Polak et al. 1982; Dupont and Drouhet 1979). Because of the slower onset of action of azole antifungals, many clinicians recommend initial therapy of serious systemic fungal infections with amphotericin B, followed by longer, follow-up treatment with an azole therapeutic protocol.

TABLE 39.1 Selected dosing protocols for amphotericin B in companion animals

Species	Formulation	Disease Treated	Dosing Protocol	Reference
Canine	Fungizone	Unspecified	Pretreatment with 0.9% sodium chloride followed by infusion of 0.5 mg/kg in 5% dextrose over 4–6 hours IV q48h; a test dose of 0.25 mg/kg is sometimes recommended.	Rubin 1986
Canine	Abelcet	Blastomycosis	1 mg/kg IV EOD to a total cumulative dose of 8–12 mg/kg.	Krawiec et al. 1996
Canine	Abelcet	Unspecified	2–3 mg/kg IV 3 times per week diluted in 5% dextrose to a concentration of 1 mg/ml for a total of 9–12 treatments (cumulative dose of 24–27 mg/kg.)	Grooters and Taboada 2003
Canine	AmBisome	Leishmaniasis	3–3.3 mg/kg IV.	Oliva et al. 1995
Canine	Fungizone 40 ml sterile water and 10 ml 10% Intralipid	Leishmaniasis	Pretreatment with 50 ml/kg of 0.9% sodium chloride followed by 10 ml/kg 20% mannitol. Drug mixture infused over 30–60 minutes at incrementally increasing dosing from 1–2.5 mg/kg IV twice a week for a minimum of 8 injections.	Lamothe 2001
Canine/Feline	Fungizone in 0.45% saline with 2.5% dextrose	Cryptococcosis	0.5–0.8 mg/kg SC in 400 ml for cats or 500 ml in dogs given twice a week for a cumulative dose of 8–26 mg/kg.	Malik et al. 1996
Feline	Abelcet	Unspecified	1 mg/kg IV 3 times per week diluted in 5% dextrose to a concentration of 1 mg/ml for a total of 12 treatments (cumulative dose of 12 mg/kg).	Grooters and Taboada 2003
Equine	Fungizone	Phycomycosis	0.38 gradually increased up to 1.47 mg/kg IV in 1 l 5% dextrose once daily.	McMullan et al. 1977
Equine	Fungizone	Pulmonary Histoplasmosis	0.3–0.6 mg/kg IV in 1 l 5% dextrose once a day or every other day.	Cornick et al. 1990
Equine	Fungizone	Systemic Candidiasis	0.1–0.5 mg/kg IV in 1 l 5% dextrose infused over 4–6 hours once daily.	Reilly and Palmer 1994
Equine	Fungizone	Candida Arthritis	0.33–0.89 mg/kg IV in 1 l 5% dextrose once a day or every other day.	Madison et al. 1995
Equine	Fungizone	Cryptococcal Pneumonia	0.5 mg/kg IV in 1 l 5% dextrose as a 1-hour infusion once a day.	Begg et al. 2004
Avian	Fungizone	Aspergillosis	1.5 mg/kg q8–12h reconstituted in sterile water and then diluted 1 : 50 with 5% dextrose for 3–7 days.	Tully 2000

ADVERSE EFFECTS. The most important clinical toxicosis associated with amphotericin B therapy is nephrotoxicity. It is a dose-related, predictable toxic effect that occurs in almost every animal treated with the conventional formulation. Direct tubular damage occurs because amphotericin B binds to cholesterol in the tubular cells, which results in electrolyte leakage from the cells (primarily K^+ loss) and renal tubular acidosis (Bennett 1990). Induced renal vasoconstriction and impaired acid excretion may also contribute to amphotericin B's renal toxicity (Greene 1990). Renal vasoconstriction may be caused by induced increases in the eicosanoid synthesis in renal blood vessels. The tubular damage, along with the renal vasoconstriction, leads to both an acute and a chronic cumulative renal toxicosis. Clinically, the signs of renal toxicosis are seen as increases in creatinine and blood urea nitrogen (BUN). Electrolyte loading, fluid diuresis, and slow infusion of amphotericin B have all been shown to decrease the severity and the rate of development of renal toxicity. Therefore, common protocols for administration of amphotericin B to animals include pretreatment with sodium chloride IV solution (Rubin 1986) with or without mannitol (Legendre 1984), and a slow infusion. Slower infusion times are associated with less kidney injury (Rubin 1986). If the dose administered during a single infusion exceeds 1 mg/kg, acute renal injury is likely (Butler and 1964).

Careful clinical monitoring will help decrease the risk of permanent renal injury. Urine sediment evaluation has been suggested to detect renal toxicity earlier than serum biochemical alterations (Greene 1990); thus, urine should be evaluated for proteinuria, cylinduria, and hematuria, as well as specific gravity. In addition, BUN, creatinine, and electrolyte concentrations should be monitored. Therapy should be temporarily discontinued when active urine sediment is detected or the serum creatinine increases. After stopping therapy, patients may undergo a fluid diuresis to decrease the azotemia. If BUN and creatinine return to near-normal reference values, treatment may be resumed. If azotemia does not improve, one should consider an alternative treatment.

Other adverse effects from amphotericin that are frequently observed in animals include phlebitis, fever, nausea, and vomiting. Measures to prevent the nausea and vomiting have included administration of antiemetic drugs such as chlorpromazine, maropitant, or metoclopramide prior to infusion (see Chapter 47 on Gastrointestinal Drugs). Hypokalemia and anemia have frequently been reported in humans and therefore should be monitored.

AZOLE ANTIFUNGAL DRUGS

The azole antifungal drugs have a high safety profile, a broad spectrum of activity and are available in topical, oral, and intravenous formulations. There are two main categories of azole antifungal drugs, the imidazoles (clotrimazole, miconazole, ketoconazole) and the triazoles (fluconazole, itraconazole, voriconazole) (Fig. 39.3). Clotrimazole and miconazole are discussed in the section on topical therapy. The important physicochemical differences between azole antifungal drugs are summarized in Table 39.2.

MECHANISM OF ACTION. All azoles exert their antifungal effect on the cell membrane of fungi by inhibiting

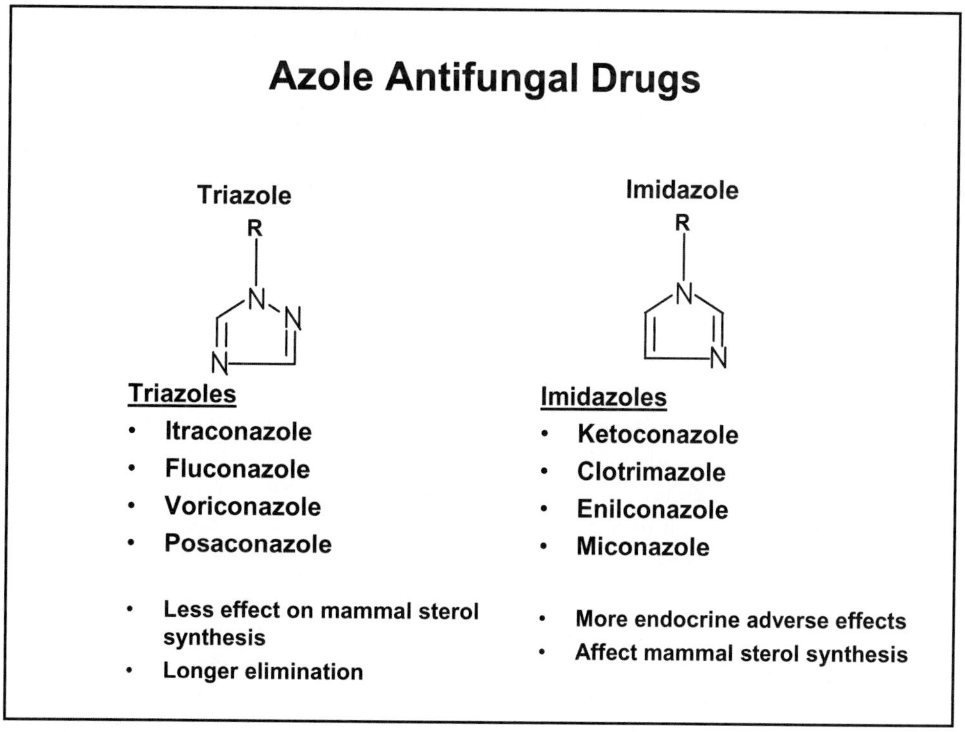

Azole Antifungal Drugs

Triazole
R
N
N
N

Triazoles
- Itraconazole
- Fluconazole
- Voriconazole
- Posaconazole

- Less effect on mammal sterol synthesis
- Longer elimination

Imidazole
R
N
N

Imidazoles
- Ketoconazole
- Clotrimazole
- Enilconazole
- Miconazole

- More endocrine adverse effects
- Affect mammal sterol synthesis

FIG. 39.3 Azole antifungal drugs.

TABLE 39.2 Comparison of the physicochemical properties and in vitro activity of commonly used azole antifungal drugs

					Activity		
Drug	Solubility	pH Dependent	LogP	Protein Binding	Yeasts	Aspergillus	Fusarium
Ketoconazole	pi	Yes	3.78	>90%	+	±	–
Fluconazole	ss	No	0.54	10–12%	+	–	–
Itraconazole	pi	Yes	5.66	>98%	+	±	–
Voriconazole	vss	No	1.81	32–58%	+	+	±

pi = practically insoluble (<0.01 mg/ml); ss = slightly soluble (1–10 mg/ml); vss = very slightly soluble (0–1 mg/ml).

synthesis of the primary sterol of the fungal cell membrane, ergosterol. Inhibition of the P450–dependent lanosterol C_{14}-demethylase enzyme results in depletion of ergosterol and accumulation of C_{14}-methyl sterols in the cytoplasmic membrane of yeasts and filamentous fungi. This enzyme is also known as CYP51A or Erg11p and is encoded by the *ERG11* gene. Inhibition of this cytochrome P450 enzyme occurs via binding of the nitrogen (N_3 of imidazoles and N_4 of triazoles) to the heme iron atom of ferric cytochrome P450. This prevents the formation of the superoxide Fe^{+3} complex ($Fe^{+3}O^-$) needed for hydroxylation of methyl sterols. The result is an inability to demethylate C_{14}-methyl sterols and reduced synthesis of ergosterol. Sterols with less planar configurations are then incorporated into the fungal cell wall, which changes membrane fluidity and interferes with the barrier function of the membrane and with membrane-bound enzymes.

Azole drugs are generally fungistatic at concentrations achieved clinically, although this may vary with the strain of fungus and with the drug. For azole drugs, the parameter that correlates best with clinical cure is the total exposure as measured by the area-under-the-curve in relation to the MIC (AUC/MIC ratio) (Goodwin and Drew 2008).

The potency of each azole drug is related to its affinity for binding the P450 enzyme. The selective toxicity of each compound is directly dependent upon its specificity for binding fungal P450 more readily than mammalian P450. Imidazoles are less specific than triazoles and produce side effects in animals attributed to inhibition of P450 enzymes that are responsible for the synthesis of cortisol and reproductive steroid hormones. Azoles may decrease cholesterol, cortisol, androgen, and testosterone biosynthesis and may interfere with several liver enzymes necessary for inactivation of toxic and carcinogenic agents (Polak 1990).

This inhibition of mammalian P450 enzymes is also responsible for drug-drug interactions that have been observed with the azole antifungals. When azoles are administered concurrently with other drugs that are metabolized by these enzymes, they can significantly increase the plasma concentrations of those drugs. Alternatively, when azoles are administered concurrently with drugs that induce the P450 enzymes, the concentrations of the azole drugs may be significantly decreased. The drug-drug interactions important to veterinary medicine are summarized in Table 39.3. The ability to inhibit mammalian P450 enzymes, and therefore the likelihood of drug-drug interactions, is greatest with ketoconazole, followed by itraconazole, voriconazole, and fluconazole.

Another method by which the azole antifungals can interfere with the absorption and pharmacokinetics of concurrently administered medications is through inhibition of the P-glycoprotein efflux pumps. These efflux pumps can be found in the intestine, where they limit the absorption of some substrates, as well as in the liver, kidney, eye, and CNS. Azole antifungals have the ability to inhibit P-glycoprotein pumps and therefore increase the oral absorption and tissue distribution of drugs within the body, particularly into protected sites, such as the blood-brain barrier and the blood-retinal barrier. The ability to inhibit P-glycoprotein is greatest with itraconazole, followed by ketoconazole and voriconazole (Wang et al. 2002). Fluconazole has little interaction with P-glycoprotein, which may explain why it has fewer significant drug interactions compared to the other azole antifungals (Yasuda et al. 2002; Wang et al. 2002).

KETOCONAZOLE. Ketoconazole (Nizoral®), one of the imidazoles, became available in 1979. The results of successful use in veterinary medicine was published shortly thereafter (Legendre et al. 1982; Medleau et al. 1985). Ketoconazole is available in 200 mg tablets, and generic formulations are inexpensive and readily available.

TABLE 39.3 Antifungal drug-drug interactions of significance in veterinary medicine*

	Drug/Drug Class	Result
Griseofulvin	Anticoagulants/Coumarin or inandione derivatives	Griseofulvin is a hepatic enzyme inducer, which may increase the metabolism of these drugs, resulting in decreased anticoagulant effects.
	Barbiturates	Impaired absorption and therefore possibly impaired effectiveness of griseofulvin.
Amphotericin B	Bone marrow depressants	Increased risk of anemia or other blood dyscrasia.
	Corticosteroids	Exacerbation of hypokalemia, particularly with those drugs that have significant mineralocorticoid activity.
	Digoxin	Hypokalemia caused by AmpB increases the potential for digitalis toxicity.
	Neuromuscular blocking agents	Hypokalemia caused by AmpB enhances the blockade of nondepolarizing agents.
	Diuretics	Potassium depleting diuretics will exacerbate hypokalemia.
	Flucytosine	Synergism of AmpB with flucytosine may decrease the dose of AmpB necessary, therefore reducing the nephrotoxicity, however AmpB-induced renal dysfunction may increase 5-FC concentrations, thus increasing the potential for blood dyscrasias.
Azole antifungals	Drugs that increase gastric pH	Decreases the absorption of those drugs with a pH-dependent solubility (ketoconazole and itraconazole only).
	Digoxin	Increased plasma concentrations of digoxin resulting from P450 inhibition may lead to increased digitalis toxicity.
	Benzodiazepines	Increased plasma concentrations of benzodiazepines, particularly midazolam, resulting from P450 inhibition may result in potentiation of the sedative effects of these drugs.
	Glipizide	Increased plasma concentrations of glipizide resulting from P450 inhibition may cause hypoglycemia.
	Second-generation antihistamines	Although identified in people, and not animals, there may be increased plasma concentrations of antihistamines resulting from P450 inhibition, which may result in cardiac arrhythmias, including ventricular tachycardia and torsades de pointes; not seen with fluconazole except at very high doses.
	Warfarin	Increased plasma concentrations of warfarin resulting from P450 inhibition may cause increased anticoagulant effects and bleeding.
	Cisapride	Although identified in people, and not animals, there may be increased plasma concentrations of cisapride resulting from P450 inhibition, which may result in ventricular arrhythmias, including torsades de pointes.
	Cyclosporine	Increased plasma concentrations of cyclosporine resulting from P450/P-gp inhibition may require adjustment of cyclosporine doses; has been used clinically to decrease the cost of cyclosporine treatment; not seen with fluconazole except at very high doses.
	Quinidine	Increased plasma concentrations of quinidine resulting from P450/P-gp inhibition may lead to increased quinidine toxicity.
	Nifedipine	Increased plasma concentrations of nifedipine resulting from P450/P-gp inhibition.
	Hydrochlorthiazide	Hydrochlorthiazide decreases the renal elimination of fluconazole, resulting in increases of fluconazole plasma concentrations.
	Carbemazapine	Induction of P450 enzymes by carbemazapine may decrease the plasma concentrations of antifungal drugs.
	Rifampin	Induction of P450 enzymes by rifampin may decrease the plasma concentrations of antifungal drugs.
	Phenytoin	Induction of P450 enzymes by phenytoin may decrease the plasma concentrations of antifungal drugs.
	Phenobarbital	Induction of P450 enzymes by phenobarbital may decrease the plasma concentrations of antifungal drugs.
Flucytosine	Bone marrow depressants	May exacerbate bone marrow toxicities.
	Nephrotoxic agents	May decrease flucytosine clearance, increasing the potential for bone marrow toxicity.
Terbinafine	*There are no reported drug-drug interactions with terbinafine.*	

*Not all of these interactions have been documented in veterinary medicine, but are present in human medicine and should be monitored for in veterinary patients.

Spectrum of Activity. Ketoconazole is most effective against yeast and dimorphic fungi such as *Candida*, *Malassezia (Pityrosporum) pachydermatis*, *C. immitis*, *H. capsulatum*, and *B. dermatitidis*, as well as most dermatophytes with MIC values less than 0.5 μg/ml. It is less effective against *C. neoformans*, *S. schenckii*, and *Aspergillus* spp., with MIC values varying from 6 to >100 μg/ml (Hume and Kerkering 1983).

Pharmacokinetics. Ketoconazole is relatively insoluble, except in an acid environment. It is not well absorbed orally unless there is acid secretion, such as after a meal. Ketoconazole is highly protein bound (>98%) and therefore does not penetrate into the cerebrospinal, seminal, or ocular fluid to a significant degree; although it is found in mother's milk. It distributes throughout the skin and subcutaneous tissue, making it effective for treatment of superficial and systemic fungal skin infections. The drug demonstrates nonlinear absorption and elimination kinetics, most probably due to saturation of metabolizing enzymes. It is biotransformed in the liver via O-dealkylation and aromatic hydroxylation and excreted mainly in the bile. Elimination half-life is approximately 2 hours in dogs.

Because ketoconazole is soluble only in acid aqueous environments (pH <3), gastric alkalizing agents (e.g., antacids, H_2 blockers, and parietal cell proton pump inhibitors) or diseases resulting in achlorhydria will decrease its dissolution and oral absorption. Because of lack of consistent gastric acidity, ketoconazole is absorbed poorly in horses. When ketoconazole was administered at 30 mg/kg to horses in corn syrup, the drug was not detected in serum; however, when it was administered with 0.2 N hydrochloric acid intragastrically, oral absorption increased but systemic availability was only 23% with peak serum concentrations of 3.76 μg/ml (Prades et al. 1989).

Clinical Use. In people, ketoconazole has been replaced in therapy by safer triazole antifungal drugs. But in veterinary medicine, owing to ketoconazole's efficacy, safety, cost, and ease of administration, it is still a popular antifungal agent. For dermatophytosis in cats, 10 mg/kg/day has been used (Medleau and Chalmers 1992). For candidiasis, 10 mg/kg/day for 6–8 weeks is recommended. For canine blastomycosis, histoplasmosis, cryptococcosis, and coccidioidomycosis, the dosage is 10–20 mg/kg every 12 hours. Ketoconazole was also effective in treating nasal cryptococcosis in a dog at a dose of 10 mg/kg/day (Noxon et al. 1986). For *Malassezia* dermatitis in dogs, dosages of 5–10 mg/kg/day have been recommended (Hill et al. 1995). The duration of treatment is highly variable. Four to six weeks is a minimum for most diseases; many patients with blastomycosis are treated for a minimum of 2 months and as long as 6 months. If there is CNS involvement, particularly with cryptococcosis, higher doses (40 mg/kg) may be necessary to improve penetration into the CNS. Cats have been successfully treated for cryptococcosis with a dosage of 10–15 mg/kg/day (Pentlarge and Martin 1986; Legendre et al. 1982; Medleau et al. 1985). As complete eradication of the fungal organism is difficult, relapse is common. For this reason, infections should be treated beyond the time clinical signs have resolved. Ketoconazole is not absorbed well orally in horses and it is not recommended. There are no approved formulations for use in food animals.

There are other uses of ketoconazole not related to the treatment of fungal infections. Because of its inhibitory effect on P450 and P-glycoprotein, administration of ketoconazole concurrently with cyclosporine for the treatment of immune diseases has been used to reduce the dose of cyclosporine by up to 75% and reduce the cost of cyclosporine therapy by 58% (Dahlinger et al. 1998).

Ketoconazole inhibits the synthesis of steroid hormones (via inhibition of the cytochrome P450 enzymes), most notably cortisol and testosterone. Although this may be a side effect of therapy, it has been exploited for the temporary management of hyperadrenocorticism in dogs (Bruyette and Feldman 1988; Feldman et al. 1990) and as an antiandrogen treatment. Steroid synthesis inhibition is only a temporary effect that persists only during dosing with ketoconazole (e.g., for up to 8 hours). Ketoconazole will not produce permanent hypoadrenocorticism.

Adverse Effects. Nausea, anorexia, and vomiting are the most common adverse effects, and may require cessation of therapy, particularly in cats (Medleau and Chalmers 1992). They are usually dose related and may be diminished by decreasing the dose, dividing the total dose into smaller doses, and administering each dose with food. With chronic therapy pruritus, alopecia, lightening and drying of the hair coat, and weight loss may occur (Greene 1990). Slight to moderate elevations of inducible hepatic enzymes are expected and may not be accompanied by hepatic injury. However, high elevations in hepatic enzymes, accompanied by other parameters (hyperbilirubinemia and clinical signs consistent with hepatic disease), may indicate hepatotoxicosis. Idiosyncratic hepatitis has been reported in animals and people (Janssen and Symoens 1983).

Ketoconazole is very potent at inhibiting fungal P450, but it also inhibits mammalian P450 at relatively low concentrations; therefore, side effects and drug interactions can occur. This includes inhibition of P450(17α) catalyzed conversion of progestins to androgens. Dose-related inhibition of testosterone has resulted in gynecomastia, sexual impotence, and azoospermia. Cats appear to be more sensitive to ketoconazole liver toxicity than are dogs but they are less sensitive to the hormonal suppressive side effects (Willard et al. 1986a,b).

Ketoconazole has been shown to be teratogenic in the rat and has resulted in mummified fetuses and stillbirths in dogs. It is therefore not recommended for use in pregnant or lactating animals. Cataracts have been reported after long-term ketoconazole therapy in dogs (de Costa et al. 1996). The average duration of therapy in affected dogs was 15 months, and dosages ranged from 6 to 31 mg/kg/day. These dogs were not diabetic. The mechanism of this reaction is not known.

FLUCONAZOLE. Fluconazole (Diflucan and generic) has replaced ketoconazole in small animals and birds for many indications. The triazole groups result in increased resistance to metabolic attack, in vivo potencies 100 times that of ketoconazole, and significantly increased aqueous solubility (8 mg/ml) (Richardson et al. 1990). Because of these properties, this compound has good efficacy in animal models and pharmacokinetics properties that are improved over other azole antifungal drugs such as ketoconazole or itraconazole. It is available in 50–200 mg tablets, powder for oral suspension, and a 2 mg/ml parenteral formulation. Compounded formulations have good oral bioavailability and can be used with a reasonable expectation of performance.

Spectrum of Activity. Fluconazole has been shown to be effective in animal models of *Blastomyces, Candida, Coccidioides, Cryptococcus*, and *Histoplasma* infections. It is not particularly active against *Aspergillus*. Resistant *Aspergillus* strains have been increasing in human medicine with MICs often >256 μg/ml. For this reason, fluconazole should not be used as a first choice for the treatment of aspergillosis unless sensitivity has been documented and can be monitored.

Efficacy of fluconazole in people has been associated with AUC/MIC ratios as being the best predictor of cures. A ratio above 25 is considered desirable for the best outcome (Goodwin and Drew 2008).

Pharmacokinetics. Fluconazole has different solubility characteristics than ketoconazole and itraconazole and is absorbed well regardless of the circumstances. Feeding or formulation (liquid versus tablet) does not affect absorption. Fluconazole demonstrates linear absorption kinetics, with bioavailability greater than 90% in most species (Brammer et al. 1990); thus, oral and IV dosages are identical. Maximum fluconazole concentrations are reached 1–4 hours after an oral dose. Unlike other azole antifungals, fluconazole is not highly protein bound. Humphrey et al. (1985) found plasma protein binding to be between 10 and 12% at concentrations of 0.1 and 1 μg/ml in mice, rats, dogs, and humans. Similar protein binding has also been documented in horses (12.3%) at a concentration of 5 μg/ml. Fluconazole's low molecular weight, water solubility, and high unbound fraction allow it to be readily distributed throughout the body, including pharmacokinetically privileged spaces. Drug concentrations in saliva, sputum, skin, nails, blister fluid, and vaginal tissue and secretions were found to be similar to plasma concentrations. The advantages of fluconazole lie in its ability to produce higher CSF concentrations than ketoconazole or itraconazole, and therefore, it may be useful for treating mycotic meningitis (Kowalsky and Dixon 1991). Fluconazole CSF/plasma or CSF/serum concentration ratios range from 0.49 in horses (Latimer et al. 2001) to 0.88 in cats (Vaden et al. 1997). The drug also penetrates well into the aqueous humor with ratios of aqueous : plasma of 0.37 in the horse and 0.79 in the cat.

Fluconazole is eliminated principally by the kidney. A unique feature of fluconazole is that this drug is the only one of the azoles that is water soluble and excreted in the urine in an active form; therefore, it may be one of the few drugs useful for treating fungal cystitis. As can be expected with a renally excreted drug, renal dysfunction affects fluconazole's elimination such that dose adjustments are necessary. When patients with normal renal function were compared with those with severe renal insufficiency, fluconazole's elimination half-life nearly tripled (from 30.1 hr to 84.5 hr) (Dudley 1990). Reduced dosages as well as extended dosing intervals have been recommended in renal insufficiency. The disparity between renal fluconazole clearance and creatinine clearance suggests that net tubular reabsorption is responsible for the extended half-life. Half-life was measured to be approximately 14 hours in dogs, 13–25 hours in cats (Vaden et al. 1997; Craig et al. 1993), and 38 hours in horses (Latimer et al. 2001). Steady-state levels are achieved in 5–7 days; thus, the manufacturer suggests a two times loading dose during the first 12–24 hours (Dudley 1990). The lack of significant hepatic metabolism allows for linear elimination kinetics; i.e., half-life is independent of dose.

Clinical Use

Small Animals. Fluconazole is most often used for treatment of dermatophytes. Although not as active against *Aspergillus* or *Penicillium* as other azoles, it has also been used to treat canine nasal aspergillosis and penicilliosis. Ten affected dogs were treated with 2.5–5 mg/kg/day fluconazole orally for 8 weeks. Six dogs became free of disease 2–4 weeks after cessation of therapy and remained free of disease for at least 6 months. Serum alkaline phosphatase and alanine transaminase activity remained within normal ranges throughout the treatment period, and adverse side effects were not noted (Sharp 1991). Doses as high as 10–12 mg/kg/day have also been recommended in dogs. For cats with systemic cryptococcosis, clinical studies have shown a benefit from a dose of 100 mg/cat/day in one or two divided doses. Other reported doses are 2.5–5 mg/kg once a day (Hill et al. 1995). Pharmacokinetic studies support a dose of 50 mg/cat per day for nasal or dermal cryptococcosis (Vaden et al. 1997).

Exotic Animals. The doses for exotic animals are listed in Table 39.4. The half-life can be prolonged in reptiles because of the dependence on renal elimination. Subsequently the half-life is 139 hours when injected SC, which allows for treatment every 5 days (Mallo et al. 2002).

Large Animals. Oral absorption in horses is reported to be greater than 100% (Latimer et al. 2001). From this cited study a dosing regimen of a loading dose of 14 mg/kg orally, followed by 5 mg/kg q24h was derived for horses to produce sufficient concentrations in plasma and tissues. This dose has been successful in treating nasal conidiobolomycosis lesions in mares (Taintor et al. 2004) as well as disseminated candidiasis in foals (Reilly and Palmer 1994).

Adverse Effects. Fluconazole has been generally well tolerated, with mild adverse effects being reported in 5–30% of cases. The GI tract was most frequently involved, followed by the CNS and skin. Mild elevations in hepatic enzymes have been observed, and two cases of hepatic necrosis and death occurred in association with fluconazole therapy (Kowalsky and Dixon 1991). Compared to ketoconazole, there is little evidence of testosterone or other steroid biosynthesis inhibition (Shaw et al. 1987) in human or animal patients (VanCauteren et al. 1987). Hematologic abnormalities, including anemia, leukopenia, neutropenia, and thrombocytopenia, have been reported in people (AHFS Drug Information 1992). In subacute toxicity studies in dogs the highest dose tested (30 mg/kg) caused slight increases in liver weight, hepatic fat, and plasma transaminase activity. Although there is no evidence of mutagenicity or carcinogenicity, its use in pregnant patients is not recommended.

ITRACONAZOLE. Itraconazole (Sporanax®) was approved for use in the United States in 1992. Of several triazole compounds screened, itraconazole, first synthesized in 1980, was selected for further clinical development due to several criteria: 1) 5–100 times better in vitro and in vivo potency than ketoconazole, 2) good activity against *Aspergillus* spp., 3) activity against meningeal cryptococcosis in animal models, 4) few adverse side effects, and 5) favorable pharmacokinetics (Cauwenbergh et al. 1987).

Itraconazole is a weak base ($pK_a = 3.7$), is highly lipophilic ($\log P = 5.66$), and is practically insoluble in water. There are several different formulations available. The intravenous formulation is rarely used in veterinary medicine due to expense as well as instability once reconstituted. There are three oral formulations available. The oral capsules were the first formulation marketed and they are still commonly used. They are available in 100 mg dose strength, and consist of drug coated onto small sugar spheres. The capsules require an acid environment for dissolution and therefore absorption is often highly variable. There is also an oral solution licensed for use in humans that contains 10 mg/ml of itraconazole complexed with hydroxypropyl-β-cyclodextrin, to increase the solubility. This product has been demonstrated to have higher, less variable absorption in humans, cats, and horses (Willems et al. 2001; Boothe et al. 1997; Davis et al. 2005). A third oral formulation is licensed for use in cats in some European countries (Itrafungol Vet®, Janssen-Cilag). This formulation is also an oral solution (10 mg/ml itraconazole) with propylene glycol, srobitol, and flavorings as excipients. Because of its low and highly pH-dependent solubility, compounded formulations of itraconazole are often not stable and not well absorbed; therefore, their use is not recommended.

Spectrum of Activity. Itraconazole has been tested both in vitro and in vivo against a wide variety of fungi (for review see Perfect et al. 1986; VanCutsem et al. 1987; VanCutsem 1990; Cauwenbergh and DeDonker 1987). It was found to be effective against virtually all medically important fungi, including *Microsporum, Trichophyton, Candida, Malassezia* (*Pityrosporum*), *Sporothrix, Pythium, Histoplasma, Aspergillus, Blastomyces, Coccidioides*, and *Cryptococcus*. It has little activity against *Fusarium* sp.

Like other azole antifungal drugs, the AUC/MIC is the best surrogate marker to predict efficacy. However, the most often reported drug concentrations from studies in humans have been the plasma concentrations measured at the lowest point (trough, or C_{MIN}) during multiple dosing. In these studies (Goodwin and Drew 2008) the trough concentrations greater than 0.5 to 1.0 µg/ml have been associated with clinical success.

Pharmacokinetics. Absorption is increased by an acid environment and when taken with meals (Graybill 1990) and is less variable than ketoconazole absorption. Bioavailability increases from 40% after fasting to 99.8% when given with a meal (VanCauteren et al. 1987), except in horses. Itraconazole is highly (99.8%) protein bound (95% to albumin and 5% to red blood cells) (Heykants et al. 1987); however, due to its lipophilicity and even higher affinity for tissue proteins, it is extensively distributed throughout the body. Tissue to plasma concentration ratios range from 1 : 1 in brain to 8 : 1 in keratin to 25 : 1 in fat stores. Highest tissue levels are seen in the liver and adrenal cortex (Heykants et al. 1987). High tissue binding also produces a very large volume of distribution (Troke et al. 1990; Heykants et al. 1990) and low plasma concentrations. Although it does not reach high concentrations in the CSF compared to fluconazole, itraconazole was found to be effective in treating meningeal cryptococcosis in both mouse and guinea pig models (Perfect et al. 1986).

Itraconazole is extensively metabolized, with less than 1% of the active drug and approximately 35% of inactive drug (as more than 10 metabolites) excreted in the urine. The major metabolite, hydroxyitraconazole, has similar antifungal activity to the parent drug, and is often found at concentrations 2–3 times higher than itraconazole in the plasma in humans (Willems et al. 2001). The metabolite to parent drug ratio is reported to be similar in dogs (Yoo et al. 2002); however, this metabolite has not been found in either cats (Itrafungol®, package insert) or horses (Davis et al. 2005). The predominant route of elimination for itraconazole is in the bile. Due to the increased metabolic stability of the triazole ring versus the imidazole ring (Richardson et al. 1990), itraconazole has a longer half-life (17–25 hr) than ketoconazole (8 hr) in humans. There is disagreement about the elimination rate since the terminal half-life in the dog has been reported to be 8–12 hours (VanCauteren et al. 1987) and 44–58 hours (Heykants et al. 1987). Differences in study methods, assay sensitivity, and pharmacokinetic analysis may account for this discrepancy. More important than plasma half-life, therapeutically active concentrations are maintained much longer in tissues than in plasma. For example, itraconazole can be detected for 4 days in vaginal epithelium and for 4 weeks in skin and nails after cessation of therapy. These long-lasting tissue concentrations account for the ability to administer this drug intermittently for some fungal infections, as will be discussed below in the dosing section. Itraconazole, like ketoconazole, exhibits nonlinear pharmacokinetics; steady-state concentrations were found to be three times higher after 14 days of therapy than those predicted by a single dose, and the half-life was seen to increase from 24 to 36 hours (Heykants et al. 1990).

Pertinent to the pharmacokinetics is the ability of itraconazole to inhibit drug metabolizing enzymes. Itraconazole and its metabolites are cytochrome P450 inhibitors (Templeton et al. 2008). Metabolizing enzymes may be saturated producing nonlinearity in elimination. In addition, repeated dosing may produce a time-dependent decrease in clearance and accumulation (Templeton et al. 2008). Therefore, with repeated dosing, the clearance may decrease and half-life increase.

Clinical Use

Small Animals. Itraconazole is considerably more potent than ketoconazole (5 to 100 times more active) and is associated with fewer side effects. It has no endocrine effects compared to ketoconazole. Itraconazole is highly bound in plasma and there is strong binding to keratin producing drug concentrations in skin that persist 2–4 weeks after cessation of drug therapy. It may be excreted into the sebum, increasing the concentrations in skin. This allows for pulse-dosing for some diseases, which is described in the dosing section.

Histoplasma, Cryptococcus, and *Blastomyces* are highly susceptible; *Candida, Aspergillus*, and *Penicillium* are less sensitive. Itraconazole also has been used to treat cutaneous Leishmaniasis because the *Leishmania* organism has ergosterol in high concentrations in its cell wall.

Cats. Itraconazole is probably better tolerated in cats than ketoconazole. Nevertheless, toxic reactions still are possible. Since most adverse effects are dose-related, one is advised to lower the dose in animals in which adverse effects are observed. One report indicated that there were dose-related GI effects of anorexia and vomiting in cats from administration of itraconazole (Mancianti et al. 1998).

The dosing regimens for cats were reviewed by Moriello (2004). Doses in cats vary from 5–10 mg/kg once a day, orally for at least 56 days, to 10 mg/kg once a day, for 28 days, followed by pulse therapy of 1 week on/1 week off. Lower doses of 1.5 to 3 mg/kg once daily for cycles of 15 days at a time are also used.

The recent addition of a commercially available registered formulation has helped to define the use in cats. As mentioned previously, itraconazole (Itrafungol) 10 mg/ml oral solution is registered for use in cats to treat dermatophytosis (not registered in the U.S.). The treatment schedule consists of once-daily doses of 5 mg/kg for three 1-week cycles. After each week of treatment, it should be followed by a week without treatment (week-on/week-off schedule). This schedule has been evaluated in cats and maintains drug concentrations in hairs during the nontreatment phase (Vlaminck and Engelen 2004).

Itraconazole has been compared to ketoconazole, with each drug administered at doses of 10 mg/kg/day for the treatment of experimentally induced feline disseminated cryptococcosis (Medleau et al. 1990). After 3 months of therapy, the infection had been cleared by both drugs as determined by cryptococcal antigen titers and CSF culture. Three months following therapy all animals remained clinically normal, and titers and CSF cultures remained negative. Although both antifungals brought about resolution of the disease, all cats receiving ketoconazole became anorectic and lost weight, requiring dosage adjustments. This was not seen with itraconazole, and in fact the animals receiving this drug gained weight during the study. Itraconazole has also been used in naturally occurring cryptococcal infections (Medleau 1990), where an increase in treatment failure was noted in cats that were seropositive for FIV or FeLV.

Dogs. In dogs, the most extensive study has been for treatment of blastomycosis (Legendre et al. 1996). In a study of 112 dogs, 5 mg/kg/day was as effective as 10 mg/kg/day. With a 60-day course of therapy, 54% of dogs were cured. Itraconazole has been used to treat ocular and systemic blastomycosis in dogs. When given 5 mg/kg itraconazole twice a day for 60 days, 76% of eyes with posterior segment disease other than optic neuritis and 18% and 13% of eyes with anterior uveitis or endophthalmitis, respectively, recovered (Brooks et al. 1992). Pulse dosing has also been evaluated in dogs. Itraconazole doses of 5 mg/kg PO q24h for 2 consecutive days per week for 3 weeks was found to be as effective as a dose of 5 mg/kg PO q24 for 21 consecutive days in the treatment of *Malassezia* dermatitis and otitis (Pinchbeck et al. 2002).

Itraconazole has been successfully used in both the prevention and the treatment of aspergillosis in caged birds. A dose of 20 mg/kg daily for at least 30 days was used to successfully treat 5 of 12 presumed cases of *Aspergillus* infections in penguins. This same author suggests its prophylactic use in penguin chicks (Shannon 1992). A different treatment protocol was recommended for aspergillosis in raptors. Birds are treated with 10 mg/kg twice daily in combination with amphotericin B nebulization three times a day for 20 minutes. Treatment for some cases lasted as long as 6 weeks. These authors also recommend the prophylactic use of itraconazole whenever the clinician expects increased risk for the disease (Forbes et al. 1992). Other antifungal dosing regimens in birds and other exotic animal species are listed in Table 39.4.

Large Animals. Itraconazole has been reported to be effective in horses for the treatment of mycotic rhinitis, osteomyelitis, and guttural pouch mycosis (Korenek et al. 1994; Foley and Legendre 1992; Davis and Legendre 1994). A recent pharmacokinetic study showed that the oral solution at a dose of 5 mg/kg q24h will produce adequate levels in blood and tissues for successful treatment (Davis et al. 2005). However, the use of the oral liquid will require large volumes—most likely requiring gastric lavage in horses—and the drug is very expensive. The oral capsules have a lower bioavailability and higher doses or more frequent dosing intervals are recommended. There are no reports of the use of this drug in food animals, and there are no approved formulations for these species.

Adverse Effects. Itraconazole is up to 125 times more selective for fungal P450 systems than mammalian liver enzymes in certain in vitro preparations (Vanden Bossche 1987). It also does not inhibit P450 systems in the testis, adrenal, or liver in vivo (Vanden Bossche et al. 1990). In clinical studies, 100 mg of itraconazole given to humans each day for 30 days had no effect on serum testosterone

TABLE 39.4 Selected systemic antifungal drugs used in exotic animal species

Species	Drug	Disease Treated	Dosing Protocol	Reference
Passerine and Softbill Birds	Fluconazole	Candidiasis	2–5 mg/kg PO q24h for 7–10 days.	Dorrestein 2000
	Griseofulvin	Dermatophytosis	20 mg/kg PO q24h for 4–6 weeks	
	Itraconazole	Aspergillosis	5–10 mg/kg PO q12–24h in orange juice or 0.1N HCl for 14 days.	
	Ketoconazole	Dermatophytosis	20–30 mg/kg PO q12h for 14–30 days.	
	Miconazole	Candidiasis or Cryptococcosis	10–20 mg/kg IM or IV q8–24h.	
	Nystatin	Intestinal candidiasis	100,000 IU/l of drinking water or 200,000 IU/kg soft food for 3–6 weeks.	
Psittacine Birds	Fluconazole	Candidiasis	2–5 mg/kg PO q24 h for 7–10 days.	Tully 2000
	Flucytosine	Aspergillosis	60–150 mg/kg PO q12h in adults; 100–250 mg/kg PO q12h in neonates. Usually given in combination with amphotericin B.	
	Itraconazole	Aspergillosis	5–10 mg/kg q12h for 4–5 weeks; 5 mg/kg q24h in African grays.	
	Ketoconazole	Candidiasis	20–30 mg/kg q12h in orange or pineapple juice, lactulose, or methylcellulose for 14–30 days.	
	Voriconazole	Asperigillosis	12–18 mg/kg oral q12h	Flammer et al. 2008
	Miconazole	Candidiasis or Cryptococcosis	20 mg/kg IV q8h.	
	Nystatin	Intestinal candidiasis	100,000–300,000 IU/kg PO q8–12h.	
Raptors	Fluconazole	Mycelial candidiasis, systemic mycosis	5–15 mg/kg PO q12h for 14–60 days.	Huckabee 2000
		Gastrointestinal and systemic candidiasis	2–5 mg/kg PO q24h for 7–10 days.	
	Flucytosine	Aspergillosis	120 mg/kg PO q6h; 20–30 mg/kg PO q6h for 60–90 days; 50–75 mg/kg PO q8h in combination with amphotericin B.	
		Candidiasis	250 mg/kg PO q12h.	
	Itraconazole	Aspergillosis	15 mg/kg PO q12h for 4–6 weeks.	
	Ketoconazole	Candidiasis	15 mg/kg PO q12h.	
		Aspergillosis	30–60 mg/kg PO q12h for 14–30 days.	
	Nystatin	Intestinal candidiasis	100,000–300,000 IU/kg PO q8–12h.	
Pet Fish	Itraconazole	Systemic Mycoses	1–5 mg/kg q24h in feed for 1–7 days.	Mashima and Lewbart 2000
	Ketoconazole	Systemic Mycoses	2.5–10 mg/kg PO, IM or ICe.	
Ferrets	Amphotericin B	Systemic mycoses	0.4–0.8 mg/kg IV once a week to a total dose of 7–25 mg.	Williams 2000
	Griseofulvin	Dermatophytosis	25 mg/kg PO q24h for 3–4 weeks.	
	Ketoconazole	Systemic mycoses	10–30 mg/kg PO q12h–24h.	
Hedgehogs	Griseofulvin	Dermatophytosis	25–50 mg/kg PO q24h	Lightfoot 2000
	Itraconazole	Systemic mycoses	5–10 mg/kg PO q12–24h.	
	Ketoconazole	Systemic yeast/fungal infections	10 mg/kg PO q24h.	
	Nystatin	Yeast infections	30,000 IU/kg PO q8–24h.	
Marsupials	Griseofulvin	Dermatophytosis	20 mg/kg PO q24h for 30–60 days.	Johnson-Delaney 2000
	Nystatin	Candidiasis	5000 IU/kg q8h for 3 days.	
Rabbits	Amphotericin B	Systemic mycoses	1 mg/kg IV q24h.	Ivey and Morrisey 2000
	Fluconazole	Systemic mycoses	25–43 mg/kg slow IV q12h.	
	Griseofulvin	Dermatophytosis	12.5–25 mg/kg PO q12–24h for 10–42 days.	
	Ketoconazole	Dermatophytosis	10–40 mg/kg PO q24h for 14 days.	

TABLE 39.4—*continued*

Species	Drug	Disease Treated	Dosing Protocol	Reference
Rodents	Amphotericin B	Candidiasis	0.43 mg/kg PO or 0.11 mg/kg SC in mice.	Adamcak and Otten 2000
	Griseofulvin	Dermatophytosis	25 mg/kg PO q24h for 14–28 days in gerbils, guinea pigs, hamsters, and rats; 14 days in mice; 28–40 days in chinchillas.	
	Itraconazole	Systemic mycoses	5 mg/kg PO q24h in guinea pigs; 50–150 mg/kg q24h in mice; 2.5–10 mg/kg PO q24 in rats.	
	Ketoconazole	Systemic mycoses/candidiasis	10–40 mg/kg PO q24h for 14 days in all species.	
Amphibians	Amphotericin B	Systemic mycoses	1 mg/kg ICe q24h for 14–28 treatments.	Walker and Whitaker 2000
	Fluconazole	Systemic mycoses	60 mg/kg PO q24h for 7 days.	
	Itraconazole	Superficial and systemic mycoses	2–10 mg/kg PO q24h for 14–28 days.	
	Ketoconazole	Systemic mycoses	10–20 mg/kg PO q24h for 14–28 days.	
Chelonians	Amphotericin B	Aspergillosis	1 mg/kg ICe q24h for 2–4 weeks.	Bonner 2000
	Griseofulvin	Dermatophytosis	20–40 mg/kg PO q72h for 5 treatments.	
	Itraconazole	*Sceloporus* sp.	20–30 mg/kg PO q6–8h in the spiny lizard.	
	Ketoconazole	Systemic mycoses	25 mg/kg PO q24h for 2–4 weeks in turtles; 15 mg/kg PO q24h (27°C) in the gopher tortoise.	
	Nystatin	Enteric fungal infections	100,000 IU/kg PO q24h for 10 days in turtles.	
Reptiles	Amphotericin B	Systemic mycoses	1 mg/kg IT q24h for 14–28 days.	Funk 2000
	Fluconazole	Systemic mycoses	2–5 mg/kg PO q24h for 5–21 days in lizards and snakes; can also mix 100 mg with 20 ml of nystatin and give PO at 0.5–0.6 ml/kg.	
	Fluconazole		For sea turtles, a loading dose of 21 mg/kg, followed by 10 mg/kg every 5 days, injected SC (Mallo et al. 2002).	
	Griseofulvin	Dermatophytosis	20–40 mg/kg PO q72h for 5 treatments in snakes.	
	Ketoconazole	Superficial and systemic mycoses	25 mg/kg PO q24h for 3 weeks in snakes.	
	Nystatin	Enteric fungal infections	100,000 IU/kg PO q24h.	

or cortisol levels (DeCoster et al. 1987). Similarly, there were no changes in testosterone and cortisol concentrations in rats and dogs receiving daily itraconazole for at least 1 month.

The biochemical basis for the specificity of itraconazole toward fungal P450 is thought to be dependent upon the hydrophobic nonligand portion of the molecule and its affinity for the apoprotein portion of the cytochrome molecule (Vanden Bossche et al. 1990). The resulting lack of significant inhibition of liver microsomal enzymes results in itraconazole's inability to affect other drugs' metabolism. Although the clinical significance is as yet unknown, drugs that can inhibit or stimulate liver degradative enzymes are able to alter the pharmacokinetics of itraconazole. Even though itraconazole is primarily cleared by hepatic metabolism, there appears to be no need for dosage adjustments in patients with liver disease (Heykants et al. 1987). As with ketoconazole, itraconazole's oral absorption is pH dependent; therefore, dosage adjustments may be necessary when gastric pH is increased.

Because itraconazole is better tolerated than ketoconazole, it is used as the drug of choice for long-term treatment. Dogs, cats, and exotic and zoo animals have received this drug for weeks without adverse effects. The capsules have been administered for up to 6 months in horses with no reported adverse effects. Nevertheless, toxic reactions are still possible. Since most adverse effects are dose related, one is advised to lower the dose in animals in which adverse effects are observed. According to Legendre (1995) about 10% of dogs receiving recommended doses develop hepatic toxicosis. Liver enzyme elevations may occur in 10–15% of dogs. Itraconazole has been well tolerated by clinically ill cats, although one case of fatal drug-induced hepatitis has been reported (Medleau 1990). Anorexia may occur as a complication of treatment, especially with high doses and high serum concentrations. It usually develops in the second month of therapy in dogs. In cats there seem to be dose-related GI effects of anorexia and vomiting (Mancianti et al. 1998). Drug-related cutaneous vasculitis has also been reported as a complication of itraconazole therapy in dogs (Nichols et al. 2001).

Dogs chronically administered itraconazole (2.5, 10, or 40 mg/kg daily for 3 months) had no significant alterations in mortality rate, behavior, appearance, food consumption, body weight, hematologic values, serum and urine chemistry, or gross pathology (VanCauteren et al. 1987b). Subacute toxicity studies in rats revealed increased adrenal gland weight and the accumulation of proteinaceous material in the mononuclear phagocyte system at doses of 40 and 160 mg/kg. Since the mononuclear phagocyte system is responsible for clearing the host of a fungal infection, the clinical importance of this toxic effect remains to be seen. Although not teratogenic at 10 mg/kg, maternal toxicity, embryo toxicity, and teratogenicity were observed at 40 and 160 mg/kg in rats (VanCauteren et al. 1987b); therefore, its use in pregnant animals is not recommended.

Postmarketing drug monitoring in humans has shown that itraconazole may cause or exacerbate underlying heart conditions. There is a dose-related negative inotropic effect seen in both healthy human volunteers and in anesthetized dogs. Owners should therefore be counseled to monitor the patients for signs of heart failure and to discontinue the drug if clinical signs are observed.

Mild to moderate renal failure has not been reported to change the pharmacokinetic clearance of itraconazole in humans. However, if the intravenous formulation or the oral Sporanox® solution is used, renal failure may decrease the elimination of the carrier molecule hydroxypropyl-β-cyclodextrin. Therefore, the oral capsules are recommended for use in these patients.

VORICONAZOLE. The newest triazole to be investigated in animals is voriconazole (Vfend®). Voriconazole is similar in structure to fluconazole (Figure 39.4); however, the substitution of a fluoropyrimidine ring for one of the triazole moieties and the additional of a methyl group to the propanol backbone increases the spectrum of activity and potency as well as the fungicidal activity against some species of molds, including *Aspergillus* and *Fusarium* spp. In a survey of fungal pathogens, itraconazole inhibited greater than 95% of *Aspergillus* with a concentration less than or equal to 1 μg/ml (Diekma et al. 2003). It is more lipophilic than fluconazole, more water soluble than itraconazole or ketoconazole, with intermediate protein binding. These properties allow for excellent oral bioavailability and tissue distribution. In people, the plasma concentrations were highly variable among individuals, which is caused by variations in hepatic metabolism, other medications coadministered, and nonlinear elimination. Such a variation is likely in animals, but there have not been enough studies reported to assess the degree of variability among patients. The concentration associated with clinical cure has been an AUC/MIC plasma concentration of 20–25, or a plasma concentration above 2 μg/ml.

Clinical Use

Dogs and Cats. Clinical experience with this drug is limited at this time. Experimental studies in dogs have shown rapid and complete absorption of the drug following oral administration (Roffey et al. 2003). Voriconazole exhibits nonlinear pharmacokinetics in this species, with a ninefold increase in plasma concentrations seen following a fourfold increase in dose. Interestingly, autoinduction of drug metabolism was shown to occur in dogs, requiring an increase in dose with multiple administrations. Its safety in cats remains to be investigated. In one anecdotal account by the authors, one cat being treated for cryptococcosis developed gastrointestinal side effects from oral voriconazole administration. The drug concentrations in this cat were extremely high and the elimination of the drug was very prolonged (half-life >4 days). Whether this caution should be extended to all cats or whether this was an idiosyncratic reaction in this individual is not known.

Horses. Recently, the pharmacokinetics of voriconazole have been studied following single and multiple dose administration in the horse (Davis et al. 2006; Colitz et al. 2007). In these cited equine studies, voriconazole had excellent oral absorption (95% and 100%) and a long half-life (8–13 hrs) following oral administration, as well as good distribution into the aqueous humor, CSF, synovial fluid, urine, and periocular tear film. The concentrations in plasma, tissues, and other fluids exceed the minimum concentration recommended for successful therapy (Goodwin and Drew 2008). The oral dose used

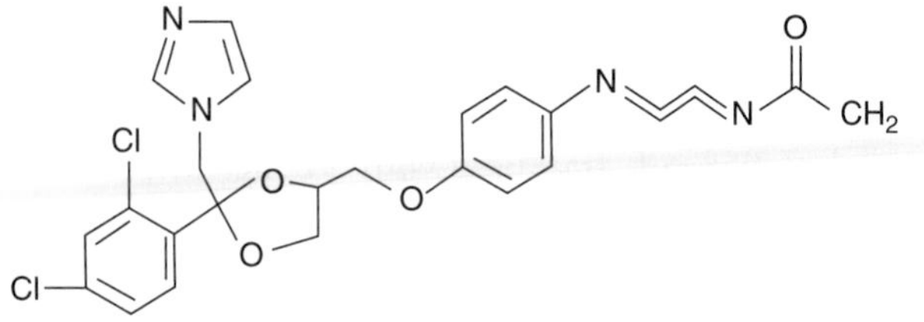

Ketoconazole

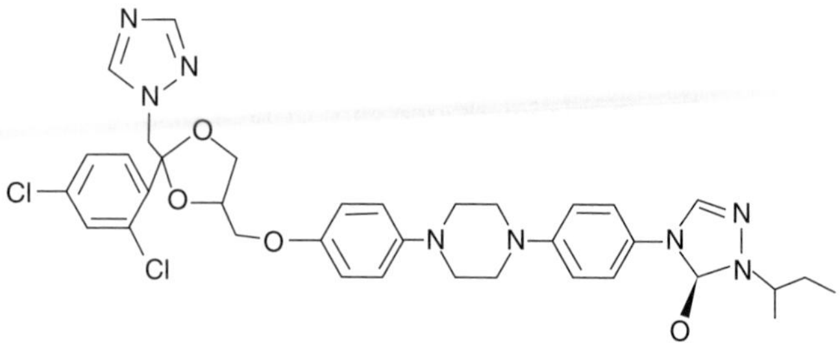

Itraconazole

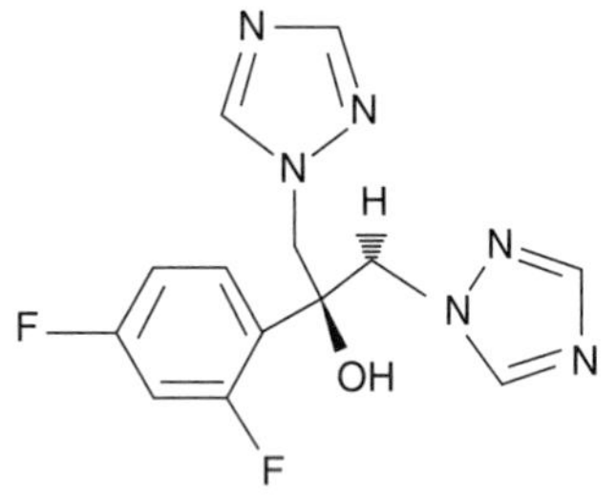

Fluconazole

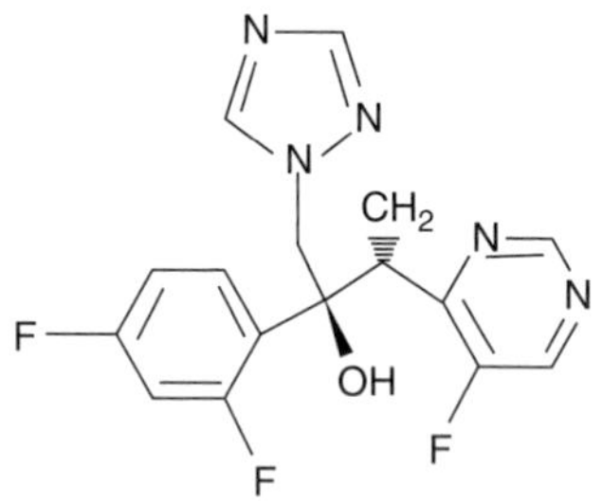

Voriconazole

FIG. 39.4 Chemical structures of commonly used systemic azole antifungal drugs.

in the study by Davis et al.(2005) was 4 mg/kg and produced plasma concentrations were higher than necessary for the treatment of most common veterinary pathogens, with the exception of *Fusarium* sp. The study by Colitz et al.(2007) used 3 mg/kg orally twice daily and produced concentrations above the minimum level necessary for successful treatment. Follow-up clinical experience with therapeutic drug monitoring by the authors cited above (Davis et al.) suggests that a dose of 2 mg/kg orally once a day would be sufficient for most fungal infections.

Birds. The experience with voriconazole in birds has been reported by Flammer et al. (2008). After oral administration of single doses ranging from 6 to 18 mg/kg in parrots, a follow-up study examined multiple doses at the highest dose (18 mg/kg every 12 hours for 9 days). Compared to mammals, the elimination half-life was short at 1.1 to 1.6 hours. With multiple doses the half-life decreased, suggesting induction of the hepatic metabolism as mentioned for dogs above. Polyuria was observed in the treated birds, but no other adverse reactions were reported. On the basis of this study, the authors concluded that 12–18 mg/kg orally twice daily would be sufficient for treatment of some *Aspergillus* infections; higher doses may be needed for some infections and to maintain concentrations during long-term treatment.

Adverse Effects. Except for the single anecdotal account in a cat cited above, and the polyuria observed in birds, there have been no other adverse effects reported for voriconazole in animals. In people, increased liver enzymes and hepatotoxicity have been observed. Liver adverse reactions are more likely in people at high plasma concentrations. In experimental animals and people, visual disturbances have been reported. In experimental dogs, the visual problems were transient. The incidence of ocular problems in people is very low.

POSACONAZOLE. Posaconazole (Noxafil®) is one of the newest azole antifungal drugs introduced. It was registered for use in people but its clinical use in animals has been limited to just a few case reports. Posaconazole resembles itraconazole in structure. It is used for invasive fungal infections, including those caused by *Aspergillus* and *Candida*. It is also active against dermatophytes, *Histoplasma capsulatum, Blastomyces dermatitidis, Coccidioides immitis*, and *Cryptococcus neoformans*. Its advantage over other azole drugs is the activity against Zygomycetes. As with other azoles, the pharmacokinetic/pharmacodynamic parameter that best correlates with clinical success is the plasma concentration AUC/MIC. For treating *Aspergillus* this ratio was above 200; for treating *Candida* the ratio was only 15. If AUC/MIC ratios cannot be monitored, it is suggested to maintain plasma concentrations above (C_{MAX}) 1.48 μg/ml or an average concentration at least 1.25 μg/ml (Goodwin and Drew 2008). Additional information has indicated that prophylactic efficacy for invasive fungal infections is optimal when plasma concentrations of posaconazole exceed 0.7 μg/ml 3–5 hours after dosing in a multiple-dose regimen. It is available as an oral suspension containing 40 mg/ml posaconazole. The dose in people is 400 mg twice a day with a meal. If not given with a meal, dosage of 200 mg four times a day is recommended.

No dose ranges have been established for animals, but in two case reports on its use in cats with successful treatment, a dose of 5 mg/kg orally, every 24 hours was used without ill effects (Wray et al. 2008). In dogs, the oral absorption is good and the half-life is 23 hours. In dogs, there is a food effect on absorption with oral systemic availability of 11% and 27% in fasted and fed dogs, respectively. It is highly protein bound with binding greater than 97% in dogs. In toxicity studies, dogs have tolerated 30 mg/kg/day for 1 year without any clinical signs. However, histologically some neuronal vacuolation was observed at this dose. It should not be used during pregnancy because of inhibition of steroidogenesis.

OTHER AZOLE ANTIFUNGAL DRUGS. There are no other azole drugs reported to be used in animals systemically. However, newer drugs are in development and may be considered in the future. Drugs currently being evaluated include triazoles such as isavuconazole, ravuconazole, and albaconazole. These drugs, with modifications of the triazole structure have advantages in pharmacokinetic properties and spectrum of action compared to older drugs.

OTHER ANTIFUNGAL AGENTS

TERBINAFINE. Terbinafine (Lamisil®) is a highly fungicidal agent. It is a synthetic drug of the allylamine class. A closely related drug of the same class is naftifine (Naftin®), which is used as a topical cream for dermatophyte infections in people. Terbinafine inhibits squalene epoxidase to decrease synthesis of ergosterol. Fungal cell death results from disruption of cell membrane (Balfour and Faulds 1992).

Spectrum of Activity. Terbinafine is active against yeasts and a wide range of dermatophytes. It is fungicidal against *Trichophyton* spp., *Microsporum* spp., and *Aspergillus* spp. It is also active against *Blastomyces dermatitidis, Cryptococcus neoformans, Sporothrix schenckii, Histoplasma capsulatum, Candida,* and *Malassezia* (*Pityrosporum*) yeast. In people, it was more effective than griseofulvin for treating dermatophytes, with fewer relapses (Hoffman et al. 1995). There may also be some activity against protozoa (e.g., *Toxoplasma*).

Pharmacokinetics. Oral bioavailability in most species is high, ranging from >46% in the dog to >85% in mice (Jensen 1989). Its lipophilic nature results in high concentrations in tissues such as stratum corneum, hair follicles, sebum-rich skin, and nails. In people, after 12 days of therapy, the concentrations in stratum corneum exceed those in plasma by a factor of 75. Concentrations in skin may be detected in people as early as 24 hours after oral administration, but maximum concentrations are reached at 7 days. Fungicidal concentrations in nails may require 3 weeks of treatment. Concentrations of terbinafine in the hair of cats being treated for dermatophytosis reach approximately 3.62 μg/g after 120 days of treatment with a dose of 30–40 mg/kg. Like itraconazole, terbinafine is highly protein bound, with values reaching >99% in dogs and rabbits (Jensen 1989).

Clinical Use. Terbinafine has been reported to be efficacious in the treatment of dermatophytosis in dogs and cats, as well as *Malassezia* dermatitis in dogs (Chen 2000). For dermatophytosis, doses of 30–40 mg/kg PO q24h are recommended (Moriello et al. 2004). In both experimental and clinical trials, terbinafine was well tolerated in dogs and cats, and the average treatment length lasted approximately 60 days. Most treatments in cats are for at least 14 days, but may extend to 60 days. For treatment of *Malassezia* dermatitis, terbinafine (30 mg/kg) is as effective as ketoconazole in reducing yeast counts on the skin (Rosales et al. 2005). There are no reports of the use of terbinafine for the treatment of systemic mycoses or of use in large animals.

It should be noted that doses in people are much different. By comparison, doses in people are only 125 mg twice daily (approx. 1.8 mg/kg q12h). Pediatric dose has been in the range of 4–8 mg/kg, once a day, but most often is at the lower dose of 4 mg/kg (Jones 1995). Terbinafine is available as a 1% topical cream (Lamisil, available over the counter) and 125 and 250 mg tablets.

Adverse Effects. In dogs treated with 30 mg/kg, serum ALT concentrations were mildly to moderately elevated in 4 of 10 dogs and ALP was increased in 2 of 10 dogs. Terbinafine does not bind to P450 enzymes as do other antifungal drugs; therefore, it does not cause drug interactions or inhibition of steroid synthesis in animals. In cats facial dermatitis and pruritus has also been reported. This reaction is a problem because it may be confused with an ongoing dermatophyte infection. In people, there is a rare incidence of severe hepatitic failure and death. No teratogenic effects of the drug have been noted in people.

LUFENURON. Lufenuron (Program®), is an orally active inhibitor of chitin synthesis that is commonly used in dogs and cats for control of flea infestations. It has recently been evaluated as an antifungal agent, since fungi also have chitin in their outer cell wall. Although there are reports of successful treatment of dermatophytosis in dogs and cats, the success of this treatment has been controversial.

In the original paper by Ben-Ziony and Arzi (2000), lufenuron provided an effective and rapid treatment of dermatophyte infections in dogs and cats. The effect on fungi is presumably because it also inhibits the cell wall of these fungi, which contains chitin, as well as other complex polysaccharides. A follow-up recommendation by Ben-Ziony and Arzi (2001) suggests that cats should be treated with a minimum dose of 100 mg/kg orally combined with environmental treatment to decrease the spread of fungal spores. House cats and dogs should be treated with 80 mg/kg. Animals that are reexposed to dermatophytes should be retreated 2 weeks after the first treatment. Lufenuron is a highly lipophilic drug and is absorbed best with a meal. If cats have free access to their food, withhold their food until such time that a meal will be consumed readily before administering the lufenuron oral dose.

The experience with lufenuron is still limited and the true efficacy still has to be determined with controlled studies. Some dermatologists are skeptical of lufenuron's efficacy for treatment of dermatophytes. Poor efficacy in some animals has been attributed to inadequate dosing or reexposure from the environment. As a pretreatment for prevention of dermatophyte infection in cats, it was not shown to be effective (Moriello et al. 2004; DeBoer et al. 2003). More recent studies have shown no effect in vitro or in vivo of lufenuron against dermatophytosis. There was a good effect of lufenuron against dermatologic disease not caused by fungi in this study, however, and an immunomodulatory effect was hypothesized (Zur and Elad 2006).

If used for dermatophyte treatment, antifungal doses of lufenuron are higher than those recommended for flea control and have ranged from 50 mg/kg to greater than 250 mg/kg. Most authors recommend treatment with 80–100 mg/kg orally, once every 2 weeks until mycological cure (Ben-Ziony and Arzi 2001).

Topical or local use of lufenuron may be more efficacious. It has been successfully used to treat fungal endometritis caused by *Candida* or *Aspergillus* spp. in horses (Hess et al. 2002). However, this too is controversial because in a study on efficacy and oral absorption (Scotty et al. 2005) lufenuron had no antifungal activity against pathogens important to horses (*Aspergillus* and *Fusarium*). If administered orally, absorption is poor and an oral dose cannot be recommended. Lufenuron may also be used in water baths for the treatment of aquatic species and amphibians (Woolfe et al. 2001).

FLUCYTOSINE. Flucytosine (5-Fluorocytosine, 5-FC, Ancobon) is a synthetic antifungal agent available as an oral preparation. Flucytosine must be taken into the fungal cell by cytosine permeate and then converted to the active form, 5-fluorouracil (5-FU), by a fungal cytosine deaminase enzyme. The 5-FU either is incorporated into RNA, disrupting protein synthesis, or is converted to a related compound that inhibits DNA synthesis. Mammalian cells do not have cytosine deaminase, which results in a selective toxicity of this compound; however, conversion to 5-FU may occur by microbes in the gastrointestinal (GI) tract resulting in 5-FU being taken up by mammalian cells, leading to anemia, leukopenia, and thrombocytopenia (Bennett 1990).

Fungal mutations leading to alterations in the permease or deaminase enzyme activity has led to the development of resistance to flucytosine, both in vitro and during therapy. As a result of this, the therapeutic indications for flucytosine are limited to adjunct therapy with amphotericin B in systemic infections caused by *Candida* or *Cryptococcus neoformans*. Synergy between these two medications, seen as a fourfold reduction in the MIC, has been demonstrated, and combination therapy has been successful, particularly in the treatment of cryptococcal meningitis (Medoff et al. 1971; Utz et al. 1975; Bennett et al. 1979). One explanation of this synergism involves the membrane-permeabilizing effects of amphotericin B facilitating flucytosine's entrance into the cell cytoplasm (Medoff et al. 1972). This combination of antifungal drugs is more effective than amphotericin B alone in the treatment of cryptococcal meningitis (Bennet et al. 1979; Utz et al. 1975). Advantages of this combination include a reduction in the amphotericin B dose, thereby limiting nephrotoxicity, as well as prevention of mutants to flucytosine (Drouhet and Dupont 1987). This combination has also been suggested for therapy of acute hematogenously disseminated candidiasis (Horn et al. 1985). Although flucytosine is synergistic with amphotericin B, there is not evidence of synergism for azole antifungal drugs and this combination should not be used. The combination of flucytosine and ketoconazole proved toxic to cats (Pukay and Dion 1984).

SODIUM OR POTASSIUM IODIDE. Iodide compounds were one of the first antifungal drugs used and they are still used today in veterinary medicine. They are inexpensive and can be administered orally which makes them useful for long-term treatment. The mechanism of action of iodide compounds against fungal organisms is largely unknown, but it may involve stimulating the host's immune response or increasing the elimination of the fungi through the skin or hair. Iodide compounds have been used to treat sporotrichosis in dogs, cats, and donkeys, as well as nasal fungal granulomas caused by *Basidiobolus*, *Conidiobolus*, and *Pseudallescheria* spp. in horses (Koehne et al. 1971; Gonzales Cabo et al. 1989; Irizarry-Rovira et al. 2000; Owens et al. 1985; Zamos et al. 1996; Davis et al. 2000). These drugs are seldom used as a sole therapy, but rather are used as an adjunct to surgical excision, intralesional injection of other antifungals, or systemic antifungal therapy. Toxic effects are possible (iodism) and may occur secondary to excessive iodide levels. Clinical signs attributable to excess iodine include lacrimation, salivation, coughing, anorexia, dry scaly skin, and tachycardia. Abortion and infertility may also be observed, therefore care should be taken when administering this drug to breeding animals. The recommended doses of 20% sodium iodide solution for dogs is 44 mg/kg PO q24h, for cats is 22 mg/kg PO q24h, and for horses is 125 ml IV q24h for 3 days followed by 30 grams PO q24h. Treatment is recommended to extend 30 days beyond the resolution of clinical signs. Iodoject IV is labeled for use in cattle for the treatment of actinomycosis and actinobacillosis at 66 mg/kg IV once a week. The use of this product for fungal infections is considered off label.

TOPICAL ANTIFUNGAL AGENTS

ENILCONAZOLE. Enilconazole (Imaverol®) is also called *imazalil* in some countries. It is an azole antifungal that has excellent activity against dermatophytes and filamentous fungi and it has a residual effect after application. It has been used in some countries for the topical treatment of dermatophyte infections in dogs and horses. For this treatment, a 10% solution is diluted 50 : 1 to form an emulsion. It may be sponged on the animal every 3 or 4 days for 4 treatments. It may be applied to the premises as well to prevent recurring infections. In an evaluation of topical therapies for treatment of dermatophyte infections in dogs and cats (White-Weithers and Medleau 1995), enilconazole was more effective than chlorhexidine, povidone iodine, ketoconazole, sodium hypochlorite, and Captan. The safety of enilconazole has been demonstrated in dogs, even at high doses. One study also showed that enilconazole is safe for treatment of dermatophytes in Persian cats (deJaham 1996). Enilconazole also has been used to treat nasal aspergillosis in dogs. It has a unique vapor effect and, if instilled into the nasal cavity of dogs, will control fungal growth (Sharp et al. 1991; Sharp and Sullivan 1992). A dose of 10 mg/kg in a volume of 5–10 ml is infused twice a day for 7–14 days. In one study using this protocol (Sharp et al. 1993) 26 of 29 affected dogs became asymptomatic. A similar protocol has been used for the successful medical treatment of guttural pouch mycosis caused by *Aspergillus* spp. in the horse (Davis and Legendre 1994).

In the United States, enilconazole is available as Clinafarm®-SG or Clinafarm®-EC. Both are approved for use in poultry hatcheries to control *Aspergillus* organisms on facilities and equipment. Clinafarm®-SG comes in a canister used for smoke generation. Clinafarm-EC is available in a 750 ml bottle containing 13.8% (138 mg/ml) enilconazole. The other ingredients listed on the Material Safety Data Sheet are benzyl alcohol and dioctyl sodium sulfosuccinate. It also contains ethoxylated castor oil. The Canadian formulation of Imaverol contains polysorbate 20 and sorbitan monolaurate as its inert ingredients with 10% enilconazole as the active drug. The Clinafarm-EC formulation is registered for controlling *Aspergillus* organisms in poultry facilities and equipment by making a 1:100 dilution and spraying or fogging the area to be treated. Although there are no published toxicology studies on this particular solution in animals, it has been used in a 50:1 dilution applied topically to dogs and cats without adverse effects. One study applied 100 ml of a 2 mg/ml formulation of Clinafarm-EC to cats and was judged to be safe (Hnilica et al. 2000). However, monitoring of liver enzymes was recommended by these authors.

CLOTRIMAZOLE. Clotrimazole (Lotrimin®) is an imidazole antifungal. It is limited to topical use because after oral administration, the metabolism produces undetectable concentrations of the drug in plasma following repeated dosing. In veterinary medicine, it has been used for treatment of nasal aspergillosis in dogs following infusion of a 1% solution over 1 hour through a nasal catheter (Matthews et al. 1998). It has also been infused into the bladder of dogs and cats with fungal candiduria (Toll et al. 2003, Forward et al. 2002). Clotrimazole can be found in combination with gentamicin sulfate and betamethasone valerate as the product Otomax® and other generic forms that are labeled for the treatment of otitis externa caused by *Malassezia pachydermatitis* or susceptible bacteria in dogs.

MICONAZOLE. Miconazole (Conofite® cream) is an imidazole antifungal effective against some fungi refractory to amphotericin B. Rapid clearance and poor oral absorption necessitated frequent IV infusions during hospitalization. In addition, the solubilizing agent in the parenteral form induces histamine-related toxic side effects, making its use hazardous. The intravenous formulation is no longer marketed in the United States. In veterinary medicine, miconazole is used as a 1% solution for topical treatment of keratomycosis. It is also available as 2% cream or 1% spray or lotion for the treatment of dermatophytosis in dogs and cats. It can also be found combined with chlorhexidine as a shampoo for the adjunct treatment of dermathophytosis in animals.

NATAMYCIN. Natamycin (Natacyn®), is a polyene antifungal with a mechanism of action similar to amphotericin B. It is approved for use in humans as a 5% ophthalmic suspension. Natamycin has excellent activity against yeasts and filamentous fungi, and it is considered the treatment of choice for *Fusarium* keratomycosis in the horse. It is most commonly used in veterinary medicine for treatment of keratomycosis in horses, although it has also been reported as a topical therapy for nasal aspergillosis as well as guttural pouch mycosis and dermatophytosis in these species (Brooks et al. 1998; Greet 1987, 1981; Oldenkamp 1979). Its systemic use is prohibited by expense, as well as toxicity.

NYSTATIN. Nystatin (Mycostatin®) is also a polyene antifungal that is limited to topical use due to systemic toxicity. Nystatin is not absorbed well from the gastrointestinal tract; therefore, it can be given orally as a "topical" treatment for oral and intestinal candidiasis, particularly in exotic animal species (see Table 39.4). In veterinary medicine, it is most commonly used in combination with antibiotics (neomycin, thiostrepton) and antiinflammatory (triamcinolone) drugs in ointments such as Panalog® and other generic formulations.

ANTIVIRAL THERAPY

The use of antiviral drugs in veterinary medicine has been limited. In human medicine, these drugs have gained greater importance and use because of treatment of human immunodeficiency virus (HIV) and associated AIDS, and for treatment of herpesvirus infections, influenza, and other diseases. In veterinary medicine, the use has primarily been limited to treatment of herpesvirus infections. Some are only used topically for treatment of ocular lesions. Consequently, compared to a human textbook, the consideration of these agents in this book is limited. Readers are encouraged to consult a human pharmacology textbook for more in-depth discussion of mechanism of action and antiviral spectrum of these agents.

The antiviral drugs are aimed at preventing or eliminating one of the steps involved in the viral replicative cycle.

IDOXURIDINE AND TRIFLURIDINE

Idoxuridine (5-iodo-2′-deoxyuridine, Herplex®, Stoxil®) and trifluridine (5-trifluoromethyl-2′-deoxyuridine, Viroptic®) are thymidine analogs that are only active against DNA viruses, primarily herpesvirus and poxvirus. The compound is phosphorylated inside the host cell and is then incorporated into growing mammalian and viral DNA strands. This DNA is thought to be more susceptible to breakage and results in faulty proteins if transcribed. Both compounds are commercially available as topical ophthalmic preparations for the treatment of herpetic keratitis. Trifluridine (also known as trifluorothymidine) is thought to have higher affinity for viral DNA than mammalian, as well as being more active; however, it also causes the most conjunctival irritation in vivo (Nasisse et al. 1989). Because of the high cost of these medications, idoxuridine should be used initially, and if no response is seen within 1 week, trifluridine therapy should be initiated (Martin 1990). Toxic side effects, including leukopenia, hepatotoxicity, and GI signs, have precluded their systemic use.

CYTARABINE AND VIDARABINE

Cytarabine (Ara-C®) and vidarabine (Ara-A®), are nucleoside analogs of cytosine and adenine, respectively. They have in vitro activity against certain DNA viruses, including herpesviruses, poxviruses, vaccinia, rabies, cytomegalovirus, and probably hepatitis B virus. Cellular enzymes convert these compounds to the triphosphate form, which then act as competitive inhibitors of DNA polymerase. Herpes-induced DNA polymerase seems to be more sensitive to this inhibition than the mammalian cellular counterpart.

Vidarabine is poorly soluble so must be given intravenously in large fluid volumes over 12 hours. Vidarabine and its active metabolite, hypoxanthine arabinoside, are widely distributed in body fluids and tissues, including the brain and cerebrospinal fluid. Cytarabine is biotransformed to an inactive metabolite and is therefore less effective than vidarabine. Major side effects include GI, neurologic, and hematologic toxicity and teratogenicity.

Vidarabine is used topically in the treatment of herpes keratitis, although it exhibits less potency against feline herpesviruses than does idoxuridine or trifluridine (Nasisse et al. 1989). Vidarabine demonstrated significant antiviral activity in vitro against the feline infectious peritonitis virus. However, this effect was seen only if the compound was used as a pre- or cotreatment with viral inoculation (Barlough and Scott 1990). It also has demonstrated in vitro activity against equine and feline rhinopneumonitis viruses (Babiuk et al. 1975).

Use of these compounds as systemic antiviral drugs in veterinary medicine is not reported. Cytarabine is used as an antineoplastic agent in dogs and cats for treatment of leukemia and lymphoma and is known to cause bone marrow suppression, which would limit its use as an antiviral agent. Its use as an anticancer drug is discussed in more detail in Chapter 45.

RIBAVIRIN

Ribavirin (Virazole®) is a triazole purine nucleoside analog that inhibits the replication of a wide range of RNA and DNA viruses in vitro. Its strongest antiviral activity is against RNA respiratory viruses (influenza A and B) and herpesviruses but also includes myxoviruses, paramyxoviruses, arenaviruses, bunyaviruses, retroviruses, adenoviruses, and poxviruses. Ribavirin is thought to have multiple sites of action. After being monophosphorylated to ribavirin 5′-monophosphate (RMP) by adenosine kinase, it is able to indirectly inhibit synthesis of guanine nucleotides. Further phosphorylation to RTP allows it to competitively inhibit ATP and GTP binding to RNA polymerase.

Ribavirin can be administered by oral, intravenous, and aerosol routes. When administered by the first two routes, anemia due to extravascular hemolysis, bone marrow suppression, GI toxicity, and central nervous signs may occur. In addition, these two routes have been shown to be ineffective in the treatment of influenza A infection (Smith et al. 1980). Aerosolized ribavirin is generally well tolerated (Hall et al. 1983) and is therefore the preferred route for treating susceptible respiratory infections.

Oral ribavirin was seen to worsen the condition of cats experimentally infected with calicivirus. Bone marrow suppression, weight loss, increased hepatic enzymes, and icterus were seen (Povey 1978). These side effects were also seen in healthy cats given the drug (Weiss et al. 1993a); however, they were not seen in dogs when given 60 mg/kg for 2 weeks (Canonico 1985). Ribavirin was shown to have in vitro antiviral activity against the FIP virus at concentrations of 150 μg/ml (Barlough and Scott 1990). Kittens experimentally infected with FIP virus had no significant difference in outcome when compared to those treated with placebo (Weiss et al. 1993b). In fact, similar to the cats infected with calicivirus, the ribavirin treated FIP kittens had a worsening of clinical signs. In vitro activity against bovine rhinotracheitis and bovine viral diarrhea has also been demonstrated, but there are no reports of the use of this compound in infected animals (Glotov et al. 2004).

ACYCLOVIR, PENCICLOVIR, AND RELATED PRODRUGS (VALACYCLOVIR AND FAMCICLOVIR)

ACYCLOVIR. Acyclovir (Zovirax®) is a synthetic nucleoside analog of the purine deoxyguanosine that has antiviral activity restricted to herpesviruses. Acyclovir is particularly active against herpes simplex 1 and 2 viruses and varicella-zoster virus but is less active against Epstein-Barr and cytomegaloviruses (CMV). Herpesvirus infections (feline herpesvirus type-1, FHV-1) in cats have been described (Thomasy et al. 2007; and in review by Gaskell et al. 2007). Infections consist of respiratory illness, upper respiratory disease, and ocular lesions. Unfortunately, some of the drugs used for herpesvirus infection in people are not as active against the feline virus (Maggs et al. 2004; Gaskell et al. 2007). Administration of valacyclovir to cats did not suppress FHV-1 and produced toxicity (see adverse effects below) (Nasisse et al. 1997).

Herpesvirus infections are particularly important in horses. In horses, the equine herpesvirus type 1 (EHV-1) causes myeloencephalopathy, respiratory disease, abortion, and neonatal infections. The sensitivity of EHV-1 to acyclovir is similar to humans with an inhibitory concentration (IC_{50}) of 0.3 μg/ml, although one study cited effective concentrations (EC_{50}) of 1.7 to 3.0 μg/ml (Garré et al. 2007).

Acyclovir is monophosphorylated by viral thymidine kinase 200 times easier than by the similar mammalian enzyme, which contributes to its good selective toxicity and high therapeutic index. Cellular enzymes then form the di- and triphosphate form, which selectively inhibit the viral DNA polymerase by competing with deoxyguanosine triphosphate. Acyclo-GTP that is incorporated into viral DNA strands causes termination of elongation. Virally infected cells are 40–100 times more efficient in converting acyclo-GMP to acyclo-GTP than are noninfected cells. Penciclovir (discussed below) and ganciclovir have similar mechanisms of action against herpesvirus. Ganciclovir has better activity than acyclovir against FHV-1 (Maggs et al. 2004) and also has activity against cytomegalovirus (CMV), but its use in animals has not been reported.

Pharmacokinetic data for acyclovir are available for horses, dogs, and cats, as well as Quaker parakeets and pheasants and other species (de Miranda et al. 1982, 1981). Oral bioavailability of the drug is high in dogs (>80%), moderate in people (10–30%), but low and variable in horses (<5%). In horses, the oral absorption was undetectable in one study (Wilkins et al. 2005), and only 2.8–4% in other studies (Garré et al. 2007; Benz et al. 2006), but when administered IV the half-life of approximately 5, 7, or 9 hours, depending on the study (Garré et al. 2007; Wilkins et al.; Bentz et al. 2006) was longer than in other species (half-life 2.3 hours in dogs and 2.6 hours in cats). An IV infusion of 10 mg/kg for 1 hour produced effective concentrations in horses for 8 hours and they concluded that this treatment could be administered twice daily for EHV-1 (Wilkins et al. 2005).

Orally administered acyclovir at 80 mg/kg IM 24 hours after herpesvirus infection in Quaker parakeets was shown to be more effective in preventing death than either low- or high-dose (40 or 250 mg/kg) intramuscular injections. At the highest dose tested, acyclovir toxicity, as seen by local muscular necrosis, was thought to contribute to bird mortality (Norton et al. 1991). Acyclovir has been shown to decrease mortality in psittacine birds with herpesviral infections if the drug is administered prior to the onset of clinical signs (Smith 1987).

Acyclovir has been used as a treatment for equine herpesvirus encephalitis. In one herd outbreak of EHV-1 neurologic disease, 7 of 19 horses were treated with acyclovir. Only one of the treated horses was euthanized; however, none of the untreated horses was euthanized (Friday et al. 2000). Given the low oral bioavailability of this drug in adult horses, its usefulness is questionable and other drugs have been considered as alternatives (see valacyclovir and penciclovir, below). Doses recommended in the literature include 10 mg/kg PO q4h and 20 mg/kg PO q8h. Acyclovir may be more useful as a treatment of neonatal herpesvirus infection. In one herd outbreak of EHV-1 in foals, 2 of 3 foals treated with acyclovir survived, whereas the 2 foals not treated died (Murray et al. 1998). Since this disease is almost universally fatal in foals, acyclovir shows promise as a therapeutic agent. The pharmacokinetics have not been studied in neonatal foals, but oral absorption may be higher, as has been seen with several other compounds.

In dogs, acyclovir is well absorbed (80–90%), but oral absorption may become saturated at high doses (Krasny et al. 1981). The elimination half-life in dogs is 2.2–3.6 hours and clearance in dogs appears to be primarily via glomerular secretion (de Miranda et al. 1981, 1982; Krasny et al. 1981).

In birds, herpesvirus infections can be an important cause of morbidity. When acyclovir was administered orally to pheasants (Rush et al. 2005), the half-life of acyclovir was approximately 3 hours. A range of doses were examined in this study, from 40 to 120 mg/kg. It was concluded that, to maintain concentrations necessary to produce antiviral effects (>1.0 μg/ml), a dose of 120 mg/kg orally every 12 hours should be used.

Valacyclovir (Valtrex). Acyclovir is absorbed poorly and inconsistently. Therefore, the prodrug valacyclovir is used to produce more effective and consistent blood concentrations. Valacyclovir (500 mg and 1 gram tablets) is much more expensive than acyclovir. As long as the expense remains high, the application for some animals, especially horses, will be uncommon. Nevertheless, valacyclovir has important advantages. It is absorbed as the prodrug, and then converted to the active drug—acyclovir—in the patient. Compared to 10–30% oral absorption of acyclovir in people, it is increased to 55% if administered as the prodrug. In horses, valacyclovir also appears to have good absorption compared to acyclovir and may potentially be used in horses to treat and prevent infections caused by EHV-1 (Garré et al. 2007). This study showed that compared to acyclovir oral absorption of 3%, oral absorption from valacyclovir was 26% in horses. These authors predicted that a dose of 40 mg/kg every 8 hours orally to horses would maintain concentrations above an effective level of 1.7 to 3.0 μg/ml for EHV-1 infections.

Valacyclovir should not be administered to cats because it does not suppress FHV-1 and is toxic, which is discussed in more detail below in the section "Adverse Effects" (Nasisse et al. 1997).

PENCICLOVIR AND FAMCICLOVIR. Penciclovir is administered topically (cream) for herpesvirus infections in people (Denavir). After topical application of the cream, the systemic absorption of penciclovir is negligible. Oral absorption of penciclovir is poor; therefore, the oral prodrug famciclovir—an ester of penciclovir—is administered instead. Penciclovir has a similar mechanism of action as acyclovir, but the half-life in virus-infected cells is 10–20 times longer (Gill and Wood 1996). In people, oral absorption of penciclovir, administered as the prodrug famciclovir, is 60% and 77% (depending on the study) (Gill and Wood 1996). After administration of famciclovir, there is extensive first-pass metabolism in people to produce the active drug. In cats, famciclovir has been used but the activity is questionable. The activity of penciclovir is not as high against the feline virus as it is against the human herpesvirus. The effective concentration (EC_{50}) has been reported as 3.5 μg/ml (Thomasy et al. 2007). When famciclovir was administered to cats at a dose of 15 mg/kg plasma concentrations were highly variable, but no adverse effects were observed. There appeared to be nonlinear (saturable) pharmacokinetics that is a potential problem for extrapolating doses and effects from multiple administrations. Plasma concentrations were much lower than reported for people, which indicates either a lack of intestinal absorption in cats, or a deficiency in cats for conversion of famciclovir to the active drug. The enzyme needed for conversion is hepatic aldehyde oxidase, which is deficient in cats (Dick et al. 2005). The half-life of penciclovir in cats was 3–4 hours and produced concentrations of 0.3 to 0.7 μg/ml (depending on the interval) but these were only 1/5 to 1/11 of the concentration needed to inhibit feline herpesvirus (Thomasy et al. 2007). Despite some of these drawbacks famciclovir has been used to treat feline herpesvirus-1 associated disease in cats (Malik et al. 2009). In the report by Malik et al. (2009) ten cats were treated with famciclovir at a dose of 62.5 mg per cat twice daily or 125 mg per cat three times daily. Although the study was not controlled, the drug was well tolerated in the cats and it appeared to have a positive effect on resolution of conjunctivitis, keratitis, rhinosinusitis and FHV-1 associated dermatitis. Absorption in dogs is higher than in cats (Filer et al. 1995). When a dose of 25 mg/kg was administered to dogs, plasma penciclovir concentrations were similar to those achieved in people. Although the conversion of famciclovir to penciclovir was slower than in other species, the pharmacokinetics are otherwise similar to people.

Adverse Effects. The adverse effects of acyclovir and related drugs have not been well-documented in animals because of their infrequent use. In people, CNS effects are the most common and consist of headache, dizziness, depression, and other CNS-related problems. When acyclovir is administered, the IV infusion should be given over 1 hour to diminish the risk of CNS problems.

When famciclovir was administered to cats, no adverse effects were reported, but absorption and conversion to the active drug was low (Thomasy et al. 2007). However, when valacyclovir was administered to cats at a dose of 60 mg/kg orally every 6 hours there were serious adverse reactions (Nasisse et al. 1997). Cats in this study became depressed and dehydrated, developed severe bone marrow suppression, and developed hepatic and renal necrosis.

ZIDOVUDINE

Zidovudine (Azidothymidine®, AZT®, Retrovir®) is a thymidine analog in which the 3′ hydroxy of the deoxyribose sugar has been replaced with an azido group. Zidovudine is more commonly known as *AZT*. AZT is phosphorylated by cellular enzymes to the triphosphate analog. This form inhibits viral reverse transcriptase (RNA-dependent DNA polymerase) as well as causing chain termination due to the unavailability of a 3′-hydroxyl moiety. AZT inhibits the viral enzyme with greater affinity (~100 times) than mammalian DNA polymerases, resulting in selective activity and low mammalian toxicity.

AZT can be given orally or IV in humans. Its oral bioavailability is 60–65%, and peak concentrations are achieved in about 1 hour. Only 25% of the drug is bound to plasma, and concentrations in the cerebrospinal fluid are similar to plasma concentrations. AZT is quickly metabolized to the 5′glucuronide, and both the metabolite and parent compound are eliminated in urine with a half-life of approximately 1 hour. The pharmacokinetics of AZT at a dose of 25 mg/kg have recently been studied in cats following IV, PO, or intragastric (IG) administration through a gastrostomy tube (Zhang et al. 2004a). Absorption following PO administration (95%) was higher than IG administration (70%), but effective plasma concentrations, as determined by the in vitro EC_{50}, were maintained for at least 12 hours following administration by all three routes. As in humans, half-life was short (1.4 hr). No adverse effects, other than hemolysis after IV injection, were observed in this study; however, only single doses were administered. These same investigators also studied the pharmacokinetics of a related compound, lamivudine, in cats (Zhang et al. 2004b). This drug was studied because it has a higher safety profile than AZT, probably because it does not get transported into the mitochondria of the cells. Additionally, lamivudine was more potent against FIV in vitro compared to other antiviral agents, including AZT. The pharmacokinetics were similar to those of AZT in cats, with a high bioavailability, short half-life, and plasma concentrations maintained above the predicted EC_{50} for 12 hours following either IV, PO, or IG dosing of 25 mg/kg.

Major toxicities of AZT include anemia and granulocytopenia, which occur in up to 45% of treated human patients (Richman et al. 1987). Dose escalation studies have demonstrated a dose-dependent and progressive anemia and neutropenia in cats chronically administered >30 mg/kg/day PO divided into three doses for 32–34 days. Marked bone marrow hypercellularity and extramedullar hematopoeisis were observed on postmortem examination (Haschek et al. 1990).

The use of AZT has been investigated in cats both as a clinical therapy for FIV and experimentally, using FIV as an animal model of HIV infection. Reverse transcriptase from FIV and HIV-1 viruses was shown to be nearly identical in sensitivity to several antiviral agents, including AZT. In addition, similar concentrations of AZT were required to inhibit replication of these viruses (North et al. 1989). Bovine leukemia virus has also been suggested as a possible animal model for investigation of retroviral infection. AZT inhibition of BLV reverse transcriptase was similar to that of FIV-RT (Reimer et al. 1989).

AZT has been shown to reduce clinical signs when given to two FIV-positive cats at a dose of 10 mg/kg twice a day subcutaneously for a period of 3 weeks (Egberink et al. 1991). Although it did not eradicate the infection, the authors suggest it is of clinical benefit and should extend the life of FIV-infected cats. In experimental FeLV infections, when treated with AZT within 1 week after virus challenge, cats are protected from bone marrow infection and viremia. Viremia persisted in cats treated between 1 and 3 weeks; however, antigen load in the blood was reduced (Tavares et al. 1987). AZT alone, or in combination with interferon or interleukin, was shown to prevent infection in cats challenged with virulent FeLV virus for a period of 6 weeks (Zeidner et al. 1989).

FOSCARNET

Foscarnet (trisodium phosphonoformate hexahydrate; PFA) is a pyrophosphate analog that exhibits antiviral activity against a variety of DNA and RNA viruses. It inhibits DNA and RNA polymerases as well as reverse transcriptase. The mechanism of foscarnet activity differs from that of the preceding antiviral agents in that it inhibits these enzymes by binding at the pyrophosphate binding site rather than at a base binding site. Thus, inhibition is noncompetitive rather than competitive (Oberg 1989).

Because phosphorylation by viral kinases is unnecessary for antiviral activity, it has potential for use in thymidine kinase-deficient herpesvirus infections (Teich et al. 1992); however, in vitro it demonstrates no antiviral activity against FHV-1 (Maggs and Clarke 2004). Viruses inhibited include avian myeloblastosis, Moloney murine leukemia, Rauscher leukemia, visna, influenza, bovine leukemia, African swine fever, baboon endogenous virus, simian sarcoma, human herpes, and human immunodeficiency viruses (Swenson et al. 1991a).

Although viral replication has been shown to be inhibited at concentrations achievable in plasma, these concentrations often vary widely. In addition, variable interindividual pharmacokinetics in humans makes optimal dosage regimens difficult to identify (Lietman 1992). The pharmacokinetics of PFA have been investigated in the cat (Straw et al. 1992). PFA was only 8% bioavailable, had a terminal half-life of approximately 3 hours, and was not metabolized, resulting in a total clearance of 1.88 ml/min/kg. The related compound thiofoscarnet (thiophosphonoformate, TPFA) had greater bioavailability (22–44%) and a shorter plasma half-life (42 minutes) and was metabolized to the active PFA, suggesting its possible use as a prodrug. The percutaneous absorption of PFA was studied in rabbits and dogs to ensure its safe topical use in herpetic mucocutaneous conditions. Systemic absorption after vaginal application was found to be 14% in the rabbit and 34% in the dog, whereas 12% (rabbit) and 3% (dog) of the dose entered the systemic circulation after topical administration (Hussain and Ritschel 1989).

The prophylactic and therapeutic use of PFA has been suggested in the cat (Swenson et al. 1991a). It is thought that long-term PFA administration to FeLV-infected cats may limit spread of infection within and between hosts via extracellular inactivation of newly produced virus particles. The authors also suggest PFA may have a role as a viral disinfectant for blood, blood products, supplies, and equipment. Toxicities associated with PFA include alterations in calcium/phosphorus homeostasis, as well as ricketslike lesions in young cats (Swenson et al. 1991b). Older cats do not show any significant changes in blood calcium levels, however osteomalacia can be seen.

AMANTADINE AND RIMANTADINE

Amantadine hydrochloride (1-adamantanamine hydrochloride, Symmetrel®) and rimantadine (Flumadine®) are water-soluble cyclic amines with antiviral activity against a narrow range of RNA viruses, including myxoviruses, paramyxoviruses, togaviruses, and most strains of influenza A virus. Rimantadine has approximately 3–4 times greater *in vitro* activity against influenza A than amantadine (Betts 1991). The mechanism of these two related compounds has been debated. They were thought at one time to prevent viral penetration and uncoating (Hoffman et al. 1965), but this was later refuted (Couch and Six 1986). Their antiviral activity is now thought to involve inhibition of late-stage assembly of the virus.

Both amantadine and rimantadine are absorbed well from the human GI tract. Serum concentrations of amantadine are greater than those of rimantadine, but the latter achieves greater concentrations in secretions (Hayden et al. 1985). The volume of distribution of amantadine is significantly less than that of rimantadine. Amantadine is excreted unchanged in urine, with an elimination half-life of ~16 hours, whereas rimantadine is 85% metabolized and eliminated with a 24–36 hour half-life. Neither agent has bone marrow, renal, or hepatic side effects, but amantadine may be neurotoxic, causing jitters, difficulty in concentrating, and seizures in certain patient populations. CNS side effects are less frequent with rimantadine. The combination of greater in vitro efficacy, greater distribution and terminal half-life, and less toxicity suggests rimantadine has greater clinical potential.

Both compounds are equally effective in the prophylactic prevention of respiratory infections caused by influenza A virus, although not as effective as vaccination. They have also been used to treat flu outbreaks, resulting in shorter duration fever and more rapid resolution of symptoms (VanVoris et al. 1981). Experimentally infected chicks that received amantadine via the drinking water were one-half as likely to die as untreated controls (Obrosova-Serova et al. 1976). However, the use of amantadine in poultry is thought to be responsible for the amantadine resistant influenza strains seen in the Chinese pandemic in 2005 (Ilyushina et al. 2005). The use of this drug in poultry should therefore be discontinued due to the potential human health risk. Amantadine had no inhibitory effect on FIP virus replication in vitro at the highest concentration tested (Barlough and Scott 1990).

These two compounds have been recently investigated for the treatment of influenza in the horse. In vitro testing suggests that amantadine suppresses viral replication at concentrations of 300 ng/ml while rimantadine is more potent and has activity at concentrations as low as 30 ng/ml (Rees et al. 1997, 1999). Amantadine caused serious adverse effects, including fatal seizures, in horses at doses of 10–15 mg/kg IV. Absorption of the drug following oral administration was highly variable between individual horses; therefore, a dose could not be recommended (Rees et al. 1997). Rimantadine shows greater promise as an antiviral drug in horses. A multiple dose study examining the effects of oral rimantadine at a dose of 30 mg/kg q12h showed adequate absorption of the drug with plasma concentrations maintained above the estimated effective concentration (30 ng/ml) throughout the dosing interval. No side effects were reported. In challenge studies using influenza virus A2, prophylactic rimantadine administration caused a significant decrease in rectal temperature and lung sounds (Rees et al. 1999).

TREATMENT OF PAIN. An additional use of amantadine is for treatment of pain syndromes in animals. The proposed mechanism of action for amantadine is via inhibiting the neurotransmitter N-methyl-D-aspartate (NMDA) (Pozzi et al. 2006). NMDA produces central sensitization and pain in animals. Blocking of the NMDA central receptor by amantadine has been associated with relief of pain syndromes. Amantadine is well absorbed orally in practically all animals, but the precise duration of action and dosing regimens have not been fully investigated in animals. In one study, it was used—in combination with nonsteroidal antiinflammatory drugs (NSAIDs)—for treatment of pain in dogs (Lascelles et al. 2007). At a dose of 3–5 mg/kg orally, once daily, with meloxicam, dogs responded better than if administered meloxicam alone. Other doses that have been cited for pain are 2–10 mg/kg orally every 8–12 hours in dogs and 2 mg/kg orally every 24 hours in cats (Pozzi et al. 2006).

INTERFERON

A complete discussion of the biochemistry, physiology, and immunological function of interferon-$\alpha_{2a,2b}$ (Roferon-A, Intron A) is beyond the scope of this chapter. Interferons are glycopolypeptide molecules produced by certain mammalian cells in response to viral infections as well as other stimuli. They are potent cytokines that possess antiviral, immunomodulating, and anticancer properties (Pestka et al. 1987). At least four classes of interferons (IFNs) exist: alpha, beta, omega, and gamma, with the last being produced solely by T lymphocytes. Subtypes can exist within each class. The antiviral activities of interferons are indirect. They cause the induction of a variety of antiviral enzyme systems within the host cells that, in turn, inhibit protein synthesis and degrade viral RNA (Moore 1996). Two of these proteins, MxA and 2′,5′ oligoadenylate synthetase, are often used as a marker protein for IFN activity, since blood concentrations of IFN may not be measurable. An interesting property of IFNs is that once they induce an antiviral state in one cell, that cell can then transfer this antiviral activity to other cells through cell-to-cell contact without requiring additional IFN. This has been demonstrated in vivo using IFN-α stimulated lymphocytes. This results in an amplification of the antiviral effect, which may explain why IFNs are efficacious despite low to undetectable plasma levels (Stanton et al. 1989). Interferons are highly conserved between species and therefore their actions are not species-specific. Natural, bacteria-derived IFNs appear to be more potent than recombinant IFNs, possibly because they contain more than one subtype, thereby providing a broader effect. In people, multiple interferons have been used for treatment of AIDS-related diseases, and cancer-associated diseases.

Interferons have been administered parenterally, intranasally, and orally. Parenteral and intranasal administration lead to an increased risk of adverse effects, including formation of neutralizing antibodies to IFN, as well as clinical signs of hyperthermia, anorexia, and malaise (Roney et al. 1985). Being peptides, interferons are inactivated by the digestive enzymes in the gastrointestinal tract, yet orally administered IFN has been shown to be an effective treatment for viral diseases in a number of species. The probable mechanism for this is uptake of IFN by the oropharyngeal-associated lympoid tissue, which sensitizes the lymphocytes in these organs. The lymphocytes are then released into the circulation where they can confer antiviral activity to cells at the site of infection (Bocci 1991).

In vitro studies have demonstrated that FHV-1 is susceptible to feline interferon or human interferon. Most of the use has been anecdotal with few clinical trials to demonstrate efficacy for treating FHV-1 infections (Gaskell et al. 2007). Interferons are licensed for use in the treatment of viral disease of dogs and cats in Japan and other countries. A summary of some of the reports of interferon use in natural and experimental viral disease of different species is presented in Table 39.5.

TABLE 39.5 Clinical and experimental uses of interferon in veterinary species

Species	Disease Treated	IFN Subtype	Dose and Route of Administration	Results	Reference
Feline	FIP (coronavirus)	Recombinant feline IFN-γ	1 million U/kg SC EOD until remission followed by weekly injections of the same dose	Produce complete remission (>2 years) in 4/12 cats, and partial remission (2–5 months) in 4/12 cats; only cats with the effusive form of FIP responded.	Ishida et al. 2004
	FeLV or FeLV/FIV coinfection	Recombinant feline IFN-ω	1 million U/kg SC q24h for 5 consecutive days in 3 series (day 0, 14, and 60)	Placebo controlled study; treated cats had significantly lower clinical scores in the first 4 months and significantly lower mortality rates at 9 and 12 months.	de Mari et al. 2004
	FeLV	Human IFN-α with or without *Staphylococcus* Protein A (SPA)	30 U/cat PO once daily on weeks 1,3,5,7, and 9	Placebo controlled study; no significant improvements seen in animals treated with IFN compared to controls; mild improvement noted based on owner perception in cats treated with SPA alone.	McCaw et al. 2001
	FIV	Natural human IFN-α	10 IU/kg PO q24h on alternating weeks for 6 months	Treated cats had a significant improvement in clinical signs and a longer survival than controls; no correlation with plasma viremia or viral load in leukocytes was noted.	Pedretti et al. 2005
Canine	Parvovirus (CPV-2)	Recombinant feline IFN-ω	1 million U/kg IV q24h for 3 consecutive days starting 4 days after viral inoculation	Placebo controlled study; treatment significantly reduced the severity of the enteritis within 12 hours of administration of the first dose; all dogs received standard supportive therapy.	Ishiwata et al. 1998
	Parvovirus	Recombinant feline IFN-ω	2.5 million U/kg IV q24h for 3 consecutive days	Multicentric, double-blind, placebo controlled field trial; treated dogs showed a significant improvement in clinical signs; mortality rate was 7% in treated dogs and 29% in controls; all dogs received standard supportive therapy.	de Mari et al. 2003
Bovine	Vaccinia (Smallpox)	Natural human IFN-α2	10 million U/kg IM q24h starting 24 hours prior to viral inoculation	Placebo controlled study; complete protection was obtained at this dose.	Werenne et al. 1985
	IBR	Recombinant human IFN-α	0.05–5 U/kg PO q24h for 4 days starting 48 hours prior to intranasal viral inoculation	Placebo controlled study; the 0.05 and 0.5 U/kg groups showed significant improvement in mean rectal temperature and duration of antibiotic therapy; the 0.05 U/kg group also had significantly better weight gain.	Cummins et al. 1993

TABLE 39.5—*continued*

Species	Disease Treated	IFN Subtype	Dose and Route of Administration	Results	Reference
	IBR	Recombinant bovine IFN-α1	10 mg/animal intranasally 48 hours prior to viral inoculation	Significant reduction in morbidity and mortality in treated animals was noted, although treatment did not prevent clinical signs or affect viral shedding.	Babiuk et al. 1987
Equine	EHV-1	Recombinant human IFN-α2a	0.22 or 2.2 U/kg PO 48 and 24 hours prior to viral inoculation and 24 hours after inoculation	No significant effects on clinical disease or duration of viral shedding were noted.	Seahorn et al. 1990
	Inflammatory airway disease	Recombinant and natural human IFN-α	90 U/horse (recombinant) or 50 U/horse (natural) PO q24h for 5 days	Placebo controlled study; all horses had a significant decrease in cough and nasal discharge; significantly fewer horses treated with either IFN product had a relapse after 4 weeks; viral etiology in this disease not proven.	Moore et al. 2004

VIRBAGEN OMEGA. Recombinant omega interferon contained in Virbagen omega is produced by silkworms previously inoculated with interferon-recombinant baculovirus resulting in the synthesis of pure interferon. Omega interferon of feline origin, produced by genetic engineering, is a type 1 interferon closely related to α interferon.

After injection, omega interferon has a half-life of 1.4 hours in dogs and 1.7 hours in cats. It is bound to receptors in cells infected by virus. Interferon has been used to stimulate immune cells in dogs with parvovirus and in cats with feline retrovirus (Feline Leukemia Virus, *FeLV*, and Feline Immunodeficiency Virus, *FIV*).

ADVERSE REACTIONS. In people, injections of interferon α have been associated with influenzalike symptoms. Other effects also have been reported in people, such as bone marrow suppression. In animals, interferon has been generally well tolerated, but may induce vomiting and nausea. In some animals it may induce hyperthermia 3–6 hours after injection. In cats, it may produce soft feces to mild diarrhea. A slight decrease in white blood cells, platelets, and red blood cells, and rise in the concentration of alanine aminotransferase may be observed. These parameters usually return to normal in the week following the last injection. In cats, it may induce transient fatigue during the treatment. Do not vaccinate dogs or cats receiving interferon.

Doses and indications for animals have primarily been based on extrapolation of human recommendations, experimental studies in animals, or specific studies in cats with viral infections.

The formulation used in veterinary medicine is available in 5 and 10 million units/vial, which is reconstituted before use. In dogs, administer 2.5 million units/kg IV once daily for 3 consecutive days. In cats, administer 1.0 million units/kg IV once daily for 5 consecutive days. Three separate 5-day treatments must be performed at day 0, day 14, and day 60.

L-LYSINE

L-lysine is an essential amino acid that blocks the availability of arginine, which is necessary for the replication of herpesviruses. In vitro testing has demonstrated an inhibitory effect of L-lysine on FHV-1 replication in the presence of arginine (Maggs et al. 2000). Additionally, a dose of 400 mg per day, given in food, reduced viral shedding following the stress of changes in housing and husbandry (Maggs et al. 2003). This beneficial effect was blocked when the cats were given methylprednisolone to induce viral shedding; however, L-lysine may also be efficacious in cases of herpesvirus keratitis in cats. When given prophylactically at a dose of 500 mg 6 hours prior to viral challenge, and then continued at 500 mg PO q12h, it decreased the severity of the ocular lesions compared to controls; however, it had no effect on virus isolation (Stiles et al. 2002). Despite the positive results cited above, a clinical study in shelter population cats did not show a benefit of treatment (Rees and Lubinski 2008). When 144 treated shelter cats were compared to 147 controls, there was no difference in prevention of upper respiratory infection or conjunctivitis when cats were supplemented with 250 or 500 mg daily oral L-lysine.

PMEA

The acyclic purine nucleoside analog 9–2(phosphonomethoxyethyl) adenine (PMEA) has been studied in the treatment of both FeLV and FIV infections in cats. PMEA was found to inhibit replication of FeLV in vitro and prevented the development of persistent antiginemia and the induction of the immunodeficiency disease in cats exposed to the virus (Hoover et al. 1991). PMEA exhibited similar effects against FIV infection. Seropositive cats with symptoms of opportunistic infection showed improvement of clinical signs during PMEA therapy at 5 mg/kg/day (Egberink et al. 1990). A comparative study on the effects of PMEA and AZT on FIV- or FeLV-positive cats showed that PMEA was superior to AZT in diminishing the clinical signs of disease; however, the adverse effects (mainly hematological) were more severe with PMEA than AZT, which would limit its use (Hartmann et al. 1992).

REFERENCES

Adamcak, A., and Otten, B. Rodent therapeutics. 2000. Vet Clin North Am Exot Anim Pract 3(1):221–37, viii.

AHFS Drug Information. Fluconazole. In McEvoy, G.K. (ed). American Society of Hospital Pharmacists pub. Bethesda, MD 1992:72–78.

Babiuk, L.A., Lawman, M.J., and Gifford, G.A. Use of recombinant bovine alpha 1 interferon in reducing respiratory disease induced by bovine herpesvirus type 1. 1987. Antimicrob Agents Chemother 31(5): 752–7.

Babiuk, L.A., Meldrum, B., Gupta, V.S., and Rouse, B.T. Comparison of the antiviral effects of 5-methoxymethyl-deoxyuridine with 5-iododeoxyuridine, cytosine arabinoside, and adenine arabinoside. 1975. Antimicrob Agents Chemother 8(6):643–50.

Balfour, J.A., and Faulds, D. Terbinafine: a review of its pharmacodynamic and pharmacokinetic properties and therapeutic potential in superficial mycoses. 1992. Drugs 43:258–284.

Barlough, J.E., and Scott, F.W. Effectiveness of three antiviral agents against FIP virus in vitro. 1989. Vet Rec 126:556–558.

Begg, L.M., Hughes, K.J., Kessell, A., Krockenberger, M.B., Wigney, D.I., and Malik, R. Successful treatment of cryptococcal pneumonia in a pony mare. 2004. Aust Vet J 82(11):686–92.

Bennett, J.E. Amphotericin B binding to serum β-lipoprotein. In Iwala, K. (ed). Recent Advances in Medical and Veterinary Mycology. Proc 6th ISHAM University Park Press, Baltimore, MD 1977;107–109.

———. Antimicrobial agents: antifungal agents. In Gilman, A.G., Rall, T.W., Nies, A.S. and Taylor, P. (eds). The Pharmacological Basis of Therapeutics. Pergamon Press, New York 1990;1165–1181.

Bennett, J.E., Dismukes, W.E., Duma, R.F., Medoff, G., Sande, M.A., Gallis, H., Leonard, J., Fields, B.T., Bradshaw, M., Haywood, H., McGee, Z.A., Cate, T.R., Cobbs, C.G., Warner, J.F., and Alling, D.W. A comparison of amphotericin B alone and combined with flucytosine in the treatment of cryptococcal meningitis. 1979. N Engl J Med 301:126–131.

Bentz, B.G., Maxwell, L.K., Erkert, R.S., Royer, C.M., Davis, M.S., MacAllister, C.G., and Clarke, C.R. Pharmacokinetics of acyclovir after single intravenous and oral administration to adult horses. 2006. J Vet Intern Med 20:589–594.

Ben-Ziony, Y., and Arzi, B. Use of lufenuron for treating fungal infections of dogs and cats: 297 cases (1997–1999). 2000. J Am Vet Med Assoc 217(10):1510–3.

———. Updated information for treatment of fungal infections in cats and dogs. 2001. J Am Vet Med Assoc 218(11):1718.

Betts, R.F. Antiviral agents in respiratory infections. 1991. Sem Resp Infect 6(3):146–157.

Bocci, V. Absorption of cytokines via oropharyngeal-associated lymphoid tissues. Does an unorthodox route improve the therapeutic index of interferon? 1991. Clin Pharmacokinet 21(6):411–7.

Bonner, B.B. Chelonian therapeutics. 2000. Vet Clin North Am Exot Anim Pract3(1):257–332, viii.

Boothe, D.M., Herring, I., Calvin, J., Way, N., and Dvorak, J. 1997. Itraconazole disposition after single oral and intravenous and multiple oral dosing in healthy cats. 1997. Am J Vet Res 58(8):872–7.

Brajtburg, J., Powderly, W.G., Kobayashi, G.S., and Medoff, G. Amphotericin B: current understanding of mechanisms of action. 1990. Antimicrob Agents Chemother 34:183–188.

Brammer, K.W., Farrow, P.R., and Faulkner, J.K. Pharmacokinetics and tissue penetration of fluconazole in humans. 1990. Rev Infect Dis 12(S3):318–326.

Brooks, D.E., Andrew, S.E., Dillavou, C.L., Ellis, G., and Kubilis, P.S. Antimicrobial susceptibility patterns of fungi isolated from horses with ulcerative keratomycosis. 1998. Am J Vet Res 59(2):138–42.

Brooks, D.E., Legendre, A.M., Gum, G.G., Laratta, L.J., Abrams, K.L., and Morgan, R.V. The treatment of canine ocular blastomycosis with systemically administered itraconazole. 1992. Prog Vet Comp Ophth 4:263–268.

Bruyette, D.S., and Feldman, E.C. Ketoconazole and its use in the management of canine Cushing's disease. 1988. Compen Contin Educ Pract Vet 10(12):1379–1386.

Butler, W.T., and Hill, G.J. Intravenous administration of amphotericin B in the dog. 1964. J Am Vet Med Assoc 144:399–402.

Canonico, P.G. Efficacy, toxicity and clinical application of ribavirin against virulent RNA viral infections. 1985. Antiviral Res (Suppl1): 75–81.

Cauwenbergh, G. and DeDoncker, P. The clinical use of itraconazole in superficial and deep mycoses. In Fromtling, R.A. (ed). Recent Trends in the Discovery, Development and Evaluation of Antifungal Agents. JR Prous Publishers, Barcelona 1987;273–284.

Cauwenbergh, G., Doncker, P.D., Stoops, K., DeDier, A.M., Goyvaerts, H. and Schuermans, V. Itraconazole in the treatment of human mycoses: Review of three years of clinical experience. 1987. Rev Infect Dis 9(S1):146–152.

Colitz, C.M.H., Latimer, F.G., Cheng, H., Chan, K.K., Reed, S.M., and Pennick, G.J. Pharmacokinetics of voriconazole following intravenous and oral administration and body fluid concentrations of voriconazole following repeated oral administration in horses. 2007. Am J Vet Res 68:1115–1121.

Cornick, J.L. Diagnosis and treatment of pulmonary histoplasmosis in a horse. 1990. Cornell Vet 80(1):97–103.

Couch, R.B., and Six, H.R. The antiviral spectrum and mechanism of action of amantadine and rimantadine. In Antiviral Chemotherapy: New Directions for Clinical Applications and Research. (Mills, J., and Corey, L., eds) Elsevier, New York 1986; 50–57.

Craig, A., Malik, R., and Ramzan, I. Pharmacokinetics of fluconazole in the cat. 1993. J Am Col Vet Int Med 7(2):137.

Cummins, J.M., Hutcheson, D.P., Cummins, M.J., Georgiades, J.A., and Richards, A.B. Oral therapy with human interferon alpha in calves experimentally injected with infectious bovine rhinotracheitis virus. 1993. Arch Immunol Ther Exp (Warsz) 41(3–4):193–7.

Dahlinger, J., Gregory, C., and Bea, J. Effect of ketoconazole on cyclosporine dose in healthy dogs. 1998. Vet Surg 27(1):64–8.

Daneshmend, T.K., and Warnock, D.W. Clinical pharmacokinetics of ketoconzole. 1988. Clin Pharmacokin 14:13–34.

Davis, E.W., and Legendre, A.M. Successful treatment of guttural pouch mycosis with itraconazole and topical enilconazole in a horse. 1994. J Vet Intern Med 8(4):304–5.

Davis, J.L., Salmon, J.H., and Papich, M.G. Pharmacokinetics and tissue distribution of itraconazole after oral and intravenous administration to horses. 2005. Am J Vet Res 66(10):1694–701.

———. Pharmacokinetics of voriconazole after oral and intravenous administration to horses. 2006. Am J Vet Res 67(6):1070–5.

Davis, P.R., Meyer, G.A., Hanson, R.R., and Stringfellow, J.S. *Pseudallescheria boydii* infection of the nasal cavity of a horse. 2000. J Am Vet Med Assoc 217(5):707–9, 674.

DeBoer, D.J., Moriello, K.A., Blum, J.L., and Volk, L.M. Effects of lufenuron treatment in cats on the establishment and course of *Microsporum canis* infection following exposure to infected cats. 2003. J Am Vet Med Assoc 222(9):1216–20.

de Costa, P.D., Merideth, R.E., and Sigler, R.L. Cataracts in dogs after long-term ketoconazole therapy. 1996. Vet Comp Ophthalmol 6:176–180.

DeCoster, R., Beerens, D., Haelterman, C., and Doolaege, R. Effects of itraconazole on the pituitary-testicular-adrenal axis: an overview of preclinical and clinical studies. In Fromtling, R.A. (ed). Recent Trends in the Discovery, Development and Evaluation of Antifungal Agents. JR Prous Publishers, Barcelona 1987;251–261.

deJaham, C. Toxicity study of enilconazole emulsion in the treatment of dermatophytosis in Persian cats. 1996. St. Hyacinthe, Quebec, Dermatology Meeting Proceedings. 3: Related Articles, Links: de Miranda, P., Krasny, H.C., Page, D.A., Elion, G.B.

deJaham, C., Paradis, M., and Papich, M.G. Antifungal therapy in small animal dermatology. 2000. Comp on Cont Educ Pract Vet 22(5):461–469.

de Mari, K., Maynard, L., Eun, H.M., and Lebreux, B. Treatment of canine parvoviral enteritis with interferon-omega in a placebo-controlled field trial. 2003. Vet Rec 152(4):105–8.

de Mari, K., Maynard, L., Sanquer, A., Lebreux, B., and Eun, H.M. Therapeutic effects of recombinant feline interferon-omega on feline leukemia virus (FeLV)-infected and FeLV/feline immunodeficiency virus (FIV)-coinfected symptomatic cats. 2004. J Vet Intern Med 18(4):477–82.

de Miranda, P., Krasny, H.C., Page, D.A., and Elion, G.B. The disposition of acyclovir in different species. 1981. J Pharmacol Exp Ther 219(2):309–15.

———. Species differences in the disposition of acyclovir. 1982. Am J Med 20;73(1A):31–5.

Dick, J.D., Merz, W.G., and Saral, R. Incidence of polyene-resistant yeasts recovered from clinical specimens. 1980. Antimicrob Agents Chemother 18:158–163.

Dick, R.A., Kanne, D.B., and Casida, J.E. Identification of aldehyde oxidase as the neonicotinoid nitroreductase. 2005. Chem Res Toxicol 18:317–323.

Diekma, D.J., Messer, S.A., Hollis, R.J., et al. Activities of caspofungin, itraconazole, posaconazole, ravuconazole, voriconazole, and amphotericin B against 448 recent clinical isolates of filamentous fungi. 2003. J Clin Microbiol 41:3623–3626.

D'mello, A., Venkataramanan, R., Satake, M., Todo, S., Takaya, S., Ptachcinski, R.J., Burckart, G.J., and Starzl, T.E. Pharmacokinetics of the cyclosporine-ketoconazole interaction in dogs. 1989. Res Commun Chem Pathol Pharmacol 64(3):441–54.

Dorrestein, G.M. Passerine and softbill therapeutics. 2003. Vet Clin North Am Exot Anim Pract 3(1):35–57, v, vi.

Drouhet, E., and Dupont, B. Evolution of antifungal agents: past, present and future. 1987. Rev Infect Dis 9(Suppl1):4–13.

Dudley, M.N. Clinical pharmacology of fluconazole. 1990. Pharmacotherapy 6(S10):141–145.

Dupont, B., and Drouhet, E. in vitro synergy and antagonism of antifungal agents against yeast-like fungi. 1979. Postgrad Med J 55:683–686.

Egberink, H., Borst, M., Niphuis, H., Balzarini, J., Neu, H., Schellekens, H., DeClerq, E., Horzinek, M., and Koolen, M. Suppression of feline immunodeficiency virus infection in vitro by 9–2(phosphonomethox yethy)ladenine. 1990. Proc Natl Acad Sci USA 87(8):3087–3091.

Egberink, H.F., Hartman, D., and Horzinek, M.C. Chemotherapy of feline immunodeficiency virus infection. 1991. J Am Vet Med Assoc 199(10):1485–1487.

Feldman, E.C., Bruyette, D.S., Nelson, R.W., and Farver, T.B. Plasma cortisol response to ketoconazole administration in dogs with hyperadrenocorticism. 1990. J Am Vet Med Assoc 197(1):71–78.

Filer, C.W., Ramji, J.V., Allen, G.D., Brown, T.A., Fowles, S.E., Hollis, F. J., and Mort, E.E. Metabolic and pharmacokinetic studies following oral administration of famciclovir to the rat and dog. 1995. Xenobiotica 25:477–490.

Flammer, K., Nettifee, Osborne, J.A., Webb, D.J., Foster, L.E., Dillard, S.L., and Davis, J.L. Pharmacokinetics of voriconazole after oral administration of single and multiple doses in African grey parrots (*Psittacus erithacus timneh*). 2008. Am J Vet Res 69:114–121.

Foley, J.P., and Legendre, A.M. Treatment of coccidioidomycosis osteomyelitis with itraconazole in a horse. A brief report. 1992. J Vet Intern Med 6(6):333–4.

Forbes, N.A., Simpson, G.N., and Goudswaard, M.F. Diagnosis of avian aspergillosis and treatment with itraconazole. 1992. Vet Rec 130(23):519–520.

Forward, Z.A., Legendre, A.M., and Khalsa, H.D. 2002. Use of intermittent bladder infusion with clotrimazole for treatment of candiduria in a dog. J Am Vet Med Assoc 220(10):1496–8, 1474–5.

Friday, P.A., Scarratt, W.K., Elvinger, F., Timoney, P.J., and Bonda, A. Ataxia and paresis with equine herpesvirus type 1 infection in a herd of riding school horses. 2000. J Vet Intern Med 14(2):197–201.

Funk, R.S. 2000. A formulary for lizards, snakes, and crocodilians. 2000. Vet Clin North Am Exot Anim Pract 3(1):333–58, viii.

Garré, B., Shebany, K., Gryspeerdt, A., Baert, K., van der Meulen, K., Nauwynck, H., Deprez, P., DeBacker, P., and Croubels, S. Pharmacokinetics of acyclovir after intravenous infusion of acyclovir and after oral administration of acyclovir and its prodrug valacyclovir in healthy adult horses. 2007. Antimicrob Agents Chemother 51:4308–4314.

Gaskell, R., Dawson, S., Radford, A., and Thiry, E. Feline herpesvirus. 2007. Vet Res 38:337–354.

Gill, K.S., and Wood, M.J. The clinical pharmacokinetics of famciclovir. 1996. Clin Pharmacokin 31:1–8.

Glotov, A.G., Glotova, T.I., Sergeev, A.A., and Sergeev, A.N. Study of antiviral activity of different drugs against bovine herpes virus and pestivirus. 2004. Antibiot Khimioter 49(6):6–9.

Gonzalez Cabo, J.F., de las Heras Guillamon, M., Latre Cequiel, M.V., and Garcia de Jalon Ciercoles, J.A. Feline sporotrichosis: a case report. 1989. Mycopathologia. 108(3):149–54.

———. Systemic azole antifungal drugs—into the 1990s. In Ryley, J.F. (ed). Handbook of Experimental Pharmacology: Chemotherapy of Fungal Diseases. Springer-Verlag, Berlin 1990;96:455–482.

Goodwin, M.L., and Drew, R.H. Antifungal serum concentration monitoring: an update. 2008. J Antimicrob Chemother 61(1):17–25.

Greene, C.E. Antifungal chemotherapy. In Greene, C.E. (ed). Infectious Diseases of the Dog and Cat. W.B. Saunders, Philadelphia 1990.

Greet, T.R. Nasal aspergillosis in three horses. 1981. Vet Rec 109(22):487–9.

———. Outcome of treatment in 35 cases of guttural pouch mycosis. 1987. Equine Vet J 19(5):483–7.

Grooters, A.M., and Taboada, J. Update on antifungal therapy. 2003. Vet Clin North Am Small Anim Pract 33(4):749–58, vi.

Gruffydd-Jones, T.J., and Wright, A.I. Deformed kittens [letter]. 1977. Vet Rec 100:206.

Guillot, J., Bensignor, E., Jankowski, F., Seewald, W., Chermette, R., and Steffan, J. Comparative efficacies of oral ketoconazole and terbinafine for reducing Malassezia population sizes on the skin of Basset Hounds. 2003. Vet Dermatol 14(3):153–7.

Hall, C.B., McBride, J.T., Walsh, E.E., Bell, D.M., Gala, C., Hildreth, S. TenEyck, L.G., and Hall, W.J. Aerosolized ribavirin treatment of infants with respiratory syncytial viral infection. 1983. N Engl J Med 308:1443–1447.

Harris, P.A., and Riegelman S. Metabolism of griseofulvin in dogs. 1969. J Pharm Sci 58:93–96.

Hartmann, K., Donath, A., Beer, B., Egberink, H.F., Horzinek, M.C., Lutz, H., Hoffmann-Fezer, G., Thum, I., and Thefeld, S. Use of two virustatica (AZT, PMEA) in the treatment of FIV and of FeLV seropositive cats with clinical symptoms. 1992. Vet Immunol Immunopathol 35(1–2):167–75.

Haschek, W.M., Weigel, R.M., Scherba, G., DeVera, M.C., Feinmehl, R., Solter, P., Tompkins, M.B., and Tompkins, W.A. Zidovudine toxicity to cats infected with feline leukemia virus. 1990. Fundam Appl Toxicol 14(4):764–75.

Hayden, F.G., Minocha, A., Spyker, D.A., and Hoffman, H.E. Comparative single-dose pharmacokinetics of amantadine hydrochloride and rimantadine hydrochoride in young and elderly adults. 1985. Antimicrob Agent Chemother 28:216–221.

Helton K.A., Nesbitt, G.H., and Caciolo, P.L. Griseofulvin toxicity in cats: literature review and report of seven cases. 1986. J Am Anim Hosp Assoc 22:453–458.

Hess, M.B., Parker, N.A., Purswell B.J., and Dascanio, J.D. 2002. Use of lufenuron as a treatment for fungal endometritis in four mares. J Am Vet Med Assoc 221(2):266–7, 240.

Heykants, J., Michiels, M., Meuldermans, W., Monbaliu, J., Lavrijsen, K., VanPeer, A., Levron, J.C., Woestenborghs, R., and Cauwenbergh, G. The pharmacokinetics of itraconazole in animals and man: an overview. In Fromtling, R.A. (ed). Recent Trends in the Discovery, Development and Evaluation of Antifungal Agents. JR Prous Publishers, Barcelona 1987.

Heykants, J., Peer, A.V., Lavrijsen, K., Meuldermans, W., Woestenborghs, R., and Cauwenbergh, G. Pharmacokinetics of oral antifungals and their clinical implications. 1990. Br J Clin Pract Sump (Suppl71):50–56.

Hiddleston, W.A. The use of Griseofulvin Mycelium in equine animals [letter]. 1970. Vet Rec 87:119.

Hiemenz, J.W., and Walsh, T.J. Lipid formulations of amphotericin B: recent progress and future directions. 1996. Clin Infect Dis 22(Suppl2): S133–S144.

Hill, P.B., Moriello, K.A., and Shaw, S.E. A review of systemic antifungal agents. 1995. Vet Derm 6:59–66.

Hnilica, K.A., Medleau, L., and Cornelius, L. Evaluation of toxicity of topical enilconazole in cats. 2000. Veterinary Dermatology 11(Suppl1):42 (Abstract P-6).

Hoover, E.A., Ebner, J.P., Zeidner, N.S. and Mullins, J.I. Early therapy of feline leukemia virus infection (FeLV-FAIDS) with 9–2(phosphonylmethoxyethyl)-adenine (PMEA). 1991. Antiviral Res 16(1):77–92.

Horn, R., Wong, B. Kiehn, T.E., and Armstrong, D. Fungemia in a cancer hospital: changing frequency, earlier onset, and results of therapy. 1985. Rev Infect Dis 7:646–655.

Huckabee, J.R. Raptor therapeutics. 2000. Vet Clin North Am Exot Anim Pract 3(1):91–116, vi.

Hume, A.L., and Kerkering, T.M. Ketoconazole 1983. Drug Intell Clin Pharm 17:169–174.

Humphrey, M.J., Jevons, S., and Tarbit, M.H. Pharmacokinetic evaluation of UK-49858, a metabolically stable trazole antifungal drug, in animals and humans. 1985. Antimicrob Agents Chemother 28(5):648–653.

Hussain, A.S., and Ritschel, W.A. "Body burden" of phophonoformic acid after topical and vaginal administration to rabbits and beagle dogs. 1989. Meth Find Exp Clin Pharm 11(2):111–114.

Ilyushina, N.A., Govorkova, E.A., and Webster, R.G. Detection of amantadine-resistant variants among avian influenza viruses isolated in North America and Asia. 2005. Virology 341(1):102–6.

Irizarry-Rovira, A.R., Kaufman, L., Christian, J.A., Reberg, S.R., Adams, S.B., DeNicola, D.B., Rivers, W., and Hawkins, J.F. Diagnosis of sporotrichosis in a donkey using direct fluorescein-labeled antibody testing. 2000. J Vet Diagn Invest 12(2):180–3.

Ishida, T., Shibanai, A., Tanaka, S., Uchida, K., and Mochizuki, M. Use of recombinant feline interferon and glucocorticoid in the treatment of feline infectious peritonitis. 2004. J Feline Med Surg 6(2):107–9.

Ishiwata, K., Minagawa, T., and Kajimoto, T. Clinical effects of the recombinant feline interferon-omega on experimental parvovirus infection in beagle dogs. 1998. J Vet Med Sci 60(8):911–7.

Ivey, E.S., and Morrisey, J.K. 2000. Therapeutics for rabbits. Vet Clin North Am Exot Anim Pract 3(1):183–220, vii.

Janssen, P.A.J., and Symoens, J.E. Hepatic reactions during ketoconazole treatment. 1983. Am J Med 74(S1B):80–85.

Jensen, J.C. Clinical pharmacokinetics of terbinafine (Lamisil). 1989. Clin Exp Dermatol 14(2):110–3.

Johnson-Delaney, C.A. Therapeutics of companion exotic marsupials. 2000. Vet Clin North Am Exot Anim Pract 3(1):173–81, vii.

Kielstein, P., and Gottschalk, C. Trichophyton metagrophytes infection in a breeding-swine herd. 1970. Mh Vet Med 25:127–130.

Koehne, G., Powell, H.S., and Hail, R.I. Sporotrichosis in a dog. 1971. J Am Vet Med Assoc159(7):892–4.

Korenek, N.L., Legendre, A.M., Andrews, F.M., et al. Treatment of mycotic rhinitis with itraconazole in three horses. 1994. J Vet Intern Med 8(3):224–7.

Kowalsky, S.F., and Dixon, D.M. Fluconazole: A new antifungal agent. 1991. Clin Pharmacy 10:179–194.

Krasny, H.C., de Miranda, P., Blum, M.R., and Elion, G.B. Pharmacokinetics and bioavailability of acyclovir in the dog. 1981. J Pharmacol Exp Ther 216(2):281–8.

Krawiec, D.R., McKiernan, B.C., Twardock, A.R., et al. Use of an amphotericin B lipid complex for treatment of blastomycosis in dogs. 1996. J Am Vet Med Assoc 209:2073–2075.

Kunkle, G.A., and Meyer, D.F. Toxicity of high doses of griseofulvin in cats. 1987. J Am Vet Med Assoc 191(3):322–323.

Lamothe J. Activity of amphotericin B in lipid emulsion in the initial treatment of canine leishmaniasis. 2001. J Small Anim Pract 42(4):170–5.

Lascelles, B.D.X., Gaynor, J., Roe, S.S., Marcellin-Little, D.J., Davidson, G., and Carr, J. Evaluation of amantadine as part of a multimodal analgesic regimen for the alleviation of refractory canine osteoarthritis pain. 2007. J Vet Intern Med [Abstract 126] Presented at the ACVIM Forum.

Latimer, F.G., Colitz, C.M.H., Campbell, N.B., et al. Pharmacokinetics of fluconazole following intravenous and oral administration and body fluid concentrations of fluconazole following repeated oral dosing in horses. 2001. Am J Vet Res. 62:1606–1611.

Legendre, A.M. Antimycotic drug therapy. In Bonagura, J.D. (ed). Current Veterinary Therapy XII. W.B. Saunders, Philadelphia 1995;327–331.

Legendre, A.M., Gompf, R., and Bone, D. Treatment of feline cryptococcosis with ketoconazole. 1982. J Am Vet Med Assoc 181:1541–1542.

Legendre, A.M., Rohrbach, B.W., Toal, R.L., et al. Treatment of blastomycosis with itraconazole in 112 dogs. 1996. J Vet Int Med 10:365–371.

Legendre, A.M., Selcer, B.A., Edwards, D.F., and Stevens, R. Treatment of canine blastomycosis with amphotericin B and ketoconazole. 1984. J Am Vet Med Assoc 184(10):1249–1254.

Levy, J.K. Ataxia in a kitten treated with griseofulvin. 1991. 198(1):105.

Lietman, P.S. Clinical pharmacology: foscarnet. 1992. Am J Med 92(2A):8S–11S.

Lightfoot, T.L. Therapeutics of African pygmy hedgehogs and prairie dogs. 2000. Vet Clin North Am Exot Anim Pract 3(1):155–72, vii.

Madison, J.B., Reid, B.V., and Raskin, R.E. 1995. Amphotericin B treatment of Candida arthritis in two horses. 1995. J Am Vet Med Assoc 206(3):338–41.

Maggs, D.J., and Clarke, H.E. In vitro efficacy of ganciclovir, cidofovir, penciclovir, foscarnet, idoxuridine, and acyclovir against feline herpesvirus type-1. 2004. Am J Vet Res 65(4):399–403.

Maggs, D.J., Collins, B.K., Thorne, J.G., and Nasisse, M.P. 2000. Effects of L-lysine and L-arginine on in vitro replication of feline herpesvirus type-1. 2000. Am J Vet Res 61(12):1474–8.

Maggs, D.J., Nasisse, M.P., and Kass, P.H. 2003. Efficacy of oral supplementation with L-lysine in cats latently infected with feline herpesvirus. 2003. Am J Vet Res 64(1):37–42.

Malik, R., Craig, A.J., Wigney, D.I., Martin, P., and Love, D.N. Combination chemotherapy of canine and feline cryptococcosis using subcutaneously administered amphotericin B. 1996. Aust Vet J 73:124–128.

Malik, R., Lessels, N.S., Webb, S., Meek, M., Norris, J.M., and Power, H. 2009. Treatment of feline herpes virus-1 associated disease in cats with famciclovir and related drugs. J Feline Med & Surg 11:40–48.

Mallo, K.M., Harms, C.A., Lewbart, G.A., and Papich, M.G. 2002. Pharmacokinetics of fluconazole in loggerhead sea turtles (*Caretta caretta*) after single intravenous and subcutaneous injections, and multiple subcutaneous injections. J Zoo & Wildlife Med 33:29–35.

Mancianti, F., Pedonese, F., and Zullino, C. Efficacy of oral administration of itraconazole to cats with dermatophytosis caused by *Microsporum canis*. 1998. J Am Vet Med Assoc 213:993–995.

Martin, C.L. Ocular infections. In Greene, C.E. (ed). Infectious diseases of the dog and cat. W.B. Saunders, Philadelphia 1990.

Mashima TY, and Lewbart GA. Pet fish formulary. 2000. Vet Clin North Am Exot Anim Pract 3(1):117–30, vi.

Mathews, K.G., Davidson, A.P., Koblik, P.D., Richardson, E.F., Komtebedde, J., Pappagianis, D., Hector, R.F., and Kass, P.H. Comparison of topical administration of clotrimazole through surgically placed versus nonsurgically placed catheters for treatment of nasal Aspergillosis in dogs: 60 cases (1990–1996). 1998. J Am Vet Med Assoc 213(4):501–6.

McCaw, D.L., Boon, G.D., Jergens, A.E., Kern, M.R., Bowles, M.H., and Johnson, J.C. Immunomodulation therapy for feline leukemia virus infection. 2001. J Am Anim Hosp Assoc 37(4):356–63.

McMullan, W.C., Joyce, J.R., Hanselka, D.V., and Heitmann, J.M. Amphotericin B for the treatment of localized subcutaneous phycomycosis in the horse. 1977. J Am Vet Med Assoc 170(11):1293–8.

Mechlinsk, W., Schaffner, C.P., Ganis, P., and Avitabile, G. Structure and absolute configuration of the polyene macrolide amphotericin B. 1970. Tetrahedron Letters 44:3873–3876.

Medleau, L. Recently described feline dermatoses. 1990. Vet Clinic North Am: Sm Anim Pract 20(6):1615–1632.

Medleau, L., and Chalmers, S.A. Ketoconazole for treatment of dermatophytosis in cats. 1992. J Am Vet Med Assoc 200(1):77–78.

Medleau, L., Greene, C.E., and Rakich, P.M. Evaluation of ketoconazole and itraconazole for treatment of disseminated cryptococcosis in cats. 1990. Am J Vet Res 51(9):1454–1458.

Medleau, L., Hall, E.J., Goldschmidt, M.H., and Irby, N. Cutaneous cryptococcosis in three cats. 1985 J Am Vet Med Assoc 187:169–170.

Medoff, G., Comfort, M., and Kobayashi, G.S. Synergistic action of amphotericin B and 5-fluorocytosin against yeast-like organisms. 1971. Proc Soc Exp Bio Med 138:571–574.

Medoff, G., Kobayashi, G.S., Kwan, C.N., Schlessinger, D., and Venkov, P. Potentiation of rifampicin and 5-fluorocytosine as antifungal antibiotics by amphotericin B. 1972. Proc Nat Acad Sci USA 69:196–199.

Moore, B.R. Clinical application of interferons in large animal medicine. 1996. J Am Vet Med Assoc 15;208(10):1711–5.

Moore, I., Horney, B., Day, K., Lofstedt, J., and Cribb, A.E. Treatment of inflammatory airway disease in young standardbreds with interferon alpha. 2004. Can Vet J 45(7):594–601.

Moriello, K.A. Ketoconazole: clinical pharmacology and therapeutic recommendations. 1986. J Am Vet Med Assoc 188(3):303–306.

———. Treatment of dermatophytosis in dogs and cats: review of published studies. 2004. Vet Dermatol 15(2):99–107.

Moriello, K.A., and DeBoer, D.J. Efficacy of griseofulvin and itraconazole in the treatment of experimentally induced dermatophytosis in cats. 1995. JAVMA 207:439–444.

Moriello, KA.,. DeBoer, D.J., Schenker, R., Blum, J.L., and Volk, L.M. Efficacy of pre-treatment with lufenuron for the prevention of *Microsporum canis* infection in a feline direct topical challenge model. 2004. Vet Dermatol 15(6):357–62.

Mundell, A.C. New therapeutic agents in veterinary dermatology. 1990. Vet Clinic North Am: Sm Anim Pract 20(6):1541–1556.

Murray, M.J., del Piero, F., Jeffrey, S.C., Davis, M.S., Furr, M.O., Dubovi, E.J., and Mayo, J.A. 1998. Neonatal equine herpesvirus type 1 infection on a thoroughbred breeding farm. 1998. J Vet Intern Med 12(1):36–41.

Nasisse, M.P., Dorman, D.C., Jamison, K.C., Weigler, B.J., Hawkins, E.C., and Stevens, J.B. Effects of valacyclovir in cats infected with feline herpesvirus 1. 1997. Am J Vet Res 58(10):1141–4.

Nasisse, M.P., Guy, J.S., Davidson, M.G., Sussman, W., and De Clercq, E. In vitro susceptibility of feline herpesvirus-1 to vidarabine, idoxuridine, trifluridine, acyclovir, or bromovinyldeoxyuridine. 1989. Am J Vet Res 50(1):158–60.

Nichols, P.R., Morris, D.O., and Beale, K.M. 2001. A retrospective study of canine and feline cutaneous vasculitis. Vet Dermatol 12(5):255–64.

North, T.W., North, G.L.T., and Pedersen, N.C. Feline immunodeficiency virus, a model for reverse transcriptase-targeted chemotherapy for acquired immune deficiency syndrome. 1989. Antimicrob Agent Chemother 33(6):915–919.

Norton, T.M., Gaskin, J., Kollias, G.V., Homer, B., Clark, C.H., and Wilson, R. Efficacy of acyclovir against herpesvirus infection in Quaker parakeets. 1991. Am J Vet Res 52(12):2007–2009.

Noxon, J.O., Monroe, W.E., and Chinn, D.R. Ketoconazole therapy in canine and feline cryptococcosis. 1986. J Am Anim Hosp Assoc 22:179–183.

Oberg, B. Antiviral effects of phosphonoformate (PFA, Foscarnet sodium). 1989. Pharmacol Ther 2:213–285.

Obrosova-Serova, N.P., Kupryasjina, L.M., Isachenko, V.A., Vorontsova, R.M., and Utkin, V.G. Experience with prevention of chicken influenza with amantadine. 1976. Veterinariia 11:62–63.

O'Day, D.M., Ray W. A., Robinson, R.D., Head, W.S. and Savage, A. The influence of yeast growth phase in vivo on the efficacy of topical polyenes. 1987. Curr Eye Res 6:363–368.

Oldenkamp, E.P. Treatment of ringworm in horses with natamycin. 1979. Equine Vet J 11(1):36–8.

Oliva, G., Gradoni, L., Ciaramella, P., et al. Activity of liposomal amphotericin B (AmBisome) in dogs naturally infected with *Leishmania infantum.* 1995. J Antimicrob Chemother 36:1013–1019.

Owens, J.G., Nasisse, M.P., Tadepalli, S.M., and Dorman, D.C. Pharmacokinetics of acyclovir in the cat. 1996. J Vet Pharmacol Ther 19(6):488–90.

Owens, W.R., Miller, R.I., Haynes, P.F., and Snider, T.G., 3rd. Phycomycosis caused by *Basidiobolus haptosporus* in two horses. 1985. J Am Vet Med Assoc 186(7):703–5.

Pedretti, E., Passeri, B., Amadori, M., Isola, P., Pede, P.D., Telera, A., Vescovini, R., Quintavalla, F., and Pistello, M. Low-dose interferon-alpha treatment for feline immunodeficiency virus infection. 2005. Vet Immunol Immunopathol [Epub ahead of print].

Pentlarge, V.W., and Martin, R.A. Treatment of cryptococcosis in three cats, using ketoconazole. 1986. J Am Vet Med Assoc 188(5):536–538.

Perfect, J.R., Savani, D.V., and Durack, D.T. Comparison of itraconazole and fluconazole in treatment of cryptococcal meningitis and candida pyelonephritis in rabbits. 1986. Antimicrob Agents Chemother 29(4):579–583.

Pestka, S., Langer, J.A., Zoon, K.C., and Samuel, S.A. Interferons and their actions. 1987. Ann Rev Biochem 56:727–777.

Pierce A.M., Pierce, H.D., Unrau, A.M. and Oehlschlger, A.C. Lipid composition and polyene antibiotic resistance of *Candida albicans* mutants. 1978. Can J Biochem 56:135–142.

Pinchbeck, L.R., Hillier, A., Kowalski, J.J., and Kwochka, K.W. Comparison of pulse administration versus once daily administration of itraconazole for the treatment of *Malassezia pachydermatis* dermatitis and otitis in dogs. 2002. J Am Vet Med Assoc 220(12):1807–12.

Plotnick, A.N. Lipid-based formulations of amphotericin B. 2000. J Am Vet Med Assoc 216:838–841.

Polak, A. Mode of action studies. In Ryley JF (ed). Handbook of Experimental Pharmacology: Chemotherapy of Fungal Diseases. Springer-Verlag, Berlin 1990;96:153–182.

Polak, A., Scholer, H.J., and Wall, M. Combination therapy of experimental candidiasis, cryptococcosis and aspergillosis in mice. 1982 Chemotherapy 28:461–479.

Povey, R.C. Effect of orally administered ribavirin on experimental feline calicivirus infection in cats. 1978. 39:1337–1341.

Powderly, W.G., Kobayashi, G.S., Herzig, G.P., and Medoff, G. Amphotericin B-resistant yeast infection in severely immunocompromised patients. 1988. Am J Med 84:826–832.

Pozzi, A., Muir, W.W., and Traverso, F. Prevention of central sensitization and pain by N-methyl-D-aspartate receptor antagonists. 2006. J Am Vet Med Assoc 228:53–60.

Prades, M., Brown, M.P., Gronwall, R., and Houston, A.E. Body fluid and endometrial concentrations of ketoconazole in mares after intravenous injection or repeated gavage. 1989. Equine Vet J 21:211–214.

Pukay, B.P. and Dion, W.M. Feline phaeohyphomycosis: treatment with ketoconazole and 5-fluorocytosine. 1984. Can Vet J 25:130–134.

Rees, T.M., and Lubinski, J.L. 2008. Oral supplementation with L-lysine did not prevent upper respiratory infection in a shelter population of cats. J Feline Medicine & Surgery 10:510–513.

Rees, W.A., Harkins, J.D., Lu, M., Holland, R.E., Jr., Lehner, A.F., Tobin, T., and Chambers, TM. 1999. Pharmacokinetics and therapeutic efficacy of rimantadine in horses experimentally infected with influenza virus A2. 1999. Am J Vet Res 60(7):888–94.

Rees, W.A., Harkins, J.D., Woods, W.E., Blouin, R.A., Lu, M., Fenger, C., Holland, R.E., Chambers, T.M., and Tobin, T. Amantadine and equine influenza: pharmacology, pharmacokinetics and neurological effects in the horse. 1997. Equine Vet J 29(2):104–10.

Reilly, L.K., and Palmer, J.E. Systemic candidiasis in four foals. 1994. J Am Vet Med Assoc 205(3):464–6.

Reimer, K., Matthes, E., Scholz, D., and Rosenthal, H.A. Effects of suramin, HPA-23 and 3′-azidothymidine triphosphate on the reverse transcriptase of bovine leukaemia virus. 1989 Acta Virologica 33(1):43–49.

Reuss, U. Management of trichophytosis in horses. 1978a. DTW 85:231.

———. Treatment of cattle trichophytosis with griseofulvin. 1978b. Tieraerztl Umschau 33:85–90.

Richardson, K., Cooper, K., Marriott, M.S., Tarbit, M.H., Troke, P.F., and Whittle P.J. Discovery of fluconazole, a novel antifungal agent. 1990. Rev Infect Dis 12(S3):267–271.

Richman, D.D. The toxicity of azidothymidine (AZT) in the treatment of patients with AIDS and AIDS-related complex. 1987. N Engl J Med 317:192–197.

Roffey, S.J., Cole, S., Comby, P., et al. The disposition of voriconazole in mouse, rat, rabbit, guinea pig, dog, and human. 2003. Drug Metab Dispos 31(6):731–41.

Roney, C.S., Rossi, C.R., Smith, P.C., Lauerman, L.C., Spano, J.S., Hanrahan, L.A., and William, J.C. Effect of human leukocyte A interferon on prevention of infectious bovine rhinotracheitis virus infection of cattle. 1985. Am J Vet Res 46(6):1251–5.

Rosales, M.S., Marsella, R., Kunkle, G., Harris, B.L., Nicklin, C.F., and Lopez, J. Comparison of the clinical efficacy of oral terbinafine and ketoconazole combined with cephalexin in the treatment of *Malassezia* dermatitis in dogs—a pilot study. 2005. Vet Dermatol 16(3):171–6.

Rottman, J.B., English, R.V., Breitschwerdt, E.B., and Duncan, D.E. Bone marrow hypoplasia in a cat treated with griseofulvin. 1991. J Am Vet Med Assoc 198(3):429.

Rubin, S.I. Nephrotoxicity of amphotericin B. In Kirk, R.W. (Ed.), Current Veterinary Therapy IX, Philadelphia: W.B. Saunders. 1986;1142–1145.

Rush, E.M., Hunter, R.P., Papich, M., Raphael, B.L., Calle, P.P., Clippinger, T.L., and Cook, R.A. Pharmacokinetics and safety of acyclovir in tragopans (*Tragopan* species). 2005. J Avian Med Surg 19:271–276.

Schutte, J.G., and van den Ingh, T.S. Microphthalmia, brachygnathia superior, and palatocheiloschisis in a foal associated with griseofulvin administration to the mare during early pregnancy. 1997. Vet Q 19(2):58–60.

Scott, D.W. Fungal disorders. Feline dermatology, 1900–1978: a monograph. 1980. J Am Anim Hosp Assoc 16:349–356.

Scott, F.W., deLahunta, A. Schultz, R.D., Bistner, S.I., and Riis, R.C. Teratogenesis in cats associated with griseofulvin therapy. 1975. Teratology 11(1):79–86.

Scotty, N.C., Evans, T.J., Giuliano, E., Johnson, P.J., Rottinghaus, G.E., Fothergill, A.W., and Cutler, T.J. In vitro efficacy of lufenuron against filamentous fungi and blood concentrations after PO administration in horses. 2005. J Vet Intern Med 19:878–882.

Seahorn, T.L., Carter, G.K., Martens, J.G., Crandell, R.A., Martin, M.T., Scrutchfield, W.L., Cummins, J.M., and Martens, R.J. Effects of human alpha interferon on experimentally induced equine herpesvirus-1 infection in horses. 1990. Am J Vet Res 51(12):2006–10.

Shah, V.P., Riegelman, S., and Epstein, W.L. Determination of griseofulvin in skin, plasma, and sweat. 1972. J Pharm Sci 61:634–636.

Shannon, D. Treatment with itraconazole of penguins suffering from aspergillosis. 1992. Vet Rec 130(21):479.

Sharp, N.J.H. Treatment of canine nasal aspergillosis/penicilliosis with fluconazole (UK-49,858). 1991. J Small Anim Pract 32:513–516.

Sharp, N.J.H., and Sullivan, M. Treatment of nasal aspergillosis. 1992. In Pract 14(1):26–31.

Sharp, N.J.H., Harvey, C.E., and Sullivan, M. Canine nasal aspergillosis and penicilliosis. 1991. Compen Contin Educ Pract Vet 13:41–49.

Sharp, N.J.H., Sullivan, M., Harvey, C.E., and Webb, T. Treatment of nasal aspergillosis with enilconazole. 1993. J Vet Int Med 7(1):40–43.

Shaw, J.T.B., Tarbit, M.H., and Troke, P.F. Cytochrome P-450 mediated sterol synthesis and metabolism: differences in sensitivity to fluconazole and other azoles. In Fromtling, R.A. (ed). Recent Trends in the Discovery, Development and Evaluation of Antifungal Agents. JR Prous Publishers, Barcelona 1987;125–139.

Shelton, G.H., Grant, C.K., Linenberger, M.L., and Abkowitz J.L. Severe neutropenia associated with griseofulvin therapy in cats with feline immunodeficiency virus infection. 1990. J Vet Int Med 4:317–319.

Shelton, G.H., Linenberger, M.L., and Abkowitz, J.L. Hematologic abnormalities in cats seropositive for feline immunodeficiency virus. 1991. J Am Vet Med Assoc 199(10):1353–1357.

Smith, C.B., Charette, R.P., Fox, J.P., Cooney, M.K., and Hall, C.E. Lack of effect of oral ribavirin in naturally occurring influenza A virus (H1N1) infection. 1980. J Infect Dis 141:548–554.

Smith, C.G. Use of acyclovir in an outbreak of Pacheco's parrot disease. 1987. Assoc Avian Vet Today 1:55–57.

Sokol-Anderson M., Sligh, J.E., Elberg, S., Brajtburg, J., Kobayashi, G.S. and Medoff, G. Role of cell defense against oxidative damage in the resistance of *Candida albicans* to the killing effect of amphotericin B. 1988. Am J Med 84:826–832.

Stanton, G.J., Lloyd, R.E., Sarzotti, M., and Blalock, J.E. Protection of mice from *Semliki Forest* virus infection by lymphocytes treated with low levels of interferon. 1989. Mol Biother 1(6):305–10.

Stiles, J., Townsend, W.M., Rogers, Q.R., and Krohne, S.G. Effect of oral administration of L-lysine on conjunctivitis caused by feline herpesvirus in cats. 2002. Am J Vet Res 63(1):99–103.

Straw, J.A., Loo, T.L., deVera, C.C., Nelson, P.D., Tompkins, W.A., and Bai, S.A. Pharmacokinetics of potential anti-AIDS agents thiofoscarnet and foscarnet in the cat. 1992. J Acquired Def Syn 5(9):936–942.

Swenson, C.L., Polas, P.J., Cheney, C.M. Kociba, G.J., and Mathes, L.E. Prophylactic and therapeutic effects of phosphonoformate against feline leukemia virus in vivo. 1991a. Am J Vet Res 52(12):2010–2015.

Swenson, C.L., Weisbrode, S.E., Nagode, L.A., Hayes, K.A., Steinmeyer, C.L., and Mathes, L.E. Age-related differences in phosphonoformate-induced bone toxicity in cats. 1991b. Calcif Tissue Int 48(5):353–61.

Taintor, J., Crowe, C., Hancock, S., Schumacher, J., and Livesey, L. Treatment of conidiobolomycosis with fluconazole in two pregnant mares. 2004. J Vet Intern Med18(3):363–4.

Tavares, L., Roneker, C., Johnston, K., Lehrman, S.N., and deNoronha, F. 3′-azido-3-deoxythymidine in feline leukemia virus-infected cats: a model for therapy and prophylaxis of AIDS. 1987. Cancer Res 47:3190–3194.

Teich, S.A., Cheung, T.W., and Friedman, A.H. Systemic antiviral drugs used in ophthalmology. 1992. Surv Ophth 37(1):19–53.

Templeton, I.E., Thummel, K.E., Kharasch, E.D., Kunze, K.L., Hoffer, C., Nelson, W.L., and Isoherranen, N. Contribution of itraconazole metabolites to inhibition of CYP3A4 in vivo. 2008. Clin Pharmacol Therapeut 83:77–85.

Thomasy, S.M., Maggs, D.J., Moulin, N.K., and Stanley, S.D. Pharmacokinetics and safety of penciclovir following oral administration of famciclovir to cats. 2007. Am J Vet Res 68:1252–1258.

Tohyama, M., Kawakami, K., and Saito, A. Anticryptococcal effect of amphotericin B is mediated through macrophage production of nitric oxide. 1996. Antimicrob Agents Chemother 40(8):1919–23.

Toll, J., Ashe, C.M., and Trepanier, L.A. Intravesicular administration of clotrimazole for treatment of candiduria in a cat with diabetes mellitus. 2003. J Am Vet Med Assoc 223(8):1156–8, 1129.

Troke, P.F., Andrews, R.J., and Pye, G.W. Fluconazole and other azoles: translation of in vitro activity to in vivo clinical efficacy. 1990. Rev Infect Dis 12(S3):276–280.

Tully, T.N., Jr. Psittacine therapeutics. 2000. Vet Clin North Am Exot Anim Pract 3(1):59–90, vi.

Utz, J.P., Garriques, I.L., Sande, M.A., Warner, J.F., Mandell, G.L., McGehee, R.F., Duma, R.J., and Shadomy, S. Therapy of cryptococcosis with a combination of flucytosine and amphotericin B. 1975. J Infect Dis 132:368–373.

Vaden, S.L., Heit, M.C., Hawkins, E.C., et al. Fluconazole in cats: pharmacokinetics following intravenous and oral administration and penetration into cerebrospinal fluid, aqueous humour and pulmonary epithelial lining fluid. 1997. J Vet Pharmacol Therap 20(3):181–186.

VanCauteren, H., Coussement, W., Vandenberghe, J., Herin, V., Vanparys, P., and Marsboom, R. The toxicological properties of itraconazole. In Fromtling, R.A. (ed). Recent Trends in the Discovery, Development and Evaluation of Antifungal agents. JR Prous Publishers, Barcelona 1987b;263–271.

VanCauteren, H., Heykants, J., DeCoster, R., and Cauwenbergh, G. Itraconazole: pharmacologic studies in animals and humans. 1987a. Rev Infect Dis 9(S1):43–46.

VanCutsem, J. Oral and parenteral treatment with itraconazole in various superficial and systemic experimental fungal infections. Comparisons with other antifungals and combination therapy. 1990. Br J Clin Pract Sump (Suppl71):32–40.

VanCutsem, J., VanGerven, F., and Janssen, P.A.J. Activity of orally, topically, and parenterally administered itraconazole in the treatment of superficial and deep mycoses: animal models. 1987. Rev Infect Dis 9(S1):15–32.

Vanden Bossche, H. Itraconazole: A selective inhibitor of the cytochrome P-450 dependent ergosterol biosynthesis. In Fromtling, R.A. (ed). Recent trends in the discovery, development and evaluation of antifungal agents. JR Prous Publishers, Barcelona 1987;207–221.

Vanden Bossche, H., Marichal, P., Gorrens, J., and Coene, M.C. Biochemical basis for the activity and selectivity of oral antifungal drugs. 1990. Br J Clin Pract (Suppl71):41–46.

VanVoris, L.P., Betts, R.F., Hayden, F.G., Christmas, W.A., and Douglas, R.G. Jr. Successful treatment of naturally occurring influenza A/USSR/77 H1N1. 1981. J Am Med Assoc 245(11):1128–1131.

Walker, I.D., and Whitaker, B.R. Amphibian therapeutics. 2000. Vet Clin North Am Exot Anim Pract3(1):239–55, viii.

Wang, E.-J., Lew, K., Casciano, C.N., Clement, R.P., and Johnson, W.W. Interaction of common azole antifungals with P glycoprotein. 2002. Antimicrob Agents Chemother.

Warnock, D.W. Amphotericin B: an introduction. 1991. J Antimicrob Chemother 28(SupplB):27–38.

Weiss, R.C., Cox, N.R., and Boudreaux, M.K. Toxicologic effects of ribavirin in cats. 1993a. J Vet Pharmacol Ther 16(3):301–16.

Weiss, R.C., Cox, N.R., and Martinez, M.L. Evaluation of free or liposome-encapsulated ribavirin for antiviral therapy of experimentally induced feline infectious peritonitis. 1993b. Res Vet Sci 55(2):162–72.

Werenne, J., Vanden Broecke, C., Schwers, A., Goossens, A., Bugyaki, L., Maenhoudt, M., and Pastoret, P.P. Antiviral effect of bacterially produced human interferon (Hu-IFN alpha 2) against experimental vaccinia infection in calves. 1985. J Interferon Res 5(1):129–36.

White-Weithers, N., and Medleau, L. Evaluation of topical therapies for the treatment of dermatophyte-infected hairs from dogs and cats. 1995. J Am Anim Hosp Assoc 31:250–252.

Wilkins, P.A., Papich, M., and Sweeney, R.W. Pharmacokinetics of acyclovir in adult horses. 2005. J Vet Emerg Crit Care 15:174–178.

Willard, M.D., Nachreiner, R., McDonald R., and Roudebush, P. Ketoconazole-induced changes in selected canine hormone concentrations. 1986a. Am J Vet Res 47:2504–2509.

Willard, M.D., Nachreiner, R.F., Howard, V.C., and Fooshee, S.K. Effect of long-term administration of ketoconazole in cats. 1986b. Am J Vet Res 47:2510–2513.

Willems, L., van der Geest, R., and de Beule, K. Itraconazole oral solution and intravenous formulations: a review of pharmacokinetics and pharmacodynamics. 2001. J Clin Pharm Ther 26(3):159–69.

Williams, B.H. Therapeutics in ferrets. 2000. Vet Clin North Am Exot Anim Pract 3(1):131–53, vi.

Wolfe, B.A., Harms, C.A., Groves, J.D., and Loomis, M.R. Treatment of *Argulus* sp. infestation of river frogs. 2001. Contemp Top Lab Anim Sci 40(6):35–6.

Wray, J.D., Sparkes, A.H., and Johnson, E.M. 2008. Infection of the subcutis of the nose in a cat caused by Mucor species: successful treatment using posaconazole. J Feline Med & Surgery 10:523–527.

Yasuda, K., Lan, L.B., Sanglard, D,. Furuya, K., Schuetz, J.D., and Schuetz, E.G. Interaction of cytochrome P450 3A inhibitors with P-glycoprotein. 2002. J Pharmacol Exp Ther 303(1):323–32.

Yoo, S.D., Kang, E., Shin, B.S., Jun, H., Lee, S.H., Lee, K.C., and Lee, K.H. Interspecies comparison of the oral absorption of itraconazole in laboratory animals. 2002. Arch Pharm Res 25(3):387–91.

Zamos, D.T., Schumacher, J., and Loy, J.K. Nasopharyngeal conidiobolomycosis in a horse. 1996. J Am Vet Med Assoc 208(1):100–1.

Zeidner, N.S., Mathiason-Dubard, C.K., Rose, L.M., et al. Zidovudine in combination with alpha interferon, interleukin-2, and activated immune lymphocytes as therapy for FeLV-induced immunodeficiency syndrome (FeLV-FAIDS). 1989. Proc XIVth Int Symp Comp Res Leukemia and Related Diseases p. 94.

Zhang, W., Mauldin, J.K., Schmiedt, C.W., Brockus, C.W., Boudinot, F.D., McCrackin, S.M., and Stevenson, M.A. Pharmacokinetics of zidovudine in cats. 2004a. Am J Vet Res 65(6):835–40.

Zhang, W., Mauldin, J.K., Schmiedt, C.W., Brockus, C.W., Boudinot, F.D., and McCrackin, S.M. Pharmacokinetics of lamivudine in cats. 2004b. Am J Vet Res 65(6):841–6.

Zur, G., and Elad, D. In vitro and in vivo effects of lufenuron on dermatophytes isolated from cases of canine and feline dermatophytoses. 2006. J Vet Med B Infect Dis Vet Public Health Apr;53(3):122–5.

SECTION 10

Chemotherapy of Parasitic Diseases

CHAPTER

40

ANTINEMATODAL DRUGS

CARLOS E. LANUSSE, LUIS I. ALVAREZ, JUAN M. SALLOVITZ, MARIA L. MOTTIER, AND SERGIO F. SANCHEZ BRUNI

The economic importance of helminth infections in livestock has long been recognized, and it is probably for this reason that the most important advances in the chemotherapy of helminthiasis have come from the animal health area (Horton 1990). Anthelmintics are used in all animal species and man. A significant part of the economic impact of parasitism in animal production is represented by the investment in control measures. Although alternative methods have been developed, chemically based treatments are the most important tool to control parasitism. A more complete understanding of the pharmacological properties of existing antiparasitic drugs should assist with more efficient parasite control both in livestock and companion animals. The development of highly efficient analytical techniques to quantify drug/metabolites concentrations in various host tissues and target parasites has significantly contributed to understanding the pharmacokinetic and metabolic features of the available anthelmintic drugs. Unfortunately, the investment in control measures does not always result in the expected therapeutic success. Among factors responsible for that therapeutic failure are 1) inadequate integration between management strategies and chemotherapy, 2) incorrect use of anthelmintic drugs due to insufficient knowledge of their pharmacological features, 3) insufficient understanding of the relationship between pharmacological properties, and 4) several host-related factors that could lead to modifications on the pharmacokinetic behavior and to a decreased antiparasite efficacy of the chosen drug. In addition, the availability of many compounds with a common mode of action and the indiscriminate use of these drugs have accounted for the widespread development of drug resistance, mainly in parasites of sheep and goats, but also in parasites of pigs, horses, and cattle. This chapter covers the information available for the different specific antinematodal drug families used in veterinary therapeutics. However, special consideration is given to the description of the large body of pharmacological knowledge generated for the benzimidazole compounds, the most intensively studied anthelmintic chemical group together with the endectocide macrocyclic lactones (see Chapter 42).

BENZIMIDAZOLES AND PROBENZIMIDAZOLES

Benzimidazole (BZD) and probenzimidazole (pro-BZD) anthelmintics are widely used in veterinary and human medicine. The pro-BZDs are inactive prodrugs metabolically converted into anthelmintically active BZD molecules in the host. The remarkable overall safety of BZD compounds has been a major factor in their successful worldwide use over 4 decades. BZDs were introduced into the animal health market primarily for the control of gastrointestinal (GI) nematodes, not only for use in livestock animals (cattle, sheep, goats, swine, and poultry), but also for horses, dogs, and cats. The use of BZD compounds quickly became widespread because they offered major advantages over previous available drugs in terms of spectrum, efficacy against immature stages, and safety for the host animal.

CHEMISTRY. Since the discovery of thiabendazole (TBZ) in 1961 (Brown et al. 1964), several thousand BZD molecules have been synthesized and screened for anthelmintic activity. However, no more than twenty of them have been commercially developed for use in domestic animals and man, either as BZD or pro-BZD. The BZD structure is a bicyclic ring system in which benzene has been fused to the 4- and 5- positions of the heterocycle (imidazole) (see Fig. 40.1). Most of the BZD compounds are white crystalline powders, with a fairly high melting point and which are insoluble or slightly soluble in water. BZD's aqueous solubility is markedly higher at low acidic pH values with the stomach/abomasum being the appropriate site for the dissolution of BZD drug particles after oral treatment. The BZD compounds can be grouped as follows:

1. *BZD thiazolyls:* thiabendazole (TBZ), cambendazole
2. *BZD methylcarbamates:* parbendazole, mebendazole (MBZ), flubendazole (FLBZ), oxibendazole (OBZ), luxabendazole, albendazole (ABZ), ABZ sulphoxide (ABZSO), also known as ricobendazole (RBZ), fenbendazole (FBZ), oxfendazole (OFZ)
3. *Halogenated BZD thiols:* triclabendazole
4. *Pro-BZDs:* thiophanate, febantel (FBT), netobimin (NTB)

Different modifications at positions 2- and 5- of the BZD ring system (see Fig. 40.1) have provided the most anthelmintically active drugs, especially with the discovery of sulfur-containing methylcarbamate derivatives such as ABZ and FBZ, which exhibit high efficacy against lungworms and inhibited larval stages of most GI nematodes. The BZD methylcarbamates are largely the most used BZD compounds. ABZ, FBZ, and their sulphoxide derivatives (ABZSO and OFZ, respectively) ruminants; FBZ and OFZ horses; FBT, FBZ, and MBZ companion animals; and FBZ and FLBZ (poultry and pigs) are currently among the most extensively used BZD methylcarbamate anthelmintics in veterinary medicine.

PHARMACODYNAMICS: MODE OF ACTION. Microtubules are hollow tubular organelles that exist in a dynamic equilibrium with tubulin, the microtubule subunit. Tubulin exists as a dimeric protein comprised of α- and β-subunits. The BZD and pro-BZD pharmacological activity is based on the binding to parasite β-tubulin, which produces subsequent disruption of the tubulin-microtubule dynamic equilibrium (see Lacey 1990 for detailed information). Competitive binding experiments using tubulin from mammalian, invertebrate, or fungal cells indicate that BZD compounds bind within the colchicine (a well-recognized microtubule inhibitor) binding domain on tubulin. Thus,

BENZIMIDAZOLE THIAZOLYLS

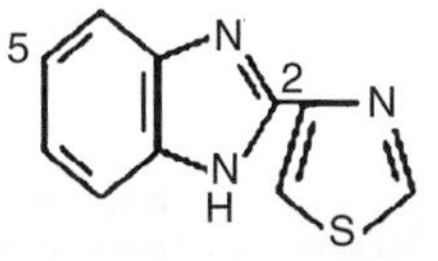

Thiabendazole (TBZ)

PRO-BENZIMIDAZOLES

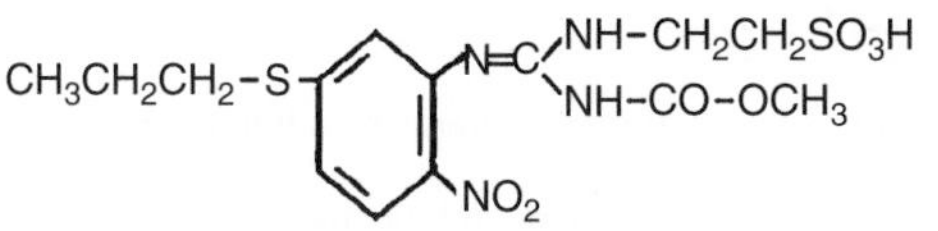

Netobimin (NTB)

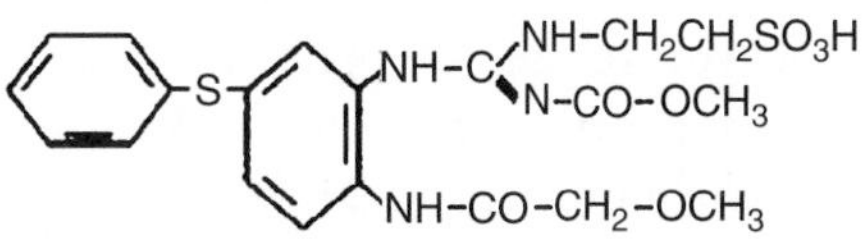

Febantel (FBT)

BENZIMIDAZOLE METHYLCARBAMATES

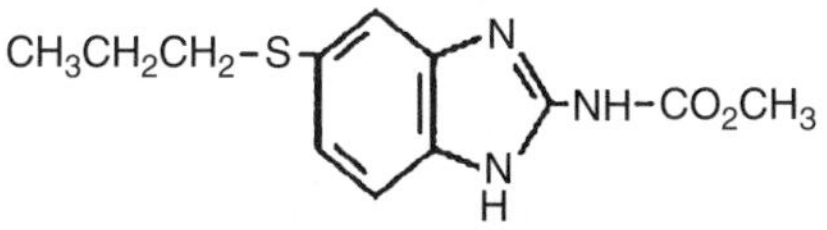

Albendazole (ABZ)

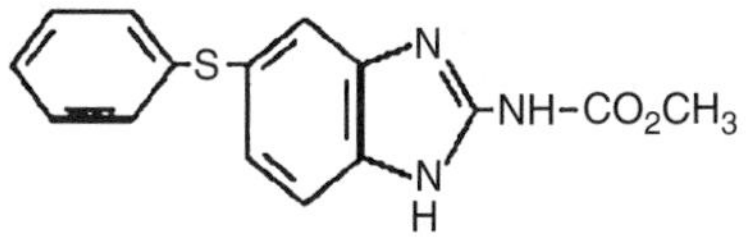

Fenbendazole (FBZ)

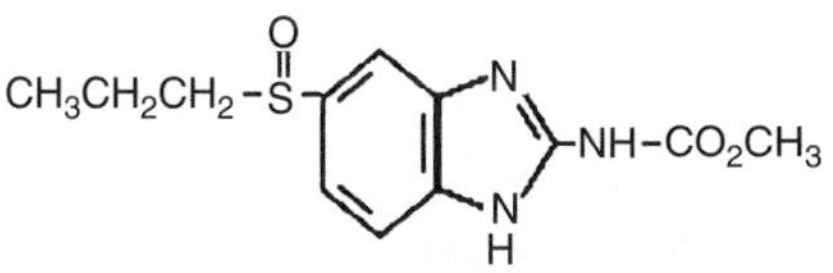

Albendazole sulphoxide (ABZSO)

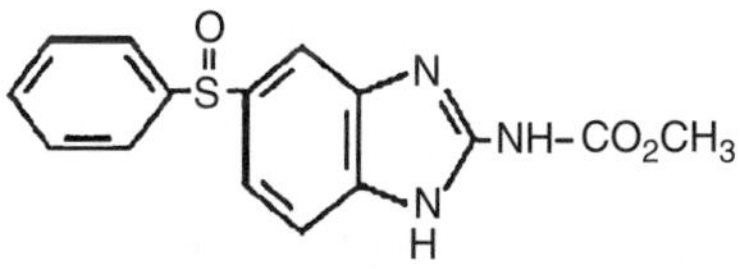

Oxfendazole (OFZ)

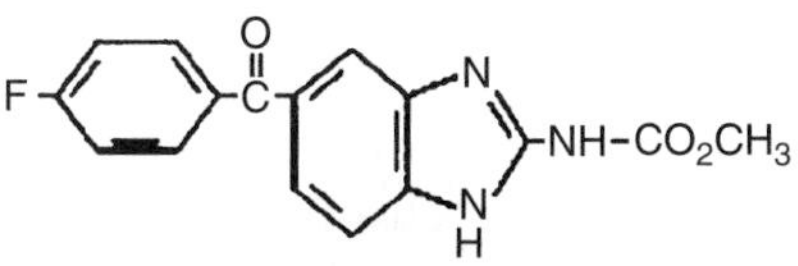

Flubendazole (FLBZ)

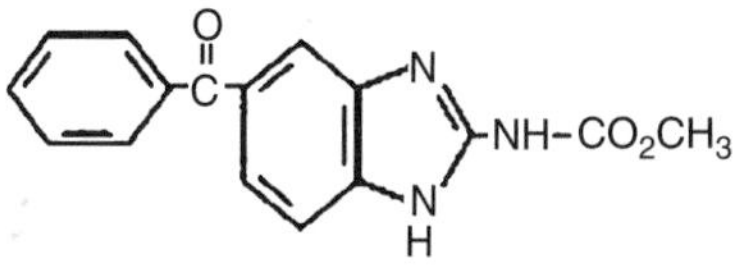

Mebendazole (MBZ)

FIG. 40.1 Chemical structures of the main benzimidazole (BZD) anthelmintics used in veterinary medicine. The positions -2 and -5 (main substitution sites) are shown in the thiabendazole structure. ABZSO is also known as *ricobendazole (RBZ)*. Triclabendazole (a halogenated flukicidal BZD) is not included here (see Chapter 41).

all the functions ascribed to microtubules at the cellular level are altered (cell division, maintenance of cell shape, cell motility, cell secretion, nutrient absorption, and intracellular transport) (Lacey 1988). Microtubules are found in animal, plant, and fungi cells. However, the rate constant for the dissociation of BZD from parasite tubulin is much lower than the rate constant for the dissociation from mammalian tubulin. These differences in dissociation rates between

BZD and tubulin in host and parasites may explain the selective toxicity of BZD compounds to parasites and its wide safety margin in the mammalian host. The microtubule loss observed at tegumental and intestinal level in cestodes and nematodes after BZD treatment is followed by loss of transport of secretory vesicles and decreased glucose uptake. A prolonged storage of secretory material within the cells is followed by cell disintegration. Cell autolysis requires a period of 15–24 hours posttreatment. Additionally, the inhibition of secretion of nematode acetylcholinesterase and inhibition of some enzymatic activities (such as fumarate reductase, malate dehydrogenase, phosphoenol pyruvate reductase, and succinate dehydrogenase) have been associated with the BZD anthelmintic action. However, all these effects may be related to the primary underlying BZD mechanism: the disruption of the tubulin-microtubules dynamic equilibrium. The effects of structural modifications to BZD-like molecules on microtubule inhibitory activity have been intensively investigated (reviewed by Lacey 1988). It has been postulated that the presence of a carbamate group in the 2- position is essential for potent microtubule inhibitory activity. Additionally, regardless of the size of the substituent in the 5- position, the pharmacological effect heavily depends on the nature of the molecule adjacent to the BZD ring system. Different studies suggest that not only the chemical substitution in the position 5- of the BZD ring, but also its conformational arrangement, are relevant in the access of the drug to the active site and in the resultant anthelmintic activity.

Benzimidazole anthelmintic activity

PK issues

- **Drug dissolution and absorption. Distribution to target tissues**
- **Drug concentrations at the site of parasite location and time of parasite exposure**
- **Mechanisms of drug transfer into target parasites**
- **Drug capacity to reach the site of action within the parasite**
- **Fate of the drug/metabolites in target parasites**

PD issues

- **Binding affinity for the parasite β-tubulin receptor**
- **Capacity to disrupt the tubulin-microtubules dynamic equilibrium**

FIG. 40.2 Relationship between the main pharmacokinetic (PK) and pharmacodynamic (PD) issues governing the anthelmintic activity of benzimidazole compounds.

Pharmacokinetic Behavior. The anthelmintic activity of BZD compounds not only depends on their binding to β-tubulin, but it also depends on the ability of the compounds to reach high and sustained concentrations at the site of parasite location that allow the delivery of effective concentrations of the compound at the receptor within the parasite cells, in sufficient time, to cause the therapeutic effect (Thompson et al. 1993) (see Fig. 40.2). As a chemical class, the BZD methylcarbamates have only limited water solubility, and small differences in drug solubility may have a major influence on their absorption and resultant pharmacokinetic behavior. The lack of water solubility is an important limitation for the formulation of BZD compounds, which mainly allows their preparation as suspensions, pastes, or granules for oral or intraruminal administration. Poor/erratic GI absorption is a common inconvenience for the systemic availability of enterally administered BZD suspensions in most species. The mucous surface in the GI tract behaves as a lipid barrier for the absorption of active substances, so absorption depends on lipid solubility and degree of ionization at GI pH levels. However, drug particles must dissolve in the enteric fluids to facilitate absorption of the BZD molecule through the GI mucosa. The dissolution rate of an enterally delivered compound influences the rate and extent of its absorption (systemic bioavailability), its maximal plasma concentration, its subsequent distribution to target tissues and its overall disposition kinetics. The BZD methylcarbamates show only limited GI absorption due to their poor solubility in water. Their dissolution rate, passage along the GI tract, and absorption into the systemic circulation are markedly slower than those observed for the more hydrosoluble BZD thiazolyls (TBZ). Such a phenomenon also results in extended residence times for the active metabolites of the BZD methylcarbamates compared to those of TBZ. This differential pharmacokinetic behavior accounts, in part, for the greater anthelmintic potency of FBZ and ABZ compared with TBZ.

PHARMACOKINETICS AND METABOLISM IN RUMINANT SPECIES

Absorption. The complexity of the ruminant digestive tract in comparison to that of the monogastric animal creates unique problems and opportunities as concerns the absorption of drugs administered orally. The rumen may substantially influence the absorption pattern and the resultant pharmacokinetics and antiparasite activity of enterally delivered BZD anthelmintics. The rumen accounts for about 20% of the animal's volume and never empties. When a BZD suspension is deposited in the rumen, solid particles mix and distribute through the digesta volume. The adsorption of BZD particles to digesta solid content, the slow mixing and long digesta residence time, and the large rumen volume assists absorption by delaying the rate of passage of drug down the GI tract (Hennessy 1993a). The rumen may act as a reservoir and prolong the duration of drug absorption and/or outflow down the GI tract. On the other hand, dissolution of BZD particles given as drug suspensions is greater at the acid abomasal pH. Thus, the time of residence of the administered BZD suspension at the abomasal level may notably affect the dissolution rate and the subsequent absorption of the drug in the gut. The rumen acts as a drug reservoir by slowing the digesta transit time throughout the abomasum, which results in improved systemic availability of BZD compounds as a consequence of a greater dissolution of drug particles in the acid pH of the abomasums (Lanusse and Prichard 1993b). The influence of the rumen on BZD absorption is evidenced by the higher and more sustained concentration of FBZ, OFZ, ABZ and their metabolites recovered in the bloodstream after oral/intraruminal treatments compared to intraabomasal administration of the same compounds in sheep (Prichard et al. 1978; Marriner and Bogan 1981).

Although the distribution of the drug in the stratified ruminal content may slow absorption and outflow down to the abomasum, the BZD methylcarbamates are less water soluble at ruminal pH than at abomasal pH. The dissolution of the sulphides ABZ and FBZ in the ruminal fluid, or at least the delay of its outflow down to the abomasum, may be important in the resultant plasma bioavailability of the sulphoxide metabolites. This relationship among drug dissolution, GI absorption, and systemic availability may be a critical issue to be considered in the development of successful BZD formulations for use in ruminants.

Metabolism and Elimination. BZD and pro-BZD anthelmintics are extensively metabolized in all mammalian species studied. As a common pattern among different BZD compounds, the parent drug is short-lived and metabolic products predominate in plasma and all tissues and excreta of the host, as well as in parasites recovered from BZD-treated animals (Fetterer and Rew 1984; Alvarez et al. 1999, 2000). The primary metabolites usually are products of oxidative and hydrolytic processes and are all more polar and water soluble than the parent drug. In addition, phase II conjugative reactions are highly important in the detoxification of BZD-derived products. The oxidized and hydrolyzed metabolites are conjugated with glucuronide and/or sulphate to increase their polarities, which facilitates urinary or biliary excretion. Since BZD anthelmintics are mainly administered by the oral route, "first-pass" metabolism is relevant in the kinetic behavior of these compounds. Intestinal, liver, and lung metabolism have been implicated in this phenomenon in most animal species. Additionally, GI metabolism is an important concern in ruminant species.

NTB (pro-BZD) is an anthelmintically inactive nitrophenylguanidine prodrug. NTB is nitroreduced and cyclized into ABZ in a microflora-mediated reductive reaction in the GI tract (Lanusse et al. 1993a). The nitroreduction and cyclization of NTB into ABZ in the host are crucial for the pharmacokinetic profile of its active metabolites and resultant anthelmintic activity. Both formulation and route of administration may dramatically affect the rate of NTB conversion and the bioavailability and disposition of its main plasma metabolites, ABZSO and $ABZSO_2$. Both sheep and cattle ruminal and ileal fluids can convert NTB into ABZ under in vitro conditions (Lanusse et al. 1992b). However, the subcutaneous administration of NTB resulted in lower plasma concentrations of active metabolites compared to those measured after oral administration of the prodrug in sheep and cattle (Lanusse et al. 1990). In conclusion, the oral administration results in an improved pharmacokinetic profile of NTB metabolites, which accounts for some advantageous anthelmintic efficacy after the oral/intraruminal compared to the parenteral treatment.

FBT is a phenylguanidine prodrug that is hydrolyzed by removal of a methoxyacetyl group and then cyclized to FBZ. FBZ is then converted to OFZ and $FBZSO_2$ in subsequent oxidative metabolic steps. Following FBT administration in both sheep and cattle, the parent drug is not found in plasma, or is detected in low concentrations for only a short period. In contrast to the extensive GI metabolism described for NTB, only a low proportion of FBT is bioconverted by sheep and cattle ruminal fluids (Beretta et al. 1987). Hepatic metabolism appears to be the main site of FBT conversion into FBZ after its oral administration to different animal species. The active molecule of the pro-BZD thiophanate is an ethyl BZD carbamate metabolite known as lobendazole (Delatour et al. 1988), formed in the liver with conversion rates of 34% (sheep), 52% (goats), and 57% (cattle).

Thiophanate is currently used as an antifungal agent (TPT-methyl) for plants.

Hepatic and Extrahepatic Oxidative Metabolism. The metabolism of BZD heavily depends on the substituent present at position 5- of the BZD ring system and involves a variety of reactions. Phase I reactions have been observed at position 5-. Hydroxylations of TBZ, ABZ, and FBZ have been demonstrated in different animal species. The sulphoxidation of ABZ and FBZ at the sulfur atom of the substituent group at the carbon 5- of the BZD nucleus have been widely investigated (see Fig. 40.1). In fact, the oxidations of ABZ to ABZSO and FBZ to OFZ have been shown to be catalyzed by the liver microsomal mixed function oxidases in different species (Galtier et al. 1986a; Souhaili El Amri et al. 1987; Montesissa et al. 1989; Lanusse et al. 1993b; Virkel et al. 2004). Additionally, the anthelmintically active sulphoxide derivatives undergo a second, slower, and irreversible oxidative step that forms the inactive sulphone ($ABZSO_2$ and $FBZSO_2$) metabolites, which are also found in the bloodstream and tissues after administration of their respective parent sulphides.

The substitution of the BZD ring in position 5- has been particularly important in determining the metabolic fate of BZD methylcarbamates. This position is metabolically labile and has permitted retardation of the biotransformation of 5-substituted BZD anthelmintics as well as improvement of their efficacy (Hennessy et al. 1989). The nature of this substitution at position 5- markedly influences the sequence of BZD liver metabolism. Aromatic BZD derivatives such as FBZ and OFZ require more extensive hepatic oxidative metabolism than aliphatic derivatives (ABZ and ABZSO) to achieve sufficient polarity for excretion (Hennessy 1993). Consequently, the rates of ABZ liver microsomal sulphoxidation in sheep and cattle were higher than those observed for FBZ (Virkel et al. 2004). Indeed, pharmacokinetic differences between ABZ and FBZ are highly based on their different oxidative metabolism. For this reason, low FBZ concentrations are recovered in plasma following its oral/intraruminal administration to sheep and cattle, while ABZ is not detected in the bloodstream after its administration as parent drug in both species. Moreover, longer plasma mean residence times and elimination half-lives for FBZ and its metabolites, compared to those of ABZ metabolites, were observed in sheep and cattle (Lanusse et al. 1995) (see Fig. 40.3).

The involvement of the cytochrome P450 (CYP) and flavin monooxygenase (FMO) systems on the liver sulphoxidation of ABZ have been demonstrated in different animal species, including sheep (Galtier et al. 1986a) and cattle (Lanusse et al. 1993b). Up to 30% of ABZ sulphoxidation in human liver is mediated by FMO, while the CYP system is the major contributor (~70%) (Rawden et al. 2000). Similarly, CYP is primarily involved (~60%) in ABZ hepatic sulphoxidation in rats, although the FMO enzymatic system is also implicated (Moroni et al. 1995). Similar in vitro studies demonstrated the relative involvement of liver FMO (~32%) and CYP (~68%) on the liver sulphoxidation of FBZ in rats (Murray et al. 1992). Inhibition of CYP-mediated sulphoxidation by piperonyl butoxide demonstrated the participation of this enzymatic system in the hepatic metabolism of FBZ in horses (McKellar et al. 2002). Conversely, it has been demonstrated that FMO is primarily involved in ABZ hepatic sulphoxidation in sheep (Galtier et al. 1986a) and cattle (Lanusse et al. 1993b). Recently, it has been demonstrated that FMO-mediated sulphoxidation accounted for up to 60% of ABZSO production from ABZ, while CYP contributed 40% in both sheep and cattle liver microsomes (Virkel et al. 2004). Similarly, FMO was estimated to be the main enzymatic system involved in the liver sulphoxidation of FBZ (~80%) in both species (Virkel et al. 2004).

Both sulphoxide metabolites (ABZSO and OFZ) have an asymmetric center in the sulfur atom of its side chain. This nucleophilic sulfur atom is attached to four different functional groups, which results in an asymmetric molecule nonsuperimposable with its mirror image. Thus, two different enantiomers of ABZSO and OFZ have been identified (by chiral separation) in the plasma of sheep and cattle treated with ABZ and FBZ (prochiral molecules), respectively (Delatour et al. 1990a; Sánchez et al. 2002) (see Fig. 40.4). It has been shown that (+)ABZSO is the main enantiomeric form recovered in plasma and tissues of parasites location (Alvarez et al. 2000) following ABZ treatment to sheep (see Fig. 40.5). The same pattern was observed after ABZSO administration to cattle (Cristofol et al. 2001). Similarly, (+)OFZ prevails in the systemic circulation after both FBZ and OFZ administrations to sheep (Delatour et al. 1990a; Sánchez et al. 2002) and cattle. The observed differences on the plasma/tissue availabilities of the (+) and (−) enantiomeric forms were attributed to the relative contribution of the FMO and CYP-dependent oxygenases to ABZ and FBZ hepatic sulphoxidation. Many steps in drug metabolism have been shown to be chiral-dependent. Enantioselectivity of

a)

b)

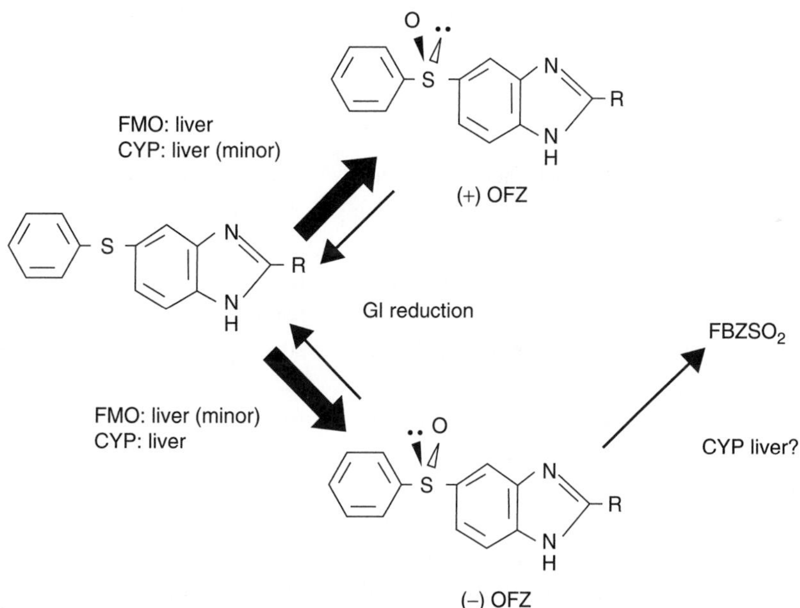

FIG. 40.3 Proposed metabolic pathways for the enantioselective sulphoxidation and sulphonation of a) albendazole (ABZ) and b) fenbendazole (FBZ). The gastrointestinal (GI) sulphoreduction of both sulphoxide enantiomers (ruminants) to form the parent thioethers (ABZ, FBZ) is also shown. The width of the arrows represents the proportional magnitude of each metabolic pathway (see the text). Data from Delatour et al. 1991; Benoit et al. 1992; Redondo et al. 1999; Virkel et al. 2002, 2004.

FMO: flavin monooxygenase; CYP: cytochrome P-450; ABZSO (ABZ sulphoxide); OFZ (oxfendazole, FBZ sulphoxide); ABZSO$_2$ (ABZ sulphone); FBZSO$_2$ (FBZ sulphone).

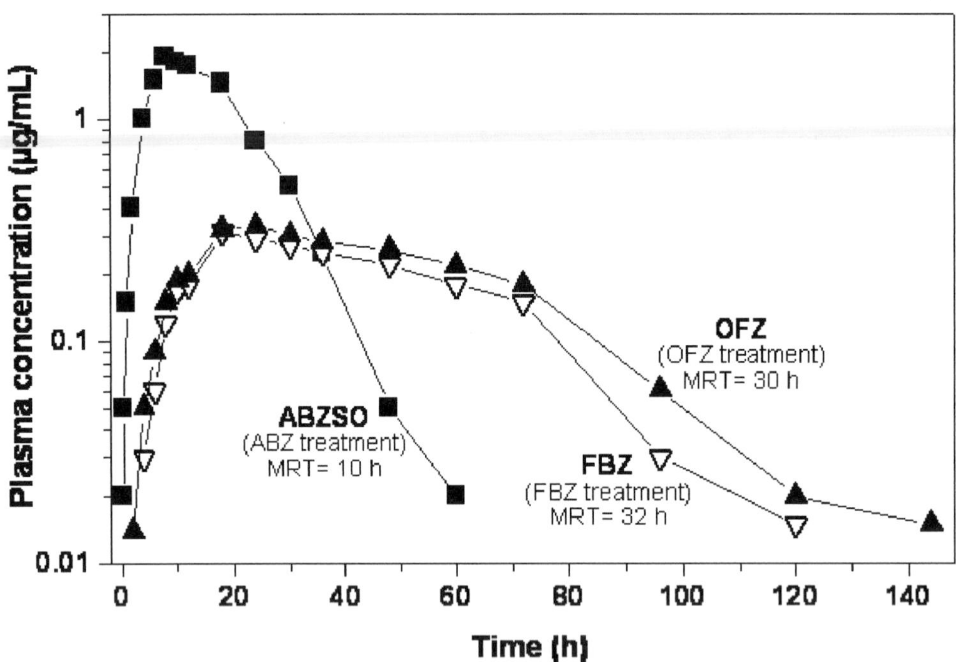

FIG. 40.4 Comparative mean (n = 5) plasma concentrations of the benzimidazole sulphoxide metabolites: albendazole sulphoxide (ABZSO) and oxfendazole (OFZ) obtained after oral administration of albendazole (ABZ), fenbendazole (FBZ), and OFZ (5 mg/kg) to adult sheep (see text for further explanation). Adapted from Lanusse et al. 1995.
MRT: mean plasma residence time (h) for each molecule.

metabolic products occurs when chiral metabolites are generated differentially (in qualitative or quantitative terms) from a single achiral substrate. Thus, two different Km values for the production of each ABZSO enantiomer have been reported after ABZ (prochiral molecule) incubation with liver microsomes obtained from rats (Moroni et al. 1995) and calves (Virkel et al. 2004). These observations are consistent with the involvement of two different enantioselective enzymatic pathways on the liver sulphoxidation of ABZ. Indeed, FMO and CYP are known to be oppositely enantioselective (Cashman 1998). FMO activity accounted for 94% (cattle) and 81% (sheep) of (+)ABZSO production in liver microsomes (Virkel et al. 2004). In both species, the enantioselectivity of the hepatic FMO system toward (+)ABZSO production was close to 100%. On the other hand, FMO-mediated sulphoxidation of FBZ generated both (+) and (−) OFZ enantiomers. FBZ oxidation was enantioselective toward the production of (+)OFZ in both sheep (65%) and cattle (79%). In conclusion, the sulphoxide metabolite recovered in plasma and target tissues after either ABZ or FBZ administration does exist as two different chemical entities: the (+) and (−) enantiomeric forms (see Figures 40.4 and 40.5).

Biotransformation takes place predominantly in the liver, although metabolic activity is apparent in extrahepatic tissues such as lung parenchyma and small intestine mucosa. Large quantities of ABZ parent drug were recovered from tissues of parasite location in both sheep and cattle. Similarly, FBZ has been recovered from tissues of parasite location following oral administration of OFZ to cattle. Altogether, these findings support the need for studying the biotransformation of BZD anthelmintics in extrahepatic tissues such as lung parenchyma and small intestinal mucosa. In fact, the relative involvement of FMO (~49–60%) and CYP (~40–51%) systems on the sulphoxidation of ABZ by gut epithelium was studied in rats (Redondo et al. 1999). The sulphoxidation of ABZ and FBZ by small intestine (cattle) and lung (sheep and cattle) microsomes was shown to be enantioselective (Virkel et al. 2004). Although the liver is the main site of ABZ and FBZ biotransformation, sulphoxidation in the intestinal mucosa and lung tissue (see Fig. 40.4) may contribute to the presystemic metabolism of both anthelmintic drugs and should not be underestimated.

The administration of TBZ results in a rapid conversion of a parent compound into a 5-hidroxy TBZ metabolite,

Ruminal enantioselective metabolism

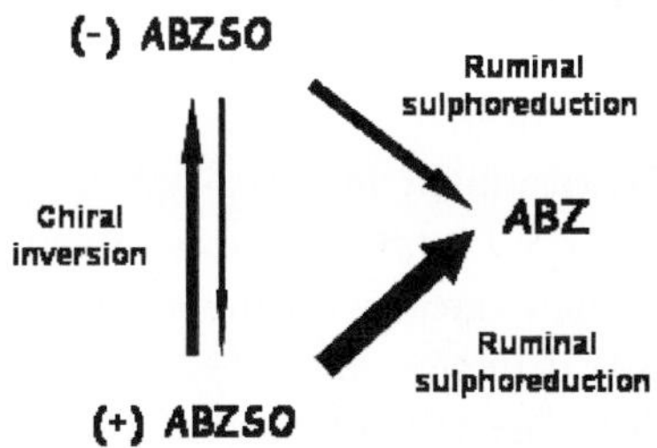

(+) sulphoxide enantiomer

- **Longer persistence in the bloodstream**
- **Higher concentrations in tissues/fluids of parasite location**
- **Higher concentration within target parasites**
- **Higher nematodicidal activity**

FIG. 40.5 Schematic representation of the ruminal biotransformation of albendazole sulphoxide (ABZSO) enantiomers. The width of the arrows indicates the magnitude of the metabolic reactions. The main pharmacological features of the (+) sulphoxide enantiomer, compared to the (–) isoform, are listed in the bottom box. The enantioselective ruminal sulphoreduction of the (+) isoform is the most relevant metabolic reaction for the formation of the parent thioether (ABZ). The same pattern is applicable to the sulphoreduction of oxfendazole (OFZ) enantiomers into fenbendazole (FBZ) (see the text for detailed explanation). Adapted from Virkel et al. 2004.

formed by aromatic ring hydroxylation. Although this metabolite is sufficiently polar for a rapid urinary excretion, both its unconjugated and sulphate or glucuronide conjugated forms have been found in urine of TBZ-treated animals (Tocco et al. 1965; Gottschall et al. 1990). MBZ is absorbed, metabolized by the liver, and excreted in bile. Following intravenous administration of [C^{14}]MBZ in bile ducts–cannulated rats, 84.3% of the total recovered radioactivity was present in the bile, whereas only 15.7% appeared in urine (Allan and Watson 1983).

After the administration of MBZ to sheep, the parent drug is rapidly absorbed and metabolized into two main metabolites, which are identified in sheep plasma after MBZ treatment (Behm et al. 1983). The main MBZ metabolite results from carbonyl reduction to the secondary alcohol, which was also identified as its glucuronide or sulphate conjugates. Although the specific enzymatic system responsible for MBZ reduction is unknown, several cytosolic ketone reductases are involved in the formation of hydrosoluble metabolites from carbonyl-containing molecules. On the other hand, combination of carbonyl reduction and carbamate hydrolysis produces the hydrolyzed metabolite of TBZ. Hydrolysis of the carbamate group eliminates both, the anthelmintic activity of the compound and its toxicity. MBZ over its metabolites appears to be the active anthelmintic molecule.

Unlike aromatic substituted methylcarbamates, 5-aliphatic substitutes such as ABZ and PBZ, when oxidized, are sufficiently polar to be largely excreted in urine rather than undergo further conjugation and secretion in bile (Hennessy et al. 1989). For instance, following ABZ treatment to sheep only 8% of the total dose was recovered in bile as unconjugated ABZSO and OH-ABZSO metabolites, and 6.3% as conjugated glucuronide and sulphate esters mainly of 2OH-ABZSO and 2OH-$ABZSO_2$ (Hennessy et al. 1989); 59% of the dose was recovered in urine of ABZ-treated cattle (Gyurik et al. 1981). On the other hand, the percentage of FBZ dose recovered in urine (2.5%) in cattle was markedly lower than that recovered from feces (42%), the latter being mainly the unchanged FBZ parent compound (Short et al. 1987).

The parent flubendazole (FLBZ) compound and its reduced (R-FLBZ) and hydrolyzed (H-FLBZ) metabolites have been identified in tissues of treated pigs, poultry, and sheep. FLBZ disposition kinetics has been recently studied in sheep (Moreno et al. 2004). After its i.v. administration, the parent drug was rapidly depleted from the bloodstream, being detectable up to 36 hours posttreatment. The metabolites R-FLBZ and H-FLBZ were rapidly detected in the bloodstream, which indicates a fast biotransformation of FLBZ to form both metabolic products. R-FLBZ was the main analyte measured in plasma for up 60 hours after the i.v. treatment. In vitro incubations with sheep liver microsomes indicate that FLBZ is biotransformed by the mixed-function oxidase system (Moreno et al. 2004). However, sheep liver microsomes failed to hydrolyze the methylcarbamate group in position -2 of the BZD ring to produce the $-NH_2$ derivative of FLBZ (H-FLBZ). The low levels of hydrolytic enzymes in the microsomal fraction may account for the lack of FLBZ conversion into H-FLBZ.

Reductive Metabolism in the Gastrointestinal Tract. In comparison to the liver where oxidative metabolism predominates, the GI microflora is very active in reductive reactions of foreign compounds, particularly those containing -nitro and -sulphoxide (Renwick et al. 1986; Rowland 1986) groups. Drug GI metabolism may be modified by the type of diet and many other factors affecting the GI bacterial reductive capacity. Orally administered compounds that are poorly absorbed from the GI tract will stand the greatest chance of undergoing metabolism by the microflora, although a large number of drug/metabolites gain entry to the gut via biliary secretion or plasma-GI distribution exchange and will also be exposed to microbial activity. Drug metabolic processes taking place in the rumen are particularly important in ruminant therapeutics.

The sequential oxidation of BZD thioether (ABZ, FBZ) compounds in the liver and extrahepatic tissues leads to the production of more polar and less anthelmintically effective sulphoxide and sulphone metabolites. However, the importance of the biotransformation of BZD and pro-BZD compounds in the lumen of the GI tract should not be underestimated. Taking into consideration the extent of the exchange surface between plasma and digestive tract in ruminants and the large volume of the forestomach, any potential bioconversion of these compounds taking place in the gut lumen could have a significant impact on both the pharmacokinetic behavior and the availability of anthelmintically active metabolites at the sites where GI and tissue-dwelling parasites are located. The metabolic sulphoreduction of the BZD sulphoxide metabolites (ABZSO and OFZ) to form the parent thioethers (ABZ and FBZ, respectively) has been shown to occur in ruminal and intestinal fluid contents from sheep and cattle (Lanusse et al. 1992b). A plasma-GI pH gradient (Lanusse et al. 1993a) and/or an active gastric secretion process (Alí and Hennessy 1995) account for the distribution of BZD metabolites from plasma to the digestive tract lumen. Therefore, ABZSO and OFZ can be reduced back to their respective thioethers by ruminal and intestinal microflora and may act as a source of ABZ and FBZ, respectively, in the GI tract. This GI metabolic reduction may be of primary importance for the antiparasitic efficacy of BZD thioethers. Since the thioethers have a greater affinity for parasite tubulin than the sulphoxides (Lacey 1990; Lubega and Prichard 1991), this bacteria-mediated reduction may have significant importance for the efficacy against GI parasites. Thus, the high efficacy of ABZSO and OFZ against GI parasites may depend on this bacterial reduction of the sulphoxide to the more pharmacologically active thioethers. The in vivo nematodicidal efficacy of ABZSO and OFZ is similar to that of ABZ or FBZ.

Undoubtedly, the plasma/GI tract distribution of the active sulphoxide metabolites is of major relevance for the efficacy of BZD anthelmintics against GI parasites. It has also been demonstrated that (+)ABZSO is the main enantiomeric form recovered in tissues of parasite location following ABZ treatment in sheep (Alvarez et al. 2000) and racemic ABZSO administration to cattle (Cristofol et al. 2001), which agrees with the lower systemic availability and faster depletion of the (−)enantiomer observed in both species. The relative contribution of the FMO and CYP-dependent oxygenases to ABZ hepatic sulphoxidation accounts for such differences in the availability of each enantiomeric form in plasma and tissues. Moreover, it has been shown that (−)ABZSO rather than its (+) antipode, would be the main substrate for the CYP-mediated formation of the inactive sulphone ($ABZSO_2$) metabolite (Delatour et al. 1991; Benoit et al. 1992). Altogether, these findings would indicate that (+)ABZSO, being predominant in the bloodstream, may be the main enantiomeric form available in the GI tract. In fact, higher availabilities of the (+)antipode, compared to that of the (−)enantiomer, were observed in plasma and GI tract after the administration of both racemic ABZSO and OFZ to cattle (Cristofol et al. 2001). Since ABZ and FBZ are formed in rumen from ABZSO and OFZ, respectively, in a bacteria-mediated sulphoreduction, the (+)enantiomers would be the main source for the parent sulphide formation (see Fig. 40.5). This is consistent with the faster depletion of the (+)ABZSO antipode incubated with ruminal fluid under anaerobic in vitro conditions (Virkel et al. 2002). The binding of BZD anthelmintics to parasite tubulin produces the subsequent disruption of the tubulin-microtubule dynamic equilibrium. It is well established that ABZ has a greater affinity for parasite tubulin than ABZSO. Although both enantiomeric forms are substrates for the formation of ABZ, the most efficient (enantioselective) sulphoreduction of (+)ABZSO to form a more pharmacologically potent product (ABZ) (Virkel at al. 2002), may greatly contribute to the pattern of efficacy of these anthelmintics against GI parasites. Indeed, these observations may suggest a lower contribution of the (−) antipode to the overall efficacy of ABZ/FBZ and related anthelmintics (see Fig. 40.5). Chiral inversion is the metabolic process by which one enantiomer is transformed into its antipode. The chiral inversions of (+) into (−) but also from (−) into (+) enantiomeric forms were observed when both enantiomers were incubated separately (as pure substrates) with ruminal fluid obtained from both sheep and cattle (Virkel et al. 2002) (Fig. 40.5). Thus, the reported data suggests that chiral inversion of RBZ and OFZ enantiomers is likely to be bidirectional and may depend on either the metabolic transformation of one enantiomer into its antipode or through the formation of parent thioether (ABZ or FBZ) as an intermediate metabolic product. Overall, the work published by Virkel et al. (2002) demonstrates that the ruminal sulphoreduction of both ABZSO and OFZ is enantioselective, with the (+) antipode being the main substrate to form the more active parent sulphide in the rumen.

Distribution to Parasite Location Tissues. Release from dosage form and absorption precede entry of any anthelmintic molecule into the bloodstream, which serves as the tissue in which drug and metabolite molecules are conducted to various parts of the body. Within the bloodstream, a fraction of most drugs binds reversibly to plasma proteins, and the remainder undergoes simultaneous distribution, metabolism and excretion. The access of BZD molecules to intracellular sites depends upon their ability to penetrate the capillary endothelium and to cross the cell membrane. Most anthelmintics are weak organic acids or bases and exist in solution, at physiological pH, as both nonionized and ionized forms; while the poor lipophilicity of the ionized molecules excludes them from passive diffusion, the lipid-soluble nonionized moieties passively diffuse across biological membranes until equilibrium is established. Once the BZD molecule has been absorbed from the GI tract, it is rapidly distributed by the circulatory system throughout the entire body. During this time, the metabolic processes necessary to facilitate its elimination commence. Extensive tissue distribution of ABZ and its metabolites in sheep (Alvarez et al. 1999) and cattle (Sánchez et al. 1997) have been reported. However, differential distribution patterns among BZD sulphides (FBZ, ABZ), sulphoxide (OFZ, ABZSO), and sulphone ($FBZSO_2$, $ABZSO_2$) metabolites, based on their differential lipophilicities, may be expected. The distribution rate, which is indicated by the apparent volume of distribution, depends on molecular weight, lipid solubility, and plasma protein binding of each drug/metabolite. The majority of BZD compounds show a binding of less than 50% to plasma protein, relatively high volume of distribution, and a relatively fast elimination rate in ruminant species.

The rate of absorption, metabolism, and excretion of BZD anthelmintics varies from drug to drug, with slower absorption and prolonged recycling between enteral and parenteral tissues being relevant to enhance efficacy. Worms attached to the lining of the gut may be more exposed to this recycling drug than to that actually passing down the GI tract in food which is being digested. Moreover, the absorbed BZD drug may be more important than unabsorbed drug passing down the gastrointestinal tract, even against gastrointestinal nematodes (Hennessy and Prichard 1981). OFZ given intravenously to sheep (5 mg/kg) has been proven to be equally or more effective than oral OFZ against BZD-resistant *Haemonchus contortus* in the abomasum and *Trichostrongylus colubriformis* in the small intestine. FBZ, OFZ, and ABZ are less water soluble than earlier members of the group and, therefore, their dissolution rate, passage along the GI tract, and absorption into the systemic circulation are markedly slower compared to TBZ. These more lipophilic substituted BZD methylcarbamate compounds remain in the bloodstream for a longer time and, since it is assumed that an equilibrium exists between plasma and GI tract, the period of exposure of GI nematodes to effective drug/metabolites concentrations is extended. In NTB treated cattle, peak concentrations of ABZSO and $ABZSO_2$ are reached at 7–10 hours (ABZSO) and at 15–22 hours ($ABZSO_2$) posttreatment followed by a well-defined decline in concentration in both plasma and GI compartments. However, whereas plasma concentration fell to undetectable levels (30–36 hours posttreatment), the profile of these metabolites in the rumen, abomasum, and ileum showed an "extra" slow elimination phase that extended to 72 hours posttreatment (see Fig. 40.6). This pharmacokinetic behavior is particularly clear for the ABZSO and $ABZSO_2$ metabolites, whose elimination half-lives in both the abomasum and ileum were significantly longer compared to plasma. This metabolite-distribution process, also described for FBZ metabolites in cattle, may be driven by a plasma/GI tract pH gradient. The ratio of nonionized to ionized forms depends upon the pKa of the drug and the pH of the fluid in which the drug is dissolved, and the pH gradient between plasma and different tissues dictates the concentrations of drug/metabolite at either side of the separating cell membranes; at equilibrium, there will be a higher total concentration of the drug on the side of the membrane where the degree of ionization is greater. For instance, the pKa for the ABZSO metabolite is 7.8, and at plasma pH, there will be an important proportion of this molecule under the nonionic form, which will facilitate its passive diffusion from plasma to parasite location tissues. A greater plasma/abomasum pH gradient compared with that of the rumen and ileum would produce a strong ionic trapping effect,

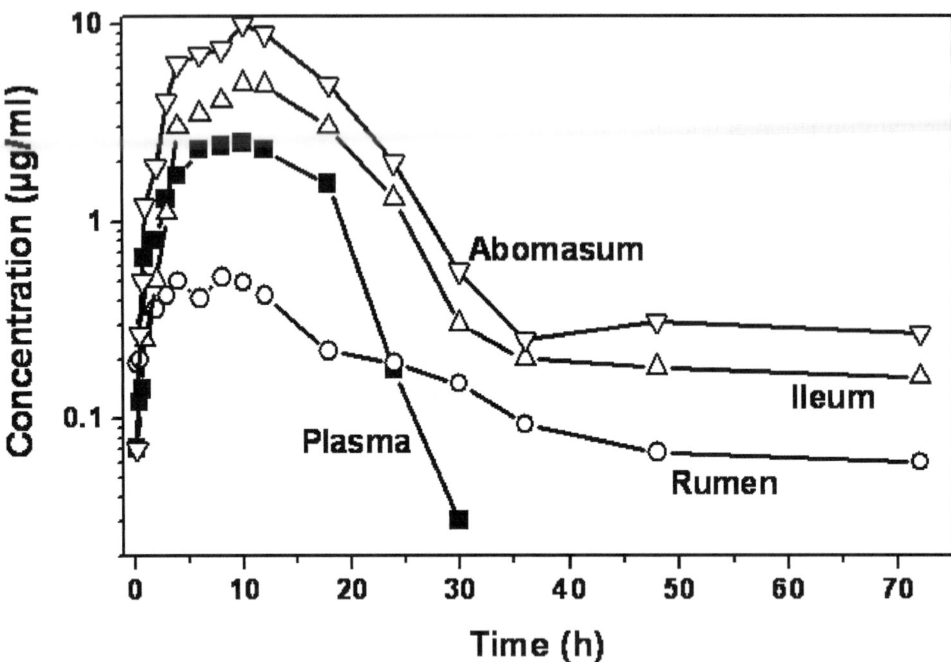

FIG. 40.6 Comparative albendazole sulphoxide (ABZSO) concentration profiles measured in the bloodstream and in different gastrointestinal compartments after the oral administration of netobimin prodrug (20 mg/kg) to cattle.

The results show the slow elimination phase observed in digestive compartments (compared to plasma), which is critical for efficacy against gastrointestinal nematodes (see the text for further explanation). ABZSO elimination half-life values were 2.29 h (plasma), 16 h (rumen), 34 h (abomasum), and 67 h (ileum). Adapted from Lanusse et al. 1993.

which would account for the significantly higher concentrations of ABZ metabolites found in the abomasum in comparison with plasma and other GI compartments. In addition, although ABZ (the most potent anthelmintic molecule) is not detected in the bloodstream, it has been recovered in different GI compartments, with particularly high concentration profiles recovered in the abomasal mucosa as well as from *Haemonchus contortus* recovered from treated sheep (see Fig. 40.7) The extensive distribution of BZD methylcarbamates from the bloodstream to the GI tract and other tissues may contribute to anthelmintic efficacy against parasites localized in body tissues, including GI mucosa and lumen, lungs, and bile ducts (Alvarez et al. 1999, 2000). The recovery of both ABZ and FBZ parent compounds from GI mucosa and lung tissue after intravenous administration of their sulphoxide derivatives to cattle (as described in the section on GI metabolism), is further evidence of the complex relationship among drug distribution, metabolism, and efficacy of BZD anthelmintics in ruminants.

Comparative studies have revealed considerable differences between ruminant species regarding the pharmacokinetics of anthelmintic drugs. Higher concentrations of TBZ have been reported in plasma of sheep compared to goats and cattle. The higher proportion of TBZ over its main metabolite 5-OH-TBZ excreted in the urine of TBZ treated sheep, compared to cattle, may be a consequence of reduced oxidative capacity of sheep liver microsomes compared to that observed for cattle and goats. The lower anthelmintic activity observed for TBZ against lung nematodes and inhibited larval stages of *Ostertagia ostertagi* in cattle, compared to that observed against lung nematodes and inhibited larval stages of *Ostertagia circumcincta* in sheep, may be related to the limited TBZ systemic availability achieved in cattle and by the fact that its main metabolite is anthelmintically inactive. On the other hand, the OFZ AUC after OFZ administration to goats was 39% smaller than that observed in sheep (Hennessy et al. 1993a). It is suggested that goats possess a faster hepatic metabolism than sheep resulting in more rapid elimination of OFZ. This lower availability may account for the poor efficacy reported for OFZ given to goats at the dose recommended for sheep. These observations suggest that extrapolated data can be

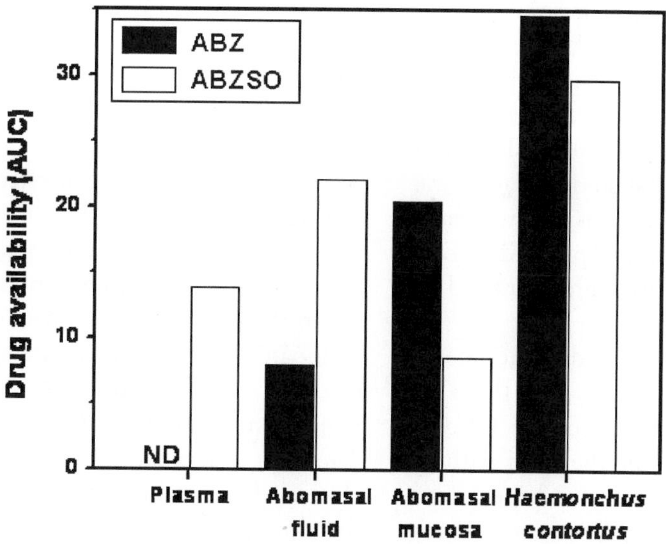

- *ABZSO was the main active molecule measured in plasma after ABZ treatment in sheep*
- *High concentrations of ABZ and ABZSO were recovered from H. contortus*
- *ABZ total availability was greater in H. contortus compared to abomasal tissue/fluid*

FIG. 40.7 Comparative albendazole (ABZ) and albendazole sulphoxide (ABZSO) availabilities (expressed as area under the concentration versus time curve, AUC) obtained in plasma, abomasal fluid, abomasal mucosa, and *Hemonchus contortus* recovered from infected sheep treated with ABZ (intraruminal at 7.5 mg/kg) (see the text for further explanation). Data adapted from Alvarez et al. 2000.
ND: not detected.
AUC values expressed in μg.h/g.

misleading in predicting adequate dosages and withdrawal times.

PHARMACOKINETICS IN NONRUMINANT SPECIES. The oral administration of BZD (FBZ, OFZ) compounds in horses demonstrated that reduced bioavailability and shorter residence times are obtained in comparison to those observed in ruminants. Following oral administration of either FBZ or OFZ (10 mg/kg) to horses, the inactive $FBZSO_2$ metabolite is the predominant analyte measured in plasma, with AUC ratios OFZ/FBZ/$FBZSO_2$ of approximately 3/1/9 (OFZ treatment) and 1/4/7 (FBZ treatment) (McKellar et al. 2002). In both cases, the time to reach the peak plasma concentration of the active OFZ metabolite was approximately 9 hours, which is earlier compared to that observed in ruminants and agrees with the reduced systemic availability observed in horses.

As described for ruminant species, ABZ is not detected in plasma after its oral administration to pigs (Alvarez et al. 1995). ABZSO and $ABZSO_2$ are the main metabolites recovered from plasma up to 48 hours posttreatment. The pattern of plasma metabolites is similar to that reported after the administration to ruminant species and there appear to be no major differences between the metabolic patterns of ABZ observed in pigs and sheep. However, marked differences in the metabolism of ABZ between cattle and pigs have been described, with predominance of the sulphoxide metabolite over $ABZSO_2$ in pig plasma, while the inverse is observed in cattle after ABZ treatment. Similar to the observations in ruminants, the time of residence of the ABZ suspension at the acidic pH of the stomach in the pig affects its dissolution rate and the subsequent absorption of the drug from the gut. Any factor that influences gastric emptying rate may have a profound effect on the rate and extent of BZD absorption in monogastric animals. After oral FBZ administration to pigs, OFZ (the main metabolite recovered) and $FBZSO_2$ are rapidly detected in plasma up to 48 hours posttreatment. OFZ reaches a Cmax value (0.7 μg/ml) at 12.5 hours posttreatment (Petersen and Friis 2000). The bioavailability of FBZ in pigs after its oral administration was estimated at about 30%. This low value is a consequence of the low water solubility of FBZ and its poor GI absorption plus the significant liver first-pass effect suffered by the drug.

The gut transit time influences the dissolution and absorption of poor water-soluble drugs such as the BZD anthelmintics. The drugs that do not dissolve in GI contents pass down and are excreted in the feces without exerting their action. The GI physiology and the digesta transit time are markedly different between monogastric species and ruminants. This is relevant for dogs and cats, whose GI transit times are significantly shorter compared to ruminant species; this has a marked effect on the absorption, kinetic behavior, and efficacy of BZD anthelmintics in companion animals. ABZ, FBZ, FBT, or MBZ formulated as tablets or suspensions for oral administration in dogs and cats must dissolve at low pH (stomach), and it has been demonstrated that the dissolution rate may be altered depending on the size of the formulation particle (Hennessy 1993). Several studies suggest that only limited rates of dissolution and absorption of BZD anthelmintics are achieved in cats, dogs, and man. Consequently, these compounds may need to be given at a higher dose or as multiple administrations in order to maintain therapeutic concentrations and, therefore, to achieve acceptable anthelmintic efficacy (Roberson and Burke 1982; Edwards and Breckenridge 1988).

MBZ is poorly absorbed after oral administration and only low concentrations (representing 10% or less of the total administered dose) of MBZ parent drug and its inactive metabolite, OH-MBZ, were recovered in plasma of humans and dogs after oral treatment (Witassek et al. 1981; Edwards and Breckenridge 1988). This observation could explain the lack of efficacy of MBZ against lung parasites in humans and dogs and the need for the design of multiple dose treatments. The pharmacokinetics of FBZ parent drug and its metabolites in dogs has been characterized (McKellar et al. 1990). FBZ parent drug, its active sulphoxide (OFZ), and inactive sulphone ($FBZSO_2$) metabolites were recovered in plasma for 48 hours after administration of a single oral dose of 20 mg/kg. Interestingly, plasma concentrations for both active molecules (FBZ and OFZ) are depleted in parallel from the body, giving an AUC ratio (FBZ:OFZ) of approximately 0.82. This may result in exposure of target parasites to the FBZ moiety (which has greater potency than OFZ), which would account for some advantageous activity against the tissue arrested larvae and other immature parasite stages (McKellar et al. 1990). When ABZ was given as a single dose in tablet form, ABZSO and $ABZSO_2$ were the main metabolites detected in plasma for up to 16 hours posttreatment (Sánchez et al. 2000a). Compared to ruminants, where the rumen acts as drug reservoir, effective treatment in dogs of monogastrics requires more prolonged, multidose regimes of at least 3 to 5 days depending on the dose used. There are conclusive pharmacokinetic results to support the concept that higher efficacy could be expected in dogs and cats by increasing the number of treatments rather than increasing the dose. In fact, the AUC of FBZ in dogs was similar after single administration of FBZ at different dose levels over a range between 2.5 and 100 mg/kg (McKellar et al. 1993). Lower FBZ plasma concentrations were achieved in dogs when FBZ was given on an empty stomach, compared with its administration in food. However, fat content in the diet does not affect the absorption of FBZ after its oral administration to dogs (McKellar et al. 1993).

After the oral administration of FBZ to chickens, the parent drug, OFZ, and $FBZSO_2$ are detected in plasma, with $FBZSO_2$, the main metabolite, recovered up to 96 hours posttreatment (Taylor et al. 1993). ABZ parent drug is absorbed slowly and detected from 1–6 hours posttreatment in chickens, with ABZSO being the main metabolite detected with a peak concentration of 0.83 μg/ml obtained at 1 hour posttreatment (Csiko et al. 1996) and low $ABZSO_2$ concentrations measured between 2.5–30 hours after ABZ administration. Data provided for chickens indicated that ABZ and FBZ are metabolized in avian species via the same metabolic pathway as in mammals (McKellar and Scott 1990). The metabolism of FBZ to its sulphoxide and sulphone metabolites appears to be much more rapid than in ruminant species. As it can be expected for dogs, cats, and man, the GI reductive metabolism of the BZD sulphoxide into the parent sulphides is markedly less relevant in poultry compared to ruminant species. FLBZ is widely used as an anthelmintic in poultry and its main metabolites, H-FLBZ and R-FLBZ, have been identified in tissues of FLBZ medicated turkeys.

MECHANISMS OF DRUG TRANSFER INTO TARGET PARASITES. Understanding the role of the cuticular/tegumental structure on the process of drug uptake by helminth parasites is a scientific area of major interest. It has been shown in ex vivo and in vivo studies that transcuticular diffusion is the predominant pathway for the entry of anthelmintic drugs into nematodes (Cross et al. 1998; Alvarez et al. 2001). Although there are relevant structural differences between the external surface of nematodes (cuticle) and cestodes/trematodes (tegument), the mechanism of drug entry to both types of helminths seems to be equally dependent on lipophilicity as a major physicochemical determinant of drug capability to reach therapeutic concentrations within the target parasite. A high correlation between the octanol-water partition coefficients for different BZD anthelmintics and their capacity to diffuse through the tegument of *Moniezia expansa* has been shown (Mottier et al. 2003). The most lipophilic BZD compounds (FBZ, ABZ, MBZ) (partition coefficients >3.7) were measured at higher concentrations within the tapeworm compared to those with the lowest lipid-water partition values (OFZ, ABZSO, TBZ, etc.). A lower diffusion of ABZ and ABZSO into *Ascaris suum* compared to *Moniezia* spp. and *Fasciola hepatica* has been demonstrated (Alvarez et al. 2001). Nematodes maintain a strongly buffered environment in the aqueous spaces of the cuticle structure, with a pH value of this compartment around 5.0 (accumulation of organic acids as products of carbohydrate metabolism). The lipid-containing region of the cuticle represents the rate-determining barrier for passive transport: the molecular size, restriction by pores, intrinsic lipid-water partition coefficient, and pH/pK_a relationship, are among the rate determining factors (Ho et al. 1992). BZD molecules are weak bases that may largely exist under their ionized form at the acidic environment of the nematode surface, which may limit their diffusion across the cuticle. This ionization-mediated impairment of drug diffusion and the complex structure of the nematode cuticle compared to the cestode/trematode tegument, may explain the drug penetration differences observed between nematode and other helminths (Alvarez et al. 2001). In fact, this work demonstrated that the diffusion of BZD molecules into *F. hepatica* and *Moniezia* spp. is markedly greater than that observed in the nematode *A. suum* maintained under the same ex vivo conditions (see Fig. 40.8).

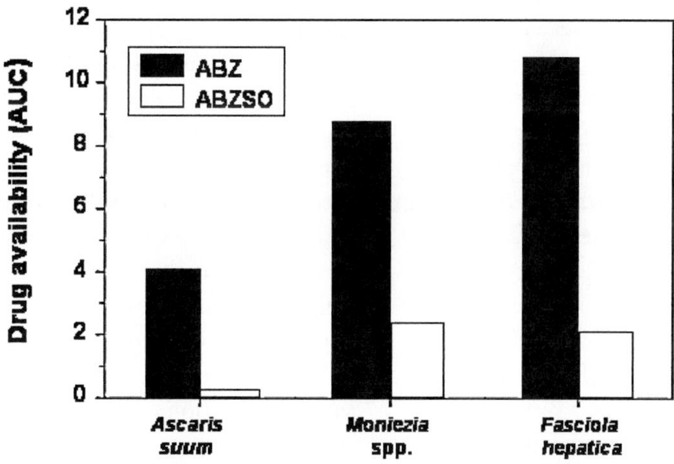

- *Greater diffusion capacity for ABZ compared to its ABZSO metabolite*
- *Lower drug diffusion into nematode compared to cestode and trematode parasites*
- *The complex external cuticule structure limits drug transfer into nematodes*

FIG. 40.8 Comparative assessment of the ex vivo transfer of albendazole (ABZ) and albendazole sulphoxide (ABZSO) into *Ascaris suum* (nematode), *Moniezia* spp. (cestode), and *Fasciola hepatica* (trematode). Values represent drug availability in the parasite tissue, expressed as area under the concentration versus time curve (AUC) (see the text for further explanation). Adapted from Alvarez et al. 2001.
AUC values expressed in µg.h/g.

The identification of the capability of different helminth parasites to biotransform anthelmintic drugs is considered as another crucial step to the overall interpretation of their pharmacological activity. It has been shown that both cytosolic and microsomal fractions obtained from different helminths are able to oxidize ABZ into its sulphoxide derivative. While this oxidative pathway is predominant in *F. hepatica*, the sulphoreduction of ABZSO into its parent sulphide compound is the main metabolic activity identified in tapeworms (Solana et al. 2001). As described above, the liver microsomal oxidation of ABZ and FBZ in sheep and cattle is enantioselective toward the (+) enantiomeric form. However, the oxidation of ABZ by helminth microsomal fractions produced equivalent proportions of both ABZSO enantiomers. Although further investigation is required to establish the pharmacological relevance of drug biotransformation in target parasites, particularly regarding its potential impact on the development of resistance, these findings are complementary to the studies addressed to understand the mechanisms of drug penetration in helminths.

Higher ABZSO and OFZ compared to ABZ and FBZ, concentrations have been reported in GI fluids of different ruminant species. However, the high lipophilicity of the parent thioethers (ABZ, FBZ) assures their penetration through the external parasite. The higher anthelmintic potency of ABZ and FBZ and their greater capability to diffuse into the parasite, suggest that the parent drug may be the main molecule responsible for the activity against GI parasites. However, a complementary effect of the sulphoxide metabolites, measured at higher concentrations in most of the parasite location tissues, may contribute to the overall anthelmintic activity of these BZD methylcarbamates. Thus, the pharmacological activity of ABZ against helminth parasites may depend on the irreversible impairment of essential microtubule-dependent cellular functions induced by an additive effect of both molecules. A similar pattern could be expected for FBZ, where the high OFZ concentration profiles recovered in tissues of the parasite location and its bacteria-mediated GI sulphoreduction into the more active FBZ parent drug could markedly contribute to its overall anthelmintic efficacy. The recovery of anthelmintically relevant concentrations of both ABZ and FBZ parent molecules in critical parasite location tissues (i.e., GI mucosa, lungs, etc.) after treating cattle with ABZSO and OFZ, respectively, strongly support the argument stated above on the relative role of the parent drug and sulphoxide metabolites on anthelmintic activity.

ANTHELMINTIC SPECTRUM. BZDs and pro-BZDs were introduced into the animal health market primarily for the control of GI nematodes, not only for use in livestock animals (cattle, sheep, goats, swine, and poultry), but also for horses, dogs, and cats. The use of BZD and pro-BZD compounds quickly became widespread because they offered major advantages over previous available drugs in terms of spectrum, efficacy against immature stages, and safety for the host animal. Additionally, BZD anthelmintics have ovicidal activity. With the exception of the halogenated BZD thiol, triclabendazole, which has only flukicidal activity against all stages of *Fasciola hepatica* (see Chapter 41), all BZDs and pro-BZDs can be classified as broad-spectrum anthelmintics. However, the substituted sulfur-containing methylcarbamates (ABZ, FBZ, etc.) and pro-BZDs (FBT, NTB) have an extended spectrum of activity compared to the earlier BZD thiazolyls (i.e., TBZ). It has been demonstrated that the greater potency and spectrum of activity of the newer BZDs are largely a function of their pharmacokinetic behavior rather than entirely due to their intrinsic differences in activity (see Fig. 40.2). Overall, the BZD methylcarbamates are broad-spectrum anthelmintics active against a variety of GI and lung nematodes, tapeworms, and trematodes (ABZ derivatives). As a consequence of their pharmacokinetic behavior in monogastric species (particularly in dogs and cats), the BZDs are more effective when they are administered for several days, over single-dose treatments. The available commercial formulations and indications for use (route of administration, dosage and target animal species), may vary among different countries. Readers interested in any specific issue on the spectrum of activity for BZD compounds are referred to the previous edition of this textbook (see Reinemeyer and Courtney 2001). Some general considerations on the spectrum of activity for the most widely used BZD and pro-BZD compounds are summarized in the following sections.

Thiabendazole. TBZ is indicated for the treatment and control of GI roundworms in horses, cattle, sheep, and goats, and the control of lungworms in sheep. TBZ is administered orally at the dose range 66 to 110 mg/kg. It is also used as a fungicide for crop protection. In horses, TBZ is used as a single oral dose administered as a drench or by stomach tube, or as an oral paste. It is usually associated with piperazine to increase the efficacy against ascarids and immature *Oxyurus* spp. TBZ is ineffective against cestodes or trematodes. In cattle, at the recommended dose rates, it is effective against adult and developing stages of *Ostertagi ostertagi* but not against EL_4. Thus, TBZ is not useful to prevent Type II ostertagiasis. In pigs, TBZ has little efficacy against *Ascaris suum* and *Trichuris suis.*

Netobimin. The pro-BZD NTB is formulated as a suspension for oral administration in cattle and sheep. It is indicated (7.5 mg/kg) for the removal and control of tapeworms (heads and segments) (*Moniezia expansa, M. benedeni*), adults and larval stages of abomasal worms (*Haemonchus contortus, H. placei, Trichostrongylus axei, Ostertagia ostertagi, Teladorsagia circumcincta, Marshallagia marshalli*), intestinal worms (*Trichostrongylus colubriformis, Chabertia ovina, Nematodirus spathiger, N. filicollis, N. helvetianus, Cooperia oncophora, C. punctata, Bunostomun phlebotomum, Oesophagostomun radiatum*), and lungworms (*Dictyocaulus filaria, D. viviparus*). Higher doses (20 mg/kg) are required for control of adult liver flukes (>14 weeks old) (*Fasciola hepatica, Fascioloides magna*) and *Thysanosoma actinioides*, and Type II ostertagiasis (cattle).

Albendazole. ABZ is formulated as a suspension for oral administration (as a drench) in cattle and sheep at the recommended dose of 7.5 and 5 mg/kg, respectively. It is indicated for the removal and control of a broad spectrum of helminth parasites, including: tapeworms (heads and segments), abomasal and intestinal nematodes (adults and 4th-stage larvae) and lungworms (adults and larval stages). Additionally, at 10 (cattle) and 7.5 mg/kg (sheep), ABZ is active against adult liver flukes (>14 weeks old). ABZ also demonstrates ovicidal activity at 8 hours posttreatment. ABZ a potential antigiardial drug to be used in farm animals (Xiao et al. 1996), appeared to be effective in suppressing cyst excretion by *Giardia*-infected calves, at the oral dose of 20 mg/kg once daily for 3 days. Similar results were observed in *Giardia*-infected dogs after its oral administration (25 mg/kg) twice a day for 2 days (Barr et al. 1993).

Ricobendazole. RBZ is the sulphoxide metabolite of ABZ and it is also available as suspension for oral administration in cattle (10 mg/kg) and sheep (7.5 mg/kg). The spectrum of activity is equivalent to that described for ABZ, including the ovicidal effect. A novel RBZ injectable solution (15%) for subcutaneous administration to cattle is available in different countries. It is successfully used to control abomasal and intestinal nematodes and lungworms. A 5 mg/kg dose rate is recommended to control the larval 4th stage of *O. ostertagi*. The formulation is not recommended for control of liver flukes or tapeworms. In Europe, RBZ is also approved for use in pheasants by feed administration (17 mg/kg during 3 days) and is mainly indicated for the control of ascarids and capillarid infections.

Febantel. FBT, a pro-BZD compound, is used in ruminants, horses, dogs, cats, and pigs. It is formulated as a paste, suspension, or tablets for oral administration. It is used at a dose of 10 (ruminants), 6 (horses), 10 (dogs and cats), and 20 (pigs) mg/kg. Dogs and cats required a 3-day period of treatment. Since FBT has no anthelmintic activity, its spectrum depends on its main active metabolites FBZ and OFZ. Consequently, its spectrum is similar to those compounds.

Fenbendazole. FBZ is formulated as a suspension for oral administration in cattle, sheep, and goats at the recommended dose of 10 (cattle) and 5 mg/kg (sheep, goats). FBZ is indicated for the removal and control of tapeworms (heads and segments), abomasal and intestinal nematodes (adults and 4th-stage larvae), and lungworms (adults and larval stages). FBZ also presents ovicidal activity. FBZ is effective for the treatment of *Giardia* infections in calves at an oral dose of 10 mg/kg administered once, or 5 mg/kg given every 24 hours for a 3-day period (O'Handley et al. 1997). FBZ is administered orally to horses at 5 mg/kg for control of large strongyles (*Strongylus vulgaris, S. edentatus, S. equinus*), small strongyles (cyathostomes), and pinworms (*Oxyuris equi*). Higher doses (10 mg/kg) are required for control of ascarids (*Parascaris equorum*). At 10 mg/kg for 5 consecutive days, FBZ is indicated for control of arteritis caused by the 4th-stage larvae of *S. vulgaris*, encysted mucosal cyathostomes larvae including early (hypobiotic), and late 3rd-stages larvae. In pigs, FBZ is used as a powder (3 mg/kg per day for 3 consecutive days), being 99% effective against *Ascaris suum* larvae migrating through the liver and lungs, and most GI nematodes (mature and immature) (*Metastrongylus apri, Oesophagostomun dentatum, O. quadrispinulatum, Hyostrongylus rubidus, Trichuris suis, Stephanurus dentatus*). FBZ is used at 50 mg/kg daily for 3 consecutive days in dogs for removal of hookworms (*Ancylostoma caninum*), ascarids (*Toxocara canis, Toxascaris leonina*), whipworms (*Trichuris vulpis*), and tapeworms (*Taenia*). However, it is not recommended for control of the cestode *Echinoccocus granulosus* or *Echinococcus multilocularis*. At a 50 mg/kg dose for 3 days, FBZ reaches good therapeutic effect against *Giardia* in dogs (Barr et al. 1993). The use of FBZ (granules) in zoo and wildlife animals has been approved by the FDA. It is used at 10 mg/kg during 3 days, orally administered with food, and is indicated for the control of nematodes (ascarids, hookworms, and tapeworms) of *Felinae* (lion, tiger, puma, cheetah, leopard) and *Ursidae* (black bear, polar bear).

Oxfendazole. OFZ is administered orally to cattle (4.5 mg/kg), sheep (5 mg/kg), and horses (10 mg/kg). Additionally, it has been used in goats, dogs, and pigs. In all cases it is recommended for the control of the same parasites as is its sulphide parent compound (FBZ). To avoid the ruminal bypass, an OFZ suspension has been approved for intraruminal administration in cattle. As described for ABZ and FBZ, OFZ can be used for the prevention and control of both Type I and Type II ostertagiasis in cattle. However, variable efficacy against EL_4 has been reported. A probable explanation for the observed variability in efficacy is the metabolic activity associated with the larval stage, where the highest efficacy could be expected during induction of inhibition and emergence of inhibited larvae and the lowest efficacy during the quiescent period. In horses, OFZ has a similar efficacy against GI nematodes to the parent FBZ.

Oxibendazole. OBZ is used in the treatment of adult and larval stages of GI nematodes of pigs, cattle, sheep, and horses. It is used orally in suspension or paste at a dosage of 10 mg/kg (sheep and cattle) or 15 mg/kg (horses). A 10 mg/kg dose in horses is sufficient for removal and control of large strongyles, small strongyles, large roundworms, and pinworms.

Mebendazole. MBZ is administered orally to horses (8.8 mg/kg), sheep, and goats (15 mg/kg). It is also used in game birds, pigs, deer, dogs, and poultry as different types of formulations: premixes for medicated feed, pastes, tablets, granules, and drenches—all for oral administration. It is indicated for the control of large strongyles, small strongyles, large roundworms, and mature and immature larval stages of pinworms in horses. Doses of 22 mg/kg for 3 consecutive days are recommended for use in dogs for the treatment of roundworms, hookworms, whipworms, and tapeworms.

Flubendazole. FLBZ is available as tablets, pastes, pellets, and premixes for oral administration in pigs, chickens, turkeys, and game birds. It is used at 5 mg/kg (single oral administration) and at 30 mg/kg in feed for 10 days in pigs, being active against lungworms, roundworms, nodular worms, and whipworms. A 10-day feed period is required for control of heavy *Trichuris suis* infestations. Oral treatment at 22 mg/kg for 3 consecutive days is recommended in dogs and cats for removal of common GI parasites and tapeworms. FLBZ is used in poultry at 60 mg/kg in feed for 7 days (equivalent to 5 mg/kg/day for broilers and 3.6 mg/kg/day for laying hens). FLBZ has ovicidal activity, and recent work done in sheep demonstrates that FLBZ has a volume of distribution higher than those reported for ABZ and OFZ (Moreno et al. 2004), which may offer a new attractive alternative for use of the drug against tissue-dwelling parasites in sheep, where the presence of high drug concentrations for an extended period of time is usually crucial to achieve optimal clinical efficacy.

ROUTES OF ADMINISTRATION AND DRUG FORMULATIONS. As expressed earlier in this chapter, BZD anthelmintic compounds are virtually insoluble in water, which limits most of the formulations to suspension, paste, granule, tablets, blocks, powder, and pellets for oral or intraruminal administration, or for administration in feed. Drench formulations are most frequently used in ruminant species, pastes are often preferred for horses, tablets for dogs and cats, and powder in feed administration for swine and poultry. BZDs are generally administered to ruminants in the form of a single oral dose. This single-dose treatment has traditionally been done by oral drench or by intraruminal injection; this latter approach is based on the design of a special syringe (intraruminal injector) that ejects the drug directly into the rumen cavity. This device is commercially available for the administration of a concentrated suspension of OFZ to cattle and was mainly designed to overcome the potential problems of the esophageal groove closure after oral treatment (see below). To reduce the cost associated with treating a large number of animals and with growing evidence that divided anthelmintic doses and prolonged administration increase anthelmintic efficacy, several methods for drug delivery have been used in the past. The incorporation of drug into feed blocks, for ingestion of small amounts over a prolonged grazing period, and the inclusion of drugs in drinking water have been used for therapeutic and prophylactic parasite control. Convenience and labor saving are obvious for these group medication systems, but at the same time no direct control is possible over the drug intake rate of individual animals.

The most versatile technology in anthelmintic drug delivery has been the development of ruminal devices that, when given to individual animals, can deliver drugs for an extended period of time. These controlled-release devices or boluses more readily provide the conditions for increased anthelmintic efficacy, such as prolonged exposure of parasites to sustained concentrations of active parent drugs or their metabolites. However, since the high selection pressure, this sustained exposure may facilitate the development of drug-resistant parasite populations. After oral administration, the boluses remain in the rumen-reticulum and release the drug over a long period of time, either in a sustained or pulsatile manner. Different controlled-release systems have been developed for the delivery of BZD anthelmintics. The OFZ pulse-release bolus (Rowlands et al. 1988) is based on the principle of releasing a series of individual therapeutic doses of OFZ at predetermined intervals (20–21 days), which approximately coincide with the prepatent period of the major redundant nematodes of cattle, and for about 4 months. This is achieved by the continuous galvanic corrosion of a magnesium alloy rod that periodically exposes an annular OFZ tablet to the ruminal fluid (Campbell 1990). An intraruminal slow-release capsule that delivers a low daily dose of ABZ for approximately 3 months has been designed. The device is a hollow cylinder of nonbiodegradable plastic that contains tablets of 3.85 g (sheep) and 18.46 g (cattle) of ABZ and two external wings. After the administration, the wings spread out while the ruminal fluid starts to dissolve the first tablet, which releases the drug slowly in the rumen; a metal spring pushes six tablets toward the pen end of the capsule. Following the administration of this device, ABZ metabolites were found in plasma for 90 days (cattle) and 105 days (sheep) postcapsule administration (Delatour et al. 1990b). ABZ is also available in controlled release capsules, which contain 2.1 and 3.85 g of ABZ/capsule for use in weaner and adult sheep, respectively, showing a sustained anthelmintic action for 90 to 100 days postadministration. Additionally, an ivermectin/ABZ capsule has been developed to assure protection against GI parasites susceptible to either compound.

Combining drugs has been used to increase anthelmintic spectrum. Furthermore, since extensive parasite resistance to different anthelmintic compounds has been reported, the use of drug combinations may be a practical approach to delay the development of resistance. Currently, there are a large number of combined anthelmintic drenches available for use in sheep. These drenches include, within the same commercial formulation, a combination of two, three, or four molecules with different mechanisms of action and spectrum. Combined preparations containing either ABZ and levamisole; FBZ and levamisole; ABZ and ivermectin or ABZ; ivermectin and levamisole; or ABZ, abamectin, levamisole, and closantel are now available in countries where anthelmintic resistance in sheep and goat nematodes is a serious problem.

FACTORS AFFECTING THE DISPOSITION KINETICS AND EFFICACY OF BENZIMIDAZOLE ANTHELMINTICS. Several *host-related factors* may affect the kinetic behavior and resultant clinical efficacy of BZD compounds. Dissolution, absorption, and biotransformation are three of the most important processes affected by a series of host-related factors. Manipulation of the pharmacokinetic and metabolic patterns and the comprehension of different factors modulating them seem to be excellent alternatives to improve the use of BZD in ruminants:

1. *Effect of ruminant esophageal groove closure:* The rumino-reticulum is usually the first enteric chamber encountered by an orally administered drug. However, ingested fluids may partially bypass the rumino-reticulum to enter the abomasum via the omasum following closure of the reticular groove, a reflex especially developed in the nursing ruminant but inconsistently active in the adult. Thus, variable portions of a drug solution or suspension administered orally may became divided between the rumino-reticulum and abomasum, resulting in a complex absorption process that may then contribute to unpredictable drug efficacy. Occasionally, reduced systemic availability and efficacy of BZD methylcarbamates have been found after oral in comparison with intraruminal administration (Prichard and Hennessy 1981). A portion of the orally administered anthelmintic may bypass the rumen and rapidly enter the abomasum by closure of the esophageal groove. As a consequence, a portion of

the dose directly enters the abomasum with resultant poor absorption due to insufficient time for dissolution of the BZD suspension's particles, which results in reduced plasma bioavailability of active BZD metabolites. Such an effect may indicate that the so called "reservoir" and "slow-delivery" effects of the rumen would be lost; although lag times between treatment and plasma detection of active metabolites could be shorter, the overall bioavailability of active BZD metabolites and their resultant efficacy are significantly reduced. In spite of conflicting results and difficulties in assessing its practical implications, it is clear that upon spontaneous closure of the esophageal groove a portion of an oral drench dose may bypass the rumen, which consequently affects the kinetic behavior and clinical efficacy. It is also likely that this phenomenon is more relevant for 1) compounds that are activated in the rumen such as netobimin prodrug, or 2) those BZD anthelmintics with a low solubility in abomasal fluid such as FBZ or ABZ. Thus, an important portion of the dose of orally administered FBZ would directly reach the abomasum, whereby FBZ insolubility and the short residence time of the digesta in this organ may account for both an inefficient and/or erratic absorption and a significant portion of the dose passing down the GI tract to be eliminated in feces.

2. *Effect of reduced GI transit time:* Modified feeding management has been recommended to restore the anthelmintic action of those BZD compounds whose potency has been compromised by resistance (Alí and Hennessy 1995). An enhanced plasma availability of OFZ induced by temporary feed restriction in sheep, accounted for increased efficacy of the drug against BZD-resistant nematode strains (Alí and Hennessy 1995). Fasting the animals prior to intraruminal treatment resulted in pronounced modifications to the absorption and disposition kinetics of ABZ metabolites in cattle, in which the administered drug appeared to be absorbed to a greater extent than in fed animals (Sánchez et al. 2000b). Starvation decreases digesta flow rates. A delayed GI transit time that decreased the rate of passage of the anthelmintic drug down the GI tract may have accounted for the enhanced ABZ absorption observed in fasted compared to fed animals (see Fig. 40.9). The fasting-induced changes to the kinetic behavior and quantitative tissue distribution of BZD methylcarbamates may have particular relevance to design strategies to increase activity against susceptible parasites and to delay the development of resistant strains. The increased concentration profiles of active drug (both parent ABZ and its sulphoxide metabolite) measured in tissues where target parasites are located (i.e., GI mucosa, lung tissue, etc.) is a strong scientific argument to recommend the "fasting approach" to improve parasite control in cattle, which is now recommended worldwide.
3. *Effect of the type of diet:* The type of feed also influences the rate of passage of digesta and that of orally administered BZD drugs in ruminants and pigs, which may in turn affect drug absorption. The binding of different BZD compounds to dietary fiber substantially modified the duration of the so-called "rumen reservoir" effect (Hennessy 1993), altering the overall bioavailability of BZDs and their metabolites in the bloodstream. Various reports using widely differing type of diets, according to local feeding conditions, have demonstrated the impact of feeding on the systemic availability of ABZ, FBZ, and OFZ in different ruminant species and pigs. The delayed GI transit time and lower abomasal pH in calves fed on a concentrate-based diet, compared to those grazing on pasture, facilitated the dissolution and absorption of ABZ administered intraruminally as a drug suspension in cattle (Sánchez et al. 1999). As a consequence, significantly higher Cmax and AUC values were obtained in calves fed on the concentrate diet compared to those grazed on pasture. Furthermore, enhanced abomasal fluid levels of ABZ and ABZSO were observed in concentrate-fed calves. Additionally, different types of diets have been shown to affect ruminal pH and to modify the microflora-mediated metabolic sulphoreduction of BZD derivatives (Virkel et al. 1997), which further impacts the disposition kinetics of these compounds in ruminants.
4. *Effect of nutritional status and parasite infection:* Because of its central position in the biotransformation and metabolic activities of the animal, the liver is vulnerable not only to damage by various foreign chemicals, microorganisms, and parasites, but also to dietary-induced metabolic disorders that may induce important changes on the pharmacokinetic behavior, side effects, and expected efficacy of the chosen anthelmintic for therapy. The results reported by Sánchez et al. (1996) showed that the poor nutritional status of feed-restricted animals induced marked modifications to the pattern of ABZ biotransformation and to its resultant disposition kinetics in cattle, which was likely produced by interference of the nutritionally induced biochemical changes on

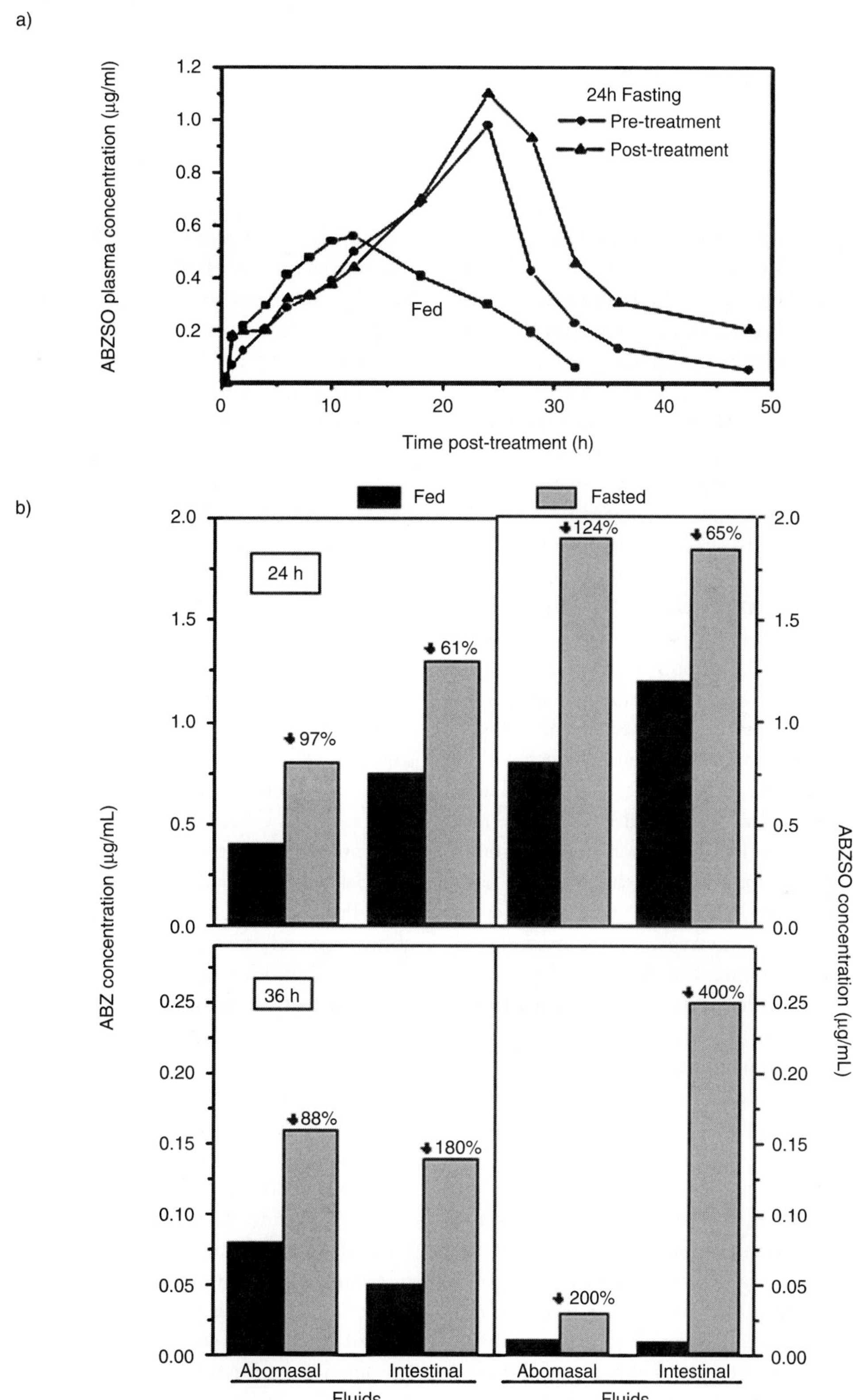

FIG. 40.9 Influence of fasting on the kinetics of albendazole in cattle. a) Mean albendazole sulphoxide (ABZSO) plasma concentrations obtained after the intraruminal administration of albendazole (ABZ) (10 mg/kg) to calves either fed ad libitum (control) or fasted during 24 h prior to or after the treatment. The systemic availability of ABZSO increased between 96% (fasting pretreatment) and 118% (fasting posttreatment) in fasted compared to calves fed ad libitum. b) Mean concentrations of ABZ (left panel) and ABZSO (right panel) obtained in abomasal and intestinal fluids at 24 and 36 h after the intraruminal administration of ABZ (10 mg/kg) to calves either fed ad libitum or fasted for 24 h pretreatment. The figures on the top of each bar represent the enhancement (percentage) on drug concentrations in the different digestive fluids observed in fasted compared to animals fed ad libitum. Adapted from Sánchez et al. 2000.

ABZ liver biotransformation. During both starvation and underfeeding in cattle, the hepatic concentrations of NADPH and ATP have been shown to decrease to about 60 and 40%, respectively, of their normal values in animals fed ad libitum. It is likely that both the decreased energy (ATP) production and the reduced NADPH availability in the liver cell may have contributed to the decreased rate of ABZ biotransformation and delayed elimination of ABZ and its metabolites observed in calves subjected to undernutrition.

The presence of the parasite itself could induce important changes to the pharmacokinetics, side effects, and expected efficacy of the chosen BZD anthelmintic for therapy. Liver disease and parasite-mediated liver damage with alteration of liver enzyme pattern could affect biotransformation and the resultant bioavailability of anthelmintically active BZD metabolites. A reduced enzymatic activity of different liver microsomal oxidases has been reported in *Fasciola hepatica*–infected sheep (Galtier et al. 1986b), which could lead to altered patterns of drug/xenobiotic metabolism and clearance. A significant decrease in the rate of both ABZ sulphonation and $ABZSO_2$ elimination has been demonstrated in sheep infected with *F. hepatica* (Galtier et al. 1991). These findings are well correlated with a 58% decrease in the rate of ABZ sulphonation by liver microsomal preparations obtained from 8-weeks–infected sheep; these authors have postulated that a decrease in the liver microsomal cytochrome P450–dependent monooxygenase activity, induced by the presence of the immature liver flukes on the hepatocyte parenchyma, could likely be the cause of such a metabolic change.

Parasite-mediated inflammatory reactions with changes in mucosal permeability and in abomasal/intestinal pHs could have an impact both on absorption and ionic-trap–mediated distribution of different BZD molecules. Elevation in abomasal pH and increased permeability of the mucosa to macromolecules has been demonstrated during abomasal parasitism. The pathophysiological changes occurring during GI parasitism may affect the absorption of BZD compounds due to modifications in the GI transit time and to the atrophy of intestinal villi. Some studies on the influence of GI parasitism on the plasma kinetics of different anthelmintic drugs have been reported. Following artificial infection with abomasal nematodes (*Ostertagia circumcincta, Haemonchus contortus*), the patterns of absorption and systemic availability of FBZ (Marriner et al. 1985), OFZ (Hennessy et al. 1993b), and FBT (Debackere et al. 1993) in sheep have been shown to be altered. On the other hand, the presence of moderate nematode infections was sufficient to identify important changes to the plasma and abomasal disposition kinetics of ABZ in both artificial and naturally infected sheep (Alvarez et al. 1997). The main modification observed in infected sheep was the elevation of the abomasal pH. The increased abomasal pH induced by the presence of the parasite, decreased the plasma/abomasum pH gradient and reduced the ionic-trapping of BZD molecules in the abomasum, which may have a relevant impact on anthelmintic efficacy.

Factors Related to Pharmaceutical Formulation. The relevance of water solubility and rates of dissolution of drug particles in the GI tract lumen on the absorption and resultant pharmacokinetic behavior of BZD compounds has been extensively demonstrated. Further evidence was obtained by altering the crystalline nature of the OFZ molecule. The production of an amorphous form of OFZ by acidic treatment has resulted in a marked change in water solubility from 4 μg/ml (crystalline form) to 11.3 μg/ml (amorphous form) at a pH of 7.6. The oral administration of amorphous OFZ resulted in a more rapid and complete absorption compared with the crystalline form. It was shown that half the dose of the amorphous OFZ produced equivalent efficacy to that of the normal crystalline OFZ. Erratic absorption and variable systemic availability can be expected after administration of low quality BZD suspensions, where large drug particle size and poor pharmacotechnical elaboration may affect the rate of dissolution and resultant absorption in the GI tract.

Different pharmaceutical strategies have been investigated to overcome the limited GI dissolution and absorption of BZD anthelmintics. An injectable formulation (solution) of ABZSO (RBZ) has been developed for use in cattle, exploiting its greater hydrosolubility compared to other BZD methylcarbamates (Lanusse et al. 1998). Development of more water-soluble prodrugs, ABZ loaded nanoparticles (Rodrigues et al. 1995), aqueous formulation of ABZ with cyclodextrins (Evrard et al. 2002), and surfactant-based ABZ suspensions (Virkel et al. 2003) are among other strategies used to enhance the GI absorption of BZD compounds. A marked enhancement in the systemic availability of ABZ metabolites has been reported after administration of an ABZ suspension prepared with sodium lauryl sulphate to cattle (Virkel et al. 2003).

WITHDRAWAL TIMES, SAFETY, AND TOXICITY. Because of tissue and milk residues of BZD compounds, slaughter clearance times are required after treatment with substituted BZD and it is recommended that milk of treated animals not be used for human consumption. Withdrawal times of 3 days (meat) and 4 days (milk) are required after TBZ treatment in cattle. When TBZ is used as a single oral dose in sheep or goats, 30 days of withdrawal time prior to slaughter is recommended. Withdrawal times are required after ABZ treatment in beef cattle (27 days) and sheep (7–10 days). For FBZ given as a suspension, a period of 8 days (cattle) and 6 days (goats) of withdrawal time is needed. However, since numerous commercial products containing BZD compounds are available around the world, it is critical to check label instructions of each formulation concerning withdrawal times before its use. BZDs are not indicated in horses to be slaughtered for food purposes. FLBZ is widely used as an anthelmintic in poultry. Its main metabolites, H-FLBZ and R-FLBZ, have been identified in tissues of FLBZ-medicated turkeys (De Ruyck et al. 2001). Concentrations of FLBZ/metabolites in eggs collected from laying hens feed with 10 and 30 mg/kg of FLBZ reached a plateau level after 10 days. The residues of FLBZ and metabolites were detected mainly in the yolk, where the metabolites, accounting for almost 60–65% of the total residue, were H-FLBZ, the main metabolite recovered (Kan et al. 1998). A 7-day withdrawal time is required for FLBZ in broiler chickens. Pigs may be slaughtered for human consumption a minimum of 7 days after FLBZ treatment.

BZDs are probably some of the least toxic of the available anthelmintics. The remarkable overall safety of BZD compounds has been a major factor in their successful worldwide use. All BZDs are extremely well tolerated by domestic animals and man, and they are usually free of side effects at therapeutic doses even when administered to young, sick, or debilitated animals. For instance, OFZ does not cause detectable toxic effects at 10 times the recommended dose or after eight successive administrations of 3 times the therapeutic dose at 4-day intervals in ruminants and horses. The high safety margins, particularly for the most potent substituted BZDs, are thought to be correlated with their low solubility in the GI fluids; this account for a low absorption rate and for insufficient drug reaching the bloodstream to induce toxic effect. Some members of the group—such as parbendazole, cambendazole, OFZ, FBT, and ABZ—have been reported to be teratogenic at approximately 4 times their recommended doses; this limits their use in the early stages of pregnancy, and sheep seem to be especially sensitive compared to other animal species (McKellar and Scott 1990). The administration of OFZ or ABZ in pregnant cows caused no increase in the incidence of congenital abnormalities in the offspring. Similar results have been reported in pigs and horses. Teratogenic effects may occur at dosages much lower than those associated with acute toxicity in target species. The observed species' differences in the sensitivity to the teratogenic activity may be related to differences in the pharmacokinetics and metabolism of BZDs among species. The main malformations observed following treatment at day 20 of pregnancy have been deformities of the limbs and overflexion of the carpal joints. In ewes treated with NTB at the 17th day of pregnancy, congenital malformations (skeletal and renal) and abortions were observed (Navarro et al. 1998). The types of malformations induced by FLBZ in rats after its oral administration (160 mg/kg/day for 7 consecutive days between days 8 through 15 of pregnancy) are similar to that described for parbendazole and cambendazole, and include encephalocele, meningocele, hydrocephaly, short tail, absent tail, fusion or agenesis of vertebrae and fused ribs. The mechanism of BZD teratogenicity seems to be related to their effects on the disruption of the tubulin-microtubules equilibrium dynamics in mammalian cells and subsequent alteration of cell division. Since the main toxic effects involve their teratogenic effect, some substituted BZD molecules are contraindicated for use in early pregnancy. ABZ is not indicated for use during the early pregnancy in cows (45 days) and ewes (30 days). The administration of FBT as tablets in dogs and cats is not recommended in pregnant animals. However, FBZ and MBZ do not appear to exert a teratogenic effect in sheep when administered in early pregnancy.

Large doses of TBZ (a more soluble BZD compound) administered for a long period has been associated with anemia in dogs. In feed, FLBZ treatment in poultry does not affect egg production, fertility, or hatchability. In spite of the antimicrotubular effect of BZD molecules, different experiments involving FBZ, ABZ, and OFZ in bulls, rams, and stallions could not demonstrate adverse effects on reproductive function, including spermatogenesis, testicular weight, and testosterone production (McKellar and Scott 1990).

IMIDAZOTHIAZOLES

CHEMISTRY. The first imidazothiazole anthelmintic introduced into the veterinary market (1967) was *tetramisole.* It is a racemic mixture of two optical isomers in equal amounts: S(−)tetramisole (*l*-tetramisole or levamisole) and R(+)tetramisole (*d*-tetramisole). Following approval and marketing of the racemic mixture, pharmaceutical scientists were able to separate *dl*-tetramisole into its two isomers. Further studies discovered that the anthelmintic activity of the racemic mixture was attributable almost solely to the *l*-isomer. Thus, by using the *l*-isomer alone, the dosage could be reduced by half. This also increased the safety margin since both components of tetramisole are similarly toxic but differ in anthelmintic efficacy. Currently, *levamisole* is the worldwide imidazothiazole compound available for use in veterinary medicine. However, in some countries, tetramisole formulations are still available. The information described below is based on the pharmacological properties of levamisole, the most extensively used drug in this chemical class. Another compound within the group, *butamisole hydrochloride,* used as an injectable anthelmintic to control whipworm (*Trichuris vulpis*) and hookworm (*Ancylostoma caninum*) infections in dogs, is no longer marketed. Interested readers are referred to earlier editions of this text (Courtney and Roberson 1995) for additional information on this molecule.

Levamisole is the *l*-isomer of tetramisole. The chemical name of levamisole is (−2,3,5,6-tetrahydro-6-phenylimidazo[2,1-*b*] thiazole) (see Fig. 40.10). Levamisole is an antinematodal drug with a broad range of activity in several host species. It is approved and marketed worldwide for use in cattle, sheep, swine, poultry, and dogs. Levamisole is a nematodicidal compound effective against lung and GI tract nematodes but not against cestode and trematode parasites. A major advantage is its formulation flexibility allowing for alternative routes of administration (oral, parenteral, topical). Depending upon formulation, the drug is marketed as levamisole hydrochloride or phosphate salts (oral drenches, feed premixes, and injectable preparations) and as levamisole base (pour-on). Levamisole hydrochloride, a white to pale cream crystalline powder, is highly soluble in water (1 g in 2 ml of water). This solubility facilitates the formulation of an injectable solution and a stable drench.

MODE OF ACTION. Levamisole acts selectively as a cholinergic agonist at the synaptic and extrasynaptic nicotinic acetylcholine receptors on nematode muscle cells. This causes a spastic paralysis of susceptible nematodes by selectively gating acetylcholine receptor ion-channels on nerve and muscle (Robertson and Martin 1993). Its uptake in helminth parasites is considered to be mainly by a transcuticular mechanism. In vitro studies have shown that levamisole (10 μM) passive transcuticular diffusion in *Trichostrongylus colubriformis* produced a plateau level after 90 minutes of incubation. Detailed information on the mechanism of anthelmintic action and resistance for levamisole can be obtained from Martin (1997), Sangster et al. (1988), and Martin and Robertson (2000).

PHARMACOKINETICS. The rate of levamisole absorption differs with the route of administration. The drug is most rapidly absorbed following intramuscular or subcutaneous injection in cattle, and the highest plasma levels (>1 μg/ml) are observed at 0.5–2 hours. Several oral formulations gave similar absorption rates (Tmax = 3 hours) and slower absorption was observed after dermal application (Bogan et al. 1982). Bioavailability differs depending on the route of administration. In sheep, the highest mean plasma concentrations were achieved after the subcutaneous (3.1 μg/ml), compared to oral (0.7 μg/ml) and intraruminal (0.8 μg/ml), administration at a dose rate of 7.5 mg/kg (Bogan et al. 1982). Following pour-on administration in cattle, plasma and GI concentrations of levamisole were lower than those measured following parenteral and oral treatments (Forsyth et al. 1983), which agrees with the limited anthelmintic efficacy reported for the topical preparation. An oral bioavailability of 44% has been demonstrated in dogs, which increased to 64% when animals were fasted for a total period of 24 hours (Watson et al. 1988). Absorption and systemic bioavailability are important since, given the mode of anthelmintic action of levamisole, the level of concentration is more important than the time of parasite exposure to drug (Lanusse and Prichard 1993b).

Once it is systemically available, levamisole is widely distributed in the organism, being recovered in tissues

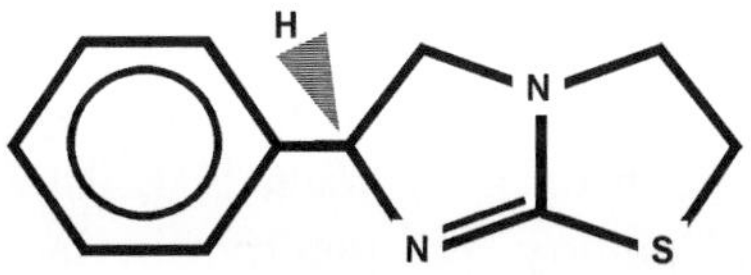

S(-) LEVAMISOLE	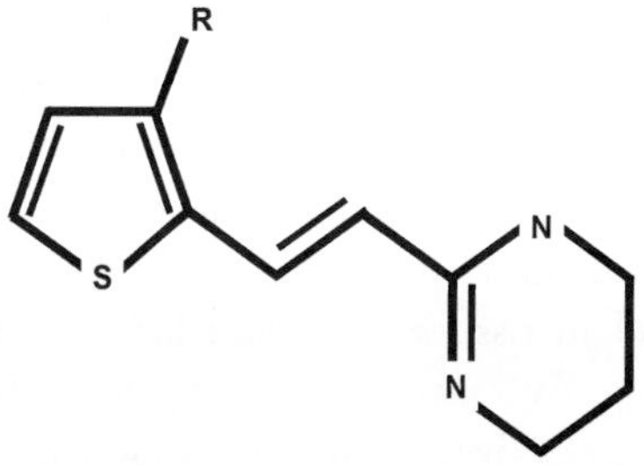	PYRANTEL: R = H MORANTEL: R = CH_3
Nicotinic receptor agonism	MODE OF ACTION	Nicotinic receptor agonism
Lung and GI nematodes (mainly adult stages)	ANTHELMINTIC SPECTRUM	GI nematodes (narrow, adult stages) Equine tapeworms (pyrantel)
Side-resistance with pyrantel and morantel	ANTHELMINTIC RESISTANCE	Side-resistance with levamisole
Rapid absorption (injectable) Limited absorption (oral, topical) Fast elimination	PHARMACOKINETICS	Poor GI absorption (ruminants) Good GI absorption (dog, pig)
Subcutaneous, Oral, Topical	ROUTES OF ADMINISTRATION	Oral (all species) Slow release bolus (cattle)
Hydrochloride, phosphate	FORMULATIONS	Pamoate, tartrate
Narrow safety margin (do not use in horses)	TOXICITY	Good safety margin

FIG. 40.10 Chemical structures and some comparative pharmacological properties of the imidazothiazole (levamisole) and tetrahydropyrimidine (pyrantel, morantel) anthelmintic compounds.
GI: gastrointestinal.

such as muscle, fat, kidney, and particularly liver, at 2 hours postadministration of an oral or subcutaneous dose. In cattle, the highest milk concentrations are achieved at 1 hour postadministration. Levamisole plasma concentrations decline over a period of 6 to 8 hours, with 90% of the total dosage being excreted in 24 hours. Levamisole is rapidly and extensively metabolized to a large number of metabolites in the liver. The main metabolizing pathways appear to be oxidation, hydrolysis, and hydroxylation. Oxidation of the imidazothiazole ring is followed by oxidation to a carbonyl and hydrolysis to a thiohydantoic acid. Excretion of both levamisole and metabolites (glucuronyl or S-cysteinyl-glycine conjugates) is mainly in the urine (about 60%) and feces (about 30%). Unchanged levamisole accounted for 5–10% of the dose in urine and feces in cattle, sheep, and swine (Nielsen and Rasmussen

1982; IPS INCHEM 2003). The reported elimination half-life values are: 4–6 hours (cattle), 1.8–4 hours (dogs), and 3.5–6.8 hours (pigs). Levamisole is fast depleted from the animal body and tissue residues of the drug are not appreciable. Approximately 0.9% of the initial dose is found in tissues (liver and kidney) at 12–24 hours after dosing. By 7 days after dosing, levamisole is not detectable in muscle, liver, kidney, fat, blood, or urine of rats or other animals tested. Unchanged levamisole accounts only for 3% of the total tissue residues measured over a 14-day period.

ANTHELMINTIC SPECTRUM. The compound has a broad spectrum of activity against mature stages of the major GI nematodes and against both mature and larval stages of lungworms. However, levamisole shows little action against arrested larval stages. Depending on the product licensed, levamisole is indicated for nematodes in cattle, sheep, goats, swine, poultry, dogs, and cats. In ruminants, levamisole has a relatively good activity against abomasal nematodes, small intestinal nematodes (not particularly good against *Strongyloides* spp.), large intestinal nematodes (except *Trichuris* spp.), and lungworms. Adult stages of the nematode that are usually covered by levamisole, include *Haemonchus* spp., *Ostertagia* spp., *Cooperia* spp., *Nematodirus* spp., *Bunostomum* spp., *Oesophagostomum* spp., *Chabertia* spp., and *Dictyocaulus vivaparus.* Levamisole is less effective against the immature forms of these parasites and is generally ineffective in cattle against arrested larval forms. In swine, levamisole is indicated for the treatment of *Ascaris suum, Oesophagostomum* spp., *Strongyloides ransomi, Stephanurus dentatus,* and *Metastrongylus* spp. Levamisole has been used in dogs against GI nematodes and as a microfilaricide to treat *Dirofilaria immitis* infection at a dosage of 5.5 mg/kg twice daily (12 hours interval) for 6 days (or up to 15 days for persistent microfilaremias). Because of its narrow safety margin and limited efficacy against many equine parasites, levamisole is not generally used in horses.

FORMULATIONS, DOSAGES, AND ROUTES OF ADMINISTRATION. Levamisole is administered as tablet, solution, oral drench, feed additive, subcutaneous injectable solution, or topical pour-on. In cattle, sheep, goats, and pigs, a dose of 8 mg/kg levamisole is recommended in a single oral or subcutaneous administration and 10 mg/kg as a pour-on for cattle. The bioavailability of levamisole in sheep was significantly lower after oral (42%) and intraruminal (45%) administration compared to the injectable treatment (Bogan et al. 1982). Administration of levamisole in drinking water is used routinely only for swine and poultry. For poultry, the medicated drinking water is prepared by calculating the total amount of drug needed to provide a dose of 40 mg/kg. As the peak concentration rather than the duration of exposure is important for the anthelmintic effect of levamisole, medicated feed should be consumed fairly rapidly; otherwise, efficacy may be reduced.

Injectable levamisole is preferred for use in cattle. The original, aqueous solution of levamisole hydrochloride was administered by intramuscular or subcutaneous injection. The hydrochloride, however, proved to be irritating to tissues, and intramuscular injection resulted in moderate to severe reactions at the injection site. The monobasic phosphoric acid salt of levamisole was found to be less irritating to tissues. Pour-on formulation for cattle contains 10–20% levamisole as base, which is absorbed through the skin following application to the midline of the back.

Levamisole is approved for use in dogs and cats in some countries. Tablets and oral solutions are used in dogs and cats at dose rates between 5 and 10 mg/kg. Oral treatment with 10 mg tetramisole/ kg/day for 2 days removed more than 95% of ascarids (*Toxocara, Toxascaris*) and hookworms (*Ancylostoma, Uncinaria*). Levamisole is not effective against canine whipworms (*Trichuris vulpis*). Overall, levamisole remains a useful nematodicidal compound as a result of an acceptable margin of safety and spectrum of activity coupled with very low cost.

IMMUNOMODULATORY EFFECTS. In addition to its anthelmintic activity, levamisole also may enhance immune responsiveness. This characteristic has caused considerable excitement in both veterinary and human medicine. Levamisole has been proven to act as an immunomodulator in experimental models and in a number of selected human and animal immunodeficiencies with related pathology. This property has been extensively reviewed (Koller 1982; Blecha 1988). The studies on its application in veterinary practice, mainly in bovine practice, have been also reviewed (Desplenter 1983). Levamisole modulates the immune function at 2–3 mg/kg of body weight, in contrast to the greater anthelmintic doses.

When administered at higher doses, levamisole may even suppress immune function. Intermittent treatment is more efficient than continuous treatment in restoring the immune responsiveness. In vitro and in vivo, levamisole is able to restore to normal the major functions of effector cells of the cell-mediated immune response. This restoration is most pronounced and consistent in compromised hosts, whose T-lymphocytes or phagocyte functions are below normal. Usually an adequate immune response is not increased. The B-lymphocyte activity is not directly stimulated: the proliferative response to mitogens is not increased and there is no direct effect on antibody production. However, it should be kept in mind that the responses to levamisole are not always predictable, even if it is used in appropriate conditions. The results are fluctuating between highly favorable and no effect. In cattle, for example, protective effects have been obtained in the prevention or reduction of complications associated with shipping fever (Desplenter 1983).

SAFETY AND TOXICITY. The pharmacodynamic actions of levamisole (or tetramisole) in the host suggest that the drug exerts both muscarinic and nicotinic effects. Signs of levamisole intoxication (salivation, defecation, and respiratory distress from smooth muscle contraction) are like those observed during organophosphate poisoning. Indeed, evidence suggests that some of the toxicity of this drug may be related to cholinesterase inhibition, leading to manifestations of the muscarinic action of acetylcholine (ACh) (i.e., constriction of pupils and respiratory bronchioles, acceleration of GI motility, slowing of the heart rate, and other autonomic actions).

Tetramisole itself has a safety margin estimated to be two to six times the therapeutic dose of 15 mg/kg. Tetramisole is lethal to sheep at a dose of 90 mg/kg. At a dose of 45 mg/kg signs of toxicity occur. Side effects or death are more likely to occur when tetramisole is administered parenterally. The safety factor of levamisole is about twice that of the parent tetramisole compound. Levamisole is considered to be more dangerous when administered parenterally than after the oral or topical treatments. Intravenous administration is particularly hazardous and is never recommended. Cattle appear to be somewhat more tolerant of parenteral administration than sheep. A twofold overdose of injectable levamisole phosphate may cause about two-thirds of treated cattle to lick their lips and to develop temporary foaming of the muzzle. The pour-on formulation has been tested on several thousand cattle with only occasional dermal irritation. When given to pigs at three times the recommended dosage, levamisole causes only occasional vomiting. In such cases, reaction is due to expulsion of the worms and should terminate in several hours. The LD_{50} of subcutaneously injected levamisole in pigs is 40 mg/kg. Simultaneous administration of pyrantel tartrate (a nicotinelike drug) enhances toxicity by lowering the levamisole LD_{50} value to 27.5 mg/kg.

Chickens tolerate tetramisole and levamisole very well. The LD_{50} for chickens is quite high (2.75 g tetramisole/kg), and minimum toxic levels of the drug in chickens exceed 640 mg/kg. In geese, however, a dosage of 300 mg/kg is known to be toxic. In chickens, therapeutic doses of levamisole (36–40 mg/kg) cause no undesirable side effects, and egg production, fertility, and hatchability are not affected adversely. Dogs and cats are much more tolerant to oral than parenteral administration of tetramisole. When given orally to dogs, doses of 20 mg/kg are well tolerated, and even 40 and 80 mg/kg are not fatal, although vomiting occurs. Subcutaneous tetramisole at 40 mg/kg is fatal to dogs in 10–15 minutes; even at 20 mg/kg, the drug causes severe reactions in dogs, although they persist for only about 20 minutes. On the basis of these findings, the oral route of administration is recommended for dogs and cats. Imidazothiazole compounds have a narrow margin of safety in horses and they are not approved for use in this species.

Levamisole should be administered within specified time periods before slaughtering swine, cattle, or sheep. A 2- to 11-day slaughter clearance time is mandated, depending on the formulation used and animal species. The identified levamisole metabolites are much less toxic than the parent compound, so the parent drug is sought in analysis of tissue samples. Since no withdrawal time is established for dairy cows, this drug should not be administered to lactating cattle producing milk for human consumption. There are no specific contraindications in administration of levamisole with other drugs. However, other nicotinelike (e.g., pyrantel, morantel) or cholinesterase-inhibitor drugs (e.g., organophosphate, neostigmine) could theoretically enhance the toxic effects of levamisole.

TETRAHYDROPYRIMIDINES

PYRANTEL. Introduced in 1966, pyrantel was the first compound within the tetrahydropyrimidine family. It was initially used as a broad-spectrum anthelmintic against GI nematodes in sheep and thereafter, developed for use in cattle, swine, horses, dogs, and cats. Subsequently, its methyl ester analogue, *morantel,* was also introduced as a nematodicidal compound in the veterinary market (see Fig. 40.10). The newest drug in this chemical family is *oxantel,* an m-oxyphenol derivative of pyrantel. However, due to its cost, it is not used in veterinary medicine.

CHEMISTRY. Pyrantel is *E*-1,4,5,6-tetrahydro-1-methyl-2 [2-(2-thienyl)vynil]-pyrimidin (Fig. 40.10). It is formulated as tartrate, citrate, or pamoate (also known as *embonate*) salts. Pyrantel pamoate is practically insoluble in water and alcohol, while the tartrate salt is more water soluble. Each gram of pyrantel pamoate is approximately equivalent to 347 mg (34.7%) of the base. Pyrantel citrate is equivalent to 410 mg (41%) of the base. Pyrantel salts are relatively stable in the solid phase. Aqueous solutions are subject to photoisomerization upon exposure to light, with loss of potency. Morantel (1,4,5,6- tetrahydro-1-methyl-2-[2-(3methyl-2-thienyl)ethenyl]pyrimidine) is mainly formulated as a tartrate salt (see Fig. 40.10). Each gram of the tartrate salt is equivalent to 59.5% of base activity. Oxantel is 1-methyl-2-(3-hydroxyphenyl-ethenyl) 1,4,5,6-tetrahydropyrimidine.

MODE OF ACTION. Tetrahydropyrimidine compounds act selectively as agonists at synaptic and extrasynaptic nicotinic acetylcholine receptors on nematode muscle cells and produce contraction and spastic paralysis. Pyrantel and morantel are 100 times more potent than acetylcholine, although slower in initiating contraction. Pharmacologic effects of pyrantel and morantel on the host are similar to the effects of levamisole. These anthelmintics share biologic properties with acetylcholine and act essentially by mimicking the paralytic effects of excessive amounts of this natural neurotransmitter. Pyrantel, morantel, levamisole, and diethylcarbamazine mimic this paralytic action, which is similar to the paralytic effect caused by nicotine; thus the action of these anthelmintics is referred to as *nicotinelike effect.* Although the chemical structures of oxantel and pyrantel are similar, oxantel offers some advantages in efficacy against *Trichuris* spp., which may be due to a difference in the cholinergic subtype selectivity between both molecules as well as to a difference in the dominant cholinergic receptor subtype present in *Trichuris* spp. compared to other intestinal nematodes (Martin et al. 2004).

PHARMACOKINETICS. The pyrantel pamoate salt is poorly absorbed from the GI tract and high concentrations of the unabsorbed drug reach the lower digestive tract in dogs, cats, and horses. Pyrantel tartrate is absorbed more readily than the pamoate salt. The tartrate salt is better absorbed in pigs and dogs compared to ruminants, with peak plasma levels occurring 3–6 hours after its oral administration. Peak plasma levels occur at highly variable times in ruminants. Absorbed drug is rapidly metabolized and excreted into the feces. Pyrantel is extensively metabolized in dogs, rats, sheep, and cattle by oxidation of the thiophene ring, oxidation of the tetrapyrimidine ring, and mercapturic acid conjugation. From the in vivo radiolabeled studies, it was shown that the thiophene ring underwent extensive degradation leading to acidic metabolites that are highly polar, eliminated mainly by urine. Urinary excretion of pyrantel accounts for about 40% of the dose in the dog and 34% in the pig, about 80% of which is excreted as metabolites. The dog is the only species excreting a larger proportion of the drug/metabolites in urine compared to feces. In ruminants, urinary excretion accounts for about 25% of the original dose, much of the remainder passing unchanged in feces. In rats, urinary excretion of the drug is minor; bile is the major route of excretion of metabolites of the absorbed drug.

Morantel is negligibly absorbed in ruminants. The drug is undetectable in the bloodstream in cattle after oral treatment. Morantel is largely excreted as the unmetabolized parent compound in the feces. In a pharmacokinetic and GI compartmental distribution study in calves treated with a morantel tartrate slow-release bolus (Lanusse et al. 1992a), it was shown that the morantel peak concentration is reached at 24 hours postadministration in all GI compartments and in feces. A steady-state concentration was reached at 7–10 days posttreatment and maintained over 84–91 days in feces and in ruminal fluid, and over 98 days in abomasal and ileal fluids. These morantel concentrations in the GI tract of cattle may account for removal of established worms with the initial high peak concentration, and prevention of establishment of incoming larvae with a plateau steady-state concentration that is desirable to minimize selection for drug resistance.

FORMULATIONS, DOSAGES, AND ROUTES OF ADMINISTRATION. Both the tartrate and pamoate salts of pyrantel are used for parasite control in horses. Pyrantel tartrate is formulated for continuous, daily administration over prolonged periods of parasite exposure. Pyrantel pamoate can be administered in suspension or paste formulations, as well as by mixing it with feed. Regardless of the method of administration, a dose of 6.6 mg pyrantel base/kg should be used. A powdered premix formulation containing 10.6% pyrantel tartrate is available for treating parasitic infections of swine via medicated feed. Overnight fasting is advised. Water should be available ad libitum during the fasting and treatment periods.

Formulations of pyrantel pamoate for dogs include suspension and tablet forms. Pyrantel pamoate is also combined with febantel and praziquantel in a tablet form for dogs. Each of the above formulations is given to dogs as a single dose. A higher dose of pyrantel pamoate (20 mg/kg) is combined with praziquantel (5 mg/kg) for cats. Administration with food delays passage through the digestive tract, prolongs contact time of the drug with parasites, and thereby increases efficacy. Mackenstedt et al. (1993) proved that preadult stages of *Toxocara canis* continuously absorbed the drug through the whole body surface and that duration of exposure to pyrantel is more important in efficacy than variations in dosage. Another formulation for dogs is a beef-based chewable form that combines ivermectin (6–12 μg/kg) for control of heartworms and pyrantel pamoate (5–10 mg/kg) for control of hookworms and ascarids. This form is administered once a month.

A sustained-release bolus of morantel tartrate for both dairy and beef cattle is widely used in Europe and has been approved in many places in America. The drug (11.8 g morantel base) is packaged in a cylindrical trilaminate cartridge, which is administered orally by a special delivery device and is retained in the rumen/reticulum. This device is known as the MSRT (morantel slow-release trilaminate bolus). The permeable wall allows continuous release of morantel tartrate (approximately 150 mg/day) into the rumen/reticulum fluid for at least 90 days (Lanusse et al. 1992a). Administration of the MSRT bolus is recommended as preventative for larvae establishing as well as to control existing adult nematode burdens in cattle. The ultimate effect is marked reduction in pasture contamination for a prolonged period, e.g., 90 days of drug release and benefits that extend for another 90 days. Inhibited *Ostertagia* larvae are not killed by this method of treatment, but lowered pasture contamination helps prevent development of type II ostertagiasis.

Dosages for pyrantel tartrate are a single therapeutic dose of 12.5 mg/kg (horses), 22 mg/kg (swine), or 25 mg/kg (sheep, cattle, goats). Dosages for pyrantel pamoate are 6.6 mg base/kg (horses), suspension and chewable form at 5 mg base/kg (dogs); tablets at 5 mg/kg for dogs over 2.2 kg, but 10–15 mg/kg for dogs less than 2.2 kg body weight. Morantel tartrate is recommended for oral treatment at 8.8–9.6 mg/kg (cattle) and at 10 mg/kg (sheep).

ANTHELMINTIC SPECTRUM. In general, activity of pyrantel on GI helminths in horses is independent of the method of administration or the salt, i.e., tartrate or pamoate. Activity of each of the two salts is characterized by consistently high efficacies. A more limited efficacy has been observed against *Strongylus edentatus*, small strongyles, and mature and immature *Oxyuris equi*. Pyrantel is >95% effective against the ileocecal tapeworm (*Anoplocephala perfoliata*) at double the regular therapeutic dosage (i.e., 13.2 mg/kg) (Reinemeyer et al. 2006).

Pyrantel is indicated for the removal or prevention of the large roundworms (*Ascaris suum*) and *Oesophagostomum* spp. in swine. It also has activity against the swine stomach worm (*Hyostrongylus rubidus*). The citrate salt of pyrantel has similar efficacy to that of pyrantel tartrate in swine. Pyrantel is used to control the following parasites in dogs: ascarids (*Toxocara cani, Toxascaris leonina*), hookworms (*Ancylostoma caninum, Uncinaria stenocephala*), and stomach worm (*Physalopter*). It is useful for similar parasites in cats and is considered to be safe to use, even in kittens.

Pyrantel tartrate is an effective nematodicidal in ruminants. It is effective in sheep, cattle, and goats against GI nematodes such as *Ostertagia* spp., *Haemonchus* spp., *Trichostrongylus* spp., *Nematodirus* spp., *Chabertia* spp., *Cooperia* spp., and *Oesophagostomum* spp. The drug is highly effective against mature worms and any immature stages that dwell in the lumen. Morantel is an effective nematodicidal drug for use in sheep and cattle. The salts of morantel have greater anthelmintic activity than the parent compound, pyrantel. Efficacy of morantel tartrate is quite good against adult and immature stages of *Haemonchus* spp., *Ostertagia* spp., *Trichostrongylus* spp., *Cooperia* spp., and *Nematodirus* spp. The MSRT (morantel bolus) has been designed for removal of established worms (initial peak concentration) and prevention of establishment of incoming larvae (plateau steady-state concentrations).

SAFETY AND TOXICITY. The salts of pyrantel are free of toxic effects in all animal hosts at doses up to approximately 7 times the therapeutic dose. The oral LD_{50} of pyrantel tartrate is 175 mg/kg in mice and 170 mg/kg in rats. In dogs, the acute oral LD_{50} for pyrantel pamoate is greater than 690 mg/kg (138 times the therapeutic dose). In chronic toxicity studies, dogs showed ill effects when administered pyrantel tartrate at 50 or more mg/kg/day for 3 months but no adverse effects when the dosage was reduced to 20 mg/kg/day for the same period. Pyrantel is safe for horses and ponies of all ages, including sucklings, weanlings, pregnant mares, and stallions. At 20 times the recommended dose in horses, ponies, and foals, pyrantel pamoate shows no adverse clinical effects or changes in blood cell values or serum chemistry parameters. Pyrantel tartrate is slightly less tolerated in horses than the pamoate salt. The tartrate salt (100 mg/kg) produced death in one of three horses. Toxic signs preceding death included a marked increase in respiration rate, profuse sweating, and incoordination. No signs of toxicosis occurred following administration of 75 mg/kg. Ataxia is seen in some cattle treated with a high dose of pyrantel tartrate (200 mg/kg). The toxic dose of the drug in pigs is not known. Pyrantel is not recommended for use in severely debilitated animals, presumably because its pharmacologic action (cholinergic) may be more pronounced in these hosts.

Withdrawal periods exist for swine and ruminants designated for slaughter. Because of lack of metabolism data in horses, the drug should not be used in horses intended for human consumption. Despite its cholinergic properties, there is no clinical evidence that simultaneous use of organophosphates increases toxicity. Thus labeling for pyrantel products indicates safety for simultaneous use with insecticides, tranquilizers, muscle relaxants, and central nervous system depressants. Pyrantel is recommended not to be used concurrently with other cholinergic agonist anthelmintics (morantel or levamisole). Piperazine and pyrantel/morantel have antagonistic mechanisms of action and their combined use should be avoided.

Morantel tartrate is a safer drug than pyrantel tartrate. The oral LD_{50} of pyrantel for mice is only 170 mg/kg while that of morantel is 5 g/kg. Chronic toxicity studies indicate that doses up to four times the therapeutic dose for sheep for 60 days and two and one-half times that for cattle for 20 days produce no toxic signs. Following a single therapeutic dose (10 mg/kg) via medicated feed, the drug is barely detectable ($\leq$0.05 mg/ml) in plasma or milk of lactating cattle and goats. Negligible levels of morantel tartrate in plasma and milk following single or sustained administration allow its use in dairy animals without a milk withdrawal restriction.

ORGANOPHOSPHATE COMPOUNDS

Organophosphate compounds had their origins as pesticides and only subsequently found use as narrow spectrum anthelmintics. Among the organosphosphates used as anthelmintics in domestic animals are dichlorvos, trichlorfon, haloxon, coumaphos, naphthalophos, and crufomate. The first two were used primarily in horses, and the latter four in ruminants. Organophosphate compounds generally remove the principal parasites of horses, pigs, and dogs but are somewhat deficient in their activity against nematodes of ruminants. Dichlorvos remains useful to control nematode parasites in monogastrics, and its spectrum includes bot flies (*Gasterophilus* spp.) in horses. Overall, the organophosphates have satisfactory efficacy for nematode parasites of the abomasum (especially *Haemonchus*) and small intestine but lack satisfactory efficacy for nematodes of the large intestine (*Oesophagostomum, Chabertia*). However nowadays, other more efficacious and safer antiparasitic drugs have replaced them. Interested readers are referred to the previous edition of this text (Reinemeyer and Courtney 2001) for additional specific information regarding the anthelmintic spectrum, mode of action and toxicity of the organosphosphate compounds. Additional information on the pharmacological properties of the organophosphate compounds can be obtained in Chapter 44.

HETEROCYCLIC COMPOUNDS

PHENOTHIAZINE. Phenothiazine was perhaps the first anthelmintic to demonstrate a fairly wide range of activity against GI nematodes. Phenothiazine was used extensively to control nematodes in sheep, cattle, goats, horses and chickens since 1938. Toxicity limited its use in swine and precluded its use in dogs, cats and humans. As stated by Reinemeyer and Courtney (2001), the emergence of phenothiazine-resistant strains of ruminant and equine nematodes in the 1960s and competition from other broad-spectrum drugs markedly reduced the utility of this compound in subsequent years. It is no longer used as an anthelmintic compound. However, readers interested in specific information on phenothiazine are referred to the previous editions of this textbook, including the 8th edition (Reinemeyer and Courtney 2001).

PIPERAZINE (DIETHYLENEDIAMINE). Discovered around 1900, piperazine was recognized as an anthelmintic moiety in 1954. It has good efficacy profiles against ascarid and nodular worm infections of all species of domestic animals, moderate for pinworm infections, and zero to variable for other veterinary helminths. Its low cost and wide safety margin in all domestic animals have been determinant for its extensive worldwide use in antiparasitic therapy. Piperazine (MW 86.14 Kda) has a relatively simple chemical structure (see Fig. 40.11). It is a strong base soluble in water (1:18), glycerol and glycols, but only sparingly soluble in alcohol and totally insoluble in ether (Pharmaceutical Codex 1979). Piperazine is relatively unstable as the free base, and to improve its stability is usually formulated as different salts such as adipate, citrate, phosphate, hexahydrate, and sulphate. Anthelmintic activity is directly related to the proportion of free base, and this varies according to the salt form (e.g., adipate, 37% free base; chloride, 48%; citrate, 35%; dihydrochloride, 50–53%; hexahydrate, 44%; phosphate, 42%; sulphate,46%) (Courtney and Roberson 1995). Most

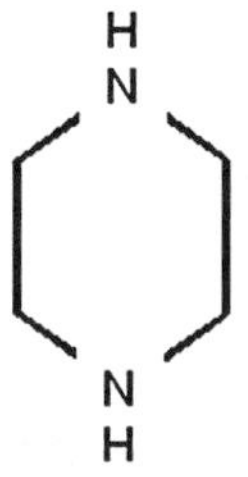

H N N H

PIPERAZINE (MW 86.1 Kda)

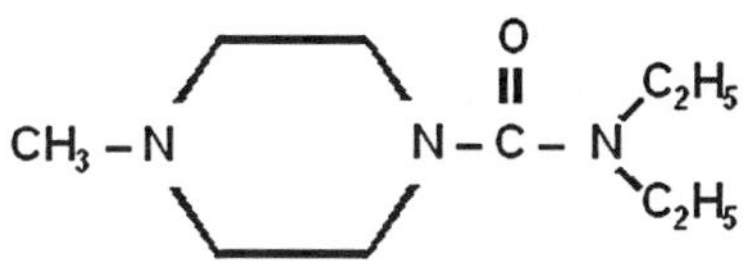

$CH_3 - N$ N – C(=O) – N(C_2H_5)(C_2H_5)

DIETHYLCARBAMAZINE (MW 391.4 Kda)

Piperazine		Diethylcarbamazine
GABA agonism. Flaccid paralysis	**MODE OF ACTION**	Inhibits cyclic peroxide generation from arachidonic acid breakdown
Narrow nematodicidal (mainly ascarids)	**ANTIPARASITIC SPECTRUM**	Only microfilaria in dogs
Horses, dogs, cats, pigs and poultry	**TARGET SPECIES**	Dogs
Formulated as various salts. Dogs-Cats 45-65 mg/kg, horse-swine 110 mg/kg, Chicken 32 mg/kg.	**FORMULATIONS - DOSES**	Tablets (6.6 mg/kg) Powder (2.5 mg/kg)

FIG. 40.11 Chemical structures and some comparative pharmacological properties of piperazine and diethylcarbamazine.

piperazine salts are white crystalline powders that are readily soluble in water. Exceptions are adipate, which dissolves to only a maximum concentration of 5% in water, and phosphate, which is insoluble.

Piperazine is classified as a narrow spectrum antinematodal drug since its efficacy has been demonstrated only against some specific nematodes in horses, pigs, dogs, cats, and chicken. In ruminants, this moiety is seldom used because of its low efficacy against the commonest sheep abomasal parasites (*Teladorsagia circumcinta*) and other parasites located in the ruminants' small intestine. Piperazine's mode of action was initially thought to involve antagonism of cholinergic receptors located on the neuromuscular membrane. However, it is now clear that piperazine blocks transmission by hyperpolarizing nerve membranes at the neuromuscular junction leading to parasite immobilization by flaccid paralysis and consequent removal from predilection site and death. The most recent studies (Martin 1997; Harder 2000) demonstrate that piperazine is a selective agonist of gamma-amino butyric acid (GABA) receptors, resulting in the opening of chloride channels and hyperpolarization of the membrane of the muscle cells of the nematode parasites. Mature worms are more susceptible to the action of piperazine than younger stages. Immature adults and lumen-dwelling larvae are sufficiently susceptible to be at least partially eliminated. Larval stages in host tissues, however, are relatively insusceptible. Because of subsequent larval development, repeated treatments are generally indicated within 2 weeks for carnivores and within 4 weeks for swine and horses.

Piperazine is readily absorbed through the GI tract and then extensively metabolized (60–70%). The remaining parent molecule is eliminated in urine over the 24-hour period following dosing. Piperazine base is detectable in urine as early as 30 minutes after the drug is administered. The therapeutic dose recommended for dogs and cats is 45–65 mg/kg of piperazine free base, given as a single oral administration. Efficacy has been demonstrated against *Toxocara* and *Toxoascaris*, although piperazine is ineffective against *Trichuris vulpis* (Jacobs 1987). Treatment of nursing pups with piperazine at 2, 4, 6, and 8 weeks of age is highly effective (over 90%) in removing prenatally acquired *Toxocara canis* infections.

The dose recommended in horses, swine, and ruminants is 110 mg/kg. In horses, different piperazine salts are highly effective against ascarids, cyathostomes, and mature pinworms (*Oxyuris equi*). In foals, treatment at 8-week intervals is recommended for prevention of patent *Parascaris equorum* populations. Retreatment within 3–4 weeks is recommended in *O. equi* infections since piperazine has not demonstrated efficacy against immature pinworms. Single doses of piperazine are also effective (approximately 100%) against ascarids and nodular worms in swine. Retreatment 1–2 months later may be desirable for optimizing the efficacy against migrating larvae from tissues after the first treatment. The drug is also recommended (2 doses of 32 mg/kg every 24 h) in two successive feedings (adipate of citrate) or drinking water (hexahydrate) as a highly effective treatment against *Ascaridia galli* in poultry. However, this treatment is apparently not effective against *Heterakis gallinarum*.

Experience over many years has confirmed the safety of piperazine; it is almost nontoxic under ordinary circumstances showing a large safety margin. However, large oral doses of piperazine produce emesis, diarrhea, incoordination, and head pressing in cats and dogs. In cats, piperazine was the anthelmintic for which toxicity (confirmed or suspected) was most frequently recorded by the Illinois Animal Poison Information Center (IAPIC) between January 1986 and August 1988 (Lovell 1990), although this may reflect its widespread use as much as its toxic potential. Symptoms of neurotoxicity in dogs and cats manifest as muscle tremors, ataxia, and alteration of the patient behavior within 24 hours after a daily dose of 100 mg/kg. No toxic effects have been reported in foals and horses after they were given six or seven times the therapeutic dose. However, four times the therapeutic dose may provoke digestive discomforts such us transitory diarrhea and excessive rumen gas accumulation in cattle. The therapeutic index of piperazine has been established as 3 (cats) to 6 (horses) (EMEA 2001). Overall, piperazine remains useful as a result of its low cost, safety, and high efficacy against ascarids in different animal species.

DIETHYLCARBAMAZINE CITRATE (DEC). DEC (MW 391.4) (see Fig. 40.11) is a derivative of piperazine, which is highly soluble in water, alcohol, and chloroform, but insoluble in organic solvents (Pharmaceutical Codex 1979); it is stable in the environment. In veterinary medicine, DEC is formulated as tablets or chewables that are sold as a preventive for heartworm disease (*Dirofilaria* *immitis*) in dogs. DEC should be administered daily throughout the mosquito vector season and continued for 2 months following. It is also used in combined commercial formulations that also contain oxibendazole, ivermectin, or milbemycin oxime. DEC has also been previously used for the treatment of lungworm infection in ruminants.

DEC appears to have a different mode of action compared with other antiparasitic molecules, since its microfilarial activity is absent in vitro but extensive in vivo. It has been shown that DEC inhibits cyclic peroxide generation from arachidonic acid (AA) breakdown, specifically through its effects on the enzymes leukotriene A4 synthetase (LTA4), prostacyclin (PGI) 2 synthetase, and prostaglandin (PG)E2 synthetase. However, DEC has no apparent inhibitory effect on thromboxane synthetase and, therefore, cannot be classified as an inhibitor of cyclooxygenase (Martin 1997). The microfilaria produces PGI2 and PGE2 within endothelial cells of blood vessels of infested patients. Since DEC can alter AA metabolism in both parasite and host, it is possible that vasoconstriction combined with amplified endothelial adhesion may be responsible for the immobilization of the microfilaria with a complementary cytotoxic action provided by host platelets and granulocytes (Martin 1997).

After oral administration, DEC is readily absorbed by the GI tract, achieving maximum plasma concentration (Cmax) at 3 hours postadministration, with a subsequent plasma detection period of approximately 48 hours. The drug is widely distributed in tissues and is metabolized in the liver by N-dealkylation and N-oxidation into four metabolites. DEC is excreted in the urine either unchanged or as the N-oxide metabolite. Urinary excretion and, consequently, plasma half-life are dependent on urinary pH (Martindale 1993). Studies with activated charcoal demonstrated that the latter significantly decreased the absorption and elimination of DEC by adsorption in the GI tract (Orisakwe et al. 2000). DEC was shown to have generally low toxicity at the therapeutic dose of 6.6 mg/kg given as oral tablets, or 2.5 mg/kg orally given in powder form once a month, although gastric irritation was observed as a side effect in a few dogs. DEC is contraindicated in dogs parasitized with adult filaria since a hypovolemic shock-type reaction may occur in a small percentage (0.3–5%) of such dogs after DEC administration, which may lead to death within in a few hours (Courtney and Roberson 1995).

HEARTWORM ADULTICIDES: ORGANIC ARSENICALS

THIACETARSAMIDE SODIUM. This compound is a disodium salt of *S,S*-diester of *p*-carbamoydithiobenearsonous acid with mercaptoacetic acid. It is recommended to evaluate the liver and kidney function before dosing since this arsenical compound has shown to be toxic. The plasma pharmacokinetics of thiacetarsamide has been reported in dogs after intravenous injection (2.2 mg/kg), displaying a two-compartment open model curve. High variation given by wide range in kinetic values, were obtained for elimination half-life (20.5 to 83.5 min) and clearance rate (80.0 to 350 ml/kg/min). The mode of action is still unclear, presumably due to the action of the arsenic on cell glycolysis. Treatments of heartworm (*Dirofilaria immitis)* is its main therapeutic use, although a potential use on chronic fatigue syndrome associated with *Staphylococcus* spp. bacteremia has recently been described (Tarello 2001). The compound has no efficacy against circulating microfilariae. Adult worms die within a week after treatment. A dose of 3.7 mg/kg daily for 3 days produced serious side effects in one-third of the dogs tested. Side effects at the standard dose increase with the clinical severity of the heartworm disease. Toxicity is revealed by vomiting, icterus, and orange-colored urine. Dimercaprol (8.8 mg/kg/day in four divided doses) is the recommended antidote when toxic signs are manifested. Cats have demonstrated sensitivity to thiacetarsamide, and its use is not recommended in this species.

MELARSOMINE. Melarsomine is a trivalent arsenical of the melanonyl thioarsenite family with activity against adult and 4-month-old heartworms (*Dirofilaria immitis*) in dogs. Melarsomine is available as a powder for mixing with sterile water before use. The FDA approved this molecule for use in dogs under a hospital setting. Its mode of action is unknown. It is rapidly absorbed after intramuscular injection (2.5 mg/kg) in dogs, achieving the Cmax at only 8 minutes postinjection. It has also been reported that melarsomine and its metabolites are free in plasma, unlike thiacetarsamide, which binds to red blood cells. Arsenic plasma levels are higher and measured for a longer time after treatment with melarsomine compared to those achieved after thiacetarsamide administration.

Melarsomine is active against immature (>4-month-old) and adult heartworms in dogs. Heartworm disease is preventable using the daily or monthly heartworm-prevention medications. It is preferred over the use of thiacetarsamide since it can be used more safely in dogs with severe heartworm disease. The side effects provoked after injection are described as pain, swelling, and tenderness at the injection site. Coughing, gagging, depression, lethargy, lack of appetite, fever, lung congestion, and vomiting may also appear as side effects. Melarsomine has a low margin of safety and it is recommended to have an accurate weight before treating. Dimercaprol can be used as a possible antidote for reversing the toxicity within 3 hours.

RESISTANCE TO ANTHELMINTIC COMPOUNDS: MOLECULAR BASIS

Perhaps it is the simplicity of treating infections with very effective drugs on a routine basis and the proven cost-effective gains in short-term productivity that has led to the predominance of chemotherapy (Zajac et al. 2000). Consequently, resistance to anthelmintic drugs has become a major problem in veterinary medicine and threatens both livestock income and animal welfare.

Resistance is present when there is a greater frequency of individuals within a population able to tolerate doses of a compound than in a normal susceptible population of the same species. The most important feature of anthelmintic resistance is that it is inherited. It is a population of worms, and not of individuals, that become resistant. Selection contributes to produce resistant populations. Once resistance is present in a population, reversion or loss of resistance has never been observed (Sangster and Dobson 2002). For each chemical class of anthelmintics, resistance to one member usually confers resistance to the other members. Genetic modifications conferring resistance are translated into different biochemical modifications that determine a reduced drug effect in the resistant cell. These molecular changes represent the pharmacological basis of the resistance phenomena. Parasites have a number of strategies to become resistant, including 1) molecular changes affecting the capacity of the drug to accumulate at intracellular site of action (reduced uptake, enhanced active efflux and metabolism); 2) modified activity of parasite enzymatic systems; 3) changes on the number, structure, and/or affinity of cellular drug receptors; and 4) amplification of target genes to overcome the effect of the anthelmintic drug. The mechanism of action determines the time of appearance of the antiparasitic effect and the potential risk for the development of resistance to a given drug chemical class. The appearance of resistance to all the major families of broad-spectrum anthelmintics—benzimidazoles, imidazothiazoles (levamisole), tetrahydropirimidines (pyrantel, morantel), and macrocyclic lactones (avermectins and milbemicyns)—has strongly motivated the development of pharmacodynamic studies in order to understand the mechanisms of drug action and resistance.

As described in this chapter, the nematodicidal action of the benzimidazole (BZD) anthelmintics is based on their selective binding to β-tubulin, which produces subsequent disruption of the tubulin-microtubule dynamic equilibrium. BZD resistance in *Haemonchus contortus* has been associated with the loss of high-affinity binding receptors and an alteration of the β-tubulin isoform pattern (Lubega and Prichard 1991) based on a well-conserved mutation at amino acids 200 or 167 (phenylalanine to tyrosine) in both β-tubulin isotypes 1 and 2 (Kwa et al. 1994; Prichard 2001).

Levamisole (LVM) acts selectively as agonist at the synaptic and extrasynaptic nicotinic acetylcholine receptors on nematode muscle cells, inducing spastic paralysis. Resistance to cholinergic agonists is produced by changes on the properties of the nicotinic receptor populations (Robertson et al. 1999) and through an alteration of the drug binding to the nicotinic receptors in the nematode muscle cells. Strains of *H. contortus, Caenorhabditis elegans,* and *Oesophagostomun dentatum* resistant to LVM presented a lower number of active receptors. Martin and Robertson (2000) reported that the normal function of the LVM receptor is modified in resistant nematodes. The active channels stay opened for a shorter amount of time, and a lower depolarization and consequently lower muscle contraction occur. In the low affinity binding site of the receptor, the resistant parasites present lower drug affinity and more binding sites (Moreno-Guzmán et al. 1998; Sangster and Gill 1999). *C. elegans*–resistant strains have a mutation at a single amino acid, replacing glutamic acid in the ion pore of the receptor with a positively charged lysine. This modification is believed to be sufficient to change the ion channel from an excitatory channel to an inhibitory one. On the hand, it has been reported that the presence of the amino acid leucine in the pore of the ion-channel is expected to produce increased desensitization and reduced affinity for the drug, rendering LVM less potent as a nicotinic agonist (Martin 1997). However, the molecular basis for the pharmacological differences between LVM-sensitive and LVM-resistant worms remains obscure (Wolstenholme et al. 2004). It is important to note that nematodes resistant to LVM are also resistant to the tetrahydropirimidine compounds (morantel, pyrantel). Although chemically different, morantel and pyrantel share the same mode of action with LVM (see Fig. 40.11) and, therefore, side resistance among them has been demonstrated and described elsewhere.

Resistance to the avermectin and milbemycin macrocyclic lactones had been related to selection of genes related to the expression of some subunits of the glutamate-gated chloride channels (GluCl) and to the drug transport P-glycoprotein (P-gp) (see Chapter 42 for detailed information). Additionally genes related to a GABA-gated chloride channel subunit and β-tubulin seem to be also associated with resistance to the macrocyclic lactone compounds (Eng and Prichard 2005). In spite of the involvement of different genes on the resistance to these molecules, not all of them may contribute to the same extent in different nematode resistant strains.

P-gp is a member of the ATP-binding cassette (ABC) group of transporters that function as an ATP-dependent efflux mechanism, enabling drugs to be expelled from cells. P-gp overexpression is a common pattern on the multidrug-resistant (MDR) phenotype in different cancer cells. Overexpression of P-gp has also been implicated in the resistance of nematodes to ivermectin and moxidectin (Pouliot et al. 1997), closantel, and BZDs, although the exact nature of the role has yet to be established. P-gp genes have been identified in *C. elegans* (at least 14 genes) (Lincke et al. 1992), in *H. contortus* (7 genes) (Sangster et al. 1999), and *Onchocerca volvulus* (2 genes) (Kwa et al. 1998). In trematodes, genes encoding ABC proteins have been identified in *Schistosoma mansoni* (Bosch et al. 1994) and *Fasciola hepatica* (Reed et al. 1998). The macrocyclic lactones interact with P-gp and ivermectin has been used as an MDR-reversing agent. It has been shown that *H. contortus* resistant to ivermectin possess an increased level of P-gp expression (Xu et al. 1998) and coadministration with verapamil (an MDR-reversing agent) increase the efficacy of ivermectin and moxidectin against resistant *H. contortus* (Molento and Prichard 1999).

Anthelmintic resistance is a worldwide problem, which mainly involves nematode parasites from sheep, goats, and horses. However, there are already cattle nematodes resistant to multiple anthelmintic classes in New Zealand and South America (Fiel et al. 2000; Mejía et al. 2003; Loveridge et al. 2003) and this will probably become more widespread. The rate at which anthelmintic resistance develops and spreads within a population is determined by the amount of parasites that survive the anthelmintic treatment and contribute their resistance genes to the next generations. This contribution is mainly influenced by parasite genetic factors, fecundity of adult parasites (generation time, offspring per generation, breeding patterns), parasites in refugia, drug features (frequency and timing of treatments, drug persistence in the host, drug dose, and efficacy), rate of consumed larvae, grazing management strategy, and climatic conditions. Refugia are subpopulations of parasites that are not selected by drug treatment. Organisms in the environment (larvae on pastures) which are not exposed to drugs are in refugia. They are important because the higher the proportion of the population in refugia, the slower the selection for resistance (Sangster 2001).

Due to the great effort that goes into the development of new anthelmintic molecules, to optimize the use of the existing ones is a high priority. Increasing drug bioavailability is a pharmacological tool that contributes to the optimization of the treatment, delaying the development of anthelmintic resistance. Any pharmacological tool that allows the enhancement of drug systemic bioavailability will facilitate higher drug concentrations reaching the sites of parasite location for sufficient time to induce the antiparasitic effect, especially on those carrying the resistant genes. This is applicable to those resistance mechanisms that depend on drug concentration. A number of strategies for optimizing the use of available anthelmintics and to delay the development of resistance are under investigation: 1) use of different pharmacotechnically based approaches to enhance drug absorption, 2) enhancement of drug systemic availability by feed management (fasting before/after treatment), 3) pharmacological interference to diminish drug efflux from resistant parasites, 4) interference on drug metabolism/elimination, etc.

The use of a drug class that has been shown to be effective, or a combination of drugs with different modes of action, combined with rotation among chemical groups and the use of as few drug treatments as possible, are the most practical and viable recommendations now to delay the development of resistance. A major challenge is to define strategies to preserve susceptibility. Monitoring parasite populations and treating the animals when numbers reach a threshold are practical options suggested to slow down the spread of resistance (Sangster 2001). Early detection of resistance and provision of information to farmers and their advisors are essential features of parasite control strategies aimed at preserving drug efficacy. In conclusion, integrated pharmaco-parasitological research is required to minimize the impact of resistance and to obtain a complete understanding of the basic biology of the parasites and the strategies they develop for becoming resistant. Such an approach may help identify solutions for delaying the development of resistance to the currently available anthelmintics.

MISCELLANEOUS AND NOVEL ANTHELMINTIC DRUGS

The development of resistance to the existing chemical classes of broad-spectrum anthelmintics is a primary challenge for discovering new drugs to assure the long-term viability of the animal health industry (Hennessy 1997). This situation highlights the need for developing new antiparasitic compounds with unique modes of action.

Nitazoxanide is a salycilanilide derivative of nithrotiazole. Nitazoxanide is effective against a broad spectrum of parasites and bacteria infecting animals and humans, including nematodes, cestodes, trematodes, coccidian, and ciliate and flagellate protozoa. Its antiparasitic activity in domestic animals was reported a long time ago (Euzeby et al. 1980) but the efficacy patterns are too low to be attractive to be marketed in veterinary medicine. The mode of action for killing worms, protozoa, and some bacteria is unknown but its comprehension may offer an opportunity to discover analogs with improved potency and efficacy (Geary et al. 1999a).

The cost of developing a new class of broad-spectrum anthelmintics for use in food-producing animals is rapidly becoming prohibitive (Hennessy 1997). However, in the last decade numerous pharmacological studies have been carried out to generate new promising molecules with potent and unique pharmacological activity: *diketopiperazines, cyclic octadepsipetides,* and *neuropeptides*. The diketopiperazines (*marcfortine* and *paraherquamide A*), cyclic octadepsipetides (*PF1022, emodepside*), and neuropeptides *(FaRP)* are among the most important novel antiparasitics. Although there is some information on the specific site of action for these novel molecules, the exact mechanism of action is not yet fully understood.

Paraherquamide (PHQ) has excellent activity against almost all the major parasites of sheep (Shoop et al. 1990). Furthermore, oxindole alkaloids in the PHQ/marcfortine family exhibit broad-spectrum anthelmintic activity including drug-resistant nematode strains (Zinser et al. 2002). PHQ and related anthelmintics act as antagonists of neuronal nicotinic cholinergic receptors in both nematodes (flaccid paralysis in vitro) and mammals, and this mechanism appears to underlie both their efficacy and toxicity. 2-Desoxoparaherquamide, known as PNU-141962, is a promising PHQ semisynthetic derivative active against both BZD- and ivermectin-resistant *H. contortus* that shows markedly lower affinity for mammalian receptors than PHQ itself (Geary and Thompson 2003).

PF1022A (Sasaki et al. 1992), the mother compound of the class of the N-methylated 24-membered cyclooctadepsipeptides obtained as a secondary metabolite of the fungus *Mycelia sterilia*, demonstrates exceptional activity against a variety of nematodes in vitro and in vivo (Conder et al. 1995; von Samson-Himmelstjerna et al. 2000). It has been reported that PF1022A paralyzes the worms by acting as GABA agonist (Chen et al. 1996) and cholinergic antagonist simultaneously (Harder et al. 2005). However, difficulties have been reported regarding its delivery to ruminant animals. *Emodepside* is a semisynthetic derivative of PF1022A, which contains a morpholine molecule attached in *para* position at each of both D-phenyllactic acids (see Fig. 40.12). This novel anthelmintic molecule is efficacious against a variety of GI nematodes. Emodepside acts presynaptically on a latrophilinlike receptor (depsiphilin, a putative G protein–coupled receptor), located in the pharynx and body wall muscle of nematodes, which induces activation of a signal transduction cascade via Gq-alfa-protein and phospolipase-C-beta causing an increase in intracellular calcium and diacylglycerol (DAG) levels. DAG activates some protein paying a relevant role in presynaptic vesicles-functioning, which leads to the release of an inhibitory neuropeptide that acts postsynaptically inducing flaccid paralysis in both pharyngeal and somatic body wall muscles of the nematode (Harder et al. 2005). Emodepside has a novel mode of anthelmintic action being fully effective against benzimidazole-, levamisole-, or ivermectin-resistant nematodes of sheep and cattle (Harder et al. 2005). Emodepside is efficacious in cats against nematodes, either following its administration alone or in combination with praziquantel, which has no nematodicidal activity. At 3.0 mg/kg emodepside (spot-on formula-

EMODEPSIDE

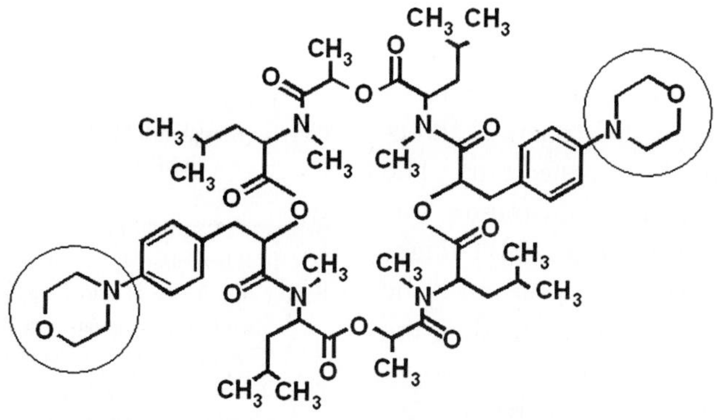

- **New anthelmintic class: N-methylated 24-membered cyclooctadepsipeptides**
- **Semi-synthetic derivative of *PF1022A*** *(circled areas represent the morpholine moiety in paraposition of the parent compound)*
- **Novel mode of action**
- **Broad nematodicidal spectrum** *(larval and adult stages)*
- **Activity against nematodes resistant to benzimidazoles, levamisole and ivermectin**
- **Anthelmintic activity assessed in various animal species** *(commercially available for use in cats)*

FIG. 40.12 Chemical structure and main pharmacological properties of emodepside, a novel anthelmintic molecule. *Emodepside* in combination with the cestodicide praziquantel is commercially available for use in cats (*Profender R Spot-on*, Bayer Health Care, Animal Health).

tion) has excellent activity against *Toxacara cati* (mature and immature adults), *Toxascaris leonina* and *Ancylostoma tubaeforme* (Altreuther et al. 2005).

The discovery of neuropeptides known as *FMRFamide-related peptides (FaRPs),* with motor-modulatory activities in both arthropods and helminths, coupled with recent progress in the characterization of invertebrate neuropeptide receptors, has demonstrated that neuropeptide signaling may be a sound approach to identify novel endectocide molecules (Mousley et al. 2004a). FaRPs play a key role in motor coordination, which has been evidenced in arthropod, flatworm, and nematode nervous systems (Geary et al. 1999b). FaRPs are the most potent peptides, supporting their selection as the strongest candidates for chemotherapy intervention (Mousley et al. 2004b). As per their marked structural diversity, FaRPs within each phylum display either myoexcitatory (flatworms) or a variety of myomodulatory effects (arthropods and nematodes) that are dependent upon peptide structure (Mousley et al. 2004a). FaRP receptors (G-protein coupled receptors) may present a suitable target for new anthelmintics (Geary et al. 1999b). FaRP receptors (or the tissues that express them) in arthropods, flatworms, and nematodes are "promiscuous" with respect to the interactive peptide ligands. In fact, an individual peptide from a nematode or arthropod source can activate receptors involved in motor function within the three phyla. The interphyla activity data support the concept of a single drug being able to interfere with FaRP signalling across the phyla that encompass metazoan parasites of importance (Mousley et al. 2004a).

The molecules described here represent encouraging classes of novel antiparasitics due to their particular mechanisms of action. They may constitute a solution to control parasites resistant to the available drugs. However, a series of difficulties (toxicity, formulation, etc.) must be overcome before most of them can reach commercial development. For instance, emodepside has been recently introduced in combination with praziquantel as a broad-spectrum anthelmintic for cats, but its use in other animal species requires further work.

CONCLUDING REMARKS

To maximize the efficacy of anthelmintic compounds against parasites difficult to control in human and veterinary medicine, while preserving an adequate margin of safety, a complete understanding of their pharmacokinetic, and metabolic patterns in the host, is necessary. The complex connections among route of administration, formulation, drug physicochemical properties, and resultant kinetic behavior need to be understood to optimize the efficacy of the existing anthelmintics. Understanding the mechanisms of drug diffusion and metabolism in target parasites is now a key issue to predict drug activity. Additionally, knowledge about the differential drug pharmacologic behavior among animal species and identification of different factors affecting drug activity is relevant for achieving optimal parasite control and avoiding selection for drug resistance. The technical information summarized in the current chapter is useful to illustrate the complexity of the pharmacology of antinematodal compounds in the different animal species. Integrated evaluation of the available knowledge regarding the pharmacological features is required to optimize their anthelmintic activity and to achieve rationale use. Considering the increasing concern for the development of resistance, the use of pharmacology-based information is critical to design successful strategies for the future of parasite control.

REFERENCES

Alí, D. and Hennessy, D. 1995. The effect of reduced feed intake on the efficacy of oxfendazole against benzimidazole resistant *Haemonchus contortus* and *Trichostrongylus colubriformis* in sheep. International Journal for Parasitology 25, 71–74.

Allan, R. and Watson, T. 1983. The metabolic and pharmacokinetic disposition of mebendazole in the rat. European Journal of Drug Metabolism and Pharmacokinetics 8, 373–381.

Altreuther, G.; Borgsteede, F.H.M.; Buch, J.; Charles, S.D.; Cruthers, L.; Epe, C.; Young, D.R. and Krieger, K.J. 2005. Efficacy of a topically administered combination of emodepside and praziquantel against mature and immature *Ancylostoma tubaeforme* in domestic cats. Parasitology Research 97, Suppl 1, S51–57.

Alvarez, L.; Saumell, C.; Sánchez, S. and Lanusse, C. 1995. Plasma disposition kinetics of albendazole metabolites in pigs fed different diets. Research in Veterinary Science 60, 152–156.

Alvarez, L.; Sánchez, S. and Lanusse, C. 1997. Modified plasma and abomasal disposition of albendazole in nematode infected-sheep. Veterinary Parasitology 69, 241–253.

Alvarez, L.; Sánchez, S. and Lanusse, C. 1999. In vivo and ex vivo uptake of albendazole and its sulphoxide metabolite by cestode parasites: relationship with their kinetic behaviour in sheep. Journal of Veterinary Pharmacology and Therapeutics 22, 77–86.

Alvarez, L.; Imperiale, F.; Sánchez, S. and Lanusse, C. 2000. Uptake of albendazole and albendazole sulphoxide by *Haemonchus contortus* and *Fasciola hepatica* in sheep. Veterinary Parasitology. 94, 75–89.

Alvarez, L.; Mottier, M.; Sánchez, S. and Lanusse; C. 2001. Ex vivo diffusion of albendazole and its sulfoxide metabolite into *Ascaris suum* and *Fasciola hepatica*. Parasitology Research 87, 929–934.

Barr, S.; Bowman, D.; Heller, R. and Erb, H. 1993. Efficacy of albendazole against giardiasis in dogs. American Journal of Veterinary Research 54, 926–928.

Behm, C.; Cornish, R. and Bryant, C. 1983. Mebendazole concentrations in sheep plasma. Research in Veterinary Science 34, 37–41.

Benoit, E.; Besse, S. and Delatour, P. 1992. Effect of repeated doses of albendazole on enantiomerism of its sulfoxide metabolite in goats. American Journal of Veterinary Research 53, 1663–1665.

Beretta, C.; Fadini, L.; Malvisi Stracciari, J. and Montesissa, C. 1987. In vitro febantel transformation by sheep and cattle ruminal fluids and metabolism by hepatic subcellular fractions from different animal species. Biochemical Pharmacology 36, 3107–3114.

Blecha, F. 1988. Immunomodulation: a means of disease prevention in stressed livestock. Journal of Animal Science 66, 2084–90.

Bogan, J.; Marriner, S. and Delatour, P. 1982. Pharmacokinetics of levamisole in sheep. Research in Veterinary Science 32, 124–126.

Bosch, I.; Wang, L. and Schoemaker, C. 1994. Two *Schistosoma mansoni* cDNAs encoding ATP-binding cassette (ABC) family proteins. Molecular and Biochemical Parasitology 65, 351–356.

Brown, H.; Matzuk, A.; Ilves, I.; Peterson, L.; Harris, S.; Sarett, L.; Egerton, J.; Yakstis, J.; Campbell, W. and Cuckler, A. 1964. Antiparasitic drugs IV. 2-(4'-thiazolyl)-benzimidazole, a new anthelmintic. Journal of the American Chemical Society 83, 1764–1765.

Campbell, W. 1990. Benzimidazoles: veterinary uses. Parasitology Today 6, 130–133.

Cashman, J. 1998. Stereoselectivity in S- and N-oxygenation by the mammalian flavin-containing and cytochrome P450 monooxygenases. Drug Metabolism Reviews 30, 675–707.

Chen, W.; Terada, M. and Cheng, J. 1996. Characterization of subtypes of gamma-aminobutyric acid receptors in an Ascaris muscle preparation by binding assays and binding of PF1022A, a new anthelmintic, on the receptors. Parasitology Research 82, 97–101.

Conder, G.; Johnson, S.; Nowakowski, D.; Blake, T.; Dutton, F.; Nelson, S.; Thomas, E.; Davis, J. and Thompson, D. 1995. Anthelmintic profile of the cyclodepsipeptide PF1022A in vitro and in vivo models. Journal of Antibiotics (Tokyo) 48, 820–823.

Courtney, C. and Roberson, E. 1995. Antinematodal drugs. In Veterinary Pharmacology and Therapeutics, 7th, edited by Adams, H. R. pp 885–1004. Ames, IA: Iowa State University Press.

Cristofol, C.; Virkel, G.; Alvarez, L.; Sánchez, S.; Arboix, M. and Lanusse, C. 2001. Albendazole sulphoxide enantiomeric ratios in plasma and target tissues after intravenous administration of ricobendazole to cattle. Journal of Veterinary Pharmacology and Therapeutics 24, 117–124.

Cross, H.; Renz, A. and Trees, A. 1998. In-vitro uptake of ivermectin by adult male *Onchocerca ochengi*. Annals of Tropical Medicine and Parasitology 92, 711–720.

Csiko, G.; Banhidi, G.; Semjen, G.; Laczay P.; Vanyine Sandor G.; Lehel J. and Fekete J. 1996. Metabolism and pharmacokinetics of albendazole after oral administration to chickens. Journal of Veterinary Pharmacology and Therapeutics 19, 322–325.

Debackere, M.; Landuyt, J.; Vercruysse, J. and McKellar, Q. 1993. The influence of *Ostertagia circumcincta* and *Trichostrongylus colubriformis* infections on the pharmacokinetics of febantel in lambs. Journal of Veterinary Pharmacology and Therapeutics 16, 261–274.

Delatour, P.; Besse, S. and Romdane, M. 1988. Pharmacokinetics and anti-Dicrocoelium activity of thiophanate and its major metabolite in ruminants. Annales de Recherches Veterinaires 19, 119–22.

Delatour, P.; Benoit, E.; Garnier, F. and Besse, S. 1990a. Chirality of the sulphoxide metabolites of fenbendazole and albendazole in sheep. Journal of Veterinary Pharmacology and Therapeutics 13, 361–366.

Delatour, P.; Benoit, E.; Lachenet, J. and Besse, S. 1990b. Pharmacokinetics in sheep and cattle of albendazole administered by an intraruminal slow release capsule. Research in Veterinary Science 48, 271–5.

Delatour, P.; Garnier, E.; Benoit, E. and Caude, I. 1991. Chiral behaviour of the metabolite albendazole sulphoxide in sheep, goats and cattle. Research in Veterinary Science 50, 134–138.

De Ruyck, H.; Daeseleire, E.; Grijspeerdt, K.; De Ridder, H.; Van Renterghem, R. and Huyghebaert, G. 2001. Determination of flubendazole and its metabolites in eggs and poultry muscle with liquid chromatography-tandem mass spectrometry. Journal of Agricultural and Food Chemistry 49, 610–617.

Desplenter, L. 1983. Levamisole as an immunomodulator in the prevention of neonatal disease. In Veterinary Pharmacology and Toxicology, edited by McDonald, L.E. pp 99–103. Lancaster, England: MTP Press Limited.

Edwards, G. and Breckenridge, A. 1988. Clinical pharmacokinetics of anthelmintic drugs. Clinical Pharmacokinetics 15, 67–93.

EMEA/MRL/807/01: http://www.emea.eu.int/pdfs/vet/mrls/080701en.pdf

Eng, J. and Prichard, R. 2005. Comparison of genetic polymorphism in populations of *Onchocerca volvulus* from untreated- and ivermectin-treated patients. Molecular and Biochemical Parasitology 142 193–202.

Euzeby, J.; Promtep, S. and Rossignol J. 1980. Experimentation des properties antihelminthiques de la nitazoxamide chez le chien, le chat et les ovines. Reveuil de Medicine Veterinaire 131, 687–696.

Evrard, B.; Chiap, P.; DeTullio, P.; Ghalmi, F.; Piel, G.; Van Hees, T.; Crommen, J.; Losson, B. and Delattre L. 2002. Oral bioavailability in sheep of albendazole from a suspension and from a solution containing hydroxypropyl-beta-cyclodextrin. Journal of Controlled Release 85, 45–50.

Fetterer, R. and Rew, R. 1984. Interaction of *Fasciola hepatica* with albendazole and its metabolites. Journal of Veterinary Pharmacology and Therapeutics 7, 113–117.

Fiel, C.; Saumell, C.; Steffan, P.; Rodriguez, E. and Salaverry, G. 2000. Resistencia de los nematodes Trichostrongylideos—Cooperia y Trichostrongylus—a Tratamientos con Avermectinas en bovinos de la pampa hmeda -Argentina-. Revista de Medicina Veterinaria 81, 310–315.

Forsyth, B.; Gibbon, A. and Prior, D. 1983. Seasonal variations in anthelmintic response by cattle to dermally applied levamisole. Australian Veterinary Journal 60, 140–141.

Galtier, P.; Alvinerie, M. and Delatour, P. 1986a. In vitro sulphoxidation of albendazole by ovine liver microsomes: assay and frequency of various xenobiotics. American Journal of Veterinary Research 47, 447–450.

Galtier, P.; Larrieu, G.; Tufenkji, A. and Franc, M. 1986b. Incidence of experimental fascioliasis on the activity of drug–metabolizing enzymes in lamb liver. Drug Metabolism and Disposition 14, 137–141.

Galtier, P.; Alvinerie, M.; Plusquellec, Y.; Tufenkji, A. and Houin, G. 1991. Decrease in albendazole sulphonation during experimental fascioliasis in sheep. Xenobiotica 21, 917–924.

Geary, T.; Sangster, N. and Thompson, D. 1999a. Frontiers in anthelmintic pharmacology. Veterinary Parasitology 84, 275–295.

Geary, T.; Marks, N.; Maule, A.; Bowman, J.; Alexander-Bowman, S.; Day, T.; Larsen, M.; Davis, J. and Thompson, D. 1999b. Pharmacology of FMRFamide-related peptides in helminths. Annals of the New York Academy of Sciences 897, 212–227.

Geary, T. and Thompson, D. 2003. Development of antiparasitic drugs in the 21st century. Veterinary Parasitology 115, 167–184.

Gottschall, D.; Theodorides, V. and Wang R. 1990. The metabolism of benzimidazole anthelmintics. Parasitology Today 6, 115–124.

Gyurik, R.; Chow, A.; Zaber, B.; Brunner, E.; Miller, J.; Villani, A.; Petka, L. and Parish R. 1981. Metabolism of albendazole in cattle, sheep, rats and mice. Drug Metabolism and Disposition 9, 503–508.

Harder, A. 2000. Chemotherapeutic approaches to nematodes: current knowledge and outlook. Parasitology Research 88, 272–277.

Harder, A.; Holden-Dye, L.; Walker, R. and Wunderlich, F. 2005. Mechanisms of action of emodepside. Parasitology Research 97, 1–10.

Hennessy, D. 1993. Pharmacokinetic disposition of benzimidazole drugs in the ruminant gastrointestinal tract. Parasitology Today 9, 329–333.

———. 1997. Modifying the formulation or delivery mechanism to increase the activity of anthelmintic compounds. Veterinary Parasitology 72, 367–390.

Hennessy, D. and Prichard, R. 1981. The role of absorbed drug in the efficacy of oxfendazole against gastrointestinal nematodes. Veterinary Research Communications 5, 45–49.

Hennessy, D.; Steel, J.; Lacey, E.; Eagleson, G. and Prichard, R. 1989. The disposition of albendazole in sheep. Journal of Veterinary Pharmacology and Therapeutics 12, 421–429.

Hennessy, D.; Sangster, N.; Steel, J. and Collins, G. 1993a. Comparative pharmacokinetic behaviour of albendazole in sheep and goats. International Journal for Parasitology 23, 321–325.

Hennessy, D.; Sangster, N.; Steel, J. and Collins, G. 1993b. Comparative kinetic disposition of oxfendazole in sheep and goats before and during infection with *Haemonchus contortus* and *Trichostrongylus colubriformis*. Journal of Veterinary Pharmacology and Therapeutics 16, 245–253.

Ho, N.; Geary, T.; Barshun, C.; Sims, S. and Thompson, D. 1992. Mechanistic studies in the transcuticular delivery of antiparasitic drugs. II: Ex vivo/in vitro correlation of solute transport by *Ascaris suum*. Molecular and Biochemical Parasitology 52, 1–14.

Horton, R. 1990. Benzimidazoles in a wormy world. Parasitology Today 6,106.

IPS NCHEM, 2003. http://www.inchem.org/documents/jecfa/jecmono/v33je02.htm

Jackson, F. and Coop, R. 2000. The development of anthelmintic resistance in sheep nematodes. Parasitology 120, 95–107.

Jacobs, D. 1987. Anthelmintics for dogs and cats. International Journal for Parasitology 17, 511–518.

Kan, C.; Keukens, H. and Tomassen, M. 1998. Flubendazole residues in eggs after oral administration to laying hens: determination with reversed phase liquid chromatography. The Analyst 123, 2525–2527.

Koller, L.D. 1982. Chemical-induced immunomodulation. Journal of the American Veterinary Medical Association 181, 1102–1106.

Kwa, M.; Veenstra, J. and Roos, M. 1994. Benzimidazole resistance in *Haemonchus contortus* is correlated with a conserved mutation at amino acid 200 in β-tubulin isotype 1. Molecular and Biochemical Parasitology 63, 299–303.

Kwa, M.; Okoli, M.; Schulz-Key, H.; Okongkwo, P. and Roos, M. 1998. Use of P-glycoprotein gene probes to investigate anthelmintic resistance in *Haemonchus contortus* and comparison with *Onchocerca volvulus*. International Journal for Parasitology 28, 1235–490.

Lacey, E. 1988. The role of the cytoskeletal protein, tubulin, in the mode of action and mechanism of drug resistance to benzimidazoles. International Journal for Parasitology 18, 885–936.

———. 1990. Mode of action of benzimidazoles. Parasitology Today 6, 112–115.

Lanusse, C.; Ranjan, S. and Prichard, R. 1990. Comparison of pharmacokinetic variables for two injectable formulations of netobimin administered to calves. American Journal of Veterinary Research 51, 1459–1453.

Lanusse, C.E.; Gascon, L.H.; Ranjan, S. and Prichard, R.K. 1992a. Morantel tartrate release from a long-acting intraruminal device in cattle: pharmacokinetics and gastrointestinal distribution. Journal of Veterinary Pharmacology and Therapeutics 15, 117–23.

Lanusse, C.; Nare, B.; Gascon, L. and Prichard, R. 1992b. Metabolism of albendazole and albendazole sulphoxide by ruminal and intestinal fluids of sheep and cattle. Xenobiotica 22, 419–426.

Lanusse, C.E. and Prichard, R.K. 1993a. Relationship between pharmacological properties and clinical efficacy of ruminant anthelmintics. Veterinary Parasitology 49, 123–58.

———. 1993b. Clinical pharmacokinetics and metabolism of benzimidazole anthelmintics in ruminants. Drug Metabolism Reviews 25, 235–279.

Lanusse, C.; Gascon, L. and Prichard, R. 1993a. Gastrointestinal distribution of albendazole metabolites following netobimin administration to cattle: relationship with plasma disposition kinetics. Journal of Veterinary Pharmacology and Therapeutics 16, 38–47.

Lanusse, C.; Nare, B. and Prichard, R. 1993b. Comparative sulphoxidation of albendazole by sheep and cattle liver microsomes and the inhibitory effect of methimazole. Xenobiotica 23, 285–295.

Lanusse, C.; Gascon, L. and Prichard, R. 1995. Comparative plasma disposition kinetics of albendazole, fenbendazole, oxfendazole and their metabolites in adult sheep. Journal of Veterinary Pharmacology and Therapeutics 18, 196–203.

Lanusse, C.; Virkel, G.; Sánchez, S.; Alvarez, L.; Lifschitz, A.; Imperiale, F. and Monfrinotti, A. 1998. Ricobendazole kinetics and availability following subcutaneous administration of a novel injectable formulation to calves. Research in Veterinary Sciences 65, 5–10.

Lincke, C.; The, I.; van Groenigen, M. and Borst, P. 1992. The P-glycoprotein gene family of *Caenorhabditis elegans*. Cloning and characterization of genomic and complementary DNA sequences. Journal of Molecular Biology 228, 701–711.

Lovell, R.A. 1990. Ivermectin and piperazine toxicoses in dogs and cats. Veterinary Clinics of North America Small Animal Practice 20, 453–468.

Loveridge, B.; McArthur, M.; McKenna, P.B. and Mariadass, B. 2003. Probable multigeneric resistance to macrocyclic lactone anthelmintics in cattle in New Zealand. New Zealand Veterinary Journal 51, 139–141.

Lubega, G. and Prichard, R. 1991. Specific interaction of benzimidazole anthelmintics with tubulin from developing stages of thiabendazole-susceptible and -resistant *Haemonchus contortus*. Biochemical Pharmacology 41, 93–101.

Mackenstedt, U.; Schmidt, S.; Mehlhorn, H.; Stoye, M. and Traeder, W. 1993. Effects of pyrantel pamote on adult and pre-adult *Toxicara canis* worms: an electron microscope and autoradiography study. Parasitology Research 79, 567–78.

Marriner, S. and Bogan, J. 1981. Pharmacokinetics of oxfendazole in sheep. American Journal of Veterinary Reserach 42, 1146–1150.

Marriner, S.; Evans, E. and Bogan, J. 1985. Effect of parasitism with *Ostertagia circumcincta* on pharmacokinetics of fenbendazole in sheep. Veterinary Parasitology 17, 239–249.

Marriner, S. 1986. Anthelmintic drugs. The Veterinary Record 118,181–184.

Martin, R. 1997. Modes of action of anthelmintic drugs. The Veterinary Journal 154, 11–34.

Martin, R. and Robertson, A. 2000. Electrophysiological investigation of anthelmintic resistance. Parasitology 120, 87–94.

Martin, R.; Clark, C.; Trailovic, S. and Robertson, A. 2004. Oxantel is an N-type (methyridine and nicotine) agonist not an L-type (levamisole and pyrantel) agonist: classification of cholinergic anthelmintics in Ascaris. International Journal for Parasitology. 34, 1083–1090.

Martindale, W. 1993. The Extra Pharmacopoeia, 30th ed. London Pharmaceutical Press.

McKellar, Q. and Scott, E. 1990. The benzimidazole anthelmintic agents—A review. Journal of Veterinary Pharmacology and Therapeutics 13, 223–247.

McKellar, Q.; Harrison, P.; Galbraith, E. and Inglis, H. 1990. Pharmacokinetics of fenbendazole in dogs. Journal of Veterinary Pharmacology and Therapeutics 13, 386–392.

McKellar, Q.; Galbraith, E. and Baxter, P. 1993. Oral absorption and bioavailability of fenbendazole in the dog and the effect of concurrent ingestion of food. Journal of Veterinary Pharmacology and Therapeutics 16, 189–198.

McKellar, Q.; Gokbulut, C.; Muzandu, K. and Benchaoui, H. 2002. Fenbendazole pharmacokinetics, metabolism, and potentiation in horses. Drug Metabolism and Disposition 30, 1230–1239.

Mejía, M.; Fernández Igartua, B.; Schmidt, E. and Cabaret, J. 2003. Multispecies and multiple anthelmintic resistance on cattle nematodes in a farm in Argentina: the beginning of high resistance. Veterinary Research 34, 461–467.

Molento, M. and Prichard, R. 1999. Effects of the multidrug-resistance-reversing agents verapamil and CL 347,099 on the efficacy of ivermectin or moxidectin against unselected and drug-selected strains of *Haemonchus contortus* in birds. Parasitology Research 85, 1007–1011.

Montesissa, C.; Malvisi Stracciari, J.; Fadini, L. and Beretta, C. 1989. Comparative microsomal oxidation of febantel and its metabolite fenbendazole in various animal species. Xenobiotica 19, 97–100.

Moreno, L.; Alvarez, L.; Mottier, L.; Virkel, G.; Sanchez Bruni, S. and Lanusse, C. 2004. Integrated pharmacological assessment of flubendazole potential for use in sheep: disposition kinetics, liver metabolism and parasite diffusion ability. Journal of Veterinary Pharmacology and Therapeutics 27, 299–308.

Moreno-Guzmán, M.; Coles, G.; Jiménez-González, A.; Criado-Fornelio, A.; Ros-Moreno, R. and Rodríguez-Caabeiro, F. 1998. Levamisole binding sites in *Haemonchus contortus*. International Journal of Parasitology 28, 413–418.

Moroni, P.; Buronfosse, T.; Longin-Sauvageon, C.; Delatour, P. and Benoit, E. 1995. Chiral sulfoxidation of albendazole by the flavin adenine dinucleotide-containing and cytochrome P450-dependent monooxygenases from rat liver microsomes. Drug Metabolism Disposition 23, 160–165.

Mottier, L.; Alvarez, L.; Pis, A. and Lanusse, C. 2003. Transtegumental diffusion of benzimidazole anthelmintics into *Moniezia benedeni:*

correlation with their octanol-water partition coefficients Experimental Parasitology 103, 1–7.

Mousley, A.; Marks, N. and Maule, A. 2004a. Neuropeptide signalling: a repository of targets for novel endectocides?. Trends in Parasitology 20, 482–487.

Mousley, A.; Marks, N.; Halton, D.; Geary, T.; Thompson, D. and Maule, A. 2004b. Arthropod FMRFamide-related peptides modulate muscle activity in helminths. International Journal for Parasitology 34, 755–768.

Murray, M.; Hudson, A. and Yassa, V. 1992. Hepatic microsomal metabolism of the anthelmintic benzimidazole fenbendazole: enhanced inhibition of cytochrome P450 reactions by oxidized metabolites of the drug. Chemical Research in Toxicology 5, 60–66.

Navarro, M.; Cristofol, C.; Carretero, A.; Arboix, M. and Ruberte, J. 1998. Anthelmintic induced congenital malformations in sheep embryos using netobimin. Veterinary Record 142, 86–90.

Nielsen, P. and Rasmussen, F. 1982. The pharmacokinetics of levamisole in goats and pigs. Pharmacologie et toxicologie veterinaire. Les colloques de l'INRA 8, 431–432.

O'Handley, R.; Olson, M.; McAllister, T.; Morck, D.; Jelinski, M.; Royan, G. and Cheng, K. 1997. Efficacy of fenbendazole for treatment of giardiasis in calves. American Journal of Veterinary Research 58, 384–388.

Orisakwe, O.E.; Ilondu, N.A.; Afonne, O.J.; Ofoefule, S.I. and Orish, C. N. 2000. Acceleration of body clearance of diethylcarbamazine by oral activated charcoal. Pharmacology Research 42, 167–70.

Petersen, M. and Friis, C. 2000. Pharmacokinetics of fenbendazole following intravenous and oral administration to pigs. American Journal of Veterinary Research 61, 573–576.

Pharmaceutical Codex. 1979. 11th ed. The Pharmaceutical Society of Great Britain.

Pouliot, J.; L'heureux, F.; Liu, Z.; Prichard, R. and Georges, E. 1997. Reversal of P-glycoprotein-associated multidrug resistance by ivermectin. Biochemical Pharmacology 53, 17–25.

Prichard, R. 2001. Genetic variability following selection of *Haemonchus contortus* with anthelmintics. Trends in Parasitology 17, 445–453.

Prichard, R.; Hennessy, D. and Steel, J. 1978. Prolonged administration: a new concept for increasing the spectrum and effectiveness of anthelmintics. Veterinary Parasitology 44, 309–315.

Prichard, R. and Hennessy, D. 1981. Effects of oesophageal groove closure on the pharmacokinetic behaviour and efficacy of oxfendazole in sheep. Research in Veterinary Science 30, 22–27.

Rawden, H.; Kokwaro, G.; Ward, S. and Edwards, G. 2000. Relative contribution of cytochromes P450 and flavin-containing monooxygenases to the metabolism of albendazole by human liver microsomes. British Journal of Clinical Pharmacology 49, 313–322.

Redondo, P.; Alvarez, A; García, J.; Larrode, O.; Merino, G. and Prieto, J. 1999. Presystemic metabolism of albendazole: experimental evidence of an efflux process of albendazole sulfoxide to intestinal lumen. Drug Metabolism and Disposition 27, 736–740.

Reed, M.; Panaccio, M.; Strugnell, R. and Spithill, T. 1998. Developmental expression of a *Fasciola hepatica* sequence homologous to ABC transporters. International Journal for Parasitology 28, 1375–1381.

Reinemeyer, C. and Courtney, C. 2001. Antinematodal drugs. In Veterinary Pharmacology and Therapeutics, 8th, edited by Adams, H.R. pp. 947–979. Ames, IA: Iowa State University Press.

Reinemeyer, C.; Hutchens, D.; Eckblad, W.; Marchiondo, A. and Shugart, J. 2006. Dose-confirmation studies of the cestocidal activity of pyrantel pamoate paste in horses. Veterinary Parasitology 138, 169–390.

Renwick, A., Strong, H. and George, C. 1986. The role of the gut flora in the reduction of sulphoxide containing drugs. Biochemical Pharmacology 35, 64–70.

Roberson, E. and Burke, T. 1982. Evaluation of granulated fenbendazole as a treatment for helminth infections in dogs. Journal of the American Veterinary Medical Association 180, 53–55.

Robertson, S.J. and Martin, R.J. 1993. Levamisole-activated single-channel currents from muscle of the nematode parasite *Ascaris suum*. British Journal of Pharmacology 108, 70–178.

Robertson, A.; Bjorn, H. and Martin, R.J. 1999. Resistance to levamisole resolved at the single-channel level. FASEB Journal 13, 749–760.

Rodrigues, J.; Bories, C.; Emery, I.; Fessi, H.; Devissaguet, J. and Liance, M. 1995. Development of an injectable formulation of albendazole and in vivo evaluation of its efficacy against *Echinococcus multilocularis* metacestode. International Journal for Parasitology 25, 1437–1441.

Rowland, I. 1986. Reduction by the gut microflora of animals and man. Biochemical Pharmacology 35, 27–32.

Rowlands, D.; Shepherd, M. and Collins, K.1988. The oxfendazole pulse release bolus. Journal of Veterinary Pharmacology and Therapeutics 11, 405–408.

Sánchez, S.; Alvarez, L. and Lanusse, C. 1996. Nutritional condition affects the disposition kinetics of albendazole in cattle. Xenobiotica 26, 307–320

Sánchez, S.; Alvarez, L. and Lanusse, C. 1997. Fasting induced changes on the pharmacokinetic behaviour of albendazole and its metabolites in cattle. Journal of Veterinary Pharmacology and Therapeutics 20, 38–47.

Sánchez, S.; Alvarez, L.; Pis, A.; Quiroga, M. and Lanusse, C. 1999. Differences in plasma and abomasal kinetics of albendazole and its metabolites in calves grazed on pasture or fed a grain-based diet. Research in Veterinary Science 66, 223–230.

Sánchez, S.; Sallovitz, J.; Savio, E.; McKellar, Q. and Lanusse, C. 2000a. Comparative availability of two oral dosage forms of albendazole in dogs. Veterinary Journal 160, 153–156.

Sánchez, S.; Alvarez, L., Sallovitz, J. and Lanusse, C. 2000b. Enhanced plasma and target tissue availabilities of albendazole and albendazole sulphoxide in fasted calves: evaluation of different fasting intervals. Journal of Veterinary Pharmacology and Therapeutics 23, 193–201.

Sánchez, S.; Small, J.; Jones, D. and McKellar, Q. 2002. Plasma achiral and chiral pharmacokinetic behaviour of intravenous oxfendazole co-administered with piperonyl butoxide in sheep. Journal of Veterinary Pharmacology and Therapeutics 25, 7–13.

Sangster, N.; Riley, F. and Collins, G. 1988. Investigation of the mechanism of levamisole resistance in trichostrongylid nematodes of sheep. International Journal for Parasitology 18, 813–818.

Sangster, N.; Bannan, S.; Weiss, A.; Nulf, S.; Klein, R. and Geary, T. 1999. *Haemonchus contortus:* Sequence heterogeneity of internucleotide binding domains from P-glycoproteins and an association with avermectin/milbemycin resistance. Experimental Parasitology 91, 250–257.

Sangster, N. and Gill, J. 1999. Pharmacology of anthelmintic resistance. Parasitology Today 15, 141–146.

Sangster, N. 2001. Managing parasiticide resistance. Veterinary Parasitology 98, 89–109.

Sangster, N. and Dobson, R. 2002. Anthelmintic resistance. In The Biology of Nematodes, edited by Lee, D.L. pp. 531–567. London: Taylor and Francis.

Sasaki, T.; Takagi, M.; Yaguchi, T.; Miyadoh, S.; Okada, T. and Koyama, M. 1992. A new anthelmintic cyclodepsipeptide, PF1022A. Journal of Antibiotics 45, 692–697.

Shoop, W.; Egerton, J.; Eary, C. and Suhayda, D. 1990. Anthelmintic activity of paraherquamide in sheep. Journal of Parasitology 76, 349–351.

Short, C.; Barker, S.; Hsieh, L.; Su-Pin, O.; McDowell, T.; Davis, L.; Neff-Davis, C.; Koritz, G.; Bevill, R. and Munsiff, I. 1987. Disposition of fenbendazole in cattle. American Journal of Veterinary Research 48, 958–961.

Solana, H.; Rodriguez, J. and Lanusse, C. 2001. Comparative metabolism of albendazole and albendazole sulphoxide by different helminth parasites. Parasitology Research 87, 275–280.

Souhaili El Amri, H.; Fargetton, X.; Delatour, P. and Batt, A. 1987. Sulphoxidation of albendazole by the FAD-containing and cytochrome P450 dependent mono-oxygenases from pig liver microsomes. Xenobiotica 17, 1159–1168.

Tarello, W. 2001. Chronic Fatigue Syndrome (CFS) in 15 dogs and cats with specific biochemical and microbiological anomalies. Compendium of Immunology and Microbiology of Infectious Diseases 24, 165–185.

Taylor, S.; Kenny, J.; Houston, A.; Smyth, W.; Kennedy, D. and Hewitt, S. 1993b. Plasma concentrations of fenbendazole and its metabolites in poultry after a single oral administration. Journal of Veterinary Pharmacology and Therapeutics 16, 377–379.

Thompson, D.; Ho, N.; Sims, S. and Geary, T. 1993. Mechanistic approaches to quantitate anthelmintic absorption by gastrointestinal nematodes. Parasitology Today 9, 31–35.

Tocco, D.; Egerton, J.; Bowers, W.; Christensen, V. and Rosenblum, C. 1965. Absorption, metabolism and elimination of thiabendazole in farm animals and a method for its estimation in biological materials. Journal of Pharmacology and Experimental Therapeutics 149, 263–265.

Virkel, G.; Lifschitz, A. ; Pis, A.; Sallovitz, J. and Lanusse, C. 1997. Diet affects the ruminal biotransformation of netobimin and albendazole sulphoxide. Journal of Veterinary Pharmacology and Therapeutics 20, 100–101.

Virkel, G.; Lifschitz, A.; Pis, A. and Lanusse, C. 2002. In vitro ruminal biotransformation of benzimidazole sulphoxide anthelmintics: enantioselective sulphoreduction in sheep and cattle. Journal of Veterinary Pharmacology and Therapeutics 25, 15–23.

Virkel, G.; Imperiale, F.; Lifschitz, A.; Pis, A.; Alvarez, A.; Merino, G.; Prieto, J. and Lanusse, C. 2003. Effect of amphiphilic surfactant agents on the gastrointestinal absorption of albendazole in cattle. Biopharmaceutics and Drug Disposition 24, 95–103.

Virkel, G.; Lifschitz, A.; Sallovitz, J.; Pis, A. and Lanusse, C. 2004. Comparative hepatic and extrahepatic enantioselective sulfoxidation of albendazole and fenbendazole in sheep and cattle. Drug Metababolism and Disposition 32, 536–544.

von Samson-Himmelstjerna, G.; Harder, A.; Schnieder, T.; Kalbe, J. and Mencke, N. 2000. In vivo activities of the new anthelmintic depsipeptide PF 1022A. Parasitology Research 86 194–199.

Watson, A.D.; Sangster, N.C.; Church, D.B. and Van Gogh, H. 1988. Levamisole pharmacokinetics and bioavailability in dogs. Research in Veterinary Science 45, 411–413.

Witassek, F.; Burkhardt, B.; Eckert, J. and Bircher, J. 1981. Chemotherapy of alveolar echinococcosis. Comparison of plasma mebendazole concentrations in animals and man. European Journal of Clinical Pharmacology 20, 427–433.

Wolstenholme, A.; Fairweather, I.; Prichard, R.; von Samson-Himmelstjerna, G. and Sangster, N. 2004. Drug resistance in veterinary parasites. Trends in Parasitology 20, 469–476.

Xiao, L.; Saeed, R. and Herd, R. 1996. Efficacy of albendazole and fenbendazole against *Giardia* infection in cattle. Veterinary Parasitology 61, 165–170.

Xu, M.; Molento, M.; Blackhall, W.; Ribeiro, P.; Beech, P. and Prichard, R. 1998. Ivermectin resistance in nematodes may be caused by alteration of P-glycoprotein homolog. Molecular and Biochemical Parasitology 91, 327–335.

Zajac, A.; Sangster, N. and Geary, T. 2000. Why veterinarians should care more about parasitology? Trends in Parasitology 16, 504–506.

Zinser, E.; Wolf, M.; Alexander-Bowman, S.; Thomas, E.; Davis, J.; Groppi, V.; Thompson, D. and Geary, T. 2002. Anthelmintic paraherquamides are cholinergic antagonists in gastrointestinal nematodes and mammals. Journal of Veterinary Pharmacology and Therapeutics 25, 241–250.

CHAPTER

41

ANTICESTODAL AND ANTITREMATODAL DRUGS

CARLOS E. LANUSSE, GUILLERMO L. VIRKEL, AND LUIS I. ALVAREZ

ANTICESTODAL DRUGS

INTRODUCTION

Anticestodal drugs used to treat tapeworm infections may act as either taeniafuges or taeniacides. The former compounds facilitate tapeworm expulsion from the host; while the latter cause the death of the tapeworm in situ. Because the cestode's scolex is capable of regenerating an entire organism, drugs that merely remove the proglottids or the whole tapeworm body but leave the scolex intact are unsatisfactory. Insufficient drug diffusion into the scolex and consecutive two or three proglottides, due to the inflammatory reaction of the intestinal mucosa, may account for such a limited cestocidal activity. The usual interval from destrobilization to patency is approximately 3 weeks, so the recommended interval for evaluating tapeworm therapy is 3 weeks after initial drug treatment. Tapeworm infection in farm animals may be a minor problem and usually does not require treatment with a specific cestocidal drug. Some of the broad-spectrum benzimidazole compounds used to control nematode infections (see Chapter 40) are also effective against tapeworms. However, special attention is given to the treatment of *Anoplocephala perfoliata* infections, the commonest tapeworm parasite in horses. This tapeworm causes erosions around the ileocecal valve and intussusception, particularly in horses chronically infected with large numbers of worms (Gasser et al. 2005). It has been shown that oral administration of a pyrantel pamoate (see Chapter 40) paste at 13.2 mg/kg resulted in effective (96%) control of this tapeworm in naturally infected horses (Reinemeyer et al. 2006). Treatment of tapeworm infections is also highly necessary in companion animals. Of greatest importance is the fact that dogs and cats are definitive hosts of tapeworms whose larval stages cause zoonosis. For example, effective treatment of *Echinococcus granulosus* in dogs is extremely important since the larval stage of this tapeworm may cause hydatidosis in the intermediate hosts, mainly sheep and humans. Environmental control of intermediate hosts is also essential to prevent reinfection after treatment. The control of fleas and lice that vector *Dipylidium caninum*, and restricted access of carnivores to mammalian intermediate hosts to preclude *Taenia* infections are essential (Reinemeyer and Courtney 2001).

Taeniafuge compounds interfere with the ability of tapeworms to maintain their site of location in the gut. They paralyze tapeworms at least temporarily, but if tapeworms recover prior to expulsion, reattachment to the gut may occur. Thus, treatment with taeniafuges has been routinely accompanied by purgation. *Arecoline,* a muscarinic agonist, induces the parasite's spastic paralysis and enhances host gut motility, which facilitates tapeworm expulsion. The search for enhanced efficacy motivated the development of synthetic taeniacidal drugs that are now widely used. Many of the older antitapeworm drugs are natural organic compounds (taeniafuges). Readers interested in specific information on those older drugs are referred to a previous edition of this textbook (Roberson and Courtney 1995).

BUNAMIDINE

Bunamidine (N,N-dibutyl-4-(hexyloxy)-1-naphthamidine) (Fig. 41.1) is a taeniacidal drug that disrupts the tapeworm's tegument and reduces glucose uptake. Consequently, subtegumental tissues are exposed and destroyed by the host's digestive enzymes. It is formulated as tablets (hydrochloride salt) or suspension (hydroxynaftoate salt) for oral administration in companion animals and ruminants, respectively. The hydrochloride salt is widely used for treatment of cestode infections in dogs and cats. Bunamidine hydrochloride exhibits >90% efficacy against *Taenia* spp., *Dipylidium* spp., *Mesocestoides* spp., and *Diphyllobothrium* spp. (oral treatment at 25–50 mg/kg). However, efficacy against *D. caninum* may be erratic. Effectiveness ranging from 85.9 to 98.8% (immature stages) and 100% (mature stages) of *E. granulosus* have been reported (Andersen et al. 1975). Bunamidine prepared as a hydroxynaftoate salt is effective against *Moniezia* spp. infections in small ruminants.

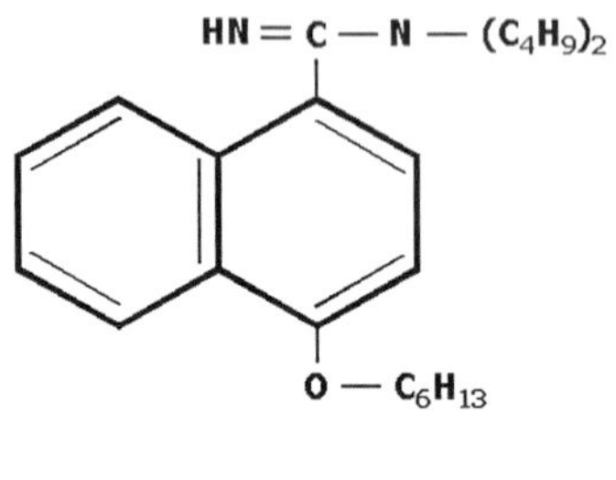

Dissolution of tablets in fasted animals is improved and, therefore, subsequent contact of the drug with the parasite in the gut is enhanced resulting in advantageous efficacy. The drug is safe because is not extensively absorbed in the duodenum and low amounts of the absorbed compound are inactivated in the liver. Administration of dissolved tablets enhances drug absorption and, consequently, the risk of systemic adverse effects such as liver damage and ventricular fibrillation. Death as consequence of cardiac failure has been sporadically reported within 24 hours posttreatment. Emesis and diarrhea are the most frequent adverse effects following bunamidine administration. More efficacious cestodicidal drugs have displaced bunamidine, which is no longer available in the U.S. market.

HN = C — N — $(C_4H_9)_2$

O — C_6H_{13}

Bunamidine

FIG. 41.1 Bunamidine chemical structure.

NICLOSAMIDE

This salicyanilide compound (5-chloro-*N*-(2-chloro-4-nitrophenyl)-2-hydroxybenzamide (Fig. 41.2) was widely used for treatment of cestode infections in dogs and cats from the 1960s to the 1980s. Niclosamide is highly effective against most of the tapeworm species in companion animals. However, it has poor efficacy against *Dipylidium* spp. and *E. granulosus.* This drug is also effective for the treatment of common tapeworms in ruminants such as *Moniezia* spp. and *Thysanosoma* spp. In horses it may be used for the treatment of *Anoplocephala* spp. Niclosamide's action involves interference with glucose absorption and

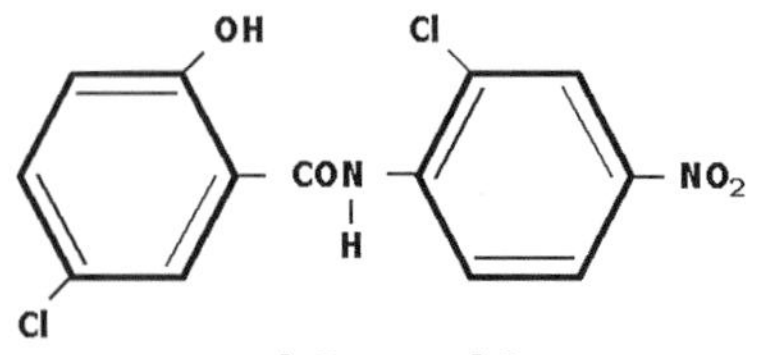

OH Cl

CON — H

NO_2

Cl

Niclosamide

FIG. 41.2 Chemical structure of the salicylanilide drug niclosamide.

oxidative phosphorylation, mechanisms that lead to the death of the parasite and its subsequent digestion within the gut. It may be administered either as suspension by oral or intraruminal routes in ruminants or as tablets for oral treatment in companion animals. Niclosamide administration in fasted animals increases its efficacy. Its oral administration at doses of 100–157 mg/kg, produced only low plasma concentrations which correlates with low GI absorption and the well-known safety of the drug. The absorbed drug is rapidly inactivated in the liver into aminoniclosamide. Similarly to bunamidine, niclosamide has been replaced in small animal practice by modern cestocides. Interested readers are referred to a previous edition of this text (Roberson and Courtney 1995) for a thorough discussion of the therapeutic properties of niclosamide.

PRAZIQUANTEL

Praziquantel is a synthetic isoquinolinepyrazine derivative: 2-(cyclohexykcarbonyl)-1,2,3,6,7,l1b-hexahydro-4*H*-pyrazino[2,1-a] isoquinolin-4-one (Fig. 41.3). Praziquantel is highly efficacious against a variety of cestode and trematode parasites and it is widely used in both veterinary and human medicine. It has extremely high activity against adult stages of all species of tapeworms in farm and companion animals (Thomas and Gonnert 1978). It also has good activity against larval forms of cestodes. Administration of praziquantel at 5 mg/kg in cats and dogs is completely effective against all stages of *Taenia hydatigena*, *T. pisiformis*, *T. ovis*, *T.taeniaeformis*, *D. caninum*, *Mesocestoides corti*, *E. multilocularis,* and *E. granulosus* (Thomas and Gonnert 1978). This dose is generally recommended for elimination of the common cestode species of dogs and cats, except *Spirometra mansonoides* and *Diphyllobothrium erinacea,* which require 25 mg/kg on each of 2 consecutive days. A 10 mg/kg dosage is required to achieve good efficacy against the juvenile forms of these parasites. The drug ensures 100% elimination of *E. granulosus* in dogs and is the unique drug recommended for the treatment of this tapeworm. A combined formulation of febantel and praziquantel is available on the veterinary market for use in the treatment of GI nematodes and cestodes. This formulation must be administered on three consecutive days, at doses of 10–15 mg/kg (febantel) and 1–1.5 mg/kg (pra-

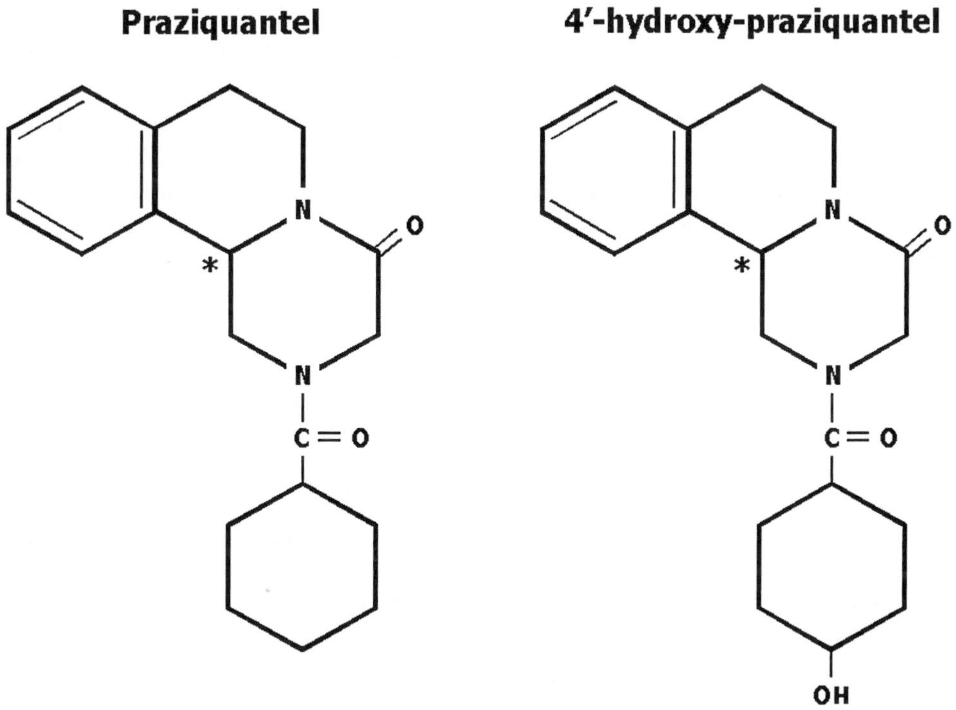

Praziquantel

4′-hydroxy-praziquantel

FIG. 41.3 Chemical structures of praziquantel and its active metabolite (4′hydroxy-praziquantel). The asterisk (*) indicates the asymmetric (chiral) center in both molecules.

ziquantel) for adult and young dogs. A triple combination of praziquantel, pyrantel, and oxantel is also marketed as a broad-spectrum dewormer for dogs and cats. Other commercial combinations used in companion animals include praziquantel plus oxibendazole, mebendazole, or fenbendazole. Recently, a combined preparation of praziquantel and emodepside (a novel nematodicidal drug) has been introduced into the market as a broad-spectrum anthelmintic for cats (see Chapter 40).

Praziquantel is also highly effective against cestodes of ruminants. All species of *Moniezia, Stilesia,* and *Avitellina* of sheep and/or goats are eliminated by a single dose of 10–15 mg/kg. Praziquantel has been approved for tapeworm treatment in horses in different countries. It has been successfully used for the treatment of the cestode *A. perfoliata* in this species (Lyons et al. 1998). Combined formulations (gel, paste) containing ivermectin plus praziquantel are marketed for use in the treatment of GI nematode and cestode infection in horses.

Most studies concerning praziquantel's mode of action have been done using the human trematode *Schistosoma mansoni* as a model parasite (Day et al. 1992). Praziquantel induces a rapid and sustained paralytic muscle contraction of the parasite and tegumental disruption. The contraction of parasite musculature is the primary effect, which is followed by a rapid vacuolization of the syncytial tegument. Muscular contraction and tegumental disruption are followed by exposure of parasite antigens, binding, and penetration of host immune cells into the parasite (Martin 1997). Metabolic changes include decrease in glucose uptake, glycogen storage, ATP content, and lactate release. All these effects are attributed either directly or indirectly to an alteration of intracellular Ca^{2+} homeostasis. Praziquantel effects are thought to be mediated by the release of intracellular stored Ca^{2+}, in addition to the increase of Ca^{2+} influx across the schistosome tegument (Day et al. 1992). Exposure and release of parasite antigens, as well as metabolic changes, are attributable to the primary effect on the tegument. The exact molecular target, as well as its location within parasite tissues remains to be completely understood. Recently, several investigations have been focused on voltage-gated Ca^{2+} channels as targets of praziquantel action (Greenberg 2005). These channels are critical sites of extracellular Ca^{2+} influx and also play an important role in regulation of intracellular Ca^{2+} homeostasis. The chiral nature of praziquantel is another feature related to its pharmacological effects on the parasite. The drug has an asymmetric center in position 11b (see Fig. 41.3) and, consequently, two enantiomeric forms: R(−) and S(+) praziquantel. Only the R(−) enantiomeric form has antiparasitic activity as shown by in vitro and in vivo experiments (Staudt et al. 1992; Cioli and Mattoccia 2003).

Praziquantel can be formulated as a tablet, paste, or suspension for oral administration, and as a solution for SC or IM injections. Commercial formulations are racemates composed of equal parts of both praziquantel enantiomers. The pharmacokinetic behavior and metabolic fate of praziquantel has been investigated in sheep and dogs (Giorgi et al. 2001, 2003). These authors used a higher oral dose (30 mg/kg) than those recommended in these species in order to generate sufficiently high plasma concentrations for analysis. In sheep, praziquantel Cmax and AUC values administered by the IM route at 15 mg/kg were sixfold higher compared to those values observed following oral treatment at 30 mg/kg (Fig. 41.4). It has been shown that praziquantel is completely absorbed in the GI tract in almost all species studied including sheep. Thus, its low oral bioavailability in sheep is not attributed to poor GI absorption but due to an extensive hepatic first-pass effect. Liver oxidative metabolism of praziquantel in sheep resulted in the production of one hydroxylated metabolite, which might be either 11b-hydroxy- or 1-hydroxy-praziquantel (Giorgi et al. 2001). A cytochrome P450 3A isoenzyme was found to be involved in praziquantel hydroxylation in sheep liver. Conversely, the metabolite formed following praziquantel administration to dogs is 4′-hydroxy-praziquantel (Giorgi et al. 2003). This is consistent with previous studies in other species such as rats, monkeys, and humans in which 4′-hydroxy-praziquantel was the main metabolite (Masimirembwa and Hasler 1994). Praziquantel and its 4′-hydroxylated metabolite were depleted in parallel from plasma in dogs, which is supported by an AUC praziquantel/4′-hydroxy-praziquantel ratio equal to 1.3 (Fig. 41.5). Increased levels of the parent drug and its metabolite following administration of liquid or dry grapefruit juice combined with praziquantel to dogs have been observed. It has been shown that grapefruit juice may be an inhibitor of the P-gp transport protein and cytochrome P450-mediated oxidative drug metabolism. Grapefruit juice may interfere with either the P-gp-mediated efflux or cytochrome P450-mediated oxidation of praziquantel. Interestingly, 4′hydroxy-praziquantel has been shown to exert roughly similar pharmacological activity compared to its parent compound (Staudt et al. 1992). Metabolism of praziquantel is also

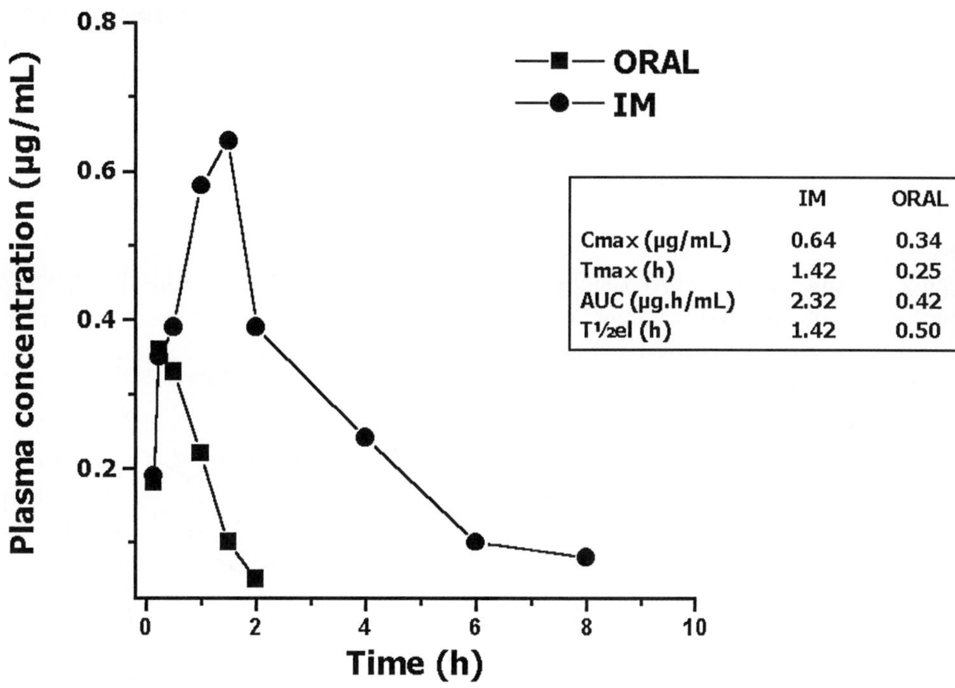

FIG. 41.4 Praziquantel plasma concentration (µg/ml) profiles measured after its oral (30 mg/kg) and intramuscular (IM) (15 mg/kg) administrations to sheep. The inserted table shows mean pharmacokinetic parameters obtained following both treatments. Adapted from Giorgi et al. (2001). Cmax: peak plasma concentration; Tmax: time to peak plasma concentration; AUC: area under concentration-time curve; T1/2el: elimination half-life.

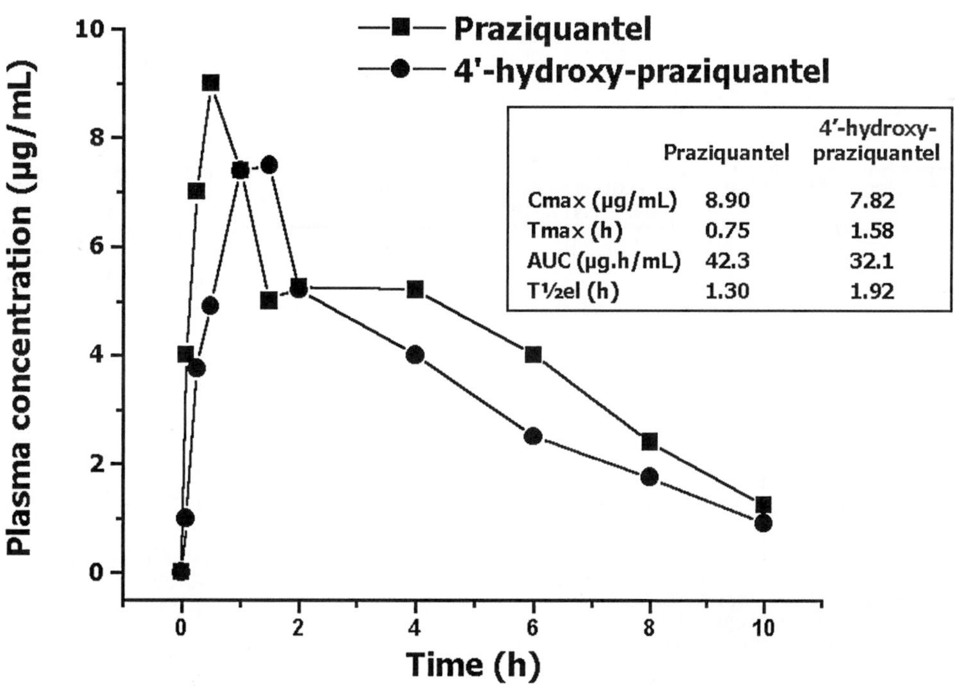

FIG. 41.5 Plasma concentration profiles of praziquantel parent drug and its main hydroxylated metabolite (4′hydroxy-praziquantel) following praziquantel administration to dogs (orally, 30 mg/kg). The inserted table shows the comparative pharmacokinetic parameters for both molecules. Adapted from Giorgi et al. (2003). Cmax: peak plasma concentration; Tmax: time to peak plasma concentration; AUC: area under concentration-time curve; T1/2el: elimination half-life.

stereoselective for the two enantiomers. Thus, two 4′-hydroxy-praziquantel isomers were identified in the plasma of human volunteers (Westhoff and Blaschke 1992). It has been shown that (−)4′-hydroxy-praziquantel is far more abundant in human plasma than its respective (+) isomer. This finding is highly relevant since, in vitro, there is no significant difference in the pharmacological effect of (−) praziquantel and its respective (−) 4′hydroxylated isomer against *S. mansoni* (Staudt et al. 1992). It has been suggested that efficacy of praziquantel in humans is mainly due to the pharmacological activity of its (−) 4′hydroxylated metabolite rather than to (−) praziquantel itself. Renal excretion is the main route of elimination of praziquantel and its metabolites.

Acute and chronic toxicity studies indicate a wide margin of safety for praziquantel. An acute, oral LD_{50} has not been established in dogs because they vomit when dosages exceed 200 mg/kg. The single therapeutic dose is 3.8–12.5 mg/kg in dogs and 4.2–12.7 mg/kg in cats. Overdoses of up to fivefold are tolerated without adverse effect. Studies in pregnant rats and rabbits detected no embryotoxic or teratogenic effects. Similar tests support the use of praziquantel in breeding and pregnant animals without restrictions.

EPSIPRANTEL

This cestocidal compound (2-(cyclohexylcarbonyl)-oxo-1,2,3,4,6,7,8,12b-octahydropyrazino[2,1-a] [2] benzazepine) (Fig. 41.6), is chemically related to praziquantel. Epsiprantel is used specifically for treatment of the common

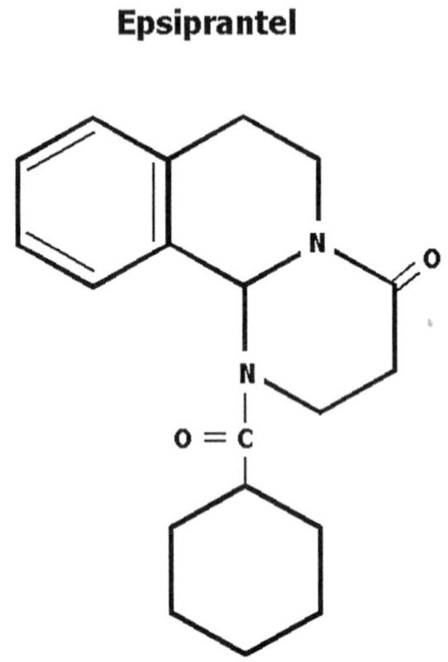

Epsiprantel

FIG. 41.6 Epsiprantel chemical structure.

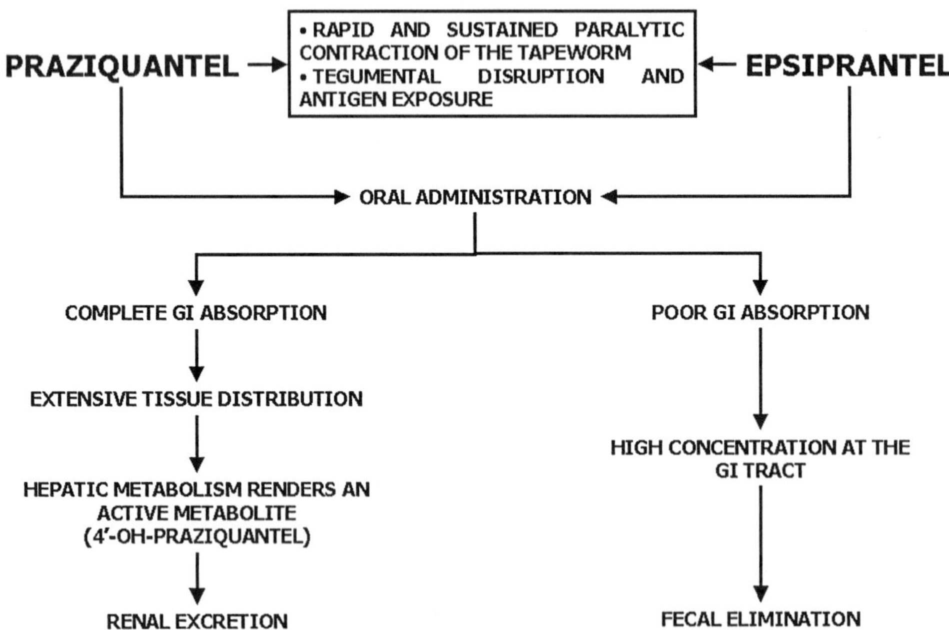

FIG. 41.7 Comparative pharmacodynamic and pharmacokinetic properties of the chemically related anticestodal drugs: praziquantel and epsiprantel. GI: gastrointestinal tract.

tapeworms of dogs (*D.caninum, T.pisiformis*) and cats (*D. caninum, T. taeniaeformis*). Recommended dosages are virtually 100% effective against those cestode parasites. Epsiprantel causes tegumental damage in larval and adult stages of *E. granulosus*. At a dosage of 5 mg/kg in dogs, the drug is 94% effective against immature (7-day-old) worms and more than 99% effective against mature stages (Thompson et al. 1991). At doses of 5.5 mg/kg in dogs and 2.5 mg/kg in cats, the drug was >99% effective against *E. multilocularis*, although residual worms may persist in some animals (Eckert et al. 2001). The recommended dose of 5.5 mg/kg is also 100% effective against *Taenia* spp. and 99.8% against *Dipylidium* (Corwin et al. 1989).

Similar to praziquantel, epsiprantel affects Ca^{2+} homeostasis within the parasite. The drug damages the tegument, making it vulnerable to lysis and digestion within the host's gut. Epsiprantel is only formulated for oral administration in dogs and cats. It is poorly absorbed in the GI tract and is thereby available to act against intestinal cestodes, being eliminated in feces. There are no metabolites and only 0.1 % of the administered drug is eliminated by urine. The comparative pharmacological properties of praziquantel and epsiprantel are summarized in Figure 41.7.

Due to its low GI absorption, epsiprantel is a safe drug. For example, cats tolerate 5 times the therapeutic dose of this cestocide once daily for 3 consecutive days. Emesis has been reported in cats administered 40 times the therapeutic dose daily for 4 days. Beagle puppies (7–10 weeks of age) given 100 mg/kg once (18 times the recommended dosage) exhibited no signs of toxicity. Adult dogs treated once with a 36 times overdose were not adversely affected. Emesis is the most commonly observed side effect of epsiprantel and may occur in prolonged treatments.

ANTITREMATODAL DRUGS

INTRODUCTION

Fasciolosis, caused by the cosmopolitan liver fluke *Fasciola hepatica*, is the most common and economically important disease caused by trematode parasites in domestic animals worldwide. Fasciolosis is an important zoonotic disease, particularly in underdeveloped countries (Mas-Coma 2004). Chemotherapy based on the use of flukicidal compounds is the main tool to control liver flukes. Most of the antitrematodal drugs discussed herein are compounds used for the treatment of fasciolosis. The tropical counterpart of *F. hepatica* is *F. gigantica* and all drugs active against one of the species are equally effective against the other (Boray 1986). Rumen fluke (*Paramphistomum* spp.) infections are common in cattle and sheep throughout the world. Adult flukes attach to the rumen wall and are of little consequence to the health of the animal. Large numbers of the immature stages, however, can be seriously pathogenic as they migrate within the gut lumen from the duodenum to the rumen. Intestinal paramphistomosis generally responds well to treatment with drugs that are effective against liver fluke and/or cestode infections in ruminants. Readers interested in specific issues regarding treatment of infections caused by either rumen flukes (*Paramphistomum* spp.) in sheep and cattle or lung flukes (*Paragonimus* spp.) in dogs and cats are referred to the previous edition of this textbook (see Reinemeyer and Courtney 2001).

The liver fluke's life cycle has several features that should be considered for a better understanding of the pharmacological properties of the antitrematodal drugs. Both immature and mature flukes damage the host liver. After the infective metacercariae are ingested by grazing sheep or cattle, the immature fluke emerges from its cyst, penetrates the wall of the small intestine, traverses the peritoneal cavity, and penetrates the liver capsule within 4 days of infection. During the next several weeks, immature flukes tunnel through liver tissues, feeding and increasing rapidly in size. Acute and subacute fasciolosis are most common in sheep. Both are characterized by the migration of a high number of immature flukes through the liver parenchyma causing severe hepatic hemorrhage, jaundice, and anemia. These stages are often fatal. Clinical signs of acute and subacute fasciolosis are presented within 6–8 weeks postinfection. Antitrematodal drugs used against immature forms must achieve effective concentrations within the liver tissue. The severity of *F. hepatica* infections in sheep may be enhanced by the fluke's potential role in disseminating enteric bacteria (*Clostridium novyi*) in the liver during migration (Reinemeyer and Courtney 2001). During the eighth week of infection, flukes begin to penetrate the main bile ducts, where they attain sexual maturity by ~10–12 weeks after infection. Adult flukes are blood-sucking parasites and penetrate within the bile ducts, causing biliary hyperplasia and progressive occlusion. The infected areas may be surrounded by connective tissue that progressively becomes calcified. Such a tissue reaction is most common in cattle where fasciolosis is typically more chronic and subclinical in nature. Although adult flukes are most susceptible (or perhaps most accessible) to fasciolicidal drugs at this stage, the affected areas of the liver tissue become progressively less penetrable by therapeutic agents and consequently more difficult to treat (Reinemeyer and Courtney 2001).

Carbohydrate and energy metabolism in helminth parasites differs from that of the mammalian host. Parasites also exhibit a wide variation in their carbohydrate breakdown pathways during their life cycle (Kita et al. 1997). Parasite metabolism uses an aerobic-anaerobic transition. In general, free-living larval stages obtain their energy from aerobic processes, whereas adult forms have mainly an anaerobic metabolism. A transition in the pathways of energy metabolism was observed in both the cytosol and mitochondria of the liver fluke *F. hepatica* (Tielens et al. 1987; Tielens 1994). Overall, energy metabolism in the adult stages is almost completely anaerobic, and aerobic processes remain only in the tegument of the parasite, which is also one of the main absorptive surfaces for drug uptake by the fluke and may be a primary target for anthelmintic action. Recent studies in *F. hepatica* have shown that the transtegumental transfer mechanism is critical to achieve sufficient drug concentration at the site of action to exert its flukicidal action (Mottier et al. 2006). Thus, adult forms in the bile ducts are exposed to anthelmintics or their metabolic products eliminated by bile excretion. Although the tegument represents only 1% of the total volume of the adult parasite, the integrity of the surface plasma membrane and the tegumental syncytium is essential for the viability of the fluke. The disruption of the tegument by different mechanisms (including those involved in energy generation) may have severe consequences for the parasite because the drug would penetrate deeper and disrupt subtegumental tissues as well. The surface damage will be exacerbated by the surfactant action of the bile. In addition, adult blood-sucking stages may uptake the anthelmintic drugs through the alimentary canal. In fact, most of the fasciolicides have high efficacy against adult flukes due to their extended residence in the systemic circulation as a consequence of their strong plasma protein binding (~98–99%).

Since the introduction of carbon tetrachloride for treatment of helminth infections of animals in the 1920s, numerous other compounds have been investigated for efficacy against *F. hepatica*. Carbon tetrachloride and other halogenated hydrocarbons have a narrow therapeutic index and their adverse effects (mainly hepatotoxicity) restrict their use for the treatment of fasciolosis. Based on their chemical structure, the fasciolicidal drugs can be classified into several groups:

1. *Halogenated hydrocarbons* (carbon tetrachloride, hexachloroethane, tetrachlorodifluoroethane, hexachloroparaxylene)
2. *Bisphenolic compounds* (hexachlorophene, bithionol)

TABLE 41.1 Comparative efficacies of the most widely used antitrematodal compounds against different stages of the liver fluke *Fasciola hepatica*

<table>
<tr><th rowspan="2">Flukicide Drugs</th><th colspan="12">Fluke's Age (in Weeks)</th></tr>
<tr><th>1</th><th>2</th><th>3</th><th>4</th><th>5</th><th>6</th><th>7</th><th>8</th><th>9</th><th>10</th><th>11</th><th>12</th></tr>
<tr><td>DIAMPHENETIDE</td><td colspan="6">90–100%</td><td colspan="6">50–80%</td></tr>
<tr><td>TRICLABENDAZOLE</td><td></td><td colspan="2">90–99%</td><td colspan="9">99–100%</td></tr>
<tr><td>RAFOXANIDE</td><td colspan="3"></td><td colspan="3">50–90%</td><td colspan="6">91–99%</td></tr>
<tr><td>CLOSANTEL</td><td colspan="6"></td><td colspan="3">50–90%</td><td colspan="3">91–99%</td></tr>
<tr><td>NITROXYNIL</td><td colspan="6"></td><td colspan="3">50–90%</td><td colspan="3">91–99%</td></tr>
<tr><td>CLORSULON (oral)</td><td colspan="7"></td><td colspan="5">90–99%</td></tr>
<tr><td>CLORSULON (SC)</td><td colspan="9"></td><td colspan="3">70–99%</td></tr>
<tr><td>ALBENDAZOLE</td><td colspan="9"></td><td colspan="3">70–99%</td></tr>
<tr><td>OXYCLOZANIDE</td><td colspan="9"></td><td colspan="3">70–99%</td></tr>
</table>

Adapted from Fairweather and Boray (1999).

3. *Nitrophenolic compounds* (nitroxynil, disophenol, niclofolan)
4. *Salicylanilides* (closantel, rafoxanide, oxyclozanide) and *brominated salicylanilides* (bromosalans)
5. *Bencenesulfonamides* (clorsulon)
6. *Benzimidazole* (albendazole, netobimin, luxabendazole) and *halogenated benzimidazole* (triclabendazole)
7. *Phenoxyalkanes* (diamphenethide)

Most of the halogenated hydrocarbons; bisphenolic compounds; the nitrophenolics, disophenol and niclofan; as well as the bromosalans are little used old drugs, which have been extensively reviewed in previous editions of this text (see Roberson and Courtney 1995). This chapter is focused on the description of the pharmacological properties of the most currently used antitrematodal drugs. A schematic representation of the efficacy of different flukicidal drugs against immature and adult stages of *F. hepatica* is shown in Table 41.1.

NITROPHENOLIC COMPOUNDS

NITROXYNIL. Nitroxynil (3-iodo-4-hydroxy-5-nitrobenzonitrile) (Fig. 41.8) was developed in the late 1960s as an injectable fasciolicide for sheep and cattle. It is a trematodicidal compound highly effective against *F. hepatica*, which also holds activity against the abomasal nematode *Haemonchus contortus*. Nitroxynil is highly effective against adult stages of *F. hepatica* (from 8 weeks postinfection) and *F. gigantica*. Activity against earlier stages is rather erratic and it is not effective for the treatment of flukes younger than 6 weeks. Moreover, this anthelmintic is used for the control of ivermectin- and benzimidazole-resistant *H. contortus* in sheep. It is also marketed for the control of *Oesophagostomum* spp. and *Bunostomum* spp. in both sheep and cattle and shows good activity against *Parafilaria bovicola* infections in cattle. On the contrary, nitroxynil is not effective for the treatment of paramphistomes in sheep and cattle.

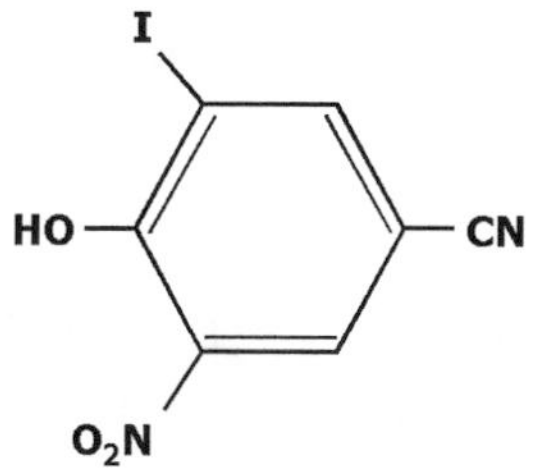

I
HO — CN
O_2N

Nitroxynil

FIG. 41.8 Chemical structure of the nitrophenolic compound nitroxynil.

Due to the structural similarity between nitrophenols and 2,4-dinitrophenol, a known uncoupler of oxidative phosphorylation, it was assumed that nitroxynil and related compounds act in a similar way in the fluke. However, there is little direct evidence showing this mechanism of action for these fasciolicides. It has been shown that nitroxynil produced a rapid spastic paralysis (within 3 h) of the fluke in vitro at similar concentrations to those found in the systemic circulation in vivo (Fairweather et al. 1984). This action was not believed to be the consequence of an uncoupling effect on the oxidative phosphorylation (Fairweather and Boray 1999). More recently, it was shown that nitroxynil causes severe disruption of the tegument of *F. hepatica*, both in vitro and in vivo (McKinstry et al. 2003). Liver flukes recovered from rats after 24 hours of nitroxynil treatment showed extensive swelling and blebbing of the tegument in both dorsal and ventral surfaces. These changes became more severe after 48 and 72 hours following nitroxynil administration, and specimens recovered following these posttreatment intervals showed more widespread tegumental loss. Although the intrinsic mechanism of nitroxynil action on the parasite has not been established as yet, it was shown that the tegument is an important target for this flukicidal drug.

Nitroxynil can be administered orally or intraruminally (IR) but is more effective when administered by parenteral routes (SC, IM). A ruminal microflora-mediated nitroreduction may account for its low efficacy after oral or IR treatments. Solutions (25% or 34%) of nitroxynil-N-alkylglucamine are available in the market to be used at 10 mg/kg. SC and IM administrations provide similar efficacy against liver flukes, but the SC route has become the method of choice in practice. Local tolerance at the site of injection is satisfactory, although transitory inflammatory swellings are occasionally observed in cattle. Nitroxynil is well absorbed after its SC administration and binds strongly to plasma proteins (~98%) mainly to albumin (Alvinerie et al. 1991). Plasma concentrations in sheep remain high within 3 days posttreatment and may be detected in the bloodstream for 60 days. Due to its high affinity for plasma proteins, nitroxynil has low tissue distribution and, consequently, the amount of drug reaching the liver parenchyma seems to be insufficient for treatment of immature flukes at the recommended dose rate.

Nitroxynil was shown to be metabolized by hydrolysis of the cyano group to produce 3-iodo-4-hydroxy-5-nitrobenzamide and 3-iodo-4-hydroxy-5-nitrobenzoic acid in rat liver. The enzyme(s) responsible for this hydrolytic reaction was primarily localized in the cytosol (Markus and Kwon 1994). Nitroxynil was also found to be nitroreduced in rat liver into 3-iodo-4-hydroxy-5-aminobenzonitrile (Maffei Facino et al. 1982). Further methylation of this metabolite into 3-iodo-4-methoxy-5-aminobenzonitrile was also shown. However, the inactive metabolites were not detected in the urine nor in the plasma of nitroxynil-treated sheep. Indeed, unchanged drug is likely to be the only source responsible for nitroxynil action. Due to its high plasma protein binding, it was suggested that the blood is the primary source of drug uptake via the fluke's digestive system. In addition, the levels of nitroxynil in bile are far lower than those observed in plasma and so, the uptake of this anthelmintic through the tegument would be limited (McKinstry et al. 2003). The urine is the primary route of nitroxynil elimination, although the drug is also excreted in feces and milk (it is not approved for use in dairy animals). Animals can be slaughtered for human consumption 60 days after nitroxynil treatment. Nitroxynil also stains wool or hair yellow; thus, care must be exercised to avoid spilling. The drug is well tolerated in cattle and sheep at the therapeutic dose of 10 mg/kg. Nitroxynil side effects in these species include hyperthermia and hyperpnea, which were associated with the uncoupling of oxidative phosphorilation in the target species and observed at higher dose levels. Doses above 40 mg/kg may be lethal.

Other nitrophenolic flukicidal compounds such as disophenol and niclofolan were replaced by nitroxynil and many other newer and safer fasciolicidal drugs.

SALICYLANILIDES

This family includes fasciolicidal drugs of similar chemical structure sharing the same mode of action. The most extensively used salicylanilides (closantel, oxyclozanide, and rafoxanide) are described here. For information on the flukicidal activity of the brominated salicylanilides (bromosdalans) readers are referred to a previous edition of this text (Roberson and Courtney 1995).

CLOSANTEL. Closantel (N-[5-chloro-4-[(4-chlorophenyl)cyanomethyl]-2-methylphenyl]-2-hydroxy-3,5-diiodobenzamide) (Fig. 41.9) is highly effective for the treatment of adult flukes and shows good activity against immature specimens aged 6–8 weeks (Table 41.1). It is not effective against earlier stages (Boray 1986). At an oral dosage of 10 mg/kg, its efficacy is more than 92% against 8-week-old and adult *F. hepatica*. It is less active against younger stages of this parasite, i.e., 70–77% efficacy for 6-week-old flukes migrating in the liver. It is also effective (94.6–97.7%) against 8-week-old *Fascioloides magna* in sheep at

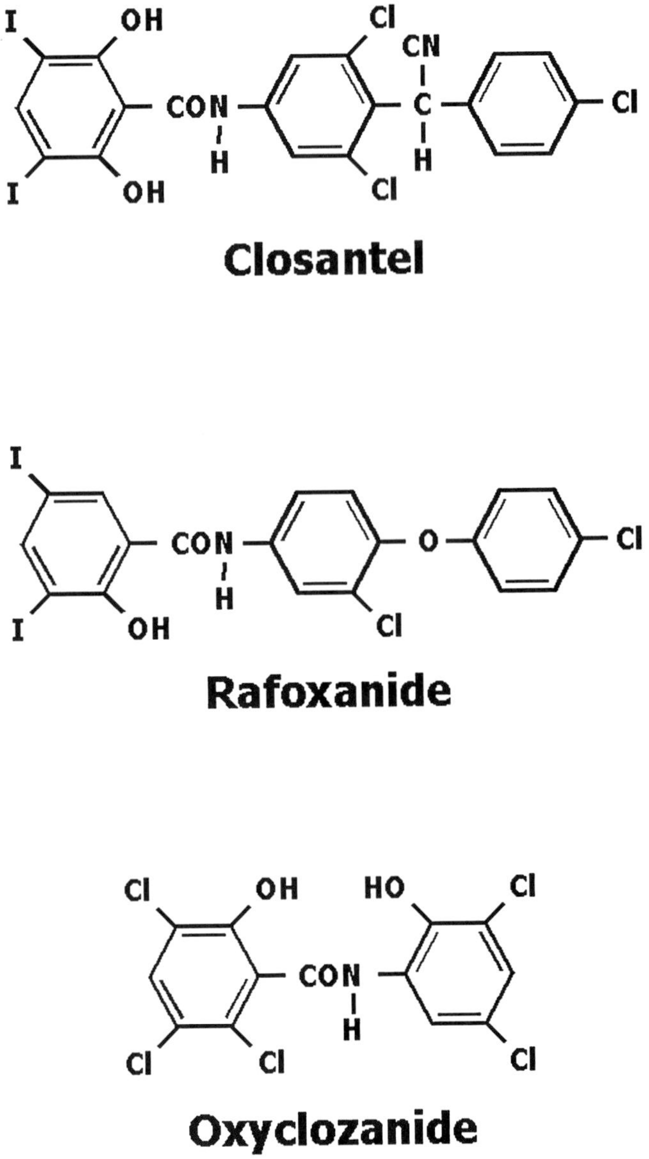

Closantel

Rafoxanide

Oxyclozanide

FIG. 41.9 Chemical structures of salicylanilide flukicidal compounds: closantel, oxyclozanide, and rafoxanide.

oral dosages of 15 mg/kg or IM dosages of 7.5 mg/kg. However, closantel is not effective against paramphistome flukes.

Closantel is also highly effective against *H. contortus* in sheep and is used as an alternative drug for the treatment of ivermectin-, benzimidazole-, levamisole- and morantel-resistant strains of this nematode. In addition, it is effective for the treatment of many other adult nematodes such as *Oesophagostomum* spp., *Bunostomum* spp. and *Ostertagia* spp. in both, sheep and cattle. Additionally, closantel is effective against certain ectoparasites such as blood-sucking lice, ticks, mites, and certain grubs of ruminants. It is also used for the treatment of the nasal bot *Oestrus ovis* in sheep. The drug can be used against the adult stage of *Ancylostoma caninum*, but is not effective against the somatic larvae of this hookworm. Closantel also has been used in horses to prevent or reduce infections of *Strongylus vulgaris* and *Gasterophilus* spp.

Closantel and other salicylanilides are uncouplers of the oxidative phosphorylation in the liver fluke. There is stronger evidence supporting this mechanism of action for these compounds than for nitrophenolic flukicides (Martin 1997). ATP production in the mitochondria is coupled to a proton (H^+) gradient across the inner mitochondrial membrane. During the oxidative phosphorylation, electrons coming from NADH or FADH are transported through a series of protein complexes on the inner mithocondrial membrane. During this process, protons (H^+) are pumped out of the mitochondrial matrix into the space between the inner and outer mitochondrial membrane, establishing a proton gradient across the inner membrane. This proton motive force is due to the pH gradient and transmembrane electric potential being critical for ATP synthesis. Salicylanilides possesse a detachable proton (H^+) that could be shuttled across the inner mitochondrial membrane, removing the proton (H^+) gradient and uncoupling oxidative phosphorilation. Metabolic changes consequently to this mechanism include increase in glucose uptake, decrease in glycogen content, changes in respiratory intermediates, and decrease in ATP synthesis (Fairweather and Boray 1999).

In addition, an alternative mechanism of action of closantel has been investigated. A significant decrease in tegumental pH (6.8 to 6.5) was observed after its in vitro incubation with *Schistosoma mansoni* and *F. hepatica* specimens (Pax and Bennett 1989). In fact, this fall occurred within 10 minutes after closantel addition and before any change in the production of ATP by the parasite. This effect was also observed at a lower concentration than that required to produce any reduction in ATP synthesis. It was concluded that the action of closantel is more complex than a conventional uncoupler of the oxidative phosphorylation. Indeed, this anthelmintic is a membrane-active molecule capable of affecting many biochemical and physiological processes within the parasite. Closantel may also shuttle protons (H^+) across the tegumental membrane leading to a disruption of the mechanisms responsible for mantaining pH homeostasis, which are likely to reside in the tegument and excretory system (Fairweather and Boray 1999). Closantel also induces spastic paralysis in *F. hepatica* at concentrations comparable to maximum blood levels attained in vivo. This effect was attributed to an increase in calcium ions in the muscle cells. It has been suggested that this neuromuscular action of closantel may take place before any disruption of energy metabolism. Consequences of the paralysis are cessation of feeding and starvation; the fluke has to draw on its energy reserves to survive, and this may account, at least in part, for some of the biochemical changes observed.

Closantel is a weak acid ($pK_a = 4.28$) molecule of high molecular weight (663 Kda) and extremely lipophilic. It is formulated for oral, IR, or parenteral (SC or IM) administration in ruminants. Closantel is marketed as 3.75 or 5% suspensions or solutions for oral drench or IR administration (solutions also may be used for parenteral administration). The pharmacokinetic behavior of a novel injectable (SC) formulation containing closantel plus ivermectin was recently studied in cattle (Cromie et al. 2006). The plasma availability of both active drugs in the combination was not affected by the presence of the other. Plasma profiles of closantel in the combined product were similar to those observed after administration of a reference product. On the contrary, ivermectin was absorbed and eliminated faster following its administration in the combined formulation compared with a reference product containing only ivermectin.

Closantel is well absorbed after either enteral or parenteral administrations in sheep and cattle. The recommended enteral dose rate in these species is 10 mg/kg; the same efficacy could be attained following its SC or IM administration at 5 mg/kg. Consequently, the oral bioavailability of closantel administered at 10 mg/kg resulted similar to that observed following its parenteral administration at 5 mg/kg (Michiels et al. 1987). It was shown that the bioavailability of closantel administered by the oral route was 50% lower compared to that observed following its parenteral administration. It has been shown that closantel is not subjected to any significant biodegradation by the ruminal fluid, but more than 80% of the drug was shown to be associated with the particulate phase of the abomasal digesta (Hennessy and Ali 1997). The strong association of closantel with the particulate digesta and the limited time available for the exchange of the drug between the particulate material and the GI fluids prior to absorption may explain its low enteral bioavailability (Hennessy and Ali 1997). In addition, closantel is a weak acid and almost 99.5% of the total drug present in the intestinal lumen may be in the ionized form at the absorption site in the intestine. Altogether these observations may help explain the incomplete GI absorption of closantel after its oral administration in ruminants. Reduction of feed intake, which slows the digesta flow rate and extends the residence of the drug within the GI's lumen, increases the plasma and GI availabilities of closantel in sheep (Hennessy and Ali 1997).

Closantel is extensively bound (>99%) to plasma proteins, mainly albumin, and has a long terminal half-life of 14.3–14.5 days in sheep (Ali and Bogan 1987; Hennessy 1993). It binds specifically to ovine serum albumin at site I, the warfarin/phenylbutazone binding site of albumin and also to invertebrate haemocyanin and haemolymph (Rothwell et al. 2000). As a consequence of its high protein binding, the duration of therapeutic levels of closantel in plasma is prolonged. Thus, a single dose of closantel protects sheep against susceptible *H. contortus* reinfection for up 28 days (Hall et al. 1981). A small apparent volume of distribution (Vd) (<0.15 l/kg) indicates that the distribution of closantel to tissues (including the liver) is limited in ruminant species (Michiels et al. 1987; Swan et al. 1999). Overall, plasma albumin constitutes a reservoir from which this anthelmintic is directly available to haematophagous helminths, such as *F. hepatica* and *H. contortus*. Indeed, the blood is the primary source for the uptake of closantel via the digestive system of the parasites.

Dehalogenation in the liver renders two inactive monoiodo metabolites (3- and 5-monoiodoclosantel), although the metabolism of closantel is poor. Approximately 80–90% of the administered drug is eliminated by biliar/fecal excretion without metabolic changes. Only 10% of the administered drug was eliminated as monoiodo metabolites in sheep. Other minor routes of elimination of closantel are urine (less than 0.5% of the administered dose) and milk. In dairy cattle, approximately 1% of the administered dose was found to be excreted with the milk per day. Residual tissue concentrations are extremely low in sheep: 7 to 21 times lower than the corresponding plasma concentrations. In cattle, closantel concentrations in milk were 45-fold lower than those observed in plasma. In addition, tissue and milk residues decline parallel to plasma levels. Animals may be slaughtered for human consumption 28 days before closantel treatment. However, the use of this anthelmintic in milk production is forbidden.

The acute toxicity resulting from single dosing of closantel in rats is characterized by hypotonia, ataxia, diarrhea and dyspnea. Clinical signs of acute toxicity in ruminants are anorexia, labored breathing, general weakness and decreased vision (or blindness) appearing approximately one week after dosing. At the lethal dose (LD_{50} in sheep = >40 mg/kg oral/IM; LD_{50} in cattle = >40 mg/kg oral and >20 mg/kg IM), anorexia, hypotonia, and quadriplegia preceded death. In short-term toxicological studies conducted in rats, male gonads and the liver were the target organs for toxicity. Some fatty deposition was observed in the liver tissue of males but not in females. Extensive reproductive studies in rams, ewes, and bulls indicate that closantel has no risk to reproductive parameters.

RAFOXANIDE. This anthelmintic is a halogenated salicylanilide. Its chemical formula is 3′-chloro-4′-(p-chlorophenoxy)-3,5-diiodosalicylanilide (Fig. 41.9). It is an off-white crystalline powder and is commercially formulated for use as a bolus or as a drenching suspension, which also may be used for IR administration. Rafoxanide was developed in 1969 and subsequently has been used extensively worldwide against fasciolosis and haemonchosis in sheep and cattle. Its principal use is as an adulticide for *F. hepatica* and *F. gigantica.* A single therapeutic dose (7.5 mg/kg) in sheep is nearly 100% effective for 12-week-old flukes of *F. hepatica*, 86–99% for 6-week-old flukes, and 50–98% for 4-week-old specimens of this parasite. At elevated doses (10–15 mg/kg), rafoxanide shows high activity against 4-week-old flukes (Boray 1986). The same dosages reach similar efficacies against *F. hepatica* in cattle. The reliable efficacy of this drug against 4- and 6-week-old flukes gives rafoxanide an advantage over strictly adulticidal drugs in the treatment of acute fasciolosis. In this case, the administration might be repeated after 3 weeks to eliminate maturing flukes that may have escaped the earlier treatment. In addition, this anthelmintic is also indicated for the treatment of haemonchosis, bunostomosis, and sheep nasal bots (*Oestrus ovis*). The mode of action of rafoxanide is similar to that described for the chemically-related salicylanilide, closantel.

Following oral dosing, rafoxanide is absorbed from the small intestine into the bloodstream. Peak plasma levels occur between 24 and 48 hours. Its bioavailability, measured as AUC and Cmax, was 2.5–3-fold greater in 5–8-week-old suckling lambs compared to weaned lambs aged 21–22 weeks (Swan and Mulders 1993). Rafoxanide is extensively bound (>99%) to plasma proteins and has a long (16.6 days) terminal half-life. The blood is the primary source for the uptake of rafoxanide via the digestive system of the haematophagous helminths. Also, the efficacy of rafoxanide against immature liver flukes is due to its prolonged persistence in the plasma, with subsequent effects on maturing flukes as they reach the bile ducts. In addition, liver fluke infection did not alter the plasma disposition of rafoxanide in sheep (Benchaoui and McKellar 1993). The drug is not metabolized to any detectable degree by cattle or sheep liver. Following a single oral dose of 15 mg/kg in cattle, no residue of the compound is detectable in edible tissues at 28 days after treatment.

OXYCLOZANIDE. Oxyclozanide (3,3′,5,5′,6-pentachloro-2′-hydroxy salicylanilide) (Fig. 41.9) was introduced over 40 years ago for use against adult fluke infections in ruminants. It has been also used against tapeworms (*Moniezia* spp.) in sheep and cattle. This anthelmintic is marketed as an oral drench (aqueous suspension) containing oxyclozanide only or in combination with levamisole hydrochloride or oxfendazole. It is also formulated as a powder to be incorporated in the feed. The recommended dose rates are 10–15 mg/kg for cattle and 15 mg/kg for sheep and goats. The mechanism of action of oxyclozanide is similar to that described for closantel. Following its oral administration to sheep, the drug is extensively (greater than 99%) bound to plasma proteins, and the plasma concentration/time curve could be best described by a tri-exponential equation. Its terminal half-life (6.4 days) is shorter compared with closantel and rafoxanide (14.5 and 16.6 days, respectively) (Ali and Bogan 1987). The drug is excreted into the bile as a glucuronide metabolite. Figure 41.10 shows the comparative plasma profiles and some pharmacokinetic parameters for closantel, rafoxanide, and oxyclozanide following their respective oral administrations to sheep.

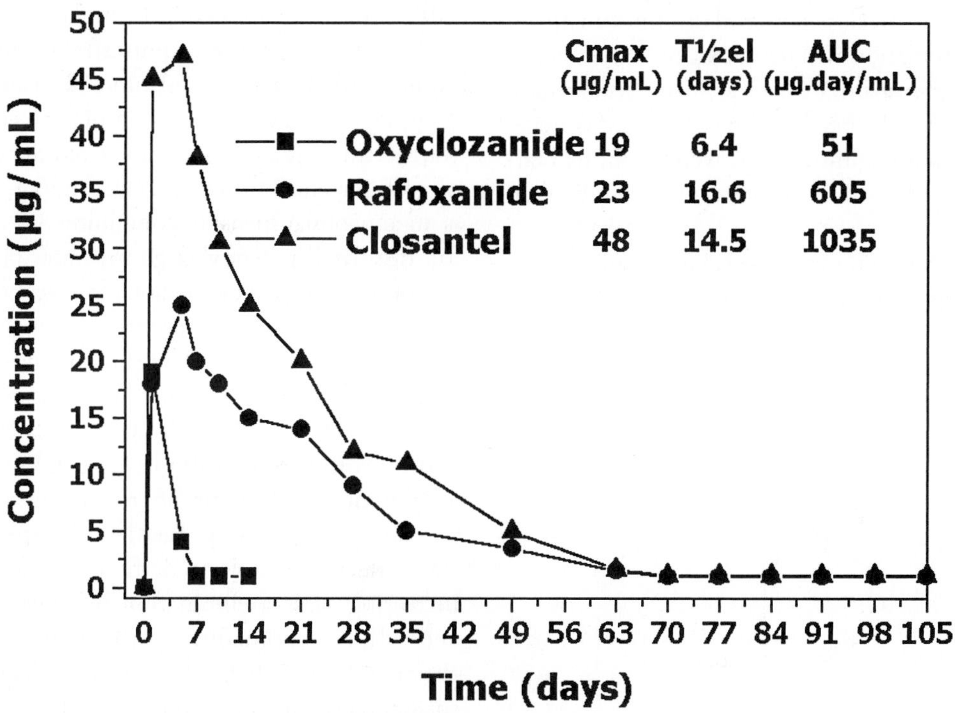

FIG. 41.10 Comparative plasma profiles of closantel (7.5 mg/kg), rafoxanide (7.5 mg/kg) and oxyclozanide (15 mg/kg) measured after their oral administration to sheep. The values of some kinetic parameters obtained for each compound are shown. Adapted from Ali and Bogan (1987). Cmax: peak plasma concentration; T1/2el: elimination half-life; AUC: area under the concentration-time curve.

BENZENESULFONAMIDES

CLORSULON. This anthelmintic is a benzenesulfonamide with the chemical formula 4-amino-6-trichloroethenyl-1,3-benzenedisulfonamide (Fig. 41.11). Clorsulon is highly effective against adult liver flukes in sheep and cattle. However, it is more effective in cattle than in sheep and goats. The recommended dose rate is 2 mg/kg body weight given by SC injection. Good efficacy against 8-week-old flukes is achieved following SC administration at 4–8 mg/kg. Oral administration at 3.75 mg/kg is effective for the treatment of adult liver flukes aged 14–16 weeks in both sheep and cattle. The recommended oral dose rate is 7 mg/kg, which is 100% effective for the treatment of 8-week-old flukes. The same dose rate is 99% effective for the treatment of adult specimens (14 weeks postinfection) in goats. The efficacy of clorsulon has been tested against infections with several other fluke species in ruminants. It was effective (>92%) against immature (8-week-old) *Fascioloides magna* in cattle and sheep at 21 mg/kg orally. Daily dosing at 7 mg/kg for 5 consecutive days has been 100% effective against adult and 92% effective against immature *Fasciola gigantica* in cattle. Clorsulon has poor efficacy against *Paramphistomum* spp.

The combination of clorsulon with ivermectin in an SC-injectable formulation was designed for simultaneous treatment of *F. hepatica* and nematode infections of cattle. The oral formulation of clorsulon also can be used concurrently with other anthelmintics (e.g., ivermectin, fenbendazole) with no reduction in efficacy of the individual products.

Chemically, clorsulon is similar to 1,3 diphosphoglycerate, an intermediary product of glycolysis. Consequently, this anthelmintic was shown to inhibit competitively the enzymes phosphoglycerate kinase and phosphoglyceromutase (Schulman and Valentino 1982). However, such disruption of glycolysis was observed in vitro with clorsulon concentrations many times greater than blood levels achieved in vivo. Thus, it is believed that clorsulon effects on the glycolitic pathway at therapeutic concentrations attained in vivo may not be relevant. Nevertheless, glycolysis is the main energy yielding pathway in the fluke and any disruption of this process would decrease glucose utilization and the production of metabolic end products (acetate and propionate) with a significant reduction in ATP levels within the parasite. Morphological changes in fluke specimens recovered from clorsulon-treated rats include severe necrosis of the gastrodermal cells and tegumental damage restricted to the cone and midbody regions of the fluke (Fairweather and Boray 1999; Meaney et al. 2003, 2004). It has also been shown that the gut was more severely affected than the tegument, which is consistent with the observation that oral ingestion is a main route of entry of clorsulon into the fluke (Meaney et al. 2005). Thus, the changes in the gut represent the direct consequence of drug action, while those observed in the tegument represent either the direct effect of transtegumental uptake of clorsulon from the bile or an indirect effect derived from gut disruption.

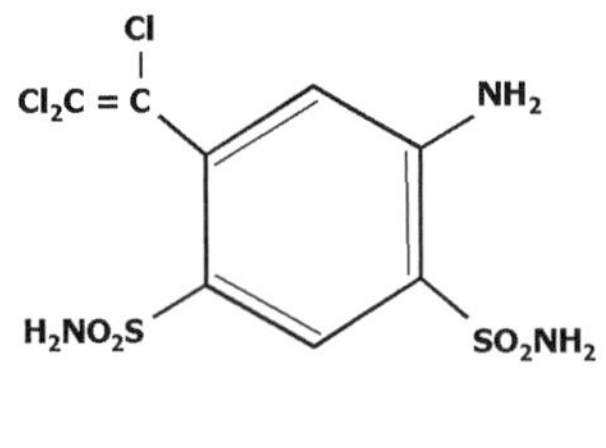

Cl
$Cl_2C = C$
NH_2
H_2NO_2S
SO_2NH_2
Clorsulon

FIG. 41.11 Chemical structure of clorsulon, a benzenesulfonamide flukicidal compound.

Clorsulon is marketed as an oral drench for sheep and cattle and as an injectable formulation (in combination with ivermectin) for SC administration to cattle. The recommended dosage of clorsulon for cattle and sheep is 7 mg/kg by oral drench. In commercial combination with ivermectin, clorsulon is administered SC to cattle at a rate of 2 mg/kg and ivermectin at 0.2 mg/kg. The oral drench is an aqueous suspension containing 8.5 mg/ml of clorsulon dissolved in propylen glycol/water (1/10). The pharmacokinetic behavior of clorsulon was studied in sheep and goats after administration of a single IV and after a single oral dose of 7 mg/kg (Sundlof and Whitlock 1992). These authors reported that the bioavailability of orally administered clorsulon was approximately 55% in goats and 60% in sheep. Peak plasma concentrations occurred at 14 hours and 15 hours after oral administration in goats and sheep, respectively. Besides, absorption from the GI tract effectively prolonged the elimination of clorsulon, increasing plasma elimination half-lives (about twofold) and MRTs (approximately three- to fourfold) in both sheep and goats. It has been shown that the rumen may substantially influence the absorption pattern and the resultant pharmacokinetic behavior and antiparasite activity of enterally delivered anthelmintic drugs. This fact has been thoroughly studied for benzimidazole anthelmintic drugs. Similarly, when a suspension of clorsulon is deposited in the rumen, the adsorption of its particles to digesta solid content, the slow mixing and long digesta residence time, and the large rumen volume assist absorption by delaying the rate of passage of drug down the GI tract (Hennessy 1993). Thus, the rumen may act as a reservoir and prolong the duration of drug absorption and/or outflow down the GI tract. Indeed, the absorption pattern of clorsulon from the GI tract influences its pharmacokinetic behavior and, consequently, its elimination from plasma is delayed. In rats, clorsulon was shown to be bounded predominately to erythrocytes at doses below 4 mg/kg. In fact, the drug is bound to red blood cell carbonic anhydrase (Schulman et al. 1982). As explained above, this is the major route of entry of clorsulon into the fluke, and drug uptake by *F. hepatica* increases in direct proportion to the blood level.

Renal excretion of the parent drug is thought to be the main route of elimination of clorsulon, accounting for approximately 50% of the IV dose at 48 hours in both sheep and goats. On the other hand, up to 30% and 41% of the orally administered dose was recovered in urine in sheep and goats, respectively (Sundlof and Whitlock 1992). The elimination rate constant (kel) in goats was nearly twice as large as the value determined in sheep, and the AUC following IV administration in goats was only 63% of the value observed in sheep, indicating that goats are more effective in their ability to eliminate clorsulon than are sheep. These differences in drug disposition between sheep and goats may account for the reduced efficacy of clorsulon reported in goats.

Clorsulon is a safe drug with high therapeutic index. Acute toxicity of this antiparasitic has been assessed in mice, rats, sheep, and cattle. The LD_{50} in mice is an intraperitoneal (IP) dose of 761 mg/kg and more than 10,000 mg/kg orally. The latter dose causes no apparent toxicity in rats. Sheep infected with flukes have been dosed repeatedly with 5 mg/kg daily for 28 days or with single doses of 100 mg/kg with no apparent effect. Uninfected sheep tolerated 200 or 400 mg/kg without adverse reactions. A toxic dosage has not been identified in cattle. Oral doses of 7 mg (recommended) and 21 mg/kg on 3 consecutive days and single oral doses of 7, 70, and 175 mg/kg (i.e., up to 25 times the label dosage) have not affected weight gains, feed consumption, or clinical or histopathologic parameters adversely. In uninfected goats, experimental dosages up to 35 mg/kg every other day for three doses did not cause adverse reactions. Clorsulon is also considered safe for use in breeding and pregnant animals. Residue studies indicate a short half-life of clorsulon in tissues and milk. Milk taken from treated animals within 72 hours (six milkings) after treatment should not be used for human consumption, and beef animals should not be slaughtered within 8 days of treatment.

BENZIMIDAZOLES

The pharmacology of the broad-spectrum benzimidazole (BZD) anthelmintic compounds has been fully described in Chapter 40. Albendazole (used at 7.5 mg/kg in sheep and at 10 mg/kg in cattle) and the pro-BZD netobimin (20 mg/kg) are active against liver flukes older than 12 weeks. Fenbendazole is not effective against *F. hepatica*, but a single treatment at 5 mg/kg reduced *F. gigantica* infection in sheep by up to 95%. Luxabendazole is also an effective flukicidal BZD, which did not reach the market. However, the halogenated BZD thiol named *triclabendazole,* which does not have nematocidal activity, is the most widely used and potent flukicidal drug active against immature and mature stages of *F. hepatica*. Its pharmacological features are described below.

TRICLABENDAZOLE. Unlike other BZD compounds, the halogenated derivative triclabendazole (5-chloro-6(2–3-dichlorophenoxy)-2-methylthio-1H-benzimidazole) (TCBZ) (Fig. 41.12) holds an excellent efficacy against the adult and juvenile stages of *F. hepatica* (down to 1-week-old flukes), which is unlike other available flukicidal drugs (Boray et al. 1983). The high activity of TCBZ against immature flukes is significant because they represent the migratory stage of the parasite, which may produce serious tissue damage in the host. However, TCBZ activity appears to be restricted to *F. hepatica*, *F. gigantica*, *Fascioloides magna* and the lung fluke, *Paragonimus* spp. (Calpoviña et al. 1988), because the drug does not show clinical efficacy against nematodes, cestodes, and other trematode (*Dicrocoelium dendriticum*, *Paramphistomun* spp., and *Schistosoma mansoni*) parasites.

The precise mode of action of TCBZ has not yet been established. BZD nematodicidal activity is based on its binding to parasite β-tubulin (Lacey 1988), which inhibits polymerization into microtubules. Thus, all the functions ascribed to microtubules at the cellular level are altered (cell division, maintenance of cell shape, cell motility, cellular secretion, nutrient absorption, and intracellular

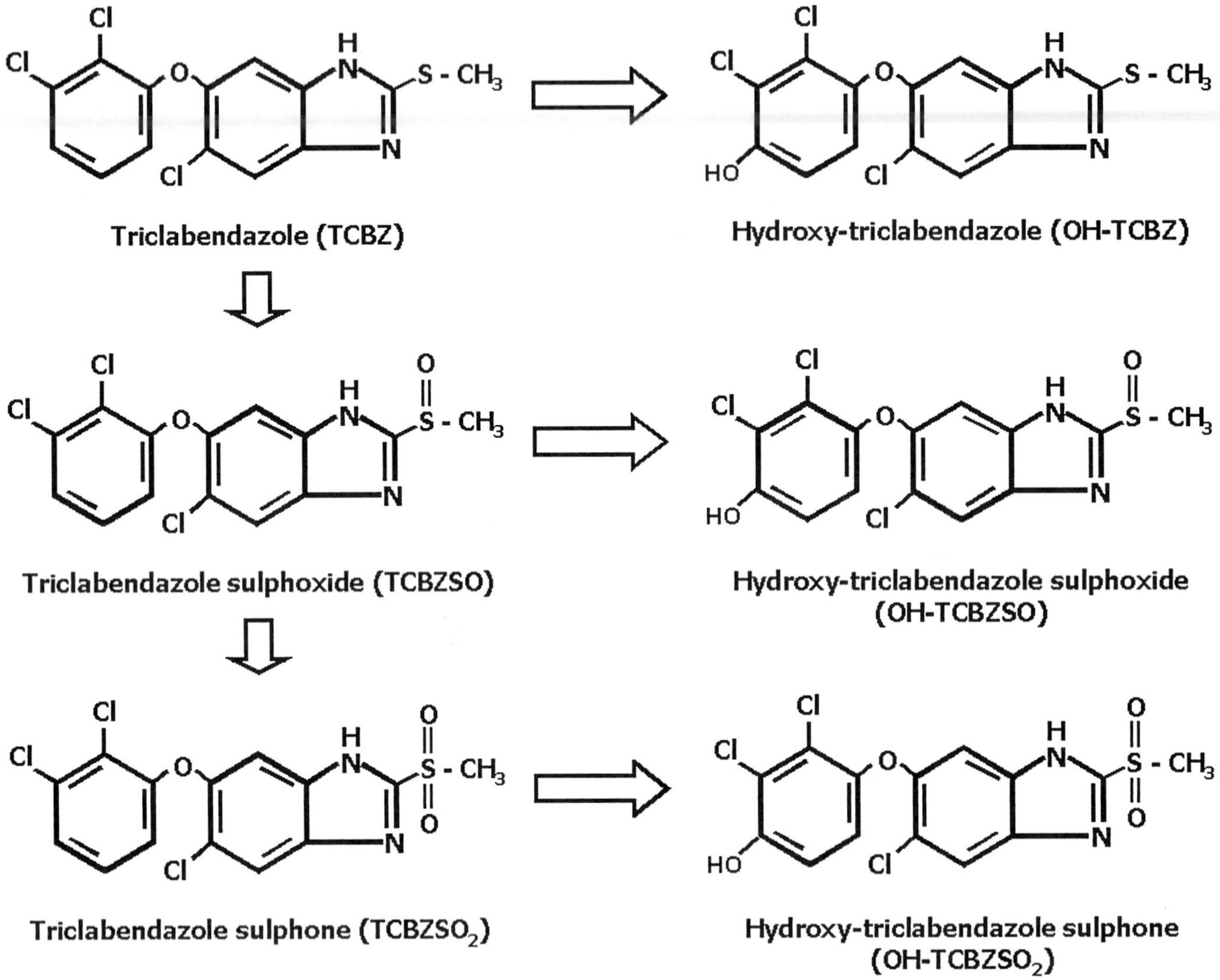

Triclabendazole (TCBZ)

Hydroxy-triclabendazole (OH-TCBZ)

Triclabendazole sulphoxide (TCBZSO)

Hydroxy-triclabendazole sulphoxide (OH-TCBZSO)

Triclabendazole sulphone ($TCBZSO_2$)

Hydroxy-triclabendazole sulphone (OH-$TCBZSO_2$)

FIG. 41.12 Triclabendazole (TCBZ) and its main metabolites: chemical structures and metabolic pathways. See the text for further explanation of TCBZ metabolism.

transport). BZD methylcarbamate molecules such as albendazole or fenbendazole act upon nematode microtubules at the tubulin colchicine binding site (Lacey 1988). It is likely that a different site of action is involved in the flukicidal activity of TCBZ, which could also explain its lack of efficacy against other helminth parasites. However, there is morphological data that support the possible binding of TCBZ to the fluke's tubulin. The TCBZ sulphoxide metabolite (TCBZSO) blocks the transport of secretory bodies from the cell body to the tegumental surface, culminating in the total loss of the tegument (Stitt and Fairweather 1994). TCBZSO also inhibits the mitotic division of spermatogenic cells and the stem vitelline cells, all changes related to microtubule inhibition. It is likely that TCBZ/metabolites may target an alternative binding site on the tubulin molecule (Fairweather 2005).

The pharmacokinetics of TCBZ has been characterized in sheep (Hennessy et al. 1987), goats (Kinabo and Bogan 1988) and cattle (Sanyal 1995). TCBZ parent drug is not detectable in plasma after its oral administration to sheep and cattle, TCBZSO and TCBZ-sulphone ($TCBZSO_2$) being the metabolites recovered from the bloodstream of treated animals (see Fig. 41.13). These metabolites reach a peak plasma concentration after 18 and 36 hours posttreatment, respectively, in sheep. Furthermore, extremely low concentrations of TCBZ were

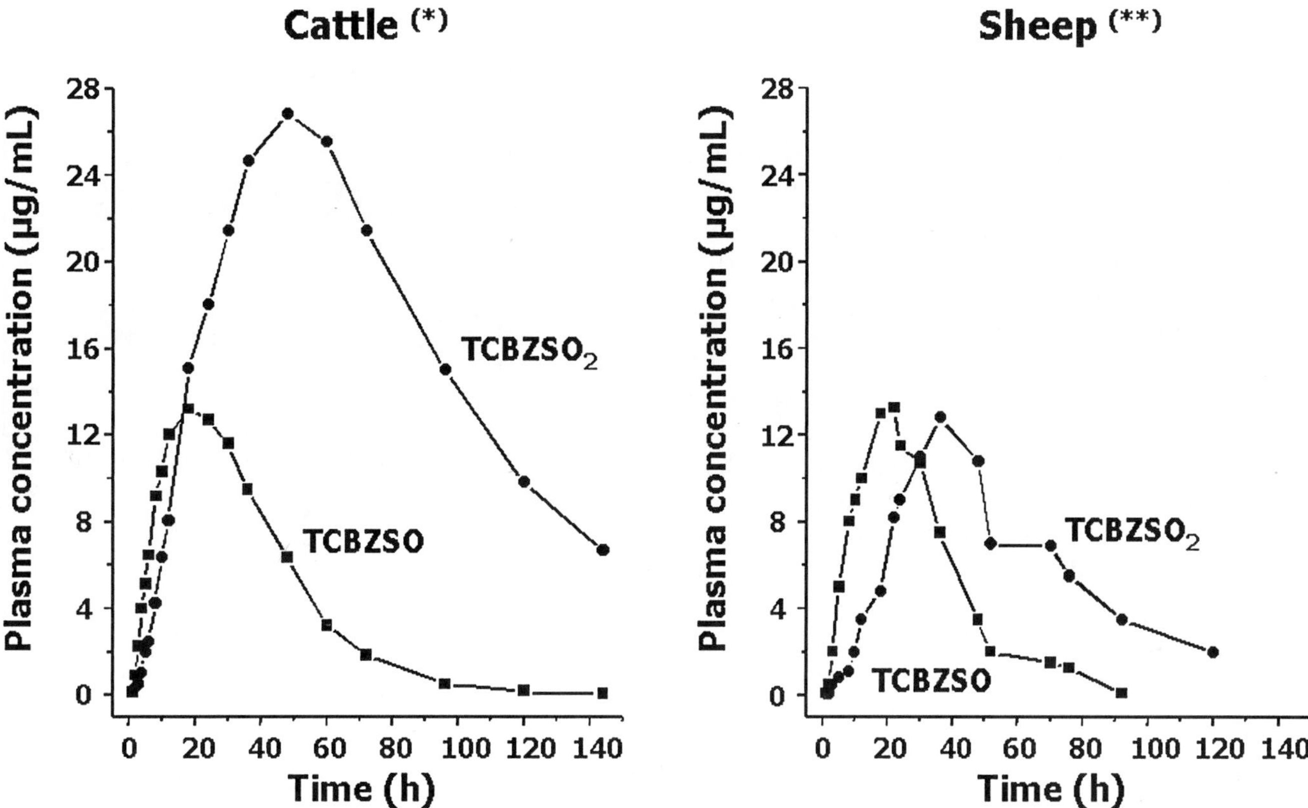

FIG. 41.13 Plasma concentration profiles of triclabendazole sulphoxide (TCBZSO) and sulphone ($TCBZSO_2$) obtained after triclabendazole administration to cattle (orally, 12 mg/kg) and sheep (intraruminal, 10 mg/kg). (*) Lanusse et al. (unpublished observations). (**) Adapted from Hennessy et al (1987).

recovered in bile; TCBZSO, $TCBZSO_2$, and the hydroxy-TCBZ derivatives were the major biliary metabolites found in sheep (Hennessy et al. 1987) (see Fig. 41.12). The metabolic fate of TCBZ and its metabolites was characterized in sheep (Virkel et al. 2006). Both FMO and cytochrome P450 enzymatic systems were found to be involved in the sulphoxidation and sulphonation of TCBZ in sheep liver. In addition, sheep ruminal microflora was able to reduce TCBZ sulphoxide derivatives, TCBZSO and hydroxy-TCBZSO, into TCBZ and hydroxy-TCBZ, respectively.

As it happens for other nematodicidal BZD sulphoxides, the sulphoxide metabolite of TCBZ is believed to have flukicidal activity. In fact, the tegument of *F. hepatica* is highly susceptible to TCBZSO, since the compound causes severe surface damage after relatively short time exposure (Stitt and Fairweather 1994). TCBZ metabolites bind strongly (>99%) to plasma proteins, specifically albumin. The long TCBZ metabolites' persistence in the bloodstream (over 120 hours posttreatment) and their high plasma concentrations compared to other BZD compounds correlate with their high plasma protein binding. These may contribute to its high flukicidal activity based on a high and prolonged drug exposure of the blood-feeding adult flukes. On the other hand, the metabolic conversion of TCBZSO into TCBZ in the rumen may give rise to a source of the main active metabolite in the liver (Virkel et al. 2006). Thus, the sulphoreduction of hydroxy-TCBZSO into hydroxy-TCBZ may be relevant as well, although the mode of action and/or the anthelmintic activity (if any) of these metabolites have not been established. Approximately 45% of the administered dose is eliminated by bile and only 6.5% is excreted in urine, mainly as TCBZSO and $TCBZSO_2$ (Hennessy et al. 1987).

Flukicidal drugs can reach target sites within *F. hepatica* either by oral ingestion of blood or by transtegumental diffusion. The large absorptive surface area of the fluke's tegument may have a major role in drug diffusion from the surrounding medium. Studies on ex vivo drug diffusion into TCBZ-susceptible *F. hepatica*, demonstrated that TCBZ, TCBZSO, and $TCBZSO_2$ have the capability to penetrate the fluke's tegument (Alvarez et al. 2004; Mottier et al. 2004). Unlike the uptake pattern previously observed for albendazole (Alvarez et al. 2001), the parent TCBZ and its sulphoxide and sulphone metabolites showed a similar ability to penetrate into the trematode parasite. However, the diffusion of the hydroxy-derivatives into the fluke was lower than that observed for TCBZ, TCBZSO, and $TCBZSO_2$ (see Fig. 41.14). These findings agree with the high correlation observed between lipophilicity and drug concentrations measured within the parasite. Those studies demonstrated that the higher the lipophilicity, the greater the ability of the BZD molecules to cross through the helminth external surfaces. These studies have also shown that the composition and physicochemical characteristics of the incubation medium drastically affect the diffusion of BZD anthelmintics into *F. hepatica*.

Since TCBZ is the most widely used flukicide due to its excellent activity against both the mature and immature stages of *F. hepatica*, the selection of TCBZ-resistant populations is now an emerging problem in several areas of the

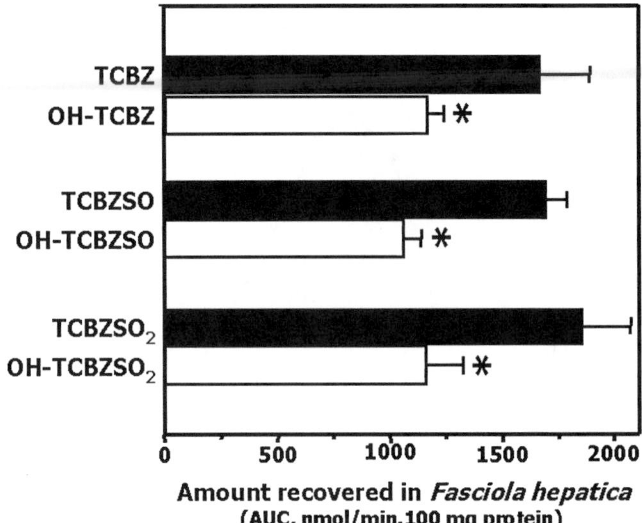

FIG. 41.14 Comparative ex vivo diffusion of triclabendazole (TCBZ), TCBZ-sulphoxide (TCBZSO), TCBZ-sulphone ($TCBZSO_2$) and its hydroxylated metabolites into adult specimens of *Fasciola hepatica*. TCBZ, TCBZSO and $TCBZSO_2$ concentrations measured within the parasite are significantly higher (*$P<0.05$) than those of their hydroxylated metabolites. See the text for further explanations. Adapted from Mottier et al. (2004).

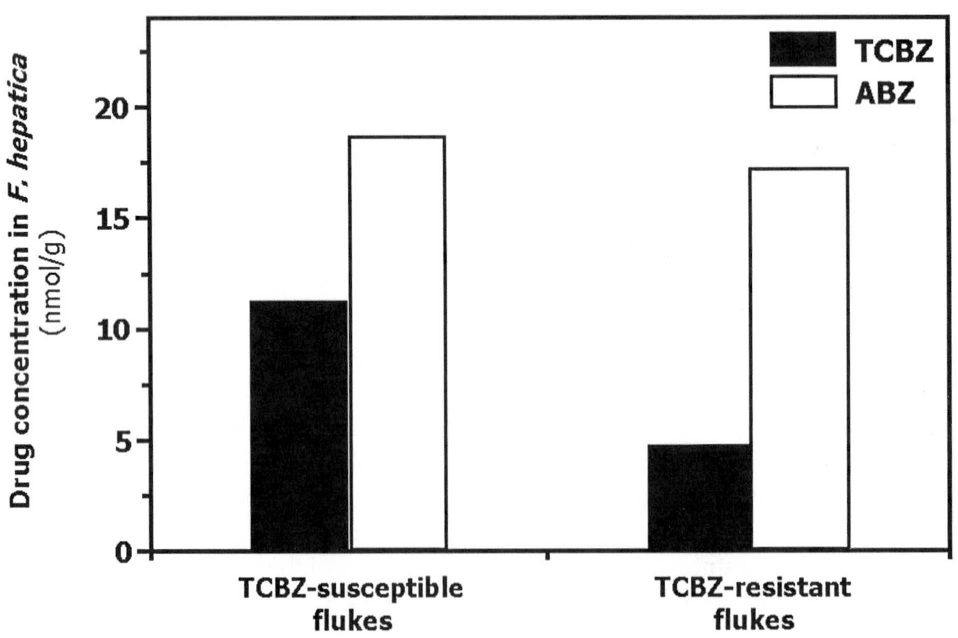

FIG. 41.15 Comparative diffusion of triclabendazole (TCBZ) and albendazole (ABZ) into adult specimens of TCBZ-susceptible and -resistant *F. hepatica*. See the text for further explanation. Adapted from Mottier et al. (2006).

world (Fairweather 2005). BZD resistance in *H. contortus* has been associated with the loss of high-affinity binding (Lubega and Prichard 1991) and an alteration of the β-tubulin isoform pattern. Although the flukicidal activity of TCBZ remains to be fully understood, there is data to support a microtubule-based action of this compound (Stitt and Fairweather 1994). However, it has been shown that the TCBZ-resistant phenotype in *F. hepatica* is not associated with residue changes in the primary amino acid sequence in β-tubulin (Robinson et al. 2002). This suggests that there may be an alternative mechanism of TCBZ resistance. In fact, the amount of TCBZ recovered from resistant flukes was significantly lower (~50%) than that measured in susceptible parasites. Increased TCBZ oxidative metabolism by the fluke and enhanced drug efflux mediated by ATP-dependent transmembrane transporters may account for the reduced drug accumulation observed in resistant flukes (Alvarez et al. 2005; Mottier et al. 2006), and have been proposed as potential mechanisms of TCBZ resistance in *F. hepatica*. Conversely, albendazole accumulation was similar in both susceptible and resistant flukes, which correlates with the observed high efficacy of this drug against TCBZ-resistant flukes in the field (Coles and Stafford 2001) (see Fig. 41.15)

TCBZ is administered orally to cattle (12 mg/kg), sheep (10 mg/kg) and goats (15 mg/kg). It is indicated for the treatment and control of all stages of TCBZ-susceptible *F. hepatica* from 2-day-old early immature to mature fluke and so is effective against both acute and chronic fasciolosis. Combined formulations containing TCBZ and different antinematodal drugs (abamectin, levamisole) are available in different countries. TCBZ is not indicated for use in lactating animals producing milk for human consumption, or in pregnant animals that are intended to produce milk for human consumption within 2 months of expected parturition. TCBZ can be administered at any stage of pregnancy. A withdrawal time of 56 days (meat) has been established for TCBZ in sheep and cattle.

PHENOXYALKANES

DIAMPHENETHIDE. This flukicidal molecule is a phenoxyalkane (N,N′-[oxybis(2,1-ethanediyloxy-4,1-phenylene)]bisacetamide) (Fig. 41.16). Diamphenethide is exceptionally effective against early immature flukes from 1 day to 6 weeks of age. Consequently, it is used for treatment of acute fasciolosis resulting from immature forms of *F. hepatica* migrating through the liver parenchyma of sheep. A dosage of 100 mg/kg is almost 100% effective against flukes from 1 to 63 days of age. However, its activity progressively decreases as the flukes develop to maturity. This is in direct contrast to other currently used fasciolicides, which tend to be less active against younger flukes. This fact could be a drawback for the clinical use of diamphenethide but the drug may be useful in prophylactic programs against liver fluke disease in sheep. A chemoprophylactic effect has been achieved as a result of strategic treatments with diamphenethide in both sheep and cattle (Enzie et al. 1980). At a dosage of 10 mg/kg of body weight (10% of the recommended dose), the drug was 87% effective in preventing establishment of *F. hepatica* infections in sheep that were given the drug daily for 14 days, and was 96% effective in sheep that were given the drug for 21 days (Enzie et al. 1980). The use of a controlled-release device of diamphenethide for the prophylaxis of fasciolosis in ruminants has also been proposed (Rew and Knight 1980).

The efficacy of diamphenethide depends upon deacetylation of the drug by liver enzymes (deacetylases) to an amine metabolite. Diamphenethide is not active in vitro, but its deacetylated (amine) metabolite, (DAMD), has flukicidal activity against liver flukes. The exact mechanism of action of DAMD remains not well established. Although it was shown that DAMD caused severe morphological damage to *F. hepatica* in vitro, energy metabolism is not the prime target for this metabolite (Fairweather and Boray 1999). DAMD-induced disruption of the tegument and osmoregulatory system of the fluke was thoroughly described using transmission electron microscopy (Anderson and Fairweather 1995). Morphological changes include swelling of the in-foldings of the basal plasma membrane leading to flooding of the syncytium and eventual sloughing of the tegument. Further information on the mode of action of DAMD can be obtained from Fairweather and Boray (1999).

Diamphenethide is administered as an oral suspension at 100 mg/kg in sheep and goats. Diamphenethide is absorbed into the blood after oral treatment and readily metabolized in the liver. High concentrations of two active deacetylated metabolites, monoamino- (MAMD) and diamino-diamphenethide (DAMD), are produced in liver parenchyma, where immature flukes are found until at least 7 weeks after infection. Metabolites reach high concentrations in the liver parenchyma but are thought to be

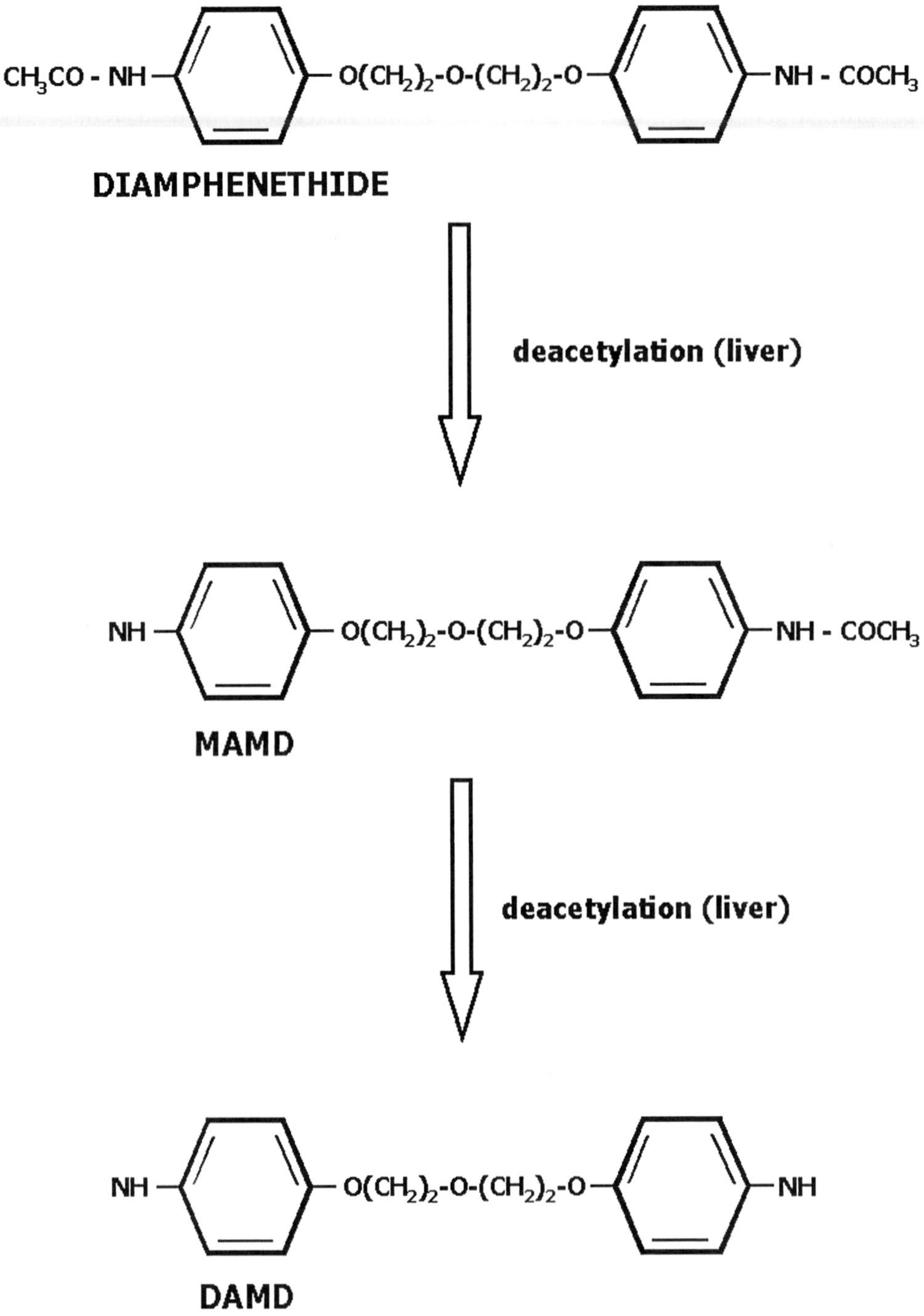

CH_3CO - NH–[benzene]–O$(CH_2)_2$-O-$(CH_2)_2$-O–[benzene]–NH - $COCH_3$

DIAMPHENETHIDE

deacetylation (liver)

NH–[benzene]–O$(CH_2)_2$-O-$(CH_2)_2$-O–[benzene]–NH - $COCH_3$

MAMD

deacetylation (liver)

NH–[benzene]–O$(CH_2)_2$-O-$(CH_2)_2$-O–[benzene]–NH

DAMD

FIG. 41.16 Diamphenethide: chemical structure and metabolic fate. Liver deacetylation of the parent drug converts it into two active diamino-metabolites: monoamino-diamphenethide (MAMD) and diamino-diamphenethide (DAMD).

rapidly biotransformed and eliminated into the bile. Only small amounts of MAMD and DAMD may escape into the bloodstream but become diluted. That is why the quantity of active metabolites reaching mature blood-sucking flukes by both oral ingestion or tegumental diffusion is small. Therefore, efficacy against adult stages located in the bile ducts is reduced.

Safety of diamphenethide for the host can be explained

on the basis of destruction of the metabolites by the liver and dilution in blood so that only small quantities reach other tissues. Its greatest concentrations are measured in the liver and gallbladder content (at 3 days posttreatment). It should be noted that adult flukes reside in intimate association with the biliary system. At 7 days after dosing, concentrations of diamphenethide in these sites are reduced approximately tenfold, to a range of only 0.1–0.5 ppm, while concentrations in the musculature are approximately 0.02 ppm. In the United Kingdom, animals intended for human consumption are permitted to be slaughtered 7 days after treatment. The usual oral dose (100 mg/kg) in sheep is apparently safe. A single oral dose four times the therapeutic dosage (400 mg/kg) produces no toxic signs. At higher dosages, toxic effects include temporary impairment of vision and loss of wool. Pastured sheep are less susceptible to toxic effects than housed sheep. There appear to be no significant contraindications for use of diamphenethide. Pregnant ewes dosed with 200 mg/kg once weekly on two, three, or four consecutive occasions during the 21-week gestation period exhibited no adverse effects on fertility or teratogenic effects in their offspring.

REFERENCES

Ali, N. and Bogan, J. 1987. The pharmacodynamics of the flukicidal salicylanilides, rafoxanide, closantel and oxyclosanide. Journal of Veterinary Pharmacology and Therapeutics 10, 127–133.

Alvarez, L.; Mottier, L.; Sánchez, S. and Lanusse, C. 2001. Ex vivo diffusion of albendazole and its sulphoxide metabolite into *Ascaris suum* and *Fasciola hepatica*. Parasitology Research 87, 929–934.

Alvarez, L.; Mottier, L. and Lanusse, C. 2004. Comparative assessment of the access of albendazole, fenbendazole and triclabendazole to *Fasciola hepatica*: effect of bile in the incubation medium. Parasitology 128, 73–81.

Alvarez, L.; Solana, H.; Mottier, L.; Virkel, G.; Fairweather, I. and Lanusse, C. 2005. Altered drug influx/efflux and enhanced metabolic activity in triclabendazole-resistant liver flukes. Parasitology 131, 501–510.

Alvinerie, M.; Floc'h, R. and Galtier, P. 1991. Plasma protein binding of nitroxynil in several species. Journal of Veterinary Pharmacology and Therapeutics 14, 170–173.

Andersen, F.; Loveless, R. and Jensen, L. 1975. Efficacy of bunamidine hydrochloride against immature and mature stages of *Echinococcus granulosus*. American Journal of Veterinary Research 36, 673–675.

Anderson, H. and Fairweather, I. 1995. *Fasciola hepatica:* ultrastructural changes to the tegument of juvenile flukes following incubation in vitro with the deacetylated (amine) metabolite of diamphenethide. International Journal for Parasitology 25, 319–333.

Benchaoui, H. and McKellar, Q. 1993. Determination of rafoxanide and closantel in ovine plasma by high performance liquid chromatography. Biomedical Chromatography 7, 181–183.

Boray, J.; Crowfoot, P.; Strong, M.; Allison, J.; Schellenbaum, M.; von Orelli, M. and Sarasin, G. 1983. Treatment of immature and mature *Fasciola hepatica* infections in sheep with triclabendazole. The Veterinary Record 113, 315–317.

Boray, J. 1986. Trematode infections of domestic animals In Chemotherapy of Parasitic Diseases, edited by Campbell, W. and Rew, R. pp. 401–426. New York: Plenum Press.

Calpoviña, M.; Guderian, R.; Paredes, W.; Chici, M. and Cooper, P. 1988. Treatment of human pulmonary paragonimiasis with triclabendazole: clinical tolerance and drug efficacy. Transactions of the Royal Society of tropical. Medicine and Hygiene 92, 566–569.

Cioli, D. and Mattoccia, L. 2003. Praziquantel. Parasitology Research 90, 83–89.

Coles, G. and Stafford, K. 2001. Activity of oxyclozanide, nitroxynil, clorsulon and albendazole against adult triclabendazole-resistant *Fasciola hepatica*. The Veterinary Record 148, 723–724.

Corwin, R.; Green, S. and Keefe, T. 1989. Dose titration and confirmation tests for determination of cestodicidal efficacy of epsiprantel in dogs. American Journal of Veterinary Research 50, 1076–1077.

Cromie, L.; Ferry, M.; Couper, A.; Fields, C. and Taylor, S. 2006. Pharmacokinetics of a novel closantel/ivermectin injection in cattle. Journal of Veterinary Pharmacology and Therapeutics 29, 205–211.

Day, T.; Bennett, J. and Pax, R. 1992. Praziquantel: The enigmatic antiparasitic. Parasitology Today 10, 342–344.

Eckert, J.; Thompson, R.; Bucklar, H.; Bilger, B. and Deplazes, P. 2001. Efficacy evaluation of epsiprantel (Cestex) against *Echinococcus mutilocularis* in dogs and cats. Berliner und Munchener Tierarztliche Wochenschrift 114, 121–126.

Enzie, F.; Rew, R. and Colglazier, M. 1980. Chemoprophylaxis with diamfenetide against experimental infections of *Fasciola hepatica* in ruminants. American Journal of Veterinary Research 41, 179–182.

Fairweather, I.; Holmes, S. and Threadgold, L. 1984. *Fasciola hepatica:* motility response to fasciolicides in vitro. Experimental Parasitology 57, 209–224.

Fairweather, I. and Boray, J. 1999. Fasciolicides: Efficacy, actions, resistance and its management. The Veterinary Journal 158, 81–112.

Fairweather, I. 2005. Triclabendazole: new skills to unravel an old(ish) enigma. Journal of Helminthology 79, 227–234.

Gasser, R.; Williamson, R. and Beveridge, I. 2005. *Anoplocephala perfoliata* of horses—significant scope for further research, improved diagnosis and control. Parasitology 131, 1–13.

Giorgi, M.; Salvatori, A.; Soldani, G.; Giusiani, M.; Longo, V.; Gervasi, P. and Mengozzi, G. 2001. Pharmacokinetics and microsomal oxidation of praziquantel and its effects on the P450 system in 3-month-old lambs infested by *Fasciola hepatica*. Journal of Veterinary Pharmacology and Therapeutics 24, 251–259.

Giorgi, M.; Meucci, E.; Vaccaro, E.; Mengozzi, G.; Giusiani, M. and Soldani, G. 2003. Effects of liquid and freeze dried grape fruit juice on the pharmacokinetics of praziquantel and its metabolite 4′-hydroxy praziquantel in beagle dogs. Pharmacological Research 47, 87–92.

Greenberg, R. 2005. Are Ca2+ channels targets of praziquantel action? International Journal for Parasitology 35, 1–9.

Hall, C.; Kelly, J.; Whitlock, H. and Ritchie, L. 1981. Prolonged anthelmintic effect of closantel and disophenol against a thiabendazole selected resistant strain of *Haemonchus contortus* in sheep. Research in Veterinary Science 31, 104–6.

Hennessy, D.; Lacey, E.; Steel, J. and Prichard, R. 1987. The kinetics of triclabendazole disposition in sheep. Journal of Veterinary Pharmacology and Therapeutics 10, 64–72.

Hennessy, D. 1993. Pharmacokinetic disposition of benzimidazole drugs in the ruminant gastrointestinal tract. Parasitology Today 9, 329–333.

Hennessy, D. and Ali, D. 1997. The effect of feed intake level on the pharmacokinetic disposition of closantel in sheep. International Journal for Parasitology 27, 1081–1086.

Kinabo, L. and Bogan, J. 1988. Pharmacokinetics and efficacy of triclabendazole in goats with induced fascioliasis. Journal of Veterinary Pharmacology and Therapeutics 11, 254–259.

Kita, K.; Hirawake, H. and Takamiya, S. 1997. Cytochromes in the respiratory chain of helminth mitochondria. International Journal for Parasitology 27, 617–630.

Lacey, E. 1988. The role of the cytoskeletal protein, tubulin, in the mode of action and mechanism of drug resistance to benzimidazoles. International Journal for Parasitology 18, 885–936.

Lubega, G. and Prichard, R. 1991. Specific interaction of benzimidazole anthelmintics with tubulin from developing stages of thiabendazole-susceptible and –resistant *Haemonchus contortus*. Biochemical Pharmacology 41, 93–101.

Lyons, E.; Tolliver, S. and Ennis, L. 1998. Efficacy of praziquantel (0.25 mg/kg) on the cecal tapeworm (*Anoplocephala perfoliata*) in horses. Veterinary Parasitology 78, 287–289.

Maffei Facino, R.; Pitre, D. and Carini, M. 1982. The reductive metabolism of the nitroaromatic flukicidal agent nitroxinil by liver microsomal cytochrome P450. Il Farmaco; Edizione Scientifica 37, 463–474.

Markus, B. and Kwon, C. 1994. In vitro metabolism of aromatic nitriles. Journal of Pharmaceutical Sciences 83, 1729–1734.

Martin, R. 1997. Modes of action of anthelmintic drugs. The Veterinary Journal 154, 11–34.

Mas-Coma S. 2004. Human fascioliasis. In Waterborne Zoonoses: Identification, Causes and Control, edited by Cotruvo, J.A.; Dufour, A.; Rees, G.; Bartram, J.; Carr, R.; Cliver, D.O.; Craun, R.; Fayer, R. and Gannon, V.P.J. pp. 305–322. London: World Health Organisation/IWA Publishing.

Masimirembwa, C. and Hasler, J. 1994. Characterization of praziquantel metabolism by rat liver microsomes using cytochrome P450 inhibitors. Biochemical Pharmacology 48, 1779–1783.

McKinstry, B.; Fairweather, I.; Brennan, G. and Forbes, A. 2003. *Fasciola hepatica:* tegumental surface alterations following treatment in vivo and in vitro with nitroxynil (Trodax). Parasitology Research 91, 251–263.

Meaney, M.; Fairweather, I.; Brennan, G.; McDowell, L. and Forbes, A. 2003. *Fasciola hepatica:* effects of the fasciolicide clorsulon in vitro and in vivo on the tegumental surface, and a comparison of the effects on young- and old-mature flukes. Parasitology Research 91, 238–250.

Meaney, M.; Fairweather, I.; Brennan, G. and Forbes, A. 2004. Transmission electron microscope study of the ultrastructural changes induced in the tegument and gut of *Fasciola hepatica* following in vivo drug treatment with clorsulon. Parasitology Research 92, 232–241.

Meaney, M.; Haughey, S.; Brennan, G. and Fairweather, I. 2005. A scanning electron microscope study on the route of entry of clorsulon into the liver fluke, *Fasciola hepatica*. Parasitology Research 96, 189–198.

Michiels, M.; Meuldermans, W. and Heykants, J. 1987. The metabolism and fate of closantel (Flukiver) in sheep and cattle. Drug Metabolism Reviews 18, 235–51.

Mottier, L.; Virkel, G.; Solana, H.; Alvarez, L.; Salles, J. and Lanusse, C. 2004. Triclabendazole biotransformation and comparative diffusion of the parent drug and its oxidized metabolites into *Fasciola hepatica*. Xenobiotica 34, 1043–1057.

Mottier, L.; Alvarez, L.; Ceballos, L. and Lanusse, C. 2006. Drug transport mechanisms in helminth parasites: passive diffusion of benzimidazole anthelmintics. Experimental Parasitology 113, 49–57.

Pax, R. and Bennett, J. 1989. Effect of closantel on intrategumental pH in *Schistosoma mansoni* and *Fasciola hepatica*. Journal of Parasitology 75, 169–171.

Reinemeyer, C. and Courtney, C. 2001. Anticestodal and Antitrematodal Drugs. In Veterinary Pharmacology and Therapeutics, 8th, edited by Adams, H. R. pp. 980–991. Ames, IA: Iowa State University Press.

Reinemeyer, C.; Hutchens, D.; Eckblad, W.; Marchiondo, A. and Shugart, J. 2006. Dose-confirmation studies of the cestocidal activity of pyrantel pamoate paste in horses. Veterinary Parasitology 138, 234–239.

Rew, R. and Knight, R. 1980. Efficacy of albendazole for prevention of fascioliasis in sheep. Journal of the American Veterinary Medical Association 176, 1353–1354.

Roberson, E. and Courtney, C. 1995. Anticestodal and Antitrematodal Drugs. In Veterinary Pharmacology and Therapeutics, 7th, edited by Adams, H. R. pp. 933–954. Ames, IA: Iowa State University Press.

Robinson, M.; Trudgett, A.; Hoey, E. and Fairweather, I. 2002. Triclabendazole-resistant *Fasciola hepatica:* β-tubulin and response to in vitro treatment with triclabendazole. Parasitology 124, 325–338.

Rothwell, J.; Lacey, E. and Sangster, N. 2000. The binding of closantel to ovine serum albumin and homogenate fractions of *Haemonchus contortus*. International Journal for Parasitology 30, 769–775.

Sanyal, P. 1995. Kinetic disposition of triclabendazole in buffalo compared to cattle. Journal of Veterinary Pharmacology and Therapeutics 18, 370–374.

Schulman, M. and Valentino, D. 1982. Purification, characterization and inhibition by MK-401 of *Fasciola hepatica* phosphoglyceromutase. Molecular and Biochemical Parasitology 5, 321–332.

Schulman, M.; Valentino, D.; Cifelli, S. and Ostlind, D. 1982. Dose-dependent pharmacokinetics and efficacy of MK-401 against old, and young-mature infections of *Fasciola hepatica* in the rat. Journal of Parasitology 68, 603–608.

Staudt, U.; Schmahl, G.; Blaschke, G. and Mehlhorn, H. 1992. Light scanning electron microscopy study on the effects of the enantiomers of praziquantel and its main metabolite on *Schistosoma mansoni* in vitro. Parasitology Research 78, 392–397.

Stitt, A. and Fairweather, I. 1994. The effect of the sulphoxide metabolite of triclabendazole (Fasinex) on the tegument of mature and immature stages of the liver fluke, *Fasciola hepatica*. Parasitology 108, 555–567.

Sundlof, S. and Whitlock, T. 1992. Clorsulon pharmacokinetics in sheep and goats following oral and intravenous administration. Journal of Veterinary Pharmacology and Therapeutics 15, 282–291.

Swan, G. and Mulders, M. 1993. Pharmacokinetics of rafoxanide in suckling and weaned lambs following oral administration. Journal of the South African Veterinary Association 64, 67–70.

Swan, G.; Koeleman, H.; Steyn, H. and Mulders, M. 1999. Intravascular plasma disposition and salivary secretion of closantel and rafoxanide in sheep. Journal of the South African Veterinary Association 70, 75–79.

Thomas, H. and Gonnert, R. 1978. The efficacy of praziquantel against cestodes in cats, dogs, and sheep. Research in Veterinary Science 24, 20–25.

Thompson, R.; Reynoldson, J. and Manger, B. 1991. In vitro and in vivo efficacy of epsiprantel against *Echinococcus granulosus*. Research in Veterinary Science 51, 332–334.

Tielens, A.; van den Heuvel, J. and van den Bergh, S. 1987. Differences in intermediary energy metabolism between juvenile and adult *Fasciola hepatica*. Molecular and Biochemical Parasitology 24, 273–281.

Tielens, A. 1994. Energy generation in parasitic helminths. Parasitology Today 10, 346–352.

Virkel, G.; Lifschitz, A.; Sallovitz, J.; Pis, A. and Lanusse, C. 2006. Assessment of the main metabolism pathways for the flukicidal compound triclabendazole in sheep. Journal of Veterinary Pharmacology and Therapeutics 29, 213–223.

Westhoff, F. and Blaschke, G. 1992. High-performance liquid chromatographic determination of the stereoselective biotransformation of the chiral drug praziquantel. Journal of Chromatography 578, 265–71.

CHAPTER

42

MACROCYCLIC LACTONES: ENDECTOCIDE COMPOUNDS

CARLOS E. LANUSSE, ADRIAN L. LIFSCHITZ, AND FERNANDA A. IMPERIALE

GENERAL PHARMACOLOGY: AVERMECTINS AND MILBEMYCINS

The integration of available information on the host-parasite–environment relationship with a more complete understanding of the pharmacological properties of existing antiparasitic drugs should assist with more efficient parasite control in domestic animals. The time of parasite exposure to active drug concentrations determines the efficacy and/or persistence of activity for most of the anthelmintic drugs used in veterinary medicine. The characterization of drug concentration profiles in tissues of parasite location and within target parasites provides a basis for understanding the differences in therapeutic and preventive efficacies observed for the different anthelmintic chemical families.

The *avermectins* and *milbemycins* are closely related 16-member macrocyclic lactones (ML), produced through fermentation by soil dwelling actinomycetes (*Streptomyces*). It was the unique combination killing of endo- and ectoparasites that gave rise to the embracing name *endectocide* by which the MLs are recognized (Shoop et al. 1995a). Information on the antiparasitic properties of the different ML compounds in all animal species has been thoroughly reviewed elsewhere (Campbell 1985; Shoop et al. 1995a; McKellar and Benchaoui 1996). The book recently edited by Vercruysse and Rew (2002), specifically devoted to the MLs, is recommended for readers interested in any further detailed issue within the topic. Enormous progress on the comprehension of the relationship among disposition kinetics, tissue distribution, and the patterns of antiparasitic persistence for the ML molecules has been

Abamectin
Avermectin B_1

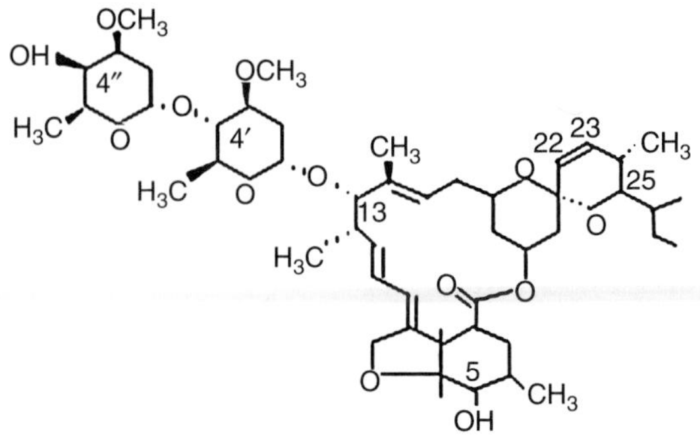

Ivermectin
22,23-Dihydro-avermectin B_1

C_{22}-C_{23}

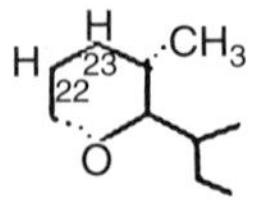

Eprinomectin
4′-epi-acetylamino-4″-deoxyavermectin B_1

$C_{4''}$

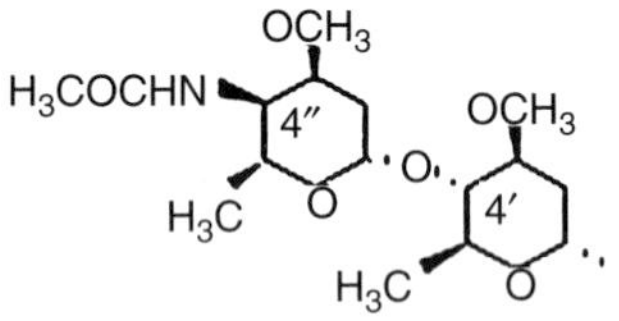

Doramectin
25-cyclohexyl-5-O-demethyl-25-de (1-methylpropyl) avermectin A_{1a}

C_{25}

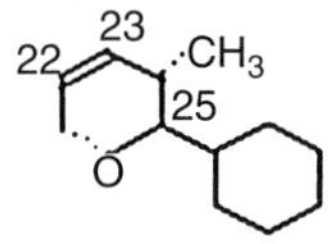

Selamectin
25-cyclohexyl-25-de (1-methylpropyl)-5-deoxy-22,23-dihydro-5-(hydroxyimino)-avermectin B_{1a}

C_{22}-C_{23}, C_{25}

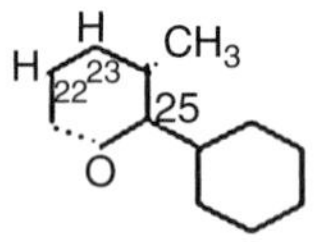

C_5

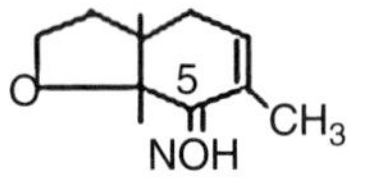

C_{13}

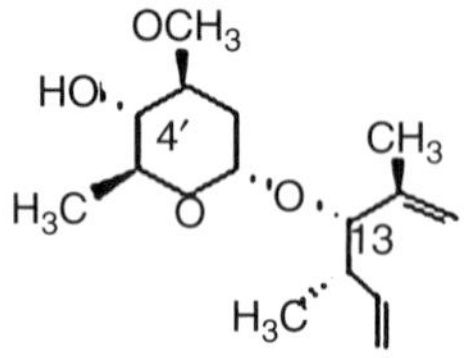

FIG. 42.1 Chemical structures of the main avermectin compounds used in veterinary medicine. The main chemical differences between abamectin (the natural fermentation product) and other avermectin-type molecules are shown. The commercially available preparations of abamectin and ivermectin contain at least 80% of the avermectin B_{1a} (the a-component has a secondary butyl side chain at the 25-position) and no more than 20% of avermectin B_{1b} (the b-component has an isopropyl substituent at the 25-position). Eprinomectin contains at least 90% of the B_{1a} and no more than 10% of the B_{1b} component.

achieved, particularly in ruminant species. The purpose of this chapter is to provide an updated and integrated overview of the main basic pharmacological features of the ML compounds, which account for their outstanding long-persistence broad-spectrum antiparasitic activity. The MLs are now considered the most widely used broad-spectrum antipararasitic drugs in veterinary medicine.

Avermectins are produced as a mixture of different components from fermentation of *Streptomyces avermitilis*. These natural products are denoted as A (those containing a methoxy group at the 5-position) and B (with a hydroxy group at the 5-position). The highest anthelmintic potency is held by the B1 homologs. The avermectin's family includes a series of natural and semisynthetic molecules, such as *abamectin, ivermectin, doramectin, eprinomectin,* and *selamectin.* Abamectin is the naturally occurring avermectin approved for animal use and the starting material for the production of ivermectin. In fact, ivermectin, the first marketed endectocide molecule, is a semisynthetic derivative of the avermectin family. Ivermectin is the generic name given to a mixture of two chemically modified avermectins containing at least 80% of 22–23-

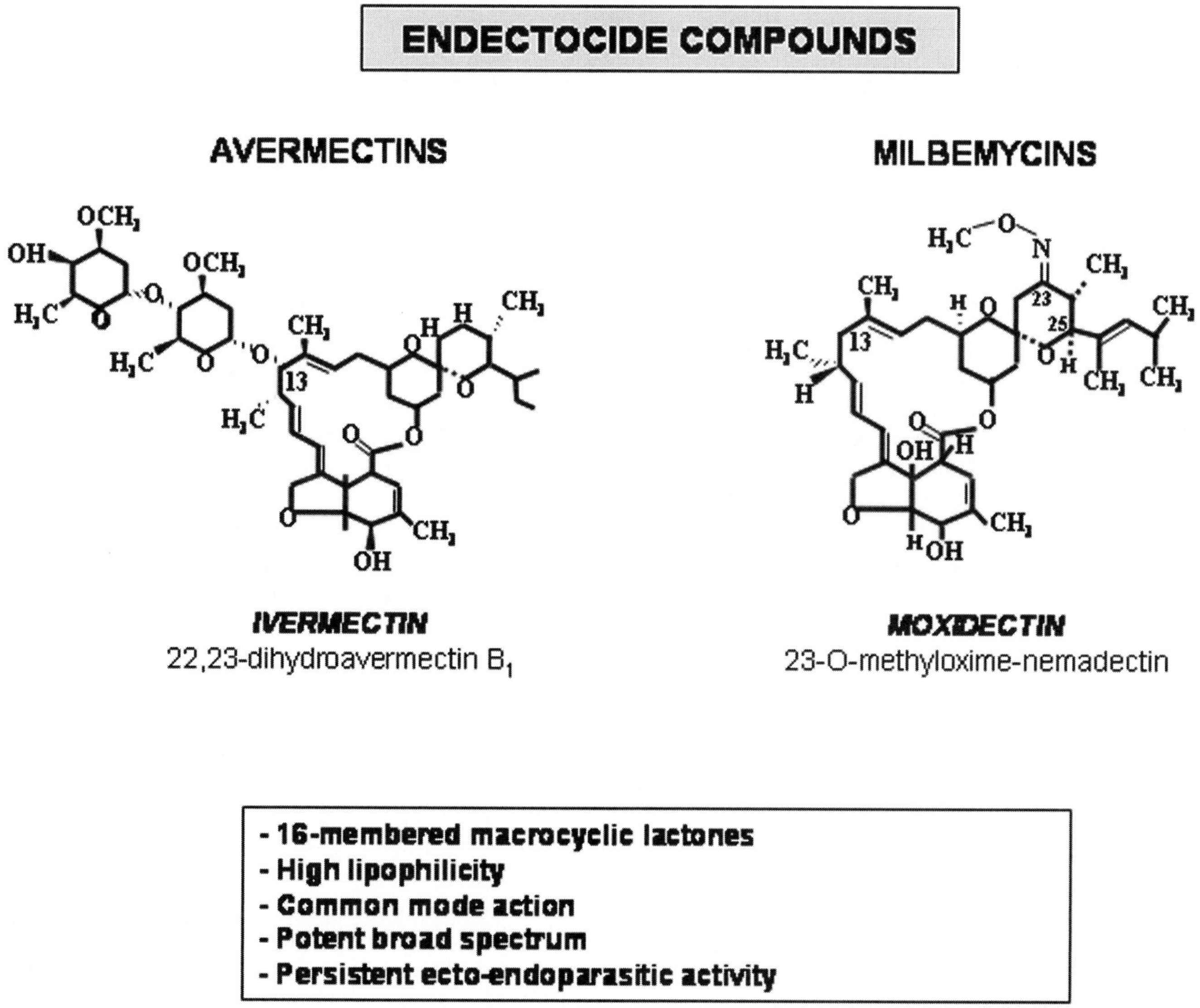

FIG. 42.2 Comparison between the avermectin (ivermectin) and milbemycin (moxidectin) molecular structures. The main pharmacological features shared by compounds in both families are listed. The main chemical differences between ivermectin and moxidectin are at the 13-, 23-, and 25-positions (see text for further explanation).

dihydroavermectin B1a and less than 20% of 22–23-dihydroavermectin B1b (Fisher and Mrozik 1989). Doramectin was obtained by mutational biosynthesis in which the precursor (cyclohexanecarboxylic acid) was fed to a mutant strain of *Streptomyces avermitilis* (Goudie et al. 1993). Eprinomectin is a semisynthetic avermectin compound, developed for topical use in cattle (Shoop et al. 1996). Selamectin is a semisynthetic monosaccaride oxime derivative of doramectin more recently introduced into the market for parasite control in dogs and cats (Bishop et al. 2000). The main chemical differences among the avermectin-type compounds are shown in Figure 42.1. It has been shown that minor chemical changes may have a profound impact on the activity of the avermectin analogs. For instance, substitution of the C-5 hydroxy with an oxo- substituent on ivermectin or doramectin monosaccharides can drastically reduce activity against *Haemonchus contortus* larvae.

Nemadectin, moxidectin, and *milbemycin oxime* belong to the *milbemycin* family. Milbemycin oxime consists of two oxime derivatives (A_4 and A_3 components) of the 5-didehydromilbemycin in a 80:20 ratio. Moxidectin is a milbemycin compound produced by a combination of fermentation and chemical synthesis. Moxidectin (23-O-methyloxime-nemadectin) is obtained by chemical modification of nemadectin, the natural compound produced when *Streptomyces cyaneogriseus* is grown under controlled culture conditions (Takiguchi et al. 1980). The molecular structures of the two endectocide families are superimposable (Shoop et al. 1995a); however, milbemycins do not have the C_{13} disaccharide substituent in the macrolide ring (Fig. 42.2). Additionally, moxidectin differs from ivermectin at the 23-position where it possesses a metoxime moiety. Moxidectin also has a differential substituted olefinic side chain at the 25-position. In spite of these chemical differences, both families share some structural and physicochemical properties and broad-spectrum antiparasitic activity against nematodes and arthropods at extremely low dosage rates (Fig. 42.2).

Various compounds from both families are used in livestock, companion animals, wildlife species, and humans (ivermectin). Ivermectin, doramectin, and moxidectin, currently marketed as injectable, pour-on (cattle), and oral (sheep, goats) formulations, are the most commonly used MLs worldwide to control endo- and ectoparasites in livestock. Exceptional potency, high lipophilicity, and the prolonged persistence of their potent broad-spectrum activity are distinctive features among antiparasitic drugs.

MECHANISM OF ACTION: ECTO-ENDOPARASITICIDAL ACTIVITY

The broad-spectrum ecto-endoparasitic activity of the MLs from both families includes selective toxic effects on insects, acarines, and nematodes. However, they do not possess efficacy against cestode and trematode parasites. The MLs induce reduction in motor activity and paralysis in both arthropods and nematodes. The paralytic effects are mediated through GABA and/or glutamate-gated chloride channels (GluCl), collectively known as *ligand-gated chloride channels*. MLs may act on both receptors, and a putative GABA-receptor subunit has been localized along the ventral nerve cord and several neurons in the head of *H. contortus* (Blackhall et al. 2003). However, considerably higher ML concentrations are required for the GABA-mediated effects than for those on the GluCl channels. In fact, a high affinity binding to GluCl channels, producing a slow and irreversible increase in chloride membrane conductance (Forrester et al. 2003), hyperpolarization, and flaccid paralysis of the invertebrate somatic muscles, is now proposed as a main mode of action (Martin et al. 2002; Geary 2005). The ML endectocides cause paralysis and death of both arthropod and nematode parasites due to their paralytic effects on the pharyngeal pump (Geary et al. 1999), which affects nutrient ingestion, and on the parasite somatic musculature limiting its ability to remain at the site of predilection in the host. In addition, inhibitory effects of the MLs on the female reproductive system may explain the observed reductions in parasite egg production (Fellowes et al. 2000). In *H. contortus*, the pharynx appears to be the most sensitive of the affected muscles (Sheriff et al. 2005). A schematic representation of the proposed main mode of action for the ML endectocides is shown in Figure 42.3.

The GluCl channels are members of the ligand-gated ion channel superfamily uniquely found in invertebrates. Some channel subunits have now been cloned from different nematode parasites, including the free-living nematodes *Caenorhabditis elegans*, *H. contortus*, and *Cooperia* spp. (Forrester et al. 2003; Njue and Prichard 2004), which has facilitated enormous progress on the understanding of the mode of action and mechanisms of resistance for the MLs. A good correlation between the presence of GluCl on neurons and muscle cells and the electrophysiological effects induced by MLs has been observed (Martin et al. 2002). Although several GluCl channel subunits have been identified, the sensitivity to these drugs

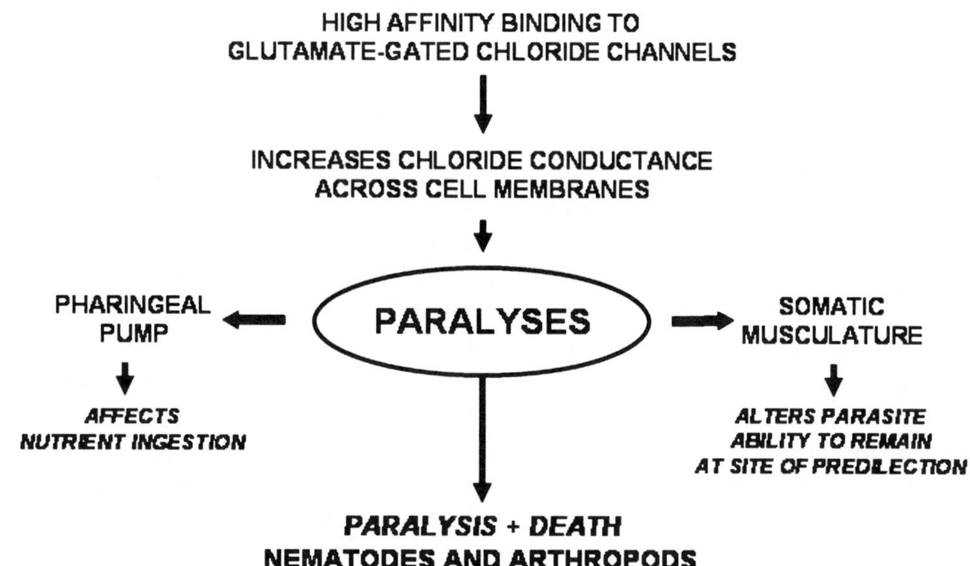

FIG. 42.3 Schematic representation of the proposed mode of action for the macrocyclic lactone endectocides.

seems to be associated with the alfa-subunit of the receptor (Arena et al. 1992; Cully et al. 1994; Njue and Prichard 2004), which is encoded by different genes indicating that nematode resistance to these compounds may be polygenic.

The different ML compounds exhibit a similar, but not identical, spectrum of activity against arthropod and nematode parasites and also show differences in the persistence of their antiparasitic activity. Even though compounds in both the avermectin and milbemycin families appear to have the same mode of action, there is now evidence of some subtle pharmacodynamic differences between families, which seem to account for a higher pharmacological potency of moxidectin compared to ivermectin, particularly evident against resistant nematode parasites. These pharmacodynamic differences have been observed at the GluCl channel where moxidectin is 2.5-fold more potent than ivermectin in terms of the required EC50 to activate this receptor expressed in *Xenopus* oocytes (reviewed by Prichard et al. 2003).

Additionally, the drug transport P-glycoprotein (P-GP) acts as an efflux pump for ML compounds lowering the local drug concentration achieved at the GluCl receptor site of action. *H. contortus* contains at least four P-GP genes (Sangster and Gill 1999) and data supporting their association with resistance to ivermectin are now available. Recently reported data indicate that a number of different P-GPs are overexpressed in resistant *H. contortus* and that ivermectin is a significantly better ligand for P-GP transport compared to moxidectin (Prichard and Roulet 2005). This enhanced ivermectin efflux may account for lower active concentrations being achieved at the receptor site in comparison to moxidectin. Overall, novel scientific data demonstrate minor pharmacodynamic differences between ivermectin and moxidectin, which could explain some differences in spectrum, potency, and the advantageous pattern of moxidectin efficacy against ivermectin-resistant nematodes of sheep, goats, and cattle.

PHARMACOKINETICS

EXCHANGE BETWEEN BLOODSTREAM AND TARGET TISSUES. The clinical efficacy of the MLs is closely related to their pharmacokinetic behavior, being the time of parasite exposure to active drug concentrations, relevant to obtain optimal and persistent antiparasitic activity. Their antiparasitic spectrum and efficacy patterns are similar; however, each compound has its own dosage limiting species. Differences in physicochemical properties among them may account for differences in formulation flexibility, kinetic behavior, and the potency/persistence of their endectocide activity. Thus, even slight modifications to the disposition kinetics or to the pattern of plasma/

tissue exchange may notably affect the persistence of their antiparasitic effect.

An enormous effort has been devoted to characterize the kinetics of the different MLs in different species. The work on the comparative plasma (Lanusse et al. 1997; Toutain et al. 1997) and target tissues (Lifschitz et al. 1999a, 2000; Sallovitz et al. 2003) disposition kinetics of ivermectin, doramectin, and moxidectin in cattle and disposition of doramectin (Hennessy et al. 2000; Carceles et al. 2001) and moxidectin (Alvinerie et al. 1998a) in sheep and goats, including evidences on their metabolic stability in the digestive tract (Lifschitz et al. 2005b) and involvement of lymphatic transport on intestinal absorption (Lespine et al. 2006) have contributed greatly to the understanding of the overall ML pharmacokinetic properties. Additionally, the characterization of the plasma/milk profiles of eprinomectin in cattle and goats (Shoop et al. 1996; Alvinerie et al. 1999b) and the studies on the comparative milk excretion patterns of different MLs in dairy sheep and their impact on drug residue profiles in milk-derived products (Imperiale et al. 2004a) have further contributed to the knowledge on ML kinetic behavior. The main pharmacokinetic features accounting for the persistent broad-spectrum antiparasitic activity of endectocides in ruminants are summarized in Figure 42.4.

Plasma concentration profiles may help predict the persistence of antiparasitic activity. However, the measurement of drug concentration profiles at the site of parasite location permits a more direct interpretation and provides a basis for understanding the differences in therapeutic and preventive efficacies observed for MLs. The characterization of drug concentrations at the sites of parasite infection for moxidectin, ivermectin, and doramectin in cattle, and the characterization of the kinetic disposition of doramectin in fluid and particulate digesta throughout the gastrointestinal tract in sheep, represent a considerable contribution to understanding the comparative persistence of activity of these compounds in ruminants. The highly lipophilic MLs are extensively distributed from the bloodstream to different tissues. Their extensive tissue distribution agrees with the large availability of these drugs in different parasite location tissues such as the gastrointestinal mucosal tissues, lungs, and skin in cattle (see Fig. 42.5), where concentrations markedly greater than those observed in plasma were measured during 50–60 days posttreatment. A strong correlation between plasma and

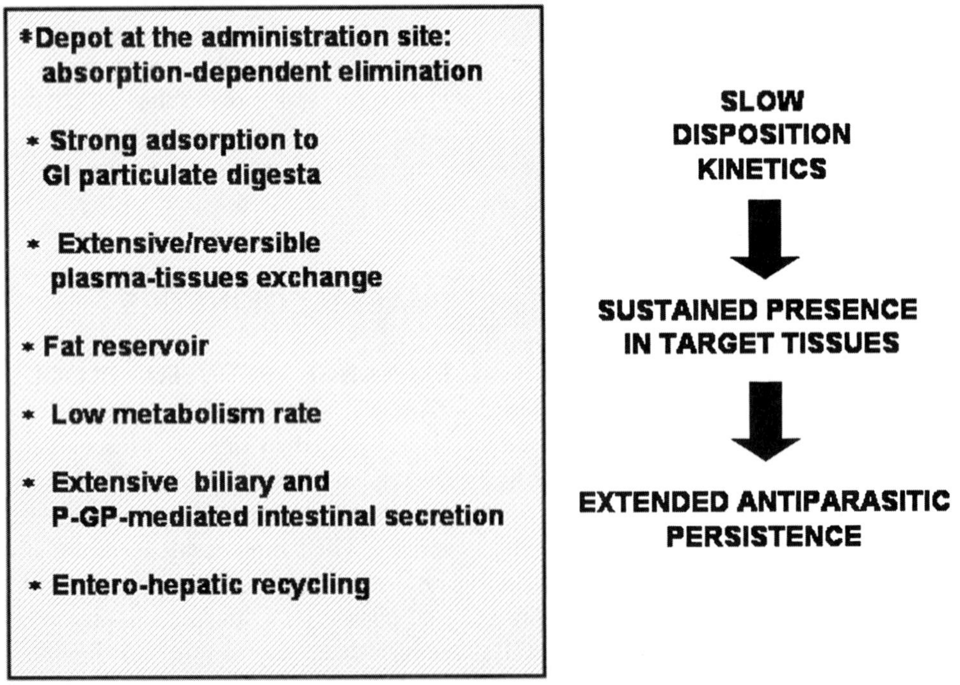

FIG. 42.4 Summary of the main pharmacokinetic features accounting for the extended broad-spectrum antiparasitic persistence of the macrocyclic lactone compounds in ruminants. GI: gastrointestinal tract; P-GP: P-glycoprotein. Adapted from Lifschitz et al. 2002a.

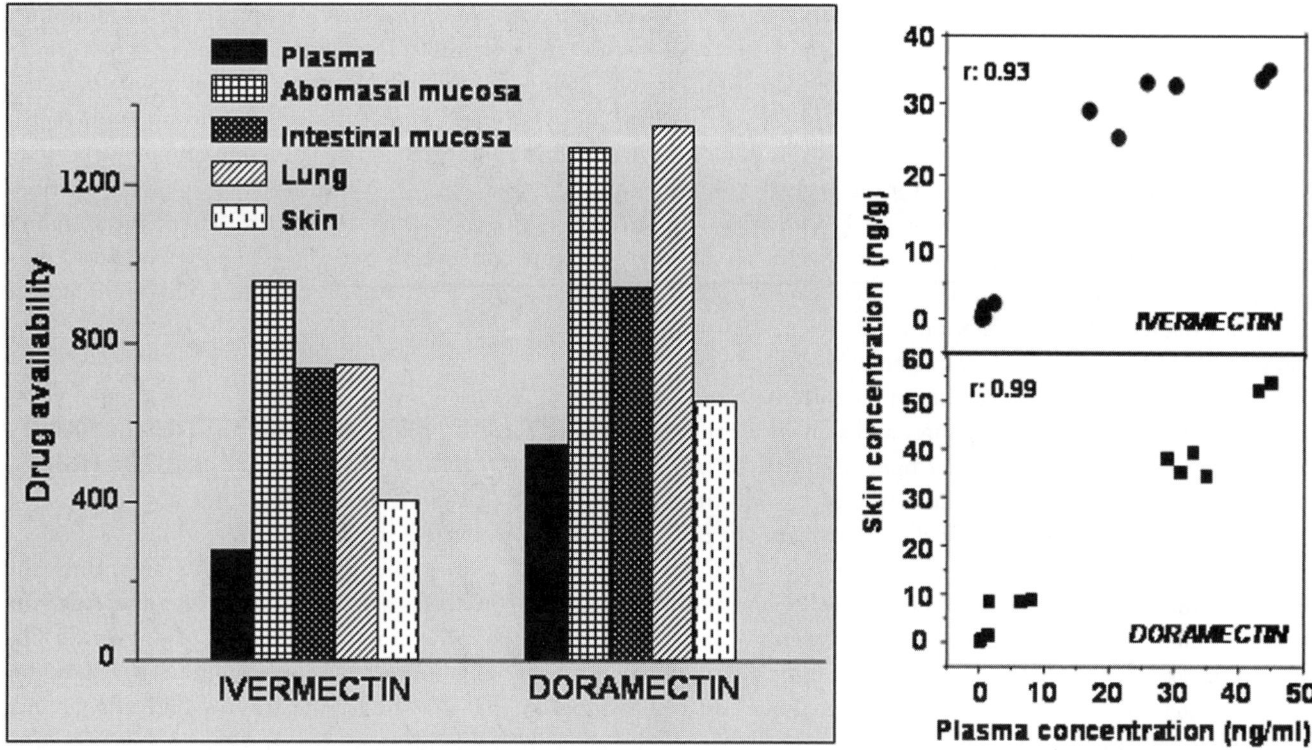

FIG. 42.5 Pattern of ivermectin and doramectin distribution to parasite location tissues in subcutaneously treated calves (0.2 mg/kg). Drug availability is expressed as area under the concentration vs. time curve (AUC) in ng.day/ml (plasma) and ng.day/g (target tissues). The correlations between drug concentrations measured in plasma and in a target tissue (skin) are shown in the right panel. r: correlation coefficient. Data from Lifschitz et al. 2000.

tissue concentration profiles for the ML compounds has been observed. The high correlation coefficients obtained showed the degree of association between ML concentrations in the bloodstream and those measured in tissues of parasite location. Despite the high correlation observed between concentrations in plasma and in tissues/fluids, ivermectin, doramectin, and moxidectin concentrations were greater in all target tissues compared to plasma.

MLs are highly effective against adult and larval stages of most gastrointestinal nematodes and *Dictyocaulus viviparus* in lung in cattle, exerting a prolonged protective effect. The achievement of high drug availability in lung tissue may explain their excellent activity against lungworms. The pulmonary tract was the target tissue in which the highest doramectin concentrations were recovered in parenterally treated cattle (Lifschitz et al. 2000). The persistence of the broad-spectrum anthelmintic activity of the MLs against adult and immature gastrointestinal parasites is facilitated by their advantageous pattern of distribution and prolonged residence in the digestive mucosal tissue. Differences in the plasma pharmacokinetic profiles between doramectin and ivermectin have been reported in cattle. Following intravenous administration of an aqueous micelle formulation to determine the intrinsic kinetic features of the compounds, higher plasma concentrations and delayed elimination of doramectin compared to ivermectin were reported (Goudie et al. 1993). After subcutaneous administration of the commercially available formulations to cattle, higher plasma profiles and extended plasma residence were observed for doramectin compared to ivermectin. The kinetic variables obtained for ivermectin and doramectin in tissues of parasite location are consistent with the described plasma kinetics data. Enhanced availability and prolonged time of residence in target tissues were observed for doramectin compared to ivermectin. The oil-based formulation of doramectin and perhaps a slowed metabolic rate based on the presence of the cyclohexyl group at C_{25} (Goudie et al. 1993) may contribute to the higher plasma and target tissues drug availability of doramectin compared to ivermectin.

Moxidectin is the most lipophilic endectocide substance; its high lipophilicity accounts for a wide tissue distribution (volume of distribution = 13.6 l/kg) and long residence in plasma, which is clearly reflected in the tissue pharmacokinetic results obtained in cattle. Distribution of the drug into adipose tissue accounts for the large distribution obtained for this compound compared to other antiparasitic drugs. The concentration of moxidectin in fat after 28 days of treatment in cattle has been shown to be ninetyfold higher than that detected in plasma (Zulalian et al. 1994). The large tissue distribution of moxidectin in cattle agrees with the high availability of moxidectin in the gastrointestinal mucosal tissues, lungs, and skin with concentrations ranging between 1 and 2 ng/g at 28 days posttreament, and with the extended detection of moxidectin concentrations >0.1 ng/g up to 58 days posttreatment in those tissues. The high Cmax values and total drug availability obtained in tissues where target parasites are located is in agreement with the extensive tissue distribution of moxidectin and may be relevant in terms of antiparasitic activity against internal and external parasites. Long residence times for moxidectin (between 6.8 and 11.3 days) were obtained in the different sites of parasite location, which agrees with the extended residence of moxidectin reported in fat and in the bloodstream (Alvinerie and Galtier 1997; Lanusse et al. 1997). Not surprisingly, moxidectin depletion half-lives in target tissues ranged from 7.73 (skin) to 11.8 (intestinal mucosa) days (Lifschitz et al. 1999a), which were significantly longer than those determined for ivermectin and doramectin in the same tissues. The deposit of moxidectin in adipose tissue may act as a drug reservoir that contributes to the long persistence of this molecule in the bloodstream and in different tissues of parasite location.

A considerable excretion of ivermectin, moxidectin, and doramectin occurs via the mammary gland, which invalidates their use in dairy animals. In an effort to identify an ML molecule that could be used in dairy cattle, the avermectin-derivative named *eprinomectin* has been introduced, which was developed for topical administration to cattle. While the milk/plasma ratio for ivermectin and moxidectin is close to 1 in sheep, goats, and cattle (Alvinerie et al. 1993, 1996; Imperiale et al. 2004b), the milk/plasma partitioning for eprinomectin in topically treated cattle falls between 0.1 and 0.2 (Shoop et al. 1996; Alvinerie et al. 1999b). These results indicate that eprinomectin, in addtion to its antiparasitic potency and broad spectrum, has a substantially reduced distribution to milk, compared to other MLs, which are probably based in some minor changes introduced to their chemical structure. In fact, changes to the milk partitioning coefficients in lactating dairy animals were achieved by manipulation of the avermectin molecule. The C4″-epi-amino analogues unsaturated at C22–23 showed that the lowest distribution into the milk is eprinomectin, 4″-epi-acetylamino-4″-deoxy avermectin B_1 (see Fig. 42.1), the best performed compound in terms of broad-spectrum antiparasitic activity.

METABOLISM, BILE AND INTESTINAL EXCRETION, AND INVOLVEMENT OF DRUG TRANSPORT SYSTEMS. Although some metabolic products have been recovered in plasma after administration of different MLs to cattle, these molecules are minimally metabolized in sheep and cattle, with bile and feces the major routes of excretion for unchanged parent drugs. The major liver metabolite of ivermectin in cattle is a 24-hydroxy-methyl-dihydroavermectin B_{1a} derivative (Chiu et al. 1987), identical to that produced by steer and rat microsomes in vitro (Miwa et al. 1982). Similarly, a doramectin metabolite accounting for 5.75% of the total recovered parent drug was detected in plasma between 8 h and 45 days postadministration of doramectin. The metabolism of moxidectin has been shown to produce the C_{29-30} and the C_{14} mono-hydroxymetyl derivatives as the main metabolic products. These and other hydroxylated metabolites have been recovered from different tissues of moxidectin-treated cattle (Zulalian et al. 1994). More extensive biotransformation of moxidectin compared to ivermectin and doramectin, would agree with the higher ratio of metabolites/parent drug recovered in plasma of moxidectin-treated animals. Interestingly, while 90% of the fat residue at 21 days posttreatment is moxidectin parent drug, ivermectin parent compound accounts for only 18% of the total fat residue at the same time posttreatment in cattle.

The avermectins are excreted in high concentration in bile and feces of treated cattle. Twenty-five % of an intraruminally administered dose of doramectin in sheep is secreted in bile, with 20% of biliary metabolites being enterohepatically recycled (Hennessy et al. 2000). Consistently, high concentrations of unchanged moxidectin are excreted in bile and feces (Zulalian et al. 1994), with concentrations greater than 2 ng/ml (ng/g) being recovered both in bile and feces up to 48 days posttreatment in cattle (Lifschitz et al. 1999a). As pointed out by Hennessy (2000), the extent to which the biliary secreted drug and metabolites are presented to the gut lumen, are reabsorbed as free compound, and participate in the enterohepatic cycle is a major contributor to parasite exposure.

The MLs abamectin, ivermectin, and moxidectin (Pouliot et al. 1997; Dupuy et al. 2001), among many other substances, have been shown to be substrates of the P-GP transport protein. In the mammalian host, P-GP participates in the mechanism of active biliary and intestinal secretion of different molecules from the bloodstream to the gastrointestinal tract. The transepithelial intestinal secretion plays a major role in the elimination of ivermectin in the rat (Laffont et al. 2002). Ivermectin clearance from the small intestine accounted for 27% of the total drug clearance, while bile secretion accounted for only 5% of the total clearance in the rat. P-GP seems to be involved in the mechanism of ivermectin and moxidectin resistance in nematodes and concurrent use of verapamil (P-GP substrate) enhanced the efficacy of ivermectin and moxidectin against resistant *H. contortus* (Molento and Prichard 1999). Some studies showed that verapamil induces a significant alteration in the plasma disposition and availability of ivermectin in sheep (Molento et al. 2004) and rats (Alvinerie et al. 1999a), and a recent report suggests that verapamil and/or its metabolites affect the P-GP–mediated efflux of moxidectin in cultured rat hepatocytes (Dupuy et al. 2001). Loperamide, an opioid derivative that reduces gastrointestinal secretions and motility, markedly enhances the systemic availability of moxidectin (cattle) and ivermectin (rat) (Lifschitz et al. 2002b, 2004b). The delayed intestinal transit caused by loperamide and a potential competition between the ML and loperamide for the P-GP–mediated bile/intestinal secretion processes, may account for the observed enhancement in MLs' availabilities. As stated here, different pharmacological approaches to delay the bile/intestinal secretions and to extend the plasma-intestine recycling time of endectocide molecules are currently being investigated and their implications on parasite control need evaluation. Recent work demonstrated that the presence of P-GP–modulating agents enhanced ivermectin accumulation in the intestinal wall and its serosal transfer both in vitro and in vivo (Ballent et al. 2006). Itraconazole, an antifungal and P-GP substrate compound, drastically affected ivermectin disposition kinetics from the bloodstream and digestive tract. The itraconazole-mediated modulation of P-GP activity induced a markedly greater effect on ivermectin kinetics in male compared to female animals (Lifschitz et al. 2005a).

PHARMACOKINETIC-PHARMACODYNAMIC RELATIONSHIP

The MLs induce a paralytic effect on the pharynx and somatic musculature of nematodes. Using in vitro assays, 1 nM ivermectin concentrations paralyze the pharynx of *H. contortus* (Geary et al. 1993) and inhibit larval development of trichotrongyloid nematodes (Gill and Lacey 1998), while much higher concentrations of ivermectin are needed to obtain an inhibitory effect of larval motility (Gill et al. 1991). The pharynx is more sensitive than axial muscle to the paralyzing action of ivermectin, suggesting that interruption of pharyngeal function, as well as nutrient ingestion and excretion, may be critical to the anthelmintic action of ivermectin and related drugs. Considering that 1 nM of ivermectin equals 0.87 ng/g, it may be possible to establish a correlation between the concentrations used in these in vitro assays with those obtained in target tissues after in vivo treatment. Therefore, it could be assumed that the period of time during which drug concentrations are above 1 ng/g in target tissues would be indicative of the period during which a paralytic effect on nematode pharyngeal pump occurs.

The ML concentrations required at the site of parasite location to inhibit parasite establishment or development have not been determined. However, it has been theoretically assumed that the period of time during which drug concentrations are above 1 ng/g (the ivermectin concentration equivalent to that required to paralyze the pharynx of *H. contortus* in different in vitro pharmacodynamic assays) in target tissues, would be indicative of the period during which the in vivo anthelmintic activity may persist. While ivermectin concentrations were >1 ng/g in gastrointestinal mucosal tissue and lung tissue for 18 days posttreatment, doramectin and moxidectin profiles remained above that level for 38 days postadministration (Lifschitz et al. 2000). The comparison between these time periods and those obtained in different persistence efficacy trials are interesting. The increase of fecal egg counts after ivermectin and doramectin administration to cattle indicate that reinfection begins 2–3 weeks and 3–4 weeks after each treatment, respectively (Ranjan et al. 1997). The characterization of drug concentrations in target tissues is useful to estimate the period of time posttreatment in which the endectocide levels at the site of parasite location remain efficacious. Understanding the relationship between drug concentrations achieved in target tissues and the persistence of activity estimated in parasitological field trials seems to be a critical step to establish the pharmacokinetic-pharmacodynamic correlation for MLs in ruminant species (see Fig. 42.6).

ML compounds have a broad spectrum of activity against adult and larval forms of many gastrointestinal nematodes in cattle. However, this pattern of efficacy varies among different nematode parasites and *Cooperia* spp. seems to be the dose-limiting nematode parasite for these compounds. While the reason for this differential susceptibility among different nematodes remains unknown, the evaluation of ML concentrations in different sections of the gastrointestinal tract provided some useful information. High moxidectin concentrations were detected in both abomasal and small intestinal mucosal tissues up to 58 days posttreatment, which accounted for the large AUC values observed in both target sites. These concentration profiles obtained in the mucosal tissue were greater than those obtained in abomasal and intestinal fluids. Only low moxidectin concentrations (below 1 ng/ml) were found in abomasal fluid following its subcutaneous administration to cattle, which is in agreement with the data previously reported for ivermectin (Bogan and McKellar 1988), where the drug was not detected in abomasal fluid, even when administered at 10 times the therapeutic dose in sheep. The greater moxidectin concentrations observed in the small intestinal fluid collected distal of the bile duct, compared with the abomasal fluid, may be associated with the biliary excretion of the drug. The higher lipid composition of the gastrointestinal mucosa compared to the fluids, considered as a more polar medium, may account for the greater moxidectin availability found in the mucosal tissues. The high availability and extended residence of moxidectin in the abomasal and intestinal mucosal tissues agree with the reported persistence of the anthelmintic effects of the drug against *Ostertagia ostertagi*, and other nematodes, for at least 35 days posttreatment (Vercruysse et al. 1997). Although differences in feeding mechanisms and site of location in the digestive tract among different nematodes should be considered to understand the overall action of the ML endectocides, the persistence of the broad-spectrum anthelmintic activity of the drug against adult and immature gastrointestinal parasites

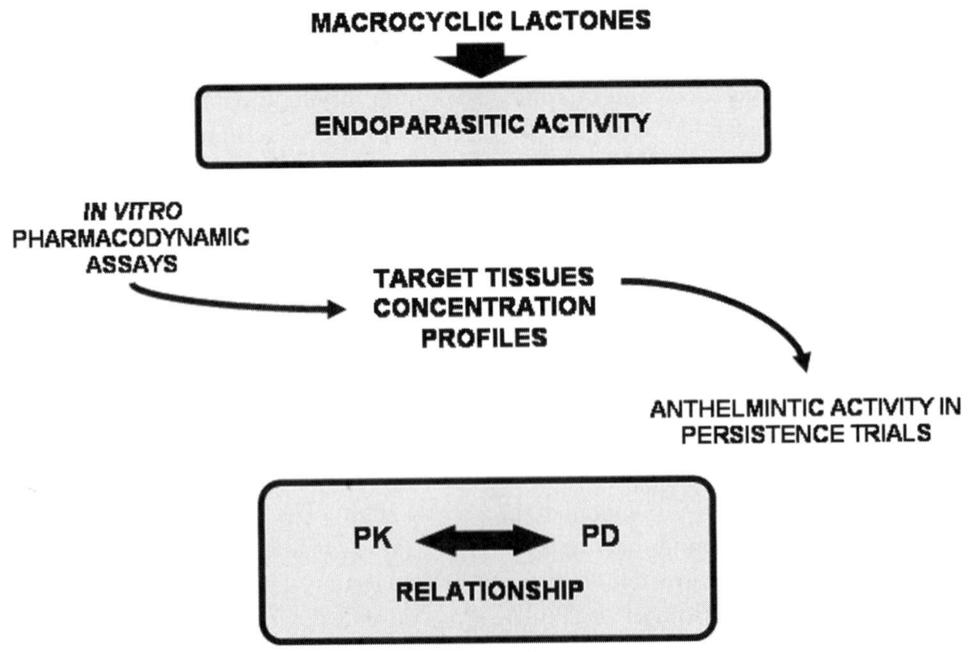

FIG. 42.6 Schematic illustration of the relationship between the pharmacokinetic (PK) behavior and pharmacodynamic (PD) endoparasitic activity for endectocide compounds in ruminants. See the text for further explanation.

is facilitated by its pattern of distribution and prolonged residence in the digestive mucosa. The described pharmacokinetic differences between moxidectin and ivermectin combined with some subtle mechanistic pharmacodynamic differences (see the section "Mechanism of Action"), are likely to be responsible for the observed differences in potency, spectrum, and expression of resistance seen between both molecules belonging to different ML families. The overall comparison of the pharmacological properties of moxidectin and ivermectin are shown in Figure 42.7.

ML endectocides are highly effective in eliminating mites and suckling lice species. The pattern of ivermectin and doramectin disposition in skin tissue showed that high concentrations of both molecules (>27 ng/g) are attained during the first 8 days posttreatment (Lifschitz et al. 2000). The sustained presence of high concentrations of ivermectin and doramectin in skin were reflected in the prolonged mean residence times values (6.8 and 9.3 days, respectively), which may also account for the efficacy of these drugs against single host ticks. The duration of effective levels of endectocide compounds in plasma may be important in the treatment of tick infestations, since this parasite can accumulate lethal drug concentrations through its feeding activity over a period of several days. Drug uptake and efficacy against arthropod ectoparasites can be markedly influenced by parasite feeding habits. Thus, the lower efficacy of the MLs against biting lice can be attributed to the lower exposure of this ectoparasite to body fluids containing drug. Moxidectin concentrations greater than 9 ng/g were detected during the first 8 days posttreatment in the skin of treated cattle (Lifschitz et al. 1999a), with a peak concentration of 84.2 ng/g achieved at day 1 postadministration. Drug concentrations in skin declined gradually with time posttreatment, as shown for other tissues, being detectable up to 58 days (>0.2 ng/g). These high moxidectin concentrations and its sustained presence in the skin account for the excellent efficacy of the drug against different ectoparasites in ruminants. Interestingly, the moxidectin and doramectin concentration profiles in the skin (dermis and epidermis) were greater than those found in the hypodermal tissue; moxidectin total availability in skin was six times greater than that observed in the subcutaneous tissue. Blood vessels in the skin are limited to the dermis, which receives the largest vascular supply. The dermis participates in the exchange of compounds between blood and tissues and as a fat reservoir (Monteiro-Riviere 1991); this physiological role of the

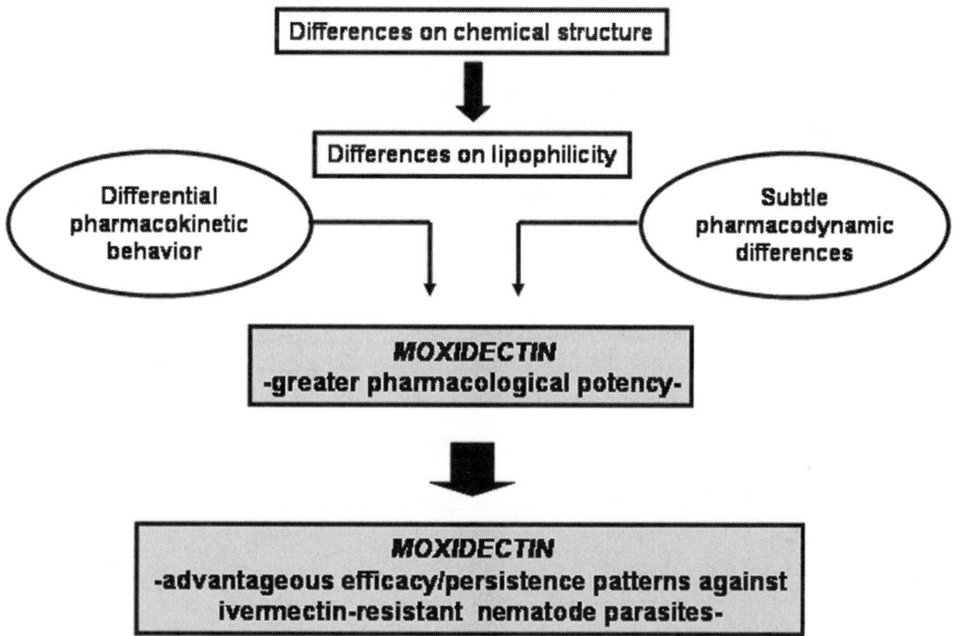

FIG. 42.7 Comparative pharmacological properties for moxidectin and ivermectin. See the text for further explanation.

dermis and the high lipophilicity of the MLs, may explain the differential distribution pattern in the skin, accounting for their higher availability in the dermis compared to the subcutaneous tissue. The arthropod ectoparasites are exposed to systemic agents during feeding; the nature of their food source, frequency and duration of feeding can have a marked influence in drug uptake and efficacy (Jackson 1989).

THERAPEUTIC USES: ANIMAL SPECIES-SPECIFIC CONSIDERATIONS

The ML compounds have exceptional potency and a broad spectrum of activity against nematodes and arthropods of different animal species. Their lack of efficacy against trematodes and cestodes may be related to the deficiency of ML specific binding sites in these parasites (Shoop et al. 1995b). Unlike benzimidazole anthelmintics, the MLs do not posses ovicidal activity. Compounds from both endectocide families share a similar broad spectrum against endo- and ectoparasites; however, some differences in activity against specific parasites may be observed among different ML molecules. A 0.2 mg/kg dose rate is required for avermectin and milbemycin compounds to eliminate their dose-limiting nematode species such as *Cooperia* spp. and *Nematodirus* spp. and to achieve the full broad-spectrum antiparasitic claim in ruminants (Shoop et al. 1995a). Extensive and detailed information on the spectrum of ecto-endoparasitic activity and on the preventive and therapeutic uses of the ML compounds in different animal species has been thoroughly reviewed elsewhere (Armour et al. 1980; Campbell 1989; McKellar and Benchaoui 1996; Vercruysse and Rew 2002). Readers are also referred to the 8th edition of this text (Reinemeyer and Courtney 2001) for additional specific information regarding the MLs' spectrum of antiparasitic activity. However, some overall concepts on the recommended use of the MLs in different animal species are summarized below.

RUMINANTS. ML compounds are available to be administered to ruminants by subcutaneous (cattle, sheep), oral (sheep and goats) (0.2 mg/kg), and topical (cattle) (0.5 mg/kg) formulations. MLs are highly effective against immature and adult stages of different gastrointestinal nematode species from ruminants such as *Ostertagia* spp. (including inhibited EL_4 in cattle), *Haemonchus* spp., *Cooperia* spp., *Nematodirus* spp., *Trichostrongylus* spp., *Strongyloides* spp., *Bunostomum* spp., *Trichuris* spp. and *Oesophagostomum* spp. and *Chabertia ovina.* MLs also possess high efficacy against lungworms (*Dictyocaulus* spp.) in sheep and cattle. The MLs are active against most of the nematode parasites affecting goats. However, the low systemic availability of some ML compounds obtained in goats (Scott et al. 1990; Alvinerie et al. 1999c) has restricted their use to extralabel prescriptions given at higher dose rates (0.3–0.4 mg/kg) for both oral and parenteral preparations.

Arthropod parasites controlled by MLs include mites (*Sarcoptes bovis, Psoroptes ovis*), oestrid larvae (*Hypoderma bovis, H. lineatum, Oestrus ovis*), and sucking lice (*Linognathus vituli, L. pedalis* and *Hematopinus eurysternus*). Ivermectin, abamectin, and doramectin are highly effective against *Dermatobia hominis* infestations. While ivermectin and abamectin aid in the control of the screwworm, *Cochliomya hominivorax*, doramectin has demonstrated a distinctive 100% protection for 21 days postinfection in calves (Moya-Borja et al. 1997). The specific distribution of the MLs in the different skin layers and their prolonged residence agree with their pattern of ectoparasiticide activity. The lower efficacy of the MLs subcutaneously administered against biting (*Damalinia* spp.) compared to sucking lices may be associated with the superficial feeding of these parasites, particularly on sloughed epidermal cells, which may contain low drug concentrations. The pour-on formulations are highly effective to control both sucking and biting lice. MLs are slightly less effective in controlling the sheep ked (*Melophagus ovinus).* MLs are highly efficacious against cattle ticks (*Boophilus microplus*). Ticks are exposed to systemic agents such as endectocides during feeding; therefore, the frequency and duration of feeding may have a marked influence in drug uptake and efficacy. The ML induces either tick mortality, lower engorgement, or fewer viable eggs. The injectable ivermectin preparation (1%) shows activity against ticks during 7 days posttreatment. Moxidectin and doramectin provide effective control of ticks for 28 days posttreatment, which is extended up to 75 days in the case of the long-acting 3.15% ivermectin formulations. The ML endectocides contribute to the control of *Haematobia irritans* (horn fly) in cattle. These compounds kill the adult flies and inhibit larval development in cattle dung. Development of the *H. irritans* fly may be reduced over 4 weeks after treatment with some ML compounds in cattle.

The concept of antiparasitic persistence acquired a great clinical significance after the discovery and commercial development of the ML endectocide compounds. The intrinsic properties of the MLs and/or their pharmacotechnical preparations allow a sustainable persistence of the active drug in the animal body, and therefore, prevent the establishment of new nematode burdens for several days after treatment. Large variations in the duration of the MLs' persistence of antiparasitic activity have been reported, particularly in cattle. The high variability is based on the parasites genera involved, the type of formulation used, different host-related factors, and the design of the experimental trials. For instance, the classic 1% ivermectin and abamectin formulations subcutaneously administered to cattle showed a persistent activity against *Cooperia* spp., *Ostertagia* spp., and *Dictyocaulus* spp. during 7, 14, and 28 days posttreatment. Longer protection periods against the same nematode parasites have been reported for moxidectin and doramectin. In fact doramectin showed a protection period between 21 and 35 days against *O. ostertagi* and 14–28 days for *Cooperia* spp. (Vercruysse et al. 2000). Moxidectin provides a protection against *Ostertagia* spp. and *Dictyocaulus* spp. during 35 and 42 days, respectively (Vercruysse et al. 1997). The ML pour-on formulations protect against nematode reinfection during the same period as that obtained after the subcutaneous treatments in cattle. The available ivermectin sustained-released bolus and the more recently introduced highly concentrated long-acting formulations (ivermectin and moxidectin) recommended for use at higher dose rates (between 0.63 and 1 mg/kg, respectively) dramatically increase the protection periods (between 60 and up to 150 days) against cattle endoparasites.

SWINE. The MLs are licensed to be used in pigs by subcutaneous (ivermectin, moxidectin), intramuscular (doramectin) administration at 0.3 mg/kg, and oral feed-formulation (ivermectin) at 0.1 mg/kg over 7 days to control endo- and ectoparasites. These compounds are active against immature and adult stages of *Ascaris suum*, *Hyostrongylus rubidus*, *Strongyloides ransomi*, *Oesophagostomum* spp., *Metastrongylus* spp., *Stephanurus dentatus*, and the intestinal (but not muscular) stages of *Trichinella spiralis*. Ivermectin efficacy against *Trichuris suis* is highly variable (between 60 and 95%). The MLs present high activity against the most common ectoparasites affecting swine herds: sucking lice (*H. suis*) and mange mites (*S. scabiei var. suis)*.

HORSES. Ivermectin (0.2 mg/kg) and moxidectin (0.4 mg/kg) are the only MLs available to be used in horses by either oral paste or gel formulations. Both compounds are highly effective against *Parascaris equorum, Oxyuris equi,* stomach worms *(Draschia megastoma, Habronema* spp., *Trichostrongylus axei), Strongyloides westeri,* and lungworms *(D. arnfieldi).* Both compounds are effective to control adult and larval stages of large strongyles *(Strongylus vulgaris, S. equinus, S. edentatus)*, adult small stronglyles *(Cyathostomes), Gasterophilus nasalis,* and *Onchocerca* spp. *microfilariae.* Consistently with the observed longer residence time in the bloodstream and tissues (Perez et al. 1999), moxidectin shows an extended period of protection against most of the target parasites in horses compared to ivermectin (Demeulenaere et al. 1997). The most important differences in the comparative efficacy of ivermectin and moxidectin in horses have been observed against mucosal larvae of *Cyathostomes* and *Gasterophilus* larvae. Ivermectin has lower efficacy than moxidectin against encysted *Cyathostomes* (Xiao et al. 1994; Monahan et al. 1996). However, while ivermectin is highly active (>99%) against all instars of *Gasterophilus intestinalis*, moxidectin shows a variable activity that ranges between 20 and 99% of efficacy when administered at recommended doses.

DOGS AND CATS. The overall efficacy and safety of the MLs designed for other species should not be assumed for dogs. It is now well known that collie dogs and other dog breeds are particularly sensitive to ivermectin (see the section "Safety and Toxicity"). Thus, ivermectin is licensed for specific therapeutic uses in dogs and cats. The available preparations are chewable formulations containing ivermectin to be administered at low doses 0.006 mg/kg (dogs) or 0.024 mg/kg (cats) as preventive against dirofilariasis. Ivermectin is effective against third and fourth stages of *Dirofilaria immitis* (Campbell 1989). Ivermectin and moxidectin approved formulations have a limited spectrum of activity against gastrointestinal nematodes in dogs and cats. However, ivermectin administered orally at higher doses (between 0.05 mg/kg and 0.2 mg/kg) may reach good efficacy against various nematode parasites (*Ancylostoma caninum, Trichuris vulpis, Toxocara canis* and *Capillaria aerophila*). Different studies have shown that two ivermectin subcutaneous doses (0.2 mg/kg) are enough to clear otodectic, sarcoptic, and notoedric mange infestations (Campbell 1989). Ivermectin is also used in the control of demodectic mange infestations in dogs at higher dosages and prolonged regimens. However, the therapeutic uses of ivermectin in dogs and cats, apart from the prevention of *D. immitis*, should be considered as an extralabel use.

Milbemycin oxime administered at 0.5 mg/kg is effective against developmental stages of *D. immitis, T. canis, T. leonina, A. caninum and T. vulpis*. Moxidectin has been introduced as a tablet (0.003 mg/kg) and long-acting sustained release injectable formulation (0.17 mg/kg) to prevent *D. immitis* infection. This injectable formulation is also useful to control *A. caninum*. Selamectin, a new avermectin compound (see Fig. 42.1) introduced as a topical formulation for dogs and cats, is active against different endo- and ectoparasites at 6 mg/kg. A greater selamectin systemic availability was observed in cats compared to that obtained in dogs (Sarasola et al. 2002). It is highly efficacious against infective stages of heartworm (*D. immitis*), *T. canis, T. leonina, A. tubaeforme,* and *T. cati.* Selamectin is also effective against ectoparasites such as fleas (*Ctenocephalides cati)*, mites (*Otodectes cynotis, S. scabiei*), and ticks (*R. sanguineous* and *Dermacentor variabilis*).

RESISTANCE

The antiparasitic strategies based almost exclusively on chemical control have been threatened by the emergence of nematode parasites resistant to the various anthelmintic chemical classes, including now the ML compounds. The increasing selection pressure on the gastrointestinal nematodes due to the high frequency of ML treatments was relevant for the development of resistance to these compounds. Changes on the glutamated-gated chloride channels structure and an increased expression of different proteins involved in drug efflux (P-GP) have been postulated as the main mechanism of resistance to the MLs in nematodes (see "Mode of Action"). It has been shown that *H. contortus* resistant to ivermectin possess an increased level of P-GP expression and that the coapplication of verapamil (a MDR-reversing agent) increased the efficacy of ivermectin and moxidectin against resistant strains of *H. contortus* (reviewed by Prichard 2002).

Initially, resistance to the MLs (largely to ivermectin) was observed in sheep and goat nematodes, particularly in *H. contortus*. However, the phenomenon has been widespread and other nematode species from small ruminants have developed resistance to the ML compounds. Field strains of *Teladorsagia circumcincta* and *T. colubriformis* resistant to ivermectin have been identified around the world. In addition, the intensive worldwide use of the different ML compounds over the last 25 years (since the introduction of ivermectin in the early '80s), has resulted in the emergence of ML resistance in cattle nematodes. In fact, different field strains of *Cooperia* spp., the dose-limiting parasite for the MLs, and *Trichostrongylus* spp. have been identified as resistant to the ML compounds (Vermunt et al. 1995; Coles et al.1998; Fiel et al. 2001). It should be noted that moxidectin conserves activity against certain ivermectin-resistant isolates, which is probably due to its differential kinetic and dynamic behavior compared to ivermectin (see Fig. 42.7).

A diminution of the selection pressure, reducing the number of treatments per year together with an integrated antiparasitic control is urgently required to prolong the usefulness of the broad-spectrum parasite control of the MLs in food-animal production. Detailed information on the parasite resistance against ML compounds in ruminant species has been reviewed by Prichard (2002) and Wolstenholme et al. (2004). Despite the widespread resistance of different equine parasites to different anthelmintics, and taking into account that ivermectin has been used in horses for 20 years, there are still no reports of *Cyathostomes* resistance (Kaplan 2002). Considering that ivermectin is the single most commonly used anthelmintic in horses, it seems that emergence of resistance would be inevitable. There are no reports of resistant heartworms, in spite of the fact that MLs have been extensively used to prevent infections in dogs on a monthly basis.

AVAILABLE PHARMACEUTICAL PREPARATIONS

Different delivery systems have been developed to administer the ML compounds to the different animal species. The available preparations include injectable solutions, oral drenches, tablets, pastes, in feed premix, pour-on formulations, and a sustained released bolus (ivermectin). An oral paste containing 1.87% of ivermectin is available for horses. In-feed formulation of ivermectin for pigs is recommended over 7 consecutive days at 0.1 mg/kg per day. Ivermectin is also formulated in a micelar solution for oral drench use in sheep and goats, and as tablet and chewable preparations for oral administration in dogs and cats. The pioneer and extensively worldwide-distributed ivermectin 1% injectable formulation for subcutaneous administration (0.2 mg/kg)in sheep and cattle (Ivomec®, Merial Ltd.) is formulated in propylene glycol (60%) and glycerol formulation (40%). A topical ivermectin formulation is also commercialized to use against the whole range of ecto- and endoparasites of cattle at 0.5 mg/kg.

Pharmaceutical technology has been applied to develop different drug formulations and delivery systems to optimize the pharmacological potency of ivermectin and other ML endectocides currently available. It has been confirmed that extended residence times of ivermectin in plasma and target tissues and the prolonged persistence of its anthelmintic activity, are obtained following the administration of an alternative oil-based formulation to cattle, compared to the standard preparation (Lifschitz et al. 1999b). Recently developed injectable long-acting formulations for cattle are essentially oil-based or thixotropic (3.15%) preparations that account for a slow absorption process from the subcutaneous space and a long persistence of active ivermectin concentrations in the bloodstream and target tissues (Lifschitz et al. 1999b, 2005c). This 3.15% ivermectin formulation (Ivomec Gold®, Merial Ltd.) given at higher doses rates (0.63 mg/kg) has persistent efficacy against cattle gastrointestinal and lung nematodes for up to 77 days and ticks for up to 75 days. Following the same concept of the extended antiparasitic persistence, other similar (generic) highly concentrated (3.15% and 3.50%) ivermectin preparations have been recently introduced into the cattle market in some countries. Another recently developed technology incorporates eprinomectin in a long-acting preparation based on poly (lactic-co-glycolic) acid copolymer, which extends its persistent activity against nematodes for up to 120 days (Marley and Tejwani 2005).

The development of the sustained-release bolus technology for the administration of antiparasitic drugs was considered an important advance for parasite control. The ivermectin sustained-release device is an osmotic bolus delivering 12.7 mg of ivermectin per day over 135 days postadministration to cattle. The excellent release performance of an ivermectin sustained-release bolus was confirmed measuring the plasma and fecal concentration profiles up to 160 days postadministration in cattle, being 90% of the total dose released from the bolus excreted in feces (Alvinerie et al. 1998b).

Controlled-release capsules providing 1.6 mg of ivermectin per day over 100 days have been commercialized for use in sheep. More recently, novel delivery technology has been applied to develop a sequential-release formulation for use in sheep, which delivers ivermectin and albendazole alternately (Gogolewsky et al. 2005). This ivermectin/albendazole sequential delivery (10 days of ivermectin followed by 20 days of albendazole release, with the same alternating release cycles for each molecule to cover 100 days posttreatment) has been designed to assure the exposure of incoming parasite larvae to two chemicals with different modes of action, which could delay the development of resistance to each of the anthelmintic agents.

Doramectin is available in an oil-based formulation containing sesame oil/ethyl oleate (90 : 10) to be administered by the subcutaneous and intramuscular routes to cattle. A doramectin pour-on preparation is licensed to be used in cattle at 0.5 mg/kg. Moxidectin is available to be administered as injectable, pour-on (cattle), and oral (sheep and horses) formulations. A 1% nonaqueous moxidectin formulation is currently available for subcutaneous injection in cattle, sheep (0.2 mg/kg), and pigs (0.3 mg/kg). Novel moxidectin long-acting preparations for use in sheep (2%) and cattle (10%) are now available for use at higher dose rates (1 mg/kg) to cover extended antiparasitic protection periods (between 60 and 150 days). A long-acting sustained release injectable formulation for dogs (0.17 mg/kg) designed to prevent *D. immitis* infection is currently available. A moxidectin gel preparation to be administered orally at 0.4 mg/kg to horses is also available in the veterinary pharmaceutical market.

Eprinomectin is approved as a topical formulation for use in beef and dairy cattle. Both the eprinomectin and moxidectin pour-on formulations are now indicated in some countries in lactating dairy cows with zero milk withdrawal time. Selamectin is formulated as a solution (6 and 12%) in an isopropyl alcohol/dipropylene glycol methyl-ether vehicle to be used in dogs and cats at a dose range between 6 and 12 mg/kg (Bishop et al. 2000). Tables 42.1 and 42.2 summarize the information on the available formulations and recommended dose rates for avermectin and milbemycin compounds, respectively, in the different animal species.

TABLE 42.1 Formulations of avermectin-type compounds commercially available for use in different animal species

Drug	Formulation and Administration Route	Dose Rate	Target Species
IVERMECTIN (Ivomec®, Merial Ltd.)	1% injectable formulation in propylene glycol/ glycerol formal (60 : 40) (SC)	0.2 mg/kg	Cattle, sheep
		0.3 mg/kg	Pigs
		0.4 mg/kg	Goats
	3.15% injectable oil-based long-acting formulation (SC)	0.63 mg/kg	Cattle
	0.5% transdermal formulation in isopropyl alcohol (pour-on)	0.5 mg/kg	Cattle
	Sustained release bolus (oral)	12 mg/day for 135 days	Cattle
	Controlled released capsules (oral)	1.6 mg/day for 100 days	Sheep
	Micelar drench formulation (oral)	0.2 mg/kg	Sheep
		0.4 mg/kg	Goats
	Liquid solution (oral)(#)	0.2 mg/kg	Horses
	1.87% paste formulation in a titanium dioxide and propylene glycol vehicle (oral) (#)	0.2 mg/kg	Horses
	In feed formulation (Premix) (oral)	0.1 mg/kg for 7 days	Pigs
	Flavored chewable and tablets formulation (oral) (##)	0.006 mg/kg	Dogs
		0.024 mg/kg	Cats
ABAMECTIN (Duotin®, Merial Ltd.)	1% injectable formulation in propylene glycol/glycerol formal (60:40) (SC)	0.2 mg/kg	Cattle, sheep
DORAMECTIN (Dectomax®, Pfizer)	1% injectable formulation in sesame oil/ethyl oleate (90:10) (SC, IM)	0.2 mg/kg	Cattle, sheep
		0.3 mg/kg	Pigs
	0.5% transdermal formulation (pour-on)	0.5 mg/kg	Cattle
EPRINOMECTIN (Eprinex®, Merial Ltd.)	0.5% transdermal formulation (pour-on)	0.5 mg/kg	Beef and dairy cattle
SELAMECTIN (Revolution®, Pfizer)	6% and 12% transdermal formulations in an isopropyl/dipropylene glycol methyl-ether vehicle (pour-on)	6 mg/kg	Dogs, cats

SC: subcutaneous; IM: intramuscular.

Trade names: (#) Eqvalan®, Merial Ltd.; (##) Heartgard®, Merial Ltd.

Table 42.2 does not include information on different ivermectin generic preparations available in some countries, particularly for the classic 1% and long-acting formulations for use in cattle.

TABLE 42.2 Formulations of milbemycin-type compounds commercially available for use in different animal species

Drug	Formulation and Administration Route	Dose Rate	Target Species
MILBEMIYCIN OXIME (Interceptor®, Novartis)	Flavor tablets (oral)	0.5 mg/kg	Dogs
		2 mg/kg	Cats
MOXIDECTIN (Cydectin®, Fort Dodge)	1% injectable formulation (SC)	0.2 mg/kg	Cattle, sheep
		0.3 mg/kg	Pigs
	10% long-acting oil- based formulation (SC in the base of the ear)	1 mg/kg	Cattle
	0.5% transdermal formulation (pour-on)	0.5 mg/kg	Beef and dairy cattle
	Drench formulation (oral)	0.2 mg/kg	Sheep
	2% long-acting oil- based formulation (SC in the base of the ear)	1 mg/kg	Sheep
	Gel formulation (oral) (#)	0.4 mg/kg	Horses
	Tablets (oral) (##)	0.003 mg/kg	Dogs
	Sustained release injectable formulation (SC) (###)	0.17 mg/kg	Dogs

SC: subcutaneous; IM: intramuscular.

Trade names: (#) Equest®, Fort Dodge; (##) ProHeart®, Fort Dodge; (###) ProHeart 6®, Fort Dodge.

DRUG AND HOST-RELATED FACTORS AFFECTING PHARMACOKINETICS AND EFFICACY IN RUMINANTS

As described in this chapter, the MLs are highly lipophilic substances that dissolve in most organic solvents. They are large molecules and despite possessing two sugar rings and two hydroxyl groups (avermectins) are relatively insoluble in water. Moxidectin solubility in water is greater than that of ivermectin and doramectin. These and other physicochemical differences between the ML molecules may account for differences in formulation flexibility and in their resultant kinetic behavior. The aqueous solubility of an active ingredient and the features of its pharmacotechnical preparation may influence the systemic availability, which relies on the rate and extent of absorption of a drug from the site of subcutaneous injection to the bloodstream. The vehicle in which the endectocide compounds are formulated may play a relevant role in their absorption kinetics and resultant plasma availability. The plasma profiles of ivermectin (Lo et al. 1985) and doramectin (Wicks et al. 1993) in cattle have been shown to be substantially affected by the composition of the administered formulation. Following parenteral administration, the low solubility of ivermectin and doramectin in water and its deposition in subcutaneous tissue favor a slow absorption from the injection site and provide prolonged duration in the bloodstream. Lanusse and co-workers (1997) characterized the comparative plasma disposition kinetics of ivermectin, moxidectin, and doramectin after their subcutaneous administration of the formulations commercially available for administration to cattle. While ivermectin was administered as the nonaqueous (60% propylene glycol/40% glycerol formal) preparation, an oil-based formulation of doramectin containing sesame oil/ethyl oleate (90 : 10) was administered to the experimental animals. The absorption of moxidectin, administered as an aqueous-based solution, from the site of subcutaneous injection was significantly faster than those of ivermectin and doramectin. Moxidectin peak plasma concentrations were achieved significantly earlier (8 h) than those of ivermectin (4 d) and doramectin (6 d posttreatment). It seems likely that moxidectin administered as an aqueous solution was more rapidly available for absorption from the subcutaneous tissue than both ivermectin and doramectin formulated in nonaqueous formulations, which agrees with the values of absorption half-lives obtained for moxidectin (1.32 h), ivermectin (39.2 h), and doramectin (56.4 h). The low solubility and the deposition of the ivermectin and doramectin nonaqueous preparations in the subcutaneous tissues favor a slow absorption from the site of injection, which may account for their prolonged residence in the bloodstream in cattle.

Several generic formulations of ivermectin have been introduced into the pharmaceutical market in different regions of the world after the expiration of the original patent of the first approved (innovator) ivermectin formulation (Ivomec®, Merial). The most of the available ivermectin generic preparations (some of them are now very well established in the pharmaceutical market) contain basically the same vehicle composition used in the innovator ivermectin formulation, but information on the comparative kinetic behavior of generic preparations in standardized pharmacokinetic trials is scarce. Lifschitz et al. (2004a) found marked differences on the absorption kinetics of ivermectin given by subcutaneous injection to cattle as four different generic (1%) formulations. The composition and quality of the vehicles and/or excipients used in the pharmacotechnical elaboration of ML formulations may be relevant to its pharmacokinetic behavior. The differences observed on the systemic availability and drug disposition kinetics among generic formulations may be reflected in the efficacy and persistence of their antiparasitic activity. Since the direct relationship between time of persistence of drug concentrations and extended efficacy against endo- and ectoparasites has been demonstrated, slight differences in formulation account for changes to the plasma kinetics and exposure of target parasites to active drug concentrations. This study was useful to build up a "conscience" on the relevance that the switchability among generic ML formulations might have on parasite control. Considering the necessary precautions to be adopted to avoid/delay the development of ML resistance in cattle nematode parasites, standardized quality control of generic formulations may greatly contribute to optimized drug use.

A number of factors affecting drug kinetics and the persistence of the antiparasitic efficacy of the ML have been identified. Among them are the animal species/breed, level of feed intake, nutritional status/body composition, influence of parasitism, formulation of dosage form, route of administration, etc. (reviewed by Lanusse and Prichard 1993; McKellar and Benchaoui 1996; Hennessy and Alvinerie 2002) (see Table 42.3). A series of relevant studies to compare the plasma profiles of MLs in different species have been reported (Alvinerie and Galtier 1997). From

TABLE 42.3 Drug and host-related factors affecting the kinetics and efficacy of the macrocyclic lactones in ruminants

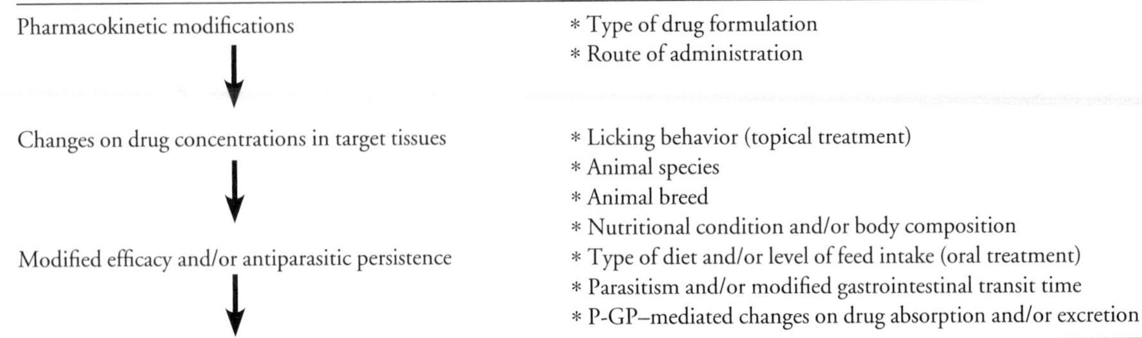

Pharmacokinetic modifications ↓	* Type of drug formulation * Route of administration
Changes on drug concentrations in target tissues ↓	* Licking behavior (topical treatment) * Animal species * Animal breed * Nutritional condition and/or body composition
Modified efficacy and/or antiparasitic persistence ↓	* Type of diet and/or level of feed intake (oral treatment) * Parasitism and/or modified gastrointestinal transit time * P-GP–mediated changes on drug absorption and/or excretion

The drug and host-related factors listed on the right may induce pharmacokinetic modifications resulting in modified drug efficacy/persistence. See the text for further explanation.

those comparisons, the consistently lower systemic availability of moxidectin (oral treatment) and ivermectin (SC treatment) observed in goats compared to sheep, emerges as a relevant finding. The influence of the route of administration on the plasma availability of the MLs has been extensively studied in ruminant species. For instance, both ivermectin and moxidectin are markedly less absorbed following oral administration to sheep compared to their subcutaneous injection. The reduced systemic availability observed following oral treatment accounted for lower milk residues excretion in orally treated dairy sheep compared to those observed after the injectable treatment (Imperiale et al. 2004b).

The ML has been traditionally administered by subcutaneous injection to cattle. However, formulations for their topical administration (pour-on) are currently marketed worldwide. Some practical advantages of the topical compared to other routes of administration have accounted for its great acceptance for parasite control in cattle. Some information is available on the plasma kinetic behavior of avermectins given topically to cattle (Gayrard et al. 1999). The plasma and tissue disposition kinetics of moxidectin and doramectin (Sallovitz et al. 2003, 2005) administered pour-on to cattle have recently been characterized. Lower moxidectin and doramectin plasma concentrations were measured following topical treatment compared to the subcutaneous injection of both compounds in cattle in spite of the use of a 2.5-fold higher dose rate for the pour-on administration (see Fig. 42.8). The absorption rate of topically administered moxidectin and its plasma availability were significantly higher in Holstein compared to Aberdeen Angus calves (Sallovitz et al. 2002), which may have considerable practical implications in terms of drug activity/persistence. Topically administered moxidectin is extensively distributed to different target tissues, including gastrointestinal mucosa, lungs, and different dermal layers. A cutaneous depot of the topically administered drug accounts for slow and sustained absorption, and agrees with the high moxidectin and doramectin concentrations measured in the epidermis and dermis of the skin from different anatomical regions.

It has been shown (Laffont et al. 2001) that the plasma and fecal disposition of ivermectin topically administered to cattle is markedly influenced by the natural licking behavior of treated animals. Higher and more variable systemic availability of ivermectin was observed in licker cattle, compared to animals whose licking behavior was prevented. These earlier results suggested that natural licking behavior may have a major influence on the kinetics of pour-on–administered MLs. More recent work (Sallovitz et al. 2005) showed that a 2-day-long licking prevention period after the pour-on treatment was sufficient to significantly reduce the doramectin concentrations measured in plasma during the first 9 days posttreatment. The animals in the free-licking group ingested topically administered doramectin by self and/or allo-licking, which accounted for the higher peak concentration observed in plasma as well as for the enhanced drug availability compared to the licking-restricted animals. As shown for moxidectin, a slow release of doramectin from the skin can be given by formation of a skin depot after the topical treatment, where the high lipophilicity facilitates drug retention in the lipid contents of the skin (fat tissue in the dermis and sebaceous secretion). Laffont et al. (2003) demonstrated that after the topical administration of ivermectin to cattle, drug absorption through the gastrointes-

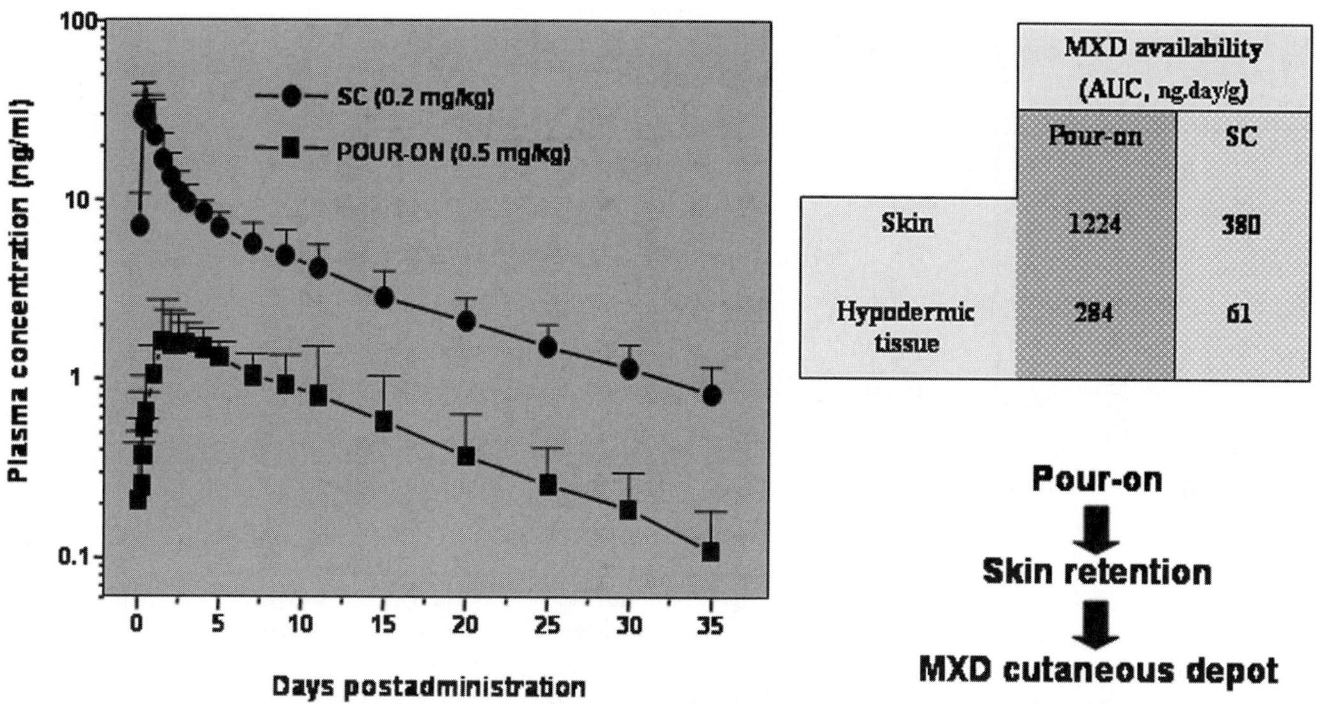

FIG. 42.8 Comparative plasma concentration profiles and total drug (expressed as AUC values) recovered in skin and hypodermic tissue after the subcutaneous (SC) and pour-on administrations of moxidectin (MXD) at recommended doses to cattle. The data illustrate the cutaneous depot of MXD after topical treatment. Data from Lifschitz et al. 1999a; Sallovitz et al. 2003.

tinal tract due to licking-induced oral ingestion is more important than the transdermal absorption in determining drug systemic concentrations. Thus, a more complete absorption of the MLs in the gastrointestinal tract following oral ingestion of the topically administered formulation, compared to the cutaneous permeation considered as the only absorption process in nonlicking animals, would explain the enhanced plasma profiles measured in calves allowed to lick freely.

Licking prevention during 10 days posttreatment permitted the identification of marked changes on the doramectin concentration profiles both systemically and, much more importantly, in the gastrointestinal tract. Doramectin concentrations in luminal contents from the intestine were markedly higher in free-licking cattle (see Fig. 42.9). Doramectin concentrations were higher in the fluid contents than in the mucosas in the licking group. Conversely, in licking-restricted calves, doramectin concentrations were higher in the mucosal tissue than in luminal content of the different gastrointestinal sections. These observations in nonlicking calves are in agreement with the data reported by Lifschitz et al. (2000) after the subcutaneous administration of doramectin, where after absorption into the systemic circulation, the drug can reach the gastrointestinal lumen by a distribution exchange between the bloodstream and the digestive compartment, which must occur through the mucosal layer of the intestine.

Considering the marked licking-induced changes observed in the concentrations of doramectin in the mucosal tissue and luminal contents from abomasum and intestine, the overall patterns of antiparasitic efficacy and persistence claimed for topically administered endectocides in cattle should be revised. On the face of the observed variations on antiparasitc response and with the threat of resistance development, the use of pour-on formulations to control endo- and ectoparasites should be carefully

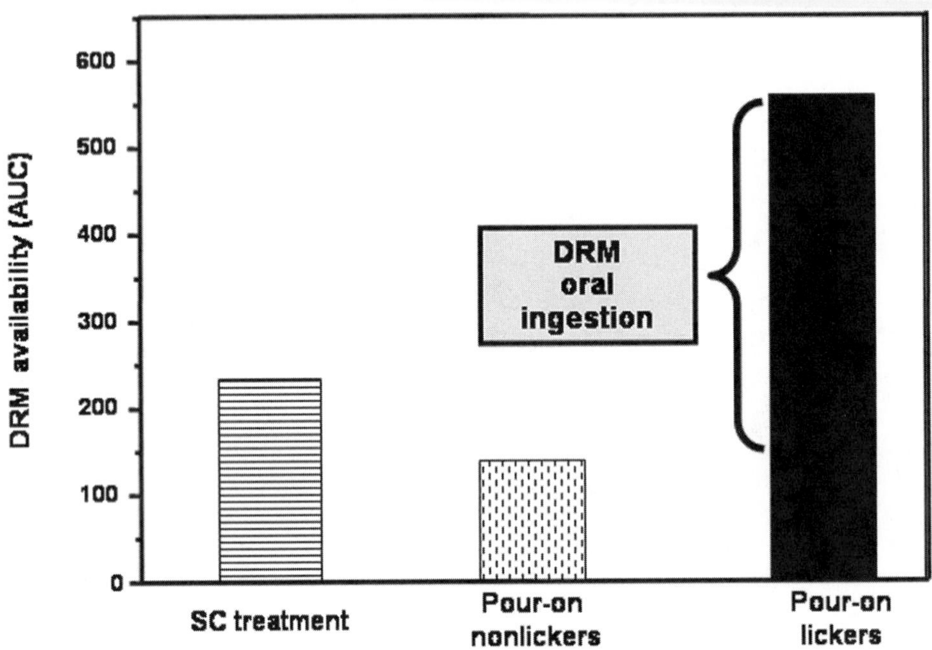

FIG. 42.9 Influence of animals' licking behavior on the intestinal availability of topically administered doramectin (DRM) in grazing cattle. The data show the AUC values obtained for DRM in the duodenal content after its topical administration (0.5 mg/kg) in both nonlicker (licking restricted over 10 days posttreatment) and free-licker calves. The comparison with the values obtained for the subcutaneous treatment (0.2 mg/kg) is included. DRM intestinal availability was significantly higher in licker calves due to licking-induced oral ingestion of the topical formulation. See the text for further explanation. AUC values are expressed in ng.day/ml. Data from Sallovitz et al. 2005.

considered. As recently pointed out by Bousquet-Mélou et al. (2004), there are many therapeutic, practical, and regulatory issues to be discussed on the basis of the altered pharmacokinetic behavior induced by the natural licking in pour-on treated cattle. While the pharmacoparasitological implications of this animal behavior need to be further evaluated, the available data on the effect of licking prevention on ML concentrations in the gastrointestinal tract illustrate the magnitude of the pharmacokinetic modifications occurring after pour-on treatments in cattle.

TISSUE RESIDUES AND WITHDRAWAL TIMES

From mouse teratogenicity studies and from multigeneration studies in rats, the no-effect levels (NOEL) of 0.2 mg/kg/day have been established. Based on the relationship of these NOEL to residue levels in edible tissues from pharmacokinetic studies, the current withholding periods for sheep and cattle have been established. However, due to their high potency and elimination through milk, the classic injectable ML formulations are contraindicated for use in animals that produce milk for human consumption. The MLs are highly lipophilic substances extensively distributed to different tissues. The highest tissue residue concentrations in food-producing animals are recovered from the liver and fat. Regulatory agencies (U.S. Food and Drug Administration, European Agency for the Evaluation of Medicinal Products) have established the maximum residue levels (MRL) in target tissues (liver and fat) for some of the ML compounds in sheep and beef cattle. A 100 μg/kg MRL value for ivermectin in liver and fat tissue has been set. The MRL values established for doramectin are 100 μg/kg (fat) and 150 μg/kg (liver). Higher MRL values were proposed for moxidectin in fat (500 μg/kg) and eprinomectin in fat (250 μg/kg) and liver (1500 μg/kg).

Posttreatment withdrawal periods have been established for the commercialized formulations in the different food-animal species. Although the established withdrawal times may vary according to the policies applied by the regulatory agencies in different countries, the classic 1% cattle injectable formulations of abamectin, ivermectin, doramectin, and moxidectin require withdrawal times ranging from 35 up to 50 days. A 120-day period is required to consume tissues from cattle treated with the 3.15% long-acting ivermectin formulation. An 84-day posttreatment period is required to deplete moxidectin below the established tolerance limits for different tissues after its administration as a long-acting preparation (10%) in cattle subcutaneously injected in the base of the ear. Withdrawal times between 10 and 15 days are required to consume meat from sheep treated with the ivermectin oral drench. In the U.S., a 45-day (35-day in Europe) withdrawal period is required for beef cattle treated with the available doramectin topical preparation. Required meat withdrawal times for doramectin in pigs parenterally treated are as follows: 24 (U.S.), 28–50 (Latin America), and 28–77 (European countries) days posttreatment. Detailed information on posttreatment withholding periods for the different ML formulations approved for use in food-producing animals in the U.S. can be found on the website for the U.S. Pharmacopeia (www.usp.org). There are no established withdrawal times for goats because MLs are not approved for use in this species. If ivermectin is administered to goats as a single extralabel oral dose of 0.2 to 0.4 mg/kg, evidence has been compiled by the Food Animal Residue Avoidance Databank (FARAD) that suggests a meat withdrawal time of 14 days and a milk withholding time of 9 days, which would be sufficient to avoid potentially harmful residues (Baynes et al. 2000).

All the ML injectable formulations are restricted for use in lactating dairy animals. However, a pour-on formulation of eprinomectin is approved for topical use in all cattle, including lactating dairy cows, without any milk withdrawal period. A moxidectin pour-on formulation is now available for use in dairy cattle with zero withdrawal time in milk. Additionally, generic ivermectin topical preparations are now approved for use in dairy cattle without milk withdrawal in some countries. Milk MRL values have been established for ivermectin (10 μg/kg), eprinomectin (20 μg/kg), and moxidectin (40 μg/kg).

SAFETY AND TOXICITY

The ML compounds given at recommended therapeutic doses are highly safe compounds in the majority of the target animal species. These large safety margins are based on the selectivity of their pharmacodynamic action. A GABA-mediated action in the mammalian central nervous system may be responsible for the neurotoxicity observed when large toxic doses of different MLs are administered (Lankas and Gordon 1989). In general, the avermectins have at least a tenfold safety margin in ruminants, horses, swine, and most dog breeds except collies and some Australian shepherds. The signs of acute toxicity include depression, ataxia, tremors, salivation, mydriasis, and in severe cases, coma and death. No effect on breeding performance, semen quality, or pregnancy was observed when bulls or cows were treated with ivermectin at 0.4 mg/kg (Campbell and Benz 1984). Avermectins are safe for use in cows during all stages of pregnancy. A twofold increase in dosage and multiple dosing have not adversely affected spermatogenesis, conception, longevity of gestation, or fetal development. Abamectin is slightly more toxic than ivermectin, with an oral LD_{50} in mice (14–24 mg/kg) higher than that of ivermectin (25–40 mg/kg). Signs of toxicosis were observed in cattle treated subcutaneously with abamectin at levels of 2–8 mg/kg. Abamectin is not recommended to be used in calves under 4 months of age (Pulliam and Preston 1989). No adverse effects were observed in different tolerance studies using up to 25-fold the therapeutic dose of doramectin injectable in cattle. Numerous field trials corroborate that eprinomectin is safe to use in cattle of all breeds and ages. Like the avermectins, milbemycin compounds have a wide therapeutic margin. No adverse effects have been observed in cattle subcutaneously treated with moxidectin up to 10 times the recommended dose (2 mg/kg). Moxidectin is safe in breeding animals. At three times the recommended dose (0.6 mg/kg), no adverse effects on reproductive performance of bulls and pregnant cows were observed.

As described, P-GP is a transport protein that acts as a multidrug efflux pump reducing intracellular concentration of different drugs, including the MLs. The activity of this transmembrane protein, located in brain capillary endothelial cells, intestinal epithelial cells, biliary canalicular cells, renal proximal tubular epithelial cells, and placental and testicular cells is related to the toxicity of the MLs. Its presence in the blood-brain barrier limits the entry of these antiparasitic molecules into the central nervous system. The accumulation of ivermectin in the brain of genetically engineered P-GP–deficient mice was 87-fold higher compared to normal mice (Schinkel et al. 1994). Certain collie dogs are more sensitive to high doses of ivermectin than other dogs and develop signs of toxicity with single doses as low as 0.1 mg/kg (Fassler et al. 1991). The higher ivermectin brain concentrations reported in the avermectin-sensitive collies versus nonsensitive dogs may be related to a limited P-GP expression (Mealey et al. 2001; Roulet et al. 2003). A 4 base-pairs deletion in the *MDR1* (multidrug resistance) gene in sensitive collie dogs seems to account for altered P-GP synthesis. Dogs homozygous for a mutant allele of *MDR1* have a nonfunctional P-GP (Mealey et al. 2001). A sample population study of 40 collie dogs in the northwestern United States found 35% to be homozygous for the mutation and 42% to be heterozygous carriers of the mutant allele (Mealey et al. 2002). A gene study of subpopulations has shown that the mutation of the *MDR1* gene can be found in members of breeds other than collie dogs (Australian shepherds, English shepherds, Shetland sheepdogs, etc.), generally at a much lower frequency (Hadrick et al. 1995).

Animals deficient in P-GP expression in the intestine may also absorb more drug after oral treatment, which may result in higher blood concentrations and enhanced potential for neurotoxicity (Shoop and Soll 2002). Additionally, limited P-GP expression in the hepatobiliary tract may result in a decreased bile excretion of the ML compounds. Selametin was evaluated in dogs and cats at 10 times the recommended doses and no adverse reactions were observed (Novotny et al. 2000; Krautmann et al. 2000). Selamectin use is also safe in ivermectin-sensitive collie dogs. No abnormalities were observed in sensitive collies treated topically with selamectin at 40 mg/kg. Milbemycin oxime is well tolerated in dogs, including collies. Clinical signs are seen only after the administration of a tenfold overdose. Overall, as suggested by Shoop and Soll (2002), the wide safety margin is based on the low therapeutically used doses and on the fact that mammals do not have glutamate-gated chloride channels (specific site of action for the MLs in target parasites). Additionally, these drugs do not cross the blood-brain barrier. The presence of P-GP in the blood-brain barrier as well as in other tissues, serves as an important protective biological barrier to any adverse effects of the MLs.

ECOTOXICOLOGICAL IMPACT

The pattern of fecal elimination of different ML compounds administered by different routes to cattle has received special attention, due to the potential negative environmental impact caused by the effect of the drugs against dung-degrading insects. This has been evaluated under different conditions, initially for ivermectin (Lumaret et al. 1993; Herd 1995) and more recently for other MLs (Suarez et al. 2003). The prolonged presence of these molecules in the feces of treated cattle produces an adverse effect against invertebrate organisms that have a relevant role on dung degradation and nutrients recycling to the soil (Strong 1993). The residues of ivermectin and abamectin in feces not only affect the development and reproduction of adult *Coleoptera* but also are toxic against larval stages between 2 and 4 weeks after an injectable treatment (Strong and Wall 1994; Herd 1995). The consequences of this toxicity over the ecosystem are not fully understood. Moxidectin has been considered as a less harmful compound compared to the avermectin-type compounds following standard injectable treatments. The lower fecal concentrations measured after moxidectin treatment in cattle compared to those obtained after ivermectin and doramectin administration (Lifschitz et al. 1999a) with a possible higher rate of environmental degradation of moxidectin may determine its lower toxicity against dung fauna. Further research is required to evaluate potential adverse environmental impact of the ML compounds under a variety of conditions. Long-term investigations under different field production systems are particularly needed.

CONCLUDING REMARKS

The avermectins' discovery and the commercial launch of ivermectin as an ecto-endoparasiticidal agent in the early 80s were a great breakthrough within veterinary therapeutics, which was successfully followed by the development of other avermectin and milbemycin compounds. The MLs from both chemical families combine excellent spectrum with safety, potency, and persistence. They are highly efficacious antiparasitic agents for use in a variety of livestock and companion animal species. The observations highlighted in this chapter on the phamacokinetic/

pharmacodynamic relationship for MLs provide pharmacological knowledge required to improve their therapeutic use. Avoiding misuse of the MLs is critical to delay the development of resistance. The integrated assessment of the drug disposition kinetics in the host, the processes of drug diffusion into different target parasites, and the use of pharmaceutical technology to improve drug delivery at the site of infection are key research areas within the pharmacology of the antiparasitic drugs.

REFERENCES

Alvinerie, M.; Sutra, J. F. and Galtier, P. 1993. Ivermectin in goat plasma and milk after subcutaneous injection. Annales de Recherches Veterinaires 24, 417–421.

Alvinerie, M.; Sutra, J. F.; Lanusse, C. and Galtier, P. 1996. Plasma profile study of moxidectin in a cow and its suckling calf. Veterinary Research 27, 545–549.

Alvinerie, M. and Galtier P. 1997. Comparative pharmacokinetic properties of moxidectin and ivermectin in different animal species. Journal of Veterinary Pharmacology and Therapeutics 20, supplement 1, 74.

Alvinerie, M.; Escudero, E.; Eeckhoutte, C. and Galtier, P. 1998a. The pharmacokinetics of moxidectin after oral and subcutaneous administration to sheep. Veterinary Research 29, 113–118.

Alvinerie, M.; Sutra, J.; Galtier, P.; Lifschitz, A.; Virkel, G.; Sallovitz, J. and Lanusse, C. 1998b. Persistence of ivermectin in plasma and faeces following administration of a sustained-release bolus to cattle. Research in Veterinary Science 66, 57–62.

Alvinerie, M.; Dupuy, J.; Eeckhoutte, C. and Sutra, J. 1999a. Enhanced absorption of pour-on ivermectin formulation in rats by coadministration of the multidrug-resistant-reversing agent verapamil. Parasitology Research 85, 920–922.

Alvinerie, M.; Sutra, J.; Galtier, P. and Mage, C. 1999b. Pharmacokinetics of eprinomectin in plasma and milk following topical administration to lactating dairy cattle. Research in Veterinary Science 67, 229–232.

Alvinerie, M.; Lacoste, E.; Sutra, J. and Chartier, C. 1999c. Some pharmacokinetic parameters of eprinomectin in goats following pour-on administration. Veterinary Research Communications 23, 449–455.

Arena, J.; Liu, K.; Paress, P.; Schaeffer, J. and Cully, D. 1992. Expression of a glutamate-activated chloride current in Xenopus oocytes injected with Caenorhabditis elegans RNA: evidence for modulation by avermectin. Brain Research. Molecular Brain Research 15, 339–48.

Armour, J.; Bairden, K. and Preston, J. 1980. Anthelmintic efficiency of ivermectin against naturally acquired bovine gastrointestinal nematode. The Veterinary Record 107, 226–227.

Ballent, M.; Lifschitz, A.; Virkel, G.; Sallovitz, J. and Lanusse, C. 2006. Modulation of P-glycoprotein-mediated intestinal secretion of ivermectin: in vivo and in vitro assessments. Drug Metabolism and Disposition 34, 3.

Baynes, R.; Payne, M. and Martin-Jimenez, T. 2000. Extralabel use of ivermectin and moxidectin in food animals. Journal of the American Veterinary Medical Association 217, 668–671.

Bishop, B.; Bruce, C.; Evans, N.; Goudie, A.; Gration, K.; Gibson, S.; Pacey, M.; Perry, D.; Walshe, N. and Witty, M. 2000. Selamectin: a novel broad-spectrum endectocide for dogs and cats. Veterinary Parasitology 91, 163–176.

Blackhall, W.; Prichard, R. and Beech, R. 2003. Selection at a gamma-aminobutyric acid receptor gene in *Haemonchus contortus* resistant to avermectins/milbemycins. Molecular and Biochemical Parasitology 131, 137–45.

Bogan, J. and McKellar, Q. 1988. The pharmacodynamics of ivermectin in sheep and cattle. Journal of Veterinary Pharmacology and Therapeutics 11, 260–268.

Bousquet-Mélou, A.; Mercadier, S.; Alvinerie, A. and Toutain, P. 2004. Endectocide exchanges between grazing cattle after pour-on administration of doramectin, ivermectin and moxidectin. International Journal for Parasitology 34, 1299–1307.

Campbell, W. 1985. Ivermectin: an update. Parasitology Today 1, 10–6.

———. 1989. Use of ivermectin in dogs and cats. In Ivermectin and Abamectin, edited by Campbell, W., pp. 245–259. Springer-Verlag, New York Inc., New York, USA.

Campbell, W. and Benz, G. 1984. Ivermectin, a review of efficacy and safety. Journal of Veterinary Pharmacology and Therapeutics 7, 1–16.

Carceles, C.; Diaz, M.; Vicente, M.; Sutra J.; Alvinerie, M. and Escudero, E. 2001. Milk kinetics of moxidectin and doramectin in goats. Research in Veterinary Science 70, 227–231.

Chiu, S.; Taub, R.; Sestokas, E.; Lu, A. and Jacob, T. 1987. Comparative in vivo and in vitro metabolism of ivermectin in steers, sheep, swine, and rat. Drug Metabolism Reviews 18, 289–302.

Coles, G.; Hillyer, M.; Taylor, F. and Parker, L. 1998. Activity of moxidectin against bots and lungworm in equids. The Veterinary Record 143, 169–170.

Cully, D.; Vassilatis, D.; Liu, K.; Paress, P.; Van der Ploeg, L.; Schaeffer, J. and Arena, J. 1994. Cloning of an avermectin-sensitive glutamate-gate chloride channel from *Caenorhabditis elegans*. Nature 371, 707–711.

Demeulenaere, D.; Vercruysse, J.; Dorny, P. and Claerebout, E. 1997. Comparative studies of ivermectin and moxidectin in the control of naturally acquired cyathostome infections in horses. The Veterinary Record 141, 383–386.

Dupuy, J.; Larrieu, G.; Sutra J.; Eeckhoutte C. and Alvinerie M. 2001. Influence of verapamil on the efflux and metabolism of 14C moxidectin in cultured rat hepatocytes. Journal of Veterinary Pharmacology and Therapeutics 24, 171–177.

Fassler, P.; Tranquilli, W.; Paul, A. et al. 1991. Evaluation of the safety of ivermectin administered in a beef-based formulation to ivermectin-sensitive collies. Journal of the American Veterinary Medical Association 199, 457–460.

Fellowes, R.; Maule, A.; Martin, R.; Geary, T.; Thompson, D.; Kimber, M.; Marks, N. and Halton, D. 2000. Classical neurotransmitters in the ovijector of *Ascaris suum*: localization and modulation of muscle activity. Parasitology 121, 325–336.

Fiel, C.; Saumell, C.; Steffan, P. and Rodriguez, E. 2001. Resistance of Cooperia to ivermectin treatments in grazing cattle of the Humid Pampa, Argentina. Veterinary Parasitology 97, 211–217.

Fisher, M. and Mrozik, H. 1989. Chemistry. In Ivermectin and Abamectin, edited by Campbell, W., pp. 1–23. Springer-Verlag, New York Inc., New York, USA.

Forrester, S.; Prichard, R.; Dent, J. and Beech, R. 2003. *Haemonchus contortus*: HcGluCla expressed in Xenopus oocytes forms a glutamate-gated ion channel that is activated by ibotenate and the antiparasitic drug ivermectin. Molecular and Biochemical Parasitology 29, 115–21.

Gayrard, V.; Alvinerie, M. and Toutain, P. 1999. Comparison of pharmacokinetic profiles of doramectin and ivermectin pour-on formulations in cattle. Veterinary Parasitology 81, 47–55.

Geary, T. 2005. Ivermectin 20 years on: maturation of a wonder drug. Trends in Parasitology 21, 530–532.

Geary, T.; Sangster, N. and Thompson D. 1999. Frontiers in anthelmintic pharmacology. Veterinary Parasitology 84, 275–295.

Geary, T.; Sims, S.; Thomas, E.; Vanover, L.; Davis, J.; Winterrowd, C.; Klein, R.; and Thompson, D. 1993. *Haemonchus contortus*: ivermectin-induced paralysis of the pharynx. Experimental Parasitology 77, 88–96.

Gill, J. and Lacey, E. 1998. Avermectin/milbemycin resistance in trichostrongyloid nematodes. International Journal for Parasitology 28, 863–877.

Gill, J.; Redwin, J.; van Wyk, J. and Lacey, E. 1991. Detection of resistance to ivermectin in *Haemonchus contortus*. International Journal for Parasitology 21, 771–776.

Gogolewsky, R.; Shiraishi, A.; Venning, M.; Chandler, D. and Hurst, J. 2005. Abstract Book Merial of the 20th International Conference of the World Association for the Advancement of Veterinary Parasitology 16–20 October. Christchurch, New Zealand.

Goudie, A.; Evans, N.; Gration, K.; Bishop, B.; Gibson, S.; Holdom, K.; Kaye, B.; Wicks, S. and Lewis, D. 1993. Doramectin a potent novel endectocide. Veterinary Parasitology 49, 5–15.

Hadrick M,; Bunch, S. and Kornegay, J. 1995. Ivermectin toxicosis in two Australian Shepherds. Journal of the American Veterinary Medical Association 206, 1147–1152.

Hennessy, D. 2000. WAAVP/Pfizer award for excellence in veterinary parasitology research. My involvement in, and some thoughts for livestock parasitological research in Australia. Veterinary Parasitology 88, 107–116.

Hennessy, D. and Alvinerie, M. 2002. Pharmacokinetics of the macrocyclic lactones: conventional wisdom and new paradigms. In Macrocyclic Lactones in Antiparasitic Therapy, edited by Vercruysse, J. and Rew, R., pp. 97–124. CAB International, Wallingford, Oxon, UK.

Hennessy, D.; Page, S. and Gottschall, D. 2000. The behaviour of doramectin in the gastrointestinal tract, its secretion in bile and pharmacokinetic disposition in the peripheral circulation after oral and intravenous administration to sheep. Journal of Veterinary Pharmacology and Therapeutics 23, 203–213.

Herd, R. 1995. Endectocidal drugs: Ecological risk and counter measures. International Journal for Parasitology 25, 875–885.

Imperiale, F.; Busetti, M.; Suárez, V. and Lanusse, C. 2004a. Milk excretion of ivermectin and moxidectin in dairy sheep: Assessment of drug residues during cheese elaboration and ripening period. Journal of Agricultural and Food Chemistry 52, 6205–6211.

Imperiale, F.; Lifschitz, A.; Sallovitz, J.; Virkel, G. and Lanusse, C. 2004b. Comparative depletion of ivermectin and moxidectin milk residues in dairy sheep after oral and subcutaneous administration. Journal of Dairy Science 71, 427–433.

Jackson, H. 1989. Ivermectin as a systemic insecticide. Parasitology Today 5, 146–155.

Kaplan, R. 2002. Anthelmintic resistance in nematodes of horses. Veterinary Research 33, 491–507.

Krautmann, M.; Novotny, M.; De Keulenaer, K.; Godin, C.; Evans, E.; McCall, J.; Wang, C.; Rowan, T. and Jernigan, A. 2000. Safety of selamectin in cats. Veterinary Parasitology 91,393–403.

Laffont, C.; Alvinerie, M.; Bousquet-Mélou, A. and Toutain P. 2001. Licking behaviour and environmental contamination arising from pour-on ivermectin for cattle. International Journal for Parasitology 31, 1687–1692.

Laffont, C.; Bousquet-Mélou, A.; Bralet, D.; Alvinerie, M.; Fink-Gremmels, J. and Toutain, P. 2003. A pharmacokinetic model to document the actual disposition of topical ivermectin in cattle. Veterinary Research 34, 445–460.

Laffont, C.; Toutain, P.; Alvinerie, M. and Bousquet-Mélou A. 2002. Intestinal secretion is a major route for parent ivermectin elimination in the rat. Drug Metabolism and Disposition 30, 626–630.

Lankas, G. and Gordon, R. 1989. Toxicology. In Ivermectin and Abamectin, edited by Campbell, W., pp. 89–112. Springer-Verlag, New York Inc., New York, USA.

Lanusse, C. and Prichard, R. 1993. Relationship between pharmacological properties and clinical efficacy of ruminant anthelmintics. Veterinary Parasitology 49, 123–158.

Lanusse, C.; Lifschitz, A.; Sanchez, S.; Sutra, J.; Galtier, P. and Alvinerie, M. 1997. Comparative plasma disposition kinetics of ivermectin, moxidectin and doramectin in cattle. Journal of Veterinary Pharmacology and Therapeutics 20, 91–99.

Lespine, A.; Chanoit, G.; Bousquet-Mélou, A; Lallemand, E. Bassissi, F.; Alvinerie, M. and Toutain, P. 2006. Contribution of lymphatic transport to the systemic exposure of orally administered moxidectin in conscious lymph duct-cannulated dogs. European Journal of Pharmaceutical Sciences 27, 37–43.

Lifschitz, A.; Virkel, G.; Imperiale, F.; Galtier, P.; Lanusse, C. and Alvinerie, M. 1999a. Moxidectin in cattle: correlation between plasma and target tissues disposition kinetics. Journal of Veterinary Pharmacology and Therapeutics 22, 266–273.

Lifschitz, A.; Virkel, G.; Pis, A.; Imperiale, F.; Alvarez, L.; Kujanek, R. and Lanusse, C. 1999b. Ivermectin disposition kinetics after subcutaneous and intramuscular administration of an oil-based formulation to cattle. Veterinary Parasitology 86, 203–215.

Lifschitz, A.; Virkel, G.; Sutra, J.; Galtier, P.; Alvinerie, M. and Lanusse, C. 2000. Comparative distribution of ivermectin and doramectin to parasite location tissues in cattle. Veterinary Parasitology 87, 327–338.

Lifschitz, A; Virkel, G.; Imperiale, F.; Pis, A. and Lanusse, C. 2002a. Fármacos endectocidas: avermectinas y milbemicinas. In Farmacología y Terapáutica Veterinaria, edited by Botana López, L.; Landoni, M. F. and Martín-Jimánez, T., pp. 545–558. McGraw-Hill Interamericana, Madrid, Spain.

Lifschitz, A; Virkel, G.; Sallovitz, J.; Imperiale, F.; Pis, A. and Lanusse, C. 2002b. Loperamide-induced enhancement of moxidectin availability in cattle. Journal of Veterinary Pharmacology and Therapeutics 25, 111–120.

Lifschitz, A.; Sallovitz, J.; Imperiale, F.; Pis, A.; Jauregui Lorda, J. and Lanusse C. 2004a. Pharmacokinetic evaluation of four ivermectin generic formulations in calves. Veterinary Parasitology 119, 247–257.

Lifschitz, A.; Virkel, G.; Sallovitz, J.; Pis, A.; Imperiale, F. and Lanusse, C. 2004b. Loperamide modifies the tissue disposition kinetics of ivermectin in rats. The Journal of Pharmacy and Pharmacology 56, 61–67.

Lifschitz, A.; Ballent, M.; Virkel; G.; Sallovitz, J. and Lanusse, C. 2005a. Involvement of p-glycoprotein on ivermectin disposition kinetics: in vitro and in vivo assessments. 14th Biennial Symposium of American Academy of Veterinary Pharmacology and Therapeutics, June. Rockville, USA.

Lifschitz, A; Virkel, G.; Ballent M.; Pis, A.; Sallovitz, J. and Lanusse, C. 2005b. Moxidectin and ivermectin metabolic stability in sheep ruminal and abomasal content. Journal of Veterinary Pharmacology and Therapeutics 28, 411–418.

Lifschitz, A.; Virkel, G.; Ballent, M.; Sallovitz, J.; Imperiale, F. and Lanusse, C. 2005c. Pharmacokinetic assessment of ivermectin (3.15%) long-acting formulations. Proceedings of the 20th International Conference of the World Association for the Advancement of Veterinary Parasitology, 16–20 October. Christchurch, New Zealand.

Lo, P.; Fink, D. W.; Williams, J. B. and Blodinger, J. 1985. Pharmacokinetic studies of ivermectin: effects of formulation. Veterinary Research Communications 9, 251–268.

Lumaret, J.; Galante, E.; Lumbreras, C.; Mena, J.; Bertrand, M; Bernal, J.; Cooper, J.; Kadiri, N. and Crowe, D. 1993. Field effects of ivermectin residues on dung beetles. Journal of Applied Ecology 30, 428–436.

Marley, S. and Tejwani, M. 2005. Abstract Book Merial of the 20th International Conference of the World Association for the Advancement of Veterinary Parasitology, 16–20 October. Christchurch, New Zealand.

Martin, J.; Robertson, A. and Wolstenholme, A. 2002. Mode of action of macrocyclic lactones. In Macrocyclic Lactones in Antiparasitic Therapy, edited by Vercruysse, J. and Rew, R. pp. 125–140. CAB International, Wallingford, Oxon, UK.

McKellar, Q. and Benchaoui, H. 1996. Avermectins and milbemycins. Journal of Veterinary Pharmacology and Therapeutics 19, 331–351.

Mealey, K.; Bentjen, S.; Gay, J. and Cantor, G. 2001. Ivermectin sensitivity in collies is associated with a deletion mutation of the mdr1 gene. Pharmacogenetics 11, 727–733.

Mealey, K.; Bentjen, S. and Waiting, D. 2002. Frequency of the mutant MDR1 allele associated with ivermectin sensitivity in a sample population of collies from the northwestern United States. American Journal of Veterinary Research 63, 479–81.

Miwa, G.; Walsh, J.; VandenHeuvel, W.; Arison, B.; Sestokas, E.; Buhs, R.; Rosegay, A.; Avermitilis, S.; Lu, A.; Walsh, M.; Walker, R.; Taub, R. and Jacob, T. 1982. The metabolism of avermectins B1a, H2B1a, and H2B1b by liver microsomes. Drug Metabolism and disposition 10, 268–274.

Molento, M.; Lifschitz, A.; Sallovitz, J.; Lanusse, C. and Prichard, R. 2004. Influence of verapamil on the pharmacokinetics of the antiparasitic drugs ivermectin and moxidectin in sheep. Parasitology Research 92, 121–127.

Molento, M. and Prichard, R. 1999. Effects of the multidrug-resistance-reversing agents verapamil and CL 347,099 on the efficacy of ivermectin or moxidectin against unselected and drug-selected strains of *Haemonchus contortus* in birds (*Meriones unguiculatus*). Parasitology Research 85, 1007–1011.

Monahan, C.; Chapman, M.; Taylor, H.; French, D. and Klei, T. 1996. Comparison of moxidectin oral gel and ivermectin oral paste against a spectrum of internal parasites of ponies with special attention to encysted cyathostome larvae. Veterinary Parasitology 63, 225–35

Monteiro Riviere, N. 1991. Comparative anatomy, physiology, and biochemistry of mammalian skin. In Dermal and Ocular Toxicology, edited by Hobson, D., pp. 3–71. CRC Press Inc., Boca Raton, USA.

Moya-Borja, G.; Muniz, R.; Umehara, O.; Goncalves, L.; Silva, D. and McKenzie, M. 1997. Protective efficacy of doramectin and ivermectin against *Cochliomyia hominivorax*. Veterinary Parasitology 72, 101–109.

Njue, A. and Prichard, R. 2004. Genetic variability of glutamate-gated chloride channel genes in ivermectin-susceptible and -resistant strains of *Cooperia oncophora*. Parasitology 129, 741–751.

Novotny, M.; Krautmann, M.; Ehrhart, J.; Godin, C.; Evans, E.; McCall, J.; Sun, F.; Rowan, T. and Jernigan, A. 2000. Safety of selamectin in dogs. Veterinary Parasitology 91, 377–391.

Perez, R.; Cabezas, I.; Garcia, M.; Rubilar, L.; Sutra, J:F.; Galtier, P. and Alvinerie, M. 1999. Comparison of the pharmacokinetics of moxidectin (Equest) and ivermectin (Eqvalan) in horses. Journal of Veterinary Pharmacology and Therapeutics 22, 174–180.

Pouliot, J.; L'Hereux, F.; Liu, Z.; Prichard, R. and Georges, E. 1997. Reversal of P-glycoprotein-associated multidrug resistance by ivermectin. Biochemical Pharmacology 53, 17–25.

Prichard, R. 2002. Resistance against macrocyclic lactones. In Macrocyclic Lactones in Antiparasitic Therapy, edited by Vercruysse, R. and Rew, R., pp. 163–182. CABI Publishing, Wallingford, UK.

Prichard, R.; Forrester, A.; Njue, A.; Feng, G. Liu, J. and Beech, R. 2003. Receptor mechanism of antiparasitics. Journal of Veterinary Pharmacology and Therapeutics. pp 29–31. Vol 26, suppl 1. Proceedings of the 9th International Congress of the European Association for Veterinary Pharmacology and Toxicology (EAVPT), 13–18 July. Lisbon, Portugal.

Prichard, R. and Roulet, A. 2005. Moxidectin pharmacodynamics, and resistance mechanisms to macrocyclic lactones in lab and field strains of nematode parasites. Proceedings of the 20th International Conference of the World Association for the Advancement of Veterinary Parasitology, 16–20 October. Christchurch, New Zealand.

Pulliam, J. and Preston, J. 1989. Safety of ivermectin in target animals. In Ivermectin and Abamectin, edited by Campbell, W., pp. 149–161. Springer-Verlag, New York Inc., New York, USA.

Ranjan, S.; Trudeau, C.; Prichard, R.; Daigneault, J. and Rew, R. 1997. Nematode reinfection following treatment of cattle with doramectin and ivermectin. Veterinary Parasitology 72, 25–31.

Reinemeyer, C. and Courtney, C. 2001. Antinematodal drugs. In Veterinary Pharmacology and Therapeutics, 8th, edited by Adams, H. R. pp. 947–979. Ames, IA: Iowa State University Press, USA.

Roulet, A.; Puel, O; Gesta, S.; Lepage, J.; Drag, M.; Soll, M.; Alvinerie, M.. and Pineau, T. 2003. MDR1-deficient genotype in collie dogs hypersensitive to the P-glycoprotein substrate ivermectin. European Journal of Pharmacology 460, 85–91.

Sallovitz, J.; Lifschitz, A.; Imperiale, F.; Pis, A.; Virkel, G. and Lanusse, C. 2002. Breed differences on the plasma availability of moxidectin administered pour-on to calves. The Veterinary Journal 164, 47–53.

Sallovitz, J.; Lifschitz, A.; Imperiale, F.; Virkel, G. and Lanusse, C. 2003. A detailed assessment of the pattern of moxidectin tissue distribution after pour-on treatment in calves. Journal of Veterinary Pharmacology and Therapeutics 26, 397–404.

Sallovitz, J.; Lifschitz, A.; Imperiale, F.; Virkel, G.; Larghi, J. and Lanusse, C. 2005. Doramectin concentration profiles in the gastrointestinal tract of topically treated calves: influence of animal licking restriction. Veterinary Parasitology 133, 61–70.

Sangster, N. and Gill, J. 1999. Pharmacology of anthelmintic resistance. Parasitology Today 15, 141–146.

Sarasola, P.; Jernigan, A.; Walker, D.; Castledine, J.; Smith, D. and Rowan, T. 2002. Pharmacokinetics of selamectin following intravenous, oral and topical administration in cats and dogs. Journal of Veterinary Pharmacology and Therapeutics 25, 265–272.

Schinkel, A.; Smit, J.; van Tellingen, O.; Beijnen, J.; Wagenaar, E.; van Deemter, L.; Mol, C.; van der Valk, M.; Robanus-Maandag, E.;

te Riele, H. et al. 1994. Disruption of the mouse mdr1a P-glycoprotein gene leads to a deficiency in the blood-brain barrier and to increased sensitivity to drugs. Cell 77, 491–502.

Scott, E.; Kinabo, L. and McKellar, Q. 1990. Pharmacokinetics of ivermectin after oral or percutaneous administration to adult milking goats. Journal of Veterinary Pharmacology and Therapeutics 13, 432–435.

Sheriff, J; Kotze, A.; Sangster, N. and Hennessy, D. 2005. Effect of ivermectin on feeding by *Haemonchus contortus* in vivo. Veterinary Parasitology 128, 341–346.

Shoop, W.; Egerton, J.; Eary, C.; Haines, H.; Michael, B.; Mrozik, H.; Eskola, P.; Fisher, M.; Slayton, L.; Ostlind, D.; Skelly, B.; Fulton, R.; Barth, D.; Costa, S.; Gregory, L.; Campbell, W.; Seward, R. and Turner, M. 1996. Eprinomectin: a novel avermectin for use as a topical endectocide for cattle. International Journal for Parasitology 26, 1227–1235.

Shoop, W.; Mrozik, H. and Fisher, M. 1995a. Structure and activity of avermectins and milbemycins in animal health. Veterinary Parasitology 59, 139–156.

Shoop, W.; Ostlind, D.; Rohrer, S.; Mickle, G.; Haines, H.; Michael, B.; Mrozik, H. and Fisher, M. 1995b. Avermectins and milbemycins against *Fasciola hepatica*: in vivo drug efficacy and in vitro receptor binding. International Journal for Parasitology 25, 923–927.

Shoop, W. and Soll, M. 2002. Chemistry, pharmacology and safety of the macrocyclic lactones: Ivermectin, abamectin and eprinomectin. In Macrocyclic Lactones in Antiparasitic Therapy, edited by Vercruysse, R. and Rew, R., pp. 1–29. CABI Publishing, Wallingford, UK.

Strong, L. 1993. Overview: the impact of avermectins on pastureland ecology. Veterinary Parasitology 48, 3–17.

Strong, L. and Wall, R. 1994. Effects of ivermectin and moxidectin on the insects of cattle dung. Bulletin of Entomological Research 84, 403–409.

Suarez, V.; Lifschitz, A.; Sallovitz, J. and Lanusse, C. 2003. Effects of ivermectin and doramectin faecal residues on the invertebrate colonization of cattle dung. Journal of Applied Entomology 127, 481–488.

Takiguchi, Y.; Mishima, H.; Okuda, M.; Terao, M.; Aoki, A.; Fukuda, R. 1980. Milbemycins, a new family of macrolide antibiotics: fermentation, isolation and physico-chemical properties. Journal of Antibiotics 33, 1120–1127.

Toutain, P.; Upson, D.; Terhune, T. and McKenzie, M. 1997. Comparative pharmacokinetics of doramectin and ivermectin in cattle. Veterinary Parasitology 72, 3–8.

Vercruysse, J.; Claerebout, E.; Dorny, P.; Demeulenaere, D. and Deroover, E. 1997. Persistence of the efficacy of pour-on and injectable moxidectin against *Ostertagia ostertagi* and *Dictyocaulus viviparus* in experimentally infected cattle. The Veterinary Record 140, 64–66.

Vercruysse, J.; Dorny, P.; Claerebout, E.; Demeulenaere, D.; Smets, K. and Agneessens, J. 2000. Evaluation of the persistent efficacy of doramectin and ivermectin injectable against *Ostertagia ostertagi* and *Cooperia oncophora* in cattle. Veterinary Parasitology 89, 63–69.

Vercruysse, J. and Rew, R. 2002. Macrocyclic Lactones in Antiparasitic Therapy, CAB International, Wallingford, Oxon, UK.

Vermunt, J.; West, D. and Pomroy, W. 1995. Multiple resistance to ivermectin and oxfendazole in *Cooperia* species of cattle in New Zealand. The Veterinary Record 137, 43–5.

Wicks, S.; Kaye, B.; Weatherley, A.; Lewis, D.; Davinson, E.; Gibson, S. and Smith, D. 1993. Effect of formulation on the pharmacokinetics and efficacy of doramectin. Veterinary Parasitology 49, 17–26.

Wolstenholme, A.; Fairweather, I.; Prichard, R.; von Samson-Himmelstjerna, G. and Sangster, N. 2004. Drug resistance in veterinary helminths. Trends in Parasitology 20, 469–476.

Xiao, L.; Herd, R. and Majewski, G. 1994. Comparative efficacy of moxidectin and ivermectin against hypobiotic and encysted cyathostomes and other equine parasites. Veterinary Parasitology 53, 83–90.

Zulalian, J.; Stout, S.; daCunha, A.; Garces, T. and Miller, P. 1994. Absorption, tissue distribution, metabolism, and excretion of moxidectin in cattle. Journal of Agricultural and Food Chemistry 42, 381–387.

CHAPTER

43

ANTIPROTOZOAN DRUGS

JENNIFER L. DAVIS AND JODY L. GOOKIN

Numerous chemotherapeutic agents are known to possess activity against parasitic protozoa (Tables 43.1 43.2). Although antiprotozoal activity is characteristic of many different chemical groups, most possess a rather narrow spectrum of activity. This is in contrast to antibacterial agents, which are effective against a wide variety of organisms. This chapter presents the clinically relevant antiprotozoan drugs used against the more important protozoal disease agents of domesticated animals.

TABLE 43.1 Summary of drugs used to treat selected protozoal diseases in animals

Protozoal Disease	Protozoa	Species	Drug Class	Drug and Dosing Regimen
Giardiasis	*Giardia duodenalis, G. intestinalis, G. lambia*	Dogs	Nitroimidazoles	Metronidazole: 12–15 mg/kg PO q12h for 8 days Tinidazole: 15 mg/kg PO q12h
			Benzimidazoles	Albendazole: 25 mg/kg q12h for 2 days Fenbendazole: 50 mg/kg q24h for 3 days Febantel, pyrantel, and praziquantal: febantel (26.8–35.2 mg/kg), pyrantel (26.8–35.2 mg/kg), praziquantel (5.4–7 mg/kg) PO q24h for 1–3 days
		Cats	Nitroimidazoles	Metronidazole: 22–25 mg/kg PO q12h for 5–7 days Tinidazole: 15 mg/kg PO q24h
			Benzimidazoles	Fenbendazole: 50 mg/kg q24h for 5 days Febantel, pyrantel, and praziquantal: febantel (56.5 mg/kg), pyrantel (11.3 mg/kg), and praziquantel (37.8 mg/kg) PO q24h for 5 days
		Horses	Nitroimidazoles	Metronidazole: 5 mg/kg PO q8h for 10 days
		Cattle	Benzimidazoles	Albendazole: 20 mg/kg PO q24h for 3 days Fenbendazole: 5–20 mg/kg PO q24h for 3 days
			Aminoglycosides	Paromomycin: 75 mg/kg PO q24h for 5 days
Trichomoniasis	*Tritrichomonas foetus, Pentatrichomonas hominis, Trichomonas gallinae*	Cats	Nitroimidazoles	Tinidazole: 30 mg/kg PO q24h for 14 days Ronidazole: 30 mg/kg PO q24h for 14 days
		Cattle	Nitroimidazoles	Metronidazole: 75 mg/kg IV q12h for 3 doses*
		Pigeons	Nitroimidazoles	Metronidazole: 40–60 mg/kg orally once a day for 5 days Ronidazole: 5 mg/kg orally once a day for 14 days Carnidazole: 20 mg/kg orally once
Trypanosomiasis	*Trypanosomas cruzi*	Dogs	Nitroimidazoles	Benznidazole: 5–7 mg/kg PO q24h for 2 months
			Nitrofurans	Nifurtimox: 2–7 mg/kg PO q6h for 3–5 months
		Cattle	Diamidene derivatives	Diminazene diaceturate: 3.5–7 mg/kg IM
Babesiosis	*Babesia divergens, B. equi, B. caballi, B. bigemini, B. canis*	Dogs	Tetracyclines	Doxycycline: 10 mg/kg PO q12h for 11 days (*B. canis*)
			Hydroxyquinolones and naphthoquinones	Atovaquone: 13.3 mg/kg PO q8h combine with azithromycin 10 mg/kg PO q24h for 10 consecutive days (*B. gibsoni*)
			Diamidene derivatives	Diminazene diaceturate: 3.5–5 mg/kg BW IM (*B. canis*); 3.5 mg/kg q12h for 2 treatments (*B. gibsoni*) Pentamidine isethionate: 16.5 mg/kg IM on 2 consecutive days Phenamidine isethionate: 15–20 mg/kg SC q24h for 2 days (*B. gibsoni*); 8–13 mg/kg SC once (*B. canis*) Imidocarb dipropionate: 7.5 mg/kg SC (*B. canis*); 3.5 mg/kg diminazene followed by 6 mg/kg imidocarb on the following day (*B. canis*)

TABLE 43.1—*continued*

Protozoal Disease	Protozoa	Species	Drug Class	Drug and Dosing Regimen
		Horses	Tetracyclines	Chlortetracycline: 0.5–2.6 mg/kg IV q24h for 6 days (*B. equi*)
			Diamidene derivatives	Diminazene diaceturate: 3–5 mg/kg IM q12h for 2 treatments (*B. caballi*); 6–12 mg/kg IM (*B. equi*); 0.5 mg/kg IM (*B. bigemina*)
				Phenamidine isethionate: 8.8 mg/kg IM q12h for 2 treatments
				Amicarbalide: 8.8 mg/kg IM q12h for 2 treatments (*B. caballi*)
				Imidocarb dipropionate: 1–2 mg/kg IM q12h for 2 treatments (*B. caballi*); 4 mg/kg IM q72h for 4 treatments (*B. equi*)
		Cattle	Tetracyclines	Oxytetracycline: 20 mg/kg IM every 4 days for 3 weeks (*B. divergens*)
			Diamidene derivatives	Diminazene diaceturate: 3–5 mg/kg IM (*B. bigemina* and *B. bovis*)
				Pentamidine isethionate: 0.5–2 mg/kg SC
				Phenamidine isethionate: 8–13 mg/kg IM q12h for 2 treatments
				Amicarbalide: 5–10 mg/kg IM
				Imidocarb dipropionate: 1–3 mg/kg IM or SC
Cryptosporidiosis	*Cryptosporidium parvum*	Cats	Aminoglycosides	Paromomycin: 165 mg/kg PO q12h for 5 days**
			Nitrothiazole derivatives	Nitazoxanide: 75 mg/kg PO once
		Cattle	Aminoglycosides	Paromomycin: 12.5–50 mg/kg PO q24h for 12 days
			Azalides	Azithromycin: 1500–2000 mg/calf/day PO for 7 days
		Goats	Aminoglycosides	Paromomycin: 50 mg/kg PO q12h for 10 days
Leishmaniasis	*Leishmania donovani, L. infantum, L. chagasi*	Dogs	Pentavalent antimonials	Sodium stibogluconate: 30–50 mg/kg pentavalent antimony IV or SC q24h for 3–4 weeks
				Meglumine antimonate: 100 mg/kg IV or SC q24h for 3–6 weeks or 75 mg/kg SC q12h
				Liposomal meglumine antimonate: 9.8 mg/kg IM or SC q24h
Hepatozoonosis	*Hepatozoon americanum*	Dogs	Aminoglycosides	Paromomycin: 20–40 mg/kg IM q24h for 15–30 days
			Hydroxyquinolones and naphthoquinones	Decoquinate: feed additive (27.2 grams/pound of pre-mix) added to moist dog food at 0.5–1.0 tablespoons per 10 kg BW twice a day
			Triazene derivatives	Toltrazuril: 5–10 mg/kg PO q12h for 5–10 days
			DHFR/TS*** inhibitors	Trimethoprim-sulfadiazine: 15 mg/kg PO q12h combined with clindamycin 10 mg/kg PO q8h and pyrimethamine 0.25 mg/kg PO q12h for 14 days****
			Diamidene derivatives	Imidocarb dipropionate: 5–6 mg/kg BW SQ or IM every 2 weeks until gamonts are no longer present in blood smears
Theileriosis	*Theileria parva*	Cattle	Hydroxyquinolones and naphthoquinones	Parvaquone: 20 mg/kg IM once
				Buparvaquone: 2.5 mg/kg IM 1–2 times
			Alkaloids	Halofuginone: 1–2 mg/kg PO once
Equine Protozoal Myelitis	*Sarcocystis neurona*	Horses	Triazene derivatives	Diclazuril: 5 mg/kg PO q24h for 30 days
				Toltrazuril: 5 mg/kg PO q24h for 28 days
				Ponazuril: 5 mg/kg PO q24h for 28 days
			DHFR/TS inhibitors	Pyrimethamine: 1 mg/kg PO q24h combined with sulfadiazine 20–30 mg/kg PO q12h for 30 days after clinical signs plateau
			Nitrothiazole derivatives	Nitazoxanide: 11.36 mg/lb PO q24h for the first 5 days, followed by 22.72 mg/lb PO q24h for 23 days

TABLE 43.1—*continued*

Protozoal Disease	Protozoa	Species	Drug Class	Drug and Dosing Regimen
Neosporosis	*Neospora caninum*	Dogs	DHFR/TS inhibitors	Pyrimethamine: 0.25–0.5 mg/kg PO q12h combined with sulfadiazine 30 mg/kg PO q12h for 2–4 weeks
			Lincosamides	Clindamycin: 12.5–18.5 mg/kg PO q12h for 2–4 weeks
		Cattle	Triazene derivatives	Ponazuril: 20 mg/kg PO q24h for 6 days
Toxoplasmosis	*Toxoplasma gondii*	Dogs	DHFR/TS inhibitors	Pyrimethamine: 0.25–0.5 mg/kg PO q12h combined with sulfadiazine 30 mg/kg PO q12h for 2–4 weeks
			Lincosamides	Clindamycin: 3–13 mg/kg PO or IM q8h for 2 weeks or 10–20 mg/kg PO or IM q12h for 2 weeks
		Cats	DHFR/TS inhibitors	Pyrimethamine: 0.25–0.5 mg/kg PO q12h combined with sulfadiazine 30 mg/kg PO q12h for 2–4 weeks
			Lincosamides	Clindamycin: 10–12 mg/kg PO q12h for 4 weeks or 12.5–25 mg/kg IM q12h for 4 weeks
Coccidiosis	*Eimeria sp., Isospora sp.*	Dogs	DHFR/TS inhibitors	Ormetoprim/sulfadimethoxine: 11 mg/kg ormetoprim combined with 55 mg/kg sulfadimethoxine PO for up to 23 days
				Trimethoprim/sulfadiazine: 5–10 mg/kg trimethoprim combined with 25–50 mg/kg sulfadiazine PO q24h for 6 days to dogs over 4 kg; dogs under 4 kg BW are given half this dosage for 6 days
			Thiamidine derivatives	Amprolium: 100–200 mg total PO q24h for 7–12 days; in drinking water (sole source) at 30 ml (9.6% solution)/gal for up to 10 days; in food at 250–300 mg (20% powder) q24h for 7–10 days
			Sulfonamides	Sulfadimethoxine: 55 mg/kg PO q24h for 1 day, then 27.5 mg/kg PO q24h for 14–20 days
		Cats	Sulfonamides	Sulfadimethoxine: 55 mg/kg PO q24h for 1 day, then 27.5 mg/kg PO q24h for 14–20 days
			DHFR/TS inhibitors	Trimethoprim/sulfadiazine: 5–10 mg/kg trimethoprim combined with 25–50 mg/kg sulfadiazine PO q24h for 6 days to cats over 4 kg; cats under 4 kg BW are given half this dosage for 6 days.
			Thiamidine derivatives	Amprolium: 110–220 mg/kg PO q24h for 7–12 days; in drinking water (sole source) at 1.5 tsp (9.6% solution)/gal for up to 10–days; 150 mg/kg PO combined with sulfadimethoxine at 25 mg/kg PO q24h for 14 days.

*The use of nitroimidazoles in food-producing animals is strictly prohibited by the US FDA. Cattle receiving metronidazole should never enter the food chain.
**See text for discussion of toxicity.
***Dihydrofolate reductase/thyamidine synthase inhibitors.
****Regimen should be followed up with decoquinate therapy.

TABLE 43.2 Drugs licensed for the treatment of coccidiosis in food animals.*

Species	Drug	Trade name	Regulatory information
Chickens	Roxarsone	Ren-O-Sal®, Roxarsone 10% Type A Medicated Article, combination products available	Not for use in laying hens; 5-day slaughter withdrawal for noncombination products
	Decoquinate	Deccox® Type A Medicated Article, combination products available	Not for use in laying hens; no withdrawal necessary for noncombination products
	Clopidol	Cloyden 25®, combination products available	Not for use in laying hens; 5-day slaughter withdrawal for noncombination products
	Robenidine	Robenz®, combination products available	Not for use in laying hens; 5-day slaughter withdrawal for noncombination products
	Amprolium	Amprol 25%, CORID 25% Type A Medicated Article, combination products available	No withdrawal necessary for noncombination products

TABLE 43.2—*continued*

Species	Drug	Trade name	Regulatory information
	Dinitolmide	Zoamix®	Not for use in laying hens; no withdrawal necessary
	Nicarbazin	Nicarbazin, combination products available	Not for use in laying hens; 4-day slaughter withdrawal for noncombination products
	Halofuginone	Stenerol®, combination products available	Not for use in laying hens; 4-day slaughter withdrawal for noncombination products
	Lasalocid	Avatec®, combination products available	Not for use in laying hens; no withdrawal necessary for noncombination products
	Maduramicin	Cygro®	Not for use in laying hens; 5-day slaughter withdrawal for noncombination products
	Monensin	Coban®, combination products available	Not for use in laying hens; no withdrawal necessary
	Narasin	Monteban®, combination products available	Not for use in laying hens; no withdrawal necessary
	Semduramicin	Aviax®, combination products available	Not for use in laying hens; no withdrawal necessary for noncombination products
	Salinomycin	Bio–Cox®, Sacox®	Not for use in laying hens; no withdrawal necessary
	Diclazuril	Clinacox®, combination products available	Not for use in laying hens; no withdrawal necessary for noncombination products
	Ormetoprim/ sulfadimethoxine	Rofenaid®, combination products available	Not for use in laying hens; 5-day slaughter withdrawal for noncombination products
	Sulfamethazine	Sulmet® Drinking Water Solution	Not for use in laying hens; 10-day slaughter withdrawal for noncombination products
Turkeys	Roxarsone	Ren-O-Sal®, Roxarsone 10% Type A Medicated Article, combination products available	Not for use in laying animals; 5-day slaughter withdrawal for most products
	Clopidol	Cloyden 25®, combination products available	Not for use in laying animals; 5-day slaughter withdrawal for noncombination products
	Amprolium	Amprol 25%, CORID 25% Type A Medicated Article, combination products available	No withdrawal necessary for noncombination products
	Dinitolmide	Zoamix®	Not for use in laying animals; no withdrawal necessary
	Halofuginone	Stenerol®, combination products available	Not for use in laying animals; 7-day slaughter withdrawal for noncombination products
	Lasalocid	Avatec®, combination products available	Not for use in laying animals; no withdrawal necessary for noncombination products
	Monensin	Coban®, combination products available	Not for use in laying animals; no withdrawal necessary for noncombination products
	Diclazuril	Clinacox®, combination products available	Not for use in laying hens; no withdrawal necessary
	Ormetoprim/ sulfadimethoxine	Rofenaid®, combination products available	Not for use in laying animals; 5-day slaughter withdrawal for noncombination products
	Sulfamethazine	Sulmet® Drinking Water Solution	Not for use in laying hens; 10-day slaughter withdrawal for noncombination products
Cattle	Decoquinate	Deccox® Type A Medicated Article, combination products available	Not for use in lactating dairy cattle; approved for preruminating calves; no withdrawal necessary for noncombination products
	Amprolium	Amprol 25%, CORID 25% Type A Medicated Article, combination products available	Not for use in preruminating calves; 1-day slaughter withdrawal
	Sulfamethazine	Sulmet® Oblets, Sulfamethazine sustained release bolus	Not for use in lactating dairy cattle; 8–10-day slaughter withdrawal for individual products
	Sulfaquinoxaline	Sulfa-nox Liquid	Not for use in lactating dairy cattle; 10-day slaughter withdrawal for noncombination products

TABLE 43.2—*continued*

Species	Drug	Trade name	Regulatory information
Sheep	Decoquinate	Deccox® Type A Medicated Article, combination products available	Not for use in lactating sheep; no withdrawal necessary for noncombination products
	Lasalocid	Bovatec®, numerous others and combination products available	Not for use in breeding animals; no withdrawal necessary for noncombination products
Goats	Decoquinate	Deccox® Type A Medicated Article, combination products available	Not for use in lactating sheep; no withdrawal necessary for noncombination products
	Monensin	Rumensin®	Not for use in lactating sheep; no withdrawal necessary
Swine	Toltrazuril	Baycox®	Extralabel drug use, contact regulatory agencies for withdrawal times
Rabbits	Diclazuril	Clinicox®	Extralabel drug use, contact regulatory agencies for withdrawal times
	Lasalocid	Avatec/Bovatec®, numerous others and combination products available	No withdrawal necessary for noncombination products
	Sulfaquinoxaline	SQ 40% Medicated feed	10-day withdrawal
Pheasants	Amprolium	Amprol 25%, CORID 25% Type A Medicated Article, numerous others and combination products available	No withdrawal necessary for noncombination products
Chukar partridges	Lasalocid	Avatec/Bovatec®	No withdrawal up to 8 weeks of age
	Ormetoprim/ sulfadimethoxine	Rofenaid®	Not released into wild before 18 weeks and can be used only up to 8 weeks of age
Bobwhite quail	Monensin	Coban®, combination products available	Not for use in laying hens; no withdrawal necessary
	Salinomycin	Bio-Cox®, Sacox®	No withdrawal necessary
Ducks	Ormetoprim/ sulfadimethoxine	Rofenaid®	Not for use in breeding animals or animals producing eggs for human consumption; 5-day slaughter withdrawal

Please see text for further explanation of dosing and toxicities. Regulatory information is applicable to drugs used in the United States, and is current only as of the writing of this chapter. Please consult the label directions on all products prior to administration because extralabel use of feed additives is prohibited by the US FDA.

NITROIMIDAZOLES

Spectrum: *Giardia, Balantidium, Entamoeba histolytica, Tritrichomonas foetus, Pentatrichomonas hominis, Trichomonas gallinae, Histomonas maleagridis, Trypanosomas sp.*

Drugs included: metronidazole, tinidazole, ronidazole, dimetridazole, ornidazole, carnidazole, benznidazole, and ipronidazole (Fig. 43.1).

Many of these important agents were used in the treatment of poultry flagellates, and all except metronidazole and tinidazole have been removed from the market in the United States. Nitroimidazoles are suspected mutagens and carcinogens; therefore their use in food-producing animals has been strictly prohibited by the US FDA. (Legal control of veterinary drugs is discussed in more detail in Chapter 56.) For companion animals, metronidazole is the most commonly used agent in this group and the most studied.

It is convenient to think of the mode of action of nitroimidazoles as occurring in four successive steps (Finegold and Mathisen 1990). First is entry into the protozoan cell, second is reductive activation, third is toxic effect of reduced intermediates, and fourth is release of inactive end products. The protozoal toxicity is due to short-lived intermediates or free radicals that produce damage by interacting with DNA and possibly other molecules. The cytotoxic intermediates decompose to nontoxic and inactive compounds.

METRONIDAZOLE. Metronidazole (Flagyl® and generic) is a weak base that is moderately lipophilic. It has a low molecular weight compared to other drugs (MW 171), which facilitates penetration across membranes. The oral absorption in most animals is almost complete and it

Name	Chemical name (Empirical formula) [Molecular weight]	Chemical structure
Dimetridazole	1,2-dimethyl-5-nitro-1*H*-imidazole ($C_5H_7N_3O_2$) [141.13]	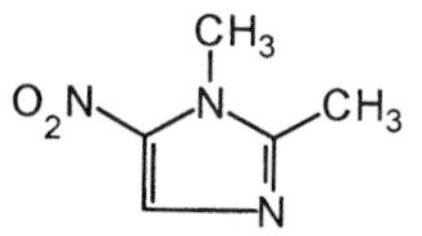
Ipronidazole	1-methyl-2-(1-methylethyl)-5-nitro-1*H*-imidazole ($C_7H_{11}N_3O_2$) [169.18]	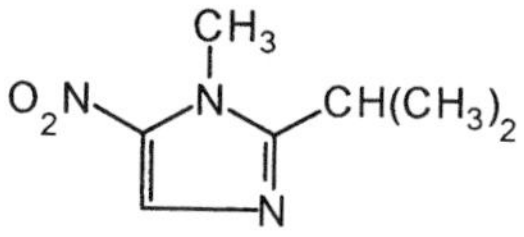
Metronidazole	1-(2-hydroxyethyl)-2-methyl-5-nitroimidazole ($C_6H_9N_3O_3$) [171.16]	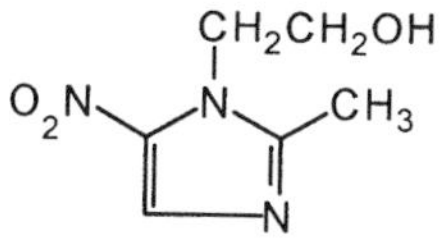
Ronidazole	1-methyl-2-[(carbamoyloxy)methyl]-5-nitroimidazole ($C_6H_8N_4O_4$) [200.16]	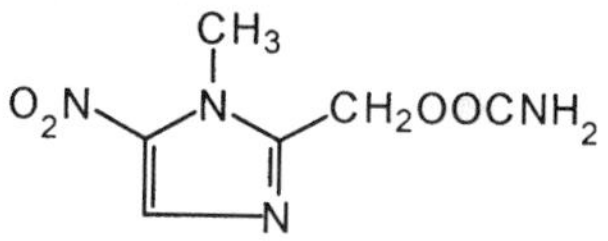
Tinidazole	1-[2-(ethylsufonyl)ethyl]-2-methyl-5-nitro-1*H*-imidazole ($C_8H_{13}N_3O_4S$) [247.26]	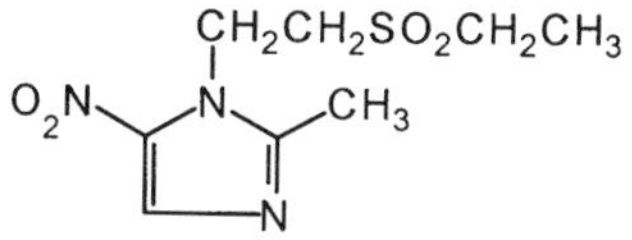

FIG. 43.1 Nitroimidazoles.

reaches high concentrations in the tissues; therefore it is active against both luminal and extraluminal protozoa (Finch and Snyder 1986). Bioavailability of metronidazole is good in most species. In the horse, the bioavailability ranges from 75–85% (Steinman et al. 2000; Sweeney et al. 1986), and in the dog, it is reported to be 60–100% (Neff-Davis et al. 1981). It has a half-life of about 6–8 hours, and less than 20% binds to plasma proteins. It is metabolized in the liver by oxidation and glucuronide formation and is excreted primarily by the kidneys. Small amounts may be found in saliva and breast milk (Finch and Snyder 1986).

Metronidazole is usually well tolerated, but potential adverse reactions include glossitis, stomatitis, and nausea.

The most important adverse effect vomiting, neurotoxicosis, and neurotoxicity (Longhofer 1988). The reactions observed appear to be caused by inhibition of the gamma-aminobutyric acid (GABA) neurotransmitter. At high doses (67–129 mg/kg/day) metronidazole has caused ataxia, lethargy, proprioceptive deficits, nystagmus, and seizurelike signs in dogs. Dogs have recovered if drug administration was discontinued, but it may require 1 to 2 weeks (Dow 1988, 1989). However, when diazepam was administered as a treatment, recovery was much faster (Evans et al. 2003). Neurotoxicosis also has been observed in cats with high doses.

Metronidazole is notoriously unpalatable. This may create difficulty for administering to difficult-to-medicate pets (cats), may be challenging to administer to horses, and the aftertaste may be accompanied by a loss of appetite.

Metronidazole Benzoate. In an attempt to provide a more palatable formulation, compounding pharmacists have provided metronidazole as an ester of benzoic acid-metronidazole benzoate, also known as *benzoylmetronidazole*. This formulation, although not registered by the FDA, is available from compounding pharmacists and has been popular for use in cats. The oral absorption is 65% and it has a half-life in cats of approximately 5 hours (Sekis et al. 2009). Metronidazole base is soluble (10 mg/ml), and has moderate lipophilicity (logP −0.02 and log D −0.27 at pH 5 and above). By contrast, the benzoate form, which is an ester, is much less soluble but more lipophilic (log P value of 2.19; log D value of 2.19 at pH 5.0 and above). The lower solubility results in less drug dissolved in the saliva of cats and therefore does not produce the degree of unpleasant taste compared to the base. The lipophilicity allows for good oral absorption from the GI tract. At a dose of 20 mg/kg of metronidazole benzoate, which is equivalent to 12.4 mg/kg of metronidazole, concentrations following the oral dose in cats were above the MIC_{90} for most anaerobic bacteria for at least 12 hours and above 1 μg/ml (for more susceptible organisms) for at least 24 hours (Sekis et al. 2009). Although cats are sensitive to benzoic acid toxicity, at these dosages it is unlikely that administration of metronidazole benzoate will produce toxicosis in cats.

Clinical Use. Metronidazole is not registered for animal use, but is available as the base in capsules (375 mg), tablets (250 and 500 mg), or for injection as metronidazole hydrochloride in 500 mg vials

Cats. Metronidazole at a dose of 25 mg/kg orally, twice daily for 7 days has been shown to completely eliminate *Giardia* cyst shedding in cats known to be chronic shedders of a human isolate of *Giardia* (Scorza and Lappin 2004). Metronidazole was also effective in eliminating cyst shedding as well as diarrhea associated with naturally occurring *Giardia* infections at a dose of 22 mg/kg orally, twice daily for 5 days (Zimmer 1987).

Dogs. Metronidazole at a dose of 12–15 mg/kg orally, twice a day for 8 days is commonly prescribed for treatment of infections caused by *Giardia*, *Balantidium*, *Entamoeba*, and *P. hominis*.

Horses. Giardia infections in horses are rarely reported to cause disease; however, successful treatment has been accomplished with 5 mg/kg of metronidazole orally, three times a day for 10 days (Kirkpatrick and Skand 1985).

Cattle. Metronidazole has been used to treat trichomoniasis in bulls at a dose of 75 mg/kg IV q12h for up to three doses. Metronidazole (and related drugs) are strictly forbidden for use in food-producing animals. Due to regulatory issues, animals treated in this manner must never enter the food chain in the United States.

TINIDAZOLE. Tinidazole (Tindamax™, Simplotan®, or Fasigyn®) is a second-generation 5-nitroimidazole that is FDA approved for use in treating *T. vaginalis*, *Giardia* spp., and *Entamoeba histolytica* infections in people. Tinidazole is completely absorbed after oral administration in cats and dogs (Sarkiala et al. 1991), and has been shown to penetrate well into various tissues where drug concentrations are found to be similar to that in plasma (Wood et al. 1973). The apparent total plasma clearance of the drug is about twofold higher in dogs than in cats, resulting in an elimination half-life that is twice as long in cats (8.4 hours) than in dogs (4.4 hours) (Sarkiala et al. 1991). It is metabolized in the liver by hydroxylation and glucuronide conjugation and is excreted into both urine and feces. Tinidazole has been administered to dogs at doses up to 150 mg/kg body weight for 24 weeks without toxic or adverse reactions. Dosages of 450 mg/kg body weight may result in liver enzyme elevations in dogs. Toxicity data in cats has not been reported.

Clinical Use

Dogs and Cats. Tinidazole at a dose of 30 mg/kg orally once a day for 14 days has been shown to suppress shedding of *T. foetus* in experimentally infected cats (Gookin 2007). Based on studies in people, tinidazole is also likely to be effective for treatment of most infections amenable to metronidazole including *Giardia* infections in dogs and cats. Pharmacokinetic studies suggest that doses of 15 mg/kg orally twice a day for dogs or once a day for cats will produce concentrations at a level that is thought to be therapeutic.

RONIDAZOLE. Ronidazole is not registered for human or veterinary use in the United States; however, it is considered an effective treatment for *T. gallinae*, *Histomonas meleagridis*, and *T. foetus* infections. It has a tenfold higher in vivo activity against trichomonal infections compared to metronidazole (Miwa et al. 1986). The susceptibility of *Tritrichomonas foetus* has been reported in two studies

(Kather et al. 2007; Gookin et al. 2006). In the study by Gookin et al. (2006) ronidazole was the most active compound tested for in vitro activity.

Clinical Use

Cats. Ronidazole at a dose of 30 mg/kg orally twice a day for 14 days has been shown to eliminate shedding of *T. foetus* in experimentally infected cats (Gookin et al. 2006). The pharmacokinetics of ronidazole has been examined in cats after IV and oral administration (LeVine et al. 2008). It was rapidly absorbed after oral administration in cats with a long terminal half-life. Although neurotoxicity has been reported from administration to cats (Rosado et al. 2007), these reactions were associated with high doses. Current recommendation are to not exceed 30 mg/kg once daily in cats. However, based on the pharmacokinetic results cited above, once-daily administration should be considered in cats at risk of neurotoxicity. In a pharmacokinetic study in which ronidazole was administered intravenously (prepared from an aqueous compounded formulation) and orally, no adverse reactions in healthy cats were observed.

Pigeons. *T. gallinae* (pigeon canker) is generally treated with ronidazole (5 mg/kg orally once a day for 14 days), carnidazole (20 mg/kg orally once) or metronidazole (40–60 mg/kg orally once a day for 5 days).

BENZNIDAZOLE. Benznidazole has been shown to produce cures of acute trypanosomiasis in dogs with fewer side effects than nifurtimox.

Clinical Use

Dogs. Dogs are treated with 5–7 mg/kg BW benznidazole orally at 24-hour intervals for 2 months (Barr 2006).

PENTAVALENT ANTIMONIALS

Spectrum: *Leishmania* spp.

Drugs included: Sodium stibogluconate, meglumine antimonate (Fig. 43.2)

Pentavalent antimonials have been shown to inhibit topoisomerase in vitro (Lucumi et al. 1998) and thereby interfere with parasite replication. They also inhibit enzymes involved in the synthesis of nucleotides and inhibit phosphofructokinases, enzymes necessary for glycolytic and fatty acid oxidation (Baneth and Shaw 2002). The in vivo mode of action of the pentavalent antimonials is still unclear. The pharmacodynamics of these drugs are still debated, and it is not known whether a better clinical response would be achieved with higher peak plasma concentrations versus prolonged time above the minimum inhibitory concentration of the protozoa (Valladares et al. 1998). Increasing resistance to pentavalent antimony compounds has been documented in recent years, and their effectiveness appears to be decreasing. In general, canine visceral leishmaniasis is more difficult to treat than the human form of the disease. The use of pentavalent antimonials is contraindicated in patients with myocarditis, hepatitis, or nephritis. Both sodium stibogluconate and meglumine antimonate are administered on the basis of their antimony content.

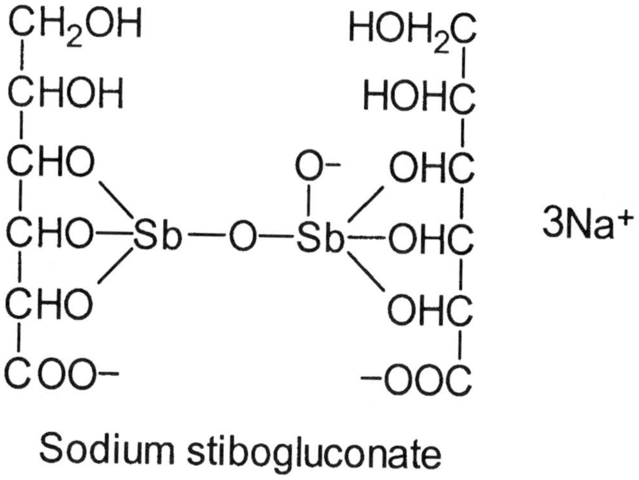

Sodium stibogluconate

FIG. 43.2

SODIUM STIBOGLUCONATE. Sodium Stibogluconate (Pentostam®) was made available in the United States from the Centers for Disease Control in 1968 for treatment of leishmaniasis in human beings (Fig. 43.2). It is in aqueous solution at a concentration of 330 mg/ml of agent, which is equivalent to 100 mg/ml pentavalent antimony. Clinical formulations consist of multiple uncharacterized molecular forms, some of which have higher molecular weights than the active compound. In human beings, most of a single dose of sodium stibogluconate is excreted by the kidneys in the urine within 24 hours regardless of whether it is given IV or IM. Antimony compounds are eliminated faster if given IM than SC or IV in dogs, and it is important to maintain serum levels of the compound to treat leishmaniasis. Pentavalent antimonials are relatively well tolerated. Adverse reactions include pain at the injection site, GI symptoms, delayed muscle pain, and joint stiffness.

Clinical Use

Dogs. Canine leishmaniasis is treated with sodium stibogluconate to deliver 30–50 mg/kg BW pentavalent antimony by either IV or SC administration at daily intervals for 3–4 weeks (Slappendel and Teske 1997). Relapses may occur a few months to a year after treatment and should be treated with another round of pentavalent antimony.

MEGLUMINE ANTIMONATE. Meglumine antimonate (Glucantime®) may be less likely to cause adverse effects than sodium stibogluconate. Adverse effects noted include lethargy, gastrointestinal disturbance, and injection site reactions, including muscle fibrosis and abscess formation with IM injection (Noli and Auxilia 2005). It is available in a solution that contains 300 mg/ml antimony. Bioavailability is approximately 92% after IM or SC administration, and 80% of the drug is excreted in the urine within the first 9 hours (Valladares et al. 1997).

Liposomal encapsulated formulations of meglumine antimonite (LMA) have also been tested in dogs. They reach higher plasma concentrations, have slower clearance, and have a higher volume of distribution than regular formulations (Valladares et al. 1997). They also reach good concentrations in the bone marrow of affected dogs. Compared to conventional formulations, a positive effect on plasma total protein and gammaglobulin concentrations was seen with the LMA formulation, with no relapses noted at 12 months after treatment. Although good results have been seen with this formulation, complete eradication of the parasite is unlikely to be achieved and the product may not be cost effective when compared to conventional formulations.

Clinical Use

Dogs. Canine leishmaniasis has been treated with meglumine antimonate given IV or SC at 100 mg/kg BW once daily for 3–6 weeks (Slappendel and Teske 1997). No advantage is provided by IV administration. Relapses will occur in long-term survivors and require retreatment. Alternatively, a dosing regimen of 75 mg/kg SC twice daily achieves higher peak concentrations and maintains detectable plasma concentrations for the entire dosing interval (Valladares et al. 1998). For liposomal encapsulated meglumine antimonite, a dose of 9.8 mg/kg q24h is recommended (Valladares et al. 2001).

ARSENICALS

Spectrum: Histomoniasis, coccidiosis

Drugs included: Arsenicals, carbarsone, nitarsone, and roxarsone

The exact antiprotozoal mechanism of action of arsenicals is not known, however these drugs are known to nonspecifically bind to disulphide moieties in proteins, thereby inhibiting many enzyme systems that use biological ligands containing available sulfhydral groups (Blum and Burri 2002). This mechanism is also thought to be related to the toxic effects of arsenic compounds on the host. These drugs continue to be administered to humans for treatment of African trypanosomiasis. These compounds were used at one time for the prevention and treatment of histomoniasis and coccidiosis in turkeys.

Clinical Use

Chickens and Turkeys. Nitarsone (Histostat-50®) is used as a feed additive for the prevention of histomoniasis in turkeys and chickens. It is not active if birds have been infected for more than 4 days. A 5-day withdrawal is required for nitarsone. Overdosing or lack of adequate water may result in leg weakness and paralysis in birds. Nitarsone is dangerous for ducks, geese, and dogs. Roxarsone is fed as a growth promotant and as a preventative for coccidiosis. A 5-day withdrawal is required for roxarsone. Like nitarsone, overdosing or lack of adequate water may result in leg weakness and paralysis in birds.

BENZIMIDAZOLES

Spectrum: Giardiasis

Drugs included: Albendazole, fenbendazole, febantel (Fig. 43.3).

The benzimidazoles are a group of agents that are widely used in the treatment of helminth parasites of large and small animals (Antihelmintics are discussed in detail in Chapters 40–42.) Some compounds in this group have excellent activity against *Giardia* spp. This group lacks or has little antibacterial activity and unlike other antigiardial agents is unlikely to interfere with intestinal microflora during treatment. The benzimidazoles are known to bind

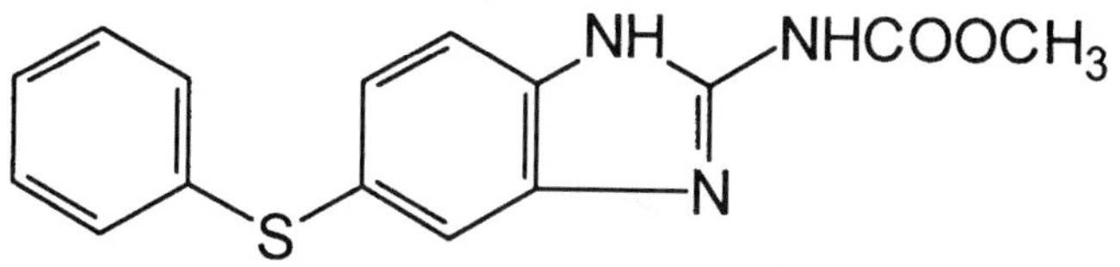

Fenbendazole
($C_{15}H_{13}N_3O_2S$)
[299.35]

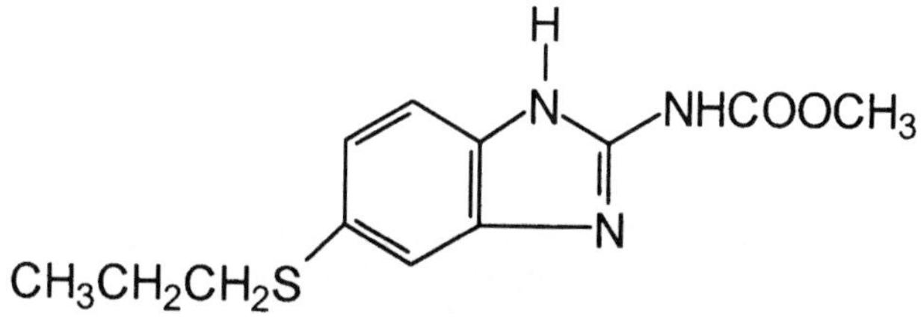

Albendazole
($C_{12}H_{15}N_3O_2S$)
[265.33]

FIG. 43.3

to β-tubulin subunits of microtubules and interfere with microtubule polymerization (Gardner and Hill 2001). This causes structural changes in *Giardia* trophozoites consistent with microtubule damage to the adhesive disk and internal microtubule cytoskeleton but not the external flagella.

ALBENDAZOLE. Albendazole (Valbazan®) is available in liquid and paste formulations. It is effective against *Giardia* sp. in human beings, mice, and dogs. Albendazole is poorly absorbed from the intestinal tract. Albendazole is potentially toxic, causing dose-dependent and idiosyncratic myelosuppression in dogs and cats respectively (Stokol et al. 1997). It is potentially teratogenic so it should not be given to pregnant animals. Its use in cats is not recommended.

Clinical Use

Dogs. Dogs treated orally with albendazole at 25 mg/kg BW every 12 hours for 2 days cleared *Giardia* cysts from their feces (Barr et al. 1993). A single oral 25 mg/kg BW treatment was not effective in clearing cysts from the feces of dogs. None of 32 dogs treated for giardiasis with albendazole developed adverse reactions (Barr et al. 1993).

Cattle. Albendazole given at 20 mg/kg BW orally for 3 days reduced *Giardia* cyst production by >90% in naturally infected calves (Xiao et al. 1996).

FENBENDAZOLE. Fenbendazole (Panacur®, Safeguard®, Axilur®) is available in numerous preparations as a paste, suspension, or granules. Side effects with this drug are rare; however, vomiting and diarrhea may occur in small animals. Pancytopenia has been reported in a dog following fenbendazole administration (Gary et al. 2004). The changes were reversible with discontinuation of therapy.

Clinical Use

Dogs. Fenbendazole is effective against *Giardia* organisms in dogs if given at 50 mg/kg BW every 24 hours for 3 days (Zajac et al. 1998). More frequent dosing at 50 mg/kg BW orally every 8 hours was as effective as every 24 hours, and no adverse effects were noted (Barr et al. 1994a).

Cats. Fenbendazole at 50 mg/kg BW every 24 hours for 5 days was effective in eliminating the shedding of *Giardia* cysts in 4/8 cats coinfected with *Cryptosporidium* (Keith et al. 2003).

Cattle. Fenbendazole is also effective against *Giardia* organisms in calves when given orally at 5–20 mg/kg BW every 24 hours for 3 days (O'Handley et al. 1997; Xiao et al. 1996).

FEBANTEL. Febantel(Drontal-Plus®) is a benzimidazole available in a combination product with pyrantel pamoate and praziquantel for the treatment of intestinal nematodes and cestodes in dogs and cats. Febantel is metabolized by the liver to fenbendazole and oxfendazole.

Clinical Use

Dogs. This combination has been shown to be effective against canine giardiasis when given orally, once daily for 1–3 days to provide praziquantel (5.4 to 7 mg/kg), pyrantel pamoate (26.8 to 35.2 mg/kg), and febantel (26.8 to 35.2 mg/kg) (Barr et al. 1998; Giangaspero et al. 2002). Strict hygiene to prevent reinfection is imperative to maximize treatment success (Payne et al. 2002).

Cats. The combination product of febantel, pyrantel, and praziquantal was shown to be effective at decreasing *Giardia* cyst shedding in naturally infected kittens at doses of 56.5 mg/kg, 11.3 mg/kg, and 37.8 mg/kg, respectively, orally once a day for 5 days (Scorza et al. 2006). In addition, kittens treated at these doses were resistant to recrudescent shedding of oocysts following administration of methylprednisolone.

AMINOGLYCOSIDES

Spectrum: Giardiasis, luminal amoebiasis, leishmaniasis, cryptosporidiosis

Drugs included: Paromomycin (Fig. 43.4).

PAROMOMYCIN. Paromomycin (Aminosidine®) is an aminoglycoside antibiotic that is produced by *Streptomyces rimosus.* Paromomycin interferes with bacterial protein synthesis by binding to 16S rRNA at the amino-acyl-tRNA binding site, which causes a conformational change and subsequent misreading of the mRNA and inhibition of translocation (Fourmy et al. 1998). Its anti-*Leishmania* mode of action is not known, but it has been suggested that it interferes with parasite mitochondrial activity (Maarouf et al. 1997).

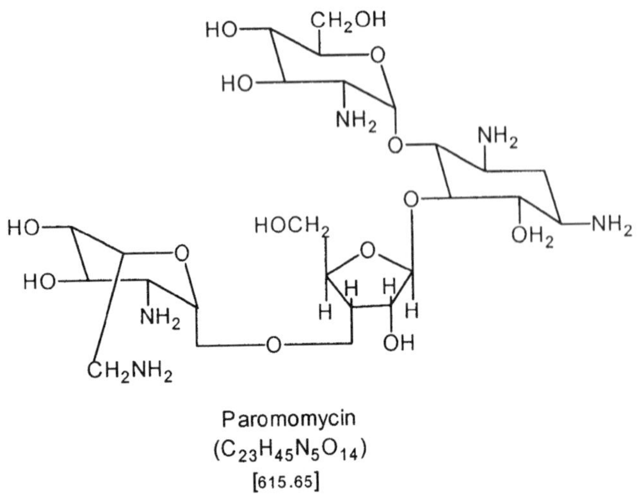

Paromomycin is used in the treatment of luminal amoebiasis, leishmaniasis, and cryptosporidiosis. It has also been used in humans for the treatment of resistant giardiasis. It is poorly absorbed following oral administration, which leads to high intestinal luminal concentrations of the drug. Paromomycin has little activity against intestinal bacteria. Side effects include nausea, vomiting, abdominal cramps, and diarrhea. Although little is absorbed from the intestinal tract, it is eliminated via the kidneys, so its use is contraindicated in patients with renal disease. It is possible that in animals with intestinal disease, the mucosal barrier may be breached to produce more systemic absorption and potential for systemic toxicity. This may have contributed to toxicity in four cats in one clinical study (Gookin et al. 1999). It also has the potential to cause reversible and irreversible vestibular, cochlear, and renal toxicity when given parenterally. Paromomycin levels peak in the serum of dogs at 30 μg/ml about 60 minutes after IM or SC administration of a 15 mg/kg BW dose (Belloli et al. 1996). About 4% is bound to serum proteins.

HO CH2OH O HO NH2 O NH2 O HO HOCH2 OH2 NH2 HO O O HO H H H H NH2 O OH CH2NH2

Paromomycin
($C_{23}H_{45}N_5O_{14}$)
[615.65]

FIG. 43.4

Clinical Use

Dogs. Paromomycin given IM at 20 mg/kg BW daily for 15 days will greatly improve clinical signs of visceral leishmaniasis in dogs (Vexenat et al. 1998). However, relapses may occur within 50–100 days. Treatment with 40 mg/kg IM once daily for 30 days may enhance the cure rate of dogs (Vexenat et al. 1998). If paromomycin is administered SC with antimony, there is no effect on the pharmacokinetics of paromomycin but there is a marked effect on the pharmacokinetics of antimony (Belloli et al. 1995). Serum levels of antimony remain higher, and the dose should be adjusted to prevent toxic levels of the metal from appearing in the blood.

Cats. A naturally infected cat with cryptosporidial diarrhea was successfully treated with oral paromomycin given at 165 mg/kg BW orally every 12 hours for 5 days (Barr et al. 1994b). As mentioned previously, it can be toxic in cats if systemic absorption occurs owing to intestinal barrier disruption. It resulted in acute renal failure, deafness, and hypermature cataract formation when given orally to four cats with *T. foetus* infection at doses as low as 70 mg/kg BW every 12 hours for 4 days (Gookin et al. 1999).

Cattle. For cryptosporidiosis, when administered at 12.5–25 mg/kg PO to calves, it delayed the onset of shedding and decreased the number of oocysts shed, while a dose of 50 mg/kg prevented oocyst shedding. Treatment of calves with oral paromomycin at 50, 25, or 12.5 mg/kg BW twice daily was effective in preventing oocyst production (50 mg/kg dose) or in delaying the onset of oocyst production and in greatly reducing the numbers of oocysts excreted (12.5–25 mg/kg BW doses) when started 1 day before inoculation and continued for 10 days after inoculation (Fayer and Ellis 1993). For giardiasis, a dose of 75 mg/kg orally, once daily for 5 days caused a 100% reduction in cyst shedding at 9 days after initiation of treatment (Geurden et al. 2006).

Goats. Treatment of 2- to 4-day-old goat kids with oral paromomycin at 50 mg/kg BW twice daily for 10 days was effective in preventing cryptosporidiosis (Mancassola et al. 1995).

Paromomycin may also have a role in treating or preventing the spread of cryptosporidiosis outbreaks in calves and goats. The anticryptosporidial activity of paromomycin apparently does not involve trafficking through the host cell cytoplasm but involves movement of the agent through altered apical membranes that surround the developing parasites (Griffiths et al. 1998). Paromomycin does not exert its effects on extracellular stages of *C. parvum* (Griffiths et al. 1998). There are no products containing paromomycin approved for use in food-producing animals in the United States; therefore, all use would be considered extralabel.

NITROFURANS

Spectrum: *Trypanosomas cruzi*

Drugs included: Nifurtimox (Fig. 43.5).

NIFURTIMOX. Nifurtimox (Lampit®) is a nitrofuran derivative that is the most widely used agent for the treatment of human *Trypanosoma cruzi* infections (Van Reken and Pearson 1990) and is effective against natural and experimental disease in dogs (Barr 2006). It is marketed as 100 mg tablets, but in the United States, must be obtained from the Centers for Disease Control. Mutagenicity and carcinogenicity of these compounds have been documented in laboratory animals; therefore, their use in food-producing animals, including the use of topical products, is strictly prohibited by the US FDA. (Legal control of veterinary drugs is discussed in Chapter 56.)

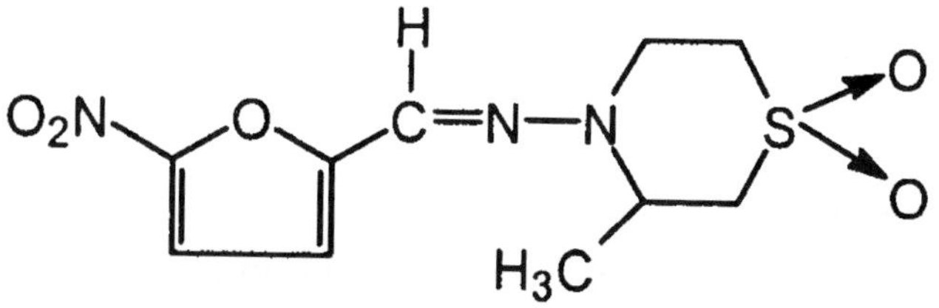

O_2N–(furan)–C(H)=N–N(thiomorpholine ring, H_3C, S→O, S→O)

Nifurtimox
($C_{10}H_{13}N_3O_5S$)
[287.29]

FIG. 43.5

Its likely mode of action is through the production of activated forms of oxygen. It is reduced to the nitro anion radical in the presence of pyridine nucleotides. The anion then reacts with oxygen to produce superoxide and regeneration of nifurtimox (Finch and Snyder 1986). This cycle continues, and the activated oxygen molecules exert their toxic effects on the parasites. This cycle is thought to be initiated by the enzyme trypanothione reductase. It has activity against amastigote and trypomastigote stages.

In human beings, nifurtimox is well absorbed after oral administration, but only low concentrations of the parent compound are found in the plasma and little is found in the tissues or urine (Webster 1990). It is excreted in the urine in the form of metabolites. Adverse side effects occur in up to 50% of human beings treated and are associated with GI and central nervous system signs.

Clinical Use

Dogs. Canine *T. cruzi* infections are treated with 2–7 mg/kg BW nifurtimox orally at 6-hour intervals for 3–5 months (Barr 2006). This is effective in preventing death from acute disease and extending life, but most dogs will still develop chronic cardiac disease, which is usually fatal (Barr 2006). Improved survival has been shown in dogs concurrently treated with antiinflammatory doses of glucocorticoids (Andrade et al. 1980).

TETRACYCLINES

Spectrum: Amoebae, flagellates, piroplasms, ciliates

Drugs included: Oxytetracycline, chlortetracycline, doxycycline

Tetracyclines represent a broad group of antiprotozoal agents, some of which have activity against amoebae, mucosal flagellates, piroplasms, and ciliates. (Chapter 35 of this book has more detailed description of the pharmacology of tetracyclines.)

Clinical Use

Cattle. A long-acting formulation of oxytetracycline (LA/200) is useful in prophylaxis of bovine *Babesia divergens* infection if 20 mg/kg BW is given IM every 4 days for 3 weeks after exposure; 10–15 mg/kg BW given IM every 4 days causes moderation in the clinical signs (Kuttler 1988). Tetracyclines can also be used to treat *Theileria* infections in cattle but are less effective and must be given in large doses early in the infection and used for longer periods of treatment. Product label for chlortracycline medicated feed includes control if active infection is caused by *Anaplasma marginale*. Oxytetracycline has been used in cattle for treatment of *Anaplasma marginale* infections. However, efficacy has been questionable. One study compared enrofloxacin (5 mg/kg IV q24h for 5 days), imidocarb (5 mg/kg IM twice, 7 days apart), or oxytetracycline (22 mg/kg IV q24h for 5 days) for elimination of persistent *Anaplasma marginale* infections in cattle. None of the tested treatments reliably eliminated persistent *A. marginale* infections in all cattle (Coetzee et al. 2006).

Horses. Chlortetracycline may be effective against *Babesia equi* infection in horses if 0.5–2.6 mg/kg BW is given IV daily for 6 days early in the infection (Kuttler 1988).

Dogs. Doxycycline is effective at preventing clinical manifestations of *Babesia canis* infection if given at 10 mg/kg BW twice daily for 11 days (Vercammen et al. 1996).

HYDROXYQUINOLONES AND NAPHTHOQUINONES

Spectrum: *Coccidia*, *Babesia* sp., *Hepatozoon americanum*, *Theileria* sp., *Cytauxzoon* sp., *T. gondii*, *Eimeria* sp., malaria, *Pneumocystis carnii*.

Drugs included: Decoquinate, atovaquone, parvaquone, buparvaquone (Fig. 43.6).

The quinolone anticoccidials inhibit coccidial respiration by interfering with cytochrome-mediated electron transport in the parasites' mitochondria. The site of action of quinolone anticoccidials is probably within the bc1 complex, where the electrons are transferred from ubiquinone to cytochrome c. These compounds are coccidiostatic and allow penetration of sporozoites, but not development. These inhibited sporozoites have the ability to resume development after the agents are removed. Little anticoccidial immunity develops in chickens on these medications.

DECOQUINATE. Decoquinate (Deccox®) is one of the quinolone (4-hydroxyquinolones) anticoccidials. It is poorly absorbed from the intestinal tract, and what is absorbed is rapidly cleared from the blood and tissues. Recent evidence indicates that decoquinate can have an anticoccidial effect on first-generation schizonts of *E. tenella*, adversely affect sporulation, and permit the development of immunity if fed at levels that are lower than its coccidiostatic levels (Williams 1997). Activity against cryptosporidium has also been demonstrated in cattle and sheep.

Clinical Use

Chickens. Decoquinate is used for prevention of coccidiosis in broilers. It should be fed for at least 28 days when development of coccidiosis is likely. Do not feed to laying chickens. No withdrawal is required.

Cattle. In cattle, decoquinate is used to prevent coccidiosis when fed for at least 28 days, but it is prohibited to feed to lactating dairy cows. In beef cattle, no withdrawal time is required.

For treatment of cryptosporidiosis, doses of 2 mg/kg were not effective at decreasing oocyst shedding or clinical signs in experimentally challenged calves (Moore et al. 2003). However, treatment of pregnant cows with 1.25 mg/kg/day in the feed for 30 days prior to and for 8 days after parturition prevented clinical signs in the calves

Sheep. Decoquinate is fed to sheep to provide 0.5 mg/kg BW for at least 28 days to prevent coccidiosis. Do not feed to sheep producing milk for human consumption. No withdrawal is required.

Goats. Decoquinate is fed to goats to provide 0.5 mg/kg BW for at least 28 days to prevent coccidiosis. Do not feed

Name	Chemical name (Empirical formula) [Molecular weight]	Chemical structure
Buquinolate	4-hydroxy-6,7-diisobutoxy-3-quinolinecarboxylic acid ethyl ester ($C_{20}H_{27}NO_5$) [361.42]	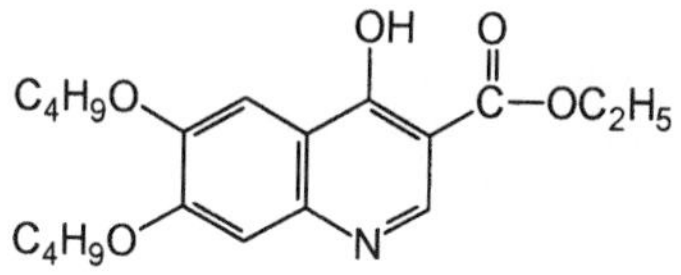
Decoquinate	6-declyoxy-ethoxy-4-hydroxy-3-quinolinecarboxylic acid ethyl ester ($C_{24}H_{35}NO_5$) [417.53]	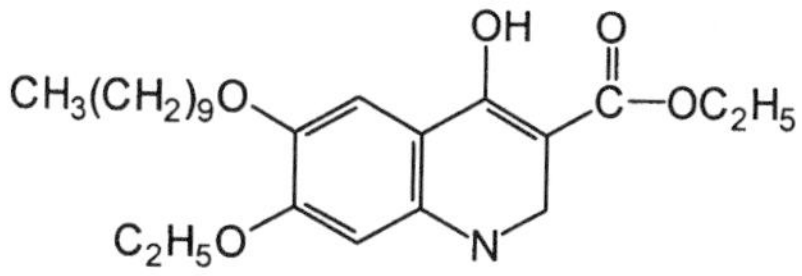
Nequinate	7-(benzyloxy)-6-*n*-butyl-1,4-dihydro-4-oxo-3-quinoline-carboxylic acid methyl ester ($C_{22}H_{23}NO_4$) [365.43]	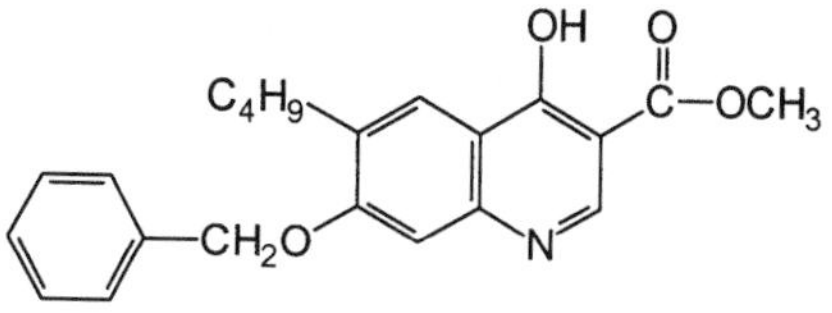
Buparvaquone	2-*trans*(4-*t*-butylcyclohexyl)methyl-3-hydroxy-1,4-naphthoquinone ($C_{21}H_{26}O_3$) [326.44]	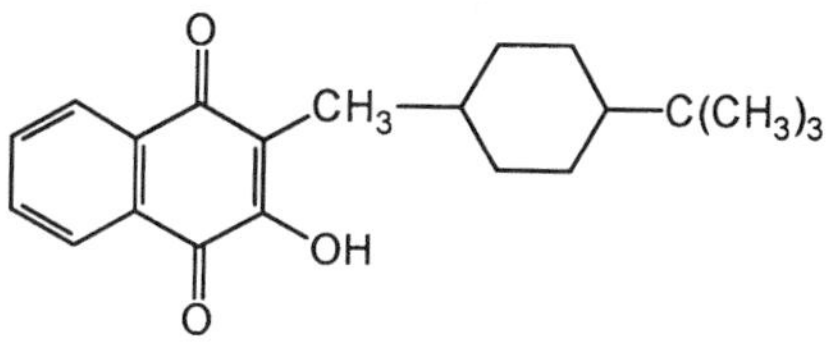
Parvaquone	2-cyclohexyl-3-hydroxy-1,4-naphthoquinone ($C_{16}H_{16}O_3$) [256.30]	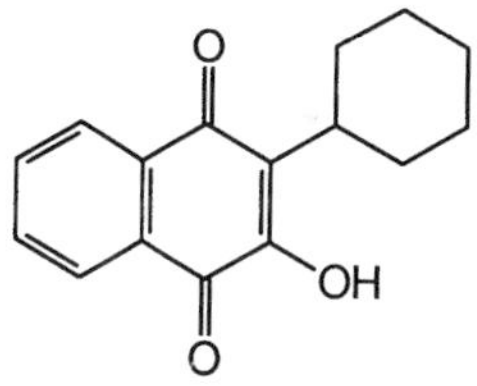
Atovaquone	2-[*trans*-4-(4-chlorophenyl)cyclohexyl]-3-hydroxy-1,4-naphthoquinone ($C_{22}H_{19}ClO_3$) [366.69]	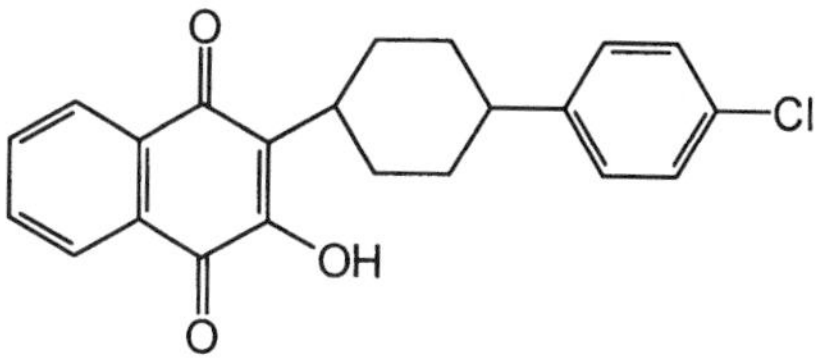

FIG. 43.6 Hydroxyquinolones and naphthoquinones.

to goats producing milk for human consumption. No withdrawal is required.

Dogs. For preventing clinical relapses of *Hepatozoon americanum* infection, decoquinate feed additive (27.2 grams decoquinate per pound of premix) can be added to moist dog food at a rate of 0.5–1.0 tablespoons per 10 kg BW twice a day (Macintire et al. 2001).

ATOVAQUONE. Atovaquone (Mepron® suspension) is a hydroxyquinolone that has broad-spectrum antiprotozoal activity. It is a yellow crystalline solid that is practically insoluble in water. Atovaquone is supplied as a bright yellow suspension of microfine particles at a concentration of 150 mg atovaquone/ml. It is highly lipophilic and administering it with food increases its absorption twofold. It was originally developed for human use to treat drug-resistant strains of malaria and *Pneumocystis carinii* pneumonia. It is discussed here because it was also found to have excellent activity against *T. gondii* and *Babesia* sp. It also has activity against *Eimeria* spp. Atovaquone is thought also to work via inhibition of electron transport at the mitochondrial bc1 complex because cross-resistance often develops between atovaquone and decoquinate (Pfefferkorn et al. 1993).

Clinical Use

Dogs. Atovaquone (13.3 mg/kg PO q8h) administered concurrently with azithromycin (10 mg/kg PO q24h) for 10 consecutive days was shown to completely eliminate *Babesia gibsoni* infection from 8 of 10 dogs treated (Birkenheuer et al. 2004). The dogs in that study had previously been treated unsuccessfully with imidocarb or diminazene.

PARVAQUONE AND BUPARVAQUONE. Parvaquone (Clexon®) and buparvaquone (Butalex®) are naphthoquinones that are used for the treatment of theileriosis. They act on the macroschizonts and intraerythrocytic piroplasms.

Theileriosis is a severe disease of cattle in Africa and is caused by *Theileria parva*, a piroplasm. Several *Theileria* spp. infect wild ruminants in the United States, but none of these causes serious illness.

Clinical Use

Cattle. Parvaquone is administered IM at 20 mg/kg BW as a single treatment for theileriosis. Buparvaquone is given IM at 2.5 mg/kg BW for 1–2 treatments. Both drugs are considered curative for *Theileria* infections in cattle.

Cats. Parvaquone and buparvaquone have been used to treat *Cytauxzoon felis* infections in cats, although their efficacy is questionable (Kier 1990).

PYRIDINOLS

Spectrum: Coccidiosis, *Leucocytozoon* sp.
Drugs included: Clopidol (Fig. 43.7)

CLOPIDOL. Clopidol (Coyden 25®) is the only pyridinol to be used as an anticoccidial. It is practically insoluble in water. It is active against the sporozoite stage, allowing host cell penetration but not parasite development. It also has activity against second-generation schizogony, gametogony, and sporulation. Sporozoites can resume development after the medication is removed. Little anticoccidial immunity develops in chickens receiving this agent. Long (1993) suggested that the mode of action of clopidol was similar to that of the quinolone anticoccidials because of similar structure and biological activity of the agents. However, cross-resistance between clopidol and quinolone anticoccidials does not occur (Long 1993).

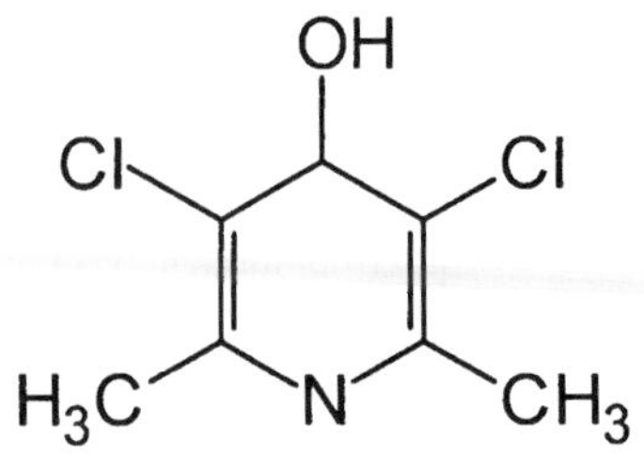

OH
Cl Cl
H_3C N CH_3

Clopidol
($C_7H_7Cl_2NO$)
[192.06]

FIG. 43.7

Clinical Use

Chickens and Turkeys. Clopidol is fed at 0.0125–0.0250% for prevention of coccidiosis. A 5-day withdrawal is required if the 0.0250% level is used. This level may be lowered to 0.0125% 5 days before withdrawal and fed. Clopidol is transmitted to the eggs of hens that are fed clopidol-containing diets (Long 1971). Clopidol is used for prevention of coccidiosis in turkeys and fed at 0.0125–0.0250%. A 5-day withdrawal is required. Clopidol is also approved for the prevention of *Leucocytozoon smithi* infections in turkeys when fed at its anticoccidial levels.

GUANIDINE DERIVATIVES

Spectrum: Coccidiosis.
Drugs included: Robenidine (Fig. 43.8).

ROBENIDINE. Robenidine (Cycostat®, Robenz®) is a synthetic anticoccidial derivative of guanidine. It is active

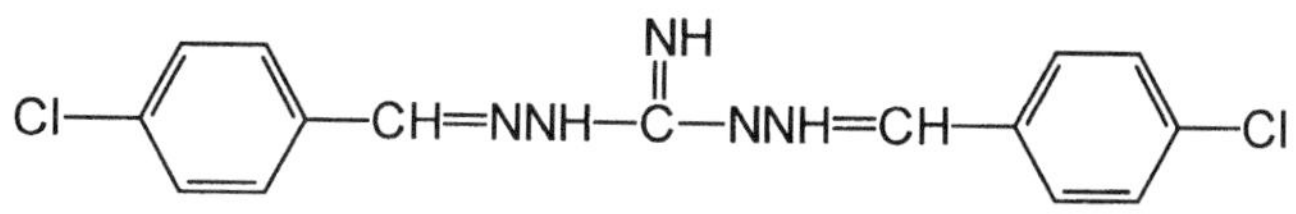

Cl—⟨benzene⟩—CH=NNH—C(=NH)—NNH=CH—⟨benzene⟩—Cl

Robenidine
($C_{15}H_{13}Cl_2N_5$)
[334.21]

FIG. 43.8

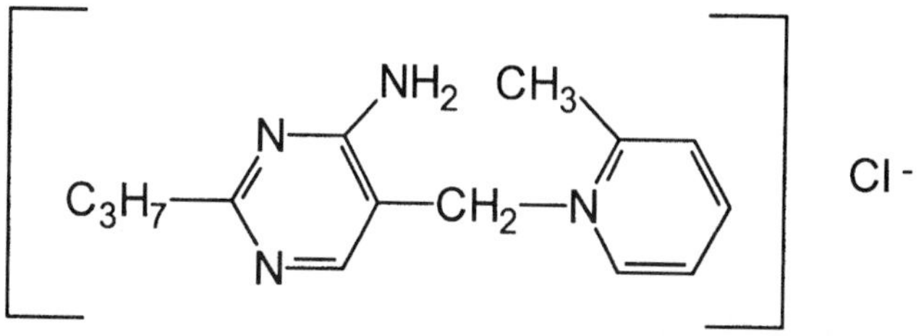

[Amprolium structure: pyrimidine ring with NH_2, C_3H_7, —CH_2—N⁺ (2-methylpyridinium, CH_3)] Cl^-

Amprolium
($C_{14}H_{19}ClN_4$)
[278.78]

FIG. 43.9

against the first-generation schizont of *E. tenella* by preventing formation of merozoites. Feeds with robenidine should not be fed to laying hens, as studies have shown that robenidine is transmitted to the eggs (Long et al. 1981), and these eggs may have an unpleasant taste even though the ability of humans to taste robenidine is apparently under genetic control. It does not have any other adverse effects on egg production or quality.

Clinical Use

Chickens. Robenidine is used for the prevention of coccidiosis in chickens. Finish feeds must be fed within 50 days of manufacture. Do not feed with bentonite clays. A 5-day withdrawal is required. If robenidine is not withdrawn 5 days before slaughter, the flesh of medicated birds will have an unpleasant taste.

THIAMINE ANALOGUES

Spectrum: Coccidiosis.
Drugs included: Amprolium (Fig. 43.9).

AMPROLIUM. Amprolium (Corid®, Amprol®) is labeled for use in the United States as a preventative and treatment of *Eimeria* infections in chickens, turkeys, pheasants, and calves. It is one of the most commonly administered anticoccidia agents in veterinary medicine. It is structurally related to the vitamin thiamine and the antiparasitic activity of the drug is thought to be related to competitive inhibition of active thiamine transport into the parasite. There is a fiftyfold greater sensitivity of the parasite system compared with the host system.

Amprolium is freely soluble in water. Because amprolium lacks the hydroxyethyl function of thiamine it is not phosphorylated to a pyrophosphate analog (Looker et al. 1986). Amprolium acts on the first-generation schizont to prevent merozoite production and has some activity against sexual stages and the sporulating oocyst. Amprolium-resistant strains of chicken and turkey *Eimeria* spp. are prevalent. Amprolium is often combined with other agents to increase activity.

Clinical Use

Chickens and Turkeys. Amprolium is used for the prevention of coccidiosis in chickens as a feed additive or in the drinking water. No withdrawal is required. Amprolium is used for the treatment and prevention of coccidiosis in turkeys when fed continuously.

Pheasants. Amprolium is approved for use in the prevention of coccidiosis in pheasants and is fed continuously. It must not be used in feeds containing bentonite.

Cattle. Amprolium is given to calves in the feed, drinking water, or orally at 5 mg/kg BW for 21 days to prevent coccidiosis or at 10 mg/kg BW for 21 days to treat coccidiosis.

Dogs. In dogs, amprolium can be used for the treatment of coccidiosis at 100–200 mg total dose (20% powder) orally once a day for 7–12 days. Amprolium is also used in the drinking water (sole source) at 30 ml (9.6% solution)/gal for up to 10 days or in the food at 250–300 mg (20% powder) once a day for 7–12 days.

Cats. Amprolium can be used for the treatment of coccidiosis at 110–220 mg/kg orally once a day for 7–12 days. Amprolium is also used in the drinking water (sole source) at 1.5 teaspoons (9.6% solution)/gal for up to 10 days.

Amprolium can be combined with sulfadimethoxine and used for the treatment of coccidiosis at 150 mg/kg BW amprolium and 25 mg/kg BW sulfadimethoxine once a day for 14 days.

NITROBENZAMIDES

Spectrum: Coccidiosis.

Drugs included: Aklomide, dinitolmide. (Fig. 43.10)

AKLOMIDE AND DINITOLMIDE. Aklomide and dinitolmide (Zoamix®) are nitrobenzamide anticoccidial agents. These agents act primarily on the first-generation schizonts, and dinitolmide inhibits sporulation of oocysts (Mathis and McDougald 1981). Dinitolmide is coccidiostatic if given for 6 days but is coccidiocidal if given for longer periods (Long 1993). Nitrobenzamide-resistant strains of coccidia are common. The anticoccidial mode of action of nitrobenzamides is not known.

Aklomide is not currently marketed as a single agent or combined with other anticoccidial drugs in the United States.

Clinical Use

Chickens and Turkeys. Dinitolmide is fed as a single agent to prevent coccidiosis in chickens. Do not feed to layers or birds over 14 weeks of age. Dinitolmide is also approved for use in nonlaying turkeys in feed in birds up to 14–16 weeks of age. Combination products are also available.

NICARBAZIN

Spectrum: Coccidiosis.

Nicarbazin (Nicarb®, Cycarb®) is an equimolecular complex of 4,4′-dinitrocarbanilide and 2-hydroxy-4,6-dimethylpyrimidine (Fig. 43.11). The agents are absorbed separately from the digestive tract, and both are needed for anticoccidial activity. Dry crystals are strongly electrostatic and present some dry-mixing problems. The precise mode of action of nicarbazin is not known. Nicarbazin causes reduced egg production, depressed egg weight, and reduced eggshell thickness and egg-yolk mottling when fed to white leghorn layers at 125 ppm (Jones et al. 1990). It also causes poor hatchability and depigmentation of brown-shelled eggs. Nicarbazin is usually restricted in use to the starting period because of potential growth-suppressing effects and to cooler months of the year because of its potential to enhance the effects of heat distress (McDougald 1993).

Clinical Use

Chickens. Nicarbazin is fed for the prevention of coccidiosis. Do not feed to laying hens. Do not use for treatment of coccidiosis. A combination of narasin and nicarbazin (Maxiban®) is available for prevention of coccidiosis in broilers. It is for broilers only and should not be fed to other types of chickens. The use of this combination has been associated with increased mortality of broilers in times of heat distress. Feed containing this combination may cause fatalities in horses that ingest it, and it should not be fed to adult turkeys.

Name	Chemical name (Empirical formula) [Molecular weight]	Chemical structure
Aklomide	2-chloro-4-nitrobenzamide ($C_7H_5ClN_2O_3$) [200.60]	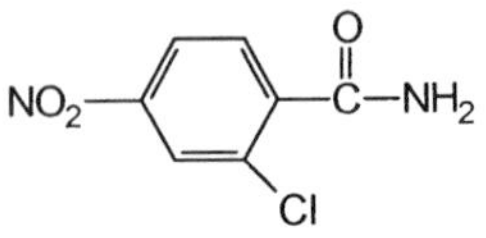 NO_2, C(=O)–NH_2, Cl
Dinitolmide	2-methyl-3,5-dinitrobenzamide ($C_8H_7N_3O_5$) [225.16]	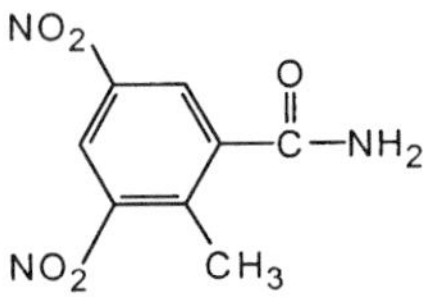 NO_2, C(=O)–NH_2, NO_2, CH_3

FIG. 43.10 Nitrobenzamides.

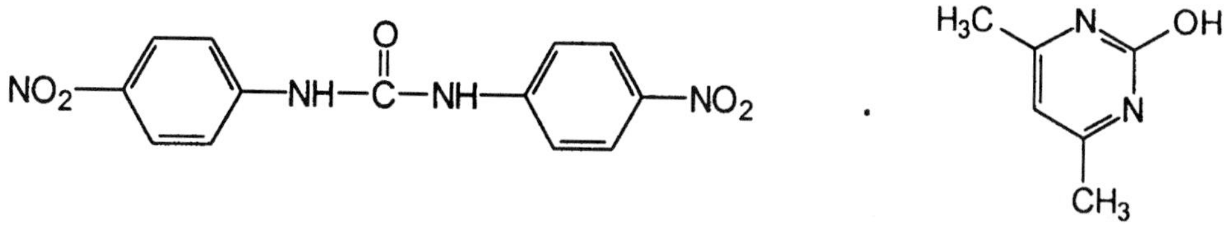

Nicarbazin
($C_{19}H_{18}N_6O_6$)
[426.38]

FIG. 43.11

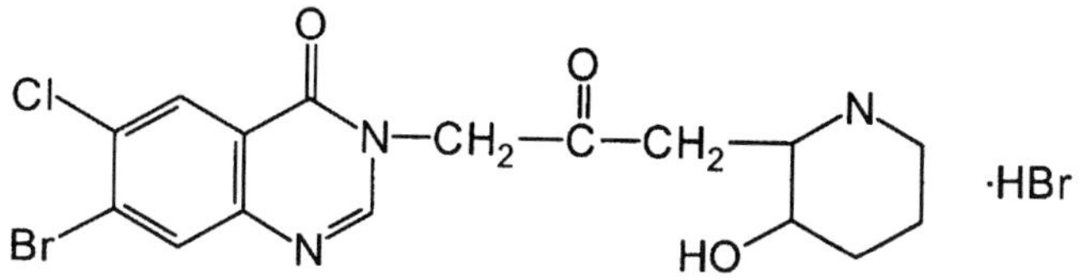

Halofuginone
($C_{16}H_{18}Br_2ClN_3O_3$)
[495.50]

FIG. 43.12

ALKALOIDS

Spectrum: Coccidiosis, theileriosis.

Drugs included: Halofuginone (Figure 43.12).

HALOFUGINONE. Halofuginone (Stenerol®) is an alkaloid originally isolated from the plant *Dichroa febrifuga.* Halofuginone is active against the asexual stages of coccidia. Its anticoccidial mode of action is not known. Halofuginone is transmitted to eggs from hens that have been fed halofuginone for 1 week (Long et al. 1981), but no adverse effects on egg production or egg quality have been associated with administration (Jones et al. 1990). Halofuginone has been associated with skin tears in chickens, and it has been shown to be an inhibitor of collagen type I synthesis in avian and mammalian cells (Granot et al. 1993). Halofuginone is toxic to fish and other aquatic life and must not be fed to waterfowl. Halofuginone is a skin and eye irritant and appropriate precautions (such as protective clothing) should be taken when handling this agent.

Clinical Use

Chickens and Turkeys. Halofuginone is used for the prevention of coccidiosis in chickens when administered in feed. Do not feed to layers. Halofuginone is also approved for the prevention of coccidiosis in growing turkeys.

Cattle. In cattle, halofuginone is given orally at 1–2 mg/kg BW for a single treatment and is curative for *Theileria* infections. At 2 mg/kg BW transient diarrhea may occur.

POLYETHER IONOPHORES

Spectrum: Coccidiosis.

Drugs included: Lasalocid, maduramicin, monensin, narasin, semduramicin, salinomycin (Fig. 43.13).

The polyether ionophore antibiotics were first discovered in the early 1950s, and their anticoccidial activities were recognized in the late 1960s. Because of their broad spectrum of activity and the development of drug resistance to other agents, the ionophores gained widespread usage in the poultry industry soon after their introduction. Polyether ionophores fall into one of five classes: monovalent, monovalent glycosides, divalent, divalent glycosides,

Name	Chemical name (Empirical formula) [Molecular weight]	Chemical structure
Lasalocid	6-[7*R*-[5*S*-Ethyl-5-(5*R*-ethyltetra-hydro-5-hydroxy-6 *S*-methyl-2*H*-pyran-2*R*-yl) tetrahydro-3*S*-methyl-2*S*-furanyl]-4*S*-hydroxy-3*R*,5*S*-dimethyl-6-oxonon-yl]-2-hydroxy-3-methylbenzoic acid ($C_{34}H_{54}O_8$) [590.80]	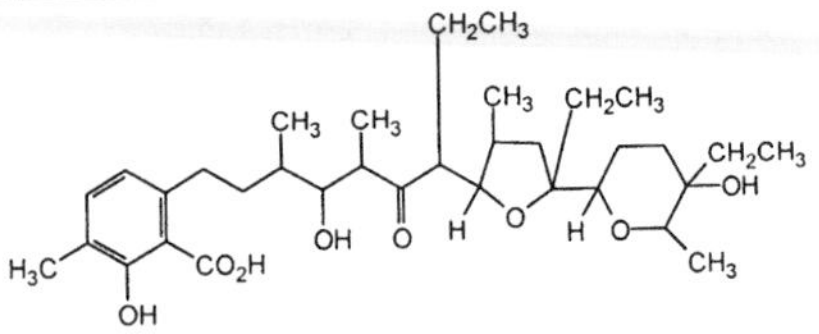
Maduramicin	(3*R*,4*S*,5*S*,6*R*,7*S*,22*S*)-23,27-Didemethoxy-2,6,22-tridemethyl-11-*O*-demethyl-22-[(2,6-dideoxy-3,4-di-*O*-methyl-β-Larabino-hexopyranosyl)oxy]-6-methyloxylonomycin A monoammonium salt ($C_{47}H_{83}NO_{17}$) [934.17]	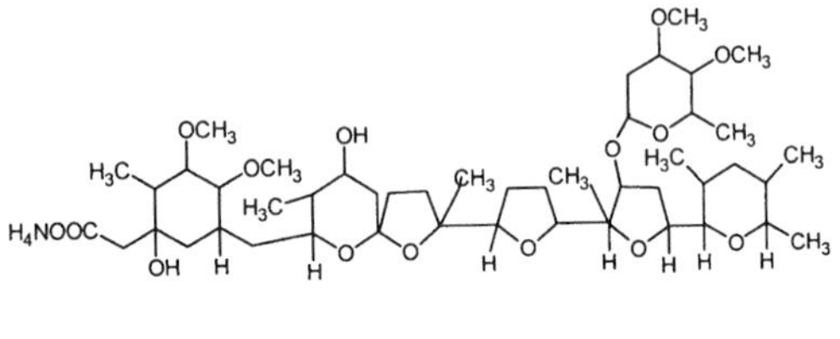
Monensin	2-[5-Ethyltetrahydro-5-[tetrahydro-3-methyl-5-[tetrahydro-6-hydroxy-6-(hydromethyl)-3,5-dimethyl-2*H* -pyran-2-yl]-2-furyl]-2-furyl]-9-hydroxy-β-methoxy-α, γ, 2,8-tetramethyl-1,6-dioxaspiro [4.5] decane-7-butyric acid ($C_{36}H_{62}O_{11}$) [670.90]	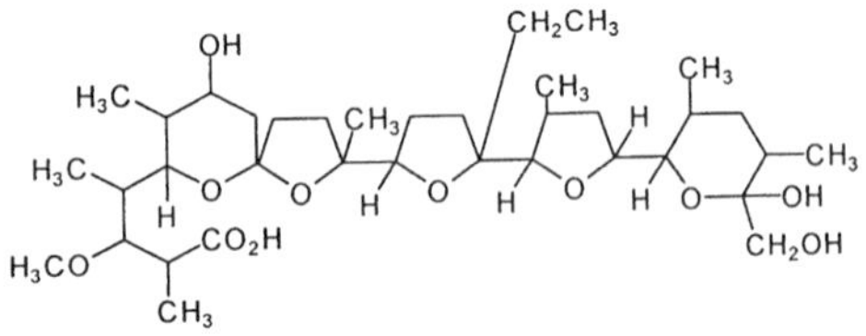
Narasin	(αβ,2β,3α,5α,6α)-α-ethyl-6-[5-[5-(5α-ethyltetrahydro-5β-hydroxy-6α-methyl-2*H*-pyran-2β-yl)-3″α,4,4″,5,5″α,6″-hexahydro-3′β-hydroxy-3″β,5α,5″β-trimethylspiro] furan-2(3*H*),2′-[2*H*]pyran-6′(3′*H*),2″-[2*H*]pyran]6″α-yl]2α-hydroxy-1α,3β-dimethyl-4-oxoheptyl]-tetrahydro-3,5-dimethyl-2*H*-pyran-2-acetic acid ($C_{43}H_{72}O_{11}$) [765.05]	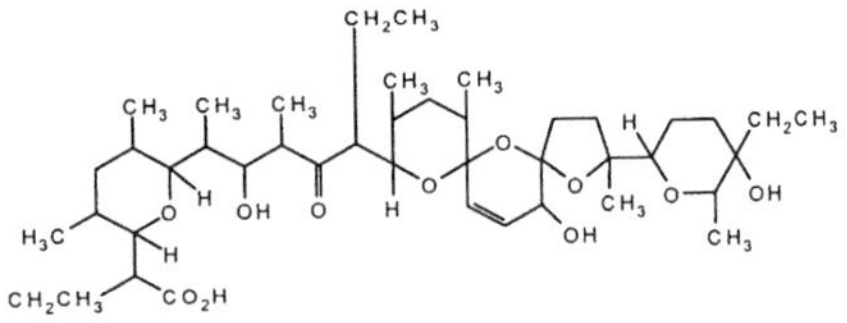
Semduramicin	(2*R*,3*S*,4*S*,5*R*,6*S*)-tetrahydro-2,4-dihydroxy-6-[(1*R*)-1-[(2*S*,5*R*,7*S*,8*R*,9*S*)-9-hydroxy-2,8-dimethyl-2-[(2*R*,6*S*)-tetrahydro-5-methyl-5-[(2*R*,3*S*,5*R*)-tetrahydro-5[(2*S*,3*S*,5*R*,6*S*)-tetrahydro-6-hydroxy-3,5,6-trimethyl-2*H*-pyran-2-yl]-3-[[(2*S*,5*S*,6*R*)-tetrahydro-5-methoxy-6-methyl-2*H*-pyran-2-yl]oxy]-2-furyl]-2-furyl]-1,6-dioxaspirol [4.5]dec-7-yl]ethyl]-5-methoxy-3-methyl-2*H*-pyran-2-acetic acid ($C_{44}H_{77}O_{16}$) [748.47]	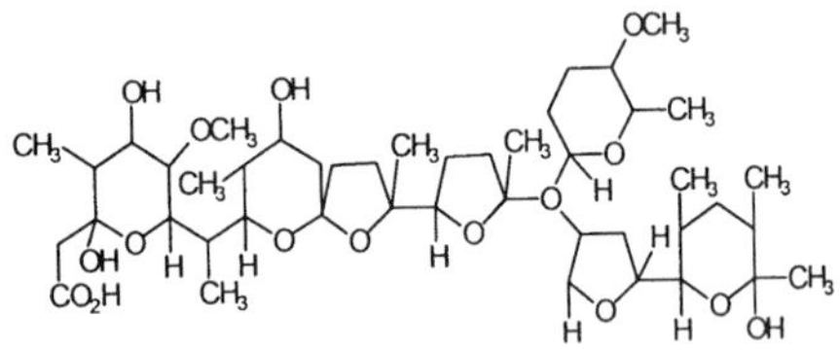

FIG. 43.13 Ionophores antibiotics.

or divalent pyrole ethers. The mode of action of ionophores is related to their ability to form lipophilic complexes with alkali metal cations and to transport these cations across biological membranes. Different ionophores may produce varying affinities for different cations. Ionophores that have anticoccidial activity are thought to act against extracellular sporozoites and merozoites. Extracellular stages develop membrane blebs indicating alterations in membrane integrity and in internal osmolality. Because coccidia have no osmoregulatory organelles, this change in internal osmotic conditions damages the parasites.

Because of the unique mode of action of ionophores, development of anticoccidial resistance to ionophores was difficult to produce under experimental conditions and slow to develop after clinical use in the field. In the mid- to late 1980s ionophore-resistant strains of chicken *Eimeria* spp. were documented in the United States, and ionophore resistance is now common. Cross-resistance between ionophores is common, although strain differences in coccidial response to specific ionophores have been demonstrated. In general, resistance to a monovalent polyether ionophore confers some cross-resistance to other monovalent polyether ionophores, but susceptibility to monovalent monoglycoside and divalent polyether ionophores may be retained.

Ionophores are potentially toxic for highly susceptible species, such as horses and other equines, and guinea fowl. Clinical signs occur from acute myocardial and muscle degeneration. Sweating, colic, and ataxia with hindlimb paresis/paralysis are also noted. Pathologically, focal degenerative cardiomyopathy, skeletal muscle necrosis, and congestive heart failure may be noted. Ionophore toxicosis can be potentiated with concurrent administration of tiamulin, chloramphenicol, macrolides, sulfonamides, and cardiac glycosides (Novilla 1992; Mitema et al. 1988). Exposure to horses is usually accidental, or resulting from horses gaining access to medicated feed. Care should always be taken to prevent highly susceptible animals from gaining access to feeds containing these products.

LASALOCID. Lasalocid (Avatec®, Bovatec®) is a divalent polyether ionophore that is a fermentation product of *Streptomyces lasaliensis* and was the second ionophore marketed in the United States. Lasalocid is well tolerated when fed with tiamulin (Meingasser et al. 1979). Lasalocid is transmitted to eggs of hens that have been fed this medication for 1 week.

Clinical Use

Chickens and Turkeys. Lasalocid is fed for the prevention of coccidiosis in chickens. Lasalocid is also approved for the prevention of coccidiosis in growing turkeys.

Chukar Partridges. Lasalocid is approved for the prevention of coccidiosis in chukar partridges and is fed until the birds are 8 weeks old.

Cattle. In cattle, lasalocid is used to prevent coccidiosis and is fed at 1 mg/kg BW, with a maximum of 360 mg/animal/day. Do not use in breeding animals.

Sheep. Lasalocid is fed in the ration to sheep to provide 15–70 mg/animal/day and is used in the prevention of coccidiosis. Do not administer to breeding animals.

Rabbits. Lasalocid is approved for use in the prevention of hepatic coccidiosis in rabbits and is fed until the rabbits are 6.5 weeks old.

MADURAMICIN. Maduramicin (Cygro®) is a monovalent monoglycoside polyether ionophore that is a fermentation product of *Actinomadura yumaense.* Maduramicin does not adversely affect egg production or egg quality (Jones et al. 1990). Maduramicin is well tolerated when fed with tiamulin (Meingasser et al. 1979). At higher doses (≥6 ppm), an adverse effect on growth and feathering may occur.

Clinical Use

Chickens. Maduramicin is used for the prevention of coccidiosis in broilers and fed at 5 ppm. It is for broilers only and should not be fed to other types of chickens.

MONENSIN. Monensin (Coban®, Rumensin®) is a monovalent polyether ionophore that is a fermentation product of *Streptomyces cinnamonensis.* Tiamulin may interfere with the metabolism of monensin in chickens and cause weight suppression (Meingasser et al. 1979). Monensin is apparently not transmitted to eggs of hens fed monensin for 1 week, nor does it adversely affect egg production or quality. Mature turkeys and guinea fowl should not have access to monensin-containing diets. Monensin will cause deaths in horses and guinea fowl that ingest feeds containing it.

Clinical Use

Chickens and Turkeys. Monensin is fed for prevention of coccidiosis in broilers. Do not feed to layers or chickens over 16 weeks of age. Monensin is used for prevention of coccidiosis in turkeys. Do not feed to turkeys over 10 weeks old.

Bobwhite Quail. Monensin is approved for use in bobwhite quail for prevention of coccidiosis and is fed at 73 g/ton from 1 day to 10 weeks old.

Cattle. In cattle, monensin is used to prevent coccidiosis and is fed to provide 100–360 mg/animal/day. It has recently been approved for use in dairy cattle as well, with a zero meat and milk withdrawal time.

Goats. Monensin is fed at 20 g/ton for the prevention of coccidiosis in confinement-reared goats. Do not feed to goats producing milk for human consumption.

NARASIN. Narasin (Monteban®) is a monovalent polyether ionophore that is a fermentation product of *Streptomyces aureofaciens.* It is structurally similar to salinomycin, differing only in the presence of a methyl group in narasin that is not present in salinomycin. It does not adversely affect egg production or egg quality. Narasin may cause fatalities in horses that ingest it, and it should not be fed to adult turkeys. Tiamulin may interfere with the metabolism of narasin in chickens and cause weight suppression (Meingasser et al. 1979).

Clinical Use

Chickens. Narasin is a feed additive for the prevention of coccidiosis in broilers. It is for broilers only and should not be fed to other types of chickens.

SEMDURAMICIN. Semduramicin (Aviax®) is a monovalent monoglycoside polyether ionophore that is a fermentation product of a mutant of *Actinomadura roseorufa* (Ricketts et al. 1992). The parent produced a diglycoside form of semduramicin that had to be semisynthetically modified. Both forms of the monoglycoside agent have identical activity. It is well tolerated when coadministered with tiamulin (Ricketts et al. 1992).

Clinical Use

Chickens. Semduramicin is used as a feed additive for prevention of coccidiosis in broiler chickens.

SALINOMYCIN. Salinomycin (Bio-Cox®) is a monovalent polyether ionophore that is a fermentation product of *Streptomyces albus* and was the third ionophore marketed in the United States. Salinomycin is active against sporozoites and early and late asexual stages of chicken coccidia (Conway et al. 1993). Salinomycin does not adversely affect egg production or egg quality. Tiamulin may interfere with the metabolism of salinomycin in chickens and cause weight suppression (Meingasser et al. 1979). It is not for use with pellet binders such as bentonite clays. Salinomycin will cause deaths in horses and adult turkeys that ingest feeds containing it.

Clinical Use

Chickens. Salinomycin is fed for prevention of coccidiosis in broilers. Do not feed to layers.

Bobwhite Quail. Salinomycin is approved for prevention of coccidiosis in bobwhite quail when administered in feed.

TRIAZINE DERIVATIVES

Spectrum: *Sarcocystis neurona*, coccidiosis, toxoplasmosis, *Neospora caninum.*

Drugs included: Diclazuril, toltrazuril, ponazuril (Figs. 43.14, 43.15).

The triazine antiprotozoal drugs act on the apicoplast, a plastid obtained by endosymbiosis that is present in apicomplexan parasites, but is not present in the vertebrate host. The exact function of the apicoplast is not known; however, it may play a vital role in biosynthesis of amino acids and fatty acids, assimilation of nitrate and sulfate, and starch storage, as has been demonstrated for other plastid organelles (Kühler et al. 1997; Fichera and Roos 1997).

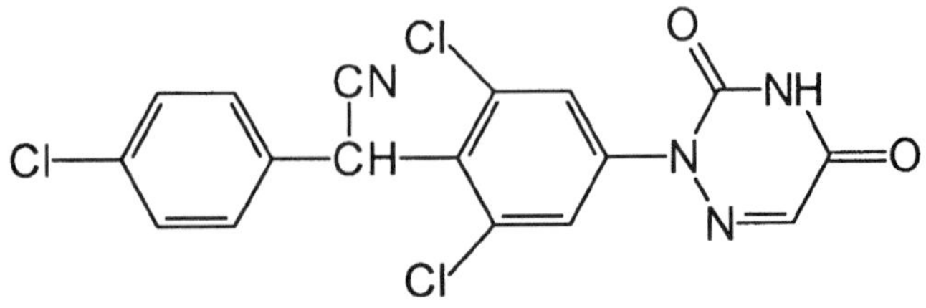

Cl CN CH Cl O NH N O N Cl

Diclazuril

($C_{17}H_9Cl_3N_4O_2$)

[407.64]

FIG. 43.14

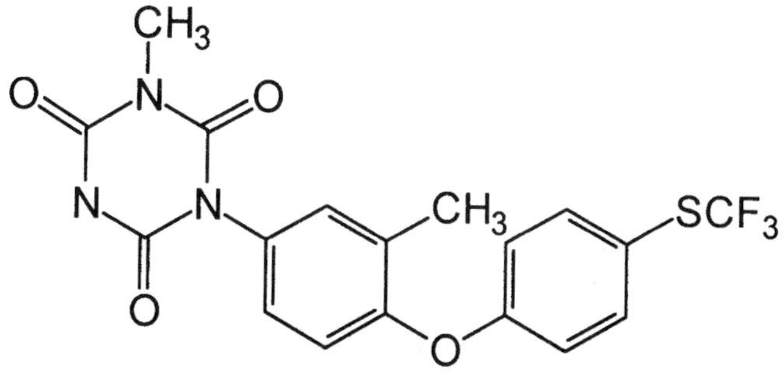

Toltrazuril

($C_{18}H_{14}F_3N_3O_4S$)

[425.38]

FIG. 43.15

DICLAZURIL. Diclazuril (Clinicox®) is a benzeneacetonitrile that has potent anticoccidial activity when fed at low levels in the feed.

Clinical Use

Horses. Diclazuril has been used as a treatment for equine protozoal myelitis (EPM). Doses of 5 mg/kg (equivalent to 500 gm Clinicox®/horse) have been successful in improving clinical signs of EPM using a shorter duration of treatment (30 days) compared to standard therapy with combinations of sulfonamides and pyrimethamine (90–120 days). Due to the large volume of drug to be administered, some horses have to be given the drug via a nasogastric tube, which makes treatment inconvenient and difficult. A recent study examined the pharmacokinetics of a sodium salt of diclazuril administered orally to horses (Dirikolu et al. 2006). This formulation had a higher oral bioavailability compared to the conventional powder or the conventional powder mixed with DMSO. This product was also able to be administered as a feed additive.

Chickens. Diclazuril is approved for use in broilers as a preventative for coccidiosis. There are several other combination products available as well. The withdrawal times can vary, depending on the product. This drug is not approved for use in laying hens.

Turkeys. Diclazuril is approved for use in the prevention of coccidiosis in turkeys. It is also available combined with bacitracin. These products should not be fed to breeding turkeys or layers.

Rabbits. When fed at 1–2 ppm continuously in pelleted feed, diclazuril was effective in controlling the clinical signs of intestinal coccidiosis in experimentally infected rabbits (Vanparijs et al. 1989).

TOLTRAZURIL. Toltrazuril (Baycox®) is a triazinon drug that has broad-spectrum anticoccidial and antiprotozoal activity. It is not commercially available in the United States. It is active against both asexual and sexual stages of coccidia by inhibiting nuclear division of schizonts and microgamonts and the wall-forming bodies of macrogamonts. It may also be useful in the treatment of neonatal porcine coccidiosis, EPM, and canine hepatozoonosis.

Clinical Use

Swine. Toltrazuril has been shown to reduce the signs of coccidiosis in naturally infected nursing pigs when a single oral 20–30 mg/kg BW dose is given to 3- to 6-day-old pigs (Driesen et al. 1995). Clinical signs were reduced from 71 to 22% of nursing pigs, and diarrhea and oocyst excretion were also decreased by the single oral treatment.

Dogs. For hepatozoonosis, toltrazuril given orally at 5 mg/kg BW every 12 hours for 5 days or given orally at 10 mg/kg BW every 12 hours for 10 days caused remission of clinical signs in naturally infected dogs in 2–3 days (Macintire et al. 2001). Unfortunately, most treated dogs relapsed and eventually died from hepatozoonosis.

Horses. Toltrazuril has also been used for the treatment of EPM. It has a better bioavailability and is easier to use when compared to diclazuril. This drug is safe, even at high doses. Current recommended treatments are 5–10 mg/kg orally for 28 days. Despite the favorable efficacy with toltrazuril, its use has diminished in horses because of better availability of other effective drugs (see Ponazuril below).

PONAZURIL. Ponazuril (Marquis®) also known as toltrazuril sulfone, is an active metabolite of toltrazuril; therefore, its mechanism of action is identical to that of toltrazuril. It is available in a paste formulation for horses.

Name	Chemical name (Empirical formula) [Molecular weight]	Chemical structure
Sulfadiazine	4-amino-*N*-2-pyrimidinylbenzenesulfonamide ($C_{10}H_{10}N_4O_2S$) [250.28]	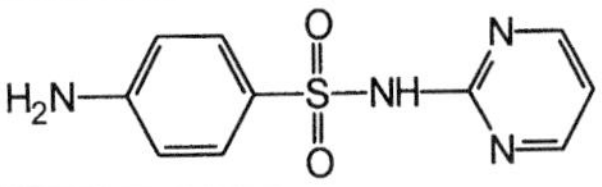
Sulfadimethoxine	4-amino-*N*-(2,6-dimethoxy-4-pyrimidinyl)-benzenesulfonamide ($C_{12}H_{14}N_4O_4S$) [310.33]	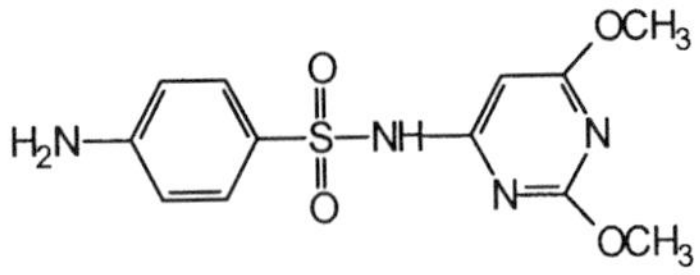
Sulfadoxine	4-amino-*N*-(5,6-dimethoxy-4-pyrimidinyl)-benzenesulfonamide ($C_{12}H_{14}N_4O_4S$) [310.34]	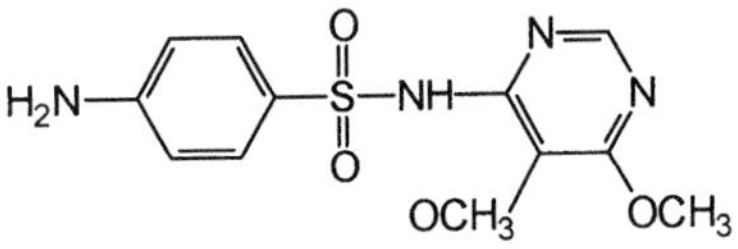
Sulfaguanidine	4-amino-*N*-(aminoiminomethyl)-benzenesulfonamide ($C_7H_{10}N_4O_2S$) [214.24]	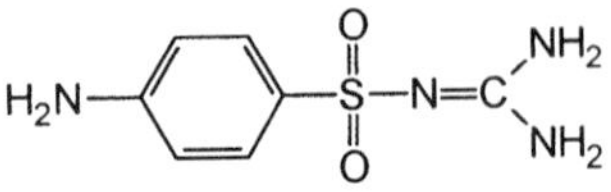
Sulfamethazine	4-amino-*N*-(4,6-dimethyl-2-pyrimidinyl)-benzenesulfonamide ($C_{12}H_{14}N_4O_2S$) [278.32]	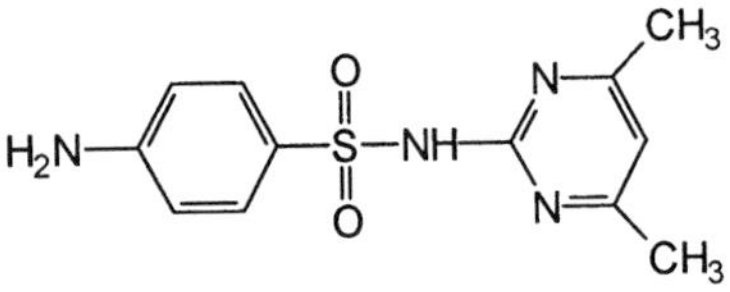
Sulfamethoxazole	4-amino-*N*-(5-methyl-3-isoxazolyl)-benzenesulfonamide ($C_{10}H_{11}N_3O_3S$) [253.31]	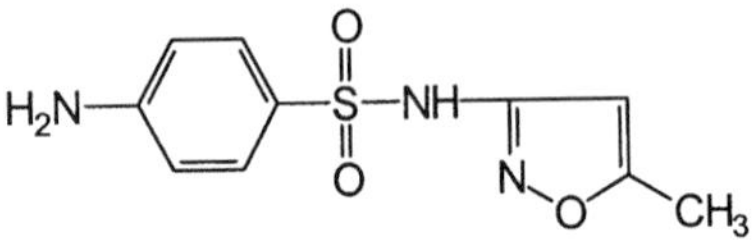
Sulfaquinoxaline	4-amino-*N*-2-quinoxalinyl-benzenesulfonamide ($C_{14}H_{12}N_4O_2S$) [300.33]	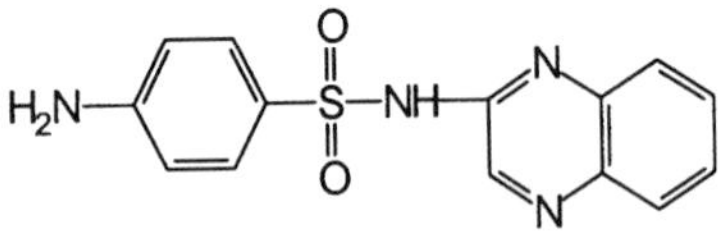
Sulfanitran	4′-[(*p*-nitrophenyl)sulfamoyl]acetanilide ($C_{14}H_{13}N_3O_5S$) [335.34]	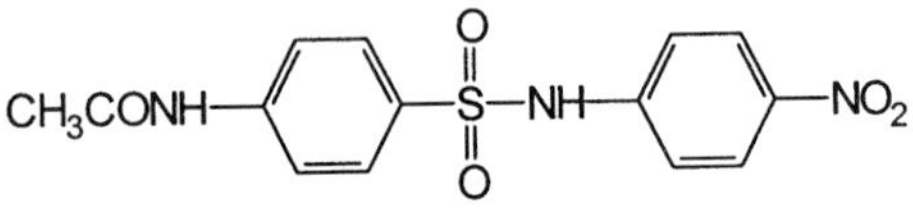

FIG. 43.16 Sulfonamides.

Clinical Use

Horses. Ponazuril is approved for use in horses as a treatment for EPM at a dose of 5 mg/kg orally for 28 days. Treatment can be extended for another 28 days if no improvement is seen. No side effects have been noted.

Cattle. Ponazuril has been shown to be effective at a dose of 20 mg/kg orally once a day for 6 days in calves experimentally infected with *Neospora caninum.*

SULFONAMIDES

Spectrum: Coccidiosis.

Drugs included: Sulfaguanidine, sulfadiazine, sulfadimethoxine, sulfadoxine, sulfamethazine (syn. sulfadimidine), sulfamethoxazole, sulfanitran, and sulfaquinoxaline (Fig. 43.16).

Sulfonamides were the first effective anticoccidials used. Sulfonamides can be either coccidiostatic or coccidiocidal. The pharmacology of sulfonamides is also discussed in Chapter 33 of this book. The structure of sulfonamides is similar to para-aminobenzoate (para-aminobenzoic acid, PABA), which is required by bacteria in the synthesis of folate (folic acid). Sulfonamides interfere in the early phases of folate synthesis. Mammalian and avian cells use preformed folate and are therefore not affected by the sulfonamide treatments. Sulfonamides are often used in combination with dihydrofolate reductase/thymidylate synthase (DHFR/TS) inhibitors because of the observed synergistic effects due to activity at two places in folate biosynthesis. Sulfonamides have most activity against the asexual stages and lesser activity against the sexual stages of coccidia.

Sulfonamides used in veterinary medicine for the treatment or prevention of coccidia and coccidialike parasites include sulfaguanidine, sulfadiazine, sulfadimethoxine, sulfadoxine, sulfamethazine (in some countries called *sulfadimidine*), sulfamethoxazole, sulfanitran, and sulfaquinoxaline. Many are used in combination with other products that have antibacterial or growth-promoting properties. Combinations with trimethoprim or ormetoprim are discussed in the next section.

Clinical Use

Chickens and Turkeys. Sulfamethazine is approved for use in chickens and turkeys for the treatment of coccidiosis when administered in drinking water. Sulfamethazine should not be administered to animals producing eggs for human consumption.

Cattle. Sulfamethazine is used to treat coccidiosis in calves by oral administration of a single dose of 100 milligrams of sulfamethazine per pound of body weight the first day and 50 milligrams per pound of body weight on each following day, not to exceed 5 days. Other formulations are also available. Do not feed to preruminating calves or lactating dairy cattle. Sulfaquinoxaline can be administered in the drinking water for 3 to 5 days. Treated animals must actually consume enough medicated water to provide 6 mg per pound body weight per day. Do not feed to calves to be slaughtered under 1 month old or use in lactating dairy cattle.

Dogs and Cats. Several agents have been used for the treatment of intestinal coccidiosis in dogs and cats (Lindsay et al. 1997a), but only sulfadimethoxine is approved by the FDA for this usage. Sulfadimethoxine is used for treatment of coccidiosis in dogs and cats at 55 mg/kg BW for 1 day, and then 27.5 mg/kg BW once a day for 14–20 days.

Rabbits. Sulfaquinoxaline is used in the feed of rabbits for 30 days for treatment of coccidiosis.

DIHYDROFOLATE REDUCTASE/ THYMIDYLATE SYNTHASE INHIBITORS

Spectrum: Coccidiosis, *Toxoplasma* sp., *Neospora* sp., *S. neurona*, leucocytozoon, *Hepatozoon americanum.*

Drugs included: trimethoprim, ormetoprim, pyrimethamine (Daraprim). (Fig. 43.17)

In protozoa, unlike other eukaryotic cells, the dihydrofolate reductase and thymidylate synthase enzymes do not exist as separate molecular entities, but instead these enzymes are part of a bifunctional DHFR/TS complex that has both DHFR and TS activity (Roos 1993). The best-known and most often used members of this group are trimethoprim, ormetoprim, and pyrimethamine.

TRIMETHOPRIM. Trimethoprim is available in several formulations, as well as in trimethoprim combinations for oral or parenteral administration. Examples include trimethoprim + sulfadiazine (Tribrissen®, Di-Trim®) and trimethoprim + sulfamethoxazole (Bactrim®, Septra®, human

Name	Chemical name (Empirical formula) [Molecular weight]	Chemical structure
Trimethoprim	2,4-diamino-5-(3,4,5-trimethoxybenzyl)pyrimidine ($C_{14}H_{18}N_4O_3$) [290.32]	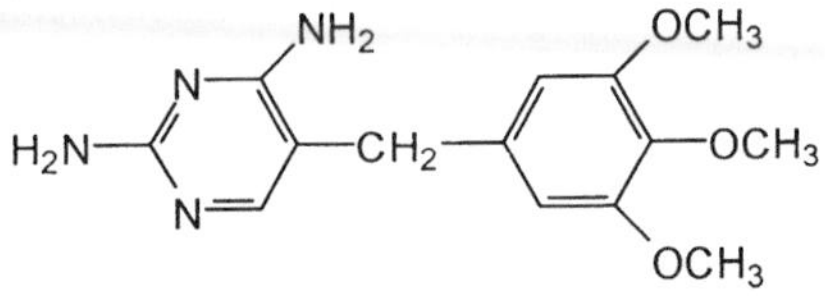
Pyrimethamine	2,4-diamino-5-(*p*-chlorophenyl)-6-ethylpyrimidine ($C_{12}H_{13}ClN_4$) [248.71]	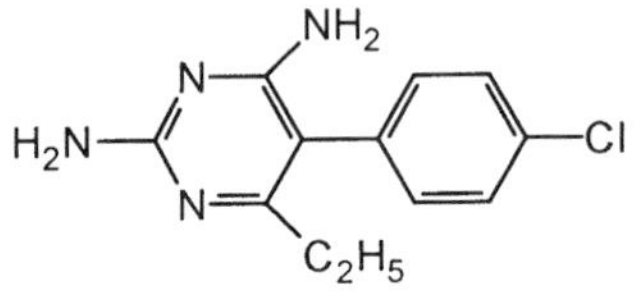
Diaveridine	2,4-diamino-5-veratrylpyrimidine ($C_{13}H_{16}N_4O_2$) [260.29]	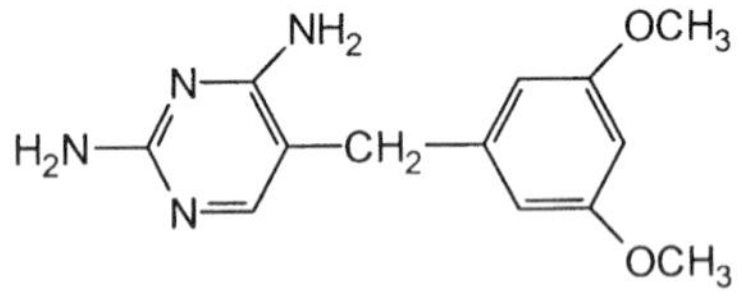
Ormetoprim	2,4-diamino-5-(4,5-dimethoxy-2-methylbenzyl)-pyrimidine ($C_{13}H_{15}N_4O_2$) [259.17]	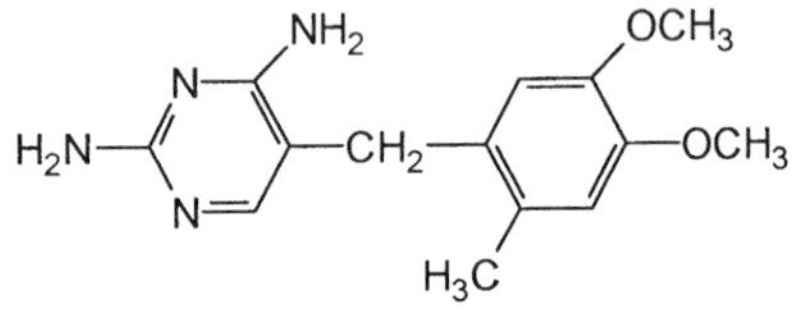

FIG. 43.17 Dihydrofolate reductase/thymidylate synthase inhibitors.

drugs). Trimethoprim also is available as a single drug (Proloprim). Pharmacology of trimethoprim is discussed in more detail in Chapter 33.

Trimethoprim is readily absorbed from the digestive tract after oral administration, and peak serum levels occur 1–4 hours later. The half-life is 3.8 hours in the horse, 3.0 hours in the dog, and 10.6 hours in human beings. Concurrent administration of sulfonamide does not affect the rate of absorption of trimethoprim. Trimethoprim is widely distributed in tissues. Levels of trimethoprim in cerebral spinal fluid are about 40% of those in the serum (Zinner and Mayer 1990). Trimethoprim is almost completely (60–80%) excreted by the kidneys within 24 hours, and some is also excreted in the bile. The remainder is excreted as metabolites by the kidneys. Use of trimethoprim and other DHFR/TS inhibitors is associated with adverse effects on bone marrow. Administration of folinic acid usually will counteract these adverse effects.

Trimethoprim is available in several tablet, liquid, and paste formulations in combination with sulfamethoxazole (Cotrimethoxazole®, Bactrim®, Septra®) or sulfadiazine (Di-Trim®) that are usually in the ratio of 1 part trimethoprim to 5 parts sulfonamide. In addition to their antibacterial use (Chapter 33), these agents are used in treatment of coccidiosis, toxoplasmosis, neosporosis, EPM, and malaria. Adverse reactions to these agents are similar to those of the individual constituents. These combinations should not be used in animals with liver disease, blood dyscrasias, or a history of sulfonamide sensitivity. Precautions normally observed when animals are taking sulfonamides should be observed. The safety of ormetoprim-sulfadimethoxine has not been established in pregnant dogs, but studies indicate that the use of trimethoprim-sulfadiazine is safe in pregnant dogs. Trimethoprim is not absorbed following oral administration in ruminating animals.

Clinical Use

Dogs. Sulfadiazine combined with trimethoprim is used as a treatment for coccidiosis at 5–10 mg/kg BW trimethoprim combined with 25–50 mg/kg BW of sulfadiazine, given for 6 days to dogs over 4 kg BW. Dogs under 4 kg BW are given half this dosage for 6 days. Remission of clinical signs of hepatozoonosis can be obtained by oral administration of a combination of trimethoprim-sulfadiazine (15 mg/kg BW every 12 hours), clindamycin (10 mg/kg every 8 hours), and pyrimethamine (0.25 mg/kg every 12 hours) for 14 days (MacIntire et al. 2001). As the therapy is ineffective in eliminating the tissue stages of the organism, clinical response is short-lived. Clinical relapses may be prevented by subsequent therapy with decoquinate (MacIntire et al. 2001).

Cats. Agents and dosages used for the treatment of canine coccidiosis are also used for the treatment of feline coccidiosis.

ORMETOPRIM. Ormetoprim combined with sulfadimethoxine (Rofenaid 40®) is the only combination DHFR/TS-sulfonamide presently available in the United States for poultry. Other combinations are intended for use in human beings, equines, and small animals. Ormetoprim is also available in combination with sulfadimethoxine in the ratio of 1 part ormetoprim plus 5 parts sulfadimethoxine (Primor®) in various size tablets.

Clinical Use

Chickens and Turkeys. Combinations are fed to chickens at 0.0075% ormetoprim and 0.0125% sulfadimethoxine to prevent coccidiosis in broiler chickens. Do not feed to birds producing eggs for food. Ormetoprim combined with sulfadimethoxine is fed to turkeys at 0.00375% ormetoprim and 0.00625% sulfadimethoxine to prevent coccidiosis. Do not feed to birds producing eggs for food.

Dogs. Sulfadimethoxine combined with ormetoprim is used as a treatment for coccidiosis in dogs at 11 mg/kg BW ormetoprim plus 55 mg/kg BW sulfadimethoxine for up to 23 days.

PYRIMETHAMINE. Pyrimethamine is available in 25 mg tablets. Pyrimethamine is well absorbed after oral administration and is slowly but extensively metabolized. Less than 3% is excreted in the urine in the first 24 hours, and the half-life is 4–6 days in human beings (Van Reken and Pearson 1990). It accumulates in the kidneys, lungs, liver, and spleen. It is excreted in urine as metabolites, but some pyrimethamine can be found in the milk. Very high doses of pyrimethamine are teratogenic in laboratory animals. Pyrimethamine is available in tablets that contain 25 mg pyrimethamine and 500 mg sulfadoxine (Fansidar®), and in tablets that contain 12.5 mg pyrimethamine and 100 mg dapsone (Maloprim®). The equine formulation is a suspension (ReBalance®) that contains pyrimethamine (12.5 mg/ml) + sulfadiazine (250 mg/ml).

Clinical Use

Avian. Pyrimethamine (1 ppm) combined with sulfadimethoxine (10 ppm) will prevent but not cure *Leu. caulleryi* infections in birds.

Dogs and Cats. For toxoplasmosis, cats and dogs are treated orally with 0.25–0.5 mg/kg BW pyrimethamine and 30 mg/kg BW sulfonamide (preferably, sulfadiazine) every 12 hours for 2–4 weeks. Canine neosporosis will also respond to the above regimens of DHFR/TS inhibitors and sulfonamides used to treat canine toxoplasmosis. Bone marrow suppression can occur with the synergistic use of pyrimethamine and sulfonamides and can be corrected by the addition of folinic acid (5 mg/day) or by the addition of yeast (100 mg/kg BW daily) to the animal's diet.

Horses. Treatment recommendations for equine protozoal myelitis include sulfadiazine at 20–30 mg/kg BW orally twice daily combined with oral pyrimethamine at 1 mg/kg BW once daily for 30 days after clinical signs have stopped improving. Twelve weeks is the average length of treatment time. Relapse is possible if horses are not treated long enough, and reactivation of the infection may occur during periods of unusual stress. It has fallen out of favor, due to the length of treatment required. The presence of food may adversely affect the absorption of DHFR/TS inhibitors, and food should be withheld 1–2 hours before and after treatment. Cell culture studies have shown that pyrimethamine kills developing *S. neurona* at 1.0 μg/ml and trimethoprim kills it at 5.0 μg/ml (Lindsay and Dubey 1999). These levels of agent probably are not reached in the treated horses. It has been suggested that intermittent (every 2 or 4 weeks) single EPM treatment may help prevent clinical relapse in horses recovering from EPM (MacKay et al. 1992). If relapse does occur, the entire treatment regimen should be repeated. A recent study of 12 horses with EPM on a farm with an EPM outbreak indicated that combination treatment with trimethoprim-sulfonamides and pyrimethamine resulted in transient fever, anorexia, and depression in 2; acute worsening of ataxia in 2; mild anemia in 4; and abortions in 3 (Fenger et al. 1997). Prolonged use of DHFR/TS inhibitors has long been known to result in bone marrow suppression. Therefore, horses should be examined periodically (about every 2 weeks) for anemia and leukopenia. If the neutrophil counts drop below 3000 cells/μL, treatment should be discontinued until the counts recover (MacKay et al. 1992). Supplementation with 40 mg/day of folinic acid is recommended in horses with bone marrow suppression. Pregnant mares should be supplemented routinely with folinic acid while on EPM treatment, and the dose of pyrimethamine should be dropped to 0.5 mg/kg BW to reduce the risks to the fetus.

LINCOSAMIDES

Spectrum: Toxoplasmosis, *Neospora* sp, hepatozoonosis.

Drugs included: Clindamycin, Lincomycin (Fig. 43.18).

CLINDAMYCIN. Clindamycin (Antirobe®, Cleocin®) has been used for treatment of disseminated toxoplasmosis in cats and dogs (Lindsay et al. 1997b). The pharmacology of lincosamides, including clindamycin, is discussed in more detail in Chapter 37 of this book. It is a semisynthetic compound produced by alteration of the parent molecule lincomycin, which is produced by *Streptomyces lincolnensis*. It differs from lincomycin in having a chlorine group at C-7 rather than a hydroxyl group. The dosages used against *T. gondii* are higher than for the treatment of the anaerobic infections for which it is marketed. Clindamycin is active against tachyzoites of *Toxoplasma gondii* and is initially coccidiostatic but becomes coccidiocidal after a few days of treatment. Oral and parenteral formulations of clindamycin have similar activity. The drug is almost completely absorbed after oral administration in both dogs and cats, and peak serum concentrations occur within 75 minutes (Harari and Lincoln 1989). The half-life is about 5 hours after oral or IV administration. Clindamycin is widely distributed in many tissues and

Name	Chemical name (Empirical formula) [Molecular weight]	Chemical structure
Clindamycin	(2*S-trans*)-methyl-7-chloro-6,7,8-trideoxy-6-[[(1-methyl-4-propyl-2-pyrrolidinyl)carbonyl]-amino]-1-thio-L-threo-α-D-galacto-octopyranoside ($C_{18}H_{33}ClN_2O_5S$) [424.98]	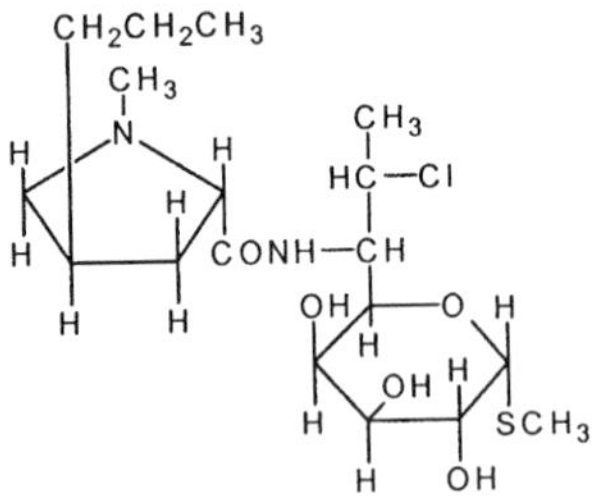
Lincomycin methyl	6,8-dideoxy-6-[[(-1-methyl-4-propyl-2-pyrrolidinyl) carbonyl]amino]-1-thio-D-erythro-α-D-galacto-octopyranoside ($C_{18}H_{34}N_2O_6S$) [406.56]	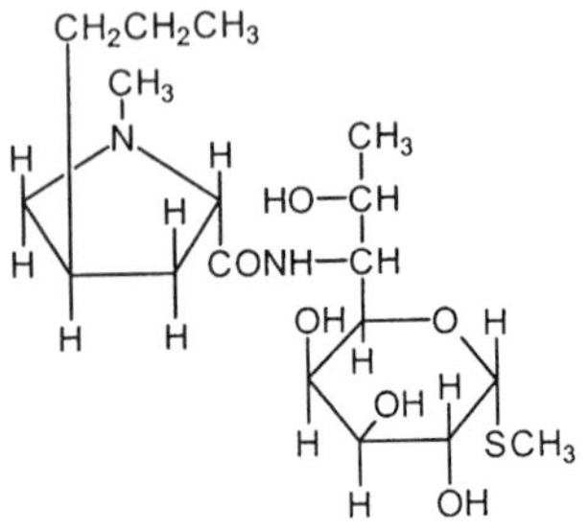

FIG. 43.18 Lincosamides.

fluids and crosses the placenta and blood-brain barrier. It is metabolized in the liver and excreted in the bile and urine as parent agent and metabolites.

Clinical Use

Dogs and Cats. For toxoplasmosis, cats are treated with clindamycin at 10–12 mg/kg BW orally every 12 hours for 4 weeks or treated with 12.5–25 mg/kg BW clindamycin IM every 12 hours for 4 weeks. Dogs are treated with 3–13 mg/kg BW orally or IM every 8 hours for 2 weeks or with 10–20 mg/kg BW orally or IM every 12 hours for 2 weeks. Clindamycin is also combined with pyrimethamine and used for the treatment of toxoplasmic encephalitis in human beings; such combinations might have applications in veterinary medicine. Neonatal canine neosporosis is treated with 12.5–18.5 mg/kg BW clindamycin orally twice daily for 2–4 weeks (Dubey and Lindsay 1998). Death may be prevented in pups with severe hindlimb involvement, but hindlimb function usually does not return to normal. The amount of clinical improvement will depend on the degree of paralysis that has occurred.

The response of *H. americanum*–infected dogs to treatment with a combination of trimethoprim plus sulfadiazine (orally 15 mg/kg BW every 12 hours) plus clindamycin (orally 10 mg/kg BW every 8 hours) plus pyrimethamine (orally 0.25 mg/kg BW daily) (TCP therapy) for 14 days demonstrated that remission of clinical signs in naturally infected dogs occurred in 2–3 days, but most treated dogs relapsed and eventually died from hepatozoonosis (Macintire et al. 2001). The best results have been seen in dogs that have undergone TCP therapy and then been placed on a daily oral treatment program with 10–20 mg/kg BW decoquinate. The decoquinate treatment must be continued because once it is stopped, relapse and clinical disease occur (Macintire et al. 2001). Dogs have tolerated this treatment and survived for over 18 months.

AZALIDES

Spectrum: Cryptosporidiosis, toxoplasmosis, babesiosis

Drugs included: Azithromycin (Zithromax®).

The azalide antimicrobials are derivatives of the macrolides. The pharmacology of the macrolides is discussed in more detail in Chapter 37 of this book. They have activity against bacteria, as well as mycoplasma. Recently, they have been investigated for the treatment of cryptosporidiosis in human patients with HIV infection, with some success (Kadappu et al. 2002). In vitro activity against *Toxoplasma gondii* has also been demonstrated. Azalides exhibit their antibacterial activity through inhibition of protein synthesis by binding to the 50S ribosomal unit of susceptible bacteria. The antiprotozoal mechanism of action is unknown.

AZITHROMYCIN. Azithromycin differs from other azalides and the macrolides by having a much higher volume of distribution and by its ability to accumulate within phagocytic cells. Concentrations are 100–200 times higher in neutrophils than in the plasma (Davis et al. 2002).

Clinical Use

Cattle. Azithromycin dihydrate given to calves naturally infected with cryptosporidiosis under field conditions, at doses of 1500 or 2000 mg per day had a lower incidence of diarrhea, decreased oocyst shedding, and increased weight gains (Elitok et al. 2005). The recommended treatment regimen is 1500 mg/calf/day for 7 days.

Dogs. Azithromycin (10 mg/kg PO q24h) administered concurrently with atovaquone (13.3 mg/kg PO q8h) for 10 consecutive days was shown to completely eliminate *Babesia gibsoni* infection from 8 of 10 dogs treated (Birkenheuer et al. 2004). The dogs in that study had previously been treated unsuccessfully with imidocarb or diminazene.

4-AMINOQUINOLINES

Spectrum: *Plasmodium* sp.

Drugs included: Chloroquine.

CHLOROQUINE. Chloroquine has been used in the treatment of avian malaria. The mechanism of action against malarial organisms involves concentration of the drug, which is a weak base, within the acidic food vacuoles of the parasites. Once inside the cell, chloroquine causes rapid clumping of heme pigments by inhibiting plasmodial heme polymerase activity (Slater and Cerami 1992). Heme then accumulates to toxic levels, causing cell death.

Clinical Use

Penguins. Clinical malaria in penguins that are kept in zoos or aquariums is caused by *Plasmodium relictum*. It is treated with an oral loading dose of 10 mg/kg BW chloroquine, followed by oral doses of 5 mg/kg BW given 6, 18, and 24 hours later (Clubb 1986).

DIAMIDINE DERIVATIVES

Spectrum: Piroplasmosis, *Hepatozoon canis*.

Drugs included: *Aromatic derivatives:* diminazene diaceturate, pentamidine isethionate, phenamidine isethionate. *Carbanilide derivatives:* amicarbalide, imidocarb dipropionate (Fig. 43.19).

These diamidine derivatives bind to DNA and interfere with parasite replication (Pilch et al. 1995; Patrick et al. 1997). This class of drugs has a tendency to accumulate in tissues; therefore, half-lives are very long, which may lead to residue problems in food-producing animals. Imidocarb was still detectable in liver samples from treated cattle 224 days after drug administration (Coldham et al. 1994). Specific drugs have been shown to cross the placenta, as well as the blood brain barrier. Toxicity may involve renal disease, hepatic disease, or pulmonary congestion and edema, and is dose-dependent. Treatment of babesiosis may produce clinical cures in some animals, but the infection is not completely cleared, leading to a carrier state in affected individuals. This depends on the susceptibility of the organism being treated.

DIMINAZENE DIACETURATE. Diminazene diaceturate (Berenil®, Ganaseg®) has a very long half-life, which is reported to be up to 29 days in the plasma of cattle, with the highest concentrations in tissues being found in the kidneys (Mdachi et al. 1995). Diminazene is excreted into the milk, with residues being reported for up to 6 days in sheep and goats (el Banna et al. 1999), and up to 21 days in cattle (Mdachi et al. 1995). Parasitic infections can alter the pharmacokinetics of this drug.

Clinical Use

Horses. *Babesia caballi* infections can be treated with 3–5 mg/kg BW IM, but 6–12 mg/kg BW is required for *B. equi* in horses. Doses as low as 0.5 mg/kg BW can be effective against *B. bigemina*. Diminazene at 5.0 mg/kg BW

Name	Chemical name (Empirical formula) [Molecular weight]	Chemical structure
Amicarbalide	3,3′-(Carbonyldiimino)*bis*-benzenecarboximidamide ($C_{15}H_{16}N_6O$) [296.34]	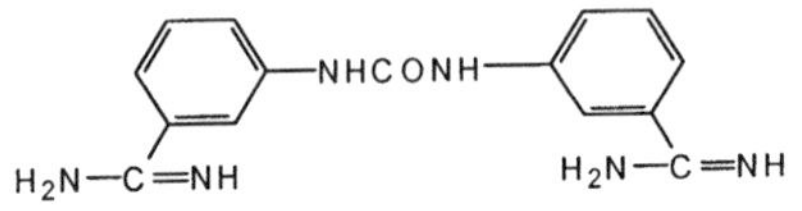 NHCONH; $H_2N-C{=}NH$; $H_2N-C{=}NH$
Diminazene	*N*-acetylglycine compounded with 4,4′-(1-triazene-1,3-diyl) *bis*-(benzenecarboximidamide) ($C_{22}H_{29}N_9O_6$) [515.54]	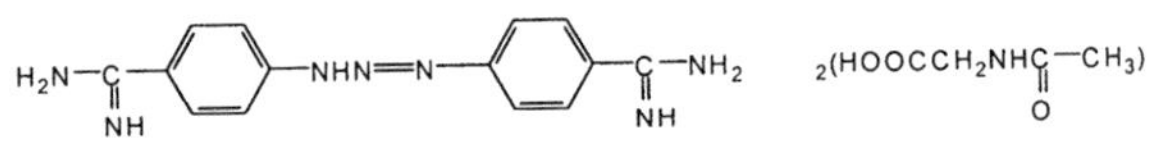 $H_2N-C(=NH)-$; NHN=N; $-C(=NH)-NH_2$; $_2(HOOCCH_2NHC(=O)-CH_3)$
Imidocarb	3,3′-di-2-imidazolin-2-yl-carbanilide ($C_{19}H_{20}N_6O$) [348.41]	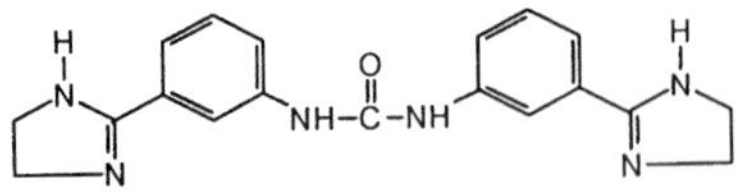 NH-C(=O)-NH
Pentamidine	4,4′-[1,5-pentanediylbis(oxy)]*bis*benzenecarboximidamide ($C_{19}H_{24}N_4O_2$) [340.43]	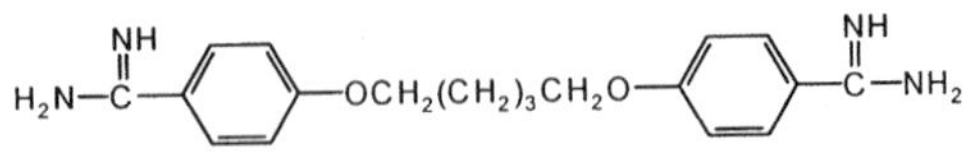 $H_2N-C(=NH)-$; $OCH_2(CH_2)_3CH_2O$; $-C(=NH)-NH_2$
Phenamidine	4,4′-oxybisbenzenecarboximidamide ($C_{14}H_{14}N_4O$) [254.29]	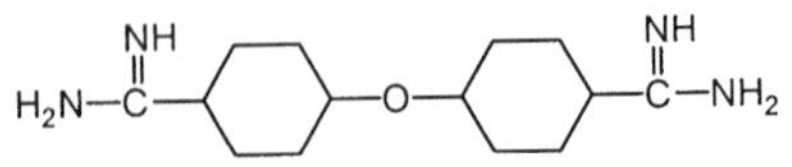 $H_2N-C(=NH)-$; O; $-C(=NH)-NH_2$

FIG. 43.19 Diamidine derivatives.

will eliminate *B. caballi* from horses if given twice during a 24-hour period (Kuttler 1988).

Cattle. Diminazene at a dose of 3–5 mg/kg IM is effective against *B. bigemina* and *B. bovis* infections (Vial and Gorenflot 2006). Doses of 3.5–7 mg/kg IM have been used for treatment of trypanosomiasis.

Dogs. A single 3.5–5 mg/kg BW IM treatment with diminazene is effective against canine babesiosis caused by *Babesia canis*, but 3.5 mg/kg BW given twice over 24 hrs is required for *B. gibsoni*. The drug may enable survival against acute hemolytic crises and clinical improvement, but is inconsistent in clearing infection. Higher cumulative doses may produce central nervous system signs.

Cats. For treatment of *Cytauxzoon* infection, two injections are given intramuscularly at 2 mg/kg BW within a 1-week interval (Greene et al. 1999). Diminazene is not effective against *B. felis* but is effective against *B. herpailuri* in cats.

PENTAMIDINE ISETHIONATE. Pentamidine isethionate (Lomidine®, Pentam 300®) is useful in programs that are attempting to produce immunity in cattle by abbreviating infections.

Clinical Use

Cattle. When given SC during the acute phase at 0.5–2 mg/kg BW, pentamidine usually produces a clinical cure, but as much as 5 mg/kg BW will not completely eradicate the parasite from cattle.

Dogs. Pentamidine is effective against canine babesiosis when given IM at 16.5 mg/kg BW on 2 consecutive days but may cause adverse reactions, including pain at the injection site, hypotension, tachycardia, and vomiting. It has also been used in the treatment of leishmaniais at a dose of 4 mg/kg BW IM twice weekly for 4 weeks. This regimen was repeated again 3 weeks later. Clinical remission was obtained in all dogs treated, and signs did not appear during a 6-month follow-up period (Noli and Auxilia 2005).

PHENAMIDINE ISETHIONATE. Phenamidine isethionate (Lomadine®) can be used to treat bovine and equine *Babesia* infections with 8–13 mg/kg BW IM. Phenamidine at 8.8 mg/kg BW will eliminate *B. caballi* from horses if given twice during a 24-hour period (Kuttler 1988).

Dogs. Phenamidine isethionate given SC at 15–20 mg/kg BW once a day for 2 days, is effective against canine babesiosis caused by *B. gibsoni*; a single dose of 8–13 mg/kg is effective against *Babesia canis*.

AMICARBALIDE. Amicarbalide (Diampron®) is effective against bovine babesiosis when given IM at 5–10 mg/kg BW. Amicarbalide at 8.8 mg/kg BW will eliminate *B. caballi* from horses if given twice during a 24-hour period but will not eliminate *B. equi* when used at levels of 22 mg/kg BW, which approaches toxic levels (Kuttler 1988).

IMIDOCARB DIPROPIONATE. Imidocarb dipropionate (Imizol®) is one of the treatments of choice for babesial infections. Also, administration of imidocarb may interfere with the efficacy of some babesial vaccines in certain species (Combrink et al. 2002). In cattle, the elimination half-life of imidocarb in liver was 48.5 days and 120 days in muscle (Coldham et al. 1995). A dose-dependent hepatic toxicity has been noted.

Clinical Use

Cattle. Imidocarb is effective against bovine babesiosis when given at 1–3 mg/kg BW IM or SC.

Horses. Imidocarb given at 1–2 mg/kg BW will eliminate *B. caballi* from horses if given twice during a 24-hour period (Kuttler 1988). When given at 4 mg/kg IM every 72 hours for a total of 4 doses, imidocarb produced a significant increase in the urine GGT:creatinine ratio, as well as mild azotemia in normal horses (Meyer et al. 2005). Liver function was not affected. This dose has been shown to be ineffective in eliminating the carrier state in *B. equi*–infected animals (Kuttler et al. 1987). At higher doses (16 and 32 mg/kg BW), renal failure, hepatic failure, and pulmonary edema were noted (Adams 1981). When administered to pregnant mares, imidocarb was detectable in fetal blood at levels similar to those found in the dam's blood (Lewis et al. 1999).

Dogs. A single 7.5 mg/kg BW SC imidocarb treatment will completely clear *Babesia canis* infections in dogs (Penzhorn et al. 1995). A single dose of 3.5 mg/kg BW SC diminazene, followed the next day by a single dose of 6 mg/kg BW SC imidocarb, will completely clear *Babesia canis* infections in dogs (Penzhorn et al. 1995). *Hepatozoon canis* infections are treated with 5–6 mg/kg BW SQ or IM every 2 weeks until gamonts are no longer present in blood smears (Baneth and Weigler 1997).

Cats. For treatment of *Cytauxzoon* infection, two injections are given intramuscularly at 5 mg/kg BW within a 1–2 week interval (Greene et al. 1999). Control of parasympathetic side effects is recommended by pretreating cats with atropine or glycopyrrolate. Feline babesiosis is refractory to treatment with imidocarb.

NITROTHIAZOLE DERIVATIVES

Spectrum: *Giardia, Coccidia,* cryptosporidiosis, *S. neurona*
Drugs included: Nitazoxanide.

The antiprotozoal action of the nitrothiazole derivatives is thought to be via interference with the pyruvate-ferredoxin oxidoreductase enzyme dependent electron transfer reaction, which is essential for anaerobic energy metabolism of the parasites (Parashar and Arya 2005). It is specific for parasites capable of intracellular reduction of the nitro group on the drug to a toxic-free radical. Nitazoxanide (NTZ) is rapidly converted to an active metabolite, deacetylnitazoxanide (also known as tizoxanide), in the horse (Navigator Paste, package insert), as well as in humans (Parashar and Arya 2005).

NITAZOXANIDE. Nitazoxanide (Navigator®) is available as a 32% paste and is registered for use in horses to treat equine protozoal myeloencephalitis (EPM). The side effects in horses are numerous and can be severe, including a fatal enterocolitis at recommended doses; therefore, its use is typically reserved for horses that have not responded to other therapies. In vitro and in vivo efficacy against *Cryptosporidium* organisms has also been demonstrated (Jenkins 2004). It is approved by the FDA as a treatment for cryptosporidial infection in children.

Clinical Use

Horses. Field trials with NTZ have shown a success rate, defined by an improvement in neurologic signs and/or conversion to a negative result on western blot of the CSF, of 57–81%. This included a 78% success rate for horses that had previously been treated with other drugs for EPM. Horses are treated for 28 days. For the first 5 days, the dose is 11.36 mg/lb orally once daily. The dose is then increased to 22.72 mg/lb orally once daily for the remaining 23 days. This drug should not be used in horses less than 1 year of age or in those horses that have concurrent disease.

Cats. Sustained inhibition of *Cryptosporidium* oocyst shedding in the feces of four naturally infected cats after a single oral dose of 75 mg/kg BW has been reported. However, reshedding of oocysts was prompted by administration of corticosteroids. NTZ is not well tolerated by cats and results in vomiting and dark, foul-smelling diarrhea (Gookin et al. 2001).

REFERENCES

Adams, L. G. 1981. Clinicopathological aspects of imidocarb dipropionate toxicity in horses. Res Vet Sci 31(1):54–61.

Andrade, S. G., Andrade, Z. A., Sadigursky, M., 1980. Combined treatment with a nitrofuranic and a corticoid in experimental Chagas' disease in the dog. Am J Trop Med Hyg 29:766–773.

Baneth, G., Weigler, B., 1997. Retrospective case-control study of hepatozoonosis in dogs in Israel. J Vet Intern Med 11:365–370.

Baneth, G., Shaw, S. E. 2002. Chemotherapy of canine leishmaniosis. Vet Parasitol 106(4):315–24.

Barr, S. C. 2006. American trypanosomiasis, In C. E. Greene, ed., Infectious Diseases of the Dog and Cat, 3rd ed., pp. 676–681. Philadelphia: W. B. Saunders.

Barr, S. C., Bowman, D. D., Heller, R. L. 1994a. Efficacy of fenbendazole against giardiasis in dogs. Am J Vet Res 55(7):988–90.

Barr, S. C., Bowman, D. D., Heller, R. L., and Erb, H. N. 1993. Efficacy of albendazole against giardiasis in dogs. Am J Vet Res 54:926–927.

Barr, S. C., Bowman, D. D., Frongillo, M. F., and Joseph, S. L. 1998. Efficacy of a drug combination of praziquantel, pyrantel pamoate, and febantel against giardiasis in dogs. Am J Vet Res 59:1134–1136.

Barr, S. C., Jamrosz, G. F., Hornbuckle, W. E., Bowman, D. D., and Fayer, R. 1994b. Use of paromomycin for treatment of cryptosporidiosis in a cat. J Am Vet Med Assoc 205:1742–1743.

Belloli, S. C., Ceci, L., Carli, S., Montesissa, C., de Natale, G., Marcotrigiano, G., and Ormas, P. 1995. Disposition of antimony and aminosidine in dogs after administration separately and together: implications for therapy of leishmaniasis. Res Vet Sci 58:123–127.

Belloli, S. C., Grescenzo, G., Carli, S., Villa, R., Sonzogni, O., Carelli, G., and Ormas, P. 1996. Pharmacokinetics and dosing regimen of aminosidine in the dog. Vet Res Com 20:533–541.

Birkenheuer, A. J., Levy, M, G., Breitschwerdt, E. B. 2004. Efficacy of combined atovaquone and azithromycin for therapy of chronic *Babesia gibsoni* (Asian genotype) infections in dogs. J Vet Intern Med 18(4):494–8.

Blum, J., Burri, C.. 2002. Treatment of late stage sleeping sickness caused by *T.b. gambiense:* a new approach to the use of an old drug. Swiss Med Wkly 132(5–6):51–6.

Clubb, S. L. 1986. Therapeutics. In G. J. Harrison and L. R. Harrison, eds., Clinical Avian Medicine and Surgery, pp. 327–355. Philadelphia: W. B. Saunders.

Coetzee, J. F., Apley, M. D., Kocan, K. M. Comparison of the efficacy of enrofloxacin, imidocarb, and oxytetracycline for clearance of persistent *Anaplasma marginale* infectins in cattle. Vet Ther 2006 Winter 7(4):347–360.

Coldham, N. G., Moore, A. S., Sivapathasundaram, S., Sauer, M. J. 1994. Imidocarb depletion from cattle liver and mechanism of retention in isolated bovine hepatocytes. Analyst 119(12):2549–52.

Coldham, N. G., Moore, A. S., Dave, M., Graham, P. J., Sivapathasundaram, S., Lake, B. G., Sauer, M. J. 1995. Imidocarb residues in edible bovine tissues and in vitro assessment of imidocarb metabolism and cytotoxicity. Drug Metab Dispos 23(4):501–5.

Combrink, M. P., Troskie, P. C., De Waal, D. T. 2002. Residual effect of antibabesial drugs on the live redwater blood vaccines. Ann NY Acad Sci 969:169–73.

Conway, D. P., Johnson, J. K., Guyonnet, V., Long, P. L., and Smothers, C. D. 1993. Efficacy of semduramicin and salinomycin against different stages of *Eimeria tenella* and *E. acervulina* in the chicken. Vet Parasitol 45:215–229.

Davis, J. L., Gardner, S. Y., Jones, S. L., Schwabenton, B. A., Papich, M. G. 2002. Pharmacokinetics of azithromycin in foals after i.v. and oral dose and disposition into phagocytes. J Vet Pharmacol Ther 25(2):99–104.

Dirikolu, L., Karpiesiuk, W., Lehner, A. F., Hughes, C., Woods, W. E., Harkins, J. D., Boyles, J., Atkinson, A., Granstrom, D. E., Tobin, T. 2006. New therapeutic approaches for equine protozoal myeloencephalitis: pharmacokinetics of diclazuril sodium salts in horses. Vet Ther 7(1):52–63.

Dow, S. W. 1988. Management of anaerobic infections. Vet Clin N Am Sm Anim Pract 18(6):1167–82.

Dow, S. W., LeCouteur, R. A., Poss, M. L., Beadleston, D. 1989. Central nervous system toxicosis associated with metronidazole treatment of dogs: five cases (1984–1987). J Am Vet Med Assoc 195(3):365–8.

Driesen, S. J., Fahy, V. A., and Carland, P. G. 1995. The use of toltrazuril for the prevention of coccidiosis in piglets. Aust Vet J 72:139–141.

Dubey, J. P., and Lindsay, D. S.. 1998. Isolation of *Sarcocystis neurona* from opossum (*Didelphis virginiana*) faeces in immunodeficient mice and its differentiation from *Sarcocystis falcatula*. Int J Parasitol 29:1823–1828.

el Banna, H. A., Abo el-Sooud, K., Soliman, G. A. 1999. Comparative pharmacokinetics of diminazene in lactating goats and sheep. Zentralbl Veterinarmed A 46(1):49–57.

Elitok, B., Elitok, O. M., Pulat, H. 2005. Efficacy of azithromycin dihydrate in treatment of cryptosporidiosis in naturally infected dairy calves. J Vet Intern Med 19(4):590–3.

Evans, J., Levesque, D., Knowles, K., Longshore, R., Plummer, S. 2003. Diazepam as a treatment for metronidazole toxicosis in dogs: a retrospective study of 21 cases. J Vet Intern Med 17(3):304–10.

Fayer, R., and Ellis, W. 1993. Paromomycin is effective as prophylaxis for cryptosporidiosis in dairy calves. J Parasitol 79:771–774.

Fenger, C. K., Granstrom, D. E., Langemeier, J. L., and Stamper, S. 1997. Epizootic of equine protozoal myeloencephalitis on a farm. J Am Vet Med Assoc 210:923–927.

Fichera, M. E., and Roos, D. S. 1997. A plastid organelle as a drug target in apicomplexan parasites. Nature 390:407–409.

Finch, R. G., and Snyder, I. S. 1986. Antiprotozoan drugs. In C. R. Craig and R. E. Stitzel, eds., Modern Pharmacology, 2nd ed., pp. 729–740. Boston: Little, Brown.

Finegold, S. M., and Mathisen, G. E. 1990. Metronidazole. In G. L. Mandell, R. G. Douglas, and J. E. Bennett, eds., Principles and Practice of Infectious Diseases, 3rd ed., pp. 303–308. New York: Churchill Livingstone.

Fourmy, D., Yoshizawa, S., and Puglis, J. D. 1998. Paromomycin binding induces a local conformational change in the A-site of the 16 S rRNA. J Mol Biol 277:333–345.

Gardner, T. B., Hill, D. R. 2001. Treatment of giardiasis. Clin Microbiol Rev 14(1):114–28.

Gary, A. T., Kerl, M. E., Wiedmeyer, C. E., Turnquist, S. E., Cohn, L. A. 2004. Bone marrow hypoplasia associated with fenbendazole administration in a dog. J Am Anim Hosp Assoc 40(3):224–9.

Geurden, T., Claerebout, E., Dursin, L., Deflandre, A., Bernay, F., Kaltsatos, V., Vercruysse, J. 2006. The efficacy of an oral treatment with paromomycin against an experimental infection with *Giardia* in calves. Vet Parasitol 135(3–4):241–7.

Giangaspero, A., Traldi, G., Paoletti, B., Traversa, D., Bianciardi, P. 2002. Efficacy of pyrantel embonate, febantel and praziquantel against *Giardia* species in naturally infected adult dogs. Vet Rec 150:184–186.

Gookin, J. L., Stauffer S. H., Coccaro M. R., Poore M. F., Levy M. G., Papich M. G. 2007. Efficacy of tinidazole for treatment of cats experimentally infected with *Tritrichomonas foetus*. AM J Vet Res 68:1085-8.

Gookin, J. L., Copple, C. N., Papich, M. G., Poore, M. F., Stauffer, S. H., Birkenheuer, A. J., Twedt, D. C., Levy, M. G. 2006. Efficacy of ronidazole for treatment of feline *Tritrichomonas foetus* infection. J Vet Intern Med 20:536–543.

Gookin, J. L., Levy, M. G., Law, J. M., Papich, M. G., Poore, M. F., Breitschwerdt, E. B. 2001. Experimental infection of cats with *Tritrichomonas foetus*. Am J Vet Res 62:1690–1697.

Gookin, J. L., Riviere, J. E., Gilger, B. C., Papich, M. G. 1999. Acute renal failure in four cats treated with paromomycin. J Am Vet Med Assoc 215:1821–1823, 1806.

Granot, I., Halevy, O., Hurwitz, S., and Pines, M. 1993. Halofuginone: an inhibitor of collagen type I synthesis. Biochem Biophys Acta 1156:107–112.

Greene, C. E., Latimer, K., Hopper, E., Shoeffler, G., Lower, K., Cullens, F. 1999. Administration of diminazene aceturate or imidocarb dipropionate for treatment of cytauxzoonosis in cats. J Am Vet Med Assoc 215:497–500, 482.

Griffiths, J. K., Balakrishnan, Widmer, G., and Tzipori, S. 1998. Paromomycin and genticin inhibit intracellular *Cryptosporidium parvum* without trafficking through the host cell cytoplasm: implications for drug delivery. Infect Immun 66:3874–3883.

Harari, J., and Lincoln, J. 1989. Pharmacologic features of clindamycin in dogs and cats. J Am Vet Med Assoc 195:124–125.

Jenkins, M. C. 2004. Present and future control of cryptospori-diosis in humans and animals. Expert Rev Vaccines 3(6):669–71.

Jones, J. E., Solis, J., Hughes, B. L., Castaldo, D. J., and Toler, J. E. 1990. Production and egg-quality responses of white leghorn layers to anticoccidial agents. Poult Sci 69:378–387.

Kadappu, K. K., Nagaraja, M. V., Rao, P. V., Shastry, B. A. 2002. Azithromycin as treatment for cryptosporidiosis in human immunodeficiency virus disease. J Postgrad Med 48(3):179–81.

Kather, E. J., Marks, S. L., Kass, P. H. 2007. Determination of the in vitro susceptibility of feline *Tritrichomonas foetus* to 5 antimicrobial agents. J Vet Intern Med 21(5):966–70.

Keith, C. L., Radecki, S. V., Lappin, M. R. 2003. Evaluation of fenbendazole for treatment of *Giardia* infection in cats concurrently infected with *Cryptosporidium parvum*. Am J Vet Res 64:1027–1029.

Kier, A. B. 1990. Cytauxzoonosis. In C. E. Greene, ed., Infectious Diseases of the Dog and Cat, pp. 792–795. Philadelphia: W. B. Saunders.

Kirkpatrick, C. E., Skand, D. L. Giardiasis in a horse. 1985. J Am Vet Med Assoc 15;187(2):163–4.

Kühler, S., Delwiche, C. F., Denny, P. W., Tilney, L. G., Webster, P., Wilson, R. M. J., Palmer, J. D., and Roos, D. S. 1997. A plastid of probable green algal origin in apicomplexan parasites. Science 275:1485–1489.

Kuttler, K. L. 1988. Chemotherapy of babesiosis. In M. Ristic, ed., Babesiosis of Domestic Animals and Man, pp. 227–243. Boca Raton, Fla.: CRC Press.

Kuttler, K. L., Zaugg, J. L., Gipson, C. A. 1987. Imidocarb and parvaquone in the treatment of piroplasmosis (*Babesia equi*) in equids. Am J Vet Res 48(11):1613–6.

LeVine, D., Papich, M. G., Gookin, J., et al. Pharmacokinetics of ronidazole in healthy cats. (2008, submitted for publication).

Lewis, B. D., Penzhorn, B. L., Volkmann, D. H. 1999. Could treatment of pregnant mares prevent abortions due to equine piroplasmosis? J S Afr Vet Assoc 70(2):90–1.

Lindsay, D. S., and Dubey, J. P. 1999. Determination of the activity of pyrimethamine, trimethoprim and sulfonamides and combinations of pyrimethamine and sulfonamides against *Sarcocystis neurona* in cell cultures. Vet Parasitol. 82:205–210.

Lindsay, D. S., Blagburn, B. L., and Dubey, J. P. 1997b. Feline toxoplasmosis and the importance of the *Toxoplasma gondii* oocyst. Comp Cont Ed Pract Vet 19:448–461.

Lindsay, D. S., Dubey, J. P., and Blagburn, B. L. 1997a. Biology of *Isospora* spp. from humans, nonhuman primates, and domestic animals. Clin Microbiol Rev 10:19–34.

Long, P. L. 1971. Maternal transfer of anticoccidial drugs in the chicken. J Comp Pathol 81:373–382.

———. 1993. Avian coccidiosis. In J. P. Kreier, ed., Parasitic Protozoa, vol. 4, 2nd ed., pp. 1–88. San Diego: Academic Press.

Long, P. L., Sheridan, K., and McDougald, L. R. 1981. Maternal transfer of some anticoccidial drugs in the chicken. Poult Sci 60:2342–2345.

Longhofer, S. L. 1988. Chemotherapy of rickettsial, protozoal, and chlamydial diseases. Vet Clin N Amer Sm Anim Pract 18:1183–1196.

Looker, D. L., Marr, J. J., and Stotish, R. L. 1986. Modes of action of antiprotozoal agents. In W. L. Campbell and R. S. Rew, eds., Chemotherapy of Parasitic Diseases, pp. 193–207. New York: Plenum Press.

Lucumi, A., Robledo, S., Gama, V., and Saravia, N. G. 1998. Sensitivity of *Leishmania viannia panamensis* to pentavalent antimony is correlated with the formation of cleavable DNA-protein complexes. Antimicrob Agents Chemother 42:1990–1995.

Maarouf, M., de Kouchkovsky, Y., Brown, S., Petit, P. X., and Robert-Gero, M. 1997. In vivo interference of paromomycin with mitochondrial activity of *Leishmania*. Exp Cell Res 232:339–348.

Macintire, D.K., Vincent-Johnson, N.A., Kane, C.W., Lindsay, D.S., Blagburn, B.L., Dillon, A.R., 2001, Treatment of dogs infected with *Hepatozoon americanum*: 53 cases (1989–1998). J Am Vet Med Assoc 218, 77–82.

MacKay, R. L., Davis, S. W., and Dubey, J. P. 1992. Equine protozoal myeloencephalitis. Comp Cont Ed Pract Vet 14:1359–1366.

Mancassola, R., Reperant, J. M., Naciri, M., and Chartier, C. 1995. Chemoprophylaxis of *Cryptosporidium parvum* infection with paromomycin in kids and immunological study. Antimicrob Agents Chemother 39:75–78.

Mathis, G. F., and McDougald, L. R. 1981. Experimental development of resistance to amprolium or dinitolmide in *Eimeria acervulina* and its effect on inhibition of sporulation of oocysts. J Parasitol 67:956–957.

McDougald, L. R. 1993. Chemotherapy of coccidiosis. Proc 6th Int Coccid Conf, Guelph, Canada, pp. 45–47.

Mdachi, R. E., Murilla, G. A., Omukuba, J. N., Cagnolati, V. 1995. Disposition of diminazene aceturate (Berenil) in trypanosome-infected pregnant and lactating cows. Vet Parasitol 58(3):215–25.

Meingasser, J. G., Schmook, F. P., Czok, R., and Meith, H. 1979. Enhancement of the anticoccidial activity of polyether antibiotics in chickens by tiamulin. Poult Sci 58:308–313.

Meyer, C., Guthrie, A. J., Stevens, K. B. 2005. Clinical and clinicopathological changes in 6 healthy ponies following intramuscular administration of multiple doses of imidocarb dipropionate. J S Afr Vet Assoc 76(1):26–32.

Mitema, E. S., Sangiah, S., Martin, T. 1988. Effects of some calcium modulators on monensin toxicity. Vet Hum Toxicol 30(5):409–13.

Miwa, G. T., Wang, R., Alvaro, R., Walsh, J. S., Lu, A. Y. 1986. The metabolic activation of ronidazole [(1-methyl-5-nitroimidazole-2-yl)-methyl carbamate] to reactive metabolites by mammalian, cecal bacterial and *T. foetus* enzymes. Biochem Pharmacol 35:33–36.

Moore, D. A., Atwill, E. R., Kirk, J. H., Brahmbhatt, D., Herrera Alonso, L., Hou, L., Singer, M. D., Miller, T. D. 2003. Prophylactic use of decoquinate for infections with *Cryptosporidium parvum* in experimentally challenged neonatal calves. J Am Vet Med Assoc 223(6):839–45.

Neff-Davis, C. A., Davis, L. E., Gillette, E. L. 1981. Metronidazole: a method for its determination in biological fluids and its disposition kinetics in the dog. J Vet Pharmacol Ther 4(2):121–7.

Noli, C., Auxilia, S. T. 2005. Treatment of canine Old World visceral leishmaniasis: a systematic review. Vet Dermatol 16(4):213–32.

Novilla, M. N. 1992. The veterinary importance of the toxic syndrome induced by ionophores. Vet Hum Toxicol 34(1):66–70.

O'Handley, R. M., Olsen, M. E., McAllister, T. A., Morck, D. W., Jelinski, M., Royan, G., and Cheng, K. J. 1997. Efficacy of fenbendazole for treatment of giardiasis in calves. Am J Vet Res 58:384–388.

Parashar, A., Arya, R. 2005. Nitazoxanide. Indian Pediatr 42(11):1161–5.

Patrick, D. A., Boykin, D. W., Wilson, D. W., Tanious, F. A., Spychala, J., Bender, B. C., Hall, J. E., Dykstra, C. C., Ohemeng, K. A., and Tidwell, R. R. 1997. Anti-*Pneumocystis carinii* pneumonia activity of dicationic carbazoles. Eur J Med Chem 32:781–783.

Payne, P. A., Ridley, R. K., Dryden, M. W., Bathgate, C., Milliken, G. A., Stewart, P. W. 2002. Efficacy of a combination febantel-praziquantel-pyrantel product, with or without vaccination with a commercial *Giardia* vaccine, for treatment of dogs with naturally occurring giardiasis. J Am Vet Med Assoc 220:330–333.

Penzhorn, B. L., Lewis, B. D., de Waal, D.T., and Lopez- Rebollar, L. M. 1995. Sterilization of *Babesia canis* infections by imidocarb alone or in combination with diminazene. J S Afr Vet Assoc 66:157–159.

Pfefferkorn, E. R., Borotz, S. E., and Nothnagal, R. F. 1993. Mutants of *Toxoplasma gondii* resistant to atovaquone (566C80) or decoquinate. J Parasitol 79:559–564.

Pilch, D. S., Kirolos, M. A., Liu, X., Plum, G. E., and Breslauer, K. J. 1995. Berenil [1,3-Bis(4′-amidinophenyl)triazene] binding to DNA duplexes and to RNA duplex: evidence for both intercalative and minor grove binding properties. Biochemistry 34:9962–9976.

Ricketts, A. P., Glazer, E. A., Migaki, T. T., and Olson, J.A. 1992. Anticoccidial efficacy of semduramicin in battery studies with laboratory isolates of coccidia. Poult Sci 71:98–103.

Roos, D. S. 1993. Primary structure of the dihydrofolate reductase-thymidylate synthase gene from *Toxoplasma gondii*. J Biol Chem 268:6269–6280.

Rosado, T. W., Specht, A., Marks, S. L. 2000. Neurotoxicosis in 4 cats receiving ronidazole. J Vet Intern Med 21(2):328–31.

Sarkiala, E., Jarvinen, A., Valttila, S., Mero, M. 1991. Pharmacokinetics of tinidazole in dogs and cats. J Vet Pharmacol Ther 14:257–262.

Scorza, A. V., Lappin, M. R. 2004. Metronidazole for the treatment of feline giardiasis. J Feline Med Surg 6(3):157–60.

Scorza, A. V., Radecki, S. V., Lappin, M. R. 2006. Efficacy of a combination of febantel, pyrantel, and praziquantel for the treatment of kittens experimentally infected with *Giardia* species. J Feline Med Surg 8(1):7–13.

Sekis, I., Ramstead, K., Rishniw, M., Schwark, W. S., McDonough SP, Goldstein RE, Papich MG, & Simpson KW. Single-dose Pharmacokinetics and Genotoxicity of Metronidazole in Cats. J Feline Medicine & Surgery (in press 2009).

Slappendel, R. J., and Teske, E. 1997. The effect of intravenous or subcutaneous administration of meglumine antimonate (Glucantime) in dogs with leishmaniasis: a randomized clinical trial. Vet Quart 19:10–13.

Slater, A. F., Cerami, A. 1992. Inhibition by chloroquine of a novel haem polymerase enzyme activity in malaria trophozoites. Nature 355(6356):167–9.

Steinman, A., Gips, M., Lavy, E., Sinay, I., Soback, S. 2000. Pharmacokinetics of metronidazole in horses after intravenous, rectal and oral administration. J Vet Pharmacol Ther 23(6):353–7.

Stokol, T., Randolph, J. F., Nachbar, S., Rodi, C., Barr, S. C. 1997. Development of bone marrow toxicosis after albendazole administration in a dog and cat. J Am Vet Med Assoc 210:1753–1756.

Sweeney, R. W., Sweeney, C. R., Soma, L. R., Woodward, C. B., Charlton, C. A. 1986. Pharmacokinetics of metronidazole given to horses by intravenous and oral routes. Am J Vet Res 47(8):1726–9.

Valladares, J. E., Freixas, J., Alberola, J., Franquelo, C., Cristofol, C., Arboix, M. 1997. Pharmacokinetics of liposome-encapsulated meglumine antimonate after intramuscular and subcutaneous administration in dogs. Am J Trop Med Hyg 57(4):403–6.

Valladares, J. E., Riera, C., Alberola, J., Gallego, M., Portus, M., Cristofol, C., Franquelo, C., Arboix, M. 1998. Pharmacokinetics of meglumine antimoniate after administration of a multiple dose in dogs experimentally infected with *Leishmania infantum*. Vet Parasitol 75(1):33–40.

Valladares, J. E., Riera, C., Gonzalez-Ensenyat, P., Diez-Cascon, A., Ramos, G., Solano-Gallego, L., Gallego, M., Portus, M., Arboix, M., Alberola, J. 2001. Long term improvement in the treatment of canine leishmaniosis using an antimony liposomal formulation. Vet Parasitol 97(1):15–21.

Vanparijs, O., Desplenter, L., Marsboom, R. 1989. Efficacy of diclazuril in the control of intestinal coccidiosis in rabbits. Vet Parasitol 34(3):185–90.

Van Reken, D. E., and Pearson, R. D. 1990. Antiparasitic agents. In G. L. Mandell, R. G. Douglas, and J. E. Bennett, eds., Principles and Practice of Infectious Diseases, 3rd ed., pp. 398–427. New York: Churchill Livingstone.

Vercammen, F., De Deken, R., and Maes, L. 1996. Prophylactic treatment of experimental canine (*Babesia canis*) with doxycycline. Vet Parasitol 66:251–255.

Vexenat, J. A., Olliaro, P. L., Castro, J. A. F., Cavalcante, R., Campus, J. H. F., Travares, J. P., and Miles, M. A. 1998. Clinical recovery and limited cure in canine visceral leishmaniasis treated with aminosidine (paromomycin). Am J Trop Med Hyg 58:448–453.

Vial, H. J., Gorenflot, A. 2006. Chemotherapy against babesiosis. Vet Parasitol 138(1–2):147–60.

Webster, L. T. 1990. Drugs used in chemotherapy of protozoal infections: leishmaniasis, trypanosomiasis, and other protozoal infections. In A. G. Gilman, T. W. Rall, A. S. Nies, and P. Taylor, eds., The Pharmacological Basis of Therapeutics, 8th ed., pp. 1008–1017. New York: Pergamon Press.

Williams, R. B. 1997. The mode of action of anticoccidial quinolones (6-decyloxy-4-hydroxyquinoline-3-carboxylates) in chickens. Int J Parasitol 27:101–111.

Wood, B. A., Rycroft, D., Monro, A. M. 1973. The metabolism of tinidazole in the rat and dog. Xenobiotica 3:801–812.

Xiao, L., Saeed, K., and Herd, R. P. 1996. Efficacy of albendazole and fenbendazole against *Giardia* infection in cattle. Vet Parasitol 61:165–170.

Zajac, A. M., LaBranche, T. P., Donoghue, A. R., and Chu, T. C. 1998. Efficacy of fenbendazole in the treatment of experimental *Giardia* infection in dogs. Am J Vet Res 59:61–63.

Zimmer, J. F. 1987. Treatment of feline giardiasis with metronidazole. Cornell Vet 77(4):383–8.

Zinner, S. H., and Mayer, K. H. 1990. Sulfonamides and trimethoprim. In G. L. Mandell, R. G. Douglas, and J. E. Bennett, eds., Principles and Practice of Infectious Diseases, 3rd ed., pp. 325–334. New York: Churchill Livingstone.

CHAPTER 44

ECTOPARASITICIDES

RONALD E. BAYNES

INTRODUCTION

The focus of this chapter is to describe the pharmacology of veterinary drugs and pesticides currently approved to control important ectoparasites that adversely affect domestic animal health and production. These ectoparasites are primarily insects (fleas, flies, lice) and ascarines (ticks and mites, flies). Effective control of these ectoparasites is not only critically important for the veterinary patients, but also from a public health perspective as several of the animal ectoparasites not only transmit disease between animals but they can also transmit major diseases to humans. Fleas are known vectors for tapeworms, *Dipylidium caninum* and humans can develop cat scratch disease when *Bartonella henselae* is transmitted from cats to humans via cat fleas. Flea allergy dermatitis (FAD) is a major concern for companion animals. These are among the most important reasons why flea control in companion animals is critical, and it explains why annual expenditures to control fleas have totaled in excess of $2 billion in the U.S. and Western Europe (Kramer and Mencke 2001). Ticks can transmit Lyme disease, Rocky Mountain spotted fever, babesia in dogs and cattle, and heartwater in ruminants to mention only a few. Mosquitoes can transmit West Nile virus to humans; heartworm diseases to pets; and malaria to birds, rodents, and primates; they also serve as biological vectors of viral encephalitides in horses. Flies not only transmit disease and cause damage to hides and coats of pets, their nuisance can result in decreased feed intake in livestock and thus reduced timely weight gain and economic loss to livestock farmers. Face flies are known to transmit the causative agent (*Moraxella bovis*) of pinkeye or infectious bovine keratoconjunctivitis in cattle. Control of myiasis-causing flies can be significantly reduced with effective ectoparasiticides.

The *feeding behaviors* of ectoparasites differ and this may be critical if the drug of choice is strictly a repellent or adulticide. Adult fleas usually engorge themselves with a blood meal from the host with 5 minutes to 1 hour of infestation of the animal, with female fleas feeding for about 25 minutes and males feeding for 11 minutes (Cadiergues et al. 2000). In order to prevent FAD, an effective ectoparasiticide should be able to prevent this feeding behavior. Comparative efficacy studies suggest that organophosphates (OPs) and/or pyrethroids, more so than the newer ectoparasiticides, may be more effective in preventing the flea from taking the first blood meal (Franc and Cadiergues 1998). Ticks feed on a blood meal for a longer period (days) before it is completed. Under these conditions pathogens such as *Borrelia burgdorferi*, which causes Lyme disease, become well adapted to this long feeding period. However, with other tickborne pathogens such as *Ehrlichia* and *Rickettsia*, transmission can occur within the first hours. For these reasons, the use of combination drugs (insecticide and repellent) will prevent ticks from attaching and feeding (Young et al. 2003). A good example of this desired combined efficacy is a drug formulation containing the repellent permethrin and the acaricide imidacloprid.

The ideal ectoparasiticide should not only be an effective repellent and adulticide, it must also be *persistent* in the blood or skin surface at therapeutic concentrations for a significantly long time, such as 1–3 months, so that there is adequate client compliance. Another challenge is the formulation of an insecticide that is *stable* to sunlight and also water/shampooing. An excellent example of this is imidacloprid, which is photostable and persistent after shampooing compared to the early generation pyrethroids that were not very stable in sunlight. Some formulations, such as Frontline Plus, contain the adulticide (fipronil) as well as an insect growth inhibitor (methoprene) because by the time pets are observed to be infested with fleas, the fleas would already have laid eggs. A final consideration in choice of therapy is whether to *treat the environment* as well as the animal. There appears to be a new paradigm within the last 10 years of treating the pet and not the environment (Rust 2005).

PHARMACEUTICS OF TOPICAL FORMULATIONS

Many of the commercial topical ectoparasiticides used to treat domestic animals are formulated to be released from 1) liquid organic/aqueous formulations and/or 2) synthetic polymers such as collars and ear tags. The rate of penetration through the skin or translocation across the skin surface is dependent on several critical pharmaceutical properties. Liquid formulations include pour-ons, topical sprays, and dips, which consist of the active ingredient and other (formerly called *inert*) ingredients that can modulate dermal pharmacokinetics. These other ingredients include mostly alcohols, oils, and spreading agents (Magnusson et al. 2001). The ear tags are composed of a solid organic polymeric macromolecule (e.g., polyvinyl chloride) and an active ingredient that are mixed with the tag being formed by injection molding. These devices are designed to slowly release the insecticide over a defined time period (e.g., Cutter Gold® lasts 5 months) as the animal moves its head, but it should be removed at the end of the fly season or before slaughter.

TRANSDERMAL DELIVERY

Topical application is more common for administration of ectoparasiticides. An understanding of the dermal pharmacokinetics of these drug and pesticide formulations will further the understanding of drug efficacy and safety. Many of these drugs and pesticides are lipophilic with large molecular weights (Table 44.1), and therefore it's not surprising that there is slow dermal absorption, low systemic *bioavailability*, large volume of distribution, and long plasma and tissue half-lives. All of these are important factors when considering repeat

TABLE 44.1 Chemical structures and physicochemical properties of common ectoparasiticides

Name	Chemical Name (Empirical Formula) [Molecular Weight] Log P	Chemical Structure
Permethrin	3-(2,2-dichloroethenyl)-2,2-dimethyl-cyclopropane-carboxylic acid (3-phenoxyphenylmethyl) ester ($C_{21}H_{20}Cl_2O_3$) [391.29] Log P = 6.10	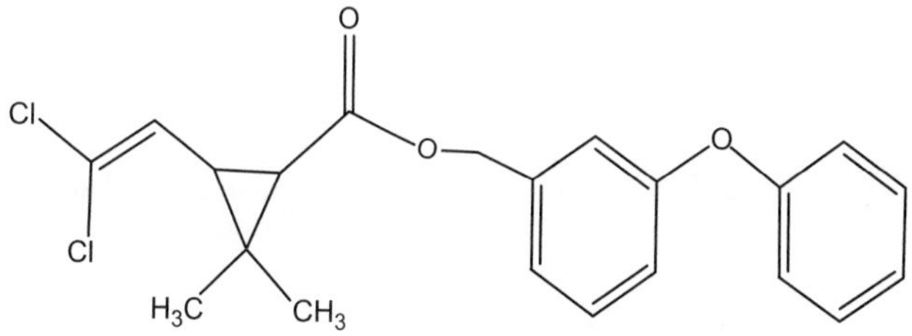
Fenthion	Phosphorothioic acid O,O-dimethyl O-[3-methyl-4-(methylthio)phenyl] ester ($C_{10}H_{15}O_3PS_2$) [278.34] Log P = 4.84	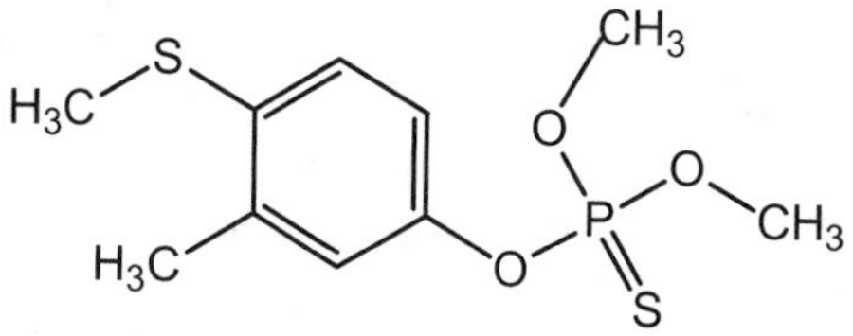
Carbaryl	1-naphthalenol methylcarbamate ($C_{12}H_{11}NO_2$) [201.22] Log P = 1.85	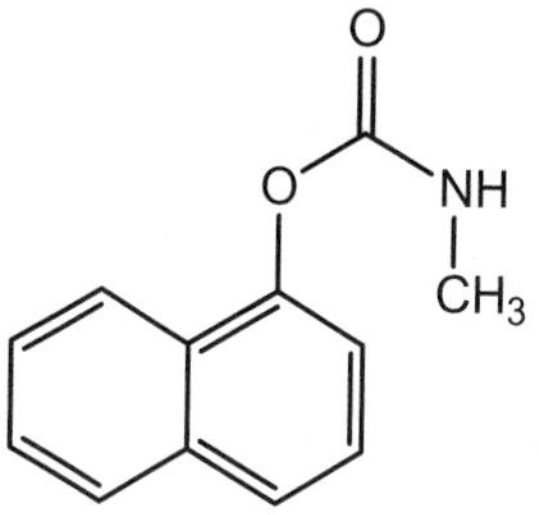
Ivermectin	22,23-dihydroavermectin B_1 ($C_{48}H_{74}O_{14}$) [875.10] Log P = 5.31	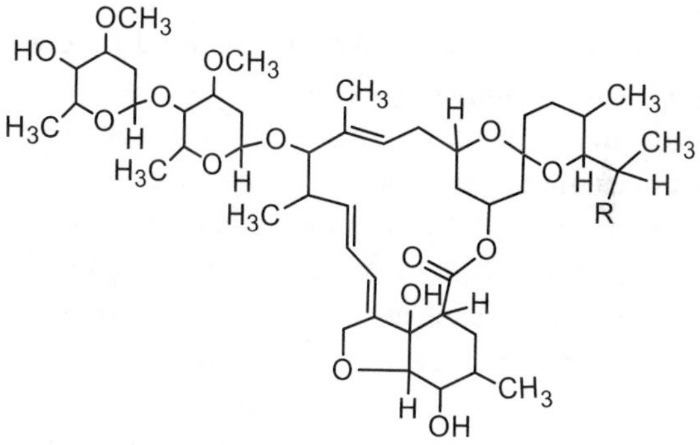
Milbemycin Oxime	5-didehydromilbemycin (oxime derivative) 80% A_4, 20% A_3 ($C_{31}H_{43}NO_7$) A_3 [541.68] ($C_{32}H_{45}NO_7$) A_4 [555.71] Log P = 5.29	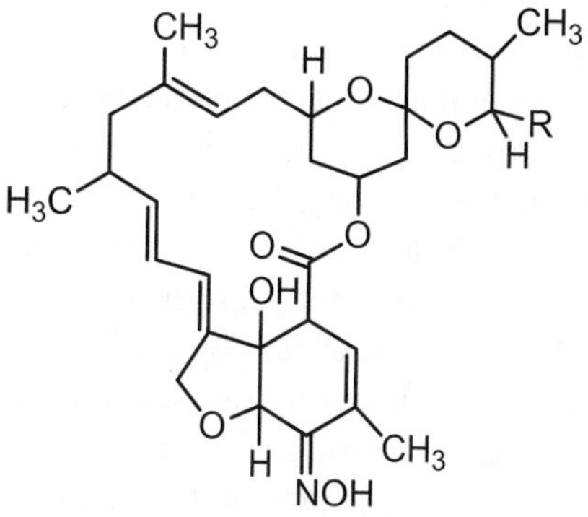

TABLE 44.1—*continued*

Name	Chemical Name (Empirical Formula) [Molecular Weight] Log P	Chemical Structure
Fipronil	5-amino-1-[2,6-dichloro-4-(trifluoromethyl)phenyl]-4-[(trifluoromethyl)sulfinyl]-1H-pyrazole-3-carbonitrile ($C_{12}H_4Cl_2F_6N_4OS$) [437.15] Log P = 4.0	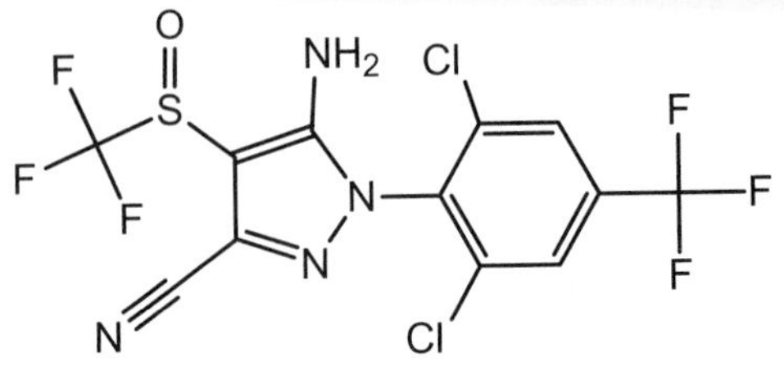
Imidacloprid	1-[(6-chloro-3-pyridinyl)methyl]-4,5-dihydro-N-nitro-1H-imidazol-2-amine ($C_9H_{10}ClN_5O_2$) [255.66] Log P = 0.57	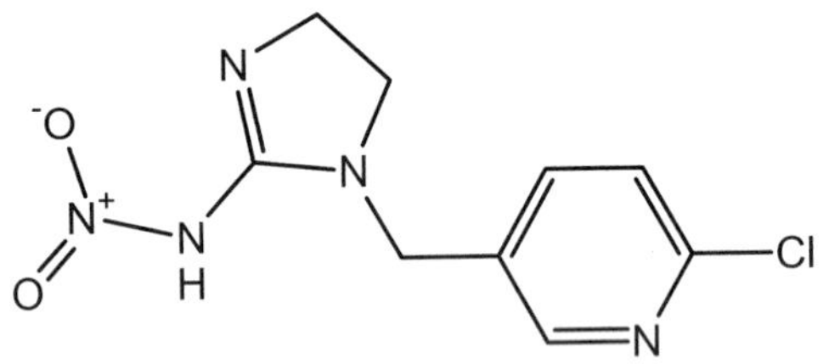

applications and strategies to minimize the emergence of pest resistance, whether it's in a house, kennel, or pasture, and also to minimize drug residues in food-producing animals.

The advantages of transdermal delivery include ease of application to the animal's coat and avoidance of the problems of first pass metabolism and gastrointestinal degradation often associated with oral administration. Some of the major disadvantages associated with this route of administration are that pet owners sometimes overdose the animal with topical sprays or pour-on formulations, which often result in toxicoses in sensitive populations such as feline species and juveniles. Licking is part of the natural grooming and social behavior of many animal species; this can result in significant oral absorption and subsequently increased systemic exposure in the treated and also untreated animals that are part of a large livestock herd (Laffont et al. 2003). Application of pour-on products to food animals can result in significantly longer withdrawal times when compared to administration by oral or injection. This is most evident with ivermectin pour-on products, which cause significant retention of ivermectin in the skin layers and thus prolong release of the drug. For example, this results in a 45-day withdrawal time for the pour-on product versus 35 days for the subcutaneous route (KuKanich et al. 2005).

ROUTES OF DERMAL ABSORPTION

There are five possible routes (Fig. 44.1) for a drug or pesticide to diffuse as it partitions from the formulation on the skin surface through the stratum corneum and viable epidermis before entering the microcapillaries at the epidermal-dermal juncture. Many if not all of the ectoparasiticides diffuse through the intercellular matrix (intercellular route) in the stratum corneum and viable epidermis. This matrix may vary biochemically between animal species, but in all species this matrix consists of varying proportions of fatty acids, ceramides, and cholesterol. The reader should also be aware that apparent epidermal thickness (Monteiro-Riviere et al. 1990) varies across animal species in the following order, thereby influencing the intercellular path length for the diffusing pesticide:

Porcine > Cattle > Canine > Feline

(52 μm) (37 μm) (21 μm) (13 μm)

The intracellular route and the sweat pores are less likely routes for these lipophilic chemicals because they have more hydrophilic properties than the intercellular matrix.

Even though light microscopy examination of skin suggests that the hair follicle extends into the dermis and

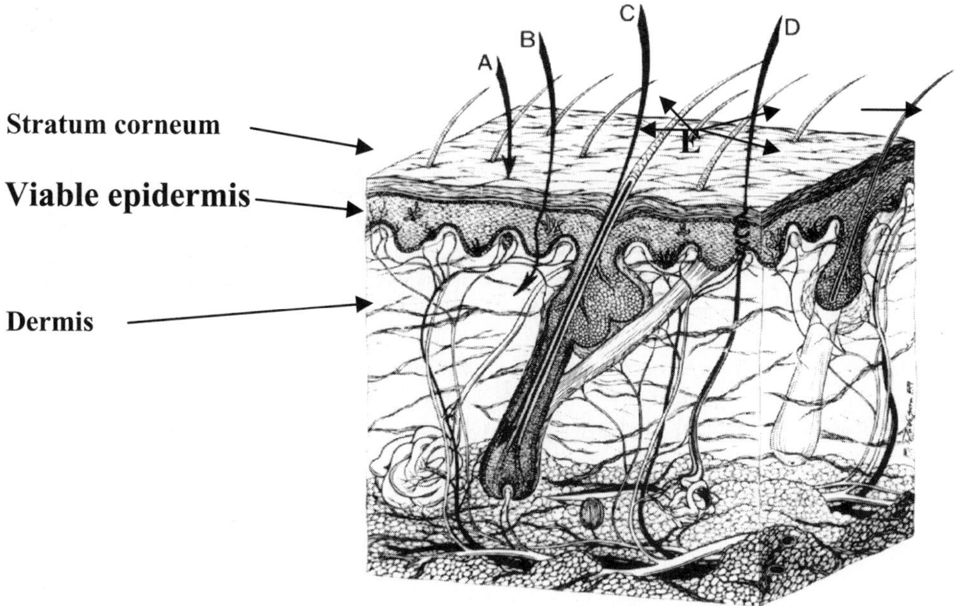

FIG 44.1 Pathways for drug and insecticide transport in mammalian skin. A = transcellular; B = intercellular; C = transfollicluar; D = sweat pore; E = lateral diffusion.

hypodermis, this is not really true. The hair follicle is really a deep invagination of the epidermis, and therefore if a drug travels down the hair follicle, it still has to cross the epidermis in order to gain access to the circulatory system. However, the presence of many hair follicles significantly increases the effective epidermal surface area and thus increased flux, although the apparent surface area may be the same. This in part explains why care must be taken when administering pour-on ectoparasiticides in an extra-label manner across species. In essence, hair follicles are arranged and distributed differently across animal species, and these differences can dictate transdermal delivery into the systemic circulation for pour-on products as well as translocation across the skin surface for topicals. The coat may contain primary and or secondary hair follicles. The former are large-diameter and deep-rooted into the dermis and associated with sebaceous and sweat glands. The secondary follicles are smaller in diameter, they are near the surface, and they have sebaceous glands but no sweat gland erector pili muscle. Horses and cattle have single hair follicles distributed evenly; pigs have single follicles grouped in clusters of 4 follicles. Dogs have primary and secondary follicles with as many as 15 hairs emerging from a single opening in the skin. Goats will have primary follicles occurring in groups of 3 with 3–6 secondary follicles associated with each group. Sheep are bit more complex. They have hair-growing regions with mostly single follicles on face, distal leg region, and ears and they have wool-growing regions over most of their body, which can be defined as mostly compound follicles. A cluster will have 3 primary follicles and several secondary follicles.

MECHANISMS OF ACTION

Ectoparasiticides can have the following broad mechanisms of action that can affect the biology of the ectoparasite. More specific examples are summarized in Table 44.2.

- Ectoparasite nervous system
  - AChE inhibitors
  - Na^+ channel blockers
  - nAChR inhibitors
  - GABA and Cl^- channel inhibitors
- Ectoparasite repellant
- Insect growth and development.

A good ectoparasiticide has a high efficacy against the ectoparasite and is not toxic to the host. Many of the organophosphate and organochlorine pesticides are very effective and have broad spectrum activity. However, because of their toxicity to mammals (Table 44.2) and the fact that there are safer pesticides available for veterinary

TABLE 44.2 Mechanisms of action of ectoparasiticides against the parasite and signs of mammalian toxicity

Drug	Mechanism of Action	Signs of Toxicity
Fipronil	Noncompetitively blocks passage of Cl ions through GABA- and glutamate-gated channels	Hyperactivity and convulsions related to GABA antagonism
Imidacloprid	Competitive inhibition at postsynaptic nicotinic acetylcholine receptors (nAChR) leads to influx of Na ions	Nicotinic effects (tremors)
Avermectins	Targets glutamate-gated chloride channels Targets GABA- and glycine-gated chloride ion channels	CNS depression and ataxia
Pyrethrins and Pyrethroids	Targets voltage-gated Na ion channels in axonal membrane	Type 1 Syndrome (tremors, hyperexcitability) Type 2 Syndrome (salivation, weakness)
Organophosphates and Carbamates	Inhibits acetylcholinesterase (AChE)	Muscarinic and nicotinic effects (miosis, tremors, depression)
Amitraz	Inhibits monamine oxidase	Activates α2-adrenergic receptors (CNS depression)
Insect Growth Regulators	Falsely signals insect to remain in immature stage Inhibits of chitin synthesis	No known toxic signs
Synergists	Inhibits cytochrome P450	Can potentiate drugs and pesticides

use, fewer chemicals from these two classes are being used in veterinary medicine. For this reason, this chapter will not discuss the organochlorines especially as they are no longer approved for veterinary use. The newer ectoparasiticides such as the neonicotinoids (e.g., imidacloprid) are more selective for certain insects such as fleas, and very few other insects. However, the term "broad spectrum" may be misleading. Recall that ivermectin which is often regarded as a broad spectrum antiparasitic drug is indeed highly effective against many nematodes and ectoparasites, but is without effect on cestodes and trematodes.

RESISTANCE TO ECTOPARASITICIDES

Resistance has been widely reported for many popular ectoparasiticides, such as the avermectins, pyrethroids, and organophosphates. Resistance also tends to occur where there is intensive use of antiparasitic drugs; even on "well managed" farms. There is some concern that as the newer insecticides, such as the neonicotinoids, become more frequently and inappropriately used, resistance can potentially emerge. However, there is little or no evidence of fleas developing resistance to the increasing use of imidacloprid (Schroeder et al. 2003). Mechanisms of resistance may be related to decreased penetration, increased detoxification enzyme activity, and decreased sensitivity of the target site. These mechanisms have been more recently elucidated from a molecular basis using annotated insect genomes and recognizing that insect resistance is mediated by complex multigene enzyme systems. Pyrethroid resistance among insects has been associated with mutations in the sodium channel genes reducing the ability of the insecticide to bind to the sodium channel. Although resistance to imidacloprid has not been demonstrated in cat fleas, mutations in nicotinic acetylcholine receptors have been associated with some agronomic insects being resistant to this new class of insecticides (Liu et al. 2005).

Cross-resistance for a specific target site is indeed very common within individual insecticide classes. However, cross-resistance across different target sites has more severe consequence and limits insect management. Detoxification mechanisms are often the source of cross-resistance between insecticides that differ in their mechanisms of action. These detoxification enzymes include the carboxylesterases, cytochrome P450 s, and glutathione-s-transferases that are often implicated in pyrethroid and OP resistance. In a more recent observation, point mutations in the *Rdl* gene in a field population of cat fleas confers cyclodiene resistance and cross-resistance to fipronil, which is one of the few new chemicals on the commercial market (Daborn et al. 2004).

Strategies that can prevent or delay resistance include 1) appropriate selection of insecticides, 2) insecticide rotations and mixtures, 3) limited interactions with agricultural pesticides, and 4) resistance monitoring. The latter is a major issue when it comes to treating fleas because there are no universally susceptible strains of cat flea known (Russ 2005). However the use of various genetic tools such as TaqMan-allele specific amplification provides a promising method for assaying large populations of insects for insecticide resistance to the newer chemistries on the commercial market. With this in mind the reader is encouraged to read recent reviews (ffrench-Constant et al. 2004) on how the new genetic tools are addressing insecticide resistance.

FIPRONIL

Fipronil was first approved in 1996 for use in dogs and cats to treat for fleas and ticks. This chemical has been marketed as Frontline® TopSpot and Frontline® Plus for dogs, puppies, cats, and kittens and Frontline® Spray Treatments for cats and dogs. The Plus product indicates that fipronil was formulated with methoprene which is an insect growth regulator (IGR), which will be discussed in more detail under IGRs. The TopSpot product contains 9.7% fipronil, and the Spray contains 0.29%.

CHEMISTRY. This insecticide is classified as phenylpyrazole with the molecular formula: $C_{12}H_4Cl_2F_6N_4OS$. Fipronil has a molecular weight of 437.15 and log P (n-octanol/water) of 4.0, and solubility of 2 mg/l in water and >10,000 mg/l in corn oil. (Merck 1996). This high affinity for oils in the skin partly explains why dermal absorption is limited.

PHARMACOKINETICS. Topical application of the fipronil formulation between the shoulder blades is believed to result in surface translocation of the chemical over the entire body with significant deposition in sebum, sebaceous glands, and hair follicles. In effect, the sebaceous glands act as a reservoir that continuously secretes fipronil out of the hair follicle forming a layer on and in the stratum corneum and fur of the animal. Recognizing that 95% effective flea control requires 0.7 μg fipronil/g fur, as much as 4.5 μg/g and 1.6 μg/g have been detected in cats at 42 days and dogs at 56 days, respectively. Dermal absorption of ^{14}C-fipronil was less than 1% of the applied dose for all doses tested (0.88–48 mg/rat) and up to 24 hours exposure (Cheng 1995).

MECHANISM OF ACTION. Fipronil acts on the central nervous system where it appears to be primarily effective in noncompetitively blocking the passage of chloride ions through GABA-gated and glutamate-gated chloride channels in ectoparasites. The latter mechanism exists in ectoparasites, but not mammals, suggesting that there are multiple insect target sites for this drug. Recent work has demonstrated that fipronil and its metabolite, fipronil sulfone, are potent inhibitors at these sites (Zhoa et al. 2005). In mammals, fipronil binding to the GABA receptor is also less effective, which also accounts for its wide margin of safety. Fipronil sulfone has a higher potency than fipronil in mammalian GABA receptors, and simultaneous exposure to other drugs that potentiate formation of the metabolite could potentially be toxic to mammals in these scenarios. However, data from the literature is conflicting as to whether metabolic conversion to the sulfone derivative represents detoxification. For example, pretreatment of mice with a cytochrome P450 oxidase inhibitor, piperonyl butoxide, increased the toxicity of fipronil by as much as sevenfold (Hainzl and Casida 1996). Prior to its veterinary approval, fipronil was and is still approved for use in plant agriculture; however, photochemical conversion can result in a desulfinylated photoproduct that is tenfold more potent than Fipronil at the mammalian chloride channel. Whether this will be a concern for livestock that forage on exposed pastures is still to be determined.

EFFICACY. Fipronil as a topical spray is effective against adult fleas, all stages of brown dog ticks, American dog tick, lone star ticks, and deer ticks. This product is approved for dogs, cats, puppies, and kittens (>8 weeks), and can provide protection for up to 30 days. The manufacturers claim that although the Topical Spot On product can be effective against fleas for as long as 3 months, they still recommend that it be applied every month. Fipronil formulated with s-methoprene (Fipronil Plus), an insect growth regulator, is not only an effective adulticide, it also kills flea eggs and flea larvae. While excellent ectoparasiticidal efficacy against fleas and ticks has been proven, there has been some concern about its repellent effects against ticks and also ticks already on the animal (Denny 2001;

Young et al. 2003). Compared to some pyrethroids and some OPs, fipronil is also not effective in preventing fleas from biting and feeding within the first hour of infestation and prior to being killed (Franc and Cadiergues 1998). Fipronil is also effective for the treatment and control of biting lice (*Trichodectes canis*) in canine infestations (Pollmeier et al. 2002, 2004), although its use to treat lice infestations is extralabel.

SAFETY/TOXICITY. Fipronil appears to have a wide margin of safety (rat dermal LD50 = 2000 mg/kg), and thus is regarded as a lower order of toxicity when used in veterinary applications. No adverse effects have been observed at five times the maximum dose rate in dogs and cats. However, slight skin or eye irritation has been observed after skin and eye exposure, respectively (Technical Information Sheet 1997). The oral and dermal LD50 in rats is 100 mg/kg and >2000 mg/kg, respectively (Merck 1996). Like the avermectins and organochlorines, fipronil's mechanism of action involves GABA receptor antagonism. At toxic doses, it can cause hyperactivity, hyperexcitability, and convulsions, which are correlated with increased spontaneous nerve activity and generation of prolonged high-frequency discharges with nerve stimulation. These symptoms are associated with blockage of the neuronal inhibition or membrane hyperpolarization because these antagonists are also blocking chloride uptake. This in effect results in stabilization of the GABA-bound form of the chloride channel (Bloomquist 2003).

There appear to be no reported interactions between fipronil and approved companion animal drugs and ectoparasiticides. Animals exposed to large doses of fipronil via accidental oral absorption are expected to display seizures, and neurological and hepatic function should be monitored (Hovda and Hooser 2002). Extralabel use in young or small rabbits can cause seizures and death. Multigenerational rat studies have concluded that this drug is not mutagenic or teratogenic.

NEONICOTINOIDS

IMIDACLOPRID. Imidacloprid has been approved for use in crop agriculture as a systemic insecticide as well as treating fleas on dogs and cats. It is available as 9.1% w/v in Advantage™ specifically to target fleas and also formulated at 8.8% w/v with permethrin (44% w/v) in K9 Advantix™ to treat for fleas as well as ticks.

Chemistry. Imidacloprid belongs to a relatively new class of synthetic insecticides known as the *neonicotinoids.* Imidacloprid (chloronicotinyl nitroguanidine) more specifically belongs to the chloronicotinyls that were first synthesized in 1985. This chemical was found to have 62-fold to greater than 3000-fold more insecticidal activity than the nicotinoids (e.g., nicotine), and was introduced into the commercial market in 1991. These chemicals are photostable, which ensures prolonged residual efficacy, and they are moderately soluble in water (0.51 gm/l). The log octanol water partition coefficient of imidacloprid is 0.57 and it has a molecular weight of 255.7. Unlike the nicotinoids, the neonicotinoids are not ionized at physiological pH. Neonicotnoids therefore more readily penetrate the CNS of insects than nicotinoids because the former has a greater hydrophobicity. This physicochemical difference in physiological conditions partly explains why the neonicotinoids have greater insecticidal activity than the nicotine-based insecticides.

Pharmacokinetics. Topical application of imidacloprid to the skin does not result in significant dermal absorption into the bloodstream, but rather surface translocation aided by body movement resulting in whole body coverage. Its efficacy is dependent on contact with the flea at the surface of the animal's skin. Results from metabolism and toxicokinetics studies in other vertebrates suggest that if this chemical becomes systemic, it is widely distributed to organs, but not to fatty tissues or the central nervous system (Sheets 2001).

Mechanism of Action. At the nicotinic cholinergic synapse, acetylcholine (ACh) is normally released from the presynaptic membrane and binding to the postsynaptic membrane results in a conformational change in the receptor molecule that leads to activation and opening of the ion channel and subsequent influx of extracellular Na^+ and efflux of K^+. This results in change in membrane potential, and propagation of nerve impulse. Imidacloprid essentially mimics the effects of ACh by competitive inhibition at the postsynaptic nicotinic acetylcholine receptors (nAChR) and it has little or no effect on muscarinic acetylcholine receptors (Buckingham et al. 1997; Tomizawa and Casida 2003). The former are widely and predominantly distributed in the neuropil regions of the CNS in insects, and imidacloprid is highly specific for nicotinic receptor subtypes unique to insects. However, instead of a depolarization of the postsynaptic neuron and transmission of the nerve impulse, as normally seen with acetylcholine, imidacloprid causes a biphasic response. This consists of increased frequency of spontaneous discharge followed by a block in nerve pulse propagation along the neurons and then insect death (Schroeder and Flattum 1984). Muscarinic receptors and other types of nicotinic receptors in mammals do not bind imidacloprid effectively, which accounts for its selectivity for insects (Kagabu 1997). There is therefore no surprise that no adverse effects are observed when dogs were topically exposed to greater than the recommended dosage. Readers should be aware that although the neonicotinoids are selective, the nicotinoids are less selective and therefore more toxic to vertebrates than the neonicotinoids.

Efficacy. Compared to fipronil and selemectin, imidacloprid appears to be more readily taken up by the flea via body contact (Mehlhorn et al. 2001). Mehlhorn and colleagues demonstrated that imidacloprid killed larvae and adult fleas within 1 hour of exposure, while similar efficacy was achieved with the other two chemicals within 24 hours. It should be noted that none of these three chemicals had any repellent activity against fleas. Imidacloprid can kill 98–100% of adult fleas for at least 4 weeks on dogs and cats. This chemical has limited activity against ticks. Imidacloprid also stops fleas from biting within 3–5 minutes after application, although the fleas do not die within this short time frame. This clearly is useful for preventing FAD. Earlier studies demonstrated that shampooing or water exposure does not significantly reduce the efficacy of imidacloprid for up to 28 days (Cunningham et al. 1997).

In Fall 2002, Bayer Corp. received registration from EPA for a topical ectoparasite K9 Advantix™, which is topical insecticide formulated with imidacloprid and permethrin to repel and kill mosquitoes, ticks, and fleas on adult dogs and puppies 7 weeks of age and older for up to 4 weeks. The product's efficacy is not affected by swimming or bathing activities. Imidacloprid acts on the postsynaptic nicotinic receptor by "locking" it in the open position, thus hyperstimulating the neuron, and permethrin keeps open the Na^+ ion exchange channels causing constant nerve impulses. Recall that these would normally close after transmitting an impulse. There is therefore a synergistic interaction on the nervous system that is associated with an overwhelmed parasite nervous system followed by rapid paralysis and death of the parasite. Due to their unique physiology and inability to metabolize certain compounds such as the pyrethroid (reduced glucuronidation activity in cats), this product must *NOT* be given to cats.

Safety/Toxicity. Clinical signs of toxicity are usually associated with nicotinic effects (e.g., tremors) and hepatic effects when dogs are exposed to 41 mg/kg in the diet high dose (Hovda and Hooser 2002). However, except for one single reported case in cats (Godfrey 1999), there are no published reports of imidacloprid causing toxicity in domestic animal species following dermal exposure. The chemical does not cause dermal irritation nor does it appear to cause dermal sensitization. Imidacloprid does not appear to be a teratogen, reproductive toxicant, mutagen, or carcinogen (Sheets 2001). The available products should not be given to puppies or kittens younger than 4 months.

NITENPYRAM. Nitenpyram (Capstar™) is in the same class as imidacloprid (i.e., chloronicotinyl), and therefore has the same mechanism of action. This is, however, not a topical application but an *oral adulticide* that is used against fleas in dogs and cats.

Chemistry. Nitenpyram, like imidacloprid, belongs to the new class of synthetic insecticides known as the *neonicotinoids*. Nitenpyram has a molecular weight of 270.72, a log octanol water partition coefficient of −0.64, and water solubility of 840 gm/l.

Pharmacokinetics. Nitenpyram is readily absorbed (bioavailability = 100%) in the gastrointestinal tract; the time to maximum blood concentration is 1.21 hours in dogs and 0.63 hours in cats. The Cmax is about 4.3 to 4.8 ppm in both dogs and cats, which is significantly greater than the blood concentration of 0.5–1.0 ppm nitenpyram required to kill 100% of the fleas. The half-life in dogs and cats is 2.8 hours and 7.7 hours, respectively, and it is primarily excreted in the urine.

Efficacy. The recommended minimum oral daily dosage is 1 mg/kg in tablet form with or without food and as often as once per day when fleas are seen on the animal. One dosage form (11 mg) is for cats and dogs up to 11 kg, and the other dosage form (57 mg) is for dogs between 11 and 57 kg. This chemical is also very effective against fleas that have become resistant to fipronil (Schenker et al. 2001). Based on the above pharmacokinetics, it is no surprise that fleas begin falling off of the coat of dogs and cats within 0.5 hours of administration of this drug (Rust et al. 2003; Rust 2005). Efficacy reaches 98.6% in dogs and 98.4% in cats within 6 hours.

Safety/Toxicity. The acute oral LD50 in male rats is 1680 mg/kg., which suggests that this chemical is very safe. Dogs and cats given 10 times the recommended dose do not appear to experience adverse health effects (7–8-month-old cats and 7-month-old dogs, Witte and Luempert 2001). In the same study, administration of one, three, or five times the recommended daily dose for 6 months resulted in no adverse health effects in dogs and cats that were initially 8 weeks old. The drug is well tolerated for daily doses in puppies and kittens that are >4 weeks. No adverse reactions were observed when used with most other drugs or ectoparasiticides such as topical carbaryl, fipronil, pyrethin, or even imidacloprid, which has a similar mechanism of action (Witte and Luempert 2001). A transient itching period observed in dogs and cats within 1–2 hours after treatment with this product appears not to be associated with the chemical irritation, but attributed to fleas displaying increased trembling activity before dying and falling off the animal (Mahoney et al. 2001).

MACROCYCLIC LACTONES

These macrolides consist of two major groups, avermectins and milbemycins, that are effective against many ectoparasites, as summarized in Table 44.3. The avermectins include ivermectin, eprinomectin, doramectin, and selamectin, and the milbemycins include moxidectin and milbemycin oxime.

CHEMISTRY. Both avermectin and milbemycin groups are 16-membered macrocyclic lactones. The avermectins are products of *Streptomyces avermitilis* that have the 16-membered macrocycle replaced by a spiroketal unit at C-17 to C-28, a hexahydrobenzofuran at C-2 to C-8a, and a bisoleadrosyloxy disaccharide at C-13. The milbemycins are also products of *Streptomyces* and are structurally similar to the avermectins, but *lack the sugars at C-13*. The latter group is believed to enhance antiectoparasite activity. The

TABLE 44.3 US FDA approved* ectoparasiticides

Drug Class	Approved Species	Approved Indications
Avermectins/Milbemycins		
Ivermectin	Cats	Ear mites
	Beef cattle	Ticks, lice, mites
	Pigs	Mites
Doramectin	Beef cattle	Lice, mites, ticks, grubs
	Pigs	Lice, mites
Eprinomectin	Dairy and beef cattle	Lice, mites, flies
Selamectin	Dogs	Fleas, mites, ticks
	Cats	Fleas, mites
Moxidectin	Dairy and beef cattle	Lice, mites, flies, grubs
Milbemycin	Cats	Ear mites
Organophosphates		
Fenthion	Beef cattle	Grubs, lice, flies
Famphur	Beef cattle	Grubs, lice, flies, ticks
Amitraz	Dogs	Mites
Nitenpyram	Dogs and cats	Fleas
Lufenuron	Dogs and cats	Fleas

*Approved as of June 2006.

nemadectins are classified as milbemycins, but differ from the milbemycins proper because they have a distributed double bond at C-26. An important nemadectin is moxidectin (e.g., Cydectin). Eprinomectin (4″-epi-acetylamino-4″-deoxy-avermectin B1) is a true second-generation macrocyclic lactone synthesized from avermectin. Doramectin differs from ivermectin in that a six-carbon ring replaces a three- or four-carbon chain at the C-25 position of the basic ivermectin. Compared to ivermectin, these molecular differences result in a more lipophilic and persistent doramectin molecule.

PHARMACOKINETICS. The oral, IV, and subQ pharmacokinetics have been described elsewhere in this book. The focus here will be to compare the dermatopharmacokinetics of topically applied avermectins. It should be first noted that eprinomectin and moxidectin pour-ons are formulated in >80% oil content. This encourages more drug depot formation on skin surface and stratum corneum, and thus *reduced bioavailability* compared to pour-on products with ivermectin and doramectin. The latter are formulated with isopropyl alcohol, which is more likely than oil to promote epidermal flux. Because of the high oil content of the eprinomectin and moxidectin formulations, there is evidence that it is rain-fast and thus impervious to rain and other forms of weather precipitation (Gogolewski et al. 1997)

The dermal bioavailability of doramectin is about 40% greater than ivermectin in cattle (Gayrard et al. 1999). The dermal bioavailability for doramectin pour-on is approximately 16% when compared to the subcutaneous route of administration. Following topical application of selamectin, this drug is slowly absorbed (flip-flop kinetics) into the bloodstream and redistributed to form reservoirs in sebaceous glands as well as the hair follicle and basal cells of the epidermis (Sarasola et al. 2002). Dermal bioavailability appears to be significantly greater in cats (74%) than in dogs (4.4%), although this may be attributed to greater self-grooming in cats than in dogs. However, selamectin flux is three times greater in cat skin (0.1 $\mu g/cm^2/hr$) than in dog skin (0.03 $\mu g/cm^2/hr$). The half-life of this drug is greater in cats (69 hours) than in dogs (14 hours), and in general, selamectin half-life is greater in cats and dogs following dermal > oral > IV administration. This demonstrates its persistence in the stratum corneum and upper epidermis. As with many of the avermectins, the dermal absorption process is the rate-limiting step, and the increased persistence in the body after dermal application should reduce reinfection rates by ectoparasites. There is also conflicting evidence of differences in selamectin disposition between male and female dogs (Sarasola et al. 2002; Dupuy et al. 2004).

MECHANISM OF ACTION. In invertebrates, the avermectins primarily target the glutamate-gated chloride channels that are close in proximity to GABA-gated sites. It is possible that these endectocides may also potentiate GABA-gated sites as well. Chloride influx lowers cell membrane resistance and causes hyperpolarization of the resting potential of postsynaptic cells. Transmission to muscles is therefore prevented. The ectoparasite therefore displays ataxia, paralysis, and death. In contrast to GABA antagonists (e.g., lindane and fipronil) that lead to convulsions, the avermectins cause a different neurological syndrome that is characterized at first by a coarse tremor followed by ataxia and comalike sedation. It should be noted that the avermectins can block GABA at low concentrations, but at high concentrations cause irreversible channel activation or enhancement of GABA effect, which is associated with the classical signs of ataxia and sedation. These endectocides have a wide margin of safety because they are very selective for the glutamate-gated channels in nematodes and arthropods but are lacking in mammals. In mammals, the avermectins primarily target the GABA- and possibly the glycine-gated chloride channels (Bloomquist 2003). Furthermore, in mammals, GABA-mediated neurotransmission occurs in the CNS, and where the blood-brain barrier (BBB) prevents uptake of the endectocides. These endectocides are also thought to interfere with parasite reproduction. It should be noted that unlike the macrolide antibiotics, these endectocides lack antibacterial and antifungal activity.

EFFICACY

Ivermectin. Injectable formulations are used to control lice (*Haematopinus suis*) and mange mites (*Sarcoptes scabiei var suis*) in *swine* and horn flies (*Haematobia irritans*); and grubs (*Hypoderma bovis*), biting and sucking lice (*Lignathus vituli, Haemaotopinus eurystemus*), and mites (*Sarcoptes scabei var bovis*) in *cattle*. Pour-on and oral formulations are also available for cattle. There is NO immediate death to ticks in cattle, but reduced reproductive potential. As these drugs are eliminated in the feces, they are effective against dung-breeding flies. Not all commercial formulations of ivermectin are approved for the treatment of the most common type of cattle mange caused by chorioptic mite. In dogs, SC doses can be effective against otodectic, sarcoptic, and notoedric mange and control of demodectic mange. A relatively new topical product (Acarexx®) is approved for treating adult ear mites (*Otodectis cynotis*) in cats and kittens 4 weeks of age and older. There is evidence that the ears do not necessarily need to be cleaned before treatment.

Eprinomectin. This is available only as a pour-on formulation (Eprinex®) and is approved only for dairy and beef cattle. It is an oil-based formulation that makes the drug "waterproof" to some extent. This broad spectrum antiparasiticide is effective against lice, horn flies, and mites. Because of its unique molecular structure, eprinomectin does not readily partition into milk and therefore is one of the two endectocides that requires NO milk withholding time. The meat withdrawal time is also zero.

Doramectin. Doramectin is available as an injectable for beef cattle (0.2 mg/kg SC and IM) and swine (0.3 mg/

kg IM) and pour-on (0.5 mg/kg) for beef cattle only. It is believed to be more efficacious than other endectocides against biting and sucking lice. This drug is not approved for dairy cattle because of the concern for significant residues in milk.

Cattle: The spectrum of activity is similar to that of ivermectin. Doramectin has activity against important sucking lice, grubs, ticks, mites, and screwworms in cattle. The latter is unique among the macrolide endectocides. Application of the pour-on can prevent reinfestation of lice for as long as 16 weeks.

Swine: Doramectin is approved for use against sucking lice and mange mites.

Moxidectin. Moxidectin products (Cydectin®, Equest®) are a new generation of milbemycins that have a broad spectrum of activity against nematode and arthropod parasites in cattle. Unlike the previously discussed endectocides, this is a single compound, and not a mixture of two compounds. The approved dose of Cydectin® pour-on is 0.5 mg/kg in cattle, and the drug has a spectrum of activity similar to ivermectin. Cydectin® *is the only pour-on endectocide labeled for control of common scab mite* (*Psoroptes ovis*), a reportable disease requiring quarantine.

Selamectin. Revolution® is a topical monthly application approved for treating dogs and cats for ear mites and adult fleas, and prevents flea eggs from hatching. In dogs, it is used in the treatment and control of sarcoptic mange (*Sarcoptes scabiei*) and control of the tick (*Dermacentor variabilis*). Selamectin is the only spot-on product approved for control of canine sarcoptic mange. There are anecdotal reports of delayed responses to this drug and a few treatment failures (Curtis 2004). However, in lieu of these situations, some veterinary dermatologists recommend that this drug be reapplied every 2–3 weeks with owner's consent as this is extralabel use of the drug.

Milbemycin Oxime. Milbemycin oxime is well known as a heartworm preventative, but it also has significant ectoparasiticidal effects. The only approved use of this chemical as an ectoparasiticide, MILBEMITE® OTIC Solution, at 0.1% is used as a treatment for ear mite (*Otodectes cynotis*) infestations in cats and kittens 4 weeks of age and older. Milbemycin oxime may also be effective in cases of amitraz-resistant demodicosis, but this is not an approved use thus far.

TABLE 44.4 Withdrawal times of pour-on macrolide endectocides

Generic Drug	Example	Approved Species	Withdrawal Times
Ivermectin	Ivomec®	Beef cattle	48 days for meat
Eprinomectin	Eprinex®	Beef and dairy cattle	0 days for meat and milk
Doramectin	Dectomax®	Beef cattle	45 days for meat
Moxidectin	Cydectin®	Beef and dairy cattle	0 days for meat and milk

SAFETY/TOXICITY. Ivermectin has a tenfold safety margin in ruminants, horses, swine, and dogs, except collies. Due to a mutation within the gene that codes for the MDR1 pump protein that normally disallows entry of ivermectin into the central nervous system, collies should not be treated with ivermectin or any other avermectin. Acute toxic signs include CNS depression, ataxia, and possible death. The principal clinical pathologic change is a decrease in serum iron values in dogs.

The meat and milk withdrawal times for this class of drugs vary across avermectins, and Table 44.4 provides clear evidence of this and why label instructions should be carefully followed. Extralabel use of doramectin or ivermectin in dairy cattle may require a milk withholding period of almost 60 days!

PYRETHRINS AND SYNTHETIC PYRETHROIDS

The pyrethrins are derived from the *Chrysanthemum* plant, but in recent years they have been slowly replaced with synthetic pyrethroids. The latter are more resistant to breakdown, which results in greater residual activity than the natural pyrethrins. Pyrethrins and pyrethroids are often formulated with insect growth regulators, synergists, and/or repellents to enhance efficacy. The more frequently used pyrethroids in veterinary formulations include permethrin, fenvalerate, cypermethrin, and phenothrin. These may be formulated as pour-ons, spray-ons, barn misters, feed-throughs, and shampoos.

CHEMISTRY. Natural pyrethrins occur as six compounds pyrethrin I, pyrethrin II, jasmolin I, jasmolin II, cinerin I, and cinerin II (Kaneko and Miyamoto 2001). The molecular weight of these insecticides ranges from 316.4 to 374.5 and log Ko/w ranges from 4.3 to 5.9. The synthetic pyrethroids are structurally similar to the natural pyrethrins, and many of those used in veterinary medicine have a wider range of molecular weights (302.4 to 416.3), logKo/w (4.6 to 7.4), and LD50 (105.8 to 4240 mg/kg). Depending on the literature reviewed, the pyrethroids can be classified in a number of ways. Some authors have grouped them into two broad generations of pyrethroids, with the first-generation being characterized as esters of chrysanthemic acid and alcohols having furan ring and terminal side-chain moieties. These pyrethroids are sensitive to light and temperature, and are therefore most effective when used indoors. The second-generation pyrethroids and for that matter, the majority of pyrethroids in veterinary use today, have a 3-phenoxybenzyl alcohol in the alcohol moiety and replacement of the photolabile moieties with dichlorovinyl, dibromovinyl substituent, and aromatic rings. These modifications provide excellent insecticidal activity and environmental stability for this class of pyrethroids.

Another classification system groups the pyrethroids into four generations, with the first generation reflecting the same properties as the first generation in the earlier classification scheme. The first-generation pyrethroids (e.g., allethrin) are similar to the natural pyrethrin, cinerin I, and therefore lack environmental stability. The second-generation pyrethroids (e.g., resmethrin and tetramethrin) are significantly more stable than the first generation and have significantly greater killing capacity than the natural pyrethrins. The third-generation pyrethroids include the ever-popular fenvalerate and permethrin, which are noted for their photostability and potency. Permethrin in particular is the most ubiquitous pyrethroid formulated with veterinary ectoparasiticidal products. The fourth-generation pyrethroids are the most potent (e.g., cypermethrin and cyfluthrin) and also the most persistent. For this reason they are most often formulated in ear-tags.

Pyrethroids are also classified as Type 2 pyrethroids (e.g., fenvalerate) because they have an alpha-cyano moiety unlike Type 1 pyrethroids (e.g., permethrin) which lack this moiety and thus are less toxic than Type 2 pyrethroids. The reader should be aware that these pyrethroid insecticides can exist as chiral and geometrical isomers, with some isomers displaying different pharmacokinetic and pharmacodynamic properties from other isomers of the same pyrethroid. Many of these chemicals are stable in weakly acidic water, but very unstable in an alkaline medium.

PHARMACOKINETICS. Dermal absorption of pyrethrins and pyrethroids is indeed very limited (<1%) across the skin of domestic and laboratory animals and humans. (Baynes and Riviere 2001). This is primarily because these chemicals are very lipophilic (Ko/w range from 4.0 to 7.4) and they have large molecular weights. There is therefore the tendency for these chemicals to reside in the outermost layer of the skin (stratum corneum) with little or no penetration into the systemic circulation. For this reason, the pyrethroids are approved by US EPA and *not* US FDA. These chemicals are also rapidly detoxified to harmless alcohol and acid metabolites and conjugates in the liver and blood, with half-lives ranging from a few minutes to typically a few hours (Ray 2005). The *trans* isomers are hydrolyzed at a faster rate than the *cis* isomers, and the presence of α-cyano group in the third- and fourth- generation pyrethroids also slows down hydrolysis and oxidation. In spite of this, many of these pyrethroids do not result in significant meat or milk withdrawal times following topical administration to food animals (Riviere and Baynes 1998). For example, there are several approved pour-on products for food animals that contain as much as 1–5% permethrin or 1% cyfluthrin but have zero meat and milk withholding times.

MECHANISM OF ACTION. Many different mechanisms of action have been proposed for this class of insecticides. Potential targets in insects include voltage-gated sodium, chloride, or calcium channels; GABA-gated chloride channels; mitochondrial ATPase; and nicotinic receptors to mention a few of the many proposed targets for pyrethroids. However, the main target is the gating kinetics of Na^+ channels in nerves, which results in repetitive discharges or membrane depolarization and ultimately death of the ectoparasite. Pyrethroids are extremely selective for insects over mammals as insect sodium channels can be as much as 100 times more sensitive than mammalian brain channels (Warmke et al. 1997). In fact, the selectivity ratio (mammalian toxicity versus insect toxicity) of most pyrethroids exceeds 1,000.

Recall that in normal voltage-gated sodium channels it is the inward sodium current that produces the action potential and then it is rapidly closed at normal resting potentials. However, with the interaction of the pyrethroid with the sodium channel this causes the sodium channel to remain open. This leads to a slowing of both the activation and inactivation process, which causes the now modified channel to be in a stable hyperexcitable state. Pyrethroid structure and stereo-specificity plays a significant role in the mechanism of action. For example, Type 2 pyrethroids such as fenvalerate keep the sodium channel open for a significantly longer period (i.e., prolongation of sodium channel current) than Type 1 pyrethroids such as permethrin, which in part explains the differential toxicity between these two classes of pyrethroids. The 1R and 1S cis isomers bind competitively while the 1R and 1S trans-isomers bind noncompetitively to another site. These insecticides, especially the Type 2 pyrethroids, could also suppress GABA and glutamate receptor-channel complexes. Pyrethroids are also classified as either Type I compounds (permethrin, resmethrin) because they cause rapid onset of hyperactivity and repetitive action potentials, or Type II compounds (fenvalerate, cypermethrin) because very low doses cause lethal effects and few behavior changes.

EFFICACY. Pyrethrins and pyrethroids are formulated in shampoos, sprays, collars, dips, dusts, and ear-tags to repel or treat for most of the known ectoparasites important to domestic animals. The discussion below attempts to review the more common applications of pyrethroid formulations used in veterinary medicine. Note that these are only examples, and that applications may vary depending on indication (spot-on versus spray) and this is related to the concentration of the pyrethroid in the formulation. These products may be formulated with synergist and/or insect growth regulators.

First-Generation Pyrethroids. Allethrin (d-trans allethrin) is most often formulated in shampoos for dogs and cats to kill fleas and/or ticks. An excellent example includes Mycodex® SensiCare™ Flea & Tick Shampoo, which has 0.12% d-trans allethrin.

Second-Generation Pyrethroids. Phenothrin (85.7%) is frequently used as a spot-on treatment for tick and fleas in dogs only. These spot-on products are *NOT* approved for cats as of 2005. There are phenothrin flea collars and a shampoo formulation available for both dogs and cats. Resmethrin (0.5%) is more often approved in foggers in stables and kennels, and it is also formulated as topical sprays for horses; there are a few shampoo formulations available for control of fleas and ticks on dogs and cats.

Third-Generation Pyrethroids. Permethrin is probably the most widely used pyrethroid in veterinary medicine. Almost all of the spot-on products are at high concentrations and are therefore approved only for dogs, and not cats, to manage fleas, ticks, and mites. The sprays, shampoos, and dusts are formulated at lower concentrations and thus approved for both species. Permethrin is also widely used in food animals as sprays and pour-ons to treat for ectoparasites and requires short withdrawal times provided the product is correctly diluted and is applied no more than every 2 weeks. For example, the Atroban spray products have a 5-day withdrawal time in swine treated with 0.11% permethrin for mange mites but 0 days in cattle treated with 0.02% pemethrin. Many products can have residual activity up to 28 days for some formulations.

Fenvalerate (8%) is formulated in ear-tags for cattle to control flies, lice, and ticks. There are no approvals for companion animals.

Fourth-Generation Pyrethroids. Cyfluthrin is approved for use as an ear-tag and as a pour-on for cattle (e.g., Cylence®, 1%) with no withdrawal time. As with other pyrethroids, there are some concentrates that are approved for use around livestock premises but not directly on animals. Cypermethrin is usually formulated as a spray and predominantly used as fly repellent around horses with some formulations marketed as being sweat resistant.

SAFETY/TOXICITY. The selectivity ratio, which compares toxicity in insects with that in mammals, is higher for pyrethrins and pyrethroids (>1000) than for organophosphates and carbamates (<100). Dermal exposure to pyrethrins and pyrethroids rarely results in systemic absorption to cause significant signs of toxicity in domestic animals, but grooming of the treated hair coat by cats can result in significant oral ingestion of pyrethroids. Cats, more so than dogs, are presented with clinical signs of toxicity, and this is often after the dog formulation was inadvertently applied topically to adult cats or kittens or the untreated cat comes into physical contact with a treated dog. Recall that cats are deficient in their ability to clear chemicals by hepatic glucuronidation. This explains why cats are more sensitive than dogs to pyrethroids. The dog-only spot-on flea and tick products can contain as much as 45–65% permethrin, which at this concentration can be very harmful to most cats (Meyer 1999). Not only is permethrin toxicity in cats a great concern, but so is phenothrin toxicity in cats. Phenothrin, a Type 1 pyrethroid similar to permethrin, was originally approved as a spot-on product with 85.7% phenothrin for cats. These products were canceled in 2005 by the manufacturer because of the adverse effects and numerous deaths in feline patients.

Clinical signs of pyrethroid toxicity may be confused with OP or carbamate toxicity, and they include nerve and muscle disorders and can be grouped in Type 1 (T) poisoning and Type 2 (CS) poisoning. The onset of signs of toxicity can occur within minutes to hours depending on the route of exposure, and the signs may resolve within 24 to 72 hours following supportive therapy. The Type 1 syndrome is similar to DDT in that it involves progressive body tremors, exaggerated startle response, hyperexcitability, and death. Type 2 syndrome is associated with induced salivation, weakness, and distinctive burrowing syndrome. These signs appear in both dogs and cats and large animals, and the prognosis is guarded to good depending on the exposure level. Readers are encouraged to refer to other texts and references on appropriate therapy (Richardson 2000).

Aquatic animals such as fish and invertebrates are highly susceptible to pyrethroids (Smith and Stratton 1986); therefore their use on and around livestock facilities should ensure that there is minimal environmental impact.

ORGANOPHOSPHATES

Organophosphates (OPs) have insecticidal, ascaricidal, and helminthicidal activity, and are thus classified as broad-spectrum ectoparaciticides, which explains why they were used in veterinary medicine for at least 4 decades since their discovery during WW II. These chemicals are becoming less popular for use in and around domestic animals as there are safer products such as the ivermectins, pyrethroids, neonicotinoids, and fipronil. Another concern is related to their persistence in the environment, which can negatively influence the ecosystem. For these and many other reasons, many of the popular organophosphates that were approved by US FDA or US EPA for use in companion or food animal species are no longer marketed or available for veterinary use. However, there is still sufficient veterinary use of OPs that are US FDA–approved (Table 44.3) and US EPA–registered that the reader should be aware of their efficacy and be able to recognize signs of organophosphate toxicity in domestic animals.

CHEMISTRY. Organophosphates are usually classified as phosphates (e.g., dichlorvos), phosphorothioates (e.g., coumaphos), or phosphorodithioates (e.g., malathion, fenthion). The term "thioates" indicates that for some OPs, the double-bonded oxygen is replaced with a sulfur molecule. They can also be classified based on when these chemicals were first developed for commercial use. The aliphatics derivatives were the first OP products and are characterized by their aliphatic-like structures (e.g., dichlorvos, malathion). These were followed by the phenyl derivatives, which contain a phenyl ring with one of the ring hydrogens displaced by Cl, NO_2, CH_3, CN, or S, (e.g., fenthion, famphur) and then the heterocyclic derivatives where the ring structures are composed of different or unlike atoms, such as N or S (e.g., diazonon, chlorpyriphos). The latter group is the longest acting OP based on chemical structure. The molecular weights of many of these chemicals used in veterinary medicine range from 257 (trichlorfon) to 384 (ethion). These chemicals can be very lipophilic with octanol-water partition coefficients ranging from 2 to 6.

MECHANISM OF ACTION. The thioate compounds ($P = S$), unlike the phosphate ($P = O$) compounds, must first be metabolized in the liver to oxy compounds before they can irreversibly inhibit acetylcholinesterase (AChE) by phosphorylation. Inhibition of AChE results in accumulation of acetylcholine (ACh) at cholinergic receptors. Recall that ACh is a normal neurotransmitter released at synapses that mediates transmission of nerve impulses to effector organs or skeletal tissues to produce a response. AChE is normally present at these nerve endings to rapidly hydrolyze ACh to control the level and duration of synaptic transmission. With OPs inhibiting AChE the resulting accumulation of ACh leads to paralysis and death to the parasite.

EFFICACY. As of 2006, there were only 10 OP generics approved for veterinary use in the U.S. Systemic bioavailability following topical application is limited, but these chemicals are distributed across the entire coat of the animal by lateral diffusion following topical application to a localized region. Several of these OPs are formulated as topical sprays and dusts or dip applications (coumaphos and phosmet), while many are formulated as ear-tags in cattle (pirimiphos and diazinon) and flea collars for dogs and cats (tetrachlorvinphos, dichlorvos, and diazinon). Chlorpyriphos and phosmet dips are the only OPs still approved for use in dogs to treat mange. Although chlorpyrifos was recently labeled for restricted use by US EPA, there are several Happy Jack products that are approved for use as shampoos and dips on dogs. These two products are indicated to kill fleas, ticks, and sarcoptic mange mites on dogs. Prior to the availability of avermectins for veterinary use, fenthion (Spotton®) and famphur (Warbex®), which are still US FDA approved drugs, were used extensively to control cattle grubs (*Hypoderma bovis* and *Hypoderma lineatum*) as well as lice. When treating for cattle grubs, the reader should be reminded that application of these therapeutics should occur soon after the heel-fly activity ceases. If the grub larvae are allowed to migrate to the esophagus or spinal canal, rapid killing of large numbers of these larvae following treatment can cause host-parasite reactions such as bloat, salivation, staggering, or paralysis.

SAFETY/TOXICITY. Inhibition of AChE can result in muscarinic and nicotinic effects. The muscarinic effects at the autonomic effector organs include miosis, lacrimation, vomiting, diarrhea, frequent urination, dypsnea, bradycardia, and hypertension. The nicotinic effects include effects at the neuromuscular junction such as muscle tremors and twitching, paresis, and possibly paralysis. Central nervous system signs may include depression, hyperactivity, and seizures, but these are rare events. Organophosphate-induced delayed neurotoxicity (clinical signs delayed for 7–21 days) may be observed in dogs and cats following exposure to some but not all OPs. The following drugs may potentiate the toxicity of OPs: phenothiazine tranquilizers, aminoglycoside antibiotics, and neuromuscular blocking agents such as levamisole and nicotine. Brahman, Charolais, and Simmental cattle are more sensitive than English breeds of cattle; greyhounds and whippets are the more sensitive dog breeds; cats are more sensitive than dogs; and poultry are more sensitive than mammals to organophosphates. Recall that several of these OPs are very lipophilic and potential residues in tissues and milk are possible. Except for fenthion and famphur, many of the currently marketed OPs approved for use in food animals as of 2006 have a very short withdrawal time or zero withdrawal times as they are less likely to cause residues in meat or milk when used according to label. These are all US EPA registered OPs, and they include coumaphos (Co-Ral®), which has a zero withdrawal time for meat and milk, and phosmet (Del-Phos® Emulsifiable Liquid Insecticide), which has a 3-day and 1-day meat withdrawal time for cattle and swine, respectively. Fenthion and famphur have very long meat withdrawal times—46 and 35 days, respectively—and are not approved for use in lactating dairy cattle.

CARBAMATES

Carbamates are cyclic or aliphatic derivatives of carbamic acid. These insecticides are generally safer than OPs, but they should be used with caution. The mechanism of action of carbamates is similar to that of OPs, except that inhibition is by carbamylation and the reaction is slowly reversible and spontaneous. The most frequently used carbamate is carbaryl, which may be formulated with pyrethrins and/or synergists. These products are approved for cats and dogs only as shampoos (0.5% carbaryl) and dusts (12.5% carbaryl). Unfortunately, these products need to be applied more often than the newer generation of veterinary insecticides and insect resistance is commonly reported. Propoxur is another carbamate that is slightly more potent than carbaryl, but it is included in flea and tick collars for dogs and cats. Toxicity associated with application of these two carbamates can be avoided if pets are not simultaneously exposed to anticholinesterase drugs or pesticides with similar mechanism of action, and exposure is limited to cats and dogs older than 12 weeks.

D-LIMONENE AND LINALOOL

These are volatile oil extracts from the peel of oranges, and it's their vapors and not necessarily direct contact that affects ectoparasites. This insecticide is formulated in shampoos and sprays. Although a relatively safe insecticide, *d-limonene* has caused *sporadic toxicoses* in cats (Hooser 1990; Lee et al. 2002). Clinical signs are not often seen at the label concentration, but they can occur at greater than five times the label dose. These signs can include excessive salivation, ataxia, and tremors as well as gross lesions in the scrotal and perineal area.

AMITRAZ

Amitraz is the only formamidine used in veterinary medicine, and is available in various formulations to treat for ticks, lice, and mites in dogs, swine, and cattle. To date, none of these approved products is labeled to repel or kill fleas. Although the mechanism of action of amitraz is not very clear, this ascaricide inhibits monamine oxidase (MAO) that normally metabolizes neurotransmitter amines present in the CNS of ticks and mites. There are no effects on cholinesterase activity.

EFFICACY. Amitraz is used as a dip (Mitaban®) to treat for generalized demodicosis (*Demodex canis*) in dogs. Amitraz can be applied as a 0.025% (250 ppm) sponge-on solution once a week (U.K.) or every 2 weeks (U.S.). However, this drug is not approved to treat localized demodicosis or scabies. There are several reports describing the use of higher concentrations (e.g., 1.25%) or more frequent applications to treat for scabies (Hugnet et al. 2001). These off-label protocols run the risk of dogs developing severe signs of amitraz-related toxicosis described below, and it's advisable to use the more safe drugs described for this condition. For example, selamectin is the only approved spot-on drug for treatment and control of scabies in dogs (Shanks et al. 2000). Amitraz is also impregnated in tick collars for dogs (Preventic®, 9% a.i.) and can kill ticks for up to 3 months, with activity beginning within 24 hours of placing the collar on the dog. These amitraz tick collars are not approved for cats.

Amitraz (e.g., Taktic® E.C., 12.5% a.i.) is approved for use in beef and dairy cattle for ticks such as *Amblyomma americanum* and *A. maculatum*; mites such as *Chorioptes bovis, Psoroptes,* and *Sarcoptes scabei;* biting louse (*Damalinia bovis*); and sucking lice *Haematopinus eurysternus, Lignathus vituli*, and *Solenoptes capillatus*. This product is also approved for use in swine to treat for mange mites and louse. *Taktic® is not approved for use in horses or dogs as it may cause death!!!* Once the spray mixture has been prepared it must be applied within 6 hours or it will lose its efficacy.

SAFETY/TOXICITY. This drug is not approved for use in cats, Chiuahuas, pregnant or nursing bitches, or puppies less than 3 months old (Curtis 2004). In mammals, Amitraz activates α_2-adrenergic receptors, and adverse effects are similar to those seen with xylazine. Signs of toxicity include CNS depression, bradycardia, polyuria, hyperglycemia, and sedation, which can last for up to 24 hours. Dogs tested with 5 or 10 times the labeled dose usually develop most of these signs; therefore, the final dip solution needs to be accurately prepared. The adverse effects from amitraz toxicosis can be reversed in dogs with a low dose of atipamezol (50 μg/kg IM), which is an α_2-antagonist (Hugnet et al. 1996). Accidental consumption of amitraz flea collars by dogs has resulted in toxicosis (Grossman 1993). Swine should not be treated more than 4 times a year and should not be treated within 3 days of slaughter. Amitraz is a potential hazard to humans (Avsarogullari et al. 2006) if they do not wear appropriate personal protection such as chemical-resistant gloves, aprons, and goggles/face shields.

INSECT GROWTH REGULATORS (IGRs)

These agents first appeared on the market in the 1980s and 1990s, and were popular because the chemicals were promoted as not being a pesticide, and therefore harmless to pets, livestock, and humans. The oral LD50 in rats for these chemicals ranges from 2 to 10 gram/kg body weight, which supports the extreme safety of these IGRs. These chemical agents affect the developing stages (eggs, pupae, and larvae) of insects and arthropods and do not affect the adult ectoparasite. Because of this, effective control is not achieved until several weeks after treatment and many of these IGRs are often formulated with adulticides described earlier in this chapter. The IGRs can be grouped as juvenile-hormone analogs (JHAs) and insect development inhibitors (IDIs).

JUVENILE HORMONE ANALOGS (JHAs). The IGRs are juvenile hormone analogs, which falsely signal organisms such as ticks, fleas, and flies to remain in their immature egg or larval stage and not develop to adult stage. In the normally developing insect, the hormone levels usually decrease prior to the adult stage. The use of these JHAs therefore falsely signals to the developing insect to remain at its immature stage. Approved JHAs include methoprene, pyriproxifen, fenoxycarb, and cyromazine, with the former two JHAs being the most frequently used in veterinary medicine. Several of these JHAs are available as individual active ingredients in several topical formulations, but they are often formulated with adulticides such as the pyrethrins and/or pyrethroids. *Methoprene* is used mainly to control horn flies in cattle by incorporating it into the cattle concentrate (0.4%) or block (0.01%). This method of application prevents the emergence of adult horn flies from cattle manure. Methoprene is formulated with adulticides for premises flea control, and also formulated with fipronil, phenothrin, and permethrin for flea and mosquito control in dogs and cats. Some of these spot-on applications may contain as much as 2–3% methoprene. *Pyriproxyfen* is often applied as a spot-on, and is effective against flea eggs in cats for up to 56 days (Rust 2005). This JHA applied every 3 months to cats significantly reduces flea numbers; 87% of the treated cats did not have fleas after 6 months (Maynard et al. 2001). As with methoprene products, pyriproxyfen is often formulated with adulticides such as permethrin and pyrethrins to be applied as sprays, spot-ons, and collars for cats and dogs.

INSECT DEVELOPMENT INHIBITORS (IDIs). The IDIs, such as the benzoylphenyl urea compounds (*diflubenzuron, lufenuron*), interfere with the development of the insect exoskeleton by inhibiting chitin synthesis or deposition pathways. Chitin is an essential constituent of flea eggshells and exoskeleton of immature fleas. Following oral ingestion of diflubenzuron, it passes unchanged in the feces where it contacts the eggs and larvae of developing flies. Lufenuron (Program®) is administered orally at monthly intervals to cats and dogs to control fleas. There is also a subcutaneous injectable (10 mg/kg) for cats that is efficacious for up to 6 months against fleas. No adverse effects have been observed in cats, but injectable lufeneron should not be given to dogs as it causes adverse local reactions at the injection sites. As this drug is lipophilic, its slow release from adipose tissues allows maintenance of effective blood levels for several weeks after administration. One of the more popular IDIs is the combination of lufenuron and milbemycin oxime that is used to control fleas on dogs as well as being a heartworm preventative.

SYNERGISTS AND REPELLENTS

Synergists such as piperonyl butoxide and N-octyl bicycloheptene dicarboximide (MGK 264) are often formulated with topical insecticide products to enhance the activity of insecticides. Almost all of the topicals formulated with these synergists contain pyrethroids and pyrethrins as the primary insecticide. These synergists inhibit oxidative and hydrolytic enzymes in the insects that are responsible for degradation of insecticides to harmless metabolites. It is believed that a carbene derivative forms and binds to the heme moiety of the cytochrome P450 enzyme making it inactive and unable to detoxify the insecticide. This then results in very high levels of the pyrethrin or pyethroid that are toxic and lethal to the ectoparasite (Murray and Reidy 1989). Synergists by themselves are less toxic than the active ingredients in a topical formulation. Owners and veterinarians should, however, be aware that when cats are exposed dermally to synergists such as piperonyl butoxide at concentrations greater that 1.5%, this may similarly reduce detoxification of pyrethrins in cats and thereby also enhance toxicity of the insecticide in cats (MacDonald and Miller 1986).

Repellents are also included in formulations to repel insects; although some repellents can be ectoparasiticidal such as permethrin, most repellents are not ectoparasiticidal. The primary advantage of the repellents is that they prevent transmission of vectorborne diseases even if these repellents are not ectoparasiticidal. A repellent can be effective via a number of mechanisms: preventing the ectoparasite from entering or landing on the hair coat, interfering with or inhibiting the ectoparasite's feeding, and causing the ectoparasite to become disoriented. Frequently used repellents include butoxypolypropylene glycol (Stabilene), di-n-propyl isocinchomeronate (MGK 326), and diethyl-m-toluamide (DEET).

DEET is an insect repellent approved by US EPA for use in dwellings; on the human body and clothing; and on cats, dogs, horses, and pet living/sleeping quarters (US EPA 1998). There are greater than 225 DEET products registered for use, with DEET concentrations ranging from 4% to 100%. However, DEET is not approved for direct application to the skin/coat of pets, and there are reports of adverse clinical signs in cats exposed to DEET topically (Dorman et al. 1990). Based on data from several experimental dermal absorption studies, DEET may influence the toxicity of insecticides by modulating insecticide dermal absorption (Baynes et al. 1997). Butoxypolypropylene glycol is usually formulated with a pyrethroid insecticide (e.g., resmethrin, permethrin) and/or a synergist (e.g., piperonyl butoxide). Most of these formulations are approved for use in horses, cats, and dogs, and formulated as sprays with concentrations ranging from 4.8 to 20%. No adverse effects in pets or laboratory animals have been

TABLE 44.5 Comparisons of US FDA CVM and US EPA with regard to ectoparasiticides

	US FDA CVM	US EPA
Mission	Approve and study effects of drugs and feed on animals Company files a New Animal Drug Application (NADA) to FDA	Preserve and improve quality of the environment and human health Registration of pesticides Company files an Application for Pesticide Registration (APR) to EPA
Scope	Concerned with drugs that work systemically in the animal Includes any route of administration to the animal	Concerned with anything that affects air, water, and soil quality Chemicals that are applied topically to animals but not absorbed systemically
Safety study requirements for FDA approval or EPA registration	Drug formulations must be evaluated in same species for which the drug is designated	Active ingredients are tested in lab animals Formulations do not have to be tested in the designated species
Efficacy	Flea control products must be at least 90% efficacious Clinical studies required	Clinical studies not required Practical efficacy in marketplace is required
Drug distribution	Often by prescription from a licensed veterinarian	Often sold over-the-counter at retail outlets

attributed to this repellent (CA EPA 2002). MGK 326 is often formulated with pyrethroids and/or synergists to be used as sprays, dips, and shampoos in horses, dogs, and cats.

ECTOPARASITICIDE APPROVAL AND REGISTRATION IN THE U.S.

Unlike other drug classes discussed in this book, either the US EPA or the US FDA Center for Veterinary Medicine (CVM) is involved in the approval of ectoparasiticides. The US FDA CVM evaluates those chemicals that are administered orally or topically but exert their effects following systemic distribution. These chemicals are classified as drugs and many of these drugs require a veterinary prescription. The US EPA evaluates those chemicals applied topically, but exert their effect on the surface of the skin or around the farm premises, and don't often require a veterinary prescription. Table 44.5 summarizes the differences in function between these two critically important federal agencies in the U.S.

In spite of these clear distinctions there is still confusion among pet owners and even some veterinarians about how flea products are marketed in the U.S. as some products can be obtained over-the-counter (OTC) in pet and feed stores while others can be obtained only from the veterinarian. The latter is often referred to as the veterinary-channel products (e.g., fipronil and imidacloprid). Even though those flea products may not require a prescription, obtaining these products from a veterinarian only ensures that a client-patient-veterinarian relationship is established, which reduces the probability of insecticide toxicoses often associated with OTC products used by pet owners. As discussed in various sections of this chapter, this has often been the problem with OTC pyrethroid and OP products used in cats and dogs.

Another issue that is of concern to the federal government is the extralabel use of ectoparasiticides. The passage of the Animal Medicinal and Drug Use and Clarification Act (AMDUCA) in 1994 allows but does not encourage the extralabel use of approved animal or human *drugs* in special circumstances. As pesticides are not approved drugs, extralabel use of these chemicals is not covered by AMDUCA and extralabel use is strongly prohibited.

REFERENCES

Avsarogullari, L., Ikizceli, I., Sungur, M., Sozuer E., Akdur O., Yucei M. (2006). Acute amitraz poisoning in adults: clinical features, laboratory findings, and management. Clin Toxicol (Phila) 44(1):19–23.

Baynes, R.E., Halling, K.B., Riviere, J.E. (1997). The influence of diethyl-m-toluamide (DEET) on the percutaneous absorption of permethrin and carbaryl. Toxicol Appl Pharmacol 144(2):332–339.

Baynes, R.E., Riviere, J.E. (2001). Pesticide Disposition: Dermal Absorption. In: Handbook of Pesticide Toxicology (Krieger R., Ed.) 2 ed., pp. 515–530. Academic Press, San Diego, CA.

Bloomquist, J.R. (2003). Chloride channels as tools for developing selective insecticides. Arch Insect Biochem Physiol 54:145–156.

Buckingham, S., Lapied, B., Corronc, H., Sattelle, F. (1997). Imidacloprid actions on insect neuronal acetylcholine receptors. J Exp Biol 200(Pt 21):2685–92.

CA EPA (2002). BUTOXYPOLYPROPYLENE GLYCOL. California Environmental Protection Agency, Department of Pesticide Regulation, Medical Toxicology Branch, Summary of Toxicology. (Stabilene®) February 5, 2002.

Cadiergues, M.C., Hourcg, P., Cantaloube, B., Franc, M. (2000). First bloodmeal of *Ctenocephalides felis felis* (*Siphonaptera: Pulicidae*) on cats: time to initiation and duration of feeding. J Med Entomol 37:634–636.

Cheng, T. (1995). Dermal absorption of 14C-fipronil REGENT 80WDG in male rats (preliminary and definitive phases). Unpublished report No. HWI 6224–210 from Hazleton Wisconsin, Inc. Submitted to WHO by Rhone-Poulenc, Inc., Research Triangle Park, NC, USA.

Cunningham et al. (1997). Effects of shampooing or water exposure on the initial and residual efficacy of imidacloprid. Supp Compend Contin Educ Vet 19:29–30.

Curtis, C.F. (2004). Current trends in the treatment of *Sarcoptes*, *Cheyletiella*, and *Otodectes* mite infestations in dogs and cats. Vet Derm 15:108–114.

Daborn, P., et al. (2004). Detection of insecticide resistance-associated mutations in the cat flea *Rdl* by TaqMan-allele specific amplification. Pest Biochem Physiol 79:25–30.

Denny, D.J. (2001). Efficacy of fipronil against ticks. Vet Rec 148(4):124.

Dorman, D.C., Buck, W.B., Trammel, H.L., Jones, R.D., Beasley, V.R. (1990). Fenvalerate/N,N-diethyl-m-toluamide (Deet) toxicosis in two cats. J Am Vet Med Assoc 196(1):100–102.

Dupuy, J., Derlon, A.L., Sutra, J.F., Cadiergues, M.C., Franc, M., Alvinerie, M. (2004). Pharmacokinetics of selamectin in dogs after topical application. Vet Res Commun 28(5):407–413.

French-Constant, R.H., Daborn, P.J., Le Goff, G. (2004). The genetics and genomics of insecticide resistance. Trends in Genetics 20(3):163–170.

Franc, M., Cadiergues, M.C. (1998). Antifeeding effect of several insecticidal formulations against *Ctenocephalides felis* on cats. Parasite 5(1):83–86.

Gayrard, V., Alvinerie, M., Toutain, P.L. (1999). Comparison of pharmacokinetic profiles of doramectin and ivermectin pour-on formulations in cattle. Vet Parasitol 81(1):47–55.

Godfrey, D.R. (1999). Dermatosis and associated systemic signs in a cat with thymoma and recently treated with an imidacloprid preparation. J Sm An Pract 40(7):333–337.

Gogolewski, R.P., Allerton, G.R., Pitt, S.R., Thompson, D.R., Langholff, W.K., Hair, J.A., Fulton, R.K., Eagleson, J.S. (1997). Effect of simulated rain, coat length and exposure to natural climatic conditions on the efficacy of a topical formulation of eprinomectin against endoparasites of cattle. Vet Parasitol 69(1–2):95–102.

Grossman, M.R. (1993). Amitraz toxicosis associated with ingestion of an acaricide collar in a dog. J Am Vet Med Assoc 203(1):55–57.

Hainzl, D., Casida, J.E. (1996). Fipronil insecticide: novel photochemical desulfinylation with retention of neurotoxicity Proc Natl Acad Sci USA Nov 12;93(23):12764–7.

Hooser, S.B. (1990). Toxicology of selected pesticides, drugs, and chemicals. D-limonene, linalool, and crude citrus oil extracts. Vet Clin N Am Sm An Pract 20(2):383–385.

Hovda, L.R., Hooser, S.B. (2002). Toxicology of newer pesticides for use in dogs and cats. Vet Clin N Am Sm An Pract 32(2):455–467.

Hugnet, C., Bruchon-Hugnet, C., Royer, H., Bourdoiseau, G. (2001). Efficacy of 1.25% amitraz solution in the treatment of generalized demodicosis (eight cases) and sarcoptic mange (five cases) in dogs. Vet Dermatol 12(2):89–92.

Hugnet, C., Buronrosse, F., Pineau, X., Cadore, J.L., Lorgue, G., Berny, P.J. (1996). Toxicity and kinetics of amitraz in dogs. Am J Vet Res 57(10):1506–1510.

Kagabu, S. (1997). Chloronicotinyl insecticides—discovery, application, and future perspectives. Rev Toxicol 1:75–129.

Kaneko, H., Miyamoto, J. (2001). Pyrethroid Chemistry and Metabolism. In: Handbook of Pesticide Toxicology Vol 2 Agents. (Krieger, R., Ed.). Academic Press, San Diego, CA.

Kramer, F., Mencke, N. (2001). Flea Biology and Control. Springer, Berlin.

KuKanich, B., Gehring, R., Webb, A.I., Craigmill, A.L., Riviere, J.E. (2005). Effect of formulation and route of administration on tissue residues and withdrawal times. J Am Vet Med Assoc 227(10):1574–1577.

Laffont, C.M., Bousquet-Melou, A., Bralet, D., Alvinerie, M., Finkgremmels, J., Toutain, P.L. (2003). A pharmacokinetic model to document the actual disposition of topical ivermectin in cattle. Vet Res 34:445–460.

Lee, L.A., Budgin, J.B., Mauldin, E.A. (2002). Acute necrotizing dermatitis and septicemia after application of a d-limonene-based insecticidal shampoo in a cat. J Am Vet Med Assoc 15;221(2):258–62, 239–40.

Liu, Z., Williamson, M.S., Lansdell, S.J., Denholm, T., Han, Z., Millar, N.S. (2005). A nicotinic acetylcholine receptor mutation conferring target-site resistance to imidacloprid in *Nilaparvata lugens* (brown planthopper). Proc Natl Acad Sci USA 102(24):8420–8425.

Macdonald, J.M., Miller, T.A. (1986). Parasiticide therapy in small animal dermatology. In: (Kirk, R.W., Ed.). Current Veterinary Therapy IX, Small Animal Practice, pp. 571–596. W.B. Saunders, Philadelphia.

Magnusson, B.M., Walters, K.A., Roberts, M.S. (2001). Veterinary drug delivery: potential for skin penetration enhancement. Adv Drug Deliv Rev 50:205–227.

Mahoney, R., Tinembart, O., Schenker, R. (2001). Flea-related itching in cats and dogs after treatment with nitenpyram. Suppl Comp Contin Educ Pract Vet 23(3A):20–23.

Maynard, L., Houffschmitt, P., Lebreux, B. (2001). Field efficacy of a 10 per cent pyriproxyfen spot-on for the prevention of flea infestations on cats. J Sm An Pract 42(10):491–494.

Mehlhorn, H., Hansen, O., Mencke, N. (2001). Comparative study on the effects of three insecticides (fipronil, imidacloprid, selamectin) on developmental stages of the cat flea (*Ctenocephalides felis* Bouché 1835): a light and electron microscopic analysis of in vivo and in vitro experiments. Parasitol Res. 87(3):198–207.

Merck & Co. (1996). The Merck Index. An Encylopedia of Chemicals, Drugs, and Biologicals, 12th Edition. (Budavari, S., Ed.). Merck & Co., Inc., Whitehouse Station, NJ.

Meyer, E.K. (1999). Toxicosis in cats erroneously treated with 45 to 65% permethrin products. J Am Vet Med Assoc 215(2):198–203.

Monteiro-Riviere, N.A., Bristol, D.G., Manning, T.O., Rogers, R.A., Riviere, J.E. (1990). Interspecies and interregional analysis of the comparative histologic thickness and laser Doppler blood flow measurements at five cutaneous sites in nine species. J Invest Dermatol 95(5):582–586.

Murray, M., Reidy, G.F. (1989). In vitro formation of an inhibitory complex between an isosafrole metabolite and rat hepatic cytochrome P450. Drug Metab Dispos 17:449–454.

Pollmeier, M., Pengo, G., Jeannin, P., Soll, M. (2002). Evaluation of the efficacy of fipronil formulations in the treatment and control of biting lice, *Trichodectes canis* (De Geer, 1778) on dogs. Vet Parasitol 107(1–2):127–36.

Pollmeier, M., Pengo, G., Longo, M., Jeannin, P. (2004). Effective treatment and control of biting lice, *Felicola subrostratus* (Nitzsch in Burmeister, 1838), on cats using fipronil formulations. Vet Parasitol. 121(1–2):157–165.

Ray, D.E. (2005). Pyrethrins/Pyrethroids. In: Encyclopedia of Toxicology, 2nd edition (Wexler, P.). Academic Press, San Diego, CA.

Richardson, J.A. (2000). Permethrin spot-on toxicoses in cats. J Vet Emerg Crit Care 10(2):103–106.

Riviere, J.E. and Baynes, R.E. (1998). Dermal absorption and toxicity assessment. In: Dermal Absorption and Toxicity Assessment, (Roberts, M.S., Walters K., Eds.), pp. 625–645. Marcel Dekker, Inc. NY, NY.

Rust, M.K. (2005). Advances in the control of *Ctenocephalides felis* (cat flea) on cats and dogs. Trends Parasitol 21(5):232–236.

Rust, M.K., Waggoner, M.M., Hinkle, N.C., Stansfield, D., Barnett, S. (2003). Efficacy and longevity of nitenpyram against adult cat fleas (*Siphonaptera: Pulicidae*). J Med Entomol 40(5):678–681.

Schenker, R., Humbert-Droz, E., Moyses, E.W., Yerly, B. (2001). Efficacy of nitenpyram against a flea strain with resistance to fipronil. Suppl Comp Contin Educ Pract Vet 23(3A):16–19.

Sarasola, P., Jernigan, A.D., Walker, K.D., Castledine J., Smith, D.G., Rowan T.G. (2002). Pharmacokinetics of selamectin following intravenous, oral and topical administration in cats and dogs. J Vet Pharmacol Therap 24:265–272.

Schroeder, I., B.L. Blagburn, D.L. Bledsoe, R. Bond, I. Denholm, M.W. Dryden, D.E. Jacobs, H., Mehlhorn, N. Mencke, P. Payne, M.K. Rust and M.B. Vaughn (2003). Progress of the international work of the imidacloprid flea susceptibility monitoring team. Parasit Res 90(3): S127–S128.

Schroeder, M.E., Flattum, R.F. (1984). The mode of action and neurotoxic properties of the nitromethylene heterocycle insecticides. Pest Biochem Physiol 22:148–160.

Shanks, D.J., McTier, T.L., Behan, S., Pengo, G., Genchi, C., Bowman, D.D., Holbert, M.S., Smith, D.G., Jernigan, A.D., Rowan, T.G. (2000). The efficacy of selamectin in the treatment of naturally acquired infestations of *Sarcoptes scabiei* on dogs. Vet Parasitol 91(3–4):269–281.

Sheets, L.P. (2001). Imidacloprid: A neonicotinoid insecticide. In: Handbook of Pesticide Toxicology, Volume 2. (Krieger, R.I., Ed.), pp. 1123–1130. Academic Press, New York.

Smith, T.M., Stratton, G.W. (1986). Effects of synthetic pyrethroid insecticides on nontarget organisms. Residue Rev 97:93–120.

Technical Information Sheet. (1997). Frontline TopSpot, Fipronil 9.7% w/w, MSDS. Rhone Merieux, Athens, GA.

Tomizawa, M., Casida, J.E. (2003). Selective toxicity of neonicotinoids attributable to specificity of insects and mammalian nicotinic receptors. Annu Rev Entomol 48:339–364.

US EPA (1998). R.E.D. Facts. DEET.

Warmke, J.W., Reenan, R.A., Wang, P., Qian, S., Arena, J.P., Wang, J., Wunderler, D., Liu, K., Kaczorowski, G.J., Van der Ploeg, L.H., Ganetzky, B., Cohen, C.J. (1997). Functional expression of Drosophila para sodium channels. Modulation by the membrane protein TipE and toxin pharmacology. J Gen Physiol 110(2):119–133.

Witte, ST., Luempert, LG. (2001). Laboratory safety studies of nitenpyram tablets for the rapid removal of fleas on cats and dogs. Suppl Comp Contin Educ Pract Vet 23(3A):7–11.

Young, D.R., Arther, R.G., Davis, W.L. (2003). Evaluation of K9 Advantix vs. Frontline Plus topical treatments to repel brown dog ticks (*Rhipicephalus sanguineus*) on dogs. Parasitol Res 90Suppl3:S116–8.

Zhao, X., Yeh, J.Z., Salgado, V.L., Narahashi, T. (2005). Sulfone metabolite of fipronil blocks gamma-aminobutyric acid- and glutamate-activated chloride channels in mammalian and insect neurons. J Pharmacol Exp Ther 314(1):363–373.

SECTION 11

Specialty Areas of Pharmacology

CHAPTER

45

CHEMOTHERAPY OF NEOPLASTIC DISEASES

GORDON L. COPPOC

Use of anticancer drugs has become an important aspect of veterinary practice that, although increasingly used in general veterinary practice, is still ideally used in specialty practices that have adequate expertise and safety facilities. Significant advances have been made in understanding the biology of cancer including the use of therapies that are more specific for certain types of tumors. Successful application of the new concepts requires in-depth understanding of the natural history of each individual type of cancer as well as knowledge of the combinations of modalities that are appropriate for each type of cancer. Application of these approaches to treatment of animal cancer is slowed by species differences, expense, and nonavailability of adequate supportive therapies in many practices. Nevertheless, veterinary cancer therapy has made tremendous strides and patient quality and/or quantity of life can be increased through rational selection of patient and therapeutic goal, therapeutic approach, and effective client education.

TREATMENT PERSPECTIVES

Cancer is defined as cured when all cancer cells have been eradicated. Cure is the ideal goal, but producing remission and/or palliation is a worthy goal. A cancer is said to be in *remission* when all clinical evidence of cancer has disappeared, but it is noteworthy that microscopic foci of cancer cells may remain. *Palliative treatment* refers to the treatment of cancer (when cure is unlikely) to reduce pain, improve the sense of well-being, or to correct some physiological malfunction insofar as possible. The therapeutic regimen selected must be consistent with the goal for the patient (i.e., cure, remission, or palliation). It is increasingly recognized that cancer is a chronic disease and that stable disease with good quality of life is an acceptable goal.

Chemotherapy may be defined as the application of drugs to kill or inhibit the growth of viruses or foreign cells, such as bacteria, in the body. Cancer cells can be

TABLE 45.1 Examples of factors affecting therapeutic strategy

Patient	Species, breed, age, sex, health status, function/role
Neoplasm	Histologic type, natural history, stage (extent), grade, location
Facilities/treatments available	Primary modalities, secondary support for follow-up care, proximity
Owner	Ability to care for animal, relationship to pet, living circumstances, commitment, financial status

considered as "foreign" in this sense. *Immunotherapy* refers to the use of specific antibodies to tumor molecules and is becoming increasingly successful. The term *targeted therapy* is increasingly used for treatment with small molecule drugs (e.g., suffix "-tinib" = suffix of tyrosine kinase inhibitors) and antibodies (e.g., "-umab" = suffix for human antibody) that are directed at very specific enzymes and receptors identified by cancer biologists as key regulators involved in cancer.

Cancer chemotherapy was first successfully practiced when nitrogen mustards used as war gases were found to inhibit tumor growth. Unfortunately, they were extremely toxic. In contrast to radiation and surgery, where the limitation is access to metastatic lesions, chemotherapy is limited by resistant cells. It is difficult to completely cure many solid tumors consisting of more than one million cells (approximately 1 mg of tissue) with chemotherapy alone. Application of new technologies and diagnostic procedures that allow identification of specific subsets of cancer types and use of special targeting mechanisms that exploit nanoparticles and other technologies promise significant improvements in the future (Service 2005).

The decision to use one or several of the treatment modalities for a patient with cancer rests on the types of factors listed in Table 45.1. Detailed recommendation of specific treatment protocols is beyond the scope of this chapter. Protocols for timing, dosage, and special precautions of certain combinations of drugs have been published (Kitchell 2003; Morrison 1998, 2002a).

CANCER BIOLOGY

A brief review of certain aspects of cancer biology is presented as background to aid in understanding the significance of various approaches and limitations of chemotherapy. Discovery of qualitative differences between normal and cancer cells that would allow more selective toxicity to the cancer cells while sparing normal tissues is a goal of current research. Although some emerging therapies that rely on specific targeting mechanisms, e.g., use of drugs linked to antibodies or to specific receptor ligands (Low and Antony 2004) are relatively specific, selectivity for the most commonly used cytotoxic agents is currently based primarily on quantitative differences. That is, both normal and cancer cells have essentially the same ongoing biochemical processes, but the rates and timing may be very different. For most tumors the success of chemotherapy depends on having drugs that are taken up more avidly, bind more tightly to some tumor cell constituent, or affect processes that occur more rapidly in tumor cells, thus enhancing their effect on cancer cells relative to normal cells.

CELL CYCLE. The *cell cycle* is the progression of a dividing cell from one mitosis to the next. Transitions between the phases of the cell cycle are controlled by the activity of specific cyclin-dependent kinases (CDKs) that are activated by cyclins, small regulatory proteins. Mutation or loss of one of these proteins or increased activity of CDKs or cyclins can lead to unrestrained cell division. Discussion of this rapidly changing field, which is beyond the scope of this chapter, can be found in a review (Deshpande et al. 2005). G_1, a presynthetic phase, immediately follows mitosis and may be extremely variable in duration depending on the cell type, presence or absence of nutrients, growth factors, and metabolic by-products. During this phase normal cellular events continue. Protein and ribonucleic acid (RNA) synthesis occur in preparation for deoxyribonucleic acid (DNA) synthesis, the S phase. The S phase may require between 8 and 20 hours for completion. The next phase is G_2, which may last 3 hours in cancer cells, during which substituents required for mitosis are synthesized. Mitosis (M phase) typically requires 1 hour for completion to end the cell cycle.

For a variety of reasons, as tumors mature, certain cells may stop traversing the cell cycle. Others may traverse it so slowly that for purposes related to cancer therapy, they are not in the population of actively dividing cells. Operationally, these cells may be grouped and referred to as being in the G_0 phase. Such cells are not part of the "growth fraction" of the tumor. However, under proper growth conditions those that were merely traversing the cycle extremely slowly may be "recruited" back into the pool of actively dividing cells.

TUMOR GROWTH RATE. The clinically apparent growth rate of a tumor does not necessarily reflect the rate at which cells traverse the cell cycle. If it did, and the tumor consisted of only one cell type that was immortal, tumor growth could be described by a simple geometric progression, i.e., the number of cells would double after an interval equal to the cell cycle time. If this were the case, and if 10^9 cells were required for diagnosis of a tumor, it would require approximately 32 cell cycle times for a single cancer cell to result in a clinically apparent tumor.

In an experimental tumor system it was observed that the time required for the number of cells to double increased from 4 days to over 100 days as the mass grew from approximately 0.3 to 10 g. The growth fraction of the tumor decreased from 80 to 10% and time required for cells to complete a cycle increased from 0.8 to 1.6 days (Frei 1977). From similar studies and much clinical experience it has been established that tumor growth rate is complex and that the "fractional" growth rate tends to decrease as the tumor matures. Models of cancer cell growth have been reviewed (Dang et al. 2003).

Depending on the tumor type and growth conditions, time required to complete a cycle may range from less than 24 hours to several days. Because of cell death, decreased growth fraction, and extended cell cycle times as tumors grow larger, cell cycle time rarely equals doubling time over the course of a tumor's lifespan. Mean clinical doubling times for some human tumors range from 2 to 5 days for Burkitt's lymphoma to 34 days for osteogenic sarcoma to 134 days for adenocarcinoma of the lung (Shackney 1993). Another level of complexity is introduced when it is appreciated that the cell population itself is likely to be quite heterogeneous (Fang et al. 2005).

The *log cell-kill* hypothesis of Skipper (1971) states that the entire population of cancer cells in a patient must be eradicated to produce a cure. A large number of experimental studies have indicated that drug-induced cell kill is a first order process; i.e., a constant proportion of the cells present, both normal and cancerous, are killed with each round of therapy. Recall that differences between cancer cells and cells of some normal tissues are not great. Yet there must be a significant difference between the proportion of cancerous and normal cells killed with each cycle of treatment. Further, normal cells must rebound more quickly than cancer cells from the therapeutic insult. The magnitude of the problem is illustrated by the fact that reduction of normal cell population by 2 to 3 log units (i.e., 99 to 99.9%) may be fatal. Realization that as many as 10^9 cancer cells may still be present after induction of remission requires that additional courses of chemotherapy be given.

CHEMOTHERAPY OF THE CANCER CELL. Increased knowledge of cell and cancer biology has increased the number of molecular targets being explored for development of anticancer drugs. These include, but are not limited to, factors involved in the cell cycle, differentiation, apoptosis, angiogenesis, signaling cell-surface receptors, ErbB family of receptors, metastasis, intracellular signaling elements, nuclear transcription factors, cell surface antigens, and other targets such as the proteasome (Frei and Eder 2003). Increasing numbers of these potential targets are entering clinical trials in people and some have entered mainstream therapy. Unfortunately, species differences and resources have slowed application to animals. This chapter focuses primarily on drugs that are used in veterinary practice.

Chemotherapeutic agents may be divided into three classes with respect to their dependence on the cell cycle. Some drugs (e.g., alkylating agents) are said to be non–cell-cycle–specific. Although they are toxic to all cells, they are especially toxic to proliferating cells. Other drugs are cell-cycle–specific. Cells must be proliferating for these drugs to be effective. Cell-cycle–specific drugs may also be cell-cycle-phase–specific; such drugs may be active only in one stage of the cell cycle.

Practical application of knowledge regarding drug activity in various phases of the cell cycle lies in providing an understanding of why tumors with large growth fractions and rapid generation times usually respond more dramatically to therapy and in guiding drug selection, sequencing, and timing in the development of new protocols (Gaffney 2004).

DRUG TOXICITY. One of the paradoxes of cancer chemotherapy is that although the drugs are most toxic to cells rapidly traversing the cell cycle, many cancers have smaller growth fractions than certain normal tissues (e.g., bone marrow and intestinal epithelium). Normal tissues typically recover more rapidly than tumor cells. Nevertheless the necessity of supportive treatment for such conditions as cytopenias and gastrointestinal disturbances cannot be overstated.

Although there are important exceptions, antitumor compounds produce characteristic toxicity to various body tissues that are related to tissue growth rate. Lymphocytes and bone marrow cells are most profoundly affected. The expected consequences are anemia, thrombocytopenia, and leukopenia. Of these the most life threatening and most common significant sequela of anticancer chemotherapy is sepsis due to neutropenia. Close monitoring of leukocyte counts is an integral and crucial aspect of chemotherapy to allow prompt cessation of anticancer drug administration and institution of appropriate antiinfective therapy if necessary.

Acceptable regimens may lower the leukocyte count significantly. In the absence of sophisticated support capability, it is not advisable to allow the count to go below 2,000/mm^3, for then the risk of infection is too great. There is some evidence that biological response modifiers such as recombinant canine granulocyte colony-stimulating factors (rcG-CSF) and agents that induce it may antagonize the myelosuppression of some anticancer agents (Ogilvie et al. 1992). They may aid in preparing cats to undergo intense radiation therapy (Obradovich et al. 1993). Because of the longevity of erythrocytes, anemia does not appear as rapidly as myelosuppression, if at all. Utility of using androgens to stimulate erythrocyte production is not unequivocally established, but such intervention is usually not needed. Infusions of platelets may be used to counteract a severe thrombocytopenia. Most cytotoxic drugs produce myelosuppression and some degree of thrombocytopenia, but L-asparaginase, vincristine, and bleomycin are minimally toxic in this regard.

Mucosal cells of the gastrointestinal tract have a turnover time on the order of 5 days and thus have a high growth fraction. Many anticancer drugs, e.g., methotrexate and 5-fluorouracil, can produce diarrhea, vomiting, and ulcerations of the mucosa (i.e., mucositis, which may manifest as ulcerative stomatitis and enteritis). These disorders can be more disconcerting to the patient and owner than the less obvious, but potentially more important effects on cells derived from the bone marrow. GI signs appear to be less prevalent in animals than humans, but should be seriously regarded when they occur. Signs of severe vomiting and diarrhea are cause for temporary cessation of therapy, because they may presage dehydration or serious mucositis, which could be life threatening.

Basal cells of the skin and especially of the hair follicle in some breeds are also highly susceptible because of high growth fraction. Hair loss, usually thinning rather than complete loss, in breeds with continuously growing hair (e.g., Poodles, Kerry Blue Terriers, and Old English Sheepdogs) may occur especially in association with doxorubicin therapy. Notable hair loss may begin 1 month after therapy. In most cases hair growth returns to normal once therapy is stopped, often beginning within 1–3 months. Change of coat color in a Standard Poodle has been reported (Simonson and Madewell 1992). Cats may lose their whiskers and outer guard hairs (Rogers and Coppoc 1991). Other toxicities related to the skin are independent of cell growth rate and include direct tissue damage as can occur on extravasation of drug during administration and hyperpigmentation. Hyperpigmentation may occur after therapy with doxorubicin, cyclophosphamide, methotrexate, and bleomycin.

Drugs such as doxorubicin, dactinomycin, mitoxantrone, vincristine, and vinblastine are notable for the severe phlebitis, cellulitis, and necrosis that follow extravasation of drug during administration. It is highly recommended that proper technique be used for intravenous injection of these drugs via an intravenous catheter. This is such a serious issue that if there is doubt as to the placement of the catheter, it should be removed and placed in a different vein before infusion is begun. If extravasation occurs, quick response, including removal of as much of the drug as possible prior to removing the needle, is paramount. Various expedients have been recommended for treating accidental extravasations, but have not proven very efficacious. Sodium bicarbonate, sodium thiosulfate, corticosteroids, hyaluronidase, dimethyl sulfoxide (DMSO), DHM3, and butylated hydroxytoluene have all been claimed to be of value for specific toxins (Dorr et al. 1990; Endicott 2003). In fact, injection of these substances may increase diffusion of the vesicant, which should be avoided at all cost. If multiple attempts to place a catheter fail, it is best to send the animal home untreated than to risk extravasation of the vesicants, especially doxorubicin (Knapp 2006).

Liver and kidney cells respond to anticancer drugs in ways frequently unrelated to proliferation. Cisplatin is directly nephrotoxic, but renal failure has also been reported following L-asparaginase, mithramycin, and high dose methotrexate therapy (Knapp et al. 1987; Endicott 2003). Acute tumor lysis syndrome which occurs in people and has been reported in dogs may lead to death due to severe metabolic imbalance (Endicott 2003). Allopurinol, to reduce uric acid formation, and fluid therapy, to produce diuresis, are prophylactic measures that reduce the risk of acute uric acid nephropathy and hyperkalemia that may result from rapid lysis of tumors during treatment. Hepatic fibrosis has been produced with folic acid antagonists such as methotrexate. The incidence may be higher when 6-mercaptopurine, daunorubicin, and cytarabine are added to methotrexate in combination chemotherapy.

As a group the cells of the central nervous system (CNS) are least affected by cytotoxic antitumor drugs because of the blood-brain barrier and their slow growth rate. Nevertheless, some of the drugs cause CNS toxicosis and it may be difficult to separate a direct drug effect on behavior from the combined effects of the tumor, debris from dying cells, poor nutritional status, and therapeutic regimen. CNS toxicity may be seen with vincristine, but peripheral neuropathies are more likely (Hamilton et al. 1991).

Allergic reactions have been reported following administration of doxorubicin, paclitaxel, etoposide, and L-asparaginase. Treatment of the reaction includes stopping administration of the drug and symptomatic therapy for allergic reactions and anaphylaxis, as appropriate. Endicott has reviewed this and other emergencies related to cancer and cancer therapy in animals (Endicott 2003).

Long-term hazards of certain anticancer drugs are their properties of oncogenesis, mutagenesis, and teratogenesis and infertility. Drugs have been categorized with respect to their carcinogenesis risk potential into four categories, but one should recognize the potential for harm with all classes of drugs. Examples of drugs in each risk category are as follows: high (mechlorethamine, nitrosoureas, etoposide); moderate (doxorubicin, cyclophosphamide, cisplatin); low (vinca alkaloids, methotrexate, L-asparaginase); and unknown (bleomycin, taxanes, mitoxantrone) (Erlichman and Moore 2001).

THERAPIST SAFETY. Anticancer drugs constitute potential hazards to those who handle and administer them, so great caution and good technique should always be observed. Accidental exposure via the skin, respiratory system, or digestive system must be prevented through the implementation of strict specific protocols. The US Department of Labor, Occupational Safety and Health Administration has issued guidelines for training of personnel in the storage, handling, and disposal of cytotoxic antineoplastic drugs (OSHA 2005). A discussion of chemotherapy safety procedures in veterinary medicine has been published (Takada 2003).

DRUG DOSAGE. Anticancer drugs are frequently dosed on the basis of surface area rather than body weight although one must be alert because there is evidence that the formula below may not be accurate for very small animals, and some anticancer drugs are dosed on the basis of weight (Frazier and Price 1998). A conversion of weight to surface area can be made with the following formula:

$$\text{Surface Area} = \frac{\text{Body weight}^{0.67} \times \text{K}}{10^4}$$

where surface area is given in square meters and body weight in grams. For cats and dogs, *K* is a constant with the value of 10.0 and 10.1, respectively. Conversion tables are widely available, but a few values may give one a perspective on the relationship. The following values list the weight in kilograms followed by the surface area in square meters: 1–0.1; 10–0.46; 20–0.74; 30–0.96; 40–1.17; and 50–1.36.

As one might predict, drug dosage, interval between doses, and duration of therapy are crucial factors in determining the success of cancer therapy (Frei and Eder 2003). It is important to realize that drugs must be used at the maximum dose possible to achieve optimum therapeutic effects. One is not justified in decreasing the dose of drug to a point that does not produce clinical toxicity, because the regimen will certainly fail.

RESISTANCE. Resistance to pharmacotherapy is a major problem in cancer chemotherapy. Resistance may result in therapeutic failure in over 90% of patients with metastatic cancer (Longley and Johnston 2005). The mass of cancer cells may be intrinsically drug-resistant or become resistant during therapy. The majority of cells in a tumor may be sensitive when therapy is begun yet the tumor may harbor a small fraction of resistant cells (innately or because of growth conditions) that become dominant as a result of selection pressure and death of sensitive cells (Goldie and Coldman 1984). According to the cancer stem cell hypothesis the cancer initiating cells may be transformed tissue stem cells (Weissman 2005). Further, there may be significant heterogeneity in these cells because of a variety of translocations that result in the development of oncogenic fusion genes (Moore 2005). The cancer stem cells may be sufficiently normal and different from the mass of the tumor that they are resistant to chemotherapeutic agents.

These may serve as a source for recurrence of a tumor that was in remission (Weissman 2005). In fact, it has been argued that the most important, and most difficult, target for cancer therapy is this stem cell population that, like all true stem cells, is normally quiescent. According to the cancer stem cell hypothesis, stem cells in such locations as the bone marrow and gut and many cancers have cells with constitutive drug resistance mediated by ABC transporters, detoxifying enzymes such as DNA repair mechanisms, and tolerance to damage (i.e., resistance to apoptosis) (Donnenberg and Donnenberg 2005).

Many tumors have a tremendous increase in mutation rate over normal cells, as much as 1 thousand to 1 million times greater in cancer cells versus normal epithelial cells (Welch 2003). This genomic instability may lead to resistance. Except in the case of multidrug resistance related to ABC transporters, such as P-glycoprotein (P-gp), mutations usually lead to resistance to a single class of agents.

Resistance can occur at many levels ranging from changes in pharmacokinetics of drugs (e.g., absorption, distribution, biotransformation, and elimination), to molecular changes in the cancer cells. Some of the mechanisms discussed below will overlap. For example, the discussion of ABC transporters is relevant to various epithelial barriers such as the blood-brain barrier and to events in organs of absorption and elimination as well as to individual cancer cells. Resistance can be due to decreased intracellular drug concentration due to decreased influx or increased efflux, decreased activation of prodrugs or increased drug inactivation in cancer cells, increased or decreased levels of target enzyme, alteration of the drug target that leads to decreased affinity for the drug, increased repair of drug damage as can occur with DNA repair systems, decreased activity of apoptotic mechanisms, decreased checkpoint function, and decreased rate of cell division as can occur as tumors outgrow their blood supply. The reader is referred to recent reviews for information on mechanisms of resistance and ways of overcoming it that are beyond the scope of this chapter (Longley and Johnston 2005; Cole and Tannock 2005; Weissman 2005; Frei and Eder 2003).

The classical mechanism of Multiple Drug Resistance (MDR) results in resistance to drugs from such structurally and mechanistically diverse classes as the vinca alkaloids and the anthracyclines. The commonality of these drugs is that they are nonpolar. MDR due to the ABC transporters is currently a major and somewhat confusing topic because of imprecise terminology. An excellent review of the ABC transporters as targets in cancer therapy has been published (Cooke et al. 2005). ABC transporters are so-called because they belong to a family of ATP-Binding Cassette transporters that use energy derived from ATP-hydrolysis to function. The first transporter to be described was the P-glycoprotein (P = *pleiotropic;* P-gp). In the new, standard terminology, this protein is encoded by the multidrug-resistance (*MDR1*) gene (gene symbol *ABCB1*). The superfamily of more than 48 proteins in humans is comprised of seven subfamilies (A through G). Other major families include "multidrug resistance protein 1" (*MRP1*; gene symbol *ABCC1*) and the "breast cancer resistance protein" (*BCRP;* gene symbol *ABCG2*). *BCRP* is also known as *MXR* for "mitoxantrone resistant protein." "Lung resistance protein" (LRP or MVP) does not belong to the ABC superfamily, but is associated with drug resistance in clinical samples. Details of the structure and mechanism of these transporters are described in reviews (Choi 2005; Cole and Tannock 2005; Dean 2002).

The physiological functions of these classes are not definitively established, but they are expressed constitutively in many normal cells such as the small and large intestine; liver and pancreas; endothelial cells; and epithelial cells of the kidneys, adrenals, brain, and testis. Absorption and secretion (excretion) of endogenous and exogenous substances are likely functions. Because a major function is to pump lipids, drugs, natural products, and peptides from cells, they have been dubbed "hydrophobic vacuum cleaners" that expel nonpolar compounds from the membrane bilayer. Of the more than 48 ABC genes reported for people, functions have been described for 16 and disease syndromes are related to 14 (Choi 2005).

Veterinary therapeutic implications of the P-gp (MDR1) have been reviewed (Mealey 2004). BCRP (ABCG2) is expressed in mammary gland alveolar epithelial cells during pregnancy and lactation. In this location it actively secretes various substances including drugs and toxins into the milk. This action has obvious ramifications for suckling babies, animals, and consumers of dairy products (van Herwaarden and Schinkel 2006). The role of biotransformation and the ABC transporters in drug delivery has been reviewed (Katragadda et al. 2005).

The ABC transporters are important modifiers of the concentration of their substrates in normal and cancerous cells by decreasing absorption from the gut and transport from the blood into the brain, hastening elimination of their substrates by the kidney and liver, and pumping drugs from cells. Implications related to absorption and elimination are that they decrease oral bioavailability of relevant drugs, requiring many of them to be intravenously administered. Even for drugs administered intravenously there can be therapeutic ramifications of genetic variation as shown by increased toxicity of doxorubicin in collies and related breeds with a deletion mutation in the canine MDR1 gene (deltaMDR1 295–298) caused by a reduced rate of drug elimination (Mealey et al. 2003). This is the same deletion mutation that leads to increased ivermectin sensitivity in collies (Mealey et al. 2002). The breed distribution and lineage of this deletion has been reviewed (Neff et al. 2004).

Intense effort is underway to find specific inhibitors of the various ABC transporters. These have been variously called *chemosensitizers*, MDR modulators, and MDR reverters (Choi 2005). A limiting caution is that results from trials in humans may not reflect results that will be obtained in animals. In a study of various substrates in an in vitro model of P-gp transmembrane flux, it was found that human and rhesus monkey membranes had binding affinities that were more similar to each other than to those of the dog. The results were consistent with gene and amino acid composition of the three species (Xia et al. 2006).

First-generation inhibitors, such as verapamil and cyclosporin A have been largely disappointing when used in conjunction with cytotoxic drugs in therapy of people because of a lack of specificity that limited dosages. A second-generation chemosensitizer is a nonimmune suppressant analog of cyclosporin A known as PSC 833 (Valspodar). PSC 833 has chemosensitivity enhancement effects on P-gp–mediated MDR about 10 times greater than that of cyclosporin A. PSC 833 reversed the P-gp–resistant phenotype in sporadic appendicular canine osteosarcoma. Simultaneous administration with doxorubicin allowed a 30% decrease in the dose of doxorubicin required to give therapeutic exposure equivalent to the nonresistant phenotype (Cagliero et al. 2004).

Concentration of reducing agents such as sulfhydryl-containing molecules in cells can provide protection against drugs that produce reactive intermediates or free radicals. Reduced glutathione (GSH) can inactivate peroxides and free radicals produced by drugs such as doxorubicin. It can also react with activated alkylating agents, cisplatin, carboplatin, and oxaloplatin to lead to conjugates that are nontoxic and that can be removed from the cell primarily by ABC transporters MRP1 and MRP2 as well as a glutathione-conjugate carrier. The conjugation reaction is catalyzed by cytosolic GSH S-transferase and glutathione peroxidase (Cole and Tannock 2005; Longley and Johnston 2005).

SELECTION OF REGIMENS. Selection of a treatment regimen for an individual patient is empirical and is based largely on the results of clinical trials of drugs in cases at a similar "stage," i.e., similar anatomic location, extent, pathologic diagnosis, and evidence of metastasis as well as local support sophistication and commitment on the part of the owner and the veterinary practice. Formal mechanisms of staging tumors have been published (Henderson et al. 1995). Histopathologic grade is an excellent prognostic tool that may provide guidance for therapeutic decisions. Significant effort to identify better predictors of success has included in vitro assays of drug effectiveness against cultured explants of the tumor. Current emphasis on the genetic and molecular basis of cancer is leading to efforts to use molecular markers as basis for predicting the course of a cancer and, hopefully, eventual success of a regimen in veterinary oncology (Mukaratirwa 2005).

MULTIMODAL THERAPY. Classical modalities of cancer therapy include surgery, radiation, and chemotherapy with surgery being the primary modality in most veterinary practices. Although techniques such as surgery and radiation have improved, it is still apparent that many patients die of cancer after the primary tumor has been "successfully" removed.

The term *adjuvant therapy* was classically used to describe chemotherapy that accompanied surgery or radiation therapy. There was controversy over the advocacy of adjuvant therapy because of the potential for producing needless toxicity in patients if no micrometastases were present and because of the carcinogenic potential of some drugs (Erlichman and Moore 2001). However, with the newer generations of therapeutic possibilities, the use of multimodal therapy has become more common. Adjuvant therapy has been successfully employed in the treatment of canine osteosarcoma in conjunction with surgery (Bergman et al. 1996).

COMBINATION CHEMOTHERAPY. A combination chemotherapy treatment regimen denotes the use of two or more chemotherapeutic agents at specified dosages and intervals. Combination protocols to be tested in clinical trials are carefully designed using knowledge of pharmacology and toxicology of drugs and their effects on tumors as individual entities.

The rationale of combination therapy is based on the facts that additive effects on tumors are frequently more pronounced than on normal tissues, there is a decreased tendency toward the development of resistance, a combination may be less toxic than an equivalently effective single agent, and heterogeneous stem cell populations usually fail to respond uniformly to a single agent. Some common-sense rules guiding selection of combinations are that each drug should be active on the tumor, drugs should have different mechanisms of action, toxicities should overlap minimally if at all, and each drug should be given at a time during the cell cycle when it will exert its maximum effect. The dosage regimen should be optimized for maximum effect on cancer cells at the shortest dosage interval that allows key normal tissues to recover.

Some success has been achieved by alternating regimens to decrease the occurrence of resistant cells during the course of therapy, but this approach has not improved long-term results against tumors that contained small numbers of genetically resistant cells at the beginning of therapy (Shackney 1993). With current advances in cancer biology, clinical trials are exploring what has been called *holotherapy*, treatment drawn from all classes of therapeutic agents, e.g., chemotherapy, immunotherapy, hormones, antibodies, antiangiogenesis, antimatrix, gene therapy, control of cell cycle (anticyclins CDK, transcriptional control, antisense), and enzyme-inhibitory drugs (Frei and Eder 2003; Varmus 2006). Cancers are increasingly being subdivided as molecular attributes are used to characterize the tumor in a specific patient, thus allowing more individualized therapy in people. These approaches will be available in clinical veterinary practice as the promises of *molecular oncology* are realized for animals.

DRUGS

Drug groups and individual drugs are discussed in this section. Extensive coverage of drugs, formulations, typical doses for dogs and cats, and specific tumor types is available in recent reviews (Morrison 2002b). Practical information on storage of these expensive drugs for veterinary medicine has been published (Rosenthal 1991).

ALKYLATING AGENTS. Alkylating agents are highly reactive molecules in their active state. Alkylating agents undergo strongly electrophilic chemical reactions through formation of carbonium ion intermediates or transition complexes with the target molecules. The intermediates then react with strongly nucleophilic substituents in the cell (e.g., phosphate, amino, sulfhydryl, hydroxyl, carboxyl, imidazole groups), to form covalent bonds. The target molecule is then said to have been alkylated. Alkylation of DNA is the effect primarily responsible for the cytotoxic activity. Such alkylation, of which the 7-nitrogen atom of guanine is an important site, may lead to covalent cross-linking of DNA strands or linking of DNA to a closely associated protein if the drug is a bifunctional alkylating agent. Alkylation of guanine may also shift its electron configuration so that it base pairs with thymine rather than cytosine, ultimately resulting in the substitution of an adenine-thymine pair in place of a guanine-cytosine pair. Labilization of the imidazole ring may cause the guanine to be lost from the DNA strand, with resultant breaking of the chain. It is not difficult to see how the alkylating agents could be mutagenic and carcinogenic.

Alkylating agents are not regarded as being cell-cycle–specific because they have more profound effects on nonproliferating cells than many of the other groups of drugs. But they are still most effective against cells rapidly traversing the cell cycle, i.e., in tumors with a high growth fraction. For this reason they are much more toxic to bone marrow than to such organs as liver and kidney. Infertility in both males and females may be a problem.

Alkylating agents are frequently referred to as radiomimetic drugs because their action in causing DNA strand breaks resembles that of radiation. Their action is also conceptually similar to that of cisplatin. Alkylating agents have a relatively wide spectrum of antitumor activity and are useful in treating tumors of lymphoreticular tissues. They have limited activity against sarcomas and carcinomas.

Tumors commonly, but slowly, develop resistance that may extend across the class of alkylating or "DNA cross-linking" agents. Several major mechanisms are involved (Cole and Tannock 2005). There may be an increase in the concentration of intracellular nucleophilic substrates (e.g., metallothionein or glutathione) that can compete with DNA for the drugs; thus, the drugs are inactivated by conjugation. There may be increased concentration of aldehyde dehydrogenase in the case of cyclophosphamide.

There may be increased activity of DNA repair systems. Reduced intracellular drug accumulation may be a factor due to decreased transport into the cell or increased removal.

Resistance to one alkylating agent does not necessarily imply resistance to the others. For example, melphalan is transported into cells by the leucine transport system whereas mechlorethamine is taken in by the choline transport system. If resistance were due to a change in one of these mechanisms, cross-resistance would be unexpected.

Nitrogen Mustards. Differences among the nitrogen mustards are primarily pharmacokinetic. The mustards are especially toxic to lymphocytes and bone marrow cells. In affected cells, mitosis is stopped and disintegration of formed elements of lymphoid tissue and bone marrow is evident within hours of a therapeutic dose. Immunosuppression and myelosuppression is profound and is a dose-limiting factor in therapy. Although large doses of the mustards can be severely toxic to the GI tract, proportionately this tendency is less severe than with other groups of drugs. The most commonly used nitrogen mustard is *cyclophosphamide.*

Cyclophosphamide, USP (Cytoxan), is widely used in veterinary medicine especially in combination with other drugs. The first of multiple steps in the activation of cyclophosphamide is accomplished by a hepatic cytochrome P450 mixed function oxidase. One of the metabolites, aldophosphamide, may be converted to the toxic compounds phosphoramide mustard and acrolein in target cells. Phosphoramide mustard alkylates and cross-links DNA strands. Increased levels of aldehyde dehydrogenase concentration have been documented in some tumors resistant to cyclophosphamide.

The important side effects of cyclophosphamide are related to myelosuppression. Neutropenia and milder thrombocytopenia are dose-limiting adverse effects with a nadir of 7–10 days. Nausea and vomiting are said to be rare, but vomiting has been observed in cats with high doses (Fetting et al. 1982). Cats given greater than 300 mg/kg exhibited reversible neurotoxicity characterized by head bobbing, broad-based stance, and falling. Alopecia may occur in continuous hair growth dogs.

Sterile necrotizing hemorrhagic cystitis, probably caused by the acrolein formed from cyclophosphamide, has been associated with administration of cyclophosphamide in both cats and dogs and is a cause for stopping therapy with the drug. To decrease the incidence of this cystitis, which is manifested by bloody urine, the drug should be administered in the morning, water intake should be high, and the animals should be encouraged to urinate frequently. Bladder irrigation with thiol compounds may help. Systemically administered N-acetylcysteine may also be of value. Mesna (sodium 2-mercaptoethanesulfonate, Mesnex) is an injectable used prophylactically and specifically to reduce the incidence of cystitis. The inert mesna disulfide (administered form) is reduced by renal tubules to mesna. Mesna binds to and detoxifies urotoxic metabolites of cyclophosphamide and ifosfamide (Elias et al. 1990).

Mechlorethamine (Mustargen) an original member of this group is rarely if ever used clinically today except, perhaps, in relapsed canine lymphoma as a member of the MOPP protocol (Mustargen, Oncovin [vincristine], procarbazine, prednisone) (Rassnick et al. 2002). It is so unstable that it must be given intravenously (IV), freshly prepared. Conversely, chlorambucil and cyclophosphamide are so stable they can be given orally. *Melphalan,* USP (L-Phenylalanine mustard, L-PAM, L-Sarcolysin, Alkeran) is used on occasion in veterinary oncology (Fujino et al. 2004). *Chlorambucil* USP (Leukeran), which is sometimes a replacement for cyclophosphamide due to its lower bladder toxicity, has been used in dogs for mast cell tumors, chronic lymphocytic leukemia, lymphoma, and some tumors in cats (Kleiter et al. 2001). *Ifosfamide* (Mitoxana, IFEX) is a structural analog of cyclophosphamide and has similar pharmacologic and toxicologic properties, including a greater tendency to produce hemorrhagic cystitis (Moore and Kitchell 2003).

Nitrosoureas. The nitrosoureas used clinically include *carmustine* and *lomustine.* A significant advantage for these drugs is their high lipid solubility that allows them to be used against tumors of the CNS. They have also been used effectively in combination protocols against relapsed canine lymphoma (LeBlanc et al. 2006). Streptozotocin, another nitrosourea, is rarely used in treatment of animal cancers. These drugs are primarily bifunctional alkylating agents that can form DNA-DNA and DNA-protein links. The O-6 methyl group of guanine is a key site of alkylation. DNA polymerase, DNA ligase, glutathione reductase, and enzymes involved in RNA synthesis and processing are also inhibited by an isocyanate produced from lomustine.

Limiting toxicities of this group are severe and include cumulative myelosuppression and thrombocytopenia that do not reach their maximum until about 7–10 days after administration of the drug in dogs. In humans the nadir is reached in 4–6 weeks! This delayed and cumulative bone marrow suppression is a noteworthy characteristic of the nitrosoureas.

There is no cross-resistance with other alkylating agents. The drugs are not cell-cycle–specific. The nitrosoureas have extremely short plasma half-lives. Lomustine is primarily biotransformed in the liver in most species. For more detailed information see Moore and Kitchell (2003).

Lomustine (cyclohexylchoroethylnitrosourea, CCNU, CeeNU) use in dogs and cats has been reviewed (Moore and Kitchell 2003). It has been used with some success in canine lymphoma, canine mast cell tumors, and possibly feline lymphoma (Fan 2003). In dogs, the half-life is approximately 15 minutes and the drug quickly enters the CSF. By 30 minutes, the plasma:CSF ratio is 1:3. Preclinical studies revealed adverse effects on the bone marrow, liver, kidneys, and gastrointestinal tract. At doses less than 100 mg/m^2, as recommended in typical clinical application, acute neutropenia was the dose-limiting toxicity with a thrombocytopenia nadir at 7 to 14 days postadministration. Lomustine is biotransformed by hepatic microsomes, so care should be observed in animals with poor liver function. Resistance is related to enhanced repair by guanine-O-6-transferase and increased glutathione concentration (Moore and Kitchell 2003).

Carmustine, N,N-bis (2-chloroethyl)-N-nitrosourea (BiCNU, BCNU), is used in humans in meningeal leukemia and other brain tumors. It has been tested in treatment of relapsed canine lymphoma as a member of a combination protocol (BOPP) that included carmustine, vincristine, procarbazine, and prednisone (LeBlanc et al. 2006). Significant neutropenia, thrombocytopenia, and gastrointestinal toxicity were observed in a promising trial, but the authors concluded that protocol needed to be optimized for the combination.

Other Alkylating Agents. *Busulfan,* USP (Myleran) is an alkylsulfonate used in people undergoing transplant surgery (Martins et al. 2005). It is seldom used in veterinary oncology. *Dacarbazine,* USP (5-(3,3-dimethyl-1-triazenyl)-1H-imidazole-4-carboxamide; DTIC, DTIC-Dome, DIC), is the only triazine compound used in tumor therapy and is rarely used in veterinary medicine.

Platinum Coordination Complexes. *Cisplatin, carboplatin, oxaliplatin,* and *lobaplatin* resemble the alkylating agents in that they form strong chemical bonds with nucleophiles such as nitrogen in nucleic acids and sulfur in proteins. Although they may be conceptually linked with alkylating agents, there are significant differences in their antitumor and toxic effects. Cisplatin is unique among anticancer drugs in being an inorganic compound; it contains two "cis-" chloride atoms and two "cis-" amino groups. The "trans-" derivatives are not effective as antitumor agents. In noncisplatin members of this group, the chloride atoms have been replaced with organic moieties that alter the toxicity pattern. For example, cisplatin produces significant renal and neurotoxicity, whereas carboplatin produces primarily hematopoietic toxicity. Lipophilicity and distribution of the various agents is determined by the substitutions on the amino groups.

Although it is possible that the chloride residues in cisplatin and the carboxyl ester groups in carboplatin and oxaliplatin can be directly replaced by nucleophiles, the reactions proceed much more rapidly if they are first replaced by water in a process called *aquation.* These aquated compounds then complete the reactions. It appears that the antitumor action of the cis-platinum agents is due to preferential reaction with the N-7 atom of deoxyguanylic acid in DNA, which results in interstrand cross-links. Intrastrand DNA cross-links may equally correlate with cytoxicity. These compounds are active against both proliferating and nonproliferating cells although cisplatin may have maximum lethal effect in late G1 phase (Boyer and Tannock 2005).

Preclinical studies of platinum complexes have been recently reviewed (Galanski et al. 2005). Cisplatin and carboplatin have been extensively used in veterinary oncology. No veterinary trials of oxaliplatin were found. Lobaplatin has been investigated as an adjuvant for therapy of canine osteosarcoma (Kirpensteijn et al. 2002) and cisplatin and carboplatin have been investigated in canine osteosarcoma (Chun and de Lorimier 2003). Resistance to platinum compounds has been linked to increased cellular concentrations of glutathione and metallothionein, presumably because of the thiol groups in the protein.

Cisplatin has been incorporated into treatment of several solid tumors including those of the testis, ovary, bladder, head, and neck in people. In dogs, activity has been demonstrated against transitional cell carcinoma, squamous cell carcinoma, osteosarcoma, and nasal adenocarcinoma (Knapp et al. 1988; Hahn et al. 1992). Because it has been so effective against a variety of tumors, there have been many investigations into reducing the adverse effects through localized, intralesional therapy. For osteosarcoma in dogs, these have included such approaches as intramedullary administration (Hahn et al. 1996b) and use of a biodegradable cisplatin-containing implant inserted into the limb-sparing surgery site at the time of surgery (Withrow et al. 2004). Intratumor administration of cisplatin was judged beneficial for cutaneous tumors of horses (Theon et al. 1999). Cisplatin is contraindicated in cats because it causes fatal pulmonary toxicity (Knapp et al. 1987), although special formulations of the drug may reduce the toxicity (Fox et al. 1999).

Cisplatin is included in many combination therapy regimens. It has been especially effective when combined with bleomycin and vinblastine against testicular tumors and with doxorubicin for ovarian tumors in humans. One especially well-known regimen for treating human testicular tumors is Einhorn, which includes cisplatin, vinblastine, and bleomycin; etoposide may or may not be included.

Cisplatin is given as a rapid IV infusion. It has a biphasic plasma-decay curve with an initial half-life of 22 minutes (probably distribution) and a terminal half-life of 5 days (probably elimination) in dogs. It is known that intracellular half-life in humans may be as long as 30 days. This presumably represents drug bound to tissue macromolecules. High tissue concentrations have been found in kidney, liver, ovary, testis, and uterus (Williams and Whitehouse 1979).

Nephrotoxicity is a dose-limiting adverse effect of cisplatin in most species, including dogs. Other major toxicities include intractable nausea and vomiting even when antiemetics are used, ototoxicity (hearing loss), anaphylactic-like reactions, and neurotoxicity. Emesis in dogs typically begins 2 hours after cisplatin administration and lasts 2–3 hours, but appears to be less severe than in people (Morrison 2002a). Myelosuppression is mild relative to alkylating agents, but thrombocytopenia and granulocytopenia may be observed by day 7–9 and 17–19 after injection, respectively. GI toxicity manifests as diarrhea and anorexia may also be observed.

Nephrotoxicity is dose-related, cumulative, apparently irreversible in some cases, and primarily affects proximal tubules in which tubular degeneration, loss of brush border, necrosis, and mineralization of tubular epithelial cells may be observed. Serum urea nitrogen may be elevated by day 7–9 after injection. Continuation of treatment should be based on evidence of suitable renal function as judged by renal concentrating ability, urine sediment, and serum creatinine concentration. Much emphasis is placed on finding ways to reduce the incidence and severity of cisplatin induced nephrotoxicosis. Hypersalination (i.e., induction of forced diuresis with infusion of hypertonic sodium chloride solution) is beneficial. Other approaches demonstrated in clinical or laboratory studies that may reduce toxicity include the use of methimazole (Vail et al. 1993), rosiglitazone (Lee et al. 2006), and L-arginine (Saleh and El-Demerdash 2005). On a practical level there is circumstantial evidence that administering cisplatin in the morning may reduce toxicity (Morrison 2002b). The mechanism of the toxic effect is uncertain.

A typical protocol for use of cisplatin in dogs is to administer 60 to 70 mg/m^2 intravenously every 3 weeks. Fasting the dog 12 hours prior to administration reduces the severity of emesis and nephrotoxicity. A recommended saline diuresis protocol in dogs is to give 18 ml/kg/hr of normal saline beginning 4 hours prior to beginning cisplatin infusion and for 2 hours after infusion (Knapp 2006). The animal should be watched carefully to ensure that it is well hydrated in the postinfusion period. Cisplatin drug should not be prepared with or administered through an aluminum needle because aluminum reacts with and inactivates the drug.

Carboplatin (CBDCA, JM-8, Paraplatin) is an analogue of cisplatin that is effective in treating human ovarian tumors. It has the same mechanism of action as cisplatin, with which cross-resistance has been reported, but is less reactive, produces a different pattern of toxicity, and can be used in cats.

It has been found to be effective in animal tumors, including post surgical osteosarcoma (Chun and de Lorimier 2003). Unlike cisplatin, carboplatin has shown no efficacy in the treatment of canine transitional cell carcinoma (Morrison 2002a). An advantage over cisplatin is that it can be used more conveniently on an outpatient basis. Its major toxicity is bone marrow depression. In dogs, leukopenia and thrombocytopenia may be severe at approximately 2 weeks after administration of high doses (Page et al. 1993). Nausea and vomiting, although common, are less severe than with cisplatin. In contrast to cisplatin, carboplatin is not regarded as nephrotoxic although it did reduce glomerular filtration rate of dogs in one study. Diuresis is not required. Because it is primarily eliminated via the kidney, preexisting renal disease can significantly increase toxicity. The dose-limiting toxicity in cats is neutropenia (Hahn et al. 1997). Pharmacokinetics of carboplatin have been studied in dogs (Page et al. 1993).

ANTIMETABOLITES. Antimetabolites resemble normal cellular substituents and either compete with them in enzymatic reactions to slow key cellular processes or replace them as substrates leading to false products that then interfere with important cellular processes. Most antimetabolites are prodrugs, i.e., they must be intracellularly converted to their active form. Clinically useful antimetabolites typically inhibit DNA synthesis as their major anticancer mechanism although their site of action may be several steps removed. In some cases, e.g., 5-FU, inhibition of RNA processing may also be important. The relative importance of altered DNA versus RNA synthesis and function may be tumor-type–dependent. Antimetabolites profoundly inhibit replication of bone marrow cells. Some cause even greater GI toxicity. As their parent category implies, these agents are highly cell-cycle–specific when inhibition of DNA synthesis is the dominant effect. Because cells are far more sensitive to some antimetabolites while in the S phase, those antimetabolites are further categorized as phase-specific.

Folic Acid Analogs. Agents that act on the folic acid pathways are used in medicine to treat cancer, infectious diseases, rheumatoid arthritis, psoriasis, and graft versus host diseases have been recently reviewed (Walling 2006). Aminopterin, the first folic acid derivative heralded the introduction of antimetabolites in cancer therapy. Aminopterin provided only brief induction of remission, but led to the development of *methotrexate* (MTX). MTX is a venerable drug that is included in cancer and nonmalignant applications in both people and animals. Members of the folic acid analog group include agents that target several key enzymes as follows: dihydrofolate reductase (DHFR) inhibitors (e.g., MTX, *edatrexate, trimetrexate,* and *PDX*), thymidylate synthase (e.g., CB3717, *raltitrexed, plevitrexed,* and AG337), purine enzymes glycinamide ribonucleotide formyl transferase (GARFT) and aminoimidazole carboxamide formyl transferase (AICARFT) (e.g., *lometrexol,* LY309887, and AG2034), and multiple folate-requiring enzymes (e.g., *pemetrexed*). Folylpolyglutamate synthase (FPGS) is a key enzyme that adds terminal glutamate residues to folic acid analogs. Reduced ability of FPGS to form polyglutamates of MTX is a mechanism of resistance to MTX; therefore, nonclassical antifolates have been developed (e.g., trimetrexate, piritrexim, plevitrexed, and AG337). These molecules are sufficiently lipid soluble that they may be effective in tumors with defective folate transport pathways. Drugs that exploit different isoforms of the folate receptor in various tissues are also being developed (e.g., LY309887) (Walling 2006). Extensive effort is being placed on covalently linking drugs that act through other pathways to folic acid to exploit the unique properties of the folic acid family receptors (Low and Antony 2004). Most of the drugs listed above are in various stages of clinical development, but MTX, trimetrexate (Neutrexin), and pemetrexed (Alimta) are marketed in the U.S. Published clinical applications in animals were found only for MTX.

Methotrexate, USP (Amethopterin), is a folic acid analog used against a wide variety of neoplasms including human choriocarcinoma. It is commonly used in combination regimens in veterinary medicine, e.g., in treatment of lymphosarcoma and osteosarcoma (Morrison 2002a). It has provided some benefit in a combination protocol in hemangiosarcoma (Smith 2003).

Methotrexate (MTX) acts as a false folate cofactor, thereby inhibiting key steps in the de novo purine and thymidylate biosynthetic pathways. After being transported into cells MTX binds strongly to dihydrofolate reductase (DHFR). The resulting inhibition of DHFR depletes cellular tetrahydrofolic acid (THF), which functions as a donor of one-carbon moieties important in the synthesis of nucleic acids. Conversion of deoxyuridylate into thymidylate by thymidylate synthase requires 5, 10-methylene tetrahydrofolate. De novo synthesis of purines requires 10-formyl tetrahydrofolate as a formyl donor. Although inhibition of DHFR is the dominant mode of action, MTX also inhibits thymidine kinase, GARFT (5-phosphoribosylglycinamide formyltransferase) and AICARFT (Aminoimidazole carboxamide ribonucleotide transferase). Inhibition of the latter two enzymes depends on the degree to which MTX is converted to the polyglutamate derivative. Increased concentration of folic acid or of the DHFR protein decreases the effectiveness of MTX. Binding of MTX increases the concentration of DHFR presumably through translational autoregulation (Walling 2006).

Methotrexate is actively transported into cells by a saturable, carrier-mediated system, so it is active at extremely low concentrations in some cell systems. It does not readily enter cells by passive diffusion and crosses the blood-brain barrier poorly. Decreased cellular accumulation of MTX due to impaired transport or decreased retention leads to resistance. Decreased retention can be caused by lack of polyglutamate formation or an increase in gamma glutamyl hydrolase activity. Two other means of resistance are production of DHF reductases that have decreased affinity for the drug and increased concentrations of the reductase through gene amplification.

The major adverse effects of methotrexate are myelosuppression and gastrointestinal mucositis at doses typically used in animals. If higher doses are used it may be advisable to monitor renal function prior to and during therapy because methotrexate produces renal tubular necrosis when given in high doses.

Pyrimidine Analogs. Because nucleic acids are involved in cell growth control, attention was given to finding analogs of natural pyrimidine and purines that could interfere with processing of DNA and/or RNA to inhibit or kill cancerous cells. The classical view is that quantitative, but not qualitative, differences exist in pathways involving the nucleic acids between normal and cancer cells providing a basis for selectivity, although emerging knowledge about single nucleotide polymorphisms (SNPs) may modify this view in the future. These "false" nucleotides may be incorporated into RNA and DNA producing nucleic acids that cannot be replicated or lead to miscoding. They may also act on regulatory processes, i.e., in feedback loops to deplete critical intermediates. Repair enzymes may negate or enhance the effect of the presence of the false nucleotides in the DNA. Nucleoside analogs may alter transport of normal nucleosides in or out of normal and cancer cells.

The natural pyrimidine cytosine is found in both DNA and RNA. Uracil is found only in RNA, but is a precursor of thymine, which occurs in DNA. Clinically used pyrimidine analogs include the uracil analog *5-fluorouracil* and cytosine analogs *cytarabine*, *5-azacytidine*, and *gemcitabine* (Pizzorno et al. 2003).

Cytarabine, USP (cytosine arabinoside, arabinosyl cytosine, Ara-C, Cytosar) differs from the endogenous nucleoside deoxycytidine only in that the sugar is arabinose instead of deoxyribose, i.e., position 2 of the sugar is hydroxylated. It is one of the most important agents in the treatment of acute myeloid leukemia in people and it also is active against other leukemias and lymphoma. It is not very effective against solid tumors (Pizzorno et al. 2003). It has been used for lymphoreticular and myeloproliferative disorders in dogs and cats.

Cytarabine enters cells via a membrane transporter and by passive diffusion at higher concentrations.

Cytoplasmic deoxycytidine kinase converts cytarabine (ara-C) to cytosine arabinoside monophosphate (ara-CMP), which is ultimately converted to cytosine arabinoside triphosphate (ara-CTP) by other enzymes. Cytidine deaminase effectively inactivates ara-C so the anticancer activity and toxicity of the drug is influenced by the relative activity of these enzymes in the tissues. Ara-CTP, a competitive inhibitor and false substrate for DNA polymerase, is the active form of the drug which causes inhibition of nuclear DNA synthesis by three mechanisms; inhibition of initiation of new replication units following incorporation of ara-C into the primer, retardation of DNA-chain elongation because of incorporation of ara-C into DNA, and inhibition of DNA primase. High concentrations of ara-CTP may increase the termination of DNA-chain elongation with chains ending in ara-C. Exonucleases, e.g., TREX 1 or 2 and p53 could remove ara-C from these terminal positions to decrease its cytotoxic effect (Pizzorno et al. 2003). The ultimate effect of the abnormal DNA produced is the induction of apoptosis.

Acquired or de novo resistance may be related to increased intracellular concentration of cytidine deaminase, which converts cytarabine to ara-U, which is less toxic. Resistant mutants that lack deoxycytidine kinase, the activating enzyme, have been identified. Some resistant mutants have been shown to have high intracellular concentrations of deoxycytidine triphosphate (dCTP) causing decreased activation (phosphorylation) of cytarabine.

Bone marrow suppression is the dose-limiting toxicity. It is manifest by leukopenia, thrombocytopenia, anemia, and megaloblastosis. It should be used with caution in animals with compromised liver function.

Intravenously administered cytarabine is included in many protocols for treatment of CNS leukemia and lymphoma in dogs and cats (Morrison 2002a). A pharmacokinetic study revealed that cytarabine did cross the blood-brain barrier and therapeutic doses could produce effective concentrations in the cerebrospinal fluid (CSF) (Scott-Moncrieff et al. 1991). The plasma elimination half-life in dogs was approximately 64 to 69 minutes, whereas the half-life of cytarabine in CSF was 165 minutes. The peak concentration of cytarabine in CSF was 29 μM.

Gemcitabine (2,2′-difluorodeoxycytidine, dFdC, Gemzar) is a cytosine analog with similarities to cytarabine except that it also has activity against solid tumors in people. It was licensed for use in people for pancreatic carcinoma and non–small-cell lung cancer, but has found application in combination therapy for other solid tumors. It has been evaluated for various tumors in dogs (Kosarek et al. 2005; Moore and Kitchell 2003). However, caution is recommended because anecdotal evidence is available that some dogs are especially sensitive and may show toxicity at doses of 675 mg/m^2 (Knapp 2006). Pharmacokinetics of gemcitabine and its primary metabolite following intravenous bolus (Freise and Martin-Jimenez 2006a) and infusion (Freise and Martin-Jimenez 2006b) to dogs have been reported.

Fluorouracil, USP (5-fluoro-2,4(1H,3H)-pyrimidinedione; 5-FU, Efudex, Adrucil), is a pyrimidine analog that resembles both uracil and thymine, components of RNA and DNA, respectively. It is used in people for carcinomas of the mammary gland and GI tract, e.g., colorectal carcinomas. Although rarely used in veterinary oncology it has shown promise in adjuvant postoperative chemotherapy of dogs with mammary cancer in combination with cyclophosphamide (Karayannopoulou et al. 2001). Topical preparation of 5-FU has been used in cutaneous squamous cell carcinomas of horses (Fortier and Mac Harg 1994).

Both DNA synthesis and RNA synthesis and function are altered by 5-FU metabolites. The prodrug, 5-FU, is metabolized intracellularly to 5′-fluorouridine monophosphate (FUMP) and then to 5′-fluorodeoxyuridine monophosphate (FdUMP). FdUMP, a potent inhibitor of thymidylate synthetase, decreases the synthesis of DNA precursors. Fluorouracil is also incorporated into RNA. It is highly cell-cycle–specific, but no clear association with a particular phase can be demonstrated. The relative importance of inhibition of DNA synthesis versus effects on RNA synthesis appears to be tumor-dependent. Severe inhibition of thymidylate synthetase in noncancer cells could lead to host toxicity due to "thymineless" death. It has been hypothesized that administration of exogenous thymidine could reverse this 5-FU induced toxicity. Unfortunately, under certain circumstances, administration of thymidine actually enhanced toxicity.

Fluorouracil is most toxic to bone marrow and oral and GI mucosa. Thus, bone marrow suppression manifested by leukopenia, thrombocytopenia, and anemia is severe and is the major dose-limiting factor. Anorexia, nausea, and vomiting are seen. Diarrhea and stomatitis are indications for the interruption of therapy. CNS toxicity is regarded as unusual in humans, but may be more common in animals. The signs include dementia, excitement, tremors, and ataxia, sometimes followed by opisthotonos, tonic-clonic convulsions, dyspnea, shock, and death. The neurotoxicity may be due to metabolites of 5-FU in the dog (Yamashita et al. 2004). Neurotoxicity contraindicates the use of 5-FU in cats (Morrison 2002a). A cream formulation has been shown to be very toxic if accidentally eaten. A 5% cream (Efudex) is intended for actinic keratoses and superficial basal cell carcinoma.

Capecitabine (pentyl[1-(3,4-dihydroxy-5-methyl-tetrahydrofuran-2-yl)-5-fluoro-2-oxo-1H-pyrimidin-4-yl]aminomethanoate, Xeloda) is an oral fluoropyrimidine derivative that facilitates administration and sustained drug exposure. Use of this drug in veterinary oncology is not established.

Purine analogs are prodrugs that must be converted to the nucleoside triphosphate to be active. Examples include *mercaptopurine,* USP (6-mercaptopurine, 6-MP, Purinethol), *thioguanine, azathioprine* (Imuran, primarily used as an immunosuppressant), and the new derivative, *fludarabine* (1-fluoro-ara-AMP, Fludara). Mercaptopurine, which is primarily used to treat lymphoreticular tumors in people, was used in older protocols for lymphosarcoma and osteosarcoma in veterinary oncology, but it and thioguanine are seldom used now.

NATURAL PRODUCTS

Microtubules. Microtubules are important for mitotic spindle formation among other important roles in normal cell structure and function. Microtubules are polymers composed of alpha- and beta-tubulin heterodimers that are dynamically assembled and disassembled as a normal aspect of cellular function and division. The mechanism of action of vinca alkaloids and taxanes is closely linked to their activity on the function and dynamics of microtubules, especially of the highly dynamic mitotic-spindle microtubules. The classical view is that these changes usually have the net effect of producing mitotic block, cell cycle arrest, and apoptosis (although some may also lead to necrosis). Potential mechanisms by which the drugs alter microtubular dynamics are complex and vary with the drug.

Three main classes of drug binding sites on tubulin have been identified: the paclitaxel site, the vinca domain, and the colchicine domain. In addition microtubule-regulatory proteins may serve as targets. Because the drugs act on different sites and have different effects on downstream signaling pathways that lead to cell death, there is potential for synergy among the drugs. Differences such as those above explain why the microtubular toxins differ in effectiveness against a variety of tumors and why significant attention is being given to development of additional drugs that alter microtubular function.

Resistance to microtubule-targeted agents may involve tubulin mutations, altered expression of tubulin isotypes, and altered expression or binding of microtubule-regulatory proteins.

A complete dissection of the complexities, including concentration effects and timing of exposure of cancer cells to these drugs, is beyond the scope of this discussion, but the reader is referred to Zhao et al. (2005).

Vinca Alkaloids. The vinca alkaloids are large, complex substances derived from the periwinkle plant (*Vinca rosea* L.). Although similar in structure, *vincristine sulfate*, USP (Oncovin), *vinblastine sulfate*, USP (Velban, Velsar), and *vinorelbine* (Navelbine) differ considerably in antitumor efficacy as well as in the doses that produce toxic effects. Vincristine is a member of many protocols used in people as well as animals. Typical indications for people include acute lymphocytic leukemia, neuroblastoma, Wilm's tumor, rhabdomyosarcoma, Hodgkin's disease, and non-Hodgkin's lymphoma. Vincristine is one of the major drugs used in veterinary oncology. It is effective against canine transmissible venereal tumor as a single agent (Nak et al. 2005). It is a member of many "named" combination protocols for lymphoreticular tumors and soft-tissue sarcomas where it is identified by the letter *O* for Oncovin, its commercial name. A vinblastine and prednisone combination has been found effective in cases of metastatic canine mast cell tumors (Govier 2003).

Vinca alkaloids are taken into cells by an energy-dependent carrier-mediated transport system. There is no cross-resistance between vincristine and vinblastine except when the tumor is multidrug-resistant due to expression of multidrug-resistance transporters (Huisman et al. 2005).

Vinblastine may produce a dose-limiting leukopenia, the nadir of which occurs at 5–10 days. Hematologic effects of vincristine are mild, but neutropenia was observed in cats treated with vincristine alone (Hahn et al. 1996a) and it can also be produced in dogs (Kanter et al. 1994). Thrombocytopenia and anemia are rare with both drugs. Vincristine induces thrombocytosis. Both are severe tissue irritants and must be administered via an indwelling catheter.

Although neither drug penetrates into the brain or CSF sufficiently for therapy, vincristine is much more likely than vinblastine to produce neurotoxicity. This difference, which may be due to differential rates of transport out of the CNS by P-gp, is paradoxical because vinblastine is more lipid soluble. One hypothetical explanation is that the slower elimination of vincristine relative to vinblastine may lead to prolonged exposure of nerve tissue to high concentrations of vincristine. The neural effect of vincristine ranges from mild to dose-limiting. A combination of vincristine, cyclophosphamide, and prednisone produced peripheral neuropathy in a dog that improved after the vincristine was removed from the protocol. Onset was sudden and included difficulty in locomotion (Hamilton et al. 1991). Neuropathy may also be manifest as paresis and voice change.

Vincristine disappears rapidly from the plasma and appears to be concentrated in platelets and cells with a large volume of distribution. Vincristine and vinblastine can be eliminated into the urine by the MDR1 gene product P-gp transporter located on the apical surface of the renal proximal tubule. Vinca alkaloids are also eliminated in the bile.

Taxanes. Plant alkaloids known as *taxanes* currently used in clinical medicine include *paclitaxel* (Taxol) and *docetaxel* (Taxotere). Paclitaxel is derived from the bark of the Pacific yew tree *Taxus brevifolia* and docetaxel is a semisynthetic derivative from the needles of the European yew tree *Taxus baccata*. These drugs have found application in treatment of ovarian, breast, lung, bladder, and head and neck cancer in people. Effectiveness of paclitaxel and docetaxel in animals is still in the early stages of evaluation, but because of their effectiveness in humans and probable eventual use in animals, some key aspects of the drugs will be covered.

The taxanes' poor water solubility requires special formulations with nonionic surfactants to allow intravenous administration. These surfactants are not pharmacologically inert and their necessary use significantly complicates both the pharmacokinetic properties and the toxicity of the commercially available forms of taxanes; therefore, their commercial names of Taxol and Taxotere will be used where appropriate. The docetaxel formulation in polysorbate 80 is commercially known as Taxotere. The commercial form of paclitaxel, Taxol, is formulated in alcohol and Cremophor EL (Cr-EL; polyoxyethylated castor oil). This has two important ramifications. First, in a dose escalation study, if was found that the Cr-EL affects the toxicity by releasing histamine following intravenous administration. Administration of antihistamines prior to infusion of Taxol is required. Despite this precaution, some dogs showed evidence of histamine release (Poirier et al. 2004). Second, the presence of the surfactant vehicle has profound effects on the pharmacokinetics of paclitaxel. Drug is entrapped in micelles, thus reducing the free fraction and altering the distribution and other pharmacokinetic parameters of the drug. In a study of a 1-hour versus a 3-hour infusion it was found that clearance and volume of distribution were significantly dependent on infusion duration. The 3-hour schedule tended to produce more hematologic toxicity "consistent with increased exposure to unbound drug." The findings help explain the fact that short-infusion schedules of Taxol lack significant myelotoxicity, but have greater potentially Cr-EL–related adverse effects, e.g., peripheral neuropathy (Gelderblom et al. 2002). Another example of the effect of the Cr-EL formulation on distribution is provided by the fact that mixing Taxol with DMSO for intravesicular instillation in dogs increased the free fraction to 92% and increased tissue penetration of paclitaxel (Chen et al. 2003).

Other potential complications for veterinary cancer studies are that interaction with other anticancer drugs can alter kinetics of paclitaxel (Kroep et al. 2006) and that there can be confusion between vehicle effects and direct effects of the drug. For example, in people, it is known that Cr-E is mainly responsible for ganglionopathy, axonopathy, and demyelination, but there is strong clinical data and data from non–Cr-EL-containing formulations that paclitaxel also produces dose-limiting neurotoxicity. This is likely due to its effects on microtubules in perikaryons, axons, and glia cells.

Taxol produced partial remission of malignant histiocytosis, mammary carcinoma, and osteosarcoma in a preliminary study in dogs that had advanced relapsed disease. Results were judged to merit further study under more optimal conditions and as part of combination protocols (Poirier et al. 2004).

Addition of cyclosporin A, an inhibitor of P-gp transporter (ABC-B1) and cytochrome P450 isoenzyme CYP3A in intestinal epithelial cells, increased oral bioavailability of docetaxel (Taxotere) from 20% to 100%. Gastrointestinal toxicity was dose-limiting in this canine study which included detailed pharmacokinetic analysis at 3 doses (McEntee et al. 2006).

Epipodophyllotoxins. Podophyllotoxin is an extract of the mandrake plant that has led to the development of two synthetic derivatives; *teniposide* (Vumon, VM-26) and *etoposide* (Etopophos, Vepesid, VP-16, VP-16–213). Teniposide and etoposide have become important in the treatment of some human tumors, e.g., Hodgkin's disease, non-Hodgkin's lymphoma, acute myelogenous leukemia, Kaposi's sarcoma and cancers of the testis, lung, and breast. They have not yet found mainline application in veterinary medicine.

Camptothecins. Two derivatives of the plant alkaloid 20(s)-camptothecin are approved for clinical use in people: *topotecan* (Hycamtin) and *irinotecan* (Campto). They are used for cancers of the ovary, lung, and colon in people. No published clinical trials of these drugs in animals were found.

Antibiotics—Topoisomerase Inhibitors. Topoisomerase enzymes control and modify the topologic states of DNA. The extremely long strands of DNA are tightly coiled in a double helical structure in the nucleus except when being transcribed or duplicated. For these processes to occur, the twisted, supercoiled DNA must be "unwound" to allow the DNA and RNA polymerases to function. Mammalian nuclei contain various isoforms of topoisomerase I and topoisomerase II. These enzymes cleave the phosphodiester backbone of DNA, form a covalent enzyme-DNA linkage that allows another single- or double-strand DNA to pass through the nick, and then reseal the backbone. Topoisomerase inhibitors prevent the religation of the DNA strands by binding to and stabilizing the DNA/topoisomerase complex to cause DNA strand breaks that are lethal to the cell. Any abnormal function of cyclins, cell- cycle–regulated kinases, or phosphatases can influence the cytotoxicity of topoisomerase I inhibitors and some dysfunctions can lead to resistance to the anticancer drugs. Doxorubicin and dactinomycin inhibit both topoisomerase I and II. Topoisomerase II is inhibited by anthracyclines and epipodophyllotoxins. The anthracyclines that inhibit topoisomerase II have long been known to intercalate between two adjacent base pairs, so it was originally thought that this was the primary means of action and, hence, of classifying them as "intercalating agents" as is common in older literature (Ratain and Plunkett 2003).

The exact mechanism by which interaction of the drugs with the topoisomerase inhibitors causes cell death is not well established. Resistance can occur when levels of topoisomerase I or II are reduced, thereby reducing the number of drug-DNA-topoisomerase complexes that can be formed. This reduces the chance that the damage will be detected to trigger an apoptotic response. Resistance can also be due to mutant, but still active, forms of topoisomerase II that have lower affinity for the drugs (Stewart and Ratain 2001). Some epigenetic mechanisms can increase the activity of the topoisomerase inhibitors. Hyperacetylated histones permit transcription to occur, e.g., treatment of leukemic cells with a histone deacetylase inhibitor increases expression of topoisomerase II thus increasing the potential target for topoisomerase inhibitors (Cole and Tannock 2005). An interesting aspect of the topoisomerase inhibitors that illustrates the complexity of the interlocking signaling pathways in cells is that they may be involved in controlling caspase-2 premessenger RNA splicing (Solier et al. 2004).

Anthracyclines. *Doxorubicin*, the first anthracycline derivative, was isolated from *Streptomyces* spp. *Daunorubicin, epirubicin,* and *idarubicin* are semisynthetic derivatives. The anthracyclines are tetracycline ring structures substituted with the sugar daunosamine. *Dactinomycin* (actinomycin D, Cosmegen) has seen little use in veterinary oncology, but a recent study found that replacing doxorubicin with it in a combination protocol for canine lymphoma warranted further investigation (Siedlecki et al. 2006). *Mitoxantrone* is often classified with the anthracyclines, but it is a synthetic anthracenedione derivative and lacks a sugar moiety.

Doxorubicin hydrochloride, USP (Adriamycin, Doxil [liposomal formulation]) is an extremely important anthracycline derivative that has antitumor activity against a wide variety of tumors in both people and animals as a single agent and in combinations. Examples of applications in people include cancers of the breast, genitourinary system, thyroid, lung and stomach; soft-tissue, osteogenic, and other sarcomas; Hodgkin's disease; non-Hodgkin's lymphoma; and acute leukemia. The list for animals is also long. It has shown activity, usually as a component of a combination, against thyroid tumors; sarcomas such as lymphosarcoma, hemangiosarcoma, and osteosarcoma; and a wide variety of carcinomas such as mammary tumors and squamous cell carcinomas, and transitional cell carcinomas (Klein 2003; Henry 2003; Sorenmo 2003; Chun and de Lorimier 2003; Kent et al. 2004). Nasal tumors were effectively treated with alternating doses of doxorubicin, carboplatin, and oral piroxicam (Langova et al. 2004). Use of doxorubicin as a sole agent in adjuvant therapy in high- grade soft-tissue sarcomas did not prove beneficial (Selting et al. 2005).

It is well established, as described above, that doxorubicin inhibits topoisomerase I and II, but it also damages DNA through free-radical generation by the electron accepting and donating quinone and p-hydroquinone moieties that cause membrane damage and DNA strand breaks. The mechanism by which doxorubicin generates free radicals has been claimed to be due to oxidation of its p-hydroquinone moiety. The resulting free radicals can cause genotoxicity and cardiotoxicity as well as participate in the anticancer action. It is likely that the carcinogenic action of doxorubicin is due to this free radical induced genotoxicity. Further, there is evidence that the critical apoptotic trigger of doxorubicin may be oxidative DNA damage by the direct H_2O_2 generation induced by doxorubicin in addition to its effects on topoisomerase II (Mizutani et al. 2005). There is also evidence that some apoptosis may be initiated by free radical independent mechanisms (Suzuki et al. 2005).

Detection of DNA damage by the cell and effective activation of apoptotic pathways is crucial to the cytotoxic effect of doxorubicin and other anticancer modalities. Dysregulation of apoptotic pathways in, e.g., breast cancers, may be due to down-regulated death receptor pathway function (Munoz-Gamez et al. 2005).

Doxorubicin enters cells by a passive process and is extensively bound in the tissues. Anthracyclines have low concentrations in the CNS either because of their low lipophilicity or because of the P-gp transporter in brain endothelial cells or both. It is biotransformed to an active metabolite (doxorubicinol) and inactive compounds in the liver and is excreted in the bile. Induction of cytochrome P450 enzymes decreases plasma doxorubicin concentration pointing to the possibility for drug interactions (Stewart and Ratain 2001).

The pharmacokinetic profile of doxorubicin in people is highly variable, with interindividual variability for most parameters ranging from 37% to 93%. Intraindividual variability ranges from 6% to 59%. Obesity has been shown to reduce clearance by approximately 50% in people, but perhaps not in dogs (see below). Pharmacokinetic variability may have a significant effect on the effects observed with doxorubicin therapy because dogs treated for lymphoma that responded to the therapy had longer terminal half-lives of the drug than dogs that did not respond (Selting et al. 2006). This study also showed that supplementation with n-3 fatty acids did not alter the doxorubicin pharmacokinetics as might have been predicted (Ogilvie et al. 2000). Pharmacokinetic values obtained after one dose were as follows: AUC = 427 ± 44 ng/ml·h, Cmax = 879 ± 83 ng/ml, Terminal $t_{1/2}$ = 8.7 ± 1.0 Vss = 703 ± 50 l/kg, CL = 83 ± 8 l/h/kg (Selting et al. 2006). The fact that no difference was found related to obesity in this study may be due to the degree of obesity as compared to some morbidly obese people.

Multidrug resistance due to the P-gp product of the MDR1 (ABCB1) gene and other members of the ATP-binding cassette (ABC) transporters was discussed previously in this chapter. Despite frequent success in in vitro studies (Page et al. 2000) attempts to use chemosensitizers, e.g., tamoxifen, cyclosporin A, and newer second-generation P-gp inhibitors such as PSC 833 (Valspodar) have produced mixed results in clinical trials. It is also likely that increased concentrations of glutathione in cells decreases the effectiveness of doxorubicin because a component of its action is to generate free radicals.

Toxicoses caused by doxorubicin have been reviewed and classified as acute, short-term, or chronic. Acute toxicosis manifests as head-shaking, localized urticaria along the course of the vein used for administration of the drug, and signs associated with histamine release including generalized blushing of the skin and acute collapse if administered too rapidly. Rapid administration may result in acute GI upset (anorexia, vomiting, and bloody diarrhea) within 12–24 hours. Histamine related signs may be decreased by pretreating dogs with diphenhydramine hydrochloride (e.g., Benadryl), 1.0 mg/kg. Improperly formulated or prepared doxorubicin may lead to increased frequency of acute reactions.

Short-term reactions include weight loss, anorexia, diarrhea, vomiting, myelosuppression, bone marrow hypoplasia, lymphoid atrophy, and alopecia. Dogs developing signs of toxicosis after their first dose of doxorubicin were 17 times more likely to develop toxicoses after the second dose (Ogilvie et al. 1989). Hematologic changes are the short-term dose-limiting manifestation of toxicity. Neutropenia is common, with a nadir at 7–10 days after treatment and returning to normal by 3 weeks. Less commonly, one may see thrombocytopenia (nadir between 3 and 8 days) and anemia that follows the same pattern. Doxorubicin produces poikilocytosis in cats (O'Keefe and Schaeffer 1992). Chronic toxicosis is associated with hair loss, testicular atrophy, and dose dependent cardiac toxicosis leading to arrhythmias and cardiomyopathy. For more details on non–cardiac-related toxicity see Ogilvie et al. (1989a).

Anthracyclines cause two types of cardiac toxicity, one immediate and the other cumulative. During IV administration, one may see cardiac arrest preceded by electrocardiographic changes such as T-wave flattening, S-T segment depression, voltage reduction, and arrhythmias. This is usually brief and is not necessarily an indication to stop using doxorubicin. If the changes are minor, some clinicians cautiously continue with slower administration of drug. Others recommend discontinuing therapy with doxorubicin until a later time. Cardiac arrest can usually be avoided by premedication with antihistamines which may be considered if an animal has previously shown a tendency to arrhythmias.

Cumulative myocardial toxicity, which ultimately manifests as congestive heart failure, is more severe and necessitates permanently stopping doxorubicin therapy. Clinical cardiac abnormalities include arrhythmias and nonspecific alterations in the R wave, ST segment, or QRS duration as well as congestive heart failure, which may be fatal. Noninflammatory myocardial degeneration was observed in the hearts of dogs that died (Mauldin et al. 1992). The risk of congestive heart failure is thought to increase sharply above 250 mg/m^2 total dose in dogs. Cats given a cumulative dose of 300 mg/m^2 had no grossly observable clinical evidence of heart disease, but some did have echocardiographic signs of heart disease and the hearts of all had myocyte vacuolization and myocytolysis as well as histological and functional evidence of renal disease (O'Keefe et al. 1993). Because of the cumulative toxicity, one should maintain a record of the total amount of doxorubicin given, stop therapy when the limit is reached, and watch carefully for signs of congestive heart failure.

The exact mechanism by which doxorubicin causes myocardial toxicity is unknown, but at least one mechanism is believed to be through the production of reactive oxygen species (ROS). ROS produced in the mitochondria and calcium may play a key role in stimulating doxorubicin-induced intrinsic (mitochondria-mediated) and extrinsic (FAS/Fas L [Fas-ligand]–mediated) forms of apoptosis in cardiac cells (Kalivendi et al. 2005). Cumulative loss of myocardial fibers may be the cause of the diffuse cardiomyopathy that is manifested by arrhythmias and congestive heart failure.

Means of decreasing the myocardial toxicity are a significant area of research. Various agents—for example, dexrazoxane (ICRF-187) tested in dogs (Imondi et al. 1996), aminoguanidine in rats (Cigremis et al. 2006), amifostine in rats (Bolaman et al. 2005), and amifostine in humans with breast cancer (Catino et al. 2003) attenuated the adverse effects. Pifithrin-alpha, a *p53* inhibitor, interferes with doxorubicin induced apoptosis in rat H9c2 cells in culture (Chua et al. 2006). Exercise has been found to reduce the cardiac toxicity induced by anthracyclines (Peng et al. 2005).

Various formulations of doxorubicin have been developed in an attempt to increase its therapeutic index. One of the more prominent is pegylated-liposomal doxorubicin (Doxil) that has been found to significantly alter the drug's pharmacokinetics. Doxil was found to be effective in reducing tumor volume and in causing apoptosis in some tumors in immune compromised mouse models with xenografts of canine transmissible venereal tumor, thus showing promise of effectiveness in dogs (Stettner et al. 2005). The relative advantages of various liposome formulations of anthracyclines such as STEALTH and DaunoXome have been reviewed (Allen and Martin 2004). Liposomes targeted with anti-CD19 antibodies may offer increased therapeutic index (Allen et al. 2005).

Doxil was found to be well tolerated and effective in dogs with cancer at doses equivalent to those of free drug. The maximally tolerated dose in these dogs was found to be 1.0 mg/kg intravenously every 3 weeks. Cutaneous toxicity that resembled palmar-plantar erythrodysesthesia was dose-limiting (Vail et al. 1997). Dosage and cautions during administration of standard doxorubicin formulations have been published (Morrison 2002a).

Doxorubicin is a severe tissue irritant (see earlier discussion of precautions regarding administration of vesicant drugs) and causes mild alopecia and hyperpigmentation in the axillary and inguinal regions. Urine may be colored red while significant quantities of the red drug and its metabolites are being eliminated. This is medically harmless and temporary.

Daunorubicin hydrochloride (daunomycin, rubidomycin, Cerubidine, DaunoXome [liposomal formulation]) differs from doxorubicin only by having a proton in place of a hydroxyl group. It is similar to doxorubicin in mechanism and toxicity except that it has more pronounced cardiomyopathic effects. It is not effective against solid tumors and seems to have primary utility in treatment of acute lymphocytic and granulocytic leukemias in combination with cytarabine. *Idarubicin* (Zavedos) is a synthetic daunorubicin analogue, with increased lipophilicity over its parent. It can be given orally and is biotransformed to an active intermediate, idarubicinol. Cardiotoxicity is less marked than with doxorubicin. Gastrointestinal toxicity and myelosuppression were observed in cats. It has been used to treat lymphosarcoma in cats. *Epirubicin* (Ellence) is a stereoisomer of doxorubicin with increased lipophilicity relative to doxorubicin and with fewer side effects. Epirubicin is administered intravenously (Ogilvie 1994; Morrison 2002a).

Anthracenediones. *Mitoxantrone* (Navatrone) is an anthracenedione that was synthesized to find a less toxic drug than the anthracyclines from which it differs by the absence of the tetracyclic ring and sugar moiety. With its three planar rings, it preferentially intercalates between guanine-cytosine base pairs of DNA. Although it is less toxic than doxorubicin, it also has a narrower spectrum of anticancer activity. Its lower cardiac toxicity as well as lower potential for nausea, vomiting, and extravasation injury may be caused by the decreased ability of mitoxantrone to participate in production of oxygen free radicals. It is an inhibitor of topoisomerase II. Mitoxantrone is subject to multidrug resistance mediated by ABC transporters BCRP (ABCG2, MXR1) and MRP2. It has activity against a variety of malignancies in dogs and cats and although less effective than doxorubicin may benefit some patients (Ogilvie et al. 1991, 1993, 1994b). Mitoxantrone was found to be effective in intracavitary treatment of carcinomatosis, sarcomatosis, and mesothelioma in dogs (Charney et al. 2005).

Enzymes. *L-Asparaginase* (L-asparagine amidohydrolase, L-asp) is an enzyme derived from bacteria that is important in treatment of lymphoid malignancies in people (Kurtzberg et al. 2003). In veterinary medicine it has primarily been used to treat canine lymphomas as a component of combination protocols (Siedlecki et al. 2006). There is evidence that L-asp should be reserved for treating relapses (MacDonald et al. 2005).

The use of L-asp stems from its asparagine amidohydrolase activity in which it hydrolyzes asparagine to aspartic acid and ammonia. In contrast to most normal cells many malignant cells have very low concentrations of L-asparagine synthetase, an enzyme that synthesizes asparagine required for cell growth. Such cancer cells survive by scavenging asparagine from the extracellular fluids. Administration of L-asp hydrolyzes circulating asparagine, thus depriving the cancer cell of an important nutrient and leading to death of the cells. This was long held to be an example of a qualitative difference between normal and susceptible cells, but it is now known that many normal tissues require preformed asparagine. Lack of asparagine impairs the synthesis of such proteins as insulin, prothrombin, albumin, and parathyroid hormone.

L-Asparaginase is derived from *E. coli* (commercially available as Elspar) and *Erwinia chrysanthemi* (Erwinia asparaginase, not officially approved by the US FDA, but available from Ogden BioServices unit, which was purchased by McKesson Corporation in 2006). Erwinia asparaginase is officially available in many European countries as Erwinase. The two preparations have generally been judged to be essentially equivalent in effectiveness, but a prospective clinical trial in human patients treated for either ALL or lymphoblastic non-Hodgkins lymphoma found that although Elspar caused slightly more coagulation related adverse effects than Erwinase, it was more effective in the treatment of these cancers (Duval et al. 2002). The *E. coli* form of the drug has been covalently linked to monomethoxy-polyethylene glycol and is known as PEG-L-asparaginase or pegasparaginase (Oncaspar). This formulation has been approved by the US FDA for treatment of people who are allergic to Elspar (Kurtzberg et al. 2003).

The main side effects of L-asp are anaphylaxis, pancreatitis, diabetes, and coagulation abnormalities that may lead to intracranial thrombosis or hemorrhage (Duval et al. 2002). The prevalence of anaphylaxis in dogs receiving L-asp for the first time is extremely low (Ogilvie et al. 1994a). It is used only once in many protocols for animals. Precautions should be taken to counteract the potential allergic reactions.

Other Natural Products. *Plicamycin,* USP (mithramycin, Mithracin) and *mitomycin* (mitomycin C, Mutamycin) have not been used much in veterinary oncology.

Sterile Bleomycin Sulfate, USP (Blenoxane) is actually a mixture of glycopeptides of which bleomycin AV2 V and BV2 V are dominant in the commercial form. This glycopeptide has an amino terminal tripeptide (S tripeptide) able to bind to DNA, and a heavy metal (copper and iron) binding component located at the opposite end. Bleomycin has produced excellent results in humans in treatment of lymphoma and embryonal testicular tumors and good results in tumors of the head, neck, and skin, including squamous cell carcinoma. It has shown activity against squamous cell carcinoma in dogs and cats. It has shown activity against confirmed canine oral melanoma when combined with electrochemotherapy (ECT). ECT combines local administration of the drug with delivery of permeabilizing electric pulses of appropriate waveform that result in increased uptake of the drug. Overall response rate of 10 treated client-owned dogs was 80% with 50% long-term control (Spugnini et al. 2006). It is highly valued in multidrug regimens because its toxicity does not overlap that of other anticancer drugs.

Bleomycin is cell-cycle-phase–specific. It is most active in G2, but is also active in late G1, early S, and M phases.

Bleomycin is unique in that although it causes chromosomal abnormalities, it causes no clinically significant toxicity to the bone marrow or GI tract. Dose-limiting toxicity of bleomycin is usually pulmonary fibrosis. Part of the explanation for this tissue selectivity may be that bleomycin is metabolized by an aminopeptidase B–like enzyme called *bleomycin hydrolase* present in most tissues except the skin and lung. Thus signs of toxicity are related to the skin and lung where drug concentration is highest.

If the endothelial lining is damaged or if the drug is given intratracheally and if significant bleomycin reaches the interstitium of the lungs or macrophages, it may be possible to produce pulmonary fibrosis with a single low dose. In dogs, bleomycin initially produces interstitial pneumonia and after intensive treatment causes pleural scarring and pulmonary fibrosis. Risk factors include total dose, age, and concomitant use of other drugs. Treatment should be stopped immediately if impairment of pulmonary function is noted. In veterinary clinical practice, a shorter duration of therapy with bleomycin lessens the likelihood of occurrence of this chronic toxicity.

Toxic effects on the skin include desquamation, hyperpigmentation, and pruritic erythema. Stomatitis, nausea, vomiting, and anorexia may be seen. Severity of reactions ranges from fever and chills to anaphylaxis. Bleomycin should be used with caution in the presence of renal or pulmonary disease. Local therapy as used in the electrochemotherapy of canine melanoma produced minimal toxicity (Spugnini et al. 2006).

Bleomycin is distributed widely throughout the body after parenteral administration, but does not enter the CSF. Decreased renal function slows elimination and necessitates dosage reduction in humans and, presumably, animals. Bleomycin is not active orally.

HORMONES AND ANTAGONISTS. Estrogens, progestins, androgens, glucocorticoids, and thyroid hormones have been used in the treatment of cancer, but are essentially only palliative. Pharmacologic doses are usually required for antitumor effects, so one should expect adverse reactions to be those of hormone excess. The spectrum of antitumor activity is limited to the usual target tissues or those that are the target of other hormones that may be affected by the hormone given. The toxicities and mechanisms of hormones are discussed in Section 8.

Estrogens. Estrogens such as *diethylstilbestrol*, USP, and *estradiol cypionate*, USP, have been used in the treatment of mammary gland cancer, prostatic hyperplasia and carcinoma, and perianal glandular neoplasms. However, the role estrogen plays in causing mammary cancer has led to a more dominant role for drugs that would decrease estrogen concentration. Toxic effects include bone marrow suppression, feminization with gynecomastia, and fluid retention.

Aromatase Inhibitors and Antiestrogens. Aromatase inhibitors and antiestrogens are used extensively in treatment of breast cancer in women. Aromatase is an enzyme that converts androstenedione and testosterone to estrone and estradiol. It is expressed in human placenta and in granulosa cells of ovarian follicles as well as in such nonglandular tissues as subcutaneous fat, liver, muscle, brain, normal breast, and breast-cancer tissue. Aromatase inhibitors currently used or in clinical trials in people include first-generation *aminoglutethimide* (Cytadren; AG), second-generation *formestane* (Lentaron) and *exemestane*, and third-generation *anastrozole* (Arimidex) and *letrozole* (Femara). Aromatase inhibitors and antiestrogens are seldom used in veterinary medicine. Consult Chabner et al. (2006) for further information.

Antiestrogens such as tamoxifen citrate (Nolvadex) may be used in the treatment of estrogen-dependent disseminated mammary gland cancer. Adverse effects of tamoxifen are mild bone marrow suppression (leukopenia, thrombocytopenia, and anemia), skin rash, alopecia, and stump pyometra. A dose escalation study of tamoxifen in dogs listed gastrointestinal toxicity and reversible neurotoxicity at doses of 600 mg/m^2 every 12 h. Detailed pharmacokinetics of tamoxifen were not reported, but peak plasma tamoxifen and its major metabolite, NDMT (N-desmethyl tamoxifen, which is active), combined was 6–11 μM at an oral dose of 600 mg/m^2 administered every 12 hours for 7 days (Waddle et al. 1999).

Adrenocorticosteroid Hormones. Adrenocorticosteroid hormones, most commonly prednisone, USP, have been used in cancer therapy for two types of action. For nonlymphoid tumors like brain tumors, they are palliative by decreasing inflammation and swelling. For lymphoreticular neoplasms and possibly mast cell tumors they may be cytotoxic. They have been shown to induce DNA fragmentation in human lymphoid leukemia cells. Resistance develops rapidly in some patients. Ideally, the glucocorticoids should be used in large doses for the minimal time required to produce remission, and then tapered as rapidly as possible. Long-term use at high doses leads to toxicity (often without benefit to the patient) and iatrogenic adrenal hypercorticism. Toxicity includes gastric ulcer, osteoporosis, and increased susceptibility to infection. Polydipsia, polyuria, polyphagia, and excessive panting are especially common and troublesome when patients are chronically maintained on these drugs. Another use of these drugs as stated above is for management of secondary complications of cancer (i.e., to elevate mood, stimulate appetite, and decrease reaction to dying cells). In addition, they are useful in the management of tumor-associated pain, hypercalcemia, hypoglycemia, and increased intracranial pressure.

Antiandrogens. Benign prostatic hypertrophy and prostate cancer of dogs have been evaluated as models of equivalent diseases in humans (Madewell et al. 2004). Few significant clinical trials in canine cancer of drugs being developed for use in people were found. Consult Chabner et al. (2006) for further information.

MISCELLANEOUS AGENTS. *Hydroxyurea*, USP (Hydrea), acts as an antimetabolite by inhibiting ribonucleotide reductase, thus limiting the availability of deoxyribonucleotides needed for DNA synthesis. Hydroxyurea is cell-cycle-phase–specific, acting on the S phase. It has been used in people for chronic myelogenous leukemia, polycythemia vera, essential thrombosis, sickle-cell disease, and as an adjunct in AIDS therapy. It is infrequently used in veterinary oncology, but has been used therapeutically in the treatment of polycythemia vera.

CYCLOOXYGENASE INHIBITORS. *Piroxicam* (Feldene) and other nonsteroidal antiinflammatory drugs have been reported to have antitumor activity against transitional cell carcinoma of the urinary bladder (Mutsaers et al. 2003) and squamous cell carcinoma of the oral cavity and skin in dogs (Schmidt et al. 2001). Although these agents have only recently received attention for the treatment or prevention of human cancer, their activity in dogs was reported several years ago (Knapp et al. 1992). Greater antitumor effects may be observed when COX inhibitors are combined with chemotherapy (Knapp et al. 2000; Boria et al. 2004). Piroxicam combined with doxorubicin was effective against multicentric lymphoma in dogs, but was not superior to doxorubicin alone (Mutsaers et al. 2002).

The mechanism of antitumor effect has not been established, but may include multiple effects. An antiangeogenesis effect has been postulated from in vitro studies of canine osteosarcoma cells (Royals et al. 2005). In vitro studies with meloxicam, a nonsteroidal COX-2 inhibitor, revealed that it caused apoptosis in canine osteosarcoma (D-17) cells (Wolfesberger et al. 2006). Increased apoptosis and reduction in urine basic fibroblast growth factor concentration has been observed (Mohammed et al. 2002). Apoptosis may be increased in oral cavity cancer cells through induction of NAG-1 (Kim et al. 2004). NAG-1 is a TGF-beta superfamily protein that has antitumorigenic activity and stimulates apoptosis in colorectal and other cancer cell lines (Baek et al. 2001). The NSAID effect on NAG-1 may be independent of an action on cyclooxygenase (Jang et al. 2004). The complexity of mechanism of nonsteroidal antitumor activity is further demonstrated by the finding that four NSAIDs, including piroxicam, given 30 minutes prior to radiation may radiosensitize tumors by increasing oxygen content in the tumors (Crokart et al. 2005).

Adverse effects of piroxicam include gastrointestinal ulceration and subclinical renal papillary necrosis (Knapp et al. 1992, 1994). Renal adverse effects may be pronounced when piroxicam is combined with cisplatin (Knapp et al. 2000).

NEW APPROACHES AND INVESTIGATIONAL COMPOUNDS. The explosion of knowledge in cancer biology and genomics has led to the development of approaches to cancer therapy that are "molecularly targeted" at specific enzymes or receptors (Adjei and Hidalgo 2005). Although a detailed discussion of these developments is beyond the scope of this chapter, the major areas will be outlined. Many of these have reached clinical use or are in clinical trials in people with cancer.

Differentiating Agents. Differentiating agents, e.g., the retinoid *tretinoin* (ATRA), are compounds that, as the name states, can facilitate induction of differentiation. Tretinoin is effective in treating acute promyelocytic leukemia.

Proteasome Inhibitors. Proteasomes process and/or degrade many regulatory proteins involved in controlling cell division, growth, and apoptosis. Chemotherapy-induced stress can activate proteasome-dependent pathways that protect a cell from apoptosis that would otherwise result from the action of the drug. By reversibly inhibiting the chymotrypsinlike activity of the proteasomes, *bortezomib* (PS-341, Velcade) decreases the protective response to the stress and enhances the activity of some chemotherapeutic agents. Because of the widespread interference in cellular regulation caused by the proteasome inhibition, bortezomib may also be an effective anticancer agent in its own right against specific tumor types. It has been approved by the FDA for use in human patients with relapsed refractory myeloma (Chabner et al. 2006).

EGFR Targets. Epidermal growth factor receptor, EGFR, is a tyrosine kinase receptor of the ErbB family that serves key roles in intracellular signaling by phosphorylating and recruiting several downstream substrates. The net effect of these changes is to promote survival of the cell, mitogenic signaling, and tumor promotion. Although normally well regulated, EGFR may be amplified or mutated in tumors. Some tumors, especially those that are more aggressive, are susceptible to inhibition of EGFR by such agents as *erlotinib* (Tarceva) and *gefitinib* (Iressa), which can prevent the ligand activation of the pathway, thereby resulting in cell cycle arrest, promotion of apoptosis, and inhibition of angiogenesis (Doroshow 2005).

Other tyrosine kinase inhibitors include *Imatinib* (Glivec, Gleevec, ST1571), the first drug introduced into clinical medicine to have such activity (Heinrich et al. 2003). Since that introduction other tyrosine kinases have entered either standard clinical use or are in clinical trials. Examples of these include *dasatinib* (Sprycel, BMS-354825) a dual SRC/ABL kinase inhibitor that is active in some cell lines resistant to imatinib, and *lapatinib* (Tykerb, GW572016, which inhibits both EGFR and ErbB-2 [HER-2] tyrosine kinases).

REFERENCES

Adjei, A.A., Hidalgo, M., 2005, Intracellular signal transduction pathway proteins as targets for cancer therapy. J Clin Oncol 23, 5386–5403.

Allen, T.M., Martin, F.J., 2004, Advantages of liposomal delivery systems for anthracyclines. Semin Oncol 31, 5–15.

Allen, T.M., Mumbengegwi, D.R., Charrois, G.J., 2005, Anti–CD19-targeted liposomal doxorubicin improves the therapeutic efficacy in murine B-cell lymphoma and ameliorates the toxicity of liposomes with varying drug release rates. Clin Cancer Res 11, 3567–3573.

Baek, S.J., Horowitz, J.M., Eling, T.E., 2001, Molecular cloning and characterization of human nonsteroidal anti-inflammatory drug-activated gene promoter. Basal transcription is mediated by Sp1 and Sp3. J Biol Chem 276, 33384–33392.

Bergman, P.J., MacEwen, E.G., Kurzman, I.D., Henry, C.J., Hammer, A. S., Knapp, D.W., Hale, A., Kruth, S.A., Klein, M.K., Klausner, J., Norris, A.M., McCaw, D., Straw, R.C., Withrow, S.J., 1996, Amputation and carboplatin for treatment of dogs with osteosarcoma: 48 cases (1991 to 1993). J Vet Intern Med 10, 76–81.

Bolaman, Z., Cicek, C., Kadikoylu, G., Barutca, S., Serter, M., Yenisey, C., Alper, G., 2005, The protective effects of amifostine on adriamycin-induced acute cardiotoxicity in rats. Tohoku J Exp Med 207, 249–253.

Boria, P.A., Murry, D.J., Bennett, P.F., Glickman, N.W., Snyder, P.W., Merkel, B.L., Schlittler, D.L., Mutsaers, A.J., Thomas, R.M., Knapp, D.W., 2004, Evaluation of cisplatin combined with piroxicam for the treatment of oral malignant melanoma and oral squamous cell carcinoma in dogs. J Am Vet Med Assoc 224, 388–394.

Boyer, M.J., Tannock, I.F., 2005, Cellular and Molecular Basis of Drug Treatment for Cancer, In: Tannock, I.F. (Ed.) The Basic Science of Oncology. McGraw-Hill, Inc., St. Louis, pp. 349–375.

Cagliero, E., Ferracini, R., Morello, E., Scotlandi, K., Manara, M.C., Buracco, P., Comandone, A., Baroetto Parisi, R., Baldini, N., 2004, Reversal of multidrug-resistance using Valspodar (PSC 833) and doxorubicin in osteosarcoma. Oncol Rep 12, 1023–1031.

Catino, A., Crucitta, E., Latorre, A., Sambiasi, D., Calabrese, P., Lorusso, V., 2003, Amifostine as chemoprotectant in metastatic breast cancer patients treated with doxorubicin. Oncol Rep 10, 163–167.

Chabner, B.A., Amrein, P.C., Druker, B.J., Michaelson, M.D., Mitsiades, C.S., Goss, P.E., Ryan, D.P., Ramachandra, S., Richardson, P.G., Supko, J.G., Wilson, W.H., 2006, Antineoplastic Agents, In: Brunton, L., Lazo, J., Parker, K. (Eds.) Goodman & Gilman's The Pharmacological Basis of Therapeutics. McGraw-Hill Medical Publishing Division, New York, pp. 1315–1403.

Charney, S., Bergman, P.J., McKnight, J., Farrelly, J., Novosad, A., Leibman, N.F., Camps-Palau, M.A., 2005, Evaluation of intracavitary mitoxantrone and carboplatin for treatment of carcinomatosis, sarcomatosis and mesothelioma, with or without malignant effusions: A retrospective analysis of 12 cases (1997–2002). Vet Comp Oncol 3, 171–181.

Chen, D., Song, D., Wientjes, M.G., Au, J.L., 2003, Effect of dimethyl sulfoxide on bladder tissue penetration of intravesical paclitaxel. Clin Cancer Res 9, 363–369.

Choi, C.H., 2005, ABC transporters as multidrug resistance mechanisms and the development of chemosensitizers for their reversal. Cancer Cell Int 5, 30.

Chua, C.C., Liu, X., Gao, J., Hamdy, R.C., Chua, B.H., 2006, Multiple actions of pifithrin-alpha on doxorubicin-induced apoptosis in rat myoblastic H9c2 cells. Am J Physiol Heart Circ Physiol 290, H2606–2613.

Chun, R., de Lorimier, L.P., 2003, Update on the biology and management of canine osteosarcoma. Vet Clin North Am Sm Anim Pract 33, 491–516, vi.

Cigremis, Y., Parlakpinar, H., Polat, A., Colak, C., Ozturk, F., Sahna, E., Ermis, N., Acet, A., 2006, Beneficial role of aminoguanidine on acute cardiomyopathy related to doxorubicin-treatment. Mol Cell Biochem 285, 149–154.

Cole, S.P.D., Tannock, I.F., 2005, Drug Resistance, In: Tannock, I.F. (Ed.) The Basic Science of Oncology. McGraw-Hill, St. Louis, pp. 376–399.

Cooke, L., Grill, M., Shirahatti, N., Mahadevan, D., 2005, MDR transporters as therapeutic targets in cancer. Science & Med 10, 30–41.

Crokart, N., Radermacher, K., Jordan, B.F., Baudelet, C., Cron, G.O., Gregoire, V., Beghein, N., Bouzin, C., Feron, O., Gallez, B., 2005, Tumor radiosensitization by antiinflammatory drugs: evidence for a new mechanism involving the oxygen effect. Cancer Res 65, 7911–7916.

Dang, C., Gilewski, T.A., Surbone, A., Norton, L., 2003, Cytokinetics, In: Kufe, D.W., Pollock, R.E., Weichselbaum, R.R., Bast, R.C., Jr., Gansler, T.S., Holland, J.F., Frei, E., III (Eds.) Cancer Medicine. BC Decker, Inc., Hamilton, Ontario, pp. 645–668.

Dean, M. 2002. The Human ATP-Binding Cassette (ABC) Transporter Superfamily. In Bethesda (MD): National Library of Medicine (US), NCBI.

Deshpande, A., Sicinski, P., Hinds, P.W., 2005, Cyclins and cdks in development and cancer: a perspective. Oncogene 24, 2909–2915.

Donnenberg, V.S., Donnenberg, A.D., 2005, Multiple drug resistance in cancer revisited: the cancer stem cell hypothesis. J Clin Pharmacol 45, 872–877.

Doroshow, J.H., 2005, Targeting EGFR in non-small-cell lung cancer. NEJM 353, 200–202.

Dorr, R.T., Averbuch, S.D., Boldt, M., Gaudiano, G., Stern, J.B., Koch, T.H., Bachur, N.R., Averbuch, S.D., Gaudiano, G., Koch, T.H., Bachur, N.R., 1990, Antidotes to vesicant chemotherapy extravasations. Blood Rev 4, 41–60.

Duval, M., Suciu, S., Ferster, A., Rialland, X., Nelken, B., Lutz, P., Benoit, Y., Robert, A., Manel, A.M., Vilmer, E., Otten, J., Philippe, N., 2002, Comparison of Escherichia coli-asparaginase with Erwinia-asparaginase in the treatment of childhood lymphoid malignancies: results of a randomized European Organisation for Research and Treatment of Cancer-Children's Leukemia Group phase 3 trial. Blood 99, 2734–2739.

Elias, A.D., Eder, J.P., Shea, T., Frei, E., III, Antman, K.H., 1990, High dose ifosfamide with mesna uroprotection: A Phase I study. J Clin Oncol 8, 170–178.

Endicott, M., 2003, Oncologic emergencies. Clin Tech Sm Anim Pract 18, 127–130.

Erlichman, C., Moore, M., 2001, Carcinogenesis: A Late Complication of Cancer Chemotherapy, In: Chabner, B.A., Longo, D.L. (Eds.) Cancer

Chemotherapy and Biotherapy: Principles and Practice. Lippincott Williams & Wilkins, Philadelphia, pp. 67–84.

Fan, T.M., 2003, Lymphoma updates. Vet Clin North Am Sm Anim Pract 33, 455–471.

Fang, B., Zheng, C., Liao, L., Han, Q., Sun, Z., Jiang, X., Zhao, R.C., 2005, Identification of human chronic myelogenous leukemia progenitor cells with hemangioblastic characteristics. Blood 105, 2733–2740.

Fetting, J.H., McCarthy, L.E., Borison, H.L., Colvin, M., 1982, Vomiting induced by cyclophosphamide and phosphoramide mustard in cats. Cancer Treat Rep 66, 1625–1629.

Fortier, L.A., Mac Harg, M.A., 1994, Topical use of 5-fluorouracil for treatment of squamous cell carcinoma of the external genitalia of horses: 11 cases (1988–1992). J Am Vet Med Assoc 205, 1183–1185.

Fox, L.E., Toshach, K., Calderwood-Mays, M., Khokhar, A.R., Kubilis, P., Perez-Soler, R., MacEwen, E.G., 1999, Evaluation of toxicosis of liposome-encapsulated cis-bis-neodecanoato-trans-R,R-1,2-diaminocyclohexane platinum (II) in clinically normal cats. Am J Vet Res 60, 257–263.

Frazier, D.L., Price, G.S., 1998, Use of body surface area to calculate chemotherapeutic drug dose in dogs: II. Limitations imposed by pharmacokinetic factors. J Vet Intern Med 12, 272–278.

Frei, E., 1977, Rationale for combined therapy. Cancer 40, 569–573.

Frei, E., III, Eder, J.P., 2003, Principles of Dose, Schedule, and Combination Therapy, In: Kufe, D.W., Pollock, R.E., Weichselbaum, R.R., Bast, R.C., Jr., Gansler, T.S., Holland, J.F., Frei, E., III (Eds.) Cancer Medicine. BC Decker, Inc., Hamilton, Ontario, pp. 669–678.

Freise, K.J., Martin-Jimenez, T., 2006a, Pharmacokinetics of gemcitabine and its primary metabolite in dogs after intravenous bolus dosing and its in vitro pharmacodynamics. J Vet Pharmacol Ther 29, 137–145.

———, 2006b, Pharmacokinetics of gemcitabine and its primary metabolite in dogs after intravenous infusion. J Vet Pharmacol Ther 29, 147–152.

Fujino, Y., Sawamura, S., Kurakawa, N., Hisasue, M., Masuda, K., Ohno, K., Tsujimoto, H., 2004, Treatment of chronic lymphocytic leukaemia in three dogs with melphalan and prednisolone. J Sm Anim Pract 45, 298–303.

Gaffney, E.A., 2004, The application of mathematical modelling to aspects of adjuvant chemotherapy scheduling. J Math Biol 48, 375–422.

Galanski, M., Jakupec, M.A., Keppler, B.K., 2005, Update of the preclinical situation of anticancer platinum complexes: novel design strategies and innovative analytical approaches. Curr Med Chem 12, 2075–2094.

Gelderblom, H., Mross, K., ten Tije, A.J., Behringer, D., Mielke, S., van Zomeren, D.M., Verweij, J., Sparreboom, A., 2002, Comparative pharmacokinetics of unbound paclitaxel during 1- and 3-hour infusions. J Clin Oncol 20, 574–581.

Goldie, J.H., Coldman, A.J., 1984, The genetic origin of drug resistance in neoplasms: implications for systemic therapy. Cancer Res 44, 3643–3653.

Govier, S.M., 2003, Principles of treatment for mast cell tumors. Clin Tech Sm Anim Pract 18, 103–106.

Hahn, K.A., Fletcher, C.M., Legendre, A.M., 1996a, Marked neutropenia in five tumor-bearing cats one week following single-agent vincristine sulfate chemotherapy. Vet Clin Pathol 25, 121–123.

Hahn, K.A., Knapp, D.W., Richardson, R.C., Matlock, C.L., 1992, Clinical response of nasal adenocarcinoma to cisplatin chemotherapy in 11 dogs. J Am Vet Med Assoc 200, 355–357.

Hahn, K.A., McEntee, M.F., Daniel, G.B., Legendre, A.M., Nolan, M.L., 1997, Hematologic and systemic toxicoses associated with carboplatin administration in cats. Am J Vet Res 58, 677–679.

Hahn, K.A., Richardson, R.C., Blevins, W.E., Lenz, S.D., Knapp, D.W., 1996b, Intramedullary cisplatin chemotherapy: experience in four dogs with osteosarcoma. J Sm Anim Pract 37, 187–192.

Hamilton, T.A., Cook, J.R., Braund, K.G., et al., 1991, Vincristine-induced peripheral neuropathy in a dog. J Am Vet Med Assoc 198, 635–638.

Heinrich, M.C., Blanke, C.D., Corless, C.L., Druker, B.J., 2003, Small-Molecule Inhibitors of Protein Kinases in the Treatment of Human Cancer, In: Kufe, D.W., Pollock, R.E., Weichselbaum, R.R., Bast, R.C., Jr., Gansler, T.S., Holland, J.F., Frei, E., III (Eds.) Cancer Medicine. BC Decker, Inc., Hamilton, Ontario, pp. 811–821.

Henderson, R.A., Brawner, W.R., Brewer, W.G., et al., 1995, Clinical Staging, In: Hahn, K., Richardson, R.C. (Eds.) Cancer Chemotherapy: A Veterinary Handbook. Williams & Wilkins, Baltimore, pp. 23–45.

Henry, C.J., 2003, Management of transitional cell carcinoma. Vet Clin North Am Sm Anim Pract 33, 597–613.

Huisman, M.T., Chhatta, A.A., van Tellingen, O., Beijnen, J.H., Schinkel, A.H., 2005, MRP2 (ABCC2) transports taxanes and confers paclitaxel resistance and both processes are stimulated by probenecid. Int J Cancer 116, 824–829.

Imondi, A.R., Della Torre, P., Mazue, G., Sullivan, T.M., Robbins, T.L., Hagerman, L.M., Podesta, A., Pinciroli, G., 1996, Dose-response relationship of dexrazoxane for prevention of doxorubicin-induced cardiotoxicity in mice, rats, and dogs. Cancer Res 56, 4200–4204.

Jang, T.J., Kang, H.J., Kim, J.R., Yang, C.H., 2004, Non-steroidal anti-inflammatory drug activated gene (NAG-1) expression is closely related to death receptor-4 and -5 induction, which may explain sulindac sulfide induced gastric cancer cell apoptosis. Carcinogenesis 25, 1853–1858.

Kalivendi, S.V., Konorev, E.A., Cunningham, S., Vanamala, S.K., Kaji, E. H., Joseph, J., Kalyanaraman, B., 2005, Doxorubicin activates nuclear factor of activated T-lymphocytes and Fas ligand transcription: role of mitochondrial reactive oxygen species and calcium. Biochem J 389, 527–539.

Kanter, P.M., Klaich, G.M., Bullard, G.A., King, J.M., Bally, M.B., Mayer, L.D., 1994, Liposome encapsulated vincristine: preclinical toxicologic and pharmacologic comparison with free vincristine and empty liposomes in mice, rats and dogs. Anticancer Drugs 5, 579–590.

Karayannopoulou, M., Kaldrymidou, E., Constantinidis, T.C., Dessiris, A., 2001, Adjuvant post-operative chemotherapy in bitches with mammary cancer. J Vet Med Series A 48, 85–96.

Katragadda, S., Budda, B., Anand, B.S., Mitra, A.K., 2005, Role of efflux pumps and metabolising enzymes in drug delivery. Expert Opin Drug Deliv 2, 683–705.

Kent, M.S., Strom, A., London, C.A., Seguin, B., 2004, Alternating carboplatin and doxorubicin as adjunctive chemotherapy to amputation or limb-sparing surgery in the treatment of appendicular osteosarcoma in dogs. J Vet Intern Med 18, 540–544.

Kim, K.S., Yoon, J.H., Kim, J.K., Baek, S.J., Eling, T.E., Lee, W.J., Ryu, J.H., Lee, J.G., Lee, J.H., Yoo, J.B., 2004, Cyclooxygenase inhibitors induce apoptosis in oral cavity cancer cells by increased expression of nonsteroidal anti-inflammatory drug-activated gene. Biochem Biophys Res Commun 325, 1298–1303.

Kirpensteijn, J., Teske, E., Kik, M., Klenner, T., Rutteman, G.R., 2002, Lobaplatin as an adjuvant chemotherapy to surgery in canine appendicular osteosarcoma: a phase II evaluation. Anticancer Res 22, 2765–2770.

Kitchell, B.E., 2003, Advances in Medical Oncology. Vet Clin North Am Sm Anim Pract 33(3):455–471.

Klein, M.K., 2003, Multimodality therapy for head and neck cancer. Vet Clin North Am Sm Anim Pract 33, 615–628.

Kleiter, M., Hirt, R., Kirtz, G., Day, M.J., 2001, Hypercalcaemia associated with chronic lymphocytic leukaemia in a Giant Schnauzer. Aust Vet J 79, 335–338.

Knapp, D.W. 2006. Personal Communication, Coppoc, G.L., ed. (West Lafayette, IN).

Knapp, D.W., Glickman, N.W., Widmer, W.R., DeNicola, D.B., Adams, L.G., Kuczek, T., Bonney, P.L., DeGortari, A.E., Han, C., Glickman, L.T., 2000, Cisplatin versus cisplatin combined with piroxicam in a canine model of human invasive urinary bladder cancer. Cancer Chemother Pharmacol 46, 221–226.

Knapp, D.W., Richardson, R.C., Bonney, P.L., Hahn, K., 1988, Cisplatin therapy in 41 dogs with malignant tumors. J Vet Intern Med 2, 41–46.

Knapp, D.W., Richardson, R.C., Bottoms, G.D., Teclaw, R., Chan, T.C., 1992, Phase I trial of piroxicam in 62 dogs bearing naturally occurring tumors. Cancer Chemother Pharmacol 29, 214–218.

Knapp, D.W., Richardson, R.C., Chan, T.C., Bottoms, G.D., Widmer, W.R., DeNicola, D.B., Teclaw, R., Bonney, P.L., Kuczek, T., 1994, Piroxicam therapy in 34 dogs with transitional cell carcinoma of the urinary bladder. J Vet Intern Med 8, 273–278.

Knapp, D.W., Richardson, R.C., DeNicola, D.B., Long, G.G., Blevins, W.E., 1987, Cisplatin toxicity in cats. J Vet Intern Med 1, 29–35.

Kosarek, C.E., Kisseberth, W.C., Gallant, S.L., Couto, C.G., 2005, Clinical evaluation of gemcitabine in dogs with spontaneously occurring malignancies. J Vet Intern Med 19, 81–86.

Kroep, J.R., Smit, E.F., Giaccone, G., Van der Born, K., Beijnen, J.H., Van Groeningen, C.J., Van der Vijgh, W.J., Postmus, P.E., Pinedo, H.M., Peters, G.J., 2006, Pharmacology of the paclitaxel-cisplatin, gemcitabine-cisplatin, and paclitaxel-gemcitabine combinations in patients with advanced non-small cell lung cancer. Cancer Chemother Pharmacol.

Kurtzberg, J., Yousem, D., Beauchamp, N., Jr., 2003, Asparaginase, In: Kufe, D.W., Pollock, R.E., Weichselbaum, R.R., Bast, R.C., Jr., Gansler, T.S., Holland, J.F., Frei, E., III (Eds.) Cancer Medicine. BC Decker, Inc., Hamilton, Ontario, pp. 823–830.

Langova, V., Mutsaers, A.J., Phillips, B., Straw, R., 2004, Treatment of eight dogs with nasal tumours with alternating doses of doxorubicin and carboplatin in conjunction with oral piroxicam. Aust Vet J 82, 676–680.

LeBlanc, A.K., Mauldin, G.E., Milner, R.J., LaDue, T.A., Mauldin, G.N., Bartges, J.W., 2006, Efficacy and toxicity of BOPP and LOPP chemotherapy for the treatment of relapsed canine lymphoma. Vet Comp Oncol 4, 21–32.

Lee, S., Kim, W., Moon, S.O., Sung, M.J., Kim, D.H., Kang, K.P., Jang, Y.B., Lee, J.E., Jang, K.Y., Park, S.K., 2006, Rosiglitazone ameliorates cisplatin-induced renal injury in mice. Nephrol Dial Transplant.

Longley, D.B., Johnston, P.G., 2005, Molecular mechanisms of drug resistance. J Pathol 205, 275–292.

Low, P.S., Antony, A.C., 2004, Folate receptor-targeted drugs for cancer and inflammatory diseases. Adv Drug Deliv Rev 56, 1055–1058.

MacDonald, V.S., Thamm, D.H., Kurzman, I.D., Turek, M.M., Vail, D. M., 2005, Does L-asparaginase influence efficacy or toxicity when added to a standard CHOP protocol for dogs with lymphoma? J Vet Intern Med 19, 732–736.

Madewell, B.R., Gandour-Edwards, R., DeVere White, R.W., 2004, Canine prostatic intraepithelial neoplasia: is the comparative model relevant? Prostate 58, 314–317.

Martins, C., Lacerda, J.F., Lourenco, F., Carmo, J.A., Lacerda, J.M., 2005, Autologous stem cell transplantation in acute myeloid leukemia. Factors influencing outcome. A 13 year single institution experience. Acta Med Port 18, 329–337.

Mauldin, G.E., Fox, P.R., Patnaik, A.K., Bond, B.R., Mooney, S.C., Matus, R.E., 1992, Doxorubicin-induced cardiotoxicosis. Clinical features in 32 dogs. J Vet Intern Med 6, 82–88.

McEntee, M.C., Rassnick, K.M., Lewis, L.D., Zgola, M.M., Beaulieu, B.B., Balkman, C.E., Page, R.L., 2006, Phase I and pharmacokinetic evaluation of the combination of orally administered docetaxel and cyclosporin A in tumor-bearing dogs. Am J Vet Res 67, 1057–1062.

Mealey, K.L., 2004, Therapeutic implications of the MDR-1 gene. J Vet Pharmacol Ther 27, 257–264.

Mealey, K.L., Bentjen, S.A., Waiting, D.K., 2002, Frequency of the mutant MDR1 allele associated with ivermectin sensitivity in a sample population of collies from the northwestern United States. Am J Vet Res 63, 479–481.

Mealey, K.L., Northrup, N.C., Bentjen, S.A., 2003, Increased toxicity of P-glycoprotein-substrate chemotherapeutic agents in a dog with the MDR1 deletion mutation associated with ivermectin sensitivity. J Am Vet Med Assoc 223, 1453–1455, 1434.

Mizutani, H., Tada-Oikawa, S., Hiraku, Y., Kojima, M., Kawanishi, S., 2005, Mechanism of apoptosis induced by doxorubicin through the generation of hydrogen peroxide. Life Sci 76, 1439–1453.

Mohammed, S.I., Bennett, P.F., Craig, B.A., Glickman, N.W., Mutsaers, A.J., Snyder, P.W., Widmer, W.R., DeGortari, A.E., Bonney, P.L., Knapp, D.W., 2002, Effects of the cyclooxygenase inhibitor, piroxicam, on tumor response, apoptosis, and angiogenesis in a canine model of human invasive urinary bladder cancer. Cancer Res 62, 356–358.

Moore, A.S., Kitchell, B.E., 2003, New chemotherapy agents in veterinary medicine. Vet Clin Sm Anim Pract 33, 629–649.

Moore, M.A., 2005, Converging pathways in leukemogenesis and stem cell self-renewal. Exp Hematol 33, 719–737.

Morrison, W.B., 1998, Chemotherapy, In: Morrison, W.B. (Ed.) Cancer in Dogs and Cats: Medical and Surgical Management. Williams & Wilkins, Baltimore, pp. 351–358.

———, 2002a, Cancer Drug Pharmacology and Clinical Experience, In: Morrison, W.B. (Ed.) Cancer in Dogs and Cats: Medical and Surgical Management. Teton NewMedia, Jackson, WY, pp. 339–358.

———, 2002b, Cancer in Dogs and Cats: Medical and Surgical Management, 2 Edition. Teton NewMedia, Jackson, WY, p. 782.

Mukaratirwa, S., 2005, Prognostic and predictive markers in canine tumours: rationale and relevance. A review. Vet Q 27, 52–64.

Munoz-Gamez, J.A., Martin-Oliva, D., Aguilar-Quesada, R., Canuelo, A., Nunez, M.I., Valenzuela, M.T., Ruiz de Almodovar, J.M., De Murcia, G., Oliver, F.J., 2005, PARP inhibition sensitizes p53-deficient breast cancer cells to doxorubicin-induced apoptosis. Biochem J 386, 119–125.

Mutsaers, A.J., Glickman, N.W., DeNicola, D.B., Widmer, W.R., Bonney, P.L., Hahn, K.A., Knapp, D.W., 2002, Evaluation of treatment with doxorubicin and piroxicam or doxorubicin alone for multicentric lymphoma in dogs. J Am Vet Med Assoc 220, 1813–1817.

Mutsaers, A.J., Widmer, W.R., Knapp, D.W., 2003, Canine transitional cell carcinoma. J Vet Intern Med 17, 136–144.

Nak, D., Nak, Y., Cangul, I.T., Tuna, B., 2005, A Clinico-pathological study on the effect of vincristine on transmissible venereal tumour in dogs. J Vet Med A Physiol Pathol Clin Med 52, 366–370.

Neff, M.W., Robertson, K.R., Wong, A.K., Safra, N., Broman, K.W., Slatkin, M., Mealey, K.L., Pedersen, N.C., 2004, Breed distribution and history of canine mdr1–1Delta, a pharmacogenetic mutation that marks the emergence of breeds from the collie lineage. Proc Natl Acad Sci U S A 101, 11725–11730.

Obradovich, J.E., Ogilvie, G.K., Stadler-Morris, S., Schmidt, B.R., Cooper, M.F., Boone, T.C., 1993, Effect of recombinant canine granulocyte colony-stimulating factor on peripheral blood neutrophil counts in normal cats. J Vet Intern Med 7, 65–67.

Ogilvie, G.K., 1994, New Chemotherapeutics: Taxol and Beyond. Proc. ACVIM 12, 866–869.

Ogilvie, G.K., Atwater, S.W., Ciekot, P.A., al., E., 1994a, Prevalence of anaphylaxis associated with the intramuscular administration of L-asparaginase to 81 dogs with cancer. J Sm Anim Hosp Assoc 30, 62–65.

Ogilvie, G.K., Fettman, M.J., Mallinckrodt, C.H., Walton, J.A., Hansen, R.A., Davenport, D.J., Gross, K.L., Richardson, K.L., Rogers, Q., Hand, M.S., 2000, Effect of fish oil, arginine, and doxorubicin chemotherapy on remission and survival time for dogs with lymphoma: a double-blind, randomized placebo-controlled study. Cancer 88, 1916–1928.

Ogilvie, G.K., Moore, A.S., Chen, C., Ciekot, P.A., Atwater, S.W., Bergman, P.J., Walters, L.M., 1994b, Toxicoses associated with the administration of mitoxantrone to dogs with malignant tumors: a dose escalation study. J Am Vet Med Assoc 205, 570–573.

Ogilvie, G.K., Moore, A.S., Obradovich, J.E., Elmslie, R.E., Vail, D.M., Straw, R.C., Salmon, M.D., Klein, M.K., Atwater, S.W., Ciekot, P.E., 1993, Toxicoses and efficacy associated with administration of mitoxantrone to cats with malignant tumors. J Am Vet Med Assoc 202, 1839–1844.

Ogilvie, G.K., Obradovich, J.E., Cooper, M.F., Walters, L.M., Salman, M.D., Boone, T.C., 1992, Use of recombinant canine granulocyte colony-stimulating factor to decrease myelosuppression associated with the administration of mitoxantrone in the dog. J Vet Intern Med 6, 44–47.

Ogilvie, G.K., Obradovich, J.E., Elmslie, R.E., Vail, D.M., Moore, A.S., Curtis, C.R., Straw, R.C., Dickinson, K., Cooper, M.F., Withrow, S.J., 1991, Toxicoses associated with administration of mitoxantrone to dogs with malignant tumors. J Am Vet Med Assoc 198, 1613–1617.

Ogilvie, G.K., Richardson, R.C., Curtis, C.R., Withrow, S.J., Reynolds, H.A., Norris, A.M., Henderson, R.A., Klausner, J.S., Fowler, J.D., McCaw, D., 1989, Acute and short-term toxicoses associated with the administration of doxorubicin to dogs with malignant tumors. J Am Vet Med Assoc 195, 1584–1587.

O'Keefe, D.A., Schaeffer, D.J., 1992, Hematologic toxicosis associated with doxorubicin administration in cats. J Vet Intern Med 6, 276–282.

O'Keefe, D.A., Sisson, D.D., Gelberg, H.B., Schaeffer, D.J., Krawiec, D. R., 1993, Systemic toxicity associated with doxorubicin administration in cats. J Vet Intern Med 7, 309–317.

OSHA 2005. OSHA Technical Manual: Controlling Occupational Exposure to Hazardous Drugs (U.S. Department of Labor, Occupational Safety & Health Administration).

Page, R.L., Hughes, C.S., Huyan, S., Sagris, J., Trogdon, M., 2000, Modulation of P-glycoprotein-mediated doxorubicin resistance in canine cell lines. Anticancer Res 20, 3533–3538.

Page, R.L., McEntee, M.C., George, S.L., Williams, P.L., Heidner, G.L., Novotney, C.A., Riviere, J.E., Dewhirst, M.W., Thrall, D.E., 1993, Pharmacokinetic and phase I evaluation of carboplatin in dogs. J Vet Intern Med 7, 235–240.

Peng, X., Chen, B., Lim, C.C., Sawyer, D.B., 2005, The cardiotoxicology of anthracycline chemotherapeutics: translating molecular mechanism into preventive medicine. Molec Interven 5, 163–171.

Pizzorno, G., Diasio, R.B., Cheng, Y.-C., 2003, Pyrimidine and Purine Antimetabolites, In: Kufe, D.W., Pollock, R.E., Weichselbaum, R.R., Bast, R.C., Jr., Gansler, T.S., Holland, J.F., Frei, E., III (Eds.) Cancer Medicine. BC Decker, Inc., Hamilton, Ontario, pp. 739–757.

Poirier, V.J., Hershey, A.E., Burgess, K.E., Phillips, B., Turek, M.M., Forrest, L.J., Beaver, L., Vail, D.M., 2004, Efficacy and toxicity of paclitaxel (Taxol) for the treatment of canine malignant tumors. J Vet Intern Med 18, 219–222.

Rassnick, K.M., Mauldin, G.E., Al-Sarraf, R., Mauldin, G.N., Moore, A.S., Mooney, S.C., 2002, MOPP chemotherapy for treatment of resistant lymphoma in dogs: a retrospective study of 117 cases (1989–2000). J Vet Intern Med 16, 576–580.

Ratain, M.J., Plunkett, W.K., Jr., 2003, Pharmacology, In: Kufe, D.W., Pollock, R.E., Weichselbaum, R.R., Bast, R.C., Jr., Gansler, T.S., Holland, J.F., Frei, E., III (Eds.) Cancer Medicine. BC Decker, Inc., Hamilton, Ontario, p. 695.

Rogers, K.S., Coppoc, G.L., 1991, Chemotherapy of Neoplastic Diseases, In: Adams, H.R. (Ed.) Veterinary Pharmacology and Therapeutics. Iowa State University Press, Ames, Iowa, pp. 1064–1083.

Rosenthal, R.C., 1991, Storage of expensive anticancer drugs. J Am Vet Med Assoc 198, 144–146.

Royals, S.R., Farese, J.P., Milner, R.J., Lee-Ambrose, L., van Gilder, J., 2005, Investigation of the effects of deracoxib and piroxicam on the in vitro viability of osteosarcoma cells from dogs. Am J Vet Res 66, 1961–1967.

Saleh, S., El-Demerdash, E., 2005, Protective effects of L-arginine against cisplatin-induced renal oxidative stress and toxicity: role of nitric oxide. Basic Clin Pharmacol Toxicol 97, 91–97.

Schmidt, B.R., Glickman, N.W., DeNicola, D.B., de Gortari, A.E., Knapp, D.W., 2001, Evaluation of piroxicam for the treatment of oral squamous cell carcinoma in dogs. J Am Vet Med Assoc 218, 1783–1786.

Scott-Moncrieff, J.D.R., Chan, T.C.K., Samuels, M.L., Cook, J.R., Coppoc, G.L., DeNicola, D.B., Richardson, R.C., 1991, Plasma and cerebrospinal fluid pharmacokinetics of cytosine arabinoside in dogs. Cancer Chemother Pharmacol 29, 13–18.

Selting, K.A., Ogilvie, G.K., Gustafson, D.L., Long, M.E., Lana, S.E., Walton, J.A., Hansen, R.A., Turner, A.S., Laible, I., Fettman, M.J., 2006, Evaluation of the effects of dietary n-3 fatty acid supplementation on the pharmacokinetics of doxorubicin in dogs with lymphoma. Am J Vet Res 67, 145–151.

Selting, K.A., Powers, B.E., Thompson, L.J., Mittleman, E., Tyler, J.W., Lafferty, M.H., Withrow, S.J., 2005, Outcome of dogs with high-grade soft tissue sarcomas treated with and without adjuvant doxorubicin chemotherapy: 39 cases (1996–2004). J Am Vet Med Assoc 227, 1442–1448.

Service, R.F., 2005, Nanotechnology takes aim at cancer. Science 310, 1132–1134.

Shackney, S.E., 1993, Tumor Growth, Cell Cycle Kinetics, and Cancer Treatment, In: Calabresi, P., Schein, P.S. (Eds.) Medical Oncology: Basic Principles and Clinical Management of Cancer. McGraw Hill, Inc., New York, pp. 43–60.

Siedlecki, C.T., Kass, P.H., Jakubiak, M.J., Dank, G., Lyons, J., Kent, M. S., 2006, Evaluation of an actinomycin-D-containing combination chemotherapy protocol with extended maintenance therapy for canine lymphoma. Can Vet J 47, 52–59.

Simonson, E., Madewell, B.R., 1992, Chemotherapy-induced change in coat color in a standard poodle dog. Vet Cancer Soc Newsletter 16, 4.

Skipper, H.E., 1971, Kinetics of mammary tumor cell growth and implications for therapy. Cancer 28, 1479–1499.

Smith, A.N., 2003, Hemangiosarcoma in dogs and cats. Vet Clin North Am Sm Anim Pract 33, 533–552, vi.

Solier, S., Lansiaux, A., Logette, E., Wu, J., Soret, J., Tazi, J., Bailly, C., Desoche, L., Solary, E., Corcos, L., 2004, Topoisomerase I and II inhibitors control caspase-2 pre-messenger RNA splicing in human cells. Mol Cancer Res 2, 53–61.

Sorenmo, K., 2003, Canine mammary gland tumors. Vet Clin North Am Sm Anim Pract 33, 573–596.

Spugnini, E.P., Dragonetti, E., Vincenzi, B., Onori, N., Citro, G., Baldi, A., 2006, Pulse-mediated chemotherapy enhances local control and survival in a spontaneous canine model of primary mucosal melanoma. Melanoma Res 16, 23–27.

Stettner, N., Brenner, O., Eilam, R., Harmelin, A., 2005, Pegylated liposomal doxorubicin as a chemotherapeutic agent for treatment of canine transmissible venereal tumor in murine models. J Vet Med Sci 67, 1133–1139.

Stewart, C.F., Ratain, M.J., 2001, Topoisomerase Interactive Agents, In: DeVita, V.T., Hellman, S., Rosenberg, S.A. (Eds.) Cancer: Principles and Practice of Oncology. Lippincott Williams & Wilkins, Philadelphia, pp. 415–431.

Suzuki, F., Hashimoto, K., Kikuchi, H., Nishikawa, H., Matsumoto, H., Shimada, J., Kawase, M., Sunaga, K., Tsuda, T., Satoh, K., Sakagami, H., 2005, Induction of tumor-specific cytotoxicity and apoptosis by doxorubicin. Anticancer Res 25, 887–893.

Takada, S., 2003, Principles of chemotherapy safety procedures. Clin Tech Sm Anim Pract 18, 73–74.

Theon, A.P., Pascoe, J.R., Galuppo, L.D., Fisher, P.E., Griffey, S.M., Madigan, J.E., 1999, Comparison of perioperative versus postoperative intratumoral administration of cisplatin for treatment of cutaneous sarcoids and squamous cell carcinomas in horses. J Am Vet Med Assoc 215, 1655–1660.

Twelves, C.W., A., Marek, M.D., et al., 2005, Capecitabine as adjuvant treatment for stage III colon cancer. NEJM 352, 2696–2704.

Vail, D.M., Elfarra, A.A., Cooley, A.J., Panciera, D.L., MacEwen, E.G., Soergel, S.A., 1993, Methimazole as a protectant against cisplatin-induced nephrotoxicity using the dog as a model. Cancer Chemother Pharmacol 33, 25–30.

Vail, D.M., Kravis, L.D., Cooley, A.J., Chun, R., MacEwen, E.G., 1997, Preclinical trial of doxorubicin entrapped in sterically stabilized liposomes in dogs with spontaneously arising malignant tumors. Cancer Chemother Pharmacol 39, 410–416.

van Herwaarden, A.E., Schinkel, A.H., 2006, The function of breast cancer resistance protein in epithelial barriers, stem cells and milk secretion of drugs and xenotoxins. Trends Pharmacol Sci 27, 10–16.

Varmus, H., 2006, The new era in cancer research. Science 312, 1162–1165.

Waddle, J.R., Fine, R.L., Case, B.C., Trogdon, M.L., Tyczkowska, K., Frazier, D., Page, R.L., 1999, Phase I and pharmacokinetic analysis of high-dose tamoxifen and chemotherapy in normal and tumor-bearing dogs. Cancer Chemother Pharmacol 44, 74–80.

Walling, J., 2006, From methotrexate to pemetrexed and beyond. A review of the pharmacodynamic and clinical properties of antifolates. Invest New Drugs 24, 37–77.

Weissman, I., 2005, Stem cell research: paths to cancer therapies and regenerative medicine. JAMA 294, 1359–1366.

Welch, D.R., 2003, Metastasis regulatory genes. Science & Med 9, 202–213.

Williams, C.J., Whitehouse, J.M.A., 1979, Cis-platinum: A new anticancer agent. Br Med J 1, 1689–1691.

Withrow, S.J., Liptak, J.M., Straw, R.C., Dernell, W.S., Jameson, V.J., Powers, B.E., Johnson, J.L., Brekke, J.H., Douple, E.B., 2004, Biodegradable cisplatin polymer in limb-sparing surgery for canine osteosarcoma. Ann Surg Oncol 11, 705–713.

Wolfesberger, B., Hoelzl, C., Walter, I., Reider, G.A., Fertl, G., Thalhammer, J.G., Skalicky, M., Egerbacher, M., 2006, In vitro effects of meloxicam with or without doxorubicin on canine osteosarcoma cells. J Vet Pharmacol Ther 29, 15–23.

Xia, C.Q., Xiao, G., Liu, N., Pimprale, S., Fox, L., Patten, C.J., Crespi, C.L., Miwa, G., Gan, L.-S., 2006, Comparison of species differences of P-glycoproteins in beagle dog, rhesus monkey, and human using ATPase activity assays. Molec Pharmaceut 3, 78–86.

Yamashita, K., Yada, H., Ariyoshi, T., 2004, Neurotoxic effects of alpha-fluoro-beta-alanine (FBAL) and fluoroacetic acid (FA) on dogs. J Toxicol Sci 29, 155–166.

Zhao, J., Kim, J.E., Reed, E., Li, Q.Q., 2005, Molecular mechanism of antitumor activity of taxanes in lung cancer (Review). Int J Oncol 27, 247–256.

CHAPTER

46

IMMUNOSUPPRESSIVE DRUGS AND CYCLOSPORINE

MARK G. PAPICH

Conditions that require immunosuppressive drugs include skin diseases such as pemphigus, pemphigoid, and lupus-like syndromes. Systemic immune-mediated diseases requiring immunosuppressive drug therapy include immune-mediated hemolytic anemia (IMHA), systemic lupus (SLE), and immune-mediated thrombocytopenia (ITP). For management of some of these disorders, corticosteroids, alkylating agents, cytotoxic drugs, cyclosporine, and gold compounds have been used. NSAIDs alone are not usually effective.

GLUCOCORTICOIDS

Glucocorticoids are usually the initial drugs used for treating immune-mediated diseases. They are consistently effective, but have multiple side effects and adverse effects, especially with long-term use. The pharmacology of glucocorticoids was discussed in detail in Chapter 30 and readers are referred to that chapter. Briefly, glucocorticoids exert their action via binding to intracellular receptors, translocating to the nucleus, and binding to receptor sites on responsive genes (Rhen and Cidlowski 2005; Boumpas et al. 1993), where they modulate the transcription of glucocorticoid-responsive genes (Barnes and Karin 1997; Barnes 2001; Hayashi et al. 2004; Rhen and Cidlowski 2005). By regulating glucocorticoid-responsive genes, protein synthesis is altered, which affects cell function.

CELLULAR EFFECTS. Corticosteroids increase the circulating numbers of mature neutrophils. There is a release of cells from the marginal pool of neutrophils and decreased migration and egress into inflammatory tissue. This effect is attributed to decreased expression of adhesion molecules, reduced adherence to the vessel endothelium, and reduced diapedesis from the vessels. Subsequently, there is decreased movement of inflammatory cells into tissues in response to chemotactic stimuli. Glucocorticoids affect leukocyte traffic more than cellular function.

Glucocorticoids also affect many functions of macrophages. They suppress the function of macrophages and decrease the inflammatory response, generation of cytokines, and the ability of macrophages to process antigens. They also inhibit phagocytosis of macrophages.

Corticosteroids decrease the numbers of lymphocytes in the peripheral circulation—caused by a redistribution of circulating lymphocytes—depress lymphocyte activation, and decrease participation of lymphocytes in inflammation. T-cells are affected more than B-cells. B-cells are generally resistant to the immunosuppressive effects of glucocorticoids, and there is minimal effect on immunoglobulin synthesis. However, high corticosteroid doses will decrease immunoglobulin levels, probably because of increased catabolism, as well as through the secondary effects to suppress accessory cells and cytokine synthesis. At antiinflammatory doses, glucocorticoids do not decrease an animal's ability to mount a normal immune response (e.g., from vaccinations) (Nara et al. 1979).

Glucocorticoids inhibit release of inflammatory cytokines from leukocytes (e.g., IL-1, TNF-α, prostaglandins). Glucocorticoids decrease expression of cytokines from lymphocytes (e.g., IL-2).

IMMUNOSUPPRESSIVE EFFECTS. It is difficult to separate the antiinflammatory from the immunosuppressive effects of glucocorticoids. For a complete review of these effects see the articles by Cohn (1991) and Barnes (2006). For severe immune-mediated disorders (e.g., autoimmune skin disease, immune-mediated hemolytic anemia and thrombocytopenia, SLE, arthritis) glucocorticoids suppress the immune system response to alleviate clinical signs. In a study in which various treatments for immune-mediated hemolytic anemia were examined, corticosteroids alone were as effective as combination treatments (for example, with azathioprine, cyclophosphamide, etc.) (Grundy and Barton 2001).

The immune-suppressing effects require higher dosages of corticosteroids than are necessary for antiinflammatory therapy (often by a factor of at least 2×). The mechanism of action for the immunosuppression caused by corticosteroids is complex. In the study by Ammersbach et al. (2006), the authors demonstrated decreased neutrophil migration and survival, decreased cytokines, decreased adhesion expression, and a decrease in the cytotoxic lymphocyte function as well as lymphocyte apoptosis. The dose used in this study in dogs was approximately 2 mg/kg per day for 3 days.

CHOICE OF DRUGS. For long-term therapy, intermediate-acting steroids (prednisone, prednisolone) are used most often because they can be administered on an every-other-day (EOD) basis. However, dexamethasone is often used for acute, short-term treatment.

DOSES. Initial (induction) dosage regimens employ daily doses of 2.2 to 6.6 mg/kg (prednisolone or prednisone). Doses greater than 6 mg/kg are rarely used in dogs. Initial doses generally are in the range of 2–4 mg/kg/day. One study reported that the optimal induction doses for skin diseases were 4.4 mg/kg/day for dogs and 6.6 mg/kg/day for cats. After an induction period, if the patient responds favorably, the dose may be decreased by a factor of 2. Eventually one should attempt to maintain the patient on this low dose on an EOD basis. Some diseases are slow to respond and a reduction of doses should be done on a gradual and prolonged schedule. For example, lowering the dose based on an evaluation every 2–4 weeks may be necessary. Eventually, for immune-mediated disease, maintenance doses of 1 mg/kg, EOD are possible but higher doses or adjunctive therapy may be necessary in individual patients. At the high dose ranges, side effects are common.

ADVERSE EFFECTS. Side effects associated with treatment—but not necessarily reasons for discontinuing therapy—include polyuria/polydipsia, increased appetite (polyphagia), and behavior changes (increased restlessness for example). Adverse effects from immunosuppressive doses of corticosteroids include risk of infectious diseases, adrenal suppression, pancreatitis, delay of healing, catabolic effects on muscle and connective tissues, and hepatopathy.

RATIONALE FOR EVERY-OTHER-DAY (EOD) THERAPY. If a glucocorticoid is used that has a duration of action of 12–36 hours (intermediate-acting), the hypothalmic-pituitary-adrenal (HPA) axis has an opportunity to recover before the next dose. It is important that one chooses a glucocorticoid that does not have a long duration of action for EOD therapy—for example, dexamethasone is unacceptable because its duration is at least 36–48 hours. After 1 mg/kg every 48 hours of prednisolone ACTH was suppressed in dogs for 18 to 24 hours, and returned to normal until the next scheduled dose (Brockus et al. 1999). EOD therapy will minimize, but *will not* prevent adrenal atrophy, and other adverse effects such as those on the immune system, and the effects on metabolism.

CYCLOSPORINE

Cyclosporine is a fat-soluble, cyclic polypeptide fungal product with immunosuppressive activity. It has been an important drug used in humans, primarily to produce immunosuppression in organ transplant patients. It has gained recognition for veterinary use because of availability of a veterinary formulation of cyclosporine (Atopica).

Cyclosporine binds to a specific cellular receptor on calcineurin and inhibits the T-cell receptor-activated signal transduction pathway (Fig. 46.1). Particularly important are its effects to suppress interleukin-2 (IL-2)

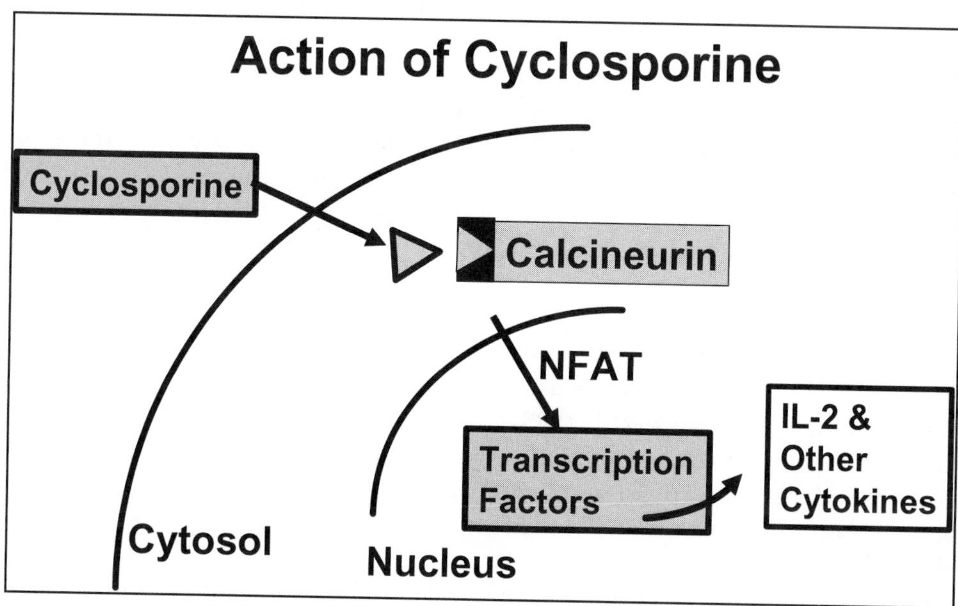

FIG. 46.1 Mechanism of action of cyclosporine. Cyclosporine enters the cytosol, where it binds and inhibits calcineurin at a specific receptor site. By inhibiting calcineurin, the movement of the nuclear factor of activated t-cells (NFAT) is prevented from entering the nucleus. Without the action of NFAT, transcription factors that produce cytokines is inhibited. (See text for additional details.) Tacrolimus is also capable of inhibiting calcineurin.

and other cytokines, and block proliferation of activated T-lymphocytes. The action of cyclosporine is more specific for T-cells as compared to B-cells. One important advantage in comparison to other immunosuppressive drugs—especially corticosteroids—is that it does not cause significant myelosuppression or suppress nonspecific immunity.

CLINICAL USE. Cyclosporine has been used for a number of diseases in veterinary medicine. Many of these diseases have been dermatologic, as reviewed by Robson and Burton (2003). In dogs, when used in the treatment of perianal fistulas, (Mathews et al. 1997; Griffiths et al. 1999) an 85% healing rate was found in one study (Mathews et al. 1997) (2.5–6 mg/kg/day); in sebaceous adenitits, good response was reported in one case (Carothers et al. 1991); and in idiopathic sterile nodular panniculitis, excellent results were seen in two reported cases which were followed for 6 months following discontinuance of the cyclosporine (Guaguère 2000).

USE FOR IMMUNE-MEDIATED DISEASES. Cyclosporine has been used for treatment of a variety of immune-mediated diseases that include immune-mediated hemolytic anemia (IMHA), inflammatory bowel disease (IBD) (Allenspach et al. 2006), immune-mediated polyarthritis, and aplastic anemia (AA). For more severe diseases that require a more consistent immunosuppressive activity, higher doses are used than for atopic dermatitis. For example, for some immune-mediated disease the dose should be in the range of at least 10 mg/kg/day, and perhaps twice a day to produce clinical effects. For these diseases, trough blood cyclosporine concentrations should be at least 600 ng/ml.

For treating immune-mediated skin diseases, the results from pilot studies for treating pemphigus foliaceous in dogs have been disappointing (Rosenkrantz et al. 1989). It did not help any patients with mycosis fungoides. In a study in which five dogs with pemphigus foliaceous were treated, there was little benefit (Olivry et al. 2003). The dogs with pemphigus foliaceous were initially treated with the "atopy dose" of 5 mg/kg/day. If there was no response the dose was increased to 10 mg/kg/day. At the end of the trial, it was concluded that at 5–10 mg/kg/day cyclosporine was unable to produce complete remission in any of the five dogs. In a case study of immune-mediated polyarthritis in dogs (Clements et al. 2004), dogs were treated with prednisolone and various other immune-modifying drugs. Three dogs treated with cyclosporine at 5 mg/kg per day did not respond.

ATOPIC DERMATITIS. In people it has been used successfully for treatment of atopic dermatitis (Camp et al. 1993). Because of this efficacy, the use of cyclosporine for treating canine atopic dermatitis has been investigated in dogs (Marsella and Olivry 2001). In a pilot study, cyclosporine was effective in 13/14 dogs with atopic dermatitis (Fontaine and Olivry 2001). In another trial of 30 dogs treated with cyclosporine (5 mg/kg/day) or prednisolone (0.5 mg/kg/day), the efficacy of cyclosporine was not statistically different than prednisolone (Olivry et al. 2000 2002). Reductions in mean lesion scores were 60% and 59% in prednisolone and cyclosporine groups, respectively. Reduction in mean pruritus scores were 81% and 78% in prednisolone and cyclosporine groups, respectively. In another published study from the same author, 91 dogs with atopic dermatitis were treated with cyclosporine. Two doses were examined, 2.5 mg/kg/day, and 5 mg/kg/day. The formulation used was *Neoral* (formulations to be discussed below). There was a dose-dependent effect. Dogs treated with 5 mg/kg had statistically significant reduction in pruritus scores (45%) and skin lesions (67%). The dose of 2.5 mg/kg was not statistically different from placebo. Some dogs may benefit from less than once-daily administration as shown in another study (Steffan et al. 2003). In this study, administration of cyclosporine (5 mg/kg) was compared to methylprednisolone (0.75 mg/kg) for treatment of canine atopic dermatitis. The response was not different between the drugs, but there was an overall better assessment of efficacy and more gastrointestinal problems in dogs treated with cyclosporine. In the cyclosporine-treated dogs, the dose was started at 5 mg/kg/day for 4 weeks, but eventually half of the dogs were adjusted to an EOD dose, and one-quarter of the dogs were given cyclosporine at 5 mg/kg only twice a week.

USE IN CATS. For organ transplantation in cats (Mathews and Gregory 1997; Kadar et al. 2005) a dose of 3 to 4 mg/kg q12h was used to achieve blood concentrations of 300–500 ng/ml. For treatment of inflammatory disease in cats, including eosinophilia granuloma complex, lower doses are possible. A good response to a dose of 25 mg/cat was seen in six cases of eosinophilic plaque and 3 cases of oral eosinophilic granuloma (Guaguère and Prèlaud 2000). In the report by Vercelli et al. 2006) cats with allergic pruritus were improved with 8 mg/kg oral q24h. Cats with plasmacytic stomatitis, and feline allergic disease have also showed improvement with oral administration of cyclosporine (Vercelli et al. 2006).

One of the capsule sizes is 25 mg and a common dosage is 25 mg/cat, once daily. (Smaller capsules are also available for veterinary use—see below.) The most common adverse effects are anorexia, vomiting, and refusal to eat their food if cyclosporine is mixed with food. Toxoplasmosis has been reported in cats treated with cyclosporine, presumably due to the immunosuppression.

FORMULATIONS AND PHARMACOKINETICS. The pharmacokinetics of cyclosporine are complicated because of the differences between dosage forms, presence of many metabolites, influence of drug interactions, and variability in oral absorption. The formulation called *Sandimmune* was used for many years but was absorbed inconsistently. A more recent human formulation is a microemulsion called *Neoral* which has a much more consistent rate and extent of absorption that is less affected by factors such as feeding than Sandimmune (Lown et al. 1997). There are now human generic equivalents of this formulation. The introduction in late 2003 of Atopica represents the first oral veterinary formulation of cyclosporine. The formulation is exactly the same as Neoral (microemulsion), except that there is a greater variety of capsule sizes available (10, 25, 50, and 100 mg). Absorption, kinetics, and dissolution are the same as for Neoral.

A human formulation called *Gengraf* is a unique formulation. Gengraf capsules have improved solubilzation by dispersing the drug in polyethylene-glycol, propylene glycol, cremophore, and polysorbate. Its interchangeability with Atopica has not been reported.

The pharmacokinetics of cyclosporine in treated animals has been examined (Steffan et al. 2004). Cyclosporine is metabolized in the intestine and liver to several metabolites. Twenty-five to thirty such metabolites have been identified. The prehepatic intestinal enzymes account for significant metabolism of cyclosporine (Wu et al. 1995), and systemic absorption in dogs is only 20–30% (Myre et al. 1991). Systemic absorption in cats is similar at 25–29% (Mehl et al. 2003). The intestinal metabolism by cytochrome P450 enzymes (CYP) and the efflux caused by intestinal p-glycoprotein (P-gp) account for most of the loss in systemic availability after oral administration. Drug enzyme inhibitors such as ketoconazole, diltiazem, or the flavonoids in grapefruit juice can inhibit the presystemic metabolism and produce a profound increase in systemic availability of cyclosporine. For example, 5–10 mg/kg of ketoconazole once daily can decrease the dose of cyclosporine because clearance is reduced by 85% (Myre et al. 1991).

ADMINISTRATION. As cited in the clinical trials above, for treating dermatitis in dogs, the effective dose has been 5 mg/kg/day. Some clinicians have been able to lower the dose, or administer the dose every other day, and still maintain clinical remission. Approximately half of treated dogs can be maintained by increasing the dose interval.

For organ transplantation in people, higher doses are used (e.g., 5–10 mg/kg/day) to achieve targeted whole blood concentrations of 150–400 ng/ml. In people, dosages are adjusted to meet the needs of the individual patient on the basis of clinical response and monitoring trough plasma concentrations. For organ transplantation in cats (Mathews and Gregory 1997) a dose of 3 mg/kg q12h of the Neoral formulation was used to achieve trough blood concentrations of 300–500 ng/ml. At NCSU we routinely administer 25 mg/cat for suppression of immunity for transplantation and modify as needed with monitoring. For organ transplant in dogs, 10 mg/kg q12h to achieve concentrations of 500–600 ng/ml has been used (Mathews et al. 2000).

A report on treating perianal fistulas in dogs (Mathews and Sukhiani 1997) found that an average dose of 6 mg/kg q12h was needed to achieve a targeted blood concentration of 400–600 ng/ml. However, this recommendation was later modified to 2.5 to 6 mg/kg/day. The most common dose for treating perianal fistulas is 3 mg/kg q12h.

MONITORING. Steffan and colleagues (2004) found that when administering approved doses to dogs with atopic dermatitis, routine monitoring of blood cyclosporine concentrations was not necessary. When animals were administered a dose of 5 mg/kg/day, there did not appear to be a strong correlation between blood concentration achieved and clinical response. However, because of wide individual variation in cyclosporine pharmacokinetics, monitoring has been used to determine the optimum dose in some patients. According to one paper, clinical benefits have not been observed when trough concentrations have fallen below 50 ng/ml; therefore, blood testing of patients failing therapy was suggested to reveal inadequate dosing (Robson and Burton 2003).

One must be cognizant of the assay used when monitoring cyclosporine. Plasma values will be lower than whole-blood assays because as much as 50–60% and 10–20% of the dose is concentrated in erythrocytes and leukocytes, respectively. Nonspecific assays will report higher values than a more specific (monoclonal or HPLC) assay. Despite the hypothesized higher specificity when using the monoclonal assay, important discrepancies between these assays and the more specific HPLC assay have been reported (Steimer 1999). For example, in people the difference between HPLC and the commonly used TDx monoclonal immunoassay was 57%. In cats, the TDx assay overestimated the true cyclosporine concentration by a factor of approximately two (that is, TDx assay reporting 500 ng/ml corresponded to an actual value of 250 ng/ml). In dogs, the TDx assay overestimates the true cyclosporine concentrations by a factor of 1.5 to 1.7 (Steffan et al. 2004). When using a specific radioimmunoassay or HPLC assay the true concentrations are measured. But, when using a TDx fluoroescence polarization assay (monoclonal whole blood), multiply the feline concentrations by 0.5 to get the true concentration, and multiply the canine concentration by 0.6 to get the true concentration.

Most current recommendations are based on trough blood sample monitoring. Trough samples are collected immediately before the next scheduled dose; therefore the sample is either 12 or 24 hours after the last dose. These recommendations are being modified in human medicine to a recommendation of a 2-hour sample (C_2). Apparently there is evidence that a C_2 blood sample value correlates better with clinical results than trough samples (Levy et al. 2002; Nashan et al. 2002). In cats, levels are approximately twice as high at 2 hours compared to the levels at 12 hours (Mehl et al. 2003).

ADVERSE EFFECTS AND PRECAUTIONS.

Cyclosporine can cause vomiting, diarrhea, anorexia, secondary infections, and gingival hyperplasia (Vaden 1995) (Table 46.1). Hyperplastic skin lesions have occasionally developed in dogs treated with cyclosporine (Favrot et al. 2005). Papillomavirus can be detected in some skin lesions. Tremors or shaking have been observed in dogs administered high doses. One reference noted few adverse effects as long as blood concentrations were kept within accepted limits (Mathews and Sukhiani 1997).

TABLE 46.1 Adverse reactions of cyclosporine (http://www.fda.gov/cvm/)

Cats: most common adverse events
- Anorexia (#1)
- Vomiting
- Weight loss, depression

Dogs: most common adverse events
- Vomiting (#1)
- Diarrhea
- Depression
- Lethargy
- Pruritus
- Anorexia
- Increased liver enzymes

The most common clinical problem with cyclosporine in dogs that has been cited in the clinical trials discussed previously (Olivry et al. 2000, 2001, 2002; Steffan et al. 2003) is gastrointestinal problems. Vomiting, anorexia, and diarrhea can be seen. When anorexia and vomiting are reported, veterinarians have tried various interventions such as lowering the dose, or administration of the dose with some food. However, whether this decreases the efficacy of the drug should be considered. Feeding will reduce the amount of cyclosporine absorbed in dogs by 15–20%, but it is unlikely that this decrease will be severe enough to affect efficacy.

Nephrotoxicity, once a problem with older forms, is rare with current formulations. Secondary malignancies are a possible complication to long-term therapy but have not been reported in dogs or cats.

DRUG INTERACTIONS.

Several drugs may interact with cyclosporine. For example, coadministration of ketoconazole to treat secondary fungal infections will decrease metabolism of cyclosporine (Myre et al. 1991). Ketoconazole has been used deliberately to reduce the need for cyclosporine in some investigations (Patricelli et al. 2002) and doses have been reduced by one-third of the original dose when administered with ketoconazole. In one study with cyclosporine in the treatment of perianal fistulae, the dose of 1 mg/kg cyclosporine combined with 10 mg/kg ketoconazole was used. The author felt that a dose of 0.5 mg/kg combined with 10 mg/kg ketoconazole also could be used (Mouatt 2002). Erythromycin, grapefruit juice, and diltiazem also may inhibit cyclosporine metabolism and increase blood concentrations.

OPHTHALMIC USE. *Keratoconjunctivitis sicca:* Cyclosporine (Optimmune) is approved to increase tear production in dogs with keratoconjunctivitis sicca (KCS). Success rates are high. Topical cyclosporine has also been used to treat other immune-mediated diseases of the eye. It is available as a 0.2% ophthalmic ointment.

Anterior uveitis: Cyclosporine intraocular implants have been developed by an ophthalmologist at NCSU (Gilger et al. 2006). These implants are administered to horses to treat anterior uveitis. This method of treatment slowly releases the medication and can produce a long-term sustained therapeutic effect.

TACROLIMUS, PIMECROLIMUS, AND SIROLIMUS

Tacrolimus (Prograf) is approved for use in people as 1 and 5 mg capsules and injection. This drug has similar immunologic effects on lymphocytes as cyclosporine. Like cyclosporine, it binds to an intracellular receptor that inhibits IL-2 gene expression in T-helper lymphocytes. It also may bind to receptors that inhibit expression of other cytokines. It has not been used systemically in veterinary medicine and may produce unacceptable adverse effects in dogs.

Tacrolimus (Protopic) has been used topically in dogs with some dermatoses. Systemic absorption is so low that it is safe for topical administration to dogs. More recently, pimecrolimus has been used in people as a topical treatment for atopic dermatitis. Pimecrolimus (Elidel) is available as a 1% cream. There is minimal systemic absorption of pimecrolimus after application.

Sirolimus (Rapamycin) is similar to tacrolimus and has been used to prevent transplant rejection in people. In dogs, sirolimus produced severe gastrointestinal toxicity with mucosa necrosis and submucosa vasculitis.

CYCLOPHOSPHAMIDE (CYTOXAN®)

Cyclophosphamide is one of the nitrogen mustards and is one of the most potent immunosuppressive drugs available. More details on the pharmacology of cyclophosphamide can be found in Chapter 45.

MECHANISM OF ACTION. The immunosuppressive effects of the nitrogen mustards can be attributed to the cytotoxic effect on lymphocytes caused by damage to DNA. Cyclophosphamide is metabolized initially to 4-hydroxyphosphamide and then at target sites metabolized spontaneously (nonenzymatically) to active compounds acrolein and phosphoramide mustard. (Fig. 46.2) Phosphoramide mustard is responsible for alkylating bases on the DNA molecule. Because of the cytotoxic action on lymphocytes, it can directly suppress B-cell activity and antibody formation. B-cells are affected more than T-cells because their rate of recovery from an alkylating agent is slower.

ADVERSE EFFECTS. Cyclophosphamide is a potent immunosuppressive drug with a high risk of myelosuppression. In dogs the most serious toxic effect is bone marrow suppression, which can lead to secondary infections, thrombocytopenia, and anemia. Another adverse effect is sterile hemorrhagic cystitis. The incidence has been estimated to be as high as 24% in treated dogs and 3.7% in treated cats. The injury to the urinary bladder is caused by the toxic effects of metabolites on the bladder epithelium (especially acrolein) that are concentrated and excreted in the urine. Various strategies have been used to decrease the injury to the bladder epithelium. Corticosteroids are usually administered with cyclophosphamide to induce polyuria and decrease the toxic effect of the drug on the epithelium. In people, and occasionally in dogs, the drug mesna (Mesnex, mercaptoethanesulfonate) has been used to prevent drug-induced cystitis. Mesna provides free active thiol groups to bind metabolites of cyclophosphamide in the urine. Another therapy that has been used to reduce hemorrhagic cystitis is the administration of furosemide. In a study of 216 cases (Charney et al. 2003), there was less hemorrhagic cystitis when furosemide was administered concurrently, compared to cyclophosphamide alone. The dose of furosemide used was 2.2 mg/kg IV administered at the time of cyclophosphamide administration.

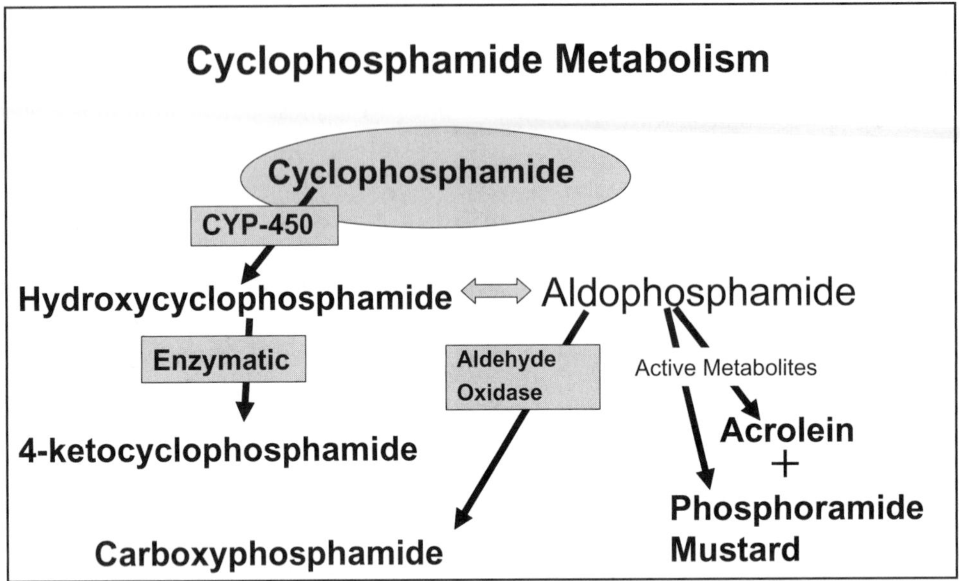

FIG. 46.2 Metabolism of cyclophosphamide. Cyclophosphamide is metabolized by cytochrome P450 enzymes to hydroxycyclophosphamide, which in turn is metabolized enzymatically to 4-ketocyclophosphamide, an inactive metabolite. Conversion of hydroxycyclophosphamide to aldophosphamide leads to nonenzymatic (spontaneous) conversion to the active metabolites, acrolein (responsible for toxicity), and phosphoramide mustard (responsible for cytotoxic, or alkylating effect).

Cats are resistant to hemorrhagic cystitis from cyclophosphamide. Gastrointestinal effects such as nausea, vomiting, and diarrhea also are possible in any species treated.

In people, long-term therapy is discouraged because of the risk that cyclophosphamide will induce secondary malignancies. Secondary malignancies have not been reported in animals that have been treated.

CLINICAL USE. The dose administered to dogs is 50 mg/m^2, which is approximately 1.5 mg/kg for large dogs and 2.5 mg/kg for small dogs. It is available in 25 and 50 mg tablets. This dose has been administered every other day (EOD) with corticosteroids administered on the alternate days. Cyclophosphamide also is administered at this dose by some clinicians as a pulse dose of 4 consecutive days/week (4 days on, 3 days off). Cats have received a total dose of 6.25–12.5 mg, once daily, 4 days per week.

For treatment of immune-mediated hemolytic anemia, the efficacy of cyclophosphamide has been questioned (Mason et al. 2003). In a study in which dogs were randomized to receive cyclophosphamide plus glucocorticoids or glucocorticoids alone, there was no added benefit from cyclophosphamide. Regeneration of red blood cells was suppressed in cyclophosphamide-treated animals.

CHLORAMBUCIL

Chlorambucil (Leukeran) also is a nitrogen mustard and is sometimes used as a substitute for cyclophosphamide. It has a similar action as cyclophosphamide, but is one of the slowest-acting of the class of nitrogen mustards. Although little has been published on the clinical use of chlorambucil, it may be effective in dogs and cats for immune-mediated disease. However, direct comparisons to other immunosuppressive drugs has not been reported. One of the most frequent uses has been for treatment of immune-mediated skin diseases of cats. In one report, cats with pemphigus and eosinophilic granuloma complex (EGC) responded favorably with few side effects (Helton-Rhodes and Shoulberg 1992).

ADVERSE EFFECTS. Chlorambucil lacks some of the adverse effects of cyclophosphamide. This drug has been administered for months to years to people safely. The bone-marrow suppressing effects are only moderate, compared to other nitrogen mustards, and are rapidly reversible. Chlorambucil has not caused cystitis, which is reported for cyclophosphamide.

CLINICAL USE. The usual dose in cats is 0.1 to 0.2 mg/kg, orally, q24h. The usual dose in dogs is 2–6 mg/m^2 q24h. After remission these doses are administered EOD. It is available as 2 mg tablets. The EOD dose may be given with oral prednisolone on alternate days.

THIOPURINES (AZATHIOPRINE)

As first-line therapy, or as an alternative to nitrogen mustard alkylating agents for treatment of immune-mediated disease, thiopurines are often administered. The most common of the thiopurines used for this purpose is azathioprine (Imuran).

MECHANISM OF ACTION. Despite the widespread use, little is known in dogs about its metabolism, risk of adverse reactions, and mechanism of immune-suppression (Rinkardt et al. 1999; Ogilvie et al. 1988). In people, azathioprine is rapidly and spontaneously metabolized to 6-mercaptopurine (6-MP). 6-mercaptopurine is further metabolized to 6-methylmercaptopurine nucleotides (6-MMPN) and 6-thioguanine nucleotides (6-TGN). (Fig. 46.3). Conversion to metabolites may occur at target cells responsible for immune effects because direct administration of 6-MP is not as effective as administration of azathioprine as a prodrug. 6-TGNs are the active cytotoxic metabolites. They are responsible for the bone-marrow toxicity, cytotoxic effects, and immunosuppression of lymphocytes (Stefan et al. 2004; Lennard et al. 1989). 6-MMPNs, on the other hand, are inactive metabolites, but can produce some adverse effects. As a consequence of the active metabolites, azathioprine interferes with lymphocyte proliferation because it inhibits de novo synthesis of purines, which is critically important for activated lymphocytes.

CLINICAL USE. In veterinary medicine, azathioprine is one of the most commonly administered drugs to suppress

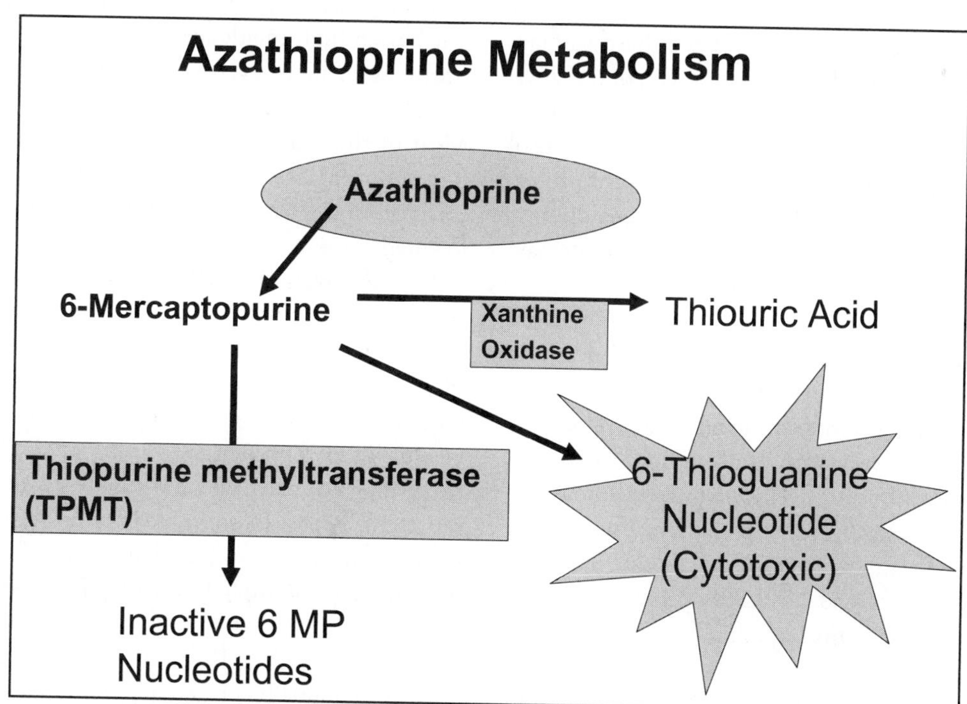

FIG. 46.3 Metabolism of azathioprine. Azathioprine is metabolized first to 6-mercaptopurine (6-MP) and then to thioguanine (6-TG) nucleotide metabolites, which produce the cytotoxic (immunosuppressive) activiy. 6-MP is also metabolized by the enzyme thiopurine methyltransferase (TPMT) to inactive metabolites. Individuals low in TPMT may have exaggerated toxic effects (myelosuppression), and individuals high in TPMT may have diminished therapeutic response. Drugs that inhibit xanthine oxidase (e.g., allopurinol) may also produce adverse effects.

immunity in dogs for treatment of dermatologic disease, immune-mediated hemolytic anemia, intestinal disease, and other immune-mediated diseases (Grundy and Barton 2001; Olivry et al. 2004; Hostutler et al. 2004; Weinkle et al. 2005).

Azathioprine is available as 50 mg tablets. It is dosed at 2 mg/kg, orally, q24h. Long-term therapy is administered at a dose of 0.5 to 1.0 mg/kg, every other day, with prednisolone administered on the alternate days. In cats, the doses are much lower, with 0.3 mg/kg being the safest (discussed below). In people there is a long lag-period before successful treatment is recognized with azathioprine, which may be as long as 2–8 months. In veterinary medicine this lag-period is probably shorter and therapeutic benefits have been observed after only 3–5 weeks, or less.

ADVERSE EFFECTS. Azathioprine myelotoxicity has been well documented in dogs (Rinkardt and Kruth 1996; Rodriguez et al. 2004). Leukopenia and thrombocytopenia can be serious. Animals that are treated with azathioprine should have the CBC monitored during therapy to identify the animals that may be at risk for toxicity and to adjust doses accordingly.

Gastrointestinal effects such as nausea and diarrhea may be only temporary and subside after several days of therapy. In people, elevated levels of 6-MMPNs are associated with hepatotoxicity (Stefan et al. 2004). Canine patients also have developed hepatic toxicity within 2–4 weeks after initiating azathioprine therapy. Signs of hepatopathy include liver enzyme increase and clinical signs that may result in discontinuation of treatment.

Long-term effects related to the immunosuppression produced by azathioprine include Demodex infection, recurrent pyoderma, and dermatophyte infections. Sterile hemorrhagic cystitis, the complication cited for cyclophosphamide, has not been seen with azathioprine. There has also been association (but not well documented) between the administration of azathioprine plus prednisolone and the development of acute pancreatitis in dogs. It has been suggested that this is caused by azathioprine's effect on decreasing pancreatic secretion in animals.

PROBLEMS IN CATS. Some veterinarians have administered azathioprine to cats at a total dose of about 6.25 mg per cat (1/8 tablet) EOD. However, doses of 2.2 mg/kg EOD produced profound neutropenia in cats (Beale et al. 1992). Although doses of 1.1 mg/kg every day, or every other day, for treatment of pemphigus have been administered to cats (Cacioloet al. 1984), other references have discouraged its use in cats because of the bone-marrow suppressing effects, even at this dose (Helton-Rhodes 1995). Differences in metabolism may explain the susceptibility in cats (discussed below under metabolism). Because of the concern for toxicity, if azathioprine is used, a recommended dose is 0.3 mg/kg once daily to every other day.

IMPORTANCE OF METABOLIC PATHWAY FOR DETERMINING TOXICITY. Azathioprine toxicity may have a genetic component. After azathioprine is converted to 6-MP, it is further metabolized by three routes to other metabolites. One metabolic route is via xanthine oxidase to inactive metabolites. Allopurinol will decrease this route because it inhibits xanthine oxidase. Another metabolic route is via thiopurine methyltransferase (TPMT), which is responsible for conversion to nontoxic 6-MP nucleotides. In people there is genetic polymorphism that determines high or low levels of TPMT. People with low TPMT activity are more responsive to therapy, but have a high incidence of toxicity (myelosuppression); people with high levels of TPMT activity have low incidence of toxicity but lower efficacy (Lennard et al. 1989). Most of the human population has high TPMT activity, but about 11% have low levels and are more prone to toxicity. In people with low TPMT activity, doses must be lowered.

In dogs, levels of TMPT also are highly variable. TPMT activity varied ninefold in a population of 177 dogs (Kidd et al. 2004). Another study with fewer dogs indicated 90% of dogs showing normal TPMT activity and 10% with low activity (White et al. 1998). The variation appears genetically determined, as it is in people. However, at this time, it is not clear whether low levels of TPMT in dogs represent a risk. In some dogs with a history of azathioprine associated myelotoxicity the animals had either intermediate or high levels of TMPT (Rodriguez et al. 2004).

Cats, as suspected because of their susceptibility to toxicity, have low TPMT activity (Foster et al. 2000). Therefore, cats are sensitive to the toxicity of azathioprine. If azathioprine is used in cats, dose should be much lower than in dogs.

MYCOPHENOLATE

Mycophenolate mofetil is metabolized to the active compound mycophenolic acid (MPA). T- and B-lymphocytes are critically dependent on de novo synthesis of purine nucleotides and mycophenolic acid is a potent inhibitor of inosine monophosphate dehydrogenate (IMPDH), an enzyme important for synthesis of purines in lymphocytes. Therefore it suppresses lymphocyte proliferation and decreases antibody synthesis by B-cells. It is available as a 250 mg capsule (CellCept). In people it is used as a replacement for azathioprine and has been primarily used for immune suppression in liver and kidney transplant patients. It is usually used in combination with glucocorticoids and/or cyclosporine.

CLINICAL USE. In dogs, mycophenolate has been used on a limited basis to treat some immume-mediated diseases. According to pharmacokinetic studies with mycophenolate in dogs, the elimination rate was rapid (half-life less than 1 hour), which may require frequent dosing in dogs to achieve successful results. For treatment of pemphigus foliaceous it was given at a dose of 22–39 mg/kg/day divided into three treatments. It was well tolerated, but only three out of eight dogs completed the study and were improved (Byrne et al. 2001). It has also been used to treat myasthenia gravis in dogs.

ADVERSE EFFECTS. The use has been uncommon and there are not many reports of adverse events in animals. In dogs, nausea, vomiting, and diarrhea have been observed, which appear dose-related.

DANAZOL

Danazol (Danocrine) is an androgenic agent that has been used for treating refractory patients with immune-mediated thrombocytopenia and immune-mediated hemolytic anemia. Its mechanism of action is not understood. It may interfere with antibody production, or interfere with the binding of complement or antibody to the platelet or red blood cell. It may also reduce receptors on monocytes for antibodies bound to platelets or red blood cells. It has been administered to dogs at a dose of 10 mg/kg q12h PO.

GOLD THERAPY (CHRYSOTHERAPY)

Drugs such as aurothioglucose (Solganal) have been used to treat some immune-mediated diseases, but its use in veterinary medicine has diminished considerably. In people, its most common use is for rheumatoid arthritis. It was originally used in the 1800s to treat tuberculosis. The exact mechanism of action is unknown but it may exert the immunomodulating through its effects on T-lymphocyte cell-mediated immunity or via inhibition of sulfhydral enzyme systems. There also may be an antiinflammatory effect on macrophages and neutrophils. A disadvantage of gold therapy is that it must be administered IM (usually once/week) and it may take several weeks for positive effects to occur. For example, in people, aurothioglucose has an onset of action of 6–8 weeks; in dogs this may be as long as 6–12 weeks.

AVAILABLE DRUGS. Gold therapy—referred to as chrysotherapy in some textbooks—includes various formulations of gold. Older formulations no longer exist commercially. Gold sodium thiomalate (Myochrysine) is available as 25 or 50 mg/ml injection in sesame oil. Aurothioglucose (Solganal) is a 50 mg/ml injection in an aqueous formulation. Oral treatment uses auranofin (Ridaura), which is available in 3 mg capsules.

CLINICAL USE. Controlled studies are lacking in veterinary medicine and case reports of successful therapy in the veterinary literature are lacking. The most common use is treatment of immune-mediated dermatologic disease unresponsive to corticosteroids alone, or in cases in which one wishes to decrease the patient's reliance on corticosteroids.

DOSES. Usually a 1 mg test dose is administered or 5 mg to larger canine patients. Doses are administered once/week until remission, and usually maintenance doses are in the range of 1–2 mg/kg every 2–4 weeks. Auranofin, an oral drug, is reported to have less efficacy in animals than injectable formulations and is not often used.

ADVERSE EFFECTS. The adverse effects are described in people, in which there is a 10–50% incidence, but they are not well documented in animals. Reported adverse effects include dermatitis (which could be confused with the underlying problem being treated), nephrotoxicity, and blood dyscrasias. When administered to animals it is recommended to monitor CBC periodically to detect drug-induced problems. Diarrhea has been reported with the oral product. In pregnant animals these drugs should not be used. They cause abortion and fetal resorption or congenital malformations in laboratory animals.

DAPSONE

Dapsone is a sulfone, which shares chemical properties with sulfonamides. It has been in use for over 50 years in human medicine. It has been used in combination with other drugs to treat leprosy in humans caused by *Mycobacterium leprae*. Other uses include prophylaxis for malaria and treatment of *Pneumocystis carinii* infections in AIDS patients. The dermatological uses include treatment of dermatitis herpetiformis, SLE, pemphigoid, subcorneal pustular dermatosis and other inflammatory dermatoses.

MECHANISM OF ACTION. For treating leprosy, dapsone acts as a folate antagonist, similar to sulfonamides. For other conditions, the mechanism is unknown, but its action appears to be attributed to a suppression of neutrophil function (Booth et al. 1992). It may suppress respiratory burst in inflammatory cells.

PHARMACOKINETICS. Similarities in metabolism to the sulfonamides are expected. It is highly absorbed with a long elimination half-life of 11–13 hrs in experimental dogs. Comparison of metabolic pathway between dogs and people and between cats and people may explain susceptibility to toxicity (see discussion of adverse effects below). In people, one pathway for metabolism is acetylation (N-acetylation). The other metabolite in people is a hydroxylamine metabolite (N-hydroxylation). This hydroxylamine metabolite is responsible for adverse effects caused by dapsone, such as methemoglobinemia (Helton-Rhodes et al. 1992). Dogs cannot acetylate drugs and a pattern of metabolism of sulfonamides has been identified in dogs that indicates that this lack of acetylation may account for a greater accumulation of toxic metabolites and increased risk of adverse effects. The same metabolic fate may explain the risk of adverse effects from dapsone in dogs.

CLINICAL USE IN ANIMALS. In animals dapsone has been used for feline leprosy, although efficacy for this disease is uncertain. In dogs, it has been used for dermatologic conditions characterized by vascular disorders, inflammatory skin disease, immune-mediated disease, and subcorneal pustular dermatosis. Since specific studies have not been performed, doses are extrapolated from humans or based on empiricism. Doses listed in textbooks are in the range of 1 mg/kg once, twice, or three times daily. It is available in 25 and 100 mg generic tablets.

ADVERSE EFFECTS. The adverse effects in animals are not well documented, but can be severe enough to discontinue therapy. In people, dapsone causes agranulocytosis, aplastic anemia, methemoglobinemia, and blood dyscrasias. Toxic dermatological reactions (e.g., toxic epidermal necrolysis) may occur. Because of the similarity to sulfonamides, do not administer to animals sensitive to sulfonamides. Since some dogs may have an inability to detoxify the hydroxylamine metabolite, this could possibly lead to a higher risk of toxicity. Cats are reported to be susceptible to hepatitis and blood dyscrasias. In people, one of the metabolites responsible for toxicity is excreted as a glucuronide metabolite. Cats may be unable to rapidly glucuronate this metabolite, which may increase a cat's risk of toxicosis compared to other animals.

REFERENCES AND ADDITIONAL READING

Allenspach K, Rüfenacht S, Sauter S, Gröne A, Steffan J, Strehlau G, Gaschen F. Pharmacokinetics and clinical efficacy of cyclosporine treatment of dogs with steroid-refractory inflammatory bowel disease. J Vet Intern Med 20:239–244, 2006.

Altman RD, Dean DD, Muniz OE, Howell DS. Prophylactic treatment of canine osteoarthritis with glycosaminoglycan oplysulfuric acid ester. Arth Rheum 32:759–766, 1989.

Ammersbach MAG, Kruth SA, Sears W, Bienzle D. The effect of glucocorticoids on canine lymphocyte marker expression and apoptosis. J Vet Intern Med 20:1166–1171, 2006.

Barnes PJ, Karin M. Nuclear factor-kB C a pivotal transcription factor in chronic inflammatory diseases. New Engl J Med 336:1066–1071, 1997.

Barnes PJ. Molecular mechanisms of corticosteroids in allergic diseases. Allergy 56:928–936, 2001.

Barnes PJ. Corticosteroids: The drugs to beat. Eur J Pharmacol 533:2–14, 2006.

Beale KM, Altman D, Clemmons RR, Bolon B. Systemic toxicosis associated with azathioprine administration in domestic cats. Am J Vet Res 53:1236–1240, 1992.

Booth SA, Moody CE, Dahl MV, et al. Dapsone suppresses integrin-mediated neutrophil adherence function. J Invest Dermatol 98:135–140, 1992.

Boumpas DT, Chrousos GP, Wilder RL, et al. Glucocorticoid therapy for immune-mediated diseases: Basic and clinical correlates. Annals of Intern Med 119:1198–1208, 1993.

Brockus CW, Dillon AR, Kemppainen RJ. Effect of alternate-day prednisolone administration on hypophyseal-adrenocortical activity in dogs. Am J Vet Res 60:698–702, 1999.

Byrne KP, Morris DO. Study to determine the usefulness of mycophenolate mofetil (MMF) for the treatment of pemphigus foliaceous in the dog. [abstract] Ann Mtg Acad of Vet Dermatol, 2001.

Caciolo PL, Nesbitt GH, Hurvitz AI. Pemphigus foliaceous in 8 cats and results of induction therapy using azathioprine. J Am Anim Hosp Assoc 20:571–577, 1984.

Camp RDR, Reitamo S, Friedmann PS, et al. Cyclosporin A in severe, therapy-resistant atopic dermatitis: Report of an international workshop. Br J Dermatol 129:217–220, 1993.

Carothers MA, Kwochka KW, Rojko JL. Cyclosporine responsive granulomatous sebaceous adenitis in a dog. J Am Vet Med Assoc 198:1645–8, 1991.

Charney SC, Bergman PJ, Hohenhaus AE, McKnight JA. Risk factors for sterile hemorrhagic cystitis in dogs with lymphoma receiving cyclophosphamide with or without concurrent administration of furosemide: 216 cases (1990–1996). J Am Vet Med Assoc 222:1388–1393, 2003.

Clements DN, Gear RN, Tattersall J, Carmichael S, Bennett D. Type I immune-mediated polyarthritis in dogs: 39 cases (1997–2002). J Am Vet Med Assoc 224:1323–7, 2004.

Cohn L. The influence of corticosteroids on host defense mechanisms. J Vet Intern Med 5:95–104, 1991.

Favrot C, Olivry T, Werner AH, Nespecca G, Utiger A, Grest P, Ackermann M. Evaluation of papillomaviruses associated with cyclosporine-induced hyperplastic verrucous lesions in dogs. Am J Vet Res 66:1764–1769, 2005.

Fontaine J, Olivry T. Cyclosporine for the management of atopic dermatitis in dogs: a pilot clinical trial. Vet Rec 148:662–3, 2001.

Fontaine J. Use of cyclosporine for the management of atopic dermatitis in dogs: a pilot trial. 16th Annual Congress, ESVD/ECVD, pp. 133, 1999.

Foster AP, Shaw SE, Duley JA, Shobowale-Bakre EM, Harbour DA. Demonstration of thiopurine methyltransferase activity in the erythrocytes of cats. J Vet Intern Med 14:552–554, 2000.

Gilger BC, Salmon JH, Wilkie DA, Cruysberg LP, Kim J, Hayat M, Kim H, Kim S, Yuan P, Lee SS, Harrington SM, Murray PR, Edelhauser HF, Csaky KG, Robinson MR. A novel bioerodible deep scleral lamellar cyclosporine implant for uveitis. Invest Ophthalmol Vis Sci. 47(6):2596–25605, 2006.

Graham-Mize CA, Rosser EJ. Bioavailability and activity of prednisone and prednisolone in the feline patient. Vet Dermatol 15:(Suppl1)9[abstract 15], 2004.

Griffiths LG, Sullivan M, Borland WW. Cyclosporine as the sole treatment for anal furnculosis: preliminary results. J Sm An Pract 40:569–72, 1999.

Grundy SA, Barton C. Influence of drug treatment on survival of dogs with immune-mediated hemolytic anemia: 88 cases (1989–1999). J Am Vet Med Assoc 218:543–546, 2001.

Guaguère E, Prèlaud P. Efficacy of cyclosporine in the treatment of 12 cases of eosinophilic granuloma complex. Vet Derm (Suppl1)11:31, 2000.

Guaguère E, Steffan J, Olivry T. Cyclospirin A: a new drug in the field of canine dermatology. Vet Derm 15:61–74, 2004.

Guaguère E. Efficacy of cyclosporine in the treatment of idiopathic sterile nodular panniculitis in two dogs. Vet Derm 11:(Suppl1)22, 2000.

Hayashi R, Wada H, Ito K, Adcock IM. Effects of glucocorticoids on gene transcription. Eur J Pharmacol 500:51–62, 2004.

Helton-Rhodes K, Shoulberg N. Chlorambucil: effective therapeutic options for treatment of feline immune-mediated dermatoses. Feline Pract 20:5, 1992.

Helton-Rhodes K. Feline immunomodulators. In Bonagura JD (ed): Current Veterinary Therapy XII. Philadelphia: WB Saunders, pp. 581–584, 1995.

Hostutler RA, Luria BJ, Johnson SE, Weisbrode SE, Sherding RG, Jaeger JQ, Guilford WG. Antibiotic-responsive histiocytic ulcerative colitis in 9 dogs. J Vet Intern Med 18(4):499–504, 2004.

Kadar E, Sykes JE, Kass PH, Bernsteen L, Gregory CR, Kyles AE. Evaluation of the prevalence of infections in cats after renal transplantation: 169 cases (1987–2003). J Am Vet Med Assoc 227(6):948–953, 2005.

Kidd LB, Salavaggione OE, Szumlanski CL, Miller JL, Weinshilboum RM, Trepanier L. Thiopurine methyltransferase activity in red blood cells of dogs. J Vet Intern Med 18:214–218, 2004.

Lennard L, Van Loon JA, Weinshilboum RM. Pharmacogenetics of acute azathioprine toxicity. Relationship to thiopurine methyltransferase genetic polymorphism. Clin Pharmacol Ther 46:149–154, 1989.

Levy G, Thervet E, Lake J, Uchida K. Consensus on Neoral C(2): Expert Review in Transplantation (CONCERT) Group. Patient management by Neoral C2 monitoring: an international consensus statement. Transplantation 73(9Suppl):S12–18, 2002.

Lown KS, Mayo RR, Leichtman AB, et al. Role of intestinal P-glycoprotein (mdr-1) in interpatient variation in the oral bioavailability of cyclosporine. Clin Pharmacol Ther 62:248–260, 1997.

Mason N, Duval D, Shofer FS, Giger U. Cyclophosphamide exerts no beneficial effect over prednisone alone in the initial treatment of acute immune-mediated hemolytic anemia in dogs: A randomized controlled clinical trial. J Vet Intern Med 17:206–212, 2003.

Mathews KA, Holmberg DL, Miller CW. Kidney transplantation in dogs with naturally occurring end-stage renal disease. J Am Anim Hosp Assoc 36:294–301, 2000.

Mathews KA, Sukhiani HR. Randomized controlled trial of cyclosporine for treatment of perianal fistulas in dogs. J Am Vet Med Assoc 211:1249–1253, 1997.

Mathews KG, Gregory CR. Renal transplants in cats: 66 cases (1987–1996). J Am Vet Med Assoc 211:1432–1436, 1997.

Mehl ML, Kyles AE, Craigmill AL, Epstein S, Gregory CR. Disposition of cyclosporine after intravenous and multi-dose oral administration in cats. J Vet Pharmacol Ther 26(5):349–54, 2003.

Moore GE, Hoenig M. Duration of pituitary and adrenocortical suppression after long-term administration of anti-inflammatory doses of prednisone in dogs. Am J Vet Res 53:716–720, 1992.

Mouatt J. Cyclosporine and ketoconazole interaction for treatment of perianal fistulas in the dog. Aust Vet J 80(4):207–11, 2002.

Myre SA, Schoeder TJ, Grund VR, Wandstrat TL, Nicely PG, Pesce AJ, First MR. Critical ketoconazole dosage range for ciclosporin clearance inhibition in the dog. Pharmacology43(5):233–41, 1991.

Nara PL, Krakowka S, Powers TE. Effects of prednisolone on the development of immune response to canine distemper virus in Beagle pups. Am J Vet Res 40:1742–1747, 1979.

Nashan B, Cole E, Levy G, Thervet E. Clinical validation studies of Neoral C2 monitoring: a review. Transplantation 73(Suppl):S3–11, 2002.

Ogilvie GK, Felsburg PJ, and Harris CW. Short-term effect of cyclophosphamide and azathioprine on selected aspects of the canine blastogenic response. Vet Immunol Immunopathol 18:119–127, 1988.

Olivry T, Rivierre C, Jackson HA, Murphy KM, Davidson G, Sousa CA. Cyclosporine decreases skin lesions and pruritus in dogs with atopic dermatitis: a blinded randomized prednisolone-controlled trial. Vet Derm 13:77–87, 2002.

Olivry T, Rivierre C, Jackson HA, Murphy KM, et al. A placebo-controlled blinded trial of misoprostol monotherapy for canine atopic dermatitis: effects on dermal cellularity and cutaneous tumor necrosis factor-alpha gene transcription. Vet Derm 11(Suppl1):47(abstract P-21), 2000.

Olivry T, Rivierre C, Jackson HA, Murphy KM, Sousa CA. Cyclosporin—A decreases skin lesions and pruritus in dogs with atopic dermatitis: a prednisolone-controlled blinded trial. Vet Derm 11(Suppl1):47(abstract P-19), 2000.

Olivry T, Rivierre C, Murphy KM. Ineffectiveness of cyclosporine for treatment induction of canine pemphigus foliaceous: a pilot clinical trial. Vet Rec 2002.

Olivry T, Rivierre C, Murphy KM. Efficacy of cyclosporine for treatment of induction of canine pemphigus foliaceous. Vet Rec 152:53–4, 2003.

Olivry T, Steffan J, Fisch RD, Prèlaud P, Guaguère E, Fontaine J, Carlotti DN. European Veterinary Dermatology Cyclosporine Group. Randomized controlled trial of the efficacy of cyclosporine in the treatment of atopic dermatitis in dogs. J Am Vet Med Assoc 221(3):370–7, 2002.

Olivry T, Mueller RS, et al. Evidence-based veterinary dermatology: a systemic review of the pharmacotherapy of canine atopic dermatitis. Vet Derm 14:121–146, 2003.

Olivry T, Bergvall KE, Atlee BA. Prolonged remission after immunosuppressive therapy in six dogs with pemphigus foliaceous. Vet Derm 15(4):245–52, 2004.

Papich MG, Davis LE. Glucocorticoid therapy. In Kirk RW (ed): Current Veterinary Therapy X. Philadelphia: WB Saunders Co., pp. 54–62, 1989.

Patricelli AJ, Hardie RJ, McAnulty JF. Cyclosporine and ketoconazole for the treatment of perianal fistulas. J Am Vet Med Assoc 220:1009–16, 2002.

Peroni DL, Stanley S, Kollias-Baker C, Robinson NE. Prednisone per os is likely to have limited efficacy in horses. Equine Vet J 34:283–287, 2002.

Rhen T and Cidlowski JA. Antiinflammatory action of glucocorticoids—new mechanisms for old drugs. New Engl J Med 353:1711–1723, 2005.

Rinkardt NE, Kruth SA. Azathioprine-induced bone marrow toxicity in four dogs. Can Vet J 37:612–613, 1996.

Robson DC, Burton GG. Cyclosporine: applications in small animal dermatology. Vet Derm 14:1–9, 2003.

Rodriguez DB, Mackin A, Easley R, Boyle CR, et al. Relationship between red blood cell thioprine methyltransferase activity and myelotoxicity in dogs receiving azathioprine. J Vet Intern Med 18:339–345, 2004.

Rosenkrantz W. Immunomodulating drugs in dermatology. In Kirk RW (ed): Current Veterinary Therapy X. Philadelphia: WB Saunders Co., pp. 570–577, 1989.

Rosenkrantz WS, Griffin CE, Barr RJ. Clinical evaluation of cyclosporine in animal models with cutaneous immune-mediated disease and epitheliotropic lymphoma. J Am Anim Hosp Assoc 25:377–84, 1989.

Scott DW, Miller WH, Griffin CE. Muller & Kirk's Small Animal Dermatology, 5th Ed. Philadelphia: WB Saunders Co., 1995.

Scott DW. Rational use of glucocorticoids in dermatology. In Bonagura JD (ed): Current Veterinary Therapy XII. Philadelphia: WB Saunders, pp. 573–580, 1995.

Stefan C, Walsh W, Banka T, Adeli K, and Verjee Z. Improved HPLC methodology for monitoring thiopurine metabolites in patients on thiopurine therapy. Clin Biochem 37:764–771, 2004.

Steffan J, Alexander D, Brovedani F, Fisch RD. Comparison of cyclosporine A with methylprednisolone for treatment of canine atopic dermatitis: a parallel, blinded, randomized controlled trial. Vet Derm 14:11–22, 2003.

Steffan J, Strehlau G, Maurer M, Rohlfs A. Cyclosporin A pharmacokinetics and efficacy in the treatment of atopic dermatitis in dogs. J Vet Pharmacol Ther 27:231–8, 2004.

Steimer W. Performance and specificity of monoclonal immunoassays for cyclosporine monitoring: How specific is specific? Clin Chem 45:371–381, 1999.

Vaden SL. Cyclosporine. In Bonagura JD (ed): Current Veterinary Therapy XII. Philadelphia: WB Saunders, 73–7, 1995.

Van den Broek AHM, Stafford WL. Epidermal and hepatic glucocorticoid receptors in cats and dogs. Res Vet Sci 52:312–315, 1992.

Vercelli A, Raviri G, Cornegliani L. The use of oral cyclosporine to treat feline dermatoses: a retrospective analysis of 23 cases. Vet Derm 17:201–206, 2006.

Weinkle TK, Center SA, Randolph JF, Warner KL, Barr SC, Erb HN. Evaluation of prognostic factors, survival rates, and treatment protocols for immune-mediated hemolytic anemia in dogs: 151 cases (1993–2002). J Am Vet Med Assoc 226(11):1869–80, 2005.

White SD, Rosychuk RAW, Scott KV. Investigation into the role of thiopurine methyltransferase in the use of azathioprine in dogs: Phase one. 14th Proceedings of AAVD/ACVD meeting, pp. 111–112, 1998.

White SD. Clinical approach to the pruritic dog: advances and basics. J Am Anim Hosp Assoc 27:489–496, 1991.

Wu, C-Y, Benet LZ, Hebert MF, Gupta SK, Rowland M, Gomez DY, Wacher VJ. Differentiation of absorption and first-pass gut and hepatic metabolism in humans: studies with cyclosporine. Clin Pharmacol Ther 58(5):492–7, 1995.

CHAPTER

47

DRUGS AFFECTING GASTROINTESTINAL FUNCTION

MARK G. PAPICH

ANTIEMETIC DRUGS

NEUROTRANSMITTERS INVOLVED IN VOMITING.

Several neurotransmitters are important for stimulating vomiting (Table 47.1) and successful therapy involves blocking one or more of the receptors for these neurotransmitters. There are differences between dogs and cats with respect to importance of various receptors, and there are also differences between dogs, cats, and people. Dogs respond readily to administration of apomorphine, which is an

TABLE 47.1 Neurotransmitters important in vomiting

- Dopamine (type 2)
- Histamine (H_1)
- Serotonin (5-HT)
- Acetylcholine (muscarinic type 1)
- Substance P (Neurokinin NK-1)

TABLE 47.2 Antiemetic drugs and doses

ANTIHISTAMINES	
diphenhydramine (Benadryl)	2–4 mg/kg, IM, PO, q8–12h
dimenhydrinate (Dramamine)	4–8 mg/kg, PO, q8–12h
promethazine (Phenergan)	0.2–0.4 mg/kg, PO,IM, q8h
PHENOTHIAZINES	
chlorpromazine (Thorazine)	0.5 mg/kg, IM,PO,q6–8h
prochlorperazine (Compazine)	0.1–0.5 mg/kg, IM, q6–8h
Acepromazine	0.1 mg/kg, IM, PO, q12h
triflupromazine (Vesprin)	0.1–0.3 mg/kg, IM, PO, q8–12h
trifluperazine (Stelazine)	0.03 mg/kg, IM, q12h
triethylperazine (Torecan)	0.13–0.2 mg/kg, IM, q8–12h
metoclopramide (Reglan)	0.1–0.3 mg/kg, IM, PO, q12h
ANTICHOLINERGIC DRUGS	
Atropine	0.02–0.04 mg/kg, IM,SC, q8–12h
methscopolamine (Pamine)	0.3–1.0 mg/kg, PO, q8h
isopropamide (Darbid)	0.2–1.0 mg/kg, PO, q12h
ANTISEROTONIN DRUGS	
ondansetron (Zofran)	0.5 to 1.0 mg/kg, IV or oral 30 min prior to administration of cancer drugs. For vomiting from other causes, 0.1–0.2 mg/kg slow IV injection and repeated every 6–12h to control vomiting.
NK-1 RECEPTOR BLOCKERS	
Aprepitant (Emend, human drug)	1 mg/kg PO, q24h.
Maropitant (Cerenia)	1 mg/kg SC, q24h, 2 mg/kg oral q24h or 8 mg/kg oral (for prevention of motion sickness).

agonist for dopamine. Cats vomit more readily from stimulation of α_2-adrenergic receptors than dogs, and respond more consistently to administration of xylazine. Histamine seems to be a more important neurotransmitter in the chemoreceptor trigger zone (CRTZ) of dogs than cats, and it is a more potent stimulant in people than in dogs. These differences and overlapping effects of neurotransmitters can be confusing, but some generalities are as follows.

In the emetic center (vomiting center), serotonin (5HT), histamine (H_1), acetylcholine (muscarinic M_1), serotonin (5-HT_3), dopamine (D_2), and neurokinin (NK-1) all play some role, although the importance may vary among species.

In the CRTZ, dopamine, serotonin, and acetylcholine (muscarinic) all play a role. Histamine is important in dogs, but less so in cats. Drugs that block dopamine can be effective antiemetics from stimulation of the CRTZ in most animals.

In the vestibular apparatus (motion sickness) acetylcholine (muscarinic receptor) and histamine (H_1) are important. Serotonin and adrenergic receptors also may play a role. Anticholinergic drugs (e.g., scopolamine) and antihistaminic drugs (e.g., diphenhydramine) can produce an antimotion sickness, antiemetic effect in people, but are less effective in dogs.

Afferents from the gastrointestinal system may mediate vomiting. Cancer drugs (e.g., cisplatin) injure the GI tract and release serotonin (5-HT_3). Cancer drugs also may stimulate the CRTZ directly.

Neurokinin (Substance P, NK-1) is a recently described neurotransmitter that stimulates vomiting from several sources. NK-1 receptors are found in the emetic center and the CRTZ, but the most important are those receptors in the emetic center. Drugs described as NK-1 receptor blockers (e.g., maropitant, aprepitant) block vomiting from several sources.

Efferents from the emetic center trigger the sequence of events that is familiar: nausea, abdominal contraction, stomach contraction, and vomiting.

PHENOTHIAZINE TRANQUILIZERS. Dopamine is one of the neurotransmitters in the emetic center and CRTZ for stimulating vomiting. Phenothiazine tranquilizers such as chlorpromazine (Thorazine®), prochlorperazine (Compazine®), promethazine, and acepromazine antagonize stimulation from dopamine in the CNS (Table 47.2). In addition to the antidopamine effects, these drugs can block alpha-adrenergic receptors (α_1) in the emetic center. Some phenothiazines also block the histaminic and muscarinic (M_1) receptors. Because of this broad action, and ability to inhibit vomiting from a variety of stimuli, this group of drugs has been called "broad-spectrum" antiemetics. Their side effects may limit clinical use in some patients. These side effects include sedation, altered involuntary motor activity (extrapyramidal signs), and peripheral α-adrenergic receptor blockade (vasodilation).

ANTIMUSCARINIC DRUGS. Drugs that block muscarinic receptors (muscarinic M_1-receptor) include atropine, scopolamine, aminopentamide (Centrine®), and isopropamide (isopropamide is combined with prochlorperazine in Darbazine®) (Table 47.2). These drugs decrease vomiting from various causes, including vomiting caused by vestibular stimulation (motion sickness) and stimulation of the CRTZ. In people, scopolamine has been one of the most effective agents for treating motion sickness (Transderm-Scop®), but it is less effective in dogs and cats. The adverse effects of anticholinergic drugs include xerostomia, decreased stomach emptying, ileus, urine retention, and constipation. These drugs should be used cautiously in patients with glaucoma because there is a risk of increased intraocular pressure. Scopolamine has produced excitement in animals, particularly cats.

ANTIHISTAMINIC DRUGS. The histamine H_1- and H_2-receptor is involved in transmission of vomiting. Histaminic nerve transmission stimulates vomiting from the CRTZ and vestibular apparatus, but apparently this effect is more prominent in dogs than cats. Antihistamines also can produce antimuscarinic (atropinelike) effects as well. Some of the phenothiazine drugs also act on histamine receptors and there is some crossover between these drug groups. Antihistamine drugs administered to control vomiting include diphenhydramine (Benadryl®), dimenhydrinate (Dramamine®), promethazine (Phenergan®, a phenothiazine with antihistamine effects), and cyclizine, (Marezine®) (Table 47.2). Diphenhydramine is the active component of dimenhydrinate. Histamine and antagonists are covered in more detail in Chapter 16.

Adverse Effects. The antihistamines are relatively safe drugs. The most significant side effect of therapy is sedation, but this usually is not undesirable in most patients being treated for vomiting. Sedation occurs because the H_1-receptor regulates sleep-wake cycles. The ethanolamines (diphenhydramine and dimenhydrinate) have the greatest sedative effects. Paradoxically, some of the antihistamines have caused excitement in cats.

METOCLOPRAMIDE (REGLAN®). This drug is also discussed later in the section on prokinetic drugs.

Metoclopramide has antiemetic effects via three mechanisms:

1. Metoclopramide (at low doses) inhibits dopaminergic (D_2) transmission in the CNS, similar to phenothiazines.
2. Metoclopramide has peripheral effects on the GI tract that increase emptying of the stomach and upper duodenum.
3. Metoclopramide (at high doses) inhibits serotonin (5-HT_3) receptors.

5-HT_3 stimulates vomiting in dogs and cats either in the CRTZ or vagal afferent neurons. Metoclopramide is a broad-spectrum antiemetic that has gained popularity in small animal medicine, particularly for animals that vomit because of drug therapy (e.g., cancer drugs). However, for control of vomiting caused by cancer drugs the results have often been disappointing (Fukui et al. 1992).

Pharmacokinetics. There is large variability in the pharmacokinetics of metoclopramide in dogs. The half-life has ranged from about 100 to 190 minutes; the systemic availability of an oral dose is only about 50%.

Adverse Effects. Metoclopramide is a dopamine antagonist and at high dosages it can produce adverse reactions that are similar to those caused by phenothiazine drugs. Adverse CNS effects from metoclopramide include excitement and behavior changes. To produce adequate antiemetic effects from blocking 5-HT receptors, often high doses are needed that increase the risk of extrapyramidal CNS effects attributed to central dopamine (D_2) antagonism.

The increase in GI motility may produce some abdominal discomfort. Because metoclopramide stimulates upper GI motility, it should not be administered if there is an obstruction. Metoclopramide produces transient endocrine changes, including an increase in prolactin.

SEROTONIN ANTAGONISTS. Specific serotonin antagonists include ondansetron (Zofran), granisetron (Kytril), palonosetron (Aloxi), and dolasetron (Anzemet). New drugs in development include tropisetron and azasetron. Of these, *ondansetron* (Zofran®) is the best known of the specific serotonin (5-HT_3) inhibitors. It is most often used as an antiemetic in cancer chemotherapy. The drugs in this group are expensive to use in veterinary patients, but have nevertheless been used to prevent vomiting associated with cancer drugs and from other gastrointestinal diseases. The doses used are 0.5 to 1.0 mg/kg, IV or oral 30 min prior to administration of cancer drugs. Serotonin and antagonists are covered in more detail in Chapter 16.

As mentioned above, metoclopramide at high doses of 1–3 mg/kg can act as a serotonin antagonist and have been used as an IV infusion during cancer chemotherapy to decrease vomiting. As mentioned above, side effects are more likely at these high doses.

GLUCOCORTICOIDS. Glucocorticoids such as dexamethasone have antiemetic properties, possibly by inhibiting prostaglandin synthesis. These drugs are used sometimes in addition to other drugs for decreasing vomiting, particularly when it is caused by cancer chemotherapy. Glucocorticoids are covered in more detail in Chapter 30.

CANNABINOIDS. Cannabinoids have been used in people who have not responded to any other antiemetic drugs (e.g., patients that are receiving anticancer drugs). They have also been used to increase the appetite in patients with terminal disease, cancer, and AIDS. Their use has not been reported in veterinary patients, but they have been used by some veterinarians to increase the appetite in cats.

The site of action for cannabinoids is unknown, but there is some evidence that the active ingredients may affect opiate receptors, or they may affect other receptors in the emetic center. Synthetic marijuana (THC) is available as a prescription drug (dronabinol) for antiemetic therapy; it is marketed as Marinol®. Cannabinoids are relatively well tolerated in people, but side effects include drowsiness, dizziness, ataxia, and disorientation. Withdrawal signs may occur after abrupt discontinuation following repeated doses. For dronabinol, the oral absorption is good, but bioavailability is low due to high first-pass effects. The volume of distribution is very high.

Suggested doses for dronabinol (Marinol) in animals (but untested in clinical trials) are 5 mg/m^2, and increased as needed up to 15 mg/m^2 for antiemetic administration prior to chemotherapy. For appetite stimulation in animals, doses start at 2.5 mg before meals. It is available as 2.5, 5, and 10 mg capsules.

NK-1 RECEPTOR ANTAGONISTS. The neurotransmitter neurokinin-1 (NK-1, also known as Substance P) has several functions (Table 47.3). A new class of antiemetics was approved for use in people for cancer chemotherapy-induced vomiting. Aprepitant (Emend) was the first substance P/neurokinin-1 (NK-1) receptor antagonist (Dando and Perry 2004). It is used primarily with drugs known to be highly emetic, such as cisplatin. This drug is effective because chemotherapy drugs release substance P, which is highly emetic. Other standard treatments for chemotherapy-induced vomiting are dexamethasone plus ondansetron. The cost of one dose of aprepitant is approximately $100 per day. The use of NK-1 receptor antagonists such as aprepitant in dogs was primarily experimental until recently (Wu et al. 2004; Watson et al. 1995; Huskey et al. 2004; Fukuda et al. 1999; de la Puente-Redondo et al. 2007; Vail et al. 2007). In 2007, a new member of this class was approved for use in animals. Maropitant (Cerenia) was registered for use in dogs. It is available as a 10 mg/ml injection to be administered 1 mg/kg once daily SC for up to 5 days, or a tablet 16, 24, 60, or 160 mg to be administered at a dose of 2 mg/kg per day, PO, for up to 5 days. The tablet can also be used to prevent vomiting caused by motion sickness (vestibulitis) at a dose of 8 mg/kg for up to 2 days. The available research has shown maropitant to be an effective antiemetic for a variety of stimuli, including cisplatin (chemotherapy)-induced vomiting, copper sulfate and apomorphine-induced vomiting, motion sickness, and ipecac-induced vomiting (Table 47.4).

TABLE 47.3 Function and location of NK-1 receptors

- Regulates vascular tone
- Regulates vascular permeability
- Respiratory tract—regulates mucus production and bronchial tone
- Tachycardia
- CNS: Locomotor activity, grooming in cats, aggression in cats
- Emetic center

TABLE 47.4 NK-1–receptor blocker (maropitant) effective for vomiting caused by

- Pancreatitis
- Enteritis (dietary indiscretion)
- Cisplatin
- Copper sulfate
- Apomorphine
- Ipecac
- Parvovirus enteritis

The efficacy of maropitant is attributed to its central site of action. It blocks neurokinin-1 (NK-1) receptors in the area of the brain called the *nucleus tractus solitarius*—the site known as the *emetic center*. Input into the emetic center may come from different sources: gastrointestinal tract, higher brain centers, chemoreceptor trigger zone (CRTZ), and vestibular apparatus (motion sickness). These inputs also utilize a variety of neurotransmitters: dopamine, histamine, acetylcholine, and serotonin. Traditionally, to block emesis from these stimuli, multiple drugs may be needed: antihistamines, antidopamine drugs (e.g., metoclopramide), dopamine antagonists (e.g., phenothiazines), and serotonin antagonists (e.g., ondansetron). Because NK-1 inhibitors—such as maropitant—block input from multiple sources regardless of the input *they are considered broad spectrum* in action.

In clinical and research trials, maropitant has been effective to treat and prevent chemotherapy-induced vomiting in dogs (Vail et al. 2007; de la Puente-Redondo 2007; Benchaoui et al. 2007) and a wide range of stimuli such as viral disease, food and toxin ingestion, enteropathy, and other diseases (de la Puente-Redondo et al. 2007). It was more effective than metoclopramide in this trial.

Pharmacokinetics. Maropitant is extensively metabolized by the liver and there is little clearance by the kidney. No dose adjustments are necessary in patients with compromised renal function. Absorption from SC administration is rapid and complete (91% absorption), but oral absorption is limited by the first-pass metabolic effects (24% at 2 mg/kg and 37% at 8 mg/kg) (Benchaoui et al. 2007). The half-life is 7.75 hours and 4–5.5 hours after SC and oral administration, respectively. However, the effects persist for at least 24 hours after a dose, presumably because of binding to the CNS NK-1 receptor that maintains the drug at the site of action. Penetration across the blood-brain barrier has been demonstrated (de la Puente-Redondo 2007), which is necessary for activity in the emetic center.

Adverse Effects. There are NK-1, -2, and -3 receptors throughout the body. Maropitant has little binding affinity to NK-receptors, other than NK-1; it also does not bind to other CNS receptors such as GABA-, opiate-, adrenergic-, serotonin-, histamine-, muscarinic-, or dopamine-receptors. Although NK-1 receptors are involved in a large number of other physiologic and behavioral responses, at doses used for antiemesis in dogs, there were no adverse effects associated with these other functions.

Compared to other antiemetic drugs, maropitant has had a good safety profile. No clinically significant adverse events have been reported in the clinical trials with maropitant conducted in dogs thus far. Maropitant studies in cats have not been reported.

GASTROINTESTINAL PROKINETIC DRUGS

Prokinetic drugs are drugs that increase gastrointestinal motility. For a review of conditions in which prokinetic drugs are used, see Washabau and Hall (1997).

METOCLOPRAMIDE, (REGLAN®, MAXERAN®).

Metoclopramide has multiple actions. It is a dopamine (D_2) antagonist, serotonin (5-HT_4) agonist and serotonin (5-HT_3) antagonist. Among the proposed mechanisms of metoclopramide is an increase in the release of acetylcholine in the GI tract, possibly via a prejunctional mechanism. It also may increase motility of gastric smooth muscle by increasing sensitivity of the cholinergic response. Since it also is a dopamine antagonist, it may antagonize dopamine's (D_2) inhibitory action on GI motility.

Metoclopramide increases gastric emptying, increases the tone of the esophageal sphincter, and stimulates motility of the duodenum. It has less effect on distal segments of the intestine. Metoclopramide acts centrally to inhibit dopamine in the CRTZ, which is responsible for antiemetic effects. In people, metoclopramide also has been used to treat hiccups and lactation deficiency.

Side effects from metoclopramide are related to CNS effects. They can include excitement (seen in horses, for example), anxiety, and involuntary muscle movements. There are also endocrine effects: There is a transient increase in prolactin and aldosterone. *Since some breast cancers are prolactin-dependent, there has been some concern about the carcinogenicity of this drug in women.*

Use in Small Animals. In dogs metoclopramide has been used as an antiemetic more commonly than other drugs. Although it has been used to promote GI motility as well, this effect is less established than previously thought. For example, it is of little benefit to increase stomach emptying in disorders of gastroparesis or chronic regurgitation. It also has been used to stimulate normal upper motility following surgery (e.g., corrective surgery for gastric dilatation), but one study showed that metoclopramide did *not* change gastric motor activity to promote gastric emptying in dogs with gastric dilatation volvulus (GDV) (Hall et al. 1996). In another study, it reduced, but did not prevent gastroesophageal reflux in anesthetized dogs at a dose of 1 mg/kg (Wilson et al. 2006). Doses are in the range of 0.25 to 0.5 mg/kg, q8–12h, but they have been increased to 1–2 mg/kg.

Use in Large Animals. The clinical use of metoclopramide in large animals has not been as common as in small animals. Metoclopramide has little usefulness in cattle, although it may increase the motility of the rumen in cattle and sheep. It has been used successfully in some cattle with functional pyloric stenosis (Braun et al. 1990), but was not effective in calves (0.1 mg/kg IM). At doses higher than 0.1 mg/kg in calves it caused severe neurologic side effects (Wittek and Constable 2005).

Use in Horses. Some equine surgeons have used infusions of metoclopramide (0.125–0.25 mg/kg/hr) added to IV fluids to reduce postoperative ileus in horses (Gerring and Hunt 1986). It may stimulate small intestine—but not large bowel—motility, but this has little benefit for horses with intestinal ileus (Sojka et al. 1988). Undesirable side effects in horses have been common, and include behavioral changes and abdominal pain. Since this drug transiently increases prolactin secretion, there has been interest in using this drug for treating agalactia in animals, but efficacy has not been determined.

DOMPERIDONE (MOTILIUM, EQUIDONE). Domperidone has been available as a 10 mg tablet outside the U.S. as a prokinetic drug. Its mechanism of action and GI prokinetic effects are similar to metoclopramide, but its efficacy has not been very impressive in animals. A difference between metoclopramide and domperidone is that the latter does not cross the blood-brain barrier. Therefore, adverse CNS effects are not as much of a problem compared to metoclopramaide in horses. It may have antiemetic properties, but only if the receptor blocked is associated with with the CRTZ. The CRTZ in the area postrema of the brain is not protected by the blood-brain barrier.

Use in Small Animals. The use is not reported, but a suggested dose is 2 to 5 mg/animal.

Use in Horses. Domperidone has been investigated for use in horses to treat fescue toxicity and agalactia. Fescue toxicosis is caused by a fungus that produces a toxin that induces reproductive problems in horses. The action of domperidone to increase lactation is through the stimulation of prolactin. Although not yet registered for use by the FDA, the equine formulation of domperidone, Equidone oral gel, 11%, is listed "for prevention and treatment of fescue toxicosis and related agalactia in periparturient mares." The dose administered to horses is 1.1 mg/kg, daily PO, starting 10 days before the scheduled foaling date. (This dose is equivalent to 5 ml per 500 kg—5 ml per horse—daily, PO of the 11% oral gel.) Administration should continue until foaling. If there is not adequate milk production after foaling, continue for 5 additional days. Do not administer with stomach antacids such as omeprazole, cimetidine, or antacids.

CISAPRIDE. In July 2000, cisapride (formerly called Propulsid®) was removed from the market because of serious cardiac adverse events, and some deaths in people. The effect is caused by cardiac arrhythmias. The drug sponsor has no plans to market this drug to veterinarians, but there is continued interest among veterinarians and it is still available via compounding pharmacists. Until other new replacement drugs become available, such as prucalopride, veterinarians will rely on compounded formulations or consider alternative drugs.

The reviews by Washabau and Hall (1995) and Van Neuten (1992) describe the details of its mechanism of action and clinical effects. Cisapride has greater prokinetic effects in comparison to the other drugs discussed thus far. Its mechanism is believed to be as an *agonist* for the 5-hydroxytryptamine (5-HT_4) receptor on myenteric neurons (5-HT_4 ordinarily stimulates cholinergic transmission in the myenteric neurons). (Serotonin and antagonists/agonists are covered in more detail in Chapter 16.) However, cisapride may also be an *antagonist* for the 5-HT_3 receptor. Via these mechanisms—or independently—cisapride may enhance release of acetylcholine at the myenteric plexus. There is evidence that, in cats, cisapride directly stimulates smooth muscle motility via an unknown noncholinergic mechanism (Washabau and Summarco 1996). Cisapride increases the motility of the stomach, small intestine, and colon. It accelerates the transit of contents in the bowel and intestines.

Pharmacokinetics. Oral absorption is variable because of extensive metabolism. The oral absorption in dogs and cats ranges from 30–60%. In horses, rectal absorption has been attempted, but the amount absorbed systemically is negligible (Cook et al. 1997).

Elimination half-life is variable, but ranges from an average of approximately 5 hours in dogs and cats to a much faster rate in large animals—2 hours or less in horses and ruminants. The volume of distribution is high in small animals (>4 l/kg) and approximately 1.5 l/kg in large animals.

Use in Dogs. In dogs at a dose of 0.1 mg/kg (range 0.08–1.25 mg/kg) orally, it stimulates the esophagus, stomach, small intestine, and colon, with a duration of effect of about 3 hours. Routine clinical doses have ranged from 0.1 to 0.5 mg/kg every 8–12 hours.

Clinical use in dogs has included treatment for gastroesophageal reflux, delayed gastric emptying, and small bowel motility disorders. Although cisapride has been used by some veterinarians for treatment of megaesophagus in dogs, the response is usually poor. The canine esophagus is striated muscle, with no smooth muscle to directly respond to the medication.

Use in Cats. Experiments have shown that cisapride will cause stimulation of the entire GI tract in cats. Of particular interest is the effect of cisapride on colonic smooth muscle. Cisapride will stimulate this motility and has been used for treating chronic constipation. By contrast, metoclopramide has no effect on colonic smooth muscle. The dose of cisapride in cats is approximately 2.5 mg per cat, two or three times daily. Doses as high as 1 mg/kg every 8 hours, or 1.5 mg/kg every 12 hours have been recommended by some investigators (LeGrange et al. 1997).

Use in Horses. In horses cisapride increases the motility of the left dorsal colon and improves ileocecocolonic junction coordination. In contrast to metoclopramide, cisapride has fewer side effects at doses needed to affect the GI tract and greater effects on the jejunum and colon than metoclopramide. Many investigators believe that it has a place in the postoperative management of horses that have undergone abdominal surgery. One dose tested to be effective was 0.1 mg/kg, IV. At this dose, the effects appear to persist for approximately 2 hours. Oral administration is usually not possible in these horses because of gastric reflux and absorption after oral administration in a horse with gastric reflux probably is questionable.

Availability of Formulations. The previously available tablet was a 10 mg tablet from Janssen Pharmaceutica. Although cisapride is insoluble in most aqueous solutions, solubility is possible in acidic solutions. An IV form may be created by preparing a 4 mg/ml solution in tartaric acid by a reputable compounding pharmacist. The preparation of this formulation was described in the publication by Cook et al. (1997). To prepare this solution, 40 mg of cisapride is combined with 1 ml of 0.4 M tartaric acid. After the cisapride is dissolved, dilute with water to obtain a total volume of 10 ml (Cook et al. 1997).

Oral formulations for cats have been prepared from the bulk powder administered in a capsule, via a suspension in a flavored vehicle or dissolved in cod liver oil.

Side Effects and Interactions. Adverse effects have not been reported in animals; however, abdominal discomfort has been observed when animals received high doses. In safety studies, dogs have tolerated high doses (40 mg/kg) for prolonged periods without problems.

In people, high plasma concentrations have caused cardiac arrhythmias. The arrhythmias are caused by prolonged QT intervals, presumably from blockade of potassium channels. This can lead to serious arrhythmias and has been responsible for deaths in people. These reactions have not been reported for animals. Nevertheless, one should be cautious about combining cisapride with drugs such as itraconazole and ketoconazole that may increase plasma concentrations by interfering with metabolism.

TEGASEROD (ZELNORM). Tegaserod use in animals has not been reported. It was removed from the human market in April 2007. It was used as a motility modifying drug to treat irritable bowel syndrome. Its action is believed to be similar to that of cisapride—a partial agonist of serotonin (5-HT_4)—but it has little effect on HT_3 or dopamine receptors. After stimulating 5-HT_4 receptors it stimulates coordinated motility by stimulating other neurons and release of other mediators. It increases gastric emptying and small bowel transit. The dose in people was 6 mg twice daily.

BETHANECHOL (URECHOLINE). Many of the formulations of bethanechol have been discontinued and are no longer marketed. Some generic forms may still remain and veterinarians have also obtained it through compounding pharmacies. This drug is a cholinergic agonist that has been used to nonspecifically stimulate smooth muscle. It binds to muscarinic receptors and initiates GI smooth muscle contractions, but its actions are nonspecific. In contrast to cisapride or metoclopramide, bethanechol has a more pronounced effect on motility of the ileocecocolic region in cattle (0.7 mg/kg). In horses, bethanechol increases gastric emptying at a dose of 0.025 mg/kg IV (Ringger et al. 1996). One of its other uses has been to stimulate contraction of bladder smooth muscle in animals that have a failure to completely empty their urinary bladder when voiding. Adverse effects are common and include diarrhea and other consequences of cholinergic stimulation.

NEOSTIGMINE (PROSTIGMIN). Neostigmine inactivates the enzyme acetylcholinesterase, which results in inhibition of degradation of acetylcholine at the synapse. It prolongs the action of acetylcholine and may directly stimulate cholinergic receptors. It is short acting. In horses, its use is discouraged because it may actually decrease intestinal propulsive contractions, delay gastric emptying, and cause abdominal discomfort.

One of the other uses of neostigmine in animals is for the treatment of neuromuscular diseases such as myasthenia gravis. Its adverse effects are significant, and include diarrhea, salivation, respiratory difficulty, vomiting, and muscle twitching. (Usually, another anticholinesterase drug, pyridostigmine is preferred for treating myasthenia gravis because it has fewer side effects.)

H_2-RECEPTOR ANTAGONISTS. H_2-receptor blockers such as ranitidine and nizatidine have prokinetic effects on intestinal smooth muscle in animals. These drugs are discussed later in the section on antiulcer drugs.

ERYTHROMYCIN. Erythromycin is a macrolide antibiotic widely used to treat bacterial infections. It has long been associated with vomiting and regurgitation in small animals as an adverse consequence of treatment. This effect on the stomach appears to be caused by stomach contraction and expulsion at high doses. But, at low doses, it can cause nonspecific stimulation of GI motility. Not all macrolide antibiotics exhibit this property because it requires a unique chemical structure that not all drugs in this class possess. In people erythromycin has been used to promote gastric motility and increase emptying in patients with diabetic gastroparesis. It also has been used in conjunction with enteral feeding in critical care patients (Hawkyard and Koerner 2007).

The action of erythromycin appears to be related to an increase in activation of motilin receptors, via release of endogenous motilin, or via cholinergic mechanisms in the upper GI tract (Hall and Washabau 1997; Lester et al. 1998; Hawkyard and Koerner 2007). (Antimicrobial details on erythromycin are covered in detail in Chapter 37.) Because most of the motilin receptors are on the stomach and proximal small intestine, responses to erythromycin may not be as profound in the distal GI tract. The dose that produces this effect in animals is in the range of 1 mg/kg or less—much lower than the antibacterial dose. In calves, doses of 8.8 mg/kg IM increased rumen motility (Wittek and Constable 2005). It was effective for stimulating motility in horses (Ringger et al. 1996) and has been examined for clinical indications, such as stimulating gastric emptying and increasing intestinal motility.

Clinical responses to erythromycin in horses have been somewhat disappointing. One study showed that responses to erythromycin in horses that had undergone surgery were different from horses that were healthy (Roussel et al. 2000). Therefore, clinical responses may not be as great in horses with motility problems as they are in normal horses. There is a concern that erythromycin may cause diarrhea in some horses through the effect on the normal bacterial flora of the intestine. An additional concern is that routine use may promote resistance.

LIDOCAINE. Lidocaine is a well-known local anesthetic. (Local anesthetics are covered in more detail in Chapter 14.) It is used for local infiltration for minor surgical procedures and to treat cardiac arrhythmias. Intravenous infusions of lidocaine also improve intestinal motility in horses (Table 47.5). Lidocaine has been used in horses

TABLE 47.5 Action of lidocaine on GI tract

- Suppresses transmission of sympathetic tone
- Prevents sympathetic reflexive spinal and peritoneal inhibition of sympathetic stimulation
- Produces direct excitatory effects on smooth muscle of intestine
- Suppresses centrally mediated hyperalgesia
- Antiendotoxin and antiinflammatory effects

TABLE 47.6 Antiulcer drugs: Clinical uses

- Gastritis
- Gastric ulcers
- Duodenal ulcers
- GI ulcer prevention
- Esophagitis
- Mast cell tumors
- Hypergastrinemic syndromes

postsurgically to reduce postoperative ileus. Postoperative ileus in horses is a widespread clinical problem that may be caused by 1) sympathetic stimulation, 2) pain, or 3) inflammation. These effects inhibit smooth muscle motility in the intestine and lidocaine may work by suppressing this transmission (see Table 47.5). Yet another view is that lidocaine does not have a direct prokinetic effect, but rather restores motility via other mechanisms (Cook and Bilkslager 2008). These authors presented evidence that in horses lidocaine restores motility by inhibiting intestinal inflammation and re-perfusion injury.

In one study (Malone et al. 2006) lidocaine administration to horses produced less reflux and shorter time of hospitalization. Infusions of lidocaine have decreased postoperative ileus either through a direct effect, or via suppression of painful stimuli. Doses in horses are 1.3 mg/kg loading dose (bolus), followed by 0.05 mg/kg/min IV infusion.

Adverse Effects. As with the other uses of lidocaine, systemic administration may produce adverse events. The most common in horses have been muscle fasciculations, ataxia, and seizures. If signs are observed, decrease rate of infusion.

NEW DRUGS TO PROMOTE INTESTINAL MOTILITY.

Mosapride is a 5-hydroxytryptamine-4 (5-HT_4) receptor agonist. It has been studied in experimental horses and demonstrated to increase motility of the small intestine and cecum at a dose of 1.5–2 mg/kg PO (Sasaki et al. 2005).

Newer approaches to treating postoperative ileus in animals has focused on blocking intestinal opiate receptors (μ-receptors). (Opiate drugs and antagonists are covered in more detail in Chapter 12.) It is well established that activation of opiate μ-receptors in the intestinal smooth muscle decreases propulsive motility. Expression of μ-opiate receptors has been found in the submucosal plexus, myenteric plexus, and longitudinal muscle of the ileum. This effect has been used to treat some forms of diarrhea with opiate-agonists (e.g., loperamide). (The role of opiates to treat diarrhea is discussed later in this chapter.) However, administration of opiate analgesics postoperatively (Boscan et al. 2006; Sojka et al. 1988), or increased levels of endogenous opioids (endorphins) stimulate these receptors to inhibit intestinal motility causing postoperative ileus (DeHaven-Hudkins et al. 2007). Opiate antagonists can restore motility to colonic intestine of ponies (Roger et al. 1985). However, use of naloxone will also cross the blood-brain barrier to diminish the analgesic effect of opioids.

Opioid antagonists are being explored for use, primarily to limit the adverse effects of opioids and pain on gastrointestinal motility. These agents are considered *peripheral* opioid antagonists, rather than *central* opioid antagonists. They do not produce a central effect because they are unable to cross the blood-brain barrier. Such agents include *alvimopan* and *methylnaltrexone*. They are being investigated to be used as therapeutic agents to treat gastrointestinal motility problems associated with opioid analgesic use as well as other stress or pain syndromes that cause a decrease in gastrointestinal motility (for example, postoperative ileus) (DeHaven-Hudkins et al. 2007; Taguchi et al. 2001). These agents are capable of restoring gastrointestinal motility, but preserving opioid-mediated analgesia. Methylnaltrexone is now registered for use in people (Relistor) as an injection. It is administered at a dose of 0.15 mg/kg SC, once every 24–28 hours. Alvimopan has advantages over methylnaltrexone with respect to potency and duration of activity.

DRUGS FOR TREATMENT OF GI ULCERS IN ANIMALS

Histamine H_2-receptor antagonists, sucralfate, proton pump inhibitors (omeprazole), and antacids remain the principal drugs used to manage gastrointestinal ulceration in small and large animals (Table 47.6; Fig. 47.1). The medical management of ulcer diseases will not be covered in this section, but readers are referred to other references for this information: The clinical description and treatment of ulcer disease in horses was thoroughly reviewed

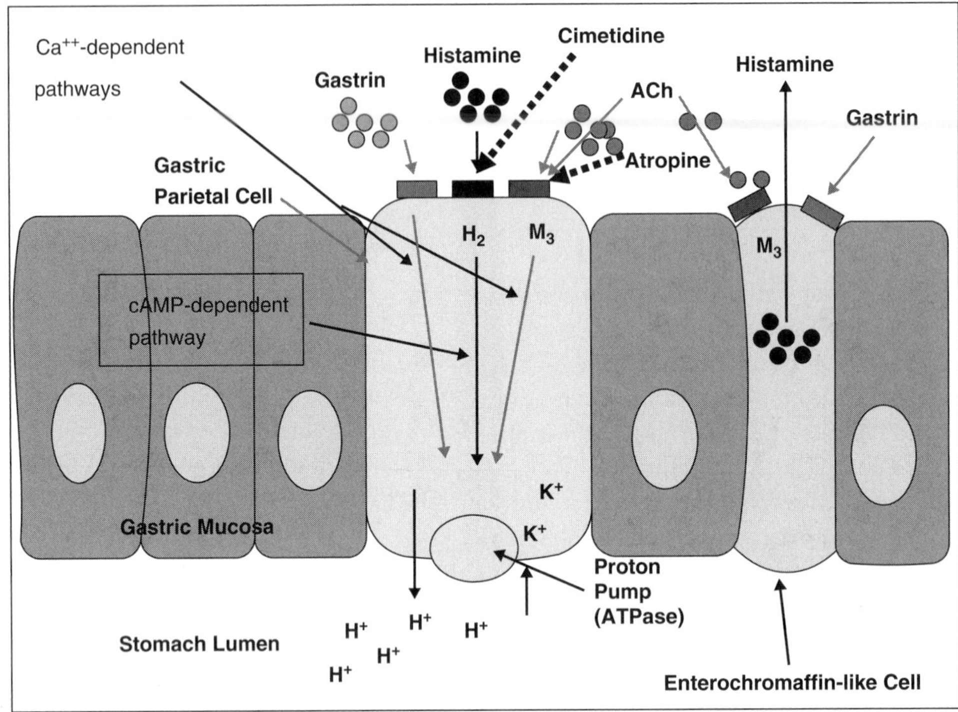

FIG. 47.1 Action of stomach antisecretory drugs. Action of H_2-receptor antagonists and proton pump inhibitors are shown. See text for details.

by Merritt (2003). Treatment in small animals was reviewed by Papich (1993) and Matz (1995). Two recent reviews on gastroprotection and ulcer treatment in dogs are available in the papers by Henderson and Webster (2006). A thorough review of H_2-receptor antagonists is found in the article by Feldman and Burton (1990).

Because many of the ulcerative diseases encountered in veterinary medicine are induced by drugs that inhibit prostaglandin synthesis (NSAIDs), one should be familiar with the role of prostaglandins in the GI tract, how their synthesis is inhibited, and treatments used to maintain the protective effect of prostaglandins in the GI tract. Veterinarians also should be familiar with the normal physiologic role of protective mucus layer in the stomach, the cytoprotective mechanisms, role of bicarbonate secretion, and the normal mechanisms that restore epithelial cells in the stomach and intestine. These factors were reviewed by Allen et al., (1993) several years ago, but are still relevant today. When these protective factors become disrupted or compromised, ulcers can occur in animals. Gastrointestinal ulcers are a major health problem in horses, pigs, dogs, cats, and zoo animals. Conditions that increase the risk of gastrointestinal ulceration are administration of ulcerogenic drugs (NSAIDs, corticosteroids, and stomach irritants), stress, disrupted mucosal blood supply, and inflammatory diseases.

Gastrointestinal ulceration is an important medical problem in horses, in which the prevalence in animals involved in showing and racing has been listed as 81–93% and as high as 100% in some studies. In Thoroughbreds and Standardbreds the prevalence is 80–95%; in show horses it may be as high as 58%. Factors such as stall confinement, intense exercise, diet (high energy concentration in diet), and racing stress may be factors. Location of ulcers in horses is primarily in the squamous epithelium (nonglandular portion). Factors that contribute to ulcers are the intermittent feeding schedule and high stomach acidity. In sick foals, ulcers are common. Factors that contribute to ulcers in foals are NSAIDs, stress, and sepsis.

ANTACIDS. The common antacids are bases of either aluminum, magnesium, or calcium. Examples include aluminum hydroxide, $Al(OH)_3$, magnesium hydroxide, $Mg(OH)_2$, and calcium carbonate, $CaCO_3$ (e.g., Tums). These drugs neutralize stomach acid to form water and a neutral salt. They have no systemic effects. In addition to their acid-neutralizing ability, antacids may benefit patients by decreasing pepsin activity, binding to bile acids in the stomach, and stimulating local prostaglandin (e.g., PGE_2) synthesis.

Formulations. Commonly available antacid preparations (e.g., Maalox, Mylanta, DiGel) are combinations of magnesium hydroxide and aluminum hydroxide to optimize the buffering abilities of each compound. These combinations balance the adverse effects of constipation from aluminum hydroxide and the laxative effect from magnesium hydroxide.

Adverse Effects. Adverse effects are rare because they are seldom administered long-term. Additionally, antacids are not absorbed and therefore lack serious systemic effects. In animals with renal failure, magnesium accumulation may be a problem. Antacids will interfere with the oral absorption of other drugs (e.g., tetracyclines, fluoroquinolones, and digoxin), if administered concurrently.

Dosing Recommendations. Dose recommendations vary, but empirically, 5–10 ml six times daily for small animals is often cited, regardless of the animal's size or product used. Doses of 180 to 250 ml have been administered to adult horses, but only suppressed acidity for 45 min to 2 hours (Murray 1997). A dose of 30–60 ml for calves and foals has been recommended. For the treatment of acid rumen, magnesium hydroxide has been administered orally at a dose of 225–440 grams per adult cow, or mineral oil at 4 liters per rumen. For the treatment of grain overload, antacids have been administered at a dose of 450 grams per rumen, repeated every 6–8 hr.

HISTAMINE H_2-RECEPTOR ANTAGONISTS. Blockade of H_2 receptors and subsequent inhibition of gastric acidity correlates with ulcer healing in the stomach and duodenum even though evidence—based on data generated from controlled studies—is lacking. The clinical impression among veterinarians indicates that cimetidine, ranitidine, and famotidine are beneficial for the treatment of gastric and duodenal ulceration, gastric erosions, esophageal reflux disease, and gastritis in animals. Drugs vary in their potency (Table 47.7) but all can effectively suppress stomach acid.

Mechanism of Action. Acid secretion is stimulated by three receptors: 1) gastrin receptor, 2) histamine type-2 (H_2 receptor), and 3) cholinergic (muscarinic) receptor (M_3). Stimulation of acid secretion occurs via stimulation of all three receptors. H_2-receptor antagonists (e.g., cimetidine, Tagamet®; ranitidine, Zantac®) effectively block gastric acid secretion from parietal cells by blocking the H_2-receptor.

TABLE 47.7 Potency of acid-suppressant drugs

Drug	Relative Potency
Cimetidine (Tagamet)	1
Ranitidine (Zantac)	4–10
Nizatidine (Axid)	4–10
Famotidine (Pepcid)	20–50

Use in Small Animals. Cimetidine at doses of 10 mg/kg (IV, IM, or orally) administered to dogs will suppress acid secretion for 3 to 5 hours. Because ranitidine has a longer half-life, it may not have to be administered as often as cimetidine. Ranitidine doses of 2 mg/kg (IV, IM, or orally) will suppress acid secretion for up to 8 hours. Famotidine (Pepcid®) has been used at 0.5 mg/kg every 12–24 hr, but doses of 0.1 to 0.2 mg/kg q12h are probably equally effective. Despite the availability of pharmacokinetic information, a precise dose interval for the drugs listed has not been established because the optimum duration or extent of acid suppression for ulcer healing to occur is not known.

Use in Horses. Suppression of gastric acidity in horses was reviewed by Murray (1997). These drugs are not absorbed orally in horses as well as in dogs (Duran and Ravis 1993), with a systemic availability of only 14 to 30%, and the high oral doses for large animals reflect this difference (Sams et al. 1997). Cimetidine is administered to horses at 40–60 mg/kg/day. Ranitidine is used in horses at a dose of 2.2 to 6.6 mg/kg q6–8h (Holland et al. 1997). In clinically normal foals, ranitidine at 6.6 mg/kg, PO, or 2 mg/kg IV suppresses acid secretion for 8 hours and 4 hours, respectively (Sanchez et al. 1998).

Use in Calves. Cimetidine and ranitidine have been used in calves to maintain the pH of the abomasum >3.5 for 75% of the dosing interval (Ahmed et al. 2001). Recommended oral doses are cimetidine 100 mg/kg q8h, or ranitidine 50 mg/kg q8h.

Adverse Effects. Generally, histamine H_2-receptor antagonists have a good safety record. Adverse effects reported in people include antiandrogenic effects, decreased reproductive performance, central nervous system toxicity, and bacterial overgrowth in the stomach. These effects are rare and have not been cited as a serious problem in veterinary patients. There have been anecdotal reports of famotidine injection producing hemolytic anemia in cats. However, the conclusion from a clinical study was that when administered IV over 5 minutes, there was not a risk (de Brito Galvao & Trepanier, 2008). Drug interactions are possible because cimetidine inhibits the clearance of other drugs via its action as a hepatic oxidation enzyme inhibitor (microsomal enzyme cytochrome P450 inhibitor). Ranitidine and others are less likely to cause such a reaction.

Other Effects of H_2-Receptor Antagonists. Histamine H_2-blocking drugs have been used for other conditions in addition to suppressing stomach acid. Some evidence suggests that cimetidine strengthens the gastric mucosal defenses against ulceration (e.g., increases bicarbonate secretion), and enhances cytoprotection, but the relationship of these effects to ulcer healing are not well understood.

Effects on Smooth Muscle Activity. Acid secretion inhibits stomach contractions. In experimental dogs, administration of cimetidine normalized the stomach contractions that were inhibited by stimulation of acid secretion in the stomach. Therefore, H_2-receptor antagonists may have a role in promoting an emptying of the stomach (Hayashi et al. 1990). In addition, ranitidine and nizatidine, but not cimetidine or famotidine, stimulate motility and increase gastric emptying and colonic motility via an anticholinesterase (AchE) action. Because of these motility effects, ranitidine has been used to stimulate GI motility as a prokinetic agent in animals. This has been more common after the prokinetic drug cisapride was withdrawn from the market. (Cisapride is discussed further earlier in this chapter.)

Immunologic Effects. Cimetidine can block H_2-receptors on suppressor T-lymphocytes, which increases lymphocyte responses to mitogen stimulation (Mavligit 1987). This effect has been applied clinically in the immunologic treatment of patients with tumors (Goetz et al. 1990), but the clinical benefit for most uses has been controversial. In people, the administration of cimetidine may accelerate healing of herpes lesions in immunocompromised patients.

Antiallergic Effects. Histamine H_2-blockers may decrease the effects of histamine on blood vessels, and may alleviate some inflammation due to allergy. However, when used as a sole treatment, the clinical response has not been encouraging. Ordinarily when antihistamine effects are desired for treating allergic conditions, histamine type 1 (H_1) antagonists are administered.

SUCRALFATE (CARAFATE®). Sucralfate dissociates in the acid milieu of the stomach to sucrose octasulfate and aluminum hydroxide (Fig. 47.2). Sucrose octasulfate polymerizes to a viscous, sticky substance that creates a protective effect by binding to ulcerated mucosa. It protects the mucosa by preventing back diffusion of hydrogen

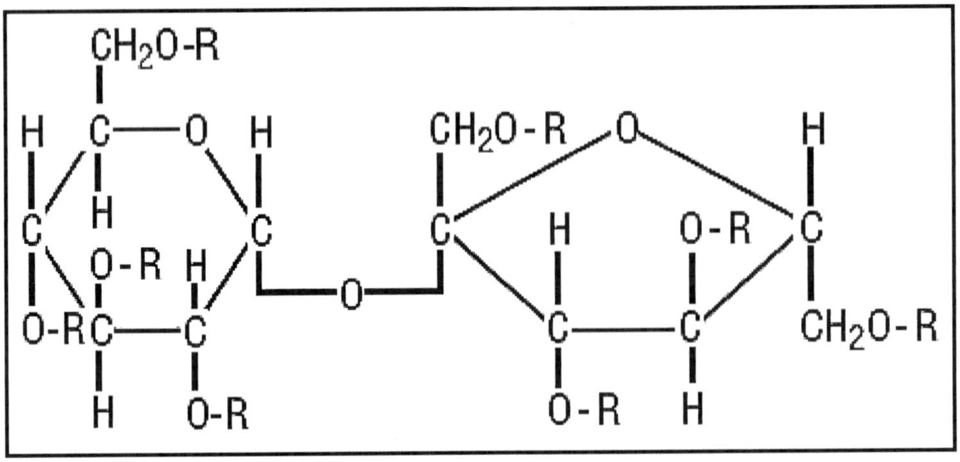

FIG. 47.2 Sucralfate structure.

ions and also inactivates pepsin and adsorbs bile acid. Additionally, sucralfate increases the mucosal synthesis of prostaglandins, which has a cytoprotective role and may promote healing. Increase in the epidermal growth factor may contribute to ulcer healing.

Clinical Use. Sucralfate has been used for the prevention and treatment of gastric and intestinal ulceration and gastritis in both small and large animals. Some veterinarians have used it to prevent or treat ulcers associated with NSAIDs. Despite this common use, there is little evidence of its efficacy for preventing NSAID-induced ulcers. Because sucralfate is not absorbed, it is virtually free of adverse effects. The most common side effect associated with its use in people has been constipation. Dosage regimens for sucralfate have been extrapolated from human dosages. Doses administered are as follows: 250 mg (one-quarter tablet) to cats two to three times daily, 500 mg to 1 gram to dogs, and 4 gm orally to foals.

Drug Interactions. Even though sucralfate has some "coating action," this does not prevent oral absorption of drugs from the intestine. However, sucralfate contains aluminum and may interfere with absorption of some drugs. For example, aluminum will chelate fluoroquinolone and tetracycline drugs and prevent absorption.

PROTON PUMP INHIBITORS (PPI). The proton pump inhibitors (PPI) inhibit the H^+/K^+ proton pump (H^+/K^+ ATP-ase) at the luminal surface of the parietal cell that secretes hydrogen ions into the stomach lumen. The most commonly used drug in this class is omeprazole (Prilosec, GastroGuard, UlcerGuard), which was registered for humans in 1989 and more recently for horses. Other drugs available are listed in Table 47.8. There are no differences in efficacy that have been reported among these drugs.

TABLE 47.8 Proton pump inhibitors (PPI)

- Omeprazole (Prilosec) 20 mg capsule
- Lansoprazole (Prevacid) 20 mg tablet
- Rabeprazole (Aciphex) 20 mg tablet and IV
- Pantoprazole (Protonix) 40 mg tablet
- Esomeprazole (Nexium) 20, 40 mg capsules

Acid Suppression and Efficacy. The proton pump inhibitors are potent acid suppressing drugs (10–20 times more than cimetidine) with effects that persist after plasma concentrations have declined. These drugs are weak bases that favor accumulation in the acidic environment of the parietal cells. After systemic absorption, they become trapped in the acidic parietal cells of the stomach (up to 1000 times) because of ionization inside the acidic parietal cell. The effect of one dose may persist for greater than 24 hours in dogs and 22 hours in foals. However, there may be a delayed onset before they achieve maximal efficacy.

There is evidence in humans that these drugs are superior to other antisecretory drugs such as H_2-antagonists for treatment and prevention of ulcers caused by NSAIDs. In human studies, omeprazole has had better healing rates in comparison to other antiulcer drugs—such as H_2-receptor blockers—for some types of ulcers and esophagitis. In addition, these drugs have an inhibitory effect on the bacteria *Helicobacter pylori*, which is a cause of gastritis and ulcers in people.

Recently, omeprazole has become available without prescription (Prilosec-OTC). There are several new drugs that produce the same action on the proton pump (see Table 47.8). One of the most popular of these drugs in human medicine is esomeprazole magnesium (Nexium). Esomeprazole is simply the S-isomer of omeprazole. Twenty mg of esomeprazole is more effective than 20 mg of omeprazole, because it essentially contains twice as much of the active drug (the S-isomer). Otherwise, there is no difference between these drugs.

Use in Small Animals. Omeprazole has been used in dogs that need potent, long-acting acid suppression, dogs with NSAID-induced ulcers, or dogs that fail to respond to other antiulcer drugs (Jenkins and DeNovo 1991). Omeprazole is available as a 20 mg capsule. A dose of 1 mg/kg q24h maintained the pH in the stomach ≥3, which is the critical range for healing ulcers (Bersenas et al. 2005). Veterinarians have used dosages of 0.7 mg/kg/day, or alternatively: dogs under 5 kg, 5 mg per dog; dogs under 20 kg, 10 mg per dog; and for dogs over 20 kg, 20 mg per dog. Each dose is administered once daily.

Omeprazole is available in capsules containing granules, which protects the drug from acid degradation. If the granules are crushed, the drug can be inactivated by stomach acid. Therefore, if the capsule is opened, one should ensure that the granules are not crushed, or administer the initial doses together with an H_2-blocker to prevent breakdown by the stomach acid. Once omeprazole has been absorbed, stomach acid will be inhibited to a sufficient extent to allow subsequent administrations.

There has been less reported on the administration to cats compared to dogs. There is no evidence published to indicate that proton pump inhibitors are unsafe in cats. Doses are similar to those used in dogs.

Use in Horses. Omeprazole suppresses acid secretion in horses and is used to treat and prevent ulcers. One mg/kg/day is needed to inhibit acid secretion (Andrews et al. 1999) and 1.4 to 2 mg/kg is needed for a more consistent effect (Baker and Gerring 1993; Murray 1997). Four mg/kg PO suppressed acid secretion in foals for 22 hours. Omeprazole (4 mg/kg PO, q24h) was significantly better than ranitidine (6.6 mg/kg PO, q8h) for healing ulcers (Lester et al. 2005).

Omeprazole is approved for this use as GastroGard®, an oral paste for horses at a dose of 4 mg/kg once daily for 4 weeks, and for prevention of ulcers the dose is 2 mg/kg once daily. Recently, an over-the-counter (OTC) form of this drug for horses has become available (UlcerGuard). The dose and concentration is the same as the prescription drug (GastroGuard). If the dosing formulation is altered by compounding, degradation may occur in the stomach, which renders the drug ineffective (Nieto et al. 2002). Three to five days of administration are required for maximal suppression of acid secretion. To promote ulcer healing in horses, the pH of the stomach should be maintained above 3.5 (Andrews et al. 1999).

Adverse Effects. The proton pump inhibitors can produce complete inhibition of acid secretion. There is no evidence that achlorhydria (lack of stomach acid) is, in itself, harmful. However, decreased stomach acid has been implicated as a cause of bacterial overgrowth in the stomach and intestines. The true cause-and-effect relationship in animals between proton pump inhibitors and gastrointestinal bacterial overgrowth has not been established. Another concern is that if bacteria are allowed to populate in the stomach as a result of stomach acid suppression, this may produce a risk if an animal aspirates stomach contents (aspiration pneumonia). Such a risk is possible if proton pump inhibitors are administered to animals prone to aspiration pneumonia, such as dogs with megaesophagus.

The long-term use (>8 weeks) of proton pump inhibitors is discouraged because of increased gastrin levels. Lack of negative feedback produces higher gastrin levels in animals. This has increased risk of gastric tumors in laboratory animals. However, there is no evidence that long-term use has been detrimental in veterinary patients.

Drug Interactions. Proton pump inhibitors are inhibitors of cytochrome P450 microsomal enzymes. This may be a problem for some drugs used in humans, but the clinical significance in veterinary medicine has not been established. Acid suppression may decrease oral availability of some oral drugs, for example, itraconazole, ketoconazole, and domperidone.

SYNTHETIC PROSTAGLANDINS. Synthetic prostaglandins—administered orally—produce many of the protective effects on the GI mucosa that natural prostaglandins have been known to achieve (Allen et al. 1993; Henderson and Webster 2006). Misoprostol (Cytotec®) is a synthetic PGE-1 analogue that has been used in people to diminish the risk of ulcers associated with NSAID therapy. In dogs, it has been shown to prevent duodenal hemorrhage and ulceration associated with aspirin therapy. Misoprostol is a better drug for preventing GI ulcers than for treating ulcers once they occur. Its use appears to be limited to NSAID therapy. Misoprostol was *not* effective for preventing gastritis, ulcers, and gastrointestinal hemorrhage associated with corticosteroid administration (Hanson et al. 1997).

Use in Small Animals. Misoprostol is available as 0.1 and 0.2 mg tablets. Dosages for dogs range from 2 to 5 μg/kg. It is absorbed and rapidly metabolized to an active metabolite. At high doses (>5 μg/kg) adverse effects of diarrhea have been reported.

Use in Horses. Misoprostol has been shown to decrease stomach acidity in horses. However, misoprostol may cause abdominal discomfort, cramping, and diarrhea. For these reasons, the use has been discouraged in horses.

Nongastrointestinal Uses for Misoprostol. Misoprostol was shown to have modest antiinflammatory effects and has been effective for some dermatoses in dogs. In these studies, 3–6 µg/kg was administered to dogs with atopic dermatitis three times daily orally. Misoprostol produced a decrease in pruritus and clinical score of 30%. Side effects may prevent more widespread use and higher doses.

Misoprostol is an effective abortifacient. It has been used as a component of medical treatment of abortion in humans—in combination with other drugs. It has not been used for this purpose in animals, but if it is administered inadvertently to a pregnant animal, abortion could occur.

DRUGS USED TO TREAT *HELICOBACTER* GASTRITIS. Treatment of gastritis and ulcers caused by the bacteria *Helicobacter pylori* and *Helicobacter*-like organisms has gained interest in veterinary medicine. This organism has been identified in biopsy specimens from dogs and cats, but its role in gastritis and ulcers has yet to be established (Yamasaki et al. 1998). Some studies have found no association between *Helicobacter* infection and gastritis (Winberg et al. 2005; Haponen et al. 1998). However, in some animals with gastritis, treatment has helped decrease signs when treatment was initiated with ampicillin, metronidazole, and famotidine (AMF). A discussion on the role of *Helicobacter* as a cause of gastritis in animals can be found in the articles by Simpson et al. (2000) and Neiger and Simpson (2000). One of the authors recommends that animals with clinical signs of gastritis and positive for *Helicobacter* or *Helicobacter*-like organisms should be treated. The oral treatment for animals that has been the most widely used is a 2-week course of the combination of metronidazole and/or clarithromycin, plus amoxicillin, and a proton-pump inhibitor, or H_2-receptor antagonist.

In people, *Helicobacter pylori* gastritis has been treated with the simultaneous use of metronidazole, omeprazole, and clarithromycin (Suerbaum and Michetti 2002). One regimen uses clarithromycin (Biaxin®) and omeprazole (Prilosec®). A product called Tritec® combines ranitidine with bismuth citrate and is designed to be administered concurrently with clarithromycin (Biaxin®). Some regimens also use amoxicillin, or metronidazole. Some synergism is achieved with these combinations. For example, H_2-antagonists or omeprazole, enhance the antibacterial activity of metronidazole and perhaps other antibiotics.

TABLE 47.9 Causes of diarrhea in animals

- Osmotic (e.g., dietary indiscretion)
- Secretory (e.g., enterotoxigenic *E. coli*)
- Increased permeability (exudative) (e.g., parvovirus diarrhea)
- Malabsorption (e.g., pancreatic insufficiency)

DRUGS FOR TREATMENT OF DIARRHEA

Therapy for diarrhea should include fluid therapy, electrolyte replenishment, maintaining acid/base balance, and control of discomfort. But drugs such as antimicrobials, motility modifiers, and intestinal protectants are sometimes used. Diarrhea caused by intestinal parasites is covered in Section 10 of this book. Common causes of diarrhea in animals is shown in Table 47.9. Many of these causes do not require drug therapy and the disease is self-limiting. In some instances, treatment may be needed to temporarily relieve clinical signs. Some of these treatments are discussed below.

MUCOSAL PROTECTANTS AND ADSORBENTS

Kaolin-Pectin Formulations. Products that are promoted as mucosal protectants such as mixtures of kaolin and pectin (Kao-Pectate®) have been popular. Kaolin is a form of aluminum silicate and pectin is a carbohydrate that is extracted from the rinds of citrus fruits. The manufacturers claim that kaolin-pectin acts as a demulcent and adsorbent in the treatment of diarrhea. The action of kaolin-pectin is believed to be related to binding of bacterial toxins (endotoxins and enterotoxins) in the GI tract. However, experimental studies have shown that kaolin-pectin is an ineffective binder of *E. coli* enterotoxin and clinical studies have failed to show a benefit from the administration of kaolin-pectin. This product may change the consistency of stools, but it will not decrease fluid or electrolyte loss, nor will it shorten the duration of illness.

Kao-Pectate formulations contain salicylate as one of the active ingredients. There is 8.7 mg/ml in the Regular Strength, and 16 mg/ml in the Extra Strength formulation. Since some animals may be sensitive to salicylates, the salicylate content of the formulation should be considered before administering the product to animals.

Clinical Use of Kaolin-Pectin. Despite the lack of clinical evidence of efficacy, some veterinarians administer this drug at a dose of 1 to 2 ml/kg, q6h. Kaolin-pectin is not absorbed, but salicylate may be absorbed in most animals (see the next section, on bismuth subsalicylate, and Papich et al. 1987). Drug interactions are also possible. Kaolin-pectin may adsorb or bind other drugs that are administered orally and decrease their effectiveness.

Bismuth Subsalicylate. The most common form of bismuth subsalicylate is Pepto Bismol®. Although other "mucosal protectants" may have questionable efficacy, this product is considered by many gastroenterologists to be the symptomatic treatment of choice for acute diarrhea. Its efficacy has been proven in controlled clinical trials in humans with acute diarrhea, particularly the form caused by enterotoxigenic *E. coli* (also known as traveler's diarrhea) (Bierer 1990). Bismuth may have some ability to adsorb bacterial enterotoxins, and it may produce some gastric or intestinal protective effect. The salicylate component is responsible for the efficacy, because it produces an antiinflammatory action. There are five sources of salicylate in this formulation accounting for approximately 9 mg of salicylate per ml. Two tablespoons (the typical human dose) contains almost 300 mg of salicylate. An "extra-strength" formulation contains twice this amount. Practically all of the salicylate from Pepto Bismol is absorbed systemically when administered to dogs and cats (Papich et al. 1987). Despite the systemic absorption, the amount is unlikely to produce salicylate toxicity. Even in cats—a species sensitive to salicylate toxicity—it is unlikely that enough would be administered from standard dosages to produce a toxic reaction.

Clinical Use of Bismuth Subsalicylate. The dose administered to animals was not derived from clinical studies, but extrapolated from human dosages. One to three ml/kg/day in divided doses have been administered safely (even to cats). Some animals may not like the taste, but otherwise there have not been serious adverse effects reported from administration of Pepto Bismol. Salicylate toxicosis is possible from overdoses, and pet owners should be advised to limit the amount administered, especially in animals with other primary diseases that may have initiated the diarrhea. Pet owners should be warned that Pepto Bismol may turn the stools black. As noted earlier, bismuth also has an anti-*Helicobacter* effect in the stomach. It has been included in many of the regimens for treating *Helicobacter*-gastritis. Therefore some benefits for treating gastritis may have been caused from the action on *Helicobacter* or *Helicobacter*-like organisms.

Pepto Bismol also has been administered for the treatment of acute diarrhea in large animals, especially foals and calves. The presumed benefit is from binding to enterotoxins or from the antiprostaglandin effect.

MOTILITY MODIFIERS FOR TREATMENT OF DIARRHEA

Anticholinergic Drugs (Antimuscarinic Drugs). Anticholinergic drugs significantly decrease intestinal motility and secretions and have been included as ingredients in antidiarrheal preparations. These drugs inhibit muscarinic action via their antagonism of either the muscarinic-M_1 or -M_3 receptor. (M_1 is a ganglionic receptor, and M_3 acts at peripheral sites.) Their parasympatholytic effects decrease segmental and propulsive intestinal smooth muscle contractions. Although they do not alter the course of the disease, anticholinergic drugs may decrease the urgency associated with some forms of diarrhea, decrease the fluid secreted into the bowel, and decrease abdominal discomfort associated with hypermotility. The limitation for the use of anticholinergic drugs lies in the questionable efficacy for most diarrhea seen in veterinary medicine (few cases of diarrhea actually can be classified as "hypermotile"). These drugs are also associated with important side effects. Anticholinergic drugs are discussed in more detail in Chapter 7.

Efficacy. Although the anticholinergic agents clearly decrease intestinal motility, there is no clear evidence that a decrease in motility is always beneficial. Intestinal motility is already impaired in many patients with some forms of diarrhea and these drugs may actually worsen the diarrhea by creating a "stovepipe" effect. The use of these drugs should be avoided if the diarrhea is infectious (e.g., caused by *Salmonella*).

Adverse Effects. Anticholinergic drugs have profound systemic pharmacological effects. If they are administered in sufficient doses to affect the bowel, side effects are possible, which include ileus, xerostomia, urine retention, cycloplegia, tachycardia, and CNS excitement. Chronic administration can lead to serious bowel atony. In addition to decreasing bowel motility, anticholinergic drugs decrease stomach emptying, which can lead to stomach distention and discomfort. This is certainly contraindicated in a

TABLE 47.10 Anticholinergic drugs used for treatment of diarrhea

Tertiary amines
- atropine
- scopolamine

Quaternary amines
- methscopolamine
- isopropamide
- propantheline
- glycopyrrolate

patient that has gastritis and is vomiting. Rumen atony is possible in cattle.

Examples of Drugs. Atropine is the best known anticholinergic drug, but because it has many other systemic effects, it is not ordinarily used for its antidiarrheal properties (Table 47.10). To avoid CNS effects, it is desirable to administer drugs that are quaternary amines. Because these drugs are charged, their lipophilicity is reduced and they do not cross the blood-brain barrier as readily as tertiary amines (see Table 47.10).

Quaternary amines used in veterinary medicine include methscopolamine, propantheline (Pro-Banthine®), and isopropamide (Darbid®). Darbazine, an old combination rarely available today, contains both isopropamide and prochlorperazine. Anticholinergic drugs have been included in formulations such as aminopentamide in Centrine® and diphemanil in Diathal®. Combination products such as Donnatal® contain scopolamine, atropine, and hyoscyamine (in addition to phenobarbital). Some of these formulations are outdated and unavailable today.

N-Butylscopolammonium Bromide (Buscopan). N-butylscopolammonium bromide is an anticholinergic drug used to treat colic in horses (0.3 mg/kg IV). Although anticholinergic drugs are not ordinarily indicated for treatment of colic in horses, this drug has FDA approval for this indication. N-butylscopolammonium bromide is considered an antispasmodic drug registered for treatment of colic associated with spasm of the intestine in horses. Within 5–10 minutes of IV injection, spasm of intestinal smooth muscle is reportedly relieved. Adverse effects from N-butylscopolammonium include other anticholinergic effects such as transient increase in heart rate lasting for approximately 30 minutes. It should not be used in horses with an impaction or in horses with ileus.

OPIOIDS. Opioids can have both antisecretory and antimotility actions as they act on the μ (mu)-opiate receptors of the GI tract. They decrease propulsive intestinal contractions and increase segmentation (an overall constipating effect) (DeHaven-Hudkins et al. 2007). They also increase the tone of GI sphincters. In addition to affecting motility, opiates have an antisecretory effect and stimulate absorption of fluid, electrolytes, and glucose. Their effects on secretory diarrhea are probably caused by inhibition of calcium influx and decreased calmodulin activity (Hedner and Cassuto 1987). These drugs can affect large animals as well as small animals. Opiates have been documented to inhibit colonic motor activity in horses (Roger et al. 1985; Boscan et al. 2006). Opiates are discussed in more detail in Chapter 12.

Examples of Drugs. The constipating effects of morphine and other opioids are well known. However, it would be irrational to administer morphine repeatedly to animals simply for the antidiarrhea effect. Instead, opioids are used that produce little systemic effect. Two synthetic opioids are known for their specificity of action on the GI tract and their effect on secretory diarrhea. They are primarily active locally on the opiate μ-receptors and they produce GI effects without other systemic side effects. Two such compounds are *diphenoxylate* (Lomotil®) and *loperamide* (Imodium®) (Johnson 1989). Diphenoxylate is a derivative of meperidine and not commonly used.

Loperamide is the most often used and is available OTC in capsules (Imodium) of 2 mg and an oral solution of 0.2 mg/ml (for dosages, see Table 47.11). The typical dose for small animals is 0.1 mg/kg, q12h, PO. Paregoric is an older compound (tincture of opium), found in many antidiarrheal products. *5 ml of paregoric corresponds to approximately 2 mg of morphine.*

Adverse Effects. Opiates can have potent effects on the GI tract and should be used cautiously. Loperamide is an over-the-counter drug available for people, often administered to animals. These drugs are generally contraindicated in infectious diarrhea because opiates may significantly slow GI transit and increase the absorption of bacterial toxins. Diphenoxylate (Lomotil) contains 25 μg of atropine per 2.5 mg tablet. The amount of atropine contained in this mixture may contribute to some inhibition of intestinal smooth muscle, but is present in the formulation primarily to discourage abuse by people.

TABLE 47.11 Antidiarrhea drugs and doses

Drug	Dose
OPIATES	
codeine	0.5–1.0 mg/kg, PO, q8–12h
morphine	0.05–0.1 mg/kg, IM, SC, q8–12h
diphenoxylate (Lomotil)	0.1–0.2 mg/kg, PO (dog), q8–12h or 0.05–0.1 mg/kg, PO (cat), q12h
loperamide (Imodium)	0.1–0.2 mg/kg, PO, q8–12h
paregoric	0.05–0.06 mg/kg, PO, q12h
ANTICHOLINERGIC DRUGS	
propantheline (Pro-Banthine)	0.25–0.5 mg/kg, PO, q8–12h
aminopentamide (Centrine)	0.01–0.03 mg/kg, q8–12h or 0.1 mg/cat PO,IM,SC, q8–12h
diphemanil (Diathal)	1.8 mg/kg, IM, q12h

Loperamide does not cause central nervous system opiate-related effects because the membrane transporter p-glycoprotein (p-gp) helps to remove this drug from the central nervous system. Dogs deficient in p-gp (e.g., Collie dogs and other herding breeds) may be prone to toxicity (Mealey 2004).

ANTIMICROBIAL THERAPY FOR TREATMENT OF DIARRHEA. The routine use of antimicrobials to treat diarrhea has been questioned by gastroenterologists. In most cases of diarrhea in small animals, a bacterial etiology cannot be identified. In large animals diarrhea is often caused by bacteria (*E. coli*, for example), but antibiotic therapy may not alter the course of the disease and there is a lack of well-controlled studies to demonstrate efficacy. Oral, nonabsorbed antibiotics are sometimes combined with motility modifiers, adsorbents, and intestinal protectants in commercial preparations, but some of these are irrational combinations. Sometimes administration of oral antibiotics can be a *cause* of diarrhea (Bartlett 2002).

For the few indications where antimicrobial therapy may be an important treatment for diarrhea, protocols are listed below. Discussions about specific drugs are provided in Chapters 33–38 of this book.

Campylobacter Enteritis. This disease is caused by *Campylobacter jejuni*, which may be transmitted to people. This organism is the most common cause of food-borne infectious diarrhea in people. The treatment is aimed primarily at maintaining fluid and electrolyte balance. If antimicrobials are considered the following have been used: erythromycin (10 to 15 mg/kg, q8h x 5 d), fluoroquinolones, tylosin, clindamycin, tetracycline, or chloramphenicol (35–45 mg/kg, q8h). Although erythromycin usually is cited as the treatment of choice, bacterial shedding may resume once therapy is stopped. (Monfort et al. 1990).

Intestinal Bacterial Overgrowth Caused by *E. coli* or *Clostridium* spp. Treatments that have been used include antimicrobial treatment and administration of probiotics. Using probiotics entails administration of bacteria that will restore a healthy population of bacteria in the intestine. When antibiotics are considered, one should administer an oral drug that is effective in the GI lumen and has activity against anaerobic bacteria. For *E. coli*, fluoroquinolones are recommended. For *C. difficile*, metronidazole or vancomycin is recommended. Other drugs to consider include amoxicillin, ampicillin, tylosin, clindamycin, or tetracyclines.

Tylosin-Responsive Diarrhea. Because some forms of chronic diarrhea in animals have been responsive to the antimicrobial tylosin (Tylan), they have been characterized as "Tylosin-Responsive Chronic Diarrhea in Dogs" (Westermarck et al. 2005). This disease, affecting both large and small bowel, is most likely caused by a bacterial pathogen, but the specific etiology has not been identified. *Campylobacter jejuni* and *Clostridium perfringens* have been identified in some animals, however. In these animals, tylosin has been effective at improving clinical signs that occur with or without organisms being identified. When administered at 12 mg/kg/day (average dose) response was prompt. Some dogs respond within 24 hours; others respond within 3 days. Other studies by the same investigators showed that a dose of 20 mg/kg/day was effective, but other drugs (metronidazole, trimethoprim-sulfonamides, doxycycline, or prednisolone) were not (Westermarck et al. 2005).

Sources of Tylosin. The powdered form for livestock (Tylan) has been mixed with the animal's food at a dosage of 40–80 mg/kg/day. One teaspoon contains approximately 3 grams (3,000 mg); therefore, 1/4 teaspoon contains 750 mg, enough for many dogs. Some animals may find the bitter taste unpleasant and refuse their food, however. Tablets for small animals are available in other countries.

METRONIDAZOLE (FLAGYL®)-RESPONSIVE DISEASES. Metronidazole is active against the protozoan *Giardia,* and it is for this use that metronidazole was first administered to treat diarrhea in small animals. (Antiprotozoan drugs are discussed in Chapter 43.) Veterinarians discovered that metronidazole also was effective in patients that did not have giardiasis. Bowel inflammation may be caused by metronidazole-sensitive bacteria, which act as a chemoattractant for neutrophils. The efficacy of metronidazole may be related to this antibacterial activity. Oral administration of metronidazole at 20 mg/kg to cats decreased the number of anaerobic and aerobic bacteria and altered the indigenous bacterial population (Johnston et al. 2000). In addition, it may have an immunosuppressive effect on the GI mucosa (decreased cell-mediated response). Metronidazole (alone and in combination with ampicillin) has been effective for histiocytic ulcerative colitis in dogs (Hostutler et al. 2004). Doses have been as high 60 mg/kg/day for 2 to 4 weeks, but many animals will respond to low doses of 30 mg/kg/day (in divided doses). Cats can receive one-quarter of a 250 mg/tablet two to three times daily (10 to 25 mg/kg). *Caution pet owners that when the tablet is broken, the exposed tablet may cause an unpleasant taste for cats.*

Adverse effects from metronidazole are primarily seen as CNS effects. Tremors, seizures, and other CNS disturbances have been documented. CNS problems are caused by inhibition of GABA. Avoid high doses to prevent the CNS adverse effects.

Salmonella. The primary goal when treating *Salmonella* is to maintain fluid balance and prevent electrolyte losses. The patients should be isolated to prevent spreading of infection, and strict containment procedures should be instituted in the hospital. Antibiotics are discouraged unless absolutely necessary for patients with salmonella. Antibiotic therapy may prolong shedding. In horses, if there is fever and neutropenia, gentamicin IV should be considered. In animals in which oral therapy is possible, drug choices include the following: fluoroquinolones, chloramphenicol, or florfenicol (depending on the species), ampicillin or amoxicillin or amoxicillin-clavulanate, trimethoprim-sulfonamide, or a cephalosporin (higher activity with third-generation cephalosporin).

Antibiotic Treatment in Calves with Diarrhea. Use of antibiotics to treat diarrhea is probably most often practiced in young ruminants. A review of this practice has summarized the relevant literature (Constable 2004). This author points out that the following antimicrobials are approved for treatment of calf diarrhea: amoxicillin, chlortetracycline, neomycin, oxytetracycline, streptomycin, sulfachloropyridazine, sulfamethazine, and tetracycline—*all* administered orally. Some of these drugs were approved many (approximately 50) years ago, before evidence was required for registration. Of all these drugs listed, only amoxicillin has been shown to be effective in well-controlled studies. Other drugs shown to be effective, (fluoroquinolones, chloramphenicol, nitrofurazone) are illegal to use for this indication in calves. If bacteremia develops as a complication of bacterial diarrhea in calves, systemic therapy is needed. Drugs most often given systemically (IM, SC, or IV) for this indication include ceftiofur and ampicillin.

Bacterial Septicemia Secondary to Diarrhea. When it is suspected that there may be a loss of the protective epithelial barrier, the intestine mucosal integrity is compromised. In these cases, bacteremia and septicemia can occur due to translocation of bacteria. Signs accompanying septicemia include a severe, bloody diarrhea, fever, and leukocytosis. This may progress to signs of endotoxic shock. If septicemia is suspected, systemic antibiotics are clearly warranted.

The choice of antibiotics will vary depending on the species and the animal's age. Some drugs are restricted in food animals. Neonates with diarrhea will deteriorate rapidly, and treatment cannot wait for culture and sensitivity results when prescribing antimicrobial therapy. Therefore, broad-spectrum antimicrobials often are used.

Recommended antibiotics include ampicillin or amoxicillin, (combined with a β-lactamase inhibitor), combination of a β-lactam (penicillin, aminopenicillin, or cephalosporin) with an aminoglycoside (gentamicin or amikacin), aminoglycoside alone, cephalosporin (extended-spectrum cephalosporin), carbapenem (meropenem or imipenem), or fluoroquinolones (enrofloxacin, marbofloxacin, difloxacin, orbifloxacin).

If the animal shows signs of sepsis, systemic antimicrobials should be used. Antibiotics that are poorly absorbed and confined to the GI lumen may be of little benefit (e.g., neomycin, ampicillin).

***Lawsonia intracellularis* (Pigs and Horses).** In horses 3–6 months old, a disease characterized as *proliferative enteropathy* is caused by the organism *Lawsonia intracellularis.* Affected animals show signs of lethargy, anorexia, depression, weight loss, colic, diarrhea, and hypoproteinemia. Treatment in horses has included erythromycin, azithromycin, chloramphenicol, clarithromycin, and doxycycline.

In pigs, *Lawsonia intracellularis* also causes intestinal disease. The recommended treatment is tetracyclines and tylosin, added to feed.

DRUGS FOR TREATMENT OF INFLAMMATORY INTESTINAL DISEASES

Intestinal inflammatory diseases cover a wide range of etiologies grouped together because they may have similar clinical signs. Among the diseases that may be included in this group are those caused by parasites, bacteria, food hypersensitivity, or immune-mediated diseases. Inflammatory bowel disease (IBD) may involve the small intestine or large intestine. There are similarities to intestinal diseases in people, which were reviewed by Hanauer (1996). For a thorough discussion of these diseases in small animals, consult reviews in clinical textbooks (Washabau & Holt 2005; Hall & German, 2005), read the chapters by Hall and German (small intestine) and Washabau and Holt (large intestine) in Ettinger and Feldman (editors, *Textbook of Veterinary Internal Medicine, 6th Edition,* Elsevier Saunders 2005; Chapter 222, page 1332, and Chapter 223, page 1378).

Inflammatory bowel disease is a collective term that describes a group of disorders characterized by persistent or recurrent signs and histologic evidence of inflammation. Inflammation may be characterized by the cells infiltrating the mucosa (lymphocytic, plasmacytic, eosinophilic, neutrophilic). In the large intestine, the disease is often referred to simply as *colitis* but also may be associated with many etiologies.

Initial therapy for inflammatory intestinal disease is aimed at managing the underlying cause. Therefore, antiparasitic therapy and dietary therapy are usually pursued initially. When these treatments have failed, or a specific etiology has not been identified, drug therapy, usually consisting of antiinflammatory drugs, is used, or added to existing treatment. Dietary management will not be discussed here. You are encouraged to consult dietary and nutrition veterinary textbooks for guidelines on diet management. Antiparasitic drugs are discussed in Section 10.

SULFASALAZINE (AZULFIDINE®). Sulfasalazine is used as an initial drug therapy for treatment of colitis. It is not as effective for inflammatory diseases of the small intestine. Sulfasalazine is a combination of sulfapyridine and 5-aminosalicylic acid (mesalamine) joined by an azo bond. The bond is broken by bacteria in the colon to release the two drugs. The sulfonamide component is absorbed into the circulation while the salicylic acid component remains active in the GI tract. Less than half of the salicylate component is absorbed systemically.

Clinical Use. Many veterinarians consider sulfasalazine to be the drug of choice for the initial treatment of ulcerative or idiopathic colitis, or plasmacytic-lymphocytic colitis after dietary therapy has been attempted. Clinical efficacy is attributed to a local antiinflammatory action from the salicylate component. There is also evidence for antilipooxygenase (LOX) activity, decreased IL-1, decreased prostaglandin synthesis, and oxygen radical scavenging activity.

Dosage recommendations start at 10–25 mg/kg q8h, PO, but have been as high as 40 mg/kg, two to three times per day. The dose is then reduced after there is an initial response to treatment.

Adverse Effects. The salicylate component is absorbed only minimally. The sulfonamide component is absorbed and can produce adverse effects in some animals, such as keratoconjunctivitis sicca in dogs (Morgan and Bachrach 1982). This drug cannot be used in patients that have allergic reactions to sulfonamides.

Other Sources of 5-Aminosalicylic Acid (Mesalamine). In people, the adverse effects associated with sulfasalazine therapy are primarily due to the sulfonamide component; therefore, drugs have been formulated to contain mesalamine (5-aminosalicylic acid) without the sulfonamide. These formulations are listed in Table 47.12. Some formulations are designed to release the active drug at the high pH of the distal intestine (Table 47.13).

ANTICHOLINERGIC DRUGS (ANTIMUSCARINIC DRUGS). As discussed previously, anticholinergic drugs (atropinelike drugs) inhibit smooth muscle and glandular secretions of the GI tract. Anticholinergic drugs occasionally have been used for the treatment of colitis. However, colitis is not ordinarily associated with hypermotility and

TABLE 47.12 Mesalamine (5-aminosalicylic acid) formulations

- Asacol®: Asacol is a tablet coated with an acrylic-based resin. The resin dissolves at a pH of 7.0 and is designed to release 5-aminosalicylic acid in the colon. It is available as a 400 mg tablet.
- Mesasal®: Mesasal is a tablet coated with an acrylic-based resin that dissolves at a pH of >6.0. It is designed to release 5-aminosalicylic acid in the terminal ileum and colon. Approximately 35% of the salicylate is absorbed systemically. It is available in 250 and 500 mg tablets. The dose in people is 1 to 1.5 g/day.
- Olsalazine sodium (Dipentum®): Olsalazine is a dimer of 2 molecules of 5-aminosalicylic acid linked by an azo bond. It is used in people who cannot tolerate sulfasalazine. Only 2% of the salicylate from this compound is absorbed systemically. It is available in 500 mg tablets. The most common adverse effect in people from this preparation has been a watery diarrhea.
- Pentasa: This formulation contains microgranules of mesalamine coated with ethyl cellulose, which releases 5-aminosalicylic acid into the small and large intestine gradually, regardless of pH.

TABLE 47.13 pH values of GI tract in small animals

	Stomach (Fasted)	Proximal S. Intestine	Distal S. Intestine	Cecum	Colon	Feces
Dog	3.4–5.5	6.2	7.5	6.4	6.5	6.2
Cat	4.2–5.0	6.2	7.6	6.0	6.2	7.0

the rationale of anticholinergic drugs should be questioned. Patients with a hypermotile or spastic bowel may have a limited benefit from these drugs.

Anticholinergic drugs also may have a role for reducing straining during the postoperative management of rectal and/or anal surgical procedures. A common drug for these indications is propantheline (Pro-Banthine®) at a dosage of 0.25 mg/kg, orally, two or three times daily.

GLUCOCORTICOIDS. The effects of glucocorticoids for treating inflammatory bowel diseases are probably related to their antiinflammatory and immunosuppressive ability (Dillon 1989). It is believed that colitis is the result of autoantibodies and T-lymphocytes directed against the colonic epithelial cells. Corticosteroids, via their ability to suppress cytokine synthesis, leukocyte migration, and lymphocyte activation suppress the activity responsible for inflammatory bowel disease clinical signs. Glucocorticoids have been used when a biopsy suggests eosinophilic colitis or lymphocytic-plasmacytic colitis (Washabau and Holt 2005; Leib et al. 1989). They are often employed when other forms of therapy (including dietary) have failed. The pharmacology of the corticosteroids was discussed in more detail in Chapter 30.

Clinical Use and Dosages. The dose of prednisolone initially is in the immunosuppressive range of 2 to 4 mg/kg per day in divided doses for dogs and cats. Although there are no comparisons between prednisone and prednisolone, it is advised to use prednisolone. Prednisone is an inactive drug that relies on the conversion to the active drug prednisolone. If a local (topical) effect is desired from an oral dose, prednisolone is preferred over prednisone. Moreover, there is evidence—at least in cats—that some animals do not convert prednisone to the active drug.

After initial response is observed, the doses are tapered to approximately 1 mg/kg every other day if there is a positive treatment response. Prednisolone may be administered with azathioprine (see next section). The magnitude of the dosage depends on the severity of the disease. Cats with severe inflammatory bowel disease have required prednisolone dosages as high as 4 mg/kg/day. Injections of corticosteroids (for example, methylprednisolone acetate DepoMedrol® at 20 mg/cat) for the control of inflammatory bowel disease has not been as successful as oral therapy. *Veterinarians should be aware that some animals develop diarrhea when treated with glucocorticoid therapy.*

Local Treatment with Budesonide (Entocort EC). Budesonide is a locally acting corticosteroid. It has been used in people, but there has been only limited use in small animals. Budesonide granules are contained in an ethylcellulose matrix that is coated with methacrylic acid polymer. This coating does not release the drug until the pH >5.5. In the proximal intestine the pH is low and it gradually increases in the distal intestine to attain a pH above 7 (see Table 47.13). Therefore, the drug is not released until it reaches the distal GI tract. If a portion of the drug is absorbed, 80–90% is inactivated by metabolism first-pass effects. Therefore, systemic glucocorticoid effects are minimized. In humans it has been as effective as other drugs for treatment of Crohn's disease. It is available in a 3 mg capsule and is used in people at a dose of 9 mg/day.

Use of Budesonide in Animals. There is only limited experience with budesonide in dogs and cats, but some animals have benefited from its administration. There is some systemic absorption as evidenced by decreased response to ACTH after 30 days of treatment to dogs at 3 mg/m^2, but other side effects were not observed (Tumulty et al. 2004).

IMMUNOSUPPRESSIVE DRUGS. Immunosuppressive drugs also have been used to manage some forms of inflammatory bowel diseases. These drugs were discussed in more detail in Chapter 46. The most commonly used immunosuppressive drug for intestinal disease is azathioprine. The use of other drugs, such as cyclosporine, has been more limited.

Azathioprine is metabolized to 6-mercaptopurine (6-MP), which inhibits de novo synthesis of purine nucleotides in activated lymphocytes thereby suppressing lymphocyte response. Azathioprine (Imuran®) has been used at dosages of 2 mg/kg once daily, to 40 mg/m^2 once daily in dogs with severe inflammatory bowel disease. The dose may be decreased to 0.5 mg/kg every other day if there is a positive initial response. Cats are more sensitive to the adverse effects than dogs. Azathioprine dosages of 2.2 mg/kg/day have produced bone marrow suppression in cats (Beale et al. 1992), but lower doses may be safe—for example 0.3 mg/kg. In one report, cats with inflammatory bowel disease responded to azathioprine at a dose of 3 mg per cat (one-eighth of a 25 mg tablet), every other day.

N-3 FATTY ACIDS FOR COLITIS. In people omega-fatty acids (n-3 fatty acids) such as eicosapentanoic acid are beneficial for the treatment of colitis. These compounds are available in veterinary medicine in products such as DermCaps®, Pet-Derm®, and others for the purpose of treating pruritic skin disease. In studies performed in people with ulcerative colitis, supplementation for 4 months with omega fatty acids reduced leukotriene levels in the colon, and improved clinical signs. The clinical efficacy of these compounds for treating small animals with colitis has not been reported.

CYCLOSPORINE. Cyclosporine (Neoral, Atopic) has been used to treat perianal fistulas, which are a component of ulcerative colitis (see Chapter 46). The treatment for this disease has been very successful. In addition, cyclosporine has been used to treat diarrhea caused by inflammatory bowel disease (Allenspach et al. 2006). At a dose of 5 mg/kg PO, q24h, ×10 weeks there was improvement in 78% of dogs. The success is attributed to the ability of cyclosporine to suppress T-cell mediated activity in the bowel, and to suppression of inflammatory cytokines.

LAXATIVES AND CATHARTICS

Laxatives and cathartics are drugs that increase the motility of bowel and change the character of the stool. Uses of these drugs are listed in Table 47.14. These drugs promote the elimination of soft-formed stool or increase fluid content of stool, which increases the bulk. Laxatives and cathartics can be divided into 1) bulk-forming laxatives, 2) stool softeners, 3) lubricants, 4) saline hyperosmotic agents, and 5) stimulants. They also may be categorized by their onset of action: The osmotic (saline) laxatives act in 1–3 hours; the direct stimulants act in 6–8 hours; the bulk laxatives and surfactants act in 1–3 days.

STIMULANT (IRRITANT) LAXATIVES. The exact mechanism of action for this group of laxatives is uncertain, but they appear to cause electrolyte loss by inhibiting Na^+/K^+-ATPase in the intestine and increasing electrolyte loss through intestinal tight junctions. These drugs are

TABLE 47.14 Use of laxatives and cathartics in veterinary medicine

- Promotes the elimination of a soft-formed stool
- Increases passage of intestinal contents to relieve an impaction (equine)
- Cleanses bowel prior to radiography or endoscopy
- Promotes the elimination of a toxin from the intestine
- Softens stools following intestinal or anal surgery (decreases straining)

among the most rapidly acting of the laxatives, with action within 6–8 hours. They can have potent effects and excessive fluid and electrolyte loss can result from overdoses. Adverse effects can result from damage to enterocytes from chronic use and abuse:

- *Diphenylmethane*: Use is not documented in veterinary medicine.
- *Phenolphthalein*: This was once an ingredient found in over-the-counter laxative preparations such as ExLax®, but is no longer available. (Other natural ingredients are used in ExLax.)
- *Anthraquinone:* These are glycoside derivatives found in bisacodyl (Dulcolax), senna (Senokot), and cascara sagrada (Nature's Remedy).

TABLE 47.15 Saline cathartics

- Sodium sulfate (Glauber's salt)
- Magnesium salts such as magnesium sulfate (Epsom Salts), magnesium hydroxide (Milk of Magnesia), and magnesium citrate (Citro-Mag)
- Nonabsorbed sugars: Lactulose, Mannitol, Polyethylene glycol (PEG)
- Lactulose also is used to treat hepatic encephalopathy. Its action lowers the bowel pH and decreases ammonia absorption by converting to NH^{+3}. The ionized form of the compound is less absorbed systemically.
- Combination products: Golytely is a strong osmotic cathartic that is a combination of sodium sulfate, potassium chloride, sodium chloride, sodium bicarbonate, and polyethylene glycol (PEG 3350). The dose is 250 ml to one liter per animal (depending on the size) and has a rapid onset of action. The most common use of this product is for bowel cleansing prior to an endoscopic procedure.

HYPEROSMOTIC CATHARTICS (SALINE CATHARTICS). The saline cathartics are nonabsorbed electrolytes that draw fluid into the bowel via osmosis. These are the most rapidly acting of the cathartics, with onset of action in 1–3 hours. The fluid content of the stool increases, which causes intestinal distention and promotes increased normal peristalsis. These have been some of the most commonly used cathartics in veterinary medicine. Most often they are dissolved in an aqueous solution (water) and administered via gastric gavage (stomach tube). These drugs have been used to prepare animals for an endoscopic procedure (*bowel cleansing)* or for cathartic treatment of poisoning. They are relatively safe drugs, but overdoses can cause fluid loss in a patient. Examples of these drugs are shown in Table 47.15.

TABLE 47.16 Bulk laxatives

- Carboxymethylcellulose
- Methylcellulose
- Psyllium (Metamucil) powder
- Prunes and wheat bran and other attempts to increase "fiber" in the diet
- For cats, canned pumpkin is a source of fiber that most cats eat readily

HYDROPHILIC COLLOIDS ("BULK LAXATIVES"). These agents are mostly natural products and dietary plant fibers. They are composed of nonabsorbed synthetic or natural polysaccharide and cellulose derivatives. These fibers are resistant to digestion and attract water into the intestine. By imbibing water, they increase the mass of nondigestible material in bowel and motility is increased through the stimulation of mechanoreceptors. They are more slowly acting than other drugs with an onset of action of 24 hours, or longer. They are relatively safe drugs with few side effects. Examples are included in Table 47.16.

LUBRICANT LAXATIVES (MINERAL OIL AND LIQUID PETROLATUM). The lubricants act by coating the surface of the stool with a water-immiscible film and increasing the water content of the stool. They also produce a lubricant action to ease passage of the stool. Lubricant laxatives usually contain mineral oil (liquid petrolatum) or white petrolatum. Many of the nonprescription products contain white petrolatum (Vaseline) as their ingredient. Administration of glycerin also has been used as a lubricant laxative. The lubricant laxatives are relatively safe because they are absorbed from the GI tract only to a small extent. The worst adverse effect is that they may possibly elicit a foreign body reaction. Chronic use may decrease the intestinal absorption of fat-soluble vitamins.

Use in Large Animals. These drugs, particularly mineral oil, are popular for several nonspecific GI problems in horses and cattle.

Use in Small Animals. Products such as Laxatone®, Felaxin®, and Kat-a-Lax® are promoted for increasing the passage of trichobezoars (hair balls) in cats. These products

TABLE 47.17 Other uses for ursodeoxycholic acid

Although listed with the laxatives, most of the use of ursodeoxycholic acid (ursodiol), in veterinary medicine is for the management of liver disease in animals, rather than for its laxative action. Ursodeoxycholic acid has an important effect in slowing progression, or improving, liver disease (Lindor 2007). Because ursodiol is a water-soluble bile acid, administration may alter the circulating pool of bile acids to replace some of the more toxic, hydrophobic bile acids from accumulating in animals with liver disease.

contain white petrolatum (Vaseline) as their active ingredient with additional flavorings.

STOOL SOFTENERS (SURFACTANTS). These drugs act to decrease surface tension and allow more water to accumulate in the stool. Their onset of action is usually 24–48 hours. They are relatively safe, except cramping pains are reported in people if they ingest high dosages.

Docusates: Dioctyl Sodium Sulfosuccinate (DSS, Colace), and Dioctyl Calcium Sulfosuccinate (Surfak, Doxidan). Also known as docusate sodium and docusate calcium, these compounds are used when there is a need to soften the stool. Efficacy in animals has not been tested.

Bile Acids. Bile acids include dehydrocholic acid and ursodeoxycholic acid (Ursodiol, Actigall). Bile acids can produce both a choleretic (increase bile flow) and laxative effect. Other uses are listed in Table 47.17.

Castor Oil. Castor oil is hydrolyzed in the bowel to release ricinoleic acid, which causes an increased secretion of water in the small intestine.

REFERENCES AND ADDITIONAL READING

Ahmed AF, Constable PD, Misk NA. Effect of orally administered cimetidine and ranitidine on abomasal luminal pH in clinically normal milk-fed calves. Am J Vet Res 62:1531–1538, 2001.

Allen A, Flemstrom G, Garner A, Kivilaakso E. Gastroduodenal mucosal protection. Physiol Rev 73:823–847, 1993.

Allenspach K, Rüfenacht S, Sauter S, Gröne A, Steffan J, Strehlau G, Gaschen F. Pharmacokinetics and clinical efficacy of cyclosporine treatment of dogs with steroid-refractory inflammatory bowel disease. J Vet Intern Med 20:239–244, 2006.

Andrews FM, Doherty TJ, Blackford JT, et al. Effects of orally administered enteric-coated omeprazole on gastric acid secretion in horses. Am J Vet Res 60:929–931, 1999.

Baker SJ, Gerring EL. Effects of single intravenously administered doses of omeprazole and ranitidine on intragastric pH and plasma gastrin concentration in nonfed ponies. Am J Vet Res 54:2068–2074, 1993.

Bartlett JG. Antibiotic-associated diarrhea. New Engl J Med 346:334–339, 2002.

Beale KM, Altman D, Clemmons RR, Bolon B. Systemic toxicosis associated with azathioprine administration in domestic cats. Am J Vet Res 53:1236–1240, 1992.

Benchaoui HA, Cox SR, Schneider RP, Boucher JF, Clemence RG. The pharmacokinetics of maropitant, a novel neurokinin type-1 receptor antagonist, in dogs. J Vet Pharmacol Ther 30(4):336–44, 2007.

Benchaoui HA, Siedek EM, De La Puente-Redondo VA, Tilt N, Rowan TG, Clemence RG. Efficacy of maropitant for preventing vomiting associated with motion sickness in dogs. Vet Rec 161(13):444–7, 2007.

Bersenas AM, Mathews KA, Allen DG, Conlon PD. Effects of ranitidine, famotidine, pantoprazole, and omeprazole on intragastric pH in dogs. Am J Vet Res 66:425–431, 2005.

Bierer DW. Bismuth subsalicylate: history, chemistry, and safety. Rev Infect Dis 12(Suppl):S3–S8, 1990

Boscan P, Van Hoogmoed LM, Farver TB, Snyder, Jr. Evaluation of the effects of the opioid agonist morphine on gastrointestinal tract function in horses. Am J Vet Res 67:992–997, 2006.

Braun U, Steiner A, Kaegi B. Clinical, haematological and biochemical findings and the results of treatment in cattle with acute functional pyloric stenosis. Vet Rec 126:107–110, 1990.

Clark ES, Becht JL. Clinical pharmacology of the gastrointestinal tract. Vet Clin North America (Eq Pract) 3:101–122, 1987.

Constable PD. Antimicrobial use in the treatment of calf diarrhea. J Vet Intern Med 18:8–17, 2004.

Cook G, Papich MG, Roberts MC, Bowman KF. Pharmacokinetics of cisapride in horses after intravenous and rectal administration. Am J Vet Res 58:1427–1430, 1997.

Cook VL, Blikslager AT. Use of systemically administered lidocaine in horses with gastrointestinal tract disease. J AM Vet Med Assoc 232:1144–1148, 2008.

Dando TM, Perry CM. Aprepitant: A review of its use in the prevention of chemotherapy-induced nausea and vomiting. ADIS drug evaluation. Drugs 64:777–794, 2004.

de Brito Galvao JF & Trepanier LA. Risk of hemolytic anemia with itravenous administration of famotidine to hospitalized cats. J Vet Intern Med 22:325–329, 2008.

DeHaven-Hudkins DL, DeHaven RN, Little PJ, Techner LM. The involvement of the mu-opioid receptor in gastrointestinal pathophysiology: Therapeutic opportunities for antagonism at this receptor. Pharmacol Therap (2007) doi: 10.1016/j.pharmthera.2007.09.007.

de la Puente-Redondo V, Tingley FD 3rd, Schneider RP, Hickman MA. The neurokinin-1 antagonist activity of maropitant, an antiemetic drug for dogs, in a gerbil model. J Vet Pharmacol Ther30(4):281–287, 2007.

de la Puente-Redondo VA, Siedek EM, Benchaoui HA, Tilt N, Rowan TG, Clemence RG. The antiemetic efficacy of maropitant (Cerenia) in the treatment of ongoing emesis caused by a wide range of underlying clinical aetiologies in canine patients in Europe. J Small Anim Pract 48(2):93–98, 2007.

de la Puente-Redondo VA, Tilt N, Rowan TG, Clemence RG. Efficacy of maropitant for treatment and prevention of emesis caused by intravenous infusion of cisplatin in dogs. Am J Vet Res 68:48–56, 2007.

DeNovo RC. Therapeutics of gastrointestinal diseases. In Kirk RW (ed), Current Veterinary Therapy IX, Philadelphia, WB Saunders Co., 1986, pp. 862–872.

Dillon R. Effects of glucocorticoids on the gastrointestinal system. In Kirk RW (ed), Current Veterinary Therapy X, Philadelphia, WB Saunders Co., 1989, pp. 897–904.

Duran SH, Ravis WR. Comparative pharmacokinetics of H_2 antagonists in horses. Proceedings of the 11th Annual Veterinary Medical Forum, American College of Veterinary Internal Medicine, May 1993, p. 687–690.

Feldman M, Burton ME. Histamine H2-receptor antagonists: Standard therapy for acid-peptic diseases. (Parts 1 and 2) New Engl J of Med 323:1672–1680, and 1749–1755, 1990.

Fukuda H, Koga T, Furukawa N, Nakamura E, Shiroshita Y. The tachykinin KN1 receptor antagonist GR205171 abolishes the retching activity of neurons comprising the central pattern generator for vomiting in dogs. Neurosci Res 33:25–32, 1999.

Fukui H, Yamamoto M, Sato S. Vagal afferent fibres and peripheral 5-HT3 receptors mediate cisplatin-induced emesis in dogs. Japan J Pharmacol 59:221–226, 1992.

Garvey MS. Fluid and electrolyte balance in critical patients. Vet Clin North America (small animal) 19:1021–1058, 1989.

Geor RJ, Papich MG. Medical therapy for gastrointestinal ulceration in foals. Comp Contin Ed 12(3):403–413, 1990.

Gerring EEL, Hunt JM. Pathophysiology of equine post-operative ileus: effects of adrenergic blockade, parasympathetic stimulation, and metoclopramide in an experimental model. Eq Vet J 18:249–253, 1986.

Goetz TE, Oglivie GK, Keegan KG, et al. Cimetidine for treatment of melanomas in three horses. J Am Vet Med Assoc 196:449–452, 1990.

Hall EJ, German AJ. Diseases of the small intestine, [Chapter 222]. In Ettinter SJ and Feldman EC. Textbook of Veterinary Internal Medicine. Diseases of the Dog and Cat, 6th Edition. Elsevier Saunders, St. Louis Missouri, 2005. 1332–1378.

Hall JA, Solie TN, Seim HB, et al. Effect of metoclopramide on fed-state gastric myoelectric and motor activity in dogs. Am J Vet Res 57:1616–1622, 1996.

Hall JA, Washabau RJ. Gastrointestinal prokinetic therapy: motilin-like drugs. Comp Contin Ed Pract Vet 19:281–288, 1997.

Hanauer SB. Inflammatory bowel disease. New Engl J Med 334: 841–848, 1996.

Hanson SM, Bostwick DR, Twedt DC, Smith MO. Clinical evaluation of cimetidine, sucralfate, and misoprostol for prevention of gastrointestinal tract bleeding in dogs undergoing spinal surgery. Am J Vet Res 58:1320–1323, 1997.

Haponen I, Linden J, Saari S, et al. Detection and effects of helicobacters in healthy dogs and dogs with signs of gastritis. J Am Vet Med Assoc 213:1767–1774, 1998.

Hawkyard CV, Koerner RJ. The use of erythromycin as a gastrointestinal prokinetic agent in adult critical care: benefits versus risks. J Antimicrob Chemother 59:347–358, 2007.

Hayashi A, Mizumoto T, Kusano T, et al. Inhibition of gastric acid secretion by H-2 receptor antagonists normalizes interdigestive motor cycle in the stomach in dog and man. Gastroenterology 98:A56, 1990.

Hedner T, Cassuto J. Opioids and opioid receptors in peripheral tissue. Scand J Gastrol 22 (Suppl):27–46, 1987.

Henderson AK, Webster CRL. Disruption of the gastric mucosal barrier in dogs. Comp Contin Ed Pract Vet 28:340–356, 2006.

———. The use of gastroprotectants in treating gastric ulceration in dogs. Comp Contin Ed Pract Vet 28(5):358–372, 2006.

Holland PS, Ruoff WW, Brumbaugh GW, et al. Plasma pharmacokinetics of ranitidine HCL in adult horses. J Vet Pharmacol Therap 20:145–152, 1997.

Hostutler RA, Luria BJ, Johnson SE, Weisbrode SE, Sherding RG, Jaeger JQ, Guilford WG. Antibiotic-responsive histiocytic ulcerative colitis in 9 dogs. J Vet Intern Med 18:499–504, 2004.

Huskey S-EW, Dean BJ, Doss GA, et al. The metabolic disposition of aprepitant, a substance P receptor antagonist, in rats and dogs. Drug Metab Dispos 32:246–258, 2004.

Jenkins CC, DeNovo RC. Omeprazole: a potent antiulcer drug. Comp Contin Ed 13:1578–1582, 1991.

Johnson SE. Loperamide: A novel antidiarrheal drug. Comp Contin Ed 11:1373–1375, 1989.

Johnston KL, Lamport AI, Ballevre OP, Batt RM. Effects of oral administration of metronidazole on small intestinal bacteria and nutrients of cats. Am J Vet Res 61:1106–1112, 2000.

King JN, Gerring EL. Actions of the novel gastrointestinal prokinetic agent cisapride on equine bowel motility. J Vet Pharmacol Ther 11:314–321, 1988.

Kohn CW, Muir WW. Selected aspects of the clinical pharmacology of visceral analgesics and gut motility modifying drugs in the horse. J Vet Int Med 2:85–91, 1988.

LeGrange SN, Boothe DM, Herndon, et al. Pharmacokinetics and suggested oral dosing regimen of cisapride: a study in healthy cats. J Am Anim Hosp Assoc 33:517–523, 1997.

Leib MS, Hay WH, Roth L. Plasmacytic-lymphocytic colitis in dogs. In Kirk RW (ed), Current Veterinary Therapy X, Philadelphia, WB Saunders Co., 1989, pp. 939–944.

Lester GD, Merritt AM, Neuwirth L. Effect of erythromycin lactobionate on myoelectric activity of ileum, and cecal emptying of radiolabeled markers in clinically normal ponies. Am J Vet Res 59:328–334, 1998.

Lester GD, Smith RL, Robertson ID. Effects of treatment with omeprazole or ranitidine on gastric squamous ulceration in racing Thoroughbreds. J Am Vet Med Assoc 227:1636–1639, 2005.

Lindor K. Ursodeoxycholic acid for the treatment of biliary cirrhosis. New Engl J Medicine 357:1524–1529, 2007.

Malone E, Ensink J, Turner T, Wilson J, Andrews F, Keegan K, Lumsden J. Intravenous continuous infusion of lidocaine for treatment of equine ileus. Veterinary Surgery 35:60–66, 2006.

Mantione NL, Otto CM. Characterization of the use of antiemetic agents in dogs with parvovirus enteritis treated at a veterinary teaching hospital: 77 cases (1997–2000). J Am Vet Med Assoc 227:1787–1793, 2005.

Matz M. Antiulcer therapy. In Bonagura JD (ed), Current Veterinary Therapy XII, Philadelphia, WB Saunders Co., 1995.

Mavligit GM. Immunologic effects of cimetidine: potential uses. Pharmacotherapy 7(Suppl):120S–124S, 1987.

Mealey KL. Therapeutic implications of the MDR-1 gene. J Vet Pharmacol Therap 27:257–264, 2004.

Merritt AM. The equine stomach: a personal perspective. AAEP Proceedings 49:75–102, 2003.

Mitchelson F. Pharmacological agents affecting emesis (two parts). Drugs 43:295–315, and 443–463, 1992.

Monfort JD, Donahoe JP, Stills HF, Bech-Nielsen S. Efficacies of erythromycin and chloramphenicol in extinguishing fecal shedding of *Campylobacter jejuni* in dogs. J Am Vet Med Assoc 196:1069–1072, 1990.

Morgan RV, Bachrach A. Keratoconjunctivitis sicca associated with sulfonamide therapy in dogs. J Am Vet Med Assoc 180:432–434, 1982.

Mullan NA, Burgess MN, Bywater RJ, et al. The ability of cholestyramine resin and other adsorbents to bind *Escherichia coli* enterotoxins. J Med Microbiol 12:487–496, 1979.

Murray MJ. Suppression of gastric acidity in horses. J Am Vet Med Assoc 211:37–40, 1997.

Neiger R, Simpson KW. *Helicobacter* infection in dogs and cats: facts and fiction. J Vet Intern Med 14:125–133, 2000.

Papich MG. Medical therapy of gastrointestinal ulceration. In Kirk RW (ed), Current Veterinary Therapy X. Philadelphia, WB Saunders Co., 911–918, 1989.

———. Toxicoses associated with human over-the-counter drugs. Vet Clin N Am (Sm Anim) 20: 431–451, 1990.

———. Antiulcer therapy. Vet Clin N Am (Sm Anim) 23:497–512, 1993.

Papich MG, Davis CA, Davis LE. Absorption of salicylate from an antidiarrheal preparation in dogs and cats. J Am Anim Hosp Assoc 23:221–226, 1987.

Ringger NC, Lester GD, Neuwirth L, et al. Effect of bethanechol or erythromycin on gastric emptying in horses. Am J Vet Res 57:1771–1775, 1996.

Roger T, Bardon T, Ruckebusch Y. Colonic motor responses in the pony: Relevance of colonic stimulation by opiate antagonists. Am J Vet Res 46:31–35, 1985.

Rollin RE, Mero KN, Kozisek PB, et al. Diarrhea and malabsorption in calves associated with therapeutic doses of antibiotics: absorptive and clinical changes. Am J Vet Res 47:987–991, 1986.

Roussel AJ, Hooper RN, Cohen ND, et al. Prokinetic effects of erythromycin on the ileum, cecum, and pelvic flexure of horses during the postoperative period. Am J Vet Res 61:420–424, 2000.

Ruckebusch Y. Pharmacology of reticulo-ruminal motor function. J Vet Pharmacol Therap. 6:245–272, 1983.

Ruckebusch Y, Merritt AM. Pharmacology of the ruminant gastroduodenal junction. J Vet Pharmacol Therap 8:339–351, 1985.

Ruckebusch Y, Roger T. Prokinetic effects of cisapride, naloxone, and parasympathetic stimulation at the equine ileo-caeco-colonic junction. J Vet Pharmacol Ther 11:322–329, 1988.

Sams RA, Gerken DF, Dyke TM, Reed SM, Ashcraft SM. Pharmacokinetics of intravenous and intragastric cimetidine in horses. 1. Effects of intravenous cimetidine on pharmacokinetics of intravenous phenylbutazone. J Vet Pharmacol Ther 20(5):355–36l, 1997.

Sanchez LC, Lester GD, Merritt AM. Effect of ranitidine on intragastric pH in clinically normal neonatal foals. Am J Vet Res 212:1407–1412, 1998.

Sasaki N, Okamura K, Yamada H. Effects of mosapride, a 5-hydroxytryptamine 4 receptor agonist, on electrical activity of the small intestine and cecum in horses. Am J Vet Res 66(8):1321–3, 2005.

Simpson KW, Neiger R, DeNovo R, Scherding. The relationship of *Helicobacter* spp. infection to gastric disease in dogs and cats. J Vet Intern Med 14:223–227, 2000.

Sojka JE, Adams SB, Lamar CH, Eller LL. Effect of butorphanol, pentazocine, meperidine, or metoclopramide on intestinal motility in female ponies. Am J Vet Res 49:527–529, 1988.

Suerbaum S, Michetti P. *Heliobacter pylori* infection. New Engl J Med 347(15):1175–1186, 2002.

Taguchi A, Sharma N, Saleem RM, Sessler DI, Carpenter RL, Seyedsadr M, Kurz A. Selective postoperative inhibition of gastrointestinal opioid receptors. New Engl J Med 345:935–940, 2001.

Tumulty JW, Broussard JD, Steiner JM, Peterson ME, Williams DA. Clinical effects of short-term oral budesonide on the hypothalamic-pituitary-adrenal axis in dogs with inflammatory bowel disease. J Am Anim Hosp Assoc 40:120–123, 2004.

Vail DM, Rodabaugh HS, Conder GA, Boucher JF, Mathur S. Efficacy of injectable maropitant (Cerenia) in a ramdomized clinical trial for prevention and treatment of cisplatin-induced emesis in dogs presented as veterinary patients. Vet Compar Oncol 5:38–46, 2007.

Van Nueten JM, Schuurkes JAJ. Development of a gastrointestinal prokinetic: pharmacology of cisapride. Front Gastrol Res 20:54–63, 1992.

Washabau RJ, Hall JA. Cisapride. J Am Vet Med Assoc 207: 1285–1288, 1995.

———. Diagnosis and management of gastrointestinal motility disorders in dogs and cats. Comp Contin Ed Pract Vet 19:721–736, 1997.

Washabau RJ, Holt DE. Diseases of the large intestine [Chapter 223]. In Ettinter SJ and Feldman EC. Textbook of Veterinary Internal Medicine. Diseases of the Dog and Cat, 6th Edition. Elsevier Saunders, St. Louis Missouri, 2005. 1378–1408.

Washabau RJ, Summarco J. Effects of cisapride on feline colonic smooth muscle function. Am J Vet Res 57:541–546, 1996.

Watson JW, Gonsalves SF, Fossa AA, McLean et al. The anti-emetic effects of CP-99,994 in the ferret and the dog: role of the NK1 receptor. Br J Pharmacol 115:84–94, 1995.

Westermarck E, Frias R, Skrzypczak T. Effect of diet and tylosin on chronic diarrhea in beagles. J Vet Intern Med 19(6):822–7, 2005.

Westermarck E, Skrzypczak T, Harmoinen J, Steiner JM, Ruaux CG, Williams DA, Eerola E, Sundback P, Rinkinen M. Tylosin-responsive chronic diarrhea in dogs. J Vet Intern Med 19(2):177–86, 2005.

Wilcke JR, Turner JC. Use of adsorbents in gastrointestinal problems in small animals. Sem Vet Med Surg (Sm Anim) 2:266–273, 1987.

Wilson DV, Evans AT, Mauer WA. Influence of metoclopramide on gastroesophageal reflux in anesthetized dogs. Am J Vet Res 67:26–31, 2006.

Winberg B, Spohr A, Dietz HH, et al. Quantitative analysis of inflammatory and immune response in dogs with gastritis and their relationship to *Helicobacter* spp. infection. J Vet Intern Med 19:4–14, 2005.

Wittek T, Constable P.D. Assessment of the effects of erythromycin, neostigmine, and metoclopramide on abomasal motility and emptying rate in calves. Am J Vet Res 66:545–552, 2005.

Wu Y, Loper A, Landis E, Hettrick I, Novak L, Lynn K, Chen C, Thompson K, Higgins R, Batra U, Shelukar S, Kwei G, Storey D. The role of biopharmaceutics in the development of a clinical nanoparticle formulation of MK 0869: a Beagle dog model predicts improved bioavailability and diminished food effect on absorption in human. Intl J Pharmaceut 285(1–2):135–146, 2004.

Yamasaki K, Suematsu H, Takahashi T. Comparison of gastric lesions in dogs and cats with and without gastric spiral organisms. J Am Vet Med Assoc 212:529–533, 1998.

CHAPTER

48

DERMATOPHARMACOLOGY: DRUGS ACTING LOCALLY ON THE SKIN

JIM E. RIVIERE

A large number of cases seen in the everyday practice of small- and large-animal veterinary medicine involve lesions of the skin or its appendages. This chapter reviews the salient features of the general anatomy, histology, and biochemistry of skin relevant to the treatment of dermatologic disease; acquaints the practitioner with the features of percutaneous drug absorption relevant to the treatment of skin disease; and discusses the categories of pharmacologic preparations available on the veterinary market to treat skin diseases in domestic animals. The specific drugs used to treat skin diseases are well covered in other chapters of this text. Chapters that should be consulted for application to skin disease include those on antimicrobials, analgesics, and antiinflammatory drugs; antipruretics and antihistamines; glucocorticoids; immunosuppressives (cyclosporine); and ectoparasiticides.

Only in the last few decades have scientists begun to understand how the skin functions in normal and diseased states, to understand the skin's barrier function in terms of water loss and drug delivery, and that attempts have been made to improve the delivery of pharmaceutical agents through the skin by temporarily adjusting that barrier to deliver the drug. In order to successfully minimize the skin's ability to block the absorption of drugs to treat dermatologic disease in domestic animals, it is imperative to understand the normal functional anatomy and biochemistry of the skin. In veterinary medicine, transdermal delivery is widely employed when pesticides are applied monthly to a single area of skin for the control of fleas and ticks over the entire body. Transdermal fentanyl patches are also widely used for postsurgical analgesia. This topical port of drug delivery will see increased use for other therapeutic indications. However, most drugs applied to the skin are not intended to be absorbed systemically but are used to elicit a local therapeutic effect in the treated skin.

The characteristic that separates dermatologic therapy from other components of veterinary pharmacology is this use of topical dosage formulations to treat surface conditions or to target the underlying skin. The drugs are not different from those used in other diseases, but they are different in the vehicles employed and mode of administration. A full understanding of the biological factors that modulate absorption and of the pharmaceutical composition of dermatologic formulations (e.g., vehicles) is essential to a proper understanding of dermatopharmacology. It must be stressed that the drugs incorporated into these formulations are the same as those used to treat diseases of other systems and thus, their descriptions will not be repeated in this chapter.

ANATOMY AND HISTOLOGY

The skin is the largest organ of the body, with the integument accounting for 24% of the overall body weight in the puppy and 12% in the adult dog (Pavletic 1991). The skin has the function of protecting the internal organs of the body from extremes in temperature fluctuations, allergens, pollutants, toxic chemicals, and organisms such as bacteria, fungi, parasites, and viruses found ubiquitously in the environment.

The skin of domestic animals is quite similar in gross and histologic morphology across species lines and is usually thickest over the head, dorsum of the neck, back, and sacrum and on the plantar and palmar surfaces of the feet. It is thinner on the ventral abdomen, the medial surfaces of the limbs, and the inner pinnae, and thinnest over the scrotum of male animals and the earlobe of the human. Perforating the skin are several types of appendages (depending on the species), such as hair follicles, sebaceous and sweat glands, spines, quills, scales, spurs, horns, claws, nails, and hooves (Montagna 1967). The specific anatomy of skin and hair has been reviewed extensively elsewhere (Monteiro-Riviere 2006; Blackburn 1965; Lloyd et al. 1979a,b; Sar and Calhoun 1966; Kozlowski and Calhoun 1969; Strickland and Calhoun 1963; Talukdar et al. 1972; Pavletic 1991; Montagna 1967; Amakiri 1973).

THE EPIDERMIS. On the histological level, the skin can be divided into two distinct units: the epidermis and the dermis. The epidermis consists of stratified squamous keratinized epithelium that undergoes a programmed proliferation and differentiation that will eventually result in the formation of the major barrier to drug penetration: the stratum corneum. Two primary cell types exist in the epidermis: those of keratinocyte origin and those of nonkeratinocyte origin.

Five distinct layers of keratinocytes can be present in the epidermis as shown in Figure 48.1. Listed from the deepest layer of the epidermis to the most superficial, they are 1) stratum basale (basal layer), 2) stratum spinosum (prickle layer), 3) stratum granulosum (granular layer), 4) stratum lucidum (clear layer), and 5) the stratum corneum (horny layer). Each cell layer has its point of origin at the stratum basale. The stratum basale is a single layer of cuboidal or columnar cells that rest on the basal lamina. These cells are attached to the basal lamina by hemidesmasomes, and to each other and to the cells of the stratum spinosum by desmasomes. The stratum basale cells continuously divide, with some remaining as basal cells and others beginning to move more superficially and mature by changing their intracellular content through the process called *keratinization*. This viable and dividing epidermal cell layer is the target for transformation into cancerous cells.

The next more superficial layer next to the stratum basale, the stratum spinosum, is composed of irregularly shaped polyhedral cells that make up much of the bulk thickness of the epidermis. The next layer composes the stratum granulosum, which consists of several layers of cells that begin to flatten horizontally. Of primary interest are the lamellated granules within these cells, which contain polar phospholipids, such as glycosphingolipids and free steroids, and numerous hydrolytic enzymes, including acid phosphatase, proteases, lipases, and glycosidases. As these intracellular products accumulate, these cells will exocytose their intracellular products and fill in the intercellular spaces, eventually forming the extracellular lipid matrix of the stratum corneum that forms the penetration

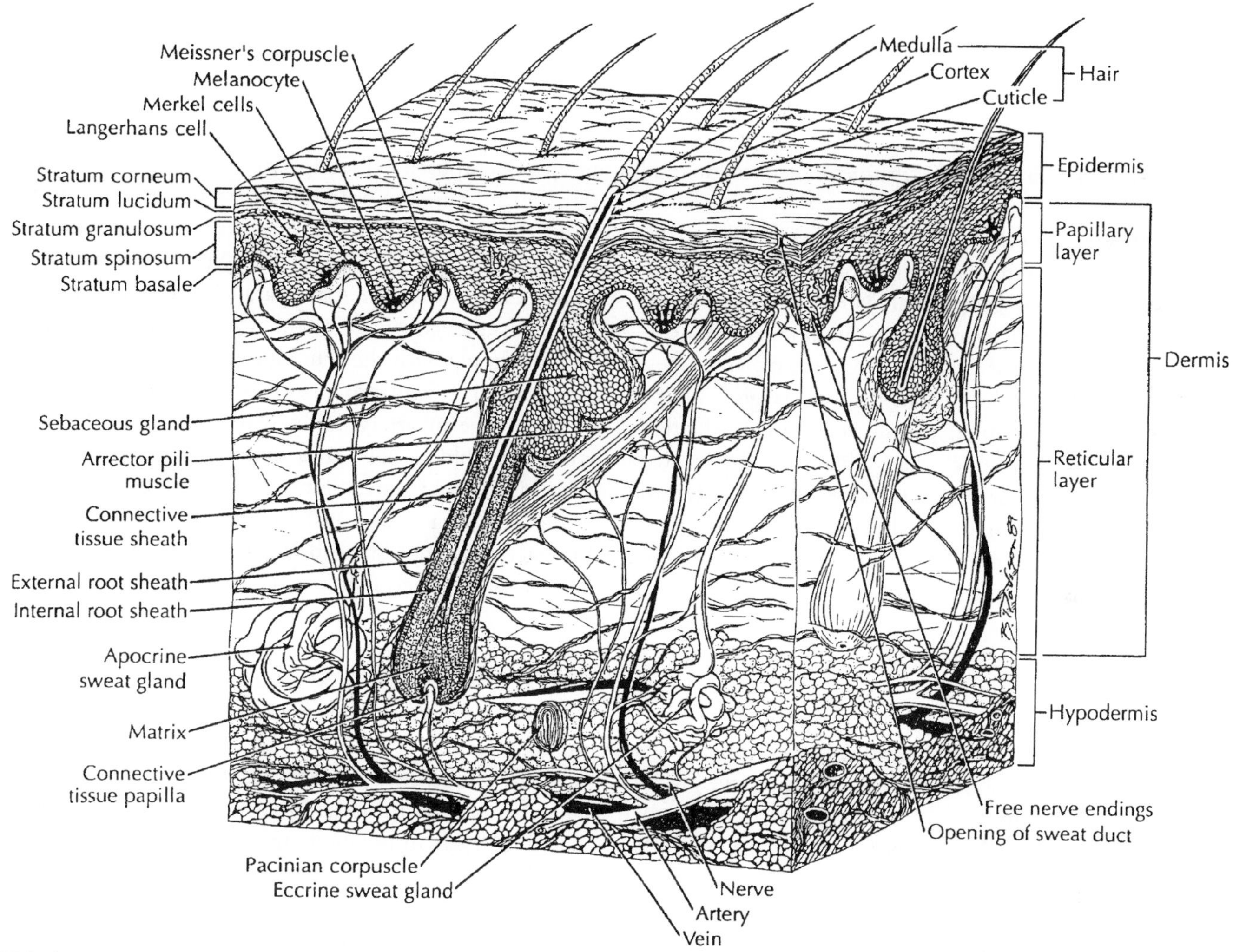

FIG. 48.1 A schematic view of the epidermis and dermis of the skin (Monteiro-Riviere 1991).

barrier of the stratum corneum. As these epidermal cells continue their migration, they form the stratum lucidum, a translucent line of cells found only in areas having very thick skin, such as plantar and palmar surfaces (footpads) and the planum nasale. These cells are translucent because both nuclei and cytoplasmic organelles are missing (Monteiro-Riviere 1991, 2006; Idsen 1975; Montagna 1967).

The stratum corneum is the final and most superficial layer of the epidermis and is its most important when considering the feasibility of topical drug therapy since it is the primary barrier to percutaneous absorption. In addition to the barrier function for xenobiotics trying to enter the body from the environment, the stratum corneum also provides a barrier to insensible water loss, an evolutionary adaptation that allows terrestial animals to exist in a nonaquatic environment. In fact, most veterinary dermatologic vehicles are targeted at this action. This layer consists of several dead layers of cells, organized into vertical columns in a tetrakaidecahedral (14-sided) configuration, the thickness of which varies depending on location (Monteiro-Riviere 1991). This particular cell shape provides a minimal surface-to-volume ratio and also minimizes systemic water loss through the skin (transepidermal water loss). Each cell is ingrained in the lipid matrix produced by the lamellated granules when the cells were still in the stratum granulosum layer. These dead cells are also surrounded by a thick plasma membrane with a submembranous layer of involucrin, also produced earlier in development. With intracellular and intercellular barriers firmly in place, the stratum corneum has the ability to constrain the passage of unwanted chemicals and toxins from the environment. Unfortunately, the stratum corneum does not discriminate between these unwanted substances and the pharmaceuticals the veterinarian may wish to penetrate the skin for topical drug therapy for the treatment of dermatologic disease.

Melanocytes are cells located in the basal layer of the epidermis and contain dark cytoplasmic granules called melanosomes. These cells impart color to the skin, the color and intensity determined by the number, size, distribution, and degree of melanization of the melanosomes. Merkel cells are also located in the basal region of the epidermis and are thought to function as slow-adapting mechanoreceptors for touch. Langerhans cells are located in the stratum spinosum but can also be present in dermal lymph vessels, lymph nodes, and dermis. The Langerhans cells' primary function is to present antigen to lymphocytes; they may also be the initial receptors for cutaneous immune responses.

THE DERMIS. The dermis is composed of connective tissue consisting of collagen, elastin, and reticular fibers dispersed in an amorphous ground substance and can be divided into two rather poorly demarcated areas. The papillary layer consists of loose connective tissue and connects the epidermis (stratum basale/basal lamina) to the deeper reticular layer of the dermis. The reticular layer consists of dense connective tissue connected to the hypodermis, which is composed mostly of fat.

Dispersed throughout both layers of the dermis is a network of arterial and venous blood vessels needed to nourish the cells of the epidermis and dermis as well as take part in the last stages of the percutaneous absorption of compounds. Lymph vessels, nerves, apocrine and eccrine sweat glands, sebaceous glands, Pacinian (pressoreceptor), Meissner's (touch receptor), and Ruffini (mechanical receptor) corpuscles, hair follicles, and smooth muscles (arrector pili) are the other major structures found in the dermis. Two types of arteries, musculocutaneous and direct cutaneous, supply the needed nutrients to the epidermis. Direct cutaneous arteries run parallel to the skin, directly supplying the skin with blood, while musculocutaneous arteries supply both the skin and underlying musculature and run perpendicular to the skin. Cutaneous blood supply by each type of artery varies with species and location. Cutaneous blood flow rates may be one of the factors affecting the passive percutaneous absorption of chemicals. Table 48.1 clearly demonstrates this by comparing laser Doppler cutaneous blood flow parameters in nine species of domestic animals (Monteiro-Riviere et al. 1990).

SPECIES DIFFERENCES. As a general rule, skin structure and function are similar across species lines. However, some minor differences are apparent.

Avian integument possesses the most profound differences in skin morphology from other domestic species. The four layers of the epidermis are, from the deepest to the most superficial, the stratum basale, the stratum intermedium (stratum spinosum), the stratum transitivum (stratum granulosum), and the stratum corneum (stratum germinativum). Unlike mammals, avians possess no skin glands (Monteiro-Riviere 2006). The skin of aquatic mammals has a very thick stratum corneum resembling

TABLE 48.1 Cutaneous blood flow measurements in nine species of domestic animals

	Buttocks	Pinnae	Humeroscapular Joint	Thoracolumbar Joint	Ventral Species Abdomen
Feline	1.82 ± 0.59	6.46 ± 2.30	1.86 ± 0.70	2.39 ± 0.35	6.19 ± 0.94
Bovine	6.03 ± 1.84	6.98 ± 2.19	5.51 ± 2.32	5.49 ± 1.49	10.5 ± 2.13
Canine	2.21 ± 0.67	5.21 ± 1.53	5.52 ± 1.31	1.94 ± 0.27	8.78 ± 1.40
Equine	3.16 ± 1.22	NA	6.76 ± 1.49	2.99 ± 0.86	8.90 ± 1.46
Primate	3.12 ± 0.58	20.9 ± 5.37	8.49 ± 3.28	2.40 ± 0.82	3.58 ± 0.41
Mouse	3.88 ± 0.92	1.41 ± 0.48	10.1 ± 3.51	20.6 ± 4.69	36.9 ± 8.14
Porcine	3.08 ± 0.48	11.7 ± 3.02	6.75 ± 2.09	2.97 ± 0.56	10.7 ± 2.14
Rabbit	3.55 ± 0.93	8.38 ± 1.53	5.38 ± 1.06	5.46 ± 0.94	17.3 ± 6.31
Rat	4.20 ± 1.05	9.13 ± 4.97	6.22 ± 1.47	9.56 ± 2.17	11.4 ± 5.53

Source: Adapted from Monteiro-Riviere et al. 1990.
Values are ml/min/100 g tissue, ± standard error of the mean.
NA = data not available.

parakeratosis and there is no stratum granulosum (Montagna 1967).

Pigskin is similar histologically to human skin (Monteiro-Riviere and Stromberg 1985) and has been used experimentally to reliably predict the percutaneous absorption of chemicals in humans (Riviere 2006). With respect to cutaneous circulation, musculocutaneous arteries are the primary vascular supply to the skin of humans, apes, and swine. Loose-skinned animals (canines and felines) lack musculocutaneous arteries; all vessels involved in cutaneous circulation travel parallel to the skin (Pavletic 1991). Recent studies of piroxicam (a nonsteroidal antiinflammatory drug) in pigs suggest that the type of cutaneous circulation may affect the local tissue concentrations of topically applied drug (Monteiro-Riviere et al. 1993). Little work has been done directly comparing the absorption of drugs and topical pesticides across veterinary species (Riviere and Papich 2001).

BIOCHEMISTRY

ENERGY PRODUCTION AND UTILIZATION. The skin, specifically the epidermis, is mostly an anaerobic organ. The absence of capillaries directly feeding oxygen to the epidermal cells makes the epidermal cells relatively oxygen poor in the normal state when compared to other tissues with a more direct blood supply. Due to this low oxygen tension, the epidermis produces 70–80% of its total energy requirements (adenosine triphosphate) through the anaerobic metabolic pathway (glycolysis), with lactic acid being the end product of glucose utilization. The epidermal cells, the most active of which are those in the single layer of the stratum basale, are the primary cells involved in this energy production, with the lactic acid end product passively diffusing into the dermis and then into the blood vasculature, eventually recycled by the liver back into glucose. Although the glycolytic pathway produces most of the energy requirements of the epidermis, other energy pathways (tricarboxylic acid cycle and pentose phosphate shunt) are also utilized to lesser degrees in some phases of epidermal growth (Freinkel 1983).

Some topically applied drugs may have an effect on energy production pathways within the epidermis. One study (Spoo et al. 1993) showed that in vitro weanling porcine skin flaps had large increases in epidermal cell glucose utilization when the skin was dosed with benzoyl peroxide. In addition to drugs, vehicles (discussed in more detail later) may also have similar effects.

DRUG BIOTRANSFORMATION. The stratum corneum is the primary line of defense to prevent percutaneous absorption of drugs. However, any drug passing through the stratum corneum may face a metabolic, rather than a physical, barrier. The skin has a remarkable ability to metabolize xenobiotics. These metabolic reactions consist mainly of oxidation, reduction, hydrolysis, and the phase I and II conjugation reactions. Enzymes present within the extracellular lipid matrix include acid lipase, phospholipase A, sphingomyelinase, glycosidases, acid phosphatases, cathepsins, and carboxypeptidases (Elias 1992). Some of these reactions are major pathways for the metabolism of topical steroids as well as other drugs such as norepinephrine, benzoyl peroxide, and benzo(a)pyrene.

Skin has been shown to metabolize organophosphate parasiticides. When parathion is topically applied to the skin and penetration through the stratum corneum occurs, it undergoes significant metabolism within the epidermis to the bioactive metabolite paraoxon and/or *p*-nitro phenol, both of which will enter the systemic circulation to possibly affect other organ systems (Riviere and Chang 1992). Additional studies have demonstrated the metabolic capabilities of skin when topically exposed to caffeine, testosterone, butylated hydroxytoluene, salicylic acid, norepinephrine, benzo(a)pyrene, and benzoyl peroxide—to name only a few—in many species of laboratory animals, as well as in human skin. Benzoyl peroxide, a popular veterinary drug used as a keratolytic and degreasing agent, is metabolized almost 100% to benzoic acid within the epidermis. In addition, the cytochrome P450 enzyme system, most commonly associated with the liver, is present and is inducible in skin (depending on the compound that was applied topically) and is the pathway that is responsible for the conversion of parathion into paraoxon in porcine skin (Riviere and Chang 1992; Mukhtar 1992; Bashir and Maibach 2005). Glutathione S-transferase, aryl hydrocarbon hydroxylase, and 7-ethoxycoumarin have also been demonstrated to exist in rat and mice epidermal cell homogenates (Raza et al. 1992). These studies all show that the skin has formidable metabolic functions as well as the traditional barrier functions.

LIPID METABOLISM. In addition to its metabolic activities, skin also has a marked ability to synthesize lipid, which is used to construct the extracellular epidermal barrier. Epidermal cells manufacture a variety of neutral lipids, ceramides, glycosylceramides, gangliosides, sterol esters, fatty acids, alkanes, and phospholipids, which are largely found in the extracellular barrier of the stratum corneum. Some of these lipids tend to be site-specific, with phospholipids and sterols residing mostly in the basal cell layers and some sterols and neutral lipids occupying the upper regions of the epidermis, mainly the stratum corneum. The effects on percutaneous absorption by the intercellular lipid structure have been discussed in greater detail elsewhere (Wertz 1992; Potts and Francoeur 1992; Hadgraft et al. 1992; Swartzendruber 1992; Elias and Feingold 1992; Monteiro-Riviere at al. 2001). It is now accepted that this complex intercellular lipid matrix provides the primary barrier to drug penetration. It is important to realize that in some skin disease states, the overall production of lipids by the epidermal cells may be altered due to altered intracellular metabolism, subsequently followed by some alterations in the percutaneous absorption patterns of many drugs. Alterations in the epidermal cells' plasma membrane (primarily composed of lipid)—whether due directly to a drug(s), by the vehicle a drug was delivered in, or due to a disease process—may incite inflammatory reactions due to the release of inflammatory mediators (eicosanoids) from the epidermal cells or from the underlying cutaneous vasculature. Eicosanoids are a group of biologically active compounds derived enzymatically from eicosatetraenoic acid (arachidonic acid). Prostaglandins, leukotrienes, thromboxanes, and hydroxyeicosatetraenoic acids can be produced in minute quantities from arachidonic acid and have powerful proinflammatory effects on skin and the surrounding tissues. Eicosanoids are found in nearly every tissue in the mammalian body (Spannhake et al. 1981; Dunn and Hood 1977; Goldyne 1986), with some cells specializing in a certain type of eicosanoid. Skin produces several prostaglandins, including PGE_2, $PGF_{2\alpha}$, and PGI_2, as well as the lipoxygenase product leukotriene B_4.

PGE_2 induces vasodilation by elevating cyclic adenosine monophosphate in vascular smooth muscle cells, while $PGF_{2\alpha}$ causes vasoconstriction of the cutaneous vasculature by elevating cyclic guanosine monophosphate levels in vascular smooth muscle cells. In contrast to PGE_2, increased $PGF_{2\alpha}$ concentrations in skin enhance the leukocytes' response to chemotactic stimuli. $PGF_{2\alpha}$ has many effects on organs other than the skin, most notably in the reproductive tract of both humans and domestic animals. PGI_2 is a potent vasodilator produced mainly by vascular endothelial cells; it also inhibits vascular platelet aggregation. PGI_2 can be released from skin in response to some vehicles—namely, alcohols such as methanol, ethanol, and 2-propanol (Landolfi and Steiner 1984; Karanian et al. 1985). Cutaneous vasodilation has been observed in humans orally consuming alcohol (ethanol), presumably due to release of PGI_2 from vascular endothelial cells in contact with the alcohol-containing blood (Landolfi and Steiner 1984).

Leukotriene B_4 (LTB_4) is an inflammatory mediator produced from arachidonic acid via 5-lipoxygenase enzyme activity (Ford-Hutchinson 1985). As with $PGF_{2\alpha}$, LTB_4 is a potent chemotactic agent (Paulissen et al. 1990; Van de Kerkhof et al. 1991) and may also be a potent vasodilator and cause significant increases in vascular permeability when coadministered with PGE_2 (Ford-Hutchinson 1985). Although LTB_4 is most commonly produced by leukocytes, skin contains some inherent 5-lipoxygenase activity as determined from studies using stimulated human keratinocytes in culture as well as human and murine epidermal homogenates (Ruzicka 1990). These inflammatory mediator-induced changes in cutaneous blood flow may impact on the absorption and cutaneous distribution of topically applied drugs.

PROTEIN METABOLISM. The primary protein product of the skin is keratin, which is the main intracellular component of the stratum corneum. In tandem with extracellular lipid, keratin forms the major component of the epidermal barrier. Keratin primarily consists of cystine, serine, glutamic acid, arginine, aspartic acid, and glycine amino acid residues. Of significance within the keratin molecule structure is the intrachain cystine disulfide bridging that further strengthens the overall keratin macrostructure. Keratin is the major protein foundation of hair (Monteiro-Riviere 1991, 2006).

PRINCIPLES OF PERCUTANEOUS ABSORPTION: SKIN PERMEABILITY

Prior to the 20th century, many scientists believed that skin was an impermeable barrier to all substances, except possibly gases. The science of dermatology has since advanced to reveal that many substances can enter the systemic circulation via the skin. Four pathways by which

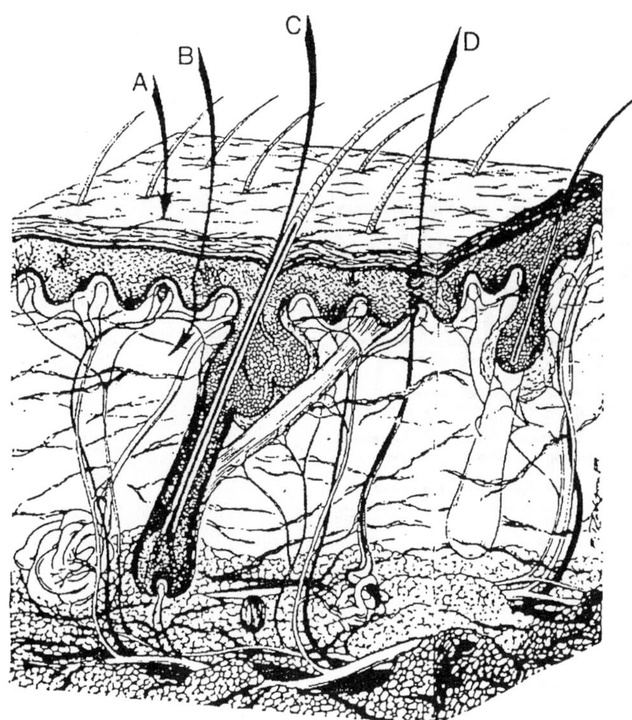

FIG. 48.2 A schematic view of the skin and the four routes of drug penetration. Drugs can penetrate through the stratum corneocytes (A), between the stratum corneocytes (B), transfollicularly via any hair follicle (C), or via an eccrine sweat gland or sebaceous gland (D).

substances can gain this access to the rest of the body have been postulated and are schematically shown in Figure 48.2.

The percutaneous absorption of drugs is important from two perspectives. Veterinary clinicians should be concerned about how much of a drug actually penetrates the skin to achieve a pharmacologic effect in treating diseases of the skin. This can be a function of several factors including vehicle selection, hydration state of the stratum corneum, partition coefficient of the drug from vehicle into the stratum corneum lipids, the integrity of the stratum corneum, and cutaneous blood flow. The other need for knowing the extent of percutaneous absorption lies in the field of public health and food consumption. Many compounds used in food animals are applied to and absorbed through the skin and enter the systemic circulation. Many of these compounds are stored in edible tissues (fat, muscle) for long periods of time, causing concern about residues in these tissues (Baynes et al. 1997; Riviere 1992).

The stratum corneum is accepted to be the major barrier, but not the only barrier, to percutaneous penetration in most species of animals. Passive diffusion is defined here as the movement of matter from one space to another space by random molecular motion. No known active transport processes are used by stratum corneum to modulate percutaneous absorption. To better understand how substances diffuse through the stratum corneum, it is convenient to think of the stratum corneum as a wall in a "brick and mortar" configuration (Elias 1983), with the bricks representing the stratum corneocytes and the mortar representing the lipid matrix around them, as shown in Figure 48.3. In this context, permeation through the stratum corneum might occur via two routes. The first involves the drug traversing through the stratum corneocytes ("bricks") and extracellular lipid matrix ("mortar"), through the cells of the deeper epidermal cells, and then into the systemic circulation. The second route involves the chemical maneuvering its way through the stratum corneum via the intercellular lipid matrix only. It is generally accepted that the primary route of penetration is via the intercellular pathway. Because of the structure of the stratum corneum and the metabolic capabilities of the lower epidermal cells, the veterinarian must be aware that only a small percentage of the drug that is topically applied is going to actually penetrate the stratum corneum. This small fraction of the total dose will need to be able to affect the disease process occurring in the underlying layers of the epidermis.

The molecular structure of the intercellular lipid matrix throughout the epidermis is in a liquid crystalline configuration, consisting of fatty acids, ceramides, triglycerides, sterols, sterol esters, cholesterol sulfate, and miscellaneous alkanes. As epidermal cells migrate superficially and transform into the cells of the stratum corneum, the lipid content surrounding these cells changes from polar to more neutral in nature. Specifically, phospholipids and triglycerides tend to decrease while fatty acids, cholesterol, cholesterol sulfate, ceramides, and sphingolipids increase as the epidermal cells differentiate (Elias 1992). Enzymes are also present within this matrix of lipid. These lipids organize themselves into a lipid bilayer structure, with the hydrophobic ends of the molecules orienting themselves with other hydrophobic ends, and the hydrophilic ends orienting themselves in a similar fashion. More than one lipid bilayer can be formed within the intercellular matrix, leading to the formation of hydrophilic and hydrophobic channels, as illustrated in Figure 48.4. One might assume

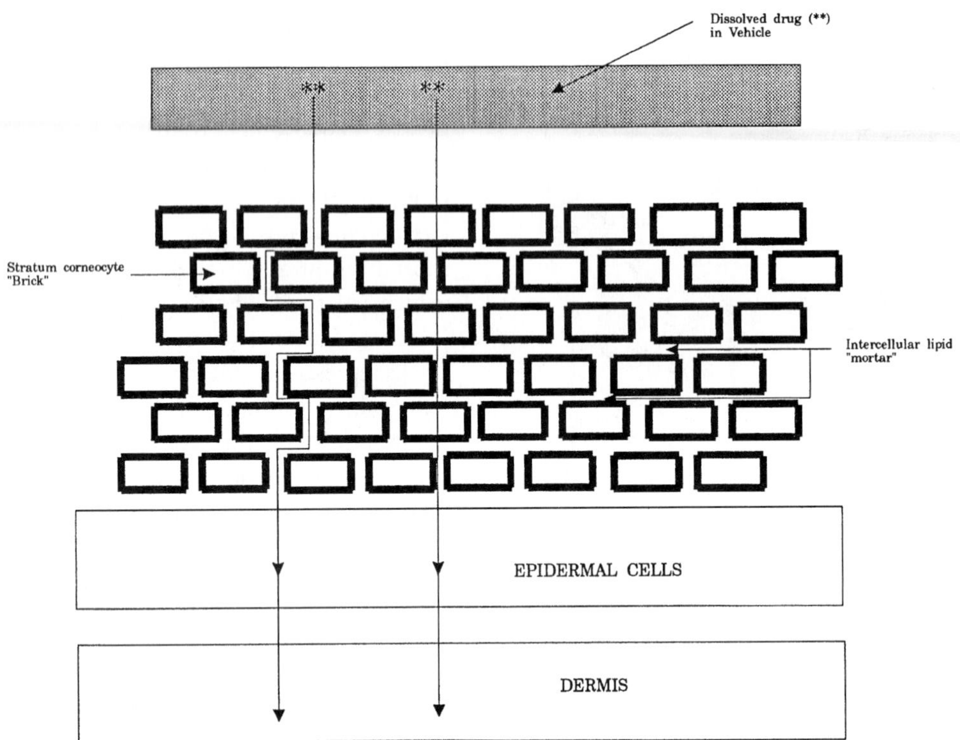

FIG. 48.3 Simplistic "brick and mortar" model of the skin. Drugs can penetrate by traveling around the stratum corneocytes through the lipid matrix, or drugs can pass through each corneocyte via the lipid matrix.

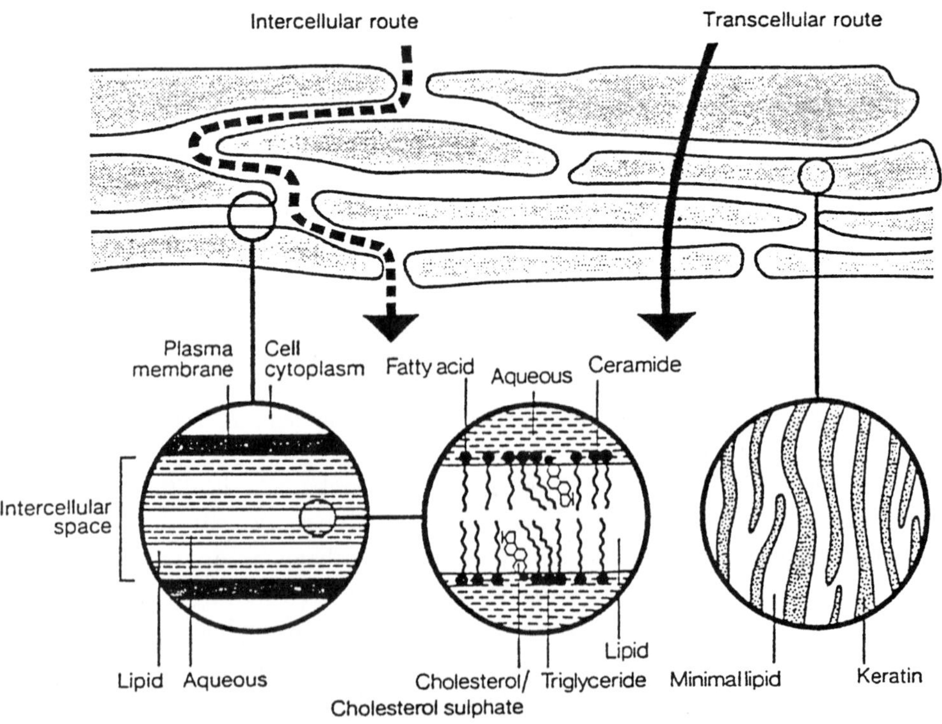

FIG. 48.4 The lipid bilayer model of the stratum corneum.

that this complex lipid barrier would result in very low absorption profiles for hydrophilic (water soluble) compounds since these molecules would have difficulty crossing a hydrophobic barrier, but some studies have shown that many hydrophilic compounds penetrate the epidermis in much higher quantities than predicted, implying that there are other mechanisms whereby hydrophilic compounds permeate the stratum corneum. The primary mechanism by which this is accomplished is for hydrophilic molecules to penetrate through fluctuations, or "kinks," in the lipid alkyl chains (Potts and Francoeur 1992; Potts et al. 1992). Further, the permeation of hydrophilic molecules (such as water, methanol, ethanol, etc.) through the lipid matrix is due to their small size and molecular weight, which aid them in traveling through the lipid matrix through passages established by the lipid alkyl chains. This view is supported by the observation that larger hydrophilic molecules have lower percutaneous absorptions than their smaller molecular weight counterparts. Alternatively, penetration may also occur through the aqueous channels formed between the polar head groups of the lipid layers.

Chemicals may also permeate the skin using the skin appendageal route, mostly by way of hair follicles and sweat ducts. The importance of the transappendageal route on percutaneous absorption is controversial, but some studies indicate that the importance of this route tends to be species-specific (Pitman and Rostas 1981). Generally, those animals possessing a sparse number of hair follicles per area of skin (humans, pigs) are considered to have little, if any, absorption of topically applied compounds via this route when compared to those animals having a high density of hair follicles (cattle, sheep). In these latter animals, the stratum corneum barrier is just as impermeable to drugs as that of their less-haired counterparts, but the drug permeates the skin barrier via the hair follicles, sweat ducts, or other openings in the stratum corneum, increasing the percutaneous absorption of the chemical. It has been demonstrated that transappendageal absorption is high initially, then becomes insignificant, due to the small surface area of follicles and glands in relation to the total surface area of the stratum corneum. Topical delivery of pesticides to domestic livestock has been used for many years for the control of external as well as internal parasites of these animals, indicating that enough of the pesticide is absorbed systemically to kill some internal parasites while not harming the host animal (Riviere 1992).

Two events must occur for a drug to be successfully delivered to the epidermis under the stratum corneum: 1) the drug must diffuse out of the vehicle and onto the surface of the stratum corneum and 2) the drug must be able to penetrate the stratum corneum (Idson 1983). Restated, the vehicle in which the topical drug is being delivered should have significantly less affinity for that drug than for the stratum corneum. In actuality, many factors enter into the release of drug from the vehicle and its penetration through the stratum corneum. These factors have been mathematically described for steady-state kinetics in Fick's first law of diffusion (Idson 1983):

$$dQ/dt = (PC)C_v\mathrm{DA}/h$$

where dQ/dt is a steady rate of penetration, PC is the drug's partition coefficient between the vehicle and the stratum corneum, C_v is the concentration of the drug dissolved in the vehicle, D is the diffusion coefficient, A is the area of skin to which the drug is applied, and h is the diffusion path length through the stratum corneum. In short, Fick's law states that the driving force causing the transfer of a drug from regions of high concentration to areas of low concentration is proportional to the concentration gradient (Idsen 1975). The diffusion coefficient is primarily correlated to the partiton coefficient of the penetrant, and can also be predicted from a knowledge of the drug's molecular volume and hydrogen bond activity (Potts and Guy 1995).

Only the nonionized moiety of a weak acid or base is available for diffusion across the stratum corneum. The pH of skin is variable and sensitive to hydration state. The typical pH of skin ranges from 4.2 to 7.3. For drugs with pK_a values within this range, the ionized fraction may vary according according to the principles governed by the Hendersen-Hasselbalch equation, which would alter the amount of drug available for absorption. This is usually controlled for in the dermatologic formulation by use of buffering systems. Theoretically, vehicles with different pH may have species-specific absorption for drugs with pKa values in this range.

TOPICAL VEHICLES

A vehicle is defined as the medium in which a medicinally active agent is topically administered. It is a gross misconception that the vehicle in which topical drugs are dissolved is inert and has little effect on the skin; in fact, the physical and chemical properties of the vehicle will largely determine how successfully the drug will penetrate the skin. This has been clearly demonstrated with the pesticide carbaryl in pigs (Baynes and Riviere 1998). The vehicle may penetrate the stratum corneum to some extent and change the solubility of the intercellular lipid matrix. A simplistic view of the fate of topically applied drugs has been outlined in Figure 48.5.

The partition coefficient is a unitless measure of the relative affinity of a compound between a highly hydrophobic phase (usually octanol) and a hydrophilic phase (water), and is a physicochemical factor that has a major role in determining the percutaneous absorption of a chemical. As the partition coefficient increases, the compound has a greater affinity for the lipid phase and less affinity for the water phase. As discussed earlier, the intercellular matrix of the skin consists of several different types of lipid, the ratios of which may vary from site to site.

Skin penetration of many chemicals has often been correlated to the partition coefficient of the penetrant. Generally, as the log of the partition coefficient increases, lipid solubility increases and there is an overall increase in the percutaneous absorption of the compound through the skin. This scenario is not always the case, however; some poorly lipid soluble compounds (i.e., low partition coefficients) sometimes penetrate the skin much more easily than compounds with higher partition coefficients. Once penetration into the skin occurs, the molecule must eventually leave the lipid phase to be able to reach the systemic circulation. Compounds with high partition coefficients tend to remain within the lipid of the skin and form a reservoir rather than pass through; this is a well-documented phenomenon in skin (Muhammad et al. 2005). It has been shown that a log partition coefficient of 1–4 is desirable for skin penetration of most compounds.

Absorption of the vehicle into the stratum corneum is another factor to consider, since the vehicle may cause some disruptions in the composition and orientation of the intercellular lipid matrix. Partition coefficients for use in predicting the percutaneous absorption of topically applied drugs should ideally measure the index of affinity of a drug between the vehicle the drug is being delivered in and the lipid/vehicle composition of the stratum corneum. Unfortunately, few measurements of this kind are in existence because interaction of the vehicle with the stratum corneum lipids invalidates its determination. The role of partition coefficients in skin has been extensively reviewed elsewhere (Surber et al. 1990a,b; Sloan et al. 1986; Aungst et al. 1990).

The optimal vehicle is one in which the drug is soluble enough to enter into solution, but has less affinity for the vehicle than the stratum corneum lipids thereby favoring partitioning from the vehicle into the epidermis. Optimal delivery for a polar drug may thus be a relatively hydrophobic vehicle that has sufficient solubility to dissolve the drug. However, if a drug is too soluble in a vehicle relative to the stratum corneum, the drug may persist in the vehicle and only slowly release drug into the skin for as long as the vehicle stays on the skin.

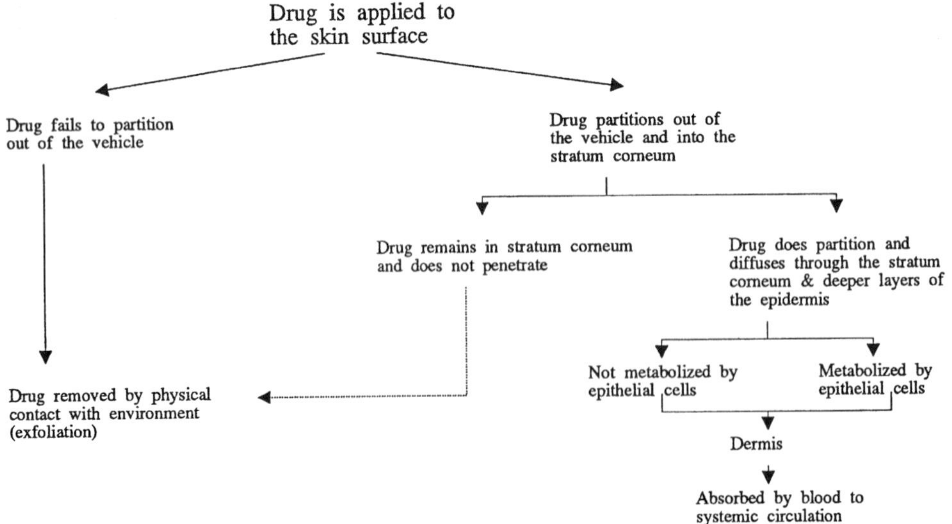

FIG. 48.5 Schematic representation of the fate of topically applied drugs.

The effect of the vehicle on chemical absorption has recently been quantitated based on competing physical chemical interactions of the drug and the vehicle versus the skin, using quantitative structure activity relationship principles (Riviere and Brooks 2005, 2007). This approach has the potential for rationally designing topical drug formulations based on physical chemical principles.

The ability of the vehicle to stay on the skin surface long enough to allow passive absorption of the drug to occur is an important factor in passive drug absorption. The vehicle can be removed by three mechanisms: 1) absorption of the vehicle through the stratum corneum, 2) evaporation from the skin surface into the surrounding air, or 3) physical removal (rubbing, licking, scratching, etc.). If the vehicle penetrates the stratum corneum more quickly than the drug, the concentration of the drug in the vehicle left on the surface of the stratum corneum will increase, which would increase the concentration of drug driving absorption, but would also have the potential of inducing precipitation of the drug onto the skin's surface. The vehicle may also change the permeability of the lipid matrix (e.g., function as an enhancer). Evaporation of the vehicle will result in a similar scenario.

Vehicles may also affect the hydration state of the stratum corneum, which in turn may affect the rate at which topically applied compounds can penetrate the stratum corneum. Occlusion of the skin significantly increases the penetration of parathion (Chang and Riviere 1993) and other compounds. The vehicle can accomplish this by modulating insensible cutaneous water loss or skin transpiration. "Transpiration" is the term used to describe the passage of water vapor from the body, through the epidermis, and out to the surrounding environment. The act of transpiration is an important factor in determining percutaneous absorption of chemicals. In the normal state, the epidermal cells below the stratum corneum are highly hydrated compared to the stratum corneum. The water in and around these epidermal cells tends to slowly "percolate" upward, following the decreasing concentration gradient of water toward the less hydrated stratum corneum, eventually passing through the stratum corneum and into the environment. This phenomenon can be noninvasively assessed by measuring transepidermal water loss (TEWL) and has been correlated to the stratum corneum permeability of hydrophilic drugs. The stratum corneum normally maintains a 10–20% hydration state. When hydration of the stratum corneum occurs, which may reach 60–80% of the total stratum corneum's mass, this water "opens" the compact substance of the stratum corneum and reduces the density of the intracellular structures, thereby decreasing the cells' resistance to passive diffusion and allowing substances to permeate more readily than in the normal, dehydrated state. Hydration of the stratum corneum can be accomplished by slowing the rate of epidermal water loss to the environment by applying occlusive emollients to the skin (petrolatum, lanolin, etc.), by applying a non–water-permeable membrane (patch), by soaking the skin in water, or by increasing the relative humidity of the air surrounding the skin (Blank et al. 1984). An increase in percent hydration from 10 to 50% in the stratum corneum can result in as much as a tenfold increase in diffusion constants (Idson 1983). This effect of environmental humidity and occlusion of the absorption of parathion through pig skin was clearly demonstrated (Chang and Riviere 1993).

Even when fully hydrated, the stratum corneum is one of the most water-impermeable biological membranes found in nature (Idsen 1975). Similarly, decreasing the hydration of the stratum corneum can decrease percutaneous absorption of substances. Dehydration of stratum corneum cells below the normal 10–15% usually results in "dry skin" and is a secondary symptom of many dermatologic diseases. Decreased stratum corneum hydration often results in a rugged and rough feeling to the skin, along with cracking, increased desquamation of the stratum corneum, and possible secondary septic or aseptic dermatitis. Dry skin can be treated by 1) treating the underlying condition causing the disease and/or 2) applying agents that will increase the hydration of the stratum corneum by slowing transepidermal water loss. Applying keratolytics (discussed later in this chapter) is also of use. This discussion should point out that selecting a vehicle that increases the amount of water in the stratum corneum will most likely result in more permeation of drug to the underlying affected tissues, an important factor in successful dermatologic therapy. In diseases involving dry skin, returning the stratum corneum to its normal hydration state should also be a goal of dermatologic therapy.

In summary, the vehicle, not just the choice of drug, plays a crucial role in determining the success or failure of dermatologic therapy. No "ideal vehicle" exists; the veterinary clinician must evaluate the patient's skin lesion and should determine what drug is indicated and which vehicle would best augment that therapy. Both factors may markedly influence the success of therapy. Pharmaceutical classifications of topical vehicles are covered at the end of this chapter.

OTHER FACTORS AFFECTING PERCUTANEOUS ABSORPTION. Other factors that may enhance or hinder percutaneous absorption are the molecular weight of the chemical, temperature, blood flow, and skin age. Increasing the blood flow through the dermis would suggest a more rapid removal of drugs absorbed from the epidermis (Riviere and Williams 1992). Vasoconstriction of these vessels has been shown to significantly decrease percutaneous absorption of 6-methylprednisolone and testosterone (Malkinson 1958). The temperature of the air surrounding the skin plays a role in blood flow, with warmer environmental temperatures or skin showing one of the cardinal signs of inflammation (heat) increasing the blood flow to the skin and cooler temperatures decreasing cutaneous blood flow. An inverse relationship appears to exist between absorption rate and the molecular weight of the drug (Idsen 1975). Although smaller molecules tend to increase total topical dose absorbed through the skin, there is considerable variability in the amounts percutaneously absorbed among compounds of similar molecular weights (Idsen 1975; Tregear 1966).

PENETRATION ENHANCERS. The stratum corneum has been portrayed as a formidable and almost impenetrable barrier to the absorption of lipophilic, hydrophilic, and amphoteric xenobiotics. Many efforts have been made to adjust the barrier of the stratum corneum to increase the percutaneous absorption of topically applied xenobiotics, for the most part with only limited success. The barrier function of the stratum corneum can be structurally modified using a relatively small class of compounds, collectively known as penetration enhancers or penetration accelerants, that increase the percutaneous absorption of many compounds.

Many reports exist in the human and veterinary literature of various agents that have been shown to accelerate penetration of compounds through the skin, but few describe the precise mechanism by which an individual penetration enhancer performs this function. One theory, the lipid-protein–partitioning concept, has been proposed for the mechanism of action of all the known penetration enhancers, including penetration via the intercellular as well as the intracellular routes (Barry 1991). For both routes, this theory acknowledges that polar (hydrophilic) molecules permeate the skin via polar channels (either by aqueous pores or by alkyl group modulation), which are different from the channels used by nonpolar (hydrophobic) molecules. After application to the skin surface, the drug molecules diffuse out of the vehicle and into the stratum corneum and begin to traverse the many aqueous and lipid barriers found in the intercellular matrix (see Fig. 48.4) in order to reach the rest of the body via the systemic circulatory system. Penetration enhancers are hypothesized to modify these lipid and aqueous bilayers of the intercellular lipid matrix and allow topically applied compounds to penetrate the stratum corneum more readily by disrupting the normally very organized structure of the lipid layers.

It is convenient to organize the known penetration enhancers into four common subgroups: azone and its derivatives, urea and its derivatives (1-dodecylurea, 1,3 didodecylurea, 1,3 diphenyl urea, propylene glycol, dimethylisosorbide), the terpenes (carvone, pulegone, piperitone, menthone, cyclohenene oxide, terpinen-4-ol, and others), and the aprotic solvents (dimethylsulfoxide, demethyl formamide, decylmethyl sulfoxide, 2-pyrrolidone, and others). At the present time, the first three groups are used almost exclusively in human pharmaceutical products and research and will not be discussed here. The most extensively used penetration enhancer in veterinary medicine is dimethylsulfoxide (DMSO).

DMSO is a product from the processing of wood pulp and is a dipolar and aprotic solvent. DMSO is also produced by phytoplankton and is present in many foods (Herschler 1982). DMSO has been used to treat a myriad of skin ailments, including otitis externa, interdigital cysts, lick granulomas, superficial burns, skin grafts, and snakebites; and to reduce the engorgement of the mammary glands of the nursing bitch (Knowles 1982). Other less common veterinary uses for DMSO have also been described (Jacob et al. 1965; Jacob 1982; Knowles 1982). In addition to penetration enhancement, DMSO is also bacteriostatic, vasodilatory, fibrinolytic, antiinflammatory, and produces some degree of topical analgesia. DMSO produces a thermal effect after direct application to the skin, which may function to alleviate pain in the skin and in the underlying muscle and bone. The transient erythema that is induced after topical administration of DMSO is due to the release of histamine (Jacob et al. 1965). These effects are considered transient and reversible and will not generally increase in severity after multiple treatments, indicating no need to discontinue therapy. Potential skin irritation occurs at concentrations of greater than 70% (see previous editons of this text for more information on DMSO).

DMSO has the potential to enhance the percutaneous absorption of a number of topically applied compounds. The exact mechanism of this percutaneous absorption enhancement has not been clearly elucidated. DMSO appears to produce only minor morphological changes in the skin. Penetration enhancement of topically applied chemicals dissolved in DMSO does not appear significant until the DMSO concentrations approach 50–60%, with overall permeability of the compound tending to increase as the concentration of DMSO applied to the skin approaches 100% (Kurihara-Bergstrom et al. 1987). Many mechanisms have been proposed to attempt to explain why DMSO enhances the percutaneous absorption of such a wide variety of compounds. Possible mechanisms include elution of stratum corneum lipids and delamination of the horny layer by stress resulting from crosscurrents of highly water interactive DMSO and water (Kurihara-Bergstrom et al. 1986). Sharata and Burnette (1988) determined that in nude mice skin, DMSO transformed the highly compact cell contents of the basal stratum corneum (keratin) into a looser meshwork of filamentous bundles, resulting in much more porous intracellular structure with an increase in intracellular surface areas, which they believed might increase percutaneous transport. Whatever the mechanism, DMSO has been shown to enhance the percutaneous absorption of many compounds, including water, hydrocortisone, salicylic acid, tubocurarine HCl, multiple glucocorticosteroids and antibiotics, estradiol, hexachlorophene, phenylbutazone, and a host of other topically applied chemicals.

Finally, recall that there is no universal penetration enhancer or vehicle, e.g., pluronic lecithin organogel (PLO) gel, that would be optimal for the delivery of all classes of topical drugs across the skin of all species. Carefully controlled studies have begun to show lack of transdermal delivery of drugs via this approach (Hoffman et al. 2002; Mealey et al. 2004). Selection of an optimal vehicle for transdermal delivery of a drug requires a close match between the physical chemical properties of the drug, vehicle, and skin lipids.

ELECTRICALLY ASSISTED TRANSDERMAL DRUG DELIVERY. An alternate approach to overcome the stratum corneum permeability barrier is by using electrical (iontophoresis) or ultrasonic (phonophoresis) energy, rather than the concentration gradient of diffusion, to drive drug through the skin (Riviere and Heit 1997). These techniques hold the most promise for delivering large drugs such as peptides and oligonucleotides that now can be administered only by intravascular injection. With these techniques, dose is based on the application surface area and the amount of energy required to actively deliver drug across the skin. In iontophoresis, this amounts to a dose being expressed in mAmps/cm^2. Formulation factors are also very different, since many of the components used are also delivered by the applied electrical current in direct molar proportion to the active drug. Finally, a recent but related strategy is to employ very short-duration high-voltage electrical pulses (electroporation) to reversibly break down the stratum corneum barrier, allowing larger peptides, and even small proteins, to be delivered systemically (Riviere et al. 1995). These approaches, if applied to veterinary medicine, could have implications for the use of controlled transdermal delivery as a viable method of drug delivery.

CLASSIFICATION OF DERMATOLOGIC VEHICLES

As discussed in the introduction to this chapter, the defining difference between dermatologic and other treatment areas of veterinary pharmacology is the topical route of administration coupled with the overriding influence that the dosage vehicle exerts on absorption and activity of the applied drug. The vehicles used as veterinary dermatologics have been historically classified into seven broad categories (Harvey 1985a,b; Block 1985; Rippie 1985; Swinyard 1985; Swinyard and Lowenthal 1985; Nairn 1985).

ADSORBENTS AND PROTECTIVES. Adsorbents and protectives are used extensively in many veterinary pharmaceutical preparations. Adsorbents act by binding gases, toxins, and some organisms (such as bacteria) to prevent exposure to the damaged skin surface. Protectives function by providing an occlusive layer of protection from the external environment or by providing mechanical support to the affected area. Protectives and adsorbents can be further subdivided into two subclasses: dusting powders and mechanical protectives.

Dusting powders are generally inert and innocuous substances. They include starch, calcium carbonate, talc, titanium dioxide, zinc oxide, and boric acid. Many are used in drug formulations alone or as a vehicle for the delivery of other drugs. If the powder particle has a smooth surface, it will act mainly to prevent friction, thus protecting abraded and raw skin surfaces; powder particles with rough or porous surfaces act on the skin by absorbing moisture. Water-absorbing powders tend to coalesce and eventually occlude the skin's surface when wetted and therefore should not be used on wet, moist, or highly exudative skin surfaces. Powders that also contain starch or other carbohydrates that are allowed to cake onto these moist skin surfaces give bacteria and fungi (mainly *Candida* spp.) a source of energy, allowing them to proliferate. This may lead to a secondary bacterial and/or fungal skin infection or exacerbation of an existing microbial skin infection. Powders should not be used within body cavities (thorax, abdomen) or in skin abscesses, especially those powders containing talc. Talc has been shown to promote severe granulomatous reactions when used in these areas but is relatively innocuous when used on intact skin surfaces.

Mechanical protectives provide an occlusive film that protects the underlying skin from irritants present in the external environment (ultraviolet radiation, contact irritants, toxins), provide mechanical support, and are popular vehicles for many drugs. Many members of this subgroup are used to treat cutaneous ulcers and other hard-to-heal cutaneous wounds. Compounds in this group include kaolin, lanolin, anhydrous lanolin, mineral oil, olive oil, peanut oil, petrolatum, zinc stearate, and recently a number of synthetic polymers.

DEMULCENTS. Demulcents are generally high molecular weight compounds that are water-soluble and function by alleviating irritation (*demulcere,* "to smooth"). Like the compounds listed in the protectives group, demulcents can coat the surface of damaged skin and protect the stratum corneum and underlying cellular structure of the epidermis by forming a protective barrier against the surrounding environment. They differ from protectives in that they inherently reduce the irritation from these external stimuli. This group comprises a large and diverse number of chemicals, including mucilages, gums, dextrins, starches, polymeric polyhydric glycols, glycerin, gelatin, hydroxypropyl cellulose, hydroxypropyl methylcellulose, hydroxyethyl cellulose, methyl cellulose, polyvinyl alcohol, and recently silicone-based polymers such as dimethicone. The dried gum extracts from the acacia and tragacanth plants can readily dissolve in water to form mucilages (see previous editions of this text for more detail). The most commonly used demulcents in veterinary dermatology today are glycerin, propylene glycol, and the polyethylene glycols.

Glycerin is a hygroscopic, trihydric alcohol prepared from propylene and has been used for many years as a suppository, with high concentrations of this vehicle relieving constipation by drawing water from the body and into the colon. Glycerin is a clear, colorless liquid that is miscible with water and alcohol and has been used neat to reduce corneal edema and to facilitate ophthalmoscopic examinations. Used in high concentrations topically on the skin, glycerin may dehydrate and irritate the skin, thereby increasing transepidermal water loss. Lower concentrations of glycerin absorbed into the skin hydrate the stratum corneum because of glycerin's hygroscopic nature. Despite its side effects, glycerin makes an excellent vehicle for topical drug delivery when used at lower concentrations.

Propylene glycol (1,2 propanediol) is a hygroscopic, colorless, odorless water-soluble liquid that is miscible with many compounds (water, alcohols, acetone, many volatile oils) and is also bacteriostatic, fungistatic, and nonocclusive. It was first considered for use in 1932 to be used with a drug to treat human syphilis and has since been used as a nontoxic antifreeze in dairies and beer breweries (Catanzaro and Smith 1991). Propylene glycol is an ideal medium for the topical delivery of many drugs in animals and humans, as well as for many oral and parenteral drug formulations, such as antitussives and shampoos. Propylene glycol spreads evenly onto the skin's surface and has a very low evaporation rate; it is not greasy to the touch, does not stain clothing or hair, and has some effect on slowing transepidermal water loss, thereby hydrating the stratum corneum to some extent. Topical hypersensitization and other toxicities are rare but have been reported (Catanzaro and Smith 1991).

Polyethylene glycols are a group of structurally similar compounds that differ in molecular weight. The larger the number, the higher the molecular weight and the more viscous the formulation becomes. At ambient temperature, polyethylene glycols 200, 300, 400, and 600 are clear viscous liquids; polyethylene glycols 900 to 9000 are semihard waxy solids at room temperature. As a group, the polyethylene glycols do not easily hydrolyze and are nontoxic, bland, highly water soluble, and nonvolatile.

EMOLLIENTS. Emollients are bland, fatty materials often used to soften or moisten the skin. Emollients are particularly useful when treating skin conditions resulting from water-soluble irritants and airborne bacteria because of their ability to act as a protectant, sequestering the damaged skin away from these noxious stimuli. When used topically, emollients soften skin by decreasing transepidermal water loss, or transpiration (discussed earlier), and increasing the hydration of the stratum corneum. Therefore, this is a useful group of compounds for treating dermatologic conditions involving dry, crusty, or flaky lesions of the epidermis. Emollients are used today as vehicles for many lipid-soluble drugs. Examples of commonly used emollients are listed in Table 48.2.

ASTRINGENTS. Astringents precipitate protein, toughen the skin, promote healing, and dry the skin when applied topically. When used to coagulate blood, astringents are said to be styptic and elicit a mildly uncomfortable sensation when applied to small open wounds. Most of the chemicals in this group are inorganic salts of aluminum, zinc, potassium, and silver, and include aluminum chloride, aluminum sulfate, calamine (a combination of Fe_2O_3 and ZnO_2), potassium permanganate, silver nitrate, zinc chloride, zinc oxide, zirconium chlorhydrate, and tannic acid. There are many germicidal agents that also have astringent activity. Other astringents are of vegetable origin, most of these preparations owing their activity to tannic acid (gallotannic acid). Astringents in the vegetable-derivative group include gallic acid, kino, krameria, and rubus (blackberry) (see previous editions of this text for more detail). Astringents have limited uses in veterinary medicine today.

RUBEFACIENTS, IRRITANTS, AND VESICANTS. Chemicals in this class are used to induce hyperemia (rubefacients), hyperemia and inflammation (irritants), or cutaneous blisters (vesicants). Heat applied to the skin via a hot-water bottle, heat lamp, moist hot pack, or an electric heating pad are acceptable rubefacients and are extensively used in human medicine. Chemical rubefacients are more commonly used in veterinary medicine, mainly due to the difficulty in applying the heat sources listed above for extended lengths of time. An abbreviated list of chemicals that are known rubefacients, irritants, or vesicants includes anthralin, camphor, coal tar, cresote, ichthamnol, menthol, methyl salicylate, resorcinol, cantharidin, black mustard, iodine, mercuric iodide, capsicum, chloroform, alcohols, turpentine, thymol, and pine tar. With the exception of coal tar, most members of the chemical group are not commonly used in modern veterinary practice because of their potential toxicity. Coal tar is a component found in many veterinary dermatology preparations (especially shampoos) and is a by-product of the distillation of bituminous coal. Photosensitization has been reported to occur. Coal tar should not be used on cats, because of frequent irritant or allergic reactions. Camphor is a rubefacient that has been used in some topical preparations and has some mild analgesic activity. It is of limited use in the treatment of mild pruritus. Similarly, menthol stimulates sensory nerve endings, inducing a feeling of coolness, induces mild analgesia, and is also a mild antipruritic (Harvey 1985).

TABLE 48.2 Emollients in use today

Official Vegetable Oils	Animal Fats	Hydrocarbons
Olive oil	Lanolin (wool fat with water added)	Paraffin
Cottonseed oil	Anhydrous wool fat (no water added)	Petrolatum
Corn oil	Lard	White petrolatum (vasoline)
Almond oil	Whale oil	Mineral oil
Peanut oil		White/yellow waxes (beeswax)
Persic oil		Spermaceti
Cocoa butter		

CAUSTICS AND ESCHAROTICS. Caustics (also known as *corrosives*) are agents that will destroy tissue after one or more applications. Escharotics are corrosive and will also precipitate proteins, leading to the formation of a scab and eventually a permanent scar. As with the rubefacient, irritant, and vesicant group, many of the caustics and escharotics have few uses in veterinary dermatology today. Historically, caustics have been used to induce desquamation of the stratum corneum (keratolytic) and to treat warts, keratoses, and other hyperplastic skin diseases. Escharotics have also been used to seal cutaneous ulcers and wounds. Examples of this group include glacial acetic acid, alum, aluminum chloride, gentian violet, phenol, potassium hydroxide, salicylic acid, and silver nitrate.

KERATOLYTICS, KERATOPLASTICS, AND ANTISEBORRHEICS. Keratolytics function by loosening keratin, which facilitates the desquamation of the stratum corneum, whereas keratoplastics attempt to "normalize" keratinization by slowing basal cell proliferation through inhibition of DNA synthesis. Other mechanisms may also contribute to this effect. Antiseborrheics attempt to modulate sebum production in the skin. Many of the keratolytics available today are also keratoplastic and/or antiseborrheic; therefore, these functions are discussed together. Most keratolytics and antiseborrheics are also cutaneous irritants, which may, in some cases, preclude their use on diseased skin in some animals (Shanley 1990). Several keratolytics and antiseborrheics used in veterinary dermatology are discussed below.

Salicylic acid (2-hydroxybenzoic acid) is used topically as a keratolytic, keratoplastic, and antiseborrheic agent and has some mild antibacterial and antifungal actions. Salicylic acid (2–10%) causes the dead or dying cells of the stratum corneum to hydrate, swell, and soften, thereby hastening their desquamation, and solubilizes the intercellular lipid layer, releasing the cells of the stratum corneum from each other. Salicylic acid is used extensively in veterinary dermatology to treat many keratoproliferative diseases. Topical use of salicylic acid may cause an irritant dermatitis in animals and has been studied extensively in both humans and many animal models (Weirich 1975; Nook 1987; deMare et al. 1988; Sloan et al. 1986; Roberts and Horlock 1978).

Benzoyl peroxide is a keratolytic and antiseborrheic agent that is also a strong oxidizer, free-radical generator, and antimicrobial and has been used in veterinary and human dermatology for many years. The majority of topically applied benzoyl peroxide is metabolized to benzoic acid by the viable epidermal cells during penetration through the skin (Holzmann et al. 1979; Nacht et al. 1981). Benzoyl peroxide in high concentrations can cause skin irritation and was identified as being a skin tumor promoter in SENCAR mice if used in tandem with 7,12-dimethylbenz(a)-anthracene (Slaga et al. 1981; Epstein 1988; Schweizer et al. 1987). The bactericidal activity associated with benzoyl peroxide comes from its ability to generate free radicals, which disrupt bacterial cell membranes. Due to its bactericidal activities, benzoyl peroxide is indicated in the treatment of pyodermas (Ihrke 1980a,b) as well as in diseases that cause keratosis. Transient stinging or burning sensations after application to the affected site have been reported in humans.

Resorcinol (*m*-dihydroxybenzene) is a keratolytic agent that also has bactericidal and fungicidal properties. Like urea (discussed below), it acts as a protein precipitant and promotes hydration of the keratin, resulting in its keratolytic function. Resorcinol may be used alone or compounded with other mild keratolytic agents, such as sulfur or salicylic acid.

Sulfur is a keratolytic, keratoplastic, and antiseborrheic agent used in a variety of topical agents. Sulfur is also antibacterial and antipruritic and has a mild follicular flushing action. The keratolytic activity of elemental sulfur is thought to be related to an inflammatory process that ultimately causes a sloughing of the stratum corneum. The formation of hydrogen sulfide and pentathionic acid is responsible for some of its keratolytic and antibacterial properties. The keratoplastic effect is most likely similar to that of the coal tars, being cytostatic (Miller 1986).

Retinoids are a class of naturally occurring or synthetically manufactured compounds that have vitamin A-like (retinoic acid) activity. Retinol (vitamin A alcohol) is the most potent analog and is metabolized to two other retinols, retinal and retinoic acid. In the early 20th century, researchers documented the importance of vitamin A in reproduction, vision, and epidermal cell growth promotion, along with its functions in differentiation and maintenance of epithelial cell surface structure, including that of the skin (Kwochka 1989). It was also found that *some* dyskeratotic skin diseases could be correlated to low levels of vitamin A, which eventually led to the therapeutic use of vitamin A to treat these skin diseases. The use of vitamin A was limited, however, as the levels needed to induce a clinical improvement of the lesions often induced signs of hypervitaminosis A. This side-effect dilemma prompted research into vitamin A substitutes, which led to the discovery and testing of over 1,500 retinoids. Three retinoids—tretinoin, isotretinoin, and etretinate—are available for clinical use today.

The retinoids, like vitamin A, act as growth and differentiation regulators in the skin when administered orally or topically. Although the exact mechanism by which the retinoids exert these effects is not completely understood, it is theorized that retinoids alter RNA synthesis within the cell, in turn altering protein synthesis and prostaglandin production, and also affecting some enzymes, such as ornithine decarboxylase and collagenase (Power and Ihrke 1990). The overall effect of the retinoids is to "normalize" the epithelium in those diseases responsive to these drugs.

In humans, the retinoids are used to treat severe recalcitrant cystic acne, psoriasis, Darier's disease, pityriasis rubra pilaris, and various other disorders of keratinization. Retinoids also have an ability to control malignant transformations in some tissues that are caused by chemical carcinogens, ionizing radiation, growth factors, and viruses. Naturally occurring retinoids have been shown to protect animals against skin papillomas and carcinomas of the skin and other organs (Griffiths and Vorhees 1994; Kwochka 1989). Numerous side effects have been associated with retinoid use in humans, including cheilitis, xerosis of the skin, pruritus, dryness of mucous membranes, epistaxis, thinning of the hair, palmoplantar desquamation, conjunctivitis, headache, ataxia, fatigue, psychologic changes, and visual disturbances. Tetragenicity is a serious problem in women who take isotretinoin during pregnancy. Symptoms of hypervitaminosis A may also occur, which is characterized by demineralization and thinning of the long bones, cortical hyperostosis, periostitis, and premature closure of the epiphyses (Kwochka 1989).

Retinoids are not used to a great extent in veterinary medicine (Werner and Power 1994). Reported uses of any of the retinoids in dogs and cats are few, and the recommendations for use and possible toxicities and side effects are based on a very small number of animals. Indications for veterinary use remain rather vague, in part because the skin diseases that retinoids may be efficacious in treating in humans do not have exact analogs in domestic animals. There is also a lack of formal studies conducted on large populations of dogs or cats. Reported uses for the retinoids in domestic animals are in disorders of keratinization, which may include primary idiopathic seborrhea in Cocker Spaniels, sebaceous adenitis, canine lamellar ichthyosis, Schnauzer comedo syndrome, and epidermal inclusion cysts, among others (Power and Ihrke 1990; Kwochka 1989). The use of retinoids in cats with neoplastic disorders, specifically squamous cell carcinoma and epidermal dysplasia, has been investigated and found to be of limited value (Evans et al. 1985). Toxicities to the retinoids in animals seem to be few, but it should be made clear that the reported side effects and toxicities are based on a small population of clinically ill animals treated for short periods of time with these compounds and these observations may prove to be inaccurate if the use of these compounds increases. Out of 29 dogs treated with isotretinoin in one study (Kwochka 1989), four dogs developed conjunctivitis that was observed to be reversible after treatments ended. There is no formal information available as to the existence of skeletal anomalies in dogs given retinoids for long periods of time (Power and Ihrke 1990). Birth defects involving the central nervous system, skeleton, thymus, and heart do occur, as seen with high doses of vitamin A during pregnancy. Cats appear to have a higher incidence of side effects associated with retinoid treatment. Cats treated with isotretinoin were observed to develop periocular erythema, periocular crusting, epiphora, and blepharospasm (Kwochka 1989).

Isotretinoin (Accutane, Roche; 13-*cis*-retinoic acid) and etretinate (Tegison, Roche) are two systemically used retinoids that also have potential veterinary applications. Power and Ihrke (1990) describe several cases where these two retinoids have been used to treat several skin diseases in dogs, with variable success. Isotretinoin is the most effective inhibitor of sebum production known (Kwochka 1989), making it potentially useful in treating primary idiopathic seborrhea and comedo syndromes. Although retinoids are associated with less toxicity than vitamin A, toxicities can occur. Etretinate may be associated with fewer toxic side effects than isotretinoin. Insufficient data are available for dogs or cats to determine its efficacy or toxicity.

Coal tar is another pharmaceutical that has keratolytic as well as keratoplastic and antiseborrheic activity. Its mechanism of action and general uses have been discussed previously. Coal tar products should not be used in the feline due to frequent irritant and allergic reactions.

Urea is a product of protein metabolism that, when used topically, acts as a protein denaturant, promoting the hydration of keratin. Once the treated areas of keratin swell, mild keratolysis ensues. The use of urea alone as a keratolytic agent is not common in veterinary dermatology today.

Selenium sulfide is an externally applied antiseborrheic, keratolytic, and keratoplastic compound that also has some antidandruff activities. Selenium sulfide exerts these actions by its antimitotic activity, slowing cell proliferation and sebum production, and tends to be irritating (especially if used in long-term treatment protocols) and also stains hair. It also causes irritation of the mucous membranes, so care should be taken to avoid contact with these tissues. Percutaneous absorption is minimal if applied to intact skin.

CLASSES OF MEDICATED APPLICATIONS

Pharmaceuticals can also be classified by the type of base in which they are formulated. There are eight classes of medicated applications (Harvey 1985; Block 1985; Rippie 1985; Swinyard 1985; Swinyard and Lowenthal 1985; Nairn 1985).

OINTMENTS. Ointments are semisolid preparations that usually (but not always) contain drugs used to treat dermatologic diseases. There are five classes of ointments commonly used in veterinary medicine.

Hydrocarbon Bases. These emollient ointment bases usually are composed of vegetable oils and animal fats. Common members of this subset include spermaceti, cetyl esters wax ("synthetic spermaceti"), oleic acid, olive oil, paraffin, petrolatum, white petrolatum, white wax, and yellow wax. Hydrocarbon base ointments are emollient and generally hydrophobic and occlusive, causing an increase in the hydration of the stratum corneum and underlying epidermal cell structure by decreasing transepidermal water loss, making them useful in rehydrating or softening the skin. Disadvantages include greasiness and their ability to stain clothing; also, they cannot be washed off in water, making them difficult to completely remove from the skin.

Anhydrous Absorption Bases. This type of ointment base contains very little (if any) water after preparation but differs from the hydrocarbon bases in that it will readily accept any water molecules it comes in contact with. Absorbent ointment bases can absorb large quantities of water and still keep their thick consistency. Examples of this subgroup include hydrophilic petrolatum and anhydrous lanolin, both of which are emollient, occlusive, and greasy.

Water-Oil Emulsion Bases. Emulsions, by definition, are oil and water combinations. Water-in-oil emulsion bases ("creams") are water-washable bases that are easily removed from the skin surface and contain more oil than water on a percentage basis. The oil phase usually consists of petrolatum or liquid petrolatum and perhaps an alcohol (cetyl or stearyl alcohol). The aqueous phase may consist of water; however, other aqueous vehicles may be used, such as propylene glycol, polyethylene glycol, or glycerin, to which various preservatives (such as paraben derivatives) are usually added. Water-in-oil bases are emollient (due to the higher percentage of oil than aqueous phase), occlusive, greasy, and may absorb some water, but not to the same degree as the anhydrous absorption bases. Other common components of water-in-oil emulsion bases include glyceryl monosterate and stearic acid.

Oil-Water Emulsion Bases. Oil-in-water emulsions are manufactured in the same manner as the water-in-oil bases, with the exception that the aqueous phase is in a higher percentage than the oil component. The same ingredients are also used to make the oil-in-water bases. Because of the higher water (or other aqueous phase) content, oil-in-water bases are water-washable, nongreasy, and nonocclusive.

Water-Soluble Bases. As the name implies, these bases have lost their hydrophobic lipid base components. These demulcent bases are primarily composed of polymers that are completely water soluble and usually anhydrous, do not easily hydrolyze, do not support mold growth, and are nongreasy, nonocclusive, and nonvolatile. If the components of a preparation contain water-soluble bases in a gelled medium, they are referred to as *gels*. Gels are a combination of propylene glycol, propylene gallate, disodium EDTA, and carboxypolymethylene that results in a clear, water-miscible, and relatively greaseless formulation. A commonly used drug in a gel formulation is DMSO (Domoso, Diamond). Glucocorticosteroids may also be formulated in this way.

POULTICES. A poultice (or cataplasm) is a soft moist mass of materials applied locally to an affected area and was historically composed of roots, herbs, seeds, and even mud in a gruellike base. The poultice was intended to be a topical wound treatment serving as a counterirritant and absorptive/adsorptive sink. Poultices are rarely used in veterinary medicine today.

PASTES. Pastes are absorptive powders placed in a gelatinous base, usually petrolatum or hydrophilic petrolatum. Pastes have been used to adhere to the skin and thereby act as a "sponge" to absorb exudates and moisture and also as a physical barrier to protect the skin from the external environment. Pastes are easily removed from the skin and can be used on moist lesions of the skin.

POWDERS. Powders have been discussed earlier in this chapter as a class of vehicle for the delivery of topical drugs to the skin. Powders are commonly used in veterinary medicine to deliver pesticides (carbaryl, permethrins, etc.) for the control of external parasites (mainly fleas) and in large animal veterinary dermatology to deliver antibiotics, such as nitrofurazone, to wounds.

DRESSINGS. Dressings are external applications of some previously discussed compounds (petrolatum, ointments) on an application device such as plastic wrap or sterile gauze and are placed over wound sites to protect the skin lesion from external environmental trauma. Dressings may also contain antimicrobial agents, such as nitrofurazone.

PLASTERS. Plasters are similar to dressings; however, they are attached to the skin via some adhesive material. They protect skin lesions from the external environment and provide an occlusive environment. Plasters have limited use in veterinary medicine today.

SUSPENSIONS. A suspension is a two-phase system composed of a finely divided solid that is dispersed in a liquid, usually water. Suspensions are not utilized to any great degree in veterinary dermatology today. They are more commonly used in oral drug preparation schemes. The most common type of suspension currently used topically is captan (Orthocide, Chevron Chemical), which is used to treat some types of superficial fungal infections and which also has some limited bacteriostatic properties.

LOTIONS. Lotions are powders dissolved in a liquid, usually water or an alcohol. Lotions, like powders, tend to be cooling, drying, and somewhat mildly antipruritic. Lotions have limited applications in veterinary medicine but are used extensively in human over-the-counter skincare products.

DERMATOTHERAPY: ATOPIC DERMATITIS

One dermatologic disease—atopic dermatitis—deserves specific mention: because it is a common clinical syndrome with various stages of presentation and potential initiating etiologies. Olivry et al. (2003) have summarized an analysis of some 40 clinical trials published in peer review journals that assessed the efficacy of 41 different drug interventions for treatment of canine atopic dermatitis. Fatty acid supplementation and allergen-specific immunotherapy were not assessed.

This analysis suggests that there was good evidence for using oral glucocorticoids and cyclosporine and fair evidence for the use of topical triamcinolone spray, topical tacrolimus lotion, oral pentoxifylline, or oral misoprostol in the treatment of canine atopy. Insufficient evidence exists for the remainder of other therapies often recommended (e.g., antihistamines, tricyclic antidepressants, etc.). However, there is evidence against the efficacy of oral arofylline, leukotriene synthesis inhibitors, and cysteinyl leukotriene receptor antagonists.

REFERENCES

Amakiri, S.F. 1973. A comparative study of the thickness of the stratum corneum in Nigerian breeds of cattle. Br Vet J 129:277–281.

Aungst, B.J., Blake, J.A., and Hussain, M.A. 1990. Contributions of drug solubilization, partitioning, barrier disruption, and solvent permeation to the enhancement of skin permeation of various compounds with fatty acids and amines. Pharm Res 7(7):712–718.

Barry, B.W. 1991. Modern methods of promoting drug absorption through the skin. Molec Aspects Med 12:195–241.

Bashir, S.J., and Maibach, H.I. 2005. Cutaneous metabolism of xenobiotics. In Percutaneous Absorption, 4th Ed. R.L. Bronaugh and H.I. Maibach, eds. pp. 51–63. New York: Taylor and Francis.

Baynes, R.E., Craigmill, A.L., and Riviere, J.E. 1997. Residue avoidance after topical application of veterinary drugs and parasiticides. J Am Vet Med Assoc 210:1288–1289.

Baynes, R.E., and Riviere, J.E. 1998. Influence of inert ingredients in pesticide formulations on dermal absorption of carbaryl. Am J Vet Res 59:168–175.

Bennett, K., ed. 1995. Compendium of Veterinary Products, 3rd Ed. Port Huron, MI: North American Compendiums and Adrian J. Bayley.

Blackburn, P.S. 1965. The hair of cattle, horse, dog and cat. In Comparative Physiology and Pathology of the Skin, A. J. Rook and G.S. Walton, eds. pp. 201–210. Oxford: Blackwell.

Blank, I.H., Moloney, J., Emslie, A.G., and Simon, I. 1984. The diffusion of water across the stratum corneum as a function of its water content. J Invest Dermatol 82(2):188–194.

Block, L.H. 1985. Medicated applications. In Remington's Pharmaceutical Sciences. 17th Ed. A.R. Gennara, ed. pp. 1567–1584. Easton, PA: Mack Publishing Co.

Catanzaro, J.M., and Smith, J.G. 1991. Propylene glycol dermatitis. J Am Acad Dermatol 24:90–95.

Chang, S.K., and Riviere, J.E. 1993. Effect of humidity and occlusion on the percutaneous absorption of parathion in vitro. Pharm Res 10(1):152–155.

deMare, S., Calis, N., den Hartog, G., van Erp, P.E.J., van de Kerkhof, P. C.M. 1988. The relevance of salicylic acid in the treatment of plaque psoriasis with dithranol creams. Skin Pharmacol 1:259–264.

Dunn, M.J., and Hood, V.L. 1977. Prostaglandins and the kidney. Am J Physiol 233(3):F169–F184.

Elias, P.M. 1983. Epidermal lipids, barrier functions and desquamation. J Invest Dermatol 80:44–47.

———. 1992. Role of lipids in barrier function of the skin. In Pharmacology of the Skin, H. Mukhtar, ed. pp. 29–40. Boca Raton, FL: CRC Press.

Elias, P.M., and Feingold, K.R. 1992. Lipids and the epidermal water barrier: metabolism, regulation, and pathophysiology. In Seminars in Dermatology 11(2):176–182. H.I. Maibach, editor in chief. Philadelphia: W.B. Saunders Co.

Epstein, J.H. 1988. Photocarcinogenesis promotion studies with benzoyl peroxide (BPO) and croton oil. J Invest Dermatol 91:114–116.

Evans, A.G., Madewell, B.R., and Stannard, A.A. 1985. A trial of 13-*cis*-retinoic acid for treatment of squamous cell carcinoma and preneoplastic lesions of the head in cats. Am J Vet Res 46(12):2553–2557.

Ford-Hutchinson, A.W. 1985. Leukotrienes: their formation and role as inflammatory mediators. Fed Proc 44(1):25–29.

Freinkel, R.K. 1983. Carbohydrate metabolism of the epidermis. In Biochemistry and Physiology of the Skin. L.A. Goldsmith, ed. pp. 328–337. New York: Oxford University Press.

Goldyne, M.E. 1986. Eicosanoids and human skin. Progr Dermatol 20: 1–8.

Griffiths, C.E.M., and Vorhees, J.J. 1994. Human in vivo pharmacology of topical retinoids. Arch Dermatol Res 287:53–60.

Hadgraft, J., Walters, K.A., and Guy, R.H. 1992. Epidermal lipids and topical drug delivery. In Seminars in Dermatology 11(2):139–144. H.I. Maibach, editor in chief. Philadelphia: W.B. Saunders Co.

Harvey, S.C. 1985. Topical drugs. In Remington's Pharmaceutical Sciences, 17th Ed. A.R. Gennara, ed. pp. 773–791. Easton, PA: Mack Publishing Co.

Herschler, R. 1982. Proceedings of the symposium on dimethyl sulfoxide: 2) Chemistry and biologic effects. VMSAC 77:367–369.

Hoffmann, S.B., Yoder, A.R., and Trepanier, L.A. 2002. Bioavailability of transdermal methimazole in a pluronic lecithin organogel (PLO) in healthy cats. J Vet Pharmacol Therap 25:189–193.

Holzmann, H., Morsches, B., and Benes, P. 1979. The absorption of benzoyl peroxide from leg ulcers. Drug Res 29(11):1180–1183.

Idsen, I. 1975. Percutaneous absorption. J Pharm Sci 64(6):901–924.

Idson, B. 1983. Vehicle effects in percutaneous absorption. Drug Metabol Rev 14(2):207–222.

Ihrke, P.J. 1980a. Topical therapy—Specific topical pharmacologic agents, dermatologic therapy (part II). J Comp Cont Ed 156(2):156–164.

———. 1980b. Topical therapy—Uses, principles and vehicles, dermatologic therapy (part I). J Comp Cont Ed 156(1):28–35.

Jacob, S. 1982. Proceedings of the symposium on dimethyl sulfoxide: 1) Mode of action and biologic effects. VMSAC 77:365–366.

Jacob, S.W., Herschler, R.J., and Rosenbaum, E.E. 1965. Dimethyl sulfoxide (DMSO): laboratory and clinical evaluation. JAVMA 147(12):1350–1359.

Karanian, J.W., Stojanov, M., and Salem, N. 1985. Effect of ethanol on prostacyclin and thromboxane A_2 synthesis in rat aortic rings in vitro. Prostagl, Leukotr and Med 20(2):175–186.

Knowles, R. 1982. Proceedings of the symposium on dimethyl sulfoxide: 3) Clinical applications in veterinary medicine. VMSAC 77:369–373.

Kozlowski, G.P., and Calhoun, M.L. 1969. Microscopic anatomy of the integument of sheep. Am J Vet Res 30(8):1267–1279.

Kunkle, G.A. 1986. Progestogens in dermatology. In Current Veterinary Therapy IX: Small Animal Practice. R.W. Kirk, ed. pp. 601–605. Philadelphia: W.B. Saunders Co.

Kurihara-Bergstrom, T., Flynn, G.L., and Higuchi, W.I. 1986. Physiochemical study of percutaneous absorption enhancement by dimethyl sulfoxide: kinetic and thermodynamic determinants of dimethyl sulfoxide mediated mass transfer of alkanols. J Pharm Sci 75(5):479–486.

———. 1987. Physicochemical study of percutaneous absorption enhancement by dimethylsulfoxide: dimethyl sulfoxide mediation of vidarabine (ara-A) permeation of hairless mouse skin. J Invest Dermatol 89:274–280.

Kwochka, K.W. 1989. Retinoids in dermatology. In Current Veterinary Therapy X: Small Animal Practice. R.W. Kirk, ed. pp. 553–560. Philadelphia: W.B. Saunders Co.

Landolfi, R., and Steiner, M. 1984. Ethanol raises prostacyclin in vivo and in vitro. Blood 64(3):679–682.

Lloyd, D.H., Amakiri, S.F., and Jenkinson, D.M. 1979a. Structure of the sheep epidermis. Res Vet Sci 26:180–182.

Lloyd, D.H., Dick, W.D.B., and Jenkinson, D.M. 1979b. Structure of the epidermis in Ayrshire bullocks. Res Vet Sci 26:172–179.

Malkinson, F.D. 1958. The percutaneous absorption of carbon-14 labeled steroids by use of the gas-flow cell. J Invest Dermatol 31:19–28.

Mealey, K.L., Peck, K.E., Bennett, B.S., Sellon, R.K., Swinney, G.R., Melzer, K., Gokhale, S.A. and Krone, T.M. 2004. Systemic absorption of amitriptyline and buspirone after oral and transdermal administration to healthy cats. J Vet Intern Med 18:43–46.

Miller, W.H. 1986. Antiseborrheic agents in dermatology. In Current Veterinary Therapy IX: Small Animal Practice. R.W. Kirk, ed. pp. 596–601. Philadelphia: W.B. Saunders Co.

Miller, W.H., Scott, D.W., and Wellington, J.R. 1992. Nonsteroidal management of canine pruritus with amitriptyline. Cornell Vet 82:53–57.

Montagna, W. 1967. Comparative anatomy and physiology of the skin. Arch Dermatol 96:357–363.

Monteiro-Riviere, N.A. 1991. Comparative anatomy, physiology, and biochemistry of mammalian skin. In Dermal and Ocular Toxicology

Fundamentals and Methods. D.W. Hobson, ed. Boca Raton, FL: CRC Press.

———. N.A. 2006. The Integument. In Delman's Textbook of Veterinary Histology, 6th Ed. J.A. Eureall and B.L. Frappier, eds. Ames, IA: Blackwell.

Monteiro-Riviere, N.A., Bristol, D.G., Manning, T.O., Rogers, R.A., and Riviere, J.E. 1990. Interspecies and interregional analysis of the comparative histologic thickness and laser Doppler blood flow measurements at five cutaneous sites in nine species. J Invest Dermatol 95(5):582–586.

Monteiro-Riviere, N.A., Inman, A.O., Mak, V., Wertz, P. and Riviere, J.E. 2001. Effects of selective lipid extraction from different body regions on epidermal barrier function. Pharm Res 18:992–998.

Monteiro-Riviere, N.A., Inman, A.O., Riviere, J.E., McNeill, S.C., and Francoeur, M.L. 1993. Topical penetration of piroxicam is dependent on the distribution of the local cutaneous vasculature. Pharm Res 10:1326–1331.

Monteiro-Riviere, N.A., and Stromberg, M.W. 1985. Ultrastructure of the integument of the domestic pig (*Sus scrofa*) from one through fourteen weeks of age. Anat Histol Embryol 14:97–115.

Muhammad, F., Monteiro-Riviere, N.A., Baynes, R.E., and Riviere, J.E. 2005. Effect of in vivo jet fuel exposure on subsequent in vitro dermal absorption of individual aromatic and aliphatic hydrocarbon fuel constituents. J Tox Environ Health Part A 68:719–737.

Mukhtar, H. 1992. Cutaneous cytochrome P-450. In Pharmacology of the Skin. Hasan Mukhtar, ed. pp. 139–150. Boca Raton, FL: CRC Press.

Nacht, S., Yeung, D., Beasley, H.N., Anjo, M.D. Benzoyl peroxide: percutaneous penetration and metabolic disposition. J Am Acad Dermatol 4:31–37.

Nairn, J.G. 1985. Solutions, emulsions, suspensions and extractives. In Remington's Pharmaceutical Sciences, 17th Ed. A.R. Gennara, ed. pp. 1492–1517. Easton, PA: Mack Publishing Co.

Nook, T.H. 1987. In vivo measurement of the keratolytic effect of salicylic acid in three ointment formulations. Br J Dermatol 117:243–245.

Olivry, T., Mueller, R.S., and The International Task Force on Canine Atopic Dermatitis. 2003. Evidence based veterinary dermatology: a systematic review of the pharmacotherapy of canine atopic dermatitis. Vet Dermatol 14:121–146.

Paulissen, M., Peereboom-Stegeman, C.P., and Van de Kerkhof, P. 1990. An ultrastructural study of transcutaneous migration of polymorphonuclear leukocytes following application of leukotriene B_4. Skin Pharmacol 3:236–247.

Pavletic, M.M. 1991. Anatomy and circulation of canine skin. Microsurgery 12:103–112.

Pitman, I.H., and Rostas, S.J. 1981. Topical drug delivery to cattle and sheep. J Pharm Sci 70(11):1181–1193.

Potts, R.O., Bommannan, D.B., and Guy, R.H. 1992. Percutaneous absorption. In Pharmacology of the Skin. Hasan Mukhtar, ed. pp. 13–28. Boca Raton, FL: CRC Press.

Potts, R.O., and Francoeur, M.L. 1992. Physical methods for studying stratum corneum lipids. In Seminars in Dermatology 11(2):129–138. H.I. Maibach, editor in chief. Philadelphia: W.B. Saunders Co.

Potts, R.O., and Guy, R.H. 1995. A predictive algorithm for skin permeability: The effects of molecular size and hydrogen bond activity. Pharm Res 12:1628–1633.

Power, H.T., and Ihrke, P.J. 1990. Synthetic retinoids in veterinary dermatology. Vet Clin N Am, Sm An Pract 20(6):1525–1539.

Raza, H., Agarwal, R., and Mukhtar, H. 1992. Cutaneous glutathione-s-transferase. In Pharmacology of the Skin. H. Mukhtar, ed. pp. 131–138. Boca Raton, FL: CRC Press.

Rippie, E.G. 1985. Powders. In Remington's Pharmaceutical Sciences. 17th Ed. A.R. Gennara, ed. pp. 1585–1602. Easton, PA: Mack Publishing Co.

Riviere, J.E. 1992. Dermal absorption and metabolism of xenobiotics in food-producing animals. In Xenobiotics and Food-Producing Animals: Metabolism and Residues. D.H. Hutson et al., eds. Chap. 7, pp. 88–97. Washington, D.C.: American Chemical Society Symposium Series 503.

———. 2006. Dermal Absorption Models in Toxicology and Pharmacology. New York: Taylor and Francis.

Riviere, J.E., and Brooks, J.D. 2005. Predicting skin permeability from complex chemical mixtures. Toxicol Appl Pharmacol 208:99–110.

———. 2007. Prediction of dermal absorption from complex chemical mixtures: Incorporation of vehicle effects and interactions into a QSPR framework. SAR QSAR Environ Res 18:31–44.

Riviere, J.E., and Chang, S.K. 1992. Transdermal penetration and metabolism of organophosphate insecticides. In Organophosphates: Chemistry, Fate, and Effects. J.E. Chambers and P.E. Levi, eds. pp. 241–253. New York: Academic Press.

Riviere, J.E., and Heit, M. 1997. Electrically-assisted transdermal drug delivery. Pharm Res 14:691–701.

Riviere, J.E., Monteiro-Riviere, N.A., Rogers, R.A., Bommannan, D., Tamada, J, and Potts, R.O. 1995. Pulsatile transdermal delivery of LHRH using electroporation. J Contr Rel 36:229–233.

Riviere, J.E., and Papich, M.L. 2001. Potential and problems of developing transdermal patches for veterinary applications. Adv Drug Deliv Rev 50:175–203.

Riviere, J.E., and Williams, P.L. 1992. Pharmacokinetic implications of changing blood flow to the skin. J Pharm Sci 81:601–602.

Roberts, M.S., and Horlock, E. 1978. Effect of repeated skin application on percutaneous absorption of salicylic acid. J Pharm Sci 67(12):1685–1687.

Ruzicka, T. 1990. Arachidonic acid metabolism in normal skin. In Eicosanoids and the Skin. Thomas Ruzicka, ed. pp. 23–31. Boca Raton, FL: CRC Press.

Sar, M., and Calhoun, M.L. 1966. Microscopic anatomy of the integument of the common American goat. Am J Vet Res 27:444–456.

Schweizer, J., Loehrke, H., Edler, L., and Goerttler, K. 1987. Benzoyl peroxide promotes the formation of melanotic tumors in the skin of 7,12-dimethylbenz[a]anthracene initiated Syrian golden hamsters. Carcinogenesis 8:479–482.

Shanley, K.J. 1990. The seborrheic disease complex: an approach to underlying causes and therapies. Vet Clin N Am, Sm An Pract 20(6):1557–1577.

Sharata, H.H., and Burnette, R.R. 1988. Effect of dipolar aprotic permeability enhancers on the basal stratum corneum. J Pharm Sci 77(1):27–32.

Slaga, T.J., Klein-Szanto, A.J.P., Triplett, L.L., and Yotti, L.P. 1981. The tumor-promoting activity of benzoyl peroxide, a widely used free radical-generating compound. Science 213:1023–1025.

Sloan, K.B., Siver, K.G., and Koch, S.A.M. 1986. The effect of vehicle on the diffusion of salicylic acid through hairless mouse skin. J Pharm Sci 75(8):744–749.

Spannhake, E.M., Hyman, A.L., and Kadowitz, P.J. 1981. Bronchoactive metabolites of arachidonic acid and their role in airway function. Prostaglandins 22(6):1013–1026.

Spoo, J.W., Rogers, R.A., and Monteiro-Riviere, N.A. 1993. Effects of formaldehyde, DMSO, benzoyl peroxide and sodium lauryl sulfate on isolated perfused porcine skin. Vitro Toxicol 5(4):251–260.

St. Omer, V.V. 1978. Efficacy and toxicity of furazolidone in veterinary medicine: a review. VMSAC, Sept. 73(9):1125–8, 1132.

Strickland, J.H., and Calhoun, M.L. 1963. The integumentary system of the cat. Am J Vet Res 24:1018–1029.

Surber, C., Wilhelm, K.P., Maibach, H.I., Hall, L.L., and Guy, R.H. 1990a. Partitioning of chemicals into human stratum corneum: implications for risk assessment following dermal exposure. Fund Appl Toxicol 15:99–107.

Surber, C., Wilhelm, K.P., Maibach, H.I., Hori, M., and Guy, R.H. 1990b. Optimization of topical therapy: partitioning of drugs into stratum corneum. Pharm Res 7(12):1320–1324.

Swartzendruber, D.C. 1992. Studies of epidermal lipids using electron microscopy. In Seminars in Dermatology 11(2):157–161. H.I. Maibach, editor in chief. Philadelphia: W.B. Saunders Co.

Swinyard, E.A. 1985. Local anesthetics. In Remington's Pharmaceutical Sciences. 17th Ed. A.R. Gennara, ed. pp. 1048–1058. Easton, PA: Mack Publishing Co.

Swinyard, E.A. and Lowenthal, W. 1985. In Remington's Pharmaceutical Sciences. 17th Ed. A.R. Gennara, ed. pp. 1278–1320. Easton, PA: Mack Publishing Co.

Talukdar, A.H., Calhoun, M.L., and Stinson, A.W. 1972. Microscopic anatomy of the skin of the horse. Am J Vet Res 33(12):2365–2390.

Tragear, R.T. 1966. The permeability of skin to albumin, dextrans, and polyvinyl pyrrolidone. J Invest Dermatol 46:24–27.

Van de Kerkhof, P., Peereboom-Stegeman, J., and Boeijen, J. 1991. An ultrastructural study of the response of normal skin to epicutaneous application of leukotriene B_4. J Dermatol 18:271–276.

Weirich, E.G. 1975. Dermatopharmacology of salicylic acid I. Range of dermatotherapeutic effects of salicylic acid. Dermatologica 151:268–273.

Werner, A.H., and Power, H.T. 1994. Retinoids in veterinary dermatology. Clin Derm 12:579–586.

Wertz, P.W. 1992. Epidermal lipids. In Seminars in Dermatology 11(2):106–113. H.I. Maibach, editor in chief. Philadelphia: W.B. Saunders Co.

CHAPTER

49

DRUGS THAT AFFECT THE RESPIRATORY SYSTEM

MARK G. PAPICH

ANTITUSSIVE DRUGS

COUGH REFLEX. The afferent arc of the cough reflex receives input from sensory nerves in the bronchial and tracheal airways. Airway irritation and inflammation stimulate the afferent nerves, which in turn activate the cough center located in the medulla oblongata.

MECHANISM OF ACTION OF ANTITUSSIVE DRUGS. The mechanism of action of antitussive drugs is not completely understood. There are both opiate and nonopiate antitussive drugs. However, there is growing evidence that the nonopiate drugs (for example, dextromethorphan) are not as effective as once thought.

The most commonly used antitussives—and apparently the most effective—are derivatives of opiate drugs. They directly depress the cough center in the medulla. The site of action may be either μ- or κ-opiate receptors. Evidence for either receptor being responsible is that both butorphanol (κ-receptor agonist) and codeine or morphine (μ-receptor agonists) can suppress cough (Takahama and Shirasaki 2007; Gingerich et al. 1983; Christie et al. 1980), and naloxone is capable of antagonizing this effect.

There may be a nonopiate mechanism for some antitussives as well. For example, dextromethorphan is an opiate derivative, but does not have activity at opiate receptors. It continues to be marketed as an over-the-counter (OTC) medication with antitussive activity for people—apparently based on early clinical trials. Its mechanism is unknown. The neurokinin receptor (NK) may play a role in antitussive activity of nonopiates, but this mechanism has not been characterized well (Takahama and Shirasaki 2007).

Beta-2 receptor agonists (β_2) will suppress cough in some animals. The effect of these drugs is mediated via bronchodilation. These drugs will be discussed in another section.

MORPHINE. Morphine and derivatives have opiate-receptor–mediated effects, but also are effective as antitussives. Morphine is a natural derivative of one of the alkaloids of opium. (Pharmacology of opiates is discussed in more detail in Chapter 12.) Morphine is the prototype of an opiate (narcotic) analgesic with good binding affinity for the μ- and κ-opiate receptors. Morphine can be administered at low doses that produce antitussive effects without causing analgesia and sedation. The antitussive dose has been reported to be approximately 0.1 mg/kg, q 6–8 h. Morphine is not regularly used as an antitussive because of the side effects and potential for abuse and addiction. Oral formulations of morphine do not have good systemic absorption in dogs.

CODEINE (METHYLMORPHINE). Codeine phosphate and codeine sulfate are found in many preparations including, tablets, liquids, and syrups. There are over 50 different combinations and preparations of codeine. Codeine oral absorption in dogs is low and inconsistent.

Codeine has analgesic effects that are approximately 1/10 that of morphine. By contrast, the antitussive potency is similar to morphine. Although codeine administered orally to dogs attains low systemic levels, other metabolites may be responsible for the antitussive effect. Its usefulness as an oral antitussive in small animals has not been measured. It is available as 15, 30, and 60 mg tablets and oral syrups (2 mg/ml). In some states (regulated by local pharmacy acts), and some countries, codeine in antitussive formulations may be obtained without prescription.

In people, the side effects of codeine at antitussive doses are significantly less than those experienced with morphine. The potential for addiction and abuse is considerably lower. Important side effects include sedation and constipation.

HYDROCODONE. Hydrocodone is similar to codeine in action, but it is more potent. Hydrocodone is combined with an anticholinergic drug (homatropine) in the preparation Hycodan®, which has been prescribed for small animals. The anticholinergic drug is added to discourage abuse rather than for a respiratory indication. In some countries (Canada) it may be obtained without the ingredient homatropine. Some veterinarians consider hydrocodone the first drug of choice for symptomatic treatment of cough in dogs.

Availability of hydrocodone tablets in the United States has diminished. Tablets are difficult to obtain, but there is an oral syrup that contains hydrocodone plus homatropine (1 mg/ml hydrocodone + 0.3 mg/ml homatropine). Although systemic availability after oral administration has not been reported, oral doses administered to dogs are approximately 0.25 mg/kg, q 6–8 h (approx. 1 tablet per 20 kg).

Hycodan bitartrate is formulated as 5 mg of hydrocodone + 1.5 mg homatropine. Only in Canada is hydrocodone available without an anticholinergic (5 mg). Hydrocodone (5 mg) + acetaminophen (500 mg) is combined in a tablet and used for analgesia (Vicodin).

DEXTROMETHORPHAN. Dextromethorphan is not a true opiate, because it does not bind μ- or κ-opiate receptors, but studies in people have supported its antitussive effects. More recent investigations have questioned the antitussive properties of over-the-counter (OTC) formulations.

Dextromethorphan is the D-isomer of levorphan (the L-isomer, levorphan is an opiate with addictive properties, but the D-isomer is not). Dextromethorphan produces mild analgesia and modulates pain via its ability to act as an NMDA (n-methyl D-aspartate) antagonist, but this is unrelated to the antitussive action (Pozzi et al. 2006).

Clinical Use. Dextromethorphan has been administered to dogs and cats, but recent pharmacokinetic studies in dogs indicated that dextromethorphan does not attain effective concentrations after oral administration (KuKanich and Papich 2004). After injections IV it produced adverse effects in dogs (vomiting after oral doses, and CNS reactions after IV administration). Even after IV administration, concentrations of the parent drug and active metabolite persisted for only a short time after dosing. Therefore, routine use in dogs is not recommended until more data are available to establish safe and effective doses.

Formulations. There are many preparations available without a prescription (over-the-counter, OTC) in liquid and tablet form. For example, *Vicks Formula 44* and *Robitussin* contain dextromethorphan as their active antitussive ingredient. OTC formulations may vary in concentration, but most contain 2 mg/ml, or 15 or 20 mg per tablet. Pet owners should be cautioned that many OTC preparations contain other drugs that may produce significant side effects. For example, some combinations also contain acetaminophen, which can be toxic to cats. Some preparations also contain a decongestant, such as pseudoephedrine, which can cause excitement and other side effects.

BUTORPHANOL (TORBUTROL®, TORBUGESIC®). Butorphanol is an opioid agonist-antagonist that has been used both as an analgesic and antitussive. It has been a potent antitussive with clinical studies that support its use in dogs (Gingerich et al. 1983; Christie et al. 1980). High doses may induce side effects such as sedation.

Butorphanol is poorly bioavailable because of oral first-pass metabolism. Therefore, in dogs the oral dose is higher (0.55 to 1.1 mg/kg) than the IV or SC dose (0.05 to 0.1 mg/kg). It is administered as frequently as needed to control cough—usually every 6 to 12 hours. In clinical studies the peak effect was rapid after the injectable formulation. After oral administration, the maximum effects were observed for 4 hours but persisted for up to 10 hours in dogs (Gingerich et al. 1983). By contrast, codeine's effect in dogs is much shorter. It is available as 1, 5, and 10 mg tablets and an injectable solution.

TRAMADOL (ULTRAM). Tramadol is an inexpensive oral drug used for analgesia. It produces opiate, serotonin, and alpha-2 activity. (The pharmacology of tramadol is discussed in more detail in Chapter 12.) The active metabolite has opiate activity and is believed to be responsible for most of the analgesia. This drug also has antitussive properties and appears to be well-tolerated in dogs and it is not a controlled substance. However, efficacy for treating cough in dogs has not been evaluated. Recommended oral dose is 5 mg/kg, every 6 hours (KuKanich and Papich 2004).

BRONCHODILATOR DRUGS (BETA-ADRENERGIC RECEPTOR AGONISTS)

The β-adrenergic receptor agonists have a beneficial effect in the treatment of some airway diseases. They are used commonly in people for the treatment of asthma. In animals, they are used for airway disease, allergic bronchitis, and similar diseases such as feline "asthma," and recurrent airway obstruction (formerly called *chronic obstructive pulmonary disease* or "*heaves*") in horses. A review of the pharmacology of this group of drugs is in the article by Nelson (1995) and the autonomic properties are discussed in more detail in Chapter 6 of this textbook.

MECHANISM OF ACTION. Bronchial smooth muscle is innervated by β_2-adrenergic receptors. Stimulation of β_2-receptors leads to increased activity of the enzyme

TABLE 49.1 Response of various organs to adrenergic receptor stimulation

Receptor Type	Organ	Response
α_1	Pilomotor smooth muscle	Contracts
α_1	Liver	Gluconeogenesis
α_1 & α_2	Peripheral and splanchnic vessels	Constricts
α_1	Sweat glands	Secretion
α_1	Urinary tract	Increases sphincter tone
$\beta 4_2$	Skeletal muscle vessels	Dilates
$\beta 4_2$	Bronchial smooth muscle	Relaxes
$\beta 4_2$	Respiratory mast cells	Stabilizes
$\beta 4 \beta_1$	Heart rate	Increases
$\beta 4_1$	Heart contraction	Increases

TABLE 49.2 Relative effects of catecholamines on adrenergic receptors

Drug	α_1	β_1	β_2	DA
Norepinephrine (Noradrenaline)	+++	1	0	0
Epinephrine (Adrenaline)	+++	+++	++	0
Ephedrine	+++	+++	+++	0
Dopamine (Intropin®)	+++	+++	+	++++
Dobutamine (Dobutrex®)	+	+++	+	0
Isoproterenol (Isuprel®)	0	+++	++++	0
Isoetharine (Bronkosol®)	0	+	+++	0
Metaproterenol (Alupent®)	0	+	++	0
Terbutaline (Bricanyl®)	0	+	+++	0
Albuterol, Salbutamol (Ventolin®)	0	+	+++	0
Clenbuterol (Ventipulmin®)	0	+	+++	0

*DA = dopamine.

adenylate cyclase, increased intracellular cyclic-adenosine monophosphate (cyclic-AMP), and relaxation of bronchial smooth muscle (Table 49.1).

Stabilize Mast Cells. Stimulation of β-receptor activity on mast cells decreases release of inflammatory mediators. The β-receptor on mast cells produces a stabilizing effect (inhibition of mediator release) (Chong et al. 2002). There is little effect on other inflammatory cells. The clinical significance of this effect has not been established.

Increased Mucociliary Clearance. There is some evidence that β-adrenergic receptor agonists increase mucociliary clearance in the respiratory tract. The clinical significance of this effect has not been established.

SHORT-ACTING NONSPECIFIC BRONCHODILATORS

Epinephrine (Adrenaline). Epinephrine stimulates α- and β-adrenergic receptors (Table 49.2). It produces pronounced vasopressive and cardiac effects. Epinephrine is considered the drug of choice for the emergency treatment of life-threatening bronchoconstriction. The nonspecific stimulation of other receptors and its short duration make it unsuitable for long-term use. The dose used in animals is 10 μg/kg IM, IV, administered as a one-time treatment, or repeated in 15 minutes. Formulations are available in either 1:10,000 concentration (0.01%, 0.1 mg/ml) or 1:1,000 concentration (0.1%, 1 mg/ml). Duration of action is short (less than 1 hr).

Norepinephrine (Levarterenol). This drug has similar β_1 effects as epinephrine but fewer α_1 and β_2 effects, and therefore is not suitable for respiratory therapy.

Isoproterenol (Isuprel). Isoproterenol is a potent β receptor agonist. It is selective for β receptors with little α-receptor–mediated effects, but the cardiac (β_1) effects make it unsuitable for long-term use. It has been administered by inhalation or injection. It has a short duration of action (<1 hr).

LONGER-ACTING β_2–SPECIFIC DRUGS. To avoid the adverse cardiac effects of β-adrenergic agonists, drugs have been developed that are more specific for the β_2-receptor. These drugs are preferred for repeated use or long-term use. These drugs are also incorporated in some of the metered-dose inhalers used to treat bronchoconstriction.

Terbutaline (Brethine, Bricanyl). Terbutaline is similar to isoproterenol for its β_2 activity, but it is longer acting (6 to 8 hours). It may be injected subcutaneously to relieve an acute episode of bronchoconstriction. (The dose in people is approx. 3.5 μg/kg, repeated once/hour.) The oral dose is 2.5 mg/dog q8h for dogs, and 0.625 mg (one-quarter of a 2.5 mg tablet) q12h for cats (e.g., cats with feline "asthma"). It is available as 2.5 and 5 mg tablets and 0.8 mg/ml (820 μ/ml) injection. The dose for injection in cats is 0.01 mg/kg IV or IM. Terbutaline has been used in horses to treat recurrent airway obstruction (RAO) (formerly called *chronic obstructive pulmonary disease, COPD*), which is a bronchoconstrictive disease in horses analogous to asthma in people. It is not absorbed after oral administration in horses; therefore, injectable preparations must be used.

Metaproterenol (Alupent®, Metaprel®). Metaproterenol is similar to terbutaline, but the duration of action is shorter (4 hours). It is available as 10 and 20 mg tablets and 2 mg/ml oral syrup. The dose in small animals is 0.325 to 0.65 mg/kg.

Albuterol (Salbutamol) (Proventil®, Ventolin®). Albuterol is similar to terbutaline and metaproterenol in its action. Doses used in small animals are 20–50 μg/kg up to 4 times/day. (Dose in people is 100–200 μg/kg 4 times daily.) It is available as 2, 4, and 5 mg tablets and 2 mg/5 ml syrup. The use of formulations for horses is discussed in another section on inhalant products (discussed with the topical agents). Levalbuterol is the R-isomer of albuterol, and is used in some products, but it has no advantage over albuterol.

Clenbuterol (Ventipulmin). Clenbuterol was approved by the FDA in 1998 for use in horses. Its use in food animals is illegal, which is discussed in a later section. Its use has not been reported in small animals. Clenbuterol has been used for the treatment of recurrent airway obstruction (RAO) (formerly called *chronic obstructive pulmonary disease, COPD*) (Table 49.3) in horses and some studies have demonstrated efficacy (Shapland et al. 1981). However, its bronchodilating ability has been questioned. Compared to other β-agonists, such as terbutaline, clenbuterol has lower clinical efficacy because it is only a partial agonist and has lower intrinsic activity (Törneke et al. 1998; Derksen et al. 1987).

TABLE 49.3 Recurrent airway obstruction (RAO) in horses

- Formerly called chronic obstructive airway disease (COPD)
- Characterized by
  - Chronic airway inflammation
  - Labored breathing
  - Bronchospasm
  - Mucus plugs
  - Tissue remodeling in airways
  - Neutrophilic inflammation in airways
  - Bronchial hyper-responsiveness
- Treatments:
  - Bronchodilators (beta-2 agonists)
  - Corticosteroids
  - Inhalant medications
  - Cromoglycate
  - Phosphodiesterase inhibitors

Clenbuterol is available as a syrup (Ventipulmin syrup, 100 ml and 33 ml bottles, 72.5 μg/ml) for horses for oral administration. The dose is 0.8 μg/kg twice daily, but can be increased to 2x, 3x, and then 4x (up to 3.2 μg/kg) if the initial dose is not effective. The duration of effect is 6–8 hours. Adverse effects in horses include sweating, muscle tremor, restlessness, and tachycardia.

Compounding of clenbuterol, especially from bulk drugs of unapproved sources, has become popular in equine medicine. Unless the source of clenbuterol for the compounding meets the criteria of the AMDUCA (FDA's Animal Medicinal Drug Use Clarification Act), this is strictly illegal.

In livestock, β_2-agonists have been used illegally as repartitioning agents. (A repartitioning agent repartitions nutrients away from adipose tissue in favor of muscle [Peters 1989].) The result is increased carcass weight, and an increased ratio of muscle to fat, while reducing the feed required per kg of gain. Because clenbuterol has not been approved for food animal use, and residues pose a threat to people (e.g. pregnant women and people with heart conditions), a "zero tolerance" level has been established for these residues. The illegal use of clenbuterol in food animals has been a concern of the FDA. Deaths in humans have been reported as a result of eating beef liver contaminated with clenbuterol residue. In the U.S., clenbuterol residues have been highest in "show animals." *There also is evidence that clenbuterol has been used for "muscle-building" in human athletes.*

Salmeterol and Formoterol. These drugs are long-acting β-agonists that have been used in human medicine, but their use in veterinary medicine has not been reported.

INHALANT FORMULATIONS: NEBULIZED β-AGONISTS.

Inhaled aerosols of β_2-agonists are important drugs for treatment of acute bronchospasm in human patients with asthma or allergic bronchitis. Nebulization is the process of creating small droplets of a drug that can be inhaled into the airways. Nebulized agents are delivered via jet nebulizers, ultrasonic nebulizers, and metered-dose inhalers. Several metered-dose inhalers are marketed for this use in people, such as albuterol (Ventolin®), bitolterol

(Tornalate®), terbutaline (Brethaire®), and pirbuterol (Maxair®).

The use of these aerosols has become more common in animals because adapters are available to allow for use by animal owners. In horses, masks are available that allow a metered-dose inhaler to be used (Derksen et al. 1996; Tesarowski et al. 1994). The AeroMask (Trudell Medical International) and Equine Haler (Equine Health Care) are two such masks. For cats, the AeroKat chamber has also been used to deliver these medications.

Albuterol (Torpex). In 2002, albuterol sulfate was approved by the US-FDA for horses, indicated for relief of bronchospasm and bronchoconstriction associated with recurrent airway obstruction (RAO). It is an aerosol formulation in a pressurized canister and delivered via a specialized nasal delivery bulb. The nasal bulb is inserted into the horse's nostril and when the horse inhales, the device is activated. Masks that fit over the horse's nose (discussed in the previous paragragh) also have been used.

In horses, doses of 360 or 720 μg delivered by aerosolization caused significant bronchodilation (Derksen et al. 1999). The same author also administered pirbuterol at 600 μg/horse with good results.

For small animals, the metered dose inhaler to deliver albuterol in people has been adapted for use. An inhalation chamber is used to deliver the drug. The use of small animal inhalers is discussed in more detail in the corticosteroid section.

ADVERSE EFFECTS FROM β-AGONISTS. The most common adverse effects from β-agonists affect the cardiovascular system (tachycardia) and skeletal muscles (muscle tremors) (Fox and Papich 1989). Cardiac effects (rapid heart rate, palpitations, tremor) can be prominent with β_1-agonists and can be produced by β_2-agonists at high doses. When high doses of β-agonists have been nebulized to horses, they produced muscle twitching, sweating, and excitement. β_2-receptor agonists also inhibit uterine motility and should not be used late in pregnancy. (However, these drugs have been used therapeutically for this purpose in situations in which it may be desirable to inhibit uterine contractions to delay labor.) High doses of β_2-agonists also can produce hypokalemia.

As noted above in the clenbuterol section, these drugs also have properties that affect skeletal muscle. These drugs have been abused in humans and animals for their muscle-building properties. High doses can cause muscle twitching and hyperthermia.

TOLERANCE WITH CHRONIC USE. Regular administration of β-agonists can produce drug tolerance, which is a loss in the sensitivity of β-adrenergic receptors owing to down-regulation of receptors. This effect occurs when β-adrenergic drugs are administered regularly for several weeks. Therefore, it is best to rely on these drugs intermittently and allow drug-free breaks in treatment. The most common use of these drugs is for short-term treatment for acute exacerbations of bronchoconstriction.

CROMOLYN (SODIUM CROMOGLYCATE) (INTAL®)

Cromoglycate is used occasionally to stabilize mast cells in animals with hypersensitive airways. It is usually administered as a 2% solution for nebulization in the treatment of bronchoconstrictive diseases. It has been used in people to treat asthma and nebulized to horses via a special mask to treat recurrent airway obstruction (RAO).

MECHANISM OF ACTION. Cromolyn inhibits mast cell release of histamine, leukotrienes, and other substances from sensitized mast cells that cause hypersensitivity reactions, probably by interfering with calcium transport across the mast cell membrane. It has no intrinsic bronchodilator action.

CLINICAL USE. Cromolyn has been used as an aerosol for treating recurrent airway obstruction (RAO) in horses (Thomson and McPherson 1981). It is administered via inhalation once daily for 1 to 4 days, which will provide a therapeutic effect for several days. In one report, nebulization of 80 mg once daily for 1–4 days prevented signs of heaves in horses for up to 3 weeks. However, other studies have produced conflicting results. The primary drawback is the route of administration and timing. To be effective, it *must* be administered before the horse is exposed to the allergen (prophylactically).

Nedocromil Sodium. Nedocromil sodium (Tilade) is a chemically unrelated drug, but has an antiinflammatory effect via a similar mechanism to chromolyn. It is approved for use in treating asthma in people but use in veterinary patients has not been reported.

METHYLXANTHINES (XANTHINES)

The methylxanthines include theobromine, caffeine, and theophylline. Pentoxifylline also is a methylxanthine, but is used for conditions other than asthma. The methylxanthines—particularly theophylline—have been used as bronchodilators, although their exact action is not understood. Once a mainstay in the therapy of human asthma, theophylline use has diminished because of a high incidence of side effects in people and because there are better-tolerated and more effective drugs available. But, in animals—particularly small animals—theophylline continues to be used because it is tolerated well and oral dosing is convenient. There are no clinical studies that have documented efficacy in small animals; the use is purely anecdotal.

PHARMACOLOGIC EFFECTS. The pharmacology of theophylline was reviewed by Weinberger and Hendeles (1996). The methylxanthines are classified as CNS stimulants, but they have a variety of pharmacological effects on various organ systems. The methylxanthines relax bronchial smooth muscle and produce antiinflammatory effects that are unrelated to the bronchodilating properties. In addition, there are nonrespiratory effects of methylxanthines, which include CNS stimulation, urinary diuresis (mild), and cardiac stimulant (mild).

Cellular Basis of Action. The cellular basis of action of the methylxanthines is still not completely understood. The effect that persists in the literature is the action to inhibit phosphodiesterase types 3 and 4. Phosphodiesterase is the enzyme that catalyzes cyclic-AMP to inactive products. Inhibition of the phosphodiesterase enzyme increases intracellular concentrations of the cyclic nucleotide cAMP. Cyclic-AMP inhibits the release of inflammatory mediators from mast cells, has antiinflammatory effects, and produces bronchial smooth muscle relaxation. More detail on the molecular mechanisms of drugs for treating asthma were discussed by Barnes (2003).

Another mechanism of action that may explain the benefits for respiratory disease is via antagonism of *adenosine* receptors. Adenosine causes bronchoconstriction in asthmatic patients, but blocking this receptor also may contribute to the adverse effects.

ANTIINFLAMMATORY EFFECTS. The antiinflammatory effects of theophylline may occur separately—and at lower concentrations—than the bronchodilating effects (Barnes 2003). This may occur by decreasing the expression of inflammatory genes. Treatment with theophylline has induced a decreased response to histamine and other inflammatory mediators in the airways. Theophylline's antiinflammatory effects include diminished activity of inflammatory and immune cells—especially eosinophils—in the airways. Eosinophils are important in the bronchial response to inhaled allergens, and they release inflammatory mediators that induce bronchoconstriction and inflammatory changes in the airways.

FORMULATIONS. Theophylline has been available in several formulations, including, injectable, aqueous solutions, elixirs, tablets, and capsules. However, the most convenient for small animal use are extended-release forms that allow for twice daily treatment in dogs and once-daily or once-every-48-hr treatment in cats. These are discussed in more detail in the section on clinical use.

Examples of other forms of theophylline are presented in Table 49.4. These salts are designed to improve solubility and decrease stomach irritation. The theophylline content of these salts must be considered when calculating a dosage regimen.

TABLE 49.4 Formulations of theophylline

	Brand Name	Percent Theophylline
Theophylline base	Many	100
Theophylline elixir	Many	100
Theophylline monohydrate		90
Theophylline ethylenediamine (aminophylline)	Many	80
Choline theophyllinate (oxtriphylline)	Choledyl	65
Theophylline sodium glycinate	Asbron	50
Theophylline calcium salicylate	Quadrinal	48

TABLE 49.5 Theophylline pharmacokinetics and doses

Species	$t^1/_2$ (Hours)	V_D (l/kg)	%F*	Suggested Dose
People	6-8	0.5	90	4 mg/kg q6h
Dog	5.7	0.82	91	9 mg/kg q6-8h, or 10 mg/kg q12h of the extended release formulations
Cat	7.8,11.7 (IV)14–18 (oral)	0.46, 0.86	96–100	4 mg/kg q8-12h or extended-release at 15 mg/kg (tab) and 19 mg/kg (cap) q24h (q48h may be possible in some cats)
Cattle	6.4	0.815	93	20 mg/kg q12h
Horse	12–15	0.85–1.02	100	5 mg/kg q12h

* %F = percent absorbed from oral administration.

PHARMACOKINETICS. After oral administration, theophylline is rapidly and completely absorbed. Systemic availability is 91%, 96–100% and 100% in dogs, cats, and horses, respectively. Theophylline is metabolized primarily by the liver in all species; only 10% of the dose is eliminated unchanged in the urine. The pharmacokinetics have been studied in several veterinary species and are listed in Table 49.5 with comparisons to people.

PLASMA CONCENTRATIONS AND CLINICAL MONITORING. Theophylline drug plasma assays are available in many laboratories. When theophylline is used long-term, monitoring is recommended to establish the optimum dose. In dogs and cats, the accepted therapeutic plasma concentration is 10 to 20 μg/kg, but these values were extrapolated from human studies. In animals, we aim for plasma concentration greater than 10 μg/ml (usually 10 to 20 μg/ml) for clinical effects. Plasma concentrations greater than 15 μg/ml have been reported to cause clinical adverse effects in horses.

Antiinflammatory action may occur in patients at concentrations that are below the concentrations usually considered for bronchodilation. For example in people, a concentration of 6.6 μg/ml theophylline caused a reduction in activated eosinophils (Sullivan et al. 1994). In the review by Barnes (2003) the antiinflammatory effects are reported to occur in people at concentrations of 5 to 10 μg/ml, which is approximately half of the concentration needed to produce bronchodilation.

SIDE EFFECTS AND ADVERSE EFFECTS. Mild adverse effects include gastrointestinal signs. Theophylline can be nauseating. The nonspecific inhibition of phosphodiesterase also can produce vomiting.

The most important side effects of theophylline are attributed to the cardiac stimulation. In this regard, theophylline is more potent than either caffeine or theobromine. The cardiac effects may be summarized as increased heart rate, increase in myocardial contractility (mild), improved right and left systolic function, vasodilation (mild), and diuretic (weak). At high doses, cardiac arrhythmias are possible.

CNS stimulation is more likely from caffeine than theophylline or theobromine. However, at high doses, theophylline also can affect the CNS. These are reported less frequently from theophylline use in small animals than in humans, but they can be common in horses. The CNS effects can be characterized by increased alertness, agitation, nervousness, increased activity, and convulsions at high doses. At high doses there is decreased cerebral blood flow (26%), which may be related to the incidence of seizures at toxic doses.

The most serious adverse effects are concentration-dependent. Caution is advised if administration is performed rapidly intravenously. These adverse effects have been described when theophylline is administered rapidly intravenously in horses and dogs. If the drug is administered orally, high peak plasma concentrations are less likely (Munsiff et al. 1988).

DRUG INTERACTIONS. Theophylline relies on hepatic metabolism by cytochrome P450 enzymes for clearance. Therefore, interactions are possible when other drugs are administered that affect these enzyme systems. The metabolism of theophylline may be inhibited by erythromycin, fluoroquinolone antibiotics (for example, enrofloxacin), and cimetidine. The metabolism may be induced by rifampin and phenobarbital, which may necessitate increasing the dose if these drugs are used together. Activated charcoal will increase the clearance of theophylline and other methylxanthines and is useful for treatment of a toxic overdose.

CLINICAL USE IN DOGS AND CATS. Theophylline has been used for the treatment of both cardiac and respiratory diseases in dogs. Some veterinarians have included theophylline in regimens for the management of congestive heart failure, although this is becoming an outdated treatment because of availability of newer cardiac drugs. Theophylline is also employed for the management of intrathoracic collapsing trachea and various forms of bronchitis.

Older sustained-release tablets have been studied in dogs and cats (Koritz et al. 1986; Dye et al. 1989). However, these formulations were recently discontinued and the dose recommendations no longer apply.

Availability of Newer Formulations. Decreased availability of older sustained-release formulations led to the use of new tablets and capsules (TheoChron 100, 200, or 300 mg tablets; or TheoCap 125 or 250 mg capsules, Inwood Laboratories). Oral administration of sustained-release formulations in dogs at a dose of 10 mg/kg, q12h will produce concentrations in dogs within a range considered to be therapeutic (Bach et al. 2004). Studies in cats (Guenther-Yenke et al. 2007), showed that a dose of 100 mg per cat of the tablet, or 125 mg/cat of the capsule (approximately 15 or 19 mg/kg, respectively) every 24–48 hours maintained plasma concentrations in a range considered to be therapeutic. (*Recently these capsule formulations have become less available, but one may continue to use the tablet form.*)

CLINICAL USE IN HORSES. Administration of theophylline to horses has a narrow therapeutic index and it is considered less effective than β-adrenergic agonists. Adverse effects have prevented more common use. Some evidence indicates that phosphodiesterase inhibitors are not effective in horses with recurrent airway obstruction (RAO) (Lavoie et al. 2006).

Despite the risk of adverse effects and questionable efficacy, theophylline has been used in the management of recurrent airway obstruction, RAO (formerly called *COPD*) in horses. Studies cited (Button et al. 1985; Errecalde et al. 1984; Ayres et al. 1985; Ingvast-Larsson et al. 1989; and Kowalczyk et al. 1984) summarize the pharmacokinetics and effects of theophylline in horses. Oral doses usually are used to avoid the high concentrations from injections. A loading dose of 12 mg/kg has been followed by maintenance doses of 5 mg/kg, every 12 hours. One study demonstrated that affected horses showed decreased wheezing, decreased respiratory effort, and an improvement in pCO_2 and blood pH following theophylline administration. However, none of the horses returned to normal. In horses there is also a positive cardiac chronotropic effect and a weak diuretic effect. Toxicosis can occur from large doses and doses administrated rapidly intravenously. Toxic signs include tremors, excitement, tachycardia, and sweating.

CLINICAL USE IN CATTLE. Although there is little clinical experience with the use of theophylline in cattle, experimental evidence suggests that it is a poor bronchodilator in this species (McKenna et al. 1989).

ANTICHOLINERGIC DRUGS

Anticholinergic (parasympatholytic/antimuscarinic) drugs such as atropine and glycopyrrolate are effective bronchodilators. (The pharmacology of anticholinergic agents was provided in more detail in Chapter 7.) Cholinergic stimulation causes bronchoconstriction. Anticholinergic drugs inhibit vagal-mediated cholinergic smooth muscle tone in the respiratory tract. Some studies suggest that asthmatic individuals have excessive stimulation of cholinergic receptors. In some people, COPD can be more effectively treated with anticholinergic drugs than by β-agonists (Barnes 2000). Although atropine will provide relief from these effects in many patients, the side effects are unacceptable for long-term use. Side effects involve the CNS and GI systems.

USE OF ANTICHOLINERGIC DRUGS IN HORSES. Pearson and Riebold (1989) compared the effects of atropine, isoproterenol, and theophylline in horses with recurrent airway obstruction (RAO, also known as *chronic obstructive pulmonary disease, COPD,* or "*heaves*"). Atropine at doses of 0.02 mg/kg, IV was better at relieving some signs of RAO (reduction in intrathoracic pressure for example) than either theophylline or isoproterenol. Isoproterenol was more effective in this study than theophylline.

DRUG CHOICES. If anticholinergic drugs are administered, the quaternary amines such as glycopyrrolate (Robinul-V®), propantheline, (ProBanthine®), and isopropamide should be used instead of atropine because quaternary amines are less likely to cross the blood-brain barrier and CNS side effects will be minimized. However, atropine is acceptable for short-term use and a 5 mg IV dose has been used as a response test in horses suspected of presenting with RAO.

Ipratropium bromide (Atrovent®) is a quaternary amine that is an effective bronchodilator in human asthmatic patients. It is administered as an aerosol and is the first anticholinergic drug to be approved as a bronchodilator. Since ipratropium is not absorbed from the airways, it is described as a "topical form of atropine." It has been administered to horses for treatment of RAO and produced effects for 6 hours at a dose of 2 μg/kg.

ADVERSE EFFECTS. The cardiac effects and inhibition of gastrointestinal function prohibit long-term use of atropine. The topical drugs (e.g., ipratropium) have less systemic effects. Anticholinergic drugs may decrease mucociliary clearance. In horses, atropine at 0.02 mg/kg decreased tracheal mucus transport rate.

GLUCOCORTICOIDS

Glucocorticoids decrease inflammation associated with inflammatory pulmonary diseases. Prednisolone has been effective for treatment of feline tracheobronchitis ("feline asthma"), nonseptic pulmonary diseases associated with pulmonary infiltrates of leukocytes (noninfectious bronchitis), allergic bronchitis, and recurrent airway obstruction (RAO) in horses. For treatment of asthma in people, inhaled corticosteroids are recognized as the most effective therapy available (Barnes 1995, 2006). In one article, they were called the "drugs to beat" (Barnes 2006).

MECHANISM OF ACTION. The pharmacology of the glucocorticoids was discussed in more detail in Chapter 30. In patients with inflammatory airway diseases, glucocorticoids have potent antiinflammatory effects on the bronchial mucosa. Glucocorticoids bind to receptors on cells and inhibit the transcription of genes for the production of mediators (cytokines, chemokines, adhesion molecules) involved in airway inflammation (Rhen and Cidlowski 2005). In horses with RAO, administration of oral dexamethasone in combination with feeding changes, decreased the gene expression of proinflammatory cytokines in bronchoalveolar cells (deLuca et al. 2008). A decrease in the synthesis of inflammatory mediators such as prostaglandins, leukotrienes, and platelet-activating factor caused by glucocorticoids also may be important (Barnes 1995a, 1989, 2006). Mast cells are not affected by glucocorticoids as much as other inflammatory cells. Glucocorticoids also enhance the action of adrenergic agonists on β_2-receptors in the bronchial smooth muscle, either by modifying the receptor or augmenting muscle relaxation after a receptor has been bound. In addition, corticosteroids may prevent down-regulation of β_2-receptors. Glucocorticoids and theophylline used together appear to be synergistic (Barnes 2003).

CLINICAL USE

Dogs. Oral prednisolone or prednisone is usually the drug of choice. A typical antiinflammatory dosage is 0.5 to 1.0 mg/kg. After an initial course of treatment many patients can be managed by administering this dose on an every-other-day (EOD) basis.

Cats. Because cats are somewhat resistant to glucocorticoids, higher doses have been used compared to doses administered to dogs. Oral prednisolone initial dosages of 2 to 4 mg/kg/day have been used for 10–14 days, followed by chronic doses of 1.0 mg/kg/day for the treatment of feline asthma (Padrid 2000). For cats, prednisolone should be used instead of prednisone because of an absorption/conversion problem similar to horses (see below) (Graham-Mize and Rosser 2004). Some veterinarians have administered 20 mg per cat of a long-acting formulation, methylprednisolone acetate (Depo Medrol®) intramuscularly. The effects of one injection may persist for 3 weeks.

Adverse effects in cats are a concern with long-term treatment (Table 49.6). Among the concerns are that corticosteroids may exacerbate or increase the risk of congestive

TABLE 49.6 Adverse effects of corticosteroids in cats

- Behavior changes
- Increased appetite
- Weight gain
- Hyperglycemia
- Increased plasma volume (secondary to hyperglycemia)
- Increased risk of heart disease (secondary to increased plasma volume)
- Hepatomegaly

heart failure in cats (Smith et al. 2004; Ployngam et al. 2006). The proposed mechanism for increasing this risk is increase in plasma glucose, volume expansion, and increase in plasma volume. The vascular volume increase may lead to an overload. To avoid systemic adverse effects, topical (inhaled) formulations have been used (see below).

Horses. In horses, corticosteroids are important for management of recurrent airway obstruction (RAO). Oral corticosteroids have been used, but there are no convenient dose formulations. In some cases tablets have been crushed and added to a drug vehicle or mixed with feed (grain). In horses, one should be cognizant of the dose form administered. Prednisone in horses is either not absorbed, and/or not converted to the active prednisolone after absorption (Peroni et al. 2002). Therefore, prednisolone tablets are the preferred drug for oral administration. The dose used initially is approximately 2 mg/kg oral, once or twice a day. Oral dexamethasone, added to the horse's feed, also can be used. In a study in which dexamethasone was effective for decreasing inflammatory cytokine expression in RAO horses, a decreasing oral dexamethasone dose of 0.165 mg/kg per day to 0.04 mg/kg per day over a course of 21 days was used (DeLuca et al. 2008). Alternatives are inhaled and injectable forms (see below).

Injections of dexamethasone have improved clinical signs of airway obstruction when administered at doses of 0.1 mg/kg (Rush et al. 1998). Despite clinical improvement, dexamethasone does not improve indicators of airway inflammation in the airways, such as AP-1, NFκB, or cytology. Dexamethasone by injection was more effective than inhaled corticosteroids in this study, but there is a concern that repeated use of injections of corticosteroids in horses may result in adverse effects, such as adrenal suppression, signs of hyperadrenocorticism, and laminitis. Nevertheless, dexamethasone can be valuable for some cases, and one of the formulations most often used is dexamethasone 21-isonicotinate suspension (Voren), which may be administered at a dose of 0.06 mg/kg IM (not intended for IV use).

INHALED CORTICOSTEROIDS. Glucocorticoids are among the most valuable drugs for managing asthma in people. For people, a metered-dose inhaler is used to deliver the drug topically in order to avoid systemic adverse effects. According to one review, Inhaled corticosteroids are the most effective agents available for the symptomatic control of asthma and improvement in pulmonary function (Busse and Lemanske 2001). Examples of aerosolized corticosteroids are listed in Table 49.7 and include beclomethasone (Beclovent®), flunisolide (Aerobid®), fluticasone (Flovent®), triamcinolone (Azmacort), and budesonide (Pulmicort). Fluticasone is the most potent (18 × dexamethasone) and is usually the one used in veterinary medicine (Table 49.7). When glucocorticoids are delivered topically with these devices, systemic adverse effects are minimized, but not eliminated. Suppression of the hypothalamic-pituitary-adrenal axis can still be observed (see also Chapter 30).

TABLE 49.7 Examples of corticosteroids available as metered-dose inhalers

Drug	Brand Name	Dose Delivered
Beclomethasone dipropionate	Vanceril	40 or 80 μg per puff
Budesonide	Pulmicort	200 μg per puff (dry powder)
Flunisolide	Aerobid	250 μg per puff
Fluticasone propionate (most potent)	Flovent	44, 110, or 220 μg per puff
Triamcinolone acetonide	Azmacort	100 μg per puff

Use in Horses. The metered-dose inhalers designed for people can be used in horses with the aid of an equine-adapted handheld metered-dose delivery device (Derksen et al. 1996; Rush et al. 2000). Delivery devices used in horses include the Equine Aeromask (Trudell Medical International), Equine Haler, (Equine Health Care), NebulalAIR (IVX Animal Health), and the 3M Equine Inhaler (3M and Boehringer Ingelheim).

Aerosolized beclomethasone dipropionate using an equine-adapted metered dose inhalation device has been effective for reducing airway inflammation in horses with recurrent airway obstruction (RAO) (Rush et al. 1998, 2000). Horses responded within 24 hours. Administration of 500 μg every 12 hours to horses was shown to produce less adrenal suppression than larger doses and still provided beneficial effects.

Use in Small Animals. Metered-dose inhalers have been successfully used in small animals, particularly cats. For this use, a chamber with a valve on one end, fitted with a mask (for example the OptiChamber by Respironics and AeroKat by Trudell Medical International) has been used to deliver the drug. Budesonide or fluticasone are most often administered because of their high potency (Table 49.7) and low systemic effects. Fluticasone has been used most often. In people it has a systemic absorption of only 18–26%, but there are extensive first-pass effects preventing systemic blood concentrations if it is swallowed after delivery. Therefore, the systemic action—and adverse effects—is expected to be small. A typical dose for fluticasone for a cat is 110 μg (one puff from a 110 μg metered dose inhaler) per day. Higher dose inhalers that deliver 220 μg are also available. In a recent study (Cohn et al. 2008) three fluticasone doses (44, 110, and 220 μg per cat) twice daily via metered dose inhaler were equivalent in an experiment model of feline asthma. When asthmatic cats were given inhaled corticosteroids twice a day and allowed 5–7 breaths (10 sec) from the chamber, it reduced the need for oral prednisolone. After 10 days, the patient may be reevaluated and frequency of administration reduced.

In one study, inhaled fluticasone reduced bronchial hyperresponsiveness and bronchoconstriction in cats with bronchitis with a dose of 250 μg per cat daily (Kirschuink et al. 2006). This dose also decreased inflammatory cells and prostaglandins in bronchoalveolar lavage fluid. In cats, flunisolide was studied for its systemic effects after administration by inhalation (Reinero et al. 2006). Although there was some suppression of the hypothalamic-pituitary-adrenal axis (indicating some systemic absorption), no systemic effects on immune cells were observed.

NONSTEROIDAL ANTIINFLAMMATORY DRUGS (NSAIDs)

NSAIDs have been administered for some types of pulmonary disease. The drug most often investigated has been flunixin meglumine. It is registered for cattle to treat inflammatory respiratory problems and as an adjunct treatment of Bovine Respiratory Disease (BRD).

Diseases in which NSAIDs may have a benefit include pulmonary thromboembolism, (for which antiplatelet doses of aspirin are used), pulmonary effects from endotoxin in horses and dogs (for which flunixin meglumine has been used) and in cattle with bovine respiratory disease, and pulmonary disease from PI-3 and 3-methyl indole in cattle.

LEUKOTRIENE INHIBITORS

Leukotrienes, such as LTD_4 contribute to airway inflammation by increasing migration of eosinophils, producing bronchoconstriction, and increasing airway wall edema. Inhibitors or blockers of leukotrienes have been used to treat these airway diseases. These were discussed in more detail by Drazen et al. (1999) and reviewed by Werz and Steinhilber (2006) and Peters-Golden and Henderson (2007). The leukotrienes have not been demonstrated to be important mediators in feline asthma (Norris et al. 2003). Therefore, these inhibitors may not have a role in feline respiratory disease. However, there is evidence that LTB_4—rather than the other leukotrienes—may contribute to airway inflammation in horses with recurrent airway obstruction (RAO) (Lindberg et al. 2004). An experimental 5-lipoxygenase inhibitor (fenleuton)—which decreases LTB_4—produced improvement in horses with RAO (Marr et al. 1998), but an LTD_4 receptor antagonist did not (Lavoie et al. 2002).

LIPOOXYGENASE INHIBITOR: ZILEUTON (ZYFLO®). Zileuton is an oral drug for treating asthma in people. It inhibits the enzyme 5-lipoxygenase and thereby inhibits synthesis of inflammatory leukotrienes. This drug has broader actions than the leukotriene receptor blockers because it inhibits effects of both LTB_4 and the cysteinyl leukotrienes (LTC_4, LTD_4, LTE_4). However, it has been less effective than leukotriene receptor blockers (see below) because, at the doses administered, it does not achieve complete suppression of the 5-lipoxygenase enzyme. In people, the safety profile has not been as good as the receptor blockers (see below). The effectiveness of zileuton for respiratory diseases in animals has not been reported. For people the dose is 600 mg, q6h and these doses have been extrapolated to animals for some studies. Treatment of other diseases in animals (e.g., allergic skin disease) have been investigated, but it has not been effective. In people it has been associated with hepatitis in some individuals.

LEUKOTRIENE RECEPTOR BLOCKERS. Zafirlukast (Accolate®), pranlukast, and montelukast (Singulair®) are leukotriene receptor blockers that have been used as oral drugs for treating asthma. They block the cysteinyl leukotriene receptor, therefore blocking the effects of LTC_4, LTD_4, and LTE_4—primarily at the $CysLT_1$ receptor site—but these drugs do not block receptors for the leukotriene LTB_4 (Drazen et al. 1999). The $CysLT_1$ receptor mediates sustained bronchoconstriction, mucus secretion, and edema in the airways (Peters-Golden and Henderson 2007). These drugs have been generally well tolerated in people, but there are some drug interactions with zafirlukast (inhibition of CYP-450 enzymes). Montelukast has fewer adverse effects in people and less risk of drug interaction than zafirlukast. The use of these drugs has not been reported to be effective for treating respiratory diseases in animals. Doses in animals are not established, but the dose in people for zafirlukast is 20 mg/person twice daily and for montelukast it is 5 mg for children and 10 mg for adults.

DUAL BLOCKERS. The only dual blocker of prostaglandins and leukotrienes (COX and LOX) is the NSAID tepoxalin (Zubrin). It is currently registered as an oral treatment for arthritis in dogs. It is not known whether the antileukotriene effect will be beneficial in patients with respiratory disease.

EXPECTORANTS AND MUCOLYTIC DRUGS

The expectorants and mucolytics comprise a diverse group of compounds, with many proposed benefits but few clinical studies that have documented efficacy. These drugs have been used to increase the output of bronchial secretions, enhance clearance of bronchial exudate, and promote a more productive cough. Some of these drugs have a traditional use in veterinary medicine and their efficacy has not been established.

SALINE EXPECTORANTS. These drugs are promoted to stimulate bronchial mucus secretions via a vagal-mediated reflex action on the gastric mucosa. Even though there are no well-designed studies that support an expectorant effect from these products, particularly the ammonium compounds, stimulating the stomach appears to trigger a reflex that stimulates bronchial secretions. However, for some of these drugs, such as potassium iodide, the dose used clinically is too low to be effective. Examples of expectorants include ammonium chloride, ammonium carbonate, potassium iodide, calcium iodide, and ethylenediamine dihydroiodide (EDDI). EDDI is the best known of these compounds by veterinarians because it is also added to the feed of cattle for the purpose of decreasing foot rot infections, lumpy jaw (*Actinomyces bovis*), woody tongue (*Actinobacillus lignieresi*), and bronchitis. There is a lack of published scientific evidence for a beneficial effect.

DIRECT STIMULANTS. Volatile oils such as eucalyptus oil (found in cough drops such as Halls Mentho-Lyptus) and oil of lemon are believed to directly increase respiratory tract secretions. Their clinical efficacy in veterinary medicine is unknown.

GUAIFENESIN (GLYCERYL GUAIACOLATE) AND GUAIACOL. Guaifenesin compounds are typically classified as muscle relaxants in anesthesia and as anesthetic adjuncts, but they also may have an expectorant effect. The anesthetic effects were discussed in Chapters 11 and 13. Their mechanism of action is uncertain, but it is possible that these compounds stimulate bronchial secretions via vagal pathways. Although guaifenesin is contained in many over-the-counter cough remedies, such as Robitussin, the efficacy is highly questionable because most preparations do not contain a dose large enough. Studies that have measured the expectorant effect of guaifenesin have noted that it does not change the volume or viscosity of bronchial secretions, but it may accelerate particle clearance from the airways.

Formulations used in people (but not evaluated in animals) employ higher doses than older over-the-counter drugs. The higher dose formulations for people include Mucinex (600 and 1200 mg tablet), Mucinex-D (with pseudoephedrine), and Mucinex-DM (with dextromethorphan). Most typical OTC older formulations contain doses of 100 mg.

ACETYLCYSTEINE (MUCOMYST®). Acetylcysteine is available as a 10% solution that can be nebulized to patients. It is used in human patients with obstructive airway disease and children with cystic fibrosis (CF) to help clear mucus. Its mucolytic effect is caused by an interaction of the exposed sulfhydral groups on the compound with disulfide bonds on mucoprotein (Ziment 1988). Acetylcysteine helps break down respiratory mucus, reduce the viscosity of mucus, and enhance the clearance. Acetylcysteine may also increase the levels of glutathione, which is a scavenger of oxygen-derived free radicals. In Europe this drug is also available as an oral formulation.

Acetylcysteine also is used to treat certain types of toxicoses. The most common condition is acetaminophen (Tylenol®) toxicosis in cats.

DEMULCENTS. Many over-the-counter preparations are formulated in an oily or syrup base to provide a demulcent action (soothing effect). They are usually used to soothe the pharynx and thus may have an antitussive effect. Home remedies such as honey mixed with herbal tea or distilled spirits probably have this effect.

DECONGESTANTS

Decongestants are used to "dry up" mucus membranes when rhinorrhea occurs (in people, caused by the common cold and allergic rhinitis). Decongestants are sympathomimetic drugs that stimulate the α-adrenergic receptors in mucus membranes and cause local vasoconstriction. The pharmacology of adrenergic agonists was discussed in more detail in Chapter 6.

TOPICAL DECONGESTANTS. Short-acting topical agents include phenylephrine and phenylpropanolamine, which are common ingredients in over-the-counter nasal sprays (e.g., NeoSynephrine®). These products also have been applied topically to decrease bleeding associated with some surgical procedures (for example, nasal turbinate surgery in horses and dogs). Some topical decongestants are particularly long-acting, such as oxymetazoline (Afrin®) and xylometazoline (Dristan®). Caution should be exercised when using the topical products chronically. Rebound inflammation and hyperemia may occur when the action of the drug diminishes, resulting in a worsening of the problem. The clinical use of these agents for nasal problems is rare in animals because they are difficult and inconvenient to administer.

SYSTEMIC DECONGESTANTS. The systemic use of adrenergic agonists as decongestants has been a common practice in medicine for decades. In human medicine, over-the-counter (nonprescription) formulations for colds and allergies have contained ephedrine, the isomer pseudoephedrine (Sudafed®), or a similar drug, phenylpropanolamine (PPA). Side effects from the orally administered drugs include vasoconstriction and increased blood pressure in susceptible individuals, and excitement. A change in heart rate is possible from direct stimulation (increased heart rate), or vasoconstriction (decreased heart rate). There are some problems with the abuse of these agents in humans, which has limited the veterinary availability of

The Controversy about Phenylpropanolamine (PPA) and Pseudoephedrine

Phenylpropanolamine was first approved in 1959 and has been widely available over-the-counter (OTC) as a nonprescription drug for many years for humans. Popular brand names were Dexatrim and Acutrim (appetite suppressants), and Propagest and Rhindecon (decongestants). A study in 2000 suggested that phenylpropanolamine in appetite suppressants, and possibly decongestants, is a risk factor for hemorrhagic stroke in women (Kernan et al. 2000). *Because of the risk of hemorrhagic stroke in women, the Food and Drug Administration (FDA), announced on November 6, 2001, that it was taking steps to remove phenylpropanolamine from all drug products and has requested that all drug companies discontinue marketing products containing phenylpropanolamine.* After this action, it created a void for veterinary prescribing because PPA has been used frequently in dogs to control incontinence. However, after the FDA action, there were soon replacement drugs on the veterinary market containing PPA. There are now several formulations that are marketed for use in dogs, even though there is not formal FDA approval.

The other major concern with over-the-counter decongestants is the diversion to manufacturing methamphetamine. Phenylpropanolamine, ephedrine, and pseudoephedrine have been used as raw ingredients to illegally manufacture methamphetamine for "street use" in the so-called "Meth Labs." Pseudoephedrine closely resembles methamphetamine in structure. Because of this diversion, the quantity of pseudoephedrine (the only one currently available OTC) that one can purchase is limited by most pharmacies. In some states, pseudoephedrine may be obtained without prescription, but it must be dispensed by the pharmacists (behind the counter). Pseudoephedrine has been eliminated from all over-the-counter medications and replaced by less effective drugs.

Sympathetic amines, such as ephedrine and ephedra alkaloids (found in herbal products), are also used and abused as CNS stimulants. Nonprescription use of so-called "herbal" products has been popular. These products contain ephedra alkaloids (also known as *ma huang*), which produces a similar effect as the drug ephedrine. Side effects are possible and fatal cardiac events and seizures have occurred in young adults consuming high doses. Adverse cardiovascular and central nervous system effects have been reported (Haller and Benowitz 2000).

these compounds (see sidebar, "The Controversy about Phenylpropanolamine (PPA) and Pseudoephedrine").

USE OF DECONGESTANTS FOR TREATMENT OF INCONTINENCE. Although these drugs are rarely used as sinus decongestants in veterinary medicine they are popular drugs for treating incontinence in dogs. The effect of phenylpropanolamine (PPA) and other sympathetic agonists, such as pseudoephedrine, for treating urinary incontinence arises from their stimulation of the alpha-receptor—to increase the tone of the urinary sphincter, and its beta-receptor effects—to relax the detrussor muscle of the bladder wall and allow more urine filling.

The most common drug used for this purpose has been phenypropanolamine (PPA) (Moreau and Lappin 1989). There is a registered formulation of phenylpropanolamine available in Europe for treatment of urinary incontinence in dogs, (Propalin syrup) which has now been marketed in the U.S. The dose is approximately 1–2 mg/kg q8 to 12 h. The PROIN phenylpropanolamine is available as 75, 50, and 25 mg liver-flavored tablets and 25 mg flavored syrup. Propalin syrup is available as a 50 mg/ml syrup.

RESPIRATORY STIMULANTS

Respiratory stimulation is due to direct effect on the chemoreceptors of carotid artery and aorta. These receptors are sensitive to changes in CO_2, which in turn stimulate the respiratory center. Doxapram (Dopram®) is used primarily in an emergency during anesthesia, or to decrease the respiratory depressant effects of certain drugs (e.g., opiates, barbiturates). In horses, doxapram will cause cardiac stimulation as well as respiratory stimulation. There have been reports that administration to neonates may increase their suckling activity shortly after birth and subsequently decrease the incidence of failure of passive transfer of immunoglobulins. Scientific studies documenting this effect are lacking. An additional use of doxapram in foals is for treatment of hypercapnia associated with hypoxic-ischemic encephalopathy (Giguere et al. 2008). This treatment with doxapram at a constant rate infusion of 0.02 to 0.05 mg/kg/hr for 8 hours, improved by restoring respiratory control and corrected hypercapnia. In this study, caffeine was not as effective.

REFERENCES AND ADDITIONAL READING

Abramowicz M (editor). Drugs for asthma. Med Letter 41:5–10, 1999.

Aubier M, Murciano P, Viires N, et al. Diaphragmatic contractility enhanced by animophylline: Role of extracellular calcium. J Appl Physiol 54:460–464, 1983.

Ayers JW, Pearson EG, Riebold TW, et al. Theophylline and dyphylline pharmacokinetics in the horse. Am J Vet Res 46:2500–2506, 1985.

Bach JE, Kukanich B, Papich MG, McKiernan BC. Evaluation of the bioavailability and pharmacokinetics of two extended-release theophylline formulations in dogs. J Am Vet Med Assoc Apr1;224(7):1113–9, 2004.

Barnes PJ. A new approach to the treatment of asthma. N Eng J Med 321:1517–1527, 1989.

———. Molecular mechanisms of antiasthma therapy. Ann Med 27:531–535, 1995a.

———. Inhaled corticosteroids for asthma. New Engl J Med 332:868–875, 1995b.

———. Chronic obstructive pulmonary disease. New Engl J Med 343:269–280, 2000.

———. Corticosteroids: The drugs to beat. Eur J Pharmacol 533:2–14, 2006.

———. Theophylline: New perspectives for an old drug. Am J Resp Crit Care Med 167:813–818, 2003.

Benowitz NL. Clinical pharmacology of caffeine. Annu Rev Med 41:277–288, 1990.

Boothe DM, McKiernan BC. Respiratory therapeutics. Vet Clin N Am Sm An 22:1231–1258, 1992.

Busse WW, Lemanske RF. Asthma. New Engl J Med 344:350–362, 2001.

Button C, Errecalde JO, Mulders SG. Loading and maintenance dosage regimens for theophylline in horses. J Vet Pharmacol Ther 8:328–330, 1985.

Chong LK, Chess-Williams R, Peachell PT. Pharmacological characterisation of the β-adrenoceptor expressed by human lung mast cells. Eur J Pharmacol 437:1–7, 2002.

Christie GJ, Strom PW, Rourke JE. Butorphanol tartrate: an new antitussive agent for use in dogs. Vet Med/Sm An Clin Oct; 75(10):1559–1562, 1980.

Cohn LA, DeClue AE, Cohen RI, Reinero CR. Dose effects of fluticasone propionate in an experimental model of feline asthma. [abstract #24] ACVIM Forum, San Antonio, Texas, 2008.

Colton T, Gosselin RE, Smith RP. The tolerance of coffee drinkers to caffeine. Clin Pharmacol Ther 9:31–39, 1968.

Colucci WS, Wright RF, Braunwald E. New positive inotropic agents in the treatment of congestive heart failure (2 parts). New Engl J Med 314:290–299, 1986, and 314:349–358, 1986.

DeLuca L, Erb HN, Yong JC, Perkins GA, Ainsworth DM. The effect of adding oral dexamethasone to feed alterations on the airway cell inflammatory gene expression in stabled horses affected with recurrent airway obstruction. J Vet Intern Med 22(2):427–435, 2008.

Derksen FJ, Olzewski M, Robinson NE, et al. Use of a hand-held, metered dose aerosol delivery device to administer pirbuterol acetate to horses with heaves. Equine Vet J 28:306–310, 1996.

———. Aerosolized albuterol sulfate used as a bronchodilator in horses with recurrent airway obstruction. Am J Vet Res 60:689–693, 1999.

Derksen FJ, Scott JS, Slocombe RF, et al. Effect of clenbuterol on histamine-induced airway obstruction in ponies. Am J Vet Res 48:423–426, 1987.

Drazen JM, Israel E, O'Byrne PM. Treatment of asthma with drugs modifying the leukotriene pathway. New Engl J Med 340:197–206, 1999.

Dye JA, McKiernan, Jones SD, et al. Sustained-release theophylline pharmacokinetics in the cat. J Vet Pharmacol Ther 12:133–140, 1989.

Errecalde JO, Button C, Baggot JD, et al. Pharmacokinetics and bioavailability of theophylline in horses. J Vet Pharmacol Ther 7:255–263, 1984.

Errecalde JO, Button C, Mulders SG. Some dynamic and toxic effects of theophylline in horses. J Vet Pharmacol Ther 8:320–327, 1985.

Forbes JA, Beaver WT, Jones KF, et al. Effect of caffeine on ibuprofen analgesia in postoperative oral surgery pain. Clin Pharmacol Ther 49:674–684, 1991.

Fox PR, Papich MG. Complications of cardiopulmonary drug therapy. In Kirk RW, Bonagura J (eds), Current Veterinary Therapy X, WB Saunders Co., Philadelphia, 1989.

Genetzky RM, Loparco FV. Chronic obstructive pulmonary disease in horses. Compend Cont Ed 7:S407–S414, 1985.

Giguère S, Slade JK, Sanchez LC. Retrospective comparison of caffeine and doxapram for the treatment of hypercapnia in foals with hypoxic-ischemc encephalopathy. J Vet Intern Med 22(2):401–405, 2008.

Gingerich DA, Rourke JE, Strom PW. Clinical efficacy of butorphanol injectable and tablets. Vet Med/Sm An Clin Feb; 78:179–182, 1983.

Graham-Mize CA, Rosser EJ. Bioavailability and activity of prednisone and prednisolone in the feline patient. [abstract] Vet Dermatol 15(Suppl1):9, 2004.

Guenther-Yenke CL, McKiernan BC, Papich MG, Powell E. Pharmacokinetics of an extended release theophylline product in cats. J Am Vet Med Assoc 231:900–906, 2007.

Haller CA, Benowitz NL. Adverse cardiovascular and central nervous system events associated with dietary supplements containing ephedra alkaloids. New Engl J Med 343:1833–1838, 2000.

Hoffman AM, Viel L, Tesarowski DB, et al. Management of severe obstructive pulmonary disease with inhaled bronchodilator treatment in a horse. Can Vet J 34:493–495, 1993.

Ingvast-Larsson C, Kallings P, et al. Pharmacokinetics and cardio-respiratory effects of oral theophylline in exercised horses. J Vet Pharmacol Ther 12:189–199, 1989.

Kernan WN, Viscoli CM, Brass LM, et al. Phenylpropanolamine and the risk of hemorrhagic stroke. New Engl J Med 343:1826–1832, 2000.

Kirschuink N, Leemans J, Delvaux F, Snaps F, Jaspart S, Evrard B, Delattre L, Cambier C, Clerex C, Gustin P. Inhaled fluticasone reduces bronchial responsiveness and airway inflammation in cats with mild chronic bronchitis. J Feline Med Surg 8:45–54, 2006.

Koritz GD, McKiernan BC, Neff-Davis CA, Munsiff IJ. Bioavailability of four slow-release theophylline formulations in the Beagle dog. J Vet Pharmacol Ther 9:293–302, 1986.

Kowalczyk DF, Beech J, Littlejohn D. Pharmacokinetic disposition of theophylline in horses after intravenous administration. Am J Vet Res 45:2272–2275, 1984.

Kukanich B, Papich MG. Plasma profile and pharmacokinetics of dextromethorphan after intravenous and oral administration in healthy dogs. J Vet Pharmacol Ther Oct; 27(5):337–41, 2004.

———. Pharmacokinetics of tramadol and the metabolite O-desmethyltramadol in dogs. J Vet Pharmacol Ther Aug; 27(4):239–46, 2004.

Lavoie J-P, Leguillette R, Pasloske K, Charette L, Sawyer N, Guay D, Murphy T, and Hickey GJ. Comparison of effects of dexamethasone and the leukotriene D4 receptor antagonist L-708,738 on lung function and airway cytologic findings in horses with recurrent airway obstruction. Am J Vet Res 63:579–585, 2002.

Lavoie J-P, Pasloske K, Joubert P, et al. Lack of clinical efficacy of a phosphodiesterase-4 inhibitor for treatment of heaves in horses. J Vet Intern Med 20:175–181, 2006.

Lindberg Å, Robinson E, Näsman-Glaser B, Jensen-Waern M, Lindgren JÅ. Assessment of leukotriene B_4 production in leukocytes from horses with recurrent airway obstruction. Am J Vet Res 65:289–295, 2004.

Marr KA, Lees P, Page CP, Cunningham FM. Effect of the 5-lipooxygenase inhibitor, fenleuton, on antigen-induced neutrophil accumulation and lung function changes in horses with chronic obstructive pulmonary disease. J Vet Pharmacol Therap 21:241–246, 1998.

McKenna DJ, Koritz GD, Neff-Davis CA, Langston VC, et al.. Field trial of theophylline in cattle with respiratory tract disease. J Am Vet Med Assoc 195:603–605, 1989.

Moreau PM, Lappin MR. Pharmacologic management of urinary incontinence. In Kirk RW (ed), Current Veterinary Therapy X. WB Saunders Co., Philadelphia, 1214–1222, 1989.

Munsiff IJ, McKiernan BC, Neff-Davis CA, Koritz GD. Determination of the acute oral toxicity of theophylline in conscious dogs. J Vet Pharm Ther 11 (4):381–389, 1988.

Nelson HS. β-adrenergic bronchodilators. New Engl J Med 333:499–506, 1995.

Norris CR, Decile KC, Berghaus LJ, Berghaus RD, Walby WF, Schelegle ES, Hyde DM, Gershwin LJ. Concentrations of cysteinyl leukotrienes in urine and bronchoalveolar lavage fluid of cats with experimentally induced asthma. Am J Vet Res 64:1449–1453, 2003.

Padrid P. CVT Update. Feline asthma. In Bonagura JD (ed), Current Veterinary Therapy XIII. WB Saunders Co., Philadelphia, 805–810, 2000.

Papich MG. Current concepts in pulmonary pharmacology. Seminars in Vet Med Surg (small animal) 1:289–301, 1986.

———. Bronchodilator therapy. In Kirk RW (ed), Current Veterinary Therapy IX, WB Saunders Co., Philadelphia, 1986.

Pearson EG, Riebold TW. Comparison of bronchodilators in alleviating clinical signs in horses with chronic obstructive pulmonary disease. J Am Vet Med Assoc 194:1287–1291, 1989.

Peroni DL, Stanley S, Kollias-Baker C, Robinson NE. Prednisone per os is likely to have limited efficacy in horses. Equine Vet J 34:283–287, 2002.

Peters AR. Beta-agonists as repartitioning agents. A review. Vet Record 124:417–420, 1989.

Peters-Golden M, Henderson WR. Leukotrienes. New Engl J Med 357:1841–1854, 2007.

Ployngam T, Tobias AH, Smith SA, Torres SM, Ross SJ. Hemodynamic effects of methylprednisolone acetate administration in cats. Am J Vet Research 67:583–587, 2006.

Pozzi A, Muir WW, Traverso F. Prevention of central sensitization and pain by N-methyl-D-aspartate receptor antagonists. J Am Vet Med Assoc 228:53–60, 2006.

Reinero CR, Brownlee L, Decile KC, Seguin B, Berghaus RD, Nelson RW, Gershwin LJ. Inhaled flunisolide suppresses the hypothalamic-pituitary-adrenal axis, but has minimal systemic immune effects in healthy cats. J Vet Intern Med 20:57–64, 2006.

Rhen T, Cidlowski JA. Antiinflammatory action of glucocorticoids—new mechanisms for old drugs. New Engl J Med 353:1711–1723, 2005.

Rosenbloom D, Sutton JR. Drugs and exercise. Med Clin N Am 69:177–186, 1985.

Rush BR, Raub ES, Rhoads WS, et al. Pulmonary function in horses with recurrent airway obstruction after aerosol and parenteral administration of beclomethasone dipropionate and dexamethasone, respectively. Am J Vet Res 59:1039–1043, 1998.

Rush BR, Raub ES, Thomsen MM, et al. Pulmonary function and adrenal gland suppression with incremental doses of aerosolized beclomethasone dipropionate in horses with recurrent airway obstruction. J Am Vet Med Assoc 217:359–364, 2000.

Sawynok J, Yaksh TL. Caffeine as an analgesic adjuvant: a review of pharmacology and mechanisms of aciton. Pharmacol Rev 45:43–85, 1993.

Shapland JE, Garner HE, Hatfield DG. Cardiopulmonary effects of clenbuterol in the horse. J Vet Pharmacol Ther 4:43–50, 1981.

Smith SA, Tobias AH, Fine DM, et al. Corticosteroid-associated congestive heart failure in 12 cats. Int J Appl Res Vet Med 2:159–170, 2004.

Sullivan P, Bekir S, Jaffar Z, et al. Anti-inflammatory effects of low-dose theophylline in atopic asthma. Lancet 343:1006–1008, 1994.

Takahama K, Shirasaki T. Central and peripheral mechanisms of narcotic antitussives: Codeine-sensitive and -resistant coughs. Cough 3:1–8, 2007.

Tesarowski DV, Viel L, McDonell WN, et al. The rapid and effective administration of a beta-2 agonist to horses with heaves using a compact inhalation device and metered dose inhalers. Can Vet J 35:170–173, 1994.

Thomson JR, McPherson EA. Prophylactic effects of sodium cromoglycate on chronic obstructive pulmonary disease in the horse. Equine Vet J 13:243–246, 1981.

Törneke K, Ingvast Larsson C, Appelgren L-E. A comparison between clenbuterol, salbutamol and terbutaline in relation to receptor binding and in vitro relaxation of equine tracheal muscle. J Vet Pharmacol Therap 21:388–392, 1998.

Turgut K, Sasse HHL. Influence of clenbuterol on mucociliary transport in healthy horses and horses with chronic obstructive pulmonary disease. Vet Rec 125:526–530, 1989.

Weinberger M, Hendeles L: Theophylline in asthma. New Engl J Med 334:1380–1388, 1996.

Werz O, Steinhilber D. Therapeutic options for 5-lipoxygenase inhibitors. Pharmacol Ther 112:701–718, 2006.

Ziment I. Acetylcysteine: A drug that is much more than a mucokinetic. Biomed Pharmacother 42:513–520, 1988.

CHAPTER

50

PHARMACOGENOMICS

KATRINA L. MEALEY

A patient's response to a drug includes both beneficial (therapeutic) effects as well as any adverse effects, including lack of therapeutic efficacy. While the goal of drug therapy is to produce a specific pharmacological effect without producing adverse effects, it is often difficult to predict how effective or how safe a medication may be for a particular patient. If 10 patients with a particular disease were administered the same drug, each might respond differently with respect to both drug efficacy and the likelihood of an adverse reaction. A number of factors may influence a patient's response to drug therapy, including the patient's age, species, concurrent medications, diet, health or disease status, and others. However, consideration of all of these factors is often not sufficient to explain the degree of interpatient variation observed. The observed interpatient variability in drug response may result primarily from genetically determined differences in drug metabolism, drug distribution, and/or receptors or drug target proteins. The branch of pharmacology that involves identifying genetic variations leading to interindividual differences in drug response is called *pharmacogenetics*. Pharmacogenetics is likely the ultimate way to establish the right drug and dose for each patient, thereby optimizing efficacy and minimizing toxicity. Despite the fact that this branch of pharmacology is still in its infancy as a science, a number of important discoveries have already contributed to improved pharmacotherapy in human and veterinary patients.

The term *pharmacogenetics* is often used interchangeably with the term *pharmacogenomics*. Strictly speaking, pharmacogenetics refers to monogenetic (single gene) variants that affect a patient's response to a particular drug. An example of a pharmacogenetic study might be one that examines the influence of mutations in the thiopurine methyl transferase gene on the response to azathioprine. Pharmacogenomics, on the other hand, refers to the entire spectrum of genes that are involved in determining a patient's response to a particular drug. An example of a pharmacogenomic study would be one that examines the interaction between cytochrome P450 genes, beta-1, beta-2, alpha-1, and alpha-2 adrenergic receptor genes, and drug transporter (i.e., MDR1) genes on the response to carvedilol. The relatively few reports of gene-drug responses in veterinary medicine are pharmacogenetic in nature.

While dramatic alterations in drug response have been identified in pharmacogenetic studies, the overall response to most drugs will likely require a pharmacogenomics approach to characterize the individual contribution of multiple genes to drug response. For the purposes of this chapter, the terms *pharmacogenetics* and *pharmacogenomics* will be used interchangeably.

The concept that inheritance might explain individual variation in susceptibility to adverse drug reactions and/or variation in drug efficacy was proposed in 1957. The term *pharmacogenetics* was coined shortly afterward, in 1959. Relatively little pharmacogenetic research occurred for the next 3 decades. A resurgence in pharmacogenetic research occurred coincidentally with the advent of the Human Genome Project in 1990. Since then, research in pharmacogenetics has expanded at a remarkable rate. There are now at least two journals exclusively devoted to pharmacogenetic/pharmacogenomic research, and many other medical and pharmacological journals encouraging submissions reporting results of pharmacogenetic research. Following completion of the Human Genome Project (announced in 2003), the National Human Genome Research Institute challenged investigators to develop genome-based approaches to predict drug response, setting the stage for continued growth in the field of pharmacogenetics.

BASIC GENETIC CONCEPTS

The human genome contains approximately 3 billion nucleotide bases, representing roughly 30,000 genes. When a gene is expressed, DNA is transcribed into RNA, which is then translated to make proteins. Three consecutive nucleotide bases form a specific codon, specifying a particular amino acid or signaling amino acid chain termination (stop codons). The genetic code is said to have redundancy, which simply means that there may be two or more different codons for the same amino acid. In humans, for example, both GGA and GGC code for the amino acid glycine. Redundancy exists in the canine genome as well, with TAA, TGA, and TAG representing stop codons. A gene is simply the DNA sequence containing a series of codons that specify a particular protein. The variation that occurs between individuals in a population is a result of differences, often the result of mutations, in specific genes.

A mutation alters the base sequence of DNA, which in turn alters the transcribed RNA creating a different codon. Some mutations, because of the redundancy described above, are silent, meaning that if the mutation results in a base change that creates a codon for the same amino acid (i.e., GGA to GGC) as specified by the original DNA sequence, there is no change in protein structure or function. However, if the mutation results in a different amino acid, or the creation of a stop codon, the change in protein structure and function can be deleterious. At each gene locus, an individual carries two alleles, one from each parent. An allele is defined as the DNA sequence at a given gene's location on the chromosome. If an individual has two identical alleles, that individual is said to have a homozygous genotype. If an individual has two different alleles, that individual is said to have a heterozygous genotype. The phenotype of each individual with regard to a specific gene is the outward, physical manifestation of a given genotype. That outward physical manifestation might be something immediately obvious in a given individual such as eye color, or it may not be apparent until a particular drug is administered to that individual.

Variations in a given gene may be present rarely in a population, or in relatively large numbers in a population. Polymorphisms are defined as genetic variations occurring at a frequency of 1% or greater in the population (species of interest). In humans, many of the genes encoding cytochrome P450 enzymes are polymorphic (specific mutations are present in greater than 1% of the population), whereas some inherited human diseases such as cystic fibrosis are caused by rare mutations occurring in less than 1% of the population. Identification of the specific mutation may be used to provide specific treatment regimens and, in the case of veterinary patients, guide breeding decisions as well. However, many common human diseases such as diabetes mellitus or hypertension are polygenic (more than one gene contributes to the disease). For diseases that are polygenic in nature, the pathophysiology of the disease is complex, and specific treatments based on particular mutations will be difficult to sort out. It is likely that many important diseases in veterinary medicine (i.e, hip dysplasia, epilepsy, most types of cancer) are polygenic also; therefore, genes linked to disease susceptibility will not be discussed in this chapter. Rather, this chapter will focus on genetic variations associated with variation in response to pharmacological agents.

APPROACHES USED TO IDENTIFY GENETIC VARIATION. In attempting to identify a molecular defect, several approaches can be used. Using the "candidate gene" approach, the researcher makes an educated guess as to which gene(s) might be involved in a particular phenotype (disease process or drug response). Candidate genes may be genes that are associated with a similar phenotype in a different species. In many instances, a molecular defect may have been identified in humans or mice, providing a reasonable candidate gene for veterinary researchers to investigate. Alternatively, a candidate gene may be selected because it encodes a protein that is structurally or functionally intimately associated with the disease process or drug response of interest. For example, cytochrome P450 enzymes are known to be involved in the metabolism of many (if not most) drugs. The genes encoding these enzymes would be logical candidate genes to investigate if attempting to identify the molecular defect associated with drug toxicities. Once a candidate gene(s) has been identified, it is then evaluated in affected and unaffected animals by one or more techniques including sequencing, Northern or Southern blot analysis, or expression arrays.

Another method, linkage analysis, can be used if the candidate gene approach was unsuccessful or in cases where a rational candidate gene is not apparent. Linkage analysis involves identifying families segregating the phenotype of interest. Linkage analysis requires well-characterized multigeneration families segregating the disease, with the likelihood of identifying true linkage increasing with larger family size, and greater numbers of families included. Once an appropriate family or families have been characterized, a set of highly polymorphic DNA markers are analyzed for each of the family members characterized (affected and unaffected). A statistical program is then used to determine the likelihood that linkage exists between the genetic markers and the phenotype of interest (disease or drug response locus).

PHARMACOGENETICS

Genetic variation can affect both the pharmacokinetics (i.e., drug absorption, distribution, metabolism, and excretion) and pharmacodynamics (i.e., interaction with drug transporters and receptors) of pharmaceutical agents. The concept of pharmacogenetics originated in the 1950s when it was discovered that the antimalarial drug primaquine caused hemolysis in a subpopulation of individuals.[1] Ultimately it was shown that the enzyme glucose 6-phosphate dehydrogenase had reduced function in affected individuals as compared to the majority of the population.[1] At the time, techniques to study molecular biology were not available, so the field of pharmacogenetics was initially based purely on phenotypic observations (measurement of enzyme function). Discovery of the specific mutation in the glucose 6-phosphate dehydrogenase gene would not occur until a few decades later.

With the rapid advancement of molecular techniques, modern pharmacogenetic research differs significantly from those initial phenotypic observations. It currently involves identifying both the phenotype and the genetic variation responsible for it. Researchers perform systematic searches to identify functionally significant variations in DNA sequences in genes that affect drug disposition. In many instances, the genetic variation in a gene is identified before the phenotypic consequence is known. Sequencing of the human, and now the canine, genome will speed the progress of pharmacogenetic discoveries, facilitating the ultimate goal of pharmacogenetics, which is individualization of drug therapy.

It is important to note that individualization of drug therapy encompasses two distinct, yet equally important, clinical implications. First is the ability to predict those patients at high risk for developing drug toxicity. These patients may have a mutation in a drug-metabolizing enzyme that results in low clearance rates for the drug. For such patients a lower drug dose or alternate drug should be administered. Second is the ability to predict those patients that are most likely to benefit from a particular drug because of appropriate receptor interactions. Patients with mutations in drug receptors may be poor responders to certain pharmaceutical agents. Rather than using a trial-and-error approach to drug therapy, a veterinarian could select the drug most likely to produce the desired pharmacological response in a particular patient, decreasing the amount of time in which the patient's disease state is poorly controlled.

Described in this chapter are several recent discoveries in veterinary pharmacogenetics and examples of pharmacogenetically based differences in drug absorption, distribution, metabolism, excretion, and drug-receptor interactions. The impact of these discoveries in clinical veterinary medicine will also be presented. To date, most of the clinically relevant pharmacogenetic discoveries involve dogs. When applicable, information about other species will also be included.

PHARMACOGENETICS OF ORAL DRUG ABSORPTION. Until recently, systemic bioavailability of orally administered drugs has been considered to be a function of physicochemical characteristics of the drug and subsequent hepatic metabolism. A number of other factors have recently been shown to impact the ability of a drug to be absorbed into the systemic circulation after oral administration. Intestinal Phase I drug metabolism and active drug extrusion by efflux transporters are now considered to be among the most important determinants of oral drug bioavailability. Consequently, genetic variation in intestinal drug metabolizing enzymes and drug transporters should dramatically affect oral drug absorption.

In people, CYP 3A is expressed at higher levels in mature villus tip enterocytes than in hepatocytes.[2] Because intestinal villi comprise such a large surface area, there is a high likelihood that absorbed drug will interact with intestinal CYP 3A enzyme, facilitating substantial first-pass metabolism. Interpatient variability in intestinal CYP3A levels has been studied in a small sample of human patients. Elevenfold variations in CYP3A protein content, and sixfold variation in enzymatic activity were identified, suggesting that CYP 3A polymorphisms exist in the human population.[3] While intestinal drug metabolism is thought to be important in veterinary patients also, relatively little is known with regard to interpatient variability in enzyme activity.

Drug transporters are also known to play an important role in drug absorption. Many drug transporters have been identified in people, but the most well-characterized drug transporter is P-glycoprotein (P-gp), the product of the MDR1 (also known as the *ABCB1*) gene. The potential impact of transporter pharmacogenetics on drug pharmacokinetics is dramatically illustrated by P-gp. P-gp is a transmembrane protein that was first described in highly resistant tumor cell lines.[4] Tumor cells expressing P-gp were cross-resistant to various anticancer agents (anthracyclines, vinca alkaloids, taxanes, and others). P-gp has since been shown to act as an ATP-dependent pump that exports drugs from nonneoplastic cells as well. In normal mammalian tissues, P-gp appears to function in a protective capacity. P-gp is expressed on bile canaliculi, renal tubular epithelial cells, the placenta, brain capillary endothelial cells, and at the luminal border of intestinal epithelial cells.[5] At these locations, P-gp pumps selected drugs either out of the body (into the bile, urine, or intestinal lumen) or away from protected sites (brain tissue, fetus).

The significant role intestinal P-gp can play in determining oral drug bioavailability has been demonstrated in rodent studies. In mdr1 (-/-) knockout mice, oral bioavailability of many P-gp substrate drugs (vinblastine, taxol, digoxin, loperamide, ivermectin, cyclosporine A, others) is substantially greater than in wildtype mice.[6,7] Similarly, MDR1 polymorphisms in people have been shown to result in altered oral bioavailability of P-gp substrate drugs. Studies have shown that oral bioavailability of digoxin, a P-gp substrate, is greater in subjects with the 3435TT MDR1 genotype compared with those with the MDR1 3435CC genotype.[8] Similarly, the P-gp substrate phenytoin has been shown to have lower oral bioavailability in subjects with the MDR1 3435 CC genotype.[9]

P-gp has been fairly well characterized in dogs. The tissue distribution of P-gp in dogs is similar to that in people,[10] and it has been shown to contribute to chemotherapeutic drug resistance in vitro and in vivo.[11–13] Although its role in determining oral drug bioavailability is not well characterized, there is some evidence that P-gp is important. Bioavailability of the anticancer agent (and P-gp substrate) docetaxel was increased seventeenfold when coadministered with a P-gp inhibitor. A polymorphism of the MDR1 gene has also been described in dogs, but results of studies investigating the effect of this polymorphism on oral drug bioavailability are not yet available.

The MDR1 polymorphism in dogs consists of a 4 base-pair deletion mutation. This deletion results in a shift of the reading frame that generates several premature stop codons.[14] Because protein synthesis is terminated before even 10% of the protein product is synthesized, dogs with two mutant alleles exhibit a P-gp null phenotype, similar to mdr1 (-/-) knockout mice. Affected dogs include many herding breeds. For example, roughly 75% of collies in the United States, France, and Australia have at least one mutant allele.[15] Other affected herding breeds, albeit at a lower frequency, include Old English Sheepdogs, Australian Shepherds, Shelties, English Shepherds, Border Collies, German Shepherds, Silken Windhounds, McNabs, and Long-haired Whippets.[16] Studies investigating the effect of the MDR1 deletion mutation on oral drug bioavailability in herding breeds are ongoing in the author's laboratory.

PHARMACOGENETICS OF DRUG DISTRIBUTION. Drug distribution, the delivery of drugs from the systemic circulation to tissues, can be dramatically affected by pharmacogenetics. The drug transporter P-gp serves as an important barrier to the distribution of substrate drugs to selected tissues. For example, P-gp is a component of the blood-brain barrier, the blood-testes barrier, and the placenta. Therefore, distribution of P-gp substrate drugs to these tissues is greatly enhanced in dogs with the MDR1 deletion mutation. Dogs homozygous for the deletion [MDR1 (mutant/mutant)] experience adverse neurological effects after a single dose of ivermectin (120 μg/kg). Heterozygous (MDR1 wildtype/mutant) or homozygous wildtype dogs are not sensitive to ivermectin neurotoxicity at the 120 μg/kg dose, but heterozygote animals may experience neurotoxicity at ivermectin doses greater than 300 μg/kg, particularly if daily doses are administered (i.e., protocols for treatment of demodectic mange). Dogs homozygous for the normal MDR1 allele (normal/normal), can receive 2000 μg/kg in a single dose without signs of toxicity, and can receive 600 μg/kg/day for months without signs of toxicity. Affected Collies also appear to have increased susceptibility to neurologic adverse effects of other avermectins including milbemycin, selamectin (Revolution® package insert), and moxidectin.[17] Interestingly, a retrospective study conducted by a national veterinary poison center reported that Collies were overrepresented in canine cases of loperamide-induced neurotoxicity.[18] Many Collies displayed signs of neurologic toxicity after administration of routinely recommended doses of the antidiarrheal agent loperamide (Imodium®). Loperamide is an opioid that is generally devoid of CNS activity because it is excluded from the brain by P-gp.[19,20] Loperamide neurotoxicity was recently reported in a Collie that had received a routine dose (0.14 mg/kg orally).[21] The dog in this report had the MDR1 (mutant/mutant) genotype. Homozygous wildtype (normal/normal) dogs do not exhibit neurologic signs after receiving even higher doses of loperamide, indicating that P-gp plays a key role in modulating distribution of substrates such as loperamide to canine brain tissue. Less information is available regarding P-gp and the blood brain barrier in cats. The author has received anecdotal reports of ivermectin toxicity in cats after standard doses, but whether the underlying cause is a result of altered P-gp expression or function is not currently known.

Distribution of some drugs to the testes and fetus may also be limited by P-gp. In human patients, this creates a problem for treating certain diseases. For example, the testes and brain are considered to be a sanctuary site for the human immunodeficiency virus (HIV).[22] Because HIV-1 protease inhibitors are substrates for P-gp, the virus can remain viable in these sanctuary sites, hampering effective therapy. Similarly, therapeutic concentrations of certain chemotherapeutic agents may not be achievable for testicular cancers because of active efflux by P-gp.[23] The effect of placental P-gp on distribution of drugs to the fetus is an area of active research in human medicine.[24] Understanding the role of pregnancy-related hormones in regulating P-gp expression and function is one possible key in developing strategies to deliver drugs to the mother with minimal fetal risk.

PHARMACOGENETICS OF DRUG METABOLISM. Presently the greatest body of knowledge with regard to pharmacogenetics involves genetic variation in drug metabolism. Pharmacogenetic variation can affect both Phase I and Phase II metabolic enzyme activity. A mutation in the pseudocholinesterase enzyme serves as an example of how pharmacogenetic variation can result in dramatic differences in drug response between patients. Patients with a normal pseudocholinesterase genotype metabolize succinylcholine and recover from neuromuscular blockade rapidly; those with the mutant genotype undergo sustained neuromuscular blockade that can result in prolonged apnea and the necessity for mechanical ventilation.[25] A number of polymorphisms have been described in human cytochrome P450 enzymes, many of these resulting in profound variations in clinical response. For example CYP2D6 is a highly variable P450 pathway in humans with individuals ranging from undetectable activity (found in 6–10% of Caucasians) to "ultrarapid" activity (found in 3–10% of Europeans and 30% of one black population).[26] The ultrarapid phenotype is due to a highly unusual gene duplication. Drugs that are substrates for CY2D6 in people include beta receptor antagonists (propranolol, timolol, metoprolol), antiarrhythmics (quinidine, flecainide), antidepressants (amitriptyline, clomoipramine, fluoxetine, imipramine), neuroleptics, and certain opioid derivatives. Depending on the patient's CYP2D6 genotype, the "typical" dose of a substrate drug may need to be decreased (poor metabolizers require 1/10 of the standard dose of nortriptyline to avoid toxicity) or increased (ultrarapid metabolizers require 5 times the standard dose to achieve therapeutic concentrations).

Relatively few polymorphisms in drug metabolizing enzymes have been described in veterinary patients, although this is likely to change as research in this area is currently in progress. However, variation in metabolism of some drugs has been documented in dogs. CYP2B11 has been shown to have at least a fourteenfold variation in activity in mixed-breed dogs.[27] Greyhounds have been shown to have particularly low CYP2B11 activity, which results in sustained plasma concentrations of propofol and delayed recovery compared to mixed-breed dogs.[28] The specific genetic alteration responsible for reduced CYP2B11 in greyhounds as compared to other canine breeds has not been determined. There is some evidence to suggest that CYP 2D15 may also be polymorphic in dogs. The NSAID celecoxib is metabolized to a large degree by CYP2D15. Clearance of celecoxib in beagles is polymorphic, with about half the population being extensive metabolizers and the remainder being poor metabolizers.[29] Celecoxib has a 1.5–2-hour half-life in extensive metabolizers and a 5-hour half-life in poor metabolizers. One pharmacogenetic variant that has been identified in the canine CYP2D15 gene, a deletion of exon 3, results in undetectable celecoxib metabolism. The frequency and breed distribution of this polymorphism has not yet been determined. However, it is likely to have clinical significance for other drugs that are CYP2D15 substrates including dextromethorphan, imipramine, and others.

A number of other mutations in drug metabolizing enzymes have been described in animals, but the clinical relevance of these mutations, if any, has yet to be determined. For example, 10% of beagles in one study were deficient in CYP1A2 because of a mutation that resulted in premature termination of protein synthesis.[30] CYP1A2 does not appear to be responsible for metabolizing clinically used drugs in veterinary medicine, but CYP1A2 is studied frequently in people with regard to susceptibility to certain types of cancers. A feline hepatic CYP 2E polymorphism has been identified, but the clinical relevance of this polymorphism has not been described.[31] Similarly, polymorphisms have been described in several drug metabolizing enzymes in cattle,[32] but these single nucleotide polymorphisms are used as molecular markers available in cattle for linkage analysis, testing of parentage, and distinction of breeds, rather than for predicting response to drug therapy.

With respect to Phase II metabolic enzymes, a panspecies defect in UDP-glucuronyl transferase exists in cats. While this is not a true example of pharmacogenetics, it serves as an example of genetic variation between species, rather than within a species, that significantly affects drug disposition. Cats have a pseudogene, rather than a functional glucuronyltransferase gene; therefore, acetaminophen and other drugs are not conjugated with glucuronide as they are in other species. Another panspecies Phase II metabolic defect occurs in dogs. N-acetyltransferase is the enzyme responsible for metabolizing sulfonamides, procainamide, hydralazine, and other drugs. Both N-acetyltransferase genes are absent in dogs, increasing the risk for hypersensitivity reactions and adverse effects from these drugs relative to other species.[33]

A true pharmacogenetic variation exists for the thiopurine methyltransferase (TPMT) enzyme. TPMT is a Phase II enzyme that is responsible for metabolizing azathioprine and its active metabolites to their inactive forms. A ninefold range in TMPT activity exists in dogs, and enzyme activity level appears to be related to breed. Giant Schnauzers had lower TPMT activity while Alaskan Malamutes had high TMT activity.[34] Decreased TPMT activity has been documented to be associated with increased susceptibility to azathioprine-induced bone marrow suppression.

PHARMACOGENETICS OF DRUG EXCRETION. Drugs are eliminated from the body either unchanged or as metabolites. Renal and biliary excretion are the most important pathways of drug elimination, but excretion may occur by other routes as well. As noted previously, P-gp is expressed on renal tubular cells and biliary canalicular cells, suggesting that it may play a role in drug excretion. Concurrent administration of a P-gp inhibitor decreases the biliary and renal clearance of doxorubicin in rats.[35] In a separate study, biliary and renal excretion of digoxin and vincristine were increased in rats after treatment with a P-gp inhibitor.[36] Further research is necessary to fully define the role of P-gp in regulating renal and biliary drug excretion in veterinary patients. However, altered biliary and/or renal excretion may play a role in the apparent increased sensitivity of herding breeds to chemotherapeutic drugs that are P-gp substrates. For example, a Collie with lymphoma developed myelosuppression and GI toxicity after treatments with vincristine or doxorubicin, even at lowered doses, but tolerated cyclophosphamide at the full dose. The patient was subsequently genotyped and was determined to have one mutant MDR1 allele and one normal MDR1 allele.[37] It is possible that deficient P-gp in this patient resulted in delayed renal and/or biliary excretion and subsequent toxicity. Other reports of severe doxorubicin and/or vincristine sensitivity in Collies and other herding breeds have surfaced on internet veterinary discussion groups. The MDR1 mutation may be a reasonable explanation for this apparent breed predilection to chemotherapeutic (vinca alkaloids; anthracyclines) drug sensitivity.

PHARMACOGENETICS OF DRUG RECEPTORS. A relatively new and important area of pharmacogenetics research involves polymorphisms in genes encoding drug receptors and effector proteins. In human patients polymorphisms have been described in angiotensin converting enzyme, beta-2 adrenergic receptors, the dopamine receptor, the estrogen receptor, and others.[38] In vitro functional studies suggest that these polymorphisms have functional significance, but reports regarding clinical effects are not available. A polymorphism in the canine dopamine receptor D4 gene has been described but its clinical implications, if any, are not yet understood.[39]

PHARMACOGENETICS AND HYPERSENSITIVITY REACTIONS. Pharmacogenetic differences in metabolic pathways can not only affect Type A adverse drug reactions (predictable; generally correlating with plasma drug concentration), but can also affect type B adverse drug reactions (idiosyncratic). Idiosyncratic toxicity to sulfonamides is similar in dogs and people and can be characterized by fever, arthropathy, blood dyscrasias (neutropenia, thrombocytopenia, or hemolytic anemia), hepatopathy consisting of cholestasis or necrosis, skin eruptions, uveitis, or keratoconjunctivitis sicca.[40] In people, slow acetylation by NAT2 has been shown to be a risk factor for sulfonamide hypersensitivity reactions. It has been proposed that the alternative metabolic pathway in these individuals produces reactive metabolites.[41] Covalent binding of reactive metabolites of these drugs to cell macromolecules results in cytotoxicity and immune response to neoantigens. Ongoing research in one veterinary pharmacology laboratory (Department of Medical Sciences, School of Veterinary Medicine, University of Wisconsin-Madison, 2015 Linden Drive, Madison, WI 53706; latrepanier@svm.vetmed.wisc.edu) is underway to characterize dogs with possible idiosyncratic sulfonamide reactions, using several methodologies including ELISA for antidrug antibodies, immunoblotting for antibodies directed against liver proteins, flow cytometry for drug-dependent antiplatelet antibodies, and in vitro cytotoxicity assays.

PHARMACOGENETICS IN CLINICAL PRACTICE. Scientific interest in the field of human pharmacogenetics has increased each year in parallel with the knowledge of the human genome. However, interest in this field by physicians has lagged significantly behind, presumably because relatively few significant clinical consequences can be correlated to the vast number of pharmacogenetic mutations described in the literature. There are two main reasons for this discrepancy. Up to this point, polymorphisms described in human patients either have had low allelic frequencies or the clinical relevance of a particular polymorphism was not significant. For example, a highly clinically relevant polymorphism in the human TPMT gene has been described. TMPT metabolic activity in affected patients is essentially absent, so these patients experience severe neutropenia after a "normal" dose of azathioprine. Because this TPMP polymorphism affects approximately 0.3% of the Caucasian population, pharmacogenetic testing is not routinely performed in clinical practice.[42] Conversely, the allelic frequency of a genetic polymorphism of the human MDR1 gene has been shown to be associated with lower levels of P-gp expression in the duodenum and other tissues. While the allelic frequency of this particular MDR1 polymorphism is relatively high (>10%), it does not appear to have an important and predictable clinical impact on drug disposition. The vast majority of pharmacogenetic research in human medicine has not extended to clinical medical practice.

In veterinary medicine, however, a commercial veterinary pharmacogenetics laboratory (Veterinary Clinical Pharmacology Laboratory, Washington State University, Pullman, WA, 99164; www.vetmed.wsu.edu/vcpl) is performing canine MDR1 genotyping for veterinarians, dog breeders, and owners. One important reason that commercial pharmacogenetic testing is readily available for canine patients, and not for human patients, is because the MDR1 mutation in dogs has a very high allelic frequency (55% in Collies; 42% in Longhaired Whippets; and roughly 20% in Australian Shepherds), and because the polymorphism is highly predictive for serious adverse drug events, not just for one drug class but for several drug classes. See Table 50.1 for a partial list of drugs that are substrates for P-gp.

FUTURE DIRECTIONS. The field of pharmacogenetics, particularly in veterinary medicine, is still in its infancy. However, we have an ever-increasing arsenal of molecular tools that can be used to expand our knowledge of pharmacogenetics. Furthermore, with the recent completion of the canine genome project, and the ongoing elucidation of its data, we may soon know the sequences of virtually all genes encoding drug metabolizing enzymes, drug trans-

TABLE 50.1 Selected P-gp substrates[43–47].

Anticancer Agents
Doxorubicin
Docetaxel*
Vincristine*
Vinblastine*
Etoposide*
Mitoxantrone
Actinomycin D
Steroid Hormones
Aldosterone
Cortisol*
Dexamethasone*
Methylprednisolone
Antimicrobial Agents
Erythromycin*
Ketoconazole
Itraconazole*
Tetracycline
Doxycycline
Levofloxacin
Sparfloxacin
Opioids
Loperamide
Morphine
Cardiac Drugs
Digoxin
Diltiazem*
Verapamil*
Talinolol
Immunosuppressants
Cyclosporine*
Tacrolimus*
Miscellaneous
Ivermectin
Amitriptyline
Terfenadine*
Ondansetron
Domperidon
Phenothiazines
Vecuronium

*Substrate of CYP 3A.

porters, receptors, and other drug targets. With this information, the traditional clinical approach to variation in drug response (phenotype-to-genotype) will likely give way to a prospective approach (genotype-to-phenotype). That is, genetic variation identified in a specific gene will be investigated to determine whether it alters pharmacological response. While the ultimate goal of modern pharmacogenomics, individualization of drug therapy, may not be achieved for all drugs, it certainly has the potential to increase both safety and efficacy of many drugs.

REFERENCES

1. Hochstein P. Glucose-6-Phosphate Dehydrogenase Deficiency: Mechanisms of Drug-Induced Hemolysis. Exp Eye Res 1971;11(3):389–95.
2. Patel J and Mitra AK. Strategies to Overcome Simultaneous P-Glycoprotein Mediated Efflux and CYP3A4 Mediated Metabolism of Drugs. Pharmacogenomics 2001;2(4):401–15.
3. Scordo MG and Spina E. Cytochrome P450 Polymorphisms and Response to Antipsychotic Therapy. Pharmacogenomics 2002;3(2):201–18.
4. Roninson IB. The Role of the MDR1 (P-Glycoprotein) Gene in Multidrug Resistance in Vitro and in Vivo. Biochem Pharmacol 1992;43(1):95–102.
5. Thiebaut F, Tsuruo T, Hamada H, Gottesman MM, Pastan I, and Willingham MC. Cellular Localization of the Multidrug-Resistance Gene Product P-Glycoprotein in Normal Human Tissues. Proc Natl Acad Sci U.S.A. 1987;84(21):7735–8.
6. Schinkel AH, Wagenaar E, van Deemter L, Mol CA, and Borst P. Absence of the Mdr1a P-Glycoprotein in Mice Affects Tissue Distribution and Pharmacokinetics of Dexamethasone, Digoxin, and Cyclosporin A. J Clin Invest 1995;96(4):1698–705.
7. Sills GJ, Kwan P, Butler E, de Lange EC, van den Berg DJ, and Brodie MJ. P-Glycoprotein-Mediated Efflux of Antiepileptic Drugs: Preliminary Studies in mdr1a Knockout Mice. In Epilepsy and Behavior. Durham, NC: Academic Press, 2000.
8. Verstuyft C, Schwab M, Schaeffeler E, Kerb R, Brinkmann U, Jaillon P, Funck-Brentano C, and Becquemont L. Digoxin Pharmacokinetics and MDR1 Genetic Polymorphisms. Eur J Clin Pharmacol 2003;58(12):809–12.
9. Kerb R, Aynacioglu AS, Brockmoller J, Schlagenhaufer R, Bauer S, Szekeres T, Hamwi A, Fritzer-Szekeres M, Baumgartner C, Ongen HZ, Guzelbey P, Roots I, and Brinkmann U. The Predictive Value of MDR1, CYP2C9, and CYP2C19 Polymorphisms for Phenytoin Plasma Levels. Pharmacogenomics J 2001;1(3):204–10.
10. Ginn PE. Immunohistochemical Detection of P-Glycoprotein in Formalin-Fixed and Paraffin-Embedded Normal and Neoplastic Canine Tissues. Vet Pathol 1996;33(5):533–41.
11. Mealey KL, Barhoumi R, Rogers K, and Kochevar DT. Doxorubicin Induced Expression of P-Glycoprotein in a Canine Osteosarcoma Cell Line. Cancer Lett 1998;126(2):187–92.
12. Page RL, Hughes CS, Huyan S, Sagris J, and Trogdon M. Modulation of P-Glycoprotein-Mediated Doxorubicin Resistance in Canine Cell Lines. Anticancer Res 2000;20(5B):3533–8.
13. McEntee M, Silverman JA, Rassnick K, Zgola M, Chan AO, Tau PT, and Page R.L. Enhanced Bioavailability of Oral Docetaxel by Co-administration of Cyclosporin A in Dogs and Rats. Vet Comp Oncol 2003;2(1):105–12.
14. Mealey KL, Bentjen SA, Gay JM, and Cantor GH. Ivermectin Sensitivity in Collies Is Associated With a Deletion Mutation of the mdr1 Gene. Pharmacogenetics 2001;11(8):727–33.
15. Mealey KL, Bentjen SA, and Waiting DK. Frequency of the Mutant MDR1 Allele Associated With Ivermectin Sensitivity in a Sample Population of Collies From the Northwestern United States. Am J Vet Res 2002;63(4):479–81.

16. Neff MW, Robertson KR, Wong AK, Safra N, Broman KW, Slatkin M, Mealey KL, and Pedersen NC. Breed Distribution and History of Canine mdr1-1{Delta}, a Pharmacogenetic Mutation That Marks the Emergence of Breeds From the Collie Lineage. Proc Natl Acad Sci U.S.A. 2004;101(32):11725–30.
17. Tranquilli WJ, Paul AJ, and Todd KS. Assessment of Toxicosis Induced by High-Dose Administration of Milbemycin Oxime in Collies. Am J Vet Res 1991;52(7):1170–2.
18. Hugnet C, Cadore JL, Buronfosse F, Pineau X, Mathet T, and Berny PJ. Loperamide Poisoning in the Dog. Vet Hum Toxicol 1996;38(1):31–3.
19. Ericsson CD and Johnson PC. Safety and Efficacy of Loperamide. Am J Med 1990;88(6A):10S–14S.
20. Wandel C, Kim R, Wood M, and Wood A. Interaction of Morphine, Fentanyl, Sufentanil, Alfentanil, and Loperamide With the Efflux Drug Transporter P-Glycoprotein. Anesthesiology 2002;96(4):913–20.
21. Sartor LL, Bentjen SA, Trepanier L, and Mealey KL. Loperamide Toxicity in a Collie With the MDR1 Mutation Associated With Ivermectin Sensitivity. J Vet Intern Med 2004;18(1):117–8.
22. Choo EF, Leake B, Wandel C, Imamura H, Wood AJ, Wilkinson GR, and Kim RB. Pharmacological Inhibition of P-Glycoprotein Transport Enhances the Distribution of HIV-1 Protease Inhibitors into Brain and Testes. Drug Metab Dispos 2000;28(6):655–60.
23. Katagiri A, Tomita Y, Nishiyama T, Kimura M, and Sato S. Immunohistochemical Detection of P-Glycoprotein and GSTP1-1 in Testis Cancer. Br J Cancer 993;68(1):125–9.
24. Young AM, Allen CE, and Audus KL. Efflux Transporters of the Human Placenta. Adv Drug Deliv Rev 2003;55(1):125–32.
25. Wing JP. Blood Protein Polymorphisms in Jewish Populations. Hum Hered 1974;24(4):323–44.
26. Cascorbi I. Pharmacogenetics of Cytochrome P4502D6: Genetic Background and Clinical Implication. Eur J Clin Invest 2003;33 Suppl 2:17–22.
27. Hay Kraus BL, Greenblatt DJ, Venkatakrishnan K, and Court MH. Evidence for Propofol Hydroxylation by Cytochrome P4502B11 in Canine Liver Microsomes: Breed and Gender Differences. Xenobiotica 2000;30(6):575–88.
28. Court MH, Hay-Kraus BL, Hill DW, Kind AJ, and Greenblatt DJ. Propofol Hydroxylation by Dog Liver Microsomes: Assay Development and Dog Breed Differences. Drug Metab Dispos 1999;27(11):1293–9.
29. Paulson SK, Engel L, Reitz B, Bolten S, Burton EG, Maziasz TJ, Yan B, and Schoenhard GL. Evidence for Polymorphism in the Canine Metabolism of the Cyclooxygenase 2 Inhibitor, Celecoxib. Drug Metab Dispos 1999;27(10):1133–42.
30. Tenmizu D, Endo Y, Noguchi K, and Kamimura H. Identification of the Novel Canine CYP1A2 1117 C > T SNP Causing Protein Deletion. Xenobiotica 2004;34(9):835–46.
31. Tanaka N, Shinkyo R, Sakaki T, Kasamastu M, Imaoka S, Funae Y, and Yokota H. Cytochrome P450 2E Polymorphism in Feline Liver. Biochim Biophys Acta 2005;1726(2):194–205.
32. Theilmann JL, Skow LC, Baker JF, and Womack JE. Restriction Fragment Length Polymorphisms for Growth Hormone, Prolactin, Osteonectin, Alpha Crystallin, Gamma Crystallin, Fibronectin and 21-Steroid Hydroxylase in Cattle. Anim Genet 1989;20(3):257–66.
33. Collins JM. Inter-Species Differences in Drug Properties. Chem Biol Interact 2001;134(3):237–42.
34. Kidd LB, Salavaggione OE, Szumlanski CL, Miller JL, Weinshilboum RM, and Trepanier L. Thiopurine Methyltransferase Activity in Red Blood Cells of Dogs. J Vet Intern Med 2004;18(2):214–8.
35. Kiso S, Cai SH, Kitaichi K, Furui N, Takagi K, Takagi K, Nabeshima T, and Hasegawa T. Inhibitory Effect of Erythromycin on P-Glycoprotein-Mediated Biliary Excretion of Doxorubicin in Rats. Anticancer Res 2000;20(5A):2827–34.
36. Song S, Suzuki H, Kawai R, and Sugiyama Y. Effect of PSC 833, a P-Glycoprotein Modulator, on the Disposition of Vincristine and Digoxin in Rats. Drug Metab Dispos 1999;27(6):689–94.
37. Mealey KL, Northrup NC, and Bentjen SA. Increased Toxicity of P-Glycoprotein-Substrate Chemotherapeutic Agents in a Dog With the MDR1 Deletion Mutation Associated With Ivermectin Sensitivity. J Am Vet Med Assoc 2003;223(10):1453–5, 1434.
38. Tribut O, Lessard Y, Reymann JM, Allain H, and Bentue-Ferrer D. Pharmacogenomics. Med Sci Monit 2002;8(7):RA152–RA163.
39. Ito H, Nara H, Inoue-Murayama M, Shimada MK, Koshimura A, Ueda Y, Kitagawa H, Takeuchi Y, Mori Y, Murayama Y, Morita M, Iwasaki T, Ota K, Tanabe Y, and Ito S. Allele Frequency Distribution of the Canine Dopamine Receptor D4 Gene Exon III and I in 23 Breeds. J Vet Med Sci 2004;66(7):815–20.
40. Trepanier LA. Idiosyncratic Toxicity Associated With Potentiated Sulfonamides in the Dog. J Vet Pharmacol Ther 2004;27(3):129–38.
41. Spielberg SP. N-Acetyltransferases: Pharmacogenetics and Clinical Consequences of Polymorphic Drug Metabolism. J Pharmacokinet Biopharm 1996;24(5):509–19.
42. Becquemont L. Clinical Relevance of Pharmacogenetics. Drug Metab Rev 2003;35(4):277–85.
43. Schwab M, Eichelbaum M, and Fromm MF. Genetic Polymorphisms of the Human MDR1 Drug Transporter. Annu Rev Pharmacol Toxicol 2003;43:285–307.
44. Fromm MF. Genetically Determined Differences in P-Glycoprotein Function: Implications for Disease Risk. Toxicology 2002;181–182: 299–303.
45. Sakaeda T, Nakamura T, and Okumura K. MDR1 Genotype-Related Pharmacokinetics and Pharmacodynamics. Biol Pharm Bull 2002;25(11):1391–400.
46. Sakaeda T, Nakamura T, and Okumura K. Pharmacogenetics of MDR1 and Its Impact on the Pharmacokinetics and Pharmacodynamics of Drugs. Pharmacogenomics. 2003;4(4):397–410.
47. Marzolini C, Paus E, Buclin T, and Kim RB. Polymorphisms in Human MDR1 (P-Glycoprotein): Recent Advances and Clinical Relevance. Clin Pharmacol Ther 2004;75(1):13–33.

CHAPTER

51

THERAPEUTIC DRUG MONITORING

MARK G. PAPICH

Methods for therapeutic drug monitoring have been published in popular textbooks. Some of the guidelines are listed the tables of this chapter. Veterinarians can find local hospitals and diagnostic laboratories that have the capability of performing drug analysis. Because of large interindividual variations in pharmacokinetics for the drugs listed, monitoring is advised for the following conditions: 1) animal refractory to medication, despite an adequate dose; 2) animal showing toxicity, despite an adequate dose; 3) assessing owner compliance; 4) switching medications (e.g., from a brand name to a generic and need to establish a baseline; 5) drug interaction (for example, to see whether or not interactions are occurring with cyclosporine administration); and 6) pharmacokinetic differences in individual patients, such as altered absorption or elimination.

THERAPEUTIC DRUG MONITORING: CONSIDERATIONS

TIMING OF SAMPLE. For short half-life drugs, more than one sample (three is ideal) is the most useful for determining individual pharmacokinetic parameters. Alternatively, a peak (C_{MAX}) and a trough (C_{MIX}) can be collected to determine the bounds of high and low concentrations at steady-state. For long half-life drugs (digoxin, bromide, phenobarbital), a single sample during the dosing interval is sufficient. If one suspects altered clearance rates, however, more samples can be collected to assess half-life. For cyclosporine, a single trough sample has been used for many years, but now recommendations are changing to a single 2-hour sample (C_2).

ASSAY. The assay will vary according to the laboratories. Many automated chemistry machines used for biochemical analysis have drug detection kits that can be added to their menus. Some laboratories use RIA methods, others use other immunoassay methods (e.g., chemiluminescence). One of the popular bench-top assay machines is the fluorescence polarization immunoassay by Abbot, known commonly as the *TDx method*. Rarely is HPLC used because of the expense and slow turnaround time, but it is still considered the gold standard for specificity.

TYPE OF SAMPLE. The type of sample will vary according to the specific assay. Most assays allow serum, some require plasma, and for some assays either is acceptable. Samples should be collected and centrifuged as soon as possible. Avoid serum-separator tubes because these may lower drug concentrations by adsorbing drug into the matrix. Some assays are specific about storage of samples. Plastic cryo-vial type tubes are acceptable for most assays. For cyclosporine, the assay specifically calls for whole blood, not plasma, collected in an EDTA tube.

Examples of drugs that can be measured in most routine clinical or diagnostic laboratories are listed in Table 51.1.

TABLE 51.1 Examples of drugs that can be measured in most clinical or diagnostic laboratories

Test	Specimen	Timing of Sample	Tube	Storage	Effect of Interference	Reference Range
Amikacin	Serum or plasma 0.5 ml	1, 2, and 4 hours after dose, preferably. Other strategies for collecting two or three samples also have been used to assess clearance.	red-top or lavender-top	30 days @ −20°C	Hemolysis: no effect Icterus: no effect Lipemia: no effect Cross-reactivity: <1% interference with other drugs and antibiotics, except tobraymycin, with which there is high cross-reactivity. Limit of detection: 0.8 μg/ml	Peak: 40 μg/ml Trough: <0.8 μg/ml Other methods to assess clearance are possible if more than two samples are collected.
Bromide (potassium or sodium bromide)	Serum 0.5 ml	Anytime during dosing interval.	red-top	60 days @ −20°C	No interference with other drugs. Bromide and phenobarbital can be analyzed in same sample. Hemolysis: no effect Icterus: no effect Lipemia: no effect	100–200 mg/dl (with phenobarbital) 200–300 mg/dl (monotherapy)
Cyclosporine	Whole blood 1.0 ml	Trough (12 hours after last dose). Alternatively, peak concentrations at 2 hours have been used.	lavender-top	30 days @ −20°C	Because of metabolites, the assay overestimates true cyclosporine concentrations by 1.5–2×. For a true level, correct result by ×0.7 in dogs; and ×0.5 in cats.	300–600 ng/ml @ 12 hr (may vary with disease)
Digoxin	Serum 0.5 ml	Anytime during dosing interval. Generally 4–6 hours after dosing.	red-top	7 days @ 2–8°C 2 months @ −20°C	Hemolysis: no effect Bilirubin: No effect Lipemia: No effect Heparin tube: decrease by 5% EDTA tube: decrease by 7% Do not use serum-separator tubes.	0.8–2.5 ng/ml

TABLE 5.1 ***continued***

Test	Specimen	Timing of Sample	Tube	Storage	Effect of Interference	Reference Range
Gentamicin	Serum or plasma 0.5 ml	1, 2, and 4 hours after dose, preferably. Other strategies for collecting two or three samples also have been used to assess clearance.	red-top or lavender-top	30 days @ −20°C	Hemolysis, Icterus, Lipemia produce <5% error in the assay. Cross-reactivity: <1% interference with other drugs and antibiotics. Limit of detection: 0.27 μg/ml	Peak: 20 μg/ml Trough: <0.27 μg/ml Other methods to assess clearance are possible if more than two samples are collected.
Phenobarbital	Serum or plasma 0.5 ml	Anytime during dosing interval.	red-top or lavender-top	2 days @ 2–8°C 1 month @ −20°C	Bilirubin: no effect Hemolysis: no effect EDTA or heparin tube: no significant effect. Do not use serum-separator tubes.	15–40 μg/ml
Theophylline	Serum 0.5 ml	Ideally, a peak and trough should be collected. If that is not possible, collect a trough immediately before the next dose.	red-top	30 days @ −20°C	Hemolysis, Icterus, produce <5% error in the assay. Lipemia produces <10% error. Cross-reactivity: <1% interference with other drugs, and 1.5% cross-reactivity with theobromine. Limit of detection: 0.82 μg/ml	10–20 μg/ml. In some patients, trough concentrations of 5 μ/ml have been effective.
Vancomycin	Serum 0.5 ml		red-top	30 days @ −20°C	Hemolysis, Icterus, Lipemia produce <5% error in the assay. Cross-reactivity: <1% interference with other drugs, and 1.5% cross-reactivity with theobromine. Limit of detection: 2.0 μg/ml	Peak: 30–40 μg/ml Trough: 5–10 μg/ml

PHENOBARBITAL

As an example of clinical therapeutic drug monitoring, specific guidelines for phenobarbital are provided: To adjust dose, monitor compliance, and assess toxicity, it is the usual practice to regularly monitor plasma or serum phenobarbital concentrations during therapy. Assays are available at most diagnostic laboratories. This can be done initially after the first 2 weeks of starting treatment and then every 6–12 months, or as needed to assess treatment.

The recommended plasma/serum therapeutic concentration for dogs is 15–40 μg/ml (65–180 mmol/l). Some textbooks list this range as 20–45 μg/ml and 15–45 μg/ml. If dogs are also receiving bromide, phenobarbital concentrations in the range of 10–36 μg/ml have been reported as therapeutic (Trepanier et al. 1998). For cats, the optimum range has been cited as 23–30 μg/ml (Quesnel et al. 1997). In the cited study, cats were more unstable than dogs, possibly because of more serious CNS disease, and required more frequent monitoring.

TIMING OF SAMPLES. Because phenobarbital has such a long half-life, fluctuations between plasma peaks and troughs are minimized when it is administered on an every 12-hour schedule. Therefore, it makes no difference when a sample is collected during a 12-hour schedule for the assessment of plasma phenobarbital concentrations (Levitski and Trepanier 2000).

BROMIDE

Bromide is the oldest of the anticonvulsants; yet, it is chemically simple. It was used in people as early as the mid-1800s and its use was first described in dogs as early as 1907. Because it is toxic in people, it was replaced by other anticonvulsants after the introduction of phenobarbital in 1918. It is now used commonly in dogs, and sometimes in cats (Podell and Fenner 1993, 1994; Trepanier 1995).

Bromide has been used in combination with phenobarbital to treat refractory seizures, and also has been used as monotherapy (single drug). When bromide is administered as a single drug, the doses may need to be higher compared to administering bromide with phenobarbital. When bromide is administered with phenobarbital, phenobarbital doses can be decreased by as much as one-half. One study reported that, in 19% of dogs receiving phenobarbital and bromide, eventually the phenobarbital was discontinued while still maintaining seizure control (Trepanier et al. 1998).

When potassium bromide (KBr) has been used to treat canine epileptics that have not responded to phenobarbital alone, success rates have been 60%, and higher. One author reported as high as 72% improvement in seizure control (Trepanier et al. 1998).

PHARMACOKINETICS. The half-life of bromide in humans is 12 days. The half-life in dogs appears to be 25 days, but can be variable and as short as 15 days. Elimination rate can vary depending on the patient's diet. Because the half-life is long, chronic daily administration will be necessary for this drug to accumulate to steady-state plasma concentrations. However, during the accumulation phase (loading dose period) the half-life is shorter (16.5 days), which results in faster accumulation. The half-life in cats appears to be a bit less than in dogs; about 14 days, and perhaps as short as 10 days.

EFFECT OF DIET. Diets high in chloride will cause bromide to be excreted more rapidly (as much as 50% decrease in half-life with high-chloride diets); therefore, keep the diet constant throughout therapy, or monitor serum bromide concentrations each time the diet is changed. Some prescription diets have either high or restricted chloride content and patients receiving these diets may need dose adjustments.

CLINICAL USE. Usually the potassium salt of bromide is used, but sodium bromide also can be substituted. Most veterinary compounding pharmacies have recipes for making up an oral solution and it is reasonably inexpensive. The typical dosage for dogs is 20 to 40 mg/kg, orally, once per day. The lower doses are more common when used with phenobarbital, while the higher doses are given when monotherapy is used.

There is high variability among animals with respect to absorption and excretion. Therefore, it is suggested that each patient be monitored for signs of toxicity (ataxia, CNS depression), as well as plasma concentration monitoring, and the dose adjusted if necessary.

LOADING DOSES. Loading doses of 600 mg/kg orally, divided over 3–4 days, have been administered in patients that need therapeutic concentrations quickly in the range of 1.0 to 1.5 mg/ml. In some cases it has been necessary to administer sodium bromide IV as a loading dose. This has been accomplished by mixing sodium bromide (potassium bromide may be too toxic if given IV), in a solution to deliver an initial dose of 600–1,200 mg/kg over approximately 8 hours. If the plasma concentration is still in the low range, an additional IV loading dose can be administered.

CLINICAL USE IN CATS. The most common dose for cats is 30 mg/kg per day. A report and accompanying review evaluated use of bromide in cats (Boothe et al. 2002). In that report, the authors identified a half-life in cats of only 11.2 days. An evaluation of the clinical use showed that there was inadequate seizure control in approximately half of the cats, despite serum concentrations that are considered effective in dogs. More importantly, there were adverse effects in approximately half of the cats. The most common adverse effect was coughing.

THERAPEUTIC MONITORING OF BROMIDE. Plasma concentrations can be measured at most veterinary diagnostic laboratories. Samples are easy to assay using a simple gold-chloride color-based (spectrophotometric) assay. Assays can be completed in less than 30 minutes. Ordinarily, effective concentrations are reported as between 1 and 2 mg/ml (100–200 mg/dl). If concentrations are less than 1.0 mg/ml, one should increase the dose. If bromide is used as the sole anticonvulsant (without phenobarbital) concentrations as high as 2–3 mg/ml (200–300 mg/dl) may be necessary.

CYCLOSPORINE

A common oral dose in people is 5–10 mg/kg/day to achieve targeted whole blood concentrations of 150–400 ng/ml. In people, dosages are adjusted to meet the needs of the individual patient on the basis of clinical response and monitoring trough plasma concentrations. For animals, doses of 10–20 mg/kg/day were frequently cited in older publications, but more recent recommendations, in which newer formulations have been used, cite lower doses. For organ transplantation in cats (Mathews and Gregory 1997) a dose of 3 mg/kg q12h of the Neoral formulation (dose was doubled for Sandimmune formulation) was used to achieve trough blood concentrations of 300–500 ng/ml. At NCSU we routinely administer 25 mg/cat for suppression of immunity for transplantation, and modify as needed with monitoring. For organ transplant in dogs, 10 mg/kg q12h to achieve concentrations of 500–600 ng/ml has been used (Mathews et al. 2000). A report on treating perianal fistulas in dogs (Mathews and Sukhiani 1997) found that an average dose of 6 mg/kg q12h was needed to achieve a targeted blood concentration of 400–600 ng/ml. However, this recommendation was later modified to 2.5 to 6 mg/kg/day (3 mg/kg q12h) to achieve an effective blood concentration of 100–300 ng/ml. When treating perianal fistulas in dogs we have achieved adequate blood concentrations, without producing toxicity, at a dose of 3 mg/kg q12h.

For treating dermatitis in dogs, the effective dose has been 5 mg/kg/day. Some clinicians have been able to lower the dose, or administer the dose every other day, and still maintain clinical remission. The pharmacokinetics of cyclosporine in treated animals has been examined by Steffan and colleagues (2004). They found that routine monitoring of cyclosporine in dogs with atopic dermatitis was not necessary. When animals were administered a dose of 5 mg/kg/day, there did not appear to be a strong correlation between blood concentration achieved and clinical response. Nevertheless, because of wide individual variation in cyclosporine pharmacokinetics, monitoring has been used to determine the optimum dose for each patient. According to one paper, clinical benefits have not been observed when trough concentrations have fallen below 50 ng/ml; therefore, blood testing of patients failing therapy was suggested to reveal inadequate dosing (Robson and Burton 2003).

Cyclosporine is available in human formulation capsules of 25 and 100 mg, 20 mg/ml oral solution, and 50 mg/ml injection. The veterinary brand (Atopica) is available as 10, 25, 50, and 100 mg. There are also generic preparations available, but their absorption and pharmacokinetics have not been reported for animals. Some comparisons have not demonstrated that the generic formulations are significantly less expensive than brand name products.

ASSAY SPECIFICITY. One must be cognizant of the assay used when monitoring cyclosporine. Plasma values will be lower than whole-blood assays because as much as 50–60%, and 10–20% of the dose is concentrated in erythrocytes and leukocytes, respectively. Nonspecific assays will report higher values than a more specific (monoclonal or HPLC) assay. Despite the hypothesized higher specificity when using the monoclonal assay, important discrepancies between these assays and the more specific HPLC assay have been reported (Steimer 1999). For example, in people the difference between HPLC and the commonly used TDx monoclonal immunoassay was 57%. In cats, we found that the TDx assay overestimated the true cyclosporine concentration by approximately twofold. (That is, TDx assay reporting 500 ng/ml corresponded to an actual value of 250 ng/ml.) In dogs, the TDx assay overestimates the true cyclosporine concentrations by a factor of 1.5 to 1.7 (Steffan et al. 2004). When using a specific radioimmunoassay or HPLC, true concentrations are measured. But, when using a TDx fluoroescence polarization assay (monoclonal whole blood) multiply the feline concentrations by 0.5 to get the true concentration, and multiply the canine concentration by 0.6 to get the true concentration.

TIMING OF SAMPLE. Most recommendations have been based on trough blood sample monitoring. Trough samples are collected immediately before the next scheduled dose; therefore, the sample is either 12 or 24 hours after the last dose. These recommendations are being modified in human medicine to a recommendation of a 2-hour sample (C_2). Apparently there is evidence that a C_2 blood sample value correlates better with clinical results than trough samples (Levy et al. 2002; Nashan et al. 2002). In cats, levels are approximately twice as high at 2 hours compared to the levels at 12 hours (Mehl et al. 2003).

AMINOGLYCOSIDES

Rational aminoglycoside dosing regimens should be based on pharmacokinetic and pharmacodynamic information derived from populations of diseased animals, and the relationship of these data to clinical outcome. Once-daily dosing regimens are the standard approach for both small animals and equine patients. In human patients, it has been shown that doses of aminoglycosides that result in peak plasma concentrations (C_{MAX}) approximately 8–10 times MIC confer optimal bactericidal effect. Aminoglycoside dosing regimens for animals also target a C_{MAX}/MIC ratio of 8 to 10. To achieve these ratios in horses, a gentamicin dose of 6.8 mg/kg and an amikacin dose of 10 mg/kg were adequate to achieve the target C_{MAX}/MIC in adult horses. For dogs and cats, the doses for gentamicin are 9–14 mg/kg and 5–8 mg/kg, respectively. For administration of amikacin in dogs and cats, the doses are 15–30 mg/kg and 10–14 mg/kg, respectively.

The aminoglycosides are distributed in the extracellular fluid (ECF) space, and neonatal foals (<4 weeks of age) have larger total body water and ECF volume compared with adult horses (see Table 51.2). Accordingly, to avoid therapeutic failure associated with inadequate peak drug concentrations, larger aminoglycoside doses are recommended for young foals. As the foals mature, the transition to adult pharmacokinetic values occurs rapidly after 6 weeks of age. The table shows recommended once-daily dosing regimens for gentamicin and amikacin in neonatal foals compared to adult horses, together with suggested target peak and trough plasma drug concentrations.

Therapeutic drug monitoring (TDM) in animals receiving aminoglycoside treatment has been used to optimize therapy. If TDM can identify situations in which the dose can be lowered, there are also cost benefits. TDM can be useful because there may be a wide variation in drug disposition among sick patients, especially in critically ill neonates. Therefore, TDM can identify those patients with parameters that do not represent the average. For example, the effective volume of distribution for the aminoglycosides is often higher in septic patients or those with a "third-space" problem (uroperitoneum, pleural effusion), necessitating a higher dose to produce the target peak plasma concentrations. Furthermore, longer clearance times for gentamicin and amikacin have been observed in premature and full-term foals with hypoxia, azotemia, and septicemia, likely the result of renal hypoperfusion and decreased glomerular filtration rate. In these cases, a longer interdose interval may be needed to reduce the risk for nephrotoxicity. Disadvantages of TDM in veterinary patients include the added expense and, particularly in field situations, the lack of access to a laboratory capable of performing the drug assays. Collecting serial blood samples after dosing in a field situation also is not often practical.

When TDM is employed, it is helpful to determine: 1) whether the target C_{MAX} is achieved, and 2) whether there is adequate clearance of the drug. (For aminoglycosides,

TABLE 51.2 Pharmacokinetic information and dosing regimens for gentamicin and amikacin in horses

	T1/2 (hr)	CL (ml/min/kg)	VD (L/kg)	C_{MAX} (μg/ml)	Dose
AMIKACIN					
Foal (<30 days old)	3.9	1.84	0.52	40	20–25 mg/kg, q24h
Adult	1.9	1.3	0.22	40	10 mg/kg, q24h
GENTAMICIN					
Foal (<30 days old)	1.6	2.7	0.356	20	10–14 mg/kg, q24h
Adult	1.70	1.5	0.18	20	4–6.8 mg/kg, q24h

T1/2: elimination half-life; CL: systemic clearance; VD: apparent volume of distribution (area method); C_{MAX}: Desired peak plasma concentration; Dose listed can be administered either IV or IM (IM absorption is nearly complete).

Pharmacokinetic values presented here are an approximation derived from several sources listed in the reference section. Values listed represent averages from more than one study.

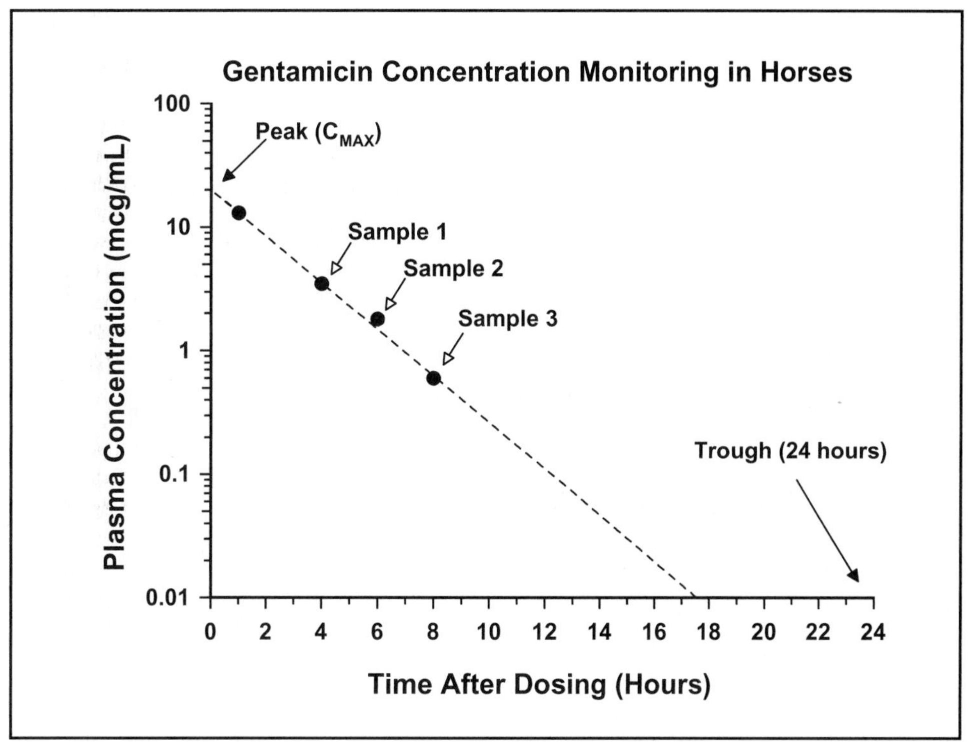

FIG. 51.1 Example of gentamicin plasma concentration monitoring. In this figure is an example in which plasma samples were collected from an adult horse given 4 mg/kg, IV, to determine gentamicin concentrations. Three strategies for plasma concentration monitoring are illustrated: (1) A single concentration, collected 1 hour after drug administration represents an approximate peak (C_{MAX}). The C_{MAX} in this case at 1 hour was 13 µg/ml, which would be adequate (i.e., 8–10 × the MIC) for organisms with an MIC of approximately 1.3 µg/ml, or less. (2) A sample collected immediately prior to the next dose (24 hours) represents the trough. The trough in this example is below the limit of detection, indicating that the risk of renal toxicity is low. If elevated trough concentrations were identified, it would increase the risk of nephrotoxicosis. (3) To estimate the half-life (T1/2) and clearance, a series of three samples can be collected approximately 1–2 hours apart, represented here by Sample 1, 2, and 3, at 4, 6, and 8 hours, respectively. In this example, the three samples were used to estimate the half-life, which was 1.6 hours—normal for an adult horse. It also can be seen that the advantage of collecting a series of three samples is that peak and trough concentrations can be extrapolated by extending the straight line to the intercepts (dashed line) to determine the true peak and trough concentrations. The true C_{MAX} in this example (y-axis intercept) was approximately 20 µg/ml. The apparent volume of distribution, calculated from VD = Dose/C_{MAX}, was approximately 0.2 l/kg—normal for an adult horse. The systemic clearance (CL) in this case, calculated from the formula: CL = (0.693 × VD)/T1/2, was 1.44 ml/kg/min—normal for an adult horse.

the systemic clearance value is a close approximation of the glomerular filtration rate (GFR) measured by creatinine clearance methods.)

To perform TDM, either a single sample can be collected 30 min to 1 hour postdosing for an estimate of the peak drug concentrations (C_{MAX}), or two or three samples can be collected at 1- or 2-hour intervals to identify the slope of the elimination curve. Analysis of a series of points requires the use of linear regression and calculation of the slope of the curve plotted on a logarithmic axis (see Fig. 51.1). From the elimination curve, an estimate of clearance, volume of distribution, and half-life (T1/2) is possible. These approaches are illustrated in Figure 51.1. Alternatively, a single trough sample can be collected immediately prior to the next scheduled dose. But as illustrated in the figure, this sample is frequently below the limit of detection of the assay, unless there is impaired clearance and drug accumulation. In situations in which TDM is not available, repeated evaluation of renal function is recommended during aminoglycoside therapy.

DIGOXIN

Digoxin is available in injectable forms (0.1 and 0.25 mg/ml Lanoxin®) and can be given IV. It is also available in

TABLE 51.3 Digoxin pharmacokinetic information

Species	Half-Life (hr)	Volume of Distribution	Recommended Dose (mg/kg)
dog	15–32	9.5–15.6 l/kg	0.01, q12h or 0.22 mg/m^2 q12h
cat	33–58	15–26 l/kg	0.01, q48h
horse	13–30	4.7–7 l/kg	0.002 IV, q12h or 0.015 oral, q12h 0.009 IV
cattle	7.8–15.2	6.4 l/kg	
man	39	3.12 l/kg	

tablet (Lanoxin®) at 0.125, 0.25, 0.5 mg, and elixir form (Cardoxin® 50 or 150 µg/ml) for oral administration.

Digoxin is eliminated approximately 15% by hepatic, and 85% by renal mechanisms. Animals with renal disease may have trouble excreting digoxin. Although digoxin has a high apparent volume of distribution, it does not distribute to fat. Therefore, when calculating doses, it often is done according to lean body weight (Table 51.3). Oral absorption is 60% and 85% for digoxin tablets and elixir, respectively (adjustments for oral absorption should be made when switching from one dosage form to another).

THERAPEUTIC MONITORING. The therapeutic serum level for most animals is believed to be 0.9 to 2.5 ng/ml (1.12–3.5 nmol/l). However, it is observed that some animals benefit from lower concentrations. In humans, it has been shown that the neurohumoral effects occur at plasma concentrations of 0.5 to 1.0 ng/ml and some of the dosing protocols are being revised to reflect this change. In veterinary medicine, there is not yet evidence relating the neuroendocrine effects with blood concentrations. Concentrations above 3.0 to 3.5 ng/ml usually will produce toxic effects.

REFERENCES AND ADDITIONAL READING

Boothe DM, George KL, Couch P. Disposition and clinical use of bromide in cats. J Am Vet Med Assoc 221:1131–1135, 2002.

Finco DR, Brown SA, Vaden SL, and Ferguson DC. Relationship between plasma creatinine concentration and glomerular filtration rate in dogs. J Vet Pharmacol Therap 18:418–421, 1995.

Levitski RE, Trepanier LA. Effect of timing of blood collection on serum phenobarbital concentrations in dogs with epilepsy. J Am Vet Med Assoc Jul15;217(2):200–4, 2000. Erratum in: J Am Vet Med Assoc Aug15;217(4):468, 2000.

Levy G, Thervet E, Lake J, Uchida K. Patient management by Neoral C2 monitoring: An international consensus statement. Transplantation. May 15; 73(9) Supplement:S12–S18, 2002.

Mathews KA, Sukhiani HR. Randomized controlled trial of cyclosporine for treatment of perianal fistulas in dogs. J Am Vet Med Assoc 211:1249–1253, 1997.

Mathews KA, Holmberg DL, Miller CW. Kidney transplantation in dogs with naturally occurring end-stage renal disease. J Am Anim Hosp Assoc 36:294–301, 2000.

Mathews KG, Gregory CR. Renal transplants in cats: 66 cases (1987–1996). J Am Vet Med Assoc 211:1432–1436, 1997.

Mehl ML, Kyles AE, Craigmill AL, et al. Disposition of cyclosporine after intravenous and multi-dose oral administration in cats. J Vet Pharmacol Therap 26:349–354, 2003.

Mouatt J. Cyclosporine and ketoconazole interaction for treatment of perianal fistulas in the dog. Austral Vet J 80:207–211, 2002.

Myre SA, Schoeder TJ, Grund VR, et al. Critical ketoconazole dosage range for cyclosporin clearance inhibition in the dog. Pharmacology 43:233–241, 1991.

Nashan B, Cole E, Levy G, Thervet E. Clinical validation studies of Neoral C2 monitoring: a review. Transplantation 73(supplement): S3–S11, 2002.

Podell M, Fenner WR. Bromide therapy in refractory canine idiopathic epilepsy. J Vet Intern Med 7:318–327, 1993.

Podell M, Fenner WR. Use of bromide as an antiepileptic drug in dogs. Compend Contin Ed Pract Vet June; 6:767–774, 1994.

Quesnel AD, Parent JM, McDonell W. Clinical management and outcome of cats with seizure disorders: 30 cases (1991–1993). J Am Vet Med Assoc 210:72–77, 1997.

Robson DC, Burton GG. Cyclosporine: applications in small animal dermatology. Vet Dermatol 14:1–9, 2003.

Schneider G, Coassolo P, Lave T. Combining in vitro and in vivo pharmacokinetic data for prediction of hepatic drug clearance in humans by artificial neural networks and multivariate statistical techniques. J Med Chem 42:5072–5076, 1999.

Steffan J, Alexander D, Brovedani F, Fisch RD. Comparison of cyclosporine A with methylprednisolone for treatment of canine atopic dermatitis: a parallel, blinded, randomized controlled trial. Vet Dermatol 14:11–22, 2003.

Steffan J, Strehlau G, Maurer M, Rohlfs A. Cyclosporin A pharmacokinetics and efficacy in the treatment of atopic dermatitis in dogs. J Vet Pharmacol Ther 27:231–238, 2004.

Steimer W. Performance and specificity of monoclonal immunoassays for cyclosporine monitoring: How specific is specific? Clin Chem 45:371–381, 1999.

Trepanier L. Optimal bromide therapy and monitoring. ACVIM Proceedings. 15th ACVIM Forum, pages 100–101, 1997.

Trepanier LA. Use of bromide as an anticonvulsant for dogs with epilepsy. J Am Vet Med Assoc Jul15;207(2):163–6, 1994.

Trepanier LA, Van Schoick A, Schwark WS, and Carrillo J. Therapeutic serum drug concentrations in epileptic dogs treated with potassium bromide alone or in combination with other anticonvulsants: 122 cases (1992–1996). J Am Vet Med Assoc 213:1449–1453, 1998.

CHAPTER

52

CONSIDERATIONS FOR TREATING MINOR FOOD-PRODUCING ANIMALS WITH VETERINARY PHARMACEUTICALS

LISA A. TELL, MARGARET OELLER, AND ARTHUR L. CRAIGMILL

THE USE OF VETERINARY PHARMACEUTICALS IN MINOR FOOD-PRODUCING ANIMALS: SPECIAL CONSIDERATIONS AND CHALLENGES

Antibiotics, antiparasitics, nonsteroidal antiinflammatory drugs, and exogenous hormones are among the essential components in the armamentarium of a food animal veterinarian to combat disease, alleviate animal pain, and minimize economic losses. In the United States, many of these veterinary products are labeled for use in a large number of major food-producing animals but not for the minor food-producing animals. According to the United States of America (USA) Food and Drug Administration (FDA), the major food-producing animals are cattle (meat and milk), swine, chickens (meat and eggs), and turkeys. The minor food-producing animals are those that do not fall into the major food-producing animal category with the most popular being goats, sheep, ranched cervids, commercially raised game birds, and nonornamental fish and shellfish. This category also includes less obvious food-producing species such as rabbits, ratites, and honey-producing bees. In the U.S., horses are a major animal species; however, they are considered companion animals and are not customarily used for human food as in some other countries. In Europe, the European Agency for the Evaluation of Medicinal Products has defined the major food-producing animals to be cattle (meat and milk), sheep (meat); pigs; chickens (meat and eggs), and salmonidae. Minor food-producing animals include minor ruminants (meat and milk), deer (including reindeer), other avian species (meat and eggs), other fish species, and other mammalian species (horse and rabbit). In other countries, the minor food-producing animals category has the potential to be considerably larger because a greater variety of species are consumed such as small rodents, canids, invertebrates, and various avian species.

In recent years there has been an increased interest in eating more meat and other products from minor food-producing animals, especially aquaculture species. As this interest grows, so will the expectations to provide safe food items for human consumption. Maintaining the overall health of minor food-producing animals is similar to managing the health of major food-producing animals, and typically requires some use of veterinary pharmaceuticals. In contrast to the major food-producing animals, few drugs have been approved for use in the minor food-producing animals.

One of the major challenges for getting veterinary products approved for use in minor food-producing animals is the minimal economic return due to small market size. Additionally, some of the minor food-producing animals are less tractable (e.g., cervids and buffalo), and there is wide variation in breeds/species with respect to size and pharmacokinetics. For aquatic species, such as finfish, mollusks, and crustaceans, there is a large number of species and incredible diversity within this category. Not only are there species differences, but environmental considerations (salinity, pH, temperature), physiologic differences (heterothermy), and management practices also impact metabolism and excretion of drugs.

This chapter addresses the availability of veterinary pharmaceuticals for use in minor food-producing animals, outlines the unique issues when considering regulatory requirements for getting a drug approved for use in a minor food-producing animal, and highlights legislation that has helped address the veterinarians' need for medications to treat these animals. In addition, government programs and scientific approaches used to meet the therapeutic needs for treating minor food-producing animals are discussed.

THE APPROVAL PROCESS FOR VETERINARY PHARMACEUTICALS FOR USE IN MINOR FOOD-PRODUCING ANIMALS

There are many veterinary pharmaceuticals marketed today that may be administered to minor food-producing animals. The ideal scenario for a veterinarian wanting to treat a minor food-producing animal is having an FDA-approved drug labeled for the intended use in question. For example, an anthelmintic approved for treating specific gastrointestinal parasites in sheep. This product will have been demonstrated to FDA's satisfaction to be safe for sheep, safe for the person administering the drug to the sheep, safe for anyone who later consumes meat from the treated sheep, and safe for the environment, both during the drug's use and its disposal. It will also have been shown to be effective for the labeled use and that it is consistently manufactured to standards of strength and purity. Such a product is labeled with intended uses, doses, and withdrawal times that are appropriate to use in sheep.

In contrast to the major food-producing animals, there are not many FDA-approved drugs labeled for use in minor food-producing animals. This is mainly because the development of new drugs for use in animals is a very expensive and time-consuming process, especially for drugs to be used in animals intended for human consumption, and the minor food-producing animal markets are too small to readily recover the pharmaceutical sponsor's investment. FDA-approved drugs for minor food-producing animals (as of September 2006) are summarized in Tables 52.1–52.5.

For a drug to be approved for use in a minor food-producing animal, the sponsor must demonstrate to the satisfaction of the scientific reviewers at FDA's Center for Veterinary Medicine (CVM) that it is safe and effective for its intended use. CVM is the part of FDA responsible for the regulation of veterinary drugs including the evaluation of such drugs prior to approval.

The information that a sponsor needs to present to support a New Animal Drug Application (NADA) includes the following as outlined in regulations published in the Code of Federal Regulations (21 CFR 514): 1) Effectiveness for the proposed use, 2) Safety to the target animal species (the animal species for which the drug is to be used) 3) Human food safety (safety to consumers of meat, milk, or eggs derived from treated animals), 4) Environmental safety, 5) Manufacturing Methods and Controls, 6) All Other Information, 7) Freedom of Information (FOI) Summary, and 8) Product labeling. These components are discussed in detail in Chapter 55 of this book. The FDA also provides a variety of guidance documents to assist sponsors in understanding the various requirements. Of particular note for sponsors seeking drug approval for a minor species use is Guidance #61 "FDA Approval of New Animal Drugs for Minor Uses and for Minor Species." These are all available on the CVM website.

Compared to the drug approval process for major food-producing animals, the drug approval process is

TABLE 52.1 Veterinary pharmaceuticals approved by the Federal Drug Administration for use in small ruminants that are considered minor food-producing animals in the United States of America as of December, 2008

Drug	Formulation	Species	Indication*
Albendazole	Liquid suspension	Sheep Goats	Internal parasites Liver Flukes
Ceftiofur sodium	Injection	Goats Sheep	Respiratory infection
Chlortetracycline	Premix (for feed)	Sheep	Vibrionic abortion Weight gain/feed efficiency
Decoquinate	Premix (for feed)	Goats Sheep	Coccidiosis
Fenbendazole	Liquid suspension	Goats	Internal parasites
Fenbendazole	Premix (for feed)	Zoo/wild Goats Bighorn Sheep	Internal parasites
Flurogestone acetate	Vaginal sponge	Sheep	Estrus synchronization
Follicle stimulating hormone	Injectable—IV, IM, SQ	Sheep	FSH deficiency
Ivermectin	Drench	Sheep	Internal parasites
Lasalocid	Premix (for feed)	Sheep	Coccidiosis
Levamisole hydrochloride	Drench Bolus Powder	Sheep	Internal parasites
Monensin sodium	Premix (for feed)	Goats	Coccidiosis
Morantel tartrate	Premix (for feed)	Goats	Internal parasites
Methoxyflurane	Inhalation	Sheep	Anesthetic
Moxidectin	Drench	Sheep	Internal parasites
Neomycin sulfate	Powder Liquid	Goats Sheep	Colibacillosis
Neomycin sulfate	Premix (for feed)	Sheep	Colibacillosis
Neostigmine methylsulfate	Injectable—SQ	Sheep	Rumen atony Curare antagonist
Oxytetracycline	Premix (for feed) Powder	Sheep	Respiratory infection Colibacillosis Weight gain/feed efficiency
Oxytetracycline hydrochloride—Polymyxin B Sulfate	Ointment	Sheep	Superficial ocular infections
Oxytocin	Injection—IM, IV, SQ	Sheep	Uterine contractions Milk letdown
Penicillin G procaine	Injectable—IM	Sheep	Respiratory infection
Pituitary luteinizing hormone	Injectable—IV, SQ	Sheep	Pituitary hypofunction
Proparacaine hydrochloride	Liquid	Sheep	Ophthalmic anesthetic
Sodium chloride gelatin	Oral liquid	Sheep	Shock/hypovolemia
Sodium selenite/ Vitamin E	Injectable—IM, SQ	Sheep	Selenium deficiency
Tetracycline	Injectable—IM	Sheep	Bacterial infection
Thiabendazole	Drench Premix (for feed) Pellet Liquid	Goats Sheep	Internal parasites
Thialbarbitone sodium	Powder—Injectable IV	Sheep	General anesthetic
Tilmicosin phosphate	Injection	Sheep	Respiratory infection
Zeranol	Implant—SQ	Sheep	Weight gain/feed efficiency

*Listed indications are broad. For specific indications, the drug label or Code of Federal Regulations should be consulted.

TABLE 52.2 Veterinary pharmaceuticals approved by the Federal Drug Administration for use in cervids/other ruminants that are considered minor food-producing animals in the United States of America as of December, 2008

Drug	Formulation	Species	Indication*
Carfentanil citrate	Injectable—IM	Deer Elk Moose	Immobilization
Ivermectin	Injection	Bison (American) Reindeer	Hypodermosis Warbles
Ivermectin	Liquid	Sheep	Internal parasites
Naltrexone hydrochloride	Injectable—IV, SQ	Elk Moose	Carfentanil antagonist
Xylazine hydrochloride	Injectable—IM, IV	Deer Elk	Sedation
Yohimbine hydrochloride	Injectable—IV	Deer Elk	Xylazine antagonist

*Listed indications are broad. For specific indications, the drug label or Code of Federal Regulations should be consulted.

TABLE 52.3 Veterinary pharmaceuticals approved by the Federal Drug Administration for use in avian species that are considered minor food-producing animals in the United States of America as of December, 2008

Drug	Formulation	Species	Indication*
Amprolium	Premix (for feed)	Pheasants	Coccidiosis
Bacitracin methylene disalicylate	Premix (for feed)	Pheasants Quail	Weight gain/feed efficiency
Bacitracin methylene disalicylate	Water-soluble powder	Quail	Ulcerative enteritis
Bacitracin zinc	Premix (for feed)	Pheasants Quail	Weight gain/feed efficiency
Bacitracin zinc	Water-soluble powder	Quail	Ulcerative enteritis
Carnidazole	Tablets	Pigeons	Trichomoniasis
Iodinated casein	Premix (for feed)	Ducks	Weight gain/feathering
Lasalocid	Premix (for feed)	Partridge (Chukar)	Coccidiosis
Monensin sodium	Premix (for feed)	Quail (Bobwhite)	Coccidiosis
Novobiocin	Premix (for feed)	Ducks	Bacterial infection
Penicillin G procaine	Premix (for feed)	Pheasants Quail	Weight gain/feed efficiency
Salinomycin sodium	Premix (for feed) Powder	Quail	Coccidiosis
Sulfadimethoxine ormetoprim	Premix (for feed)	Ducks Partridge (Chukar)	Bacterial infection Coccidiosis
Thiabendazole	Premix (for feed)	Pheasants	Gapeworm

*Listed indications are broad. For specific indications, the drug label or Code of Federal Regulations should be consulted.

not significantly easier for products intended for use in a minor food-producing species. However, there are a few advantages afforded to products intended for use in a minor food-producing animal. These include the possibility of a waiver from user fees, the ability to apply conclusions reached from the radiolabeled residue study in the major food-producing animal to the human food safety evaluation for the minor food-producing animal, the possibility of a categorical exclusion from the need to provide an environmental assessment, and the possibility that fewer sites will be needed for effectiveness clinical trials.

TABLE 52.4 Veterinary pharmaceuticals approved by the Federal Drug Administration for use in aquaculture species in the United States of America as of December, 2008

Drug	Formulation	Species	Indication*
Florfenicol	Premix (for feed)	Catfish	Enteric septicemia of catfish
Florfenicol	Premix (for feed)	Freshwater-reared Salmonids	Coldwater disease Furunculosis
Florfenicol (conditional Approval)	Premix (for feed)	Catfish	Columnaris disease
Formalin	Water treatment	Finfish eggs Shrimp (Penaeid)	Antiprotozoal Antifungal
Human chorionic gonadotropin	Injection	Finfish (male & female broodstock)	Spawning aid
35% Hydrogen peroxide	Water treatment	Freshwater-reared Salmonids	Bacterial gill disease
35% Hydrogen peroxide	Water treatment	Freshwater-reared finfish eggs	Saprolegniasis
35% Hydrogen peroxide	Water treatment	Freshwater-reared cool water finfish and channel catfish	External columnaris disease
Oxytetracycline dihydrate	Premix (for feed)	Lobsters	Gaffkemia
Oxytetracycline dihydrate	Premix (for feed)	Salmonids	Ulcer diseases
Oxytetracycline dihydrate	Premix (for feed)	Salmonids and catfish	Bacterial hemorrhagic septicemia and Pseudomonas disease
Oxytetracycline hydrochloride	Water treatment	Finfish	Skeletal marking
Sulfadimethoxine ormetoprim	Premix (for feed)	Catfish Salmonids	Enteric septicemia of catfish Furuncluosis
Sulfamerazine	Premix (for feed)	Trout	Furunculosis
Tricaine methanesulfonate	Water treatment	Fish	Temporary immobilization

*Listed indications are broad. For specific indications, the drug label or Code of Federal Regulations should be consulted.

TABLE 52.5 Veterinary pharmaceuticals approved by the Federal Drug Administration for use in miscellaneous minor food-producing animals as of December, 2008

Drug	Formulation	Species	Indication*
Bicyclohexyl ammonium (Fumagillin)	Powder	Bees	Nosema
Lasalocid	Premix (for feed)	Rabbits	Coccidiosis
Oxytetracycline	Premix (for feed) Water soluble powder	Bees	American foulbrood
Sulfaquinoxaline	Premix (for feed)	Rabbits	Coccidiosis
Tricaine methanesulfonate	Water Tx	Amphibians	Temporary immobilization
Tylosin tartrate	Water soluble powder	Bees	American foulbrood

*Listed indications are broad. For specific indications, the drug label or Code of Federal Regulations should be consulted.

LEGISLATION AND POLICIES SUPPORTING THE USE OF VETERINARY PHARMACEUTICALS IN MINOR FOOD-PRODUCING ANIMALS

ANIMAL MEDICINAL DRUG USE CLARIFICATION ACT (AMDUCA). The U.S. Congress recognized the drug availability problem for both major and minor animal species when it passed the Animal Medicinal Drug Use Clarification Act (AMDUCA) in 1994 (Public Law No. 103–396; Monti 2000). This law addressed the fact that FDA generally approves veterinary drugs for narrow intended uses. For example, a broad-spectrum antibiotic that would be safe and effective for the treatment of a wide variety of bacterial infections may only be *approved* for use in cattle for the treatment of respiratory disease caused by specific bacteria. From a practical standpoint, the pharmaceutical sponsor cannot demonstrate safety and effectiveness for every possible intended use of the product. This means that veterinarians frequently administer the drug for indications that are not on the label. In other words, they use the drug for different diseases, at different doses, by different routes of administration, and in different animal species than what is indicated on the label. AMDUCA legalized this practice for veterinarians within a set of limitations described in the Code of Federal Regulations (21 CFR 530). In general, veterinarians, within the context of a valid veterinarian-client-patient relationship, may use approved dosage form products (but not medicated feeds) outside their labeling. This is allowed only when there is no approved drug for the intended use; other approved drugs are not effective for such use, when the dose is not effective for that use, or in cases where an approved formulation is not appropriate. When using a drug outside of its labeling for a food-producing animal, the veterinarian is responsible for using the drug in a manner that will not result in a violative residue in any food product derived from that animal. The veterinarian must establish a withdrawal period based on some scientific information although resources for establishing such times are few. The withdrawal period may be based on data in published literature, extrapolated from the pharmacokinetic profile of the drug, or determined through consultation with organizations such as the Food Animal Residue Avoidance Databank (FARAD).

COMPLIANCE POLICY GUIDE 615.115. Because the extralabel use of medicated feeds is prohibited by law, an undue hardship was placed on minor food-producing animals that could not be practically medicated in any other way. An example would be commercially raised game birds, such as pheasants, that are raised in very large outdoor pens. If these birds become ill, they cannot be dosed individually and they will drink water from puddles rather than medicated water. Therefore, they are most often treated via the feed. Aquaculture species are another group of animals best treated with medicated feed. Given that there are few drugs approved for these species (and some of these not marketed) a means of relief was provided through a compliance policy guide (CPG). This CPG is FDA's direction to field investigators to exercise enforcement discretion in these cases. This does not make extralabel use of medicated feed legal and a CPG can be rescinded at any time. It simply means that if veterinarians and producers follow the parameters laid out in the guide, no action will be taken against them. In effect, this guide allows veterinarians to recommend approved medicated feeds to be fed to minor food-producing animals in an extralabel manner. For example, pheasants can be fed medicated feed that is labeled for chickens. However, the formulation of the feed cannot be altered to accommodate the dietary requirements of the pheasants. The CPG is not the answer to the issue of drug availability, but is a temporary solution that should someday be made unnecessary by drug approvals.

MINOR USE AND MINOR SPECIES ANIMAL HEALTH ACT. In 2004, the Minor Use and Minor Species (MUMS) Animal Health Act was passed giving the United States Food and Drug Administration the opportunity to encourage the approval of drugs for minor animal species and for minor uses in major animal species (Haley 2006). The MUMS legislation modified the Federal Food, Drug and Cosmetic Act in three significant ways; by providing the options of conditional approval, indexing, and designation for veterinary drugs used in minor animal species (Public Law 108–282).

Conditional Approval. The MUMS Act provides an opportunity for drugs that will be used for minor uses in major species and for minor species, including minor food-producing animals to be conditionally approved. Conditional approval allows drug sponsors to market the product on a yearly renewal basis for up to 5 years while gathering effectiveness data. All other requirements for a conditional approval (e.g., human food safety) are the same as for a full approval. The standard for conditional approval is "a reasonable expectation of effectiveness" rather than "substantial evidence." Within the 5 years allowed for conditional approval, the sponsor must provide effectiveness data to the full approval standard. Conditionally approved new animal drugs must be so labeled and are not eligible for extralabel use.

Indexing. Indexing will not apply to minor food-producing animals as indexing is reserved for drugs to treat diseases or conditions in animals where human food safety is not a concern. It is also limited to minor species exclusively. The intent of the Legally Marketed Unapproved New Animal Drug Index is to provide a means for sponsors to make products available for markets that cannot meet requirements of the new animal drug application (NADA) due to small populations, intrinsic value of the animals, wide variety of species, etc. The index is intended to serve laboratory animals, zoological animals, companion rodents, ornamental fish, etc.

Designation. The designation portion of the MUMS legislation created a program for veterinary medicine that somewhat mirrors what has been done with the orphan drug program in human medicine. Designation is intended to create incentives to encourage pharmaceutical companies to support drug development for minor species and minor uses. Designated drugs are granted 7 years of marketing exclusivity beginning on the date of approval or conditional approval. The MUMS Act also authorizes future availability of grants to support safety and effectiveness testing of designated new animal drugs.

PROGRAMS SUPPORTING THE USE OF VETERINARY PHARMACEUTICALS IN MINOR FOOD-PRODUCING ANIMALS

NATIONAL RESEARCH SUPPORT PROJECT #7 (NRSP-7). As already noted, the small market size for therapeutic veterinary products for minor food-producing animals makes the time and expense of drug approval unattractive to pharmaceutical companies. To assist and increase drug availability for minor food-producing animals, the United States Department of Agriculture (USDA) sponsors a program to generate data to support such drug approvals.

The National Research Support Project #7 (NRSP-7) is a USDA-supported program for minor use of drugs in major food-producing animals and primary use of drugs in minor food-producing animals of agricultural importance. This encompasses animals used to produce food or fiber. This program is intended to help fill the need for effective and safe drugs for use in minor food-producing animals, such as sheep, goats, rabbits, game birds, bison, deer, bees, and aquaculture species. A review of this program has been published by Ringer et al. (1999). The program accepts requests for needed drugs from a wide range of stakeholders, including veterinarians, producers, and pharmaceutical companies. In most cases the program funds studies to complete data requirements for effectiveness, target animal safety, human food safety, and environmental safety. Once these requirements have been reviewed and accepted by CVM, the data are gathered into a Public Master File, and a notice of availability of the data is published in the Federal Register. Because public money was used to conduct these studies, the data are all publicly available. A pharmaceutical sponsor can use these data in conjunction with its own manufacturing and labeling information to file an NADA for the product. In this way, costs to the pharmaceutical company are drastically reduced.

Because the NRSP-7 program has a limited budget, it generally, but not always, selects projects for minor food-producing animals that will be supplemental to existing products that are already labeled for use in major food-producing animals. The toxicology part of the human food safety technical section of an NADA is much too expensive for the program to fund for each minor food-producing animal. If this was already done by the pharmaceutical sponsor to support a cattle or swine approval, for example, it does not need to be repeated for the minor food-producing animal. Residue depletion and antimicrobial resistance issues still need to be addressed. Effectiveness and target animal safety need to be demonstrated in the minor food-producing animals and the environmental component must be addressed. Again, if an approval for a major food-producing animal already exists, a categorical exclusion from the requirement to provide an environmental assessment is a likely option, unless the new approval is for an aquaculture use.

At any given time, the NRSP-7 program is sponsoring 15 to 20 active projects. Working in cooperation with universities, producers, veterinarians, and government agencies, the program leverages a small budget into many studies. Since its inception in the early 1980s, the program has been successful in supporting over 25 drug approvals for a wide range of species. Information about the program and its projects can be found at http://www.nrsp7.org.

THE FOOD ANIMAL RESIDUE AVOIDANCE DATABANK (FARAD). The Food Animal Residue Avoidance Databank (FARAD) assists veterinarians in the establishment of scientifically based withdrawal intervals (not withdrawal times) that will prevent the occurrence of illegal residues in edible products derived from food-producing animals treated in an extralabel manner (Payne et al. 1999). (A *withdrawal time* is a legal requirement established by the FDA/CVM as part of the drug approval process. A *withdrawal interval* is a recommended preslaughter or milk discard time provided by FARAD to veterinarians in support of the AMDUCA requirement for an extended withdrawal interval for extralabel drug use in food animals.)

FARAD utilizes a decision tree approach to the problem and uses all available published data (and unpublished confidential data from pharmaceutical firms whenever possible) to guide the establishment of a withdrawal interval. When tissue or milk data are not available, the establishment of withdrawal intervals sometimes relies on blood (and serum or plasma) pharmacokinetic data to help define the final phase elimination of a drug. In such cases where serum or plasma data are used for estimating tissue residue depletion, it is assumed that the final edible tissue elimination phase will be at least as long as that seen in plasma. All possible data are used to help in this estimation, and whenever a recommendation is made, withdrawal estimations are increased to provide a wider margin of safety. In this way, "safety factors" are built in when assumptions must be made to help ensure that the estimated withdrawal interval will be sufficient. In many cases, data do not exist that can be used to make a withdrawal interval estimation, and the practitioner is advised to consider a different drug for treatment.

Recently, a patented algorithm called the Extended Withdrawal Estimator (EWE) has been established to help automate this process. The EWE utilizes data in the FARAD pharmacokinetic database, residue tolerances from the FARAD tolerance database, and a sophisticated mathematical procedure to calculate the best estimate for a withdrawal interval following a specific dose, via a specific route to a species (Martin-Jimenez et al. 2002). Allometric comparisons between species are built into the EWE as a subroutine that can be used if there are data-gaps for a particular species. Newly published data on the pharmacokinetics of drugs in food-producing animals are constantly being added to the FARAD pharmacokinetic files, and as the knowledge base increases, so will the predictive capability of the EWE. Additionally, new algorithms will be established and linked to the EWE based on in vitro and in vivo data from minor food-producing animals.

METHODS FOR ESTIMATING WITHDRAWAL INTERVALS FOR VETERINARY PHARMACEUTICALS ADMINISTERED TO MINOR FOOD-PRODUCING ANIMALS IN AN EXTRALABEL MANNER

When drugs are used in an extralabel manner in food animals, veterinarians need to determine withdrawal intervals to prevent the occurrence of illegal drug residues. FARAD uses several methods to establish withdrawal intervals for drugs administered to minor food-producing animals in an extralabel fashion. All of the methods are dependent in some way on pharmacokinetic and tissue residue data to estimate withdrawal intervals after extralabel use. When pharmacokinetic data are lacking in a minor species, these data may be estimated using allometric scaling techniques, species grouping, and in vitro and molecular techniques.

PHARMACOKINETIC STUDIES. Drug absorption, distribution, metabolism, and excretion (pharmacokinetics of a drug) in minor food-producing animals are the key factors for determining withdrawal intervals for drugs used in an extralabel manner. A traditional pharmacokinetic study carried out in small groups of individual animals is the "standard" method. Additionally, tissue residue studies are carried out in a similar manner, with a small number of animals serially slaughtered at various times after drug treatment allowing the establishment of the kinetics of residue depletion.

Pharmacokinetic Studies Using Individual Animal Subjects. Pharmacokinetic studies using individual animals have been the cornerstone in the study of comparative pharmacology to elucidate interspecies differences in drug response. Thousands of manuscripts have been published on the pharmacokinetics of drugs in food-producing animals. Some of the studies focus on just one species whereas others are more helpful in that they compare the pharmacokinetics of drugs between major and minor food-producing animals (Modric et al. 1998; Craigmill et al. 2000; Lanusse 2003). When using pharmacokinetic data from a major food-producing animal to predict drug pharmacokinetics in a minor food-producing animal, it is important to consider factors that will impact absorption, distribution, metabolism, and excretion of a drug before determining whether extrapolation is feasible. The potential for one species of animal (e.g., a major food-producing animal) to help predict the pharmacokinetics of a drug in a minor food-producing animal depends on a number of factors. These include similarities and differences in absorption (e.g., intrinsic absorption of a given drug across the gastrointestinal wall mucosa, gastric pH, first-pass metabolism, etc.), elimination (e.g., glomerular filtration, hepatic blood flow if the drug is excreted primarily through the liver, etc.), and biochemical factors (e.g., protein binding, drug metabolism, etc.) (Lin 1995).

For major and minor food animals, there do not appear to be species differences in the types of metabolites formed; however, there may be differences in the ratios of these metabolites formed. Juskevich published a review of comparative food animal drug metabolism that provides an excellent overview covering important factors that must be considered when comparing drug metabolism between species (Juskevich 1987). Short (1994) published a review comparing factors that impact drug metabolism and disposition in sheep and other domestic ruminants to demonstrate whether pharmacokinetic profiles could be predicted for antimicrobials used in these animal species.

FARAD has been collecting pharmacokinetic data from the published literature since 1982 and currently has 8,280 citations that contain pharmacokinetic data on chemical or drug residues for a variety of animal species. The data from numerous food-producing animals have been compiled and published as a reference textbook (Craigmill et al. 2006). Data are available for minor food-producing animals for comparison to those from major food-producing animals. In comparison to the major food-producing animals, the minor food-producing animals have considerably fewer published pharmacokinetic studies for the various categories of antibiotics, anthelmintics, nonsteroidal antiinflammatories and exogenous hormones. Using ruminants as an example, Table 52.6 demonstrates the preponderance of pharmacokinetic-based publications in the FARAD database for cattle versus some of the minor food-producing animals. While the focus of the FARAD data collection has been residue avoidance, considerable data are also available on serum/plasma pharmacokinetics of drugs that can be useful for therapeutic purposes as well.

Population Pharmacokinetics and Meta-Analysis. One of the limitations of most comparative pharmacokinetic studies that have been done to date is the small number of animals of each species used. In most studies, all of the animals representing a species have been obtained from one supplier and are of one breed or strain. Therefore, the variability in parameters within a species (intraspecific variability) cannot be assessed. Such unknown variability within a species makes it even more difficult to evaluate variability between species (interspecies). The use of population-based pharmacokinetic modeling procedures will help to define this, but these methods require substantial amounts of data to give the best results. Martin-Jiminez and Riviere defined population pharmacokinetics as "a study of the basic features of drug disposition in a population, accounting for the influence of diverse pathophysiological factors on pharmacokinetics, and explicitly estimating the magnitude of the interindividual and intraindividual variability" (Martin-Jimenez and Riviere 1998). The advantage to this technique is that it allows for assessment of how clinical factors (age, gender, renal and hepatic function, etc.) impact the pharmacokinetic parameter estimate. Another proposed benefit is that population pharmacokinetic studies could be conducted using a multicompartment experimental protocol to predict food animal residue avoidance. The application of such a methodology would greatly benefit minor food-producing animals because collective sampling might ultimately establish significant baseline data reflecting the pharmacokinetic parameters of a drug in a field or production setting.

Another approach is meta-analysis, in which data from multiple studies are carefully combined to increase the number of subjects. This approach was applied to procaine penicillin G and oxytetracycline using data from FARAD to look at the intramuscular pharmacokinetics in nonlactating cattle (Craigmill et al. 2004) and to ampicillin trihydrate in cattle (Gehring et al. 2005). Meta-analysis requires careful selection of data according to predetermined standards to ensure data quality, including such factors as analytical methodology and study design. Under optimal conditions, the meta-analysis is conducted using population pharmacokinetic modeling procedures when individual animal pharmacokinetic data from multiple studies and individual animal covariate data (sex, weight, age, health, etc.) are available.

TABLE 52.6 Comparison of numbers of Food Animal Residue Avoidance Databank publications with drug concentration versus time dependent data for ruminants as of December, 2008

Drug Category	Cattle	Buffalo	Cervids	Sheep	Goats
Aminoglycosides	164	11	2	48	48
Cephalosporins	144	5	1	32	17
Fluoroquinilones	82	6	0	17	32
Macrolides	87	2	1	20	8
Penicillins	448	13	0	59	40
Sulfonimides	284	47	0	79	111
Tetracyclines	212	8	2	52	37
Anthelmintics	270	33	6	312	75
Hormones	161	0	0	37	4
Nonsteroidal Antiinflammatories	115	3	0	33	29

Physiologically Based Pharmacokinetic (PBPK) Modeling. Physiologically based pharmacokinetic (PBPK) modeling might prove a very effective method for making interspecies comparisons for drugs. Physiologically based pharmacokinetics (PBPK) offers another way to study interspecies relationships, and has been used extensively for predicting human tissue concentrations of toxicants using animal data. PBPK also offers researchers the opportunity to utilize in vitro metabolism data (K_m and V_{max}) to help predict clearance rates of chemicals in multiple species. PBPK modeling uses physiological and biochemical parameters, therefore this method can be mechanistic as well as predictive. Physiological parameters used in PBPK models may be measured directly or derived from allometric equations. PBPK models have been developed for fish (Law 1999), turkeys (Pollet et al. 1985), cattle (Achenbach et al. 1998), horses (Trachsel et al. 2004; Knobloch et al. 2006), swine (Buur et al. 2006), rabbits (Tsuji et al. 1985), and sheep (Craigmill 2003). PBPK modeling has been used to evaluate oxytetracycline residues in cattle, sheep, and fish and may prove useful for predicting the depletion of drug residues in the tissues of other minor food-producing animals in the future (Achenbach et al. 1998; Law 1999; Craigmill 2003).

ALLOMETRIC SCALING. For decades, veterinary medicine has used allometric scaling to ascertain effective doses and dosage regimens for a variety of animals. For a detailed presentation of the use of allometry for interspecies pharmacokinetic parameter scaling, readers are referred to recent published review manuscripts (Mahmood et al. 2006; Martinez et al. 2006). Riviere and colleagues (1997) gathered pharmacokinetic parameter data for 44 drugs using the Food Animal Residue Avoidance Databank and found that 11 of the 44 drugs showed significant allometric relationships of their pharmacokinetic parameters for extrapolation between veterinary species. Nine of these eleven drugs were antibiotics. Some of the drugs that did not demonstrate allometric relationships with respect to their pharmacokinetic parameters were low hepatic excretion drugs. For the other drugs, the results were equivocal.

These pharmacokinetic allometric studies can also be used to estimate withdrawal intervals using kinetic parameter data for drugs in blood, serum or plasma. For unmetabolized drugs (e.g., ones that are not highly protein bound in plasma and are not specifically bound by tissue components), one could expect that tissue residue parameters would mirror blood kinetic parameters. Tissue residue elimination would then be dependent on blood flow and the tissue/plasma partition coefficient, and drugs that are highly fat soluble would be removed from fat depots slowly. This slow removal would subsequently be seen as a prolonged elimination phase.

SPECIES GROUPING. Researchers within and external to the NRSP-7 program have been working collaboratively to develop approaches to group minor food-producing animals by doing studies in an "indicator" species for that group. Animal categories that have been considered for such grouping include avian species, cervids, and fish. The primary focus has been on aquaculture species due to the large number of aquatic species that are in need of drugs to treat diseases and parasites that are often caused by the same organism in multiple species. Several possible ways to achieve this goal include grouping of species based on physiology, drug delivery mechanism, target pathogen, culture system, economic importance, and human food safety concerns (Greenlees and Bell 1998). Sources of variability in the pharmacokinetics of drugs in aquaculture species include interspecific variability, intraspecific variability, habitat variability, temperature, size/age, and sexual maturity (Gingerich et al. 1998). Poikilothermic animals present a greater challenge than homeothermic animals because the environmental temperature has such a great effect on their physiology. Therefore, studies focusing on poikilothermic animals should consider environmental temperature as a mixed "physiological" and environmental variable.

For grouping of the minor aquatic and avian species, two approaches are being used by the NRSP-7 program. The first is to explore species grouping of finfish for drugs that are not significantly metabolized and thus are excreted unchanged. The primary method being used for this aspect is the development of pharmacokinetic data for serum and tissues in several fish species at different temperatures. A second approach is focusing on establishing in vitro drug metabolism parameters in avian species and linking them with pharmacokinetic serum and tissue data using physiologically based pharmacokinetic modeling.

FUTURE DIRECTIONS: IN VITRO AND MOLECULAR STUDIES. **In vitro** and molecular based research might help establish some differences in drug metabolism before going to whole animal models. **In vitro** methods for exploring comparative metabolism include P450 assays, microsomes, tissue slices, isolated cells, and cell culture. P450 assays have been used to evaluate species differences for major and minor food-producing animals (Dalvi et al. 1987; Nebbia et al. 2001; Machala et al. 2003; Dacasto et al. 2005). Microsomes from food-producing animals have been used to evaluate gender and breed differences (Dacasto et al. 2005). Another study evaluated the biotransformation of cultured hepatocytes from goats, sheep, and cattle using five different test substrates and determined that cultured hepatocytes appeared to be a good in vitro model to study comparative metabolism of veterinary drugs in these animal species (van 't Klooster et al. 1994).

Genomic and proteomic methods to evaluate interspecies differences in drug metabolizing enzymes might also be useful for minor food-producing animals. Examination of DNA using Southern blot analysis can be used to determine if genes exist that code for specific drug metabolizing enzymes. Northern blots may be used to find mRNA transcripts of genes that code for drug metabolism enzymes. For minor food-producing animals, this investigation could start by using cDNA probes for a subfamily of P450 enzymes that are extensively involved in drug metabolism, such as the CYP3 family. Hepatic mRNA from a minor food-producing animal of interest could also be evaluated using commercially available P450 cDNA probes. Using this approach, one could establish only that probe hybridization patterns were similar between the minor food-producing animals being considered. If similar hybridization patterns existed, one could hypothesize that those species evaluated might be similar in drug metabolic capability, at least on a qualitative basis. This hypothesis could then be tested using in vitro (including expression vectors and drug substrate assays) or in vivo methods.

Immunoblotting would be another approach to assess similarities or differences between minor food-producing animals. For this approach, antibodies for the specific protein of interest would need to be developed for minor food-producing animals because most of the commercial probes/antibodies are usually from non–food-producing animals (e.g., mouse, rat, monkey, human). Therefore, the use of the commercial antibodies in such assays would be limited for interspecies analysis because the metabolic enzymes from different species cannot be assumed identical. In addition, structural homology does not guarantee functional homology. Nevertheless, because there is considerable sequence conservation across species in the cytochrome P450 enzyme superfamily and metabolic enzymes in general, such studies may be quite useful to characterize potential metabolic enzyme capacities of minor food-producing animals.

As the field of proteomics expands and protein sequence methods become quicker, the identification and characterization of drug-metabolizing enzymes for minor food-producing animals will be easier and more economical. Progress in this area is dependent on increased funding for such research, which may result from growing concern over therapeutic drug residues in food-producing animals.

SUMMARY

Improving drug availability for food-producing minor species is proceeding on several fronts. It will still take time for the various incentive programs and research programs to have a noticeable effect. With the great variety of diseases and species that this group represents, every possible incentive must be exploited and every research option explored. Veterinarians, researchers, pharmaceutical companies, governmental agencies, producers, and consumers all have a stake in the success of this work.

REFERENCES

Achenbach, T., Abedini, S., Cox, W., Law, F.C.P. 1998. Development of a physiologically based pharmacokinetic (PBPK) model for oxytetracycline in cattle. Toxicol Sci 42:140.

Buur, J., Baynes, R., Smith, G., Riviere, J. 2006. Use of probabilistic modeling within a physiologically based pharmacokinetic model to predict sulfamethazine residue withdrawal times in edible tissues in swine. Antimicrob Agents Chemother 50:2344–2351.

Craigmill, A.L. 2003. A physiologically based pharmacokinetic model for oxytetracycline residues in sheep. J Vet Pharmacol Ther 26:55–63.

Craigmill, A.L., Holland, R.E., Robinson, D., Wetzlich, S., Arndt, T. 2000. Serum pharmacokinetics of oxytetracycline in sheep and calves and tissue residues in sheep following a single intramuscular injection of a long-acting preparation. J Vet Pharmacol Ther 23:345–352.

Craigmill, A.L., Miller, G.R., Gehring, R., Pierce, A.N., Riviere, J.E. 2004. Meta-analysis of pharmacokinetic data of veterinary drugs using the Food Animal Residue Avoidance Databank: oxytetracycline and procaine penicillin G. J Vet Pharmacol Ther 27:343–353.

Craigmill, A.L., Riviere, J.E., Webb, A.I. 2006. Tabulation of FARAD Comparative and Veterinary Pharmacokinetic Data. Ames, Blackwell Publishing.

Dacasto, M., Eeckhoutte, C., Capolongoa, F., Dupuy, J., Carletti, M., Calleja, C., Nebbia, C., Alvinerie, M., Galtier, P. 2005. Effect of breed and gender on bovine liver cytochrome P450 3A (CYP3A) expression and inter-species comparison with other domestic ruminants. Vet Res 36:179–190.

Dalvi, R.R., Nunn, V.A., Juskevich, J. 1987. Studies on comparative drug metabolism by hepatic cytochrome P-450–containing microsomal enzymes in quail, ducks, geese, chickens, turkeys and rats. Comp Biochem Physiol C 87:421–424.

Gehring, R., van der Merwe, D., Pierce, A.N., Baynes, R.E., Craigmill, A.L., Riviere, J.E. 2005. Multivariate meta-analysis of pharmacokinetic studies of ampicillin trihydrate in cattle. Am J Vet Res 66:108–112.

Gingerich, W.H., Stehly, G.R., Clark, K.J., Hayton, W.L. 1998. Crop grouping: a proposal for public aquaculture. Vet Hum Toxicol 40 Suppl 2:24–31.

Greenlees, K.J., Bell, T.A. 1998. Aquaculture crop grouping and new animal drug approvals: a CVM perspective. Vet Hum Toxicol 40 Suppl 2:19–23.

Haley, C.J. 2006. The Minor Use and Minor Species Animal Health Act: past, present, and future. Food Drug Law J 61:13–43.

Juskevich, J.C. 1987. Comparative metabolism in food-producing animals: programs sponsored by the Center for Veterinary Medicine. Drug Metab Rev 18:345–362.

Knobloch, M., Portier, C.J., Levionnois, O.L., Theurillat, R., Thormann, W., Spadavecchia, C., Mevissen, M. 2006. Antinociceptive effects, metabolism and disposition of ketamine in ponies under target-controlled drug infusion. Toxicol Appl Pharmacol 216(3):373–86.

Lanusse, C.E. 2003. Comparative pharmacokinetics of anthelmintic drugs in ruminants: Updated integration of current knowledge. J Vet Pharmacol Ther 26:42–47.

Law, F. 1999. A physiologically based pharmacokinetic model for predicting the withdrawal period of oxytetracycline in cultured Chinook salmon (*Onchorhynchus tshawytscha*), in Smith, D., Gingerich, W.H., and Beconi-Barker, M.G., (ed): Xenobiotics in Fish, pp. 105–121, New York, Kluwer Academic/Plenum Publishers.

Lin, J.H. 1995. Species similarities and differences in pharmacokinetics. Drug Metab Dispos 23:1008–1021.

Machala, M., Soucek, P., Neca, J., Ulrich, R., Lamka, J., Szotakova, B., Skalova, L. 2003. Inter-species comparisons of hepatic cytochrome P450 enzyme levels in male ruminants. Arch Toxicol 77:555–560.

Mahmood, I., Martinez, M., Hunter, R.P. 2006. Interspecies allometric scaling. Part I: prediction of clearance in large animals. J Vet Pharmacol Ther 29:415–423.

Martin-Jimenez, T., Baynes, R.E., Craigmill, A., Riviere, J.E. 2002. Extrapolated withdrawal-interval estimator (EWE) algorithm: a quantitative approach to establishing extralabel withdrawal times. Regul Toxicol Pharmacol 36:131–137.

Martin-Jimenez, T. and Riviere, J.E. 1998. Population pharmacokinetics in veterinary medicine: potential use for therapeutic drug monitoring and prediction of tissue residues. J Vet Pharmacol Ther 21:167–189.

Martinez, M., Mahmood, I, Hunter, R.P. 2006. Interspecies allometric scaling: prediction of clearance in large animal species: Part II: mathematical considerations. J Vet Pharmacol Ther 29:425–432.

Modric, S., Webb, A.I., Derendorf, H. 1998. Pharmacokinetics and pharmacodynamics of tilmicosin in sheep and cattle. J Vet Pharmacol Ther 21:444–452.

Monti, D.J. 2000. AMDUCA regulates small and large animal practice. J Am Vet Med Assoc 216:1889.

Nebbia, C., Ceppa, L., Dacasto, M., Nachtmann, C., Carletti, M. 2001. Oxidative monensin metabolism and cytochrome P450 3A content and functions in liver microsomes from horses, pigs, broiler chicks, cattle and rats. J Vet Pharmacol Ther 24:399–403.

Payne, M.A., Craigmill, A.L., Riviere, J.E., Baynes, R.E., Webb, A.I., Sundlof, S.F. 1999. The Food Animal Residue Avoidance Databank (FARAD). Past, present and future. Vet Clin North Am Food Anim Pract 15:75–88.

Pollet, R.A, Glatz, C.E., Dyer, D.C. 1985. The pharmacokinetics of chlortetracycline orally administered to turkeys: Influence of citric acid and *Pasteurella multocida* infection. J Pharmacokin Biopharm 13:243–264.

Ringer, R.K., Miller, L.R., Saylor, W.W. 1999. Minor-use animal drug program—A national agricultural program to approve animal drugs for minor species and uses. J Am Vet Med Assoc 214:1636–1637.

Riviere, J.E., Martin-Jimenez, T., Sundlof, S.F., Craigmill, A.L. 1997. Interspecies allometric analysis of the comparative pharmacokinetics of 44 drugs across veterinary and laboratory animal species. J Vet Pharmacol Ther 20:453–463.

Short, C.R. 1994. Consideration of sheep as a minor species: comparison of drug metabolism and disposition with other domestic ruminants. Vet Hum Toxicol 36:24–40.

Trachsel, D., Tschudi, P., Portier, C.J., Kuhn, M., Thormann, W., Scholtysik, G., Mevissen, M. 2004. Pharmacokinetics and pharmacodynamic effects of amiodarone in plasma of ponies after single intravenous administration. Toxicol Appl Pharmacol 195:113–125.

Tsuji, A., Nishide, K., Minami, H., Nakashima, E., Terasaki, T., Yamana, T. 1985. Physiologically based pharmacokinetic model for cefazolin in rabbits and its preliminary extrapolation to man. Drug Metab Dispos 13:729–739.

van 't Klooster, G.A., Woutersen-van Nijnanten, F.M., Blaauboer, B.J., Noordhoek, J., van Miert, A.S. 1994. Applicability of cultured hepatocytes derived from goat, sheep and cattle in comparative drug metabolism studies. Xenobiotica 24:417–428.

CHAPTER

53

ZOOLOGICAL PHARMACOLOGY

ROBERT P. HUNTER

INTRODUCTION

Species differences in drug absorption, distribution, metabolism, and excretion (ADME) for numerous pharmaceutical agents have been well documented for domestic species; however, there is limited information concerning the ADME of drugs in nondomestic species. Lack of approved pharmaceutical agents and/or pharmacokinetic data in the literature for exotic, wildlife, and zoo species is a major issue for veterinarians attempting to treat these animals. Under the Animal Medicinal Drug Use Clarification Act (AMDUCA), practitioners take approved agents (veterinary or human) and extrapolate their use to nonapproved species, often with little scientific basis to support this decision. To further complicate treatment, zoo veterinarians often have to formulate the medication(s) into a meal or treat, hoping that the animal will ingest it. Due to lack of patient compliance, the clinician may have to resort to other means of drug administration. Additionally, due to the value of these animals or their status as threatened or endangered species, the traditional method of trial and error for treatment selection is inappropriate. This results in a mentality where no zoo veterinarian wants to be the first to administer an agent/formulation in an untested species.

The range of animals a zoo veterinarian cares for varies from very small invertebrates (honeybees) to megavertebrates such as elephants and whales. There is currently only one United States approval for the class amphibians, four agents approved for use in invertebrates, and eight to ten compounds for mammalian zoo and wildlife species compared to almost 300 for domestic cattle. Various methods have been used to extrapolate/predict safe and effective dosage regimens. No attempt will be made to turn this chapter into a formulary. Excellent formularies already exist to provide for that need (Antinoff et al. 1999; Carpenter 2005; Hawk and Leary 1999; Kreeger et al. 2002; Nielsen 1999). This chapter provides information and guidance on comparative physiology, formulation considerations, and dosage scaling across wide and varied species.

SPECIES GROUPS

Working with exotic animals, even during routine daily care, can be very dangerous. This is magnified when working around sick or injured animals where the patient is subject to increased stress, pain, and deviations from the usual routine—for example, those associated with treatment and drug administration. If given the opportunity, most animals can inflict injury to humans using almost any body part. They can crush with the body or head; kick with exceptional force; or grasp with their hands, body, tail, or trunk. During medication attempts, the individuals administering the treatment are at great risk because they are close to the animal and often working near the head, teeth, fangs, or hands. Safety precautions must be considered prior to treating any animal.

INVERTEBRATES. The numbers of invertebrate zoos and species within those facilities are increasing rapidly. The main concern when treating these species is that they typically lack the membrane barriers that are foundations for therapeutic choices in domestic mammalian species. This likely makes them more susceptible to serious adverse events from agents that are considered safe in mammals, especially anthelmentics or neuro-acting agents.

There are only four agents approved for use in invertebrates (shellfish, shrimp, lobsters, or honeybees): bicyclohexylammonium, formalin, oxytetracycline, and tylosin. All of these species are treated as food animals and residues are of concern. These agents have specific approvals in one or more of these species.

Another consideration is the use of invertebrates as drug delivery devices. This is typically done for insectivores or marine mammals (squid to sperm whales). The book *Eat this Bug*, by Davis (1996) may be useful for assisting veterinarians in selecting appropriate "treat" species to use as drug vehicles. This concept is similar to the use of rodents as dosage forms ("fuzzy" dosage forms) for raptors or reptiles. This concept of using insects as dosage forms is commonly used clinically to increase calcium in the diet of insect-eating reptiles (Donoghue and Langenberg 1996).

VERTEBRATES

Reptile and Amphibian. With over 4,000 amphibian species, 3,750 species of lizards, 2,500 species of snakes, 270 species of turtles, and 22 species of crocodilians there is currently only one approval in the U.S. for this group. Tricaine methanesulfonate (MS-222) is a Na^+-channel–blocking local anesthetic. It is used for temporary immobilization to aid in handling during weighing, measuring, marking, surgical operations, transport, photography, and research.

Route of administration is especially challenging in these species. For amphibians, oral, topical, and injectable routes are common. Topical baths can be very beneficial since the skin of amphibians has similar properties to mammalian mucosal surfaces. The pH and temperature of the bath must be appropriate for the treated species (Mader et al. 1985; Walker and Whitaker 2000). This can also allow for group treatment of animals that are on display or for treatment off-exhibit in special treatment tanks. As with all treatments, the animals must be monitored so that they are not harmed or injured in the bath (Walker and Whitaker 2000).

Routes of drug delivery are similar between reptiles and amphibians. Several studies have been done investigating the pharmacokinetics of various agents in all four groups of reptiles: snakes, turtles, lizards, and crocodilians.

Drug metabolism may be affected by prandial state in the snake and other sporadic feeding reptiles. This mechanism allows for minor metabolic investment of digestion to occur after a period of fasting and energy reserve depletion; thus nutrient metabolism peaks about 1 week after feeding. With variable physiological states, drug metabolism and elimination could be affected by feeding intervals. Thus, the effect of feeding could greatly affect the way orally administered pharmacologic agents are absorbed by snakes. When a snake consumes a meal, the small intestinal mucosa will increase in thickness at least three times while total length of the small intestine does not change. Correspondingly, villi length is two times prefeeding length, resulting in an increase in small intestine surface area as a result of feeding. Azithromycin absorption in ball pythons was prolonged, compared to all mammalian species reported, based on relatively large mean absorption time (MAT) and T_{max} values.

Four of the fifteen circulating azithromycin metabolites: 3′-desamine-3-ene-azithromycin, descladinose dehydroxy-2-ene-azithromycin, 3′-desamine-3-ene descladinose-azithromycin, and 3′-*N*-nitroso,9a-*N*-desmethylazithromycin are unique to the ball python. As azithromycin metabolism in mammals is mediated by several cytochrome P450 isoforms, it is possible that these systemic metabolites are a result of novel cytochrome P450 isoforms, the unique gastrointestinal physiology of the ball python, or some combination of both. The unique gastrointestinal physiology of the snake does appear to lend itself to increased metabolism of xenobiotics. Due to the long GI transit times of boid snakes of >1 week, this presents the opportunity for a xenobiotic, such as azithromycin, to undergo repeated enterohepatic recirculation during the course of a single drug administration. This provides an effect similar to that produced by sustained-release oral formulations in mammals. The percentage of each plasma metabolite differed for only a few metabolites when comparing i.v. with p.o. administration results from this study (Hunter et al. 2003b). This phenomenon would be expected to correspondingly prolong tissue concentrations of the parent compound and its metabolites. These factors are also likely to have an impact on bioavailability relative to time of feeding in snakes. This would likely make prediction of oral drug absorption dependent, to some extent, on time after feeding.

Reptiles have a renal portal system. This means that a first-pass effect of renally cleared drugs can take place if the animal is injected in the posterior half of the body. This system is not fully understood, and it may not be as restrictive as once believed. However, until definitive data are available, reptiles should be injected in the anterior portion of the body when agents dependent upon renal clearance are administered.

The rehabilitation of wild reptiles, such as sea turtles, requires the use of a variety of different medications; most have never undergone any pharmacokinetic studies in the target species to establish a basis for a safe and efficacious dose. Many of the commonly used treatments have had few studies (pharmacokinetic or efficacy) in any reptile species. This makes use of these drugs guesswork at best and dangerous at worst. For instance, when antimicrobials are underdosed this may not only lead to ineffective treatment of bacterial infections but may also lead to the development of resistant strains of bacteria. Likewise, overdosing may lead to adverse effects. The low basal metabolic rate of reptiles, in general, may correlate to the overall metabolism and distribution of drugs; this, along with the variation in metabolic rates among reptile species, makes dosage determination from dramatically different reptile species far less than desirable—let alone when extrapolation from mammalians species is done. The extent of plasma protein binding varies between species and is temperature-dependent. This is a key point to remember when treating poikilothermic species.

Avian. Avian medicine is a field of rapid growth in veterinary medicine. Greater than 95% of all pharmaceuticals used in clinical practice to treat various avian species are based upon empirical doses and the personal experiences of the attending clinician. This raises issues concerning the health of the animals being treated. Therefore, the pharmacokinetics of pharmaceutical agents used to treat avian species is an area of research that is needed to ensure the safe and proper dosing of these animals. However, there is limited information on the pharmacokinetics of agents used to treat psittacines, anseriforms, galiforms, passerines, softbills, and raptors. As a result of the lack of pharmacokinetic data, dosage regimens are designed using linear extrapolation from doses approved in domestic species, such as poultry (Baert and De Backer 2003). It is possible that use of linear extrapolation could lead to the development of toxicity or lack of efficacy in the treated animal(s) as a result of inaccurate dosing.

Extrapolation of doses is difficult between mammalian and avian species, both qualitatively and quantitatively. The avian renal cortex is more similar to the reptile cortex than the mammalian cortex. Glomerular filtration is not constant in birds, as it is in mammals, and likely has an impact on the pharmacokinetics of pharmaceuticals in avian species (Frazier et al. 1995). Avian species appear to be more susceptible to the renal ischemia and tissue damage of nonsteroidal antiinflammatory drugs (NSAIDs) than the gastrointestinal side effects (Paul-Murphy and Ludders 2001). While avian cytochrome P450 activities have been reported, their expression and role in avian drug metabolism is not well documented (Walker 1998).

All of the approvals in this group are for species used as food animals (poultry and galliforms). While it would seem logical to extrapolate a dose from a chicken to an ostrich, this could be equated to extrapolating a dose in horses to elephants.

The concept of "fuzzy" (use of rodents) dosage forms for raptors has been mentioned previously. While rodents can be viewed in many ways (pets, pests, or research test subjects), to the avian (and reptile) veterinarian they are a drug delivery device. In red-tailed hawks, the extent of oral bioavailability of enrofloxacin between intramuscular and "fuzzy" oral dosing was not different, even though the oral T_{max} was five times the intramuscular route (Harrenstien et al. 2000). The difference in T_{max} appears logical when considering dissolution and gastrointestinal transit in these animals.

Mammalian. Oral absorption has been shown to vary within a species. Within domestic dog breeds (Beagle and mongrel), different gastrointestinal transit times and mouth-to-small-intestine transit times have been reported (Sagara et al. 1995). When one considers the anatomical differences between true monogastrics (canine or feline species), hindgut fermentors (rodents, rabbits, horses, or elephants), foregut fermentors (Colobus monkeys, camelids, and kangaroos), and ruminants (cattle, goats, sheep, or antelope), the potential differences are staggering and support the concept that bioavailability is not scalable across mammalian species (Mahmood 2000, 2002). The large body sizes of some mammalian species produces problems for treatment and places significant limitations on drug delivery. Aside from the weight of the animal, the size, thickness, and density of various anatomical structures can physically hinder drug administration.

Small/Pocket Pets/Rodents. There is a wealth of data in the literature concerning the pharmacokinetics and safety of almost every human drug in rodents, such as mice and rats and often for rabbits as well. While ferrets are a laboratory species, research is narrower in scope, but could still be useful in treating these small mammal species. While the doses may be above that needed for efficacy, safety is well understood. The issue is typically formulating the agent into a dosage form that can be used clinically. With the Internet and various medical literature search tools, such as Medline, PubMed, and Highwire, the busy clinician can find information for treating just about any disease in small mammals.

However, there is no published, peer-reviewed information concerning the pharmacokinetics of drugs used in more exotic small mammals, such as hedgehogs, sugar gliders, and honey bears. Historically, mite infestations (*Chorioptic* sp.) in hedgehogs have been treated with either ivermectin or amitraz (Lightfoot 2000). This treatment has been shown to be effective, but requires weeks or months of therapy. Fleas and lungworms also infest these animals, and with a broad-spectrum, topical endectocide, such as selamectin, treatment could be carried out easily and rapidly, allowing for treatment of both the mite and flea infestations with a single compound (Fig. 53.1).

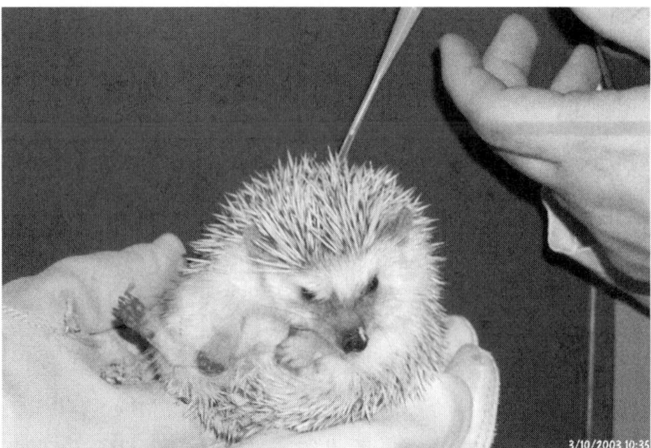

FIG. 53.1 Topical dose administration to an African hedgehog.

Farmed/Domestic Species. There are ≤50 compounds approved in the United States for sheep, ≤12 for goats, and none for New World camelids (Sundlof et al. 1992). As producers and veterinarians have taken approved agents for cattle, sheep, or goats and extrapolated their use to exotic domestic species, such as New World camelids, safety and efficacy have been the main issues. There are many different species-related factors, such as absorption, elimination, and metabolism, that could lead to variation in the pharmacokinetic parameters between species and possibly decrease the efficacy or increase the toxicity of a compound (Hunter and Isaza 2002; Short 1994; Xia et al. 2006). These differences make extrapolation very difficult from one species to another.

An example of species differences in pharmacokinetics is the data for topical doramectin. The mean C_{max} and AUC values for llamas and alpaca was approximately 33% less than that reported for cattle using the same dose and formulation. The mean T_{max} values for both species were 1 day longer than reported in cattle. It appears that the extent of absorption, as evaluated by C_{max} and AUC, is much less than that reported for cattle (Hunter et al. 2004a). This was also the case for moxidectin in these two species (Hunter et al. 2004b).

Zoo/Marine Mammals. All of the routes and issues discussed previously apply to this group of patients. If a well-trained animal can be difficult to treat (which they are), an uncooperative animal can easily prevent almost any unwanted medication from being administered. This is especially true of large carnivores, primates, and megavertabrates (elephants). The animal's combined size, strength, and/or intelligence effectively precludes forcing it to ingest medication or allowing someone to get close enough to manually administer medication.

The capture and chemical immobilization of a variety of zoo and wildlife species has been enhanced with the use of potent synthetic opiates, such as carfentanil (Haigh 1990). These opiates generally provide rapid induction and relatively long-lasting immobilization. They are usually administered parenterally, the small volumes required making them ideally suited for use in remote delivery systems such as darts (Fowler 1995). Furthermore, immobilization by these drugs can be completely reversed by the administration of specific opioid antagonists. This is particularly important for immobilization of free-living wildlife, which cannot be closely monitored after the immobilization period. These opioid anesthetic agents have provided zoo veterinarians and wildlife researchers not only a method to restrain animals for a variety of medical and research procedures, but have become an indispensable tool to the practice of zoological veterinary medicine.

Carfentanil has become the drug of choice for a wide variety of non–domestic animal immobilizations, particularly for hoofstock, and has been used either alone or in combination with sedatives for rapid immobilization of captive and free-ranging wildlife. The potency and formulation of this drug allow for a small volume to be administered, which is ideal for remote delivery systems (darts). Naltrexone is the antagonist used routinely in carfentanil immobilization procedures, because it has a longer half-life than other antagonists such as naloxone or nalorphine in domestic species. One adverse effect with the use of carfentanil is that of renarcotization. This is the reoccurrence of the effects of the opioid agonists up to 72 hours after apparent full recovery from the drug. The effect varies in severity from mild sedation to full immobilization and has also been associated with a high incidence of mortality. The choice of antagonist and dose used are important factors in the incidence of renarcotization. Also, certain species appear to have a higher tendency to develop renarcotization than others. Possible mechanisms for renarcotization are listed by Haigh (1990): enterohepatic recycling, metabolism of antagonist to form a metabolite with agonist properties, release of the agonist from body depots after the antagonist has been eliminated, antagonist underdosing, and metabolism of a short-acting antagonist and reestablishment of a longer-acting agonist. Studies are needed to assist with determining the actual cause(s) but there are currently no published PK/PD studies of any opioid agonist or antagonists in exotic ungulates.

Anesthesia of nonhuman primates is risky and stressful. Squeeze cages and darts have been used for administration of parenteral anesthetic agents, and various anesthetics have been administered orally using treat or food items. Although these formulations work well for these primate species, care should be taken to avoid conditioning the animal to associate the treat or personnel with the procedure (Hunter and Isaza 2002). Transmucosal fentanyl is approved for use in the United States as a preanesthetic agent in humans in a lollipop formulation. When this preparation of fentanyl is chewed and swallowed, it still results in a sedative effect with a corresponding longer T_{max} when compared to true transmucosal absorption. When this formulation was used in a study on great apes (Figs. 53.2, 53.3), nine chimpanzees were evaluated with only one being successfully offered a dose after having refused

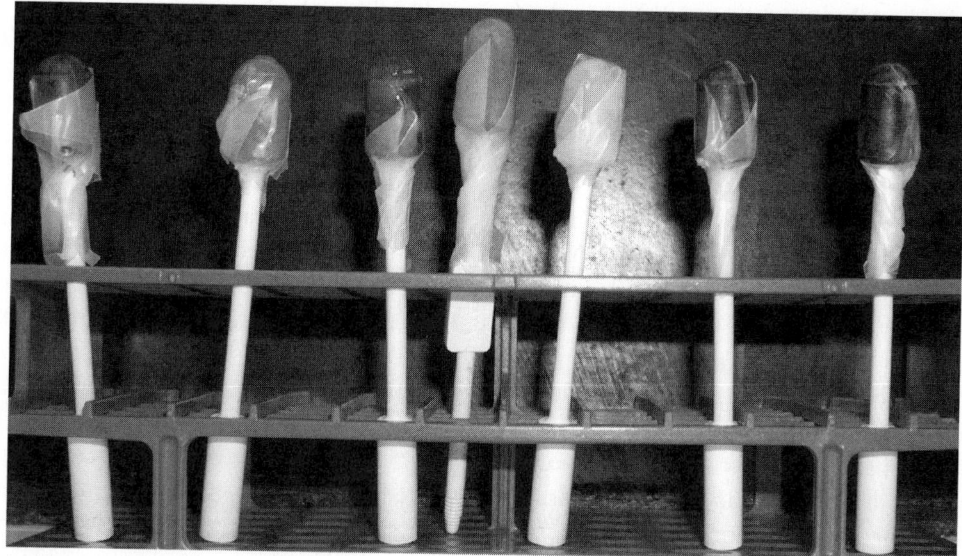

FIG. 53.2 The white fentanyl (Actiq®) lollipops were painted with candy coloring to match the colors of the placebo lollipops.

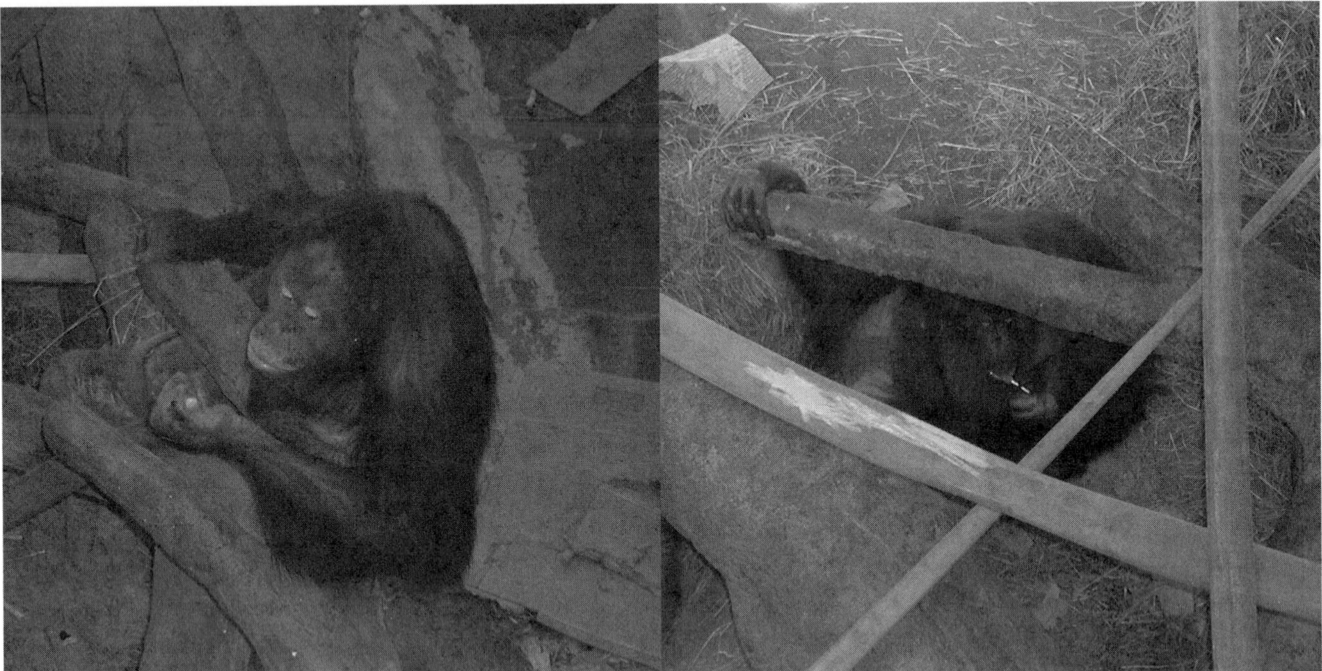

FIG. 53.3 Use of fentanyl lollipops to sedate an orangutan.

the lollipop on an earlier attempt; two other animals also refused to ingest their lollipops. All orangutans accepted at least one dose with several accepting two or more. The gorillas accepted multiple lollipops. The orangutans and gorillas demonstrated less stress when darted and showed signs of sedation after fentanyl administration. The main metabolite in humans, norfentanyl, was identified in only one of the test subjects, an orangutan. An effective dosage of fentanyl for orangutans and gorillas was dependent on an effective training program; cooperation of the keeper staff and zoo administration; and facilities that allow for individual, overnight housing of animals. In contrast, chimpanzees were suboptimally sedated with transmucosal fentanyl (Hunter et al. 2004c).

Foot problems affect over 50% of the captive elephant population. These problems may progress to arthritis, a debilitating condition often resulting in euthanasia of the animal. Arthritic elephants are typically treated with a wide variety of antiinflammatory and analgesic drugs, which offer only palliative treatment. Due to the side effects of these agents in domestic species, accurate therapeutic regimens are critical to properly treating diseased elephants. Simply guessing at a dosage can have disastrous consequences, as was illustrated in a case report where lysergic acid diethylamide (LSD) was tested in an elephant and the animal died violently within minutes (West et al. 1962).

The lack of pharmacokinetic data is reflected in the sparse number of published studies in elephants. Almost all of these studies have focused on antimicrobials, with little data being reported for analgesic and/or antiinflammatory agents. As a result of the lack of pharmacokinetic data, dosage regimens are designed using the assumption that pharmaceuticals administered to the elephant are absorbed, distributed, metabolized, and excreted in approximately the same manner as horses (Page et al. 1991). However, at least one example exists in the published literature to contradict this statement. For the chiral NSAID ketoprofen, the *S*-enantiomer is cleared from elephant plasma much more rapidly than the *R*-form. This is different than the domestic horse where the *R*-form is cleared more rapidly. This was explained as either selective clearance from plasma in the Asian elephants or as chiral inversion. Also in this study a possible novel metabolite, a Phase II glycine conjugate, was reported (Hunter et al. 2003a).

ALLOMETRY IN ZOO MEDICINE

Allometric scaling of pharmaceuticals to predict pharmacokinetics in zoo/exotic animals has considerable benefit for zoological veterinarians. This tool, when used appropriately, can provide an *estimate* for designing dosage regimens. The example of differences in ketoprofen inversion across species emphasizes the need to understand and be aware of the assumptions when designing treatment regimens based on allometric scaling data.

Just as mammals can range from a few grams to thousands of kilograms, reptiles and birds can also vary in body weight across a wide range. It has been suggested that it is impossible to derive a single equation correlating body mass to metabolic rate for all 6,000 species of reptiles (Funk 2000). Without knowledge as to the extent and route of elimination of an administered pharmaceutical agent, extrapolation of dosage regimens from one class to another is difficult, if not impossible, with any certainty. It is apparent that more research is needed on the drug metabolism and excretion capabilities in snakes, let alone reptiles in general. This type of research would increase the ability of clinicians to determine more effective and safe dosage regimens for their patients. Another consideration when using allometry is the nonlinearity of pharmacokinetics in some species (Manire et al. 2003; Rush et al. 2005).

There are two major components of hepatic clearance of xenobiotics: hepatic blood flow and enzymatic metabolism. Renal clearance is the other major route by which drugs are excreted. Renal clearance is composed of three parts: glomerular filtration, active tubular secretion, and tubular reabsorption. Glomerular filtration rate is allometrically scalable in mammalian species, as is *p*-aminohippuric acid clearance (Edwards 1975; Holt and Rhode 1976). However, allometric scaling of active tubular secretion and tubular reabsorption have not been reported in the published literature.

The concept of metabolic or allometric scaling has been used as the basis for comparison across species since the 1930s. Benedict's *Vital Energetics* appears to be the first comprehensive discussion on the topic of metabolic scaling. Benedict's work laid the foundation for scaling of metabolic rates across a wide range of species. Metabolic rate for mammals was described by Kleiber (1932, 1961). Various physiologic processes such as heart rate, blood volume, and glomerular filtration rates can be predicted reasonably accurately for a wide variety of species based solely on the weight of the animal.

Linear extrapolation is the use of a single mg/kg dose across all species, so that the total amount of drug increases in a linear fashion as body weight increases. When dosages are extrapolated to other species of different weights, this method assumes that dosage versus weight is directly (linearly) proportional. This method assumes that differences in weight and in species pharmacokinetics are not clinically relevant. Although this is the simplest and most common method of extrapolation, it may overdose large animals and underdose small animals.

Metabolic scaling uses the ratio of a known physiologic process (i.e., metabolic rate) of two species to estimate a dosage in a species where there are no measured pharmacokinetic data. This method uses the dosage in a specific species and links the dosage to a physiological function instead of the animal's body weight (Dorrestein 2000; Mortenson 2001; Sedgwick 1993; Sedgwick and Borkowski 1996). In this method the chosen function forces an allometric (log-log) relationship, usually with an exponent of 0.6–0.8. The key assumption is that since most physiological functions follow allometric equations relative to body weight, pharmacological parameters must also follow similar allometric relationships, and to this end, basal metabolic rate is used as the universal scaling factor. This method of dose extrapolation provides a relatively smaller dose for large animals and a higher dose for small animals. A specific method for interspecies extrapolation of drug dosages used in the zoological medicine field is metabolic scaling as described by Sedgwick and others (Dorrestein 2000; Mortenson 2001; Sedgwick 1993; Sedgwick and Borkowski 1996). All species are placed in one of five groups, termed *Hainsworth's energy groups:* passerine birds, nonpasserine birds, placental mammals, marsupial mammals, or reptiles. Using a predetermined K value, a specific minimum energy cost (SMEC) value is calculated and the ratio of the target species SMEC to the SMEC of a safe effective dose in a known species is calculated to achieve that appropriate dosage regimen (Dorrestein 2000; Mortenson 2001; Sedgwick 1993; Sedgwick and Borkowski 1996). This method is simple in that the metabolic rate can be estimated for most species and applied to any pharmaceutical agent. A known drug dosage is multiplied by the ratio of metabolic rate of a known, similar species and the new species. Unfortunately, this method has not been well validated and several pharmacologic papers have illustrated specific failures in this method of extrapolation.

The allometric approach is to measure a pharmacokinetic parameter in multiple species and to plot the data against weight to derive a new allometric equation that can be used to estimate the pharmacokinetic parameter in an unknown species. Similar to its use for selecting the first time dose in humans (Boxenbaum and DiLea 1995), interspecies extrapolation serves an important function within the framework of veterinary medicine. In this regard, among its uses, it is especially important for estimating an appropriate dose in large animal species for which there does not exist pharmacokinetic or clinical information to support dose estimation. The caveat is that where first dose in humans is a prediction of a safe dose, in zoological medicine, the extrapolated dose in nonapproved species must be *both* safe and efficacious. Despite the potential for extrapolation error, the reality is that allometric scaling is needed across many veterinary practice situations and therefore will be used. For this reason, it is important to consider mechanisms for reducing the risk of extrapolation errors that can seriously affect target animal safety, therapeutic response, or the accuracy of withdrawal time predictions. Based upon this analysis, it appears that inclusion of at least one large animal in the scaling (with or without human data) can improve predictions (Mahmood et al. personal communication). In large animals, correction factors could not be applied because there was no trend seen between the exponents of the simple allometry and the appropriate correction factor for improving our predictions (Mahmood et al. personal communication). In addition, the vast majority of large animals for which pharmacokinetic data are available are herbivores. Conversely, the smaller animal species are either omnivores (mouse, rat, monkey, and human) or carnivores (dogs and cats). This difference in feeding behavior itself can influence drug metabolism and renal elimination. While large carnivore data (lion, tiger, polar bear, etc.) would be helpful, the obvious dangers hinder this area of research. Some marine mammal species may be worthy of consideration, but due to body fat composition of species, such as killer whales (*Orcinus orca*), the results would be of limited use. There is little way to predict, a priori, which animal species will be best suited for inclusion in the interspecies predictions. Another point of consideration is the interspecies differences in the contribution of various organ systems and differences in body composition as it pertains to the body weight estimates.

All extrapolation methods assume that the route of elimination is similar across all species used in the extrapolation and this is simply not true. The reality is that most drugs, 75% in Riviere's published data (Riviere et al. 1997) are not scalable across multiple species and that allometric scaling of pharmacokinetic parameters, while useful, has limitations. It is necessary, for the best therapeutic outcome, to have pharmacokinetic and efficacy data in each species that is treated in zoological medicine. The use of the available literature to understand the route of elimination and the extent of metabolism of therapeutic agents will greatly assist in determining allometric relationships of pharmacokinetic parameters. This should lead to more realistic and rational design of dosage regimens in zoological medicine.

"No presently available chemical restraint agent is equally effective and safe for use with all 45,000+ vertebrate species" (Fowler 1995). This statement relates not just to chemical restraint, but to therapeutic use in general within zoological medicine. Changes in minor species drug approval could make it easier for the needed information to get into the hands of veterinarians. The Minor Use and Minor Species Animal Health Act of 2004 (MUMS) has been enacted to address the lack of drug availability for minor species. This includes food animals, companion pets, wildlife, and zoo species. An increase in basic pharmacokinetic parameters in zoological species will increase the therapeutic options for veterinarians. Any pharmacokinetic or pharmacodynamic studies in these species would be welcomed.

Some of the specific needs for zoological medicine are formulations that would allow for administration of therapeutic agents via the drinking water or milled into the feed. Other routes of administration that have not been used to their full extent in zoological medicine are rectal, sustained or controlled release, and topical. Increased information and formulations that would allow for administration of appropriate therapeutic agents would be of great benefit. This chapter brings to light some of the issues that face veterinarians on a daily basis when they deal with nontraditional species. Clearly it is not economically feasible to develop every drug for every species. However, targeted approvals or research could greatly increase the efficacy and safety of current and future therapeutics. Also, this type of approach would increase the quality of care provided to zoological species.

REFERENCES

Antinoff, N., Bauck, L., Boyer, T., Brown, S., Harkness, J., and Sakas, P. (1999) Exotic Formulary, 2nd Edition, AAHA Press, Lakewood, CO.

Baert, K. and De Backer, P. (2003) Comparative pharmacokinetics of three non-steroidal anti-inflammatory drugs in five bird species. Comparative Biochemistry and Physiology Part C, 134, 25–33.

Boxenbaum, H. and DiLea, C. (1995) First-time-in-human dose selection: allometric thoughts and perspectives. Journal of Clinical Pharmacology, 35, 957–966.

Carpenter, J.W. (2005) Exotic Animal Formulary, 3rd Edition, Elsevier, Inc., St. Louis, MO.

Davis, L. (1996) Eat This Bug: A Guide to Invertebrate Live Foods for Reptiles & Amphibians, Hillview Press, Redwood City, CA.

Donoghue, S. and Langenberg, J. (1996) Nutrition. In D.R. Mader, (Ed.), Reptile Medicine and Surgery, W.B. Saunders Company, Philadelphia, PA., pp.148–174.

Dorrestein, G.M. (2000) Quick reference for drug dosing. In T.N. Tully, M.P.C. Lawton, G.M. Dorrestein (Eds.), Avian Medicine, Butterworth Heinemann, Oxford, United Kingdom, pp. 386–390.

Edwards, N.A. (1975) Scaling of renal functions in mammals. Comparative Biochemistry and Physiology, 52A, 63–66.

Fowler, M.E. (1995) Restraint and Handling of Wild and Domestic Animals, 2nd Edition, Iowa State University Press, Ames, IA.

Frazier, D.L., Jones, M.P., and Orosz, S.E. (1995) Pharmacokinetic considerations of the renal system in birds: Part I. Anatomic and physiologic principles of allometric scaling. Journal of Avian Medicine and Surgery, 9, 92–103.

Funk, R.S. (2000) A formulary for lizards, snakes, and crocodilians. Veterinary Clinics of North America: Exotic Animal Practice, 3, 333–358.

Haigh, J.C. (1990) Opioids in zoological medicine. Journal of Zoo and Wildlife Medicine, 21, 391–413.

Harrenstien, L.A., Tell, L.A., Vulliet, R., Needham, M., Brandt, C.M., Brondos, A., Stedman, B., and Kass, P.H. (2000) Disposition of enrofloxacin in red-tailed hawks (*Buteo jamaicensis*) and great horned owls (*Bubo virginianus*) after a single oral, intramuscular, or intravenous dose. Journal of Avian Medicine and Surgery, 14, 228–236.

Hawk, C.T. and Leary, S.L. (1999) Formulary for Laboratory Animals, 2nd Edition, Iowa State University Press, Ames, IA.

Holt, J.P. and Rhode, E.A. (1976) Similarity of renal glomerular hemodynamics in mammals. American Heart Journal, 92, 465–472.

Hunter, R.P. and Isaza, R. (2002) Zoological pharmacology: current status, issues, and potential. Advanced Drug Delivery Reviews, 54, 787–793.

Hunter, R.P., Isaza, R., and Koch, D.E. (2003a) The pharmacokinetics and oral bioavailability of racemic ketoprofen in Asian elephants (*Elephas maximus*). American Journal of Veterinary Research, 64, 109–114.

Hunter, R.P., Koch, D.E., Coke, R.L., Goatley, M.A., Isaza, and R. (2003b) Azithromycin metabolite identification in plasma, bile and tissues of the ball python (*Python regius*). Journal of Veterinary Pharmacology and Therapeutics, 26, 117–121.

Hunter, R.P., Isaza, R., Koch, D.E., Dodd, C.C., and Goatley, M.A. (2004a) The pharmacokinetics of topical doramectin in llamas (*Lama glama*) and alpacas (*Lama pacos*). Journal of Veterinary Pharmacology and Therapeutics, 27, 187–189.

———. (2004b) Moxidectin plasma concentrations following topical administration to llamas (*Lama glama*) and alpacas (*Lama pacos*). Small Ruminant Research, 52, 275–279.

Hunter, R.P., Isaza, R., Carpenter, J.W., and Koch, D.E. (2004c) Clinical effects and plasma concentrations of fentanyl after transmucosal administration in three species of great ape. Journal of Zoo & Wildlife Medicine, 35, 162–166.

Kleiber, M. (1932) Body size and metabolism. Hilgarida, 6, 315–353.

———. (1961) The fire of life. An introduction to animal energetics, Wiley, New York, NY.

Kreeger, T.J., Arnemo, J.M., and Raath, J.P. (2002) Handbook of Wildlife Chemical Immobilization, International Edition, Wildlife Pharmaceuticals, Inc., Fort Collins, CO.

Lightfoot, T.L. (2000) Therapeutics of African pygmy hedgehogs and prairie dogs. Veterinary Clinics of North America: Exotic Animal Practice, 3, 155–172.

Mader, D.R., Conzelman, G.M., and Baggot, J.D. (1985) Effects of ambient temperature on the half-life and dosage regimen of amikacin in the gopher snake. Journal of the American Veterinary Medical Association, 187, 1134–1136.

Mahmood, I. (2000) Can absolute oral bioavailability in humans be predicted from animals? A comparison of allometry and different indirect methods. Drug Metabolism and Drug Interactions, 16, 143–155.

———. (2002) Interspecies scaling: predicting oral clearance in humans. American Journal of Therapeutics, 9, 35–42.

Manire, C.A., Rhinehart, H.L., Pennick, G.J., Sutton, D.A., Hunter, R.P., and Rinaldi, M.G. (2003) Steady-state plasma concentrations of itraconazole following oral administration in Kemp's Ridley sea turtles, *Lepidochelys kempi*. Journal of Zoo & Wildlife Medicine, 34, 171–178.

Mortenson, J. (2001) Determining dosages for antibiotic and anti-inflammatory agents. In B. Csuti, E.L. Sargent, U.S. Bechert (Eds.), The Elephant's Foot: Prevention and Care of Foot Conditions in Captive Asian and African Elephants, Iowa State University Press, Ames, IA, pp. 141–144.

Nielsen, L. (1999) Chemical Immobilization of Wild and Exotic Animals, Iowa State University Press, Ames, IA.

Page, C.D., Mautino, M., Derendorf, H.D., and Anhalt, J.P. (1991) Comparative pharmacokinetics of trimethoprim-sulfamethoxazole administered intravenously and orally to captive elephants. Journal of Zoo and Wildlife Medicine, 22, 409–416.

Paul-Murphy, J. and Ludders, J.W. (2001) Avian analgesia. Veterinary Clinics of North America: Exotic Animal Practice, 4, 35–45.

Riviere, J.E., Martin-Jimenez, T., Sundlof, S.F., and Craigmill, A.L. (1997) Interspecies allometric analysis of the comparative pharmacokinetics of 44 drugs across veterinary and laboratory animal species. Journal of Veterinary Pharmacology & Therapeutics, 20, 453–463.

Rush, E.M., Hunter, R.P., Papich, M., Calle, P., Clippinger, T., Raphael, B., and Cook, R. (2005) Pharmacokinetics and safety of acyclovir in tragopans (*Tragopan* sp.). Journal of Avian Medicine & Surgery, 19, 271–276.

Sagara, K., Mizuta, H., Ohshiko, M., Shibata, M., and Haga, K. (1995) Relationship between the phasic period of interdigestive migrating contraction and the systemic bioavailability of acetaminophen in dogs. Pharmaceutical Research, 12, 594–598.

Sedgwick, C.J. (1993) Allometric scaling and emergency care: the importance of body size. In M.E. Fowler (Ed.), Zoo & Wild Animal Medicine, 3rd edition, W.B. Saunders Company, Philadelphia, PA, pp. 34–37.

Sedgwick, C.J. and Borkowski, R. (1996) Allometric scaling: extrapolating treatment regimens for reptiles. In D.R. Mader (Ed.), Reptile Medicine and Surgery, W.B. Saunders Company, Philadelphia, PA, pp. 235–241.

Short, C.R. (1994) Consideration of sheep as a minor species: comparison of drug metabolism and disposition with other domestic ruminants. Veterinary and Human Toxicology, 36, 24–40.

Sundlof, S.F., Riviere, J.E., and Craigmill, A.L. (1992) Food Animal Residue Avoidance Databank Trade Name File, 8th Edition, University of Florida, Gainesville, FL.

Walker, C.H. (1998) Avian forms of cytochrome P450. Comparative Biochemistry and Physiology Part C, 121, 65–72.

Walker, I.D.F. and Whitaker, B.R. (2000) Amphibian therapeutics. Veterinary Clinics of North America: Exotic Animal Practice, 3, 239–255.

West, L.J., Pierce, C.M., and Thomas, W.D. (1962) Lysergic acid diethylamide: its effects on a male Asiatic elephant. Science, 138, 1100–1103.

Xia, C.Q., Xiao, G., Liu, N., Pimprale, S., Fox, L., Patten, C.J., Crespi, C.L., Miwa, G., and Gan, L.-S. (2006) Comparison of species differences of p-glycoproteins in beagle dog, rhesus monkey, and human using ATPase activity assays. Molecular Pharmaceutics, 3, 78–86.

WEBSITES OF INTEREST

FARAD: http://www.farad.org

MUMsR$_x$: http://www.nrsp-7.org/mumsrx/

Elephant Care International: http://www.elephantcare.org/

Association of Reptilian and Amphibian Veterinarians: http://www.arav.org/Default.htm

American Association of Zoo Veterinarians: http://www.aazv.org/

Association of Avian Veterinarians: http://www.aav.org/

International Association for Aquatic Animal Medicine: http://www.iaaam.org/

MUMS act: http://www.fda.gov/cvm/minortoc.htm

SECTION 12

Regulatory Considerations

CHAPTER

54

LEGAL CONTROL OF VETERINARY DRUGS

STEPHEN F. SUNDLOF

LEGISLATIVE MILESTONES IN THE DEVELOPMENT OF LAWS PERTAINING TO THE REGULATION OF ANIMAL DRUGS

There are indications that the regulation of drugs in America began with the earliest colonies. For example, records of the Massachusetts Bay Colony tell of Nicholas Knopf, who in 1630 was sentenced to pay a fine or be whipped for selling "a water of no worth nor value" as a cure for scurvy. However, federal controls over drugs did not begin until 1848, when the Import Drug Act was passed to stop the adulteration of quinine used to treat American troops who had contracted malaria in Mexico. The Import Drug Act was the first federal statute to guarantee the quality of medicines, and US Customs laboratories were established to administer the law. The mission of the new Customs laboratories was to enforce the purity and potency standards of the *US Pharmacopeia,* which had been compiled in 1820 by trade and professional leaders. Subsequently support dwindled and the program gradually faded away. There was no organizational connection with the agency now known as the Food and Drug Administration.

The first state pure food and drug law was passed by California in 1850. During subsequent years many other states enacted similar legislation, but the need for regulation on an interstate basis was becoming more and more evident.

In 1880, Peter Collier, chief of the Division of Chemistry, US Department of Agriculture (USDA), began advocating enactment of a national food and drug law. In 1883 Dr. Harvey W. Wiley succeeded Collier as chief chemist and continued and broadened his efforts advocating a national food and drug law. Initially there was little interest in this kind of reform. Advocates were generally regarded as cranks and radicals. Over 100 bills were to be introduced in the US Congress before the first Federal Food and Drugs Act (and the Meat Inspection Act) of 1906 was enacted.

Conditions in the drug industry can scarcely be imagined today. The great advances in bacteriology were just beginning to have an impact on infectious diseases. Milk was still unpasteurized and cows were not tested for tuberculosis. Thousands of so-called patent medicines such as Kickapoo Sagwa Renovator for Stomach, Liver, and Kidney; Dr. Shreve's Anti-Gallstone Remedy; and Hamlin's Wizard Oil—Cures All Pain in Man or Beast flooded the marketplace. "Medicine-men" competed with circuses, minstrel shows, and "Wild West" shows to entertain the public and sell their products. Medicines containing opium, morphine, heroin, and cocaine were sold without restriction and without even any indication of the presence of the drugs in the product. Preparations that were otherwise harmless, other perhaps than being alcohol based, were labeled for the cure of every disease or symptom of man and beast. Labels did not list ingredients, and warnings against misuse were virtually nonexistent. Of course, such practices were by no means universal, and many firms were producing reliable and wholesome products. However, there was no lack of material for investigation and disclosure by Dr. Wiley's chemists. In order to generate support for his cause, Dr. Wiley took their findings to the public, speaking frequently at women's clubs and civic and business organizations. Crusading reporters (muckrakers), organized women's clubs, and farsighted businessmen became his strong supporters. In 1903, Dr. Wiley captured the attention of the public by establishing his now famous volunteer "poison squad" of young men who agreed to eat only foods treated with measured amounts of chemical preservatives, in order to evaluate the safety of such products. Thanks to the publicity engendered by Dr. Wiley's work, public concern began to build. It reached a climax with the publication of Upton Sinclair's book *The Jungle,* a brutally graphic novel, which focused national attention on the unsanitary conditions in U.S. meat packing plants. As a result the first federal food and drug law, the Food and Drugs Act of 1906, was passed by Congress and signed into law by President Theodore Roosevelt on June 30, 1906.

Basically the law banned from interstate commerce any traffic in adulterated or misbranded food or drugs. The act defined "drug" to include all medicines and preparations recognized in the *US Pharmacopeia* or *National Formulary* for internal or external use and any substance or mixture of substances intended to be used for the cure, mitigation, or prevention of disease in either humans or other animals.

Drugs were to be deemed "adulterated" if they were sold under or by a name recognized in the official compendia (the *US Pharmacopeia* and the *National Formulary*) but failed to meet the standards set forth therein, except that a recognized drug not meeting the official standard would not be deemed adulterated if it met its own standard of strength, quality, and purity as stated on the container. A drug was deemed "misbranded" if the label bore any statement, design, or device regarding the contents which was false or misleading, or if the drug was falsely branded as to the state, territory, or country in which it was manufactured. Drugs would also be misbranded if they were an imitation of, or offered for sale under the name of, another article or if the original contents had been removed in whole or in part and/or other contents added. Drugs would also be misbranded if their labels failed to disclose any quantities of alcohol, narcotics, and other specified substances present in the product.

Although the 1906 law represented a great step forward, there were obvious weaknesses. In 1911, the Supreme Court ruled that the labeling provisions of the act prohibited *only* false statements about the identity of the drug product but not false therapeutic claims. The Congress responded by passing the Shirley Amendment of 1912, which outlawed false *and fraudulent* curative or therapeutic claims. Under the Shirley Amendment, the government was required to prove that a false claim was also fraudulent, that is, that the promoter *intended* to deceive the purchaser. A defendant had only to show that he personally believed in his patent medicine to escape prosecution. This remained a major weakness in the law for 26 years.

The USDA's Bureau of Chemistry enforced the law until 1927, when the bureau was reorganized in order to separate law enforcement functions from agricultural research and development. The Food, Drug, and Insecticide Administration was formed. It was renamed the Food and Drug Administration (FDA) in 1931, and in 1940 the FDA was transferred from the USDA to the Federal Security Agency, in order to eliminate recurring conflicts between consumer interests and producer interests. In 1953, the Federal Security Agency became the Department of Health, Education. and Welfare—now the Department of Health and Human Services (DHHS).

An interesting side note: FDA's budget (appropriations), because of its origins in the USDA, comes through the House and Senate Agricultural Appropriations committees. Amendments to the Federal Food, Drug, and Cosmetic Act, however, come under the jurisdiction of the Senate Committee on Labor and Human Resources and the House Committee on Energy and Commerce.

By the early 1930s it was evident that there were serious shortcomings in the 1906 act. False advertising in print and on the radio was blatant, and manufacturers had found many ways to circumvent the law. Technological advancements were revolutionizing the production and marketing of foods, drugs, and related products, making the 1906 law obsolete.

In 1933 Walter Campbell, then chief of the FDA, seized an opportunity to work with Rexford Tugwell a member of newly elected president Franklin D. Roosevelt's "brain trust" who had been appointed assistant secretary of agriculture, in developing a complete revision of the Food and Drugs Act. When the resulting "Tugwell bill" was introduced in Congress, it was a legislative disaster. Opposition to this New Deal legislation by industry and advertising interests was total. This was due in part to Rexford Tugwell's reputation in the business community and to some extent in Congress. The Columbia University economics professor, who believed in and advocated a planned economy, was greatly feared in business circles. The Senate sponsor of the bill, Royal S. Copeland, M.D., of New York, aided by FDA officials, consumer-minded congressmen, attorneys, and staffers, began the laborious process that was to become a bitter 5-year battle for new legislation.

As before, public opinion was to play a major role in pushing Congress to act, and again organized clubwomen were very important in generating and molding public support. Public opinion was aroused by a shocking and tragic drug disaster that resulted in more than 100 deaths. The drug involved was "Elixir of Sulfanilamide," sulfanilamide dissolved in diethylene glycol. Sulfanilamide had only recently become available, and salesmen reported that there was a demand for a liquid form. Since sulfanilamide is poorly soluble in water. The manufacturer dissolved the drug in diethylene glycol and added coloring and flavoring. The solution was tested for flavor, appearance, and fragrance, but since existing laws did not require manufacturers to demonstrate that their products were safe, no safety or toxicity testing was done. Before the product could be identified and recalled it had claimed 107 lives in 15 states from Virginia to California.

Shortly after the sulfanilamide disaster, Congress adopted portions of the Copeland bill and it was passed as the Federal Food, Drug, and Cosmetic Act (FFD&C Act) of 1938, also referred to as the Copeland Act. Under the 1938 act, interstate commerce in a new drug (for humans or animals) was prohibited unless it had been adequately tested to show that it was safe for use under the conditions of use prescribed on its label. Thus, it was illegal to ship a drug across state lines unless it had been shown to be safe. An exemption to this requirement was provided for a drug intended solely for investigational use by qualified scientific experts.

The 1938 act also required labels to bear adequate directions for use and to include warnings against unsafe use, where drugs (or devices) might be injurious to health. It required official drugs to be packaged and labeled as prescribed by the official compendia; required the labels of nonofficial drugs to list active ingredients; and required precautionary labeling of drugs subject to deterioration. Note that the 1938 act still did not require demonstrated proof of effectiveness of drugs.

The new law, and World War II, greatly expanded the FDA's workload. This period was characterized by the development of many new "wonder drugs," especially antibiotics, which were made subject to FDA testing beginning with penicillin in 1945. Fortunately the law required premarket approval of new drugs, but there were no premarket clearance requirements for a host of new chemicals of unknown safety. The law prohibited poisonous substances but provided no requirement that food ingredients be shown to be safe. The law did provide for exemptions and establishment of safe tolerances for unavoidable or necessary poisons such as pesticides, but when the FDA attempted to set a pesticide tolerance, the courts ruled that the lengthy procedure required by law was unworkable. The FDA was able to stop the use of known poisons where they posed a hazard (and did so in many cases) but the vast research effort needed to ensure that all food chemicals were safe was clearly beyond available resources. During the 1940s there was a substantial increase in the use of commercial pesticides in the growing of agricultural products and in the use of chemicals for flavoring, coloring, preserving, and packaging of processed foods. In 1950, the House of Representatives adopted a resolution creating a Select Committee to Investigate the Use of Chemicals in Foods. Representative James T. Delaney of New York served as its chairman. The committee began extensive hearings that were to go on for 2 years. As a result of the committee's work and the work of the FDA and others, three very significant amendments to the FFD&C Act were enacted: the Pesticide Amendment (1954), the Food Additives Amendment (1958), and the Color Additives Amendment (1960).

The Food Additives Amendment of 1958 was particularly significant in terms of its impact on the regulation of animal drugs since animal drugs approved for use in food animals were considered to be food additives and thus had to meet not only the drug standards of the act but also the food additive standards. Further, since the 1958 amendment required the pre-market clearance of food additives, this meant that for the first time, sponsors of drugs indicated for use in food animals were required to demonstrate, as a condition of approval, the safety to humans of any residues present in food products derived from treated animals. A direct result of this provision has been the development, within veterinary pharmacology and toxicology, of a whole new subdiscipline, that of residue sciences.

This was also significant because it brought animal drugs for use in food animals under the provisions of the "Delaney anticancer clause," which provided that no additive will be deemed to be safe if it is found to induce cancer in humans or animals. The Delaney anticancer clause as it applied to animal drugs was amended in 1962 to include a provision that permits administration of a compound known to induce cancer in humans or animals to food-producing animals when it has been shown that "no residue" will occur in food products. Specifically, this exception, known as the DES Proviso required that no residue will be found by methods of examination prescribed or approved by the secretary of the DHHS. Initially, the "no residue" provision was met simply by applying the most sensitive analytical methods available. However, it was recognized in doing so that "no residue" did not mean "zero residue" but rather was defined by the sensitivity of the analytical method employed. This was unacceptable. As a result, FDA developed a regulation commonly referred to as the Sensitivity-of-Method procedure, or SOM, now known as the animal drug safety policy, which defined "no residue" in terms of the level of residue that presents an insignificant risk of cancer to the consuming public. The safe level is then described with a finite number in parts per million (ppm) or parts per billion (ppb).

The regulation defines an insignificant risk of cancer as a 1 in 1 million increase in risk over the normal lifetime risk of cancer. Further, the regulation spells out how the level of residue that represents an insignificant risk of cancer is determined. The method to be used in monitoring for residues of the compound then must be sensitive enough to detect the level of residue determined to represent an insignificant risk.

During this period two other amendments to the FFD&C Act were to have a significant impact on veterinary medicine. The first was the Durham-Humphrey Amendment of 1951, which for the first time defined the kinds of drugs for human use that may be dispensed by a pharmacist only upon the prescription of a "practitioner licensed by law to administer such drugs." This was very significant because it created and defined the category of prescription drugs. Under previous law, a drug manufacturer decided whether a given drug would be available by prescription or over the counter. The language of the Durham-Humphrey Amendment specifically restricted the term "prescription" to drugs and medical devices for human use by replacing a section of the 1938 FFD&C Act that contained explicit reference to a "prescription signed by a physician, dentist, or veterinarian." Language in both the Senate and House reports that accompanied the amendment, however, recognized the need for a similar category of "prescription" animal drugs, which the FDA had established by regulation. The FDA's authority to restrict a drug to use "by or on the order of a licensed veterinarian" has been upheld by the courts on several occasions, but statutory recognition of the prescription provision pertaining to animal drugs was not codified in the law until the enactment of the Generic Animal Drug Patent Term Restoration Act of 1988.

The Kefauver-Hams Drug Amendments of 1962 were also to have a significant impact on veterinary medicine. The Drug Amendments of 1962, like the 1938 act, were enacted into law following a disaster involving drugs: the "thalidomide disaster." Thalidomide, a sedative that was prescribed to pregnant women, is a potent teratogen causing severe deformities called phocomelia. Although the FDA never approved thalidomide for commercial marketing in the United States, it was distributed to selected doctors for experimental purposes, and it was approved and widely used in Europe.

The 1962 amendments extended, expanded, and strengthened the FDA's regulatory authority with respect to drugs. For the first time manufacturers were required to provide "substantial evidence" of the effectiveness of new drugs, as well as of their safety, as a condition of approval. Labeling now had a material bearing on the matter of new drug approval in that it must not be false or misleading in any particular. With respect to drugs already on the market, the manufacturer was required to report promptly to the FDA any information concerning adverse effects and other clinical experience or data relating in any way to safety and effectiveness.

Relative to effectiveness, the amendments also included a provision that enabled the FDA to require an effectiveness review of every new drug introduced between 1938 and 1962. The program, which began in the late 1960s, was called the Drug Efficacy Study Implementation (DESI) program. As a result of the DESI program, many older products, particularly those with multiple ingredients, were removed from the market. Those products remaining had labeling claims that could be substantiated through adequate studies and thus met the FDA standard for effectiveness. In 1968, legislation was passed to consolidate provisions of the FFD&C Act with respect to the regulation of animal drugs. Prior to 1968 the act generally did not distinguish between human drugs and animal drugs. Both the House and the Senate reports on the amendment pointed out that, in many cases, the requirements for clearance of new animal drugs were more complicated than the clearance procedures for drugs for humans. This was because animal drugs indicated for use in food animals were required to meet not only the drug standards of the act but also the food additives standards. In fact, ensuring that food products from animals treated with a particular animal drug pose no risk to public health is often the most expensive and time-consuming part of the developmental process for a new animal drug intended for use in food animals.

It is important to note two additional aspects of food and drug legislation. First, the Food Additive Amendments of 1958 included language prohibiting the use of an animal drug other than in accord with its approved uses. This reflected congressional concern for human food safety, but it also made extralabel drug use in animals illegal under the act. At the same time Congress was operating on the principle that animal drugs should be routinely available to farmers to treat their animals, i.e., to protect their property. The act requires that for an animal drug to be legally marketed in the United States, it must bear adequate directions for use by a layperson. Animal drugs that do not or cannot bear such directions for use are considered to be misbranded. The FDA, as noted above had recognized the need for an exception to this requirement and had, by regulation, provided for the marketing of "prescription" animal drugs which could be used safely by or on the order of a licensed veterinarian, but for which adequate directions for lay use cannot be written.

The congressional bias in favor of the availability of animal drugs direct to farmers was to have a profound effect on the drug development and approval process and ultimately on veterinary pharmacology in the United States. It is reflected in the history of the FDA approvals of drugs for food animals. Even after establishing a category of prescription animal drugs in 1988, most drugs approved for food animals, with the exception of therapeutic antimicrobial agents, are classified as over-the-counter (OTC), whereas most drugs approved for companion animals are classified as prescription.

This focus on OTC drugs (and the attendant need to be able to provide labeling that can be reasonably followed by laypersons) has led to the approval of OTC drugs that are labeled for very specific and limited indications and that have directions for use which provide little or no flexibility in how the product can be used. As a result, there are many animal species for which there are no drugs approved, and for others the number of approved drugs is very limited and may not include drugs such as anesthetics, antiinflammatory agents, or other drugs with low market potential.

Faced with an insufficient armamentarium of drugs approved for all of the various animal species-disease combinations encountered in veterinary practice, veterinarians historically have exercised considerable judgment in utilizing therapeutic agents, often going beyond the limits of approved labeling. Prior to 1994, veterinarians who engaged in extralabel drug use technically were in violation of federal law, unlike their physician counterparts, who were not prohibited by the act from using or prescribing drugs for use in humans as they deemed appropriate. In spite of the fact that the act clearly specifies that an animal drug must be used in strict accordance with the indications and directions for use contained in its labeling, FDA policy was very permissive in this regard.

During the late 1970s and early 1980s the FDA recognized the need for a more structured policy regarding such use, one that would define the conditions under which such use would not ordinarily result in regulatory action while at the same time drawing attention to the responsibilities incurred by the veterinary practitioner electing to use a drug in an extralabel fashion, especially in a food-producing animal. The policy took the form of a Compliance Policy Guide (CPG). CPGs are used to provide guidance regarding regulatory initiatives and enforcement priorities to FDA field and headquarters personnel. CPG 7125.06, titled "Extra-Label Use of New Animal Drugs in Food-Producing Animals," communicated the FDA's recognition that the extralabel use of a drug in food-producing animals may be considered by a veterinarian when the health of animals is immediately threatened and suffering or death would result from failure to treat the affected animal(s). In instances of this nature, regulatory action would not ordinarily be considered provided that several criteria were met (see Chapter 61).

The FDA also recognized that in the case of companion animals (nonfood animals) veterinarians had become reliant on a number of drugs approved for use in humans but for which no counterparts were approved for use in animals. Examples of human drugs widely used in companion animals include digitalis derivatives, insulin, and anticancer drugs. CPG 7125.35, "Human Drugs Distributed to Veterinarians for Use in Animals," basically provides that as long as such distribution of a human drug is initiated (ordered) by a licensed veterinarian and is *not* intended for use in food-producing animals, the FDA would *not* ordinarily consider regulatory action. However, it should be noted that the manufacturers are *not* permitted to advertise or otherwise promote the use of human-labeled drugs for use in animals.

Although CPGs generally discourage the use of human drugs in food animals, certain exceptions are recognized. These include certain poison antidotes, insulin for use in the treatment of ketosis, and certain anesthetics and analgesics for use in surgical cases and for relief of pain and suffering.

Despite the efforts of the FDA to establish policies that recognized the needs of animals while protecting the public's health, such policies were based on the agency's authority to exercise discretion in deciding whether to enforce certain provisions of the act. The fact that the FDA elected not to take enforcement actions against veterinarians who administered drugs in an extralabel manner in no way conferred legal status to such practices. Concerned by the notion that veterinarians, unlike the members of any other licensed profession, were forced to repeatedly break the law in order to responsibly carry out their professional duties, the American Veterinary Medical Association actively petitioned Congress to amend the act.

In 1994, Congress, in an effort to decriminalize the everyday practice of veterinary medicine, passed the Animal Medicinal Drug Use Clarification Act of 1994. This law allows licensed veterinarians to use and prescribe, under specified conditions, animal and human drugs for extralabel purposes. In general the law is intended to codify in law and regulations the conditions and restrictions for extralabel use provided in CPG 7125.06 and CPG 7125.35 as outlined above. It also recognized compounding of animal drugs from FDA-approved human or animal drugs as a form of extralabel drug use. Such compounding is permissible by a veterinarian or a pharmacist on the order of a veterinarian provided that 1) there is no approved new animal or new human drug that, when used as labeled and in the available dosage form and concentration, appropriately treats the condition diagnosed; 2) the compounding is performed by a licensed pharmacist or veterinarian within the scope of a professional practice; 3) adequate procedures and processes are followed that ensure the safety and effectiveness of the compounded product; 4) the scale of the compounding operation is commensurate with the established need for compounded products (e.g., similar to that of comparable practices); and 5) all relevant state laws relating to the compounding of drugs for use in animals are followed. Compounding from a human drug for use in food-producing animals is not permitted if an approved animal drug can be used for compounding. Compounding from bulk drugs is not permitted under the act; however, the FDA on occasion has exercised regulatory discretion in allowing compounding from bulk drugs where the need was great and the risk to animals and the public was small. Additional information on compounding of drugs for use in animals is published in CPG 7125.40.

Although the Animal Medicinal Drug Use Clarification Act provided psychological relief to veterinarians by codifying into law practices previously permitted by the FDA under more tenuous compliance policy guides, it did not address the underlying problem that necessitated extralabel use: the insufficiency of drugs available to treat animals. This sentiment was reflected in the Congressional Record immediately following passage of the bill in the Senate. At that time Senator Coates of Indiana stated that the bill "does nothing to expedite the review process of the FDA and CVM. Through future legislative initiatives, we now need to address the animal drug availability deficiencies." Shortly after the passage of the Animal Medicinal Drug Use Clarification Act, the Coalition for Animal Health formed with the purpose of increasing the availability of animal drugs through statutory changes to the FFD&C Act. The Coalition, made up of veterinarians, animal producer organizations, the animal feed industry, and the animal drug industry, drafted proposed legislation, which eventually was signed into law on October 9, 1996. The Animal Drug Availability Act (ADAA) introduced major reforms in the way that the FDA evaluates and approves new animal drugs. These reforms are intended to facilitate the approval of new animal drugs and medicated feeds by building greater flexibility into the existing animal drug review processes. Such flexibility does not compromise the FDA's authority to ensure that animal drugs are safe for the animal patient and for the public consuming animal-derived foods.

Most of the reform measures brought about by the ADAA addressed the standard for determining whether a new animal drug is effective for its specified conditions of use. The FFD&C Act provides that the FDA may refuse to approve a new animal drug if it finds that there is a lack of *substantial evidence* that the drug will have the effect it claims under the conditions of use prescribed recommended. or suggested in the proposed labeling. Prior to ADAA the FDA had interpreted the phrase *substantial evidence* in fairly rigid terms, requiring a fixed minimum number of field studies (generally three) conducted at geographically distinct locations. (Field studies are clinical studies conducted under conditions that closely approximate the condition under which the new animal drug, if approved, is intended to be applied or administered.) With the changes effected by the ADAA it is now possible that even a single *adequate and well-controlled* study may provide substantial evidence of effectiveness. Furthermore in certain cases a field investigation may not be necessary to allow the FDA to conclude that the drug is effective.

The ADAA further allowed the FDA to redefine the phrase "adequate and well-controlled" as it applies to field investigations. Because field studies are conducted under field conditions (e.g., on farms or commercial livestock production facilities) it is recognized that the level of control over some study conditions need not or should not be the same as the level of control in laboratory studies. Under the ADAA, the FDA will balance the need to control study conditions with the need to observe the true effect of the drug under closely approximated actual-use conditions in determining whether a field study is adequate and well controlled.

Prior to the ADAA, products containing two or more drugs (combination drugs) were required to meet the same rigorous standard for effectiveness as products containing a single drug, even when the individual drugs in the combination product had been previously proven to be effective. The ADAA streamlined the process for approving a combination new animal drug if each of the drugs used in the combination has been previously approved separately for the uses for which it is intended in the combination. In such cases, additional studies for effectiveness and animal safety are often not required.

The FFD&C Act required that the FDA approve new animal drugs based on the concept of a single optimal dose (i.e., a single dosage that does not exceed the amount reasonably required to accomplish the drug's intended effect). This "optimal dose" concept left little flexibility for veterinarians to exercise professional judgment in the treatment of their patients. Furthermore, for certain drugs such as antimicrobial and antiparasitic agents, the approved "optimal dose" may become ineffective over time. Determining the optimal dose is a time-consuming and costly practice requiring pharmaceutical companies to conduct dose titration studies. The ADAA amended the FFD&C Act to allow the FDA to approve any effective dosage regimen as long as it is safe for the patient and does not result in a residue that exceeds the tolerance (see Chapter 61 on Chemical Residues in Tissues of Food Animals). Labeling animal drug products with dosage ranges rather than a single fixed dose allows veterinarians to select a dosing regimen tailored to the specific needs of each patient.

The ADAA defined an entirely new class of drugs differentiating them from over-the-counter and prescription classifications. Veterinary Feed Directive (VFD) drugs are intended for use in or on animal feed and are limited by approved application to use under the professional supervision of a licensed veterinarian. Previously, all feed additive drugs were available through over-the-counter channels. VFD drugs and animal feeds containing them must be labeled with a cautionary statement, and an animal feed containing a VFD drug can be used only by a licensed veterinarian or upon the lawful VFD issued by a licensed veterinarian. Because veterinary supervision is required the VFD classification allows the FDA to approve potent new therapeutic drugs for administration to animals via feed.

The Animal Drug User Fee Act of 2003 (ADUFA) authorized FDA to collect fees from pharmaceutical firms in support of the review of new animal drugs. The law authorizes the collection of fees to enable FDA to hire and train additional scientific reviewers and implement enhanced processes to accelerate and improve the review process. This law is intended to help FDA expedite and improve its review of applications for new animal drugs so that safe and effective new products will be available more quickly. Specifically, the law requires the FDA to continuously reduce the time it takes to review drug applications.

FDA anticipates that ADUFA will bring substantial savings to the animal drug industry in regulatory review and developmental expenses. A faster, more predictable review process is expected to spur more research and development by the animal drug industry.

The law also requires the agency to adopt administrative processes to ensure that review times for generic animal drugs (which are not assessed user fees) do not increase due to activities under ADUFA.

The Minor Use and Minor Species Animal Health Act of 2004 (MUMS) provides innovative, flexible ways to make drugs available to treat minor animal species as well as uncommon diseases in the major animal species. It is designed to help pharmaceutical companies overcome the financial burdens they face in providing limited-demand animal drugs. By making more drugs available for minor species, the law is expected to benefit certain agricultural groups, zoo and wildlife veterinarians, and owners of pets other than cats and dogs. The new law modifies provisions of the Federal Food, Drug, and Cosmetic Act in three key ways, providing for the following:

1. *Conditional Approval:* The sponsor of a minor use or minor species veterinary drug can ask FDA for "conditional approval," which allows the sponsor to market the drug after that proving the drug is safe and establishing a reasonable expectation of effectiveness, but before collecting all the effectiveness data needed to support a full approval. The drug sponsor can keep the product on the market for up to 5 years, through annual renewals, while gathering the required effectiveness data for full approval.
2. *Indexing:* The law gives FDA authority to add a minor species drug to an index of unapproved new animal drugs that may be legally marketed when the potential market for the drug is too small to support the costs of the drug approval process, even under a conditional approval. This provision will be especially helpful to veterinarians treating zoo or endangered animals, and to owners of minor pet species such as ornamental fish or caged reptiles, birds, or mammals.
3. *Designation:* This aspect of the law provides incentives for minor use or minor species drug approvals, such as grants to support safety and effectiveness testing. Sponsors must apply for designation prior to filing a new animal drug application for FDA approval. At the time that a designated drug gains approval or conditional approval, it is awarded 7 years of exclusive marketing rights, which means that FDA will not approve another application for the same drug in the same dosage form for the same intended use until after the 7 years have elapsed. This is 2–4 years longer than the protection provided from generic copying of nondesignated drugs.

Another area of drug regulation directly affecting the veterinarian is the Comprehensive Drug Abuse Prevention and Control Act of 1970 commonly called the Controlled Substances Act (CSA). At the turn of the century in the United States, opium, morphine, cocaine, and other such drugs were freely available to the public. In fact, as noted previously, many of the nostrums and patent medicines available at that time contained such drugs even though labels gave no hint of their presence. Although the Food and Drugs Act of 1906 required that the presence of such substances be specified on labels, it was clear that the ready availability of such substances had to be restricted. Thus, in 1914, the Congress enacted the Harrison Narcotic Act, which restricted narcotic drugs such as the opiates, cocaine, and ecgonine and any substances containing such compounds to legitimate medical uses. These drugs could be dispensed by pharmacists only on the basis of a prescription written by a veterinarian, physician, or dentist who was registered with the US Treasury Department. It later became apparent that there were dangers inherent in the distribution and use of many nonnarcotic drugs. Accordingly, in 1965, drug abuse amendments to control traffic in barbiturates, amphetamines, and other abused drugs were added to the FFD&C Act. In 1968, the FDA's Bureau of Drug Abuse Control was transferred to the Department of Justice, where it was consolidated, along with the Treasury Department's Bureau of Narcotics, into the current Drug Enforcement Administration (DEA).

Under the 1970 act, controlled substances include opiates, barbiturates, hallucinogens. methadone, stimulants such as amphetamines, and other addictive or habituating drugs. This act regulates the manufacturing, distribution, and dispensing of controlled substances by providing for a closed system of registered people (manufacturers and distributors, pharmacists, licensed practitioners, and others) authorized to handle such compounds. A veterinarian licensed to practice by a state and wishing to use or prescribe controlled substances must register annually with the DEA. Controlled drugs and drug products are categorized in five schedules, and an applicant requests certification for those schedules or categories of drugs that he or she expects to purchase, store, dispense, and use. The registered person or hospital is given a DEA certificate for display, a registration number, and official forms that must be used in ordering and purchasing controlled substances. The registration number must be used on all prescriptions and order forms. Registrants (and those authorized under a registration) must keep accurate records of orders, receipts, and uses of controlled substances. Current inventory must be reconcilable with amounts received and used or dispensed. All records and activities are subject to inspection by DEA personnel at any time. Both the veterinarian and the pharmacist are legally responsible for the proper prescribing and dispensing of drugs covered by the CSA. Further, controlled substances must be stored in a locked cabinet or preferably in a safe secured to a concrete floor.

The manufacturers and distributors are required to identify a controlled substance on the label of original containers by a symbol corresponding to the schedules specified by DEA for each controlled substance. The symbol is a capital C (for controlled substance), followed by the Roman numeral (I–V) corresponding to the schedule to which the substance is assigned.

Schedule I drugs have a high abuse potential and are not currently accepted in the United States for use in any practice situation, although they may be obtained for research or instructional use. Examples are heroin, LSD, mescaline, marijuana, methaqualone, and peyote.

Schedule II drugs have a high abuse potential, their use can produce severe psychic or physical dependence in humans, and they apparently have similar effects in animals. These are the former Class A narcotic drugs plus certain stimulant drugs. Examples are opium, morphine, hydromorphone (Dilaudid), cocaine, methadone, meperidine (Demerol), fentanyl, and cocaine; and the barbiturates amobarbital (Amytal), pentobarbital (Nembutal), and secobarbital (Seconal) and their salts. The amphetamines are no longer available under Schedule II for veterinary use.

Schedule III drugs have less abuse potential than those in Schedules I and II. Abusive use of Schedule III drugs leads to moderate or low physical dependence but often high psychological dependence in humans. Examples of Schedule III drugs include anabolic steroids such as stanozolol (Winstrol), trenbolone (Finaplix), and testosterone; some opioids such as nalorphine (Nalline) and opium combination products (e.g., Paregoric); some barbiturates that are not classified in Schedule I or II such as thiamylal (Surital) and thiopental (Pentothal); and some nonnarcotic drugs such as tiletamine and zolazepam combination products (e.g., Telazol), phencyclidine, ketamine, and benzphetamine.

Schedule IV drugs have a low abuse potential that can lead to limited physical or psychological dependence in humans. Included here are barbital, phenobarbital, methylphenobarbital, chloral hydrate, butorphanol, meprobamate (Miltown, Equanil), chlordiazepoxide (Librium), and diazepam (Valium).

Schedule V drugs have a lesser abuse potential and include some codeine and dihydrocodeine preparations (Robitussin A, Cophene-S), diphenoxylate preparations (Lomotil), and others.

Anabolic steroids were added to the list of controlled substances in 1991 under the Anabolic Steroids Control Act (ASCA). Certain veterinary products fall under the ASCA and have been classified as Schedule III drugs under the CSA. These products include boldenone, mibolerone, stanozolol, testosterone, and trenbolone and their salts, esters, and isomers. Estrogens and progesterones are not subject to the ASCA or the CSA.

Anabolic steroid implants in the final dosage form, if expressly intended for use in cattle or other nonhuman species in accordance with their approvals under the FFD&C Act, are exempted from the scheduling requirements. However, any person or firm engaged or proposing to engage in the production of such implants must comply with the Schedule III requirements of the CSA and must register with the DEA.

DRUG COMPENDIA

It is critically important to the veterinarian, pharmacist, and physician and their patients and clients that the drugs they employ are of uniform potency, purity, and quality. Without such standardization, rational pharmacotherapy would be impossible. Such assurance is a basic objective of the laws and regulations described above and is the purpose of the *US Pharmacopoeia* (USP)-*National Formulary* (NF). The USP-NF is the legally recognized drug compendium for the United States. The USP was originally compiled and first published in 1820 and has been regularly and continuously revised by the US Pharmacopeial Convention, which is composed of elected delegates representing human medicine, pharmacy, veterinary medicine, dentistry, and nursing. The National Formulary was a separate official compendium published by the American Pharmaceutical Association to serve the need of pharmacists for standardization of certain pure drugs that were not used widely enough to be included in the USP. During the 1975–80 USP revision period these two official compendia were "unified" into a single USP-NF compendium. At that time the scope of the two components was changed in that the USP covered all drug substances and drug products, while the NF was devoted exclusively to pharmaceutic ingredients.

In addition to USP and NF designations, a drug may be given an International Nonproprietary Name (INN).

The USP and NF derive their official status from the FFD&C Act. Standards promulgated by the Committee of Revision of the USP Convention are enforceable by the FDA.

CHAPTER

55

DRUG APPROVAL PROCESS

MARILYN MARTINEZ, MELANIE BERSON, BERNADETTE DUNHAM, JOAN GOTTHARDT, AND LAURA HUNGERFORD

INTRODUCTION

The availability of new animal drugs for use in livestock, poultry, pets, and other animals is vital to protecting the health of animals, increasing the efficiency of food production, and protecting the health of humans who consume the products of food-producing animals. Appropriate use of animal drugs also enhances human health through prevention of zoonotic disease transmission, protection of the food supply, and preservation of the human-animal bond. Practical application of the principles of pharmacology is important for development of safe and effective animal drugs and for making the best use of these products during clinical practice. An understanding of considerations and regulatory constraints that guide the evaluation of veterinary pharmaceutical products by the US Food and Drug Administration (FDA) is vital for optimizing the animal drug development process and for using label information to customize treatments to match patient needs.

Section 512 of the Federal Food Drug and Cosmetic Act (FFDCA) provides the statutory provisions governing the regulation of veterinary products. Through this act, a new animal drug is considered to be unsafe unless there is in effect an approval of a New Animal Drug Application (NADA) and unless the use of a drug and its labeling conform to the approved application. The term *adulterated* can also apply to new animal drug products that are not the subject of an approved NADA or an Abbreviated NADA (ANADA). Virtually all animal drugs are *new animal drugs* within the meaning of the FFDCA, and are therefore subject to Section 512 (http://www.fda.gov/opacom/laws/fdcact/fdcact5a1.htm).

The url for the FDA home page is http://www.fda.gov and access to the Center for Veterinary Medicine (CVM) home page is obtained by selecting the **Animal & Veterinary** header located in the left column of the FDA website. Alternatively, you can go directly to the CVM home page using http://www.fda.gov/cvm. The regulations and policies governing FDA activities are published in the Federal Register. All FDA regulations are codified in Title 21 of the Code of Federal Regulations (CFR), which can be accessed from the FDA website at http://www.accessdata.fda.gov/scripts/cdrh/cfdocs/cfcfr/cfrsearch.cfm. The booklet *FDA and the Veterinarian,* published by CVM, provides additional details on some of the legal aspects of FDA activities (http://www.fda.gov/cvm/3047.htm). Essential laws, regulations, and guidance applicable to the animal drug approval process are provided as active links [note: forthcoming changes to the FDA website are anticipated in 2009]. Concise summaries are displayed with each link. The CVM home page also provides links to the Freedom of Information (FOI) summaries for NADAs, Supplemental NADAs, and ANADAs. These summaries provide valuable information on the data submitted to support the approval of the application.

This chapter describes the regulatory framework that guides animal drug approval within the United States. This process provides exciting career opportunities for veterinarians, pharmacologists, and others in both industry and the federal government. The efficiency and success of drug development directly impacts the availability and approved uses of drugs for veterinary practitioners. Through the use of published literature and simulated examples, this chapter covers the use and application of the pharmacokinetic principles described in Chapters 2 and 3 of this book.

HISTORY OF THE FDA AND ITS RELATIONSHIP TO VETERINARY MEDICINE

Although veterinarians have been a part of the FDA since it was formed in 1927, regulation of veterinary pharmaceuticals was not initiated until the 1950s. When the FDA was divided into five bureaus in 1954, a branch dedicated to the evaluation of veterinary medicine was created within the Bureau of Medicine. This branch became a bureau of its own in 1965, and in 1984, the Bureau of Veterinary Medicine became the current Center for Veterinary Medicine (CVM). A brief chronology of FDA history is provided in Table 55.1. Additional information on the history and current responsibilities of the FDA and CVM is available on the web (www.fda.gov and www.fda.gov/cvm).

TABLE 55.1 Historical overview of the US FDA

http://www.fda.gov/cvm/aboutcvm/aboutbeg.htm

1848: Import Drugs Act was enacted (first federal statute for guaranteeing quality of medicines).
1862: President Lincoln created the Department of Agriculture (USDA).
1880: After a year's investigation into food and drug adulteration, USDA began advocating enactment of a national food and drug law.
1906: First Federal Food and Drug Act was signed into law and was administered by USDA's Bureau of Chemistry after studying food and drug adulteration.
1927: The Food, Drug, and Insecticide Administration was formed.
1938: Due to deaths from a sulfanilamide elixir containing an antifreeze analogue, the Federal Food, Drug, and Cosmetic Act (FFDCA) was enacted, requiring manufacturers to provide evidence of product safety.
1951: The Durham-Humphrey Amendment initiated prescription requirements for certain human drugs. The veterinary Rx legend was effected through rulemaking.
1953: The FDA was transferred to the Department of Health, Education and Welfare.
1954: The FDA was organized into five bureaus, including a Bureau of Medicine, within which was a Veterinary Medical Branch.
1959: The Veterinary Medical Branch became a Division due to extensive use of animal drugs and medicated feeds.
1962: The Kefauver-Harris Drug Amendments resulted from the thalidomide disaster, requiring that drugs show both safety and effectiveness, and establishing GMPs.
1965: The Bureau of Veterinary Medicine (BVM) was established.
1984: The BVM became the Center for Veterinary Medicine (CVM).

Today, veterinary products are regulated by the FDA, USDA, and Environmental Protection Agency (EPA). FDA/CVM regulates the manufacture and distribution of drugs, food additives, and medical devices used in veterinary species. This includes both product approval and postapproval monitoring to ensure continued product safety and effectiveness. According to the Act, a *device* is an instrument, apparatus, implement, machine, contrivance, implant, *in vitro* reagent, or other similar or related article, including any component, part, or accessory, which is intended for use in the diagnosis of disease or other conditions, or in the cure, mitigation, treatment, or prevention of disease, in man or other animals, or intended to affect the structure or any function of the body of man or other animals, and which does not achieve any of its principal intended purposes through chemical action within or on the body of man or other animals and which is not dependent upon being metabolized for the achievement of any of its principal intended purposes. Currently, there are no FDA premarketing approval requirements for medical devices intended for animal use. However, veterinary medical devices are subject to the general provisions of the Act that relate to misbranding and adulteration (Sections 501 and 502 of the FFDCA).

Veterinary biologics (such as vaccines, antitoxins, and diagnostics that are used to prevent, treat, or diagnose animal diseases) are regulated by the USDA Animal and Plant Health Inspection Service, Center for Veterinary Biologics under the Virus Serum Toxin Act of 1913 (http://www.aphis.usda.gov/animal_health/vet_biologics/). Pesticides (e.g., including preparations for use on inanimate objects, rodenticides, and most insecticides) are subject to the Federal Insecticide, Fungicide, and Rodenticide Act, administered by the Pesticide Regulation Division of the EPA (http://www.epa.gov/pesticides/). Animal grooming aids are currently not regulated by these agencies, unless the products are intended for any therapeutic purpose or are intended to affect the structure or function of the animal (FDA) or contain pesticides (EPA).

CHALLENGES IN VETERINARY DRUG EVALUATION

The process leading to the approval and marketing of a new animal drug product is similar to that associated with human pharmaceuticals (Fig. 55.1). In fact, many animal drugs were initially developed for potential use in humans. However, veterinary pharmaceutical development encounters numerous complexities that are not faced by our human health counterparts. In addition to the challenges associated with between-individual variability (which is seen both in human and veterinary medicine), the development of new animal drugs also contends with such issues as the following:

- The enormous diversity in size, behavior, metabolic needs, and lifespan between animal species
- Species and breed differences in both pharmacokinetic and toxicity profiles
- A wide spectrum of disease agents that produce different disease manifestations under different conditions
- A range of husbandry practices, which include the array of settings in which animals are kept—ranging from animal companions in the home to large livestock operations
- Inability to communicate directly with the animal patient
- Public health concerns, including environmental safety, human food safety, and the potential influence of veterinary antimicrobial use on development of resistance in bacteria of concern to both veterinary and human medicine

There are also differences in the use of drug products in food-producing animal species versus companion animal species. The focus of diagnostics, drug therapy, and monitoring of treatment response is on the individual companion animal. The goals of therapy are to prevent, treat, or manage a disease or to improve the quality of life for the individual animal. Some therapies may be continued throughout the life of the companion animal. For food-producing animals, the focus is generally on the health of an entire group (herd or flock) of animals instead of an individual animal. Although food-producing animals may be individually dosed using injectable or topical products to treat or control certain diseases, group dosing via medicated drinking water or feed is often used in order to minimize handling stress and to allow for a more efficient means of dosing a large number of animals during a disease outbreak. The goal in food animal medicine is to manage the health of the herd.

A further challenge to animal drug development is the low cost and narrow profit margin of veterinary pharmaceuticals. During the development of animal drug products, the process of product development to marketing approval by the FDA takes, on the average, 10 years and costs about $40 million (http://www.ahi.org/content.asp?contentid=692). In contrast, a 2004 survey estimated that for human pharmaceuticals, it takes on the average of 12 to 15 years to bring a new prescription product to market at an average cost of $800 million dollars (http://www.phrma.org/files/Cost_of_Prescription_Drugs.pdf). Public spending on products used to treat and prevent disease in both companion animals and farm animals in the United States in 2004 reached nearly $5 billion (http://www.ahi.org/content.asp?contentid=692). By comparison, in 2004, U.S. retail prescription sales totaled $168 billion in 2004 (Kaiser Family Foundation: http://www.kff.org/insurance/7031/ti2004-1-19.cfm). Animal Health Institute (AHI) member companies spent $618 million in 2006 to research and develop potential new products and

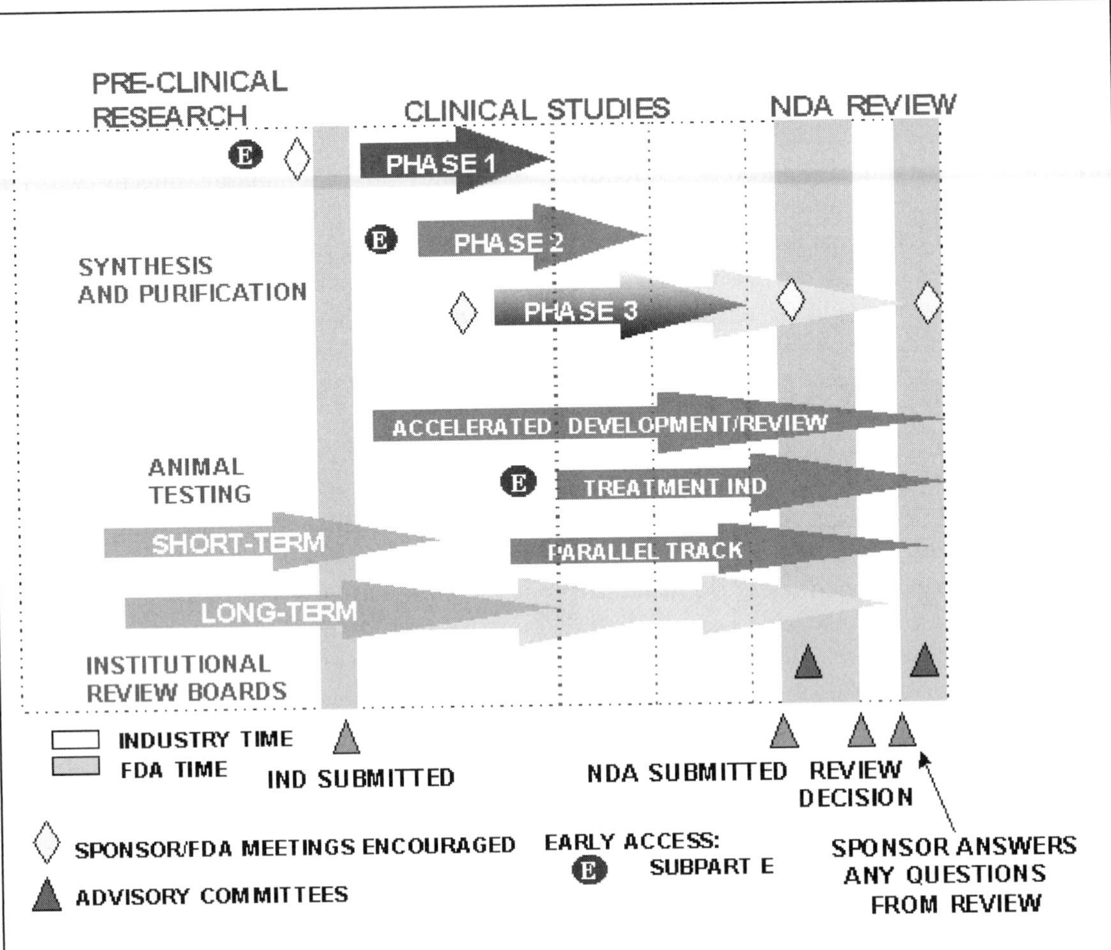

<u>Short-term testing</u> in animals ranges in duration from 2 weeks to 3 months. <u>Long-term testing</u> in animals ranges in duration from a few weeks to several years. Some animal testing continues after human tests begin to learn whether long-term use of a drug may cause cancer or birth defects.

<u>Phase 1</u> includes the initial introduction of an investigational new drug into humans. During Phase 1, sufficient information about the drug's pharmacokinetics and pharmacological effects should be obtained to permit the design of well-controlled, scientifically valid, Phase 2 studies.

<u>Phase 2</u> includes the early controlled clinical studies conducted to obtain some preliminary data on the effectiveness of the drug for a particular indication or indications in patients with the disease or condition. This phase of testing also helps determine the common short-term side effects and risks associated with the drug. Phase 2 studies are typically well-controlled, closely monitored, and conducted in a relatively small number of patients, usually involving several hundred people.

<u>Phase 3</u> studies are intended to gather the additional information about effectiveness and safety that is needed to evaluate the overall benefit-risk relationship of the drug. Phase 3 studies also provide an adequate basis for extrapolating the results to the general population and transmitting that information in the physician labeling. Phase 3 studies usually include several hundred to several thousand people.

FIG. 55.1 A flow diagram of the informational paradigm supporting human drug approvals is accessible online at the website of the Center for Drug Evaluation and Research (CDER) (http://www.fda.gov/cder/handbook).

to ensure the safety and effectiveness of existing products, according to AHI's latest Research and Development Survey (http://www.ahi.org/content.asp?contentid=692). In comparison, with respect to human pharmaceutical product research and development, the Pharmaceutical Research and Manufacturers of America (PhRMA), which represents the country's leading pharmaceutical research and biotechnology companies, have invested an estimated $44.5 billion in 2007 in discovering and developing new medicines. Industrywide research and investment reached a record $58.8 billion in 2007 (http://www.phrma.org/about_phrma/).

The limited opportunity for cost recovery forms a barrier to increasing the availability of new animal products. As a practical matter, the amount of data contained in a New Animal Drug Application (NADA) is substantially less than that submitted to support a New Drug Application (NDA) for human use. For example, the number of patients enrolled in clinical trials of new animal drugs is substantially smaller than the thousands of patients generally enrolled in trials submitted in support of human NDAs.

Despite these constraints, the same statutory requirements regarding the demonstration of product safety and effectiveness apply to the regulation of both human and veterinary drug products. Therefore, innovative application of the principles of pharmacology and research study design is important in meeting the challenge of developing cost-effective ways to generate the data necessary to meet the statutory requirements of the FFDCA. Pharmaceutical companies are encouraged to consult closely with CVM to develop study designs and assays that maximize the value of the collected data to support their drug applications.

REGULATORY BASIS OF VETERINARY DRUG EVALUATION

The approval process is linked to the legal prohibition of adulteration or misbranding of food, drugs, or devices in interstate commerce. The specific requirements for gaining an approval are in Sections 512 (New Animal Drugs) and 571-573 (New Animal Drugs for Minor Use and Minor Species) of the FFDCA.

RECENT AMENDMENTS TO THE FFDCA

The Animal Medicinal Drug Use Clarification Act of 1994 (AMDUCA). Prior to the enactment of the AMDUCA of 1994, the FFDCA prohibited veterinarians from prescribing new animal drugs for any indications other than the specific conditions of use on the approved labeling. This extralabel use restriction precluded veterinarians from using an approved new animal drug for an unapproved animal species, for an unapproved indication, or for an approved species at dosage levels higher than that stated on the label. Prior to 1994, the use of human drugs for treating animals was also illegal.

In 1996, Title 21 of the Code of Federal Regulations was amended to add part 530, entitled "Extralabel Drug Use in Animals." This action served to implement AMDUCA to permit veterinarians to prescribe extralabel uses of certain approved animal and human drugs to treat animals under certain conditions. These regulations gave veterinarians the flexibility to meet patient needs in the practice of veterinary medicine (21 CFR §530; http://www.fda.gov/cvm/Images/530.pdf). Under AMDUCA, the key constraints are that any extralabel use must be by or on the order of a veterinarian within the context of a veterinarian-client-patient relationship; the use must not result in violative residues in food-producing animals; and certain listed compounds are prohibited from extralabel use in food-producing animals (http://www.fda.gov/ohrms/dockets/98fr/020602b.htm). The Agency may establish safe and violative levels for residues for extralabel use and may require development of analytical methods for residue detection. If, after affording an opportunity for public comment, FDA finds that an extralabel animal drug use presents a risk to public health or that no analytical method has been developed and submitted, the Agency may prohibit the extralabel use. The Agency has prohibited the extralabel use of the following drugs in food-producing animals:

- Chloramphenicol
- Clenbuterol
- Diethylstilbestrol (DES)
- Dimetridazole
- Ipronidazole
- Other nitroimidazoles
- Furazolidone (except for approved topical use)
- Nitrofurazone (except for approved topical use)
- Sulfonamide drugs in lactating dairy cattle (except approved use of sulfadimethoxine, sulfabromomethazine, and sulfaethoxypyridazine)

Neither AMDUCA nor the implementing regulations lessen the responsibility of the manufacturer, the veterinarian, or the food producer to prevent risks to public health from drug residues in animal-derived foods.

Updates on issues pertaining to the Animal Medicinal Drug Use Clarification Act of 1994 and its implementation by CVM can be found at http://www.fda.gov/cvm/amducatoc.htm.

The Animal Drug Availability Act of 1996 (ADAA). In an effort to increase the number of animal drugs on the market and to reduce regulatory burdens on the animal health industry without undermining the safety of animal drug products, the ADAA was signed into law on October, 1996 (http://www.fda.gov/cvm/adaatoc.html). The current study requirements associated with NADAs reflect changes instituted by this Act. In brief, the ADAA provides for the following (Annon 1996):

- An amendment to the definition of substantial evidence of effectiveness that provided CVM with greater flexibility to make case-specific scientific determinations regarding the number and types of adequate and well-controlled studies that will provide, in an efficient manner, substantial evidence that a new animal drug is effective (21 CFR Part 514 [Docket No. 97N-0435] Substantial Evidence of Effectiveness of New Animal Drugs. Notice of proposed rulemaking. http://www.fda.gov/cvm/Regulatory_Notice_Letters/fr971105.pdf).
- Greater direct interaction between animal drug sponsors and the FDA during the drug development process. The law requires a presubmission conference, held at the sponsor's discretion, to discuss the drug development at its earliest stages. The goal is for the FDA and the manufacturers to reach a common understanding regarding what data will be needed to establish safety and effectiveness, and what types of studies can be conducted to generate such data.
- The ability to market an animal drug with a range of acceptable/recommended doses on animal drug product labeling, rather than as one optimum dose. In addition, the law directs FDA to broaden the approval process to make available more animal drugs to treat minor species.
- A new category of drugs, "Veterinary Feed Directive Drugs" (VFD), that allows approval and use of new animal drugs in animal feed, on a veterinarian's order, while incorporating safeguards to ensure the safe use of such drugs. This new category of drug is discussed below.

The Veterinary Feed Directive (VFD). Before the passage of the ADAA, the FFDCA provided FDA only two options for regulating the distribution of animal drugs: over-the-counter (OTC) and prescription (Rx). A product can be approved as OTC if adequate directions for use can be written for the layperson. In contrast, use of Rx products requires veterinary intervention with respect to diagnosing the disease and monitoring the response to therapy, as well as monitoring the potential for adverse effects in the patient.

The prescription legend invoked the application of state pharmacy laws, and the pharmacy laws in a significant number of states prohibited feed manufacturers from possessing and dispensing prescription animal drugs and medicated feed containing those drugs. Pharmacy laws in other states required the presence of a pharmacist at the feed manufacturing facility that uses prescription drugs in the manufacture of medicated feeds. As a practical matter, the application of state pharmacy laws to medicated feeds would burden state pharmacy boards and impose costs on animal feed manufacturers to such an extent that it would be impractical to make these critically needed new animal drugs available for animal therapy. For this reason, through the ADAA, Congress enacted legislation to create the VFD, providing a new class of restricted feed use drugs that may be distributed without invoking state pharmacy laws. Although statutory controls on the distribution and use of VFD drugs are similar to those for prescription animal drugs regulated under section 503(f) of the FFDCA (21 U.S.C. 353(f)), the VFD regulations are tailored to the unique circumstances relating to the distribution of animal feeds containing a VFD drug. Unlike prescription drugs, VFD drugs are not be regulated by state pharmacy bodies (page 35966 Federal Register/Vol. 64, No. 127/ Friday, July 2, 1999). No extralabel use of a VFD drug is permitted, and a veterinarian may issue a VFD only if a valid veterinarian-client-patient relationship exists, as defined in 21 CFR §530.3(i). More information regarding VFD is available from the FDA on the web (http://www.fda.gov/cvm/vfd.html).

COMPONENTS OF NADAs AND ANADAs

Regulatory Overview. The legal requirements for NADAs are detailed in 21 CFR §514.1. Required information for evaluation of the NADA is grouped into technical sections listed on Form FDA 356V (Figs. 55.2A, B) and includes the following:

- Target Animal Safety
- Effectiveness
- Human Food Safety
- Chemistry, Manufacturing, and Controls
- Environmental Impact
- All Other Information
- Labeling

The Office of New Animal Drug Evaluation (ONADE) within CVM is responsible for the review of information submitted by drug sponsors to obtain approval to manufacture and market animal drugs. Highlights for each of these technical sections are provided in the next several sections of this chapter.

Technical Sections of NADAs

Target Animal Safety (TAS). The purpose of the TAS studies is to evaluate potential harmful effects associated with use of a new animal drug in a controlled setting, as a prediction of product safety in the larger patient population. The regulation for TAS, 21 CFR §514.1(b)(8)(i), requires "adequate tests by all methods reasonably applicable to show whether or not the new animal drug is safe and effective for use as suggested in the proposed labeling." The FDA develops guidance documents (http://www.fda.gov/cvm/Guidance/published.htm) to summarize recommendations and suggestions for efficiently carrying out these studies. The FDA is also currently participating in the international harmonization of guidelines for TAS testing.

As with human pharmaceuticals, published literature, preliminary studies (including pharmacokinetics and pharmacodynamics, and extrapolation from toxicity testing in laboratory animals), and safety observations in clinical effectiveness trials are considered in the safety evaluation. But for new animal drugs, safety is also directly assessed in the target species through laboratory-based (overdose) studies. These nonclinical laboratory studies must be conducted in accordance with Good Laboratory Practices (GLP) regulations (21 CFR Part 58). FDA does not require that domestic animals be maintained under the conditions required for laboratory animals during GLP testing. Although clinical effectiveness studies contribute data to the overall safety assessment of a drug, GLP regulations do not apply to clinical studies. Furthermore, the product evaluated in the TAS studies should be identical to the product intended to be marketed, i.e., same chemical, same particle size and formulation, and manufactured in conformity with the principles of Good Manufacturing Practices (GMP).

Although the specific information needed to assess TAS in a particular NADA depends on a variety of factors (e.g., proposed usage regimen and dose, type of drug, pharmacokinetics, chemistry and manufacturing considerations, claims, previous use history, and animal species including class and breed), the underlying scientific approach, as outlined in FDA guidance documents, is common to all. Studies generally compare healthy control animals with small numbers of healthy animals of the target species treated with multiples of both the recommended dose and duration of administration of the product. Appropriate observations, physical examinations, clinical pathology tests (hematology, blood chemistry, urinalysis, fecal analysis, etc.), necropsy, and histopathology should be conducted to identify possible adverse effects. Additional specialized studies, such as evaluation of injection sites, topical administration sites, reproductive safety, and mammary gland safety, may be needed depending on the conditions of use and the characteristics of the drug. There may also be additional species-specific study requirements based upon unique physiology and or husbandry practices. For example in fish, target animal safety can change as a function of water temperature, ionic strength and composition, and life stage (Storey 2006).

Effectiveness. 21 CFR §514.4(b)(2) requires that a sponsor submit data generated from well-controlled studies of a new animal drug to distinguish the effect of the new animal drug from other influences, such as spontaneous change in the course of the disease, normal animal production performance, or biased observation. The data provided for substantial evidence of effectiveness must permit qualified experts to conclude that a new animal drug will have the effect it purports or is represented to have under the conditions of use suggested in the proposed labeling (21 CFR §514.4(b)(3)(i)(C)). Generation of these data represents a significant component of drug development time and cost such that the amount and nature of the evidence needed can be an important determinant of whether and when new animal drugs become available to the public. If there is a lack of substantial evidence that the new animal drug will have the effect it purports or if the proposed labeling is false or misleading as it relates to

Form Approved: OMB No. 0910-0032; Expiration Date: 4/30/2011
See OMB Statement on Page 3.

DEPARTMENT OF HEALTH AND HUMAN SERVICES
FOOD AND DRUG ADMINISTRATION

APPLICATION FOR APPROVAL OF A NEW ANIMAL DRUG
(OR SUBMISSION TO SUPPORT NEW ANIMAL DRUG APPROVAL)
(Sections 512 and 571 of FFDCA and Title 21, Code of Federal Regulations, Part 514)

APPLICATION OR INVESTIGATIONAL FILE NUMBER

DATE OF SUBMISSION

APPLICANT INFORMATION

APPLICANT NAME		CONTACT NAME *(authorized representative or U.S. agent)*	
APPLICANT ADDRESS *(Number, Street, City, State, Country, and ZIP or Mail Code)*		CONTACT ADDRESS *(Number, Street, City, State and ZIP Code)*	
		E-MAIL ADDRESS:	
TELEPHONE NUMBER	FACSIMILE (FAX) NUMBER	TELEPHONE NUMBER	FACSIMILE (FAX) NUMBER

PRODUCT DESCRIPTION

ESTABLISHED NAME *(e.g., USAN name)*

PROPRIETARY NAME *(trade name)*, IF ANY

DOSAGE FORM:

DOSE or DOSE RANGE:

ROUTE(S) OF ADMINISTRATION

SPECIES AND, IF APPLICABLE, CLASS

PROPOSED MARKETING STATUS *(check one)*

- ☐ Prescription (Rx) *(section 503(f)(1) of FFDCA)*
- ☐ Over-the-Counter (OTC) *(section 502(f)(1) of FFDCA)*
- ☐ Veterinary Feed Directive (VFD) *(section 504 of FFDCA)*

DESIGNATED NEW ANIMAL DRUG? ☐ Yes ☐ No

DATE OF DESIGNATION:

PROPOSED INDICATION(S) FOR USE

APPLICATION DESCRIPTION

TYPE OF APPLICATION *(check one, if applicable)*

- ☐ New Animal Drug Application (NADA) *(section 512(b)(1) of FFDCA)*
- ☐ Abbreviated New Animal Drug Application (ANADA) *(section 512(b)(2) of FFDCA)*
- ☐ Application for Conditional Approval *(section 571(a) of FFDCA)*

Administrative Application? ☐ Yes ☐ No

FOR AN ANADA, IDENTIFY THE FOLLOWING INFORMATION FOR THE REFERENCE LISTED DRUG

Proprietary Name

Application Number

Holder of Approved Application

TYPE OF SUBMISSION *(check one)*

- ☐ Submission of data or information to an Investigational File (and Amending Submissions)
- ☐ Submission to a Master File
- ☐ Original Application
- ☐ Supplement requiring review of safety or effectiveness data *(21 CFR § 14.8(c)(1))*
- ☐ Chemistry, Manufacturing and Controls: Supplement or Report *(also check specific type)*
  - ☐ Prior Approval *(21 CFR § 14.8(b)(2))*
  - ☐ Changes Being Effected (CBE) - 30 day *(21 CFR § 14.8(b)(3)(i))*
  - ☐ CBE - Immediate *(21 CFR § 14.8(b)(3)(vi))*
  - ☐ Minor Changes and Stability Report (MCSR) *(21 CFR § 14.8(b)(4))*
- ☐ Labeling Supplement *(also check specific type)*
  - ☐ Prior approval *(21 CFR § 14.8(c)(2))*
  - ☐ CBE *(21 CFR § 14.8(c)(3))*
- ☐ Amendment to Pending Application, Supplement or MCSR
- ☐ Reactivation of Application, Supplement, or MCSR
- ☐ Request for renewal of conditionally approved Application *(section 571(d)(1) of FFDCA)*
- ☐ Other *(please describe)*:

FORM FDA 356v (4/08) PSC Graphics (301) 443-1090 EF **Page 1 of 6**

FIG. 55.2 Form FDA 356V. A: front view; B: back view.

SUBMISSION CONTENT *(Check each box that describes a type of information included in your submission)*

To support an NADA or application for conditional approval	***To support an ANADA***
☐ 1. Identification *(21 CFR § 14.1(b)(1))*	☐ 9. Identification
☐ 2. Table of contents and summary *(21 CFR § 14.1(b)(2))*	☐ 10. Table of contents and summary
☐ 3. Technical sections	☐ 11. Technical sections
☐ a. Labeling *(21 CFR § 14.1(b)(3)) (check one)* ☐ Draft (facsimile) labeling ☐ Final printed labeling	☐ a. Withdrawal period information *(section 512(n)(1)(A)(ii) of FFDCA)*
☐ b. Chemistry, manufacturing, and controls *(21 CFR § 14.1(b)(4) and (5))*	☐ b. Bioequivalence *(section 512(n)(1)(E) of FFDCA) (check one)* ☐ Documentation supporting a request for waiver ☐ Bioequivalence study or information
☐ c. Human food safety *(21 CFR § 14.1(b)(7) and (8))*	☐ c. Labeling *(sections 512(n)(1)(F) and (G) of FFDCA) (check one)* ☐ Draft (facsimile) labeling ☐ Final printed labeling
☐ d. Target animal safety (TAS) (21 CFR § 14.1(b)(8))	
☐ e. Effectiveness *(check one)* ☐ Substantial evidence of effectiveness (21 CFR § 14.1(b)(8)) ☐ Reasonable expectation of effectiveness (section 571(a)(2)(B) of FFDCA)	☐ d. Chemistry, manufacturing, and controls *(section 512(n)(1)(G) of FFDCA)* ☐ e. Patent certification *(section 512(n)(1)(H) of FFDCA)*
☐ f. Environmental impact *(21 CFR § 14.1(b)(14))*	☐ f. Environmental impact *(21 CFR § 5.15)*
☐ g. All other information *(21 CFR § 14.1(b)(8)(iv))*	☐ g. Freedom of information summary *(21 CFR § 14.11) (for administrative application, submit FOI TSC letter)*
☐ h. Freedom of information summary *(21 CFR § 14.11) (for administrative application, submit FOI TSC letter)*	☐ Other *(please describe)*:
☐ 4. Samples *(21 CFR § 14.1(b)(6)) (submit only on the request of FDA)*	
☐ 5. For VFD drugs, submit copies of the VFD *(21 CFR § 14.1(b)(9))*	
☐ 6. Commitments required by 21 CFR § 14.1(b)(11) and (12)	
☐ a. Labeling and advertising *(21 CFR § 14.1(b)(11))*	
☐ b. Shipping of approved drug intended for use in the manufacture of animal feeds *(21 CFR § 14.1(b)(12)(i))*	
☐ c. Good manufacturing practices *(21 CFR § 14.1(b)(12)(ii))*	
☐ d. Good laboratory practice compliance statement *(21 CFR § 14.1(b)(12)(iii))*	
☐ 7. Patent information on any patent which claims the drug or a method of using the drug *(section 512(b)(1) of FFDCA)*	
☐ 8. User fee cover sheet *(Form FDA 3546)*	

NUMBER OF VOLUMES SUBMITTED	DESCRIPTION OF ANY ELECTRONIC MEDIA SUBMITTED

CROSS REFERENCES *(list applications or files, (e.g.. investigational new animal drug files (INADs), generic INADs (JINADs), NADAs. and master files) referenced in the current application, including by right(s) of reference)*

FORM FDA 356v (4/08) **Page 2 of 6**

FIG. 55.2—*continued*

CERTIFICATIONS

I certify that:

- I have personally reviewed this submission (or received assurances from qualified personnel) and determined that this submission and all supporting data, to the best of my knowledge and belief, are true, accurate, and complete,
- All copies (paper or electronic) of the submission are identical,
- For any information submitted by reference to a master file, investigational file, or application, the reference was made with the belief that the information contained in the referenced file is true, accurate, and complete,
- The services of any person debarred under section 306(a) or (b) of FFDCA have not been used in any capacity related to this submission, and
- I am aware that there are significant penalties for submitting false information, including the possibility of fine and imprisonment for knowing and willful violations (18 U.S.C. § 1001).

If this application is approved, I agree:

- To submit safety update reports as requested by FDA under its statutory authority or as provided for by regulation,
- To comply with all applicable statutes and regulations that apply to approved applications,
- Not to market this drug product until the Drug Enforcement Administration makes a final scheduling decision if this application applies to a drug product that FDA has proposed for scheduling under the Controlled Substances Act, and
- To notify FDA of any change to the conditions established in this approval.

SIGNATURE OF RESPONSIBLE OFFICIAL	NAME AND TITLE *(Printed or Typed)*	DATE
SIGNATURE OF U.S. AGENT *(if applicable)*	NAME AND TITLE *(Printed or Typed)*	DATE

Paperwork Reduction Act Statement - A Federal agency may not conduct or sponsor, and a person is not required to respond to a collection of information unless it displays a currently valid OMB control number. Public reporting burden for this collection of information averages 5 hours per response, including time for reviewing instructions and completing the form. Send comments regarding the burden estimate or any other aspect of this collection of information to: Food and Drug Administration, Office of Chief Information Officer (HFA-250), 5600 Fishers Lane, Rockville, MD 20857.

This space intentionally left blank.

FORM FDA 356v (4/08) **Page 3 of 6**

FIG. 55.2—*continued*

INSTRUCTIONS FOR COMPLETING AND SUBMITTING FORM FDA 356v

GENERAL INSTRUCTIONS

Applicant Information

Provide your name, address, and telephone and facsimile numbers (including the country code if needed). This address will be the address of record we use for all contacts initiated by us and not directly related to a submission. Also provide the name of the individual who will serve as your contact (i.e., your authorized representative or U.S. agent). If you or your authorized representative do not reside or have a place of business within the United States, you must provide the name and address of a U.S. agent as your contact. A U.S. agent is a person who is a permanent resident of the United States and acts as your agent. Your U.S. agent must also sign your application (see 21 CFR § 14.1(a)).

Product Description

Include all of the information necessary to identify the drug product that is the subject of your submission. The manufacturer or sponsor of a new animal drug for a minor use or use in a minor species may request designation under section 573(a) of FFDCA. Indicate whether your drug has been declared a designated new animal drug and, if so, the date of designation.

Application Description

Type of Application:

- If you are submitting an application, check the appropriate box to identify whether you are submitting a new animal drug application (NADA), an abbreviated NADA (ANADA), or application for conditional approval. Please check whether the application is an administrative application. If this is an ANADA, identify, for the reference listed new animal drug, the proprietary name of the reference listed drug, its NADA number, and the name of the holder of the approved NADA for the referenced listed drug.

- **DO NOT** check a box under Type of Application if you are submitting information or data to an investigational file or master file. Instead, check the "submission of data or information to an investigational file," "submission to a master file," or "other" under type of submission and the appropriate item(s) from the Submission Content list of items.

Type of Submission: Check the appropriate box.

- **Submission of Data or Information to an Investigational File:** Data or information (including amending data or information) supporting a single technical section submitted for phased review. This submission should include labeling language, and may include Freedom of Information (FOI) information, relevant to the specific technical section.

- **Submission to a Master File:** Data or information submitted to a master file that may be referenced (by the owner or a person granted a right of reference) to support the approval of a new animal drug.

- **Original Application:** A complete application (i.e., containing all applicable technical sections or copies of technical section complete letters for all applicable technical sections) that you have not submitted before.

- **Supplement Requiring Review of Safety or Effectiveness Data:** A supplemental application (21 CFR § 14.8(a)) requesting a change to an approved application that requires FDA to review safety or effectiveness data (e.g., the addition of a new claim or species). Note: An applicant may not supplement an application for conditional approval to add indications of use (section 571(g) of FFDCA).

- **Chemistry, Manufacturing, and Controls - Supplement or Report:**

  – **Prior approval:** A supplemental application for any change in the drug, production process, quality controls, equipment, or facilities that has a substantial potential to have an adverse effect on the identity, strength, quality, purity, or potency of the drug as these factors may relate to the safety or effectiveness of the drug (21 CFR § 514.8(b)(2)).

  – **Changes being effected (CBE) in 30 days**: A supplemental application for any change in the drug, production process, quality controls, equipment, or facilities that has a moderate potential to have an adverse effect on the identity, strength, quality, purity, or potency of the drug as these factors may relate to the safety or effectiveness of the drug. (See examples in 21 CFR § 14.8(b)(3)(ii)). You may commercially distribute the drug made using the change 30 or more days after FDA receives your supplemental application unless FDA informs you otherwise within 30 days of its receipt of the application.

  – **Changes being effected (CBE):** A supplemental application for certain changes in the drug, production process, quality controls, equipment, or facilities that have a moderate potential to have an adverse effect on the identity, strength, quality, purity, or potency of the drug as these factors may relate to the safety or effectiveness of the drug (for examples, see 21 CFR § 514.8(b)(3)(vi)). You may

FIG. 55.2—*continued*

commercially distribute the drug when FDA receives your supplemental application.

– **Minor changes and stability report (MCSR):** An annual report that documents changes in the drug, production process, quality controls, equipment, or facilities that have a minimal potential to have an adverse effect on the identity, strength, quality, purity, or potency of the drug as these factors may relate to the safety or effectiveness of the drug (21 CFR § 14.8(b)(4)).

- **Labeling Supplement:**
  - **Prior approval:** A supplemental application requesting labeling changes that requires approval before the drug may be distributed (for examples, see 21 CFR § 14.8(c)(2)).
  - **Changes being effected (CBE):** A supplemental application requesting labeling changes that can be placed into effect before approval. These supplements request changes in labeling that increase the assurance of drug safety (21 CFR § 14.8(c)(3)(i)) or that do not decrease the safety of drug use (21 CFR § 14.8(c)(3)(ii)).

- **Amendment to a Pending Application, Supplement, or MCSR:** Any submission that provides additional information to an application or report while it is under review.

- **Reactivation of an Application, Supplement, or MCSR:** Resubmission of an application or report to address the deficiencies described in an incomplete letter from FDA.

- **Other:** Any submission that does not fit within one of the types of submissions described above.

Submission Content: Please check each box that describes a type of information that is included in your submission. Note that items 1-7 apply to the submission of NADAs and applications for conditional approval (or to their supporting investigational files), item 8 applies specifically to NADAs, and items 9-11 apply to ANADAs (or to their supporting investigational files).

- A complete NADA and application for conditional approval must include information and any right(s) of reference to information for items 1-7 (21 CFR § 14.1; section 571(a)(2)(A), (B) and (C) of FFDCA). A supplemental NADA may omit statements made in the application concerning which no change is made. If you are submitting information required by sections 571(a)(2)(D) - (F) of FFDCA to support conditional approval, check "other" and describe the information you are submitting. Indicate the order in which these sections appear in your submission in your table of contents. A completed User Fee Cover Sheet (item 8) should accompany each NADA and supplemental NADA subject to fees. To determine if your NADA or supplemental NADA is subject to an application fee, see section 740(a)(1) of FFDCA.

- For submissions other than applications (e.g., a submission to an investigational file for phased review), check only those items that apply and indicate the order in which these sections appear in your submission in your table of contents. Do not check Labeling or Freedom of Information Summary if the submission contains such information only as it relates to a technical section. For administrative applications, submit a copy of your FOI technical section complete letter.

- A complete ANADA should include items 9-11. A supplemental ANADA may omit statements made in the approved application concerning which no change is made.

- The "other" category should be checked and include a description of the submission when you are submitting certain information supporting a conditional approval (see instructions above) or when your submission does not fall into the above categories.

Description of Submission

Enter the number of volumes you are submitting. Describe any electronic media in your submission.

Cross References

List all investigational new animal drug files (INADs, JINADs), new animal drug applications (NADAs, ANADAs, applications for conditional approval), master files (VMFs, DMFs, PMFs), or other applications or files referenced in your current submission, including by "right of reference." If you reference data or information in any file you don't own, make sure a copy of your authorization to reference such data or information is included with your submission or has already been submitted to the file in which you referenced it.

Signature

After carefully reading the certifications, sign and date the form. Ordinarily only one person must sign the form, i.e., the applicant, or the applicant's attorney, agent, or other authorized official. However, if you do not reside or have a place of business within the United States, your U.S. agent must also sign the application.

INSTRUCTIONS FOR SUBMITTING AN APPLICATION

1. Include a completed and signed Form FDA 356v (pages 1 through 3) with all submissions relating to

FIG. 55.2—*continued*

new animal drug approval (i.e., NADAs, ANADAs, applications for conditional approval, submissions of data or information to an investigational file, supplements, amendments, reactivations, and MCSRs). The completed form should be placed before the cover letter, table of contents, and submission.

2. Submit three identical copies of your submission (21 CFR § 14.1(b)). A copy of the Form FDA 356v should accompany each copy of your submission.

3. Place the applicant's name and address and the proprietary name(s) (if available) and established name(s) of the new animal drug on the front cover of each copy of your submission (21 CFR § 14.1(b)).

4. Fully describe the submission in your cover letter (e.g., for a supplemental application, describe the change(s) you are seeking to the approved application).

5. Include a comprehensive table of contents in your submission (21 CFR § 14.1(b)(2)).

6. Format your submission so each of your sections begins on a new page.

7. Sequentially number the pages of the submission.

8. Send your submission and copies to:

   Document Control Unit (HFV-199)
   Center for Veterinary Medicine
   Food and Drug Administration
   7500 Standish Place
   Rockville, MD 20855

This space intentionally left blank.

FORM FDA 356v (4/08) **Page 6 of 6**

FIG. 55.2—*continued*

the demonstration of effectiveness of the new animal drug, CVM is required to issue an order refusing to approve the NADA (21 CFR §514.4; [Docket No. 97N-0435] Substantial Evidence of Effectiveness of New Animal Drugs. Notice of proposed rulemaking. http://www.fda.gov/cvm/Regulatory_Notice_Letters/fr971105.pdf).

The availability of certain approved new animal drugs for use in livestock, poultry, pets, and other animals is vital to protecting the health of animals and the health of humans who consume the products of food-producing animals. The availability of other approved new animal drugs is vital to increasing the efficiency of food production in the United States. The changes made to the definition of *substantial evidence* by the ADAA and by the further definition of that term provided CVM with greater flexibility to make case-specific scientific determinations regarding the number and types of adequate and well-controlled studies that will provide, in an efficient manner, substantial evidence that a new animal drug is effective.

One or more adequate and well-controlled studies are required to establish, by substantial evidence, that a new animal drug is effective. These trials are intended to demonstrate that a new animal drug is effective for each proposed intended use and the associated conditions of use (21 CFR §514.4). The intended use includes the dose or dose range, frequency, duration, timing (e.g., in relation to the onset of clinical signs), animal species, age, gender, class, and breed of animal for which the new animal drug is intended for use. Subsequent to the enactment of the ADAA, the specific number and types of adequate and well-controlled studies for providing substantial evidence of effectiveness depend upon the number of intended uses, how narrowly or broadly each intended use is defined, and the conditions of use in the proposed labeling. When a proposed therapeutic indication is associated with a dose range, substantial evidence of effectiveness is demonstrated for the lowest proposed dose. The highest dose within the dose range is contingent upon a demonstration of target animal safety (FR Notice Vol. 64, No. 144, July 28, 1999, Substantial Evidence of Effectiveness of New Animal Drugs. Docket Number 97N-0435. http://www.fda.gov/ohrms/dockets/98fr/072899a.pdf). Sponsors also need to justify the intended dose. The basis of this justification can include pharmacokinetic/pharmacodynamic relationships, literature, and laboratory tests.

The effectiveness studies are designed to test the product under actual conditions of use. In contrast to studies conducted under controlled laboratory settings, the clinical trial provides information pertaining to how the product will perform under real-world conditions in the patient population. The effectiveness studies are typically designed with a negative (placebo) control or an active control. An active control is an approved product of established effectiveness for the same indications as the proposed product under development, with a known margin of superiority relative to a placebo (Piaggio et al. 2006). The evaluation of the active control study should explain why the new animal drugs should be considered effective in the study, for example, by reference to results in previous placebo-controlled studies of the active control (21 CFR §514.117(b)(3)(iii)). The study is typically masked, and patients are randomized to treatment groups. In so doing, the investigator can evaluate the drug effects with minimal bias. The study is typically a multicenter and multiinvestigator design to increase the likelihood that the product will perform as expected in the broader population postapproval. The study is testing whether the product will perform in the hands of multiple investigators under a variety of husbandry conditions, clinical practice settings, different breeds and ages of the patient populations, and perhaps different stages of the disease or condition. The proposed indication drives the design of the effectiveness study. Likewise, the results of the effectiveness study drive the wording of the indication. The final approved indication and dosage are confirmed by the results of the effectiveness studies. The effectiveness studies also provide important safety information about the use of the product in the patient population.

The manufacturing characteristics of the product used in the efficacy study must be provided as part of the study results in order to provide CVM with an assurance that the test article used is representative of the product intended for marketing (21 CFR §514.117).

Human Food Safety (HFS). By the general safety provisions of Sections 409, 512, and 706 of the Federal Food, Drug, and Cosmetic Act (http://www.accessdata.fda.gov/scripts/cdrh/cfdocs/cfcfr/cfrsearch.cfm), FDA must determine for each food additive, new animal drug, or color additive proposed for use in food-producing animals whether the edible products derived from treated animals are safe for human consumption. Accordingly, the sponsor must demonstrate *reasonable certainty of no harm* to human health for all drug products intended for use in food-producing animals.

A human food safety evaluation focuses on residues that are present in the intended type of food animal following intended use of the drug. A *residue* is "any compound present in the edible tissues of the target animal which results from the use of the sponsored compound, including the sponsored compound, its metabolites, and any other substances formed in or on food because of the sponsored compound's use" (21 CFR §500.82 (B)).

The information needed to demonstrate human food safety for a NADA generally includes the following:

- *Evaluation of carcinogenicity:* To establish the safety of veterinary drug residues in human food, a number of toxicological evaluations are recommended, including an assessment of the potential to induce neoplasia. Exposure to residues of veterinary drugs will usually occur at extremely low levels, but for potentially long periods. To ensure that substances that could pose carcinogenic potential at relevant exposure levels are adequately assessed, a number of issues should be considered, including genotoxicity, metabolic fate, species differences, and cellular changes. As part of the human food safety package, sponsors must determine whether carcinogenicity testing should be conducted. The decision to undertake carcinogenicity testing should take into consideration 1) the results of genotoxicity tests, 2) structure-activity relationships, and 3) findings in systemic toxicity tests that may be relevant to neoplasia in longer-term studies. It should also take into consideration any known species specificity of the mechanism of toxicity. Any differences in metabolism between the test species, target animal species, and human beings should be taken into consideration. For additional information, refer to CVM Guidance #141 (http://www.fda.gov/cvm/Guidance/guide141.pdf).
- *Toxicological assessment:* Toxicology tests are conducted in laboratory animals to determine the dose at which the compound produces an adverse effect and a dose that produces a no observed effect level (NOEL).
- *Determination of an Acceptable Daily Intake (ADI):* The acceptable daily intake (ADI) is derived from the results of the study illustrating the most sensitive endpoint in the most appropriate species. The ADI is the highest dose used in the study that demonstrates a no-observed-effect-level (NOEL) divided by an appropriate safety factor. As a general rule, CVM will use the safety factors indicated below for the various types of studies

TABLE 55.2 Safety factors associated with the different kinds of toxicology investigations

Type of Study	Safety Factor
Chronic	100
Reproduction/Teratology	100 or 1000; 100 for a clear indication of maternal toxicity, 1000 for other effects
90-Day	1000

The ADI is estimated as

$$\text{ADI}\,(\mu g/kg/day) = [(\text{NOEL}\,(\mu g/kg))/(\text{Safety Factor}\,(day^{-1}))]$$

The appropriate safety factor depends upon the type of study being used for establishing the ADI, as described in Table 55.2.

- *Determination of a safe concentration:* The safe concentration is, by definition, the amount of residue that can be eaten in any edible tissue each day for an entire lifetime without exposing the consumer to residues in excess of the ADI. To estimate the safe concentration, FDA considers the ADI, the weight in kg of an average adult human (60 kg), and the amount of the product that may be consumed in grams per day (where consumption values, in grams consumed per day, are 300 for muscle, 100 for liver, 50 for kidney and 50 for fat):

$$\text{safe concentration}\,(\mu g/g) = \frac{\text{ADI}\,(\mu g/kg/day) \times 60\,kg}{\text{grams consumed per day}}$$

Once a safe concentration has been determined, methods are developed and validated that will allow future testing of animal tissues to monitor for residues. Withdrawal times are determined to allow use of the drug, with any residues expected to be below the safe concentration.

- *Selection of a marker residue:* The marker residue is a residue used to monitor the depletion of total residues in edible tissues in a food animal. The marker residue must have a demonstrated relationship with the total radiolabel drug residues such that when the concentration of the marker residue is less than a specific value (the tolerance) in the target tissue, the total residues in all the edible tissues are less than their respective safe concentrations.
- *Development and validation of an analytical method to measure the marker residue:* This method serves as the

regulatory method for determining the withdrawal time and for assessing whether animal-derived products contain residue concentrations in excess of the established limit (violative residues of meats and animal-derived food products). This method will be used after a drug is approved by validated analytical laboratories during inspections, insuring the absence of violative residues in marketed human food products derived from animal sources.

- *Establishment of a tolerance:* A tolerance (the FDA maximum concentration of the marker residues within the target tissue) or the European version of a tolerance, the maximum residue limit (MRL) is determined based on the marker residue (http://www.fda.gov/cvm/index/vmac/fried_files/fried_text.htm). The target tissue for the tolerance is generally the edible tissue from which residues most slowly deplete.
- *Establishment of a withdrawal time:* The withdrawal time is the time interval between the last administration of the drug to the food animal and the time when the animal can be slaughtered, or products, such as milk or eggs, can be used for food, without incurring violative drug residues in the food product. The regulatory objective of the FDA is to predict a time when we can be 95% certain that the tissue residue concentrations in 99% of the animal population receiving the drug product (when dosed in accordance to the approved product label) will be at or below tolerance. Generally, multiple animals are sampled across at least four time points and regression methods with tolerance limits are used to set the withdrawal time. Concentrations of the marker residue must be measured with the same FDA-approved analytical method that will be used for the regulatory inspections.

  For antibacterial drugs, additional information is assessed as part of the human food safety section. Two types of potential effects of the new animal drug on bacteria of human health concern are considered (see below).
- *Microbiological Effects on Bacteria of Human Health Concern:* The level of antimicrobial residues present in food should not have clinically relevant effects on the human intestinal microflora. In addition, consideration is given to potential microbiological effects on foodborne bacteria of human health concern (FDA/CVM Guidance for Industry [#144], Pre-Approval Information for Registration of New Veterinary Medicinal Products for Food-Producing Animals with Respect to Antimicrobial Resistance VICH GL27. Finalized 04-27-04. http://www.fda.gov/cvm/guidance/guide144.doc). FDA/CVM has published a guidance document (#152) that serves as an initial step in developing internationally harmonized technical guidance for characterization of antimicrobial resistance selection in bacteria of human health concern in the European Union, Japan, and the United States. This includes a qualitative risk assessment approach for characterizing the potential risk to human health of a proposed use of the antimicrobial new animal drug. FDA/CVM then uses the resulting risk estimation ranking, along with other data and information submitted in support of the NADA, to determine if the drug is approvable under specific risk management conditions.

Details regarding human food safety assessments are provided in CVM Guidance #3 (*General Principles for Evaluating the Safety of Compounds Used in Food-Producing Animals,* http://www.fda.gov/cvm/Guidance/GFI003.htm) For more information on issues pertaining to HFS, the reader is referred to Chapter 61 of this textbook.

Chemistry, Manufacturing, and Controls. Several pivotal considerations go into the evaluation of the chemistry and manufacturing of a new animal drug product. These considerations are intended to ensure the quality and performance of the product, both prior to and subsequent to marketing. CVM requires that sponsors provide the information needed to ensure that each lot of the product released to consumers performs in a consistent manner, and that consumers have the necessary information with regard to product storage conditions so that product quality and performance are maintained (21 CFR §514.1).

A full description of the methods used in, and the facilities and controls used for, the manufacture, processing, and packaging of the new animal drug must be provided in the new animal drug application. This description should include full information with respect to any new animal drug in sufficient detail to permit an evaluation of the adequacy of the described methods of manufacture, processing, and packing, and the described facilities and controls. This information is evaluated by CVM's Division of Manufacturing Technologies to determine the identity, strength, quality, and purity of the new animal drug. Information is also needed with regard to the methods used in the synthesis, extraction, isolation, or purification of any new animal drug and the precautions being taken to ensure proper identity, strength, quality, and purity of the raw materials, whether active or not. Sponsors must provide

CVM with the instructions used in the manufacturing, processing, packaging, and labeling of each dosage form of the new animal drug, and precautions being taken to ensure batch-to-batch product uniformity.

To ensure adequate performance as the product ages, the sponsor also must conduct studies of the stability of the new animal drug in the final dosage form. Expiry dates represent the duration of time for which product quality and performance can be assured if the product is stored in accordance with label recommendations. The time for expiry is based upon extensive stability testing that is conducted by the drug sponsor on the product intended for marketing, and these data are evaluated by the Division of Manufacturing Technologies at CVM.

Additional information pertaining to current good manufacturing practices (cGMPs), including a listing of current guidance documents on this subject, can be obtained at http://www.fda.gov/cder/gmp/. Pertinent guidance documents include

Guidance for Industry #42: Animal Drug Manufacturing Guidelines, Dated 1994. http://www.fda.gov/cvm/Guidance/Guideline42.htm

Guidance for Industry #48: Guidance for Industry: Submission Documentation for Sterilization Process Validation in Applications for Human and Veterinary Drug Products, Dated 1994. http://www.fda.gov/cvm/Guidance/cmc2.pdf

Guidance for Industry #57: Guidance for Industry for the Preparation and Submission of Veterinary Master Files, Dated 1995. http://www.fda.gov/cvm/Guidance/Guideline57.htm

Environmental Impact. Statutory data requirements associated with Environmental Impact are defined in 21 CFR §514.50(D)(8). Every application or supplemental application must contain either an environmental assessment under 21 CFR §25.31, or a request for categorical exclusion under 21 CFR §25.24. Categorical exclusions are generally granted for ANADAs and for NADAs intended for use in companion animals.

Environmental documentation addresses the potential impact of the manufacturing and use of the product if the application were approved. The FDA *Environmental Assessment Technical Handbook* is available through the National Technical Information Service (NTIS) to assist in determining the contents of environmental documents (NTIS, 5285 Port Royal Road, Springfield, VA 22161, (703) 605-6000; order number PB 87-175345/AS; http://www.ntis.gov). GLP compliance is required for all environmental laboratory studies. Preapproval GMP inspections are used to confirm the contents of environmental documents that apply to manufacturing environmental permits and controls.

The overall target of the assessment is the protection of ecosystems. The field of ecotoxicology is a complex science and gaps in data and knowledge exist. Nevertheless, CVM and the International Veterinary Cooperative and Harmonization (VICH) have developed guidance (CVM Guidance #166 dated 1/09/2006) that describes the kinds of information needed as part of the Environmental Impact Assessment (EIA) of veterinary medicinal products (VMPs).

The goal of the EIA is to assess the potential for VMPs to affect nontarget species in the environment, including both aquatic and terrestrial species. It is not possible to evaluate the effects of VMPs on every species in the environment that may be exposed to the VMP following its administration to the target species. The taxonomic levels tested are intended to serve as surrogates or indicators for the range of species present in the environment. Impacts of greatest potential concern are usually those at community and ecosystem function levels, with the aim being to protect most species. However, it may be important to distinguish between local and landscape effects. There may be some instances where the impact of a VMP at a single location may be of significant concern, for example, for endangered species or a species with key ecosystem functions. These issues are handled by risk management at that specific location, which may even include restriction or prohibition of use of the product of concern in that specific local area. Additionally, issues associated with cumulative impact of some VMPs may be appropriate at a landscape level.

The route and quantity of a VMP entering the environment determines the risk assessment scenarios that are applicable and the extent of the risk assessment. The EIA is based on the accepted principle that risk is a function of the exposure, fate, and effects assessments of the VMP for the environmental compartments of concern. While emission can occur at various stages in the life cycle of the product, with the exception of certain topicals or those added directly to water, most VMPs first pass through the animal to which it is administered. Generally the most significant environmental exposure results from excretion of the active substance(s).

All Other Information. The *All Other Information* section must include all other information, not included in any of the other technical sections, that is pertinent to an evaluation of the safety or effectiveness of the new animal drug for which approval is sought, 21 CFR §514.1(b)(8)(iv). All other information includes, but is not limited to, any information derived from other marketing (domestic or foreign) and favorable and unfavorable reports in the scientific literature.

Product Labeling. The ability to interpret and understand drug labels is essential in ensuring that use of a particular drug achieves the intended outcome and minimizes unintended effects. The product labeling is the avenue through which CVM communicates instructions about product use and storage conditions to veterinarians, as well as communicating the benefits and risks associated with the use of a drug product.

Section 201K of the FFDCA defines *label* as a display of written, printed, or graphic matter upon the immediate container of any article. A drug's "labeling" includes all labels and other written, printed, or graphic matter, such as package inserts, on the drug, its containers or wrappers, or accompanying the drug. Labeling information is derived from studies submitted by the pharmaceutical sponsor to the FDA to support new animal drug approval and is developed as a collaboration between FDA and the drug sponsor.

Through the product label, the FDA provides the practitioner with a thorough understanding of the benefits and risks associated with the use of a drug product in the animal patient. The concept of "safe use" includes safety to the animal patient, safety to the person administering the product, the safety of food derived from the treated animal, and environmental safety issues associated with use or disposal of the product. Safety information on the labeling can be derived from studies conducted by the pharmaceutical sponsor, studies from peer-reviewed scientific literature, or from extrapolation from human drug labeling information that reasonably applies to the target species. Safety information is provided throughout the package insert under several different headings, including Contraindications, Warnings, Precautions, Adverse Reactions, and Animal Safety. No doubt, each veterinary student has heard the advice, "Above all, do no harm." Therefore, it is extremely important that the practitioner become familiar with all sections of the package insert in order to better understand both the risks and benefits associated with use of the product. The safety information can be viewed from the perspective of a hierarchy of severity, with Contraindications being the most serious, followed by Warnings and Precautions. The Animal Safety section is generally derived directly from laboratory target animal safety studies. The Adverse Reactions section is developed directly from the preapproval field effectiveness studies and the postapproval experience after the drug is marketed to the larger population. The Contraindications, Warnings, and Precautions statements can be modified by new findings from the postapproval surveillance of product use. The following are typical sections/information found on a package insert:

- Product identification, description, and prescription legend
- Indications
- Dosage and administration
- Contraindications
- Warnings
- Precautions
- Adverse reactions
- Information for the owner or person treating the animal
- Clinical pharmacology
- Effectiveness
- Target animal safety
- Storage information
- How the product is supplied
- NADA or ANADA number and FDA approval statement

The following describes these sections in detail:

- **Product Identification, Description and Prescription Legend** provides the product's brand name (often indicated by ®), generic name (the name give to the chemical entity), the dosage form (e.g., tablet, sterile solution, oral suspension, etc.), and the prescription legend (OTC, Rx, or VFD). The regulatory decision for designating a product as Rx, OTC, or VFD takes into consideration the need for veterinary involvement in the safe and effective use of the product. Considerations include the potential toxicity or other harmful effects of the product, its method of administration, collateral measures necessary for its use (e.g., accurate diagnosis of a disease with reasonable certainty), and all types of potential safety risks. The labeling for all veterinary prescription products contains the following statement: "Caution: Federal law restricts this drug to use by or on the order of a licensed veterinarian.

- **Indications** lists the specific disease(s) or conditions(s) for which a particular drug product is approved. The specific wording in this section depends upon the data contained in the effectiveness technical section of the approved new animal drug application.
- **Contraindications** defines the known circumstances under which a product should not be used because the risk associated with drug use clearly outweighs the possible benefit. Contraindications are based upon reasonable evidence that a drug caused a specific adverse reaction. Use of the drug in the situations described in the Contraindications section is likely to result in a serious adverse event that is fatal; life-threatening; requires professional intervention; or causes an abortion, stillbirth, infertility, congenital anomaly, or prolonged or permanent disability or disfigurement to the treated animal.
- **Warnings** describes serious adverse reactions and potential safety hazards to the animal being treated. Although the adverse reactions may be serious, FDA has determined that the benefit of using the drug outweighs the risk of the adverse event.

  The Warnings section may also describe potential actions that could be taken by the veterinarian to mitigate the adverse reaction should it occur, or to decrease the likelihood of the adverse reaction occurring, such as avoiding use in a predefined high-risk population. Warning statements are based on evidence indicating an association of a serious hazard with a drug, but not necessarily proof that the drug caused the reaction. Significant problems that may lead to death or serious injury may require a "boxed warning" on the package insert.

  The Warnings section may also include a user safety (Human Warnings) or human food safety section. The user safety section provides information regarding hazards to human health by contact, inhalation, ingestion, injection, or by other exposure to the product. The human food safety (Residue Warnings) section states the withdrawal time for use of the product in a food animal species. This section also warns against use of the drug in animals for which a withdrawal time has not been determined.
- **Precautions** includes additional information to enhance the safe use of the product by the practitioner. The Precautions section includes any additional information that is important for the safe use of the product that has not been included in the Contraindications or Warnings sections. The Precautions section may include recommendations for screening or diagnostic tests, information about drug-drug interactions, carcinogenesis, reproductive safety, adverse reactions in species other than the target species, or use in particular subpopulations of the target species, such as pediatric, geriatric, or animals with a particular disease.
- **Adverse Reactions** lists undesirable effects reasonably associated with the use of the drug that may occur as part of the pharmacological action of the drug or that may be unpredictable in their occurrence. The Adverse Reactions section is developed from the field effectiveness studies conducted by the pharmaceutical sponsor to support new animal drug approval. This section may also include a postapproval experience section, reporting any additional undesirable effects reported from the postapproval surveillance of the product in the larger population. The Adverse Reactions section includes a toll-free number for the practitioner to call for technical assistance from the pharmaceutical sponsor.
- **Information for Owner or Person Treating Animal** contains specific information for the owner or person treating the animal regarding the safe and effective use of the product. This information is designed to be conveyed by the prescribing veterinarian to the animal owner. Some products have a separate client information sheet (CIS) in addition to the package insert. The CIS sheet is designed to be given to the animal owner every time the product is dispensed. The CIS is typically required by the FDA when there is a need to give the animal owner detailed information about the potential for serious adverse reactions from the drug. The CIS may include information to help the animal owner recognize and report to the veterinarian any early signs of problems following the use of the product in the individual patient.
- **Clinical Pharmacology** is a concise summary of the pharmacology, pharmacokinetics, and pharmacodynamics of the drug in the target species. This section may also provide information about the drug class, potential drug-drug interactions, and the effect of food on product

bioavailability. For an antimicrobial agent, this section often includes a microbiology section with susceptibility data for the specific pathogens for which the product is approved.

- **Effectiveness** contains an abstract of the results from the effectiveness studies published in the FOI summary. The abstract provides a concise summary of the pivotal effectiveness studies and includes information such as the number and geographic location of study sites; the age, sex, and total number, etc., of animals in the study; a brief description of the study design; and the study results. The abstract describes how the effectiveness studies were conducted and how well the treated animals fared as compared to the control animals. This information can be considered from the perspective of the similarity between the study population versus the potential patient undergoing treatment (where the "patient" can represent an individual animal or a group of animals). For example, relevant questions may include whether the patient and the study population are of a similar age, class, and level of morbidity. This kind of information may be particularly useful when choosing between similar products that are approved and available for the same indications.With regard to the database supporting product approvals, more detailed information than provided by the abstract can be obtained in the FOI summary. These summaries are easily accessed from CVM's website (http://www.fda.gov/cvm/FOI/efoi.html) by simply inserting the NADA or ANADA number (another piece of information found on the package insert) for that product.
- **Animal Safety** provides an abstract of the results from the TAS studies that are required for FDA approval of the new animal drug. This information demonstrates the margin of safety for the drug. It also allows the reader to see what types of signs were observed in animals that received the drug at higher doses and for longer times than the intended dosage. It should help the practitioner decide whether to use the drug in animals that may be old or young or have compromised organ function. If adverse signs in a treated animal are observed, the package insert provides information regarding whether similar signs were noted during the safety testing of this application.
- **Storage Information** describes the recommended storage conditions that are needed to maintain the potency of the drug within acceptable limits before the established expiration date. When applicable, this includes practical information for shipping, warehouse storage, and storage by the user. Any mandatory storage conditions are described, e.g., "Store at controlled room temperature, 20–25°C (68–77°F)". When the drug is to be mixed with a diluent before use, this section describes the storage conditions for the diluted drug and also the time limitations for use of the diluted drug.
- **How the Product Is Supplied** can include a description of the delivery device, the number of units per package, and the dosage strengths.
- **NADA or ANADA Number** and **FDA Approval Statement:** The NADA or ANADA number can be used for searching the FDA/CVM website or for reporting product-specific adverse reactions.

The ANADA. In 1984, Congress signed into law the Drug Price Competition and Patent Term Restoration Act (Waxman Hatch Act, Public Law #98-14). This legislation created a system for the review and approval of generic versions of post-1962 human "pioneer" drug products through the use of ANADAs. In 1988, the Generic Animal Drug and Patent Term Restoration Act (GADPTRA) was signed into law (Public Law #100-670), amending section 512 of the FFDCA (21 U.S.C. 360b). GADPTRA provides statutory authority to approve ANADAs for generic copies of off-patent animal drugs approved for safety and efficacy.

Prior to GADPTRA, the FDA could approve abbreviated applications only for copies of animal drugs approved prior to 1962 and found to be effective under the DESI (drug efficacy study implementation) program. The intent of GADPTRA was to encourage competition and lower animal drug prices by allowing abbreviated applications for copies of previously approved drugs, without the generic drug sponsor duplicating the safety and efficacy studies that were required for the original NADA approval. GADPTRA permits an ANADA for an animal drug product that is the same as an animal drug product listed in the approved animal drug product list published by the Agency (listed new animal drug) with respect to conditions of use recommended in the product labeling, active ingredient(s), dosage form, strength, and route of administration.

An ANADA applicant may petition the Agency under Section 512(n)(3) of the FFDCA for permission to file an ANADA for a new animal drug product with certain defined changes from an approved pioneer product. The changes are limited to the following:

- A change of one active ingredient in an approved combination product
- A change in dosage form
- A change in dosage strength
- A change in route of administration
- A change in one active ingredient in a feed mixed combination

A generic sponsor may file a suitability petition to request that the specific change in the pioneer product be allowed. The petition must follow the format and content described for a Citizen Petition (21 CFR §10.20), which is a public document filed with the FDA. The FDA response to the petition is also a public document. The Agency determines whether to deny or approve the petition.

ANADAs need to address all the technical sections applicable to NADAs, but in some cases, the information needed to fulfill these requirements is different. For example, target animal safety and effectiveness are evaluated through the demonstration of product bioequivalence between the pioneer and generic products. The focus of bioequivalence studies is to determine whether differences in product manufacturing and formulation will affect the rate and extent of drug absorption. The fundamental assumption of all bioequivalence testing is if the rate and extent of drug absorption are comparable, the products will be medically indistinguishable and therefore interchangeable. Bioequivalence studies (i.e., blood level, pharmacologic endpoint, and clinical endpoint studies) and tissue residue depletion studies are conducted in accordance with GLP regulations (21 CFR Part 58). When absorption of the drug is sufficient to enable the quantification of drug concentrations in the blood (or other appropriate biological fluid or tissue) and if systemic absorption is relevant to drug action, a blood (or other biological fluid or tissue) level bioequivalence study should be conducted.

For certain generic drug products, the Agency may waive the requirement for demonstration of bioequivalence to the pioneer product. In general, the bioequivalence between solutions is considered to be self-evident for solutions with the same active and inactive ingredients in the same concentrations and with the same pH and physicochemical characteristics as the pioneer product. Categories of products that may be eligible for waivers include parenteral solutions intended for injection by the intravenous, subcutaneous, or intramuscular routes of administration, oral solutions or other solubilized forms, topically applied solutions intended to produce local therapeutic effects, and inhalant volatile anesthetic solutions.

When using serum or blood concentrations of drug in the evaluation of product bioequivalence, the principles underlying this assessment reflect a blending of pharmacokinetics and biostatistics. In addition to its use in generic drug product applications, bioequivalence studies may be used to support the approval of proposed changes in the manufacturing of a generic version of an approved off-patent product or to cover the safety and/or effectiveness of a sponsor's own drug. Blood level bioequivalence studies compare a test formulation to a reference formulation using parameters derived from the concentrations of the drug moiety and/or its metabolites (as a function of time) in the plasma, serum, or other appropriate biological fluid. This approach is applicable to dosage forms intended to deliver the active drug ingredient(s) to the site of action by way of the systemic circulation. Although usually conducted as a comparison of blood levels following single-dose administration, a multiple-dose study may be appropriate when there are concerns regarding poorly predictable drug accumulation. For details regarding the assessment of product bioequivalence, readers are referred to CVM Guidance #35 (*Bioequivalence Guidance*). Further discussion of the pharmacokinetic and statistical basis for bioequivalence determinations are provided later in this chapter in the section "The Use and Application of Pharmacokinetic Information."

Since veterinary generic drug products must contain all the same indications, warnings, cautions, directions for use, etc., that are associated with the approved pioneer product (except as deemed appropriate on the basis of the Suitability Petition, 21 CFR §512(n)(1)(F)), a bioequivalence study is generally needed for each species for which the pioneer product is approved (with the exception of "minor" species. See the section "The Office of Minor Use and Minor Species Animal Drug Development" of this chapter for additional information).When the product in question is a generic product intended for use in a food-producing animal, sponsors are required to conduct both bioequivalence and tissue residue studies unless blood concentrations of the active drug can be measured out to the withdrawal time of the pioneer product. The requirement is based upon the conclusion that tissue residue depletion of generic products is not adequately addressed through blood level bioequivalence studies. Differences that may go undetected in a blood level study (and which would be without clinical significance) could impact the withdrawal time because the latter is based on extremely low drug concentrations in the tissue (see earlier section, Human Food Safety [HFS]). A tissue residue study should generally accompany clinical endpoint and pharmacologic endpoint bioequivalence studies, 21 USC 360 b (n) (1) (A) (ii).

The sponsor of the generic product application uses the existing tolerance, marker residue, target tissue, and analytical method (as contained within the pioneer product's approved NADA) to determine the withdrawal time for the generic product (FDA/CVM Guidance For Industry [#35]). Accordingly, generic sponsors need only monitor the depletion of the unlabeled marker residue in the target tissue to establish a withdrawal time for the generic product. However, for reasons explained above, there is a risk that the generic formulation will be associated with a withdrawal time that differs (longer or shorter) from that of the pioneer product. For this reason, the end users of generic products should carefully read each product label to avoid the potential for incurring violative residues.

The Phased Review Process. Sponsors may submit a complete technical section for review during the investigation of the new animal drug under a process called *phased review*. The same requirements under 21 CFR §514.1 apply to all NADAs whether for phased review or not. Phasing of NADA submissions is a voluntary program. The option to phase the review of data submissions applies to all original NADAs and ANADAs and can be exercised up to the point at which the sponsor submits an NADA or ANADA. If a sponsor exercises the option to use the phased review process:

- Submissions relating to technical sections should be submitted during the investigation of the new animal drug and filed in an Investigational New Animal Drug (INAD) file established by CVM for the new animal drug.
- Each submission should contain information and data relating to only one technical section and should be under a separate cover. Sponsors are encouraged to contact the reviewing division regarding what information and data should be submitted together.

For additional information about the Administrative NADA process, refer to CVM Guidance #132 (*Guidance for Industry:* FDA/CVM Guidance for Industry, *The Administrative New Animal Drug Application Process*).

THE OFFICE OF MINOR USE AND MINOR SPECIES ANIMAL DRUG DEVELOPMENT

OVERVIEW. The Minor Use and Minor Species Animal Health Act of 2004 (the MUMS Act) provided for the establishment of the Office of Minor Use and Minor Species Animal Drug Development (OMUMS) (refer to FFDCA Title 21, Section 571, Subchapter F—New Animal Drugs for Minor Use and Minor Species). OMUMS reports directly to the director of CVM, and is responsible for overseeing the development and legal marketing of new animal drugs for minor uses (disease conditions that are rare) in major species (cattle, swine, chickens, turkeys, dogs, cats, and horses) and for minor species that fall under the category of "all other animals," including sheep, goats, game birds, emus, ranched deer, alpacas, llamas, deer, elk, rabbits, guinea pigs, pet birds, reptiles, ornamental and other fish, shellfish, wildlife, zoo animals, aquarium animals, and bees.

Because the markets are small and profit margins low for new animal drugs intended for minor uses in major species or for minor species, there are often insufficient economic incentives to motivate sponsors to develop the data necessary to support FDA approvals. In addition, some minor species populations are too small or their management systems too diverse to make it practical to conduct traditional studies to demonstrate safety and effectiveness. Consequently, manufacturers have not, in many cases, been willing to fund research to collect these data. Accordingly, very few new animal drugs intended for minor uses or for minor species have been approved and are legally marketed.

The limited availability of approved new animal drugs intended for minor uses or minor species has limited the availability of options for treating these sick animals. In many cases, the choices are to leave a sick animal untreated or to treat the animal with an unapproved drug. Failure to treat sick animals appropriately may increase public health hazards. For example, the transmission of disease from animals to humans or the shedding of disease-producing organisms by untreated animals into the environment may increase health risks to humans as well as to other animals. Treating an animal with an unapproved drug introduces questions of effectiveness and safety to the animal, to the environment, and to the public (e.g., human food safety).

Enactment of the 1996 ADAA reflected Congress' concerns about the lack of availability of approved new animal drugs. Among other things, the legislation recognized particular problems relating to the availability of approved new animal drugs for minor uses in major species and for use in minor species. The ADAA directed the Secretary of Health and Human Services to consider legislative and regulatory options for facilitating approval under section 512 of the Federal Food Drug and Cosmetic Act (FFDCA) (21 U.S.C. 360b) of new animal drugs intended for use in minor species or for minor uses. The ADAA further required the secretary to announce proposals for legislative or regulatory change to the approval process for new animal drugs intended for use in minor species or for minor uses. The MUMS Act is intended to amend the FFDCA to address the critical shortage of approved animal drugs for minor species and for minor uses in major species. It is intended to increase the availability of new animal drugs for minor species and for minor uses, while still ensuring appropriate safeguards for animal and human health.

The MUMS legislation modifies provisions of the FFDCA in three key ways, providing for

- **Conditional Approval**: The sponsor of a veterinary drug can ask CVM for conditional approval, which allows the sponsor to market the drug after proving the drug is safe and establishing a reasonable expectation of effectiveness, but before collecting all of the effectiveness data needed to support a full approval. The drug sponsor can keep the product on the market for up to 5 years, through annual reviews, while gathering the required effectiveness data.
- **Indexing:** The implementation of this regulation allows the FDA to add a minor species drug to an index of unapproved new animal drugs that may be legally marketed when the potential market for the drug is too small to support the costs of the drug approval process, even under a conditional approval. This provision is especially helpful to veterinarians treating zoo or endangered animals, and to owners of minor pet species such as ornamental fish or caged reptiles, birds, or mammals.
- **Designation**: This legislation provides incentives for approvals, such as grants to support safety and effectiveness testing. Sponsors must apply for designation prior to filing a new animal drug application for FDA approval. At the time that a designated drug gains approval or conditional approval, it is awarded 7 years of exclusive marketing rights. This means that FDA will not approve another application for the same drug in the same dosage form for the same intended use until after the 7 years have elapsed. This is 2 to 4 years longer than the protection provided from generic copying of nondesignated drugs. The MUMS marketing exclusivity also protects against approval of another pioneer (nongeneric) application for the same drug, in the same dosage form, for the same intended use.

GRANTS. The legislation also includes a provision that will allow Congress to appropriate funds for grants to defray the costs of safety and effectiveness testing for designated drugs.

IMPLEMENTING REGULATIONS FOR THE MUMS ACT. Both designation and conditional approval became available to sponsors when the bill was signed. Drugs could not be indexed until regulations implementing that provision were finalized (http://www.fda.gov/cvm/CVM_Updates/proMumsDes.htm). Those regulations were published December 6, 2007, and the agency started accepting indexing submissions in February 2008.

ADDITIONAL INFORMATION. For additional information regarding drug use in minor species, the reader is referred to Chapters 52 and 53 of this book.

INTERNATIONAL HARMONIZATION

Historically, the FDA has been concerned with the safety and effectiveness of animal drugs produced or marketed within the U.S. The FFDCA requires that exported pharmaceuticals meet or exceed the standards for approval in the U.S. *or* for the country to which they are being exported. It also requires that animal drugs marketed in interstate commerce in the U.S. be approved through the same process by the FDA, regardless of where they are manufactured. In addition to the US FDA, other countries have independently developed regulations and regulatory agencies that review safety, effectiveness, and purity of drugs that are intended for marketing within their specific jurisdiction for use in humans and/or animals. Although, internationally, the regulations share the common goal of protection of public health, the specific requirements and methodologies used in the evaluations of these products may diverge.When pursuing a broad international market, products may undergo multiple complete and autonomous reviews by regulating agencies in different countries or regions, and differences in the regulatory requirements between these agencies can retard the development of new drugs and drug products. Regulatory differences can also increase product development expenses, complicate international trade (both of products and of foods derived from animals consuming these products), and lead to duplication of animal studies. Growing globalization, emergence and spread of new animal diseases, and the international nature of the scientific community make it important to share innovation in animal treatment across borders, while maintaining standards for safety, quality, and effectiveness.

Internationally, formation of the European Community (EC) and later the European Union (EU) served as an impetus for the development of a shared regional process for the approval of new animal drugs. This set a pattern for harmonizing separate and diverse regulations among member countries. In 1990, the International Conference on Harmonisation of Technical Requirements for Registration of Pharmaceuticals for Human Use (ICH) was formed. This was followed by formation of the VICH in 1996. The VICH initially included the U.S., EU, and Japan, with the addition of Canada and New Zealand/ Australia as observers.The objectives of the VICH (http:// vich.eudra.org/htm/what.htm) are to:

- Establish and monitor harmonized regulatory requirements for veterinary medicinal products in the VICH regions, which meet high quality, safety, and efficacy standards and minimize the use of test animals and costs of product development.
- Provide a basis for wider international harmonization of registration requirements.
- Monitor and maintain existing VICH guidelines, taking particular note of the ICH work program and, where necessary, update these VICH guidelines.
- Ensure efficient processes for maintaining and monitoring consistent interpretation of data requirements following the implementation of VICH guidelines.
- By means of a constructive dialogue between regulatory authorities and industry, provide technical guidance enabling response to significant emerging global issues and science that impact on regulatory requirements within the VICH regions.

VICH Expert Working Groups, composed of scientific and technical experts representing each region, meet regularly to develop recommendations for more uniform standards for collection of preapproval and postapproval safety, purity, and effectiveness data. The goals of these working groups are to evaluate requirements of member agencies (within the context of current and emerging scientific knowledge), and to craft harmonized, science-based standards wherever possible. These standards are intended to maintain or enhance animal and public health and wellbeing. Despite the challenges of reaching scientific and regulatory harmony, this process has led to a long list of approved and draft guidances (http://vich.eudra.org/htm/ guidelines.htm), with more documents currently in development. These guidances are intended to allow the same studies to be used during the animal drug approval process of different regulatory agencies.

The FDA also participates in other international activities with a goal of protecting human and animal health in the global economy. During the early 1960s, the Food and Agriculture Organization (FAO) Conference and the World Health Organization (WHO) launched a joint effort to "protect the health of the consumers and ensure fair practices in the food trade." The primary product resulting from this program is the *Codex Alimentarius*, which literally means the food code (http://www.cfsan.fda. gov/~cjm/codex.html). This code represents a collection of food standards and guidance documents published jointly by the FAO and the WHO. Among these standards are maximum residual limits (MRLs) for veterinary drugs (MRLVD), as well as documents related to their use and control. The Codex Committee on Residues of Veterinary Drugs in Foods (CCRVDF) is specifically responsible for addressing the MRLVD (http://www.codexalimentarius. net/web/index_en.jsp). Additional information pertaining to WHO initiatives can be found elsewhere (Martinez et al. 2004).

The FDA also participates in General Subject Committees, Commodity Committees and Task Forces that determine standards and codes of practice for international trade (http://vich.eudra.org/htm/what.htm.; Castle 2005).

ADVERSE DRUG EXPERIENCE REPORTS

The primary purpose for maintaining the Food and Drug Administration—Center for Veterinary Medicine (FDA/CVM) Adverse Drug Experience (ADE) database is to provide an early warning or signaling system for adverse effects not detected during premarket testing of FDA-approved animal drugs and for monitoring the performance of drugs not approved for use in animals. The FDA/CVM ADE reporting system depends on the detection of an adverse clinical event by veterinarians and animal owners, the attribution of the clinical event to the use of a particular drug ("suspect" drug), and the reporting of the ADE to the manufacturer of the suspected drug or directly to FDA. Data from these ADE reports are coded and entered into the computerized FDA/CVM ADE database.

It is important to remember certain caveats when using data from the FDA/CVM ADE database:

- For any given ADE report, there is no certainty that the suspected drug caused the adverse event. This is because veterinarians and animal owners are encouraged to report all suspected ADEs, not just those that are already known to be caused by the drug. The adverse event may have been related primarily to an underlying disease for which the drug was given or to other concomitant drugs, or may have occurred by chance at the same time the suspect drug was administered.
- Accumulated ADE reports should not be used to calculate incidence rates or estimates of drug risk. The Division of Surveillance is responsible for consolidation of all drug experience reports, necessary referrals and consultations, and preparation of the summary reports. The division's ADE scoring system uses a modified Kramer scoring system (Bataller and Keller 1999). In this system, each sign is separated from the other signs and scored according to previous experience with the drug, alternative etiologic candidates (other causes), timing of the event, whether there was an overdose, whether the reaction continued or subsided with withdrawal of the drug, and whether a reaction recurred on reintroduction of a drug. Additional information on the criteria and responsibilities for the consolidation, screening, review, and evaluation of drug experience reports is further detailed in the CVM Program Policy and Procedures Manual section 1240.3522, Review and Evaluation of Drug Experience Reports (http://www.fda.gov/cvm/Policy_Procedures/3522.pdf).

Veterinarians and animal owners are encouraged to report adverse experiences and product failures to the government Agency that regulates the product in question. To access the FDA/CVM website for information and forms that are needed to report adverse experience with veterinary drugs, the reader is referred to http://www.fda.gov/cvm/adereporting.htm. Pretesting by the manufacturer and review of the data by the government does not guarantee absolute safety and effectiveness due to the inherent limitation imposed by testing the product on a limited population of animals. CVM encourages veterinarians and animal owners to contact the manufacturer of a suspect product. Withdrawal of an approved drug may be recommended if it is determined to be unsafe or ineffective.

The drug company marketing the drug product in question should be notified of the need to report an ADE for an FDA-approved animal drug. Drug company phone numbers can usually be obtained from product labeling. Technical services will ask a series of questions about the event, complete the FDA 1932 form, and forward the report to CVM. Alternatively, the report may be submitted directly to the FDA on Form 1932a.

Reports should preferably include a good medical history, all concomitant drugs the animal has been given, any recent surgical procedures, and as much in the way of clinical findings as is possible. Clinical findings may include veterinary exam, clinical chemistries, complete blood counts, urinalysis, fecal exams, radiographic results, and hemodynamic data such as blood pressure, any other pressure measurements in or around the heart, and neurological assessments.

"Veterinary Adverse Experience, Lack of Effectiveness or Product Defect Report," form *FDA 1932a*, is a preaddressed, prepaid postage form (Figs. 55.3A, B) that can be completed and dropped in the mail. This form may be

A

FOLD, SEAL, AND RETURN

VETERINARY ADVERSE DRUG REACTION, LACK OF EFFECTIVENESS OR PRODUCT DEFECT REPORT

DATE REPORTED

Form Approved: OMB No. 0910-0284
Expiration Date: January 31, 2010

NOTE: This report is authorized by 21 U.S.C 352(a) and (f). While you are not required to report, your cooperation is needed to assure comprehensive and timely assessment of product labeling.

If you do NOT want your identity disclosed to the manufacturer, place an "X" in this box. ☐

1. VETERINARIAN'S NAME AND ADDRESS

TELEPHONE (Include Area Code) ___ — ___ — ____

2. OWNER'S NAME OR CASE ID *(In Confidence)*

3. NADA NUMBER (For FDA Use)

4. SUSPECTED DRUG AND DOSAGE FORM

5. MANUFACTURER'S NAME

6. DIAGNOSIS AND / OR REASON FOR USE OF DRUG

7. ADMINISTERED BY
☐ VETERINARIAN
☐ OWNER

8. DOSAGE ADMINISTERED AND ROUTE *(Ex. 250 mg. q 12h, 5 days, orally)*

9. DATE(S) OF ADMINISTRATION

10. SPECIES	11. BREED	12. AGE	13. SEX	14. WEIGHT
				____ LBS.

15. CONCURRENT CLINICAL PROBLEMS
☐ NONE

OVERALL STATE OF HEALTH WHEN SUSPECTED DRUG GIVEN:
☐ GOOD ☐ FAIR ☐ POOR ☐ CRITICAL

16. CONCURRENT DRUGS ADMINISTERED
☐ NONE

17. REACTION INFORMATION

a. TIME BETWEEN INITIATION OF THERAPY WITH SUSPECTED DRUG AND ONSET OF REACTION WAS ____

b. TIME BETWEEN LAST ADMINISTRATION OF SUSPECTED DRUG AND ONSET OF REACTION WAS ____

c. OUTCOME: ☐ RECOVERED FROM REACTION ☐ DIED FROM REACTION ☐ OTHER *(Comment Below)*

d. WAS THE REACTION TREATED? ☐ NO ☐ YES *(Comment Below)*

e. WHEN THE REACTION APPEARED, TREATMENT WITH SUSPECTED DRUG:

☐ HAD ALREADY BEEN COMPLETED
☐ WAS DISCONTINUED DUE TO REACTION
☐ WAS DISCONTINUED AND REPLACED WITH ANOTHER DRUG
☐ WAS DISCONTINUED AND REINTRODUCED LATER
☐ WAS CONTINUED AT ALTERED DOSE
☐ OTHER *(Comment Below)*

AND THE REACTION

☐ CONTINUED
☐ STOPPED
☐ RECURRED
☐ OTHER *(Comment Below)*

f. LEVEL OF SUSPICION THAT DRUG CAUSED THE REACTION: ☐ HIGH ☐ MEDIUM ☐ LOW

18. DESCRIBE THE REACTION, ADD DETAILS ABOUT CASE HISTORY AND OUTCOME *(Include numbers if group of animals involved)*, GIVE COMMENT ON POSSIBLE CONTRIBUTING FACTORS. DESCRIBE LACK OF EFFECTIVENESS OR PRODUCT DEFECT *(Include Expiration Date and Lot No.)*

NOTE: Triple fold as marked, seal with tape, no postage required, additional space on back, if needed.

FORM FDA 1932a (3/07)

PSC Graphics: (301) 443-1090 EF

FIG. 55.3 Form FDA 1932A. A: front view; B: back view.

B

Public reporting burden for this collection of information is estimated to average 1 hour per response, including the time for reviewing instructions, searching existing data sources, gathering and maintaining the data needed, and completing and reviewing the collection of information. Send comments regarding this burden estimate or any other aspect of this collection of information, including suggestions for reducing this burden to:

Department of Health and Human Services
Food and Drug Administration
CVM, HFV-210 (0910-0012)
7500 Standish Place
Rockville, MD 20855

An agency may not conduct or sponsor, and a person is not required to respond to, a collection of information unless it displays a currently valid OMB control number.

FOLD

DEPARTMENT OF
HEALTH & HUMAN SERVICES

Public Health Service
Food and Drug Administration
Rockville MD 20857

Official Business
Penalty for Private use $300

NO POSTAGE NECESSARY IF MAILED IN THE UNITED STATES

BUSINESS REPLY MAIL

FIRST CLASS PERMIT NO. 946 ROCKVILLE MD

POSTAGE WILL BE PAID BY FOOD AND DRUG ADMINISTRATION

Department of Health and Human Services
Food and Drug Administration
CVM, HFV-210 (0910-0012)
7500 Standish Place
Rockville MD 20855

FOLD

THANK YOU FOR SHARING YOUR CONCERN ABOUT ANIMAL DRUG EFFECTS

18. *(Continued)*

FOR FDA USE ONLY

1. ______	☐ D	☐ NAI	**Confidentiality:** The owner's identity is held in strict confidence by FDA and protected to the fullest extent of the law. The reporter's identity, including the identity of self-reporter, may be shared with the manufacturer unless requested otherwise. However, FDA will not disclose the reporter's identity in response to a request from the public, pursuant to the Freedom of Information Act.	COMMENT
2. ______	☐ PR	☐ AI		
3. ______	☐ PO	☐ AP		
4. ______	☐ R	☐ AL		
5. ______	☐ NC			
6. ______				
T. ______				
☐ I.L.	☐ CR	☐ CONT		

WHEN MAILING FOLD THIS SECTION INSIDE

FIG. 55.3—*continued*

obtained by accessing the following web url: http://www.fda.gov/opacom/morechoices/fdaforms/FDA-1932a.pdf or by writing to

ADE Reporting System
Center for Veterinary Medicine
U.S. Food & Drug Administration
7500 Standish Place
Rockville, MD 20855-2773

The CVM can also be reached by phone at 800-FDA-VETS.

The Center may occasionally need more detailed information about an incident and the reporter may be called by a CVM staff veterinarian. The identities of all persons and animals is held in strict confidence by FDA and protected to the fullest extent of the law. The reporter's identity may be shared with the manufacturer or distributor unless requested otherwise. However, FDA will not disclose the reporter's identity to a request from the public, pursuant to the Freedom of Information Act. Information requested includes the reporter's name, address, phone number and the brand name of the drug involved. For information regarding CVM's surveillance program, the reader is referred to Chapter 58 of this textbook.

Additional contact information includes:

- Animal biologics: vaccines, bacterins and diagnostic kits: U.S. Department of Agriculture. 800-752-6255.
- Pesticides: topically applied external parasiticides: U.S. Environmental Protection Agency, 800-858-PEST.

LEVERAGING WITH THE FDA

Over the last few years, the FDA has emphasized the value of collaborating or partnering with outside parties as a primary strategy to more effectively accomplish its mission of promoting and protecting the public health. This concept of collaboration and partnership in FDA is generally known as *leveraging*. Within the framework of leveraging activities, collaborators work synergistically to achieve goals that neither party could achieve on its own. Examples include joint workshops to assess particular public health challenges, cosponsored training sessions, consensus standard setting, and mission-related research (Batson and Starinsky 2002).FDA/CVM partnerships reflect the creative thinking and initiative of our outside stakeholders, frontline employees, managers, and others. It is from these ideas that formal agreements and informal collaborative relationships have flourished. Formal agreements may include the following (Batson and Starinsky 2002):

- **Cooperative Agreement:** This involves a collaborative effort between the FDA and the partner in which substantial technical expertise is anticipated between both parties and FDA will provide at least part of the funding for the project.
- **Cost-Sharing Contract:** A cost-sharing contract is one under which the federal government contracts for goods or services and the contractor absorbs a portion of the total cost of the effort. These arrangements are usually appropriate when the contractor is able to apply or market the developed product for the benefit of their business.
- **Cooperative Research And Development Agreement (CRADA):** CRADAs involve collaborative efforts between the FDA and one or more partners (academia, industry, not-for-profit, for-profit, and state and local government organizations). From the FDA perspective, the CRADA is intended to help develop FDA technology, inventions, training programs, etc., that will facilitate achievement of mission-related goals. The CRADA partner, in return, receives some benefit from the establishment of this collaboration. The CRADA partner may provide funds to be used for the CRADA project. FDA and the partner may each contribute staff time and expertise, equipment, supplies, and facilities. Both parties are expected to make significant intellectual contributions to the objectives of the project.
- **Interagency Agreement (IAG):** The purpose of the collaboration is the sharing of knowledge, personnel, or other resources to strengthen programs of mutual concern between two or more federal agencies. It is also used as a mechanism for eliminating overlap or duplication of effort. Within the framework of the IAG, the parties may either contribute or receive funds, services, staff, property, facilities, or equipment, or exchange information to forward the common project goal.
- **Cosponsorship Agreement:** This can involve activities such as the joint development of a conference, seminar, symposium, educational program, or public information campaign that is related to the mission of the Agency. This kind of cooperative agreement involves the FDA and one or more nonfederal entities that share a mutual interest in the subject matter. As part of this cooperation, each party provides its own funding or staffing.

Potential leveraging opportunities should be brought to the attention of FDA/CVM program personnel or CVM Leveraging Points of Contact. After the idea or concept is discussed and a decision made with respect to moving forward, the appropriate mechanism for implementing the collaboration can be determined. Additional information on FDA leveraging activities can be obtained from the FDA's Leveraging Handbook, which is available on the FDA website http://www.fda.gov/oc/leveraging/default.htm

THE USE AND APPLICATION OF PHARMACOKINETIC INFORMATION

Since this is a pharmacology textbook, we would like to take this opportunity to discuss the potential value of pharmacokinetics for understanding product *in vivo* performance characteristics and how use of the pharmacokinetic information provided on a product label can address questions that may arise within the context of clinical practice situations. The basic pharmacokinetic principles being applied in this section have been discussed elsewhere in this textbook. Readers are referred to Chapters 2 and 3 for in-depth discussions of these basic pharmacokinetic principles. Many animal drug labels contain specific pharmacokinetic information that can assist veterinarians in their judgments regarding drug selection and dosage. Furthermore, there is a growing effort to characterize the impact of variables such as age, weight, gender, breed, diet, etc., on the rate and extent of systemic drug exposure. Therefore, to efficiently use such information, it is important that veterinarians understand how to interpret and apply this information and such variables as terminal elimination half-life, bioavailability, systemic clearance, and volume of distribution.

Pharmacokinetics has been used in many different aspects of drug development. Examples of possible uses of pharmacokinetics in the new animal drug development process are provided in Table 55.3. In some circumstances, drug concentrations in other matrices (such as

TABLE 55.3 Applications of pharmacokinetics in a regulatory environment

Purpose	Type of Studies	Relevant Examples or Published Guidance Documents
Bridging between formulations	Bioequivalence studies for generic drug approvals	CVM Bioequivalence Guidance (Guidance #35)
	Relative bioavailability studies to bridge between safety and/or effectiveness data contained in a sponsor's NADA	CVM Guidance #82 (Development of Supplemental Applications for Approved New Animal Drugs)
Bridging between animal species	Relative bioavailability studies to provide substantial evidence of effectiveness for minor species	CVM Guidance #61 (Guidance for industry: FDA approval of new animal drugs for minor uses and for minor species)
Dose justification/dose rationale	Blood levels that may help in dose selection when there is information available on pharmacokinetic-pharmacodynamic relationships	e.g., FOI for NADA 141-081; NADA 141-232
Information to assist in protocol development	Target animal safety and/or clinical effectiveness studies	e.g., Guidance 123 (Development of target animal safety and effectiveness data to support approval of nonsteroidal antiinflammatory drugs (NSAIDS) for use in animals)
For setting *in vitro* release specifications	Correlation of *in vitro* release characteristics with *in vivo* bioavailability.	e.g., see Shah 2005
For conveying information to the veterinarian on variables that may affect systemic drug exposure	Studies to characterize the drug's pharmacokinetics (e.g., clearance, volume of distribution, protein binding, metabolism, and route of elimination). Additional information may include dose proportionality, potential food effects or drug/drug interactions, and influence of age, gender or disease on dose-exposure relationships.	See discussion on pharmacokinetic information that may be provided in the package insert.

cerebrospinal fluid, bronchial secretions and urine) may provide valuable information regarding in vivo product performance.

Pharmacokinetic information is only as good as the experimental design and analytical method used to generate these data. For example, in the 1970s a pharmacokinetic study was conducted to determine whether cephalothin might be a good candidate for the treatment of bacterial meningitis in humans. Based on bacterial susceptibility and drug concentrations achieved in cerebrospinal fluids (CSF), as measured by bioassay, cephalothin appeared to achieve the concentrations in the CSF needed to treat bacterial meningitis. However, this drug was a clinical failure. The reason for this conflict was that the bioassay of CSF drug concentrations was actually measuring the cephalothin metabolite, desacetylcephalothin. Although the organism used in the bioassay, *Sarcina lutea,* was highly susceptible to both the parent and the metabolite, the targeted pathogens, *S. pneumoniae* and *N. meningitidis* were resistant to the metabolite (Nolan and Ulmer 1980). Because of the importance of using a validated analytical method for assaying drug concentrations in biological matrices, CVM provides recommendations on the methods assessments that should accompany the submission of pharmacokinetic datasets (FDA/CDER/CVM Guidance for Industry: Bioanalytical Method Validation Dated 05-2001. http://www.fda.gov/cder/guidance/4252fnl.htm).

Examples of other points that may be important during analysis of pharmacokinetic data include the following:

- Did animals vomit following administration and when did the event occur relative to dosing?
- Were the pharmacokinetic data generated with the final product formulation?
- Were animals fed or fasted prior to dosing?
- For some topically administered products, were the animals able to lick the product? (Laffont et al. 2003; Bousquet-Melou et al. 2004).
- Are there active metabolites?
- Does the drug exhibit stereospecific pharmacokinetics? For example, ketoprofen has been shown to have stereospecific pharmacokinetics (Lees al. 2003; Landoni et al. 2003).
- What is the magnitude of protein binding?

Table 55.3 provides examples of how pharmacokinetics has been applied in the evaluation of animal drug products.

In determining what type of studies may be appropriate, CVM recommends that factors such as the proposed conditions of use, release characteristics of the dosage form, the intended target animal species, and the drug's therapeutic uses be considered.

INTERPRETING THE PHARMACOKINETIC INFORMATION PROVIDED IN THE PACKAGE INSERT.

Types of pharmacokinetic information that a sponsor may choose to convey in the clinical pharmacology portion of the package insert include the basic pharmacokinetic parameters such as volume of distribution (V), systemic clearance (CL), terminal elimination half-life (T1/2), AUC, Cmax, time to Cmax (Tmax), mechanisms of elimination, magnitude of protein binding, and factors that may influence systemic drug exposure (e.g., food effects, influence of age, gender, altered hepatic or renal function). By the inclusion of labeling information on these variables, the veterinarian is informed of those clinical factors that may necessitate dose adjustments.

Terminal Elimination Half-life (T1/2). The T1/2 provides a clinician with an estimate of the time it will take to totally eliminate the drug from the body or the duration of dosing needed to attain steady-state conditions. As a general rule of thumb, when there are no saturable kinetic processes, veterinarians can multiply the half-life by 10 to estimate the duration of time it will take to effectively eliminate the active moiety from the systemic circulation. From a regulatory perspective, this information can be used when evaluating protocols for clinical safety and/or effectiveness studies, as well as for estimating the duration of washout needed between periods of a bioequivalence trial employing a crossover study design. It should be noted that 10 times the plasma or serum half-life value often differs from the withdrawal time established for human food safety. This difference may be because the tissue half-life and blood half-life differ, because the moiety being measured may differ, or because the endpoint (time to some established tolerance, as previously defined) differs. Furthermore, withdrawal time includes an additional factor to account for population variability. As previously mentioned, it is a statistical calculation of the time it takes to be 95% certain that 99% of the animals will have tissue concentrations of the marker residue that are at or below tolerance. There are some additional rules of thumb that can be applied to predict a likely withdrawal time for many compounds, as discussed in Chapter 61.

T1/2 can also be a valuable tool for estimating the time it will take to reach 90% steady-state blood levels of the drug (e.g., approximately 4 times the T1/2 under conditions of linear pharmacokinetics). When a drug can be described by a single exponential and it is administered via intravenous injection (or when the product is rapidly absorbed relative to the time it takes to eliminate the compound from the blood), T1/2 can be used to estimate the accumulation at steady-state using this equation (Gibaldi and Perrier 1982):

$$R = \frac{1}{1 - \exp^{-\lambda_z \times \tau}}$$

where R = the accumulation index, λ_z = the slope of the depletion phase (also referred to as *Kel* for a one-compartment model), and τ = the dosing interval (e.g., q24hr, q12hr, etc.).

Therefore, if we are dosing once daily (i.e., τ = 24 hr) and the half-life for that compound is 15 hr, then

$$\lambda_z = 0.693/15 \text{ hr} = 0.0413 \text{ hr}^{-1}, \text{ and}$$

$$\text{R} = \frac{1}{1 - \exp^{-0.0413 \times 24}} = 1.49$$

The accumulation index provides information on the ratio of Cmax values (comparing steady-state Cmax values to that observed following a single dose). It can also be used to predict the Cmin ratios (steady-state versus dose 1) or the ratio of AUC values estimated over a single dosing interval at steady-state versus the AUC estimated over the first dosing interval ($AUC_{0-\tau ss}/AUC_{0-\tau dose1}$) (Gibaldi and Perrier 1982).

This equation can also be used to provide a close approximation of the magnitude of accumulation that will occur for drugs that follow a two-compartment open body model. Errors can occur when there is a deep peripheral compartment. An important caveat is that this equation provides a good approximation of the magnitude of accumulation at steady-state primarily when the rate-controlling step in drug elimination is its CL. Overestimation of the magnitude of drug accumulation is likely to occur when the rate of absorption is slower than the rate of elimination. Situations that fall within this category include sustained-release products. To illustrate this point, we provide the following example of the relationship between estimates of T1/2 (based on the use of noncompartmental methods), dosing interval, and predicted versus actual level of drug accumulation. Drug profiles were simulated under a variety of conditions, including a drug that follows a one-compartment body model (i.e., the rate of depletion is best described by a single exponential), a drug that follows a two-compartment model and the majority of the AUC is associated with the β elimination phase, and a third compound exhibiting a slowly depleting compartment that is responsible for only a small portion of the overall AUC value (refer to Chapter 2 of this book for information on the pharmacokinetic characteristics of drug absorption, metabolism, distribution, and clearance). A comparison of the single dose profiles for these drugs is provided in Figure 55.4.

In this example, the fundamental difference in the profiles of the compounds following a one- versus two-compartment model is the "nose" representing the distribution phase of the drug associated with two compartments. In the case of the deep compartment, there is a very rapid initial distribution phase (α), a slower secondary depletion phase (β) and a very slow third depletion phase (γ). The vast majority of the profile is associated with the β elimination phase. Therefore, marked overestimations will occur if the γ elimination phase is used to estimate the magnitude of accumulation at steady-state. Although kinetic distinctions can be readily identified in these simulated examples, factors such as within and between subject pharmacokinetic variability, the selection of blood sampling times, and analytical method limitations can occasionally obstruct the identification of drug kinetic properties from actual datasets.

Another factor that can influence our ability to predict steady-state concentrations is the presence of an absorption rate constant that is less than the elimination rate constant of a drug when that drug is administered in an immediate release dosage form. This phenomenon is coined "flip-flop kinetics." Thus, as the absorption rate constant approaches or is less than the elimination rate constant, there is an increase in the magnitude of error associated with the predictions or *R*. The influence of pharmacokinetic model or rate of absorption on the accuracy of our estimates of steady-state drug concentrations is provided in Table 55.4.

The estimates for $AUC_{0-\tau ss}/AUC_{0-\tau dose1}$ and Cmax ratios were generally similar (except for the very slow absorption situation where there was a marked underestimation of the amount of drug absorbed after dose 1). However, dissimilar conclusions were derived from steady-state versus dose

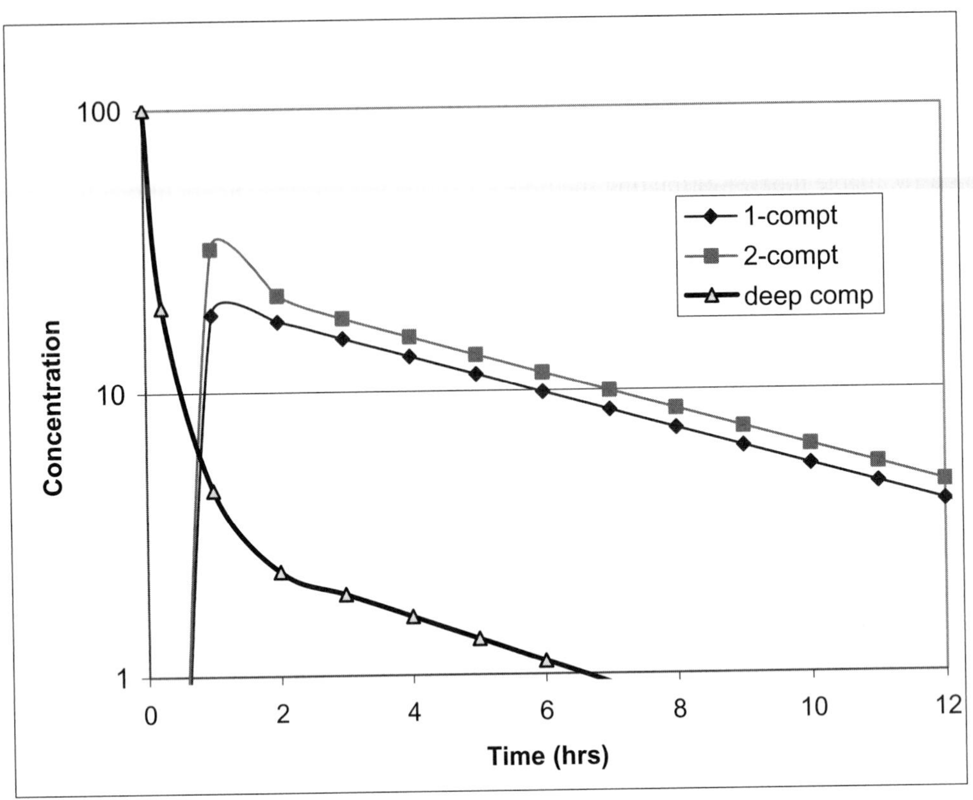

FIG. 55.4 Profile of the three kinds of compounds used in these simulations.

TABLE 55.4 Accuracy of estimating steady-state drug concentrations based upon the arithmetic estimate of R when applied to various pharmacokinetic situations. Doses were administered either once daily (two-compartment drug) or every 6 hours (deep-compartment drug)

Model	Absorption Rate Constant, Ka (hr^{-1})	Estimated Terminal Slope (λ_z), Dose 1 (hr^{-1})	Estimated Terminal Slope at Steady-State (λ_z, hr^{-1})	R-Estimated	Observed Accumulation Based upon Observed Parameter Values: AUC Ratios*	Cmin Ratios**	Cmax Ratios***
1-compt	0.01	0.0036		11.95	6.25	4.78	5.18
			0.0084	5.48			
	0.149	0.0986		1.10	1.15	1.06	1.14
			0.1057	1.09			
	0.5	0.149		1.03	1.04	1.03	1.04
	2.5	0.149		1.03	1.03	1.03	1.03
2-compt	0.01	0.0043		10.20	6.08	4.80	5.22
			0.0087	5.30			
	0.149	0.1008		1.10	1.13	1.06	1.14
			0.1024	1.09			
	0.5	0.149		1.03	1.04	1.03	1.04
	2.5	0.149		1.03	1.03	1.03	1.03
Deep-compt	Rapid input	0.185		1.49	1.00	1.49	1.02

*AUC ratio = $AUC_{0-\tau}/AUC_{0-24}$.
**Cmin ratios = Cmin at steady-state versus the concentration at hr 24 postdose. ***Cmax ratios = Cmax at steady-state versus Cmax after dose 1.

1 ratios based upon AUC and Cmax versus Cmin values when there was a deep compartment or when the absorption phase encompasses a large portion of the dosing interval. When there is a deep compartment, slow depletion from the deep compartment will have a substantial effect on Cmin values. However, if this deep compartment provides only a small contribution to the total AUC (e.g., less than 10%), this accumulation will have negligible impact on either steady-state AUC or Cmax values. This is graphically shown for the simulated example in Figure 55.5. In this case, $AUC_{0-\tau ss}/AUC_{0-\tau dose1})$ ~1.0 and only minimal accumulation was seen in Cmax (due to the slight elevation in Cmin values relative to Cmax), despite the substantial increase in Cmin.

Assessments of the likely magnitude of prediction error should be based on our understanding of the pharmacokinetics of the drug in question. When absorption is rapid and the majority of the AUC is associated with the depletion phase being used in our estimates of λ_z, R can serve as a valuable tool for predicting steady-state drug exposure.

The accuracy of our predictions of time to at least 90% steady-state concentrations was likewise dependent upon our ability to accurately capture half-life. The presence of flip-flop kinetics of a deep tissue compartment influences the accuracy not only of the predictions of steady-state drug accumulation but also the time to reach steady-state (Table 55.5).

Food Effects. Numerous products, when administered orally to monogastric species, have been found to have altered bioavailability when administered with food (Persson et al. 2005; Kung et al. 1995). This can be both drug-specific and formulation-specific (Jinno et al. 2006). For example, highly lipophilic compounds may have enhanced bioavailability when administered with food.

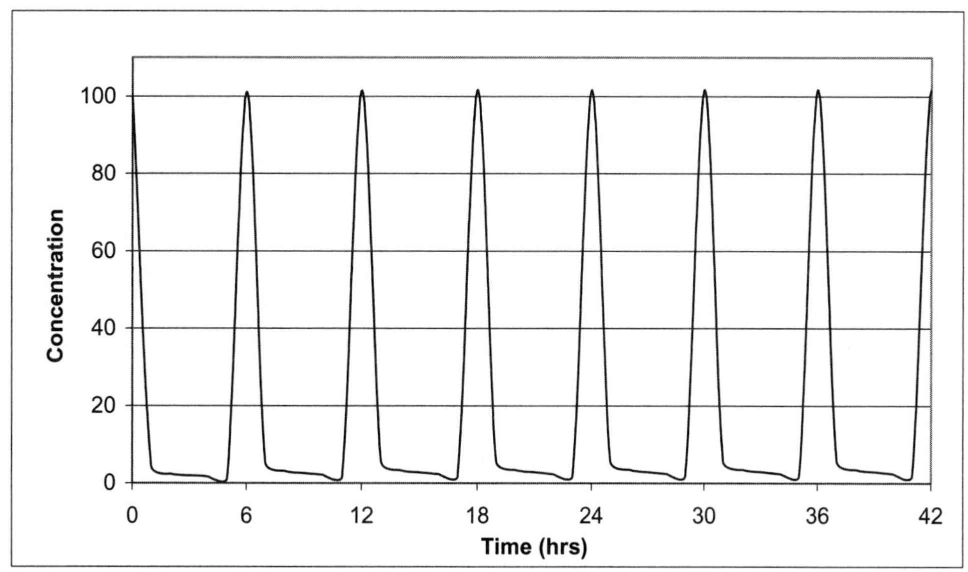

FIG. 55.5 Accumulation with repeated administrations.

TABLE 55.5 Accuracy of estimating time to at least 90% steady-state concentrations estimated on the basis of T1/2 values (where time to 90% accumulation is approximately equal to 4 × T1/2)

Model	Absorption Rate Constant, Ka (hr^{-1})	Using First Dose T1/2 (hr)	Using Last Dose T1/2 (hr)	Actual Dose When $AUC_{0-\tau}/AUC_{0-inf} > 0.9$
2-compartment	0.01	644 (dose 27)	311 (dose 13)	216 hr (dose 9)
	0.149	35	34	By dose 2
	0.5	23	—	By dose 2
	2.5	23	—	By dose 2
Deep compartment		19	—	By dose 2 (hr 12)

Acid labile products may be degraded by stomach acids when retention time is increased due to the intake of a meal. Changes in retention time are likely to influence the dissolution and hence alter drug absorption for drugs with either pH-dependent dissolution or for those compounds for which absorption rate is determined by the rate of gastric emptying. Information on the product package insert will indicate whether an effect of food has been evaluated and needs to be considered when the drug is being administered (e.g., NADA 141-151).

Effect of Age. There is little published information available on the influence of age on drug pharmacokinetics in veterinary species. The age of animal for which the product can be labeled is usually determined on the basis of the population of animals evaluated in the target animal safety and effectiveness studies. The package insert will indicate whether there are recommended age restrictions in product use due to lack of adequate safety information in that age group (e.g., NADA #111-798), whether there are recognized safety concerns associated with its use in very young animals (e.g., NADA #141-081), whether there are use restrictions due to the absence of a withdrawal period established in very young animals (e.g., preruminating calves) (e.g., NADA #141-061).

It is only recently that age has been an important focus within the context of human pharmaceutics (de Zwart et al. 2002). Certain differences, such as those seen in preruminating versus ruminating calves, bring obvious differences in drug bioavailability. Other less obvious differences are seen in drug metabolism. Renwick (1998) observed the following general trends in humans:

- Children tend to eliminate drugs more rapidly than do adults.
- For renally cleared compounds, elimination is markedly slower in neonates as compared to other age groups.
- There are some drugs that show age-related shifts in body weight adjusted clearance (such as amrinone, meropenen, midazolam, and cefotaxime). However, other drugs reach adultlike clearance values after the first few months of life (such as zidovudine, amikacin, and ketamine).

Clark University, in cooperation with the Connecticut Department of Public Health, created an extensive pediatric database containing published information across a wide range of pharmaceutical substances (Hattis et al. 2001).

In veterinary medicine, Sequin et al. (2004) observed that feline enrofloxacin pharmacokinetics was markedly influenced by animal age. They noted that the T1/2 was shorter in kittens 2 to 8 weeks of age as compared to adult cats and that the apparent volumes of distribution were lower at 2 to 4 weeks of age and greater at 6 to 8 weeks of age. The greater volume of distribution and clearance in kittens 6 to 8 weeks of age resulted in lower plasma concentrations, and the authors concluded that doses may need to be increased to achieve therapeutic drug concentrations when enrofloxacin is administered to kittens 6 to 8 weeks of age. In terms of geriatric animals, practitioners need to consider the possible decrease in renal and/or hepatic function as these could lead to substantial increases in drug exposure (remember that $AUC = Dose \times F/CL$. Therefore, a change in CL is equivalent to a commensurate change in dose). Similarly, old age may be associated with changes in volume of distribution, thus influencing free drug concentrations (Crome 2003; Steinmetz et al. 2005).

Effect of Body Weight. For highly lipophilic compounds, animal weight may influence volume of distribution and therefore T1/2. In dogs, the proportion of body adipose tissue per unit body weight was significantly increased in animals less than 4 weeks of age as compared to adults (Kienzle et al. 1998). Gender differences may occasionally be attributable to differences in the proportion of body fat per unit weight. For example, significant weight effects were observed when oral moxidectin was administered to beagle dogs (Vanapalli et al. 2002). Along with this finding, the terminal half-life was statistically significantly longer in females as compared to males. To some degree, this problem is less dramatic in veterinary medicine as compared to human medicine because most veterinary compounds are prescribed on a mg/kg basis. Nevertheless, practitioners may find it helpful to consider the potential impact of body composition when prescribing medications.

Gender Effects. For some compounds, differences have been observed between the pharmacokinetics in males versus females (Harris et al.. 1995; Lin et al. 1996; Parkinson et al. 2004; Ohhira et al. 2006). Related concerns associated with gender effects in human medicine can be found at the CDER website (http://www.fda.gov/cder/reports/womens_health/women_clin_trials.htm). If present, the label will indicate whether the dosing recommendations differ between males and females.

Change of Pharmacokinetics in Pregnancy and Lactation. Numerous changes in pharmacokinetics can occur during pregnancy (FDA/CDER Draft Guidance for Industry: Pharmacokinetics in Pregnancy—Study Design, Data Analysis, and Impact on Dosing and Labeling: Draft dated 10/2004). These pharmacokinetic alterations can be due to such factors as the following:

- Changes in total body weight and body fat composition
- Delayed gastric emptying and prolonged gastrointestinal transit time
- Increased extracellular fluid and total body water
- Increased cardiac output, increased stroke volume, and elevated maternal heart rate
- Decreased albumin concentration with reduced protein binding
- Increased blood flow to the various organs (e.g., kidneys, uterus)
- Increased glomerular filtration rate
- Changed hepatic enzyme activity, including phase I CYP450 metabolic pathways (e.g., increased CYP2D6 activity), xanthine oxidase, and phase II metabolic pathways (e.g., N-acetyltransferase)

Clinically important changes in drug pharmacokinetics can also occur during lactation (Petracca et al. 1993; Hossaini-Hilali and Olsson 1993; Soback et al. 1994; Cao et al. 2001; Mottino et al. 2002). These changes may be the result of extensive partitioning of the drug into milk (increasing drug clearance and, if there is transfer between milk and blood, increasing the volume of distribution), differences in transporter activity or metabolism caused by endogenous hormonal changes, altered body fat proportion, and changes in weight or muscle mass (FDA/CDER Guidance for Industry: Clinical Lactation Studies—Study Design, Data Analysis, and Recommendations for Labeling. *Draft Guidance* dated 02/2005). These changes may influence the safety and effectiveness of the drug in the patient or, if pregnant or nursing, may pose risks in the fetuses/nursing animals. Therefore, the product label will generally state whether CVM has evaluated the safety and effectiveness of that product for use in reproducing and lactating animals (e.g., NADA #141-075). In terms of lactating dairy cattle, it is important not to use a product that has not been approved for this purpose as violative residues in milk may result (e.g., June 21 2004 CVM update http://www.fda.gov/cvm/CVM_Updates/milkresup.htm).

Breed Effects. There are recognized breed differences in metabolism, disease response and kinetics in cattle (Elsasser et al. 2005). Similarly, metabolic differences have been observed across breeds of dogs (http://omia.angis.org.au/). There are over 350 inherited disorders that have been described in the purebred dog population (Patterson et al. 1988). Breed-related differences in drug absorption have been correlated with differences in intestinal transit time (Meyer et al. 1993; Weber et al. 2002, 2003) and potential differences in intestinal permeability (Randell et al. 2001; Weber et al. 2002). An example of breed effect that has been included in product labeling is the warning associated with use of ivermectin-containing compounds in some sensitive collies (e.g., NADA 140-971). An extensive review of breed effects in dogs has recently been published elsewhere (Fleischer et al. 2008).

Protein Binding. For certain compounds (specifically, those associated with low renal or hepatic extraction ratios), protein binding can significantly affect the total systemic clearance. Furthermore, when evaluating the pharmacokinetic-pharmacodynamic relationship of antimicrobial compounds, it is generally appropriate to base these evaluations on free (unbound) rather than total (free plus bound) drug concentrations (Liu et al. 2002; Drusano 2004; Müller et al. 2004). This is because the pharmacodynamic component is expressed relative to drug antimicrobial activity that is usually estimated in protein-free media. In disease states associated with altered plasma protein binding, changes in total drug concentrations may occur for highly protein bound drugs (e.g., >90%). For certain drug moieties, such as propofol, altered protein binding can have clinically relevant effects (Hiraoka et al. 2004). However, in most cases, altered protein binding will not influence the AUC of the free drug moiety, although total drug concentrations may change (Benet and Hoener 2002; Toutain and Bousquet-Melou 2002). The potential disparity between free and total drug concentrations should be considered if one is doing therapeutic drug monitoring because in many situations, adjustments in dose, when based solely upon total plasma concentrations, can lead to higher than desired free drug concentrations and, possibly, drug toxicity. For additional information on therapeutic drug monitoring, the reader is referred to Chapter 51 in this textbook.

Protein binding information can be found in the clinical pharmacology portion of the product label (e.g., see NADA # 140-684).

Michaelis Menton Kinetics. When there are saturable processes associated with either the absorption or elimination of a compound, it is no longer appropriate to predict dose-proportional changes in drug exposure with changes in a dosage regimen. When there are saturable absorption processes, the increase in drug exposure will be less than that expected on the basis of the magnitude of increase in administered dose. This may impact product effectiveness. Conversely, if there are nonlinear elimination processes, the increase in drug exposure will exceed what is anticipated on the basis of the increase in delivered dose. This may impact target animal safety. Therefore, any known information regarding nonlinear kinetics will be described on the package insert (e.g., NADA # 141-075).

TYPES OF MEANS USED IN PRODUCT LABELING.

An aspect of pharmacokinetic information that may be unfamiliar to users is that parameter values provided in the package insert are listed as arithmetic means, least square (LS) means, harmonic means, or geometric means (Zar 1998). The question is how do these various means differ? To address this question, Table 55.6 lists 10 estimates of half-life. These initial values are then manipulated as indicated in this table. From the change in the value associated with each mean, we see that identical values can result in differing mean estimates, depending on how these means were calculated.

Another question pertains to the difference between LS means and arithmetic means. Arithmetic means and LS means are identical when groups contain an identical number of observations across animals with differing characteristics. However, when there are inequalities in the numbers of these disparate subjects, the arithmetic and LS means can differ. For example, if the half-life of a drug is longer in females than males, the arithmetic means would be higher for a group composed of 7 females and 3 males than for a group containing 5 females and 5 males. In contrast, the LS means would adjust for the differences in these ratios. This point is illustrated in Table 55.7.

To provide an example of how the method of calculation can influence our interpretation of the study data, let's consider the following hypothetical everyday situation:

A survey was being conducted to determine the number of individuals that arrived by bus or by car to a particular tourist destination and to determine whether the duration of the journey was generally shorter when the travelers arrived by car or by bus. The survey resulted in the following table of values (Table 55.8).

The tourist company found that only slightly more people arrived by bus (73) as compared to by car (70) and that most of the tourists lived more than 300 miles away. When examining the arithmetic mean, they concluded that the time for arrival to destination was similar when the tourists arrived by car or by bus. While that was a true

TABLE 55.6 Comparison of various kinds of means used with pharmacokinetic data

	T1/2	Ln-Transformed	Reciprocal T1/2	0.693/T1/2 (= λ_z)
	5.00	1.61	0.20	0.14
	8.00	2.08	0.13	0.09
	9.00	2.20	0.11	0.08
	4.00	1.39	0.25	0.17
	4.00	1.39	0.25	0.17
	6.00	1.79	0.17	0.12
	7.00	1.95	0.14	0.10
	7.00	1.95	0.14	0.10
	8.00	2.08	0.13	0.09
Arithmetic mean	6.44	1.83	0.17	0.12
Geometric mean[1] [exp (Ln T1/2)]		6.21		
Harmonic mean[2]			5.95	
T1/2 based on 0.693/λ_z[3]				5.95

[1]Geometric mean = the back-transformed mean of the log-transformed variables
[2]Harmonic mean = the reciprocal of the arithmetic mean of reciprocals
[3]$T1/2 = Ln(2)/\lambda_z = 0.693/\lambda_z$. T1/2 can also be expressed as $Ln(1/2)/-\lambda_z = -0.693/-\lambda_z$.

TABLE 55.7 An example of differences in the LS mean versus the arithmetic mean

Subject #	Gender	$T^{1/2}$ (hr)
1	Male	2
2	Male	3
3	Male	4
4	Female	7
5	Female	8
6	Female	9
7	Female	9
8	Female	7
9	Female	6
10	Female	8
Arithmetic mean		6.3
LS mean		5.3

TABLE 55.8 Survey results from a tourist company

Length of Journey	Bus	Car
>300 miles	38 travelers, average = 7.9 hr	22 travelers, average = 9.7 hr
200 to 300 miles	28 travelers, average = 6.3 hr	12 travelers, average = 7.7 hr
<200 miles	7 travelers, average = 3.4 hr	36 travelers, average = 4.8 hr
Arithmetic mean	6.64 hr	6.56 hr
LS means	5.86 hr	7.37 hr

statement, it is also evident that there is bias in the arithmetic mean. When considering that more folks used the bus when traveling from further distances, it became clear that in part, the arithmetic mean was confounded by the distance traveled. To correct for this imbalance, the LS mean was evaluated. When corrected for distance, the conclusion was actually quite different, and it was evident that the trip was generally more rapid when individuals took the bus (5.86 hr) as compared to the car (7.37 hr).

ASSESSING PRODUCT RELATIVE BIOAVAILABILITY. The pharmacokinetic and statistical considerations that are involved in the design and analysis of in vivo bioequivalence trials are described in CVM's Guidance #35 (Bioequivalence Guidance). The pivotal blood level parameters for supporting product comparability are the AUC measured from time zero to the last quantifiable drug concentration (for a single dose study), and the Cmax (FDA/CVM Guidance #35). When blood levels are measured under steady-state conditions, the AUC is measured over a single dosing interval (AUC $_{0-\tau}$). Prior to initiating any bioequivalence trial, CVM protocol concurrence is always strongly encouraged.

Ordinarily, studies are conducted with healthy animals that are representative of the species, class, gender, and physiological maturity for which the pioneer drug product is approved. The assumption is that the potential for formulation effects on drug absorption will be the same in the healthy animal and in the targeted patient population.

When using a bioequivalence trial to compare formulation effects, a basic tenant is that there is no difference in either the volume of distribution or the clearance of drug between administrations. For example, when comparing estimates of AUC, we are actually comparing the following:

$$\text{Relative bioavailability} = \frac{\dfrac{F_{test} \times D_{test}}{CL_{test}}}{\dfrac{F_{ref} \times D_{ref}}{CL_{ref}}}$$

where D_{test} = dose of the test product; D_{ref} = dose of the reference product; F_{test} = fraction absorbed of the test product; F_{ref} = fraction absorbed of the reference product; CL_{test} = total systemic clearance of the test product; CL_{ref} = total systemic clearance of the reference product.

It is only when $D_{test} = D_{ref}$ and $CL_{test} = CL_{ref}$ that our comparisons provide an unbiased estimate of the product ratio of fraction absorbed. Therefore, we cannot use traditional *in vivo* bioequivalence studies to compare two dosage forms that may differ in terms of the actual dose administered to or consumed by the patient. For example, a product approved for administration in drinking water may have a different pattern of intake as compared to the same drug in medicated feed. Therefore, even if the two dosage forms are found to have no pharmacokinetic differences (e.g., as shown by a comparison of equal gavage doses), potential differences in "D" under clinical conditions confound our ability to declare the two dosage forms as being bioequivalent.

Cmax is a parameter that reflects both the rate and extent of absorption. This point can be seen in the equation that describes Cmax for a drug that follows a one-compartment body model:

$$C\max = \frac{Ka \times F \times D}{V(Ka - Kel)} \times \left(e^{-Kel \times T\max} - e^{-Ka \times T\max}\right)$$

where Ka = the absorption rate constant, $Kel = \lambda_z$ = the terminal elimination rate constant (where Kel = CL/V), $Tmax$ = the time to Cmax, and V = the volume of distribution. Therefore, any change in F will influence both AUC and Cmax. However, changes in Ka affect only Cmax values.

Similar to AUC, to obtain an unbiased estimate of the influence of formulation on Cmax, we need to have a comparison where the values of D, V, and Kel are equal across treatments.

The ability to declare products as equivalent depends upon the number of subjects included in the investigation, the magnitude of difference in the pharmacokinetic parameter, and the variability associated with that parameter. When a crossover design is used, intersubject variability is removed from the statistical model, leaving only the variability that cannot be explained by either period or treatment effects. When a parallel study design is used, intersubject variability cannot be removed from the effects associated with treatment effects. Since between-subject variability is generally larger than within-subject variability, it is frequently more difficult to determine product bioequivalence when using a parallel as compared to crossover study design.

Statistically, CVM advocates use of the 90% confidence intervals (the one-sided test procedure originally described by Schuirrman (1987)). Within the U.S., the limits necessary to define bioequivalence are generally 0.80–1.20 (untransformed data, based upon treatment differences and expressed relative to the reference mean) or 0.80–1.25 (Ln-transformed data, expressed as the ratio of the test/reference means). While alternative statistical methods are described in CDER guidance documents (FDA/CDER Guidance for Industry, Statistical Approaches To Establishing Bioequivalence, Finalized 01/2001), use of these alternative methods has not been described in CVM's Guidance #35. When using the 90% confidence interval approach to declare two products as being bioequivalent, we are stating that we are 90% certain that the interval from X to Y contains the true ratio of treatment means across the population of individuals. For any level of certainty, the width of the interval can decrease by the following:

- Decreasing the variability in estimates of the treatment means. Therefore, study design and analytical method are important points of consideration. Whenever possible, crossover studies are generally preferred to parallel designs.
- An increase in subject numbers. The larger the sample size, the greater the representation of the true population. The better the representation of the population, the smaller the intervals need to be to achieve the same level of certainty.

To demonstrate the latter point, we simulated a parallel study that employed two identical populations of subjects. The parameter values for the two treatments were identical and each input parameter was generated with identical amounts of variability. In this simulation, the distribution of AUC values for the test and reference products were identical (and therefore, the two products were in fact equivalent). However, the AUC values for these two products had a coefficient of variation equal to ~30%. Using this information, we explored the frequency of simulating a bioequivalence trial that succeeded in demonstrating that the two products were indeed bioequivalent as a function of the number of subjects included in the study. The result of this exercise is provided in Table 55.9.

From this table, it is seen that despite the large variability, as study size increases, there is an increase in ability to accurately declare these two products as bioequivalent. With very large sample sizes, bioequivalence is declared despite the high level of variability associated with these two simulated datasets.

In a typical two-period crossover design, subjects are randomly assigned to either sequence A or sequence B with the restriction that equal numbers of subjects are initially assigned to each sequence. The design is as follows:

TABLE 55.9 Relationship between the numbers of subjects included in a simulated bioequivalence trial versus the frequency of correctly declaring these two products as being bioequivalent (e.g., 0.48 means that equivalence criteria were met in 48% of the simulations)

# Subjects	10	15	20	24	30	40	100	1000
Declare equivalence	0.48	0.57	0.65	0.70	0.73	0.78	0.97	1.00

Sequence A	Sequence B
Period 1 Test	Reference
Period 2 Reference	Test

A critical assumption in the two-period crossover design is that there is an equal magnitude of physiological and pharmacological carryover between periods 1 and 2, regardless of the order of treatment administration. This carryover is also termed *residuals* or *residual effects*. Unequal residual effects may result, for example, from an inadequate washout period. A one-period parallel design may be preferable when the drug induces physiological changes in the animal (causing a physiological carryover effect); when the drug has a very long terminal elimination half-life, creating a risk of residual drug present in the animal at the time of the second period dosing; and when the duration of the washout time for the two-period cross-over study is so long as to result in significant maturational changes in the study subjects.

Another assumption inherent in bioequivalence trials is that there is no subject by formulation interaction. In other words, the assumption is that the population of all potential drug recipients will exhibit similar relative bioavailability of the test and reference products. If this is not the case, it would be possible to overlook the presence of a small subpopulation for which the two products may not perform in an equivalent manner (Meyer 1995). Fortunately, subject-by-formulation interactions are rarely observed.

When a generic drug sponsor seeks the approval of a multistrength solid oral dosage form product, waiver of *in vivo* bioequivalence study requirements may be granted if *in vivo* bioequivalence has been demonstrated between the highest strengths of the generic and pioneer products, the lower dosage strengths exhibit in *vitro* dissolution characteristics comparable to that of the corresponding strength of the pioneer product, and the generic product formulations are dose-proportional with respect to the ratio of active and inactive ingredients. In cases where the active drug has poor water solubility, manufacturing and tableting conditions may alter product bioavailability and *in vivo* bioequivalence studies of both the highest and lowest dosage strengths may be needed. A bioequivalence waiver may be granted on the basis of *in vitro* dissolution if minor changes in the composition or manufacturing method of an approved product are proposed (refer to FDA/CVM Guidance #83: Chemistry, Manufacturing and Controls Changes to an Approved NADA or ANADA: Guidance). Most recently, the mechanism for granting waivers for Type A medicated articles has been established for active ingredients that are soluble in aqueous fluids across a pH range of 1.2 (0.1N HCl) to 7.5 (FDA/CVM Guidance for Industry #171).

UNDERSTANDING THE RELATIONSHIP BETWEEN DOSE AND DRUG EXPOSURE. Examples of the many variables that can potentially influence drug exposure were described in the previous section "Interpreting the Pharmacokinetic Information Provided in the Package Insert."

Much of the information generated on the safety of products under the intended dosing conditions are derived from the TAS study (refer to the previous section "Technical Sections of NADAs/Target Animal Safety (TAS)." The use of exaggerated doses and duration of dosing during the TAS study accommodates the variability in animal sensitivity to the drug and its metabolites. In addition to difference in kinetics that can occur across animal breeds, there can also be changes in CL that occur as a consequence of disease (Kraemer et al. 1982; Abdullah and Baggot 1986, 1988; Monshouwer et al. 1996a,b; Renton 2001). Since TAS studies are typically conducted in healthy animals, blood samples taken during the TAS study can help identify the potential risk of toxicity if/when some pharmacokinetic parameters change under disease conditions.

To illustrate how blood level data may be helpful in the interpretation of target animal safety data, let's take a hypothetical example of a drug that exhibits nonlinear absorption. For simplicity, let's assume that our orally administered drug follows a one-compartment open body model with the following mean pharmacokinetic parameters: ka = 1.25 hr^{-1}, kel = 0.05 hr^{-1}, and V/kg = 1.0 l. In this example, F is ~100% below a 100 mg dose, but declines to ~28% at a 500 mg dose. The actual mg dose absorbed in this example is provided in Figure 55.6.

Although we administered a 1X, 3X, 5X dose (100, 300, and 500 mg dose), the drug exposure reflected the absorption of only a 90 mg, 132 mg, and 140 mg dose (i.e., F = 0.9, 0.44, and 0.28 for a 1X, 3X, and 5X dose, respectively). Such nonlinearity may occur with some drugs, particularly those orally administered drugs that either are absorbed via carrier-mediated pathways or are highly lipophilic in nature (therefore, in vitro dissolution may be problematic at exaggerated doses). Generally, the animals

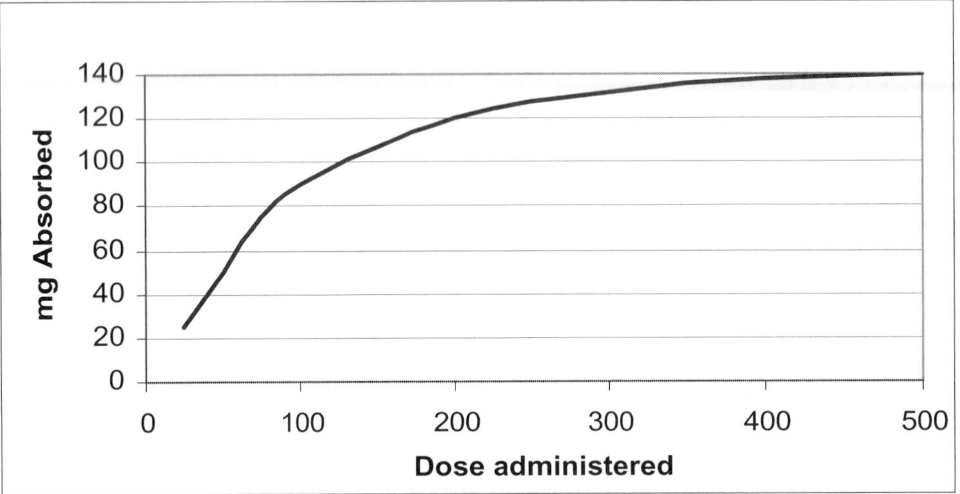

FIG. 55.6 Nonlinear absorption.

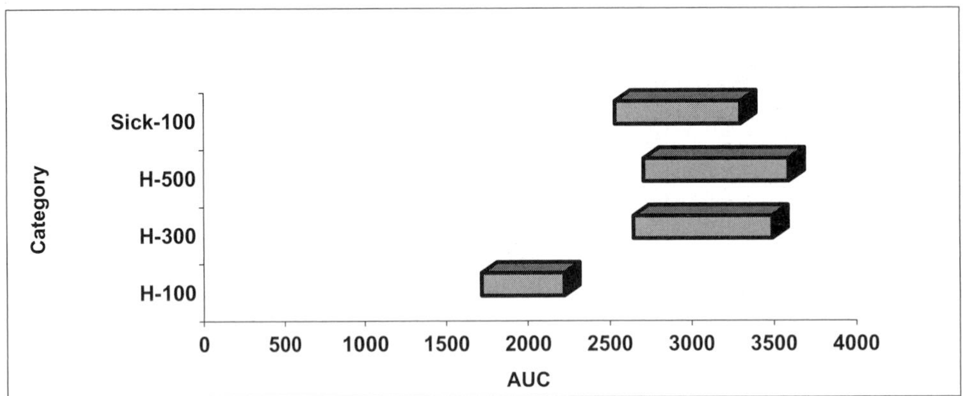

FIG. 55.7 Simulated example of a potential relationship between dose and AUC in healthy versus diseased animals.

enrolled in the TAS trial are of a single breed, healthy, and are maintained under well-controlled conditions. The laboratory setting tends to minimize between-subject variation. To accommodate the potential differences in pharmacokinetics in laboratory animals versus the targeted animal patient, our simulations include a 50% reduction in CL and an increase in the variability of that CL to 40% CV. For the sake of simplicity, we will assume that there is no change in either F, Ka, or V. The resulting AUC values (mean ±1 standard deviation) are provided in Figure 55.7.

In this illustration, there is a substantial difference in the AUC of the 1X versus the 3X and 5X groups during the TAS study. However, under the simulated conditions for diseased animals, there is an overlap between the AUCs associated with a 1X dose in diseased subjects versus the 3X and 5X drug exposure generated with parameters representing laboratory animals. Thus, in this example, it would be preferable to consider the margin of safety from a perspective of drug exposure rather than of dose.

CONCLUSION

The Center for Veterinary Medicine is a consumer protection agency, fostering public and animal health by approving safe and effective products for animals and by enforcing other applicable provisions of the Federal Food, Drug, and Cosmetic Act and other authorities. CVM works to safeguard the health and increase productivity of food-producing animals in the United States—97 million cattle,

59 million pigs, 8.8 billion chickens, 272 million turkeys, and 7 million sheep. CVM also evaluates the safety and effectiveness of drugs used to treat more than 100 million companion animals (http://www.fda.gov/opacom/factsheets/justthefacts/6cvm.html). The regulation of new animal drugs represents an interaction of science, statistics, veterinary practice, and law. These efforts are complicated by an ever-changing scientific, political, and veterinary medical landscape. As these changes occur, regulators work diligently in an effort to accommodate new issues, concerns, and technologies.

ACKNOWLEDGMENTS

The authors would like to thank the following individuals for sharing their expertise on the following sections:

Manufacturing Chemistry: Mr. William Marnane
Human Food Safety: Dr. Mark Robinson
Environmental Safety: Dr. Charles Eirkson

REFERENCES

Abdullah, A.S. and Baggot, J.D. 1986. Influence of *Escherichia coli* endotoxin-induced fever on pharmacokinetics of imidocarb in dogs and goats. American Journal of Veterinary Research 45:2645–2648.

———. 1988. The effect of food deprivation on the rate of sulfamethazine elimination in goats. Veterinary Research Communications 12:441–446.

Annon. 1996. CVM Update: October 18, 1996 President Signs Animal Drug Availability Act. http://www.fda.gov/cvm/CVM_Updates/adaa.html. Accessed 06-30-06.

Bataller, N. and Keller, W.C. 1999. Monitoring adverse reactions to veterinary drugs. Pharmacovigilance. Veterinary Clinics North America, Food Animal Practice 15:13–30.

Batson, D. and Starinsky, M. 2002. FDA leveraging initiative in line with President's management agenda. FDA Veterinarian Newsletter, July/August Vol 17.

Benet, L.Z. and Hoener, B.A. 2002. Changes in plasma protein binding have little clinical relevance. Clinical Pharmacology and Therapeutics 71:115–121.

Bousquet-Melou, A., Mercadier, S., Alvinerie, M., and Toutain, P.L. 2004. Endectocide exchanges between grazing cattle after pour-on administration of doramectin, ivermectin and moxidectin. International Journal of Parasitology 34:1299–1307.

Cao, J., Huang, L., Liu, Y., Hoffman, T., Stieger, B., Meier, P.J., and Vore M. 2001. Differential regulation of hepatic bile salt and organic anion transporters in pregnant and postpartum rats and the role of prolactin. Hepatology 33:140–147.

Castle, P. 2005. European Pharmacopoeia (EP), USDA and MAFF standards—Will they ever be harmonised under the VICH umbrella? Developments in Biologicals (Basel) 121:227–234.

Crome, P. 2003. What's different about older people. Toxicology 192: 49–54.

De Zwart, L.L., Haenen H.E.M.G., Versantvoort, C.H.M., and Sips A. J.A.M. 2002. Pharmacokinetics of ingested xenobiotics in children: a comparison with adults. RIVM report #623860011/2002.

Drusano, G.L. 2004. Antimicrobial pharmacodynamics: critical interactions of "bug and drug." Nature Reviews. Microbiology 4:289–300.

Elsasser, T.H., Blum, J.W., and Kahl, S. 2005. Characterization of calves exhibiting a novel inheritable TNF-α hyperresponsiveness to endotoxin: associations with increased pathophysiological complications. Journal of Applied Physiology 98:2045–2055.

Fleischer, S., Sharkey, M., Mealey, K., Ostrander, E.A., and Martinez M. 2008. Pharmacogenetic and metabolic differences between dog breeds: their impact on canine medicine and the use of the dog as a preclinical animal model. AAPS Journal 10:110–119.

Gibaldi, M. and Perrier, D. 1982. Pharmacokinetics, 2nd edition. Marcel Decker, Inc., New York. pp. 113–141.

Harris, R.Z., Benet, L.Z., and Schwartz, J.B. 1995. Gender effects in pharmacokinetics and pharmacodynamics. Drugs 50:222–239.

Hattis, D., Russ, A., Banati, P., Kozlak, M., Goble, R., Ginsberg, G., and Smolenski, S. 2001. Background and User's Guide: Comparative Child/Adult Pharmacokinetic Database based upon the Therapeutic Drug Literature, September, 2001, http://www2.clarku.edu/faculty/dhattis/CHLDPKDATABASE-USERGUIDE.DOC

Hiraoka, H., Yamamoto, K., Okano, N., Morita, T., Goto, F., and Horiuchi, R. 2004. Changes in drug plasma concentrations of an extensively bound and highly extracted drug, propofol, in response to altered plasma binding. Clinical Pharmacology and Therapeutics 75:324–330.

Hossaini-Hilali, J. and Olsson, K. 1993. Lactation affects pressor, volumetric and natriuretic responses to angiotensin II in goats. Acta Physiologica Scandinavica 147:499–156.

Jinno, J., Kamada, N., Miyake, M., Yamada, K., Mukai, T., Odomi, M., Toguchi, H., Liversidge, G.G., Higaki, K., and Kimura, T. 2006. Effect of particle size reduction on dissolution and oral absorption of a poorly water-soluble drug, cilostazol, in beagle dogs. Journal of Controlled Release 111:56–64.

Kienzle, E., Zentek, J., and Meyer, H. 1998. Body composition of puppies and young dogs. Journal of Nutrition 128:2680S–2683S.

Kraemer, M.J., Furukawa, C.T., Koup, J.R., Shapiro, G.G., Pierson, W.E., and Bierman, C.W. 1982. Altered theophylline clearance during an influenza B outbreak. Pediatrics 69:476–480.

Kung, K., Hauser, B.R., and Wanner, M. 1995. Effect of the interval between feeding and drug administration on oral ampicillin absorption in dogs. Journal of Small Animal Practice 36:65–68.

Laffont, C.M., Bousquet-Melou, A., Bralet, D., Alvinerie, M., Fink-Gremmels, J., and Toutain, P.L. 2003. A pharmacokinetic model to document the actual disposition of topical ivermectin in cattle. Veterinary Research 34:445–460.

Landoni, M.F., Comas, W., Mucci, N., Anglarilli, G., Bidal, D., Lees, P. 2003. Enantiospecific pharmacokinetics and pharmacodynamics of ketoprofen in sheep. Journal of Veterinary Pharmacology and Therapeutics 22:349–359.

Lees, P., Taylor, P.M., Landoni, F.M., Arifah, A.K., and Waters, C. 2003. Ketoprofen in the cat: pharmacodynamics and chiral pharmacokinetics. Veterinary Journal 165:21–35.

Lin, J.H., Chiba, M., Chen, I.W., Nishime, J.A., and Vastag, K.J. 1996. Sex-dependent pharmacokinetics of indinavir: in vivo and in vitro evidence. Drug Metabolism and Disposition 24:1298–1306.

Liu, P., Müüller, M., Grant, M., Webb, A.I., Obermann, B., and Derendorf, H. 2002. Interstitial tissue concentrations of cefpodoxime. Journal of Antimicrobial Chemotherapy 50 Suppl:19–22.

Martinez, M.N., Hungerford, L., and Papich, M. 2004. Veterinary pharmaceuticals: Factors influencing their development and use. In: Encyclopedia of Pharmaceutical Technology, James Swarbrick and James C. Boylan (eds). Marcel Dekker, New York: pp. 1–24.

Meyer, H., Kienzle E., Zentek J. 1993. Body size and relative weights of gastrointestinal tract and liver in dogs. Journal of Veterinary Nutrition 2:31–35.

Meyer, M. 1995. Current scientific issues regarding bioavailability/bioequivalence trials: an academic view. Drug Information Journal 29:805–812.

Monshouwer, M., Witkamp, R.F., Nijmeijer, S.M., Van Leengoed, L.A., Vernooy, H.C., Verheijden, J.H., and Van Miert, A.S. 1996a. A lipopolysaccharide-induced acute phase response in the pig is associated with a decrease in hepatic cytochrome P450-mediated drug metabolism. Journal of Veterinary Pharmacology and Therapeutics 19:382–388.

Monshouwer, M., Witkamp, R.F., Nijmeijer, S.M., Van Amsterdam, J.G., and Van Miert, A.S. 1996b. Suppression of cytochrome P450- and UDP glucuronosyl transferase-dependent enzyme activities by proinflammatory cytokines and possible role of nitric oxide in primary cultures of pig hepatocytes. Toxicology and Applied Pharmacology 137:237–244.

Mottino, A.D., Hoffman, T., Dawson, P.A., Luquita, M.G, Monti, J.A., and Sanchez Pozzi, E.J. 2002. Increased expression of ileal apical sodium-dependent bile acid transporter in postpartum rats. American Journal of Physiology. Gastrointestinal and Liver Physiology 282:G41–50.

Müller, M., dela Peňa, A., and Derendorf, H. 2004. Minireview: Issues in pharmacokinetics and pharmacodynamics of antiinfective agents: distribution in tissue. Antimicrobial Agents and Chemotherapy 48:1441–1453.

Nolan, C.M. and Ulmer, W.C. 1980. A study of cephalothin and desacetylcephalothin in cerebrospinal fluid in therapy for experimental pneumococcal meningitis. Journal of Infectious Diseases 141:326–330.

Ohhira, S., Enomoto, M., and Matsui, H. 2006. Sex difference in the principal cytochrome P450 for tributyltin metabolism in rats. Toxicology and Applied Pharmacology 210:32–38.

Parkinson, A., Mudra, D.R., Johnson, C., Dwyer, A., and Carroll, K.M. 2004. The effects of gender, age, ethnicity, and liver cirrhosis on cytochrome P450 enzyme activity in human liver microsomes and inducibility in cultured hepatocytes. Toxicology and Applied Pharmacology 199:193–209.

Patterson, D.F., Haskins, M.E., Jezyk, P.F., Giger, U., Meyers-Wallen, V.N., Aguirre, G., Fyfe, J.C., and Wolfe, J.H. 1988. Research on genetic diseases: reciprocal benefits to animals and man. Journal of the American Veterinary Medical Association 193:1131–1144.

Perrson, E.M., Gustafsson, A.-S., Carlsson, A.S., Nilsson, R.G., Knutson, L., Forsell, P., Hanisch, G., Lennernas, H., and Abrahamsson, B. 2005. The effects of food on the dissolution of poorly soluble drugs in human and in model small intestinal fluids. Pharmaceutical Research 22:2141–2151.

Petracca, K., Riond, J.L., Graser, T., and Wanner, M. 1993. Pharmacokinetics of the gyrase inhibitor marbofloxacin: influence of pregnancy and lactation in sows. Zentralblatt für Veterinärmedizin. Reihe A. 40:73–79.

Piaggio, G., Elbourne, D.R., Altman, D.G., Pocock, S.J., and Evans, S.J.W. 2006. Reporting of noninferiority and equivalence randomized trials: an extension of the CONSORT statement. Journal of the American Medical Association 295:1152–1160.

Randell, S.C., Hill, R.C., Scott, K.C., Omori, M., and Burrows, C.F. 2001. Intestinal permeability testing using lactulose and rhamnose: a comparison between clinically normal cats and dogs and between dogs of different breeds. Research in Veterinary Science 71:45–49.

Renton, K.W. 2001. Alteration of drug biotransformation and elimination during infection and inflammation. Pharmacology and Therapeutics 92:147–163.

Renwick, A.G. 1998. Toxicokinetics in infants and children in relation to the ADI and TDI. Food Additives and Contaminants 15 Suppl:17–35.

Schuirmann, D.J. 1987. A comparison of the two one-sided tests procedure and the power approach for assessing the equivalence of average bioavailability. Journal Pharmacokinetics and Biopharmaceutics 15:657–680.

Sequin, M.A., Papich, M.G., Sigle, K.J., Gibson, N.M., and Levy, J.K. 2004. Pharmacokinetics of enrofloxacin in neonatal kittens. American Journal of Veterinary Research 65:350–356.

Shah, J.C. 2005. Developing in vivo/in vitro correlations for parenteral products. In Proceedings, 14th Biennial Symposium of the American Association of Veterinary Pharmacology and Therapeutics. Internet publisher International Veterinary Information Service, Ithaca, New York. www.ivis.org/aavpt/2005/shah/chapter.asp?LA=1. Accessed 03-06-06.

Soback, S., Gips, M., Bialer, M., and Bor, A. 1994. Effect of lactation on single-dose pharmacokinetics of norfloxacin nicotinate in ewes. Antimicrobial Agents and Chemotherapy 38:2336–2339.

Steinmetz, K.L., Coley, K.C., and Pollock, B.G. 2005. Assessment of geriatric information on the drug label for commonly prescribed drugs in older people. Journal of the American Geriatrics Society 53:891–894.

Storey, S. 2005. Challenges with the development and approval of pharmaceuticals for fish. The AAPS Journal 7(2):E335–43.

Toutain, P.L. and Bousquet-Melou, A. 2002. Free drug fraction vs. free drug concentration: a matter of frequent confusion. Journal of Veterinary Pharmacology and Therapeutics 25:460–463.

Vanapalli, S.R., Hung, Y.P., Fleckenstein, L., Dzimianski, M.T., and McCall, J.W. 2002. Pharmacokinetics and dose proportionality of oral moxidectin in beagle dogs. Biopharmaceutics and Drug Disposition 23:263–272.

Weber, M.P., Martin, L.J., Biourge, V.C., Nguyen, P.G., and Dumon, H. J. 2003. Influence of age and body size on orocecal transit time as assessed by use of the sulfasalazine method in healthy dogs. American Journal of Veterinary Research 64:1105–1109.

Weber, M.P., Martin, L.J., Dumon, H.J., Biourge, V.C., and Nguyen, P.G. 2002. Influence of age and body size on intestinal permeability and absorption in healthy dogs. American Journal of Veterinary Research 63:1323–1328.

Weber, M.P., Stambouli, F., Martin, L.J., Dumon, H.J., Biourge, V.C., and Nguyen, P.G. 2002. Influence of age and body size on gastrointestinal transit time of radiopaque markers in healthy dogs. American Journal of Veterinary Research 63:677–682.

Zar, JH. 1998. Biostatistical Analysis (4th Edition). Prentice-Hall, Englewood Cliffs, New Jersey, pp. 20–29.

CHAPTER

56

VETERINARY PHARMACY

GIGI DAVIDSON, BSPh

INTRODUCTION

A pharmacist's responsibility for providing patients with high-quality pharmaceutical care extends beyond the human species. Although colleges of pharmacy and licensing boards have focused almost exclusively on human pharmacotherapy, society expects an equally competent quality of pharmaceutical care and products to be provided for non-human family members. Veterinarians are well schooled in providing quality care and products to animal patients, but few pharmacists are. It behooves all pharmacists to be equipped with a working knowledge of veterinary pharmacotherapy and to develop a clinically and legally sound algorithm for processing veterinary prescriptions. Because this process is very slowly evolving in the pharmacy profession, veterinarians should be well versed in pharmacy issues related to veterinary medical therapy. Although several of these issues have been introduced or discussed in previous chapters, this chapter describes a variety of pharmacy-related topics of which all veterinarians should be aware.

REGULATORY REQUIREMENTS FOR USE OF DRUGS IN ANIMAL PATIENTS

Unlike human patients, some animals or their by-products have potential to end up in the human food chain. Drug use and consequential drug residues in animal tissue pose a human health hazard through allergic reactions, bacterial resistance due to chronic exposure to drugs, and carcinogenicity. Because of these hazards, the Animal Drug Amendment to the Food Drug and Cosmetic Act imposed a strict regulation on the use of drugs in animal patients stating that drugs must be used as labeled in the approved species, for the approved indication, and at the approved dose. All animal patients were included in this ruling because it was increasingly difficult to categorize food animals strictly by species. Traditional food animals in the United States include cattle, pigs, poultry, fish, shellfish and their meat, milk, and eggs. However, animals such as dogs, rabbits, ostriches, and alligators can be considered pets, food animals, or exotic animals, depending on cultural or philosophical preference.

REGULATORY DISCRETION FOR EXTRALABEL USE

Advances in medical knowledge occur at a much faster rate than do drug product approvals. Since it is impossible for a drug company to test marketed drugs in all species at all doses and for all indications, very few approved drug products can be used by veterinarians to achieve therapeutic successes strictly as described on the product label. Passage of the Animal Drug Amendment in 1968 significantly restricted use of drugs in animals to use only in those species for which the product was labeled with strict adherence to the labeled indication, dose, route of administration, and duration of therapy. Any use of a human-labeled drug in animals, for example, would be illegal. Pursuant to enactment of this legislation, veterinarians were forced to break the law most of the time when using drugs in their patients. Physicians, on the other hand, were still allowed to use any drug at any dose for any indication in human patients.

Realizing the impracticality of strict interpretation of this law for veterinarians, the Food and Drug Administration published compliance policy guidelines (CPGs) in 1993 to show veterinarians the boundaries for regulatory discretion by FDA inspectors. Four main CPGs provided the boundaries for drug use by veterinarians: Extralabel Drug Use, Human Label Drug Use, Use of Drugs in Food Producing Animals, and Compounding for Animals (see www.fda.gov for summaries of these CPGs).

NEED FOR LEGAL EXTRALABEL USE—AMDUCA

Although these CPGs provided veterinarians with a higher comfort level for using drugs in animal patients, extralabel use of drugs in animals was still illegal. The law did not change. CPGs only informed veterinarians of occasions when FDA inspectors would exercise regulatory discretion with respect to interpreting and enforcing extralabel drug use. In 1993, veterinarians, tired of being forced to break the law, demanded the same legal right physicians had in treating their patients. On October 22, 1994, the Animal Medicinal Drug Use Clarification Act (AMDUCA) was passed allowing veterinarians to legally use drugs off label under certain circumstances. AMDUCA went into effect December 9, 1996. Concurrently, Congress passed the Animal Drug Availability Act, significantly expediting the process by which FDA approved products intended for use in animals. Passage of both laws was intended to significantly improve the ability of veterinarians to best treat nonfood-producing animal patients.

ANIMAL MEDICINAL DRUG USE CLARIFICATION ACT. On October 22, 1996, the Animal Medicinal Drug Use Clarification Act of 1994 was enacted into law, allowing veterinarians to prescribe extralabel use of veterinary and human drugs for animals under specific circumstances

TABLE 56.1 Requirements for extralabel drug use (ELDU) in animals

- ELDU is permitted only by or under the supervision of a veterinarian.
- ELDU is allowed only for FDA-approved animal and human drugs.
- A valid veterinarian/client/patient relationship is a prerequisite for all ELDU.
- ELDU is for therapeutic purposes only (animal's health is suffering or threatened), not for production use.
- Rules apply to dosage for drugs and drugs administered in water. ELDU in feed is prohibited.
- ELDU is not permitted if it results in a violative food residue, or any residue that may present a risk to public health. FDA prohibition of a specific ELDU precludes such use (Table 56.2).

TABLE 56.2 Drugs prohibited for extralabel use in food animals

- Chloramphenicol
- Clenbuterol
- Diethylstilbestrol (DES)
- Dimetridazole
- Ipronidazole
- Other Nitroimidazoles
- Furazolidone (except for approved topical use)
- Nitrofurazone (except for approved topical use)
- Sulfonamide drugs in lactating dairy cows (except approved use of sulfadimethoxine, sulfabromomethazine, and sulfaethoxypyridazine)
- Fluoroquinolones
- Glycopeptides (example: vancomycin)
- Phenylbutazone for female dairy cattle over 20 months of age

TABLE 56.3 Record requirements for drugs dispensed for animals

- Identify the animals, either as individuals or a group.
- Animal species treated.
- Numbers of animals treated.
- Condition being treated.
- The established name of the drug and active ingredient.
- Dosage prescribed or used.
- Duration of treatment.
- Specified withdrawal, withholding, or discard time(s), if applicable, for meat, milk, eggs, or animal-derived food.
- Keep records for 2 years.
- FDA may have access to these records to estimate risk to public health.

TABLE 56.4 Label requirements for drugs prescribed for animals

Name and address of the prescribing veterinarian.
Established name of the drug.
Any specified directions for use including the class/species or identification of the animal or herd, flock, pen, lot, or other group; the dosage frequency and route of administration; and the duration of therapy.
Any cautionary statements.
Your specified withdrawal, withholding, or discard time for meat, milk, eggs, or any other food.

and also codified compounding for animal patients provided the starting ingredients were FDA-approved drug products. The key extra-label provisions of the Animal Medicinal Clarification Act are provided in Table 56.1. (A copy of the AMDUCA Extra Label Drug Use Guidelines Brochure is available in the February 15, 1998, issue of JAVMA or may be obtained from the AVMA website: www.avma.org.) Some drugs are strictly prohibited from administration to food animals because a safe level of residue in food products cannot be identified (Table 56.2).

Additional provisions of the AMDUCA legislation require proper dispensing and labeling of prescribed drugs for animals (Tables 56.3 and 56.4).

CLASSIFICATION OF DRUGS

DRUG. A chemical can be considered a drug if is meets one of the following criteria:

1. It is an article recognized in one of the official compendia, i.e., the *United States Pharmacopoeia/National Formulary* or the official *Homeopathic Pharmacopoeia* of the United States or their supplements.

TABLE 56.5 A valid veterinarian-client-patient relationship (VCPR)

- The veterinarian has assumed the responsibility of making medical judgments regarding the health of the animal(s) and the need for medical treatment, and the client (owner or other caretaker) has agreed to follow the instructions of the veterinarian.
- There is sufficient knowledge of the animal(s) by the veterinarian to initiate at least a general or preliminary diagnosis of the medical condition of the animal(s). This means that the veterinarian has recently seen and is personally acquainted with the keeping and care of the animal(s) by virtue of an examination of the animal(s), and/or by medically appropriate and timely visits to the premises where the animal(s) are kept.
- The practicing veterinarian is readily available for follow-up in case of adverse reactions or failure of the regimen of therapy.

2. It is an article intended for use in the diagnosis, cure, mitigation, treatment, or prevention of disease in man or other animals.
3. It is an article other than food intended to affect the structure or any function of the body of man or other animals.
4. It is an article that is intended to be used as a component of an item falling into one of the three categories above.

This definition does not differentiate between prescription drugs and nonprescription drugs, nor does it distinguish legal or lawful drugs from illicit ones. Because of this broad definition, *any substance that is used to treat an animal can be ultimately considered to be a drug and can be regulated and actionable as such.*

LEGEND ("PRESCRIPTION") DRUGS. Prescription drugs are limited to dispensing by or upon the order of a licensed prescriber ("prescription") because they are habit forming, are toxic, or have potential for harm. These drug labels contain the following warnings identifying them as legend drugs:

- *Veterinary Legend*: "Caution: Federal law restricts this drug to use by or on the order of a licensed veterinarian."
- *Human Legend:* "Rx only."

Legend (prescription) drugs *cannot* be dispensed without a prescription and may only be prescribed and dispensed within the confines of a valid veterinarian-client-patient relationship (VCPR) (Table 56.5). Because of the requirement of a valid VCPR, if a veterinarian has not examined the animal, he/she cannot prescribe legend drugs for use in that animal. Likewise, a veterinarian cannot "fill a prescription" for an animal unless he/she has a valid veterinarian-client-patient relationship with that animal. Veterinarians filling prescriptions for other veterinarians are considered to be practicing "pharmacy" and are subsequently subject to action by state pharmacy regulatory boards.

OVER-THE-COUNTER ("NONPRESCRIPTION") DRUGS. Over-the-counter (OTC) drugs are also considered "nonprescription" drugs. These are familiar to veterinarians and pet owners because they are available for human use in retail outlets such as pharmacies, markets and grocery stores. Such OTC products can also be found for animals in the same retail outlets as for humans as well as in pet and feed stores. These drugs have been recognized by experts as safe and effective and bear extensive labeling which renders them safe for use by laypersons and are sold "over the counter," without a prescription.

All OTC products must be used *precisely* as labeled just as legend drugs. Use outside of these specifications constitutes extralabel use and the aforementioned guidelines should govern this use. Veterinarians should avoid repackaging OTC medications for dispensing because reproducing the required labeling that is comprehensive enough for safe use by a layperson is difficult and dangerous.

CONTROLLED SUBSTANCES. Controlled substances ("narcotics") are defined and monitored by the Drug Enforcement Authority (under jurisdiction of the Controlled Substances Act of 1970) and are divided into five schedules according to potential for abuse. An example of the schedules used for opiate drugs is provided in Chapter 12. These drugs are strictly controlled by federal and state law and specific requirements for administering, dispensing, and prescribing are addressed later in this chapter.

COMPOUNDED DRUGS. Compounded drugs are mixtures of approved dosage forms or drugs formulated from bulk chemicals that are not approved by FDA for use as drugs in the United States. Veterinarians may compound items for their own use or write prescriptions for their patients for some of these chemicals to be filled by licensed pharmacists. These chemicals (e.g., potassium bromide, cisapride, phenylpropanolamine, diethylstilbestrol) are recognized by FDA to be essential in the treatment of some companion, nonfood animals. As many of these chemicals have been withdrawn from the market due to human hazards, the FDA has published a "negative" list for human compounding describing the chemicals that are either prohibited for use in humans or are restricted to small dosages. Note that some of the chemicals (e.g. cisapride and diethylstilbestrol) may still be compounded for nonfood animals such as companion animal pets but never for food animals or humans.

CURRENT STATUS OF COMPOUNDED VETERINARY DRUGS

Drug compounding has always been an important component of veterinary medicine. Historically, veterinarians have prepared concoctions, mixtures, and remedies for their patients because there were few approved formulations on the market for animals. Now, there are more available drugs for animals, and pharmaceutical science has provided for a better understanding of the risk factors contributing to poor drug bioavailability, instability and physical incompatibility. Over the last several years, questions concerning the practice of compounding have been raised, particularly with respect to stability, purity, and potency when the original dosage form of the drug is altered.

Compounding is the alteration of the original drug dosage form for the purposes of ease of administration or because the original dosage form is unsuitable for the purpose intended. According to the *United States Pharmacopeia* (USP), compounding involves the preparation, mixing, assembling, packaging, and labeling of a drug or device in accordance with a licensed practitioner's prescription. The USP chapter on pharmacy compounding states that "compounding is an integral part of pharmacy practice and is essential to the provision of health care" (USP [795]).

Further defined by the FDA in an early Compliance Policy Guideline (FDA-CVM 1996), "compounding is any manipulation to produce a dosage form drug other than that manipulation that is provided for in the directions for use on the labeling of the approved drug product." Compounding does not include the preparation of a drug by reconstitution or mixing that is according to the manufacturer's instructions on an approved human or veterinary drug product.

In 1993, a symposium on compounding in veterinary medicine was held by the American Academy of Veterinary Pharmacology and Therapeutics (AAVPT) (JAVMA 1994). This symposium had representatives from AVMA, FDA/CVM, pharmacology and pharmacy groups, and USP. From this symposium emerged a Task Force Report

TABLE 56.6 Compounding Compliance Policy Guideline (Federal Register, July 3, 1996)

1. The FDA lists three criteria that must be met before compounding is deemed necessary and acceptable.
   (1) A legitimate medial need is identified (the health of animals is threatened and suffering or death would result from failure to treat the affected animals),
   (2) There is a need for an appropriate dosage regimen for the species, age, size, or medical condition of the patient, and
   (3) There is no marketed approved animal drug which when used as labeled (or in an extra-label manner in conformity with criteria listed in CPG 615.100, or human-label drug, when used in conformity with criteria listed in CPG 608.100) may treat the condition diagnosed in the available dosage form, or there is some other rare extenuating circumstance. (For example the approved drug cannot be obtained in time to treat the animals in a timely manner, or there is a medical need for different excipients.)
2. All drugs dispensed to the animal owner by the veterinarian or pharmacist bear labeling information which is adequate to assure proper use of the product. The following label information should be included:
   (a) name and address of the veterinary practitioner;
   (b) active ingredient(s) or ingredient(s),
   (c) the date dispensed and the expiration date, which should not exceed the length of the prescribed treatment except in cases where the veterinarian can establish a rationale for a later expiration date,
   (d) directions for use specified by the practitioner, including the class/species or identification of animals; and the dosage, frequency, route of administration, and duration of therapy,
   (e) cautionary statements specified by the veterinarian and/or pharmacist (this would include all appropriate warnings necessary to ensure safety of human operators handling the finished drug, especially if there are potential hazards of exposure to any components,
   (f) the veterinarian's specified withdrawal/discard time(s) for meat, milk, eggs or any food which might be derived from the treated animal(s). (While the veterinarian must set the withdrawal time, he may in doing so use relevant information provided by a dispensing pharmacist although the veterinarian retains the ultimate responsibility),
   (g) if dispensed by a licensed pharmacist, the name and address of the dispenser, serial number and date of order or its filling,
   (h) if dispensed by a veterinarian, the serial number, and
   (i) any other applicable requirements of state or federal law.

that summarized the presentations and resulted in the Compliance Policy Guide published in 1996, summarized in Table 56.6 (FDA 1996). The proceedings from this symposium are very informative and contain 115 pages of presentations, which cannot be adequately summarized here. The FDA revised this Compliance Policy Guide (CPG) for compounding drugs for use in animals in 2003 (FDA-CVM 2003). The 2003 version of the CPG provides guidance to FDA's staff with regard to the compounding of animal drugs by veterinarians and pharmacists for use in animals. This CPG is available from the FDA, or on the Internet at this address: http://www.fda.gov/ora/compliance_ref/cpg/default.htm or http://www.fda.gov/OHRMS/DOCKETS/98fr/03d-0290-gd10001.pdf. At the time of this writing, the FDA is apparently revising the CPG for a third iteration, but that document is not yet available for public view.

The FDA recognizes the importance of compounding in veterinary practice, but also must ensure that compounded drugs do not cause harm to the treated animals or their caregivers, that compounded preparations are bioavailable, effective, stable and potent, and that compounded preparations do not cause drug residues in food animals. FDA regulations permit the compounding of formulations from approved animal or human drugs under the current federal code: 21 *CFR* 530.13 (AMDUCA). The FDA is concerned that some compounding by veterinarians and pharmacists is performed to circumvent the usual drug approval process. Some activities performed under the guise of compounding (e.g., mass preparation of compounds that are wholesaled to veterinarians with no patient identified at the time of compounding, *dispensing* of compounds intended only for *administration* by the veterinarian in the office, or compounding less expensive copies of commercially available approved drugs) mimics exactly the manufacturing and distribution of what FDA defines as "new animal drugs." A court ruling by the 5th Circuit of Appeals (*Medical Center Pharmacy vs. Mukasey*, July 2008) reasserted that compounds prepared for animals outside of the provisions of AMUDCA definitely fit the description of new animal drugs. New animal drugs must undergo the long and arduous FDA approval process to ensure the safety of the public health. Compounds have clearly not undergone this scrutiny to determine the safety, efficacy, potency, purity, and stability required of drug manufacturers in order to receive FDA approval for marketing. Pharmacies are held to Good Compounding Practices as adopted by their state boards of pharmacy; however, compounds, under no circumstances, can be manufactured or wholesaled. Licensed veterinary distributors who wholesale compounds from compounding pharmacies are in direct violation with licensure as granted by state licensing agencies (usually the Department of Agriculture). Compounds must be prepared pursuant to a valid prescription order for an individual patient or for use in a veterinary practice ("office use") in the few states where this is permitted according to state law. At the time of this writing, only 20 states allow compounding for office use and all 20 states specifically prohibit dispensing of "office use" compounds to be used outside of the veterinary practice.

The CPG published in July 2003 specifically was intended to clarify the regulations on compounding from unapproved or bulk chemicals. *Bulk chemicals* are defined as active ingredients used in the manufacture of finished dosage forms of the drug. Bulk chemicals are also referred to as *active pharmaceutical ingredients (APIs)*. Compounding from APIs or unapproved drug substances is not allowed except for a few chemicals provided in Appendix A of the 2003 version CPG for Compounding For Animals. Compounding with these chemicals is allowed in instances where the health of the animal is at risk and there are no other remedies. The list includes antidotes such as methylene blue, sodium thiosulfate, or sodium nitrite. (A complete list of bulk chemicals tolerated for animal compounding is listed in the FDA document cited earlier.) Chemicals used for compounding that are not listed in Appendix A are subject to FDA regulatory discretion. The FDA has seized compounds prepared from bulk chemicals and issued warnings to pharmacies when there have been violations (http://www.fda.gov/foi/warning.htm). At the time of this writing, a legal battle initiated by compounding pharmacies challenging FDA's right to regulate compounding pharmacies has been heard and successfully appealed in the 5th District Circuit of Appeals. While this ruling is in direct conflict with a previous ruling by the 9th Circuit Court of Appeals in 2001 regarding compounding for humans, the legality of compounding with bulk chemicals for human patients must be decided by either the Supreme Court or codified through legislation. As the rulings by the 5th and 9th Circuit Courts of Appeals did not apply to compounding for animals, this too must be challenged at the level of the Supreme Court or codified through legislation.

POTENTIAL PROBLEMS FROM COMPOUNDED DRUGS

Because many drugs are not in a form that is ideal for the species being treated, either due to body size, taste preferences, or species-specific metabolic intolerances, commercially available drug products have been altered to make a more convenient and palatable oral dose form. However, when protective coatings on tablets or capsules are disrupted, and suspending or solubilizing vehicles are diluted or changed, the bioavailability and stability of the product may be compromised. In some instances, the only change is a slight alteration of pH. But, according to the USP (2008), "improper pH ranks with exposure to elevated temperature as a factor most likely to cause a clinically significant loss of drug. A drug solution or suspension may be stable for days, weeks, or even years in its original formulation, but when mixed with another liquid that changes the pH, it degrades in minutes or days. It is possible that a pH change of only one unit could decrease drug stability by a factor of ten or greater." Addition of a water-based solution to a product to make a liquid solution or suspension can hydrolyze some drugs (beta-lactams, esters). Some drugs undergo epimerization (steric rearrangement) when exposed to a pH range higher than what is optimum for the drug (for example, this occurs with tetracycline at a pH higher than 3). Other drugs are oxidized, catalyzed by high pH, which renders the drug inactive. Drugs most likely to be subject to oxidation are those with a hydroxyl group bonded to an aromatic ring structure. Oxidation may occur from exposure to light and oxygen during reformulation and mixing. Oxidation is catalyzed by high pH and usually leads to drug inactivation. Other factors contributing to instability and decrease in bioavailability may be through the addition of sugars and starches to an oral suspension. For example, it is well documented that the presence of sugar significantly decreases the stability of oral suspensions of atenolol and pyrimethamine, and the addition of methylcellulose to solutions of pyridostigmine will significantly decrease the oral bioavailability of pyridostigmine resulting in potential harm to the patient receiving these medications.

Veterinarians and pharmacists are obligated to be cognizant of the potential for interactions and interference with stability (Table 56.7). Oxidation is often visible through a color change (color change to pink or amber, for example). Loss of solubility may be observed through precipitation. Some drugs are prone to hydrolysis from moisture. A rule-of-thumb for veterinarians is that if a drug is packaged in blister packs or moisture-proof barrier, it is probably subject to loss of stability and potency if mixed with aqueous vehicles. If compounded formulations of solid dose forms show cracking or "caking," or swelling, the formulation has probably accumulated moisture and may have lost potency. Another rule-of-thumb is that if the original packaging of a drug is in a light-resistant or amber container it is prob-

TABLE 56.7 Signs of drug instability of compounded formulations

Liquid Dose Forms
Color change (pink or amber)
Signs of microbial growth
Cloudiness, haze, flocculent or film formation
Separation of phases (e.g., oil and water, emulsion)
Precipitation, clumping, crystal formation
Droplets or fog forming on inside of container
Gas or odor release
Swelling of container
Solid Dose Forms
Odor (sulfur or vinegar odor)
Excessive powder or crumbling
Cracks or chips in tablets
Swelling of tablets or capsules
Sticking together of capsules or tablets
Tackiness of the covering of tablets or capsules

ably prone to inactivation by light. Vitamins, cardiovascular drugs, and phenothiazines are labile to oxidation from light during compounding. Also, as a general rule, if an antibiotic is available in a powder that must be reconstituted in a vial or oral dispensing bottle prior to administration, it is probably unstable for long periods of time and should also not be mixed with other drugs.

EXAMPLES OF POTENTIAL PROBLEMS. There are very few published studies in which drugs for veterinary patients have been tested for stability under the conditions used during compounding. In a commercial formulation, the inactive ingredients and excipients added to drug formulations are done so as to ensure the stability of the drug; provide an optimum chemical environment, pH; or increase the ease of packaging or handling. However, adding other chemicals, flavorings, or vehicles, or interfering with protective coatings of tablets may affect the stability of the drug, decreasing potency, oral absorption, and efficacy. There are published formulas in compounding journals, and texts, but few of these formulations have been tested for safety, efficacy, bioavailability, stability, potency, and purity for use in the target species. As the responsibility for risk when using compounded preparations rests squarely on the shoulders of prescribing veterinarians, they have an obligation to request evidence from compounding pharmacists about the stability and potency of formulations prepared for their patients. When veterinarians compound formulations in their own practices, they should be cognizant of the potential interactions and alterations that may compromise the stability and potency of the active ingredient and should not attempt compounding without proper training, equipment, and quality assurance techniques.

There are published examples in which drug stability and efficacy have been compromised through compounding. For example, when omeprazole was compounded for oral use in horses, it was not as effective for treating gastric ulcers as the commercial formulation registered for horses (Gastroguard) (Nieto et al. 2002). Systemic bioavailability and potency of the compounded formulation was not as high as for the proprietary product. Omeprazole is known for its instability unless administered in the original formulation intended for horses or people.

Fluoroquinolone antibiotics are frequently modified for administration to exotic animals and horses. The compatibility of enrofloxacin and orbifloxacin with flavorings, vehicles, and other ingredients has been evaluated. With few exceptions, this class of drugs is compatible with most mixtures and remarkably stable. A notable exception is the chelation of enrofloxacin with iron and aluminum-containing products (e.g., antacids, sucralfate, mineral supplements, iron-containing molasses), in which a significant portion of the medication may become unavailable for absorption. It has also been observed that certain mixtures and flavorings may be incompatible with fluoroquinolones if they contain metal ions that are known to cause chelation. For example, when crushed orbifloxacin tablets were mixed with a vitamin and mineral supplement (Lixotinic) that is sometimes used as a flavored vehicle for oral administration of drugs, the potency of orbifloxacin was decreased from its original concentration by 50%. (Lixotinic contains 2.5 mg/ml iron.) Other flavorings and vehicles (for example, corn syrup, regular molasses, fish sauce, and Syrpalta) had no effect.

Antifungal drugs are subject to instability if not maintained at an optimum pH and formulation conditions. Itraconazole is frequently compounded from the bulk chemical or the proprietary capsules. However, itraconazole must be complexed onto cyclodextran in order to be orally bioavailable, and as bulk chemical preparations of itraconazole are not complexed in this fashion, they have not been found to be orally bioavailable in animal patients. Itraconazole may also adsorb to plastic and glassware during compounding, decreasing the predicted potency of the finished preparation.

Aminoglycoside antibiotics (gentamicin, tobramycin, kanamycin) are inactivated when admixed with other antibiotics, particularly beta-lactams. This interaction is greatest from carbenicillin, followed by ticarcillin, penicillin G, and ampicillin. Loss of potency by as much as 50% can occur within 4 to 6 hours. This interaction is a potential problem when antibiotic mixtures are prepared in a vial or fluid administration set and dispensed to be used several hours later. This interaction does not occur intravascularly at therapeutic concentrations in the patient because the drugs are diluted out in plasma and body fluids, but visual precipitation of these agents in IV administration sets is commonly reported when they are mixed.

Drugs formulated as acids—such as the hydrochloride form of basic drugs—are formulated to maintain their solubility in aqueous solutions. However, when these formulations are mixed with other drugs that are more basic, or added to basic vehicles, drug precipitation may occur.

Several drugs are not soluble in aqueous vehicles. Therefore they are dissolved in organic solvents (propylene or ethylene glycol, for example) or alcohols. These are notoriously unpalatable to some animals, particularly cats. However, if these formulations are diluted in aqueous fluids, precipitation may occur. When these are stored at home by the pet owner, precipitation of the drug to the bottom of the container results in dilute oral dosing when the container is sampled from the top, and highly concentrated formulation when the container is sampled from the bottom (assuming that the precipitate at the bottom can be resuspended). This also may be observed when mixing some drugs in aqueous fluids. For example, if diazepam solution (which contains propylene glycol and alcohols) is diluted in saline solution or Lactated Ringer's solution, precipitation occurs.

COMPOUNDED TRANSDERMAL MEDICATIONS FOR PETS. Because of convenience, ease of administration, and therapeutic success with some transdermal drugs (antiparasitic agents and fentanyl), there is considerable interest in formulating a wide range of other drugs for use by this route. Historically, transdermally administered drugs were formulated for single-dose delivery in a liquid preparation, or for continuous delivery out of a drug-releasing matrix or "patch." A compounding pharmacist (Marty Jones, PharmD) discovered a penetration-enhancing drug vehicle in the 1990s, and application of this delivery system to drugs used in animals rapidly caught on. A quick Internet search of "compounding pharmacy + transdermal" will reveal over 11,000 advertisements from compounding pharmacies who provide drugs in transdermal delivery gels. Noninvasive, nonstressful, palatable drug delivery is ideal for many veterinary patients, especially cats. Consequently, many veterinarians are eager to try this dosage form on fractious or fragile patients who should not be (or do not want to be) stressed during medication. While transdermal drug delivery is appealing, there are still many questions to be resolved regarding its use in veterinary medicine. The skin is a formidable barrier to drug penetration, and drug absorption into systemic circulation is a predictably tricky feat. In order to facilitate drug transport across skin, drugs need to be small in molecular weight and placed in a biphasic vehicle that can propel the drug across the various lipophilic and hydrophilic layers of the skin. Passage of the drug across the skin relies on the thickness of the skin, the partition coefficient of the drug, the diffusion coefficient of the skin, and the concentration of drug in solution. The partition coefficient, the diffusion coefficient, and the thickness of the skin are not alterable, so transdermally applied drugs must be placed in high concentrations in vehicles that accommodate the various coefficients of diffusion. Drugs have been combined with penetration enhancers to facilitate transdermal absorption. One commonly used penetration enhancer is pleuronic lecithin organogel (PLO), which is lecithin (derived from eggs or soybeans) mixed with isopropyl palmitate and a poloxamer (Pluronic). The ingredients in PLO act as surfactants, emulsifiers, and solubilizing agents to escort drug across the skin into systemic vasculature. There are many other penetration-enhancing vehicles (e.g., Lipoderm, Van Penn) utilized to compound transdermal preparations, but at the time of writing, there are no commercially available formulations that utilize these penetration-enhancing vehicles to deliver systemic drugs. Most commercially available transdermal drugs are available as patch delivery systems or are single-dose applications of parasiticides. Compounded transdermal preparations are formulated in high concentrations so that a therapeutic dose may be delivered in 0.1–0.2 ml, which is applied to a hairless area and rubbed in until no residue remains on the skin surface. Because the drug must be in solution in order to penetrate skin, many drugs are logically precluded from transdermal administration because they are not soluble in concentrations high enough to deliver a dose in 0.1–0.2 ml (e.g., any drug dosed at 10 mg/kg requires a transdermal concentration of at least 500 mg/ml to deliver a 0.1 ml dose to a 5 kg cat). The majority of drugs are not soluble at these high concentrations.

At the time of this writing, there have been few published reports regarding compounded transdermally administered drugs. Single-dose pharmacokinetic studies for transdermally administered drugs have demonstrated that absorption was incomplete, nonexistent, or highly inconsistent among study cats, and that after single doses, bioavailability was low compared to a single oral dose. There have been an even smaller number of chronic dosing safety and efficacy studies for transdermally administered drugs, and few of those demonstrated positive evidence of efficacy. Incredibly, the stability or potency of the transdermal formulated for the study was not determined except in only two of the investigations, so it is difficult to draw conclusions from any study where the potency of the study drug was undetermined. Transdermally administered drugs examined so far have included methimazole, amlodipine, glipizide, dexamethasone, buspirone, amitriptyline, metoclopramide, atenolol, fentanyl, morphine, fluoxetine, and diltiazem. Methimazole was not absorbed well according to a pharmacokinetic study (Hoffman et al. 2002; Trepanier 2002), but produced clinical efficacy with repeated transdermal application in other studies (Hoffman et al. 2001). Transdermally administered amlodipine did effect a decrease in blood pressure in hypertensive cats and was found to be stable for at least 60 days when formulated in a transdermal gel (Helms 2007). Absorption of atenolol from a transdermal preparation in cats was low and inconsistent and did not produce therapeutic blood levels of atenolol after a week of chronic dosing at an equivalent oral dose. (MacGregor et al. 2008). The remaining drugs were examined as single-dose pharmacokinetic studies and showed poor bioavailability as compared to oral dosing and a high degree of intrasubject variation in drug absorption.

A major concern for use of transdermally administered drugs, for which there is no safety, efficacy, or potency evidence, is the risk of poor absorption or decreased stability of the formulated drug. For example, unstable or poorly absorbed transdermal antibiotics will surely result in subtherapeutic drug concentrations leading to therapeutic failure, and even worse, the development of antimicrobial drug resistance. Increased risk of toxicity also is a potential problem. Misinterpretation of single-dose pharmacokinetic studies might lead prescribers to increase transdermally administered drug doses, leading to accumulation of drug and severe toxicity. For example, the transdermal bioavailability of amitriptyline was 10% compared to oral dosing in a single dose pharmacokinetic study. Several veterinarians erroneously interpreted these results to mean that transdermal amitriptyline should effectively be administered at 10 times the oral dose. Obviously, there also is considerable risk for absorption by the human caregiver. Drugs toxic to humans (e.g., chloramphenicol, carprofen, digoxin) are extremely poor candidates for transdermal drug administration. Similarly, caregiver health and lifestyle must also be considered when prescribing transdermal drugs for pets. For example, a hypothyroid owner is a poor candidate to administer transdermal methimazole to her hyperthyroid cat, and a long-distance truck driver subject to periodic drug testing is a poor candidate for administration of transdermal opiates to his pet in pain.

COMPOUNDING GUIDELINES FOR VETERINARIANS AND VETERINARY PHARMACISTS. The FDA-CVM uses regulatory discretion to allow veterinary drug compounding within the scope of clinical veterinary practice through the Compliance Policy Guideline. However, there are still some restrictions that apply, and each state may have more restrictive requirements than federal law. The purity standard of the bulk chemical should be that of a USP- or an NF-grade substance. Compounded therapies should be prepared from a commercially available formulation, if a suitable approved product exists. Compounding from bulk chemicals is not allowed if a proprietary registered formulation is available unless the veterinarian can document a medically necessary reason (economic reasons are not valid) why the commercially available product is not appropriate. If bulk chemicals are utilized because there is no commercially available form (e.g., pergolide, potassium bromide, cisapride, or diethylstilbestrol), the pharmacist should use bulk chemicals obtained through an FDA-registered chemical supplier and accompanied by a valid certificate of analysis for that specific batch and lot number of chemical. It is absolutely critical that compounders examine the certificate of analysis for potency, because many bulk chemicals (e.g., aluminum hydroxide, doxycycline, and chloramphenicol palmitate) are not supplied as 100% potent powders and potency may be as low as 57% for some of these chemicals. If these bulk chemicals are used in compounding, appropriate mathematical conversions must be calculated to ensure expected potency of the final preparation.

It is the responsibility of the veterinarian and pharmacist to ensure that regulations and guidelines are being followed to ensure confidence in the compounded medication. The FDA website cited above lists the labeling requirements for compounded drugs. The United States Pharmacopeia (USP), a national standard-setting organization for pharmaceuticals, lists specific guidelines for pharmaceutical compounding in Chapters 795 Pharmaceutical Compounding—Non-Sterile Preparations, and 797 Pharmaceutical Compounding—Sterile Preparations,

(USP-NF 2008, http://www.usp.org). One important guideline for compounded preparations is that the final potency of the finished preparation is not less than 90.0% and not more than 110% of the theoretically calculated and labeled quantity of active ingredient per unit weight or volume. This is also the requirement for FDA-approved commercially available drugs, so the pharmacist may be starting with more or less of the active ingredient than is labeled on the commercially available product when utilizing approved products to compound. There are also guidelines available for stability considerations in the chapter on Observing Products for Evidence of Instability (Chapter 1191) (USP-NF 2008). Generally, the beyond-use dating (BUD) for a nonaqueous solid compounded dosage form should not be later than 25% of the time remaining until the expiration date of the shortest-dated ingredient or 6 months, whichever is shorter. For water-containing formulations the beyond-use date is not later than 14 days stored at cold temperatures, and for nonaqueous liquid formulations USP Chapter 795 allows for the beyond-use date to be no later than the intended duration of therapy or 180 days, whichever is earlier. These limits may be exceeded when there is supporting valid scientific data that applies to the specific compounded formulation.

The Society of Veterinary Hospital Pharmacists, an organization of academic veterinary teaching hospital pharmacists, has published a position statement on Compounding For Animal Patients that may be consulted by pharmacists or veterinarians for further guidance (http://www.svhp.org.).

Finally, veterinarians should seek the services of a Pharmacy Compounding Accreditation Board (PCAB) accredited pharmacy when prescribing compounds. Formed in 2004 by eight national pharmacy organizations, the nonprofit PCAB runs a voluntary accreditation program to ensure quality standards for compounding pharmacies. PCAB currently represents the only validated set of professional and ethical standards for compounding pharmacies. Once a pharmacy applies for PCAB accreditation, they must undergo a rigorous standards evaluation that is then validated by multiple site visits and inspections by PCAB surveyors. If a pharmacy meets the incredibly rigorous accreditation standards, a veterinarian can be assured that the pharmacy is legally and ethically impeccable and that its compounds are of the highest possible quality. At the time of this writing, PCAB has accredited 46 pharmacies in 40 states, and 40 more pharmacies are awaiting accreditation. PCAB maintains an interactive map of accredited pharmacies in each state list of accredited compounding pharmacies on their website, or veterinarians can contact PCAB's executive director to find an accredited pharmacy in their state. Further information regarding PCAB can be reached at http://www.pcab.org.

UNAPPROVED DRUGS AVAILABLE BY IMPORTATION

When a veterinarian requires a drug that is not approved for use in this country, but is available as an approved dosage form in other countries, he may obtain it through FDA's personal importation policy. These dosage forms may be obtained through importation from other countries by filing a Medically Necessary Personal Veterinary Import form with FDA CVM. This form may be obtained by contacting the FDA. The requesting veterinarian must complete information regarding intended use of the drug and quantities imported. Filing this form alerts the FDA to the fact that a veterinarian is importing a drug from out of the U.S. and will prevent the drug from being seized by U.S. Customs officials upon entry to the United States. Drugs deemed hazardous by FDA may still be seized.

PRESCRIBING CONTROLLED SUBSTANCES

A veterinarian who administers, dispenses, or prescribes controlled substances in the course of his practice *MUST* register with the Drug Enforcement Authority (DEA). This requires submission of an application, which may be obtained from the DEA. Practitioners must have a separate registration for every practice site employed. State regulations also must be followed and practitioners must contact their state authorities to determine the requirements.

Prescribing controlled substances requires submission of appropriate forms and maintaining records for controlled substances. Documentation must be made in the patient's medical record of all controlled substances administered, and such records must be stored in a readily retrievable fashion for 3 years. Appropriate entries must be made for waste or disposal of unused portions of controlled substance and witness is required for disposal. Records must be kept of all controlled substances dispensed, and such records must be stored in a readily retrievable fashion for 3 years. While the law does not specifically require a dispensing record separate from the medical record, a separate record-keeping system provides more readily retrievable dispensing records than does the patient's medical record. A separate dispensing log does *NOT* replace the need to document dispensing of drugs in the medical record because these drugs are still restricted to the order of a licensed practitioner. It is also recommended that Schedule II dispensing records be maintained separately from other records.

PRESCRIBING RECORDS. Practitioners are not required to keep records of prescriptions written for controlled substances, but it is in the best interest of the veterinarian to make a note of such prescriptions in the patient's medical record to provide for a complete patient medical profile.

INVENTORY RECORDS. All DEA 222 order forms for Schedule II orders as well as other commercial invoices accompanying controlled drugs must be signed and dated, and items must be counted, noted, and stored in a readily retrievable file for 3 years. Schedule II records must be stored separately from Schedule III-V records.

A complete and accurate inventory of all stocks of all controlled substances must be taken every 2 years on the anniversary of the practitioner's initial DEA registration. The written inventory should contain the following information:

- The name, address, and DEA registration number of the registrant
- The date and time the inventory is taken
- The signature of the person taking inventory
- An indication that the inventory is maintained for at least 2 years at the location appearing on the registration
- An indication that inventory and other records of Schedule II drugs are maintained separately from other drugs

STORAGE AND SECURITY OF CONTROLLED SUBSTANCES. Controlled substances "must be stored in a securely locked, substantially constructed cabinet." If there is loss or theft, upon discovery of loss of theft of controlled substances, the registrant must immediately notify the region office of the DEA and then must complete DEA form 106 describing the loss. If a theft is verified, the local police department must also be notified.

DISPENSING MEDICATIONS INTENDED TO GO HOME WITH A PATIENT

Many state and federal legal requirements exist for the act of dispensing a drug to go home with a patient. Any prescription medications that leave a practice to go home with a patient must be labeled with the information indicated in Table 56.8.

Any medications that leave a practice to go home with a patient must be packaged in a child-resistant container

TABLE 56.8 Drug dispensing labeling requirements

- name, address, and phone number of the dispensing facility
- name of client
- animal identification (name and species)
- date dispensed
- full directions for use
- name, strength, and quantity of drug dispensed
- name of prescribing veterinarian
- for controlled substances, the label must also contain the message "Caution: Federal law prohibits transfer of this drug to any person other than the patient for whom it was prescribed."

TABLE 56.9 Requirements for writing a prescription for noncontrolled substances

The elements listed below are required by law to be included on the written prescription document:

- printed or stamped name, address, and telephone number of the licensed practitioner
- DEA registration number of the licensed practitioner
- legal signature of the licensed practitioner
- name and strength of drug
- directions for use
- full name and address of the client
- animal identification (name and/or species)
- cautionary statements including, if applicable, withdrawal times for food animals
- number of refills, if any

TABLE 56.10 Requirements for writing a prescription for controlled substances

The elements listed below are required by law to be included on the written prescription document:

- printed or stamped name, address, and telephone number of the licensed practitioner
- DEA registration number of the licensed practitioner
- legal signature of the licensed practitioner followed by printed name of the practitioner
- name and strength of drug
- directions for use
- full name and address of client
- animal identification (name and/or species)
- cautionary statements including, if applicable, withdrawal times for food animals

Note: No refills are allowed on Schedule II prescriptions and refills are limited to 5 times or 6. months (whichever comes first) on prescriptions for drugs in Schedules III–V.

TABLE 56.11 Officially recognized Latin abbreviations used in prescription writing

a.c.	before meals	ml	milliliter
a.d.	right ear	o.d.	right eye
a.s.	left ear	o.s.	left eye
a.u.	both ears	o.u.	both eyes
amp	ampoule	p.c.	after meals
b.i.d.	twice daily	p.o.	by mouth
cc	cubic centimeter	p.r.n.	as needed
c	with	q.	every
cap	capsule	q4h	every 4 hours, etc.
disp	dispense	q.i.d.	four times daily
g or gm	gram	q.s.	a sufficient quantity
gtt(s)	drop(s)	Sig.	directions to patient
h	hour	SQ	subcutaneously
h.s.	at bedtime	stat	immediately
IM	intramuscularly	susp	suspension
IP	intraperitoneally	tab	tablet
IV	intravenous	TBSP	tablespoonful (15 ml)
kg	kilogram	t.i.d.	three times daily
lb	pound	tsp	teaspoonful (5 ml)
m^2	meter squared	Ut. dict	as directed
mg	milligram		

Note: Do not use q.d., q.o.d., and s.i.d. because they are confused with other abbreviations. S.I.D. is unknown to health professionals outside of veterinary medicine. If in doubt about an abbreviation, write out the directions in plain English. Also, avoid using abbreviations such as b.i.d., t.i.d., q.i.d., as they are confusing to clients. Abbreviations such as q12h, q8h and q6h are much clearer.

as described by the Poison Prevention Packaging Act. Medications dispensed in non–child-resistant containers should be adequately labeled with auxiliary labels indicating "Caution: Package not child resistant" and "Keep out of reach of children." Other auxiliary labels detailing important information such as "shake well," "refrigerate," "not for injection," etc. should also be affixed to the container.

PRESCRIPTION WRITING

A prescription is a written order or other order, which is promptly reduced to writing for a controlled substance or for a preparation, combination, or mixture thereof, issued by a practitioner who is licensed in his state to administer and prescribe drugs in the course of his professional practice. A prescription does not include an order entered in a chart or other medical record for drugs administered. Always store blank prescription pads in a secure place with access limited to minimal personnel. The elements required in a valid prescription are provide in Tables 56.9 and 56.10. When writing a prescription, abbreviations are allowed. Some commonly accepted and recognized abbreviations are listed in Table 56.11. When in doubt about an abbreviation, *spell it out.*

REFERENCES AND ADDITIONAL READINGS

AVMA Guidelines for Supervising Use and Distribution of Veterinary Prescription Drugs (http://www.avma.org).

Center for Veterinary Medicine of the Food and Drug Administration (http://www.fda.gov). This site is maintained for veterinary professionals and pet owners. Supported by veterinary specialists, it is an excellent source of drug and regulatory information.

FDA-CVM. FDA/CVM's Compliance policy guide on compounding of drugs. J Am Vet Med Assoc 209:2025–2029, 1996.

———. FDA seeks to clear up confusion about compounding. J Am Vet Med Assoc 223:1103–1106, 2003.

———. Compliance Policy Guide: Compliance Policy Guidance for FDA Staff and Industry. Chapter 6, Subchapter 600, Sec. 608.400—Compounding of Drugs for Use in Animals, July 2003. Food and Drug Administration, 5600 Fishers Lane, Rockville MD. http://www.fda.gov/ora/compliance_ref/cpg/default.htm or http://www.fda.gov/OHRMS/DOCKETS/98fr/03d-0290-gd10001.pdf.

Helms SR. Treatment of feline hypertension with transdermal amlodipine: a pilot study. J Am An Hosp Assoc 43:149–156, 2007.

Hoffman G, Marks SL, Taboada J, et al. Topical methimazole treatment of cats with hyperthyroidism. J Vet Intern Med 15:299, 2001.

Hoffman SB, Yoder AR, Trepanier LA. Bioavailability of transdermal methimazole in a pluronic lecithin organogel (PLO) in healthy cats. J Vet Pharmacol Therap 25:189–193, 2002.

MacGregor JM, Rush JE, Rozanski EA, Boothe DM, Belmonte AA, and Freeman LM. Comparison of pharmacodynamic variables following oral versus transdermal administration of atenolol to healthy cats. Am J Vet Res 69(1):39–44, 2008.

Nieto JE, Spier S, Pipers FS, Stanley S, Aleman MR, Smith DC, and Snyder JR. Comparison of paste and suspension formulations of omeprazole in the healing of gastric ulcers in racehorses in active training. J Am Vet Med Assoc 221(8):1139–1143, 2002.

Trepanier LA: Transdermal formulations: which ones are effective? ACVIM Proceedings, 2002, pages 463–464.

USP 31, NF 26. The United States Pharmacopeia and The National Formulary. Chapter ⟨795⟩ Pharmaceutical Compounding. United States Pharmacopeial Convention Inc., Rockville Maryland: 2008.

———. The United States Pharmacopeia and The National Formulary. Chapter ⟨1191⟩ Stability Considerations in Dispensing Practice. United States Pharmacopeial Convention Inc., Rockville Maryland: 2008.

———. The United States Pharmacopeia and The National Formulary. Chapter ⟨1075⟩ Good Compounding Practices. United States Pharmacopeial Convention Inc., Rockville Maryland: 2008.

Willis-Goulet HS, Schmidt BA, Nicklin CF, et al. Comparison of serum dexamethasone concentrations in cats after oral or transdermal administration using Pluronic Lecithin Organogel (PLO): a pilot study. Vet Dermatol 14:83–89, 2003.

CHAPTER

57

REGULATION OF DRUG AND MEDICATION USE IN PERFORMANCE ANIMALS

CYNTHIA A. COLE AND KEITH ZIENTEK

Horses and greyhounds frequently compete in athletic events in which the use of drugs and medications are regulated. The goals of these medication control programs are threefold: 1) assure a fair and level playing field for the competitors, 2) protect the health and welfare of the animal and human participants, and 3) safeguard the public interest whenever parimutuel wagering is involved. The actual rules for these programs can vary widely depending on the type of competition and the philosophy of the regulating authority. For example, some programs, such as that administered by the Fédération Equestre Internationale (FEI), which is considered to have one of the strictest rules, permit no medications to be present in the horse's system at the time of competition except for approved antiulcer therapies. Other programs allow horses to compete with pharmacologically significant concentrations of a limited number of therapeutic medications in their system. These permitted or authorized medications may include various nonsteroidal antiinflammatory drugs (NSAIDs), muscle relaxants such as methocarbamol, and corticosteroids such as dexamethasone. These rules usually limit the amount of a drug that can be administered to the horse by stipulating a maximum permitted serum concentration; the presence of the drug above that concentration is considered a violation of the rule. By most rules unless a medication is expressly authorized, its mere presence in any detectable amount is considered a violation. Regardless of their specifics, most regulations are enforced by collecting urine and/or blood samples from animals participating in a competition and testing those fluids for the presence of unauthorized drugs and medications and overages of permitted medications in forensic drug testing laboratories. Violations of the rules can be punishable by fines, suspensions, and in severe cases expulsion from the sport.

The testing process itself involves two steps. First, all samples are subjected to a series of screening tests. If the results of any of the screening tests suggest the presence of a drug or an unauthorized medication or indicate an overage of a permitted medication, the sample in question undergoes a second confirmatory testing process. Because of recent advances in analytical chemistry it is now possible to detect drug substances that the animal may have been exposed to through its environment, as well as therapeutic medications at concentrations that could be considered pharmacologically insignificant. This has led many regulatory authorities to move toward the adoption of thresholds or regulatory limits for some environmental contaminants and therapeutic medications. If a substance is present in the serum or urine at a concentration below the regulatory limit or threshold, no action is taken by the regulatory authority (Table 57.1).

TABLE 57.1 Internationally accepted serum or urine threshold concentrations

Dimethyl sulfoxide	15 μg/ml in urine or 1 μg/ml in plasma
Arsenic	3 μg/ml in urine
Hydrocortisone	1 μg/ml in urine
Salicylic acid	625 μg/ml in urine or 5.4 μg/ml in plasma
Testosterone	0.02 μg (free and conjugated)/ml in urine from geldings, and 0.055 μg (free and conjugated)/ml in fillies and mares (unless in foal)
Theobromine	2 μg/ml in urine
Total carbon dioxide	36 millimoles/l in plasma
Boldenone (other than geldings)	Free and conjugated boldenone 0.015 μg/ml in urine or 1 μg/ml in plasma
Estranediol in male horses (other than geldings)	The ratio of the mass of 5a-estrane-3b,17a-diol (free and conjugated) and the mass of 5(10)-estrene-3b-17a-diol (free and conjugated) in urine must be less than 1.
Methoxytyramine	4 μg (free and conjugated) 3-methoxytyramine/ml in urine

DRUG AND MEDICATION RULES

THE RACING COMMISSIONER'S INTERNATIONAL (RCI). The Racing Commissioner's International (RCI) is an organization consisting of racing regulators primarily from the U.S., Canada, and the Caribbean. Although it has no direct role in enforcement of racing regulations, the organization encourages standardization within the industry by developing model rules and penalty guidelines covering a broad range of violations (Racing Commissioner's International Model Rules). The organization, which currently lists over 800 agents, has also adopted a Uniform Classification Guideline for Foreign Substances that consists of five classes (Racing Commissioner's International Model Rules). The classification scheme is based on a number of factors, including the potential for the agent to affect a horse's athletic performance, whether it has a recognized therapeutic use, and the frequency of that use in normal veterinary practice. Drugs listed in the Class 1 category are considered to have the most potential to affect racing performance and have no accepted medical use in racing animals. As shown in Table 57.2, this would include many agents that are also listed as Schedule 1 drugs in the U.S. Drug Enforcement Agency's drug classification system. Class 2 agents also have the potential to affect the performance of an animal, but less so than Class 1 agents. While some Class 2 agents have no recognized therapeutic use in veterinary medicine, others are therapeutic agents that have a high abuse potential in athletic competition. They include drugs used in human medicine as antipsychotics and antidepressants, as well as those used in veterinary medicine as general and local anesthetics (Table 57.2). The difference between drugs in Class 2 and Class 3 is often a question of the frequency of their use in veterinary medicine. For example, while most local anesthetics are in Class 2, the local anesthetic procaine is a Class 3 agent

TABLE 57.2 Examples of drugs and medications categorized in the Association of Racing Commissioner's Drug Classification Guideline

Class 1	Class 2	Class 3	Class 4	Class 5
Amphetamines	Barbiturates	Clenbuterol	Aspirin	Cromolyn
Apomorphine	Benzodiazepines	Detomidine	Betamethasone	Dicumarol
Cocaine	Fluphenazine	Glycopyrrolate	Boldenone	Dimethylsulfoxide
Etorphine	Ketamine	Ipratropium	Carprofen	Famotidine
Fentanyl	Lidocaine	Procaine	Flunixin	Nedocromil
Heroin	Mepivacine	Salmeterol	Stanozolol	Omeprazole
Morphine	Paroxetine	Xylazine	Prednisolone	Warfarin

primarily because it is commonly used in the slow release formulation of penicillin (procaine penicillin). Other Class 3 agents include bronchodilators and sedatives, such as acepromazine and detomidine that are commonly used in veterinary medicine (Table 57.2). Class 4 agents are commonly used therapeutic agents that have a limited capacity to affect racing performance such as isoxsuprine and methocarbamol. Class 5 agents are those that have very specific actions with little potential to alter athletic performance and include antiulcer medications, mast cell stabilizers, and anticoagulants (Table 57.2).

There are several controversial aspects to the RCI classification system. For example, one limitation of the classification system is that it is based on the effects of the drugs on healthy horses. Because of this approach the corticosteroid agents, such as methylprednisolone and triamcinolone, which are commonly used as intraarticular medications are listed in Class 4 indicating that they are therapeutic agents with limited ability to influence performance. While intraarticular administration of corticosteroids may have limited potential to alter the performance of a normal sound horse, they have enormous potential to alter the performance of a horse with an inflamed, arthritic joint (Shoemaker et al. 1992; Carter et al. 1996). In a similar manner NSAIDs, such as flunixin and naproxen, are included in Class 4, despite their significant analgesic and antiinflammatory effects. Finally, anabolic steroids, which are prohibited substances in most human athletic competitions, are also Class 4 agents. Several anabolic steroids are approved by the FDA for use in dogs and horses and some practitioners contend that there are legitimate therapeutic uses for these compounds. Whether anabolic steroids can alter athletic performance in horses and dogs has not been determined, and their class 4 designation reflects this uncertainty.

FÉDÉRATION EQUESTRE INTERNATIONALE (FEI).

The FEI is the governing body recognized by the International Olympic Committee. It establishes the rules and regulations, including those for medication use, under which a number of different international equestrian disciplines compete, including Jumping, Dressage, Eventing, and Endurance Riding. The FEI drug and medication rule is one of the most conservative in equine sports and reflects the philosophy that the horse should compete on its own merits without any unfair advantage that might follow the use of drugs (FEI Veterinary Regulations 2005). The FEI considers a prohibitive substance as any agent capable at any time of acting on one or more of the following mammalian body systems: the nervous system, the cardiovascular system, the urinary system, the reproductive system, the musculoskeletal system, the blood system, the endocrine system, the immune system (other than licensed vaccines against infectious agents), the digestive system (other than orally administrated antiulcer medications) and the skin. An extensive list of specific prohibited agents is approved each year. The medication rule states that the finding of a prohibited substance means the detecting of the substance itself, a metabolite of the substance, an isomer of the substance, or an isomer of a metabolite (FEI Veterinary Regulations 2005). In addition, the finding of any biological or scientific indicator of administration or other exposure to a substance is equivalent to the detection of the substance itself. This latter aspect of the rule allows for methods of detection that do not specifically identify the substance itself, but rather detect some secondary physiological change that occurs following its administration. The list of medications not considered prohibited substances is quite short and includes antibiotics, with the exception of procaine penicillin; antiparasite drugs, with the exception of levamisole; and three agents commonly used to prevent or treat gastric ulcers—omeprazole, ranitidine, and cimetidine. In addition, mares with estrus-related behavioral problems can be treated with the substance altrenogest with certain limitations (FEI Veterinary Regulations 2005). Although the FEI has adopted thresholds on a number of different substances, unlike many other drug and medication rules, the FEI strictly limits the type of substances for which thresholds may be adopted. Their rule states that thresholds can be adopted only for substances endogenous to the horse, substances arising from plants traditionally grazed or harvested as equine feeds, and substances in equine feed arising from contamination during cultivation, processing, treatment, storage, or transportation (FEI Veterinary Regulations 2005).

UNITED STATES EQUESTRIAN FEDERATION (USEF).

Formerly known as the American Horse Show Association, the U.S. Equestrian Federation (USEF) is the largest regulatory organization for show horses in the U.S. Numerous riding and breed disciplines compete under the USEF umbrella, including Arabian, Eventing, Connemaras, Reining, Vaulting, etc. USEF has two drug and medication rules and each discipline chooses under which rule they want to compete (USEF 2005 General Rules). The No Foreign Substance Rule is very similar to the FEI medication rule, and currently only FEI and Endurance Riding events are conducted according to its provisions. The remaining disciplines compete under the Therapeutic Substance Rule, which is considered the more permissive of the two. Under this rule, forbidden substances are any stimulant, depressant, tranquilizer, local anesthetic, or psychotropic agent and/or drug that might affect the performance of a horse and/or pony or any metabolite and/or analogue of any such substance except where expressly permitted (USEF 2005 General Rules). The premise of the Therapeutic Substance Rule is that any drug or medication administered to a competing horse is to be used only for a legitimate, therapeutic purpose. This means that the drug is deemed to be necessary for the proper diagnosis and treatment of an existing illness or injury (USEF 2005 General Rules). Under the Therapeutic Substance Rule some medications are permitted to be present at concentrations likely to be pharmacologically significant. For example, the NSAIDs that are currently permitted and their respective maximum allowed plasma concentrations are shown in Table 57.3. Up to two of the NSAIDs listed may be present in a single plasma or urine sample, except the combination of flunixin and phenylbutazone, which is not permitted. NSAIDs other than those expressly allowed are considered prohibited substances and their presence in a sample collected during a competition would be considered a violation. The Therapeutic Substance Rule also allows the use of the muscle relaxant methocarbamol and the corticosteroid dexamethasone, as long as their plasma concentrations do not exceed 4.0 μg/ml and 0.003 μg/ml, respectively.

DRUG AND MEDICATION RULES IN RACING DOGS AND HORSES IN THE U.S. In the United States each racing jurisdiction adopts its own rules and regulations. Because parimutuel wagering is involved, it is the state governments that hold the ultimate authority, but that authority is often delegated to racing commissions or boards that are appointed by the governor of the respective state. In addition, there may be multiple boards within one state or racing jurisdiction. For example, different boards may oversee horse versus dog racing and/or Thoroughbred versus Standardbred racing. As mentioned previously the ARCI is a voluntary organization of racing commissioners that has attempted to standardize rules and regulations between the various jurisdictions without much success. In the U.S. there is little consistency in drug and medication rules and penalties among the different states, and therefore veterinarians need to familiarize themselves with the specific regulations in each jurisdiction in which they practice.

TABLE 57.3 Maximum permitted plasma concentrations of nonsteroidal antiinflammatory agents allowed by USEF under the Therapeutic Substance Rule

Diclofenac	0.005 μg/ml
Phenylbutazone	15 μg/ml
Ketoprofen	0.25 μg/ml
Meclofenamic Acid	2.5 μg/ml
Naproxen	40 μg/ml
Flunixin	1.0 μg/ml

In horseracing there are two medications that are regulated across the U.S. in a fairly consistent manner, the NSAID phenylbutazone and the diuretic furosemide. For example, in most jurisdictions phenylbutazone can be administered up to 24 hours before the post time of the race in which the horse is entered. Although doses and specific routes of administration are not mandated, most rules stipulate that the concentration of phenylbutazone cannot exceed 5 μg/ml in serum samples collected immediately following the race. In addition, other NSAIDs, such as flunixin meglumine and ketoprofen, are permitted by few racing jurisdictions as alternatives to phenylbutazone. The presence of more than one permitted NSAID in a single serum sample would be considered a violation in most jurisdictions.

In addition to phenylbutazone, most racing jurisdictions in the U.S. permit the administration of the diuretic furosemide to racehorses suffering from exercise-induced pulmonary hemorrhage (EIPH). Furosemide is a loop diuretic that induces natriuresis, chloruresis, increased hydrogen ion excretion, and a profound diuresis (Hinchcliff and Muir 1991). These effects are mediated by the inhibition of Na^+-K^+-$2Cl^-$ transporters in the thick ascending limb of the loop of Henle, although furosemide also has important extrarenal effects, including venodilation and prevention of bronchoconstriction (Broadstone et al. 1991; Wiemer et al. 1994). Whether or not furosemide is an effective therapy for EIPH, has not been proven. For example, Pascoe and colleagues (1985) concluded that furosemide decreased the severity of EIPH in racehorses. That study, however, used an admittedly subjective grading scale to judge the severity of the disease, and therefore, the results were not considered conclusive. Nevertheless, if the pathogenesis of EIPH is associated with the unusually high pulmonary arterial pressures (>70 mm Hg) that develop in the horse during intense exercise, as has been proposed, there is evidence that furosemide may be effective at decreasing those pressures and thus could be therapeutic for EIPH (Manohar 1993; Gleed et al. 1999; Magid et al. 2000).

Even though furosemide is permitted in every racing jurisdiction in the U.S. its use remains controversial, primarily because there is some evidence that it can enhance the athletic performance of horses apart from any effects on EIPH. For example, it has been hypothesized that the diuretic-induced fluid losses associated with furosemide administration result in a moderate, but significant weight loss in the horse, which could enhance its athletic performance (Hinchcliff et al. 1993; Hinchcliff and McKeever 1998). In addition to the controversy regarding the effects of furosemide on equine athletic performance, it has been proposed that the dilute urine that follows furosemide administration may interfere with the detection of other drugs (Soma et al. 1984; Stevenson et al. 1990). For this reason, the dose and timing of furosemide administration are regulated to minimize the chance that that urine samples collected postrace will be dilute (i.e., urine specific gravity <1.010). Most commonly, furosemide administration is restricted to 250 to 500 mg, administered intravenously no closer than 4 hours before post time.

Unlike racing horses, there are no commonly accepted permitted medications for greyhounds racing in the U.S. Although there are many NSAIDs approved by the FDA for use in dogs, the detection of any of these medications in urine samples collected following a race would be considered a violation of most medication rules. In addition, because dogs do not suffer from EIPH to any significant degree, the administration of furosemide is also not permitted. Some states, however, do allow the administration of anabolic steroids to intact female greyhounds to prevent the onset of estrus.

THE DRUG TESTING PROCESS

The drug testing process aims to separate and identify nonendogenous components or drugs in biological matrixes, such as urine and plasma. The analytic process used to accomplish this goal can be separated into three components: extraction of the drug from the biological matrix, separation of the drug from other compounds, and detection and identification of the drug.

ANALYTICAL METHODS FOR EXTRACTION. The goal of the extraction process is to isolate and concentrate the drug, often referred to as an *analyte*, from the sample while removing endogenous matrix materials that could interfere with the detection process. One of the simplest and most traditional methods of sample preparation is liquid-liquid extraction (LLE). In LLE, an aqueous sample such as plasma or urine is mixed with an organic solvent that is not miscible with the sample. Most drugs are more soluble in the organic solvent than in the aqueous media of the sample, and therefore, they partition into and concentrate in the organic phase during the mixing process. The selection of optimal conditions, such as pH and solvent polarity, will result in the majority of any analyte present being extracted into the chosen solvent. To complete LLE, the two liquid layers are separated and the solvent layer is kept for further manipulation, such as concentration through evaporation and reconstitution, which improves the sensitivity of the method.

Solid-phase extraction (SPE) is another technique used to separate and concentrate analytes from aqueous samples. Where LLE uses a liquid solvent to separate the analytes from the sample matrix, SPE uses adsorption to a solid surface to achieve this same separation. Most commonly, SPE methods use prepackaged columns containing bonded silica sorbents to which functional groups, such as hydrocarbons or ion exchange groups have been bound. First, the column of material is washed and buffered to the desired pH to facilitate analyte binding, and then the liquid sample is passed through the bed of adsorbent particles. While the analytes are retained on the column, contaminating matrix material is removed by washing the column with water, buffer, or other solvents. In the final step the column is buffered to a specific pH to facilitate release of the analytes, which are then removed from the column with a small amount of elution solvent. The sample is then evaporated and reconstituted in a solvent amenable to analysis.

The third type of extraction process commonly used in forensic drug testing laboratories is separation by precipitation. This method relies on differences in the solubility of the analytes and the other compounds in the matrix. This method is commonly used to precipitate proteins from plasma or serum samples after which the resulting supernatant is analyzed directly. This extraction method does not involve a concentration step, so the sensitivity is generally less than LLE or SPE.

ANALYTICAL METHODS OF SEPARATION. The goal of the sample separation process is to isolate analytes from each other after extraction and prior to the detection process. The most common method used in forensic drug testing laboratories for separation of analytes is chromatography. For a chromatographic separation, the analytes are dissolved in a mobile phase and passed through an immiscible stationary phase. Differences in the chemical characteristics, such as the polarity, size, and charge state of the analytes, will cause them to have different rates of migration through the stationary phase. These differences in migration rates result in separation of the components in time into a series of discrete bands or peaks that can be collected for further analysis. The two types of chromatography commonly used in forensic drug testing are planar and column chromatography.

One of the simplest types of chromatography is planar chromatography, where the stationary phase is bonded to a piece of paper or glass, and the mobile phase passes over it by either gravity or capillary action. One of the most common types of planar chromatography is thin layer chromatography (TLC), which utilizes a very thin coating of stationary phase on a flat surface called a *plate*. Because it is possible for different analytes to have very similar migration patterns, TLC provides only presumptive qualitative identification of the analyte. In addition, because it is difficult to completely recover the analyte from the plate, quantitative analysis is also problematic. Therefore, TLC is used as a general screening technique and the putative detection of any drug in a sample using TLC would be confirmed by a second analytical method that provides more definitive identification, such as mass spectroscopy.

In column chromatography, the stationary phase is contained within a tubular container (i.e., a column) and the mobile phase, either liquid or gas, is passed through it by either gravity or positive pressure. Liquid chromatography (LC) and gas chromatography (GC) are the two most common column chromatography techniques currently utilized by forensic drug testing laboratories.

In gas chromatography, samples are vaporized in a heated inlet kept in excess of 200°C and moved through the column by an inert carrier gas, such as argon, helium, or nitrogen. The carrier gas acts as the mobile phase and the stationary phase is contained within the column. Typical GC columns are several meters long with an internal diameter of 1 mm or less. One disadvantage of GC is that the majority of analytes of interest to forensic drug testing laboratories require a lengthy derivatization step before analysis. Derivatization is the process by which an analyte is modified by a chemical reaction to produce a new compound that is more amenable to separation by GC. Derivatization is used to increase the volatility and stability of compounds of interest. The advantages of using GC are that the systems are fairly simple to operate and the methods are relatively straightforward because few modifications of the stationary and mobile phases are possible.

In liquid chromatography, compounds in a sample are separated by utilizing the differences in polarity of the analytes, the liquid mobile phase, and the solid stationary phase contained within the column. Typical LC columns are 100–500 mm long with an internal diameter of 3 mm or less. Unlike GC, in LC the composition of both the mobile and stationary phases can be modified to optimize the analytical separation. Another advantage of LC separation methods is that they are accomplished using aqueous mobile phases at room temperature. Therefore, LC methods are not limited by the thermal stability or volatility of the compound, because vaporization of the sample is not required. Together these factors have made LC an increasingly popular technique for separation in forensic drug testing laboratories.

ANALYTICAL METHODS FOR DETECTION. While extraction and separation are essential components of the analysis, it is important to note that neither of these processes provide data sufficient to definitively identify a drug. The two most common methods used in forensic drug testing laboratories to identify analytes are absorption spectroscopy and mass spectrometry.

Absorption spectroscopy detection methods employ ultraviolet or visible light, utilizing the property that many molecules are capable of absorbing certain frequencies of light. The degree of absorbance for a molecule is generally directly proportional to the concentration of that molecule in solution at concentrations in the range of 10^{-2} to 10^{-6} M. Because most absorption spectroscopic methods are very robust and relatively inexpensive, they are commonly used for quantitative analysis in forensic drug testing laboratories. One of the limitations of absorption spectroscopy, however, is that two analytes with overlapping absorption spectra and with similar elution times will be difficult to differentiate. In addition, the presence of chemical and/or spectral interferences can cause erroneous detector responses resulting in quantitation errors.

In mass spectrometry (MS), following the extraction and separation process the analytes in the sample are serially injected into the mass spectrometer for identification. While many different types of mass spectrometers are commercially available, in the type most commonly used in forensic drug testing laboratories analytes are bombarded with a beam of electrons, which causes the molecules to become ionized. While some of these ions will remain intact, many will fragment into smaller ions and neutral fragments. The original ionized precursor molecules and the product fragments are then separated in electric or magnetic fields based on their mass to charge ratio and then serially passed into a detector that measures the abundance of each ion. A plot of the abundances of the precursor and productions versus their mass : charge ratios is referred to as the compound's *mass spectrum* (Fig. 57.1). The highest molecular weight peak in a spectrum will usually represent the parent molecule minus a single electron (ionized), and is referred to as the *molecular ion*. The mass spectrum of the analyte is compared to a computerized database of mass spectra referred to as a *library* or an *authenticated standard* of a known compound. Because the fragmentation pathways for many molecules are well characterized and extremely reproducible, unambiguous identification of a compound can be achieved. Even analytes with the same nominal mass can be differentiated, because they usually produce very different fragmentation ions. Because the abundance of the ions is directly proportional to the concentration of the analyte in the solution, extremely accurate quantitation is possible using MS methods. One of the disadvantages of mass spectrometry is that it requires a highly trained analyst to develop the methods and interpret the data. Nevertheless, because of the high degree of specificity inherent in the results, mass spectrometry has become the de facto standard method for drug identification in forensic drug testing programs.

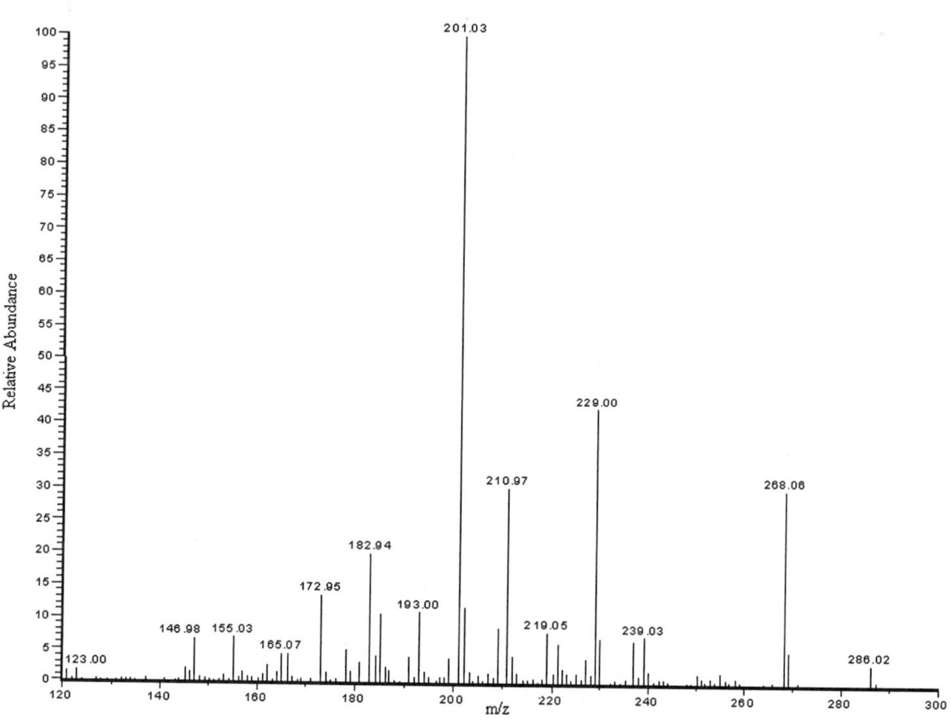

FIG. 57.1 Mass spectrum of morphine obtained by liquid chromatography mass spectrometry. Sample concentration was 50 pg/ml and the flow rate was 0.2 ml/min. Thirty-two scans were signal-averaged to produce the resultant mass spectrum.

SAMPLING, SCREENING, AND CONFIRMATION IN THE RACING LABORATORY

Sample Type and Collection. Drug and medication rules are generally enforced by the collection and testing of blood and urine samples from animals performing in athletic competitions. Sample collecting procedures must take into consideration both scientific and legal issuees. An important legal aspect of the process is chain-of-custody documentation, which is a tamper-resistant paper or electronic trail indicating where the sample has been and who has had custody of it at all times. For this reason the actual drug testing process begins when a sample is collected. In addition, because many modern mass spectrometric techniques can detect quantities of drugs or medications in the picogram to femtogram range, special care must be taken by the sampling personnel to prevent contamination from environmental sources during the collection process. Only clean sample collection vessels should be used, and personnel should wear the appropriate attire, such as disposable gloves, and should refrain from eating, drinking, and smoking during the process. Once collected, the samples are sealed with tamperproof evidence tape and secured in locked containers or coolers for transport to the testing laboratory. To prevent degradation of the samples, nonfrozen samples should be kept cold and shipped overnight. Otherwise the samples should be frozen and kept frozen until immediately prior to analysis.

Urine is the primary bodily fluid used for drug testing in most programs because it is relatively easy to obtain, and because most drugs and their metabolites are present in urine in higher concentrations than in blood. Generally, urine samples are collected from the animals following competitive events. In some programs blood, plasma, or serum samples are also collected, although this is done more commonly in horses than dogs. Plasma or serum samples are primarily used to regulate authorized or permitted medications, such as NSAIDs, where maximum serum/plasma concentrations have been adopted by the regulatory agency.

Occasionally other bodily fluids or tissues are collected for drug analysis. For example, in the past decade interest in the analysis of hair for drug detection has increased in forensic sciences. However, not all drugs administered to the horse will be incorporated into growing hair. In addition, when a drug is detected in hair it can be difficult to determine when the animal was actually exposed to the compound. For example, a sample of a horse's mane positive for the bronchodilating agent clenbuterol could be the result of an administration 6 or more months previously. For this reason, the usefulness of hair analysis and the legal and ethical ramifications of proceeding with regulatory action against an owner or trainer based on a positive hair test, remain to be determined. Saliva samples have also been tested for the presence of unauthorized medications. The principal value of testing saliva samples is the ability to detect agents recently administered by the oral route due to residual contamination of the mouth and pharyngeal area. Saliva is collected by swabbing the animal's mouth with a cotton gauze held in forceps. One of the principal disadvantages of saliva testing is that it is difficult to obtain a useful volume of fluid.

Testing Scheme Overview. Over the years, the drug testing process has evolved into a two-step procedure. When the samples arrive at the laboratory, small aliquots of each are subjected to multiple screening tests. In North America, thin layer chromatography (TLC), enzyme-linked immunosorbent assays (ELISAs) and instrumental techniques employing mass spectrometry are the most common methods used for sample screening. If the results of all the screening tests are negative, the sample is declared negative and no further action is taken. However, if the results of one or more of the screening tests are suspicious, the sample undergoes a second round of testing to confirm the presence of, and definitively identify, the substance. The results of the confirmation test must be able to withstand legal challenge and intense scientific scrutiny, making the identification of the compound by mass spectrometry essential. Although gas chromatography-mass spectrometry (GC-MS) has been the most commonly used method of confirmation, liquid chromatography-mass spectrometry (LC-MS) is rapidly becoming the method of choice in most forensic drug testing laboratories.

Screening Methods. The ideal screening test should be rapid, sensitive, and inexpensive. Specificity is not a necessity because the results are only preliminary and will be confirmed in a second round of testing that is highly specific. TLC has been used in forensic drug testing laboratories for over five decades and it remains one of the most common screening methods used in North America despite numerous disadvantages. For example, TLC methods require large volumes of both sample and solvent, they involve subjective interpretation of the results by the chromatographer, and their sensitivity is often not adequate to detect many of the more potent drugs in use today. The TLC limit of detection (LOD), which is the lowest concentration of a drug that can be reliably detected by an analytical method, is usually in the range of 100 nanograms per milliliter (ng/ml) or parts per billion (ppb) for most analytes. TLC remains in use primarily because of its simplicity (technicians can be trained in a few weeks), dependability (complex instrumentation is not required), and capacity to simultaneously detect a wide range of substances in a single analysis.

ELISA testing is an integral component of most screening programs in forensic drug analysis, primarily because of its simplicity and sensitivity. The majority of laboratories use ELISA in conjunction with TLC or instrumental methods. In its simplest form the method has three primary components: an antibody specific for the drug or class of drugs, drug molecules labeled with an enzyme conjugate, and a substrate that will produce a measurable color change when the enzyme conjugate binds to the antibody. Drug molecules in the sample compete with enzyme-labeled drug molecules for binding sites on the antibodies. Enzyme-labeled drug bound to the antibody will react with the added substrate to produce a color change in the solution. Therefore, when unlabeled drug molecules are present in the sample, there is a decrease in color due to the competitive binding and this change can be measured by optical spectroscopy.

As mentioned previously, one of the advantages of the use of ELISA testing is its superior sensitivity. The LODs for most ELISAs are in the range of 1–10 ng/ml. ELISAs are generally designed to be very specific, detecting either an individual drug or a class of drugs that are structurally similar. Because there are a limited number of commercially available ELISA tests kits, however, the breadth of coverage that can be provided by these kits is limited. Most programs combine ELISA testing with other screening methods in order to increase the number of drugs that can be detected. Because they are an immune-based test, there is always the potential for nonspecific cross-reactions to occur. Therefore, like TLC, the results of ELISA tests are only presumptive and confirmation of those test results using a method with a higher degree of specificity is required for definitive identification.

In recent years, screening tests have been developed using GC/MS and LC/MS methods. As their names imply, these instrumentally based methods utilize either gas or liquid chromatography to separate any compounds of interest in a sample, which are then serially injected into the mass spectrometer for identification. In general these methods are equal to or more sensitive than ELISA testing, with LODs commonly in the range of 0.01–1 ng/ml. However, in a manner more similar to TLC analysis, they can detect a wide range of substances simultaneously in a single analysis. The primary limitations to these instrumentally based screening approaches are the initial costs of the instruments as well as the need for highly trained analysts, making the initial implementation of these methods expensive.

Confirmation Methods. If one or more of the screening tests gives results suggestive of the presence of a nonauthorized drug or medication, the sample undergoes a second round of testing, the purpose of which is to definitively confirm the presence and identity of the drug. The method used for confirmation must be highly specific and sensitive. The two most common methods used are GC/MS and LC/MS. Confirmational analysis is usually performed on only one sample at a time, as the extraction, separation, and detection steps are labor-intensive and may require one or more days of sample preparation. Traditionally the process has been only qualitative in nature, as the presence alone of a nonpermitted substance is considered a violation by most drug and medication rules, regardless of the amount in the sample. However, because improvements in analytical methods have resulted in the detection of smaller and smaller amounts of drugs, quantitative information can be useful in differentiating residues of therapeutic agents administered days or even weeks before the race from pharmacologically significant concentrations more indicative of race-day administrations.

REFEREE SAMPLE ANALYSIS. As described above, before a reputable laboratory reports that a sample contains an unauthorized drug or an overage of an authorized medication, the sample has undergone multiple screening and confirmation tests using several different analytical methods. Nevertheless, a split or referee sample analysis is permitted by many drug and medication rules. In the split sample process, an aliquot or small portion of the original sample is reanalyzed at a second laboratory to verify the positive test. The purpose of the split sample analysis is to verify the results of the original laboratory and, in so doing, guard against laboratory mistakes or contamination of the original sample during the collection process. If the second laboratory does not confirm the presence of the unauthorized substance found by the primary laboratory, no regulatory action is taken.

There are several variations in split sample analysis programs. For example, under FEI regulations a split sample analysis is automatically conducted by a second FEI-associated laboratory following any finding of a violation of its drug and medication rule (FEI Veterinary Regulations 2005). Should the second analysis fail to confirm the original finding, however, the rule does not stipulate whether regulatory actions will or will not be taken. The USEF recently implemented a program that allows for collection of a split sample and testing of that sample at a second referee laboratory (USEF 2005 General Rules).

FACTORS AFFECTING WITHDRAWAL TIMES

Veterinary practitioners often want to know withdrawal times or how long before an event or race they should discontinue treatment with a particular medication in order to avoid having an animal test positive for that agent. Unfortunately, it is very difficult for laboratories to generate accurate withdrawal times for therapeutic medications because many different factors can affect how long a drug remains detectable after administration. Probably the most important factor is the sensitivity of the testing method used by the laboratory. As discussed previously, the LODs for different analytical methods vary widely. For example, in general, TLC is much less sensitive than instrumental or ELISA analysis. Therefore, the withdrawal time for a medication tested by ELISA in one laboratory would be significantly longer than the withdrawal time determined by another laboratory using TLC analysis as its testing method. Even if the same method of analysis is used, differences in sample preparation can result in higher or lower analyte recoveries that can ultimately affect withdrawal time.

Many other factors outside of the laboratory may also affect withdrawal times. For example, the higher the administered dose, generally the longer the withdrawal time. The route of drug administration is also important. Intravenous administration generally results in the shortest withdrawal time compared to oral or other parenteral forms of dosing, such as intramuscular or subcutaneous. In addition, some drugs, such as clenbuterol and isoxsuprine, accumulate in the body with repeated dosing, and drug residues can persist in urine samples for 30 days or longer after the medications are withdrawn. There can also be large variations in the clearance rates of many medications among different horses. Because of all of these factors, in order to generate an accurate withdrawal time each laboratory may need to administer the medication in question at the highest dose commonly used for a prolonged period of time to a large number of horses. The laboratory must then collect and analyze samples from these horses using the same methods that they would use to screen their regulatory samples. Due to time constraints and financial limitations few laboratories have completed this process with more than a handful of medications.

THRESHOLDS, REPORTING LEVELS, AND CUTOFFS

As analytical chemistry methodology has improved, the smallest amount of a drug or medication that can be detected in bodily fluids has progressively decreased. Currently the LOD in urine for most substances of concern are in the low ng/ml range. As a result of this sensitive testing the use of drugs and medications in equine sports is considered by many to be well controlled. The side effect of this sensitive testing, however, can be the detection of substances that were not purposely administered to the horse. In some situations these agents are contaminants in the horse's environment. For example, theobromine can be found in cocoa husks, and scopolamine and atropine occur naturally in many plants in the genus *Datura*. In addition, it is now recognized that some substances thought to be exogenous synthetic agents are actually endogenous, albeit usually produced only in very small amounts. For example, both hydrocortisone and nandrolone are now recognized as occurring naturally in animals. In addition, as previously discussed, some medications can be detected in urine days or even weeks following the last administration.

As a result of the sensitive testing and the recognition that some substances may be endogenous to the horse or contaminants in its environment, almost every organizational body that regulates equestrian activities has adopted thresholds or cutoffs for a number of substances. Horses may compete in sanctioned events with the presence of these substances in their tissues, bodily fluids, or excreta, provided the concentration of the substance does not exceed the predetermined threshold value. Table 57.1 lists a number of thresholds accepted by many regulatory agencies.

SUMMARY

Drug testing programs are implemented in order to enforce drug and medication rules. Most programs consist of a two-part testing process that utilizes urine as the primary sample type. All samples are tested in a preliminary screening process, and any samples with suspicious results undergo an additional round of confirmatory testing. Veterinarians need to be aware of the drug and medication rules under which their clients compete, and because detection periods have not been determined for many therapeutic substances they should allow for extended withdrawal times in order to avoid inadvertent positive tests.

REFERENCES

Broadstone, R. V., N. E. Robinson et al. (1991). Effects of furosemide on ponies with recurrent airway obstruction. Pulm Pharmacol 4(4):203–8.

Carter, B. G., A. L. Bertone et al. (1996). Influence of methylprednisolone acetate on osteochondral healing in exercised tarsocrural joints of horses. Am J Vet Res 57(6):914–22.

Fédération Equestre Internationale Veterinary Regulations. 9th edition (2005). Effective 1st January 2002, revised 2005. Available at www.horsesports.org.

Gleed, F. D., N. G. Ducharme et al. (1999). Effects of frusemide on pulmonary capillary pressure in horses exercising on a treadmill. Equine Vet J Suppl 30:102–6.

Gowen, R. and J. Lengel, Eds. (1993). Regulatory Aspects of Drug Use in Performance Horses. In: Drug Use in Performance Horses. Philadelphia: WB Saunders.

Hinchcliff, K. W. and K. H. McKeever (1998). Fluid administration attenuates the haemodynamic effect of frusemide in running horses. Equine Vet J 30(3):246–50.

Hinchcliff, K. W., K. H. McKeever, et al. (1993). Effect of furosemide and weight carriage on energetic responses of horses to incremental exertion. Am J Vet Res 54(9):1500–4.

Hinchcliff, K. W. and W. W. Muir, 3rd (1991). Pharmacology of furosemide in the horse: a review. J Vet Intern Med 5(4):211–8.

Magid, J. H., M. Manohar, et al. (2000). Pulmonary vascular pressures of thoroughbred horses exercised 1, 2, 3 and 4 h after furosemide administration. J Vet Pharmacol Ther 23(2):81–9.

Manohar, M. (1993). Pulmonary artery wedge pressure increases with high-intensity exercise in horses. Am J Vet Res 54(1):142–6.

Pascoe, J. R., A. E. McCabe, et al. (1985). Efficacy of furosemide in the treatment of exercise-induced pulmonary hemorrhage in Thoroughbred racehorses. Am J Vet Res 46(9):2000–3.

Racing Commissioner's International Model Rules and Uniform Classification Guideline for Foreign Substances, available at www.arci.com.

Shoemaker, R. S., A. L. Bertone, et al. (1992). Effects of intra-articular administration of methylprednisolone acetate on normal articular cartilage and on healing of experimentally induced osteochondral defects in horses. Am J Vet Res 53(8):1446–53.

Soma, L. R., K. Korber, et al. (1984). Effects of furosemide on the plasma and urinary concentrations and the excretion of fentanyl: model for the study of drug interaction in the horse. Am J Vet Res 45(9):1743–9.

Stevenson, A. J., M. P. Weber, et al. (1990). The influence of furosemide on plasma elimination and urinary excretion of drugs in Standardbred horses. J Vet Pharmacol Ther 13(1):93–104.

United States Equestrian Federation (2005). 2005 General Rules. Available at www.usef.org.

Wiemer, G., E. Fink, et al. (1994). Furosemide enhances the release of endothelial kinins, nitric oxide and prostacyclin. J Pharmacol Exp Ther 271(3):1611–5.

CHAPTER

58

ADVERSE DRUG REACTIONS

VICTORIA HAMPSHIRE AND MARGARITA A. BROWN

Veterinarians are overwhelmingly successful in the use of pharmaceuticals to prevent and treat disease. Occasionally, veterinarians and animal owners observe adverse drug reactions. These may be associated with failures in the safety and efficacy of commercially marketed drugs. To this end, regulators in most western countries have developed and refined adverse drug event reporting systems. The stakeholders in this process are animal owners, veterinarians, drug sponsors, and regulators. Adverse drug event reporting has been a growing aspect of veterinary medicine, and practitioners are increasingly concerned with issues of informed consent.[4,5,10,11,15,16,21,31] The process of monitoring for drug risks and conveying ways to optimize benefit and minimize risk is called *pharmacovigilance*. The World Health Organization (WHO) defines pharmacovigilance as the science and activities relating to the detection, assessment, understanding, and prevention of adverse effects or any other drug-related problems.[30]

For most of the history of modern veterinary medicine, drugs approved for human use have been prescribed in an extralabel manner (that is, the indication for treatment of the subject species is not on the label). Since the United States Food and Drug Administration (FDA) established a veterinary bureau and subsequently since the formation of a Center for Veterinary Medicine (CVM) in 1984, growing numbers of drugs are specifically approved by FDA for use in animals. These approvals are based on review and assessment of carefully designed animal studies that specifically address safety and efficacy in the target species. For drugs that are approved for use in animals used for human food, a human food safety assessment is also done as delineated in the Code of Federal Regulations, Analytical Methods for Residues (21CFR§514.1 9b [7]).[25] Similarly, the United States Department of Agriculture regulates veterinary biologics, including vaccines (Virus-Serum-Toxin Act, Chapter 5)[26] The United States Environmental Protection Agency (EPA) regulates pesticides, such as topical flea and tick products (Federal Insecticide, Fungicide and Rodenticide Act, Section 3).[27] This chapter focuses on the regulation of postapproval animal drug risk information by the FDA CVM, with attention to the key aspects of the reporting process and basic methods of adverse drug event assessment that will be useful to veterinary students, academicians, and practicing veterinarians.

When a new drug is approved for veterinary use, it is given a new animal drug application number (NADA number) by which the postapproval information can be archived. The labeling includes the primary container label, package inserts, packaging of any secondary containers, and any accompanying consumer information that was required at product launch. The labeling contains information about side effects, precautions, warnings, and contraindications that were discovered in preapproval studies. Labeling may also include promotion and advertising materials and client education sheets.

A marketed drug product may expand the number of times a drug is administered from what was observed in a relatively small number of animals utilized for preapproval studies. In the veterinary world, average clinical studies range from 30 or 40 in the target animal safety studies to 300 or 400 in clinical efficacy studies.[8] After approval, the number of doses sold can reach a treatment subpopulation within the estimated 62 million owned dogs and 76 million owned cats that exist in America.[1,28] There is no reliable nonproprietary data for exact numbers of prescriptions administered to dogs or cats. However, depending on the popularity of a new drug and the prevalence of a commonly diagnosed condition, such as arthritis, one can easily see the potential growth from several hundred animals dosed to several million. Thus, clinical manifestations that are too infrequent to be detected in relatively small preapproval studies begin to emerge in this period. Additionally, conditions of use that were not predicted in the preapproval period and other confounding factors, such as the possibility of targeted use in a particular age group, may influence the emergence of new clinical manifestations. The purpose of veterinary adverse drug event monitoring is to assess the frequency, similarity, and severity of such signs so that regulators can consider the possibility of drug association.

In the United States, postapproval monitoring for adverse drug events, ineffectiveness, and product defects falls under regulations promulgated in the Code of Federal Regulations. 21CFR§514.3 describes the reporting requirements to veterinary drug companies and contains important definitions:

An *adverse drug experience (ADE)* is any adverse event associated with the use of a new animal drug, whether or not considered to be drug-related, and whether or not the new animal drug was used in accordance with the approved labeling (i.e., used according to label directions or used in an extralabel manner, including but not limited to different route of administration, different species, different indications, or other than labeled dosage). Adverse drug experience includes, but is not limited to

1. An adverse event occurring in animals in the course of the use of an animal drug product by a veterinarian or by a livestock producer or other animal owner or caretaker.
2. Failure of a new animal drug to produce its expected pharmacological or clinical effect (lack of expected effectiveness).
3. An adverse event occurring in humans from exposure during manufacture, testing, handling, or use of a new animal drug.

The term *adverse drug event* is often used interchangeably with *adverse drug experience*. The regulations also distinguish *serious* ADEs as "an adverse event that is fatal, or life threatening, or requires professional intervention, or causes an abortion, or stillbirth, or infertility, or congenital anomaly, or prolonged or permanent disability, or disfigurement."

The definition of an *unexpected* adverse drug experience is "an adverse event that is not listed in the current labeling for the new drug and includes any event that may be symptomatically and pathophysiologically related to an event listed on the labeling, but differs from the event because of greater severity or specificity."

In the United States, the reporting of suspect veterinary drug reactions is initiated as a passive, or voluntary, process. This is important because most experts estimate that only a fraction of the real occurrences of adverse events are reported.[3,9,18,22,23,24] An adverse event may occur whether or not a drug is used according to its label, and regardless of regulatory labeling for that species as "FDA approved." Extralabel use should not be a deterrent to reporting an adverse event. The condition of use is important to CVM in evaluating what might be future supplemental claims, or in assisting CVM in noting conditions of use that should be placed as warnings or precautionary statements on a modified label.

Sponsors of new animal drug applications must report timely information regarding drug side effects after approval. Once a veterinary drug firm becomes aware of a voluntary report (either from the veterinarian or animal owner) there is a legal requirement for the firm to report serious and unexpected signs (those signs not presently on the label as side effects) to FDA CVM within 15 working days and to follow up on outstanding or unresolved cases, regardless of any opinion of causality. Other reports are submitted in the semiannual or annual reports that sponsors send to FDA CVM. Current regulations require that the sponsor submit a summary report every 6 months for the first 2 years of marketing and annually thereafter.

Nearly all the reports that FDA CVM receives come directly from the drug sponsor on FDA CVM forms that contain key data elements describing the reaction and the context of the reaction.[7] Approximately 1% of reports come directly to FDA CVM from the animal owner or veterinarian and bypass the sponsor and/or request confidentiality from the sponsor.[6]

METHOD

FDA CVM monitors the frequency, severity, and similarity of clinical signs reported as adverse drug events. The *frequency* of an ADE clinical sign or syndrome is the number of times it or any other sign or syndrome is reported to the FDA CVM. The *severity* of the reaction or event includes the evaluation of individual reports that contain one or more clinical signs associated with death or serious clinical pathology that could be reasonably expected to end in death or serious debilitation (such as blindness, deafness, etc.) if intervention was not provided in a timely or aggressive manner. The *similarity* of the reactions or events refers to the situation where the reports in the database for a single drug are similar in onset, severity, and clinical signs.

If the frequency, severity, and/or clinical similarity of reports reach a level of concern that is observably or interpretively (as judged by the majority of the reviewers) occurring more than clinically expected in a population of similar size, age, and health status, the generated signal must be examined in greater depth, even if it represents a small number of reports.[17]

Identification of a signal generated for a particular sign or syndrome may result in a label change. Significant changes to the label are supplied in the form of a "Dear Doctor" letter mailed to veterinary practitioners across the nation, alerting veterinarians to an increase in frequency, similarity, or severity of drug-associated signs. In some cases there may be a recall or withdrawal of the drug. Clinicians should acquaint themselves and office staff with the appearance of these critical communiqués so that they are not discarded unread.

ALGORITHMS. FDA CVM utilizes a modified Kramer algorithm to assess whether an observed ADE is drug-related (Fig. 58.1). The algorithm has standardized criteria to facilitate an objective review process.[2,1.14]

There are six axes or criteria that are used together with an accompanying questionnaire and provide guidance. The basic tenet is to assess the occurrence of a clinical sign as a causally related clinical sign. Thus, the causal relationship is based on established knowledge—previous documentation of the clinical sign, alternative explanations for the clinical sign, timing of events, dosage given, diminution of the clinical sign when the influence of the drug passes (dechallenge), and reappearance of the clinical sign when the drug is given again (rechallenge).[17]

The algorithm is applied to each clinical manifestation in an adverse event report. The scores for each axis of the algorithm are summed to arrive at a causality assessment score for each clinical sign. General categories of drug-related association are

Remotely
Possibly
Probably
Definitely

All clinical manifestations with causality assessment scores of Possibly, Probably, or Definitely drug-related are included in the monthly update of the cumulative summary on the FDA CVM website.

Since the inception of the FDA CVM's ADE system, the development of new types of drugs has required closer attention to its application.[11,12,13] Take as an example the macrocyclic lactone heartworm preventives, which are given monthly or at even longer intervals. Since these drugs are reapplied at such long intervals, it can take a while for an association to be realized if an adverse drug event occurs.[12] Consider this analogy: clinical manifestations from agents such as *Campylobacter* and *Salmonella* can take days to appear, but most people blame their most recent meal for their gastrointestinal upset. Similarly, recurrence of the adverse event may not be recognized until after several rechallenges due to the length of time between applications.

It can be very difficult to determine the appropriate designation for dechallenge with a drug that can remain in the body for a month or longer. Typically, toxicologists use seven terminal half-lives as a timeframe for calculating drug disappearance where 99% of the drug is eliminated from the body.[19] Although for the most part events are expected to occur during times of peak serum concentration, reviewers should also consider chronic syndromes

Elements of Adverse Clinical Manifestation (CM) Algorithm

1. **Previous Experience With Drug:**
   - **+1** CM generally recognized to occur in this species at the dosage received.
   - **0** CM is not generally recognized to occur in this species at the dosage received but has been previously reported in veterinary and/or human medicine.

     Drug has limited accumulated clinical experience (time and/or quantity marketed).
   - **–1** CM previously unreported and drug has substantial accumulated clinical experience (time and/or quantity marketed).
2. **Alternative Etiologic Candidates:**
   - **+2** There is **no** good candidate or no change in a candidate which can explain the CM, exclusive of drug administration.
   - **0** An alternative candidate(s) exists, but not a good one(s) which can well explain the CM.

     CM commonly occurs spontaneously in this type of patient and situation, usually in the absence of any recognizable alternative candidate(s).
   - **–1** There is a good candidate or a change in a candidate which can well explain the CM, exclusive of drug administration.
3. **Timing of Events:**
   - **+1** Timing was consistent and as expected for this type of CM to this drug.
   - **0** Do not know what timing to expect.
   - **–2** Timing was inconsistent for this type of CM to this drug.
4. **Evidence of Overdose:**
   - **+1** CM is clearly a dose-related type of manifestation, **and** there is unequivocal evidence that the amount of drug received was an overdose for this animal.
   - **0** CM is not a dose-related type of manifestation **or** there is no evidence of an overdose.
5. **Dechallenge:**
   - **+1** CM diminished or disappeared after discontinuation of suspect drug or administration of **a specific** antidote.

     CM is known to be dose-related, and CM diminished or disappeared after dosage reduction.
   - **0** Dechallenge difficult, impossible, or inappropriate to assess.

     A non-specific agent or maneuver (non-antidotal) was administered that was directed against the CM and that usually produced the degree and rate of improvement observed in the case.

     CM characteristically transient and episodic, and there is no established pattern episodes (regardless of what occurs after discontinuing the drug).

     CM known to be dose-related, and CM did not diminish or disappear after dosage was reduced.
   - **–1** CM did **not** diminich or disappear after discontinuation of suspect drug.

     CM improved without dechallenge **and** the improvement **cannot** be attributed to the development of tolerance.
6. **Rechallenge:**
   - **+1** CM unequivocally recurred or exacerbated after rechallenge.
   - **0** There was no rechallenge attempted.

     A non-specific agent or maneuver (non-antidotal) was administered that obscured the response of the CM.

     CM failed to recur or exacerbate on rechallenge, **but** the dosage or duration of drug administration on rechallenge was substantially less than that suspected of causing the original CM.

     Recurrence or exacerbation of CM was impossible to assess because it was progressing or was at a level of severity that any further increase would be difficult to appreciate.
   - **–1** CM failed to recur or exacerbate on rechallenge.

FIG. 58.1 Elements of adverse clinical manifestation (CM) algorithm.

that might emerge from residual drug or drug product, such as cachexia or neoplasia. Such syndromes might be attributed to the "background" frequency of disease occurrence and could easily be missed.

The effect on the algorithm in these situations is to skew the summed causality assessment lower (to the level of "Possibly" or "Remotely" drug-related), since it is difficult to assign a positive number to represent a strong association in time, recognition of rechallenge, or a definite result of dechallenge. This means that the signal of an emerging adverse event could be overlooked. This will be an ongoing consideration as new types of drugs are developed.

STRENGTHS OF ADE REPORTING SYSTEMS

Strengths of the ADE reporting systems include

1. ADE reporting provides a cost-effective way to study the safety and effectiveness of drugs in large, heterogeneous animal populations, compared to the animals in preapproval studies; thus, signals may be evaluated with greater correlation to context of use.[22]
2. The FDA CVM can monitor early risk signals and maintain ongoing surveillance.

Signals generated by evaluation of ADE reports can be used to generate hypotheses and can serve as the foundation for postapproval safety studies by the manufacturer.[20]

LIMITATIONS OF ADE REPORTING SYSTEMS

Limitations of the ADE reporting systems include

1. *Underreporting.* Spontaneously reported ADEs represent only a small portion of the number of ADEs that have actually occurred, resulting in an underestimate of the number of suspected ADEs.
2. *Lack of accurate exposure data.* In most cases in veterinary medicine, precise information related to doses sold and/or administered is not available. For this reason, it is not always possible to calculate the number of dogs affected by the drug compared to the number that actually received the drug (incidence). Likewise, it is usually not possible to calculate the number of those suspected to have reacted to the drug compared to the number of those suspect drug reactions that were actually reported to CVM (reporting rates).
3. *Report quality is often lacking.* Reports relying solely on contact with the animal owner often lack medical information such as laboratory test values, concomitant medications administered, and preexisting medical conditions. Attempts to collect information from veterinarians may be incomplete due to reliance on lay staff to complete the report form. Sometimes the attending veterinarian is too busy to discuss the case. Follow-up information about the outcome of the event may be lost when owners change veterinarians, move, or simply never bring the animal back for reexamination.
4. *Potential bias.* Media coverage, including direct-to-consumer advertising, and internet access have greatly increased consumer awareness in general. If a product receives media attention or becomes the subject of an internet website, there may be a flurry of reports from the public. The number of ADEs submitted for a drug is at its highest by the end of the first 2 years of its marketing.[29] Drug manufacturers with sophisticated pharmacovigilance programs are more likely to provide greater numbers of timely and accurate ADE reports than those without these systems. Another source of bias may be the failure to recognize a problem in a product due to a high level of comfort with its use, such as with a product that has been marketed for years or a new product perceived as having no side effects. Still another source could be failure to recognize a timely association of the event with a drug that has a sustained or chronic effect.

Still, despite these limitations, CVM and other FDA centers have found pharmacovigilance a valuable tool for communicating drug risk to the health professional and consumer.[10,17,20]

TRENDS IN PHARMACOVIGILANCE AT FDA CVM. Currently, the FDA CVM receives more than 30,000 ADE reports each year. There has been a steady increase from the approximately 4,500 received at the inception of the current ADE program in 1997. Figure 58.2 demonstrates the growth in adverse experience reporting to CVM over time.

The ADE reports sent to the CVM primarily represent adverse events occurring in the U.S.A., but may include foreign reports if the suspect product carries the same label used in the U.S. This means that adverse events are not reported for the same product that carries a different brand name in another country, although such events may be known to the regulatory authority of that country. As a result, a single report of a serious adverse event may seem insignificant in one country but, if it were known that similar events had been reported in other countries, this "isolated" event might be viewed with more importance.

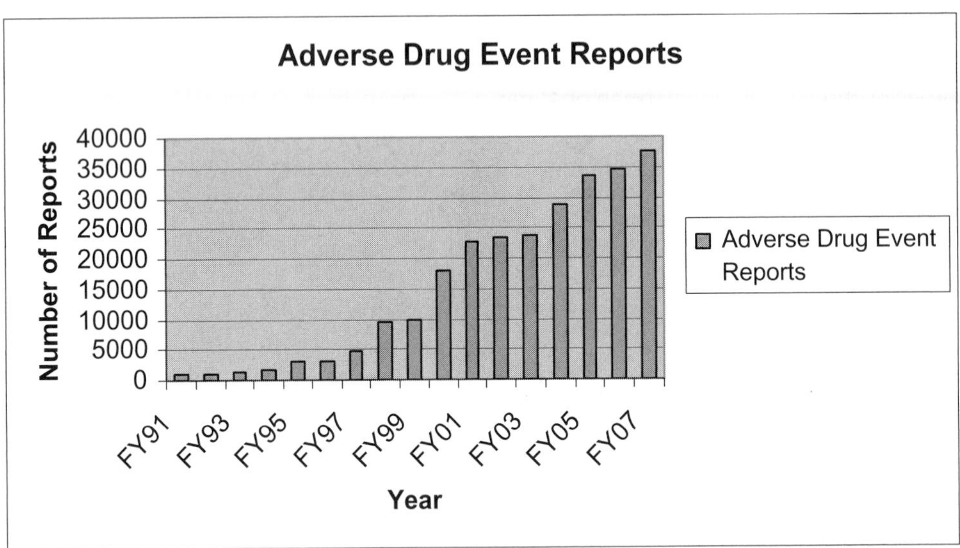

FIG. 58.2 The number of veterinary adverse drug events filed with the U.S. Food and Drug Administration Center for Veterinary Medicine by fiscal year.

The number of veterinary adverse drug events in a foreign country also depends on such factors as the market size of the drug in that country, consumer awareness and tendency to report, and existence of an established reporting program.

The effort to allow such important information to reach the countries in which the same product is marketed (albeit under different names) is being addressed by the Expert Working Group for Pharmacovigilance of the International Cooperation on Harmonization of Technical Requirements for Registration of Veterinary Medicinal Products (VICH). Regulators from global regions and representatives from industry and observer countries are arriving at agreements that will allow some expedited reports of adverse events to be sent to all participating countries.

Standardization of information submitted by VICH regions will help to maximize the quality of the adverse event reports, providing more complete data for analysis.

Paper submissions of adverse events are bulky and labor-intensive to process and store. As international sharing of information progresses, electronic submissions will be increasingly important. An electronic submissions system common to the FDA CVM and the major pharmaceutical companies will minimize the clerical effort of receiving, tracking, entering, and analyzing adverse event information; this is already in the testing phase and should be established within the next year. Web-based forms are being investigated for ease of submission that should make reporting more practical for today's busy professional. The integrated result of the informed client, the attentive clinician, the detailed adverse event report, and vigilant surveillance activity by pharmaceutical firms and regulatory authorities should result in timely, user-friendly web postings of accumulated ADE information as well as rapid identification and correction of emerging safety issues.

REFERENCES

1. American Pet Association. http://www.apapets.org.oetstats2.htm.
2. Bataller N, Keller WC. 1999. Monitoring adverse reactions to veterinary drugs. Pharmacovigilance. Vet Clin N Am Food Anim Pract 15(1):13–30.
3. Brown SD. 2001. Recognizing, reporting and reducing adverse drug reactions. South Med J 94(4):370–373.
4. Fettman MJ, Rollin BE. 2002. Modern elements of informed consent for general veterinary practitioners. J Am Vet Med Assoc Nov15;221(10):1386–93.
5. Flemming DD, Scott JF. 2004. The informed consent doctrine: What veterinarians should tell their clients. J Am Vet Med Assoc May1;224(9):1436–9.
6. Form 1932A. U.S. Government Printing Office. Washington, D.C.
7. Form 1932. U.S. Government Printing Office. Washington, D.C.
8. FDA Summary of Safety and Effectiveness Studies. http://www.fda.gov/cvm/FOI/foiabst2.html.
9. Funmilayo O. 2000. Adverse drug reactions, a review of relevant factors J Clin Pharmacol 40:1093–1101.
10. Hampshire V. 2004 Emerging issues regarding informed consent. J Am Vet Med Assoc Jan15;224(2):177.

11. Hampshire VA, Doddy FM, Post LO, et al. 2004. Adverse drug event reports at the United States Food and Drug Administration Center for Veterinary Medicine. J Am Vet Med Assoc 225(4):533–536.
12. Hampshire, VA. 2005. Evaluation of efficacy of heartworm preventative products at the FDA. Vet Parasitol 133:191–195.
13. Hutchinson TA, Leventhal JM, Kramer MS, et al. 1979. An algorithm for the operational assessment of adverse drug reactions. I. Background, description and instructions for use. J Am Med Assoc 242(7): 623–632.
14. Hutchinson TA, Leventhal JM, Kramer MS, et al. 1979. An algorithm for the operational assessment of adverse drug reactions. II. Demonstration of reproducibility and validity. J Am Med Assoc 242(7): 633–638.
15. Ingwersen W. 2004. Your client credibility: Are your pharmacy practices helping or hindering? Can Vet J Aug;45(8):695–9.
16. Kahler SC. 2003. Is AMDUCA enough? Animal Medicinal Drug Use Clarification Act. J Am Vet Med Assoc Feb15; 222(4):423–4. No abstract available.
17. Keller WC, Bataller N, Oeller DS. 1998. Processing and evaluation of adverse drug experience reports at the Food and Drug Administration Center for Veterinary Medicine. J Am Vet Med Assoc 213(2): 208–211.
18. Kimmel SE, Sekeres MA, Berlin JA, et al. 1998. Adverse events after protamine administration in patients undergoing cardiopulmonary bypass: risks and predictors of under-reviewing. J Clin Epidemiol 51(1):1–10
19. Klaassen, CD. 2001. Casarett & Doull's Toxicology—The Basic Science of Poisons (6th ed). McGraw Hill. 2001.
20, Medwatch: The Clinical Impact of Adverse Drug Event Reporting. PDF article download from http://www.fda.gov/medwatch/articles/medcont/medcont.htm. Accession date 12–29–05.
21. Osborne CA. 2002. Client confidence in veterinarians: how can it be sustained? J Am Vet Med Assoc Oct1;221(7): 936–8.
22. Sgro C, Clinard F, Ouazir K, et al. 2002. Incidence of drug-induced hepatic injuries: A French population-based study. Hepatology 36(2):451–5.
23. Strom BL, Tugwell P. 1990. Pharmacoepidemiology: current status, prospects, and problems. Ann Intern Med 113:179–181.
24. Trontell A. 2004. Expecting the unexpected—drug safety, pharmacovigilance, and the prepared mind. NE J Med 351:1385–1387.
25. United States Code of Federal Regulations, 21, Part 500–599. 2004. Office of the Federal Register, National Archives and Records Administration, U.S. Government Printing Office, Washington, D.C. Vet Rec Sep20;153(12):370–1.
26. United States Code of Federal Regulations, Title 9, Parts 101–123. 2004. 37 Stat. 832–833; as amended December 23, 1985, Pub. L. 99–198, 99 Stat.1654–1655; 21 U.S.C. 151–159, National Archives and Records Administration, U.S. Government Printing Office, Washington, D.C. Web accession site: http://www.aphis.usda.gov/vs/cvb/vsta.htm
27. United States Code of Federal Regulations, Title 7, Parts 150 to 189. 2005. National Archives and Records Administration, U.S. Government Printing Office, Washington, D.C. Web Access: http://www.epa.gov/pesticides/regulating/laws.htm#fifra
28. United States Pet Ownership and Demographics Sourcebook. 2002 Edition. American Veterinary Medical Association. Schaumberg, IL. Accession via AVMA website at http://www.avma.org/membshp/marketstats/sourcebook.asp Contents Accession Date 2–6-06.
29. Weber JCP. 1984. Epidemiology of adverse reactions to nonsteroidal antiinflammatory drugs. In: Rainsford KD, Velo GP, eds. Advances in Inflammation Research. Vol 6. New York: Raven Press, pp. 1–7.
30. World Health Organization. 2002. The importance of pharmacovigilance: safety monitoring of medicinal products. http://www.who.int/medicines/library/qsm/ip_booklet.pdf
31. Wray, JG. 2003. Veterinary surveillance and client consent. Vet Rec Sep20;153(12):370–1.

CHAPTER

59

DOSAGE FORMS AND VETERINARY FEED DIRECTIVES

JIM E. RIVIERE AND GEOF W. SMITH

One of the primary differences between human and veterinary pharmacology is the wide range of dosage forms available to the veterinarian that occurs as a direct consequence of significant differences in the way drugs are administered to animals and humans. These differences are a consequence of obvious dissimilarity in anatomy and physiology, but also are a direct consequence of variations in behavior, husbandry practices, and inability to verbally communicate with animal versus human patients. Additionally, as discussed in Chapter 61, some animals are raised for human food production and thus drug delivery strategies that result in so-called injection-site residues may not be acceptable solely due to possible human consumption of the delivery device or its residues. Different dosage forms are employed for three main reasons: ease of administration and thus compliance, controlled rate of drug delivery, and husbandry constraints in treating populations of animals in a production environment.

The focus of this chapter is to introduce the reader to the wide variety of dosage forms encountered in veterinary medicine. Specifics on most of these formulations can be found in the individual therapeutic chapters or the introductory chapters on pharmacokinetics and ADME.

PHARMACOKINETIC CONSIDERATIONS AND CONTROLLED-DRUG DELIVERY

By far, the dosage form has the greatest influence on the rate and extent of absorption of drugs. The physiology behind these factors was discussed in Chapter 2 and their resulting effects on a drug's plasma concentration-time profile were presented in Chapter 3. The development and impact of these formulations has been extensively reviewed elsewhere (Hardee and Baggot 1998; Baggot 2002; Martinez et al. 2002). When the absorption characteristics of a drug formulation become rate limiting, and flip-flop pharmacokinetics becomes operative, the shape of the drug's concentration-time profile, and thus pharmacologic effect, is in control of the formulation and not the animal's ability to clear the drug. Secondly, innovations in drug delivery allow existing drugs to be more effectively used and provide extension of the commercial life of the product for a manufacturer.

The classic example of the effect of formulation is seen with the plasma concentration-time profiles of potassium, procaine, and benzathine penicillin G (Fig. 59.1). The formulation strategy is to complex the active drug (e.g., penicillin G) with a moiety that delays its release to the

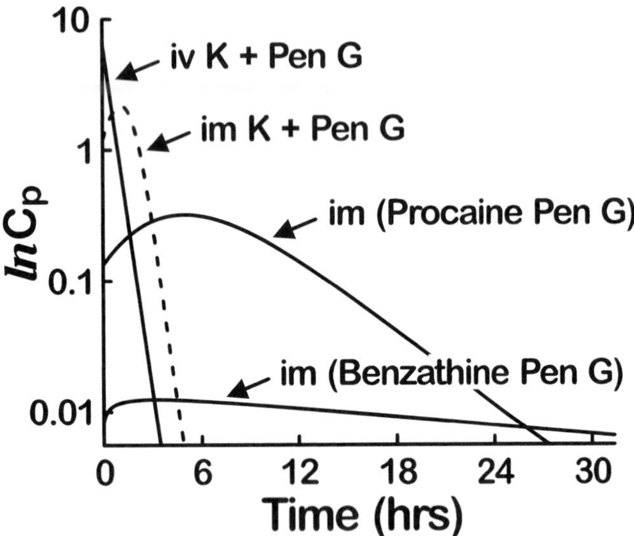

FIG. 59.1 Effects of formulation and route of administration on the plasma concentration versus time profiles of penicillin G.

surrounding capillary beds by modulating the drug's solubility. A pharmaceutics text should be consulted for the chemistry of these processes. The result is that the rate of release of the compound from the dosing formulation becomes slower than that of the drug's elimination, making it rate limiting.

The potential problems with these strategies are twofold. If one considers antimicrobial therapy, for bacteria with very high therapeutic thresholds (e.g., minimum inhibitory concentrations, MICs), the prolonged release formulations may never provide effective therapeutic drug concentrations. Second, such so-called "depot" preparations in food animals may result in persistent drug concentrations in tissues, thereby prolonging the withdrawal time (see Chapter 61). Drug depots at injection sites may persist much longer than effective blood concentrations and may be easily detected at slaughter. One must exhibit care to differentiate drug tissue concentrations at injection sites from those achieved after absorption and systemic distribution (Sanquer et al. 2006).

This scenario also nicely illustrates the reason that knowledge of both the extent and rate of drug absorption are needed to adequately describe the absorption of a drug and underscores why determination of drug bioequivalence (e.g., dosage form interchangeability) requires assessing both metrics related to rate (peak, time to peak) and extent (AUC) of drug absorption. The importance of these factors was also discussed in Chapter 3 under dosage regimen construction.

Approved dosages are very dependent upon the formulation of the drug utilized, a factor that must be considered when using any drug in a veterinary patient. This approach has recently been taken advantage of to develop other once-daily dosing of drugs such as antibiotics in veterinary species, the increased dosing interval being due either to the use of drugs with inherently long half-lives or depot release characteristics. These formulations stress the necessity of knowing the dosage form used when conducting any pharmacokinetic analysis as it may modulate the rate-controlling factor in drug disposition. In many cases, this can be detected only from intravenous pharmacokinetic experiments.

The development of depot preparations has received a great deal of attention by pharmaceutical industries. Some contraceptives in humans achieve monthly dosing intervals through injection in the subcutaneous tissue of insoluble tablets, which results in very slow drug release; the best example is the use of levonorgestrel implanted capsules (Norplant®). Similar strategies have been employed in veterinary medicine for the administration of growth promotants. These include estradiol formulated in rubber implants (Compudose®), progesterone and estradiol pellets (Implant-C®), and zeranol (Ralgro®). Newer approaches include use of biodegradable gels that may be injected as a liquid through a syringe; these gels form a slowly degrading solid once in the tissue. Temperature-sensitive thermogels can also be used to control release of drug once in the body at physiological temperatures. A great deal of new technology is being developed for such formulations that promises more sophisticated dosage forms in the future.

Oral drug dosage forms achieve control of release through modulation of the surface area of dissolving drug particles, through the size of particles that alter their gastrointestinal transit time, or through the use of multiple layers in the formulation that control the rate and extent of drug release and dissolution. The simplest example is to coat a drug to prevent its dissolution in the acid environment of the stomach. These formulations are specifically designed for specific species, due to differences in gastrointestinal content and motility, as well as issues that include palatability. Capsules can be designed that initially release a bolus of readily soluble drug that functions as a loading dose into the animal. This is then followed by slower release of drug that maintains effective levels. For some compounds, only local delivery is needed to the gastrointestinal tract (e.g., certain antiparasitics), and the formulation can be designed for such activity. Work has occurred in humans to specifically deliver drug to the colon for localized effect. Again, it must be stressed that many of these controlled-release dosage formulations are specifically designed for species-specific anatomical (size of pyloris), biochemical (cellulose based for nonruminants), and/or physiological (pH, transit time) factors that prevent easy use in other species.

A truly unique aspect of dosage form not seen in human medicine are those employed in ruminants that take advantage of the observation that heavy materials sink in the rumen and are not passed further along the digestive tract. This has resulted in the design of mechanical dosage devices that infuse drug into the rumen for specific durations. Some materials are formulated to be flocculent and float in gastrointestinal contents allowing controlled passage though the stomach. Finally, slow-release osmotic pumps may be implanted in animals to achieve controlled drug infusions.

A major variable concerning parenteral injections relates to the physiology of the injection site. For a drug to be adequately absorbed from a depot preparation, there must be access to the perfusing capillaries and an adequate rate of tissue perfusion. A major source of variability is the muscle into which intramuscular injections are made. Studies have elegantly demonstrated in horses that if the injection is made between the fascial tissue bundles of a muscle group, less systemic absorption will occur than if the injection is in the muscle mass. Similarly, if the muscle group, or more likely, the SC injection site, has poor blood perfusion, less absorption may occur. If the injection results in a local tissue reaction, subsequent inflammation and fibrosis may "wall off" the drug formulation preventing absorption. Changes in ambient temperature, with compensatory changes in skin blood perfusion, may modulate absorption rate. There are numerous variables in these processes, and it is often only through the use of careful pharmacokinetic analyses that their influence on drug absorption cause can be ascertained.

Topical dosage forms include gels and patches that control diffusion from the dosage form to be rate limiting for dermal absorption. These products have been discussed in Chapter 2 and are fully reviewed elsewhere (Riviere and Papich 2001). The advantage of dermal over oral or parenteral controlled-released approaches is that the topical gel or patch can be removed should cessation of dosing be required. Transdermal fentanyl patches for analgesia in dogs has been a particularly successful story for using human patches. However, these cannot be easily transferred between species as the rate-limiting barrier may be species- and site-specific. As of this time, specific patches for animals have not been marketed.

In contrast, there are numerous topical spot-on, pour-on, collars, dip, and shampoo formulations for topical pesticides, often focusing on flea control. Some of these have resulted in once-monthly dose administration and increased owner compliance. These preparations are fully covered in Chapters 44 and 48 of the present text. In addition to these unique pour-on applications, large-animal veterinary medicine also employs ear-tags and dust-bags that allow topical drug delivery in cattle and swine in a rate- and dose-controlled fashion.

PALATABILITY AND EASE OF DRUG ADMINISTRATION

Another factor relatively unique to veterinary medicine relates to the ease of drug administration to animals that might present danger to the individual administering the drug. This has resulted in formulating drugs in dosage vehicles that are palatable and will be easily eaten by the animal, but made of ingredients that do not alter drug absorption properties. A great deal of information is available from the pet food and vitamin industry that provides quantitative approaches to assess factors such as taste preferences and palatability (Ahmed et al. 2002; Thombre 2004). This has resulted in the development of chewable drug formulations as well as flavor ingredients that mask bitter taste or odors that animals refuse to eat. In contrast to human medicine, where sight and verbal cues may allow administering distasteful drugs to adults, animals rely on senses of taste and smell to determine whether a drug-containing formulation will be consumed. Other approaches to oral drug administration under consideration include use of dissolvable films and oral sprays for targeting the buccal cavity of patients. These are particularly being developed for cats where owners often have difficulty in administering other oral drug formulations.

A final approach that is relatively unique to veterinary medicine includes the direct administration of drug into drinking water, into lick-tanks, or on feed for use in large production settings (e.g., cattle, swine, poultry). An important distinction with this continuous form of drug administration is that, unlike the bolus effect seen with individual liquid dosing or rapidly dissolving tablets, absorption may not be first-order. If administration is constant in water or feed, absorption may be zero-order and have pharmacokinetic behavior resembling an infusion. Finally, drugs may be administered in medicated blocks, which results in ease of administration but little control of individual animal dosage.

VETERINARY FEED ADDITIVES

One strategy for administering drugs to animals that is unique to veterinary medicine is oral dosing via feed. This is often necessary due to the need to treat a large number of animals in a production environment. Unlike individual animal dosing, this approach does not assure that a specific dose of drug reaches each animal, since drug dosage is now a function of food consumption. As mentioned above, issues of palatability and odor also must be taken into consideration.

The legal control of feed additives is also different than other drug formulations. The Veterinary Feed Directive (VFD) refers to a relatively new category of medicated feeds created by the Animal Drug Availability Act of 1996. Prior to this time, the Food and Drug Administration (FDA) had only two options for regulating the distribution of animal drugs: over-the-counter or prescription. The primary purpose of the VFD was to provide an alternative to these categories for certain therapeutic drugs that are mixed in feed. A VFD drug still ensures the participation of a veterinarian, but it allows producers to acquire medicated feeds through traditional manufacturers without involving a pharmacist or having to follow state pharmacy laws.

In 1996 the Center for Veterinary Medicine (CVM) of the FDA expressed a greater need for control over the use of certain antimicrobial agents in medicated feeds. Initially it was suggested to mandate all new therapeutic agents approved for use in feed be for use by prescription only. However, having additive drugs approved as prescription-only was unacceptable to the animal agriculture and feed industry. Requiring these drugs to be for use by prescription only would have turned feed mills into drug stores because they would be forced to mix a new batch of feed each time a prescription was written. Studies done by the American Feed Industry Association (AFIA) in the 1990s estimated the average feed costs in the swine industry would have risen from \$36 to \$100 per ton because of additional costs associated with special ordering and the need to mix only small volumes of feed at once. These prescription drugs would also fall under the direction of most state pharmacy regulations, which would further complicate the ability to manufacture and distribute medicated feed.

The VFD was therefore created to be an alternative to the traditional prescription classification. It places a much greater emphasis on professional control as compared to over-the-counter medications while still allowing agricultural producers to obtain medicated feeds efficiently and cost effectively. This classification applies only to drugs that are newly approved as VFD medicated feeds. As of 2006, the two drugs that have been approved in this category are tilmicosin (Pulmotil®), which is approved for control of swine respiratory disease associated with *Actinobacillus pleuropneumoniae*, and *Pasteurella multocida* and florfenicol (Aquaflor®), which is indicated for the control of mortality in catfish due to enteric septicemia associated with *Edwardsiella ictaluri*. As with other medicated feeds, the extralabel use of any VFD drugs is prohibited.

The initial requirement of using a VFD medicated feed is a valid veterinarian-client-patient relationship. As defined by the American Veterinary Medical Association (AVMA), this relationship exists when

1. The veterinarian has the responsibility for making medical judgment regarding the health of the animal(s) and the need for medical treatment, and the client has agreed to follow the instructions of the veterinarian.
2. There is sufficient knowledge of the animal(s) by the veterinarian to initiate at least a general or preliminary diagnosis of the medical condition of the animal(s). This means the veterinarian has recently seen and is personally acquainted with the keeping and care of all the animal(s), and/or by medically appropriate and timely visits to the premises where the animals are kept.
3. The practicing veterinarian is readily available, or has arranged for emergency coverage, for follow-up in case of adverse reactions or failure of the therapeutic regimen to solve the problem.

Once a veterinarian has made an initial diagnosis, he/she can issue a signed VFD on a preprinted, multipart form. The veterinarian gives the form to the producer, who then orders the medicated feed from the feed supplier. A VFD feed may not be distributed to a producer without a signed VFD form. Three groups are involved:

1. The person or firm supplying a VFD drug to a producer must receive and retain a copy of the signed VFD form issued by the veterinarian.
2. Licensed feed manufacturers and distributors who ship VFD feed to a downstream distributor or retailer for inventory must receive and retain a copy of written acknowledgement stating that the VFD feed will be further distributed only in accordance with FDA requirements.
3. All distributors and retailers who do not hold a feed mill license must notify the FDA within 30 days of their initial VFD feed shipment.

The form for Veterinary Feed Directive products should be provided to the veterinarian by the manufacturer of the specific therapeutic agent (Fig. 59.2). This form must be completed by the veterinarian and should normally include the following information:

1. The name, address, and telephone number of the producer
2. The species, location, number of, and description of animals being treated
3. The date(s) of treatment (if different from the date on the VFD form)
4. The name of the drug to be used, the concentration of the drug to be included in the feed, and the amount of feed to be manufactured
5. The directions for mixing and feeding (including dilution) and duration of treatment, including appropriate withdrawal times. The expiration date of the feed

ELANCO Pulmotil

PULMOTIL® (tilmicosin) Veterinary Feed Directive

EP140751

Client: See More Swine
Address: 123 Pig Lane
Sample City, NC 20060

Phone #: 919-539-8177

Fax #:

Veterinarian: Jim Smith
Address: Hog and Dog Veterinary Services
2625 N Loop Drive
Sample City, NC 20060

Phone #: 919-123-4567

Fax #: 919-123-4678

Swine to be treated (number and location):
Count: 2500 Group Name: Barn 2

Mix into Type C Medicated Feed to provide: 181 g/ton [ ] 272 g/ton [x] 363 g/ton [ ]

Warning: Feeds containing tilmicosin must be withdrawn 7 days prior to slaughter.

Feeding Directions: Feed continuously as the sole ration for 21 days beginning approximately 7 days before an expected outbreak of swine respiratory disease.

Special Instructions:
Feed for 21 days/18 tons of feed

Expiration Date: 11/22/2006
Month/Day/Year (Not to exceed 90 days)

Amount of final (Type C) feed: 18.0 tons

Veterinarian's Signature: Sample DVM

Date: 8/22/2006

License Number and State: 00000 North Carolina

FIG. 59.2 Sample Veterinary Feed Directive form for tilmicosin (reprinted with permission from Elanco Animal Health).

7. The veterinarian's name, address, license number, state of licensing, and signature

The form is the most significant component of using VFD approved medications. A VFD order cannot be issued by telephone. If the form cannot be hand-delivered, it can be faxed or sent via an email attachment; however, the original form must be received by the distributor within 5 working days. VFD forms have to be retained for a minimum of 2 years by all three parties involved (the veterinarian, the producer, and the feed mill) and should be available for review by the FDA.

Only vendors with a valid feed mill license are authorized to store VFD products, which means that a producer is not allowed to keep a surplus of medicated feed on the farm. However licensed veterinarians are allowed to act as distributors of VFD feeds by notifying the FDA once, in writing, 30 days before the first anticipated distribution of medicated feed.

SITE-DIRECTED THERAPY

The final consideration related to veterinary dosage forms are those drugs specifically designed for local effects. These include intramammary and intrauterine formulations, and ophthalmic and otic drugs. Examples of these are discussed under the individual drug sections and special therapy chapters of this text.

REFERENCES

Ahmed, I., and K. Kasrarian. 2002. Pharmaceutical challenges in veterinary product development. Adv Drug Deliv Rev 54:871–882.

Baggot, J.D. 2002. Veterinary Dosage Forms. Encyclopedia of Pharmaceutical Technology. New York: Marcel Dekker.

Hardee, G.E., and J.D. Baggot, eds. 1998. Development and Formulation of Veterinary Dosage Forms, 2nd Ed., New York: Marcel Dekker.

Martinez, M., G. Amidon, L. Clark, W.W. Jones, A. Mitra, and J.E. Riviere. 2002. Applying the biopharmaceutics classification system to veterinary pharmaceutical products. Part II. Physiological considerations. Adv Drug Deliv Rev 54:825–850.

Riviere, J.E. and M. Papich. 2001. Potential and problems of developing transdermal patches for veterinary applications. Adv Drug Deliv Rev 50:175–203.

Sanquer, A., G. Wackoweiz, and B. Havrileck. 2006. Critical review on the withdrawal period calculation for injection site residues. J Vet Pharmacol Therap 29:355–364.

Thombre, A.G. 2004. Oral delivery of medications to companion animals: palatability considerations. Adv Drug Deliv Rev 56:1399–1413.

CHAPTER

60

USP'S ROLE IN VETERINARY PHARMACOLOGY AND EVIDENCE-BASED INFORMATION

CORY LANGSTON, STEFAN SCHUBER, AND IAN F. DEVEAU

The *United States Pharmacopeia (USP)* is a nonprofit organization that few veterinary practitioners are familiar with; yet it plays important roles in maintaining drug quality and promoting the proper use of medications. There are two sections to this chapter, the first, "*USP* and Its Compendia," explains the history of the organization, its continuing mission, and its publications. The second section, "*USP* Evidence-Based Pharmacotherapy," details the evidence-based approaches used by *USP* in creating its veterinary drug information monographs and how these are increasingly finding utility by veterinarians, particularly relative to extralabel drug use.

USP AND ITS COMPENDIA

As stated in the preface to the first *USP* of 1820, *USP*'s mission was and continues to be

> . . . to select from among substances which possess medicinal power, those, the utility of which is most fully established and best understood and to form from them preparations and compositions, in which their powers may be exerted to the greatest advantage. It should likewise distinguish those articles by convenient and definite names, such as may prevent trouble or uncertainty in the intercourse of physicians and apothecaries.[1]

There are many important words in this brief text, but the first two (*to select*) are among the most important. *USP* was not intended to be simply a listing of all available drugs but rather a selection of the *best* drugs, which came to be termed *official drugs*. The first *USP* of 1820 also provided a list of the *Materia Medica* of the time (". . . simple medicines, together with some prepared medicines, which are kept in the shop of the apothecary, but not necessarily prepared by him") and a third list of secondary drugs—"the claims of which [were] of a more uncertain kind." These three categories duplicate remarkably the items now available in a modern pharmacy: 1) the best drugs (now mostly manufactured and FDA-approved, including safe and effective OTC products usually marketed subject to FDA and *USP* monographs), 2) a secondary list (some dietary supplements), and 3) routine items of health care not requiring preparation on the part of the pharmacist. The first *USP* in principle was thus based on the idea of a national formulary composed of the best drugs, drawing them out of a sea of nostrums of uncertain safety, efficacy, and quality.

After *USP*'s first convention in 1820, the selection of the best or official drugs for subsequent editions of *USP* was directed by the Committee on Scope (now the Council of Experts). Historically, physicians held a majority on the Committee of Revision, and pharmacists constituted a minority. This dichotomy at times sparked debate between physicians and pharmacists about appropriate admissions of the best drugs to *USP*. For example, during the 19th century, physicians but not pharmacists resisted the inclusion of hydroalcoholic patent medicines of dubious provenance and value that entered commerce around the Civil War. As a general approach, the Committee of Revision tended to select single-entity therapeutics for inclusion in *USP*, advancing the science of therapeutics from use of crude mixtures to pure moieties.[2] In a development that in many ways parallels that of *USP*, pharmacists increasingly relied on the American Pharmaceutical Association's *National Formulary* (*NF*), first published in 1888. The early *NF* attempted to provide standardized recipes for compounded preparations—in fact, the full title of the first *NF* was *The National Formulary of Unofficinal Preparations,* the word *unofficinal* alluding to the acts of compounding and dispensing of prescriptions from ingredients (many of which were included in *USP*) and standard preparations made and kept by pharmacists.[3]

In 1985, *USP* ended the Committee on Scope (as it came to be known) with the preparation of *USP XXI,* which became official in 1985.[4] This occurred for good reason: *USP* no longer selected the best drugs for the U.S. marketplace. During the 20th century, FDA had taken on the task of approving all new drugs in the U.S. based on a determination of both safety and efficacy relative to benefit. These then were the best drugs. *USP*'s role became one of providing public quality monographs for these drugs, which also includes monographs for a small number of pre-1938 "grandfathered" drugs (i.e., certain drugs that were marketed before the passage of the 1938 Federal Food, Drug, and Cosmetic Act; see below). As a result of the long and illustrious scientific history of work by dedicated compendial scientists, government regulators and policymakers, pharmaceutical manufacturers, compounding professionals, and many others, a robust set of good-quality drugs now is available to practitioners and patients in the U.S.

***USP* AND FDA.** Spurred by stories of U.S. soldiers dying because of substandard drugs during the Mexican War (1846–1848), the U.S. government recognized *USP* and some European pharmacopeias in the 1848 Drug Import Act,[5] which sought to control the quality of drugs moving in commerce at the time. *USP* was officially incorporated as a nonprofit organization in Washington, D.C., in 1900. Six years later the Federal Food and Drugs Act of 1906, signed by President Theodore Roosevelt, declared that drugs were adulterated if they differed "from the standard of strength, quality, or purity, as determined by the test set down in the *United States Pharmacopeia* or *National Formulary* . . .".[6] In 1938, 105 people died of diethylene glycol poisoning after consuming Massengill's Elixir Sulfanilamide.[7] In response, that same year Congress passed the Federal Food, Drug, and Cosmetic (FD&C) Act, which preserved and strengthened the recognition of *USP* in federal law, prevented the Secretary of Agriculture (now the Secretary of Health and Human Services) from unilaterally amending *USP* tests or methods of assay, and recognized *USP* packaging and labeling requirements as federal requirements.[8]

In 1974 *USP* acquired *NF* and since 1975 has published the two compendia as one volume, *USP–NF.* Publication now occurs annually with two *Supplements,* reflective of continuing advances in new therapies and in the science of metrology. From provisions in the 1938 FD&C Act, *USP* and *NF* are designated official compendia of the U.S. and are recognized as well in other national and international laws for enforcement and other purposes.[9] *USP*'s volunteer bodies consist of convention delegates who meet at 5-year intervals, an 11-member Board of Trustees, and the Council of Experts, the standards-setting arm of the organization. In its 2000–2005 cycle, the Council of Experts was composed of the chairs of 31 Expert Committees that created standards for *USP–NF.* An additional 28 Expert Committees created value-added content for the *USP–Drug Information* (*USP–DI*) series[10] and an additional three (Safe Medication Use, Information Development and Dissemination, and Therapeutic Decision-Making) focused on special topics. The chairs of the Council are responsible for electing membership of each Expert Committee, which numbers usually between 5 and 20 members. All are assisted by a staff of approximately 400 in *USP*'s Rockville, MD, offices.

USP reengaged in the provision of drug information in 1970 with publication of the *USP–DI* series (*Volume I: Drug Information for the Health Care Professional, USP–DI Volume II: Advice for the Patient,* and *Volume III: Approved Drug Products and Legal Requirements*), which provided value-added information (off-label uses, safety, dosing, and other information) to supplement FDA-approved labeling. In 1998, *USP* sold rights to *Volumes I* and *II* to Thomson Publishing Company, retaining editorial control for value-added content. However, the agreement between *USP* and Thomson was that Thomson would abandon the publication of veterinary drug information monographs, allowing *USP* to seek other venues for publication.

USP EVIDENCE-BASED PHARMACOTHERAPY

INTRODUCTION. Veterinarians traditionally obtain their knowledge from subject-matter experts via lectures, textbook chapters, journal articles, web resources, or personal consultations. Although this approach will always have a place in teaching medicine, obtaining knowledge from a single expert has potential drawbacks: experts may have their own biases, unevaluated dogmas may be perpetuated, and opinions may differ among experts. Most importantly, when relying solely on expert opinion clinicians have no basis on which to make their own determinations about the best approach for their particular patients.

In the 1990s a paradigm shift began in human medicine that concentrated less on authority-based expertise and instead emphasized the critical review of the scientific literature. This approach became known as evidence-based medicine (EBM). EBM has been defined as the "conscientious, explicit, and judicious use of current best evidence in making decisions about the care of individual patients. This means integrating individual clinical expertise with the best available external clinical evidence from systematic research."[11] To those unfamiliar with EBM, it might seem that this approach offers nothing new. Although it is true that the literature has been used to guide medical decisions for as long as we can remember, EBM formalizes that process and filters the literature so that clinicians are aware of the evidence that influences their decisions and the strength of that evidence. It should be pointed out that EBM does not ignore expert opinion altogether; it does, however, relegate its importance to a much lower level of influence than other recognized resources.

Because an exhaustive analysis of the literature can be quite time consuming, physicians rely on what are commonly known as "systematic reviews" instead of performing their own EBM synopses. "Systematic reviews comprehensively examine the literature, seeking to identify and synthesize all relevant information to formulate the best approach to diagnosis or treatment."[12] An example of a systematic review conducted in human medicine might include a topic such as "What is the role of estrogen exposure and the risk of breast cancer?"[13]

EBM is well entrenched in human medicine and many resources exist for the physician. Databases devoted exclusively to systematic reviews in human medicine include the *Cochrane Collaboration* and the *British Medical Journal's Clinical Evidence Compendium.* The extent to which this approach has been adopted is further demonstrated in that a search of the *PubMed* online database for articles containing the words "Systematic review" in their title produced 4,178 articles. This abundance of literature is not, however, the case with evidence-based veterinary medicine (EBVM). A similar *PubMed* search restricted to contain the word *veterinary* in the title, abstract, or key words produced only 6 journal articles.

An exception to this paucity of EBVM is the veterinary drug information monographs published by the *United States Pharmacopeia (USP).* The method whereby these monographs are produced is unique in veterinary medicine because it incorporates evidence-based approaches, but interpretation of that evidence takes place via consensus of the members of the Veterinary Medicine Information Expert Committee with an opportunity for public review and comments before the information is authorized by the *USP.* Over the years since its inception, this committee has been composed of 8 to 15 veterinary pharmacologists, clinical pharmacologists, pharmacists, and species experts. The *USP* veterinary drug information monographs are at present freely available to the public at the *USP* website www.usp.org/audiences/veterinary/monographs/registration.html (complimentary registration required).

A hard-copy publication, the Veterinary Pharmacopeia, is under development by *USP* and will contain the information monographs along with additional pharmaceutical information of veterinary importance.

THE VETERINARY PHARMACEUTICAL INFORMATION MONOGRAPH CREATION PROCESS. The process of monograph creation begins with a *USP* staff veterinarian obtaining information available on the drugs for review, including U.S. and Canadian label information, FDA Freedom of Information documents, foreign drug labels, and journal articles. Careful attention is paid to species-specific information. This information is then arranged into a specified format containing commonly used brand names, category of drug, indications, regulatory considerations, chemistry, pharmacology/pharmacokinetics (i.e., mechanism of action/effect, absorption, distribution, protein binding, biotransformation, elimination), precautions to consider, side/adverse effects, overdose treatment, client consultation, and veterinary dosing information.

Many sections, such as chemistry and regulatory considerations, are noncontentious and are merely formatted to fit the monograph layout. Any pharmacokinetic information gathered is added, regardless of species. Dosage recommendations, label and extralabel, are based on Expert Committee consensus. When an extralabel dosage recommendation is made for a food animal, the Food Animal Residue Avoidance Database provides an associated recommended withdrawal time. The indications section, however, requires the greatest effort and is the section to which the EBVM approach is most obviously applied.

For all extralabel indications and for any label indication that is viewed as contentious by an Expert Committee member, evidence tables are generated relative to that indication. Each table contains the citation information, the type of study (e.g., case report[s], clinical trial, disease model, in vitro study, meta-analysis, pharmacokinetic study without surrogate endpoints, pharmacokinetic study with surrogate endpoints), whether treatments were randomized, type of control used (e.g., positive, negative, uncontrolled), and the type of masking used (e.g., single-masked, double-masked, nonmasked). A synopsis of the methods used, doses and duration of therapy studied, results, author conclusions, and limitations noted by *USP* staff are included. This is repeated for each item of litera-

Title: Efficacy of Doxycycline, Azithromycin, or Trovafloxacin for Treatment of Experimental Rocky Mountain Spotted Fever in Dogs

Breitschwerdt, EB, Papich, MG, Hegarty, BC, Gilger, B, Hancock, SI and Davidson, MG. Efficacy of Doxycycline, Azithromycin, or Trovafloxacin for Treatment of Experimental Rocky Mountain Spotted Fever in Dogs. *Antimicrobial Agents and Chemotherapy*, Vol, 43, no 4, April 1999. (813–821).

Author Year (Ref.) Sponsor(s)	**Design Methods Goal**	**Dose Duration N**	**Results Conclusions**	**Limitations of Study/DID Staff Comment**
Breit-schwerdt, EB Papich, MG Hegarty, BC Gilger, B Hancock, SI Davidson, MG 1999	**Design:** -in vivo study -R, C **Methods:** -Vero cell culture-grown *R rickettsii* were inoculated into egg yolk sacs to produce an infective inocubim. A Guinea pig model was used to optimize the inoculum given to the test dogs -Sixteen 4- to 5-month-old female laboratory-raised beagles were randomly divided into	**Dose:** -Group 1 served as untreated controls -Groups 2 through 4 received doxycycline hyclate (5 mg/kg of body weight given orally, at 12-h intervals), azithromycin (3 mg/kg orally, once daily), or trovafloxacin (5 mg/kg orally, at 12-h intervals), respectively. **Duration:** -began on PID 5 and continued for 7 days for doxycycline and trovafloxacin, and for 3	**Results:** -All dogs were febrile and positive for circulting rickettsiae in blood as detected by tissue culture and/or PCR by PID 5, at which time treatments were begun for the three treatment groups. Compared to the infection control group, treatment groups experienced a statistically significant improvement in attitudinal scores (P = 0.0003) by 48 h after the initiation of treatments. Following the initiation of antimicrobial therapy, rectal temperatures nonmalized after 12 h in	Short duration of azithromycin treatment may have decreased the efficacy of the drug.

FIG. 60.1 Example evidence table.

ture relevant to the proposed indication for that drug. A portion of an example evidence table is given in Figure 60.1.

The available information about the indications, all of which are species-specific, is placed into one of three categories. "Accepted" indications are those that have substantial data supporting them and are in common use. The majority of these indications are labeled indications, but extralabel indications also are included if they rise to the required level of evidence. The next indications category is "Potentially effective" (analogous to "Acceptance not established" in earlier published monographs). These are indications with moderate evidence to support a particular use. Last, an indication may be deemed "Unaccepted," meaning the drug should not be used for a given purpose. This latter categorization is most often applied to older drugs that have been rendered obsolete by newer treatments. In addition, beginning in 2005 all new monographs and periodic revisions of older monographs include evidence ratings for each indication. Each rating is composed of one overall Evidence Quality indicator and one or more Evidence Type indicators (see Table 60.1 and Figure 60.2). The monograph identifies into which of the three categories an indication falls, combined with the drug product's evidence ratings, thereby providing an evidentiary basis to support an indicated use.

The initial draft, evidence tables, references, and specific questions or problems obvious to the staff are sent to Expert Committee members, ad hoc reviewers with selected expertise, and manufacturers of the drug under review.

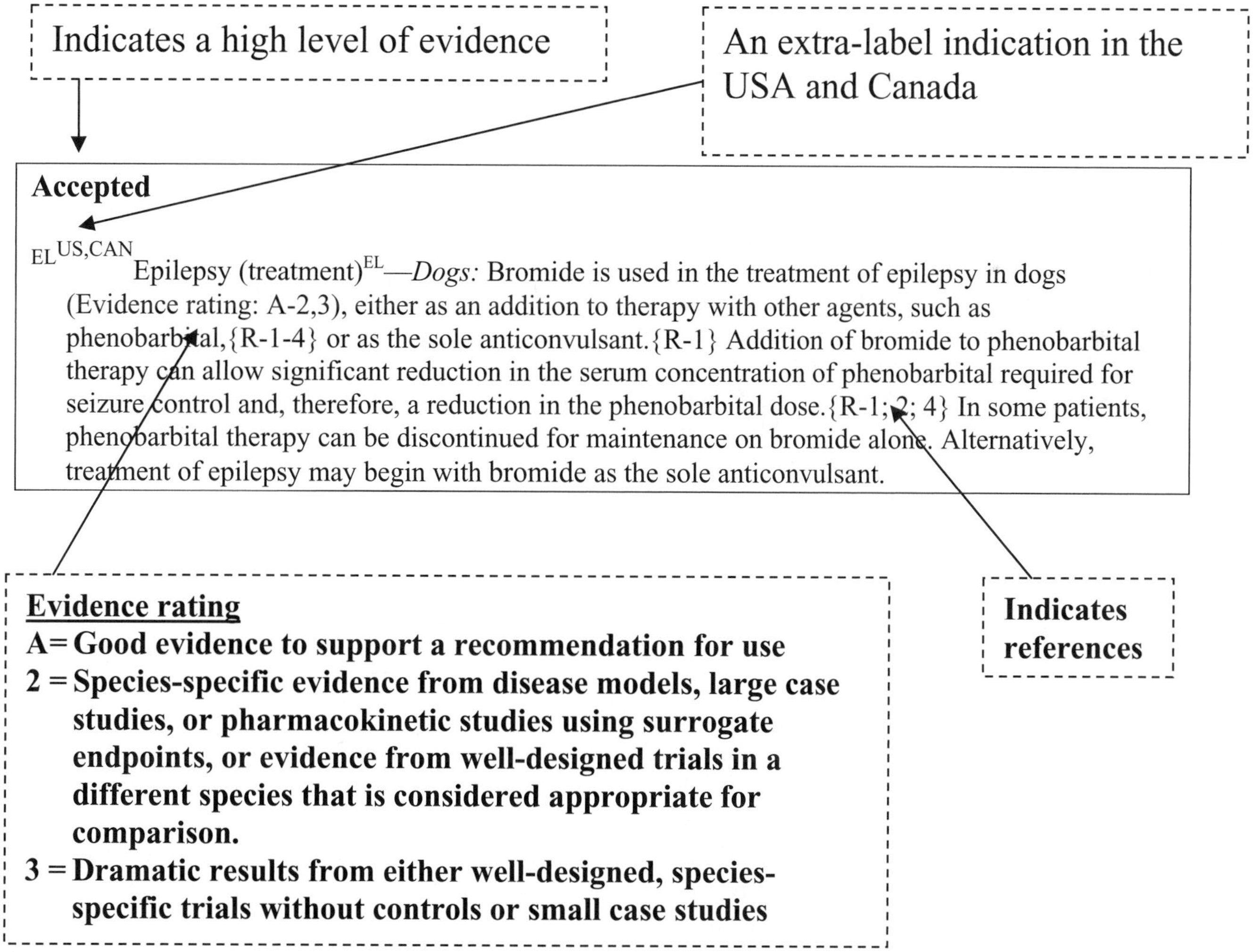

FIG. 60.2 How to read a USP indication (the same nomenclature applies to dosage sections).

TABLE 60.1 Evidence ratings

Evidence Quality

A. Good evidence to support a recommendation for use
B. Moderate evidence to support a recommendation for use
C. Insufficient evidence to support a recommendation for use
D. Moderate evidence to support a recommendation against use
E. Good evidence to support a recommendation against use

Evidence Type

1. Species-specific evidence from at least one large randomized and controlled trial (RCT) or multiple small RCTs
2. Species-specific evidence from a small RCT, disease models, large case studies, or pharmacokinetic studies using surrogate endpoints or evidence from well-designed trials in a different species that is considered appropriate for comparison.
3. Dramatic results from either well-designed, species-specific trials without controls or small case studies.
4. Pharmacokinetic studies without surrogate endpoints
5. In vitro studies
6. Opinions of respected authorities on the basis of clinical experience or reports of expert committees.

Comments and concerns are then addressed in revised monographs and ballots. Monograph revision and Expert Committee review continue as many times as needed by means of an iterative process until a consensus is reached. Before the monograph is finalized it is listed for public review on *USP*'s website, during which time copies of draft text are made available on request to all interested parties for review and comment. Following public review the monograph is finalized, becomes a part of *USP*'s authorized text, and is published (Fig. 60.3). Monographs undergo periodic updates at 2- to 4-year intervals or more often, if needed. At present, *USP* monographs are the only drug information source in veterinary medicine undergoing such extensive evidence-based evaluation coupled with expert panel review, a process by which the scientific credibility of the information is maintained.

- The incorporation of extra-label and label indications and dosages for all domestic species.
- The inclusion of slaughter and milk withdrawals when extra-label drug use in food animals is considered an acceptable option for therapy. (Withdrawal times provided by FARAD for the specified conditions noted.)
- The inclusion of information for U.S. and Canadian veterinary drugs.
- The grouping of indications into three categories. The "Accepted" category indicates that clear evidence exists to support use of the drug for a particular purpose. "Potentially effective" (formerly "Acceptance not established") indicates that use of the drug for an indication may be worthy of consideration if superior therapies do not exist, but the evidence is either scant or subject to concern based on experimental design. If a use is viewed as ineffective or has been replaced by clearly superior therapies, the indication is deemed "Unaccepted." These categorizations are applied to label and extra-label uses.
- The inclusion of evidence levels (flags) in newer and revised monographs for each indication.
- The use of evidence tables to address controversial issues, particularly relative to extra-label drug use.
- The U.S. Food and Drug Administration and product manufacturers are included in the review cycle. (Although comments made by FDA are considered, those opinions are nonbinding on USP. The information contained in these monographs should not be considered an endorsement or "acceptance" by FDA regarding a given use or dosage.)
- The review of each monograph by the USP Veterinary Medicine Drug Information Expert Committee. This committee consists of 10 to 15 volunteers recognized as experts in pharmacology, internal medicine, or species discipline.

FIG. 60.3 Unique features of a USP Drug Information Monograph.

DRAWBACKS TO THE *USP* MONOGRAPH CREATION PROCESS. The same process that creates the *USP* information monographs, which may be the best compilation of drug information in veterinary medicine, also creates its drawbacks. Because *USP* information monographs seek to be the most comprehensive single source of veterinary information about a drug, the vast amount of information can be overwhelming to new users. Because of this information overload, users experience a learning curve while they gain experience in knowing how to quickly find the information needed.

When the *USP* Veterinary Medicine Expert Committee was first formed, its members made an attempt to create the monographs. Unfortunately, the use of volunteer experts produced a limited number of monographs that displayed variable quality. The addition of a full-time *USP* staff veterinarian to create the draft monographs resulted in a dramatic improvement in both quality and quantity of monographs produced. Because of the amount of information that must be amassed and filtered, evidence tables created, and the multiple reviews involved, a tremendous amount of time is required to produce a monograph. This effort coupled with the time required to revise older monographs every 2 to 4 years limits the number of new monographs that can be produced in a year.

Perhaps the most serious drawback to the *USP* approach to monograph creation is the cost involved. Though the committee members volunteer their services, the overhead for *USP* staff salaries, meetings, and publications can be quite large. Hard-copy publication costs are why evidence tables are for internal use rather than being released with the monograph. Nevertheless, work continues to address new families of pharmaceuticals while updating existing monographs.

For those who are familiar with the monographs created by *USP* there is little doubt that they represent the most complete source of veterinary pharmaceutical information and the only evidence-based resource. The degree to which the veterinary profession will embrace and volunteer to support and enhance these efforts will determine the future of the program.

REFERENCES

1. USP. The Pharmacopoeia of the United States of America. Boston: Charles Ewer; 1820, p. 3.
2. Kremers E, Urdang G. History of pharmacy. Sonnedecker GA, ed., 4th ed. Philadelphia: J.B. Lippincott Company; 1976.
3. Sonnedecker G. The changing character of the National Formulary (1890–1970). In One Hundred Years of the National Formulary: A Symposium. Higby GJ, ed. Madison, WI: American Institute of the History of Pharmacy; 1989.
4. Anderson L, Higby GJ. The spirit of voluntarism: a legacy of commitment and contribution—the United States Pharmacopeia 1820–1995. Rockville, MD: The United States Pharmacopeial Convention; 1995;432.
5. 9 Stat. 237 (1848).
6. 34 Stat. 768 (1906).
7. Wax, PM. Elixirs, diluents, and the passage of the 1938 Federal Food, Drug, and Cosmetic Act. Ann Intern Med 1995;122(6):456–461.
8. 52 Stat. 1040 (1938), codified at 21 USC 301 et seq.
9. Council of Experts Executive Committee, Ad Hoc Council of Experts Committee, and USP Staff. Development of a new official compendium, separate from *USP–NF*, for articles not legally marketed in the US. Pharm Forum 2004;30(5):1877–1883.
10. USP–DI Volume I: Drug information for the health care professional. USP–DI Volume II: advice for the patient. USP–DI: Volume III: approved drug products and legal requirements. Greenwood Village, CO: Thomson Publishing–Micromedex.
11. Sackett DL, Rosenberg WMC, Gray JAM., Haynes RB, Richardson WC. Evidence based medicine: what it is and what it isn't. Brit Med J 1996;312:71–72.
12. Siwek J, Gourlay ML, Slawson DC, Shaughnessy AF. How to write an evidence-based clinical review article. Am Fam Phys 2002;Jan 15;65(2):251–8.
13. Yager JD, Davidson NE. Estrogen carcinogenesis in breast cancer. NE J Med 2006;354:270–282.

CHAPTER

61

CHEMICAL RESIDUES IN TISSUES OF FOOD ANIMALS

JIM E. RIVIERE AND STEPHEN F. SUNDLOF

Most of this textbook has focused on describing the pharmacodynamics and pharmacokinetics of drugs in animals. In both human medical and companion-animal veterinary practice, the primary concern in drug selection and use is the therapeutic end point, whether or not the drug is efficacious against the disease being treated. Doses are usually administered at label recommendations, and if greater than label doses are administered, only potential toxicity is of concern. While this line of reasoning is also true to a large degree in food-animal production, veterinarians and producers involved in the treatment of disease in food animals bear the additional concern of the persistence of drug residues in the edible tissues after the disease process has been treated. Adulteration of the food supply with antimicrobial agents, pesticides, environmental contaminants, and other chemicals has been a growing source of concern to the general public and special-interest groups in recent years.

The importance of chemical residues in the edible tissues of food-producing animals has been thoroughly reviewed elsewhere (Sundlof 1989; Riviere 1991, 1992a; Van Dresser and Wilcke 1989; Mercer 1990; Kindred and Hubbert 1993; Bevill 1989). The purpose of this chapter is to acquaint the veterinarian with the legal and regulatory issues concerning the control of drug and other chemical residues in the United States, and to review some of the pharmacokinetic parameters used to determine withdrawal times for drugs and other chemicals in food animals. The primary parameter used by veterinarians to prevent violative tissue residues is the length of the withdrawal time, or the time required for a drug to be depleted from the animal before the animal's meat can be marketed for human consumption. In dairy practice, this is the milk discard time. Recently, government regulation and control have necessitated more stringent adherence to withdrawal times, and on-site monitoring for many drugs has been instituted. This may have an economic impact on production costs. Unlike in previous editions of this text, withdrawal times will not be tabulated, because they are subject to constant regulatory revision. Extensive tables of tissue depletion pharmacokinetic data are published elsewhere (Craigmill et al. 2006).

THE CONCERN OVER RESIDUES IN FOOD

A great deal of concern has been demonstrated over the last 40 years about the presence of chemical adulterants or residues, mainly antimicrobials and pesticides, in the meat, poultry, and milk supplies of the United States. By definition, a chemical residue is either the parent compound or metabolite of that parent compound that may accumulate, deposit, or otherwise be stored within the cells, tissues, organs, or edible products (e.g., milk, eggs) of an animal following its use to prevent, control, or treat animal disease, or to enhance production. Residues can also result from unintentional administration of drugs, or food additives. Finally, accidental exposure to chemicals in the environment can also result in tissue residues.

Concerns over food residues are economic as well as public health related. For example, the contamination of milk with antibiotics, most commonly penicillin, can affect starter cultures used to make fermented milk products such as cheeses, buttermilk, sour cream, etc., which can result in economic losses to those processors. From a public-health viewpoint, both the U.S. government and producer associations have taken active roles in minimizing antibiotic residues in meats and milk. Penicillin, for example, is known to induce allergic reactions in some sensitive people, and therefore, penicillin-tainted milk poses a health risk for these individuals. Similarly, chloramphenicol has been reported to induce blood dyscrasias that may lead to death; hence, its use in food-producing animals has been prohibited by the Food and Drug Administration (FDA). The FDA has also prohibited the use of nitrofurans in food-producing animals (excluding the topical routes for administration) because studies have shown them to be carcinogenic. Not only therapeutic drugs but pesticides create residue problems. Most pesticides are administered topically, allowing some amount of percutaneous absorption and sequestration in edible tissues. Lindane has been detected in the fat deposits of sheep dipped in a 0.0125% lindane emulsion 12 weeks after topical exposure (Collett and Harrison 1963). Other studies have shown lindane residues in sheep, goats (Jackson et al. 1959), and lactating cows (Oehler et al. 1969). In addition to lindane, many common pesticides (organochlorines, organophosphates, botanicals, pyrethrins, etc.) and herbicides used in agriculture today that are applied topically have been shown to produce residues in food-producing animals. Environmental contaminants (e.g., heavy metals, PCB, dioxins, mycotoxins) are also of major concern today. Tissue residue violations detected by governmental monitoring programs have been summarized by Sundlof (1989). More information on xenobiotics in food-producing animals is available in Riviere (1992a). Both public-health and economic concerns have been the major driving forces in the United States and in other countries behind the search for ways to minimize the threat of residue contamination of the public food supply.

Contamination of the food supply with chemical residues is rarely an intentional act and usually results either from failure to observe the correct meat withdrawal or milk discard time for a drug after it has been used to treat a disease process in food animals or from accidental contamination of feed by chemicals or drugs. A study by Van Dresser and Wilcke (1989) provides some interesting insight on drug residue problems in food-producing animals. In that study, streptomycin, penicillin, sulfamethazine, and oxytetracycline were the four most common antibiotics found in tissues, with sulfamethazine being the most commonly found sulfonamide in animal tissues. Long-acting formulations of these drugs (i.e., penicillin and oxytetracycline) had the highest association with violative residues in the animals involved in the study. Injectable drugs were more likely to be associated with residue problems than were feed additives and boluses. Most of these residues were found in veal calves, cows, and market barrows and gilts. The most frequently cited reason for violative residues was failure to observe the correct withdrawal time for the drug. Failure to observe the correct withdrawal time was cited as the most common reason for violative drug residue levels in a study performed by the FDA in the 1970s (Bevill 1984) and continued to be the most common cause of residue violations in the 1990s. Interestingly, in this study the producer was found to be the responsible party in 80% of the cases investigated for violative levels of drug found in edible tissues (when the responsible party could be identified); unapproved drug use (extralabel drugs) is not considered a major cause of drug residues in animals. Ways to prevent drug residues will be discussed later in this chapter.

The FDA and Environmental Protection Agency (EPA) establish tolerances for a drug, pesticide, or other chemical in the relevant tissues of the food-producing animals. The tolerance is the tissue concentration below which a marker residue for the drug or chemical must fall in the target tissue before that animal's edible tissues(s) (meat, milk, or eggs) are considered safe for human consumption (Riviere 1991). The marker residue may be the parent compound, or a metabolite, and reflects a known relationship to the total residues of the drug or chemical (parent and all metabolites). The target tissue is an edible tissue, frequently liver or kidney which, when the compound has depleted below the tolerance, assures that all edible tissues are safe for human consumption. Tolerances for different tissues are considered legal end points for which drug withdrawal times are established. Tolerances are established based on assessment of potential hazard of consumption to humans, a topic extensively reviewed elsewhere (Gehring et al. 2006). Oral toxicity studies are conducted in animals leading to the determination of an acceptable daily intake (ADI) for the compound in the human diet. These studies consider the compound's carcinogenic potential, systemic, reproductive, and developmental toxicity, and incorporate various safety factors. Recently, the potential for an antimicrobial compound to induce resistance in bacteria is also factored in. A safe concentration for human consumption is calculated using an equation which accounts for the amount of a specific food consumed by a person representing a high-consuming population (e.g., 19-year-old males) so that a safe concentration of the drug in this food (e.g., meat, milk, eggs) can be established. Various safety factors and statistical considerations are built into these determinations, and a tolerance for this drug in the specific tissue is established where appropriate and published. For example, safety factors reflect the duration of exposure and the nature of the toxic effects associated with the chemical. A teratogen requires a larger safety factor than a nonteratogen, and ADIs based on a short-term subchronic study use a larger safety factor than ADIs based on chronic studies. The tolerance is for a specific drug or chemical entity and reflects both the inherent toxicity of the chemical as well as assumptions about the human consumption of the tissue for which the tolerance is established. Tolerances are determined for the active ingredient (the drug substance or its metabolite) and are not established for the specific formulation of the commercial drug product. A full discussion of this process has recently been reviewed (Baynes et al. 1999) and can be found in toxicology or risk assessment texts. It is important for the veterinarian to realize that the end point for determining withdrawal times, the tolerance, is a combined scientific and legal concept and therefore *is* ultimately controlled by regulatory and not medical practices.

The actual withdrawal time appearing on a drug label is also a function of the experimental design that the manufacturer used in the research studies submitted to the FDA for approval. Thus, although the science governing the withdrawal time is based on the pharmacokinetic principles discussed below, the withdrawal time is actually determined based on experimental data. Generally, a drug is administered to healthy animals, groups of the animals are slaughtered at sequential time intervals, and their edible tissues are analyzed for drug concentrations. The withdrawal time is the time from cessation of treatment to the time it takes for the residues of the drug to deplete below the safe concentration. A statistical method is used to determine the time at which the marker residue depletes to the tolerance in the target tissue. The method determines the time, rounded to the next whole day, at which the upper bound of the marker residue tissue concentration is below the established tolerance in the target tissue (where the upper bound is statistically determined to represent with 95% confidence the 99th percentile of the population). Withdrawal times for the FDA-approved drugs for use in food animals are only valid for the specified species, dose, route, and frequency of administration. They are also specific to the manufacturer's product and formulation; thus, a drug substance (the active ingredient) may have different withdrawal times when present in differently formulated drug products. An analogous process occurs in establishing milk discard times and in determining the withdrawal times for drugs administered to egg-laying poultry (although presently, all drugs approved in the U.S. for use in laying hens have a 0-day withdrawal).

REGULATION OF DRUG RESIDUES IN ANIMALS

Producers, veterinarians, and other persons involved with chemicals and food-animal production should be acquainted with a few terms and the agencies involved in drug residue control in order to better understand the drug residue problem and how withdrawal times are determined.

The use of drugs in veterinary medicine especially in food-producing animals is closely regulated in the United States by the FDA under the Department of Health and Human Services. The FDA is charged, through the Federal Food, Drug and Cosmetic Act, with regulating the use of drugs in humans and in animals as well as requiring that the safety and efficacy of a drug be established before the product can be approved for use in animals, including those drugs added to animal feeds. The FDA also regulates human biologics, medical devices, drugs, and food safety. The FDA's Center for Veterinary Medicine (FDA-CVM) is responsible for the regulation of drugs, medical devices, and feeds intended for animals. The FDA is charged with the responsibility for establishing withdrawal times for drugs and the tolerances of drugs. The FDA and the EPA share responsibility for establishing tolerances for pesticide residues in animal-derived foods.

Whereas the FDA establishes safety guidelines for drug use in food animals, it is the responsibility of the USDA to enforce the standards established by the FDA and the EPA. The USDA, through authorization by the Federal Meat Inspection Act and the Poultry Inspection Act, inspects meat and poultry for sale through interstate commerce. The USDA is also authorized to test the tissues of food-producing animals through provisions in the Federal Insecticide, Fungicide and Rodenticide Act to determine whether violative levels of residues of chemicals and drugs are present. The Food Safety Inspection Service (FSIS), a division of the USDA, monitors these tissues through the National Residue Program (NRP) and identifies problems with drug and chemical residues. The NRP has been in existance for over 25 years and has concentrated on individual as well as population sampling for monitoring and surveying possible residue problems in slaughter animals. In 1992, the NRP estimated they would collect some 350,000 specimens that year to analyze for antimicrobial and pesticide residues (Kindred and Hubbert 1993). The FSIS is the largest safety inspection force in the federal government (Norcross and Post 1990).

The FSIS uses several rapid tests for determining contamination of animal products. Among these are the Swab Test on Premises (STOP) for antibiotic and sulfonamide residues, the Overnight Rapid Beef Identification Test (ORBIT) for species identification of meat, the Calf Antibiotic and Sulfa Test (CAST), the Sulfa-on-Site (SOS), and a variety of Enzyme-Linked Immunosorbant Assays (ELISAs) (Norcross and Post 1990). Rapid screening tests for residues have been summarized (Sundlof 1989). Milk in bulk tanks and from individual animals is assayed for antibiotic residues using various testing strategies: Penzyme III (SmithKline Beecham Animal Health), Spot Test (Cambridge Biotech Corp.), Charm Tests (Charm Sciences, Inc.), and Delvo tests (Gist-Brocades Food Ingredients, Inc.), to name only a few. This area is difficult to adequately summarize because rapid advances in analytical screening methodologies have led to the rapid development of new tests.

Other federal government agencies have defined roles in regulating the sale and use of drugs in animals, including the Drug Enforcement Agency (a division of the Department of Justice), the Animal and Plant Health Inspection Service (a part of the USDA), the EPA (mainly for pesticides), and the Department of Transportation. On a state level, the Department of Public Safety, Department of Health, the Animal Health Commission, Boards of Veterinary Medical Licensing, and Pharmacy Boards all have some regulatory influence over the use of drugs in food-producing as well as companion animals.

THE VETERINARIAN AND EXTRALABEL DRUG USE. The FDA approves new animal drugs for specific indications in a particular species or subclass of animals (e.g., dairy cattle, weanling pigs, etc.). Occasionally, veterinarians may encounter diseases or conditions in animals for which there are no FDA approved drugs. Under such circumstances, veterinarians often administer drugs that are not approved for use in food animals or they administer approved drugs in nonapproved ways, practices commonly referred to as "extralabel" usage. Extralabel drug use is defined as the use of a drug in a manner that is inconsistent with its FDA-approved labeling, a practice that, until 1994, was technically illegal. Recognizing that the Food, Drug and Cosmetic Act (FD&C) placed veterinarians in an untenable position of having to choose between providing for relief of animal suffering or complying with the law, the U.S. Congress passed the Animal Medicinal Drug Use Clarification Act (AMDUCA) in 1994. AMDUCA amended the FD&C Act to allow veterinarians under specific conditions to prescribe and administer drugs in an extralabel manner. Table 61.1 lists drugs specifically prohibited from extralabel use in food animals. Under AMDUCA, veterinarians may resort to the extralabel use of approved animal and human pharmaceuticals provided that the following conditions are met:

1. There is no approved new animal drug that is labeled for the intended use and that contains the same active ingredient which is in the required dosage form and concentration, except where a veterinarian finds, within the context of a valid veterinarian-client-patient relationship, that the approved new animal drug is clinically ineffective for its intended use.
2. Prior to prescribing or dispensing an approved new animal or human drug for an extralabel use in food animals, the veterinarian must
   - Make a careful diagnosis and evaluation of the conditions for which the drug is to be used;

TABLE 61.1 Drugs prohibited from extralabel use in food animals

Chloramphenicol
Clenbuterol
Diethylstilbestrol (DES)
Dipyrone*
Gentian Violet
Nitroimidazoles (including dimetridazole, metronidazole, and ipronidazole)
Nitrofurans (including nitrofurazone and furazolidone; topical use prohibited as well)
Phenylbutazone use in adult dairy cattle
Sulfonamide drugs in lactating cows**
Fluoroquinolones*
Glycopeptides

*Prohibition does not apply to approved uses.

**Prohibition does not apply to approved uses of sulfadimethoxine, sulfabromomethazine, and sulfaethoxypyridazine.

- Establish a substantially extended withdrawal period prior to marketing of milk, meat, eggs, or other edible products supported by appropriate scientific information, if applicable;
- Institute procedures to assure that the identity of the treated animal or animals is carefully maintained; and
- Take appropriate measures to assure that assigned timeframes for withdrawal are met and no illegal drug residues occur in any food-producing animal subjected to extralabel treatment.

The following additional conditions must be met for a permitted extralabel use of in food-producing animals of an approved *human* drug, or of an animal drug approved only for use in animals not intended for human consumption:

1. Such use must be accomplished in accordance with an appropriate medical rationale.
2. If scientific information on the human food safety aspect of the use of the drug in food-producing animals is not available, the veterinarian must take appropriate measures to assure that the animal and its food products will not enter the human food supply.
3. Extralabel use of an approved human drug in a food-producing animal is not permitted if an animal drug approved for use in food-producing animals can be used in an extralabel manner for the particular use.

Implicit in these regulations are that the veterinarian makes every effort to first use an approved drug at an approved dosage, that an individual veterinarian-client-patient relationship exists between the producer and the veterinarian, that proper animal identification and documentation be maintained, and that the veterinarian makes every effort to determine an extended withdrawal time for this usage (e.g., consult with a databank such as the Food Animal Residue Avoidance Databank, FARAD), which the producer must adhere to. The regulation prohibits extralabel use for routine production purposes, routine disease prevention, or as feed additives.

PHARMACOKINETICS AND RESIDUES

Pharmacokinetics is the science of quantitating the change in drug concentration in the body over time as a function of the administered dose. Although this discipline has been covered in Chapters 2 and 3 of this text and elsewhere (Riviere 1992b, 1999), it is important to review some principles here since it serves as the basis for understanding withdrawal times.

How a drug or combination of drugs behaves in the body after administration not only is important from a therapeutic point of view but is of paramount importance to the producer and veterinarian in order to prevent residues in the edible tissues after the disease process has been resolved and the animal is slaughtered. For therapeutic usefulness and drug residue determinations, a known amount of drug is administered to a healthy animal. Serum concentration data are collected and mathematical models are created so that the overall disposition of the drug in the body can be evaluated in relation to absorption, distribution, metabolism, and elimination. Parameters for these models are estimated by fitting regression lines to the observed serum concentration versus time profiles, an example of which was shown in Chapter 3, Figure 3.15.

The slopes of the three lines shown in Figure 3.15, when plotted on a semilogarithmic plot, represent distribution (λ_1), short-term elimination (λ_2), and long-term elimination (λ_3) from the body. The λ_1 (or α) and λ_2 (or β) phases of the serum concentration versus time profile are the only phases that are usually present when serum concentrations are monitored over a short period of time after dosing and are typically used to predict therapeutic drug concentrations. When serum concentrations are monitored for longer periods of time after drug administration using more sensitive assay methods, however, the λ_3 (or γ) phase of elimination appears for certain compounds. This can be present for several days or several months after the last administered dose depending on the drug's physicochemical properties, the amount of drug administered, and the species in which it was administered. This λ_3 phase reflects drug disposition in the so-called "deep compartments." Alternatively, for prolonged-action depot preparations (e.g., benzathine penicillin), this terminal phase may actually reflect the rate-limiting absorption phase ("flip-flop" phase). For purposes of determining withdrawal times of drugs that may be used in food-producing animals, we will focus our discussion on the terminal phase of drug elimination to determine the half-life ($t_{1/2}$) of the drug in the body, since this is the measurement that is relevant in determining drug withdrawal times.

In the actual research studies conducted to determine a withdrawal time, it is the half-life of drug in the specific tissue that is of paramount importance. This information is not available to the veterinarian. Additionally, tissue pharmacokinetics are exceedingly complex, and a discussion here of terminal half-lives will be sufficient to illustrate the concepts involved. For more in-depth information on the clinical application of pharmacokinetics and how pharmacokinetic parameters can affect clinical parameters, readers should consult Chapters 3 and 51 of this textbook.

The half-life of the drug or chemical in the body is the primary biological measurement used to determine withdrawal times of drugs and chemicals in food-producing animals; however, this parameter can be influenced by many biological factors. The $t_{1/2}$ of a drug by definition is the time is takes for 50% of the drug in the animal to be eliminated from the body and is based on the terminal slope of the elimination curve used to determine the withdrawal time of a drug. The $t_{1/2}$ is calculated using the equation

$$t_{1/2} = \ln 2/\text{slope or } t_{1/2} = 0.693/\text{slope}$$

If the concentration of a drug in the muscle of a food animal after dosing is 100 parts per million (ppm), then the time it takes for the concentration in the muscle to decrease to 50 ppm would be the biological half-life of the drug in the muscle. Extrapolated out, the amount of drug in the muscle after 10 half-lives would be 0.1 ppm, or, put in other terms, 99.9% of the drug would have been eliminated from the muscle after 10 half-lives. If the dose is doubled and the beginning concentration in the muscle is now 200 ppm, only 1 additional half-life would be required to reach the 0.1 ppm concentration. On the other hand, if the half-life of the drug in the muscle is doubled, perhaps due to a disease state, then the elimination half-life would also double, thereby increasing the risk of violative drug residues in the edible tissues of that animal.

As stated above, the elimination half-life can be influenced by many biological factors. The half-life of a drug or chemical in the body is influenced by how well it distributes in the body and how quickly it is eliminated from the body. The physicochemical properties of a drug can influence its disposition in the body—in particular, how well it distributes into certain tissues, whether or not it penetrates intracellularly, or whether it permeates the blood-brain barrier. The volume of distribution (V_d) is the quantitative estimate of the extent of the distribution of the drug in the body and can therefore directly influence the $t_{1/2}$ of the drug. It is a proportionality constant relating the concentration of drug in the serum to the total amount of drug in the body. For an intravenous injection of a drug, the equation for calculating V_d is

$$V_d = \text{amount of drug in the body}/\text{serum drug concentration}$$

It is important to point out that the V_d, typically reported in l/kg, does not actually refer to any specific physiologic space or body area; rather, it gives a good indication of how well a drug in general distributes throughout the body. A drug that has a large V_d typically has good tissue distribution throughout the body (e.g., tetracyclines), while a drug with a small V_d has less penetration into the body tissues as whole, perhaps being confined to the extracellular spaces due to one or more of its physicochemical properties (not lipid soluble, fixed charge). While V_d may give an indication of the overall distribution of a drug, some drugs may not be uniformly distributed throughout the body. In this case, a drug may seek specific cells or organs or be bound to tissue macromolecules, resulting in a large V_d measurement and yet a relatively poor overall distribution in a majority of the body's tissues. Some drugs may have prolonged withdrawal times due to a large V_d.

In addition to V_d, the clearance (Cl) of the drug also plays an important part in determining the withdrawal time of the drug. Clearance quantitates the efficiency of the elimination processes and is defined as the rate of drug elimination from the body relative to the concentration of drug in the serum by the equation

$$Cl = \text{rate of elimination}/\text{serum drug concentration}$$

Drugs that have a slow rate of elimination from the body will tend to have protracted half-lives, while those that are eliminated quickly will have shorter half-lives.

The $t_{1/2}$ is dependent on two functions: V_d and Cl. By combining terms, an equation can be derived that reflects the influence of V_d and Cl on the $t_{1/2}$ of a drug:

$$t_{1/2} = \ln 2V_d/Cl \text{ or } t_{1/2} = 0.693\ V_d/Cl$$

Several physiologic events can occur to change V_d or Cl and can therefore influence the $t_{1/2}$ of the drug in the body. For example, if renal function is impaired, the drug's clearance may be reduced and the $t_{1/2}$ prolonged by several hours or several days, in turn prolonging the withdrawal time of the drug. If the animal's fluid balance changes, the V_d may change accordingly. Factors such as the age, nutritional status, percentage of body fat, species, presence of other drugs, extent of protein binding can all have a significant role in determining the V_d and Cl and hence the $t_{1/2}$ of any drug introduced into the body. For more information on the pharmacokinetics, readers are encouraged to consult Chapters 2 and 3.

Recent work has used physiologically based pharmacokinetic modeling (similar to Fig. 3.18) to develop models that incorporate tissue compartment measurements into their structure (Craigmill 2003; Buur et al. 2005, 2006). These models also allow direct incorporation of statistical estimates of population variability in all processes impacting on residue depletion to be included in the modeling. Their downside is that significant data are required for their solution.

The pharmacokinetic behavior and efficacy of the drug or chemical used to treat a disease process are of major concern early on in the successful management of herd health in food animals. For residue control in food-animal species, the primary purpose of knowing the pharmacokinetic behavior of the drug (i.e., the terminal elimination half-life) is to determine the withdrawal time to avoid residue accumulation in those tissues consumed by humans. A knowledge of what physiological processes affect the half-life is thus essential to determine when a withdrawal time might need to be modified due to disease-induced prolongation of the withdrawal time.

Theoretically, if a tissue tolerance and the dose of drug were known, pharmacokinetic techniques could be used to calculate an individual withdrawal time. For an oral drug, this requires knowing the fraction of the dose administered which is absorbed into the body (e.g., bioavailability). This amount, divided by the V_d, is the initial concentration of drug in the body (C^0). If one were to assume that the loss of drug from the body were only dependent upon the terminal withdrawal time, then adjusting equation 3.10 by solving for T as the withdrawal time, and substituting K as 1.44 $t_{1/2}$, the following relationship can be derived as

$$\text{withdrawal time} = 1.44 \ln\left(C^0/\text{tolerance}\right)\left(t_{1/2}\right).$$

Of course, this is an oversimplification. In reality, this equation would work if C^0 were the concentration of drug in the target tissue at the end of drug administration, as this amount is dependent upon the λ_2-phase elimination processes. Complex pharmacokinetic models can be used to calculate this number. Then the above equation would be valid. Officially established withdrawal times must take into account all interanimal variability, and thus statistical processing of these data establishes the withdrawal time for the worst-case scenario.

The above equation is useful to gain a perspective on what the withdrawal time is relative to the terminal half-life. Assume that for most antibiotics a "therapeutic" concentration is 10 μg/ml and the tissue tolerance is 0.01 ppm (0.01 μg/ml). One also must assume homogeneous distribution of the drug throughout the body. Thus, withdrawal time equals 1.44 [ln (10/0.01)] $t_{1/2}$, or 9.94 $t_{1/2}$. A withdrawal time for this drug would be equal to 10 half-lives. If the drug has a short half-life (e.g., penicillin), the withdrawal time is short. However, if the drug has a prolonged tissue half-life (e.g., an aminoglycoside), the withdrawal time could exceed a year in the target tissue. Similarly, a drug with a very low tissue tolerance has a longer withdrawal time because ln (C^0/tolerance) is now greater. If a drug is metabolized, the metabolite may determine the withdrawal time ("marker residue") since its half-life is rate limiting.

This "rule of 10" can be derived by assuming that 10 half-lives are required to eliminate 99.9% of an administered dose, as discussed earlier in this section. An examination of half-lives and withdrawal times for a number of approved pharmaceutics confirms this relation as being very conservative relative to human food safety endpoints (Gehring et al. 2004). In fact, these so-called "half-life multipliers" of 4–5 were often sufficient since the target tolerance for drugs with minimal adverse effects was not at very low concentrations reflective of complete drug elimination. Using a divisor of 5 could actually be considered even more conservative since the additional time added to the withdrawal time would be longer.

This relationship is important to consider when one administers an increased dose of drug. If the dose is doubled, withdrawal time should just be increased by a single half-life. In the above example, the calculation would 1.44 ln (20/0.01), or 10.94 half-lives, which confirms this concept. However, if a disease process changed the half-life by either increasing volume of distribution or decreasing clearance (e.g., kidney disease) causing the half-life to double, withdrawal time should be doubled. This phenomenon supports the observation that seriously ill animals with altered pharmacokinetics deserve increased attention to ensure complete drug withdrawal. It is also important to note that withdrawal time is determined in healthy animals, and thus serious disease conditions may cause residues even when the approved dose and official withdrawal time are used. *It is critical for a veterinarian to have a conceptual understanding of this relationship between withdrawal time and half-life before doses are modified in food-producing animals.* When such a withdrawal time is calculated, the animal should be checked with the appropriate rapid screening test.

For lactating dairy cows and goats, the identical principles apply to determining the milk discard times. The milk discard or withholding time is the time after drug administration when the milk cannot be used for human consumption. This is determined by administering the drug and collecting and analyzing milk until drug concentrations are below the milk tolerance established for that drug. Like withdrawal times, the discard time is product and species-dependent. In this case, it is based on the half-life of the drug in the milk. If one knows the concentration of the drug in the milk at the end of drug administration, the milk half-life, and the milk tolerance, the above equation can be used to precisely calculate withdrawal. This has been particularly useful when valuable dairy cows have been accidentally exposed to pesticides (e.g., heptachlor) and pharmacokinetic data were used to determine milk discard times since approved withdrawal times do not exist. In this case, the relevant parameter is the half-life of drug in milk. All of the principles discussed above relative to meat withdrawal apply. The half-life in milk is a function of how the drug is excreted into the milk after systemic administration (or oral or interuterine) or is retained in the udder after intramammary infusion. For example, basic drugs such as erythromycin have longer discard times than acidic drugs such as penicillin because the former tend to distribute more readily into milk due to the pH partitioning phenomenon. Similarly, lipophilic drugs will tend to have longer milk discard times. Discard times are different for these different routes of administration. One must be sure that a drug used as dry cow therapy is not inadvertently administered to a lactating cow, because the residue concerns are different since most dry cow formulations are long-acting preparations.

DRUGS PROHIBITED FROM EXTRALABEL USE

Certain drugs are prohibited from extralabel use in food animals under AMDUCA (Table 61.1). The FDA may prohibit the extralabel use of an approved new animal or human drug or class of drugs in food animals if FDA determines that the extralabel use of the drug or class of drugs presents a risk to the public health, or an acceptable analytical method needs to be established but such method has not been established. A prohibition may be a general ban on the extralabel use of the drug or class of drugs or may be limited to a specific species, indication, dosage form, route of administration, or combination of factors.

RESIDUE PREVENTION

Although public awareness of the drug residue problem in food is high and several governmental agencies spend large amounts of time attempting to control this problem, residues in animal tissues are still an important concern today. The responsibility for residue control and prevention cannot lie solely within a governmental agency; rather, the responsibility must be shared by the government, producers, veterinarians, teachers and academicians, marketing associations, and other interested parties, who must strive for both healthy and efficiently grown animals as well as a safe food supply. Several approaches can be taken to achieve this goal.

The first step in residue prevention is to make individuals and organizations aware of the problem through education. Education of laypersons can be accomplished through a variety of mechanisms: available open lay and veterinary medical literature, computer databases, consultations with veterinary medical personnel, or the efforts of national organizations. A number of national producer organizations have firm initiatives in place to prevent harmful residues in food-producing animals, including dairy (Adams 1993), beef (Wilkes 1993), pork (Lautner 1993), and veal (Wilson and Dietrich 1993) organizations. Awareness has also been raised concerning some species of companion animals (Macomber 1993; Kay 1993).

Failure to observe the correct withdrawal time of a drug was the leading cause of tissue residue violations in two studies (Van Dresser and Wilckie 1989; Bevill 1984). Once the importance of residue control in the U.S. food supply is made clear and the importance of observing the correct legal withdrawal times for the drugs used in food-producing animals is understood, the incidence of tissue residue violations will (theoretically) decrease dramatically. Many have reported on other possible ways to reduce or prevent residues from occurring in food animals (Gehring et al. 2006; Riviere 1991; Marteniuk et al. 1988; Sundlof 1989; Kindred and Hubbert 1993; Mercer 1990). Rapid screening test technology has advanced significantly in the past few years and has been used to detect low levels of residue contamination in slaughtered animals in a quick manner. As these tests become more sensitive and more widely used, animals with residue contamination can be isolated and removed before reaching the end consumer, further decreasing the residue problem.

Several rapid screening tests are available. They are powerful tools for the veterinarian using a drug in an extralabel manner or in a seriously diseased animal. Once the veterinarian establishes a putative withdrawal time using the principles discussed above, the animal should be tested with the appropriate rapid screening assay to ensure that the prediction is accurate. If a residue is detected, a prolonged withdrawal time should be recommended until a negative screening value is observed. If this practice is followed, the veterinarian will have done everything possible to ensure a residue-free product.

FARAD is a USDA-supported computerized databank of scientific and regulatory information, established in 1982 and reauthorized by the U.S. Congress in 1998, that can assist the veterinarian, producer, or other individuals in making rational choices in preventing drug and pesticide residues in food animals. It is a collaboration of North Carolina State University, University of California at Davis, and University of Florida at Gainesville. FARAD contains information on veterinary drug registration information; current label information; foreign registration and safety data; tolerances for drugs and pesticides for tissues, eggs, and milk; withdrawal information; physicochemical properties; pharmacokinetic and toxicokinetic information; residue test information; bibliographic citations; and other information useful in preventing drug residues in food animals. The database is regularly updated to provide users with the most current information available. FARAD is easily accessed by voice telephone (888-USFARAD), fax, and electronic mail at two regional access centers (North Carolina State University and University of California Davis). By contacting an access center, users can obtain any of the current information listed above. FARAD services are free to clientele. FARAD also publishes periodic updates on extralabel drug withdrawal time estimates and other issues as a regular feature in the *Journal of the American Veterinary Medical Association* (FARAD DIGESTS). The program's website (www.farad.org) should be consulted for orientation to its services and current access information. More information on FARAD is available elsewhere (Riviere et al. 1986; Payne et al. 1999).

Other sources of drug information pertaining to residues in food animals are also available. The FARAD pharmacokinetic data have been published in book form (Craigmill et al. 2006). The Food and Agriculture Organization (FAO) and World Health Association (WHO) Joint Expert Committee on Food Additives (JECFA) has evaluated several drugs and has published monographs that list toxicity, metabolism, acceptable daily intakes, maximum residue levels permitted for different tissues, and biological fate of drugs in food-producing animals. The *United States Pharmacopoeia* (USP) also publishes monographs (similar to the monographs for human drugs) that go into more depth about expanded (extralabel) pharmaceutical usage and pharmacokinetic variables that can alter withdrawal times in food-producing animals (Sundlof 1993).

The prevention of harmful residues in the edible tissues of our food-producing animals is the responsibility of many producers, veterinarians, professional and layperson associations, and governmental agencies. All of these groups must continue to strive to regulate and utilize the drugs used to prevent or cure animal diseases in a responsible manner in order to prevent the accumulation of harmful amounts of residues in the food supply.

REFERENCES

Adams, J.B. 1993. Assuring a residue-free food supply: milk. JAVMA 202(10):1723–1725.

Baynes, R.A., Martin, T., Craigmill, A.L., and Riviere, J.E. 1999. Strategies for estimating provisional acceptable residues (PAR) for extralabel drug use in livestock. Reg Toxicol Pharmacol 29:287–299.

Bevill, R.F. 1984. Factors influencing the occurrence of drug residues in animal tissues after the use of antimicrobial agents in animal feeds. JAVMA 185(10):1124–1126.

———. 1989. Sulfonamide residues in domestic animals. J Vet Pharmacol Therap 12:241–252.

Buur, J., Baynes, R., Smith, G., and Riviere, J.E. 2006. The use of probabilistic modeling within a physiological based pharmacokinetic model to predict drug residue withdrawal times in edible tissue: sulfamethazine in swine. Antimicrob Agents Chemother 50:2344–2351.

Buur, J.L., Baynes, R.E. Craigmill, A.L., Riviere, J.E. 2005. A physiological based pharmacokinetic model of sulfamethazine in swine applied to tissue residues. Am J Vet Res 66:1686–1693.

Collett, J.N., and Harrison, D.L. 1963. Lindane residues in sheep following dipping. NZ J Agricul Res 6:39–42.

Craigmill, A.L. 2003. A physiological based pharmacokinetic model for oxytetracycline residues in sheep. J Vet Pharmacol Therap 26:55–63.

Craigmill, A.L., Riviere, J.E., and Webb A.I. 2006. Tabulation of FARAD Comparative and Veterinary Pharmacokinetic Data. Ames, IA: Blackwell Press.

Freese, W.R. 1993. Responsibilities of food animal practitioner regarding extra-label use of drugs. JAVMA 202(10):1733–1734.

Gehring, R., Baynes, R.E., Craigmill, A.L., and Riviere, A.L. 2004. Feasibility of using half-life multipliers to estimate extended withdrawal intervals following the extralabel use of drugs in food producing animals. J Food Protect 67:555–560.

Gehring, R., Baynes, R.E. and Riviere, J.E. 2006. Risk assessment and management principles and their application to the extralabel use of drugs in food producing animals. J Vet Pharmacol Therap 29:5–14.

Geyer, R.E. 1993. Implications for the FDA/Center for Veterinary Medicine (CVM). JAVMA 202(10):1718–1719.

Guest, G.B., and Solomon S.M. 1993. FDA extra-label use policy: 1992 revisions. JAVMA 202(10):1620–1623.

Jackson, J.B., Ivey, M.C., Roberts, R.H., and Radeleff, R.D. 1959. Residue studies in sheep and goats dipped in 0.025% lindane. J Econ Entomol 52(5):1031–1032.

Jenkins, W.L. 1993. Professional responsibilities. JAVMA 202(10): 1742–1743.

Kay, W.J. 1993. Responsibilities under an amended Food, Drug and Cosmetic Act: companion animal practitioners. JAVMA 202(10): 1736–1737.

Kindred, T.P., and Hubbert, W.T. 1993. Residue prevention strategies in the United States. JAVMA 202(1):46–49.

Lautner, B. 1993. Assuring a residue-free food supply: pork. JAVMA 202(10):1727–1729.

Macomber, L.E. 1993. Responsibilities under an amended Food, Drug and Cosmetic Act: equine practitioners. JAVMA 202(10):1735.

Marteniuk, J.V., Alwynelle, S.A., and Bartlett, P.C. 1988. Compliance with recommended drug withdrawal requirements for dairy cows sent to market in Michigan. JAVMA 193(4):404–407.

Mercer, H.D. 1990. How to avoid the drug residue problem in cattle. Comp Contin Educ Pract Vet-Food Animal 12(1):124–126.

Norcross, M.A., and Post, A.R. 1990. New food safety initiatives in the Food Safety and Inspection Service, US Department of Agriculture. J An Sci 68:863–869.

Oehler, D.D., Eschle, J.L., Miller, J.A., Claborn, H.V., and Ivey, M.C. 1969. Residues in milk resulting from ultra-low volume sprays of malathion, methoxychlor, coumaphos, ronnel, or gardona for control of the horn fly. J Econ Ento 62(6):1481–1483.

Payne, M.A. 1991. Extralabel drug use and withdrawal times in dairy cattle. Comp Contin Educ Prac Vet (Food Animal) 13:1341–1351.

Payne, M.A., Craigmill, A.L., Riviere, J.E., Webb, A., Baynes, R.A., and Sundlof, S.F. 1999. Food Animal Residue Avoidance Databank. Vet Clin N Am 15:75–88.

Riviere, J.E. 1988. Veterinary clinical pharmacokinetics. Part I. Fundamental concepts. Compend Contin Educ Pract Vet 10:24–30.

———. 1991. Pharmacologic principles of residue avoidance for veterinary practitioners. JAVMA 198(5):809–815.

———. 1992a. Dermal absorption and metabolism of xenobiotics in food-producing animals. In Xenobiotics and Food-Producing Animals: Metabolism and Residues, ed. D.H. Hutson et al., Chap. 7, pp. 88–97. Washington, D.C.: American Chemical Society Symposium Series 503.

———. 1992b. Practical aspects of the pharmacology and antimicrobial drug residues in food animals. Agri-Practice 13(6):11–16.

———. 1999. Comparative Pharmacokinetics: Principles, Techniques and Applications. Ames: Iowa State University Press.

Riviere, J.E., Craigmill, A.L., and Sundlof, S.F. 1986. Food Animal Residue Avoidance Databank (FARAD): an automated pharmacologic databank for drug and chemical residue avoidance. J Food Protection 49(10):826–830.

Sundlof, S.F. 1989. Drug and chemical residues in livestock. Vet Clin N Am, Food An Pract 5(2):411–449.

———. 1993. Availability and use of existing scientific information for responsible drug prescribing. JAVMA 202(10):1696–1699.

Teske, R.H. 1993. Current FDA policy on use of human-labeled drugs in animals. JAVMA 202(10):1632–1633.

Van Dresser, W.R., and Wilcke, J.R. 1989. Drug residues in food animals. JAVMA 194(12):1700–1710.

Wilkes, D. 1993. Assuring a residue-free food supply: beef. JAVMA 202(10):1725–1727.

Wilson, L.L., and Dietrich, J.R. 1993. Assuring a residue-free food supply: special-fed veal. JAVMA 202(10):1730–1733.

INDEX